FOREWORD

The mobility of doctors is again illustrated in this edition which contains the usual extensive revisions.

The publication of a Directory for the Canadian medical profession was assumed by this publishing house out of necessity. We consistently keep in mind the needs for accuracy and usefulness. From year to year the staff grows and the active research staff has increased considerably in the past 12 yrs.

Grateful acknowledgment is made to the thousands of physicians who return questionnaires promptly and accurately. The Registrars, the Medical Council of Canada, the College of General Practice, the Royal College of Physicians and Surgeons, the Medical Associations, Health Department and others are thanked for their contributions to the effectiveness of the Directory.

Once again those who may use the Directory as a check on possible improper use of a medical name to endorse a prescription for narcotic drugs, are WARNED that the Directory can accept no responsibility and that the final authority of a licence to practice rests with the Registrar in each of the ten provinces.

Subscribers may notice, in some cases, that the doctor's residence address does not appear. Where there has been a change in the doctor's residence address since 1966 this information has been omitted. This is the first step in the elimination of all residence addresses, except where it coincides with the doctor's office address. This is done because of the wishes of many physicians and also to streamline the Directory, growing longer by the year, so that it contains only significant information.

Physicians are again reminded, when they receive their questionnaires for the 1968 edition, that the accuracy of their answers is the single most important factor influencing the accuracy of the Directory.

This edition has been compiled by Mrs. Anne Newcombe, with the assistance of Miss Frieda Hamilton.

HOW TO USE THE DIRECTORY with abbreviations

Please note that over 75% of the listings were compiled or approved by the doctors themselves during a six month period. However, some doctors may have changed address, etc., during that time.

The Directory contains three sections: the white pages, which contain the biographical listings of physicians; the blue pages, listing physicians by province and town; and the buff pages, containing miscellaneous information.

In the white pages will be found biographical listings, in alphabetical order, for every qualified doctor known to be in Canada at the time of publication, with the exception of those doctors who graduated from Canadian medical schools in 1966. Their names will be found in the buff pages.

For each doctor the following information is given, as appropriate: name; first name and initials; office address (if in private practice); home address, if different; university and year of graduation; other degrees, including specialist certificates and appointments.

Canadian universities are abbreviated to the first three letters, as follows. Other universities are shown in full.

Dal—Dalhousie
McG—McGill
Ott—Ottawa
Tor—Toronto
Man—Manitoba
Lav—Laval
Mon—Montreal
Qns—Queens
Wes—Western Ontario
Alb—Alberta
UBC—British Columbia
Sask—Saskatchewan

Degrees are abbreviated as follows:

A.A.C.P.—Assoc. American College of Physicians
A.A.C.S.—Assoc. Amer. College of Surgeons
A.A.O.O.—Amer. Academy of Ophthalmology & Otol.
A.A.P.C.C.—American Assoc. of Psychiatric Clinics for Children
A.B.A.—American Board of Anaesthesia
AB.Av.M.—American Board of Aviation Medicine
A.B.D.R.—American Board of Diag. Radiology
A.B.D.S.—Amer. Board of Dermatology and Syph.
A.B.I.M.—American Board of Internal Medicine
A.B.N.P.—American Board of Neurology & Psychiatry.
A.B.N.S.—American Board of Neurosurgery.
A.B.O.G.—American Board of Obstetrics and Gynaecology
A.B.O.M.—American Board of Occupational Medicine
A.B.O.S.—American Board of Orthopaedic Surgery
A.B.Ot.—American Board of Otolaryngology
A.B.P.—American Board of Paediatrics
A.B.P.M.R.—American Board of Physical Med. and Rehab.
A.B.Prev.Med.—American Board of Preventive Medicine
A.B.T.S.—American Board of Thoracic Surgery
A.F.A.C.C.—Assoc. Fell. Amer. Coll. Cardiol.
A.F.A.C.C.P.—Assoc. Fellow, American College of Chest Physicians
A.C.C.P.—American College Chest Physicians
A.I.C.S.—Assoc. Intern. College of Surgeons
A.M.A.A.N.—Assoc. Memb., American Academy of Neurology
A.M.A.C.C.P.—Assoc. Member American College of Chest Physicians
A.M.C.A.A.—Assoc. Member Can. Acad. Allergy.
A.M.C.G.P.—Assoc. Member, College of General Practice of Canada
A.M.L.F.C.—Assoc. Medecin Langue Francais du Canada
A.P.A.—American Psychiatric Assoc.
A.R.I.C.—Assoc., Royal Institute of Chemistry
A.S.F.P.S.—American Society of Facial Plastic Surgery
B.A.O.—Bachelor of the Art of Obstetrics
B.Chir.—Bachelor of Chirurgie
B.Pharm.—Bachelor of Pharmacy
C.H.A.—Certificate, Hospital Administration
Ch.B.—Bachelor of Chirurgie
C.M., Ch.M.—Master of Surgery
C.M.H.A.—Certificate, Mental Health Assoc.
C.P.A.—Canadian Psychiatric Association
C.P.H.—Certificate in Public Health
D.A.—Diploma in Anaesthesia
D.A.B.A.—Diploma, American Board of Anaesthesia
D.A.B.D.—Diploma, American Board of Dermatology
D.A.B.D.S.—Diploma, American Board of Dermatology and Syphilology
D.A.B.I.M.—Diploma, American Board of Internal Medicine
D.A.B.I.M.C.—Diploma, American Board of Internal Medicine (Cardiology)
D.A.B.N.—Diploma, American Board of Neurology
D.A.B.N.S.—Diploma, American Board of Neurosurgery
D.A.B. Op.—Diploma, American Board of Ophthalmology
D.A.B.Ot.—Diploma, American Board of Otolaryngology
D.A.B.O.G.—Diploma, American Board of Obstetrics and Gynaecology
D.A.B.O.S.—Diploma, American Board of Orthopaedic Surgery
D.A.B.P.—Diploma, American Board of Paediatrics
D.A.B.Path.—Diploma, American Board of Pathology
D.A.B. Path. Anat.—Diploma, American Board of Pathological Anatomy
D.A.B.Path. & M.A.—Diploma, American Board of Pathology and Morbid Anatomy
D.A.B.P.H.—Diploma, American Board of Public Health
D.A.B.P.M.—Diploma, American Board of Physical Medicine
D.A.B.P.M.R.—Diploma, American Board of Physical Med. and Rehab.
D.A.B.P.S.—Diploma, American Board of Plastic Surgery
D.A.B.P.N.—Diploma, American Board of Psychiatry and Neurology; Psy; Neuro; NeurPsy; Chi.P.
D.A.B.Prev.Med.—Diploma, American Board. Preventive Medicine
D.A.B.R.—Diploma, American Board of Radiology
D.A.B.T.R.—Diploma, American Board of Therap. Radiology
D.A.B.T.S.—Diploma, American Board of Thoracic Surgery
D.A.B.S.—Diploma, American Board of Surgery
D.A.B.U.—Diploma, American Board of Urology
D.A.I.P.—Dip. American Inst. of Psychoanalysis
D.C.H.—Diploma, Child Health
D.D.R.—Diploma, Diagnostic Radiology
D.D.S.—Doctor of Dental Surgery
D.G.O.—Diploma, Gynaecology and Obstetrics
D.G.S.—Diploma, General Surgery
D.H.A.—Diploma, Hospital Administration
D.I.F.A.—Diploma, International Fertility Assoc.
D.I.H.—Diploma, Industrial Health
D.I.M.—Diploma, Internal Medicine
D.L.I.M.—Dip. in Life Ins. Medicine
D.L.O.—Diploma, Laryngology and Otolaryngology
D.M.R.E.—Diploma, Medical Radiology and Electrology
D.M.R.T.—Diploma, Medical Radiotherapy
D.N.—Diploma—Neurology
D.N.B.M.E.—Dip. National Board of Med. Exam. (U.S.)
D.N.S.—Diploma Neurosurgery
D.O.M.S.—Diploma, Ophth. Med. and Surgery
D.P.—Diploma in Psychiatry
D.P.A.—Diploma, Pathological Anatomy
D.P.H.—Diploma, Public Health
D.P.M.—Diploma, Psychological Medicine
D.R.—Diploma, Radiology

(continued on page 4)

Thirteenth Annual

CANADIAN MEDICAL DIRECTORY

Published at SECCOMBE HOUSE
443 Mount Pleasant Road, Toronto 7, Canada
Telephone: Area Code 416 : 487-1191

D.R.C.O.G.—Diploma, Royal College of Obstetricians and Gynaecologists
D.O.—Diploma in Ophthalmology
D.O.G.—Diploma ObstGyn.
D.S.—Diploma in Surgery
D.S.C.—Doctor, Surgical Chiropody
D.Sc.—Doctor of Science
D.S.Sc.—Diploma, Sanitary Science
D.T.D.—Diploma in Tuberculous Diseases
D.T.H.—Diploma, Tropical Hygiene
D.T.M.—Diploma, Tropical Medicine
D.U.—Diploma, Urology
F.A.A.A.—Fellow, American Academy of Allergy
F.A.A.A.S.—Fellow, American Assoc. for Advancement of Science
F.A.A.D.S.—Fellow, American Academy of Dermatology & Syphilology
F.A.A.M.D.—Fellow, American Assoc. on Mental Deficiency
F.A.A.O.O.—Fellow, American Academy of Ophthalmology and Otolaryngology
F.A.A.O.S.—Fellow, American Academy of Orth-Surgery
F.A.A.P.—Fellow, American Academy of Paediatrics
F.A.A.O.S.—Fellow, American Academy of Orthopaedic Surgeons
F.A.A.S.T.—Fellow, American Academy of Surgery of Trauma
F.A.A.T.S.—Fellow, American Academy of Thoracic Surgeons
F.A.B.A.S.—Fell. American Bd. of Abdominal Surg.
F.A.B. Prev. M.—Fellow, American Board of Preventive Medicine
F.A.C.A.—Fellow, American College of Anaesthesia
F.A.C.C.—Fellow, American College of Cardiology
F.A.C.C.P.—Fellow, American College of Clin. Pharm & Chemotherapy.
F.A.C.D.—Fellow, American College of Dermatology
F.A.C.G.—Fellow, American College of Gastroenterology
F.A.C.H.A.—Fellow, American College of Hospital Administration
F.A.C.O.G.—Fellow, American College of Gynecologists
F.A.C.O.N.—Fellow, Am. College of Neuropsychopharm
F.A.C.P.—Fellow, American College of Physicians
F.A.C.Path.—Fellow, American College of Pathology
F.A.C.P.T.—Fellow, American College of Physical Therapy
F.A.C.R.—Fellow, American College of Radiology
F.A.C.S.—Fellow, American College of Surgeons
F.A.G.S.—Fellow, American Geriatric Society
F.A.M.W.A.—Fellow, American Medical Writer's Assoc.
F.A.P.A.—Fellow, American Paediatric Ass'n.
F.A.P.A.—Fellow, American Psychiatric Association
F.A.P.H.A.—Fellow, American Public Health Ass'n.
F.A.P.M.—Fellow Acad. of Psychosomatic Medicine.
F.A.S.A.S.—Fellow, American Soc. Abdominal Surgeons.
F.A.S.E.A.—Fellow, Assoc. of Surgeons of East Africa
F.A.S.C.P.—Fellow, American Society of Clinical Pathologists
F.A.S.H.A.—Fellow, American Surgery of Hand Assoc.
F.A.S.O.O.—Fellow, American Society of Ophthalmologists and Otolaryngologists
F.B.L.I.M.—Fellow, Bd. of Life Insurance Medicine
F.C.Path.—Fellow of the College of Pathologists
F.C.C.P.—Fellow, College of Chest Physicians
F.C.R.A.—Fellow, College Radiologists (Australia)
F.C.S.E.—Fell. Can. Soc. Electroencephalographers
F.F.A.R.C.S.—Fellow, Fac. of Anaesthesia, Royal College of Surgeons (Eng.)
F.F.R.—Fellow, Faculty of Radiology
F.H.C.S.—Fellow, Hungarian College of Surgeons
F.I.A.A.—Fellow, International Ass'n. Allergists
F.I.A.P.—Fellow, International Association of Proctology
F.I.C.A.—Fellow, International College of Anaesthestists
F.I.C.A. (An.)—Fellow, Int'l. College of Anatomists.
F.I.C.A. (Ang.)—Fellow, Int'l. College of Angiology.
F.I.C.S.—Fellow, International College of Surgery
F.I.M.—Fellow, Industrial Medicine
F.I.M.A.—Fellow, Industrial Medical Association
F.I.S.C.E.H.—Fellow, Int'l. Soc. for Clin. & Experimental Hypnosis.
F.I.S.H.—Fellow, Internat. Soc. Haematology
F.N.A.P.—Fellow, International Gastroenterologists' Society
F.N.G.S.—Fellow National Gastroenterologists Soc.
F.R.A.C.P.S.—Fellow, Royal Austral. College of Physicians & Surgeons
F.R.A.C.S.—Fellow, Royal Australian College of Surgeons
F.R.A.I.—Fellow, Royal Anthropological Institute
F.R.C.P.—Fellow, Royal College of Physicians
F.R.C.S.—Fellow, Royal College of Surgeons
F.R.F.P.S.—Fellow, Royal Faculty of Physicians and Surgeons
F.R.C.M.—Fellow, Royal College Medicine
F.R.C.O.G.—Fellow, Royal College Obstetrics & Gyn.
F.R.S.—Fellow of the Royal Society
F.R.S.C.—Fellow, Royal Society of Canada
F.R.S.H.—Fellow, Royal Soc. of Health
F.R.S.M.—Fellow, Royal Society of Medicine
F.R.S.T.M.—Fellow, Royal Soc. Trop. Med. (Lond.)
F.S.C.E.H.—Fellow, Society for Clinical & Experimental Hypnosis
F.S.I.H.—Fellow, Society of Industrial Hygiene
L.A.B.O.—Licentiate, Amer. Board of Ophthamology
L.G.M.C.U.K.—Lic. Gen. Med. Council, of the United Kingdom
L.A.B.I.M.—Licentiate, American Board of Internal Medicine
L.A.B.P.—Licentiate, American Board of Paediatrics
L.A.B.R.—Licentiate, American Board of Radiology
L.I.C.A.—Licentiate, International College of Anaesthestists
Ll.D.—Doctor of Laws
L.M.—Licentiate in Midwifery
L.M.C.C.—Licentiate Med. Council of Canada.
L.M.S.S.A.—Licentiate in Medicine and Surgery Society of Apothecaries
L.Ps.—Licentiate in Psychiatry
L.R.C.P.—Licentiate, Royal College of Physicians
L.R.C.S.—Licentiate, Royal College of Surgeons
L.R.F.P.S.—Licent. of Royal Faculty of Physicians & Surgeons
M.A.A.G.P.—Member, American Academy of General Practice
M.A.A.P.—Member, American Assoc. of Physicians
M.A.B.I.M.—Member. American Board of Internal Medicine
M.A.B.R.—Member, American Board of Radiologists
M.A.C.H.A.—Member, American College of Hospital Administration
M.A.C.R.—Member, Australian College of Radiology
M.A.I.S.—Member Assoc. Industrial Surgeons
M.A.O.—Master, Art of Obstetrics
M.A.R.S.—Member Assoc. Railway Surgeons
M.B.—Bachelor of Medicine
M.C.A.A.—Member Can. Acad. Allergy
M.C.G.P.—Member of College of General Practice of Canada
M.Ch. Orth.—Master of Orthopaedic Surgery
M.C.N.S.—Member, Congress of Neurological Surgeons

CONTENTS

GENERAL

M.I.M.A.—Member, Industrial Medical Assoc.
M.M.S.A.—Member, Medical Specialists' Assoc.
M.P.H.—Master of Public Health
M.R.A.C.P.—Memb. Royal Australian College of Physicians
M.R.C.O.G.—Member, Royal College of Obstetricians and Gynaecologists
M.R.C.P.—Member, Royal College of Physicians
M.R.C.S.—Member, Royal College of Surgeons
M.R.S.H.—Member, Royal Society of Hygiene
M.S.—Master of Surgery
N.P.—Not Practising
Phm.B.—Bachelor of Pharmacy
Ph.D.—Doctor of Philosophy
P.&O.T.—Phys. & Occup. Therapy
T.D.D.—Tuberculosis Diseases, Diploma
T.T.C.—Toronto Transit Commission

APPOINTMENTS

Assoc.—Associate
Ass't.—Assistant
Att.—Attending
Chm.—Chairman
Clin.—Clinical
C.F.M.C.—Canadian Forces Medical Council
C.F.M.S.—Canadian Forces Medical Service
C.N.R.—Canadian National Railways
Comm.—Commission
Cons.—Consultant
C.O.—Commanding Officer
Court—Courtesy
C.P.R.—Canadian Pacific Railways
Dem.—Demonstrator
Dir.—Director
Dist.—District
D.M.S.—Director of Medical Services
D.V.A.—Department of Veterans Affairs
Edin.—Edinburgh
Extn.—Externe
Fell.—Fellow
Fr.—France
Gen. General
Germ.—Germany
Hon.—Honorary
Hosp.—Hospital
Hung.—Hungary
Ins.—Insurance
Intn.—Interne
Inst.—Institute
Instr.—Instructor
Ire.—Ireland
It.—Italy
Jr.—Junior
Lect.—Lecturer
Lit.—Lithuania
Mem.—Memorial
Mil.—Military
M.O.H.—Medical Officer of Health
Mun.—Municipal
M.P.—Member of Parliament
M.P.P.—Member of Provincial Parliament
M.H.O.—Medical Officer of Health
Neth.—Netherlands
O.P.D.—Outpatient Dept.
P.G.—Postgraduate
Phys.—Physician
Pres.—President
Prof.—Professor
Prov.—Provincial
P.S.I.—Physicians' Services, Inc.
Q.C.—Queen's Counsel
Q.H.P.—Queen's Honorary Physician
Q.H.S.—Queen's Honorary Surgeon
R.C.A.F.—Royal Can. Air Force
R.C.A.M.C.—Royal Can. Army Med. Corps
R.C.A.S.C.—Royal Canadian Army Service Corps
R.C.N.—Royal Can. Navy
(res)—Residence
Res.—Resident
San.—Sanitorium
S.Afr.—South Africa
Sec.—Secretary
Serv.—Service
Scot.—Scotland
Spec.—Specialist
Sr.—Senior
S.M.O.—Senior Medical Officer
Supt.—Superintendent
Switz.—Switzerland
T.C.A.—TransCanada Airlines
T.D.—Territorial Decoration
T.T.C.—Toronto Transit Commission
Twp.—Township
U.—University
Vis.—Visiting
Vol.—Voluntary
W.C.B.—Workmen's Compensation Board
W.H.O.—World Health Organization
W.M.A.—World Medical Association

CERTIFICATION

Certification by the Royal College of Physicians and Surgeons of Canada is shown as below. Certification by a provincial body is distinguished by the addition of the recognized abbreviation for that province, e.g., IntMed (P.Q.)—certified in internal medicine by the College of Physicians and Surgeons of the Province of Quebec.

A doctor certified nationally and provincially in one specialty is shown with the national symbol only. If he is so certified in different specialties, the provincial certification is shown first.

Anaesthesia
Bacteriology
Cardiovascular & Thoracic Surgery
Dermatology
General Surgery
Internal Medicine
Neurology
Neurosurgery
Obstetrics
Gynaecology
Obstetrics and Gynaecology
Ophthalmology
Otolaryngology
Orthopaedic Surgery
Paediatrics
Pathology
Physical Medicine & Rehabilitation
Psychiatry
Plastic Surgery
Public Health
Radiology — Diagnostic
Radiology — Therapeutic
Thoracic Surgery
Urology

CANADIAN MEDICAL DIRECTORY 1967

PHYSICIANS OF CANADA

The publishers of the Canadian Medical Directory make every effort to ensure accuracy, but they do not hold themselves responsible for any consequences that may arise from errors or omissions.

DECORATIONS AND MEDALS

A.F.C.—Air Force Cross
A.M.—Albert Medal (Gold)
B.E.M.—British Empire Medal
C.B.—Companion, Order of the Bath
C.B.E.—Commander, Order of British Empire
C.D.—Canadian Forces Decoration
C.H.—Companion of Honour
C.M.G.—Companion, Order of St. Michael and St. George
D.F.C.—Distinguished Flying Cross
D.S.C.—Distinguished Service Cross
D.S.O.—Distinguished Service Order
E.D.—Efficiency Decoration
G.B.E.—Knight Grand Cross, Order of British Empire
G.C.—George Cross
G.C.V.O.—Knight Grand Cross, Royal Victorian Order
G.M.—George Medal
K.B.E.—Knight Commander of British Empire
K.C.B.—Knight Commander, Order of Bath
K.St.J.—Knight Commander, Order of St. John of Jerusalem
M.B.E.—Member, Order of British Empire
M.C.—Military Cross
M.M.—Military Medal
O.B.E.—Officer, Order of the British Empire
O.M.—Order of Merit
Q.H.P.—Queen's Honorary Physician
Q.H.S.—Queen's Honorary Surgeon
V.C.—Victoria Cross
V.D.—Veteran's Decoration

BLUE PAGES

In the blue pages active civilian doctors are listed by province and town, and specialty is shown as applicable, using the abbreviations above. Interns, hospital residents and medical officers of the armed forces have been excluded from this list, but appear individually in the white pages.

BUFF PAGES

In these pages will be found lists of the medical officers of the armed forces (excluded from the blue pages) and the members of the 1965 classes in medicine at Canadian universities, excluded from the white and blue pages, as well as information about hospitals, health departments, universities, etc. At the back of this section is the Medical Journals' Guide, a handy index designed to aid in selecting current medical Journals.

PLEASE NOTE

- **that over 95% of doctors approved their own listings between March 1955 and December 1st, 1966.**
- **but that changes of address, etc., occurring thereafter have not been incorporated.**
- **and that in the next year at least 10,000 more changes will be made in the Directory records.**
- **so that the annual editions of the Directory will be necessary to provide an up-to-date reference source.**
- **The initials M.C.G.P. appearing in the alphabetic listings indicate membership in the College of General Practice.**
- **The alphabetic listing of M's, Mc's, Mac's follows procedure of the Bell Telephone Company — i.e. all names are listed in strictly alphabetic order, with no separate division of Mac's and Mc's.**

The preparation of the next edition of the Directory will be much simplified if doctors will notify all changes of address to the Canadian Medical Directory, Seccombe House, 443 Mount Pleasant Rd., Toronto 7, Canada.

Each doctor who can be contacted will be given the opportunity of revising his listing for the next edition.

AALL-JILEK, Louise M.; Zurich (Switz.) '58; Psy; Staff, Hop. St. Charles, Joliette, P.Q. Tel. 766-1681, Ext. 440.

AARON, Theodore H.; 221 Med. Arts Bldg., 11010 Jasper Ave., Edmonton, Alta.; Alb'42; FACP; FAAA; FCCP; IntMed; Lect. (Med.), U. of Alberta; Tel. 488-0141.

ABBATT, John D.; Edinburgh (Scot.) '45; DMRT(Ed.); Ass't. Chief, Rad. Protection Div., Dept. of National Health & Welfare, Brookfield Rd., Ottawa 8, Ont.

ABBE, Robert L.; Mon'51; D&TRad; Staff, Dept. of Rad., Hop. Gen. Fleury, Montreal 12, P.Q.

ABBOTT, A. Clifford; Abbott Clinic, 274 Osborne St. N., Winnipeg, Man.; 130 Handsart Blvd., Wpg. 29 (res); Man '21; FRCS(Edin.), FACS, FICS, FRCS(C), GenSurg; Urol; Cons. Surg. St. Boniface Hosp. & Dept. of Research, U. of Manitoba; Tel. 786-5481.

ABBOTT, Albert P.; Bristol (Eng.) '63; M.B., Ch.B.; Res., Child Guidance Clinic, Winnipeg, Man.

ABBOTT, Caroline M.; Dal'62; Staff, Ontario Hosp., 999 Queen St. W., Toronto, Ont.; Tel. LE 3-8501.

ABBOTT, C. Edward; Abbott Clinic, 274 Osborne St. N., Winnipeg, Man.; 283 Carpathia Rd. (res); Man '55; GenSurg; DABU; Active. Staff, (Urol), St. Boniface Hosp.; Dem. (Urol.), U. of Manitoba; Tel. 774-4567.

ABBOTT, Derrick; Sheffield (Eng.) '54; MC(Path); Hd., Div. of Haem., New Mount Sinai Hosp., Toronto, Ont.; Lect., Dept. of Path., U. of Toronto.

ABBOTT, E. Carl; Dal '59; FRCP(C), IntMed; Staff, Victoria Gen. Hosp., Halifax, N.S. Abroad.

ABBOTT, Edwin V.; Municipal Offices, 2001 Eglinton Ave. E., Scarborough, Ont.; Tor'49; DPH; Ass't. MOH, Scarborough Health Dept.; Tel. 759-4747.

ABBOTT, Mark O.; Man'64; Jr. Int., St. Boniface Hosp., St. Boniface, Man.

ABBOTT, Michael M.; 250 St. Clair W., Toronto 7, Ont.; Tor '51; FACP; FCCP; IntMed; Tel. WA 1-1592.

ABBOTT, Ronald T.; Assoc. Med. Clinic, The Pas, Man.; 727 **Taylor** Ave. (res); Glasgow (Scot.) '56; Staff, St. Anthony's Hosp.; Tel. 3-3291.

ABBOTT, S. Frank; 179 Dowling Ave., Toronto 3, Ont.; Wes '03, M.R.C.S.(E), L.R.C.P. (Lond.); Assoc. Staff Toronto Western Hosp.; Tel. LE 2-0263.

ABBOTT, William E.; Abbott Clinic, 274 Osborne St. N., Winnipeg 1, Man.; 536 Cordova St., Wpg. 9 (res); Man '56; DABOG; ObstGyn; Staff (ObstGyn), Wpg. Gen. & Grace Hosp's.; Dem., U. of Manitoba; Tel. SP 4-4567.

ABBOTT, William F.; Abbott Clinic Bldg., Winnipeg, Man.; 203 Grenfell Blvd., (res); Man '16; F.A.C.S.; ObstGyn.; Tel. SP 4-4567.

ABBOTT-SMITH, Charles W.; McG '63; Jr. Ass't. Res., Montreal Gen. Hosp., Montreal, P.Q.; Abroad.

ABEAR, Peter T.; London (Eng.)'54; Staff, c/o Regional Dir., European Reg., Dept. of National Health & Welfare, 38 Grosvenor St., London, W.1., England; Abroad.

ABEL, Robert B.; Birch Crescent, Kinghurst, **N.B. (res); McG'48; DAB (Path. Anat.); FASCP;** MCAP; Founding Memb., British College of Pathologists (M.C. Path); Pathol., Dir. of Labs., Lancaster Hosp., Lancaster, N.B.; Tel. 694-2651.

ABELL, Norman H.; House 32, 1400 Winding Trail, Cooksville, Ont.; Tor'56; FRCS(C), OrthSurg.

ABELSON, Stanley J.; 232 Metcalfe St., Ottawa, Ont.; 676 Highland (res); Ott '51; Psy; Att'd. Staff, Ottawa Civic Hosp.; Lectr., (ClinPsy), U. of Ottawa; Tel. CE 3-4009.

ABER, Samuel; 345 Sydney St., Cornwall, Ont.; McG '40; M.C.G.P.; Staff, Cornwall Gen. and Hotel Dieu Hosps.; Tel. WE 2-1623.

ABERHART, William R.; 303 Huron St., London, Ont.; Tor '27.

ABLENAS, Vytautas A.; 86 Division St., Kingsville, Ont.; 8 Spruce St. (res); Vytautas the **Great, (Lit.) '41; Tel. RE 3-4213.**

ABOU-SHABANAH, Elsayed H.; Edinburgh (Scot.)'42; FRCS, MRCOG; Staff, Royal Victoria Hospital, Montreal 2, P.Q.

ABRAHAM, Alexander J.; 227 N. Mitton St., Sarnia, Ont.; London (Eng.) '39 LRCP (Lond.), MRCS (Eng.), FRCS (Eng.), PlasSurg; OrthSurg; Chief of Surg., Sarnia Gen. Hosp.; Staff, St. Joseph's Hosp., & Sydenham & Dist. Hosp., Wallaceburg; Tel. ED 7-7125.

ABRAHAM, Guy; Mon '61; Res., Hop. Ste-Justine, Montreal 26, P.Q.

ABRAHAM, John A.; 500 Parliament St., Toronto, Ont.; 25 Brunswick Ave.; London (Eng.) '56; M.B., B.S., B.Pharm., ARIC; FRSH; Dir. of Personal Health & Physio., Doctor's Hosp.; Tel. WA 5-4381.

ABRAHAMS, Vivian; Edinburgh (Scot.) '52; Staff, Dept. of Physiol., Queen's U., Kingston, Ont.

ABRAM, August J.; Hemmingford, P.Q.; Mon '22.

ABRAMOVITCH, Henry; 4907 MacDonald Ave., Montreal 29, P.Q.; McG'56; IntMed.

ABRAMS, Marvin J.; 294 Bayview Plaza, Richmond Hill, Ont.; Tor '62.

ABRAMSON, Harry; Ste. 206, 262 Wilson Ave., Downsview, Ont.; Tor'54; IntMed; Research Assoc., New Mount Sinai Hosp., Toronto; Staff, North York Branson & Doctor's Hosp's.; Tel. ME 5-0148.

ACHESON, Hugh F.; 1132-100th St., North Battleford, Sask.; Edinburgh (Scot.)'50; Tel. 445-3706.

ACHESON, Thomas W.; Ste. 460, 2184 W. Broadway, Vancouver 9, B.C.; 4850 Fannin (res); Man '49; Tel. RE 1-6010.

ACHIM, Roland; 119 Green, St. Lambert, P.Q.; Mon '33.

ACHONG, Eamon H.; 4771 Lacombe Ave., Montreal 26, P.Q.; McG'60; Psy.

ACHPISE, Alexandre; 1438 rue MacKay, Montreal, P.Q.; Paris (France) '20; GenSurg; Phys., French Consulate; Tel. WE 7-4919.

ACKAD, Emile; Beyrouth (Lebanon) '44; Staff, Hop. St-Charles, Joliette, P.Q.

ACKER, John C. Sr.; 14 Med. Arts Bldg., 5880 Spring Garden Rd., Halifax, N.S.; 6913 Tupper Gr. (res); McG '23; OrthSurg; Chief OrthSurg., Children's Hosp.; Cons., OrthSurg., Victoria Gen., Grace Maternity & Rehabil. Centre; Assoc. Prof. (OrthSurg), Dalhousie U.; Tel. 423-6588.

ACKER, John C. Jr.; 371 Brunswick St., Fredericton, N.B.; Dal'65, AMCGP; Staff, Victoria Pub. Hosp.; Tel. 454-5220.

ACKER, Melvin I.; 5 Water St., St. Stephen, N. B.; Dal '48; IntMed; Anaes. Tel. 466-1695.

ACKER, Murray S.; Tor'43; DPH; PH; Staff, Clarke Inst. of Psy., 250 College St., Toronto 2B, Ont.

ACKER, Thomas B.; 14 Med. Arts Bldg., 5880 Spring Garden Rd., Halifax, N.S.; 108 Henry St. (res); Dal'21; OrthSurg; Cons. OrthSurg., Victoria Gen. Hosp.; Emer. Prof. (OrthSurg.), Dalhousie U.; Tel. 423-6588.

ACKMAN, Charles F. D.; 4690 Westmount Ave., Westmount 6, P.Q.; '61; Urol (P.Q.).

ACKMAN, F. Douglas, C. D.; 600 Seaforth Med. Bldg., 3550 Cote des Neiges Rd., Montreal 25, P.Q.; 4690 Westmount Ave., Westmount (res); McG'23; FACS; FRCS(C); GenSurg; ThorSurg (P.Q.); Hon. Att'd, Surg., Montreal Gen. & Royal Edward Chest Hosp.; Chief Surgeon, Grace Dart Hosp.; Tel. 932-7241.

ACRES, Stanley E.; 57 Birch Ave., Ottawa 7, Ont. (res); Qns '57; DPH; M.O., Epidemiology Div., Dept. Nat. Health & Welfare; Tel 992-6868.

ACTON, William C.; Provost Medical Centre, Provost, Alb.; Alb '44; M.C.G.P.

ADAIR, Ross K.; McG '64; Res., Montreal Gen. Hosp., Montreal, P.Q.

ADAM, Baker H.; Box 937, Beausejour Clinic, Beausejour, Man.; Ankara (Turkey)'53.

ADAM, John E.; Ste. 301, 267 O'Connor St., Ottawa 4, Ont.; Qns'61; FRCP(C), Derm.

ADAM, Kenneth S.; Tor'61; Res., Allan Mem. Inst., Montreal 2, P.Q.

ADAM, Robert A.; Lav'65; Res., Hop., Hotel-Dieu, Quebec, P.Q.

ADAMKIEWICZ, Lidia M. (Gowor); 5507 Cote St. Antoine, Montreal 28, P.Q.; Lausanne (Switz.) '47; IntMed (P.Q.); Tel. HU 8-4163.

ADAMS, Arthur R. F.; The Glades, N.B.; R.C.P. &S (Dublin, Ire.) '37; Ass't. Supt., Jordan Mem. San.; M.O., Dept. of Health, N.B.; Tel. 756-3355.

ADAMS, **Barrett R.**; 164 Metcalfe St., Ottawa, Ont.; Ott'59; Paed; Staff, Ottawa Gen. Hosp. Tel. CE 6-0333.

ADAMS, Carl R.; 527 Admiral St., Woodstock, Ont.; Dal '44; FIAP; GenSurg; Staff, Woodstock Gen. Hosp.; Tel. 537-7921.

ADAMS, **Douglas G.**; 4772 Spring Rd., Victoria, B.C.; McG '52; Tel. EV 2-9464.

ADAMS, **Grenfell**; McG '64; Res., Royal Victoria Hosp., Montreal 2, P.Q.

ADAMS, G. T.; McG '31; DiagRad; Dir. Radiology, Dept. Veterans Affairs, Queen Mary Vet. Hosp., Montreal 26, P.Q.; Tel. RE 8-9481.

ADAMS, **James F.**; Med. Arts Bldg., 1011 Ouellette Ave., Windsor, Ont.; 1929 Ontario St., Walkerville (res); Tor '17; L.R.C.P. (Lond.), M.R.C.S.(Eng.), GenSurg; Surg Cons., Grace Hosp.; Tel. CL 4-1222.

ADAMS, **John W.**; 904A Cavalier Towers, Saskatoon, Sask. (res); **Tor '39; Path; Ass't. Pathol., University Hosp.; Prof. Path., U. of Saskatchewan; Tel. CH 2-7641; CH 2-7671.**

ADAMS, Kenneth M.; 115 Lower Union St., Kingston, Ont.; 25 Copperfield Dr. (res); Qns '54; Preceptor Dept. of Prev. Med., Queen's U.; Med. Examiner ALCAN, Kingston; Tel. 542-5088.

ADAMS, **Kenneth W.**; 402 Metro, Pointe Claire, P.Q.; Wes'55; Ophth; Teach. Fell., Mtl. Children's Hosp.; Att'd. Staff, Lakeshore Gen. Hosp.; Clin. Ass't. Retina Clin., Mtl. Gen. Hosp.; Tel. 695-3866.

ADAMS, **Leyland J.**; Ste 212, 1414 Drummond, Montreal 24, P.Q.; 612 Victoria Ave. (res); McG '27; F.A.C.P., F.R.C.P.(C), IntMed; Assoc. Phys. **Montreal Gen. Hosp.; Tel. VI 2-1523.**

ADAMS, Michael B.; 1208 Main St. E., Hamilton, Ont.; Qns '37; M.C.G.P.; Tel. LI 4-9151.

ADAMS, **Myles D.**; Kerrobert Clinic, Kerrobert, Sask.; Univ. Coll. (Dublin, Ire.) '52; MAO; DRCOG; Tel. 834-2412.

ADAMS, **Paul V. C.**; 526 Med. Arts Bldg., 404-406 Graham Ave., Winnipeg 1, Man.; Man '52; FRCS(C), ObstGyn; Active Teach. Staff, St. Boniface & Misericordia Hosp's.; Clin. Tutor (Med.), U. of Manitoba; Tel. WH 3-5416.

ADAMS, Ralph E.; 924 McClune, Victoria B. C.; U. of Oregon (U.S.A.) '56; Med. Dir., St. Joseph's Hosp.; Tel. 384-1131.

ADAMS, **Samuel T.**; Room 269, Mtl. Gen. Hosp., Montreal 25, P.Q.; McG'42; DABO; Ophth; Dir., **Dept. of Ophth, Montreal Gen. & Children's Hosp's; Ass't. Prof. (Ophth), McGill U. Tel. WE 2-3026.**

ADAMS, Winston E.; National Univ. (Ireland) '52; M. B., B.CH.; B.A.O.; D.C.H.; L.M., (Dublin); D.P.H; Davson Silver & Gold Medalist for Medical Research, Whitewood, Sask.

ADAMSON, **David H.**; Edinburgh (Scot.)'52; Res., Westminster Hosp., London, Ont.

ADAMSON, **David P.**; 379 Bendamere Ave., Hamilton, Ont.; London (Eng.) '53.

ADAMSON, Donald N.; 12918-127th St., Edmonton, Alta.; 11524-135th St. (res); Alb '51; MCGP; Active Staff, Royal Alexandra Hosp.; Tel. GL 5-1616.

ADAMSON, Douglas L.; 312 Medical Arts Bldg., Hamilton, Ont.; 69 Amelia St. (res); Tor '32; F.A.C.O.G.; F.I.C.S., F.R.C.S.; ObstGyn; Staff, (ObstGyn), Hamilton Civic Hosp's; Tel. JA 2-0444.

ADAMSON, Gilbert L.; Winnipeg Clinic, Winnipeg 1, Man.; 727 South Dr., Wpg. 9 (res); Man '21; F.R.C.P. (Edin.), F.R.C.P.(C), NeurPsy; Neur. & Assoc. Psy., Winnipeg Gen. Hosp.; Cons. (Psy.), RCAF; Assoc. Prof. (Emer.), U. of Manitoba; Tel. 942-0551.

ADAMSON, James W.; Shaunavon Clinic, Shaunavon, Sask.; Edinburgh (Scot.) '54; Staff, Shaunavon Union Hosp.; District Coroner; Aviation Med. Examiner; Tel. 297-2625.

ADAMSON, John D.; 110 Med. College, Bannatyne & Emily, Winnipeg 3, Man.; 367 Oak St. Wpg. 9 (res); Man '56 FRCP(C), Psy; Staff, Winnipeg Gen. Hosp., Ass't. Prof., (Psy.), U. of Manitoba; Co-ordinator Psy Research. Prov. of Man.; Tel. 786-3645.

ADAMSON, Morris C.; Man '17; Staff, University Hosp., Edmonton, Alta.

ADDERLEY, Francis G.; 799A Brimley Rd., **Scarborough, Ont.**; 56 Rossander Ct. (res); **Qns '52; M.C.G.P.; Active Staff, Scarborough Gen. Hosp.; Assoc. Staff, Toronto East Gen.** Hosp. Tel. 261-6171

ADDISON, David J.; Edinburgh (Scot.)'64; Res., Ottawa Gen. Hosp., Ottawa, Ont.

ADDISON, Joseph A.; Box 130, 140 Townsend St., Clinton, Ont.; Wes'37; MCGP; Tel. 482-9694.

ADDLEMAN, William; 1390 Sherbrooke St. W., **Montreal 25, P.Q., 5 Severn (res); McG '27; IntMed; Gastroent. (P.Q.); Chief (Gastroent.),** Jewish Gen. Hosp.; Tel. VI 2-5994.

ADELBERG, Jacob L.; 749 King St. W., Kitchener, Ont.; Tor '53.

ADELMAN, Allan G.; Tor'61; Res., Toronto Gen. Hosp., Toronto 2, Ont.

ADELMAN, David A.; Man '62; Jr. Intn., Winnipeg Gen. Hosp., Winnipeg 3, Man.

ADEVOSO, Lauro L.; Santo Thomas, (Philip), '54, Jr. Intn., Royal Alexandra Hosp., Edmonton, Alta.

ADEY, Andrew B.; Atikokan Clinic, 123 Marks, Atikokan, Ont.; 120 Willow Rd. (res); Man '45; M.C.G.P.; Tel. 2721.

ADHIKARI, Kiran C.; Medical Arts Clinic, Regina, Sask.; Assam Med. Coll. (India)'54; IntMed.

ADHIKARI, Prasant; Calcutta (India) '52; MRCP (Edin); FRCP(C), IntMed; Staff, Children's Hosp., Winnipeg, Man.; Ass't. Prof., U. of Manitoba; Tel. SP 5-8311.

ADILMAN, Bernard; Alb '45; Path; Pathol., St. Thomas Elgin General Hosp., St. Thomas, Ont.; Tel. ME 1-2020.

ADILMAN, Philip H.; 1175 Denman St., Vancouver, B.C.; **5650 Heather St.** (res); Sask '59; **MCGP; Vis. Staff, Vancouver Gen., St. Paul's Grace & Children's Hosp.; Tel. MU 5-0161.**

ADLER, Allan; Qns'65; Res., Douglas Hosp., Montreal 19, P.Q.

ADLER, Herbert G.; 520-17th St., West Vancouver, B.C.; Man '57; Psy; Staff (Psy.), Provincial Mental Hosp., Essondale; Tel. 926-1717.

ADLER, Kay; 2621 Hastings, Vancouver 6, B.C.; Apt. 203, 1025 W. 13th Ave. (res); Belgrade (Yugoslavia) '38; Tel. AL 3-1636.

ADLER, Kurt; Chinook Health Clinic, Fort MacLeod, Alta.; Dublin (Ire.) '47; DPH; M.O.H. & Dir., Chinook Health Clinic; Advisor, Public Health, Pincher Creek Hosp., Claresholm Hosp. & Crow's Nest Pass Hosp.; Tel. 234-3588.

ADLER, Oscar J.; Ste. 209, 280 Bloor St. W., Toronto 5, Ont.; Budapest (Hung.)'52; MCGP; Court. Staff, New Mount Sinai Hosp.; Tel. EM 6-7361.

ADLER, William; 168 Oakwood Ave., Toronto 10, Ont.; 460 Winona (res); Budapest (Hung.) '52; Tel. LE 1-6897.

ADOLPH, Inge S.; 791 Albion Rd., Rexdale, Ont. (res); Germ '49; Staff, Dept. of Health, Toronto. Tel. EM 3-1211.

ADOLPH, Jack; 421-15th St. N.E., Swift Current, Sask.; **Alb '55; Path; Staff, Swift Current** Union Hosp.; Tel. 773-4641.

ADRIAN, **Alfred**; 755 W. Broadway, Vancouver 9, B. C.; **Man '57; MCGP; Tel 738-5512.**

ADRIAN, John J.; 755 W. Broadway, Vancouver 9, B. C.; 2237-W. 33rd (res); UBC '54; MCGP; Tel. TR 2-2558.

ADSETT, C. Alexander; 5205 Byron Rd., Oklahoma City, Okla, U.S.A.; Wes '54; FRCP (C); IntMed; Psy; Ass't. Prof. (Med & Psychiatry), Univ. of Oklahoma; Abroad.

AEBERLI, E. W.; Department of National Health & Welfare, c/o Regional Superintendent, European Region. Abroad.

AERICHIDE, Nicholas; 1431 McKay, Montreal, P.Q. (res); Paris (Fr.) '53; IntMed (Cardiol.) (P.Q.); Staff, Inst. of Cardiol.

AFAGANIS, Harry E.; 721 Fairfax Apts., 43rd & Locust, Philadelphia, Pa., U.S.A.; Alb'61; Otol.

AFRUKHTEH, Djamal; 837 Valley Way, Niagara Falls, Ont.; Germany '56; D.Pharm (Teheran); Tel. 354-1211.

AFTAHI, Farhang; Med. Arts Clinic, 2125-11th Ave., Regina, Sask.; Teheran U. (Iran) '55; AAP; Paed; Staff, Regina Gen. & Grey Nuns Hosp's.; Tel. 523-0691.

AGARWALA, Vinod K.; Lucknow (India) '61; Res., Ottawa Gen. Hosp., Ottawa, Ont.

AGBEBIYI, Adeyinka B.; London (Eng.)'64; Staff, Dept. of Anat., U. of Toronto, Toronto, Ont.

AGELOPOULOS, Theodor; Qns'64; Res., Toronto East Gen. Hosp., Toronto 6, Ont.

AGNEW, Glenn A.; Ste. 350, 5780 Cambie St., Vancouver 15, B.C.; Alb '43; MCGP; Tel. TR 4-0641.

AGNEW, G. Harvey; 44 Jackes Ave., Toronto 7, Ont.; Tor'18; FACP; LLD; FACHA; Prof. (Emer.), Hosp. Admin., U. of Toronto; N.I.P.

AGNEW, Terence J.; 208-1669 Victoria St., Prince George, B.C.; 675 Patricia Blvd. (res); Alb. '28.

AGNOS, John W.; 230 Richmond St., London, Ont.; Wes '52; DMR; DABM; DABR; DiagRad; Radiol, Westminster Hosp.; Lect. (Rad.), U. of Western Ont.; Tel. GE 2-6711.

AGRAS, W. Stewart; 4052 Grey Ave., Montreal 28, P.Q. (res); London (Eng.) '55; Psy; Staff, **Montreal Gen. Hosp.; Tel. WE 7-6011.**

AGRO, Charles F.; 78 Barton St. W., Hamilton, Ont.; 401 Hess St. S. (res); Qns'41; MCGP; Staff, St. Joseph's & Gen. Hosp's.; Tel. JA 2-4632.

AGUAYO, Alberto J.; Cardoba (Argentine) '59; FRCP(C) Neur; Staff, Montreal Gen. Hosp., Montreal 25, P.Q.; Tel. 937-6011.

AGUIRRE-FERRO, Jose; 92 Woodland Ave., St. Catharines, Ont.; Granada (Spain) '51; Tel. 684-7329.

AGUZZI, Gastone; 600 Caledonia Rd., Toronto 10, Ont;. Florence (Italy) '53; Tel. 783-5929.

AHAD, Victor; 1259 B. Est. St. Zotique, Montreal 35, P.Q.; Cairo (Egypt)'56.

AHIER, Alexandre; 287 St. Jerome, Matane, P.Q.; Lav '35; OphthOtol (P.Q.); Tel. 562-0282.

AHMAD, Salaruddin; Kettle Valley Clinic, Grand Forks, B.C.; Patna (India) '55.

AHMAD, Shafi; Patna (India)'56; Staff, Riverview Hosp., Essondale, B.C.

AHMED, M. Nisar; '55; Res. Royal Victoria Hosp., Montreal 2, P.Q.

AHSAN, Amir; 208 Edmonton St., Winnipeg 2, Man.; Dacca (E. Pakistan) '56; OrthSurg; Cons. Staff, Deer Lodge Hosp.; Tel. 942-6391.

AHUJA, Suraj P.; Nagpur (India)'56; DTM&H (Eng.); Staff, Victoria Hosp., London, Ont.; Cardiac Cons., Westminster Hosp.; Sr. Research Fell., Ont. Heart Fdn.; Instr., U. of Western Ont.; Tel. 432-5261, Loc. 287.

AICHROTH, Paul M.; Val Marie, Sask.; London U. (Westminster H.) '59.

AIDUN, Jamshid S.; The Brandon Clinic, P.O. Box 280, Brandon, Man.; Karachi (Pakistan)'57; Dip. Surg.; Urol; Att'd. Staff, Brandon Gen. & Assiniboine Hosp's.; Tel. PA 9-6444.

AIELLO, Albert L.: Box 560, 135—3rd Ave. W., Drumheller, Alta.; 435—4th Ave. W. (res); Alb 36; Anaes.; Tel. 823-3345.

AIELLO, Emil; C.N.P. Clinic, Blairmore, Alta.; Alb'35; Tel. 562-2243.

AIKEN, David A.; 2011 Victoria Pk. Ave., Scarborough, Ont.; Ire'52; A.M.C.G.P.; Abroad.

AIKEN, Joseph B.; 205 Medical Centre, 8th Ave. & 8th St. S.W., Calgary, Alta.; 620 Crescent Blvd. S.W. (res); Tor '33; IntMed.; Med. Dir. Western Co-op., Fertilizer Co.; Tel. 263-3764.

AIKENHEAD, David C.; 5088 Lakeshore Rd. E., R.R. 2, Burlington, Ont. (res); Man '16; FRCP (C); Anaes; Retired.

AIKENHEAD, David E.; Victoria Med. Centre, 111 Waterloo St., London, Ont.; Man'46; MRCP (Lond.); FRCP(C), IntMed; Staff, Victoria Hosp.; Cons. (Med.), Westminster Hosp.; Instr. (Med.), U. of Western Ontario; Tel. 432-9102.

AIKENHEAD, Donald H.; Box 28, Milton, Ont; UBC'55; MCGP; Tel. 3-2702.

AIKENHEAD, John F.; 214-6th Ave., S.W., Calgary, Alta.; Alb'43; OphthOtol; Cons., Col. Belcher D.V.A. Hosp.; Tel. AM 3-7120.

AIKENHEAD, J. William; 232 Indian Rd., Toronto, Ont.; 2 High Park Gdns. (res); Wes '13; M C.G.P.; Tel. RO 6-1414.

AIKENS, Helen B.; Lincoln Co. Health Unit, Box 13, 23 Centre St., St. Catharines, Ont.; Tor'44.

AIKENS, Robert L.; Med. Arts Bldg., 5880 Spring Garden Rd., Halifax, N.S.; 1050 Bellevue Ave. (res); Dal '39; FRCP(C), FCCP; IntMed; Cons. Phys., Camp Hill, Grace & Cd'n. Forces Hosp's; Assoc. Prof. (Med.), Dalhousie U.; Tel. 423-8843.

AIKINS, Joseph A.; Medical Arts Bldg., 121 Wellington St. W., Barrie, Ont.; McG '52; Tel. 728-2618.

AINLIE, William E.; 1865 Barclay St., Vancouver, B C. (res); McG '04; OphthOtol; Retired.

AINSCOUGH, G. Alan; 501 Hunt Bldg., Lethbridge, Alta.; 1103—13 St. S. (res); Alb '54; Assoc. Staff, St. Michael's & Lethbridge Mun. Hosp's; Tel. 327-3184.

AINSLIE, Everett H.; 35 Morewood Cr., Willowdale, Ont. (res); Wes '33; M.Sc.; DIM; DA (Eng.); FRCP (C); Anaes; IntMed; Hd. of Serv. Chron. Treatment, Sunnybrook Hosp., Toronto; Tel. 485-8651.

AINSLIE, James D.; Private Phys., Ste. 3, 825 Coxwell Ave., Toronto, Ont.; Tor'55; FRCS(C); GenSurg; Urol; Staff, Hosp. for Sick Children; Tel. 461-1537.

AINSLIE, Robert D, 2933 Lundy's Lane, Niagara Falls, Ont.; Tor '54; M.C.G.P.; Staff, Greater **Niagara Gen. Hosp.; Tel. EL 6-2229.**

AINSLIE, Wm. H.; 2933 Lundy's Lane, Niagara Ont.; 2954 Lundy's Lane (res); Tor '54 DABS; FICS; FRCS(C), GenSurg; Staff, Gtr. Niag. Gen. Hosp.; Tel. EL 6-2220.

AIRD, Georges; Mon '63; Int., Inst. Albert-Prevost, Montreal, P.Q.; Abroad.

AIRLIE-BROWN, Thomas (see Brown, T. Airlie)

AITCHISON, David B.; Box 590, Hamilton Health Assoc., Hamilton, Ont.; R.R. No. 1., Jerseyville (res); Tor '24; FACCP; FICS; GenSurg; Tel. 385-5341.

AITCHISON, William S.; Apt. 303, 2313 Lakeshore Blvd. W., Toronto 14, Ont. (res); Tor '18; PH; M. O. H., Village of Swansea, Toronto 3.

AITKEN, Donald M.; 150 St. George St., Toronto 5, Ont.; Dal'61; Ass't. Sec., C.M.A.; Tel. 924-0751.

AITKEN, Donald W.; 452 Charlotte St., Peterborough, Ont.; 475 Gilmour St. (res); Tor'42; Anaes; Tel. RI 5-2491.

AITKEN, Elizabeth H. P. (Johnson); 283 Queen's Ave., London, Ont.; Man '46; Anaes; Court. Staff, Victoria & St. Joseph's Hosp's.; Tel. 438-5143.

AITKEN, George W.A.; 414 Wortley Rd., London, Ont.; Wes '14; Anaes.; Retired.

AITKEN, Harold E.; No. 8 Highway, Winona, Ont.; McG '55; MCGP; Tel. 643-1755.

AITKEN, James A.; 2564 Lake Shore Blvd. W. Toronto 14, Ont.; 41 Lakeshore Rd. (res); Glasgow (Scot.) '47; Tel. 251-0991.

AITKEN, Ronald R.; 287 Queen's Ave., London, Ont.; Wes '43; Anaes; Ass't. Clin. Prof. (Anaes.), U. of Western Ontario; Teach. Staff, Victoria Hosp.; Tel. 438-5143.

AIYEDE, Adebayo O.; 291 King St., Powassan, Ont.; Man'60; Court. Staff, North Bay Civic Hosp. & St. Joseph's Hosp., North Bay; Tel. 724-2734.

AKHTAR, Syer N.; 8 Rodney Rd., Dartmouth, N.S.; Punjab (India)'59.

AKIN, Frederick L.; 5 Clifton Ave., Windsor, N.S.; Dal '45; MCGP; Staff, Payzant Mem. Hosp; MOH; Tel. 798-2234.

AKINS, Keith B.; 714 Fairmont Med. Bldg., 750 W. Broadway, Vancouver 9, B.C.; Qns '57; ABNP; Psy; Cons., Children's Fdn.; Att'd. Staff, Vancouver Gen. Hosp.; Clin. Instr. (Psy.), U. of British Columbia; Tel. 874-2523.

AKKERMAN, Otto S.; Box 788, 575 Queen St., Chatham, Ont.; Utrecht (Neth.)'50; Vice Consul of the Netherlands; Tel. 352-1250.

AKRIOTIS, Dimitrios J.; Ste. 110, 400 Walmer Rd., Toronto 10, Ont.; Athens (Greece) '39; Staff, Doctor's Hosp.

ALABY, Antoine G.; 415 Ste Helene, Longueuil, P.Q.; Cairo (Egypt)'49; Otol.

ALARIE, Roger; 3423 rue St.-Denis, Montreal, 18, P.Q.; 7200 des Erables (res); Lille (Fr.) '54; Tel. VI 2-4892.

ALARIE, Sylva; 635-20E rue, Charny, P.Q.; Lav'64.

ALATON, Aneta; Istanbul (Turk.) '48; Staff, **Princess Margaret Hosp., Toronto 5, Ont.**

ALATON, Isak; Ste. 307, 2045 Dufferin St., Toronto 10, Ont.; Istanbul (Turk)'48; **Ophth**; Tel. 651-1210.

ALBELDA, Jose L. S.; Valencia (Spain)'58; ObstGyn; Staff, Women's College Hosp., Toronto 5, Ont.

ALBERGA, Vincent H.; Tor '58; AMCGP; Jr. Ass't. Res. (Ophth), Montreal Gen. Hosp., Montreal, P. Q.

ALBERS, Henry J.; 450 Central Ave., London, Ont.; Dusseldorf (Germ.)'58; Derm; Tel. 432-3968.

ALBERT, Darius J.; 25 Canada Rd., Edmundston, N.B. (res); Lav '40; D&T Rad; Staff, Hotel Dieu Hosp.; Tel. RE 5-3361.

ALBERT, Guy; Lav'62; IntMed; Staff, Hop. Hotel Dieu, Gaspé, P.Q.

ALBERT, Jean; 1185 rue Hart, Trois Rivieres, P.Q.; Lav '58; Anaes; Staff, Hop. Ste-Marie; Tel. FR 5-7191.

ALBERT, John R.; 780 Lakeshore Dr., Dorval, P.Q. (res); Brussels (Belg.) '51; DIM; IntMed; Haematol, (P.Q.); Att'd. Staff, Lachine Gen. & Lakeshore Gen. Hosp's.; Cons. (Haem.), DVA Hosp., Ste-Anne-de-Bellevue; Tel. 631-9687.

ALBERT, Moss; 428 Professional Bldg., 10830 Jasper Ave., Edmonton, Alta.; 14011-88th Ave. (res); London (Eng.) '37; LRCP, MRCS; FRCS (Eng.), FRCS(C), OrthSurg; Staff, Misericordia & Glenrose Prov. Gen. Hosp.; Tel. 429-1144.

ALBERT, Philippe; 3999 Montee St.-Hubert, St.-Hubert, P. Q.; Mon '42.

ALBERT, Roland; Lav'65; Res., Hop. St. Francis d'Assise, Quebec 3, P.Q.

ALBERT-GRAVEL, Colette Y.; **605, boul. Leblanc, Duvernay, Laval-des-Rapides, P. Q.; Lav** '62; Tel. 677-1828.

ALBERTON, Rina M. (See D'Amico, Rina M.)

ALBERTS, Johannes J.; Cannon Clinic, McCallum Rd., Abbotsford, B.C.; Fraser St. (res); **Groningen (Neth.) '35; Tel. 853-2291.**

ALBERTSON, David B.; 501 Kerr Bldg., 1864 Scarth St., Regina, Sask.; 241 Leopold Cres. (res); Tor '41; NeurSurg; Chief, Dept. Neur. Surg., Regina Gen. & Regina Grey Nuns' Hosp's.; Cons. (NeurSurg), Sask. Cancer Comm. & Regina D.V.A.; Tel. 523-0320.

ALBERTSON, Mary E.; (Mrs. H. M. Saul); 930 Med. Arts Bldg., 170 St. George St., Toronto 5, Ont.; Tor '38; Ophth; Chief of Ophth., Women's College & St. Joseph's Hosp's.; Tel. WA 3-7467.

ALBI, Frank; St. Boniface Clinic, 343 Tache Ave., St. Boniface, Man.; Man '58; MCGP; Tel. WH 7-1581.

ALBI, Wilfred N.; 343 Tache Ave., St. Boniface, Man.; 111 Eastgate, Wpg. (res); Ott '51; MCGP; Court. Staff, St. Boniface Hosp.; Tel. WH 7-1581.

ALCANTARA, Eladio N.; Manila (Philipp.)'54; Path; Staff, Regional Lab., Campbellton, N.B.

ALCINDOR, J. A.; Haiti '58; FRCP(C), Path; Staff, Hop. St. Joseph de Rosemont, Montreal, P.Q.; Tel. 256-2681.

ALCOCK, A. John; Winnipeg Municipal Hosp's., Winnipeg 13, Man.; 297 Overdale, St. James 12 (res); **Man '45; IntMed; Med. Dir., Wpg.** Mun. Hosp.; Tel. 452-3411.

ALCORN, Douglas E.; Ste. 325-327, 645 Fort St., Victoria, B.C.; McG '31; FAPA; FAGS; FAAAS; NeurPsy; Lect., Royal Jubilee Hosp., School of Nursing, Hollywood San., Queen Alexandra Solarium, Veteran's Hosp. & U. of Victoria; Tel. 382-3236.

ALDERMAN, Philip M.; 2906 Westlynn Shopping Centre, North Vancouver, B.C.; 2140 Grand Blvd. (res); Tor '53; Tel. YU 8-4744.

ALDERTON, Harvey R.; 22 Everingham Ct., Willowdale, Ont. (res); London(Eng.) '50; D.P.M.; Psy; Clin. Dir., Thistletown Hosp.; Assoc. Psy., U. of Toronto; Tel. 741-1210.

ALDIS, John S. W.; Wes'50; MCGP; Exec. Dir., Ontario Med. Serv. Insurance Div., 135 St. Clair Ave. W., Toronto 7, Ont.; Tel. 365-5506.

ALDIS, Pamela W.; Med. Clinic, 710 Seymour St., Vancouver 2, B.C.; London (Eng.)'63; MRCS; LRCP; Tel. MU 4-1511.

ALDIS, Robert M.; 24 St. Andrew St., Stratford, Ont.; Wes'45; DPH; Dir. & M.O.H., Perth Co. Health Unit; Cons. Staff, Stratford Gen. & Listowel Mem. Hosp's.; Tel. 271-7600.

ALDOUS, N. Ronald; 1024 Med. Arts Bldg., 1538 Sherbrooke St. W., Montreal 25, P. Q.; Qns '57; Psy; Clin. Ass't. (O.P.D.), Dept. of Psy., Mtl. Gen. Hosp.; Lect. (Psy.), McGill U.; Tel. 935-8004.

ALDRIDGE, Douglas; 235 Church St., Oakville, Ont.; Sheffield (Eng.)'55; FRCS (C), GenSurg; Cons., Oakville-Trafalgar Mem. Hosp.; Tel. 845-3614.

ALDRIDGE, Harold E.; 101 College St., Toronto **2, Ont.; 16 Malabar Pl., Don Mills (res)**; London **(Eng) '54; M.B., B.S. (Lond.); IntMed; Staff** Phys., Toronto Gen. Hosp.; Clin. Teach., U. of Toronto; Tel. EM 6-8211.

ALEIXANDRE, Luis E.; 995 Queen St. E., Sault Ste. Marie, Ont.; Valencia (Spain) '56; MCGP; Officer in Charge of Treaty Indians.

ALEWICK, N. A.; 920 Ouellette Ave., Windsor, Ont.; Wes '40; Tel. 254-6977.

ALEXANDER, Angus F.; Grand Falls Clin., Grand Falls, Nfld.; 37 Carmelite Rd. (res); Edinburgh (Scot.) '42; FRCS(E); Assoc. Chief (Surg.), Central Nfld. Hosp.; Vis. Cons. Surg., Springdale Hosp. & M. J. Boylen Hosp., Baie Verte; Tel. 2185.

ALEXANDER, Benjamin; 919 Medical Arts Bldg., 1538 Sherbrooke St. W., Montreal, P.Q.; 1606 Seaforth Ave. (res); McG '25; D.O.M.S. (Eng), Ophth; Ophth. in Chief, Montreal Gen. Hosp.; Cons. (Ophth.), Montreal Children's Hosp.; Assoc. Prof. Ophth., McGill U.; Tel. WE 5-3688.

ALEXANDER, Charles J.; Dal '50; Staff (Path), Saint John Gen. Hosp., Saint John, N.B.; Tel. 693-3351.

ALEXANDER, David S.; 221 King St. E., Kingston, Ont.; 12 Jorene Dr. (res); Edinburgh (Scot.); '50; M.B., Ch. B.; Paed; Att'd. Staff (Paed.), Kingston Gen. Hosp.; Lect. (Paed.), Queen's U.; Tel. 542-2677.

ALEXANDER, E. H.; 2890 Pt. Grey, Vancouver, B.C.; Ophth, Otol; Clin. Instr. (Otol.), U. of British Columbia; Retired.

ALEXANDER, Eileen; 52 Regent St., Welland, Ont.; Ott'65; Assoc. Staff (G.P.), Welland County Gen. Hosp.

ALEXANDER, H. Douglas; 135 St. Clair Ave. W., Toronto 5, Ont.; Tor'35; FACS; Gen Surg; Obst Gyn; Med. Cons., Ont. Med. Serv. Ins. Plan; Tel. 365-5557.

ALEXANDER, Howard J.; 5 Ridout St. E., Tillsonburg, Ont.; 11 Concession St. E. (res); Tor '25; MCGP; Coroner, Oxford Co.; Tel. VI 2-4231.

ALEXANDER, Hugh J.; The Medical Clinic, 3009-31st. Ave., Vernon, B.C.; 2501-23rd Ave., (res.); McG. '35; Gen. Surg.; Tel. 542-4321.

ALEXANDER, James F.; McG'63; Res., Montreal Gen. Hosp., Montreal, P.Q.; Abroad.

ALEXANDER, John C.; 331 Sheddon Ave., Oakville, Ont.; Tor'58; Ophth; Active Cons., Oakville-Trafalgar Mem. Hosp. & Joseph Brant Hosp., Burlington; Tel. 845-7841.

ALEXANDER, John D. F.; Ste. 305, 1701 West 9th Ave., Vancouver 9, B.C.; 1519 West 35th (res); McG '34; F.R.C.S.(C), GenSurg; Att'd. Staff, Vancouver Gen. Hosp.; Vis. Staff, St. Paul's & Children's Hosp's.; Clin. Instr. (Surg.), U. of British Columbia; Tel. RE 3-3133.

ALEXANDER, John F.; Sask'65; Res., Ste. 311, University of Alberta Hosp., Edmonton, Alta.

ALEXANDER, Joseph F.; Dublin (Ireland) '50; BAO; Staff, Brandon Mental Hosp., Brandon, Man.; Tel. PA 6-2321.
ALEXANDER, Laurence G.; 203 Fitzpatrick Bldg., Calgary, Alta.; 1306 Scotland St. (res); Man '25; M.C.G.P.; Retired.
ALEXANDER, Marilyn G.; Wes '60; Jr. Int'n., Vancouver Gen. Hosp., Vancouver 9, B.C.
ALEXANDER, Nancy; Wes'54; Res., Addiction Research Fdn., 477 Waterloo St., London, Ont.
ALEXANDER, N. E.; 201 CNR Bldg., Edmonton, **Alta.; 10955-85th Ave. (res); Alb '29; GenSurg; Hon. Staff (Surg.), U. of Alberta; Tel 422-4880.**
ALEXANDER, Robert L.; Tor'61; Ophth; Staff, Toronto Western Hosp., Toronto 2B, Ont.
ALEXANDER, Sara K. (Mitchell); Medical Arts **Bldg., Oakville, Ont.; 163 Dianne Dr. (res); Dublin (Ire.) '50; BAO; Tel. VI 4-2381.**
ALEXANDER, Walter; 206 Medical Arts Bldg., Winnipeg 1, Man.; 150 Oak St. (res); Man '38; D.A.B.O., OphthOtol; **Head (Otol.), Winnipeg Gen. Hosp.; Chm. (Otol.), U. of Manitoba; Tel. WH 2-3864.**
ALEXANDER, **Walter J.;** McG '60 FRCP(C), DiagRad; Staff, Dept. of Rad., Montreal Children's Hosp., Montreal 25, P.Q.; Tel. 937-8511, Loc. 255.
ALEXANDER, **William H.;** Man '49; Diag Rad; Dir., Dept. of Rad., Trenton Mem. Hosp., Trenton, Ont.; Tel. EX 2-3526, Ext. 6.
ALEXANDRIS, Athina; Apt. 44, 3330 Ridgewood, Montreal 26, P.Q.; Athens (Greece); Psy.
ALEXANDROFF, Max; 127 Queenston St., St. Catharines, Ont.; 9 Forest Hill Rd. (res); Tor '43; A.I.C.S.; M.C.G.P.; Staff, St. Catharines Gen. Hosp.; Tel. MU 4-4802.
ALFORD, Lloyd; Box 100, 302 Morin, Ste. Adele-En-Haut, P.Q.; 104 Dufresne Ave. (res); McG '40.
ALFORD, Malcolm A.; Prince Albert Clinic, 49-13th W., Prince Albert, Sask.; Man '64.
ALGIE, Gordon H.; 43 Oak Park Cr., Sault Ste. Marie, Ont.; Dal '49; DiagRad; Rad., Plummer Mem. Hosp. & St. Joseph's Hosp., Blind River; Rad., Lady Dunn Hosp., Wawa; Tel. AL 4-5166.
ALI, Muntaz; 6291 Coburg Rd., Halifax, N.S.; Dal'66.
ALI, Syed H.; 107 Church St., Amherst, N.S.; Patna (India)'58; Ophth.
ALI, Unus O.; see OMARALI, U.
ALISON, Ruth E.; 35 St. Germain Ave., Toronto 12, Ont.; Tor '51; FRCP (C); IntMed; Staff, Princess Margaret Hosp.; Clin. Teach., U. of Toronto; Tel. 924-0671, Loc. 420.
AL-KATIB, Fatih M.; Medical Centre, Meadow Lake, Sask.; London (Eng.)'64; MRCS; LRCP.
ALLADIN, Herman U.; Raxlen Clinic, 500 Parliament St., Toronto 5, Ont.; 81 Frost St., Rexdale (res); Tor '62; Tel. WA 5-4381.
ALLAIRE, Andre; 122 rue St-Jean, Drummondville, Quebec 6, P.Q.; Mon '60; OrthSurg (P.Q.); Staff, Hop. Maisonneuve, Quebec; Tel. 254-8341.
ALLAIRE, Jacques; Box 460, Richibucto, N.B.; Lav '51; Tel. 523-4382.
ALLAIRE, J. Neree; 300 Carre St. Louis, Montreal, P.Q.; 621 Cote St. Antoine (res); Mon '37; DiagRad.; Tel. VI 5-0679.
ALLAIRE, Louis R. E.; Ogema, Sask.; Lav '20; Dist. Coroner.
ALLAN, Barbara M.—see—Garrow, Barbara M.
ALLAN, Blandford M. E.; 312 Toronto Western Medical Bldg., 25 Leonard Ave., Toronto 2B, Ont.; 64 Hillholm Rd. (res); Tor '33; NeurPsy; Staff Phys. Toronto Western Hosp.; Tel. EM 4-0805.
ALLAN, **Charles M.;** 5025 Sherbrooke St. W., Ste. 415, Montreal, P.Q.; McG '52; M.Sc.; FACS; GenSurg; Surg., Queen Elizabeth Hosp.; Tel. HU 1-1503.
ALLAN, **Douglas J. M.;** 386 Cambria St., **Stratford, Ont.; Denison Ave. (res); Edinburgh (Scot.) '50; LRCP & S (Edin.); DRCOG; ObstGyn; Staff, (ObstGyn), Stratford Gen. Hosp.; Tel. 271-0337.**
ALLAN, George G. S/L; Box 1038, C.F.B., Cold Lake, Alta.; Glasgow (Scot.)'48; ObstGyn; ObstGyn., Base Hosp.; Tel. 248-3311, Loc. 192.
ALLAN, Leslie C.; 933 Lansdowne Ave., Calgary, **Alta.; Aberdeen (Scot.) '38; D.P.H.;** Med. **Health** Officer, City of Calgary; Tel. 269-0397.
ALLAN, Malcolm L.; Chest Clinic, 53-Sixth St., New Westminster, B.C.; Tor'39; ThorSurg; Dir., New Westminster Chest Clinic; Tel. 526-3634.
ALLAN, Margaret D.; 386 Cambria St., Stratford, Ont.; Edin. (Scot.) '52; Tel. 271-3200.
ALLAN, Norman J.; 400 Med. & Dental Bldg., Rose St. & 11th Ave., Regina, Sask.; Glasgow (Scot.)'45; DRCOG; MRCOG; FRCS(C), ObstGyn; ObstGyn., Regina Gen. & Grey Nuns Hosp's.; Tel. 527-7877.
ALLAN, William K. G.; County Health Unit, 16 Lynch St., Brampton, Ont.; Glasgow (Scot.)'56; DPH; Med. Dir. & MOH, Peel County Health Unit; Tel. 451-2150.
ALLAN, William S.; 808 Medical Dental Bldg., 1825-11th. Ave., Regina, Sask.; McG '28; Tel. 522-4264.
ALLANACH, J. Ralph; 321 Orange St., Woodstock, N.B. (res); Tor '43; **D.P.H.;** Dist. M.O.H., **York, Carleton & Victoria Counties;** Dept. of **Health & Social Services, New Brunswick. Tel. 328-3336.**
ALLANACH, William G.; 14 Church St., Moncton, N.B.; 18 John St., (res); Tor '43; Urol.; Tel. EV 2-5746.
ALLARD, Albert; 80A Puyjalon, Hauterive, Cte. Saguenay, P.Q.; Lav'45; GenSurg (P.Q.); Surg., Hotel-Dieu; Tel. 589-2021.
ALLARD, Antonio; 2122 Centre St., Montreal, P. Q., Mon '31; Tel. WE 5-8090.
ALLARD, Charles A.; 10118-111th St., Edmonton, Alta.; 11405-100th Ave. (res); Alb '43; DABS; FRCS(C), GenSurg; Lect. U. of Alberta; Tel. 422-8207.
ALLARD, Ernest; 76 Rue St. Jean Baptiste, Baie **St. Paul, Co. Charlevoix, P.Q.; Lav '03.**
ALLARD, Eugene; 1970 rue Vitre, Quebec 3, P.Q. (res); Lav'31; FICA, FACA; Anaes; Chief of Anaes., Hop.-de-l'Enfant-Jesus; Ass't. Prof., Laval U.; Tel. LA 9-4511.
ALLARD, J. Pierre, Capt.; Lav'64; Staff, Military Hosp., 2705 Blvd. Laurier, Quebec 10, P.Q.
ALLARD, J. Theophile; Richibucto, N.B.; Lav '34.
ALLARD, Pierre P. Capt.; 2 RCHACFPO 505 Can. Armed Forces, Germany; Ott '55; IntMed (Cardiol.) (P.Q.). Abroad.
ALLARD, Raymond; 133 Thornton, Montreal 16, **P.Q. (res); Lav '55; Anaes; Staff, Hop.-St.-Luc; Tel. UN 1-7261.**
ALLARD, Rene; 79 rue Logan, St.-Lambert, P.Q. (res); Mon '53; PhysMed (P.Q.); Staff, Hotel-Dieu Hosp. & Hop. Ste. Justine; Tel. VI 4-0161.
ALLARDYCE, D. Bruce; UBC'62; Res., Vancouver Gen. Hosp., Vancouver 9, B.C.
ALLARY, Bruno; 545 Auger, Alma, Cte. Lac St. Jean, P.Q.; Lav'33; PH (P.Q.).
ALLCOCK, John M.; 3 Foxchapel Rd., London, Ont. (res); London (Eng.)'47; MRCS (Eng.), LRCP (Lond.); DMRD; FFR; DiagRad; Assoc. Rad., Victoria Hosp.; Sr. Teach. Fell., (DiagRad), U. of Western Ont.; Tel. GE 2-5261.
ALLEMANG, William H.; 134 Private Patient's Pav., Toronto Gen. Hosp., Toronto, Ont.; Tor'46; FRCS(C), ObstGyn; Clin & Instr. (ObstGyn.) Toronto Gen. Hosp. & U. of Toronto; Tel. EM 6-8211.
ALLEN, A. G.; 258 Brenda Cres., Woodstock, Ont.; Tor '31; D.Psy., Psy; Ass't. Supt., Epilepsy Dir., Ontario Hosp., Woodstock; Tel. LE 9-1251.
ALLEN, A. Gibson; Box 10, 100 Victoria St., Tweed, Ont.; 32 Colborne (res); McG '50; M.C.-G.P.; Active Staff, Belleville Gen. Hosp.; Coroner, Hastings, Lennox & Addington Co's.; Tel. 478- 3315.
ALLEN, Alexander; McG '59; Research, Neonatal Unit, Women's Pavilion, Royal Victoria Hosp., Montreal, P.Q.
ALLEN, Anthony B.; 303 Goldstream, Colwood, Victoria, B.C.; 553 View Royal (res); St. Bart's (London, Eng.) '54; Tel. GR 8-1744.

ALLEN, A. Stewart; Lewis St., Cardinal, Ont.; Joseph St. (res); McG '29; F.I.C.S., F.R.C.S.(C), GenSurg; TB & Pulm. Dis. (P.Q.); Staff, Brockville Gen. & St. Vincent de Paul Hosp's.; Tel. 657-3483.
ALLEN, Betty J.; London (Eng.)'61; Res., Sunnybrook Hosp., Toronto, Ont.
ALLEN, Cameron S.; Ste. 60, 3195 Granville St., Vancouver 9, B.C.; Man '39; Ch.M., FRCS(C), GenSurg; OrthSurg; M.S. (Orth.) (Minn.); FACS; Att'd. Staff, Vancouver Gen. Hosp.; Clin. Instr. (Orth.), U. of British Columbia; Tel. RE 1-4611.
ALLEN, D. Reg.; Colborne St., Walkerton, Ont. (res); Tor '40; D.P.H.; M.O.H., Bruce County Health Unit; Tel. 881-1920.
ALLEN, Edward A.; 1139 Yates St., Victoria, B.C.; Cape Town (S. Africa) '53; FCCP; FRCP (C), IntMed; Court. Staff, St. Joseph's & Royal Jubilee Hosp's; Tel. 388-4211.
ALLEN, George G.; Box 66, Lanigan, Sask.; Qns '51.
ALLEN, H. Hugh; Ste. 102, 450 Central Ave., London, Ont.; 736 Springbank Dr. (res); Wes '48; FRCS (C); FACS; ObstGyn; Ass't. Prof. (ObstGyn) U. of Western Ont.; Tel. 433-0134.
ALLEN, Hugh W., 64B Front St., Sioux Lookout, Ont.; Man '39; M.C.G.P.; Dist. Coroner.
ALLEN, Irene V.; Dal '29; F.A.C.P., F.C.C.P., IntMed (TB); Sr. Res. Phys., St. John T.B. Hosp., East St. John, N.B.; Med Cons. in T.B., St. John Gen. Hosp.; Tel. 693-6551.
ALLEN, James R. A., St. George, N.B.; Tor '39.
ALLEN, J. Donald; 232 Metcalfe St., Ottawa, Ont.; Qns '31; Ophth; Acting Hd., Dept. of Ophth., Ottawa Gen. Hosp.; Assoc. Prof. (Ophth.), U. of Ottawa; Tel. 232-5949.
ALLEN, Lloyd S.; Harshman Blk., Sydney, N.S.; 81 Park (res); Dal '48; M.Sc.; GenSurg; Staff, Sydney City & St. Rita's Hosp's.; Cons. Phys., Dosco; Tel. 564-8105.
ALLEN, L. Phillipe; 902 rue St.-Jean, Quebec 4, P.Q.; Lav'43; F.A.C.O.G.; Gyn (P.Q.); Staff, Hop-St.-Francois-d'Assise; Teach. Ass't., Laval U.; Tel. 525-6875.
ALLEN, Marc.; 1005 St. Prosper, Trois Rivieres, P.Q.; 3200 Neree-Beauchemin (res); Lav '44; Anaes.; Tel. FR 5-2211.
ALLEN, Michael S.; 688 Coxwell Ave., Ste. 210, Toronto, Ont.; Tor'59; FRCS(C); GenSurg; Paed. Surg., Toronto East Gen. Hosp.
ALLEN, Murray E.; 384 Tranquille Rd., N. Kamloops, B.C.; Alb'64; Tel. 376-3135.
ALLEN, Peter; Ste. 814, 750 W. Broadway, Vancouver 9, B.C.; 2858 W. 49th Ave. (res); Tor '46; F.R.C.S.(C), GenSurg; ThorSurg; Clin. Instr. (Cardiovas.), U. of British Columbia; Tel. 876-6828.
ALLEN, Peter B.; Ste. 520, 8409-112th St., Edmonton, Alta.; Alb'56; FRCS(C); NeurSurg; Cons. NeurSurg., Alberta, Royal Columbian, Edmonton Gen., Misericordia & Charles Camsell Hosp's; Clin. Instr., U. of Alberta; Tel. 439-1124.
ALLEN, Rovelle H.; Laboratory of Hygiene, Dept. Nat'l. Health & Welfare, Ottawa, Ont.; U. of Wisc. (U.S.A.)'41; Ph.D. (Biochem.)
ALLEN, William A.; 212 Canada Bldg., Saskatoon, Sask.; Tor'40; Vis. Phys., University Hosp.; Protem. Acting Chief of Med., City Hosp.; Clin. Assoc. (Med.), U. of Saskatchewan; Tel. 244-1161.
ALLFREE, A. John; Roberts Med. Bldg., 95 Le Marchant Rd., St. John's, Nfld.; Sheffield (Eng.) '62; Tel. 579-0240.
ALLIN, Eardley S.; 10155-120th St., Edmonton, Alta.; 8808-111th St. (res); Tor '31; FRCS (Eng.); FRCS (C); GenSurg; Pres. Staff, Royal Alexandra Hosp. & Chief Surg., Misericordia Hosp.; Instr., (Surg.), U. of Alberta; Tel. 488-7271.
ALLIN, George E.; 10155-120 St., Edmonton, Alta.; 9711-143A St. (res); Alb '51; F.R.C.S. (Eng.), GenSurg; Surg. Staff, Royal Alexandra Hosp.; Clin. Instr. (Surg.), U. of Alberta; Tel. 488-7271.
ALLIN, J. Drew; 208 St. Clair Ave. W., Toronto, Ont.; 294 Oriole Parkway (res); Tor '51; FRCS(C); ObstGyn; Staff, Grace Hosp.; Tel. WA 2-7281,
ALLIN, Robert C.; Tor'65; Res., Shaughnessy Hosp., Vancouver 9, B.C.
ALLIN, Robert W.; P.O. Box 100, Clarksburg, Ont.; Qns '53; M.C.G.P.; M.O.H., Collingwood Twp.
ALLIN, Warren D.; Tor'63; Ass't. Res. (Ophth.), U. of Toronto, Toronto, Ont.
ALLISON, F. Gerard; 417 Medical Arts Bldg., Winnipeg, Man.; Man '29; M.R.C.P. (Lond), F.R.C.P.(C), F.A.C.P., IntMed, Cardiol., Children's and Grace Hosps.; Assoc. Phys., Winnipeg Gen. Hosp.; Assoc. Prof. (Med.), U. of Manitoba; Tel. WH 2- 3846.
ALLISON, Gerda E. (Fremming); 73 Kingsway, Winnipeg, Man. (res); Man '37; F.R.C.P.(C), Psy; Staff, Winnipeg Gen. & Children's Hosp's.; Ass't. Prof. (Psy), U. of Manitoba; Lectr. Grad. Schl. of Social Work; Tel. 786-3645.
ALLISON, Gerald; 61 Main St., Picton, Ont.; Tor '15; GenSurg; Active Staff, Prince Edward Co. Mem. Hosp.; Tel. GR 6-3035.
ALLISON, James C.; 9 Garrick Rd., Scarborough, Ont. (res); Tor'43; Chief, Medical Rehabilitation and Chronic Care Services, Ont. Dept. of Health, Toronto.
ALLISON, Richard G.; Man'65; Jr. Int., Winnipeg General Hosp., Winnipeg 3, Man.
ALLISON, Wilma G.; (See Stewart, Wilma G.)
ALLMAN, Reginald G.; 31 Centre St. S., Brampton, Ont.; Tor '50; IntMed; Cons. Med., Peel Mem., Northwestern Gen. & Branson Hosp's., Toronto; Tel. 677-3113.
ALLODI, Federico A.; Madrid (Spain)'57; FRCP(C), Psy; Staff, Clarke Inst. of Psy., 250 College St., Toronto 2B, Ont.
ALLORE, Robert L. W.; 276 Charles St., Belleville, Ont.; 45 Victoria Ave. (res); Tor '47; ObstGyn; Chief of Obst., Belleville Gen. Hosp.; Cons. Staff, Trenton Memorial Hosp.; Trenton & Prince Edward County Mem. Hosp., Picton; Tel. 962-0200.
ALLOUCHERIE, Marthe (Pelland); 935 St. John, Quebec, P.Q.; 1475 Blvd. Laurier, Sillery (res); Mon '30; Neurol.; Tel. 527-1935.
ALLT, William E. C.; 149 Admiral Rd., Toronto 5, Ont.; Dublin (Ire.) '43; DMRT (Eng.); FFR; TherRad; Sr., Rad., Ont. Cancer Inst. & Princess Margaret Hosp.; Cons. (Rad.), Sunnybrook DVA Hosp.; Ass't. Prof. (Rad. & Biophysics), U. of Toronto; Tel. 924-0671, Local 295.
ALMEIDA, Jose G. D.; 94 Compton Rd., Regina, Sask.
ALMOND, W. W.; Vulcan, Alta.; McG '21.
ALMS, Michael; Ste. 121, Med. Arts Bldg., Saskatoon, Sask.; Bristol (Eng.)'45; FRCS (Eng.), M.Ch. Orth (Liverpool); OrthSurg; Clin. Instr. (Orth), U. of Saskatchewan; Tel. 244-0994.
ALMUDEVAR, Manuel; Zaragoza (Spain)'50; Staff, Douglas Hosp., Montreal 19, P.Q.
ALP, Necati M.; Istanbul (Turk.) '47; Sr. Res., Hosp. for Mental & Nervous Dis., St. John's Nfld.
ALPORT, P. Jill (Lockley); P. O. Box 523, Regina, Sask.; 35 Academy Park Rd. (res); London (Eng.) '47; Anaes; Staff, Regina Gen. & Grey Nuns Hosp.; Tel. LA 2-1811.
ALPORT, W. E. H.; 812 Medical-Dental Bldg., Regina, Sask.; Tor '49; M.C.G.P.; Tel. LA 2-4515.
ALT, Kuno; 1434 Queen St. W., Toronto 3, Ont.; Tor '55.
ALTER, Charles; 262 Wilson Ave., Downsview, Ont.; Tor '44; FRCP (C); IntMed; Phys., Diabetic Clin., Toronto Gen. Hosp.; Fell., U. of Toronto; Tel. WA 2-7855.
ALTER-KOWALEWSKI, Jan E.; 48 Joicey Blvd., Toronto 12, Ont. (res); Liege (Belg.) '31; Warsaw '33; Staff, Dept. of Health, Toronto; Tel. 366-8411.
ALTON, Douglas J.; Tor '56; DMR; Diag Rad; Staff, Toronto Western Hosp., Toronto 2B, Ont.; Tel. 368-2581; Abroad.
ALTON, J. D. McGregor; 430 Phys. & Surg. Bldg., 8409-112th St., Edmonton, Alta.; Alb '51; FRCS (C), GenSurg; PlasSurg; Instr., U. of Alberta.
ALTOSE, Murray D.; Man'65; Jr. Int., Winnipeg General Hosp., Winnipeg 3, Man.

ALTSCHUL, Rudolph; 224 Cumberland Ave., N., Saskatoon, Sask.; Prague (Czecho-Slovakia) '25; **Prof. of Anatomy, U. of Saskatchewan;** Tel. CH 2-7671.

ALVAREZ, Arthur F.; 815 Victoria St., Trail, B.C.; 305 Kootenay (res); Birmingham (Eng.) '45; MRCS, LRCP, FRCS(Eng.), FICS; GenSurg; Cons. Surg., Trail-Tadenac Hosp. & Mater Misericordia (Rosslands) & Castelgar & Dist. Hosp.; Chmn., Med. Assoc. Clin.; Tel. 364-1234.

ALVAREZ, Eduardo B.; Med. Arts Clinic, 2125-11th Ave, Regina, Sask.; Valladoid (Spain) '53; FRCS(C), Plas Surg.

ALVAREZ, German; 465 Scott St., St. Catharines, Ont.; Lav'58; **Teach. Psy.,** Mack School of Nursing; Tel. 682-6021.

ALVAREZ, Joaquin A.; '62; Int., Queen Mary Vet's. Hosp., Montreal 26, P.Q.

ALVI, Abdul W.; 12 Victoria Cres., Winnipeg 8, Man. (res); Punjab (India) '53; IntMed.; Staff, St. Boniface Hosp.; Lect. (IntMed.), U. of Manitoba; Tel. WH 3-0311.

ALWAY, Alan E.; 762 Commissioner's Rd., London, Ont.; Wes '43; M.Sc., F.R.C.P.(C), IntMed.; Staff, Westminster DVA Hosp.; Clin. Lect., Med., U. of Western Ont.; Tel. GE 2-6711.

ALYANAK, N. B. Oz; 99 Avenue Rd., Ste. 205, **Toronto 5, Ont.; 456 Merton St., Toronto 7 (res); Istanbul (Turkey) '42; IntMed (Turkey); Tel.** 924-7851.

AMACHER, A. Loren; Wes'62; Res., Victoria Hosp., London, Ont.

AMAL, Swarnamanickam; 9291 Central Ave., Apt. 4, Lasalle, P.Q.; Madras (India)'56; FRCP(C), IntMed.

AMANN, Eric W.; Lockwood Clin., 300 Bloor St. E., Toronto 5, Ont.; Man'61.

AMAR, Jagdish C.; Punjab (India) '58; FRCP (C), IntMed; Staff, Vancouver Gen. Hosp., Vancouver, B.C.

AMERONGEN, Leo J.; Calwood Clinic, 11816-124th St., Edmonton, Alta.; 11516-140th St. (res); Alb '56; Tel. 454-6571.

AMES, Harold D.; Box 219, Beaverton, Ont.; **Morrison Ave. (res); McG '47; MCGP; Staff,, Soldiers' Mem. Hosp., Orillia; MOH, Beaverton;** Reg. M.O., CNR & Bell Telephone Co.; Tel. 426-7331.

AMIES, Cleeve R.; Public Health Lab., Box 9000A, Toronto 1, Ont.; London (Eng.)'26; BS; MRCP(Lond.); DTM&H; FC(Path); **Bact; Chief Bact.,** Public Health Lab., Ontario Dept. of Health.

AMIES, David R.; Moose Jaw Clinic, 200 Scott Bldg., Moose Jaw, Sask.; U. of Witwatersrand (S. Africa)'52; Alb'54; MB., B.Ch., IntMed; Tel. 692-2373.

AMIN, Thakor C.; Killam, Alta.; '57.

AMIREAULT, Gilles; Mon '63; **Res., Hop. Notre-**Dame, Montreal 24, P.Q.

AMIR-JAHED, Abasali K.; Lausanne (Switz.) '57; FRCS(C), GenSurg; **Research & Teach. Staff,** Card. Vasc. Research Lab., Dept. of Physiol., U. of Montreal, Montreal, P.Q.

AMODEO, William; 229 Brock St., Ste. 1, Kingston, Ont.; Qns '40; MCGP; Assoc. Staff, Kingston Gen. & Hotel-Dieu Hosp's.; Att'd. Staff, St. Mary's of the Lake Hosp.; Phys., Kingston Penitentiary; Tel. 548-4756.

AMOOZEGAR-FARD, Ezatollah; 106 Med. Arts Bldg., Saskatoon, Sask.; Tehran (Iran)'57; Psy; Tel. 653-3737.

AMORUSO, Frank; Brunswick Diagnosic Group, 25 Brunswick Ave., Toronto 4, Ont.; 485 Spadina Rd. (res); Bari (Italy) '39; GenSurg; Staff, Doctors' Hosp.; Tel. 925-8588.

AMOS, E. A.; 1414 Drummond Bldg., Montreal, P.Q.; 561 Roslyn (res); Mon '25; Ophth; Tel. AV 8-1571.

AMOURS, Claude; 1207 ave Rousseau, Quebec 6, P.Q.; Lav'52; Path(P.Q.).

AMOURS, Marcel D.; Lav '60; Res., Saint-Sacrement Hosp., Quebec 6, P.Q.

AMOURS, Olier D.; 256 blvd St. Joseph, Hull, P.Q.; Lav'38; Pulm. Dis. & T.B. (P.Q.).

AMUNSDEN, L. Roy; Blairmore, Alberta; Alb'44; LMCC; MCGP; Tel. 562-2243.

AMUNDSON, Clifford S.; P.O. Box 1000, Tisdale, Sask.; Man '51; Tel. 2151.

AMY, John V.; 22 Central Ave. W., Brockville, Ont.; Ott'65.

AMYOT, Arthur; Mon'64; Int., Inst. Albert Prevost, Montreal, P.Q.

AMYOT, Gilles; 4135 Ave. Papineau, Montreal 24, P.Q.; Mon '56; Obst; Tel. 526-7656.

AMYOT, Gregoire F.; 2675 Queenswood Dr., R.R. No. 5, Victoria, B.C. (res); Tor '25; **DPH; PH; Deputy Minister of Health, Dept. of Health Serv. & Hosp Ins. (BC), Hon. Lectr. Pub. Health Admin., U. of British Columbia; Retired.**

AMYOT-LEGAULT, Arlette; Mon '64; **Res., Hop.** St. Luc, Montreal, P.Q.

AMYOT, Lucien; 1694 Blvd. Pie IX, Montreal, **P.Q.; Mon '30; A.M.C.G.P.**

AMYOT, Marcel; Mon '58; **Int., Hop. Maison-**neuve, Montreal, P. Q.

AMYOT, Raymond; 564 Blvd. Manseau, Joliette, **P.Q.; 1114 Notre-Dame (res); Mon '54; M.C.-G.P.; Tel. PL 3-5562.**

AMYOT, Roma; 389 est Blvd. St. Joseph, Montreal, P.Q.; 1120 St. Clare Rd., Ville Mont Royal (res); Mon '24; M.D. (Paris), F.R.C.P.(C), NeurPsy; Chief of Neur. Psy. Serv., Hop. Notre Dame; Assoc. Prof., U. of Montreal; Tel. RE 3-9951.

AN, Song-Hi; Soeul (Korea)'49; AB (Path & Clin. Path); Pathology Inst., Halifax, N.S.; Ass't. Prof. Path., Dalhousie U.; Dir., Diag. Cytol. Lab., Pathology Inst.; Tel. 422-9661, Ext. 213.

ANAND, Sundaram; 2 Med. Arts Bldg., 12 Master Ave., Kentville, N.S.; Agra (India) '53; FRCS (Eng.); DLO (Lond.); GenSurg; **Staff,** B.F.M. Hosp.; Tel. 678-4779.

ANAND, Saroj; 2 Med. Arts Bldg., Masters Ave., Kentville, N.S.; R.C.S. (Ireland) '58.

ANAWATI, Naguid K.; Med. Clin., Tracadie, N.B.; Alexandria (Egypt) '55; Urol; Assoc. Phys., Hotel-Dieu-St. Joseph; Tel. 395-2268.

ANAYA, Jacinto M.; Madrid (Spain) '53; Jr. Intn., Metropolitan Gen. Hosp., Windsor, Ont.

ANBIN, Gilles; R.R. No. 2, Sainte-Sophie, Terrebonne, P.Q.; Mon '60.

ANCHELSON, Arnold A.; Ste. 201, 1200 Lawrence Ave. E., Don Mills, Ont.; Tor'58; **Staff, New Mount Sinai, Toronto East Gen. & Grace** Hosp's.

ANCTIL, Marc-Andre; 1500 18th. St., Quebec 3, P.Q.; Lav '64.

ANDERMAN, Eva — see **DEUTCH-ANDERMAN,** Eva.

ANDERMANN, Frederick; 1400 Pine Ave. W., Montreal, P.Q.; Mon'57; Neur; **Staff, Montreal Children's & Mtl.Neur. Inst. Tel. WE 7-3884.**

ANDERSEN, Armand; Poly Clinique Gravel, 66 rue St-Jean Baptiste, Victoriaville, P.Q.; Lav '43; Otol (P.Q.)

ANDERSEN, Melvin A.; Man'62; Res., Vancouver General Hospital, Vancouver 9, B.C.

ANDERSEN, Richard G.; 520-17th St., West Vancouver, B.C.; 1460 Esquimalt Ave., Apt. 12A, West. Van. (res); McG'60; MCGP; Tel. WA 2-2112.

ANDERSON, Alliston; 69 Carleton St., S., Thorold, Ont.; 51 Welland St. S. (res); Tor '36; Chief, Dept. Gen. Pract., St. Catharines Gen Hosp.; Tel. 227-1851.

ANDERSON, Alvin J.; 123 Edward St., Toronto 2, Ont.; 8 Edgehill Rd., Islington, Ont. (res); Wes '52; GenSurg; Att'd. Staff, Doctor's, Central & Grace Hosp's.; Tel. 366-3836.

ANDERSON, Andrew J.; 604-4th St. E., Cornwall, Ont.; Rome (Italy)'52; Urol; Chief Urol., Hotel-Dieu Hosp.; Cons. Urol., Cornwall Gen. Hosp., St. Lawrence San., McDonell Mem. Hosp., Cornwall, & Glengarry Mem. Hosp., Alexandria; Tel. WE 3-1610.

ANDERSON, Cameron D.; 1428 Ouellette Ave., Windsor, Ont.; 841 Kildare Rd. (res); Tor '55; FRCP (C); IntMed.; Active Staff, Hotel-Dieu of St. Joseph, Metropolitan, Grace, & I.O.D.E. Mem. Hosp's; Tel. 256-0551.

ANDERSON, Clare L.; 42 Forest Hill Rd., St. Catharines, Ont. (res); Tor '32; Anaes; Chief, Dept. of Anaes., St. Catharines Gen. Hosp.; Tel. MU 2-4612.

ANDERSON, David M.; Ott'65; Res., Montreal General Hosp., Montreal 25, P.Q.

ANDERSON, Donald N.; 19 Pettit Dr., Weston, Ont. (res); Tor '52; D.Psy; Psy; Ass't. Supt., Ontario Hosp., 999 Queen St. W., Toronto 3, Ont.; Clin. Instr. (Psy), U. of Toronto; Tel. LE 3-8501.

ANDERSON, Donald O.; Room 300, Westbrook Bldg., U. of British Columbia, Vancouver 8, B.C.; UBC'54; S.M. (Hygiene) (Harvard); FRCP(C); IntMed; Assoc. Prof. (PrevMed); U. of British Columbia; Tel. 228-2772.

ANDERSON, Douglas L.; 630 Professional Bldg., 10830 Jasper Ave., Edmonton, Alta.; Sask '57; Ophth Otol; Active Staff Royal Alexandra Hosp.; Tel. 422-6363.

ANDERSON, Eric S.; Box 40, 81 Bruce Ave., South Porcupine, Ont.; Dublin (Ire.)'52; LRCP & LRCS(I); L.M.; MPH (Yale).

ANDERSON, Ernest J.; Woodville, Ont.; Qns'28; Dist. Coroner; Tel. 439-2411.

ANDERSON, Ernest J.; Box 70, Main St., Lucan, Ont.; Wes'65.

ANDERSON, Frank H.; UBC '63; Ass't. Res. (Med.), Vancouver Gen. Hosp., Vancouver, B. C.

ANDERSON, George H.; Dept. of Path., Ottawa Civic Hosp., Ottawa, Ont.; 121 Iona St. (res); London (Eng.) '54; Path; Ass't. Path. Ottawa Civic Hosp.; Med.Dir., Red Cross Blood Trans. Service, Ottawa; Lect., U. of Ottawa; Tel. PA 9-2511, Local 244.

ANDERSON, Gordon L.; 333 George St., Sarnia, Ont.; McG '34; DPH; PH; Dir., Lambton Health Unit; Cons., Sarnia Gen. & St. Joseph's Hosp's.; Lect., U. of Western Ontario & Michigan U.; Tel. DI 4-8809.

ANDERSON, Harry M.; 99 Avenue Rd., Ste. 405, Toronto 5, Ont.; Tor'58; D.Psy; Psy; Staff, O.P.D., Ontario Hosp.; Tel. 927-6820.

ANDERSON, I. H., S/L; Aberdeen(Scot.) '52; MIH; SMO, 2nd Fighter Wing, c/o Air Off. Command., 1 Air Div., HQ., RCAF, CAP 5052, CAF, Europe: Att'nd. SOMS.

ANDERSON, Jack B.; 1026 Cook St., Victoria, B.C.; 805 Dereen Pl. (Res); **McG '50;** M.C.G.P.; **Staff, St. Joseph's Hosp., Court. Staff, Jubilee Hosp.; Tel. EV 6-4341.**

ANDERSON, James E.; 5133 Bayfield Cresc., Burlington, Ont.; Tor'53.

ANDERSON, James L.; 1436 Kingsway, Vancouver 12, B.C.; Sask '59.

ANDERSON, James O.; 406 Scarboro Ave., Calgary, Alta. (res); Alb. '39; Anaes; Colonel **Belcher Hosp., Calgary; Tel. AM 6-7001.**

ANDERSON, James R.; 150 St. George St., Toronto, Ont.; Tor'43; DPH; Assoc. Edit., Cdn. Med. Assoc. Journal; Tel. 924-0751.

ANDERSON, James W.; Med. Arts Bldg., 1105 Pandora Ave., Victoria, B. C.; 3026 McAnally **(res); Edinburgh (Scot.) '22;** FRCS (Ed.); GenSurg; Active Staff, Royal Jubilee Hosp.; Court. Staff, St. Joseph's Hosp.; Tel. EV 3-8322.

ANDERSON, Joe G. D.; Tor '62; Res., St. Michael's Hosp., Toronto, Ont.; Abroad.

ANDERSON, J. Larry; 213 Victoria Quay, Alberni, B.C.; Sask '59; Tel. 723-8141.

ANDERSON, J. L. Murray; 3523 Redwood Ave., Victoria, B.C. (res); Tor '29; D.P.H.; Med. Admin., Royal **Jubilee Hosp.;** Tel. 386-3131.

ANDERSON, John B.; Wes '57; Res., Westminster Hosp., London, Ont.

ANDERSON, John D.; Medical Arts Clinic, Regina, Sask.; 3540 Albert St. **(res); Tor '36;** D.A.B. Ot; Ophth, Otol; Sr. Staff, Regina Gen. & Regina Grey Nun's Hosp's; Cons. (Ophth), **University Hosp.; Clin. Instr. U. of Saskatchewan;** Tel. 523-0691.

ANDERSON, John E.; 311 Main St., Picton, Ont.; 28 Paul St. (res); Qns '61; Tel. GR 6-5744.

ANDERSON, John F. C.; 502 Queen St., Saskatoon, Sask.; 710-8th Ave. N. (res); Tor '29; Ll.D. (Sask); IntMed; Assoc. Prof. (IntMed), U. of Saskatchewan; Tel. 242-1293.

ANDERSON, John O.; Oshawa Clinic, 117 King St. E., Oshawa, Ont.; 976 Mohawk St. (res); Tor **'47;** ObstGyn.; **Tel. 728-1661.**

ANDERSON, John S.; 200 St. Clair W., Toronto, Ont.; Man '34; Tel. WA 1-7557.

ANDERSON, Joseph C.; Ste. 540, 2184 W. Broadway, Vancouver 9, B.C.; Glasgow (Scot.)'44; MCGP; Tel. 736-4911.

ANDERSON, Julius; Apt. 401, Sussex House, 230 Roslyn Rd., Winnipeg 13, Man.; Man'36; Retired.

ANDERSON, Kenneth; Dal'65; Staff, Come-by-Chance Hosp., Come-by-Chance, Nfld.

ANDERSON, Lewis S.; 253 E. 14th St., North Vancouver, B. C.; 13048 Lowood Rd. (res); Manchester (Eng.) '37; B. Sc.; DPH (Edin.); PH; Dir., The North Shore Health Unit, North Vancouver; Tel. 988-5231. Abroad.

ANDERSON, L. M.; UBC '63; Int. Vancouver Gen. Hosp., Vancouver, B. C.

ANDERSON, Oswald W.; Bancroft, Ont.; Tor **'24; M.O.H., Village of Bancroft; Coroner, Hastings County.**

ANDERSON, Ralph Joseph; Wes'64; Res., Victoria Hosp., London, Ont.

ANDERSON, R. E. C.; Medical Arts Bldg., Windsor, Ont.; R.R. No. 1, Belle River (res), **Qns '35; Urol.; Tel. 252-7284.**

ANDERSON, Reginald M.; 111 St. Clair Ave W., Toronto 7, Ont.; 192-8th Line, Oakville (res); McG'36; MCGP; Vice-Pres. & Med. Dir., Clin. Research, Mead Johnson of Canada Ltd.; Tel. 921-4184.

ANDERSON, Robert C.; 502 Queen St., Saskatoon, Sask.; Sask '58; FRCP(C); IntMed; Clin. Teach. (Med.), U. of Saskatchewan; Tel. 242-1293.

ANDERSON, Robert N.; 526 Westminster, Ladner, B.C. **(res); McG '33; Dist Coroner.**

ANDERSON, Robert N.; 5880 Spring Garden Rd., Halifax, N.S.; 1641 Vernon St. (res); Dal'54; **FRCP(C), IntMed (Cardiol.); Ass't. Phys., Vic**toria Gen. Hosp.; Ass't. Prof. (Med.), Dalhousie U.; Tel. 423-7417.

ANDERSON, Ronald I.; Box 1138, Banff, Alta.; Glasgow (Scot.)'64.

ANDERSON, Roy L.; Physicians & Surgeons Bldgd., 11154—84th St., Edmonton, Alta.; Alb '27; F.A.C.S., F.R.C.S.(C), **GenSurg;** Retired.

ANDERSON, Rudolph C.; 701 Campbell Bldg., 1029 Douglas St., Victoria, B.C.; Ste. 450, 1105 Pandora Ave.; **Man '35;** M.Ch., OrthSurg; Staff, St. Joseph's, Veteran's & Jubillee Hosp's.; Tel. 384-4121 & 383-4151.

ANDERSON, Terence W.; 179 Glengrove Ave. W., Toronto 12, **Ont. (res); Oxford (Eng.) '55;** DIH; **AMCGP; Lec., School of Hygience, U. of** Toronto; Editor, Applied Therapeutics, Seccombe House, 443 Mt. Pleasant Rd., Toronto 7; Tel. 483-5644.

ANDERSON, Thomas A.; 3 Burns Dr., Armdale, Halifax Co., N.S. (res); Dal '43; Anaes; Staff (Anaes), Children's Hosp.; Instr. Anaes., Dal**housie U.; Tel. 422-8441.**

ANDERSON, Thomas B.; Ott'63; Int., Ottawa Civic Hosp., Ottawa 3, Ont.

ANDERSON, T. G.; 9 Monkstown, St. John's, Nfld.; U.K. '33; Paed.; Tel. 578-3421.

ANDERSON, Theodore A.; 131 Park W., Windsor, Ont.; 2643 Turner Rd. (res); Qns '50; Tel. 253-5711.

ANDERSON, T. Stuart; Man'57; Res., University Hosp., Edmonton, Alta.

ANDERSON, Walter F.; 1635 Abbott St., Kelowna, B.C.; 2302 Abbott St. (res); McG '35; FACOG; MCGP; Med. Staff, Kelowna Gen. Hosp.; Tel. 762-2740.

ANDERSON, Walter S.; 1004-105th St., Edmonton, Alta.; 13723 Summit Pt. (res); Tor '34; M.S. (Tor.); FRCS(C); FACS; DABS; GenSurg; Hd., Dept. of Surg., Royal Alexandra Hosp.; Prof. Surg., U. of Alberta; Tel. GA. 4-2121.

ANDERSON, Wilford L.; 331 Sheddon Ave., **Oakville, Ont.; 294 - 8th Line N. (res); Tor '51; MCGP; Staff, Oakville Mem. Hosp.; Tel. VI 5-1281.**

ANDERSON, William; 56 Baby Pt. Rd., Toronto, Ont. (res); Edinburgh (Scot.) '41; Path; Surg. Path., Toronto Gen. Hosp.; Ass't. Prof. of Path., **U. of Toronto; Tel. EM 6-8211.**

ANDISON, Alexander W.; Winnipeg Clinic, Winnipeg, Man.; 115 Brock St. (res); Man '35; F.R.C.O.G., F.R.C.S.(C), ObstGyn; Assoc. Prof. Obst.Gyn., U. of Manitoba; Assoc Obst. Gyn., Winnipeg Gen. Hosp.; Tel. 942-0551.

ANDRACHUK, John J.; 960 Dundas St. W., Toronto, Ont.; 148 Old Forest Hill Rd. (res); Tor **'33; Tel. 531-6929.**

ANDRACHUK, Wilbur W.; Box 231, 404 Cody Hall, U. of Windsor, Windsor, Ont.; Leeds (Eng.) '50.

ANDRADE, Elmer M.; Santo Tomas (Philipp.)'58; ObstGyn; Staff, Saint John Gen. Hosp., Saint John, N.B.

ANDREE, Peggy (See Ross)

ANDREIU, Liviu; 238 Notre-Dame S., Thetford Mines, Co. Megantic, P.Q.; 97 Notre Dame (res); Cluj (Roumania) '42; Otol (P.Q.); Staff, St. Joseph's Hosp.; Tel. 388-1121.

ANDRES, Edward J.; 837-8th Ave. N., Saskatoon, Sask.; Tor '48; D.A.B.P.; Staff, Saskatoon City Hosp.; Tel. 242-0030.

ANDREW, Archibald; Edinburgh(Scot.) '61; Jr. Intn., St. John's Gen. Hosp., St. John's, Nfld.

ANDREW, Daniel E.; Tor'61; Res., Hotel-Dieu de Quebec, Quebec 4, P.Q.

ANDREW, Robert B.; 1016 Wyandotte, Riverside, Ont.; 241 Rossini Blvd., Windsor (res); Tor '47; FACS; FRCS (C); GenSurg; Chief of Surg., Grace Hosp.; Surg. Staff, Metropolitan & Hotel-Dieu Hosp's.; Cons., Riverview Hosp.; Tel. 945-6562.

ANDREW, Rodney F.; Box 311, Red Lake Med. Group, Red Lake, Ont.; London (Eng.)'62; M.B.; BS.; MRCS; LRCP; Tel. 200.

ANDREWS, Arnold J.; 23 Kingsdale Ave., Willowdale, Ont. (res); Tor '39; DABR; DR; Diag-Rad; MCGP; Chief Rad., North York Branson Gen. Hosp.; Tel. BA 5-9276.

ANDREWS, C. Herbert, 302 Med. Bldg., Prince Albert, Sask.; 157-19th St. W. (res); Rush Med. Coll (Chicago **U.S.A.) '24; OphthOtol; Vis. Cons. (Ophth.), Union Hosp.; Tel. 763-3186.**

ANDREWS, John L.; 1207 Douglas, Victoria, B.C.; 1946 Mayfair Dr. (res); Tor '42; Anaes; **Att. Staff, Royal Jubilee Hosp.; Tel. EV 3-3261.**

ANDREWS, John W. S/L; 1 CBMU Iserlohn, CFPO 5050, CAF, Europe; London (Eng)'54; FRCS(C), ObstGyn; Abroad.

ANDREWS, Leslie G.; G. F. Strong Rehab. Centre, 900W 27th Ave., Vancouver 9, B.C.; 4549 Connaught Dr. (res); London (Eng.) '52; M.B., B.S. (Lond.); LRCP (Lond.); MRCS (Eng); DCH (Eng.); D. Phys. Med. (Eng.); PhysMed & Rehab; **Paed; Ass't Med. Dir., G. F.** Strong Rehab. & Childrens' Rehab. Cerebral Palsy Assoc.; Att'd. Phys., Sunnyhill Childrens' Hosp.; Vis. Phys., Vancouver Gen, Hosp.; Pres. North West Assoc. PhysMed & Rehab.; Lect. (Rehab Med.), U. of British Columbia; Tel. RE 1-3111.

ANDREWS, Phillip; The Medical Arts Bldg., 260 Cedar St., Sudbury, Ont.; Tor '55; F.R.C.S.-(C), Otol.; Tel. 673-3695.

ANDREWS, Robin H.; Western Med. Clinic, 111-9th St., Brandon, Man.; London (Eng.)'54; MCGP.

ANDREWS, Thomas C.; The Med. Centre, Sackville, N.B.; Cambridge (Eng.) '61; D.Obst-RCOG; DA (Eng.); Anaes., Sackville Mem. Hosp.; Tel. 536-0567.

ANDREWS, Warwick N.; 15 Deerwood Cr., Yorkton, Sask. (res); New Zealand '47; DPM (Eng.); Psy; Deputy Sup., Yorkton Psy. Centre; Tel. 783-2491.

ANDRIASCHUK, Sophie M.; Alb'65; Res., Women's College Hosp., Toronto 5, Ont.

ANDRUCSON, Victor M.; Smith Clinic, 4815-51st St., Camrose, Alta.; Sask'61; Tel. 672-2424.

ANDRUKAITIS, Edward V.; 956 Sherbrooke East, Montreal, P.Q.; 1325 Dutrisac, Ville St. Laurent (res); Mon '43; Neur; Staff, St.-Jean-de-Dieu & Notre Dame Hosp's.; Tel LA 2-7236.

ANDRY, Harold P.; 212 James St. S., Hamilton, Ont.; 118 Mt. Brow Blvd. (res); Wes '56; Anaes; Staff, St. Joseph's Hosp.; Tel. 528-8437.

ANFOSSI, Harold C.; 11 Argyle St., Bowmanville, Ont.; Qns '58; Staff, Bowmanville Mem. Hosp.; Tel. 623-2552.

ANGEL, Aubie; 3775 University St., Montreal 2, P.Q.; Man'59; FRCP(C), IntMed; Clin. Ass't. Royal Victoria Hosp.; Ass't. Prof. Path., & Lect. Med., McGill U.; Tel. VI 2-1251.

ANGEL, Norman; Apt 605, 2500 Bathurst St., Toronto 19, Ont.; Birmingham (Eng.) '34; M.B., Ch.B., MRCS; LRCP; DPH; Med. Dir., Queen Elizabeth Hosp.; Spec. Lect. in Chronic Diseases, Dept. of Biometrics, School of Hygiene, U. of Toronto; Tel. 366-8411.

ANGELOMATIS, Stanley G.; 1744 W. Broadway, Vancouver 9, B.C.; 3992 W. 13th St. (res); Vienna (Austria) '34; M.C.G.P.; Vis. Staff, Vancouver **Gen., St. Paul's & Grace Hosp's.; Tel. RE 8-3813.**

ANGELOPOULOS, Theodor M.; 1421 Danforth Ave., Toronto 6, Ont.; Qns'64.

ANGERS, Benoit; 475 Boul. Talbot, Chicoutimi, P.Q.; 227 Racine E. (res); Lav '42; FACC; Int-Med; Cardiol. (P.Q.); Tel. 549-1920.

ANGERS, Charles E.; Neuville Co. Pt. Neuf, P.Q.; Lav '51.

ANGHELIS, Basil; Athens (Greece) '52; Staff, **Hosp. for Mental Diseases, Selkirk, Man.**

ANGIOLI, Guido; 6872 St.-Denis, Montreal 10, **P.Q.; 50 Dobie, Twn. of Mt. Royal (res); Rome (Italy) '53; Gyn (PQ); Tel. CR 2-7733.**

ANGLIN, Adrian F. W.; Ste 1202, 123 Edward St., Toronto 2, Ont.; 51 Castle Frank Rd. (res); Tor. **'33; F.A.C.C.P.; IntMed; Att'd. Phys., St. Michael's Hosp.; Phys., Chest Clin., Hosp. for Sick Children & St. Michael's Hosp.; Assoc. Prof.** (Med.), U. of Toronto; M.O.; Shell Oil Co. of Canada; Tel. 363-3861.

ANGLIN, Crawford S.; East York Med. Centre, 901 O'Connor Dr., Toronto 16, Ont.; 144 Glenrose Ave. (res); Tor '43; Paed; Assoc. Phys., Hosp. for Sick Children; Assoc. (Paed), U. of Toronto; Tel. PL 7-6269.

ANGLIN, John V.; Coronation, Alta.; McG '53; GenSurg.

ANGLIN, Ruth C. C. (nee Cale); 9 Governor's Rd., Toronto 5, Ont. (res); Tor '17; Retired.

ANGROVE, Richard H.; 24 Elmwood Ave., Senneville, P.Q. (res); Qns '16; Psy., D.V.A., Hosp., St. Anne de Bellevue, P.O.; Retired.

ANGUS, Elizabeth H.; 1199 Austin Ave., Coquitlam, New Westminster, B.C.; 925 Austin Ave. (res); Edinburgh (Scot.) '55; Tel. WE 9-7345.

ANGUS, George A. W.; Western Nova Scotia Clin. 36 Forest St., Yarmouth N.S; Edinburgh **(Scot.) '40; DPM (Lond.); Med. Dir., Western** N.S. Med. Centre & Hd. Sub. Dept. of Psy., Yarmouth Reg. Gen. Hosp.; Tel. 742-3611.

ANGUS, Michael F.; Leigh Square Med. Centre, Port Coquitlam, B.C.; McG '51; GenSurg; Surg Staff, Royal Columbia Hosp.; Court. Staff, St. Mary's Hosp.; New Westminster; Tel. 942-7227.

ANGUS, Robert J.; 324 Prince Edward Dr., Toronto 18, Ont.; Tor'52; Staff, Queen Elizabeth Hosp.; Tel. BE 1-5720.

ANHALT, Arthur W.; Winnipeg Clinic, Winnipeg 1, Man.; 676 Ingersoll St. (res); Man '45; Derm-Syph; Hon. Att. Staff, Winnipeg Gen & Children's Hosp's.; Assoc. Att. Staff, Misericordia Hosp.; Lect. (Derm.), U. of Manitoba; Tel. 942-0551.

ANHALT, Edward F.; Winnipeg Clinic, N.E. St. Mary's & Vaughan, Winnipeg 1, Man.; Man '56; Ophth.; AB (Ophth); Active Staff, Wgp. Gen. & Children's Hosp's.; Court. Staff, St. Boniface & Misericordia Hosp's.; Dir. Retina Clinic & Dem., U. of Manitoba; Tel. 942-0551.

ANHOLT, L. M., S/L; Nat. Defence Med. Centre, Ottawa, Ont.; Alb '58.

ANJILVEL, George M.; Madras (India) '54; FRCS(C), GenSurg; Staff, Pathological Inst., McGill U., Montreal, P.Q.

ANKENMAN, G. John; 1210-750 W. Broadway, Vancouver 9, B.C.; 6455 Marguerite St. (res); **Qns '49; FRCS(C), Urol; Att'd. Staff, Vancouver Gen. & Shaughnessy Hosp's.; Clin. Instr., U. of** British Columbia; Tel. TR 2-2595.

ANNAND, Robert T.; Queen St., Bridgetown, N.S.; Dal '51.

ANNEAR, W. Cameron; Med. Arts Bldg., 420 East St. N., Sarnia, Ont.; 142 Norman (res); Dal '42; GenSurg; Staff, Sarnia Gen. & St. Joseph's Hosp's.; Tel. DI 4-8283.
ANNETT, Robert K.; 408-450 Central Ave., London, Ont.; 106 Iroquois St. (res); Wes '46; MCGP; Tel. GE 8-7771.
ANNIS, Lloyd H.; 555—4th Ave. W., Owen Sound, Ont. (res); Qns '47; D.Rad; DiaRad., Rad., General & Marine Hosp.; Tel. FR 6-2121.
ANNIS, Robert V.; 314 Kerr St., Oakville, Ont.; Tor'65.
ANQUIST, Kenneth A.; 214-6th Ave. S.W., Calgary, Alta.; Alb '57; FRCS(C), OrthSurg; Abroad.
ANSARI, Amir H.; Teheran (Iran)'56; FRCS(C), ObstGyn.; Staff, Univ. Hosp., Edmonton, Alta.
ANSELMO, John E.; 9918-114th St., Edmonton, Alta.; Alb'58; FRCS(C), GenSurg; Teach. Fell., U. of Alberta Hosp.; Tel. 439-5911.
ANSELMO, Romualdo S.; Santo Tomas (Philipp.) '57; Staff, Nova Scotia Hosp., Dartmouth, N.S.
ANSLEY, Harold A.; 216 Heath St. W., Toronto 9, Ont.; Tor'29; DPH; PathBact; Retired.
ANTEN, Edward V.; 69 N. Court St., Port Arthur, Ont.; Tor '37.
ANTHONISEN, Nicholas; Harvard (U.S.A.)'58; Staff, Royal Victoria Hosp., Montreal 2, P.Q.
ANTHONY, Alan R.; 2932 Marine Dr. West Vancouver, B.C.; (res); McG '33; FICS, FRCS-(C); Ophth; Chief of Ophth., St. Paul's & Children's Hosp's.; Tel. MU 5-0454.
ANTHONY, Anwar; Lausanne (Switz.)'45; Staff, Hop. Mont Providence, Montreal 5, P.Q.
ANTHONY, G. Philip; 849 Oxford St., Winnipeg, Man.; London (Eng.) '55; M.B., B.S.; DCH; DA (Eng.); Anaes; Staff (Anaes.), St. Boniface Hosp.; Tel. 943-0311, Loc. 209.
ANTHONY, Louis; 786 Eglinton Ave. E., Toronto, Ont.; 35 Glenvale Blvd. (res); Tor '44; Vis. Staff, St. Michael's Hosp.; Tel. HU 5-6692.
ANTIC, Branislava; 3380 Maplewood, App. 406, Montreal 26, P.Q.; Yugoslavia'52; Paed.
ANTOCHIN, Michael D.; Workmen's Comp. Bd., P.O. Box 68, Elliot Lake, Ont.; Belgrade (Yugo.)'32; Staff, Chest Serv., W.C.B.; Dir., Miner's Chest Exam. Station; Tel. 848-2492.
ANTONEVYCH, Danilo; 828 Juniper St., Oshawa, Ont. (res); Tubingen (Germ.) '49; Anaes; Hd., Dept. of Anaes., Oshawa Gen. Hosp.; Tel. RA 8-6124.
ANTONIK, Ladislav; 550 Clark Rd., New Westminster, B.C. (res); Qns '46; MCGP; Tel. WE 9-1212.
ANTONUK. Philippe; Ste. 713, 30 est, boul. St. Joseph, Montreal 14, P.Q.; Mon '59; ObstGyn (P.Q.)
APARICIO, Carlos; Mon'56; DiagRad; Staff, Hop. Hotel-Dieu, Gaspe, P.Q.
APARICIO, Oscar; Valladolid (Spain) '56; Jr. Int., Hamilton Gen. Hosp., Hamilton, Ont.
APEN, Edward M.; McG '61; Jr. Intn., Montreal Gen. Hosp., Montreal 25, P.Q.
APPEL, Bernard; Glace Bay, N.S.; U.K. '41.
APPELL, Adolph A.; 99 Avenue Rd., Toronto 5, Ont.; 6 Forest Wood Dr. (res); Tor '29; M.S., GenSurg; Sr. Att. Surg., Mt. Sinai Hosp.; Tel. 924-1489.
APPEN, Ursula J.; Marburg (Germ.) '48; Staff, Ontario Hosp., Port Arthur, Ont.
APPLEBY, John; 1543 Victoria Pk. Ave., Scarborough, Ont.; 28 Nightingale Pl. (res); Alb '48; Psy; Staff, Scarborough Gen. Hosp.; Cons. (Psy), Toronto Family Serv. Centres; Tel. PL 9-5281.
APPLEBY, Kenneth G.; 3863 E. Hastings St., Burnaby 2, B.C.; Qns '54; Tel. CY 9-3457.
APPLEBY, Lyon H.; 2184 W. Broadway, Vancouver 9, B.C.; 1584 W. 29th Ave. (res); Qns '19; F.R.C.S. (Eng.), F.R.C.S.(C), F.A.C.S., F.I.C.S., GenSurg; Surg.-in-Chief, St. Paul's Hosp.; Cons. Surg., Children's Hosp.; Clin. Assoc. Prof. (Surg.), U. of British Columbia; Tel. RE 3-1101.
APPLEBY, Lyon M.; Box 1329, Quesnel, B.C.; Box 37 (res); Qns '50; Tel. 992-2171.
APPLEBY, Shirley V.; Brimley Rd. & Finch, R.R. No. 1, Agincourt, Ont.; Alb '48; Staff, Scarborough Gen. Hosp.; Tel. AX 3-8181.
APPLEFORD, Robert D.; 155 Aberdeen Ave., Hamilton, Ont. (res); Tor '36; D.P.H., Occ. Med.; Plant Phys., Steel Co. of Canada; Tel.
APPLETON, Sherwood S.; 101 Ridelle Ave., Toronto 19, Ont.; Tor'60; Psy.
APPLEYARD, Herbert E.; Ont. Hosp. Services Comm., 2195 Yonge St., Toronto 7, Ont.; Wes '30; M.Sc. (Columbia); MRCP (Lond.), FACHA; FRCP(C), IntMed.
APRIL, Jacques; 551-24th Ave., Lachine, Montreal 32, P.Q.; Mon '53; Paed (P.Q.); Tel. 634-1151.
APTED, William E.; Ste. 205, 280 Bloor St. W., Toronto, Ont.; 20 Ava Rd. (res); Tor '38; ObstGyn; Dem. Obst. Gyn., U. of Toronto; Tel. WA 2-7484.
AQUINO, Andres D.; Div. of Labs., Charlottetown, P.E.I.; Santo Tomas (Philipp.)'55; DABP; Tel. 892-1228.
AQUINO, Jose; 1 Swallow St., Rockingham N. S.; Santo Tomas. Manila (Philippines) '53; TherRad; Ass't. Rad., Victoria Gen. Hosp.; Lect., Dalhousie U.; Tel. 422-7371.
AQUINO, Lilia; Santo Tomas (Philipp.) '55; Staff, Sydney City Hosp., Sydney, N.S.; Tel. 564-5507.
ARAI, Arnold T.; Ste. 205, 59 Yonge St., Richmond Hill, Ont.; 232 Rosemar Gdns.(res); Tor'56; GenSurg; Active Cons., York Central Hosp.; Tel. TU 4-7616.
ARANAS, Arturo L.; Mental Health Centre, 1904 Fort St., Victoria, B.C.; Santo Tomas (Philipp.)' '56.
ARBER, Frederick W.; 1940 Lonsdale Ave., North Vancouver, B.C.; 4018 Bayridge (res); Qns '46; FACS, FICS, FRCS(C), GenSurg.; Tel. YU 7-6940.
ARBER, Sidney R.; Box 220, Haney, B.C.; River Rd. (res); Qns '40; Dist. Coroner; Tel. IN 5-1621.
ARBOUR, Jean C.; 240 rue Elm, St. Lambert, P.Q.; Mon '54; DiagRad; Chief of Rad. Serv., Hop. Gen. de St-Lambert & Hop. Charles, Le Moyne, Greenfield Park; Tel. 671-3781.
ARBOUR, Pierre; 1102 Francis, Jacques-Cartier, P.Q.; Mon'58; FRCS(C), Otol.
ARBUCKLE, John William Jr.; 1214-750 W. Broadway, Vancouver 9, B. C.; 1387 Minto Cres. (res); McG '41; FRCS (C); Urol; Clin. Staff, Shaughnessy Hosp. & Children's Hosp.; Clin. Instr., Dept. of Surg., Vancouver Gen. Hosp.; and U. of British Columbia; Tel. TR 2-2816.
ARBUCKLE, J. W., Sr.; 990 Lagoon Dr., Vancouver, B.C. (res); McG '08; ObstGyn; Retired.
ARBUS, Gerald S.; Tor '63; Int., New Mount Sinai Hosp., Toronto 2, Ont.
ARCHAMBAULT, Adrien D.; 4600 Lasalle Blvd., Verdun, Montreal 19, P.Q.; Mon '29; M.C.G.P.; Anaes; Tel. PO 9-5151.
ARCHAMBAULT, Andre; 178-12th Ave., Villes des Laurentides, P.Q.; Mon'55; Tel. 223-2504.
ARCHAMBAULT, Andre; Mon'61; FRCP(C), Int.Med; Staff, Hop. Notre Dame, Montreal; Abroad.
ARCHAMBAULT, G.; 472 Laurier St., St. Jean, P.Q.; 75 Blvd. St. Joseph (res); Lav '32; Dist Coroner.
ARCHAMBAULT, Hugues; Ste. Catherine, Cté Portneuf, P.Q.; '53; DiagRad (P.Q.).
ARCHAMBAULT, Jacques; 125 des Braves, Sept. Iles, P.Q.; Lav'61; GenSurg (P.Q.).
ARCHAMBAULT, Jean; 37 Thornton, Montreal 16, P.Q.; Mon '49; Anaes; Staff, Hop.-Ste-Jeanne-d'Arc; Tel. VI 2-5201.
ARCHAMBAULT, Jean P. E.; 542 Sherbrooke W., Montreal, P.Q.; Mon '19; Med. Exam. Army, 4 P.D., 772 Sherbrooke St. W.
ARCHAMBAULT, J. Raymond; 421 Apple Tree Lane, Ottawa 7, Ont.; Ott'59; Diag Rad.
ARCHAMBAULT, Jules; 35 Sunset Ave., Outremont, Montreal 8, P.Q. (res); Mon '09; Derm (Paris); Syph & Serol. P.G. N.Y.; Former Minister of Health, P.Q.; Retired.
ARCHAMBAULT, Lambert; 10353 Blvd. St. Laurent, Montreal, P.Q.; 11 D'Avaugour Duvernay; Mon '51; Tel. DU 8-6915.

ARCHAMBAULT, Laurent G.; Ste. 201, 1656 est rue Sherbrooke, Montreal 24, P.Q.; 754 Ave. Pratt, Outremont (res); Mon '43; F.R.C.S.(C), GenSurg; GenSurg., Hop.-Notre-Dame; Tel. 521-2116.

ARCHAMBAULT, L. P.; 408 Laurier, St. Jean, P.Q. (res); Lav '13.

ARCHAMBAULT, Luc; Mon '63, Intn., Hotel-Dieu-de-Montreal, Montreal, P.Q.

ARCHAMBAULT, Luc F.; 4104 ouest, St-Jacques, Montreal 30, P.Q.; Mon '64; Tel. 932-5560.

ARCHAMBAULT, Paul; 835 Blvd. St. Joseph Est, Montreal, P.Q.; 228 ave. Simcoe, Ville Mt. Royal (res); Mon '34; Tel. VI 5-1134.

ARCHAMBAULT, Paul A.; 225 est rue Sherbrooke, Montreal, 18, P.Q. (res); Mon '32; Staff, Hop.-St.-Luc; Tel. UN 1-7261.

ARCHAMBAULT, Paul R.; 300 Carre St. Louis, Ste. 9, Montreal, P.Q.; 41 Ave. Sunset, Outremont (res); Mon '25; IntMed (TB); Pulm. Dis & TB (P.Q.); M.C.G.P.; Phys., Hop. Maisonneuve; Cons. Hop. St. Luc; Tel. AV 8-4710.

ARCHAMBAULT, Pierre; 553-12th Ave., Ville LaSalle, P.Q.; Mon'61; DiagRad; Staff, Hop. Hotel-Dieu.

ARCHAMBAULT, Raymond J.; Ott '59; Diag Rad; Staff, Hop.-Notre-Dame, Montreal 24, P.Q.

ARCHAMBAULT, Reginald A.; 835 Blvd. St. Joseph Est, Montreal, P.Q.; 207 Ave. Simcoe, Ville Mt. Royal (res); Lav '35; Tel. VI 5-1134.

ARCHAMBAULT, Remi; 55 Ave de l'Eglise, Montreal 19, P.Q.; 928 est Boul. St. Joseph, Montreal 34; Mon'42; Paed (P.Q.); Ass't., Verdun Gen. Hosp.; Phys., Bruchesi Inst.; Tel. LA 1-3836 & PO 6-3593.

ARCHAMBAULT, Roland; 12774 ouest boul. Gouin, Pierrefonds, P.Q.; Mon '54; AMCGP; Tel. 626-5441.

ARCHAMBAULT, Romeo; Clinique Med.-Chir., 2775 rue Bourdages, St.-Hyacinthe, P.Q.; 2789 Girouard (res); Lav '46; ObstGyn.; Tel. PR 3-1663.

ARCHAMBAULT, Viateur; 3662 Adam St., Montreal 4, P.Q.; 5105 Des Melezes (res); Mon '34; MCGP; Tel. LA 3-9855.

ARCHDEKIN, Fennell F.; Port Carling, Ont.; Wes '57; M.C.G.P.; Tel. 764-1123.

ARCHER, Leonard T.; UBC'59; Assoc. Res. (Anaes.), Vancouver Gen. Hosp., Vancouver, B.C.

ARCHIBALD, A. M. S.; 391 Old Orchard Grove Toronto, Ont. (res); Man '37; Part-time staff, U. of Toronto.

ARCHIBALD, David B.; 342 Charlotte St., Sydney, N.S.; Shore Rd., Sydney Mines (res); Dal '43; Urol; Staff, City of Sydney & St. Rita Hosp's., Sydney, Hamilton Memorial Hosp., North Sydney, Harbour View Hosp., Sydney Mines; Tel. 564-8436.

ARCHIBALD, David M.; P.O. Box 33, Kingston, N.S.; Dal '47; Active Staff, Soldier's Mem. Hosp., Middleton; Tel. 765-4044.

ARCHIBALD, Donald A.; Port Rowan, Ont.; Tor '27; M.O.H., Port Rowan; Dist. Coroner; Tel. 586-3912.

ARCHIBALD, Douglas W.; Eriksdale, Man.; Dal'60; MCGP.

ARCHIBALD, Gerald W.; 98 Guestville Ave., Toronto 9, Ont.; 17 Del Ria Dr. Tor. 15 (res); Dal '55; Staff, Humber Mem. Hosp., Weston; Tel. RO 3-1171.

ARCHIBALD, William S.; 221 Birks Bldg., Jasper Ave. & 104th St., Edmonton, Alta.; 12620-104th Ave. (res); McG '32; GenSurg; Tel. GA 2-2663.

ARCHIBALD, Willis M.; Anesthesia Assoc., 900 King St. W., Kitchener, Ont.; Dal'53; Anaes; Staff, Kitchener-Waterloo & St. Mary's Hosp's.; Tel. SH 4-7361.

ARCHIBALD, W. Stanley; Ste. 3, Gower Bldg., Dawson Creek, B. C.; McG '39; M. C. G. P.; Tel. ST 2-4323.

ARDITTI, Joseph; 115 Hazen St., Saint John, N.B.; Istanbul (Turk.)'54; ABNS; Active Staff, (NeurSurg), St. Joseph's Hosp. & Saint John Gen. Hosp.; Tel. 693-2837.

ARDOUIN, Graham J.; Bentley, Alta.; London (Eng.) '57; MCGP; Staff, Bentley Mun. Hosp.; Assoc. Staff, Rimbey Mun. Hosp.; Vis. Staff, Red Deer Mun. Hosp.; Tel. 64.

ARENA, Ugo; 5470 Victoria Dr., Vancouver 16, B.C.; Milan (Italy) '42; Tel. 325-4514.

ARENAS, Arnolfo A.; Manila Central (Philipp.) '55; Staff, Riverview Hosp., Esondale, B.C.; Tel. LA 1-1911.

ARENDT, Eva C. see Racine, Eva C.

ARFAI, Esmail K.; Staff, Brandon Mental Hosp., Box 420, Brandon, Man.

ARGUE, F. J.; 188 Joicey Blvd., Toronto 12, Ont. Man '34; Tel. HU 8-8355.

ARGUE, Robert L.; Man '60; DiagRad; Staff, St. Boniface Hosp., Winnipeg, Man. Abroad.

ARGUE, Stanley E. C.; 3451 Cardiff Pl., Victoria, B.C.; Man '23; GenSurg; Pt.-time Metropolitan Health Bd.; Tel. EV 2-4953.

ARGYROPOULOS, Nicholas; Athens (Greece) '52; Jr. Intn., St. Catharines Gen. Hosp., St. Catharines, Ont.

ARHANIC, Milivoj C.; Zagreb (Yugo.)'59; Sr. Res., Sunnybrook Hosp., Toronto, Ont.

ARJONA, Manuel Q.; 26 Roche St., St. John's, Nfld.; Manila (Philipp.)'55.

ARKINSTALL, Margaret (Smith); 628 Davis Dr., Newmarket, Ont.; Tor '30; Phys., York Manor Home for the Aged; Tel. 895-6461.

ARKINSTALL, William C.; 106 Med. Arts Bldg., 628 Davis Dr., Newmarket, Ont.; Qns '30; Med. Surg. & Cons. Surg., York Co. Hosp.; Tel. 895-6461.

ARKLIE, Daphne W.; 69 Monkstown Rd., St. John's, Nfld. (res); Dal '50; Ass't. to Dir., T.B. Dispensary, Dept. of Health.

ARMANIOUS, Finley; Medical Arts Clinic, Swift Current, Sask.; Cairo, (Egypt) & London (Eng.) '62; Int Med.

ARMBRUST, Nancy E.; 143 Peter St. N., Orillia, Ont. (res); Qns '50; DPH; M.O.H., Orillia Br., Simcoe Health Unit; Tel. 326-2141.

ARMBRUSTER, Robert; Man'65; Jr. Int., St. Boniface Hosp., St. Boniface 6, Man.

ARMETT, Vera (See Gellman).

ARMIT, J. Conn; 330 Medical Dental Bldg., Regina, Sask.; 2905 McCallum Ave. (res); Man '40; Tel. 527-8561.

ARMITAGE, Donald P.; Tor'63; Ass't. Res. (Med.), Toronto Western Hosp., Toronto, Ont.

ARMITAGE, George C.; Med. Arts Bldg., 31 Centre St. S., Brampton, Ont.; Tor '31; MCGP; Chief, Dept. of Anaes., Peel Mem. Hosp.; Tel. 451-2922.

ARMITAGE, John; Med. Arts Clinic, 51-6th St. S. E., Medicine Hat, Alta.; 52-1st St. S. W. (res); St. Andrews (Scot.) '56; Staff, Medicine Hat Gen. Hosp.; Tel. 527-2281.

ARMITAGE, T. F. Harvey; 136 E. 15th St., North Vancouver, B.C.; Alb '38; IntMed; Tel. YU 8-0330.

ARMOUR, John A.; Wes'63; Res., Hosp. for Sick Children, Toronto 2, Ont.; Abroad.

ARMOUR, W. Edward; 60 Russel Hill Rd., Toronto 7, Ont. (res); Tor '41; MCGP; Ass't. Sec., Ont. Med. Assoc., 244 St. George St., Tor. 5; Chmn., Ont. Bd. of Rad. Technicians; Sec't., Ont. Committee on Children; Tel. WA 5-3264.

ARMSTRONG, Alan H.; 55 Avondale Blvd., Bramalea, Ont. Queen's U. (Belfast, N. Ire.) '56; M.B., B.Ch., BAO; Act. Med. Staff, Peel Mem. Hosp.; Tel. 451-7575.

ARMSTRONG, Allan I.; 2 South Dr., St. Catharines, Ont.; Tor '50; DPM (Eng), DABPN (P); Psy; Tel. 685-8523.

ARMSTRONG, Arthur R.; Tor'30; Bact; Dir., Dept. of Labs., Hamilton Health Assoc., Box 590, Hamilton, Ont.; Tel. 385-5341.

ARMSTRONG, Bruce P.; Ste. 101, 5890 Monkland, Montreal, P.Q.; 4582 Melrose (res); McG '56; M.C.G.P.; Ass't. Phys., Queen Elizabeth Hosp.; Tel. HU 6-9542.

ARMSTRONG, Charles A.; Ste 506, 625-5th Ave., New Westminster, B.C.; 519 Second St. (res); Tor '33; FICS, FRCS(C), GenSurg; Tel. LA 1-5121.

ARMSTRONG, Dawna (Duncan); Man '61; Jr. Intn., Winnipeg Gen. Hosp., Winnipeg 3, Man.

ARMSTRONG, Donald J.; Qns'60; Ass't. Res., Dept. of Anaes., U. of Toronto, Toronto, Ont.

ARMSTRONG, Francis B.; 12815-116th Ave,. Edmonton, Alta. (res); Dal '55; M.O., Charles Camsell Indian Hosp.

ARMSTRONG, George W.; 406 Medical Arts Bldg., 180 Metcalfe St., Ottawa, Ont.; 50 Carling Ave. (res); Tor '22; D.A.B.O.S., F.A.C.S., F.R.C.S.(C), OrthSurg; Cons., OrthSurg, Ottawa Civic Hosp., Royal Ottawa San. & D.V.A.; Tel. 233-1139.

ARMSTRONG, Gordon W. D.; 406 Med. Arts Bldg,. 180 Metcalfe St., Ottawa 4, Ont.; 513 Mayfair Ave. (res); Qns '47; DABOS; OrthSurg., Ottawa Civic Hosp.; Clin. Instr. (OrthSurg), U. of Ottawa; Tel. 233-1139.

ARMSTRONG, Harvey A.; P.O. Box 880, Wabush, Labrador; Tor'64; M.O.H.; Industrial Health Officer, Scully Mine; School Health Officer, J. R. Smallwood Collegiate; Tel. 282-6701.

ARMSTRONG, H. Brock; 314 Medical Arts Bldg., Edmonton, Alta.; 10915-85th Ave. (res); Alb '43; Paed; Ass't. Clin. Prof. (Paed.), U. of Alberta; Tel. 422-3213.

ARMSTRONG, Ida M.; 113 Medical Arts Bldg., Winnipeg, Man.; 344 Yale Ave. (res); Man '36; MCGP; Retired.

ARMSTRONG, Irvin; 15 Woodlawn Place, Brockville, Ont.; Qns '22; MCGP; Act. Staff, Brockville Gen. & St. Vincent de Paul Hosp's.; Tel. 345-5645.

ARMSTRONG, J. Kent; Ste. 300, 955 Queen St. E., Sault Ste. Marie, Ont.; Tor'49; FRCS(C); GenSurg; Cons. Staff, Plummer Mem. & Gen. Hosp's.; Tel. AL 6-5574.

ARMSTRONG, John B.; McG'65; Res., St. Paul's Hosp., Vancouver, B.C.

ARMSTRONG, John B.; 1130 Bay St., Toronto 5, Ont.; 273 Yonge Blvd., Tor. 12 (res); Tor '43; FACC; FRCP(C), IntMed; Exec. Dir., Cdn. Heart Fdn.; Ass't. Tor. Gen. Hosp.; Assoc. Prof. (Pharmacol.) & Research Assoc. Med., U. of Toronto; Tel. 924-1411.

ARMSTRONG, John D.; 280 Bloor St. W., Ste. 101, Toronto Ont.; 47 Lower Links Rd., Willowdale (res); Tor'43; D.Psy; Psy; Dir., Mental Health Clin., North York Gen. Hosp., Willowdale; Tel. WA 1-0014.

ARMSTRONG, L. Noble; Ste. 205, 10 Montreal St., Kingston, Ont.; 110 Bagot St., Apt. 1 (res); Qns'16; FRCS; OphthOtol; Att. Staff, Kingston Gen. & Hotel Dieu Hosp's.; Hon. Cons., Ontario Hosp. Servs.; Tel. 548-8373.

ARMSTRONG, Margaret I.; 207 Owen Blvd., Willowdale, Ont. (res); Tor '43; Retired.

ARMSTRONG, Mary (See Hall)

ARMSTRONG, M. Patricia (See White)

ARMSTRONG, Richard M.; Man '61; Jr. Intn., Winnipeg Gen. Hosp., Winnipeg 3, Man.

ARMSTRONG, Richard P., Capt.; c/o MIR, Cdn. Forces Base, Westwin, Winnipeg, Man.; Man'63.

ARMSTRONG, Robert A.; 1482 Portal Ave., Ottawa, Ont. (res); Tor '49; M.O., Dept. Nat. Health and Welfare; Tel. CE 2-8211.

ARMSTRONG, Roderick A.; Digby Community Mental Health Centre, Box 249, Digby, N.S.; London (Eng.) '46; BA(Oxon.); LMSSA(Lond.); Exec. Dir., Digby Annapolis Mental Health Serv. Bd.; Instr., (Clin.Psy.), Research Cons. (Social Psy.), School of P.H., Harvard U., Boston, Mass.; Tel. 425-2498.

ARMSTRONG, Ronald D.; Apt. 1203, 3 Goldfinch Court, Willowdale, Ont.; Wes'57; DiagRad; Staff, Dept. of Rad., Toronto Gen. Hosp.

ARMSTRONG, Ross F.; Lamont Clinic, Lamont, Alta.; Tor'59; MCGP; Tel. 895-5534.

ARMSTRONG, Thomas K.; Medical Arts Bldg., 2150 Valley Way, Niagara Falls, Ont; 1257 Drummond Rd. (res); Tor '48; Med. Staff, Greater Niagara Gen. Hosp.; Tel. EL 8-3838.

ARMSTRONG, Thomas W.; 11 Kirkland St.,Kirkland Lake, Ont.; 8 Porteous Ave. (res); Tor' 42; MCGP; Coroner Dist. of Timiskiming; Tel. 567-3217.

ARMSTRONG, Walter J.; 23 Vista Cres., Kitchener, Ont. (res); Tor '36; PathBact; Path., St. Mary's Hosp., Kitchener; Reg. Path., Attorney Gens. Dept., Prov. of Ont.; Tel. 744-3311.

ARMSTRONG, W. Frank; Box 165, North Bay, Ont.; Tor '57; MCGP; Tel. 472-3660.

ARMSTRONG, William S.; 408 McLeod Bldg., 100th St., Edmonton, Alta.; McG '24; Otol; Ass't. Clin. Prof. (Otol), U. of Alberta.

ARMSTRONG, W. T.; Box 480, Revelstoke, B. C.; Alb '49; MCGP; Staff, Queen Victoria Hosp.; Tel. 837-3131.

ARNEIL, Allan S.; 9757 Carlton St., Chilliwack, B.C. (res); Glasgow(Scot.) '47; D.R.C.O.G.; PH; D.P.H.; Dir., Upper Fraser Valley Health Unit (Kootenay Lake Gen. Hosp., Nelson; Chilliwack Gen., Fraser Canyon & Abbottsford Hosp's); Tel. SY 2-3411.

ARNOLD, Craig R.; 750 W. Broadway, Vancouver 9, B.C.; Wes '50; IntMed; Att'd. Staff, Vancouver Gen. Hosp.; Cons. Med., Shaughnessy Hosp.; Instr. (Med.), U. of British Columbia; Tel. TR 4-4321.

ARNOLD, Hugh A.; Haig Clinic, 601-6th Ave. S., Lethbridge, Alta.; 2871 Parkside Dr. (res); Alb '38; FACP; IntMed; Chief of Med., St. Michael's Hosp.; Tel. 328-6641.

ARNOLD, John C.; R.R. 1, Peterborough, Ont.; Wes '35; Retired.

ARNOLD, Robin A.; 3481 Danforth Avenue, Toronto 13, Ont.; Tor '56; Tel. OX 4-6488.

ARNOLD, Walter C.; 572 Lake Shore Rd., Haileybury, Ont.; Tor '10.

ARNOLD, William J. D.; 122—2nd Ave. W., Prince Rupert, B.C.; UBC '55; M.C.G.P. Abroad.

ARNOT, Richards G. S/L; R.C.A.F. Station, Lancaster Park, Alta.; Alb '62.

ARNOTT, David C.; St. Joseph's Hosp., Port Arthur, Ont.; 96 South High St. (res); St. Thomas' H. (London, Eng.) '38; DCH; D.Phys-Med.; PhysMed. & Rehab; Med. Dir., Lakehead Rehab. Centre; Tel. DI 4-2431.

ARNOTT, James H.; Tor'61; FRCP(C), IntMed; Staff, Sunnybrook Hosp., Toronto 12, Ont.

ARNOTT, Janet E.; Royal Free Hosp. (London, Eng.) '53; FRCP(C); Path; Staff, Dept of Path., Winnipeg Gen. Hosp., Winnipeg 3, Man.; Tel. SP 4-6511.

ARNOTT, Ruth M.; 96 South High St., Port Arthur, Ont.; London (Eng.) '42.

ARNUP, William B.; 237 Kent St. W., Lindsay, Ont.; 110 Adelaide St. N. (res); Tor '44; Int Med.; Tel. 324-5321.

ARONOFF, Alexander; 4119 Sherbrooke St. W., Westmount, Montreal 6, P.Q.; McG '49; B.Sc., FACP; FRCP(C), IntMed; Cons. (Med.) & Ass't. Chief of Med., Queen Mary Vet's. Hosp.; Dir. of Hepatic & GI Serv., Queen Mary Vet's. Hosp.; Clin. Ass't., Royal Victoria Hosp.; Cons. (Med.), Montreal Rehab. Inst.; Lect. (Clin.Med.), McGill U.; Tel. WE 2-1053.

ARONOFF, Morton; Catalina Med. Centre, 2222 N. Craycroft Ste 1-8, Tuscon, Arizona, 85716, U.S.A.; Dal '56; PlasSurg; Abroad.

ARONOVITCH, Michael; 4119 Sherbrooke W., Westmount, P.Q.; 1530 Dumfries Rd., Mount Royal (res); McG '35; F.A.C.P., F.C.C.P., Pulm. Dis. & TB (P.Q.), F.R.C.P.(C), IntMed; Med. Dir., Mt. Sinai San., Prefontaine; Assoc. Phys. Royal Victoria Hosp., Cons., Queen Mary Vet's., Royal Edward Laurentian, Grace Dart and Herbert Reddy Mem. Hosp's.; Ass't. Prof., (Med.), McGill U.; Tel. WE 2-0834.

ARONSON, Andres; Tartu (Estonia) '41; Staff, Provincial Hosp., Lancaster, N.B.; Tel. 694-4481.

ARRANZ, Carlos C.; 691 Main St., Moncton, N.B.; Madrid (Spain)'52; Anaes; Staff, Moncton Hosp.; Tel. 389-9467.

ARRO, Endel; 183 James St. S., Hamilton, Ont.; Tartu (Estonia) '43; Staff (Med.), Hamilton Civic & St. Joseph's Hosp's.; Tel. 528-5427.

ARRONET, George H.; 4751 Sherbrooke St. W., Montreal 15, P.Q.; 4765 Grosvenor (res); Berlin (Germ.) '39; ObstGyn; Dir. Infertility Centre, Royal Victoria Hosp.; Instr. McGill U.; Tel. WE 3-3505.

ARROWSMITH, Ralph C.; Ste. 502, 101 Royal Ave., New Westminster, B.C. (res); UBC'54; Psy; Staff, Riverview Hosp., Essondale; Tel. LA 1-1911.

ARSCOTT, Allan G.; Box 550, Marathon, Ont.; Tor '54.

ARSENAULT, Armand; 1150 est. boul. St-Joseph, Montreal, P.Q.; Lav'50; DABOt; FAAO; FACS; Otol.; Tel. LA 7-1241.
ARSENAULT, Charles; C.P. 87, Squatteck, Co. Temiscouata, P.Q.; Lav '59.
ARSENAULT, Gatien; 1230 Blv. Mercure, Drummondville, P.Q.; Lav '60.
ARSENAULT, J. Theodore; Lav '60; Res., Royal Victoria Hosp., Montreal 2, P.Q.
ARSENAULT, Lorne J. A.; Lav'60; GenSurg; Staff, Hop. d'Amqui, Amqui, P.Q.
ARSENAULT, Marc; Lebel Sur Quevillon, Cte. Abitibi Est., P.Q.; Lav'48.
ARSENAULT, Raymond; 142 est Notre-Dame, Victoriaville, P.Q.; Lav '55; MCGP.
ARSHAWSKY, Pearl R.; 2901 Lawrence Ave. E., Scarborough, Ont.; McG '55; MCGP; Staff, Scarborough Gen. Hosp.; Tel. AX 3-7551.
ARSTIKAITIS, Maria J. (Uleckas); Ste. 1116, 123 Edward St., Toronto 2, Ont.; Innsbruck (Austria) '47; Ophth; Staff, Hosp. for Sick Children; Cons. Ophth., Toronto Dept. of Public Health; Tel. 368-2661.
ARTES, Waldemar E.; Box 190, Dominion City, Man.; Albert St. (res); Donetz Med. Coll. (U.S.S.R.) '36; M.C.G.P.; M.O.H.
ARTHUR, Charles L. T.; 6275 Nelson Dr., Gleneagles, West Vancouver, B.C.; Man '15; F.R.C.S.-(C); Retired.
ARTHUR, Geraldine M.; Tor'53; Staff, Toronto Dept. of Health, 358 Keele St., Toronto 9, Ont.; Tel. 367-9111.
ARTHUR, John F.; 4027 E. Hastings, N. Burnaby, B.C.; 301 North Hythe (res); Man '40; Vis. Staff, Vancouver Gen., St. Paul's, St. Vincent's, St. Joseph's Hosp's.; Att. Staff, Burnaby Gen. & Grace Hosp's.; Tel. CY 9-2677.
ARTHURS, James; Qns '36; Staff, Queen Elizabeth Hosp., Toronto 3, Ont.; Tel. 534-7513.
ARTHURS, James; 89A Lake Promenade, Toronto 14, Ont.; Qns'47.
ARTHURS, James E.; 375 Main St. E., Hamilton, Ont.; 210 St. Clair Blvd. (res); Tor '45; Staff, St. Joseph's Hosp.; Tel. JA 9-2423.
ARTHURS, Robert G. S.; Clarke Inst. of Psy., 250 College St., Toronto, Ont.; 64 Russell Hill Rd. (res); Tor'43; D. Psy.; Psy; Clin. Teacher, U. of Toronto; Cons. (Psy.), Sunnybrook Hosp.; Tel. WA 1-7625.
ARUNDELL, Faye D.; Wes '56; FRCP(C), Derm; Staff, Cleveland Clinic, 2020 E. 93rd. St., Cleveland 6, Ohio, U.S.A.; Abroad.
ARVANITAKIS, Constantinos J.; McG'65; Jr. Int., Ottawa Civic Hosp., Ottawa, Ont.
ARWA, Eleonore (See Schumacher)
ASA, Morris; 1428 Ouellette Ave., Windsor, Ont.; 8465 Glenwood Ave. (res); Istanbul (Turkey) '48; FACS; FRCS (C); GenSurg; ThorSurg; Active Staff, Hotel-Dieu, Grace & Metropolitan Hosp's.; Tel. 253-4032.
ASANO, Kouichi; 2615-E 49th, Vancouver 16, B.C.; Tokyo (Japan)'57.
ASCAH, Geoffrey M.; 77A Main St., Huntsville, Ont.; 29 Brunel Rd. (res); McG '44; Tel. 789-2345.
ASCHE, Gerd A.; Hope Medical Dental Centre, Hope, B.C.; Bonn (Germ.) '51.
ASCHE-QUINT, Ursula; Box 400, Hope, B.C.; Bonn (W. Germ.) '51.
ASGHAR, Mohammed I.; Lahore (India)'55; FRCS(C); GenSurg; Staff, Victoria Hosp., London, Ont.; Abroad.
ASH, Clifford L.; 500 Sherbourne St., Toronto 5, Ont.; 258 Warren Rd. (res); Tor '34; D.M.R., F.A.C.R., FRCP(C), D&TRad; Rad-in-Chief, Toronto Gen. Hosp.; Dir., Ontario Cancer Inst. & Princess Margaret Hosp.; Prof. of TherRad, U. of Toronto; Tel. 924-0671.
ASH, Daniel G. G.; Clarence & 8th St. E., Saskatoon, Sask.; Sask'64.
ASH, Leslie C.; Tor'63; Staff, Ontario Hosp., Whitby, Ont.
ASHBY, J. Gary; Tor'62; Ass't. Res., Montreal Neurolog. Inst., 3801 University St., Montreal 28, P.Q.
ASHBY, Roy M.; 1436 Kingsway, Vancouver 12, B.C.; Man'53; MCGP; Tel. TR 9-1501.
ASHENHURST, Alex W.; 34 Main St., Georgetown, Ont.; Tor'64.
ASHENHURST, Alexander E.; 232 High Park Ave., Toronto, Ont.; Tor '29; M.C.G.P.; Tel. RO 7-4147.
ASHENHURST, Edward M.; 1133 Elliott St., Saskatoon, Sask (res); Queens U. (Belfast, N. Ireland)'53; BAO; MRCP (Edin.); FRCP(C); Neur.; Assoc. Prof. Med., U. of Saskatchewan; Tel. CH 2-7641.
ASHFORD, David R.; Alb'61; Path; Staff, University Hosp., Edmonton, Alta.
ASHFORTH, Ian; Box 620, St. Paul, Alta.; Sheffield (Eng.)'51.
ASHKENAZY, William; 5845 Cote-des-Neiges Rd., Montreal 25, P.Q.; McG '41; B.Sc.; Radiol., Protestant School Bd.; Tel. 739-1904.
ASHLEY, Evelyn P.; 1125 Islington Ave. N., Rexdale, Ont.; Man '54; Part-time, Dept. of Health, Toronto; Tel. CH 7-8253.
ASHLEY, Harold I.; 1125 Islington Ave. N., Rexdale, Ont.; Tor'48; M.C.G.P.; Active Staff, Queensway Gen. Hosp.; Tel. CH 7-8253.
ASHLEY, Mary J.; 188 Mill St. South, Brampton, Ont.; Tor'63.
ASHMORE, Phillip G.; Ste. 1204, 750 W. Broadway, Vancouver 9, B.C.; 6287 Marguerite St. (res); Tor '48; F.R.C.S.(C), GenSurg; ThorSurg; Staff (Surg.), Vancouver Gen. Hosp. Clin. Ass't. Prof. (Dept. of Surg.), U. of British Columbia; Tel. TR 9-4324.
ASHRAFI, Massoud; Tehran (Iran)'54; Res., Children's Hosp., Halifax, N.S.
ASHWELL, Thomas O.; Med. Arts Bldg., 22 William St. W., Smiths Falls, Ont.; Tor '56; Staff, St. Francis Gen. & Public Hosp's.; Staff, Smith Falls Ontario Hosp.; Tel. 283-0710.
ASHWORTH, E. John; 183 James St. S., Hamilton, Ont.; London (Eng.) '55; Anaes; Staff (Anaes), Hamilton Gen. Hosp.; Tel. JA 9-8875.
ASHWORTH, Lyn (See Robinson)
ASHWORTH, Murray A.; 217 Glenclair Ave., Toronto, Ont. (res); Tor '41; B.Sc. (Med.), Ph.D.; Assoc. Prof. (Physiol.), U. of Toronto; Tel. HU 8-2860.
ASKEY, Alan W.; 45-9th Ave., Cranbrook, B.C.; 122-9th Ave. (res); Alb '60; Staff, St. Eugene & Kimberley Dist. Hosp's.; Tel. 426-4231.
ASP, Douglas M.; 4231 Gloucester Dr., Calgary, Alta. (res); Alb '52; Path; Staff, Holy Cross Hosp.; Tel. AM 6-7231.
ASPINALL, Roy J.; UBC '55; PathBact; Staff, Dept. of Path., St. Paul's Hosp., Vancouver, B.C.; Tel. MU 3-2211.
ASQUITH, Eric; 235 Medical Dental Bldg., Rose St. & 11th Ave., Regina, Sask.; 3480 Angus St. (res); London(Eng.) '42; D.A., F.F.A.R.C.S.; Staff (Anaes), Regina Gen. and Grey Nuns Hosp's; Tel. 527-6762.
ASQUITH, Raymond; Med. Arts Bldg., 121 Wellington St. W., Barrie, Ont.; (London (Eng.) '39; DCH(Lond.); Paed; Chief of Paed., Royal Victoria Hosp.; Court. Cons., St. Andrew's Hosp., Midland, Soldier's Mem. Hosp., Orillia, & Stevenson Mem. Hosp., Allison.
ASREGADOO, Edward R.; 153 Pinnacle St., Belleville, Ont.; Boston (U.S.A.) '51.
ASSELIN, J. Nelson; 1379 rue St-Martial, Quebec 3, P.Q.; Lav '37.
ASSELIN, Jean Paul; 6719-43e ave., Rosemont, Montreal 36, P.Q.; FRCS(C) GenSurg; Staff, Hop. Hotel-Dieu; Tel. VI 4-0161.
ASSELIN, Paul E.; Lav '58; Res., Hop. Notre-Dame, Montreal 24, P.Q.
ASSELSTINE, Albert P.; 10 Egerton St., Kapuskasing, Ont. (res); Qns '35; Med. Dir., Spruce Falls Power & Paper Co., Kapuskasing; Tel. 335-2311.
ASSELSTINE, Harold S.; 1219 Devonshire Rd., Windsor, Ont. (res); McG '43; Path; Staff, Grace Hosp.; Tel. CL 6-2361.
ASSELSTINE, James L.; 700 Elgin Ave., Winnipeg 3, Man.; Tor'44; Psy; Hon. Att'd. Phys., Wpg. Children's Hosp.; Dir. Child Guidance Clin. of Gtr. Winnipeg; Assoc. Prof. (Psy.), U. of Manitoba; Tel. SP 5-7101.

ASSELSTINE, Kenneth M.; 181 McIntyre St. W., North Bay, Ont.; 1548 Pinewood Cres. (res); Tor '55; GenSurg; Surg., Staff, St. Joseph's & Civic Hosp's.; Tel. 472-3660.

ASSELSTINE, Stanley M.; 1466 Ouellette Ave., Windsor, Ont.; 3563 Ouellette Ave., Sandwich W. (res); Qns'13; PathBact; IntMed; Cons. (IntMed), Hotel-Dieu, IODE, Grace & Metropolitan Gen. Hosp's.; Tel. 256-7453.

AST, Helga; 11613 Joly St., Pierrefonds, P.Q.; McG '57; Psy(P.Q.); Staff, Verdun Gen. Hosp., Montreal; Dem. (Psy.), McGill U.; Tel. 766-8511.

ASUNCION, Jacobo R. Jr.; Sir Charles Tupper Med. Bldg., Rm. 14A-1, Faculty of Med., Dalhousie U., Halifax, N.S.; Santo Tomas (Philipp.) '56; Ass't. Prof., Dept. of Anat., Dalhousie U., Halifax, N.S.

ATACK, Edward A.; 300 Cooper St., Ste. 2, Ottawa, Ont.; Qns'49; FACP; FRCP(C); Neur; Chief of Neurol. & NeurSurg., Ottawa Civic Hosp.; Ass't. Prof. Med. (Neur.), U. of Ottawa; Tel. 236-5170.

ATACK, Mary H. G.; 123 Edward St., Toronto, Ont.; **228 Glengrove W. (res); Tor '30; Staff, Women's College Hosp.;** Tel. **WA 1-4313.**

ATCHESON, John D.; 82 Ravensbourne Cres., Islington, Ont. (res); **Wes '41;** D.Psy., Psy; Supt., Thistletown Hosp.; Assoc., Dept. of Psy., **U. of Toronto; Lect., School of Nursing; Tel.** 724-1210.

ATERMAN, Kurt; 69 Shirley St., Halifax, N.S. (res); Queen's U. (Belfast, Ire.) '42; **Ph.D., M.R.C.P., D.C.M.; Assoc. Prof. (Path.), Dalhousie U.;** Tel. 2-4406.

ATHANS, George; Knox Clinic, 1605 Glenmore St., Kelowna, B.C.; McG'48; MCGP; Tel. 762-2002.

ATHANS, Tino; '60; Res. Winnipeg Gen. Hosp., Winnipeg, Man.

ATHLEY, Prabhakar A.; Box 258, Oxford, N.S.; Calcutta (India) '49.

ATIN, Harvey L.; Ste. 202, 25 Brunswick Ave., Toronto 4, Ont.; 138 Kilbarry Rd. (res); Tor'53; IntMed; Active Staff, Doctor's Hosp.; Tel. 924-9741.

ATKINS, Ainsley S.; 101 Pacific Medical Bldg., 1665 West Broadway, Vancouver, B.C.; 1915 Drummond Dr. (res); Dal '47; F.R.C.P.(C), Int Med; **Attend. Staff, Vancouver Gen. Hosp.; Tel. RE 1-4144.**

ATKINS, E. Laurence; 5 Academy Med. Bldg., 1812-4th St., S.W. Calgary, **Alta.;** 36 Grafton Dr. (res); Alb '55; M.Sc.; FRCP(C); IntMed; Reg. Phys., Imperial Oil Company; Tel. 266-3211.

ATKINS, John L.; 300 St. Clair Ave. W., Toronto 7, Ont.; Tor'31; M.Sc. (Med.) (Penn.); DABOT; FICS; Otol; Sr. Att'd. Otol., Northwestern Gen.; Att'd. Otol., New Mt. Sinai Hosp.; Cons. (Otol.), Baycrest & Doctors' Hosp's.; Tel. WA 2-5414.

ATKINSON, Anson R.; Peterboro St., Norwood, Ont.; McG '35; M.C.G.P.

ATKINSON, David I.; Wes'65; Res., Hosp. for Sick Children, Toronto, Ont.

ATKINSON, Hubert H.; 610 Medical Centre, 8th St. & 8th Ave. S.W., Calgary, Alta.; London (Eng.)'35; MRCS; LRCP; FRCS(Ed.); Tel. 262-9128.

ATKINSON, Joan M.; Pickering Med. Centre, Pickering, Ont.; Tor '59.

ATKINSON John W.; 440 Hinton Ave., Ottawa, Ont.; 1950 Bromley Rd. (res); Qns '59; Anaes; Staff (Anaes), Ottawa Civic Hosp.: Tel. 728-6914.

ATKINSON Kenneth G.; 817 Medical Dental Bldg., 925 W. Georgia St., Vancouver 1, B.C.; UBC '55; GenSurg; Tel. MU 4-6477.

ATKINSON, Margaret (See Horne).

ATKINSON, Martin H.; Alb '64; Res. University Hosp., Edmonton, Alta.

ATKINSON, Peter I.; Mount Pearl, Box 100, Nfld. (Calcutta, India) '45.

ATKINSON, Reginald D.; 92 Margaret Ave. N., Waterloo, Ont. (res); Tor'51; MCGP; Assoc. Med. Dir., Mutual Life Assurance Co. of Canada; Tel. 745-6181.

ATKINSON, Theodore E.; 77 Main St., Salisbury, N.B.; Dal'62; AMCGP.

ATKINSON, Walter L.; 465 Duchess Ave., Ottawa 2, Ont. (res); Tor '24; Med. Adv. Cdn. Pensions Comm., Daly Bldg.; Retired.

ATKINSON, William H.; 153 McNaughton St., Sudbury, Ont.; Tor '33; Temp. Retired.

ATNIKOV, Murray G.; 713 Columbia, New Westminster, B.C.; 42 Royal Ave. (res); Man '50; Anaes; Tel. LA 2-4241.

ATLEE, Harold B.; Box 556, Bedford, N. S.; Dal' 11; FACOG; FICS; FRCS (Edin.); FRCS (C); **ObstGyn; Obst., Grace Maternity Hosp.; Gyn., Victoria Gen. Hosp.; Prof. Emer. (ObstGyn.),** Dalhousie U.; Tel. 423-6566.

ATTARIWALA, Gurcharanjit S.; 505 Med. Centre Bldg., 906-8th Ave. S.W., Calgary, Alta.; Madras (India) '55; FRCS(C), Ophth.

ATTENBOROUGH, Richard G.; Box 177, Vermilion, Alta.; London (Eng.) '53; MRCS (Eng.); LRCP (Lond.).

ATTENDU, Charles A.; 10470, Papineau, Montreal 12, P.Q.; Mon '37; Obst; Staff, Hop. Notre Dame; Tel. AV 8-2383.

ATTIE, Henriette; Geneva (Switz.) '53; Res., Hop. Ste-Justine, Montreal, P. Q.

ATTRIDGE, Frank R.; Ste. 1303. 750 W. Broadway, Vancouver 9, B.C.; Man '29; F.A.A.O.O., Otol; Vis, Staff, Vancouver Gen., St. Paul's, **Children's and Burnaby Gen. Hosp's; Memb., Pan-Pacific Surg. Asoc.; Tel. TR 4-5611.**

ATWOOD, Hugh K.; Williams Lake, B.C.; Tor '42

ATYEO, Ralph D.; Medical Arts Bldg., Hamilton, Ont.; Qns '49; M.R.C.O.G.; ObstGyn; Staff, Hamilton **Gen. Hosp.; Tel. JA 8-2441.**

AUBE, Laurent; 65 est Grande-Allee, Quebec 4, P.Q.; Lav '57; DiagRad; Staff, Hop. Hotel-Dieu.

AUBE, Louis A.; 14 Lobban Ave., Chatham, N.B.; Church St. (res); McG '43; DABOph; Tel. PR 3-5437.

AUBE, L. Remi; 414 rue Commerciale, Alma, P.Q.; Lav '43; MCGP; M.O., Aluminum Co. of Canada.

AUBE, Marc; Mon'65; Staff, Hop. Manicouagan, Cte. Saguenay, P.Q.

AUBIN, Gervais; Lav '60; Paed; Staff, Institut Medical, 475 boul. Talbot, Chicoutimi, P.Q.; Tel. 549-1034.

AUBIN, Gilles; 614 rue St.-Georges, St.-Jerome, Cte. Terrebonne, P.Q.; Mon '60; Tel. GE 2-7982.

AUBIN, Jean; Ott '62; Res., Hosp. for Sick Children, Toronto, Ont.

AUBIN, Raymond; 219 Baldwin St., Cornwall, Ont.; 131 rue Jarvis (res); Lav '57; GenSurg.; Tel. WE 3-3350.

AUBRY, Andre; 55a Fusey, Cap-de-la-Madeleine, P.Q.; Lav'60; ObstGyn; Tel. 378-2514.

AUBRY, Ubald; 170 rue First, St. Lambert, Cite-Jacques-Cartier, P.Q.; Lav '54; Anaes; Staff, Hop.-Notre-Dame, Mtl.; Tel. LA 5-6363.

AUBUT, J. E.; rue Lauzon, Lac Megantic, **Cte. Frontenac, P.Q.; Lav '40; Anaes.** (P.Q.) Dist. Coroner; Tel. 583-0232.

AUCKLAND, Norman L. D.; Ste. 1114, Fairmont **Medical Bldg., 750 W. Broadway, Vancouver, B.C.; 2114 W. 53rd (res); Man '41, Neur; Assoc. (Neur) & Dir. Electro-Encephalographic Dept., Vancouver Gen. Hosp.; Cons. (Neur), (Part-time), Electro-Encephalographer, Shaughnessy Hosp., D.V.A.; Clin. Instr., (Neur.), U. of British Columbia; Tel. TR 6-2281.**

AUCLAIR, Paul; 8892 St. Hubert, Montreal 11, P Q.; Mon '65.

AUDE, Salim; Bay l'Argent, Nfld.; '50.

AUDET, Blaise; Lav '63; Res., Dept. of Neurosurg., U. of Laval, Quebec, P.Q.; Abroad.

AUDET, Irenee; 317A boul St-Joseph, Roberval, P.Q.; Lav '52; Tel. 275-1116.

AUDET, Jacques; 655 Grande-Allee, Quebec, P.Q.; Lav '35; Ophth, Otol; Hd. Dept. of Ophth., Assoc. Prof. Laval U.; Tel. 523-6585.

AUDET, Jacques; Mon '61; Anaes; Staff, Hop.-Notre-Dame, Montreal, P.Q.; Abroad.

AUDET, Jean C.; Lav '52; M.C.G.P.; C.P. 157, Mistassini, Co. Lac St. Jean, P.Q.

AUDET, J. Romuald; Lav '60; Res., Hop. de l'Enfant-Jesus, Quebec, P.Q.

AUDET, Luc; 1872 Blvd. Laurier, Sillery, Quebec, P.Q. (res); Lav '48; D&TRad; Staff, Hop. St. **Sacrement, Chief of Rad., Laval U.; Tel. LA 7-3461.**

AUDET, Wilfrid; 3777 Lacombe, Montreal 26, P. Q.; Lav '30; Tel. RE 8-3336.
AUDET-LAPOINTE, Jean; 5757 Decelles Ave., Montreal 26, P.Q.; 16 Springrove, Outremont (res); Mon '25; C. Op. Tech. Paris; F.A.A.O.O., Ophth, Otol; Ass't. Chief (Ophth., Otol.), Hop. Ste. Justine; Tel. RE 9-4055.
AUDET-LAPOINTE, Pierre; Mon'60; ObstGyn; Staff, Hop.-Notre Dame, Montreal, P.Q.
AUER, J.; 405 Huron Ave., Ottawa 3, Ont. (res); Leiden (Neth) '39; D.Sc. (Leiden); Ass't. Dean & Prof. & Hd. Dept. of Anat., U. of Ottawa; Tel. CE 5-6751.
AUFFREY, Paul E.; 640 Chemin Mountain, Moncton, N.B.; Mon '55; Tel. 389-9808.
AUFREITER, Gottfriede; 22 Sunnyside Ave., Westmount, Montreal 6, P.Q. (res); Vienna (Austria) '39; Neurol. & Psy. (Vienna); Psy (P.Q.); Lect., McGill U.; Tel. HU 6-3917.
AUFREITER, Johann; 22 Sunnyside Ave., Westmount 6, P.Q. (res); Vienna (Austria)'39; Psy (P.Q.); Assoc. Psy., Royal Victoria Hosp.; Training Analyst, Cdn. Inst. of Psychoanalysis; Assoc. Prof. (Psy.) McGill U.; Tel. VI 2-1251, Loc. 619.
AUGER, Antonio, M.P.P.; 159 St. Joseph, St. Joseph D'Alma, P.Q.; **Lav '26; Memb. Legislative Council (P.Q.).**
AUGER, Carleton; 1323 Lemoine, Sillery, Quebec, P.Q. (res); **Lav '38; F.R.C.P.(C), PathBact; Cons. Path., Hotel-Dieu, Hop.-Ste-Foy & Hop.-St. Francois-d'Assise; Prof. (Path). Laval U.; Tel. LA 9-4511.**
AUGER, Eugene; 382 McGill, Hawkesbury, Ont.; Mon '40.
AUGER, Gustave L.; 1061 Des Erables, Quebec, P.Q.; Lav '33; GenSurg; Prof. Surg., Laval U.; Surg. & Chief of Clinic, Hotel-Dieu de Quebec; Tel. 529-9151.
AUGER, Henri-R.; 5689 Rosemont, Montreal, P.Q.; 4430 Pie IX Blvd. (res); Mon '48; Pulm. **Dis. & TB (P.Q.); Ass't., St. Joseph San.; Tel. CL 6-2681**
AUGER, L. Desire; 992 de la Mine, Acton Vale, P.Q.; Lav '35; PH(P.Q.); Tel. 546-2695.
AUGER, Michel; 88 Iles Percees, Boucherville, P.Q.; Mon'62.
AUGER, Paul; 1000 Chemin Ste.-Foy, Quebec, P.Q.; 1345 Ave. Pasteur, Sillery (res); Lav '46; GenSurg; (P.Q.); Asst. Surg., Hop. St. Sacrement & Laval U.; Tel. 681-6241.
AUGER, Paul; 74 Principale, Granby, P.Q.; 48 rue Elgin (res); Lav '37; D.P.H.
AUGER, Paul; 270 Brassard, Nicolet, P.Q.; Lav'51.
AUGER, P. Claude; 191-14eme Ave. St-Lin-des-Laurentides, Cte L'Assomption, P.Q.; Mon '61; Tel. 223-2020
AUGER, Pierre; Lav'62; Res. (Cardiol.), Toronto Gen. Hosp., Toronto, Ont.
AUGER, Rene; App. 8, 2208, Chemin-Ste-Foy, Quebec 10, P.Q.; Lav '50; Anaes.; Tel. 527-4049.
AUGER, Sylvain; 7 St. Joseph, Levis, P.Q.; Lav '34; Tel. 837-4254.
AUGER, Wilfred J.; 25 Brentcliffe Rd., Leaside, Ont.; 37 Rumsey Rd. (res); Tor '35; Tel. HU 8-6300.
AUGUSTINE, John R.; 910 Ridgeway St., Fort William, Ont.; 416 Catherine St. (res); Wes '52; F.A.C.P.; IntMed; Staff, McKellar Gen. Hosp.; Chmn., Prof. Advisory Comm., Lakehead Branch, Addiction Research Fdn. Tel. MA 2-5301.
AUGUSTT-MOFFATT, Solomon E.; 41 Carluke Cr., Apt. 414, Willowdale, Ont.; London (Eng.) '57; ObstGyn; Staff, Mount Sinai Hosp.
AULD, C. R. Benson; 679 Quinpool Rd., Halifax, N.S.; 10 Rosemount Ave. (res); McG '49; GenSurg; Instr., Dalhousie U.; Tel. 455-3122.
AULD, Peter A.; McG '52; F.R.C.P.(C), Paed; Staff, Montreal Children's Hosp., Montreal 25, P.Q.; Tel. WE 7-8511.
AULD, R. Waldron; Kensington, P.E.I.; Dal '49; M.C.G.P.; Tel. 267-3300.
AUM, Eull N.; Box 416, Elliot Lake, Ont. (res); Seoul (Korea) '45; Anaes; Staff, St. Joseph's Hosp.; Tel. VI 8-7181.
AUMONT, Gerald; 1051 St. Denis St., Montreal, P. Q.; Mon '36; Tel. 861-3040.
AUMONT, Marcel; Eastern Med. Center, 5965 est, rue Sherbrooke, Montreal 5, P.Q.; Mon '56; MCGP; Tel. CL 4-5394.
AUMONT, Robert; Napierville, P.Q.; McG '57.
AUNS, Zanis; 260 St. Patrick St., Ottawa 2, Ont.; Riga (Latvia)'32; MCGP; Tel. CE 4-2800.
AUSTIN, Charles J.; 46 Division, Bowmanville, Ont.; Qns '37; Dist. Coroner; Tel. 623-5584.
AUSTIN, Martin; 214-6th Ave. S.W., Calgary, Alta.; London (Eng.)'57; DA (Eng.); Tel. 263-7120.
AUSTIN, Robert R.; 186 Broadway, Orangeville, Ont.; Wes '50; M.C.G.P.; Tel. 941-0161.
AUSTIN, Thomas W.; West'65; Jr. Int., Vancouver General Hosp., Vancouver, B.C.
AUSTIN, W. Eric; 750 W. Broadway, Vancouver, B.C.; Man '32; F.R.C.S. (Ed), F.R.C.S.-(C), F.A.C.S., GenSurg; Att. Staff, Vancouver Gen. Hosp.; Instr. (Surg.), U. of British Columbia.; Tel. 874-8914.
AUSTMANN, Kristjan J.; 403 Cordova St., Winnipeg, Man. (res); Man '21; Ophth, Otol; Cons. Otol., DVA Deer Lodge Hosp.; Retired.
AUSTRUP, Margaret J.; 749 King St. W., Kitchener, Ont.; Madras (India)'53; ObstGyn.
AUSTRUP, Roland H.; 200 King St. W., Waterloo, Ont.; Muenster (Germ.) '52; AMCGP; Active Staff, St. Mary's & Kitchener-Waterloo Gen. Hosp's.; Tel. SH 3-6328.
AUTHIER, Richard (Joseph Rene); 250 est St. Cyrille, Quebec 4, P.Q.; Lav'59; Path.; Tel. 529-9611, Loc. 230.
AUTOTTE, Esdras E.; 6507 Molson St., Montreal, P.Q.; Mon '34; Paed (P.Q.); Ass't. Serv. Paed., Hop. Notre Dame; **Dir. Clin. Paed., & Dir. Medical Health Unit, Bruchesi Inst.; Tel. RA 2-6261.**
AVANZADO, Elena B.; Manila (Philipp.)'59; Res., Hop. St. Jeanne d'Arc, Montreal 18, P.Q.
AVERY, Calvin R.; Dal'56; Res., Dept. of Obst Gyn, Dalhousie U., Halifax, N.S.
AVERY, J. Frank; Ste. 120, Oakridge Plaza, 5780 Cambie St., Vancouver 15, B.C. 6448 Macdonald St., Van. 13 (res); Tor '38; Tel. FA 7-1716.
AVERY, Lawrence E.; 3524 West-21st Ave., Vancouver 8, B.C.; Qns '43; GenSurg.
AVON, Jean C.; 2600 Louisbourg Terr., Montreal 12, P.Q.; Mon'61; DiagRad (P.Q.); Staff, Hop. Notre-Dame; Tel. 525-6363.
AVREN, Max; Westbrook Med. Centre, 1800 **Logan Ave., Winnipeg 23, Man.; 150 Westgate (res); Man '52; MCGP; Tel. SP 2-9453.**
AVRUSKIN, Theodore W.; 300 Longwood Ave., Boston, Mass., U.S.A.; Tor '60; Paed; Abroad.
AW, Chawl F.; Path; Staff, University Hosp., Saskatoon, Sask.
AWAD, Said; Cairo (Egypt)'59; FRCS(C), Urol; Staff, Hosp. for Sick Children, Toronto, Ont.
AWAIS, Jirius J.; Tor'60; ObstGyn; Staff, St. Michael's Hosp., Toronto, Ont.
AWDE, Charles M.; 14 Main St., Hagersville, Ont.; Tor'46; Active Staff, West Haldimand Hosp.; Court. Staff, Hamilton Gen. & Chedoke Hosp's., Hamilton; Tel. 768-3052.
AWERBUCK, Bernard G.; 106 Tor. Western Med. Bldg., 25 Leonard Ave., Toronto 2B, Ont.; 81 Ridge Hill Dr. (res); Tor '54; DMR; DiagRad; Staff, Toronto Western Hosp.; Clin. Instr., U. of Toronto; Tel. EM 3-1197.
AWREY, William R.; 1658 King St. E., Hamilton, Ont.; Qns. '61; AMCGP; Tel. LI 4-7477.
AXELRAD, Arthur A.; 3 Troon Ct., Willowdale, Ont.; McG '49; Ph.D. (Anat.); Scien. Div. of Biological Research, Ont. Cancer Inst., Princess Margaret Hosp.; Assoc. Prof. Med. & Biophysics Ass't. Prof. Anat., U. of Toronto; Tel 924-0671.
AXELROD, Haim I.; 31 Hilltop Rd., Toronto 10, Ont. (res); Tor '51; D.N.B.M.E., D.A., F.A.C.A.; Anaes; Att. Staff (Anaes.), New Mount Sinai Hosp.; Tel. RU 2-7877.
AXMITH, David; Ste. 808, 99 Avenue Rd., Toronto 5, Ont.; 4 Forest Ridge Rd. (res); **Tor '37; MCGP; Staff, Mount Sinai Hosp.; Tel. 921-3671.**
AXMITH, Kenneth T.; 2 Norelco Dr., Weston, Ont.; Qns'62; Med. Dir., Wm. S. Merrell Co.; Staff, St. Michael's Hosp.; Tel. 749-2550.

AYDIN, Mustafa; Istanbul (Turk.) '51; Staff, Provincial Hosp., Lancaster, N.B.
AYER, Isabel; 202 Medical Arts Bldg., Toronto, Ont.; 30 Oriole Rd., (res); Tor '21; ObstGyn; Tel. WA 2-1902.
AYERS, Thomas N.; Man'57; GenSurg; Staff, (NeurSurg.), University Hosp., Edmonton, Alta.
AYLESWORTH, J. A.; Aberhart Memorial San., University Ave., Edmonton, Alta.; 11327—75th Ave. (res); Alb '32; T.B. Off. Dept. of Health, Prov. of Alberta; Tel. GE 9-0051.
AYLLON-GALVAN, Rafael; 3755 Cote St. Catherine, Montreal, P.Q.; Mexico'54.
AYLWARD, Bedford Z.; Dal'57; Res., University Hosp., Edmonton, Alta.
AYLWARD, Gerald F.; 582 Goldstream Ave., Victoria, B.C.; McG '23; Anaes; Retired.
AYOTTE, Louis G.; 9921—110th St., Edmonton, Alta. (res); Lav '40; ObstGyn.
AYRE, W. Burton; 1333 Laird Blvd., Mount Royal, Montreal 16, P.Q.; Alb '43; MCGP; Assoc. Med. Dir., Canada Group, Continental Ins. Co's.; Tel. RE 7-6937.

AZAUSTRE, Jesus S. — See (Silva-Azaustre).

AZIM, Hassan F. A.; Allan Mem. Inst., Montreal, P. Q.; 3625 Ridgewood Ave., Apt. 303 (res); Cairo (Egypt) '55; DIM; D.Psy; Psy; Sr. Psy., Douglas Hosp.; Ass't. to Outdoor Clinics, Royal Victoria Hosp.; Lect. (Psy.), McGill U.; Tel. VI 2-1251, Local 444.
AZIZ, Yousef; Wright Clinic, Parry Sound, Ont.; Cairo Egypt '53; FRCS(C), GenSurg; FRCS (Eng.); Surg., Parry Sound Gen. & St. Joseph's Hosp's.; Tel. 746-2181.
AZOULAY, Leon-J. L.; 5240 Van Horne Ave., Apt. 3, Montreal 26, P.Q.; Mon '23; Tel. RE 9-8225.
AZZOPARDI, Paul; 2865 Lawrence Ave. E., Scarborough, Ont.; Royal Malta U. '46; D.C.H. (Lond.); Paed; Staff, Hosp. for Sick Children; Tel. AM 6-2741.
BAAR, Frederick; 955 Queen St. E., Sault Ste. Marie, Ont.; Prague (Czech.)'37; LRCS(Edin.), FRCS(Edin.); GenSurg; Staff, Plummer Mem. & Sault Ste. Marie Gen. Hosp's.; Tel. AL 6-7156.
BAARS, Cornelius, Capt.; McG'64; RCAMC, Box 471, Petawawa, Ont.
BABATZANIS, John; 2272 W. 7th Ave., Ste 206, Vancouver 9, B.C.; Greece '55; Psy; Tel. 521-3080.
BABB, I. Louis; 262 St. Clair Ave. W., Toronto 7, Ont.; 2191A Queen St. E.; 81 Riddelle Ave. (res); Tor '50; GenSurg; Staff, Doctors Hosp.; Tel. WA 2-0562.
BABB, John W.; 330 Queen's Ave., London, Ont.; Wes '41; D.A.B.Ot.; Otol; Staff, Royal Victoria & Westminster Hosp's; Cons. Beck Mem. San., & RCAF Stn.; Assoc. Clin. Prof., (Otol.), U. of Western Ont.; Tel. 439-8211.
BABCHUK, Robert B.; Broadway Med. Clin., 1319 Broadway, Regina, Sask.; Tor '60; Tel. 527-3793.
BABIAK, Walter; Kiel (Germ.) '49; D. Psy.; Psy; Staff, Ont. Hosp., St. Thomas, Ont.; Tel. ME 1-8510.
BABIN, Charles E.; Mica Med. Clinic, Mica Creek, B.C.; Ott'60.
BABINEAU, Georges, Major; Valcartier Camp, Quebec, P.Q.; Lav '45.
BABINEAU, Maurice J.; Medical Arts Bldg., 171 Montreal Rd., Cornwall, Ont.; 720 Guy St. (res); Ott '54; Paed; Staff, Cornwall Gen. & Hotel Dieu Hosp's.; Tel. WE 2-5582.

BABIUK, Marshal E.; 8225-105th St., Edmonton, Alta.; Alb'58.
BABIUK, Myron J.; 11227-59th Ave., Edmonton, Alta.; Alb'59.

BABYN, Roman B.; 576 Christie St., Toronto 4, Ont.; Lemburg (Poland) '37; OrthSurg; Staff, Queensway Gen. Hosp.; Tel. LE 2-4000.

BABYN, Mrs. R. (See Sheppard, Dorothy A.).

BACAL, Harry L.; 4640 Stanley Weir St., Montreal 29, P.Q.; 4636 Stanley Weir St. (res); McG '30; Paed All. (P.Q.); Phys. and Dir. All. Dept., Montreal Children's Hosp.; Assoc. Phys., Royal Victoria and Jewish Gen. Hosp's.; Cons. (All.), Queen Mary Vets' Hosp., Lect. Paed., McGill U.; Tel. RE 1-4006.

BACH, Rolf K.; Corner Water & Bridge St., Almonte, Ont.; 240 King St. (res); Heidelberg (Germ.) '49; Pt.-time M.O.H. Almonte & Huntley; Tel. 721.

BACH, William G.; 209 Menagen Rd., Fort Ord, California, U.S.A.; Alb'60; Psy; Abroad.

BACHAND, Andre J.; Mon'61; Haem(P.Q.); Staff, Hop. Jean Talon, Montreal 35, P.Q.

BACHAND, Jean P.; Lav'63; Res., Hop. St. Francois d'Assise, Quebec 3, P.Q.
BACHAND, L. J.; St. Joseph du Lac, Co. Deux Montagnes, P.Q.; Mon '33; M.C.G.P.; Tel 473-5013.

BACHAND, Lucien; 141 rue Noel, Asbestos, P.Q.; Lav '62; Tel. 879-2212.

BACHAND, Robert; 375 Boul. Laurier, Beloiel, P.Q.; Mon'61; Tel. 467-4935.

BACHAND, S. Martial; 912 est Sherbrooke, Montreal 24, P.Q.; Lav'49; F.R.C.S.(C), ObstGyn; Ass't. Obst. Gyn., Hop de la Misericorde; Tel. 525-2637.

BACHMANN, Fritz H.; 7145 Quinpool Rd., Halifax, N.S.; Munich (Germ.) '24; LRCP; LRCS (Ed.); LRFPS(Glasg.); M.O., C.S.S. "Baffin"; Tel. 454-4574.

BACHOP, David, M.; 1410-750 W. Broadway, Vancouver 9, B. C.; 1837 W. 36th (res); Edinburgh (Scot.) '55; M.B., Ch.B.; MCGP; Att'd. Staff, Vancouver Gen. Hosp.; Tel. TR 2-5601.

BACHYNSKI, Borden; 2125-11th Ave., Regina, Sask.; Tor'47; FAAOS; DABOS; FACS; FRCS(C); OrthSurg; Hd. Orthopaed. Sect., Med. Arts Clinic; Chief Orthopaed. Sect., Regina Gen. Hosp.; Cons. Orthopaed., Sask. Crippled Children & Adults Soc. & D.V.A.; Tel. 523-0691.

BACHYNSKI, John E.; Man '62; Res., Royal Victoria Hosp., Montreal, P.Q.

BACHYNSKI, Vladimer F.; 263 Broadway Ave., Winnipeg 1, Man.; 115 Grenfell Blvd., Tuxedo 9 (res); Man '35; F.A.G.S., F.I.C.S., M.C.G.P.; Tel. WH 3-5474.
BACKER, David R.; Ste. 215, 4560 Decarie Blvd., Montreal 29, P.Q.; McG '26.
BACKMAN, Keith M.; Box 1239, Kimberley, B.C.; Alb'55.
BACKSTROM, Alvin R.; Alb'56; B.Sc. (Pharm.); Res., Royal Victoria Hosp., Montreal 2, P.Q.
BACKUS, Allin B.; Medical Centre, Ponoka, Alta.; London (Eng.) '41; M.R.C.S., L.R.C.P.; D. Obst., R.C.O.G.; M.R.C.O.G.; Ass't. Lect., Ponoka Mental Hosp.; Tel. 783-3306.
BACKUS, Winston O.; 9905-101st Ave., Grande Prairie, Alta.; London (Eng.)'46; MRCS; LRCP; MCGP; Staff, Grande Prairie Mem. Hosp.; Tel. 532-5511.
BACON, Hugh M.; Dal'60; Psy; Staff, U. of Alberta Hosp., Edmonton, Alta.
BACON, Thomas N.; 1 Oriole Rd., Toronto 7, Ont.; Tor '61; Staff, OPD, St. Michael's Hosp.; Tel. 921-8638.
BACONGALLO, Ben E.; Soeul (Korea)'57; Res., Hotel-Dieu Hosp., Moncton, N.B.
BADEAUX, Georges; 502 Cherrier St., Montreal, P.Q.; 42 Holyrood (res); Mon '11.
BADEAUX, Jacques; 534 Cherrier St., Montreal, P.Q.; 61 Thornhill, Westmount; Mon '40; Otol (P.Q.); Staff, Hotel Dieu; Tel. VI 2-2580.
BADENOCH, A. Guthrie; Aberdeen (Scot.) '23; D.P.H.; Staff, Nova Scotia Hosp., Dartmouth, N.S.
BADGER, Garnet A.; Ste 615, 925 W. Georgia St., Vancouver 1, B.C.; 946 Groveland Rd. (res); Alb '39; D.A.B.Ot; Otol; Att'd. Staff, Vancouver Gen., Shaughnessy DVA & Children's Hosp's; Clin. Instr., U. of British Columbia; Tel. MU 1-1010.
BADRE, Emile J. P.; 380 Oakridge Plaza, 5780 Cambie St., Vancouver 15, B.C.; Qns'43; GenSurg; PlasSurg; Hd. Plas Surg. Children's Hosp.; Active Staff, Van. Gen.; Att'd. Staff, St. Vincent's Hosp.; Vis. Staff, St. Paul's & Mt. St. Joseph's Hosp's.; Cons. Staff, St. Mary's Hosp., N. Westminster; Tel. RE 3-2710.

BAER, Richard A.; Med. Art Bldg., 2150 Valley Way, Niagara Falls, Ont.; 3903 Lewiston Rd., N.F., N.Y. (res); Buffalo (N.Y.) '46; FACS, DABU; Urol; Court. Staff, (Urol.), Gtr. Niagara Gen. Hos.; Att'd. (Urol.), Mem. Hosp., N.F., N.Y.; Cons. Urol., Mt. St. Mary's Hosp., N.F., N.Y.; Tel. EL 6-2030.

BAERG, Peter J.; Fernie, B.C.; UBC '55; Staff, Leroux Clin.

BAERGEN, Ernest **H.;** 932 Spadina Cr. E., **Saskatoon, Sask.; 2514 Jarvis Dr. (res); Sask** '57; MCGP; Tel. **652-6066.**

BAGGS, Cecil R.; 584 Jones Ave., Toronto, Ont.; 1 Hill Cres., R.R. No. 2, Scarborough; Tor '35; Urol; Staff, Toronto East Gen. Hosp. Tel. 461-9211.

BAGLIERI, John A.; 2489 Bloor St. W., Toronto, **Ont.; 15 Ridge Valley Cr., (res); Tor '46;** Obst. Gyn; Active Staff, St. Joseph's Hosp.; Tel. RO 6-4501.

BAGNALL, Arthur W.; 115—3195 Granville St., Vancouver, B.C.; 4337 Pine Cres. (res); Tor '37; F.R.C.P.(C), M.R.C.P. (Lond.), IntMed; **Assoc. Clin. Prof. of Medicine, U. of British** Columbia; Hon. Medicine, Shaughnessy Hosp.; **Sr. Phys. (Med.), Vancouver Gen. Hosp.; Tel. RE** 3-7540.

BAGNALL, Howard J.; Ste. 307, 1105 Carling **Ave., Ottawa 3, Ont.; 161 Billings Ave., Ott. 1 (res); Birmingham (Eng.) '45; F.R.C.S. (Eng.), F.A.C.S.; NeurSurg; Sr. NeurSurg., Ottawa Civic Hosp.; NeurSurg., Ottawa Gen. Hosp.; Cons. (NeurSurg), Ottawa Mental Health Clin., Tri-Service & DVA and Kemptville Hosp's.; Clin. Lect., Ottawa U.; Tel. PA 9-2881.**

BAGRATION, Alexander; (See DVALI, Alexander).

BAGSHAW, Elizabeth C.; 608 King St. E., Hamilton, Ont.; Tor '05; M.C.G.P.

BAGSHAW, John I.; 608 King St. E., Hamilton, Ont.; 60 Wexford S. (res); Wes '53; MCGP; Tel. JA 9-8740.

BAHMANN, Henry J.; 755 Brimley Rd., Scarborough, Ont.; Tor '63.

BAICHWAL, Krishna S.; Cook Med. Bldg., 1175 Cook St., Victoria, B.C.; Bombay (India)'52; MB; BS; FRCS(Ed.); ThorSurg.

BAIDA, Michael; 280 Bloor St. W., Ste. 208, Toronto 5, Ont.; Tor'57; FRCS(C), GenSurg; Active Staff, GenSurg & Paed. Surg., St. Joseph's Hosp.; Tel. 925-2693.

BAILEY, Allan A.; Dept. of Med., U. of Saskatchewan, Saskatoon, Sask.; Tor '35; M.S. (NeurPsy., Minn.); FRCP(C), NeurPsy; Prof. & Hd., Dept. of Med., U. of Saskatchewan; Tel. 242-7641, Loc. 461.

BAILEY, Alan J.; 2927 Angus St., Regina, Sask. (res); Sheffield '39; MRCP (Lond.); Sr. Clin. Assoc., Allan Blair Mem. Clinic, Regina Grey Nuns' Hosp.; Tel. JO 9-9621.

BAILEY, Gaston; 401 rue Queen, Rawdon, P. Q.; Mon '60; Tel. 834-2404.

BAILEY, Graeme M.; 5300 Cote des Neiges Rd., Montreal 26, P.Q.; 60 Granville (res); McG '41; **ObstGyn (P.Q.); Tel. RE 1-3357.**

BAILEY, John D.; Hosp. for Sick Children, Room 116, 555 University Ave., Toronto 2, Ont.; Tor '47; FRCP(C), Paed; FAAP; Ass't. Phys. (Paed.), Hosp. for Sick Children; Dir. of Med. OPD., Hosp. for Sick Children & Research Inst., Hosp. for Sick Children; Assoc. Prof. (Paed.), U. of Toronto; Tel. EM 6-7242, loc. 2164.

BAILEY, John F.; Box 219, Little Current, Ont.; Tor'47; Active Staff, St. Joseph's Gen. Hosp.

BAILEY, Mamie E.; Box 667, Prince Albert, **Sask. (res); Alb '49; Path; Staff, Victoria & Holy Family Hosp's.; Tel. 763-8325.**

BAILEY, Marguerite E., 256 Oriole Pkwy., Toronto 7, Ont.; Tor '30; Med. Dept., Women's College Hosp.; (Part-time) Dept. of Public Health, Toronto; Tel. HU 5-5722.

BAILEY, Norman L.; Ste. 340, Med. Arts Bdlg., 1105 Pandora, Victoria, B.C.; Liverpool (Eng.) '45; DOMS; Ophth; Tel. EV 4-2622.

BAILEY, Paul; 123 Edward St., Toronto, Ont.; 98 Bideford Ave. (res); Tor '47; Anaes; **Staff (Anaes),** St. Michael's Hosp.; Clin. Teach. **(Anaes),** U. of Toronto; **Tel. EM 8-3439.**

BAILEY, Ralph A.; 202 Southgate Apts., **10405** Saskatchewan Dr., Edmonton, Alta.; **McG'35;** FRCS(C) NeurSurg; M.O., Veteran's Affairs, University Hosp.; Tel. 439-5911, Ext. 367.

BAILEY, Ronald A.; Box 160, Flin Flon Clinic, Flin Flon, Man.; Edinburgh (Scot.)'62; **FRSM;** Mem. BMA.

BAILEY, Thomas J.; Health & Welfare Centre, 1947 Cook St., Victoria, B.C.; Edinburgh (Scot.) '55; DPH; Dir. School Med. Serv.; Tel. 384-0571.

BAILEY, Warwick; Sydney (Australia) '33; FRCS(Ed); Staff, James Paton Mem. Hosp., Gander, Nfld.; Abroad.

BAILEY, W. Harvey; 450 Central Ave., London, Ont.; Wes'58; FRCS(C), GenSurg; OrthSurg.

BAILEY, William J.; Medical Arts Bldg., 121 Wellington St. W., Barrie, Ont.; Tor '51.

BAILEY, W. Stuart; 24 Catherine St., Trenton, **Ont.; 33 Fairview Cresc. (res); Qns '52; Tel. EX 2-4325.**

BAILLARGEON, Bernard; 30 boul. St. Joseph, est, Montreal 14, P.Q.; Mon'38; F.R.C.P.(C), IntMed; Ass't. (Med.), Hop.-Notre-Dame; Cons., Queen Mary Vet's. Hosp.; Med. Dir., Alliance Mutual Life Assur. Co.; Assoc. Prof., U. of Montreal; Tel. LA 6-4441; RE 3-9951.

BAILLARGEON, Jacques; 1560 est rue Sherbrooke, Montreal 24, P.Q.; Lav'53; FRCP(C); IntMed; Gastroent (P.Q.); Staff, Hop. Notre-Dame; Ass't. Prof. (Med.), U. of Montreal; Tel. LA 4-0986.

BAILLARGEON, Thomas-Ls.; 2404 St. Marc, Shawinigan Falls, P.Q.; 352-9th St. (res); Lav '43; Staff, Hop. Ste. Therese, Shawinigan Falls **and Hop. Lafleche, Grand'Mere; Tel. LE 9-4524.**

BAILLARGEON, Yvon; 3447 St. Hubert, Montreal, P.Q.; 3 Logan St., Apt. 5, St. Lambert **(res); Mon '50; DermSyph (P.Q.); Ass't. (Derm.), Hop. Hotel Dieu; Tel. 523-2503.**

BAILLIE, Alexander C.; 40 Coldwater St., Orillia, **Ont.;** 187 **Peter St. N. (res); Tor '32; Dist** Coroner.

BAILLIE, David M.; 5451 Alderley Rd., Victoria, B.C. (res); Aberdeen (Scot.) '09; D.P.H.; Int Med; Retired.

BAILLIE, James H.; Bell Telephone Co., **393** University Ave., Toronto, Ont.; Tor'38; **D.P.H.,** D.A.B. Prev. M., PH; Regional Medical Dir., **Bell** Telephone Co. of Canada; Tel. 929-7033.

BAILLIE, Nigel M.; Caledonia, Ont.; **London** (Eng) '63.

BAILLIE, William H. T.; 152 Stibbard Ave., Toronto 12, Ont. (res); Tor '15; Prof. Mammalian Anatomy, U. of Toronto.

BAILLY, Roland; 4339 Delorimier, **Montreal, P.Q.; Lav '37; M.C.G.P.; Tel. 525-6411.**

BAIMAKOS, Demetrius G.; '57; Staff, Harbour Breton Hosp., Harbour Breton, Nfld.

BAIN, Gordon O.; 13007-63rd. Ave., Edmonton, Alta.; Alb '51; Path; Staff (Path.), U. of Alberta Hosp. and Prov. Lab. of Public Health; Assoc. Prof. (Path.), U. of Alberta; Tel. 439-5911.

BAIN, Harry W.; 555 University Ave., Toronto, **Ont.; 19 York Valley Cr., Willowdale (res);** Tor'44; FRCP(C), Paed; Chief of Paed., Hosp. for **Sick Children; Assoc. Prof. (Paed.), U. of Tor**onto; Tel. EM 6-7242.

BAIN, James A.; Wes '59; Anaes; **Med. Research** Fell. (Physiol.), U. of Western Ontario, **London,** Ont.

BAIN, Jerald; Wes'65; Ass't. Res., New Mount Sinai Hosp., Toronto, Ont.

BAIN, Joan E.; 939 Lawrence Ave. E., Don Mills, Ont.; 26 Denewood Cres. (res); Tor '55 MCGP; Tel. HI 4-2291.

BAIN, John A.; Porcupine Medical Clinic, Porcupine Plain, Sask.; Edinburgh (Scot.)'52; Tel. 73 & 23.

BAIN, Stanley T.; 939 Lawrence Ave. E., **Don** Mills P.O., Ont.; Apt. 4, 1216 Don Mills Rd (res); Tor '53; MCGP; Tel. HI 4-2291.

BAIN, Theodore D.; 1933 West King **Edward** Ave., Vancouver 9, B.C.; Tor '26; Hosp. Supt. **and Sr. Treatment M.O., Shaughnessy Hosp., D.V.A.; Tel. TR 6-6767.**

BAINBOROUGH, A. Raymond; 966-13th St. S. Lethbridge, Alta (res); Wes '46; Path; Path. and Dir. of Labs., Lethbridge Municipal & St. Michael's Gen. Hosp's.; Tel. FA 7-8591.

BAINES, Andrew D.; Tor '59; Research, Banting Inst., U. of Toronto, Toronto 5, Ont.

BAINES, Cornelia J. (Van Erk); 183 Berry Rd., Apt. 9, Toronto, Ont.; Tor '60; Research Fell., Toronto Western Hosp.; Tel. 368-2581.

BAINES, Heather; 81 Bruce Ave., South Porcupine, Ont.; Liverpool (Eng.) '62.

BAIRD, Arthur G.; 1544 Dundas St., London, Ont.; Wes '48; Tel. 451-1200.

BAIRD, Charles D.; 43 Victoria Ave., Chatham, Ont.; Qns'41; Ophth; Chief, Dept. of Ophth., St. Joseph's & Chatham Gen. Hosps.; Tel. 354-4700.

BAIRD, D. Alastair; 428 Med. Arts Bldg., 404-406 Graham Ave., Winnipeg 1, Man.; Edinburgh (Scot.) '51; M.B., Ch.B., DRCOG; FRCS(C), PlasSurg; GenSurg; Cons. Plastic & Recons. Surg., St. Boniface, Children's & Deer Lodge Hosp's.; Lect. (Surg.), U. of Manitoba; Tel. WH 2-5632.

BAIRD, Douglas A.; Tor '61; Res. Toronto East Gen. Hosp.. Toronto 6, Ont.

BAIRD, Ellice A.; (See Parmenter, Ellice A.).

BAIRD, James A.; Leigh Square Medical Centre, Port Coquitlam, B.C.; 4614 N.W. Marine Dr., Vancouver, B.C. (res); Qns '54; Dist. Coroner.

BAIRD, James C.; Box 530, Wadena, Sask.; Glasgow (Scot.) '52; M.B., Ch.B., DPH; Tel. 82546.

BAIRD, James T.; 119 Sydney St., Cornwall, Ont.; 1613 Jane St., (res); Glasgow (Scot.) '42; DOMS (Eng.); Ophth; Chief of Ophth., Hotel-Dieu Hosp.; Staff, Cornwall & Ottawa Gen. Hosp's.; Cons. (Ophth), St. Lawrence San., Cornwall; Lect'r. (Ophth), U. of Ottawa; Tel. WE 2-0524.

BAIRD, John D. B.; 11B Monkstown Rd., St. John's Nfld.; 15 Glenridge Cres. (res.); Tor '43; F.R.C.S.(C), GenSurg; Jr. Surg., St. John's Gen Hosp.; Tel. 578-6325.

BAIRD, Kenneth A.; 562 Dunn Ave., Lancaster, N.B.; FACA; MAAA; FAGS; FAACIA; FCAA; DermSyph; Cons., Saint John's Gen. & St. Joseph's Hosp's., Saint John; Tel. 694-1681.

BAIRD, Murray M.; Ste. 370, 5780 Cambie St., Vancouver 15, B. C.; 5809 Cartier St., (res); Oxford (Eng.) '24; F.R.C.P. (Lond.), F.R.C.P.-(C), IntMed; Chief of Serv. (Med.) Shaughnessy Hosp.; Clin. Assoc. Prof. of Med., U. of British Columbia.; Tel. FA 1-1112.

BAIRD, Patricia A. (Holt); McG '63; Res., Vancouver Gen. Hosp., Vancouver, B. C.

BAIRD, Robert D.; 176 York St., Fredericton, N.B.; Dal '33; F.R.C.S. (Edin.), F.R.C.S.(C), GenSurg; Staff (Surg.), Victoria Public Hosp.; Tel. GR 5-8421.

BAIRD, Robert M.; Ste. 417, 925 W. Georgia St., Vancouver 1, B.C.; UBC '57; M.Sc. (McGill); FRCS(C); GenSurg; Staff, Dept. of Surg., St. Paul's Hosp. & Shaughnessy Hosp.; Clin. Instr. Surg., U. of British Columbia; Tel. MU 5-7201.

BAIRD, Ronald J.; 399 Bathurst St., Ste. 305, Toronto 2B Ont.; 28 Summerhill Ave. (res); Tor '54; M.S.(Tor); FACS; FRCS(C); GenSurg; FRCS(C), Cardiovasc. & Thor Surg; Cardiovasc. Surg., Toronto Western Hosp.; Research Assoc. Ontario Heart Fdn.; Assoc. Surg., U. of Toronto; Tel. 364-9491.

BAIRD, Ronald P.; 230 Frederick St., Kitchener, Ont.; Dal '37; D.O.M.S., Ophth.; Staff (Ophth.), Kitchener-Waterloo & St. Mary's Hosps.; Tel. 742-3811.

BAITZ, Thomas; 404-8½ Ave. N.W., Rochester, Minn. 55901, U.S.A.; Alb'61; FRCP(C), IntMed.

BAJUSZ, Eors; 3520 Maplewood Ave., Montreal, P.Q. (res); Budapest (Hung.) '50; Ph.D. (Exper. Med. & Surg); FACC, FICS, FAGS; Cons. & Research Assoc. Cardio-vasc. Unit, U. of Vermont, Burlington, Va., U.S.A.; Ass't. Prof. (Exper. Path.), U. of Montreal; Tel. RE 3-9951.

BAK, Zonko; Ste. 1216, 123 Edward St., Toronto 2, Ont.; Tor '54; Anaes; Staff, St. Michael's Hosp.; Tel. 362-4461.

BAKAR, Nadir J.; McG'64; Res., Royal Victoria Hosp., Montreal 2, P.Q.

BAKER, Alvin A.; 704 Coxwell Ave., Toronto 6, Ont.; 42 Braeside Rd. (res); Tor '42; Otol; Staff, Toronto E. Gen. Hosp.; Cons.-in-Hearing, Dept. of Health, City of Toronto. Tel. 465-8056.

BAKER, A. R.; 1151 Lorne Park Rd., Port Credit, Ont.; Tor '64.

BAKER, Brian; Box 298, Arborfield, Sask.; Birmingham (Eng.)'55; Tel. 769-8711.

BAKER, Bryan L.; Box 2378, Kittimat, B.C.; London (Eng.)'60; MB; BS; MRCS; LRCP.

BAKER, Charles E.; 403 Waverley St., Port Arthur, Ont.; Man '39; F.R.C.S. (Eng.); Gen Surg.; Tel. DI 4-6021.

BAKER, C. Harold; 8 Crest Rd., Rockingham, Halifax Co., N.S. (res); Dal '35; Anaes; Staff, Halifax Infirm.; Assoc. Prof. (Anaes), Dalhousie U.; Tel. 422-1511.

BAKER, Clare B.; Ste 1220, 123 Edward St, Toronto 2, Ont.; 5 Peebles Ave., Don Mills, (res); Tor '46; FACS, FRCS(C), GenSurg; ThorSurg (Cardiovas.); Staff, St. Michael's Hosp.; Ass't. Prof. (Surg.), U. of Toronto; Tel. 366-3216.

BAKER, Clarice A.; Oxford (Eng.)'58; FRCS (Eng.); D.Obst RCOG; Res., Wpg. Gen. Hosp., Winnipeg 3, Man.

BAKER, Donald B.; Smith Clinic, Camrose, Alta.; 4411-52A St. (res); Alb '50; IntMed.; Tel. 672-2424.

BAKER, Earle F.; 63 Snowdon Ave., Toronto 12, Ont. (res); Tor '51; D.Psy; F.R.C.P.(C), Psy; Att'd. Staff, Toronto Western Hosp.; Clin. Instr. (Psy), U. of Toronto; Tel. 369-5742.

BAKER, Eric J.; Cereal, Alta.; Alb '50; M.C.G.P.; Tel. 55.

BAKER, Frederick W.; 710 Canada Bldg., Saskatoon, Sask; 21 Rutter Cres. (res); Alb '56; Paed; Clin. Ass't. (Paed.), U. of Sask.; Tel. 244-1116.

BAKER, Gordon A.; Ste. 809, 99 Avenue Rd., Toronto 5, Ont.; Tor'58; Psy; Staff Psy., New Mount Sinai Hosp.; Tel. 445-1548.

BAKER, Harold E.; 53 Harvie Ave., Toronto, Ont.; Tor '20; AICS; Tel. LE 3-5662.

BAKER, Harry; 2152 W. 41st St., Vancouver 13, B.C.; 1868 Acadia Rd., Van. 8, (res); Tor '33; Paed; Att'd. Staff, Children's Hosp. & Health Centre for Children; Clin. Ass't. Prof. (Paed.), U. of British Columbia.; Tel. AM 6-8555.

BAKER, H. Gordon; 119-16th St., West Vancouver, B.C.; 1381-27th St. (res); McG '36; DPH; IntMed; Cons. Staff, Lions Gate Hosp.; Tel. WA 2-2020.

BAKER, James R. W/C; Dal'53; GenSurg; Chief of Surg., RCN Hosp., Canadian Forces Base, Esquimalt, B.C.; Reg. Cons., Gen. Surg., Pacific Reg. Maritime Command, Cdn. Armed Forces.

BAKER, John B.; Med. Arts Bldg., 335-339-6th Ave. S. W., Calgary, Alta.; 3406-10th St. S. W. (res); Man '43; DiagRad; Tel. 262-9183.

BAKER, John E.; 211 Third Ave., Ottawa 1, Ont. (res); Qns '34; Phys., Civil Serv. Health Centre, Dept. Nat. Health & Welfare; Tel. CE 2-8211.

BAKER, Kathleen T. (McCurley;) 12920-102nd Ave., Edmonton, Alta.; Liverpool (Eng.) '53; M.O., Oliver Mental Hosp.

BAKER, Kenneth; Guys Hosp. (London, Eng.) '48; Staff, Union Hosp., Mossbank, Sask.

BAKER, Kenneth; Baker Clinic, 10004-105th St., Edmonton, Alta.; 12920-102nd Ave. (res); Liverpool (Eng.) '45; M.R.C.O.G., F.R.C.S.(C), Obst Gyn; Active Staff, University Hosp; Att'd. Staff, Royal Alexandra Hosp.; Tel. 424-2121.

BAKER, Louis K.; 2775 W. Broadway, Vancouver, B. C.; 2387 Eddington Dr. (res); Qns '34; Staff, Van. Gen., St. Paul's, Grace & Mt. St. Joseph's Hosp's.; Tel. RE 3-6512.

BAKER, Robert S.; Ste. 4, 360 The West Mall, Etobicoke, Ont.; Tor'60; FRCP(C); Anaes; Staff, South Peel Hosp., Cooksville; Tel. 621-4238.

BAKER, Samuel W.; Ste. 508, 718 Granville St., Vancouver 2, B. C.; Man '25; Tel MU 5-5524.

BAKER, Stanley E.; 1434 King W., Toronto 3, Ont.; Tor '23; Tel. LE 2-0871.

BAKER-THOMAS, Shirley M.; 7250 Arbutus Place, W., Vancouver, B.C. (Res.); Tor'52.

BAKER, Vivian; Bristol (Eng.) '54; DPH (Tor.); Res., Vancouver Gen. Hosp., Vancouver, B.C.
BAKER, William A.; Keewatin, Ont.; Qns '42; F.R.C.S. (Edin.), F.R.C.S. (Eng.), F.A.S.A.S, Tel. KI 7-2222.
BAKER, William E; Belmont Bldg., Government St., Victoria, B.C.; McG '24; Otol; Med.Exam., Cdn. Pensions Comm.
BAKER, W. Ward; 62 Bridge St. W., Campbellford, Ont.; Tor '32; Staff, Campbellford Mem. Hosp.; Tel. 653-2310.
BAKISH, Mark; 3805 Van Horne Ave., Montreal 26, P.Q.; 3820 Plamondon Ave. (res); Sofia (Bulgaria) '37; Tel. RE 7-4933.

BAKKER, Johan P.; 2 Underhill Dr., Don Mills, Ont.; Amsterdam (Neth.) '53. Tel. 444-1623.

BAKO, Erwin E.; 216 Le Marchand Mansions, Edmonton, Alta.; **13608-109A Ave.** (res); Berlin (Germ.) '35; OrthSurg (Berlin); M.C.G.P.; **Assoc. Staff, Edmonton Gen. Hosp.; Court. Staff, Misericordia Hosp.; Tel. 488-5382.**
BAKOS, Leslie D.; Med. Arts Clinic, 2125-11th Ave., Regina, Sask.; 70 Lake St. (res); Budapest (Hung.) '52; DiagRad; Tel. 523-0691.
BALA, Roman M.; Mall Med. Group, Winnipeg, Man.; Alb'58; FRCP(C); Int-Med; Lect., U. of Manitoba; Tel. SP 4-2411.
BALANGERO, Eugene F.; 485 Blvd. St. Joseph E., Montreal, P. Q.; 2020 Louisbourg (res); Lav '42; FICS; FACS; GenSurg; Surg. Staff, Ste-Jeanne d'Arc, St. Michel & St. Joseph de Rosemont Hosp's.; Tel. VI 5-7094.
BALATON, Joseph; 1108 Central Ave., Saskatoon, Sask.; Budapest (Hung.) '53; Staff, Saskatoon City & St. Paul's Hosp's.; Tel. 343-0212.

BALDWIN, John H.; Caledonia Medical Bldg., 340 Campbell St., Nanaimo, B.C.; 210 Stewart Ave. (res); Dal '41.
BALDWIN, S. G.; 801-5805 Balsam St., Vancouver, B.C.; 5062 Granville (res); McG '14; ObstGyn; Retired.
BALDWIN, William E.; Tor'62; Res., Toronto Gen. Hosp., Toronto, Ont.
BALDWIN, William F.; Ste. 301, 4900 Kingsway, South Burnaby, B.C.; Deer Lake Dr., North Burnaby (res); McG '49; ObstGyn; Chief (Obst. Gyn.), Burnaby Gen. Hosp., Assoc. Staff, Grace Hosp.; Vis. Staff, Vancouver Gen., St. Vincent's, Mt. St. Joseph's and St. Paul's Hosp's.; Tel. 434-1211.

BALDWIN, William W.; Brooklin Medical Centre, Brooklin, Ont.; Tor '34; M.C.G.P.; Board of Directors, Ont. Med. Assoc.

BALFE, John W.; Qns '62; Ass't. Res., Hosp. for Sick Children, Toronto, Ont.; Abroad.

BALFOUR, G. Rupert; 178 St. George St., Toronto 5, Ont.; 307 Warren Rd. (res); Tor '26; Anaes; Sr. Anaes., Toronto Gen. Hosp.; Assoc. Anaes., U. of Toronto.; Tel. EM 6-8211; WA 3-1154.
BALFOUR, G. Sigurd; Campbell Clinic, 430 Mayor Magrath Dr., Lethbridge, Alta.; 2105-17th Ave. S. (res); Alb'43; D.I.M., F.A.C.P., F.R.C.P.(C), IntMed; Staff Phys., Lethbridge Mun. & St. Michael's Hosp's.; Tel. FA 7-5737.
BALFOUR, John; 815 Fairmont Med. Bldg., 750 W. Broadway, Vancouver 9, B. C.; 2015 S. W. Marine Dr. (res); Alb '35; FRCS (C); Urol; Hd., Dept. of Urol, Vancouver Gen. Hosp.; Assoc. Prof. Surg. (Urol.), U.B.C.; Tel. TR 6-1820.
BALFOUR, John E.; Tor '62; Intn., Shaughnessy Hosp., Vancouver, B.C.; Abroad.
BALINSON, Robert H.; P.O. Box 396, Hamilton, Ont.; Tor'39; MCGP; Ass't. to S.T.M.O. "Hm" District D.V.A. Hamilton, Sr. Active Staff, St. Joseph's Hosp.; Court. Staff, Ham. Civic & Chedoke Children's Hosp's.; Tel. JA 2-3522.
BALIS, George U.; 66 Spadina Rd., Apt. 602, Toronto 4, Ont. (res); Athens (Greece) '54; Psy; Staff, Ontario Hosp., Whitby; Sr. Active Staff, St. Joseph's; Court. Staff, Hamilton Civic Chedoke & Gen. Hosp's.; Tel. 668-5881.
BALISKY, Larry; R.R. 1., Sexsmith, Alta.; Alb '63. Abroad.
BALKANY, Andrew F.; Box 760, North Fraser Health Unit, Mission, B.C.; Sydney (Australia) '46; PH.
BALKANY, Michael S.; 252 Oriole Pkwy., Toronto 7, Ont.; Budapest (Hung.) '14; ObstGyn; Tel. 488-7841.

BALKISSOON, M.; 605 McCowan Rd., Scarborough, Ont.; Tor'65.

BALL, George H.; 770 City Hall, Edmonton, Alta.; 11683-72nd Ave. (res); Liverpool (Eng.) '41; DPH; MOH, City of Edmonton; Sr. Lect., (PrevMed), U. of Alberta; Tel. 424-0211.
BALL, Harold D.; Ste. 782 Physicians & Surgeons Bldg., 86 Bloor St. W., Toronto, Ont.; 16 Castle Frank Cresc. (res); Tor '10; Court. Staff, Wellesley Hosp.; Tel. WA 2-1449.

BALL, John C.; 131 Ontario St., St. Catharines, Ont.; McG'49; Ophth; Chief, Dept. of Ophth., Hotel-Dieu Hosp.; Deputy Chief Ophth. St. Catharines Gen. Hosp.; Cons. Ophth., Niagara Peninsular San.; Tel. 682-8186.
BALL, Melvyn; Tor '63; Res., Toronto Gen. Hosp., Toronto, Ont.
BALL, Norbert J.; 105 W. 6th St., Oliver, B.C.; Tor'29; M.C.G.P.; Dist. Coroner; Tel. 498-2343.
BALL, Norman J.; 203 Professional Bldg., Jasper Ave., Edmonton, Alta.; Trinity Coll. (Dublin, Ire.) '53; B.A., B.Ch., BAO; Ass't. Path., Edmonton Gen. Hosp.; Cons. Path., St. Mary's Hosp., Camrose; Tel. 424-0061.
BALL, Roger J.; Tor'63; P.G., ObstGyn., U. of Toronto & St. Michael's Hosp., Toronto, Ont.
BALL, Roy B.; 68 Belvedere Ave., Toronto, Ont.; Tor '15; Tel. RU 1-9729.
BALL, W. Mansell; 197 Dundas St. E., Toronto 2, Ont.; Tor '25; Tel. EM 4-9834.

BALLAGH, Robert G.; 399-10th St., Hanover, Ont.; Tor'63; DPH; Active Staff, Hanover Mem. Hosp.; Tel. 364-2820.

BALLAM, Charles F.; UBC'54; Med. Cons., B.C. Hosp. Insurance Service, Parliament Bldgs., Victoria, B.C.

BALLANTYNE, Gwyneth J.; 2656 Heather St., Vancouver 9, B.C.; Man '52; Staff, B.C. Cancer Inst.

BALLANTYNE, James F.; 326 Queens Ave., London, Ont.; 430 St. George St. (res); Tor **'49; FRCS(C); Ophth; Chief of Staff, St. Joseph's & Cons., Westminster Hosp's; Ass't. Prof. (Ophth.), U. of Western Ontario; Tel. GE 4-9761.**

BALLANTYNE, Peter M.; The Port Arthur Clinic, Port Arthur, Ont.; 84 South High St. (res); Tor '23; F.R.C.S. (Edin.) & (C), F.A.C.S.; GenSurg; Chief, (Surg.) St. Joseph's and Gen. Hosp's.; Tel. 344-7271.

BALLARD, Emeric J.; Yellowknife, N.W.T.; Bologna (Italy)'34; LDS; Staff, Stanton Yellowknife Hosp.; Tel. Y.K. 4456.

BALLARD, James Howard; Glenridge Plaza, Glenridge Ave., St. Catharines, Ont.; Wes'64; Staff, Hotel-Dieu & Gen. Hosp's., St. Catharines; Tel. 227-5255.

BALLEM, C. Miller; Ste. 8A, 1374 Sherbrooke St. W., Montreal, P.Q. 147 Portland Ave., Town of Mount Royal (res); Dal '43; Gastroent, (P.Q.), Int Med; Lect. (Med. & Clin Med.), McGill U.; staff, Royal Victoria Hosp.; Tel. VI 4-6513.
BALLEM, Ralph W.; 5871 Spring Garden Rd., Halifax, N.S.; 29 Doug Smith Dr. (res); Dal '44; F.A.C.A., D.A.B.A., F.I.C.A.; Anaes; Staff (Anaes.), Victoria Gen. Hosp.; Ass't. Prof. (Anaes.), Dalhousie U.; Tel. 2-4406.

BALLON, David H.; 1538 Sherbrooke St. W., Montreal, P.Q.; 4300 Western Ave., Apt. 905, Westmount (res); McG '09; F.A.C.S., F.R.C.S.(C), Otol; Cons. Otol., Royal Victoria, Lake Placid Hosp., Lake Placid, N.Y. & Jewish Gen. Hosp.; Emer. Prof. (Otol.), McGill U.; Tel. WE 5-3454.
BALLON, Harry C.; 1414 Drummond St., Montreal, P.Q.; 3980 Cote-des-Neiges, Apt. C58 (res); McG '23; FACS; FRCS(C), GenSurg; Hon. Cons. Surg., Jewish Gen. Hosp.; Fd. Memb. A.B. **ThorSurg; Tel. VI 9-7927.**
BALLON, Henry; Geneva (Switz.) '62; Jr. Int., Shaughnessy Hosp., Vancouver 9, B.C.; Abroad.

BALLON, Jonathan D.; Ste 520, 600 Cote des Neiges Rd., Montreal 26, P.Q.; McG'52; B.A., MDCM (McG); FCCP; AFACC; IntMed; Cardiol (P.Q.); Staff, The Jewish Gen. & Reddy Mem. Hosp's.; Chm., Med. Bd., Montreal Conv. Hosp.; Tel. 739 3566.
BALLYK, Donald D.; 162 York St., St. Catharines, Ont.; 107 Queen St. (res); St. Louis U. Med. School (Mo., U.S.A.); Tel. MU 4-7431.
BALMANNO, James T.; 508 Main St., Yarmouth, N.S.; 28 Elm St. (res); Dal '49; GenSurg; Surg., Yarmouth Reg. Hosp.; Tel. 742-5134.
BALMER, H. Clark; Box 139, Kleinburg, Ont. (res); Tor'37; Anaes; Anaes. Staff, St. Joseph's Hosp.; Pres. & Med. Dir., Glaxo-Allenbury's (Canada) Ltd., 52 Bartor Rd., Weston; Tel. 247-6163.
BALMER, Ian A.; 736 Granville St., Vancouver 2, B.C.; 1970 W. 41st Ave., Van. 13 (res); McG '31; MCGP; Vis. Staff, Van. Mun. Hosp's.; Tel. MU 1-2937.
BALOGH, Lajos; 236 Ridout St. S., London, Ont.; Pecs (Hung.) '53; Tel. 432-0266.
BALSDON, Lewis A.; 2 Princess St., St. Thomas, Ont; Wes '62.
BALSHIN, Bernard; 6 Strathern Rd., Toronto 10, **Ont.; Tor '52; Path; Dir. of Labs. & Path., Doctor's Hosp.; Tel. WA 3-5411.**

BALTHAZARD, Jean G.; Ste 521, 30 est, St-Joseph, Montreal 14, P.Q.; Mon '59: Otol.
BALTHAZARD, Leopold; Mon'24; Staff, Sanatorium St. Jean, Macamic, P.Q.
BALTHAZARD, Yves; 50-4ieme rue, La Sarre, Cte. Abitibi, **P.Q. (res.); Mon '55; Staff, Hop St. Francois.**

BALTRUSAITIS, Jonas; 269 Main St. W., North Bay, Ont.; Kaunas (Lith.) '42; FCCP; Staff, Chest Clin., Ontario Dept. of Health, Div. of TB Prev.; Tel. 472-8090.
BALTRUSAITIS, Victor P.; 38 Division St. S., Kingsville, Ont.; Kaunas (Lithuania) '40; Tel. RE 3-4042.

BALTZAN, Betty L. (Roy); 408 MacMillan Bldg., 135-21st St. E., Saskatoon, Sask.; Johns Hopkins (U.S.A.)'58; Tel. 653-1855.
BALTZAN, David M.; 404-8 MacMillan Bldg., Saskatoon, Sask.; 219 Sask. Cres. W. (res); McG '20; F.R.C.P.(C), F.A.C.P., D.A.B.I.M.; Int-Med.; Chief of Med., St. Paul's Hosp.; Med & Clin Med. Prof., U. of Saskatchewan; Cons. Staff, Dept. of Med., University Hosp.; Tel. 653-1855.
BALTZAN, Donald M.; 408 MacMillan Bldg., 135-21st St. E., Saskatoon, Sask.; McG'57; Chief Res. Surg., Baltimore City Hosp. (On leave of absence). Active Staff, St. Paul's Hosp.; Tel. 653-1855.
BALTZAN, Marcel A.; 408 MacMillan Bldg., 135-21st St. E., Saskatoon, Sask.; McG'53; FRCP(C), IntMed; Att'd. Phys., St. Paul's Saskatoon City & University Hosp's., Ass't. Clin. Prof. (Med.), U. of Saskatchewan; Tel. 653-1855.
BALTZAN, Richard B.; 402-408 MacMillan Bldg., 135-21st St. E., Saskatoon, Sask.; McG '59; FRCP(C) IntMed; Assoc. Staff, St. Paul's & University Hosp's.; Tel. 242-0271.

BAMBRIDGE, Honore E. (see Munro-Faure)

BAMSHAD, Jalal; Med. Arts Bldg., 2125-11th Ave., Regina, Sask.; Shiraz (Iran) '56; Derm; Tel. 522-1651; Abroad.
BAN, Thomas A.; 3221 Forest Hill, Apt. 41, Montreal, P.Q.; Budapest (Hung.)'54; .D.Psy; Psy; Ass't. Dir., (Research), Douglas Hosp.; Ass't. Prof. (Psy.), McGill U.; Tel. 766-8511.
BANASSE, J. Edgar; 461 Ave. Brochu, St. Sept. Iles, P.Q.; Lav '30; ObstGyn (P.Q.).
BANDEEN, J. Catherine; 83 Curtis St., St. Thomas, Ont.; 63 St. Catherine St. (res); Wes '51; ObstGyn.; Tel. ME 1-3594.
BANDURA, Walter P.; 7 Welland Ave., St. Catharines, Ont.; 10 Champa Dr. (res); Ott '55; GenSurg.: Tel. MU 4-8555.
BANERJEE, Prabhat; Ontario Cancer Fdn., Victoria Hosp., London, Ont.; Calcutta (India)'52; MB; BS; DMRT(Eng.); FFR(Eng.); TherRad; TherRad., London Clinic, Ont. Cancer Fdn.; Instr. (TherRad.), U. of Western Ont.; Tel. 432-5261.

BANERJEE, Samarendranath; 1592 Pine Ave W., Montreal 25, P.Q.; Calcutta (India) '56; FRCS(C), OrthSurg.
BANFILL, S. Martin, MBE; 87 Percival Ave., Montreal West, P.Q. (res); McG'33; Prof. **(Anat.) & Assoc. Dean of Med. Fac., McGill U.; Tel. VI 4-6311.**
BANISTER, Philip G.; Ste. 12, 174 Dufferin Rd., Ottawa 2, Ont.; Edinburgh (Scot.)'51; Paed; M.O., Dept. of National Health & Welfare.
BANKIER, Robert G.; Box 9600, Selkirk, Man.; Glasgow (Scot.)'49; D.Psy; FRCP(C); Psy; Ass't. Research (Psy.) & Lect. (Psy.), U. of Manitoba.
BANKS, Bligh W.; 318 Alberta Corner, 804-**1st St. S. W., Calgary, Alta.; Man '37.**
BANKS, Peter J.; 360 Medical Arts Bldg., 1105 Pandora Ave., Victoria, B.C.; 2997 Seaview Rd. **(res); London (Eng.) '46; M.R.C.P. (Eng.), M.R.C.S., L.R.C.P., F.R.C.P.(C), IntMed; Chief of Med. & Tutor to Intns., St. Joseph Hosp.; Tel. EV 2-8570.**

BANNATYNE, M. Muriel see Wilson.

BANNO, M. Patrick; 4900 Kingsway, South **Burnaby, B.C.; UBC '58; Otol; Tel. 433-5610.**
BANTING, Henrietta E. (Ball); 150 Farnham Ave., Toronto 7, Ont. (res); Tor '45; MRCOG; FRCOG; ObstGyn; Dir., Cancer Detection Clinic, Women's College Hosp.; Tel. WA 3-7381 Ext. 364.
BANVILLE, Paul; 6370 des Angevins, Ville dAnjou, Montreal 5, P.Q.; Lav '52.
BANVILLE, Roch; 307 Arnaud, Sept-Iles, P.Q.; Lav '60; Tel. 942-4597.
BANVILLE, Romeo; St. Felicien, P.Q.; 98 Blvd. Sacre Coeur (res); Lav '32.
BAPTY, Leonard; 202 Cook Med. Bldg., 1175 Cook St., Victoria, B.C.; Aberdeen (Scot.) '36; GenSurg; Staff, St. Joseph's Hosp.; Vis. Staff, Royal Jubilee Hosp.; Tel. EV 4-2213.
BAPTY, Walter; Bonnie Brae Farm, R.R. 2, Royal Oak, Victoria, B.C.; Wes '06; GenSurg; Sr. Memb. C.M.A.; Retired.
BARAGAR, Fletcher D.; 800 Sherbrook St., Winnipeg 2, Man.; 10 Waterford Bay, Wpg. 19 (res); Man '55; FRCP(C), IntMed; Active Staff, St. Boniface & Man. Rehab. Hosp.; Cons. (Rheum.), Wpg. Mun. Hosp. & Cdn. Arthritis Soc.; Spec. Lect. & Dem., U. of Manitoba; Tel. SP 5-0181.
BARBEAU, Andre; 3769 Ave. Wilson, Montreal 28, P.Q. (res); McG '56; F.R.C.P.(C), Neur; Staff, Montreal Neurol. Inst.; Ass't. Prof. (Neur. Sciences), U. of Montreal; Tel. 488-8952.
BARBEAU, Eugene; 700 Cremazie E., Montreal, **P.Q.; 55 Spring Grove Cres. (res); Mon '35; Anaes.; Tel. DU 8-3263.**

BARBER, Albert S.; West'65; Res., Royal Victoria Hosp., Montreal 2, P.Q.
BARBER, G. Stuart; 35 Charlotte St., Brantford, Ont.; 21 Riverview Dr. (res); Tor '34; F.R.C.S.-(C), F.I.C.S., GenSurg; ObstGyn; Staff, Brantford Gen. & St. Joseph's Hosp's. & Willett Hosp., Paris; Tel. 752-7871.
BARBER, Hugh O.; Suite 330, Medical Arts Bldg., 170 St. George St., Toronto 5, Ont.; 206 Cortleigh Rd. (res); Tor '45; F.R.C.S.(C), Otol; Clin. Teacher, U. of Toronto; Att. Otol., Toronto Gen. Hosp.; Tel. WA 2-7258.
BARBER, John R.; 420 Med. Arts Bldg., Windsor, Ont.; 3730 Ouellette Ave. (res); Wes '47; M.S. (OrthSurg.); FACS; FICS; OrthSurg; Chief of OrthSurg., Metropolitan Gen. Hosp.; Att'd. Staff, Hotel-Dieu Hosp.; Cons., Essex City San. & Riverview Hosp.; Tel. 253-5900.

BARBER, Gwendolyn F. (See Service)

BARBER, Neil C.; Box 1329, Avery Clinic, Quesnel, B.C.; Cambridge (Eng.)'59.
BARBER, Philip A.; 6236 Fraser St., Vancouver 15, B.C.; Man '57; MCGP; Vis. Staff, Vancouver Gen., St. Vincent's, Grace, & St. Joseph's Hosp's.; Insurance Examiner, Crown Life, Dominion Life & Mutual of New York; Tel. FA 5-4011.

BARCELO, Maurice; 700 Main St., Waterloo, Co. Shefford, P.Q.; Mon '52.
BARCELO, Raymond; 1150 est, boul St.-Joseph, Montreal 34, P. Q.; 6722-10th Ave., Rosemont (res); Mon '57; FRCP(C); IntMed; Staff, Hop. Maisonneuve; Tel. LA 7-1241.

BARCLAY, Ian H. G/C; Durham (Eng.) '38; DTM&H (McG.); Regional CFMS HQTS, 5217 South St., Halifax, N.S.

BARCLAY, John A.; 256 Golfdale Rd., Toronto 12, Ont. (res); Glasgow (Scot.) '43; F.R.F.P.S. (Glas.), F.R.C.S. (Ed.); GenSurg; Staff, Workman's Comp. Bd., 90 Harbour St., Toronto, Ont.; Tel. 362-3411.

BARCLAY, Lyman T.; The Mill, Greenwood, Ont. (res); Tor '26; F.R.C.S. (Edin.), F.R.C.S.(C), PlasSurg; Retired.

BARCLAY, Thomas H. C.; Allan Blair Mem. Clinic, Regina, Sask.; 2355 Cross Pl. (res); **Glasgow (Scot.) '40; M.B., Ch.B., Ch.M., (Hons.);** FRCS (Glasg.) FRFPS; Sr. Clin. Assoc., Saskatchewan Cancer Commission; Tel. 527-9651.

BARCLAY, William S.; 1110 W. Georgia St., Vancouver 5, B. C.; 3606 Point Grey Rd. (res); Man '24; FCCP; IntMed (T.B.); Reg. Supt., Pacific Region Indian Health Services. Retired.

BARD, Harry; Lausanne (Switz.) '62; Res., Children's Hosp., Montreal 25, P.Q.

BARD, Jean L.; 229 St. Joseph, Lauzon, P.Q.; Lav'65.

BARD, Martin G.; 1222 Bonnie Cres., City View, Ottawa 5, Ont. (res); Tor '57; Anaes; Staff, Ottawa Civic Hosp.; Tel. 729-7247.

BARDAL, Sigurgeir; Shoal Lake Hosp., Shoal Lake, Man.; Jane St. (res); Man'17; Memb. Advisory Comm. Minister of Health, Birtle-Shoal Lake Health Unit; Tel. 40.

BARDARI, A.; 5514 Laurendeau, Montreal, P.Q.; Mon'48; GenSurg (P.Q.); MCGP.

BARDAWILL, Charles J.; 30 Bond St., Toronto, Ont.; 88 Sutherland Dr. (res); Tor '43; M.A. (Clin. Path.); Dir., Dept. of Haem., & Dir. Research Lab., St. Michael's Hosp.; Assoc. (Med.), U. of Toronto; Tel. EM 2-4461.

BARDINS, Peter; 33 Dalton Rd., Toronto 4, Ont.; 375 Brock Ave. (res); Latvia '31. Tel. WA 1-7203.

BARENDS, Howard A.; 938 Killeen Ave., Ottawa 13, Ont.; Qns '44; Anaes; Active Staff, Ottawa Civic Hosp.; Tel. 728-2100.

BARETTE, Rosaire; Ste. Genevieve, Co. Champlain, P.Q.; Mon'42.

BARG, Peter; 214 Margaret Ave., Wallaceburg, Ont.; 20 Grand Ave. (res); McG '44; MCGP; MOH, Lambton Co.; Tel. 627-5711.

BARI, Mohammed; 465 King St., Bridgewater, N.S.; Karachi (Pakistan)'57.

BARIBEAU, Claude; Lav '62; P.G. University of Toronto, Toronto, Ont.

BARIBEAU, Gaetan; 1005 St. Prosper, Trois Rivieres, P.Q.; Lav'53; Haem (P.Q.); Staff, Hop. St-Joseph.

BARIBEAU, Leo; 230 Longueuil, St-Jean, P.Q.; Lav '59; ObstGyn.

BARIBEAU, Michel; Lav '62; Res., Hop. St-Joseph, Trois-Rivieres, P.Q.; Abroad.

BARIL, Edmond; 301 Carre-St-Louis, Montreal, P.Q.; Mon '41; Paed (P.Q.); Cons., Gen. Cigar Co; Tel. AV 8-7580.

BARIL, Henry P.; Man'54; MCGP; Res., Rehab. Inst., 6300 Darlington, Montreal 26, P.Q.

BARKAUSKAS, Antanas; Staff, Ontario Hosp. School, Smith's Falls, Ontario. '40; Tel. 283-2990.

BARKER, Arthur J.; Ste. 5.-285-17th St., West Vancouver, B. C.; 1337 Mathers (res); UBC '59; Tel. 922-0155.

BARKER, C. Scott; 1538 Sherbrooke W., Montreal, P.Q.; 203 Ballantyne N. (res); McG '32; F.R.C.P.(C), F.A.C.P., IntMed.; Lect. Dept. of Med., McGill U.; Assoc. Phys., Royal Victoria Hosp.; Tel. WE 2-7024.

BARKER, Elliott T.; 75 Willingdon Blvd., Toronto 18, Ont.; Tor '58; Psy; Staff, Toronto Psych. Hosp.; Tel. WA 5-6371. Abroad.

BARKER, Harold M.; Ste. 422 Med. Arts Bldg., 11010 Jasper Ave., Edmonton, Alta.; Wes '50; B.Sc., D.Psy; Psy; AAPCC (Paed. Psych.); Cons. Child Psy., Our Lady of Charity School for Girls, Prov. of Alberta, Dept. of Child Welfare, City of Edmonton, Kiwanis Teen House & Kiwanis Children's Home; Act. Staff, Royal Alexandra Hosp.; Lect. Psy., U. of Alberta; Tel. 424-8474.

BARKER, John H.; 1186 Cloverbrae Cres., Port Credit, Ont. (res); Tor'49; Cons. (Perm. Disability Dept.), WCB; Tel. CR 4-3439.

BARKER, Leslie K.; 518 Brant St., Burlington, Ont.; London (Eng.) '57; Tel. NE 4-5033.

BARKER, William E.; 532 Med. Arts Bldg., 404-6 Graham Ave., Winnipeg 1, Man.; Man'49; OrthSurg; Staff, University of Manitoba; Retired.

BARKIN, Martin; 85 Prue Ave., Toronto 19, Ont. (res); Tor'60; FRCS(C), Urol; Staff Research, Banting Inst.; Tel. 781-5014.

BARKMAN, Bernard G.; Drawer 130, Abbotsford, B.C.; Man '45; MCGP; Staff, M.S.A. Gen. Hosp.; Tel. 859-5401.

BARKUN, Harvey; France '57; Ass't. Supt., Queen Mary Veteran's Hosp., Montreal 26, P. Q.: Tel. 738-9481.

BARLASS, Jack L.; 214-6th Ave. W., Calgary, Alta.; 3435-62nd Ave. S. W. (res); Alb '52; FRCS (C) NeurSurg; Staff, Dept. NeurSurg., Calgary Gen., Holy Cross & Childrens' Hosp's.; Cons. Foothill Hosp.; Tel. 263-7120.

BARLOW, H. S.; 11 Victoria Ave., Chatham, Ont.; 142 Victoria (res); Tor '24; M.C.G.P.; **Cons. Staff Public Gen. & St. Joseph's Hosp's.**

BARLOW, R. Blake; 143 Thames St., Chatham, Ont.; 81 Dunn (res); Wes '50; M.C.G.P.; Staff, Chatham Gen. & St. Joseph's Hosp's.; Tel. 352-5050.

BARLOW, William R.; Lake Echo, Halifax Co., N.S.; London (Eng.) '11; Tel. 469-2994.

BARNABE, Gerard; 2775 rue Bourdages, St. Hyacinthe, P.Q.; Mon '58; Paed.; Staff, Hop. Ste. Justine.

BARNABY, Henry C.; 115 Woolwich St., Guelph, Ont.; 35 Tiffany St. W. (res); Dal '29; DABOt; Otol; Active Staff, Guelph Gen. & St. Joseph's Hosp's.; Tel. TA 2-7506.

BARNARD, James E.; 299 King St. W., Beamsville, Ont.; McG '40; DPH; DTM; ABOM; Staff, Hotel-Dieu & St. Catharines Gen. Hosp's.; Med. Dir., McKinnon Industries Ltd.; Tel. MU 4-7211.

BARNBROOK, Douglas H.; 518 Med. Arts Bldg., Hamilton, Ont.; Birmingham (Eng.) '45; FRCS (Eng.); FICS; GenSurg; Active Staff (Surg.), Hamilton Gen. & St. Joseph's Hosp's.; Tel. JA 7-5693.

BARNBROOK, Robert B.; 2907 W. 29th Ave., Vancouver 8, B.C.; London (Eng.)'59; MB; MRCS(Eng.); LRCP (Lond.); Anaes; Staff, St. Vincents Hosp.

BARNBY, T. Ivison; Medical Arts Bldg., Windsor, Ont.; 1909 Verdun Ave. (res); Wes '25; Tel. 254-6277.

BARNER, Herbert D.; 5798 Victoria Dr., Vancouver 16, B.C.; 1375 W. King Edward Ave., (res); Tor '32; A.M.C.G.P.; Staff, Grace & Burnaby Gen. Hosp's.; Tel. FA 5-1288.

BARNES, Adam G.; Dal '65; Staff, Cottage Hosp., Channel-Port aux Basques, Nfld.

BARNES, David S.; 742 King St. W., Kitchener, Ont.; 109 Hickory, Waterloo (res); Wes '57; Psy; Adjunct. Prof. (Psychol.), U. of Waterloo; Tel. 745-0711.

BARNES, Francis E.; Wes '60; Jr. Int'n., Victoria Hosp., London, Ont.

BARNES, Guy W.; 713 Columbia St., New Westminster, B.C.; 1731 Dublin St. (res); Tor '42; Anaes.; Tel. LA 2-4241.

BARNES, H. M.; 184-2nd Ave., Ottawa 2, Ont. (res); Qns '16; Staff, DVA; Retired.

BARNES, Lancelot S.; 170 St. George St., Toronto 5, Ont.; 41 Ridge Dr. (res); Tor '23; A.B.-Op., Ophth,Otol; Dept. Otol., Toronto Western Hosp. Tel. WA 2-1829.

BARNES, Michael J.; Box 1000, Estevan, Sask.; London (Eng.) '61.

BARNES, Philip H.; Mall Med. Bldg., Northwest St. Mary's & Memorial Blvd., Winnipeg 1, Man.; 644 Niagara St., Wpg. 9. (res); Man '52; FRCS (C); ObstGyn; Active Staff, St. Boniface & Misericordia Hosp's.; Dem. (ObstGyn.) U. of Man.; Tel. SP 4-2411.

BARNES, Priscilla A. (Ridge); 2104-2nd St. S.W., Calgary, Alta.; London (Eng.) '53; MB., BS., MRCS., LRCP; DMRT (Eng.); Radiother., Cancer Clin; Tel. AM 3-0770.

BARNES, R. Randolph; 145 Carling Ave., Ottawa, Ont.; 25 Madawaska Dr. (res); Qns '30; F.I.C.S., ObstGyn; Cons. ObstGyn, Ottawa Civic & Grace Hosp's.; Tel. CE 2-5284.
BARNES, W. Bruce; 1247 King St. W., Toronto, Ont.; Tor '18; Tel. LE 2-0228.
BARNES, William H.; 66 Charleton St. W., Hamilton, Ont.; Qns '51; M.Sc. (Surg.); FACS; DABS; FRCS(C), GenSurg; Cons. Staff, Hamilton Gen. Hosp.; Tel. 522-7835.
BARNETT, George D.; Fort San, Sask.; Man '44; D.H.A.; Gen. Supt. & Dir. Med. Services, Sask. Anti-TB League; Tel. 332-5785.
BARNETT, Henry J M.; 624 Medical Arts Bldg., 170 St. George St., Toronto 5, Ont.; Tor '44; FRCP(C); Neur; Phys., Toronto Gen. Hosp.; Ass't. Prof. (Med.), U. of Toronto; Tel. WA 2-4705.
BARNETT, R. Douglas; Ste. 205, 4900 Kingsway, Burnaby, B.C.; UBC '56 Tel. HE 1-6696.
BARNHILL, B. Edward W.; Sackville Medical Centre, Sackville, N.B.; 79 Lansdowne St. (res); Dal '38.
BARNHOUSE, L. Dorothy (Mrs. G. H. Yates); R. R. No.1, Tappen, B. C.; Alb '37; Anaes; Staff, Shuswap Gen. Hosp., Salmon Arm, B. C.
BARON, Henry A.; 6000 Cote des Neiges Rd., Ste. 345, Montreal 26, P.Q.; McG'28; DNB; FACOG; FACS; ObstGyn; Sr. ObstGyn., Jewish Gen. Hosp.; Cons. ObstGyn., Mt. Sinai Hosp., Jewish Hosp. of Hope & Maimonides Hosp.; Tel. RE 3-4311.
BARON, Paul J.; Ste. 101, 1541 W. Broadway, Vancouver 9, B.C.; Man '44; GenSurg.
BARON, Robert H.; Ott'60; IntMed; Staff, Cardiovasc. Serv., Ottawa Gen. Hosp., Ottawa 2, Ont.; Clin. Ass't., Dept. of Med., U. of Ottawa; Tel. CE 6-0333, Ext. 409.
BAROOTES, E. William; 802 Medical & Dental Bldg., Regina, Sask.; 2805 McCallum Ave., (res); Tor '43; F.R.C.S.(C), Urol; Staff, Gen. & Grey Nuns' Hosps. Tel. LA 2-6649.
BARR, Andrew S.; Civic Serv. Health Centre. Parliament Bldgs., Toronto 5, Ont.; Glasgow (Scot.) '55; Tel. EM 3-1211.
BARR, Donald A.; 6 Glengrove Ave. W., Toronto 12, Ont. (res); Tor '53; M.C.G.P.; Active Staff North-York Branson Hosp; O.P.D. Staff, Toronto Western Hosp; Staff Phys., Health Serv. Ryerson Inst. of Technology; Tel. 635-6211.
BARR, Elizabeth B. (Sheppard); 6 Glengrove Ave. W., Toronto 12, Ont. (res); Tor '53; Retired.
BARR, Elsie; See (Culliton).
BARR, Hugh P.; 383 Ellis St., Penticton, B.C.; Man '43; MCGP; DO; Vis. Staff, Penticton Gen. Hosp.; Tel 492-3024.
BARR, Hugh W.; Ste. 211, 111 Waterloo St., London, Ont.; Wes'59; FRCS(C), NeurSurg.
BARR, James A.; Medical Clinic, 3009-31st Ave., Vernon, B.C.; Alb'64.
BARR, James S.; 330 Phys. & Surg. Bldg., 8409-112th St., Edmonton, Alta.; Glasgow (Scot.) '45; FRCOG; FRCS(C), ObstGyn; Instr. (ObstGyn.), U. of Alberta; Tel. 439-1672.
BARR, John W. B. Brig.; Cdn. Forces Headquarters, 48 Rideau St., Ottawa, Ont.; Qns'40; Deputy Surg. Gen., Cdn. Forces; Tel. 992-5227.
BARR, Johnston R.; Glasgow (Scot.) '50; M.B., Ch.B.; Path; Ass't Path., Ottawa Civic Hosp., Ottawa, Ont.; Regional Path., County of Carleton; Tel. 729-2511, Ext. 254.
BARR, Margaret N.; 8 Mutchmor Rd., Ottawa 1, Ont. Edinburgh **(Scot.) '51; FFARCS (Eng.)**; DRCOG; Anaes; Civilian M.O., Dept. of National Defence; Cons. Anaes., Royal Ottawa San.; Phys. Alcoholism & Drug Addict. Research Fdn.; Tel. 232-2363.
BARR, Robert M.; Wes. '63; Int., Victoria Hosp., London, Ont.; Abroad.
BARR, Murray L.; 149 Windsor Ave., London, Ont. (res); Wes '33; M.Sc., LI.D.; FRSC; FRCP (C); Prof. & Hd. Dept., Microscopic Anat. U. of Western Ontario; Tel. GE 9-1681.
BARRERA, Alberto M.; The Purdue Frederick Co. & Affiliates, 99 Saw Mill River Rd., Yonkers, N.Y., U.S.A.; Shanghai (China) '41; MCGP; Med. Dir., Purdue Frederick Co.; Abroad.

BARRETT, Ann (Stillapere); Ste. 201, 1482 Bathhurst St.,Toronto 10, Ont.; Tartu, (Estonia) '44; Assoc. Staff, Women's College Hosp.; Court Staff, Salvation Army Grace Hosp.; Tel. LE 2-0331.
BARRETT, Connor; Ste. 210, 4900 Kingsway, South Burnaby, B.C.; Dublin (Ire.) '52; BAO; FRCS(I); GenSurg; Vis. Staff, Burnaby Gen. Hosp.; Abroad.
BARRETT, George R.; 405 Hendryx St., Nelson, B.C.; 303 Silica St. (res); Man '33; M.C.G.P.; Chief, Dept. Med., Kootenay Lake Gen. Hosp.; **Tel. 352-6611.**
BARRETT, Kevin A.; 2411-26th Ave. N.W., Calgary, Alta. (res); Dublin (Ire.) '52; D.P.H.; Ass't. M.O., City Hall.
BARRETTE, Andre; 602 Boul. Senecal, Chambly, P.Q.; Mon '54; Tel. 658-2280.
BARRETTE, Elzear; 2995 Ave. Royale, Gifford, Quebec 5, P.Q.; Lav '38; Tel. 663-6533.
BARRETT, G. A. David; UBC'62; Res., Alberta Hosp., Box 1000, Ponoka, Alta.
BARRETTE, Gaston; 4 Main Rd., Hudson Co., Vaudreuil, P.Q.; Mon '56.
BARRETTE, J. Arthur; Ste. 12 ,12245 rue Grenet, Montreal 9, P.Q.; Ott'57; Ophth.
BARRETTE, J. P. Jacques; 517 Station, Shawinigan, P.Q.; 362 Blvd. St. Maurice (res); Lav '32; GenSurg (P.Q.); Surg., Hop. Ste. Therese, Shawinigan; Tel. LE 6-3681.
BARRETTE, Louis-Rene; Lav'65; Res., Hotel-Dieu, St. Vallier, Chicoutimi, P.Q.
BARRETTE, Marcel; 35rue Legault, St.-Jerome, P.Q.; Mon '53; IntMed, Cardiol (P.Q.); Tel. GE 8-8739.
BARRETTE, Marcel F.; 31 Montcalm, Hull, P.Q.; Ott '58; MCGP; Tel. 771-6345.
BARRETTE, Rosaire; Mattagami, Cte Abitibi Est, P.Q.; Mon '42.
BARRIE, Howard J.; R.R. No. 1, Schomberg, Ont.; Oxford (Eng.) '33; Path; Dir. of Path., Sunnybrook Hosp., Toronto, Ont.; Tel. 485-8651.
BARRIE, Michael O.L.; 395 College St., Cobourg, Ont. (res); Qns '32; D.Psy; Psy; Med. Supt., Ontario Hosp., Cobourg; Tel. 372-3341.
BARRINGTON, Thomas W.; One Medical Place, 20 Wynford Dr., Don Mills, Ont.; Tor '56; FRCS (C); OrthSurg; Staff, Toronto East Gen. Hosp.; Cons. (Orth.), Sunnybrook Hosp.; Tel. 922-3368.
BARRIT, Derek S.; Box 9, Goodsoil, Sask.; Aberdeen (Scot.)'59.
BARRON, Beverley G. (Nelems); 2 Core Cres., Brampton, Ont.; Tor '61. Retired.
BARRON, L. Robert; 20802 Lakeshore Rd., Baie D'Urfe, P.Q.; Dorval Shopping Centre, Dorval; 860 Decarie, St. Laurent; McG '50; B.Sc.; ObstGyn; Staff, Catherine Booth, Lakeshore Gen. & Lachine Gen. Hosp's.; **Tel. 631-8530, 453-5510 & 747-3288.**
BARRON, Robert D.; 209 Glen Rd., Toronto 5, Ont.; Tor'39; DPH; DIH.
BARRY, Agathe; 2015 Bourbonniere, Quebec 6, P.Q.; Lav '58; Haem (P.Q.). Abroad.
BARRY, Antoine; Lav'60; Res., Hop. de l'Enfant Jesus, Quebec 3, P.Q.
BARRY, A. Wayne; McG'65; Res., Ottawa Civic Hosp., Ottawa, Ont.
BARRY, Gladys N.; (Mrs. Donesky); 1624 Jackson Ave., Saskatoon, Sask.; Loma Linda (Calif., U.S.A.) '52; Active Staff (GP), Saskatoon City Hosp.; Assoc. Staff, St. Paul's Hosp.; Clin. Fell. (Psy), University Hosp.; Tel. 949-3040.
BARRY, James E.; 14 Pine St. S., Timmins, Ont.; 16 Mattagami (res); Tor '16; GenSurg; ObstGyn; Tel. AM 4-7100.
BARRY, John M.; 182 Princess St., Saint John, N.B. (res); Baltimore, U.S.A. '01; Retired.
BARRY, Macdonald L.; Med. Arts Bldg., 626 Main St., Penticton, B.C.; 1082 Ross Ave. (res); McG '52; GenSurg; Staff, Penticton Hosp.; Tel. HY 2-8017.
BARRY, Michael P.; 17 Academy Park Rd., Regina, Sask. (res); Man. '48; DiagRad; Staff, Anti-TB League; Tel. LA 7-4007.
BARRY, Michael; Tor'61; Res., Clarke Inst. of Psy., Toronto 2B, Ont.
BARRY, Murray P.; Qns'65; Jr. Int., Vancouver General Hosp., Vancouver, B.C.

BARRY, Nicole; Lav'65; Res., Hotel-Dieu, Sherbrooke, P.Q.
BARRY, Pierre P.; 5691 Place Donat, Ville-d'Anjou, Montreal, P.Q.; Lav '57; Anaes; Staff, Hop. Maisonneuve; Tel. 254-8341.
BARRY, Richard E.; 132 Parkdale Ave. S., Hamilton, Ont.; Qns'63; AMCGP; Tel. 547-0218.
BARRY, Thomas L. J.; 3503 Grey Ave., Montreal 28, P.Q. (res); National U. of Ire. (Cork) '25; F.R.C.S. (Eng.); Exec. Dir., Reddy Mem. Hosp. Tel. WE 5-9641.
BARSKEY, Simon; 1431 Bishop St., Montreal, P.Q.; 719 Wiseman Ave.; **Outremont (res)**; Mon '31; **IntMed & Cardiol (P.Q.); Ass't. Phys. Jewish Gen. Hosp; Tel. VI 9-2700.**
BARSKY, Morley; 203 Edmonton St., Winnipeg, Man.; Apt. 7P-525 Lanark St. Wpg. 9 (res); Man '55; GenSurg; **Assoc. Staff, Misericordia Hosp**; Court. **Staff, St. Boniface & Victoria Hosp's.**; Tel. **SP 4-6581.**

BARSKY, Percy; 1459 Main St., Winnipeg, Man.; 6 Greenmor Apts., 1311 Main St. (res); Man '49; FAAP; Paed; Paed. Staff, St. Boniface & Children's Hosp's.; Lect., Dept of Paed., Man. Med. Coll.; Med. Dir. CAS of Winnipeg; Tel. JU 6-5002.
BARSONY, Bela; 602 Med. Arts Bldg., Saskatoon, Sask.; Budapest (Hung.) '53; LRCP (Lond.); LRCS (Edin.); LRFPS (Glasgow); Anaes; Staff, Saskatoon City Hosp.; Tel. 224-6681.
BARSONY, Peter; 170 The Donway West, Don Mills, Ont.; Budapest (Hung.)'50; D. Psy; Psy.
BARSS, Allison H.; Rose Bay, N.S.; Dal '44; MCGP.
BARSS, Geoffrey A.; Rose Bay, N.S.; Dal '13. Retired.
BARTE, Paul; 90 Mary St., New Liskeard, '55 Ont.
BARTEAUX, John W.; Woodlawn Medical Clinic, 110 Woodlawn Dr., **Dartmouth, N.S.; Dal '60;** AMCGP. Tel. 469-1563.
BARTELINK, Dirk L.; Amsterdam (Neth) Research Prof. (Rad. Anat.), U. of Western Ont., London, Ont.; Tel. GE 9-1681.
BARTHA, Julius; 466 Oakwood Ave., Toronto 10, Ont.; Debrecen (Hung.) '43; Tel. RU 3-4318.

BARTLETT, Glen S.; 688 Coxwell Ave., Toronto 13, Ont.; Tor '58; FRCS(C), GenSurg; Att'd. Surg., Toronto East General Hosp.; Tel. 699-5290.
BARTLETT, Leslie H.; Ste. 108, 1940 Lonsdale Ave., North Vancouver, B.C.; 487 Gordon Ave., W. Vancouver, (res); McG'52; FRCS(C), OrthSurg; Tel. YU 7-1711.
BARTLETT, Lloyd C.; 507 Med. Arts Bldg., Winnipeg 1, Man.; 97 Yale Ave., Wpg. 9 (res); Wes '41; FRCS(C), GenSurg; Dir. PG Surg. Educ., U. of Manitoba; Tel. WH 2-8388.
BARTLETT, O. Russell; 5020 Riverside Dr., Riverside, Ont. (res); Wes '41; Anaes; Retired.
BARTLETT, Wilbert W.; 51 Queen St. E., Brampton, Ont.; 90 Elizabeth St. S. (res); Tor '31; Chief of Surg., Peel Mem. Hosp.; Tel. GL 1-0241.
BARTLEY, Alfred H.; 90 Main St. West, Grimsby, Ont.; London (Eng.)'34; MRCS(Eng.); LRCP (Lon.); MRSH(Eng.).
BARTMAN, Eugene; Man '58; AMCGP; Res., Winnipeg Gen. Hosp., Winnipeg 3, Man.

BARTON, E. Lawrence; Wes '37; PactBact; Dir. of Labs., Guelph Gen. Hosp., Guelph, Ont.; Tel. TA 2-5350.
BARTON, Frederick C.; 10 Tecumseh St., Orillia, Ont.; Tor'38; Staff, Ont. Hosp. Schl.; Tel. **326-7361.**
BARTON, Frederick J.; 180 Portland St., Dartmouth, N.S. (res); Dal '41; FACS; GenSurg; Chief of Staff, Assoc. Surg., Hlfx. Infirmary; Ass't. Prof. (Surg.), Dalhousie U.; Tel. 466-7471.
BARTON, H. Gerald; Winchester, Ont.; Qns'43; Staff, Winchester Dist. Mem. Hosp.; Tel. 613-774-2121.
BARTON, Michael C. R.; Ste 203, Med. Centre, 10006-149th St., Edmonton, Alta.; Alb '61; Staff, Phys., Northern Transportation Co.; Tel. 489-7931.

BARTON, Robert C.; Clarenville, Nfld.; Trinity Coll. (Dublin, Ire.) '60.
BARTON, Robert S.; Tor '49; D.Psy., Psy; **Staff, Ontario Hosp., Whitby, Ont.; Tel. MO 8-5881.**
BARTON, Robert W.; Baden, Ont.; Tor '48; M.C.G.P.
BARTON, W. Bruce; Victoria Hosp. London, Ont.; Wes '45; FRCP(C), IntMed; Assoc. Prof. (PathChem), Ass't. Prof. (ClinMed.), & Hon. Lect. (TherRad.), U. of Western Ontario; Tel. 432-5261.

BARTRAM, Edward A.; 462 Wellington St., London, Ont.; 431 Regent St. **(res); Wes '28; IntMed; Ass't. Prof. Med., U. of Western Ontario; Chief, Dept. Cardiol., Victoria & St. Joseph's Hosp's., London; Tel. GE 4-7608.**
BARTULICA, Nicolas; Yugoslavia '53; Staff, Hop. Pierre Janet, 20 Pharand, Hull, P.Q.
BARWELL-CLARKE, Ivor F.; Ste. 607, 625-5th Ave., New Westminster, B.C.; Wales'44; FRCS (Eng.); FRCS(C); PlasSurg; GenSurg.
BARWICK, Peter E.; McG '62; Res., Royal Victoria Hosp., Montreal, P.Q.
BARWINSKY Jaroslaw; 301 Med. Arts Bldg., 404-406 Graham Ave., Winnipeg 1, Man.; Man '55; Dip. Surg. (Man.); DABS; DABTS; FACS; FRCS(C), GenSurg; ThorSurg; Active Staff (Surg.), St. Boniface Gen. Hosp.; Court. Staff, (Surg.), Wpg. Gen., Wpg. Children's & Misericordia Hosp's.; Dir. Surg. Research Lab., St. Boniface Hosp.; Lect. Surg., U. of Manitoba; Tel. 947-1737.

BARYLUK, Victor L.; 618 Church St., Toronto 5, Ont.; Man '60.
BARZA, David; 548 Cote-St-Catherine Rd., Montreal 8, P.Q.; McG '31; IntMed; Clin. Ass't., Royal Victoria Hosp.; Assoc. Phys., Jewish Gen. Hosp.; Clin. Ass't. McGill U.; Phys-in-Charge Simon Cigar Co., Ville St. Laurent; Tel. CR 9-7253.

BARZA, Michaeal J.; McG '64; Res., Royal Victoria Hosp., Montreal 2, P.Q.
BARZA, Sidney; 3545 Cote des Neiges Rd., Ste. 105, Montreal 25, P.Q.; McG'49; D.Psy; Psy; Sr. Psy., Mental Hygiene Inst.; Ass't. Psy., Allan Mem. Inst.; Ass't. Prof. McGill U.; Tel. 935-8415.

BASCO, Vivien E.; B.C. Cancer Inst., 2656 Heather St., Vancouver 9, B.C.; Birmingham (Eng.), '58; FFR; DMRT; Ther Rad.
BASE, Gerald S.; Box 275, 235 Church St., Oakville, Ont.; Qns '52; Anaes; Chief of Anaes., Oakville-Trafalgar Mem. Hosp.
BASECQZ, Guy; Louvain (Belgium)'61; Staff, Hop. St.-Jean-de-Dieu, Montreal 5, P.Q.
BASHOW, Lynn E.; Dal'43; PhysMed. & Rehab.; Staff, Ridgewood Rehab Centre, Lancaster, N.B.
BASHUCKY, William; Winnipegosis, Man.; Man '45; Dist. Coroner.
BASIAN, Herbert; Suite 808, 99 Avenue Rd., Toronto 5, Ont.; 174 Roywood Dr., Don Mills (res); Tor '54; DABS; FRCS(C); GenSurg; Vol. Ass't., Toronto Gen. Hosp.; Court. Staff, Doctor's Hosp.; Tel. WA 3-9318.
BASIOR, Rajzla; 121 Stafford Rd., Willowdale, Ont.; Basle (Switz.) '35; Tel. 225-1350.
BASMAJIAN, John V.; 55 Jane Ave., Kingston, Ont. (res); Tor '45; Prof. and Head, Dept. of Anat., Queen's U.; Tel. LI 6-1731.
BASRUR, Vasanth R.; Tor'61; Res., Hamilton Gen. Hosp., Hamilton, Ont.
BASSER, W. V.; Tor '63; Int., Wellesley Hosp., Toronto 5, Ont.

BASSETT, Alan A.; 158 St. George St., Toronto 5, Ont.; 7 Westgate Cres. (res); Tor '39; FACS, GenSurg; Sr. Att'd. Surg.; Dir. Tumour Clin. & Chm. Tumour Comm. New Mt. Sinai Hosp.; Sr. Cons. (Surg.), Baycrest Home & Hosp. for the Aged; Tel. 924-2249.
BASSETT, Byron C.; 4049 Kensington Ave., Montreal, P.Q.; Cardiff (Wales) '58.
BASSETT, Lloyd; 318 Cook Medical Bldg., 1175 Cook St., Victoria, B.C.; 3040 Beach Dr. (res); Alb '36; Staff, Dept. of Obst. (ObstGyn.), Royal Jubilee & St. Joseph's Hosp's.; Tel. EV 3-3114.

BASSETT, Terence H.; Purity Dairy Bldg., Lethbridge, Alta.; 1106—7th Ave. S. (res); London (Eng.) '39; M.R.C.S. (Eng.), L.R.C.P. (Lond.), D.Ophth.; Tel. FA 7-2510.
BASTA, **Domenico**; 600 Caledonia Rd., Toronto 10, Ont.; Naples (Italy) '54; Tel. 781-7262. 781-7262.
BASTARACHE, Alfred; 58 Peter St., Moncton, N.B. (res); Lav '46; Path; Pathol., Regional Labs.; Tel. 389-9141.
BASTARACHE, Marie S. (St-Jacques); C.P. 578, La Pocatiere, Kamouraska, P.Q.; Lav'59.
BASTARACHE, Rene; 1010 Chemin St-Roch, Tracy, P.Q.; Lav '59; IntMed.
BASTARACHE, **William**; Centre Medicale, La Pocatiere, Cte Kamouraska, P.Q.; Lav'59; GenSurg.
BASTED, Robert M.; (See BAIRD, Robert M.)
BASTEDO, Donald L.A.; 9 Margaret Ave., Kitchener, Ont.; **6 Maple Hill Dr. (res); Tor '45**; ABP; Paed; **Active Staff, Kitchener-Waterloo Hosp.; Cons. Staff, St. Mary's Hosp.; Vol. Ass't., OPD, Hosp. for Sick Children, Toronto**; Tel. SH 3-1486.
BASTEDO, George M., D.S.O., 15 Forest Glen Cres., Toronto 12, Ont. (res); Tor '31; GenSurg; Surg. Cons., W.C.B.; Tel. 362-3411.
BASTER, Norman; 420 B.C. Trust Bldg., Lethbridge, Alta.; Leeds (Eng.)'37; DPH; PH; Dir., Barnes Health Unit; M.O.H., Lethbridge; Dist. Coroner; Tel. 318-4203.
BASTIAN, Frank O.; Estevan Med. Assoc., Estevan, Sask.; Sask'64.
BASTIEN, Edouard; Mon'64; Res., Hop. Maisonneuve, Montreal 36, P.Q.
BASTIEN, **Godfrey P.**; 50 Cremazie Ouest., Montreal 11, P.Q.; 12265 Guertin (res); Mon **'47; GenSurg (P.Q.); Surg., Hotel Dieu, Mtl. & Hop. Notre Dame de l'Esperance, St. Laurent.** Tel. 384-0244.
BASTIEN, Jean C.; 241 ouest Fleury, Montreal 12, P.Q.; Mon '63; Tel. DU 1-7281.
BASTIEN, Marcel; 7820 Marquette, Montreal 35, P.Q.; Mon '60; Tel. RA 5-3636.
BASTIEN, Pierre; 241 ouest, Fleury, Montreal 12, P.Q.; Mon '63.
BASTOMSKY, Charles H.; Witwatersrand (S. Africa)'57; MRCP(Ed.); Fell(Med.), Royal Victoria Hosp., Montreal 2, P.Q.
BASTOW, Douglas C.; 183 St. Clair Ave. W., Toronto, Ont.; 30 Riverview Dr. (res); Tor '21; Anaes.; Tel. HU 9-5754.
BASTRASH, **Normand**; C. P. 1240, Louisville, Co. Maskinonge, P.Q.; Lav '53.
BASU, Prasanta K.; 19 Ringwood Cr., Willowdale, Ont.; Calcutta (India) '46; DOMS; Assoc. Prof. & Dir. of Ophth. Research, U. of Toronto; Sr. Ophth., Toronto Gen. Hosp.; Med. Research Assoc., M.R.C.; Tel. WA 5-7487.
BASUALDO-VIDELA, Carlos A.; Cordoba (Argentina) '58; Jr. Intn., Hamilton Gen. Hosp., Hamilton, Ont.
BATALION, Hyman; 4932 Carlton Ave., Montreal 29, P.Q.; McG'61; Staff, Queen Mary Vet's Hosp.; Tel. 733-4184.
BATANOFF, Katherine (see Cross)
BATE, George W.; 115 Hazen St., Saint John, N.B.; 239 Princess St. (res); Dal '51; DABS; FACS; GenSurg; Ass't. Surg., Saint John Gen. Hosp.; Surg., St. Joseph's Hosp.; Tel. 693-2449.
BATE, John T.; Ste. 34, 31 Yonge St. N., Richmond Hill, Ont.; Tor '57; FRCS(C), ObstGyn; Chief, ObstGyn., York Central Hosp.; Tel. TU 4-3498.
BATEMAN, Beverly M.; 151 Forest Hill Rd., Toronto, Ont. (res); Tor '42; Retired.
BATEMAN, Charles L. F/L; RCAF Station, Cold Lake, Alta.; Qns'63.
BATEMAN, Charles R.; Tor '59; AMCGP; Res., Royal Victoria Hosp., Montreal 2, P.Q.
BATEMAN Evelyn (Tattersall); Women's College Anaes., Ste. 15, 501 Yonge St., Toronto, Ont.; Tor '34; Anaes; Chief Dept. of Anaes., Women's College Hosp.; Clin. Teach, Dept. of Anaes., U. of Toronto; Tel. WA 2-0244.
BATEMAN, George L.; 402 Pitt St., Cornwall, Ont.; Qns '41; Tel. WE 2-2061.
BATEMAN, H. E. D.; 217 Second St. E., Cornwall, Ont.; Qns '34; M.C.G.P.; Staff, Cornwall Gen. & Hotel Dieu Hosp's.; Tel. WE 3-4165.
BATEMAN, James E.; 422 Med. Arts Bldg., 170 St. George St., Toronto 5, Ont.; 151 Forest Hill Rd. (res); Tor '38; DABOS; FRCS(C); Orth-Surg.; Chief of Staff, Orth. & Arthritic Hosp.; **Tel. 922-2525.**
BATEMAN, James H.; 217 Pinnacle St., Belleville, Ont.; 155 Bleecker St. (res); Qns '35; F.R.C.S.(C); GenSurg; Surg., Belleville Gen. Hosp.; Tel. 962-4221.
BATEMAN, **Russel**; 278 Charles St., Belleville, Ont.; Qns '42.
BATEMAN, William E.; Ste. 202, 98 Guestville Ave., Toronto 9, Ont.; 171 Hillhurst Blvd. (res); Tor '43; FACOG; ObstGyn; Staff, Humber Mem. Hosp.; Tel. RO 3-1171.
BATEMAN, **W. R.**; 250 Lawrence Ave. W., Toronto 12, Ont.; Qns'11; Tel. 787-2323.
BATES, Clarence L.; 85 King St. W., Dundas, Ont.; 87 King St. W. (res); McG'34; MCGP; Chmn. Med. Advisory Bd., Alcoholism & Drug Addict. Research Fdn.; Tel. MA 8-2721.
BATES, David V.; 470 Portland Ave., Twn, of Mount Royal Montreal 16, P.Q.; Cambridge (Eng.) '44; MRCS; LRCP; MRCP (Lond.); M.D. (Cambridge); FRCP(C); Dir., Respiratory Div., Joint Cardioresp. Serv., Montreal Children's & Royal Victoria Hosp's.; Prof. of Experim. Med. & Assoc. Dean for Grad. Studies & Research, McGill U.; Tel. VI 2-1251.
BATES, Gordon A.; 111 Avenue Rd., Toronto 5, Ont.; Tor '07; Dir., Health League of Canada & Editor "Health" Magazine; Retired.
BATES, J. F.; 258-4th Ave., Ottawa, Ont. (res); GenSurg; Staff, Pensions' Branch Dept., D.V.A., Ottawa; Tel. CE 2-8211.
BATES, Kendal; 519 Jarvis St., Toronto, Ont.; Tor '08. Tel. WA 1-3488.
BATES, Millie V.; 1550 Glenwatson Dr., Port Credit, Ont. (res); Tor '32; Anaes.; Hon. Staff, Women's College Hosp., Toronto; Temp. Ret.
BATES, Robert W.; 194 Fenn Ave., Willowdale, Ont. (res); Tor '50; FRCP(C), IntMed; Staff, St. Michael's Hosp.; Tel. 362-4461.
BATES, **William F.**; 247 John St., Belleville, Ont.; Qns'64; Active Staff, Belleville Gen. Hosp.; Tel. 962-7500.
BATOL, Zenaida G.; 5th Floor Wesley Bldg., 120 Holland Ave., Ottawa 3, Ont.; Santo Tomas (Manila, Philipp.)'57.
BATSHAW, Anne T.; 4336 Montrose Ave., Montreal, (Westmount) P.Q.; McG '24; Staff, Jewish Gen. Hosp.; Tel. WE 5-9002.
BATSON, Herbert H.; Otterville, Ont.; Tor '23.
BATSTONE, Harry L.; Ontario Hosp., Kingston, Ont.; Qns '32; Psy; Phys., Ontario Hosp.; Tel. 546-1101.
BATT, C. Margaret F.; 141 Carter Ave., Noranda, P.Q.; Tor '29; Retired.
BATTCOCK, George W.; Cornwall Drug Bldg., 323 Hamilton Ave., St. John's, Nfld.; 4 Bonaventure Ave. (res); Dal '50; GenSurg; Tel. 579-3305.
BATTERSBY, Geoffrey S.; Alaska Dr., Burns Lake, B.C.; Wes'61; Staff, Burns Lake & Dist. Hosp.; AMCGP; Tel. 9.
BATTERSBY, Lawrence H.; 2165 Wellington St., Montreal 22, P.Q.; McG '42; Tel. WE 2-8201.
BATTERSHILL, James H.; 338 Rouge Rd., Winnipeg 22, Man.; Man'51; IntMed; Research Fell., (Physiol.), Winnipeg Gen. Hosp. & U. of Manitoba.
BATTLE, Frederick G.; 19 Dunlop Blk., Yorkton, Sask.; 19 Logan Cres. W. (res); Man '57; Tel. 783-2294.
BATTY, David M.; 2255 Elgin St., Port Coquitlam, B.C.; Birmingham (Eng.)'60; Tel. 942-7292.
BAUCKHAM, John F.; 34 Sheppard Ave. E., Willowdale, Ont.; 84 Heathcote Ave. (res); Tor '47.
BAUGH, Chas. W.; 49 Broad St., Brockville, Ont,; Qns '53; M.Sc. (Med.); IntMed; Staff, St. Vincent de Paul & Brockville Gen. Hosp's.; Tel. 342-0430.
BAULD, Elro D.; Box 510, Fort Saskatchewan, Alta.; Edinburgh (Scot.)'57.

BAUMAL, Allen; 1054 Gerrard St. E., Toronto 6, Ont.; Tor '58; FRCP(C), Derm.
BAUMAL, Reuben; Tor'63; Int., Toronto Western Hosp., Toronto, Ont.
BAUMAN, John C.; Man '59; Jr. Int'n., St. Boniface Hosp., St. Boniface, Man.
BAUMAN, Laszlo; 2002 Bathurst St., Toronto, Ont.; 20 Fraserwood Ave., Tor. 19 (res); Budapest (Hung.) '51; DiagRad; Tel. RU 9-2929.
BAUNEMANN, Heiko; Muenster (Germ.) '60; Jr. Intn., University Hosp., Saskatoon, Sask.
BAUTISTA, Juanito S.; Santo Tomas (Philippines) '56; Res., St. John's Sanatorium, St. John's, Nfld.; Abroad.
BAWDEN, John W.; 306 Medical-Dental Bldg., Regina, Sask.; 2258 Montague St. (res); Man '45; Ther Rad; Dir., Dept. of Rad., Grey Nun's Hosp.; Hon. Cons. Rad., Allan Blair Memorial Clinic, Regina; Tel. LA 3-7653.
BAXTER, Charles R.; 230 Highfield St., Moncton, N.B.; Dal'25; FACS; FICS; GenSurg; Cons. Moncton Hosp.; Reg. M.O., Dept. of Transport, Immig. Med. Serv.; Tel. 855-3110.
BAXTER, Donald W.; Montreal Gen. Hosp., Montreal 25, P.Q.; 177 Jasper Ave. (res); Qns '51; M.Sc. (Neurol.); ABNP; FRCP(C); Neur; Dir., Div. of Neurol., Montreal Gen. Hosp.; Assoc. Prof. (Neurol.), McGill U.; Tel. 937-6011.
BAXTER, Hamilton; Ste. 714, Medical Arts Bldg., 1538 Sherbrooke St. W., Montreal 25, P.Q.; 68 Belvedere Rd., Westmount (res); McG '36; M.Sc., D.D.S., F.A.C.S., D.A.B.P.S.; GenSurg; PlasSurg; Chief, Dept. of PlasSurg., Royal Victoria Hosp.; Assoc. Prof., Plas Surg., McGill U.; Tel. WE 5-3323.
BAXTER, James D.; Linton Apts., Ste. 12, 1509 Sherbrooke St. W., Montreal, P.Q.; 74 Fernley Cr., Town of Mt. Royal (res); McG '47; FRCS-(C), Otol; Staff, (Otol), Royal Victoria and Montreal Children's Hosp's.; Staff, McGill U.; Tel. 937-9926.
BAXTER, Kemlo R.; Apt. 331, 40 Glen Rd., Toronto 5, Ont.; Tor '29; Dist. Coroner.
BAXTER, Kenneth L.; Muskoka Lakes Clinic, Manitoba St., Bracebridge, Ont.; 286 Hiram St. (res); Tor '60; AMCGP; Tel. 645-4457.
BAXTER, Robert; 112 Victoria St. E., Alliston, Ont.; Cambridge (Eng.) '52; M.R.C.S. (Eng.), L.R.C.P. (Lond.); B.Ch; Staff, Stevenson Mem. Hosp.; Tel. HE 5-6282.
BAXTER, Robert G.; 4492 Sherbrooke St. W., Montreal, P.Q.; McG '38; IntMed (P.Q.); Ass't. Phys., Royal Victoria Hosp.; Dem. (Med.), McGill U.; Cons. (Metab.), Royal Edward Laurentian Hosp.; Tel. WE 5-8222.
BAXTER, William J.; 649 Manawagonish Rd., Lancaster, N.B.; 80 Douglas Ave. (res); McG '29; GenSurg; Staff (Surg.), Saint John Gen. Hosp.; Tel. 694-1631.
BAYATPOUR, Mahin; Shiraz (Iran)'58; Staff, University Hosp., Saskatoon, Sask.
BAYDUZA, Jeanette D.; Alb '64; Res., Hosp. for Sick Children, Toronto, Ont.
BAYENS, Johannes H.; 1495 Kipling Ave. N., Rexdale, Ont.; Amsterdam (Neth.)'56; MCGP.
BAYES, Beverley J.; Tor '61; Res. Hosp. for Sick Children, Toronto, Ont.
BAYLEY, T. Arnold; 208 St. Clair Ave. W., Toronto 7, Ont.; Tor '55; FRCP(C), IntMed; Staff (OPD), St. Michael's & Sunnybrook Hosp's.; Tel. 925-6042.
BAYLISS, Colin E.; Tor'61; Res., Toronto West. Hosp., Toronto, Ont.
BAYLY, Peter L.; Main St., Lively, Ont.; Tor '63; Tel. 692-4774.
BAYNE, Archibald R.; 288 St. Joseph St., La Tuque, P.Q. (res); McG '15; Retired.
BAYNE, H. Douglas; Box 120, Melbourne, P.Q.; McG '14; Retired.
BAYNE, James R.; Oshawa Clinic, 117 King St. E., Oshawa, Ont.; 290 Mary St. (res); Tor '32; Tel. 728-1661.
BAYNE, Ronald D.; 6 Winchester Ave., Montreal 6, P.Q.; McG '47; FACP; IntMed; Phys. I/C Geron. Serv., D.V.A.; Lect. Psy., McGill U.; Tel. HU 9-8381.
BAYROKAL, Sadt.; Istanbul (Turk.) '53; Staff, Hop. Mont Providence, 7200 Gouin Blvd. E., Montreal 39, P.Q.
BAZANT, Francis J.; 10 Academy Med. Bldg., 1812-4th St. S.W., Calgary, Alta.; 2005-26th Ave. N.W. (res); Qns '57; FRSC(C); OrthSurg; Staff (OrthSurg.), Alberta Childrens', Holy Cross & Calgary Gen. Hosp's.; Tel. 263-1736.
BAZIN, A. R.; 1414 Drummond, Montreal, P.Q.; 55 Merton Rd. Hampstead, Que. (res); Edinburgh (Scot.) '32; GenSurg; Ass't. Surg., Montreal Gen. Hosp.; Tel. AV 8-4931.
BAZIN, Yvon; Lav '64; Res., Hop. L'Enfant Jesus, Quebec 3, P.Q.
BAZINET, Denis; Mon'61; Anaes; Staff, Hop. Santa Cabrini, Montreal, P.Q.
BAZINET, Henri-P.; 12245 rue Grenet, Montreal 9, P.Q.; 11285 Drouart (Bordeaux) (res); Ott '53; Paed; Active Staff, Sacred Heart Hosp.; Tel. DU 1-7281.
BAZINET, Rene E.; Ott '63; Res., Ottawa Gen. Hosp., Ottawa, Ont.
BAZOIAN, Matthew; 212 James St. S., Hamilton, Ont.; Tor '51; Anaes; Staff, St. Joseph's Hosp.; Tel. 528-8437.
BAZZARD, Paul M.; Parsons Clinic, 4826 Ross St., Red Deer, Alta.; Wales'61.
BEACH, Albert M., DFC & Bar, G/C; Inst. of Aviation Med., 1107 Avenue Rd., Toronto 12, Ont.; McG '49; D.Psy; Psy.
BEACH, Donald W.; 7085 Victoria Dr., Vancouver 16, B.C.; Ste. 5, 1025 E (res); Yale (New Haven, U.S.A.) '34; D.N.B.; Tel. FA 1-8712.
BEACH, John K.; 5 James St., Frankford, Ont.; Qns'43; AMCGP; Active Staff, Trenton Mem. Hosp., Trenton; Tel. 398-6761.
BEACH, Michael A.; 168 Charlotte St., Ottawa 2, Ont.; Qns '62; AMCGP; Tel. 234-8513.
BEACOCK, Grant C.; Ste. 800, 143 James St. S., Hamilton, Ont.; 128 Chedoke Ave. (res); Qns '41; D.Psy.; Psy; Chief, Dept. of Psy. & Dir. Psy. Unit, Hamilton Civic Hosp.; Cons. Psy., DVA, CPC, St. Joseph's & Chedoke Gen. Hosp's.; Tel. 528-9793.
BEACOCK, Peter R.; 64 Taylor, Thessalon, Ont.; Tor '51; M.O.H., Five Twnps.; Tel. 785-3758.
BEADOIN, J. Edmond; 221 est, rue Laurier, Ottawa 2, Ont.; Lav '48; ObstGyn; Clin. Ass't. (Gyn.), U. of Ottawa; Tel. CE 5-4498.
BEADSWORTH, Barrington J.; 2150 Valley Way, Niagara Falls, Ont.; Glasgow (Scot.)'58.
BEAGLEHOLE, Peter; 2363 McIntyre St., Regina, Sask.; Apt. 15, 2240 Robinson St. (res); Edinburgh (Scot.) '57; Assoc. Memb. (G.P.), Regina Gen. & Grey Nun's Hosp's.; Tel. 527-0641.
BEAIRSTO, Arthur W.; 150 Metcalfe St., Ottawa 4, Ont.; Tor '43; Tel. 232-8396.
BEALE, Francis A.; Princess Margaret Hosp., 500 Sherbourne St., Toronto 5, Ont.; Edinburgh (Scot.) '46; FFR; DMRT; TherRad; Rad., Princess Margaret Hosp.; Assoc., Dept. of Rad., U. of Toronto; Tel. WA 4-0671; Loc. 343.
BEALE, Lillias E.; 70 Dunvegan Rd., Toronto 7, Ont.; Edinburgh (Scot.) '48; Staff, P.H., York Twp.; Tel. 766-3481.
BEALL, George M.; 1101 Munroe Ave., Saskatoon, Sask.; Tor '39; Dist. Coroner; Clin. Instr., Obst Gyn., U. of Saskatchewan; Tel. 343-2512.
BEAMISH, Oswald F.; Kemptville, Ont.; McG '21; MCGP; Staff, Kemptville Dist. Hosp.; Tel. 258-2214.
BEAMISH, Robert E.; Manitoba Clinic, 790 Sherbrook St., Winnipeg 2, Man.; 176 Oxford St., Wpg. 9 (res); Man '42; MRCP (Lond.); FRCP (Edin.); FACP, FACC, FCCP, FRCP(C), IntMed (Cardiol.); Assoc. Phys., Hon. Att'd. Staff, Wpg. Gen. Hosp.; Assoc. Prof. (Med.), U. of Manitoba; Tel. SP 4-6541.
BEAMISH, William E.; Alb'56; Res., University Hosp., Saskatoon, Sask.
BEAN, David M.; 80 Queen St. N., Kitchener, Ont.; Tor '41; FACS; FCCP; FRCS(C); GenSurg; Surg-in-Chief, Kitchener-Waterloo Gen. Hosp.; Cons. Gen. Surg., St. Mary's Hosp.; Cons. ThorSurg., Freeport San.; Lect. (Anat.) U. of Waterloo; Tel. 742-6104.
BEAN, Douglas E.; 765 King St. W., Kitchener, Ont.; Qns'60; AMCGP; Chmn. Emergency Committ., Memb. Admission & Discharge Committ. & Sec., Dept. of Med., Kitchener-Waterloo Hosp.; Tel. 576-4410.

BEAN, Helen A. (Stutt); Allan Blair Mem. Clinic, Regina, Sask.; 60 Academy Park (res); Man '45; TherRad; Radiotherapist, Allan Blair Mem. Clin.; Tel. 527-9651.
BEAN, Irwin W.; Medical Arts Clinic, Regina, Sask.; Qns '43; MCGP; Memb., Sask. Care Ins. Comm.; Med. Dir. Sask. Government Ins.; Tel. 523-0691.
BEAN, John L. M.; 702 Med. Arts Bldg., 170 St. George St., Toronto 5, Ont.; Tor '45; FRCOG; FRCS(C), ObstGyn; Staff ObstGyn., Toronto Gen. Hosp.; Cons. Gyn., Princess Margaret Hosp. & Ontario Crippled Children's Centre; Assoc. Dept. of ObstGyn., U. of Toronto; Tel. WA 1-4774.
BEAN, Samuel J. T.; 527 English St., London, Ont. (res); Wes '14; Retired.
BEANLANDS, Donald S.; 20 Glentworth Rd., Willowdale, Ont. (res); Dal '58; FRCP(C); IntMed; Staff, Toronto Western Hosp.; Tel. 368-2581.
BEARDALL, Peter J.; McLeod Med. Bldg., 340 McLeod St., Ottawa 4, Ont.; 1311 Morley Blvd.; Witwatersrand (S. Africa)'56; FRCS(C), ObstGyn; Tel. 232-9058.
BEARDEN, William A.; Box 509, 401 Johnston Rd., Port Alberni, B.C.; Qns'37.
BEARDMORE, Harvey E.; 2300 Tupper St., Ste. 1130, Montreal, P.Q.; 3186 The Blvd., Westmount (res); McG '48; FAAP; FACS; FRCS(C), GenSurg; Assoc. Surg., Mtl. Children's Hosp.; Lect. (Surg.), McGill U.; Tel. WE 7-8511.
BEARDMORE, M. Beatrice; 68 Eastbourne Ave., Toronto, Ont. (res); Tor '17; Retired.
BEARDSWORTH, John H.; Associate Clinic, Innisfail, Alta.; McG '55; MCGP; Tel. 227-3741.
BEARE, Maurice S.; Med. Arts Clinic, Bradbrooke Block, Swift Current, Sask.; National U. (Ire.)'42; BAO; FRCS(Eng.).
BEATON, Anita C.; 121 Wellington St. W., Barrie, Ont.; Tor '51; Anaes.
BEATON, B. Wayne; 109 King St. E., Oshawa, Ont.; Loma Linda (Calif., U.S.A.)'64.
BEATON, Edward J.; Med Arts Bldg., 121 Wellington St. W., Barrie, Ont.; Tor '51; FRCS(C); GenSurg; Cons. Surg., Royal Victoria Hosp.; Tel. PA 8-7271.
BEATON, James M.; 7184 King George Hwy., North Surrey, B.C.; 13578—61A Ave. (res); Man '57; Tel. 596-6201.
BEATTIE, Adam N.; 1745 St. Ann St., Victoria, B.C.; Wes'31; DPH; Tel. 383-6381.
BEATTIE, B. Lynn; UBC'65; Res., Sunnybrook Hosp., Toronto 12, Ont.
BEATTIE, George E. S.; 274 King St. W., Chatham, Ont.; 201 Victoria Ave. (res); Wes '31; LM (Rotunda); Staff, St. Joseph's & Public Gen. Hosp's.; M.O., Victoria Home for Aged; Tel. EL 4-3121.
BEATTIE, Homer W.; 66 Charleton St. W., Hamilton, Ont.; McG'49; FACC; FRCS(C), GenSurg (Cardiovasc.); Chief (ThorSurg), Joseph Brant Mem. Hosp.; Active Staff (Cardiovasc. & ThorSurg), Hamilton Gen. Hosp.; Cons. Staff, St. Joseph's Hosp.; Tel. JA 9-4793.
BEATTIE, Howard A.; 839 Edgeworth Ave., Ottawa 14, Ont. '40; Tel. 729-8402.
BEATTIE, Joan K.; Qns'65; Res., Shaughnessy Hosp., Vancouver 9, B.C.
BEATTIE, John H.; 283 Cathcart St., London, Ont.; Wes'35; Cons. Staff, St. Thomas Elgin Hosp.; Tel. 471-1440.
BEATTIE, Lillian M.; International Grenfell Mission, St. Anthony, Nfld.; Wes'54; FRCS(C); ObstGyn; Ass't. Surg. & Chief ObstGyn., Int. Grenfell Mission.
BEATTIE, Nancy M.; 8 Hillcrest Ave., Hamilton, Ont. (res); St. Andrews (Scot.) '39; FCCP; Dir. TB Control, Hamilton Health Dept., 74 Hughson St. S.; Tel. 528-1441.
BEATTIE, Walter H.; 74 Johnston St., Kingston, Ont.; 315 McMahon Ave. (res); Wes '52; DMRD (D); DiagRad; Assoc. Rad. Hotel-Dieu Hosp.; Clin. Ass't. Queen's U.; Tel. LI 6-1151.
BEATTIE, William B.; 6 Catherine St., Belleville, Ont.; Qns'49; MCGP; Hd. Dept. of G.P., Belleville Gen. Hosp.; Tel. WO 2-3080.
BEATTIE, W. Gordon; Ottawa Civic Hosp., Ottawa 3, Ont.; Tor'44; FACS; FRCS(C), GenSurg; Chmn., Div. of Surg. & Chief, Dept. of Gen.Surg., Ottawa Civic Hosp.; Prof. of Clin. Surg., U. of Ottawa; Tel. 729-2511, Loc. 537.
BEATTY, E. Geoffrey; 4 Turner Ave., Hamilton, Ont. (res); Tor '53; Path; Staff (Path.), Hamilton Gen. Hosp.; Tel. 527-0271.
BEATTY, Helen S. (nee Robinson); 537 Markham St., Toronto 4, Ont. (res); Tor '26; Retired.
BEATTY, Samuel R.; Durham St., Madoc, Ont.; Tor '25; Dist. Coroner; Tel. 473-2355.
BEAUBIEN, Fernand; 201 est, boul. Cremazie, Montreal 11, P.Q.; Lav'43.
BEAUBIEN, Jacques F.; 900 Sherbrooke St. West, Montreal 2, P.Q.; 460 Lakeshore Rd., Beaurepaire (res); McG '40; Psy (P.Q.); Ass't. Psy., Royal Victoria Hosp.; Psy. Cons. D.V.A. & Royal Edward Laurentian Hosp.; Tel. VI 5-3809.
BEAUBIEN, Miriam F.; 900 Sherbrooke St. W., Montreal, P.Q.; 460 Lakeshore Rd., Beauprairie (res); McG '41; D.Psy.; Psy (P.Q.); Staff, Royal Victoria & Laurentides Hosp's.; Tel. VI 5-3809.
BEAUCHAMP, Arthur J.; 405 Hendryx St., Nelson, B.C.; 909-9th St. (res); Alb '42; MCGP; Staff, Kootenay Lake Gen. Hosp.; Tel. 352-6611.
BEAUCHAMP, Louis E.; 707 Professional Bldg., 10830 Jasper Ave., Edmonton, Alta.; 13833 Summit Dr. (res); Alb'46; F.A.A.P.; Paed; Chief Paed., Edmonton Gen. Hosp.; Lect. (Paed.), U. of Alberta; Tel. 422-3354.
BEAUCHAMP, Marcel; 4373 rue St. Hubert, Montreal, P.Q.; Mon '45; F.I.C.S., F.A.C.S., GenSurg (P.Q.); Ass't. Surg., Hosp. Ste. Jeanne d'Arc & St. Jean de Dieu; Tel. LA 2-0807.
BEAUCHEMIN, Andre; 641 Place Publique, Ste Dorothee, P.Q.; Mon '65.
BEAUCHEMIN, Jacques; 8601 est, Sherbrooke, Montreal 5, P.Q.; Mon'61.
BEAUCHEMIN, J. Charles; 6975-43E Ave., Montreal 36, P.Q.; Mon'62; GenSurg.
BEAUCHEMIN, Jean M.; 100—16th Ave., Lachine, P.Q.; Mon '54; Staff, Hop. St. Joseph; Tel. 637-9921.
BEAUCHEMIN, L. O.; 208 Grain Exchange Bldg., Calgary, Alta.; Lav '13; Tel. 262-2011.
BEAUCHEMIN, Marc; 11305 rue Meunier Montreal 12, P.Q.; Mon '61; Anaes.
BEAUCHESNE, Andre; 2145 Marie-Victorin, Quebec 6, P.Q.; Lav '50; Pulm Dis & TB (P.Q.); MAHP; FCCP; Tel. 681-8577.
BEAUCHESNE, Claude; Mon '59; AMCGP; Res., Hop.-Maison-neuve, Montreal, P.Q.
BEAUCHESNE, Georges; 492 Lindsay, Drummondville, P.Q.; Lav '40; Ophth, Otol (PQ); Tel. GR 2-3933.
BEAUDET, Adelard; 1816 Blvd. Laird Mont Royal, Montreal 16 P.Q. (res); Mon '40; Anaes (P.Q.); Anaes., Hop. Notre Dame; Tel. LA 5-6363.
BADUDET, Alexandre; 605-6th Ave., Grand'mere, Cte. Laviolette, P.Q. (res); Lav '43; M.O.H., Unité Sanitaire.
BEAUDET, Gustave; 8290 Trait Carre E., Charlesbourg, Quebec 3, P.Q., Lav '10; Gov., Coll. of Phys.; Pres., Quebec Co. Med. Assoc.; Tel. 623-2332.
BEAUDET, Hector J.; 1500-18th rue, Quebec 3, P.Q.; 8 Terrasse Dufferin (res); Lav '39; F.A.C.S,. F.R.C.S.(C), GenSurg; ThorSurg (P.Q.); Hd. Surg. Serv., Hop-de-l'Enfant-Jesus; Ass't. Prof. Laval U.; Tel. 525-8116.
BEAUDET, Jean-Charles; St. Nicholas Station, P.Q.; Lav '25.
BEAUDET, Jean P.; 987 St. Prosper, Trois Rivieres, P.Q.; 1941 Blvd. St. Louis (res); Lav '36; D.P.H., All (P.Q.), Paed. (P.Q.); Head of Dept. of Paed., Hop. St. Joseph; Tel. FR 5-4945.
BEAUDET, Marc; 438 Thibeau, Cap de la Madeleine, P.Q.; Lav'53; GenSurg (P.Q.); Staff, Hop. Cloutier; Tel. 378-1753.
BEAUDET, Paul E.; Unite Sanitaire, Gaspe, P.Q. Lav '46.
BEAUDET, Regent; Mon.'65; Res., Hotel-Dieu-Montreal, Montreal 18, P.Q.; Abroad.
BEAUDIN, Adjutor; R.R. No. 1, Loretteville, P.Q. (res); Lav '18; Retired.

BEAUDIN, Gaetan; Mon '55; RCAF Station, St. Jean, P.Q.
BEAUDIN, Jean; Napierville, P.Q.; Mon '30; Dist. Coroner. Temp. Retired.
BEAUDIN, Rouville; 274 Principale, Farnham, Cte. Missisquoi, P.Q.; Lav '45.
BEAUDOIN, Andre; Lav '57; Res., Hop.-St.-Michel-Archange, Quebec, P.Q.
BEAUDOIN, Eddy; 1640 Tillemont, **Montreal, P.Q.; Mon '53; Tel. RA 9-6371.**
BEAUDOIN, Gaston L.; 7373A, St.-Denis, Montreal 10, P.Q.; Mon '24; Tel. 276-0551.
BEAUDOIN, Gerard; 4000 boul. Lasalle, Verdun, P.Q.; 3731 Hochelaga (res); Mon '48; Psy (P.Q.); Head, Psy. Dept., Verdun Gen. Hosp.; Tel. 766-9070.
BEAUDOIN, Gerard L.; 420 Jean Talon E., Montreal 34, P.Q.; Mon '24.
BEAUDOIN, Ghislain; 541 de l'Hopital, Jonquiere, P.Q.; 626 Iberville (res); Lav '52; GenSurg; Tel. 547-9341.
BEAUDOIN, Hermann; Ste. Claire, Co. Dorchester, P.Q.; Lav '59; Tel. 645-3329.
BEAUDOIN, Herve; 499 Bonaventure, Trois **Rivieres, P.Q.; Mon '23; F.A.C.P.; Pulm. Dis. & TB (P.Q.), IntMed (TB); Med. Dir., Cooke Hop-San; Tel. FR 6-3721.**
BEAUDOIN, Jean G.; Mon'63; Res., Royal Victoria Hosp., Montreal 2, P.Q.
BEAUDOIN, Jean L.; C.P. 68, Haute-ville, Quebec 4, P.Q.; Lav'51; FRCP(C), IntMed; Cardiol (P.Q.); Dir., Med. Interns, Hotel-Dieu Hosp.; Staff, Laval U.; Tel. 523-5863.
BEAUDOIN, J. Edmond; 221 est rue Laurier, Ottawa, Ont.; Lav '48; ObstGyn; Clin. Ass't. (Gyn.), U. of Ottawa; Tel. 232-4843.
BEAUDOIN, Louis A.; Centre Medical St.-Urbain, 3875 rue St.-Urbain, Montreal 18, P.Q.; 432 Ave. Ardwell Ville-Mt.-Royal (res); Mon '49; FRCS(C), GenSurg; Surg; Hop.-Hotel-Dieu; Ass't Prof. Surg., U. of Mtl.; Tel. VI 4-0161.
BEAUDOIN, Louis P.; 3919 Blvd. Lasalle, Verdun, Montreal 19, P.Q.; Lav '45; Staff, Hotel-Dieu, Montreal, P.Q.; Tel. 766-0121.
BEAUDOIN, Marc; Mon'65; Res., Hop. Notre Dame, Montreal 24, P.Q.
BEAUDOIN, Real; 51A Ouest, St-Charles, Longueuil, P.Q.; Man'61; Tel. 677-8981.
BEAUDOIN, Roger; 10728 Grande-Alle, Montreal 12, P.Q.; Mon '27; Tel. DU 1-7110.
BEAUDOING, Roger J.; 904B Brunette St., New Westminster, B.C.; Ott '57; Tel. LA 6-5501.
BEAUDRY, Claude; 1150 est, boul. St-Joseph, Montreal 34, P.Q.; Mon '59; FRCP(C), IntMed; Chief of Health Serv., Hop. Maisonneuve; Dem., U. of Montreal; Tel. LA 7-1241.
BEAUDRY, Edouard L.; 469 Jacques-Cartier E., **Chicoutimi, P.Q.; 454 Ave. de Sales (res); Lav '46; F.R.C.S.(C), GenSurg; Surg., Hotel-Dieu St.-Vallier, Chicoutimi & Staff, Laval U.; Tel. 549-0434.**
BEAUDRY, Gerald; 31 King St. W. Sherbrooke, P.Q.; Lav '49; FACOG; ObstGyn; Tel. LO 2-7066.
BEAUDRY, Jacques; 1720 De Fondville, Quebec 3, P.Q.; Mon'36; Anaes.
BEAUDRY, Jacques F.; 31 King St. W., Sherbrooke, P.Q.; 189 Heneker (res); Lav '48; ObstGyn (P.Q.); Ass't (ObstGyn) Hop. St. Vincent-de-Paul; Tel. LO 7-5737.
BEAUDRY, Jean-L.; 985 Laviolette, Trois Rivieres, P.Q.; 987 Laviolette (res); Lav '40; Obst. (P.Q.); Chief of Obst., Hop. Ste-Marie; Tel. FR 5-1444.
BEAUDRY, Jean M.; 32 Croissant d'Avaugour, Duvernay, Montreal 40, P.Q.; Mon '50; D.P.H.; PH(P.Q.); Med. Instr., Montreal Health Serv.
BEAUDRY, J. L. Stanislas; 7184 Bordeaux, **Montreal 36, P.Q.; Lav '15; Retired.**
BEAUDRY, Maurice; 240 rue St.-Jean, Quebec 4, P.Q.; 1720 Blvd. Sir Wilfred Laurier, Sillery (res); Lav '30; DermSyph; Chief of Derm., Hops. St. Francois-d'Assise, & de-l'Enfant-Jesus; Assoc. Prof. **Laval U.; Tel. 524-3456.**
BEAUDRY, Paul E.; 1113 St. Denis, Montreal, P.Q.; Mon '25; Tel VI 5-3505.
BEAUDRY, Pierre H.; 2300 Tupper St., Montreal 25, P.Q.; Mon '54; Paed; Ass't. Dir., Resp. Function Serv. & Ass't. Phys. (Paed.), Mtl. Children's Hosp.; Lect. (Paed.), McGill U.; Tel. WE 7-8511.
BEAUDRY, Raphael; 324 rue Main, Magog, P.Q.; Lav '34; GenSurg (P.Q.); Tel. 843-4491.
BEAUDRY-REMILLARD, Janine; C.P. 2280, Outardes 4, Cte Saguenay, P.Q.; Ott'63; Tel. 734-2250.
BEAUDRY, Rene; Mon'61; FRCP(C), IntMed; Staff, Toronto Gen. Hosp., Toronto 2, Ont.
BEAUDRY, Roland H.; Ott '57; GenSurg; Active **Staff, Franklin Hosp., Franklin, N.H., U.S.A.; Abroad.**
BEAULAC, Joseph; 1350 Waterloo, Ville Mont Royal, P.Q. (res); Mon '24; Retired.
BEAULAC, Gilsele; Ste. 812, 30, boul. St. Joseph est, Montreal 14, P.Q.; Mon '55; Paed (P.Q.).
BEAULE, Andre; 341 de la Couronne, Quebec 2, P.Q.; Lav '45; GenSurg (P.Q.); Tel. 524-6704.
BEAULE, Jean-Luc; 820 Dupre, Beloeil, P.Q.; Mon' 60; Tel. 467-6994.
BEAULIEU, David; Lav '31; Med. Dir., Hop. St-Joseph, La Tuque, P.Q.; Tel. 523-4581.
BEAULIEU, Elphege; Lav'62; DiagRad; Staff, Hop. Maisonneuve, Montreal 36, P.Q.
BEAULIEU, Emile; 70-2nd St., Port Alfred, P.Q. (res); Lav '28; FIMA; MCGP; Phys., Consol. Paper Corp. Ltd., Saguenay Terminals Ltd.; Tel. Pt. Alfred, 544-3233.
minals Ltd; Tel. Pt. Alfred, 544-3233.
BEAULIEU, F. Xavier; 181 rue Lindsay, Mont-Joli, P.Q.; Lav '46; Pulm. Dis. & TB (P.Q.); Staff, San. St-George, Mont-Joli; Tel. PR 5-4335.
BEAULIEU, Gerard; Sept-Iles, Saguenay Co., P.Q.; 735 Arnaud St. (res); '36.
BEAULIEU, Jacques; 188 Boul. d'Iberville, Repentigny, P.Q. (res); Mon '58; DiagRad; Staff, Hop.-Notre-Dame; Tel. LA 5-6363.
BEAULIEU, Jean-Charles; Tring-Jonction, Beauce, P.Q.; Lav'57; Tel. 426-2026.
BEAULIEU, Leon; 10 rue Petit, St.-Honore, **Co. Chicoutimi, P.Q.; Lav '60; AMCGP; Tel. 673-4862.**
BEAULIEU, Maurice; 1281 Bishop, Ste. Foy, P.Q.; Lav'45; ThorSurg; ThorSurg., Hop. Laval.
BEAULIEU, Origene; 126 Rue Commercial, Cabano, P.Q.; Lav'53; Tel. 854-2442.
BEAULIEU, Richard; Ste. 304, 1248 Chemin St-Foy, Quebec 6, P.Q.; Lav '51; AICS (PlasSurg.); Otol (P.Q.); Chief of Otol. & PlasSurg. Dept's., Jeffrey Hale's Hosp.; Tel. 681-3477.
BEAULIEU, Robert W.; 9531 Central, Ville LaSalle, Lachine, P.Q.; Lav '55.
BEAULIEU, Rodolphe P.; 123 Walsh, Moncton, N.B. (res); Lav '57; DiagRad; Staff, Hotel-Dieu-Reine-Marie, Montreal 26, P.Q. (res); Mon '33; Staff, Dept. of Health.
BEAULIEU, Roger; 5170 des Sorbiers Ave., Montreal, P.Q. (res); Mon '42; Clin. Path. (P.Q.); Dir. of Labs., Notre Dame de l'Esperance Hosp., Ville St. Laurent; Dir. School of Med., Technology and Ass't. Prof Physiol., U. of Montreal; Tel. RI 7-4771.
BEAULNES, Aurele; 5260 ave Durocher, Outremont, Montreal, P.Q.; Mon '53; Assoc. Prof. & Dir., Dept. of Pharm., U. of Montreal; Tel. RE 3-9951.
BEAUMONT, Edmond J.; 50 Avenue de Rouville, Baie Comeau, Cte. Saguenay, P.Q.; Lav'57.
BEAUMONT, Henry W.; Box 38, Pinawa, Man.; RCP & S. (Dublin, Ire.)'55; Tel. 753-2969.
BEAUMONT, Louis; Mon'65; Res., Hop. Notre Dame, Montreal 24, P.Q.
BEAUMONT, Margaret (Reynolds); Lac du Bonnet, Man.; Leeds (Eng.) '52; Ass't. M.O.H., Selkirk Health Unit; Tel. 345-2551.
BEAUPRE, Jacques; Box 8100, C.N.R. Medical, Montreal 3, P.Q.; Mon'45; MCGP; Staff, C.N.R. Med. Dept.
BEAUREGARD, C. Germain, Capt.; National Defence Med. Centre, Ottawa, Ont.; Mon'63.
BEAUREGARD, Gerard; St. Jude, Cte. St. Hyacinthe, P.Q.; Mon '38; Staff, Hop. St. Charles; Tel. PR 4-5331.

BEAUREGARD, Jean M.; Faculte de Medecine, Univ. de Sherbrooke, Sherbrooke, P.Q.; Mon'45; FRCP(C); IntMed; Vice Dean, Faculty of Med., Sherbrooke U.; Tel. 567-3901.
BEAUREGARD, Leon; 2215 Parc Lotbiniere, Sillery, P.Q. (res); Lav '43; D&T Rad; Staff, Hop. du St. Sacrement; Tel. LA 7-3461.
BEAUREGARD, Lorenzo; 106 Ramsay N., Marieville, P.Q.; Lav '31; Tel. LU 9-7461.
BEAUREGARD, Pierre; 50 ouest Blvd. Cremazie, Ste. 507B, Montreal, P.Q.; Mon '57; FACS; FRCS(C), GenSurg; Staff, Hop. Fleury Gen. & Hop. Notre-Dame de l'Esperance; Tel. 384-0244.
BEAUREGARD, William L.; McG '58; FRCS(C), GenSurg; Staff, Wellesley Hosp., Toronto, Ont.; Tel. 921-4111.
BEAUSEJOUR, Andre; Lav'58; Res., Dept. of Psy., Laval U., Quebec, P.Q.
BEAUVILLIERS, Jules; 4962, Cote des Neiges, Montreal 26, P.Q.; Mon '33; PH (P.Q.); Staff, Dept. of Health.
BEAUVILLIERS, Roger; 3270 Lacombe, Montreal 26, P.Q. (res); Mon '39; PH(P.Q.); M.O. Dept. Health, Montreal.
BEAZLEY, Gary G.; 311 Day St., Winnipeg 25, Man.; Ste. 10, 128 Kildare Ave. E., Transcona (res); Man '61; Tel. CA 2-4259.
BEAZLEY, Ronald W.; 34 Pleasant St., Dartmouth, N.S.; Shannon Med. Clinic, Dartmouth, N.S.; Dal'65; AMCGP; Tel. 469-2445 & 469-9261.
BEAZLEY, Gerald P.; 6 Fairlawn Ave., Toronto 12, Ont.; Dublin (Ire.) '41; L.M. (Rotunda). Tel. HU 1-9731.
BEBB, Douglas E.; 350-5780 Cambie St. Van. 15; 1226 W. 26th Ave., Van. 9 (res); UBC '56; M.C.G.P.; Tel. FA 7-6533.
BEBCHUK, William; Psychiatric Inst., Winnipeg 3, Man.; Man'59; Psy; Dir. O.P.D., Psy. Inst.; Ass't. Prof. (Psy.), U. of Manitoba.
BEBENSEE, D. L.; Massey, Ont.; Wes '55.
BEBLIS, Ishoona; Box 1570, Williams Lake, B.C.; Tehran (Iran)'56.
BECCAT, Nicole; Mon'65; Res., Hop. St. Luc, Montreal 18, P.Q.
BECHARD, Bendit; Lav '64; Res., Toronto Gen. Hosp., Toronto 2, Ont.
BECHARD, J. C. Leonard; 107 rue St.-Louis, Warwick, P.Q.; Lav '39; Med. Staff, Hotel-Dieu, Arthabaska, P.Q.
BECHARD, Jean Benoit; 143 Champlain, Valleyfield, P.Q.; Mon'41; GenSurg (P.Q.); Tel. 373-7070.
BECHARD, Michel; 7227 St. Denis, Montreal 10, P.Q.; Mon '44; Ophth (P.Q.); Tel. 274-6472.
BECHER, John C.; 6669 Jubilee Ave., Burnaby 1, B.C.; 4916 Rowan Ave. (res); Wes '41; Active Staff, Burnaby Gen. Hosp.; Visiting Staff, Vancouver Gen., Grace & Mt. St. Joseph's Hosp's; Tel. HE 3-8241.
BECK, C. Adeline; Alb'65; Staff, Ontario Hosp., Hamilton, Ont.
BECK, Henry O.; 100 Sheppard Ave. W., Willowdale, Ont.; Heidelberg (Germ.)'50; ObstGyn; Active Staff, North York Branson Hosp.; Court. Staff, St. Michael's Hosp., O.P.D. (ObstGyn); Tel. 221-4181.
BECK, Ivan T.; Division of Gastroenterology, Hotel-Dieu, Hosp., Kingston, Ont.; Geneva (Switz.)'49; PhD; FACP; FRCP(C); IntMed; Gastroent (P.Q.); Gastroent-in-Charge, Hotel-Dieu Hosp.; Assoc. Prof. Med., Queen's U.; Tel. 546-1151.
BECK, John C.; 592 Kenaston Ave., Montreal 16, P.Q. (res); McG '47; FACP; FRCP(C); IntMed; Chief, Endocrine-Metabolic Unit & Phys., Royal Victoria Hosp.; Assoc. Prof. (Med.), McGill U.; Tel. VI 2-1251, Ext. 1579.
BECK, Malcolm N.; P.O. Box 3000, Charlottetown, PEI; 35 Ambrose St. (res); McG '49; Psy; Dir., Mental Health Clinic & Sherwood Hosp.; Tel. 894-3187.
BECK, Philip R.; McG'64; Res. (Psy.), Jewish Gen. Hosp., Montreal, P.Q.
BECK, Richard E.; 750 W. Broadway, Vancouver 9, B.C.; 2575 W. 37th Ave. (res); Qns '47; F.R.C.P.(C), IntMed; Clin. Instr. (Med.), U. of British Columbia; Tel. TR 4-4922.
BECK, R. Neil; 860 University Dr., Saskatoon, Sask. (res); Queen's U. (Belfast, N. Ire.) '48; M.B., B.A.O., B.Ch., M.D., M.R.C.P. (Lond.); F.R.C.P.(C), IntMed; Ass't. Prof. of Med. (Endo-crin.), U. of Saskatchewan; Tel. 242-7641, Ext. 293.
BECK, R. Peter; Dept. of ObstGyn., University Hosp., Edmonton, Alta.; Qns'55; FACOG; FRCOG; FACS; FRCS(C); ObstGyn; Prof. & Hd., Dept. of ObstGyn., University Hosp. & U. of Alberta; Tel. 439-5911.
BECKER, Anthony; 227 Med. Arts Bldg., Saskatoon, Sask.; 619-7th Ave. N. (res); McG '40; D.A.B.R.; D & T Rad., St. Paul's Hosp.; Clin. Instr., Diag Rad. U. of Saskatchewan; Tel. 244-1169.
BECKETT, Donal P.; Innisfail, Alta.; Dublin (Ire.) '37; F.R.C.S.(I.).
BECKETT, Matthew C.; Ste. 380, 5655 Cambie St., Vancouver 15, B.C.; 6908 Ash St. Van. 14 (res); UBC '54; MCGP; Tel. 261-8655.
BECKETT, Roy F.; Oshawa Clinic, 117 King St. E., Oshawa, Ont.; Liverpool (Eng.) '56; M.B., B.Ch.; ObstGyn; Tel. 728-1661.
BECKETT, Trevor R.; Apt. 810, 16 Rosedale Rd., Toronto 5, Ont.; Tor '30; FACA; Anaes.
BECKHAM, L. Maurice; 900 King St. W., Kit-chener, Ont.; Wes'52; DABA; FACA; Anaes; Chief, Dept. of Anaes., Kitchener-Waterloo Hosp.; Active Staff, St. Mary's Hosp.; Tel. 744-7361.
BECKLAKE-McGREGOR, Margaret; Royal Victoria Hosp., Montreal, P.Q.; Witwatersrand (S. Africa)'44; MRCP (Lond.); Pulm Dis. & TB (P.Q.); Ass't. Phys., Royal Victoria Hosp.; Assoc. Prof. (Exp. Med.), McGill U.; Tel. VI 2-1251, Loc. 1738.
BECKMAN, I. H.; 601 Boyd Bldg., Winnipeg, Man.; 330 Montrose Ave. (res); Man '24; Ophth. Otol.; Tel. WH 2-8703.
BECKSTEAD, James Lewis; 407 Medical Arts Bldg., 404 Graham Ave., Winnipeg, Man.; 543 Waverley St. (res); Man '41; IntMed; Med. Staff, St. Boniface, Grace & Deer Lodge Hosp's.; Ass't. Prof. (Med.), U. of Manitoba; Tel. 943-8008.
BECKWITH, Charles J. W.; Dalhousie Public Health Clinic, University Ave., Halifax, N.S.; 5785 Harrington Dr. (res); Dal '27; DPH; Int Med (TB); PH; FCCP; Cons. Dis. of Chest, Victoria Gen. & Cdn. Forces Hosp.; Assoc. Prof. (Med.) & Ass't. Prof. Prev. Med., Dalhousie U.; Exec. Sec., Med. Soc. of N.S.; Tel. 423-1216.
BECOTTE, Jean-M; 19 Laurier, Arthabaska, P.Q.; Lav '33; F.R.S.C.(C), F.I.C.S., GenSurg; Tel. 357-2422.
BEDARD, Andre; Lav'65; Res., Hop. L'Enfant-Jesus, Quebec 3, P.Q.; Abroad.
BEDARD, Arthur; 370 St. Cyrille W., Quebec 6, P.Q.; 1935 St. Cyrille, Sillery (res); Lav '34; Urol; M.C.G.P.; Hd. Dept. (Urol.), Hop-Hotel-Dieu; Cons. (Urol.), Ste. Foy Vet's Hosp.; Assoc. Prof. (Med.) & Hd. Dept. (Urol.), Laval U.; Tel. 681-3633.
BEDARD, Conrad; St.-Perpetue, P.Q.; Lav '56; A.M.C.G.P.
BEDARD, Dominique; 1135 Ave. Belvedere, Quebec, P.Q. (res); Lav'50; Psy; Dir. Psy. Serv., Dept. of Health (P.Q.); Tel. LA 4-8411.
BEDARD, Emillien; 4193 Lasalle, Verdun, P.Q.; Mon '28; Anaes.
BEDARD, Georges; 4 Taschereau, Hull, P.Q.; Lav '52; FACS; FRCS(C), GenSurg; Tel. 771-8215.
BEDARD, Gilles; 775 rue St.-Germain, Rimouski-Est, P.Q. (res); Lav '54; Dir. Med. Hop-St. Jospeh; Tel. 723-7851.
BEDARD, Guy; 437-lere rue, Iberville, P.Q.; Mon '50.
BEDARD, Guy; Lav'62; Res., Hop. Hotel-Dieu, Quebec 4, P.Q.
BEDARD, J. Alexandre; 1165 rue Claire Fontaine, Quebec 4, P.Q.; Lac Beauport (res); Lav '36; MCGP; Med. Dir., Clinique Bedard & Metropolitan Police, City of Quebec; Tel. 525-7164.
BEDARD, Jean P.; Sutton, Cte. Brome, P.Q.; Mon '61.
BEDARD, Jean P.; Polyclinique de Sherbrooke, 31 rue King ouest, Sherbrooke, P.Q.; Lav'57; FRCS(C), OrthSurg; Tel. 567-8844.

BEDARD, J. Henri; 573, rue St. Valier ouest, Quebec 8, P.Q.; Lav '36; Med. Dir., W.C.B. (P.Q.)

BEDARD, John E.; 196 E. Main St., Welland, Ont.; 182 Church St. W. (res); Qns '36; MCGP; Cons. Staff, Welland Co. Gen. Hosp.; Tel. RE 5-5075.

BEDARD, J. Paul; Lav'65; Res., Hop. du Sacrement, Quebec 6, P.Q.

BEDARD, J. Urbain; 625—1st Ave., Charlesbourg, Quebec 7, P.Q.; Lav '29.

BEDARD, Lucien; 122 Radisson, Trois-Rivieres, P.Q.; 575 des Volontaires (res); Mon '43; Gen Surg (P.Q.); Tel. FR 4-4637.

BEDARD, Nicolas; Lav'63; Res., Hop. Notre-Dame, Montreal 24, P.Q.

BEDARD, Pierre; C.P. 205, 630 - 6eme. rue, Grand'Mere, P.Q.; Lav'60; Anaes; Staff, Hop. Lafleche; Tel. LE 8-3381.

BEDARD, Pierre; Mon'61; FRCS(C) GenSurg; Staff, Hop. St. Luc, Montreal, P.Q.

BEDARD, Pierre; Lav'64; Res., Toronto Gen. Hosp., Toronto, Ont.

BEDARD, Raymond; 360 Richileu, Quebec 4, P.Q.; Lav '55.

BEDARD, Yvan; Lav'65; Res., Hop. St. Sacrement, Quebec 6, P.Q.

BEDDIE, Allastair J.; Aberdeen (Scot.) '34; **Supt., Saskatchewan Training Schl., Moose Jaw, Sask.; Clin. Instr. (Psy)**, U. of Saskatchewan; Tel. CH 2-7671.

BEDER, Edward; 62 Matson Rd., Downsview, Ont.; Tor '60. Tel. CH 7-9661.

BEDFORD, Ronald F.; 4 Harrogate Pl., S.S. 4, Ottawa, Ont.; Alb '52; Staff, Dept. of Veteran's Affairs; Tel. CE 2-8211.

BEDNARD, Dorothy E.; Man'61; Sr. Ass't. Res., Royal Victoria Hosp., Montreal, P.Q.

BEDWELL, Stephen F.; 407 Med. Arts Bldg., 5880 Spring Garden Rd., Halifax, N.S.; Tor '55; FRCP(C), Neurol; Ass't. Phys., Victoria Gen. Hosp.; Cons. (Neurol.), Halifax Infirmary, Cdn. Forces & Blanchard-Fraser Mem. Hosp., Electroenceph., Halifax Infirmary; Lect. (Med. Neurol.); Dalhousie U.; Tel. 423-8753.

BEECROFT, John D.; 2 Fourth Ave., Trenton, Ont.; London (Eng.)'49; MRCS; LRCP; Plant Phys., Domtar Newsprint Ltd. & Pyrotewax Co. of Canada; Tel. EX 2-3062.

BEER, Agnes (See SOMLO)

BEER, John K.; 5 Central St., Summerside, P.E.I.; 161 Fitzroy St. (res); **Dal '41**; GenSurg; **Staff, Prince County Hosp., Summerside; Tel.** 436-2277.

BEESLEY, J. Bernard; Irving Clinic, 74 W. Seymour St., Kamloops, B.C.; 133 W. Nicola St. (res); McG '53; MCGP; Indus. First Aid Examin.; M.O. Cdn. Forces Reserve; Tel. 1090.

BEESLEY, Mary G.; 200 St. Clair Ave. W., Toronto 7, Ont.; Apt. 12, 494 Avenue Rd. **(res); Tor '57; D. Psy; Psy; Active OPD**, Women's College Hosp.; Tel. 921-7674.

BEEVOR-POTTS, Charles H.; 149 Ingram St., Duncan, B.C.; 2889 Phillip St. (res); Tor '32; M.C.G.P.; Tel. 746-4401.

BEGG, Douglas C.; 818-9th Ave. N., Port Alberni, B.C.; Edinburgh (Scot.)'51.

BEGG, Herbert N.C.; 435 Tegler Bldg., 10189-101st St., Edmonton, Alta.; 10952-125th St. (res); Alb'28; AMCGP; Health Officer Royal Alexandra & Glenrose Hosp's.; Tel. 422-1568.

BEGG, Robert W.; 522 Lake Cres., Saskatoon, Sask. (res); Dal '42; M.Sc., D.Phil.; FRCP(C); Dean of Med. & Prof. of Chemical Path., U. of Saskatchewan; Tel. 242-7641.

BEGGS, John A.; 296 Metcalfe St., Ottawa 4, Ont.; 95 Reid Ave. (res); Qns '42; LM (Rotunda); DGO (TCD); FACOG, FASAS; FICS; ObstGyn; Sr. Obst., Grace Hosp.; Att'd. ObstGyn., Ottawa Civic Hosp.; Clin. Instr. U. of Ottawa; Tel. 232-1154.

BEGIN, B. Guy; 12075 Pasteur, Montreal 12, P.Q.; Mon '41; FCCP; ThorSurg (P.Q.); Surg., Hop. Sacre-Coeur; Cons., St-Jean San., Macamic; Vis. Staff, Hop. St. Joseph de Rosemont; Exec. Ass't., Assoc. des Medecins de Langue Francaise; Gov. (P.Q.); Amer. College of Chest Physicians; Tel. 331-3032.

BEGIN, Gregoire; 164 est, McLaren, Buckingham, P.Q.; Lav '58; GenSurg; LMCC; Surg., Hop. St-Michel; Tel. 986-3341.

BEGIN, Michel; P.O. Bolduc, Beauce, P.Q.; Lav '50.

BEIGHTON, Thomas E.; 104 Norlyn Med. Bldg., 309 Hargrave St., Winnipeg 2, Man.; 34 Thatcher Dr., Fort Garry (res); Man '49; Tel. WH 3-7596.

BEIQUE, Claude; 1150 est boul. St-Joseph, Montreal 34, P.Q.; Mon'57; Paed (P.Q.); Allergy (P.Q.); Cons. Hop. Maisonneuve; Tel. LA 7-1551.

BEIQUE, Leon; Ste. 201, 1656 Est, Rue Sherbrooke, Montreal 24, P.Q.; 3980 est rue Sherbrooke (res); Mon '42; FRCS(C); GenSurg; Surg., Hop-Notre-Dame; Tel. 521-2116.

BEIRNE, Patrick F.; Ste 1212, Toronto Professional Bldg., 123 Edward St., Toronto, Ont.; 108 Roxborough Dr. (res); National U. (Ire.) '46; BAO; FRCS(C) ObstGyn; Active Staff, St. Michael's Hosp.; Assoc. (Med.), **U. of Toronto;** Tel. 368-5423.

BEISER, Morton; 921 West 38th Ave., Vancouver, B.C. (res); UBC '60.

BEITINS, Inese Z.; Tor '62; Intn., Hosp. for Sick Children, Toronto 2, Ont. Abroad.

BELAIR, Antonin; 222 est Henri-Bourassa, Montreal 12, P.Q.; 2280 de Montreuil (res); Mon '50; Urol; Staff, Sacred Heart Hosp., Cartierville; Tel. DU 8-7608.

BELAK, Zenon D.; Assiniboia, Sask.; Sask '62; Tel. 642-4284.

BELAND, Anicet; 12 Elm Ave., New Liskeard, **Ont.; Lav '52**; MCGP; **Staff, Misericordia Hosp.; Tel. 647-5334.**

BELAND, Charles; 444 Laviolette, Trois Rivieres, P.Q.; 2060 Lajoie (res); **Lav '45; Paed (P.Q.); Chief (Paed), Hop. Ste-Marie; Tel. FR 5-7796.**

BELAND, Claude, Major; Lav '45; Psy; Staff, Quebec Military Hosp., Quebec, P.Q.; Tel. 653-7201.

BELAND, Gilles A.; Ste. 204, 30 Est Boul. **St.** Joseph, Montreal 14, P.Q.; Mon'57; FRCS(C); Urol; GenSurg (P.Q.); Tel. 845-4241.

BELAND, Guy; 200 St-Aime, Louiseville, P.Q.; Lav'63; Tel. 228-5025.

BELAND, Jean E., Lav '54; Path (P.Q.); Staff, Santa Cabrini Hosp., Montreal 36, P.Q.; Tel. 254-8311.

BELAND, Leonard; Lac Bouchete, P.Q.; Lav '53.

BELANGER, Albert; Lav'62; Res., Hop. Notre-Dame, Montreal 24, P.Q.

BELANGER, Andre; 301 rue Dufort, Laprairie, P.Q.; Lav'61.

BELANGER, Claude; 2290 Angers, Sillery, Quebec, P.Q. (res); Lav'51; FRCP(C); Neurol; Chief of Neurol. Services, Hop-de-l'Enfant-Jesus; Prof., Laval U.; Tel. 525-4643.

BELANGER, Georges; 1063 St-Denis, Montreal 18, P.Q.; Mon '58; NeurSurg (P.Q.); Tel. 842-4816.

BELANGER, Gerard A.; Lav '57; MCGP; Res., Hop. St-Francois d'Aissise, Montreal, P.Q.

BELANGER, Gilles; 475 boul. Talbot, Chicoutimi, P.Q.; Lav '59; Ophth.

BELANGER, Henri; 541 rue de l'Hopital, Jonquiere, P.Q.; 639 rue Pasteur (res); Lav '49; F.R.C.S.(C), ObstGyn; Chief, Dept. of ObstGyn, Hotel-Dieu Notre Dame de l'Assomption; Tel. 547-9341.

BELANGER, Jacques; Lav '60; Anaes; Staff, Hop. Hotel-Dieu, Sorel, **P.Q.**; Tel. RI 3-5521.

BELANGER, Jean M.; 2157 Fleury E., Montreal 12, P.Q.; 12145 Blvd. Taylor (res); Lav '50; GenSurg; Tel. DU 1-2581.

BELANGER, Jean-M.; 802 Chanoine Scott, Quebec, P.Q.; Lav '40; Tel. 653-4931.

BELANGER, J. Edward; 328 Somerset St. W., Ottawa 4, Ont.; Mon '28; Ph.D.; FACP, FAGS, FCIA, FAPM; Tel. CE 3-1353.

BELANGER, J. Francois; 800 ouest, boul. Gouin, Montreal 12, P.Q.; **Mon '43; Staff, Hop.** Bordeaux.

BELANGER, Joseph-A.; 4 Morin, Levis, P.Q.; 15 Guenette (res); Lav '24; Paed (P.Q.); Chief of Paed. Serv., Hotel Dieu de Levis; Tel. 837-9341.

BELANGER, Joseph E.; 2037 St. Denis St., Montreal, P.Q. (res); **Mon '24. Retired.**

BELANGER, Leo; Mont Joli, P.Q. (res); Lav '49; Pulm. Dis. & TB (P.Q.); Staff, San. St. Georges; Tel. PR 5-4355.
BELANGER, Leonard F.; 395 Templeton St., Ottawa 2, Ont.; Mon '37; M.A.(Med.Sc.), Harvard; F.R.S.C.; Prof. & Head, Histol & Embryol., U. of Ottawa. Tel. 235-6751, Loc. 289.
BELANGER, Marc; 127 rue du Prince, Sorel, P.Q.; Lav'60; FRCS(C); ObstGyn.
BELANGER, Maurice; 444 de la Salle Ave., Chicoutimi, P.Q. (res); Lav '42; Biochem, (P.Q.); Path (P.Q.); Phys., Hop. Hotel Dieu; Tel. 549-1588.
BELANGER, P.A.; Department of National Health & Welfare, c/o Regional Superintendent, European Region. Abroad.
BELANGER, Paul L. R.; Hemmingford, P.Q.; Mon '54.
BELANGER, P. B.; 217 Laurier Ave. E., Ottawa, Ont.; McG '15; GenSurg; Staff, Ottawa Gen. Hosp. Tel. CE 4-0117.
BELANGER, Pierre Y.; 15 ouest Prefontaine, Ste-Agathe-des-Monts, P.Q.; Mon'63.
BELANGER P. Marcel; 4395 ave Verdun, Ste. 17, Montreal 19, P.Q.; 2375 Bord du Lac (res); Mon '49; Urol; Chief of Serv. (Urol.), Hop. General Christ-Roi de Verdun; Tel. PO 9-5222.
BELANGER, Raoul; 30 Lepage, Rimouski, P.Q.; Lav '20; Dist. Coroner.
BELANGER, Raymond; 18-3rd Ave. E., La-Sarre, Abitibi, P.Q.; Lav '50; M.C.G.P.; Staff, Hop.-St.-Francois-de-La-Sarre; Tel. 333-2545.
BELANGER, Raymond; Leger & Associes, 1656 est rue Sherbrooke, Montreal 24, P.Q.; Mon'56; D&TRad; Staff, Hop.-Notre-Dame; Tel. LA 5-6363.
BELANGER, Rene, Capt.; 1 RCHA, Camp Gagetown, Oromocto, N.B.; Mon'65.
BELANGER, Ronaldo; Ste-Martine, P.Q.; Lav '45.
BELANGER, Yvon; 1670 Blvd. Pie IX, Montreal, P.Q.; Mon '41; Ass't. Prof. Histology & Embryology, U. of Montreal; Tel. RE 3-9951.
BELCH, Lindsay A.; 2221 Keele St., Toronto 15, Ont.; 18 Thornbank Rd., Thornhill (res); Tor '55; FRCS(C); ObstGyn; Active Staff (ObstGyn.), Toronto Northwestern & Toronto Western Hosp's; Court. Staff (ObstGyn.), North York Branson Hosp.; Tel. CH 4-1000.
BELCH, Thomas N.; Tor'53; Res., Ontario Hosp., 999 Queen St., Toronto 3, Ont.
BELCH, Willoughby W.; 584 Charlotte St., Peterborough, Ont.; Tor'51; FACS; FRCS(C); GenSurg; Active Staff, Peterborough Civic & Chief of Staff, St. Joseph's Hosp.; Tel. 742-6812.
BELCOURT, Christian L.; London (Eng.) '52; LRCP (Lond.); MRCS (Eng.); Diag Rad; Staff, Ottawa Civic Hosp., Ottawa, Ont.; Tel. 729-2511.
BELCOURT, Denis; Ste. 12, 222 Henri Bourassa, Montreal, P.Q.; 1414 Prieur E. (res); Mon '51; GenSurg (PQ); Tel. DU 7-9609.
BELCOURT, Louis E.; 1036 Main St. N., Moose Jaw, Sask.; Man '15.
BELCOURT, Roger J-P.; 1 Snowcrest Ave., Willowdale, Ont.; Lav' 42; B.A., M.A., Bact; Research Memb., Connaught Med. Research Labs., U. of Toronto; Tel. 633-8700.
BELDAVS, Jaseps T.; 5305 des Sapins Ave., Montreal 36, P.Q. (res); Riga (Latvia) '40; Anaes; Staff, Hop.-Maisonneuve; Tel. 254-8341.
BELEN, Jaime O.; Santo Tomas (Phillipp.)'62; Ass't. Res., Saint John Gen. Hosp., Saint John, N.B.
BELHUMEUR, Jean; 1210 lere Ave., Quebec 3, P.Q.; Lav '57; FRCS(C), ObstGyn; Staff, Hop.-de-l'Enfant-Jesus. Tel. 524-4972.
BELICK, J. B.; Tor'65; Res., Ross Pavillion, Royal Victoria Hosp., Montreal 2, P.Q.
BELISLE, Ferdinand; 6293 Cartier St., Montreal 35. P.Q.: Mon '48.
BELISLE, Gillies; 111 des Iris, Chicoutimi-Nord, P.Q.; Lav '54; Staff, Hop. Hotel-Dieu-St-Vallier, Chicoutimi; Tel. 543-2552.
BELISLE, Leo G.; 11 Bellingham, Outremont 8, P.Q.; Mon'53; Psy; Dir. Internal Clinic, Dept. of Child Psy., Hop. Ste Justine; Tel. 738-8761.
BELISLE, Louis P.; Ste 509, 801 est rue Sherbrooke, Montreal 24, P.Q.; 1555 Bernard W. (res); Mon '33; DiagRad; Cons. Anti TB Assoc. & Hop. & Prison de Bordeaux; Tel. VI 5-8998.
BELISLE, Maurice; 1801 Sherbrooke E., Montreal, P.Q.; 482 Blvd. Marie Victorin, Boucherville (res); Mon '44; F.R.C.P.(C), IntMed; Ass't., Hop. Notre Dame; Cons., Hop. Misericorde: In charge of Dept. Radioisotopes, Inst. Radium; Ass't. Prof., U. of Montreal; Tel. LA 2-1728.
BELISLE, Paul E.; 639 Principale, Buckingham, P.Q.; Mon '40; Tel. 986-3670.
BELIVEAU, Denis; 1150 Blvd. St. Joseph, Montreal, 34, P.Q.; Mon'49; GenSurg (P.Q.); Staff (Surg) Hop. Maisonneuve; Tel. LA 7-1241.
BELIVEAU, Lionel; 1297 St. Viateur, Outremont, P.Q.; Mon'60; Psy(P.Q.); Tel. 274-1608.
BELIVEAU, Pierre; Lav'65; Res., Hop. St. Sacrement, Quebec 4, P.Q.
BELKIN, Alex; 400 Med. Centre, 906-8th Ave. S. W., Calgary, Alta.; 408 Cumberland House, Rideau Towers (res.); Man. '28; FACP; IntMed; Tel. AM 3-1326.
BELL, Adelaine; 48 Irwin Ave., Sault-Ste.-Marie, Ont. (res); Qns '59; School M.O., Bd. of Education; Tel. AL 6-7466. Temporarily retired.
BELL, Aletta G.; Wes '61; Jr. Intn., Victoria Hosp., London, Ont.
BELL, Alexander G.; Tor '53; M.A.; Dept. of Path., Toronto Gen. Hosp., Toronto 2, Ont.; Ass't. Prof., (Depts. of Path. & Zool.) & Research Assoc. (Med.), U. of Toronto; Tel. EM 6-8211, Loc. 2008 or 2750.
BELL, Cecil D.; Tor'64; Res., Hosp. for Sick Children, Toronto 2, Ont.
BELL, Charles G.; 95 Hanna E., Windsor, Ont. (res); Wes '11; Staff, DVA; Retired.
BELL, Clinton A.; Port Stanley, Ont.; Tor '41; Dist. Coroner.
BELL, David A.; Wes '63; Int., Sunnybrook Hosp., Toronto, Ont.
BELL, David M.; 521 Med. Arts Bldg., 1110 Jasper Ave., Edmonton, Alta.; 8404-118th St. (res); Alb '43; IntMed; Att'd. Staff, Royal Alexandra & Univ. Hosp's.; Clin. Instr. (Med.), U. of Alberta; Med. Dir., Alcoholism Fdn. of Alberta; Tel. 422-6222.
BELL, David N.; 440 Hinton Ave., Ottawa 3, Ont.; 2121 Killarney Dr. Ott. 13 (res); Tor '53; Anaes; Staff (Anaes), Ottawa Civic Hosp.; Tel. 725-1163.
BELL, Delos E.; Workmen's Compensation Board, 90 Harbour St., Toronto; 1476 Carmen Dr., Port Credit (res); Qns '14; Med. Cons., Workmen's Compensation Board; Tel. 362-3411.
BELL, Donald; Binbrook, Ont.; Qns '55; MCGP; Staff, Hamilton Gen., St. Joseph's & Chedoke Hosp's.; Tel. 692-4449.
BELL, Donald M.; 10011-103rd St., Edmonton, Alta.; 13809-Summit Dr. (res); Alb '44; FACS; FRCS(C), ObstGyn; Att'd. Phys., University Royal Alexandra & Gen. Hosp's; Lect., U. of Alberta; Tel. GA 2-2223.
BELL, Douglas N.; 6668 Fraser St., Vancouver 15, B.C.; McG '55; MCGP; Tel. FA 7-4252.
BELL, E. G.; Tor'65; Res., Princess Margaret Hosp., Toronto 5, Ont.
BELL, Frank G.; 144 Main St., Liverpool, N.S., Dal'55; Staff, Queens Gen. Hosp.; Tel. 354-4458.
BELL, Fred C.; 6015 Eagleridge Dr., Eagle Harbour, B.C. (res); Man '09; Retired.
BELL, George A.; Man'60; Res., Shaughnessy Hosp., Vancouver, B.C.
BELL, Gordon I.; 409 Medical Arts Bldg., Edmonton, Alta.; 11135 Sask Dr. (res); Alb '40; F.A.C.P. IntMed; Lect. (Med.), U. of Alberta; Tel. GA 2-1431.
BELL, Harold E.; 7504-118th St., Edmonton, Alta.; Alb '49; B.Sc.; Path; Ass't. Dir., Clin. Labs., University Hosp.; Ass't. Prof. (Pathol.), U. of Alberta; Tel. 439-5911 Loc. 453.
BELL, H. Michael; UBC '59; FRCS(C), OrthSurg; Staff, Hosp. for Sick Children, Toronto, Ont.: Tel. 366-7242.
BELL, Ian; Wes '61; Jr; Jr. Intn., Hamilton Gen. Hosp., Hamilton, Ont.
BELL-IRVING, Peter; 119 Hycroft Med. Bldg., 3195 Granville St., Vancouver, B.C.; Tor '46; FRCP(C), IntMed; Tel. RE 8-9511.

BELL-IRVING, Robin W.; 520-17th St., West Vancouver B.C.; Tor '46; FRCP(C); IntMed; Att. Staff, Vancouver Gen. & Lions Gate Hosp's.; Vis. Staff, St. Paul's & Active Cons. Staff, N. Vancouver Gen. Hosp's.; Tel. WA 2-6410.

BELL, James F.; Valleyview, Alta.; Tor' 59.

BELL, James M.; 1105 Pandora Ave, Victoria, B.C.; 1988 Woodley Rd. (res); Glasgow (Scot.) '51; Active Staff, Royal Jubilee & Victoria Hosp's.; Tel. 385-7441.

BELL, James S.; 8 Glen Robert Dr., Toronto 16, Ont.; Tor'44; DPH; PH; Chief Epidem., Ontario Dept. of Health; Ass't. Prof. (Epidem.), School of Hygiene, U. of Toronto.

BELL, James W.; 1143 Mississauga Rd., Port Credit, Ont. (res); Tor '22; PathBact; Bact., **Ont. Dept. Health, Toronto, Ont.; Tel. EM** 3-1211.

BELL, J. Douglas; 196 George St., Hamilton, Ont.; Qns '57; M.C.G.P.; Staff, Mountain San.; Tel. JA 7-1545.

BELL, J. Kenneth; 10 Willowdale Ave., St. Catharines, Ont. (res); **Wes '37; FIM; Med. Dir.** Ontario Paper Co., Thorold; Tel. CA 7-1121.

BELL, J. K. Stuart; Edinburgh (Scot.)'63; Res., Ottawa Civic Hosp., Ottawa 3, Ont.

BELL, John N.; 6920 Isleview Rd., West Vancouver, B.C.; McG '53; Path; Staff, Shaughnessy Hosp., Vancouver; Tel. TR 6-6767.

BELL, Lennox G.; Manitoba Med. College, 750 Bannatyne Ave., Winnipeg 3, Man.; Ste. 2, 64 Nassau St., Wpg. 13 (res); Man '28; FRCP (Lond.), FRCP(C); FACP; IntMed; Hon. Att'd., Staff, Wpg. Gen. Hosp.; Dean & Prof. (Med.), U. of Man.; Tel. 786-3557.

BELL, M. E. Adeline (Bouck); 40 Tadcaster Place, Sault Ste. Marie, Ontario (res); Qns '59; Temporarily retired.

BELL, M. Ruth; (See Tatham)

BELL, Munroe C.; Brookfield, Colchester Co., N.S.; Edinburgh (Scot.)'40; Staff, Colchester County Hosp., Truro; Tel. 893-9425.

BELL, O. Gwyneth (Jones); Haig Clinic, 601-6th Ave. S., Lethbridge, Alta.; Birmingham (Eng.) '52; M.B., Ch.B.; Tel. 327-3171.

BELL, R. Edward; University Hosp., Edmonton, Alta.; 11607-78th Ave. (res); Alb '42; D.A.B.C.-P., F.C.A.P.; Path; Dir. Clin. Lab. Serv., U. of Alta. Hosp.; Prof. (Path), U. of Alberta; Tel. 439-5911.

BELL, R. Glen; 117 King St. E., Oshawa, Ont.; 309 Golf St. (res); Qns '39; M.P.H.; Tel. 728-1661.

BELL, R. Gordon; Donwood Fdn., 175 Brentcliffe Rd., Toronto 17, Ont.; Tor'43; Spec. Lect., Dept. of Pharm., U. of Toronto; Tel. 425-3930.

BELL, Robert; 2117 Pelissier, Windsor, Ont.; 2282 Chilver (res); Qns '56; Tel. 254-9294.

BELL, Robert D.; 408 Toronto Western Medical Bldg., 25 Leonard Ave., Toronto 2B, Ont.; 67 Twyford Rd. (res); Tor '42; D.L.O., F.R.C.S.(C), Otol; Att. Staff, (Otol), Toronto Western & Sunnybrook Hosp's.; Clin. Instr., (Otol), U. of Toronto. Tel. EM 3-3918.

BELL, Robert H.; 483 George St. S., Peterborough, Ont.; 191 O'Carroll Ave. (res); Tor **'41; M.C.G.P.; Tel. 742-0461.**

BELL, Ross H.; 541 Sammon Ave., Toronto, Ont.; Tor '44; DTM&H; Med. Missionary, Nigeria (on leave 1 year).

BELL-SMITH, Donald; Tor '31; Psy; Hd. of Male Serv., Ontario Hosp., Brockville, Ont.; Tel. DI 5-1461.

BELL, Thomas J.; 58 St. Mary St., Toronto 5, Ont. (res); Tor '55; Part-time staff, Toronto Gen. Hosp. & Lyndhurst Lodge; Tel. EM 6-8211.

BELL, William J.; 1139 Yates St., Victoria, B.C.; UBC '54; MCGP; Active Staff, St. Joseph's Hosp.; Tel. EV 8-4211.

BELL, William P.; 3013 Bathurst St., Toronto, Ont.; 27 Fairholme Ave. Tor. 19 (res); Tor '58; Court. Staff, New Mount Sinai & North York Branson Hosp's. Tel. 782-9672.

BELL, W. Robert; 14 Parkwood Dr., Galt, Ont.; **(res); Alb '41; DMR; DABR; D & T Rad; Radiol., S. Waterloo Mem. Hosp. & Milton Dist. Hosp., Milton; Cons. Georgetown & Dist. Mem. Hosp.; Tel. 621-2330.**

BELL, W. W.; Lantzville, B.C.; McG '23; Retired.

BELLAMY, Brenda; Sheffield (Eng.) '61; Jr. Intn., Winnipeg Gen. Hosp., Winnipeg 3, Man.

BELLAMY, Jean G., 404 Greyhound Bldg., Calgary, Alta.; 21 Kendell Pl. (res); Tor'47; MCGP; Tel. 262-2517.

BELLAMY, Lorna E.; Wetaskiwin, Alta.; Tor '42; Retired.

BELLAMY, Kenneth E.; 381 Churchill, Ottawa, Ont.; 650 Keenan St. (res); Qns '29.

BELLAMY, Richard P.; Box 1868, Wetaskiwin, Alta.; Man '44; M.C.G.P.

BELLAN, Samuel; 284 Salter St., Winnipeg, Man.; 320 Bredin Dr. (res); Man '40; M.C.G.P.; Tel. JU 2-5786.

BELLEAU, Louis P. G.; La Sarre, Abitibi, P.Q.; Geneva (Switz.) '34; Coroner, Abitibi Ouest.

BELLEAU, Paul E.; 1089-4th Ave., Quebec 3, P.Q.; Lav '30; IntMed; Tel. 524-5430.

BELLEFEUILLE, Francois L.; 9320 Place du Berger, Charlesbourg, P.Q.; Lav'65.

BELLEFEUILLE, Phillippe; 2960 Neree Beauchemin, Trois Rivieres, **P.Q. (res); Lav '48; MCGP; Med. Dir., Hop. St. Joseph; Tel. FR 4-3013.**

BELLEGARDE, J. O. Vilbon; 194 Saguenay, Noranda, P.Q. (res); Lav'47; DHA; MACHA; Med., Hop.-Youville; Tel. 762-7070.

BELLE-ISLE, Jean; 31 ouest rue King, Sherbrooke, P.Q.; Lav '60; Derm.

BELLEMARE, F. Bertrand; 225 Grande-Allee, Quebec, P.Q.; 575-1057 Ave. Demontigny, Sillery (res); Lav '43; M.P.H., F.A.P.H.A., F.A.A.C.M., F.I.M.A., PH(P.Q.); Med. Dir., Indus. & Prev. Med., Dept. of Labour, Workmen's Comp. Bd., (P.Q.); Prof. Laval U.; Tel. 693-5995.

BELLEMARE, Fernand; 425 Blvd. Charest, Que. 2, P.Q.; Lav '44; OphthOtol (P.Q.); Chief of Serv., Hop. St-Ambroise-de-Lorettville; **Tel. 529-3694.**

BELLEMARE, Gaston; 911 Cherrier, Montreal, P.Q.; 4821 Upper Roslyn (res); Mon '40; Derm Syph (P.Q.); Tel. LA 4-7717.

BELLEMARE, Henri; 222 est, Boul. Henri- Bourassa, Montreal 12, P.Q.; 12215 Ave. de Poutrincourt (res); Mon '55; IntMed; Staff Phys., Hop.-Sacre-Coeur; Tel. 381-7177.

BELLEMARE, Jean A.; 30 est, boul. St-Joseph, Montreal 14, P.Q.; Mon '55; MCGP.

BELLEMARE, Jean L.; 339A boul, Ste-Madeleine, Cap-de-la-Madeleine, P.Q.; Lav '58.

BELLEMARE, Joachim; 1485 Chemin-Ste-Foy, Quebec, P.Q.; Lav '42; Tel. 527-3163.

BELLEMARE, Marcel; 444 Laviolette, Trois-Rivieres, P.Q.; Lav'55; GenSurg (PQ); Tel. 378-2121.

BELLEMARE, Maurice; 965 Royale, Trois Rivieres, P.Q.; Lav '36; Ophth; OphthOtol (P.Q.); Staff, Hop. St. Joseph; Tel. FR 4-9262.

BELLERIVE, R.; 1840 St.-Marc, Shawinigan Fall, P.Q.; Lav '56; Tel. LE 7-1587.

BELLEY, Jacques; Mon'64; Res., Mtl. Children's Hosp., Montreal 25, P.Q.

BELLEY, Maurice; 1500-18eme rue, Quebec, P.Q.; Lav '60; Otol; Staff, Hop. Enfant-Jesus, Quebec, P.Q.; Tel. 529-8711.

BELLIVEAU, Gerald D.; 253 Main St., Yarmouth, N.S.; 11 Highland Ave. (res); Lav '54. Tel. 742-7184.

BELLIVEAU, Normand J.; Ste 1931, No. 1, place ville Marie, Montreal 2, P.Q.; **505 Champagneur, Outremont, Montreal 8 (res); Lav '46; F.A.C.S., F.C.C.P., GenSurg; Staff, Royal Victoria & St. Joseph de Rosemont Hosp's.; Tel. VI 2-9497.**

BELLIVEAU, Robert P.; P.O. Box 130, Meteghan,, Cte. Digby, N.S.; Lav '52; Tel. 200.

BELLMAN, Agnes M.; 17 Rivercrest Rd., Toronto 9, Ont.; Tor '36; Staff, O.P.D. (Obst.), Women's College Hosp. Tel. RO 7-6203.

BELMONTE, Jose F.; 625 Queenston St., Winnipeg 9, Man.; Santo Tomas (Manilla, Philipp.) '54; Dip. Anaes.

BELMONTE, Mimi M.; 2300 Tupper St., Montreal, P.Q.; 418 Pine Ave. W. (res); McG '52; F.R.C.P.(C), Paed; Clin. Ass't., Royal Victoria Hosp.; Ass't. (Metabolism), Montreal Children's Hosp.; Dem. (Paed.), McGill U.; Tel. WE 7-8511, Loc. 495.

BELTEN, M. K.; 975—11th St., Hollyburn, B.C. (res); McG '41; Anaes; Staff, Vancouver Gen. Hosp., Vancouver; Tel. TR 6-3211.

BELTON, John H.; 168 Ontario St., St. Catharines, Ont.; Tor'39; FACOG; ObstGyn; Staff (ObstGyn) & Memb. Bd. of Governors, St. Catharines Gen. Hosp.; Staff (ObstGyn), Hotel-Dieu Hosp.; Tel. MU 4-6977.

BELTRAMI, Edouard; Mon'63; Res., Jewish Gen. Hosp., Montreal, P.Q.

BELYEA, Clifford C.; 28 Weber St. W., Kitchener, Ont.; Tor '23; M.C.G.P.; Staff, Kitchener-Waterloo & St. Mary's Hosp's.; Dist. Coroner; Tel. 744-3311.

BELYEA, George N.; 395 Regent St., Woodstock, N.B.; McG '19; F.A.C.S., GenSurg; Chief Staff Surg., Carleton Memorial Hosp.; Tel. 328-3391.

BELZIL, Benoit; 17 Ave. Begin, Levis, P.Q.; Lav '46; OphthOtol (P.Q.); Tel. 837-5917.

BELZILE, Andre; Lav '61; Res., Toronto Gen. Hosp., Toronto 2, Ont.

BELZILE, Andre; 186 Burma St., Arvida, P.Q.; Lav'58.

BELZILE, Gabriel; Lav'58; Res., Hop. Notre-Dame, Montreal 24, P.Q.

BELZILE, Marcel J.J.; 822 est, rue Sherbrooke, Montreal, P.Q.; Lav '52; Otol; Staff (Otol.), Notre Dame Hosp.; Tel. LA 5-6363.

BEN, John H.; Suite 15, 2917 Bloor St. W., Toronto 18, Ont.; Tor'58; MCGP; Staff, St. Joseph's & Queensway Gen. Hosp's.; Indust. Phys., Consumer's Gas; Tel. 233-3343.

BENARD, Bernard; 23 Silvia Crt., Hyde Park, Boston, Mass. 02136, U.S.A.; Mon'60; FRCP(C), IntMed; Abroad.

BENCOSME, Sergio A.; 37 Jorine Dr., Kingston, Ont.; Mon '47; M.Sc., Ph.D.; Att'd. Staff, Kingston Gen. Hosp.; Assoc. Prof. (Path.), Queen's U.; Tel. LI 6-1731.

BENDER, Frank J.; Budapest (Hung.) '37; Ph.D., IntMed.; Staff, Mountain San., Hamilton, Ont.; Tel. 385-5341.

BENDETH, Basil S.; 79 Underhill Dr., Don Mills, Ont.; London (Eng.) '49; M.B., B.S., LRCP; MRCS; Court. Staff, Scarborough Gen. Hosp.; Tel 447-6171.

BENDING, Glenville C.; 319 Speedvale Ave. E., Guelph, Ont.; 14 Fairview Blvd. (res); Wes '52; F.A.A.O.O.; D.A.B.Oph; Ophth; Active Staff, Guelph Gen. & St. Joseph's Hosp's.; Tel. TA 2-5500. Abroad.

BENDKOWSKI, Boleslaw; 501 Med. Arts Bldg., 1 Young St., Hamilton, Ont.; Edinburgh (Scot.) '49.

BENDOR-SAMUEL, John E. L.; Winnipeg Clinic, Wpg. 1, Man.; 604-811 Grosvenor Ave., Wpg. 9 (res); London (Eng.) '30; LRCP; MRCS; DOMS (Eng.); Ophth; Ass't. Ophth., Winnipeg Gen. & Children's Hosp's.; Tel. 942-0551.

BENFEY, B. G.; Hamburg (Germ.) '48; Assoc. Prof. Pharm., U. of McGill, Montreal, P.Q.

BENIANS, Mary E. (Mrs. Smits); 61 Kensington Ave., Kingston, Ont.; London (Eng.) '47; LRCP; FRCS; Psy; M.O., Ontario Hosp., Kingston.

BENIERAKIS, Constantine; Trinity Coll. (Dublin, Ire.) '57; Psy; Pt-time Staff, Royal Victoria Hosp., Children's Psychiatric Clinic, 505 Pine Ave. W., Montreal, P.Q.; Tel. VI 2-1251, loc. 728.

BENJAMIN, Peter; 3550 Cote des Neiges Rd., Ste. 450, Montreal 25, P.Q.; McG '55; FRCP(C), Paed; Dir., Teen Age Clinic, Montreal Children's Hosp.; Dir. of Nursery, Bellechasse Hosp.; Staff Phys., Montreal Children's & Jewish Gen. Hosp's.; Tel. 932-5852.

BENNEE, A. John; 3703 Pleasant Valley Rd., Vernon, B.C.; Witwatersrand (S. Africa)'41; Psy.; Abroad.

BENNETT, Edward J.; 100 Osborne Med. Bldg., 190 Osborne St. N., Winnipeg 1, Man.; 10B Colonial House (res); Man '25; Phm.B., MCGP; Tel. 783-7085.

BENNETT, George; Ste. 6, 220-4th Ave., Kamloops, B.C.; Manchester (Eng.) '44; DOMS (Eng.); Ophth; Opth Surg., Royal Inland Hosp.; Tel 372-8323.

BENNETT, Ian; Durham (Eng.) '62; Res., Staff, Lucky Lake Union Hosp., Lucky Lake, Sask.

BENNETT, Ilo M. F. (Fraser); 672 Oriole Pkwy., Toronto 12, Ont. (res); Tor '27; Phys., Cdn. Baptist Mission; Tel. HU 1-1597.

BENNETT, James E.; 110 Ridgedale Cr., Winnipeg 20, Man. (res); Glasgow (Scot.)'45; DMRT; TherRad; Sr. TherRad., St. Boniface Hosp., St. Boniface; Lectr. (Rad.), U. of Manitoba; Tel. CH 7-9742.

BENNETT, John S.; Knox Clinic, 1605 Glenmore St., Kelowna, B.C.; 309 Poplar Pt. Dr. (res); U. of London, St. Mary's H. (Eng.) '53; MB., BS., MRCS, LRCP; LMSSA; FASAS; ObstGyn; Chief (ObstGyn), Kelowna Gen. Hosp.; Tel. 762-2002.

BENNETT, Keith T. F.; 1928 Eglinton Ave. W., Toronto 10, Ont.; 64 Greenbrook Dr. (res); Tor '52; M.C.G.P.; Staff, Northwestern, St. Joseph's (GenSurg), University Hosp., Saskatoon, Sask. & St. John's Convalescent Hosp's. Tel. RU 3-3503.

BENNETT, Marjorie R.; 321 Medical Arts Bldg., 404-406 Graham Ave., Winnipeg 1, Man.; 1194 Kildonan Dr., East Kildonan (res); Man '35; Anaes; Chief Anaes., St. Boniface Hosp.; Lectr. (Anaes), U. of Manitoba; Tel. WH 3-0311.

BENNETT, Michael F.; 534 Valleyfield Dr., Sarnia, Ont.; Ire '52; D & T Rad; Staff, St. Joseph's Hosp.; Tel. ED 6-6121.

BENNETT, Norman T.; Madrona Bldg., 140 Wallace St., Nanaimo, B.C.; Alb '46.

BENNETT, Richard B.; 2489 Bellevue Ave., West Vancouver, B.C.; UBC'58.

BENNETT, Ronald; 722-13th St. N., Lethbridge, Alta.; Man '54; MCGP; Staff, Lethbridge Municipal, Lethbridge Auxiliary & St. Michael's Hosp's.; Tel. 327-0522.

BENNETT, Ross C.; 350 Beech Ave., Toronto 13, Ont.; 1 Faircroft Blvd. (res); Wes '54. Tel. 694-1126.

BENNETT, S. R.; 1 Serpentine St., Copper Cliff, Ont.; Tor '26; Ophth, Otol.

BENNETT, Stafford Z.; Alexander Ave., Salmon Arm, B.C.; Lakeshore Terrace (res); Man '30; M.C.G.P.; Staff, Shuswap Lake Gen. Hosp., Salmon Arm; Retired.

BENNETT, T. D.; 174-25th St. W., Prince Albert, Sask.; Qns '16; L.R.C.P. (Lond.), M.R.S.C. (Eng.), Dist. Coroner; Temp Retired.

BENNETT, W. Douglas; 59 Rose Park Dr., Toronto 7, Ont. (res); Tor '45; Clin. Phys. Gage Inst. Tel. HU 9-5380.

BENNETT, Wilfred H.; District Health Unit, Box 1019, Bracebridge, Ont.; Tor'41; MCGP.

BENNETT, William E. J.; 408 Hammond Bldg., Moose Jaw, Sask.; 1026 Henry St. (res); King's Coll. Hosp. (London, Eng.) '43; M.R.C.S.(Eng.), L.R.C.P.(Lond.), F.R.S.C.(Eng.), F.R.C.S(C), GenSurg; Staff, Moose Jaw Union & Providence Hosp's.; Tel. 692-1812.

BENNETT, W. J.; 7A Town House Apts., 346 Broadway, Winnipeg, Man. (res); Man '38; Int Med; Staff, Deer Lodge Hosp.; Lect. (Med.), U. of Manitoba; Tel. GR 4-9110.

BENNETT, William L. L., Lt.-Col.; Base Surg., Cdn. Forces Base Toronto, Downsview, Ont.; Alb'46; Psy; Tel. 633-6200, Loc. 401.

BENNETT, William W.; 27 Pleasant St., Bridgewater, N.S.; Dal '33; Staff, Dawson Mem. Hosp.; Tel. 543-2360.

BENNETTO, Frederick R.; 88 Wentworth S., Hamilton, Ont.; 51 Claremont Dr. (res); Tor '07; OphthOtol.; Tel. 383-2481.

BENNETTS, R. Carlton; 4250 Sherbrooke St. W., Westmount 6, Montreal, P.Q.; McG '33; IntMed; Assoc. Phys., Montreal Gen. Hosp.; Ass't. Prof. (Med.), McGill U.; Tel. 935-5563.

BENOIT, Alphonse; Mon '58; Res., Hop. Notre-Dame, Montreal 24, P.Q.

BENOIT, Brien G.; Ott'62; Ass't. Res. Surg., Ottawa Civic Hosp., Ottawa, Ont.

BENOIT, Clair F.; Ste. 203, 419 Graham Ave., Winnipeg 1, Man.; 625 Niakwa Rd. St. Boniface (res); Man '43; D.A.B.O., M.Sc., Ophth (Minn.); Tel. WH 3-6930.

BENOIT, Ivan; 3545 Hochelaga, Montreal 4, P.Q.; 10917 St. Denis (res); Mon '55; Tel. LA 3-5848.

BENOIT, Jacques; Mon'61; FRCP(C); IntMed; Staff, Montreal Gen. Hosp., Montreal 25, P.Q.

BENOIT, Joseph; 725 Couvent, Montreal 30, P.Q.; Mon '21; Tel. WE 3-4010.
BENOIT, Leo; 775 Laframboise, Saint Hyacinthe, P.Q.; 2790 Girouard (res); Lav '31; Anaes., Hop. St. Charles; Dist. Coroner; Tel. PR 4-7144.
BENOIT, Michel; 7680-9th Ave., Ville St. Michel, Montreal 38, P.Q.; 10917 St. Denis (res); Mon '57; A.M.C.G.P.; Tel. 721-4333.
BENOIT, Paul; 11907 James-Morrice, Montreal 12, P.Q. (res); Lav '59; FRCP(C), Paed (P.Q.). Abroad.
BENOIT, Raymond; St. Zotique, Co. Soulanges, P.Q.; Mon '55.
BENOIT, Rene H.; Ste. 812, 30 est, boul St. Joseph, Montreal 14, P.Q.; Mon'38; FAAP; Paed., Hd. of Paed., Hop. Misericorde; Ass't. Paed., Hop. St. Luc. & Ass't. Prof. (Paed.), U. of Montreal; Tel. 842-1996.
BENOIT, Yvon; Mon '64; Res., Hop. Hotel-Dieu, Montreal 18, P.Q.
BENSIMON, Joseph R.; 1734 W. Broadway, Vancouver, B.C.; Paris (France)'56; Paed; Research Fell., U. of British Columbia.
BENSLEY, Edward H., MBE; 157 Morrison Ave., Montreal 16, P.Q.; Tor '30; D.Sc. (Acadia); FRCP (C), FCIC, FACP; IntMed; Hon. Cons., Montreal Gen. & Royal Victoria Hosp's.; Prof. (Med.), & Hon. Lect. (Biochem.) & Vice Dean, Fac. of Med., McGill U.; Tel. 844-6311, Ext. 1450.
BENSLEY, Sylvia H. (Holton); 7 Balmuto St., Toronto 5, Ont. (res); Chicago (USA) '29; Assoc. Prof. Anatomy (Histol.) U. of Toronto; Hon. Cons. (Histol.), Hosp. for Sick Children; Tel. WA 3-6611.
BENSON, Cyril K.; 947 Woodbine Ave., Toronto 13, Ont.; Qns '40; FRCS(C); GenSurg; Staff, Toronto East Gen. Hosp.; Tel. OX 4-9366.
BENSON, Eric; 513 Med. Dental Bldg., Regina, Sask.; 3916 Princess Dr. (res); UK '53; Tel. LA 2-6541; Abroad.
BENSON, John B.; 126 Walton St., Port Hope, Ont., Tor '43; Tel. 885-5823.
BENSON, Kenneth I.; 2073 Renfrew Rd., Victoria, B.C. (res); Edinburgh (Scot.) '51; D.P.H.; PH; Ass't. Prov. Health Off., & Dir., Bureau of Local Health Serv., Dept. of Health, (B.C.); Tel. EV 2-3193.
BENSON, R. Ashley; 1833 Riverside Dr., Apt. 516, Ottawa 8, Ont. (res); Tor '32; IntMed (T.B.); Med. Dir., Metropolitan Life Ins. Co.; Tel. 232-2631.
BENT, Maurice A.; Tor'62; Res., Toronto Western Hosp., Toronto 2B, Ont.
BENT, Wilfrid I.; Dal'36; DPH; Dir., Lunenburg-Queens Health Unit, 399 King St., Bridgewater, N.S.; Tel. 543-3234.
BENTHAM, William H.; 3000 Lawrence Ave. E., Scarborough, Ont.; McG'55; Anaes; MCGP; Staff, Scar. Gen. Hosp.; Tel. AX 3-8681.
BENTLEY, Charles H.; 14 Louise Ave., Dartmouth, N.S. (res); Edinburgh (Scot) '31; Ass't. Supt., Nova Scotia Hosp.; Tel. 469-7500.
BENTLEY, Dorothy C.; Room 930, Bell Telephone Co., 1050 Beaver Hall Hill, Montreal 1, P.Q.; McG'42; IntMed (P.Q.); Staff Phys., Bell Telephone Co.; Tel. 870-2976.
BENTLEY, Kenneth C.; McG '62; Jr. Intn., Montreal Gen. Hosp., Montreal 25, P.Q.
BENTZ, J. Barrie; 1199 Austin Ave., Coquitlam, New Westminster, B.C.; 1839 Harbour Dr. (res); UBC '61; AMCGP; Tel. WE 9-7345.
BENTZ, Peter E.; Port Arthur Clinic, 194 Northcourt St., Port Arthur, Ont.; 101 Regent St. (res); Tor '61; AMCGP; Active Staff, Port Arthur Gen. & St. Joseph's Hosp's.; Tel. 344-7271.
BENTZON, Johanne W.; 1849 Yonge St., Toronto 7, Ont.; Copenhagen (Denmark) '48; Paed; Staff, Hosp. for Sick Children; Cons. Paed., Scarborough Gen. Hosp.; Tel. HU 1-0059.
BENWELL, Charles E.; 321 Agnes St., New Westminster, B.C. (res); Tor '18; Psy; Retired.
BERANKOVA, Vera; 585 Ingrid St., Fabreville, P.Q.; Prague (Czech.) '35.
BERARD, Michel J.; 3785 Ave. Harvard, Montreal 28, P.Q. (res); Mon'53; FACS, FACOG; FRCOG; FRCS(C); ObstGyn; Chief, (ObstGyn) Hop.-Notre-Dame, Prof. & Dir. Dept. of Obst Gyn, U. of Montreal; Tel. 523-8469.
BERARD, Paul E.; 48 St. Michel, Mistassini, Co. Lac St. Jean, P.Q.; Mon '48; M.C.G.P.
BERARD, Rosario; 415 Blvd. St. Joseph Est, Montreal 34, P.Q.; Mon '27; Staff, Dept. of Health Montreal; Tel. VI 5-9798.
BERBRAYER, Peter; 604 Boyd Bldg., Winnipeg, Man.; 687 Niagara St. (res); Man '34; F.R.C.S. (Eng.); Cons. OrthSurg., Deer Lodge Hosp.; Ass't. Surg., Wpg. Gen. Hosp.; Lect. OrthSurg; U. of Manitoba; Tel. WH 2-5337.
BERCOV, H. A.; 112 Medical Arts Bldg., Calgary, Alta.; 3641—13th St. S.W. (res); Alb '25; M.C.G.P.; Tel. 263-3404.
BERCOVICI, Jean T.; 250 Ellendale Med. Bldg., 5845 Cote-Des-Neiges Rd., Montreal 26, P.Q.; 3400 Ridgewood Ave. (res); Cluj (Roumania) '45; Otol; Cons., Queen Mary Vet's. Hosp.; Vis. Phys., Hop.-Maisonneuve; Tel. 735-1852.
BERCOVITCH, David D.; 6650 Wilderton Ave., Montreal 26, P.Q.; McG'58; Int. Med.
BERDALA, Jesus; Zaragoza (Spain) '53; Staff, Riverside Hosp., Charlottetown, P.E.I.; Tel. 4-5581; Abroad.
BERDNIKOFF, George; 3175 Chemin Ste-Catherine, Montreal 26, P.Q.; 486 Oakdale Ave., Twn. of Mt. Royal (res); Aurora U. (Shanghai, China) '48; Path; Assoc. Dir. Pathol., Hop.-Ste-Justine; Ass't. Prof. (Path), U. of Montreal; Tel. RE 1-4931, Loc. 320; RE 3-9951, Loc. 422.
BERDNIKOFF, Katherine (Golubyatnikoff); Apt. 23, 2850 Kent Ave., Montreal 26, P.Q.; Aurora (Shanghai, China)'48; Paed; Staff, Ste. Justine Hosp.
BERDUSCO, Arthur S.; Wes'61; Otol; Staff, Victoria Hosp., London, Ont.
BERECZ, Jospeh R.; Mon '63; Jr. Ass't. Res., (Surg.), Royal Victoria Hosp., Montreal, P.Q.
BEREGOFF-GILLOW, Pauline; 3295 Beach Dr., Oak Bay, Victoria, B.C.; Cartagena (Columbia, S. America) '25; Retired.
BERENYI, Veronica (See Halmos)
BERESFORD, James M.; 1105 Carling Ave., Ottawa 3, Ont.; Liverpool (Eng.)'58; MRCOG; FRCS(C); ObstGyn; Tel. 728-1713.
BEREZAN, David; Box 1210, Stettler, Alta.; Alb '43; MCGP.
BEREZNAY, Ivan; Box 370, Fisher Branch, Man.; U. of Pecs. (Hungary) '53; DTM; Tel. 372-6258.
BEREZOWSKI, Hector V.; Apt. 2, 300 Cooper St., Ottawa, Ont.; McG '54; FRCS(C); NeurSurg; Staff, NeurSurg, Ottawa Gen. Hosp., Tel CE 6-4592. Abroad.
BERG, C. Douglas; Dept. of Surg., University Hosp., Saskatoon, Sask.; Man'54; DABS; FRCS(C), GenSurg; Vis. Phys., St. Paul's & City Hosp's.; Ass't. Prof. Surg., U. of Saskatchewan; Tel. 652-8221.
BERG, Morton D.; 4 Deer Park Cr., Toronto 7, Ont.; 27 Rosemary Lane (res); Tor '50; DAPA; Research Assoc., New Mt. Sinai Hosp.; Tel. 921-0781.
BERGAL, Joseph; Westbrook Med. Centre, 1800 Logan Ave., Winnipeg 23, Man.; 416 Kelvin Blvd., Wpg. 29 (res); Man '50; MCGP; Tel. SP 2-9453.
BERGEN, Peter C.; RR. 1, Galt, Ont.; Tor '55.
BERGER, Benjamin; 1541 W. Broadway, Vancouver 9, B.C.; 2662 W. King Edward, Van. 8 (res); Man '45; Ophth; Att'd. Staff, Van. Gen. & Shaughnessy DVA Hosp's.; Tel. RE 1-3258.
BERGER, David M.; Tor'61; Psy; Staff, New Mount Sinai Hosp., Toronto 2, Ont.
BERGER, David; Ste. 103, 3545 Cote des Neiges Rd., Montreal 25, P.Q.; Krakow (Poland) '27; D&TRad; Rad., Royal Edward Chest Hosp.; Cons. Rad., Jewish Hosp. of Hope & Laurentian Chest Hosp.; Dem., McGill U.; Tel. 937-6321.
BERGER, Emile C.; Ste. 300, 6000 Cote des Neiges Rd., Montreal 26, P.Q.; 4888 Grosvenor Ave. (res.); Vienna (Austria) '51; NeurSurg; Tel. RE 1-0559.
BERGER, Martin; 1401 W. Broadway, Vancouver 9, B.C.; Tor'57; FRCP(C), Paed.; Abroad.
BERGER, Maurice; 1348 Main St., Winnipeg, Man.; 704 Oak St., (res); Man '42; Paed; Hon. Staff, Grace, Winnipeg Gen., & Children's Hosp's.; Lect'r. (Paed), U. of Manitoba; Tel. JU 6-3792.

BERGER, Saul S.; 901 Boyd Bldg., Winnipeg 6, Man.; Tor '43; FABDS; DermSyph; Chief of Derm., St. Boniface & Deer Lodge Vet's. Hosp's; Lect. (Med.), U. of Manitoba; Tel. WH 3-1387.
BERGERON, Armand; 2785 Boul. Laurier, Ste-Foy, Quebec, P.Q.; Lav'59.
BERGERON, Claude; Inst. Med. Clinic, 475 boul. Talbot, Chicoutimi, P.Q.; Lav '56; FACS; FRCS(C), GenSurg; Gyn (P.Q.); Staff, Hop. Hotel-Dieu-St. Vallier; Tel. 549-0023.
BERGERON, Dollard; Lav'58; Staff, (Pulm. Dis. & TB), Roberval San, Roberval, P.Q.
BERGERON, Fernand; 207 Richelieu, St-Jean, P.Q.; Mon '59.
BERGERON, George H.; 313 Perreault St. E., Rouyn. P.Q.; Mon '33; DiagRad; Staff, Youville Hosp.; Tel. RO 2-2301.
BERGERON, Georges-A.; 965 Rue Ernest-Gagnon, Quebec, P.Q. (res); Lav '42; FRCP(C); IntMed; Vice Dean Med., Laval U.; Tel. 656-2400.
BERGERON, Hugues; C.P. 1310, Outardes-3, Co. Saguenay, P.Q.; Lav'65.
BERGERON, Jacques; 970 ave. Cartier, Quebec, P.Q.; Lav '51; IntMed (P.Q.); Cons. (IntMed.), Hop. Ste. Foy; Phys., Bell Telephone Co. of Canada; Med. Dir., Domrency Clinic Quebec Inc.; Internist., Hop. St. Augustin, Courville; Prof. (Fac. of Science), Laval U.; Tel. 529-4678.
BERGERON, J. Adelard; Causapscal Stn., P.Q.; Lav '21.
BERGERON, J. Andre; C.P. 604, 794-5e rue, Shawinigan, P.Q.; Lav '61; Paed.
BERGERON, J. Aurele; 15 Balsam S., Timmins, Ont.; 131-3rd, Schumacher (res); Lav '55; MCGP; Tel. AM 4-1711.
BERGERON, J. Baptiste; 177 St. Etienne, La Malbaie, Cte. Charlevoix, P.Q.; Lav '50.
BERGERON, J. Claude; 520, boul. Deschenes, Beloeil, Co. Vercheres, P.Q.; Mon '57; DiagRad (P.Q.)
BERGERON, Jean; Lav '63; Res., Hop. Notre-Dame, Montreal 24, P.Q.
BERGERON, Jean-L.; 360 Main West, Magog, P.Q.; Lav '51.
BERGERON, Jean-M.; 1564—5th Ave., Shawinigan S., P.Q.; 2000—5th Ave. (res); Lav '49; Anaes (P.Q.); Tel. LE 6-4073.
BERGERON, Laurent; 1656 est rue Sherbrooke, Montreal 24, P.Q.; Mon '36; GenSurg; Staff, Hop.-Notre-Dame; Tel. 526-3783.
BERGERON, Leo; 225 Grande Allee E., Quebec 4, P.Q.; Lav '32; M.O., W.C.P. (P.Q.); Tel. 522-4751.
BERGERON, Lionel; 2839-1st Ave., Quebec, P.Q.; 215-78th St. E.; Charlesbourg (res); Lav '48; M.C.G.P.; Tel. 623-1688.
BERGERON, Marc; 1150 rue Ste Anne St-Hyacinthe, P.Q.; 2325 rue Moreau (res); Mon '35; DPH; PH(P.Q.); Med. Dir., Sherbrooke Dist. Health Unit & Hotel-Dieu-de-St. Hyacinthe; Tel. PR 3-9715.
BERGERON, Omer; 3548 Ontario E, Montreal, P.Q.; Mon '48; Tel. LA 4-5509.
BERGERON, Pierre; 565 rue Commerciale, La Tuque, P.Q.; Lav '60; Tel. 523-5125.
BERGERON, Raymond; Lav '60; Res., Hop. Notre-Dame, Montreal 24, P.Q.
BERGERON, Roland; 1740 Bardy, Quebec 3, P.Q.; Lav'33; FICS; GenSurg.
BERGH, Rodney M.; 206 Rookwood Ave., Fredericton, N.B.; Dal '57; Paed; Active Staff, Victoria Public Hosp.; Tel. 475-7701.
BERGHUIS, Sybolt H.; 4390 Valencia Ave., North Vancouver, B.C. (res); Amsterdam (Neth.) '40; Staff, St. Paul's Hosp.
BERGMAN, Bergthor J.; Man '57; Path; Staff, Kitchener-Waterloo Hosp., Kitchener, Ont.; Tel. 745-9451, Ext. 251.
BERGMANN-PORTER, Eleonore; 12 Vancouver St., Yarmouth, N.S.; Munich (Germ.)'33; Edinburgh (Scot.)'34; MCGP; Staff, Yarmouth Hosp.; Tel. 742-3471.
BERGSAGEL, Daniel E.; 500 Sherbourne St., Toronto, Ont.; Man '49; D.Phil. (Oxon.); ABIM; Assoc. Prof. (Med.), U. of Toronto; Chief of Med., Princess Margaret Hosp.; Tel. 924-0671, Ext. 419.
BERGNER, Harvey A.; Man '61; Res., Winnipeg Gen. Hosp., Winnipeg, Man.
BERGSTROME, Brant E.; 172 East St., Napanee, Ont.; McG '52; Court. Staff, Kingston Gen. & Hotel-Dieu Hosp's.; Chmn., Bd. of Dir., Lennox & Aldington County Gen. Hosp., Napanee; Tel. 354-4661.
BERILGEN, Abuzer; Ankara (Turkey) '56; Jr. Int.. St. Paul's Hosp., Saskatoon, Sask.
BERKELEY, James A.; 2523 St. John St., Port Moody, B.C.; Qns'45; M.C.G.P.
BERKELEY, Joseph; 1273 Ouellette Ave., Windsor, Ont.; Glasgow (Scot.) '43; DPH; PhysMed; Chief Cons. (PhysMed.), Windsor Hosp's.; Red Cross Centre & Cedar Springs Ontario Hosp.; Tel. CL 6-4692.
BERKELEY, Kenneth H.; 203 Water St. N., Galt, Ont.; 37 Parkwood Dr. (res); Qns '53; M.C.G.P.; Tel. 623-0271.
BERKMAN, Emily J. (Gear); 217 Melrose, Ottawa 3, Ont.; Tor '49; ObstGyn; Att'd. Staff, Ottawa Civic Hosp., & Ont. Cancer Clinic; Clin Instr. Ottawa U.; Tel. PA 9-7903.
BERKMAN, Franklin; 217 Melrose Ave., Ottawa, Ont.; (res); Qns '49; M.Sc.; FRCP(C); IntMed (Cardiol); Dir. Card. Unit., Ottawa Gen. Hosp.; Assoc. Prof. Med. Ottawa U.; Tel. 236-0333.
BERKMAN, Paul; 437 Grosvenor Ave., Montreal 6, P.Q.; Basel (Switz.) '27; Staff Anaes., Doctor's Hospital; Tel. RE 9-7771.
BERKS, Gerald; 1590 Ouellette Ave., Windsor, Ont.; 3510 Ouellette Ave. (res); Lon. U. (Eng.) '54; Phys., Riverview Hosp.; Tel. 256-4155.
BERKSON, Nathan; Rm. 201, 352 Dorval Ave., Dorval, Lachine, P.Q.; 5603 Westminster Ave., Mtl. 28 (res); McG '49; GenSurg; Staff, Lachine Gen. Hosp.; Cons., Sherwin-Williams Co.; Tel. 631-8530.
BERLAS, Naeema (See Matuk)
BERLIN, Seymour; 895 Bloor St. W., Toronto 4, Ont.; 526 Briar Hill Ave. (res); Tor '62; Staff, Mount Sinai & Doctor's Hosp's.; Tel. 537-2527.
BERLINGUET, Lorne; 747 Laviolette St., Three Rivers, P.Q.; McG '37.
BERMAN, Bennie; 25 Brunswick Ave., Toronto 4, Ont.; 1 Chadwick Ave., Tor. 10 (res); Tor '53; Urol; Staff (Urol.), Doctors' Hosp.; Tel. WA 3-5541.
BERMAN, Graham; 7040 Chester Ave., Montreal 29, P.Q.; Otago (N. Zealand) '60; FRCP(C), Psy; Staff, Children's Hosp.; Tel. WE 7-8511.
BERNARD, Albert; Ste. 519, 30 est Boul. St. Joseph, Montreal 14, P.Q.; 2445 rue Haig (res); Mon '51 FRCP(C); IntMed; Cardiol (P.Q.); Staff, Hop. Ste Jeanne d'Arc.; Tel. 845-4251.
BERNARD, Denis; Man '63; Res. Hop. Maisonneuvre, Montreal, P.Q.
BERNARD, Fernand; St. Joseph de Beauce, P.Q.; Lav '53.
BERNARD, Gilles; 306 E. Boulv. St. Joseph, Mtl. 14, P.Q.; 550 Davaar Ave., Outremont 8 (res); Paris (Fr.) '54; ObstGyn (P.Q.); Ass't., Hop.-de-la-Misericorde; Tel. 849-9865.
BERNARD, Gilles; C.P. 31, Ste. 216, 129 Principale, Rouyn, P.Q.; Lav '54.
BERNARD, J. Andre; 87 Montenach, Longueuil, Montreal 23, P.Q.; Mon '57; Tel. 677-1936.
BERNARD, Jean-Guy; 372-lere ave., St-Georges Est, P.Q.; Lav '65.
BERNARD, Louis-C.; 1058 St. Denis, Montreal, P.Q.; Mon'29; GenSurg; Gyn(P.Q.); Dir., Hop. St. Luc.; Tel. 861-7321.
BERNARD, Louis E.; Lav'64; Res., Hop. Ste Justine, Montreal 9, P.Q.
BERNARD, P. Louis; 800 Cherrier, Montreal 24, P.Q.; Mon '45; GenSurg (P.Q.); Tel. LA 3-2883.
BERNARD, Real; C.P. 128, Beauceville Ouest, P.Q.; Lav '63.
BERNARD, Renald M.; 670-1ere Ave. est, St. Georges, P.Q.; Lav'65.
BERNARDO, Isagni R.; Santo Tomas '60; Jr. Intn., Ottawa Civic Hosp., Ottawa, Ont.
BERNATCHEZ, Jean P.; Lav'65; Res., Hop. St. Michel Archange, Quebec 5, P.Q.
BERNATH, Joseph G.; 306 Boul. St. Joseph E., Montreal 14, P.Q.; 11405 Frigon (res); Munich (Germ.) '52; Cardiol. (PQ); Cardiol., Hop.-St.-Luc; Ass't. Prof., U. of Montreal; Tel. 844-4114.

BERNDT, Peter U.; 331-3rd Line, Oakville, Ont.; Tor '62; Staff, Oakville-Trafalgar, Mem. Hosp.; Tel. VA 7-4144.
BERNE, Maurice; 368 Redfern Ave., Montreal 6, P.Q.; Mon '28; Otol, (P.Q.); Ass't. (ORL), Reddy Mem. Hosp.; Tel. WE 2-5800.
BERNECHE, Roland; Maskinonge, P.Q.; Lav '34;
BERNER, Cecil A.; 438 Professional Bldg., 10830 Jasper Ave., Edmonton, Alta.; 13644 Ravine Dr. (res); Man'39; Staff, Royal Alexandra Hosp.; Tel. 422-8581.
BERNER, George; 400 Spadina Ave., Toronto 2B, Ont.; Tor '60; Court. Staff, Toronto Western & Doctor's Hosp's.; Pt.-time Instr. (Russian), U. of Toronto; Tel. EM 6-5152.
BERNER, M. Barbara (Richards); 2007 Danforth Ave., Toronto 6, Ont.; 27 Restwell Cres., Willowdale (res); Tor '54; M.C.G.P.; Tel. OX 9-3396.
BERNESKE, Gerald M.; 19 Dundas St. W., Waterdown, Ont.; Tor '39; Coroner, Twp. of East Flamboro.
BERNIER, Andre G.; C.P. 68, 95 Ave. Principale, Amos, P.Q.; 192-12th Ave. (res); Lav '54; A.M.C.G.P.; Anaes., Hotel Dieu d'Amos.
BERNIER, Andre H.; 298 St-Germain, Rimouski, P.Q.; Lav '55; FRCS(C); ObstGyn; Tel. 723-2180.
BERNIER, Gilles; 1150 Est Boul. St. Joseph, Montreal 34, P.Q.; Mon'58; FRCS(C); ObstGyn; Staff, Hop. Maisonneuve.
BERNIER, Gilles; Mon '64; Int., Hop. Maisonneuve, Montreal, P.Q.
BERNIER, Jacques; 3990 Lacombe, Montreal, P.Q. (res); Mon '44; FRCP(C), IntMed; Dir. Dept. of Med., Hop. St.-Luc; Tel. UN 1-7261.
BERNIER, Jacques Major; RCAF Station Namao, Lancaster Park, Edmonton, Alta.; Lav'56; DMRD; DiagRad.
BERNIER, Jean J.; Box 158, Noranda, P.Q.; Lav '50; GenSurg (P.Q.).
BERNIER, J. M. Wellie; 248 Principale, La Sarre P.Q.; 17 Blvd. Allard (res); Lav '34; Med. Dir., Hop. St. Francois; Tel. FE 3-2311.
BERNIER, Leonard; 901 Ave Rochette, Quebec 10, P.Q.; Lav '53; Path; Staff, Hop. Hotel Dieu, Quebec: Tel. 529-9151.
BERNIER, Louis J.; Benito, Man.; Man '57.
BERNIER, Marcel; 825 est Blvd. St. Joseph Montreal, P.Q.; Mon '27; Tel. VI 4-1668.
BERNIER, Maurice; 31 Brooks S., Sherbrooke, P.Q Lav '50; OrthSurg (P.Q.); Tel. 567-7252.
BERNIER, Paul E.; 6701 Delorimier Ave., Montreal 35, P.Q.; Mon'48; Staff, Dept. of Health, City of Montreal.
BERNIER, Raymond; 2725 Chemin-Ste.-Foy, Quebec 10, P.Q.; 3004 La Promenade (res); Lav '55; DABR; D & T Rad; Radiol., Hop-Laval & Cardiol. Inst.; Tel. 653-5251.
BERNO, Ernesto; 815 Victoria St., Trail, B.C.; UBC'63.
BERNSTEIN, Aaron D.; McG '61; M.O., Sioux Lookout Indian Hosp., Sioux Lookout, Ont.
BERNSTEIN, Abraham; 158 St. George St., Toronto, Ont.; 54 Old Park Rd. (res); Tor '51; F.R.C.S.(C), ObstGyn; Att. Staff, New Mount Sinai Hosp. Tel. WA 3-4234.
BERNSTEIN, Felix; 320 Ellendale Med. Bldg., 5845 Cote-des-Neiges Rd., Montreal 26, P.Q.; 6275 Northwest Pl. Apt 721 (res); McG '21; IntMed. (P.Q.); Hon. Att'd. Staff, Montreal Gen. Hosp.; Att. Staff, Jewish Gen. Hosp.; Court. Staff, Royal Victoria Hosp.; Tel. RE 1-1000.
BERNSTEIN, George I.; 1428 Ouellette Ave., Windsor, Ont.; 930 Riverside Dr., Riverside (res); Tor '50; F.A.C.S., F.A.A.O.S., D.A.B.O.S, F.I.C.S.; Orth Surg; Chief, (Orth Sect.) Grace Hosp.; Att'd. Staff, Metropolitan & Hotel-Dieu Hosp's; Cons. Orth., Riverview Hosp.; Tel. 253-4673.
BERNSTEIN, Merton; 220 Tecumseh Rd. W., Windsor, Ont.; Tor'50; Ophth; Tel. 256-3386.
BERNSTEIN, Philip H.; 135-6th Ave., Cochrane, Ont.; 171-7th Ave. (res); Qns '34; M.C.G.P.; Staff, Lady Minto Hosp.; Dist. Coroner; Tel. 272-3276.
BERRIS, Barnet; 550 University Ave., Toronto 2, Ont.; Tor '44; M.S., FRCP(C), IntMed; Chief of Med., New Mount Sinai Hosp.; Tel. 366-7171.
BERRY, Arthur G.; 73 Mandeville Dr., St. Thomas, Ont. (res); Qns '32; Staff, Ontario Hosp., St. Thomas; Tel. ME 1-8510.
BERRY, Brian H.; 240 Duplex Ave., Toronto, Ont.; Tor '27; M.C.G.P. Tel. HU 9-4221.
BERRY, Gerald R.; Dal '59; AMCGP; Res., Montreal Gen. Hosp., Montreal 25, P.Q.
BERRY, Frank; Liverpool (Eng.)'52; Ass't. Path., Providence Hosp. & Union Hosp.; Moose Jaw, Sask.; Tel. 692-1841.
BERRY, Henry; 170 St. George St., Ste. 407, Toronto 5, Ont.; Tor '54; D.Psy; FRCP(C), IntMed; Neurol; MRCP (Lond); Clin. Teach. (Med.), U. of Toronto Tel. 921-4903.
BERRY, James W.; 240 Brock St., Kingston, Ont.; Qns '58; Tel. 542-5810.
BERRY, J. Ralph; 101 Rideau Medical Centre, 1711-4th St. S.W., Calgary, Alta; 4427 Britania Dr. (res); Alta '39; OphthOtol; Staff, Calgary Gen., Holy Cross & Children's Hosp's.; Cons. RCAF; Tel 262-3240 & 269-3440.
BERRY, J. Victor; Ste. 505, 267 O'Connor St., Ottawa 4, Ont.; 39 Buena Vista Rd., Rockcliffe (res); Qns'31; FACS; Urol; Assoc. Chief (Urol), Ottawa Civic Hosp.; Sr. Lect. (Urol.), U. of Ottawa; Tel. 722-8536.
BERRY, Kenneth; 1081 Burrard St., Vancouver 1, B.C.; UBC'56; FRCP(C); Neurol; Chief, Div. of Neurol., St. Paul's Hosp.; Chief Instr., (Neurol.) & Paed., U. of British Columbia; Tel. MU 2-2344.
BERRY, Marion; Ste. 204, 1160 W. 13th Ave., Vancouver 9, B.C.; London (Eng.) '50; DA (Eng.); FRCP(C); Anaes; Staff, St. Paul's Hosp.; Tel. RE 1-1882.
BERRY, Nathan E.; 119 Queen's Cres., Kingston, Ont. (res); Qns '26; Urol; Prof. of Urol., Queen's U.; Retired.
BERRY, Ronald E.; 266 Oxford St., London, Ont.; Wes'57; MCGP; Staff, St. Joseph's, St. Mary's & Victoria Hosps.
BERRY, R. Staveley; Box 10, Tweed, Ont.; McG'52; M.C.G.P.; Active Staff, Belleville Gen. Hosp.; Coroner, Hastings and Lennox & Addington Counties; M.O.H., Hungerford Twp.; Tel. 478-3315.
BERRY, William E.; Wallace St., Woodbridge, Ont.; Qns '14.
BERTALANFFY, Felix D.; 886 Lindsay St., Winnipeg 9, Man. (res); McG '54; Assoc. Prof. Anat., Fac. of Med. & Dentistry, U. of Man.; Tel. 786-3651.
BERTHIAUME, Charles A.; 433 Blvd. St. Joseph E., Montreal 34, P.Q.; Mon '38; OphthOtol; Tel. VI 9-5122.
BERTHIAUME, Jogues; 3220 Louis Dantin, Montreal 9, P.Q. (res); Mon '54; Anaes (P.Q.); Staff, Hop.-Sacre-Coeur, Cartierville; Tel. 334-1210.
BERTHIAUME, J. Pierre; Mon'65; Res., Inst. Albert Prevost, Montreal, P.Q.
BERTHIAUME, Lorenzo; 2802 Blvd. Rosemont, Montreal, P.Q.; Mon '28; Tel. 721-5046.
BERTHIAUME, Marcel; 1037 Est, Boul. St-Joseph, Montreal 34, P.Q.; Mon '49; Psy; Scien. Dir., Hop.-St-Jean-de-Dieu; Tel. VI 1-7804.
BERTHO, Emile M.; 446 rue de Tilly Chicoutimi, P.Q. (res); Paris (Fr.) '50; FACS, FACG, FACCP, FACAS, AFACC, FICS, FICA, FRCS(C), GenSurg; ThorSurg (PQ); Chief, Cardiovas. & Thor. Surg. (Clin. & Experim.), Hotel-Dieu-St.-Vallier; Tel. 549-1312.
BERTRAM, Alice W.; 32 Cross St., Dundas, Ont. (res); Qns '48; Retired.
BERTRAM, Lee I.; 11655-73rd Ave., Edmonton, Alta.; Wes '48; Staff, Dept. of Health, Edmonton: Tel. 439-6149.
BERTRAND, Charles; 233 Ch. Ste. Catherine, Montreal, P.Q.; Lav '15; Tel. 272-7337.
BERTRAND, Claude; 1392 Sherbrooke St. E., Montreal 24, P.Q.; 15 Springrove Cres., Outremont (res); Mon '40; F.R.C.S.(C), NeurSurg; Chief of Neur. Surg., Hop. Notre Dame; Ass't. Prof. Surg., U. of Montreal; Tel. LA 6-0491.
BERTRAND, Giguere; 238 sud, Notre-Dame, Thetford Mines, P.Q.; Lav '53; IntMed.

BERTRAND, Gilles G. P.; 3801 University, Montreal, P.Q.; 385 Lethbridge (res); Mon '49; F.R.C.S.(C), NeurSurg; Assoc. NeurSurg. & Ass't. Neurpath., Montreal Neurol. Inst.; Head, Dept. of NeurSurg., McGill U.; Tel. AV 8-7064.
BERTRAND, Guy; 3125 rue de Galais, Ste. Foy, Quebec 10, P.Q.; Lav'53; Gastroent (P.Q.); Staff, Hop. de l'Enfant-Jesus & Laval U.; Tel. 653-7753.
BERTRAND, Guy L.; 126 rue Brooks Sud., Sherbrooke, P.Q.; Mon '34; FACS; FICS; GenSurg; Chief Surg., Hotel-Dieu Hosp.; Tel. LO 2-7975.
BERTRAND, J. Albert; 6275 Northcrest Pl., Montreal 8, P.Q.; Mon '19; Bact; Bacteriol., Hop.-Notre-Dame; Prof. Emerit., U. of Montreal; Tel. 525-6363, Loc. 572.
BERTRAND, J. H., 476 St. Cyrille, Quebec, P.Q.; Mon '22.
BERTRAND, Leopold R.; 440 Beaubien E.; Montreal 10, P.Q.; 10407 Grande Allee (res); Mon '41; Tel. 277-4094.
BERTRAND, Marc; Lav'55; Res., Hop. Sacre-Coeur, Montreal 9, P.Q.; Lav'55.
BERTRAND, Maurice; 241 Fleury St. W., Montreal, P.Q.; Mon '56; A.M.C.G.P.; Tel. 381-7281.
BERTRAND, Norris R.; 65 Academy Med. Bldg., 1812-4th St. W., Calgary, Alta.; Alb'48; St. (res); Alb '48; FACOG;ObstGyn; Tel. 262-3872.
BERTRAND, Paul-E.; 770-1ere Ave., Quebec 3, P.Q.; 5945-3ere Ave. E. (res); Lav '54; Tel. 529-0042.
BERTRAND, Pierre; Mon '58; FRCS(C), OrthSurg; Staff, Hop. Jean-Talon, Montreal 35, P.Q.
BERTRAND, Pierre; 30 est Boul. St.-Joseph, Montreal 14, P.Q.; 10055 Verville (res); Mon '53; PulmDis & TB. (P.Q.); Tel. 845-4241.
BERTRAND, Pierre E.; Mon '60; FRCS(C), Urol; Staff, Hop. Maisonneuve, Montreal, P.Q.; Tel. 254-8341.
BERTRAND, Robert; 156 Rue Ashton, Ville St. Laurent, Montreal, P.Q.; Mon '59; DiagRad; Staff, Hop. Ste. Justine; Tel. RE 1-4931.
BERTRAND, Robert A.; Ste. 301, 801 est rue Sherbrooke, Montreal, P.Q.: Mon'58; FRCS(C); Otol; McLaughlin Fell.

BERUBE, Adrien; 82 Brooks St. S., Sherbrooke, P.Q.; Lav '20; GenSurg (P.Q.); Surg., St. Vincent de Paul Hosp.; Assoc. Surg., Sherbrooke & Hotel Dieu Hosp's; Tel. LO 2-1414.
BERUBE, Gaeton; 294 St. Germain, Rimouski, P. Q.; Lav '52; Tel. 723-3461.
BERUBE, Gilbert Sg/Lt; Lav '64; RCNH, Cornwallis, N.S.
BERUBE, Guy; 298 rue St.-Germain, Rimouski, P.Q.; Lav '49; Ophth (PQ); Otol; Tel. 723-2361.
BERUBE, Marius; Compton, Cte Compton, P.Q.; Lav '58; Tel. 835-5408.
BERUBE, Medard; 8 Court, Edmundston, N.B.; Lav '64.
BERUBE, Rosaire; C.P. 1150 Amos, Co. Abitibi, P.Q.; Lav '41; DPH; PH(P.Q.); Tel. 732-3537.

BESANT, Donald F.; 211 Med. Arts Bldg., 404 Graham Ave., Winnipeg 1, Man.; 31 Cascade Bay, St. Boniface 6 (res); Man '54; Paed; Staff, Wpg. Children's, St. Boniface Gen. & Grace Hosp's.; Lect. (Paed.), U. of Manitoba; Tel. 942-5912.

BESECKER, Lester D.; Kaslo, B.C.

BESLEY, J. Keith, Lt.Col.; Nat. Defence Med. Centre, Smyth & Alta Vista, Ottawa 8, Ont.; Tor '50; GenSurg; Tel. 733-6600.

BESMARGIAN, Marie J.; 80, Brooks, Sherbrooke, P.Q.; Lav '56; Paed (P.Q.).
BESNER, Claude; 191 Commerciale, Maniwaki, P.Q.; Ott'64.
BESNEY, Morris; 6414-118th Ave., Edmonton, Alta.; 9302 Edinboro Rd. (res); Alb '48; F.A.C.S., F.R.C.S.(C) GenSurg; Att'd. Staff, Royal Alexandra & Misericordia Hosp's.; Instr., U. of Alberta; Tel. GR 7-8827.

BESSELL, John A.; The Rowell Clinic, Carbonear, Nfld.; Cambridge (Eng.)'56; DObstRCOG.

BESSETTE, Gerard; 4395 Verdun, Montreal 19, P.Q.; 2A Sioux St., Log Village, Fabreville (res); Lav '49; D & T Rad; Staff, Hop.-Maisonneuve; Tel. VI 2-4892.
BESSETTE, Jean; 336 Hall St., St. Lambert, P.Q.; Lav '57; Anaes; Staff, Hop. St-Lambert; Tel. 677-7227.
BESSETTE, Marcel; 129 Peres Eudistes, Chandler, Cte Gaspe, P.Q.; Mon '51; GenSurg (P.Q.); Staff Hop. de la Providence; Tel. 516.
BESSONETTE, John; Shannon Med. Clinic, 34 Pleasant St., Dartmouth, N.S.; Dal'65.
BEST, Brian D.; The Winnipeg Clinic, Winnipeg, Man.; 133 Montrose St. (res); Man '34; F.R.C.S. (E), F.R.C.S. (C), ObstGyn; Assoc. Obst. Gyn., Winnipeg Gen. Hosp.; Prof. Obst. Gyn., U. of Manitoba; Obst. Gyn., Winnipeg Clinic; Tel. 942-0551.
BEST, Charles H., CBE; Chas. H. Best Inst., 112 College St., Toronto 2, Ont.; 105 Woodlawn Ave. W. (res); Tor '25; M.A., M.D. (Tor.), D.Sc. (Lond., Chic., Oxford, Cantab., Laval); M.D. (Hon.) (Paris, Amsterdam, Louvain, Liege); Ll.D. (Dalhousie, Queens, Melbourne, Edinburgh); F.R.C.S., F.R.S., F.R.C.P. (Eng.), F.R.C.P.(C); Dir., Banting & Best, Dept. of Med. Research & Dept. of Physiol., U. of Toronto; Tel. 928-2586.
BEST, Christopher N.; Port Arthur Clinic, Port Arthur, Ont.; London (Eng.) '50; M.R.C.P. (Edin.), F.R.C.P. (C), IntMed.; Tel. 344-7271.
BEST, Douglas W. S.; 2066 Blairholm Ave., Burlington, Ont. (res); Tor '43; Anaes; Active Staff, St. Joseph's Hosp., Hamilton, Ont.; Tel. 522-4941.
BEST, Edward W.; 735 Highland Ave., Ottawa 13, (res); Tor '44; D.P.H., PH.; Chief Epidemiology Div. Dept. of Nat'l. Health & Welfare; Tel. CE 2-8211.
BEST, Ray G.; 405 Canada Bldg., Ouellette Ave., Windsor, Ont.; 1210 Dougall Rd. (res); Tor '50; Ophth; Surg. Staff, Metropolitan & Hotel Dieu Hosp's.; Teach. Staff, Grace Hosp.; Tel. 253-6355.
BEST, Stanley C.; 2945 Rae St., Regina, Sask. (res); Tor '43; M.P.H., F.A.P.H.A., F.A.A.P.; Paed; Dir. Div. of Child Health, Dept. of Public Health; Lectr., U. of Saskatchewan; Tel. LA 3-0611. Abroad.
BESWICK, John A. Lt. Col.; 1842 Playfair Dr., Ottawa 8, Ont.; Tor '50; Ophth; Hd., Dept. of Ophth., National Defence Med. Centre; Hon. Cons. (Ophth.), Ottawa Gen. Hosp.
BETHUME, Clarence M., M.B.E.; 1597 Oxford St., Halifax, N.S. (res); Dal '31; Anaes, Admin., Victoria Gen. Hosp.; Prof. (Admin.), Dalhousie U.; Tel. 422-7371.
BETHUNE, Gordon W.; Med. Arts Bldg., 5880 Spring Garden Rd., Halifax, N.S.; 100 Oxford St. (res); Dal '43; F.R.C.S.(C), GenSurg; Assoc. Surg., Victoria Gen. Hosp.; Ass't. Prof., Dalhousie U.; Tel. 2-4406.
BETHUNE, Richard D.; 57 Wilson St., Ancaster, Ont.; Tor'58; AMCGP; Active Staff, Chedoke Gen., Hamilton Gen. & St. Joseph's Hosp's., Hamilton; Tel. MI 8-1111.
BETKOWSKI, Jerzy P.; Jasper Med. Group, 517 Geikie St., Jasper, Alta.; Polish Med. Schl. (Edinburgh, Scot.) '47; L.R.C.P. (Lond.), M.R.C.S. (Eng.); GenSurg; Dist. Coroner; Tel. 852-3434.
BETTER, Ned; Linton Clinic, 6000 Cote des Neiges Rd., Montreal 26, P.Q.; 3127 Brighton Ave. (res); Geneva (Switz.) '54; GenSurg; Jr. Ass't Dept. of Surg., Jewish Gen. Hosp., Vis. Staff, Bellechase Hosp.; Tel. 739-4546.
BETTEZ, Paul; 16 Place Le Roy, Repentigny, P.Q.; Lav'55; FRCP(C), Path.
BETTS, Douglas H.; Dal '61; Res. (Psy.), Montreal Children's Hosp., Montreal, P.Q.
BETZNER, Norman E.; 213 Hammond Bldg.; Moose Jaw, Sask; 1030—1st St. N. E. (res); Tor '15; M.R.C.S. (Eng.), L.R.C.P. (Lond.); Tel. 692-5119.
BEUGLET, Ernest; 605 Med. Arts Bldg., 1011 Ouellette Ave., Windsor, Ont.; 6280 Riverside Dr. (res); Wes '28; Otol; Sr. Active Staff (Otol.), Hotel-Dieu Hosp.; Tel. 256-9598.
BEVER, Jurgen G. F.; 114 Medical Arts Bldg., Fort William, Ont.; 410 Oakdale Cres. (res); Goettingen (Germ.) '47; MCGP; Tel MA 2-6459.
BEVERIDGE, George; 261 Talbot St. E., Aylmer, Ont.; Edinburgh (Scot.) '52; MCGP; Active Staff, St. Thomas Elgin Gen. Hosp.; Tel. 773-8406.

BEVERIDGE, James M.; Wes '50; Ph.D., FRSC; President Acadia Univ., Wolfville, N.S.
BEVERIDGE, Kenneth; 32 Wellington St. E.; Aurora, Ont.; Durham (Eng.)'59.
BEVERIDGE, Thomas F.; Carberry Med Centre, Carberry, Man.; Glasgow (Scot.)'57; Chief of Staff, Fox Mem. Hosp.; Tel. 133.
BEVERSTEIN, Jacob; 1758A Victoria Pk. Ave., Scarborough, Ont.; 60 Amsterdam Ave. (res); **Bologna (Italy) '38; A.M.C.G.P.; Tel. PL 5-3422.**
BEWICK, John B.; 115 Hazen St., Saint John, N.B.; 24 Seely St. (res); McG '51; IntMed; Staff, Saint John Gen. St. Joseph's & Lancaster DVA Hosp's; Tel. 692-1311.
BEWS, Donald C.; 41 Tunstall Ave., Senneville, P.Q. (res); **Qns '35; D.P.H., D.T.M., D.A.B.** PrevMed, Med. Dir. Bell Telephone Co. of Canada —1050 Beaver Hall Hill, Rm. 800, Montreal; Lect. **Dept. of Health & Soc. Med. McGill U.; Tel. 870-2903.**
BEZEREDI, Tibor; 4400 Grandview H'way, Burnaby 2, B.C.; UBC'60; Psy.
BEZNAK, Aladar B. L.; 15 Boucherville Ave., Hull, P.Q.; Debrecen (Hung.) '24; Prof. Emer. (Physiol.), U. of Ottawa, Ottawa, Ont.
BEZNAK, Margaret (Hortobagyi); 61 Reid Ave., Ottawa 3, Ont. (res); Budapest (Hung.)'39; Prof. Physiology & Hd. Dept., U. of Ottawa; Tel. PR 1-2349.
BHALA, Ram P.; Punjab (India)'59; PhysMed. & Rehab.; Staff, Toronto East Gen. Hosp., Toronto 6, Ont.; Abroad.
BHALLA, Shri K.; Panjab (India)'58; GenSurg; Staff, Toronto East Gen. Hosp., Toronto, Ont.
BHAMBHANI, Madhu D.; Agra (India)'55; Anaes; Staff, Royal Victoria Hosp., Mtl. 2, P.Q.
BHARADWAJ, Baikunta B.; Nagpur (India) '59; Int., Hosp. for Sick Children, Toronto, Ont.
BHARGAVA, Usha; 417 Billings Ave., Ottawa 8, Ont.; Lucknow (India) '56; M.O., Dept. of National Health & Welfare.
BHATIA, Mahomedali G.; Birmingham (Eng.)'54; Res., Calgary Gen. Hosp., Calgary, Alta.
BHATTACHARYYA, Amal; Calcutta (India)'59; Staff, Nova Scotia Hosp., Dartmouth, N.S.
BHAVAKULA, Kalapangha; 180 Madison Ave., Toronto 5, Ont.; Thailand'56; FRCP(C), Anaes.
BHAVNANI, Mulchand J.; Breton, Alta.; London (Eng.) '48; Tel. 696-3676.
BHERER, Robert; St. Cesaire, Cte. Rouville, P.Q.; Lay '51; M.C.G.P.
BIANCHI, Fernando A.; Ste. 700A, 155 St. James St. S., Hamilton, Ont.; Ott'59; IntMed.
BIANCO, Mario A.; 10 Mountain Ash Court, Etobicoke, Ont. (res); Rome (Italy) '53; Anaes; Staff, St. Joseph's Hosp.; Tel. 255-1252.
BIBAUD, Barthelemi; 65 rue Nicholson, Valleyfield, P.Q.; 110 rue St. Jean-Baptiste (res); Mon **'17; DiagRad (P.Q.); Tel. 373-2123.**
BICE, William K.; Wes '30; Staff, Ont. Hosp., St. Thomas, Ont.; Tel. ME 1-8510.
BICKFORD, Frederick L.; 607 Dawson St., Port Arthur, Ont.; 133 Hill St. S. (res); Man '24.
BICKLE, Graham S.; 960 Eagle Cr., London, Ont.; Wes'61.
BICKLE, John A.; Workmen's Comp. Bd., 737 W. 37th Ave., Vancouver, B.C.; 1056 W. 46th **Ave. (res); McG '29; Tel. AM 6-0211.**
BICKLE, Margaret E.; 2058 Culp St., Niagara Falls, Ont.; Tor '35; DMRT; Diag Rad; Rad., **Greater Niagara Gen. Hosp.; Tel. EL 8-3611.**
BICUM, G.; Elstow, Sask.; Qns '22; M.C.G.P.; Dist. Coroner.
BIDWELL, Peter A.; 26 Water St., Chippawa, Ont.; Wes'65.
BIE, William F.; Ste. 1013, 750 W. Broadway, **Vancouver, B.C.; 719 Eyremount Dr., W. Vanc.** (res); McG '39; ObstGyn; Sr. (ObstGyn), Vancouver Gen. Hosp; **Clin. Assoc. Prof. (ObstGyn), U. of British Columbia; Tel. TR 2-5484.**
BIECHL-O'Neill, Anna see O'NEILL (Biechl), Anna.
BIEHN, John T.; Medical Centre, 168 Essex St., Sarnia, Ont.; Wes'62; AMCGP; Tel. 337-8566.
BIEHN, J. Telford; 282 Wellington St., Sarnia, Ont.; 327 N. Brock St. (res); Tor '30; Ophth, Otol; Tel. ED 7-2242.
BIELY, G. Gordon; 3485 Atwater Ave., Montreal 25, P.Q.; UBC **'58; D. Psy;** Psy; Sr. Instr. (Psy.), Montreal Gen. Hosp.; Dem. (Psy.) & Lect. (Phys. & Occ. Ther.), **McGill U.; Tel.** 937-7057. Abroad.
BIEN, Ernest; 4790 Cote des Neiges, Montreal, P.Q.; Vienna (Austria) '23; Tel. 737-9985.
BIER, N. B.; Tor '63; Staff, St. Anthony Hosp., St. Anthony, Nfld.; Abroad.
BIEZUNER, John J.; 69 Sherman Ave. S., Hamilton, Ont.; 53 Colquhoun Cres. (res); **Paris (Fr.) '39; F.C.C.P., F.A.C.P., M.C.G.P.; Staff (Indoor Med.), Hamilton Gen. Hosp.; Tel. LI 5-3288.**
BIGELOW, D. R.; 325 Med. Arts Bldg., Winnipeg, Man.; 152 Leighton Ave. (res); Man '48; Am. Bd. P.T.I. (Orth); OrthSurg; Assoc. Staff, St. Boniface Hosp.; Temp. (Orth) Staff, Deer Lodge Mil. Hosp.; Lect. (Orth), U. of Manitoba; **Tel. WH 3-8853.**
BIGELOW, George B.; 1121 Yates St., Victoria, B.C.; 995 Terrace Ave. (res); Edinburgh (Scot.) '32; Anaes; Chief Anaes., Victoria Vet's. Hosp.; Tel. EV 5-3465.
BIGELOW, H. M.; 4462 W—10th Ave., Vancouver 8, B.C. (res); Man '34; Tel. CA 8-8333.
BIGELOW, Jesse K.; Bigelow Fowler Clinic 1605-9th Ave. S., Lethbridge, Alta.; Qns '24.
BIGELOW, L. H.; 39 Owen St., Barrie, Ont.; Tor '24.
BIGELOW, Wilfred A.; 41 Clement Bldg., Brandon, Man.; **Man '03;** F.A.C.S., GenSurg.
BIGELOW, Wilfred G.; 709 Med. Arts Bldg., 170 St. George St., Toronto 5, Ont.; 137 Douglas Dr. (res); Tor '38; M.S., F.A.C.S., F.R.C.S.(C), Gen-**Surg; Sr. Surg; Hd. Div. of Cardiovasc. Surg.,** Toronto Gen. Hosp.; Cons. (Cardio-Vasc. Surg.) Women's College Hosp. & Sunnybrook Hosp.; Bd. of Dir. Ont. Heart Fdn. & Memb. Defence Research Bd.; Assoc. Prof. (Surg.), U. of Toronto; Tel. 923-9784.
BIGELOW, William L.; Main St., Atwood, Ont.; Tor '56; Staff, Listowel Mem. Hosp.; Court. Staff, Stratford Gen. Hosp.; Tel. Area 519; 356-2642.
BIGFORD, Ray A.; Maple, Ont.; Qns '23; M.C.G.P.
BIGONESE, Pierre; 722 Chanoine Scott, nord, Ste. Foy, Quebec 10, P.Q.; '62; Paed(P.Q.).
BIGORNIA, Generoso V.; 15 Eastgate, Winnipeg 1, Man. (res); Santo Tomas (Philippines) '54; **Anaes; Staff, Winnipeg Gen. Hosp.; Tel. SP 4-6511.**
BIGRAS, Jean M.; 61 Guigues St., Ottawa, Ont. (res); Mon'32; Staff, Ottawa Gen. Hosp.; Tel. CE 4-2509.
BIGRAS, Julien; 3100 Ellendale, Montreal 26, P.Q.; Mon'58; Psy.
BIGUE, Germain; 1076-7eme rue, Val d'Or, P.Q.; 980 Blvd. Forest (res); Lav '38; FICS; GenSurg; Chief Surg., Hop.-St.Sauveur; Tel. 824-6823.
BIGUE, Paul; 449-3rd Ave., Quebec, P.Q.; 1070-de Montigny (res); Lav '38; Ophth Otol (P.Q.); Tel. 529-1765.
BIKADOROFF, Serge; 5025 Sherbrooke St. W., Montreal 6, P.Q.; **McG '58; Psy; Staff,** Jewish Gen. & **Queen Elizabeth Hosp's.; Clin.** Instr. (Psy.) McGill U.; Tel. 488-5774.
BILBEY, Douglas L. J.; Box 608, 100 Mile House, B.C.; London (Eng.)'63; Ph.D.
BILDFELL, John A.; Lansdowne, Ont.; Man '33; Tel. 274.
BILEFSKY, Ralph; McG '61; Res. (Path.), Royal Victoria Hosp., Montreal, P.Q.
BILLARD, Albert C.; 269 King Avenue, Bathurst, N.B.; Dal'51; GenSurg; Tel. 546-6794.
BILLETTE, Jacques; Mon'65; Res., Dept. of Psy., Univ. of Montreal, Montreal, P.Q.
BILLINGS, Roger M.; 401 Earl St., Kingston, Ont. (res); Qns '38; D.Psy., Psy.; Dir. Provincial Mental Health Clinic, Kingston; **Clin. Lect. Psy., Queen's U.; Cons., Kingston Gen., Belleville &** Pembroke Hosp's; Tel. 546-1101.
BILLINGS, Ronald F.; 901 O'Connor Dr., Toronto 16, Ont.; 31 Denver Cres., Willowdale (res); Tor '54; D.Psy: Psy; Staff, Tor. East Gen. Hosp.; Tel. 759-9521.

BILLUNG-MEYER, Wiechmann; 505 Campbell Bldg., 1029 Douglas St., Victoria, B.C.; UBC '62; AMCGP; Tel. EV 6-3561.
BILODEAU, Henri P.; 465-5eme rue, Shawinigan, P.Q.; Lav '53. Cardiol. (P.Q.).
BILODEAU, Marcel; 73 de l'Eglise, Windsor, P.Q.; Lav '60.
BILODEAU, Marcel; Lav '60; Staff, Hop. Laval, Quebec 10, P.Q.
BILODEAU, Rolland; Ste. 320, 30 est boul. St. Joseph, Montreal 14, P.Q.; Mon'60; Obst; Staff, Hop. Maisonneuve; Tel. 845-4241.
BILSBARROW, Georges; 53 White St., Dryden, Ont.; Earl St. (res); Liverpool (Eng.) '48; M.C.G.P.
BILSKI, Stanislaw T.; 42 Barton Ave., Toronto 4,Ont.; Vilna **(Poland) '38.**
BILYNSKY, Wolodymyr; Whitemouth, Man.; 5 Henderson Ave. (res); Innsbruck (Aust.) '47; MCGP; Med. Supt., Whitemouth Hosp.; MOH & Dist. Coroner; Tel. 348-2226.
BIMPEH-SEGU, Michael; Box 670, Fort Qu'-Appelle, Sask.; Royal College (Ireland)'64; Staff, Fort Qu'Appelle Indian Hosp.; Tel. 332-5550.
BINDA, Antoine; 6302 rue St.-Denis, Montreal, P.Q.; 865 **Des Ecores St. (res); Mon '50;** M.C.G.P. Tel. 272-9857.
BINDA, Jean; 150 est, Jarry, Montreal 11, P.Q.; Mon '64.
BINDING, David G.; 4 Ockley Close, Oriole Park, Red Deer, Alta.; Wales'62; DObstRCOG.
BINET, Edwin E.; 1375, Sherwood Cres., Montreal 16, P.Q.; Lav '30; Tel. 737-0619.
BINETTE, Claude; 41 St. Eustache, St. Eustache, P.Q.: Mon '51.
BINETTE, Marcel; Lav'65; Res., Hop. St. Michel Archange, Quebec 5, P.Q.
BINGHAM, Dermid L. C.; 203 Professional Bldg., 11 Princess St., Kingston, Ont. (res); Edinburgh (Scot.) '34; Ch.B., FRCS(E), FACS, FICS, FRCS (C), Gen-Surg; Surg., Kingston Gen. & DVA Hosp's.; Cons. Surg. & ThorSurg., Hotel-Dieu Hosp.; Emer. Prof. (Surg.), Queen's U.; Tel. LI 2-2821.
BINGHAM, John M.; Tor '57; Psy; Staff, Ont. Hosp., Hamilton, Ont. Tel. 385-5361.
BINGHAM, John R.; 212 Western Med. Bldg., 25 Leonard Ave., Toronto 2B, Ont.; Man '40; FRCP(C), IntMed; Staff, Toronto Western Hosp.; Assoc. (Med.), U. of Toronto; Tel. 366-6091.
BINHAMMER, Harold E. W.; Reddendale Med. Centre, Lakeview Ave., Kingston, Ont.; Qns '57; M.Sc. (Med); MCGP; Assoc. Staff, Kingston Gen. & Hotel-Dieu Hosp's.; Tel. 389-1604.
BINKLEY, W. E.; 56 Robert St. W., Penetanguishene, Ont.; Tor '36; M.C.G.P.; Dist. Coroner; Tel. 549-2444.
BINNEY, John C.; McG'64; Res. (Psy.), Allan Mem. Inst., Montreal, P.Q.
BINNS SMITH, Malcolm; 74 Cassandra Blvd., Ste 2, Don Mills, Ont.; Edinburgh (Scot.) '58; Path.
BINNINGTON, Vera I.; Tor '39; D.P.H., Paed.: Staff, Ontario Hosp. School, Orillia, Ont.; Tel. 326-7361.
BINSTED, Anthony H.; Acadia-Fairview Med. Bldg., 8330 Fairmount Dr. S.E.; Calgary, Alta.; London (Eng.)'62.
BIRCH, D.M.; Tor'63; Res., St. Michael's Hosp., Toronto, Ont.
BIRCH, John R.; UBC'59; FRCS(C), PlasSurg; Staff, Hosp. for Sick Children, Toronto 2, Ont.
BIRCHARD, Edna L.; 503 Medical Arts Bldg., Hamilton, Ont.; 335 Shoreview Dr., Burlington (res); McG '52; Paed; Staff Paed., Hamilton Gen. & St. Joseph's Hosp's.; Med. Dir., Cerebral Palsy Center; Tel. JA 9-4412.
BIRCHARD, James R.; 225 Bridge St. E., Belleville, Ont.; Qns'54; FACOG; FRCS(C); ObstGyn; Cons. ObstGyn., Belleville Gen. Hosp., Trenton Mem. Hosp. & Prince Edward County Mem. Hosp.; Tel. 962-8055.
BIRCHWOOD, Barbara L.; 617 Merton St., Toronto 7, Ont.; Leiden (Holland)'58; M.S. (Nutr.); Research Ass't., St. Michael's Hosp. & U. of Toronto; Tel. 362-4461.

BIRD, Bruce L.; 101 Post Rd., Don Mills, Ont.; Tor '52; F.R.C.P.(C), DiagRad; Staff (Rad), St. Michael's Hosp.; Clin. Instr. (Rad.), U. of Toronto; Tel. WA 3-6611.
BIRD, Charles E.; Etherington Hall, Stuart St., Kingston, Ont.; Qns '56; FRCP(C), IntMed; Ass't. Prof. (Med.), Queen's U.; Tel. 546-9553.
BIRD, F. V.; Boissevain, Man.; Man '13; Dist. Coroner.
BIRD, Gordon S.; Ste. 201, Glenwood Medical Centre, Brockville, Ont.; Qns'54; M.Sc.; Paed; Chief of Paed., Brockville Gen. Hosp.; Staff, St. Vincent-de-Paul Hosp.; Tel. DI 2-6569.
BIRD, Grant S.; 160 Wellesley St. E., Toronto 5, Ont;. 30 York Valley Cr., Willowdale (res); Tor '51; DiagRad; Radiol., Wellesley Hosp.; Cons. (Rad.), Princess Margaret Hosp.; Assoc. (Rad.), U. of Toronto; Tel. WA 1-4111.
BIRD, H. Arthur; 139 Douglas Ave., Saint John, N.B. (res); Dal '43; Path; Ass't. Path., St. John Gen. Hosp.; Pathol., St. Joseph's Hosp.; Tel. 693-3351; OX 2-2621.
BIRD, H. Godfrey; 134 Pine St., Gananoque, Ont.; Tor '22; MRCP(Lond.), FRCP(C), IntMed; Tel. 382-3361.
BIRD, Josephine N.; 101 Post. Rd., Don Mills, Ont. (res); McG '53; IntMed; Retired.
BIRD, Ralph L.; Qns '31; Med. Advisor, Canadian Pensions Commission, 2110 Veterans' Mem. Bldg., Ottawa, Ont.; Tel. CE 2-8211.
BIRD, Stephen B.; 128 Main St., Liverpool, N.S.; Dal '41; Indust.Phys., Bowaters Mersey Paper Co.; Tel. 354-4414.
BIRDSELL, Dale C.; Alb '61; Research Fell. (Surg.), Hosp. for Sick Children, Toronto, Ont.
BIRENBAUM, Samuel J.; 3042 Keele St., Downsview, Ont.; 1 Viamede Cr., Willowdale (res); **Tor '56; MCGP; Staff, North York Branson Hosp.; Tel. ME 3-6560.**
BIRKBECK, John A.; Health Centre for Children, 715 W. 12 Ave., Vancouver 9, B.C.; 2886 W. 30th Ave., Van. 8 (res); Edinburgh (Scot.) **'57; Paed; Att'd. Staff, Vancouver Gen. Hosp.;** Vis. Staff, Children's Hosp.; Ass't Prof. (Paed.), U. of British Columbia; Tel. TR 6-3211, Loc. 2693.
BIRKETT, Barbara M. (Davison); 331 Sheddon Ave., Oakville, Ont.; McG'58; Derm; Cons. Staff, Oakville-Trafalgar Mem. Hosp.; Court. Staff, Joseph Brant Hosp., Burlington; Active outdoor Staff, Women's College Hosp., Toronto; Tel. 845-6891.
BIRKETT, Charles W.; 8 Welton St., Maple, Ont.; Tor '59.
BIRKETT, David P.; 250-6th Ave. E., Owen Sound, Ont.; Wales (U.K.)'57; MRCP(Ed.); Staff, Ontario Hosp.; Tel. 376-6130.
BIRKS, Richard S.; 4138 Girouard, Montreal, P.Q.; McG '42; M.C.G.P.; Tel. 484-3927.
BIRMINGHAM, Lloyd W.; Box 6090, Aluminum Co. of Canada, Montreal 3, P.Q.; McG '45; Gen Surg; M.O., Aluminum Co. of Canada; Clin. Ass't., O.P.D., Montreal Gen. Hosp.; Tel. WE 2-8825.
BIRNBAUM, Frank M.; 1353 Dundas St. W., Toronto, Ont.; **10 Austin Cres. (res); Tor '36; M.C.G.P.; Assoc. Staff, Mount Sinai Hosp.; Tel. LE 3-8722.**
BIRNBAUM, Jacob; 62 Mattson Rd., Crang Plaza, Downsview, Ont.; 65 Whitburn Cres. (res); Tor '52; Tel. CH 1-7413.
BIRNBOIM, Hymie; Ste. 4, 725 Sherbrooke St., Winnipeg 2, Man. (res); Man '60; Research, U. of Manitoba.
BIRO, Charles; 508 Canada Bldg., Saskatoon, Sask.; 912 Queen's St. (res); Budapest (Hung) '26; FIAP; FACG; FICS; GenSurg; Active Staff, City & University Hosp's.; Court Staff, St. Paul's Hosp.; Tel. 242-2724.
BIRO, George; 1163 Bloor St. W., Toronto 4, Ont.; Vienna (Aust.) '37; Court. Staff, Toronto Western Hosp.; Tel. LE 5-5292.
BIRO, George P.; Qns'63; Staff, Dept. of Physiol., Queen's U., Kingston, Ont.
BIRO, Louis; 202 Plaza Bldg., 1538 Foster St., White Rock, B.C.; 13357 Marine Dr. (res); **McG '52; Med. Staff, White Rock Hosp.; Tel. 531-4393.**

BIRON, Guy; Mon'65; Res., Hop. du Sacre Coeur, Montreal 9, P.Q.
BIRON-SUTTO, Madeleine; 4617 Vezina, Montreal 29, P.Q.; Mon'65.
BIRON, Peter E.; 62A Lakeshore Dr., North Bay, Ont.; Apt. 18, 40 Judge (res); Ott '57.
BIRON, Pierre; Mon '58; Staff, Dept. of Pharm, U. of Montreal, Montreal, P.Q.
BIRON-BEAUDRY, Pauline; C.P. 97, Station Delorimier, Montreal 34, P.Q.; 1481 est, boul. St.-Joseph, Apt. 2 (res); Mon '54; Anaes; Staff, Hop. Sacre-Coeur; Tel. FE 4-1210.
BIRRELL, John D.; Calgary Associate Clinic, 214 —6 Ave. W., Calgary, Alta.; Tor'39; Paed; Tel. 263-7120.
BIRRELL, Russell G.; 24 Harbord St., Toronto, Ont.; 192 Owen Blvd. Willowdale (res); Tor '21; Occ. Med.; Pt.-time Addiction Research Fdn.; Tel. 365-4523.
BIRSE, Sheila H.; Kirkham's Rd., P.O. Box 70, West Hill, Ont. (res); Edinburgh (Scot.) '52; Retired.

BIRSEL, N.; Freeport, Digby Co, N.S.; '47.

BIRT, Arthur R.; 429 Medical Arts Bldg., Winnipeg, Man.; Man'30; FRCP(C); DermSyph; Chief Derm., Winnipeg Gen. & Children's Hosps.; Assoc. Prof. Med., U .of Manitoba; Tel. 942-2979.

BISHOP, Agnes J.; Dal'64; Res. (Paed.), Winnipeg Children's Hospital, Winnipeg, Man.
BISHOP, Beryl (Rathjev); Teulon, Man.; Man '61; Tel. 67.
BISHOP, Duane S.; Ste. 300, Med. Arts Bldg., Calgary, Alta.; Alb'65.
BISHOP, J. Arthur; Dal'62; AMCGP; Res., Victoria Gen. Hosp., Halifax, N.S.
BISHOP, James R.; 513 Med. Dental Bldg., Rose St. & 11th Ave., Regina, Sask.; 2512 Grant Rd. (res); Leeds (Eng.) '56; AMCGP; Tel. LA 2-8541.
BISHOP, Jeffrey W.; National Health & Welfare, Tunney's Pasture, Ottawa, Ont.; London (Eng.) '51; MRCS (Eng.); LRCP (Lond.).
BISHOP, M. A., Trenton, Ont.; Tor '42; Tel. 392-6114.
BISHOP, Maurice L.; Teulon, Man.; Manchester (Eng.) '53. Tel. Teulon 67.
BISHOP, Michael B., Miles Hood Bldg., 219-1st St., Kamsack, Sask.; London (Eng.) '61; DA (Eng.); D.ObstRCOG; Staff, Kamsack Union Hosp.; Tel. 542-2623.

BISKUPSKI, Jan S.; Aguathuna, Nfld.; Polish School of Med. (Edinburgh, Scot.) '49; M.O.H.; Tel. 8-2465.
BISMANIS, Jekabs E.; 4306 W. 8th Ave., Vancouver 8, B.C.; Riga (Latvia) '35; Bact; Assoc. Prof. Microbiol, U. of British Columbia; Tel. 224-0811.
BISMILLAH, Abdul H.; 350 St. Andrew St., Fergus, Ont.; Witwatersrand (S. Africa)'49; Tel. 843-1844.
BISSELL, Erwyn W.; 421 Professional Bldg., 10830 Jasper Ave., Edmonton, Alta.; 12803-63rd Ave. (res); Alb '50; FACS; PlasSurg; Clin. Instr,. U. of Alberta; Tel. GA 4-2088.
BISSET, John G. V.; 5020 Grosvenor Rd., Montreal 6, P.Q.; Glasgow (Scot.) '51; M.B., Ch.B.; Ophth; Tel. RE 9-4013.
BISSET, John M. C.; Box 577, Preeceville, Sask.; St. Andrews (Scot.) '52; M.B.; Ch.B., DTM; DABS; FRCS(C), GenSurg; Staff, Preeceville Union Hosp.; Cons. Canora Union Hosp., Canora; Tel. 547-2027.
BISSON, Christophe; 428 est, Boul. St. Joseph E., Montreal 34, P.Q.; Mon '36; FACS; FICS; GenSurg; Hd. Dept. of Surg., Hop.-Ste.-Justine; Tel. VI 4-3446.
BISSON, D. Romeo; 9697 est rue Notre-Dame, Montreal 5, P.Q.; Lav '17; M.C.G.P.; M.O.H., Montreal East. Tel. CL. 5-6488.
BISSON, Francois R.; 855 boul. Laurentien, Chambre 103, St. Laurent, Montreal 9, P.Q.; Mon '52; Psy; Dir., Dept. of Psy., Hop. Gen. Fleury; Tel. 744-2217.
BISSON, G. Ernest; 1005 Main St., Cowansville, P.Q.; McG'49; Gen. Surg.
BISSON, J. Robert; 33 Montcalm, Hull, P.Q.; Ott '51; M.C.G.P.
BISSON, Lise; Lav'60; Anaes; Staff, Hop. Cloutier, Cap-de-Madeleine, P.Q.; Tel. FR 4-6261.
BISSON, Marcel; 444, Laviolette, Trois-Rivieres, P.Q.; Lav '62; Tel. FR 5-0577.
BISSON, R. D. A.; 718 Granville St., Vancouver, B.C. 1883 W. 41st. (res); McG '31; M.C.G.P.; Tel. MU 3-3918.
BISSONNETTE, Andre G.; Mon'62; Res., Hop. Notre-Dame, Montreal 24, P.Q.
BISSONNETTE, Gilles; 2157 Fleury E., Montreal 12, P.Q.; Mon'60; Tel. DU 1-2581.
BISSONNETTE, Jean; 1402 Boul. Pie IX, Montreal 4, P.Q.; Bordeaux (Fr.) '54; Tel. 521-6611.
BISSONNETTE, Jean P.; 71 Ste. Anne, Quebec, P.Q.; Lav '49; GenSurg (P.Q.); Tel. 522-1501.
BISSONNETTE, J. Eugene; 388 ouest, St. Vallier, Quebec 8, P.Q.; Lav '18; Vice. Pres. Admin., Hop. Christ-Roi; Tel. 529-4187.
BISSONNETTE, Marcel X.; Ott '60; GenSurg; Staff, Argenteuil Hosp., Lachute, P.Q.; Tel. LO 2-5211.
BISSONNETTE, Michel; 388 St. Valliere Ouest, Quebec 8, P.Q.; 676 Chouinard (res); Lav '57; Tel. 529-4187.
BISSONNETTE, Raymond G.; 146, boul. Leger, Pont Viau, P.Q.; Mon '58; GenSurg.
BISSONNETTE, Robert N.; 117 Waterloo St. S., Stratford, Ont.; R.R. 5 (res); Wes '49; Tel. 271-3280.
BISSYLAS, Savas J.; 36 Thorncliffe Ave., Toronto 6, Ont. (res); Athens (Greece) '49; D&TRad; Staff, Toronto Gen. Hosp.; Tel. EM 6-8211.
BISTEVINS, Rita (Rieksts); 58 King St., Dartmouth, N.S.; 64a Hazelhurst St. (res); Dal '60; MCGP; Tel. 466-7511.
BITENC, Igor A. S.; 1374 Sherbrooke St. W., Montreal 25, P.Q.; Vienna (Austria) '51; F.R.C.S. (C), OrthSurg; Staff, Royal Victoria Hosp. & Shriner's Hosp.; Teach, Fell., McGill U.; Tel. VI 9-5165.
BITNUM, Samson; Med. Assoc. Clin., 405 Hendrix St., Nelson, B.C.; Cape Town (S.Africa)'54; M.B., Ch.B., Paed; Tel. 352-6611.
BITTAR, Neville; McG'61; Int., Montreal Gen. Hosp., Montreal, P.Q.
BJARNASON, Arlan E.; 6470 Victoria Dr., Vancouver, B.C.; 3013 Beresford St., S. Burnaby (res); McG '53; M.C.G.P.; Tel. FA 5-2314.
BJORNSON, S. E.; 1080 Dorchester Ave., Winnipeg, Man. (res); Man '16; Retired.
BLACHFORD, Jean; London (Eng.)'62; Staff, Children's Psy. Inst., Sanitorium Rd., London, Ont.
BLACK, Boris; 614 Boyd Bldg., Winnipeg, Man.; 306 Queenston St. (res); Man '20; M.C.G.P.; Tel. WH 2-5670.
BLACK, Brian O.; 1010—13th St. S., Lethbridge, Alta. (res); Dal '41; DiagRad; Rad., St. Michael's Gen. Hosp., Lethbridge, Alta.; Tel. FA 7-1531.
BLACK, Charles R.; Ste. 3, 77 Upper Middle Rd., Cooksville, Ont.; Qns '44; DLO (Eng.); Otol; Tel. 277-4180.
BLACK, Davidson; 226 Med. Arts Bldg., Toronto, Ont.; Tor '46; Ophth. Tel. WA 1-8527.
BLACK, Donald K.; C.P. 95, Hudson Heights, P.Q.; McG'52; FRCS(C); GenSurg.
BLACK, Donald M.; 3348 Edgemont Blvd., N. Vancouver, B.C. (res); Man '24; D.P.H.; PH; Dir. North Shore Health Unit, 253 E.-14th St. N., Vancouver; Retired.
BLACK, Douglas G.; Digby, N.S.; Queen St. (res); Dal '44; M.C.G.P.; Tel. 245-2299.
BLACK, Douglas P.; UBC '61; AMCGP; Staff, M. J. Boylen Hosp., Baie Verte, Nfld.
BLACK, Duncan M.; 7406 Horne St., Mission City, B.C.; Queen's U. (Belfast, Ire.)'36; DPH; PH; Dir. Central Fraser Valley Health Unit; Tel. 826-7166.
BLACK, Elinor F. E.; Ste. 22, 30 Spence St., Wpg. 1 Man. (res); Man '30; FICS, FRCOG, FACS, FACOG, FRCS(C), ObstGyn; ObstGyn-in-Chief, Wpg. Gen. Hosp.; Head & Prof. (ObstGyn), U. of Manitoba; Retired.
BLACK, George A.; Apt. 67, 146 Stewart St., Ottawa 2, Ont. (res); Wes '30; F.C.C.P.; IntMed; Adm. Dept. Nat. Health & Welfare; Tel. 234-5782.

BLACK, George M.; 32 Tupper St. N., Portage-la-Prairie, Man.; 560 Crescent Rd. W. (res); Man '38; FACS; GenSurg; Tel. 857-4660.

BLACK, Harvey H.; 27 Academy Med. Bldg., 1812-4th St. W., Calgary, Alta.; 1143 39th Ave. S.W., (res); McG '43; MCGP; Tel. 263-7240.

BLACK, Ian; 1265 West-15th Ave., Vancouver 9, B.C.; Edinburgh (Scot.) '51; Path; Ass't. Path., Vancouver Gen. Hosp.; Clin. Inst'r., U. of British Columbia; Tel. TR 6-3211.

BLACK, James H. S.; Medical Arts Bldg., Aspen Hill, Grand Falls, Nfld.; Aberdeen (Scot.)'64; MB; ChB; Tel. 2136, 2137, 2185.

BLACK, J. E. R.; c/o Chief Civil Service Health Div., Dept. Nat'l. Health and Welfare, No. 3 Temporary Bldg., Ottawa, Ont.; Tel. CE 2-8211.

BLACK, John D.; 157 Ontario St., St. Catharines, Ont.; 6 Swan Dr. (res); Tor '45; GenSurg; Staff, St. Catharines Gen. & Hotel Dieu Hosp's.; Tel. MU 2-8238.

BLACK, John H.; 925 W. Georgia St., Vancouver, B.C.; Tor'36; M.C.G.P.; Tel. MU 1-9454.

BLACK, Leslie W.; 825 Coxwell Ave., Toronto 6, Ont.; 64 Rosedale Hts. Dr. (res); Tor '26; F.A.C.S.; GenSurg; OrthSurg; Chief Orth.Surg., Gen. Surg. Toronto East Gen. & Orth. Hosp. Tel. HO 3-2244.

BLACK, Lyall M.; Box 130, Fort Churchill, Man.; Edinburgh (Scot.)'56; Area Dir., Keewatin Area, Dept. of National Health & Welfare; Tel. 444.

BLACK, Max W.; Neudorf, Sask.; London (Eng.) '54; Tel. 160.

BLACK, N. S.; Dept. of National Health & Welfare, c/o Regional Superintendent, European Region; Dal '50. Abroad.

BLACK, Thomas H.; 955 Queen St. E., Sault Ste. Marie, Ont.; 45 Ford St. (res); Tor '41 Cons. (Obst Gyn), Sault Ste. Marie Gen. Hosp.; Chief, Obst. Gyn., Plummer Mem. Hosp.; Dist. Coroner; Tel. AL 4-2821.

BLACK, T. M.; 108 Medical Dental Bldg., Regina, Sask.; 89 Calder Cres. (res); Qns '49; Obst Gyn.; Tel. LE 3-7631.

BLACK, William A.; Ste. 100, 219 Kennedy St., Winnipeg 1, Man.; 272 Cordova (res); Man '27.

BLACK, Wm. Lyle; The Greig Med. Group, 44 Kimberley Ave., Bracebridge, Ont.; Tor '53; MCGP Staff, South Muskoka Mem. Hosp.; Med. Advisor, The Muskoka Dist. Home for the Aged; Tel. 645-2281.

BLACK, William R.; 10155-120th St., Edmonton, Alta.; Alb '56; FRCP(C) IntMed.; Tel. 488-7271.

BLACK, William W.; 2 Spruce Terr., Fredericton, N.B.; St. Andrews (Scot.) '42; B.Sc., M.B., Ch.B.; DPM; Psy; Dir., Fredericton Mental Health Clin; Cons. Psy., Victoria Public Hosp. & U. of New Brunswick; Tel.454-4792.

BLACKBURN, Georges-H.; Saint Ambroise, Chicoutimi, P.Q.; Lav '50.

BLACKBURN, Gerard; Apt. 4, 3780 Maplewood Ave., Montreal 26, P.Q. (res); Mon '51; Path., Verdun Gen. Hosp., Verdun; Tel. PO 6-3551.

BLACKBURN, Gilles; Lav'65; Res., Boisvert Mem. Hosp., Baie Comeau, P.Q.

BLACKBURN, Robert; 1190 rue Portland, Sherbrooke, P.Q.; Lav'53; D & T Rad; Staff, Hop.-Hotel-Dieu; Tel. LO 2-5444.

BLACKIE, Peter B.; Dal'61; Staff, James Paton Mem. Hosp., Gander, Nfld.

BLACKLER, A. William J.; 30 London Rd., St. John's, Nfld.; Qns '26; F.I.C.S., OphthOtol; Surg.-(E.E.N.T.), St. John's Gen. Hosp.; Tel. 578-2730.

BLACKSTOCK, Ross E.; 3269 Norwood Ave., North Vancouver, B.C.; Alb '48.

BLACKWELL, Frederick N.; Cobourg Medical Centre, 68 King St. E., Cobourg, Ont.; 380 George St. (res); Tor '31; Dist. Coroner; Tel. FR 2-5494.

BLACKWELL, Gilbert L.; P.O. Box 730, Bradford, Ont.; Tor'44; Chief of Staff, York County Hosp., Newmarket; District Coroner, Simcoe County; Tel. 775-2302.

BLACKWELL, William C.; Box 240, 155 Durham St. W., Lindsay, Ont.; Qns'32; MCGP; Chief of Staff, Ross Mem. Hosp.; Dist. Coroner; Tel. 324-5211.

BLACKWOOD, H. John; 215 LeMarchant Rd., St. John's, Nfld.; 8 Falkland St. (res); Dal '51; GenSurg; Tel. 578-7957.

BLACKWOOD, John R.; 498 Adelaide St., Woodstock, Ont.; Wes '42; MCGP; Chief of Surg., Woodstock Gen. Hosp.; Coroner Oxford Co.; Tel. 537-3361.

BLADEK, Roman; 302 Toronto Western Medical Bldg., 25 Leonard Ave., Toronto 2B, Ont.; 25 Hampshire Hgts. (res); Tor '53; MA; FRCP(C), IntMed; Att'd Staff (Med.), Tor. Western Hosp.; Clin. Ass't., U. of Toronto; Tel. 363-0988.

BLADES, Thomas R.; 15496 North Bluff Rd., White Rock, B.C.; Alb '40; MCGP; Dist. Coroner; Tel. 531-5595.

BLAGDON, Georges; Ste. 304, 1000 Ste. Foy Rd., Quebec, P.Q.; Lav'60; ObstGyn (P.Q.); Staff, Hop. St. Sacrement.

BLAHEY, Peter R.; Ste. 1005, 1414 Drummond St., Montreal 25, P.Q.; 141 Radcliffe Ave. Mtl. West (res); Tor '41; D.A.B.O.G., F.A.C.O.G., F.R.C.O.G., F.R.C.S.(C), ObstGyn; Ass't. ObstGyn., Mtl. Gen. Hosp.; Clin. Ass't. (ObstGyn), Royal Victoria Hosp.; Lect. (ObstGyn), McGill U.; Tel. VI 4-1865.

BLAIKIE, William D.; 117 Buckingham Dr., Sydney, N.S.; Glasgow (Scot.)'58.

BLAIN, Emile; 400 est Sherbrooke, Montreal, P.Q.; 1804 Lajoie, Outremont (res); Mon '24; Ophth; Staff, Hop.-Notre-Dame; Cons., WCB (P.Q.); Assoc. Prof. (Ophth), U. of Montreal; Exec. Dir., Assoc. des Medecins de Langue Francaise du Canada — 5064 Ave.-du-Parc, Mtl. 8; Tel. 273-2321.

BLAIN, Gilbert; 738 McEachran, Montreal 8, P.Q.; Mon '55; MAH; Dir. of Hosp. Admin., University of Montreal; Tel. 733-9951.

BLAIN, Julien; 1740 Girouard, St. Hyacinthe, P.Q.; Mon '53; Tel. PR 4-7430.

BLAIN, Rene; 2033 Blvd. St. Joseph E., Montreal 34, P.Q.; Mon '33; Tel. 522-0733.

BLAINE, J. Delmar; 5 Med. Centre, 8th Ave. & 8th St. S.W., Calgary, Alta.; 19 Malibou Rd. (res); Qns 40; Urol; Active Staff, Calgary Gen. & Holy Cross Hosp's.; Tel. 262-6266; Abroad.

BLAIR, David C.; 1712-12th St. S.W., Calgary Alta. (res); McG '52; PhysMed & Rehab; Dir. PhysMed & Rehab., Calgary Gen. Hosp; Dir. PhysMed., Col. Belcher (D.V.A.) Hosp.; Tel. AM 6-7541, Loc. 477.

BLAIR, Edward J.; 193 Ontario St., St. Catharines, Ont.; Wes '54; D.A.B.O.S.; OrthSurg; Vice Chmn. Staff, Hotel-Dieu Hosp; Assoc. Staff, St. Catharines Gen. Hosp.; Court. Staff, Gtr. Niagara Hosp.; Tel. MU 4-8441.

BLAIR, E. Murray; 2772 Spruce St., Vancouver, B.C.; McG '17; ObstGyn; Hon. Cons. Vancouver Gen. Hosp.; Semi-retired.

BLAIR, John H.; 2221 Keele St., Toronto 15, Ont.; 11 Greenbrook Dr., (res); Wes '49; F.A.C.A., F.I.C.S.; Anaes; Chief, Dept. of Anaes., Northwestern Gen. Hosp.; Tel. 249-1555.

BLAIR, Nathaniel J.; 1734 W. Broadway, Vancouver 9, B.C.; 1122 W. 40th Van. 13 (res); Man '38; Otol; Att'd. Staff, Vancouver Gen. Hosp.; Teach. Staff, (Otol.), U. of British Columbia; Tel. RE 6-0331.

BLAIR, R. Gordon; Dal'65; Res., St. John's Gen. Hosp., St. John's, Nfld.

BLAIR, T. A.; UBC '63; Int., Shaughnessy Hosp., Vancouver, B.C.

BLAIR, W. Arthur; 435 Piccadilly Ave., Ottawa 3, Ont. (res); Qns '50; Psy; Chief, Dept. of Psy., Ottawa Civic Hosp.; Cons. Ottawa Gen., Dept. of Justice & DVA; Assoc. Prof., Ottawa U.; Tel. 729-2511, Loc. 580.

BLAIR, Wilfred E.; Apt. 1108, 5950 Bathurst St., Willowadale, Ont.; Qns '30; Anaes; Staff, Branson Hosp., Toronto; Tel. 633-9420.

BLAIR, William H.; 8152 Wedgewood St., S. Burnaby, B.C. (res); Man '50; Anaes; Staff, Royal Columbian Hosp., Vancouver; Tel. LA 2-2771.

BLAIR, William K.; 109 King St. E., Oshawa, Ont.; 290 Mary St., Apt. 305; Tor'34; Tel. 723-4541.
BLAIS, Alphonse M.; 2134 Alta Vista Dr., Ottawa, Ont. (res); Lav '54; D.Psy; Psy; Dir., Psy. Unit, Ottawa Gen. Hosp.; Tel. CE 6-4592.
BLAIS, Antoni; Lav'30; Staff, Pavillion Dufrost, Hop. St-Michel Archange, Mastai, P.Q.
BLAIS, E. Rolland; 1779 ave-de-l'Eglise, Montreal 20, P.Q.; 3591 Lacombe (res); Mon '28; DermSyph (P.Q.); Sec-Treas., Assoc-des-Medecins-de-langue-Francaise-du Canada; President Aeturna Life; Tel. 273-2321.
BLAIS, Guy; 30 est boul St.-Joseph, Montreal 14, P.Q. 2302 E. Ontario (res); Mon '54; Obst (P.Q.); Tel. 845-4241.
BLAIS, J. Antoine; 52 Lockhart, Montreal 16, P.Q. (res); Mon '42; IntMed (P.Q.); Assoc. Prof., U. of Montreal; Cons., Northern Electric Co.
BLAIS, J. Camille; 2302 est, rue Ontario, Montreal 24, P.Q.; Mon '25; Staff, Bruchesi Inst.; Cons. Liquor Comm. (P.Q.); Tel. LA 1-1650.
BLAIS, Jean-M.; 137 Blvd. Quinn, Longueuil, P.Q. (res); Mon '43; Prof. & Dir. Dept. Microscopic Anatomy, U. of Montreal; Tel. RE 3-9951.
BLAIS, Leo E.; 845 Belvidere S., Sherbrooke, P.Q.; 830 Cambrai (res); Lav '37; A.I.C.S., GenSurg (P.Q.); Tel. LO 9-1414.
BLAIS, Louis-P.; La Trappe, Cte. Deux-Montagnes, P.O. (res); Lav '26; Retired.
BLAIS, Madeleine; Mon '63; Sr. Int., Hop. Notre-Dame, Montreal, P.Q.
BLAIS, Mathieu; 17 Ste-Catherine, Longueuil, Cite-Jacques-Cartier, P.Q.; Lav '51.
BLAIS, Noel; 290 Montcalm, Granby, P.Q.; Lav '43; D.P.H., GenSurg (P.Q.); Tel. 372-7773.
BLAIS, Paul E.; 50 Riv. du Moulin, Chicoutimi, P.Q.; Lav '40; Anaes.; Tel. 543-4274.
BLAIS, Raymond; 837 Cherrier St., Montreal, P.Q.; 34 Ouest Fleury (res); Lav '39; Otol; Staff Notre Dame & Queen Mary Veterans' Hosp's.; Staff U. of Montreal; Tel. LA 2-1105.
BLAIS, Richard; 3719 Fleury E., Montreal Nord, P.Q.; 10526 St. Vital (res); Mon '60; A.M.C.G.P.; Tel. 321-5124.
BLAIS, Robert; Gracefield, Cte. Gatineau, P.Q.; Lav '63.
BLAIS, Yves; 2106 rue St. Marc, Shawinigan Falls, P.Q.; Lav '51.
BLAKE, Barbara J. (McCallum); 509 Island Pk. Dr., Ottawa 3, Ont. (res.); Tor '48; D.P.H.; Lect. Dept. of Prev. Med., U. of Ottawa; Tel. CE 5-6751.
BLAKE, Earl M.; Box 110, 1 Shaw St. E., Waterloo, P.Q.; 200 Main St. (res); McG'34; MCGP.
BLAKE, J. Desmond; 6014 Yonge St., Willowdale, Ont.; Nat. U. (Ire.) '47; DPH, MCGP; Staff Branson North York Hosp. & St. Michael's Hosp.; Tel. 221-8162.
BLAKE, J. Maurice; 507 Querbes Ave., Outremont, P.Q.; Lav '58; IndustMed; MCGP; Ass't. Med. Dir. Hoechst Pharmaceuticals; Tel. 739-2701.
BLAKE, Roy M.; 1640-16th Ave. N. W., Calgary, Alta.; McG '59; Paed.
BLAKE-KNOX, Peter E. A., S/L: Trinity Coll. Dublin (Ire.) '50; MB., B.Ch., BAO; DTM&H; Anaes; Ass't Chief Anaes, National Defence Med. Centre, Ottawa; Tel. 733-6600; Loc. 216.
BLAKELY, Arthur M.; 286 Rossini Blvd., Windsor, Ont.; Tor '16; Retired.
BLAKELY, John A.; 191 Yonge St. S., Richmond Hill, Ont.; 81 Arnold Ave., Thornhill (res); Sask '58; FRCP(C); IntMed; Phys., York Central Hosp.; Research Cons., Sunnybrook Hosp.; Tel. TU 4-7581.
BLAKSLEE, V.; 111 Victoria Ave., Belleville, Ont.; Qns '13.
BLANCHAER, Marcel C.; 961 Dorchester Ave., Winnipeg, Man. (res); Qns'46; Prof. of Biochem., U. of Manitoba; Dir. Biochemistry, St. Boniface Hosp.; Tel. 786-3501.
BLANCHARD, Antonin; Box 430, Chatham, N.B.; Lav'53; MCGP.
BLANCHARD, Bernard; Ste. 204, 4050 Blvd. Rosemont, Montreal 36, P.Q.; Mon'56; FRCS(C); OrthSurg.
BLANCHARD, George A.; Ste. 301, 3875 rue St. Urbain, Montreal 18, P.Q.; 773 ave Stuart, Outremont (res); Mon'37; F.I.C.S. Ophth, Otol (P.Q.); Staff, Ste-Justine & Ste-Jeanne-d'Arc; Tel. VI 4-3186.
BLANCHARD, Guy A.; Ste. 204, 4050 Blvd. Rosemont, Montreal 36, P.Q.; Ott'56; FRCS(C); OrthSurg.
BLANCHARD, Hervé; Port-Au-Prince (Haiti)'58; FRCS(C), GenSurg; Staff, Hop. Ste-Justine, Montreal 26, P.Q.
BLANCHARD, J. Donald; 1314 Fairmont Med. Bldg., 750 West Broadway, Vancouver 1, B.C.; 5762 Highbury St. (res); Tor '53; Vis. Staff, Van. Gen., Grace & St. Vincent's Hosp's.; Tel. MU 4-6308.
BLANCHARD, Kenneth R.; Cannon Clinic, McCallum Rd., Abbotsford, B.C.; Tor '42.
BLANCHARD, Pierre L.; 12774 boul. Gouin ouest, Pierrefonds, P.Q.; Ott'58; FRCS(C); ObstGyn; Tel. 684-8460.
BLANCHARD, Richard; 31 St. Germain Ave., Toronto, Ont.; Tor'11; Retired.
BLANCHARD, Robert J.; Man '59; FRCS(C), GenSurg; Staff, Winnipeg Gen. Hosp., Winnipeg 3, Man.; Tel. SP 4-6511; Abroad.
BLANCHARD, Roger; 259 St. Georges, St. Jerome, P.Q.; Mon '53; FAAP; Paed; Dir., Paed. Serv., Hotel-Dieu de St-Jerome; Tel. GE 8-8519.
BLANCHET, Georges; Lav '60; Staff, Hop. St-Francois d'Assise, Quebec 3, P.Q.; Tel. 529-7311.
BLANCHET, Gerald L.; Ste. 2, 2461 Bloor St. W., Toronto 9, Ont.; Tor '46; Chief, Dept. of G.P., Queensway Gen. Hosp.; Assoc. Coroner, York County; Tel. RO 6-2252.
BLANCHET, Jean; 500 Seaforth Med. Bldg., 3550 Cote des Neiges Rd., Montreal 25, P.Q.; Lav'60; FRCS(C); ObstGyn.
BLANCHET-PATRY, Madeleine; Unite San Hochelaga, 8616 boul. Gouin est, Montreal, P.Q.; Lav'57; PH (P.Q.).
BLANCHETTE, Claude; 21 rue Cote, Roberval, P.Q.; Lav '58; Paed; Staff, Hop. Hotel-Dieu St. Michel; Tel. 275-0640.
BLANCHETTE, Gilles; Lav '63; Int. Hop. St-Luc, Montreal, P.Q.
BLANCHETTE, Michel; Mon '63; Res., Hop. Notre-Dame, Montreal 24, P.Q.
BLANCHETTE, Oscar; Lemieux, Co. Nicolet, P.Q.; Mon'37.
BLANCHETTE, Roger; Mon'59; Res., Hop. Notre-Dame, Montreal 24, P.Q.
BLANCK, Julius A.; Waskada, Man.; Tartu (Estonia) '27; M.O.H.
BLANCO, Ramon; Philippines '58; Jr. Intn., Victoria Gen. Hosp., Halifax, N.S.
BLAND, Henry J.; Med. Centre, Canso, N.S.; Bristol (Eng.) '50; DRCOG (Lond.); MCGP; M.O.H. & Port M.O., Canso; Tel. 150.
BLAND, J. Stewart; Woodlands School, New Westminster, B.C.; Camb. & Birm. (Eng.)'46; MRCS(Eng.); LRCP(Lond.); DPM(Eng.); Psy.
BLAND, Roger C.; Flin Flon Clinic, Box 160, Flin Flon, Man.; Liverpool (Eng.)'60; MRCS (Eng.); LRCP (Lond.); D.ObstRCOG.
BLAND, S. Scott; 59 King St. W., Ingersoll, Ont.; Dal '43; Pres. Med. Staff, Alexandra Hosp.; Tel. 485-0550.
BLANK, Tibor; 817A George St., Hearst, Ont.; Budapest (Hung.) '52; FICS; ObstGyn; Chief (ObstGyn), Notre-Dam Hosp.; Tel. 362-4797.
BLASTORAH, William D. J., 334 Charlotte St., Peterborough, Ont.; 1107 Closilla Ave. (res); Tor '46; GenSurg; Surg. Staff, Peterborough Civic & St. Joseph's Hosp's.; Tel. RI 2-6141.
BLATCHFORD, Ellen H. (Comisky); Rm. 15, 501 Yonge St., Toronto, Ont.; Tor'23; Anaes; Active Cons. (Anaes.), Women's College Hosp.; Tel. WA 2-0244.
BLAU, Alexander; 605 Bloor St. W., Toronto 4, Ont.; Bologna (Italy) '39; IntMed. Tel. 531-6996.
BLAYNEY, E. Bruce; Box 429, High River, Alta.; Alb'50; MCGP.
BLAYNEY, Margery M.; Box 429, High River, Alta.; Alb'49.

BLAYNEY, R. York; Thistletown Plaza, 964 Albion Rd., Rexdale, Ont.; 2 Parkchester Rd., Tor. 15 (res); Tor '55; M.C.G.P.; Active Staff, Queensway Gen. Hosp. Tel. 741-2930.

BLAYNEY, York; Box 279, High River, Alta; Tor '17; M.C.G.P.; Tel 652-2492.

BLAZIC, Charles; 7 Allison Dr., Toronto 18, Ont. (res); Tor '53; Psy; Staff, Ontario Hosp., New Toronto; Tel. CL 9-8291.

BLEEKS, Cherry K.; 227 Med. Arts Bldg., 404 Graham Ave., Winnipeg 1, Man.; 561 Academy Road, Winnipeg, 9. (res); Man '30; ObstGyn; Ass't. Obst Gyn., Winnipeg Gen. Hosp.; Ass't. Prof. ObstGyn., U. of Manitoba; Tel. WH 2-0633.

BLEJER, Hector; 111 Queen St. E., Toronto, Ont.; McG '58; DIH; Staff, St. Michael's Hosp.; Med. Dir., Imperial Life Assur. Co.; Tel. 364-8211.

BLENKINSOP, Edwin I.; Canwood Community Clinic, Canwood, Sask.; Durham (Eng.)'51; DPH; Tel. 120.

BLENKINSOP, Gavin W.; 221 King St. E., Kingston, Ont.; Lakeland Pt. (res); Qns '36; MCGP; Assoc. Staff, Kingston Gen. & Hotel Dieu Hosp's.; Tel. 548-3898.

BLENKINSOP, Jean A.; 508 Medical Centre, 906-8th Ave. S.W., Calgary, Alta.; Liverpool (Eng.) '57; Tel. 269-7154.

BLENKINSOP, Peter R.; 508 Med. Centre, 914-8th Ave. S.W., Calgary, Alta.; 4011 Comanche Rd. N.W., (res); Liverpool (Eng.) '57; DLO; Otol; Staff, Calgary Gen., Children's & Holy Cross Hosp's.; Tel. AM 3-1340.

BLENNERHASSETT, George H.; Dublin (Ire.) '39; Med. Supt., Jordan Mem. San., The Glades, N.B.; Tel. 756-3355.

BLEVIS, Leon S.; 174 Fenn Ave., Willowdale, Ont.; Tor'54; Path; Assoc. Path., Doctors' Hosp., 45 Brunswick Ave., Toronto 4, Ont.; Tel. WA 3-5411.

BLEW, Douglas R.; Tor'65; Res., Montreal Gen. Hosp., Montreal 25, P.Q.

BLEZARD, John A.; 1101 The Parkway, London, Ont. (res); Qns '14; Anaes; Chief, (Anaes), Victoria, St. Joseph's Hosp's & Beck Mem. San.; Prof. & Hd. Dept. of Anaes., U. of Western Ont.; Retired.

BLIEK, Abraham J.; 6319 Browness Rd. N.W., Calgary, Alta.; 6023 Bow Cres. (res); Utrecht (Neth.)'48; Tel. 288-2495.

BLIGHT, William J.; 660 Elizabeth Rd., St. Boniface 6, Man.; 94 Blackberry Bay; Sask.'59; A.M.C.G.P.; Tel. AL 3-5609.

BLINKHORN, David H., Fergus Clinic, Box 29, Fergus, Ont.; Dal '54; DABS; Chmn., Med. Staff, Groves Mem. Community Hosp.; Tel. 843-3210.

BLISS, James Q.; 3475 Ridgewood Rd., Montreal 26, P.Q. (res); Tor '56; Ph.D. (Physiol); Ass't. Prof. (Physiol.), McGill U.; Tel. VI 4-6311.

BLITZ, Alfred E.; Lloydminster Clinic, Lloydminster, Sask.; Glasgow (Scot.)'59.

BLIZZARD, Stephen V. F/L; Wes'63; Mir. RCAF Station, Rockcliffe, Ottawa, Ont.

BLOCK, Erwin W.; Spirit River, Alta.; Alb '62; Tel. 864-3962.

BLOCK, Henry J. 1221 Ave. J. N., Saskatoon, Sask. (res); Tor '52; Path; Dir. of Labs. & Chief (Path), Saskatoon City Hosp.; Sess. Lect. (Path), U. of Saskatchewan; Tel. CH 2-6681.

BLODGETT, A. L. Nelson; Aldershot, Ont.; Tor '52.

BLOEMHOF, Bauke; 4900 Kingsway, South Burnaby, B.C.; Groningen (Neth.)'48; Otol; Cons. Otol., Burnaby Gen. Hosp.; Tel. 433-3414.

BLOIS, George M.; 1856 Bloor St. W., Toronto 9, Ont.; 19 Baby Point Rd. (res); Tor '31. Tel. RO. 7-2424.

BLONDAL, Harold; Man '49; Assoc. Med. Dir., Charles E. Frosst & Co., P.O. Box 247, Montreal, P.Q.; Tel. WE 2-7111.

BLONDIN, Claude; Mon '62; Res., Hop. Hotel-Dieu, Montreal, P.Q.

BLOOM, David S.; Man '61; Jr. Intn., Winnipeg Gen. Hosp., Winnipeg 3, Man.

BLOOM, Howard W.; 99 Avenue Rd., Ste. 409, Toronto 5, Ont.; 58 Wembely Rd. (res); Tor '55; FRCP(C); IntMed; Staff, New Mount Sinai Hosp.; Tel. 922-0417.

BLOOM, Joseph; 175 Ellendale Med. Bldg., 5845 Cote-des-Neiges Rd., Montreal 26, P.Q.; 160 Maplewood Ave., Outremont (res); McG '34; DiagRad (P.Q.); Assoc. Rad., Jewish Gen. Hosp.; Tel. VI 5-9105.

BLOOM, Leon; 99 Avenue Rd., Toronto, Ont.; 308 Finch Ave. W., Toronto, Ont.; Tor'56; FRCS(C); OrthSurg; Court. Staff, North York Branson & Doctor Hosp's.; Tel. 921-0731.

BLOOMBERG, Max-Louis; 3235 Granby Ave., Domaine Shopping Centre, Montreal 5, P.Q.; 8100 Dalkeith, Ville D'Anjou (res); Geneva (Switz) '52; FRCS(C), GenSurg; Vis. Phys., Jean Talon, Maisonneuve, & Eastern Hosp's.; Tel. CL 9-4039.

BLOOMER, Earl; 16 Margaret St., St. Thomas, Ont. (res); Harvard (U.S.A.) '17; Part-time Staff, Ontario Hosp., St. Thomas.

BLOOMFIELD, Michael A.; Ste. 100, Victoria Med. Centre, 111 Waterloo St., London, Ont.; Manchester (Eng.) '54; DMRD; DiagRad; Assoc. Rad., Victoria Hosp.; Instr. (Rad.), U. of Western Ontario.

BLOOMFIELD, Robert C.; 3331 Bloor W., Toronto 18, Ont.; 10 Appleby Ct., Islington (res); Queen's U. (Belfast, N. Ire.) '52; DLO (Eng.); DRCOG (Eng.); Otol; Active Staff, Queensway Gen. & Bethesda Hosp's.; Cons. S. Peel Gen. Hosp.; Tel. 239-7751.

BLOOMFIELD, Saul S.; 819 Decarie Blvd., St. Laurent, Montreal 9, P.Q.; 553 Algonquin Ave. (res); Geneva (Switz.) '53; MCGP; Ass't. Phys. Jewish Gen. Hosp.; Court. Staff, Jean Talon & Queen Elizabeth Hosp's.; Lect. U. of Montreal; Phys., Thrift Stores Ltd. Abroad.

BLOTT, Gordon R.; Ste. 3, Madrona Bldg., 140 Wallace St., Nanaimo, B.C.; Rockoak, R.R. 4, Wellington (res); Alb' 41; FACOG; Tel. SK 3-4251.

BLOTT, R. D.; R.R. 7, Dunnville, Ont.; Tor'23; Dist. Coroner.

BLOUIN, Claude; 132 Lowring, Drummondville, P.Q.; Lav'65.

BLOUIN, Louis C.; Amqui, P.Q.; Lav '37; Dir. Gen. Med., Hop. d'Amqui; Tel. 16.

BLOUIN, Reginald; Rm. 81, La Sauvegarde Assce. Co., 152 Notre Dame St. E., Montreal 1, P.Q.; 150 Somerville (res); Mon '24; Med. Dir., La Sauvegarde Assce. Co.; Med. Cons., Montreal Transport Commission; Retired.

BLOUIN, R. Hugues; C.P.367, Magog, P.Q.; Lav '54; GenSurg (P.Q.).

BLOUIN, Yvan; 519 rue Meilleur, Sherbrooke, P.Q.; GenSurg(P.Q.).

BLOUW, Dirk; Doctor's Bldg., 394 Graham Ave., Winnipeg 1, Man.; 68 Niagara, Wpg. 9 (res); Groningen (Neth.) '43; MCGP; Tel. 942-1610.

BLOUW, Hendrik; 124 Frederica St. E., Fort William, Ont.; 313 Catherine St. (res); Groningen (Neth.) '47; Tel. MA 2-3346.

BLOYARD, George J.; 1384 Jean-Talon E., Montreal 10, P.Q.; Paris (Fr.) '44; M.C.G.P.

BLUE, Gordon D.; 537 Medical Arts Bldg., Saskatoon, Sask.; 1402-14th St. E. (res); Tor '43; F.A.C.S., F.R.C.S.(C), Urol; Staff Surg. (Urol.), Saskatoon City, St. Paul's & University Hosp's.; Cons. (Urol.), D.V.A.; Ass't. Prof. in Surg. (Urol.), U. of Saskatchewan; Tel. 652-0531.

BLUE, William W.; 28, Court St., St. Catharines, Ont.; London (Eng.) '54; M.B., B.S.; NeurSurg; NeurSurg., St. Catharines Gen. & Hotel-Dieu Hosp's.; Court. Staff, Gtr. Niagara Gen. Hosp.; Tel. 682-8582.

BLUM, Jack; Sask '60; Ass't. Res. (Otol.), Royal Victoria Hosp., Montreal, P.Q.

BLUMBERGER, Samuel; 193 Hastings St. E., Vancouver 4, B.C.; Tor '05.

BLUME, Warren T.; McG '62; Int., Montreal Children's Hosp., Montreal, P.Q.; Abroad.

BLUMENSTEIN, Janos; 15 Newgate Rd., Toronto 19, Ont.; Tor '58; Ph.D., Staff, New Mount Sinai Hosp.; Tel. EM 6-7361.

BLUMENTHAL, Sidney; Mall Med. Group, 280 Osborne St. N., Winnipeg 1, Man.; 583 Queenston (res); Birmingham (Eng.) '53; D.R.C.O.G.; FRCP(C), IntMed; Dem. (Med.), U. of Manitoba; Tel. SP 4-2411.

BLUMER, Herbert M.; Ste 330, 6000 Cote-des-Neiges Rd., Montreal 26, P.Q.; 5620 Cork Ave.. Mtl. 29 (res); McG '56; M.Sc., DIM; FRCP(C), IntMed; Allerg. (PQ); Active Staff, Jewish Gen. & Bellechase Hosp's. Tel. RE 3-7381.

BLUMES, Abie B.; 307 Alberta Corner, Calgary, Alta.; Man '32; MCGP; Tel. 262-2328.

BLUNDELL, John E.; 2300 Tupper St., Montreal, P.Q.; 3644 Ontario Ave., Apt. 62 (res); Cambridge (Eng.) '40; M.A., M.D., B.Chir., MRCP (Lond.); FRCS (Eng.); Neur (P.Q.); Dir. Dept. of Neurosurg., Mtl. Children's Hosp., Assoc. NeurSurg. Montreal Gen. Hosp., Adjunct NeuroSurg. Mon. Neurological Inst., & Ass't. Prof. Neurol. & NeurSurg., McGill U.; Tel. WE 7-8511.

BLUNDELL, Peter E.; Tor '54; FRCS(C), ThorSurg. (Cardiovasc.); Staff, Montreal Gen. Hosp., Montreal 25, P.Q.; Tel. 937-6011.

BLUNDELL, Stanley F.; McG '40; Med. Services Clinic Dept of National Health & Welfare, Immigration Bldg., Burrard St., Vancouver 1, B.C.; Tel. MU 3-1937.

BLUNDEN, Anthony G.; 11666-95th St., Edmonton, Alta.; 13655-108th Ave. (res); London (Eng.) '57; MCGP; Active Staff, Royal Alexanda, St. Joseph's & Good Samaritan Hosp's.; Tel. 474-3481.

BLUESTEIN, Joseph E.; McG'61; FRCP(C), Psy; Staff, Royal Victoria Hosp., Montreal 2, P.Q.

BLUTEAU, Paul E.; Lav '57; FRCP(C); Path; Staff, Hop. General-de-Verdun, Montreal 19, P.Q.; Tel. 766-8511.

BLYE, Ross A.; 370 Dundas E., Toronto, Ont.; Tor '21. Tel. WA 1-1343.

BOAKE, H. Kenneth; Box 608, Parsons Clinic, Red Deer, Alta.; Alb'60; AMCGP; Tel. 347-2308.

BOAKE, Rex C.; Alb. '61; Res., University Hosp., Edmonton, Alta.

BOAN, D. Bruce; 755 Quilchena Cres., Wellington, B.C.; Sask'65.

BOARD, Harry K.; 5 Young St., Hamilton, Ont.; 40 Robinson St. (res); Qns '28; Urol.; Tel. JA 7-3344.

BOBECHKO, Walter P.; 178 St. George St., Toronto 5, Ont.; Tor'57; B.Sc. (Med.); FRCS(C); OrthSurg; OrthSurg., Hosp. for Sick Children; Cons., Bloorview Children's Hosp.; Clin. Teach. (Surg.), U. of Toronto; Cons. Ont. Crippled Children's Centre; Tel. 923-4471.

BOBEY, William; 11120-102nd St., Edmonton, Alta.; Alb'60; Child Psy., Alberta Guidance Clinic; Tel. 424-0571.

BOBRA, Stanislaw T.; 525 Alfred St., Pembroke, Ont. (res); Lwow (Poland) '39; Path., Pembroke Gen. Hosp.; Tel. RE 2-2811.

BOBYN, Patrick; 341 Medical Arts Bldg., Saskatoon, Sask.; 1326-11th St. E. (res); Sask '59; Assoc. Staff, St. Paul's & City Hosp's.; Tel. 652-5414.

BOCCACCIO, Jack G.; 297 James St. N., Hamilton, Ont.; Wes '58; AMCGP; Staff, Hamilton Civic, St. Joseph's & Chedoke Gen. Hosp's.; Tel. JA 2-2171.

BOCHNER, Maxwell K.; 170 Bloor St. W., Toronto 5, Ont.; Park Plaza Hotel (res); Tor '23; F.A.A.O., A.B. Ophth., Ophth; Chief of Staff, New Mt. Sinai & Scarborough Gen. Hosps.; Chief, Dept. of Ophth. Mt. Sinai & Scarborough Hosps. Tel. WA. 1-2131.

BOCIEK, Robert C.; Central Med. Bldg., 440 Hinton Ave., Ste. B-6, Ottawa 3, Ont.; Ott'55; DABR; D&TRad; Cons., N.D.M.C.; Tel. 725-2125.

BOCKING, Douglas; 429 Averill Cr., London, Ont. (Res.); Wes'43; DABIM; DPM; FRCP(C); IntMed; FACP; Dean, Faculty of Med., U. of Western Ontario; Tel. GE 9-3861.

BOCTOR, Zaher N.; Cairo (Egypt) '57; FRCS (C), Urol; Staff, Royal Victoria Hosp., Montreal, P.Q.; Tel. 842-1251.

BODDIE, Charles A.; Med. Arts Bldg., Empire Ave., St. John's, Nfld.; Queen's U. (Belfast, Ire.) '52; Psy; Dir., Psy. Clinic for Children; Lect. (Child Development), Memorial U.; Tel. 8-3428.

BODDINGTON, George D. M.; Anaes. Assoc., Med. Arts Bldg., Toronto, Ont.; 167 Rosedale Heights Dr. (res); Tor '37; Anaes; Sr. Anaes., Toronto Gen. Hosp.; Clin. Teacher (Anaes.), U. of Toronto; Tel. EM 6-8211.

BODE, Otto B.; 9—10011—123 St., Edmonton, Alta. (res); Berlin (Germ.) '31; M.R.C.S., L.R.C.P. (Lond.) IntMed; Staff, IntMed., Edmonton Gen. Hosp.; School M.O., Board of Health, Edmonton; Tel. GA 2-2032.

BODNAR Stephen; 3465 Cote des Neiges, Montreal, P.Q.; 3221 Forest Hill (res); Debrecan (Hung.) '51; ObstGyn; Staff, Royal Victoria, Reddy Mem., Catherine Booth & Queen Elizabeth Hosp's.; Tel. 935-4477.

BODRUG, Andrew G.; 792A Gerrard St. E., Toronto, Ont.; 28 Meadowacres Dr., Agincourt (res); Tor '54. Tel. HO 6-6844.

BOESKE, Margaret (Ziegenbein); 6414-118th Ave., Edmonton, Alta.; 11161-96th St. (res); Goettingen (Germ.) '44; MCGP; Tel. GR 7-8227.

BOETTGER, R. F.; 195 King St. N., Waterloo, Ont.; Tor '40; M.C.G.P.; Active Staff, Kitchener-Waterloo & St. Mary's Hosp's; Tel. SH 5-9451.

BOFFA, Nicola; Box 600, Louisdale, N.S.; Bologna (Italy)'47.

BOGERT, John R.; 350 Selby Ave., Westmount, P.Q.; 465 Clarke (res); McG '43; GenSurg (P.Q.); Anaes; Assoc. Med. Dir., Charles E. Frosst & Co.; Tel. WE 2-7111.

BOGGIE, Alexander; 3009-31st Ave., Vernon, B.C.; 2202-26th St. (res); UBC '54; MCGP; Tel. 542-4321.

BOGHEN, Dan; Mon'63; Res., Hop. Hotel-Dieu, Montreal 18, P.Q.; Abroad.

BOGO, Norman H.; McG'65; Res., Allan Mem. Inst., Montreal 2, P.Q.

BOGOCH, Abraham; 3195 Granville St., Vancouver 9 ,B.C.; Tor'46; B.Sc., D.Sc., FRCP(C); FACP; IntMed; Chief (Gastroent.) Shaughnessy Hosp. & Vancouver Gen. Hosp.; Hon. Cons., St. Paul's Hosp. & Crease Clinic; Clin. Ass't. Prof. (Med.) U. of B.C.; Tel. RE 8-4246.

BOGOCH, Margaret A. (Mullinger); Health Centre for Children, U. of B.C.; 715 W. 12th, Vancouver, B.C.; Tor'46; A.B.P., Paed; Clin. Inst'r. (Paed.), U. of British Columbia; Tel. CA 4-1111.

BOGORUS, Murray S.; Alb'65; Jr. Int., Royal Alexandra Hosp., Edmonton, Alta.; Abroad.

BOHATIRCHUK, Fedor; Dept. of Anatomy, Ottawa U., Ottawa, Ont.; 500 Driveway (res); Kiev (USSR) '17; D.Sc.; Assoc. Prof., Ottawa U.; Tel. CE 5-6751.

BOHEMIER, Anatole; 3425 St. Hubert, Montreal, P.Q.; Mon '24; IntMed (P.Q.); Staff, Hop. St. Jeanne D'Arc; Retired.

BOHEMIER, Charles A.; 3427 rue St. Hubert, Montreal, P.Q. (res); Lav '18; F.A.C.S., F.I.C.S.; GenSurg (P.Q.); Chief Surg., Hop.-Ste-Jeanne-d'Arc; Retired; Tel. LA 3-7974.

BOHEMIER, J. A.; 688 Blvd. Manseau, Joliette, P.Q.; Mon '32; OphthOtol (P.Q.); Tel. 756-6226.

BOHLIG, Gustav K.; 999 Merivale Rd., Ottawa 3. Ont.; 152 Ruskin Ave. (res); Munich (Bavaria) '48; Tel. PA 8-4380.

BOHNEN, David R.; 550 University Ave., Toronto 2, Ont.; Tor '42; FACS; FRCS(C), GenSurg; Surg-in-Chief, New Mount Sinai & Baycrest Hosp's.; Assoc. Prof. (Surg.), U. of Toronto; Tel. EM 6-7905.

BOIES, Ernest; C.P. 1450, Hop. Schefferville, Schefferville, P.Q.; Lav'61; GenSurg.

BOILARD, Charles A.; 65 Grande Allee E., Quebec 4, P.Q.; 8155 - 1st Ave., Charlesbourg (res); Lav '49; ObstGyn (P.Q.); Staff (ObstGyn), Hop. Hotel Dieu; Tel. 529-9691.

BOILEAU, Georges; 10932 Armand-Lavergne, Montreal-Nord, P.Q.; Mon '58; Chief, Dept. of Med., Fleury Gen. Hosp.; Med. Exam., Metropolitan & Mutual Life Ins. Co's.; Staff, Hop. Mont. Providence; Tel. DA 2-6440.

BOILEAU, G. Rene; 10118-111th St., Edmonton, Alta.; Alb'46; FRCS(C), DABS, FACS; Gen Surg; Att'd. Surg., Edmonton Gen. & Misericordia Hosp's.; Co-ordinator of Intern's Training, Edmonton Gen. Hosp.; Clin. Instr. (Surg.), U. of Alberta; Tel. 422-8207.

BOILEAU, Herve-Jos.; Mon'21; Staff, Notre-Dame de Stanbridge, Bedford, Co. Missisquoi, P.Q.; Tel. 296-4322.

BOILEAU, J. A. Guy; Mon'63; Res., Hop. Hotel-Dieu, Montreal 18, P.Q.

BOILEAU, James R. E.; New Richmond, P.Q.; Lav '18.

BOILEAU, Jean G.; Clinique Medicale Ahuntsic, 241 Fleury St. W., Montreal 12, P.Q.; Mon '59.

BOILEAU, Paul A.; 1150 est boul. St.-Joseph, Montreal 24, P.Q.; Mon'52; Obst; Court. Staff (Obst.), Hop. Maisonneuve.

BOILEAU, Wilfrid; 353 Blvd. St.-Joseph E., Montreal, P.Q.; Mon '33; ClinPath (P.Q.); Phys., "La Presse". Tel. 845-4821.

BOILLAT, Joyce E. L. (Cridland); 541A St. George Blvd., Moncton, N.B.; Tor'54; MCGP; Active Staff, Moncton City & Hotel Dieu Hosps.; Tel. 24280.

BOILY, G. Marcel; 320 de Lavaltrie, Trois Rivieres, P.Q.; Lav'55; PhysMed & Rehab.

BOILY, Jean; 5 rue Laurier, Magog, P.Q.; Mon '62.

BOILY, Laval; 79 Sacre-Coeur, St. Felicien, P.Q.; 60 Sacre-Coeur (res); Lav '63; B.A.; B.Ch.; Tel. 679-0943.

BOILY, Raymond; Lav'59; Res., Hotel Dieu De Montreal, Montreal 18, P.Q.

BOIS, Marc A.; Institut de Cardiologie, 5000 est rue Boulanger, Montreal 36, P.Q.; Mon'57; Cardiol (P.Q.); Tel. 376-3330.

BOIS, Pierre; Mon '53; Ph.D. (Experim [illegible] Assoc. Prof. & Dir. Anat., U. of Montreal, Montreal, P.Q.; Tel. RE 3-9951.

BOISSIERE, Gaston De La; (See De-La-Boissiere)

BOISSONNEAULT, Emile; 247 Birks Bldg., Edmonton, Alta.; Ste O, Westminster Apts. (res); Lav '11; M.C.G.P.; Retired.

BOISSONNEAULT, Yvon; 16 rue Lizotte, Roberval, P.Q.; Lav '60; Anaes.

BOISVERT, Jacques; Mon'65; Res., Hop. Notre Dame, Montreal 24, P.Q.

BOISVERT, Jules; 1628 rue St.-Louis, Plessisville, Co. Megantic, P.Q.; Lav '57.

BOISVERT, Leo P.; 212 Principale, St.-Basile-le-Grand, Cte. Chambly, P.Q.; Mon '55.

BOISVERT, Marcel; 4384 ave. Harvard, Montreal 28, P.Q. (res); McG '61; Research, Royal Victoria Hosp.; Tel. VI 2-1251.

BOISVERT, Marcel; 315 Stuart Ave., Outremont, Montreal 8, P.Q.; Lav '50; Psy; Cons., Hop. Sacre Coeur, Cartierville; Clin. Ass't. Inst. of Psychotherapy; Tel. 277-0404.

BOISVERT, Michel J. G.; Lav '58; Anaes; Staff (Anaes), Hop.-St.-Ambroise, Loretteville, P.Q.; Tel. 842-3651.

BOISVERT, Paul R.; 550 Sacre-Coeur, St.-Hyacinthe, P. Q.; Lav '42; Ophth (P.Q.); Otol; Tel. PR 4-8154.

BOISVERT, Raymond; Med. Dir., Sanatorium St-Francois, Sherbrooke, P.Q.; Lav '37; Pulm. Dis & T.B. (P.Q.); Tel. 569-2551.

BOISVERT, Rene, Sg. Lt.; Lav'65; 11 Detach. RCAMC, 4050-4th Ave. W., Vancouver 8, B.C.

BOISVERT-THEORET, Suzanne; 3715 Beaumont, Southgate, Ville Brossard Co., Laprairie, P.Q.; Mon '57; Path (PQ).

BOITEAU, Guy M.; 2725 Chemin Ste-Foy, Quebec 10, P.Q.; Lav '55; Cardiol (P.Q.); Staff, Hop. Laval; Tel. 653-5251.

BOIVIN, Germain L.; Lav'57; Phys Med. & Rehab; Staff, Hotel-Dieu de Sherbrooke, Sherbrooke, P.Q.; Tel. 569-2551, Ext. 335.

BOIVIN, J. Claude; 430 Monique, St. Jerome, P.Q.; Mon '54; FRCP(C), Path; Staff, Hotel-Dieu; Tel. GE 8-4886.

BOIVIN, Jean L.; 3901 des Champs, Trois Rivieres, P.Q.; Lav '53; FRCP(C), Anaes.

BOIVIN, Roch; 2651 Roussel, Chicoutimi, Nord P.Q.; Lav '41; Anaes (P.Q.); Anaes., Hotel Dieu, St. Vallier de Chicoutimi; Tel. 549-1452.

BOIVIN, Yvan; 3840 St. Urbain, Montreal 18, P.Q.; Ott '58; Path (P.Q.).

BOJKO, Myron; 145 Wellington St., Sarnia, Ont.; Germany '45.

BOLAND, Katherine E.; 1125 East Hastings St., Vancouver 6, B.C.; Tor'65.

BOLDT, Werner; Alb '61; Res., Vancouver Gen. Hosp., Vancouver, B.C.

BOLDUC, Jean P.; Mon'65; Res., Hop. Maisonneuve, Montreal 36, P.Q.

BOLDUC, Louis deG.; 650-10th Ave. Senneterre, P.Q. Lav '33; Tel. 737-2111.

BOLDUC, Philippe; Mon'65; Res., Hop. Hotel-Dieu, Montreal 18, P.Q.

BOLDUC, William L.; 1009 No. 3 Rd., Richmond, B.C.; Alb'61; MCGP.

BOLEY, John P.; 1279 Ouellette Ave., Windsor, Ont.; 1432 Victoria Ave. (res); Tor '23; D.A.B. Op., FRCS(C), Ophth.; Tel. 254-4433.

BOLLAND, Peter G.; 1265 Clarkson Rd. N., Clarkson, Ont.; Tor'57; M.C.G.P.; Staff, Oakville-Trafalgar Hosp. & South Peel Hosp.; Tel. 822-9171.

BOLTE, Edouard; 5623 ave. Darlington, Montreal, P.Q.; Mon'56; IntMed(P.Q.); Staff, Hop. Hotel Dieu, Montreal & Dept. of Physiol., U. of Montreal; Tel. VI 4-0161.

BOLTON, Charles F.; University Hosp., Saskatoon, Sask.; Qns'56; FRCP(C), Neur; Lect. (Neur.), U. of Saskatchewan.

BOLTON, Peter S.; McGregor Clinic, 250 Main St. E., Hamilton, Ont.; Qns'58; FRCP(C), Derm; Active Staff, Hamilton Gen. & Henderson Gen. Hosps.; Court. Staff, Chedoke Gen. & Children's Hosps.; Tel. 527-2711.

BOLTON, Robin J.; Qns '61; Jr. Intn., Victoria Hosp., London, Ont.

BOMBARDIER, Jean P.; 55 Ave. de l'Eglise, Verdun, Montreal 19, P.Q.; 4375 Ave. Coolbrook (res); Mon '37; F.A.A.P.; Paed (P.Q.); Chief, Paed Serv., Verdun Gen. Hosp.; Assoc. Prof. (Paed), Montreal U.; Tel. RE 3-9951.

BOMBARDIER, Romuald; 10759 Grande Allee, Montreal 12, P.Q. (res); Mon '36.

BONACCORSI, Maria T.; 266 Cote St. Catherine, Montreal, P.Q.; Pavia (Italy) '55; Paed (Italy); Psy; Dir. Dept. of Psy., Hop. Mont Providence; Tel. 665-4971.

BONAR, James G.; Deloraine, Man.; Man '53; M.C.G.P.; Tel. 277.

BOND, Alan F.; Box 280, Brooks, Alta.; Ott '54; GenSurg.

BOND, Archibald W.; Box 129, Smithville, Ont.; Wes'48; M.C.G.P.; Tel. 957-7025.

BOND, Ian K.; 55 Elderwood Drive, Toronto 10, Ont. Edin. (Scot.) '52; D.Psy; Psy; Staff, Ont. Hosp., New Toronto. Tel. CL 9-8291.

BOND, Solomon C.; 937 Broadview Ave., Toronto, Ont.; Tor '43; M.C.G.P.; Staff, O.P.D., New Mount Sinai Hosp.; Tel. HO 6-7185.

BONDAR, George F., 305 Professional Bldg., 10830 Jasper Ave., Edmonton, Alta.; McG '57; FRCS(C), GenSurg; FACS; DABS; Att'd. Staff, Edmonton Gen. Hosp.; Court. Cons. Misercordia Hosp.; Clin. Cons. Cancer Clin., Gov't. of Alberta; Research Fell., S.M.R. Inst. of Alta.; Instr., U. of Alberta; Tel. 424-6606.

BONDY, Donald C.; 291 Dundas St., London, Ont.; 26 St. Neots Dr. (res); Wes '56; FRCP(C); IntMed; Staff, & Exec. Officer Clin. Invest. Unit., Westminster DVA Hosp; Lect. (Med.) Western U.; Tel. GE 4-2683.

BONELL, J. Douglas; Arnprior Med. Centre, 104 Daniel St., Arnprior, Ont.; Qns '50; GenSurg; Staff, Arnprior & Dist. Mem. Hosp.; Tel. 623-3131.

BONENFANT, Guy; 5 rue St-Jacques, St-Bruno, P.Q.; Mon'61; Tel. 677-6262.

BONENFANT, Jean L.; 1017 Forget, Sillery, Quebec, P.Q.; (res); Lav '46; F.R.C.P.(C), Path; Ass't. Path., Hotel-Dieu; Path., Hotel Dieu de la Beauce, St. Georges; Assoc. Prof. Pathological Anat., Laval U.; Tel. LA 9-4511.

BONFIELD, J. P.; 163 Laurier Ave. E., Ottawa 2, Ont.; Qns '29; Anaes; Staff, Ottawa Gen. Hosp.; Tel. CE 6-0333.

BONFIELD, John P.; 497 Somerset St. W., Ottawa, Ont.; Qns '16; M.R.C.S., L.R.C.P.; GenSurg; Staff, Ottawa Gen. Hosp.; Lect., (Anaes.), U. of Ottawa; Tel. CE 2-2366.

BONGA, Agatha C. (Van Vierssen Trip); R.R. No. 3, Mouth of Keswick, N.B.; Sask '58; Court. Staff, Victoria Public Hosp., Fredericton.

BONHAM, Gerald H.; North Shore Health Unit, 253 E. 14th St., North Vancouver, B.C.; Man '56; DPH; PH; Tel. 988-5231.
BONHOMME, P. E.; 196 rue St. Catherine, Beauharnois, P.Q.; McG '48; Tel. 268-3433.
BONIN, Andre; Mon'62; Path(P.Q.); Staff, Hop. Ste-Justine, Montreal, P.Q.
BONIN, Gerard; 489 Blvd. Ste-Anne, Joliette, P.Q.; 919 Bordeleau (res); Mon '54; GenSurg; Tel. 756-8073.
BONIN, Marcel; 119 Dufferin, Stanstead, P.Q.; Mon '54; MCGP; Tel. 876-2172.
BONIN, Raymond; 14 Severn St., Sudbury, Ont.; Lav'61; Path.; Staff, Hop. St. Joseph.
BONIN, Rolland J.; 42 Pare, Granby, P.Q.; 165 boul. Leclerc (res); Mon '58; Chief of Med. Serv., St. Joseph's Hosp.; Tel. 372-4454.
BONKALO, Alexander; 2 Surrey Pl., Toronto 5, **Ont.; 12 Fidelia Ave., Tor. 12 (res); Budapest (Hung.) '37; Psy; Staff, Tor. Psy. Hosp.; Ass't. Prof. (Psy), U. of Toronto; Tel. WA 5-6371.**
BONNELL, Frederick H.; 700 Campbell Bldg., Victoria, B.C.; 1910 **Watson St. (res); Qns '35; D.M.R., D & TRad.; Tel. EV 2-9104.**
BONNELL, George E.; Fredericton Med. Clinic, **206 Rookwood Ave., Fredericton, N.B.; 404 Albert St. (res); Dal '53; Urol; Tel. 475-7701.**
BONNELL, John C.; Dal'60; Res., Royal Victoria Hosp., Montreal 2, P.Q.
BONNELL, Lorne; Murray River, P.E.I.
BONNELL, Ronald R.; 3195 Granville St., Vancouver, B.C.; 4537 Haggart St. (res); Qns '51; DiagRad; Staff (Rad.), Burnaby Gen. & White Rock Dist. Hosp's.; Tel. RE 1-5241.
BONNELL, Saul; 925 W. Georgia St., Vancouver, B.C.; 1445 Marpole St. (res); McG '46; GenSurg; Tel 733-6913.
BONNER, Keith P.; 200 St. Clair Ave. W., Toronto 7, Ont.; 20 Ardmore Rd. (res); Tor '34; D.D.R.; DiagRad., Grace **Hosp. & Workman's** Compensation Board; Tel. WA 3-5148.
BONNER, Kevin J.; 36 Coburg St., Saint John, N.B.; 253 Somerset St. (res); Ott'52; FACS; GenSurg; Surg Cons., Lancaster DVA Hosp.; **Surg. Staff, St. John's Gen. & St. Joseph's Hosp's.; Tel. 693-2341.**
BONNEY, W. Robert; 40 George St. N. Galt, Ont.; 187 West River Rd. (res); Tor '46; B.Sc. (Med.); IntMed; Staff, South Waterloo Mem. Hosp.; Tel. 623-1756.
BONNIER, Jean G.; 13 Strathyre, Ville-La-Salle, Lachine, P.Q.; 769-40th Ave. (res); Mon '56; PH (P.Q.); D.P.H.; F.A.G.S.; A.M.C.G.P.; Med. Dir., Dept: of Health Ville-La-Salle & Hop.-Gen.; I/C PrevMed., U. of Mtl.; Tel. DO 6-7110.
BONSER, Frank H.; 4528A Kingston Rd., West Hill, Ont.; 93 Pegasus Trail, Scarborough (res); Tor '61; Tel. 282-1573.
BOODOOSINGH, Ram S.; River Hebert, N.S.; Dal '64.; Tel. 153 Exchange 133.
BOOK, Howard E.; Man'65; Res., St. Boniface Hosp., St. Boniface 6, Man.
BOOK, Noel A.; 814 Boyd Bldg., Winnipeg 1, **Man.; 764 Montrose St. (res); Man. '51; Ophth; Tel. WH 3-0148.**
BOON, Alfred H.; Birch River, Man.; Northwestern U. (Chicago, Ill.) '11; M.R.C.S.(Eng.), L.R.C.P. (Lond.); Tel. AD 6-4333.
BOON, David A.; Ste. 202, 141 Victoria St., Kamloops, B.C.; UBC'56; Otol.
BOONE, Frank H.; 705 Medical Arts Bldg., Hamilton, Ont.; 137 Mountain Park (res); Tor '17; **FAAP, Paed.; Tel. TA 8-7663.**
BOONE, James E.; 555 University Ave., Toronto 2, Ont.; 225 Harborn Rd., Cooksville (res); Tor '51; FRCP(C); Paed; Staff, Hosp. for Sick Children; Ass't. Prof. (Paed.), U. of Toronto; Tel. EM 6-7242.
BOONE, John A.; UBC'62; Res., Royal Victoria Hosp., Montreal 2, P.Q.
BOORMAN, G. C.; Rimbey, Alta.; Alb '45; MCGP Dist. Coroner; Tel. 843-2180.
BOORMAN, Samuel T.; Dawson Creek Med. Clin., 816-103rd Ave., Dawson Creek, B.C.; 1320-93rd Ave. (res); **Alb '51; F.R.C.S.** (C), Gen-Surg; Tel. ST 2-4848.
BOOTH, Denton H.; 8 Kingston Row, Winnipeg 8, Man.; Man '45; Pension Med. Examiner, Cdn. Pension Commission; Tel. CH 7-2539.
BOOTH, George H.; Pioneer St., Agassiz, B.C.; 7291 Morrow Rd. (res); Victoria U. (Manchester, Eng.) '25; Tel. 796-9120.
BOOTH, John F.; 280 Marlborough Pl., Niagara **Falls, Ont. (res)**; Belfast (N.Ire.) '45; B.A.O.; Path.; Dir. of Labs., Greater Niagara Gen. Hosp.; **Reg. Path. Attorney-General's Dept.**; Tel. EL 8-3611.
BOOTH, John H.; Box 129, Agassiz, B.C.; UBC'60; FRCS(C), ObstGyn; Abroad.
BOOTH, L. Isabel; 250 Lawrence Ave. W., Toronto 12, Ont.; 114 Inglewod Dr. (res); Tor '39; Paed; Staff, Hosp. for Sick Children & Women's College Hosp.; Tel. RU 7-1082.
BOOTH, Marvin L.; 305 Nelson St., Wallaceburg, Ont.; 48 Dundas St. (res); Wes '32. Tel. 627-2442.
BOOTH, Patricia M. (Bradford); 196 Valley Rd., Willowdale (res.); London (Eng.) '58; LRCP (Lond.); MRCS (Eng.); Staff, W.C.B.
BOOTHROYD, Lawrence S.A.; 520-17th St., West Vancouver, B.C.; 1940 Lonsdale, N. Van.; 2976 Mathers Ave. West Van. (res); St. Thomas (London, Eng.) '43; M.B., B.S., M.R.C.S. (Eng.), L.R.C.P. (Lond.), F.R.C.S. (Eng.), F.A.C.S., F.R.C.S.(C), GenSurg; Urol; Cons. Surg., Lion's Gate Hosp., N. Van.; Tel. WA 2-2531; YU 5-5015.
BOOTHROYD, Margaret D. (Findlay); 2976 Mathers Ave., West Vancouver, B.C. (res); London (Eng.) '50; D.R.C.O.G.; Retired.
BOOTHROYD, Wilfred E.; 15 York Downs Dr., Downsview, Ont. (res); Dal '40; Psy; Hd. Div. of Psy., Sunnybrook D.V.A. Hosp.; Cons. Dept. of Reform Inst. (Ont.); Ass't. Prof. (Psy), U. of Toronto; Tel. 485-8651.
BORCENA, Herminia C.; Santo Tomas (Philipp.) '50; Staff, Regina Gen. Hosp., Regina, Sask.
BORDELEAU, Jean-M.; 3423 St.-Denis, Montreal 18, P.Q.; 6227 Deacon Rd. (res); Mon '51; Psy (P.Q.); IntMed (P.Q.); Dir. Research, Inst., Albert Prevost; Ass't Prof. (Psy), U. of Montreal; Tel. VI 2-4892.
BORDELEAU, Normand J.; 304 St. Odilon, Proulxville, Champlain, P.Q.; Lav'65.
BORDEN, Harry A.; 730 King St., Preston, Ont.; 666 Queen St. (res); Tor '32; Indus. Phys., General Foods & Savage Shoe Co.; Tel. 653-6833.
BORDEN, Russell P.; 22853 MacDonald Rd., Langley, B.C.; **Harvard (Yale) '15; Retired.**
BORDUAS, A. Guy; 94 Ouest Blainville, Ste-Therese, Co. Terrebonne, **P.Q.; Mon'64.**
BORDUAS, Jean L. S.; 8415 St-Denis, Montreal, P.Q.; 265 Chemin St. Catherine, Outremont (res); Mon'50; Cardiol (P.Q.); Chief Cardiol., Hop. Jean Talon; Tel DU 1-5311.
BORESKIE, Joseph P.; Box 95, Gretna, Man.; Man '48; MCGP; Public Health Officer; Tel. 327-5555.
BORETSKY, Peter; 5253 Decarie Blvd., Ste. 202, Montreal, P.Q.; 5285 Mayfair (res); Qns '45; Pt.-time Staff, Queen Mary Vet's Hosp.; Tel. 484-5575.
BORG, Francis X.; 3564 Dufferin St., Downsview, Ont.; **Royal Malta U. '49;** D.A.R.C.S. (Eng.); Ph.C. (Malta); Anaes; Chief Dept. of Anaes., Humber Mem. Hosp.; Tel. ME 5-6556.
BORGAONKAR, Ram D.; Vikram '59; FRCP(C), IntMed; Staff, Ottawa Civic Hosp., Ottawa, Ont.
BORGIEL, Alexander E. H.; 3394 Grand Forks **Rd.**, Cooksville, Ont.; Tor '64.
BORIGHT, H. Angus; 4491 Sherbrooke St. W., Montreal 6, P.Q.; McG '55; IntMed (P.Q.); Tel. 935-7892.
BORIGHT, Robert R.; 596 Cote St-Antoine Rd., Westmount 6, P.Q.; McG'44; Anaes; Jr. Ass't. Anaes., Montreal Gen. Hosp.
BORINS, Elaine F. (Manace); Ste. 106, 400 Walmer Rd., Toronto 10, Ont.; Tor'62.
BORLAND, Kyle R.; 4204 Sheppard Ave., Agincourt, Ont.; Tor '44; MCGP; Vis. Staff, Toronto East Gen. & Scarborough Gen. Hosp's.; Tel. 293-4121.
BORLAND, N. Joan (Farquharson); Tor '44; DPH; Staff, School of Hygiene, U. of Toronto; Toronto, Ont.; Tel. WA 3-6611.

BORN, Gunter; 411 Med. Arts. Bldg., 1 Young St., Hamilton, Ont.; Bern (Switz.) '52; FRCS(C), PlasSurg; Active Staff, Hamilton Civic & St. Joseph's Hosp's.; Court. Staff, Chedoke Gen., Children's & Joseph Brant Hosp's.; Tel. 525-0560.
BOROWY, Zenan J.; Ste. 402 Medical Arts Bldg., 170 St. George St., Toronto 5, Ont.; 26 Ballantyne Ct. (res); Tor '49; F.R.C.S.(C), GenSurg; Staff (Surg.), St. Joseph's Hosp.; Assoc. Staff (Surg.), Queensway Gen. Hosp.; Tel. WA 2-1737.
BORRAJO, Cesareo P.; 88 Berbard Ave., Apt. 1007, Toronto 5, Ont.; Santiago (Spain)'57; Paed.
BORRON, Randolph W. J.; 272 Roncesvalles Ave., Toronto, Ont.; 1 Kingsmill (res); Tor '26; DiagRad.; Tel. LE 6-6023.
BORROWMAN, Almer M. W.; 291 Wellington St., Sarnia, Ont.; 860 Lakeshore Rd. (res); Alb '30; ObstGyn; Chief (ObstGyn), Sarnia Gen. Hosp.; Tel. ED 7-3771.
BORSCH, Roman N.; 400 Walmer Rd., Toronto 10, Ont.; Tor'57; Psy.
BORSCHNECK, Anthony G.; 208 Mary St., Chilliwack, B.C.; UBC'64; Tel. 795-7228.
BORSI, Mario R.; 158 Lake St., St. Catharines, Ont.; Rome (Italy) '44; Cert. Chest Dis. (Rome), F.C.C.P.; Tel. 684-6728.
BORSMAN, Charles H.; 260 Bentall Bldg., 1070 Douglas St., Victoria, B.C.; McG '48; MRCOG; ObstGyn; Chief, ObstGyn., St. Joseph's Hosp.; Court. Cons. Staff. Royal Jubilee Hosp.; Tel. EV 3-7624.
BORSOOK, Dorothy H.; 99 Avenue Rd., Toronto 5, Ont.; 324 Glenayr Rd. (res); Tor '31; ObstGyn; Staff (Obst. Gyn), Women's College & Toronto Gen. Hosp's.; Tel. 924-3743.
BORZECKI, Julita L. (Staweno); 30 Trinity Circle, Dollard-des-Ormeaux, P.Q.; Brussels (Belg.) '49; Anaes.
BOS, Carlo G.; 1538 Sherbrooke St. W., Montreal, P.Q.; 3605 Marlowe Ave., N.D.G. (res); McG '43; Psy; Assoc. Psy., Royal Victoria Hosp.; Assoc. Prof. (Psy.), McGill U.; Tel. WE 2-6842.
BOSCH, Jan W.; 226 Harwood Ave. N., Ajax, Ont.; 70 Hill's Rd. (res); Leiden (Netherlands) '46; MCGP; Tel. 942-2100.
BOSCO, Francesco; 4346 St.-Denis, Montreal, P.Q.; Qns '30; Tel. VI 4-3945.
BOSLEY, Eliska M. (Soulova); Geneva (Switz) '60; Staff, (Phys. Med. & Rehab.), Manitoba Rehab. Hosp., Winnipeg, Man.; Tel. SP 5-0181.
BOSS, Mark M.; 49 Broad St., Brockville, Ont.; McG '49 ;MCGP; Active Staff, St. Vincent de Paul Hosp., & Brockville Gen. Hosp.; Med. Dir., Henry K. Wampole Co. Ltd., Perth; Tel. 342-7650.
BOSSE, Jean; 3100 rue Ellendale, Montreal, P.Q.; Mon'59; Psy(P.Q.).
BOSSE, Jean-Paul; 30 St. Joseph Boul. est, Montreal 14, P.Q.; Mon'59; FRSC(C), Plas Surg; Staff, Hop. Hotel-Dieu, Montreal 36, P.Q.
BOSSINOTTE, Antonio; Parliament Bldgs., Quebec City, P.Q.; 1224 Preston Ave. (res); Lav '20; Chief, Public Charities & Assistance Div., Dept. of Health, P.Q.; Retired.
BOSTOCK, Douglas; Thorhild, Alta.; Sheffield (Eng.)'60; MB; ChB.
BOSTON, R. Wesley; 318 Palace Rd., Kingston, Ont.; Qns'57; FRCP(C), Paed; Staff, Dept. of Paed., Kingston Gen. Hosp.; Ass't. Prof. (Paed.), Queen's U.
BOSWELL, Gerald C.; 2020 Mountainside Dr., Burlington, Ont.; Tor '58.
BOTA, William; 41 Braemar Place, Hamilton, Ont.; Wes '55; Anaes; Active Staff, St. Joseph's Hosp.; Tel. 522-4941.
BOTTERELL, E. Harry, O.B.E.; 2 Lakeshore Blvd., Kingston, Ont. (res); Man '30; M.S., F.R.C.S. (C), GenSurg; NeurSurg; Cons. (ex Off.), Hotel-Dieu Hosp.; Cons. C.F.M.C.; Hon. Cons., Tor. Gen. Hosp. & Memb. Advis. Bd., Lyndhurst Lodge; Dean, Fac. of Med., & Prof. (NeurSurg), Queen's U.; Tel. 546-3871.
BOTTOMLEY, H. W.; Winnipeg Clinic, Winnipeg 1, Man.; 627 South Dr. (res); Man '43; FACP; IntMed (Allerg.); Dir. of Allergy Clinic, Winnipeg Chidren's Hosp.; Te 942-0551.
BOUAZIZ, Ali; 1105 ave Belvedere, App. 124, Quebec 6, P.Q.; Paris (France)'60; FRCS(C), GenSurg.
BOUCHARD, Adrien J. G.; 1044 Riviera Dr., Ottawa 7, Ont.; Ott'59; GenSurg.
BOUCHARD, Gilles; 101 rue Principale, Rock Island, P.Q.; Mon '63.
BOUCHARD, Guy R.; 541 rue de l'hopital, Jonquiere, P.Q.; Lav '55; Otol (P.Q.); Staff, Hop. Notre-Dame de l'Assomption; Tel. 547-9341.
BOUCHARD, Henri L.; Lav'65; Res., Hotel-Dieu de Quebec, Quebec 4, P.Q.
BOUCHARD, Jean; Hop. Royal Victoria, Montreal, P.Q.; Lav'34; DABR; DMR (Cantab.); FACR; FRCP(C), D&TRad; Chief Rad., Royal Victoria Hosp.; Prof. & Dir. Dept. of Rad., McGill U.; Tel. 842-1251, Loc. 771.
BOUCHARD, Jean P.; Lav'57; Psy (P.Q.); Staff, Hop. Pierre Janet, 20 rue Pharand, Hull, P.Q.
BOUCHARD, Jean P.; Lav'65; Res., Hop. l'Enfant Jesus, Quebec 3, P.Q.
BOUCHARD, Joachim; 106 St. Edouard St., Urbain, Cte. Charlevoix, P.Q.; Lav '60.
BOUCHARD, Laurier; 9320 est, rue Notre-Dame, Montreal 5, P.Q.; Lav '52.
BOUCHARD, Marc; 1321 Nelles, Quebec 10, P.Q.; Lav'61; Biochem(P.Q.); Research, Laval Univ., Quebec, P.Q.; Tel. 681-7987.
BOUCHARD, Marcel; 38 de la Colombiere, Mastai, P.Q. (res); Lav '49; Psy; Staff Psy., Hop.-St-Michel & Hop.-Ste-Foy (DVA); Lect., Laval U.; Tel. 661-7781.
BOUCHARD, Maurice; Centre Medical Jeffery Hale, 1248 Chemin Ste-Foy, Ste. 103, Quebec, P.Q.; Lav '60; Paed; Chief of Paed., Jeffery Hale's Hosp.; Tel. 681-0833.
BOUCHARD, Remi; Lav '53; F.R.C.S.(C), GenSurg; Staff, Hop. Hotel Dieu St. Michel, Roberval, P.Q.; Tel. 275-0110.
BOUCHARD, Reynald; 209 boul. Dequen, Alma, Lac-St-Jean, P.Q.; Lav '65.
BOUCHARD, Toussaint; Lav '51; Res., Hop.-St.-Vincent-de-Paul, Sherbrooke, P.Q.
BOUCHARD LEBEL, Jean; 4065 rue Saint-Hubert, Montreal, P.Q.; Mon '37.
BOUCHER, Andre J.; Richibucto, N.B.; Lav'65.
BOUCHER, Benoit; 120 Ste-Anne, Quebec 4, P.Q.; Lav '45; IntMed (P.Q.); Med. Dir., Hop.-St.-Augustine, Ancienne-Lorette; Med. Ass't., Hop.-Ste-Foy (DVA); Cons. Quebec Rehab. Clin., Hop.-Laval; Prof. PhysMed & Rehab & Pedagogie, Laval U.; Ass't Med. Dir., Indus. Assur. Co.; Tel. 524-8501.
BOUCHER, Bertrand; Ste. Croix, Co. Lotbiniere, P.Q.; Lav '58.
BOUCHER, Clement; 5181 rue Notre Dame, Banlieue, Trois-Rivieres, P.Q.; Lav '46, Staff Anaes., St. Joseph's Hosp.; Tel. FR 4-6211.
BOUCHER, Daniel; Box 817, Jonquiere, Co. Lapointe, P.Q.; Lav. '55.
BOUCHER, Denis; Mon '48; Pulm. Dis. & TB (P.Q.); Chief Phys., San. St. Georges, Mont Joli, P.Q.; Tel. PR 5-4355.
BOUCHER, Duncan W.; 102 Wellington St., Kingston, Ont.; 96 Hill St. (res); Qns '28; F.R.C.S. (Edin.), F.R.C.S.(C), GenSurg; Assoc. Prof. Surg., Queen's U.; Chief of Surg., Hotel Dieu; Att. Surg., Kingston Gen. Hosp.; Tel. 548-4750.
BOUCHER, Georges H.; 6907 10eme ave., Rosemont, Montreal, P.Q.; Lav '53; AMCGP.
BOUCHER, Harold H.; 925 W. Georgia St., Vancouver, B.C.; 6025 Angus Dr. (res); McG '26; M.Sc., OrthSurg; Hon. Cons., Shaughnessy Hosp. & Vancouver Gen. Hosp.; Clinical Asst. Prof. (Orth. Surg.), U. of British Columbia; Tel. 683-3381.
BOUCHER, Jacques R.; 5180 Ave Des Sorbiers, Montreal 36, P.Q.; Lav '57; Anaes; Staff, Hop. Notre-Dame; Tel. LA 5-6363.
BOUCHER, Jean L.; Lav'52; Res., Hop. Maisonneuve, Montreal 36, P.Q.
BOUCHER, Joseph H.; St-Jean-Baptiste, Man.; Lav '49; M.C.G.P.
BOUCHER, Louis A.; Irving Clinic, 74 Seymour St. W., Kamloops, B.C.; Alb'62.
BOUCHER, Marcel F.; St. Bruno, Co. Lac., St. Jean, P.Q.; Lav'60.

BOUCHER, Marcel H.; Lav '60; Anaes (P.Q.); Staff, Hop. St-Francois-d'Assise, Quebec 3, P.Q.; Tel. 529-7311.
BOUCHER, Peter R.; Ott'63; Res., Vancouver Gen. Hosp., Vancouver, B.C.
BOUCHER, Raymond R.; Lav '54; DiagRad; Staff, Hotel-Dieu, Notre-Dame-de-l'Assomption, Jonquiere, P.Q.; Tel. 542-4124.
BOUCHER, Roland; 5790 Maricourt, Montreal-Nord, P.Q.; Man '44; Staff (Admin) Hop. Notre-Dame; Tel. 523-5656.
BOUCHER, Thomas; 3350 de Courual, Trois-Rivieres, P.Q.; Lav'59; IntMed.(P.Q.); Pulm. Dis. & TB(P.Q.).
BOUCHER, Yvon; 2465 rue Sicotte, St. Hyacinthe, P.Q.; Mon'61; GenSurg.
BOUCK, Adeline (see Bell, M. E. Adeline)
BOUDREAU, Andre; 969 Route De L'Eglise, Quebec 10, P.Q.; Lav'54; Dir., Alcoholism Div., Prov. Dept. of Health.
BOUDREAU, A. T.; 830—3e Ave., Quebec, P.Q.; Lav '31; MCGP.
BOUDREAU, Claude; 5137 Clairewood Terr., Pointe-Claire, P.Q.; '60; Gastroent(P.Q.).
BOUDREAU, Gabriel; Cheticamp, Inverness Co., N.S.; Dal '35; Tel. 28.
BOUDREAU, Germain P.; Mon'62; Res., Hop. du Christ-Roi, Montreal 19, P.Q.
BOUDREAU, J. Donald; 90 Charlotte St., Saint John, N.B.; Ott'53; M.O., W.C.B.; Tel. 692-0181.
BOUDREAU, John F.; 2022 Robie St., Halifax, N.S.; 146 Oxford (res); Dal'51; AMCGP.
BOUDREAU, Marcel A.; Amqui, P.Q.; Lav '40.
BOUDREAU, Romeo; Bonaventure, P.Q.; Lav '53.
BOUDREAULT, Gerard; C.P. 292, 475 Boul. Talbot, Chicoutimi, P.Q.; 223 Boul.-St.-Sacrement (res); Lav'44; IntMed (Cardiol)(P.Q.); Chief, Cardiol., Hotel-Dieu-St.-Vallier; Tel. 549-3313.
BOUDREAULT, Wilfrid; C.P. 129, 18 rue Bergeron, Roberval, P.Q.; Mon '28.
BOUDRIAS, Jean; P.O. Box 79, Cookshire, P.Q.; P.O. Box 10, Waterville (res); Mon '44; D.P.H.
BOUDRIAU, Albert; 1625 Blvd. Morgan, Montreal 4, P.Q.; Mon. '41; Tel. 255-2147.
BOUFFARD, Marcel; Hauterive, Co. Saguenay P.Q.; Lav '46; Dist. Coroner.
BOUGHEN, Frederick L.; 110 Harvie St., Gravenhurst, Ont.; 120 Harvie St. (res); Tor '53; MCGP; Chief of Staff, South Muskoka Mem. Hosp., Bracebridge; Coroner Muskoka; Tel. 687-2266.
BOUGHNER, Derek R.; West'65; Jr. Int., Victoria Hosp., London, Ont.
BOUGHTON, Harvey C.; 623 Rusholme Rd., Saskatoon, Sask. (res); Man '14; IntMed (TB); Hon. Cons. (Med.), University Hosp.; Retired.
BOUJOFF, George V.; Tor'62; Res., New Mount Sinai Hosp., Toronto 2, Ont.
BOULAIS, Claude N.; 240 rue Elm, St. Lambert, P.Q.; Mon'58; FRCS(C), ObstGyn; Staff, Hop. Charles Le Moyne; Tel. 671-3086.
BOULAIS, Frederick L.; 6565 Boul Pie IX, Montreal 36, P.Q. (res); Mon '24; DermSyph; M.O., Health Dept.
BOULANGER, Jacques; 45 Ste.-Ursule, Quebec, P.Q.; Lav '42; Ophth, Otol (P.Q.); Ass't. Ophth, Hop.-Ste-Foy; Chief, Ophth,Otol., Hop.-St.-Francis-d'Assise; Assoc. Prof., Laval U.; Tel. 525-6272.
BOULANGER, Jean-B; 3610 ave. Atwater, Montreal 25, P.Q.; Mon'48; M.A.; L.Psy.; D.I.P. (Paris); FRCP(C); FAPA; NeurPsy (P.Q.); Psy; Cons. Psy., Inst. Albert-Prevost, Hop. Gen. Verdun & Lakeshore Gen. Hosp.; Cons. (Child Psy.) & Dir., Group Psycotherapy, Hop. Ste-Justine; Training Analyst, Can. Inst. Psychoanalysis; Lect. (Psycopath.), Laval U.; Assoc. Prof. (Psy.), U. of Montreal; Tel. 932-4562.
BOULANGER, Lionel; St.-Pascal, Cte. Kamouraska, P.Q.; Lav '53; M.C.G.P.
BOULANGER, Marcel L.; 752 Bloomfield, Montreal 8, P.Q.; Lav'54; Anaes; MCGP; Staff, Hop. Notre-Dame, Montreal 24, P.Q.; Tel. 525-6363.
BOULANGER, Michel J.; 10018-102 A Ave., Edmonton, Alta.; Ott '51; Tel. 424-4959.
BOULARD, Gilles; 371 rue Flamand, Joliette, P.Q.; Mon '54; DiagRad; Staff, Hop.-St.-Eusebe; Tel. PL 6-8041.
BOULAY, Gaspard; 151 rue King O., Sherbrooke, P.Q.; 1501 rue Leclerc (res); Mon '39; IntMed (P.Q.); Head of Dept. of Med., Hop. Gen., St. Vincent de Paul; Tel. LO 2-7533.
BOULAY, Jacques; 299-5eme rue, Quebec 3, P.Q.; 857 rue Chanoine Martin, Ste.-Foy (res); Lav '53; F.R.C.P. (C), IntMed; Haem (P.Q.); Haematol., Hop.-St. Francois-d'Assise & Hop.-Laval; Med. Dir., Red Cross Blood Transfusion Centre; Tel. 529-7311.
BOULAY, J. Raymond; 18 O'Leary St., Campbellton, N.B.; Lav '51; ObstGyn; Tel. PL 3-4431.
BOULAY, Leo; 1150 St. Joseph Blvd. E., Montreal 34, P.Q.; Mon'50; GenSurg (P.Q.); Surg., Hop. Maisonneuve; Tel. LA 7-1241.
BOULAY, R.; Kedgewick, N.B.; Lav '26; Dist. Coroner.
BOULDING, C. R.; Tor '23; House Phys., Home for the Aged, Greenacres, Newmarket, Ont.
BOULDING, Joseph E.; Ste. 2, 140 Wallace St., Nanaimo, B.C.; McGill'53; Psy.; Tel. 753-1175.
BOULET, Maurice; 39 rue St-Louis, Quebec 4, P.Q.; Lav '32; Staff, Allocation-Sociales-de-Quebec.
BOULET, Roland; Mon'58; Res., Hop. St. Jean De Dieu, Montreal 5, P.Q.
BOULIANE, Roland J.; 300 Boul. Wilfrid-Hamel, Quebec 8, P.Q.; Lav '49; D.M.R.E. (France); D & T Rad.
BOULIANE, Philippe; Lav'52; Res., Dept. of Anthropol., U. of Toronto, Toronto, Ont.
BOULIANNE, Jean C. Capt.; 891 ave Laurier, Quebec 4, P.Q.; Lav'65.
BOULOS, Anthony N.; 33 Beaverbrook Ave., Saint John, N.B.; Damascus (Syria)'57; Gen Surg; Staff, Saint John Gen. & St. Joseph's Hosp's.; Tel. 693-9372.
BOULOS, Joseph B.; Le Marchant Drug Bldg., 8 Campbell Ave., St. John's, Nfld.; National U. (Galway, Ire.) '54; M.B., B.Ch., BAO; FACOG; Staff, St. Clare's Mercy, St. John's Gen., Grace Maternity & Hosp. for Mental & Nervous Diseases; Tel. 579-8807.
BOULT, G. Frank; 25 Medical Arts Bldg., Winnipeg, Man.; 238 Oxford St. (res); Man '39; D.A.B.R., D & T Rad; Staff, Winnipeg Gen. & Children's Hosp's.; Tel. WH 2-6345.
BOULTER, W. Leland; 1935 W. 13th Ave., Vancouver 9, B.C. (res); Tor '23; ObstGyn; Tel RE 8-7995.
BOULTON, Basil C.; UBC '63; Jr. Int., Montreal Gen. Hosp., Montreal, P.Q.
BOULTON, James J.; Alb'65; Jr. Res., Edmonton Gen. Hosp., Edmonton, Alta.
BOULTON, Kenneth A.; Cannon Clinic, Abbotsford, B.C.; Bristol (Eng.)'51; FRCS(Eng.).
BOURASSA, J. Yves; Lav'61; Cardiol.(P.Q.); Staff, Hop. Hotel-Dieu, Montreal 18, P.Q.
BOURASSA, Marcel; 26 Leblanc, L'Epiphanie, Co. L'Assomption, P.Q.; Mon '52.
BOURASSA, Martial G.; 4 ave. Georges Vanier Ile Bigras, Ville de Laval, P.Q.; Lav'59; IntMed (Cardiol.) (P.Q.); Staff, Institut de Cardiologie de Montreal.
BOURASSA, Roland; 1570 rue St. Hubert, Montreal, P.Q.; Lav '31.
BOURBEAU, Jean-M.; 1255 Rosseau, Quebec 6, P.Q.; Lav'54; Med. Staff, Hop. Christ-Roi & Notre-Dame de l'Esperance; Vis. Phys., Hop. St. Sacrement, Hop. de l'Enfant Jesus & Hop. St. Francois d'Assise; Tel. 681-3222.
BOURBONNAIS, Andre; 89 rue Larente, La-Salle, P.Q.; Mon '62.
BOURBONNAIS, Arthur J. H.; 5813 Bannantyne **Ave., Verdun, Montreal 19, P.Q.; Mon '50. MC-GP; Tel. PO 8-1443.**
BOURBONNAIS, Earl; 52 Grande-Ile, Valleyfield, **P.Q.; 123 Blvd. du Havre (res); Mon '42.**
BOURBONNIERE, Gerald; 78 Blainville W., Ste-Therese, P.Q.; McG '49; M.C.G.P.; Tel. 435-3179.
BOURDEAU, Yvon; 103 St. George St., Alexandria, Ont.; Ott'64; AMCGP; Staff, Glengarry & Hotel-Dieu Hosp's.; Tel. 842.

BOURDUA, Serge; Fort Chimo, Nouveau, P.Q.; Mon'64.

BOURGAULT, Jean M.; 5229 rue Brillon, Montreal 28, P.Q. (res); Mon '51; Biochem.; (P.Q.); Staff, Hop. Notre-Dame, Ass't Prof. (Biochem.), U. of Montreal; Tel. RE 3-9951.

BOURGAULT, Lucien; St. Andre Avellin, Co. Papineau, P.Q.; Mon '30; Dist. Coroner.

BOURGAULT, Norbert; Room 719, 30 Blvd. St. Joseph E., Montreal 34, P.Q.; 237 Stanstead Ave., Ville Mt. Royal (res); Lav '33; Ophth.Otol; Staff, Hop. Ste. Jeanne d'Arc; Tel. VI 2-1356.

BOURGAULT, Reginald; St-Francois-du-Lac, P.Q. Lav '36.

BOURGEAU, Denis; Ste. 1014, 30 est Boul. St. Joseph, Montreal 14, P.Q.; Mon'58; FRCS(C), OrthSurg.

BOURGEAU, P. E.; Ste 406, 2950 Masson St., Montreal, P.Q.; Mon '31; M.C.G.P.

BOURGEOIS, Camille M.; 180 Archibald St., Moncton, N.B.; Lav '30.

BOURGEOIS, Didace; 127 de-l'Hopital, Amqui, P.Q.; Lav'56; F.R.C.S.(C), GenSurg; Tel. 651.

BOURGEOIS, Jean G.; 28 rue Charles, St.-Eustache, P.Q.; Mon '58.

BOURGEOIS, Jeanne; 411 est Blvd. St. Joseph, Montreal, P.Q.; Mon '51; Path (P.Q.).

BOURGEOIS, Paul; 1560 rue Sherbrooke E., Montreal 24, P.Q.; Mon '28; F.R.C.S. (C); F.I.-C.S. (Hon.); GenSurg; Urol; Director General Hop.Notre-Dame; Tel. 525-6363. Loc. 567.

BOURGEOIS, R. Clifford; 188 St. George St., Moncton, N.B.; Lav '42; Ophth; Cons. Staff, Hotel-Dieu & Moncton Gen. Hosp's.; Tel. 855-5987.

BOURGEOIS, Ulysse J.; Tracadie, N.B.; Lav '25; Staff, Hotel Dieu St. Joseph.

BOURGEOIS-SAVOIE, Isabelle Y.; Caraquet, N.B. (res); Lav '50; Not practising.

BOURGET, Joachim E.; 3819 ave. Marlowe, Montreal 28, P.Q.; Mon '12.

BOURGET, J. O. R.; 42 St. Joseph, Bienville, P.Q.; Lav '19.

BOURGET, Paul; Ste. Perpetue, Co. L'Islet, P.Q.; Lav '19.

BOURGIE, Berthol; 832 Blvd. St. Joseph E., Montreal 34, P.Q.; 6362 Louis-Hebert (res); Mon '48; Obst. (P.Q.); Staff, Hop. de la Misericorde; Tel. LA 1-3431.

BOURGOIN, Louis P.; 918 ave-de-la-Colline, Ste-Foy, Quebec 10, P.Q., Mon '45; Psy; Ass't Psy., Roy Rousseau Cons. Psy., Soc. Rehab. Serv., Quebec; Staff, Laval U.; Tel. LA 9-4511.

BOURGOUIN, Jean J.; 301 Medical Arts Bldg., Winnipeg, Man.; 190 Cambridge St. (res); Man '25; D.A.B.U., Urol; Urol., St. Boniface Hosp.; Lect. Urol., U. of Manitoba; Nat'l Board Med. Examiners; Tel. WH 2-8941.

BOURGOUIN, Maurice; 415 Ave. Barton, Montreal 16, P.Q.; Mon'43.

BOURKE, Geoffrey J.; Wainwright Clinic, 401— 10th St., Wainwright, Alta.; Nat. U. (Dublin, Ire.) '53; L.M., D.C.H., D.P.H.; Tel. 842-3341.

BOURNE, F. Munroe; 1414 Drummond St., Montreal, P.Q.; 604 Victoria Ave., Westmount (res); McG '37; MA (Oxon); F.A.C.P., F.R.C.P. (C), IntMed; Assoc. Phys., Mtl. Gen. Hosp.; Cons. (Med.), Queen Mary Vet's. Hosp.; Ass't. Prof. (Med.), McGill U.; Tel. VI 9-6848.

BOURNE, G. Ronald; 25 St. Clair Ave. E., Toronto 7, Ont. Wes '38; DGO; D.ObstRCOG; Reg. Aviation M.O., Med. Serv., Dept. of National Health & Welfare; Abroad.

BOURNE, Hilary B.; 680 Seaforth Med. Bldg., 3550 Cote des Neiges, Montreal, P.Q.; 630 Victoria Ave., Westmount (res); McG '45; FRCS (C); ObstGyn; Assoc. Staff (ObstGyn) Royal Victoria & Montreal Gen. Hosp's; Lect. (ObstGyn) McGill U.; Tel. 937-3546.

BOURNE, R. Alan; Ste. 150, 3550 Cote des Neiges, Montreal 25, P.Q.; 73 Rosemount Cres., Mtl. 6 (res); McG'41; FACS; FAAOO; Ophth; Ass't. Ophth., Mtl. Children's & Cons. Ophth., Grace Dart & Alexandra Hosp's.; Assoc. Ophth., Mtl. Gen.; Lect. McGill U.; Tel. 849-7111.

BOURNE, Robert H.; Ste. 405, 5025 Sherbrooke St. W., Montreal 28, P.Q.; McG '49; Gastroent (P.Q.); IntMed; Ass't. Phys., Queen Elizabeth Hosp.; Cons., O.P.D., Royal Victoria Hosp.; Tel. HU 8-7797.

BOURNIVAL, Jacques; 2541 Belanger est, Montreal, P.Q.; 6827 15ieme Ave. Rosemont (res); Lav '53; Otol.; Tel. 727-6823.

BOURQUE, Henri; 150 rue Metcalfe, Ottawa, Ont.; 351 Main St. (res); Lav '43; Paed; Staff, Ottawa Gen. Hosp.; Lect. (Paed.), U. of Ottawa; Tel. CE 5-5485.

BOURQUE, Jacques; 300 King est, Sherbrooke, **P.Q. (res); Lav '53; DiagRad; Staff, Hop-St-Vin-**cent-de-Paul; Tel. LO 9-6381.

BOURQUE, Jean C.; 35 rue Lynott, Edmunston, N.B.; 15-18eme Ave. (res); Lav '46; Psy; Dir. & Phys. (Psy.) Mental Hygiene Clinic; Tel. 735-5529.

BOURQUE, Jean C.; Apt. 1, 2925 Fleury E., Montreal 12, P.Q.; Mon '60.

BOURQUE, Jean J., Capt.; Werl Dependent Clinic, 1 CBMU, CFPO 5050, Cdn. Air Force, Europe; Lav'64; Abroad.

BOURQUE, Jean M.; 55 ave-de-l'Eglise, Verdun, Montreal 19, P.Q.; 355 Grenfell (res); Mon '42; GenSurg (P.Q.); Surg. Staff, Hop.-Gen.-de-Verdun; Tel. 766-6130.

BOURQUE, R. Claude; 875 des Recollets, Trois **Rivieres, P.Q.; 2990 St. Julie (res); Lav '52; FRCP(C), IntMed., Cardiol. (P.Q); Tel. FR 5-4313.**

BOURQUE, Robert; 3244 Beaubien est, Montreal 36, P.Q.; Mon '58; MCGP; Med. Staff, Santa Cabrini Hosp.; Phys., Montreal Home for Alcholism; Tel. RA 9-1891.

BOURQUE, Roch A.; 802 Chanoine Scott, Ste Foy, P.Q.; Lav'59; FRCS(C), GenSurg; Staff, Hop. Laval; Tel. 653-4931.

BOURRET, Andre; 378 rue Cartier, Laval-des-Rapides, P.Q.; Mon'63.

BOURRET, Robert; 3886 Ave. Verdun, Verdun, Montreal 19, P.Q.; Mon '59.

BOUSQUET, HorMisdas; 22 rue Quintal, St-Liboire, P.Q.; Lav '12.

BOUSQUET, J. Ernest; 369 Redfern Ave., Montreal, P.Q.; Mon '36; GenSurg (P.Q.), ThorSurg (P.Q.), Pulm. Dis. & TB (P.Q.), IntMed (T.B.); Dir., Surg. Serv. & Thor Surg., Hop. San. St. Joseph; Tel. CL 6-2681.

BOUSQUET, Jean-P; 300 Carre St. Louis, Montreal, P.Q.; Varennes, Co. Richelieu-Vercheres (res); Mon'44; Tel. VI 5-9085.

BOUSSENS, Jean; 480 est, Boul. St.-Joseph, Montreal 34, P.Q.; Bordeaux (Fr.) '55; Otol; Chief (Otol.), hop.-Santa-Cabrini; Staff Ass't. Hop.-St-Luc; Tel. VI 9-6543.

BOUTET, Claude; 978 Ave. Moncton, Quebec 6, P.Q.; Lav '50; Tel. 681-5900.

BOUTET, Laurier; St. Gabriel de Brandon, Co. Berthier, P.Q.; Mon '45.

BOUTHILLETTE, Michel, Capt.; Station Hosp., Camp Borden, Ont.; Lav'65.

BOUTIN, Georges J.; 230 Longueuil, St. Jean, P.Q.; Ott'60; FRCS(C), OrthSurg.

BOUTIN, J. Ralph; App. 2008, 4530 Cote des Neiges, Montreal 26, P.Q.; Mon '37; F.A.C.H.A.; Med. Dir., Hop. Notre Dame; Tel. LA 5-6363.

BOUTIN, Paul; 230-5th Ave., Timmins, Ont.; 296 Lakeshore (res); Mon '32.

BOUTIN, Roger; 4994 Victoria, Montreal 29, P.Q.; Mon '52; Psy (PQ); Ass't. (Psy), Jewish Gen. Hosp. & Hop. Notre-Dame; Tel. RE 5-1895.

BOUVIER, D.D.; Box 22, Lac La Biche, Alta.; Alb'54; Tel. 623-4421.

BOUVIER, Guy; Mon'65; Res., Univ. of Laval, Quebec, P.Q.

BOUWMAN, Henry W.; 336 Professional Bldg., 10830 Jasper Ave., Edmonton, Alta.; 14412-87th Ave. (res); Alb '53; OrthSurg; Teach. Staff, U. of Alberta & Royal Alexandra Hosp's.; Cons. Staff, Misericordia Hosp.; Tel. 424-4352.

BOUX, Pierre A.; 215 rue Chasse, Asbestos, P.Q.; Lav'65.

BOUZIANE, N. R.; 3115 St. Zotique E., Montreal 36, P.Q. (res); Mon '35; M.Sc.; Ph.D.; FCIC, FISH; Cert. AACS; Clin Path (P.Q.); Haem (P.Q.); Bact; Dir. Labs. & Research & Dir. Radioisotopes DiagRad. Lab. Hop-Ste-Jeanne-d'Arc; Prof. Clin. Path & Assoc. Prof. Biochem. U. of Mtl.; Tel. RE 3-9951.

BOW, Leonard W.; 1153 Carey Rd., Oakville, Ont. (res); Tor '52; D.Psy; Psy; Dir., Mental Health Clin. & Day Hosp., New Toronto; Electroenceph., Ont. Hosp's., New Toronto & Hamilton; Cons. Psy., Oakville-Trafalgar Mem. Hosp.; Tel. 259-8291.

BOW, Malcolm R.; 9315-149th St., Edmonton, Alta. (res); Qns '11; A.P.H.A., DPH; PH; Chief, M.O.H., Dept. of Health, Yukon Terr.; Retired.

BOWDEN, Drummond H.; Dept. of Path., U. of Manitoba, Winnipeg, Man.; Bristol (Eng.) '48; MRCP (Lond.); M.C. (Path.); Path; Cons. Path., Wpg. Gen. Hosp.; Assoc. Prof. (Path.), U. of Manitoba; Tel. GR 4-9110.

BOWDEN, Nicholas; 115 Palliser Ave., St. James, Winnipeg 12, Man. (res); Man '31.

BOWE, Vincent J.; McG '60; Res., Queen Elizabeth Hosp., Montreal 28, P.Q.

BOWEN, Herbert M.; 302 Bloor St. W., Toronto, Ont.; Qns '09; New York '11; OphthOtol; Cons. Toronto Western & Queen Elizabeth Hosp's.; Tel. WA 2-2965.

BOWEN, Michael D.; 2633 Portage Ave., St. James 12, Man.; Edinburgh (Scot.) '40; M.B., Ch.B.; M.O., Fort Osborne Barracks; Vis. Staff, Deer Lodge Veterans Hosp., Winnipeg; Tel. 837-5772.

BOWEN, Peter; University of Alberta Hosp., Edmonton, Alta.; Tor'56; FRCP(C), IntMed; Active Staff, (Paed.), U. of Alberta Hosp.; Assoc. Prof. (Human Geneticist), U. of Alberta; Tel. 439-5911.

BOWEN, Richard A., Capt.; Camp Chilliwack, Vedder Crossing, B.C.; Alb '64.

BOWEN, R. J.; 268 Ridout St. S., London, Ont.; Wes '31.

BOWER, Campbell M.; 364 E. Plains Rd., Burlington, Ont.; Tor '43; Court. Staff; Hamilton Gen. Hosp.

BOWER, David; Apt. 218, 103 Lakeshore Rd., Toronto, Ont.; M.B., B.Ch. (Cantab.) '53; F.R.C.S. (Eng.), D. Obst., R.C.O.G. (Lond.); Research Fell. (ObstGyn), U. of Toronto; Tel. 255-7804.

BOWER, Harry L.; Main St., Monkton, Ont.; Wes'46; FAGS; MCGP; Staff, Listowel Hosp.; Tel. 347-2284.

BOWER, John; 1210-4th Ave. S., Lethbridge, Alta.; Dublin (Ire.) '46; DPM; Psy., St. Michael's & Municipal Hosp's; Dir. Provincial Guidance Clinic; Cons. Family Court; Tel. FA 8-4092.

BOWER, Robert R.; 103 Renfrew St., Pembroke, Ont.; 268 Rosewood Ave. (res); McG '52; Tel. RE 2-7762.

BOWERING, Melvin W.; 1010 McCallum Hill Bldg., 1874 Scarth St., Regina Sask.; Man '38; Anaes; Dir. Anaes., Regina Gen. Hosp.; Clin. Assoc., University Hosp.; Tel. 522-0704.

BOWERMAN, Derek; 142 Simcoe St. N., Oshawa, Ont.; 300 Mary St., Apt. 404 (res); London (Eng.) '51; D.O.; Ophth; Tel. 728-2311.

BOWERS, Brian S.; Lampman Clinic, Lampman, Sask.; London (Eng.) '61; M.B., B Chir (Cantab); LRCP; MRCS; Staff, Lampman Hosp.; Tel. 487-2488.

BOWERS, Dorrance; Knox Clinic, 1605 Glenmore St., Kelowna, B.C.; 2405 Abbott St. (res); Tor '49; M.Sc. (Med., Minn.); D.A.B.I.M., F.A.C.P., F.R.C.P.(C), IntMed; Att'd. Staff, Kelowna Gen. Hosp.; Tel. 762-2002.

BOWERS, J. David; 116 Elm St. E., Sudbury, Ont.; Ott '63.

BOWERS, N. Herbert; 348 Fraser St., North Bay, Ont.; Tor '27; Hd., Dept. of Med., North Bay Civic Hosp.; Tel. 474-3150.

BOWERS, Norman S.; 16 Ontario St., Grimsby, Ont.; 6 Kingsway Cres. (res); Qns '42; M.C.G.P.

BOWES, Gerald C.; Grenville, P.Q.; McG '40.

BOWES, Kenneth L.; Qns '62; Res. (Surg.), University Hosp., Edmonton, Alta.

BOWIE, Iain A.; 7375 Kingsway, Burnaby, B.C.; Glasgow (Scot.) '52; MCGP.

BOWKER, Howard A.; High St., Ladysmith, B.C.; Gill Rd. (res); Man '36; GenSurg; Tel. 245-3413.

BOWLES, A. Webster; 601-511 Ash St., New Westminster, B.C.; McG'19; FRCS (Edin.); OphthOtol; Hd., Dept. of EENT, St. Mary's Hosp.; Tel. LA 1-5232.

BOWLES, Howard E.; 132 Med. Arts Bldg., 404-406 Graham Ave., Winnipeg, Man.; 355 Kingston Cres. (res); Man '45; MCGP; Tel. GR 5-5750.

BOWLSBY, Cleve S.; 3195 Granville St., Vancouver 9, B.C.; Alb '48; DiagRad; Ass't. Rad., Vancouver Gen. Hosp.; Tel. RE 1-5241.

BOWMAN, Basil; 520 Med. Arts. Bldg., Hamilton, Ont.; McG'26; DABDS; DermSyph; Chief of Serv. (Derm.), Hamilton Gen. Hosp.; Hon. Cons., Chedoke Gen. & Children's Hosp's.; Tel. JA. 2-6184.

BOWMAN, Frederick B.; 615 Med. Arts Bldg., Hamilton, Ont.; 260 Bay St. S. (res); Tor '06; FRCP(C); Proct; Hon. Cons. Staff, Hamilton Gen., Chedoke & St. Joseph's Hosp's.; Tel. JA 7-4561.

BOWMAN, Graham R.; 519 Med. Arts Bldg., 11010 Jasper Ave., Edmonton, Alta.; Ste. A, 14230-85th Ave. (res); Sask. '59; MCGP; Tel. 488-0670.

BOWMAN, Helen C. (Wright); Apt. 1507, 1400 Pine Ave. W., Montreal, P.Q.; Glasgow (Scot.)'50; Dip. Anaes (McGill); Anaes; Ass't. Anaes., Dr. W. G. Cullen & Associates; Dem. (Anaes.), McGill U.; Tel. 845-3604.

BOWMAN, John M.; Manitoba Clinic, 790 Sherbrook St., Winnipeg, Man.; 257 Harvard (res); Man '49; Paed; Active Att'd Staff, Children's Grace & Gen. Hosp's.; Clin. Dir. RH Lab & Ass't. Prof. (Paed.), U. of Man.; Tel. SP 4-6541.

BOWMAN, Lesley R.; Qns'62; Res., Toronto Gen. Hosp., Toronto, Ont.

BOWMAN, William D.; Manitoba Clinic, 790 Sherbrooke St., Winnipeg, Man.; 328 Oxford St., (res); Man '49; Paed; Ass't. Paed., Wpg. Gen. & Children's Hosp's.; Chief Paed.Serv., Grace Hosp.; Lect. (Paed), U. of Manitoba; Tel. SP 4-6541.

BOWMER, Ernest J.; Division of Labs., 828 W. 10th Ave., Vancouver 9, B.C.; Liverpool (Eng.) '38; MRCS; LRCP; DTM&H; MC Path; Bact; Dir., Div. of Labs., Health Branch, Vancouver; Tel. TR 4-2331.

BOWYER, John H.; 6 George St. S., Brampton, Ont.; Tor '56; Paed; Cons. Paed., Peel Mem. Hosp., Georgetown & Dist. Hosp. & Dufferin Area Gen. Hosp., Orangeville; Tel. 459-3170.

BOX, Donald E.; Qns'55; Staff, General Hosp., Frobisher Bay, N.W.T.

BOX, John H.; Arnprior, Ont.; Qns '15; M.C.G.P.

BOX, T. Rodney H.; 170 The Donway W., Ste. 405, Don Mills, Ont.; 7 Lacewood Cr. (res); Tor '52; IntMed; Ass't: Phys., Toronto East Gen. Hosp.; O.P.D. Staff, Sunnybrook Hosp.; M.O., The Acadia Life Insurance Co. & Allstate Assur., Dow Brewery Ltd. & Int. Business Machines Co.; Tel. 447-9441.

BOXALL, Ernest A.; Ste. B.10, 750 W. Broadway, Vancouver 9, B.C.; Qns's44; FRCP(C), IntMed; Cons. Int. Med., Shaughnessy Hosp.; Clin. Instr., Dept. of Med., U. of British Columbia; Ass't. Dir. Med. Services, Med. Serv. Assoc. of B.C.; Att. Staff, Vancouver Gen. Hosp.; Tel. RE 8-0214.

BOXALL, John O.; Manitou, Man.; Man '49; Dist. Coroner; Tel. 25; Abroad.

BOXALL, Lionel B.; London (Eng.)'56; DCH; Res. (Derm.), Sunnybrook Hosp., Toronto, Ont.

BOXER, Alvin; 2660 E. Hastings St., Vancouver 6, B.C.; 855 W. 10th (res); UBC '60; AMCGP.

BOXER, Louis; 440 Seaforth Med. Bldg., 3550 Cote des Neiges Rd., Montreal 25, P.Q.; 4375 Grand Boul. (res); Man '32; Ophth; Chief (Ophth.) Reddy Mem. Hosp.; Assoc. Staff, Jewish Gen.; Tel. 932-9411.

BOYANER, Don.; Ste 490, 6000 Cote des Neiges Rd., Montreal, P.Q.; McG'51; DAB Ophth; Ophth; Att. Staff, Jewish Gen. Hosp.; Tel. RE 9-1011.

BOYAR, William T.; 47 Academy Medical Bldg., 1812-4th St. W., Calgary, Alta.; Alb '50; Gen-Surg.; Tel. 262-4229.

BOYCE, H. A.; 56 Hill, Kingston, Ont. (res); Qns '16; Dept. of Nat. Health & Welfare; Retired.

BOYCE, Kenneth C.; 4625 Clovelly Walk, W. Van., B.C. (res); Qns'45; IntMed; Att'd. Staff, Van. Gen. Holy Family & Shaughnessy Hosp's.; Cons. (Med.) Cdn., Arthritis & Rheum. Soc.; Lect. (Med.), U. of British Columbia; Tel. TR 4-2211.

BOYCE, R. Murray; 129 Hunt Club Dr., London, Ont. (res); Wes '49; D.Psy; Psy; Dir. Out-Patients Serv., Victoria Hosp.; Instr. (Psy), Western U.; Tel. GE 2-5261. Local 343.

BOYD, A. R. J.; 84 Colin Ave., Toronto, Ont. (res); McG '31; PH; Dept. of Health, Toronto.

BOYD, Barry A.; Tor '45; D. Psy; Psy; Supt., Ont. Hosp., Penetanguishene, Ont.; Tel. 549-7437.

BOYD, Carl E.; 985 Mountainview Ave., Ottawa 14, Ont. (res); Qns'59; Pharmacol., Food & Drug Dir., Dept. of Nat. Health & Welfare; Tel. CE 2-8211.

BOYD, David C.; Medical Arts Bldg., 626 Main St., Penticton, B.C.; 948 Fairview Rd. (res); Edinburgh (Scot.) '43; M.B., Ch.B.; Med. Staff, Penticton Gen. Hosp.; Tel. 492-2742.

BOYD, David M.; 220 Yarrow Bldg., 645 Fort St., Victoria, B.C.; 644 Beach Dr. (res); Tor '43; Paed; Med. Supt., Queen Alexandra Solarium for Crippled Children, 2400 Arbutus Rd., Active Staff (Paed), Royal Jubilee Hosp.; Vis & Cons., St. Joseph's Hosp.; Tel. EV 2-2711.

BOYD, Donald M.; 712 Canada Bldg., Saskatoon, Sask.; Man '46; FRCS (Eng.); GenSurg; Staff, St. Paul's & City Hosp's.; Tel. 652-9166.

BOYD, Douglas L.; 183 James St. S., Hamilton, Ont.; 121 Hunter St. W., (res); Qns '59; Anaes; Staff (Anaes) Hamilton Gen. Hosp.; Tel. JA 9-8875.

BOYD, Edmond A.; 135 St. Clair Ave. W., Toronto 7, Ont.; Cambridge (Eng.)'46; Med. Research Cons., Ontario Dept. of Health.

BOYD, Eldon M.; 211 Union St. W., Kingston, Ont. (res); Qns '32; FACCPC; Prof. & Head, Dept. of Pharamacology, Queen's U.; Cons. Kingston Gen. Hosp.; Tel. 546-1731, Local 407.

BOYD, George E.; Dal'64; Res., Victoria Gen. Hosp., Halifax, N.S.

BOYD, Gordon E.; Box 1150, Terrace, B.C.; Man '57; ObstGyn; Staff, Mills Mem. Hosp.; Court. Staff, Kitimat Gen. Hosp., Kitimat; Tel. 843-5444.

BOYD, H. Neil J.; 2nd St. S.W. & 22nd Ave., Calgary, Alta.; 2911 Lyndon Dr. (res); Wes '47; Path; Dir. of Labs., Holy Cross Hosp.; Tel. AM 6-7231, Loc. 241.

BOYD, James; 607 Main St. E., Hamilton, Ont.; Tor'25; Court. Staff, Hamilton Gen. Hosp.; Tel. JA 2-4718.

BOYD, J. Aubrey; 2547 Danforth Ave., Toronto, Ont.; 22 Old Yonge St. (res); Tor '40; DiagRad.; Tel. OX 4-4434.

BOYD, John A.; 2 LeMarchand Bldg., Edmonton, Alta.; Man '45; FRCS(C), ObstGyn.; Lect., U. of Alberta; Tel. 488-1620.

BOYD, John R.; 1665 W. Broadway, Vancouver, B.C.; 3864 Osler (res); McG '50; F.R.C.S.(C), Obst. Gyn.; Ass't. Prof., U. of British Columbia; Tel. RE 8-7511.

BOYD, Kenneth D.; 1151 Lorne Pk., Port Credit, Ont.; 1357 Birchview Dr. (res); Glasgow (Scot.) '52; DCH; (Lond.); AMCGP; Assoc. Staff, South Peel Hosp.; Tel. 278-2565.

BOYD, Lucy (See Duncan).

BOYD, Mark E.; 102 Le Marchand Apts., 116th St. & 100th Ave., Edmonton, Alta.; Sask'57; FRCS(C), ObstGyn.

BOYD, Martin S.; Swift Current Clinic, Swift Current, Sask.; St. Andrew's (Scot.)'48.

BOYD, Norman O.; 618 Lincoln Rd., Windsor, Ont.; 1175 Kildare Rd. (res); Wes '39; M.C.G.P.

BOYD, R. P.; Edinburgh (Scot.)'39; L.R.C.P. (Edin.), L.R.C.S. (Edin.), L.R.F.P.S. (Glas.), D.P.H.; Staff, Baker Mem. San., Calgary, Alta. Tel. BU 8-2311.

BOYD, R. Wallace; 4287 Angus Dr., Vancouver, B.C. (res); McG '31; F.A.C.R., D & TRad; Dir. of Rad., Vancouver Gen. Hosp.; Clin. Assoc. Prof. of Med. (Rad.), U. of British Columbia; Tel. TR 6-3211.

BOYD, Samuel A.; 211 Medical Arts Bldg., Winnipeg, Man; 299 Oakwood Ave. (res); Man '31; Paed Paed., Children's, Winnipeg Gen., Grace and Shriners Hosp's.; Assoc. Prof. (Paed.), U. of Manitoba.; Tel. WH 2-5912.

BOYD, T. Arthurs B.; Med. Arts Bldg., 2125-11th Ave., Regina, Sask.; 3068-25th Ave. (res); Tor '43; F.A.C.S., F.R.C.S.(C), GenSurg; ThorSurg; Surg., Regina Gen. & Grey Nun's Hosp's.; Tel. 523-0691.

BOYD, Thomas A. S.; 202, University Hosp., Edmonton, Alta.; 7118-119th St. (res); Glasgow (Scot.) '42; DOMS (Eng.); FRCS (Eng.); Ophth; Assoc. Prof. (Ophth), Dir. Div. of Ophth., U. of Alberta; Tel. 439-5911.

BOYD, William; 40 Arjay Cres., Willowdale, Ont. (res); Edinburgh (Scot.) '08; D.Psy; M.R.C.P. (Edin.), F.R.C.S.(C), Path; F.R.C.P. (Hon.) (Edin. & Lond.), M.D. (Hon.) (Oslo), D.Sc.(Hon.) (Manitoba), LL.D. (Hon.) (Sask. & Queen's); F.R.S.(C); Prof. Emerit. (Path), U. of Toronto; Tel. HI 4-8690.

BOYD, William J.; 430 Besserer St., Ottawa 2, Ont.; Man'24.

BOYD, William J.; 132 Medical Arts Bldg.; Winnipeg, Man.; 108 Chataway Blvd. (res); Man '35; M.C.G.P.; Court Staff, Grace, Winnipeg Gen., Misericordia & Children's Hosp's.; Tel. WH 3-2364.

BOYD, William T.; 62A Lake Shore Dr., North Bay, Ont., Tor'46; MCGP; Staff, North Bay Civic & St. Joseph's Hosp's; Tel. 474-8090.

BOYD, W. Kendall; 2 Baby Pt. Rd., Toronto, Ont.; Tor '36; Phys., Swift Canadian Co.; Dist. Coroner; Tel. RO 7-4943.

BOYDEN, Raymond W.; 94 Cumberland St., Toronto, Ont.; 282 Lawrence Ave. E. (res); Tor'24; Tel. WA 2-3087.

BOYER, Claude L.; 75 St. Jean Baptiste, Chateauguay, P.Q.; 298 Fairmount (res); Mon '60; Tel. 692-6701.

BOYER, Claude M.; 713 Manseau, Joliette, P.Q.; Mon '60.

BOYER, Donald E.; 1712 Alberta St., Windsor, Ont.; Tor'54; Anaes; Chief, Dept. of Anaes., Metropolitan Hosp.; Tel. 969-6456.

BOYER, J. Andre; 241 ouest, Fleury, Montreal, P.Q.; Ott '64; Tel. DU 9-7281.

BOYER, J. Maurice; 50 rue Jacques Cartier, Valleyfield, P.Q.; Mon. '49; Anaes (P.Q.); Tel. 373-8181.

BOYER, Leo; 241 Fleury W., Montreal 12, P.Q.; Mon '56.

BOYER, Rene; App 2, 2625 Boul. de Varennes, Trois Rivieres, P.Q.; Mon'61; GenSurg.

BOYES, David A.; Qns '49; ObstGyn; TherRad; Staff, B.C. Cancer Inst., 2656 Heather, Vancouver 9, B.C.; Clin. Instr., U. of British Columbia; Tel. CA 4-1111.

BOYES, Fred F.; Parkhill, Ont.: '36; M.C.G.P.; M.O.H., Parkhill, Grand Bend, McGillivary Twp.; Dist. Coroner.

BOYES, Harold W.; 417 Rosemary Rd., Toronto 10, Ont.; Wes '42; Anaes; Anaes.-in-Chief, Toronto Western Hosp.; Ass't. Prof., (Anaes), U. of Toronto; Tel. HU 1-2941.

BOYLAN, Terence M.; 1155 Oxford St. W., London, Ont.; National U. (Ire.)'58.

BOYLE, Edward J.; Ste. 221, One Medical Place, 20 Wyndford Dr., Don Mills, Ont.; McG '54; FRCS(C), GenSurg; Staff, Surg., Scarborough Gen. Hosp.

BOYLE, Ernest S.; 3375 Ridgewood, Apt. 222, Montreal 26, P.Q.; McG '23; M.O., CPR; Tel. UN 1-6811.

BOYLE, Patrick J.; National U. (Dublin, Ire.) '50; M.B., B.Ch., BAO; DA; FFA; M.Sc., Ph.D., LAH; Staff, James Paton Mem. Hosp., Gander, Nfld.; Tel. 3961.

BOYLE, William G.; Fort Frances Clinic, 301 Victoria, Fort Frances, Ont.; Tor '28; Dist. Coroner; Tel. 274-3287.

BOZYK, Alexander J.; Box 311, Marathon, Ont.; Vienna (Austria) '44.

BRAATEN, Vergil F.; 205-1669 Victoria St., Prince George, B.C.; Alb'51; Paed; Tel. 564-7475.

BRABANDER, Joachim O. W.; 1390 Sherbrooke St. W., Montreal 25, P.Q.; 4705 Roslyn Ave. (res); McG '32; F.A.C.P., IntMed; Assoc. Phys., Royal Victoria Hosp.; Lect. in Med., McGill U.; Tel. AV 8-2095.

BRACALENTI, Ivan A.; 38 Kenilworth Ave. S., Hamilton, Ont.; Wes'61; MCGP; Tel. 545-6947.

BRACHMAN, Edwin F.; 127 Church St., Chilliwack, B.C.; **Apt. 10, 7 Mellard St. (res); Man '54.**

BRACKEN, A. Douglas; 209 Med. Arts Bldg., Winnipeg, Man.; 234 Oxford St. (res); Man '39; Ophth; Staff, Deer Lodge Hosp.; Tel. WH 2-5826.

BRADEN, Donald H.; 567 Earl St., Kingston, Ont.; Qns'59; FRCP(C); Psy; Staff, Ontario Hosp.; Assoc. Staff, Kingston Gen. & Hotel-Dieu Hosp's; Lect., Dept. of Psy., Queen's U.

BRADFORD, C. Ronald; 227 Med. Arts Bldg., 404 Graham Ave., Winnipeg 1, Man.; 1 Fidler Ave., St. James **(res)**; Man '51; F.R.C.S.(C), ObstGyn; Ass't. Gyn., Wpg. Gen. Hosp.; Ass't. Prof. (ObstGyn), I/C PG & Research Co-ord., U. of Manitoba; Tel. WH 3-6033.

BRADFORD, John G.; 32 St. Margaret's Rd., Ancaster, Ont.; London (Eng.) '52; M.B., B.S.; Active G.P. Staff, Hamilton Health Assoc. & Gen. Hosp.; Tel. MI 8-4483.

BRADFORD, Norman W.; 148 Underhill Dr., Don Mills, Ont. (res); **Qns. '52; Ass't. Supt.,** Sunnybrook Hosp., Toronto; Tel. 485-8651.

BRADLEY, Brian M.; 139 Wellington St., Sarnia, Ont.; 1254 Ridgewood Dr. (res); Wes '54; Ophth.; Tel. ED 6-6732.

BRADLEY, George C.; 350 Medical Dental Bldg., Regina, Sask.; 3208 College Ave. (res); Alb '28; M.C.G.P.

BRADLEY, J. C.; 316 Maple Ave., Pembroke, Ont. (res); Tor '11; Coroner, Renfrew Co.; Retired.

BRADLEY, John; Box 38, North Battleford, Sask.; 1142-105th St. (res); Cracow (Pol.)'38; DOMS (Eng.); Ophth; Staff (Ophth), Union Hosp.; Tel. 445-3261.

BRADLEY, John E.; 7214-119th St., Edmonton, Alta. (res); Alb '40; MCGP; Exec. Dir., Glenrose Provincial Hosp.; Tel. 474-2451.

BRADLEY, Katharine F. (Wilson); St. Andrew's (Scot.) '48; M.O., Prov. Mental Hosp., Ponoka, Alta.; Tel. 3-3301.

BRADLEY, Kenneth J.; Qns'63; Ass't. Res. (Surg.), Toronto Western Hosp., Toronto, Ont.

BRADLEY, Leonard O.; 2575 Assiniboine Cres., St. James, Winnipeg 12, Man.; Alb '38; Exec. Dir., Winnipeg Gen. Hosp.; Tel. SP 4-6511.

BRADLEY, Robert; Otago (New Zealand) '45; DPH (Lond.); DIH; DTM&H (Eng.); PH; Staff, La Ronge Hosp., La Ronge, Sask.; M.O., Dept. of Transport; Tel. 2231.

BRADLEY, Robert Colin P.; Trinity College (Dublin) University C. (Ire); B.A.O., M.B., Bch.; M.O.H., Provincial Mental Hospital, Ponoka, Alta.; Tel. 783-3301.

BRADLEY, Robert E.; McG '62; Jr. Intn., Montreal Gen. Hosp., Montreal 25, P.Q.

BRADSHAW, Phyllis E.; 1374 Pelissier St., Windsor, Ont.; 1432 Victoria Ave. (res); Tor '30; Schl. M.O., Bd. of Health; Active Med. Staff, Metropolitan Gen. Hosp.; Tel. 253-1701.

BRADY, Arthur J.; 6411 Quinpool Rd., Halifax, N.S.; Edinburgh (Scot.) '31; M.B., Ch.B., MCGP; Court. Staff, Victoria Gen. Hosp.; Halifax Infirmary, Children's & Grace Maternity Hosp's.; Active Staff, Halifax Civic Hosp.; Ass't. M.O., U.S.P.H.S., Halifax; Tel. 422-4565.

BRADY, F. Alfred; 206 Bloor St. W., Toronto 5, Ont.; 229 Dunvegan Rd. (res); Tor '32; School M.O.; Tel. 924-1794.

BRADY, Harry; 201 Med. Centre, Calgary, Alta.; 316-47th Ave. S.W. (res); Alb '55.

BRADY, Paul L.; Medical Clinic, Goderich St. W., Seaforth, Ont.; Tor'38; MCGP; **Teach. Staff, St. Joseph's Hosp., London; Tel. 527-1770.**

BRAHAM, John K.; 31 Centre St. S., Brampton, Ont.; Qns '56; D.Psy; Psy; Staff, Mental Health Dept., Thistletown Hosp.; Tel. 459-2420.

BRAHY, Jules; Apt. 1610, 2150 St. Luke St., Montreal, P.Q.; Mon'23; Ophth & ORL(Paris), FAAOO, OphthOtol; Head of EENT Dept., Rosemont San.; Staff, E.N.T. Dept., Notre Dame Hosp.; Ass't. Prof. (ORL), U. of Montreal; Retired.

BRAIDA, R. L.; Tor'64; Res., Ontario Hosp., 999 Queen St. W., Toronto, Ont.

BRAIDEN, Robert S.; Ste. 6, 2917 Bloor St. W., Toronto 9, Ont.; 88 The Kingsway, Tor. 18 (res); Tor'39; MCGP; Assoc. Staff, Toronto Western Hosp.; Tel. RO 2-3395.

BRAIL, J. N.; 1495 Kipling Ave. N., Rexdale, Ont.; UBC'64.

BRAIS, E. Paul; App. 48, 55, de l'Eglise, Montreal 19, P.Q.; 4061 ave. Marlowe, N.D.G., Montreal; Mon '39; IntMed; (P.Q.); Ass't Staff, Hop. Gen. de Verdun; Tel. PO 9-3044.

BRAIS, Pierre M.; Mon'65; Res., Hop. Notre Dame, Montreal 24, P.Q.

BRAITHWAITE, Desmond L.; McG '62; Res. Mtl. Gen. Hosp., Montreal 25, P.Q.

BRAJAC, Josip; 137 Wellington St., Sarnia, Ont.; 764 Lakeshore Rd. (res); Zagreb (Yugoslavia) '53; Tel. DI 4-5261.

BRAMLEY-MOORE, W.; College of Phys. & Surg., 9901-108th St., Edmonton, Alta.; 9218-117th St. (res); Alb'31; Registrar, College of Physicians & Surgeons of Alberta; Sec., C.M.A. (Alta. Div.); Lectr. (Med. Econom.), U. of Alberta; Tel. 422-6184.

BRAMSTRUP, Peter A.; Otis, Lower Southampton, N.B.; Copenhagen (Den.) '39; Tel. 88.

BRANCH, Charles L.; 3801 University St., Montreal, P.Q.; 319 Monmouth Ave., Twn. of Mt. Royal (res); Vanderbilt U. (Nashville, Tenn.) '53; M.Sc.; FACS; (McGill-Neurophysiol.); Ass't. NeurSurg., Montreal Neurol. Inst.; Clin. Ass't (NeurSurg.), Royal Victoria Hosp.; Lect. (Neur & NeurSurg.), McGill U.; Tel. VI 2-1251; AV 8-7320.

BRANCH, E. Arnold G.; Box 25, Rothesay, N.B.; McG '20; DAB Path., PathBact; Chief Lab. Serv., Lancaster Hosp., Lancaster, N.B.; Prov. Med. Dir., Red Cross Blood Transfusion Service; Tel. 694-2651.

BRAND, Clarence W.; 113 Pacific Ave., Toronto, Ont.; Tor '00; Retired.

BRAND, J. David; Tor'62; AMCGP; Res., Sunnybrook Hosp., Toronto 12, Ont.

BRAND, Lewis M., M.P.; House of Commons, Ottawa, Ont.; 220 Poplar Cr., Saskatoon, Sask. (res); Man'49.

BRAND, Maurice H.; 735 Professional Bldg., **10830 Jasper Ave., Edmonton, Alta.; 82 Westmount, Shoppers Park; 10567-45th St. (res); Durham (Eng.) '47; MCGP; Staff, Misericordia Hosp.; Sess. Instr. (PrevMed.), U. of Alberta; Tel. 429-3351.**

BRAND, T. Malcolm; 210E - 50th Ave., Vancouver 15, B.C.; Manchester (Eng.)'39; M.R.C.P., IntMed; Att. Staff, Vancouver Gen. Hosp.; Tel. TR 4-6723.

BRANDER, James A.; Dal'54; DiagRad; Staff, X-Ray Dept., Halifax Infirmary, Halifax, N.S.

BRANDER, James F.; 10936-68th Ave., Edmonton, Alta; Qns '06; Part-time practice.

BRANDER, J. Wesley E.; 3331 Bloor St. W., Toronto 18, Ont.; 186 Humbervale Blvd. (res); Tor '46; F.R.C.S.(C), GenSurg; Att. Surg., Queensway Gen. Hosp.; Assoc., Toronto Western Hosp.; Tel. BE 3-0841.

BRANDER, Margaret R. (Rae); Ste. 2, Applewood Acres Shopping Centre, 23 Applewood Village, Cooksville, Ont.; Tor '46; MCGP; Active Staff, South Peele Hosp. & Queensway Gen. Hosp.; Court. Staff, Toronto Western & Women's College Hosp's; Tel. 277-9311.

BRANDL, Thomas; 40 Coldwater St. E., Orillia, Ont.; 357 Highland Ave. (res); Middlesex (Eng.) '46; L.R.C.P., M.R.C.S.; GenSurg; FACS; Surg. Staff, Orillia Soldiers' Hosp.; Tel. 326-3541.

BRANDT, J. Leonard; 4252 Isabella Ave., Montreal 26, P.Q. (res); Long Island Coll. of Med. (N.Y., U.S.A.) '43; D.A.B.I.M.; Phys.-in-Chief, Jewish Gen. Hosp.; Ass't. Phys., Royal Victoria Hosp.; Lect. (Med.), McGill U.; Tel. 735-3771.

BRANDT, Marvin K.; 18-3rd Ave. N.W., Dauphin, Man.; Man '36; Tel. 638-3332.

BRANIGAN, Donald W.; Box 757, Manning, Alta.; Alb'63.

BRANOVACKY, Eugene; Belgrade (Yugo.)'54; Staff, Mont. Providence Hosp., Montreal, P.Q.

BRANNEN, Ronald E.; 36, Fairknowe Dr., **Brockville, Ont. (res); Dal '44; DiagRad; Hd. Dept of Rad., Brockville Gen. Hosp.;** Cons. **Rad., Ontario Hosp.; Tel. 345-5645.**

BRANT, Clare C.; Qns'65; Res., Kingston Gen. Hosp., Kingston, Ont.

BRANT, David J.; Merritt, B.C.; MCGP; Alb '52; Temporarily Retired.

BRAS, Annabelle M.; Med. Arts Clinic, 51-6th St. S.E., Medicine Hat, Alta.; Aberdeen (Scot.) '53. Abroad.

BRAS, Jan F.; Med. Arts Clinic, 51-6th St. S.E., Medicine Hat, Alta.; 245-2nd St. S.W., (res); Glasgow (Scot.) '58; FRCS (Edin.); DO (Lond.); Ophth; Staff, Medicine Hat Gen. Hosp.; Tel. 527-2281. Abroad.

BRASCH, Harold A.; 1371 Centre Rd., Port Credit, Ont.; McG '45; D. Psy; Active Cons. & Hd. Dept. of Psy., South Peel Hosp., Cooksville; Staff, Humber Mem. & Queensway Gen. Hosp's.; Med. Dir. Lord Simcoe Hotel & Scottish & York Ins. Co. Tor.; Coroner County of Peel; Tel. CR 8-4021.

BRASHER, Irene M. (Watts); 279 Sixth St., Midland, Ont.; Cambridge (Eng.)'51; Tel. 526-5408.

BRASHER, Peter H.; 279 Sixth St., Midland, Ont.; London (Eng.) '47; FRCS (Eng.); GenSurg; Cons. Surg., St. Andrews Hosp., Midland, & Penetang Gen. Hosp., Penetanguishene; Tel. 526-5408.

BRASSARD, Gaston; 227 Blvd. St. Joseph, Roberval, P.Q.; Lav'51; GenSurg (P.Q.); Chief, Dept. of Surg, Hotel-Dieu St-Michel de Roberval; Tel. 275-0503.

BRASSARD, Georges R.; 34 rue St.-Pierre, Metabetchouan, P.Q.; Lav '56; Anaes.

BRASSARD, J. Emile; 129 St-Dominique, Jonquiere, Co. Chicoutimi, P.Q.; Lav '24.

BRASSARD, Raymond; 227 Blvd. St-Joseph, Roberval, P.Q.; Lav '46; GenSurg.; Tel. 275-0503.

BRASSARD, Roger; 454 Chapais, Chicoutimi, P.Q. (res); Lav '56; FRCP(C), Anaes; Staff, Hop. Hotel Dieu St. Vallier.

BRASSARD, Victor N.; 520—8eme rue, Grand'-Mere, P.Q.; 1260-2eme rue (res); Mon '34; Anaes; Chief Anaes., Hop. Lafleche, Grand'Mere; Tel. 538-3660.

BRASSARD, Yvan; 50 Jacques Cartier, Valleyfield, P.Q.; 21 rue Bay (res); Mon'37; DiagRad; MCGP; Chief Rad., Hotel Dieu & Valleyfield Med. Centre; Tel. 373-3162.

BRATINA, Gloria S. (CERAR); 983A College St., Toronto 4, Ont.; Graz (Austria) '59; Tel. 537-5791.

BRATJAKIN, Anna A.; (Shwidkova); 760 Rockland Ave., Outremont, Montreal, P.Q. (res); Jusowka (Ukraine) '40; IntMed (P.Q.); Staff Phys. (IntMed.), St. Anne's D.V.A. & Reddy Mem. Hosp's.; Tel. 271-8665.

BRATTMAN, David P.; Trinity Coll. (Dublin, Ire.) '57; DiagRad; Staff, Reddy Mem. Hosp., Montreal, P.Q.; Tel. WE 5-9641.

BRATTY, Paul J.; 204-3195 Granville St., Vancouver 9, B.C.; Tor '55; FRCP(C), Neurol; Att'd. Staff, Vancouver Gen. Hosp.; Cons. Staff, Shaughnessy Hosp.; Cons., Riverview Hosp., Essondale; Tel. 736-5310.

BRAUDO, Michael; Ste. 113, 170 Donway W., Don Mills, Ont.; **Witwatersrand (S. Africa) '50;** MRCP (Edin.); **FAAP; DCH (Lond.); DABP; Paed; Staff, Hosp. for Sick Children; Clin. Instr.,** U. of Toronto; Tel. 444-2425.

BRAUL, William; Golden, B.C.; Alb'64.

BRAULT, Jean-Paul; 1656 est, rue Sherbrooke, Montreal, P.Q.; Mon '44; FRCS(C), Urol; Chief of Urol. Serv., Hop. Notre-Dame & Hop. Ste-Justine; Cons., Queen Mary Vet's. Hosp.; Adv., W.C.B.; Tel. 526-3783.

BRAULT, Jules; 418 est, rue Sherbrooke, Montreal 24, P.Q.; 1330 St-Viateur ouest, Outremont (res); Mon '21; F.R.C.S.(C), F.A.A. Ophth. Otol; Ophth; Sr. Ophth., Hop-Notre-Dame; Cons. Ophth., I.N.C.A.; Assoc. Prof. (Ophth), U. of **Montreal; Tel. AV 8-3327.**

BRAULT, Norman; 949 Galt St. W., Sherbrooke, P.Q.; Lav '55.

BRAULT, Roger; 1715 1ere avenue, Quebec 3, P.Q.; 944 Adolphe Routhier (res); Lav '40; ObstGyn (P.Q.); Staff Hop.-St.-Francois-d'Assise; Prof (Obst.) Laval U.; Tel. 523-9429.

BRAULT, Roger B.; Medical Arts Bldg., Ponoka, Alta.; Ott '57; Abroad.

BRAULT, Thomas; 6731 St. Denis, Montreal, P.Q.; Lav '05; Retired.

BRAUN, Walter; 1955 W. Broadway, Vancouver 9, B.C.; Graz (Austria) '19; Vis. Staff, Vancouver Gen. & St. Paul's Hosp's.; Vis. Staff, St. Vincent's Hosp.; Tel. 733-8211.

BRAUND, Margaret R.; 605 Rossland Rd. E., Whitby, Ont.; Ott '55; DPH; M.O.H. & Dir., Ontario County Health Unit; Tel. 668-8843.

BRAUNSTEIN, David; 970 St. Mary's Rd., St. Vital, Man.; 755 Waterloo (res); Man '29; Court Staff, St. Boniface, Misericordia, Victoria, Grace & Municipal Hosp's.; Tel. AL 3-4911.

BRAUNSTEIN, M. M.; Ste. 39, The Sherbrooke, 1390 Sherbrooke St. W., Montreal, P.Q.; 4808 Roslyn Ave. (res); McG '30; Phys-in-charge of **Sterility Clin., Jewish Gen. Hosp.; Tel. VI 4-9259.**

BRAUNSTEIN, Philip; Durham (Eng.) '54; Res., New Mount Sinai Hosp., Toronto, Ont.

BRAUNSTEIN, Ronald E.; Man'65; **Jr. Int., St.** Boniface Hosp., St. Boniface 6, Man.

BRAWLEY, G. Peter; Tor '60; P.G. (Psy.), U. of Toronto, Toronto 5, Ont.

BRAY, Gordon; 227 Med. Arts Bldg., 102 Canada Bldg., Saskatoon, Sask; Tor '49; D.A.B.R.; DiagRad; Active Staff, Saskatoon City & St. Paul's Hosp's.; Assoc. Staff, University Hosp.; Tel. 244-1167-9.

BRAY, Lloyd G.; Moose Jaw Clinic, 200 Scott Blk., Moose Jaw, Sask.; 105 Hall St. E. (res); Man '38; Paed; Chief of Staff, Providence Hosp.; Clin. Assoc. (Paed.), U. of Saskatchewan; Tel. 692-2373.

BRAYLEY, James L.; 77 Upper Middle Rd., South Peel Med. Arts, Cooksville, Ont.; Tor '51; ObstGyn; Chief of ObstGyn., South Peel Hosp.; Tel. 279-6430.

BRAYTON, Merritt J.; 132-16th Ave, N. E., Calgary, Alta.; McG '24.

BRAZEAU, Michel; Mon'65; Res., Hop. Notre Dame, Montreal 24, P.Q.

BREAKWELL, William G.; Markdale, Ont.; Tor '45; MCGP; Tel. 140.

BREARLEY, Guy G.; P.O. Box 317, Belleville, Ont.; 236 McDonald Ave. (res); Alb '30; Dir., Provincial Chest Clinic; Tel. WO 2-0211.

BREAULT, Henri J.; 1011 Ouellette, Windsor, Ont.; 36 Reedmere, Riverside (res); Wes '36; D.A.B.P., F.A.A.P., Paed; Chief Paed., Hotel Dieu; Paed., Grace, Metropolitan, Fred Adams Hosp's., Detroit Children's Hosp. & Well Baby **Paed. Clinic, Bd. of Health, Windsor; Tel. 254-5282.**

BREAULT, Jacques; Mon'65; Res., Hop. St. Charles, Joliette, P.Q.

BREAULT, Yves; Mon'57; MCGP; Anaes(P.Q.); Staff, Hop. Vincent de Paul, Sherbrooke, P.Q.

BREBNER, Colin N.; 11 Kirkland St., Kirkland Lake, Ont.; 99 First St. (res); Tor '38; GenSurg.

BREBNER, John; Tor'62; Res., rotating at various Toronto Hospitals.

BREDO, Gerald A.; Med. Clinic, Powell River, B.C.; Alb'64.
BREEN, Harvey; 956 Westview Cr., North Vancouver, B.C.; UBC'59; Psy.
BREITHAUPT, David J.; 200 Bloor St. E., Toronto, Ont.; 86 Brenda Cres., Scarborough (res); Tor'41; D.P.H., F.R.C.P.(C), IntMed; Med. Dir., Manufacturers Life Ins. Co.; Tel. 928-4252.
BREITKREUTZ, Herbert E.; Alb'64; Res., University of Alberta Hosp., Edmonton, Alta.
BREITMAN, Reuben; 716 Medical Arts Bldg., Montreal, P.Q.; 4609 Hutchinson St. (res); McG '29; A.B.O.S., OrthSurg.; Tel. WE 5-5652.
BREMNER, J. Murray; 37 Glenwood Ave., Toronto 9, Ont. (res); Tor '14; Retired.
BREMNER, John E.; Apt. 37, 4351 Bloor St. W., Etobicoke, Ont.; Ott'55; Path.
BREMNER, R. Gordon; 27 Anglesey Blvd., Islington, Ont.; Tor '50; M.C.G.P.; Tel. BE 1-6843.
BREMNER, Ronald M.; 404 Medical Arts, Saskatoon, Sask.; Tor'45; F.A.A.D.S., DermSyph; Ass't. Clin. Prof., Dept. of Med., U. of Sask.; Chief of Serv., (Derm) University Hosp.; Cons. (Derm.) Dept. of Veterans Affairs; Tel. 242-0580.
BREMNER, Walter V.; 208 St. Clair Ave. W., Toronto 7, Ont.; 414 Glengarry Ave. (res); Tor '37; DPM. (Eng.); NeurPsy; Staff, O.P.D. (Psy.), Toronto Western Hosp.; Tel. WA 1-4545.
BRENNAN, Charles F.; Med. Arts Bldg., 336 Kings Rd., Sydney, N.S.; Dal '55; ObstGyn.
BRENNAN, Donald S.; Bear River, N.S.; Dal '49; Staff, Digby Gen. Hosp. & Annapolis Gen. Hosp.; Tel. 467-3524.
BRENNAN, Edward J.; Angus Block, 374 Fraser St., North Bay, Ont.; 859 Main St. W. (res); Qns '16; Coroner, North Bay; Med. Off. Casselholme of Aged & Children's Welfare; Tel. 474-2250.
BRENNAN, Francis J.; Box 130, Paille Block, Melville, Sask.; Ire. '42.
BRENNAN, James C.; 38 Shea St., St. John's, Nfld. (res); Dublin (Ire.) '50; Ass't. Dir. Med. Service, Nfld.; Path., St. John's Gen. Hosp.; Tel. 8-0471.
BRENNAN, J. H. Lawrence; Tor '31; F.A.C.C.P., IntMed (TB); M.O., Workmen's Compensation Board, in Charge of Industrial Dis., 90 Harbour St., Toronto, Ont.; Tel. 362-3411.
BRENNAN, Joseph W.; 218 Hanna Rd., Leaside, Ont. (res); Tor'32; GenSurg; Surg. Staff, St. Michael's Hosp.; Assoc. (Surg.), U. of Toronto; Tel. WA 2-6327.
BRENNAN, Kieran S.; Belfast (N. Ire.) '57; Staff, Psychiatric Centre, Yorkton Hosp., Yorkton, Sask.; Tel. 783-2401.
BRENNAN, Maxwell D.; 180 Portland St., Dartmouth, N.S.; 3 Tulip St. (res); Edinburgh (Scot.) '36; GenSurg; Staff, Halifax Infirmary, Victoria Gen., Childrens' & Grace Maternity Hosp's.; Tel. 466-7471.
BRENNAN, Michael; 39 Russell St. E., Smiths Falls, Ont.; Dublin (Ire.)'54; MCGP.
BRENNAN, R. Lyle; 108 Oakridge Ave., Pointe Claire, Lachine, P.Q.; McG'50; MCGP; Med. Dir., Avon Cosmetics (Canada), Pulp & Paper Research Inst. (of Canada) & Noranda Research Inst.; Registra. Phys., Emergency Serv. & Sect., Dept. of G.P., Lakeshore Gen. Hosp.; Exec. Comm. P.G., Bd., Royal Victoria Hosp.
BRENNAND, Shirley Z.; 132 Dawson Ave., Dorval Lachine, P.Q. (res); Ott '50; Paed.
BRENNER, C. Gloria; (See Jacobs, C. Gloria).
BRENT, Florence; Ste. 1215, 8510-111th St., Edmonton, Alta.; Alb'42; FACOG; FACS; DABOG.
BRENT, Frank de Niord; 30 Alcan N., Place Ville Marie, Montreal, P.Q.; Wes'38; MIH (Harvard); Occ. Health (AB PrevMed); PH (P.Q.); FACPM; Dir. of Health Serv., Aluminum Co. of Canada; Chief Health Serv., Aluminum Fiduciaries Ltd.; Tel. 877-3374.
BRENT, Henry P.; Ste. 202, 250 Lawrence Ave. W., Toronto 12, Ont.; 38 Castleknock Rd. (res); Tor '54 M. A. (Physiol.); Ophth; Clin, Ass't., Hosp. for Sick Children; Assoc. Staff, Tor. Western Hosp.; Cons. (Ophth), Queen Elizabeth Hosp.; Tel. 787-3777.
BRERETON, Charles H.; 168 Oakwood Ave., Toronto, Ont.; Wes '13; Tel. RU 2-1414.
BRERETON, Donald C.; 209 Medical Arts Bldg., Winnipeg, Man.; Man '42; IntMed; Staff, Deer Lodge, DVA & Winnipeg Mun. Hosp's.; Tel. 942-6018.
BRERETON, Frank W.; Royal York Plaza Med. Centre, 1500 Royal York Rd., Weston, Ont.; 23 Westmount Pk. Rd. (res); Tor '46; M.C.G.P.; Staff (Med.) Northwestern Gen. Hosp.; Tel. CH 4-6153.
BRERETON, William J.; Group Health Assoc., 240 McNabb St., Sault Ste Marie, Ont. R.C. (Ire) '55; Tel. 254-6421.
BRESLIN, Rueben H.; 66 Spadina Rd., Toronto 4, Ont.; Tor '26; Tel. WA 1-2998.
BRESNAHAN, T. James; 190 MacLaren St., Ottawa 4, Ont.; 1890 Wembley Ave., Ott. 13 (res); Qns '47; MRCP (Lond.); IntMed; Tel. 236-5581.
BRETON, F; 222 est, Henri Bourassa, Montreal 12, P.Q.; Mon '53; MCGP; Tel. DU 1-3800.
BRETON, Gerard J.; Breton Clinic, 1261-101st St., North Battleford, Sask.; 1072 Henry St. (res); Alb '45; FICS; GenSurg; Tel. 445-4422.
BRETON, Jean P.; 55 rue Champagnat, Levis, P.Q.; Lav'54; PH (P.Q.).
BRETON, J. Jacques; Lav'65; Res., Hop. St. Michel Archange, Quebec, P.Q.
BRETON, Liguori J. F.; 306 Rue St. Louis, Warwick, Cte. Arthabaska, P.Q.; 346 Rue St. Louis (res); Lav '36; Staff, Hotel Dieu, Arthabaska.
BRETON, T. A.; 316 Wellington St. W., Sault Ste. Marie, Ont.; 125 Wellington St. W. (res); McG '38.
BRETT, Frederick; Green's Harbour, Trinity Bay, Nfld.; Tor '54; M.O.H.; Tel. 13F41.
BRETT, H. Brian; Wes '56; Zone Supt., MacKenzie Zone, Northern Health Serv., 12702-114th Ave., Edmonton, Alta.; Tel. 454-3670.
BRETTLER, Adolf; 398 Bloor St. W., Toronto 4, Ont.; 239½ Lonsmount Dr. (res); Berlin (Germ.) '31; Urol; Tel. WA 1-7671.
BREULS, Alexander M.; 695 Markham Rd., Scarborough, Ont.; 46 Felicity Dr. (res); Tor '46; DPH; MCGP; Ass't. MOH, Scarborough Twp.; Tel. AT 2-6301.
BREULS, Robert W.; Sharon P.O., Ont.; Tor '09; Retired.
BREWER, Jack R.; McG '61; Jr. Intn., Royal Victoria Hosp., Montreal 2, P.Q.
BREWER, Lloyd M.; 9 Talbot St. E., Leamington, Ont.; 4 Smith St. (res); McG '48; IntMed; Tel. FA 6-4421.
BREWERTON, Steele C.; Raymond Magrath Clinic, Magrath, Alta.; Alb'48; Tel. 758-3134.
BREWSTER, Francis A.; 895-4th Ave. E., Owen Sound, Ont. (res); Tor '10; Retired.
BREWSTER, James M.; 405 Ninth St. E., Owen Sound, Ont.; 435 Ninth St. E. (res); Qns '43; IntMed.; Chief of Med., Owen Sound Gen. & Marine Hosp.; Tel. 376-7644.
BREWSTER, John M.; 291-9th St. E., Owen Sound, Ont.; 664-2nd Ave. W. (res); Qns '41; FACS; GenSurg; Staff, Gen. & Marine Hosp.; Tel. FR 6-4606.
BREWSTER, Ormond M.; 77 Westmount Rd., Guelph, Ont.; 22 Maple St. (res); Glasgow (Scot.) '41; B.Sc., M.B., Ch.B., F.R.C.S. (Ed.); Gen-Surg; Surg. Guelph Gen., & St. Joseph's, Guelph, Georgetown & Milton District Hosp's.; Tel. TA 4-5460.
BREWSTER, Walter R.; 713 Columbia St., New Westminster, B.C.; Tor '19.
BRIANT, T. David; 320 Med. Arts Bldg., 170 St. George St., Toronto 5, Ont.; Tor '55; FRCS(C); Otol; Active Staff, Toronto Gen. Hosp.; Court. Staff, Central Hosp.; Cons. Staff, Princess Margaret Hosp.; Tel. 922-7751.
BRIANT, Thomas E.; 23 Division St., Welland, Ont.; Tor'24; FACS; AB OphthOtol; Ophth, Otol; Chief, Dept. of Ophth & Otol., Welland Gen. Hosp.; Cons. Plas. Surg. (Head & Neck); Hotel-Dieu Hosp., St. Catharines; Cons. Otol., Niagara Pen. San.; Tel. 735-5294.
BRICK, Miriam A.; 55 Woodlawn Ave. W., Toronto 7, Ont. (res); Tor '30; Paed; OPD., Chest Clin., Hosp. for Sick Children; Ass't. Phys., IODE San.; Retired.

BRICKENDEN, Arthur W.; 1960A Eglinton Ave. W., Toronto 10, Ont.; 240 Northcliffe Blvd. (res); Tor '50; M.C.G.P.; O.P.D., St. Michael's Hosp.; Tel. RU 7-1391.

BRICKER, James D.; 705 Medical Arts Bldg., Windsor, Ont.; 2496 Gladstone Ave. (res); Tor '51; DiagRad.; Tel. 254-7551.

BRICKLEY, J. R.; 331 Sheddon Ave., Oakville, Ont.; McG '57; MCGP; Tel. 844-3561.

BRICKMAN, Helen (Friedman); 5031 Ponsard Ave., Montreal 29, P.Q.; Man '41; Paed; Ass't. Phys., Mtl. Children's Hosp.; Assoc. Phys., Jewish Gen. & Royal Edward Laurentian Hosp's.; Tel. 484-3348.

BRIDGE, H. William; Ass't. Dir., Mental Health Services, 828 W. 10th Ave., Vancouver 9, B.C.; Dublin (Ire.)'52; BAO; M.Sc. (Admin. Med. Columb.); CMHA (APA); Psy.

BRIDGE, Robert W.; Sask'60; Res., Regina Gen. Hosp., Regina, Sask.

BRIDGE, Tom; Room 211, 925 W. Georgia St., Vancouver 1, B.C.; McG'47; DiagRad; Staff, Shaughnessy Hosp.; Tel. MU 4-4177.

BRIDGER, Spencer M.; Dal'60; Res., Mtl. Gen. Hosp., Montreal 25, P.Q.

BRIDGMAN, Morley C.; Box 847, Oliver, B.C.; Man '09; Tel. HY 3328; Semi-Retired.

BRIEN, Francis S.; 144 Iroquois Ave., London, Ont. (res); Tor '33; FRCP (Lond.), FACP; MCGP (Hon.); FRCP(C); IntMed; **Phys-in-Chief, Victoria Hosp.; Cons., Westminster DVA, Beck Mem. San., Ont. Hosp., St. Thomas, & RCAF; Prof. & Hd. Dept. of Med., U. of Western Ont.; Tel. GE 2-5261, Loc. 285.**

BRIEN, Louis; Lav '64; Res., Inst. Albert-Prevost, Montreal, P.Q.; Abroad.

BRIEN, Wilbert P.; 806 Ouellette Ave., Windsor, Ont.; 2177 Chilver Rd., (res); Tor '40; M.C.G.P.; Staff, Metropolitan Gen. & Grace Hosp's.; Tel. 254-9227.

BRIERE, Claude R.; Lav'63; Res., Hotel-Dieu de Quebec, Quebec 4, P.Q.

BRIERE, Jacques; 1150 est, Boul-St-Joseph, Montreal 34, P.Q.; Mon'57; FRCS(C); GenSurg; Staff, Hop. Maisonneuve; Lect. U. of Montreal; Tel. LA 7-1241.

BRIERE, Jean P.; Lav'55; MCGP; Physiat. (P.Q.); Staff, Queen Mary Veteran's Hosp., Montreal, P.Q.

BRIESKORN, Hans H.; 38 Victor St., London, Ont. (res); Heidelberg (Germ.) '46.

BRIFFETT, Ralph L.; Springdale, Nfld.; Dal '64.

BRIGGS, Alice E.; Ste. 206, 250 Lawrence Ave. W., Toronto 12, Ont.; 478 Oriole Parkway, Tor. 7 (res); Tor '55; IntMed; Teach. Staff, O.P.D., **Toronto Western Hosp. & Bethesda Hosp.; Tel. 789-5581.**

BRIGGS, E. J. Nixon; Winnipeg Clinic, Man.; 118 Westgate (res); London (Eng.) '45; MRCP; AKC; DCH; FAAP; Paed; Cons., St. Boniface, Misericordia & Children's Hosp's.; Ass't. Prof. **(Paed.), U. of Manitoba; Tel. 942-0551.**

BRIGGS, James A. D.; 250 Lawrence Ave. W., Toronto 12, Ont.; Cambridge (Eng.) '53; DMRD **(Eng.); DiagRad; Staff, York County & York Central Hosp's.; Tel. RU 7-0229.**

BRIGGS, Peter D.; Box 126, 108 Henry St., Stirling, Ont.; 172 Edward St. (res); Cambridge (Eng.) '58; MA; MB; B.Chir. (Cambridge); **MRCS (Eng.); LRCP (Lond.); Tel. 395-2588.**

BRIGGS, Robert F.; 49 Dickens Dr., Kingston, Ont. (res); McG '55; D. Psy; Psy; Dir. Child & Adoles. Psy. Clinic. & Lect. Child Psy., Dept. of Psy & Paed., Kingston Gen. Hosp. Ass't. Prof. **(Psy & Paed.), Queen's U.; Tel. 546-3841, Loc. 320.**

BRIGHT, Bertha G.; 42 Hillendale Ave., Kingston, Ont. (res); Wes '37; Temp. Ret.

BRIGHT, Hugh J.; 447 Thessaly Circle, Ottawa 8, Ont.; (res); Tor '36; DPH; DHA; FABPM; (Av.Med); Deputy Med. Officer of Health for City of Ottawa.

BRIGHT, Ray C.; Minnedosa Med. Group, Minnedosa, Man.; Man'65.

BRILLINGER, H. Roy; 67 Bond St. S., Hamilton, Ont. (res); Tor '31; Psy; Dir., Mental Health Clin., Ontario Hosp., Hamilton; Tel. 385-5361.

BRILLON, Germain; Mon '63; Int. Hop. Ste-Justine, Montreal 26, P.Q.

BRINDLE, George F.; 3801 University St., Montreal, P.Q.; McG'52; FRCP(C), Anaes; Joint Chief of Staff, Queen Mary Vet's. Hosp.; Anaes., Mtl. Neurol Inst. & Royal Edward Laurentian Hosp.; Ass't. Prof. (Anaes), McGill U.; Tel. 849-4955.

BRINDLE, Michael J.; c/o Dr. S. C. Windle & Assoc., 105-10049 Jasper Ave., Edmonton, Alta.; Liverpool (Eng.)'58; DiagRad.

BRINK, G. Clair; 49 St. Leonard's Cres., Toronto 12, Ont. (res); Tor '13; IntMed (TB); Dir. TB Prev., Dept. of Health, Ont.; Retired.

BRINKOP, Hanna (See LITTLE, Hanna).

BRINSMEAD, Alan N.; Col. Mewburn Pavilion, **112th St. & 87th Ave., Edmonton, Alta.; Man'43;** Att'd Staff, Misericordia Hosp.

BRISBY, James M.; 2374 Eglinton Ave. E., Scarborough, Ont.; **82 Rossander Crt. (res); Tor '53; M.C.G.P.; Tel. PL 7-3217.**

BRISCOE, Maureen (see Maxwell)

BRISEBOIS, Maxime P.; 816 Sherbrooke E., Montreal, P.Q.; Mon'21; FRCS(C); Retired.

BRISEBOIS, Rolland C.; 951 Aime Bibeau, St. Vincent-de-Paul, Montreal, P.Q. (res); Mon '45; Psy (P.Q.); Staff, Hop. St. Jean de Dieu; Tel. CL 4-5361.

BRISSET DES NOS, Louis; 3470 Dezery, Montreal, P.Q.; Mon '21.

BRISSETTE, Yvette B. (Larochelle); 80 rue St.-Louis, Quebec, P.Q. (res); Lav '41.

BRISSON, Bernard P.; Chibougamau, P.Q.; Ott '52; Coroner, Abitibi East.

BRISSON, Dennis A.; 1361 Ouelette Ave., Windsor, Ont.; Ott '57; FRCS(C), Otol.

BRISSON, Francois X.; P.O. Box 444, Chicoutimi, P.Q. (res); Lav '46; GenSurg (P.Q.); Surg., Hotel Dieu St. Vallier Hosp., Chicoutimi; Coroner, Dist. of Chicoutimi; Clin. Ass't., Laval U.; Tel. 549-0598.

BRISSON, Gerald; 175 Champlain, Hull, P.Q.; Mon '25; GenSurg, ObstGyn (P.Q.); Chief of Obst. Gyn., Hop du Sacre Coeur; Instr., Obst. Gyn., U. of Ottawa; Vis. Surg., Ottawa Gen. Hosp.; Dist. Coroner; Tel. PR 7-6440.

BRISSON, Jean M.; 4 Taschereau, Hull, P.Q.; 190 Ste.-Marie (res); Lav '55; FRCS(C), Otol; Active Med. Staff, Hop-Sacre-Coeur; Tel. PR 1-9392.

BRISSON, John E.; 2095 Wyandotte St. W., Windsor, Ont.; Ott '55; Tel. 252-4042.

BRISTOW, Morval E.; Man '30; DABPM; Psy; Med. Supt., Hosp. for Mental Diseases, Box 420, Brandon, Man.; Tel. PA 6-2321.

BRISTOW, R. J.; 291 Talbot St., St. Thomas, Ont.; 21 Farley Place (res); Wes '29; GenSurg; Chief of Surg., St. Thomas Elgin Hosp.; **Cons. (Surg.), Ontario Hosp.; Tel. ME 1-0226.**

BRITT, Beverley A.; Tor'56; FRCP(C), Anaes; Staff, U. of Toronto, Toronto 5, Ont.

BRITTEN, Stanley E.; Ste 11A-12, 3108 Oak St., Vancouver, B.C.; 57 W. 41st Ave. (res); McG '51; Tel. TR 6-2145.

BRITTON, H. E.; 54 Highfield St., Moncton, N.B.; McG '18; FACS, GenSurg.; MCGP; Tel. EV 4-4534.

BRITTON, Michael H.; McG'65; Jr. Int., Royal Victoria Hosp., Montreal 2, P.Q.

BRITTON, William A.; Ste. 401, 1105 Carling Ave., Ottawa 3, Ont.; Qns '56; FRCS(C), Ophth; Dir. & Staff, Strobis. Clinic, Ottawa Civic Hosp.; Lect. (Ophth.), Ottawa U.; Tel. 722-7649.

BROADFOOT, Thomas W.; 237 Kent St. W., Lindsay, Ont.; Tor '40; Tel. 324-3193.

BROADHURST, Carole A.; Tor '58; Res., St. Michael's Hosp., Toronto 2, Ont.

BROADWELL, Douglas J.; 2085 Tecumseh Rd., East Windsor, Ont.; Qns'43; Staff (ObstGyn) & Chm. Adm. & Disch. Comm., Metropolitan Gen. Hosp.; Dist. Coroner; Memb. Bd. of Dir., Windsor Med. Ser.; Plant Phys., Dominion Forge Ltd.; Tel. 256-7281.

BROCHU, Donald; Cap St-Ignace, Cte Montmagny, P. Q.; Lav '63.

BROCHU, Gaston; Lav'65; Res., Hotel-Dieu Hosp., Montreal, P.Q.

BROCHU, Jean; 1500-181eme rue, Quebec 3, P.Q.; **582 Ave. Mont-Marie Ste. Foy, Quebec 10 (res); Lav '49; GenSurg(P.Q.), M.Sc. (Surg.), Penn.; Ass't. (Surg.), Hop. de l'Enfant-Jesus; Tel. 524-6132.**

BROCHU, Jean L.; 770 1ere Ave., Quebec 3, P. Q.; 325-70th rue E., Quebec 7 (res); Lav '58; Tel. 523-8500.

BROCHU, Louis A.; 225 Grande Allee E., Quebec 4, P.Q.; 999 Bougainville (res); Lav '26; M.O., W.C.B., (P.Q.); Tel. 522-4751.

BROCHU, Omer; Cap aux Meules, Isles de la Madeleine, P.Q.; Lav '39; GenSurg (P.Q.); Surg., Hop. Notre-Dame-de-la-Garde & Phys., Isles de la Madeleine.

BROCHU, Paul-E.; 2839-1st Ave., Quebec, P.Q.; **2835—1st Ave. (res); Lav '41; GenSurg (P.Q.); Ass't. Surg., Hop. St. Francois d'Assise; Tel. 623-1065.**

BROCHU, Raoul; 1105 St. Jean St., Quebec, P.Q.; 178 Murray St. (res); Lav '18.

BROCK, W. George; 432 Medical Arts Bldg., Winnipeg 1, Man.; Man'25; MS (Derm.); DermSyph; Cons. & Hon. Att'd. Staff, Winnipeg Gen. Hosp.; Assoc. Prof. Med. (Derm.), U. of Manitoba; Tel. 943-7208.

BROCKINGTON, Colin W. M.; 17-11th Ave. S., Cranbrooke, B.C.; McG'43; DPH; MCGP; Tel. **426-2201.**

BROCKLEHURST, John C.; c/o I.G.A., North West River, Labrador (res); Glasgow (Scot.) '47; M.O. Internat. Grenfell Assoc., Labrador, Nfld.

BROCKWAY, Eric N.; 901 Helena, Trail, B.C.; London (Eng.) '34; FRCS (Edin.); OrthSurg; Tel. 368-5211.

BRODER, Elsa A.; 324 Glen Ayr Rd., Toronto **10, Ont.;** Tor'58; Psy; Staff, Thistletown Hosp., Thistletown; Tel. 741-1210.

BRODER, Irvin; 324 Glenayr Rd., Toronto 10, Ont. (res); Tor '55; **FRCP** (C); IntMed; Active Staff, Toronto Western Hosp.; Clin. Teach., U. of Toronto; Tel. 368-2581.

BRODER, Morris H.; 208 Doctor's Bldg., Winnipeg, Man.; 1 Crocus (res); Man '52; FRCS(C), GenSurg; Tel. 943-8954.

BRODEUR, Gilles; 2055 Girouard, St. Hyacinthe, P.Q.; Mon'59; Tel. 773-0225.

BRODEUR, Jules; Mon '61; M.S.C. (Pharm.), Ph.D. (Pharm.); Staff, Dept. of Pharm., U. of Montreal, Montreal, P.Q.; Tel. RE 3-9951, Ext. 275.

BRODEUR, Michael T.; McG '56; Res., Royal Victoria Hosp., Montreal 2, P.Q.

BRODEUR, Pierre; 426 St. Joseph Blvd. E., Montreal 34, P.Q.; Mon '51; Paed.; Tel. VI 4-7383.

BRODEUR, Roger; Mon '63; Res., Hop. Ste-Justine, Montreal 26, P.Q.

BRODEUR, Yvan; 2128 Blvd. Laframboise, St. Hyacinthe, P.Q.; 1745 rue Nelson (res); Lav '51; MCGP; Staff, Hop. St. Charles; Tel. PR 4-8242.

BRODEY, Abraham; 1711 Bathurst St., Toronto 10, Ont.; 54 Avenue Rd. (res); Tor '14; Tel. HU 5-5500.

BRODEY, Joshua B.; Ste 414, 1849 Yonge St., Toronto 7, Ont.; Qns '59; Psy.

BRODIE, Douglas W.; Stouffville Med. Centre, **200 Main St. W., Stouffville, Ont.; 365 Glad Park Ave (res); Tor '54; MCGP; Staff, Uxbridge Cottage & Scarborough Gen. Hosp's.; Tel. 640-3100.**

BRODIE, Elizabeth; 174 St. George St., Toronto 7, Ont. (res); Vienna (Austria) '57; D. Psy; Psy; U. of T. Fell; Staff, Toronto Psy. Hosp.; Tel. WA 5-6371.

BRODIE, Hugh R.; 2300 Tupper St., Montreal 25, **P.Q.; 600 Lansdowne Ave. (res); McG '51;** DCH (Eng.), D.A.B.Paed; **Paed (P.Q.); Ass't. Phys., Montreal Children's Hosp.; Paed., Queen Elizabeth Hosp.; Dem., (Paed.), McGill U.; Tel.** WE 7-8511.

BRODIE, Ian H.; 202 Underwood Bldg., 1311-1st St. S.W., Calgary, Alta.; 703-32nd Ave. S.W. (res); McG '23; GenSurg (Alb); Staff, Calgary Gen., Holy Cross & Grace Hosp's.; Retired.

BRODIE, Robert B.; 2620 Eglinton Ave. E., Scarborough, Ont.; 95 Confederation Dr. (res); Tor '53; M.C.G.P.; Staff, Scarborough Gen. Hosp.; Tel. AM 7-6961.

BRODKIN, Elliot; McG'58; Path; Ph.D.; Path. & Dir. of Labs., Bellechasse Hosp., Montreal, P.Q.

BRODOVSKY, David M.; 627 Med. Arts Bldg., 404 Graham Ave., Winnipeg, Man.; 836 Brock St. (res); Man '57; FRCS(C); DABO; Otol; Active **Staff, St. Boniface, Wpg. Children's, Deer Lodge,** & Man. Rehab. Hosp's.; **Tel. 943-0629.**

BRODRICK, Robert J.; Ste. 455, 5025 Sherbrooke St. W., Montreal, P.Q.; McG'47; FCCP; DABIM; IntMed; Assoc. Phys. (Med.), St. Mary's & Queen Elizabeth Hosp's; Tel. HU 8-3878.

BRODY, Gary S.; Alb '56; Research, McGill U., Montreal 2, P.Q.

BRODY, Harry; Foothills Hospital, Calgary, Alta.; Alb'56; FACOG; FRCS(C), ObstGyn; Dir. Dept. of ObstGyn., Foothills Hosp.; Tel. 283-0751.

BROGDEN, Lawrence F.; 3585 West 43rd Ave., Vancouver, B.C. (res); **Tor '11; Retired.**

BROKOVSKI, Ellen J. (Lewinsohn); 582 Waverley St.. Winnipeg 9, Man. (res); Welsh Nat. U. (Cardiff) '41; LRCP, MRCS; Phys., City Health Dept.; Retired.

BROMAGE, Philip R.; 3235 Ridgewood, Apt. 209, Montreal, P.Q. (res); London (Eng.) '44; M.B., B.S., DA., FFARCS; Anaes; Anaes., Royal Victoria Hosp.; Ass't. Prof. (Anaes), Mc-Gill U.; Tel. VI 2-1251. Loc. 724.

BROMAN, Roy D.; Ste. 107, 1940 Lonsdale Ave. North Vancouver, B.C.; **UBC '62.**

BROMLEY, A. J.; 16 Sunnylea Ave., Toronto 18, Ont.; Tor '21; Staff, D.V.A.

BROMLEY, Alfred T.; 410 Hammond Bldg., 310 Main St. N., Moose Jaw, Sask.; Madras (India) '47; D.Obst RCOG; LMSSA (Lond.); Staff, Moose Jaw Union & Providence Hosp's.; Tel. 693-3661.

BROMLEY, K. J.; 470 Paris, Sudbury, Ont.; Qns '29; Anaes.

BRONSTEIN, Gregor; 102 Baltimore Rd., Winnipeg 13, Man.; L'Aurore, Shanghai & Aix Marseille (France)'35 & '41.

BRONSTEIN, Seymour B.; Box 45, Bolton, Ont.; Qns '55; Staff, Dufferin Area Hosp., Orangeville; Assoc. Staff, **Peel Mem. Hosp., Brampton; Tel.** 941-2410.

BRONSTONE, Robert F.; Man '61; Jr. Intn., Winnipeg Gen. Hosp., Winnipeg 3, Man.

BROOK, John R.; 156 St. Paul Cres., St. Catharines, Ont.; 110 Rivercrest Blvd. (res); London (Eng.) '53; MRCS, LRCP; Tel. 684-8507.

BROOK, Joseph; 505 Canada Bldg., Saskatoon, Sask.; 825 University Dr. (res); Man '41; M.C.G.P.; Staff, Saskatoon City, University & St. Paul's Hosp's.; Clin. Instr., ObstGyn., U. of Saskatchewan; Tel. 242-0213.

BROOK, Morris H.; 505 Canada Bldg., Saskatoon, Sask.; Ste. 9, Parklane Apts. (res); Man'35; M.C.G.P.; Staff, (GP), University, St. Paul's & City Hosp's; Clin. Instr. (ObstGyn), U. of Saskatchewan; Tel. 242-0213.

BROOKE, Hewitt H. W.; 20 Hycroft Med. Bldg., 3195 Granville St., Vancouver, B.C.; 1619 King Edward Ave., Van. 9 (res); McG '39; DABR; D & T Rad; Chief Rad., Burnaby Gen. Hosp.; Cons. Rad. 4000 RMU 19th Wing RCAF & Other Armed Services, Van.; Tel. RE 1-5241.

BROOKS, Alfred J.; McG '55; DiagRad; Staff, Metro. X-Ray Assoc., 1849 Yonge St., Toronto 7, Ont.

BROOKS, Carman H. Capt.; RCAF Station, Trenton, Ont.; Alta'65.

BROOKS, David H.; Box 1690, Edson, Alta.; Sheffield (Eng.)'62; Tel. 723-3366.

BROOKS, David Hall; Forest Hill Rehab. Centre, Box 265, Woodbridge St., Fredericton, N.B.; Oxford & St. Bart's (Lond., Eng.) '46; B.A., B.M., B.Ch. (Oxon.), M.A. (Sc.); FRSM, MRCS (Eng.), LRCP (Lond.), MCMG; MCGP; PhysMed & Rehab; Med. Dir. & Physiatrist, Forest Hill Rehab. Centre; Cons. PhysMed., Rehab. Div., Prov. Dept. of Health; Cons. PhysMed. & Rehab., W.C.B. & Ridgwood Rehab. Centre, Lancaster; Tel. 475-3309.

BROOKS, Donald W.; 356 Woodroffe Ave., Ottawa 3, Ont.; 688 Mansfield (res); Tor '50; IntMed; Staff, Ottawa Gen. Hosp.; Lect., U. of Ottawa; Tel. 729-8307.

BROOKS, Edward F. J.; Ste. 513, Medical Arts Bldg., 170 St. George St., Toronto 5, Ont.; 28 Millbank Ave. (res); Tor '28; F.R.C.P.(Lond.), F.R.C.P.(C), IntMed, Neur; **Phys.-in-Chief, St. Michael's Hosp.; Prof., Dept. of Med., U. of Toronto; Tel. WA 1-7474.**

BROOKS, Harvie C.; 1849 Yonge St., Ste. 509, Toronto 7, Ont.; 45 Donegall Dr. (res); Tor '55; MCGP; Court. Staff, Wellesley & Grace Hosp's.; Tel. HU 5-5222.

BROOKS, Henry J.; Leeds (Eng.)'42; DCH (Eng.); Paed; Staff, Woodlands Hosp., Kingsway, New Westminster, B.C.

BROOKS, James S.; 366 Vaughan Road, Toronto 10, Ont.; Tor'64; Tel. 651-0211.

BROOKS, Ralph W.; Hatfield Pt., Kings County, N.B.; Dal '52; Tel. Springfield 23.

BROOKS, Theodore H.; 101 Fir St., Sherwood Park, Alta.; 408 Oak St. (res); London (Eng.) '25; LRCP (Lond.); MCGP; Tel. 699-5671.

BROOKSBANK, Ronald C.; Wellington St. Clinic, 510 Wellington St., Wallaceburg, Ont.; Wes'63; Tel. 627-3306.

BROOME, Thomas P.; Links Associate Clinic, 10951-124th St., Edmonton, Alta.; Qns '56; FRCP (C); IntMed; Active Staff, Royal Alexandra Hosp.; Assoc. Teach. Staff, U. of Alberta; Tel. 454-4551.

BROOMHEAD, Edward A.; Sheffield (Eng.)'42; Staff, Tobique Valley Hosp., Plaster Rock, N.B.

BROSNAN, Morgan L.; 131 Ontario St., St. Catharines, Ont.; Dublin (Ire.) '50 L.R.C.P. & S. **(I.); Otol.; Tel. MU 4-9663.**

BROSSARD, Claude L.; Mon '61; Res. Hop. Hotel-Dieu, Montreal 18, P. Q.

BROSSARD-DAIGNEAULT, Paulette; St. Philippe, Cte La Prairie, P.Q.; Mon '63.

BROSSEAU, Andre; 3244 Beaubien St. E., Montreal, P. Q.; Mon '53; Tel. RA 9-1891.

BROSSEAU, Bernard E.; Bonnyville, Alta.; Alb '60.

BROSSEAU, Bernard L. P.; Canadian Hosp. Assoc., 25 Imperial St., Toronto 7, Ont.; Mon'41; DTM&H; Exec. Dir., Cdn. Hospital Assoc.; Tel. HU 1-2244.

BROSSEAU, Claude R.; 763 ave Chevremont, Quebec 10, P. Q. (res); Lav '54; FRCP (C); IntMed; Haem; Dir. Haematology Lab., Hop-de-l'enfant Jesus; Tel. 529-8711.

BROSSEAU, Emile; St. Stanislas de Kostka, P.Q.; Lav '13.

BROSSEAU, Maurice; 11610 Tanguay, Ahuntsic, Montreal 12, P.Q.; Mon '51; Psy; Psy., Hop. Maisonneuve; Ass't. Prof. (Psy.), U. of Montreal; Tel. VI 2-5141.

BROSSEAU, Raymond; Ste. 344, 3600 Barclay Ave., Montreal 26, P.Q.

BROSSEAU, Victor; San Begin, Co. Dorchester, P.Q. (res); **Mon '40; Pulm.Dis. & TB (P.Q.);** Chief of Staff, San Begin; Tel. 3-1011.

BROSSEAU, Wilfrid; 4164 Parc LaFontaine, **Montreal, P.Q.; Mon '23; Obst (P.Q.); Staff (Obst.), Hop. Ste. Jeanne d'Arc; Tel. 524-2944.**

BROTMAN, Ervin H.; Mall Medical Bldg., Winnipeg, Man.; 266 Elm St. (res); Man '36; Tel. SP 4-2411.

BROTMAN, Herbert L.; 6000 Cote des Neiges Rd., Montreal 26, P.Q.; McG'30; GenSurg; Sr. Surg., Jewish Gen. Hosp.; Tel. 342-2912.

BROTMAN, Martin; Man '62; Jr. Intn., Winnipeg Gen. Hosp., Winnipeg, Man.

BROUGH, William J.; 140 Markland, Hamilton, Ont.; Qns '22.

BROUGHTON, Florence E. (McKim); 6863 Laurel St., Vancouver 14, B.C.; Man'39; Psy.

BROUGHTON, Roger J.; Qns '60; Staff, Montreal Neurological Inst., Montreal 2, P.Q.; Tel. 842-1251.

BROUILLE, Raynald; Mon '61; Res. Ste-Jeanne d'Arc, Montreal 18, P.Q.

BROUILLET, Joffre; 2647 Pl. Joseph-Casavant, Montreal 12, P. Q.; Mon '56; Dir. Lab. Endocrin., Hotel-Dieu Hosp.; Ass't. Prof. (Med.), U. of Montreal; Tel. VI 4-0161.

BROUILLETTE, Gilles; 30 est, boul St-Joseph, Montreal 14, P.Q.; Mon '63.

BROUILLETTE, Jean; 875 des Recollets, Trois-**Rivieres, P.Q.; 3900 Neree Beauchemin (res); Lav** '55; OrthSurg; Tel. 378-3365.

BROUILLETTE. Maurice; Mon '49 DiagRad; Staff, Brome Missisquoi Perkins Hosp., Sweetsburg, P.Q.; Tel. 263-1333.

BROUSSEAU, Jean-Guy; 4647 Ave. Verdun, Verdun, Montreal 19, P. Q.; Mon '59; Tel. 767-5304.

BROW, George R.; Ste 7, 1374 Sherbrooke St. **W., Montreal 25, P.Q.; 619 Murray Hill, Westmount (res); McG '20; F.A.C.P., F.R.C.P.(C), IntMed; Cardiol. (P.Q.); Hon. Cons., Royal Victoria Hosp.; Emer. Prof. (Med.),** McGill U.; Tel. **VI 2-3355.**

BROW, James R.; Wes '60; FRCP(C), IntMed; Staff, Royal Victoria Hosp., Montreal 2, P.Q.; Abroad.

BROWETT, Robert J.; 4794A Joyce Ave., Powell River, B.C. (Mailing Address); Med. Clinic, 5885 Arbutus St. (Office); Alb '62; Tel. 485-6261.

BROWMAN, Mark; 7841-2nd Ave., Ville-St.-Michel, Montreal 38, P.Q.; 60 Summit Circ., **Westmount (res); McG '49; GenSurg (P.Q.); Sr. Staff Memb., Bellechasse Hosp.; Tel. RA 7-5305.**

BROWN, Albert B.; 222 Sask. Cres. W., Saskatoon, Sask. (res); Qns '43; FACOG; FRCS(C), ObstGyn; Dept. Head (ObstGyn), University Hosp.; Prof. (ObstGyn), U. of Saskatchewan; Tel. 652-6078.

BROWN, Albert S.; Tor '37; Staff, Toronto Hosp., Weston, Ont.; Tel. RO 9-1161.

BROWN, Alexander P.; 2495 Commercial Dr., Vancouver, B.C.; **2365 West 19th Ave. (res);** Qns '46; M.C.G.P.; **Vis. Staff, Burnaby, Vancouver Gen., St. Vincent's & Grace Hosps.; Tel. TR 4-6431.**

BROWN, Allan T.; 4 Wychwood Rd., St. Catharines, Ont. (res); McG '37; Anaes; Dir. Dept. of Anaes, St. Catharines Gen. Hosp.; Anaes., Hotel-Dieu Hosp; Dir. Poison Control Centre; Tel. MU 2-5300.

BROWN, Alice A. R.; 15 Coburg St., Saint John, **N.B.; Tufts (U.S.A.) '35; Anaes; Staff, St. John Gen. & St. Joseph's Hosp's.; Tel. 693-4622.**

BROWN, A. W.; 543 Lawrence Ave., Kelowna, B.C.; McG'24; Ophth; Ophth., Kelowna Gen. Hosp.; Tel. 762-2003.

BROWN, Basil St. J.; Montreal Children's Hosp., 2300 Tupper St., Montreal, P.Q.; London (Eng.) '51; M.B., B.Sc.; FRCP(C); DiagRad; TherRad; Ass't. Rad., Montreal Children's & Catherine Booth Hosp's.; Dem. (Med.), McGill U.; Tel. 937-8511, Loc. 255, 256.

BROWN, Berkeley C.; Ste. 460, 1105 Pandora Ave., Victoria, B.C.; Wes '40; MRCP (Lond.); Cons. (Med.), Vet's. Hosp.; Tel. 388-5145.

BROWN, Bernard J.; 815c Park Rd., Richmond, B.C.; Queen U. (Belfast, Ire.)'61; MCGP; Tel. 278-9505.

BROWN, Brock R.; National Defence Med. Centre, Ottawa, Ont.; 289 Clemow Ave., (res); Tor '30; B.Sc. (Med.), M.I.H. (Harvard); F.A.C.P.M. (Av. Med.); Sr. Treatment Med. Officer, Ottawa District DVA.; Tel. 733-6600 Ext. 35.

BROWN, Bryce A.; 141 Simcoe St. S., Oshawa, Ont.; 1110 Simcoe St. S., (res); McG '18; MCGP; Active Staff, Oshawa Gen. Hosp.; Tel. 723-7063.

BROWN, B. Stanley W.; 23 Drummond St. Granby, P.Q.; McG '35; M.C.G.P.; Med. Dir., Protective Assur. of Canada.

BROWN, Carl M.; Dal'58; AMCGP; DiagRad; Staff, Ottawa Civic Hosp., Ottawa, Ont.

BROWN, Charles A.; Dal'65; Res., Children's Hosp., Halifax, N.S.

BROWN, Charles B.; 700 Medical Arts Bldg., 170 St. George St., Toronto 5, Ont.; 89 Riverwood Pkwy., Tor. 18 (res); Tor '39; F.R.C.P.(C), IntMed; Cons., Sunnybrook & Wellesley Hosp's.; Assoc. Prof. Med., U. of Toronto; Tel. WA 2-5036.

BROWN, Charles C.; 1710 Dufferin St., Toronto 10, Ont.; 40 Glen Rd. (res); Tor '18; Tel. LE 4-3202.

BROWN, Charles Y.; 460 Med. Arts Bldg., 1105 Pandora Ave., Victoria, B.C.; 3480 Upper Terrace, (res); Wes'46; IntMed; Med. Dir., CARS Clinic; Med. Advisory Bd., George Rd. Rehab. Hosp.; Tel. 388-5145.

BROWN, Claude B.; McAdam, N.B.

BROWN, Colin J.; 1256 Victoria Ave., Niagara Falls, Ont.; Wes '31; Obst.

BROWN, David N.; 625-5th Ave., New Westminster, B.C.; Man'57; FRCS(C), NeurSurg; Tel. 526-4481.

BROWN, David R.; 1427 Prince Rd., Windsor, Ont. (res); Glasgow (Scot.) '35; M.B., Ch.B., DPH; DPA; FCCP; Admin. & Med. Supt., IODE Mem. Hosp. & Essex Co. San.; Tel. CL 2-2771.

BROWN, Donald A.; 3516 Manitoba St., Vancouver 10, B.C.; Alb'57; FRCS(C) GenSurg.

BROWN, Donald C.; 49½ Victoria St. E., Amherst, N.S.; Dal '59; MCGP; Active Med. Staff Pres., Amherst Med. Soc.; Phys., Sifta Salt Ltd.; Tel. 279-7330.

BROWN, Donald C.; 1477 Mildmay Court, Clarkson, Ont. (res); Tor'52; DABR; DiagRad; Staff,.. Rad., South Peele Hosp., Cooksville; Tel. 277-2761

BROWN, Donald R.; McLeod Med. Bldg., 340 McLeod St., Ottawa 4, Ont.; McG'48; D.A.B.S., F.A.C.S., F.R.C.S.(C), GenSurg; Staff, Ottawa Civic Hosp.; Lect., (Clin. Surg.), U. of Ottawa; Tel. CE 6-2455.

BROWN, Douglas C. S.; 6067 Inglis St., Halifax, N.S.; Dal'57; FRCS(C), OrthSurg.

BROWN, Duncan; Alb '64; Res., University Hosp., Edmonton, Alta.

BROWN, E. Earle; 751 King St. W., Kitchener, **Ont.; 45 Westmount Rd. N., Waterloo (res), Wes '56; FRCP(C), IntMed; Dir., Radioiso. Lab.,** St. Mary's Hosp.; 745-3821.

BROWN, E. Clifford; 540 Notre Dame Ave., St. Lambert, P.Q.; 538 Notre Dame Ave. (res); McG **'18; Phys., Chambly Co. Prot. Schl.; Tel. 671-** 7366.

BROWN, Edwin J.; **Ste. 6, 8-45th Ave., Lachine, P.Q.;** 791-37th **Ave. (res); McG '48;** GenSurg; Att'd. Surg. Staff, **Lachine Gen. Hosp.;** Court. Surg. Staff, St. **Joseph's Hosp. & Reddy Mem. Hosp., Mtl.; Tel. 637-8741.**

BROWN, Edwin L.; 14 Hincks St., St. Thomas, Ont.; 6 Scott St. (res); Wes '40; M.C.G.P.; Chief of Staff, St. Thomas-Elgin Gen. Hosp.; Med. Dir., **Vick Chemical Clevite Ltd.; Tel. ME 1-8680.**

BROWN, E. Gibson; 21 Seventh St., Chatham, Ont.; Man '42; DPH; Med. Dir., Kent County Health Unit; Tel. 352-6960.

BROWN, E. James; 302 Med. Arts Bldg., 1 Yonge St., Hamilton, Ont.; Wes '55; MRCOG; FACOG; FRCS(C); ObstGyn; Act. Staff (ObstGyn.), Hamilton Civic Hosp's.; Clin. Assoc. ObstGyn, McMaster U.; Cons., McMaster Univ. Clin., Henderson Gen. Hosp.; Tel. 522-1562.

BROWN, Ernest W.; Ste. 111, 21 Upper Middle Rd., Cooksville, Ont.; Tor'55; D.Psy; Psy; Tel. 277-3583.

BROWN, Esther M.; 1402—14th St. E. Saskatoon, Sask. (res); Man '45; D.A.B.T.R., TherRad; Sr. **Assoc., Saskatoon Cancer Clin.; Ass't. Prof. (Ther Rad) & Clin. Instr. (Med.), U. of Saskatchewan. Tel. 652-3850.**

BROWN, F. Norman; Ste. 402, 1105 Carling Ave., Ottawa 3, Ont.; 402-3rd Ave. (res); Qns '47; FACS; FRCS(C), GenSurg; Surg., Ottawa Civic Hosp.; Lect. (ClinSurg.), U. of Ottawa; Tel. 728-3563.

BROWN, Frederick W.; Wes'63; Jr. Int., Toronto Gen. Hosp., Toronto 2, Ont.

BROWN, Giles W.; Athens, Ont. (res); Tor '24; Retired.

BROWN, G. Malcolm; Med. Research Council, Montreal Rd., Ottawa 7, Ont.; Qns '38; D.Phil. (Oxon); FRCP (Lond.); FACP; FRCP(C), Int Med.; Chmn. Med. Research Council; Prof. Med., U. of Ottawa; Tel. 993-2375.

BROWN, Gordon D.; 536 Professional Bldg., 10830 Jasper Ave., Edmonton, Alta.; Alb'48; IntMed; Cons. Diabetes, University & Edmonton Gen. Hosp's.; Lect. (Med.), U. of Alberta; Tel. 427-7011.

BROWN, Gregory M.; 40 Summerhill Ave., Toronto 7, Ont. (res); Tor '59; D.Psy; Psy; P.G., Toronto Psychiatric Hosp.; Tel. 365-1511. Abroad.

BROWN, Harry M.; 350 Wellington St., Sarnia, Ont.; 1232 Marcin Rd. (res); Wes '52; MCGP; Tel. ED 7-3221.

BROWN, Harvey A.; 5889 Bathurst St., Willowdale, Ont.; Qns '29; Tel. 222-6761.

BROWN, Harvey C.; Qns '62; Res., Mtl. Gen. Hosp., Montreal 25, P.Q.

BROWN, Helen R.; Ste. 6D, 9820-104th St., Edmonton, Alta.; London (Eng.) '56; IntMed; Staff, Aberhart Mem. San.; Retired.

BROWN, Henry I.; Box 760, Langley, B.C.; Tor'46; DiagRad.

BROWN, Henry M. O.; 9933 Elbow Dr., Calgary, Alta.; 19 Sydney Dr. (res); Dublin (Ire.) '53; MB., B.Ch., BAO; MCGP; Active Staff, Calgary Gen. Hosp., Holy Cross & Alberta Children's Hosp's.; Tel. 252-1168.

BROWN, Hugh A.; McG '59; Anaes; Staff, St. Mary's Hosp., Montreal 26, P.Q.

BROWN, Hugh J.; 2946 Parkdale Ave., Pinewood Acres, Halifax, N. S., (res); Dal '58; Dir. Halifax Children's Hosp.; Tel. 422-8441.

BROWN, Hugh M.; Dir., Stony Plain-Lac Ste. Anne Health Unit, Box 210, Stony Plain, Alta.; Durham (Eng.) '28; DPH; Tel. 777-2206.

BROWN, Ian S.; Cancer Clinic, 11250-84th Ave., Edmonton, Alta.; Durham (Eng.)'50; FRCS(E), FFR; DMRT; Tel. 433-5807.

BROWN, Ian D.; 550 Ingersoll Ave., Woodstock, Ont.; 131 Light St. (res); Glasgow (Scot.) '49; Tel. 539-3031.

BROWN, I. Patricia; 550 Ingersoll Ave., Woodstock, Ont.; Glasgow (Scot.) '46; Tel. 539-3031.

BROWN, James H.; Edinburgh (Scot.)'49; MRCP(Ed.); DPM(Lond.); Psy; Staff, Dept. of Psy. Med. Coll., Winnipeg 3, Man.

BROWN, James J.; 69 Kirkland St., Guelph, Ont.; 128 London Rd. (res); Wes '50; F.A.A.P.; Paed; Chief of Paed., St. Joseph's & Guelph Gen. **Hosp's.; Tel. TA 2-7581.**

BROWN, James R.; 53 King St., Dartmouth, N.S.; 32 Queen St. (res); Dal '50.

BROWN, James S.; Brown Clinic Bldg., 700-8th St. S.W., Calgary, Alta.; Man '49; B.Sc.; DO; DLO; FACS; FRCS (Eng.); Otol; Cons. (Otol.), Calgary Gen., Calgary Children's & Holy Cross Hosp's.; Chief of Otol., Alberta Children's Hosp.; Tel. AM 3-1340.

BROWN, J. Donovan; Avon Med. Clinic, 2715 Avonhurst Dr., Regina, Sask.; Belfast (N. Ire.) '56.

BROWN, J. Ernest; 214 Jarvis St., P.O. Box 98, Fort Erie, Ont.; Qns'43; Active Staff & Chief Anaes., Douglas Mem. Hosp.; Tel. 871-2991.

BROWN, John D.; Ste. 4, 888 Grosvenor Ave., Winnipeg 9, Man.; Man'64.

BROWN, John F.; 7B Church Rd., Grand Falls, Nfld. (res); Dal '24; Staff, Lady Northcliffe Hosp., Grand Falls.

BROWN, John M.; Edson Health Unit, Edson, Alta.; Glasgow (Scot.) '37; CPH; DPH; Staff, Hinton Municipal Hosp., St. John's Hosp., Edson, & Municipal Hosp., Drayton Valley; Tel. 723-4128.

BROWN, John R.; 150 College St., Toronto 5, Ont.; London (Eng.)'52; Ph.D. (Lond.); Prof. & Head., Dept. of Physiol. Hygiene, School of Hygiene, U. of Toronto; Hon. Phys., Soc. for Crippel Civilians; Tel. 928-2746.

BROWN, Joseph A.; Med. Arts Clinic, Regina, Sask.; 3270 Albert St. (res); Tor '27; ObstGyn; Chief, Dept. of ObstGyn., Regina Gen. Hosp.; Chm., Med. Arts Clinic; Tel. LA 2-1651.

BROWN, Josephine M.; Athabaska, Alta.; Alb '46.

BROWN, Kenneth A.; 1121 O'Connor Dr., Toronto 16, Ont.; 86 Elvaston Dr. (res); Tor '45; GenSurg, Tel. PL 5-1031.

BROWN, Kenneth B.; Ste. 206, Med-Dental Centre, 1221 Algonquin Ave., North Bay, Ont.; 797 McIntyre St. W. (res); McG'51; GenSurg; Chm. Dept. of Surg., St. Joseph's Hosp.; Att'd Staff (Surg.), Civic Hosp.; Tel. GR 2-5510.

BROWN, Kenneth R.; 2878 Ness Ave., Winnipeg 12, Man.; Wes'62; Staff, Winnipeg Gen. Hosp., Winnipeg 3, Man.

BROWN, Kenneth W. G.; 922 Med. Arts Bldg., 170 St. George St., Toronto 5, Ont.; 39 Douglas Dr. (res); Tor '46; B.Sc. (Med.), F.A.C.P.; FACC; F.R.C.P.(C), IntMed; Cons. (Med.), Sunnybrook Hosp.; Ass't. Phys., Toronto Gen. Hosp.; Rykert Research Cardiol; Assoc. Staff (Med.), U. of Toronto; Tel. WA 3-3397.

BROWN, Laurie M.; 1746 Jane St., Weston, Ont.; Dal'52; Anaes.

BROWN, Laurence W.; 633 Fraser Ave., Ottawa 3, Ont. (res); McG '25; AACP; IntMed; Deputy Chief Med. Adviser, Cnd. Pension Comm.; Tel. CE 2-8211.

BROWN, Lee M.; 307 Bruce Ave., Windsor, Ont.; 1156 Ouellette Ave. (res); Qns '56; M.C.G.P.

BROWN, Leigh B.; 320 Med. Arts Bldg., 11010 Jasper Ave., Edmonton, Alta.; Alb'44; FRCS(C), ObstGyn; Att'd. Staff, University Hosp.; Instr., Dept. of ObstGyn., U. of Alberta; Tel. 424-1284.

BROWN, Lieselotte (See HOLLAND, Lieselotte.).

BROWN, Lyla I.; 904 Med. Arts Bldg., 1538 Sherbrooke W., Montreal 25, P.Q.; McG '30; AMCGP; Staff (Med.), Reddy Mem. Hosp.; Tel. WE 2-6822.

BROWN, Michael; Ste. 402, Med. Arts Bldg., Metcalfe St., Ottawa 4, Ont.; Qns '59; IntMed; Staff, Ottawa Civic Hosp.; Tel. 729-2511.

BROWN, Milton H., OBE; 42 McRae Dr., Toronto 17, Ont.; Tor '24; DPH; DAB (PrevMed.); FCCP; Bact; PH; Staff, Chest Clinic, Toronto Western Hosp.; Ass't. Dir., Connaught Labs.; Assoc. Dir. School of Hygiene; Prof. (PrevMed.), U. of Toronto; Tel. 928-2743.

BROWN, Norman; 2035 Crescent St., Montreal, P.Q.

BROWN, Norman M.; 1414 Drummond St., Montreal, P.Q.; 32 Franklin Ave., Town of Mt. Royal (res); McG'40; D & TRrad; Rad., Catherine Booth Mothers' Hosp.; Cons. Rad., Shriners Hosp. for Crippled Children; Staff, Lakeshore Gen. Hosp., Pointe Claire; Tel. VI 4-2672.

BROWN, Patrick B.; 13665-96th Ave., North Surrey, B.C.; Cambridge (Eng.) '50; Tel. 581-4611.

BROWN, P. Beckett; 62 Richmond St. W., Toronto 1, Ont.; 7 Thornwood Rd., Tor. 5 (res); Tor '16; Indus. Ins. Exam.; Tel. EM 4-4886.

BROWN, P. Staples; 940 Sifton Blvd., Calgary, Alta.; McG '24; Anaes.

BROWN, R., S/L; Aberdeen (Scot.)'51; D. Psy; Psy; Dep. Hd., Dept. of Psy., Nat. Defence Med. Centre, Smyth Rd., Ottawa 8, Ont.

BROWN, Rennie; Durham (Eng.)'53; D.Obst RCOG; Staff, James Paton Hosp., Gander, Nfld.; Tel. 256-8221.

BROWN, Robert; Aberdeen (Scot.) '51; Psy; Dept. of Psy., National Defence Med. Centre, Ottawa 8, Ont.

BROWN, Robert D.; 2109 Woodcrest Rd., Ottawa, Ont. (res); Tor '39; D.P.H., D.I.H.; Ass't. Surg. Gen., Prev. & Ind. Med., C.F.M.S.

BROWN, Robert F.; Main St. N. Coldwater, Ont.; **Tor '52; Phm.B.; Dist. Coroner.**

BROWN, Robert J.; Terminal Bldg., Moncton, N.B.; 162 Portledge Ave. (res); Alb '31; DAB-PM; FACPM (Occ.Med.); PH; Reg. M.O., Atlantic Reg., CNR & Air Canada; Tel. 382-0551, Loc. 286.

BROWN, Robert L.; 5691 Duffus St., Halifax, N.S.; Dal '63; AMCGP; Tel. 454-3728.

BROWN, Ronald E.; 1705-3rd Ave., Prince George, B.C.; McG '27; AICS; Staff, Prince George Reg. Hosp.; Tel. 4-4133.

BROWN, Ross E.; Man '61; Res., Winnipeg Gen. Hosp., Winnipeg, Man.

BROWN, Roy P.; 501 Sargent Ave., Winnipeg, Man.; 241 Brock (res); Man '39; M.C.G.P.

BROWN (Airlie-Brown), Thomas; 411 Portland Ave., Montreal 16, P.Q.; Edinburgh (Scot.) '49; F.R.C.P.(C), IntMed; Clin. Ass't., Mtl. Gen. Hosp.; Med. Dem., McGill U.; Dir. Clin. Research Merck, Sharp & Dohme Canada; Abroad.

BROWN, Thomas C.; 500 Sherbourne St., Toronto 5, Ont.; Tor '43; FACP; Path; Chief Pathol., Princess Margaret Hosp.; Dir., Clin. Path., Wellesley Hosp.; Assoc. Prof., Dept. of Path., U. of Toronto; Tel. WA 4-0671.

BROWN, Thomas C.; Wes'60; Res., Toronto Gen. Hosp., Toronto 2, Ont.

BROWN, Thomas E.; Campbell Clinic, 329—7th St. S., Lethbridge, Alta.; 604—15th St. S. (res); Qns '26; Chief, Obst. Gyn., St. Michael's Hosp.; Staff, Galt Hosp.; Tel. FA 7-5737.

BROWN, Thomas L.; 6070 Yonge St., Wilowdale, Ont., 5 Dallas Rd. (res); Coll. of Medical Evangelists, California (U.S.A.)'53; MCGP; Tel. BA 1-3431.

BROWN, Thomas M. D.; 180 Metcalfe St., Ste. 402, Ottawa, Ont.; Qns'59; FRCP(C), IntMed.

BROWN, Walter A.; 114 Renfrew Ave. E., Renfrew, Ont.; McG '14; Tel. 432-2424.

BROWN, W. Gordon; 162 Rosedale Hgts. Dr., Toronto, Ont. (res); Tor '28; DPH; PH; Depty. Minister of Health, Ont.; Spec. Lect. (PH), U. of Toronto; Tel EM 3-1211.

BROWN, Wilber F.; 2056 Veterans Affairs Bldg., Ottawa, Ont.; 68 Renfrew Ave. (res); Tor '31; M.R.C.P. (Edin.), F.R.C.P. (Edin.); IntMed; Chief Med. Adv., Cdn. Pension Comm.; Tel. CE 2-8211.

BROWN, Willa M.; Qns'65; Res., Toronto Gen. Hosp., Toronto, Ont.

BROWN, William A.; 311 Toronto Western Med. Bldg., 25 Leonard Ave., Toronto 2B, Ont.; 41 Whitney Ave., Tor. 5 (res); Tor '43; F.A.C.S., F.R.C.S.(C), GenSurg; PlasSurg; Att'd. Surg. **Staff, Toronto Western Hosp.; Ass't. Prof. Surg.,** U. of Toronto; Tel. EM 6-2109.

BROWN, William G.; 306 Med. & Dental Bldg., Regina, Sask.; Qns '58; FRCP(C); DiagRad; Staff, Regina Grey Nun's Hosp.; Tel. 523-7653.

BROWN, William T.; 750 W. Broadway, Vancouver, B.C.; 3863 W. 11th Ave., Vancouver, B.C. (res); UBC '58; B.Sc., Ph.D., Psy; Cons., Riverview Hosp., Essondale; Instr. Dept. of Psy., UBC; Tel. LA 1-1911.

BROWNE, Alfred F.; 618 Church St., Toronto 5, Ont.; Tor '51; Tel. WA 3-3507.

BROWNE, Carman C.; Caledonia Medical Bldg., 340 Campbell St., Nanaimo, B.C.; 297 Machleary Rd. (res); Dal '29.

BROWNE, John S. L.; Dept. of Investigative Med., McGill U., Montreal, P.Q.; McG '29; LL.D. (Qns), PH.D. (McG); F.A.C.P., F.R.S.C., F.R.C.P.(C), IntMed; Tel. VI 4-6311.

BROWNE, John K.; Dublin (Ire.)'57; FRCS(C), OrthSurg; Staff, Shaughnessy Hosp., Vancouver 9, B.C.

BROWNE, N. L. Mason; 3195 Granville St., **Vancouver 9, B.C.; 2640 Rosebery Ave., West Van. (res); Edinburgh (Scot.) '51; Psy; Tel.** RE 3-5515.

BROWNE, Robert C.; 114 Med. Arts Bldg., 100 May St. S., Fort William, Ont.; 1747 Isabella **(res); Man '30; Paed; Tel. MA 2-6459.**

BROWNE, Ronald A.; Camelot Towers, Apt. 402, 1001 Main St. W., Hamilton, Ont.; Aberdeen (Scot.) '53; M.B., Ch.B., Anaes; Staff, Hamilton Civic Hosp., Hamilton, Ont.; Tel. 527-0271.

BROWNELL, A. Keith; Irving Clinic, 74 W. Seymour St., Kamloops, B.C.; Qns '64.

BROWNELL, Edward G.; Winnipeg Clinic, St. Mary's & Vaughan, Winnipeg, Man.; 291 Kingsway Ave., (res); Man '46; FACP; FRCP(C); MRCP (Lond.); AACP; IntMed; Ass't. Phys, Wpg. Gen. Hosp.; Cons. (Cardiol.), Children's Hosp.; Staff, O. P. D. (Cardiol.), Wpg. Gen. Hosp.; Assoc. Prof. (Med.), U. of Man.; Tel. 942-0551.

BROWNLEE, John G.; 308 St. Clair Ave. W., Toronto 10, Ont.; Qns '31; Assoc. Staff, Toronto Western Hosp.; Tel. WA 1-2525.

BROWNLEE, Robert W.; McG '59; Staff, Riverview Hosp., Windsor, Ont.

BROWNLEE, Richard T.; Alb'63; Jr. Int., University Hosp., Edmonton, Alta.; Abroad.

BROWNLEE, Thomas I.; P.O. Box 65, Russell, Man.; Man'21; Tel. 22.

BROWNRIDGE, Thos. R.; 2905 McCallum Ave., Regina, Sask.; Man '16.

BROWNRIGG, Garrett M., C.B.E.; 47 Queen's Rd., St. John's, Nfld.; McG '32; F.A.C.S., GenSurg; Chief, Surg. Serv. 3, St. John's Gen. Hosp.; Chief of Serv. (Surg.), D.V.A., Nfld.; Chief, ThorSurg Unit, T.B. San.; Chief of Staff, St. Clare's Mercy Hosp.; Cons. Surg., Grace & Janeway Children's Hosp's.; Tel. 726-5083.

BROWNRIGG, Leslie W.; 24 Marks St., St. Stephen, N.B.; McG '32; GenSurg; Tel. 466-3749.

BROWNSTEIN, Seymour; McG'65; Res., Jewish Gen. Hosp., Montreal 26, P.Q.

BRUBACHER, Lloyd E.; 216 Wharncliffe Rd., London, Ont.; Wes'65.

BRUCE, Andrew W.; Etherington Hall, Stuart St., Kingston, Ont.; Aberdeen (Scot.)'47; FRCS (Edin.); FRCS (Eng.); FRCS(C), Urol; Chief of Urol., Kingston Gen. Hosp.; Assoc. Prof. & Hd., Dept. of Urol.; Queen's U.; Tel. 546-3361.

BRUCE, Ian F.; 253 Main St., Yarmouth, N.S.; Edinburgh (Scot.) '47; Staff, E.E.N.T., Yarmouth Reg. Hosp.; Tel. 742-3577.

BRUCE, John D.; Mitton-Essex Med. Bldg., 168 Essex St., Sarnia, Ont.; 552 Cathcart Blvd. (res); Man '41; MCGP; Chief Dept. of G. P., St. Joseph's Hosp.; Active Staff, Sarnia Gen. Hosp.; Tel. DI 4-7131.

BRUCE-LOCKHART, Patrick; 289 Cedar St., Sudbury, Ont.; Edinburgh (Scot.) '41; MRCOG; FRCOG; ObstGyn; Chief Obst., Sudbury Mem. Hosp.; Deputy Chief Gyn., Sudbury Gen. & Mem. Hosp's.; Tel. OS 4-3131.

BRUCE, Malcolm M.; 8 Arlington Pl., Truro, N.S. 90 Smith Ave. (res); Dal '59; MCGP; Tel. 893-7460.

BRUCE-ROBERTSON, Alan; 47 Harper Ave., Toronto 7, Ont.; Tor '50; Research Fell., Ontario Cancer Inst., Princess Margaret Hosp.; Fell Med., U. of Toronto; Tel. 924-0671, Loc. 316.

BRUCE, Stuart B.; 289 Dufferin Ave., London, Ont.; Qns '56; Ophth.; Tel. 434-0581.

BRUCE, Thomas A.; Dal '56; Res., University Hosp., Edmonton, Alta.

BRUCE, W. Robert; 294 Belsize Dr., Toronto 7, Ont. (res); Chicago (U.S.A.) '58; Ph.D.; Med. Research, Dept. of Med. Biophysics, Ontario Cancer Inst., Princess Margaret Hosp.; Ass't. Prof. Med. Biophys., U. of Toronto; Tel. 924-0671; WA 3-6611.

BRUCHOVSKY, Nicholas S.; 28 Lynd Ave., Toronto 3, Ont.; Tor'61.

BRUCKSCHWAIGER, Irene (Wehner); 1661 Trafalgar St., London, Ont. (res); Rostock (Germ.) '40; Retired.

BRUCKSCHWAIGER, Otto; 1661 Trafalgar St., London, Ont. (res); Vienna (Aust.) '40; F.A.C.S., F.I.C.S., F.R.C.S.(C), GenSurg; Urol; Court. Staff, Victoria & St. Joseph's Hosp's.; Tel. 451-4810.

BRUDER, Alfred; 350 King St. W., Kitchener, Ont.; Wes'58.

BRUECKNER, Joseph B.; Prov. Laboratories Castle St., Saint John, N.B.; Budapest (Hun.) '36; Tel. 692-2644.

BRUEHLER, Gustav; 321 E. Columbia St., New Westminster, B.C.; UBC'59; MCGP; Vist. Staff, Royal Columbia & St. Mary's Hosp's.; Tel. 524-3621.

BRUMMITT, John R.; 209 Westbrook Bldg., U. of British Columbia, Vancouver 8, B.C.; UBC '57; Paed; Ass't. Prof. (Paed.), U. of British Columbia; Dir. Child Health Programme, U.B.C.; Tel. 228-3149.

BRUMMITT, Redvers B.; Medical Assoc. Clin., 405 Hendryx St., Nelson, B.C.; 820 Davies St. (res); Tor '25; M.C.G.P.; Staff, Kootenay Lake Gen. Hosp.; Tel. 352-6611.

BRUMMITT, William M.; 44 Denver Cres., Willowdale, Ont.; Tor '52; FRCP(C); Anaes; Staff, Hosp. for Sick Children, Toronto; Clin. Teach. (Anaes.), U. of Toronto; Tel. EM 6-7242.

BRUMWELL, Charles A.; 4326 W. 10th Ave., Vancouver 8, B.C.; 5888 Wiltshire St., Van. 13 (res); UBC '58; MCGP; Phys., U. of British Columbia Health Serv.; Att'd GP Staff, Vancouver Gen. Hosp.; Tel. CA 4-1355.

BRUNEAU, Emile F.; 165 King East, Sherbrooke, P.Q.; 636 Ontario (res); Mon '39; GenSurg (P.Q.); Pres., Med. Bureau, Hotel Dieu Hosp., Sec., Sherbrooke Surg. Soc.; Tel. LO 2-2755.

BRUNEAU, I. Edgar; 3544 Park Ave., Montreal, P.Q.; McG '13; Retired.

BRUNEAU, Jacques; Ste. 307, 3875, St-Urbain, Montreal 18, P.Q.; Mon '38; GenSurg; ThorSurg (P.Q.); Surg., Hop. Hotel-Dieu; Prof. & Derm., Dept. of Surg., U. of Montreal.

BRUNEAU, Joseph; 121 des Glaieuls St., Chicoutimi Nord, P.Q. (res); Mon '47; Path.(P.Q.); Path., Hotel Dieu St. Vallier; Tel. 549-1452.

BRUNEAU, Luc; Mon '58; GenSurg (P.Q.); Staff, Hop. Hotel Dieu, Montreal 18, P.Q.; Tel. RI 4-0161.

BRUNEAU, Rene F.; 9 Rue Dufferin, Granby, P. Q.; Lav '33; D. P. H. (Tor.).

BRUNELLE, Jacques; 7522 Champagneur Ave., Montreal 15, P.Q.; Mon'65.

BRUNELLE, Jean P.; 5555 Ave. des Cedres, Montreal 36, P.Q. (res); Mon '49; Anaes; Staff, Anaes., Hop. Notre Dame; Tel. LA 5-6363.

BRUNELLE, Paul, D.F.C.; 1260, boul. St. Joseph est, Montreal, P.Q.; Mon '51; DAB Ophth; FAAOO; Otol (P.Q.); Ass't. (Otol.), Hop. Notre-Dame; Ass't. Prof. (Med.), U. of Montreal; Tel. LA 6-6608.

BRUNELLE, Simon; 129 rue Principale, Granby, P.Q.; 130 Rue Sherbrooke (res); Mon '43; M.C.G.P.; Staff (Med.) Hop. St. Joseph; Tel. FR 2-5491.

BRUNER, George W.; 36 Main St. E., Kingsville, Ont.; Thorncrest St. (res); Wes '53.

BRUNET, Andre; Mon'62; Res., Hop. Maisonneuve, Montreal 36, P.Q.

BRUNET, Armand J.; Dept. of Veterans Affairs (DVA), Ottawa 4, Ont.; Mon '36; F.A.H.A., Dir. Hospital Accommodation, Medical Research & Educ. & Prosthetic Services; Tel. 992-3801.

BRUNET, Claude; 1500-18eme rue, Quebec 4, P.Q.; Lav '54; F.R.C.S.(C), GenSurg; Staff, Hop.-de-l'Enfant-Jesus; Lect., Laval U.; Tel. LA 5-8116.

BRUNET, Ernest, Sr.; 546 St. Patrick St., Ottawa, Ont.; Qns '09; Assoc. Staff, Ottawa Gen. Hosp.; Tel. CE 6-6592.

BRUNET, Gilles; 48 Ste-Trinite, Contrecoeur, P.Q.; 55 Ste-Trinite (res); Mon '54; Tel. 786-2121.

BRUNET, Jacques; 1000 Chemin Ste-Foy, Quebec 10, P. Q.; Lav '52; FRCP(C); IntMed; Staff, Hop. Ste Sacrement, Laval U.; Tel. 683-4481.

BRUNET, J. A. David; 310-6th Ave., Grand'Mere, P.Q.; McG'52; MCGP; Admin. Grand'Mere Gen. Hosp.; Dir. Med. Serv., Consolidated Paper Corp. Ltd.; Med. Exam., Dept. of Transport Air Services; Tel. 538-9533.

BRUNET, Jean C.; 490 Venise, Ville Brossard, C.J.C., P.Q.; OrthSurg (P.Q.); Staff, Hop. Ste-Justine; Tel. RE 1-4931.

BRUNET, Jean L.; 405 Ave. Woodlea, Mont Royal, Montreal 16, P.Q. (res); Mon '44; Anaes; Staff, Hop. Hotel Dieu; Tel. VI 4-0161.

BRUNET, J. Ernest D.; 223 Echo Dr., Ottawa, Ont.; Revelstoke Dr. (res); Mon '41; Staff, Ottawa Gen. Hosp., Tel. CE 5-8342.

BRUNET, Joseph; 299 St. Jean, Quebec, P.Q.; Lav '43; GenSurg (P.Q.); Te.525-5507.

BRUNET, J. Maurice; 100 Erables, Laval sur-le-Lac, Co. Laval, P.Q. (res); Lav '32; Ass't. Med. Supt., Queen Mary Vet's. Hosp.; Tel. RE 8-9481.

BRUNET, J. P. Ernest; 5180 Cote St. Antoine, Montreal, P.Q. (res); Mon '17; Psy; Psy., St. Jean de Dieu Hosp. & Inst. Albert Prevost; Tel. CL 4-5361.

BRUNET, Michel R. P.; Mon'59; Ophth; Staff, Hop. Maisonneuve, Montreal, P.Q.

BRUNET, Suzanne; Centre Medicale St-Laurent, 960 boul. Ste. Croix, Ville St. Laurent, Montreal 9, P.Q.; Mon'60; Paed.

BRUNET, Treffle; 27 Laniel, Ste. Genevieve, d'Pierre Fonds, P.Q.; Mon '58.

BRUNET, Willie, Jr.; 1098 Ave de la Tour, Quebec 4, P. Q.; Lav '51; Tel. 529-7540.

BRUNET, Willie E.; 600 Ave. Laurier, Quebec 4, P.Q.; Lav '26; Tel. 523-2743.

BRUNETTE, Jean Real; 30 boul. St. Joseph est, Montreal 14, P.Q.; Mon'57; **FRCS(C),** Ophth; **Ass't. Serv. (Ophth) Hop. Maisonneuve;** I/C Basic Science Courses (Ophth) affil., U. of Montreal; Tel. RE 1-9458.

BRUNETTE (Gagnand), Michele; Mon '57; P.G., University of Montreal, P. Q.

BRUNNELLE, G.; 2464 rue St. Marc, Shawinigan Falls, P.Q.; Mon '35.

BRUNSDON, David F.V.; 118 Springhill Dr., Lorne Park, Port Credit, Ont.; Guy's Hosp. (London, Eng.) '46; M.B., B.S., MC (Path); Path; Dir. of Labs., South Peel Hosp., Cooksville; Tel. 279-7330.

BRUNTON, Elizabeth; Apt. 202, 1020 Park Blvd., Victoria, B.C. (res); Alb '26; Retired.

BRUNTON, J. E.; 68 Symons St., Toronto 14, **Ont.; Tor '52; MCGP; Tel. CL 1-6901.**

BRUNTON, James F.; Apt. 202, 1020 Park Blvd., Victoria, B.C. (res); Alb '28; F.A.C.S., Urol; Retired.

BRUNTON, Lauder; 4500 Sherbrooke St. W., Montreal, P.Q.; 3182 The Boulevard, Westmount (res); McG '42; Haem (P.Q.); FACP; IntMed; Assoc. Phys., Royal Victoria Hosp.; Cons. (Haem.), Queen Mary Vet's. Hosp.; Ass't. Prof. (Med.), McGill U.; Tel. WE 7-8893.

BRUNTON, Lawrence J.; Sydney (Australia) '45; Phys Med. & Rehab; Staff, G. F. Strong Rehab. Centre, 900 W. 28th Ave., Vancouver 9, B.C.; Tel. RE 1-3111.

BRUSER, David M., MBE; 280 Osborne St. N., Winnipeg 1, Man.; 300 Montrose St., Wpg. 9 (res); Man '36; FRCS(C), GenSurg; OrthSurg; Chief, OrthSurg., Deer Lodge DVA Hosp.; Ass't. Orthopaed., Wpg. Gen.; Cons. OrthSurg., Wpg. Mun. Hosp's.; Ass't. Prof. Surg., (Orthopaed.), U. of Manitoba; Tel. SP 4-2411.

BRUSER, Harry H.; Rapid City, Man.; Man'17.

BRUSER, Michael; Mall Med. Bldg., 280 Memorial Blvd., Winnipeg 1, Man.; Alb '39; ObstGyn; Active Staff, Misericordia Gen. Hosp.; Cons. Staff, Women's Pavilion, St. Boniface & Grace Hosp's.; Tel. SP 4-2411.

BRUVELS, Nikolajs R.; P.O. Box 238, O'Leary, P.E.I. (res); Latvia '39; Gen. Surg. (Latvia); Surg.; Community Hosp., O'Leary & Western Hosp., Alberton.

BRUYERE, Jean C., Sg/Lt.; Ott'61; Cdn. Forces Base, Uplands, Ottawa, Ont.

BRUYERE, Rodrigue; 3875 St-Urbain, Ste. 203, Montreal 18, P.Q.; Lav '46; FACOG; FRCS(C), ObstGyn; Staff (ObstGyn.), Hotel-Dieu Hosp.; Staff (ObstGyn.), St. Mary's Hosp.; Ass't. Prof., U. of Montreal; Tel. 845-7545.

BRYAN, Clayton G.; 540 Mt. Pleasant Rd., Toronto, Ont.; Tor '22; D.A.(Eng.); Anaes, Tel. HU 9-5996.

BRYAN, Lawrence E.; 100 Church Ave., Chilliwack, B.C.; 46293 Brooks Ave. (res); Alb '61; MCGP; Tel. SY 3-7271.

BRYANS, Alexander M.; Dept. of Paed., Queen's U.; Kingston, Ont.; Tor'44; FRCP(C); FAAP; Paed.; Chief of Paed., Kingston Gen. Hosp.; Prof. **& Hd. Dept. of Paed., Queen's U.; Tel. 546-2566.**

BRYANS, Frederick E.; Willow Pavilion, Vancouver Gen. Hosp., Vancouver, B.C.; 2098 W. **46th Ave. (res);** Tor '46; F.R.C.S.(C), ObstGyn; **Prof. & Head (ObstGyn), U. of British Columbia; Tel. TR 6-3211.**

BRYANT, Arthur J. S.; 3014 Witmore Ave., Regina, Sask. (res); Tor '40; TherRad, IntMed; Dir., Allan Blair Memorial Clinic, Sask. Cancer Comm., Grey Nuns' Hosp., Regina; Tel. 527-9651, Loc. 207.

BRYANT, E. Cullen; 825 Coxwell Ave., Toronto 6, Ont.; 10 Taylor Dr. (res); Tor '29; L.M. (Dublin), F.R.C.S.(C), M.R.C.O.G.(Lond.); ObstGyn; Chief-of-Staff, Obst. Gyn., Toronto East Gen. Hosp. Tel. HO. 5-2910.

BRYANT, H. Russell; Sussex, N.B.; Dal '39; M.C.G.P.; Staff, Kings County Memorial Hosp.

BRYANT, John A.; 22 Laurier, Magog, P.Q.; Cedar House, R.R. No. 3 (res); McG '51; Staff, Hop. La Providence; Tel. VI 3-3543.

BRYANT, Margaret E. E.; R.R. No. 2, Fulford Harbour, B.C. (res); London (Eng.) '15; D.T.M. & H. (Cantab); Retired.

BRYANT, Marie; 21 Ottawa St. S., Kitchener, Ont.; Tor '50; Paed; Tel. 744-9113.

BRYANT, Murray E.; 955 Woodbine Ave., Toronto 13, Ont.; 20 Barbara Cres., Toronto 6 (res); Wes '49; F.R.C.S.(C), ObstGyn; Staff (ObstGyn), Toronto East Gen. Hosp. Tel. HO 5-2910.

BRYANT, William E.; Medical Centre, Kirkland Lake, Ont.; 88-1st St. (res); Wes '35; M.C.G.P.; Active Staff, Kirkland Dist. Hosp.; Memb. Sect. of G.P., Ontario Med. Assoc.; Tel. 567-5709.

BRYANT, William H.; 751 King St. W., Kitchener, Ont.; Wes'64; Active Staff, Kitchener-Waterloo & St. Mary's Hosp's.; Tel. 576-4910.

BRYCE, Douglas P.; 320 Med. Arts Bldg., 170 St. George St., Toronto 5, Ont.; 19 Plymbridge Cres. (res); Tor '42; F.A.C.S., A.B.Ot., F.R.C.S.(C), Otol; Staff, Otol., Toronto Gen. & Sunnybrook Hosp's.; Assoc. Staff (Otol.), U. of Toronto; Tel. WA 2-7676.

BRYCE, James C.; London (Eng.)'40; MRCS (Eng.); LRCP (Lond.); DRCOG; Psy; Staff, Dept. of Psy., Union Hosp., Moose Jaw, Sask.

BRYDON, Alan W.; UBC. '61; Res., Shaughnessy Hosp. Vancouver, B.C.

BRYK, Wladimir S.; 11029-127th St., Edmonton, Alta.; Vienna (Austria) '49; Tel. 454-8808.

BRYNGELSON, Earl S.; Lake of the Woods Clinic, 112 Matheson St. S., Kenora, Ont.; 834-4th Ave. S. (res); Man '51; M.C.G.P.; Tel. HO 8-6423.

BRYSON, Bruce F.; 104 Rickman Pl., New Westminster, **B.C. (res); McG '37; APA (Cert. Mental** Hosp. Admin); Med. Supt. Riverview Hosp., Essondale, B.C.; Tel. LA 1-1911.

BRYSON, William; Grantham Shopping Plaza, Scott St., St. Catharines, Ont.; St. Andrews (Scot.) '45; **M.B., Ch.B.,** Tel. 684-8061.

BRYTOW, Praxeda; Apt. 1, 4921 Sherbrooke St. W., Montreal 6, P.Q.; Wilno (Poland) '34; Tel. 482-6325.

BRZEZINA, Jeanie (Shkimba); 500 Parliament St., Toronto 5, Ont.; 51 Alexander St., Apt. 108 (res); Tor '62; Staff, Raxlen Clinic; Tel. WA 5-4381.

BUCHAN, Douglas J.; 15 Moxon Cres., Saskatoon, Sask. (res); Man '46; FACP, FRCP(C), IntMed; Staff, University Hosp.; Assoc. Prof. (Med.), U. of Saskatchewan; Tel. 242-7641.

BUCHAN, James K.; 40 Cambridge St. N., Lindsay, Ont.; Tor'62.

BUCHANAN, Bruce H.; Tor '51; Res., Hosp. for Sick Children, Toronto 2, Ont.

BUCHANAN, Charles A.; 223 Highland Rd., London, Ont.; Wes '34; Ophth.; Tel. 432-1767.

BUCHANAN, David M.; 8225-105th St., Edmonton, Alta.; Alb'57; MRCOG; FACOG; DABOG; FRCS(C), ObstGyn; Clin. Instr., U. of Alberta; Tel. GA 4-2121.

BUCHANAN, Donald I.; Blood Transfusion Serv., 9941-106 St., Edmonton, Alta.; 9134-117th (res); Glasgow U. (Scot.) '40; M.D., (Glas.), DPH (Glas.); Med. Dir., Blood Trans. Serv., University Hosp.; Lect. (Path), U. of Alberta; Tel. GA 4-5134.

BUCHANAN, Douglas R.; 21 Academy Medical Bldg., 1812-4th W., Calgary, Alta.; 4507 Coronation Dr. (res); Alb'42; ObstGyn.; Dir. Dept. of ObstGyn., Calgary Gen. Hosp.; Tel. 266-4555.

BUCHANAN, Ian; The Shopping Centre, 26 Meadow Lark Pk., Edmonton, Alta.; 11304-109A Avenue, (res), Edinburgh (Scotland) '32; Dist. Coroner; Tel. 489-2374.

BUCHANAN, Isabel J.; 17 Stanley Grove Apts., 2170 Portage Ave., Winnipeg 12, Man. (res); Edin. (Scot) '52; Retired.

BUCHOK, Roman W.; 561 Machray Ave., Winnipeg 4, Man.; Madrid (Spain) '50; Ph.D.; MCGP; Active Staff, Misericordia Hosp.; Court. Staff, Children's & Winnipeg Gen. Hosp's.; Tel. 586-8076.

BUCK, Carol W. (Whitlaw); 181 Elmwood Ave., London, Ont. (res); Wes '47; Ph.D., D.P.H.; Prof. Prev. Med., U. of Western Ontario; Tel. 679-3858.

BUCK, Clarence A.; 100 Roehampton, Toronto 12, Ont.; Qns '31; Psy; Dir., Ontario Mental Hosp's.; Tel. 485-6284.

BUCK, H. William; 614 Fairmont Med. Bldg., 750 W. Broadway, Vancouver 9, B.C.; 1220 Dogwood Cres., N. Van (res); Alb '55; FRCP(C), Derm; Att'd. Staff, Van. Gen. Hosp.; Cons. (Derm.), Shaughnessy Hosp.; Tel. TR 2-2814.
BUCK, J. Donald; 632 King St. E., Hamilton, Ont.; 103 Inverness (res); Wes '60; AMCGP: ; Tel. JA 8-5926.
BUCK, Robert C.; 181 Elmwood Ave., London, Ont. (res); Wes '47; M.Sc., Ph.D.; Prof. Microscopic Anatomy, U. of Western Ontario; Tel. 679-3745.
BUCKIEWICZ, Petronela L.; 922 Decarie Blvd., Ville-St.-Laurent, Montreal 9, P.Q.; 570 Cardinal (res); Edinburgh (Scot.) '48; Med. Examin. Protestant Schl. Bd., Greater Mtl.; Staff, PH, City, St-Laurent; Tel. RI 7-6627.
BUCKINGHAM, Gerard A.; 82 Elizabeth Ave., St. John's, Nfld.; Ire. '55.
BUCKLER, William St. J.; 4518 Marine Dr., W. Vancouver, B.C.; London (Eng.) '43; D. Phys. Med.; Dir. (PhysMed.), Vancouver Gen. Hosp.; Tel. TR 6-3211.
BUCKLEY, Francis J.; Leoville, Sask.; McG '23; Staff, Union Hosp.; Coroner.
BUCKLEY, George F.; 291 Colbourne St. W., Orillia, Ont. (res); Tor '52; B.Sc. (Med.); Path; Staff, Soldiers' Mem. Hosp., Orillia, South Muskoka Mem. Hosp., Bracebridge, & Huntsville Dist. Mem. Hosp.; Tel. 325-2201, Ext. 243.
BUCKNER, Robert D.; 39 Wellington St., Acton, Ont. (res); Edinburgh (Scot.) '28; LRCP; LRCS; LRPS; DPM; Coroner, Halton County; Tel. 853-1240.
BUCKRIDAN, Latif; 1684 Queen St. W., Toronto 3, Ont.; 7 Crownhill Place, Apt. B7, Etobicoke (res); Tor '62; Tel. 537-2042.
BUDA, Yvonne; 191 Westminster Ave., Toronto, Ont. (res); Vienna (Aust.) '48; Jr. Staff, Women's College (Hosp. Tel. RO 2-4498.
BUDZINSKI, M. G., Capt.; 1st Field Ambulance RCAMC, CFPO. 5050, Can. Armed Forces, Europe; Sask '63.
BUELL, Arthur L.; ..960 Brentwood, 4567 Lougheed Hwy., North Burnaby, B.C.; McG '27; Retired.
BUENTIPO, Benigno V.; Med. Group., Box 400, Rosetown, Sask.; Philippines '56; GenSurg; Active Staff, Union Hosp.; Tel. 882-2644.
BUFFAM, G. B. Bonar; 645 Fort St., Victoria, B.C.; 2855 Beach Dr. (res); McG '35; MCGP; Staff, Royal Jubilee & St. Joseph's Hosp's.; Tel. EV 3-0215.
BUFFETT, Lawrence M.; Dal'63; Res., Nova Scotia Hosp., Dartmouth, N.S.
BUGDEN, Claude; Jeffrey S., West Coast, Nfld.; Dal'65.
BUGDEN, Cyril W.; Woodlawn Medical Clinic, 110 Woodlawn Road, Dartmouth, N.S.; Dal'59; AMCGP.
BUGDEN, Raymond L.; Medical Centre, West St., Corner Brook, Nfld.; 38 Brookfield St. (res); Dal '53.
BUGEAUD, Jean P.; Bonnyville Med. Centre, Bonnyville, Alta.; Ott '53; M.H.O.; Dist. Coroner; Tel. 826-3320.
BUGG, Thomas E.; 502 Med. Dental Bldg., Rose St. & 11th Ave., Regina, Sask.; 2947 Grant Rd. (res); Sask'61; MCGP; Active Med. Staff, Regina General & Grey Nun's Hosp's.; Tel. 522-8541.
BUGG, William J.; Westminster Hosp., London, Ont. (res); Wes'38; GenSurg; Supt. and Sr. Treatment M.O., DVA Westminster Hosp.; Tel. GE 2-6711, Loc. 341.
BUGIS, Joseph; 320 Medical Arts Bldg., 11010 Jasper Ave., Edmonton, Alta.; Alb '42; FACOG; ObstGyn; Lect. (ObstGyn.), U. of Alberta; Tel. GA 4-6319.
BUHR, Alvin J.; Medical Arts Bldg., 5880 Spring Garden Rd., Halifax, N.S.; Wes '49; OrthSurg; Tel. 423-6042.
BUHR, Lois M.; Qns'65; Rotating Int., Toronto Western Hosp., Toronto, Ont.
BUICK, Robert J. W.; New Zealand '52; MCRA; DiagRad; Staff, Sunnybrook Hosp., Toronto, Ont.; Tel. 485-8651.
BUIE, William J.; 2940-17th Ave. S.W., Calgary, Alta.; 5-4020 Glenpark Cres. (res); Alb. '54; F.R.C.S.(C), GenSurg. Tel. CH 9-5566.
BUIES, Robert; 5757 ave. Decelles, Montreal 26, P. Q.; 4914 Kent, Apt.2, (res); Lav '53. D.Psy; Psy (P.Q.); Staff, Inst., Albert Prevost & Hop.-Ste.- Justine; Tel. 739-6416.
BUIRS, E. John; Box 220, Abbotsford, B.C.; Groninger (Neth.)'50.
BUISSON, Jacques; 490 - 17eme rue, Grand'Mere, P. Q.; Mon '63.
BUIST, Thomas A.; 15 Church Hill, St. John's, Nfld.; 320 Hamilton Ave. (res); Edinburgh (Scot.) '55; D.R.C.O.G.; Assoc. Staff, St. Clares Mercy & Grace Hosp's.; Tel. 80421.
BUJOLD, Gustave; Res. Hopital Hotel-Dieu, Quebec, P.Q. Lav '60.
BUJOLD, J. Edese; 276 rue Victoria, Dalhousie, N.B.; Lav '49 M.C.G.P.; Staff, Hop. St. Joseph.
BUKA, Norman; Seaforth Medical Bldg., 3550 Cote des Neiges, Montreal 25, P.Q.; McG'60; FRCS(C), ObstGyn; Staff, Montreal Gen. Hosp.
BUKSA, Eddy S.; 1669 Victoria St., Prince George, B.C. Alb '58; Tel. 564-5511.
BULAJIC, Bozo; 722 Tegler Bldg., Edmonton, Alta.; Prague (Czech.) '25.
BULFORD, Harold E.; 1403 Main St. E., Hamilton, Ont.; Pottruff Park, R.R. No. 3; Qns '33; M.C.G.P.; Staff, Hamilton Gen. Hosp.; Dist. Coroner; Tel. LI 4-1400.
BULL, Andrew L.; 194 Court St. N., Port Arthur, Ont.; 403 Ford St. N., Fort William (res); Tor'57; FRCS(C); ObstGyn; FACS; FACOG; Att'd. Staff, Port Arthur Gen. & St. Joseph's Hosp's.; Court. Staff, McKellar Hosp.; Tel. 344-7271.
BULL, Archie F.; 2130 Gary Cres., Burlington, Ont. (res); Wes '50; D.H.P.; Dir. & M.O.H., Halton County Health Unit, Milton; Tel. 878-2801.
BULL, J. Alan; 2001 Eglinton Ave. E., Scarborough, Ont.; 41 Agincourt Dr., Agincourt (res); Tor '31; DPH; Ass't., MOH., Scarborough Twp.; Tel. 757-4747.
BULL, Maurice H.; 1590 Ouellette Ave., Windsor, Ont.; Cambridge (Eng.) '61; LRCP (Lond.); MRCS (Eng.); AMCGP; Tel. CL 6-0617.
BULL, R. Charles; 1920 Weston Rd., Weston, Ont.; 22 Yorkleigh Ave. (res); Tor'58; B.Sc. (Med); FRCS(C); GenSurg; Staff, Surg., Humber Mem. Hosp.; Dem. (Anat.), U. of Toronto; Tel. 241-1254.
BULL, Robert C.; Thunder Bay Clinic, 2829 Victoria Ave., Fort William, Ont.; 1730 Isabella St. (res); Tor '22; MCGP; Active Staff (GP), McKellar Gen. Hosp.; Coroner, Dist. of Thunder Bay; Phys. & Surg., C.P.R.; Tel. 622-9637.
BULLARD, John A. A.; Assoc. Clin., 214-6th Ave. S.W., Calgary, Alta.; London (Eng.)'54; MCGP.
BULLEN, Arthur E.; 63 Paget St., New Liskeard, Ont.; McG '47; Staff, Misericordia Hosp., Haileybury.
BULLER, Frederick J.; 1149 W. 39th, Vancouver, B.C. (res); Tor '05; F.R.C.P.(C); Retired.
BULLER, William K.; 96 Erie Ave., Brantford, Ont.; 17 White Oaks Ave. (res); Wes '51; GenSurg; Att'd. Surg., Brantford Gen. & St. Joseph's Hosp's.; Tel. 756-6511.
BULMER, Fred. M. R.; 100 Eastbourne Ave., Toronto, Ont.; Hd. Dept. of Indus. Hygiene, Ontario Dept. of Health, Parliament Bldgs.; Tel. EM 3-1211.
BULMER, Harry R.; Toronto Int'l. Airport, Malton, Ont.; 51 Humber Blvd. W., Rexdale (res); Tor '21; PH; Retired.
BULLOCH, Colin; Box 30, Rainy River, Ont.; London (Eng.)'63.
BULLOCK, B. J.; Public Welfare Dept., 1631 Queen St. E., Toronto 8, Ont.; Tor'65.
BUNCIC, J. Raymond; McG'65; Res., Royal Victoria Hosp., Montreal, P.Q.
BULLOCK, Michael; Alb '60; Jr. Intn., University Hosp., Saskatoon, Sask.
BUNDOCK, Jean B.; Brooke-Claxton Bldg., Tunney's Pasture, Ottawa, Ont.; Lav'38; Princ. M.O., Special Projects, Dept. of National Health & Welfare. Tel. 992-7753.

BUNKER, Manzer L.; 305 Toronto Western Med. Bldg., 25 Leonard Ave., Toronto 2B, Ont.; 303 Lytton Blvd., Tor. 12 (res); Tor '49; F.R.C.S.(C), ObstGyn; Att'd. Staff, Toronto Western Hosp.; Cons. (Gyn) Princess Margaret Hosp.; Clin. Instr. (ObstGyn), U. of Toronto. Tel. EM 6-1045.

BUNT, Donald G.; 2009 Danforth Ave., Toronto 6, Ont.; Tor '51; MCGP; Tel. OX 8-5565.

BUNTAIN, **John H.;** 11 Webster St., Kentville, N.S.; 14 Academy St. (res); Dal '35; Staff, Blanchard Fraser Memorial Hosp.

BUNTON, Peter; 2690 Mathers, West Vancouver, B.C.; London (Eng.)'57; LRCP(Lond.); MRCS (Eng.) Psy.

BUONINSEGNI, **Franco;** Rome (Italy) '49; Staff, Aberhart Mem. San., Edmonton, Alta.; Tel. GE 9-0051.

BURAK, Michael A.; 740 Brimley Rd., Scarborough, Ont.; Tor '58. Tel. AM 1-0722.

BURCH, John E.; Winnipeg Clinic, Winnipeg, Man.; 445 Kingston Cres. (res); Man '33; Psy; **Ass't. Psy., Winnipeg Gen. Hosp.; Lect. (Psy.), U. of Manitoba; Tel. 942-0551.**

BURCH, Jean L. (Fyfe); Apt. 1204, 200 Rideau Terrace, Ottawa, Ont. (res); Birmingham (Eng.) '44; Court Staff, Grace Hosp.

BURCHAK, E. **Carl; Alb '61;** Staff, Charles Camsell Hosp., Edmonton, Alta.

BURCHILL, W. Charles; 229C Woolwich St., Guelph, Ont.; 90 Marlborough Rd. (res); Tor '46; IntMed; Active Staff, Guelph Gen. & St. Joseph's Hosp's.; Tel. TA 2-5342.

BURDEN, R. Arnold; Springhill Med. Centre, Springhill, N.S.; 21 MacFarlane St. (res); Dal **'52; M.C.G.P.; Med. Staff, All Saints Hosp.; Tel.** 597-3615.

BURDETT, Lorne H.; 267 O'Connor, Ottawa, Ont.; 150 Driveway (res); Dal '48; Ass't (Plas-**Surg.), Ottawa Civic Hosp.; Tel. CE 4-4800.**

BURDITT, Anna Mary; 5 Park Ave., East St. John, N.B.; 25 Spruce Ave. (res); Qns '61; AMCGP; Active Staff, St. John's Gen. & St. Joseph's Hosp's.; Tel. 692-6500.

BUREAU, Jules; 825 sud, rue Belvedere, Sherbrooke, P.Q.; Mon '56; GenSurg; Tel. 567-4357.

BUREAU-BLOUIN, Liliane; 730 rue Olive, Magog, Quebec, P.Q.; Lav '62.

BURFOOT, Michael F.; 40 Roxton Cres., Montreal 29, P.Q. (res); Oxford (Eng.) '58; MA; DA; Anaes; Research Ass't. (Anaes); Royal Victoria Hosp.; Dem. (Anaes.), McGill U.; Tel. VI 2-1251.

BURGE, Elizabeth; Ste. 100, 219 Kennedy St., Winnipeg 1, Man.; Bristol (Eng.) '55. Abroad.

BURGE, J. L. F.; 123 Kent St., Charlottetown, P.E.I.; 4 Queen's Ct. (res); M.C.G.P.

BURGEN, Arnold S.; 4823 Roslyn Ave., Montreal 29, P.Q. (res); London (Eng.) '45; Teach. U. Med. Clinic & Montreal Gen. Hosp.

BURGER, Edward G.; 180 Ross St., St. Thomas, Ont.; 67 Wilson (res); Dal '49; Tel. ME 1-8810.

BURGER, Jack S.; Res., Hosp. for Sick Children, Toronto, Ont.; Tor '59.

BURGESS, Beverley A. (Clark); 44 Lake Ave. N., Stoney Creek, Ont.; Tor '54; DOMS (Eng.); FAAOO; Hon. Cons., Milton Dist. Hosp.; Staff, Hamilton Gen. & Henderson Hosp's; Tel. 664-4031.

BURGESS, David W.; 97 Bridge St. E., Campbellford, Ont.; Saskatoon Ave. (res); Guy's (London, Eng.) '41; Staff, Campbellford Mem. Hosp.; Tel. 653-3430.

BURGESS, F. Joseph; Abbott Clinic, 274 Osborne N., Winnipeg 1, Man.; Man '50; IntMed; Staff, Mun. Hosp's.; Tel. SP 4-4567.

BURGESS, Geoffrey W.; McGregor Clinic, 250 Main St. E., Hamilton, Ont.; Sydney (Australia) '54; FRCS (Ed.); M.Ch. (Gold Medal, Liverpool); FRACS; FRCS(C); OrthSurg; OrthSurg., St. Joseph's Hosp.; Court. Staff, Hamilton Civic & Hamilton Health Assoc.; Tel. 527-2711.

BURGESS, George H.; 55 Humewood Dr., Toronto 10, Ont.; Man '50.

BURGESS, Glenn N.; 10516 Xavia St. N.W., Coon Rapids, Minn., U.S.A.; Wes'57; Psy; Abroad.

BURGESS, Ian R.; Man '59; Res., Children's Hosp., Winnipeg 3, Man.

BURGESS, John H.; McG'58; Cardiol,(P.Q.); FRCP(C), IntMed; Staff, Montreal Gen. Hosp., Montreal 25, P.Q.

BURGESS, Robert M.; 123 Edward W. Toronto 13, Ont.; Wes '52; Psy; Staff, Ontario **Hosp., New Toronto; Tel.** 259-8291.

BURGESS, William J.; Tor'59; Res., St. Joseph's Hosp., Toronto 3, Ont.

BURGOYNE, Bud R.; UBC '58; Intn., Shaughnessy Hosp., Vancouver 9, B.C.

BURGOYNE, Frederick H.; 308 Lamont Blvd., Winnipeg, Man.; Man '45; F.A.C.P., F.I.C.S., Path; Chief (Path.), St. Boniface Hosp.; Ass't. **Prof. (Path.), U. of Manitoba; Tel. WH 3-0311.**

BURK, Lawrence A.; 102 Hamilton Rd., Dorchester, Ont.; Wes'59; Tel. 268-7391.

BURKE, Clarence L.; 909 Royal York Rd., Toronto 18, Ont.; Tor '37; Assoc. Staff, Tor. Western Hosp.; OPD, Sunnybrook Hosp.; M.O., CPR; Med. Exam., Fed. Dept. of Transport (Civil **Aviation); Tel. BE 1-2000.**

BURKE, Desmond T.; 2286 Lakeshore, Oakville, Ont.; Qns '32; D.R.M., DiagRad; Staff, Oakville-Trafalgar Mem. Hosp.; Ass't. Prof. (Rad.) & Dir. Radiog. Course, Extens. Dept., U. of Toronto; Tel. VI 5-2571.

BURKE, Frank A.; Box 552, Charlottetown, P.E.I.; Dal'65; Staff, Charlottetown Hosp.; Court. Staff, P.E.I. Hosp.; Med. Cons., Riverside Gen. Hosp.; Tel. 894-5209.

BURKE, Gerald L.; Ste. 330, 5780 Cambie St., Vancouver 15, B.C.; Alb '35; FICS; OrthSurg; Cons., Burnaby Gen. Hosp., Children's, & Chilliwack Gen. Hosp.; Vis. Staff, Royal Columbian, Squamish Gen., St. Paul's, St. Vincent's & Vancouver Gen. Hosp's.; Tel. FA 5-5533.

BURKE, Hugh E.; Royal Edward Chest Hosp., 3650 St. Urbain St., Montreal 18, P.Q.; McG'23; MSc; PhD.; Pulm. Dis. & TB (P.Q.); IntMed (TB) (P.Q.); Cons. Advisor, Royal Edward Chest Hosp. & Laurentian Chest Hosp., Ste. Agathe des Monts; Tel. VI 9-5201.

BURKE, Jerome S.; Tor'65; Res., Toronto Gen. Hosp., Toronto 2, Ont.

BURKE, John, C.B.E.; Grand Bank, Nfld.; Dal '19; M.C.G.P.; M.H.O., Grand Bank Cottage Hosp.

BURKE, J. Peter; 235 Springfield Rd., Ottawa 2, **Ont. (res); Ott '51; Staff (Path.), St.-Louis-Marie-de-Montfort Hosp.; Ass't. Prof. (Path), Ottawa U.; Tel. CE 5-6751.**

BURKE, Margaret G. M.; 1105 Carling Ave., Ottawa, Ont.; National U. (Ireland) '45; BAO; Psy; Pt-time Staff, Royal Ottawa San.; Tel. 725-1353.

BURKE, Morris E.; 712 Watt St., Winnipeg 5, **Man.; 23 Pearce Ave., Wpg. 17 (res); Man '51; MCGP; Tel. ED 4-7514.**

BURKE, Nathy F.; 192 Camden Rd., Napanee, **Ont.; 209 East St. (res); National U. (Ire.) '52; Tel. 354-4521.**

BURKE, W. Desmond; 1019 Pinewood Ave., Oakville, Ont.; Tor '57; DiagRad; Staff, Oakville-Trafalgar Mem. Hosp.; Tel. VI 5-2571.

BURKELL, Chas. C.; Cancer Clinic, University Hosp., Saskatoon, Sask.; 109 Temperance St. (res); Tor '41; DMRT (Eng.); TherRad; Ass't. Dir., Sask. Cancer Clin.; Clin. Med. Assoc. & Assoc. Prof., TherRad, U. of Saskatchewan; Tel. 652-3850.

BURKHARDT, Lore (Maksymiuk); Box 307, Alberta Hosp., Edmonton, Alta.; Tubingen (W.-Germ.) '49.

BURKHOLDER, Joseph N.; R.R. No. 2, Markham, Ont.; Tor '53.

BURLAND, George R.; Olds, Alta.; Man '48; F.R.C.S.(C), GenSurg.

BURLEIGH, H. C.; Bath, Ont.; Qns '26.

BURLEIGH, William A.; Dal'53; Res. Ottawa Civic Hosp., Ottawa 3, Ont.

BURLEY, John S.; Bristol, N.B.; Dal '39; A.M.C.G.P.

BURLEY, Malcolm P.; Chipman, N.B.; Dal '50; Dist. Coroner.

BURMEISTER, Richard F.; Ste. 230, 5780 Cambie St., Vancouver 15, B.C.; Germ. '24.
BURNES, John S. D.; 3195 Granville St., Vancouver, B.C.; 2003 W. 20th (res); Man '45; F.A.C.S., Gen. Surg; Cons. Surg., Shaughnessy Hosp.; Vis. Staff, Vancouver Gen., St. Paul's, St. Vincent & Burnaby Gen. Hosp's.; Clin. Instr., U. of British Columbia; Tel. RE 3-0411.
BURNETT, Denis J.; 119 Gertrude St., Alberni, B.C.; 17th Ave. N. Port Alberni (res); Med. Coll. (Calcutta, India) '31; Lond. U. (Eng.) '46; D.R.C.O.G.; Staff, West Coast Gen. Hosp.; Tel. 723-2401.
BURNETT, H. Allan; Ste 906, 1849 Yonge St., Toronto 12, Ont.; 117 Dawlish Ave. (res); Tor '32; IntMed.; Tel. 483-3589.
BURNETT, R.R.; Durham, Ont.; Wes '30.
BURNETT, W. Hilson; 241 Queens Ave., London, Ont.; 893 Waterloo St. (res); Tor '41; Otol; Chief (Otol.), Westminster DVA Hosp.; Instr. (Otol.), U. of Western Ontario; Tel. GE 2-1275.
BURNFIELD, Clifford R.; 560 O'Connor Dr., Toronto, Ont.; Qne '30; Tel. GA 1-6767.
BURNFORD, David W.; Medical Arts Bldg., Port Arthur, Ont., & Ridgeway Clinic Bldg., Fort William; 28 Winnipeg Ave., Port Arthur (res); Cambridge (Eng.) '40; D.C.H. (Eng.); Paed.; Tel. DI 4-3291.
BURNIE, Ruth M.; 98 Guestville Ave., Toronto 9, Ont.; 3532 Eglinton Ave. W.; Tor '47. Tel. RO 3-1171.
BURNS, Charles M.; 221 Medical Arts Bldg., Winnipeg, Man.; 247 Niagara St. (res); Man '51; F.R.C.S.(C); GenSurg; Lect'r. (Surg) U. of Manitoba; Tel. WH 2-1614.
BURNS, Charles W.; 232 Medical Arts Bldg., Winnipeg, Man.; 139 Grenfell Blvd. (res); Man '16; F.R.C.S.(C), F.A.C.S., F.I.C.S., L.L.D. (Hon.) U. of Man.; GenSurg; Prof Emer (Surg), U of Manitoba; Cons. Surg., Winnipeg, Gen. Hosp.; Tel. WH 3-5495.
BURNS, Gerrard, F/L; Lav'64; National Defence Med. Centre, Ottawa 8, Ont.
BURNS, James H.; 803 Second St. E., Cornwall Ont.; RCS (Ireland)'52.
BURNS, J. Lloyd Jr.; 825 Coxwell Ave., Toronto 6, Ont.; 65 Rollscourt Dr., Willowdale (res); Tor '41; Ophth; Chief Dept. of Ophth., Toronto East Gen. Hosp. & Orthopaedic Hosp.; Tel. HO 6-7321.
BURNS, J. Lloyd; 693 Broadview Ave., Toronto, Ont.; ObstGyn; Retired.
BURNS, Orland G.; 11-14 Wing Bldg., 220 Third Ave., Kamloops, B.C.; Man '50; MCGP; Tel. 372-5022.
BURNS, Stuart J.; 419 Dundas St., London, Ont.; 1033 Richmond St. (res); Wes '56; M.C. G.P.; Tel. 433-3946.
BURNS, William E.; 89 Dundas St. W., Napanee, Ont.; 91 Dundas St. W. (res); Qns'43; Tel. 354-5233.
BURNSTEIN, Mendel E.; The Park Victoria, 1333 South Park St., Halifax, N.S.; Dal'52; AMCGP.
BURR, Lawrence H.; Box 69, Princeton, B.C.; UBC '64.
BURR, Ronald C.; 74 Johnson St., Kingston, Ont.; Qns '32; FRCS (Ed.); FRCS(C); FACR; D&TRad; Dir., Ont. Cancer Fdn., Kingston Clinic; Chief, Dept. of TherRad., Kingston Gen. Hosp.; Staff, Hotel-Dieu Hosp.; Emer. Prof. (Rad.), Queen's U.; Tel. 542-2791.
BURRAN, Edward L.; 543 Lawrence Ave., Kelowna, B.C.; Wes '59; Ophth.
BURREL, Archie P.; 2 Tollerton Ave., Willowdale, Ont.; Tor '54; Tel. 225-1626.
BURRELL, Richard H.; New Zealand '51; Psy; Staff, Saskatchewan Hosp., Weyburn, Sask.; Tel. 842-3812.
BURRELL, Richard O.; 218 Medical Arts Bldg., Winnipeg, Man.; 115 Westgate (res); Man '32; Ch.M., F.I.C.S., F.R.C.S.(Ed.), F.R.C.S.(C), Gen Surg; Chief, Dept. Surg., St. Boniface Hosp.; Assoc. Prof. Surg., U. of Manitoba, Winnipeg, Man.; Tel. WH 2-2329.
BURRINGTON, John D.; 2911 Bayview Ave., Bayview Mews, Apt. 106, Willowdale, Ont.; Harvard (U.S.A.); **FRCS(C), GenSurg.**
BURRIS, D. Stewart; Burris Clinic, Kamloops B.C.; 503 Bluff Ave. res) McG '47; M.R. C.O.G., FRCOG; ObstGyn; Cons. Gyn. Tranquille San.; Tel. 372-2143.
BURRIS, H. L.; c/o Burris Clinic, Kamloops, B.C.; Tor '04.
BURRIS, John M.; Elmsdale, N.S.; Dal '54. Tel. 883-2216.
BURRIS, Samuel M.; 203-1st St. S., Kenora, Ont.; 512-2 Ave. S. (res); Alb '31; Dist. Coroner; Tel. HO 8-7152.
BURROUGHS, Ralph B.; 159-1st Ave. N.E., Swift Current, Sask.; Man '44; Ophth (U.S.A.); Active Staff, Swift Current Union Hosp.; Tel. 773-4320.
BURROWS, Derek S.; Burlington X-Ray Centre, 672 Brant St., Burlington, Ont.; Ireland'45; MRCP; DMRD; FFR; DiagRad; Hd. Dept. of Rad., Brant Mem. Hosp.; Radiol., West Lincoln Mem. Hosp.; Tel. 637-7155.
BURROWS, George M.; Sutton West, Ont.; Tor '54; **M.C.G.P.; Staff, York Co. Hosp. Tel. PA 2-3251.**
BURROWS, James W.; Spence Clinic, 910 Ridgeway St., Fort William, Ont.; 2621 Park Row, (res); **Qns '54; FRCP(C), IntMed.; Tel. MA 2-5301.**
BURROWS, John F.; 30 Bursthall St., Marmora, Ont.; Qns '57; Tel. 472-2417.
BURROWS, W. G.; Dept. of National Health & Welfare, c/o Regional Superintendent, European Region; Tor '43; DPM (Trin.); FAPA; FRCP (C); Psy; Overseas Psy. Cons., Dept. of National Health & Welfare; Hon. Cons. (Psy.), London Marriage Council. Abroad.
BURSEWICZ, Anne M. (McCartney); Prov. Lab. of PH, Edmonton, Alta.; Edinburgh (Scot.) '47; DPH (Tor); Research Assoc., University Hosp.; Ass't. Prof. (Bact), U. of Alberta; Ass't. Prov. Bact., Prov. Lab., Edmonton; Tel. 433-5811.
BURT, Robert K.; 4822-51st St., Red Deer, Alta.; 4745-56th St. (res); Glasgow (Scot.) '49; MRCOG; FRCS(C), ObstGyn; Chief of Obst., Red Deer Gen.; Tel. 347-4484.
BURT-GERRANS, Norman E.; 520 Vincent St., Woodstock, Ont.; Wes '57; MCGP; Staff, Woodstock Gen. & St. Joseph's Hosp's.; Tel. 537-6554.
BURTNICK, Walter; Box 371, Sechelt, B.C.; UBC'57.
BURTON, Blanche; 2135 Gerrard E., Toronto, Ont.; Tor '29; Phys., Dept. of Health; Tel. OX 4-6490.
BURTON, Carl R.; 932 Med. Arts Bldg., 170 St. George St., Toronto 5, Ont.; **25 Old Forest** Hill Rd. (res); **Tor '36;** M.R.C.P.(Lond.), F.A.C.P., F.R.C.P.(C), IntMed; Sr. Phys., Toronto Gen. Hosp.; **Assoc. Prof. (Med.), U. of** Toronto; Tel. **WA 3-1674.**
BURTON, Dorothy F.; 16 Tranquil Dr., Toronto 18, Ont.; (res); Tor '53; Staff Phys., Workmen's Comp. Bd.; Tel. 362-3411 Loc. 359.
BURTON, George V.; 508 Main St., Yarmouth, N.S.; McG '49.
BURTON, Glenn S.; 150 Delhi St., Guelph, Ont.; Qns '31; Psy; Med. Supt., Homewood San.; Tel. 824-1010.
BURTON, Jeffrey D.; UBC '56; Res., Vancouver Gen. Hosp., Vancouver, B. C.
BURTON, Peter M.; 180 Metcalfe St., Ottawa, Ont.; London U. (Eng.) '40; M.B., B.S., MRCS, LRCP; 'A' Staff (Med.), Ottawa Civic Hosp.; Tel CE 3-9572.
BURTON-STEWART, Ann — see **STEWART-BURTON, Ann.**
BURWELL, G. B.; 57 Renfrew, Ont.; Qnb '51.
BURWELL, Robert B.; 140 Brown's Line, Toronto 14, Ont.; **1628 Rometown Dr., Port Credit (res); McG '48, IntMed; Staff, Queensway Gen.** & South Peel Hosp's.; Cons. Med. Ontario Hosp., New Toronto; Phys. Ont. Hydro; Tel. CI 1-2841.
BURWELL, William B.; 66 Quarry St., Renfrew, Ont.; 187 Stevenson Cres. (res); McG '53; Tel. HE 2-4616.
BURWELL, W. Keith; 718 Granville St., Vancouver, B.C., & 4291 Charles; 1949 Beach (res); McG '26; **ObstGyn; Tel. MU 1-9704.**

BURY, John D.; Med. Clin. Group, Community Health Serv., Avenue Bldg., Saskatoon, Sask.; London (Eng.) '48; M.B., B.S., MRCS; LRCP; MRCOG; DObstRCOG; Assoc. Staff, University, St. Paul's & City Hosp's.; Tel. 652-0300.
BURY, Katherine D.; Tor'62; Res., Wellesley Hosp., Toronto, Ont.
BURY, Robert J.; 203 Med. Arts Bldg., 11010 Jasper Ave., Edmonton, Alta.; 14015-85th Ave. (res); Wes '46; FACS; GenSurg; Att'd. Staff, (Surg.), Royal Alexander Hosp.; Assoc. Clin Prof. (Anat.) U. of Alta.; Tel. GA 4-7433.

BUS, Ilona (Szterszky) Debregen (Hung.) '52; Res. Vancouver Gen. Hosp., Vancouver, B. C.
BUS, Mhaly; 550 Clarke Rd., Coquitlam, New Westminster, B.C.; UBC '63; Tel WE 9-1212.

BUSBY, Stuart M.; 562 Wellington St., London, Ont.; Wes '43; Urol; Chief Cons. Urol., Westminister Hosp.; Cons. Urol., Victoria Hosp. & Beck Mem. San.; Tel. 434-8602.
BUSCHLEN, Walter J.; 1770 Paris St., Sudbury, Ont.; Tor '48.
BUSH, Arthur J.; 211 Victoria Pk. Ave., Scarborough, Ont.; 140 Fallingbrook Rd. (res); Tor '50; FRCS(C), ObstGyn; MCGP; Tel. 699-2034.
BUSH, Raymond S.; Tor '61; FRCP(C), Ther Rad; Staff, Princess Margaret Hosp., Toronto, Ont.; Abroad.
BUSHEIKIN, Joseph B.; 1401 W. Broadway, Vancouver 9, B.C.; Alb '61; Abroad.
BUSHEIKIN, Theodore M.; Alb'59; ObstGyn; Staff, Shaughnessy Hosp., Vancouver, B.C.
BUSQUE, Denis; 310-6 1eme Ave., Grand'mere, P.Q.; Lav'65.
BUSQUE, Lionel; Lav'62; Anaes; Staff, Hop. St-Francois d'Assise, Quebec, P.Q.
BUSSE, Edward F.; Johns Hopkins (Baltimore, U.S.A.) '61; Res, Royal Edward Chest Hosp., Montreal 18, P.Q.
BUSSIERE, Henry C.; 415 Medical Arts Bldg., Montreal, P.Q.; Mon '20; Paed. (P.Q.); Tel. WE 5-1500.
BUSSIERES, J. Donat; 10365 Ave. d'Auteuil, Montreal, P.Q.; **Mon '20; O.R.L. (Lond.), Otol (P.Q.); Chief of Otol., Hop-Ste-Justine; Tel. DU 8-2374.**
BUSTARD, Victor W.; 11 Med. Centre, 331 Sheddon Ave., Oakville, Ont.; Dal '56; FRCS(C); ObstGyn; Assoc. Staff, Oakville-Trafalgar Mem. Hosp.; Cons. Staff, Milton & Georgetown Dist. Hosp's.; Tel. 845-7751.
BUSTEED, Daniel F.; 4176 Selkirk St., Vancouver, B.C. (res); McG '13; Retired.
BUSTILLO, Jose L.; 605 Professional Bldg., 10830 Jasper Ave., Edmonton, Alta.; Salamanca (Spain)'57; OphthOtol.
BUSTIN, Howard B.; McG '24; Pension Med. Examiner, Can. Pension Comm., Lancaster Hosp., St. John, N.B.; Tel. 694-2651.
BUTAS, Constandina; 3555 Atwater Ave., Montreal 25, P.Q. (res); Roumania '39; Bact (P.Q.); Ass't. Prof. Bact., McGill U.; Tel. WE 7-0461.
BUTAS, Nerva; 7497 St.-Denis, Montreal 10, P.Q.; Cluj (Roum.)'45; MCGP; Tel. 277-3053.
BUTCHER, John J.; 300 St. Clair Ave. W. Toronto, Ont.; Tor '44; DPH; DPsy.; Tel. 924-5563.
BUTLER, Albert A.; 1538 Sherbrooke St., Ste. 320, Montreal 25, P.Q.; 5630 Queen Mary Rd., Hampstead, Mtl. 29 (res); McG '35; FACS; OrthSurg; OrthSurg., Royal Victoria & Reddy Mem. Hosp's.; Cons. (Orth.), Queen Mary Vet's. Hosp.; Lect. (Orth.), McGill U.; Tel. WE 5-1661.
BUTLER, Douglas E.; Dal'58; Res., St. Johns Gen. Hosp., St. Johns, Nfld.
BUTLER, Gordon C.; 10145-121st St., Edmonton, Alta.; Dublin (Ire.)'44; MB, BCh, BAO, DPH; Reg. Dir., Northern Region Med. Serv.
BUTLER, H. Roy; 168 Essex St., Sarnia, Ont.; Wes '63.
BUTLER, James A.; McG '59; Jr. Int'n., Royal Victoria Hosp., Montreal, P.Q.
BUTLER, John F.; Manuels, Nfld.; R.C.P.S. (Dublin, Ire.) '59; AMCGP.
BUTLER, Kenneth C.; 1273 Terrebonne Dr., Ottawa, Ont. (res); Qns'32; AFACC; Hon. Cons. Staff (Med.), Ottawa Civic Hosp.; Tel. PA 9-2511.
BUTLER, Kenneth F.; 12702-114th Ave., Edmonton, Alta.; 11502-128th St. (res); Dublin (Ire.) '52; Zone Supt., Mackenzie & Western Arctic Northern Health Serv.
BUTLER, Kenneth R.; 507 Med. Arts Bldg., 170 St. George St., Toronto 5, Ont.; Tor'50; FRCP(C); IntMed; Assoc. Haem., St. Michael's Hosp.; Chmn., O.M.A. Section of Haem.; Clin. Teach. (Med) U. of Toronto; Tel. 366-3316.
BUTLER, Pieter O.; Ste. 203, 280 Bloor St. W., Toronto 5, Ont.; London (Eng.)'48; M.R.C.S., L.R.C.P.; D.Psy; Psy; Ass't. Cons. (Psy), U. of Toronto; Tel. WA 1-4313.
BUTLER, R. Hearder; Med. Centre, 12 West St., Corner Brook, Nfld.; Highland Ave. (res); Dal '50; GenSurg; Tel. 634-6363.
BUTLER, V. John; Tor'55; D.Psy; FRCP(C), Psy; Staff, Psy. Unit, Toronto Gen. Hosp., Toronto 2, Ont.
BUTLER, William E.; 35 Frank St., Strathroy, Ont.; Wes '57; MCGP.
BUTLER, William S.; 348 Fraser St., North Bay, Ont., 770 Reynolds (res); McG '25; GenSurg; Dist. Surg., Bell Telephone Co., International Harvester Co., A. & P. Stores & Northern Electric Co.; Tel. 474-0320.
BUTLIN, Jorge R.; 1647 Kathryn Dr., London, Ont.; Litoral (Argent.)'55; Staff, Victoria Hosp.; Teach. Fell. Med., U. of Western Ontario; Tel. GE 9-1681.
BUTSON, A Richard C.; Med. Arts Bldg., 1 Young St., Hamilton, Ont.; 20 Glenwood Cres. (res); Cambridge (Eng.) '45; M.A., M.D., F.R.C.S.(Eng.), F.R.C.S.(C), GenSurg; Surg., **St. Joseph's & Hamilton Gen. Hosp's.; Tel. JA 9-9665**
BUTSON, Franklin J.; 216 Wharncliffe N., London, Ont.; 858 Riverside Dr. (res); Wes '50; M.C.G.P.; Court. Staff, Victoria & St. Joseph's Hosp's.; Tel. 433-3167.
BUTT, Donald F.; Tor'60; MCGP; Med. Supt., M. J. Boylen Hosp., Baie Verte, Nfld.
BUTT, E. G.; Med. Arts Bldg., Windsor, Ont.; R.R. 3, Amherstburg (res); Wes '43; DiagRad; Cons. Rad., Metropolitan & Grace Hosp's.; Tel. 254-7551.
BUTT, John A.; 397 Reid Street, Peterborough, Ont.; Tor '48; F.R.C.S.(C), ObstGyn; Staff & Cons. Peterborough Civic & St. Joseph's Hosp's.; Tel. RI 2-4893.
BUTT, John C.; Alb '60; Ass't. Res. (Neurol), Vancouver Gen. Hosp., Vancouver, B.C. Abroad.
BUTT, Robert M.; Med. Arts Clinic, West Valley Rd., Corner Brook, Nfld.; McG '54; GenSurg; Surg., Serv., **Western Mem. Hosp.; Tel 4-3734.**
BUTT, Ronald B.; 948 Main St. E., Hamilton, Ont.; Wes '56.
BUTT, William A.; 7 Conrad Avenue, Toronto 10, Ont.; Tor '40; FACA; FICA; Anaes.; Anaes, Toronto Western Hosp.; Assoc. (Anaes.), U. of Toronto; Tel. LE 3-7081.
BUTT, William D.; Ste. 535, Medical Arts Bldg., **Toronto 5, Ont.; Tor '46; PlasSurg. Tel. WA 1-4943.**
BUTT, William J.; 361 Dundas St., Woodstock, Ont.; 325 Ingersoll Ave., (res); Wes '49; M.C.G.P.; Indus.Phys., Canada Cement Co. Tel. LE 7-6501.
BUTT, William P.; Tor'59; FFR; FRCP(C), DiagRad; Staff, Toronto East Gen. Hosp., Toronto 13, Ont.
BUTTOO, Ajit S.; 625 Beaton Ave., Sudbury, Ont.; Manchester (Eng.)'63.
BUTTON, F. John; 200 Main St. W., Stouffville, Ont.; Tor '40.
BUTTON, James R.; 51 Main St. E., Ridgetown, Ont.; Wes '49; MCGP; Tel. GR 4-2882.
BUTTS, M. Wilfrid; 200 Brock St. N., Whitby, Ont.; 345 Fairview Dr. (res); Dal '59; Staff, Oshawa Gen. Hosp.; Tel. 668-3378.
BUXTON, Elmira M. (Richli); 14 Virgilwood Dr. Willowdale, Ont.; (res); Loma Linda (Calif., U.S.A.) '41; DNBME; Tel. 636-5317.
BUXTON, Nigel A.; 14 Virgilwood Dr., Willowdale, Ont.; Cambridge (Eng.)'37; MRCS (Eng.); LRCP (Lond.); Tel. 636-5317.

BYERS, James M.; Alberta Hosp., Box 1000, Ponoka, Alta.; Alb'35; MSc; CMHA; Psy; Med. Supt., Alberta Hosp.; Tel. 783-3351.
BYERS, John R.; Gananoque, Ont.; Glasgow (Scot.) '04; L.R.C.P., L.R.C.S. (Edin.), F.R.C.P.(C); Retired.
BYERS, John N.C.; Ponoka, Alta.; McG '30.
BYERS, S. John; Box 340, Ponoka, Alta.; Alb '57; Tel. 783-3527.
BYERS, Wilmer M.; Winchester, Ont.; Qns '41.
BYK, Adolf; 3400 Bohle, Montreal 9, P.Q. (res); Italy '39; M.C.G.P.; Anaes; Staff, Hop. Sacre Coeur; Tel. FE 4-1210.
BYKERK, Henry; 331 Sheddon Ave., Oakville, Ont.; Amsterdam (Neth), MCGP; Phys., St Lawrence Cement, Clarkson & Shell Oil Co., Oakville; Tel. 845-7577.
BYKOWSKI, Orest M.; 10006-149 St., Edmonton, Alta.; Alb '64; Tel. 489-4948.
BYRNE, Aidan A.; Lethbridge Health Unit, 909 4th Ave. S., Lethbridge, Alta.; Roy. Coll. Surg. (Ire.)'39; DPH; MOH, Lethbridge Health Unit.
BYRNE, Alexander, Major; Sheffield (Eng.)'57; Ass't. Res. Path., St. Michael's Hosp., Toronto, Ont.
BYRNE, Ernest H.; 1088 Fennel Ave. E., Hamilton, Ont.; Ott '61; AMCGP; Tel. 389-2244.
BYRNE, John V.; 24 Catherine St., Trenton, Ont.; **Qns '35; MCGP; Sec. of Med. Staff, Trenton Mem. Hosp.; Chairman Dist. No. 6. CMA; Tel.** EX 2-6226.
BYRNES, Michael C.; Tor'60; Psy; Staff, Ont. Hosp., Toronto, Ont.
CABANA, Hubert; c/o M. M. Vallee, Causapscal, Co. Matapedia, **P.Q. (res); Retired.**
CABANA, J Ernest; App 2, 83 eme Ave., Chomedy, P.Q.; 3968 rue du Havre (res); Mon '36; FACS; FICS; GenSurg; Gen. Surg in Chief, Hop. St. Jean-de-Dieu; Chief Ass't Surg., Hop Ste-Justine; Ass't. Prof., U. of Montreal; Tel. RE 3-9951.
CABANA, Marc; La Patrie (Compton), P.Q.; Mon '49; **M.C.G.P.; Vis. Phys., Hop. Hotel Dieu** de Sherbrooke; Tel. 888-2288.
CABATU, Moises D.; Fredericton Medical Clinic, 206 Rookwood Ave., Fredericton, N.B.; Santo Tomas (Philipp.)'52; MCGP; Active Staff, Victoria Public Hosp. & Forest Hill Rehab. Centre; Tel. 475-7701.
CABLE, Ralph M.; Box 56, Rimbey, Alta., Alb '52; MCGP.
CABLE, Ronald; 122 Commercial St., Middleton. N.S. (res); St. Andrews (Scot.) '52; DMRD (Eng.); DiagRad; Staff, Soldiers' Mem. Hosp. & Western Kings Mem., Berwick; Tel. 825-3411.
CADGER, Douglas; 65 Academy Medical Bldg., 1812-4th St. W., Calgary, Alta.; 102 Waterloo Dr., Wildwood (res); Edinburg (Scot.) '52; IntMed. Tel. AM 2-1013.
CADHAM, Roper G.; City Health Dept., Civic Centre, Winnipeg, Man.; Man '38; D.P.H.; PH; Med. Health Off. Winnipeg; Ass't. Prof. (Dept. Soc. & Prev. Med.), U. of Manitoba; Tel. GR 4-9110.
CADIEUX, Andre; 1952 Jean-Talon E., Montreal, P.Q.; Mon '53; Tel. 728-4221.
CADIEUX, Jean P.; Ste. 303, 50 Place Cremazie, Montreal, P.Q.; Mon. '47; IntMed (P.Q.).
CADIEUX, Roger; 3886 Ave. Verdun, Verdun, Montreal 19, P.Q.; Mon '59.
CADIEUX, Roland; 10320 Verville, Montreal, P.Q.; Mon '40; Tel. 381-6435.
CADMAN, Thomas A.; 220 Moore St., Sherbrooke, P.Q.; McG'41; Otol(P.Q.); Tel. 562-4033.
CADOGAN, George I.; Alb '58; Ass't. Res. (Rad.), Toronto Gen. Hosp., Toronto, Ont.
CADORET, Remi j.; 56 Riverside Dr., Fort Garry, Man. (res); Yale U. (New Haven, Conn.) '53; Ass't. Prof. & Research, Dept. of Physiol., **U. of Manitoba, Winnipeg; Tel. GR 4-9110.**
CADOTTE, J. Marcel; 2345 Etienne-Parent, Montreal 12, P.Q.; Mon'62; Path(P.Q.).
CADOTTE, M. Lucie C.; 12092 rue Pasteur, Montreal 12, P.Q.; Mon'52; DHP; Staff, Dept. of Health; Tel. FE 4-3626.
CADRIN, Gilles P.; 190 rue Wolfe, Levis, P.Q.; Lav'60; ObstGyn (P.Q.); Tel. 837-8859.
CADZOW, William J.; Box 510, Lac La Biche, Alta.; Alb '41; Tel. 623-4421.
CAESAR, John J.; UBC '55; FRCP(C), Anaes; Staff, University Hosp., Philadelphia, P.A., U.S.A. Abroad.
CAGEORGE, John D.; 3925 Broadway, Lachine. P.Q.; McG '44; Tel. 637-8222.
CAHILL, Claude F.; 286 Hunter St. W., Peterborough, Ont.; Qns '38.
CAHILL Cyril F.; 3690 Peel St., Montreal, P.Q.; Heidelberg (Germ.) '55; D. Psy (McG); Psy (P.Q.); Staff Mental Hygiene Inst.; Lect. (Psy.), McGill U.; Tel. UN 6-9581.
CAHILL, Joan F.; 3643 Dutch Village Rd., Halifax, N.S.; 1264 Seymour St. (res); Dal '63; M.Sc. (Pharm.); AMCGP; Instr., Dalhousie Med. School; Tel. 454-1379.
CAHN, Charles H.; 6875 Lasalle Blvd., Verdun, **Montreal 19, P.Q.; Tor '45; Psy; Ass't. Med.** Supt., Douglas Hosp.; Lect. (Psy), McGill U.; Tel. 766-8511.
CAHOON, Erroll B.; 2917 Bloor St. W., Toronto 18, Ont.; 35 Pinehurst Cres., Islington (res); Tor'43; D. Psy.; Psy; Staff, St. Joseph's, Sunnybrook, South Peele, Northwestern & Queen Elizabeth Hosp's; Tel. 233-3111.
CAILLE, Jacques; 2, St-Michel, Vaudreuil, P.Q.; Lav '54; MCGP; Tel. 234-2012.
CAILLOUX, Robert; 3423 rue St. Denis, Montreal 18, P.Q.; Mon '40; Obst. (P.Q.): Staff Phys., Hop. Gen. de la Misericordia; Tel. VI 2-5141.
CAIN, Douglas R.; Spence Clinic, 910 Ridgeway St., Fort William, Ont.; Man'59; Urol.
CAIN, Molson C.; 1053 Avenue Rd. N.. Toronto, Ont. (res); Tor '26; Staff D.V.A.; Tel. HU 3-3333.
CAIRA, Eugene G.; Thorold Med. Clinic, 60 Albert St. W., **Thorold, Ont.; R.R. 3., St.** Catharines (res); **Glasgow (Scot.) '49; M.Sc.;** GenSurg; **LRCP & S. (Edin.); Tel. CA 7-5211.**
CAIRNS, Alexander R. M.; 6730 Churchill St., West Vancouver, B.C. (res); UBC'56; FRCP(C), IntMed; Staff, Van. Gen. Hosp.; Ass't. Prof. (Med.), U. of British Columbia; Tel. TR 6-3211.
CAIRNS, Andrew; 10155-120th St., Edmonton, Alta.; 7606-119th St. (res); Alb '45; IntMed; Instr. (ClinMed), **U. of Alberta; Tel. 488-7271.**
CAIRNS, Edmund A. M.; Haig Clinic, Lethbridge, Alta.; 1415—10th Avenue A. (res); Alb '34; F.A.A.P., Paed.; Chief, Dept. Paed, Lethbridge Mun. Hosp.; Tel. 328-6641.
CAIRNS, James W.; Pipestone, Man.; Man 15, Phm.B.; Indian Health Service; Dist. Coroner.
CAIRNS, John A.; Room 307, 736 Granville St., Vancouver 2, B.C.; Alb'59; Ophth; Tel. 681-1515.
CAIRNS, John D.; 2516 Bayview Ave., Willowdale, Ont.; **412 St. Clements, Tor. 12 (res); Oxford (Eng.) '50; MA; FRCS(C), FACS; Obst**Gyn; Staff, ObstGyn., Toronto East Gen. Hosp.; Tel. HI 7-7188.
CAIRNS, Joseph M.; 6183 Cedar St., Halifax, N.S.; Dal'54; IntMed; Staff, Camp Hill Hosp.; Tel. 423-1371.
CAISSE, J-J. Gaston; 901 est Boul. St. Joseph, App. 1, Montreal, P.Q.; Mon'27; OrthSurg; Dir. Gen., Can. Disability Assoc.; Tel. 271-6583.
CAKULS, Pavils; Leeds (Eng.)'56; Res. (Psy.), Ontario Hosp., London, Ont.
CALARCO, J. A.; 1800 Bloor St. W., Toronto, Ont.; Tor '41; Anaes. Tel. RO 6-3179.
CALARSU, Franco R.; Milan (Italy)'53; PhD; Ass't. Prof. (Physiol.), University of Alberta, Edmonton, Alta.; Scholar Med. Research Council of Canada.
CALDBICK, George G.D. A/C; 39 Dunvegan Rd., Ottawa, Ont. (res); **Qns '37; D.P.H., F.A.C.P.M.** (Avia. Med.); Derm; Hd. of Med. Sect., Defence Research Bd.; Tel. 992-4958.
CALDER, Aileen A. (Morrison); Cottage Hosp., Burgeo, S.W. Coast, Nfld.; Jersey Lodge (res); **Edinburgh (Scot.) '55; Ass't. M.O., Cottage** Hosp., & Schls. M.O.; D.M.O., Grand Bruit.
CALDER, Alexander McP.; Box 89, Forest, Ont. Wes '28; M.C.G.P.; M.O.H., Forest, Ont.; Dist. Coroner: Tel. 873-2433.
CALDER, Allister; 3 York St., Glace Bay, N.S.; Dal '09; F.A.C.S.; Staff, Glace Bay Gen. Hosp. (T.B. Unit); Retired.

CALDER, Alistair D.; Box 30, Coronach Clinic, Coronach, Sask.; Aberdeen (Scot) '52; Tel. 95.

CALDER, A. Louise; Alb '63; Res. Hosp. for Sick Children, Toronto, Ont.

CALDER, Alvinus; Bishop Block, Sydney, N.S.; Qns '19.

CALDER, Colin M. S.; Cottage Hosp., Burgeo, Nfld.; Jersey Lodge (res); Edinburgh (Scot.) '52; M.O.H.; Tel. 3131.

CALDER, Gordon; 321 Dufferin Ave., London, Ont.; Wes '30.

CALDER, James; 210 McLeod Bldg., Edmonton, Alta.; 11631 Saskatchewan Dr. (res); Alb '30; Paed; Clin. Prof. (Paed.), U. of Alberta Hosp.; Cons. (Paed.), Charles Camsell Indian Hosp.; Tel. GA 2-7412.

CALDER, John R.; 20 Dundas St., Brantford, Ont.; McG '18; Anaes; Staff, Brantford Gen., St. Joseph's & Willett Hosp., Paris, Ont.; Tel. 752-1142.

CALDER, Mary; Glasgow (Scot.) '49; **Sr. Ass't. Med. Res. (Paed.), Montreal Children's Hosp., Montreal, P.Q.**

CALDER, Norma M.; 2595 Lawson Ave., Hollyburn, B.C. (res); McG '53.

CALDER, Thomas L.; 2489 Bellevue Ave., West Vancouver, B.C.; McG '53; MCGP; Chief, Div. of GP. Lions Gate Hosp.; Tel. WA 2-9397.

CALDERBANK, Arthur D.; Eatonia Med.-Dental Clinic, Eatonia, Sask.; 5th Ave. E. (res); Manchester (Eng.) '55; Abroad. Tel. 159.

CALDWELL, Albert E.; Viking, Alta.; Alb '41; M.C.G.P.; Dist. Coroner; Tel. 336-3311.

CALDWELL, Douglas Y.; Ste. 103, 688 Coxwell Ave., Toronto 13, Ont.; Tor'52; Anaes; Anaes., Toronto East Gen. Hosp.; Tel. 465-7533.

CALDWELL, J. Donald; Ste 205, 1105 Carling Ave., Ottawa, Ont.; 356 First Ave. (res); Tor '37; GenSurg; F.I.C.S.; AMCGP; Tel. CE 4-6451.

CALDWELL, Lorne A.; 328 Second St. W., Cornwall, Ont.; Tor '31; GenSurg; Staff, Cornwall Gen. & Hotel Dieu Hosp's.; Tel. 932-1252.

CALDWELL, Robert J.; Petitcodiac, N.B.; McG '27.

CALDWELL, Robert M.; Main St., Yarmouth, N.S.; 18 Brunswick St. (res); Dal '32.

CALDWELL, William S.; 73 Queen St. E., Brampton, Ont.; 84 Main St. S. (res); Tor '24; MCGP; Hon. Acting Staff, Peel Mem. Hosp.; Tel. GL 1-1244.

CALLAGHAN, James E.; Wes'63; Res., Montreal Gen. Hosp., Montreal 25, P.Q.

CALLAGHAN, James L.; 89 Cross St., Chatham, Ont. (res); Wes'28; DiagRad; Chief, Dept. of Rad., St. Joseph's Hosp.; Tel. EL 2-2500.

CALLAGHAN, John C.; 550 Physc. & Surgs. Bldg., 8409-112th St., Edmonton, Alta.; Tor '46; F.A.C.S., F.R.C.S.(C), GenSurg, ThorSurg; Clin. Prof. or Sur. & Dir. Cardio-Vasc. & ThorSurg., University of Alberta Hosp.; Cons. Cardio-Vasc. & ThorSurg., D.V.A.; Tel. GA 4-7460.

CALLAGHAN, Wilfred E.; Box 1542, 295 Church St., Summerside, P.E.I.; 257 Central St. S. (res); Dal'41; Dist. Coroner; Tel. 436-2352.

CALLAGHAN, William J. O.; Dal'61; Res., Hosp. for Sick Children, Toronto 2, Ont.

CALLAHAN, George A.; Ste. 102, 215 Victoria St., Toronto 2, Ont.; 402 Vesta Drive (res); Tor '50; M.C.G.P.; Staff, O.P.D., St. Michael's Hosp. Tel. 364-5325.

CALLAHAN, William P.; 183 St. Clair Ave. W., Toronto 7, Ont.; 109 Warren Rd. (res); Tor '45; F.R.C.S.(C), Ophth; Staff, Hosp. for Sick Children & St. Michael's; Assoc. (Ophth), U. of **Toronto; Tel. 924-2424.**

CALLBECK, Gordon R. M.; P. O. Drawer 426, Duncan, B.C.; Alb '44.

CALLEGARINI, Umberto; Ste. 610, 5300 Cote-des-Neiges, Montreal 26, P.Q.; 3770 Maplewood No. 2 (res); Padua (Italy)'52; FAAP; Paed. (P.Q.); Jr. Clin. Ass't. (Paed.), St. Mary's Hosp. & Mtl. Children's Hosp.; Ass't. Paed., Santa Cabrini Hosp.; Tel. 733-0681.

CALLEIA, Sarah G.;Tahsis, B.C.; McG'62; Tel. 934-2121.

CALO, Romuald; Holden, Alta.; Bologna (Italy) '48; L.R.C.P. & S. (Ire.), D.L.M.

CALLOC'H, Jean P.; 5537 Cote des Neiges, **Montreal 26, P.Q.; Mon '57; Tel. RE 3-1912.**

CALVERLEY, Milton O.; Ste. 501, 625 - 5th Ave., New Westminster, B.C.; Man'53; Psy; Hd., Dept. of Psy., Royal Columbian Hosp.; Staff, St. Mary's & Surrey Mem. Hosp's.; Tel. 526-6422.

CALVERT, Kenneth G.; 406 Rideau Medical-Dental Centre, 1711-4th St. S.W., Calgary, Alta.; 2917 Wolfe St., S.W. (res); Wes '39; DABOG; **FACS; Cons. (ObstGyn), Holy Cross Hosp.,** Dept. Head. & Cons. (Gyn.), Grace Hosp.; Tel. 263-2737.

CALVERT, Leslie J.; Med. Centre, 707 Charlotte St., Peterborough, Ont.; Wes '42; F.A.C.S.; GenSurg; Urol.; Tel. 742-3871.

CAMBON, Eileen S. (Nason); Ste. 201, 1701 W. Broadway, Vancouver 9, B.C.; McG '51; DAB (Ophth.); Ophth; Cons., Shaughnessy Vet's Hosp.; Tel. RE 1-1241.

CAMBON, Kenneth G.; Ste. 201, 1701 W. Broadway, Vancouver 9, B.C.; McG '51; Otol; Att'd. Staff, Vancouver Gen. Hosp.; Phys-in-Charge, Otol. & Audiology Unit, Children's Health Centre; Clin. Instr. (Otol.), U. of British Columbia; Tel. RE 1-1241.

CAMERON, Archie P.; Box 178, Swan River, Man.; Man '16.

CAMERON, Campbell G.; The Spence Clinic, 910 Ridgeway St., Fort William, Ont.; 512 S. Selkirk Ave. (res); Qns '52; IntMed; Staff, McKellar **Gen. Hosp.; Tel. MA 2-5301.**

CAMERON, C. Gordon; 3000 Lawrence Ave. E., Scarborough, Ont.; 35 Bendale Blvd. (res); Tor **'44; FRCP(C), IntMed; Chief (Med.), Scarborough Gen. Hosp.; Tel. 291-0351.**

CAMERON, D. Ewen; 1025 Pine Ave. W., Montreal, P.Q.; Mt. Whitney Rd., Lake Placid, N.Y. (res); Glasgow (Scot.) '24; D.P.M.(Lond.); D.A.B.P.N.; F.R.C.P.(C), Psy; Psy-in-Chief, Royal Victoria Hosp., Dir., Allan Mem. Inst. of Psy.; Prof. & Chm., Dept. of Psy., McGill U., **Pres. World Psy. Assoc.; Tel. VI 2-1251, Loc. 382.** Abroad.

CAMERON, D. Murray; Man '55; Res., Vancouver Gen. Hosp., Vancouver, B.C.

CAMERON Donald A.; 1050 Queen's Blvd., Kitchener, Ont.; Tor '51; A.M.C.G.P.; Med. Dir., Dominion Electrohome Indust.; C.O., 12th Med. Co., R.C.A.M.C. (Militia). Tel. SH 2-6612.

CAMERON, Donald F.; Faculty of Medicine, University of Alberta, Edmonton, Alta.; Alb'49; FACA; Anaes; Assoc. Dean, Faculty of Med.; Assoc. Prof. Anaes. & Pharm.; Tel. 439-8721, Ext. 354.

CAMERON, Donald J.; 38 Mount Hope St., Kitchener, Ont.; Ott '57; GenSurg; Active Staff, Kitchener-Waterloo & St. Mary's Hosp's.; Tel. 743-8001.

CAMERON, Donald M.; 5876 Adera St., Vancouver 13, B.C.; Man'55; DiagRad.

CAMERON, Douglas G., MC; Montreal General Hosp., 1650 Cedar Ave., Montreal 25, P.Q.; McG '40; B.Sc. (Oxon.); MRCP (Lond.); FACP; Haem (P.Q.); FRCP(C), IntMed; Phys-in-Chief & Dir., McGill U. Med. Clinic, Montreal Gen. Hosp.; Prof. of Med. & Chmn., McGill U.; Tel. WE 7-6011, Loc. 375.

CAMERON, D. S.; P.O. Box 566, Station Q, Toronto, Ont.; McG '55.

CAMERON, Evan G.; Ste. 404, Central Med. Bldg., 1105 Carling Ave., Ottawa 3, Ont.; Box 237 Riverside Dr., Billings Bridge P.O. (res); Qns'44; ObstGyn; Staff, Ottawa Civic & Grace Hosp's. & Cons. (Gyn), Ontario Cancer Fdn.; Tel. PA 8-1713.

CAMERON, G. D. W.; 432 Daly Ave., Ottawa, Ont. (res); Qns '27; D.P.H., F.R.C.P. (Lond.), Hon. LL.D. (Qns); PH; Dept. Minister of Nat. Health & Welfare (Health); Retired.

CAMERON, George J.; 417 Pitt St., Cornwall, Ont.; Alb '29; Staff, Hotel Dieu & Cornwall Gen. Hosp's.; Tel. WE 2-4630.

CAMERON, Gordon S.; 507 Medical Arts Bldg., Hamilton, Ont.; 15 W. 34th St. (res); Tor '51; F.R.C.S.(C), GenSurg; Staff, Hamilton Gen. & St. Joseph's, Chedoke; Court Staff, Brant Mem. Hosp.; Tel. JA 9-5023.

CAMERON, Gordon W.; 108 Med. Arts Bldg., 11010 Jasper Ave., Edmonton, Alta.; 11108-90th Ave. (res); McG '45; F.A.C.S., F.R.C.S.(C), OrthSurg; Att'd. Staff, U. of Alberta Hosp.; Lect. (OrthSurg), U. of Alberta; Tel. GA 2-6216.

CAMERON, G. Stewart; 318 Stewart St., Peterborough, Ont. (res); Tor '96; F.R.C.S.; Cons. Emer.; Retired.

CAMERON, G. Stuart; Drayton Valley, Alta.; Sask '61; Staff, Drayton Valley & Breton Hosp's.; Tel. 542-3475.

CAMERON, Harold; Westminster Hosp., London, Ont. (res); Edinburgh (Scot.) '48; F.A.C.A.; Anaes; Chief Anaes., Westminster Hosp.; Instr. (Anaes), U. of Western Ont.; Tel. GE 9-1681.

CAMERON, Helen C. (See Cohoe, Helen C.).

CAMERON, Howard S.; Ste. 211, 450 Central Ave., London, Ont.; Wes'50; FACS; FRCS(C), OrthSurg; GenSurg; Cons. (OrthSurg), St. Joseph's & Westminster DVA Hosp's.; Cons., St. Mary's, Parkwood & Ontario Hosp's. (London & Cedar Springs); Teach. Fell. (Surg.), U. of Western Ontario; Tel. 433-2912.

CAMERON, Hugh C.; 559 O'Connor Dr., Toronto 6, Ont.; 15 Strathgowan Cres. Tor 12 (res); Qns '54; FAAP; Paed; Att'd., Paed., Toronto E. Gen. Hosp. & The Crippled Children's Centre; Tel. 421-4972.

CAMERON, J. A. Maxwell, CD; 200 Med. Centre Bldg., 906-8th Ave. S.W., Calgary, Alta.; Man '34; FRCS (Edin.); FRCS(C), GenSurg; Tel. 262-6361.

CAMERON, John D.; 55 Kingsmount Blvd., Sudbury, Ont.; Tor'39; Anaes; Active Staff, (Anaes.) St. Joseph's, Sudbury Gen. & Mem. Hosp's.; Tel. 674-0140.

CAMERON, Kenneth G.; 15 King St., Huntingdon, P.Q.; Fairview Rd. (res); McG '49; Staff, Huntingdon County Hosp. & Barrie Memorial Hosp., Ormstown; Tel. 264-5334.

CAMERON, M. G. Peter; 101 Normandy Gdns, London, Ont. (res); Tor '42; FRCP(C); IntMed; Phys. Med. & Rehab; Dir. PhysMed & Rehab., Victoria Hosp.; Prof. & Hd. (Phys. Med.), U. of Western Ont.: Tel. 432-5261.

CAMERON, Paul M.; Tor'65; Res., Royal Victoria Hosp., Montreal 2, P.Q.

CAMERON, Roderick J. R.; 19 Limardo Dr., Dartmouth, N.S.; Dal'40; DPH; Dir., Atlantic Health Unit; Tel. 469-6430.

CAMERON, Sheldon R.; Med. Centre, 5 Central St., Summerside, PEI; Dal '55; MCGP; Tel. 436-2277.

CAMERON, Stewart H.; Med. Hall Bldg., Stellarton, N.S.; McG'51; Tel. 752-6114.

CAMERON, William G.; Dingwall Clinic, Dryden, Ont.; 42 Victoria St. (res); Dal'51; M.C.G.P.; M.O., Dryden Chemical Plant; Tel. 223-2258.

CAMERON, William H.; 2315 Weston Rd., Weston, Ont.; 20 Browside Ave., Toronto (res); Tor '25; M.R.C.S., L.R.C.P.(Lond.). Tel. CH 1-2301.

CAMERON, William J. M.; 1448 Corley Dr., London, Ont. (res); Wes'39; FCCP; FRCP(C); IntMed; Cardiol., Westminster DVA Hosp.; Staff, Victoria Hosp.; Cons., Ontario Hosp.; Clin. Lect., U. of Western Ontario; Tel. 432-6282.

CAMERON, William K.; 2315 Weston Rd., Weston Ont.; Tor '44; A.M.C.G.P. Tel. CH 1-2301.

CAMERON, William M.; Winnipeg Clinic, St. Mary's & Vaughan Streets. Winnipeg, Man.; Qns '60; FRCP(C), IntMed; Tel. 942-0551.

CAMERON, William R.; Ste. 111, 108 Isabella St., Toronto 5, Ont.; Tor'35; MCGP; Tel. WA. 1-3203.

CAMGOZ, Hulusi T.; Sask'59; Staff, Kipling Mem. Union Hosp., Kipling, Sask.

CAMIL, Victor S.; 914 St. Clair Ave. W., Toronto 10, Ont.; 578 Castlefield Ave.(res); Yassy (Roumania) '31; LCMC; ObstGyn (Roumania); Staff, Doctor's Hosp.; Tel. LE 5-4759.

CAMINETSKY, Sydney; 104 Norlyn Bldg., 309 Hargrave St., Winnipeg 2, Man.; 894 Corydon Ave. (res); Man '48; M.C.G.P.; Tel. WH 2-4184.

CAMPAIGNE, Margaret Y. (Senior); 378 Oriole Court, Burlington, Ont. (res); Tor '49; Part-time School M.O., Hamilton.

CAMPBELL, A. Craig; 20 Abercrombie Rd., New Glasgow, N.S.; Dal '51.

CAMPBELL, Alexander A.; 95 Sherbrook St., Winnipeg 1, Man.; Man '50; MCGP; Chmn., Med. Staff, Misericordia Hosp.; Tel. SP 5-4471.

CAMPBELL, Alexander D.; 900 King St. W., Kitchener, Ont.; Tor'39; Anaes.

CAMPBELL, Alexander N., Major; Dal'54; GenSurg; Staff, Canadian Forces Hosp., Halifax, N.S.

CAMPBELL, Andrew H.; Broadview, Sask.; Qns '15; GenSurg.

CAMPBELL, Angus; Workmen's Compensation Board, 657-W. 37th Ave., Vancouver 13, B.C.; 4837 Angus Dr. Van. 9 (res); Edinburgh (Scot.) '23; D.R. (Edin.); Radiol., WCB of B.C.; Tel. AM 6-0211.

CAMPBELL, Angus J.; Dal '52; AMCGP; Res., Victoria Gen. Hosp., Halifax, H.S.

CAMPBELL, Archibald D.; 1414 Drummond St., Montreal, P.Q.; 54 Forden Cres., Westmount (res); McG '20; F.R.C.O.G., F.A.C.S., F.R.C.S.-(C), ObstGyn; Const. Staff, Montreal Gen. Hosp.; Retired.

CAMPBELL-BROWN, Hugh I.; 3009-1st Ave., Vernon, B.C.; McG. '29.

CAMPBELL, Bruce A.; 42 Albert St., Stratford, Ont.; Wes'39; FRCS(C); FACS, GenSurg; Surg. Staff, Stratford Gen. Hosp.; Tel. 271-3532.

CAMPBELL, Byron A.; 50 Lauder Ave., Toronto, Ont.; Tor '94.

CAMPBELL, Charles S.; Oshawa Clinic, 117 King St. E., Oshawa, Ont.; 943 Chevrolet St. (res); Man '51; FRCS(C), GenSurg; Staff, Oshawa Gen. Hosp.; Tel. 728-1661.

CAMPBELL, Clarence M., F/L; Dal '65; Staff, Camp. Hosp., Gagetown, N.B.

CAMPBELL, Clifford G.; 395—7th St. E., Owen Sound, Ont.; 853-5th Ave. E. (res); Qns '38; Anaes.; Tel. 376-6553.

CAMPBELL, Colin A.; 1541 W. Broadway, Vancouver 9, B.C.; Man '55; DiagRad.

CAMPBELL, David; 10 Stavebank Rd. N., Port Credit, Ont.; Indian Valley Trail (res); Cambridge (Eng.) '53; M.B., B.Chir.; MCGP; Staff, South Peele Hosp.; Tel. CR 8-0121.

CAMPBELL, Donald A.; Man '35; Staff, Pearson T.B., 700 W. 57th Ave., Vancouver 15, B.C.

CAMPBELL, Donald; Bigelow-Fowler Clinic, Lethbridge, Alta.; 3 Belmont Apts. (res); Glasgow (Scot.) '52; Active, Staff, Galt & St. Michael's Hosp's., Lethbridge; Tel. FA 7-3121.

CAMPBELL, Donald B.; 331 Sheddon Ave., Oakville, Ont.; 60 Barringham Dr. (res); Tor '48; FACOG; FRCS(C), ObstGyn; Staff, Oakville-Trafalgar, South Peel & Milton Dist. Hosp's.; Tel. 844-6902.

CAMPBELL, Donald C.; Main St., Dutton, Ont.; Nancy St. (res); Wes '57; Staff, St. Thomas-Elgin Gen. Hosp., St. Thomas; Tel. 369.

CAMPBELL, Donald D.; McGregor Clinic, 250 Main St. E., Hamilton, Ont.; Man. '34; FRCS (Ed.); FRCS(C); GenSurg; Chief of Surg., Chedoke Gen. Hosp.; Active Staff, Hamilton Civic Hosp.; Tel. JA 7-2711.

CAMPBELL, Donald K.; 270 Moore St., Sherbrooke, P.Q.; McG '62.

CAMPBELL, Don L.; 2769 Lundy's Lane, Niagara Falls, Ont.; Tor '39.

CAMPBELL, Douglas B.; 922 Med. Arts Bldg., 170 St. George St., Toronto 5, Ont.; Tor '44; Tel. WA 1-3019.

CAMPBELL, D. Robert; King St., Shelburne, N.S.; Dal '55.

CAMPBELL, D. Ross; Qns '24; Med. Supt., Nanaimo Indian Hosp., Nanaimo, B.C. Retired.

CAMPBELL, Duncan A.; Hillcrest Clinic, Bridgewater, N.S.; Dal'50; Med. Staff, Dawson Mem. Hosp.; Tel. 543-4343.

CAMPBELL, Duncan E. M.; 24 Catherine St., Trenton, Ont.; 281 Dundas W. (res.); Qns's45; Tel. 392-3212.

CAMPBELL, Edward B.; Ste. 105, 262 St. Clair Ave. W., Toronto 7, Ont.; 158 Kenilworth Ave. (res); Tor '43; GenSurg; Surg. Cons., Sunnybrook Hosp. Tel. 924-4055.

CAMPBELL, Elspeth S. K.; (See Kay, Elspeth).

CAMPBELL, Eric O'F.; Tor '37; IntMed; Clin. Dir., Addiction Research Fdn., 1206 Bank St., Ottawa, Ont.; Tel. 733-8343.

CAMPBELL-FOWLER, Colin; Box 300, Falher, Alta.; Glasgow (Scot.)'42; Tel. 86.

CAMPBELL, Frank M.; 1548 Lonsdale Ave., North Vancouver, B.C.; 1239 W. 22nd St. (res); Man '59; Tel. 985-5381.

CAMPBELL, Frederick J. H.; Apt. 415, Park Towers, 10 Beechwood Pl., London, Ont.; Wes '17; M.R.C.P. (Lond.), F.R.C.P.(C), IntMed; Retired.

CAMPBELL, Gordon E.; 1062 Dovercourt Rd., Toronto, Ont.; Tor '24, Tel. LE 6-9914.

CAMPBELL, H. Hoyle; 215 Victoria St., Toronto 5, Ont.; Tor '36; PlasSurg; Assoc. Surg., U. of Toronto; Tel. 364-5325.

CAMPBELL, Hudson M.; 126 Sydenham St., Kingston, Ont.; 334 Victoria St. (res); Qns '42; M.C.G.P.; Phys., Health Serv., Kingston Gen. Hosp.; Tel. 546-0192.

CAMPBELL, Hugh C.; 815 Victoria St., Trail, B.C.; 135 Oxford Rd. (res); Qns '52; Tel. 364-1944.

CAMPBELL, Iivi (Ratas); Tor'62; Jr. Ass't. Res., New Mount Sinai Hosp., Toronto, Ont.

CAMPBELL, Irwin P.; 352 McGill St., Peterborough, Ont.; Tor '31.

CAMPBELL, James D.; Calgary Assoc. Clinic, 214-6th Ave., S.W., Calgary, Alta.; 708 Crescent Rd. N.W. (res); Wes'54; Otol; Tel. 269-1796.

CAMPBELL, James M.; 812 Cook Rd., Richmond, B.C.; Trinity Coll. (Dublin, Ire.)'56; MCGP; Tel. CR 8-5191.

CAMPBELL, James M.; 309 Lancaster Ave. W., Kitchener, Ont.; Wes'60; AMCGP; Tel. 744-4221.

CAMPBELL, James M.; 537 Medical Arts Bldg., Saskatoon, Sask.; 218 Poplar Cres. (res); Man '34; F.A.C.S., Urol; Att'd. Urol., University, City & St. Paul's Hosp's.; Assoc. Clin. Prof. (Surg.), U. of Saskatchewan; Tel. 652-0531.

CAMPBELL, James S.; 101 Dominion Bank Bldg., Fort William, Ont.; Man. '46; Ophth.; Tel. 623-8113.

CAMPBELL, James S.; Med. Arts Clinic, 2125-11th Ave., Regina, Sask.; Glasgow (Scot.)'51; Urol; Staff, Regina Gen., Grey Nuns & D.V.A. Hosp's.; Tel. 523-0691.

CAMPBELL, James S.; 327 Marshall Ct., Ottawa 8, Ont. (res); Dal '47; DABP; Path; Pathol., Ottawa Gen. Hosp.; Cons. Path., NDMC & Nat. Cancer Inst.; Prof. (Pathol.), U. of Ottawa; Tel. 236-0333; CE 5-6751.

CAMPBELL, Janet E.; Box 160, Hastings, Ont.; McG '51; Paed; Tel. 696-2461.

CAMPBELL, J. C. Maurice; 122 rue Radisson, Trois Rivieres, P.Q.; 384 rue Notre-Dame, Cap-de-la-Madeleine (res.); Mon '45; IntMed.; Chief Dept. of Med. & IntMed., Hop. St. Joseph de Trois Rivieres; Tel. FR 4-4637.

CAMPBELL, Jean F.; 893 Richmond St., London, Ont.; R.R. No. 3 (res); Wes '33; D.R.C.O.G., L.M. Rotunda, D.A.B.O.G., F.A.C.O.G.; ObstGyn; Tel. GE 4-1291.

CAMPBELL, John D.; 1814A Eglinton Ave. E., Scarborough, Ont.; 15 Foxhill Rd., Agincourt (res); Tor'57; Tel. PL 5-1431.

CAMPBELL, John E.; 6695 Fielding Ave., Apt. 19, Montreal, P.Q.; Dal '58, FRCP(C), DiagRad; Staff, Royal Victoria Hosp.; Tel. VI 2-1251. Abroad.

CAMPBELL, John G.; 13 Randolph St., Fleming Hgts., Armdale, N.S.; Dal '16; Sr. Pension Examiner, St. John's; Retired; Tel. 477-3721.

CAMPBELL, John S.; 234 Lawrence Ave., Kelowna, B.C.; 1033 Harvey Ave. (res); Queen's U. (Belfast, N. Ire.) '38; D.M.R.D.; DiagRad; Radiol., Kelowna Gen. Hosp.; Tel. 762-4455.

CAMPBELL, J. Michael; 32 Lawrence Cr., Toronto 12, Ont. (res); Queens (Belfast, Ire.) '50; FRCP(C); Anaes; Staff Anaes., Toronto Western Hosp.; Clin. Teach. (Anaes.), U. of Toronto; Tel. 485-5034.

CAMPBELL, Keith D.; 221 Brant Avenue Brantford, Ont.; 692 Colborne St., (res); Wes '58; ObstGyn.; Staff, Brantford Gen. Hosp.; Tel. 752-6625.

CAMPBELL, Kenneth A.; Ste. 40, 3195 Granville St., Vancouver 9, B.C.; McG '42; Paed; Staff, St. Paul's & Children's Hosp's.; Clin. Instr., U. of British Columbia, Tel. RE 1-2155.

CAMPBELL, Margaret K. (Patterson); 1039 Richmond St., London, Ont.; Tor '30; A.B.P., Paed; Staff, Victoria & St. Joseph's Hosp's.; Ass't. Prof. (Paed.), U. of Western Ontario; Tel. 432-8672.

CAMPBELL, Margaret M. (Kennedy); George St., Shelburne, N.S. (res); St. Andrews (Scot.) '49; M.H.O.

CAMPBELL, Margo H. (See Summerer).

CAMPBELL, Murray H.; 95 Sherbrooke St., Winnipeg, Man.; 954 Dorchester Ave. (res); Man '33; Hon. Att. Staff, Winnipeg Gen. Hosp.; Lect., U. of Manitoba; M.O., Christie's Biscuits; Tel. SP 4-6511.

CAMPBELL, Norman J.; Alb'48; Anaes; Staff, Vancouver Gen. Hosp., Vancouver, B.C.

CAMPBELL, P. L.; Tor'65; Res., Shaughnessy Hosp., Vancouver 9, B.C.

CAMPBELL, Robert; 2015 Girouard, St-Hyacinthe P.Q.; Mon '58; Tel. PR 3-1963.

CAMPBELL, Ronald W.; Canadian Pension Commission, Ottawa, Ont.; Glasgow (Scot) '46; D. Obst., RCOG; MCGP; Tel. 992-7978.

CAMPBELL, Ross D.; Box 999, Taber, Alta.; 5215-51st St. (res); Man '54; Tel. 223-3525.

CAMPBELL, S. Hardie; 1710 Ottawa St., Windsor, Ont.; 1128 Kildare Rd. (res); McG'23; Tel. 256-3456.

CAMPBELL, Stanley M.; 178 St. George St., Toronto 5, Ont.; 365 Glencairn Ave. (res); Tor '24; D.A. (Eng.), F.F.A.R.C.S. (Eng.), F.R.C.P.-(C), Anaes; Cons. Anaes., Toronto Gen., Hosp. for Sick Children, Women's College, Wellesley and Princess Margaret Hosp's.; Sec. Treas., Cdn. Arthritis Soc.; Tel. WA 3-1154.

CAMPBELL, V. Joseph; 10004 - 105th St. Edmonton, Alta.; 9721 - 100A St. (res); Alb '53; Int-Med.; Tel. GA 4-2121.

CAMPBELL, Walter R.; 101 Douglas Dr., Toronto 5, Ont. (res); Tor '15; F.R.S.C., F.R.C.P.-(C), IntMed; Retired.

CAMPBELL, W. Graham; Box 130, Main St., Vineland, Ont.; Qns '58; Coroner, Lincoln Co.; Tel. LO 2-4152.

CAMPBELL, Wilfred C.; Medical Arts Clinic, 51—6th St. S.E., Medicine Hat, Alta.; 330—1st St. S.E. (res); Man '28; F.A.C.S.; Staff, Medicine Hat Mun. Hosp.; Tel. JA 7-2211.

CAMPBELL, William A.; 123 College St., Kingston, Ont. (res); Qns '24; Anaes.; Ass't. Prof. Dept. Anaes., Queen's U.; Chief of Staff, Kingston Gen. Hosp., Tel. 546-1731.

CAMPBELL, William D.; 2221 Keele St., Toronto 15, Ont. (res); Qns '59; Anaes; Staff, North Western Gen. Hosp.; Tel. 762-3641.

CAMPBELL, William N.; Bridge St., Hastings, Ont.; McG '19; Tel. 696-2461.

CAMPBELL, W. N.; Alb '61; Jr. Intn., Royal Alexandra Hosp., Edmonton, Alta.

CAMPEAU, Alphonse; Clinique Medicale, 166 Brunelle, Beloeil, P.Q.; Mon '48.

CAMPEAU, Lucien; 6895 rue Viau, Montreal 36, P.Q.; Lav'53; F.R.C.P.(C), IntMed, Cardiol (P.Q.); Staff, Inst. de Cardiologie; Tel. 637-5382.

CAMPEAU, Paul; 55, ave. de l'Eglise, Verdun, Montreal 19, P.Q.; 550 Osborne, St. Lambert (res); Mon '48.

CAMPIN, Colin R.; London (Eng.) '61; Res., St. Michael's Hosp., Toronto 2, Ont.

CAMPION, George F.; 102 Queen St., St. Catharines, Ont.; Tor '48.

CAMPIONI, Emile C.; Woodview Park Med. Centre, 3236 Weston Rd., Weston, Ont.; Leyden (Netherlands)'57; MCGP; Court. Staff, Humber Mem. Hosp.; Tel. 636-6825.

CAMPOLONGO, Joseph T.; 222 Eramosa Rd., Guelph, Ont. 15 Sherwood Dr. (res); Tor '49; MCGP; Tel. TA 4-1507.

CAMPSALL, E. W. Robert; 513 Oak Ridge Dr., Suburban Serv. No. 1, London, Ont.; Qns '49; Staff, Victoria Hosp.; Ass't Prof. (Bact & Immunol.), U. of Western Ontario; Tel. GE 9-1681.

CAMRASS, Hugh P.; 160-14th St., Brandon, Man.; 26 Almond Cres. (res); Glasgow (Scot.) '55; Anaes; Active Staff, Brandon Gen.; Cons. Staff (Anaes.), Assiniboine Hosp., Man. San. & Brandon Hosp. for Mental Dis.; Tel. PA 6-2086.

CAMUNIAS, **Eulogio R.;** Manila Central (Philipp.)'58; Staff, Saskatchewan Hosp., Box 700, Weyburn, Sask.

CANAKIS, Andre I. P.; 240 Elm, St.-Lambert, Cite Jacques-Cartier, P.Q.; Paris (France) '58; OrthSurg; Tel. OR 2-1212.

CANAVAN, **Bernard;** Ste. 108, 688 Coxwell Ave., Toronto 13, Ont.; Edinburgh (Scot.)'60.

CANCILLA, Pasquale A.; Box 160, Flin Flon, Man.; 43 Hapnot (res); Man '56.

CANDLISH, Henry M.; 5782 Mountain Sights Ave., Montreal, P.Q.; McG'23; Tel. RE 3-6488.

CANGE, Rigaud; 415 Ste-Helene, Longueuil, P.Q. 251 de Chateauguay (res); Mon '45; IntMed (Cardiol) (P.Q.); Staff, Inst. de Cardiologie, Mtl., & Hop-Gen. St. Lambert; Vist. Staff, St. Joseph **de Rosemont; Tel. OR 4-6281.**

CANILANG, Enrique P.; Dept. of PhysMed., St. John's Gen. Hosp., St. John's, Nfld.; Manila (Philippines) '55; ABPMR; Sr.-Cons. PhysMed., Dept. of Health, Prov. of Newfoundland; Cons. PhysMed., St. John's Gen. Hosp., St. John's San., Children's Rehab. Centre & Hosp. for Mental & Nervous Diseases.

CANNELL, Douglas E.; 69 Bloor St. E., Toronto 5, Ont.; 371 Walmer Rd., Toronto 4, Ont. (res); Tor '27; B.Sc. (Med); FRCS(C); FACOG; ObstGyn; Med. Dir., Ont. Cancer Treatment & Research Fdn.; Tel. 923-1830.

CANNON, B. W.; 401—6th Ave., New Westminster, B.C. (res); Qns '17; Retired.

CANNON, Harry E.; Cannon Clinic, McCallum Rd., Abbotsford, B.C.; Man '33.

CANNON, Peter J. S.; Box 90, Mayerthorpe, Alta.; London (Eng.) '55; D.Obst, R.C.O.G.

CANT, Donald; Medical Centre, Corner Brook, Nfld.; 23 Farm Rd. (res); Durham (Eng.) '39; **F.A.C.S., F.C.C.P., F.I.C.S., GenSurg; ThorSurg; Tel. 634-2819.**

CANTELON, C. Bruce; West Lorne, Ont.; Wes '46.

CANTELON, Gerald W.; 290 Giles Blvd. E., Windsor, Ont.; 1191 Kildare Rd. (res); Wes '42; Psy; Ass't. Dir. (Psy.), Metropolitan Hosp.; Tel. 253-5908.

CANTELON, J. Frank; 411 Med. Arts Bldg., 170 St. George St., Toronto 5, Ont.; 90 Lawrence Cres (res); Wes '32; FACP, IntMed; Dir. Diabetes Clinic (OPD), Tor. Western Hosp.; Cons. Geriatric Centre; Cons. Phys., Orthopaedic & Rheumatic Hosp.; Tel. WA 1-7990.

CANTELOPE, Douglas C.; Pelham St., Lunenburg, N.S.; Dal'42; GenSurg (N.S.); Active Staff, Dawson Mem., Fishermen's Mem. & Lunenburg Mun. Hosp's.; Port Phys.; District Coroner; Tel. 634-4454.

CANTERO, Antonio; 1396 St. Catherine St. W., Room 417, Montreal, P.Q.; 98 Elmwood Pl., Outremont (res); McG '27; M.Sc., Gastroent. (P.Q.), IntMed; Research Dir., Montreal Cancer Inst., Notre Dame Hosp.; **Assoc.-in-Int. Med., Hubert Reddy Memorial Hosp.: Co. Dir., Cancer Inst., Rio de Janeio, Brazil; Tel. LA 5-6363.**

CANTIN, Austin; 365 rue Tait, Ville Saint-Laurent, **P.Q. (res); Lav '31; D.P.H.; Div. of** Quarantine, Immigration & Seamen, Dept. of National Health & Welfare.

CANTIN, Georges; 100 Jeannotte, Mascouche, Cte L' Assomption, P. Q.; Lav '49.

CANTIN, **Jacques;** Mon'59; FRCS(C), GenSurg; Staff, Hop. Hotel Dieu, Montreal, P.Q.

CANTIN, Jules; C.P. 55, 1661 rue St-Calixte, Plessisville, Meg., P.Q.; Lav '39; Med. Dir., Hop. du Sacre-Coeur; Tel. 362-2224.

CANTIN, Marc; Apt. 7, 4820 Cote St. Catharine Rd., Montreal 26, P.Q. (res); Lav '58; Research, Inst. Experim. Surg.

CANTIN, Marcel; 143 Ave. Giroux, Laval des Rapides, Montreal 40, P.Q. (res); Lav '50; D.P.H., PH(P.Q.); Med. Health Serv. U. of **Montreal; Tel. RE 3-9951.**

CANTIN, P. F. Roland; St. Pierre, Man.; London (Eng.) '55; MRCS (Eng.); LRCP (Lond.); MCGP; Dist. Coroner; Med. Staff, De Salaberry Hosp.; Tel. 202.

CANTIN, Raymond; 268 rue Notre Dame, Donnacona, Cte. Portneuf, P.Q.; Lav '54.

CANTIN, Real; 2665 Chemin des Quatre-Bougeois, Quebec 10, P.Q.; Lav '60.

CANTIN, **Robert;** Lav'65; Res., Hop. Hotel Dieu, Quebec, P.Q.

CANTLIE, George S.; Royal Victoria Hosp., Montreal 2, P.Q.; McG'60; FRCP(C), IntMed; Research Fell. (Haem.); Tel. VI 2-1251, **Ext. 397.**

CANTLIE, Helene B.; 4918 Piedmont St., Montreal 26, P.Q.; McG'65.

CANTOR, Hymie; Cor. 3rd Ave. & High St., Drawer 198, Ladysmith, B.C.; Man '37.

CANTOR, Kenneth Z.; McG '63; Res., Montreal Gen. Hosp., Montreal, P.Q.

CANTOR, Max. M.; 510 Tegler Bldg., Edmonton, Alta.; 8003 Saskatchewan Dr. (res); Man '29; **F.A.C.P.; IntMed; Assoc. Phys. (Emer.), U. of** Alberta Hosp.; Ass't. Clin. Prof. Path. (Med. Jurisprudence & Toxicol.), U. of Alberta; Coroner, **N.W.T. & Yukon T.; Chief Prov. Coroner, Al**berta; Tel. 424-5877; 229-3355.

CANTWELL, Joseph F.; 5760 Inglis St., Halifax, **N.S.; Dal '49; FAGS; Tel. 423-8538.**

CAOUETTE, J. Guy; 1000 Chemin Ste.-Foy, Quebec 6, P.Q.; Lav '57; Otol.; Tel. 683-3092.

CAOUETTE, Maurice G.; 401 est, Grande-Allee, Quebec 4, P.Q.; 1276 Ave.-des-Pins, Sillery, (res); Lav '46; FRCS(C), ObstGyn; Ass't. (ObstGyn), Hotel-Dieu-de-Quebec; Assoc. Prof., Laval U.; **Tel. 525-5675.**

CAOUETTE, Robert; 1026 rue St. Jean, Quebec 4, P.Q.; 920 Adolphe Routhier (res); Lav '42; F.A.C.P., F.R.C.P.(C) IntMed; Assoc. Prof. **(Clin. Med.), Hotel Dieu de Quebec; Tel. 522-4236.**

CAOUETTE, Suzanne; App. 2, 3158 rue Hochelaga, Quebec 10, P.Q.; **Lav '60. Retired.**

CAPARAS, **Virginia P.;** Santo Tomas (Philipp.) '56; Staff, Saskatchewan Hosp., Box 700, Weyburn, Sask.; Tel. 842-3812.

CAPE, David G. M.; 85 Gables Ct., Beaconsfield, Montreal 33, P.Q. (res); McG '50; Anaes; Staff, **Lachine Gen. Hosp.; Tel. ME 7-1161.**

CAPELLO, Peter J.; 420 Central Med. Bldg., 1105 Carling Ave., Ottawa 3, Ont.; Ott '56; FRCS(C); GenSurg; Active Staff (Surg.), Ottawa Civic Hosp.; Lect., U. of Ottawa; Tel. 728-3563.

CAPLAN, Barry; 310 Boyd Bldg., 388 Portage Ave., Winnipeg 1, Man.; Man' 57; FRCS(C); Urol; Active Staff, St. Boniface Gen. & Victoria Gen. Hosp's.; Court. Staff, Winnipeg Gen., Misercordia & Children's Hosp's.; Tel. 943-2162.

CAPLAN, Barry L.; Alb'65; Jr. Ass't. Res., University of Alberta Hosp., Edmonton, Alta.

CAPLAN, Harvey; 4119 Sherbrooke St. W., Montreal, P.Q.; 3115 Lacombe Ave. (res); McG **'44; Otol; Tel. 935-9126.**

CAPLAN, Hyman; 4631 Sherbrooke St. W., Montreal, P.Q.; 2082 Fulton Rd. Twn. of Mt. Royal (res); McG '44; D.A.B.P.N. (Child Psy); Psy; Ass't. Dir. Dept. of Psy., Montreal Children's Hosp.; Assoc. Prof. (Psy.), McGill U.; Tel. WE 2-9069.

CAPLAN, Joseph; Ste. 416, 1849 Yonge St., Toronto 7, Ont.; Glasgow (Scot.)'57; D.Psy; Psy; Active Staff, Lakeshore Psy Hosp.; Tel. 483-5858.

CAPLAN, Murray C.; Sask'65; Res., Jewish Gen. Hosp., Montreal 26, P.Q.

CAPLAN, Ronald M.; McG '62; Res., Royal Victoria Hosp., Montreal, P.Q.

CAPLE, Harold H.; Highcroft Med. Bldg., 319 Granville St., Vancouver 9, B.C.; 6044 Collingwood St. (res); Tor '24; DPH; FRCOG; ObstGyn; Hd., Dept. of ObstGyn., St. Vincent's Hosp.; Tel. RE 8-5313.

CAPLIN, Doreen F.; 32 Forest Wood, Toronto 12, Ont.; Tor '49; Anaes; Staff, New Mt. Sinai Hosp.; Tel. EM 6-7361.

CAPLING, Lloyd C.; Ste. 14, 22707 Loughheed Hwy Haney, B.C. 21775 Ridgeway Cr. (res); Alb '48; MCGP; Active Staff, Maple Leaf Hosp.; Tel. 463-4102.

CAPOMBASSIS, Panos A.; 5025 Sherbrooke St. W., Ste. 355, Montreal, P.Q.; Athens (Greece) '55; Ophth (P.Q.); Teach. Staff, McGill U.; Tel. 488-5669.
CAPON, Alec W.; 200 St. Clair W. Ave., Toronto,, Ont.; Cambridge (Eng.) '42; M.R.C.P. (Lond.), F.C.C.P.; IntMed.; Staff, O.P.D., Toronto Western Hosp.; CMO, Canada Mercantile & Gen. Re-Ins. Co., London Assur. Co. & Royal Ins. Co.; Tel. WA 1-1550.
CAPPE, Solomon; 395 College St., Toronto, Ont.; 57 Old Park Rd. (res); Tor '34; M.C.G.P.; Med. Staff, New Mt. Sinai Hosp.; Tel. WA. 2-2254.
CAPPON, Daniel; 516 Medical Arts Bldg., 170 St. George St., Toronto 5,, Ont.; London (Eng.) '44; MRCP (Eng.); DPH; FRCP (Edin.); Psy; Research Assoc., Toronto Gen. Hosp.; Head, Perceptual Research Lab., Dept. of Psy., U. of Toronto; Tel. WA 1-6653.
CARBALLO, Arthur S.; 8353-11th Ave., Ste. N 106, Burnaby 3, B.C.; Barcelona (Spain)'57; Anaes.
CARBALLO, Arthur S.; Ste. N-106, 8353-11th Ave., Burnaby, B.C.; Barcelona (Spain)'57.
CARBIN, Robert J.; Tor '62; Intn., Hosp. for Sick Children, Toronto 2, Ont.
CARBONE, Renzo; Bologna (Italy) '50; Res. Ontario Hosp., Toronto 2, Ont.
CARBONIN, George; Padua (Italy)'46; Res., Mtl. Neurol. Hosp., 3801 University St., Montreal 2, P.Q.
CARBONNEAU, Marcel; 3070 Le Chasseur, Ste Foy, P.Q.; Lav'59; OrthSurg (P.Q.).
CARBOTTE, Marcel N. N.; 1000 Chm. Ste.-Foy, Quebec 6, P.Q.; 305 Grande Allee (res); Lav '41; ObstGyn (P.Q.); Ass't. Gyn., Hop. St. Sacrement; Tel. 681-6241.
CARD, John R. J.; 452 Main St. E., Hamilton, Ont.; Qns '37; DermSyph; Tel. JA 9-3240.
CARD, Lawrence W. B.; 1726 W. Broadway, Vancouver 9, B.C.; 1178 W. 38th, Vancouver 13 (res); Tor '38; D.Rad., D&TRad; Staff, St. Vincent's Grace & Children's Hosp's.; Tel. RE 8-5118.
CARD, Lorne C.; Apt. 107, 697 Eglinton Ave. W., Toronto 10, Ont. (res); McG '31; M.O., Workmen's Comp. Bd., Malton Rehab. Centre; Tel. 244-1761.
CARDARELLI, Giovanni G.; 600 Caledonia Rd., Toronto 10, Ont.; Rome (Italy) '51; Tel. RU 7-9131.
CARDEN, Roger D.; London (Eng.) '52; M.H.O., Rose Blanche, Nfld.
CARDILLO, Peter J.; Workmen's Comp. Bd., 115 Torbarrie Rd., Downsview, Ont.; Wes'59; GenSurg.
CARDIN, Jean L.; 477 Principale, Farnham, Co. Mississquoi, P.Q.; Mon '47.
CARDIN, Laurent; Mon'65; Res., Hop. Maisonneuve, Montreal 36, P.Q.
CARDINAL, Guy; 1021 Bar Le Duc, Ste. Foy, Quebec, P.Q.; Mon'59; Pum. Dis. & TB (P.Q.).
CARDISH, Albert A.; 1 Old Park Rd., Toronto 10, Ont.; 37 Elm Ridge Dr. (res); Tor '32; M.C.G.P.; Staff, New Mt. Sinai Hosp.; Tel. RU 2-6781.
CARDWELL, Henry A.; 13 Linwood Dr., Welland, Ont.; Wes '47; D.Psy.; Psy; Dir. Welland County Mental Health Clinic, Welland County Gen. Hosp.; Tel. RE 2-6111.
CARDWELL, Robert J.; 279 King St., Midland, Ont.; 171 Hugel Ave. E. (res); Tor '50; Tel. 526-5408.
CARERE, Romulus P.; Ste. 202, 77 Westmount Rd., Guelph, Ont.; 16 Caledonia Ave. (res); Ott'54; Vice Pres., St. Joseph's Hosp. Med. Staff; Tel. TA 2-9492.
CARETTE, J. Paul; Box 217, Sillery, P.Q.; Lav'32; GenSurg.
CARETTE, Laval; 801 Cardinal Rouleau, Quebec 6, P.Q.; Lav '33.
CAREY, Thomas M., S/L; Queen's U. (Belfast, Ire.) '48; Anaes; RCAF Station, Cold Lake, Alta.
CARGILL, Lorne G.; Box 40, Thornbury, Ont.; Wes '23; Staff (Ophth), Meaford Gen. Hosp.; Tel. 599-5932.
CARGILL, Richard E. D.; 953 Garwood Ave., Ottawa, Ont.; Oxford (Eng.) '24; LRCP (Lond.); MRCS (Eng.); FRCS (Edin.); FRCS(C); Obst-Gyn. Retired.
CARIGNAN, Andre; 97 Notre Dame E., Victoriaville, P.Q.; 82 Notre Dame E. (res); Lav '44; Tel. 752-2350.
CARIGNAN, A. Pierre; 1773 de l'Eglise, Montreal 20, P.Q.; Mon '59.
CARIGNAN, Gaston; 10595 Hamel, Montreal 12, P.Q.; 11803 Pontrincourt (res); Lav '50; Anaes; Staff, Hop.-Notre-Dame & Hop.-Le-Gardeur, Repentigny; Tel. LA 5-6363, Local 306.
CARIGNAN, Leopold; C.P. 189, 14A Richardson, Beauharnois, P.Q.; Lav '50.
CARIGNAN, Louis; 215 rue Chasse, Asbestos, P.Q.; Lav'65.
CARIGAN, Raymond; 522 Notre-Dame, Repentigny,, P.Q.; Mon '61.
CARLE, Alfred; 1780 Amherst St., Montreal, P.Q.; Mon '34; Tel. LA 8-1521.
CARLE, J. Aime; 5005 Ave. Delorimier, Montreal 35, P.Q.; Mon '38; MCGP; Tel. 721-1361.
CARLE, Leopold; 2650 Beaubien St. E., Montreal, P.Q.; Mon '32; M.C.G.P.; Tel. 721-4400.
CARLE, Robert; Mon'62; Paed(P.Q.); Staff, Hop. Ste. Jeanne d'Arc, Montreal, P.Q.
CARLE, Roger; Lav'64; Res., Hop. St-Michel-Archange, Quebec 5, P.Q.; Abroad.
CARLEN, Sidney A.; Ste. 310, 99 Avenue Rd., Toronto 5, Ont.; 16 Highland Cres. (res); Tor '36; A.A.C.P.; Int Med.; Tel. WA 1-6245.
CARLETON, Barry M.; 510 Main St. N., Dauphin, Man.; Man'62; Tel. 638-6611.
CARLETON, G. Wylie; 721 Coxwell Ave., Toronto, Ont.; 100 Hudson Dr. (res); Tor'11; MCGP(Hon.); Tel. HO 1-6000.
CARLETON, Merrell; 513 Medical Arts Bldg., Winnipeg, Man.; 383 Overdale St., St. James (res.); Man '31; MCGP; (Hon.); Tel. WH 2-8063.
CARLISLE, Andrew M.; Grande Prairie, Alta.; Tor '21; Dist. Coroner; Retired.
CARLISLE, James S.; 223 Echo Dr., Ottawa, Ont.; Alb '53; DTM & H (Lond); Assoc. Staff, Ott. Gen. Hosp.; Pt-time Phys., Addiction Research Fdn., Ottawa Br.; Tel. CE 5-8342.
CARLISLE, Robert V.; 437 Highland Rd. E., Kitchener, Ont.; Tor '59; AMCGP; Ass't. Med. Dir., Mutual Life Assur. Co., Waterloo; Tel. 744-2592.
CARLOW, Donald R.; 1175 Cook St., Victoria, B.C.; 710 Chesterlea Rd. (res); U.B.C. '60 AMCGP; Active Staff, St. Joseph's Hosp.; Tel. EV 8-5577.
CARLSEN, Lloyd N.; One Medical Place, 20 Wynford Dr., Don Mills, Ont.; 2901 Lawrence Ave. E., Scarborough, Ont.; Qns'57; FRCS(C); PlasSurg; Staff, Scarborough Gen. & Toronto East Gen. Hosp's.; Tel. 759-2172.
CARLSON, Glen C.; Box 998, Merritt, B.C.; UBC'60; Vis. Staff, Nicola Valley Gen. Hosp.; Tel. 378-2286.
CARLSON, Jacqueline A.; '56; Res., Hosp. for Sick Children, Toronto 2, Ont.
CARLSON, Kenneth M.; 279 King St., Midland, Ont.; Man '61.
CARLSON, Margaret; Box 2090, Merritt, B.C.; UBC'64.
CARLSON, Robert J.; 7937 Granville St., Vancouver 14, B.C.; 3953 W. King Edward Ave. (res); Tor '58; Vis. Staff, St. Paul's, Vancouver Gen., St. Vincent's & Grace Hosp's; Tel. AM 1-1730.
CARLYLE, R. W. Capt.; CFPO 5050 Cdn. Armed Forces, Europe; Tor '63; Abroad.
CARMICHAEL, John A.; 35 Copperfield Dr., Kingston, Ont.; Qns'53; FRCS(C), ObstGyn.
CARMONA, Robert A.; Man'63; Res. (Anaes.), St. Boniface Gen. Hosp., Winnipeg, Man.
CARNAGHAN, William C.; Forestburg, Alta.; Wes '33; MCGP.
CARNAHAN, Clifford J.; Box 100, Langton, Ont.; Qns '50.

CARNAT, Morris; 406 Medical Centre, 906-8th Ave. S.W., Calgary, Alta.; Alb'34; Psy; Dir. of Psy., Calgary Gen. Hosp.; Staff, DVA Colonel Belcher Hosp.; Cons. Calgary School Bd.; Cons. Attorney General Dept., Govt. of Alberta; Tel. 266-1988.

CARNDUFF, Donald W.; Med. Arts Clinic, Regina, Sask.; 30 Langley St. (res); Qns '51; GenSurg; Sr. Active Staff, Regina Gen. & Grey Nun's Hosp's; Tel. LA 2-1651.

CARNEY, Leonard R.; 13634 Grosvenor Rd., North Surrey, B.C.; Edinburgh (Scot.) '58.

CARNOVALE, Benjamin V.; Qns'62; Res., c/o 986 Falcon Blvd., Burlington, Ont.

CAROM, Donald P.; Ste. 504, Med. Arts Bldg., Windsor, Ont.; Tor'63; Tel. 256-0382.

CARON, Claude; Mon'65; Res., Hop. Gen. du Christ Roi, Montreal 19, P.Q.

CARON, Claude H.; 1848, Chemin Gomin, Quebec 6, P.Q.; Lav '63. Abroad.

CARON, E. Sylvio; 2965 Ave. Royale, Quebec 5, P.Q.; Lav '19; F.R.C.P.(C), NeurPsy; Med. Dir., Roy-Rousseau Clin.; Cons. Neur., Hop.-Ste-Foy; Prof. Neur, Laval U.; Tel. LA 9-4511.

CARON, Florent; St. Ursule; Co. Maskinonge, P.Q.; Lav '56.

CARON, Gaetan; St. Raymond, Co. Portneuf, P.Q.; Lav '62.

CARON, Gerald; 30 est, boul St-Joseph, Montreal 14, P.Q.; Mon '50; MCGP.

CARON, Gerard; 73, King George St., Kenogami, P.Q.; 23 rue Fortier (res); Lav '34.

CARON, Jacques; Lav '57; Otol; Staff, Jeffery Hale's Hosp., Quebec 6, P.Q.; Tel. 681-0943.

CARON, Jean; 2944 Les Grondines, Ste-Foy, Quebec 10, P.Q.; Lav '49; Anaes (P.Q.); Staff, Hop. St-Francois d'Assises; Tel. 529-7311.

CARON, Jean; Res. c/o 52-19th Ave., Roxboro, P.Q.; Abroad.

CARON, Jean-Guy; 595 est, Boul. Charest, Quebec 2, P.Q.; 2394 St-Georges, Apt. 3, Giffard **(res); Lav '61; Tel. 529-9721.**

CARON, Jean M.; 14 est, Dumais, Thetford Mines, P.Q.; 10-9th rue (res); Lav '50.

CARON, Jean M.; Main St., Mattawa, Ont.; Ott '52; M.O.H. & Coroner, Dist. Nipissing; Sup't., **Mattawa Gen. Hosp; M.O., C.P.R.; Tel. 744-5331.**

CARON, Joseph O. Jean; 210 St. George St., Bathurst, N.B.; Princess Dr. (res); McG '52; F.R.C.P.(C), Anaes; Staff, Hotel-Dieu-de-St.-Joseph; Tel. 546-5622.

CARON, Lorenzo; Sayabec, Co. Matapedia, P.Q.; Lav'57; MCGP.

CARON, Marie; Lav '64; Res., Hop. Notre Dame, Montreal 24, P.Q.

CARON, Maurice; 5088 Blvd. Langelier, Montreal 5, P.Q.; Mon '31; PulmDis & TB (P.Q.); Staff, Dept. of National Health & Welfare; Tel. 256-3880.

CARON, Paul; Lav '60; Anaes; Staff, Hop. Notre-Dame-de-Beauce, St. Georges, P.Q.; Tel. 228-4831.

CARON, Pierre; Ste. 519, 30 est Boul. St. Joseph, Montreal 14, P.Q.; Mon'57; FRCP(C); IntMed; Staff, Hop. Ste-Jeanne d'Arc; Cons. (Endocrin & IntMed.), Hop. St-Michel; Tel. 845-4241.

CARON, Pierre; 215 ouest, Des Chenes, Quebec 3, P.Q.; 7320 Germain, Charlesbourg (res); Lav '58; IntMed. (P.Q.); Tel. 626-0464.

CARON, Placide; 24, St. Joseph, Bromptonville, P.Q.; Lav '63.

CARON, Raymond; 159 ouest rue Craig, Montreal, P.Q.; Mon'44; Med. Dir., Montreal Transport Commiss.; M.O., British American Oil Co. & Shawinigan Chemicals; Tel. 877-6021.

CARON, Real R.; 1307 Boul. Masson, Les Saules, P.Q.; Lav'53; Tel. 683-9966.

CARON, Richard E.; 15 Prefontaine W., Ste.-Agathe-des-Monts, P.Q.; Mon '45; MPH (Yale); **MCGP; Tel. 326-2715.**

CARON, Roger; 11769 Pasteur, Montreal 12, P.Q. (res); Lav '49; Anaes; Staff, Sacred Heart Hosp.; Tel. 334-1210.

CARON, Roger; 595 Charest Blvd. E., Quebec 2, **P.Q.; 75½ Charleroi St., Giffard; Lav '50; Tel. 529-9721.**

CARON, Roger; 168 Cuting, Coaticook, P.Q.; Lav '62.

CARON, Roger A.; 1447 Laverendrye, Trois-Rivieres, P.Q.; Lav '52; MCGP; Tel. FR 6-6611.

CARON-SMITH, Ginette; 2300 Goyer St., Montreal 26, P.Q.; Mon'65.

CARON, Wilfrid M.; 1000 Chemin-Ste.-Foy, Quebec, P.Q.; 137 St. Felix, Cap Rouge (res); Lav '39; FACS, FRCS(C), GenSurg; ThorSurg (P.Q.); Prof. & Hd. Dept. of Surg., U. of Laval; Tel. 683-4481.

CARPENDALE, Michael T.; 11416-73rd. Ave., Edmonton, Alta. (res); St. Thomas' Hosp. (London, Eng.) '47; M.Sc. (Minn.), L.R.C.P. (Lond.), M.R.C.S.(Eng.); **PhysMed & Rehab; Dir., Rehab., U. of Alberta Hosp.; Ass't. Prof. (Med.), U. of Alberta; Abroad.**

CARPENTER, Charles W.; 608 Fairmont Med. Bldg., 750 W. Broadway, Vancouver 9, B.C.; Qns '54; M.Sc., FRCS(C), ObstGyn; Staff, Vancouver Gen. Hosp.; Ass't. Prof. (ObstGyn.), U. of British Columbia; Tel. 876-1415.

CARPENTER, John C.; Med. Assoc. Clinic, 405 Hendryx St., Nelson, B.C.; 1413 Front St. (res); Alb '52; Tel. 352-6611.

CARPENTER, Lorne E.; 310 Toronto Western Medical Bldg., 25 Leonard Ave, Toronto 2B, Ont.; **26 Pinehurst Cres. (res); Tor '42; D.Psy; Psy; Assoc. Staff (Psy), Toronto Western Hosp.** Tel. EM 3-0773.

CARPENTER, William B.; 1623-3rd St. N.W., Calgary, Alta.; Alb'56.

CARPENTIER, Paul A.; Lav'65; Res., Hop. Hotel-Dieu, Quebec 4, P.Q.

CARR, A. Michael; Box 40, Catalina, Trinity Bay, Nfld (res); Durham (Eng.) '59; M.B., B.S.; MCGP; Dist. Med. Health Officer; Tel. Catalina 2222.

CARR, Charles W.; 9 Colindale St., Fleming Heights, Armdale, N.S. (res); Tor '26; Anaes; M.O. Camp Hill Hosp., Halifax, N.S.; Tel. 423-1371.

CARR, David H.; 649 Viscount Rd., London, Ont.; **(res); Liverpool (Eng.)'40; Ph.D. (Anat.) Assoc.** Prof., Micro. Anat., U. of Western Ont.; Tel. GE 9-1681.

CARR, Donald M.; Alb'65; Res., University Hosp., Edmonton, Alta.

CARR, Gerald R.; 289 McArthur Rd., Ottawa 7, Ont.; Ott'63; AMCGP; Tel. 749-4956.

CARR, Meyer; 452 Main St. E., Hamilton, Ont.; 40 Amelia St. (res); Tor '33; DCH (Lond.). M.R.C.P. (Edin.); F.A.A.P.; Paed; Chief of **Paed., St. Joseph's Hosp.; Tel. JA 7-3821.**

CARR, Stephen F.; Bow Island, Alta.; Alb '35; Tel. Area 403; 545-2477.

CARR, William G.; Man'60; Paed; Staff, Winnipeg Children's Hosp., Winnipeg, Man.

CARRENO-SEGURA, Luis; 3495 Tecumseh E., Windsor, Ont.; Madrid (Spain)'51; GenSurg.

CARRERAS, Pedro; Mental Health Clinic, Swift Current, Sask.; Barcelona (Spain) '48.

CARRIE, Alan W.; 2221 Keele St., Toronto 15, Ont.; 27 Westmount Pk. Rd. Weston (res); Tor '46; F.A.C.S., F.R.C.S.(C), GenSurg; Active Surg. Staff, Northwestern Gen. & North York Branson Hosp's.; Tel. 247-7010.

CARRIER, Charles; 40 ave Lamontagne, Quebec 3, P.Q.; Lav'57; FAAP; FRCP(C); Paed; Ass't. Dept. of Paed., Hop. St. Francois d'Assise; Prof. Dept. of Paed., Laval U.; Tel. 523-2412.

CARRIER, G. Robert; 746 Avenue Dalquier, Quebec 10, P.Q.; Lav'60; Biochem. (P.Q.); Admin. Staff, Faculty of Med., U. of Laval.

CARRIER, Henri; 285 Ave. Begin, Chicoutimi, P.Q.; 225 Delisle, Chicoutimi Nord (res); Lav '50; M.Ch.Orth. (Liverpool); OrthSurg (P.Q.); Staff, Hop. Hotel Dieu St. Vallier; Tel. 549-3051.

CARRIER, J. Gaetan; 159A St.-Damase, Drummondville, P.Q.; 552 Ferland (Res); Lav '59; Tel. GR 8-2454.

CARRIER Ovila; St. Edouard, Cte. Lotbiniere, P.Q.; Lav '45.

CARRIER, Rene E.; Lav'57; Res. (Rad.), Royal Victoria Hosp., Montreal, P.Q.

CARRIERE, J. Serge; Mon '59; FRCP(C); IntMed; Staff, Hop. Maisonneuve, Montreal 36, P.Q.

CARRIERE, N. J., S/L; Royal Ottawa San., Ottawa 8, Ont.; Alb'54.

CARRIGAN, Edward P.; Liverpool (Eng.)'52; Res., Ottawa Civic Hosp., Ottawa, Ont.
CARROLL, Brooke P.; London (Eng.)'55; MRCS (Eng.); LRCP (Lond.); AMCGP; Res., Vancouver General Hosp., Vancouver 9, B.C.
CARROLL, James J.; P. O. Box 111, Bay St., Antigonish, N.S.; Hillcrest St. (res); Dal '24; MCGP; Vis. Staff, St. Martha's Hosp.; Tel. 863-4727.
CARROLL, James R.; 25 Hillside Dr., Brampton, Ont.; Alb'59; Flight-Surg., Air Canada; Assoc. Staff, Peel Mem. Hosp.; Tel. 459-3013.
CARROLL, John J.; 6325 Fraser St., Vancouver 15, B.C.; 1530 W. 37th Ave. (res); McG '40; FACA; Anaes; Dir. Anaes., Grace Hosp., Richmond Gen. & Riverview Hosp's.; Clin. Ass't., U. of British Columbia; Tel. FA 5-4040.
CARROLL, Joseph; Fort Garry Med. Centre, 1288 **Pembina Hwy., Winnipeg 9, Man.; Nat. U. (Dublin, Ire.) '48; Staff Off., Med. Serv., R.C.A.F., Winnipeg; Tel. GR 4-1351.**
CARROLL, Joseph J.; 707 Med. Arts Bldg., 1 Young St., Hamilton, Ont.; Dal'53; DABS; GenSurg; Staff, Hamilton Gen. & St. Joseph's Hosp's; Court. Staff, Chedoke Gen. Hosp.; Tel. JA 9-6355.
CARROLL, Louis H.; Box 300, Haliburton, Ont.; Tor '33; MOH, Dysart et al; Dist. Coroner, Co. of Haliburton; Tel. 178.
CARROLL, Norris C.; Dal '60; Res., Hosp. for Sick Children, Toronto, Ont.
CARROLL, S. Edwin; Surgery Office, St. Joseph's Hosp., London, Ont.; Wes'53; FRCS(C); Cardiovasc. & ThorSurg; GenSurg; Chief Surg., St. Joseph's Hosp.; Tel. 439-1121.
CARROW, Glenford W.; 2700 Dundas St. W., Toronto 9, Ont.; Tor '22; M.S., F.R.C.S.(C), GenSurg; Tel. RO 9-5755.
CARRUTHERS, Bruce M.; 4460 W. 6th. Ave., Vancouver 8, B.C. (res.); Qns. '56; FRCP(C), Int. Med.; Staff, Shaughnessy Hosp.; Tel. 6-6767.
CARRUTHERS, Calvert M.; 369 London Rd., Apt. 302, Sarnia, Ont. (res); Qns '21; L.R.C.P. (Lond.), M.R.C.S. (Eng.), F.A.C.S., F.I.C.S., F.R.C.S. (Eng.), F.R.C.S.(C), GenSurg; Chief of Staff, St. Joseph's Hosp.; Cons. Surg., Sarnia Gen. Hosp.; Retired.
CARRUTHERS, Ewen P.; 1635 Abbott St., Kelowna, B.C.; 1847 Maple St. (res); McG '41; FCCP, **AACP; IntMed; Phys., Kelowna & Vice-Pres. Med. Staff, Kelowna Gen. Hosp.; Phys. (Cardiovasc. & Respirat.) Underhill Clinic; Tel. 762-2740.**
CARRUTHERS, Grace F.; 442 N. Christina St., Sarnia, Ont.; Wes'56; Staff, Lambton Health Unit; Tel. 336-3046.
CARRUTHERS, Howard C.; 841 Collinson St., Victoria, B.C.; 2233 Cadboro Bay Rd. (res); Man '48; Anaes; Staff, (Anaes.), St. Joseph's Hosp.; Tel. 384-1131.
CARRUTHERS, John; 92 Otter Cres., Toronto 12, Ont. **(res); Wes '55; Path; Staff, Banting** Inst.; Tel. 928-2011.
CARRUTHERS, Walter B.; 137 Wellington St., Sarnia, Ont.; 1428 Lakeshore Rd. (res); Qns '20; FRCP(C); **IntMed; Tel. 344-5261.**
CARRUTHERS, Walter L.; Mount Albert, Ont.; **Tor '22; Retired.**
CARSCADDEN, Terence R.; Med. Centre, Lively, Ontario; Qns'64; Tel. 692-4774.
CARSCADDEN, Walter G.; 170 St. George St., Toronto, Ont.; Tor'25; F.A.C.S.; GenSurg; Assoc. in Gen. Surg. U. of Toronto; Att. Surg., St. Michael's Hosp.; Tel. WA 3-5053.
CARSCALLEN, Howard B.; 97 Kingsford Cres., London, Ont. (res); Wes '35; D.Psy., Psy; Med. Spec. (Psy.), Westminster D.V.A. Hosp.; Instr. (Psy.), Dept. of Psy., U. of Western Ontario **Med. School; Tel. 432-6711.**
CARSCALLEN, W. Franklin; 209 Renfrew House, Rideau Towers, Calgary, Alta. (res); McG '22; Retired.
CARSON, G. Donald; Ste. 460, 8409-112th St., Edmonton, Alta.; 7310-118 St. (res); Alb '42; Psy; Staff, University Hosp.; Cons. Psy., Alberta Alcoholism Fdn.; Instr. (Psy.) U of Alberta; Tel. GE 9-1732.
CARSON, George M.; 2008 Park Ave., Bowness, Alta. (res); Tor '11; Retired.
CARSON, George T.; 340 McLeod St., Ottawa, Ont.; Qns'41; FACOG; FRCOG; ObstGyn; Att'd. Staff, (ObstGyn.), Ottawa Civic Hosp.; Chief ObstGyn., Riverside Hosp.
CARSON, James D.; 200 St. Clair Ave. W., Toronto 7, Ont.; 280 Hollywood Ave., Willowdale (res); Tor '56; MCGP; Tel. WA 2-8464.
CARSON, James H.; 221 Brant Ave., Brantford, Ont.; Mt. Pleasant (res); Tor'45; MCGP; Staff, Brantford Gen. & St. Joseph's Hosp's.; Tel. 753-8666.
CARSON, J. Donald; 229 King Ave., Bathurst, N.B.; Dal '55; MCGP; Active Staff, Hotel-Dieu Hosp.; Tel. 65256.
CARSON, J. Elmer; 221 Brant Ave., Brantford, Ont.; Tel. PL 3-8666.
CARSON, Max M.; 418A Parliament St., Toronto, Ont.; Tor '53; Staff, New Mt. Sinai Hosp., Wellesley & Doctor's Hosp's.; Tel. 924-6116.
CARSON, Palmer S.; 490 Huron St., Toronto, **Ont.; Tor '31; Tel. WA 1-0134.**
CARSON, Patrick J.; 1669 Victoria, Prince George, B.C.; UBC '55; Tel. 564-9311.
CARTER, Arnold K.; 2115 Gladstone Ave., Windsor, Ont.; 1538 Victoria Ave., (res); Wes '47; M.C.G.P.; Staff (IntMed & G.P.), Grace Hosp.; Staff (ObstGyn & G.P.), Metropolitan Hosp.; Court. Staff, Hotel Dieu Hosp.; Tel. 252-8261.
CARTER, Clement J. O.; 930 Chemin Ste Foy, Quebec 6, P.Q.; Lav'56.
CARTER, Gordon W.; Lockwood Clinic, 300 Bloor St. E., Toronto 5, Ont.; Tor'53; Tel. 921-2121.
CARTER, Guy; 2091 Chemin Ste-Foy, Quebec 10, P.Q.; Lav '57.
CARTER, Harold R.; 701 Campbell Bldg., 1029 Douglas St., Victoria, B.C.; Ste. 450, 1105 Pandora Ave.; UBC '54; FACS; OrthSurg; Tel. 384-4121.
CARTER, Ivan E.; London (Eng.)'62; Caledonia, Ont.
CARTER, Jean; Mon'64; Res., Verdun Gen. Hosp., Montreal 19, P.Q.
CARTER, Stefan A.; 234 Elm St., Winnipeg 9, Man. (res); Man '54; M.Sc.; Dir., Cardiovas. **St. Boniface Hosp.; Ass't. Prof. (Physiol.), U. of Manitoba; Tel. GR 4-9110.**
CARTER, William A.; Associate Clinic, Red Deer, Alta.; 4410—43 Ave. (res); Tor '42; Dist. Coroner; Tel. 346-2057.
CARTER, Yale K. W/C; Dept. of Rad., National Defence, Med. Centre, Ottawa, Ont.; Qns '53; Diag Rad.
CARTIER, George E.; Ste. 309, 3875 St-Urbain, Montreal 18, P.Q.; Mon '34; GenSurg; Head (Vasc.), Dept. of Surg., Hotel-Dieu Hosp.; Ass't. Prof., U. of Montreal; Tel. 845-4925.
CARTIER, Jacques; C.P. 250, 120 Rue Principal, **L'Annonciation, P.Q.; Mon '34; Dist. Coroner.**
CARTIER, Jacques Jr.; C.P. 248, L'Annonciation, P.Q.; Mon'62.
CARTIER, Jules J. Sg/Lt.; 1509 Des Oblats, Chambly, P.Q.; Lav'64; Tel. 346-4411, Ext. 233.
CARTIER, Paul; Ste. 403, 3875, rue St-Urbain, Montreal 18, P.Q.; Mon '47; CardiovascSurg (P.Q.); Surg. I/C (Cardiovasc.) Hop. Ste. Justine; Ass't. Surg. (Cardiovasc.), Hop. Hotel-dieu.
CARTIER, Paul H.; Box 247, Thetford Mines, **P.Q. (res); Mon '34; D.P.H., F.A.P.H.A., Pulm.** Dis. & TB (P.Q.): Med. Dir., Thetford Indus**trial Clinic Inc.; Tel. 335-7159.**
CARTIER, Therese D.; 769 Dunlop Ave., Outremont, Montreal 8, P.Q. (res); Mon '45; Anaes; Anaes., Hotel Dieu de Montreal; Tel. VI 4-0161.
CARTMILL, Thomas; Med. Arts Clinic, Regina, Sask.; Glasgow (Scot.) '44; FRCS (Ed.); DLO (Lond.); Otol; Staff, Regina Gen. & Grey Nun's Hosp's.; Tel. 523-0691.
CARTWRIGHT, David B. M.; 314 Kerr St., Oakville, Ont.; 251 Riverside Dr. (res); Tor '57; Staff, Oakville-Trafalgar Mem. Hosp.; Tel. VI 5-4213.
CARVER, John B.; 6411 Quinpool Rd., Halifax, N.S.; Cambridge (Eng.)'53; Tel. 422-4526.
CARVETH, Richard W. J.; 1680 St. Clair Ave. W., Toronto, Ont.; Tor. '33; Tel. RO 9-3652.

CARVETH, W. Herbert; 100 Roxborough St. W., Toronto, Ont.; Tor '04; Retired.
CASE, George E.; 435 Park Ave., Newmarket, Ont.; Tor '22; M.C.G.P.
CASE, George L.; 150 Dublin St., Guelph, Ont. (res); Tor '28; A.C.R., Diag Rad; Staff, St. **Joseph's Hosp., Guelph; Tel. TA 4-2620.**
CASE, George R.; Medical Arts Bldg., 121 Wellington St., Barrie, Ont.; Tor'56; IntMed.
CASELLA, Luigi; 123 Edward St., Toronto 2, Ont.: Naples (Italy) '53; FRCP(C) IntMed; Staff, St. Michael's Hosp., Toronto, Ont.; Tel. 362-4461.
CASEY, John H.; Queensland (Australia) '56; Staff, Royal Victoria Hosp., Montreal, P.Q.; Research Fell. (Endocrin.), McGill U.; Tel. VI 2-1251.
CASEY, M. Thomas; 5880 Spring Garden Rd., Halifax, N.S.; 1607 Edward St. (res); Dal '53; DABS; FRCS(C); FACS; FICS; GenSurg; Active Staff (Surg.), Halifax Infirmary & Victoria Gen. Hosp.; Cons. Surg., Cdn. Forces Hosp.; Ass't. Prof. Surg., Dalhousie U.; Tel. 422-4529.
CASEY, R. Jack; Box 490, Didsbury, Alta.; Alb '57; MCGP.
CASEY, Stephen; 5417-44th Ave., Wetaskiwin, Alta. (res); Queen's U.(Belfast, Ire.) '45; B.A.O., **D.P.H. (Eng.); M.O.H., Wetoka Health Unit; Tel. 352-2578.**
CASHMAN, Edward F.; Windsor Towers Ouellette Ave., Windsor, Ont.; Ott '58; ObstGyn; Tel. 254-4041.
CASHMAN, T. Leo; 177 Alexander St., Pembroke, Ont.; Ott'53; AMCGP; Tel. RE 2-9362.
CASHMORE, Alan A.; Mental Health Centre, 4400W. Grandview-Douglas H'way, Burnaby 2, B.C.; London (Eng.) '45; M.B., B.S., M.D. (Psychol. Med. London); Sr., Child Psy., Burnaby Mental Health Centre; Clin. Instr. (Psy.), Vancouver Gen. Hosp.; Tel. HE 4-4247.
CASHMORE, Philip; Hamiota Medical Group, Hamiota, Man.; London (Eng.)'49; Tel. 220.
CASKEY, John A.; Rothesay, King's Co., N.B.; Edinburgh (Scot.) '43; DMRT; TherRad; Dir. (TherRad), Saint John Gen. & Victoria Hosp's.; Cons. (TherRad), Lancaster DVA Hosp.; Tel. 693-3351.
CASPER, George F.; 114 Conifer St., Sherwood Park, Alta.; Alb'40.
CASPERS, Anthony P.; 122 Norfolk St., Guelph, Ont.; London (Eng.) '49; M.R.C.S. (Eng.), L.R.-C.P. (Lond.); Cons. (Derm.), Guelph Gen. & St. Joseph's Hosp's.; Tel. TA 4-5200.
CASS, Emily E.; London (Eng.) '27; M.B., B.S.; MRCS (Eng.); LRCP (Lond.); Ophth. Surg., Indian Northern Health Services, Dept. of Nat. Health & Welfare, Fort Smith, N.W.T.
CASS, Elie; 648 Bathurst St., Toronto 4, Ont.; Tor '53; MCGP; Coroner, Toronto & York County; Staff, New Mount Sinai Hosp.; Tel LE 5-5053.
CASS, Isadore M.; 42 Purdon Dr., Downsview, Ont.; Tor '40; Path; Pathol., Ajax & Pickering Gen. Hosp.
CASSAN, Stanley; McG '62; Jr. Intn., Jewish Gen. Hosp., Montreal 26, P.Q.
CASSAR, Louis; Elliot Lake Med. Centre, Box 520, 134 Spruce Ave., Elliot Lake, Ont.; 55 Bouck Rd. (res); McG '53.
CASSELL, Wilfred A.; Qns'58; Res., Saskatchewan Hosp., Box 39, North Battleford, Sask.
CASSELLS, Irene M. (McAndrew); 10 Beacon St., Yarmouth, N.S. (res); London (Eng.) '54; DA; MRCS; LRCP; Staff (Anaes.), Yarmouth Reg. Hosp.; Tel. 742-3541.
CASSELLS, Michael J.; 10 Beacon St., Yarmouth, N.S. (res); London (Eng.) '51; MRCS; LRCP; Path; Path., Yarmouth Reg. Hosp.; Tel. 742-3541.
CASSELMAN, B. W.; 316 Wellington St. W., Sault Ste. Marie, Ont.; Qns '33.
CASSELMAN, Juanita E. (Wood); Tor'52; Ass't. Psy., Allan Mem. Inst.; Lect. McGill U.; Tel. 844-6311, Loc. 524.
CASSELMAN, W. G. Bruce; 171 Brittany Ave., Montreal 16, P.Q., res.; Tor'49; PhD; Medical Director, Geigy (Canada) Ltd., 4948 Place de la Savane, Montreal 9, P.Q.
CASSERLY, James G.; Ott'65; Res., Hosp. for Sick Children, Toronto, Ont.
CASSIDY, Douglas M.; Calgary Assoc. Clinic, 214-6th Ave. S.W., Calgary, Alta.; 615-49th **Ave. S.W. (res); Dublin (Ire.) '48; Staff, Holy Cross & Calgary Gen. Hosp's.; Tel. AM 3-7120.**
CASSIDY, Frank R.; Ste. 501, 215 Victoria St., Toronto 2, Ont.; Wes '54; FRCP(C), IntMed; Staff, OPD, St. Michael's Hosp.; Research Fell., Banting Inst.; Tel. EM 8-6535.
CASSIDY, Gordon J.; 900 Sherbrooke W., Apt. 2, Montreal, P.Q.; 5215 Victoria Ave., Apt. 15 (res); McG '21; M.Sc. Med, IntMed; Phys.-in-Charge, St. Mary's Hosp.; Tel. 735-3511.
CASSIDY, Lorne E.; 2 Desaulniers Blvd., St. Lambert, Cite Jacques Cartier, P.Q.; Ott'57; IntMed (P.Q.); Staff Montreal Gen. Hosp.; Dem. Med. & Clin. Med., McGill U.; Tel. 671-5124.
CASSIMJEE, Mahomed I.; 395 Tower St. S., Fergus, Ont.; Witwatersrand (S.Africa) '49; M.B., Ch.B., D.ObstRCOG; MRCOG; ObstGyn; Tel. 843-1844.
CASSIN, Stanley B.; 1343B Northmount Drive N.W., Calgary, Alberta; Tor'63; AMCGP; Staff, Calgary Gen., Grace & Foot Hills Hosp's.; Tel. 289-9268.
CASSIN, Teresa (See Gurrin).
CASTAGNER, Jacques; 298 Labelle, St.-Jerome, **P.Q. Mon '48; M.C.G.P.; Tel. GE 2-4301.**
CASTANEDA, Jose D.; 276 Duncan Rd., Estevan, Sask.; Santo Tomas (Philipp.)'57; DR; DiagRad.
CASTONGUAY, Bruno; 4231 Est rue St-Catherine, Montreal 4, P.Q.; Mon '55; Tel. CL 5-4467.
CASTONGUAY, Denise; 4231 Ste. Catherine E. Montreal 4, P.Q.; Mon '56; Staff, Dept. of Health, Montreal.
CASTONGUAY, E. J.; 4231 St. Catherine St. E., Montreal, P.Q.; Lav '11.
CASTONGUAY, Michel; 150 Jarry est, Montreal, P.Q.; Mon'57; FRCS(C); ObstGyn; Staff, Hop. St.-Michel; Tel. 722-2571.
CASTONGUAY, Yves R.; 5000 est Rue Belanger, Montreal 26, P.Q.; Mon'55; GenSurg (P.Q.); Cardiovasc & ThorSurg (P.Q.); Active Staff, St. Joseph De Rosemont Hosp.; Assoc. Staff, Inst. De Cardiologie; Tel. 376-3330.
CASTONGUAY, Yvon; Lav '61; Res., Hop. Hotel-Dieu, Montreal, P.Q.
CASTOR, William R.; 1021 Huron Ave., Port Arthur, Ont.; Alb'60; D&TRad.
CASWELL, Clive B.; 14 Crestview Rd., Toronto 12, Ont. (res); Qns '36; DPH; DIH; Clin. Phys., WCB Rehab. Centre; Tel. 244-1761, Ext. 256.
CASWELL, Lloyd A.; 1610 Pine Ave. W., Montreal, P.Q.; 3588 Marlowe Ave. (res); Qns '41; **FAGS, FCCP, FACP; Pulm. Dis. and TB** (P.Q.), IntMed; DTM; Assoc. Phys., O.P.D., & Assoc. Dir., Cardio-resp. Dept., Montreal Gen. Hosp.; Assoc. Phys., Herbert Reddy Mem. Hosp.; Chief Phys., Grace Dart Hosp.; Lect. (Med.), McGill U.; Tel. WE 7-4659.
CATELLIER, Claude R.; 298 boul. St-Germain, Rimouski, P.Q.; Lav '57; IntMed; Staff, Hop. St-Joseph; Tel. 742-4555.
CATENACCI, Victoria M.; 3040 Don Mills Rd. E., Willowdale, Ont.; Tor'64.
CATES, Bruce A.; 13665-96th Ave., North Surrey, B.C.; 3491 W. 35th Ave. (res); Man '44; GenSurg.; Tel. 581-6755.
CATES, Geoffrey W.; 2413 Lansdown Ave., Saskatoon, Sask. (res); Tor'47; Path; Path., University Hosp.; Lect. (Path.), Sask. U.; Tel. CH 2-6681.
CATHCART, Bessie C.; 124 Duncan, Wallaceburg, Ont.; Tor '15.
CATHCART, John P. S.; 183 Metcalfe St. Ottawa, Ont.; 223 Somerset St. W. (res); Tor '11; F.A.P.A., NeurPsy; Active Cons. Neur. & Psy., Ottawa Civic Hosp.; Active Cons. Psy., Ottawa Gen. Hosp.; Tel. CE 2-3273.
CATHCART, L. M.; 812 Cook Rd., Richmond, **Vancouver 14, B.C.; Alb '53; M.C.G.P.; Tel. 278-5191.**
CATLING, Joy; London (Eng.)'63; Staff, I.G.A. Hosp., North West River, Labrador.
CATTERALL, Sydney; 529 Tegler Bldg., Edmonton, Alta.; 1176 **University Ave. (res);** Aberdeen (Scot.) '40; M.B.; Ch.B.; DPM; AMBPS; Psy; Tel. 424-3215.

CATTERILL, T. Brian; Ste. 640, 5025 Sherbrooke St. W., Montreal, P.Q.; McG'54; MRCOG; FRCS(C), ObstGyn; Obst-Gyn-in-Chief, Queen Elizabeth Hosp.; Tel. 489-9713.

CATTERSON, Alistair G.; Apt. 106, 810 Edgeworth Ave., Ottawa, Ont.; McG'56; Psy.

CATTON, Donald V.; 24 West 33rd. St., Hamilton, Ont. (res); Wes'56; **FRCP(C),** Anaes; Staff (Anaes.), Hamilton Civic Hosp's.; Tel. 527-0271.

CATTON, Gordon E.; 81 Irving Pl., Ottawa, Ont. (res); London (Eng.) '44; **D.M.R.T.(Eng.);** TherRad; Sr. RadTher., Ont. Cancer Fdn., Ottawa **Clin.; Lect.-(TherRad.), U. of Ottawa; Cons.** (TherRad.) NDMC; Lect. (Rad.), U. of Ottawa; Tel. 728-3745.

CATURAY, Gregorio; 5175 Rumble St., South Burnaby, B.C.; Santa Tomas (Philipp.) '56.

CAUCHON, Roland; Clinique-Medicale-St.-Francois-d'Assise, 1210-1ere Ave., Quebec 3, P.Q.; 820 Cardinal Rouleau (res); Lav '34; FACS; **Urol; GenSurg (P.Q.); Chief Surg., Hop.-St.-Francois-d'Assise; Prof., Laval U.,** Tel. 522-4677.

CAUCHON, Rosaire; 333 rue Notre-Dame, Donnacona, P.Q.; Donnacona Co. Portneuf (res); Lav '32; M.C.G.P.; Tel. 285-3535.

CAUDWELL, Gordon G.; Tor '43; F.R.C.S.(C), GenSurg; Med. Cons., Ontario Hosp. Serv., 2195 Yonge St., Toronto 7, Ont.; Tel. 487-1711.

CAUGHEY, Gordon C.; 43 King St., Picton, Ont.; Qns'37; Staff, Prince Edward County Mem. Hosp.; Tel. GR 6-6464.

CAULEY, Albyn A.; 375 Main St. E., Hamilton. Ont.; 232 Mountain Brow Dr. (res); Qns '18; Tel. 522-2600.

CAUMARTIN, Armand; 300 Carre St-Louis, Montreal 18, P.Q.; Mon '52; GenSurg. (P.Q.); Tel. VI 5-0376.

CAUMARTIN, Paul; 300 Carre St. Louis, Montreal 18, P.Q.; Mon '29; GenSurg (P.Q.).

CAUNT, Thomas G. B.; 221—6th Ave., New Westminster, B.C. (res); Man '34; F.A.P.A., M.H.A.; Psy; Med. Supt., Crease Clinic & Prov. **Mental Hosp., Essondale, B.C.; Tel. LA 1-1911.**

CAUSING, Sergio S.; Eastern Passage, N.S.; Santo Tomas (Manila)'53; AMCGP.

CAUX, Daniel; C.P. 338, 43A St-Jean Baptiste, Victoriaville, P.Q.; Lav'61; Otol.

CAUX, J. Arthur; St. Flavien, Lotbiniere, P.Q. (res); Lav '29; D.P.H., PH(P.Q.); M.O.H., Health Unit, Lotbiniere.

CAUX, J. Norbert; Lav'62; Res., Hop. Notre-Dame, Montreal, P.Q.

CAUX, Majella; 75 rue-St.-Louis, Quebec, P.Q.; 208 rue Frontenac (res); Lav '43; Ophth, Otol (P.Q.); Ass't. Otol., Hop.-St.-Sacrement; Chief, Ophth, Otol. Serv., San Begin, Ste-Germaine; **Staff, Laval U.; Tel.: 523-5605.**

CAUX, Real; 52, rue St-Georges, Windsor, Cte. Richmond, P. Q.; **Lav '64.**

CAVANAGH, J. V. A.; 145 Main St., Aylmer, P.Q.; Qns '30.

CAVE, George D.; 608 Fairmont Med. Bldg., 750 W. Broadway, Vancouver 9, B.C.; UBC '55; DABOS; FRCS(C); GenSurg; Att'd. Staff, Vancouver Gen. Hosp.; Tel. TR 4-0441.

CAVE, William S.; 1605 Glenmore St., Kelowna, B.C.; 2425 Taylor Cres. (res); McG '51; **F.R.C.S.(C). FACS; GenSurg; Hd. Dept. of Surg., Kelowna Gen. Hosp.; Tel. 762-2002.**

CAVEN, W. H.; 267 O'Connor Dr., Ottawa, Ont.; **109 Helena St. (res); Tor '40; GenSurg.; Sr. Lect., (Clin. Surg), U. of Ottawa; Tel. PA 2-6327.**

CAVEN, W. Robertson; 502, Medical Arts Bldg., Toronto, Ont.; Tor'23; IntMed; Court. Staff, Toronto Gen. & Wellesley Hosp's.; Tel. WA 1-0700.

CAVERHILL, John W.; 98 Earl St., Kingston, Ont.; Tor'60; Psy; Staff, Ontario Hosp., Kingston, Ont.; Tel. 546-1101.

CAWKER, C. Agnew M.; 407-1541 W. Broadway, Vancouver 9, B.C.; 2462 Edgar Cr. (res); Alb '37; FRCS(C); FACS; FICS; DABU; Urol; Active Staff, St. Paul's Hosp.; Tel. 731-2218.

CAWSEY, Lewis A.; 502 Med. & Dental Bldg., Regina, Sask.; Man'49; MCGP; Tel. 522-8541.

CAWSON, Helen A.; 421 Eglinton Ave. E., Toronto 12, Ont. (res); **Liverpool** (Eng.) '45; M.R.C.O.G., D.C.H., **D.P.H.;** Staff, Women's **College Hosp.; Tel. WA 3-7381.**

CAWTHORPE, Harriett A.; Box 1063 Sudbury, Ont. (res); McG '43; **Anaes;** Staff, Sudbury Gen.

CAYER, J. Lomer; App. 1, 880, ave Calixa-Lavallee, Quebec 6, **P.Q.; 1135 de Montigny** (res); Lav '40; ObstGyn (P.Q.); Tel. 523-1150.

CAYFORD, E. Howard; 287 Lakeshore Rd., Strathmore, P.Q. (res); McG '26; GenSurg; **Ass't. Surg. & Dem. Surg., Montreal Gen. Hosp.; Retired.**

CAYOUETTE, Paul E.; 3960 Parc Lafontaine, Montreal, P.Q. (res); Lav '54; Psy (P.Q.); Staff, Hop.-Ste.-Jeanne-d'Arc; Tel. VI 2-5201.

CAYS, Fred A.; 124 Wellington St., Kingston, Ont.; 18 Wellington St. (res); Qns '08; F.R.C.-S.(C), Ophth, Otol; Emer. Prof. (Ophth, Otol), **Queen's U.; Tel. 548-4366.**

CAZA, MacDonald; 50 rue Jacques Cartier, Valleyfield, P.Q.; **Wes** '52; GenSurg (P.Q.).

CAZABON, Alcide A.; 45 Elm St. E., Sudbury, Ont.; Lav '50; Tel. 673-9301.

CECILIONI, Victor A.; 740 Barton St. E., Hamilton, **Ont.; 122 Barnesdale N. (res); Qns '34;** Tel. LI 4-1321.

CECUTTI, Albert G.; 289 Cedar St., Sudbury, Ont.; Tor '59; MCGP; Tel. 674-3131.

CECUTTI, Antonio; One Medical Place, 20 Wynford Dr., Don Mills, Ont.; Tor '51; ObstGyn; Tel. 429-1766.

CENAIKO, Frederick T.; Wakaw, Sask.; Alb '54; MCGP; Staff, Wakaw Union Hosp.; Tel. 233-4411.

CERA, Alvin E.; Osborne Med. Bldg., 190 Osborne St. N., Winnipeg, Man.; Man '57; AMCGP.

CERA, Gerald; Doctor's Bldg., 394 Graham Ave., Winnipeg, Man.; Man '57. Abroad.

CERA, Leslie J.; 203 Edmonton St., Winnipeg, Man.; 815 Campbell St. (res); Man '49; M.Sc., F.A.C.P.; F.R.C.P.(C), IntMed; Staff, St. Boniface Hosp.; Dir. Anticoag. Clin., Deer Lodge Hosp.; Lect. Med. U. of Manitoba; Tel. WH 2-5647.

CERAT, Jacques; 1252 Boulanger E., Montreal 35, P.Q.; **Apt. 3,** 3940 St.-Zotique E. (res); Mon **'55; M.C.G.P.; Tel. 274-7076.**

CERESNEY, Fred P.; 20571 Douglas Cres., Langley, B.C.; 6877-202nd. (res); Tor '54; Tel. 534-4713.

CEREZO, Paula B.; Manila Central (Philipp.) '58; Res., The Provincial Hosp., Lancaster, N.B.

CERNAVSKIS, Velta J. (Oss); Ste. 201, 1482 Bathurst St., Toronto 10, **Ont.;** Wes '55; Fell., Dept. of Path. Chem., U. of Toronto; Tel. 533-2072.

CERVENKO, Francis W.; Qns'61; FRCP(C), Anaes.; Dept. of Anaes., Royal College of Surg. of England, London W.C. 2, Eng.; Abroad.

CHABLANI, Gope V.; 204 Med. Centre, 906-8th Ave. S.W., Calgary, Alta.; Bombay (India)'56; Psy.

CHABOT, Charles E.; Ste. Rose, Temiscouata, P.Q.; Lav '44; GenSurg (P.Q.).

CHABOT, Claude; 6500 Place Bonaparte, Charlesbourg 7, P.Q.; Lav'58; Psy(P.Q.).

CHABOT, Emilien J. E.; Lambton, Cte. Frontenac, P.Q.; Lav '30; Tel. 12.

CHABOT, Felix; 229 St.-Joseph, Lauzon, P.Q.; Lav '58; MCGP.

CHABOT, Joseph-Alphee; 1605-1ere Ave., Quebec 3, P.Q.; Lav '32; DPH; FAPHA; PH; Med. Dir., Hop. St-Francois d'Assise; Tel. 529-7311.

CHABOT, J. A. N.; Ste. Claire, Co. Dorchester, P.Q.; Lav '01.

CHABOT, Jean A.; 3264 Carre Bochart, Quebec 10, P.Q.; Lav'60; Neur(P.Q.); Staff, Hop. St-Michel Archange.

CHABOT, Marcel; South Durham, Co. Drummond, **P.Q.; Lav '48; Tel. 826-2844.**

CHABOT, Maurice; 522 Ave. Royale, Beauport, Quebec 5, P.Q.; Lav '55.

CHABOT, Michel; Man '58; IntMed; **Staff, Inst de Cardiologie, 5415 boul, l'assomption, Mon**treal 36, P.Q.

CHABOT, Oscar; Lav '35; Unite Santaire, Shawinigan Falls, P.Q.
CHACKO, John; Box 557, Medical Arts Clinic, Regina, Sask.; Harvard (U.S.A.)'60; FRCS(C), GenSurg.
CHADSEY, Donald E.; Qns '63; Res. (Obst-Gyn.), University Hosp., Edmonton, Alta.
CHADSEY, Louis C.; 1 Court House Square, Brockville, Ont.; McG'24; MCGP; Att'd. Staff, Brockville Gen. & St. Vincent de Paul Hosp's.; Tel. 342-3262.
CHADWICK, John A. Capt.; HMCS Stadacona, Naval Hosp., Halifax, N.S.; McG'65.
CHADWICK, Paul; London (Eng.)'48; Staff, Dept. of Microbiol., Queen's U., Kingston, Ont.
CHADWICK, Rodney N.; Associate Clin., 4820 Gaetz Ave., Red Deer, Alta; 4750-56th St. (res); Man '41; IntMed.; Tel. 346-2057.
CHAGNON, Edward C.; 17 King St. W., Stoney Creek, Ont.; 113 Margaret St. S., Fruitland (res); Wes '55; Tel. 662-4995.
CHAGNON, Gerard; 2255 Etienne Parent, Montreal 12, P.Q.; Mon'38.
CHAGNON, Germaine E.; 66 St. Jean Baptiste, Victoriaville, P.Q.; Lav'65.
CHAGNON, Jacques, Capt.; Cdn. Forces Base, St. Jean, P.Q.; Mon'65.
CHAGNON, Jean; 822 Sherbrooke St. E., Montreal 24, P.Q.; Mon '54; Paed; Tel. 523-1137.
CHAGNON, Jean P.; 135 Main St., Aylmer, P.Q.; Ott '54; M.C.G.P.; Tel. 684-5679.
CHAGNON, Rene; 418 Grand Allee, St. Jerome, P.Q. (res); Lav '50; D & TRad; Staff, Hop. Hotel-Dieu; Tel. GE 2-9711.
CHAI, Kyong S.; Seoul (Korea)'53; Jr. Int., Misericordia Hosp., Winnipeg 1, Man.
CHAIKOF, Leo; 25 Brunswick Ave., Toronto 4, Ont.; 324 Richview Ave., Tor. 10 (res); Tor'56; M.S. (Surg., Ann Arbor); FACS; DABS; FRCS(C), GenSurg; Staff, Doctors' Hosp.; Tel. 927-3041.
CHAIKOFF, Joseph S.; 9 Fairholme Ave., Toronto 19, Ont.; 41 Strathearn Rd. (res); Tor '26; F.A.C.A.; Anaes; Chief, Dept. Anaes., Bethesda Gen. Hosp.; Court. Staff, Doctors' Hosp.; Tel. RU 1-8433.
CHAIKOFF, Ronald H.; 500 Parliament St., Toronto 5, Ont.; Tor '55; FRCP(C), IntMed; Cons., Raxlen Clinic; Assoc. Staff (IntMed.), Doctor's Hosp.; Vol. Ass't., O.P.D., Toronto Gen. Hosp.; Tel. WA 5-4381, Ext. 34.
CHAKRABARTI, Gobinda L.; Calcutta (India)'53; FRFPS(Glas.); MRCP(Ed.); Res. (Path.), Winnipeg Gen. Hosp., Winnipeg, Man.
CHALKE, F. Rhodes; 48 Powell Ave. Ottawa 1, Ont. (res); Man '43; M.Sc. (Med.); Psy; Staff, Mental Health Div., Royal Ottawa San.; Prof. & Exec. Dir. (Psy.), U. of Ottawa; Tel. PA 2-6521.
CHALLENGER, N. E.; 107 Hollyburn Medical Centre, 520—17th St., West Vancouver, B.C. McG '19; Tel. WA 2-7733.
CHALLIS, Albert H.; Fort Francis Clinic, 301 Victoria, Fort Francis, Ont.; 203 Armit (res); **London (Eng.) '42; MRCS; LRCP; Res. Med.** Staff, La Verendrye Hosp.; Tel. 274-6549.
CHALLIS, E. Bruce; Beech Clinic, 350 Beech Ave., Toronto 8, Ont.; 8 Romana Dr. (res); Tor '56; Tel. 694-1126.
CHALLIS, Thomas W.; 74 Johnson St., Kingston, Ont.; McG'51; FRCP(C); GenSurg; DiagRad; Staff, Kingston Gen. Hosp.; Ass't. Prof. (Rad.), Queen's U.; Tel. 542-2791.
CHALMERS, Alistair C.; Manitoba Clinic, Winnipeg, Man.; 1208 Lorette St. (res); Glasgow (Scot.) '55; Tel. 774-6541.
CHALMERS, G. Everett; MPP; 206 Rookwood **Ave., Fredericton, N.B.; 63 Grey St. (res); McG '33; FACS; GenSurg; Surg.-in-Chief, Victoria Public Hosp.; Tel. 475-7701.**
CHALMERS, Robert H.; Fredericton Med. Clinic, 206 Rookwood Ave., Fredericton, N.B.; 334 University Ave. (res); McG '41; ObstGyn.; Tel. 475-7701.
CHALOULT, Louis; Lav'60; Res., Hop. Maisonneuve, Montreal 36, P.Q.
CHALUT, Fernand; 4572 Wellington, Verdun, Mtl. 19, P.Q.; 557 Carroll, Lasalle (res); Mon '47; Assoc. Staff, Hop.-St.-Luc; Vis. Staff, Hop. Gen. de Verdun; Med. Dir. Hop.-Ste-Therese & Biermans Rest Home; Tel. 769-1941.
CHALUT, Pierre; Mon'53; GenSurg; Staff, Hop. Charles Lemoyne, 121 Blvd. Taschereau, Greenfield Park, P.Q.; Tel. 671-3811.
CHAM, Max; 148 McAdam Ave., Winnipeg 4, Man. (res); Man '45; FICS; Anaes; Staff, St. Boniface & Victoria Hosp's.; Lect. (Anaes.), U. of Manitoba; Tel. WH 3-0311.
CHAMBERLAIN, Clive G.; Tor '61; Res., Mental Health Clinic, 514 Jarvis St., Toronto 5, Ont.
CHAMBERLAIN, Dean W.; 172 Queen St. W., Brampton, Ont.; Tor'64; Tel. 451-1262.
CHAMBERLAIN, George E.; Chatsworth, Ont.; Wes'65.
CHAMBERLAIN, John H.; 17 Mill St., Georgetown, Ont.; Alb'42; MCGP; Dist. Coroner; Tel. TR 7-2972.
CHAMBERLAND, J. Adelard; St. Basile, Co. Port Neuf, P.Q.; Lav '54.
CHAMBERLAND, Jean M.; 111-23 rue E., St. Georges, Co. Beauce, P.Q.; Lav'51; Med. Staff, Hop. Notre Dame de Beauce.
CHAMBERS, A. L.; Ste. 203, 1705—3rd Ave., Prince George, B.C.; 1386 Third Ave. (res); Alb '32; GenSurg; Dist. Coroner.
CHAMBERS, Gordon B.; Ste. 107, 688 Coxwell Ave., Toronto 13; 4 O'Connor Dr. (res); Tor '43; ObstGyn.; Staff, Tor. E. Gen. Hosp.; Tel. 924-3464.
CHAMBERS, Graham L.; 17 Queen E., Toronto 1, Ont.; 86 Wells Hill Ave. (res); Tor '21; Tel. EM 4-1919.
CHAMBERS, Harold L. H.; 710 Seymour St., Vancouver, B.C.; **1859 Allison Rd. (res); Tor** '42; Urol; Ass't., Dept. Surg., U. of British **Columbia; Tel. MU 4-1511.**
CHAMBERS, Hugh R.; 60 Bessborough Dr., Toronto 17, Ont.; Tor '59; Assoc. Staff, Tor. E. **Gen. & Bethesda Gen. Hosp's.; Tel. 425-0021.**
CHAMBERS, Margaret C.; 4 O'Connor Dr., Toronto, Ont.; Man '43; Anaes.; Tel. HO 3-3122.
CHAMBERS, Philip J.; 340 Campbell St., Nanaimo, B.C.; London (Eng.)'56.
CHAMPAGNE, Edward B.; Ste. 500, 5300 Cote **des Neiges Rd., Montreal 26, P.Q.; France '54;** Jr. Clin. Ass't., St. Mary's Hosp.; Clin. Ass't., Jewish Gen. Hosp.; Tel. RE 1-3141.
CHAMPAGNE, Fortunat A.; St. Claude, Man.; Man '52; M.C.G.P.
CHAMPAGNE, Jacques; 259 St-Georges, St-Jerome, P. Q.; Mon '45; Obst (P.Q.); Chief (ObstGyn.), Hop. Hotel-Dieu de St-Jerome; Tel. GE 8-2051.
CHAMPAGNE, Reginald; Main St., Elie, Man; Lav'60; Coroner; Tel. 3252.
CHAMPEAU, Jean; 1180 Sherbrooke St. E., **Montreal, P.Q.; Mon '27; Obst; Tel. LA 2-0896.**
CHAMPION, Glen; Oliver, B.C.; London (Eng.) '60; M.S., B.S.; MRCS (Eng), LRCP (Lond.); Tel. 498-2343.
CHAMPOUX, Gatien; 4105 St. Zotique E., Montreal 36, P.Q.; Lav '50; Tel. 722-6708.
CHAMPOUX, Hughes P.; Clin. Med. Fleury, 2157 Fleury est, Montreal 12, P.Q.; Lav'65.
CHAMPOUX, Marcel 1229 Notre-Dame, Lachine, P.Q.; Mon '40.
CHAMPOUX, Roger; Ste. 201, 1656 est rue Sherbrooke, Montreal 24, P.Q.; 5530 rue Isabella (res); Mon '43; F.R.C.S.(C), GenSurg; Surg., Hop.-Notre-Dame; Tel. 525-6363.
CHAN, Alice M.; McG '62; Sr. Ass't. Res., Hosp. for Sick Children, Toronto, Ont.
CHAN, Edward S.; 212-4900 Kingsway, South Burnaby, B.C.; Shanghai (China) '48.
CHAN, Eugene J.; 543 Main St., Vancouver 4, B.C.; UBC'58; Derm.
CHAN, Ger Au; 30 Windemere Cres., Woodstock, Ont. (res); Lingnan U. (China) '42; M.P.H.; **F.C.C.P.; Staff Phys., Ontario Hosp., Woodstock; Tel. LE 9-1251.**
CHAN, Guy H.; 543 Main St., Vancouver 4 B.C.; Northwestern (U.S.A.) '21; Tel. MU 4-2824.

CHAN, Ngai T.; 1119 Victoria Ave., Fort William, Ont.; National Med. College (Shanghai) '48; Psy; Tel. DI 4-2431.
CHAN, Norman Y. H.; 5104-5th Ave., Bonnyville, Alta.; Taiwan (Formosa) '57; M.B.; Tel. 826-3152.
CHAN, Pablo L.; Santo Tomas (Phillip.) '54; Staff Central Hosp., Toronto 2, Ont.; Tel. WA 5-8991.
CHAN, Pang L.; McG '62; Jr. Intn., Royal Victoria Hosp., Montreal 2, P.Q.
CHAN, Paulino S.; Ste. 2, Millar Block, North Battleford, Sask.; Santo Tomas (Philipp.) '56; Tel. 445-3551.
CHAN, Philip W. C.; Manila (Phillipines) '58; Sr. Res. (Derm.), Montreal Convalescent Hosp., Montreal, P.Q.; Tel. 737-3661.
CHAN, Shiu F.; 85 Wellesley St., Apt. 811, Toronto, Ont.; Taiwan (China)'59; IntMed.
CHAN, Tin S.; 5175 Rumble St., Burnaby 1, B.C.; Nat. Defence Med. Centre (Taiwan, Formosa)'58.
CHAN, William K.; McG'65; Res., Montreal Gen. Hosp., Montreal 25, P.Q.
CHAN, William S.; Ott'60; Staff, Dept. of Anaes., Grace Hosp., Windsor, Ont.
CHAN, William Y.; Box 400, Rosetown, Sask.; Taiwan (Formosa)'52.
CHANDER, Vinay; Delhi (India) '56; Anaes; Staff, Montreal Children's Hosp., Montreal, P.Q.
CHANDLER, Brian M.; Victoria Gen. Hosp., Halifax, N.S.; Dal'61; FRCP(C), IntMed; Ass't. Phys., Victoria Gen. & Dalhousie U.; Tel. 422-7371.
CHANDLER, Colin R.; 31 Academy Med. Bldg., 1812-4th St. S.W., Calgary, Alta.; Leeds (Eng.) '56; M.B., Ch.B., DIH (Lond.); Med. Advis., City of Calgary; Tel. 266-4001.
CHANDLER, Margaret R.; St. Bart's H. (London, Eng.) '53; Fell. (Ophth), Dalhousie U., Halifax, N.S.; Tel. 2-4406.
CHANG, Chung A.; 200 Scott Bldg., Moose Jaw, Sask.; 579 Vaughan St. (res); Sun Yet Sen U. (Canton, China) '43; Anaes; Tel. 692-1841.
CHANG, In W.; 2633 Portage Ave., Winnipeg, Man.; Soeul (Korea)'57; FRCS(C), ObstGyn; Staff, Winnipeg Gen. Hosp.
CHANG, Jone; 829 W. Broadway, Vancouver 9, B.C.; 6875 Tisdall St., Van. 14 (res); Tor '49; FRCP(C), Anaes; Att'd. Staff, Van. Gen. Hosp.; Clin. Ass't. Prof. (Surg.), UBC; Tel. TR 4-5291.
CHANG, Keun H.; Box 370, Sidney, B.C.; Seoul Nat. (Korea) '55.
CHANG, Seg-Kin; 2790 East 1st Ave., Vancouver, B.C.; National Defence Med. College (Formosa)'58.
CHANG, Theodore Y.; 193 E. Hastings St., Vancouver, B.C.; Tor '46; GenSurg; Chief of Staff, Mt. St. Joseph's Hosp.; Vis. Staff, Vancouver Gen. Hosp.; Tel. MU 5-7516.
CHANG, Thomas M.; Apt. 48, 3524 Hutchison, Montreal 18, P.Q.; (res); McG '61; Att'd. Staff, Montreal Chinese Hosp.; Lect. (Physiol.) McGill U.; Research Fell. (Physiol.), McGill U.; Tel. VI 5-3552.
CHANGFOOT, George H.; Capetown (S. Africa) '64; Res., St. Paul's Hosp., Vancouver 1, B.C.
CHANT, Elizabeth (See Robertson, Elizabeth).
CHANT, George N.; 29 Dickson St., Galt, Ont.; Wes '59; AMCGP; Tel. 623-1925.
CHAPADOS, Roger; Mon '60; Anaes; Staff, Hop. Maisonneuve, Montreal 36, P.Q.; Tel. 254-8431.
CHAPDELAINE, Alcide; Mon'58; FRCP(C), IntMed; Staff, Hop. Maisonneuve, Montreal 36, P.Q.
CHAPDELAINE, Pierre; 40 rue Ste-Anne, Ste-Anne de Bellevue, P.Q.; Mon '61.
CHAPESKIE, Andrew H.; Box 238, Barry's Bay, Ont.; Ott '55; Tel. 170.
CHAPLIN, G. Eleanor (Bean); 65 Pepler Ave., Toronto 6, Ont.; Wes '43; Retired.
CHAPLIN, Robert A; 65 Pepler Ave., Toronto 6, Ont.; Wes '43; F.A.C.A.; Anaes; Anaes.-in-Chief, Toronto East Gen. Hosp.; Clin. Instr. (Anaes), U. of Toronto; Tel. HO 5-1469.
CHAPMAN, C. W.; Major; Nat. Defence Med. Centre, Ottawa, Ont.; U.S.A. '44.
CHAPMAN, David J.; 20 Arcade Cres., Hamilton, Ont. (res); London (Eng.) '45; DMRD; DiagRad; Dir. of Rad., Henderson Gen. Hosp.; Tel. JA 7-0271.
CHAPMAN, Eric F.; Esterhazy, Sask.; Man '40; **M.C.G.P.; Dist. Coroner.**
CHAPMAN, George Watt, Lt.-Col.; National Defence Med. Centre, Ottawa, Ont.; Stanford U. (California, U.S.A.)'44; GenSurg; Clin. Asst'. Surg., U. of Ottawa; Tel. 733-6600.
CHAPMAN, G. William; 3556 Kelsey Pl., Victoria, B.C.; Tor'35; Anaes.; Court. Staff, Royal Jubilee Hosp.; Tel. 388-4652.
CHAPMAN, Harry L.; 109 Medical Arts Bldg., Port Arthur, Ont.; 120 S. High St. (res); Man '30; ObstGyn: Chief of Obst. Staff, Port Arthur **Gen. Hosp.; Tel. DI 4-6621.**
CHAPMAN, Marion Elizabeth; Apt. 207, 124 St. James St., London, Ont. (res); Tor '48; Psy; Staff, Ontario Hosp.; Tel. 455-5110.
CHAPMAN, Neil H.; Ste. 640, 5025 Sherbrooke St. W., Montreal 28, P.Q.; McG'49; FACOG; ObstGyn (P.Q.); Staff, Queen Elizabeth Hosp.; Tel. 489-9713.
CHAPNIK, Jerry S.; Tor '62; Res., St. Michael's Hosp., Toronto 2, Ont.
CHAPPEL, John N.; Medico Malayan Team, Kuala Lipis, Pahang, Malaya; Alb '60; Abroad.
CHAPPELLE, Gerard F.; 14625 Stoney Plain Rd., Edmonton, Alta.; Alb '28.
CHAPUT, Jean M.; 225 Notre Dame, St. Pie, Co. Bagot, P.Q.; Mon '50.
CHAPUT, Marcel; 263 College St., Richmond, P.Q.; Mon '40
CHAPUT, Noel; 335 rue Provost, Lachine, P.Q.; 761—13ieme Ave. (res); Mon '49; Med. & Obst. Staff, Hop. St. Joseph de Lachine; Tel. 637-2772.
CHAPUT, Normand; 415 Ste.-Helene, Longueuil, **Montreal S., P.Q.; 276 de Chateauguay (res); Mon '50; Tel. CR 4-6281.**
CHAPUT, Yves; 958 est Sherbrooke, Montreal, P.Q.; 5535 Cote Saint Antoine (res); Mon '37; F.A.C.G., Gastroent (P.Q.), IntMed; Phys., **Hop. Notre Dame; Assoc. Prof. U. of Montreal; Tel. 525-6363.**
CHARBONNEAU, Aubin; 883 Pierre Bedard, Chicoutimi, P.Q.; Lav '49; DABS; DABTS; GenSurg (P.Q.); ThorSurg (P.Q.); Surg. Staff, Hotel-Dieu-de-St-Vallier; Tel. 549-2432.
CHARBONNEAU, Edgar; 277 Montreal Rd., **Eastview, Ottawa 2, Ont.; Qns '55; M.C.G.P.; Tel. 749-5121.**
CHARBONNEAU, Fernand; Mon'65; Res., Hop. Maisonneuve, Montreal 36, P.Q.
CHARBONNEAU, Ivan; Mon'65; Res., Hop. Notre Dame, Montreal 24, P.Q.
CHARBONNEAU, Jean; Centre Medical-St.-Urbain, 3875 rue St.-Urbain, Montreal 18, P.Q.; 2903 Fendall (res); Mon '42; FRCS(C), FICS; Urol; Tel. VI 9-2911.
CHARBONNEAU, J. Henri; 3095 Sherbrooke St. E., Montreal, P.Q.; 7, ave Touzin, Dorval (res); Mon '27; Paed; Med. Dir., Hop. Pasteur; Tel. LA 3-1173.
CHARBONNEAU, J. Paul; 335 Williams St., Hawkesbury, Ont.; Mon '50; M.C.G.P.
CHARBONNEAU, Louis P.; 217 Laurier Ave. E., Ottawa 1, Ont.; 2063 Chalmers Rd. (res); Lav '46; FRCS(C), Otol; Clin. Ass't., Ottawa Gen. Hosp.; Tel. 236-3797.
CHARBONNEAU-PANISSET, Louise; Mon'65; Res., Hop. Notre Dame, Montreal 24, P.Q.
CHARBONNEAU, Paul E.; 30 Blvd. St. Joseph E., Montreal, P.Q.; 678 rue Chatelain (res); Mon '50; FRCS(C); GenSurg; Staff, Hop. Maisonneuve & Hop. St. Luc; Tel. 254-8341.
CHARBONNEAU, Rene; 1260 est, Boul. St.-Joseph, Montreal 34, P.Q.; 2903 Fendall (res); Mon '41; Ophth; Otol (P.Q.); Ass't. Ophth, Notre-Dame Hosp.; Cons., Ophth., Queen Mary Vet's.; Ass't. Prof. (Ophth), U. of Montreal; Tel. RE 3-9951.
CHARBONNEAU, Rene; 11807 Alfred Laliberte, Montreal 12, P.Q.; Mon '58; Psy.

CHARBONNEAU, Roland; 1058 St. Denis, Montreal 18, P.Q.; Mon '52; FCCP; FRCP(C), IntMed; Pulm Dis & TB(P.Q.); Ass't. (Med.), Hop. St. Luc; Ass't. Prof. (Med.), U. of Montreal; Tel. 861-8087.

CHARBONNEAU, Romeo; 372 Sir George Etienne Cartier, Montreal, P.Q.; Mon '42; Tel. 932-5652.

CHARENDOFF, Morris D.; Ste. 208, 4949 Bathurst St., Willowdale, Ont.; Tor'47; FRCS(C), OrthSurg; Surg. Staff, New Mt. Sinai Hosp.; Tel. 921-0731.

CHAREST, Fernand; 3620 Ontario St. E., Montreal, P.Q.; Mon '39; FRCS(C); NeurSurg; I/C Dept. of Neur. Surg., Hop. du Sacre-Cœur, Cartierville; Tel. **WA 3-9376.**

CHAREST, Georges-A.; Dept. of Physical Education, U. of Montreal, 250 ouest Mont Royal, Montreal, P.Q.; Lav'50; Tel. RE 3-9951.

CHAREST, Gustave; 1124 est, Ontario, Montreal 24, P.Q.; Mon '34; PH (P.Q.); DPH; MPH; Supt. Spec. Div. of Contagious Diseases, Dept. of Health, 700 Craig St. E.

CHAREST, Yvan; 11 ouest, Boul. St.-Joseph, Montreal 14, P.Q.; Lav '48; Otol (P.Q.); Cons. (Otol.), **Hop.-Ste-Justine & Hop.-St. Michel, Ville-St.-Michel; Tel. RE 1-4931.**

CHARETTE, Denis; Ste. 1016, 30 est Boul. St. Joseph, Montreal 14, P.Q.; Mon'52; FRCS(C), GenSurg.

CHARETTE, Henry; Ste. 140, **4 rue Taschereau,** Hull, P.Q.; Mon'48; DiagRad; Hd. Dept. of Rad., Hop-du-Sacre-Coeur; Tel. PR 1-4021.

CHARETTE, Jean J.; 30 est, boul St-Joseph, Montreal 14, P.Q.; 310 E. Legendre, App. 8 (res); Mon '57; Cons., Montreal Post-Natal **Clin.; M.O., R.C.A.S.C.**

CHARETTE, Robert; 6335 de Carignan, Montreal, P.Q.; '62; Psy(P.Q.).

CHARGHI, Ali; Geneva (Switz.) '57; FRCS(C), Urol; Staff, Hotel-Dieu, Montreal, P.Q.; Tel. VI 4-0161.

CHARLAND, Raymond; Mon'65; Res., Hop. Hotel Dieu, Montreal 18, P.Q.

CHARLAND, Renee; Mon'65; Res., Hop. Hotel Dieu, Montreal 18, P.Q.

CHARLAND, Richard; Centre Medical-St.-Urbain, **3875 rue St.-Urbain, Montreal 18, P.Q.; 46 Kenwood Rd., Beaconsfield (res); Mon '47; FICS; Otol; Active Staff (Otol.), Hotel-Dieu; Clin. Ass't., U. of Mtl; Tel. VI 2-9958.**

CHARLEBOIS, Benoit; 8170 Ave du Mail, Anjou, Montreal 4, P.Q.; Lav'37; Dir. (Home Care), **Hop.-Ste.-Jeanne-d'Arc; Tel. VI 2-5201.**

CHARLEBOIS, Jean; 3211 Chemin Ste-Foy, Ste-Foy, Quebec 10, P.Q.; Lav'65.

CHARLEBOIS, Peter A.; 3000 Lawrence Ave. E., Scarborough, Ont.; Tor '56; Anaes; Staff, Scarborough Gen. Hosp.; Tel. AX 3-8681.

CHARLES, David; Maple Creek Clinic, Maple Creek, Sask.; 301 Sidney St. (res); London (Eng.) '49; M.R.C.O.G., ObstGyn.

CHARLES, Laerte; 7301 rue Cellier, Ville d'Anjou, Montreal 5, P.Q.; Haiti '55; Anaes; Staff, Hop. Notre-Dame.

CHARLES, W. Bruce; Ste. 5, 825 Coxwell Ave., Toronto 13, Ont.; 115 Rochester Ave. (res); Tor '38; D.A.B.I.M., F.R.C.P.(C), IntMed; Phys.-in-Chief, Toronto East Gen. Hosp.; Cons. Phys., Sunnybrook D.V.A. Hosp.; Tel. HO 5-8682.

CHARLESWORTH, Gerald, S.; 250 Birks Bldg., Edmonton, Alta.; 10220—133 St. (res); Tor '26; Obst.; Retired.

CHARLTON, Marion E.; (See Dennis, Marion E.)

CHARLTON, Ronald W.; 4537 Kingston Rd., West Hill, Ont.; Tor '58; Tel. 284-4901.

CHARLTON, William H. M.; 4 King Cres., Weston, Ont.; 2 King Cres. (res); Tor '24; M.C.G.P.; **Dist. Coroner; Tel. 249-3995.**

CHARLTON, William J.; Room 107, 736 Granville St., Vancouver, B.C.; 1781 W. 60th Ave. (res); Man '45: F.R.C.S.(C), GenSurg; Instr. (Surg.), U. of British Columbia; Att. Staff, Shaughnessy Hosp.; Vis. Staff, Vancouver Gen., **St. Paul's & St. Vincent's Hosp's.; Tel. MU 2-4840.**

CHARLWOOD, Ronald R.; Tusket, N.S.; Oxford (Eng.)'54; DObstRCOG.

CHARMAN, John H.; 5991 Spring Garden Rd., Halifax, N.S.; 6990 Armview Ave. (res); Dal '43; FRCS(C), GenSurg; Ass't. Surg., Victoria **Gen. Hosp.; Assoc. Prof. (Surg.), Dalhousie U.; Tel. 423-7578.**

CHARRETTE, Edward; Ott'59; Res., Montreal Gen. Hosp., Montreal, P.Q.

CHARROIS, Marie — see DUBREUIL-CHARROIS, Marie.

CHARROIS, Romeo; 1345 ave. William, Quebec, P.Q.; Lav'61; FRCS(C), Urol; Travelling McLaughlin Fell. in 1967.

CHARRON, Jules; 1656 est Sherbrooke, Montreal 24, P.Q.; 355 Leacross (res); Mon '55; FRCS(C); Urol; Staff, Hop. Notre-Dame; Tel. 526-3783.

CHARRON, Kenneth C.; 735 Avenue Rd., Toronto 7, Ont.; Tor '34. Deputy Minister of Health, Ont. Dept. of Health.

CHARRON, Raymond; 1836 Ste. Calixte, Plessisville, P.Q.; Lav '32; M.C.G.P.; Med. Dir., Hop. **Sacre Coeur; Dist. Coroner; Tel. 362-7351.**

CHARRON, Richard C.; 735 Avenue Rd., Toronto, Ont.; Tor'61; FRCP(C), IntMed.

CHARTERIS, Richard W.; 65-6th St., Chatham, Ont.; Wes '55; Tel. 354-1511.

CHARTERS, James W.; Steel Co. of Canada, Hilton Works, Wilcox Ave., Hamilton, Ont.; Qns'52; Active Staff, Hamilton Civic & St. Joseph's Hosp's.; Tel. JA 8-2511.

CHARTERS, J. Ewart; 112 Victoria St. E., Alliston, Ont.; Doner St. (res); Tor '54; Staff, Stevenson Mem. Hosp.; Tel. 435-6225.

CHARTERS, John S.; 10 Touzin Ave., Dorval, P.Q.; McG '44; Paed.; Ass't. Phys., Montreal **Children's Hosp.; Dem. (Paed.), McGill U.; Tel. WE 7-8511.**

CHARTIER, Aime; 716 Medical Arts Bldg., 1538 ouest rue Sherbrooke, Montreal 25, P.Q.; Lav '12; Retired.

CHARTIER, Jean; Mon '39; Staff, Queen Mary Vet's Hosp., Montreal 26, P.Q.; Tel. 738-9481.

CHARTIER, Marcel; 2282 rue Ste. Anne, St. Hyacinthe, P.Q.; 2595 Laframboise St. (res); Mon '49; Tel. PR 4-7313.

CHARTIER, Maurice G.; 12245 rue Grenet, Montreal 9, P.Q.; Mon'54; FRCP(C), IntMed; Teach., Hop. Notre Dame; Tel. LA 5-6363.

CHARTRAND, Claude; 10454 Blvd. Gouin W., Roxboro, P.Q.; 20B-8th Ave. (res); Mon '60; Tel. 684-4330.

CHARTRAND, Florian; 56 Church, Verdun, P.Q.; Mon '50; A.M.C.G.P.; Tel. 769-7211.

CHARTRAND, Gilles; 240 Elm St., St. Lambert, P. Q.; 105 De Toraine, Preville (res); Mon'60; Staff, Hop. Charles Le Moyne; Tel. 671-5411.

CHARTRAND, Jean L.; 7630 Central, Ville la Salle, Montreal 32, P.Q.; Mon '51; Chief of Obst., Hop. Gen. La Salle; Tel. 366-0122.

CHARTRAND, Raymonde; Mon'65; Res., Hop. St Luc, Montreal 18, P.Q.

CHARTRAND, Rene; 8455 Ave. Henri Julien, Montreal, P.Q. (res); Mon '36.

CHARTRAND, Yolande; 6768 rue St. Denis, Montreal 10, P.Q.; '52.

CHARTRAND, Yvon; 12245 Grenet, Montreal 9, P.Q.; Mon'53; GenSurg; Staff, Hop. Sacre Coeur, Montreal, P.Q.; Tel. 334-1210.

CHASE, Lillian; 228 Medical Arts Bldg., 170 St. George St., Toronto, Ont.; 3112 Yonge St. (res); Tor '22; IntMed; Staff, Women's College Hosp; O.P.D. & Sunnybrook Hosp.; Tel. WA 1-3617.

CHASE, N. Douglas; 2007 Danforth Ave., Toronto 6, Ont.; 236 Donway E., Apt. 5, Don Mills (res); Tor '54; Assoc. & OPD Staff, Toronto E. Gen. Hosp.; Assoc. GP Staff, Scarborough Gen. Hosp.; Tel. OX 9-3937.

CHASE, Victor E.; 209 Melrose Ave., Ottawa 3, **Ont.; Manchester (Eng.) '52; Psy.; Lect., (Clin-**Psy), U. of Ottawa; Tel. GE 5-6751. Abroad.

CHASE, William H.; McG'52; Path; Assoc. **Prof., Dept. of Path, U. of British Columbia, Vancouver 9, B.C.; Tel. CA 4-1111.**

CHASMAR, Leslie R.; 606 Medical Arts Bldg., Saskatoon, Sask.; McG'51; FRCS(C), GenSurg; PlasSurg; Active Staff, University, City & St. Paul's Hosp's.; Clin. Ass't. Prof., U. of Saskatchewan; Tel. 242-8082.
CHASSE, Andrée; 5351 boul. Rosemont, app. 2, Montreal, P.Q.; '62; Paed(P.Q.).
CHASSE, N. J.; St. Jean Port Joli, P.Q.; Lav '43; Dist. Coroner.
CHASSE, Reynald; 857 Puy Jalon, Hauterive, P.Q.; Lav'63.
CHASSELS, John; 2714 Dorset Rd., Victoria, B.C. (res); Tor '15; Anaes; Retired.
CHATTERJEE, Kam; 163 Laurier Ave. E., Ottawa 2, Ont.; Calcutta (India) '52; M.B., B.S.; Anaes; Lect. (Anaes.), Ottawa U.; Tel RE 3-1930.
CHATTERJEE, Maureen; Dunlop Block, Broadway Ave., Yorkton, Sask.; Durham (Eng.)'61.
CHATTERS, Othello P.; 309 Wyandotte St. E., Windsor, Ont.; 804 Giles Blvd E. (res); McG '23.
CHATTERTON, Roy T. Capt.; Wes'65; Shilo Military Hosp., Nr. Brandon, Man.
CHATWIN, James C.; Med. Arts Clinic, Regina, Sask.; 3100 Retallack St. (res); Ott '54; MCGP; Tel LA 2-1651.
CHAUDHARI, Jagat M.; Panjab (India)'56; Res., Pathology Inst., 5800 University Ave., Halifax, N.S.
CHAUDHARY, Basudeo; Patna (India)'57; Res., St. Boniface Gen. Hosp., St. Boniface, Man.
CHAUDHURI, Asim K.; Apt. 41, 131 Parkdale Ave., Ottawa, Ont.; Calcutta (India)'55; ObstGyn.
CHAURETTE, Gilles; 55 rue de l'Eglise, Verdun, Montreal 19, P.Q.; 5408 Coolbrook (res); Mon '51; IntMed; Ass't. Med. Serv., University & Verdun Gen. Hosp's.; Tel. 766-4897.
CHAUVEAU, Pierre; St. Barthelmy, Cte. Berthier, P.Q.; Mon '36; Staff, Hop. Comotois, Louisville; Tel. 885-3232.
CHAUVIN, Russel G.; Ott '63; (Intern) c/o 701 Bedford, Windsor, Ont.
CHEESMAN, Frederick J.; 239 Princess St., Saint John, N.B.; Dal '31; GenSurg; Surg., St. John Gen. & St. Joseph's Hosp's.; Tel. 693-3351.
CHEESEMAN, Norman H.; 194 King St. S., Waterloo, Ont.; Ott '57; Tel. SH 4-3721.
CHEIFETZ, Philip N.; McG '60; Res., Royal Victoria Hosp., Montreal, P.Q.
CHEN, Chijen; Apt. 413, 730 Ontario St., Toronto 5, Ont.; Taiwan (Formosa)'58; GenSurg.
CHEN, Larry T.; Box 6900, Campbell River, B.C.; UBC '62; Tel. 287-6228.
CHEN, Nora P.; Santo Tomas (Philipp.)'57; Res., St. Paul's Hosp., Vancouver 1, B.C.
CHEN, Patricia P.; Box 6900, Campbell River, B.C.; UBC '63; Tel. 287-6883.
CHEN, Robert; Royal Alexandra Hosp., Edmonton, Alta.; R.C.S. (Dublin, Ire.)'60; DCH; Paed; Teach. Fell., U. of Alberta.
CHEN, Tah Y.; 354 Hinton Ave., Ottawa 3, Ont.; Yat-Sen (China)'42; TherRad.
CHEN, Walter T.; Ste. 212, 1669 Victoria St., Prince George, B.C.; Shanghai (China) '49.
CHENARD, Georges E.; Man'59; Res., Ottawa Civic Hosp., Ottawa 3, Ont.
CHENARD, Jacques P.; 1301 Pelletier, Quebec 6, P.Q. (res); Lav '56; FRCP(C), Path; Staff, Hop.-Laval; Tel. 653-5251.
CHENEL, J. Leon; 380—18e Rue, Quebec, P.Q.: Lav '34; D.P.H.; Tel. 523-0324.
CHENG, Huo; Box 187, Portage Health Unit, Portage Le Prairie, Man.: Berlin (Germ.) '37; Honan (China)'35; DPH (Tor.).
CHENG, M. C.; 132 Sheraton Dr., Montreal, P.Q. (res); Nanking (China) '49; Anaes; Staff, Royal Victoria Hosp.; Tel. VI 2-1251.
CHENG, Patricia P. N.; Bonnyville, Alta.; Taiwan (China)'57; Tel. 826-1352.
CHENIER, Real; 960, boul Ste-Croix, Montreal 9, P.Q.; Apt. 17, 3445 Papineau (res); Mon '49; Gyn (P.Q.); Tel. 747-3501.
CHENOWETH, Rodger S.; Medical Centre, 707 Charlotte St., Peterborough, Ont.; Tor'35; F.A.C.S., F.I.C.S., GenSurg; Surg. Serv., Peterborough Civic & St. Joseph's Hosp., & The Medical Centre, Tel. RI 2-3871.
CHENOWETH, T. Oswald; 1 St. Edmund's Dr., Toronto 12, Ont.; Melbourne (Aus.) '10; F.R.C.S. (Edin.), GenSurg; Retired.
CHEPEHA, Nicholas; Cuthbertson Clinic, 11666-95th St., Edmonton, Alta.; Alb '58; MCGP; Tel. 474-3481.
CHEPESIUK, Martin W.; 92 Roncesvalles Ave., Toronto, Ont.; Qns '47; D.P.H.; M.C.G.P.; Assoc. (Med.) St. Joseph's Hosp.; Dist. Phys. Health Dept,. Toronto, Tel. LE 4-2115.
CHEPESIUK, Maurice W.; 3410 W - 42nd Ave., Vancouver, B.C. (res); Qns '43; Phys Med & Rehab; Chief of Serv. & Dir. (Phys Med.), Shaughnessy Hosp.; Tel. TR 6-6767.
CHEREWATY, Theodore W.; 211 Simcoe St. S., Oshawa, Ont.; Tor '63; Staff, Ontario Hosp., Whitby; Staff, Oshawa Gen. Hosp.; Tel. 3-2211.
CHERKEZOFF, Alexander; 2493 Commercial Dr., Vancouver 12, B.C.; 3577 W. 35th (res); UBC '57; MCGP; Tel. TR 4-8919.
CHERNENKOFF, Ralph M.; 40 Dolphin Bay., Regina, Sask.; Sask '63.
CHERNENKOFF, William; 631 Med. Arts Bldg., 750 Spadina Cr. W., Saskatoon, Sask.; Sask'63; AMCGP; Staff, City & St. Paul's Hosp.; Staff (ObstGyn.), University Hosp.; Tel. 244-2951.
CHERNIACK, Louis Winnipeg Clinic, St. Mary's & Vaughan St., Winnipeg 1, Man.; 206 Hampton House, 333 Wellington Cr. (res); Man '32; B.Sc. (Med.); MRCP (Lond.); FACP; FCCP; FRCP(C); IntMed; Assoc. Phys. (Med.), Winnipeg Gen. Hosp.; Assoc. Prof. (Med.), U. of Man.; Tel 942-0551
CHERNIAK, Morris M.; 5456A Westminster Ave., Montreal 29, P.Q.; 4640 Bourret (res); Tor '52; Paed; Tel. HU 1-7167.
CHERNIAK, Reuben M.; Cardio-Resp. Unit, Winnipeg Gen. Hosp., Winnipeg 3, Man.; Man'48; MSc(Med.); FACP; FRCP(C), IntMed; Dir. Cardio-Resp Unit & Intensive Care Unit, Winnipeg Gen. Hosp.; Assoc. Prof. Med., U. of Manitoba; Tel. SP 4-6511, ext. 234.
CHERNIAK, Avinoam B.; (Intern) c/o Apt. 1105, 518 Mohawk Rd. E., Hamilton, Ont.; Wes'62.
CHERNICK, Beryl A. (Wilensky); Wes '62; Res., Med. Research, Dept. of ObstGyn. & Pharm., U. of Western Ontario, London, Ont.
CHERNICK, Victor; 23 Peony Ave., Winnipeg 17, Man.; Man'59.
CHERRY, Richard R.; Devon Clinic, Devon, Alta.; McG'50; Tel. 447-3798.
CHERTKOW, Gerald; 519 Med. Arts Bldg., Saskatoon, Sask.; Tor '50; FRCP(C), IntMed; Active Clin. Staff, University, City & St. Paul's Hosp's.; Med. Dir., Saskatoon Depot Cdn. Red Cross Transfusion Serv.; Ass't Clin. Prof. (Med.), U. of Saskatchewan; Tel. 242-5132.
CHESEBROUGH, John N.; 847 Princess St., Kingston, Ont. (res); Qns '59; Research, Queen's U.
CHESKES, Albert; Ste. 210, 170 Bloor St. W., Toronto 5, Ont.; Tor'61; Ophth.
CHESLER, Abraham L.; 2080 Willistead Cr., Windsor Ont.; Witwatersrand (S. Africa) '52; DiagRad.
CHESLEY, Arthur E.; 246 Princess St., Saint John, N.B.; 99 Wentworth St. (res); Dal '55; FRCS(C), Urol; Urol., Saint John Gen. & Saint Joseph's Hosp's.; Tel. 692-0601.
CHESNEY, D. Desmond; Box 639, Ponoka, Alta.; Trinity C. (Dublin, Ire.) '52; Tel. 783-3306.
CHESNEY, L. Parker; 1414 Drummond St., Montreal 25, P.Q.; 3455 Glencoe Ave. Mtl. 16 (res); McG'40; M.C.G.P.; Assoc. Phys., OPD, Mtl. Gen. Hosp.; Dem. Med., McGill U.; Med. Dir. Health Serv., Imperial Tobacco Co.; Tel. AV 8-7430.
CHESNEY, Robert; Dublin (Ire.) '54; Res. (Rad.), Toronto Gen. Hosp., Toronto, Ont.
CHESNIE, Joshua J.; 316 St. Clair Ave. W., Toronto 10, Ont.; 349 Courtleigh Blvd., Tor 12 (res); Tor '43; IntMed; Att'd. Phys., New Mt. Sinai Hosp.; & Baycrest Home for the Aged; Vol. Clin. Ass't., U. of Toronto; Tel. 922-6104.
CHESTNUT, Harold W.; Box 207, Moosomin, Sask.; Man '40; GenSurg; Tel. 435-2500.

CHESTNUT, Walter O.; Box 199, Hartland, N.B.; McG '23; M.C.G.P.; Staff, Carleton Mem. Hosp.; Dist. Coroner; Tel. 375-4334.

CHETWYND, John B.; 20 Edgewood Cres., Toronto 5, Ont. (res); Edinburgh (Scot.) '43; D.M.-R.D. (Eng.), DiagRad; Sr. Ass't. Rad., Toronto East Gen. Hosp.; Tel. 461-8272.

CHEUK, Shu Kwan; Man '61; Jr. Intn., St. Boniface Hosp., St. Boniface, Man.

CHEUNG, On T.; Lingnan (China) '48; DPH; FCCP; Staff, Phys., Toronto Hosp. for TB, Weston, Ont.; Tel. 769-1161.

CHEVALIER, Louise M.; Room 402, Montreal Children's Hosp., Montreal 25, P.Q.; Tor'57; Paed (P.Q.); Staff, Mtl. Children's Hosp.; Fell., Tumour Serv; Tel. WE 7-8511.

CHEVALIER, Paul A.; Edifice Continental, 111 King St. W., Sherbrooke, P.Q.; 411 Liege (res); Lav '51; FRCS(C), GenSurg.; Surg., Hop.-St.-Vincent-de-Paul; Tel. LO 9-4022.

CHEVALIER, P. M.; Department of National Health & Welfare, c/o Regional Superintendent, European Region. Abroad.

CHEVALIER, Veronique; Mon '64; Res., Inst. Albert-Prevost, Montreal, P.Q.; Abroad.

CHEVREFILS, Paul E.; 7960A St. Denis, Montreal, P.Q.; Mon '47; Tel. 387-6448.

CHEVRETTE, Georges A.; 554 Blvd. Manseau, Joliette, P.Q.; Mon '50; Teacher, School of Nursing.

CHEVRETTE, Line; 344 Chemin-Ste-Catherine, Montreal, P.Q.; Mon'58; Ophth.

CHEW, C. Ken; 340 McLeod St., Ottawa 4, Ont.; Adelaide (Aust.)'56; FRCP(C), IntMed; Staff, Ottawa Gen. Hosp.; Lect. Med., U. of Ottawa; Tel. 731-9425.

CHIANG, James B.; 1530 Albion Rd., Rexdale, Ont.; Tor '62.

CHIANG, Patrick J.; McG'65; Jr. Int., St. Marys Memorial Hosp., Montreal 26, P.Q.; Abroad.

CHIANG, Thomas H.; 327 Erie Ave., Brantford, Ont.; Shanghai (China) '35; D.T.M. (Calcutta); D.P.H.

CHIAO, John T. Y.; Peiking (China) '49; Dir. Dept. of Health, Regina, 1910 McIntyre St., Regina, Sask.; Tel. 522-1621, Ext. 277.

CHIASSON, Armand; C.P. 1570, 368-3eme Ave., Amos, P.Q.; Lav '59; GenSurg (P.Q.); Staff, Hop. d'Amos; Tel. 732-3341.

CHIASSON, Edgar; Grand Falls, N.B.; Mon '25.

CHIASSON, Jean P.; 505 de Lanaudiere, Joliette, P.Q.; Lav'46; Psy(P.Q.); Staff, Rehab. Clinic for Alcoholism.

CHIASSON, Marcelle; Box 2049, 4444 Lakelse Ave,. Terrace, B.C.; Ott '62.

CHICK, John M.; Ott'63; Res., Hosp. for Sick Children, Toronto 2, Ont.

CHICOINE, F. Luc.; Hop. Ste-Justine, Montreal, P.Q.; Mon'53; DABP; FRCP(C), Paed; Assoc. Prof. (Paed.), U. of Montreal; Tel. 731-4931.

CHICOINE, Jean M.; Mon '63; Res., Hop. Notre-Dame, Montreal, P.Q.

CHICOINE, Paul E.; 1251 St.-Denis, Montreal 18, P.Q.; Vercheres (res); Mon '37; Tel. VI 4-5402.

CHICOINE, Raymond; 1150 Blvd. St. Joseph E., Montreal 34, P.Q.; Mon '54; Paed; Tel. LA 7-1551.

CHILD, Barry G.; London (Eng.) '56; Staff, Grenfell Hosp., St. Anthony, Nfld.

CHILDE, Arthur E.; 25 Medical Arts Bldg., Winnipeg 1, Man.; 62 Mount Royal Cres., St. James, Winnipeg 12 (res); Man '25; A.C.R., Diag. Roent., F.A.C.R.; DiagRad; Rad., Children's Hosp.; Assoc. Rad., Winnipeg Gen. Hosp.; Assoc. Prof. (Rad.), U. of Manitoba; Tel. GR 4-9110.

CHILDS, Mary C.; 14 Lakeside Rd., Valois, P.Q. (res); McG '22; Paed; Retired.

CHIN, Edward J.; 50 Larkfield Dr., Don Mills, Ont.; McG'59.

CHIN, Wilfred C.; 74 W. Seymour, Irving Clinic, Kamloops, B.C.; 657 Tunstall Cres. (res); McG '54; Paed; Staff, Royal Inland Hosp.; Tel. 372-5251.

CHINN, Betty C. (See DEWICK)

CHIONG, Miguel A.; Etherington Hall, Queen's U., Kingston, Ont.; Havana (Cuba)'50; MSc (Med); PhD; FRCP(C), IntMed; Ass't. Prof. (Med. & Phys.), Queen's U.

CHIPMAN, Charles D.; 1735 Beech Ave., Halifax, N.S.; Dal '53; F.R.C.P.(C), Path; Staff, Path. Inst. Halifax, Ass't. Prof. Dalhousie U., Tel. 24406.

CHIPPERFIELD, D. V.; Prince Albert Clinic, 49-13th St. W., Prince Albert, Sask.; 244-19th St. W. (res); Man '43; MCGP; Tel. 764-4241.

CHIPPERFIELD, Lawrence S.; Ste. 600, 713 Columbia St., New Westminster, B.C.; 413 Queens Ave. (res); Man '35; M.C.G.P.; Chief, Med. Staff, St. Mary's Hosp.; Tel. LA 1-5941.

CHIPPERFIELD, W. Gordon; Man'52; GenSurg; Staff, Colonel Belcher Hosp., Calgary, Alta.

CHIRICOSTA, Albert A.; Ott '64; Jr. Int., St. Mary's Hosp., Montreal, P.Q.

CHISHOLM, A. Roy; 1841 Bush St., Nanaimo, B.C.; Dal '25.

CHISHOLM, Arthur W.; Sunnybrook Hosp., Toronto, Ont.; Tor'49; FRCP(C), IntMed; Dir., Div. of Cardiovasc Dis., Sunnybrook Hosp.; Ass't. Prof., U. of Toronto.

CHISHOLM, Brock; West Coast Rd., Sooke, Victoria, B.C.; Tel. 472-5974.

CHISHOLM, David M.; 904A Brunette St., New Westminster, B.C.; Sask '64.

CHISHOLM, Hugh A.; 812 Fairmont Med. Bldg., 750 W. Broadway, Vancouver 9, B.C.; 6727 Marine Cres. (res); Dal '41; GenSurg; Tel. TR 4-6633.

CHISHOLM, J. Ian; Dal '52; Med. Supt., R. W. Large Mem. Hosp., Bella Bella, B.C.

CHISHOLM, Laurence W. L.; 818-9th Ave. N., Port Alberni, B.C.; Alb '39; MCGP; Tel. 723-2111.

CHISHOLM, Lionel D.; 503 Medical Dental Bld., 1849 Yonge St., Toronto, Ont.; Tor'59; FRCS(C), Ophth.

CHISHOLM, Malcolm J.; New Waterford Medical Clinic, New Waterford, Cape Breton, N.S.; Gibbon St. (res); Dal '34; Staff, New Waterford Gen. Hosp.

CHISHOLM, Mary (See MacLaren, Mary).

CHISHOLM, Robert A.; Dal'62; Res., Victoria Gen. Hosp., Halifax, N.S.

CHISHOLM, W. Laurie; Port Alberni Med. Bldg., 818-9th Ave. N., Port Alberni, B.C.; 207-7th Ave. S. (res); Alb '39; MCGP; Tel. 623-2111.

CHISHOLM, W. Murdoch; 41 Academy Med. Bldg., 1812—4th St. W., Calgary, Alta. 1122 Levis Ave. (res); Dal '52; MCGP; Tel. 263-6262.

CHITTICK, William J.; Muskoka St., Gravenhurst, Ont.; John St. (res); Tor '50.

CHIU, Sylvester S.; McG'64; Res., Royal Victoria Hosp., Montreal 2, P.Q.; Abroad.

CHIU, Wing G.; 193 E. Hastings St., Vancouver 4, B.C.; UBC '60; Tel. 683-4020.

CHLEBUS, Andrew; 1908 Weston Rd., Weston, Ont.; Tor '57; FRCP(C), Paed; D&TRad; Chief of Paed., Humber Mem. Hosp.; Clin. Ass't., Hosp. for Sick Children; Tel. 241-3461.

CHMARA, John; 464 King St. E., Oshawa, Ont. (res); Tor '42; D.I.M.; Med. Dir., General Motors of Canada, Oshawa; Tel. 725-7311.

CHOATE, John F.; Box 849, Steinbach Clin., Steinbach, Man.; Man '55; Dist. Coroner.

CHOCHINOV, Harvey; 401 Med. Arts Bldg., 404-406 Graham Ave., Winnipeg 1, Man.; Man '51; B.Sc. (Med.); Dip.Surg. (U. of Man.); DABS; FACS; FRCS(C), GenSurg; Active Staff, Wpg. Gen & Grace Hosp's.; Cons. Staff, Manitoba Rehab. Hosp.; Court Staff, Children's, St. Boniface & Misericordia Hosp's.; Lect. (Surg.), Dental Fac. & Dem. (Surg.), U. of Manitoba; Tel. 943-6996.

CHO-CHU, Claude B.; Arnprior Med. Centre, 104 Daniel St., Arnprior, Ont.; McG'65.

CHODIRKER, William B.; 304 Suburban Crt., Apt. 13, Rochester, N.Y., U.S.A. 14620; Man '59; FRCP(C), IntMed; Abroad.

CHODOS, Hedgwige E.; Ste. 904, 750 W. Broadway, Vancouver 9, B.C.; U. de Genève (Switz.) '50; F.R.C.S.(C), Ophth.; Tel. TR 2-2601.

CHODOS, Joel B.; Ste. 904, 750 W. Broadway, Vancouver 9, B.C.; U. de Genève (Switz.) '53; F.R.C.S.(C), Ophth.; Tel. TR 2-2601.
CHODYNIECKI, Carl P.; 171 Montreal Road, Cornwall, Ont.; Lav'49; AMCGP; Tel. WE. 2-3354.
CHOI, Jae K.; Kunyngpook (N. Korea); Staff, Saskatchewan Hosp., Weyburn, Sask.
CHOI, Joseph H.; Chonnam (Korea)'57; Staff, Dept. of Path., Queen's U., Kingston, Ont.
CHOI, Ock Soon; 35 Woodridge Cr., Apt. 112, Ottawa 14, Ont.; Soeul (Korea)'55; IntMed.
CHOI, Soon M.; Seoul (Korea)'55; Psy; Staff, Provincial Hosp., Campbellton, N.B.
CHOINERE, Jacques A.; 1 Ave. Lorrain, Iberville, P.Q.; Mon '54; Path (PQ).
CHOINIERE, Jacques A.; 217 rue Longueuil, St. Jean, P.Q.; Mon'54; Path(P.Q.).
CHOINIERE, Jean L.; Mon '63; Sr.Int., Hop. Hotel-Dieu, Montreal 18, P.Q.
CHOLETTE, Albert M.; 1451 Blvd. St. Joseph E., Montreal, P.Q.; Lav '11; Tel. LA 1-9630.
CHOLETTE, Claude; 1457 est, Boul. St-Joseph, Montreal 34, P.Q.; Mon '48; F.R.C.S.(C), GenSurg; Tel. LA 2-7195.
CHOLETTE, Gilles; 1133 Blvd. St. Joseph E., Montreal 34, P.Q.; Mon '53; F.R.C.S.(C), GenSurg.; Tel. 272-8229.
CHOLETTE, Jean P.; Ste. 307, 3875, St-Urbain, Montreal 18, P.Q.; Mon '41; FRCS(C); GenSurg; Surg., Hop. Hotel-Dieu de Montreal; Ass't. Prof. (Surg.), U. of Montreal.
CHOLETTE, J. Rene; P.O. Box 480, Sturgeon Falls, Ont.; Lav '45; MCGP; M.O.H., Sturgeon Falls.
CHOLOD, Eugene J.; Alb'62; Res., Victoria Hosp., London, Ont.
CHOLOD, Steven; Myrnam, Alta.; Qns '44; M.C.-G.P.; Dist. Coroner.
CHONG, Henry K. H.; 4582 W. 10th, Vancouver B.C.; 5826 Tisdall No. 9 (res); UBC'56; AMCGP; Tel. CA 4-0480.
CHONG, Ming; (See Yao, Ming).
CHONG, Paul; Ott '60; Res., Kingston Gen. Hosp., Kingston, Ont.
CHONG, Pook C. Li; National U. (Ire.)'56; Staff, Bingham Mem. Hosp., Matheson, Ont.; Abroad.
CHONKO, Michael E.; Two Hills, Alta.; Alb '48; M.C.G.P.
CHOQUET, Jean; 4395 Verdun Avenue, Verdun, P.Q.; Mon '46; Gyn. (P.Q.).
CHOQUET, Marcel; 307 St- Jacques, St- Scholastique, Cte Deux-Montagnes, P.Q.; Mon '60.
CHOQUETTE, Gaston; 2260 Blvd. Pie IX, Montreal 4, P.Q.; 1826 rue Lajoie, Outremont (res); Mon '50; IntMed (Cardiol.) (PQ); Staff, Inst.-de- Cardiol. & Hop.-Jean-Talon; Teach. Staff, U. of Montreal; Tel. CL 5-9989.
CHOQUETTE, Gaudias; 1570, rue St.-Hubert, Montreal 24, P.Q.; Mon '24; Staff, Dept. of Health; Retired.
CHOQUETTE, J. Luc; 3720-2e rue, Chomedey, P.Q.; Mon '60; Tel. 681-0539.
CHOQUETTE, Pierre; Mon '64; Int., Hop. Maisonneuve, Montreal, P.Q.
CHOQUETTE, Rene; 8415 St.-Denis, Montreal 11, P.Q. Mon '54; Tel. DU 1-1801.
CHOQUETTE, Stanislas; 2260 Blvd. Pie IX, Montreal 4, P.Q.; Lav '16; Tel. CL 5-9989.
CHORAS, Peter T.; McG'59; Psy(P.Q.); Res., Children's Psych. Clinic, Royal Victoria Hosp., Montreal 2, P.Q.
CHORLEY, Gordon E.; 2402-5th Ave. S., Lethbridge, Alta.; London (Eng.) '50; M.R.S.C. (Eng.), L.R.C.P. (Lond.), D.A.(Eng.), Anaes.
CHORNEY, Joseph K.; Lab., St. Paul's Hosp., Saskatoon, Sask.; Alb '56; Path; Assoc. Path., St. Paul's Hosp.; Sess. Lect. (Path.), U. of Saskatchewan; Tel. 652-8220.
CHORNOBAY, William; Ste. 104, 634 3rd. Road, Richmond, B.C.; Man'49.
CHOU, Chun L.; Box 730, North Battleford, Sask. (res); National Central U. (Nanking, China) '45; DPH; MCGP; M. O., Dept. of National Health & Welfare.
CHOU, Liang-Ying; 208—1541 W. Broadway, Vancouver, B.C.; 1925 W. 12th (res); Lingnan **(China) '45; Paed.; Tel. RE 3-0911.**
CHOU, Wei H.; Taiwan (Formosa) '51; Path; Staff, St. Martha's Hosp., Antigonish, N.S.; Tel. 863-2830.
CHOUDHRI, Fiaz A.; Punjab, (Pakistan) '60; Res. Victoria Gen. Hosp., **Halifax, N.S.**
CHOUINARD, Alphonse M.; 307 Ave. Arnaud, Sept-Iles, Cte. Saguenay, P.Q.; **Lav '50.**
CHOUINARD, Clarence J.; 127 Church Ave., Chilliwack, B.C.; Alb'49; DiagRad.; DABR; Staff, Chilliwack Gen. Hosp., Langley Mem. Hosp., Langley, Mission Mem. Hosp., Mission City & M.S.A. Hosp., Abbotsford; Tel. 795-7205.
CHOUINARD, Crescent; Lav'64; Res., Hop. St. Justine, Montreal 26, P.Q.
CHOUINARD, Jean; 630, Baillarge, Quebec, P.Q.; Lav '49; Anaes.
CHOUINARD, Pierre P.; 2 de l'Eglise, St- Romauld, Cte Levis, P.Q.; Lav '58; AMCGP.
CHOVIL, Alan C.; Shouldice Clinic, 618 Church St., Toronto 5, Ont.; Cambridge (Eng.)'50; MCGP; Tel. WA 3-3507.
CHOW, Kenneth C.; Sask'64; Res. (Rad.), University Hosp., Saskatoon, Sask.
CHOWDHARY, Bharat L.; Bihar (India)'57; Staff, RCAF Hosp., Portage La Prairie, Man.
CHOWN, Bruce, M.C.; 735 Notre-Dame, Winnipeg 3, Man.; 147 East Gate (res); Man '22; Paed; Cons. Paed., Winnipeg Children's, Grace & St. Boniface Hosp's.; Prof. (Paed), U. of Manitoba; Tel. GR 4-9110.
CHRETIEN, J. F. Maurice; 537 Station, Shawinigan Falls, P.Q.; 842 rue St-Hubert (res); Lav '37; F.R.C.S.(C), ObstGyn; Chief of ObstGyn., **Hop. Ste. Therese; Tel. LE 6-2020.**
CHRETIEN, Louis; Lav'62; GenSurg; Staff, Hotel-Dieu de Quebec, Quebec, P.Q.
CHRETIEN, Michel; Mon '60; Res. Hop. Hotel Dieu, Montreal, P.Q.
CHRIS, Samuel M.; Ste 606, 99 Avenue Rd., Toronto 5, Ont.; 67 Hillhurst Blvd., Tor. 12 (res); London (Eng.) '43; FRCS (Eng.) GenSurg; Active Surg., Staff, New Mt. Sinai Hosp.; Teach (Surg.), U. of Toronto; Tel. WA 1-1993.
CHRIST, Elly; Central Butte, Sask.; Amsterdam; **(Holl) '52.**
CHRIST, George J.; 892 Queen's Blvd., Kitchener, Ont.; St. Andrews (Scot.) '49.
CHRIST, Louis W.; Central Butte, Sask.; Amsterdam (Neth.) '52.
CHRISTENSEN, H. F.; 3596 W. 27th Ave., Vancouver, B.C.; 3328 Point Grey (res); Alb '42; M.C.G.P.; Tel. RE 3-7112.
CHRISTENSEN, Kenneth H.; Box 2049, 4444 Lakelse Ave., Terrace, B.C.; 4828 Davis Rd. (res); Tor '57; MCGP; Sec., Med. Staff, Mills Mem. Hosp.; Tel. VI 3-2273. Abroad.
CHRISTENSEN, Ralph M.; 711-750 W. Broadway, Vancouver 9, B.C.; 5970 Hudson St. (res); UBC '54; FRCS(C); GenSurg; Att'd. Surg., Vancouver Gen. Hosp.; Clin. Instr. (Surg), U.B. C.; Tel. 874-3611
CHRISTIANSEN, Harvey; Box 1925, Nipawin, Sask.; Wes '56.
CHRISTIE, Clara; 140-2nd Ave. W., Calgary, Alta.; McG '25; Retired.
CHRISTIE, David; Apt. 2102, 1450 W. Georgia St. Vancouver 5, B.C. (res); Man '29; IntMed; Staff, St. Paul's Hosp.; Part-time Cons. (Med.), Shaughnessy Hosp., D.V.A.; Tel. MU 1-9924.
CHRISTIE-DOWLING Pearl; Sub. P.O. 13, Calgary, Alta. (res); McG '27; Paed; Retired.
CHRISTIE, Francis M.; Campbell Clinic, Lethbridge, Alta., 2839 Parkside (res); Alb '41; Chief of Surg., Lethbridge Mun. Hosp.; Cons. Surg., Prov. Cancer Clin.; Tel. FA 7-5737.
CHRISTIE, Garth B.; 225 Main St., Nashwaksis, N.B.; Dal'65.
CHRISTIE, Henry R.; 901 Helena St., Trail, B.C.; 27 Hazlewood Dr. (res); McG '28; ObstGyn.
CHRISTIE, Hugh E.; 107 Church St., Amherst, N.S.; 195 Victoria St. E. (res); Dal '39; D.I.M., F.R.C.P.(C), IntMed; Staff, Highland View Hosp.

CHRISTIE, John E.; 20 Harriet, Lachute, P.Q.; McG'19.
CHRISTIE, Keith A.; Winnipeg Clinic, St. Mary's Ave. & Vaughan St., Winnipeg 1, Man.; Ste. 306, 491 Stradbrook Ave. (res); Man '57; Paed, Active Staff, Winnipeg Children's Hosp.; Tel. WH 2-0551.
CHRISTIE, Paul; Ontario Hospital, 999 Queen St. W., Toronto 3, Ont.; McG'51; D.Psy; Psy; Supt. Ontario Hosp.; Ass't. Prof. (Psy.) U. of Toronto; Central Reg. Rep., Mental Health Div., Ont. Dept. of Health; Tel. LE 3-8501, Loc. 241.
CHRISTIE, R. George; Ste 1302, 750 W. Broadway, Vancouver 9, B.C.; Alb'45; Psy; DPH; Tel. 876-6921.
CHRISTIE, Ronald J.; 4 King Cres., Weston, Ont.; 146 Queenslea Ave. (res); Tor '57; MCGP; Staff, Humber Mem. Hosp.; Tel. 248-1712.
CHRISTIE, Ronald V.; Edinburgh (Scot.) '25; D.Sc. (Lond.); FRCP (London); FACP; FRCP(C); IntMed; Prof. & Dean, Faculty of Med., McGill U., Montreal, P.Q.; Psy.-in-Chief, Royal Victoria Hosp.; Tel. VI 2-1251.
CHRISTIE, Thomas A.; 1010 McCallum Hill Bldg., Regina, Sask.; 3808 Lakeview Ave. (res); Queen's U. (Belfast, N. Ire.) '52; Anaes; Sr. Anaes., Regina Gen. & Grey Nuns Hosp's.; Tel. LA 2-0704.
CHRISTIN, Rolland; 2260 E. Boul. St.-Joseph, Montreal 34, P.Q.; Mon '34; Tel. 526-7588.
CHRISTOPHERSON, E.; Ste. 813-4, 750 W. Broadway, Vancouver 9, B.C.; 4712 W. 6th Ave. (res); Man '36; F.A.C.P., F.R.C.P.(C), IntMed; Att'd. Staff, Shaughnessy DVA Hosp. & Vancouver Gen. Hosp.; Clin. Instr. U. of British Columbia; Tel. TR 9-5744.
CHRISTY, Nicholas G.; Tor'61; Res., Hosp. for Sick Children, Toronto 2, Ont.
CHRITCHLEY, John H.; Wes'65; Res., University of Alberta Hosp., Edmonton, Alta.
CHROM, Vivian H.; 695 Markham Rd., Scarborough, Ont.; 23 Wetherfield Pl. Don Mills (res); Tor'58; AMCGP; Tel. AT 4-4441.
CHRZAN, B. George; 241 Colborne St., London, Ont.; 183 Cathcart St. (res); Poznan (Poland) '38; M.C.G.P.
CHRZANOWSKI, Zbigniew P.; 8225-105th St., Edmonton, Alta.; Alb'62; Court. Staff, Edmonton Gen. & St. Joseph's Hosp's.; Tel. 433-1402.
CHU D. Donald; McG'65; Jr. Int., St. Michael's Hosp., Toronto 2, Ont.; Abroad.
CHU, Dodd, Q.; Ste. 215, 4900 Kingsway, South Burnaby, B.C.; 642-W. 51st Ave. (res); McG '49; DIM; IntMed; Cons. (Med), St. Mary's, Royal Columbian, Burnaby Gen., Mt. St. Joseph's & Surrey Mem. Hosp's.; Vis. Staff, Vancouver Gen. Hosp.; Tel. HE 3-0545.
CHU, Frederick S.; Ste 304, 16 E. Hastings St., Vancouver, B.C.; 610 Esquimalt Ave., West Vancouver (res); McG '39; Tel. MU 3-2053.
CHU, J. Thomas; Stonegate Plaza, 150 Berry Rd., Toronto 18, Ont.; 79 Jameson Ave. (res); UBC '62; Staff, St. Joseph's & St. Michael's Hosp's.; Tel. 239-9292.
CHU, Ming; Manchuria '45; Staff, Yorkton Union Hosp., Yorkton, Sask.
CHU, Peggy S.; Tsingtao (China)'62; Res., Royal Alexandra Hosp., Edmonton, Alta.
CHUBB, David; Tor'64; Res. (Ophth.), U. of Toronto, Toronto, Ont.
CHUGHTAI, Mohammad S.; 3622 Durocher St., Apt. 401, Montreal, P.Q.; Punjab (India)'57; FRCS(C), GenSurg.
CHUI, David H. K.; McG '63; Jr. Ass't. Res., Royal Victoria Hosp., Montreal, P.Q. Abroad.
CHUN, Won C.; Box 488, Prince Rupert, B.C.; Seoul Women's Med. Coll. (Korea)'55; DABP; M.O., Dept. of National Health & Welfare; Tel. 624-1817.
CHUNG, Hiyoung; '57; Channel Port aux Basques, Nfld.
CHUNG, M. H.; 222 E. Broadway, Vancouver, B.C.; Yale (China) '48; ObstGyn.; Tel. TR 6-2618.
CHUNG, Wallace B.; 1538 W. 40th Ave., Vancouver 13, B.C. (res); McG '53; F.R.C.S.(C), GenSurg; Staff (Surg.), Vancouver Gen. Hosp.; Ass't. Prof. (Surg.), U. of British Columbia; Tel. TR 6-3211.
CHURCH, Athol C.; 74 Hughson St. S., Hamilton, Ont.; 110 Terrace Dr. (res); McG '39; D. Psy.; Dir., Mental Health Clinic, Dept. of Public Health, Hamilton. Retired.
CHURCH, C. B. G.; 10 Wilson W., Perth, Ont.; R.R. No. 5 (res); McG '33; M.C.G.P.; Tel. 267-3500.
CHURCH, J. Peter; Box 260, 282 Byrne Rd., Temiscaming, P.Q.; McG '51; Staff, Temiscaming Hosp.; Tel. GE 7-3251.
CHURCHILL, Bernard M.; Alb '63; Res. (GenSurg.), University Hosp., Edmonton, Alta.
CHURCHILL, Lewis P.; Shelburne, N.S.; McG '09; Roseway Hosp. Pres. Med. Bd.; M.O.H., Sherbourne; Retired.
CHURCHILL, Margaret E.; 253 Main St., Yarmouth, N.S.; Dal '60; Paed.
CHUTE, Andrew L., O.B.E.; 78B Crescent Rd., Toronto 5, Ont. (res); Tor'35; PhD.; FRCP(C), Paed; Prof. Dept. of Paed., Hosp. for Sick Children; Dean, Faculty of Med., U. of Toronto; Tel. 928-2710.
CHUTE, Helen Evans Reid; 77 Golfdale Rd., Toronto, Ont. (res); Alb '35; Paed; Retired.
CHWELOS, Nicholas; Ste. 502 Britannia, 800 Elbow Dr. - 50th Ave. S.W., Calgary, Alta.; UBC'55; Psy.
CIABURRO, Hugo E.; Mon '62; Res., Hop. Notre-Dame, Montreal 24, P.Q.
CIANFLONE, Carlo G.; 4130 Decarie Blvd., Montreal 28, P.Q.; Ott '54; DiagRad; Staff, Queen Elizabeth Hosp.; Tel. 738-9481.
CIOTOLA, Georges J.; 7229 St. Denis, Montreal, P.Q.; McG '64; Tel. 277-0644.
CIPRICK, William J.; 148 Reynolds Ave., Oakville, Ont.; McG '58; Anaes; Tel. 845-8701.
CIPYWNYK, Dmytro; Cumberland Square Shopping Centre, Saskatoon, Sask.; Sask'64; AMCGP; Active Staff, St. Paul's & Saskatoon City Hosp's.; Tel. 343-1631.
CIRKOVIC, Miodrag; 9648 boul La Salle, Cite Lasalle, P.Q.; Paris (France) '56; Anaes; Hop.-Gen.-La-Salle; Tel. DO 5-1510.
CITRON, Sidney P.; 62 Matson Rd., Downsview, Ont.; Tor '60; Tel. CH 7-9661.
CITRY, Edgar; 1 Croydon Rd., Toronto 10, Ont. (res); Bologna (Italy) '37; D.Psy; Psy; Clin. Dir. (Male Serv.) Ontario Hosp., Whitby, Ont.; Tel. RU 7-7676.
CIVKIN, Sidney W.; Ste. 702, 625 - 5th Ave., New Westminster, B.C.; 6922 Laurel, Van. 14 (res); Man'42; Otol; Hd. Dept. Ophth, Otol, Royal Columbian Hosp.; Tel. LA 2-4434.
CLAMAN, A. David; 302, 720 W. Broadway, Vancouver 9, B.C.; 3374 Osler St. (res); Qns '46; FRCS(C), ObstGyn; Ass't. Prof. (ObstGyn.), & Dir. of P.G. Educ., U. of British Columbia; Tel. TR 6-2626.
CLAMEN, Marvin; Ste 265, 6000 Cote des Neiges Rd., Montreal, P.Q.; 4991 Circle Rd. (res); McG '52; F.R.C.P.(C), IntMed; Ass't. Phys., Jewish Gen. Hosp.; Tel. RE 9-8651.
CLANCEY, Ian L. W.; 1259 Meadowlands Dr. E., Ottawa, Ont. (res); London (Eng.) '40; MRCS (Eng.); LRCP (Lond.); DPM (Lond.); Psy; Med. Supt. (Psy. Div.), Royal Ottawa San.; Ass't. Prof. (Psy.), U. of Ottawa; Tel.PA 2-9047.
CLANCY, Patrick R.; 287 Queen's Ave., London, Ont.; Wes '53; Anaes; Staff, St. Joseph's & Victoria Hosp's.; Instr. (Anaes.), U. of Western Ont.; Tel. GE 8-5143.
CLAPPERTON, Gage; Grande-Riviere, P.Q.; Lav '53; Pres. Med. Staff, Hop.-de-la-Providence, Chandler; Tel. 33.
CLAPPERTON, James A.; 9 Stadium Shopping Centre, Calgary, Alta.; Wes'63; AMCGP.
CLAPPERTON, Joyce C.; Ste. 207, 1632-14th Ave. N.W., Calgary, Alta.; R.R. 4, (res); Edinburgh (Scot.) '57; MCGP; Tel. AV 9-7394.
CLARE, David W.; DVA Clinic, 185 Ouellette Ave., Windsor, Ont.; Qns'40; MCGP.

CLARE, Rupert M.; 308 Professional Bldg., 10830 Jasper Ave., Edmonton, Alta.; 13830 Ravine Dr. (res); Alb '38; DABR; D & T Rad; Dir. Dept. of Rad., Edmonton Gen. Hosp.; Lect., U. of Alberta; Tel. 422-1390.
CLARE, W. Harvey; Ste. 220, Med. Arts Bldg., Hamilton, Ont.; 36 Searle St. (res.); Wes. '41; D. Psy; Psy; Chief of Psy., St. Joseph's Hosp.; Tel. JA 9-2004.
CLAREMONT, Peter F.; Sydney (Australia) '56; DMRD (Lond.); DiagRad; Rad., St. Joseph's Hosp., Dawson Creek, B.C.; Staff, Providence Hosp., Fort St. John.
CLARK, Alexander M.; Pubnico, N.S.; Birmingham (Eng.)'47.
CLARK, Arthur; Tofield, Alta.; London (Eng.) '55; M.B., B.S., Tel. 662-3242. Abroad.
CLARK, Barry L.; Qns '58; Res., Royal Victoria Hosp., Montreal, P.Q.
CLARK, Cecil W.; Manitoba Clinic, 790 Sherbrook St., Winnipeg, Man.; 140 Waterloo St., (res); Man '31; F.R.C.S. (Edin.), F.A.C.S., F.R.C.S.(C), GenSurg; Cons. Surg; Deer Lodge DVA Hosp.; Assoc. Surg., Winnipeg Gen. Hosp.; Surg., Children's Hosp.; Assoc. Prof. (Surg.), U. of Manitoba; Tel GR 4-9110.
CLARK, David B.; McG'56; Psy; Staff Psy., Royal Victoria Hosp., Barrie, Ont.
CLARK, Dennis M.; 1669 Victoria St., Prince George, B.C.; UBC'56; Hd. Anaes. Serv., Prince George Reg. Hosp.; Tel. LO 4-7007.
CLARK, Donald R.; 707 Charlotte St., Peterborough, Ont.; 634 Weller St. (res); Tor '42; Paed; Staff, Peterborough Civic & St. Joseph's Hosp's; O.P.D. Staff, Hosp. for Sick Children, Toronto; Tel. 742-3871.
CLARK, Donald S.; Waverley, N.S.
CLARK, Douglas; Glazier Med. Centre, 136 Simcoe St. N., Oshawa, Ont.; Glasgow (Scot.)'46.
CLARK, Ernest A.; 116 Chapman St. W., Port Dover, Ont.; Qns '24; Psy; Psy., Ontario Hosp., Woodstock; Tel. 537-5511.
CLARK, George C.; 110 Med. Arts Bldg., 73 Cumberland St. N., Port Arthur, Ont.; Qns '49; Anaes; Active Staff, St. Joseph's, Gen. & McKellar Gen. Hosp., Fort William; Tel. 344-1813.
CLARK, George N.; Morinville, Alta.; Aberdeen (Scot.) '27; F.R.C.S.
CLARK, Gordon A.; 241 Colborne St., London, Ont.; 79 Centre St. (res); Wes '43; FRCS (Edin.); FRFPS (Glasgow); Pt.-time Cons. Surg., Westminster DVA Hosp.; Tel. 432-1536.
CLARK, Gordon F.; Box 182, Vancouver, B.C.; Alb'48; Anaes; Tel. WA 2-8690.
CLARK, James M.; 235 Church St., Box 275, Oakville, Ont.; Guy's Hosp. (London, Eng.) '55; M.B., B.S., D.A., Anaes; Active Cons., Oakville Trafalgar Mem. Hosp.; Tel. 844-6005.
CLARK, James V.; Mayo, Yukon T.; McG '50; Public Health Officer; Tel. 3201.
CLARK, John A.; UBC'60; FRCP(C), Derm; Staff, Dept. of Derm., Mayo Clinic, Rochester, Minn. 55901, U.S.A.; Abroad.
CLARK, John C.; 276 Elgin St., Ottawa 4, Ont.; Wes '41; FACS; FICS; GenSurg; Att'd. Surg. & Gastroscopist, Ottawa Civic Hosp.; Cons., E. B. Eddy Co.; Tel. CE 2-2027.
CLARK, John W.; Medical Arts Bldg., 2150 Valley Way, Niagara Falls, Ont.; 3071 Brookfield Ave. (res); Qns '41; GenSurg.; Tel. EL 4-4761.
CLARK, J. Ralph; 291 Charlotte St., Peterborough, Ont.; 319 Stewart St. (res); Qns '39; Tel. 742-8866.
CLARK, Kenneth L.; 33 White St., St. Thomas, Ont.; 77 Mandeville Rd. (res); Qns '44; IntMed; Head of Dept. of Med., St. Thomas Elgin Gen. Hosp.; Cons. Staff, Ont. Hosp., St. Thomas; Tel. 631-4320.
CLARK, Lillian (nee Sugarman); 1793 North Main St., Niagara Falls, Ont.; 3071 Brookfield Ave. (res); Tor '41; Paed; Staff, Greater Niagara Gen. Hosp.; Tel. EL 4-4664.
CLARK, Marvin R.; P.O. Box 9, Kensington, PEI; Dal '61; MCGP; Tel. 267-3137.
CLARK, Michael D.; Box 250, Lillooet, B.C.; UBC '57; Tel. 62.
CLARK, Nigel H.; Ste. 270, 809 W-41st St., Vancouver 13, B.C.; UBC'54; MCGP; Assoc. Staff, St. Vincent's Hosp.; Tel. 327-7511.
CLARK, Nigel W.; UBC '56; Res., Vancouver Gen. Hosp., Vancouver 9, B.C.
CLARK, Richard L.; Wes'64; Res., Dept. of Anat., U. of Western Ontario, London, Ont.
CLARK, Robert F.; 406 Med. Arts Bldg., 750 Spadina Cr. E., Saskatoon, Sask.; Alb '57; Clin. Teach. (ObstGyn.), U. of Saskatchewan; Tel. 242-0522.
CLARK, Roland M.; 220 Woodlea Cres., Oshawa, Ont.; Tor '50; Path; Pathol., Oshawa Gen. Hosp. & Oshawa Clinic; Tel. 723-2211.
CLARK, Roy G.; 10 George St. N., Galt, Ont.; Tor'35; Staff, South Waterloo Mem. Hosp.; Tel. 621-783.
CLARK, Roy F.; C. S. William Clinic, 901 Helena St., Trail, B.C.; Alb '50; Anaes; Tel. 368-5211.
CLARK, Roy G.; 50 Ainslie St. N., Galt, Ont.; R. R. 4. (res;) Tor 35; 'Tel. 621-2330.
CLARK, Roy M.; London (Eng.)'54; MRCS (Eng.); LRCP(Lond.); FFR; DMRT(Eng.); DObstRCOG; TherRad; Staff, Princess Margaret Hosp., Toronto, Ont.
CLARK, Samuel; McG '58; Res., Royal Victoria Hosp., Montreal, P.Q.
CLARK, Stanley K.; 267 Russell Hill Rd., Toronto, Ont.; McG '22; Int Med; Retired.
CLARK, Stephen D.; 131 Main St., Lancaster, N.B.; 351 Lancaster Ave (res); McG '42; MCGP; Chief, (GP), Saint John Gen. Hosp.; Active Staff, St. Joseph's Hosp.; Acting Dist. M.O.H.; Tel. 694-1382
CLARK, T. Crossan; 51 Herkimer St., Hamilton, Ont.; Tor '13; Paed; Hon. Staff, Hamilton Gen., St. Joseph's & Civic Hosp's.; Tel. JA 2-9266.
CLARK, William N.; 170 Donway W., Don Mills, Ont.; 77 Banbury Rd. (res); Tor '52; Paed; Staff, Tor. E. Gen. Hosp.; Tel. HI 7-1031.
CLARKE, Austin M.; 120 MacBeath Ave., Moncton, N.B. (res); McG '25; IntMed (TB). D.P.H., PH; Exec. Dir., Moncton Hosp.; Tel. 384-4421.
CLARKE, David A.; 390 Queensway Ave., Kelowna, B.C.; 1935 McDougall St. (res); Wes '50; MPH (Harvard); PH; Med. Dir., S. Okanagan Health Unit; Schl. MO; Tel. PO 2-2704.
CLARKE, E. Aileen; 14 Oneida Ave., Algonquin Island, Toronto 2, Ont.; London (Eng.) 56; Staff, Workmens Comp. Bd.; Tel. 362-3411.
CLARKE, Frank D.; 37 Dundas St., Brantford, Ont.; Tor '30; Dist. Coroner; Tel. 752-7631.
CLARKE, George L.; 309 Lancaster St. W., Kitchener, Ont.; Wes'52; MRCOG; FACS; ObstGyn; Active Med. Staff, St. Mary's Gen. & Kitchener-Waterloo Hosp's.; Tel. 744-4552.
CLARKE, Haldane D.; London (Eng.) '56; Staff, Cornwall Gen. Hosp., Cornwall, Ont.; Tel. WE 2-3300.
CLARKE, Joe T. R.; Alb'65; Ass't. Res., Hosp. for Sick Children, Toronto, Ont.
CLARKE, June M.; Georgian Apt., 295 Dale Cr., Waterloo, Ont.; Tor'61; Psy.
CLARKE, Kenneth A. C.; 305 Medical Arts Bldg., Edmonton, Alta.; 10731—86 Ave. (res); Alb '40; A.B.Ot., Otol; Att. Staff, U. of Alberta Hosp. & Royal Alexandra Hosp.; Clin. Prof. (Otol.), U. of Alberta; Tel. GA 4-1354.
CLARKE, Kenneth S.; 408 Med. Arts Bldg., 11010 Jasper Ave., Edmonton, Alta.; Qns '43; FRCS (Ed.); FRCS (Eng.); FRCS(C); PlasSurg; Active Staff, Misericordia Hosp. Court. Cons., Royal Alexandra Hosp.; Sess. Instr., Dept. of Surg. (Div. of PlasSurg.), U. of Alberta; Tel. 424-6575.
CLARKE, Margaret E.; 408 Med. Arts Bldg., 11010 Jasper Ave., Edmonton, Alta.; UBC '55; Tel. 424-6475.
CLARKE, Paul D.; Tor '58; Res. (Neurpath), Banting Inst., U. of Toronto, Toronto 2, Ont.
CLARKE, Robert S.; Tor '42; Path; Staff, Nanaimo Gen. Hosp., Nanaimo, B.C.; Tel. 753-4321.
CLARKE, Thomas R.; 10011-103rd St., Edmonton, Alta.; Alb '35; MRCOG; FRCOG; ObstGyn; Att'd. Staff, U. of Alberta, Royal Alexandra & Edmonton Gen. Hosp's.; Ass't. Prof. (ObstGyn), U. of Alberta; Tel. 422-2223.

CLARKE, William A.; 411 Queens Ave., New Westminster, B.C. (res); Tor '10; Retired.
CLARKE, William T.; 300 Med. Arts Bldg., 170 St. George St., Toronto 5, Ont.; 119 Roxborough Dr. (res); Tor '44; FRCP(C), IntMed; Phys. (Med.), Toronto Gen. Hosp.; Ass't. Prof. (Med.), U. of Toronto; Tel. WA 1-2205.
CLARKSON, J. Graham; 29 Haultain Cr., Regina, Sask. (res); Glasgow (Scot.) '52; MPH (Yale); Deputy Minister of Health, Province of Saskatchewan; Tel. 522-1448.
CLARKSON, Maurice F.; 327 Charlotte St., Peterborough, Ont.; Weller St. W. (res); Tor '43; IntMed; Dir. Trent U. Health Serv.; Tel. 743-2040.
CLAVEAU, Cleophas; 53B Bagot St., Bagotville, P.Q.; Lav '49; M.C.G.P.
CLAVEAU, J. Charles; Institute Medical de Chicoutimi, 475, boul. Talbot, Chicoutimi, P.Q.; Lav '51; Paed; Staff, Hop.-Hotel-Dieu-St-Vallier.
CLAVEAU, Paul; 2152 Parc Bourbonniere, Sillery, Quebec 6, P.Q.; Lav '36; D.P.H., PH; Dir., Div. of Health Services, Dept. of Health, P.Q.; Prof. Hyg. & Prev. Med., Laval U.; Tel. 693-6430.
CLAVEAU, Robert; 282 St.-Vallier, Chicoutimi, P.Q.; Lav '45; M.C.G.P.; Staff (ObstGyn), Hotel-Dieu-St. Vallier.
CLAVEAU, Rosario; 359, de l'Assomption, Chicoutimi, P.Q.; Lav '50; Haem (P.Q.); FRCP(C); IntMed; Hd., Dept. of Haem. (Clin. & Lab.), Hotel-Dieu-St-Vallier; Tel. 549-2195.
CLAVET, Marcel; 419 Chantal Ave., Quebec 5, P.Q. (res); Lav '48; Anaes; Staff, Hop.-Hotel-Dieu & Laval U.; Tel. LA 9-4511.
CLAY, M. Graham; Ste. 608, 750 W. Broadway, Vancouver 9, B.C.; 3438 Cedar Cr. (res); UBC '56; FRCS(C); GenSurg; Vis. Staff, Vancouver Gen. Hosp.; Tel. TR 9-5622.
CLAYDEN, Gerald R.; Dept. of Rad., Victoria Public Hosp., Fredericton, N.B.; Dal '49; DABR; D&TRad; Dir., Dept. of Rad., Victoria Public Hosp.; Tel. 475-3351.
CLAYTON, Alastair J. W. S/L; Commanding Officer, Base Hosp., Cdn. Forces Base, Borden, Ont.; St. Andrew's (Scot.)'58.
CLAYTON, John K.; Qns '51; D. Psy; Psy; Unit Dir., Ont. Hosp., 999 Queen St. W., Toronto 3, Ont.; Clin. Instr., U. of Toronto; Tel. LE 3-8501.
CLEARIHUE, Irene M.; 2445 Lansdowne Rd., Victoria, B.C. (res) London (Eng.) '22; M.R.C.S., L.R.C.P.; Anaes; Retired.
CLEARIHUE, Joyce G.; 102 Campbell Bldg., 1029 Douglas St., Victoria, B.C.; 2445 Lansdowne Rd. (res); McG '53; DABDS; Derm; Active Staff, Royal Jubilee Hosp.; Cons. Staff, St. Joseph's Hosp .; Tel. 384-0011.
CLEARY, T. Emmett; 248 Brant Ave., Brantford, Ont.; 22 Maple Ave. (res); Qns '53; Paed; Chief, Dept. of Paed., St. Joseph's Hosp.; Tel. PL 3-4973.
CLEAVE, Russell J.; 191 Inkster Blvd., Winnipeg 4, Man.; 324 Scotia St., W. Kildonan (res); Man '24; L.M.C.C.(Man.); M.C.G.P.; Court. Staff, Grace, Misericordia, St. Boniface & Victoria Hosp's.; Tel. JU 6-3762.
CLEGG, John W.; London (Eng.) '36; Staff, Kirkland & District Hosp., Kirkland Lake, Ont.
CLEGHORN, Gordon M.; 108 Med. Arts Bldg., 404-406 Graham Ave., Winnipeg 12, Man.; 522 Laidlaw, Tuxedo (res); Man '55; DABR; DiagRad; Active Staff (Rad.), Misericordia Hosp.; Tel. 943-7301.
CLEGHORN, John M.; Allan Mem. Inst., 1025 Pine Ave. W., Montreal 2, P.Q.; McG '58; Psy; Ass't. Psy., Royal Victoria Hosp.; Clin. Ass't., Jewish Gen. Hosp.; Lect. Psy., McGill U.
CLEGHORN, Robert A.; 1025 Pine Ave. W., Montreal, P.Q.; 3160 St. Sulpice Rd., Mtl. 6 (res); Tor '28; D.Sc., IntMed; Psy (P.Q.); Dir., Experm. Therapeutics Lab., Allan Mem. Inst.; Psy-in-Chief, Royal Victoria Hosp.; Prof. (Psy.), McGill U.; Tel. VI 2-1251, Loc. 1609.
CLEIN, Lawrence J.; London (Eng.) '58; B.Sc. (Med.) (Alta.); FRCS(C), NeurSurg; Staff, (Neurosurg.), University of Alberta Hosp., Edmonton, Alta.; Tel. 439-5911.
CLELAND, Charles A.; 351 Sunset Dr., St. Thomas, Ont. (res); Qns '30; F.A.P.A.; Psy; Supt., Ontario Hosp., St. Thomas; Cons. Psy., St. Thomas-Elgin Hosp.; Lect. (Psy), U. of Western Ontario, London; Tel. ME 1-8510, Loc. 1.
CLEMENGER, Allan K.; 363 Markham Rd., Richmond Hill, Ont.; Alb '56.
CLEMENT, A. B.; Les Cedres, P.Q.; Mon '21; Dist. Coroner.
CLEMENT, Douglas B.; 686 No. 3 Rd., Richmond, B.C.; 753 Greenlees Rd. (res); UBC '59; AMCGP; Tel. CR 8-8435.
CLEMENT, George F.; 2250 Haines Rd., Cooksville, Ont.; Wes '52; Anaes; Active Staff, South Peel Mem. Hosp.; Tel. 277-3734.
CLEMENT, George H.; 1410-750 W. Broadway, Vancouver 9, B.C.; 1545-14th St. W. (res); Tor '11; F.A.C.S.; GenSurg; Cons. Surg., Vancouver Gen. Hosp.; Att'd. Staff, B.C. Cancer Inst.; Tel. TR 2-5025.
CLEMENT, Howard F.; 2880 Lundy's Lane, Niagara Falls, Ont.; Qns '56; GenSurg; Staff, Gtr. Niagara Gen. Hosp.; Tel. 356-0922.
CLEMENT, Jules; 1120 Clemenceau, Verdun, Montreal, P.Q.; Geneva (Switz) '53; Tel. 568-5126.
CLEMENT, Marcel; 260 Beique, Dorion, Cte. Vaudreuil, P.Q. (res); Mon '50; Chief M.O. Quarantine & Immig. Div. Dept. Nat. Health & Welfare, Dorval Airport, Dorval, P.Q.; Tel. 861-8811.
CLEMENT, P. Andre, Capt.; Med. Militaire, RCAF Base, North Bay, Ont.; Mon'65.
CLEMENTI, Kenneth J.; Medicine Hat Health Unit, 770-1st St. S.E., Medicine Hat, Alta.; London (Eng.)'40; MRCS(Lond.); LRCP(Eng.).
CLEMENTS, Daphne I. (Lingas); 11626-71st Ave., Edmonton, Alta.; Alb '55; MOH, Edmonton Bd. of Health. Abroad.
CLEMENTS, Duaine A. (Peacock); 601 Centre St. S., Whitby, Ont.; Tor '57; Staff, Ont. Hosp.; Tel. MO 8-8274.
CLEMENTS, M. Keith; Alb '55; FRCS(C), ObstGyn; Staff, University Hosp., Edmonton, Alta. Abroad.
CLEMES, Ian L.; 222 Eramosa Rd., Guelph, Ont.; 37 Lynwood Pl. (res); Tor '49; GenSurg; Chief of Surg., St. Joseph's Hosp.; Staff, Guelph Gen. Hosp.; Tel. TA 4-2920.
CLEMETSON, C. Alan B.; University Hosp., Saskatoon, Sask.; 816 Ave. C. N. (res); Oxford (Eng.) '48; M.R.C.O.G.; ObstGyn; Ass't. Prof. (ObstGyn.), U. of Saskatchewan; Tel. CH 2-7641.
CLEMIS, Jack D.; 6530 Drake, Lincolnwood, Ill., U.S.A.; Alb '58; Otol. Abroad.
CLERMONT, Andre; 301 Dufort, Laprairie, P.Q.; Mon '59.
CLERMONT, Joseph; 8493 Boul. St.-Laurent, Montreal 11, P.Q.; 2170 Ave. Laure Conan, Mtl. 12 (res); Haiti '50; GenSurg (P.Q.); Surg. Staff, Hop.-Ste-Justine; Tel. DU 7-6134.
CLEROUX, Alfred; 266 St. Louis Sq., Montreal, P.Q.; 3447 St. Hubert (res); Mon '47; IntMed (P.Q.); Ass't. Prof. Med. U. of Montreal, Phys., Hotel-Dieu; Tel. VI 4-0161
CLEVELAND, Eric J.; Earnscliffe Ave., Wolfville, N.S.; Dal '48; D. Psy; Psy; Exec. Dir., Fundy Mental Health Centre, Staff, Eastern Kings Mem., Blanchard-Fraser Mem. & N.S. San., Kentville; Assoc. Prof., Acadia U.; Tel. 542-2325.
CLEWS, Alan G.; Kerrobert Clinic, Kerrobert, Sask.; Birmingham (Eng.) '52; M.B., ChB., DRCOG (Lond.); MCGP; Chief Of Med. Staff, Kerrobert Union Hosp.; Tel. 834-2412.
CLICHE, Francois; 1795 - 10e Ave., St. Georges-Ouest, P.Q.; Lav'48; Anaes; Staff, Hotel-Dieu de Notre Dame; Tel. 228-4831.
CLICHE, Pierre-A.; 1045 Chemin-Ste-Foy, Quebec 6, P.Q.; Lav '38; GenSurg (PQ); Pt-time Med. Dir., Hop.-St.-Ambroise-de-Loretteville; Tel. 842-3651.
CLIFFORD, Douglas J.; 119 Gertrude St., Alberni, B.C.; 165 Elizabeth St. (res); Otago (N. Zealand) '43; Active Staff, (G.P.) West Coast Gen. Hosp.; Tel. 723-5822.
CLIFFORD, Ernest J.; 928 Medical Arts Bldg. 170 St. George St., Toronto, Ont.; 23 Shields Ave. (res); Tor '14; IntMed.; Tel. WA 1-7841.

CLIFT, Allan M.; Med. Arts Bldg., 420 East St. N., Sarnia, Ont.; Wes'53; MCGP; Tel. DI 4-0582.

CLINCKETT, Fred R.; 267 O'Connor St., Ottawa 4, Ont.; 714 Parkdale Ave. (res); Tor '43; Ophth; **Att. Staff, Ottawa Civic Hosp. Sr. Lect. (Clin. Ophth), Ottawa U.; Tel. CE 5-0725.**

CLINE, Chas. A.; 325 Queen's Ave., London, Ont.; Wes '22; Cons. Neurol., Westminster Hosp.; Sr. Assoc. (Med.), U. of Western Ontario. Retired.

CLINE, D. Aileen F.; 325 Queens Ave., London, Ont. (res); Wes '31; Part-time Teaching, Neuroanat. Dept., U. of Western Ontario; Retired.

CLINTON-Thomas, Chas. L.; 97 Dunlop St. W., Barrie, Ont.; London (Eng) '37; F.R.C.S. (Eng); GenSurg.

CLOGG, Donald K.; 5025 Sherbrooke St. W., Westmount, Montreal, P.Q.; McG '49; Paed; Dir., Isotope Lab., Montreal Children's Hosp.; Staff, Queen Elizabeth Hosp.; Lect., McGill U.; Tel. 935-9893.

CLOKIE, J. Kenneth; 4298 Dunbar St., Vancouver 9, B.C.; **360 E. Blvd. (res); Man '48; MCGP; Staff Phys., University Hosp., Att. Staff, Van. Gen.; Vis. Staff, Grace & St. Vincent's Hosp's.; Tel. RE 1-3612**

CLOUATRE, Andre; C.P. 940, Farnham, P.Q.; Mon '64.

CLOUGH-ORMISTON, Michael W.; 107 Park St., Kingston, Ont. (res); London (Eng.) '46; Phys., Ongwanada San., Kingston.

CLOUTIER, Alphonse; Bromptonville, P.Q.; Lav '18.

CLOUTIER, A. MacLeod; 1509 Sherbrooke St. W., Montreal, P.Q.; **506 Mountain Ave., Montreal 6 (res); McG '51; PlasSurg (P.Q.), Staff, Montreal** Children's & Reddy Mem. Hosp's.; Tel. 927-3861.

CLOUTIER, Benoit F.; 23 Avenue Laporte, Edmundston, N.B.; Lav '50; GenSurg; Tel. 735-6215.

CLOUTIER, Denys; Lav'62; Res., Hop. de la Misericorde, Quebec 6, P.Q.

CLOUTIER, Diogene, Capt.; Nat. Defence Med. Centre, Camp Valcartier, P.Q.; Lav '65.

CLOUTIER, Edward J.; 77A Main St., Huntsville, Ont.; **41 Lansdowne St. (res); Tor '35.**

CLOUTIER, Francois; Ste. 226, 5757 Ave. Decelles, Montreal 26, P.Q.; **Lav'48**; Psy.

CLOUTIER, Georges-E.; 1656 Sherbrooke E., Montreal, P.Q.; Apt. 12, 2475 Maplewood (res); Mon '38; FACS; FRCS(C), PlasSurg; Chief Dept. **PlasSurg., Notre-Dame, Queen Mary Vet's., St.-**Jean, & Ste-Justine Hosp's.; Ass't. Prof. (Surg.), **U. of Montreal; Tel. RE 3-9951.**

CLOUTIER, Gilles; 910 St. Joseph Boul. E., Montreal 34, P.Q.; 8150 Du Mail-Ville, D'Anjou (res); Mon '53; Tel. 524-0493.

CLOUTIER, Jean M.; Ste. 204, 30 est boul. St. Joseph, Montreal 14, P.Q.; Ott'54; FRCS(C), OrthSurg.

CLOUTIER, Joseph R. P.; 864 ave Bégin, Quebec, P.Q.; Lav'60; FRCS(C), GenSurg.

CLOUTIER-LAMBIN, Louise; Lav'65; Res., Hop. St Sacrement, Quebec 6, P.Q.

CLOUTIER, Leo; St. Ours, P.Q.; Mon '37.

CLOUTIER, Louis G.; Lav'65; Res., Hotel-Dieu St. Vallier, Chicoutimi, P.Q.

CLOUTIER, Louis V.; St. Georges, Beauce Co., P.Q.; Lav '27; IntMed (P.Q.); Med. Staff, Hop. Notre Dame de Beauce.

CLOUTIER, L. Paul; 419, boul. St-Joseph ouest, Montreal 8, P.Q.; Mon '40.

CLOUTIER, Marcel; 150 Sanborn, Sherbrooke, P.Q.; 1206 Dominion St. (res); Lav '48; Orth Surg; Tel. 569-3130.

CLOUTIER, Paul-Emile; 351 rue Labelle, St. Jerome, P.Q.; 13 rue St-Georges (res); Lav '51; DPH; PH(P.Q.); MOH, Prov. Dept. of Health; Tel. GE 2-7432.

CLOUTIER, Roland; Ste. 600, 1538 ouest, rue Sherbrooke, Montreal, P.Q.; 2325 Dover, Ville Mt-Royal (res); Mon'40; DABO; Ophth; Ass't. (Ophth.), Hop. Notre-Dame; Hd. Dept. (Ophth.), U. of Montreal; Tel. 935-3181.

CLOW, L. Roberts; Ste. 2057, Etherington Hall, Kingston, Ont.; 41 Copperfield Dr., Woodlands (res); Qns'45; FRCS(C), ObstGyn; Active Staff (ObstGyn), Hotel-Dieu Hosp.; Assoc. Staff, Kingston Gen. Hosp.; Clin. Ass't. & Lect. (ObstGyn), Queen's U.; Tel. 542-6512.

CLUFF, Joseph W.; 750 W. Broadway, Vancouver, B.C.; 1271 W. 32nd Ave. (res); Man '42; F.R.C.S.(C) NeurSurg; Hd. Dept. of NeurSurg., St. Paul's Hosp.; Clin. Ass't. Prof., Surg., U. of British Columbia; Tel. TR 2-5544.

CLUNAS, Daniel R.; Wes '57; Ass't. Res. (Anaes), St. Michael's Hosp., Toronto 2, Ont.

CLUNAS, Duke E.; Harrison, Ont.; Wes '46.; MCGP.

CLUTE, Kenneth F.; 9 Cortleigh Blvd., Toronto 12 (res); Tor '45; F.R.C.P.(C), Paed; Assoc. Prof., Med. Care, Dept. of Schl. of Hygiene, U. of Toronto; Albert G. Milbank Fell., in Law & Public Health; Tel. 928-2742.

CLYSDALE, Earle S.; Alvinston, Ont.; Tor '24; M.O.H.; Coroner, Lampton & Middlesex Cos.

CO, Pedro C.; Santo Tomas (Philippines) '59; Jr. Intn., Lancaster Hosp., Lancaster, N.B.

COAD, Ralph L.; 2161 Danforth Ave., Toronto 13, Ont.; Tor'53; Court. Staff, St. Michael's Hosp.; Tel. 691-9401.

COADY, Basil K.; 5880 Spring Garden Rd., Halifax, N.S.; Dal '38; F.A.C.S.; GenSurg; Assoc. Surg., Victoria Gen. Hosp.; Cons. Surg. RCN Hosp.; Chief, Dept. of Surg., Halifax Infirmary; Assoc. Prof. (Surg.), Dalhousie U.; Tel. 423-8514.

COADY, C. A.; Charlottetown Clinic, Charlottetown, P.E.I.; **65 McGill Ave. (res); Qns '46; M.C.G.P.; Staff, Charlottetown Hosp.; Assoc. Staff, P.E.I. Hosp.; Dist. Coroner.**

COADY, Campbell J.; 8889-10th Ave., New Westminster, B.C.; McG '49; F.R.C.P(C), Path; Dir. of Labs., Royal Columbian Hosp.; Clin. Instr. (Path), U. of British Columbia; Tel. CA 4-1111.

COALLIER, Gabriel; 1876 Rosemont Blvd., Montreal 35, P.Q.; Mon '60; Tel. 277-1982.

COALLIER, Joseph A.; 147 St-Trinite, Contrecoeur, P.Q.; Lav '16.

COALLIER, Rene; 2295 est, Ontario, Montreal, 24 P.Q.; Mon '47; MCGP.

COALS, John T.; Virden Clinic, Virden, Man.; **London (Eng.) '53; M.B., B.S., LRCP (Lond.);** FRCS (Eng.); GenSurg; Med. Staff, Virden Dist. Hosp.; Tel. 477.

COATES, Donald B.; Clarke Inst. of Psychiatry, 250 College St. W., Toronto, Ont.; Tor'54; D.Psy; FRCP(C), Psy; Research Assoc., Clarke Inst. & Dept. of Psy., U. of Toronto; Tel. 924-6811.

COATES, Geoffrey; 89 Ambridge Dr., Ansonville, Ont.; Durham (Eng.) '63; Staff, Anson Gen. Hosp.; Tel. 1043.

COATES, Kenneth J.; Man'37; DPH; DIH; Staff, M.O., The Workmen's Comp. Bd., Hospital & Rehab. Centre, 115 Torbarrie Rd., Downsview, Ont.

COATES, William O.; 72 Church St., Amherst, **N.S; Man '29; GenSurg; Board of Comm.** Highland View Hosp., Amherst, N.S.; Dist. Coroner.

COATES, William Robert; 135 Clarkson Ave. S., Port Arthur, Ont.; Tor 54; D'. Psy.; Psy; Clin. Dir., Ontario Hosp.; Tel. DI 4-3571.

COBB, George M.; 77 Westmount Rd., Ste. 208, Guelph, Ont.; Dal'58; **FRCS(C), Ophth.**

COBBAN, Andrew C.; Box 928, Assoc. Med. Clinic, Westlock, Alta.; Aberdeen (Scot.)'44; Active Staff, Imaculata & Auxiliary Hosp's.; Tel. 342-3341.

COBURN, Frank E., 1302 Colony St., Saskatoon, Sask.; Tor'39; DAPB & N; Psy; Prof. (Psy.), U. **of Saskatchewan; Clin. Dir. (Psy.), University Hosp.; Tel. 242-7641, Loc. 382.**

COBURN, J. Blair; Qns '49; DPH; M.O., Bell Telephone Co., 161 Laurier Ave., Ottawa 4, Ont.; Tel. 239-5353.

COBURN, Wallace A.; 674 Kingsway, Vancouver 10, B.C.; 1012 Balfour Ave., Vancouver 9 (res); Tor '26; Tel. TR 6-7511.

COCCO, John M.; McG '63; Res., Royal Victoria Hosp., Montreal, P.Q.

COCHEN, A. Ronald; 21 Upper Middle Rd., Ste. 107, Cooksville, Ont.; Tor'59; FRCS(C), ObstGyn; Staff, South Peel Hosp. & Queensway Gen. Hosp., Toronto; Tel. 279-1782.

COCHEN, Sandra J.; Apt. 115, 51 Alexander St., Toronto 5, Ont.; Qns '57; FRCP(C), Anaes; Tel. WA 5-3713.

COCHRANE, R. Cameron; 312 Glen Manor Dr., Toronto 13, Ont.; London (Eng.) '52; DRCOG; D.Psy.; Psy; Staff, Clarke Inst. of Psy.; Associate U. of Toronto; Tel. 698-3092.

COCHRANE, William A.; The Children's Hosp., Halifax, N.S.; Tor'49; FAAP; FRCP(C), Paed; DABP; Phys-in-Chief, Children's Hosp.; Prof. & Hd., Dept. of Paed., Dalhousie U.; Tel. 422-8441.

COCHRANE, William H.; 13907-92nd Ave., Edmonton, Alta.; Queen's U. (Belfast, N. Ire.) '49; DA (Eng.); FFARCS (Eng.); Anaes; Att'd. Staff, Royal Alexandra Hosp.; Tel. HU 8-7994.

COCK, J. Gordon; 438 Botsford St., Newmarket, Ont.; Tor '37; Chief of Anaes., York Co. Hosp.; Tel. TW 5-4521.

COCKBURN, D. G.; Flin Flon Clinic, 82 Church St., Flin Flon, Man.; Tor'64.

COCKBURN, Douglas W.; 479 Highland Ave., Ottawa 13, Ont. (res); Qns '43; D&TRad; Ass't. Dir. (Rad.), Ottawa Civic Hosp.; Tel. 729-2511, Ext. 357.

COCKCROFT, Denis; 35 Scholfield Ave., Port Colborne, Ont. (res); Middlesex Hosp. (Lond.) '45; M.R.C.S. (Eng.), L.R.C.P. (Lond.), D.M.-R.D., DiagRad; Staff, Port Colborne Gen. Hosp.; Tel. TE 4-4501.

COCKCROFT, William H.; 750 W. Broadway, Vancouver 9, B.C.; 5611 Highbury (res); Tor '42; D.P.H., Bact; Staff, Vancouver Gen. Hosp. & U. of British Columbia; Tel. TR 6-3211.

COCKER, W. John B., Capt.; Ste. 108-2515 Portage Ave., Winnipeg 12, Man. (res); London (Eng.) '58; Staff, Fort Osborne Barracks.

COCKFIELD, Richard L.; 630 St. Clair Ave. W., Toronto 10, Ont.; Qns'31; MCGP; Tel. LE 2-7773.

COCKINGS, Edward C.; Dept. of Anaes., University Hosp., Saskatoon, Sask.; Manchester (Eng.) '55; DRCOG; FACA; DABA; FRCP(C); Anaes; Staff, University Hosp.; Assoc. Prof. (Anaes.), U. of Saskatchewan; Tel. 652-8821, Ext. 413.

CODDINGTON, Rupert D.; 106 Birks Bldg., 718 Granville St., Vancouver 2, B.C.; McG '30; GenSurg; Surg. Staff, St. Paul's Hosp., Miller Bay Hosp., Prince Rupert, & Coqualeetza Hosp., Sardis; Tel. MU 3-1422.

CODE, Thomas G.; Box 725, Brockville, Ont. (res); Wes'57; MCGP; Chief (G.P.), Brockville Gen. Hosp.; Sec. Med. Staff, St. Vincent de Paul Hosp.; Tel. 345-1458.

CODERE-ROBERGE, Gertrude (Mrs.); 3rd Range, Thetford Mines, P.Q. (res); Mon '50; Retired.

CODERQUE, Juan A.; 541 College St., Toronto 5, Ont.; 328 The Heights Dr., Don Mills (res); Saragossa (Spain) '53; Otol; Staff, New Mt. Sinai & St. Joseph's Hosp's.; Cons. (Otol.), Lambert Lodge; Tel. 924-3281.

CODRINGTON, Walter R.; 90 The West Mall, Etobicoke, Ont.; McG '58.

CODY, Alan C.; 415 Greyhound Bldg., Calgary, Alta.; 1202 Lansdowne Ave. (res); Tor '42; Paed; Tel. 266-3920.

CODY, Duncan B.; 1904a-20th Ave. N.W., Calgary, Alta.; 3032 Capitol Hill Cr. (res); Alb '51; Staff, Calgary Gen., Holy Cross & Grace Hosp's.; Tel. 289-1116.

CODY, D. Thane; Dal '57; Res., Prov. Labs., Saint John, N.B.

CODY, Michael C.; Alb'65; Cdn. Forces Base, Portage la Prairie, Man.

CODY, Philip C.; 1021-925 Georgia St. W., Vancouver, B.C.; Tor'53; OphthOtol; DOMS.

COFFEY, J. Edwin; 370 Seaforth Med. Bldg., 3550 Cote des Neiges Rd., Montreal 25, P.Q.; 115 Aberdeen Ave., Wesmount 6 (res); McG 52; FRCS(C); ObstGyn; FACOG; Att'd. Staff, Catherine Booth Hosp.; Dem., McGill U.; Att'd. Staff, Montreal Gen. Hosp.; Tel. 932-8601.

COFFEY, Owen F.; 714 Boyd Bldg., Winnipeg 1, Man.; Dublin (Ire.) '48.

COFFEY, Patrick G.; 399 Dibble St., Prescott, Ont.; Edinburgh (Scot.)'54; DRCOG(Lond.); GenSurg.

COFFIN, Everett; Box 467, Gaspe, P.Q.; Lav '56. ObstGyn (P.Q.);

COGAN, Roy; 6014 Yonge St., Willowdale, Ont.; Tor '47; AMCGP; Tel. 221-0887.

COGGINS, Brian H.; Ste. 103, 688 Coxwell Ave., Toronto 6, Ont.; Tor'55; Anaes; Staff, Toronto East Gen. Hosp.; Tel. 461-8272.

COGHLAN, Robert O.; P.O. Box 216, Glaslyn, Sask.; Tor '06; Dist. Coroner.

COGLON, Russel B.; 10004-105th St., Edmonton, Alta.; Alb '54; FRCP(C), IntMed; Clin. Instr., U. of Alberta; Tel. GA 4-2121.

COGSWELL, David L.; Box 107, Aylesford, N.S.; Dal '60; MCGP; Vis. Phys., Kings County Hosp. & Mountain View Home, Waterville; Tel. 427-3770.

COGSWELL, Eric E.; Dal'62; Res., Camp Hill Hosp., Halifax, N.S.

COGSWELL, Laverne E.; Berwick, N.S.; Dal '32; Dist. Coroner.

COHANIM, Moussa; Tehran'52; Staff, Clin. Invest., Toronto Gen. Hosp., Toronto 2, Ont.

COHEN, Alvin; 720 W. Broadway, Vancouver, B.C.; 1541 W. King Edward (res); Man '36; D.O.M.S. (Lond.); **Ophth; Att'd. Staff, Van**couver Gen. Hosp.; Cons. Staff, Shaughnessy Hosp.; Clin. Instr. (Opth), **U. of British Columbia; Tel. TR 4-8711.**

COHEN, Arthur; 415 Ellendale Med. Bldg., 5845. Cote des Neiges Rd., Montreal 26, P. Q.; 280 Dufferin Rd., Hamstead (res); McG '40; DABU; Otol; Assoc. (Otol.), Children's Hosp.; Ass't. Otol., Jewish Gen. Hosp.; Cons. Otol., Royal Edward Laurentian & Verdun Protestant Hosp's.; Tel. 735-3111.

COHEN, Gerald S.; 39 Blueforest Dr., Downs**view, Ont.; Tor '55; MCGP; OPD Staff, Toronto** Gen. Hosp., **Court. Staff, Branson & Mount Sinai Hosp's.; Tel. 633-4984.**

COHEN, Goodman; Ste. 101, 199 Holland Ave., Ottawa 3, Ont.; McG'47; FRCPC; IntMed (Cardiol); Chief, Cardiopulm. Unit, Cardiol. Serv. & Cardiac. Clinic, Ottawa Civic Hosp.; Lect. Med. Ottawa U.; Tel. 725-2159.

COHEN, Harry; Professional Arts Bldg. Ste. 725, 155 James St. S., Hamilton, Ont.; 52 Dromore Cres. (res); Montpellier (Fr.) '57; Staff, Hamilton Civic, Henderson Gen. & St. Joseph's Hosp's.; Tel. 527-7781.

COHEN, Herman; 6000 Cote des Neiges Rd., Montreal 26, P.Q.; McG '49; GenSurg; Tel. RE 3-2363.

COHEN, Jack; McG'59; FRCS(C), PlasSurg; Staff, Jewish Gen. Hosp., Montreal, P.Q.; Abroad.

COHEN, Joan K. P. (Crane); 1200 Grosvenor Ave., Winnipeg, Man. (res); Man '48; Temp. Retired.

COHEN, Leslie G.; 790 E. Hastings St., Vancouver 4, B.C.; Man'51; MCGP; Vis. Staff, Vancouver Gen., Grace, Mount St. Joseph's & St. Paul's Hosp's.; Tel. 254-4755.

COHEN, Maurice S.; 5757 Decelles Ave., Montreal 26, P.Q.; McG '34; Derm Syph; Staff. Royal Victoria Hosp., Montreal; Tel. RE 7-3424.

COHEN, Max; 4975 Lacombe Ave., **Montreal,** P.Q. (res); McG '40; **Anaes; Anaes-in-Chief, Jewish Gen. Hosp.; Tel. 735-3771.**

COHEN, May (Lipman); 120 Overbrook Place, Downsview, Ont.; **Tor '55; MCGP; Research** Fell., **U. of Toronto; Tel. 633-4984.**

COHEN, Minnie W. (Wladowsky); Tor '22; Staff (Paed.), O.P.D., New Mount Sinai Hosp., Toronto, Ont.

COHEN, Morley; 218 Med. Arts Bldg., Winnipeg, Man.; 1200 Grosvenor Ave. (res); Man '48; Ph.D. (Minn.); DABS; FACS; F.R.C.S.(C), GenSurg; Active Staff, & Dir. Cardiopulm. Surg. Unit, St. Boniface Hosp.; Assoc. Prof. Surg. & Dir. Div. of Cardiovasc Surg., U. of Manitoba; Tel. WH 2-2379.

COHEN, Peter W.; Ste. 500, Chinook Prof. Bldg., Calgary, Alta.; Amsterdam (Neth.)'58; MCGP.

COHEN, Saul; Regina Med. Centre, 1847 Rose St., Regina, Sask.; 2811—24th Ave. (res); Tor '43; M.C.G.P.
COHEN, Seymour; 1404 Webb Ave., Chomedy, P.Q.; Mon'56; Paed.
COHEN, William; Ste. 712, 1414 Drummond St., Montreal, P.Q.; 10 Aberdeen Ave., Westmount (res); McG '33; IntMed; Assoc. Phys., Montreal Gen. Hosp.; Phys., Royal Edward Laurentian Hosp.; Cons. (Med.), D.V.A.; Clin. Ass't., Jewish Gen. Hosp.; Lect. (Med.), McGill U.; Tel. VI 2-1371.
COHOE, Clarence E. K.; Pilot Mound, Man.; **Man '51; M O.H.; Pilot Mound & Louise; Tel. 222.**
COHOE, Helen C. (Cameron); P.O. Box 46, Pilot Mound, Man.; Man '51; Temp. Ret.
COHOLAN, Francis G.; 175 Russell Ave., St. Catharines, Ont.; Ott '53.
COHOON, W. J.; Tor'65; Res., Toronto Western Hosp., Toronto 2B, Ont.
COITEUX, Carl; 5079 est Ste Catharine, Montreal 4, P.Q.; Mon '65.
COJOACRU, Nicolas; 1000 Chemin Ste-Foy, Quebec 6, P.Q.; Lav'54; FRCS(C), Urol.; Tel. 681-1122.
COKE, Lawrence R.; 432 Med. Arts Bldg., Winnipeg 1, Man.; Man '36; FCCP; FACP; IntMed; Active Staff, Deer Lodge, St. Boniface & Grace Hosp's.; Assoc. Prof. (Med.), U. of Manitoba; Tel. WH 2-1893.
COKE, William L.; 2834 Murray Dr., Victoria, B.C.; Wes '28; Supt., Veteran's Hosp.; Tel. 382-4221.
COLANTONIO, Aldo F.; Tor'55; DiagRad; Staff, Hosp. for Sick Children, Toronto, Ont.
COLAPINTO, Ronald F.; 9 Cottonwood Dr., **Don Mills, Ont. (res); Tor '55; DMR; FRCP(C), DiagRad; Ass't. Rad., Toronto Gen. Hosp.; Clin. Instr. (Rad.), U. of Toronto; Tel. EM 6-8211.**
COLAPINTO, Vincent; Ste. 627, 170 St. George St., Toronto 5, Ont.; Tor'52; F.R.S.C.(C), GenSurg; Urol; Staff, St. Michael's Hosp.; Cons. (Urol), **Sunnybrook DVA & Cons. (GU), Princess Margaret Hosp's.; Clin. Instr., (Surg), U. of Toronto; Tel. WA 2-7703.**
COLBERT, John G.; C. S. Williams Clinic, 901 Helena St., Trail, B.C.; Man '46; PlasSurg; Staff, Trail-Tadanac Hosp. & Mater Misericordia Hosp., Rossland; Tel. 368-5211.
COLE, Anne R.; 955 Queen St. E., Sault Ste. Marie, Ont.; 3 Fauguier Ave. (res); Birmingham (Eng.)'46; Paed; Tel. 254-5521.
COLE, Arthur H.; 123 Edward St., Toronto, Ont.; Tor '55; Anaes; Staff, St. Michael's Hosp.; Clin. Ass't., U. of Toronto.
COLE, Arthur R.C.; 250 Lawrence Ave. W., Toronto 12, Ont.; 72 Alexandra Blvd., Tor. 12 (res); Tor '43; Paed; Clin. Ass't., Hosp. for Sick Children; Paed. I/C, (Paed.), Princess Margaret Hosp.; Tel. RU 1-4341.
COLE, C. E. Cooper; OBE; 705 Med. Arts Bldg., 170 St. George St., Toronto 5, Ont.; 273 Poplar Plains Rd. (res); Tor '07; F.A.C.P., F.R.C.P.(C), IntMed; Med. Ref., Ont. Blue Cross; Retired.
COLE, John E. C.; 705 Medical Arts Bldg., 170 St. George St., Toronto 5, Ont.; 12 Clarendon Ave. (res); Tor'44; FRCP(C), IntMed; Clin. Teach., U. of Toronto; Ass't. Phys., Tor. Gen. Hosp.; Assoc. Med. Dir., North American Life Assur. Co.; Tel. 362-6011.
COLE, Louis J.; 99 Avenue Rd., Toronto 5, **Ont.; 17 Browside Ave., (res); Tor '40; D.A.B.-I.M., F.A.C.P., F.R.C.P. (C), IntMed; Att. Staff, & Chief G.I. Clin., New Mt. Sinai Hosp.; Ass't. Prof., (Med.), U. of Toronto; Tel. WA 1-0222.**
COLE, Murray S.; 119 Brant Ave., Brantford, Ont.; Tor '23; GenSurg; Med. Dir., Can. Order **of Foresters; Tel. 752-7421.**
COLE, Philip; Peterborough Clinic, 327 Charlotte St., Peterborough, Ont.; 125 Roper Dr. **(res); Manchester (Eng.) '51; DLO; Otol; Staff, Peterborough Civic & St. Joseph's Hosp's.; Tel.** 743-2040.
COLE, Philip A.; Hubbards, N.S.; Dal '45; Staff, Grace Maternity Hosp., Halifax; Tel. 29.
COLE, Philip T.; USA'65; Jr. Int., Royal Victoria Hosp., Montreal 2, P.Q.

COLE, Robert H.; 531 Highcroft Ave., Ottawa 3, **Ont.; Man '45; D.A., Anaes.**
COLE, Sholto F.; Trinity Coll. (Dublin, Ire.)'60; FRCS(C), GenSurg; Staff, Royal Victoria Hosp., Montreal, P.Q.; Abroad.
COLE, William S.; 30 Tacoma Dr., Westphal, **Dartmouth, N.S.; London (Eng.) '56.**
COLEMAN, Dennis C.; Box 280, Courtenay, B.C.; Glacier Dr., Comox (res); McG '52; Tel. 334-2445.
COLEMAN, Gerald; Box 1180, Duncan, B.C.; UBC'64.
COLEMAN, Herbert M.; Private Physicians Ste., Ste. 10, 825 Coxwell Ave., Toronto 13, Ont.; 15 Wychwood Pk. **(res); Tor '34; F.R.S.C.(Edin.),** F.R.C.S.(C), OrthSurg; Chief of OrthSurg., Toronto East Gen. & Orthopaedic Hosp's.; Tel. HO 6-7626.
COLEMAN, Isobel M.; Apt. 402, 263 Russell Hill Rd., Toronto 7, Ont.; Queen's U. (Belfast, Ire.) '44; DPH; Public Health Officer, City of Toronto.
COLEMAN, John U.; P.O. Box 1180, Duncan, **B.C.; Lakes Rd. (res); Tor '35; GenSurg; MCGP; Staff, King's Daughters Hosp.; Tel. 746-4102.**
COLEMAN, Laura I. M. (See Forgues).
COLEMAN, W. Roy, Major; Tor '50; DMR; DiagRad; Dept'y., Chief of Rad., NDMC, Ottawa, Canada; Tel. 733-6600, Ext. 206.
COLERT, Walter M.; Morden, Man.; Man '36; Coroner; Tel. 822-4474.
COLES, Bonar C.; 254—13th Ave., Richelieu, P.Q. (res); Tor '35; **D.P.H.; A.B. Prev. Med. (Av. Med.).**
COLES, John C.; 209 Med. Dental Bldg., 450 Central Ave., London, Ont.; Wes'48; FACC; FACS; F.R.C.S.(C), GenSurg; ThorSurg; Card. & ThorSurg., Victoria Hosp.; Card. & Vasc. Surg., Westminster Hosp.; Cons. Cardiovasc. & ThorSurg., St. Joseph's Hosp.; Ass't. Prof. (Surg.), U. of Western Ont.; Tel. 432-2878.
COLES, John M.; 1103-750 W. Broadway, Vancouver 9, B.C.; Tor'51; Psy; Staff, Dept. of Med., St. Vincent's Hosp.; Tel. 266-7033.
COLEY, Charles E.; West Park Med. Clinic, Red Deer, Alta.; 9 Savoy Cr. (res); Glasgow (Scot.) '55; M.B., Ch.B.; Tel. 347-3586.
COLFORD, Horace B.; 22 Piers Ave., Armdale, Halifax Co., N.S. (res); Dal '51.
COLIN, Anne Marie; 12016 Lachapelle, Montreal 9, P.Q.; Lav '42.
COLLEDGE, A. Douglas; 110-3rd St. N.E., Weyburn, Sask.; Edinburgh (Scot.)'56; AMCGP.
COLLETT, Elizabeth (See Schwab)
COLLEY, R. Q.; 2525 Pine St., Vancouver 9, B.C.; 6926 Laburnum (res); Alb '44; Ophth; Vis. **Staff, Vancouver Gen. Hosp.; Tel. TR 6-3211.**
COLLIER, Hugh N.; 3236 Weston Rd., Weston, Ont.; Queens U. (Belfast, N. Ire.)'64; Abroad.
COLLIER, Kenneth J.; 6th St. S.E. & Queen, Portage La Prairie, Man.; Man '64; Tel. 857-6873.
COLLIN, Louis D., M.M. (Medaille d'Honneur, Fr.); 149 Dollard Blvd., St. Boniface, Man.; '11; F.R.C.S.(C), GenSurg; Retired.
COLLIN, Pierre-Paul; 30 est, boul. St. Joseph, Apt. 806, Montreal 14, P.Q.; Mon '48; GenSurg (P.Q.); Chief of Surg., Hop. Ste-Justine; Ass't. Prof. (Surg.), U. of Montreal; Tel. 845-4241, Loc. 52.
COLLING, John F.; 8 Talbot Rd. N., Lambeth, Ont.; Wes '18; M.C.G.P.; M.O.H., Westminster Twp., Coroner Middlesex Co.
COLLING, Kenneth G.; 995 Main St. E., Hamilton, Ont.; 6 Ravenscliffe Ave. (res); Wes '45; **FAADS; DABDS; DermSyph; Staff, Hamilton Gen. Hosp; Tel. LI 9-4361.**
COLLINGWOOD, William P.; 38 Circular Rd., St. John's, Nfld. (res); Edinburgh (Scot.) '38; Cons., Treatment Serv., Dept. of Health, St. John's; Tel. 951578.
COLLINS, Arthur L.; 10111 Richmond Ave., Grande Prairie, Alta.; London (Eng.)'38; MRCS(Eng.); LRCP(Lond.).
COLLINS, Bridget M.; London (Eng.)'54; **Staff, Hosp. for Mental & Nervous Diseases, St. John's, Nfld.**

COLLINS, David L.; 750 W. Broadway, Vancouver 9, B.C.; 6242 Alma St. (res); McG '54; FACS; FRCS(C); GenSurg; Att'd Staff, Vancouver Gen. Hosp.; Vis. Staff, Lions Gate, Burnaby, St. Paul's & St. Vincent's Hosp's.; Teach. Fell. (Surg.), U. of British Columbia; Tel. TR 9-4324. Abroad.

COLLINS, Donald R.; Medical Clinic, 4794A Joyce Ave., Powell River, B.C.; Man '43; MCGP; Deputy Coroner; Anaes., Powell River Gen. Hosp.; Chm., Med. Clinic, Powell River; Tel. 483-3241.

COLLINS, George F.; Res., Hosp. for Sick Children, Toronto 2, Ont.

COLLINS, Harry A.; 538 Dundas St., London, Ont. (res); Wes '44; D.P.H.; M.C.G.P.; Ass't. M.O.H., London.

COLLINS, Harry M.; 301 Canada Bldg., Saskatoon, Sask.; 1904-14th St. E. (res); Tor '47; Tel. 653-1543.

COLLINS, John A.; 8 Briar Hill Place, London, Ont.; Wes'60; FRCS(C), ObstGyn; Staff, Victoria Hosp.; Abroad.

COLLINS, John F.; Ste. 4., Med. Arts Bldg., Empire Ave., St. John's, Nfld; 4 Bonaventure Ave. (res); Edinburgh (Scot.) '50; MRCP (Edin.); DCH (Lond.); Paed; Active Staff, Grace & St. Clare's Mercy Hosp's.; Assoc. Staff, Gen. Hosp.; Tel. 579-6070.

COLLINS, K. G.; Department of National Health & Welfare, c/o Regional Superintendent, European Region. Abroad.

COLLINS, Lorne B.; The Associate Clinic, Box 549, Pincher Creek, Alta.; Man'41; MCGP; Chief of Staff, St. Vincent's Hosp.; Tel. 627-3321.

COLLINS, Margaret R.; 11124-84th Ave., Edmonton, Alta.; Dal '23; Retired.

COLLINS, Rhonda M.; Pincher Creek Associate Clinic, Pincher Creek, Alta.; Man '43.

COLLINS, Russell J., Hardings Point, R.R. No. 2, Kings Co., N.B.; Western Reserve School of Med. (Cleveland, U.S.A.) '15; F.R.C.P. (Edin.), M.R.C.P., F.A.C.P., F.R.C.P. (C), IntMed (TB), Cons. Phys. (Diseases of the Chest), Lancaster DVA Hosp.; Retired.

COLLINS, S. Burritt; Dept. of National Health & Welfare, Brooke Claxton Bldg., Ottawa 3, Ont.; Qns'49; Tel. 992-6286.

COLLINS, Selwyn; 4852A Yonge St., Willowdale, Ont.; R.C.S. (Dublin, Ire.) '56; LRCP, LRCSI, DPA; LM; Staff, Branson & Grace Hosp's.; Tel. 223-1030.

COLLINS, Thos. M.; 76 Cochrane St., St. John's, Nfld. (res); Dublin (Ire.)'57; M.O., Dept. of Health, St. John's; Tel. 578-0454.

COLLINS, William E.; Ste. 207, 1105 Carling Ave., Ottawa 3, Ont.; Qns'38; FACS; FRCS(C); Urol; Chief Urol., Ottawa Civic Hosp.; Cons. Urol., Royal Ottawa San.; Prof. of Surg. & Hd. Sub., Dept. of Urol., Ottawa U.; Tel. 729-1848.

COLLINS-WILLIAMS, Cecil; Toronto Professional Bldg., 123 Edward St., Toronto, Ont.; 39 Bennington Heights Dr. (res); Tor '44; FRCP (C); Paed; Dir., Allergy Clin., Hosp. for Sick Children; Assoc. Prof. (Paed.), U. of Toronto; Tel. 363-8225.

COLLIOU, Louis L.; Manitoba Clinic, 790 Sherbrook St., Winnipeg 2, Man.; 1070 Notre Dame Ave. (res); Ott '57; Tel. 774-6541.

COLLIP, John B.; 9244-116 Street, Edmonton, Alta.; Alb'50.

COLLISON, David B.; Fairmont Med. Bldg., 750 W. Broadway, Vancouver 9, B.C.; 4388 Angus Dr. (res); McG '33; ObstGyn; Clin. Instr., U. of British Columbia; Tel. 874-1323.

COLLYER, James A.; 33 John St., Leamington, Ont.; Wes '57; MCGP; Tel. 326-2151.

COLLYER, John E.; Ste. 101, 396 Queens Ave., London, Ont.; 1571 Ryersie Rd. (res) Wes '57; MCGP; Active Staff, Victoria & Parkwood Hosp's.; Court. Staff, St. Joseph's & St. Mary's Hosp's.; Tel. 432-8593.

COLLYER, Robert T.; 326 Queens Ave., London, Ont.; 7 Chalmers Ave. (res); Wes '55; FRCS(C); Ophth; Staff, Westminster Hosp.; Instr. (Ophth.), U. of Western Ontario; Tel. 433-4101.

COLMAN, Harry; Ste. 203, 333 Wilson Ave., Downsview, Ont.; 413 Rosemary Rd. (res); **Man '38; FRCS (Edin.), GenSurg; Urol; Active Staff, North York Branson Hosp.; Tel. 636-0661.**

COLOHAN, Austin B.; Queen's U. (Belfast, N. Ire.) '40; Med. Supt., St. John's San., St. John's, Nfld.; Tel. 579-2081.

COLONNIER, Marc L.; 729 Cote Ste-Catherine, Outremont, Montreal 8, P.Q.; Ott'59.

COLPITTS, Grant A.; Man '46; DAB; Path; Staff, Union Hosp., Moose Jaw, Sask.

COLPRON, Guy; 3423, rue St.-Denis, Montreal 18, P.Q.; Mon '61; Tel. 842-4892.

COLQUHOUN, James T.; Port Arthur Clinic, 194 North Court St., Port Arthur, Ont.; Tor '51; MCGP; Active Staff, Port Arthur Gen. & St. Joseph's Hosp's.; Tel. DI 4-7271.

COLQUHOUN, Philip; Waterville, P.Q. (res); McG '96; Retired.

COLTART, James L.; 2812 W. 16th Ave., Vancouver 8, B.C.; 3404 Cedar Crescent (res); Man '39; M.C.G.P.; Tel. RE 1-3154.

COLTER, Donald R.; 100 Med. Dental Bldg., 10603-100th Ave., Edmonton, Alta.; 8934-120th St. (res); Alb '49; OrthSurg; Teach. Staff, Royal Alexandra Hosp.; Tel. 424-1617.

COLTHART, John M.; 393 University Ave., Toronto 1, Ont.; 64 Harrison Rd., Willowdale (res); Wes '42; DABPrevMed; Sr. M.O., Bell Telephone Co. (Tor.); Tel. 929-2811. Abroad.

COLTHART, Shirley M.; 350 Christie St., Toronto, Ont.; 64 Harrison Rd., Willowdale (res); Wes '42; Cons. (Psy.), Metro Toronto Dept's. of Welfare, Homes for the Aged; Tel. HI 4-3818. Abroad.

COLTMAN, Rodney; Essex Medical Group, Essex, Ont.; London (Eng.)'55; MRCS(Eng.); LRCP (Eng.).

COLWELL, Bruce T.; 74 Johnson St., Kingston, Ont.; 2 Park Cres. (res); Wes '45; DMR; D & T Rad; Chief (Rad., Hotel-Dieu Hosp.; Ass't. Prof. (Rad), Queen's U.; Tel. 542-2791.

COLWELL, Garnet J.; Ste. 302, 5880 Spring Garden Rd., Halifax, N.S.; 1920 Connaught Ave. (res); Dal'50; PhysMed; Hd. PhysMed., Victoria Gen. & Camp Hill Hosp's.; Co-Dir., PhysMed., Halifax Infirmary; Assoc. Prof. Dalhousie U.; Tel. 422-5989.

COLWELL, Murray C.; 214-6th Ave. S.W., Calgary, Alta.; 1605 Shelbourne St. (res); Alb '54; Paed; Tel. AM 3-7120.

COLWILL, John C.; Ste. 209, Med. Arts Bldg., 170 St. George St., Toronto 5, Ont.; Tor'54; FRCS(C), OrthSurg; Tel. 921-1455.

COMEAU, Adeline E.; 770 King St., Bathurst, N.B. (res); Staff, Hotel Dieu.

COMEAU, Maurice; Clinique Lavoisier, 5136 rue Bellechasse, Montreal 36, P.Q.; 885 rue St. Aubin, Ville St-Laurent (res); Mon '49; Pulm. Dis. & T.B. (P.Q.); FRCP(C); IntMed; Chief (Med.), Hop. St. Joseph de Rosemont & Inst. Lavoisier; Tel. 254-4583.

COMEAU, Richard E.; 179 Water, Campbellton, N.B.; Dal '62.

COMPTON, Stephen F.; 412 Roslyn Ave., Westmount, P.Q.; Glasgow & Edinburgh (Scot.)'20; M.D. Berlin (Germ.); Staff, Royal Edward Laurentian Hosp.; Tel. 866-5410.

COMRIE, Clifford L.; 318 Medical-Dental Bldg., Regina, Sask.; 2555 Lindsay St. (res); Man '42; IntMed; Cons. to Outdoor Clinic, D.V.A. Wing, Regina; Tel. 536-2420.

COMTOIS, Gaston; 190 Blvd. St. Sacrement, Chicoutimi, P.Q.; Lav '46; Anaes (P.Q.); Chief Anaes., Hotel Dieu St. Vallier; Tel. 549-1452.

COMTOIS, J. Bernard; 36 Elm St. E., Sudbury, Ont.; 273 Elm St. W. (res); Mon. '43; Anaes.; Tel. 675-5833.

COMTOIS, Marcel; 5631-11eme Ave., Rosemont, Montreal 36, P.Q.; Mon '54; M.C.G.P.; Tel. RA 2-5713

COMTOIS, Max; 169 Labonte, Longueuil, Montreal, P.Q.; 166 St. Laurent (res); Mon '22.

COMTOIS, Robert; Mon'65; Res., Hop. Hotel-Dieu, Montreal 18, P.Q.

CONDE, Arthur B.; Philippines'57; Res., Brandon Mental Hosp., Brandon, Man.; Abroad.

CONDON, Cyril; Med. Centre, Corner Brook, Nfld.; 40 Brookfield Ave. (res); Nat. U. (Dublin, Ire) '52; Anaes; Chief Anaes., Western Mem. Hosp.; Anaes., West Coast San.; MO, Corner Brook; Tel. 4-7107.

CONDY, William A.; 2027 Parker St., Halifax, N.S.; Dal '54; MCGP; Tel. 423-6613.

CONEGHAN, Catherine; Cabri, Sask.; Anderson College, Glasgow (Scotland) '49; Tel. 587-2288.

CONEGHAN, John L.; Wascana Medical Assoc., 3831 Albert St., Regina, Sask.; Glasgow (Scot.) '58.

CONEN, Patrick E.; 10 Sussex Ave., Toronto 5, Ont.; London (Eng.)'51; MRCP(Lon.); Path; MC Path.; Assoc. Scientist, Research Inst.; Research Pathol., Hosp. for Sick Children; Ass't. Prof. (Path.), U. of Toronto; Tel. 922-5536.

CONKLIN, Francis J., 217 Laurier E., Ottawa 2, Ont.; 330 Metcalfe St. Apt. 110, Ott. 4 (res); Ott '53; F.R.C.S.(C), ObstGyn.; Tel. CE 5-8107.

CONLEY, A. E.; 75 Pine St. N., Thorold, Ont.; Wes '39; Dist. Coroner.

CONLON, Ellen M.; (SEE VAN DER HOEVEN, Ellen M.).

CONLON, Michael P. R.; Avondale, Nfld.; R.C.S. (Dublin, Ire.) '50.

CONLIN, Thomas B.; Dublin (Ire.)'64; Res., Gen. Hosp., St. John's, Nfld.

CONLY, D. Bryan, F/L; C.F.B., Summerside, P.E.I.; Man'63.

CONN, Alan W.; 2615 Lake Shore Blvd W., Toronto 14, Ont.; Tor '48; F.R.C.P.(C), Anaes; Staff, (Anaes), Hosp. for Sick Children; Clin Instr. (Anaes), U. of Toronto; Tel CL 9-2967.

CONN, E. Bert; 216 Macdonald Ave., Belleville, Ont.; Qns'57; D.Psy; Psy; Dir., Mental Health Clinic, Belleville, Gen. Hosp.; Tel. 962-8088.

CONN, Garson S.; 24 Old Park Rd., Toronto 10, Ont.; Tor'58; FRCS(C), OrthSurg; Staff, St. Joseph's Hosp.; Tel. 923-5618.

CONN, R. S.; 1230 Esquimalt Rd., Victoria B.C.; 645 Lampson St. (res); McG '27; M.C.G.P.

CONNELL, F. Ralph; Assoc. Anaesthetists, 15 Coburg St., Saint John, N.B.; 177 Princess St. (res); McG '31; Anaes; Anaes., St. Joseph's Hosp.; Staff Anaes., Saint John Gen. Hosp.; Tel. 692-6658.

CONNELL, George, F.; 674 Fennel Ave. E., Hamilton, Ont.; 29 Endfield Ave. (res); Tor '57.

CONNELL, W. Bruce; Qns'62; Chief Res. (Med.), Ottawa Civic Hosp., Ottawa, Ont.

CONNELL, W. Ford; Etherington Hall, Stuart St., Kingston, Ont.; 11 Arch St. (res) Qns '29; FRCP (Lond.); FACC; FACP; MABIM; FRCP (C); IntMed; Chief of Med. & Dir. of Cardiol. Dept., Kingston Gen. Hosp.; Dir., Anticoagulant Serv., Kingston Gen. Hosp.; Prof. & Hd. (Med.), Queen's U.; Tel. 546-3092.

CONNELL, Walter T.; 11 Arch St., Kingston, Ont. (res); Qns '49; LL.D., M.R.C.S. (Eng.), L.R.C.P. (Lond.), F.A.C.P., F.R.C.P.(C); Emer. Prof. (Med.), **Queen's U.; Retired.**

CONNELL, William S. T.; 433-1/2 Kings St. E., Hamilton, Ont.; 31 Claremont Dr. (res); Qns '14; FAAIS; MCGP; Staff, Hamilton Civic,, St. Joseph's & Chedoke Hosp's.; Div. Surg., C.N.R., **Hamilton & Med. Dir., Republic Iron & Steel; District Coroner; Tel. JA 2-2042.**

CONNELLY, Peter; Assiniboine Clinic, 633 Lodge Ave., Winnipeg 12, Man.; Glasgow (Scot.)'56; MCGP; Tel. 837-1363.

CONNELLY, William J.; 881 Maitland Ave., Ottawa 3, Ont. (res); Glasgow (Scot.) '45; D.P.H.; PH; Med. Cons. (Div. of Child & Maternal Health), Dept. of National Health & Welfare; Tel. CE 2-8211.

CONNERS, Charles E.; Listowel Clinic, Listowel, Ont.; Main St. (res); Qns '35; Dist. Coroner.

CONNOLLY, Bernard M.; 237 Geneva St., St. Catharines, Ont.; Qns '40.

CONNOLLY, James; Ituna, Sask.; Dublin (Ire.) '50.

CONNOLLY, James F.; Ste. 103, 356 Woodroffe Ave., Ottawa 3, Ont.; 2308 Dobson Rd. (res); Ott '55. Abroad.

CONNOLLY, John F.; 1541 W. Broadway, Vancouver, B.C.; 3183 S.W. Marine Dr. (res); Trinity C. (Dublin, Ire.) '48; DRCOG; ObstGyn; Active Staff (ObstGyn), St. Paul's & Mt. St. Joseph's Hosp's.; Tel. RE 3-7312.

CONNOLLY, John G.; Etherington Hall, Stuart St., Kingston, Ont.; Tor'49; FRCS(Ed); FRCS(C), Urol; Att'd. Urol., Kingston Gen. Hosp. & Hotel-Dieu Hosp.; Tel. LI 6-1731.

CONNOLLY, Leonard J.; Sussex, N.B.; Tor '53; M.C.G.P.

CONNOLLY, Valentine P. L.; Sq. Cdr.; Nat. Defence Med. Ctr., Ottawa 8, Ont.; 2072 Palmer Ave. (res); Birmingham (Eng.)'42; M.B., Ch.B.; Derm; Chief Derm., NDMC; Court. Staff, Ottawa Civic Hosp.; Tel. 733-6600.

CONNOP, Peter J.; Birmingham (Eng.) '60; M.O., RCAF Station, Portage La Prairie, Man.

CONNOR, Terrence P.; Apt. 406, 3625 Ridgewood Ave., Montreal 26, P.Q.; London (Eng.) '54; M.B., B.S.; DiagRad.

CONRADI, Gerhard J.; 327 LeMarchand Bldg., Edmonton, Alta.; 6304-129th St. (res); **Jena (Germ.) '42; Paed; Chief of Paed.,** Misericordia Hosp.; Att'd. Staff, Royal Alexandra Hosp.; Clin. Instr., U. of Alberta; Tel. HU 8-3656.

CONRAN, Helen J.; '63; Res., St. John's Gen. Hosp., St. John's, Nfld.

CONROY, Frederick D.; 462 Professional Bldg., 10830 Jasper Ave., Edmonton, Alta.; 13016-104th Ave. (res); **Alb '38; Urol; Chief of Urol., Edmonton Gen. & Misericordia Hosp's.; Instr. (Urol.), U. of Alberta; Tel. GA 2-6271.**

CONROY, James B.; 4769 Sherbrooke St. W. Westmount, P.Q.; McG '39; Ophth; Clin. Ass't., Montreal Gen. Hosp.; Dem., Path. of the Eye, McGill U.; Tel. 933-2291.

CONSTABLE, William C.; Halifax Infirmary, Halifax, N.S.; Edinburgh (Scot.) '55; DMRT; Dir., Dept. of Rad., Halifax Infirmary; Cons. Rad., Victoria Gen. Hosp.; Instr., Dalhousie U.; Tel. 422-1511.

CONSTANTIN, Laurent; 101A, rue Principale, Rouyn, P.Q.; Lav '59; Paed.

CONSTANTINE, Rodric R.; M.O.H., Dept. of Health & Welfare, Princess St. & 6th Ave., Dawson City, Yukon; Budapest (Hung.)'46; MCGP; Phys. & Surg. & G.P., Dawson City & Klondike Valley Reg.; Phys., Yukon Consolidated Gold Corp.; Phys., Cassiar Asbestos Corp. Ltd., Clinton Creek; Tel. 2121.

CONSTANTINI, Giovanni; Radway, Alta.

CONSTANDINES, Paris; 658 School Rd., Winnipeg 22, Man.; M.D. (Vienna & Austria) '43; Ph.D. (Montreal); Abroad.

CONSTANTINIDIS, Peter; 658 School Rd., Kirkfield Park, Winnipeg 22, Man. (res); Alexandria **(Egypt) '57; IntMed; Deputy M.O., Dept. of** Health, Wpg.; Lect., Dept. of Social & PrevMed., Manitoba Med. College; Tel. WH 6-0415.

CONSTANTINIDIS, Stamatios; Greece '53; GenSurg; Staff, Halifax Infirmary, Halifax, N.S.; Tel. 422-1511.

CONTWAY, M. Alan; 717 Coxwell Ave., Toronto, Ont.; 21 Garfield Ave. (res); Tor '34; FICS; GenSurg; Surg. Staff, Scarborough Gen. Hosp.; Cons. Surg., Sunnybrook Hosp.; Assoc. Surg. Staff, Toronto East Gen. & St. Michael's Hosp's.; Tel. HO 5-2272.

CONVERY, Ernest B.; 226 Clemow Ave., Ottawa, Ont. (res); McG '14; F.I.C.A., Anaes; Med. Adviser, War Veterans Allowance Bd.; Advisor in Geriatrics, D.V.A.; Retired.

CONWAY, Bernard B.; 345 Bloor St. W., Toronto 5, Ont.; 4101 Bathurst St. (res); Tor '32; F.A.A.P.; Paed; Jr. Att'd. (Paed) New Mt. Sinai Hosp.; Tel. ME 5-0373.

CONWAY, Dominick J.; 84 Rebecca Cres., Box 598, R.R. 1, Ottawa, Ont. (res); Cambridge (Eng.) '42; D.C.H., D.T.M. & H., M.R.C.P., F.R.C.P.(C), Paed; Chief (Dept. of Paed), Ottawa Gen. Hosp.; Prof. (Paed), Ottawa U.; Tel. SH 6-8944.

CONWAY, Donal F.; Yorkton-Melville, Health Reg. No. 10, Yorkton, Sask.; National U. (Ireland)'50; DPH(Lond.); DTM&H(Eng.); Tel. 783-3647.

CONWAY, Patrick F.; 209 Rideau Med. Dental Centre, 1711-4th St. S.W., Calgary, Alta.; Dublin (Ire.) '51; Psy; Tel. 263-1498.

COODIN, Fischel J.; 805 Boyd Bldg., 388 Portage Ave., Winnipeg 1, Man.; 8 Primrose Cres., Wpg. 17 (res); Qns '47; F.A.A.P.; Paed; Att'd. Paed., St. Boniface & Children's Hosp's.; Chief of Paed., Misericordia Hosp.; Lect. (Paed), U. of Manitoba; Tel. WH 3-0641.

COODIN, Pesach; 805 Boyd Bldg., 388 Portage Ave., Winnipeg 1, Man.; 34 Carman Ave. (res); Man '27; M.C.G.P.; Tel. WH 2-1424.

COOK, Arlen; 2514 St. John St., Port Moody, B.C.; Sask'65.

COOK, Barry W.; 145 Wellington St., Sarnia, Ont.; Sask'60; FRCS(C), Urol.

COOK, Clarence E.; Ste. 350, 2184 W. Broadway, Vancouver 9, B.C.; Alb '35; F.R.C.S.(C), OrthSurg; Active Staff, Children's Hosp.; Lect., B.C. Med. School; Vis. Staff, St. Paul's Hosp.; Tel. RE 8-7612.

COOK, David F.; Tor'62; D.Psy; Res., Clarke Inst. of Psy., Toronto 5, Ont.

COOK, Edward G.; Woodlands School, New Westminster, B.C.; 923-2nd St. (res); London (Eng.) '42; MRCS; LRCP; MRCP (Lond.); DCH; Paed; Staff, Royal Columbian & St. Mary's Hosp's.; Tel. LA 1-2611.

COOK, Faustina A. (Kelly); 137 Cedar St., Apt. 6, Sudbury, Ont. (res); Tor '20; Retired.

COOK, George H.; 515 Prince St., Truro, N.S.; Dal '54; GenSurg.; Tel. 893-3410.

COOK, Gerald T.; Ste. 301, Toronto Western Hosp., Toronto 2B, Ont.; Wes'56; FRCS(C), Urol; Att'd. Staff, Toronto Western & Hosp. for Sick Children; Clin. Teach., U. of Toronto; Tel. 364-4694.

COOK, John B.; 50 Cedar St., Sudbury, Ont.; McG '38; D.P.H.; PH; M.O.H. & Dir., Sudbury & Dist. Health Unit; Tel. 674-0776.

COOK, Maynard S.; 7 Burton Ave., Westmount, Montreal 6, P.Q.; McG '28.

COOK, Norman C.; Med. Arts Bldg., 1105 Pandora Ave., Victoria, B.C.; 2925 Tudor Rd. (Res): Man '30; Otol; Tel. EV 3-5033.

COOKE, George L.; Lloydminster Clinic, Lloydminster, Sask; 5101—49 St. (res); Qns '10; Dist. Coroner.

COOKE, Joseph F.; 51 King St. E., Brockville, Ont.; 5 Fairknowle Dr. (res); Qns '55; ObstGyn; Tel. DI 2-4017.

COOKE, Robert L.; Manitoba Clinic, 790 Sherbrook, Winnipeg, Man.; 37 Kingsway (res); Man '39; F.R.C.S. (Eng.), D.A.B.S.; F.R.C.S.(C), GenSurg; Ass't. Surg., Winnipeg Gen. & Grace Hosp's.; Ass't. Prof. & Lect. (Anat.), U. of Manitoba; Tel. SP 4-6541.

COOKE, W. A. Ralph; Ste. 625, 5025 Sherbrooke St. W., Montreal, P.Q.; McG '57; FACOG; FRCS (C), ObstGyn; Att'd. Staff, Queen Elizabeth & Catherine Booth Hosp's.; Tel. 482-8523.

COOKE, William J. D.; Tor '50; Res., Ottawa Civic Hosp., Ottawa, Ont.

COOKSON, Brian A.; 6 Fordham Pl., Don Mills, Ont. (res); Edinburgh (Scot.) '45; D. Psy; Psy; Staff, Tor. Gen. & Ont. Hosp's.; Tel. 924-3553.

COOKSON, Francis B.; Dept. of Anat., U. of Alberta, Edmonton, Alta.; Manchester (Eng.)'56; B.Sc., DObstRCOG.

COOKSON, Thomas S.; Box 480, McCutcheon Bldg., Sylvan Lake, Alta.; London (Eng.)'52; MRCS, LRCP; Med. Staff, Red Deer & Eckville Mun. Hosp's.; Tel. 887-2370.

COOKSON, Wm. H.; 5891 Arbutus St., Powell River, B.C.; Liverpool (Eng) '55; M.B., Ch.B., FRCS(Eng.); FRCS(Edin.); FRCS(C), GenSurg; Staff, Powell River Gen. Hosp.; Tel. 483-4112.

COOMBES, Archibald C.; 188 Prince St., Pembroke, Ont.; 522 Fraser St. (res); Tor '42; Att. Staff, Pembroke Gen. & Cottage Hosp's.; Tel. 732-7351.

COOMBES, Wilfred N.; Tilden Bldg., 347 Sherbrooke St., North Bay, Ont.; 635 Baywood St. (res); Cambridge (Eng.) '43; F.R.C.S. (Eng.), GenSurg.; OrthSurg; Cons. OrthSurg., North Bay; Tel. 472-1331.

COOMEY, Ernest J.; 3571 Sheppard Ave. E., Agincourt. Ont.; London (Eng.) '57; Tel. AX 3-4171.

COOP, C. W. A.; 277 Main St. N., Brampton, Ont.; Tor'50.

COOPER, Alfred J.; 27 Cedar St. N., Timmins, Ont.; Ott '58; Staff, St. Mary's & Porcupine Gen. Hosp.; Tel. 264-1234.

COOPER, Basil J.; Arnprior Med. Centre, Arnprior, Ont.; McG '58.

COOPER, Bernard A.; 32 Arlington Ave., Montreal 6, P.Q. (res); McG '53; FRCP(C); IntMed; Staff, Royal Victoria Hosp.; Ass't. Prof., Med. & Clin. Med., McGill U.; Tel. VI 2-1251.

COOPER, Bruce M.; 110 Bathurst Ave., Pointe Claire, P.Q.; McG '43; Staff, Lachine Gen. & Lakeshore Gen. Hosp's.; Tel. 697-1961.

COOPER, Donald A.; 1428 Ouellette Ave., Windsor, Ont.; UBC '55; IntMed; Chief, Dept. of Med., IODE Hosp.; Ass't. Instr. (Med.), Wayne State U., Detroit, U.S.A.; Tel. 252-7757.

COOPER, Eric; 350 Albert St., Nanaimo, B.C.; Liverpool (Eng.) '44; M.B., Ch.B., GenSurg; Staff, Nanaimo Reg. Hosp.; Tel. SK 3-3431.

COOPER, Everett A.; 422 London, Sherbrooke, P.Q.; 233 Howard Ave. (res); McG '41; FACS; FACOG; ObstGyn; Chmn., Dept. of Obst Gyn., Sherbrooke Hosp.; Tel. 562-9386.

COOPER, Frank C. T.; Box 40, Mount Albert, Ont.; Royal College Phys. & Surg. (London, Eng.)'57; Staff, York County Hosp.; Tel. 473-2443.

COOPER, Gardner E.; 604 Med. Arts Bldg., Hamilton, Ont.; 8 Searle St. (res); Tor'40; FRCS(C); GenSurg; OrthSurg; Head, Dept. of Surg., Hamilton Civic Hosp's. Tel. JA 9-4331.

COOPER, Harold G.; 141 Hawthorne Ave., Kingston, Ont. (res); Birmingham (Eng.) '50; M.R.-C.S., L.R.C.P., D.Psy.; Psy; Staff Psy., Ontario Hosp., Kingston; Tel. LI 6-1101.

COOPER, H. G.; 925 W. George St., Vancouver, B.C.; Alb '40; Urol; Clin. Instr. (Urol), U. of British Columbia; Tel. MU 5-5460.

COOPER, Jerry J.; Tor'62; Res., St. Michael's Hosp., Toronto 2, Ont.

COOPER, John H.; Pathol. Inst., 5880 University Ave., Halifax, N.S.; 3196 Mayfield Ave. (res); Glasgow (Scot.)'45; Path; Admin. Pathol., Path Inst.; Assoc. Prof. (Path.), Dalhousie U.; Tel. 422-9661.

COOPER, John W.; 645 Fort St., Victoria, B.C.; Alb '51; Staff, St. Joseph's Hosp.

COOPER, Michael A.; 360 Beach Dr., Victoria, B.C.; London (Eng.)'55; AMCGP; Court. Staff, St. Joseph's Hosp.; Assoc. Staff, Royal Jubilee Hosp.; Tel. 385-2535.

COOPER, Michael T.; King St., Shelburne, N.S.; Sheffield (Eng.)'59; Med. Exam., Fatalities Enquiry Act; Pres. Med. Staff, Roseway Hosp.; Tel. 511.

COOPER, Pamela E.; 35 Alwington Ave., Kingston, Ont. (res); Birmingham (Eng.) '51; M.R.-C.S. (Eng.); L.R.C.P.(Lond.); Temp. Retired.

COOPER, Perry; Tor'63; Res., Jewish Gen. Hosp., Montreal 26, P.Q.

COOPER, Robert C.; 4728 Ross St., Red Deer, Atla.; Sask '57; MCGP.

COOPER, Robert M.; 337 Donlands Ave., Toronto, Ont.; McG '49; M.C.G.P.; Exam. Phys., Prudential Ins. Co. of America; Tel. GA 1-4545.

COOPER, Ross H.; 326 Medical Arts Bldg., Winnipeg, Man.; 288 Waverley St. (res); Man '30; Tel. WH 2-7978.

COOPER, Stewart R.; 4333 Western Ave., Montreal 6, P.Q.; 4199 Northcliffe Ave. (res); McG '43; IntMed; Tel. VI 5-9889.

COOPER, William E.; Ste. 8 Medical Arts Bldg., 2150 Valley Way, Niagara Falls, Ont.; London (Eng.) '48; M.R.C.S. (Eng.), L.R.C.P. (Lond.); IntMed; Chm. Dept. IntMed., Gtr. Niagara Gen. Hosp.; Hon. Cons. Phys., Douglas Mem. Hosp., Fort Erie; Tel. EL 4-7332.

COOPER, William L.; Saint Martin's, N.B.; Kansas City U. (Kansas, U.S.A.) '32; Ophth; Att. Staff, St. John Gen. Hosp., St. John, N.B.

COOPERBERG, A. A.; 670 Ellendale Med. Bldg., 5845 Cote-des-Neiges Rd., Montreal 26, P.Q.; 395 St. Catherine Rd. (res); McG '42; Haem. (P.Q.); IntMed; Tel. RE 1-9811.

COOPERMAN, Earl M.; Qns'61; Paed; Staff, Kingston Gen. Hosp., Kingston, Ont.

COOPERSMITH, Harvey; Tor'55; MCGP; Res., Toronto Western Hosp., Toronto 2B, Ont.

COOPLAND, Ashley T.; UBC '58; Res. Winnipeg Gen. Hosp., Winnipeg, Man.

COPAS, Desmond E.; Psychiatric Centre, Yorkton, Sask.; Wales'50; M.B., B.Ch., DPM; Tel. 783-2491.

COPE, G. W.; 5507 Columbia St., Vancouver, B.C. (res); **Man '30; Workmen's Compensation Bd.,** 707 W. 37th Ave., Vancouver, B.C.

COPE, R. Alun; Med. Clinic, Innisfail, Alta.; Cardiff (Wales) '61; M.B., Ch.B.; Tel. 227-3419.

COPELAND, George G.; 288 Queen's Ave., London, Ont.; 862 Waterloo St., **Wes '43;** ObstGyn; **Staff, Victoria & St. Joseph's Hosp's.; Teach.** Staff, U. of Western Ontario; Tel. 434-1542.

COPEMAN, John W.; 262 Essex Ave., Richmond Hill, Ont.; Tor '55; Anaes; Staff (Anaes.), York Central Hosp.; Tel. 884-3647; Abroad.

COPEMAN, William J.; P.O. Box 40, Sundridge, Ont.; Tor '47; M.C.G.P.; M.O.H., Sundridge, South River & Twps. of Strong & Joly; Coroner, **Parry Sound Dist.; Tel. 384-5384.**

COPESTAKE, Gerald G.; 263 Regent St., London, Ont. (res); Cambridge & St. Bart's (London, Eng.) '43; DMRD (Ed.), DABR; DiagRad; Dir. DiagRad., Victoria Hosp.; Assoc. Prof. & Acting Hd. Dept. of DiagRad., U. of Western Ont.; Tel. GE 2-5261.

COP-HODJERA, Branislava M.; 4734 Alexander Ave., Pierrefonds, P.Q.; Belgrade (Yugo.) '52; Anaes; Staff, Lakeshore Gen. Hosp., Beaconsfield, LaSalle Gen. Hosp., Ville LaSalle & Hop. Notre-Dame de l'Esperance, Ville St. Laurent; Tel. 684-2201.

COPLAND, Graeme M.; 60 Northdale Rd., Willowdale, Ont.; Aberdeen (Scot.)'56; FRCP(C), IntMed; Cons. Dept. of Med., Sunnybrook Hosp.; Assoc. (Med.), University of Toronto.

COPLEY, Donald R.; Canada Pension's Commission, Sunnybrook Hosp., Toronto 12, Ont.; McG'60; Pension Med. Exam.; Tel. 485-8651, Loc. 562.

COPP, Arthur G. B.; 34 Kensington Ave., London, Ont.; 91 Elworthy Ave. (res); **Wes '33; MCGP; Tel. GE 4-3889.**

COPP, Douglas H.; 4755 Belmont Ave., Vancouver 8, B.C. (res); **Tor '39; Ph.D.; FRSC; Prof. & Head, Dept. of Physiol., U. of British Columbia;** Tel. CA 4-4111. Loc. 264.

COPP, Joseph C.; 490 Runnymede Rd., Toronto, Ont.; Tor '18; O.P.D., Toronto Western Hosp.; Tel. RO 7-2217.

COPP, Stephen E.; 131 Grove St., Danville, P.Q.; Dal '52; F.C.C.P.; Tel. TE 9-2158. Abroad.

COPP, Walter F.; 190 High St., London, Ont.; **Wes '38; M.C.G.P.; Tel. 434-0721.**

COPPING, Gordon A.; 4485 Sherbrooke St. W., Montreal, P.Q.; **803 Upper Belmont Ave. West-**mount (res); McG '30; MRCP(L); F.R.C.P.(C), IntMed Sr. Phys, The Mtl Gen Hosp. Med. Cons., Queen Mary Vet's. Hosp., (DVA) Assoc. Prof. (Med.), McGill U.; Tel. WE 7-3028.

COPPING, John D.; 23A Mowhawk, Port Credit, Ont.; Tor '53; Staff, St. Michael's & Queen Elizabeth Hosp's., **Toronto; Tel. 278-8311.**

COPPING, Winona M. (Rostocky); 23A Mohawk Ave., Port Credit, Ont.; **Tor '51; Staff, Queen Elizabeth & Toronto Western Hosp's.;** Tel. 278-8311.

COPPINGER, Harry; 626 Wardlaw Ave., Winnipeg 13, Man.; Man '16.

COPPINGER, William W.; 868 Waterloo St., London, Ont.; Oxford U. & London U. (Eng.); **'37;** M R.C.O.G.; **ObstGyn; Tel. GE 3-3713.**

COPPOLINO, Andrew G.; 97 Frederick St., Kitchener, Ont.; Tor'57; Psy.; Tel 745-6641.

CORBEIL, Claude; 719 2nd St. E., Cornwall, Ont.; Lav '51.

CORBEIL, Jacques; 55 Church Ave., Verdun, Montreal 19, P.Q.; Mon '54; FRCS(C); FACS; FACOG; ObstGyn; Chief of Obst., Hop. General de Verdun; Tel. PO 6-0115.

CORBEIL, Jerome, Jr.; Rockland, Ont.; **Ott '53;** M.C.G.P.

CORBER, A. Alan; 802 Rockland Ave., Outremont, **Montreal, P.Q.; McG '40; Tel. 277-7773.**

CORBET, Richard C. B.; 401 Rideau-Medical-Dental Centre, 1711-4th St. S.W., Calgary Alta.; 2105-7th St. S.W. (res); Alb'46; Paed; Att'd. Staff, Calgary Gen., Holy Cross & Alberta Children's Hosp's.; **Tel. 266-4464.**

CORBETT, Brian N.; 18-3rd Ave. W., Dauphin, Man.; Man'65.

CORBETT-DALY, Carmel P.; Box 1588, Lloydminster, Sask.; Nat. U. (Ire.)'56; Abroad.

CORBETT, Herbert R.; 172 South Bentinck St., Sydney, N.S. (res); **Dal '23; DiagRad; Rad., City & St. Rita Hosp's.; Cons. Rad., Dosco Emergency** Hosp.

CORBETT, John R.; Clark's Harbour, N.S.; **McG '21; Port Phys. & M.O.H.,** Clark's Harbour; Coroner, Shelburne Co.; Tel. 70.

CORBETT, William E. N.; 300 Norman Rogers Dr., Kingston, Ont.; (res); **Qns '56;** FRCP(C) Path; Pathol., Kingston Gen. Hosp.; Ass't. Prof (Path.), Queen's U.; Tel. 546-3841, Ext. 277.

CORBETT, W. E. P.; L.M.S.S.A. (Lond.); 513[illegible] Cordova Bay Rd., Victoria, B.C. (res); Retired.

CORBETT, W. J.; 1146 Marine Dr., North Vancouver, B.C.; 1795—15th St. W., Norgate Par[illegible] **(res); Tor '52; MCGP; Tel. YU 8-5291.**

CORBIN, Emmett N.R.; P.O. Box 430 Gran[illegible] Falls, N.B.; Lav'49; MCGP; Sec. Med. Staf[illegible] Grand Falls Gen. Hosp.; Tel. 78.

CORBIN, Mark F.; 1367 Tatra Dr., Bay Ridge[illegible] Ont.; Tor '40; Outdoor Staff, New Mt. Sin[illegible] Hosp.; Tel. 839-3353.

CORCORAN, Michael; 4 Sussex Ave., Toronto [illegible] Ont.; Tor '47; MA; MRSH; FRIPHH; FRMS (Psychol.); Tel. WA 2-2078.

CORCORAN, Timothy V.; Staff, Colonel Belch[illegible] Hosp., Calgary, Alta.; Dublin (Ire.) '52; Tel. A[illegible] 6-7001.

CORDEAU, Claire; 1133 Blvd. St. Joseph E[illegible] Montreal 34, P.Q.; Mon '53; F.R.C.S.(C), Obs[illegible] Gyn; Tel. 272-8229.

CORDEAU, Jean M.; Mon '58; Intn., Hop. Hot[illegible] Dieu, Montreal, P.Q.

CORDEAU, J. Pierre; 644 Stuart, Outremon[illegible] Montreal, P.Q. (res); Mon '54; B.Sc.; Vice-De[illegible] (Med.) & Prof. & Hd. Dept. of Neurophysiol., [illegible] of Montreal; Tel. RE 3-9951.

CORDEAU, Luc J.; 12405 rue Crevier, Montr[illegible] 9, P.Q.; Mon'60; Psy; Staff, Inst. Albert P[illegible] vost.

CORK, John F.; 2025 W. Broadway, Ave., Va[illegible] couver 9, B.C.; 7250 Arbutus St., Van. 14 (res[illegible] **Tor '39; Ass't. Med. Dir., Med. Serv. Asso[illegible] Tel. RE 3-8141.**

CORK, S. B. F/L; National Defence Med. Cent[illegible] Smyth Rd. & Alta Vista Dr., Ottawa, Ont.; [illegible] '64.

CORKRAN, R. Gerald; 1248 Chemin Ste-F[illegible] Quebec, P.Q.; McG '45; GenSurg; Staff, Jeff[illegible] Hale's Hosp.; Tel. 681-0228.

CORKUM, T. P.; Tor '64; Res., Banting In[illegible] Toronto 2, Ont.

CORLESS, John R.; Tor'62; Res., Hosp. for S[illegible] Children, Toronto 2, Ont.

CORLEY, John B.; Chinook Shopping Cen[illegible] McLeod Trail, Calgary, Alta.; Alb'42; MC[illegible] Dir. Gen. Practice Res., College of G.P.; Ch[illegible] Ethics Comm., American Soc. Clinical Hypno[illegible] Tel. AL. 5-5566.

CORMACK, Gary D.; Tor '54; D. Psy; P[illegible] Staff, Ontario Hosp., Toronto 14, Ont.; Tel. **3-8501.**

CORMACK, George N.; 10515-133rd St., Edm[illegible] ton, Alta.; Alb '44; Tel. 488-6434.

CORMACK, John J.; North West River, Lab[illegible] dor; Edinburgh (Scot.) '55.

CORMIER, Andre; 1656 est rue Sherbro[illegible] Montreal 24, P.Q.; 2640 Prieur (res); Mon '[illegible] F.R.C.S.(C), ObstGyn; Vol. Ass't. ObstG[illegible] Hop.-Notre-Dame.; Tel. LA 5-6363.

CORMIER, Bruno M.; 509 Pine Ave. W., Montreal, P.Q.; 506 Pine Ave. W. (res); Mon '48; D.Psy., Psy. (P.Q.); Lect., McGill U.; Ass't. Psy., Royal Victoria Hosp.; Psy., St. Vincent de Paul Penitentiary; Tel. 489-7570.

CORMIER, Dollard; 232 St. George St., Moncton, N.B.; Lav '50; ObstGyn; Tel. 384-7991.

CORMIER, Eugene J.; 640 Chemin Mountain, Moncton, N.B.; Lav '46.

CORMIER, Jean G.; Box 537, Dorchester St., Sydney, N.S.; Lav '28; OphthOtol.

CORMIER, Paul E.; 1835 Sir Mathias, Tellier, P.Q.; Lav '57; Psy; Staff, Hop. St-Michel-Archange; Tel. 663-7151.

CORMIER, Rene J. G.; 3026 Le Chasseur, app 7, Ste-Foy, Quebec, P.Q.; Lav'57; GenSurg; Urol.

CORMIER, Wilbrod F.; Montreal Rd., Ottawa 7, Ont.; 344 Grandmaitre, Ott. 7 (res); Lav '43; FCCP(A); IntMed (PQ); PulmDis & TB (PQ); DHA; Med. Dir., Hop.-St.-Louis-de-Montfort; Pt.-time Field Rep. CCAH; Lt.-Col. 10th Med. Unit; Pres. Health Office, Eastview; Tel. SH 6-4621.

CORNE, Norman I.; 302 Boyd Bldg., Winnipeg, Man. 555 Niagara St. (res); Man '40; ChM.; M.C.G.P.; Assoc. Staff, Misericordia & Winnipeg Gen. Hosp's; Courtesy Staff, St. Boniface, Grace & Children's Hosp's; Tel SP 4-6581.

CORNE, Robert A.; 302 Boyd Bldg., 388 Portage Ave., Winnipeg 1, Man.; Man'59; FRCP(C), IntMed; Dem. (IntMed.), U. of Manitoba Med. Coll.; Tel. 943-6437.

CORNELIS, Johan M.; Louvain (Belgium)'61; PlasSurg; Staff, Saint John Gen. Hosp., Saint John, N.B.

CORNELIUS, Leigh R.; 1139 Yates St., Victoria, B.C.; Brentwood Bay Rd. (res); UBC '60.

CORNELL, James M.; Osoyoos, B.C.; Qns '51.

CORNER, F. David; Dinsmore, Sask.; Durham (Eng.)'56; Tel. 64.

CORNETT, J. William D.; 19 Greenbelt Dr., Don Mills, Ont.; 20 Berkindale Dr., Willowdale (res); Qns '45; M.C.G.P.; Med. Dir., Ortho Pharmaceutical (Can.) Ltd.; Tel. HI 4-4461.

CORNETT, Robert W.; 408 Med. Arts Bldg., Hamilton, Ont.; 182 Buckingham Dr. (res); Qns '52; M.Sc.; FRCP(C); IntMed; Active Staff, Hamilton Civic & Hamilton Health Assoc.; Hon. Cons. Staff, St. Joseph's Hosp.; Tel. 528-1961.

CORNFORD, Stanley E., F/L; Leeds (Eng.) '57; Sr. MO, RCAF Stn., Winnipeg, Man.

CORNISH, Arthur L.; Hazel Dr., Coquitlam, B.C.; Man'30; Retired.

CORNISH, David R.; Apt. 704, 12207 Jasper Ave., Edmonton, Alta.; Alb'58; D.Psy; Psy; Staff, Alberta Hosp.

CORNISH, Sidney J.; Box 8, Claresholm, Alta.; Alb '50; M.C.G.P.; Dist. Coroner; Tel. 235-3411.

CORNOCK, William Y.; 424-7th St. S., Lethbridge, Alta.; 618-29th St. S. (res); Glasgow (Scot.) '37; FRCS(Edin), FRCS(Glas.); GenSurg; Active Staff, St. Michael's & Mun. Hosp's.; Tel. 7-4781.

CORR, John J.; 2085 Tecumseh Rd. E., Windsor, Ont.; 1128 Devonshire Rd. (res); Qns '56 MCGP; Tel. 252-7289.

CORRIGAN, Cameron; 13904-92nd Ave., Edmonton, Alta. (res); Man '37; Act. T.B. Control Off., Charles Camsell Hosp.

CORRIGAN, Cecil E., DSO; 428 Med. Arts Bldg., Winnipeg, Man.; 203 Montrose St. (res); Man '25; FRCS (Eng.); FRCS(C), GenSurg; Cons. Gen. Surg., Deer Lodge DVA Hosp.; Pt.-time M.O., W.C.B.; Tel. 942-5632.

CORRIGAN, John A.; Apt. 11, 4320 Delorimier Ave., Montreal 34, P.Q.; Mon'23; Phys., C.P.R., Fry-Cadbury Ltd., Confederation Life Ins. & Bruchesne Inst.; Tel. LA 1-6481.

CORRIGAN, Vincent A.; 1085 Queen's Blvd., Kitchener, Ont. (res); Qns '38; Urol; Tel. 742-7611.

CORRIN, Bernard N.; 253 Josephine St., Wingham, Ont.; 112 Diagonal Rd., (res); Wes '46; MCGP; Active Staff, Wingham Gen. Hosp.; Tel. 357-2500.

CORRIN, Melvin H.; Lucknow, Ont.; Wes '47; MCGP; Pres. Med. Staff, Wingham Dist. Hosp.; Member, Bd. of Governors; Tel. 528-2907.

CORRIN, Roger C.; Wes '61; Res., Tor. Psychiatric Hosp., Toronto 2, Ont.

CORRIVEAU, A. R.; 150 Metcalfe St., Ottawa, Ont.; 748 Parkdale St. (res); Lav '43; Ophth, Otol; Staff, Ottawa, Gen. Hosp.; Tel. PA 2-6253.

CORRIVEAU, Gerald; 150 St. Georges, Levis, P.Q.; Lav '54; M.C.G.P.

CORRIVEAU, Robert A.; 168 rue St. Georges, Levis, P.Q.; Lav'65.

CORRIVEAU, Yvon; 64 rue St-Eustache, St. Eustache, P.Q.; 68 rue St-Eustache (res); Mon '35; Vis. Phys., Hop. du Sacre-Coeur, Cartierville; Tel. 473-3221.

CORSILLI, Mario; 6809, boul. St-Laurent, Montreal 10, P.Q.; Geneva (Switz.) '57.

CORSON, J. A.; 4614 Kingston Rd., West Hill, Ont.; Tor '41; M.C.G.P.; Tel. AT 2-2282.

CORSTON, James M.; 5750 South St., Halifax, N.S.; 5865 Inglis St. (res); Edinburgh (Scot.) '41; FICS; FACOG; FRCOG; ObstGyn; Assoc. Gyn., Victoria Gen. Hosp.; Obst., Grace Maternity Hosp.; Assoc. Prof. (ObstGyn),Dalhousie U.; Tel. 422-5802.

CORTES, Julio P.; Santiago (Spain) '53; Jr. Intn., Winnipeg Children's Hosp., Winnipeg, Man.

COSBIE, W. Gerald, MC, ED; 537 Med. Arts Bldg., 170 St. George St., Toronto 5, Ont.; 12 Dunloe Rd. (res); Tor '15; F.R.C.O.G., F.R.C.S (C), ObstGyn; Med. Dir., Ont. Cancer Treatment & Research Fdn.; Cons., ObstGyn, Toronto Gen. Hosp.; Lect. P.G., U. of Toronto; Retired.

COSENS, Mary; 360 Christie St., Toronto, Ont.; Tor '29; Bact; Lab. Scientist, Prov. of Ont. Govt., Dept. of Health Central Lab.; Not Practising.

COSENTINO, Francis V.; Lac La Biche, Alta; Tor '31.

COSETTE, Rene; 824 St. Ursule, Three Rivers, P.Q.; Lav '51.

COSGRAVE, J. J.; 40 Cambridge St. S., Lindsay, Ont.; Tor'62.

COSGROVE, James B. R.; Montreal Neurological Inst., 3801 University St., Montreal, P.Q.; 455 Barton Ave. Twn. of Mt. Royal (res); Man '44; M.Sc. (Cantab.); Neur; Dir. Multiple Sclerosis Research Lab., Montreal Neurol, Inst.; Ass't. Neurol, Royal Victoria Hosp.; Ass't. Prof. (Dept. Neurol. & NeurSurg.), McGill U.; Tel. 845-8672.

COSHAN, Angus W.; 61 Phipps St., Fort Erie, Ont.; Madras (India) '45; MB; BS; GenSurg; Sec. Hosp. Staff, Douglas Mem. Hosp.; Tel. 871-1220.

COSKUN, Nejat; 48 Queen St., Dartmouth, N.S.; Istanbul (Turkey) '50.

COSMAN, H. Herbert; Ste. 305, 340 McLeod St., Ottawa 4, Ont.; 1987 Bel Air Dr., Ott. 5 (res); Man'49; FRCP(C), IntMed; Act. Sr. Phys., Ottawa Civic Hosp.; Clin. Ass't. (Med.), U. of Ottawa; Cons. Med. National Defence H.Q.; Tel. 722-3635.

COSSETTE, Albert; 105 rue Rochefort, Cap-de-la-Madeleine, P.Q.; Lav '50; Anaes (P.Q.).

COSSETTE, Gilles; 11890, boul. L'Acadie, Montreal 12, P.Q.; Lav '54; Anaes; Chief Anaes., Hop. Hotel-Dieu, St. Jerome; Tel. GE 2-9711.

COSSETTE, Honore; 470 Notre-Dame, Charette, Co. St. Maurice, P.Q.; Lav'50; Tel. 221-2104.

COSSETTE, Jacquelin; Amos, P.Q.; Mon '60; AMCGP; Tel. 732-4644.

COSSETTE, Rene; 383-6th Ave., Grand'Mere, P.Q.; 80-10th Ave. (res); Lav '51; GenSurg (P.Q.); Ass't. (Surg.), Hop Lafleche.

COSSETTE, Robert; Mon '64; Res., Hop. Maisonneuve, Montreal, P.Q.

COSSETTE, Yves, 1840 St. Marc, Shawinigan Falls, P.Q.; Lav '52; Paed (P.Q.)

COSTAIN, William A.; 1567 Bathurst St., Toronto, Ont.; 244 Lonsmount Dr. (res); Tor '11; GenSurg; Assoc. Staff, Toronto Western Hosp. Retired.

COSTANTINI, W. Anthoni; 403 Rideau Med. Centre, 1711-4th St. S.W., Calgary, Alta.; 2220 Capitol Hill Cr. (res); Man '44; OrthSurg; Assoc. Staff, Calgary Gen., Holy Cross & Alberta Children's Hosp's.; Tel. 263-2070.

COSTANZO, John E.; Medical Arts Bldg., 2150 Valley Way, Niagara Falls, Ont.; 2968 Gordon St. (res); Qns '56.
COSTELLO, Bernard G.; Ott '64; Res., Royal Victoria Hosp., Montreal 2, P.Q.
COSTELLO, J. Bernard; Ste. 370, 5655 Cambie St., Vancouver 15, B.C.; 4850 Selkirk St., Van. 9 (res); McG'49; ObstGyn; Acting Chief, Dept. of ObstGyn, St. Vincent's Hosp.; Cons. Staff, Mt. St. Joseph's Hosp.; Tel. 263-3810.
COSTIGAN, Patrick G.; Box 1080, Banff, Alta., Alb '43; Dist. Coroner.
COSTIN, Philippe A.; Lav'41; Med. Dir., Hosp. St. Luc, 1038 St. Denis St., Montreal 18, P.Q.; Tel. 861-7321, Ext. 291.
COSTIN, Saul J.; 1538 Sherbrooke St. W., Ste. 1002, Montreal 25, P.Q.; McG '49; MCGP; Att'd. Staff, Reddy Mem. & Jewish Gen. Hosp's.; Tel. 935-5161.
COSTIN, T. Blair; 316 White Pines Dr., Burlington, Ont.; Tor '61; Active Staff, Joseph Brant Mem. Hosp.; Tel. 634-1544.
COSTLEY, Samuel R.; Rynard Clinic, 11 Coldwater St., Orillia, Ont.; London (Eng.) '57; M.B., B.S., Staff, Orillia Soldiers Mem. Hosp.; Tel. 325-2711.
COSTLEY-WHITE, Katherine; London (Eng.) '65; Res., Shaughnessy Hosp., Vancouver 9, B.C.
COSTOM, David; 3455 Cote des Neiges Rd., Ste. 110, Montreal 25, P.Q.; 4617 Michel Bibaud (res); McG '30; IntMed (P.Q.); **Ass't. Phys., Montreal** Jewish Gen; Assoc. Phys., Montreal **Jewish Hosp. of Hope; Tel. CL 5-2847.**
COSTOPOULOS, Lambros B.; Athens (Greece) '52; DiagRad; Staff, University Hosp., Edmonton, Alta.
COTE, Albert R.; Brownsburg, P.Q.; Mon '31; Part-time Phys., **Canadian Industries** Ltd., Ammunition Div.
COTE, Alexandre; Lav'53; Res., Hop. St. Michel Archange, Quebec 5, P.Q.
COTE, A. Luc; 5970-21st Ave., Rosemont, Montreal 36, P.Q.; Lav '57.
COTE, Aurelien; 863 ave. Rochette, Ste-Foy, Quebec 10, P.Q.; Lav '50; PulmDis&TB (P.Q.); Ass't. Serv. (Pneumo-Phthisiology), Hop. Laval; Clin., Quebec Anti-Tuberculan League; Lect. (Resp. Infections), U. of Laval; Tel. 683-0641.
COTE, Bernard M.; 1618 King Ouest, Sherbrooke, P.Q.; Mon'62; AMCGP; Tel. 569-9151.
COTE, Carol; 384 Chatelaine, Apt. 4, Sherbrooke, P.Q.; Lav '57; GenSurg.; Tel. 562-4804.
COTE, Chas. A.; 12273 Laurentian, Montreal, **P.Q.; Mon '56; Tel. FE 4-7474.**
COTE, Charles E.; 85 St. Vallier ouest, Quebec, **P.Q.; Lav '37; Ophth, Otol (P.Q.); Tel. 525-8304.**
COTE, Donald P.; Mon '64; Sr. Int., Notre Dame Hosp., Montreal 24, P.Q.
COTE, Edouard; 61 Notre Dame W., Victoriaville, P.Q.; 449 Notre-Dame W. (res); Lav '35; **GenSurg; Surg-in-chief, Hotel Dieu Arthabaska, P.Q.; Tel. 752-2750.**
COTE, Fernand; 483 Blvd. St. Joseph E., Montreal, P.Q.; 770 Wiseman, Outremont (res); Mon '43; Neur. Psy. (P.Q.); F.R.C.P.(C), Psy; Chief, Dept. of Psy., Hop. Maisonneuve; Assoc. Prof. (Psy.), U. of Montreal; Tel. VI 2-2691.
COTE, Fernand; 292 Ave. Michaud, Rimouski, P.Q.; Lav'62.
COTE, Francois H.; 225 Metcalfe St., Ottawa, Ont.; 540 Fairview, Rockcliffe (res); Tor '35; F.I.C.S., F.A.C.S., F.R.C.S.(C) GenSurg; Gyn; Assoc. Prof. Surg., **Ottawa U.; Tel SH 9-5173.**
COTE, Gaston; 115-1ere rue, St.-Fabien, P.Q.; Lav '63.
COTE, Georges; Blvd. Talbot, Laterriere, Co. Chicoutimi, P.Q. (res); Lav '49; PH (P.Q.).
COTE, Gilles; Lav '63; Res., Hop. St-Sacrement, Quebec 6, P.Q.
COTE, Gilles A.; 3422 St. Hubert, **Montreal, P.Q.; Mon'56; Psy; Staff, Hop. Notre-Dame.**
COTE, Gregoire; Lav '59; Staff, Domremy Quebec Inc., 610 Calixa-Lavallee, Quebec 6, P.Q.
COTE, Guy; 728 Wallberg, Dolbeau, Co. Lac-St.-Jean, P.Q.; Lav '60.
COTE, Henri, Capt.; 2 R22R, CAPO 5050, Cdn. Armed Forces, Europe; Lav'64; **Abroad.**
COTE, Jacques C.; 240 rue St.-Jean, Quebec 4. P.Q.; 3815 Place Toulouse, Ste.-Foye (res); Lav '51; M.S. (Mayo); GenSurg (PQ); Surg. Staff, Hop-de-l'Enfant-Jesus; Tel. 523-8049.
COTE, J. Alexandre; St. Come, Cte. Beauce, P.Q.; Lav '53.
COTE, J. Marie; Robertsonville Co. Megantic, P.Q.; Lav'50; Tel. 335-7808.
COTE, Jean; 11061 rue Hotel-de-Ville, Beaupre, P.Q.; Lav '58.
COTE, Jean M.; C.P. 188, L'Isletville, P.Q.; Lav '60.
COTE, Jean M.; 870, ave. Royale, St. Jean 10, P.Q.; Lav '55; Staff, Hop. St. Jean.
COTE, Jean-P.; Polyclinique Gravel, 56 St. Jean Baptiste, Victoriaville, P.Q.; Lav'62; OrthSurg (P.Q.).
COTE, J-Henri G.; Lav'64; 2 R22R CAPO, 5050, Cdn. Armed Forces, Europe; Abroad.
COTE, Leo; 779 ave de Longpre, St. Foy, Quebec, 10, P.Q.; Lav'40; GenSurg(P.Q.).
COTE, Louis; Lav'53; MCGP; Res., **c/o Apt. 4,** 89 Roywood **Terrace, Ville-Lemoyne, P.Q.**
COTE, Marcel; 643 Carre Dufault, Ste. Therese-en-Haut, P.Q.; Lav'61; Anaes(P.Q.).
COTE, Maurice; '61; Sr. Int., Hop. St-Sacrement, Quebec, P.Q.
COTE, Napoleon; 725 Boul. Hamel, Quebec 4, **P.Q.; Lav'36; MCGP; Phys., W.C.B.; Tel. 693-2985.**
CO-TE, Pacita; Santo Tomas (Philippines) '56; Paed; Staff, The Woodlands School, New Westminster, B.C.
COTE, Patrice; 698 Ave. Royale, Quebec 5, P.Q.; Lav'62.
COTE, Paul E.; 1500-18eme rue, Quebec 3, P.Q.; Lav'41; **D.M.R.T.(Lond.); D&T Rad; Ass't. Rad.,** Hop de Enfant-Jesus; Chief Rad., Jeffrey Hale's & Hop. Ste. Foy; **Cons., R.C.A.M.C. (Quebec) & Hop. St. Augustin; Staff, Laval U.; Tel. 523-5077.**
COTE, Pierre; App. 1, 5020 Drolet, Montreal 14, P.Q.; Mon '52; Tel. 842-3620.
COTE, Raymond; 1563 Notre Dame, Ancienne **Lorette, P.Q.; Lav '50; Tel. 872-2244.**
COTE, Raymond M.; 119 De L'Eglise, B.P. Calliere, Beauport, P.Q.; Lav'60.
COTE, Raynald; Lav'62; Psy; Staff, Hop. St-Michel Archange, Quebec 5, P.Q.
COTE. Richard; 8 du Rocher. Riviere-du-Loup, P.Q.; Lav '58; Tel. 562-6528.
COTE, Robert; 214 Laurier Blvd., Beloeil, P.Q.; Mon '43.
COTE, Robert; 1000, Chemin Ste-Foy, Quebec 6, P.Q.; Lav '51; M.S. (Surg.); FACS; FRCS(C), GenSurg; Ass't. Surg., Hop. du St. Sacrement; Assoc. Prof., Laval U.; Tel. 681-0175.
COTE, Roland; 260 Ball St., Sherbrooke, P.Q.; **415 Vimy (res); Lav '46; GenSurg (P.Q.); Tel. 562-4844.**
COTE, Rolland; 2047 Parc Gomin, Sillery, **P.Q.; Lav '48; FRCP(C); IntMed; Staff, Hop.** St. Michel-Archange; I/C **Ther.** Course, Laval U.; Tel. 663-3571.
COTE, Sarto G.; 177 rue Empire, Granby, P.Q.; 166 rue Dufferin (res): McG '43; M.C.G.P.
COTE, Yves; 415 ouest rue Fleury, Montreal 12, P.Q.; Mon'59; Tel. 381-8761.
COTE, Zepherin; 825 Belvedere S., Sherbrook, **P.Q.; Lav '49; M.C.G.P.; Tel. 562-3434.**
COTNAM, H. Beatty; 897 Bay St., Toronto 5, Ont.; 20 Brian Cliff Dr., Don Mills (res); McG '41; Supervising Coroner, & Gen. Inspect. of Anatomy, Prov. of Ontario; Local Insp., Anat., County of York; Tel. 365-2565.
COTTON, Anthony M.; Assoc. Med. Clinic, 320 Fischer Ave., The Pas, Man.; 601 Edwards Ave. (res); London (Eng.) '59; **LRCP; MRCS;** DRCOG; Staff, St. Anthony's Hosp.; Tel. MA 3-3291.
COTTON, Odilon; Gaspe, P.Q., **Lav '49;** GenSurg (P.Q.).
COTTREAU, Thomas; Lav'65; Res., Royal Victoria Hosp., Montreal, P.Q.
COTTRELL, Donald G.; Central Bldg., **Richmond** Ave., Grande Prairie, Alta.; **Manchester** (Eng.) '49; Active Staff, Grande Prairie Mun. Hosp.; Tel. 532-2480.

COTTRELL, Jack D.; 2113-2nd St. S.W., Calgary, Alta.; Alb'44; IntMed.
COTTRELL, Leonard G.; Clarke Inst. of Psy., 250 College St., Toronto, Ont.; Birmingham (Eng.)'54; DPM; Psy; Assoc. Psy., Clarke Inst.
COUCH, Albert E. H.; Kincardine, Ont.; Tor 18.
COUCH, J. Harold; 1341 Lakeshore E., Oakville, Ont. (res); Tor'25; FRCS(Ed.), FRCS(C), GenSurg; OrthSurg; Lect. PG (Surg.), U. of Toronto.
COUILLARD, Auguste C.; Vegreville, Alta.; Qns '06; Retired.
COUILLARD, Edgar; 64 Ste. Ursule St., Quebec, P.Q.; Lav '04; Retired.
COUILLARD, Fernand; St. Adelphe, Champlain, P.Q.; Lav '65.
COUILLARD, J. A.; La Patrie, Compton County, P.Q. (res); McG '14; A.C.C.P., IntMed (TB); Retired.
COUILLARD, Jean M.; Lav '22; Staff, Hop.-de-l'Immigration, Quebec, P.Q.
COUILLARD, Philippe; Mon '61; Res. Hop. Ste-Justine, Montreal 26, P.Q.
COUILLARD, Theodore J.; 10951-124th St., Edmonton, Alta.; 11311-110 Ave. (res); Alb '53; MCGP; Tel. GL 4-4551.
COULAS, Leonard G.; 3535 Lakeshore Blvd. W., Toronto 14, Ont.; Tor'57; Ophth; Active Staff, Queensway Gen. Hosp.; Assoc. Staff, St. Joseph's Hosp.; Tel. 255-2947.
COULDWELL, William J.; Ste. 706, 625 - 5th Ave., New Westminster, B.C.; McG'50; Ophth; Tel. LA 2-8638.
COULOMBE, Albert; 17 rue Fusey, Cap-de-la-Madeleine, P.Q.; 278 St. Georges (res); Mon '48; Tel. 378-2022; Abroad.
COULOMBE, Claude; 1010 Chemin St Roch, Tracy, P.Q.; Mon '65.
COULOMBE, Gisele; 1563 Notre Dame, Ancienne Lorette, P.Q.; Lav '50.
COULOMBE, Jean-Louis; Lav '64; Res., Notre-Dame Hosp., Montreal 24, P.Q.
COULOMBE, Leo; 4090 Old Orchard, Montreal, P.Q.; Mon '31.
COULOMBE, Maurice; 1451, rue Dobell, Quebec 6, P.Q.; Lav '49; Psy; Ass't. (NeurPsy.), Hop.-de-l'Enfant-Jesus & Hop. St-Michel-Archange; Lect., Laval U.; Tel. LA 9-4511.
COULOMBE, Paul; St-Cyprien, Cte, Riviere du Loup, P.Q.; Lav'64.
COULOMBE, Pierre; 1500, 18eme rue, Quebec 3, P.Q.; Lav '55; PlasSurg (P.Q.); Staff, Hop. Enfant Jesus & Hop. Christ-Roi; Tel. 525-8117.
COULOMBE, Rene; Ste. Marthe, P.Q.; Mon '31
COULOMBE, Roland; Lav '59; Res. (Psy), Hop.-St-Michel-Archange, Quebec, P.Q.
COULONVAL, Louis F.; 35 Ste-Ursule St., Quebec, P.Q.; 1369 Marechal-Foch **(res); Lav** '46; F.R.C.S.(C), Urol; Ass't. Urol., **Hop.-Hotel-Dieu; Staff, Laval U.; Tel. 522-4259.**
COULSON, David B.; Port Arthur Clinic, Port Arthur, Ont.; 156 Robinson Dr. (res); Qns '55; M.C.G.P.; Staff, Port Arthur Gen. & St. Joseph's Gen. Hosp's; Tel. DI 4-7271.
COULSON, Earl G.; 9 Tally Lane, Willowdale, Ont. (res); M.D., M.B. (U. of T); D.R., FAGS; DRO; Tor '18; DiagRad; Rad., W.C.B., Toronto; Tel. 362-3411.
COULSON, Gordon M.; Ste. 2, 1862 W. Broadway, Vancouver 9, **B.C.; Dal '61; Tel. 733-6818.**
COULTER, George F.; 584 Jones Ave., Toronto 6, Ont.; 364 Mt. Pleasant Rd., Toronto 7 (res); Tor '57; Tel. 461-9211.
COULTER, Hugh B.; 15108 Rio Terrace Dr., Edmonton, Alta. (res); Queens U. (Belfast, N. Ire.) '55; DA (Eng.); FFA (Ire.); Anaes; Court. Staff (Anaes.), Royal Alexandra Hosp.; Tel. GR 4-3431.
COULTER, James G.; 775 Earlscourt Dr., Sarnia, Ont.; Tor '54; DiagRad; Staff, Sarnia Gen. Hosp.; Tel. DI 4-3661.
COULTER, Patrick T.; 72 Victoria Ave., Chatham, Ont.; Qns '43; Urol.; Tel. 354-0232.
COULTER, S. G.; 584 Jones Ave., Toronto 6, Ont.; Qns '45; M.C.G.P.; Tel. 461-9211.
COULTER, W. Keith; Ste. 312, 450 Central Ave., London, Ont.; Wes '56; FRCP(C), IntMed; Cons. (Arth.), Victoria & Westminster Hosp's.; Instr. (Med.), U. of Western Ontario; Tel. 439-0798.
COULTHARD, Hugh S.; 57 John St., Weston, Ont. (res); Tor'26; IntMed (T.B.); Ass't. Supt. Toronto Hosp. for T.B.; Clin. Teacher, Faculty of **Med., U. of Toronto; Tel. 769-1161.**
COUPAL, J. Albert; 30 est, Boul. St.-Joseph, Montreal 14, P.Q.; Mon '35.
COUPAL, Jean L.; Med. Arts Bldg., 180 Metcalfe St., Ottawa, Ont.; 221 River Rd., Eastview (res); Mon'24; Ophth; Otol; Hon. Cons., Ottawa Gen. Hosp.; **Emer. Prof. (Otol.), Ottawa U.; Tel. CE 2-7411.**
COUPAL, Jean-Paul; 180 avenue du Parc, Gatineau, P.Q.; Bordeau (France) '57; Paed; Staff, Hop. St-Michel, Buckingham, & Hop. Sacre-Coeur, Hull; Tel. 663-2274.
COUPAL, Yves; 20 Rue Bourdages, Sept-Iles, P.Q.; Mon'61.
COUPE, Robert L.; 140 E. 14th St., North Vancouver, B.C.; Liverpool (Eng.) '58; FRCP(C), Derm.; Instr. Dept. of Derm., U. of British Columbia; Tel. 987-4814.
COUPER, Edward H.; Nipawin Medical Clinic, Nipawin, Sask.; London (Eng.) '54.
COUPER, W. Mason; 202 Medical Arts Bldg., 1538 Sherbrooke St., Montreal, P.Q.; 11 Grove **Park, Westmount (res); McG '34; F.R.C S. (Edin.)** & (C) GenSurg; Assoc. Surg., Royal Victoria Hosp.; **Cons. Surg., Queen Mary Veterans' Hosp.; Ass't. Prof. (Surg.), McGill U.; Tel. WE 5-4482.**
COUPLAND, Douglas C. T.; 3260 Edgemont Blvd., North Vancouver, B.C.; Qns '58.
COURCHESNE, Georges H.; 1280 de Callieres, Quebec 6, P.Q.; Lav '20; Anaes; Staff, Hop. Notre-Dame-de-l'Esperance & Hop. St-Joseph-de-Bellevue; Tel. 527-3183.
COURCY, Gilbert; L'Islet, Co. L'Islet, P.Q.; Lav '52; M.C.G.P.; Med. Staff, Hop.-Hotel-Dieu-de-Montmagny & Hop.-St.-Jean, Port-Joli.
COURSLEY, Gerald; Ste. 303, 625 - 5th Ave., New Westminster, B.C.; Mon'50; D.A.B.S., F.R.C.S.(C), GenSurg; Cardiovasc. & ThorSurg.; Tel. LA 4-3133.
COURTEAU, Roger; 1150 Blvd. St. Joseph E., Montreal 34, P.Q.; 2170 Capitaine Bernier (res); Mon '48; Urol; Head (Urol.), Maisonneuve Hosp.; Staff, St. Joseph de Rosemount & Jean Talon **Hosp's.; Tel. 254-8341.**
COURTEMANCHE, A. Douglas; 706-750 W. Broadway, Vancouver 9, B.C.; 1163 W. 29th Ave. **(res); Tor '55; FRCS(C); PlasSurg; Active** Staff, Vancouver Gen. Hosp.; Clin. Instr., Dept. **of Surg., U. of British Columbia; Tel. 879-4020.**
COURTEMANCHE, Leonard; Clinique Medicale de l'Ouest, 4647, Avenue Verdun, Verdun, P.Q.; Mon '64; Tel. PO 7-5304.
COURTENAY, Harold D.; 222 Elgin St., Ottawa, Ont.; Tor '15; OphthOtol; Tel. 235-5587.
COURTENAY, Peter H. E.; Cook Med. Bldg., 1175 Cook St., Victoria, B.C.; London (Eng.)'51; MRCS; LRCP; FRCS(Eng.); FRCS(C), OrthSurg.
COURTOIS, Guy A.; 5570 Canterbury, Montreal 26, P.Q. (res); Mon '48; Neur; **Chief, Electroenceph. Lab., Hop.-Hotel-Dieu; Ass't. Prof. (Neur.), U. of Montreal; Tel. VI 4-0161.**
COURTRIGHT, Lucy; Ott'65; Jr. Int., Ottawa Civic Hosp., Ottawa 3, Ont.
COUSINEAU, C. Russell; Athabaska, Alta.; Alb'33.
COUSINEAU, George; 5700 Blvd. Gouin W., **Montreal 9, P.Q.; Mon '33; Anaes; Tel. FE 4-5950.**
COUSINEAU, Gilles G.; 78 St. Joseph Blvd. W., Laurent (res); Mon '48; Ophth (P.Q.); Ass't. Ophth., Hotel-Dieu de Montreal, Hop Ste- Justine; Tel. VI 4-0161.
COUSINEAU, Guy; 4920 Adam, Montreal 4, P.Q.; Mon '40 Tel. CL 5-1041.
COUSINEAU, Guy C.; Ott '58; Res., Ottawa Gen. Hosp., Ottawa 2, Ont.
COUSINEAU, Jean; 85 Poplar, Gatineau, P.Q. (res); Mon '24; Phys., Can. International Paper Co., Gatineau.

COUSINEAU, Leo E.; 9363 Greenfeld Terrace, Ville Lasalle, P.Q.; Mon'58; Haem(P.Q.).
COUSINEAU, Michelle; 10782 Blvd. St.-Laurent, Montreal 12, P.Q.; Mon '60; Tel. 331-1851.
COUSINEAU, Pierre E.; Mon '63; Res., Verdun Gen. Hop., Montreal 19, P.Q.
COUSINS, James A.; Ste. 216, 1900 Lonsdale **Ave, N. Vancouver, B.C.; 234 W. Braemar Rd., N. Van. (res); UBC '57; Staff, Lion's Gate Hosp.; Tel. 988-4710.**
COUSINS, R. J.; Leader, Sask.
COUSLAND, P. A. Clyde; 1029 Douglas St., **Victoria, B.C.; 1040 Hulford St. (res); Tor '24; IntMed; Chief, Sub-dept. Cardiol., Royal Jubilee Hosp.; Retired.**
COUTU, Albert H.; 1070 Rielle St., Verdun, P.Q.; Mon '35; F.R.C.S.(C), GenSurg; Surg.-in-Chief, Hop. Gen. de Verdun; Tel. 766-8511.
COUTU, Gilles; Lav'58; Psy(P.Q.); Phys., Reynolds Aluminium Co. of Canada, St.-Laurent Blvd., Cap-de-la-Madeleine, P.Q.
COUTU, Luciene; 3003 Chemin de la Cote Ste. Catherine, Montreal, P.Q. (res); **Mon '26**; Paed; **Staff Hop. Ste. Justine, Tel. RE 1-4931.**
COUTU, Lucien L., 2900 Bl. Mt.-Royal, Montreal, P.Q.; 592 est, rue Liege, Mtl. 11 (res); **Mon '48; FRCP(C), IntMed; Dean U. of Montreal; Tel. RE 3-9951.**
COUTU, Noel; 31 rue Montcalm, Hull, P.Q.; Mon '37; GenSurg (P.Q.); Tel. 777-6522.
COUTURE, Andre; 297 Boul. Ste-Genevieve, Chicoutimi, Nord, P.Q.; Lav'56.
COUTURE, Ernest; 161 Laurier Ave. E., Ottawa, Ont.; McG '16; Obst; Med. Staff, Ottawa Gen. Hosp.; Tel. CE 6-4592.
COUTURE, Francois; 1000 Chemin Ste-Foy, Quebec 6, P.Q.; Lav'59; FRCP(C), IntMed; Cardiol (P.Q.); Ass't. Dept. of Med., Hop. du St-Sacrement; Prof. Med., Laval U.; Tel. 681-1066.
COUTURE, Jean A.; Mon'60; Res., Hop. Maisonneuve, Montreal 36, P.Q.
COUTURE, Jean G.; 1000 Chemin-Ste.-Foye, Quebec, P.Q.; 2040 Chemin St.-Louis, Sillery (res); Lav '49; FACS; FRCS(C), GenSurg; Assoc. Prof., U. of Laval; Tel. 681-0175.
COUTURE, J. F. P. Capt.; 2421 Carlsen St., Ottawa 8, Ont. (res); Staff, NDMC, Ottawa.
COUTURE, Jean P.; Imperial Oil Ltd., 10510 Notre Dame St. E., Montreal 5, P.Q.; Mon'48; IntMed(P.Q.); MCGP.
COUTURE, Jean-P.; 17 Charles Edouard, Levis, P.Q.; Lav '57; Anaes (PQ); Staff, Hop.-Hotel-Dieu; Tel. 837-9341.
COUTURE, J. Pierre; 669 ave. Mille-Isles ouest, Ste-Therese-en-Haut, P.Q.; Lav '60.
COUTURE, Magelli; 22 rue Sacre-coeur, Alma, Cte Lac St-Jean, P. Q.; 769 Jeanne d'Arc (res); Lav '55; FACS; FRCS(C); GenSurg; Staff, Hotel-Dieu d'Alma; Tel. 662-3421.
COUTURE, Richard; St.-Hugues, P.Q.; Lav '52.
COUTURE, Roger A.; McG '57; FRCP(C); IntMed; Staff, Ottawa Gen. Hosp., Ottawa, Ont.; Lect., U. of Ottawa; Tel. 236-0333.
COUTURIER, Alphonse, The Hon., M.P.; 500 Lafontaine St., **Riviere-du-Loup, P.Q.; 127 Temiscouata St. (res); Lav '30; GenSurg; Minister of Health, Province of Quebec, Parliament Bldgs., Quebec City, P.Q.; Tel. UN 2-3563 & Quebec — LA 4-8411.**
COUTURIER, Albert; 301 Carre Saint-Louis, Montreal, P.Q.; 5596 Stirling (res); Lav '29; OrthSurg; **Assoc. Prof., U. of Montreal;** Chief of Orth. Serv., Hop. St. Luc; Tel. 845-7272.
COUVES, Cecil M.; 241, University of Alberta Hosp., Edmonton, Alta.; Man '45; FRCS(Ed), FRCS(C), FACS; GenSurg; ThorSurg (Cardiovasc.); Assoc. Prof. (Surg.), U. of Alberta; Tel. GE 3-6237.
COVERT, Earle L.; Box 126, Hay River, N. W. T.; Qns '63. Area M.O.H.; Tel. 2496.
COVERNTON, Carleton C.; Suite 120, 3195 Granville St., Vancouver, B.C.; McG'40; IntMed; Att. Staff, Vancouver Gen. & Ass't. Supt. Shaughnessy Hosp's.; Clin. Instr., U. of British Columbia; Tel. RE 8-6822.
COVILL, Frank J.; Vermillion Health Unit, Vermillion, Alta.; London (Eng.)'50.
COW, David N.; 548 King St., Port Colborne, Ont.; 64 Steele St., (res); London (Eng.) '49; MRCS, LRCP, MCGP; Coroner Welland Co.; Med. Staff, Port Colborne Gen. Hosp.; Tel. 834-3684.
COWAN, Agnes I. C.; 55 Anderson Ave., Toronto, Ont.; Tor '24; Retired.
COWAN, Barbara W. (Dean); 81 Cornwall Ave., Town of Mount Royal, Montreal 16, P.Q. (res); McG '47.
COWAN, David K.; 68 Madeleine St., Sault-Ste.-Marie, Ont.; Edinburgh (Scot.) '31; DIH; Med. Dir., Algoma Steel Corp. Ltd.; Tel. AL 6-2261.
COWAN, Davina (Van Weel); 1220 Colony St., Saskatoon, Sask. **(res); Edinburgh (Scot.) '41; D.A. (Lond.); Anaes., City and St. Paul's Hosp's.; Tel. 653-0362.**
COWAN, Donald H.; Room 136, Private Patients' Pavilion, Toronto Gen. Hosp., Toronto, Ont.; Tor '56; FRCP(C), IntMed, Ass't. Phys., Toronto Gen. Hosp.; Clin. Teach., (Med.), U. of Toronto; Tel. EM 6-8211, Loc. 2389.
COWAN, George A.; 1220 Colony St., Saskatoon, Sask. (res); Glasgow (Scot.) '44 DMRT (Lond.); TherRad; Sr. Clin. Assoc., Saskatoon Cancer Clin., University Hosp.; Ass't. Prof. (TherRad), U. of Saskatchewan; Tel. CH 2-7671.
COWAN, J. Earle; P.O. Box 4208, O'Mara-Martin Bldg., St. John's Nfld.; 33 Monkstown Rd. (res); Dal '51; OrthSurg; Active Staff, St. John's Gen., St. Clare's Mercy & Grace Hosp's.; Cons. Staff, **Hosp. for Mental & Nervous Dis. & St. John's** San.; Tel. 726-8123.
COWAN, John M.; Med. Arts Clinic, 51-6th St. S.E., Medicine Hat, Alta.; 412 Prospect Dr. (res); Alb '48; GenSurg; Staff, Medicine Hat Gen. Hosp.; Tel. JA 7-2281.
COWAN, John M.; Manchester (Eng.)'65; Res., Kingston Gen. Hosp., Kingston, Ont.
COWAN, Larry H.; 575 Upper James St., Hamilton, Ont.; 500 Mountain Park Ave. Unit 6, Apt. 401 (res); Wes '51; Tel. 389-1328.
COWAN, Leonard E.; Box 557, Med. Arts Clinic, Regina, Sask.; Qns'36; FACOG; DRCOG; FICS; Chmn., Dept. of ObstGyn, Regina Gen. & Grey Nuns Hosp's.; Cons., Sask. Cancer Commission; Clin. Instr., U. of Saskatchewan; Tel. 523-0691.
COWAN, Lorraine Y.; Alb '56; Staff, Box 307, Alberta Hosp., Edmonton, Alta.; Tel. 7-0221.
COWAN, Marjorie D. (See FISH)
COWAN, Robert; 181 Queen St. N., Kitchener, Ont.; 246 Stanley Dr., Waterloo (res); Wes '42; F.R.C.S.(Ed), GenSurg.; Tel. 742-6722.
COWAN, Robert J.; 925 W. Georgia St., Vancouver 1, B.C.; 4184 East Blvd. (res); Tor '41; F.R.C.S.(C), GenSurg; PlasSurg; Att'd. Staff, Shaughnessy, Vancouver Gen., St. Paul's & Chil-dren's Hosp's.; Hd. Sub. Dept. PlasSurg., Vancouver Gen. Hosp.; Clin. Ass't. Prof., U. of British Columbia; Tel. 681-4622.
COWAN, Royden; 560 Bathurst St., Toronto 4, Ont.; Tor '34; MCGP; Active Staff, Doctor's Hosp.; Court. Staff (Obst.), Toronto Gen. Hosp.; Tel. 922-6033.
COWAN, T. Archibald; 81 Cornwall Ave., Mount Royal, Montreal 16, P.Q.; McG '47; Paed; Att. Staff, Montreal Children's & Catherine Booth **Hosp's.; Dem. (Paed.), McGill U.; Tel. 737-9070**
COWAN, W. Cameron; 4 Church St. E., Richmond Hill, Ont.; Tor'41; M.C.G.P.; Tel. 884-4471.
COWAN, William E.; 19 Rosebery Ave., Ottawa 1, Ont.; McG '26; GenSurg; Att'd. Surg. Staff, Ottawa Civic Hosp.; **Tel. CE 2-6345.**
COWARD, N. Barrie; 1649 Oxford St., Halifax, N.S.; Dal '28; F.A.A.P.; Paed; Phys.-in-Chief, Children's Hosp.; Paed.-in-Chief, Grace Maternity **Hosp. & Halifax Infirmary; Prof. (Paed.), Dalhousie U.; Tel. 423-8590.**
COWELL, Carol A.; Alb '62; Res., Toronto Gen. Hosp., Toronto 2, Ont.
COWEN, June (Woods); 33 Ridgehill Dr., Brampton, Ont.; Qns '55. Retired.
COWEN, Robert H.; 31 Centre St. S., Brampton, Ont.; Qns '55; GenSurg; Cons. Staff, Peel Mem. Hosp.; Tel. 451-8080.

COWLE, Joseph E.; Rm. 212, Prov. Health Dept., 67 College St., Toronto 2, Ont.; 181 Broadlands Blvd., Don Mills (res); Tor '42; MO, I/C Indus. Chest Unit, Indust. Hyg. Br., Ont. Dept of Health; Sec., Silicosis Referee Bd.; Tel. EM 3-1211.

COWLEY, Frank C.; Shawville, Co. Pontiac, **P.Q.; McG '43; Dist. Coroner; Tel. 647-2520.**

COWMAN, David R.; Brooklin Med. Centre, Brooklin, Ont.; Birmingham (Eng.)'56; Tel. 655-3321.

COX, Alan J.; 108 Scott Bldg., Moose Jaw, Sask.; 1037 Simcoe St. (res); Man '57; MCGP; Active Staff, Moose Jaw Union & Providence Hosp's.; Tel. 692-1827.

COX, Albert R.; 6050 Alma Rd., Vancouver 13, B.C. (res); UBC '54; FRCP(C), IntMed (Cardiol.); Att'd. Staff, Vancouver Gen. Hosp.; Assoc. **Prof., Dept. of Med., U. of British Columbia; Tel. TR 6-3211.**

COX, Andrew D.; 232 Metcalfe St., Ottawa 4, Ont.; Qns '27; Tel. CE 2-3112.

COX, Felicity C.; 2800 Lundy's Lane, Niagara Falls, Ont.; London (Eng.)'59; Tel. 358-7840.

COX, Gordon E.; 250 Med. Arts Bldg., 1105 Pandora Ave., Victoria, B.C.; 1751 Cedar Hill X Rd. (res); UBC'55; MCGP; Tel. EV 6-2621.

COX, Kenneth G.; Qns '53; Admin. Staff, Dept. of Health & Welfare, Burrard St., Vancouver, B.C.; Tel. MU 3-1937.

COX, Lloyd S.; 170-172 Fitzroy St., Charlottetown, **PEI; 71 Goodwill Ave. (res); Dal '48; DABS; FACS; GenSurg; Att'd. Staff, PEI Hosp.; Court. Staff, Charlottetown Hosp.; Tel. 894-7325.**

COX, Margaret (DOBSON); Dept. of Paed., 715 W. 12th Ave., Vancouver 9, B.C.; UBC'55. Tel. TR 6-3211, Loc. 2683.

COX, M. Armacost; Ste. 107, **250 Lawrence Ave. W., Toronto 12, Ont.; 488 Avenue Rd. (res); Tor '18; Paed; Phys.-in-Chief, O.P.D. (Med.), Hosp. for Sick Children; Chief Paed., St. Mary's Home; Prof., Preventive Dentistry (Fac. of Dent.), & Assoc. Paed. (Fac. of Med.), U. of Toronto; Tel. RU 1-4224.**

COX, Phoebe L.; 3430 McTavish, Apt. 202, Montreal 2, P.Q. (res); McG '47; Ph.D.

COX, Robert H.; Nyanza, Co. Cape Breton, N.S.; McG '40; AICS.

COXON, Melville G.; 14 Brochen St., Gander, Nfld. (res); Tor '37; MCGP; Sr. M.O. & Supt., Sir Frederick Banting Mem. Hosp.; Tel. 8-2211.

COY, Filmer E.; Invermere, B.C. (res); McG '14; Retired.

COY, Peter; 2656 Heather St., Vancouver 9, B.C.; Wales (U.K.)'56; DMRT; TherRad; Staff, B.C. Cancer Inst.; Att'd. Staff, Vancouver Gen. Hosp.; Clin. Instr. Dept. of Surg., U. of British Columbia; Tel. TR 4-9321.

COYLE, James H.; Qns'63; D.Psy; Res., Ontario Hosp., Toronto, Ont.

COYLE, John V.; 221 New Gower St., St. John's, Nfld., 7 Dover Pl. (res); Glasgow (Scot.) '43; Tel. 9-1570.

CRABB, Alfred M.; 88 Wentworth St. S., Hamilton, Ont.; 17 Fiddler's Green Rd., Ancaster (res); Wes '47; Ophth; Assoc. Staff, Hamilton Gen. St. Joseph's and Chedoke Gen. Hosp's.; Tel. 522-3563.

CRACK, Isaac E.; 970 King St. E., Hamilton, Ont.; McG '04; Coroner, Hamilton & Wentworth County.

CRADDOCK, Arthur B.; 722-23rd St. N., Lethbridge, Alta.; Edinburgh (Scot.)'59; Tel. 327-1071.

CRADDOCK, Shirley R.; 1605-15th St. S., Lethbridge, Alta.; Edinburgh (Scot.) '59; DA; Tel. 328-5749.

CRAFT, George; 355 Ellendale Med. Bldg., 5845 Cote-des-Neiges Rd., Montreal 26, P.Q.; 4869 Jean Brillant, Mtl. 26 (res); Mon '38; MCGP; Clin. Ass't. Jewish Gen. Hosp.; Tel. 735-0161.

CRAGG, Bruce E.; 2765 Sea View Rd., Victoria, B.C. (res); McG '43; F.A.C.A., Anaes; Tel. GR 7-1626.

CRAGG, C. Edward A.; The Peterborough Clinic, 327 Charlotte St., Peterborough, Ont.; 230 Geraldine Ave. (res); Qns '43; D.O.M.S. (Eng.); F.R.C.S. (Eng.); F.R.C.S.(C), Ophth; Staff, **Peterborough Civic & St. Joseph's Hosp's.; Tel. 742-3401.**

CRAGG, George E; 1146 Marine Dr., North Vancouver, B.C.; 1185-W. 26th St. (res); Qns '50; MCGP; Active Staff, Lions Gate Hosp.; Tel. YU 8-5291.

CRAIG, Barbara J.; Tor '63; Research Fell. (Ophth.), Canadian National Inst. for the Blind, Toronto, Ont.

CRAIG, Cecil R.; 2085 Tecumseh St. E., Windsor, Ont; 1551 Victoria Ave (res); Wes '49; MCGP; Tel. 252-8886.

CRAIG, G. Gardner; Assoc. Clinic, 4728 Ross St., Red Deer, Alta.; Alb '42.

CRAIG, David O.; 10 Gore St. W., Perth, Ont.; Aberdeen (Scot.) '46; D.Obst, RCOG; Tel. 267-3737.

CRAIG, C. B.; 2045 Dufferin St., Toronto 10, Ont.; Tor'65.

CRAIG, Gibson E.; 1414 Drummond St., Montreal, P.Q.; McG '43; DTM; DermSyph; Derm-in-Chief, Royal Victoria Hosp.; Cons., Royal Edward & Shriners Hosp's.; Assoc. Prof. (Med.), McGill U.; Tel. VI 9-3735.

CRAIG, J. David; Liverpool (Eng.)'57; MRCS; LRCP; Res., U. of Alberta Hosp., Edmonton, Alta.

CRAIG, John; 48 St. Claire Ave., Charlottetown, P.E.I. (res); Glasgow (Scot.)'47; MC(Path); Path., Charlottetown & P.E.I. Hosp's.; **Dir., Div.** of Labs., Dept. of Health; Dir., P.E.I. Cdn. Red Cross Blood Transfusion Serv.; Tel. 892-1277.

CRAIG, John M.; 206 Rideau Med. Bldg., 1711-4th St. S.W., Calgary, Alta.; 2317 Carlton St. (res); Aberdeen (Scot.) '50; MRCOG; FACOG; ObstGyn; Tel. AM 2-5006.

CRAIG, John S.; 206 Rideau Medical-Dental Centre, 1711-4th St. S.W., Calgary, Alta.; Glasgow (Scot.) '17; Tel. 262-5006.

CRAIG, Joseph; Liverpool (Eng.) '57; Staff, St. John's Gen. Hosp., St. John's, Nfld.; Tel. 8-0471.

CRAIG, Robert E.; McG '62; Jr. Intn., Royal Victoria Hosp., Montreal 2, P.Q.

CRAIG, Ronald T.; 33 Beaverbrook Ave., Saint John, N.B.; Dal'65; Tel. 687-3920.

CRAIG, Ross H.; 267 O'Connor St., Ottawa, Ont.; **50 Hutchison Ave., Ottawa 3, (res); Qns '52; GenSurg; Tel. 235-8466.**

CRAIG, William F.; 42 Northside Rd., Ottawa 6, Ont.; 39 Mowhawk Cr. (res); Ott '58; Tel. 828-9117.

CRAIGEN, Daniel; Glasgow (Scot.)'52; DPM (Lond.); Staff, Matsqui Inst., Abbotsford, B.C.

CRAIGIE, Andrew; Plaza Med. Office, Red Deer, Alta.; Glasgow (Scot.)'54; MB; ChB; Tel. 347-5300.

CRAM, Douglas M.; 231 Base Line Rd., London, Ont.; Wes '45; Paed; Clin. Ass't. Prof. (Paed.), U. of Western Ontario; Tel. 433-1781.

CRAM, E. John; Dept. of National Health & Welfare, 89 Canterbury St., Saint John, N.B.; McG '32; DPH; Med. Officer-In-Charge, Quarantine, Immigration Med., & Sick Mariner's Serv.

CRAM, Gordon A.; Ste. 203, 299 Main St., Chilliwack, B.C.; Tor'48; DABOG; FRCS(C), ObstGyn.

CRAM, Robert W.; 602 Medical Arts Bldg., Saskatoon, Sask.; Tor'43; F.R.C.S.(C), D.A.B.S., GenSurg; Dept. of Surg., University, Saskatoon City & St Paul's Hosp's.; Ass't. Prof. U. of Sask.; Tel. Area 306; 244-6818.

CRAMER, Joseph B.; Woodville, Ont.; Qns '28; MCGP.

CRAMER, Joseph E.; Box 488, High River, Alta.; Alb '58; Tel. 652-2682.

CRANDALL, R. Gordon; 12 Vista Dr., Lewisville, N.B.; Dal'56; MS; Psy; Med. Dir., Moncton Mental Health Clinic; Staff, Moncton Hosp.; Teach. Staff, U. of Moncton; Tel. 389-2987.

CRANE, H. Grahame; 111 York Mills Rd., Willowdale, Ont.; Sydney (Australia)'51; DPM (Eng.); Psy; Staff, Thistletown Hosp., Rexdale; Tel. 922-3443.

CRANE, K. P. Joan; (See COHEN, K. P. Joan).

CRANFIELD, Harold V.; 331 Sheddon Ave., Oakville, Ont.; Tor'34; PhysMed; Cons. Rehab., Oakville & Trafalgar, Mem. Hosp., Scarborough Gen. Hosp., Hosp. for Sick Children, Bloorview Home, Our Lady of Mercy, C.P. Workshop & Providence Villa Hosp's.; Adv. (Rehab.), Prov. Dept. of Welfare; Tel. VI 5-0724.

CRANG, Charles L.; 155 Kingsmount Blvd., Sudbury, Ont. (res); Tor '31; D.A.B. Roent., DiagRad; Staff (Rad.), St. Joseph's, Sudbury Gen., Sudbury Mem. and Copper Cliff Hosp's.; Tel. 054-3101.

CRANG, Donald F.; 155 Kingsmount Blvd., Sudbury, Ont.; Wes'53; DiagRad; DMR; Staff, Sudbury Gen. Hosp.; Tel. 673-3601.

CRANLEY, William J.; Ste. 118, 517-4th Ave, S., Lethbridge, Alta.; Nat. U. (Dublin, Ire.) '39; Staff, St. Michael's & Lethbridge Mun. Hosp's.; Tel. 327-7222.

CRANN, George R.; 603 Ludgate St., Peterborough, Ont. (res); Tor '07; Retired.

CRANSTON, Gerald P.; 3094 Danforth Ave., Scarborough, Ont.; Qns '54; Tel. 691-7710.

CRANSTON, James A.; Med. Arts Clinic, 51-6th St. S.E., Medicine Hat, Alta.; **165-8th St. N.E. (res); Wes '50; Staff, Medicine Hat Gen. Hosp.; Tel. 527-2281.**

CRANSTON, J. Robert; 39 Charlton St. E., Hamilton, Ont.; Qns'59; FRCS(C), Otol.; Court. Staff, St. Joseph's, Hamilton Gen., Chedoke & Joseph Brant Hosp's.

CRANSTON, Thomas R.; Calgary Assoc. Clinic, 214 - 6th Ave. S.W., Calgary, Alta.; 1923 - 10A St. S.W. (res); McG'53; MCGP; Tel. 263-7120.

CRANZ, Harro J. A.; 540 Tegler Bldg., Edmonton, Alta.; Freiburg (Germ.)'45; DiagRad.

CRAPNELL, Victor E.; Box 250, Picture Butte Med. Clinic, Picture Butte, Alta.; London (Eng.) '54; MRCS; LRCP; Staff, Picture Butte Municipal Hosp. & Lethbridge Auxiliary Hosp.; Anaes., Carmangay Hosp.; Tel. 732-4221.

CRAPPER, Donald R.; 58 Grenoble Dr., Apt. 48, Don Mills, Ont.; Tor'57; FRCP(C), Neur.

CRASSWELLER, Henry; 405 Med. Arts Bldg., **Windsor, Ont.; 2014 Willstead Cr. (res);** Tor '08; GenSurg; Chief of Staff, Grace Hosp.; Retired.

CRASSWELLER, Peter O.; 204 Toronto Western Med. Bldg., 25 Leonard Ave., Toronto 2B, Ont.; 281 Russell Hill Rd., Tor 7 (res); Tor '45; FACS; FRCS(C), GenSurg; Urol; Urol.-in-Chief, Tor. Western Hosp.; Cons., Queensway Gen. & Oakville-Trafalgar Hosp.; Prof. (Surg.), U. of Toronto; Tel. EM 4-9828.

CRAVEN, Austin J.; 63 Brant Ave., Brantford, **Ont.; Tor '28; GenSurg.; Dist. Coroner;** Tel. **752-2342.**

CRAW, Helen (See Mitchell)

CRAWFORD, Charles S.; Ste. 415, 6450 East Blvd., Vancouver 13, B.C. (res); Man '26; GenSurg; **Retired.**

CRAWFORD, Clarence M.; 4015 W. 20th Ave., Vancouver, B.C.; Qns '11; F.A.C.P.; Psy; Retired.

CRAWFORD, Derek C.; 311 Day St., Transcona, Man.; 606 Coldstream Ave. (res); Birmingham (Eng.)'58; Active Staff, St. Boniface & Concordia Hosp's.; Tel. 222-4259.

CRAWFORD, D. J. McGregor; 901 Helena St., Trail, B.C.; 209 Kootenay Ave. (res); Alb '27; IntMed; Staff (Med.), Trail Tadanac & Mater-Missericordia **Hosp's., Rossland; Dist. Coroner.**

CRAWFORD, Edwin M.; 43 Waverley Rd., Pointe-Claire, Lachine, P.Q.; Mon '26; F.A.C.R., F.F.R.; D & T Rad; Dir. Dept. of Rad., Queen Elizabeth Hosp.; Retired.

CRAWFORD, Elsie M. (Hoffman); Sudbury & Dist. Health Unit, Ste. 3, 50 Cedar St., Sudbury, Ont.; 110 Hyland Dr. (res); Tor '49; MCGP; **Clinic., Sud. & Dist. Health Unit; Tel. 674-0776.**

CRAWFORD, Erwin A.; 305 Finch Ave. W., Willowdale, Ont.; College of Med. Evangelists (Loma Linda, Calif.) '44; F.A.C.S., F.I.C.S., F.A.C.O.G.; ObstGyn; Chief of ObstGyn, Northwestern & North York Branson Hosp's.; Tel. **ME 5-0626.**

CRAWFORD, Glen M.; B.C. Cancer Inst., 2656 Heather St., Vancouver 9, B.C.; 4015 W. 20th Ave. (res); Wes'47; TherRad; DMRT; Staff, B.C. Cancer Inst. & Vancouver Gen. Hosp.; Clin. Instr., U. of B.C.; Tel. TR 4-9321.

CRAWFORD, James E.; Edson, Alta.; Alb '52; MCGP; Dist. Coroner; Tel. 723-3366.

CRAWFORD, James S.; 151 Marion St., Toronto, **Ont.; 28 Grenadier Heights (res); Tor '17; Tel.** LE 2-2902.

CRAWFORD, John N.; Dept. of Veteran's Affairs, Wellington St., Ottawa, Ont.; Man '30; Paed; Ass't. Deputy Minister (Treatment), DVA; Tel. 992-5679.

CRAWFORD, John S.; Room 119, 555 University Ave., Toronto 2, Ont.; Qns '39; DOMS (Eng.); ABO; Ophth; Chief, Dept. of Ophth., Hosp. for Sick Children; Ass't. Prof. (Ophth.), U. of Toronto; Tel. 366-7242, ext. 1621.

CRAWFORD, John S.; 70 Sir William's Lane, Islington, Ont. (res); Tor'44; FRCP(C); IntMed; PhysMed & Rehab; Dir. (PhysMed & Rehab.) & Att'd. Phys. Toronto Western Hosp.; Ass't. Dir., Phys. & Occupational Therapy, U. of Toronto; Ass't. Prof. Med., U. of Toronto; Chmn. Med. Advis. Bd., Toronto Rehab. Centre; Tel. 368-4335.

CRAWFORD, Lois D. (Wright); 620 King George's Way, West Vancouver, B.C.; Tor '49; Anaes; Vis. Staff (Assoc.), Lion's Gate, North Vancouver & St. Paul's Hosp.; Hon. Vis. Staff, Vanc. Gen. Hosp.; Tel. WA 2-2040.

CRAWFORD, Vinton A.; Tor'65; Res., Ottawa Civic Hosp., Ottawa 3, Ont.

CRAWFORD, Wallace A.; 194 E. King Edward Ave., Vancouver, B.C.; 553 W. 63rd Ave. (res); Alb '56; MCGP; Tel. TR 6-8414.

CRAWFORD, Wilfred A.; Patrick St., Wingham, Ont.; Tor '27; MCGP; Chief of Staff, Wingham Dist. Hosp.; Tel. 357-3800.

CRAWFORD, William J.; 3434 Lane Cresc., Lakeview, Calgary S.W., Alta.; Queen's (Belfast, N. Ire.)'50; Anaes.

CRAWFORD, William S.; 2621 - 10th Ave. A South, Lethbridge, Alta.; Dublin (Ire.)'54; DTM&H; BAO; MRCOG.

CRAWSHAW, E. Douglas; Edinburgh (Scot.)'62; Res., Royal Victoria Hosp., Montreal 2, P.Q.

CRAY, J. F.; 265 Woolwich St., Guelph, Ont.; Tor '26.

CRAYMER, William J.; 44 Kimberley Ave., Bracebridge, Ont.; McG '54; MCGP; Staff, South Muskoka Mem. Hosp., & Orillia Soldier's Hosp.; Tel. 645-2281.

CRAYTHORNE, Norman W.; 30 Sheraton Dr., Montreal West, P.Q. (res); **Queen's U. (Belfast, Ire.) '54; Anaes; Staff, Montreal Neurol. Inst.; Tel. VI 2-1251.**

CREAGHAN, Mark; Box 269, 396 Water St., Newcastle, N.B. (res); Tor'51; GenSurg; Tel. 622-1110.

CREAMER, Alice M.; Dublin (Ire.) '42; Psy; Staff, Riverview Hosp., Essondale, B.C.

CREAMER, Thomas L.; 115 Hazen St., Saint John, N.B.; 117 Harbary Terr., Lancaster (res); Ott '52; ObstGyn; Active Staff, Saint John Gen. & St. Joseph's Hosp's.; Tel. 693-1574.

CREASE, Arthur L.; Ocean Park Rd., White Rock, B.C.; McG '10; **Psy; Retired.**

CREASY, Gerald J.; Box 9600, Selkirk, Man.; Man '30; M.O.H.; Coroner.

CREE, Ian C.; Dept. of Surg., New York Med. College, Flower & Fifth Ave. Hosp's., New York, N.Y., U.S.A.; London (Eng.)'54; MS; MRCS; LRCP; FRCS(Eng.); FRCS(C), GenSurg.; Assoc. Prof. (Surg.), New York Med. College; Abroad.

CREIGHTON, Austin M.; Tatamagouche, N.S.; Dal '45; M.C.G.P.

CREIGHTON, Howard A.; Box 520, 120 Pelham St., Lunenburg, N.S.; **70 Cumberland St. (res);** Dal '24; GenSurg; **Vis. Staff, Fishermen's Mem.** Hosp.; Tel. 634-8866.

CREIGHTON, John O.; 107 Elizabeth St. W., Welland, Ont.; 225 Aqueduct St. (res); London (Eng.) '36; MRCS, LRCP; MCGP; **Staff Welland Co. & Pt. Colborne Gen. Hosp's.; Tel. RE 5-5005.**

CREIGHTON, Robert E.; Tor '59; FRCP(C), Anaes; Staff, Hosp. for Sick Children, Toronto, Ont.; Tel. EM 6-7242. Abroad.
CREIGHTON, Robert J.; Box 160, Clifford, Ont.; Tor '57; Tel. 88.
CREIGHTON, William; 195 Waverley St., Winnipeg 9, Man.; Man'08; Retired.
CRENNELL, E. H.; Centre Bldg., St. John's, Nfld.; Ire '55.
CREPEAU, C. Andre; 761 Stuart Ave., Outremont, Montreal 8, P.Q.; Lille (France)'59; Anaes.
CREPEAU, G. Andre; 259 King Edward, Ottawa 2, Ont.; 2212 Carnegie St. (res); Lav '55; FRCS(C); ThorSurg; (Cardiovasc) OrthSurg (P.Q.); Staff, Ottawa Gen. Hosp.; Cons. Staff (ThorSurg., Cardiovasc) Montford Hosp., Eastview & Sacre-Coeur Hosp's., Hull; Lect. (Cardio-Thoracic Surg.) U. of Ottawa; Tel. 236-4344.
CREPEAU, Jacques; 825 sud, Belvedere, Sherbrooke, P.Q.; Lav '54; FRCP(C), IntMed; Cardiol (P.Q.): Staff (Med. & Cardiol.), Hotel-Dieu Hosp.; Tel. 569-5078.
CREPEAU, Maurice; 541 rue de l'Hopital, Jonquiere, P.Q.; 80 Maisonneuve (res); Lav '53; F.R.C.S.(C). OrthSurg.; Tel. 547-9341.
CREPIN, Gilles; 2259 Royale, Quebec 5, P.Q.; Lav'61; Paed.
CRETE, Charles; C.P. 786, 332 St. Joseph, La Tuque, P.Q.; 505 St. Joseph (res); Lav '49; Dist. Coroner; Tel. LA 3-2566.
CREURER, Maurice; Med. Clin., C.N.R. Tower, Edmonton, Alta.; Lav'58; MCGP.
CREVIER, Paul H.; Centre-Medical-St-Urbain, 3875 St.-Urbain, Montreal 18, P.Q.; 436 rue Melbourne Mon. 16 (res); Mon '47; FRCS(C), NeurSurg; Ass't. NeurSurg., Hotel-Dieu-de-Mtl.; Chief of NeurSurg. Dept., Hop.-St.-Jean-de-Dieu; Cons. NeurSurg., Hop.-Ste-Jeanne- d'Arc & Notre-Dame-de-l'Esperance; Tel. CL 4-5361.
CREWSON, Arthur L.; 132 Second St. W., Cornwall. Ont.; 136 Second St. E. (res); McG '23; OphthOtol; Staff, Hotel Dieu & Cornwall Gen. Hosp's.; Tel. WE 2-3232.
CREWSON, Walter L.; 5 Young St., Hamilton, Ont.; 310 North Shore Blvd. W. Burlington (res); McG'21; Ophth; Retired.
CRICHTON, Erica P.; Provincial Lab. of Public Health, Calgary, Alta.; Glasgow (Scot.)'48; Path; Bact. & Assoc. Pathol.; Tel. 288-2604.
CRICHTON, John U.; Department of Paed., University of British Columbia, Vancouver, B.C.; Edinburgh (Scot.)'44; MRCP(E); DCH(Lond.); Paed.
CRIDLAND, Joyce; (See BOILLAT, Joyce E.L.).
CRIMP, Leonard H.; Moose Jaw Clinic, 200 Scott Blk., Moose Jaw, Sask.; 1072-5th N.W. (res); Tor '46; FRCS(C), Urol; Staff, Moose Jaw Union & Providence Hosp's.; Tel. 692-2373.
CRISP, Allan G.; Ste. 609, 99 Avenue Rd., Toronto 5, Ont.; 1 Clarenden Ave., Apt. 502 (res); Tor '34; DPM (Lond.); NeurPsy; Cons. (Neur. & Psy.) Sunnybrook Hosp.; Tel. WA 1-8801.
CRISPIN, Edward J.; 137 Norfolk St., Guelph, Ont.; 17 Wolfond Cr. (res); Wes '55; Pres. (Med. Staff), Guelph Gen. Hosp.; Tel. TA 2-4423.
CRISPIN, John S.; Man'55; 37 Tod Drive, Winnipeg, Man.; Man'55; FRCS(C), GenSurg.
CRISWICK, Valentine G.; Sask '63; Res., Dept. of Ophth., Vancouver Gen. Hosp., Vancouver 9, B.C.
CRITCHLEY, James D.; 5122 Cordova Bay Rd., Victoria, B.C.; 4474 Saanich Rd.; London (Eng.)'57; Tel. 658-5414 & 479-4931.
CROAL, Albert E.; 26 Belhome Ave., Brantford, Ont. (res); Tor '56; Path; Assoc. Pathol., Brantford Gen. Hosp.; Tel. 752-7871.
CROCKER, Audrey N.; (Mrs. Bishop) Ste 1, 2221 Keele St.,, Toronto 15, Ont. 99-9th St., **Tor 14 (res); Tor '52; DRCOG; Active Staff** North-western Gen. & Court. Staff, Humber Mem. Hosp's.; Tel. CH 9-3787.
CROCKER, Keith M.; 456 Med. Arts Bldg., Saskatoon, Sask.; 510 Garrisson Cr. (res); McG '48; DRCOG; MRCOG; ObstGyn; Ass't. Prof. (ObstGyn.), U. of Sask.; Tel. 242-2429.
CROCKFORD, Peter M.; Alb '59; FRCP(C), Int-Med. Staff, University Hosp., Edmonton, Alta.; Tel. 439-5911.
CROFT, John H.; 6913 Livingstone Dr., Calgary, Alta.; Birmingham (Eng.)'56; DA(Eng.); Anaes; Med. Staff, Holy Cross & Alberta Children's Hosp's.
CROFTON, Francis D.; 323 E. Columbia St., New Westminster, B.C.; McG '43; DiagRad.; Tel. FA 5-3244.
CROISETIERE, Fernand; 176 St. Joseph's Blvd. E., Montreal 14, P.Q.; Mon '42; OphthOtol **(P.Q.) Ass't. (Ophth.), Hop. Ste Justine; Tel. RE 1-4931.**
CROLL, L. Duncan; 216 Doctors Bldg., 394 Graham Ave., Winnipeg 1, Man.; 93 Harrow St. (res); McG '27; F.A.C.S.; OrthSurg; Cons. (Orth), Municipal Hosp.; Active Staff (OrthSurg), Misericordia Gen. Hosp.; Court. Staff, (OrthSurg), Winnipeg Gen. & Grace Hosp's.; Tel. WH 2-6325.
CROMARTY, Raymond; 35 Swordhill Dr., Islington, Ont. (res); McG'53; Path; Dir. Path. Labs., Humber Mem. Hosp.; Tel. 249-8111.
CROMARTY, Robert P., ED; The Bigelow Clinic, 41 Clement Bl., Brandon, Man.; 119-19th St. (res); Tor '18; M.Sc., FRCS(C), GenSurg; Surg. Staff, Brandon Gen. Hosp.; Cons. (Urol.), Manitoba Mental Hosp. & Assiniboine Hosp.; Tel. PA 9-1469.
CROMBY, James W.; 605 Mc Cowan Ave., Scarborough, Ont.; Durham (Eng.)'56; Tel. 267-3772.
CROMPTON, Charles P.; 71 Valecrest Dr., Islington, Ont. (res); Tor '51; Anaes; Staff (Anaes), Toronto Western Hosp.; Clin. Ass't., U. of Toronto; **Tel. 368-2581.**
CROMPTON, Charles R. B.; 49 Glen Elm Ave., Toronto 5, Ont.; Tor '15; M.S. (Minn.); F.R.-**C.S. (C). Urol; Tel. WA 5-1222.**
CRONHELM, Claude H.; 750 W. Broadway, Vancouver, B.C.; Queen's U. (Belfast, Ire.) '57; FRCS(C), ObstGyn; Att'd. Staff, Vancouver Gen. Hosp.; Tel. TR 2-5484.
CRONIN, Robert F. P.; 1650 Cedar Ave., Montreal 25, P.Q.; 762 Lansdowne Ave. (res); McG '53; M.Sc.; MRCP (Lond.); FRCP(C); IntMed (Cardiol); Assoc. Phys., Montreal Gen. Hosp.; Cons. (Cardiol.) DVA; Ass't. Prof. (Med. & Physiol.) McGill U.; Tel. WE 7-6011, Loc. 686.
CRONK, George S.; 216 MacDonald Ave., Belleville, Ont.; 220 MacDonald Ave. (res); Qns '15; GenSurg; Surg. Staff, Belleville Gen. Hosp.; Cons., Trenton Mem. Hosp.; District Coroner; **Tel. WO 2-1515.**
CRONK, L. Bruce; 216 MacDonald Ave., Belleville, Ont.; 221 MacDonald Ave. (res); Qns '46; F.R.C.P.(C), IntMed; Active & Cons. Staff, Belleville Gen. Hosp.; Cons., Trenton Memorial Hosp., Prince Edward County & Campbellford Memorial Hosp.; Lect., (Med.), Queen's U.; Tel. WO 2-4210.
CROOK, Alfred F.; 1527 Kilborn Ave., Ottawa, **Ont. (res); Queens U. (Belfast N. Ire.) '39;** D.M.R.T. (Lond.), F.R.C.S. (Edin.); TherRad; Cons., Ontario Cancer Fdn.; Ottawa Civic & Ottawa Gen. Hosp's.; Lect. (TherRad), Ottawa U.; **Tel. RE 3-4662.**
CROOK, Raymond A.; 330 Medical Dental Bldg., Regina, Sask.; 9 Newlands St., (res); London (Eng.) '49; L.R.C.P., M.R.C.S. (Eng.), D.L.O. (Eng); Otol; Med. Staff, Regina Gen. & Grey Nuns' Hosp's.; Tel. 527-8561.
CROOKS, H. James; 10951-124th St., Edmonton, Alta.; 9134-118th St. (res); Alb'54; DABOG; FACOG; ObstGyn; Active Staff, Royal Alexandra Hosp.; Clin. Instr., ObstGyn., U. of Alberta; Tel. GL 4-4551.
CROOKS, William L.; 214-6th Ave. S.W., Calgary, Alta.; Alb '57; OrthSurg; Staff, Holy Cross, Alberta Children's, Foothills, Calgary Gen. & Auxiliary Hosp's.; Cons., Cerebral Palsy Clinic; Tel. 263-7120.
CROOKSTON, John H.; 246 Russell Hill Rd., Toronto 7, Ont.; Tor '47; Ph.D. (Cantab.); Hd., Div. of Haem. & Blood Transfusion, Toronto Gen. Hosp.; Phys., Toronto Gen. Hosp.; Lect., Dept. of Path., & Ass't. Prof. (Med.), U. of Toronto; Tel. EM 6-8211.
CROOME, Robert R.; 24 Grasspoint Cres., Markland Woods, Etobicoke, Ont. (res); Tor '43; GenSurg; Staff, Sunnybrook Hosp.; Tel. 485-8651.

CROSBIE, Jack C.; 84 Lincoln Rd., Grand Falls, Nfld.; Dal '57; Paed; Chief of Staff, Central Nfld. Hosp.; Tel. 4844.
CROSBIE, Pierce D.; 005 Ridean Med. Dent. Centre, 1711-4th St. S.W., Calgary, Alta.; Dublin (Ire.)'41; MRCS; LRCP.
CROSBY, Adam B.; 203 Med. Arts Bldg., 5880 Spring Garden Rd., Halifax, N.S.; 12 Inglewood Dr. (res); Dal '42.
CROSBY, Clayton H.; Medical Arts Clinic, 2125-11th Ave., Regina, Sask.; McG '37; FACS, FRCS (C), GenSurg; ThorSurg; Chief of Surg., Regina Gen. Hosp.; Sr. Surg., Regina Grey Nun's Hosp.; Cons. Surg., University Hosp.; Clin. Assoc. Surg., U. of Saskatchewan; Tel. 523-0691.
CROSBY, David R.; Wes '63; Staff, Bella Coola **Gen. Hosp., Bella Coola, B.C.**
CROSBY, Joan M.; 6156 Quinpool Rd., Halifax, N.S.; Dal '51; Paed; Active Staff, Halifax Children's, Grace Maternity & Halifax Infirmary; Lect. (Paed.), Dalhousie U.; Tel. 422-5943.
CROSKERY, W. Howard, A/Col; Tor '43; IntMed; Staff, Toronto Military Hosp., Toronto 12, Ont.
CROSS, Carleton E.; 311 Frontenac St., Sherbrooke, P.Q.; McG '09; F.R.C.S. (Edin.), F.R.C.S.(C), GenSurg; Retired.
CROSS, Dezso F.; 137 Wellington St., Sarnia, Ont.; 233 North Brock St. (res); Budapest (Hungary) '25; Paed; Staff (Paed.), St. Joseph's & Sarnia Gen. Hosp's.; Tel. DI 4-5261.
CROSS, Edgar G.; Ste. 3, Toronto East Gen. **Hosp., Toronto 6, Ont.; Medalist Rd., Willowdale (res); Tor '48; F.R.C.P.(C), IntMed; Att'd. Phys., Toronto E. Gen. & Sunnybrook Hosp's.; Tel. 461-8685.**
CROSS, Hector C.; 2 Rex Gate, Rexdale, Ont.; Glasgow (Scot.) '51; IntMed; Tel. CH 4-0431.
CROSS, John M.; Quill Lake, Sask.; Alb'62.
CROSS, John P.; 1343 Kilborn, Ottawa, Ont.; **McG '52; Tel. 733-7965.**
CROSS, John S.; 31 Sweetland Ave., Ottawa, Ont.; McG. '19; Cons. Staff, Ottawa Gen Hosp.; "B" Staff, Ottawa Civic Hosp.; Courtesy Staff, Grace & St. Louis Marie de Montford Hosp's; Dist. Coroner; Tel. 233-8725.
CROSS, Katherine Batanoff; P.G. Pub. Health, U. of T., Toronto, Ont.; Tor '49.
CROSS, William D. S.; Tor '20; Psy; Ass't. Hosp. Supt., Westminster Hosp., London, Ont.; Retired.
CROSS, William H.; 4 Humber Ridge, Toronto 18, Ont.; Wes '49; DPH; Hd. Diagnostic Serv., Dept. of Health, Queen's Park; Tel. 365-2404.
CROSS, W. W.; Dept. of Pub. Health, Edmonton, **Alta.; 10939—86th Ave. (res); Dist. Coroner;** Retired.
CROSSFIELD, Paul O.; 203 Medical Centre, Calgary, Alta.; 2201—7th St. S.W. (res); Royal U. of Malta '47; D.C.H. (Eng.), M.R.C.P. (Ed.), F.A.C.P.; IntMed; Cons. Staff, Holy Cross Hosp. & Calgary Gen. Hosp's., Phys., Prov. Dept. Child **Welfare; Tel. AM 3-3320.**
CROSSLAND, Alfred M.; 201 Simcoe Med. Group, 121 Wellington W., Barrie, Ont.; Tor '40; FRCS (C); GenSurg; Active Staff, Royal Victoria Hosp.; Tel. PA 8-2476.
CROSSLEY, Harry; 11 Dunlop Bl., Yorkton, Sask.; 225-5th Ave. S. (res); Man '51; MCGP; Tel. 783-2279.
CROSSLEY, Stanley G.; Radway, Alta.; Alb'62; Tel. 27.
CROSSON, Ernest W.; 20 Fielding Ave., Kentville, N.S. (res); Dal '57; Staff, Nova Scotia San.
CROTEAU, J. Rene; 2539 Belanger E., Montreal 36, P.Q.; Lav '57; Tel. 727-1500.
CROTEAU, Laurent; C. P. 401, Grand'Mere, P.Q.; Lav '50.
CROTIN, Abraham M.; Apt. 5, 31 Meadowbrook, Toronto, Ont.; Tor'59; Otol.
CROWE, Francis; 84 Dieppe Ave., Riverside, Windsor, Ont.; London (Eng.)'60; D.Obst. RCOG; DA; Tel. 948-1147.
CROWE, J. Bruce; New Germany, N.S.; Dal '43; Vis. Staff Dawson Mem. Hosp., Bridgewater.
CROWE, L. L.; 181 McIntyre W., North Bay, Ont.; 753 McLaren St. (res); Tor '23; M.C.G.P.; **MOH, City of North Bay; Dist. Surg., CPR; Tel. 472-3660.**
CROWE, Wilfred R.; 228 Kent St. W., Lindsay, Ont.; Qns '22; Dist. Coroner; Staff, Ross Mem. Hosp.; Tel. 324-5352.
CROWELL, Douglas E.; 47 Thicket Rd., Etobicoke, Ont.; McG'57; FRCP(C); Anaes; Staff, St. Joseph's Hosp., Toronto 3, Ont.; Tel. LE 4-9531, Loc. 601.
CROWLEY, Patrick C.; 35 Frank St., Strathroy, Ont.; Wes '53; GenSurg.; Tel. 245-2960.
CROWSON, Charles N.; 507-8 Boyd Bldg., 388 Portage Ave., Winnipeg 1, Man.; 143 Kane Ave. St. James (res); McG '49; Ph.D.; Path (Edin.); Path; Dir. of Labs., Misericordia Hosp.; Ass't. Prof. (Path.), U. of Manitoba; Tel. WH 2-1710.
CROWTHER, T. Albert; 1004 Med. Arts Bldg., Toronto 5, Ont.; Tor'27; IntMed; Cons. Med., **Tor. Gen. Hosp.; Assoc. Prof. (Med.), U. of** Toronto; Tel. 923-3221.
CROZIER, Douglas N.; 1849 Yonge St., Toronto **7, Ont.; 81 Hudson Dr. (res); Tor '52; Paed;** Med. Supv., Bloorview Hosp., Home & School; Paed., Ont. Crippled Children's Hosp.; Dir., Cystic Fibrosis Clinic, Hosp. for Sick Children; Clin. Teach., U. of Toronto; Tel. HU 3-3105.
CROZIER, I. M.; Avery Clinic, 644 Front, Quesnel, B.C.; Tor'64; Abroad.
CROZIER, P. Grant; 2005 Amiens Ave., Wind**sor, Ont.; Wes '47; Full-time Indus. Phys., Chrysler Canada Ltd.; Tel. 252-3651.**
CRUESS, Richard L.; 526 Mount Pleasant Ave., Montreal 6, P.Q.; Columbia (N.Y., U.S.A.)'55; FRCS(C), OrthSurg; Staff, Royal Victoria Hosp.; Ass't. Surg., Mtl. Shriner's Hosp.; Ass't. Prof. (OrthSurg.), McGill U.
CRUICKSHANK, Donald A.; 2160 Weston Rd., Weston, Ont.; 20 Palace Arch Dr., Islington (res); **Tor '51; Active Staff, Humber Mem. Hosp.; Tel.** CH 4-5566.
CRUICKSHANK, Frederick D.; 2160 Weston Rd., Weston, Ont.; Tor '22; **Staff Phys., Humber Mem. & Toronto Western Hosp's.; Tel. CH 4-5566.**
CRUIKSHANK, George H.; Lyndock St., Corunna, Ont.; Wes '50; MCGP; Tel. 862-1155.
CRUICKSHANK, James W.; Simcoe St., Angus Ont. (res); Dal '56.
CRUICKSHANK, Jane E.; 2160 Weston Rd., Weston, Ont.; 1061 Main St. N. (res); Tor '54; Tel. CH 4-5566.
CRUICKSHANK, Lionel F. G.; 320 Dromore Ave., Winnipeg 9, **Man. (res); Edinburgh (Scot.) '45; D.A.R.C.S.(E), F.F.A.R.C.S. (E), Anaes.; Hon. Anaes., Winnipeg Gen. Hosp.; Lect.** (Anaes.), U. of Manitoba; Tel. GL 3-7022.
CRUICKSHANK, W. Harvey; 1050 Beaver Hall Hill, Montreal, P.Q.; Tor '36; D.Psy; DPH; PH; Vice-Pres. (PR), Bell Telephone Co. Canada; **Tel. 870-1511.**
CRUISE, John T.; 818 Douglas St., **Victoria, B.C.; 1520 Regents (res); Man '31; Ophth; Tel. EV 3-8312**
CRUMMEY, Arthur S.; 607 Medical Arts Bldg., 180 Metcalfe St., Ottawa, Ont.; Qns'54; Otol; Att'd. Staff, Ottawa Civic Hosp.; Tel. 232-0626.
CRUMMEY, Clarence B.; 98 Guestville Ave., Toronto 9, Ont.; Dal '32; MCGP; Active Staff, Humber Mem. Hosp.; Tel. RO 3-1171.
CRUSE, Peter J. E.; 404 Rideau Medical Centre, **1711-4th St. S.W., Calgary, Alta.; 856 Hillcrest Ave. (res); Capetown (S. Africa) '51; FRCS** (Edin.); FRCS(C), GenSurg; GenSurg., Colonel Belcher DVA, Holy Cross & Foothills Hosp's.; Tel. 262-4923.
CRUST, Joseph H.; 1088 Pembina Hwy., Fort Garry, Winnipeg 19, Man.; 560 South Dr., Wpg. 19 (res); Man '51; MCGP; Dem. (Anat.), U. of Manitoba; Tel. 453-3303.
CRUX, Norman W.; Rabbit Lake, Sask. Alb '43.
CRUZ, Amelia M.; Ste. 805, 64 Pepperrell, St. John's, Nfld.; Philippines'54; Staff, St. John's Gen. Hosp.
CRUZ, Arturo A.; Medical Bldg., West St., Cor**ner Brook, Nfld.; Santo Tomas (Philipp.) '54.**

CRYDERMAN, Wilbur J.; 106 Toronto Western Medical Bldg., 25 **Leonard** Ave., Toronto **2B,** Ont.; 292 The Kingsway, **Islington, Ont. (res);** Tor '21; F.F.R. (Lond), **DiagRad; Cons. Rad.,** Toronto Western Hosp. & Hosp. for **Consumptives,** Weston; Retired.

CRYSDALE, W. S.; Tor'64; Res., Sunnybrook Hosp., Toronto 12, Ont.

CRYSLER, W. Elgin; 145 Dufferin Ave., Brantford, Ont.; Wes '38; D. Rad; DABR; FACR; D & T Rad; Phys-I/C Dept. of Rad., Brantford Gen. Hosp.; Staff, Willet Hosp., **Paris & Lady Willingdon Hosp., Ohsweken;** Tel. 752-7871.

CRYSTAL, Harvey; Tor '60; Jr. Int'n., Toronto Gen. Hosp., Toronto 2, Ont.

CSEREPES, Alexander O.; McG'55; GenSurg; Staff, Shaughnessy Hosp., Vancouver 9, B.C.

CSEREPKA, Margaret I.; 350 Bellamy Rd., Scarborough, Ont.; Tel. 266-2509.

CSERHALMI, Elmer D.; 2 Park Ave., Elmira, Ont.; Budapest (Hung.) '51; Staff (Surg.), Kitchener-Waterloo & St. Mary's Hosp's.; Tel. 668-5471.

CSOKA, Alice; 115 Queen St., St. Catharines, Ont.; Debrecen (Hung.) '44; Staff, Lincon Health Unit.

CSONT, Eva; — See DEKANY Eva.

CSONT, Lewis; 13 McDougal, Ottawa, Ont. (res); **Budapest (Hung.) '51.**

CUBBAGE, John S.; Box 130, Cumberland, B.C.; UBC '59; Active Staff, **Cumberland Gen. Hosp.;** Court. Staff, **St. Joseph's Hosp., Comox.**

CUDDY, Frederick A. B.; 201 Byron St. S., Whitby, Ont.; Tor '30; **Dist. Coroner.**

CUDDY, Thomas E.; 969 Sherburn St., **Winnipeg 3, Man. (res); Man '54; FRCP(C); IntMed (Car**diol; Ass't Dir., Cardio-Respiratory Unit. & Dir., Electrocardiograph Dept., Winnipeg Gen. Hosp.; Ass't Prof. (Med.), U. of Manitoba; Tel. SP 4-6511, Local 234.

CUDKOWICZ, Leon; 5849 University Ave., Halifax, N.S.; London (Eng.)'46; MRCP (Lond.); **FACP; Ass't. Phys., Victoria Gen. Hosp., Halifax; Dir. Cardio-Pulm. Lab.** & Assoc. Prof. **Med. & Physiol,** Dalhousie U.; Tel. 423-7483.

CUDMORE, Douglas W.; Dal'62; FRCS(C), ObstGyn; ObstGyn., Victoria Gen. & Grace Maternity Hosp's., Halifax, N.S.

CUDMORE, D. Paul; 660 South St., Halifax, N.S.; Dal '59; MCGP; Dir., Student Health Serv. & Ass't. Dir., P.G. Div., Dalhousie U.; Tel. 429-1420, Ext. 261; Abroad.

CUILLERIER, Jean F.; 235, des Cedres, Dorion, Cte. Vaudreuil, P.Q.; Mon '48.

CULL, James S.; 4829 Blenheim St., Van. 8 (res); Tor '31; DPH; PH; Dir., Metropolitan Health Unit, No. 1; Tel. MU 4-2377.

CULLEN, Edwin S.; Manning, Alta.; Edinburgh (Scot.) '57.

CULLEN, Frank R., Col.; 14 Grosvenor Ave., Rockingham, N.S. (res); Tor '50; Anaes; Chief-of-Anaes., Cdn. Forces Hosp., Halifax; Tel. 423-1161, Ext. 369.

CULLEN, Gerald C. R.; Dal'63; Res., Dept. of Ophth., University of British Columbia, Vancouver, B.C.

CULLEN, James B.; Tor'63; Res., Toronto Western Hosp., Toronto 2B, Ont.

CULLEN, Phillip J.; 703 Robinson Dr., Sudbury, Ont. (res); Tor '52; DiagRad; Staff, Sudbury Mem. Hosp.; Tel. 4-4903.

CULLEN, William G.; 2121 Northcliffe Ave., **Montreal 28, P.Q.; 226 Ballantyne Ave. N.** (res); **Tor '32; DABA, FACS, FFARCS(Eng.); Anaes; Anaes-in-Chief, Queen Elizabeth Hosp.; Ass't. Prof. (Anaes), McGill U.; Tel. 484-3221.**

CULLIGAN, John D.; 6 Aldershot Blvd., Winnipeg 29, Man.; Dublin (Ire.)'48; FACA; Anaes; Active Staff, St. Boniface & Winnipeg Children's Hosp's.; Dem. (Anaes.), Dept. of Surg., U. of Man.; Tel. SU 3-7271.

CULLIMORE, Dora (Polynchuck); 1415 Victoria Ave., Niagara **Falls,** Ont.; 408 Sarah **Ave.,** Chippewa (res); Tor '43; F.A.A.P.; **Paed.**

CULLINAN, Louis V.; Ste. B-4, 440 **Hinton Ave., Ottawa 3, Ont.; 1975 Bel-Air Dr., Ottawa 5 (res); Dal '54; Anaes., Ottawa Civic Hosp.; Tel. 722-3027.**

CULLITON, Elsie I. (Barr); 31 James St., Parry Sound, Ont.; Man'51; B.Sc.

CULNAN, George F.; 1576 Weston Rd., Weston, Ont.; 90 Dunvegan Rd., **Toronto (res); Tor '48;** F.R.C.S.(C), F.I.C.S., **GenSurg.; Tel. CH 1-2441.**

CULP, Edward M.; 840 Glenwood Crt., Oshawa, Ont.; Tor'54; Med. Staff & Sec. Treas., Oshawa Gen. Hosp.; Tel. 728-3694.

CULVER, Ronald L.; 8941-82nd Ave., Edmonton, Alta.; Alb'65.

CULVER, Roy W.; 205 Med. Arts Bldg., Calgary, Alta.; 3010-8th St. S.W., (res); Tor '31; Ophth, Otol; Staff, Holy Cross, Calgary Gen. & Alberta Children's Hosp.'s.; Tel. 269-4883.

CULVERHOUSE, John K. H.; Box 225, Burlington, Ont.; 3052 New St. (res); London (Eng.) '52; Anaes.; Chief of Anaes., Joseph Brant Hosp.; Tel. NE 7-6298.

CUMBERLAND, June R.; 2300 Tupper St., Montreal 25, **P.Q.; 3600 Ridgewood Ave. Apt. 401** (res); **McG '55; Psy; Dir., Day Treatment** Centre, Montreal Children's Hosp.; Lect., McGill **U.; Tel. WE 7-8511, Loc. 401.**

CUMMING, George A.; 156 St. Paul Cr., St. Catharines, Ont.; Manchester (Eng.) '59; M.B., Ch.B.; Tel. 684-8507.

CUMMING, Gordon R.; 440 Cordova St., Winnipeg 9, Man. (res); Man '53; B.Sc. (Med.), **FRCP(C), FACC; IntMed. (Cardiol.); Cardiol. & Dir. Cardiac Lab., Wpg. Children's Hosp.; Att'd-**Phys., Wpg. Gen. Hosp.; **Lect. (Med.), U. of** Manitoba; Tel. SP 5-8311.

CUMMING, Harold W.; 104 Johnson St., Kingston, Ont.; 309 Union St. W. (res); Qns '51; MCGP; Assoc. Staff, Kingston Gen. & Hotel Dieu Hosp's.; Preceptor Dept. of Preventive Med., Queen's U.; Tel. 542-1988.

CUMMING, James D. A.; Parsons Clinic, Red Deer, Alta.; 5055-45th Ave. (res); Alb '51; MCGP; Staff, Red Deer Mun. Hosp.; Tel. 346-3321.

CUMMING, James F.; 304 Birks Bldg., Saskatoon, Sask.; 1018 Victoria Ave. (res); Tor '47; Staff, Saskatoon City, **St. Paul's Hosp's.**

CUMMING, Roger A., Fl/Lt; Alb'63; National Defence Med. Centre, Ottawa 8, Ont.

CUMMING, Ronald K.; 22 Lynwood Ave., Ottawa, Ont.; McG '45; F.I.C.A., Anaes; Anaes., Ottawa Civic Hosp.; Tel. PA 9-2511.

CUMMING, Wilfred S.; Alb '64; Sr. Int., Edmonton Gen. Hosp., Edmonton, Alta.

CUMMING, Wilfred T.; Three Hills, Alta.; Edinburgh (Scot.) '35; FRCS (Edin.); Staff, Three Hills Mun. Hosp.; Tel. 443-5244.

CUMMING, William A.; Tor'58; Staff, Toronto Western Hosp., Toronto 2B, Ont.; Tel. 368-2581.

CUMMINGS, E. Arthur; 192 Bayview Heights Dr., Toronto 17, Ont.; Tor '28; Anaes; Staff, Toronto East Gen. Hosp.

CUMMINGS, Ina E.; McG '64; Res., Montreal Gen. Hosp., Montreal 25, P.Q.

CUMMINGS, Robert H.; 300 King St. W., Oshawa, Ont.; Ott '59; IntMed.

CUNDY, Richard R.; Box 760, **Salmon Arm, B.C.; London (Eng.) '54; L.R.C.P., M.R.C.S.;** Staff, Salmon Arm Gen. Hosp. & Shuswap Lake Gen. Hosp.; Tel. 832-2051.

CUNNING, Clive L.; 812 Medical & Dental Bldg., Regina, **Sask.; Ste. 24, Chateau Apts. (res);** UBC '56; Tel. 536-2202.

CUNNINGHAM, A. Ian; 23 Centre St., St. Catharines, Ont.; Tor'23; DPH; DTM&H; MOH, St. Catharines & Lincoln Health Unit.

CUNNINGHAM, Allister L.; Workmen's Comp. Bd., Sydney, N.S.; McG'38; Tel. 564-6426.

CUNNINGHAM, Augustine; 5899B Arbutus St., Powell River, B.C.; 7147 Huntingdon St. (res); Liverpool (Eng.)'49; DTM & H; DPA; PH; Dir., Powell River Health Unit.

CUNNINGHAM, Edison; 1215 W. 13th Ave., Vancouver, B.C. (res); Man '21; F.A.C.S., **F.I.C.S.; D.O.M.S. (Eng.), Ophth, Otol; Retired.**

CUNNINGHAM, Ernest K.; Box 340, 72 Villard Ave., Carman, Man.; 157 Villard (res); McG'27; **MCGP; Tel. SH 5-3509**

CUNNINGHAM, Gladys (Story); 1215 W. 13th Ave., Vancouver, B.C. (res); **Man '23; F.R.C.O.G.** (Lond.), F.I.C.S.; ObstGyn; **Retired.**

CUNNINGHAM, Helen M.; 71 Johnstone Ave., Dartmouth, N.S.; Tor'47.
CUNNINGHAM, H. Patrick; Lynden, Ont.; McG '61; GP Staff, Brantford Gen. & St. Joseph's Hosp's., Brantford & Willett Mem. Hosp., Paris; Tel. 647-3422.
CUNNINGHAM, J. I.; Department of National Health & Welfare, c/o Regional Superintendent, European Region. Abroad.
CUNNINGHAM, James B.; Bengough Sask.; Durham (Eng.) '60; Staff Bengough Union Hosp.; Tel. 18.
CUNNINGHAM, Janet B.; Bengough, Sask.; Glasgow (Scot.) '26.
CUNNINGHAM, J. Nelson; 410 Toronto Western Med. Bldg., 25 Leonard Ave., Toronto 2B, Ont.; 12 Blythwood Cres. (res); Tor '42; IntMed; Dir. O.P.D., Toronto Western Hosp.; Clin. Teach. (Med.), U. of Toronto; Tel. 363-**9721.**
CUNNINGHAM, R. Murray; 71 Johnstone Ave., Dartmouth, N.S.; Tor'48; DMRT; D&TRad; Hd. Dept. of Rad., Victoria Gen. Hosp.; Assoc. Prof. (Rad.) Dalhousie U.; Tel. 422-7371, Loc. 781.
CUNNINGHAM, Roy; UBC '64; Res., Vancouver Gen. Hosp., Vancouver, B.C.; Abroad.
CUNNINGHAM, Stella H.; 1073 Bay St., Toronto, Ont.; Tor '11; Tel. WA 2-1575.
CUNNINGHAM, Thomas A.; Campbellford Clinic, 49 Doxee Ave. S., Campbellford, Ont.; RCS (Dublin, Ire.)'53; Staff, Campbellford Mem. Hosp.; Tel. 653-3550.
CUNNINGHAM, Thomas A.; 43 MacDermid Cres., Saskatoon, Sask. (res); Glasgow (Scot.) '49; MRCP (Edin.); IntMed; Path; Ass't. Pathol., University Hosp.; Ass't. Prof., Path. & Lect. Med., U. of Saskatchewan; Tel. CH 2-7641.
CUNNINGHAM, Wallace H.; 109¼ Church St., St. Catharines, Ont.; Tor '18.
CUNNINGHAM, Warren J.: 3009-31st Ave., Vernon, B.C.; R.R. No. 2 (res); UBC '58; MCGP; Tel. 542-4321.
CUPPLES, James F.; 304 Cook Medical Bldg. **1175 Cook St., Victoria, B.C.; 2833 Dufferin** Ave. (res); **McG '51;** MCGP; Tel. EV 3-7431.
CURKOWSKYJ, Roman N.; 25 Brunswick Ave., Ste. 402, Toronto, Ont.; 72 Baby Point Rd., Toronto 9 (res); Franz Joseph U. (Graz, Austria) '42; OrthSurg; Tel. 925-1013.
CURRAN, Christina A.; 401 Med. Arts Bldg., 404-406 Graham Ave., Winnipeg 1, Man.; 178 **Garrioch (res); Man '43; Paed; Teach. Staff, Children's Hosp.; Att'd. Staff, Grace Hosp.; Tel. WH 3-3031.**
CURRAN, Daniel D. G.; 267 O'Connor St., Ottawa, Ont.; 497 Mayfair Ave. (res); University Coll. (Dublin, Ire.); '43 F.R.C.S. (Ed.), Gen-**Surg; Active Staff, (Surg) Ottawa Gen.** Hosp.; Court. Staff, Ottawa Civic Hosp., Assoc. Prof. (Surg.), U. of Ottawa; Tel. CE 5-6385.
CURREY, Douglas V.; 69 South Drive, St. Catharines, Ont. (res); **Tor '09; DPH; PH;** Examin. in PH Can. Med. Council; Retired.
CURRIE, Byron M.; Ste. 205, 1640-16th Ave. N.W., Calgary, Alta.; Alb '58; MCGP.
CURRIE, Donald J.; 123 Edward St., Toronto, Ont.; 122 Alexandra Blvd., Tor 12 (res); Tor '47; D.S., M.Sc., FRCS(E), FRCS(C), GenSurg; FACS; Att'd. Staff, St. Michael's Hosp.; Assoc. Dept. of Surg., U. of Toronto; Tel. EM 8-9223.
CURRIE, Edmond V.; 26 Rodney Ave., Valois, P.Q. (res); Tor '49; D.P.H.; Phys. Northern Electric Co. Ltd., 1261 Shearer St., Montreal, P.Q.: Tel. WE 7-6071.
CURRIE, Eoin A.; 12 Rochelle Cres., Don Valley Village, Willowdale, Ont.; Wes '43; M.O. I/C Dist. Admiss. Serv., Sunnybrook Hosp., Tor. 12; Tel. 485-8651.
CURRIE, George C.; 2401 Bloor W., Toronto, Ont.; 290 Riverside Dr. (res); Tor '24; Otol., **Retired; Tel. RO 7-3171.**
CURRIE, Gordon; London (Eng.)'53; M.O., Dept. of National Health & Welfare, Miller Bay Indian Hosp., Prince Rupert, B.C.
CURRIE, Helen M.; Qns'63; Res., Women's College Hosp., Toronto 5, Ont.
CURRIE, Ross E.; 6 George St. N., Galt, Ont.; Wes '61.
CURRIE, Roy S.; 245 Marion St., Norwood, Man.; Man '55; MCGP; Active Staff, St. Boniface San; Court. Staff, St. Boniface Gen., Victoria, Misericordia & Grace Hosp's.; Tel. 233-1476.
CURRIER, Thos. E.; 277 Stewart St., Peterborough, Ont.; 54 Edgewood Rd. (res); Qns '40; IntMed; **Staff, Peterborough Civic & St. Joseph's** Hosp's; Pres. Peterborough County Med. Soc.; Tel. 742-5841.
CURRY, B. H. Gaylord; 49 Rochester Ave., Toronto 12, Ont. (res); Man '37; F.R.C.S.(C) OrthSurg; Med. Dir., Hosp. & Rehab. Centre, Workmen's Comp. Board., 115 Torbarrie Rd., Downsview, Ont.; Tel. 244-1761.
CURRY, Fabien D.; Oakridge Rd. At Bay, Parry Sound, Ont. (res); Wes '49; DiagRad; Radiol., Parry Sound & St. Joseph's Gen. Hosp's.; Tel. RI 6-2925.
CURRY, Richard H.; 51 Lawrence Cr., Toronto 12, Ont.; Tor'59; Path.
CURTIN, A. Ann; 826 Medical Arts Bldg., 170 St. George St., Toronto 5, Ont.; Tor '20; D.P.H.
CURTIN, James J.; Med. Arts Bldg., 420 East St. N., Sarnia, Ont.; National U. (Dublin, Ire.) '51; D. Psy; Psy; Tel. ED 7-3112.
CURTIS, Arthur; Dal '60; DiagRad; Staff, Kingston Gen. Hosp., Kingston, Ont.; Tel. 546-3842.
CURTIS, Donald D.; 327 Charlotte St., Peterborough, Ont.; Tor '59; Tel. 742-3401.
CURTIS, Frederic W.; 742 Waterloo St., London, Ont.; Wes '43; Tel. 439-4051.
CURTIS, James Dowler; Wes '64; Res., Royal Victoria Hosp., Montreal 2, P.Q.
CURTIS, J. Eric; 23 Mapledawn Rd., Etobicoke, Ont. (res); Qns '50; Anaes; Staff Anaes., Queensway Gen. Hosp., Toronto; Tel. 233-7500.
CURTIS, John E.; Dal '63; Res., Toronto Gen. Hosp., Toronto 2, Ont.
CURTIS, John F.; 548 Talbot St., St. Thomas, **Ont.; Tor '30.**
CURTIS, Owen H.; Box 3000, 188 Prince St., Charlottetown, P.E.I.; 90 Greenfield Ave. (res); Dal'40; D.P.H.; Dep. Min. Health; Exec. Dir., Hosp. Services Comm.; Tel. 894-1293.
CURTIS, Ronald B.; Qns '58; Psy; Staff, Mental Health Clinic, Carling Ave., Ottawa, Ont.; Tel. PA 2-6521.
CUSACK, C. Albert; Lestock, Sask.; R.C.S. (Ireland)'49; Tel. Lestock 27.
CUSHING, Marian C.; McG '64; Res., Hosp. for Sick Children, Toronto 2, Ont.; Abroad.
CUSSON, Andre H.; 8415 St. Denis, Montreal, P.Q.; 6935 Jean Bourdon (res); Mon '43; OrthSurg (P.Q.); Ass't. Orth. Surg., Hop. de Sacre Coeur, Cartierville; Tel. 381-5311.
CUSSON, Leon; 7400 Fabre, Montreal, P.Q.; Mon '49; M.C.G.P.; Tel. 721-1531.
CUSTEAU, Pierre; Mon'62; Anaes; Staff, Hotel-Dieu-Montreal, Montreal, P.Q.
CUTHBERTSON, A. Neil; 11666-95 St., Edmonton, Alta.; 9007-120 St. (res); Wes '45; M.Sc., GenSurg; Surg. Staff, Royal Alexandra Hosp.; Tel. 474-3481.
CUTHILL, John D.; Box 225, Bella Coola, B.C.; UBC'65.
CUTLER, Barry K.; Tor '62; Ass't. Res., St. Michael's Hosp., Toronto 7, Ont.
CUTLER, Judith H.; 475 Oriole Pkwy., Toronto 7, Ont.; Tor '62; Research, Best Inst.
CUTLER, Noel M.; 1847 Rose St., Regina, Sask.; 2100 Cross Pl. (res); Man '53; GenSurg; Staff, Regina Gen. & Grey Nuns' Hosp's.; Tel. LA 2-6661.
CUYLITS, M. Helen; Apt. 17, 1390 W. 14th Ave., Vancouver 10, B.C.; Leiden (Neth.)'40; Parttime Public Health.
CYNBERG, David; Ste. 128, 3545 Cote des Neiges Road, Montreal, P.Q.; 5801 Cote St. Luc Rd. (res); McG'48; IntMed (P.Q.); Staff, Reddy Mem. Hosp.; Tel. 935-5585.
CYR, Claire; 8415 rue St-Denis, Montreal 11, P.Q.; 3815 Van Horne (res); Mon'56; **DABOph; Ophth; Assoc. Staff (Ophth), Hop.-du-Sacre-Coeur; Tel. 288-7533.**

CYR, Honore; St. Basil, N.B.; Lav '17: Anaes.
CYR, Joseph G.; Box 600, Grand Falls, N.B.; Lav'50.
CYR, Rene; 169 Charron St. Ville Lemoye, Co. Chambly, P.Q.; Mon '49.
CYR, Romeo; C.P. 148, 110 Deslauriers, Ste. Rose, Co. Laval, P.Q.; Mon'34; Staff, Dept. of Health, Montreal.
CZEREVKO, Jaroslaus Z.; Stone Rd., Virgil, Ont.; Innisbruck (Austria) '48.
CZIGLER, Paul H.; 11 Clarissa St., Brockville, **Ont.; '33; MCGP;** Tel. DI 2-9573.
CZILLER, Elizabeth; Royal Hungarian Elizabeth U. (Hung.) '26; A.B.P.N.; Staff, Brandon Mental Hosp., **Brandon, Man.**
CZITROM, Andre; 38 ave Little, Chandler, P.Q.; **Paris (France) '50; Staff, Hop. de la Province; Tel. 219.**
CZUBA, Ted; Wawa, Ont.; Tor'61; Staff, Lady Dunn Gen. Hosp.; Tel. 856-2231.
CZUBATY, Wolodymyr; 291 Burrows Ave., Winnipeg, Man.; Prague (Czech.) '29.
D'ABADIE, Frank A.; Ste 455, 5025 Sherbrooke St. W., Montreal, P.Q.; 3600 Ridgewood (res); McG'56; Cardiol(P.Q.); **FRCP(C),** IntMed; Jr. Clin. Ass't., St. Mary's Hosp.; Staff, OPD, Mtl. Gen. Hosp.; Tel. WE 5-8824.
da COSTA, Granville A.; UBC'60; Psy; Staff, Clarke Inst. of Psy., 250 College St., Toronto, Ont.
DADMARZ, Kewmars E.; Tehran (Iran) '53; Res. ThorSurg., U. of Alberta Hosp., Edmonton, Alta.
DAFOE, Charlotte S. (Small); 8731 Sask Dr., Edmonton, Alta. (res); Tor'36; DA(Eng.); Anaes; M.O., Dept. of Public Health; Tel. CA 9-3550.
DAFOE, Colin S.; 508 Medical Arts Bldg., Edmonton, Alta.; 11067-82 Ave. (res); Qns '36; F.A.C.S., F.C.C.P., F.R.C.S.(Edin.), ThorSurg; FACCP; Head Dept. of ThorSurg., Royal Alexandra Hosp.; ThorSurg., Aberhart San. & Edmonton Gen. & Misericordia Hosp's; Lect. (ThorSurg), U. of Alberta; Tel. GA 4-6242.
DAFOE, William A.; 627 Medical Arts Bldg., 170 St. George St., **Toronto 5,** Ont.; **41 Glen Rd.** (res); **Tor '20; F.R.C.O.G., F.R.C.S.(C) Obst-**Gyn; Assoc. **Prof. Obst.Gyn.,** U. of Toronto; Sr. Obst. Gyn, & Chief, Wellesley Div., Toronto Gen. Hosp.; Retired.
D'AGATA, Giuseppe; 671 Lansdowne Ave., Toronto 4, Ont.; Rome (Italy) '59; Tel. 533-4257.
D'AGATA, Victor P.; 106 Le Marchand Mans., Edmonton, Alta.; Cairo (Egypt)'49; Staff, Edmonton Gen. Hosp.; Tel. 488-5932.
DAGENAIS, Fernand; 11 de Tilly, Boucherville, P.Q.; Mon '55.
DAGENAIS, Gilles R.; Mon '64; Int., Hop. Hotel-Dieu, Montreal 18, P.Q.
DAGENAIS, Guy; 7775 rue Delorimier, Montreal 35, P.Q.; Mon'62; Anaes.
DAGENAIS, Maurice; 8001 St.-Denis St., Montreal, P.Q.; Mon '45; Tel. DU 8-2888.
DAGENAIS, Rene; Mon '64; Res., Hop. Notre-Dame, Montreal, P.Q.
DAGENAIS, Yves-M.; 3875 St.-Urbain, Montreal, P.Q.; 820 Hartland, Outremont (res); Mon '53; F.R.C.P.(C), IntMed; Clin. Hotel-Dieu & Cons. Hop Ste-Justine; Ass't. Prof., U. of Montreal; Tel. 842-3865.
DAGENAIS-PERUSSE, Paul; 301 **Carre-St.-Louis, Montreal, P.Q.; Mon '48;** F.A.A.P.; **Paed; Chief-of-Paed, Hop-Ste-Jeanne-d'Arc; Ass't. Prof. (Paed), U. of Montreal; Tel. VI 2-5201.**
D'AGINCOURT, Raymond Gouges; (See GOUGES).
DAGLISH, George H.; Liverpool (Eng.)'40; MRCS(Eng.); LRCP(Lond.); Staff, Dept. of Anat., U. of Manitoba, Winnipeg 3, Man.
DAGMAR, Kindy; McG **'60; Res., Montreal Children's Hosp., Montreal, P.Q.**
DAGNEAU, Clovis J.; 33 Brooks St. S., Sherbrooke, P.Q.; 386 Vimy (res); Lav '39; FICS, GenSurg (PQ); Med. Dir., Hotel-Dieu; Tel. 569-3311.
DAHL, Ralph G.; Calgary Assoc. Clinic, 214-6th Ave. S.W., **Calgary, Alta.;** 3031 Beil Ave. (res); **Alb '56; Tel. 263-7120.**
DAHL, R. Mark; Staff, Raymond Magrath Clinic, Magrath, **Alta.; Alb '53.**
DAICAR, Anthony O.; 115 Lower Union St., Kingston, Ont.; Qns'57; FRCS(C); ObstGyn; Att'd. Staff, Kingston Gen. Hosp.; Assoc. Staff, Hotel-Dieu Hosp.; Lect., Queen's U.; Tel. 546-4124.
DAIGLE, Emilien; Lav'65; Res., Hops. St. Sacrement, Quebec 6, P.Q.
DAIGLE, Georges A.; 106 ave.-Mont-Marie, Levis, P.Q.; Lav '50; FACS; OrthSurg; Hd. Dept. of OrthSurg., Hotel-Dieu; Tel. 837-9341.
DAIGLE, Gerald E.; Maple St., **Brownsburg, P.Q.; Mon '59.**
DAIGLE, Jean M.; 401 rue Sud, Cowansville, P.Q.; Mon'65.
DAIGLE, J. Egbert; 691 Main St., Moncton, N.B.; Lav '56; Anaes.
DAIGLE, M. Joffre; Box 709, Dalhousie, N.B.; Lav'54; Tel. SK 4-2394.
DAIGLE-LOCK, Rita; 4957 Prince St., Pierrefonds, P.Q.; Lav '58; Paed; Pt-time Staff (Paed.), Hop. Mont Providence, Riviere des Praires; Dir. Cerebral Palsy Clin., Hop. Ste Justine, Montreal; Tel. 684-8262.
DAIGLE, Robert C.; Pfizer Co. Ltd., 50 Place Cremazie, Montreal 11, **P.Q.; Lav'53.**
DAIGNEAULT, Bernard; St-Philippe, Cte. Laprairie, P.Q.; Mon '62.
DAIGNAULT, Gerard; 300 ouest Commerciale, Chandler, P.Q.; Mon'32; MCGP; Med. Dir., Hop.-de-la-Providence; Cons. Gaspesia Sulphite Co. Ltd.
DAIGNEAULT, Leo R.; 171 Montreal Rd., Cornwall, Ont.; 626 Guy (res); Lav '49; MCGP; Tel. WE 2-1261.
DAIN, Irving; 210, castle Bldg., 1 Duke St. Hamilton, Ont.; 69 Pleasant Ave. (res); Qns '56; D. Psy., Psy; Staff, Ontario Hosp.; Cons., Mount St. Joseph Res. Treatment Centre; Tel. JA 2- 7844.
DAINARD, Grace L.; 117 John St. S., **Fort** William, Ont. (res); Man '42; **Temp.; Retired.**
DAINARD, R. Bruce; Crease Clinic Essondale, **B.C.; 802-1095 Bute St. (res); Ott '57; Tel. 521 1911, Loc. 458.**
DAKIN, Warren A.; Medical Arts Bldg., **2125-11th Ave., Regina, Sask.; 303 Angus St. (res);** McG '10; Urol.
DALAL, Ajit; Med. Arts Bldg., 1255-100th St., North Battleford, Sask.; Bombay (India) '55; IntMed.
DALBY, Clive D.; Barrington Passage, N.S.; Birmingham (Eng.)'58; Tel. 43.
DALBY, Richard W.; Ridout St., Tillsonburg, Ont.; Wes '63; AMCGP; Tel. 842-8805.
DALCOURT, A.; Louiseville, Co. Maskinonge, **P.Q.; 4 St. Laurent (res); Mon '35.**
DALE, Albert D.; National Health & Welfare, Ottawa, Ont.; McG'53.
DALE, B. T.; 9 Vardon Dr., Guelph, Ont.; Lwow **(Poland) '31.**
DALE, Colin C.; Brown Clinic, 700-8th St. S.W., Calgary, Alta.; London (Eng.)'58; Otol.
DALE, Gordon G.; 5150 Dundas St. W., Islington, Ont.; 18 Boxwood Rd., Etobicoke (res); Tor '54; FRCS(C); OrthSurg; Staff, St. Joseph's & Queensway Gen. Hosp's.; Tel. 239-9932.
DALE, Gordon M.; 84 Woodlawn Ave. E., Toronto, **Ont.; Tor '15; OrthSurg.**
DALE, J. Peter; Ste. 706, 625-Fifth Ave., New Westminster, B.C.; McG'50; **Ophth.**
DALE, William N.; Tor'61; Res., Toronto East Gen. Hosp., Toronto 13, Ont.
DALES, C. W.; 66 Glenwood Ave., Toronto 9, **Ont. (res); Tor '24; Staff, Phys. Workmen's Compensation Board, 90 Harbour St.; Tel. 362-3411.**
DALES, John W.; R.R. 2, 1889 Blythe Rd., **Clarkson, Ont.; Tor '48; Anaes; Staff, Queensway Gen. Hosp., Toronto; Tel. CL 9-6671.**
DALES, Merrill G.; Victoria St., Tweed, Ont.; Tor '21; Coroner, Hastings County; M.O., C.P.R.; Phys. Nichols Chemical Co., Sulphide, Ont.; Retired.
DALES, Michael; 55 Avondale Blvd., Bramalea, Ont.; UBC'59.
DALES, Walter; 214 Larch St., Sudbury, Ont. (res); Tor '05; Retired.
DALEY, Daniel A.; 75A James St., Parry Sound, Ont.; Tor '52; MCGP; Tel. 746-2181.

DALEY, Dorothy; O.M.S.I.P., 135 St. Clair Ave. W., Toronto 7, Ont.; Tor'39; Tel. 365-5559.
DALGLEISH, Harold D.; 514 Medical Arts Bldg., Saskatoon, Sask.; 920 University Dr. (res); Man '36; GenSurg; Clin. Teach. (GenSurg.), U. of Saskatchewan; Tel. 242-1263.
DALGLEISH, P. Douglas; Ste. 101, 688 Coxwell Ave., Toronto 13, Ont.; Tor'56; Tel. 466-0592.
DALLAIRE, Gerard; 902 Poire, Ste-Anne-de-la-Pocatiere, P.Q.; Lav '39; M.P.P.
DALLAIRE, Henri; 2517 ave Royale, Quebec 5, P.Q.; Lav '48; Tel. 663-9344.
DALLAIRE, Louis; Douglas Hosp., 6875 Lasalle Blvd., Verdun, P.Q.; Lav'60; PhD.; Scientific Dir., Children's Serv., Douglas Hosp.; Lect. McGill U.; Tel. 769-9691, Loc. 35.
DALLAIRE, Michel E.; Lav'65; Res., Hop. Hotel-Dieu, Quebec 4, P.Q.
DALLAIRE, Michel H.; Lav'65; Res., Hop. Enfant Jesus, Quebec 3, P.Q.
DALLAIRE, Roger R. D.; St. Benoit Labre, Beauce, P.Q.; Lav '55; Vis. Phys. Hops. St. Georges & Beauceville.
DALLA-VEDOVA, Giuseppe; 37 Duke St., St. Catharines, Ont.; Naples (Italy) '53; IntMed.
DALLIMORE, Sydney T.; 26 Water St. Chippawa, Ont.; Qns. '50; MOH, Chippawa; Phys., Norton Co.; Tel. AX 5-4323.
DALLING, John; 106-9th St., Brandon, Man.; Glasgow (Scot.)'56; MB; Ch.B.; FRCS(Glas.).
DALLISON, Frank L. Capt.; Alb'64; Staff, Alberta Military Hosp., Cdn. Forces Base, Calgary, Alta.
D'ALMEIDA, Jose G.; 1010 McCallum Hill Bldg., 1874 Scarth St., Regina, Sask.; Hong Kong (China) '53; Staff, Assoc. Anaes.; Tel. 522-0704.
D'ALOISIO, Joseph F.; 83 Larch St., Sudbury, Ont.; Ott'58; Urol.; Tel. 674-6987.
DALPE, Candide; 2801 boul. Rosemont, Montreal 36, P.Q.; Mon '43.
DALRYMPLE, Sydney J. V.; Tor '38; Staff, Niagara Peninsula San., St. Catharines, Ont.
DALRYMPLE, Thomas; 175 E. Broadway, Vancouver, B.C.; McG '33; MCGP; Tel. TR 4-7233.
DALTON, Eric G.; 2800 Lundy's Lane, Niagara Falls, Ont.; Wes '58. Abroad.
DALTON, John B.; 327 Charlotte St., Peterborough, Ont.; Wes '60; IntMed.
DALTON, Roberta D.; Man'65; Staff, R. W. Large Mem. Hosp., Bella Bella, B.C.
DALY, J. Stuart; 901 Helena St., Trail, B.C.; 31 Hazlewood Dr. (res); Qns '27; FACP; IntMed; Cons. (Med.), Trail-Tadanac Hosp. & Mater Misericordia Hosp., Rossland; Tel. 368-5211.
DALY, Nicholas; Roberts Med. Group, 95 LeMarchant Rd., St. John's, Nfld.; 19 Falkland St. (res); Nat. U. (Cork, Ire.) '50; BAO; ObstGyn; Staff, St. John's, St. Clare's Mercy & Grace Hosp's.; Tel. 8-2230; 8-4487.
DALY, Patrick; Prelate, Sask.; RCP & S (Dublin, Ire.)'28; LRCP(I); LRCS(I); Med. Supt., Prelate Union Hosp.
DALY, Patrick H.; Norwood Professional Bldg., 11664-95th St., Edmonton, Alta.; 13104-104th (res); St. Mary's Hosp. (London, Eng.) '32; MRCS (Eng.), LRCP (Lond.); Tel. GR 7-5271.
DALY, Patrick J.; National U. (Ire.) '55; Staff, Community Health Services Assoc., Beaver Hotel Bldg. North Battleford, Sask.
DALY, Patrick J.; Security Trust Bldg., Lloydminster, Alta.; National U. (Ire.) '38.
DALY, Timothy; 605 Professional Bldg., 10830 Jasper Ave., Edmonton, Alta.; 4615-106B Ave. (res); National U. (Dublin, Ire.) '45; D.O.M.S. (Lond.), Ophth; Staff, Edmonton Gen., Misericordia & Royal Alexandra Hosp's.; Tel. 422-4536.
DALZELL, Robert T.; Man'56; Path; Staff, Dept. of Path., St. Paul's Hosp., Vancouver 1, B.C.
D'AMICO, Rina M. (Alberton); 2493 Commercial Dr., Vancouver, B.C.; 795 W.-41st St. (res); Rome (Italy) '47; Tel. TR 2-2821.
D'AMOURS, Claude; Lav'52; Path(P.Q.); Staff, Hop.-de-l'Enfant-Jesus, Quebec, P.Q.; Tel. 529-8711.
D'AMOURS, Claude; Lav '57; Res., Hop. Hotel-Dieu, Quebec, P.Q.
D'AMOURS, Oliver; 16 Bisson, Hull, P.Q. (res); Lav '38; Pulm. Dis. & TB (PQ); Med. Supt., St. Laurent San.; Tel. PR 7-5245.
D'AMOURS, Marcel; Lav '60; Res., Hop. Ste-Foy, Quebec 10, P.Q.
DAMPHOUSSE, J. B. Alban; 452 Mercier, Shawinigan, P.Q.; 1259 rue Hart, Trois-Rivieres; 600-114eme rue, Shawinigan Sud (res); Lav '44; GenSurg; Surg., Hop-Ste-Marie, Trois-Rivieres; Tel. LE 6-2092.
DANAIS, Remi; Lav '62; Res., Hop.-St.Sacrement, Quebec, P.Q.
DANAIS, Remi; Lav '54; Res., Hop-St-Ambroise, Loretteville, P.Q.
DANAIS, Slevin; 401 Queen, Rawdon, P.Q.; 145 Metcalfe (res); Lav '61; Tel. 834-2304.
DANAK, Manubhai T.; Medical Clinic, Sydney Mines, N.S.; '46.
DANBY, Charles W.; Box 383, 253 Ontario St., Kingston, Ont.; 465 King W. (res); Qns '40; FRCP(C); DermSyph; Att'd. Phys. I/C Derm. Clinics, Kingston Gen. & Hotel-Dieu Hosp's.; Cons. (Derm.), Cdn. Forces Hosp., Dept. of Justice; Ass't. Prof. (DermSyph.), Queen's U.; Tel. 542-4337.
DANBY, John H.; 602 Med. Dental Bldg., Regina, Sask.; 6 Bole Pl. (res); Leeds (Eng.) '56; MCGP; Med. Staff, Regina Gen. & Grey Nuns Hosp.; M.O., Cdn. Pacific Railways; Tel. 522-8579.
DANBY, S. L. Everett; 180 Metcalfe St., Ottawa 4, Ont.; 330 Metcalfe St., Ott 4 (res); Tor '21; FACS; GenSurg; Cons. (GenSurg), Ottawa Civic Hosp.; Tel. 234-1750.
DANCEY, John T.; McG'65; Res., Montreal Gen. Hosp., Montreal 25, P.Q.
DANCEY, Travis E.; 4015 Wilson Ave., Montreal 28, P.Q.; McG '34; Psy; Psy.-in-Chief, Queen Mary Vets. Hosp.; Assoc. (Psy.), Montreal Gen. Hosp.; Assoc. Prof. (Psy.), McGill U.; Adv. (Psy.), Dir. Gen. Treatment Servs., D.V.A.; Tel. HU 4-5761.
DANDENAULT, Augustus G.; 126 Medical Arts Bldg., Winnipeg, Man.; 363 Kingston Cres., St. Vital (res); Man '26; F.A.C.S.
DANDENAULT, J. Yves; 52 Grande-Ile, Valleyfield, P.Q.; 254 Salabery (res); Lav '43;
DANDURAND, Bruno; Mon'65; Res., Hop. Hotel-Dieu, Montreal 18, P.Q.
DANDURAND, J. Emilien; 10147 Peloquin, Montreal 12, P.Q.; Mon '23.
DANEAU, Jacques; 145 Blvd. Laurentian, Shawinigan Sud., P.Q.; Lav'37; D&TRad; Rad., Hop. Ste. Therese & Hop. Joyce Mem.; Tel. 537-8587.
DANGOR, Abdulla I.; 2nd Floor, Avenue Bldg., 220-3rd Ave. S., Saskatoon, Sask.; Royal College of Surg. (Ire.) '60; LRCP; LRCS; LM; ECFMG; MCGP; Tel. 652-0300.
DANIEL, Alexander; 1028 Drouillard Rd., Windsor, Ont.; 1630 Ypres Blvd. (res); Vienna (Aust.) '41; McG '52; Tel. 256-4463.
DANIEL, Emil; Box 3004, Dryden, Ont.; Man'41; Tel. 223-2258.
DANIEL, George A.; 5757 Decelles Ave., Ste. 511, Montreal 26, P.Q.; Budapest (Hung.) '50; GenSurg; Jr. Ass't. Surg., Reddy Mem. Hosp.; Cons. Surg., Jewish Convalescent Hosp.; (Experim. Surg.), McGill U.; Tel. 739-5408.
DANIEL, Maurice A.; 13774 St. Gregory Rd., St. Clair Beach, Windsor, Ont.; Ott '55.
DANIEL, Susan; 28 St. Andrews Gardens, Toronto 5, Ont.; Budapest (Hung.) '54; Anaes; Staff, St. Michael's Hosp.; Tel. 372-4461.
DANIEL, Philippe; Paris (Fr.) '51; Ass't. Prof. (Microbiol.), Laval U., Quebec, P.Q.
DANIELS, James H.; 125 Montrose St., Winnipeg 9, Man.; Qns'52; DA; FACA; FICS; Anaes.
DANIELS, Roy K.; Man '49; Staff, Aberhart Mem. San., Edmonton, Alta.
DANILOV, George; Belgrade (Yugo.) '34; Staff, Ongwanada San., Kingston, Ont.; Clin. Ass't., Queen's U.; Tel. 548-4417.
DANIS, James T.; 507 Medical Arts Bldg., 170 St. George St., Toronto 5, Ont.; 300 Glencairn (res); Tor '21; F.A.C.S., F.R.C.S. (Edin.), GenSurg (Proct.); Cons. Surg., St. Michael's Hosp.; Retired.

DANIS, Joseph J.; Horseshoe Lane, Lakeville, Conn., U.S.A.; Tor'59; Psy; Abroad.
d'ANNA, Antonino; 6818 St. Denis St., Montreal 10, P.Q.; Bologna (Italy) '27, Mon '31; Tel. 271-9412.
DANSEREAU, Alphonse; 832 Blvd. St. Joseph Est, Montreal, P.Q.; Mon '41; Obst (P.Q.); Chief of Obst., Hop de la Misericorde; Ass't. Prof. of Obst., U. of Montreal; Tel. VI 2-5141.
DANSEREAU, Jacques; 1150 est, boul. St-Joseph, Montreal 34, P.Q.; Mon '58; FRCS(C), PlasSurg; Tel. LA 7-1241.
DANSEREAU, Michel; 80 Ave Hollyrood, Outremont, Montreal 8, P.Q.; Mon '50; Staff, U. of Montreal; Tel. 735-0163.
DANSEREAU, Remi; 166 Brunelle, Beloeil, P.Q.; McG '43.
DANTO, Julius L.; 745 West Broadway, Vancouver 9, B.C.; 2350 W. 39th Ave. (res); Loyola (U.S.A.) '45; A.B.D.S., DermSyph; Vis. Staff, Vancouver Gen. & St. Paul's Hosp's.; Phys., V.D. Control, Public Health Dept. of B.C.; Tel. TR 4-8138.
DANTOW, James E. F/L.; MIR, Armed Forces Hosp., Kingston, Ont.; Sask'65.
DANTOW, Matthew; Library Bldg., Saskatoon, Sask.; 933 University Dr. (res); Glasgow (Scot.) '36; DPH; PH; MOH, Saskatoon; Clin. Prof. (Soc. & Prev. Med.), U. of Saskatchewan; Tel. CH 2-7671.
DANYLCHUK, Alexander; 220 Main St., Canora, Sask.; Man '41; Chief of Surg., Canora Union Hosp.; District Coroner; Tel. 563-5633.
DANYLUK, John; Alb'65; Jr. Int., Misericordia Hosp., Edmonton, Alta.
DANZIGER, Hans G. U.; 5 Maplewood Cres., Welland, Ont.; Leipzig (Germ.) '30; D.T.M. (Hamburg); Path; Path. & Dir. of Labs., Welland Co. Gen. Hosp.; Tel. RE 2-6111.
DANZIGER, R.; 540 Mountain Ave., Winnipeg, Man.; Man '30; Tel. JU 9-4397.
DANZINGER, Rudolph G.; Man '64; Res., Wpg. Gen. Hosp., Winnipeg, Man.
DAOUST, Jean P.; 222 Henri Bourrassa est, Montreal, P.Q.; 1135 Drovoit (res); Mon '56; FRCP (C); IntMed; Tel. 387-6556.
DAOUST, Louis C.; 4725 Chemin Cote-Ste-Catherine, Montreal 26, P.Q.; Mon '52; Psy; Staff, Hop.-de-Bordeaux; Tel. DU 9-1321.
DAOUST, Pierre; 1 Golf Ave., Pte-Claire, **Lachine, P.Q.; Mon '52; FRCP(C), IntMed.; Tel. 695-3844.**
D'APPOLONIA, Gino L.; 815 Victoria St., Trail, B.C.; Alta'54.
DARAMOLA, Florence G.; Apt. 209, 1862 Bathurst St., Toronto 10, Ont. (res); Research, Banting Inst., Toronto; Tel. WA 3-6611.
DARAMOLA, Taiwd; Apt. 209, 1862 Bathurst St., Toronto 10, Ont.; Tor '61; P.G., U. of Toronto.
DARBY, George E.; 4702 W. 7th Ave., Vancouver 8, B.C. (res); Tor '13; FRAI; Co-ordinator, United Church Hosp's.; Retired.
DARBY, George H.; Tor'52; D.Psy; Dir., Oak Ridge Div., Ontario Hosp., Penetanguishene, Ont.
DARCHE, Jean H.; 1385 Jean Talon E., Montreal, P.Q.; 12412 Olivier St. Mtl. 9 (res); McG '39; GenSurg (P.Q.); Chief Surg., Jean Talon; Tel. CR 3-5151.
DARCHE, J. Lionel; 1618 King W., Sherbrooke, P.Q.; Mon '62; AMCGP; Tel. LO 2-0654.
DARCHE, Lionel; 166 King Ouest, Sherbrooke, P.Q.; 604 Ontario (res); Mon '22; Ophth; Tel. 562-0654.
DARDICK, Irving; 2286 Carling, Ottawa 14, Ont.; Qns'57; MCGP; Tel. 729-8241.
DARE, Norman; 45 Sumner Rd., London, Ont.; Cheeloo (China)'47; ABDR; Staff Rad., Westminster Hosp.; Fell. (DiagRad.), U. of Western Ont.
d'ARGENCOURT, Guy; 360 rue Marchand, Drummondville, P.Q.; Mon '30; **F.R.C.S.(C), Gen** Surg; ObstGyn; Tel. GR 2-3858.
DARGIS, Gaston; P. O. Box 550, Malartic, P.Q.; Lav '51.
DARGIS, Jean; Lav '43; DPH; PH (P.Q.); Staff, Hop. Maisonneuve, Montreal 36, P.Q.; Tel. 254-3341.
DARIS, J. A.; Beaubien, Riviere du Loup, P.Q.; Lav '31; Gyn. (P.Q.).
DARJA, Maria; 515-9th St. E., Saskatoon, Sask. (res); Graz (Austria) **'30; Staff, University** Hosp.
DARKE, Trevlyn V.; 1010 McCallum Hill Bldg., 1874 Scarth St., **Regina, Sask.; Royal College** (Edinburgh, Scot.) '51; Tel. 522-0704.
DARRAGH, James H.; 1414 Drummond St., Montreal 25, P.Q.; 645 Belmont Ave., Westmount 6 (res); McG '48; M.Sc. (Experi. Med.); DABIM; FRCP(C), IntMed; Ass't. Phys., Mtl. Gen.; Cons. (Endocrin.), Queen Mary Vet's. Hosp.; Lect. (Med.), McGill U.; Tel. VI 5-8677.
DARTE, John M. M.; 555 University Ave., Toronto 2, Ont.; 105 Bernard Ave., Tor. 5 (res); Tor '44; DMRT (Eng.), FRCP(C), Paed.; TherRad; Phys. & Assoc. Path. (Haem.), Hosp. for Sick Children; Cons. Paed., Princess Margaret Hosp.; Assoc. Prof. (Paed.), U. of Toronto; Tel. EM 6-7242.
DARVEAU, Claude; Lav '63; Res., Hop. Ste-Justine-Montreal, Montreal, P.Q.
DARVEAU, Jean C.; 79 St. Thomas, Montmagny, P.Q.; Lav '32; Pres. Bureau Medical, Hotel Dieu, **Montmagny; Tel. 636.**
DARVEAU, Robert; 2075 Parc Gamior, Quebec, **P.Q. 2200 Dickson, Sillery, P.Q. (res); Lav '49, Ass't. Anaes., Hop. St. Sacrement; Tel. 522-4329.**
DARVEAU, Roger; 1624 Notre Dame, Ancienne Lorette, P.Q.; Lav '49.
DAS, Esmaralda; 546 Pharmacy Ave., Scarborough, Ont.; 20 Doris Ave. (res); Tor '57.
DAS, Kshitish C.; Calcutta (India) '56; DABPN; Staff Saskatchewan Hosp., Box 39, North Battleford, Sask.; Tel. 445-2421; Abroad.
DAS, Jagessar; 11967-88th Ave., North Surrey, B.C.; UBC '62.
DAS VARMA, Ranendra L.; Patna (India)'59; IntMed; Staff, Westminster Hosp., London, Ont.
DaSILVA, Guy; 756 Rockland Ave., Outremont, Montreal 8, P.Q.; Mon '57; Psy (P.Q.); DABPN; Ass't. O.P.D. & Supervisor of Group Therapy, Inst. Albert Prevost; Mental Hygiene Cons., Sir. George William U.; Tel. 271-6281.
DaSILVA, Thos.; 65 Bruyere St., Ottawa, 2, Ont. (res); Porto (Portugal) '42; GenSurg.
DaSYLVA, Normand P.; 3244 Beaubien E., Montreal 36, P.Q.; 911, Aime Bibeau Mtl. 40 (res); McG '54; MCGP Sec. (Quebec Chapter), College of G.P. of Canada; Tel. RA 9-1891.
DATZEFF, G. A.; 3111 Sheppard Ave. E., Agincourt, Ont.; 8 Walgreen (res); **Wes '51; A.M.-C.G.P.;** Tel. HI 4-2459.
DAUDELIN, Andre; 645 St. Pierre, La Providence Co., St. Hyacinthe, P.Q.; Mon '57; Tel. 774-8863.
DAUGAVIETIS, Hugo E.; St. Catharines Med. Centre, 292 Oakdale Ave., St. Catharines, Ont.; 27 West Hampton Rd. (res); U. of Latvia)Riga) '44; IntMed; Active Staff, St. Catharines Gen. Hosp.; Court. Staff, Hotel-Dieu Hosp.; Tel. MU 2-8344.
DAUNAIS Gilles; Central Medical, 86 rue St. Vincent, St. Agathe, P.Q.; 31 Principale (res); Mon '51; Tel. 326-1122.
DAUNAIS, Guy; 537-16th Ave., Pointe-aux-Trembles, P.Q.; Lav '65.
DAUNAIS, Jean A.; 6380 Blvd. Jos. Renaud, Ville d'Anjou, P..Q; Mon'51; GenSurg(P.Q.).
DAUNT, Ivan E.; 208 Medical Arts Bldg., Saskatoon, Sask.; National U. (Cork, Ire.)'50; MB; BCh; BAO; DRCOG; Staff, St. Paul's & City Hosp's.; Tel. 244-1137.
DAUPHINAIS, Joseph L.; Arnprior Medical Centre, Arnprior, Ont.; **Lav '48; Dist. Coroner.**
DAUPHINEE, James A. OBE; 214 Inglewood Dr., Toronto 7, **Ont. (res); Tor '30; Ph.D.,** F.R.S.C., F.R.C.P.(C), IntMed; **Prof. & Hd.** Dept. (PathChem) **& Assoc. (Med.), U. of Toronto; Att'd. Phys., Toronto Gen. Hosp.; Pt-time** Cons. (Med.), **Sunnybrook (DVA) Hosp.; Tel. 928-2663.**
DAUPHINEE, W. Dale; Dal'64; Res., Royal Victoria Hosp., Montreal, P.Q.
D'AUTEUIL, Pierre; 6615-lere Ave., Quebec 7, P.Q. (res); Lav '55; Haem (P.Q.); F.R.C.P.(C), IntMed; Staff, Hop. Hotel-Dieu; Tel. 529-9151.

DAVEY, Eric L.; 100 Acacia Ave., Rockcliffe Park, Ont. (res); Tor '35; D.P.H., P.H.; Chief, Civil Service Health Div., Dept. Nat. Health & Welfare, No. 3 Temporary Bldg., Ottawa, Ont.; Med. Adv., Carleton U.; Tel. 992-3418.

DAVEY, James E.; 2 Ray St. S., Hamilton, Ont.; Tor '02; Court. Med. Staff, Hamilton Med. Assoc. Hosp's & St. Joseph's Hosp.; Med. Exam., Hamilton Dept. of Public Welfare; Retired.

DAVEY, Jean F., OBE; 280 Bloor Street West, Toronto 5, Ont.; Tor'36; FACP; FRCP(C); IntMed; Dir. of Medical Teaching in Outpatient Dept., Women's College Hosp.; Assoc. Prof. of Medicine, Univ. of Toronto; Tel. 921-2818.

DAVEY, Jean M. (nee Meiners); 100 Acacia Ave., Ottawa 2, Ont. (res); Tor '41; Paed; Semi-retired.

DAVEY, Lloyd M.; 224 Alfred Ave., Willowdale, Ont. (res); Tor '42; D.P.H.; M.O., W.C.B., Ont.

DAVEY, Peter W.; 6004-109B Ave., Edmonton, Alta. (res); Qns '49; Path; Dir. of Labs., Royal Alexandra Hosp.; Ass't. Prof. Path), U. of Alberta; Tel. GR 4-3431.

DAVID, Andre V.; 822 rue Sherbrooke est, Montreal, P.Q.; 5900 rue de Verneuil, Ville d'Anjou (res); Mon '52; Cardiol (P.Q.); IntMed; Tel. 526-3788.

DAVID, Claude; 5330 Duquette, Montreal, P.Q.; Mon '55; GenSurg.

DAVID, Claytus J.; 3844 E. Pender St., Vancouver, B.C. (res); UBC '60.

DAVID, Clive M.; Birmingham (Eng.)'56; Staff, Indian Hosp., Nanaimo, B.C.

DAVID, Donald; 398 Commerciale ouest, Chandler, P.Q.; Mon'65.

DAVID, J. Raymond; 8162 Mirepoix, St. Leonard, P.Q.; Mon'57; DiagRad.

DAVID, Paul; 5330 Duquette, Montreal, P.Q.; Mon'59; IntMed; Cardiol(P.Q.).

DAVID, Paul; 5000 est, rue Belanger, Montreal 36, P.Q.; Mon '44; IntMed (P.Q.); Cardiol. (P.Q.); Dir., Montreal Cardiological Inst.; Assoc. Prof., U. of Montreal; Tel. 376-3330.

DAVID, Pierre C.; Ste. 444, 5757 Decelles, Montreal, P.Q.; Mon'60; FRCP(C), Neur.

DAVID, Pierre-Paul; 960 Ste Croix, St. Laurent, P.Q.; 3198 St. Charles, St. Laurent (res); Mon '63; Tel. 747-3501.

DAVIDMAN, Morris; Alb'62; Res., University Hosp., Edmonton, Alta.

DAVIDSON, Alan S.; 24 Harbord St., Toronto, **Ont.; Tor '56; Psy; Staff, Ont. Hospital, Toronto; Tel. 481-5916.**

DAVIDSON, Alexander L.; 1088 Pembina Hwy., Winnipeg 19, Man.; St. Andrews (Scot.) '47; GenSurg; Tel. GL 3-3303.

DAVIDSON, Allan M., LT/COL; Man '46; GenSurg; FACS; Head, Dept. of Surg., Cdn. Forces Hosp., Kingston, Ont.; Lect. (Surg.), Queen's U.; Tel. 546-3811.

DAVIDSON, Allen E.; 828 W. 10th Ave., Vancouver, B.C.; 629-4th St., New Westminster (res); Alb '31; FAPA; Psy; Dep. Minister & Dir. Mental Health Serv. BC; Clin. Ass't. Prof. (Psy.), U. of British Columbia; Tel. TR 4-2331.

DAVIDSON, Andrew M.; 504 Medical Dental Bldg., 925 West Georgia St., Vancouver 1, B.C.; 3950 Hudson St. (res); Edinburgh (Scot.) '12; M.R.C.P. (Edin.), D.A.B.D., F.R.C.P.(C), Derm Syph; Cons. Derm, St. Paul's Hosp.; Tel. MU 5-9018.

DAVIDSON, Barrie D.; Moosomin, Sask.; Man '60.

DAVIDSON, C. Roderick S.; 384 Queen St. S., Kitchener, Ont.; Tor '40; F.R.C.S. (Edin.); Tel. 742-7722.

DAVIDSON, C. Ronald; Box 1079, Sussex, N.B.; Dal'52; AMCGP.

DAVIDSON, D. A.; Tor '63; Res., Toronto Western Hosp., Toronto 2B, Ont.

DAVIDSON, David A.; Cartwright, Man.; Man '30; Dist. Coroner.

DAVIDSON, Derek A.; Tor'63; Ass't. Res., (Med.), Toronto Gen. Hosp., Toronto, Ont.

DAVIDSON, Donald A.; Medical Arts Bldg., 1011 Ouellette Ave., Windsor, Ont.; 49 Jefferson Blvd., Riverside (res); Tor '35.

DAVIDSON, George A.; Ste 204, 3195 Granville St., Vancouver 8, B.C.; 315 Stevens Dr., West Vancouver (res); Man '22; MRCP (Lond.); FACP; FRCP(C); NeurPsy; Hon. Att'd. Staff, Vancouver Gen. Hosp.; Clin. Prof. (Med.), UBC; Tel. RE 3-1080.

DAVIDSON, Harold J.; 224 Charlotte St., Sydney, N.S.; 6 Howe St. (res); Dal '35; B.Sc., F.I.C.S.; Staff, (Ophth,Otol), City of Sydney, St. Rita, Harbour View & St. Elizabeth's Hosp's.; Tel. 564-8312.

DAVIDSON, Harry A.; 480 Guelph Line, Burl**ington Ont.; 3398 Regal Rd. (res); Tor '59; Active Staff, Joseph Brant Mem. Hosp.; Court. Staff, St. Joseph's, Hamilton Gen. & Chedoke Hosp's., Hamilton; Tel. 637-2349.**

DAVIDSON, Hugh D.; 226 Harwood Ave., Ajax, **Ont.; 7 Preston Ct. (res); Qns '57; Tel. 924-1090.**

DAVIDSON, Jack W.; 15 Limerick Ave., Weston, Ont. (res); Tor'51; Anaes; Staff, Ontario Hosp., Hamilton; Phys., Ont. Dept. of Health.

DAVIDSON, James D.; 923 Main St. E., Hamil**ton, Ont.; Qns '59; MCGP; Tel. LI 4-5241.**

DAVIDSON, James H.; 1234 Victoria Ave., Niagara Falls, Ont.; **Tor '27; Obst.**

DAVIDSON, James W.; Aberdeen (Scot.)'53; DiagRad; Staff, X-Ray Dept., Princess Margaret Hosp., Toronto 5, Ont.

DAVIDSON, John A.; 37 Bridge St., Ormstown, P.Q.; 39 Bridge St. (res); McG '33; GenSurg (P.Q.); MCGP; Surg. Staff, Barrie Mem. Hosp.; Tel. 829-2234.

DAVIDSON, J. Peter; 1234 Victoria Ave., Niagara Falls, Ont.; 636 Sheppard Ave. (res); Tor '60; Tel. EL 8-5708.

DAVIDSON, J. Ross; 707 W. 37th Ave., Vancouver 13, B.C.; Ste. 203, 2155 W. 38th Ave., Van. 13 (res); McG '29; GenSurg; Chief M.O., WCB (BC); Tel. AM 6-0211.

DAVIDSON, Kenneth; 1694 Fort St., Victoria, B.C.; St. Andrews (Scot.) '60.

DAVIDSON, Kenneth G. S.; 504-925 W. Georgia St., Vancouver 1, B.C.; 5837 Angus Dr., Vancouver 13 (res); Edinburgh (Scot.) '43; D.T.M., DermSyph; Cons., Pearson T.B. Hosp.; Vis. Staff, Vancouver Gen. & Children's Hosp's.; Cons. Derm. HMCS "Naden"; Tel. MU 5-9018 & 278-5822.

DAVIDSON, Murray; Tor'61; Res., Toronto Western Hosp., Toronto 2B, Ont.

DAVIDSON, R. Edward; 993 Kingston, Road, Toronto 8, Ont.; Tor '08; Sr. Cons. (Med.) Toronto East Gen. Hosp.; Tel. OX 1-0522.

DAVIDSON, R. Glenn; 326-3rd St. S., Kenora, Ont. (res); Qns '23; Retired.

DAVIDSON, Richard; Lav'43; Res., Hop. Maisonneuve, Montreal 36, P.Q.

DAVIDSON, Russell W.; 1625 Oak Bay Ave., Victoria, B.C.; Edinburgh (Scot.)'54; MCGP.

DAVIDSON, Victor D.; 34 Cobourg St., St. John, N.B.; Rothesay (res); Dal '15; FACS; GenSurg; Retired.

DAVIDSON, William; Glasgow (Scot.) '59; Paed; Staff, Hosp. for Sick Children, Toronto 2, Ont.

DAVIDSON, William Robert; 34 Erie St. E., Windsor, Ont.; 12408 Riverside Dr., Tecumseh, **Ont. (res); Wes '35; Otol.; Tel. 253-1532.**

DAVIES, Allan J.; Box 280, Unity, Sask.; London (Eng.)'62; Tel. 228-2638.

DAVIES, Alan J. M.; Indian Head, Sask.; Man '42; GenSurg; Tel. 695-3422.

DAVIES, Charles E.; 2525 Pine St., Vancouver 9, B.C.; 4050 Pine Cres. (res); Alb '27; DABO; Ophth; **Clin. Instr. (Ophth), U. of British Col**umbia; Retired.

DAVIES, David W.; Cabri, Sask.; Sheffield (Eng.) '61.

DAVIES, Dewi R.; Duke St., Oxford, N.S.; London (Eng.) '36; MRCS (Eng.); LRCP (Lond.); Med. Staff, All Saints Hosp., Springhill; Tel. OXford 147.

DAVIES, Edward G.; 2200 Dixie Rd., Cooksville, Ont.; Tor'64; Staff, South Peel & Queensway Gen. Hosp's.; Tel. 279-1700.

DAVIES, Eleanor M. (Setterington); Northcrest Dr., R.R. 2., London, Ont. (res); Tor '51; Path; Pathol., St. Joseph's Hosp.; Tel. GE 9-3271.

DAVIES, Elspa; Durham (Eng.)'59; Res., St. Paul's Hosp., Vancouver 1, B.C.
DAVIES, E. Mary; Apt. 701, 54050 Vine St., Vancouver 13, B.C.; Bristol (Eng.)'47; Phys.Med. & Rehab.; Dir. Activation Unit, Lions Gate Hosp.

DAVIES, Eudora (See Rees-Davies).

DAVIES, G. J. Llewelyn; May Court Chest Clinic, 374 Besserer St., Ottawa, Ont.; 743 Eastbourne Ave. (res); **Guys Hosp. (London, Eng.) '41;** M.R.C.S., L.R.C.P., D.P.H.; Dir., May Court **Chest Clinic; Tel. 749-2098.**
DAVIES, Gordon R.; Irving Clinic. 74 W. Seymour, Kamloops, B.C.; 642 Tunstall Cr. (res); McG '53; FRCS(C), GenSurg; Surg., Royal Inland Hosp.; Tel. 372-5251.
DAVIES, Harold L.; 190 Tache Ave., St. Boniface, Winnipeg 6, Man.; Man '46; Paed; Staff, St. Boniface Hosp.; Tel. WH 3-0311.
DAVIES, Helen I.; 142 Queenston St., St. Catharines, Ont.; Tor'54; D.Psy.; Psy; Staff, St. Catharines Gen. Hosp.; Tel. **MU 4-7271.**
DAVIES, Hugh R.; 87 Adelaide St. N., Lindsay, Ont.; Tor '49; MCGP; Staff, Ross Mem. Hosp.; Tel. 324-2561.
DAVIES, James H.; 674 Kingston Rd., Toronto 13, Ont.; 62 Beaufort Rd. (res); Tor '47; M.C. G.P.; Tel. OX 1-1718.
DAVIES, John E.; 1897 Portage Ave., St. James, Winnipeg 12, Man.; 177 Campbell Ave. (res); Dal '16; London (Eng.) '44; MRCS, LRCP; M.P.H.(Harvard); **Cons. Epidem., Children's Hosp.;** Tel. SP 5-8311.
DAVIES, John S.; 717 Coxwell Ave., Toronto, Ont.; 21 Rosedale Heights Dr. (res); Qns '36; FICS; GenSurg; Cons., Pension Commission, Sunnybrook DVA Hosp.; O.P.D., Surg., Toronto East Gen. & Scarborough Gen. Hosp's.; Court. Staff Grace Hosp.; Tel. HO 5-2272.
DAVIES, John W.; Dept. of National Health & Welfare, Brooke Claxton Bldg., Ottawa, Ont.; London (Eng.) '50; Med. Cons. (Epidem.), Dept. of National Health & Welfare; Tel. CE 2-8211.
DAVIES, Kenneth J.; 5479 Greenleaf Rd., West Vancouver, B.C. (res); Man'54; Psy; Dir., Mental Health Centre, Burnaby; Ass't. Prof. (Psy.), U. of British Columbia.
DAVIES, L. E. Charles; Canadian Immigration Bldg., Burrard St., Vancouver 1, B.C.; Oxford (Eng.)'39; MRCS; LRCP; MA(Oxon.).
DAVIES, Lewis E. C.; 11319 Groat Rd., Edmonton, Alta.; Oxford (Eng.) '39; MRCS; LRCP; M.A. (Oxon.); Zone Supt., Northern Alberta, c/o Indian Health Services, Dept. of National Health & Welfare.
DAVIES, Leonard S.; 99 Avenue Rd., Toronto 5, Ont.; 11 Park Lane Circle, Tor. (res); Tor'44; F.R.C.S.(C), OrthSurg; OrthSurg., New Mt. **Sinai, Scarborough Gen. & Toronto Gen Hosp's.;** Tel. WA 1-8443.
DAVIES, Lois E.; 829 W. Broadway, Vancouver, B.C.; Tor '46; **Anaes; Staff, Vancouver Gen.** Hosp.; Clin. Instr. **(Anaes), U. of British Columbia; Tel. TR 6-3211.**
DAVIES, Nans E.; Medical Arts Clinic, Regina, Sask.; Alb '54; Abroad.
DAVIES, Richard O.; 145 Cresswell St., Beaconsfield, P.Q.; Tor'62; B.Sc. (Pharm); M.A.; Ph.D.; Clin. Pharm., Montreal Gen. Hosp.; Ass't. Med. Dir., Ayerst Laboratories Ltd.
DAVIES W. Fred A.; 267 O'Connor St., Ottawa 4, Ont.; 469 Piccadilly Ave., Ott. 3 (res); McG **'42; Staff, Ottawa Civic & Grace Hosp's.; Tel.** 232-2655.

DAVIGNON, Andre; 3175 Chemin St. Catherine, Montreal 26, P.Q.; Mon'54; Cardiol (P.Q.); Paed; Chief of Hemodynamique Lab., Hop. Ste Justine; Teach. Staff, (Paed.), U. of Montreal; Tel. RE 1-4931.

DAVIS, Albert J.; Medical Centre, West Street, Corner Brook, Nfld.; Dal'55; Paed; Hd. Dept. of Paed., Western Mem. Hosp.; Tel. 634-7476.
DAVIS, Bernard A.; 5845 Cote des Neiges Rd., Montreal 26, P.Q.; McG'53; FACOG; FRCS(C), ObstGyn; Att'd. Staff, Jewish Gen. Hosp.; Tel. 735-3122.
DAVIS, Claytus J.; 4027 E. **Hastings** St., North **Burnaby, B.C. UBC '60.**
DAVIS, Colmer B.; 19 Geneva Ct., Brockville, Ont.; Qns '34.
DAVIS, Eli R.; 96 Coburg St., Saint John, N.B.; **Dal '42; Anaes; Dir. of Med. Educ., Saint John Gen. Hosp., Staff, St. Joseph's Hosp.; Tel. 692-6658.**
DAVIS, F. Andrews; McG'63; Res., Shaughnessy Hosp., Vancouver 9, B.C.
DAVIS, F. H.; 292 St. Clair Ave. W., Toronto, Ont.; Tor '43; Psy.
DAVIS, Frederick G.; Main St., Sundridge, Ont.; Tor '14.
DAVIS, G. Albert; 12 Belsize Dr., Toronto, Ont.; 9 Hycrest Ave., Willowdale (res); Tor '16; Paed.; Tel. HU 9-1520
DAVIS, G. E. Donald; 217 St. Clair Ave. W., Toronto 7, Ont.; 152 Forest Hill Rd. (res); Tor '50; D.Psy; Psy; Staff, O.P.D., Toronto Western Hosp.; Tel. WA 1-3231.

DAVIS, George W.; Sydenham, Ont.; Qns '33.

DAVIS, Gerald E.; 1090 Ridgewood Dr., Halifax, N.S. (res); Dal'49; DiagRad; Assoc. Rad., Victoria Gen. Hosp.; Assoc. Prof. (Rad.), Dalhousie U.; Tel. 422-7371.
DAVIS, Henry R.; 1313 Fairmont Medical Bldg., 750 W. Broadway, Vancouver 9, B.C.; 4645 W. 9th Ave., Vancouver 8 (res); McG '28; Vis. Staff, **Vancouver Gen., St. Paul's & Grace Hosp's.; Tel.** TR 6-2717.
DAVIS, John F.; 498 Beaumont E., St. Bruno, Co. Chambly, P.Q.; McG '50.
DAVIS, Leonard; Box 486, Nanaimo, B.C.; UBC '62. Abroad.
DAVIS, Lyle A. Capt.; AMH(S), Currie Barracks, RCAMC, Calgary, Alta.; Sask'63; Tel. 242-1161, Loc. 593.
DAVIS, Marjorie I.; 321 Med. Arts Bldg., 170 St. George St., Toronto 5, Ont.; 5 Glen Edith Pl. (res; Tor'35; FRCS(C); GenSurg; Assoc. Chief of Surg., Women's College Hosp.; Assoc. Prof. (Surg.), U. of Toronto; Tel. WA 1-6843.
DAVIS, Matthew; Medical Arts Clinic, 51-6th St. S.E., Medicine Hat, Alta.; 9-1st St. S.W. (res); Alb '43; ObstGyn; Staff, Medicine Hat Mun. **Hosp.; Tel. 527-2281.**
DAVIS, Michael L.; River Pk. Med. Centre, 14th St. & 34th Ave. S.W., Calgary, Alta.; 3014-5A St. S.W. (res); St. Mary's Hosp., London U. (Eng.)'52; Assoc. (G.P. Dept.), Holy Cross & **Calgary Gen. Hosp's.; Tel. 243-0626.**
DAVIS, Murray M.; 1585 South Park St., Halifax, N.S.; **6452 Jubilee Rd. (res); Dal '44; FACS, FICS; FACOG; ObstGyn; Active Staff, Halifax Infirmary, Grace Maternity & Victoria Hosp's.; Clin. Instr., Dalhousie U.; Tel. 423-6640.**
DAVIS, M. William; Humboldt Clinic, Humboldt, Sask.; Cambridge (Eng.)'55; DA(Eng.); Tel. 682-2618.
DAVIS, Pamela M.; 44 Swordfish Dr., Shearwater, N.S.; London (Eng.) '60; Staff, Dept. of Health, Halifax, N.S.
DAVIS, Peter L.; McG '60; Ophth; Staff, Royal Victoria Hosp., Montreal, P.Q. Abroad.
DAVIS, Ray G.; 339 Professional Bldg., 10830 Jasper Ave., Edmonton, Alta.; Alb '52; FACS; FRCS(C), GenSurg; Surg. Staff, Royal Alexandra Hosp.; Instr. (Surg.), U. of Alberta, Tel. 422-2709.
DAVIS Richard N.; 3745 Southridge Ave., West Vancouver, B.C.; London (Eng.) '54; M.B., B.S.; DPM; Psy; Staff (Psy.), Childrens' Clinic, Mental Health Centre, Burnaby; Tel. 434-4247.
DAVIS, Robert E.; 72 Dominion Ave., Kapuskasing, Ont.; Tor '10.
DAVIS, Royden A.; Manitoba Clinic, 790 Sherbrook St., Winnipeg 2, Man.; 226 Oxford St., Wpg. 9 (res); King's College (Lond., England) '50; MRCS; LRCP; Derm; Ass't Derm., **Winnipeg Gen. Hosp.; Cons. (Derm.), Manitoba** Rehab. Hosp.; Lect. (Derm.), U. of Manitoba; Tel. SP 4-6541.
DAVIS, Ruth M.; 152 Forest Hill Rd., Toronto 7, Ont.; Tor '51.
DAVIS, Sidney; 418A Parliament St., Toronto 2, Ont.; 660 Eglinton Ave. W., Apt. 504 (res); Tor'53; MCGP; Staff, New Mt. Sinai, Wellesley & Doctors' Hosp's.; Tel. 924-6116.

DAVIS, Thomas G.; 130 Pine St., Gananoque, Ont.; Qns '39.
DAVIS, Thomas W.; 2828 Waterloo St., Vancouver 8, B.C. UBC '56; FRCP(C); IntMed; Staff, St. Paul's Hospital; Tel. MU 3-2311.
DAVIS, William J.; Box 1120, St. Mary's, Ont.; Wes '49; MCGP; Tel. 284-3450.
DAVIDSON, Barbara (See BIRKETT)
DAVISON, David L.; Linden Bldg., Wolfville, N.S.; Dal '52; Active Staff, Eastern Kings Mem. Hosp.; Tel. 542-3422.
DAVISON, Donald H.; Box 179, Orangeville, Ont.; McG '57; DPH; Staff, Dufferin Area Hosp.; Phys., McCord Corp., Tel. 941-3950.
DAVISON, Glen R.; 10945-89th Ave., Edmonton, Alta. (res); Qns '21; IntMed; Dir. Div. of TB Control (Alta.), Aberhart Mem. San.; Chest Cons., WCB; Chm. Silicosis Med. Bd.; Tel. GE 9-0051.
DAVISON, Roderick C.; 428 Med. Arts Bldg., 404 Graham St., Winnipeg 1, Man.; 60 Queenston St. (res); Man '50; Otol; Staff, Wpg., Gen., Grace, Misericordia, Children's Hosp's. & U. of Manitoba; Tel. WH 3-7760.
DAVISON, William E.; 1364 Islington Ave. N., Rexdale, Ont.; Tor '61; AMCGP; Staff, Humber Mem. Hosp.; Tel. 741-2020.
DAWE, Gerald A.; Medical Centre, Virgil, Ont.; Dal '47.
DAWE, Jean (See Griffin)
DAWKINS, Oswald S.; U.B.C. '57; FRCP(C), Anaes; Staff, Univ. Coll. Hosp. of W. Indies, Mona, St. Andrew, Jamaica, W.I.; Abroad.
DAWKINS, William A.; 1206 Freeman, Prince George, B.C.; London (Eng.) '54; Path.
DAWOSYR, Irene (Jaworowsky); 131 Ibbetson St., Port Arthur, Ont. (res); Innsbruck (Aust.) '48; Assoc. Pathol., St. Joseph's Gen. Hosp.; Tel. DI 4-2431.
DAWSON, Arthur D.; 7515 Cabrillo Ave., La Jolla, Calif.; McG '56; MRCP; FRCP(C); IntMed; Cardiol; Assoc. Staff, Scripps Clinic & Research Fdn., La Jolla; Abroad.
DAWSON, David T. P.; Alb'65; Res., Royal Alexandra Hosp., Edmonton, Alta.
DAWSON, Howard L.; Ste. 704, Medical Arts Bldg., 1538 Sherbrooke St. W., Montreal, P.Q.; 14 Bellevue Ave., Westmount (res); McG '21; GenSurg; Surg., Royal Victoria Hosp.; Retired.
DAWSON, John W.; Foothills Hosp., Calgary, Alta.; Tor'53; FRCP(C), IntMed; Dir. Dept. of Med., Foothills Hosp.; Tel. 283-0751.
DAWSON, Joseph C. C.; 64 Prince Arthur Ave., Toronto 5, Ont.; Tor '33; DRCOG; Obst; Registrar-Treas., College of Phys. & Surg. of Ont.; Exec. Comm., Med. Council of Canada; Tel. 924-2577.
DAWSON, K.; Chesley, Ont.; **Qns '26.**
DAWSON, Keith G.; Ste. 25, 1390 Sherbrooke St. W., Montreal 25, P.Q.; Columbia U. (New York, U.S.A.) '56; ABIM; FRCP(C), IntMed; Research Ass't. Royal Victoria Hosp.; Lect. (Med.), McGill U.; Industrial M.O., Twn. of Mount Royal; Tel. 845-4848.
DAWSON, L. E.; South River, Ont.; Tor '21.
DAWSON, Peter S.; 20 Lakeshore Dr., Morrisburg, Ont.; McG'64.
DAY, Albert; Ste. 4, 890 Blvd. Decarie, St. Laurent, P.Q.; 5385 Place d'Argenteuin, Cartierville (res); Mon '53; Staff, Hop. Notre Dame de l'Esperance, St. Laurent; Tel. RI 7-4771.
DAY, Clarence S.; 518 Med. Arts Bldg., 170 St. George St., Toronto 5, Ont.; **109 Dunvegan Rd. (res); Tor '32; FRCS, FACS; FRCS(C), GenSurg; Staff, St. Michael's Hosp.; Cons. Surg.,** Sunnybrook Hosp.; **Ass't. Prof. (Surg.), U. of Toronto; Tel. WA 2-7036.**
DAY, Edmund A.; 27 Cedar St. N., Timmins, Ont.; 184 Hemlock St. (res); Wes '20; Indus. Phys. & M.O., C.N.R.; Tel. AM 4-1234.
DAY, Edwin E.; 925 W. Georgia St., Vancouver 1, B.C.; 8515 Wiltshire St., Vancouver 14 (res); McG '24; D.L.O., Ophth, Otol; Cons., Vancouver Gen. Hosp.; Tel. MU 5-5943.
DAY, Frank E. H.; 1116 Barton St. E., Hamilton, Ont.; 66 London St. S. (res); Tor '36; O.P. Staff, (Obst.), Mt. Hamilton Hosp.
DAY, Frederick G.; 100 Medical Dental Bldg., Edmonton, Alta.; Helenslea Farm, Winterburn (res); Alb '42; M.Ch.Orth. (Liverpool), F.R.F.P.-S. (Glasgow), F.I.C.S., F.A.A.C.P., FRCS (Scot.); OrthSurg; Chief, Orth., Royal Alexandra Hosp.; Assoc. Staff, University Hosp.; Prov. Dir. for Cerebral Palsy; Lect. (OrthSurg), U. of Alberta; Tel. 424-1617.
DAY, Harrison G.; Verona, Ont.; Qns '56; Court. Staff, Kingston Gen. & Hotel-Dieu Hosp's., Kingston; Tel. 118.
DAY, J. Albert; 960 boul Ste-Croix, Montreal 9, P.Q.; 5385 Place D'Argenteuil (res); Man '53; Staff, Hop. de l'Esperance, St. Laurent.; Tel. 747-3501.
DAY, James H.;McG '59; Res., Kingston Gen. Hosp., Kingston, Ont.
DAY, John C.; 407 Professional Bldg., 10830 Jasper Ave., Edmonton, Alta.; 9119-118th St. (res); Alb '43; ObstGyn; Att'd. Staff, Royal Alexandria & Misericordia Hosp's.; Tel. 424-7423.
DAY, John J.; R.R. 3, Manotick, Ont. (res); McG'31; D.P.H.; Prof. Preventive Med., & Sec., Fac. of Med., U. of Ottawa; Tel. GE 5-6751, Ext. 296.
DAY, Ralph R. J.; Clarenville Nfld.; Dal '54; MCGP; Anaes., Come-by-Chance Hosp.; Att'd. Staff, University & Royal Alexandra Hosp's.; Instr. (ObstGyn.), U. of Alberta; Tel. GA 2-7221.
DAY, Richard A.; 10011-103rd St., Edmonton, Alta.; Tor '57; FRCS(C), ObstGyn; Tel. 424-1617.
DAY, Stacey B.; 1415 Sherwood Cr., Town of Mount Royal, Montreal P.Q.; Ire. '55; LRCP(I), LRCS(I); Ph.D. (Experim. Surg.); Prof. (Ex-perim. Surg.), McGill U.; Tel. RE 1-8832; Abroad.
DAYA, Fillmore; '55; Staff, Burin Cottage Hosp., Burin, Nfld.
DAYAL, Susheela; 5142 Patricia Ave., Montreal, P.Q.; Patna (India)'59; ObstGyn.
DAYAL, Vijay S.; Dept. of Otol., Royal Victoria Hosp., Montreal, P.Q.; Patna (India)'59; MSc (McG); DABOt; FRCS(C), Otol; Research Ass't., Otol. Inst., Royal Victoria Hosp. & McGill U.; Tel. VI 2-1251.
DAYAP, Felicisimo D.; Manilla (Philipp.) '57; Staff, Saskatchewan Hosp., North Battleford, Sask.; Tel. 445-2421.
DAYKIN, Charles E.; Carp, Ont.; McG '34; Tel. 839-2847.
DAZE, Fernand; 1824 Rachel Est., Montreal, P.Q.; Mon '29; IntMed (P.Q.); Staff, Hotel-Dieu; Tel. VI 4-0161.
DEACON, Alfred E.; 532 Medical Arts Bldg., Winnipeg, Man.; **353 Cambridge St. (res); Man '29; M.Sc., OrthSurg; Chief of Orth. Serv., Children's Hosp.; Assoc. Orth., Winnipeg Gen. Hosp.; Ass't. Chief Surg., Shriner's Hosp.; Ass't. Prof. (Orth.), U. of Manitoba; Tel. WH 2-2493.**
DEACON, Arthur S.; 172 Oakwood Ave., Toronto, Ont.; 17 St. Leonard's Ave. (res); Tor '43; Staff, O.P.D., St. Michael's Hosp.; Tel. LE 6-0880.
DEACON, Crosby B.; 1542 Westbrook Dr., Peterborough, Ont. (res); Tor '46; DABP; Paed; Derm; Staff, Peterborough Civic & St. Joseph's Hosp's.; Retired.
DEACON, John K.; Box 115, Westlock, Alta.; Durham (Eng.) '51; M.C.G.P.; Tel. 342-3341.
DEADMAN, Albert C.; 308 Med. Dental Bldg., 450 Central Ave., **London, Ont.; 536 Canterbury** Rd. (res); Wes '49; OrthSurg; **Instr. (Anat. &** Phys. Educ.), U. of **Western Ontario; Tel. GE** 8-3643.
DEADMAN, John C.; 185 Cottonwood Dr., Don Mills, Ont. (res); Tor '57; D.Psy; Psy; Staff, O.P.D. Lakeshore Psychiatric Hosp.; Tel. 365-1511.
DEAKIN, Barry; Box 730, Salmon Arm B.C.; Manchester (Eng.) '58; Tel. 832-2191.
DEAN, James F. B.; 322 Wellington St., Sarnia, Ont.; 850 Charlesworth Dr. (res); Man '51; M.C.G.P.

DEAN, John; 3195 Granville St., Vancouver, B.C.; 1320 Nanton Ave. (res); **Cambridge (Eng.) '42; MRCP (Lond.); Paed; Clin. Ass't. Prof. (Paed.), U. of British Columbia; Tel. 731-2155.**

DEAN, Thomas W.; 47 Cait Cres., Ancaster, Ont. (res); Tor '33; **D&TRad; Staff, Joseph Brant** Mem. Hosp., Burlington; Tel. 637-2361.

De ANDRADE, John R.; Bombay (India)'56; FRCS(C), OrthSurg; Staff, Sunnybrook Hosp., Toronto 12, Ont.

DEANE, Diane H. (Johnston); Ste. 320, 5780 Cambie St., Vancouver 15, B.C.; Manchester (Eng.) '62; Tel. FA 1- 8822.

DEANE, Lawrence S.; Ste. 110, 5780 Cambie St., Vancouver 15, B.C.; Manchester (Eng.)'53; D.ObstRCOG; MRCOG; FRCS(C), ObstGyn; Staff, Royal Columbian Hosp., New Westminster.

DEANE, William J.; 696 Waterloo St., Apt. C.; London, Ont. (res); Wes '48; ObstGyn; Staff, Victoria Hosp.; Tel. 432-5261.

de ARAGON, Jose M.; Madrid (Spain) '48; ACCP; Staff, Freeport San., Kitchener, Ont.; Tel. SH 5-4797.

DEBAS, Haile T.; McG '63; Int., Vancouver Gen. Hosp., Vancouver, B.C.

de BEAUPRE, Ernest J.; 659 Hamilton Rd., London, Ont.; 336 Ridout St. (res); Qns '15.

de BELLEFEUILLE, Paul; 65 rue Bruyere Ottawa 2, Ont.; Mon '47; FRCP(C) Paed; Form. Ass't. Paed. (Paris, France); Staff, Ottawa Gen., Ottawa Civic, Grace & Riverside Hosp's.; Cons. Paed., Hop. Saint-Coeur-de-Marie, Hawkesbury, Ont.; Assoc. Prof. (Paed.), U. of Ottawa; Tel. 236-1333

DEBENHAM, Guy P.; Thorold Med Clinic, 60 Albert W., Thorold, Ont.; Edinburgh (Scot.) '45; FRCS (Eng.); FRCS(C), GenSurg.; Tel. 227-5525.

DEBENHAM, Patrick A.; Box 818, New Westminster, B.C.; Ste. 401, 411 Agnes St. (res); Middlesex H. (London, Eng.)'57; Anaes; Cons. Anaes., Royal Columbian Hosp.; Tel. LA 2-4241.

DeBERA, Vladimir; 312 Bathurst St., Toronto 2B, Ont.; Tel. EM 4-8532.

deBLOIS, Pierre; 802 Chanoine-Scott, Quebec 10, P.Q.; 482 Robertson, Ville St-Laurent (res); Lav '55; Otol (P.Q.); Tel. 681-3162.

De BOISSIERE, Vernon R.; Ste. 112, 520-17th St., West Vancouver, B.C.; Guys Hosp. (London, Eng.) '23; FICS; LRCP; MRCS; Otol; Cons. Staff, Lions Gate Hosp., West Vancouver & North Vancouver; Tel. 922-4525.

DEBOW, S. Lawrence; Tor'64; Res., Douglas Hosp., Montreal, P.Q.

de BUDA, Yvonne E. G. (KOWARIK); 276 Runnymede Rd., Toronto 9, Ont.; Vienna (Aust.) '48; MCGP; Active Staff, Women's College Hosp.; Tel. RO 2-4498.

De CANDOLE, Corry A.; R.R. 2, Qualicum Beach, B.C.; **Cambridge (Eng.)'30;** MRCS(Eng.); MRCP(Lond); Retired.

DECARIE, John O.; 598 Montreal St., Sherbrooke, P.Q.; Ott '58; ObstGyn. (P.Q.); Assoc. Staff, Sherbrooke Hosp.; **Tel. 567-2555.**

DECARIE, Leandre; 55 Ave. de l'Eglise, Verdun, Montreal 19, P.Q.; 5383 Grovehill Pl. (res); Mon '51; F.R.C.P.(C), IntMed; Cardiol (P.Q.); Ass't. **Med. & Cardiol., Verdun Gen. Hosp.; Tel. 766-8511.**

DECARIE, Michel; Mon'60; 11282 De Saint Real, Montreal 12, P.Q.; NeurSurg(P.Q.).

DECARIE, Pierre A.; 3871 est, rue Belanger, Montreal 36, P.Q.; Lille (France) '62.

DECARIE, Roland; 524 est, Sherbrooke, Montreal, P.Q.; Mon '30; GenSurg; Ass't. Surg. Clin., U. of Montreal & Hop. Notre-Dame; Tel. VI 4-1355.

DE CARVALHO, Luis M.; Lisbon (Portugal) '56; Res., Hamilton Gen. Hosp., Hamilton, Ont.

DE CARVALHO, Roberto M.; Brazil '59; Res., Ottawa Civic Hosp., Ottawa, Ont.

DECARY, Charles; 1229 Notre-Dame, Lachine, P.Q.; 4801 St-Joseph (res); Mon '40; IntMed **(P.Q.); Chief (Med.), Hop. St. Joseph; Tel. 637-7284.**

DECARY Paul; 2852 blvd. St. Joseph, Montreal, P.Q. (res); Mon '23; Anaes. (P.Q.); **Psy; Anaes., Hop. St. Jean de Dieu; Tel. CL 4-5361.**

de CHARETTE, Benoit; 186 Bonaventure, Trois-Rivieres, P.Q.; 2323 Blvd. Laviolette (res); Lav **'39; M.C.G.P.; Staff, Hop. St-Joseph; Tel. FR 4-6211.**

De CHARETTE, Louis G.; Pointe du Lac, P.Q.; Lav'27; Gyn(France); Tel. FR 4-1500.

DECHENE, Euclide; 314 du Roi, Quebec, P.Q.; 871 Ave., **Moncton (res); Lav '37; FAAP; Paed; Chief of Paed. Serv., Hop.-St.-Francois-d'Assise; Chief of Clin., St.-Vincent-de-Paul Creche; Assoc. Prof. (Paed), Laval U.; Tel. 525-7825.**

DECHENE, Jean-Paul; 828 ave de la Colline, Ste. Foy, P.Q. (res); Lav '48; Anaes; Chief Anaes., Hop. Laval & Assoc. Prof. (Anaes.), U. of Laval; Tel. 653-3875 .

DECHERT, Kenneth I.; Tor'53; Chief Res., Hamilton Civic Hosp., Hamilton, Ont.

DECK, John H.; Tor'56; Path; Staff, Toronto Gen. Hosp., Toronto, Ont.

DECK, Josephine; St. Clair-Dufferin Med. Centre, 1268 St. Clair W., Toronto 10, Ont.; Liverpool (Eng.) '62; Tel. LE 6-2128.

DECOSSE, Roland F.; St. Paul, Alta.; **Man '46; FRCS(C), Orth Surg; Dist. Coroner; Tel. 645-3311.**

De COUTERE, Ivan A. A.; Guidance Clinic, 11120-102nd St., Edmonton, Alta.; London (Eng.)'57; DTM&H; Psy; Tel. GA 4-0571.

de CSILLERY, Andre; 260 rue Lefebvre, Drummondville Ouest, P.Q.; Budapest (Hung.) '08; Retired.

DECTER, Oscar; 416 Souris, Weyburn, Sask.; Man '46.

DECTER, P.H.; Manitoba Clinic, Sherbrook Ave., Winnipeg, Man. 234 Elm St. **(res); Man '42;** F.R.C.S(E) **& (C), OrthSurg; Lect. (Anat.), U. of Manitoba; Tel. SP 4-6541.**

de DOMENICO, Ivan J.; 327 Dorval Ave., Ste. 16, Dorval, P.Q.; Royal U. (Malta)'52; DABU; FACS; FRCS(C), Urol; **Dir.,** Dept. of Urol., Montreal Children's Hosp.; Urol., Lakeshore Gen. & Lachine Gen. Hosp's.; Tel. 453-3748.

DEEGAN, Francis K.; 51 King St. E., Brock-ville, Ont.; Ott'55; FACS; GenSurg; Chief Surg., Brockville Gen. Hosp.; Cons. Staff, St. Vincent de Paul Hosp.; Cons. Staff, (Active), Kemptville & Dist. Hosp.; Tel. 342-2231.

DEEP, Albert R.; Qns '59; FRCP(C), IntMed; Fell. (Cardiol.), Montreal Gen. Hosp., Montreal 25, P.Q. Abroad.

DEETH, John H.; 5052 Dundas St. W., Islington, Toronto 18, Ont.; Tor '33; M.C.G.P.; Assoc. Staff, St. Joseph's & Queensway Gen. Hosp's.; Tel. BE 1-0411.

DEFILLO, Mariano; Santo Domingo '58; **Jr.** Intn., Ottawa Gen. Hosp., Ottawa, Ont.

DE FREITAS, Andre; Apt. 10, 33 Ocean Court, Lancaster, N.B.; Lisbon (Portugal)'55.

DEFRIES, Robert D., C.B.E; 186 Dawlish Ave., Toronto 12, Ont.; Tor '11; DPH; PH; Bact; Dir., Emer. & Cons., Connaught Med. Research Labs.; Retired.

De GRACE Marc; 360 L'Ange Gardien, L'Assomp-tion, P.Q.; Mon '59.

de GRANDPRE, Lorenzo; 128 Nicholson, Valleyfield, P.Q.; 209 Salaberry (res); Mon'28; Staff, Hotel-Dieu Hosp.; Tel. 373-4422.

de GRANDPRE, Romeo; 10690 Ave. d'Auteuil, **Montreal 12, P.Q.; Mon '47; Ph.D.; Dir. Inst. d'Endocrin. et Gerontologie Inc.; Tel. DU 1-6291.**

De GROOT, Genevieve; Mon'62; Res., (PlasSurg.), Hotel-Dieu, Montreal, P.Q.

De GROOT, Jean A.; Mon'65; Intern. c/o Apt. 17, 5255 Cote St-Luc, Montreal 28, P.Q.

DE GROOT, Lambertus C.; Amsterdam (Neth.) '59; Paed; Staff, Vancouver Gen. Hosp., Vancouver 9, B.C.

DeGROOT, Walter P.; 13620 Grosvenor Rd., North Surrey, B.C.; Amsterdam (Neth.) '59.

DE GROSBOIS, Paul S.; Ott '52; DPH; Admin., North Bay Health Unit, 1850 Cassells St., North Bay, Ont.; Tel. 474-1400.

de GUISE, Clement; Apt. 79, 3525 Durocher, Montreal 18, P.Q.; Mon '25; M.P.H., PH **(Johns** Hopkins); Chief M.O., N.D.G. Dist., Montreal Dept. of Health; Tel. VI 9-3460.

de HAAS, William G.; 603 Medical Centre, 906-8th Ave. S.W., Calgary, Alta.; Pretoria (S. Africa) '50; FRCS (Edin.), FRCS(C), OrthSurg; Cons. OrthSurg., Calgary Gen., Holy Cross & Alberta Children's Hosp's.; Tel. 266-5931.
DEHNEL, M. K.; 2936 McCallum Ave., Regina, Sask. (res); Poland '34; Regional M.O.H., Regina.
DE HOSTOS, Gustav A.; 14 rue Elgin, Quebec 4, P.Q.; Mon'44.
DEINUM, E. Jeanne; 284 Sunset Dr., St. Thomas, Ont. (res); Wes '55; D.Psy; FRCP(C), Psy; Staff, Ont. Hosp., London, Ont.; Tel. 455-5110.
DEITCHER, Joseph; Apt. 204, Widdicombe Hill, Weston, Ont.; UBC'62.
DeJAIFFE, Guy S.; Louvain (Belgium)'59; Psy; Staff, Hop. St-Jean-de-Dieu, Montreal, P.Q.
De JONG, Bernard P.; Medical Clinic, 4794A Joyce Ave., Powell River, B.C.; UBC '57; Tel. HU 5-6261; Abroad.
De JONG, David; Ste. 101, 4643, Sherbrooke St. W., **Westmount, Montreal 6, P.Q.; 361 Roslyn Ave., Westmount (res); McG '50; M.R.C.P., F.R.C.P.(C), IntMed; Tel. 935-6007.**
de JONG, Pieter; 533 Brant St., Burlington, Ont.; Leiden (Neth.) '50; Tel. 637-3522.
de JONGH, Herman J.; 11208-70th Ave., Edmonton, Alta.; Amsterdam (Neth.)'47; Anaes; Court. Staff, Royal Alexandra Hosp.; Tel. 434-2733.
DEKABAN, Anatole S.; Warsaw (Poland) '41; Neur; Staff, **Shaughnessy (DVA), Vancouver, B.C.; Tel. TR 6-6767.**
DEKANY, Eva (Csont): 300 King St., Oshawa, Ont.; Budapest (Hung.) '53; Ophth; Staff, Oshawa Gen. Hosp.; Tel. 723-9101.
de KENEDY, Geyza L.; Prince Albert Clinic, 49-13th St. W., Prince Albert, Sask.; 565-20th St. W. (res); Franz Joseph (Szeged, Hung.) '38; FRCS(H); FICS; Urol; Staff, Victoria Union & Holy Family Hosp's.; Tel. 764-4241.
DEKKER, A. Albert; 350 Albert St., Nanaimo, B.C.; **30 Prideaux (res); Groningen (Neth.) '49.**
DeKOVEN, Maurice J.; 706 Commercial Bldg., **169 Pioneer Ave., Winnipeg 1, Man.; Man '33; FRSH; DPH (Tor.); Reg. M.O., Dept. of National Health & Welfare & Civic Aviation Med.;** Tel. 489-8875.
DeKOVEN, Percy; 396 Francis Rd., Richmond, B.C.; 726 Gilhurst Cres. (res); Man '52; MCGP; Tel. BR 7-7166.
DE LA BASTIDE, Yves H.; Nat. Defence Med. Centre, Alta Vista Dr., Ottawa, Ont.; London (Eng.) '52; LRCP (Lond.); MRCS (Eng.); Otol; Chief Otol., NDMC; Tel. RE 3-6600, Loc. 251.
De La BOISSIERE, Gaston; Lav '56; MCGP; Res., Maisonneuve Hosp., Montreal 36, P.Q
DELAGE, Claude; Lav'65; Res., Hop. L'Enfant-Jesus, Quebec 3, P.Q.
DELAGE, Jean; Lav '48; Psy; Dir., Social Medical Centre for Children, 898 Richelieu, Quebec 4, P.Q.; Assoc. Prof. (Psy.), Laval U.
DELAGE, Jean-M.; 895 Dessane, Quebec, P.Q. (res); Lav '46; Haem (P.Q.); FRCP(C), IntMed; Haem., Hop-St.-Sacrament; Cons. Haem., Hotel Dieu & Ste-Foy DVA Hop.; Assoc. Prof. (IntMed), Laval U.; Tel. LA 9-4511.
DELAGE, Marc; 180 Notre Dame N., Thetford Mines, P.Q.; Lav '46; GenSurg (P.Q.); Tel. 335-5382.
DELAGE, Maurice; Centre des Readaption, 854 ave Bellevue, Quebec 10, P.Q.; Lav'42; PhysMed; Staff, Hotel-Dieu; Ass't. Prof., Laval U.; Tel. LA 9-4511.
DELAHAY, J. Reginald; Medical Arts Bldg., Ottawa, Ont.; 379 Huron Ave. (res); McG '25; **D.L.O., Otol; Sr. Otol., Ottawa Civic Hosp.; Tel. PA 9-2511.**
DELAHAYE, Donald J.; Etherington Hall, Queen's University, Kingston, Ont.; Qns'50; Paed; Ass't Prof., Dept. of Paed., Queen's University; Tel. 542-8074.
DELAHAYE, John S.; 305 King St. W., Kingston, Ont.; Qns '27; Paed; Med. Referee, Empire Life Ins. Co.; Tel. 548-7525.
DELAHUNT, J. Austin; 6086 Quinpool Rd., Halifax, N.S.; 5894 Rogers Dr. (res); **Dal'53;** AMCGP; Tel. 423-7400.
DELAHUNTY, James M.; Medical Centre, West St., Corner Brook, Nfld.; National U. (Ire.)'59.
DELAMERE, Peter M.; Medical Dental Bldg., 112 Mathison St. S., Kenora, Ont.; Qns'59; MCGP; Tel. 648-6423.
DELANEY F. George; Box 274, Balmertown, Ont.; Lav '51
DELANEY, J. A.; 78 Botsford St. Moncton, N.B.; Mon '43; ObstGyn.; Tel. EV 2-8167.
DELANEY, Robert J.; Medical Arts Bldg., 121 Wellington St. W., Barrie, Ont.; Tor '44; FACS; FRCS(C), GenSurg; Chief of Surg., Royal Victoria Hosp.; Tel. 728-5909.
DELANEY, Thomas F.; 622 Somerset St. W., Ottawa, Ont.; Qns '15.
DELANEY, William L.; 30 Des Jardins, Quebec, P.Q.; McG '42; Staff, Jeffrey Hale's Hosp.; Tel. 683-4471.
DELAQUERRIERE, Liliane; 1251 Saint-Marc, Apt. 24, Montreal 25, P.Q.; Mon '57.
DELAQUIS, Hubert; Notre Dame de Lourdes, Man.; Mon **'47; Dist. Coroner.**
DELAQUIS, Roger; 960 Boul Ste. Croix, Montreal, P.Q.; Mon'53.
de la RIVA, Ricardo; 115 Cedar St., Sudbury, Ont.; Valladolid (Spain) '54; Tel. 675-2712.
DELARUE, Norman C.; 530 Medical Arts Bldg., 170 St. George St., Toronto 5, Ont.; 25 Donlea Dr., Toronto 17 (res); Tor '39; M.S. (Tor.), F.A.C.S., F.C.C.P., F.R.C.S.(C), GenSurg, ThorSurg; Surg., Toronto Gen. Hosp.; Sr. **Cons.** (ThorSurg), Toronto Hosp. for TB, Weston; **Sr.** Cons. Surg. (Cancer of Breast & Lung), Ontario Cancer Inst., Princess Margaret Hosp.; **Cons.** Surg., Toronto Psychiatric Hosp.; Cons. (Chest Surg.), Women's College Hosp.; Cons. (ThorSurg), Niagara Penin. San. Assoc., St. Catharines; **Ass't.** Prof. (Surg.), U. of Toronto; Tel. WA 2-8444.
de LAUNIERE, Henri; 914 des Erables, Quebec 6, P.Q.; Lav '60; **Tel. 527-0187.**
de LEEUW, Nannie K. M.; 3610 McTavish St., Apt. 12, Montreal, P.Q. (res); Ryks U. (Leiden, Neth.)'45; M.Sc. (Exp.Med.); Haem.(P.Q.); IntMed (Haem.); Clin. Ass't., Royal Victoria Hosp.; Ass't. Prof. (Med.), McGill U.; Tel. VI 2-1251, Loc. 1636.
DE LEON-LAURENZA, Alberto; McG'64; Res., Royal Victoria Hosp., Montreal 2, P.Q.
DELGADO, Alfonso; Colombia (S. America)'62; Staff, Universite Laval, Quebec, P.Q.
DELISLE, Andree E.; 11824 Alexandre-Lacoste, Montreal 12, P.Q.; Lav '59; Anaes (P.Q.); Pt-time Staff, Hop. St-Joseph de Rosemont; Tel. 334-2891.
DELISLE, Georges; Lav'65; Res. Hop. de l'Enfant Jesus, Quebec 3, P.Q.
DELISLE, J. Claude; 1500-18e rue, Quebec 3, **P.Q.; 1215 de Luxemborg (res); Lav '49.**
DELISLE, Michel; Res. Hosp. for Sick Children, **Toronto 2, Ont.; Lav '63.**
DELISLE, Remi; 541 rue de l'Hopital, Jonquiere, P.Q.; 635 rue Pasteur (res); Lav '50; IntMed; Chief of Med., Hop. Jonquiere; Tel. 547-9341.
DELORME, Alexandre; St. Isidore Laprairie, P.Q.; Mon '34; Tel. 454-9922.
DELORME, Fernand; 113, Boul.-Ste-Anne, Ste-Anne-des-Plaines, Cte. Terrebonne, P.Q.; Mon '62; Tel. 435-2673.
DELMORE, Pierre J.; Ste. 217, 3875 rue St-Urbain, Montreal 18 P.Q.; 12169 James-Morrice (res); Mon '56; M.Sc.; FRCP(C); IntMed; Allerg (P.Q.); Staff, Hotel-Dieu; Ass't. Prof., U. of Montreal; Tel. 288-1652.
DELORY, Maurice E.; Hillcrest Clinic, Bridgewater, N.S.; Dal '55; GenSurg.
de Los SANTOS, Justiniano M.; Beechy, Sask. Manila (Philipp.) '59.
DELPORTE, Gabriel A. D.; 4251 rue St.-Hubert, Montreal 34, P.Q.; Lav '11; Staff, Queen Elizabeth Hosp.; Tel. 524-1222.
DEL ROSARIO, Pedro G.; Box 39, Saskatchewan Hosp., North Battleford, Sask.; Santo Tomas (Manila) '56; Tel. 5-2421.
DELVA, Pierre L.; London (Eng.) '48; Paed; Staff, Dept. of PrevMed., Queen's U., Kingston, Ont.

del VALLE, Ramon; 314-8th St. S., Lethbridge, Alta.; Madrid (Spain)'55; Med. Staff, Lethbridge Mun. & St. Michael's Hosp's.; Tel. 328-4941.

DELVECCHIO, Marc; 294 Carre St. Louis, Montreal, P.Q.; 617 Rockland (res); Mon '39; Diag-Rad; Tel. 279-9049.

DEMANUELE, Frederick; 2936 Dundas St. W., Toronto 9, Ont.; 228 St. Marks Rd. (res); Malta '55; Tel. RO 2-6631.

de MARGERIE, Jean-Marie; Lav'52; D.Phil. (Oxon.); FRCS(C), Ophth; Staff, Centre Hosp. U., Sherbrooke, P.Q.

De MARCO, Frank F.; 929 Wyandotte St. E., Windsor, Ont.; Wes '43; MCGP; Chief, Dept. of G.P., Hotel-Dieu Hosp.; Tel. 253-9116.

De MARIA, F. John; Dept. of ObstGyn., Vancouver Gen. Hosp., Vancouver, B.C.; Malta'52; MRCOG; FACOG; FRCS(C), ObstGyn; Cons. Gyn., Vancouver Gen. Hosp.; Ass't. Prof. U. of British Columbia; Tel. TR 6-3211, Ext. 2588.

DEMAY, Maurice; Lav '41; M.H.A.(A.P.A.), Psy; Supt., Saskatchewan Hosp., North Battleford, Sask.; Vis. Cons., University Hosp., Saskatoon; Tel. 445-2421.

DEMARY, Robert F.; 751 King St. W., Kitchener, Ont.; Tor'41; MCGP; Tel. 742-0423.

DEMERS, Antonio; 32 Boul. St.-Joseph Ouest, Montreal, P.Q.; 6801 Boul. Pie IX (res); Lav '43; Ophth; Staff (Ophth), Hotel-Dieu; Ass't. Prof. (Ophth), U. of Montreal; Tel. AV 8-4873.

DEMERS, Francois X.; 234 St.-Jean, Quebec 4, P.Q.; Lav '33; FACS; FACOG; Obst-Gyn; Chief, Dept. ObstGyn., Hop.-de-l'Enfant-Jesus; Prof. (Gyn), Laval U.; Tel. LA 5-7782.

DEMERS, Gaston; Lav'60; Res., Hop. L'Enfant Jesus, Quebec 3, P.Q.

DEMERS, Gerald; 9A Commercial, Roxboro, P.Q.; 4825 Millette, **Pierrefonds (res); Mon '61.**

DEMERS, Jacques, Capt.; Fort Garry Horse MIR, Sarcee Barracks, Calgary, Alta.; Lav'65.

DEMERS, Jacques; Lav '64; Res., Hop. Hotel-Dieu, Quebec, P.Q.

DEMERS, Jean-P.; 30 est, boul. St-Joseph, Montreal 14, P.Q.; Mon '58; Ophth; Tel. 845-4241.

DEMERS, Jocelyn; Mon'65; Res., Hop. St. Vincent de Paul, Sherbrooke, P.Q.

DEMERS, Leon; Ste. 202, 825 sud, Belevedere, Sherbrooke, P.Q.; Lav '53; FACS; FICS; FICA; FRCS(C), GenSurg; Tel. 562-4521.

DEMERS, Louis P.; 260 Ball St., Sherbrooke, P.Q.; 120 Vimy N., Apt. No. 8 (res); Mon '33.

DEMERS, Marc A.; 192 Principale, Hull, P.Q.; Lav '50; ObstGyn; Tel. 777-9502.

DEMERS, Paul A.; 4453 Ste Catharine St. W., Montreal 6, P.Q.; Mon '39.

DEMERS, Paul-Eugène; 7045 ave. Fielding, Montreal 29, P.Q.; '60; Ophth(P.Q.).

DEMERS, Percy T.; 3225 Wyandotte St., Riverside, Ont.; 145 Homedale (res); Ott '55; IntMed; Tel. 948-3712.

DEMERS, Pierre P.; 1000 Chemin-Ste.-Foy, Quebec 6, P.Q.; 1764 Pl. Philippe (res); Lav '53; FRCP(C), Paed; Staff, Hop.-St.-Sacrement; Tel. LA 7-3461.

DEMERS, Roger; 303 Centre-Medical-St.-Urbain, 3875 St.-Urbain, Montreal 18, P.Q.; Mon '48; FRCP(C), IntMed; Cons. (IntMed.), Hotel-Dieu Hosp.; Tel. VI 4-0161.

DEMERS, Yvon; Lav '61; Res., Hop-du-St-Sacrement, Quebec, P.Q.

DEMIRSAR, Aydin; Istanbul (Turk)'50; Staff, Douglas Hosp., Verdun, P.Q.; Abroad.

DEMMER, Hans T.; Main St., Mount Forest, Ont.; Frankfort (Germ.)'48; Tel. 860.

DEMONE, Agnes W.; (See Threlkfeld, Agnes W.)

deMONTIGNY, J. L. Pol; 102 Med. Dental Bldg., 299 Main St., Chilliwack, B.C.; Ott '55; MCGP; Tel. 792-1722.

DEMONTIGNY, Pierre D.; 513 Ste-Cecile, Trois-Rivieres, P.Q.; Lav '65.

DEMPSEY, Ethel A. (Noble); P.O. Box 181, Belleville, Ont.; Tor '33; Anaes; Cons. Staff (Anaes.), Belleville Gen., Trenton Mem. & Prince Edward County Mem. Hosp's.; Staff, Lennox & Addington County Hosp's.; Tel. WO 8-7238.

DEMPSTER, George; 222 Poplar Cres., Saskatoon, Sask. (res); Edinburgh (Scot.) '40; M.D. (Bact.); MC(Path); Prof. & Head, Dept. of Bact., U. of Saskatchewan; Dir. of Bact., University Hosp.; Tel. CH 2-7641.

DENEKA (Platt), Shirley I.; Alb'58; Res., Victoria Hosp., London, Ont.

DENFIELD, Avery S.; 49 Sanders Blvd., Hamilton, Ont.; London (Eng.) '59; MRCS; LRCP; Dip. Child Health (Eng.); Tel. JA 8-0136.

DENHEZ, Julien; 4207 Old Orchard, Montreal, P.Q. (res); Mon '53; PH (P.Q.); DPH; Adm. Health Serv., & Prof., Schl. of Hygiene, U. of Montreal; Tel. RE 3-9951.

DENHOLM, Kenneth A.; 11 James Street, Parry Sound, Ont.; Qns'15; Tel. 746-2139.

DENIS, Bernard; 21 Ave. Ste.-Genevieve, Berthierville, Cte. Berthier, P.Q.; Mon '62.

DENIS, Claude; St. Raymond, Cte. Portneuf, P.Q.; **Lav '56.**

DENIS, Gustave; Ott '58; Ass't. Prof., Dept. of Physiol., U. of Montreal, Montreal, P.Q.; Tel. RE 3-9951.

DENIS, Jean; 3447 St. Hubert, Montreal, **P.Q.; 901 Canora Rd. (res); Mon '38; All. (P.Q.), IntMed (P.Q.); Chief Serv. (All.), Ste. Justine Hosp.; Cons. St. Jeanne d'Arc, & Notre Dame de L'Esperance Hosp's.; Dem. (Bact.), U. of Montreal; Tel. RE 1-4931.**

DENIS, J. P. Rosario; 5625 Ave.-des-Chenes, Montreal 36, P.Q.; (res); Lav '51; Anaes; Staff, Hop.-Notre-Dame; Tel. LA 5-6363.

DENIS, Marius; 9269 Berri St., Montreal 12, P.Q.; Mon '44; Tel. 388-7903.

DENISON, Archibald G.; 201 Medical Dental **Bldg., 450 Central Ave., London, Ont.; 234 Sherwood Ave. (res); Wes '34; D.C.H.(Eng.), F.A.-A.P., Paed; Ass't. Prof. of Paed., U. of Western Ontario; Tel. 439-5781.**

DENNE, A. John; Ste. 303, 111 Queen St. E., Toronto, Ont.; 15 Evergreen Gdns., Tor. 17 (res); Tor '41; DPH; Indust. Phys., MacLean Hunter **Publishing Co., Rolph Clark & Stone, Ltd., Texaco, & Cdn. Imperial Bank of Commerce; Tel. 368-1828.**

DENNE, Doris H.; 98½ Waverley Rd., Toronto, **Ont.; 242 Glen Manor Dr. (res); Tor '40; Tel. OX 4-3329.**

DENNERY, Jean M.; Ste. 303, 100 Gloucester St., Ottawa 4, Ont.; Haiti '56; FRCS(C); NeurSurg; Staff, Ottawa Gen. Hosp.; Cons. Staff, Ottawa Civic, St. Louis de Monfort, Sacre Coeur, Hull, & St. Vincent Hosp's.; Clin. Ass't. (NeurSurg.), Ottawa U.; Tel. 232-1549.

DENNERY, Mona L.; Haiti '56; FRCP(C), Path; Staff, Ottawa Civic Hosp., Ottawa, Ont.; Tel. 729-2511.

DENNEY, William S.; 548 Mohawk E., Hamilton, Ont.; Ott'55; Staff, Chedoke Gen. & **Children's** Hosp's.; Div. Surg., **St. John's Ambulance Brigade.**

DENNIS, Frederick T.; 187 Arthur St., Port Arthur, Ont.; 100 Summit Ave. (res); Tor '48; Anaes; Chief Anaes., Port Arthur Gen. & St. Joseph's Gen. Hosp's.; Tel. DI 4-6621.

DENNIS, John W.; Ste. 5, 6325 Fraser St., Vancouver 15, B.C.; Man'45; Anaes; Anaes. Staff, Burnaby Gen. Hosp., Burnaby; Tel. HE 4-4211.

DENNIS, Leslie R.; 1223 Sayers Rd., Clarkson, Ont.; London (Eng.)'50; DCH; DRCOG; Active Staff, Oakville-Trafalgar Mem. Hosp.; Tel. 822-0412.

DENNIS, Marion E. (Charlton); 404 Wortley Rd., London, Ont. (res); Wes '53; MCGP; Staff, Victoria & St. Joseph's Hosp's.; Staff (G.P.), Victoria Hosp., London.

DENNIS, Stephen M.; Ste. 903, 24 Queen St. E., Brampton, Ont.; Wes'63.

DENNIS, William F.; 537 Mountain Rd., Moncton, N.B.; Dal '61.

DENNISON, Alfred H.; Durham (Eng.) '54; M.B., B.S.; Med. Supt., Notre-Dame Bay Mem., Hosp., Twillingate, Nfld.; Tel. 2212.

DENNY, Douglas A.; 4900 Kingsway, South Burnaby, B.C.; 2540 Dunblane Ave. (res); Qns '53.

DENNY, Wilmer L.; 26 Alma St., London, Ont. (res); Wes '17; Paed; Retired.

DENONCOURT, J. Avila; 329 Laviolette St., Trois-Rivieres, P.Q.; Lav '28; GenSurg; **Orth-Surg; Chief, Dept. of Surg., Hop.-St.-Joseph; Assoc. Prof. Laval U.; Tel. FR 4-6211.**

DENSMORE, Lambert **D.;** 197 St. George St., **Bathurst, N.B.; Qns '01; GenSurg; Dist. Coroner; LI 6-4755.**

DENSON, Raymond; 1232 Elliott St., Saska-toon, Sask.; McG '56; FRCP(C), Psy; Sr. Psy., Sask. Dept. of Public Health; Clin. Instr., University Hosp.; Tel. 242-7641.

DENT, Lionel R.; 190 MacLaren St., Ottawa, Ont.; 297 Sherwood Dr. (res); Tor '42.

DENT, Orlo V.; 67 College St., Room 203, Toronto 2, Ont.; 2 Burnelin Dr., Islington (res); **Wes '33; IntMed (TB); Tel. BE 1-4860.**

DENT, Peter B.; Tor '60; Paed; Dept. of Paed., U. of Minn. Minneapolis, Minn, U.S.A.; Abroad.

DENTON-CARDEW, Roger; Cambridge & London (Eng.)'46; Res., Vancouver Gen. Hosp., Vancouver 9, B.C.

DENTON, Daphne F.; Bank of Montreal, Main Office, Calgary, Alta.; McG'53; Anaes.

DENTON, G. Douglas; 384 Main St., Wolfville, N.S.; 7 Chestnut Ave. (res); McG '45; IntMed; Active Staff, Eastern King's Mem. Hosp.; Cons. (IntMed), Payzant Mem. Hosp., Windsor, N.S., Blanchard-Fraser Mem. Hosp., Kentville, West King's Mem. Hosp., Berwich, N.S.; Tel. 542-3424.

DENTON, Ronald L.; 2300 Tupper St., Montreal, P.Q.; McG. '37 Haem (P.Q.); F.R.C.P.(C), Paed; Staff, Montreal Children's Hosp.; Assoc. Prof. of Paed., McGill U.; Tel. WE 7-8511.

d'ENTREMONT, Felicien; Anse St-Jean, Cte. Chicoutimi, P.Q.; Lav '64.

d'ENTREMONT, Philippe; 640 Chemin Mountain, Moncton, N.B.; 140 rue Church (res); Lav '44; FACS, GenSurg.; Tel. 384-7080.

DEOM, Pierre; Centre Psycho. Social, 412 boul. du Havre, Valleyfield, P.Q.; Mon '55; Psy.

D'EON, Benedict J.; Dept. of National Health & Welfare, c/o Regional Superintendent, European Region; Lav '43. Abroad.

DE PAPE, Albert D. J.; 243 Marion St., Norwood, Man.; 124 Lawndale (res); Man '48; F.R.-C.P.(C), Paed; Paed.-in-Chief, St. Boniface Hosp.; Att. Staff, Winnipeg Children's Hosp.; Ass't. Prof. (Paed.), U. of Manitoba; Tel. 233-3557.

DEPEW, John G.; Campbell River, B.C.; Alb '49.

DEPOCAS, Pierre; 8415 St. Denis, Montreal 11, P.Q.; France '54.

DEPOT, Rene; 191 boul. Ste-Rose, Ste-Rose-de-Laval, P.Q.; Mon '61; Tel. 625-0701.

DEPOW, C Wilfred; Woodstock Med. Clinic, Chapel St., Woodstock, N.B.; McG '47; GenSurg; Staff, Carleton Mem. Hosp.; Tel. 328-6403.

DERBACH, Bernard; 633 Lodge Ave., Winnipeg 12, Man.; 1 Bruce Ave. (res); Ott'52; MCGP.

DERBAWKA, Allen J.; Sask '60; Res., Royal Alexandra Hosp., Edmonton, Alta.

DERBY, A. Campbell; McG '41; FACS; FRCS(C); GenSurg; Surg-in-Chief, Queen Elizabeth Hosp., Montreal, P.Q.; Cons. Surg., Mtl. Gen. Hosp.; Tel. 488-2311, Ext. 395.

DERBY, James H.; McG '60; Res., Royal Victoria Hosp., Montreal 2, P.Q.

DERBYSHIRE, Wilfred; CD; 70 Princess St., Fort Erie, Ont.; Tor '26; FAGS; Staff Anaes., Douglas Mem. Hosp.; Tel. 416-871-5540.

DERECHIN, William; Porcupine Clinic, Box 490, Porcupine Plain, Sask; Man '52; Dist. Coroner.

DERJANECZ, Brenda; Alliston Clinic, 132 Victoria St. W., Alliston, Ont.; Sheffield (Eng.)'61.

DERJANECZ, John J.; Alliston Clinic, 132 Victoria St. W., Alliston, Ont.; Pecs (Hung.)'54; LRCP & LRCS (Edin.); LRFPS (Glas.); FRCS(C), GenSurg.

DERKSEN, Cornelius; 171 Donald St., Winnipeg 1, Man.; **Man '57; A.M.C.G.P.; Tel. ED 9-2658.**

deROCHE, James E.; Ste. 2, 8 George St. N., Galt, Ont.; Ott '58; Urol; Staff, South Waterloo Mem. Hosp., Galt; Tel. 621-0490.

DEROME, Albert; Unite Sanitaire, 18 Centre, Granby, P.Q.; Mon '35.

DEROME, Andre; 3875 St. Urbain P.Q.; 10773 Waverley (res); Mon '48; OrthSurg; Ass't., Hotel-Dieu, Montreal, & Hop. Sacre-Coeur, Cartierville; Cons. Hosp. St. Charles St. Hyacinthe; Tel. 524-1119.

DEROME, Armand; 4032, ave. Marcil, Montreal 28, P.Q.; Mon '24; IntMed.

DEROME, Gilles; 800 est, boul. St-Joseph, Montreal 34, P.Q.; Mon '53; ObstGyn; Staff, Hop. Ste-Jeanne d'Arc; Cons., Hop. Fleury & Hop. St. Michel; Tel. LA 6-5555.

DEROME, Leo; C.P. 579, Amos, P.Q.; 31-5th Ave. (res); Mon '54; Tel. 732-2911.

DEROME, Leon; Centre-Medical-St.-Urbain, 3875 rue St.-Urbain, Montreal 18, P.Q.; Mon '43; FRCP(C), IntMed; Tel. 849-6680.

de ROOS, Thomas; Ste. 125, 624-6th St. New Westminster, B.C.; Utrecht (Holland) '47; MCGP; Tel. 526-7871.

de ROOY, Gerrit; 8821-120th St. North Surrey, B.C.; Amsterdam (Neth.) '47; FCCP (Holland); Tel. 594-9812.

De ROSARIO, John Laurence O.; 1669 Victoria St., Prince George, B.C.; 59A Watrous St. (res); Madras (India) '47; FRCS(C); FRSACS (Hon.); GenSurg; Med. Staff, Prince George Regional Hosp.; Tel. LO 4-4411.

DERRY, C. Clifford; 55 Russell St., Madoc, Ontario; Qns'63; Coroner Hastings County; M.O.H., Twsps. of Limerick, Tudor & Cashel; Tel. 473-4236.

DERRY, David M.; 3575 University Ave., Apt. 415, Montreal, P.Q.; UBC'62.

DERY, Andre; 3545 Hochelaga, Montreal, P.Q.; **Mon '55; Tel. LA 3-5848.**

DERY, Leo; 912 Sherbrooke St. est, Montreal 24, P.Q.; Mon'52; ObstGyn(P.Q.).

DERY, Paul R.; 1535 rue Quebec, Chomedey, P.Q.; Lav '54.

DERY, Raynald; 1825 rue DesRoches, Quebec 3, P.Q.; Lav '58; FRCP(C), Anaes; Staff, Hotel-Dieu; Tel. 529-9151.

DERY, Talbot; Lav '55; Path(P.Q.); Staff, Hop. St-Sacrement, Quebec 6, P.Q.; Tel. LA 7-3461.

DESAI, Urmila R.; Dept. of National Health & Welfare, Tunney's Pasture, Ottawa 4, Ont.; Bombay (India)'54; M.Sc(Clin. Gyn.).

DE SAINT VICTOR, Henri R.; 222 Daly, Ottawa, Ont.; 217 River Rd., Ottawa 2 (res); Lav '33; ObstGyn; Prof. (Obst.), Fac. of Med., U. of Ottawa; Tel. 235-7131.

de SAINT-VICTOR, Jean; App. 1, 945 ave Juttre, Quebec, P.Q. 1218 Preston Ave., Sillery, P.Q.; Lav '35; ObstGyn; Assoc. Prof. (Obst.), Laval U.; Chief of Gyn. Clinic, Hop. St. Sacrement; Cons. (Obst. Gyn.), Hop. D.V.A., Quebec; Tel. 522-2998.

DESAULNIERS, Andre Gelinas (see GELINAS-DESAULNIERS)

DESAULNIERS, Rene L.; 3488 Laval Ave., **Montreal, P.Q.; Lav '18; IntMed; Tel. AV 8-2078.**

DESAULTELS, J. Leo; 245 Marion St., St. Boniface, Man.; 55 Victoria Cres., St. Vital (res); Ott '55; MCGP; Assoc. Staff, Misericordia Gen. Hosp.; Court. Staff, St. Boniface Gen. Hosp., Winnipeg; Tel. CH 7-4572.

DESAUTELS, Paul G.; Standon, Cte. Dorchester, P.Q.; Lav '51.

DESAUTELS, Sylvio; 239 Chemin Cote-Ste-Catherine, Montreal 8, P.Q.; 3812 Northcliffe (res); Mon '51; IntMed. (Cardiol.) (P.Q.); Tel. 272-5446.

DESBIENS, Andre; 229 boul St-Joseph, Roberval, P.Q.; Lav '63.

DESBIENS, Paul E.; Lav'65; Res., Hop. Hotel-Dieu St. Vallier, Chicoutimi, P.Q.

DESBIENS, Rene; Lav'65; Res., Hop. Hotel-Dieu, Montreal 18, P.Q.

DESBRISAY, Harold A.; 925 Georgia St. W., Vancouver, B.C.; 1208 W. 47th Ave. (res); McG '17; F.A.C.P., IntMed; Cons. Dept. Med., Vancouver Gen. Hosp.; Clin. Instr. (Med.), U. of **British Columbia; Tel. MU 1-2642; Abroad.**

DESBRISAY, William M.; Apt. 307, 229 Edmund St., Sudbury, Ont.; McG'53.

DESCARREAUX, Gregoire; Lav '34; Pulm. Dis. & TB (P.Q.); IntMed (TB); Staff, San Lac Edouard, Lac Edouard, P.Q.; Dist. Coroner.
DESCARREAUX, Jacques; 350 - 51st St. W.; Quebec 7, P.Q.; Lav'62.
DESCARRIES, Laurent; Mon'61; FRCP(C) Neur; Staff, Hop. Maisonneuve, Montreal 36, P.Q.
DESCARY, Lucien; 5662 Queen Mary Rd., Hampstead, Montreal 29, P.Q.; 45 Stirling (res); Mon '33.
DESCARY, Marie C.; Mon'65; Res., Hop. Notre-Dame, Montreal 24, P.Q.
DESCHAMBAULT, Jacques; 23 Ouest, Boul. Desjardins, Ste. Therese de Blainville, P.Q.; Mon '42.
DESCHAMPS, Rene; Mon '55; Res. St-Jean-de-Dieu, Montreal 5, P.Q.
DESCHENES, Aurele; Lav'62; Ophth; Staff, Hop. Hotel Dieu St. Vallier, Chicoutimi, P.Q.
DESCHENES, Jos. A.; 572 rue Dufferin, Sherbrooke, P.Q. (res); Lav '10; M.O.H., Dept of Health, Quebec; Tel. LA 4-8411.
DESCHENES, Luc; Lav '61; FRCS(C), GenSurg; Staff, Hop-du-St-Sacrement, Quebec, P.Q.; Tel. 681-7211.
DESCHENES, Lucien; 960 boul. Ste. Croix, Montreal 9, P.Q.; Mon'58; Paed; Staff, Hop. **Ste-Justine; Tel. RE 1-4931.**
DESCORMIERS, Antonio; App. 305, 4444 Sherbrooke St. Ouest, Montreal 6, P.Q.; Mon '24; Surg (Paris); GenSurg; Cons., W.C.B., P.Q.; Tel. 381-9211.
DESCOTEAUX, Wilfrid; 4474 ave de Lorimier, Montreal, P.Q.; Mon '22; Tel. LA 3-8689.
DE SERRES, Guy; Jacques Cartier Med. Clinic, 1926 St. Helene, Cite Jacques Cartier, P.Q.; 373 **De Lorraine, Longueuil (res); Mon '59.**
de SEVE, Alain; 843 Est. Blvd. Gouin, Montreal, P.Q.; Mon'34; Tel. DU 8-2202.
DESFORGES, Aime; 300 St. Louis Sq., Montreal, P.Q.; 5625 Darlington (res); Mon '28; Derm Syph; Tel. VI 9-9093.
DESGAGNES, J. R.; Baie St.-Paul, Cte. Charlevoix, **P.Q.; Lav '45.**
DESGROSEILLIERS, Irenee; 24 rue de-l'Eglise, Lacolle, P.Q.; Mon '63; Tel. CH 6-3900.
DESGROSEILLIERS, Jean P.; Ott'65; Res., Ottawa Gen. Hosp., Ottawa 2, Ont.
DESHAIES, Benoit; 230 ouest boul Gouin, Montreal 12, P.Q.; 11375 Meunier (res); Mon '55; GenSurg; Staff, Hop-St-Michel; Tel. RA 2-2571.
DESHAIES, Gaetan; Lav' 61; Res., Notre Dame Hosp., Montreal 24, P.Q.
DESHARNAIS, Benoit E.; Lav'60; Res., Mtl. Children's Hosp., Montreal 25, P.Q.
DESHAYE, Jean V.; 42 rue Champlain, St. Boniface, Man. (res); Lav '49; D.P.H.; Health Off. & Med. Dir. for Red River, Prov. Dept. of Health.
DESILETS, Roland G.; 1150 Blvd. St. Joseph, Montreal 34, P.Q.; 5095 rue Lacordaire (res); Mon '49; F.R.C.S.(C), GenSurg; Staff (Surg), **Hop. Maisonneuve; Ass't. Prof. Mtl. U.; Tel. LA 7-1241.**
DESJARDINS, Albert E.; 711 Cherrier, Montreal **24, P.Q.; 913 Cherrier (res); Mon '28; Urol; Chief of Serv. (Urol.), Hop. Ste. Jeanne d'Arc;** Tel. VI 2-5201.
DESJARDINS, Alex; 2816 Willowdale, Outremont, P.Q.; Lav'26.
DESJARDINS, Andre; 184 Iberville, Repentigny, P.Q.; Lav '62.
DESJARDINS, Andre; Mon'65; Res., Hop. Notre Dame, Montreal 24, P.Q.
DESJARDINS, Bernard; Clinique-Medicale-Belanger, 3871 Belanger E., **Montreal 36, P.Q.; Mon '58; MCGP; Tel. RA 9-5231.**
DESJARDINS, Claude; Petit-Rocher, N.B.; Lav '51.
DESJARDINS, Denis R.; 178 Laurier Ave. E., Ottawa 2, Ont.; Ott '55; FACS; FRCS(C), Orth-Surg; Active Staff, Ottawa Gen.; Cons. St. Vincent's Hosp.; Court. Staff, St.-Louis-Marie-de-Montfort Hosp.; Lect., U. of Ottawa; Tel. 236-0586.
DESJARDINS, Edouard L.; 138 rue Wellington, Hull, P.Q.; Mon '43.
DESJARDINS, Edouard; 279 ave de l'Epee, Outremont, P.Q. (res); Mon '22; FACS; FRCS (C); GenSurg; Ass't. Med. Dir., Hotel-Dieu Hosp.; Prof. (Surg.), U. of Montreal; Tel. VI 4-0161.
DESJARDINS, F. Rosaire; 29 rue Turgeon, Ste. Therese de Blainville, P.Q.; Mon'48; Tel. 435-7545.
DESJARDINS, Jacques; Mon'65; Res., Hop. Notre-Dame, Montreal 24, P.Q.
DESJARDINS, Jean G.; 3142 Marie-Guyard, Montreal 26, **P.Q.; Mon '56; FRCS(C), GenSurg;** Tel. 737-8040.
DESJARDINS, Jean-Pierre; Ott'64; Ass't. Res. (OrthSurg.), Ottawa Gen. Hosp., Ottawa, Ont.
DESJARDINS, O. E.; 336 Bonaventure, Trois-Rivieres, **P.Q.; Lav '04; Retired.**
DESJARDINS, Origene; 556 Lafontaine, Riviere du Loup, P.Q.; **Lav '51; Med. Staff & Teach.** Staff, Student Nurses, Hop. St. Joseph; Tel. 862-5201.
DESJARDINS, Paul; 4240 Powell, Montreal 9, P.Q.; Mon'61; ObstGyn.
DESJARDINS, Raoul; 6 Montcalm N., Candiac, Co. Laprairie, **P.Q.; Mon '58; Phys., Iroquois** Glass Co.
DESJARDINS, Rene; 16-231 eme Rue, St.-Georges Est, Beauce, P.Q.; Lac Poulin, Beauce (Res); Lav '41; Otol (P.Q.); Head, Dept. ORL Hotel-**Dieu Notre-Dame de Beauce & St. George Ouest; Tel. 228-4831.**
DESJARDINS, Roger B.; 8415 St. Denis, Montreal 11, P.Q.; 28 Hazelwood, Outremont (res); Mon **'48; Otol;** D.Ph., Tel. DU 1-5311.
DESJARDINS-McMILLAN, Helene; 128 Jasper Ave., Town of Mt. Royal, Montreal 16, P.Q.; McG '56; Clin. Ass't. Med., Royal Victoria Hosp.; Tel. RE 1-6961.
DESJARLAIS, Etienne; 1275 Laviolette, Trois Rivieres, P.Q.; Lav '57.
DESLAURIERS, Gabriel; 133 rue Messier, St-Hilaire Cte. Rouville, P.Q.; Mon '50; Ther-Rad.
DESLAURIERS, Jean-Jacques; 2701 Allard, Montreal 20, P.Q.; Mon '55; A.M.C.G.P.
DESLAURIERS, Joseph A.; 1251 Jean Talon, Montreal, P.Q.; Mon '18.
DESLAURIERS, S. Denis.; 834 Pitt St., Cornwall, Ont.; 1112-5th St. E.(res); Ott'60; AMCGP Tel. WE 3-4064.
DESLIPPE, Gaston; 250 Lavoie, Laprairie, P.Q.; Lav '42.
DESLIPPE, G. Wilfrid; Mon '63; Res., Hop. Hotel-Dieu, Montreal, P.Q.
DESLIPPE, Paul A.; 710, boul. Houde, St. Lambert, P.Q.; Mon '58; Anaes; Staff, Hop. Jean Talon.
DESLOGES, Alfred; 1321 ouest Sherbrooke, **Montreal, P.Q.; Mon '23; Ophth; Tel. 842-6372.**
DESMARAIS, Bernard; Ste. 903, 30 est Boul. St-Joseph, Montreal 14, P.Q.; Mon'49.
DEMARAIS, Claude; Mon'64; Sr. Int., Hotel-Dieu de Montreal, Montreal 18, P.Q.
Des MARAIS, Gabriel; 14 ave. Green, St. Lambert, P.Q.; Mon'49; ObstGyn; FACOG; FAGS; Chief of Serv. (ObstGyn.), Hop. Gen. de St. Lambert & Hop. Charles Lemoyne; Tel. 672-2211.
DESMARAIS, Gilles; 4 Durham St. N., Sudbury, Ont.; 210 Cedar St. (res); Mon '32; Gyn; Dist. **Coroner; Tel. 674-4011.**
DESMARAIS, Jean N.; 279 Wembley Dr., Sudbury, Ont. (res); Ott '51; D.A.B.R., D & T Rad; Staff, St. Joseph's, Sudbury Gen. & Sudbury Mem. Hosp's., Sudbury & Copper Cliff Hosp., Copper **Cliff; Tel. 674-3101.**
DESMARAIS, Marcel; 52 Ste-Trinite, Contrecoeur. P.Q.; Mon '43.
DESMARAIS, Max H. L.; 401 Medical Arts Bldgs., Winnipeg, Man.; 14 Roslyn Cres. (res); London (Eng.) '39; M.R.C.S., L.R.C.P., D. PhysMed.; Dir. (PhysMed), Municipal Hosp.; **Cons. (Phys. Med.), Children's Hosp.; Tel. GL 2-3411.**

DESMARAIS, Ovila; 2389 rue Girouard, St. Hyacinthe, P.Q. (res); Mon '24; Anaes; Anaes., Hop.-St. Charles; Tel. PR 4-5331.
DESMARAIS, Roland; 21 Leblanc, L'Epiphanie, Co. L'Assomption, P.Q.: Mon '45; Dist. Coroner.
DESMEULES, Henri; Lav'65; Res., Hop. Hotel-Dieu, Quebec 4, P.Q.
DESMEULES, Jean; 1005 Principale, Cowansville, P.Q.; Lav'65.
DESMEULES, Marc; Lav'65; Res., Hop. Hotel-Dieu St. Vallier, Chicoutimi, P.Q.
DESMEULES, Paul; Lav '64; Res., Hotel-Dieu Hosp., Montreal, P.Q.
DESMEULES, Roland; 525 Grande Allee, Quebec, P.Q.; Lav '22; F.R.C.P.(C); IntMed; Pulm. Dis. & TB (P.Q.), Prof. of T.B. Clinic; Chief, Dept. Med., Hop. Laval; Chief Dept. Phys., Hop. Ste. Foy; Tel. 525-6952.
DESMOND, John W.; 181 Poplar Plains Rd., Toronto 7, Ont. (res); Madras (India) '51; DA (Lond.); FRCS(C), Anaes.; Staff, Toronto Gen. Hosp.; Tel. 923-6002.
DESNOYERS, Danielle; Mon'65; Res., Hop. Notre Dame, Montreal, P.Q.
DESNOYERS, Yvon; Mon'62; Anaes; Staff, Hop. Ste. Jeanne d'Arc, Montreal 18, P.Q.
DESORMIERS, Yvan; Saint-Lin, Cte. L'Assomption, P.Q.; Mon '48.
DESPARTS, Francois; 9 rue Dufferin, Granby, P.Q.; Lav '51.
DESPINS, Clement; Lav '57; Haem (P.Q.); Staff, Hop.-du-Sacre-Coeur, Hull, P.Q.
DESPINS, Richard; 11, rue Notre-Dame, Ville-Marie, Cte Temiscaming, P.Q.; Lav '52.
DESPRES, Jean P.; Hop. Laval, Quebec, P.Q.; Lav'54; FRCS(C), GenSurg; ThorSurg(P.Q.); Tel. 653-5251, Ext. 395.
DESROBERTS, Yvon; 122 Ball, Sherbrooke, P.Q.; Lav '59.
DESROCHERS, Denis P.; Lav'65; Res., Hop. St. Sacrement, Quebec 6, P.Q.
DESROCHERS, Gerald; 75 St. Jean Baptiste, Chateauguay, P.Q.; 94 Giroux (res); Mon'62; Tel. 692-6701.
DESROCHERS, G.; Hop.-St.-Michel-Archange, Mastai, P.Q.; Lav '22; FRCP(C), NeurPsy; Prof. (Toxicol. & Med. Juris.), Laval U.; Tel. LA 9-4511.
DESROCHERS, Jacques B.; 30 est, boul St-Joseph, Montreal 14, P.Q.; 6797-19th Ave. (res); Mon '49; Tel. 845-9884.
DESROCHERS, Jean L.; Centre-Medical-St.-Urbain, 3875 St.-Urbain, Montreal 18, P.Q.; 10635 St. Denis (res); Mon '41; Neur Psy (P.Q.); FRCP(C), Neurol; Chief of Serv. (NeurPsy.), Hop.-Ste-Justine; NeurPsy., Hotel-Dieu; Assoc. Prof. (Neur). Montreal U.; Tel. RE 1-4931.
DESROCHERS, Jules B.; 30 est Boul. St. Joseph, Montreal 34, P.Q.; Mon '49; Tel. 845-9884.
DESROCHERS, Louis P.; 1570, St- Hubert, Montreal 24, P.Q.; Mon '38.
DesROCHERS, Marcel; Lav'57; DiagRad(P.Q.); Staff, Hop. Christ-Roi, Quebec 8, P.Q.
DESROCHERS, Paul E., S/L; No. 1 Air Div. RCAF, CFPO 5052, Can. Armed Forces, Europe; Lav '57. Abroad.
DESROCHERS, Yves; 340 Kindersley, Montreal 16, P.Q. (res); Mon '51; Cardiol (P.Q.); Staff, Inst.-de-Cardiology; Tel. 254-8341.
DESROCHES, Francois; 2157 Fleury E., Montreal 12, P.Q.; Mon'65; Tel. 381-2581.
DESROCHES, Jean-Marie; 8097 St.-Hubert, Montreal 10, P.Q.; 9822 St.-Denis (res); Mon '59; Tel. CR 2-0835.
DESROSIERS, Bernard; 167 Blvd. Maloney Gatineau, P.Q.; Mon '45.
DESROSIERS, Deliphat; St. Anselme, Co. Dorchester, P.Q.; 925 Bourgainville, Quebec 6, (res); Lav '30; D.P.H., P.H.(P.Q.); M.O.H., Dorchester Co.
DESROSIERS, Georges; 2257 est, Fleury, Montreal 12, P.Q.; 1720 Dauphin, Duvernay (res); Mon '54; MCGP; Tel. DU 9-5973.
DESROSIERS, Gerard; St. Narcisse, Cte. Champlain, P.Q.; Lav '46.
DESROSIERS, Gilles; 2257 est Fleury, Montreal 12, P.Q.; 282 Toulon, Pont-Viau (res); Mon '58; AMCGP; Tel. 389-5973.
DESROSIERS, Hector; 2174 Centre St., Montreal, P.Q.; 3525 Vendome (res); Mon '25; Anaes; Tel. WE 2-0477.
DESROSIERS, Henri; 734 Gadoury, Joliette, P.Q. (res); Mon '48; Path (P.Q.); Staff, Hop. St. Eusebe, Joliette; Tel. PL 6-8021.
DESROSIERS, Jean L.; 222 Henri Bourassa est, Montreal, P.Q.; Mon '51; Paed; Chief of Paed., Hop. Sacre-Coeur, Cartierville; Tel. DU 7-0924.
DESROSIERS, J. Jacques; Clinique Metropolitaine, 1150 est, boul St-Joseph, Montreal 34, P.Q.; Lav '55; ObstGyn.; Tel. 527-1241.
DESROSIERS, J. R. Fernand; 11 de l'Hopital, Loretteville, P.Q.; Lav'55; FACS; FRCS(C), GenSurg; Sr. Ass't. (Surg.), St. Ambroise Hop.; Tel. 842-4086.
DESROSIERS, Louis; 2880 Masson, Montreal, P.Q.; 5404 Bld. Rosemont (res); Mon '43; Obst.; Ass't. (Obst.), Maisonneuve Hosp.; Tel. 254-8341.
DESROSIERS, Michel; Mon'65; Res., Hop. Maisonneuve, Montreal 36, P.Q.
DESROSIERS, Pierre; Centre Medical Laval, 915 Ave Suzanne, St. Vincent de Paul, P.Q.; Mon '65.
DESROSIERS, Roland; Lav'61; Anaes; Staff, Hop. Laval, Ste-Foy, P.Q.
DES ROSIERS, Saint-Jean; 929 rue Cherrier, Montreal 24, P.Q.; Mon '27; Gastroent (P.Q.); Tel. LA 7-0111.
DESROSIERS, Suzanne; Mon '64; Res., Hop. Notre-Dame, Montreal, P.Q.
DES RUISSEAUX, Paul Wintle; 1010 St. Cyrille W., Sillery, Quebec 6, P.Q.; Ott '57.
DESSUREAULT, Paul; 1150 St. Joseph Blvd. E., Montreal 34, P.Q.; Mon'49; FRCS(C), Urol; Staff, Maisonneuve Hosp.; Cons., Valleyfield Hosp., Valleyfield & Hop. Notre-Dame L'Esperance, St. Laurent; Tel. LA 7-1241.
DESSUREAULT, Richard; 940—12th Ave., Grand'mere, P.Q. (res) Lav '48; Path & Clin. Path. (P.Q.); Dir. of Lab. Hop. La Fleche; Tel. LE 8-3381.
DESTOUNIS, Nikolas; 6209 University Ave., Halifax, N.S.; Athens (Greece) '53; Research, Dalhousie U.
DESTROISMAISONS, Roland; 400 Blvd. St. Joseph E., Montreal 34, P.Q.; Mon'38; OphthOtol (P.Q.); Chief O.R.L. Serv., Hop. Ste. Justine; Tel. RE 1-4931.
DESTRUBE, Ilse F. (Cloos); Ste. 410, 1207 Douglas St., Victoria, B.C.; 766 Sea Dr., Brentwood Bay (res); Munich (Germ.)'43; MCGP; Tel. EV 2-8691.
D'ESTRUBE, Pierre-F.; Mental Health Centre, Victoria, B.C.; Alb '52; Psy.
DESY, Antonio; 241 rue Principale, St. Sauveur des Monts, P.Q.; Mon '53.
de TAVEL, Franz E.; Berne (Switz.) '34; M.C. (Zurich); Med. Adviser, Internat. Civil Aviation Org., Internat. Aviation Bldg., Montreal, P.Q.
D'ETCHEVERRY, Andre; 1531 Garand, Sherbrooke, P.Q.; Lav '43; D & T Rad; Rad., Hop.-Hotel-Dieu; Tel. LO 9-2551.
De TORREGROSA Navarro Carlos; 1140 Jean Talon E., Montreal, P.Q.; Madrid (Spain) '45; GenSurg; Tel. 274-4461.
DETWEILER, Herbert K.; Suite 1007, Medical Arts Bldg., Toronto, Ont.; R.R. No. 4, Bolton (res); Tor '14; Hon. Fell., C.A.A., M.A.C.P., F.R.C.P.(C), IntMed; Cons. Phys., Toronto Gen., Toronto Western & Wellesley Hosp's.; Retired.
DETWILER, Robert C.; 68 Charlton W., Hamilton, Ont.; 1 Rosscliffe Dr. (res); Wes '50; DABOS; FRCS(C), OrthSurg.; Tel. JA 8-8563.
DEUTCH-ANDERMAN, Eva; McG'63; Research Fell. (Med. Genetics), Montreal Children's Hosp., Montreal, P.Q.
DEUTSCH, Leon; 2038 Norway Rd., Montreal 9, P.Q.; Prague (Czechoslovakia) '37; Psy (P.Q.);
de VARENNES, Paul H.; 692 Cartier St. E., Chicoutimi, P.Q. (res); Lav '31; D&T Rad; Hd., Dept. of Rad., Hop. Hotel-Dieu; & Staff, Laval U.; Tel. 549-1452.
DEVEAU, George R.; Apt 207, 5959 Spring Garden Rd., Halifax, N.S.; Lav '18.
DEVEBER, George A.; Tor'56; IntMed; Staff, Toronto Western Hosp., Toronto 2B, Ont.

deVEBER, Leverett L.; 392 South St., London, Ont.; Tor'53; FRCP(C), Paed; Ass't. Prof. (Path.Chem.) & Lect. (Paed.), U. of Western Ontario; Dir., Immunol. Serv. & Ass't. Dir. Blood Bank, Victoria Hosp.; Tel. GE 2-5261.

DEVENYI, Paul; 119 Elmhurst Dr., Hamilton, Ont.; 45 Fennell Ave. E. (res); Budapest (Hung.) '54; Fell., Alcoholism Research Fdn.; Tel. 389-1525.

DEVEREUX, Harold J.; 56 Inglis St., Sydney, N.S.; Dal'36; MCGP; Staff, St. Rita & Sydney City Hosp's.; Memb. N.S., Hosp. Ins. Commiss.; Tel. 564-6149.

De VERTEUIL, Roger L.; 6615 LaSalle Blvd., Verdun, Montreal 19, P.Q.; McG '48; Psy (P.Q.); Psy., Verdun Protestant Hosp.; Tel. 766-8511.

de VILLIERS, Arnoldus J.; Guy's Hosp. (London, Eng.) '48; MRCS(Eng.); LRCP(Lond.); DIH (Eng.); D.Sc. (Pittsburgh); ABPM; Sr. Clin. Cons. & Dir., Biomedical Unit, Occupational Health Div., Dept. of National Health & Welfare, Ottawa, Ont.

DEVILLY, Daniel J.; Box 371, Drake-Merritt, Goose Bay, Labrador; Ire. '50.

DEVINE, Stewart W.; 10155-120th St., Edmonton, Alta.; Sask '58; FRCS(C), ObstGyn; Clin. Instr. (ObstGyn.), U. of Alberta; Tel. HU 8-7271.

DEVINS, M. Audrey C.; 21 Wellington St. E., Aurora, Ont.; Tor '18; Retired.

DEVITO, W. Peter; Box 274, Qualicum Beach, B.C.; UBC'54; DiagRad.

DEVITT, James E.; 402 Central Med. Bldg., 1105 Carling Ave., Ottawa 3, Ont.; 243 Irving Ave. (res); Qns '50; M.Sc., FRCS (Ed.), FRCS (C), GenSurg; Surg., Ottawa Civic Hosp.; Lect. (Clin. Surg.), Ottawa U.; Tel. 728-3563.

DEVLIN, Henry; 2172 Eglinton Ave. W., Toronto 10, Ont.; 470 Coldstream Ave. (res); Tor '40; Tel. RU 3-2370.

DEVLIN, Henry E.; 94 Highbourne Rd., Toronto 7, Ont.; Trinity Coll. (Dublin, Ire.) '44; Anaes; Staff Anaes., Humber Mem. Hosp.; Tel. HU 9-7911.

DEVLIN, J. Desmond; Ste. 301, 4900 Kingsway, South Burnaby, B.C.; 1764 W. 57th Ave., Van. 14 (res); Man '51; IntMed; Staff, Van. Gen., Shaughnessy & Burnaby Hosp's.; Tel. 434-1211.

DEVLIN, John T.; Baie Verte, Nfld.; Dublin (Ire.) '53.

DEVLIN, Roger J.; Indian River, Ont.; Qns '21.

DE VRIES, Joan A.; Ste 220, 3550 Cote des Neiges Rd., Montreal 25, P.Q.; McG '32, Bact (P.Q.).

DE VRIES, Johannes D.; Leiden (Neth.) '60; Res., Ottawa San., Ottawa 3, Ont.

DE VRIES, Johannes D.; Amsterdam (Neth.) '57; Res., Royal Ottawa San., Ottawa, Ont.

DEWAJI, V. R.; 2332 Angus St., Regina, Sask.; M.O., Dept. of Public Health, Golden Mile Plaza, Regina, Sask.; Tel. 523-0410.

DEWAN, John G.; Ste. D., 6 Crescent Rd., Toronto 5, Ont.; Wes'32; DPM(Eng.); Ph.D. (Cantab.); FACP; FAPA; FRCP(C), NeurPsy; Exec. Cons., Ontario Mental Health Fdn.; Cons. Psy., Sunnybrook Hosp. & U. of Toronto Health Serv.; Prof. (Psy.), U. of Toronto.

DEWAN, Margaret T.; (See SPENCE).

DEWAR, Charles M.; O'Leary, P.E.I.; Dal '54; M.C.G.P.; Dist. Coroner.

DEWAR, Frederick P.; 706 Med. Arts Bldg., 170 St. George St., Toronto 5, Ont.; 122 Inglewood Dr., Apt. 2, Tor. 7 (res); Tor '36; FRCS (Eng.), FRCS(C), OrthSurg; GenSurg; Sr. Surg., (OrthSurg.), Tor. Gen. Hosp.; Cons (OrthSurg.), Women's College & Sunnybrook Hosp's.; Med. Bd. St. John's Conval. Hosp.; Assoc. Prof. (Surg.), U. of Toronto; Tel. WA 2-4919.

DEWAR, James D.; 97 Charlotte St., Port Colborne, Ont.; 152 Rose Mount (res); Wes '63 MCGP;

DEWAR, James W.; Irving Clinic, Box 150, Kamloops, B.C.; Glasgow (Scot.)'51; MCGP; Assoc. Med. Staff, Royal Indian Hosp.; Tel. 372-5251.

DEWAR, L. George, The Hon., MPP; O'Leary, P.E.I.; Dal '43; DPH; MCGP; Staff, Community Hosp.; Court. Staff, Prince County Hosp., Sunnyside & Western Hosp, Alberton; Minister, Educ., Prov. of P.E.I.; Tel. 15

DEWAR, Ranald S.; 4623 Banff Coach Rd., Calgary, Alta.; Aberdeen (Scot.) '39; Abroad.

DEWDNEY, Alice W.; Wes '64; Jr. Int., Montreal Gen. Hosp., Montreal 25, P.Q.

DEWICK, Betty C. (Chinn); Willow Chest Centre, 2647 Willow St., Vancouver 9, B.C.; Qns '54; Phys., Dept. of Health & Welfare; Tel. TR 4-2331.

deWIT, Sharon A. M. (O'Rourke); UBC'64; Res. (Path.), Vancouver Gen. Hosp., Vancouver, B.C.

DeWITT, C. E. Avery; 6 Park St., Wolfville, N.S.; McG '09; Retired.

DEXTER, Derrick; 2155 Cross Place, Regina, Sask. (res); Sheffield (Eng.)'46; MC(Path); Path; Dir. of Path., Grey Nuns Hosp.; Tel. 527-9641.

DEYELL, J. Arthur; 165 Plymouth Rd., Welland, Ont.; Tor '50; GenSurg.

DEYO, Gerald M.; 333 Reid St., Peterborough, Ont.; Tor'54; MCGP; Active Staff, Peterborough Civic & St. Joseph's Hosp's.; Hon. Staff, Porcupine Gen. Hosp.

DEYOUNG, George G.; 20 Olie St., Spryfield, N.S.; Wes'63.

DEZA, Plaridel C.; Santa Tomas (Manila, Philipp.)'56; Psy; Sr. Psy., Saskatchewan Hosp., North Battleford, Sask.; Abroad.

DEZIEL, Jean; 1366 est Laurier, Montreal 34, P.Q.; 2200 Dudemaine (res); Mon '57; FRCS(C); GenSurg; Ass't Prof., U. of Montreal; Tel. 521-6645.

DHAITI, Jean J. G.; Haiti'55; IntMed; Staff, Hop. St. Charles, Joliette, P.Q.

DHALLA, Said N.; 1136 W. 10th St., Vancouver 9, B.C.; Tehran (Iran)'55; GenSurg.

DHUNDSHY, Sarvotham S.; Bombay (India)'54; Res., University Hosp., Edmonton, Alta.

DIACK, Helen (Brown); R.R. 2, Brampton, Ont.; Aberdeen (Scot.) '21; Pt-time, Dept. of Health.

DIAMAND, Salim; 651 College St., Toronto, Ont.; 277 Russell Hill Rd. (res); Naples (Italy) '39; M.C.G.P.; Tel. LE 4-4463.

DIAMANT, Nicholas E.; Qns '60; FRCP(C), IntMed Research, Western Hosp., Toronto 2B, Ont. Abroad.

DIAMOND, A. William; 110 Yonge St. S., Aurora, Ont., Tor '61; AMCGP; Tel. 727-4245.

DIAMOND, Edgar G.; 1407-70th. Ave. S. W., Calgary, Alta.; Alb '54; Anaes; Staff, Calgary Gen. Hosp.

DIAMOND, John (Jack); Medical Centre, Queen St., Port Perry, Ont.; Glasgow (Scot.) '52; M.C.G.P.; Staff, Port Perry Community Mem. Hosp. & Uxbridge Cottage Hosp.; Tel. 985-7301.

DIAMOND, Michael J.; Anesthesia Assoc., 892 Queens Blvd., Kitchener, Ont.; Leeds (Eng.) '53; D.A. (Eng.); Anaes; Staff, Kitchener-Waterloo & St. Mary's Hosp's.; Tel. 744-7361.

DIAZ, Jose M.; 725 Churchill Ave., Ottawa 3, Ont.; Madrid (Spain) '51.

DIBAJI, S. Nasser; 1136 West 10th Ave., Vancouver 9, B.C.; Tehran (Iran)'55; GenSurg.

DiCESARE, John N.; 1069 Ronlea Ave., Oshawa, Ont.; Ott'60; DiagRad.

DICK, Abram; 631 Med. Arts Bldg., 750 Spadina Cr. E., Saskatoon, Sask.; Tor'47; FRCS(C), GenSurg; Active Staff, Saskatoon City & St. Paul's Hosp.; Vis. Phys., University Hosp.; Tel. 244-2951.

DICK, Arthur; 1605 Glenmore St., Kelowna, B.C.; Man'59; MCGP; Tel. 762-2002.

DICK, Clifford J. W.; 5016-48th Ave., Taber, Alta.; 5003-52nd Ave. (res); Man '45; GenSurg.; Tel. 223-3525.

DICK, Donald A.; 11426-74th Ave., Edmonton, Alta. (res); Edinburgh (Scot.) '48; D.M.R.T.; F.F.R.; TherRad; Assoc. Dir. Cancer Clin., 11250 —84th Ave., Edmonton, Alta.

DICK, Jacob A.; 631 Medical Arts Bldg., 750 Spadina Cres. E., Saskatoon, Sask.; Man '56.; Tel. 244-8106.

DICK, Jacob J.; 121 Wellington St. W., Barrie, Ont.; Tor'63; Staff, Royal Victoria Hosp.; Tel. 728-2476.

DICK, John; 750 West 9th., Vancouver, B.C.; 5838 Adera St. (res); Glasgow (Scot.)'44; FACP; IntMed; Att. Staff, Vancouver Gen. Hosp.; Med. Dir., B.C. Epilepsy Centre; Clin. Instr. (Med.), U.B.C.; Tel. TR 2-2711.

DICK, John B.; 242 Main St., Steinbach, Man.; Man'55; MCGP; Med. Staff, Bethesda Hosp.; Tel. DA 6-3476.

DICK, John J.; 69 Eglinton Ave. E., Toronto 12, Ont.; 650 Briar Hill Ave., Apt. 509 (res); Tor '35; Co. Phys., Tip Top Tailors Co. Ltd.; Med. Exam., Equitable Life Ins. Co.; Tel. 488-8932.

DICK, Kenneth D.; Medical Arts Bldg., 1105 Pandora, Victoria, B.C.; UBC '57.

DICK, Robert N.; Chemainus, B.C.; McG '32; M.C.G.P. Retired.

DICK, Victor; Box 129, Manitou, Man.; Man'58; AMCGP.

DICKER, Robert; 30 Sheppard Ave. E., Willowdale, Ont.; Apt. 210, 30 Vinci Cres., Downsview (res); Tor '52; MCGP; Adj. Clin. Phys., Mt. Sinai Hosp.; Tel. 225-3781.

DICKEY, Marvin R.; 925 West Georgia St., Vancouver, B.C.; 1683 W. 60th Ave. (res); Man '34; D.A.B.R., DiagRad; Part-time Rad., Shaughnessy Hosp. + DVA; Tel. MU 4-4177; RE 8-3188.

DICKIE, Albert W.; 214 Avenue Bldg., 220-3rd Ave. S. Saskatoon, Sask. (Queens, N. Ire.) '48.

DICKINSON, Gordon T.; 150 St. George St., Toronto 5, Ont.; 9 Kendal Ave. (res); McG '58; Editor, CMA Publications; Tel. 924-0751.

DICKINSON, Howard J.; Oxford & London (Eng.) '37; Res., Victoria Gen. Hosp., Halifax, N.S.

DICKINSON, John H.; 710 Seymour St., Vancouver 2, B.C.; Tor '49; F.R.C.S.(C), ObstGyn; Staff, Vancouver Gen. & Grace Hosp's.; Clin. Instr., U. of British Columbia; Tel. MU 4-1511.

DICKINSON, O. B.; 28 Inniswood Dr., Scarborough, Ont.; Qns '35; F.R.C.S. (Eng.), F.I.-A.P., F.R.C.S.(C), GenSurg; Tel. PL 5-1613.

DICKINSON, P. Taylor; McG '62; Res., Montreal Gen. Hosp., Montreal, P.Q.

DICKINSON, Thurston E.; 2150 Valley Way, Niagara Falls, Ont.

DICKISON, J. Campbell; 1414 Drummond St., Montreal, P.Q.; 12 Stratford Rd., Hampstead (res); McG '40; FRCS(C), GenSurg; Ass't. Surg., Mtl. Gen. Hosp.; Assoc. Surg., Reddy Mem. Hosp.; Cons. Surg., Queen Mary Vet's. & Catharine Booth Hosp's. & Cons. Cdn. Seafarer's Welfare; Lect. (Surg.), McGill U.; Tel. WE 7-6011.

DICKOUT, John M.; Drawer 890, Lloydminster, Sask.; Alb '43; Tel. 4240.

DICKS, Royal E.; 31-3rd Ave. N.E., Dauphin, Man.; 213 McLeod Ave. (res); Man '19; M.C.-G.P.; Obst., Dauphin Gen. Hosp.; Dist. Coroner.

DICKSON, Adolph D.; 427 Willowdale Ave., Willowdale, Ont.; Kaunas (Lithuania)'43; MCGP; Staff, Gage Inst., College St., Toronto; Tel. 225-5971.

DICKSON, David H.; 90 Wilton Dr., Brampton, Ont.; Wes '62; Research, Banting Inst., Toronto.

DICKSON, Garnet D.; 359 Lytton Blvd., Toronto, Ont.; Tor '36; Anaes; Staff, Toronto Western Hosp.; Dept. of Med. (Anaes.) U. of Toronto; Tel. HU 9-3633.

DICKSON, James; 95 Le Marchant Rd., St. John's Nfld.; Glasgow (Scot.) '51; FRCP(C), Anaes; Staff, St. John's Gen. Hosp.; Anaes., Grace & St. Clare's Mercy Hosp's.; Tel. 578-7909.

DICKSON, John H.; 1139 Yates St., Victoria, B.C.; Cambridge (Eng.)'51; D. ObstRCOG; ObstGyn.

DICKSON, John T.; Tor'62; Res. (Otol.), Toronto Western Hosp., Toronto, Ont.

DICKSON, M. Elizabeth; 359 Lytton Blvd., Toronto 7, Ont. (res); Tor '37; Retired.

DICKSON, Robert C., OBE; Ste. 206, O.P. Bldg., Victoria Gen. Hosp., Halifax, N.S. (res); Tor'34; FACP; FRCP(C); IntMed; Phys-in-Chief, Victoria Gen. Hosp.; Cons. (Med.), Camp Hill DVA, Cdn. Forces & Children's Hosp's. & Halifax Infirmary; Prof. (Med.), Dalhousie U.; Tel. 429-5151.

DICKSON Robert I.; Man '64; Res., Deer Lodge Hosp., Winnipeg 12, Man.

DICKSON, R. Robert K.; 176 King St., St. Catharines, Ont.; 13 Marlene Dr. (res); Wes '44; A.A.C.P.; IntMed; Staff, St. Catharines Gen. Hosp. & Hotel-Dieu; Cottage Hosp., Niagara-on-the-Lake; Tel. 682-8638.

DICKSON, W. Lorne C.; 630 St. Clair Ave. W., Toronto, Ont.; 192 Pinewood Ave. (res); Qns '37; AMCGP; Tel. LE 2-7773.

DICUM, Frank J.; Tor '62; Res., New Mount Sinai Hosp., Toronto, Ont.

DIDCOTT, P. Ralph; 1548 Lonsdale Ave., North Vancouver, B.C.; UBC'62.

DIDUCH, Lawrence T.; 229 Professional Bldg., 10830 Jasper Ave., Edmonton, Alta.; 14240 Laurier Dr. (res); Alb '56; Otol; Active Staff, **Royal Alexandra & Edmonton Gen. Hosp's.; Tel. 424-9919.**

DIEHL, Garth R.; 332 Med. Arts Bldg., Winnipeg 1, Man.; 564 Niagara St., Wpg. 9 (res) Man '46; MCGP; Pres. Elect., College of General Practice; Pres., Med. Staff, Grace Hosp.; Court. Staff, Winnipeg Gen., Misericordia, Childrens, St. Boniface & Municipal Hosp's.; Tel. WH 2-8038 & WH 2-2159.

DIESCH, Richard; 62 Avondale Blvd., Bramalea, Ont.; Teubingen (Germ.) '47; Staff, Peel Mem. Hosp.; Tel. 459-1812.

DIETRICH, Michael; 72 Altadore Cr., Woodstock, Ont. (res); Wes'54; Path; Pathol., Woodstock Gen. & Alexandra Hosp., Ingersoll; Cons., Ontario Hosp., Woodstock; Instr., Dept. of Path., U. of Western Ontario, London; Tel. 537-5511, Ext. 228.

DIEZ, Pablo; Valladolid (Spain)'58; Staff, Hop. Mont Providence, Montreal 39, P.Q.

DI GASPARI, Joseph; 57 Champlain, Baie Comeau, Co. Saguenay, P.Q.; McG '47; M.O., Quebec North Shore Paper Co.; Tel. 584-3401.

DIGBY, James R.; 221 Brant Ave., Brantford, Ont.; **53 Franklin St. (res); McG '52; FACS; FRCS(C); GenSurg; Acting Staff, Brant**ford Gen. Hosp.; Court, Staff, St. Joseph's Hosp.; Med. Dir., Cockshutt Farm Equipment (Can.) & Brantford Coach & Body Ltd.; Tel. 756-5311.

DIGBY, John W.; 222 Med. Arts Bldg., 170 St. George St., **Toronto 5. Ont.; 44 Douglas Dr.** Tor-17 (res); Tor '54; FRCP(C), IntMed.; Clin. Inst., St. Michael's Hosp. and U. of Toronto; Editor, Modern Medicine of Canada, Seccombe House, 443 Mount Pleasant Rd., Toronto 7; Tel. 921-2712.

DIGGINS, William L.; Bay Cities Mall, Port Arthur, Ont.; McG '58.

DIGNAN, John G.; 4675 Tecumseh Rd. E., Windsor, Ont.; 1089 Victoria Ave. (res); Tor '42; M.C.G.P.; Staff, Grace, Hotel Dieu & Metropolitan Gen. Hosp's.; Tel. 945-5261.

DIGOUT, Joseph H.; Box 148 St. Peters, N.S.; Lav'25; Reserve Phys., Micmac Indians; Port Phys., Dept. of National Health & Welfare; Tel. 17.

DIKE, Anna I. (Murray); 86 Bloor St. W., Toronto, Ont.; 8 Astley Ave. (res); Dal '29; Med. Service & Dir. Spec. Clinic, Women's College Hosp.; Tel. WA 2-8855. Retired.

DILISI. Joseph; 611 Bloor St. W., Toronto 4, **Ont.; Tel. LE 7-3967.**

DILLABOUGH, Charles D.; 51-6th St. S.E., Medicine Hat, Alta.

DILLANE, J. E.; Powassan, Ont.; Wes '32.

DILLANE, James G. R.; Medical Arts Bldg., James St. S., Hamilton, Ont.; Tor '28; D.O.M.S. (Eng.), Ophth; Chief of Ophth., Hamilton Gen. Hospital; Tel. JA 7-6517.

DILLANE, W. Edward; 613 Medical Arts Bldg., Hamilton, Ont.; 36 Duke St., Apt. 203 (res); Tor '37; DermSyph; Head (Derm.), Hamilton Gen. Hosp.; Retired.

DILLENBERG, Hermann O.; 231 College Ave. E. Regina, Sask.; Berlin (Germ.) '38; Prov. Epidermiologist, Dept. of P.H.; Clin. Assoc., U. of Saskatchewan.

DILLON, Jeremiah J.; 117 King St. E., Oshawa Ont.; 355 Elizabeth St. (res); Nat. U. (Ire.) '46 B.A.O.; Anaes; Staff (Anaes.), Oshawa Gen Hosp.; Tel. 728-1661.

DILLON, Michael T.; 1629 Dundas St. E.; London, Ont.; Wes '52 MCGP. ;
DIMARUCOT, Avelina B.; Santo Tomas (Philip.) '55; Staff, Saskatchewan Hosp., Weyburn, Sask.; Tel. VI 2-3812.
DIMILILER, Ismail; Dept. of Surg., University of Sask. Med. College, Saskatoon, Sask.; Istanbul (Turkey)'47.
DIMITRIADIS, George; 6267 Quinpool Rd., Halifax, N.S.; 5523 Inglis St. (res); Athens (Greece) '47; Tel. 423-7652.
DIMITROFF, Daniel C.; Ste. 413, 1849 Yonge St., Toronto 7, Ont.; Tor '60; Court. Staff, Toronto East Gen. Hosp.; Tel. 488-2215.
DIMITROV, Sacha; 907 rue Cherrier, Montreal 24, P.Q.; Paris (Fr.) '51; F.R.C.S.(C), GenSurg; Surg., Hop. Ste. Jeanne d'Arc; Tel. VI 2-5201.
DIMOCK, Gordon K.; Blacks Harbour, N.B., Dal '56; MCGP; P.G. GenSurg., St. John's Gen. Hosp.; Tel. 693-3351.
DIMOCK, H. Barss; 901 Helena St., Trail, B.C.; 3505 Aster Dr. (res); Alb '48; IntMed; Tel. 368-5211.
DIMOCK, Homer C.; 306 McLeod Bldg., Edmonton, Alta. Alb '31; M.C.G.P.; Tel. GA 4-3391.
DIMOFF, Stephanie S.; Tor'65; Res., Shaughnessy Hosp., Vancouver 9, B.C.
DIN, Ghulam; New Germany, N.S.; '30.
DINAN, John J.; Ste. 200, 5300 Cote des Neiges Rd., Montreal 26, P.Q.; 150 Portland, Town of Mount Royal (res); McG '34; GenSurg; F.A.S.C.; Surg., Ste. Mary's Hosp.; Med. Dir., Canadair; Tel. RI 4-1511.
DINCSOY, Mehmet Y.; 1061 Wellington St., Apt. 5, Halifax, N.S.; Istanbul (Turk.) '55; Paed; Staff, Halifax Children's Hosp.; Tel. 422-8441.
DINCSOY, Hosoon P.; Soeul (Korea)'49; Path; Staff, Dept. of Path., Dalhousie U., Pathol. Inst., Halifax, N.S.
DINELLE, Jacques; 3244 Beaubien E., Rosemont, Montreal 36, P.Q.; 8180 Ave. du Mail (res); Mon '53; MC.G.P.; Tel. RA 9-1891.
DINGLE, Donald M.; Come-By-Chance, Nfld.; London (Eng.) '57; Supt., Come-By-Chance Hosp.
DINGLE, Russell T.; 1457 Ontario St., Burlington, Ont.; Wes'26; Dist. Coroner; Tel. NE 4-3770.
DINGLE, William Thomas; 4 Academy Med. Bldg., Calgary, Alta.; Man '36; MRCOG; MACR; ObstGyn; D&TRad; Rad., Grace & Alberta Children's Hosp's.; Assoc. Rad., Calgary Gen. Hosp.; Tel. 263-3770.
DINGWALL, Donald G.; Dingwall Med. Clinic, Dryden, Ont.; **87 Princess St. (res); Qns '06.**
DINGWALL, Malcolm; 21 East Ave. S., Hamilton, Ont.; 50 Auchmar Rd. (res); Qns '40; Paed; Active Staff, Hamilton Gen. & St. Joseph's Hosp's.; Tel. JA 2-3924.
DINGWALL, Roderick W.; 221 King St. E., Kingston, Ont.; 32 Macdonnell St. (res); Qns '43; IntMed; A.M.C.G.P.; Att. Staff, Kingston Gen. Hosp.; Clin. Ass't. (Med.), Queen's U.; Tel. 546-0174.
DINIZ, Anthony P.; 1682A Victoria Pk. Ave., Scarborough, Ont.; 79 Glenwood Cres., Tor. 16 (res); Aurore U. (Shanghai, China) '35; MCGP; Indoor Staff, Scarborough Gen. Hosp.; OPD Staff, St. Michael's Hosp.; Tel. PL 5-3287.
DINSDALE, Henry B.; Etherington Hall, Stuart St., Kingston, Ont.; Qns'55; FRCP(C), Neur; Att'd. Phys., Kingston Gen. & Hotel-Dieu Hosp's.; Cons. (Neurol.), Ont. Hosp., Kingston & Smiths Falls; Ass't. Prof. (Neurol.) Queen's U.; Tel. 546-6013.
DINSDALE, Sidney M.; Qns '63; Res., Sunnybrook Hosp., Toronto, Ont.; Abroad.
d'INTINO, Carmen A.; 133 Bay St., Sydney, N.S.; 110 James St. (res); Dal '45; M.C.G.P.; Staff, Sydney City & St. Rita Hosp's.
DION, Charles; 506 rue La Fontaine, Riviere-du-Loup, P.Q.; 8 ave de Gaspe (res); Lav '26; OphthOtol; Staff (OphthOtol.), Hop-St-Joseph; Tel. UN 2-4993.
DION, Claude; McG '62; Res., Hop. St-Michel-Archange, Quebec, P.Q.
DION, Claude; 1301 ave. Leblanc, Sillery, Quebec 6, P.Q.; Lav '60; Psy; Staff, Clinique Roy-Rousseau; Tel. 661-7735.
DION, Gerard; 298 St.-Germain, Rimouski, P.Q.; 17 Lavoie (res); Lav '46; FRCP(C), IntMed; Staff, Hop.-St.-Joseph, Rimouski & San.-St.-Georges, Mt. Joli; Tel. 723-3461.
DION, J. A.; L'Islet, P.Q.; Lav '98; Retired.
DION, J. Albert; 28 Brooks St. S., Sherbrooke, P.Q.; 30 Brooks (res) Mon '28; Gyn (P.Q.); Tel. 562-3134.
DION, Joseph; Premiere rue ouest, Amos, P.Q.; GenSurg.
DION, Marcel; 8415 St. Denis, Montreal 11, P.Q.; Lav ' 53; Anaes.
DION, Marcel A.; 1150 Blvd. St. Joseph E., Montreal, P.Q.; Mon '57; FRCS(C), PlasSurg; Tel. LA 7-1241.
DION, Raymond M.; 4 Taschereau, Ste. 370, Hull, P.Q.; 30 Lacasse (res); Lav '52; FRCS(C); GenSurg; Chief of Surg. Serv., Hop. Sacre-Coeur; Tel. 771-0332.
DION, Robert; 261 St. Vallier-Ouest, Quebec 8, P.Q.; Lav'48; Pulm Dis. & TB(P.Q.); Tel. 529-4121.
DION, Yvan; 960 boul Ste-Croix, Montreal 9, P.Q.; 364 Ave. Wiseman (res); Mon '48; GenSurg (P.Q.); Surg., Hop. Ste. Justine; Tel. RE 1-4931.
DIONNE, Andre; 2717 Davidson, Montreal 4, P.Q.; Mon'54; MCGP; Vis. Staff, Hop. Santa Cabrini; Tel. 525-7711.
DIONNE, Gilles; Sillery Plaza, app 319, 2590 rue Plaza, Quebec, P.Q.; Lav'61; DiagRad.
DIONNE, J. A.; 406 Boulevard St. Joseph est, Montreal 34, P.Q.; Mon '45; ObstGyn (P.Q.); Med. Dir. & Admin., Fleury Gen. Hosp.; Tel. DU 1-6235.
DIONNE, Jacques; Lav'65; Res., Hop. Hotel-Dieu, Quebec 4, P.Q.
DIONNE, J. Denis; Windsor Towers, Windsor, Ont.; Ott'57.
DIONNE, Jean; 222 Henri Bourassa E., Montreal 12, P.Q.; Mon '50; GenSurg (P.Q.).
DIONNE, Jean M.; Blvd. Walberg, Dolbeau, P.Q.; Lav '40.
DIONNE, Louis J.; 1002 des Gouverneurs, Quebec 6, P.Q.; Lav'57; FRCS(C), GenSurg; Staff, Hop. Hotel-Dieu; Tel. 529-9151.
DIONNE, L-Rene; 4380 Boul. Pius IX, Montreal, P.Q.; Mon '27; GenSurg; Ass't. Prof. (Clin.Surg.) & Ass't. Staff (GenSurg.), Hop. Notre-Dame; Tel. 259-1571.
DIONNE, Louis P.; 200 Notre Dame, St. Marie de Beauce, P.Q.; Lav '36.
DIONNE, Paul; 222 est, Henri-Bourassa, Montreal 12, P.Q.; 945 Gauthier Ave., St. Laurent, Mtl. 9 (res); Mon '44; Bact (P.Q.); Bact. Hop.-du-Sacre-Coeur; Tel. FE 4-1210.
DIONNE, Paul E.; 3449 Appleton, Montreal 26, P.Q.; Man '57; Tel. 738-4300.
DIONNE, Philippe; 31 King St. W., Sherbrooke, P.Q.; 1380 Simard (res); Lav '46; GenSurg; Ass't. Surg., Hop. St. Vincent de Paul; Tel. 567-4663.
DIOSI, Ida (See Kovacs)
DIOSY, Andrew; Warner-Lambert Research Inst. of Canada Ltd., Sheridan Park, Clarkson, Ontario; Szeged (Hung.)'50; FRCP(C), IntMed; Ass't. Dir. (Clin. Research), Warner-Lambert Research Inst. of Canada Ltd.; Staff (O.P.D.), Toronto Gen. Hosp.; Tel. 274-3601.
DI PROFIO, Charles F.; 1108 Exmouth, Sarnia, Ont. (res); Dal '54; Path; Staff, Sarnia Gen. Hosp.; Tel. DI 4-3661.
DIRAUF, John; McCreary, Man.; Germany'31.
DIREN, Gultekin; 106 McIntyre St. E, North Bay, Ont.; Istanbul (Turk.) '52; Paed; Staff. St. Joseph's & Civic Hosp's.; Tel. 474-2210.
DIRKS, Henry; 440 Desalaberry, Winnipeg 5, Man.; 54 Eastgate (res); Man'59; MCGP; Tel. JU 9-5306.
DIRKS, John H.; 59 Cleve Rd., Montreal 29, P.Q.; Man'57; FRCP(C), IntMed; Dir. Renal Lab., Royal Victoria Hosp.

DIRNBERGER, Walter; Anaes; Staff, Toronto Hosp., Weston, Ont.; Tel. 259-8291.
DIRNFELD, Victor; Man '61; Jr. Intn., St. Boniface Hosp., St. Boniface, Man.
DISENHAUS, Edward I.; Ste. 203, 688 Coxwell Ave., Toronto, Ont.; 161 Brookbanks Dr., Don Mills, Ont. (res); Tor'55; MCGP; Assoc. Staff, Toronto East Gen. & Doctor's Hosp's.; Tel. HO 6-3431.
DISENHOUSE, Robert B.; 100 Sheppard Ave. W., Willowdale, Ont.; 31 Acton Ave., Downsview (res); Tor '49; Paed; Clin. Ass't., Hosp. for Sick Children; Cons. (Paed.), North York Branson Hosp.; Court. Staff, New Mount Sinai Hosp.; Clin Teach., U. of Toronto; Tel. 225-1677.
DISHER, Irwin S.; McG '51; Psy; Staff, Montreal Children's Hosp., Montreal, P.Q.; Tel. WE 7-8511.
DISLER, Elizabeth; Ste. 907, 1849 Yonge St., Toronto 7, Ont.; Tor '62; Assoc. Staff, Women's College Hosp.; Tel. 481-5943.
DISNEY, Thomas F.; Qns '64; Res., Kingston Gen. Hosp., Kingston, Ont.; Abroad.
DITCHBURN, Frederick G.; 487 Roslyn Blvd., North Vancouver, B.C. (res); Tor '52; Staff, Workmen's Comp. Bd.; Tel. 929-3130.
DITOR, Allan S.; Brandon Clinic, Brandon Man.; Man '61; Tel. PA 9-6444. Abroad.
DIVIC, Josif.; Belgrade (Yugo) '58; D.Psy; Staff, Allan Mem. Inst., Montreal 2, P.Q.
DIVIS, Boris O.; Box 100, Chesley, Ont.; St. Andrew's (Scot.)'58.
DIX, G. Wesley; 117 Laurentide Dr., Don Mills, Ont. (res); Tor '43; Anaes; Staff Anaes., Hosp. for Sick Children, Toronto; Clin. Instr. (Anaes.), U. of Toronto; Tel. EM 6-7242.
DIXON, Allan A.; 119 Medical Arts Bldg., Calgary, Alta.; Alb '45; DermSyph.; Lect., U. of Alberta; Tel. 262-1451.
DIXON, Allen E.; Box 490, Enderby, B.C.; Alb '48; MCGP.
DIXON, Austin L.; 1173 Tecumseh Rd. E., Windsor, Ont.; 3620 Ouellette Ave. (res); St. Louis U. (U.S.A.) '53; Staff, (Dept. of Surg.), Metropolitan Hosp.; Tel. CL 3-6027.
DIXON, Desmond H.; Medical Arts Bldg., Oakville, Ont.; "Willowstream Farm", R.R. 1, Oakville, (res); Qns '42; M.C.G.P.; Staff, Oakville-Trafalgar Mem. Hosp.; Tel. VI 5-4221.
DIXON, Edward R.; Box 10, Ganges, B.C.; London (Eng.)'60; M.B., B.S., MRCS; LRCP.
DIXON, F. O.; 109 Cedar St., Sudbury, Ont.; 68 Kingsmount (res); Tor '32; Paed.; Tel. 673-9524.
DIXON, Garnett D.; 259 Lytton Blvd., Toronto, Ont.; Tor '36; Anaes; Staff, Toronto Western Hosp.; Lect. U. of Toronto, Dept. of Med. (Anaes.).; Tel. 368-2581.
DIXON, James F.; Wes '60; Res., Victoria Hosp., London, Ont.
DIXON, John H.; 24 Academy Medical Bldg., 1812-4th St. W., Calgary, Alta.; 4551 Stanley Dr. (res); McG '44; GenSurg.; Tel. 266-4337.
DIXON, Keith W.; Alb '55; Res. Royal Victoria Hosp., Montreal, P.Q.
DIXON, Margaret J.; 3440 Durocher St., Apt. 712, Montreal, P.Q.; London (Eng.)'61; Anaes.
DIXON, M. Elizabeth; 259 Lytton Blvd., Toronto, Ont.; Tor '37; Retired.
DIXON, Michael E.; McG'60; FRCP(C), IntMed; Staff, Queen Mary Vet's Hosp., Montreal, P.Q.
DIXON, Thomas P.; 59 Durham St. S., Sudbury, Ont.; Tor '43; Dip. Psy; Psy; Dir. Dept. of Psy., Sudbury Gen. Hosp.; Cons. Sudbury Algoma San; Tel. 674-0749.
DIXON, William G.; Ste 9, 45th Ave., Lachine, P.Q.; 24 Ducharme Ave., Dorval (res); McG '45; Obst Gyn; Staff, Lachine Gen. & Catherine Booth Hosp's.; Tel. 637-5383.
DIXON-WARREN, Brian C.; Med. Centre, Meadow Lake, Sask.; London U. (Eng.) '57; DRCOG; LRCP; MRCS; Att'd. Staff, Meadow Lake & Union Hosp's.; Tel. 236-5635.
DIXON, W. S.; Tor'64; Res., Shaughnessy Hosp., Vancouver, B.C.
DLIN, Barney M.; Ste. 504-1541 West Broadway, Vancouver 9, B.C.; 4784 Angus Dr. (res); Alb '49; Psy.
DOBAI, Bela; 465 Bloor St. W., Toronto, Ont.; 2603 Bathurst St., Apt. 307 (res); Czecho-Slavakia & Hungary '20; Tel. WA 3-8821.
DOANE, Benjamin K.; 1339 Edward St., Halifax, N.S.; Dal'62.
DOBB, Clifford A.; 153 Bridge St., Carleton Place, Ont.; Lake Ave. E. (res); McG '49; Staff, Carleton Pl. Mem. & Almonte Gen. Hosp's.; Tel. 526.
DOBBIN, Gordon M.; 22 Rose Park Cres., Toronto, Ont. (res); Tor '17; D.P.H.; Retired.
DOBBIN, M. Campbell; 901 O'Connor Dr., Toronto 16, Ont.; Tor '52; Ophth; Staff, Toronto East Gen. Hosp.; Tel. 759-3417.
DOBBS, Eric H.; 512 Herald Bldg., S.W., Calgary, Alta. (res); Man '44; Anaes; Dir. of Anaes., Calgary Gen. Hosp.; Tel. AM 6-7541.
DOBBS, Kenneth; 2221 Keele St., Toronto, Ont.; Tor '54; Tel. RU 1-3028.
DOBELL, Anthony R.; Royal Victoria Hosp., 687 Pine Ave. Montreal 2, P.Q.; 361 Lazard Ave. (res); McG '51; DABS; DABTS(C); FACS; FRCS(C); GenSurg; ThorSurg; Ass't. Surg., Mtl. Children's, Royal Victoria & Mtl. Gen. Hosp's.; Ass't. Prof., McGill U.; Tel. VI 2-1251.
DOBIE, Frederick C.; 812 Medical-Dental Bldg., Regina, Sask.; 2876 Albert St. (res); Qns '40; GenSurg; M.C.G.P.; Tel. LA 2-5629.
DOBIJA-DOMARADZKI, Maria; 5601 Ave des Cedres, Rosemount, Montreal 36, P.Q. (res); Beirut (Lebanon) '50; Bact (P.Q.); Staff, Hop.-St.-Joseph de Rosemont; Tel. CL 6-2681.
DOBREVA-Kamburoff, Tonka S.; See Kamburoff, Tonka S.
DOBREY, Austin N.; 1687 W. Broadway, Vancouver 9, B.C.; 5375 Angus Dr. Van. 13 (res); Alb '35; FACA, FCAA, Anaes; MCGP; Med. Advis. Bd. & Att'd. Staff, St. Vincent's Hosp.; Tel. FA 1-1010.
DOBRINOFF, Michael; Gottingen (Germ.) '50; M.O., Lady Willingdon Hosp., Ohswekan, Ont.
DOBROWOLSKI, Kazlimierz; 350 Christina St. N., Sarnia, Ont.; Warsaw (Poland) '32; Staff, Sarnia Gen. & St. Joseph's Hosp's.
DOBRY, Edwin J.; 3118-32nd Ave., Vernon, B.C.; Alb'57; Ophth.; Tel. 542-5915.
DOBRY, Joseph J.; 604 Bamlett Bldg., Calgary, Alta.; 1119 Premier Way (res); Alb '28; M.C.-G.P.; Chief of Med., Sarcree Hosp's.; Tel. AM 6-4105.
DOBSON, Clare W.; Ste. 309, Toronto Western Med. Bldg., 25 Leonard Ave., Toronto 2B, Ont.; 1908 Weston Rd., Weston; 23 Queensborough Cres. (res); Tor'51; FRCS(C), Otol; Att'd. Staff, Toronto Western Hosp.; Cons. (Otol.), Princess Margaret Hosp. & Humber Mem. Hosp., Weston; Clin. Instr., (Otol.), U. of Toronto; Tel. EM 4-4855.
DOBSON, Creighton R.; 401 Medical Arts Bldg., Edmonton, Alta.; 10750-125 St. (res); Alb '32; Gen Surg; Att. Surg., Royal Alexandra Hosp.; Clin. Instr., U. of Alberta; Tel. 422-6201.
DOBSON, Dennis; Shellbrook Clinic, Shellbrook, Sask.; Sask'65.
DOBSON, Donald; Med. Centre, Stettler, Alta.; Sheffield (Eng.) '54; MRCS(Eng.); LRCP(Lond.); MCGP; Staff, Stettler Municipal Hosp.; Tel. 742-3441.
DOBSON, Edmund A.; 65 Balsam St. S., Timmins, Ont.; 451 Patricia Blvd. (res); Tor'38; F.R.C.S.(C), GenSurg; Chief Surg., St. Mary's Hosp.; Tel. 264-1357.
DOBSON, Herbert V.; Peterborough Clinic, 327 Charlotte St., Peterborough, Ont.; Tor '19; M.S.; FACP; FAGS; IntMed; Staff, St. Joseph's & Peterborough Civic Hosp's.; Tel. RI 2-3401.
DOBSON, H. Lionel; 10102-101st St., Grande-Prairie, Alta.; 10134-90th Ave. (res); Alb '41; Tel. 532-4444.
DOBSON, J. Arthur; Moncton Anaes. Serv., P.O. Box 892, Moncton, N.B.; McG'49; Anaes; Active Staff (Anaes.), Moncton Hospital; Tel. 389-9467.
DOBSON, John B.; 131 Ontario St., St. Catharines, Ont.; 8 Ridgewood Rd. (res); Wes '51; Paed; Staff (Paed.), St. Catharines Gen. Hosp.; Chief of Paed., Hotel-Dieu Hosp.; Tel. MU 4-9201.

DOBSON, Jos. W.; 106 Alma St., Moncton, N.B.; McG'25; FACS, FRCS(C), GenSurg; Tel. 855-3266.
DOBSON, Margaret (see Cox).
DOBSON, Marion C. (Kerr); Box 70, Winfield, B.C.; R.R. 1 (res); St. Andrew's (Scot.) '50; Schl. Med. Inspector, S. Okanagan Health Unit; Tel 766-2777.
DOBSON, Ross A.; Ste 206, 3000 Lawrence Ave. E., Scarborough, Ont.; Tor '49; M.S. (Surg.), Minn.; **F.R.C.S.(C),** GenSurg; **Att. Staff, Scarborough Gen. Hosp.; Tel. 291-0201.**
DOBSON, T. Albert; Lamont, Alta.; Alta'41; FRCS(C), GenSurg; Staff, Archer Mem. Hosp.; Tel. 895-5522.
DOBSON, Thomas B.; 412 Mountain Ave., Neepewa, Man.; R.C.S. (Dublin, Ire.) '54; LRCP & S. (Ire.); Tel. 380.
DOBSON, William G.; Box 11, Vineland, Ont.; Vineland Stn. (res); Wes '51; MCGP; Assoc. Staff (ObstGyn), St. Catharines Gen. Hosp.; Tel. LO 2-4511.
DOBSON, W. J.; c/o Chief Medical Officer, Dept. **Nat'l. Health & Welfare, 61 Green St., London, W.1, England.**

DOCHERTY, Denis F.; 518 Ridge Rd., Ridgeway, Ont.; Ont.; **Dublin (Ire.) '46; F.I.C.S., F.A.C.S., F.R.C.S. (Ire); Tel. 869-3603.**
DOCHERTY, John A.; Box 39, Saskatchewan Hosp., North Battleford, Sask.; Glasgow (Scot.) '52.
DOCKRILL, Lionel G.; 5 Fairfield, Picton, Ontario; Dal '54.
DOCRAT, Kassim; 45 Brunswick Ave., Toronto 4, Ont.; RCS (Dublin, Ire.)'58; DA; Assoc. Anaes., Doctor's Hosp.; Tel. WA 3-5411.

DODD, I. Norma; 2121 Hope St. S.W., Calgary, Alta.; Durham (Newcastle-on-tyne, Eng.) '48; Ass't. M.O., City of Calgary.
DODD, Thomas P.; Lav'46; Res., Ottawa Civic Hosp., Ottawa 3, Ont.
DODD, W. Alan; Ste. 901, 750 W. Broadway, Vancouver 9, B.C.; UBC'60; FRCP(C), Derm.

DODDS, Donald J.; Ste. 205, 5150 Dundas St. W., **Islington, Ont.; McG '53; MCGP;** Active Staff, Queensway Gen. & Court. Staff, St. Joseph's Hosp's; **Tel. 231-1623.**
DODDS, James R.; 1414 Drummond St., Montreal, P.Q.; 23 Brock Ave. S., Mtl. W. (res); McG '40; ObstGyn; Clin. Ass't., **Royal Victoria & Montreal Gen. Hosp's.; Dem., McGill U.; Tel. VI 2-1251.**
DODDS, John K.; 250 Church St., Streetsville **Ont.; Tor '55; Active Staff, South Peel Hosp.,** Cooksville; Court, Staff, Queensway Hosp., Etobicoke; Tel. 826-1108.
DODDS, William A.; 410-750 W. Broadway, Vancouver 9, B.C.; Tor'44; Anaes; Staff Anaes., Vancouver Gen. Hosp.; Clin. Ass't. Prof. (Anaes), U. of British Columbia; Tel. 879-5355.

DODEK, Morton; 2660 E. Hastings St., Vancouver 6, B.C.; UBC '54; MCGP; Tel. AL 3-3166.

DODICK, Cecil; 1119 Victoria Ave., Fort William, Ont.; **420 Oakdale Cres. (res); Wes '54;** Staff, McKellar Gen. Hosp., **Fort William & St. Joseph's & Port Arthur Gen. Hosp's., Port Arthur;** Tel. 622-7729.
DODICK, Joe L.; 3225 Wyandotte St., Riverside, Ont.; Wes '57.

DOEL, Michael L.; 204 Professional Bldg., 407 Graham Ave., Winnipeg 2, Man.; 189 Elm St., Wpg. 9 (res); The Middlesex Hosp. (London, Eng.) '51; Tel. WH 2-2431. Abroad.
DOENNE, Annamarie E. M.; (Weitz); R.R.1. Priceville, Ont.; **Frankfurt (Germ.) '50; AMCAA; MCGP; Tel. Flesherton 115 J. 4.**
DOERFFER, Frederick R.; Med. Arts Bldg., Hamilton, Ont.; 765 Mohawk Rd. (res); Qns '46; FRCS(C); ObstGyn; Staff, Hamilton Gen. Hosp.; Cons. Staff, West Lincoln Mem. Hosp.; Tel. JA 7-0006.
DOERR, R. Seldon; 213 Medical Arts Bldg., 170 St. George St., **Toronto 5, Ont.; Tor '42;** Tel. WA 2-0645.
DOGAN, Kutas; Istanbul (Turkey) '60; Staff, Regina Gen. Hosp., Regina, Sask.; Tel. 522-1811, Ext. 313.

DOHAN, Charlotte B.; 37 Beach Dr., Victoria, B.C. (res); Glasgow (Scot.) '38; Retired.
DOHERTY, Brian G.; 118 Simcoe St. N., Oshawa, Ont.; 235 Woodlea Cres. (res); McG '50; MCGP; Tel. 723-4195.
DOHERTY, Christopher J.; National U. (Ire.) '38; BAO; FCCP; FAGS; Med. Supt., Sudbury-Algoma Sanatorium, Sudbury, Ont.; Tel. OS 5-8351.
DOHERTY, Elisabeth M.; Lloydminster Clinic, Lloydminster, Sask.; RCS&P. (Dublin, Ire.)'48; DCH; Tel. 875-2221.
DOHERTY, G Harvey; Tor '61; Res., Toronto **Western Hosp., Toronto, Ont.**
DOHERTY, John M. L.; 1539 Erie St. E., Windsor, Ont.; 1805 Riverside Dr. W., Apt. 304 (res); Wes '62; Tel. 252-2733.
DOIDGE, William A.; 121 Wellington St. W., Barrie, Ont.; Tor '33; MCGP; Staff, Royal Victoria Hosp.
DOIG, John N.; 212 First Ave. S., Saskatoon, Sask.; 315 Garrison Cres. (res); Oxford (Eng.) '52; M.A.(Oxon); Assoc. Staff, Saskatoon City & St. Paul's Hosp's.; Clin. Fell. University Hosp.; Tel. 652-4261.
DOIRON, Leo; 172 Victoria St., Moncton, N.B.; **Lav '26; Tel. 382-7452.**

DOLAN, Dominic J.; 37 Main St., Alexandria, Ont.; Kenyon St. (res); Qns '21; Dist. Coronor.
DOLAN, F. Gerard; 5750 South St., Halifax, N.S.; 25 Wenlock Cr., Boulderwood (res); Dal '51; FRCS(C); GenSurg; Ass't. Surg., Victoria Gen., Childrens' & Camp Hill Hosp's.; Ass't. Prof. **(Surg.), Dalhousie U.; Tel. 422-4578.**
DOLAN, Harold S.; 1509 Sherbrooke St. W., Montreal 25, P.Q.; 69 Rosemount Cres. (res); Dal '23; F.A.C.S., GenSurg; Surg-in-Chief, St. Mary's Hosp.; Clin. Ass't., Royal Victoria Hosp.; **Ass't. Prof. Surg., McGill U.; Tel. 735-3511.**
DOLAN, James; Glasgow (Scot.)'40; MRCP; DPM; DPH; FRCP(C), Psy; Staff, Ontario Hosp., St. Thomas, Ont.; Tel. 631-8510.
DOLAN, James D. F/L; Trenton RCAF Hosp., Trenton, Ont.; Qns'64.
DOLAN, Raymond J.; 280 Aberdeen St., Fredericton, N.B. (res); Qns '19; Dir., Cancer Control, Dept. of Health (N.B.); Tel. GR 5-7711.
DOLAN, Ronald A.; 214 Med. Arts Bldg., Hamilton, Ont.; 838 Danforth Pl., Burlington (res); Qns '44; FACS; NeurSurg; Chief of NeurSurg., Hamilton Civic Hosp's; Cons. NeurSurg., St. Joseph's Hosp.; Active Staff, Joseph Brant Hosp., Burlington; Court. Staff, Chedoke Gen. & Children's Hosp's.; Tel. 528-9801.

DOLGOY, Max; 707 Tegler Bldg., 10189-101st St., Edmonton, Alta.; 10233-125th St. (res); Alb '36; MCGP; Tel. 422-2025.

DOLL, William A.; 829 West Broadway, Vancouver, B.C.; Alb'53; Anaes; Staff, Dept. of Anaes., Vancouver Gen. Hosp.; Tel. TR 6-3211.
DOLLFUSS, Rudolf; McG '62; Res., Montreal Gen. Hosp., Montreal, P.Q.

DOLMAN, Clarissa L. (Aszkanazy); 1611 Cedar **Cres., Vancouver 9, B.C.; Tor '47; Path; Staff (Path), Vancouver Gen. Hosp.; Assoc. Clin. Prof.,** U. of British Columbia; Tel. CA 4-1111.
DOLMAN, Claude E.; 1611 Cedar Cr., Vancouver 9, B.C.; London (Eng.) '30; DPH; Ph.D. (Bact. Lond.); MRCS (Eng.); FRCP (Lond.); FRSC; FAPHA; FRCP(C); Bact; Hon. Cons., Vancouver Gen. Hosp.; Research Member, Connaught Med. Research Labs., Toronto, Ont.; Prof. & Hd. Dept. of Bact. & Immunol., U. of British Columbia; Tel. CA 4-1111.
DOLMAN, Mortimer; Qns'63; Res., c/o 3133 Van Horne Ave., Montreal 26, P.Q.
DOLMAN, Robert S.; 3650 Danforth Ave, Toronto 6, Ont.; Qns '52; MCGP; Med. Dir., Eli Lilly & Co.; Tel. 694-3221.

DOLOVITCH, Jerry; Ste 217, 3787 Cote des Neiges Rd., Montreal 25, P.Q.; Man '59; FRCP (C), IntMed; Staff, Montreal General Hosp., Montreal, P.Q.; Tel. WE 7-6011. Abroad.
DOLSON, Ernest; 16 Ontario St., Grimsby, Ont.; 75 Livingstone (res); Wes '52; MCGP; Tel. WH 5-2144.

DOMBROWSKI, Simon; 2960 rue Gentilly, Ste. Foy, Quebec 10, P.Q. (res); Lav '51; Anaes (P.Q.); Staff, Hop. de l'Enfant Jesus; Tel. 529-8711.

DOMBSKY, Victor M.; 13665-96th Ave., North Surrey, B.C.; 11075-136th St. (res); Aurora (Shanghai, China) '42; Tel. 581-2727.

DOMEGAN, Patrick R.; Box 999, Neepawa, Man.; Dublin (Ire.)'54; DCH; DPH.

DOMINGUE, Albert C.; 1570, St. Hubert, Montreal 24, P.Q.; Lav '28, OphthOtol.

DOMINGUE, Guy; 9765 rue Sackville, Montreal 12, P.Q.; Mon '50; DiagRad; Tel. 381-3668.

DOMINGUEZ, Antonio; Box 1098 Camp Petawawa, Petawawa, Ont.; Madrid (Spain) '54; Tel. 687-2111.

DOMINIC, Rufus G.; National U. (Dublin, Ire.) '54; Paed; Staff, Children's Med. Centre, St. John's, Nfld.

DOMKE, Oscar; 232 Medical Arts Bldg., Winnipeg, Man.; Ste. 3, 808 Sherbrooke St. (res); Man '2 M.C.G.P.; Tel. WH 3-5495.

DOMOSZLAI, Emma I.; Peter Pazmany U. (Budapest, Hung.)'55; Res., Hosp. for Sick Children, Toronto 2, Ont.

DON, Conway J.; Box 598, 34 Rebecca Cres., R.R. No. 1, Ottawa, Ont. (res.); London (Eng.) '46; M.R.C.P. (Lond.), D.M.R.D., F.F.R., DiagRad; Dir. (Rad.), Ottawa Gen. Hosp.; Prof. & Head (Rad.), U. of Ottawa; Tel. SH 9-3767.

DON, Hillary F.; 3635 Ridgewood Ave., Montreal 26, P.Q.; Cambridge (Eng.) '58; FRCP(C); Anaes; Staff, Royal Victoria Hosp.; Tel. 739-9833.

DONACHIE, Joseph P.; 1 Church St., Amherst, N.S.; Glasgow (Scot.) '60; DObstRCOG; DA; Anaes., Highland View Hosp.; Tel. 667-7125.

DONAHOE, J. Emmett; 5441 Bannantyne Ave., Verdun, Montreal, P.Q.; 36 Finchley Rd., Hampstead (res); Dal '37; GenSurg (P.Q.); Surg. Staff, St. Mary's Hosp.; Tel. PO 6-2151.

DONALD, Dominic M.; Man'63; Res., Vancouver Gen. Hosp., Vancouver 9, B.C.

DONALD, Edward F.; 510 Medical Arts Bldg., Edmonton, Alta.; Alb'35; AMCAA, IntMed; Med. Staff, U. of Alberta Hosp.; Clin. Instr., (IntMed), U. of Alberta; Tel. GA 4-1465.

DONALD, John P.; Box 700, Hanna, Alta.; Glasgow (Scot.) '60; Staff, Hanna Municipal Hosp.; Tel. 854-3351.

DONALD, Paul J., Capt.; UBC '64; Staff, RCN Hosp., HMCS Naden, Victoria, B.C.

DONALD, William A.; 207 The Med. Centre, 908 - 8th Ave. S.W., Calgary, Alta.; Glasgow (Scot.)'41; FRCS (Ed.); GenSurg; MCGP; Vis. Staff, Calgary Gen., Holy Cross, Alberta Children's & Grace Hosp's.; Tel. 262-1858.

DONALDSON, George D.; Mahone Bay, N.S.; Dal '36; Anaes; Chief Anaes., Fisherman's Mem. Hosp., Lunenburg & Dawson Mem. Hosp., Bridgewater; Tel. Lunenburg - 634-8801.

DONALDSON, Harry V.; 512 Herald Bldg., 206 - 7th Ave. S.W., Calgary, Alta.; Alb'56; Anaes; Dir. (Anaes.) Calgary Gen. Hosp.; Tel. 262-4742.

DONATI, Serge; Chambre 1305, 1150 Chemin St-Louis, Quebec 6, P.Q.; Lav'49.

DONATO, George; 1384 Jean Talon E., Montreal 35, P.Q.; Mon '62; Tel. 274-5583.

DONEGAN, Edmond A.; 256 Med. Arts Bldg., Saskatoon, Sask.; Glasgow (Scot.) '37; DOMS (Lond.); Ophth.; Tel. 653-0011.

DONEVAN, David F.; 131 Ontario St., St. Catharines, Ont.; 17 Forest Hill Rd. (res); Qns '56; FRCS(C), ObstGyn; Tel. MU 2-1332..

DONEVAN, Richard E.; 3650 St. Urbain St. Montreal, P.Q.; Qns '54; Pulm. Dis & T.B. (P.Q.); FRCP(C), IntMed; Ass't. Phys., Royal Victoria Hosp.; Phys., Royal Edward Chest Hosp.; Cons. Phys., Queen Mary Vet's Hosp., Lect. McGill U.; Tel. 849-8563.

DONEVAN, William J.; 11 Coldwater St. E., Orillia, Ont.; 108 Penetang St. (res); Qns '46.

DONEY, E. Harvey; 2590 Midland Ave., Agincourt, Ont. (res); Tor '31; Dir., Med. Rehab. Unit, Hosp. & Rehab. Centre, W.C.B., Ont.; Assoc. Staff (Med.), Toronto Western Hosp.; Tel. 244-1761.

DONIGIEWICZ, Stanislaw B.; 108 Church St., Antigonish, N.S. (res); Leeds (Eng.) '50; LRCP(Lond.), MRCS(Eng.); FACA; Anaes; Chief Anaes., St. Martha's Hosp.; Tel. 10.

DONIN, Jerry F.; 101 Oak St., Winnipeg, Man.; Man '50; Ophth.

DONISCH, Eric W.; 1064 Dearness Dr., London, Ont. (res); Bonn (Germ.)'47; Ass't. Prof. (Anat.), U. of Western Ont.

DONISCH, Valentina (Deinihovskaya); 1064 Dearness Dr., London, Ont. (res); Bonn (Germ.) '47; PhD; Research Staff, U. of Western Ont.

DONNELL, James M.; 230 St. Charles Rd., Beaconsfield, P.Q.; McG '55; FACS; DABS; GenSurg; Att'd. Staff, Reddy Mem. Hosp.; Staff Surg., Bell Telephone Co. Tel. 697-3383.

DONNELL, Margaret M.; Ste. 203, 310 Bloor St., W., Toronto 4, Ont.; 852 Mt. Pleasant Rd. (res); Tor '39; MCGP; Staff, OPD Women's College Hosp.; Tel. WA 2-8171.

DONNELLY, Andrew; 159 Ontario St., St. Catharines, Ont.; 31 Parnell Rd. (res); Glasgow (Scot.) '53; Urol; Tel. 684-7345.

DONNELLY, C. W.; 7575 Cambie St., Vancouver, B.C.; Man '46; M.C.G.P.; Tel. FA 7-6318.

DONNELLY, Grace C.; 1414 Drummond St., Montreal, P.Q.; 1009 Laird (res); McG '41; ObstGyn; Staff, Royal Victoria Hosp.; Tel. VI 2-1251.

DONNELLY, J. Brendan; Box 4, Erickson, Man.; Ireland '44.

DONNELLY, Kenneth R.; 3996 Rumble St., Burnaby, B.C. (res); UBC '55; Ass't. Prof. Anat., U. of British Columbia; Tel. 228-2586.

DONNELLY, Thomas H.; McG '42; Staff, Canadian Pension Commiss., Shaughnessy Hosp., Vancouver, B.C.; Tel. TR 6-6767.

DONOHUE, William L.; 71 DeVere Gdns., Toronto, Ont. (res); Tor '32; M.A., FRCP(C); PathBact; Dir. of Path., Hosp. for Sick Children; Assoc. Prof. (Path), U. of Toronto; Tel. EM 6-7242.

DONOVAN, A. L.; 41 Orange St., St. John, N.B.; McG '29; F.A.C.P., IntMed.; Chief Dept. Med., St. John Gen. Hosp.; Tel. 693-2123.

DONOVAN, Cornelius; Cork (Ire.) '48; Psy; Dir., Cape Breton Mental Health Clinic, Sydney, N.S.; Lect. (Psy), St. Francis-Xavier College; Tel. 562-3202.

DONOVAN, C. R.; 410 Oxford St., Winnipeg, Man.; Qns '15; D.P.H.; Retired.

DONOVAN, Edward G.; 505 Fairmont Medical Bldg., 750 W. Broadway, Vancouver 9, B.C.; Liverpool (Eng.)'43; MRCP (Lond.); DMRD, DCH; DiagRad; Ass't. Rad., Vancouver Gen. Hosp.; Tel. TR 9-4177.

DONOVAN, S. Georgina; Ott'64; Res. (Rad.), Royal Victoria Hosp., Montreal, P.Q.

DONSKY, Gordon J.; Tor'61; FRCP(C) Paed; Staff, Toronto East Gen. Hosp., Toronto, Ont.; Abroad.

DONSKY, Howard J.; 2901 Lawrence Ave. E., Scarborough, Ont.; Tor'60; FRCP(C), Derm; Clin. Teach. (Derm.), Toronto Gen. Hosp. & U. of Toronto; Tel. 266-4497.

DONTIGNY, Gilles; 1681 Parc Lafontaine, Montreal, P.Q.; Mon '49.; Tel. 526-6482.

DONTIGNY, Leon; Mon '64; Res., Notre-Dame Hosp., Montreal 24, P.Q.

DONTIGNY, Paul; 1681 Parc Lafontaine, Montreal, P.Q.; 53 ave. Oakland, Westmount (res); Mon '42; Ph.D.; IntMed (P.Q.); Staff, Hop.-Notre-Dame; Ass't. Prof., Montreal U.; Tel. RE 3-9951.

DONTIGNY, Yvon M.; 411 rue Laviolette, Trois Rivieres, P.Q.; 3108 Faucher (res); Lav '55 ObstGyn (P.Q.).

DONWORTH, John J.; 28 Montebello Place, St. Catharines. Ont.; National U. (Ire.) '45; Anaes; Chief Anaes, Hotel-Dieu Hosp.; Tel. MU 4-9201.

DOOLEY, Patrick E.; Box 180, Petawawa, Ont.: Ott '52; Tel. 687-4691.

DOOLEY, Robert J.; 151 Holland Ave., Ottawa, Ont.; Qns '37; M.C.G.P.; Staff, Ottawa Civic & Grace Hosp's.; Tel. PA 8-3788.

DORAN, Morton L.; Box 2058, Whitehorse, Y.T.; Tor'64; Staff, Whitehorse Gen. Hosp.

DORAN, Terence A.; 714 Med. Arts Bldg., 170 St. George St., Toronto 5, Ont.; 939 Lawrence Ave. E., Don Mills; 78 Golfdale Ave. (res); Tor '53; FRCS(C), ObstGyn; Staff, Tor. Gen. Hosp. & Dept. of ObstGyn., U. of Toronto; Tel. WA 2-0850.

DORAY, Bernard; 3175 Cote St. Catherine, Montreal 26, P.Q.; 10980 Pasteur (res); Mon '54; **FRCP(C), Paed; Ass't. Hop-Ste-Justine; Tel.** RE 1-4931.

DORAY, Jacques E.; 222 est, Henri Bourassa, Montreal 12, P.Q.; Mon '57; FRCS(C), GenSurg; PlasSurg; Tel. 384-9361.

DORAY, Maurice; 222 est, Henri Bourassa, Montreal, P.Q.; Mon '49; FCCP; Pulm. Dis. & TB (P.Q.); Cardiol. (P.Q.); Staff, Hop. du Sacre-Coeur, Cartierville; Tel. JU 8-9019.

DORCAS, Phyllis; (see Bursey).

DORE, Bruno; 259 rue St. Georges, St. Jerome, P.Q.; 535 du Palais (res); Lav '45; Ophth, Otol (P.Q.); Tel. GE 8-8632.

DORE, Louis J.; Mon'61; Res., Montreal Children's Hosp., Montreal, P.Q.

DORFMAN, Lionel E.; Tor '60; Res., Sunnybrook Hosp., Toronto 12, Ont.

DORFMAN, Sheila; 1200 Pembina, Winnipeg 19, Man.; Alb'63.

DORGELO, Gerhard H.; 901 Helena St., Trail, B.C.; 21 Hazelwood Dr. (res); Amsterdam (Neth.); '50; DABP; Paed; Phys. I/C Newborn Nurseries Trail-Tadanac Hosp.; Cons., Mater Misericordiae & Castlegar & Dist. Hosp's.; Tel. 368-9881.

DORIAN, William; 245 Victoria Ave., Montreal, P.Q.; Cluj (Rumania) '48; IntMed; Assoc. Dir., Med. Research, Merck, Sharp & Dohme of Canada; Tel. WE 3-7371.

DORION, Jules-E.; 609E. Blvd. Charest, Quebec, P.Q.; 1330, Ave. Lemoine, Sillery (res); Lav '26; Med. Dir., Quebec Health Services; Tel. 523-1153.

DORION, Marc; Lav'62; DiagRad; Staff, Hop. Hotel-Dieu, Quebec 4, P.Q.

DORION, Marie M.; Dept. of National Health & Welfare, Brooke Claxton Bldg., Tunney's Pasture, Ottawa, Ont.; Lav '51; M.Sc. (Harvard); DPH; PH (P.Q.); Med. Cons., Maternal & Children's Hygiene; Tel. 922-7995.

DORION, Marguerite; 1650 Laurier, Sillery, P.Q.; Lav '48; P.H. (P.Q.).

DORION, Roger; 262 St. Joseph W., Alma, Co. Lac St. Jean, P.Q.; Lav '56; A.M.C.G.P.; Tel. 662-3632.

DORMAAR, Nicholaas G.; Box 1570, Williams Lake, B.C.; Holland '55.

DORMAN, J. Garth; 3579 W. 41st Ave., Vancouver 13, B.C.; 6875 Angus Dr. (res); UBC '61. Tel. 261-6361.

DORR, H. Patrick; Ste. 430, 5300 Cote-des-Neiges, Montreal, P.Q.; McG'56; FRCS(C), ObstGyn; Staff, St. Mary's Hosp.; Tel. 731-5227.

DORRAN, Brian W.; Box 800, Roblin, **Man.;** London (Eng.)'59; MRCS(Eng.), LRCP(Lond.).

DORRANCE, Frank S., M.M.; Ste. 1023, 1538 Sherbrooke W., Montreal 25, P.Q.; McG'24; MCGP (Hon.); Hon. Att'd. Staff, Montreal Gen. Hosp.; Tel. 935-3235.

DORRANCE, Wallace J.; 925 W. Georgia St., Vancouver, B.C.; McG '21; GenSurg; Tel. MU 1-5471.

DORSEY, Douglas M.; 154 James St. S., Hamil-ton, Ont.; Qns'58; Ophth; Tel. JA 7-3724.

DORSEY, Frank R. J.; 208 Medical Arts Bldg., Edmonton, Alta.; 5322-111 Ave. (res); Alb '43; **ObstGyn.; Instr., U. of Alberta; Tel. 424-1273.**

DORSEY, Mallory C. C.; 154 James S., Hamil-ton, Ont.; 87 Flatt Ave. (res); Tor '26; Ophth, **Otol; Tel. JA 7-3724.**

DORVAL, Charles H.; 1750 Blvd. Benoit XV, Quebec 3, P.Q.; Lav '42; Cert. Ass't. TB (Paris, **Fr.); Pulm. Dis. & TB (PQ); Hd. Pulm. Serv. & IntMed. Clin., Hop.-Laval; Registrar, Anti-TB League (PQ); Assoc Prof., Laval U.; Tel. 523-7647.**

DOSMAN, James A.; 301 Canada Bldg., Saskatoon, Sask.; Sask '63.

DOSSETOR, John B.; Royal Victoria Hosp., Montreal, P.Q.; Oxford (Eng.)'50; Ph.D., MRCP (Lond.); FACP; **FRCP(C), IntMed; Dir. of Renal & Urol. Research, & Ass't Phys., Dept. of Med., Royal Victoria Hosp.; Ass't. Prof. of Med. & Experim. Surg., McGill U.; Tel. VI 2-**1251.

DOSTALER, A. Pierre; 513 Ste. Cecile, Trois Rivieres, P.Q.; 650 Des Commissaires (res); Mon '54; M.C.G.P.

DOTTEN, Dale A.; Tor '62; Intn., Banting Inst., Toronto, Ont.

DOUBEK, Ladislav; 340 McLeod St., Ste. 404, Ottawa, Ont.; 874 Kirkwood Ave. (res); Prague (Czech.)'49; Surg., Ottawa Civic Hosp.; Tel. PA 9-2511.

DOUBILET, Sidney I.; 5441 Bannantyne Ave., Verdun, Montreal, P.Q.; McG '25; A.A.P., Paed: **Hon. Staff, Royal Victoria, Montreal Children's & Jewish Gen. Hosp's.; Dem. in Paed., McGill U.;** Tel. 761-7746.

DOUBROVINE, Violet D. (See SMALL)

DOUCET, Calixte; Campbellton, N.B.; 18 O'Leary St. (res); Lav '34; GenSurg; Tel. PL 3-4431.

DOUCET, Felix J.; P.O. Box 113 Weymouth, Digby Co., N.S.; Lav '57.

DOUCET, Louis-Pierre; 5 ave. Peronne, Outremont 8, P.Q.; Mon '57; Psy; Staff, Inst. Albert Prevost; Tel. RE 1-0417.

DOUCET, Noel; 1010 Chemin St Rock, Tracy, **P.Q.; Lav '57. Gen Surg. (P.Q.);**

DOUCET, Pierre; 195 boul. du Havre, Valleyfield, P.Q.; Mon'61; Cardiol(P.Q.).

DOUCHET, George L.; Box 550, Peace River, Alta.; **Alb '61; Tel. 624-2969.**

DOUGALL, Donald R.; Petrolia, Ont.

DOUGALL, Marion; Petrolia, Ont.; **Wes '27.**

DOUGALL, Robert H.; 1004-105th St., Edmonton Alta.; 7923-94th Ave. (res) Alb '53 IntMed; Instr. (Med.), U. of Alberta; Tel. Ga 4-2121.

DOUGAN, Alfred A.; 33 Clough Ave., Lennoxville, P.Q. (res); McG '42; Anaes; Med. Dir. & **Hd. of Anaes., Sherbrooke Gen. Hosp.; Tel. LO 9-3661.**

DOUGAN, John McD., M.C.; Manitoba Clinic, 790 Sherbrook St., Winnipeg 2, Man.; Trinity Coll. (Dublin, Ire.) '39; BAO; Psy; Tel. SP 4-6541.

DOUGHTY, William; 814 Cook Rd., Richmond, B.C.; 768 Garden City Rd. (res); Man '54; Tel. CR 8-2191.

DOUGLAS, Allan B.; Qns'60; Res., Toronto Gen. Hosp., Toronto 2, Ont.

DOUGLAS, Eustace S. M.; 160 Queen St. E., Brampton, Ont.; Edinburgh (Scot.) '42; Staff, Peel Mem. Hosp.; Tel. GL 1-1645.

DOUGLAS, Frederick G.; Tor'61; FRCP(C), IntMed; Staff, Royal Victoria Hosp., Montreal, P.Q.

DOUGLAS, G. David; Dal'65; Res., Victoria Gen. Hosp., Halifax, N.S.

DOUGLAS, G. Ritchie; 100 Provost St., New Glasgow, N.S.; 79 Mountain Rd. (res); Dal '39; F.R.C.S.(C), F.A.C.S., GenSurg; Surg-in-chief, Aberdeen Hosp.; Tel. 752-8311.

DOUGLAS, H. Townley; 212 Rideau Terrace, Ottawa, Ont.; McG '12; Retired.

DOUGLAS, John C.; 289 Dufferin Ave., London, Ont.; 85 Regent St. (res); Wes '43; IntMed; Med. Staff, Victoria Hosp.; Fell. (Med.), U. of **Western Ontario Med. School; Tel. GE 2-3552.**

DOUGLAS, Kenneth M.; 248 Bridge St. E., Belleville, Ont.; **Edinburgh (Scot.) '45; F.R.C.S. (Ed.); FACS, GenSurg; Cons. Surg., Belleville Gen. & Trenton Mem. Hosp's.; Tel. WO 8-7940.**

DOUGLAS, Leith G.; Dal'62; Res. (PlasSurg.), Toronto Gen. Hosp., Toronto, Ont.

DOUGLAS, Louis H.; 14 Okanagan Dr., Ottawa 6, Ont.; Tor'43; DPH; Dir., Carleton Health Unit.

DOUGLAS, Mary C.; Sutton, Ont.; Qns '60.

DOUGLAS, Richard P.; 3906-4A St., S.W., Calgary, Alta.; **Tor '35; Anaes; Staff, Holy Cross,** Alberta Children's & Calgary Gen. Hosp's.; **Tel.** 243-0026.

DOUGLAS, Robert W.; 6238 Fraser St., Vancouver 15, B.C.; 4649 Osler St., Van. 29 (res); Edinburgh (Scot.) '55; Tel. FA 7-6637.

DOUGLAS, Roy G.; 435 Tegler Bldg., 10189-101st St., Edmonton, Alta.; Tor '11; MCGP; Staff, Royal Alexandra Hosp.; Tel. 422-1568.
DOUGLAS-MURRAY, Gael M.; 104 Johnson St., Kingston, Ont.; Qns'57; FRCS(C), ObstGyn; Clin. Teach. (Obst.), Queen's U.; Tel. 546-5873.
DOUGLASS, Arthur S.; Knowlton, P.Q.; Dal '32; Chairman, Med. Board, Brome Missiquoi Perkins Hosp., Sweetsburgh, P.Q.
DOUKETIS, John; 344 Bloor St. W., Ste. 204, Toronto 5, Ont.; 11 Walmer Rd., Apt. 506 (res); Athens (Gr.) '36; Tel. 925-7023.
DOUPE, Nona E. (Wright); Psychiatric Inst., 75 Emily St., Winnipeg 3, Man.; London (Eng.) '40; Psy; Sr. Psy., Prov. of Man.; Lect. (Psy.), U. of Manitoba; Tel. SP 4-6511.
DOUST, John W. L.; (See LOVETT-DOUST, John W.).
DOUVILLE, Elmer Louis; 259 King Edward, Ottawa, Ont.; Ott '51; M.Sc. (Minn); DABS; FACP; FICS; FACG; FICA; ThorSurg; Active Staff, Hop. St. Louise de Montfort; Cons. Staff, Hop. Sacre-Coeur, Hull & Hop. St. Vincent, Hull: Tel. CE 5-0350.
DOUVILLE, Gedeon J. T.; 1314 Lemoine Quebec 4, P.Q.; Lav '50; Anaes (P.Q.); Tel. 524-6831.
DOUVILLE, Joseph; St. Stanislas Cte. Champlain, P.Q.; Lav '42; Vis. Phys., Hop. Lafleche, Grandmere; Tel. 17.
DOVE, Robert F.; 2 Marcelle Ave., Corner Brook, Nfld. (res); Dal '36; GenSurg; M.O. Bowaters Pulp & Paper Mills; Tel. 634-5151.
DOVER, Mark R.; Ste. 901, 199 Holland Ave., **Ottawa 3, Ont.; Ott '55; DABS; FACS; FRCS-(C), GenSurg; Staff Ottawa Civic Hosp.; Clin. Ass't., U. of Ottawa;** Tel. 729-8112.
DOVEY, Bruce B.; Aspen Med. Centre, 425 Tranquille Rd., North Kamloops, B.C.; UBC'58; Tel. 376-7242.
D'OVIDIO, Vincent; 1267A St. Clair Ave. W., Toronto 10, Ont.; Bologna (Italy) '57; Tel. 536-5711.
DOW, Edward W.; 18 Crown St., Trenton, Ont.; Qns'50; Active Staff, Trenton Mem. Hosp.; MOH, Town of Trenton & Twp. Sidney, Village of Frankford; Tel. 392-4741.
DOW, Edward W. Jr.; 18 Crown St., Trenton, Ont.; Qns'64; Quarantine Officer, C.F.B., Tel. 392-4741.
DOW, George E.; Killarney Med. Centre, Killarney, Man.; Man '55; M.C.G.P.; M.O.H.; Dist. Coroner; Tel. 523-4241.
DOWD, Ainslie H.; 500 Deschenes, Box 125, Beloeil, P.Q.; Qns '52; Plant Phys., C.I.L., Mc-Masterville; Tel. 467-2491.
DOWD, Emerson C.; 90 Harbour St., Toronto 1, Ont.; 636 Pharmacy Ave., Scarborough, Ont. (res); Qns'47; Gen. Surg.; Staff, WCB; Court. Surg. Staff, Scarborough Gen. Hosp.; Tel. 362-3411, Loc. 445 or 446.
DOWD, J. E.; Fenwick, Ont.; McG '26.
DOWD, Jean (See O'Heany)
DOWD, J. Ronald; Qns'61; FRCS(C), ObstGyn; Staff, St. Michael's Hosp., Toronto 2, Ont.
DOWD, Judith A.; Qns'65; Staff, Government Hosp., Sioux Lookout, Ont.
DOWD, K. E.; Box 8100, 935 Lagauchetiere W., Montreal 3, P.Q.; 59 Balfour Ave. Mtl. 16 (res); **McG '25; F.A.C.S., A.B.P.M., (Avia. Med.),** F.A.M. (Aero-Med. Assoc.), Chief Med. Off., Air Canada & C.N.R.; Retired.
DOWD, Robert A.; Osgoode, Ont.; Qns '16; Tel. 489-3554.
DOWD, William R.; Kinburn, Ont.; McG '18; MCGP; Dist. Coroner; Tel. 839-2156.
DOWER, Gordon E.; 4640 N.W. Marine Dr., Vancouver 8, B.C. (res); St. Bart's, London (Eng.) 49; M.R.C.S., L.R.C.P.; Cons. Shaughnessy Hosp.; **Research (Electrocardiol.) & Ass't. Prof. (Pharmacol.), U. of British Columbia; Tel. CA 4-1111.**
DOWLING, Harvey E.; 315 Greyhound Bldg., Calgary, Alta.; Sub P.O. No. 13 (res); McG '25; **Ophth, Otol; AAO & O; Tel. 269-4838.**
DOWLING, Sterling O.; 217 Medical Arts Bldg., Winnipeg, Man.; 530 Basswood Rd. (res); Man **'38; O.P. Staff, Winnipeg Gen. Hosp; Tel. SP 4-6511.**
DOWNE, William N.; 1053 Talbot St., London, Ont. (res); Wes '50; Psy; Psy. Staff, St. Joseph's Hosp.; Cons., Westminster Hosp.; Instr. (Psy), U. of Western Ont.; Cons. Dept. of Reform Institutions; Tel. GE 9-3271.
DOWNES, William P.; 849 Main St. E., Hamilton, Ont.; Qns '18.
DOWNEY, Joe L.; 630 Med. Arts Bldg., Winnipeg, Man.; 307 Waverley St. (res); Man '35; FCCP; FACCP; IntMed; Active Med. Staff, St. Boniface Hosp.; Ass't. Prof., U. of Manitoba; Tel. WH 2-7706.
DOWNIE, Donald M.; 25 St. Michael St., St. Albert, Alta.; Alb'55.
DOWNIE, Frederick J.; 36 River Rd. E., Kitchener, Ont.; **London (Eng.) '62; AMCGP; Active Staff, Kitchener-Waterloo & St. Mary's Hosp's.;** Tel. 745-6128.
DOWNING, G. Murray; Otterville, Ont.; Tor '40; MCGP; Tel. 879-6939.
DOWNING, John B.; The Medical Centre, 5 Central St., Summerside, P.E.I.; 92 Summer St. (res); Dal '43; IntMed; Chief Med., Prince County **Hosp.; Tel. 2246.**
DOWNS, Allan R.; 790 Sherbrooke St., Winnipeg 2, Man.; 261 Rita St. (res); Man '54; FRCS (C); GenSurg; Pt.-time Clin. Tutor, Wpg. Gen. Hosp. Lect., U. of Man; Tel. SP 4-6541.
DOWNS, William J.; 10308-133rd St., Edmonton, Alta.; McG '34;; IntMed (T.B.); Sr. Phys., Aberhart Mem. San.; Instr. (Med.), U. of Alta.; Staff, W.C.B.; Tel. GE 9-0051.
DOWSLEY, G. A.; 710 Seymour St., Vancouver. **B.C.; 5711 Marguerite St. (res); Tor '26; Tel. MU 4-1511.**
DOYLE, Arthur M., MBE; Med. Arts Bldg., 280 Bloor W., Toronto 5, Ont.; 24 Forest Glen Cres. (res); Tor'31; DABPN; NeurPsy; Chief of Psy., St. Michael's Hosp.; Assoc. Prof. (Med. & Psy.), U. of Toronto; Tel. WA 2-5588.
DOYLE, Brian P.; c/o Camp Borden Stn. Hosp., Camp Borden, Ont.; London (Eng.) '48; M.B., B.S.; GenSurg.
DOYLE, Charles E.; 380 St. George St., Moncton, N.B.; 500 Yale Ave., Riverview Hgts. (res); Dal '45; F.A.C.S., GenSurg; Sr. Att. Surg., Moncton Hosp.; Court. Surg. Staff, Hotel Dieu Hosp.; Tel. 384-8604.
DOYLE, F. Patrick; Ste.-Anne, Man.; Lav '48; **MCGP; Dist. Coroner; Memb. Man. Hosp. Comm.; Tel. GA 2-5377.**
DOYLE, Guy; 6412 rue Langelier, Montreal 36, P.Q.; '60; TherRad(P.Q.).
DOYLE, Henry S.; 52 Walmsley Blvd., Toronto, Ont. (res); Tor '36; Ass't. Supt. (Med.), Toronto Gen. Hosp.; Tel. GA 2-5377.
DOYLE, John A.; 164 Metcalfe St., Ottawa, Ont.; 1054 Chelsea Dr. (res); Ott '51; Paed; Staff, Ottawa Gen. Hosp.; Court. Staff, St. Louis-Marie-de-Montfort, Eastview & Grace Hosp.; Lect. (Paed), U. of Ottawa; Tel. CE 3-1166.
DOYLE, Lewis J.; Lav '35; Pulm. Dis. & TB (P.Q.), Staff, Indian Hosp., Fort Qu'Appelle, Sask.; Tel. 332-5785.
DOYLE, Michael; Lav '61; Res., Queen Mary Vet's. Hosp., Montreal 26, P.Q.; Abroad.
DOYLE, Patrick E.; 5 Ave. N., Swan River, **Man.; National U. (Ire) '54.**
DOYLE, Patrick J.; 5780 Cambie St., Vancouver **15, B.C.; 1428 W. 40th (res); Alb '49; DABOt; Otol; Att'd. Staff, St. Vincent's, Children's & Shaughnessy Hosp's.; Clin. Insr. (Otol.), U. of** British Columbia; Tel. FA 1-0522. Abroad.
DOYLE, Phillip E.; 267 O'Connor St., Ottawa 4, Ont.; McG '37; FRCP(C), IntMed; Staff, Ottawa Civic Hosp.; Ass't. Prof. (Ther.), U. of Ottawa; Tel. 234-8526.
DOYLE, Philip John; 80 Hunter St. E., Peterborough; Kawartha Heights (res); Qns '53; Tel. 745-3215.
DOYLE, William J.; Unity, Sask.; Tor '45; M.C.-G.P.; Dist. Coroner.
DOYON, Denis; 2788 Willowdale, Montreal, 26, **P.Q.;** Lav'52; Psy; Chief of Psy., Hop. Notre-Dame; Tel. 731-5556.
DOYON, Maurice; C.P. 1928 Amos, P.Q.; Lav '60; FRCS(C); GenSurg.

DOZIOS, Jaques; 5 Blvd. Des Laurentides Pont Viau, Laval-des-Rapides, P.Q.; 54 Conrad (res); Mon '53 MCGP; Tl. 669-6701.
DOZOIS, Roger; Lav'65; Res., Hop. St. Francis d'Assise, Quebec 3, P.Q.; Abroad.
DRABITT, T. Sylvester; Man'61; Res., St. Boniface Hosp., Winnipeg 6, Man.
DRACHE, Victor; Medical Bldg., 5780 Cambie St., Vancouver 15, B.C.; 1308 W. 46th (res); Man '25; F.R.C.S.(Ed.), GenSurg; Vis. Staff, Vancouver Gen., St. Vincent's, St. Paul's & Children's Hosp's.; Tel. FA 5-4232.
DRAGANIC, Rudolph; 669 Barton St. E., Hamilton, Ont.; Zagreb (Yugoslavia) '44; Tel. 544-9283.
DRAISEY, Tom F.; Bristol (Eng.)'60; Path; Staff, Grace Hosp., Windsor, Ont.
DRAKE, Charles G.; Ste. 211, Victoria Bldg., 111 Waterloo St., London, Ont.; 1545 Gloucester **Pl. (res); Wes '44; M.Sc., FRCS(C); FACS; M.S. (Tor.); NeurSurg; Staff, (NeurSurg.), Victoria Hosp.; Assoc. Prof. (NeurSurg.), U. of Western Ont.; Tel. 439-7881.**
DRAKE, H. Martyn; Oxford (Eng.) '59; Ass't. M.O., Grand Bank Cottage Hosp., Grand Bank, Nfld.; Tel. PG 1941.
DRAKE, Leslie J.; Ste. 400, 5300 Cote des Neiges Rd, Montreal 26, P.Q.; 4660 Doherty (res); McG '53; DABS; FRCS(C); FACS; GenSurg; Ass't. Surg., St. Mary's Hosp.; Tel. RE 7-3575.
DRAKE, Robert M.; London (Eng.) '61; Staff, Muskoka Lake Clinic, Bracebridge, Ont.; Tel. 645-4457.
DRANCE, Stephen M.; 2550 Willow St. Vancouver 9, B.C.; 1561 Westbrook Cr., Van. 8 (res); Edinburgh (Scot.) '48; D.O.; FRCS (Eng.) Ophth; Assoc. Prof. (Ophth.), U.B.C.; Dir., Glaucoma Serv., U.B.C.; Tel. TR 6-3211, Local 2431.
DRAPEAU, Blaise; 166 King St. W., Sherbrooke, P.Q.; 223 Heneker St. (res); Lav '50; O.R.L. (New York), Otol; Chief (Otol), Hop. **St. Vincent de Paul; Tel. LO 9-6381.**
DRAPEAU, Joseph O.; 124 St. Germain, Rimouski, P.Q.; Lav '24; Surg., Hop. St. Joseph.
DRAPEAU, Napoleon; Isle Verte, P.Q.; Lav '16.
DRAPEAU, Pierre; Lav'62; Psy; Staff, Hop. Ste-Justine, Montreal 26, P.Q.
DRAPER, Dennis C.; 309 Med. Arts Bldg., 1 Young St., Hamilton, Ont.; McG '45; GenSurg; Staff, Hamilton Gen. & Chedoke Gen. Hosp's.; Tel. JA 9-3070.
DRESSLER, Joachim A.; 114 Purcell's Cove Rd., Armdale, Halifax, N.S. (res); Mainz (Germ.) '47; **Lect., Pathol. Inst., Dalhousie U.**
DREW, George W.; Qns'63; Staff, M. J. Boylen Hosp., Baie Verte, Nfld.
DREYFUS, Michel A.; 470 Wilbrod, Ottawa, Ont.; Paris (Fr.) '42; D.I.H. (Fr.), U.N.R.R.A. Med. Off.; Staff (Paed.), Hop. St.-Louis-Marie-de-Montfort; Tel. CE 3-9161.
DRIEDGER, Gerhard; Haig Clinic, 601-6th Ave. S., Lethbridge, Alta.; Kiel(Germ.) '48; FACS; FRCS(C), OrthSurg; Active Staff, Lethbridge Mun. & St. Michael's Hosp's. Staff, Lethbridge Auxiliary Hosp. & Little Bow Hosp.; Cons. Staff, Taber Mem. Hosp., Taber; Tel. 328-6641.
DRIEMEN, Pearl M. (Sures); 403 Doctor's Bldg., 267 O'Connor, Ottawa, Ont.; 85 Range Rd. (res); **Ott '55; A.M.C.G.P.; Staff. Ottawa Civic Hosp.; Tel. PA 9-2511.**
DRIESSEN, Henri E.; 724-736 Granville St., Vancouver 2, B.C.; Amsterdam (Netherlands)'40.
DRILLIS, G. Linard; 939 Lawrence Ave. E., Don Mills, Ont.; 9 Roanoke Rd. (res); Riga (Latvia) '44; Staff, Wellesley Hosp., Toronto; Tel. 444-1781.
DRKULEC, Vladimir; 41 Giles Blvd. E., Windsor, Ont.; Wes '60; Tel. 252-1943.
DROLET, Conrad; Lav '48; Psy; Staff, Clinique Roy Rousseau, Chemin-de-la-Canardiere, Mastai, Quebec 5, P.Q.; Tel. 661-7735.
DROLET, Gilles P.; Ott '59; Staff. Sanatorium St.-Jean, Macamic, P.Q.
DROLET, Henri; 15 Louis Hebert, Loretteville, P.Q.; Lav '56; Anaes (P.Q.); Anaes-in-Chief, Hop.-St.-Ambroise; Tel. 842-7749.
DROLET, J. E.; Val Brilliant, P.Q.; Lav '12.
DROLET, Marcel; 31 King St. W., Sherbrooke, P.Q.; 150 rue Vimy (res); Lav '49; IntMed; Dir. Radioisoptope Lab.; Tel. LO 9-1234.
DROLET, Maurice; 1301 ave. Fitzpatrick, Quebec 6, P.Q. Lav '51; D & T Rad.; Tel. 527-9970.
DROLET, Michel E.; Lav'63; Res., Mtl. Neurological Inst., Montreal 2, P.Q.
DROLET, Michel J.; 1000 Chemin Ste-Foy, Quebec 6, P.Q.; Lav '64.
DROLET, Terrence A.; Ghitter Clinic, Box 1569, Wetaskiwin, Alta.; **Alb '60; Tel. 352-3661 .**
DROLET, Yvan; Lav'65; Res., Hop. Notre-Dame, Montreal 24, P.Q.
DROLET, Yvon C.; Ott'53; Res., c/o Apt. 804, 3645 Sherbrooke Est., Montreal 4, P.Q.
DROUIN, Bernard; 1562 Ave. Notre-Dame, Ancienne-Lorette, P.Q.; Lav '62.
DROUIN, Claude; 750 St-Vallier ouest; Quebec 8, **P.Q.; 2008 Louis Jette, Ste Foy (res); Lav '58;** Dist. Coroner; Tel. 527-5533.
DROUIN, Georges; 1185 Chemin-Ste-Foy, Quebec 6, P.Q.; 945 ave. Brown, Que. 6 (res); Lav '48; Obst (PQ); Clin. Ass't. & Instr. (Obst.), Hop.-de-la-Misericorde; Cons. Matern. & Child Welfare, P.Q.; Staff (Path.), Dept. of Obst., U. of Laval; Tel. 683-7924.
DROUIN, Gilles; St-Andre-Avellin, Cte Papineau, P.Q.; Lav'55.
DROUIN, Guy; Hop. St. Sacrement, Quebec 6, P.Q.; Lav'32; Cardiol (P.Q.); FACC; FACP; IntMed; Chief, Dept. of Med., Hop. St. Sacrement; Assoc. Prof. (Med.), Laval U.
DROUIN, Guy; Mon' 62; Res., Hotel-Dieu, Montreal 18, P.Q.
DROUIN, J. Guy; 1307, Boul. Masson, Les Saules, Quebec, P.Q.; Lav'62.
DROUIN, Jacques; 960 Boul. Ste-Croix, St. Laurent, P.Q.; Mon'59; Psy(P.Q.); Dir., (Home Care), Inst. Albert-Prevost; Tel. 747-3501.
DROUIN, Jean; 700 ave Laure, Sept-Iles, P.Q.; Lav'53; Tel. 942-4218.
DROUIN, Jean-E.; 164 MacLaren E., Buckingham, P.Q.; 579 rue David (res); Ott '57; MCGP; Tel. 986-5415.
DROUIN, J. Paul; 428 Rideau, Ottawa 2, Ont.; Box 424, R.R. No. 1, Rothwell Hts. (res); Alb '46; F.A.C.S., F.R.C.S.(C), GenSurg; Staff, St. **Louis-Marie-de-Montfort; Assoc. Prof. Clin. Surg., U. of Ottawa; Tel. CE 4-9695.**
DROUIN, Michel; Lav '64; Res., Hop. Hotel-Dieu, Quebec 4, P.Q.; Abroad.
DROUIN, Noel H.; C.P. 177, Limoilou, Quebec 3, P.Q.; Lav'49.
DROUIN, Patrice; Lav '60; FRCP(C), Neur; Staff, Hop. St-Sacrement, Quebec 6, P.Q.; Tel. 681-7211.
DROUIN, Rene; 1000, Chemin Ste-Foy, Quebec 6, P.Q.; Lav '51; D & TRad; Rad., Hop. St. Sacrement; Tel. 681-5242.
DROUIN, Raynald; Lav'65; Res., Hop. Maisonneuve, Montreal 36, P.Q.
DROUIN, Rosaire; 1787 Jacques Lemaistre, Montreal 11, P.Q.; Lav'51; Anaes.; Tel. 387-7247.
DROVER, Wilfred H.; O'Mara-Martin Bldg., St. John's, Nfld.; Dal 35; MCGP.
DRUCKER, William R.; 15 Purling Place, Willowdale, Ont.; U.S.A.'46; Chief, Dept. of Surg., Univ. of Toronto; Tel. 928-2710.
DRUCKMAN, Paul B.; Tor '61; Jr. Intn., Toronto Gen. Hosp., Toronto 2, Ont.
DRUITT, A. W. Nigel; Box 150, 260 Black Mt. Rd., Rutland, B.C.; R.R. 5, Jose Rich Rd., Kelowna (res); St. Bart's (London Eng.) '42; MCGP; Tel. 765-5335.
DRULAK, Stephen L.; 609 Boyd Bldg., Winnipeg, Man.; 308 Boreham Blvd. (res); McG '43; Anaese; Staff Anaes.. Misericordia Gen. Hosp.; Tel. SP 4-6581.
DRUMMOND, Denis S.; McG'62; Res., Toronto East Gen. Hosp., Toronto 13, Ont.
DRUMMOND, George; Glasgow (Scot.)'56; FRCP(C), Anaes; Staff, (Anaes.), Foothills Hosp., Calgary, Alta.

DRUMMOND, John A.; Ste. 322, 1414 Drummond St., Montreal 25, P.Q.; 3042 Trafalgar (res); **McG '43; DDS; FACS; FRCS(C); PlasSurg;** Surg. I/C. Sub. Dept. PlastSurg., Royal Victoria Hosp.; Cons. Plas. Surg., Queen Elizabeth Hosp.; Cons., Queen Mary Vet's Hosp.; Ass't. Prof. (PlasSurg.), McGill U.; Tel. 845-6910.

DRUMMOND, John C.; 2 South Dr., St. Catharines, Ont.; 28 Belton Blvd. (res); Liverpool (Eng.) '23; M.Ch.Orth., F.R.C.S.(Edin.), Orth-Surg; OrthSurg., St. Catharines Gen. & Hotel **Dieu; Gtr. Niagara Gen. & San.; Tel. MU 4-3556.**

DRUMMOND, Keith A.; Oxbow, Sask.; Sask '59.

DRUMMOND, Keith N.; Room S215, Montreal Children's Hosp., 2300 Tupper St., Montreal, P.Q.; McG '55; FRCP(C), Paed; Assoc. Phys. & Dir., Renal Lab., Montreal Children's Hosp.; Ass't. Prof. (Paed.), McGill U.; Tel. WE 7-8511, Area 514.

DRUMMOND, Kenneth L.; Elbow, Sask.; Tor'43.

DRUMMOND, Mabel M.; 32 Irwin Ave., Toronto 5, Ont.; Liverpool (Eng.) '36; Tel. 921-6242.

DRUMMOND, William A.; Sorrento, B.C.; Alb '32; C.P.R.

DRUMMOND-HAY, Malcolm J.; Tor '60; Res., Westminster Hosp., London, Ont.

DRURY, David; 156 Victoria E., Amherst, N.S., Dal '18; Staff, Highland View Hosp.

DRUTZ, Myer G.; 1623 Keele St., Toronto 15. Ont.; 392 Glencairn Ave. (res); Tor '36; M.C.-G.P.; Sr. Phys., Dept. Med., Northwestern Gen. Hosp.; Tel. RO 9-8967.

DRYER, Ellice A. (Parmenter); 501 Yonge St., Toronto 5, Ont.; St. Andrew's (Scot.)'44; Anaes; Staff, Anaes., Women's College Hosp.

DRYSDALE, Alan A.; 2390 Armcrescent W., Halifax, N.S. (res); Dal '55; Anaes; Staff (Anaes.), Victoria Gen. Hosp.; Ass't. Prof., (Anaes.), Dalhousie U. & Lect. (Anaes.), Fac. of Dentistry; Tel. 423-8484.

DRYSDALE, Ian A.; 123 Erie Ave., Brantford, Ont.; Durham (Eng.)'59.

DRYSDALE, Ian O.; Dal'61; Ophth; Staff, Banting Inst., U. of Toronto, Toronto, Ont.

DRYSDALE, Ronald D.; The Polyclinic, 170-172 Fitzroy St., Charlottetown, P.E.I.; 78 Goodwill Ave. (res); Dal '48; F.R.C.P.(C), IntMed; Staff, P.E.I. Hosp.; Tel. 894-7325.

DRZEWICKA-KUBINSKI, Halina M.; 210 Hammond Bldg., Moose Jaw, Sask.; 1113 Grafton (res); Brussels (Belg.) '49.

DU, Nhac H.; Taiwan (China) '61; Jr. Intn., Wpg. Children's Hosp., Winnipeg, Man.

DUBE, Claude B.; 9 Jacques Cartier, Valleyfield, P.Q.; Lav '45; OphthOtol (P.Q.); Tel. 373-0255.

DUBE, Edgar; 6340 Des Angevins, Montreal 5, P.Q.; Lav'59.

DUBE, Francois J.; 136 Laval St., Ottawa 7, Ont.; Ott '61; Staff, Dept. of National Health & Welfare.

DUBE, Gaetan; 163 Jeanbaptiste Jobin, Boucherville, Cte. Chambly, P.Q.; Lav'57.

DUBE Gilles; 371A Boul St.-Joseph, Roberval, P.Q.; Lav '63.

DUBE, Ide; Lav '62; Res., Hop. L'Enfant Jesus, Quebec 3, P.Q.

DUBE, Jacques; Notre-Dame-du-Lac, Temiscouata, P.Q.; Lav '43; GenSurg (P.Q.); Surg., Hop. Notre-Dame-du-Detour; Tel. 899-6812.

DUBE, Jacques; Lav '61; FRCP(C), IntMed; Staff, Hop. Hotel-Dieu, Montreal 18, P.Q.; Tel. VI 4-0161.

DUBE, Jean; Mon '56; FRCP(C), PhysMed & Rehab; Staff, Hotel-Dieu Hosp., Levis, P.Q.; Tel. 837-9341.

DUBE, Louiselle; Unite Sanitaire, New-Carlisle, Quebec, P.Q.; Lav '56; PH.

DUBE, Louis-P.; St. Sylvester, P.Q.; Lav '24. Tel.11.

DUBE, Marie J.; 180 Dufferin St., Granby, P.Q.; Mon '31. Retired.

DUBE, Marius; 280-56eme rue ouest, Quebec 7, P.Q.; '62; GenSurg(P.Q.).

DUBE, Paul C.; Algonquin Dr., Lucerne, P.Q.; Lav'51; Staff, Dept. of National Health & Welfare, Brooke Claxton Bldg., Ottawa, Ont.; Abroad.

DUBE, Roch; Clinique Centrale, 210 Principale, Granby, P.Q.; Mon'60; Tel. 372-5401.

DUBE, William J.; UBC '63 Res., Vancouver Gen. Hosp., Vancouver, B.C.; Abroad.

DUBE, Yvon; 523 est rue Labrecque, Alma, P.Q.; Lav'62; Anaes.

DUBEAU, J. A. Marius; 777 Blvd. St. Joseph E., Montreal 34, P.Q.; 1600 Mattawa, Fabreville (res); Mon '40; FACA; FICS; Anaes; Dir. Anaes., Hop. Maisonneuve; Ass't. Prof (Anaes.) U. of Mtl.; Tel. 273-2854.

DUBELSTEIN, Peter A.; 189 Third Line Rd., Oakville, Ont.; Tor '62; Staff, St. Joseph's Hosp., Toronto, & Oakville Trafalgar Mem. Hosp.

Du BERGER, Pierre; 7662 rue St.-Denis, Montreal 10, P.Q.; 11387 rue de-St.-Real (res); Mon '62; Tel. CR 4-9286.

DuBERGER, Rene L.; 1054 Prospect, Sherbrooke, P.Q.; McG '23; DiagRad; Chief Radiol., Hop.-St.-Vincent-de-Paul; Tel. 562-7592.

DUBICANAC, Stefan T.; 1578 Jean-Talon E., Montreal 35, P.Q.; 2010 Ekers Ave. (res); Yugoslavia '39; M.C.G.P.; Tel. 728-9203.

DUBICKI, Carl B.; Dal '62; Res., Wellesley Hosp., Toronto, Ont.

DUBO, Hyman I.; Man '63; Res., Manitoba Rehab. Hosp., Winnipeg 2, Man.; Abroad.

DUBOIS, Gaston G., Sg/Lcdr; National Defence Medical Centre, Ottawa, Ont.; Ott'58.

DUBOIS, Georges H.; 26 rue Demers, Victoriaville, P.Q.; Lav '53; Path; Dir of Labs., Hotel-Dieu, Arthabaska; Tel. 357-2031.

DUBOIS. Guy; 5965 est, rue Sherbrooke, Montreal 5, P.Q; Lav '62; Tel. 254-5394.

DUBOIS, Jacques D.; 258 Crowland, Welland, Ont.; 7 Susan (res); Mon '49; MCGP; Staff, Welland Gen. Hosp.; Tel. 732-5912.

DUBOIS, Jacques M.; 29, ave-du-Lac, Dorval, P.Q.; Mon '52; Psy; Ass't. Supt., Hop. Saint-Jean-de-Dieu, Gamelin; Tel. 631-1709.

DUBOIS, J. Maurice; 67 Main St. E., Hawkesbury, Ont.; Lav '50.

DUBOIS, John R. Jr.; 534 Queens Ave., London, Ont.; Michigan (U.S.A.)'56.

DUBOIS, Paul F.; Boyd Bldg., Gore Ave. & Young St., Chilliwack, B.C.; 104 Gore Ave. (res); Amsterdam (Neth.) '47; M.C.G.P.; Staff, Chilliwack Gen. Hosp.

DuBOULAY, Maurice R.; Ste. 7, 1658 Victoria Pk. Ave., Scarborough, Ont.; 2303 Eglinton Ave. E. Apt. 427 (res); Tor '53; Tel. PL 7-3237.

DUBOW, Harry I.; Ste. 460, 5845 Cote des Neiges Rd., Montreal 26, P.Q.; McG '58; FRCS(C), Orth-Surg.

DUBRAVCIK, Paul; Czechoslovakia '55; Res. (OrthSurg.), Montreal Children's Hosp., Montreal, P.Q.

DUBREUIL-CHARROIS, Marie; Lav'61; Staff, Dept. of Path., U. of Laval, Quebec, P.Q.

DUBREUIL, Lucien; 685 ave. Rockland, Montreal 8, P.Q. (res); Mon '30; MPH; P.H. (PQ); Supt. Div. of Child Welfare, Health Serv., Mtl.

DUBREUIL, Paul; 238 Sud, Notre-Dame, Thetford Mines, P.Q.; Lav '53. Paed (P.Q.);

DUBREUIL, Richard; Disraeli, Co. Wolfe, P.Q.; Lav '46; P.H. (P.Q.).

DUBSKY, Frederick; Prague (Czech.) '34; F.C.-C.P.; Staff Phys., Fort William San., Fort William, Ont.; Tel. MA 3-7493.

DUBUC, Charles Yves; 2815 boul de la Concorde, **Durvenay, P.Q.; 580 rue Franchere (res); Lille (France) '55; Tel. 663-1671.**

DUBUC. Francois L.; Mon '62; Res., Hop. St. Luc, Montreal, P.Q.; Abroad.

DUBUC, Gustave; 176A Church Ave., Verdun, Montreal 19. P.Q.; Mon '41; Ophth.Otol (P.Q.); Tel. 769-7911.

DUBUC, Gustave; 53 Chemin St.-Louis, Beauharnois, P.Q. (res); McG '37; M.O. Aluminum Co. of Canada.

DUBUC, Hector; 1953 Blvd. Rosemont, Montreal, P.Q.; 159 Dufferin Rd. (res); Mon '32; Ophth, Otol; Tel. 271-5604.

DUBUC, L.; St. Remi, P.Q.; Mon '34.
DUCHAINE, Prime; 1010 St.-Cyrille ouest, Quebec 6, P.Q.; 61 Pierre Maufay (res); Lav '49; Obst-Gyn (PQ); Staff, Hop. Misericorde & Laval U.; Tel. 681-2837.
DUCHARME, Alfred; 366 rue Manseau, Joliette, P.Q.; St. Felix de Valois (res); Lav 21; Phys. Hop. St. Felix de Valois.
DUCHARME, Fergus A.; 195 Laurier Ave. E., Ottawa 2, Ont.; Ott'52; M.Ch.Orth. (Liverpool); FRSC(C), OrthSurg; FACS; Staff, Ottawa Gen. Hosp.; Ass't Prof. (OrthSurg.), U. of Ottawa; Tel. CE 5-4123.
DUCHARME, George P.; Ste 502, 45 Elm St. E., Sudbury, Ont.; Ott'52; FACOG; ObstGyn; Chief of Obst. & Deputy Chief (Gyn.), St. Joseph's Hosp.; Clin. Teach, School of Nursing; Tel. 674-3863.
DUCHARME, Gerard; 426 est boul St-Joseph, Montreal 34, P.Q.; 5710 Wilderton, Mtl. 26 (res); Mon '38; Obst (P.Q.); Clin. Ass't. (Obst.), Hop-Ste-Jeanne-d'Arc; Ass't. Prof. (Obst.), U. of Montreal; Tel. VI 5-0701.
DUCHARME, Guy; 36, ave. Hotel-Dieu, Sorel, P.Q.; Mon '60.
DUCHARME, Jacques C.; 640 Dawson Ave., Montreal, P.Q.; Mon '54; M.Sc. (Med.); GenSurg; Staff Surg., Hop. Ste-Justine; Tel. DU 1-5311.
DUCHARME, Jacques R.; 3175 Chemin-Ste.-Catherine, Montreal 26, P.Q.; 505 rue Stuart, Outremont 8 (res); Mon '54; DABP; FAAP; Paed. (PQ); Dir. Paed. (Endocrin. Research) Lab., Hop.-Ste.-Justine; Assoc. Prof. (Paed.), U. of Mtl.; Tel. RE 1-4931, Loc 467.
DUCHASTEL, Yves J.; Centre medical Henri-Bourassa, 222 est, boul. Henri-Bourassa, Montreal, P.Q.; Mon '59; Neur (P.Q.); Active Staff, Hop. du Sacre-Coeur, Cartierville; Cons. Neur., Hop. Notre Dame de l'Esperance & Hop. de St-Eustache; Research Staff (Neuro-Genet.), U. of Montreal; Tel. 731-5263.
DUCHENSE, Antonio; 129 Principale, Granby, P.Q.; 248 Savage, Granby (res); Lav '46; Anaes (P.Q.); Chief Anaes., Hop. St. Joseph; Tel. FR 2-5491.
DUCHESNE, Claude; Mon '61; Res., Hop. Maisonneuve, Montreal 36, P.Q.
DUCHESNE, Gerard; Lav '64; Res., Dept of Rad., Hop. Hotel-Dieu, Montreal 18, P.Q.
DUCHESNE, Guy; Mon '60; Res., Hop.-Notre-Dame, Montreal 24, P.Q.
DUCHESNE, Laurent; 75 ouest, Dorchester, Montreal, P.Q.; 517 N.D. de Fatima, Durvenay (res); Mon '47; Med. Dir., Hydro, Quebec; Tel. 875-4311.
DUCHESNE, Roland; 2484 des-Hospitalieres, Sillery, Quebec 6, P.Q. (res); Lav '42; DABA; Anaes; Dir., Anaes. Serv., Hop.-St.-Francois-d'Assise; Ass't Prof., Laval U.; Tel. 527-7914.
DUCKETT, Guy; 1365 est Jean Talon, Montreal, P.Q.; Lav'50; D&TRad; Staff, Hop. Hotel-Dieu; Tel. CR 3-5151.
DUCKWORTH, Dyce A.; 1576 Weston Rd., Weston, Ont.; Tor'35; Med.Sc.D. (Columbia); Urol; Staff (Urol), St. Michael's Hosp.; Cons. (Urol), Humber Memorial Hosp.; Teach. Staff, U. of Toronto; Tel. WA 2-6749.
DUCKWORTH, G. S.; Albany Clinic, 200 Danforth Ave., Toronto 6, Ont.; Tor'65.
DUCKWORTH, John W. A.; 50 Lawton Blvd., Toronto 7, Ont. (res); Edinburgh (Scot.) '36; Prof. of Anat. & Head of Dept., U. of Toronto; Principal M.O., H.M.C.S. York; Surg. Capt., R.C.N.(R); Tel. WA 3-6611.
DUCLOS, Gaston R.; 707 Medical Arts Bldg., 1538 Sherbrooke St. W., Montreal, P.Q.; 4017 Lacombe Ave. (res); Lav '40; F.A.C.S., F.A.-A.O., Ophth; Ophth-in-Charge, St. Mary's Hosp.; Dir. of Ophth., Queen Mary Vets' Hosp.; Tel. 735-3511; RE 8-9481.
DUDAR, W. J.; 1523 Dupont St., Toronto, Ont.; 12 Herne Hill Rd. (res); Tor. '47; Tel. LE 2-8997.
DUDLEY, John H.; 340 Campbell St., Nanaimo, B.C.; 941 Malaspine Cr. (res); UBC '54; MCGP; Tel. 753-3202.
DUFAULT, Camille A.; Mon '55; FRCP(C), IntMed; Staff, Hopital-St.Luc, Montreal 18, P.Q., Tel. 861-7321.
DUFEUTRELLE, Henri; 3516 Park Ave., Montreal, P.Q.; Lav '02.
DUFF, Anne M. (Elwood); 84 Colleen Cres., Chinook Pk., Calgary, Alta.; Belfast U. (N. Ire.) '56; Staff, Col. Belcher Hosp.
DUFF, Bruce R.; 65 Rameau Dr., Ste. 106, Willowdale, Ont.; Wes'61; GenSurg.
DUFF, Francis P.; Dal'57; FRCS(C), OrthSurg; 10 Circular Rd., St. John's, Nfld.
DUFF, Frank; 25 Academy Med. Bldg., 1812-4th St. S.W., Calgary, Alta.; 84 Colleen Cres., Chinook Pk. (res); Queen's U. (Belfast, N. Ire.) '48; FRCS(Ed.), GenSurg; Staff, Colonel Belcher Hosp.; Tel. AM 6-5313.
DUFF, John H.; Tor '57; A.M.C.G.P.; FRCS(C), GenSurg; Staff, Royal Victoria Hosp., Montreal, P.Q.; Dem.(Surg.), McGill U.; Tel. VI 2-1251.
DUFFETT, William H.; Box 45, 171 Dundas St. W., Napanee, Ont.; Qns '16; M.O.H., Deseronto.
DUFFIELD, Anne; The Edgemont, Apt. 804, 1949 Barclay St., Vancouver 5, B.C. (res); Queen's (Belfast, N. Ire.) '56; MB, B.Ch; Anaes; Staff, Burnaby Gen. Hosp.; Tel. HE 4-4211.
DUFFIN, Donald F.; 11 Viola Ct., Stratford, Ont. (res); Wes '50; DMRD; DiagRad; Ass't. Rad., Stratford Gen. Hosp.; Tel. 271-2120; Loc. 249.
DUFFIN, Grant W.; 271 Pillette Rd., Windsor, Ont.; 1985 Lorraine (res); Wes '21.
DUFFIN, John D.; 26 Academy Med. Bldg., Calgary, Alta.; Box 24, Midanpore (res); Tor'38; PathBact; Chief of Lab. Services, Holy Cross & Col. Belcher Hosp's.; Tel. 236-2396.
DUFFY, James C.; 187 Wellington St., Chatham, N.B.; Dal '39; Tel. PR 3-4316.
DUFFY, Mary H.; Tor '53; M.O., Industrial Hygiene Branch, Parliament Bldgs., Toronto 2, Ont.
DUFFY, Raymond A.; 95 Le Marchant Rd., St. John's, Nfld.; Dublin (Ire.) '53; Staff (Anaes.), St. John's Gen., St. Clare's Mercy, Grace, St. John's Mental & St. John's San. Hosp's.; Tel. 726-5233.
DUFFY, St. Clair; B. 26, 3980 Cote-des-Neiges, Montreal 25, P.Q.; McG '26; GenSurg. (P.Q.); Tel. WE 2-7626.
DUFOUR, Andre; 2180 Blvd. Ste. Anne, Quebec 4, P.Q.; Lav '57.
DUFOUR, Fernard; 222 Beaucage, Quebec 8, P.Q.; Lav '54; Tel. 681-4165.
DUFOUR, Francois; Labelle, Co. Labelle, P.Q.; Mon'65.
DUFOUR, Georges; Lav'65; Res., Hop. Hotel-Dieu, Quebec 4, P.Q.
DUFOUR, Georges E.; Mon'63; Res., Inst. Albert Prevost, Montreal 9, P.Q.
DUFOUR, Jacques; Lav'62; Psy(P.Q.); Staff, Hop. St. Justine, Montreal 26, P.Q.
DUFOUR, Ladislas; Lav '45; Anaes; Pt.-time Med. Dir., Hop. St. Joseph, Riviere-du-Loup, P.Q.
DUFOUR, Thomas T.; Ott'64; Jr. Int., University Hosp., Edmonton, Alta.
DUFOUR, Thomas T.; 222 Daly Ave., Ottawa, Ont.; Qns'28; MCGP; Staff, Ottawa Gen. & St. Louis Marie de Montfort Hosp's.; Tel. 234-3873.
DUFOUR, Victorin; Lav'63; Res., Hop. du St. Sacrement, Quebec 6, P.Q.
DUFRESNE, Albert; 1155—117th St., Shawinigan Falls, P.Q.; Mon '11.
DUFRESNE, Irenee; 528 St. Jean, Ville St. Joseph, Co. Drummond, P.Q.; Mon '48; F.R.-C.P.(C), D & TRad.
DUFRESNE, Jacques; (Intern) c/o Ste. 117, 207 Richelieu, St. Jean, P.Q.; Mon'65.
DUFRESNE, J. Armand; 785 Montreal Rd., Forbes P.O., Ottawa, Ont. (res.); Lav '38; Anaes; Chief, Dept. of Anaes. & Sec. Med. Staff, Hop.-St.-Louis-Marie-de-Montfort; Cons. Hydro (P.Q.); Tel. SH 6-4621.
DUFRESNE, J. Arthur; 407 Blvd. St. Joseph E., Montreal, P.Q.; Lav'18; Retired.
DUFRESNE, Jean D.; Lav'61; Res., Hop. St. Vincent de Paul, Sherbrooke, P.Q.
DUFRESNE, J. Paul; 975 St. Prosper St., Trois Rivieres, P.Q.; 3381 Neree Beauchemin (res); Lav '41; F.A.A.D.; DermSyph; Chief, DermSyph, Serv. Hop.-St. Joseph; Tel. FR 4-2479.

DUFRESNE, Louis R.; Mon '63; Res., Montreal Gen. Hosp., Montreal 25, P.Q.
DUFRESNE, Marc G.; Lav'62; Res., Hop. Hotel-Dieu, Montreal 18, P.Q.
DUFRESNE, Marc H.; Mon'60; FRCS(C), GenSurg; Urol; Staff, Hop. du Sacre-Coeur de Cartierville, Montreal, P.Q.
DUFRESNE, Maurice; 1275 Hodge Ave., Ville St. Laurent, Montreal 9, **P.Q. (res); Mon '51; D&T Rad; Staff, Dept. of Rad. Hop. Notre Dame; Tel. LA 5-6363.**
DUFRESNE, Maurice R.; 773 Wilder Ave., Outremont, **P.Q. (res); McG '50; Med. Dir., Ayerst,** McKenna & Harrison, Montreal; Tel. 272-5559.
DUFRESNE, Origene; 5559 Canterbury, Montreal 26, P.Q.; Mon'25; FACR, FRCP(C), D&T-Rad; PhysMed(P.Q.); Dir., Med. & Scien. Inst.-du-Radium; Assoc. Prof. (Rad.), U. of Montreal; Tel. LA 3-3151.
DUFRESNE, Oscar; Mon '64; Res., Hop. Notre-Dame, Montreal, P.Q.
DUFRESNE, Roger; 515 Frechette St., Sherbrooke, P.Q.; Mon'36; FRCP(C) Gastroent(P.Q.).
DUFRESNE, Yves; Lav '46; Staff, Hop. St-Charles, Joliette, P.Q.
DUGAL, Jean P.; 370 St. Cyrille W., Quebec 6, P.Q.; 370 Fraser (res); Lav '34; All. (P.Q.), Gastroent, (P.Q.); IntMed; Staff, Hotel Dieu de Quebec; Assoc. Prof., Gastroent., Laval U.; Tel. 681-3179.
DUGAL, Leon; 3034 rue Chambalon, Ste. Foy, Quebec 10, P.Q. (res); Mon'40; Phys., Alcoholism Rehab. Clinic; Assoc. Dir., Studies on Alcoholism —Dept. of Health (P.Q.), Hotel-du-Gouvernement; Tel. 681-7848.
DUGAL, Pierre; 945 ave. Myrand, Quebec 10, P.Q.; '62; GenSurg(P.Q.).
DUGAS, Andre; Lav '60; Anaes; Staff, Hotel-Dieu St. Vallier, Chicoutimi, P.Q.; Tel. 549-2195.
DUGAS, Paul A.; Lav '59; Res. Hop. Notre-Dame, Montreal 24, P.Q.
DUGAS, Yves; 1058 rue St-Denis, Montreal 18, P.Q.; 299 Notre Dame de Fatima, Duvernay (res); Mon '53; Anaes (P.Q.); Anaes., Hop-St.-**Luc; Tel. UN 1-7261.**
DUGGAN, Francis A.; 2056 Chalmers Rd., Ottawa 1, Ont.; Tor '45; Anaes; Staff, Ottawa Civic Hosp.; Tel. PA 9-2511.
DUGGAN, H. Ewart; Alb '38; DABR; FACR; D&TRad; Staff, Foothills Prov. Hosp., Calgary, Alta.
DUGGAN, J. Winston; Security Bldg., 10023-103rd St., Edmonton, Alta.; 11803-91st **Ave.** (res); **Alb '43; MMS (Tulane); DABOphth; FACS; FRCS(C), Ophth; Assoc. Prof. (Ophth), U. of Alberta; Tel. GA 4-1426; GE 9-4951.**
DUGGAN, Richard S.; Medical Arts Bldg., 2150 Valley Way, Niagara Falls, Ont.; St. Davids (res); Qns '41; Lect. Nursing School, Gen. Hosp.; Memb. Bd. of Directors, O.M.A.; Tel. 354-4444.
DUGGLEBY, Henry E.; 102 The Med. Bldg., 217-3rd Ave. N., Saskatoon, Sask.; Alb. '52; Active Staff, City, St. Paul's & University Hosp's.; Dem. (Med.), U. of Saskatchewan; Tel. 652-1020.
DUGRE, Jacques; 1000 Chemin-Ste-Foy, Quebec 6, P.Q.; 950 Ave. Gatineau, Ste Foy (res); Lav '51; Ophth; Ass't. Ophth., Hop. St. Sacrement; Cons. Ophth., Hop. Laval; Tel. 681-1586.
DUGRE, J. Rodrigue; Lav '40; Staff San. Begin, Lac Etchem'n, P.Q.
DUGRE, Rodrigue; 444 Laviolette, Trois Rivieres, P.Q.; La Pointe-du-Lac, Co. St. Maurice (res); Mon '21; GenSurg; Staff, Hop. St. Joseph.; Tel. FR 6-6778.
DUGRE, Yves; 836 des Ursulines, Trois-Rivieres, P.Q.; Lav '65.
DUGUAY, Claude; Grande Riviere, Cte Gaspe Sud, P.Q.; Lav '64.
DUGUAY, Georges H.; C.P. 577, Gaspe, P.Q.; Lav '60; Otol.
DUGUAY, J. Etienne; Box 484, Bathurst, N.B.; Mon '43; Cons., Regional Hygiene; Tel. 546-4226.
DUGUAY, Martin R.; 367 Est. Boul. St. Joseph, Montreal 14, P.Q.; Mon'59; Psy(P.Q.); Tel. 844-5554.
DUHAIME. Constance; 3514 Marcil Ave., Montreal 28, P.Q.; Leiden (Neth.) '33; Dir. Child Guidance Clin., St. Mary's Hosp.; Tel. 735-3511.
DUHAIME, L. J. Henri; 513 Ave. Montcalm. Chicoutimi, P.Q.; Lav '02; Ophth, Otol. Retired.
DUHAIME, Maurice; 444 Laviolette, Trois-Rivieres, P.Q.; 2005 Victoria **(res); Lav '49; F.R.-C.S. (C). GenSurg; Tel. FR 5-8100.**
DUHAIME, Morris; Mon'61; OrthSurg(P.Q.); Staff, Hop. Ste. Justine, Montreal 26, P.Q.
du HEAUME, Brian; 10951-124th St., Edmonton, Alta.; London (Eng.)'48; MRCS; LRCP; D.Obst RCOG; Assoc. Staff, Royal Alexandra Hosp.; Tel. 454-4551.
DUHAMEL, G. Henri; 4367 St. Hubert St., Montreal, P.Q.; Mon '34.
DUKAY, Alexander C.; Ste 515, 5025 Sherbrooke **St. W., Montreal 28, P.Q.; Budapest (Hungary) '46; Tel. HU 9-8070.**
DUKE, Elgin E.; Tor'64; Res., Winchester Mem. Hosp., Winchester, Ont.
DUKE, Peter C.; Man '64; Res., Winnipeg Children's Hosp., Winnipeg 3, Man.; Abroad.
DUKELOW, James B.; The Underhill Clinic; 1635 Abbott St., Kelowna, B.C.; Man '52; FRCS (C), ObstGyn; Tel. 762-2740.
DUKSZTA, Janusz R.; 18 Park Rd., Toronto **4, Ont; Nat. Univ. (Ire.) '56; Psy; Staff, Ontario Hosp., New Toronto; Tel. WA 2-9791.**
DULAY, Juan R.; Santo Tomas (Manila, Philipp.) '57; Staff, Riverview Hosp., Essondale, B.C.
DUMAINE, Leon; Geneva (Switzerland) '57; **GenSurg; Staff, Whissell Clinic, Westtlock, Alta.**
DUMAINE, Marcel; 52 ave Grande Ile, Valleyfield, P.Q.; Mon'65.
DUMAIS, Bertrand G.; 55 Church, Verdun, Montreal 19, P.Q.; 9003 boul La Salle, La Salle (res); Mon '58; Cardiol (P.Q.); Tel. 366-1979.
DUMAIS, Gaston J. R.; 5787 boul. Gouin ouest, Montreal 9, P.Q.; Mon '58; FRCP(C); Derm; **Staff, Hop. Ste. Justine & Sacre-Coeur, Cartierville; Con s. Derm., Hop. Notre-Dame & Hop.** Bellechasse; Tel. 331-4890.
DUMAIS, J. A. Roger; St. Charles-de-Caplan, Cte., Bonaventure, P.Q.; Lav '47.
DUMAIS, Jean; 204-2eme Ave., La Pocatiere, Co. Kamouraska, P.Q.; Lav '58; Tel. 208.
DUMAS, Albert; 821 Place Rougemont, Quebec 10, P.Q.; Lav '36; PH (P.Q.).
DUMAS, Charles; 1414 Drummond, Montreal, P.Q.; **3145 avenue Van Horne (res); Mon '45;** F.R.C.P.(C), Neurol; Psy; Phys. (NeurPsy), **Hotel-Dieu; Ass't. Prof (Psy.), U. of Montreal; Tel. VI 4-0161.**
DUMAS, Jean; 30 boul. St. Joseph est, Montreal 14, P.Q.; Lav'55; FRCS(C), Ophth; I/C Basic Science Courses (Ophth) Affil., U. of Montreal; Tel. 845-0274.
DUMAS, Jean M.; Lav'65; Res., Royal Victoria Hosp., Montreal 2, P.Q.
DUMAS, Paul; 418 W. rue Prince Arthur, Montreal, P.Q.; 3678 rue Ste. Famille (res); Mon '34; IntMed; Chief (Endocrin.), Hop. Hotel Dieu de Montreal; Cons., Hop. de St-Jean de Dieu; Prof., U. of Montreal; Tel. VI 4-0161.
DUMAS, Wilfrid; 79 Blvd. Sacre-Coeur, St. Felicien, Co. Lac St. Jean; P.Q.; Lav '50; M.C.-G.P.; Staff, Hop. St. Michel, Roberval.; Tel. 679-0943.
DUMONT, Andre L., Capt.; Officers Mess, Cdn. Forces Base, Lancaster Park, Alta.
DUMONT, Felix; C.P. 218, Campbellton, N.B.; Lav '26.
DUMONT, Fernand; 126 Brooks, Sherbrooke, P.Q.; Mon '47; **IntMed (P.Q.); Chief of Med. Serv.,** Hop. Hotel-Dieu; Tel. 562-9042.
DUMONT, Guy R.; 305 ave. Glengarry, Ville Mont Royal, P.Q.; Mon '56; FRCP(C), IntMed; Cardiol **(P.Q.); Staff, Hop. Notre-Dame; Teach. Staff,** U. of Montreal; Tel. LA 5-6363.
DUMONT, Hubert; 2185 W. 4th Ave., Vancouver, B.C.; Alb'35; Anaes; Tel. 733-3010.
DUMONT, J. Andre; 655 St. Aubin, St. Laurent, Montreal 9, P.Q.; Path(P.Q.); Staff, Hop. Hotel-Dieu.
DUMONT, J. Felix E.; 46 rue Rosebery, Campbellton, N.B.; 34 rue Stanley (res); Lav '26. Retired.

DUMONT, Paul; 231 St. Philippe, Arvida, P.Q.; Lav'62; FRCS(C), ObstGyn.

DUMOUCHEL, Jean-P.; 152 Blvd. Leclerc, Granby P.Q. (res); Mon '49; D & TRad; Rad., Hop. St. Joseph; Tel. FR 2-5491.

DUMOULIN, Guy; Mon'63; Res., Hop. Maisonneuve, Montreal 36, P.Q.

DUMOULIN, Pierre; 329 Laviolette, Trois Rivieres, **P.Q.; Mon '47; Paed (P.Q.); Chief of Paed. Serv., Hop. St. Joseph; Tel. FR 5-1005.**

DUNBAR, David A.; 2508 Nelson Ave., West Vancouver, B.C. **(res); McG '10; Retired.**

DUNBAR, J. Scott; 2300 Tupper St., Montreal, P.Q.; 247 Ballantyne St. N. (res); Tor '45; FRCP(C), Diag Rad; Dir., Dept. of Rad., Montreal Children's Hosp.; Rad., Alexandra Hosp., for Infectious Dis.; Assoc. Rad., Royal Victoria Hosp.; Assoc. Prof. (Rad.), McGill U.; Tel. WE 7-8511.

DUNBAR, Lawrence G.; Man'53; Ass't. Res. (Rad.), Toronto Gen. Hosp., Toronto, Ont.

DUNCAN A. Gordon; 211 Rideau Med. Centre, 1711-4th St. S.W., Calgary, Alta.; 4235 Britannia Dr. (res); Man '34; Derm Syph; Cons. (Derm.). D.V.A. Colonel Belcher Hosp.; Cons. (Syph.), Div. Social Hyg., Prov. of Alta.; Tel. AM 2-2572.

DUNCAN, Alexander H.; 963 Owenwood Dr., Lorne Park, Port Credit, Ont.; Tor'29.

DUNCAN, Allan C.; 1309-925 W. Georgia St., Vancouver, B.C.; 6088 Marguerite St. (res); Man '31; FRCS (Edin.); GenSurg; Tel. MU 5-5041.

DUNCAN, Barrie P.; 108 Medical Dental Bldg., Regina, Sask.; **3100 Retallack St., (res); Man '39; Paed; Sr. Staff Memb., Regina Gen. & Grey Nuns Hosp's; Hon. Att. Staff, University Hosp., Saskatoon; Tel. LA 3-7633.**

DUNCAN, Clifford W.; 124 Harbison Ave., Winnipeg, 5, Man.; Qns '26; Tel. LE 3-2100.

DUNCAN, David; 168 Essex St., Sarnia, Ont.; 583 Berkshire Rd. (res); Edinburgh (Scot.) '46; FRCS (Ed.); GenSurg; Active Staff, Sarnia Gen., & St. Joseph's Hosp's.; Tel. 337-3244.

DUNCAN, Dawna L.; (See Armstrong).

DUNCAN, E. Howard; 502 Med. & Dental Bldg., Regina, Sask.; Sask '34; GenSurg; Tel. LA 2-8541.

DUNCAN, Gordon B.; 8311-153rd St., Jasper Place, Alta. (res); Alb '59; Staff, Aberhart Mem. **San., Edmonton; Tel. GE 9-0051.**

DUNCAN, Hugh A. G.; Ste. 508, 1538 Sherbrooke St. W., Montreal 25, P.Q.; McG'42; Ophth; Ass't. Ophth., Royal Victoria Hosp.; Dem Ophth., McGill U.; Tel. VI 2-1251.

DUNCAN, Ian B. R.; 488 Lawson Rd., London, Ont. (res); Glasgow (Scot.) '51; M.B., Ch.B., M.D. (Glas.); M.C. (Path.); FRCP(C), Bact: Dir. Microbiol., St. Joseph's Hosp.; Cons. Bact., Westminster Hosp.; Assoc. Prof. Bact., U. of Western Ont.; Tel. 439-3271.

DUNCAN, J. Donald; Med. Dental Bldg., Box 760, Nechako Centre, Kitimat, B.C.; Man '48; MCGP; Tel. 2102.

DUNCAN, Kenneth B.; Box 880, Campbell River, B.C.; Man'50; Active Staff, Campbell River District Hosp.; Tel. 287-7441.

DUNCAN, Lucy M. C. (Boyd); 583 Berkshire Rd., Sarnia, Ont. **(res)**; Glasgow (Scot.) '49; D.P.H. (Edin.), D.C.H. (Eng.); Temp. Retired.

DUNCAN, MacAdam; 6389 Coburg Rd., Halifax, N.S.; Glasgow (Scot.) '58.

DUNCAN, Neil F.; 10004—105th St., Edmonton, Alta.; 9647—85th St. (res); Alb '49; F.A.A.P., Paed.; **Staff, Royal Alexandra & University Hosp's. Ass't. Clin. Prof. (Paed.), U. of Alberta; Tel. GA 4-2121.**

DUNCAN, Phyllis (Jewitt); Dept. of Health, St. John's, Nfld.; 38 Le Marchant Rd. (res); St. Andrew's (Scot.) '48; School M.H.O., Prov. of Nfld.; Retired.

DUNCAN, Raymond; Dept. of Social Welfare, 800 Cassiar St., Vancouver 6, B.C.; Alb'46; DABS; FRCS(C), GenSurg; Ass't. Dir., Med. Serv. Div.; Tel. 299-9131.

DUNCAN, Robert A.; 227 Administration Bldg., 109th & 98th Ave., Edmonton, Alta.; 11819-73rd Ave. (res); Qns '51; DPH (Tor.); Dir., Emergency Health Services, Alta.; Tel. CA 9-3034.

DUNCAN, Yvonne E., see DUNDEE, Yvonne E.

DUNCANSON, Don A.; 2 Princess Ave., St. Thomas, Ont.; **Wes '50.**

DUNCE, Sidney H.; Moose Jaw Clinic, 200 Scott Bldg., Moose Jaw, Sask.; '51.

DUNDAS, J. Brock; 6000 Cote des Neiges Rd., Montreal 26, P.Q.; McG'59; FRCP(C), Paed.; Att'd. Staff, Mtl. Children's Hosp.; Tel. 737-5120.

DUNDEE, Douglas J.; Med. Dental Bldg., Box 760 Nechako Centre. Kitimat, B.C.; Man '54; FRCS(Eng.); MCGP; Tel. 2102.

DUNDEE, Yvonne E. (Duncan); Box 760, Kitimat, B.C.; Man'54; MCGP; Tel. 2102.

DUNDON, Charles; 38 Mount Hope St., Kitchener, Ont.; Cork (Ire.)'43; M.Ch; FRCS(Eng.); GenSurg; Urol; Chief of Surg., Kitchener-Waterloo Hosp.; Urol., Kitchener-Waterloo & St. Mary's Hosp's.; Tel. 743-9781.

DUNFIELD, James C., Major; 1 CBMU, CFPO 5050, Cdn. Armed Forces, Europe; Tor'53; GenSurg; Abroad.

DUNHAM, Burtt T.; 925 W. Georgia St., Vancouver, B.C.; 2993 W. 44 Ave. (res); Alb '34; MCGP; Tel. MU 1-8633.

DUNHAM, Henry S.; 727 King St. W., Toronto 2B. Ont.; Tor '35; MCGP; Vice Pres., & Med. Dir., Warner-Lambert Canada; Tel. 362-5792.

DUNKLEY, E. Malcolm; 4652 Victoria Ave., Montreal 29, P.Q.; Wales'55; DABA; FACA; FRCP(C), Anaes; Att'd. Staff, Montreal Gen. Hosp., Montreal, P.Q.; Lect., McGill U.

DUNLOP, Donald L.; Bigelow Fowler Clinic, 1605-9th Ave. S., Lethbridge, Alta.; Man'52; FRCS(C), ObstGyn.

DUNLOP, Harold W.; 221 King St. E., Kingston, Ont.; 185 College St. (res); Qns '43; GenSurg.; Tel. 546-0291.

DUNLOP, Ivor H.; 506 Professional Bldg., Chinook Centre, Calgary, Alta.; London (Eng.)'56; MRCS; LRCP; Med. Staff, Holy Cross, Foothill's, Grace & Alberta Children's Hosp's.; Tel. 252-6271.

DUNLOP, Monique L.; 327 Waverley St., Winnipeg 9, Man.; Queens (Belfast, Ire.)'46.

DUNLOP, Peter E.; 420 Lock St. W., Dunnville, Ont.; Qns'63; AMCGP.

DUNLOP, Thomas C.; 200 Bloor St. E., Toronto, Ont.; 29 Hopperton Dr., Willowdale (res); Tor '37; DPH; Chief Med. Dir., Manufacturer's Life Ins. Co.; Tel. 928-4251.

DUNN, Anthony A.; 22 Central Ave., Brockville, Ont.; 166 Hartley St. (res); Ott '55; MCGP; Chief (GP), Brockville Gen Hosp.; Staff, St. Vincent de Paul Hosp.; Tel. 342-6272.

DUNN, Arthur J.; 215 Victoria St., Toronto 1, Ont.; 20 Rumsey Rd. (res); Tor '47; Anaes., Staff, Anaes, St. Michael's Hosp.; Clin. Ass't., Toronto University; Tel. 368-3439.

DUNN, Benjamin H.; 339 Crawford Ave., Windsor Ont.; Qns '52; Path; Path. & Dir. of Labs., Grace Hosp.; Tel. 256-2361. Loc. 24.

DUNN, Donald H.; Med. Dental Bldg., 1151 Lorne Pk. Rd., Port Credit, Ont.; 1189 Queen Victoria Ave. (res); Tor '44; MCGP; Tel. CR 8-2565.

DUNN, Earl V.; Kilmar, P.Q.; McG '60; Tel. ME 2-6018.

DUNN, Effie; 8958 Windsor Rd., Edmonton, Alta.; Alb '40; Anaes; Retired.

DUNN, F. Gordon C.; 2184 W. Broadway, Vancouver, B.C.; 100-1220 Cardero (res); Qns '54; **GenSurg; Tel. RE 6-4451; Abroad.**

DUNN, Henry G.; 715 W. 12th. Ave. **Vancouver 9, B.C.;** 4088 East Blvd. (res); **Cambridge (Eng.); '42; MRCP (Lond.); DCH; Paed; Att'd. Phys., Health Centre for Children, Vancouver Gen. Hosp.; Assoc. Prof. (Paed.)** U. of B.C.; Tel. TR 6-3211, Loc. 2678.

DUNN, John F.; 410 Scott Block, Moose Jaw, Sask.; Glasgow (Scot.)'48; DPM; Tel. 692-1911.

DUNN, N. Elliott; 1166 Henleaze Ave., Moose Jaw, Sask. (res); Tor '33; D.M.R.D. (Lond.), Diag Rad; Rad., Moose Jaw Union Hosp.; Tel. 692-1841.
DUNN, Percy R.; 1538 Sherbrooke St. W., Suite 10, Montreal, P.Q.; 4655 Bonavista Ave., Apt. 404 (res); McG '28; F.A.C.G.; Gastroent, (P.Q.), IntMed; Gastrointestinal Clin. & Phys., St. Mary's Hosp.; Tel. 735-3511.
DUNN, Roy E.; 289 Cedar St., Sudbury, Ont.; 49 Windsor Cr. (res); Wes '60; Tel. 674-3131.
DUNN, R. Walter; Ste. 380, 403-6th St., New Westminster, B.C.; Cambridge (Eng.) '42; LRCP; MRCS; MRCOG; ObstGyn; Active Staff, Royal Columbian & St. Mary's Hosp's.; Vis. Cons. Staff, Surrey Mem., Grace & Burnaby Gen. Hosp's.; Tel. 522-6855.
DUNN, Stuart D.; 4 George St., Pictou, N.S. (res); Dal '43; D.P.H.; Dir. M.H.O., Northumberland Div., N.S. Dept. of Health; Tel. 485-4119.
DUNN, William F.; Ste. 5, 4825 Maplewood Ave., Montreal, 26, P.Q. (res); McG '28; F.R.-C.P.(C), IntMed.; Chief of Serv. (Med.), Ste. Anne's Hosp., D.V.A.
DUNN, William L.; Cancer Research Centre, U. of British Columbia, Vancouver, B.C.; Wes '54; Ph.D(Path.) (London, Eng.); Path; Ass't. Pathol., Vancouver Gen. Hosp.; Ass't. Prof. (Path.), U. of British Columbia; Tel. 224-1111.
DUNNE, James T.; Dal'64; Res., Grace Maternity Hosp., Halifax, N.S.
DUNNE, Roger F.; 1048 St.-Jean, Quebec 4, P.Q.; 220 Grande-Allee (res); Lav '41; IntMed. (PQ); Staff, Hop.-Ste.-Foy & St. Augustin; Cons. RCAF; Tel. 524-9919.
DUNNETT, Ian P.; 105-3195 Granville St., Vancouver, B.C.; Edinburgh (Scot.) '49; M.B., Ch.B., M.R.C.O.G. (Eng.); F.R.C.S.(C), ObstGyn; Staff (ObstGyn), Vancouver Gen. Hosp.; Tel. RE 8-5313.
DUNNING, G. Willard; 401 Medical Arts Bldg., 180 Metcalfe St., Ottawa, Ont.; 730 Parkdale Ave. (res); Tor '23; F.A.C.S., GenSurg; Cons. Surg., Ottawa Civic Hosp. & Ont. Cancer Foundation; Tel. CE 2-3151.
DUNNING, H. A.; 38 Silver St., Cobalt, Ont.; 58 Nickel St. (res); McG '33; Chief of Surg., Misericordia Hosp., Haileybury; Tel. 679-4666.
DUNPHY, A. Emerson; 36 Hillcrest St., Antigonish, N.S. (res); McG '51; FACS; GenSurg; Surg. Staff, St. Martha's Hosp.; Tel. 863-4308.
DUNSEATH, Barry; 137 Wellington St., Sarnia, Ont. McG '63.
DUNSMORE, Joseph M.; 21 Dale Ave., Toronto 5, Ont. (res); Tor '34; DiagRad; Staff, Humber Mem. Hosp.; Tel. 249-8111.
DUNSTER, Brian J.; Wes'65; Res., St. Paul's Hosp., Vancouver, B.C.
DUNSWORTH, Francis A.; 5570 South St., Halifax, N.S.; 561 Young Ave. (res); Dal '43; DAB-Psy; Assoc. Prof. (Psy), & Dir., Child Guidance Clinic, Dalhousie U.; Tel. 423-8866.
DUNTON, Austin S.; 138 Grand River St. N., Paris, Ont.; 209 Grand River St. N. (res); Tor '23; M.C.G.P.; Staff, Willett Hosp.; District Coroner; Tel. 442-3842.
DUNTON, E. Aenid (Jones); McG '49; D.P.H; Staff, County Health Unit, Brantford, Ont.; Tel. 753-7377.
DUPAL, Marie F.; 5574, Canterbury, Montreal 26, P.Q.; Louvain (France) '60; Paed; Staff, Hop. Ste. Justine; Tel. RE 1-4931.
DUPLANTIS, Fernand; 593, 31e avenue, LaSalle, P.Q.; Mon'61; FRCP(C), Neur.
DUPLESSIS, Joseph, 4020 Adam St., Montreal, P.Q.; Mon '36; Paed. (P.Q.).; Tel. 521-1271.
DUPLESSIS, L. Gerard; 8470 boul. Lacordaire, Montreal-Nord, P.Q.; Mon '57; Tel. 321-3364.
DUPONT, Charles A.; C.P. 158, Grenville, P.Q.; Lav '18.
DUPONT, Claude G.; 1656 est, rue Sherbrooke, Montreal 24, P.Q.; 8121 de Gaspe (res); Mon '52; F.R.C.S.(C), GenSurg; PlasSurg; Staff, (PlasSurg), Hop.-Notre-Dame; Tel. LA 5-6363.
DUPONT, Denyse; Lav '61; Research, Dept. of Bacteriol., McGill Univ., Montreal, P.Q.
DUPONT, Gerald; 1230 rue Notre-Dame, St-Cesaire, P.Q.; Mon'52; MCGP; Tel. 536-2822.
DUPONT, Jean A.; 1244 Brooke Claxton Bldg., Ottawa 3, Ont.; Lav'53; D.P.H.(Tor.).
DUPONT, Jean R.; 695 Notre-Dame, Repentigny, P.Q.; Lav '56.
DUPONT, Joseph A., Capt.; Hop. St. Foy, Quebec 10, P.Q.; Lav'65.
DUPONT, Richard; 210 Main St., Granby, P.Q.; Mon '60.
DUPONT-LEGAULT, Micheline; 1553 Viel, Montreal 12, P.Q.; 2255 Mesplet, Mtl. 12 (res); Mon '60; Tel. FE 4-3470.
DUPRAT, Gerard E.; 401 Sud., Cowansville, P.Q.; Lav '44; GenSurg.; Tel. 263-0774.
DUPRE-STRACHAN, A. Suzanne; 64 rue Principale, Vercheres, P.Q. (res); Lav '56; D. Bact (Tor.); Staff (Bact.), Dept. of Health, Montreal.
DUPRE, Georges H.; 127 Prince, Sorel, P.Q.; Lav '43.
DUPRE, John; IntMed(P.Q.); Staff, Royal Victoria Hosp., Montreal, P.Q.
DUPRE, Raymond N.; C.P. 250, 1004 rue Ouimet, St.-Jovite, P.Q.; Mon'47; MCGP; Staff, Hop. St. Paul; Tel. 425-2741.
du PREEZ, Jacobus J.; Pretoria (S. Africa) '60; Jr. Intn., Joseph Brant Mem. Hosp., Burlington, Ont.
DUPUIS, Chanel; 170 Notre Dame St. W., Trois Pistoles, P.Q.; Mon '61. Abroad.
DUPUIS, Gaston; 11 rue St. Zotique Est, Montreal, P.Q.; Mon '40; Tel. 277-6255.
DUPUIS, Gilbert J.O.; 150 Jarry est, Montreal 11, P.Q.; 4574 Marquette (res); Mon '59; Tel. 381-2312.
DUPUIS, Guy; Lav '59; Res., Hop. St-Francois d'Assise, Quebec, P.Q.
DUPUIS, Michel; 6300 Darlington Ave., Montreal, P.Q.; Mon'60; D.PhysMed. (Eng.); FRCP(C), PhysMed. & Rehab; Tel. 735-3741.
DUPUIS, Paul C.; 133 St-Jean Baptiste, Montmagny, P.Q.; McG '29; IntMed (P.Q.); Dist. Coroner.
DUPUIS, Paule (Ladouceur); 570 du Roi, Quebec, P.Q.; 1465 Ave. Charles Huot, Quebec, P.Q. (Res.); Lav'45; Staff, Dept. of Health, Quebec; Tel. 523-5305.
DUPUIS, Pierre; 1744 St. Pascal, Quebec, P.Q.; Lav '44; GenSurg (P.Q.), ThorSurg (P.Q.); Ass't. Surg., Hop de l'Enfant-Jesus; Ass't., Dept. Exp. Phys., Laval U.; Tel. 661-2031.
DUPUIS, Roland; 4801 boul. Lasalle, Verdun, Montreal 19, P.Q.; Mon '24; GenSurg; Tel. 769-3511.
DUPUIS, Ronald; 4395 Ave. Verdun, Verdun, Montreal 19, P.Q.; 460 Villeneuve (res); Mon '37; GenSurg; Staff, Verdun Gen. Hosp.; Tel. 766-8511.
DUPUIS, Z.; c/o Chief Medical Officer, Dept. Nat'l. Health & Welfare, 61 Green St., London W1, England.
DUPUY, Jean E.; 260 St. Patrick St., Ottawa 2, Ont.; '44; Anaes.
DUQUETTE, Claude; Lav'65; Res., Hop. L'Enfant-Jesus, Quebec 3, P.Q.
DUQUETTE, Jacques; Ste. 219, 3875 St-Urbain, Montreal 18, P.Q.; Mon '49; IntMed (P.Q.); Tel. 844-7020.
DURAND, Georges A.; 8639 St. Denis St., Montreal 11, P.Q.; Mon '53.
DURAND, Georges E.; 4 rue Agnes, Lac Megantic, Co. Frontenac, P.Q.; Lav '48; Tel. 583-1922.
DURAND, Henri; 6630 Isaac-Bedard, Charlesbourg, P.Q. (res); Lav '50; Anaes; Anaes., Hop.-St.-Sacrement & Staff, Laval U.; Tel LA 9-4511.
DURAND, Laurier; 1204 Visitation, Montreal, P.Q.; Mon '45; Tel. LA 2-4464.
DURAND, Lucien; 51A St.-Charles Ouest, Longueuil, Cite-Jacques-Cartier, P.Q.; 91A rue Guillaume (res); Lav '57; DPH; Tel. OR 7-8981.
DURCAN, Dermot J.; Brown Clinic, 700-8th St. S.W., Calgary, Alta.; London (Eng.) '51; M.B., B.S.; D.L.O.; FRCS (Eng.); Abroad.
DURITY, Joyce V. (Archer); 396 Francis Rd., Richmond, B.C.; UBC'65.

DURIVAGE, Jacques; 1290 est Sherbrooke, Montreal, P.Q.; 8 ave Glencoe, Outremont (res); Mon '44; IntMed (P.Q.); Staff, Hop. Hotel Dieu; **Ass't. Prof. IntMed., U. of Montreal; Tel. VI 4-0161.**

DURNIN, Robert A.; 605 McCowan Rd., Scarborough, Ont.; 27 Cliffside Dr., Apt. 31 (res); Qns '60; Tel. AM 7-3772.

DUROCHER, Evarist; 606 Med. Arts Bldg., Windsor, Ont.; Wes '32; Hon. Cons. Staff, Metropolitan & Grace Hosp's.; Chief of ObstGyn. Dept., Hop. Hotel-Dieu; Tel. 253-7745.

DUROCHER, Juliette; 163 ave. Laurier, Ottawa 2, Ont.; Mon '43; Anaes; Staff, Ottawa Gen. & Notre Dame Hosp's.

DUROST, Henry B.; Ste. 15A, 4328 Sherbrooke W., Montreal 6, P.Q. (res); McG '50; D.Psy; Psy; Exec. Dir., Douglas Hosp.; Assoc. Prof. (Psy.), McGill U.; Tel. 932-0382.

DuSABLON, Guy; 6447 Delorimier, Montreal 35, P.Q.; 7339 Blvd.-Pie IX (res); Mon '60.

DUSEVIC, Joseph; Leader, Sask.; 1440 Robinson (res); Graz (Austria) **'47;** Staff, Grey Nuns & Gen. Hosp's., Regina; **Dist.** Coroner.

DUSHENSKI, Ladimer A.; 6908-92A Ave., Edmonton, Alta.; Alb **'57; IntMed;** Staff, **University** Hosp.; Tel. 439-5911. Abroad.

DUSHINSKI, Leslie M.; 10004-105th St., Edmonton, Alta.; Alb'60; FRCS(C), Urol.; Staff, Royal Alexandra Hosp.

DUSSAULT, Andre; Ott '58; AMCGP; Res., Hop. St-Jean-de-Dieu, Montreal, P.Q.

DUSSAULT, Antoine B.; St. Marc-des-Carrieres, P.Q.; Lav'39; Tel. 268-3306.

DUSSAULT, Charles; 805 Commerciale, St. David, Co. Levis, P.Q.; Lav '31; GenSurg (P.Q.).

DUSSAULT, Fernand; 537 Curzon Ave., St. Lambert, Montreal 23; P.Q.; Mon '35.

DUSSAULT, Gerard; 240 rue Elm, St.-Lambert, **Cite-Jacques-Cartier, P.Q.; 210 Blvd. Desaulniers** (res); Mon'37; M.O., City of St. Lambert; Tel. 671-4567.

DUSSAULT, Jean O.; 547 St. Jean, Quebec 4, P.Q.; Lav '12.

DUSSAULT, Jean; Lav'65; Res., Hop. L'Enfant-Jesus, Quebec 3, P.Q.

DUSSAULT, Jeanne M.; App. 11, 3360 Cote Ste-Catherine, Montreal 26, P.Q.; Mon '47; Staff, Hop. Mont Providence; Tel. 665-3801.

DUSSAULT, J. F.; 131 Fraser St., Levis, P.Q.; Lav '32.

DUSSAULT, J. Jacques; Clinique Industrielle-de-Thetford, Inc., Thetford Mines, P.Q.; 472 Bennett N. (res); Lav '52; Pulm. Dis. & TB (PQ); Tel. FE 5-3989.

DUSSAULT, Louis; Dept. of National Health & Welfare, Halifax, N.S.; Mon '46; GenSurg (P.Q.).

DUSSAULT, Pierre; Lav '63 Res., Hop. Ste-Justine, Montreal 26, P.Q.

DUSSAULT, Roland; Apt. 1, 8255 boul. l'Acadie, Montreal 15, P.Q. (res); Mon'35; Haem(P.Q.); IntMed; Staff, Hop. Hotel-Dieu; Prof. (Med.), U. of Montreal.

DUTHIE, Cameron S.; 77 Westmount Rd., Guelph, Ont.; Wes'60; Tel. TA 4-5392.

DUTHIE, George A.; Box 127, Invermere, B.C.; Tor '52; M.C.G.P.; Staff, Windermere Dist. Hosp.

DUTKEVICH, Eudoxia; 123 Tivey St., Peterborough, Ont. (res); USSR '28; Path; Dir. of Labs. (Path), St. Joseph's Hosp.; Tel. 742-3425.

DUTTA, Paritosh C.; Medical Clinic, Box 2058, Whitehorse, Yukon; Patna (India)'59; FRCP(C), IntMed.

DUTTON, Peter W.; 219-1st Street, Kamsack, Sask.; Cambridge (Eng.)'60; MA; MB; B.Chir; D.ObstRCOG; Active Staff, Kamsack Union Hosp.; Tel. 542-2623.

DUTTON, William A. W.; The MacGregor Clinic, 250 Main St. E., Hamilton, Ont.; Bristol (Eng.) '50; MRCS (Eng.); LRCP (Lond.); MMSA (Lond.); MRCOG; FRCS(C); FACOG; ObstGyn; Active Staff, Hamilton Civic Hosp.; ObstGyn., MacGregor Clinic; Tel. JA 7-2711; Abroad.

DuVAL, Frederick W.; 325 Med. Arts Bldg., Winnipeg, Man.; 255 Waverley St.(res); Man '50; DAVS; FRCS(C); GenSurg; Att'd. Surg., Winnipeg Childrens' & Deer Lodge Vet's Hosp's.; Ass't. Surg., Winnipeg Gen. Hosp.; Ass't. Prof., U. of Manitoba; **Tel. WH 3-7145.**

DUVAL, Laurent; 17 Des Forges, Victoriaville, P.Q.; Lav '43 DPH; PH (P.Q); M.O., Health Unit, Victoriaville; Med. Dir., Hotel-Dieu d'Arthabaska; Tel 752-9725.

DUVAL, Luc; 150 Est Jarry St., Montreal 11, P.Q.; Mon'57; FRCS(C), GenSurg.

DUVAL, P. Claude; 1365 Jean Talon est, Montreal, P.Q.; Mon '54; Anaes (P.Q.); Staff, Hop. Jean Talon; Tel. 273-5151.

DUVAL Philippe E.; 34 Gamble St. E., Rouyn, P.Q.; Lav '43; FACCP; PulmDis&TB(P.Q.).

DUVENCI, Jale; Apt. 300, 3404 Prud'homme Ave., Montreal 28, P.Q.; Istanbul (Turk.) '54.

DUVERNET, Edward O.; 8584 Granville St., Vancouver 14, B.C.; McG '21; Anaes; Tel. 266-0723.

DUXBURY, J.; 59 Worthington Ave., St. Vital, Winnipeg 8, Man. (res); Man '05; Retired.

DUXBURY, James H.; 1121 Yates St., Victoria, B.C.; 3270 Woodburne Ave. (res); McG '53; FRCS(C), Urol; Staff, Royal Jubilee Hosp.; Tel. EV 6-6151.

DVALI, Alexander; 1047 Main St. E., Hamilton, Ont.; Tiflis (USSR) '39; Tel. LI 9-5019.

DVORKIN, Joseph; 506 Med. Arts Bldg., 11010 Jasper Ave., Edmonton, Alta.; 7 Valleyview Cres. (res); Alb '43; FACC; FACP; IntMed; Att'd. Staff. U. of Alberta Hosp.; Ass's. Clin. Prof. (Med.), U. of Alberta; Tel. 424-5070.

DWAN, David; 203 Fitzpatrick Bldg., Calgary, **Alta.; Dublin (Ire.) '48; Tel. 262-1400.**

DWERSTEG, Ewald V.; 556 Med. Arts Bldg., 750 Spadina Cr. E., Saskatoon, Sask.; Mainz (Germ.) '55; Otol; Tel. 244-2979.

DWORATZEK, Lucian G.; 4208 Bathurst St., Downsview, Ont.; Tor '63; Tel. ME 3-9090.

DWORKIN, Howard J.; Albany Med. Coll. (New York)'59; Staff, Princess Margaret Hosp., 500 Sherbourne St., Toronto 5, Ont.

DWORKIN, Simon; 417 Med. Arts Bldg., 1538 Sherbrooke St. W., Montreal 25, P.Q.; McG '27; FACP; IntMed; Hon. Att'd. Staff, Royal Victoria Hosp.; Cons. (Arthritis), Queen Mary Vet's. Hosp.; Ass't. Prof. (Physiol.), McGill U.; Tel. 937-6720.

DWORSCHAK, Francis; 327 Frank St., Ottawa 4, Ont.; 33 Lynwood Ave. (res); Vienna (Austria) '48; AMCGP; Tel. 723-9444.

DWYER, Charles H.; Ste. 308, 1541 W. Broadway, Vancouver 9, B.C.; 1276 W. 26th Ave. (res); Wes '31; Tel. RE 3-0117.

DWYER, Daniel E.; 522 Medical Arts Bldg., Hamilton, Ont.; Tor'57; FRCP(C), IntMed; Tel. Ja. 8-6531.

DWYER, Emmet; C.N. Station. Winnipeg, Man.; 118 Chataway Blvd.. Wpg. 29 (res); Man '29; ABPM (Occup. Med.); FACPM; Reg. **M.O.,** CN Rlwys. & Air Canada; **Tel. WH 6.2491.**

DWYER, Joseph; Ott '55; Diag Rad; Staff, Greater Niagara Gen. Hosp., **Niagara Falls, Ont.;** Tel. EL 8-3611.

DWYER, Mary M. O.; 1159 Tattersall Dr., Victoria, B.C.; Wes'64.

DWYER, William F.; 735 Colborne St. E., Brantford, Ont.; Tor '50; Staff, Brantford Gen. & St. Joseph's Hosp's; Tel. 752-3446.

DYAKOWSKI, Stefan; 1740 Davie St., Vancouver 5, B.C.; Polish School of Med., Edinburgh (Scot.) '46.

DYBLE, Richard H.; U.S. Consulate General, 1558 McGregor Ave., Montreal 25, P.Q.; Tor '30.

DYCK, Frank; 414 Med. Arts Bldg., Spadina Cr. & 23rd St., Saskatoon, Sask.; Sask '58; FRCS(C), ObstGyn; Assoc. Staff, University Hosp.; Active Staff, St. Paul's & City Hosp's.; Clin. Assoc. (Obst Gyn), U. of Saskatchewan; Tel. 244-6144.

DYCK, Helmut H.; 465 Scott St., St Catharines, Ont.; Tor'64; Staff, St. Catharines Gen. & Hotel-Dieu Hosp's.; Tel. 684-1022.

DYCK, Jacob; Westbrook Med. Centre, S.W. Keewatin & Logan Ave., Brooklands, Winnipeg 23, Man.; 868 Lindsay St. (res); Man '55; Gen-Surg; Active Staff, Misericordia Hosp.; Tel. SP 2-9453.

DYCK, Victor J.; 100 Church Ave., Chilliwack, B.C.; 418 William St. N. (res); Man '52; MCGP; Staff, Chilliwack Gen. Hosp.; Tel. 795-7271.

DYCKHOFF, Pauline R.; Manchester (Eng.) '53; Anaes; Staff, Brant Mem. Hosp., Burlington, Ont.; Tel. 637-2361.

DYE, Geneva (See Turner)

DYER, Alan M.; Medical Arts Clinic, 51 6th St. S.E., Medicine Hat, Alta.; Glasgow (Scot.)'60; D.O.(Eng.); Staff, Medicine Hat Gen. Hosp.; Tel. 527-2281.

DYER, Clark W.; Ste 7, 2221 Keele St., Toronto 15, Ont.; 11 Paulson Rd. (res); Tor '43; FICS; GenSurg; Active Staff Surg., Northwestern Toronto Hosp.; Cons. Surg. Staff, North York Branson Hosp.; Tel. 247-3348.

DYER, Douglas W.; Tor '47; Staff, Workmen's Comp. Board, Toronto 1, Ont.; Tel. 362-3411.

DYER, Harold; 464—E. 17th St., North Vancouver, B.C. (res); London (Eng.) '98; M.R.C.S. (Eng.), L.R.C.P. (Lond.), F.R.C.S. (Edin.); Coroner, North Shore of Burrard Inlet; Retired.

DYER, H. Floyd; 422 Medical Arts Arts Bldg., Hamilton, Ont.; Indian Point, Burlington (res); Tor '24; M.C.G.P.

DYER, Justin; 2171 **Queen St. E., Toronto 13, Ont.; Ott '60; Tel. 699-9823.**

DYER, Natalie M.; 26 Taylorwood Dr., Islington, Ont.; Tor '47; Staff (Anaes.), Humber Mem. Hosp.; Tel. 248-1215.

DYER, Thomas M.; 11442-76th Ave., Edmonton, Alta. (res); **McG '23; I/C, OP Clin., DVA.**

DYER, Wilfred J.; 14A Trafalgar Apts., 3010 The Boulevard, Montreal 25, P.Q.; Dal '36; Research.

DYKE, Elgin E.; Tor'64; Staff, Winchester Mem. Hosp., Winchester, Ont.

DYKE, John L.; Acadia Fairview Clinic, 8330 Fairmount Dr. S.E., Calgary, Alta.; Birmingham (Eng.)'55; Tel. 252-1161.

DYKEMAN, Douglas L.; 320 College St., Richmond, P.Q; **McG '53; MCGP; Assoc. Staff, Sherbrooke Hosp., Sherbrooke; Reg. M.O., C.N.R.;** M.O.H. Hussars, M.O., D.V.A.; Tel. 826-3443.

DYKER, Gordon R.; 206 Medical Bldg., Prince Albert, Sask.; 545—20th St. W. (res); Man '42; IntMed; Staff, Victoria Union & Holy Family Hosp's.; Tel. 763-6401.

DYKES, R. Murray; Box 9, Wetaskiwin, Alta.; Edinburgh (Scot.) '46; LRCP; LRCS (Edin.); LRFPVS (Glasgow); Staff, Wetaskiwin Mun. Hosp.; Tel. 352-2511.

DYLOWNA, Lucyna M.; (See Matzinger, Lucy M.).

DYMOND, Hon. Mathew B.; M.P.P.; Parliament Bldgs., Toronto, Ont.; **Qns '41; M.C.G.P.; Minister of Health, Ontario; Tel. EM 3-1211.**

DYMOND, Richard F.; 303 Fifth Ave., Timmins, Ont.; Qns'60; AMCGP; Staff, St. Mary's Hosp.; Tel. 264-8320.

DYRDA, Ihor; 2420 Moreau, Brossardville, P.Q.; Mon'59.

DYSART, Robert M.; 25 John St., Moncton, N.B.; McG '47; F.R.C.P.(C), IntMed; F.R.C.S.(C), GenSurg; Staff, Moncton & Hotel-Dieu Hosp's.; Tel. EV 2-8548.

DYSON, Charles; 280 Queens Ave., London, Ont.; 1587 Gloucester Rd. (res); **Wes '43;** DABOph; Ophth; Hd. Dept. of **Ophthal.,** Victoria Gen. Hosp.; Clin. Prof. (Ophth), U. of Western Ont.; Tel. GE 2-6921.

DZIUBA, Rollie J.; 42 Northside Rd., Ottawa 6, Ont.; Ott '59; Tel. 828-9117.

DZIUBANOWSKY, Teodor B.; 833 Ottawa St., Windsor, Ont.; **2561 Windermere Rd. (res); Cracow (Poland) '36; MCGP; Tel. 254-1777.**

DZIURDZY, S. A.; Tor '63; Int., Ontario Hosp., Hamilton, Ont.

EADE, Norman R.; McG '64; Res., Dept. of Pharmacology, McGill U., Montreal, P.Q.

EADIE, John A.; Room 311, Norquay Bldg. 401 York Ave., Winnipeg 1, Man.; Edinburgh (Scot.) '44; DPH(Edin.); Dir., V.D. Control, Prov. of Manitoba; Tel. WH 6-7746.

EADIE, W. W.; 11752—81st St., Edmonton, Alta.; Alb'25; MCGP(Hon.); Att'd. Staff, Royal Alexandra Hosp.; Tel. GR 7-8446.

EAGER, Richard F. R.; 1827 Main St., Niagara Falls, Ont.; 1550 McGrail Ave., Apt. 2 (res.), McG'24; Otol; Staff, Gtr. Niagara Gen. Hosp.; Tel. EL 8-8717.

EAGLES, Allan M.; Trowbridge St., Meaford, **Ont.; Syke St. (res); Wes '46.**

EAGLES, Eldon L.; 12 Rockwood Ave., Armdale, Halifax Co., N.S. (res); Dal '36; D.P.H., PH; Dir. Child & Maternal Health & Communicable Disease Control; Dept. of Public Health of Nova Scotia; Tel. 5-8271.

EAGLES, George H.; 431-2nd Ave. E., Owen Sound, Ont., Tor '20; DPH; Path., General & Marine Hosp.; Reg. Path., Attorney General's Dept.; Cons. Path., Ontario Hosp.

EAGLESHAM, Douglas C.; 66 Grange St., Guelph, Ont. (res); Man '32; DABR; D & T Rad; Dir., Dept. of Rad., Guelph Gen. Hosp.; Tel. TA 2-5350.

EAGLESHAM, Fergus C.; Box 1418, 110-3rd St., Weyburn, Sask.; 607-4th (res); **McG '36; Staff,** Weyburn Union Hosp.; Tel. 842-5404.

EAGLESHAM, H.; Sask'64; Res., St. Boniface Hosp., Winnipeg 6, Man.

EAGLESON, William M.; Medical Arts Bldg., 31 Centre St. S., Brampton, Ont.; 6 John Beck Cres. (res); Tor '47; F.R.C.S.(C), GenSurg; Cons. (Surg.), Peel Mem. Hosp.; Cons. Surg., South Peel Hosp.; Tel. GL 1-5641.

EAID, Charles R. M.; 316 Wellington St. W., Sault Ste. Marie, Ont.; 1570 Queen St. E. (res); Qns '43; M.C.G.P.; Tel. 256-6313.

EAKIN, William W.; 704 Medical Arts Bldg., 1538 Sherbrooke St. W., Montreal 25, P.Q.; 736 Lexington Ave., Westmount (res); McG '21; F.R.C.P.(C), IntMed; Cardiol. (P.Q.); Assoc. Phys., Royal Victoria Hosp.; Cons. Cardiol., Montreal Children's, Queen Elizabeth & Verdun Protestant Hosp's.; Tel. WE 5-2723.

EAKINS, George E.; 167 Summit Ave., Port Arthur, Ont. (res); Tor '04; Retired.

EAMAN, Stanley G.; McG'65; Res., Royal Victoria Hosp., Montreal 2, P.Q.

EARL, Thomas J.; Port Elgin, Ont.; Qns'44; MCGP.

EARLE, Anne M.; Prov. Bldg., Prince St., Sydney, N.S.; Bristol (Eng.) '49.

EARLE, Brian V.; Seven Mile Bridge House, R.R. No. 3, Sydney, N.S.; Dublin (Ire.) '44; M.R.C.P. (Lond.), D.P.M.; Dir., Cape Breton Mental Health Centre.

EARLE, Frank E.; 267 O'Connor St., Ottawa 4, Ont.; 15 Crescent Hgts. (res); **Qns '36; MCGP; Staff. Ottawa Civic & Grace Hosp's.; Tel. PA 9-2511.**

EARLE, Max R.; 1022 Med. Dental Bldg., 925 W. Georgia St., Vancouver 1, B.C.; 838 Esquimalt W. Van. (res); Alb '41; D.A.B.O.; ObstGyn.; Tel. MU 4-8623.

EARLE, Richard W. L.; Main St., Perth, N.B.; Dal '03.

EARLE, Thomas H.; Middle Musquodoboit, Halifax, Co., N.S.; Dal '48; Att. Phys., Musquodoboit Valley Mem. Red Cross Hosp.; Courtesy Staff, Colchester Co. Hosp., Truro, N.S.; Dist. Coroner

EARN, Albert Abraham; 203 Edmonton St., Winnipeg 1, Man.; 126 Machray Ave., Wpg. 4. (res); Man '36; M.Sc.; MRCOG; FICS; FACOG; ObstGyn Chm. & Hd., Dept. of ObstGyn., Misericordia Gen. Hosp.; Staff, St. Boniface Gen. Hosp. & Women's Pavilion; Lect. (ObstGyn.), U. of **Manitoba; Tel. WH 2-1420.**

EASON, M.; 1209 College St., Toronto, Ont.; 81 Ridelle (res); Tor '38; Tel. LE 6-2434.

EAST, Harold M.; 459 Broadview Ave., Toronto, Ont.; Tor '05; Tel. HO 6-5313.

EAST, W. H. Sparling; Fernie, B.C.; Man '41; M.C.G.P.

EASTERBROOK, W. M.; Tor'65; Res., Montreal Gen. Hosp., Montreal 25, P.Q.

EASTON, Donald R.; 11135-105th St., Edmonton, Alta.; 11902-89th Ave. (res); Tor '33; FACHA: MRSH; FAGS; Psy; Exec. Dir. Edmonton & Rural Norwood Auxiliary Hosp.; Tel. GR 4-5441.
EASTON, Elinor J.; Dal '64; Res., Halifax Infirmary, Halifax, N.S.
EASTON, Jessie K.; Alb '57; PhysMed. & Rehab; Staff, University Hosp., Edmonton, Alta.; Tel. 439-5911.
EASTON, Norman L.; 3131 Lake Shore Blvd. **W., Toronto 14, Ont. (res); Tor '26; Psy; Sr.** Med. Spec., Ontario Hosp., New Toronto; Tel. CL 9-8291.
EASTON, Sam; Mall Med. Bldg., Memorial Blvd., Winnipeg, Man.; Apt. 301, 71 Roslyn Rd. (res); Man'26; Tel. SP 4-2411.
EASTON, William I.; 371 Eveline St., Selkirk, Man.; 278 Eveline St. (res); Man '34; M.C.G.P.
EASTWOOD, Sybil B.; (see Fowlow Sybil B.).
EATON, A. T.; Medical Arts Bldg., 1 Young St., Hamilton, Ont.; Winona (res); Qns '19; F.I.C.S., GenSurg; Chief of Serv. (Colon & Rectal Surg.), **Hamilton Gen. Hosp.; Tel. JA 7-0271.**
EATON, David B.; Box 8080, Weyburn, Sask.; Edinburgh (Scot.)'51; FRCS(Edin.); FRCS(C), GenSurg; Abroad.
EATON, Douglas H.; Greig Clinic, 44 Kimberley Ave., Bracebridge, Ont.; Oxford (Eng.)'51; DIH.
EATON, Gerald D.; Box 604, 91 Tudhope St., Espanola, Ont.; 197 Sheppard St. (res.); Qns '56; AMCGP; Sr. Active Staff, Espanola Gen. Hosp.; Tel. 869-2620.
EATON, John L.; Box 788, Estevan, Sask.; U.K. '51.
EATON, Reginald C.; Provincial Hosp., Campbellton, N.B.; Dal'49; Psy.; Tel. 753-4461.
EATON, Richard D.; Manchester (Eng.) '47; DTM&H; DPH; Staff, Indian Hosp., North Battleford, Sask.
EATON, Robert B.; Ste. 202, 1111 Main St., Moncton, N.B.; 234 Cameron St. (res); Dal '32; F.R.C.S. (Edin.), F.A.C.S., F.R.C.S.(C), GenSurg; Sr. Surg., Moncton Gen. & Hotel Dieu Hosp's.; Tel. EV 2-3615.
EBACHER, Roch; 27 Presbytere, Pierreville, Co. Yamaska, P.Q.; Lav '51; Tel. 568-2133.
EBBS, J. Harry; 555 University Ave., Toronto 2, Ont.; 72 St. Leonards Ave., Tor. 12 (res); Tor '31; M.D. (Birm.), MRCP (Lond.), DCH (Lond.), FRCP(C), Paed; Phys., Hosp. for Sick Children; Assoc. Prof. (Paed), U. of Toronto; Tel. EM 6-7242.
EBERLIE, William J.; Box 370, Colborne, Ont.; London (Eng.)'44; MRCP; MRCS; LRCB; DTM & H (Eng.).
EBY, Wilbert H.; 1516 Bathurst St., Toronto 10, Ont.; Tor '13; Retired.
ECCLESTONE, Edward R.; Wes'62; Res., Hosp. for Sick Children, Toronto 2, Ont.
ECCLESTONE, Robert C.; McG'65; Res., Montreal Gen. Hosp., Montreal 25, P.Q.
ECHENBERG, Isidore; 4620 Decarie Blvd., Montreal 29, P.Q.; 4809 Wilson Ave. (res); McG '27.
ECHLIN, Thomas H.; 2115 Pelissier St., Windsor, Ont.; 2754 Buckingham (res); Qns '56; MCGP; Tel. 254-3794.
ECK, Christie A. Barr; Tor '24; Staff, Beck Memorial San., **London, Ont.**
ECKER, Donald A.; 496 Main St., Exeter, Ont.; 490 Main St. (res); **Wes '56; M.C.G.P.; Staff, S. Huron Hosp., Exeter. & St. Joseph's & Victoria Hosp's, London; Tel. 235-0910.**
ECKERT, Grant H.; Tor'52; Ass't. Res. (Anaes.), Toronto Gen. Hosp., Toronto, Ont.; AMCGP.
ECKERT, Lawrence A.; 2489 Bloor St. W., Toronto 9, Ont.; 1630 Pinetree Cres., Port Credit, Ont. (res); Tor '45; FRCS(Eng.), GenSurg; Att. Surg., Queensway & South Peel Hosp's., Assoc. Surg., St. Joseph's Hosp.; Tel. RO 9-8142.
EDDIE, Edouard S.; 215 Main St., Bathurst, N.B.; Paris (Fr.) '53; FCCP, FICP; Cons. (Cardiol.), Hotel-Dieu, Bathurst & Campbellton & Hop. St. Joseph, Dalhousie; Tel. 546-5361.
EDDIS, Mary J.; 24 Harbord St., Toronto 5, Ont.; Tor. '25; D.Psy.
EDDY, George E.; 10004-105th St., Edmonton, Alta.; 12 Wellington Cr. (res); Dal '54; DABP; **FRCP(C); Paed; Active Staff, Royal Alexandra** Hosp.; Court. Staff, University Hosp.; Chief Med. Staff & Paed., Glenrose Hosp.; Instr. **(Paed.), U. of Alta.; Tel. GA 4-2121.**
EDDY, Robert G.; 171 Brant Ave., Brantford, Ont.; 25 Forsythe Ave. (res); Wes '55; MCGP; Tel. 752-7470.
EDE, William O. M.; 4 Thornbank Rd., Thornhill, Ont.; Cambridge (Eng.) '32; D.A.; Chief-of-Anaes., York Central Hosp., Richmond Hill; Tel. 889-6751.
EDELIST, G. J.; Tor '59; Jr. Int'n., New Mount Sinai Hosp., Toronto, Ont.
EDELSTEIN, Eugene; 6000 Cote des Neiges, **Rd., Montreal 26, P.Q.; Alb '60; AMCGP; Tel. 739-5348.**
EDEN, John; Ste. 514-750 W. Broadway, **Vancouver 9, B.C.; 6506 Angus Dr. (res); Durham** (Eng.) '37; D.A.B.C.P., D.A.B.C.C.; Path (Clin-**Path.). Vancouver Gen. Hosp.; Clin. Assoc. Prof. (Path), U. of British Columbia; Tel. TR 2-2696.**
EDEN, Joseph D.; Med. Centre, Virgil, Ont.; Durham (Eng.) '57.
EDES, Andrew O.; Prince Albert Clinic, Prince Albert, Sask.; **225-21st St. W. (res); Budapest (Hungary) '44; IntMed.**
EDEY, R. Bruce; 272 Runnymede Ave., Toronto 9, Ont.; Tor'65.
EDGAR, Arthur B.; Lancaster Med. Centre, 131 Main St., Lancaster, N.B.; 514 Earl Ave. (res); McG '51.
EDGAR, Hugh W.; Ste. 103, 450 Central Ave., London, Ont.; Wes '58; Dip.Rad.(McG.) DiagRad; Staff, St. Joseph's Hosp.; Lect. (DiagRad.), U. of Western Ontario; Tel. 433-2841.
EDGAR, Murray L.; Ste. 240, 5780 Cambie St., Vancouver 15, B.C.; **4583 Connaught Dr., Vancouver 9 (res); Qns '43; MCGP; Tel. FA 5-7434.**
EDGECOMBE, John M.; Dal '58; Res., Sunnybrook Hosp., Toronto, Ont.
EDGELL, Peter G.; 570 Seaforth Med. Bldg., 3550 Cote des Neiges Rd., Montreal 25, P.Q.; McG '43; DIM; FAPA; Psy; Att'd. Psy., Montreal Gen. Hosp.; Assoc. Psy., Reddy Mem. Hosp.; Assoc. Prof. (Psy.), McGill U.; Tel. WE 3-0994.
EDGETT, J. Thomas; 272 St. George St., Moncton, N.B.; Dal'55; IntMed.; Tel. 384-7654.
EDIE, James C.; Box 370, 20 Main St. S., Kenora, Ont.; 3241-3rd St. S. (res); Edinburgh (Scot.) **'48; Tel. HO 8-8642.**
EDINGTON, Archibald M.; 23 Kingsdale Ave., Willowdale, Ont.; McG'36; DABR; D&TRad; Active Staff, North York Branson Hosp.; Tel. 225-9276.
EDINGTON, Robert F.; 60 Drinkwater St., Sudbury, Ont.; Glasgow (Scot.) '50; M.B., Ch.B., M.D. (Glas.); FRCS(C), ObstGyn.; Chief Obst-Gyn., Sudbury Mem. and Chief Gyn., St. Joseph's Hosp's; Tel. 673-2781.
EDMEADS, John G.; Tor '59; FRCP(C), Neur; Staff, Sunnybrook Hosp., Toronto 12, Ont.; Tel. 485-8651.
EDMISON, Henry M.; 777 Mount Joy, Victoria, B.C. (res); Man '31; D. & TRad; Dir. Rad. Royal Jubilee Hosp., Victoria; Tel. EV 6-3131.
EDMISON, Jack N.; Ste 30, Medical Arts Bldg., 1105 Pandora Ave., Victoria, B.C.; 1940 Mayfair Dr. (res); Man '44; DiagRad; Staff, D.V.A. Hosp.; Tel. EV 5-1481.
EDMISON, Ross E.; 812 Fisher Ave., Ottawa, Ont. (res); Tor '35; M.O., Dept. Nat'l. Health & Welfare; Tel. 992-4841.
EDMONDS, Charles B.; Tor'62; Res., Toronto Western Hosp., Toronto 2B, Ont.
EDMONDS, Edward P.; 92 Mary St., Orillia, Ont.; Tor '54; Tel. 325-5632.
EDMONDS, Lewis C.; 1983 Queen St. E., Toronto, Ont.; 273 Lawrence Ave. E. (res); Tor '18; Retired.
EDMONDS, W. B.; 930 Medical Arts Bldg., 170 St. George St., Toronto, Ont.; 11 Bombay Ave., Downsview P.O.; Tor '21; Neur.; Retired.
EDMUND, Ed; Omenica Clinic, Columbia St., Vanderhoof, B.C.; Tor'61; Abroad.

EDMUNDS, Lawrence M.; 5112-50th St., Vegreville, Alta.; 5006 Huyke Ave. (res); Alb '44; MCGP; Dist. Coroner; Tel. 632-2822.

EDOUARD, Julio; Port-Au-Prince (Haiti) '54; Jr. Int., Royal Ottawa San., Ottawa, Ont.

EDSALL, Milton C.; Box 98, Wheatley, Ont.; Tor '29; Tel. 825-4153.

EDSON, Irvin; 2390 Eglinton Ave. E., Scarborough, Ont.; Tor '58; AMCGP; Tel. 757-2854.

EDWARD, James F.; 615 Medical Arts Bldg., Winnipeg, Man.; 175 Lenore St. (res); Man '44; FASCH M.C.G.P.; Courtesy Staff, Grace Gen. Hosp.; Tel. WH 2-8729.

EDWARDS, Allan M.; Ste. 420, 8409-112th St., Edmonton, Alta.; Alb '50; FRCP(C); IntMed; Cons., Charles Campsell Indian Hosp.; Att'd. Staff, University Hosp.; Clin. Instr. (Med.), U. of Alberta.

EDWARDS, Frank J.; 304 Admin. Bldg., 109th St. & 98th Ave., Edmonton, Alta.; McG'43; Psy.

EDWARDS, G. Keith; McLeod Med. Bldg., 340 McLeod St., Ottawa, Ont.; Wes'54; Ophth; Active Staff, Ottawa Civic Hosp., Lect., U. of Ottawa; Tel. 232-7385.

EDWARDS, Glen E.; 10 Academy Med. Bldg., 1812-4th St. W., Calgary, Alta.; 1004 Kerfoot Cr. (res); Alb '54; FRCS(C); FACS; OrthSurg; Staff Calgary Gen., Holy Cross, Children's, & Col. Belcher Hosp's.; Tel. 263-1736.

EDWARDS, Harold E.; 688 Coxwell Ave., Ste. 205, Toronto 13, Ont.; Tor'27; FASHA; FAAP; Paed; Active Cons., Hosp. for Sick Children; Paed I/C Paed., Toronto East Gen. & Orthopaedic Hosp's.; Assoc. Prof. (Emer.), U. of Toronto; Tel. 465-8308.

EDWARDS, H. L.; Main St., Birtle, Man; Qns '24.

EDWARDS, Hollis A.; Man'64; Res., Allan Mem. Inst., Montreal, P.Q.

EDWARDS, Jack L.; Medical Arts Clinic, 51—6th St. S.E., Medicine Hat, Alta.; 438 Prospect Dr. (res); Alb '46; IntMed; Staff, Medicine Hat Mun. Hosp.; Tel. 527-2281.

EDWARDS, J. Chas. R.; 291 Stewart St., Newmarket, Ont.; Box 10 (res); Tor '21; GenSurg; Cons. Surg., York County Hosp.; Dist. Coroner.

EDWARDS, John M; 92 Mary St., Orillia, Ont.; 46 Heyden Ave. (res); Wes '55; Tel. 325-2622.

EDWARDS, Kenneth F.; Box 250, Collins Bay, Ont. (res); Tor '49; Anaes; Att. Staff, Kingston Gen. Hosp.; Clin. Ass't. (Anaes.), Queen's U.; Kingston; Tel. 542-2821.

EDWARDS, Kenneth N.; Box 40, Lytton, B.C.; Man '43; MCGP; Chief of Staff, St. Bartholomew's Hosp.; Tel. 455-2332.

EDWARDS, Larry A.; Tor '61; Res., Sunnybrook Hosp., Toronto, Ont.

EDWARDS, L. Homer, A/Col.; Nat. Defence Med. Centre, Ottawa, Canada; Alb '46; Anaes; Chief of Anaes., NDMC.

EDWARDS, Philip A.; R.R. 1, Dorion, P.Q.; McG '36; D.T.M., F.C.C.P., Pulm. Dis. & TB (P.Q.); Att. Staff, & Clin. Parasitologist (Hon.), Royal Victoria Hosp., Montreal; Med. Spec., D.V.A.; Lect. (Med.), McGill U.; Tel. VI 2-1251.

EDWARDS, Richard B.; 181 Main St. E., Milton, Ont.; 360 Martin St. (res); Tor '57; MCGP; Chief of Anaes., Milton Dist. Hosp.; Tel. TR 8-2383.

EDWARDS, William F.; 4035 Braefoot Rd., Victoria B.C. (res); Alb '48; Adm., Dept. Health & Welfare. Victoria, B.C.; Tel. EV 2-6211.

EDWARDS, William S.; Ste. 203, 267 O'Connor St., Ottawa, Ont.; 485 Mansfield Ave. (res); Tor '35; F.I.C.S., ObstGyn; Att. Staff, Ottawa Civic & Grace Hosp's.; Tel. CE 4-3693.

EDWORTHY, James M.; Irving Clinic, Woodward Towers, Kamloops, B.C.; 187 St. Paul W. (res); Wes '44; DABP; Paed; Staff, Royal Inland Hosp.; Tel. 372-5251.

EDWORTHY, Murray A.; Ste. 203, 625-5th Ave., New Westminster, B.C.; 311-6th Ave. E. (res); McG '51; M.C.G.P.; Staff, Royal Columbian & St. Mary's Hosp's; Tel. 521-4020.

EFFER, Sidney B.; 459 Soudan Ave., Toronto 7, Ont.; Tor'57; FRCS(C), ObstGyn; Abroad.

EFFORD, Robert J.; Ste. 502, 625-5th Ave., New Westminster, B.C.; Washington (Seattle, U.S.A.) '56; M.A., Ph.D., FRCP(C), IntMed; Cons. & Active Staff, Royal Columbian Hosp.; Cons. Staff, St. Mary's Hosp., Surrey Mem. Hosp., Maple Ridge & Langley Mem. Hosp's.; Tel. 522-7511.

EFTHIMIOU, Hippocrates; 1828 Union St., Windsor, Ont.; Paris (Fr.) '57.

EFTIHIADES, Theodore D.; Centre-Psycho-Social; 412 boul. du Havre, Valleyfield, P.Q.; Athens (Greece) '56.

EGAN, Bernard J.; 224 Regent Ave. W., Transcona, Man; 536 Rosseau Ave. W. (res); Nat. U. (Ire.) '46; L.M., D.C.H; Tel. CA 2-8366.

EGAN, Charles; 562 Johnson St., Kingston, Ont.; Qns '41; D.T.M. & H. (Eng.), D.A.; Anaes.

EGAN, John M.; Medical Centre, Stettler, Alta.; U. College (Dublin, Ire.) '51; B.A.O., D.P.H. Abroad.

EGAN, Kerry J.; Tor'63; Res., Toronto Gen. Hosp., Toronto 2, Ont.

EGELI, C. Nevzat; Ste. 27, 55 Church St., Verdun, Montreal 19, P.Q.; Istanbul (Turk.)'52; ObstGyn; Staff, Verdun Protestant Hosp. & Hop. LaSalle; Tel. 767-5192.

EGGERT, Frederick W.; Killaloe, Ont.; Qns '34.

EGGERTSON, S. H. Octavius; C.N.R. Clinic, Union Station, Winnipeg, Man.; 633 Viscount Pl., Fort Garry (res); Man '46; Tel. WH 6-2491.

EGGLETON, G. Frederick; 614 Medical Arts Bldg., 1 Young St., Hamilton, Ont.; 16 Pinehurst Dr. (res); Tor '51; Phys., Steel Co. of Canada; Tel. JA 8-3904.

EGIER, Arthur I.; Ste. 305, 99 Avenue Rd., Toronto 5, Ont.; 131 Sultana Ave. (res); Wes '47; ObstGyn; Adj., Dept. Obst. Gyn., New Mt. Sinai Hosp.; Tel. WA 2-2711.

EHLERS, Eginhart O.; 2 Marcia Ave., Toronto 19, Ont.; Heidelberg (Germ.) '51; Treatment M.O., Workmen's Comp. Bd.

EHRENREICH, Karl A.; 216 Lynedock Cr., Don Mills, Ont.; Vienna (Aust.)'60; AMCGP; Phys., Alcoholism & Drug Addiction Fdn.; Staff (G.P.), Scarborough Gen. Hosp.; Tel. 751-0955.

EHRLICH, Baruch; 130 Ellesmere Rd., Scarborough, Ont.; Sheffield (Eng.) '60; AMCGP; Staff, Scarborough Gen., Toronto East Gen. & York Central Hosp's.; Tel. 447-5531.

EHRLICH, Bernard; 1350 Main St., Winnipeg 4, Man.; Royal Forest, Ste-208, 1880 Main St. (res); Durham (Eng.) '56; M.B., B.S., B.Sc. (Hons.), Physiol.

EHRLICH, Robert M.; Ste. 702, 1849 Yonge St., Toronto 7, Ont.; Tor'55; FRCP(C), Paed; Staff, Hosp. for Sick Children; Clin. Ass't. Paed., U. of Toronto; Tel. 455-4419.

EHRLICH, Seweryn K.; 447 Parr St., Winnipeg 4, Man.; Lwow (Poland) '31. Retired.

EIBEL, Philip; 370 Ellendale Med. Bldg., 5845 Cote-des-Neiges Rd., Montreal 26, P.Q.; McG'33; OrthSurg; Clin. Ass't. OrthSurg., Reddy Mem. Hosp. & Jewish Gen. Hosp.; Tel. 375-0421.

EID, Frederick L.; Macklin, Sask.; Heidelberg (Germ.) '21; GenSurg; MCGP; Chief of Staff, St. Joseph's Hosp.; Cons. Surg., Provost Mun. Hosp.; Tel. 220.

EID, Thomas C.; Ste. 340, 8409-112th St., Edmonton, Alta.; Tor'56; FRCS(C), Urol; Staff, University Hosp.; Instr.(Urol.), U. of Alberta; Tel. 433-0982.

EIDEM, Rodney; 205 Northgate Bldg., 10049 Jasper Ave., Edmonton, Alta.; Alb '55 FRCP(C), IntMed; Staff, University Hosp.; Tel. 439-5911.

EIDINGER, Samuel L.; 1437 MacKay St., Montreal, P.Q.; 30 Oakland Ave., Westmount (res); McG '35; AMCAA, DACA; Allerg. (PQ); MCGP; Staff, Reddy Mem. & Jewish Gen. Hosp.'s.; Tel. VI 2-6528.

EIDINGER, Stanley L.; 240 Seaforth Med. Bldg., 3550 Cote des Neiges Rd., Montreal 25, P.Q.; 15 Renfrew Ave., Westmount (res); McG '49; Pulm Dis & TB(P.Q.); DABIM; FCCP; FRCP(C); IntMed; Staff, Montreal Gen., Jewish Gen., & Royal Edward Laurentian Hosp's.; Cons. (IntMed.), Mount Sinai Hosp.; Dem. (Med.), McGill U.; Tel 935-3975.

EINARSON, Dawson W.; Qns'52; FRCP(C), Anaes; Staff, Kingston Gen. Hosp., Kingston, Ont.

EINBINDER, H.; 337 Dufferin, Sherbrooke, P.Q.; McG '37; M.C.G.P.

EINHORN, Roman; Ste. 1005, 143 James St. S., Hamilton, Ont.; Tor'56; FRCP(C); Neur.; Active Staff, Hamilton Gen. Hosp.; Court. Staff, St. Joseph's & Chedoke Hosp's.; Tel. JA 2-8425.

EISDORFER, Maximillian; 5440 Park Ave., Montreal, P.Q. (res); Budapest (Hung.)'13; MCGP; Tel. 271-5161.

EISEN, Abraham; 158 St. George St., Toronto 5, Ont.; Tor '51; FRCS(C); ObstGyn; Active Staff, New Mt. Sinai Hosp.; Tel. WA 3-4234.

EISEN, Abraham H.; Ste. 434, Montreal Children's Hosp., Montreal 25, P.Q.; 3982 Maplewood Ave. (res); Tor '56; Allergy (P.Q.); FRCP(C); Paed; Clin. Ass't., Dept. of Paed., Allergy & Clin. Immunol., Montreal Children's Hosp.; Tel. WE 7-8511, Loc 369.

EISEN, David; 200 Danforth Ave., Toronto, Ont.; 630 Vesta Dr. (res); Tor '22; M.Sc(Med.), D.A.-B.R., DiagRad.; Tel. 924-2700.

EISEN, Isadore M.; 250 St. Clair Ave. W., Toronto 7, Ont.; 1884 Eglinton Ave. E.; Tor'51; FACOG; FRCS(C), ObstGyn; Staff Phys., New Mt. Sinai, Toronto Gen. & Doctor's Hosp's.; Tel. 924-8009.

EISEN, Saul M.; 105 Dewbourne Ave., Toronto 10, Ont (res); Tor '42; Anaes; Chief Anaes., New Mount Sinai Hosp.; Tel. EM 6-7361.

EISTETTER, Alfred E.; 550 Med. & Dental Bldg., Rose St. & 11th Ave., Regina, Sask.; Wes '55; MRCOG; FRCS(C), ObstGyn; Staff, Regina Gen. & Bd. of Directors, Grey Nuns Hosp's.; Tel. 527-6606.

EITCHIS, Sara; 774 McEachran, Montreal, P.Q.; Prague (Cezch.) '25; Tel. 271-7123.

EKAIREB, Saul Y.; 13656-102nd Ave., North Surrey, B.C.; Cairo (Egypt) '49; Paed.; Tel. 581-7212.

EKINS, William E. J.; 210 Beechwood, Victoria, B.C. (res); Tor '03; Ophth, Otol; Retired.

EL DEIRY, Sameer K.; 31 Betts Ave., Yorkton, Sask.; 128 Logan Cr. W. (res); Cairo (Egypt) '47; DRCOG; MRCOG; Staff, Yorkton Union Hosp.; Tel. 783-3430.

ELDER, Arthur M.; Ste. G.01, 3000 Lawrence Ave. E., Scarborough, Ont.; 250 Ridgewood Rd., West Rouge, West Hill (res); Tor '54; DiagRad; Staff, Scarborough Gen. Hosp.; Tel. 291-1121.

ELDER, Henry W.; Wes'50; MCGP; Fell. (Clin. Allergy), Toronto Western Hosp., Toronto, Ont.

ELDER, John M.; 4569 Sherbrooke St. W., Montreal 6, P.Q.; 588 Lansdowne Ave., Westmount (res); McG '51; Paed; Ass't. Phys., Mtl. Gen., Mtl. Children's & Catherine Booth Hosp's.; Tel. WE 3-8437.

ELDER, John R.; Tor '61; Res., Hosp. for Sick Children, Toronto, Ont.

ELDER, Lawrence J.; 1499 Pharmacy Ave., Scarborough, Ont.; 105 Rexleigh Dr., Toronto 13 (res); Tor '53; Assoc., Toronto Gen. & Scarborough Gen. Hosp's.; Tel. HI 4-2971.

ELDER, Robert H.; 7 Commanche Dr., Ottawa 5, Ont.; Wes '49; Bact; Cons. Bact., Ottawa Civic Hosp.; Chief, Bact. Labs., Lab. of Hygiene; Lect. (Bact.), U. of Ottawa; Tel. PA 9-2511.

ELDER, Thomas R.; 1216 Douglas St., Victoria, B.C.; 373 Richmond Ave. (res); St. Andrew's (Scot.) '52.

ELDERKIN, Robert E.; 190 King St., St. Catharines, Ont.; McG '24; GenSurg; MCGP; Hon. Cons., (Surg.), St. Catharines Gen. & Hotel-Dieu Hosp's.; Tel. MU 2-4701.

ELEK, Dezso; 42 Giles Blvd. E., Windsor, Ont.; 1195 Bruce (res); Budapest (Hung.) '38; MCGP; Tel. 252-2611.

ELEK, Michael; 1983 Queen St. E., Toronto 8, Ont.; Tel. 691-8383.

ELEK, Susanne; 1983 Queen St. E., Toronto 8, Ont.; Tel. 691-8383.

ELGIE, Richard W.; 955 Queen St. E., Sault Ste. Marie, Ont.; 37 Summit Ave. (res); Tor '46.

ELGIE, Robert G.; Etherington Hall, Queen's University, Kingston, Ont.; Ott'59; FRCP(C), NeurSurg; Ass't. Prof. Surg., Div. of NeurSurg, Queen's U.

ELIAS, George L.; McG '57; M.Sc. (Experm. Surg.); FRCS(C), GenSurg; Teach. Fell. (1963-64), Mtl. Gen. Hosp., Montreal, P.Q.; Tel. WE 7-6011.

ELIAS, John C.; Dept. of Health, 411 Norquay Bldg., Winnipeg 1, Man.; Man '40.

ELIE, Jean C.; Paris (Fr.) '60; Jr. Intn., Hotel Dieu Hosp., Windsor, Ont.

ELKERTON, Lionel E.; 71 Sutherland Dr., Toronto, Ont. (res); Tor '33; D.P.H., Bact; Dir., Div. of Labs., Ontario Dept. of Health; Sp. Lect., School of Hyg., U. of Toronto; Tel. LE 4-3511.

EL-KHATIB, Abdallah; 1618 Camille-Paquet, Montreal 12, P.Q.; Bordeaux (France)'54; GenSurg(P.Q.).

ELKIN, David; Ste 120, 6000 Cote-des-Neiges Rd., Montreal 26, P.Q.; 5606 Eldridge Ave., Cote-St.-Luc (res); McG '52; FACS; FRCS(C), PlasSurg; Att'd. Staff. Jewish Gen. Hosp.; Tel. 735-3771.

ELKINGTON, Andrew R.; North West River, Labrador; Cambridge (Eng.) '60; M.B.(Camb.), B.Chir.

ELKINGTON, Eric H. W.; Medical Arts Bldg., 1105 Pandora Ave., Victoria, B.C.; 572 Island Rd. (res); McG '18; D.O.M.S., Ophth., Royal Jubilee Hosp.; Tel. EV 4-2622.

ELKUN, Leonard D.; Man'65; Jr. Int., Winnipeg Gen. Hosp., Winnipeg 3, Man.

ELLENBERGER, Henri F.; 5744 ave. Northmount, Montreal 26, P.Q. (res); Paris (Fr.) '34; Prof. (Soc. Sc.), U. of Mtl.; Tel. RE 3-9951.

ELLENBURGH, Nicholas; Ste. 6, 1855 Rose St., Regina, Sask.; Oxford (Eng.)'45; FRCS(Eng.); GenSurg; Surg., Regina Gen. & Grey Nuns Hosp's.; Tel. 522-1334.

ELLERKER, Alan R.; P.O. Box 266, Sydney, N.S.; Guys Hosp. (London, Eng.) '47; Staff, (Anaes.), Sydney City & St. Rita's Hosp's.; Tel. 562-1200.

ELLICOTT, Ernest R.; Bridge St., Napanee, Ont.; Qns '31.

ELLINGHAM, Frank H.; Federal Bldg., 150 Main St. W., Hamilton, Ont.; Tor '50; MCGP; Pension Med; Examiner, Cdn. Pension Commission; Tel. 522-3522.

ELLIOT, Alfred J.; 1108 Fairmont Med. Bldg., 750 W. Broadway, Vancouver 9, B.C.; 6012 Newton Wynd, Van. 8 (res); Tor '37; Med. Sc.D. (Columbia); DOMS (Lond.); Ophth; Hd. Subd-Dept. Ophth., Van. Gen. Hosp.; Hd. Dept. of Ophth, Shaughnessy DVA Hosp.; Prof. Surg. (Ophth.), U. of British Columbia; Tel. TR 4-7533.

ELLIOT, Arthur W.; 65 Dufferin Ave., Brantford, Ont. (res); Dal '51; DiagRad; Dir. of Radiology, St. Joseph's Hosp.; Tel. PL 3-3461, Ext. 28.

ELLIOT, George R.; 828 W. 10th Ave., Vancouver 9, B.C.; 7390 Hudson St. (res); Qns '35; DPH; DABPH; PH; Deputy Minister of Health, & Dir. of Bureau of Special Prev. & Treatment Serv. (B.C.); Prof. (Prev.Med.), U. of British Columbia; Tel. TR 4-2331.

ELLIOT, John A. F.; Ste 1404, 750 W. Broadway, Vancouver 9, B.C.; Tor '33; FRCS (Edin.), FACS; GenSurg., Surg., Vancouver Gen. Hosp.; Cons. Surg., D.V.A. Hosp.; Clin. Ass't. Prof. (Surg.), U. of British Columbia; Tel. TR 2-5733.

ELLIOT, S. Graham; 1826 W. Broadway, Vancouver 9, B.C.; 1610 Wesbrook Cres., Van. 8 (res); McG '24; ORL; Otol; Tel. 731-1826.

ELLIOT, Walter J., Sg. Radm., CD, QHS; 1449 Palen Ave., Ottawa 8, Ont. (res); Qns '37; Ophth; Surgeon-General, Canadian Forces; Tel. 992-0431.

ELLIOTT, Alan M.; Medical Centre, 707 Charlotte St., Peterborough, Ont.; Qns'56; AMCGP; Tel. 742-3871.

ELLIOTT, Alistair J. K.; Medical Arts Bldg., Ponoka, Alta.; Alb '42; Tel. 783-3306.

ELLIOTT, Alvin J.; The Brandon Clinic, Box 280, Dennis & McTavish, Brandon, Man.; 713-22nd St. (res); Man'50; IntMed; Att'd. Staff, Brandon Gen. & Assiniboine Hosp's.; Tel. PA 9-6441.
ELLIOTT, Carl M.; 1192 Weston Rd., Toronto 15, Ont.: Tor '51; Tel. RO 6-7611.
ELLIOTT, Donald W.; 216 Wharncliffe Rd. N., London, Ont.; Wes'64; AMCGP; Courtesy Staff, Victoria & St. Joseph's Hosp's.; Tel. 433-3167.
ELLIOTT, Fred W.; Ste. 607, 110 Georgia St. W., Vancouver, B.C.; UBC'62.
ELLIOTT, George B.; Dept of Surgical Path., Vancouver Gen. Hosp., Vancouver, B.C.; Durham (Eng.) '40; MRCS (Eng.) LRCP(Lond.); FC (Path.); **FACP; Path; Chief of Surg. Path.,** Vancouver Gen. Hosp.; Assoc. Clin. Prof.(Path.), U. of British Columbia; Tel. 876-3211.
ELLIOTT, George F.; Med. Arts Clinic, Regina, Sask.; Sask '58; MCGP; Active Staff, Regina Gen. & Grey Nuns Hosp's; Tel. 523-0691.
ELLIOTT, Harold W.; Turtle Pond Farm, Como, P.Q. (res); McG '36; FACS; NeurSurg; Cons., Montreal Gen., Cornwall Gen., Lachine Gen., Lakeshore Gen. & Hotel-Dieu, Cornwall; Ass't. Prof., McGill U.; Tel. WE 7-1604.
ELLIOTT, Harry R.; 250 Main St. E., Hamilton, Ont.; 39 Oak Knoll Dr. (res); Tor '27; F.R.-C.S.(C) Urol; Staff (Urol), Hamilton Gen. & St. Joseph's Hosp's.; Lect. (Urol.) to Nurses, Mc-Master U.; Tel. JA 7-2711.
ELLIOTT, H. Noel; 2578 Lake Shore Blvd. W., Toronto 14, Ont.; Wes '37; M.C.G.P.; Assoc. **Staff, St. Joseph's Hosp.; Tel. 251-9551.**
ELLIOTT, James F.; Ste. 420, 8409-112th St., Edmonton, Alta.; Alb '36; FACP; FRCP(C), Int-Med; Clin. Prof. (Med.) & Dir., Student Med. Service, U. of Alberta.
ELLIOTT, James M.; 1248 St-Foy Rd., Quebec 6, P.Q.; McG '27; FICS; GenSurg.
ELLIOTT, John T.; 2405 Lake Shore Blvd. W., Toronto 14, Ont.; 34 Saybrook Ave., Tor. 18 (res); Tor '52; M.C.G.P.; Tel. CL 9-4711.
ELLIOTT, Kathleen A. (Grant); Calgary Medical Centre, 8th Ave. & 8th St. W., Calgary, Alta.; **822 Hillcrest Ave. (res); Durham (Eng.) '42;** M.R.C.S. (Eng.), L.R.C.P. (Lond.), D.M.R.D. (Eng). DiagRad.; Tel. AM 3-6850.
ELLIOTT, L.; 428½ Talbot St., **St. Thomas, Ont.; Sparta, Ont. (res); Wes '13.**
ELLIOTT, Morley R., OBE; 1207 Goodacres Towers N., 360 Douglas St., Victoria, B.C.; Man'26; DPH; PH; Retired.
ELLIOTT, Robert C., A/Col.; Cdn. Forces Med. Serv., 48 Rideau St., Ottawa, Ont.; Qns'44; GenSurg; Dir. of Treatment Serv.; Tel. 992-6228.
ELLIOTT, Ronald; 10 Main St., Dundas, Ont.; McG '51.
ELLIOTT, S. Margarett; see Jenkner.
ELLIOTT, William J.; 25 Medical Arts Bldg., Winnipeg, Man; 109 Parkside Dr., St. James (res); Man '40; D.A.B.R., D&TRad.; Dem. Rad., U. of Manitoba; Tel. WH 2-6453.
ELLIOTT, W. Ord; 111 Main St., Brighton, Ont.; Dal '54; MCGP; Active Staff, Trenton Mem. Hosp.; Tel. 475-2100.
ELLIS, Alan C.; Leeds (Eng.) '51; DPH (Lond.); MOH., Foothills Health Unit, Box 638, High River, Alta.; Tel. 652-2341.
ELLIS, Christopher F. G.; Ste. 405, 340 McLeod St., Ottawa 4, Ont.; Wes'56; FRCS(C), **OrthSurg; Staff, Ottawa Civic Hosp.; Cons. Orth., Perley Hosp.; Hon. Cons. Lachine Gen. Hosp.,** Lachine, P.Q.; Clin. Ass't. (OrthSurg.) Ottawa U.; Tel. 729-0531.
ELLIS, Claude D.; 205 Doctors Bldg., 394 Graham Ave., Winnipeg, Man.; Academy Rd. (res); Man '44; MCGP; Court. Staff, Children's, Misericordia & Victoria Hosp's.; Tel. WH 2-4653.
ELLIS, Donald G.; Greene Clinic, 122-2nd Ave. W., Prince Rupert, B.C.; Liverpool (Eng.)'58.
ELLIS, George H.; 1468 St. Clair W., Toronto, Ont.; 63 High Park Ave. **(res); McG '35; Dist. Coroner;** Tel. LE 1-6089.
ELLIS, Gordon N.; 408 Medical Arts Bldg., Edmonton, Alta.; 52 St. George's Cres. (res); Qns '26; F.A.C.S., Urol.; **Assoc. Prof. Surg. (Urol.), U. of Alberta; Tel. GE 9-8721.**
ELLIS, John P.; 7182 Saanich Rd. W., Brentwood Bay, B.C.; Man'30; MCGP; Staff, Royal Jubilee Hosp., Victoria & Rosehaven Hosp's., Sidney; Tel. 652-2212.
ELLIS, Kent G.; Hunter River, P.E.I.; Dal'59; MCGP; Tel. 45.
ELLIS, Mildred C.; 719 Clarke Rd., Coquitlam, New Westminster, B.C. (res); Dal '53; Admin. M.O., Shaughnessy Hosp., Vancouver; Tel. TR 6-6767.
ELLIS, Peter M.; Oshawa Clinic, 117 King St. E., Oshawa, Ont.; Birmingham (Eng.)'60; M.B., Ch.B.
ELLIS, Ronald D.; The Underhill Clinic, 1635 Abbott St., Kelowna, B.C.; Man '52; IntMed; Staff, Kelowna Gen. Hosp.; Tel. 762-2740.
ELLIS, Vernon G.; 132 Parkdale Ave S., Hamilton, Ont.; Wes'64; AMCGP; Tel. 545-3059.
ELLISON, Gladys (Nitikman); 1545 McGregor St., Montreal 25, P.Q.; Man '36; Anaes; Staff Anaes., Royal Victoria Hosp.; Ass't Prof., McGill U.; Tel. VI 2-1251; Loc. 530.
ELLISON, Lucille G.; 2656 Heather St., Vancouver, B.C.; 1207 W. 40th, Van. 13 (res); Man '45; **Staff, B.C. Cancer Inst.; Clin. Instr. (Surg.), U. of British Columbia; Tel. CA 4-1111.**
ELLISON, Norman P.; 1054A Wilson Ave., Downsview, Ont.; 80 Clearview Hgts. (res); Belfast (Ire.) '50; **MCGP; Tel. ME 3-3711.**
ELLTOFT, J. David; Virgil Medical Centre, Virgil, Ont.; London (Eng.)'64.
ELLYATT, William G.; 381 Dieppe St., London, Ont.; Wes '58; MCGP; Staff, Victoria. St. Joseph's. St. Mary's & Parkwood Hosp's.; Tel. 439-6035.
ELMIK, Arno; Bass River, N.S.; Tartu (Estonia) '44; Tel. 14.
ELNES, Nyla R.; 3744 Cote des Neiges Rd., Montreal 25, P.Q.; 122 Lockhart, Town of Mt. Royal (res), Woman's Med. Coll. (Penn., U.S.A.) '45; Clin. Ass't., O.P.D.. Montreal Gen. Hosp.; Tel. 932-1732.
ELPHINSTONE, Norah C.; 222 Le Merchant Rd., St. John's Nfld., 46 Linden Court Apts. (res); London (Eng) '46; M.B., B.S. (Lond.); DCH (Eng.); Paed; Staff (Paed.), St. John's Gen., St. Clare's & Grace Hosp's.; Tel. 579-7807.
EL-RAREI, Nabil H.; Alexandria (Egypt)'57; Res., Winnipeg Gen. Hosp., Winnipeg, Man.
ELSE, David G.; Hudson Bay, Sask.; Oxford (Eng.)'61.
ELTON, Charles D.; 12316-66A Ave., Edmonton, Alta.; London (Eng.)'51; MRCS; LRCP; DA (Eng. & C.); Anaes; Staff, University Hosp.; Sessional Instr., U. of Alberta; Tel. 439-5911.
ELVIDGE, Arthur R.; 3801 University St., Montreal, P.Q.; 1465 Bernard Ave. W., Outremont (res); McG '24; M.Sc., Ph.D., D.A.B.N., F.R.-C.S.(C), NeurSurg; LLD; Hd. Div. of Neur-Surg., Queen Mary Vet's. Hosp.; NeurSurg., Montreal Neurol. Inst. & Royal Victoria Hosp.; Cons. NeurSurg., St. Mary's, Verdun Protestant & Montreal Children's Hosp's.; Tel. AV 8-4083.
ELVIN, Norman L., OBE; 309 Med. Arts Bldg., Winnipeg, Man.; 102 Chataway Blvd. (res); Man '27; Ophth; Hd. Dept. of Ophth.. Wpg. Gen. & Deerlodge DVA Hosp's.; Tel. WH 3-0507.
ELWOOD, T. Neville; 1359 Barrington St., Halifax, N.S.; Queen's U. (Belfast, N. Ire.)'52; M.B., B.Ch., BAO; Tel. 423-7463.
EMANUEL, Elliott; 352 Dorval Rd., Dorval, P.Q. 2055 Lakeshore Dr. (res); Oxford (Eng.) '41; MRCP (Eng.); DCH; DPM; FAPA; Psy; MCGP; Chm., Dept. of Med., Lachine Gen. and Lakeshore Hosp's.; Tel. 631-3021.
EMANUELE, Hugo; 626 Main St., Penticton, B.C.; 798 Argyle St. (res); McG '37; Tel. 492-4242.
EMANUELS, Eddy J.; Ste. 11, 13656-102nd Ave., North Surrey, B.C.; 10879 Oriole Dr. (res); **Amsterdam (Neth.) '51; Staff, Royal Columbian & St. Mary's Hosp's., New Westminster, & Surrey Mem. Hosp., North Surrey; Tel. 581-1711.**
EMARD, Elzear; 425—2nd St. W., Cornwall, Ont.; Mon '25; ObstGyn.

EMARD, Ladislas M.; 119 Marlborough N., Cornwall, Ont. (res); Mon '27; M.C.G.P.
EMBREE, Garth H.; Ste. 303, 100 Gloucester St., Ottawa 4, Ont.; Dal '57; FRCP(C); Neurol; Instr. (Neurol.), U. of Ottawa.
EMERY, Arnold W.; 815C Park Rd., Richmond, B.C.; UBC'63; AMCGP; Tel. CR 8-5191.
EMERY, E. Douglas; 2311 Oak Bay Ave., Victoria, B.C.; Alb '31; Ophth; Tel. 385-6011.
EMERY, George H.; 19 King St. W., Ingersoll, Ont.; 264 Oxford St. (res); Qns '39; Dist. Coroner.
EMERY, Guy N.; Apt. 2, 13 Bayview Court, Willowdale, Ont.; Qns'60; FRCP(C), IntMed.
EMERY, John E.; 215 Victoria St., Toronto 2, Ont.; Qns '57; FRCS(C), PlasSurg;
EMERY, Michael A.; 308 Med. Arts Bldg., 11010 Jasper Ave., Edmonton, Alta.; McG '57; FRCS(C), OrthSurg; Active Staff, University Hosp.; Cons., Misericordia & Royal Alexandra Hosp's.; Sessional Instr., U. of Alberta; Tel. 429-1883.
EMMETT, James C.; 95 St. Clair Ave. W., Toronto 7, Ont.; Tor'40; Med. Dir., The Imperial Life Assur. Co.; Tel. 364-8211.
EMMONS, Helen J.; UBC '61; Jr. Intn., St. Joseph's Hosp., Victoria, B.C.
EMMONS, W. Frank; 4786 Drummond Dr., Vancouver, B.C. (res); McG '24; M.Sc., Ph.D. (Physiol.), Neur; NeurSurg; Tel. CA 4-3050.
EMMONS, William F., Jr.; UBC'64; Res., St. Paul's Hosp., Vancouver 1, B.C.
EMO, Ralph G.; 508 St. John S. Rd., Pointe Claire, P.Q.; McG'58; IntMed.
EMOND, Georges V.; 55 ave. de l'Eglise, Montreal 19, P.Q.; Mon '39; MCGP.
EMOND, Jacqueline; Mon'65; Res. (Path.), Hop. Maisonneuve, Montreal, P.Q.
EMOND, Jean; Lav'65; Res., Hop. Notre-Dame, Montreal 24, P.Q.
EMOND, Michel; App. 2, 2201 Maplewood, Montreal 26, P.Q.; Mon'60; IntMed; Staff, Hop. Notre-Dame.
EMPEY, Reginald L.; Hamilton Health Assoc., Box 590, Hamilton, Ont.; Qns'32; FCCP.
EMPSON, John D.; 86 Selena Ave., Belleville, Ont.; Qns '40; Tel. WO 2-8811.
EMSON, Harry E.; 23 Weir Cres., Saskatoon, Sask.; Oxford (Eng.) '52; Path; Dir. of Labs., St. Paul's Hosp.; Lectr. Path., U. of Saskatchewan; Tel. 382-3220.
ENDELMAN, A. Andrzej; R.C.S. (Ireland)'54; Res., Vancouver Gen. Hosp., Vancouver 9, B.C.
ENDICOTT. William J.; 901 Helena St.. Trail, B.C.; 1350-3rd. Ave. (res); Tor '32; MCGP; Staff, Trail-Tadanac Hosp. & Mater-Misericordiae Hosp., Rossland; Tel. 368-3311.
ENESCO, Mircea; 12245 Grenet, Montreal 9, P.Q.; Jassy (Roum.)'42; L.Sc. (France); Ph.D. McGill; FRCP(C); IntMed; Tel. CR 4-2511.
ENG, F.W.H.T.; 73 Glengrove W., Toronto 12, Ont. (res); Philippines '61; Staff, Dept. of Biochemistry, U. of Toronto.
ENG, Ah-Yin; Taiwan (Formosa)'59; Staff, Fisher River Indian Hosp., Hodgson, Man.
ENGELBRECHT, Evelyn R.; Sask'62; Res., Vancouver Gen. Hosp., Vancouver, B.C.
ENGELBRECHT, Florence M. (Hanna); 36 Main St. S., Georgetown, Ont.; Tor'65; Tel. 877-4216.
ENGELBRECHT, Rodney O.; 36 Main St. S., Georgetown, Ont.; Tor'64.
ENGELS, W. Dennis; 1025 Pine Ave. W., Montreal, P.Q.; 3221 Forest Hill Ave. (res); Alb '56; Psy; Clin. Ass't., Royal Victoria Hosp.; Lect. (Psy.), McGill U.; Tel. VI 2-1251, Ext. 212.
ENGEN, Elgin S.; Apt. 907, 550 West 12th Ave., Vancouver 9, B.C.; Man'58.
ENGLAND, Harold H.; 14616-88 Ave., Edmonton, Alta.; Alb. '52; Anaes; Staff, Edmonton Gen. Hosp.; Tel. HU 8-8181.
ENGLAND, Nelles J., MBE; 450 Central Ave., Ste. 412, London, Ont.; 429 Wortley Rd. (res); Wes '39; FACP, FCCP, FRCP(C), IntMed; Chest Cons., Westminster DVA Hosp.; Cons., Ontario Hosp. & Beck Mem. San.; Instr. (Med.), U. of Western Ontario; Tel. GE 8-0105.
ENGLISH, Roderick A.; McG '55; Path; Staff, Dept. of Path., St. Paul's Hosp., Vancouver, B.C.; Tel. MU 3-2211.
ENKIN, Murray W.; 452 Main St. E., Hamilton, Ont.; 47 Bowman (res); Tor '47; FRCS(C), ObstGyn; Ass't. Hd., (ObstGyn Dept.), St. Joseph's Hosp.; Tel. JA 2-9412.
ENNALS, Addie C.; UBC '62; Jr. Intn., St. Joseph's Hosp., Victoria, B.C.
ENNIS, Julius M.; 21 Division St., Welland, Ont.; 164 Parkway (res); Tor '43; Paed.; Tel. 734-6780.
ENNS, Gerhard F.; 299 Main St., Chilliwack, B.C.; Man '39; MCGP; **Active Staff, Chilliwack Gen. Hosp.; Tel. 795-5774.**
ENNS, James W.; Rose Ave., Grandview, Man.; Man '59.
ENNS, Peter P.; 440 Desalaberry St., Winnipeg, Man.; 130 Dunvegan St. (res); **Man '48; M.C.-G.P.; Tel. 334-1096.**
ENRIGHT, Thomas J.; 208 Catalina Dr., Scarborough, Ont.; Tor '57; D.Psy; Psy; Dir., Mental Health Clinic, Whitby; Tel. 466-8985.
ENTA, Thomas; 200 Scott Bldg., Moose Jaw, Sask.; UBC'58; Derm; Abroad.
ENTIN, Martin A.; 1538 Sherbrooke St. W., Montreal, P.Q.; McG '45; Psy(P.Q.); FACS; PlasSurg; Assoc. Surg., (PlasSurg.), Royal Victoria Hosp.; Chief Cons., (PlasSurg.), Shriner's Hosp.; Ass't. Prof.(Surg.), McGill U.; Tel. WE 2-8413.
EPP, David L.; 750 W. Broadway, Vancouver 9, **B.C.; 1290 W-25th St. (res); Man '32; MCGP; Tel. 879-3919.**
EPP, Frank, L.; 755 W. Broadway, Vancouver 9, B.C.; 2171 Marine Dr. (res); Alb '50 D.D.S. Tel. TR 2-5844.
EPPING, John R.; Med. Centre, 707 Charlotte St., Peterborough, Ont.; Tor '40; Tel. 742-3871.
EPSTEIN, Arnold A.; 99 Avenue Rd., Toronto 5, Ont.; 174 Old Forest Hill Rd. (res); Dal '39; D&TRad.; Ass't. Rad., St. Joseph's Hosp.; Sr. Att. Rad., New Mt. Sinai Hosp.; Tel. WA 1-4757.
EPSTEIN, B. John; 7 Willow Rd., Grandfalls, Nfld.; Dal'58; ObstGyn.
EPSTEIN, Hans H.; Woodstock Med. Clinic, Woodstock, N.B.; Dal '56; IntMed; Tel. 328-6553.
EPSTEIN, Menu; Ste. 3, 914 St. Clair Ave. W., Toronto 10, Ont.; 44 Glengrove Ave. W. (res); Bucharest (Roumania) '51; Tel. LE 6-0371.
EPSTEIN, Nathan B.; 764 Upper Belmont, Westmount (P.Q.) (res); Dal'48; D. Psy; Psy; Cert. in Psychoanalytic Med. (Columbia); Psy-in-Chief, Jewish Gen. Hosp.; Dir. of Psy. Research., Chmn. Med. Bd. & Assoc. Prof. Psy., McGill U.; Tel. RE 1-1814.
EPSTEIN, Norman; Ste. 203, 158 St. George St., Toronto 5, Ont.; **173 Old Yonge St.,** Willowdale (res); Dal '53; M.C.A.A., Paed; Dir., Allergy Clin., St. Joseph's Hosp.; Hon. Cons. (All.), Queensway Gen. & South Peel Hosp's.; Tel. WA 1-8073.
EPSTEIN, Stanley W.; Dal'62; FRCP(C), IntMed; Staff, Toronto Western Hosp., Toronto 2B, Ont.
ERALP, M. S.; Istanbul (Turk.)'56; Res., Winnipeg Gen. Hosp., Winnipeg 3, Man.
ERB, John T.; 15 Braemore Gdns.,, Toronto 4, Ont.; Tor '45; Staff, Riverdale Hosp.
ERB, L. Jean; 15 Braemore Gardens, Toronto 4, Ont.; Tor '45; Pt-time Phys., Dept. of Health, City of Toronto.
ERB, R. Gordon; 22 King St. E., Hespeler, Ont.; Ont.; 469 Victoria Ave., Preston (res); Tor '50; Tel. 658-4271.
ERDEI, Alexander; 288 St. Clair Ave. W., Toronto 7, Ont.; 76 Burnaby Blvd. (res); Vienna (Austria) '25; **M.R.C.P.(Lond.), IntMed.**
ERDOGAN, Mehmet; Medical Arts Bldg., 5880 Spring Garden Rd., Halifax, N.S.; Istanbul (Turkey) '54; FRCS(C), OrthSurg; Staff, Camp Hill Hosp.; Tel. 422-6398.
EREAUX, Lemuel P.; 1414 Drummond St., Ste. 722, Montreal 25, P.Q.; McG '23; FRCP(C), DermSyph.
ERENBERG, Morris; 784 Ash St., Winnipeg 9, **Man.; 285 Bonnerman (res); Man '51; Tel. HU 9-8293.**

ERENST, Michael M.; 394 Bloor St. W., Toronto, Ont.; Berlin (Germ.) '39; GenSurg; Dem. (Anat.), U. of Toronto; Tel. WA 2-6593.

ERICKSON, Einar H.; Box 580, Can. Bank of Commerce Bldg., Mission City, B.C.; 33583 Main St. (res); Man '28; Pt-time M.O., Indian Health Serv., & CPR; Tel. 826-6011.

ERICKSON, E. Ralph; 692 Latchford St., Haileybury, Ont.; Wes '54; Path.

ERICKSON, Le Roy M.; Alb '64; Medical Clinic, Box 190, Fort St. John, B.C.; Tel. 785-6677.

ERITSLAND, O. B.; 530 Tegler Bldg., Edmonton, Alta.; 11649-77nd St. (res); Alb '54.

ERJAVEC, Bogdan; Weymouth, N.S.; Paris (Fr.) '50.

ERLICH, Baruch; 81 Elmsley St. N., Smith Falls, Ont.; Durham (Eng.) '56.

ERNEST, Maurice; London U. & St. Bart's Hosp. (London, Eng.)'47; MB; BS; MRCS; LRCP; Path; Staff, Toronto North Western Hosp., Toronto, Ont.

ERNST, David S.; 749 King St. W., Kitchener, Ont.; Tor '43; FRCS(C), ObstGyn; Staff (ObstGyn), St. Mary's Hosp.; Cons., ObstGyn., South Waterloo Mem. Hosp.; Tel. 743-3162.

ERNST, W. Alan; 5991 Spring Garden Rd., Halifax, N.S.; 5960 Inglis St. (res); Dal. '51; Urol; Ass't. Urol., Victoria Gen. & Camp Hill DVA Hosp's.; Staff (Urol), Children's & Hlfx. Infirmary; Ass't. Prof. (Urol.), Dalhousie U.; Tel. 422-6376.

ERYILMAZ, Kemal; Istanbul (Turkey) '49; Staff, Saskatoon San., Saskatoon, Sask.

ESCOTT-BEAL, Mary E. (See Young).

ESDALE, William L.; 4487 Townley St., Vancouver 8, B.C.; Alb '50; FACA; Anaes; Att'd. Staff, St. Paul's Hosp.; Instr. (Anaes), U. of British Columbia; Tel. RE 3-9240; MU 5-8623.

ESHER, Frederick J. S.; Birmingham (Eng.)'26; MB; ChB.; DPM; MRCS; LRCP; Staff, Dept. of Psy., Room 533, University Hosp., Saskatoon, Sask.

ESHOO, Homer; 31 Kingston Row, Winnipeg 8, Man. (res); Man '41; Anaes; Assoc. Anaes., Winnipeg Gen. Hosp.; Hon. Att. Staff, Children's, King George Isolation Winnipeg Gen. Hosp's; Dem., Dept. of Surg. Anaes.), U. of Manitoba; Tel. SP 4-6511

ESPERANCA, Manuel J.; 630 Bathurst St., Toronto, Ont.; Lisbon (Port.) '56; DPH; ABP; Paed; Att'd. Staff, St. Joseph's Hosp.; Tel. 534-8711.

ESSER, Irving O.; 2818 Keele St., Downsview, Ont.; 54 Grace St. (res); Tor '58; A.M.C.G.P.; Staff, New Mt. Sinai Hosp., Toronto; Tel. ME 6-2211.

ESSIG, Karl H.; Ste. 400, 5300 Cote-des-Neiges Rd., Montreal 26, P.Q.; 370 Wood Ave., Westmount (res); Tuebingen (Germ.) '43; Staff, St. Mary's Hosp.; Tel. RE 7-3812.

ESTEY, Harold W.; Ste. 537, Med. Arts Bldg., Saskatoon, Sask.; 20 Weir Cr. (res); Tor '49; FRCS(C); Urol; FACS; Staff, University Hosp., St. Paul's. & Saskatoon City Hosp's.; Lect., U. of Saskatchewan; Tel. 652-0531.

ESTRADA, Roberto L.; 1414 Drummond St., Ste. 906, Montreal 25, P.Q.; 4375 Oxford Ave., Mtl. 28 (res); McG '43; D.Surg; FACS, FRCS(C), GenSurg; Ass't. Surg., Mtl. Gen. & Att'd. Surg., Reddy Mem. Hosp's.; Ass't Prof. (Surg), McGill U.; Tel. AV 8-1724.

ESTRELLA, Fernando I.; 230-5th Ave., Timmins, Ont.; Santo Domingo '48; GenSurg.; Tel. 264-6326.

ETELE, Julius; 214 Greyhound Bldg., 622—1st St. W., Calgary, Alta.; 3822—8th St. S.W. (res); Budapest (Hung.) '42; AMCGP; Tel. 269-2918.

ETHANS, Constantine T.; 501 Cordova St., Winnipeg, Man.; Man'60; Anaes.

ETHERINGTON, Elizabeth M. B. (Fletcher-Barret); Haig Clinic, Lethbridge, Alta.; Durham (Eng.)'51; Staff, Lethbridge Municipal, St. Michael's & Lethbridge Aux. Hosp's.; Tel. 328-6642.

ETHERINGTON, John S.; Haig Clinic, Lethbridge, Alta.; Durham (Eng.) '52; M.B., B.S., MCGP; Staff, Lethbridge Municipal, Lethbridge Aux. & St. Michael's Gen. Hosp's.; Tel. 328-6641.

ETHIER, Fernand; 700-lere Rue, Iberville, P.Q.; Mon '35; Head Dept. Obst. & Mem. Exc., Med. Staff, St. Jean Hosp, Que.

ETHIER, Jacques P.; 324 est boul. St. Joseph, Montreal 14, P.Q.; Mon'42.

ETHIER, Jean G.; Ott '55; MCGP; Res., Hop. St. Luc, Montreal, P.Q.

ETHIER, Jean L.; 5381 Viau, Montreal 36, P.Q.; Mon '61; Staff, Mtl. Transport Comm; Tel. 254-9829.

ETHIER, Romeo; 55 Lockhart, Montreal 16, P.Q. (res); Mon '55; DiagRad; Ass't. Rad., Montreal Neurol. Inst.; Tel. VI 2-1251.

ETTINGER, G. Harold, MBE; 67 Queen's Cres., Kingston, Ont. (res); Qns '20; D.Sc., FRCS; M.D. (Hon. U of O.); Dean Emeritus, Fac. of Med., Queen's U.; Chm. Med. Advisory Bd., & Dir. Med. Planning, Alcoholism & Drug Addiction Research Fdn., Toronto 5, Tel. 365-4507.

ETZIONY, Mordecai; 4765 Maplewood Ave., Montreal 26, P.Q.; McG '38; IntMed (P.Q.); Ass't. Phys., Montreal Jewish Gen. Hosp.; Assoc. Phys., Jewish Hosp. of Hope.; Tel. 735-2112.

ETZKORN, Kenneth R.; 401 Med. Centre, 906-8th Ave. S.W., Calgary, Alta.; Alb '51; Psy. Cons. City Welfare Dept. & U. of Calgary Student Health Serv.; Tel. 269-2242.

EUSTACE, Thomas H.; Drayton Valley, Alta.; London (Eng.)'44; DObstRCOG.

EVANS, A. Maxwell; 6209 Elm St., Vancouver, B.C. (res); McG '32; D.M.R.E. (Camb.), TherRad; Dir., B.C. Cancer Inst., 2656 Heather St.; Med. Dir., B.C. Cancer Fdn.; Clin. Ass't. Prof. (Dept. of Surg.), U. of British Columbia; Tel. TR 4-9321.

EVANS, Barry V.; 105 Northgate Bldg., Edmonton, Alta.; 7508-139th St. (res); Man '55; DABDR; DiagRad; Active Staff, Royal Alexandra Hosp.; Tel. 429-2508.

EVANS, Clarence C.; 70 Cedar St., Sudbury, Ont.; 147 McNaughton St. (res); Tor '31; ObstGyn; Tel. OS 5-8386.

EVANS, C. Edward; Box 1060, Wainwright, Alta.; King's College Med. Schl. (London, Eng.) '60; M.B., B.S., MRCS(Eng), LRCP(Lond.); MCGP; Tel. 842-4333.

EVANS, Daniel; 181 Russell Ave., St. Catharines, Ont.; Ott'51; FACS; Tel. 684-2619.

EVANS, David; 16 Wells Hill Ave., Toronto, Ont; Birmingham (Eng.) '56; FRCP(C), Anaes; Staff, Toronto Western Hospital; Tel. EM 8-2581.

EVANS, David T. R.; 221 Brant Ave., Brantford, Ont.; London (Eng.) '42; MRCS; LRCP; FRCS (Eng.); GenSurg; Surg. Staff, Brantford Gen., St. Joseph's & Willett Hosp., Paris; Tel. 753-6050.

EVANS, Dennis C.; Ste. 109, 1 Medical Place, 20 Wynford Dr., Don Mills, Ont.; Cape Town (S. Africa)'51; FRCS (Eng.); FRCS (Ed.); FRCS(C), OrthSurg; OrthSurg., Toronto East Gen. Hosp.; Tel. 429-0787.

EVANS, Dennis W.; Atomic Energy Canada Ltd., Chalk River, Ont.; Liverpool & Birmingham (Eng.)'47.

EVANS, Dita M. (Williams); Box 279, Hanna, Alta.; Aberdeen (Scot.)'57; DPH; M.O.H., Sig County Health Unit; Tel. 854-3055.

EVANS, E. Hugh; 11 Tremont Dr., Rockingham, N.S.; London (Eng.) '35; M.R.C.S., L.R.C.P.

EVANS, Ella C.; 740 Evelyn Dr., Hollyburn, B.C. (res); Alb '37; Retired.

EVANS, Enos; 800 Wilton Pl., Woodstock, Ont. (res); Tor '39; IntMed.; Staff, Ont. Hosp.; Tel. 539-1251.

EVANS, Esther M.; 2545 Virginia Pk., South Windsor, Ont.; Man '44: Retired.

EVANS, Francis J., Major; RCAMC, National Defence Med. Centre, Ottawa, Ont.; Ott '54; Tel. 733-6600.

EVANS, George P.; 1947 Cook St., Victoria, B.C.; Liverpool (Eng.)'55; DPH; PH; Dir., Saanich & South Vancouver Island Health Unit; Deputy M.O., Greater Victoria Met. Bd. of Health; Research Fell., Dept. of PrevMed; Tel. EV 5-5711.

EVANS, Gerald E.; Ste 203, 299 Main St., Chilliwack, B.C.; Alb '50; Paed.

EVANS, Griffith H.; 45 Cheltenham Ave., Toronto 12, Ont. (res); London (Eng.) '33; DiagRad; Staff, Sunnybrook Hosp.; Tel. HU 1-8224.
EVANS, Gwilyn; No. 7 1108 Williams Rd., Richmond, B.C.; Liverpool (Eng.)'55; DMRD; DiagRad; Tel. 277-3181.
EVANS, Harold S.; Brandon Clinic, Box 280, Brandon, Man.; 355-22nd St. (res); Man'28; FACS, FRCS(E) & (C), GenSurg; Chief of Staff, Brandon Gen. Hosp.; Cons. Surg., Brandon Hosp. for Mental Dis. & San. Bd. of Manitoba; Tel. PA 9-6444.
EVANS, Harvey A.; Tor'62; Res., Jewish Gen. Hosp., Montreal, P.Q.
EVANS, Hugh S.; Box 247, Rockglen, Sask.; Liverpool (Eng.) '50; DPH Tel. Rockglen 7.
EVANS, James C.; Box 305, Bradford, Ont.; Tor '59;
EVANS, John F., Lt/Col; Qns'45; Psy; Chief, Dept. of Psy., RCN Hosp., C.F.B., Esquimalt, FMO, Victoria, B.C.; Tel. 382-9211.
EVANS, John G.; One Medical Place, 20 Wynford Dr., Don Mills, Ont.; Tor '52; FRCS(C), OrthSurg; Staff, (OrthSurg.), St. Michael's Hosp.; Ass't. Prof., (Surg.), U. of Toronto; Tel. 429-0673.
EVANS, John R.; Faculty of Medicine, McMaster U., Hamilton, Ont.; Tor '52; D.Phil. (Oxon); FRCP(C), IntMed; Dean, Faculty of Med., Principal, College of Health Sciences, & Prof. Dept. of Med., McMaster U.; Tel. 522-4971.
EVANS, Joseph A.; 309 Avenue Rd., Toronto, Ont.; Tor '07; L.R.C.P., L.R.C.S. (Ire.), L.M.; MCGP; Assoc., Phys., Toronto Western Hosp.; Tel. WA 3-5692.
EVANS, O. B.; 112 Waterloo St., Saint John, N.B.; McG '23 FACS, GenSurg; Tel. 693-2987.
EVANS, Ramon J.; Ste. 10, 6 Vendome Place, Don Mills, Ont.; London (Eng.)'58; GenSurg; Research Fell., Toronto Gen. Hosp. & University of Toronto; Tel. EM 6-8211, Ext. 2774.
EVANS, S. Courtenay; 267 O'Connor St., Ottawa, Ont.; 20 Clemow Ave. (res); McG '39; IntMed; Att. Phys., Ottawa Civic Hosp.; Clin. Ass't (Med.), U. of Ottawa; Tel. CE 2-1773.
EVANS, Sidney E.; 925 W. Georgia St., Vancouver 1, B.C.; Hollyburn Med. Centre, West Van.; 740 Evelyn Dr., Hollyburn (res); Alb '39; MRCOG, ObstGyn.; Tel. MU 4-3942; WA 2-2912.
EVANS, Wilford G.; Box 719. West Summerland, B.C.; Man '46.
EVANS, Wilfred M.; St. Bart's (London, Eng.) '40 M.R.C.S. (Eng.), L.R.C.P. (Lond.); Supt., Springdale Hosp., Springdale, Nfld.; Tel. 6913.
EVELYN, Kenneth A.; G. F. Strong Lab. for Med. Research, 10th Ave. & Heather St., Vancouver 9, B.C.; 5510 Chancellor Blvd. (res); McG '38; F.A.C.P., F.R.C.P.(C), IntMed; Dir., G. F. Strong Lab. of Med. Research; Sr. Phys., Vancouver Gen. Hosp.; Prof. (Med.), U. of British Columbia; Tel. CA 4-1111.
EVELYN, Stephen J.; 377 Vaughan Rd., Toronto, Ont.; Tor '19; Anaes; Cons. (Anaes.), Toronto Gen. & Wellesley Hosp's.; Tel. RU 7-4011.
EVENSON, Leonard G. Capt.; 1 CBMU, CFPO 5050, Canadian Armed Forces, Europe; Sask'64.
EVERARD, Elizabeth P.; 4 Lynndale Rd., Toronto 13, Ont.; London (Eng.) '46; ObstGyn; Retired.
EVERETT, Herbert S.; 12 Water St., St. Stephen, N.B.; McG '23; GenSurg; Staff, Charlotte County & Regional County Hosp's.; Tel. 466-1799.
EVERIST, Wilfred C.; 39 Birchleaf Cr., Weston, Ont.; Tor '24.
EVIS, Frederick A., Q.C.; 2195 Yonge St., Toronto 7, Ont.; 25 Russell Hill Rd., Tor. 7 (res); Tor '49; DPH; FASCH; MCGP; Medico-Legal Cons., Ontario Hosp. Services Comm.; Tel. 487-1711.
EWART, Douglas M.; 200 Scott Block, Moose Jaw, Sask.; 1146—2nd Ave., N.W. (res); Qns '41; Anaes; Chief of Anaes., Moose Jaw Clinic; Tel. 692-2373.
EWART, E. Wilson; 83 Alma St., Moncton, N.B.; Tor '21; D.A.B.O.S., F.A.A.O.S., OrthSurg; Att. Orth.Surg., Moncton & Hotel Dieu de l'Assomption Hosp's; Cons. Orth. Surg., Moncton Tuberculosis Hosp.; Tel. EV 4-3650.
EWART, Hugo T.; Qns '35; FACHA; Med. Supt., The Hamilton Health Assoc., Box 590, Hamilton, Ont.; Tel. 385-5341.
EWART, William B.; Winnipeg Clinic, Winnipeg 1, Man.; 948 McMillan, Wpg. 9 (res); Man '52; IntMed; Dem. (Med.), U. of Manitoba; Tel. WH 2-6441.
EWASEW, Leo M.; 1407 W. Broadway, Vancouver 9, B.C.; Ste. 304, 1235 Comox St. (res); **McG '56; MCGP; Vis. Staff. Vancouver Gen., Grace, St. Vincent's & St. Paul's Hosp's.; Tel. RE 1-1717.**
EWASEW, Walter T.; 1407 W. Broadway, Vancouver 9, B.C.; Sask'61; AMCGP; Active Staff, Vancouver Gen., St. Vincent's & Grace Hosp's.; Tel. RE 1-1717.
EWENER, William A.; 1281 Dundas St., London, Ont.; Wes '48; MCGP; O.C., Med. Sec., Manning Depot, S.W. Ont., Area Comm., St. John's Ambulance; Tel. 451-3410.
EWERT, Arnold; 273 Scott St., St. Catharines, Ont.; Freiburg (W. Germ.) '40; GenSurg.; Tel. 684-1482.
EWERT, Edwin L.; 103 King St. E., Bowmanville, Ont.; 3 Frederick Ave. (res); Qns'43; Tel. 623-7261.
EWERT, George W.; 309 Medical Centre Bldg., Calgary, Alta.; Poznan (Poland) '36.
EWERT, Gertrude M. (Schindler); 273 Scott St., St. Catharines, Ont.; Munich (Germ.) '50.
EWERT, Robert A.; 1669 Victoria, Prince George, B.C.; 3100 Nechako Dr. (res); McG '53; GenSurg; Tel. LO 3-3411.
EWING, Cecil C.; 1222 Elliott St., Saskatoon, Sask. (res); Bristol (Eng.) '50; DO (Lond.); Ophth; Staff, University Hosp.; Ass't Prof., (Ophth), U. of Saskatchewan; Tel. 242-7641, Loc. 477.
EWING, Donald; 750 King St. W., Kitchener, Ont.; Wes '36; F.I.C.S., F.A.C.O.G., ObstGyn; Staff, St. Mary's Hosp.; Cons. Staff, ObstGyn., Kitchener Waterloo Hosp.; Tel. SH 5-5112.
EWING, Gerald H.; Medical Arts Clinic, 2125-11th Ave., Regina, Sask.; Edinburgh (Scot.) '55. IntMed; Tel. 523-0691.
EWING, J. Burke; 106 Med. Arts Bldg., 180 Metcalfe St., Ottawa 4, Ont.; 368 Lisgar Rd., Rockcliffe (res); Qns '32; FRCS(Edin.), FRCS(C), FICS, FACS, GenSurg; Surg.-in-Chief Ottawa Gen. Hosp.; Cons. Surg., Ottawa Civic & St. Louis-Marie-de-Montfort Hosp's.; Prof & Hd. Dept. of Surg., U. of Ottawa; Cons. Surg., Dept. of National Defence Med. Centre; Tel. 236-7257.
EWING, Margaret L.; McG'65; Jr. Int., Royal Victoria Hosp., Montreal 2, P.Q.
EWING, R. Dennis; Churchill St., Hudson Bay, Sask.; Cambridge (Eng.) '35; M.R.C.S., L.R.C.P. (Lond.), F.R.C.S. (Eng.), F.I.C.S., F.R.S.T.M. (Lond.), F.A.S.P., F.A.G.S.; Staff, Hudson Bay Hosp.; Tel. 865-2414.
EYDT, John N.; 452 Main St. E., Hamilton, Ont.; 28 Searle St. (res); Wes '44; IntMed; Active Staff, St. Joseph's Hosp.; Tel. 529-1222.
EYRES, Herbert H.; 211 Main St. N., Weston, Ont. (res); Tor '10; Retired.
EZERS, Inara A.; Tor'63; Res., Toronto Western Hosp., Toronto 2, Ont.
EZRIN, Calvin; 4 Ava Crescent, Toronto, Ont.; Tor '49; FRCP(C), IntMed; Phys., Toronto Gen. Hosp.; Ass't.Prof., Dept. of Path., U. of Toronto; Tel. WA 3-1404.
FABI, Robert; Mon '60; Sr. Int'n., Hop. Maisonneuve, Montreal, P.Q.
FABRIGAR, Carmelo; Arcola, Sask.; Manila (Philippines)'54; FICS; FICA; Tel. 455-2288; Abroad.
FADER, William H.; 395 Brooke Ave., Toronto 12 Ont.; 38 Howard Dr., Willowdale (res); Tor '48; MCGP; Court. Staff, St. Michael's Hosp.; Active Staff Grace Hosp.; Med. Dir., Canadian National Inst. for the Blind; Tel. 783-7500.

FAFARD, Andre; Lav '63; Ass't. Res., Notre Dame Hosp., Montreal, P.Q.
FAFARD, Arthur; 27 Guenette, Levis, P.Q.; 29 Guenette (res); Lav '19; Ophth. Otol; Tel. 837-5029.
FAGAN, Joel E.; Tor'65; Res., Hosp. for Sick Children, Toronto, Ont.
FAHEY, John J.; Marysville, Ont.; Ott. '52.
FAHEY, Philip J.; 323 Hamilton Ave., St. John's, Nfld.; Dublin (Ire.)'55; Urol.
FAHLMAN, John J.; Box No. 214, Kinistino, Sask.; Sask '37; Staff, Union Hosp.
FAHMI, Nihad; French Faculty of Medicine '61; Jr. Intn., University Hosp., Saskatoon, Sask.
FAHMY, Nishat; 152 Ochterloney St., Dartmouth, N.S.; Punjab (India) '53; Tel. 466-2742.
FAHRNI, Brock M.; 1665 W. Broadway, Vancouver, B.C.; 1761 Drummond Dr. (res); Man '38; F.R.C.P.(C), IntMed; Att'd. Staff, Vancouver Gen. Hosp.; Prof. & Hd. Schl. of Rehab Med., U. of British Columbia; Tel. CA 4-1432.
FAHRNI, Gordon P.; D.S.C.; 423 Med. Arts Bldg., Winnipeg, Man.; 1338 Wolseley Ave. (res); Man '40; FACS, FRCS(C), GenSurg; Staff, Winnipeg Gen. Hosp.; Chief of Surg., Municipal Hosp. & Grace Hosp.; Ass't. Prof. (Surg.), U. of Manitoba; Tel. 942-6389.
FAHRNI, Gordon S.; 2191 W. 39th Ave., Apt. 1001, Vancouver 13, B.C.; Man'11; FACS; DABS; FRCS(C); FICS; (Hon.) GenSurg; Prof. Emer. (Med.), U. of British Columbia; Retired.
FAHRNI, W. Harry; Ste. 1316, 750 W. Broadway, Vancouver 9, B.C.; Man'40; FRCS(Ed.), M. Ch. Orth. (Liverpool), FRCS(C), OrthSurg; Ass't. Orth. Surg., U. of British Columbia; Attend. Staff (Orth.), Vancouver Gen. & Children's Hosp's.; Orth., Cons., Shaughnessy Hosp.; Tel. RE 1-1410.
FAIGEN, Morris; 4037 Oak St., Vancouver, B.C.; Tor '38; Derm.
FAILLE, Roland; 30 est, boul St-Joseph, Montreal 14 P.Q.; 209-300 Blvd. Graham (res); Mon '48 DABS; GenSurg., Surg., Hop. Ste. Jeanne d'Arc; Tel. LA 6-6000.
FAINMAN, Jack; 310 Boyd Bldg., 388 Portage Ave., Winnipeg 1, Man.; Man '54; FRCS(C); ObstGyn; Clin. Tutor, St. Boniface Hosp.; Teach. Staff, St. Boniface & Grace Hosp's.; Tel. 947-1815.
FAINSTEIN, Saul B.; 2461 Bloor St. W., Toronto 9, Ont.; 219 Richview Ave. (res); Man '42; Ophth; Staff, Queensway Gen. & North Western Hosp's.; Tel. RO 6-6332.
FAIR, John W.; Ste. 208, Rideau Med. Dental Centre 1711-4th St. S.W., Calgary, Alta.; Alb '54; Psy; AAPCC; Cons. Psy., William Roper Hull Home, Prov. Welfare Dept., Catholic Family Service Bureau & Calgary Family Service Bureau; Tel. 262-3616.
FAIR, Michael A.; 4151 Sheppard Ave., Agincourt, Ont.; Tor '53; MCGP; Att'd. (G.P.) Staff, Scarborough Gen. Hosp.; Tel. 293-4189.
FAIRBAIRN, Logan M.; 48 Academy Med. Bldg., 1812-4th St. W., Calgary, Alta.; Man '27; GenSurg; Staff, Calgary Gen., Holy Cross, & Colonel Belcher Hosp's.; Tel. AM 6-6426.
FAIRBAIRN, Robert F.; Box 8, 12-3rd. St. S. E., Redcliff, Alta.; Alb '58; MCGP; M.O.H., Dom. Glass Co. Ltd.; Tel. 548-3467.
FAIRBANK, William H.; Ste. 302, 625-5th Ave., New Westminster, B.C.; Oxford (Eng.)'47; MCGP; Tel. 522-7730.
FAIRBANKS, C. Joseph; 307 N.W. Prof. Centre, 1640-16th Ave. N.W., Calgary, Alta.; Alb'58; FRCS(C), OrthSurg.
FAIRCHILD, William G.; Elliot Lake Clinic, 46 Ontario Ave., Elliot Lake, Ont.; St. Andrews (Scot.)'55; M.B., Ch.B.; Active Staff & Hd. Dept. of ObstGyn., St. Joseph's Gen. Hosp.; Tel. 848-7176.
FAIRFIELD, Finlay M.; Box 1868, Wetaskiwin, Alta.; Alb'61; AMCGP.
FAIRFIELD, George C.; Box 460, Portage-la-Prairie, Man.; Man'36.
FAIRHURST, Kenneth W.; Edinburgh (Scot.)'60; FRCP(C), Anaes; Staff, Toronto Gen. Hosp., Toronto, Ont.
FAIRLEY, H. Barrie; Dept. of Anaes., Toronto Gen. Hosp., Toronto 2, Ont.; London (Eng.)'49; MRCS; LRCP; DA; FFARCS; Anaes; Sr. Anaes., Toronto Gen. Hosp.; Assoc. Prof., U. of Toronto; Tel. EM 6-8211.
FAIRLEY, John; Box 400, Comox, B.C.; Cambridge (Eng.) '52; DA; DRCOG; Tel. 339-2266.
FALARDEAU, Ivy F.; 847 Spruce St., Winnipeg 10, Man.; Man '25; Phys., Sunset Lodge; Prov. Coroner; Tel. 783-5318.
FALARDEAU, Jean J.; 31 Cartier, St. Iamé, Cte. Richelieu, P.Q.; Lav'53; Tel. St. Iamé 50.
FALARDEAU, Maurice; 7472 Montpetit, Montreal 35, P.Q.; Mon'59; FRCS(C); GenSurg; Staff, Hop. Notre-Dame.
FALCKH, Robert C. F.; Port Arthur Clinic, 194 North Court St., Port Arthur, Ont.; 141 Winnipeg Ave. (res); Durham (Eng.) '54; Ophth; Active Staff, Port Arthur Gen & St. Joseph's Hosp's.; Tel. DI 4-7271.
FALCONER, J. Gilbert; 232 Forest Hill Rd., Toronto, Ont. (res); Tor '25; M.R.C.P.(Lond.), F.R.C.P.(C), IntMed; Med. Director North American Life Assurance Co., Toronto; Tel. EM 2-6011.
FALCONER, William L.; 14415-94th Ave., Edmonton, Alta. (res); Man '26; Reg. Sup't Indian Health Services, Dept. of N.H. & W., Charles Camsell Indian Hosp., Edmonton; Tel. GL 5-7141. Retired.
FALK, Robert C.; Port Arthur Clinic; 194 Court St., Port Arthur, Ont.; Tel. 344-7271.
FALK, Rudolf E.; Man '60; Res., Toronto East General Hosp., Toronto 2B, Ont.
FALK, William A.; 1730 Richmond Ave., Victoria, B.C.; 1950 Waterloo Rd. (res); Alb '49; MCGP; Staff, Royal Jubilee Hosp.; Tel. EV 5-4434.
FALK, William M.; 6325 Fraser St., Vancouver, B.C.; Dublin (Ire.)'57; M.B.; BCh; BAO; Anaes.; Staff, Grace Hosp. & Richmond Gen. Hosp., Richmond; Tel. FA 5-4040.
FALKINGHAM, John P.; Carmel Clinic, 124-1st Ave. N.W., Swift Current, Sask.; Leeds (Eng.) '48; MB., BCh.; Tel. 773-8333.
FALKNER, Charles F.; Box 290, Tisdale, Sask.; Man'52.
FALLIS, Fred B.; 2135 Avenue Rd., Toronto 12, Ont.; 128 Ridley Blvd., Tor. 12 (res); Tor '53; MCGP; Vol. Ass't. Med., O.P.D., Spec. Treatment Clinic, Toronto Gen. Hosp.; Tel. HU 5-0725.
FALLIS, James C.; Ste 114, 250 Lawrence Ave. W., Toronto 12, Ont.; Tor '55; FRCS(C), GenSurg; FACS; Ass't. Surg., Staff, Hosp. for Sick Children & Clin. Instr. (Surg.), U. of Toronto; Tel. 789-5961.
FAMINOW, Wm. S.; Box 147, Bassano, Alta.; Alb '55.
FANJOY, Roy W.; 2 Germain St., Saint John, N.B.; Rothesay, P.O. Box 90 (res); Dal '48; D.A.B.Otol., Otol; Staff (E N.T.), Saint John Gen., St. Joseph's & Lancaster (D.V.A.) Hosp's.; Cons., Provincial Hosp., Lancaster.; Tel. 692-1498.
FANNING, E. Anne; Wes'63; Res., Royal Alexandra Hosp., Edmonton, Alta.
FANNING, Vern R.; 8330 Fairmont Dr., Calgary, Alta.; Alb'57; AMCGP; Abroad.
FANNING, William J.; Roberts Medical Group, 95 Lemarchant Rd., St. John's, Nfld.; Dal'57; Tel. 579-0055.
FARAH-LAJOIE, Claude; 12245 rue Grenet, Montreal 9, P.Q.; Mon'65.
FARBER, Earl P.; 31 Yonge St. N., Richmond Hill; Med. Arts Bldg., Newmarket; Tor'57; FRCS(C) GenSurg; PlasSurg; Tel. 884-6251.
FARBER, Robert; Ste. 702, 1849 Yonge St., Toronto 7, Ont.; 21 Hedgewood Rd. (res); Tor '48; FRCP(C), Paed; Fell., Hosp. for Sick Children; Adjunct, New Mt. Sinai Hosp.; Lect. (Paed), U. of Toronto; Tel. WA 3-4113.
FAREWELL, Anna E. (Bryce); Man '44; Paed; Staff, Coqualeetza Indian Hosp., Sardis, B.C.; Tel. SY 3-7212.

FARFAN, Henry F.; 5300 Cote-des-Neiges Rd., Montreal '26; P.Q.; 404 Dulwich Ave., St. Lambert (res); McG '51; F.R.C.S.(C), OrthSurg; Staff, Montreal Children's, St. Mary's & Reddy Mem. Hosp's.; Tel. 733-3861.

FARIBAULT, Claude; 361 Wiseman Ave., Outremont, Montreal 8, P.Q. (res); Mon '50; D&T-Rad; Rad., Hop. Notre Dame; Tel. LA 5-6363.

FARIS, John W.; 1116 Barton St. E., Hamilton, Ont.; 49 Edgwood Ave. (res); Wes '49; Tel. 547-2544.

FARISH, James R.; Ste. 220, 5780 Cambie St., Vancouver 15, B.C.; 4666 Bellevue Dr. Van. 8 (res); McG '43; F.R.C.S.(C), GenSurg; Att'd. Surg. Staff, St. Vincent's & Shaughnessy Hosp's; Cons. Staff, B.C. Cancer Inst.; Clin. Instr. Dept. of Surg., U. of British Columbia; Tel. FA 5-8311.

FARIVAR, Iraj; 100 Rowena Dr., Apt. 919, Don Mills, Ont.; Brussels (Belgium)'59; Paed.

FARKAS, Eric J.; 120 Lake Shore Rd. W., Port Credit, Ont.; Budapest (Hung.) '39; MCGP; Tel. CR 8-1551.

FARKAS, Nicholas, 3741 Ouellete Ave., Windsor, Ont.; 3945 Tecumseh E. (res); Florence (Italy) '30; Anaes; Tel. 945-9135.

FARKAS, Tibor; Budapest (Hung) '56; Res., Verdun Protestant Hosp., Montreal, P.Q.

FARKASHIDY, Joseph; 288 St. Clair Ave. W. Toronto 7, Ont.; Budapest (Hung.) '39; FRCS(C), Otol; Clin. Ass't. (Otol.), Toronto Gen. Hosp.; Clin. Teach., U. of Toronto; Tel. 925-5884.

FARKOUH, Edward F.; Cairo (Egypt)'57; FRCS(Ed); FRCS(Eng.); FRCS(C), GenSurg; Staff (GenSurg), Lakeshore Gen. Hosp., Pointe Claire, P.Q.

FARLEY, John F.; 6319-111th Ave., Edmonton, Alta. (res); Alb '54; Anaes; Staff, Royal Alexandra Hosp.; Tel. GR 4-3431.

FARLEY, John W.; 141 Dundas St. W., Trenton, Ont.; Tor '23; Dist. Coroner; Tel. EX 2-3601.

FARLEY, Louis V.; 4373 St. Hubert St., Montreal P.Q.; Mon '34; IntMed.; Tel. LA 3-8856.

FARLEY, Richard G.; 32 West St., Brantford, Ont.; 85 Parkside Dr. (res); Wes '51; Tel. 753-0445.

FARLEY, Robert O.; 232 Elm St., St. Thomas, Ont.; 124½ St. George St. (res); Wes '54; F.R.-C.S.(C), GenSurg; Cons. Staff, St. Thomas Elgin Gen. Hosp.; Instr. (Anat.), U. of Western Ontario.; Tel. 631-0567.

FARLEY, Robert W.; 32 West St., Brantford, Ont.; 59 Queensway Dr. (res); Wes '54; MCGP; Tel. 752-6523.

FARLEY, William J.; 46 Radcliffe Rd., Montreal West, P.Q.; Qns' 59; FRCP(C), Anaes; Staff, Queen Elizabeth Hosp., Montreal, P.Q.; Dem. (Anaes.), McGill U.; Tel. 488-2311.

FARLINGER, Fraser A.; 16 Paget St., New Liskeard, Ont.; McG '47; MCGP; Chief of Surg, New Liskeard & Dist. Hosp.; Court. Staff, Misericordia Hosp., Haileybury; Tel. MI 7-5111.

FARMER, Alfred W., MBE, QHS; 325 Med. Arts Bldg., 170 St. George St., Toronto 5, Ont.; 7 Thornwood Rd., Apt. 309, (res); Tor'27; FRCS-(C); PlasSurg, OrthSurg; GenSurg; Surg.-in-Chief, Hosp. for Sick Children; Prof. of Surg., U. of Toronto; Tel. WA 2-7714.

FARMER, G. Richard D., CBE, ED; 18 Maple Lane, Ottawa, Ont. (res); Tor '18; Med. Adviser, War Veterans Allowance Bd., DVA; Tel. CE 2-8211.

FARMER, H. Frank; 222 Eramosa Rd., Guelph, Ont.; McG '45; FACS; GenSurg; Staff, Guelph Gen. & St. Joseph's Hosp's.; Cons., Groves Mem. Hosp., Fergus; Tel. TA 2-1871.

FARMER, Louis; 5441 Bannantyne E., Verdun, Montreal 19, P.Q.; Mon '53; Paed.

FARMER, Raymond; 10616 Grande'Allee, Montreal 12, P.Q. (res); Mon '58; Path Anat (P.Q.); Staff, Hop.-St.-Jean-de-Dieu; Tel. CL 4-5361.

FARMER, Richard H.; McGregor Clinic, 250 Main St. E., Hamilton, Ont.; Oakridge, Ancaster (res); Tor '52 Plas Surg; Staff, Hamilton Gen., Chedoke Gen. & Brant Hosp., Burlington; Staff, Hamilton Civic & Children's Hosp's.; Court. Staff, St. Joseph's Hosp.; Tel. JA 7-2711.

FARMER, Ronald A.; Mental Health Div., Dept. of Health, Prov. of Ontario, Queen's Park, Toronto, Ont.; Tor'58; MBA; DHA; Dir. Hosp. Management Serv. Branch.

FARMER, T. Leonard; 162 Great George St., Charlottetown, P.E.I.; Dal '32; MCGP; Staff, P.E.I. & Charlottetown Hosp's.; Tel. 894-9723.

FARNALLS, Raymond B.; 118 11th Ave. S.E., Calgary, Alta.; Alb'60; Psy.

FARQUHAR, David I.; Box 280, The Brandon Clinic, Brandon, Man.; Manchester (Eng.)'57; Active Med. Staff, Brandon Gen. & Assiniboine Hosp's.; Tel. PA 9-6444.

FARQUHAR, Donald J.; 2356 W. 41st Ave., Vancouver 13, B.C.; 1320 W. 45th St. (res); UBC '58; MCGP; Tel. AM 1-5626.

FARQUHARSON, Charles D.; 4204 Sheppard Ave. E., Agincourt, Ont. (res); Tor'16; F.A.P.H.A., **F.R.C.P.(C), PH, IntMed; MO.H., Scarborough Twp.; Tel. AX 3-5753.**

FARQUHARSON, N. Joan (See Borland)

FARQUHARSON, Richard A.; 3310 Boundary Rd., Vancouver 12, B.C.; 5016 Grafton St., South Burnaby (res); Tor '44; GenSurg; Tel. 434-3131.

FARR, James A.; Qns '63; M.O., Fourth Field Ambulance, CAPO 5050, Germany; Abroad.

FARR, John; Winnipeg Clinic, St. Mary & Vaughan, Winnipeg, Man.; 35 Roslyn Cres. (res); Man '33; FRCS(Ed), FRCS(C), GenSurg; Assoc. Surg., Wpg. Gen. Hosp.; Ass't Prof. (Surg.), U. of Manitoba; Tel. 942-0551.

FARR, Russell H.; Workmen's Compensation Board, 90 Harbour St., Toronto 1, Ont.; Tor'52.

FARRAR, Clarence B.; 20 Oriole Rd., Toronto 7, Ont. (res); Johns Hopkins (USA) '00; ABP&N, D.Sc. (McGill); FRCP(C), NeurPsy; Editor, Am. Jrl. of Psychiatry; N.I.P.; Tel. WA 1-3849.

FARREHI, Cyrus; 11005-98th Ave., Apt. 409, Edmonton, Alta.; Tehran (Iran)'58; FRCP(C), IntMed.; Staff, Dept. of Med., University Hosp.

FARRELL, Hugh S.; 5590 St. Urbain St., Montreal, P.Q. (res); McG '42; GenSurg.

FARRELL, Jean C. (Roche); 683 Main St. E., Hamilton, Ont.; St. Andrew's (Scot.) '51; D.A. (Eng.); Dist. M.O., Hamilton Dept. of Health; Tel. LI 4-4242.

FARRELL, Maurice J.; Qns'55; FRCS(C), ObstGyn; Staff, St. Michael's Hosp., Toronto 2, Ont.

FARRELL, Patrick J.; 110 Larch St., Sudbury, Ont.; 217 Wembley Dr. (res); Qns '49; ObstGyn; Chief of Obst., Sudbury Gen. Hosp.; Tel. 673-4208.

FARRELL, Thomas C.; Med. Centre, West St., Corner Brook, Nfld.; 11 Marcelle Ave. (res); Dublin (Ire.) '49; Staff, Western Mem. & Christopher Fisher Hosp's.; Port Phys., Corner Brook; Tel. 47780.

FARRELL, William A.; 48 Blueridge Ave., Kitchener, Ont. (res); Tor '32; D.Rad., D.A.B.R., D&T Rad; Rad.-in-Chief, St. Mary's Hosp.; Tel. 744-3311.

FARRELL, William J.; 212 James St. S., Hamilton, Ont.; 104 Inverness Court (res); Tor '50; Anaes; Staff, St. Joseph's Hosp. & Assoc. Anaes., Hamilton; Tel. 528-8437.

FARRINGTON, William C.; Med. Arts Bldg., 121 Wellington St. W., Barrie, Ont.; Wes '60; Dist. Coroner, County of Simcoe; Tel. 726-6061.

FARROW, Grant A.; 407 Medical Arts Bldg., 170 St. George St., Toronto 5, Ont.; Tor'58; FRCS(C); Urol.

FASSAERT, Hubert A.; 3920 Smith Ave., South Burnaby, B.C.; 796 W. 42nd Ave. (res); Amsterdam (Neth) '53; Tel. HE 1-1929.

FAST, Bernhard B.; Winnipeg Clinic, St. Mary's **Ave. & Vaughan St., Winnipeg 1, Man.; 1131 Wellington Cres. (res); Man '51; FRCP(C); FACP; IntMed; Active Staff, Wpg. Gen. Hosp.;** Chief, Dept. of Med., Concordia Hosp.; Ass't. Prof. **(Med.), U. of Manitoba; Tel. 942-0551.**

FAST, Cornelius W.; Man'61; IntMed; Staff, Shaughnessy Hosp., Vancouver 9, B.C.

FAST, Isaac M.; 2463 Pauline St., Abbotsford, B.C.; Man'51; Tel. 853-2918.

FATTAL, Garabed A.; 26 Wardsworth Way, Winnipeg 22, Man. (res); Beirut (Lebanon) '53; Path; Chief of Labs., Deer Lodge DVA Hosp.; Ass't. Prof. (Path), U. of Manitoba; Tel. TU 8-4861.

FAUBERT, Gilles C.; 10 rue Talon, Hull, P.Q.; OrthSurg.(P.Q.).

FAUCHER, C. Raymond; Mon '63; Res., Albany Med. Centre Hosp., Montreal, P.Q.

FAUCHER, Euclide; 147 Chemin Ste. Foy, Quebec, **P.Q.; Lav '22; GenSurg (P.Q.); Tel. 525-8331.**

FAUCHER, Guy L.; 1150 Blvd. St. Joseph E., Montreal 34, P.Q.; Mon'59; ObstGyn.

FAUDEMER, W.A.; 110 Younge St. S., Aurora, Ont.; Tor'62; Tel. 727-4245.

FAUGHT, Kenneth A.; 1105 Carling Ave., Ottawa 1, Ont.; Tor'59; Paed.; Tel. 729-5194.

FAULCONBRIDGE, A. James; Whissell Clinic, Westlock, Alta.; McG '60; FAGS.

FAULDS, George E.; 524 William St., London, Ont.; 17 Harrison Cres. (res); Wes '37; MCGP; Pt-time Phys., Bell Tel. Co.; Instr. (PrevMed.), **U. of Western Ontario; Tel. 439-4641.**

FAUTEUX, Gerald; 1681 Parc Lafontaine, Montreal 34, P.Q.; Ott'57; IntMed (P.Q.); Pt-time Cons. (Med.), Alcan & Co.; Tel. 744-4318.

FAUTEUX, Henri; 745-5th St., Shawinigan Falls, P.Q.; 5ieme Ave (res); Lav '36.

FAUTEUX, Jean-P.; 1457 est Blvd. St. Joseph, Montreal, P.Q.; 3027 Lacombe (res); Mon '50; FRCS(C), GenSurg; Cons., Standard Paper Box Ltd.; Tel. LA 2-7195.

FAUTEUX, Pierre; 169 est, Fleury, Montreal 12, P.Q. (res); Mon '56; DiagRad; Staff, Hop.-Hotel-Dieu; Tel. VI 4-0161.

FAVREAU, Gautier L.; Ste. 1, 240 rue Court, Sherbrooke, P.Q.; Mon '25; Prison M.O.; Dir., No. 5 V.D. Dispensary, Hop. Gen. St.-Vincent-de-Paul; Tel. Area 819; 569-1560.

FAVREAU, J. Calixte; 32 ouest, Blvd. St. Joseph, Montreal 14, P.Q.; 228 Chemin Ste. Catherine (res); **Mon '28; FRCS(C); OrthSurg; Chief of Serv. (Orth.), Hop. Ste. Justine; Med. Dir., Ecole Enfants Infirmes; Prof. of Orth U. of Montreal; Tel. RE 1-4931.**

FAVREAU, Jean; 1150 est, boul. St-Joseph, Montreal 34, P.Q.; Mon'51; Derm.

FAVREAU, Robert; 525 est rue Sherbrooke, Montreal, P.Q.; Mon'43; FICS; ObstGyn; Staff **(Gyn.), Hop. Jean-Talon; Tel. 842-3905.**

FAVREAU-ETHIER, Martine F.; Apt. 2, 3156 Maplewood Ave., Montreal 26, P.Q. (res); Mon **'55; DiagRad; Staff, Hop. Ste.-Justine; Tel. RE 1-4931.**

FAWCETT, David M.; University of Alberta Hosp., Dept. of Med., Edmonton, Alta.; Alb'59; PhD; Med. Research Council Scholar; Ass't. Prof. (Med.), U. of Alberta; Tel. 439-5911, Loc. 259.

FAWCETT, John P.; 206 Main St., Hamilton, Ont.; McG '18; ObstGyn.

FAWCETT, John S.; Durham (Eng.)'56; Path (P.Q.); Staff, Dept. of Path., Montreal Children's Hosp., Montreal, P.Q.; Tel. WE 7-8511.

FAY, John E.; Etherington Hall, Stuart St., Kingston, Ont.; London (Eng.) '49; FACC; FRCP(C), IntMed; Ass't. Prof., Queen's U.; Tel. 546-1731, Loc. 604.

FAYERMAN, Jack; 309A Medical Centre, 906-8th Ave. S.W., Calgary, Alta.; Man'55; Otol.; Tel. 262-4030.

FAYERMAN, Joseph W.; 801 Fairmont Med. Bldg., 750 W. Broadway, Vancouver 9, B.C.; 7845 Cambia St. (res); Man '48; Otol; Tel. TR 6-0828.

FAYLE, Brian W. K.; 18 Corwin Blvd., Galt, Ont. **(res); Cambridge (Eng.) '56; B. Chir., M.B., DMR; DiagRad; Staff, South Waterloo Mem. Hosp., Galt; Milton & District Hosp.; Milton & Georgetown; Tel. 621-2330.**

FAZZARI, Frank; 539 Cassell St., North Bay, Ont.; Ott'52; Paed; Staff, St. Joseph's Gen. Hosp. & North Bay Civic Hosp.; Tel. 472-4050.

FEARON, Blair; Suite No. 308, Medical Arts **Bldg., Toronto 5, Ont.; 13 Douglas Cres. (res);** Tor '44; F.R.C.S.(C) Otol; Clin. Teacher, (Otol.), U. of Toronto; **Ass't. Surg., Hosp. for Sick Children; Cons. Otol., Oakville-Trafalgar Memorial** Hosp., Oakville, & Cons. Broncho-Esophag., Women's College Hosp.; Pres. Am. Broncho-Esoph. Soc.; Tel. WA 1-4091.

FEARON, John D.; 628 Davis Dr., Newmarket, Ont.; 220 Millard Ave. (res); Tor '58; AMCGP; Sr. Active Staff, York County Hosp.; Tel. 895-5941.

FEASBY, William R.; Queen Elizabeth Hosp., 130 Dunn Ave., Toronto, Ont.; Tor'37; IntMed; Med. Dir., Queen Elizabeth Hosp.; Lect. Med. History, Fac. of Med., U. of Toronto; Tel. 534-7513.

FEATHERSTONE, Hector; 54 Reid Ave., Ottawa, Ont. (res); Qns '21; Ass't. Supt., Ottawa Civic Hosp.; Tel. 729-1611. Retired.

FEAVER, Bruce D.; Wes'59; AMCGP; Res., Winnipeg Gen. Hosp., Winnipeg, Man.

FEDDER, Jack; 398 Bloor St. W., Toronto 5, **Ont.; 846 Duplex Ave., Tor. 12 (res); Tor '42;** FACOG; ObstGyn; Active Staff, New Mt. Sinai Hosp.; Tel. 924-1224.

FEDEROFF, Paul; 1007 Colony St., Saskatoon, Sask.; Petrograd (Russia) '18; Retired.

FEDYNA, Andrij; 288 Bathurst St., Toronto 2B, Ont.; '44; MCGP; Tel. EM 3-3661.

FEE, D. A.; 2234 Broadway Ave., Saskatoon, **Sask.; Tor '46; TherRad; Tel. 652-8851.**

FEE, G. Alexander; 307 Toronto Western Med. Bldg., 25 Leonard Ave., Toronto 2B, Ont.; 4111 Yonge St. (res); Tor '35; FAAOO, Otol; Staff (Otol), Toronto Western Hosp.; Clin. Instr. (Otol.), U. of Toronto; Tel. EM. 3-4712.

FEENER, Melvin G.; 284 Main St., Middleton, N.S.; 7 Riverside Dr. (res); Dal '52; GenSurg; **Cons. (Surg.) Soldier's Mem. Hosp.; Tel. 825-4544.**

FEENEY, Neil; 1414 Drummond St., Montreal, P.Q.; McG '27; F.A.C.P.; Cardiol. (P.Q.), Int-**Med; Memb. Bd., Montreal Gen. Hosp.; Tel. AV 8-7732.**

FEGLER, John G.; Box 1210, Med. Centre, Stettler, Alta.; Edinburgh (Scot.)'58; Tel. 742-3441.

FEHER, Peter J.; McG'59; Derm; Staff, Queen Mary Vet's Hosp., Montreal, P.Q.

FEHN, Franklin; Edmonton Cancer Clin., 11250-84th Ave., Edmonton, Alta.; Oslo (Norway)'40.

FEHRMANN, Anne M.; 24 Wells Hill Ave., Toronto 4, Ont. (res); Germany '48; Staff, Grace Hosp.; Tel. WA 5-2251.

FEINBERG, Jonathon F.; 154 Old Forest Hill Rd., Toronto 10, Ont. (res); Tor '60; Abroad.

FEINDEL, James R.; Dal '42; Dir. Commun. Dis. & Cancer, Dept. of Health, Fredericton, N.B.; Tel. 475-7711.

FEINDEL, John H.; 2320 Armcrest W., Halifax, N.S. (res); McG '56; Anaes; Staff, Halifax Infirmary; Lect., Dalhousie U.; Tel. 422-1511, Loc. 333.

FEINDEL, William H.; 3801 University St., Montreal 2, P.Q.; McG '45; DABN; D.Phil. (Neuroanat., Oxon.); FRCS(C), NeurSurg; Neurosurg.-in-Chief, Montreal Neurological Hosp.; Att'd. Staff, Catherine Booth, Royal Victoria, & Sherbrooke Gen. Hosp., Sherbrooke; Dir., Cone Lab. for NeuroSurg. Research, Montreal Neurological Inst.; Wm. Cone Prof. (NeuroSurg.), McGill U.; Tel. AV 8-4705.

FEINMAN, Saya V.; 187 St. Clair Ave. W., Toronto, Ont.; 117 Ava Rd. (res); Vienna (Austria) '48; FRCP(C); IntMed; Attending Staff (Med.), New Mount Sinai Hosp.; Clin. Teach., U. of Toronto; Tel. WA 2-6022.

FEIR, Terence C.; Ste. 1208; 750 W. Broadway, Vancouver 9, B.C.; Ste. 1, 3870 Cambie St. (res); Alb '54; Psy; Adm. Mental Health Centre, Vancouver; Tel. TR 6-5015.

FEITELSOHN, Madeleine L.; 115 Queen St., St. Catharines, Ont.; Bucharest (Roum.) '56; Tel. 682-8344.

FEJER, Imre F.; 2605 Eglinton Ave. E., Scarborough, Ont.; Cluj (Roumania) '39; IntMed (Hungary); Staff, Geriatric Unit, Ontario Hosp., Whitby; Tel. 267-3115.

FEJES, Deszo; Herzl Health Centre, 5780 Decelles Ave., Montreal 26, P.Q. Budapest (Hung.) '19.

FEKETE, John F.; Regional Lab., 71 Brunswick St., Fredericton, N.B.; Budapest (Hung.)'51; Path; Dir. Regional Lab. & Chief Pathol., Victoria Hosp.; Tel. 475-9944.

FEKETE, Zoltan C.; 300 King St. W., Oshawa, Ont.; 2374 Eglinton Ave. E., Scarborough (Branch Office); Debrecen (Hung.) '48; Derm; Staff, Oshawa Gen. & Ajax Pickering Hosp's.; Tel. 728-6266 & 757-3575.

FELD, Ronald; 1192 Queen St. E., Toronto 8, Ont.; 680 Roselawn Ave., Apt. 104 (res); Ott '57; MCGP; Att'd. Staff, Central Hosp.; Court. Staff, Doctors' & Tor. E. Gen. Hosp's.; Vol. Ass't. New Mt. Sinai Hosp.; Tel. 463-4878.

FELDERHOF, Herman H.; 303 Maritime Bldg., New Glasgow, N.S.; Utrecht (Neth.) '33.

FELDMAN, Allan; 5778 Smart Ave., Cote-St.-Luc, Montreal 29, P.Q.; Montpellier (Fr.) '56; Paed. (P.Q.); Tel. 489-4770.

FELDMAN, Edward D. A.; 3310 Yonge St., Toronto 12, Ont.; 631 Briar Hill Ave. (res.); Tor '43; MCGP; Staff, New Mount Sinai & Baycrest Hosp's.; Tel. HU 7-4747.

FELDMAN, Fredrick; Tor '60; AMCGP; Res., Banting Inst., Toronto 2, Ont.

FELDMAN, Ronald B.; 3755 Cote Ste. Catherine Rd., Montreal 26, P.Q.; Apt. 101, 5160 Macdonald Ave., Montreal 29, P.Q. (res); Tor'58; D.Psy; Psy; Assoc. Dir., Clin., Dept. of Family Psy., Jewish Gen. Hosp.; Tel. 735-3771, Loc. 588.

FELDMAN, Rubin M.; 3205 Notre Dame Blvd., Chomedy, P.Q.; Montpellier (France)'57; Med. Dir., Jewish Convalescent Hosp.; Tel. 681-2800.

FELDMAN, Sidney; 6000 Cote des Neiges Rd., Montreal 26, P.Q.; Paris (France)'55; Int.Med.; Cons. Med., Bellechasse & Jewish Convalescent Hosp's.; Att'd. Staff, Jewish Gen. Hosp.; Tel. 731-7121.

FELDMAN, Stephan; 320 Riverside Dr., Toronto 3, Ont. (res); Prague (Czecho-Slov.) '46; Psy; Staff, Ontario Hosp., N. Toronto; Tel. GL 9-8291.

FELDMAN, William; McG'61; FRCP(C), Paed; Staff, Children's Hosp., Montreal 25, P.Q.

FELIX, Cornelius H.; 1029 Douglas, Victoria, B.C.; Leiden (Neth.) '46; Surg (Neth); Tel. EV 3-6587.

FELIX, John L.; 459 Bloor St. W., Toronto, Ont.; 1042 Davenport Rd. (res); Budapest (Hun.) '50; IntMed (Bud.); Tel. WA 5-0411.

FELLEGI, Anita (See Jarvis).

FELLENZ, Klaus-Peter; Burris Clinic, 242 Victoria, Kamloops, B.C.; 601 Brandon Ave., N. Kam. (res); Marburg (Germ.) '55; DABPaed; **Paed; Chief Paed., Royal Inland Hosp.; Tel. 372-3303.**

FELLER, Jacob; 267 O'Connor St., Ottawa 4, Ont.; 85 Range Rd. (res); McG '33; IntMed; **Staff, Ottawa Civic Hosp.; Cons. (IntMed, Metabol.), Dept. of Nat. Defence; Cons. (IntMed),** Dept. of Nat. Health & Welfare; Tel. CE 5-8282.

FELLOWS, Robert E.; McG '59 Res., Royal Victoria Hosp., Montreal 2, P.Q.

FELTON, Richard; 2812 Cadboro Bay Rd., Victoria, B.C. (res); Guy's (London, Eng.) '02; M.R.C.S., L.R.C.P., D.PH.; Retired

FENESS, Joseph Z.; 739A The Queensway, Toronto 18, Ont.; 22 Baliacaine Dr., Tor. 18 (res); Tor '57; Staff, St. Joseph's Hosp.; Tel. 255-4511.

FENIGSTEIN, Henry; 2787 Bathurst St., Toronto 19, Ont.; Warsaw (Poland) '38; MCGP; D.Psy; Staff, Toronto Psychiatric Hosp., Toronto, Ont.

FENN, John E.; Ste 903, 1849 Yonge St., Toronto, Ont.; 904 Avenue Rd. (res); Tor '47; ObstGyn; Tel. 488-1778.

FENN, William E.; Ste. 903, 1849 Yonge St., Toronto 7, Ont.; Ott'52; FRCS(C); GenSurg; Tel. 488-1151.

FENNESSY, Thomas J.; Prelate, Sask; National U. (Ire.) '51; Tel. 15.

FENTON, David B.; 5150 Dundas St. W., Islington, Ont.; Tor '55; Tel. BE 1-3355.

FENTON, Frederick R.; Qns '64; Res., Montreal Gen. Hosp., Montreal 25, P.Q.

FENTON, Godfrey M. J.; 111 Huron St., Woodstock, Ont.; Sheffield (Eng.) '58; Assoc. Staff, Woodstock Gen. Hosp.; Tel. 539-2973.

FENTON, Joseph A.; 620 Bathurst St., Toronto, Ont.; 23 Ridelle (res); Tor '49; MCGP; Court. Staff, (Obst.), Toronto Gen. Hosp.; Staff (G.P.), Doctor's Hosp.; Tel. LE 1-7200.

FENTON, Lawrence G.; Chemainus, B.C.; UBC '59.

FENWICK, John B.; 814 Fairmont Med. Bldg., 750 W. Broadway, Vancouver 9, B.C.; Man '43; IntMed; Att'd. Staff, Vancouver Gen. & St. Vincent's Hosp's.; Cons. (Med.), Shaughnessy Hosp. & Cdn. Arthritis & Rheum. Soc.; Tel. TR 4-0512.

FENYVESSY, Joseph Z. (See Feness, Joseph Z.).

FEORE, Dermot R.; 33 Jefferson Blvd., Riverside, Ont. (res); Dublin (Ire.)'55; DABR; FRCP(C); DiagRad; Staff, Hotel-Dieu Hosp., Windsor, Ont.; Tel. 945-1910.

FERDAIS, Jean P.; Clinique Med. St. Remi, St. Remi, P.Q.; Mon'40.

FERG, Edwin J.; 899 Palmerston Ave., Winnipeg, Man.; Man '13; GenSurg; Retired.

FERGUS, Allan; Ott '61; Res., Ontario Hosp., 999 Queen St. W., **Toronto 3, Ontario.**

FERGUSON, Charles A.; McG '57; Res., Children's Hosp., Winnipeg 3, Man.

FERGUSON, Colin C.; Dept. of Surg., U. of Manitoba, Winnipeg 3, Man.; 167 Waverly St., Wpg. 9 (res); Man'45; D.S. (McG); FACS, FAAP, **FRCS(C), GenSurg; Surg.-in-Chief, The Children's Hosp.; Prof. & Hd., Dept. of Surg., U. of Manitoba; Tel. 786-3575.**

FERGUSON, Colin G.; 100 Main St., Toronto 13, Ont.; 6 Enderby Rd. (res); Tor '41; D.P.H.; Tel. OX 9-3619.

FERGUSON, C. Ross; Copper Cliff Int. Nickel Co. Hosp., Copper Cliff, Ont.; 3 School St. (res); Tor '27; GenSurg; **Pres., Med. Soc., Sudbury Mem. Hosp.; Court. Staff, Sudbury Gen. & St. Joseph's Hosp's.; Dist. Coroner; Tel. OS 3-3601.**

FERGUSON, Donald B.; 186 Wortley Rd., London, Ont.; 149 Elworthy Ave. (res); Wes '46; FAGS; Staff, Victoria, St. Joseph's & St. Mary's Hosp.'s.; Tel. 434-3694.

FERGUSON, Donald H.; Box 1540, Carleton Place, Ont.; Qns' 64.

FERGUSON, Gary G.; West'65; Res., Victoria Hosp., London, Ont.

FERGUSON, George C.; Port Arthur Clinic, Port **Arthur, Ont., 186 Summit Ave., (res); Tor '30;** FRCS(C), IntMed.; Tel. DI 4-7271.

FERGUSON, George G.; The Medical Centre, Sackville, N.B.; 32 Charles St. (res); Nat. U. (Dublin, Ire.) '42; F.R.C.S. (Eng.). FACS; Surg., Sackville Mem. Hosp.; Tel. 536-0770.

FERGUSON, Harold; Box 159, 117 Queen St., Bowmanville, Ont.; Tor'20; AMCGP; Tel. 623-5789.

FERGUSON, Hugh; 253 Davis St. Sarnia, Ont.; 132 Euphemia St. (res); Glasgow (Scot.) '41; D.P.H., M.R.C.O.G., ObstGyn; Active Staff, St. Joseph's & City Gen. Hosp's.; Tel. DI 4-3661.

FERGUSON, Ian A.; Medical Arts Clinic, 51-6th. St. E., Medicine Hat, Alta.; Alb'55; ObstGyn; Staff, Medicine Hat Gen. Hosp.

FERGUSON, James G.; 46 Robina Ave., Toronto, Ont. (res); Tor '26; Chief Med. Exam., Cdn. Pension Comm., 55 York St., Toronto.

FERGUSON, James H.; Room 4073 Med. Science Bldg., U. of Alberta, Edmonton, Alta.; Glasgow (Scot.)'60.

FERGUSON, James K. W., MBE; 56 Clarkehaven St., Thornhill, Ont. (res); Tor'32; MA; FRSC; **Dir., Connaught Med. Research Labs., U. of Toronto; Tel. 928-2046.**

FERGUSON, John M.; 444 Beaconsfield Blvd., Beaurepaire, P.Q.; 426 Edgewood Rd. (res); McG '53; GenSurg; Active Staff, Lachine Gen. & Lakeshore Gen. Hosp's.; Tel. 695-6302.

FERGUSON, J. S.; 47 King St. W.; Chatham, Ont.; 522 King W. (res); Tor '21.

FERGUSON, Kenneth R.; 6875 Lasalle Blvd., Verdun, P.Q.; Qns'52; Psy; Sr. Psy., Douglas Hosp. & Lakeshore Gen. Hosp.; Dem. McGill U.; Tel. 766-8516.

FERGUSON, Kerry G.; Wes'60; IntMed; Staff, Westminster Hosp., London, Ont.
FERGUSON, Peter D.; Staff, Nova Scotia Hosp., Dartmouth, N.S.; Dal '42.
FERGUSON, **Pierre J.**; 13 Tulip St., Dartmouth, N.S.; 18 Carver St. (res); Dal '56; AMCGP.
FERGUSON, Robert, M.B.E.; 838-1650 Cedar Ave. W., Montreal 25, P.Q.; 739 Upper Belmont Ave. Westmount (res); Tor '33; Anaes; Dir., Dept. of Anaes., Montreal Gen. Hosp.; Cons. Anaes., Montreal Children's Hosp.; Ass't. Prof. (Anaes.), McGill U.; Lect. (Anaes.), School of Dentistry; Tel. 937-1732.
FERGUSON, Robert H.; 440 Hinton Ave., Ottawa 3, Ont.; 5 Bayswater Pl. (res); Tor '42; DA; Anaes; Att'd. Staff, Ottawa Civic Hosp.; Tel. 725-1163.
FERGUSON, Robert S.; 141 Wortley Rd., London, Ont.; Wes '31; MCGP; FAGS, Staff, Victoria, St. Joseph's & Parkwood Hosp's.; Tel. GE 2-6631.
FERGUSON, Russell B.; 1737 Pandosy St., Kelowna, B.C.; Man '61; Tel. 762-4212.
FERGUSON, **Thomas B.**; Diagnostic Lab., 906-8th Ave. S.W., Calgary, Alta.; Glasgow (Scot.)'48; DiagRad; DPH; DMRD(Eng.).
FERGUSON, William F.; 208 Medical Arts Bldg., 11010 Jasper Ave., Edmonton, Alta.; 10418-139th St. (res); Alb '50; ObstGyn; Ass't. Prof., U. of Alberta; Teach. Appt. & Active Staff, U. of Alberta & Royal Alexandra Hosp.; Tel. 424-1273.
FERGUSSON, Ewart A.; Edinburgh (Scot.) '27; GenSurg; Sup't., Westminster Hosp., London, Ont.; Tel. GE 2-6711.
FERGUSSON, Roslyn M.; 30 Maple St. N., Smith's Falls, Ont.; Qns '10; F.A.C.S.
FERGUSSON-STEWART, **G. J.**; Tor'65; Res., Toronto Gen. Hosp., Toronto 2, Ont.
FERLAND, Hugues; Lav'54; Anaes; Staff, Hop. Gen. de Fleury, Montreal, P.Q.
FERLAND, J. A.; 5801 Blvd. Monk, Montreal 20, P.Q. (res); Mon '37; M.C.G.P. Tel. 766-7054.
FERLAND, Jean J.; 1500-18e rue, Quebec 4, P.Q.; Lav '55; FRCS(C), OrthSurg.; Tel. 523-8008.
FERLAND. Lucian; Ste. Emelie de l'Energie, Joliette, P.Q.; Mon '43.
FERLAND, Marcelle; 1823 ave Nord, Montreal 8, P.Q.; Mon'52; Health Serv., Montreal, P.Q.; Tel. 735-2060.
FERLAND, Sylvio; 489 Boul. Ste-Anne, Joliette, P.Q.; Mon '38; GenSurg (P.Q.); Staff Surg., Hop-St-Eusebe; Tel. PL 6-8041.
FERN, Brian J.; Box 280, Milden, Sask.; Manchester (Eng.)'61; D.Obst RCOG.
FERNANDEZ, **Emilio M.**; Madrid (Spain)'56; Path; Staff, St. Joseph's Hosp., Guelph, Ont.
FERNANDEZ, Gabriel; Box 308 Val Caron, Ont.; Valladolid (Spain) '56.
FERNANDO, **B. Aaron**; Box 459, Radville, Sask.; Ceylon '52.
FERNANDO, **Oscar**; Santo Tomas (Philipp.)'58; Staff, International Grenfell Assoc., St. Anthony, Nfld.; Abroad.
FERNET, Pierre Y.; Lav '58; Path; Staff, (Path), Hotel-Dieu, Chicoutimi, P.Q.; Tel. 549-1452.
FERNS, James M.; 350 Beach Ave., Toronto, Ont.; 90 Pine Cres. (res); Tor '51; Assoc. Staff, Toronto East Gen. Hosp.; Tel. 694-1126.
FERRARI, Remo L.; Box 99, 228 Fir St., Sherwood Park, Alta.; London (Eng.); '44 MRCS; LRCP; Tel. 699-5410.
FERRE, Alexander F.; Emerson, Man.; Voronezh. (U.S.S.R.) '41; MCGP.
FERRE, Norbert J.; 403 Hinton Ave., Ottawa, Ont.; Ott'62.
FERREIRA, Bernard E.; 391 Wellington St., Sarnia, Ont.; Tor'60; ObstGyn.
FERRIE, Alan S.; 40 Harvey St., Tillsonburg, Ont.; 23 Lisgar Ave. (res); Glasgow (Scot.) '51; MCGP; Staff, Tillsonburg Mem. Hosp.; Tel. VI 2-3682.
FERRIE, Kenneth E.; 107 Medical Arts Bldg., 280 Bloor St. W., Toronto 5, Ont., 25 Coulson (res); Tor'29; MRCP (Edin.), IntMed.; Hon. Staff, Toronto Gen. Hosp.; Tel. WA 2-2093.
FERRIE, Robert K.; Tor'62; Res., St. Michael's Hosp., Toronto 2, Ont.
FERRIER, C. W.; 103 King St. E., Oshawa, Ont.; Phys., Oshawa Gen. Hosp.; **Tel. 723-3943.**
FERRIER, George C.; Box 930, Port Arthur, Ont.; Tor '36; D.Psy;Psy; Supt., Ontario Hosp., **Port Arthur; Tel. DI 4-3571.**
FERRIER, Gordon J.; 167 Royal York Rd., Toronto 14, Ont.; Tor'15; Staff, St. Joseph's Hosp.; Tel. 251-9711.
FERRIER, Robert A.; 214 Med. Arts Bldg., 335-6th Ave. S.W., Calgary, Alta.; 2444 Sovereign Cres. (res); Man '45; Tel. 262-2608.
FERRIER, Thompson A.; Sault Ste. Marie Dist. Health Group Assoc., 240 McNabb St., Sault Ste Marie, Ont.; '47; MCGP; MPH; Tel. AL 4-6421.
FERRIES, John M.; 1940 Lonsdale Ave., North Vancouver, B.C.; 6009 Eagleridge Dr., West Van. (res); Aberdeen (Scot.) '48; D. Ophth (Lond.); Ophth; Cons. Staff, Lion's Gate Hosp.; Tel. YU 7-8233.
FERRILL, Chas. W.; Carleton Place, Ont.; Qns '20; D.Ophth. Otol. (Manhattan, N.Y.).
FERRIS, Paul W.; 60 De Vere Gdns., Toronto 12, Ont.; Tor '36; Anaes; Staff, St. Joseph's Hosp.; Tel. 364-5325.
FERRO, **Jose Aguirre**; Apt. 2, 456 Carlton St., St. Catharines, Ont.
FERRON, Guy; 30 est, boul. St-Joseph, Montreal 14, P.Q.; Mon '43; Staff, Hop-St-Jean-de-Dieu & Aide-a-la Femme.
FERRON, Jacques; 1285 Chemin Chambly, Cite Jacques-Cartier, P.Q.; Mon'50; Tel. OR 4-8111.
FERRON, Jean P.; Mon'65; Res., Hop. Maisonneuve, Montreal 36, P.Q.
FERRON, L. Paul; 1285 Chemin Chambly, Longueuil, Cite-Jacques-Cartier; Mon '50; Psy(P.Q.); Staff, Hop.-St.-Jean-de-Dieu; Tel. CL 4-5361.
FERRON, Marcel; 1150 boul. St. Joseph, Montreal 34, P.Q.; Mon'44; FACOG; FICS; Obst (PQ); Hd. Dept. of Obst., Hop.-Maisonneuve; Prof. Obst., U. of Mtl.; Tel. AV 8-9221.
FERRON, Pierre; Mon '64; Int., Hop. Notre-Dame, Montreal 24, P.Q.
FESSLER, Alfred; McG '62; Res., Royal Victoria Hosp., Montreal 2, P.Q.
FETTERLY, John C. M.; Ontario Cancer Foundation, London Clin., Victoria Hosp., London, Ont; 34 Bromleigh Ave., London (res); Qns '46; D.M.R.T. (Eng.), TherRad; Teaching Staff, Victoria Hosp. & Ass't Prof., U. of Western Ontario; Tel. GE 2-5261.
FEUER, Steven I.; Ste. 4., 394 Bloor St. W., Toronto 4, Ont.; Szeged (Hungary) '49; AMCGP; Tel. 927-0633.
FEUILTAULT, Robert; 1320 Jean Dequen, Ste-Foy, P.Q.; Lav '43; IntMed; Staff, Clinique Domrency; **Tel. 527-0678.**
FEYERER, Edward J.; Medical Arts Bldg., Hamilton, Ont.; North Shore Blvd. (res); Tor **'46; Urol; Att. Urol., Hamilton Gen. Hosp.; Tel. JA 8-4332.**
FIALKOV, Gershon J.; Ste. 11, 605 Bloor St. W., Toronto 4, Ont.; Hebrew U. (Jerusalem)'54; Otol.; Tel. LE 2-6845.
FICHMAN, Stephen H.; McG '63; Int., Queen Mary Vet's Hosp., Montreal, P.Q. Abroad.
FICKE, Karl H.; Ste. 37, 3930 Robinson St., Regina, Sask. (res); Muenster (Germ.) '49; DiagRad; Staff, Regina Gen. Hosp.; Tel. LA 2-1811.
FICZYCZ, Nestor; Med. Arts Clinic, Regina, Sask.; Sask'65.
FIDDES, Gladstone W. J.; 346-4th Ave. W., Prince Rupert, B.C. (res); Qns'40; FCCP; DPH; Supt. Miller Bay Hosp.; Cons. Staff, Prince Rupert Gen. Hosp. & Kitimat Gen. Hosp.; Tel. 624-1850.
FIDDESS, James; 605 Campbell Bldg., 1029 Douglas St., Victoria, B.C.; 1915 Fairfield Rd. (res); Cambridge (Eng.) '47; Active Staff, St. Joseph's Hosp.; Court. Staff, Royal Jubilee Hosp.; Tel. EV 3-6311.
FIDLAR, Edward; 38 Admiral Rd., Toronto 5, Ont. (res); Tor '07; Retired.
FIDLER, Antony; Ste 101, 27 Henderson, Ottawa 2, Ont.; Warsaw (Poland) '27; IntMed; Phys.-in-Chief, Ottawa Gen. Hosp.; Prof. (Med.), U. of Ottawa.

FIDLER, Herbert K.; 5612 Laburnum St., Vancouver 13, B.C. (res); Man '34; Path Bact; Dir., Dept. of Path., Vancouver Gen. Hosp.; Clin. Prof., Path., U. of British Columbia; Tel. TR 6-3211.
FIDLER, Keith E.; Wes '62; Umri Mission Hosp., Yoetmal District, Mahurashtra State, India; Abroad.
FIELD, Paul; 225 Larch St., Sudbury, Ont.; 79 Windsor Cr. (res); London (Eng.)'54; LRCP (Lond.); MRCS(Eng.); FACS; FRCS(Edin.); FRCS(C); GenSurg; Cardiovasc & ThorSurg; Active Staff (Surg.), Sudbury Mem. Hosp.; Research Assoc., Laurentian Univ.; Tel. 675-3374.
FIELDEN, Edgar C.; 131 Manor Rd. E., Toronto, Ont.; Tor'25; MCGP; PathBact; Phys. Isabel & Arthur Meighen Lodge; Court. Staff, St. Michael's Hosp.; Tel. HU 9-2767.
FIELDEN, Robert H. N.; 272 Bloor St. W., Toronto 5, Ont.; Tor'55; FRCS(C), OrthSurg; Staff, & Clin. Teach., St. Michael's Hosp.; Tel. 922-9160.
FIELDING, E. Mack V.; 1105 Valley Way, Niagara Falls, Ont.; Tor '26; Anaes; M.C.G.P.; Staff, Greater Niagara Gen. & Niagara Hosp's., Niagara-on-the-Lake; Dist. M.O., C.N.R.; Coroner, Welland Co.; Tel. EL 4-6731.
FIELDING, John F.; 340 McLeod, Ottawa, Ont.; Wes '54; FACS; FRCS(C), PlasSurg; Att'd. Staff, Ottawa Civic Hosp.; Cons. PlasSurg., N.D.M.C.; Lect. (Surg.), U. of Ottawa; Tel. CE 3-9811.
FIELDMAN, Joseph D.; 1369 St. Catherine St. W., Montreal 25, P.Q.; 5181 Cote St. Antoine (res); Man '22; Hon. Phys., Reddy Memorial Hosp.; Tel. 866-6185.
FIELDS, Harold; Ste. 1228, 123 Edward St., Toronto 2, Ont.; 100 Gloucester St., Apt. 1010 **(res); Tor '53; FRCP(C), IntMed; Staff, St.** Michael's Hosp.; Tel. 366-3454.
FIFE, Brenda C.; Med. Centre, 5027-52nd St., Warburg, Alta.; Birmingham (Eng.) '34; DTM& H; AMCGP; Tel. 848-2268.
FIGLIOLI, Guiseppe; Italy '45; Psy; Staff, St-Jean-de-Dieu Hosp., Montreal 5, P.Q.; Tel. 254-8381.
FILBEE, John F.; 6064 Oakland Rd., Halifax, N.S. (res): London (Eng.) '49; MRCS, LRCP, D.M.R.T. (Lond.); TherRad; Ass't. TherRad., **Victoria Gen. Hosp.; Ass't. Prof. (TherRad), Dalhousie U.; Tel. 422-7371.**
FILDERMAN, Ronald B.; Tor'64; Res., Hosp. for Sick Children, Toronto 2, Ont.
FILIATRAULT, Claude; Lav '60; Anaes; Staff, Hop. St. Joseph, Rimouski, P.Q.; Tel. 723-7851.
FILIATRAULT, Jacques; 51 Tache, Rimouski, P.Q;. Lav '54; GenSurg (P.Q.).
FILIATRAULT, Jean-M.; 127 Highfield, Montreal, P.Q.; Mon '38; Plum. Dis. & TB (P.Q.). Tel. RE 8-6102.
FILION-LAPORTE, Liliane; 864 Stuart Ave., Montreal 8, P.Q.; Lav '60; Staff, Children's Hosp., Montreal 25, P.Q.; Tel. WE 7-8511.
FILION, Michel; Mon'65; Res., Univ. of Montreal, Montreal, P.Q.
FILION Yvan; Centre Med., St-Polycarpe, Cte., **Vandreuil-Soulanges, P.Q.; Mon '60; Tel. 265-3271.**
FILIP, Juretic; Perugia (Italy)'54; Staff, Provincial Hosp., Campbellton, N.B.
FILIPICH, Rudy L.; Wes '64; Res., St. Joseph's Hosp., Hamilton, Ont.
FILL, Helen L. (see RUFF)
FILLMORE, Eric E.; 71-17th Ave., Roxboro, P.Q.; McG '43; Staff, Lachine Gen. Hosp., M.O., Cdn. Vickers Ltd.; Tel. 684-3651. Abroad.
FILOTTO, Jean; Mon '64; Res., Hop. Notre-Dame Montreal 24, P.Q.
FILTEAU, Charles; 285A St. Georges, St. Jerome, P.Q.; Lav '48; F.R.C.P.(C), IntMed.; Tel. GE 2-7722.
FILTEAU, Maurice M.; Mon'62; Anaes; Staff, Hop. Hotel Dieu, Montreal, P.Q.
FINCH, Graham C.; 820 Victoria Rd., Sydney, N.S.; Dal'65.
FINCH, John A.; Main St., Milk River, Alta.; Glasgow (Scot.)'47.
FINCH, Peter G.; 155 Howard St., Kimberley, B.C.; London (Eng.)'44; MB; BS; DCH.
FINDLAY, Charles A.; 1718-25th St. S.W., Calgary, Alta. (res); Admin. Col. Belcher Hosp.; Retired.
FINDLAY, Douglas; 1270 Regent Rd., Montreal 16, P.Q.; McG '41.
FINDLAY, Douglas; R.R. No. 4, Rockwood, Ont. (res); Tor '17; Retired.
FINDLAY, Ian D.; 525 Columbia St., Kamloops, B.C.; 179 Connaught Rd. (res); Aberdeen (Scot.) '46; DPH; PH; Dir. South Central Health Unit; Tel. 372-5212.
FINDLAY, John A.; Box 280, Brandon Clinic, Brandon, Man.; 349-22nd St. (res); Man '39; ObstGyn; Chief of ObstGyn., Brandon Gen. Hosp.; Cons. (ObstGyn), Brandon Hosp. for Mental Dis.; Tel. PA 9-6444.
FINDLAY, Margaret (See Boothroyd)
FINDLAY-KITZ, Alice D.; see KITZ, Alice D.
FINDLAY, Stanley P.; 27,124 Trans Canada Hwy., Aldergrove, B.C.; 2917 Jackman Rd. (res); McG '25; Anaes.; Med. Staff, Langley Mem. Hosp., Murrayville, New Westminster, B.C.; Dist. Coroner; Tel. 856-2313.
FINE, Barry N.; 330 Spadina Rd., Apt. 2001, Toronto, Ont.; Tor'64; MBA; Tel. 782-0494.
FINE, Harold; 99 Avenue Rd., Toronto 5, Ont.; 19 Elderwood Dr. (res); Tor '39; IntMed; Att'd. Phys., New Mt. Sinai Hosp.; Pt.-time Cons., Chest Clinic, Gage Inst.; Tel. 924-3500.
FINE, Sylvia; (See FISHBEIN, Sylvia).
FINES, Simon G.; 842 Wilson Ave., Downsview, Ont.; 557 Roselawn Ave. (res); Tor '30; M.C.-G.P.; Staff, New Mt. Sinai Hosp.; Court Staff, Doctor's Hosp.; M.O., Dept. of Welfare & Housing, Metro Toronto; Tel. ME 5-8551.
FINK, Alois; Links Associate Clin., 124th St., **109A Ave., Edmonton, Alta.; 10751—107th St. (res); Berlin (Germ.) '44; Ph.D. (Vienna); MCGP; Tel. GL 4-4551.**
FINK, N. R., Major; McG '53; Staff, Military Hosp., Camp Petawawa, Ont.; Tel. 687-5511, Loc. 410.
FINK, Stanley M.; 1495 Kipling Ave. N., Rexdale, Ont.; UBC '63; Staff, Humber Mem. Hosp.; Tel. 241-5264.
FINKEL, Kenneth C.; Winnipeg Clinic, N.E. St. Mary's & Vaughan, Winnipeg 1, Man.; Trinity Coll. (Dublin, Ire.)'50; DCH; MRCP(I); Paed; Active Staff & Dir. Home Care Program, Children's Hosp.; Ass't. Prof. (Paed.), U. of Manitoba; Tel. WH 2-0551.
FINKELSTEIN, Benjamin; 49 Dow Ave., Hamilton, Ont.; 31 London St. (res); Qns '41; M.C.-G.P.; Staff, Hamilton Gen. Hosp.; Phys., Canada Iron Foundries; Tel. 527-5105.
FINKELSTEIN, Jerry Z.; McG'63; Res., Montreal Children's Hosp.; Montreal, P.Q.; Abroad.
FINKELSTEIN, Moses N.; 360 Pine Ave. W., Montreal, P.Q.; 406 Pine Ave. W. (res); McG '27; Med. Staff, Jewish Gen. Hosp.; Tel. VI 5-7311.
FINKLESTEIN, Marcus P.; 5045 Park Ave., Montreal, P.Q.; McG '19; Tel. 277-9000.
FINKLESTEIN, Mitchell; Regina Med. Centre, 1847 Rose St., Regina, Sask.; **3451 Rae St. (res); Tor '42; M.C.G.P.; Sr., Dept. of G.P., Regina** Gen. & Regina Grey Nuns' Hosp's.; Tel. 522-6661.
FINLAY, John M.; Ste. 426 Med. Arts Bldg., 170 St. George St., **Toronto 5, Ont.; 30 Chatsworth** Dr. (res); Tor '47; FACP, FRCP(C), IntMed; Staff Phys., Toronto Gen. Hosp.; Assoc. Med. U. of Toronto; Tel. WA 2-1690.
FINLAYSON, Alexander; 221 Brant Ave., Brantford, Ont. Glasgow (Scot.) '42 D.Psy; Psy; Staff, Brantford Gen. Hosp.; Tel. 752-4849.
FINLAYSON, Alexander J.; 268 Brant Ave., Brantford, Ont.; R.R. 1. Paris (res); Tor '38; ObstGyn; Staff, Brantford Gen. & St. Joseph's Hosp's.; Tel. 752-7321.
FINLAYSON, Christopher M.; 108 Canaoda Bldg., Prince Albert, Sask.; 103-12th St. W .(res); Qns '16; Urol; Dist. Coroner; Tel. 763-2110.
FINLAYSON, Donald C.; 106 Banstock Rd., Willowdale, Ont.; Tor'52; FRCP(C), Anaes; Clin. Teach., St. Michael's Hosp. & U. of Toronto.

FINLAYSON, Donald M.; 801 Med. Arts Bldg., 170 St. George St., Toronto 5, Ont.; 103 Alexandra Blvd. (res); Tor '46; B.Sc. (Med.); FRCP (C), FACP; FCCP; IntMed; Indoor Staff, St. Michael's Hosp.; Assoc. (Med.), U. of Toronto; Tel. WA 2-8577.

FINLAYSON, Morrison H., Montreal Gen. Hosp., 1650 Cedar Ave., Montreal 25, P.Q.; Edinburgh (Scot.) '58; M.B., B.Ch.; FRCP(C); Neur; Path; Tel. 937-6011.

FINLAYSON, Roderick A.; 188 Cline St. N. Hamilton, Ont.; (res); Tor '27; Psy.; Tel. JA 7-4713.

FINLEY, Alan H.; Ste. 101, The Abbey Apts., 4643 Sherbrooke St. W., Montreal 6, P.Q.; 53 Thornton Ave., Twn. of Mt. Royal, Mtl. 16 (res); McG '53; F.R.C.P.(C), Paed; Att'd. Staff, Montreal Children's, Reddy Mem. & Alexandra Hosp's; Phys., Dept. of Health, Twn. of Mount Royal; Hosmer Teach. Fell. (Paed), McGill U.; Tel. WE 2-8226. Abroad.

FINLEY, Gordon R.; 13620 Grosvenor Rd., N. Surrey, B.C.; 9709 Scott Rd., R.R. 7, New Westminster (res); Alb '48.; Tel. 584-5242.

FINLEY, John A.; 115 Hazen St., Saint John, N.B.; 90 Sunset Dr. (res); McG '37; FAGS: GenSurg; Att'd Surg., Saint John Gen. & St. Joseph's Hosp's.; Chief of Surg., Lancaster DVA Hosp.; ThorSurg., St. John's T.B. Hosp.; Tel. 693-3528.

FINLEY, John C.; Box 448, Meaford, Ont.; Qns'35; MCGP.

FINN, J. H.; Wellesley, Ont.; Tor '51.

FINN, William P.; 66 Charlton Ave. W., Hamilton, Ont.; Tor'59; FRCS(C), GenSurg; Assoc. Surg., Hamilton Civic Hosp.; Court. Staff, Chedoke Gen. & Children's Hosp.

FINNIE, Jerrold N.; Alb '63; Jr. Int., Montreal Gen. Hosp., Montreal 25, P.Q.

FINNEMORE, Brian I.; Box 100, Westbank, B.C.; UBC'57; Staff, Kelowna Gen. Hosp.; Tel. 768-5561.

FINNIGAN, Moira A. see **SCOTT, Moira A.** (Finnigan)

FINZER, Karl H.; Heidelberg (Germ.) '54; Res., University Hosp., Edmonton, Alta.

FIORINI, Godfrey; 671 Lansdowne Ave., Toronto 4, Ont.; '55; MCGP; Tel. LE 5-8152.

FIRCKSER, Boris; Ste. 18, 22707 Lougheed Hwy., Haney, B.C.; Germany' 35; Tel. 942-4018.

FIREMAN, Harold H.; 334 Kent St., Ottawa 4, Ont.; 190 Buena Vista Rd., Rockcliffe Pk. (res); Tor '42; FRCP(C), IntMed; Phys., Ottawa Civic Hosp.; Cons. (Med.), National Defence Med. Centre; Lect. (Med.), U. of Ottawa; Tel. 233-3030.

FIRLOTTE, Robert W.; 242 Murdoch Ave., Noranda, P.Q.; Ott '55; Tel. 762-1490.

FIRME, Florencio N.; '52; Staff, General Hosp., St. Johns, **Nfld.**

FIROR, Whitmer B.; Johns Hopkins (Baltimore, USA)'57; FRCS(C) Cardiovasc & ThorSurg; Staff, University Hosp., Saskatoon, Sask.

FIRSTBROOK, John B.; 68 Kensington Ave., **Kingston, Ont.; Tor 45; Ph.D.; IntMed; Assoc.** Dean of Med., Lect. in Med. & Physiol., Queen's U.; Tel. LI 6-1731.

FIRTH, John D. A.; Apt. 33, 3644 Ontario Ave., Montreal 25, P.Q. (res); Tor '40; Anaes; Assoc. **Anaes., Royal Victoria Hosp.; Tel. VI 2-1251.**

FIRTH, S. Terry; Qns'65; Res., (Psy.), The Douglas & Allan Mem. Hosp's., Montreal, P.Q.

FISCH, Christian; Mon '55; Res., Montreal Children's Hosp., Montreal 25, P.Q.; Abroad.

FISCHER, Elsbeth (Ramcke); 90 Harbour St., Toronto 1, Ont.; Hamburg (Germ.) '42; MCGP; Staff, W.C.B.

FISCHER, Gerhardt E.; Alb '61; Res., Royal Alexandra Hosp., Edmonton, Alta.

FISCHER, Herman R.; Box 129, Vernon, B.C.; Utrecht (Neth.)'52; DiagRad.; Tel. 2-7526.

FISCHER, Martin A.; 99 Avenue Rd., Toronto 5, Ont.; 94 Cortleigh Blvd. (res); Tor '43; D.A.B.-P.N., D.Psy., Psy; Chief Psy. & Sr. Att. Phys., New Mt. Sinai Hosp.; Clin Teach. (Psy.), U. of Toronto; Cons. Psy., Metro Children's Aid Soc., & Warrendale Residential Treatment Centre for Emotionally Disturbed Girls; Tel. WA 1-0636.

FISCHER, Phyllis V. (Brown); McG '55; Path; Staff, Toronto Gen. Hosp., Toronto 2, Ont.; Tel. 2-7526.

FISCHER, Richard M.; 241 Colborne St., London, Ont.; Pisa (Italy) '40; M.C.G.P.

FISET, P. E. Armand; 15 St. Jean Baptiste, Baie St-Paul, Cte. Charlevoix, P.Q.; Lav '43; MCGP; Med. Dir., Hop. Ste-Anne; Staff, Hop. St-Foy & Laval U.

FISET, Raymond; Lav '60; FRCS(C), ObstGyn; Staff, Hop. de L'Enfant Jesus, Quebec 3, P.Q.; Tel. 529-8711; Abroad.

FISH, Edward B.; 321 Med. Arts Bldg., 170 St. George St., Toronto 5, Ont.; Tor'49; DABS; FRCS(C); GenSurg; Surg. Staff, Women's College Hosp.; Clin. Teach. (Surg.), U. of Toronto; Tel. 922-1902.

FISH, E. Laurence; 503 Chinook Prof. Bldg., Macleod Trail, Calgary, Alta.; Alb'54; ObstGyn.

FISH, Frank H.; 201-33rd Ave. S.W., Calgary, Alta. (res); McG '21; Anaes; Retired.

FISH, Harvey W.; McLennan, Alta.; Alb '36; Dist. Coroner.

FISH, Margaret I. (Trotter); Dept of Anat., U. of Ottawa, Ottawa, Ont.; Alb '55; M.Sc; AMCGP; Ass't. Prof. (Anat.), U. of Ottawa; Research **Assoc., Ontario Heart Fdn.; Tel. 235-6751, Loc. 294.**

FISH, Marjorie D. (Cowan); Tor'57; MCGP; Staff, International Grenfell Assoc., St. Anthony, Nfld.

FISHAUT, S. H.; 1892 Acadia Rd., Vancouver 8, B.C. (res); Warsaw (Pol.) '30; IntMed; Staff, Pearson's Hosp., Vancouver; Tel. 224-3924.

FISHBEIN, Gerald D.; 983 Pape Ave., Toronto, Ont.; 248 Howland Ave. (res); Tor '60; AMCGP. Staff, Diabetic Clinic, Toronto East Gen. Hosp.; Tel. HO 1-8163.

FISHBEIN, Sylvia (Fine); 1097A Victoria Pk. Ave., Scarborough, Ont.; 12 Sandalwood Pl. Don Mills (res); Tor '60; AMCGP; Retired.

FISHELL, Eve; 678 Kennedy Rd., Scarborough, **Ont. '55; Tel. 261-5512.**

FISHER, Andrew A.; 1397 Spring St., Niagara Falls, Ont.; Qns'60; ObstGyn; Tel. 358-5234.

FISHER, Benjamin K.; 409 Med. Centre, 8th Ave. & 8th St. S.W., Calgary, Alta.; Geneva (Switzerland)'54; FRCP(C); Derm; Tel. 262-6766.

FISHER, Charles F.; 290 Huron St., London, **Ont.; Wes '43; M.Sc., IntMed; Staff, Victoria St. Joseph's, Parkwood & St. Mary's Hosp's.; Teach. Staff (Med.), St. Joseph's Schl. of Nursing & U. of Western Ont.; Tel. 439-6831.**

FISHER, DeWenten H.; Med. Centre, Springhill, N.S.; 169 Main St. (res); Dal '52; Tel. 597-3614.

FISHER, D. Gwendoline (Calvert); 511 Central Ave., Sutherland, Sask. (res); Wes '52; Retired.

FISHER, Florence M.; Wes'64; Res., St. Joseph's Hosp., London, Ont.

FISHER, Frederick; Leigh Sq. Med Centre, Port Coquitlam, B.C.; Vienna (Aust.)'37; MCGP; Active Staff Royal Columbian Hosp. & St. Mary's Hosp., New Westminster; Tel. 942-7227.

FISHER, G. E.; Alb '61; Jr. Intn., Calgary Gen. Hosp., Calgary, Alta.

FISHER, J. Gordon; 751 King St. W., Kitchener, Ont.; Wes'65.

FISHER, J. H.; 524 Princess St., Kingston, Ont.; Qns '15.

FISHER, John E.; Grand Falls, Nfld.; National U. (Ire.)'57; MB; ChB; BAO.

FISHER, John G.; 101 St. Anne St., Apt. 4, Quebec 4, P.Q.; Lav '29; FICS; Urol Ass't. (Urol.), Hop.-de-l'Enfant-Jesus; Ass't. Prof., U. of Laval; Tel. 522-4536.

FISHER, John H.; 383 Huron St., London, Ont. (res); **Wes '22; M.Sc., F.R.C.P.(C), PathBact; Path-in-Chief, Victoria Hosp.; Dist. Path., Attorney Gen. Dept., Prov. of Ont.; Cons. Path., Westminster D.V.A. Hosp.; Prof. of Path., U. of Western Ontario; Tel. GE 2-5261.**

FISHER, John K.; 90 Woodstock St. N. Tavistock, Ont.; Wes '37.

FISHER, Margaret C.; (See Mahood, Margaret C.).

FISHER, Mark M.; Qns'65; Res., Kingston Gen. Hosp., Kingston, Ont.
FISHER, M. Malcolm; 2 Burnham Rd., Toronto 7, Ont.; Tor'58; FRCP(C), IntMed; Staff, Toronto Gen. Hosp., Toronto 2, Ont.
FISHER, Murray M.; 260 Muskoka St. S., Gravenhurst, Ont.; 385 Sarah St. N. (res); Tor '23; M.C.G.P.; Staff Bracebridge Mem. Hosp.; Tel. 687-2271.
FISHER, Paul W.; 1657 Truscott Dr., Clarkson, Ont.; Wes'63; M.O., C.N.R. Med. Clin., Toronto; Tel. 822-1032.
FISHER, Ralph E.; 5885 Arbutus St., Powell River, B.C.; Alb'42; GenSurg; Chief of Surg., Powell River Gen. Hosp.; Tel. 483-9362.
FISHER, Samuel A.; 1812 Buchanan Ave., Niagara Falls, Ont.; 50 Rolling Acres Dr. (res); Qns '29; GenSurg; M.C.G.P.; Tel. EL 8-9223.
FISHER, Trenholm L.; 728 Parkdale Ave., Ottawa 3, Ont.; McG '27; FACP; IntMed; Pres. Med. Staff, Perley Hosp.; Sec-Treas., Cdn. Medical Protective Assoc., 26 Nepean St., Ste. 115; Tel. 234-3589.
FISHER, Walter J.; 11 Clear View Cres., Dartmouth, N.S.; Breslau (Germ.) '24; NeurPsy; Chief, Female Serv., Nova Scotia Hosp., Dartmouth, N.S.; Tel. 466-7411.
FISHER, William F.; 6 Lorne St. W., Thessalon, Ont.; Qns '45.
FISHMAN, Sherold; Ste. 408, 750 W. Broadway, Vancouver 9, B.C.; UBC'59; PhD(BioChem.); FRCP(C); IntMed; Dir. & Cons.(ClinChem), Isotope Unit, Shaughnessy Hosp.; Clin. Instr., Faculty of Med., UBC; Tel. TR 4-1333.
FISK, Guy H.; 814 Med. Arts Bldg., 1538 Sherbrooke St. W., Montreal 25, P.Q.; 565 Portland Ave., (res); McG '33; DTM & H; FRCP(C); PhysMed; Phys-in-Chief, Montreal Gen. Hosp.; Assoc. Prof. (PhysMed), McGill U.; Dir. Schl. Phys.Med. & Occup. Therapy, McGill; Cons. Armstrong Cork & Chas. E. Frosst Co.; Tel. 933-2111.
FISK, R. Leighton; Alb'65; Res., University Hosp., Edmonton, Alta.
FISK, Murray K.; 40 George St. N., Galt, Ont.; 155 Salisbury (res); Tor '47; ObstGyn; Chief of Obst., South Waterloo Mem. Hosp.; Tel. 623-0865.
FITCH, Frederick F.; 439 Magnolia Cr., London, Ont. (res) Tor '29; Tel. 455-4971.
FITCH, Maxwell, Col.; National Defence Med. Centre, Smyth Rd. & Alta Vista, Ottawa 8, Ont.; McG'43; DPH; DIH; PH; Dir., PrevMed., Cdn. Forces; Tel. 992-2521.
FITCH, Ralph H.; 541 B. St. George Blvd., Moncton, N.B.; Dal'45; Paed; Sr. Paed., Moncton Hosp.; Staff, Paed., Hotel-Dieu Hosp.; Tel. EV 4-3965.
FITCH, Shirley M. (see Colthart).
FITTERMAN, Herbert N.; Ste. 105, 2096 W. 41st Ave., Vancouver 13, B.C.; Man '57; Ophth; Tel. AM 1-0811.
FITTON, Harry; Centre Blvd., Nipawin, Sask.; 4th Ave. (res); Man '36.
FITTON, John H.; 4027 E. Hastings St., North Burnaby, B.C.; Sask '62.
FITZ-GERALD, B. Reginald; Minden, Ont.; McG'53; GenSurg.
FITZ-GERALD, Conrad T.; Apt. 63, 110 Stewart St., Ottawa, Ont.; McG '99; Retired.
FITZGERALD, David P.; 2 George St., Stratford, Ont.; Birmingham (Eng.)'46; MRCS; LRCP; Tel. 271-5831.
FITZGERALD, Edward J.; Alb'56; Res., Royal Alexandra Hosp., Edmonton, Alta.
FITZGERALD, Ernest K., Lt/Col; Cdn. Forces Hosp., Kingston, Ont.; Tor'50.
FITZGERALD, G. Walker; 214 Med. Arts Bldg., 170 St. George St., Toronto 5, Ont.; 660 Eglinton Ave. W. (res); Tor '43; F.R.P.C.(C), Neurol; Att'd. Staff (Neurol.), St. Joseph's Hosp.; Cons. (Neurol.), Northwestern & N. York Branson Hosp's. & Ont. Dept. of Health; Tel. WA 1-3733.
FITZGERALD, Jeremiah J.; Associated Med. Clinic, Moose Jaw, Sask.; Nat. U. (Cork, Ire.)'50.
FITZGERALD, John D.; 407, Toronto Western Med. Bldg., 25 Leonard Ave., Toronto 2B, Ont.; 75 Dunvegan Rd. (res); Tor '42; FAAA; FRCP (C), IntMed; Dir. Allerg Clin. & Att'd. Staff (Med.), Toronto Western Hosp.; Ass't. Prof. (Med.), U. of Toronto; Tel. EM 6-5505.
FITZGERALD, Maurice; 105 Northgate Bldg., 10049 Jasper Ave., Edmonton, Alta.; Nat. U. (Ire.)'49; MB; BCh; D&T Rad.
FITZGERALD, Maurice F.; MacLeod Bldg., New Glasgow, N.S.; McG '43; M.C.G.P.; Tel. 752-3251.
FITZGERALD, Patrick J.; Nat. U. (Ire.) '48; DiagRad; Staff, Lakeshore Gen. Hosp., Pointe Claire, P.Q.; Tel. 636-0364.
FITZGIBBON, Gerald M.; W/C; 1891 Florida Ave., Ottawa, Ont. (res); Dublin (Ire) '52; IntMed; Chief Cardio-Pulm. Unit., National Defence Med. Centre, Ottawa 8, Ont.; Clin. Ass't. (Med.), U. of Ottawa; Tel. 733-6600.
FITZGIBBON, Henry; 54 Brant Ave., Brantford, Ont.; 35 Toll Gate Rd. (res); Dublin (Ireland) '40; L.M. (Rotunda), M.A.O., FACOG; ObstGyn; Cons. Staff, Brantford Gen. & Willet Hosp., Paris; Chief of Obst., St. Joseph's Hosp.; Tel. 756-6333; Abroad.
FITZHARDINGE, Pamela M.; 100 Seaforth Med. Bldg. 3550 Cote des Neiges Rd., Montreal 25. P.Q.; 194 Betournay Ave., St. Lambert (res); McG '56; F.R.C.P.(C.) Paed; Staff, Royal Vic. & Montreal Childrens' Hosp's.; Dem. McGill U.; Tel. 937-0937.
FITZHENRY. E. M. J.; Ste. 110, 688 Coxwell Ave., Toronto 13, Ont.; Tor'40; Otol.
FITZ-JAMES, Philip C.; Dept. of Bact., Med. Sciences Centre, U. of Western Ontario, London, Ont.; Wes'49; Ph.D. (Bact. & Biochem.); Assoc. Prof. (Bact.), U. of Western Ontario; Lect. Biochem; Research Assoc., Med. Research Council; Tel. 679-3757.
FITZMAURICE, Lawrence W.; WHO, Ministry of Public Health Devavesm Palace, Bangkok, Thailand; McG'25; F.A.C.S., F.I.C.S.; PH; Abroad.
FITZOSBORNE, Donald J.; 1810 Kingsway, Vancouver, B.C.; 427 W. 49 Ave. (res); Alb '33; Staff, DVA, Shaughnessy Military Hosp.; Tel. TR 6-8010.
FITZPATRICK, David P.; 2 George St., Stratford, Ont.; '46.
FITZPATRICK, Garry F.; McG'65; Jr. Int., Montreal Gen. Hosp., Montreal 26, P.Q.; Abroad.
FITZPATRICK, Peter James; 500 Sherbourne St., Toronto 5, Ont.; 50 Heathcote Ave., Willowdale (res); London (Eng.) '54; M.B., B.S.; D.M.R.T.; D.R.C.O.G.; F.F.R.; TherRad; Cons (TherRad.), Princess Margaret Hosp. & Ontario Cancer Inst.; Clin. Teach., U. of Toronto; Tel. 445-1502.
FITZPATRICK, W. S.; 335 Stewart St., Peterborough, Ont.; Qns '26; Paed.; Tel. 743-3219.
FITZSIMMONS, Sylvia M.; Qns'60; Staff, (Psy.), Ontario Hospital, Hamilton, Ont.
FIVIE, J. N.; 11511—80th Ave., Edmonton, Alta.; Staff, Dept. of Nat. Health & Welfare.
FJELDSTED, Fridrik; 106-9th St., Brandon, Man.; 1530 Victoria Ave. (res); Man '32; Staff, Brandon Gen. & Assiniboine Hosp's. Tel. PA 6-4509.
FLAK; Edgar A.; Med. Centre, 707 Charlotte St., Peterborough, Ont.; 639 Walkerfield Ave. (res); Heidelberg (Germ.) '46; DMD; Otol., (Facial Maxillary Surg.); Staff, Civic & St. Joseph's Hosp's; Tel. 742-3871.
FLAK, Ludmila; 639 Walkerfield Ave., Peterborough, Ont. (res); Heidelberg (Germ.) '50; Staff, Dept. of Health, Peterborough. Phys-in-Charge, Civic Hosp. School of Nursing.
FLAMANK, J. Peter; Box 33,000, Seven Islands, P.Q.; University College Hospital, (London) '51.
FLANAGAN, John R.; 1730 Richmond Rd., Victoria, B.C. (res); Alb '48; M.C.G.P.; Dept. Health & Welfare; Tel. EV 5-4434.
FLATH, Everon; 54 The Kingsway, Toronto 18, Ont. (res); Tor '00; Retired.
FLATHER, Barrie C.; 7159 King George Hwy., North Surrey, B.C.; UBC'59; MCGP.
FLATHER, L. Elwood; Ste 408, 3635 Ridgewood Ave., Montreal 26, P.Q.; UBC'55; Psy.; Abroad.

FLATHER, Verne D.; Ste. 102, 1940 Lonsdale Ave., North Vancouver, B.C.; 1054 Mountain Highway (res); UBC'62; Tel. 987-3357.

FLATMAN, J.G.; London (Eng.) '57; M.B.; B.S.; DiagRad; Staff, Yorkton Union Hosp., Yorkton, Sask.; Tel. 783-2401.

FLATT, W. D.; 228 Medical Arts Bldg., 170 St George St., Toronto 5, Ont.; 30 Ava Rd. (res); Tor '34; ObstGyn.; Tel. WA 1-9292.

FLAY, W. Jackson; Kemptville, Ont.; Qns '41; MCGP; Staff, Kemptville Dist. Hosp.; Tel. 258-2454.

FLECK, Elizabeth B.; 6336 Wiltshire St., Vancouver 13, B.C.; Wes'46; Tel. AM 1-6690.

FLECK, William W.; 213 Renfrew St., Dalhousie, N.B.; McG '19; GenSurg; Surg Staff, St. Joseph's Hosp., Dalhousie; Soldiers Memorial Hosp; Campbellton; Med. Staff, St. Joseph's Hosp.; Port Phys.; Tel. SK 4-2173.

FLEGEL, Helen M.; 604 Canada Bldg., 21st. St. E. & 1st Ave. S., Saskatoon, Sask.; Wes'54; Tel. 242-1333.

FLEGG, Keith R. Sg/Lcdr; National Defence Med. Centre, Ottawa, Ont.; Qns '56; Ophth.

FLEMING, Adelaide L. (McLeese); 88 Dunvegan Rd., Toronto 7, Ont.; Dal'44; Paed; Staff, Hosp. for Sick Children; Clin. Instr. (Paed.), U. of Toronto; Tel. HU 5-0981.

FLEMING, Daniel M.; Sault Ste. Marie Dist. Health Group Assoc., 240 McNabb St., Sault Ste. Marie, Ont., 119 Princess Cres. (res); Wes '61; AMCGP; Staff, Sault Ste. Marie & Dist. Health Clinic; Tel. AL 4-6421.

FLEMING, Donald S.; 5540 Queen Mary Rd., Montreal 29, P.Q.; McG '36; DPH; PH; Bact; Sr. Bact., Montreal Gen. Hosp.; Lect., Dept of Epidem. & Health, McGill U. Tel. 937-6011, Loc. 294.

FLEMING, John H.; SG/Capt.; Tor '41 Principal M.O., RCN Hosp., HMCS Naden, Esquimalt, B.C.

FLEMING, John M.; 2 Windridge Dr., Markham, Ont.; Tor '29; M.C.G.P.; Dist. Coroner. Staff, Scarborough Gen. Hosp. Tel. 294-3322.

FLEMING, Joseph P.; 750 W. Broadway, Ste. 1415, Vancouver 9, B.C.; Dublin (Ire.) '53; MB., B.Ch; FRCS(C), PlasSurg.; Tel. 874-4824.

FLEMING, J. Pliny; 49 McRae Dr., Toronto, Ont.; Tor. '30; Indus. Phys.; Tel. HU 8-0605.

FLEMING, J. F. Ross; Western Med. Bldg., 25 Leonard Ave., Toronto 2B, Ont.; Tor'47; M.S. (Tor.); FRCS(C); NeurSurg; Active Att'd Staff, Toronto Western Hosp.; Ass't. Prof. (Surg.), U. of Toronto; Tel. EM 6-1311.

FLEMING, Karl F.; 48 George St. N., Galt, Ont.; 42 Highland Cres. (res); Ott '51; FRCS(C), GenSurg; Tel. 621-5365.

FLEMING, Kelvin O.; 721 Medical Dental Bldg., 925 W. Georgia, Vancouver 1, B.C.; 5788 Cypress St. (res); McG '45; D.A.B.O., Ophth; Ass't. (O.P.D.), Vancouver Gen. Hosp.; Clin. Lect. Ophth., U. of British Columbia; Tel. MU 4-8915.

FLEMING, Peter C.; 1607 Kenmuir Ave., Port Credit, Ont. (res); London (Eng.) '50 MRCS; LRCP; M.B., B.S.; MCP; Assoc. Bact., Hosp. for Sick Children, Toronto; Tel. EM 6-7242 Loc. 1173.

FLEMING, R. A. Paul; 5871 Spring Garden Rd., Halifax, N.S.; 361 Crows Nest Dr. (res); Qns '43; DA (McG); FACA; FICA; Anaes; Ass't. Anaes., Victoria Gen. Hosp.; Ass't. Prof. (Anaes), Dalhousie U.; Tel. 422-7371.

FLEMING, Raymond W.; Box 897 Banff Clin., Banff, Alta.; Alb '52; M.O.H., Banff Yoho Nat. Pks.; Tel. 762-2233.

FLEMING, Robert A., OBE (Mil.); Durham (Eng.)'39; FICS; FRCS(Edin.); Staff, Indian Hosp., Fort Qu'Appelle, Sask.

FLEMING, Sandford R.; Qns'65; Staff, Inuvik Gen. Hosp., Inuvik, N.W.T.

FLEMING, Sandford T.; Mall Med. Bldg., 280 Memorial Blvd., Winnipeg 1, Man.; Ste. 8, 2425 Portage Ave. Man 12 (res); Man '57; F.R.C.P.-(C), IntMed; Research, Deer Lodge Hosp.; Tel. SP 4-2411.

FLEMING, Shirley A.; 346 Glengrove Ave. W., Toronto 12, Ont.; '31; DA(Eng.); FFARCS; Anaes; Staff, Toronto Gen. Hosp.; Tel. EM 6-8211.

FLETCHER, Calvin M.; 8715-120 St., Edmonton, Alta. (res); Alb '46; Anaes.; Tel. GE 3-6283.

FLETCHER, Donald L.; Wes'49; MCGP; Ass't. Res. (DiagRad.); Toronto Gen. Hosp., Toronto 2, Ont.

FLETCHER, Duncan A.; 56 Broadway, Standard, Alta.; 110 Frederick (res); Wes '12; Tel. 53.

FLETCHER, George E.; Harvey Station, N.B.; Dal '51; M.C.G.P.; Dist. Coroner.

FLETCHER, Grant M.; 233 Annette St., Toronto 9, Ont.; Tor '28; Staff, Ont. Hosp.; Tel. RO 9-0607.

FLETCHER, H. Bruce; 478 Argyle St., Sherbrooke, P.Q.; McG'43; Staff, Sherbrooke Hosp.; Tel. 569-1565.

FLETCHER, Harold W.; Abbott Clinic, 274 Osborne St. N., Winnipeg 1, Man.; 907 Beaverbrook St., Wpg 9 (res); Man '53; IntMed; Assoc. Staff St. Boniface Hosp., Lect., U. of Man.; Tel. 774-4567.

FLETCHER, Hugh G.; 1135 Richmond St., London, Ont.; Arva, Ont. (res); Wes '23; M.C.G.P.; Chief, Dept. of G.P., Victoria Hosp.; Chief of Staff, Parkwood Hosp. (Chron. Ill); M.O.H., London Twp.; Tel. 439-9871.

FLETCHER, James D.; 4900 Kingsway, S. Burnaby, B.C.; 4371 Greta (res); Manchester (Eng.) '52.; Tel. HE 3-0564.

FLETCHER, Joan (See Harrison).

FLETCHER, John P.; 215 Cooper St., Ottawa, Ont.; 15 Clemow Ave. (res); Tor '37; Paed; Staff, Civic Hosp.; Tel. CE 2-4424.

FLETCHER, Malcolm C.; 420 Main St., Exeter, Ont.; 60 Victoria St. W. (res); Wes '23.

FLETCHER, Marwood D.; 25 Centre St., Strathroy, Ont.; 141 Kittridge Ave. (res); Wes '23; MCGP; MOH; Tel. 245-0232.

FLETCHER, Maurice M.; Tor'34; DPH; M.O.H. & Dir. Wentworth County Health Unit, 50 Main St. E., Hamilton, Ont.

FLETCHER, Walter R.; 33 Glendonwynne Rd., Toronto 9, Ont.; 21 King George's Rd. (res); McG '25; Obst.; Tel. RO 9-7882.

FLETT, Robert O.; 632 Medical Arts Bldg., Winnipeg, Man.; 68 Kingston Row, St. Vital (res); Man '39; M.C.G.P.; Clin. Ass't., O.P.D., Med., Winnipeg Gen. Hosp.; Tel. WH 2-2549.

FLETT, Ross H.; 405 Medical Arts Bldg., 170 St. George St., Toronto 5, Ont.; 168 Hudson Dr. (res); Tor '33; Urol; Tel. WA 2-8276.

FLEURENT, Bernard; Intern c/o, 7743 Place Pigeon, Ville d'Anjou, P.Q.; Mon '60.

FLEURY, Benoit; 234 Marie Incarnation, Quebec, P.Q.; 238 Marie Incarnation (res); Lav '53; Tel. 527-9437.

FLEURY, Pierre H.; 4521 rue Orlean, Montreal, P.Q.; 5240 Boul. Pie IX (res); Mon '53; Vis. Phys., Hop. Maisonneuve; Tel. 352-6450.

FLEWELLING, William H.; Seaforth Clinic, Seaforth, Ont.; Qns '54.

FLIGHT, George H.; Med. Arts Bldg., 5880 Spring Garden Rd., Halifax, N.S.; 1791 Rosebank Ave., (res); Dal '50; FRCS(C), ObstGyn; Active Staff, Victoria Gen. & Grace Matern. Hosp's Lect. (ObstGyn), Dalhousie U.; Tel. 423-6821.

FLINDALL, Richard J.; Qns '63; Int., Vancouver Gen. Hosp., Vancouver, B.C.

FLINT; Anna; 715 Medical Arts Bldg., 1538 Sherbrooke St. W., Montreal 25, P.Q.; 4111 Beaconsfield (res); Paris (Fr.) '47; DermSyph; Jr. Ass't. Derm., Mtl. Gen. & Montreal Childrens Hosp., Dem. McGill U.; Tel. WE 3-8052.

FLINT, Clare M.; 222 Edison Ave., St. Lambert, Cite-Jacques-Cartier, P.Q.; McG '42; Ass't. Phys., OPD, Mtl. Gen. Hosp.; Dem. (IntMed), McGill U.; Tel. OR 1-7887.

FLINT, John R.; 5175 Rumble St., Burnaby 1, B.C.; 3940 Sperling (res); Tor '49; Tel. HE 1-4733.

FLINT, W. Frame; M.O., Dept. of Public Health, 2363 McIntyre St., Regina, Sask.

FLOCK, G. M.; 1402 Ouellette Ave., Windsor, Ont.; Tor '14.

FLOCK, Murray A.; Box 90, Southampton, Ont.; Tor '45; Tel. 797-3242.
FLOMMERFELT, Thomas E.; 1207 King St. W., Toronto, Ont.; 8 Woodhaven Heights (res); Tor '28; GenSurg; Assoc. Staff, Wellesley Hosp.; Dist. Coroner; Tel. LE 2-3715.
FLOOD, Francis P.; Ste. 530, 5300 Cotes des Neiges, Montreal 26, P.Q.; McG'38; FRCS(C), GenSurg; Cons. Mtl. Locomotive Works.
FLOOD, Henry J.; McG '55; DiagRad; Staff, X-Ray Dept., St. Joseph's Hosp., Saint John, N.B.; Tel. 692-2691.
FLORENCE, Joseph; 703 Spadina Ave., Toronto, Ont.; 322 Lytton Blvd. (res); Tor '38; IntMed.; Tel. WA 2-8697.
FLORENCE, Ralph; 99 Avenue Rd., Toronto, Ont.; 11 Wilket Rd., Willowdale (res); Tor '55; P.G.U. of Penn.; Derm; Att'd. Phys., New Mt. Sinai Hosp.; Tel. WA 3-9809.
FLORENDINE, Douglas G.; 501 Chinook Prof. Bldg., Calgary, Alta.; 802 Prospect Ave. (res); Alb'42; DABR; MACR; D & T Rad; Chief Rad., Holy Cross Hosp.; Tel. 262-9183.
FLORENT, Hughes V., F/L; C.F.B., RCAF Station, Clinton, Ont.; Lav'65.
FLOR-HENRY, Pierre; Raxlen Clinic, 500 Parliament St., Toronto 5, Ont. Edinburgh (Scot.) '57; Tel. WA 5-4381.
FLOWER, Christopher D.; Med. Assoc., 112 Victoria St. E., Alliston, Ont.; Cambridge (Eng.)'63.
FLOWERS, Raymond W.; 139 High St., Clinton, Ont.; Wes'56; Int. Med.; Staff, Clinton Public Hosp., Alexander & Marine Gen. Hosp's., Goderich & Wingham & Dist. Hosp.; Tel. 482-7743.
FLOYD, Robert J.; 130 Ross St., St. Thomas, Ont.; Qns '64.
FLYNN, Kevin; 62 King St., Trenton, Ont., Dublin (Ire.) '57; M.B., B.Ch.; Med. Staff, Trenton Mem. Hosp.; Tel. 392-7470.
FLYNN, Patrick; 5770 South St., Halifax, N.S.; National U. (Ire.) '57; Psy.
FOERSTER, Alfred R.; 289 Cedar St., Sudbury, Ont., Qns '43; M.C.G.P.; Tel. 674-3131.
FOERSTER, Darryl K.; 383 Ellis St., Penticton, B.C.; 1325 Kendall Cres. (res); Tor '51; IntMed; Tel. 492-3024.
FOEX, Harold E.; 195 Wellington St. W., Chatham, Ont.; 500 King St., W. (res); Tor '32; Gen Surg; Surg., St. Joseph's & Chatham Gen. Hosps.; Tel. 354-3430.
FOGEL, Bernard; 609 Bloor St. W., Toronto 4, Ont.; Tor 61; AMCGP; Staff, Doctor's Hosp.; Mount Sinai & Baycrest Hosp's.; M.O.H., Juvenile Court of Toronto; Tel. LE 4-4214.
FOGEL, Sydney; 807 Canada Bldg., Saskatoon, Sask.; Edinburgh (Scot.)'52; MCGP; Active Med. Staff, St. Paul's & City Hosp's.; Tel. 242-4243.
FOGG, Norman W.; 366 Korah Rd., Sault-Ste-Marie, Ont.; Harry Yates Farm (res); Cambridge (Eng.) '54; Tel. 3-7245.
FOGO, Edward M.; Halifax Health Centre, 5970 University Ave., Halifax, N.S.; Dal'42; DPH; Dir. of Communicable Dis. Control; Tel. 422-8571.
FOISY, Jean P.; 1871 est, rue Sherbrooke, Montreal, P.Q.; Mon '38; DermSyph; Ass't. Prof., Derm. Syph., U. of Montreal; Ass't. Derm.Syph. Clinic. Hop. Notre-Dame; Tel. RE 3-9951.
FOJCIK de ARAGON, Hilary A.; 21 Pandora Ave. S., Kitchener, Ont.; R.R. 3., Kitchener- Freeport San. (res); Poland '55; Tel. 744-9791.
FOLDES, Erik G.; 700 Coxwell Ave., Toronto 6, Ont.; Budapest (Hung.) '50; IntMed. (Budapest); Assoc. Staff, Toronto E. Gen. Hosp.; Court. Staff, Lockwood Clinic, Central Hosp. & Grace Hosp.; Research Fell., Lakeshore Psy. Hosp.; Tel. HO 5-3082.
FOLEY, Adrien-Roger; Dept. of Health, Parliament Bldgs., Quebec, P.Q.; 1080 Ave. Ploermel, Sillery, 6 (res); Lav '22; M.P.H., D.P.H. (Johns Hopkins); PH; Chief (Div. of Epidemiology), Dept. of Health, P.Q.; Assoc. Prof., Laval U.; Tel. LA 4-8411.
FOLEY, Horace A.; Canning, N.S.; Dal '41.
FOLEY, Marc; Lav '60; Res., Hop.-Hotel-Dieu, Quebec, P.Q.
FOLINSBEE, Mildred; (see Newell).
FOLKINS, Donald F.; Dal'61; IntMed; Staff, Children's Hosp., Halifax, N.S.
FOLKINS, Horace G.; Chauvin, Alta, (res); McG '02; Retired.
FOLLETT, Arthur V.; 218 Medical Arts Bldg., Calgary, Alta.; 2415-30th Ave. S.W. (res); Alb '48; Tel. 262-5339.
FONG, Amy; 10022—103rd St., Edmonton, Alta.; 12908—120th Ave. (res); Alb '50; M.C.G.P. Tel. GA 4-8076.
FONG, W. C. Philip; Medical Dental Bldg., 24 Fourth St., Weyburn, Sask.; National U. (Ireland)'58; Staff, Weyburn Union Hosp.; Tel. 842-4542.
FONTAINE, Andre; 565 rue Ste. Anne, St. Hyacinthe, P.Q.; Lav '53.
FONTAINE, Andre; Mon '61; DiagRad; Staff, Christ-Roi Verdun Hop., Montreal 19, P.Q.
FONTAINE, Francine; Mon'65; Res., Hop. Maisonneuve, Montreal 36, P.Q.
FONTAINE, Jean G.; Lav'65; Allan Mem. Inst., Montreal 2, P.Q.
FONTAINE, Jean M.; Lyon (France)'51; Bact; Staff, Dept. of Microbiol., Hop. Notre Dame, Montreal, P.Q.; Ass't. Prof. U. of Montreal.
FONTAINE, Gustave; 272 St. Vallier, Quebec 8, P.Q.; Lav '50; Tel. 524-7904.
FONTAINE, Leonard; Box 668, Beauceville Est, P.Q.; Lav '46.
FONTAINE, Roger; Lav '57; Staff, c/o 930 Bell Telephone Co., 1050 Beaver Hall Hill, Montreal 1, P.Q.
FONTAINE, Rosario; 443 St. Vincent St., Montreal, P.Q.; 221 McDougall (res); Mon '18.
FONTAINE, Valmore; Lav'57; Bact. (P.Q.); Staff, Hop. St. Vincent de Paul, Sherbrooke, P.Q.; Tel. 569-6381.
FOOHEY, J. O.; 610 Pembroke St. W., Pembroke, Ont.; 247 Victoria St. (res); Lav '46; D.O.G. (Dublin); L.M. (Rotunda); M.C.G.P.; Chief of Obst., Pembroke Gen. & Cottage Hosp's.; Tel. RE 2-3101.
FOOKS, J. Anthony; 10 Stavebank Rd. N., Port Credit, Ont.; London (Eng.)57.
FOOTE, John W.; McG'62; Res., Kingston Gen. Hosp., Kingston, Ont.
FOOTE, Reginald E.; 98 Sherman Ave. S., Hamilton, Ont.; McG '57; Tel. LI 4-1067.
FOOTE, Ronald J.; Tor '57; Res., New Mount Sinai Hosp., Toronto 2, Ont.
FOOTE, William R.; 1390 Sherbrooke St. W., Montreal, P.Q.; 1409 St. Clare Rd., Twn. of Mont Royal (res); McG '34; F.R.C.O.G., F.A.C.S., F.R.C.S.(C), ObstGyn; Staff, Royal Victoria & Montreal Gen Hosp's.; Ass't Prof. (ObstGyn), McGill U.; Tel. VI 2-9791.
FOOTE, W. S.; 174 Grand River, Paris, Ont.; Tor '16.
FORBATH, Nicholas F.; Toronto Gen. Hosp., Private Patients Pavilion, Toronto 2, Ont.; Budapest (Hung.)'53; FRCP(C), IntMed; Staff, Toronto Gen. & U. of Toronto; Tel. EM 6-8211, Ext. 2378.
FORBATH, Peter G.; 288 St. Clair Ave. W., Toronto 7, Ont.; 2 Austin Terr. (res); Peter Pazmany U. (Budapest, Hung.) '48; Paed; Staff, St. Michael's Hosp. & St. Joseph's Hosp.; Research Assoc., U. of Toronto; Tel. WA 2-2983.
FORBES, David B.; 5300 Cote des Neiges Rd., Montreal, P.Q.; FRCS(C), OrthSurg; Staff, Montreal Children's, Reddy Mem. & Lakeshore Gen. Hosp's.; Tel. 737-4672.
FORBES, Donald E.; 13656—102nd Ave., North Surrey, B.C.; Dal '51; M.C.G.P.
FORBES, F. D.; Department of National Health & Welfare, c/o Regional Superintendent, European Region; UBC '57. Abroad.
FORBES, Frederick; 5262 Ave. Papineau, Montreal 34, P.Q.; Lav '11; Tel. 521-8028.
FORBES, Gerard; 154 Boul. Sacre-Coeur, Rimouski, P.Q. (res); Lav '48; Staff, St. Joseph Hosp.; Tel. 723-2393.
FORBES, G. Ronald; 454 Main St., Kentville, N.S.; 36 Highland Ave. (res); Dal '26; M.C.G.P.
FORBES, M. Elizabeth; 76 Grenville St., Toronto, Ont.; Apt. 742, 21 Dale Ave. Tor. 5 (res); Wes '42; D.A.B.D.R.; DiagRad; Chief Rad., Women's College Hosp.; Tel. WA 3-7381.

FORBES, Patricia A.; 4747 Dornal Ave., Montreal 26, P.Q.; Manchester (Eng) '58; Paed. Staff, Mtl. Children's Hosp.; Tel. 937-8511.
FORBES, Robert A.; Queen's U. (Belfast, N. Ire.) '39; Clin. Dir., St. John's San., St. John's, Nfld.; Tel. 92081.
FORBES, Robert D.; Oshawa Clinic, 117 King St. W., Oshawa, Ont.; Qns'63.
FORBES, Ronald I.; 57 Berczy St., Barrie, Ont. London (Eng.) '54; Dir. of Labs., Royal Victoria Hosp.; Dir. of Lab., Med. Arts Bldg.; Tel. 728-5951, Loc. 278.
FORBES, William D.; 4865 Blenheim St., Vancouver, B.C.; Edinburgh (Scot.)'55; FRCS(C), GenSurg.
FORBES-WINSLOW, Vivian F.; London (Eng.) '33; M.O., Dept. of Health, Box 306, Corner Brook, Nfld.
FORCIER, Pierre; Lav' 62; Res., Toronto Gen. Hosp., Toronto 2, Ont.
FORD, Bruce F.; 198 Bagot St., Cobourg, Ont.; Wes'63; AMCGP.
FORD, Denys K.; 4380 Locarno Cres., Vancouver 8, B.C. (res); Cambridge (Eng.) '47; M.R.C.P. (Lond.), F.R.C.P.(C), IntMed; Att'd. Med. Staff, Vancouver Gen. Hosp.; Assoc. Prof. (Med.), U. of British Columbia; Dir., Cdn. Arthritis & Rheumatism Soc.; Tel. TR 6-3211.
FORD, Edmund R.; Box 610, Portage Clinic, Portage La Prairie, Man.; Birmingham (Eng.)'51; MCGP; D.Obst.RCOG.
FORD, Hugh S.; Med. Arts Bldg., 1105 Pandora Ave., Victoria, B.C.; 2540 Cotswold Rd. (res); Tor '43; FRCS(C), GenSurg; Chief of Surg., Royal Jubilee Hosp.; Tel. EV 5-1614.
FORD, Joan J.; 7375 Kingsway, Burnaby 3, B.C.; Sheffield (Eng.) '48; DRCOG; DCH; MCGP; Active Staff, Royal Columbian & St. Mary's Hosp's.; Vis. Staff, Burnaby Gen.; Tel. LA 2-3738.
FORD, Kevin J.; Winnipeg Clinic, Winnipeg, Man.; 226 Oak Ave. (res); Manchester (Eng.) '45; M.R.C.S.(Eng.), L.R.C.P.(Lond.); D.P.M. (Manch); Psy; Lect. U. of Manitoba; Telephone WH 2-6441.
FORD, Robert M.; Montreal Gen. Hosp., Montreal, P.Q.; 4808 Grosvenor Ave., Westmount, P.Q. (res); Mon'58; FRCS(C), NeurSurg; Cons. (NeurSurg), Mtl. Gen. & Queen Mary Vet's Hosp's.; Tel. WE 7-6011, Loc. 577.
FORD, Ronald; UBC'65; Res., Dept. Neurophysiology, Univ. of British Columbia, Vancouver, B.C.
FORD, Stuart E.; Box 1090, Medical Dental Clinic, Dryden, Ont.; Birmingham (Eng.) '62; D.Obst RCOG; Tel. 223-2287.
FORD, Wilson H.; Keene, Ont.; Qns '40.
FORDE, John D.; Qns '41; Staff, Ontario Hosp. Schl., Cedar Springs, Blenheim, Ont.; Tel. 676-5431.
FOREMAN, John A.; 209 Medical Arts Bldg., 1538 Sherbrooke St. W., Montreal 25, P.Q.; No. 83—3510 Mountain St. (res); Wes '51; Ophth; Att. Staff, Royal Victoria Hosp.; Lect. (Eye Path.), McGill U.; Tel. WE 5-2188.
FOREST, Jean P.; 4872 Papineau, Montreal 34, P.Q.; Mon '50; Gyn (P.Q.); Tel. 524-5718.
FOREST, J. Elisee; 489 Boul. Ste-Anne, Joliette, P.Q., Lav '27; GenSurg (P.Q.); Tel. 756-8073.
FOREST, Leo; 8410 Chartrand, St-Francois, P.Q.; Mon '47; Anaes.
FORGACS, Paul; 127 rue Prince, Sorel, P.Q.; 118 Chemin Ste-Anne (res); Milan (Italy) '36; Tel. RI 3-9333.
FORGET, Gaston; 259 St.-Georges, St. Jerome, P.Q.; 401 Laviolette (res); Mon '54; FRCS(C); FABAS; FACS; GenSurg; Active Surg. Staff, Hotel-Dieu. Tel. GE 8-2774.
FORGET, Gerard; Mon'56; Res., Hop. St. Jean de Dieu, Montreal, P.Q.
FORGET, Guy; Mon '62; Res., Hop.-Maisonneuve, Montreal, P.Q.
FORGET, Jean P.; 11015, Boul. L'Archeveque, Montreal-Nord, P.Q.; Mon '63; Tel. DA 2-2591.
FORGET, Yvon; Intern c/o 6667 De Lanaudiere, Montreal 35, P.Q.; Mon '62.
FORGIE, Robert E. S/L.; Staff, Cdn Forces Hosp., Halifax, N.S.; London (Eng.)'54; FRCS(C), Ophth; Instr. (Ophth.), Dalhousie U.
FORGIE, Ronald R.; Ste. 406, 645 Fort St., Victoria, B.C.; 1108 Bewdley St. (res); Alb '59; Tel. EV 4-7106.
FORGIEL, Walter J.; Med. Dir., Calmic Ltd., 16 Curity Ave., Toronto 16, Ont.; Tor '61; Tel. 755-7718.
FORGUES, Laura I. M. (Coleman); 230 Clemow Ave., Ottawa 1, Ont. (res); McG '47; Psy; Dir., Children's Psychiatric Services, Royal Ottawa San.; Assoc. Staff, Ottawa Civic Hosp.; Lect. (Med. & Psy.), U. of Ottawa; Abroad.
FORGUES, Richard P.; Ste. 507B, 50 ouest, boul. Cremazie, Montreal 11, P.Q.; Lav '59; FRCS(C); GenSurg.; Surg. Staff, Hop. Gen. Fleury; Tel. 384-0244.
FORMAN, Dayton M.; 507 Medical Arts Bldg., 170 St. George St., Toronto 5, Ont.; 45 Glengowan Rd. (res); Tor '49; F.R.C.P.(C), IntMed; D.Psy; Att'd. Phys., Toronto Gen. Hosp.; Cons. (Psy), Sunnybrook DVA Hosp., Ass't. Prof. (Psy.) & Assoc. Prof. (Med.), U. of Toronto; Cons. Psy., Ontario Div. CNIB & CARS; Tel. WA 1-6027.
FORMAN, Edward T.; 25 Brunswick Ave., Toronto 4, Ont.; Tor'52; MCGP.
FORNASIER, Victor L.; Tor'62; Res., Princess Margaret Hosp., Toronto 5, Ont.
FORREST, James R.; 4847 Westmount Ave., Montreal 6, P.Q.; 635 Lansdowne Ave., Westmount (res); McG '25; Ass't. Med. Mtl. Gen. Hosp.; Cons. Phys., Jenkins Bros.; Tel. HU 1-7645.
FORREST, Samuel J.; 262 St. Clair Ave. W., Toronto, Ont.; 61 Braemore Gdns. (res); Tor '25; F.C.C.P., IntMed; Chief, Chest Clinic & Staff Phys., St. Joseph's Hosp.; Clin., Chest Clinic, Toronto Western Hosp.; Tel. WA 3-8079.
FORREST, William J.; Dept. of Anat., Queen's U., Kingston, Ont.; Qns'63; MSc(Med.); Ass't. Prof. Anat.; Tel. 546-3871, Loc. 406.
FORRESTER, James A.; 400 Wood Ave., Rockcliffe Park, Ont. (res); Tor '50; MCGP; Admin. Staff, Canadian Pension Commission, Ottawa; Tel. CE2-8211.
FORRESTER, James H.; 65 Bridge St. E. Belleville, Ont.; Tor '30; Ophth, Otol; Cons. Staff (Ophth), Otol), Belleville Gen. & Trenton Mem. Hosp's.; R.C.A.F. Trenton; Tel. WO 2-4069.
FORRESTER, Roland A.; Ste. 104, 400 Walmer Rd., Toronto, Ont.; 400 Avenue Rd., Apt. 108 (res); London (Eng.)'50; D. Psy; Memb. Cdn. & British Psycho-Analytic Societies; Tel. 925-7223.
FORSE, R. Armour; 250 Percival St., Montreal, P.Q. (res); McG '47; M.Sc. (Surg.), D.Surg. (McGill); GenSurg; Jr. Ass't. (Surg.), Reddy Mem. Hosp.; Surg. Outdoor Indus. Ass't., Montreal Gen. Hosp.; M.O. C.N.R.; Tel. HU 6-1757.
FORSENG, Evan G.; Ste. 5, 6325 Fraser St., Vancouver, B.C.; UBC '58; FRCP(C), Anaes; Assoc. Staff, Burnaby Gen. Hosp.; Tel. FA 5-4040.
FORSEY, R. Roy P.; Drummond Medical Bldg., 1414 Drummond St., Montreal 25, P.Q.; 24 Willow Ave., Westmount (res); Tor '41; FRCP-(C) Derm Syph; Assoc. Prof. Med., McGill U.; Derm.-in-chief, Chairman of Dept., Montreal Gen. Hosp.; Cons. Derm.; Queen Mary Veterans' Hosp.; Hon. Cons., Reddy Mem. Hosp. & Barrie Mem. Hosp., Ormstown; Tel. VI 4-5647; WE 7-6011.
FORSHNER, Reginald S.; Preeceville, Sask.; Man '53; Tel. 547-2011.
FORSSANDER, C. A.; Department of National Health & Welfare, c/o Regional Superintendent, European Region. Abroad.
FORSSELL, P. G.; Department of National Health & Welfare, c/o Regional Superintendent, European Region. Abroad.
FORSTER, Douglas S.; 44 Argyle St., Simcoe, Ont.; Qns '33.
FORSTER, Elliot D.; Box 100, Belleoram, Fortune Bay, Nfld.; Cambridge (Eng.)'45; MRCS; LRCP; District M.O., Fortune Bay; Tel. 2291.
FORSTER, Fred J. R.; 63 Front St. N., Stratford, Ont. (res); Tor '97; F.A.C.S., Ophth, Otol; Retired.

FORSTER, John M.; 17673-58th Ave., Box 370, Cloverdale, B.C.; Middlesex (London, Eng.) '55; Active Staff, Surrey Mem., St. Mary's & Royal Columbian Hosp's.; Tel. 574-4321.

FORSTER, Margaret; (see Sylling).

FORSTER, William; Peterborough Civic Hosp., Peterborough, Ont.; Durham (Eng.)'41; LRCP (Ed.), LRCS (Ed.), LRFP&S (Glas.), DPM (Eng.); Psy; Dir. of Psy., Peterborough Clin.; Tel. 742-6548.

FORSTNER, Gordon G.; 17 Hudson Dr., Toronto 7, Ont.; Tor'58; FRCP(C), IntMed; Staff, St. Michael's Hosp., Toronto 2, Ont.

FORSTNER, Janet F.; UBC '62; Jr. Intn., Toronto Gen. Hosp., Toronto 2, Ont.; MCGP;

FORSYTH, Clifford W.; Qns '38; MCGP; Staff, Col. Belcher Hospital, Calgary, Alta.; Tel. AM 6-7001.

FORSYTH, Donald A.; Dominion Public Bldg., 150 Main St. W., Hamilton, Ont.; 49 Cayley St., Dundas (res); Dal '31; Staff, Canadian Pension Commission.

FORSYTHE, Robert G.; 25 Prince Charles Dr., **Charlottetown, PEI (res); Dal '53; Psy; Supt.,** Riverside Hosp., Box 4000; Dir. Mental Health **for PEI; Tel. 4-5581.**

FORT, Thomas C.; 1877 Seldon St., Halifax, N.S.; Cambridge (Eng.)'43; MRCS; LRCP; DLO(Eng.); Otol; Hd. Dept. of Otol., Halifax Infirmary; Cons. Camphill DVA Hosp.; Cons. Cdn. Forces Hosp.

FORTIER, A. Guy; Gaspe, P.Q.; Lav '37; Gen Surg; Surg., Hotel Dieu de Gaspe; M.P.P.; Tel. 400.

FORTIER, Claude; 1014 de Grenoble, Ste-Foy, Quebec 10, P.Q. (res); Mon '48; Ph.D., FRSC; FRCP(C); Prof. & Dir., Dept. of Physiol., U. of Laval; Vice Pres., Med. Research Council of Canada; Tel. LA 9-4511.

FORTIER, Claude; Mon '62; Res., Inst., Albert Prevost, Montreal, P.Q.

FORTIER, Clement; 34 Lacasse St., Hull, P.Q.; Mon'52; D&T Rad; Staff, Hop. Sacre-Coeur; Tel. 777-2721.

FORTIER, Clement; 358 St. Louis, Black Lake, P.Q.; 356 St. Louis (res); Lav '55; AMCGP; Tel. 423-5040.

FORTIER, de la Broquerie; 1004 Mont-Ste.-Denis, Quebec 6, P.Q. (res); Lav '32; F.A.A.P.; Paed; **Hd. (Paed.), Hop-de-l'Enfant-Jesus; Prof. Paed., Laval U.; Tel. LA 9-4511.**

FORTIER, George L.; 63 Devon Rd., Baie d'Urfe, P.Q.; McG '52; M.C.G.P.; Staff, Lachine Gen. Hosp., Lachine, & Queen Elizabeth Hosp., Montreal; **Tel. 488-2311.**

FORTIER, J. A. Bernard; 3 Fairmont Ave., Ottawa, Ont.; 222 Sherwood Dr. (res); Mon '38; Tel. 728-3337.

FORTIER, Jacques; 3425 Ave. Papineau, Montreal 24, P.Q.; 4614 Michel Bibaud (res); Mon '29; D. Puericulture (Paris); Obst; Chief Obst., Hop. Notre Dame; Assoc. Prof. Obst., U. of Montreal; Dir. Maternal Aid, Montreal; Tel. LA 6-8523.

FORTIER, Jean-P.; 30 Gordon, Sherbrooke, P.Q.; 1327 rue Bradley (res); Lav '46; A.I.C.S.; Ophth Otol. (P.Q.); Chief Ophth., Hotel-Dieu Hosp.; Cons., Ophth, Otol, St. Francis San.; **Tel. 562-2888.**

FORTIER, Jean R.; 1715-1eme Ave., Quebec, P.Q.; 32 ave Begin (res); Lav '40; IntMed (Cardiol.) (P.Q.); Cardiol., Dept. of Pensions, Quebec Veterans' Hosp.; Ass't. Med., Hop.-St.-Francois d'Assise; Assoc. Prof. (Int.Path), Laval U.; Tel. 529-4478.

FORTIER, L. E.; 418 Sherbrooke St. E., Montreal, P.Q. ; Mon '27; IntMed.; Tel. VI 4-7614.

FORTIER, Lise; 812 Rockland Ave., Outremont, Montreal 8, P.Q.; 15 de Vimy (res); Mon '50; FRCS(C), ObstGyn; Clin. Ass't. (Gyn), Hop.-Notre-Dame; Ass't. Prof. (Gyn.), U. of Montreal. Tel. CR 6-6894.

FORTIER, Marcel; 837 rue Cherrier, Montreal **24, P.Q.; Mon '41; OrthSurg; Tel. VI 4-9280.**

FORTIER, Maurice; Ste. 8, 222 Blvd. Henri Bourassa E., Montreal 12, P.Q.; Mon '33; OrthSurg; Chief, Serv. Traumat. & Ass't. (OrthSurg), Hop. du Sacre-Coeur; Tel. 387-8787.

FORTIER, Paul E.; 286 Dorchester, Quebec 2, P.Q.; Lav'41; Staff, Hop. St. Francois d'Assise; Tel. 523-0800.

FORTIER, Yvon; 89 rue Larente, Lasalle, P.Q.; Mon'65.

FORTIN, Antonio; 228 Querbes, Montreal, P.Q.; Mon '26; Tel. 274-7054. Abroad.

FORTIN, Armand; Ste. 716, 30 est boul, St-Joseph, Montreal 14, P.Q.; 60 Nelson, Outremont (res); Mon'52; FRCP(C); Neurol; Att'd. Staff, **Hop. Notre-Dame; Ass't. Prof. (Med.), U. of Montreal; Tel. 845-4241.**

FORTIN, Benoit; 738 Jacques Cartier Est., Chicoutimi, P.Q. (res); Lav '33; D.P.H., P.H. **(P.Q.); M.O.H., Chicoutimi, P.Q.; Tel 549-2633.**

FORTIN, Benoit; Lav '57; Res. Hop. de l'Enfant Jesus, Quebec 3, P.Q.

FORTIN, Claude; 1 Lemoine, Port Cartier, Co. Saguenay, P.Q.; Lav'41.

FORTIN, Claude; Lav'57; OrthSurg; Chief of OrthSurg., Hotel-Dieu St. Michel, Roberval, P.Q.; Tel. 275-0110.

FORTIN, Claude L.; 1000 Chemin Ste-Foy, Quebec, P.Q.; Lav'58; FRCS(C), GenSurg; Ass't. Surg., Hop. St. Sacrement; Tel. 683-4481.

FORTIN, E.; St. Victor, Co. Beauce, P.Q.; Lav '27.

FORTIN, Germain; 750 St. Vallier ouest, Quebec 8, P.Q.; Lav'46; GenSurg(P.Q.).

FORTIN, Gilles; 771-10eme Ave., Senneteere, **Cte. Abitibi, P.Q.; Lav '63.**

FORTIN, Gilles A.; 57, Vieux Chemin, Cabano, Cte. Temiscouata, P.Q.; Lav '51; Tel. 854-2303.

FORTIN, Guy; 215 **Richelieu S., St.-Hilaire,** P.Q.; Lav '43; **DA; Anaes; Staff (Anaes), Hop.-**Notre-Dame, Mtl.; **Cons. (Anaes), Queen Mary Vet's; Hosp.; Ass't. Prof. (Anaes), U. of Montreal; Tel. LA 5-6363; FO 7-4020.**

FORTIN, Jacques; Lav'61; PhysMed & Rehab (P.Q.); Staff, Hop. Sacre-Coeur, Montreal, P.Q.

FORTIN, Jean; 1195 Frigon, Shawinigan Falls, P.Q.; Lav '48; Att. Staff, Hop. Ste. Therese, Shawinigan & Hop. Lafleche, Grand'Mere. (P.Q.); **Clin. (T.B.), Ministry of Health P.Q.; Tel. LE 9-9333.**

FORTIN, Jean N.; 718 ave Hartland, Montreal 8, P.Q.; 5576 Canterbury Ave. (res); Mon'50; Psy; Head, Dept. of Psy., Hop-Notre-Dame; Ass't. Prof. (Psy.), U. of Montreal; Tel. RE 3-6016.

FORTIN, Jean P.; 2065 Brulart, Sillery, Quebec 6, P.Q.; Lav '43; Tel. 527-3715.

FORTIN, Jean P.; 55 de l'Eglise, Kenogami, P.Q.; Lav '58; M.C.G.P.

FORTIN, J. E. Richard; 2103-10th Ave., St. Georges Ouest, Co. Beauce, P.Q.; Lav '42; ObstGyn (P.Q.); Chief, (ObstGyn) Serv., Hotel Dieu, Notre-Dame de Beauce; **Tel. 228-4831.**

FORTIN, Joseph L.; Lav '31; PulmDis & T.B. (P.Q.); Staff, Unite Sanitaire, 1150 Ste-Anne, St-Hyacinthe, P.Q.; Tel. 773-9715.

FORTIN, Joseph M.; Lav '53; DPH; Staff, Accidents du Travail, 50 ouest boul. Cremazie, Montreal 11, P.Q.

FORTIN, J. P.; 126 Brooks South, Sherbrooke, P.Q.; Lav '37; M.C.G.P.; Tel. 562-9007.

FORTIN, Justin; Lav '55; Diag Rad(P.Q.); Staff, Hop.-Hotel-Dieu-St.-Vallier, Chicoutimi, P.Q.; Tel. 549-1452.

FORTIN, Louis J.; 290 Chartier, Sherbrooke, P.Q.; McG'50; Court. Staff, Sherbrooke Hosp. & St. Vincent de Paul Hosp.

FORTIN, Luc; 8322 rue Viau, St. Leonard, P.Q.; Mon'53; Psy; Staff, Hop. Gen. Fleury; Tel. DU 1-9311.

FORTIN, Michel; 1012-3eme Ave., Val-d'Or, P.Q.; Lav '57. GenSurg (P.Q.)

FORTIN, Paul; 420 Chomedy, Charlesbourg P.Q. (res); Lav '55; FRCP(C); Path; Staff Path., Hop. de-l'Enfant-Jesus; Tel. 529-8711.

FORTIN, Paul E.; 1185 Chemin Ste.-Foy, Quebec 6, P.Q.; Lav '54; ObstGyn; Staff, Hop.-de-**la-Misericorde & Laval U.; Tel. 683-7924.**

FORTIN, Paul H.; 195 Laurier Ave., Ottawa, **Ont.; Lav '49; Otol.; Tel. 233-6144.**

FORTIN, Robert; 355 rue Labrecque, Alma, P. Q.; Lav '59.

FORTIN, Robert; 6230-40th Ave., Montreal 36, P.Q.; Mon '53; DPH; Staff, Dept. of Health, Montreal; Tel. 254-5677.
FORTIN, Robert J. C.; 3015 La Retraite, Quebec 10, P.Q. (res); Lav '54; D.A.B.R., D&TRad; Staff, Hop. Hotel Dieu, Quebec; Tel. 529-9151.
FORTIN, Zamilda, Capt.; Mont Apica, Parc des Laurentides, P.Q.; Lav '65.
FORTYE, Robert A.; 1207 Douglas St., Victoria, B.C.; 1045 Belmont Ave. (res); Qns '40; Anaes; Anaes. Staff, Royal Jubilee Hosp.; Tel. EV 6-3131.
FORWARD, Alan D.; Ste. 711, 750 W. Broadway, Vancouver, B.C.; UBC '57; FRCS(C), GenSurg; Att'd. Staff, Vancouver Gen. & Shaughnessy Hosp's.; Clin. Instr., U. of British Columbia; Tel. 874-3611.
FORWARD, Jas. D.; 904 Greyhound Bldg., Calgary, Alta.; Tor '56; AMCGP; Tel. 262-3534.
FORWARD, Robert B.; 217 Bath Rd., Apt. 501, Kingston, Ont. (res); Tor '60; Ass't. Prof. (Anat.), Queen's U.; Tel. LI 6-1731.
FOSTER, Archibald D.; 2401 Bloor St. W., Toronto, Ont.; 447 The Kingsway (res); Tor '43; ObstGyn; Staff, St. Joseph's Hosp.; Head, Dept. Obst. Gyn., Queensway Gen. Hosp.; Tel. RO 7-2145.
FOSTER, Arthur O.; Ferryland, Nfld.; London (Eng.)'42; MRCS; LRCP; Tel. 88.
FOSTER, David D.; 16 Talbot St., Essex, Ont.; 22 Iler Ave. (res); Birmingham (Eng.) '53; FRCS(Eng.); Tel. 776-7347.
FOSTER, Dwight L.; 1684 Queen St. W., Toronto 3, Ont.; Meharry Med. Coll (Nashville, Tenn., U S.A.) '56; M.Sc., Ph.D. (Cornell); Anaes; Staff Anaes., Central Hosp.; Tel. WA 5-8991.
FOSTER, Edward A.; 2221 Keele St., Toronto 15, Ont.; Tor '39; AICS; Staff (Anaes.), Northwestern Gen. Hosp.; Tel. CH 9-3232.
FOSTER, George E.; Castor, Alta.; McG '38; MCGP; Chief of Staff, Our Lady of the Rosary Hosp.; Tel. 882-3940.
FOSTER, H. E.; 8 George St. N., Galt, Ont.; 48 Brant St. N. (res); Man '36; MCGP; GenSurg; Staff, South Waterloo Mem. Hosp.; Tel. 621-4720.
FOSTER, Herbert L.; 3087 South Dr., Burlington, Ont. (res); Tor '38; PathBact; Dir. of Labs., Hamilton Gen. Hosp.; Tel. JA 7-0271.
FOSTER, H. Lee; Medical Arts Bldg., Hamilton, Ont.; 15 Wycliffe Ave. (res); Qns '40; D.A.B.A., F.A.C.A., Anaes; Staff (Anaes.), Hamilton Gen. Hosp.; Tel. JA 7-0271.
FOSTER, K. H.; 636 Kildare Rd., Windsor, Ont.; Wes '35.
FOSTER, Norman E.; 117 Superior Ave., Calgary, Alta. (res); McG '38; Anaes.; Staff, Calgary Gen. Hosp.; Tel. AM 6-7541.
FOSTER, Peter; 122A—16th Ave. N.E., Calgary, Alta.; Liverpool (Eng.) '45; Tel. 277-5566.
FOSTER, Thomas A.; 115 Hazen St., Saint John, N.B.; 977 Kennebacasis Dr. (res); Dal '50; F.A.C.S., ObstGyn; Active Staff (ObstGyn), Saint John Gen. & St Joseph's Hosp's.; Tel. 2-6631.
FOSTER, William; 1721 Hillside Ave., Victoria, B.C.; Leeds (Eng.)'53; MMSA; DCH; DA; DRCOG; Staff, Royal Jubilee & St. Joseph's Hosp's.; Tel. EV 5-4121.
FOSTIAK, Michael; 51 Elgin St. N., Sudbury, Ont.; Cardiff (Wales) '55; Staff, Copper Cliff Hosp.; Tel. MU 2-4421.
FOTHERINGHAM, John B.; 127 Elgin St., Thornhill, Ont.; McG'54; D. Psy; Psy; Clin. Dir. Mental Retardation Centre; Clin. Instr. (Psy.), U. of Toronto; Tel. WA 3-6611.
FOUCAR, H. Olding; 484 Waterloo St., London, Ont.; Wes '17; F.I.C.S., GenSurg, PlasSurg; Chief of Med. Staff, St. Mary's Hosp.; Sr. Surg. Cons., St. Joseph's Hosp.; Surg. Cons., Ontario Hosp.; Surg. Cons., Pitts Insce. Co.; Tel. 432-1032.
FOUCHER, Armand; 7820 Marquette, Montreal 35, P.Q.; Mon '61; Staff, Hop.-Jeanne-Mance; Tel. CR 3-5151.
FOUCHER, Emile; 7963 Notre Dame est, Montreal 5, P.Q.; Mon'64.
FOULDES, Helen (See Wilson).
FOULKES, Richard G.; 833 Cumberland St., New Westminster, B.C.; UBC'54; Med. Dir., Royal Columbian Hosp.; Tel. 521-2611.
FOUND, Eric M.; McGill Ave., Charlottetown, P.E.I.; 107 North River Rd. (res); Dal '35; F.C.C.P.; Med. Dir., Chest Clinics, Dept. of Health Welfare, P.E.I.; Supt. Provincial San.; Exec. Advisor P.E.I. T.B. League; Tel. 894-7124.
FOUND, Norman; 2212 Queen St. E., Toronto 8, Ont.; 1 Sprucehill Rd. (res); Tor '19; Tel. OX 1-2453.
FOUND, N. Paul; 543 Lawrence Ave., Kelowna, B.C.; 1445 Glenview Ave. (res); Tor '45; Otol; Tel. 762-2003.
FOURNELLE-LE BUIS, Flore; 51 rue Beloeil, Montreal, P.Q.; Mon'62; TherRad.
FOURNIER, Antonin; 271 ouest, St.-Vallier, Quebec, P.Q.; Lav '59; Tel. 525-6811.
FOURNIER, Antonio R.; 243 Bellevue Dr., Pincourt, P.Q.; GenSurg(P.Q.).
FOURNIER, Claude; Ste. 603-606, 925 West Georgia St., Vancouver, B.C.; 6212 Angus Dr., (res); McG'32; DermSyph; Assoc. Staff, St. Paul's Hosp.; Tel. MU 1-6036.
FOURNIER, Emery; Irving Clinic, 74 Seymour St. W., Kamloops, B.C.; Ott '52.
FOURNIER, Ferdinand E.; 219 Vansittart Ave., Woodstock, Ont. (res); Budapest (Hung.) '39; Staff, Ont. Hosp.; Tel. LE 9-1251.
FOURNIER, Flavien; 65 Notre-Dame, St.-Pie, Cte. Bagot, P.Q.; Mon '61.
FOURNIER, Georges E.; 858, Terrasse Turcotte, Trois Rivieres, P.Q.; Lav '33; Med.Dir., Unite Sanataire.
FOURNIER, Jacques; 317-10e rue, Quebec 3, P.Q. (res); Lav '50; Anaes.; Anaes., Hotel Dieu; Tel. 529-9151.
FOURNIER, J. Donat; 1649 Montarville, St. Bruno, Co Chambly, P.Q.; Mon '32.
FOURNIER, Jean-Marie; Ste. 117-119, 207 Richelieu, St-Jean, P.Q.; Mon '65.
FOURNIER, Lionel E.; 1656 est rue Sherbrooke, Montreal 24, P.Q.; 10370 Berri (res); Mon '37; F.I.C.S.; Urol; Staff (Urol), Hop.-Notre-Dame; Ass't. Prof. (Urol.), U. of Montreal; Tel. 526-3783.
FOURNIER, Louis; Lav '59; Res., Hop. Hotel-Dieu, Quebec, P.Q.
FOURNIER, Lucien; 6984 ave. Papineau, Montreal 35, P.Q.; Mon '51; Staff, Hop. Ste-Justine; Tel. 729-2311.
FOURNIER, Marcien; Lav'61; Path(P.Q.); Staff, Hop. St. Joseph. Rimouski, P.Q.
FOURNIER, Maurice; 1820 Est Boul. St. Joseph E., Montreal 34, P.Q.; 6548 Chauvin (res); Ott '59; Tel. LA 3-3563.
FOURNIER, Pierre W.; Dept. of Path., Promendae Riverside, Ottawa 8, Ont.; Ott'53; Path; Dir. of Labs., Hop. Riverside; Ass't. Prof. (Path.), U. of Ottawa; Tel. 236-0333, Loc. 234.
FOURNIER, Rene Lt-Col.; Admin., Secteur Medical de l'est du Quebec, 891 Ave. Laurier, Quebec, P.Q.; Lav '46; DPH.
FOURNIER, Rino; 2 Sormany St., Edmundston, N.B. (res); Lav '46.
FOURON, Jean-C.; Hop. Ste.-Justine, 3175 Chemin Ste-Catherine, Montreal 26, P.Q.; Haiti '58; FRCP(C), Paed; Tel. RE 1-4931. Abroad.
FOURON, Paul; Centre Medical, 55 rue Emerson, Edmunston, N.B.; Haiti'57; Ophth.
FOWLER, Alan F.; 232 Portland Ave., Mount Royal, Montreal 16, P.Q.; McG '27; IntMed; Dir., Div. of Metabolic Dis., Montreal Gen. Hosp.; Assoc. Prof. (Med.), McGill U.; Tel. RE 8-7587.
FOWLER, Arthur C.; 22 Wilson St. W., Perth, Ont.; Tor'26; MCGP; Tel. 267-2181.
FOWLER, Charles S.; Box 669, Castelgar, B.C.; Washington (USA) '51; Chm., Castelgar & Dist. Hosp.; Court. Staff, Trail-Tadenac Hosp.; Tel. 365-9952.
FOWLER, Jack L. A.; 263 Riverside Dr., Oakville, Ont.; Tor '37; IntMed; Vol. Ass't., O.P.D., Tor. Gen. Hosp.; Ass't Med. Dir., Imperial Oil Ltd.; Clin. Ass't., U. of Toronto; Tel. 924-9111, Loc. 2101.

FOWLER, James A.; Ste. 214, 1175 Cook St., Victoria, B.C.; Aberdeen (Scot.) '53; MCGP; Vice Chief of Staff, St. Joseph's Hosp.; Tel. 385-4723.
FOWLER, John H.; Tor '58; Sr. Int., Princess Margaret Hosp., Toronto 5, Ont.; Abroad.
FOWLER, John R.; 7123-119th St., Edmonton, Alta.; 11681-72nd St. (res); Alb '42; FRCP(C); PhysMed. & Rehab; Dir., WCB Rehab. Clinic; Tel. 433-4321.
FOWLER, Lillian E.; 1320 W. 48th Ave., Vancouver 13, B.C. (res); Rush Med. Coll. (Chicago) '13; M.S.; Anaes; Retired.
FOWLER, R. N.; 4 King Cres., Weston Ont.; Tor '64; Assoc. Staff, Humber Mem. Hosp.; Tel. 248-1712.
FOWLER, Rodney S.; 555 University Ave., Toronto 2, Ont.; 15 Duncannon Dr., Tor. 7 (res); Tor '51; Paed; Clin. Ass't. Hosp. for Sick Children; Assoc. (Paed). U. of Toronto; Telephone EM 6-7242, Loc. 1323.
FOWLER, Victor B.; McG'51; Path; Lab. Dir., Dept. of Path., Joseph Brant Mem. Hosp., 1240 Lake Shore Rd., Burlington, Ont.; Tel. 637-2361.
FOWLER, William; 10 Beechwood Pl., London, Ont. (res); Tor '33; DPH; Prin. Med. Exam. Cdn. Pension Comm. (DVA); Tel. GE 4-7321, Loc. 25.
FOWLER, William G.; Acme, Alta.; Tor '08; Dist. Coroner.
FOWLER, William J.; Ste. 1114, 750 W. Broadway, Vancouver 9, B.C.; Tor '34; DABNS; NeurSurg; Staff, Vancouver Gen., St. Pauls & Children's Hosp's.; Tel. 872-2210.
FOWLOW, S. Beatrice (Eastwood); 352 Wildwood Dr., Calgary, Alta.; Tor '49.
FOWLOW, William A.; Ste. 25, Academy Med. Bldg., 1812-4th St. S.W., Calgary, Alta.; Wes'49; PlasSurg; Tel. 266-5343.
FOWNES, John A.; 71 Church St., Moncton, N.B.; Dal '42; FRCP(C), IntMed; Staff (Med.), Moncton Hosp.; Tel. EV 4-5516.
FOX, Gordon S.; 6862 Kildare Rd., Montreal 29, P.Q.; Tor'60; FRCP(C); Anaes; Ass't. Anaes., Royal Victoria Hosp.; Tel. 842-1251, Local 530.
FOX, John E.; 3000 Lawrence Ave. E., Scarborough, Ont.; 1300 York Mills Rd., No. 801, Don Mills (res); Wes '51; Anaes; Active Staff, Scarborough Gen. Hosp.; Tel. AX 3-8681.
FOX, John G.; 1123 Rothesay St., North Kildonan, Winnipeg 16, Man.; Man'49; Dip. Bact., (Tor.); Path; Cons. Path., Winnipeg Municipal Hosp. & Man. Rehab. Hosp.; Ass't. Prof. (Bact. & Immunol.), U. of Manitoba; Dir. Lab. Serv., Manitoba Government; Tel. SP 5-4456.
FOX, Maurice; 208 Hastings St. E., Vancouver, B.C.; Man '24; M.C.G.P.
FOX, Terrence W.; 693 McCowan Rd., Scarborough, Ont.; Tor'55; FRCP(C), IntMed; Att'd. Staff (Med.), Scarborough Gen. Hosp.; Dir. of Health Serv., Scarborough College, U. of Toronto; Tel. 267-1605.
FOX, Zelda R. see **ROTHBART-FOX, Zelda R.**
FOXGORD, Raymond N.; 790 E. Hastings St., Vancouver 4, B.C.; 3508 S.W. Marine Dr. (res); Qns '44; Tel. MU 4-7557.
FOXWELL, Rodney B.; Ste. 601, 625-5th Ave., New Westminster, B.C.; University Coll. (Cork, Ire.)'55; OrthSurg; Tel. 521-6346.
FOY, Edward; 405 Professional Bldg., 10830 Jasper Ave., Edmonton, Alta.; 13806-101st Ave. (res); Alb '35; Ophth.; Tel. 422-2257.
FOY, Georges; 870 Sir Adolphe Routhier, Quebec, P.Q.; Lav '24; Dist. Coroner.
FRACKOWIAK, John T.; 2605 Eglinton Ave. E., Scarborough, Ont.; Cracow (Poland)'52; GenSurg; Urol; Staff, Toronto East Gen. Hosp.; Tel. 266-6491.
FRACKSON, S. Harry; 2660 E. Hastings St., Vancouver, B.C.; UBC '55 MCGP; Vis. Staff, Vancouver Gen., Grace, Children's, St. Paul's & St. Vincent's Hosp's; Tel. AL 3-3166.
FRADETTE, Arthur; 188 St. Jerome Avenue, Matane, P.Q.; Lav '43.
FRADETTE, Clermont; Lav'65; Res., Hop. Hotel-Dieu, Chicoutimi, P.Q.
FRAIN, J. Bruce; Winnipeg Clinic, St. Mary's & Vaughan, Winnipeg, Man.; Tor '44; FACP; FRCP(C), IntMed; Active Staff, Wpg. Gen. & Man. Rehab. Hosp's.; Cons. Rheumatol., Wpg. Municipal Hosp.; Lect. (Med.), U. of Man.; Tel. 942-0551.
FRALEIGH, Sydney B.; Main St., Petrolia, Ont.; Wes '27; M.O.H., Petrolia.
FRAME, James; Box 300, R.R. 1, Kingston, Ont. (res); Glasgow (Scot.) '53; DMRT (Eng.); TherRad; Att'd. Staff, Kingston Gen. Hosp.; Radiother., Ont. Cancer Found., Kingston Clinic; Clin. Ass't. (TherRad), Queen's U.; Tel. 613:-542-2877.
FRANCE, K. Alan; Knox Clinic, 1605 Glenmore St., Kelowna, B.C.; Qns'54; MCGP.
FRANCIS, Arnold; Ganges, Salt Spring Island, B.C.; Tor '22; M.C.G.P.
FRANCIS, Gerald J.; Alb'54; FRCS(C), Gen Surg; Staff, University Hosp., Edmonton, Alta.; Tel. 439-5911; Abroad.
FRANCIS, Gordon H.; 925 W. Georgia St., Vancouver, B.C.; 4592 W. 2nd Ave (res); Wes '36; Otol; Clin. Assoc. Prof., & Head of Dept. of Otol., U. of British Columbia & Vancouver Gen. Hosp.; Chief of Serv. (Otol.), Shaughnessy DVA Hosp.; Tel. MU 5-0040.
FRANCIS, James R.; 35 Academy Med. Bldg., 1812-4th St. W., Calgary, Alta.; 4719 Coronation Dr. (res); Alb '40; F.A.C.S.; F.R.C.S.(C), GenSurg; Chief of Staff, Calgary Gen. Hosp.; Tel. AM 6-7541.
FRANCIS-KELEN, Marian; 17 Church St., Ormstown, P.Q.; McG'45.
FRANCIS, Milton A.; 303 - 5th Ave., Timmins, Ont.; 661 Patricia Blvd. (res); Tor '52; MCGP; Staff, St. Mary's & Porcupine Gen. Hosp.'s.; Tel. AM 4-3920.
FRANCIS, Robert R.; 302 Medical Arts Bldg., Edmonton, Alta.; 11528—78 Ave. (res); Alb '42; FACS, F.R.C.S.(C), Urol.; Ass't. Clin. Prof. (Urol.), U. of Alberta; Tel. GA 2-6531.
FRANCIS, William G.; 202 St. Clair Ave. W., Toronto 7, Ont.; 177 Glencairn Ave., Tor. 12 (res); Tor '54; FICS; FACOG; FRCS(C), ObstGyn; Active Cons. Staff, Toronto Grace Hosp.; Assoc. Staff, Tor. Western Hosp.; Tel. WA 3-7182.
FRANCOEUR, Francois; 1510-5th ave, Shawinigan Sud, P.Q.; 675-119th rue (res); Lav '53; Tel. LE 7-1393.
FRANCOEUR, Jacques R.; Lav'60; 150 Donway West, Apt. 605, Don Mills, Ont.; P.G. (NeurSurg.), Toronto Gen. Hosp., Toronto, Ont.
FRANCOEUR, Jean; 1000 Chemin Ste-Foy, Quebec, P.Q. (res.); Lav '50; FRCS(C), ObstGyn; Tel. LA 7-3461.
FRANCOEUR, Jules A.; 351 Desoblats, Maniwaki, P.Q.; Ott'58; Tel. 449-1282.
FRANCOEUR, Leonide; St. Tite de Champlain, P.Q.; Lav '24.
FRANCOEUR, Nicolas; 227 rue Notre Dame, St. Tite, Co. Champlain, P.Q.; 225 rue Notre Dame (res); Lav '53.
FRANCOIS, Gerard; Haiti '54; FRCP(C), IntMed; Staff, Hop. Jean Talon, Montreal 35, P.Q.; Tel. 273-5151.
FRANCOMBE, William H.; Wes '58; FRCP(C), IntMed; Staff, Dept. of Haem., Toronto Gen. Hosp., Toronto 2, Ont.; Tel. EM 6-8211.
FRANK, Frances J. (Baker); 108 Glendonwynne Rd., Toronto 9, Ont.; Dublin (Ire.) '51; D.A. (R.C.S. Eng.); Tel. RO 3-3036.
FRANK, Frederick W.; 512 Catharine St. N., Hamilton, Ont.; Tor '23; Tel. JA 2-7022.
FRANK, Harold; 5560 Campden Place, Montreal 26, P.Q. (res); Mon '57; Pulm. Dis & T.B. (P.Q.); FRCP(C); IntMed; Staff, Jewish Gen. Hosp.; Tel. 735-3771.
FRANK, Harold F.; 14 Jasper Ave., Smith's Falls, Ont. (res); McG'35; D.Psy; Neur Psy; Staff, Ontario Hosp.; Tel. 283-2990.
FRANK, William; 108 Glendonwynne Rd., Toronto 9, Ont.; Glasgow (Scot.) '56; D.P.H.; Dist. M.O.; Tel. RO 3-3036.
FRANKLIN, Yvette A. P. (Bennett); 408 Hammond Bldg., Moose Jaw, Sask.; 1026 Henry St. (res); London (Eng.) '49; MRCP (Lond.); DCH; Tel. 693-1812.

FRANKLING, Samuel R.; Ste. 106, Med. Arts Bldg., 77 Upper Middle Rd., Cooksville, Ont.; Tor '49; Ophth; Cons., South Peel Hosp.; Cons., Sunnybrook DVA Hosp., Toronto; Tel. 279-1800.
FRANKO, George; Qns'65; Res., Kingston Gen. Hosp., Kingston, Ont.
FRANKS, Frederick J.; Gilbert Plains, Man.; Man '42.
FRANKS, Wilbur R., OBE, Legion of Merit (USA); 71 Crescent Rd., Toronto 5, Ont. (res); Tor '28; Avia. Med. (U.S.A.); Prof. Dept. of Med. Research, Banting & Best Inst., U. of Toronto; Sci. Adviser, (Avia. Med.) RCAF; Tel. WA 2-1438.
FRANKS, William M.; Tor'60; FRCP(C) Phys. Med. & Rehab.; Staff, Toronto Western Hosp., Toronto 2B, Ont.
FRANSMAN, Salomon L.; 64 Hill St., Kingston, Ont.; Amsterdam (Neth.) '36; FCCP; FRCP(C); DiagRad; Head, Dept of Rad., Kingston Gen. Hosp. & Queen's U.; Sr. Cons., Cdn. Forces Hosp. for Rad; Tel. 546-5101.
FRAPPIER, Armand, OBE; 558 ave. Rockland, Outremont, Montreal, P.Q. (res); Mon '30; Dip. TB (Trudeau); Bact; F.R.S.C.; Dean & Dir. of Studies, Schl. of Hygiene & Prof. of Bact., U. of Montreal; Tel. 3-9951.
FRAPPIER, Guy; 191 Boul. Ste-Rose, Ste-Rose-de-Laval, P.Q.
FRAPPIER, Jean; 3189 Lacombe Ave., Montreal, P.Q. (res); Mon '39; Assoc. Prof., Histol. & Embryol. & Registrar, & Ass't. to Dean of the Faculty of Med., U. of Montreal; Tel. RE 3-9951.
FRAPPIER, Jean R.; 561 est Cremazie, Montreal 11, P.Q.; Mon '59; Tel. 388-8810.
FRAPPIER, Sylvio; 127 Du Prince, Sorel, P.Q.; Mon '29.
FRAPPIER-DAVIGNON, Lise; 745 Hartland Ave., Outremont, Montreal 8, P.Q. (res); Mon '54; Ass't. Prof., School of Hygiene, U. of Montreal; Tel. RE 3-9951.
FRASER, A. A.; Lakefield, Ont.; McG '20; Retired.
FRASER, Bridget A.; 233 Pathfinder Dr., R.R. 1, Cooksville, Ont.; Edinburgh (Scot.) '48; Anaes; Staff, South Peel Hosp.; Tel. 277-2761.
FRASER, Christina A.; 4365 Erwin Dr., West Vancouver, B.C. (res); Tor '32; D&T Rad; Rad., Children's Hosp. & Med. Clinic, 710 Seymour St.; Tel. MU 4-1511.
FRASER, David B.; Dal'58; MCGP; Res., Victoria Gen. Hosp., Halifax, N.S.
FRASER, David C. E.; 5025 Sherbrooke St. W., Ste. 405, Westmount 28, P.Q.; McG '51; FCCP; IntMed(P.Q.); Phys., Queen Elizabeth Hosp.; Assoc. Phys., Royal Edward Hosp.; Tel. 488-8031.
FRASER, D. George; McG'65; Res., Royal Victoria Hosp., Montreal 2, P.Q.
FRASER, Donald; 24 Wychwood Park, Toronto 4, Ont.; Tor'44; PhD; Paed; Assoc. Phys., Hosp. for Sick Children; Assoc. Scientist, Research Inst., H.S.C.; Ass't. Prof. (Physiol. & Paed.), U. of Toronto; Tel. EM 6-7242; Loc. 1755.
FRASER, Donald G.; 319 Speedvale Ave. E., Guelph, Ont.; UBC '56; Tel. 824-8610.
FRASER, Donald J.; Ste. 120, Shorecrest Pl., 81 Roslyn Rd., Winnipeg 13, Man. (res); Man '21; Retired.
FRASER, Donald M.; 121 Oakdale Ave., St. Catharines, Ont.; 14 Elm Ridge Dr. (res); Tor '51; M.C.G.P.; Active Staff, St. Catharines Gen. & Hotel-Dieu Hosp's.; Tel. MU 5-8700.
FRASER, F. Clarke; 124 Percival Ave., Montreal West, P.Q. (res); McG '50; Ph.D. (Genetics); Dir. Dept. of Med. Genetics, Mtl. Children's Hosp.; Prof. Med. Genetics, McGill U.; Tel. WE 7-8511.
FRASER, F. Murray; 7193 Quinpool Rd., Halifax, N.S.; 1980 Prince Arthur St. (res); Dal '32; MCGP; Tel. 454-1547.
FRASER, Frieda H.; 28 Burlington Cres., Toronto 4, Ont. (res); Tor '25; Bact., PH; Research Assoc., Connaught Med. Research Labs., Prof., Hygiene & Prev. Med., U. of Toronto; Tel. WA 1-8911.
FRASER, G. D.; 406, 1541 W. Broadway, Vancouver 9, B.C.; 1070 27th Ave. (res); Man '46; M.C.G.P.
FRASER, George A.; 290 Giles Blvd. E., Windsor, Ont.; 2360 Chilver Rd. (res); Edinburgh (Scot.)'40; Paed; Chief, Dept. of Paed., Grace Hosp.; Tel. CL 3-6177.
FRASER, George M.; 23 Clearview Cres., Dartmouth, N.S.; Dal '50.
FRASER, Ilo (See Bennett).
FRASER, James; Box 704, Sunnyside Shopping Plaza, Bedford, N.S.; London (Eng.)'59; MRCS; LRCP; AMCGP; Court. Staff, Victoria Gen., Grace & Children's Hosp's.; Tel. 835-3361.
FRASER, James E.; Port Elgin, Ont.; Qns '16; M.C.G.P.; Dist. Coroner.
FRASER, James J. A.; Thorold Med. Clinic, Thorold, Ont.; 29 Claremont St. (res); Qns '55; FRCS(C), Obst Gyn; Tel. CA 7-5255.
FRASER, James O.; 284 Duckworth St., St. John's, Nfld.; 60 Cornwall Ave., (res); McG '24; MCGP; Cons. Staff, Grace & St. Clare's Hosp's.; Hon. Staff, St. John's Gen. Hosp.; Tel. 578-2494.
FRASER, J. Gregory; 24 Harbord St., Toronto 5, Ont.; Man'57; FRCP(C), IntMed; Clin. Dir., The Alcoholism & Drug Addiction Research Fdn.; Tel. 365-4545.
FRASER, John; Westminster Med. Bldg., 625-5th Ave., New Westminster, B.C.; 5245 Keith Rd., West Van. (res); London (Eng.) '50; MRCP (Lond.), DMRD (Eng.); DiagRad; Rad., St. Paul's Hosp.; Tel. LA 2-6818.
FRASER, John H.; Med. Centre, 707 Charlotte St., Peterborough, Ont.; 987 Weller St. (res); Tor '42; F.R.C.S.(C) ObstGyn; Staff, Peterborough Civic & St. Joseph's Hosp's.; Tel. RI 2-3871.
FRASER, John H.; North St., Westville, N.S.; Dal '52; M.C.G.P.; Staff, Aberdeen Hosp., New Glasgow; Tel. 752-8311.
FRASER, John L.; Ste. 12, 324 Prince Edward Dr., Toronto 18, Ont.; London (Eng.) '52; FRCS(C); ObstGyn; Active Staff, St. Joseph's & Queensway Gen. Hosp's.; Tel. 233-6885.
FRASER, John M.; Empress, Alta.
FRASER, John Roger; Almonte, Ont.; F.A.C.S., F.R.C.O.G., F.R.C.S.(C), ObstGyn.
FRASER, John T. M.; 180 Metcalfe St., Ottawa, Ont.; 646 Island Park Dr. (res); Qns '43; F.A.C.P., F.A.C.C., F.C.C.P., FAIM.; Int Med; Chief of Med, Grace Hosp.; Phys., Ottawa Civic Hosp.; Cons. Med. Smiths Falls Public Hosp., Victoria Hosp., Renfrew & Hosp's. in Winchester, Kemptville, Shawville, etc.; Lect (Med), U. of Ottawa; Tel. 232-4256.
FRASER, J. S. Gordon; 120-3rd St., Rainy River, Ont.; Man'42; Tel. 852-3215.
FRASER, Kenneth A.; Box 880, Main St., Sydney Mines, N.S.; Dal'43; Staff, Med. Surg. Clinic; Dist. Coroner.
FRASER, Murray M.; Med. Arts Clinic, Regina, Sask.; 33 Academy Pk. Rd. (res); Qns '45; FRCS(C), GenSurg; Pres. Med. Staff & Chief of Surg., Regina Grey Nuns' Hosp.; Tel. 523-0691.
FRASER, Norman L.; 1961 Gerrard St. E., Toronto 13, Ont.; Tor '62; Tel. 694-1171.
FRASER, Raymond H.; Bay St., Antigonish Hosp., Antigonish, N.S.; Dal'32.
FRASER, Robert C.; Dal '61; AMCGP; Res., Grace Maternity Hosp., Halifax, N.S.
FRASER, Robert G.; Dept. of DiagRad., Royal Victoria Hosp., Pine Ave. W., Montreal, P.Q.; Man '45; DABR; DR; FRCP(C), D&TRad; Diag-Rad-in-Chief, Royal Victoria Hosp.; Cons. Rad., RCAF, St. Hubert; Cons., Montreal Children's & Mtl. Neurological Hosp's.; Cons., C.N.R.; Assoc. Prof. (Rad.), McGill U; Tel. 842-1251, Loc. 326 & 771.
FRASER, Robert S.; 7426-118a St., Edmonton, Alta. (res); Alb '46; M.Sc. (Biochem.); FACP; FACC; FRCP(C), IntMed (Cardiol.); Dir. Div. of Cardiol., University Hosp.; Prof. (Med.), U. of Alberta; Tel. 439-5911.
FRASER, Ronald L.; 4611 Howard Ave., Windsor, Ont.; Ott'60; FRCS(C), OrthSurg.
FRASER, Ronald M.; Box 2327, Hinton, Alta.; Aberdeen (Scot.)'54.

FRASER, Russell J.; 125 South Oval, Hamilton, Ont. (res); Wes '28; Anaes; Head of Dept., Anaes., St. Joseph's Hosp., Hamilton; Retired.
FRASER, Simon B.; 224-2nd St. E., Cornwall, Ont.; McG '28; M.C.G.P.; Staff, Cornwall Gen. & Hotel Dieu Hosp's.; Tel. WE 3-1330.
FRASER, Thomas.; S/L; 21 Indian Mound Cres., Scarborough, Ont. (res); Edinburgh (Scot.) '44; M.Sc., DABPrevMed; O/C Schl. of Aviation Med., RCAF, Toronto; Tel. 633-6200.
FRASER, Vernon M.; Tor'54; Res., New Mount Sinai Hosp., Toronto 2, Ont.
FRASER, W. Allan, O.B.E.; 2535 Cotswold Rd., Victoria B.C.; McG '23; FACS; Urol; Cons. Staff, Provincial, Royal Jubliee, St. Joseph's & Victoria Veterans Hosp's.; Cons., B.C. Hosp. Insurance Scheme; Tel. EV 3-3050.
FRASER, W. Dennis; 1390 Sherbrooke St. W., Ste. 2, Montreal 25, P.Q.; 2265 Hanover Rd., Twn. of Mt. Royal (res); Tor '53; M.R.C.O.G.; F.R.C.S.(C); ObstGyn; Staff, Royal Victoria Hosp.; **Chief, Obst., Chinese Hosp.; Lect. McGill U.;** Tel. 842-9791.
FRASER, Wilbert G.; 180 Metcalfe St., Ottawa, Ont.; 12 Lakeview Terr. (res); McG '10; F.A.-C.S., A.B.O., Ophth; Cons. Ophth., Ottawa Civic **Hosp.; Tel. 233-1818.**
FRASER, William P.; 6 George St. N., Galt, Ont.; 184 Salisbury Ave. (res); McG '56; MCGP; Staff, South Waterloo Mem. Hosp.; Pres., South Water-loo Med. Soc.; Med. Dir., Dobbie Industries and Mosport; Tel. 621-3680.
FRASER, William R.; 42 Wharncliffe Rd. N., London, Ont.; 292 Victoria St. (res); Wes '34; MCGP; Chief, Dept. of GP, St. Joseph's Hosp.; Court. Staff, Victoria Hosp.; Tel. GE 2-6786.
FRASER, Wilmur F.; McLeod Med. Bldg., 340 McLeod St., Ottawa 4, Ont.; McG'48; Ophth; **Ass't. Surg. (Ophth.), Ottawa Civic Hosp.; Lect., Clin. Ophth, U. of Ottawa; Tel. CE 5-3932.**

FRATKIN, Leonard B.; Ste. 510, 750 W. Broad-way, Vancouver 9, B.C.; 1645 W. 25th (res); Alb'42; FACS; FRCS(C); GenSurg; Att'd. Staff, Vancouver Gen. & Shaughnessy Hosp. & B.C. Cancer Institute; Instr. (Dept. of Surg.), U. of British Columbia; Tel. 879-5791.

FRAWLEY, N. D'Arcy; 31 Hillholme Rd., Toronto, Ont. (res); Tor '06; F.R.C.P.(C), ObstGyn; Retired; Tel. HU 3-6201.

FRAYN, Douglas H.; Qns'61; Psy; Staff, Dept. of Psy., Queen's U., Kingston, Ont.
FRAYWORTH, Eric A.; 95 Le Marchant Rd., St. John's, Nfld.; **Edinburgh (Scot.) '47; DTM&H;** DA (Eng.).
FRAZEE, James L.; Ste. 21, 659 Clyde Ave., **West Vancouver, B.C.; Dal '49; D.Psy; Psy; Tel.** 922-3110.

FRECHETTE, Antonin; 1259 Hart St., Trois Rivieres, P.Q.; Lav '53; F.R.C.S.(C), Neur-Surg; Staff, Hop-Ste-Marie; Tel. FR 5-3104.
FRECHETTE, Gerard; 75, de l'Eglise, Windsor, P.Q.; Lav '51.
FRECKER, G. Allan; 213 Lemarchant Rd., St. John's, Nfld.; Dal'59; Psy; Staff, Hosp. for Mental & Nervous Dis., Tel. 9-5061.
FRECKER, Richard C.; Dal'66; Staff, Botwood Hosp., Botwood, Nfld.
FREDERICK, Alexander; 820 St. Joseph Blvd. E., Montreal 34, P.Q.; Mon '24.
FREDETTE, Jean M.; Ministry of Health, 960 Chemin Ste-Foy, Quebec 6, P.Q.; Lav'60; DPH; PH(P.Q.).
FREEBURY, David R.; Wales (U.K.)'58; D.Obst-RCOG; Res. (Psy.), New Mount Sinai Hosp., Toronto, Ont.
FREEBURY, William H.; Tofield, Alta.; Alb '48; MCGP; Chief of Staff, Tofield Mun. Hosp.; Dist. Coroner; Tel. 34.
FREED, Bruce D.; 172 Queen St. W., Brampton, Ont.; Tor '38; Chief Obst., Peel Memorial Hosp.; Tel. 451-1262.
FREEDMAN, Arthur N.; Ste 210, 3550 Cote des Neiges Rd., Montreal 25, P.Q.; McG '55; M.Sc., FRCS(C), GenSurg; DABS; FACS; Staff, Jewish Gen., Royal Victoria, Queen Mary Vet's. & Jewish Hosp. of Hope; Dem., McGill U.; Tel. 932-5529.
FREEDMAN, Giselle; 1538 Sherbrooke St. W., Montreal, P.Q.; 4145 Blueridge .Cr., (res); Sorbonne (Fr.) '25; ObstGyn; Ass't, Jewish Gen. Hosp.; Tel. WE 3-3326.
FREEDMAN, Harvey B.; 24 Silverton Ave., Downsview, Ont. (res); Tor '54; Psy; Staff, Clarke Inst. of Psy., 250 College St., Toronto 5, Ont.
FREEDMAN, Hyman Michael; 3414 Park Ave., Montreal 18, P.Q.; 5724 Kincourt, Cote St. Luc. (res); Mon'36; Abroad.
FREEDMAN, Hymie; McG'65; Res., Jewish Gen. Hosp., Montreal 26, P.Q.; Abroad.
FREEDMAN, Lewis H.; 108 Waterloo St., Saint John, N.B.; Dal'48; Assoc. Staff, Anaes., Saint John Gen. Hosp.; Staff, St. Joseph's & Evangeline Maternity Hosp's.; Tel. 693-2033.
FREEDMAN, Nathan; Ste. 360, 6000 Cote des Neiges Rd., Montreal 26, P.Q.; McG'19; Obst (P.Q.); Ass't. Obst. & Gyn., Jewish Gen. Hosp.; Cytol. Jewish Gen. Hosp.; Tel. RE 1-4224.
FREEDMAN, Newman B.; 807 Med. Arts Bldg., 1538 Sherbrooke St. W., Montreal 25, P.Q.; Apt. 12, 1520 McGregor (res); McG '25; GenSurg (P.Q.); Ass't. (Surg.), Jewish Gen. Hosp.; Tel. WE 5-5000.
FREEDMAN, Ralph E.; 3000 Lawrence Ave. E., Scarborough, Ont.; 7 Montressor Dr., Willowdale (res); Tor '55; DABR; DiagRad; Att'd. Radiol., Scarborough Gen. Hosp.; Tel. 225-1896.
FREEDMAN, Samuel O.; 1650 Cedar Avenue, Montreal 25, P.Q.; McG '53; FACP; FRCP(C), IntMed; Allergy(P.Q.); Dir. of Clin. Immunol. & Allergy, Montreal Gen. Hosp.; Assoc. Prof. (Med.); McGill U.; Tel. 937-6011, Ext. 368.

FREEL, Herbert B.; 83 Main St. W., Stouffville, Ont.; 155 Birkholder St. (res); Tor '16; Tel. 640-2310.

FREEMAN, Arnold I.; Tor'62; Res., Sunnybrook Hosp., Toronto 12, Ont.; Abroad.
FREEMAN, Daniel M. A.; Tor '62; Jr. Intn., Toronto Gen. Hosp., Toronto, Ont.
FREEMAN, Edward O'B.; 213 Le Marchant Rd., St. John's, Nfld.; National U. (Dublin, Ire.) **'52; Psy; Ass't. Supt., Hosp. for Mental & Nervous Dis.; Tel. 94465.**
FREEMAN, Gladys D.; see **MARSHALL, Gladys D.**
FREEMAN, Kenneth I.; 895 Bloor St. W., Toronto 4, Ont.; 2917 Bloor St. W., Tor. 18; Tor'31; DermSyph; Hd. O.P.D., Derm. Clinic, New Mount Sinai Hosp.; Tel. 533-0777 & 239-3252.
FREEMAN, Lincoln C.; Geneva (Switz.) '52; Res., Hop., Maisonneuve, Montreal, P.Q.
FREEMAN, Norman V.; Battersea, Ont.; R.R. 5, Kingston (res); Qns '22; M.O.H., Twp. Kingston and Storrington; Dist. Coroner.
FREEMAN, Stanley J. J.; 250 College St., Toronto 2B, Ont.; Tor'53; MA(Physiol.); D.Psy; Psy; Chief of Serv., (Community Psy.) Clarke Inst. of Psy.; Assoc. Dept. of Psy., U. of Toronto.

FREEMESSER, George F.; 2990 Riverside Dr. W., Windsor, Ont.; Ott'60.
FREI, Jaroslav V.; Cancer Research Lab., U. of Western Ont., London, Ont.; Qns'56; M.Sc. (Path); Ph.D. (Path); Path(P.Q.).
FREIBERG, Arnis; Tor'61; Res., Toronto Western Hosp., Toronto 2B, Ont.
FREIER, Andrew A.; Med. Centre, 1428 Ouellete Ave., Windsor, Ont.; London (Eng.) '47; MRCOG; FACS; FACOG; FRCS(C); ObstGyn; Sr. Active Staff (ObstGyn.), Grace Hosp.; Ac-tive Staff, ObstGyn., Hotel-Dieu; Teach. Staff, Harper Hosp., Detroit, Mich.; Ass't. Clin. Prof., Wayne State U., Detroit; Tel. 253-5543.
FREIGANG, Bruno; 66 Academy Med. Bldg., 1812 4th Ave. S.W., Calgary, Alta.; Alb'60; Paed; Active Staff, Holy Cross Hosp.
FREIMANIS, Natalie; 49 Hallowell Ave., Westmount, Montreal 6, P.Q. (res); Res., Alexandra Hosp.
FREITAG, Leopold; 798 Main St. E., Hamilton, Ont. Graz (Aust.) '49; Staff, St. Joseph's Hosp.; Tel. 499-9635.
FRELICK, Linden F.; Qns'64; Res., Kingston Gen. Hosp., Kingston, Ont.

FREMES, I. Arthur; 250 Lawrence Ave. W., Toronto 12, Ont.; Tor '40; AMCAA; Paed; Clin., Hosp. for Sick Children; Instr. (Paed.), U. of Toronto; Tel. 782-3203.

FREMES, Norman E.; 4761 Yonge St., Willowdale, Ont.; 3106 Bayview (res); Tor '49; IntMed; Chief (IntMed), N.York Branson Hosp.; Tel. BA 1-4741.

FREMING, Gerda E. (See Allison).

FRENCH, Arthur D.; 5025 Sherbrooke St. W., Montreal 28, P.Q.; McG '50; DiagRad; Rad., Queen Elizabeth Hosp.; Tel. 488-2311.

FRENCH, Derek L.; 918 Esquimalt Rd., Victoria, B.C.; 896 Admirals Rd. (res); London (Eng.) '54; DA; Tel. 382-6013.

FRENCH, Donald B.; 409 Toronto Western Medical Bldg., 25 Leonard Ave., Toronto 2B, Ont.; 9 The Kingsway (res); Tor '34; Otol; Staff, Toronto Western Hosp.; Ass't. Prof. (Otol.), U. of Toronto; Tel. EM 6-1877.

FRENCH, E. Thomas; 534 Medical Arts Bldg., 170 St. George St., Toronto 5, Ont.; Tor '43; F.R.C.S. (Eng.), & (C), GenSurg; ThorSurg; Tel. WA 1-1353.

FRENCH, Gordon S.; 190-4th St. W., Owen Sound Ont.; Tor '32; FFR (Eng.); DABR; D&TRad; Dir., Dept. of Rad., Gen & Marine Hosp's., Owen Sound; Cons., all Grey County Hosp's.; Tel. FR 6-2121.

FRENCH, William E.; 242 Victoria St., Kamloops, B.C.; 171 Battle St. W. (res); Alb '44; GenSurg; Med. Staff, Royal Inland Hosp.; Tel. 372-3303.

FRENCH, William G.; 135 Ashdale Ave., St. Boniface 6, Man. (res); Anderson College of Med. Glasgow (Scot.)'50; DPH (Tor.); Med. Dir., St. Boniface Health Unit; Tel. 233-2464.

FRENETTE, Edmour; 263 ave Labonte, Longueuil (res); Mon '30; P.H. (P.Q.); Hyg., Unite San., Vercheres, P.Q.; Tel. OR 4-7683.

FRENETTE, Francis F.; Plaster Rock, N.B.; Dal '57.

FRENETTE, H. Claude; 358 Boul-des-Prairies, Laval-des-Rapides, P.Q.; Mon '55; Tel. 669-9100.

FRENETTE, Louis A.; 490-17eme rue, Grand 'Mere, P.Q.; Lac-a-la-Tortue (res); Lav '38; FRCP(C); FACS; FICS; GenSurg; Surg-in-Chief, Hop-Lafleche; Tel. LE 8-8635.

FRENETTE, Louis; 2590 Mousseau, Montreal, P.Q.; Mon '40; Tel. CL 5-4913.

FRENETTE, Rene G.; 163 King St. E., Sherbrooke, P.Q.; Mon'53; Urol. (P.Q.); Med. Dir., Hop. La Providence, Magog; Tel. 562-8123.

FRENETTE, Rolland; 492 rue St. Joseph, Laurentides, P.Q.; Mon '38.

FRENETTE, Ronald; Ham Nord, Cte. Wolfe, P.Q.; Lav '63.

FRENETTE, Ulric; 12245 Grenet St., Montreal, P.Q.; Lav '30; FRCS(C), OrthSurg; Tel. WE 2-3113.

FRETZ, Norman A.; 1453 Prince Rd., Windsor, Ont.; Wes '59; Psy; Dir., In-Patient Serv., I.O.D.E. Community Psy. Hosp.; Med. Staff, Metropolitan Gen. Hosp.; Tel: 252-2771.

FREUND, Gertrude J.; 61 Grosvenor St., Toronto, Ont.; 31 Alexander St., Apt. 1214 (res); Prague (Czech.) '45; Anaes; Staff, Women's College Hosp., **Toronto; Tel. WA 3-7381.**

FREVE, Leonard; Les Eboulements, P.Q.; Lav '40; MCGP; Tel. 635-2444.

FREW, W. Douglas; Ste. 330, Phys. & Surgeons Bldg., 8409-112th St., Edmonton, Alta.; Edinburgh (Scot.) '41; DRCOG; FACS; FRCS(C), ObstGyn; Active Staff, University Hosp.; Cons. Staff, Edmonton Gen. & Misericordia Hosp's.; Ass't Clin. Prof. (ObstGyn.), U. of Alberta; Tel. 439-1672.

FREYGOOD, (See Wilson, Rolla E.).

FRID, James G.; Med. Centre, 707 Charlotte St., Peterborough, Ont.; 633 Gilmour (res); Wes '50; DABP; FAAP; Paed; Staff (Med.), St. Joseph's Hosp.; Staff (Paed.), Peterborough Civic Hosp.; Staff (OPD), Sick Children's Hosp., Toronto; Tel. RI 2-3871.

FRID, John I.; McGregor Clinic, 250 Main St. E., Hamilton, Ont.; 170 Dufferin St. (res); Wes '52; IntMed; Med. Dir., Hamilton & Dist. Rheumatic Dis. Unit, Medical Advisory Bd., Hamilton Health Assoc.; Staff, Chedoke Gen. Hosp.; Court. Staff, St. Joseph's & Hamilton Civic Hosp's.; Tel. JA 7-2711.

FRIDAY, Winston H.; 9 Margaret Ave., Kitchener, Ont.; 134 Stirling Ave. N. (res); Tor '46; Phm. B.; Paed; Active Staff, St. Mary's & Kitchener-Waterloo Hosp's.; Ass't. O.P.D., Toronto Hosp. for Sick Children; Tel. SH 3-1486.

FRIED, Isaac; Dal'58; Res., Royal Victoria Hosp., Montreal, P.Q.

FRIED, Thomas; 1838 Bathurst St., Toronto, Ont. (res); Budapest (Hung.) '50; M.O., Workmen's Comp. Bd. Hosp. & Rehab. Center, Downsview; Tel. 244-1761.

FRIEDBERG, Jacob; Tor'63; Res., Toronto East Gen. Hosp., Toronto 13, Ont.

FRIEDE, Hans; 780 Eglinton Ave. W., Toronto 10, Ont.; Berlin (Germ.) '30; Rome (Italy) '34; NeurPsy; Clin. Instr., Dept. of Psy., U. of Toronto; Tel. RU 2-4567.

FRIEDLICH, Thomas L.; Lockwood Clinic, 300 Bloor St. E., Toronto 5, Ont.; Tor'60; Tel. 921-2121.

FRIEDMAN, Leon; 240 McNabb St., Sault Ste Marie, Ont.; Qns '59; Assoc. Staff, Plummer Mem. & Sault Ste. Marie Gen. Hosp's.; Tel. 254-6421.

FRIEDMAN, Manuel W.; 1022-103rd St.. Edmonton, Alta.; 11219-100th Ave. (res); Alb '55; MCGP; Staff, Misericordia & Royal Alexandra Hosp's.; Tel. 429-3781.

FRIEDMAN, Morris H.; 401 Birks Bldg., Jasper Ave. & 104th St., Edmonton, Alta.; 11219-100th Ave (res); Alb '54; GenSurg; Staff, University Hosp's.; Tel. 429-3781.

FRIEDMAN, Reuben; 5835 Verdun Ave., Verdun, P.Q.; 1617 Norway Rd. (res); McG '42; MCGP; Staff, Jewish Gen. Hosp.; Tel. 735-3771.

FRIEDMAN, Shulmon; Ste 255. 6000 Cote des Neiges Rd., Montreal 26, P.Q.; Ott'58; Ophth. (P.Q.); Clin. Ass't. Jewish Gen. & Reddy Mem. Hosp's.; Staff, Maimonidis Hosp.; Tel. 737-2982.

FRIEDMAN, Sydney M.; 4916 Chancellor Blvd., Vancouver 8, B.C. (res); McG '40; Ph.D.; Prof. and Head, Dept. of Anat., U. of British Columbia; Tel. CA 4-1111, Loc. 260.

FRIEDRICH, Stefan K.; 88 Blake St., Barrie, Ont.; Vienna (Austria) '39.

FRIEFELD, Harry; 3581 Ste-Famille, Montreal 18, P.Q.; 3261 Cedar Ave. Westmount (res); McG '19; Tel. VI 2-4945.

FRIEND, William D.; 246 Linwood, Burlington, Ont. (res); Tor '52; DiagRad; Rad., St. Joseph's Hosp., Hamilton, Ont.; Tel. 522-4941.

FRIERI, Andrew; 600 Caledonia Rd., Toronto 10, Ont.; 46 Calvington Dr., Downsview (res); Naples (Italy) '52; Tel. 781-3496.

FRIESEN, Alvin T.; Box 627, Meadow Lake, Sask.; Man '57. Abroad.

FRIESEN, Gerhard; 901 Helena St., Trail, B.C.; Man '51; M.S. (Minn.); DABS; FACS; FRCS(C), GenSurg; Surg.Staff, Trail Tadanac & Mater Misericordia Hosp's.; Cons., Castlegar Hosp.; Tel. 368-5211.

FRIESEN, H. Edward; Box 640, Rosthern, Sask.; Sask '57.

FRIESEN, Henry G.; Man'58; FRCP(C), IntMed; Staff, Royal Victoria Hosp., Montreal 2, P.Q.; Ass't. Prof. Med., McGill U.; Tel. 842-1251, Ext. 729.

FRIESEN, Leo V. C.; 3237 Fraser St., Vancouver, B.C.; Man'45.

FRIESEN, Peter H.; 440 Desalaberry St., Winnipeg 5, Man.; 111 Oakview Ave. (res); Man '51; M.C.G.P.; Tel. JU 9-5306.

FRIESEN, Rhinehart F.; 409 Med. Arts Bldg., 404-406 Graham Ave., Winnipeg 1, Man.; 280 Yale Ave., Wpg. 9 (res); Man '44; FRCS(C), ObstGyn; Ass't. ObstGyn., Wpg. Gen., St. Boniface & Grace Maternity Hosp's.; Cons. Obst. Gyn., Man. Rehab. Hosp.; Lect. (ObstGyn), U. of Manitoba; Tel. WH 3-5976.

FRIESEN, W. Glenn; 321 E. Columbia St., New Westminster, B.C.; UBC '61; Tel. 524-3621.
FRIESEN, William J.; Manitoba Clinic, 790 Sherbrook St., Winnipeg, Man.; Man'43; FRCS(C), ObstGyn; Ass't. ObstGyn; Wpg. Gen. & Grace Hosp's.; Assoc. Prof. (ObstGyn), U. of Manitoba; Tel. SP 4-6541.
FRIGON, Jean L.; 5597 Laurendeau, Montreal **20, P.Q.; 444 Moffat, Verdun (res); Lav '50; Tel. 768-6300.**
FRIHAGEN, Lloyd M.; Man '57; Res., Hosp. for Mental Diseases, Selkirk, Man.
FRINTON, Ernst; Westminster Med. Bldg., B-1, 625-5th Ave., New Westminster, B.C.; 138 Stevens Dr., W. Van. (res); St. Mungo's Coll. (Glasgow, Scot.) '43; L.R.C.P.&S. (Edin.), LRFP&S (Glas.) DiagRad.; Chief Rad. Surrey Mem. Hosp.; Active Staff, Royal Columbian Hosp.; Tel. LA 2-6818.
FRISHETTE, William A.; Wes'60; Staff, Victoria Hosp., London, Ont.
FRITSCHE, Wolfgang; 209 Garrison Cres., Saskatoon, Sask. (res); Germ. '50; Prof. (Anat.), U. of Saskatchewan; Tel. CH 2-7671.
FRKOVICH, George; 1903 E. Hastings St., Vancouver 6, B.C.; Qns '50; GenSurg; Staff, Van. Gen. Hosp.; Tel. AL 5-9020.
FROBB, Paul W.; Vilna, Alta.; **Alb '44; M.O.H.,** Vilna; Dist. Coroner.
FROESE, Abram D.; 15 John St., Leamington, Ont.; Tor '32; Chief, Dept. of G.P., Leamington Dist. Mem. Hosp.; Res. Phys., Leamington Mennonite Home for the Aged; Tel. 326-6621.
FROESE, Arthur P.; Man'64; Res., Hosp. for Mental Diseases, Selkirk, Man.
FROESE, Bernard J.; 963 Henderson H'way, East Kildonan, Man.; Man'56.
FROESE, Daniel W.; 755 W. Broadway, Vancouver 9, B.C., **4439 Cambie St. (res); UBC '57;** MCGP· Att'd Staff, Vancouver Gen. Hosp.; Visiting Staff, St. Paul's, St. Vincent's, St. Joseph's & Grace **Hosp's.; Tel. TR 2-2541.**
FROESE, Gerhard J.; 397 Beverly St., Winnipeg 10, Man.; Man '53.
FROGGATT, James R.; Med. Arts Clinic, 2125-11th Ave., Regina, Sask.; Alb'60; FRCS(C), OrthSurg; Staff, Regina Gen. & Grey Nun's Hosp.; Tel. 523-0691.
FROHLICH, Louis I.; 3850 Van Horne Ave., Montreal, P.Q.; McG '29; M.C.G.P.; Ass't. Phys. (Med.), Jewish Gen. Hosp.; Tel. RE 8-7862.
FROHWEIN, Gottfried E.; 24 Peach Tree Park, Fonthill, Ont. (res); Berlin (Germ.) '30; Staff, Welland & Dist. Health Unit; Tel. 892-6275.
FROM, George L.; Tor'61; FRCP(C), IntMed; Staff, Charles H. Best Inst., Toronto 2, Ont.
FROST, A. C. Gardner; 3195 Granville St., Vancouver 9, B.C.; 1537 W. 40th Ave. (res); McG **'32; MRCOG; FRCOG; DABOG; ObstGyn; ObstGyn., Staff St. Paul's Hosp.; Tel. RE 8-7118.**
FROST, H. Maxwell; 207 Hycroft Medical Bldg., 3195 Granville St., Vancouver 9, B.C.; 4362 Angus Dr. (res); McG '41; ObstGyn; Active Staff, St. Paul's Hosp.; Tel. RE 8-7118.
FROST, John W.; 3195 Granville St., Vancouver 9, B.C.; 1498 Laurier Ave. (res); McG '36; F.R.C.S.(Edin.), F.R.C.S.(C), GenSurg; Att'd. Staff, St. Paul's Hosp.; Clin. Instr., U. of British Columbia; Tel. RE 8-7118.
FROST, Louis J.; Ste. 401, 340 McLeod St., Ottawa 4, Ont.; Dal'62; DDS; OralSurg.
FROST, William H.; 218 Roger Rd., Ottawa, Ont. (res); Dal '39; D.P.H.; Chief, Quarantine Immigration Med. & Sick Mariners Service Div., Dept. of Nat., Health & Welfare; Tel. CE 2-8211.
FRUHLING, George; Bucharest (Roum.) '41; Res., Ontario Hosp., Kingston, Ont.
FRY, John; 1466 Ouellette Ave., Windsor, Ont.; 44 Jefferson Blvd., Riverside (res); Tor '47; ObstGyn; Staff, ObstGyn; Grace, Hotel-Dieu & Metropolitan Hosp's.; Tel. 254-3261.
FRY, William H.; 201 Medical Bldg., Prince Albert, Sask.; 302-19th W. (res); Tor'45; FACS; FACOG; Obst Gyn; Tel. 763-2681.
FRY, W. Rowe; Westminster Hosp., London, Ont.; Wes '37; FAGS; Staff, Westminster Hosp.; Sr. Pension Med.Exam., C.P.C.; Tel. 432-6711.
FRYER, Avard I.; Fort William Clinic, 117 John St. S., Fort William, Ont.; 224 Summit Ave. (res); **Man '42; M.C.G.P.**
FRYER, Gordon E.; American Cyanamid, North Middletown Road, Pearl River, New York, U.S.A.; Man '39; Medical Research, Lederle Laboratories. Abroad.
FRYER, Irvin O.; 530 Somerset Block, Winnipeg, Man.; Suite 12, Gloucester Apts.; 28 Woodlow Pl. (res.); Man'13; Inspector of Anat., Manitoba U.; **Dist. Coroner; Tel. WH 2-8824.**
FRYER-MANACKI, Ruth E.; 33 Edgemore Dr., Toronto 18, Ont. (res);Man'49; D.P.H.; M.O., Village of Forest Hill; Tel. HU 1-5918.
FUERST, Heinrich J.; 329 Le Marchand Mansions, 116th-100th Ave., Edmonton, Alta.; Munich (Germ.)'39; D. Psy (McG); Psy; Att'd. Staff, University & Misericorde Hosp's.; Clin. Instr., U. of Alberta; Tel. 488-6160.
FUGERE, Louis; 2938 Coin des Caps, Quebec 10, P.Q.; Lav '59; Anaes; Staff, Jeffery Hale' Notre Dame de L'Esperance, La Misericorde & St. Joseph de Bellevue Hosp's.; Tel. 653-7720.
FUGERE, Paul; 1120 Bougainville, Quebec 6, P.Q.; Lav '43; FAAOO; Otol; Dir. Speech & Hearing Centre, Hotel-Dieu; Assoc. Prof. ORL, U. of Laval; Tel. 527-3252.
FUGERE, Pierre; Ste. 208, 30 boul. St. Joseph est, Montreal, P.Q.; Mon'59; FRCS(C), ObstGyn; Staff, Hop. St. Luc.; Teach. Staff, U. of Montreal; Tel. 521-8585.
FUJIMAGARI, Tak; McG '56; DiagRad; Staff, St. Catharines Gen. Hosp., St. Catharines, Ont.; Tel. MU 4-7271.
FUJINO, Donald S.; 331 Sheddon Ave., Oakville, Ont.; Tor'58; Anaes; Active Staff, Oakville-Trafalgar Mem. Hosp.; Tel. 844-6960.
FUJIWARA, MISAO (Yoneyama); 1849 Yonge St., Toronto 7, Ont.; Alb'43; Obst Gyn; Staff, Women's College Hosp.; Tel. 485-8912.
FUJIWARA, M. Wesley; 1195 Sheppard Ave. E., Willowdale, Ont.; Tor '46; FRCP(C), Paed; Ass't. Phys., Hosp. for Sick Children; Clin. Instr. (Paed.), U. of Toronto; Tel. 223-0616.
FULFORD, Robert A.; Qns'61; FRCS(C), OrthSurg; Staff, Montreal Gen. Hosp., Montreal 25, P.Q.
FULLER, Charles K.; Medical Arts Bldg., 253 Main St., Yarmouth, N.S.; Tor '16; F.R.C.S. (Edin.), **F.R.C.S.(C), Ophth, Otol; Chief of Staff (Ophth, Otol) Yarmouth Gen. Hosp.; Tel.** 742-3451.
FULLER, Donald R.; 24 Hope St. W., Tavistock, Ont.; 23 William St. (res); Tor '58; MCGP; Active Staff, Dept. of Med., Stratford Gen. Hosp.; Court. Staff, Woodstock Gen. Hosp.; Tel. 655-2322.
FULLER, Stewart C.; Bedford, N.S.; Dal'49; MCGP.
FULLERTON, Charles W.; 1414 Drummond St., Montreal, P.Q.; 473 Strathcona Ave. (res); McG '26; F.A.C.P., IntMed; Sr. Phys., Montreal Gen. Hosp.; Prof. of Med., McGill U.; Tel. VI 4-3595.
FULLERTON, Kathleen A.; 55A Yonge St. S., Richmond Hill, Ont. (res); Tor '53; FRCP(C); Paed; Staff, York Central Hosp., Richmond Hill; Clin. Ass't., Hosp. for Sick Children; Assoc. Staff, York County Hosp.; Tel. 884-4732.
FULLERTON, Samuel G. B.; 6044 Quinpool Rd., Halifax, N.S.; 108 Preston St. (res); Dal '52; M.C.G.P.; Tel. 423-8678.
FULTHORPE, Gordon H.; 25 Lake Avenue Dr., Stoney Creek, Ont.; London (Eng.) '63; M.B., B.S.
FULTON, A. L.; Tor'64; Int., c/o 96 Walker Ave., Toronto 7, Ont.
FULTON, Alan P.; Oshawa Clinic, 117 King St. E., Oshawa, Ont.; 191 Woodlea Cres. (res); McG '42; F.R.C.S.(C), F.A.C.S., GenSurg; Staff, Gen. Surg., Oshawa Gen. Hosp.; Chmn., Reg. Comm. on Trauma, Amer. College of Surgeons; Tel. 728-1661.
FULTON, Gerald A.; Wes'63; Res., Toronto Western Hosp., Toronto 2B, Ont.
FULTON, J. Blair; 2315 W. 18 Ave., Vancouver, B.C. (res.); Alb '44; Anaes; Staff (Anaes.), Vancouver Gen. Hosp. U. of British Columbia; Tel. TR 6-3211.

FULTON, Joseph R. W.; 379 O'Connor Dr., Toronto 6, Ont.; 2557 St. Clair Ave. E. (res); Tor '43; F.R.C.S.(C), GenSurg.; Tel. GA 1-6633.
FULTZ, Wm. E.; 29½ Commercial St., Glace Bay, N.S.; Upper Main St. (res); Dal '25; Ophth.
FUMERTON, John L.; 2117 Departure Bay Rd., Nanaimo, B.C.; Man'55; Paed; ABP; Chief, Dept. of Paed., Nanaimo Reg. Hosp.; Cons. Ladysmith, Chemainus & Port Alberni Gen' Hosp's.; Tel. 758-6022.
FUNG, Franklin K.; McG'65; Res., Vancouver Gen. Hosp., Vancouver 9, B.C.
FUNG, Kee-Wai; National Defence Med. Centre (Taiwan)'60; Res. (Cardiol.) Sunnybrook Hosp., Toronto, Ont.
FUNG, Wing K.; Community Health Clinic, Eston, Sask.; Taiwan (Formosa) '60.
FUNG, Robert H. P.; McG'60; FRCP(C), Paed; Staff, Montreal Children's Hospital, Montreal, P.Q.
FUNK, Edwin H.; 904-W. 16th Ave., Vancouver 9, B.C.; McG '09; DABS; GenSurg; Semi-retired.
FUNK, Karin M.; 68 Langbourne Pl., Don Mills, Ont. (res); Heidelberg (Germ.) '51; MCGP; Temp. Retired.
FURESZ, Eva B.; 1207 Evans Blvd., Ottawa 8, **Ont.; 2247 Courtice Ave. (res); Budapest (Hung.)** '51; IntMed. (Budapest); AMCGP; Tel. RE 3-2361.
FURESZ, John; Budapest (Hung.)'51; Med. Virologist, Staff, Lab. of Hygiene, Dept. of National Health & Welfare, Ottawa 4, Ont.; Tel. 922-0873.
FURLONG, F. W.; Tor '64; Jr. Int., Toronto Gen. Hosp., Toronto 2, Ont. Abroad.
FURNESS, A.; 172 Queen St. West, Brampton, Ont.; Tor'11.
FURUYE, Hisashi; Kumamuto (Japan) '54; Jr. Intn., Winnipeg Gen. Hosp., Winnipeg 3, Man.
FUTERNAN, Bernard R.; 2175 Victoria Park Ave., Scarborough, Ont.; Tor'60; AMCGP; Staff, Toronto East Gen. & Scarborough Gen. Hosp's.; Tel. 447-9621.
FUZI, Andrew; 900 Wingate Dr., Ottawa, Ont.; Germ. 4'9; M.C.G.P.; Tel. 733-0317.
FYFE, F. W.; 69 Edward St., Halifax, N.S.; Aberdeen (Scot.) '37; M.A., M.B., Ch.B.; Assoc. Prof. (Anat.), Dalhousie U.; Tel. 2-4406.
FYFE, Harry W/C; St. Andrews' U. (Scot.) '50; Psy; Cons. Psy., Queen Mary Vet's Hosp.; Dem. (Psy.), McGill U.; M.O., RCAF Med. Serv., NDMC, Ottawa, Ont.; Tel. CE 2-8211.
FYFE, James G.; 2000A Veteran Mem. Bldg., Ottawa, Ont.; Man'38.
FYFE, Joseph W.; 30 Lambton Court, Sudbury, Ont.; Tor '46; Anaes; Chief, Dept. of Anaes., **Sudbury Gen. Hosp.; Tel. OS 3-3601.**
FYFE, Patrick R.; 139 Mark St., Sault Ste. Marie, Ont.; Tor'49; FRCS(C), Orth Surg.
FYFE, Ronald M.; 242 Stanstead Ave., Mount Royal, Montreal 16, P.Q.; McG '43; Clin. Ass't., Royal Victoria Hosp.; Med. Dir., Hoffmann-La Roche Ltd.; Tel. 748-8751.
FYFFE, Gordon J.; 107 Queens Ave., New Westminster, B.C.; Tor'53; Anaes.
FYLES, Shirley M.; 393 Roslyn Ave., Westmount, Montreal, P.Q.; Qns '54; Neur; Staff, Royal Victoria Hosp.; Tel. WE 7-8325.
FYLES, T. William; 232 Yale Ave., Winnipeg 9, Man. (res); Man '49; M.Sc. (Man.); F.R.C.P.(C), IntMed; Dir. OPD, Wpg. Gen. Hosp.; Ass't. Dean, Fac. of Med., U. of Manitoba; Telephone GR 4-9110.
FYSHE, Thomas G.; 418 Med. Arts Bldg., 1 Yonge St., Hamilton, Ont.; 123 Amelia St. (res); McG '36; FRCS(C); FRCS (Edin.); GenSurg; Staff, Surg., St. Joseph's, Chedoke Gen. & Hamilton Gen. Hosp's.; Tel. JA 7-1992.
FYVIE, James N.; 5116 Elbow Dr. S.W., Calgary, Alta.; Alb '55; B.Sc., MCGP; Ass't. Dir., Dept. of G.P., Calgary Gen. Hosp.; Act. Staff, Alberta Children's Hosp.; Tel. 255-6647.
GABATIN, Jose Q.; Santo Tomas (Philipp.)'55; Jr. Int., Victoria Gen. Hosp., Halifax, N.S.
GABEL, Frederick E. J.; 31 Betts Ave., Yorkton, Sask.; Man'43; FRCS(C) GenSurg; Staff, Yorkton Union Hosp.; Tel. 783-3430.
GABERT, Harvey A.; Alb '62; Res., University Hosp., Edmonton, Alta.
GABOR, Andrew; 5845 Cote des Neiges Rd., Montreal 26, P.Q.; Budapest (Hung.) '49; Obst-Gyn (Budapest); Staff, Catherine Booth & Doctor's Hosp's.; Tel. RE 7-3782.
GABOR, E. Peter; McG '59; Research, Dept. of Hematology, Royal Victoria Hosp., Montreal 2, P.Q.; Tel. VI 2-1251. Abroad.
GABOR, Ivan R.; McG '64; Res., Montreal Gen. Hosp., Montreal 25, P.Q.; Abroad.
GABOURY, Hector, P.O. Box 179, Plantagenet, Ont.; McG '21; Tel. 673-4877.
GABOURY, Jacques; 7820 rue Marquette, Montreal 35, P.Q.; Mon '56. GenSurg; Tel. 729-6371.
GABOURY, Pierre; 46 Ste. Anne, Ville Marie, Co. Temiscamingue, P.Q.; Mon '59.
GADBOIS, Andre; 1965 est, Belanger, Montreal 35, P.Q.; Mon '31; GenSurg (PQ); Surg., Victoria Gen. Hosp.; Tel. VI 2-1251.
GADBOIS, Jacques; 175 St. Ephrem, Chicoutimi Nord, P.Q.; Mon'53; MCGP.
GADBOIS, Yves; 6 Brook St. S., Sherbrooke, P.Q.; 1690 White (res); Lav '41; Ophth, Otol **(P.Q.); Chief (Otol.), Hotel Dieu; Tel. 562-0615.**
GAERBER, Bernard J.; 418-925 W. Georgia St., Vancouver, B.C.; 4684 Granville St. (res); Vienna (Austria) '23; Psy; Att. Staff, Vancouver **Gen. Hosp.; Vis. Staff, St. Paul's Hosp.; Tel. MU 4-8846.**
GAGLIANO, Anthony; 2427 Mississauga Rd. W., Port Credit, Ont. (res); Messina '49; Anaes; Staff, South Peel Hosp., Cooksville; Tel. 279-7330.
GAGLIANO, Elio; Palermo (Italy)'30; Dept. of Pathology, Grace Hosp., Winnipeg 10, Man.; Tel. SU 3-7271, Ext. 354.
GAGNAN-BRUNETTE, Michele; 731 Chemin Dumfries, Montreal, 16, P.Q.; Mon '60; FRCP(C), Paed.
GAGNE, A. Aime; 41 Gendron, Hull, P.Q.; Lav '53; Anaes; Staff, Hop.-Sacre-Coeur; Tel. 777-2721.
GAGNE, Claude A.; Lav '59; Res., Centre d'Ophtalmologie, Hop. Maissonneuve, Montreal 36, P.Q.
GAGNE-DESROSIERS, Rita; 1275 Cote Vertu, St-Laurent, P.Q.; Lav '57; Anaes.
GAGNE, Ernest; 87 Jacques Cartier est, Chicoutimi, P.Q.; Lav '20.
GAGNE, J. Gerard; 142 Champlain, Hull, P.Q.; Lav'36; GenSurg (PQ); Surg., Hop.-du-Sacre-Coeur; Cons. Surg., San. St. Laurent; Tel. Area 819; 771-6239.
GAGNE, J. Guy; Lav'57; Anaes; Staff, Hotel-Dieu d'Athabaska, Arthabaska, P.Q.
GAGNE, L. Francois; 1320 Carroll, Que. 6, **P.Q. (res); Lav '48; F.R.C.P.(C), Path; Dir., Dept. Path. Anat., Hop. de l'Enfant-Jesus; Ass't. Prof., Dept. Path. Anat., Laval U.; Tel. 529-8711.**
GAGNE, Pierre P.; Mon'65; Res., Hop. Notre Dame, Montreal 24, P.Q.
GAGNE, Raymond; Lav '61; Res., Hop. Enfant-Jesus, Quebec 3, P.Q.
GAGNE, Roger; Centre Medical Fleury, 2157 est rue Fleury, Montreal 12, P.Q.; Mon'61; Tel. DU 1-2581.
GAGNE, Roland; 222 Daly Ave., Ottawa, Ont.; 389 Roxborough Rd., Rockcliffe (res); Mon'33; Tel. CE 4-1611.
GAGNE, Serge P.; 1500 18 rue, Quebec 3, P.Q.; Lav'61; Cardiol(P.Q.).
GAGNER, Raymond; 31, ouest, King. Sherbrooke, P.Q.; Mon '58. FRCS(C), ObstGyn; Tel. 567-8666.
GAGNIER, Leglius A.; 3484 Laval, Montreal, P.Q.; 62 Beloeil Ave (res); Mon '27; D & TRad; **Staff, Hop. St.-Jean-de-Dieu; Tel. CL 4-5361.**
GAGNIER, Maurice; 1202 est Blvd. St. Joseph, Montreal, P.Q.; 37 Kelvin Ave., Outremont (res); Mon '48; Obst. (P.Q.); Chief of Obst., Misericordia Hosp.; Assoc. Prof. (Obst.), U. of Montreal; **Tel. LA 6-1420.**
GAGNON, Alban J.; Med. Centre, Maria, P.Q.; Lav '55; GenSurg (P.Q.); Chief, Dept. of Surg., Notre-Dame de Chartres Hosp.; Med. Dir., Bathurst Paper Ltd., New Richmond; **Tel. 759-3481.**

GAGNON, Andre; 1063 ave.-St-Denis Montreal, P.Q.; 1283 Ave. St. Viateur, Outremont, Mtl. 8 (res); Lav '48; Ophth, Otol; Assoc. Staff (ORL), Hop.-St.-Luc; Cons. Hop.-Le Gardeur, Repentigny; Tel. 842-4816.

GAGNON, Andre; 3139 ave Royale, Quebec 5, P.Q.; Lav '59; Tel. 663-0889.

GAGNON, Armand J.; Elgin St., Bagotville, P.Q.; Lav '55; A.M.C.G.P.

GAGNON, Arthur P.; 5610 Plantagenet, Montreal, P.Q. (res); Mon '39; Biochem. (P.Q.); **Prof. of Biochemistry, U. of Montreal**; Tel. RE 3-9951.

GAGNON, Bernard; 391 Blvd. St. Madeleine, Cap-De-La Madeleine, P.Q.; Lav'51.

GAGNON, Camille; Macamic, P.Q. (res); Lav '50; Tel. 747-3230.

GAGNON, Charles; 1493 Mt. Royal Ave. E., Montreal, P.Q.; 757 Davaar Ave., Outremont (res); Mon '28; Pres. & Med. Dir., Hop. Crescent Inc.; **Pres., Quebec Private Hosp's.; Tel.** VI 9-4501.

GAGNON, Conrad; Ste 445, 3440 rue Ontario est, Montreal 4, P.Q.; 3163 rue Dickson (res); Mon '41; Pres., Assoc. Gen. Pract., Montreal; Tel. LA 2-3523.

GAGNON, Donat; Lav'62; Anaes; Staff, Hop. St. Joseph, Riviere-du-Loup, P.Q.

GAGNON, Edouard D.; C.P. 1003, 30 est Boul. St. Joseph, Montreal 14, P.Q.; Mon'42; M.S., FCCP, FRCS(C), GenSurg, ThorSurg; Head, Dept. of ThorSurg & Cardio. Vasc. Surg., Hop. Notre Dame; Cons. ThorSurg. & Head, Cardiac Surg., Queen Mary Vets' Hosp.; Cons. Surg. (Chest Dis.), Bruchesi Inst.; Assoc. Prof. Surg., U. of Montreal; Tel. LA 6-4441.

GAGNON, Fernand; 79 Blvd. Sacre-Coeur, St. Felicien, Co. Roberval, P.Q.; Lav '50; M.C.G.P.; Ass't. Med., St. Michel-de-Roberval.

GAGNON, Francois; 4413 ave des Roses, Orsainville, P.Q.; Lav'63.

GAGNON, Fraser; Inst. Med.-de-Chicoutimi, 475 Boul. Talbot, Chicoutimi, P.Q.; Lav '55; Int-Med. & Cardiol, (P.Q.).

GAGNON, Gabriel; Lav'61; Cardiol(P.Q.); Staff, Inst. de Cardiologie, 5415, boul. l'Assomption, Montreal 26, P.Q.

GAGNON, Georges; 37 Ave. Glencoe, Outremont, **Montreal 8, P.Q.; Mon '39; Ph.D.; Psy.; Tel. WE 2-0486.**

GAGNON, Georges H.; 3 ave Cote, Rimouski, P.Q.; Lav '60.

GAGNON, Gerard; Hotel Dieu St. Vallier, Chicoutimi, **P.Q.; 306 Ave. Labrecque (res); Lav '39;** D.A.B.S., F.A.C.S., F.I.C.S, GenSurg (P.Q.), ThorSurg (P.Q.), Gyn (P.Q.); Chief Surg., **Hotel-Dieu-St-Vallier; Assoc. Prof., Laval U.;** Tel. 549-1224.

GAGNON, Gilles; 1255 est Beaubien, Montreal 35, P.Q.; Lav '61.

GAGNON, Herve; 1645 Girouard, St.-Hyacinthe, P.Q.; 620-23rd St. (res); Lav '27; IntMed; M.C.-G.P.; 2nd. Vice President Coll. P. & S., (P.Q.); Dir. Indus. Med. Assoc. (P.Q.); Phys. Goodyear Tire & Rubber Co. & Kimberlyclark Can. Ltd.; Tel. PR 4-6060.

GAGNON, Irenee; Sayabac, Cte. Matapedia, P.Q.; Lav '40.

GAGNON, Jacques; Mon'65; Res., Hop. St. Jean de Dieu, Montreal 5, P.Q.

GAGNON, Jacques A.; 3025 Ouest, Boul. Gouin, Montreal 9, P.Q. (res); Mon '52; Path (P.Q.); Chief of Path, Hop.-Ste. Justine; Assoc. Prof. (Path), U. of Montreal; Tel. FE 4-3607 & 731-4931.

GAGNON, Jacques B.; 490-17eme rue, Grand-'Mere, P.Q.; Ott '54; FRCS(C); GenSurg.; Tel. LE 8-8740.

GAGNON, Jacques N.; 1264 Est Boul. St. Joseph, Montreal 34, P.Q.; Mon '43; F.I.C.S.; Obst. (P.Q.); Head of Dept. of Obst., & Cons., Hop. Misericorde; Ass't. Prof. (Obst.), U. of Montreal; Tel. LA 3-6835.

GAGNON, Jacques O.; 4395 Verdun Ave., Ver-**dun, Montreal 19, P.Q.; Mon '51; Gastroent (P. Q.); Tel. 769-4962.**

GAGNON, Jacques S.; 541 rue de l'Hopital, Jonquiere, P.Q.; Lav '52; GenSurg; Staff, Hop. Gen. **de Jonquiere; Tel. 547-9341.**

GAGNON, J. Anatole; St. Pamphile, Co. L'Islet, P.Q.; Lav '57.

GAGNON, J. Antoine; Lav'46; Intern c/o 5857 Chardin, St. Leonard Pt. Maurice, Montreal, P.Q.

GAGNON, Jean; Lav '60; Sr. Int'n., Hop-St-Sacrement, Quebec 6, P.Q.

GAGNON, Jean B.; 475 Blvd. Talbot, Chicoutimi, P.Q.; 799 rue Marie Victorin (res); Lav '49; IntMed (PQ); Hd. (Rheum.), Hotel-Dieu St.-Vallier; Tel. 549-0090.

GAGNON, Jean J.; 8415 St.-Denis, Montreal 11, **P.Q.; 1687 Charles-Falkner (res); Mon '54; Gen-Surg (P.Q.); Tel. DU 1-1801.**

GAGNON, Jean H.; Lav '60; DiagRad; Staff, Royal Victoria Hosp., Montreal, P.Q.; Dem. Mc-Gill U.; Tel. 842-1251.

GAGNON, Jean L.; 2319 Roussel, Chicoutimi-Nord, P.Q.; Lav '54; FRCS(C), GenSurg.

GAGNON, Jean L.; Lav '60; Anaes; Staff, Hop. Hotel-Dieu-St-Vallier, Chicoutimi, P.Q.; Tel. 549-1452.

GAGNON, Jean-Marcel; 21 Johnson, Granby, **P.Q.; 70 Grove (res); Lav '52; Cardiol (P.Q.);** Tel. FR 2-3211.

GAGNON, Joseph A.; Dal '58; Jr. Ass't. Res. (Path), Pathological Inst., Montreal, P.Q.

GAGNON, J. Raoul; 12 Ave. Desjardins, Matane, P.Q.; Lav '25; Dist. Coroner.

GAGNON, J. R. Paul; 2157 est Fleury, Montreal 12, P.Q.; 11305 rue Pasteur (res); Lav '42; MCGP;

GAGNON, Jules; 58 rue, Sacre-Coeur, Alma, P.Q.; Lav'57; Otol. (P.Q.); Tel. 662-7305.

GAGNON, Louis; 661 rue Murray, Sherbrooke, P.Q.; Lav '37 Coroner, Dist. St. Francis.

GAGNON, Louis; 1239-3ieme Ave., Quebec, P.Q.; Lav '43; Tel. 525-5248.

GAGNON, Louis F.; 402 St. Jean, Quebec, P.Q.; 220 Grande Allee (res); Lav '22; Prof. Gyn. Clinic, & Head of Dept. (Obst. Gyn.), Hop. St. **Sacrement; Tel. LA 7-3461.**

GAGNON, Marc; Mon '63; Res., Hop. Ste-Justine, Montreal 26, P.Q.

GAGNON, Marc A.; Lav '64; Res., Dept. of Pharmacology, Laval U., Quebec 10, P.Q.

GAGNON, Marc G.; 960 boul. Ste-Croix, Montreal 9, P.Q.; Mon '51; Obst; Staff, Ste-Justine Hop.; Tel. 747-3501.

GAGNON, Maurice; 110 boul Laurentides, Pont-Viau, Laval-des-Rapides, P.Q.; Mon '63; Tel. 663-4014.

GAGNON, Maurice; 355 rue Labrecque, Alma, Cte Lac-St-Jean, P.Q.; 290 rue Boivin (res); **Lav '50; Staff, Hotel-Dieu-du-Christ-Roi & Price** Brothers; Tel. 2-2713.

GAGNON, Michel; Lav'64; Res., Hop. Hotel-Dieu, Quebec 4, P.Q.

GAGNON, Michel; Mon '60; FRCP(C), Int-Med.; Staff, Hop.-Notre-Dame, Montreal, P.Q.

GAGNON, M. Paule; (See Tourillon, M. Paule).

GAGNON, Normand B.; 425 ave. Stuart, Montreal 8, P.Q.; Mon'58; Otol.

GAGNON, Normand; Lav'65; Res., Hop. L'Enfant-Jesus, Quebec 3, P.Q.

GAGNON, Omer; 3335 rue Montpetit, App. 1, Ste. Foy, P.Q.; IntMed(P.Q.); Gastroent(P.Q.).

GAGNON, Paul A.; Ste. 8, 222 Blvd. Henri **Bourassa, Montreal 12, P.Q.; Mon '52; Orth-Surg; Tel. DU 1-3380.**

GAGNON, Paul-Alcide; 3221 Place Helen-Boullé, Montreal, P.Q.; Mon'58; FRCS(C), OrthSurg.

GAGNON, Paul E.; 127 Grande Allee, Quebec, P.Q.; Lav '51.

GAGNON, Paul M.; 431 Durvenay, Sherbrooke, P.Q.; Lav'51; D.Sc. (Laval); FRCP(C), Path.

GAGNON, Pierre; Lav'65; Res., Hop. Jeffery Hale, Quebec 6, P.Q.

GAGNON, Pierre P.; 65 Grande Allee E., Quebec 4, P.Q.; Lav '50; GenSurg (P.Q.); FRCS(C), PlasSurg.; Tel. 529-9691.

GAGNON, Pierre-Paul; 22 rue Sacre-Coeur est, Alma, P.Q.; 153, boul Auger (res); Lav '58; Otol.; Tel. 662-4062.

GAGNON, Raymond M.; Sault au Mouton, Co. Saguenay, P.Q.; Lav '55.
GAGNON, Real; 1170 Champigny, St. Laurent, Montreal 9, P.Q. (res); Mon '51; Ph. D. (Mich.); **Prof., U. of Montreal; Tel. RE 3-9951.**
GAGNON, Robert F.; 72 Milford, Waterloo, Ont. (res); Lav '50; D & T Rad; Staff, St. Mary's Hosp.; Tel. 744-3311.
GAGNON, Roch; 600 Med. Arts Bldg., 1538 ouest, rue Sherbrooke, Montreal 25, P.Q.; Mon '60; Ophth; Ophth., Hop. Notre-Dame; Tel. 937-9296.
GAGNON, Rogath; 2421 boul du Carmel, Trois-Rivieres, P.Q.; Mon '58; Staff, Hop. Ste-Marie.
GAGNON, Roger; 138 King St., Thetford Mines, P.Q. (res); Lav '48; DiagRad; Rad., St. Joseph's **Hosp.; Tel. 418-2971.**
GAGNON, Roger; Ste. 201, 1656 est rue Sherbrooke. Montreal 24, P.Q.; Mon '51; GenSurg.; Tel. 521-2116.
GAGNON, Roger; 5593 Blvd. Gouin W., Montreal, P.Q.; 504 Blvd. des Rapides, Laval des Rapides (res); Mon '48; Anaes; Chief Anaes., Hop. du Sacre-Coeur; Prof. of Physiol., P. G. Course in **Anaes. & Ass't. Prof. of Anaes., U. of Montreal; Tel. FE 4-1210.**
GAGNON, Romeo; 921 Moissan St., Arvida, P.Q. (res); Lav '37; GenSurg (P.Q.); Chief of Surg., **Saguenay Gen. Hosp.; Tel. 548-8231.**
GAGNON, Romuald; 25 rue Elgin, Bagotville, P.Q.; 179A-8th Ave. (res); Lav '61; AMCGP.
GAHUNIA, Udhe S.; Manila (Philipp.)'62; Res., Winnipeg Gen. Hosp., Winnipeg, Man.
GAILIUS, Anselm T.; 9217 Glover, Fort Langley, B.C.; Alb '44; Tel. 534-5515. Abroad.
GAILLARD, Claude; 1265 est Boul. St. Joseph, **Montreal, P.Q.; Lav '40; GenSurg (P.Q.); Tel. LA 1-4464.**
GAIN, Donald B.; 1199 Austin Ave., New Westminster, B.C.; 945 Canyon Ct. (res); UBC'56; MCGP; Staff, Royal Columbian Hosp.; Tel. 939-7345.
GAIN, Edward A.; 8919-140th St., Edmonton, **Alta. (res); Alb '43; FACA; FRCP(C); Anaes Dir. (Dept. of Anaes), University Hosp.; Clin.** Prof. (Anaes), U. of Alberta; Tel. GE 9-5911. Ext. 473.
GAL, Kamill; Dept. of Path., New Mount Sinai Hosp., 550 University Ave., Toronto, Ont.; Budapest (Hung.) '52; Bact; Assoc. Dir. of Labs., New Mount Sinai Hosp.; Dem. (Path.), U. of Toronto; Abroad.
GAL, Stephen; Ottewell Plaza, 6138-90th Ave., Edmonton, Alta.; Budapest (Hung.)'52; Research Staff, U. of Alberta Hosp.
GAL, Veronica (Katona); Res. (Bact.), Hosp. for Sick Children, Toronto 2, Ont.; Abroad.
GALAMBOS, Michael; Budapest (Hung.) '55; Phys.-in-Charge, Saskatchewan Training School, P.O. Box 1240, Prince Albert, Sask.; Tel. 763-7401.
GALANTI, Arnaldo; Rome (Italy) '37; DiagRad; Staff, Dept. of Radiol., University Hosp., Edmonton, Alta.; Tel. 439-5911, Ext. 465.
GALARDO, Anthony T.; Mon '61; Res., Albert Prevost Inst., Montreal, P.Q.
GALBRAITH, Craig L.T.; 3091 W. Broadway, Vancouver 8, B.C.; UBC '56; MCGP; Att'd. Staff, Vancouver Gen. Hosp.; Tel. RE 3-7226.
GALBRAITH, Donald A.; Wes'61; Psy; Staff, Ontario Hosp., London, Ont.
GALBRAITH, Frank O.; Calgary Assoc. Clinic, 214-6th Ave. S.W., Calgary, Alta.; McG '29; FICS; GenSurg; MCGP; Tel. 263-7120.
GALBRAITH, H. Claire; Wes '50; Psy; Ass't. Supt., Ontario Hosp., London, Ont.; Instr. (Psy), **U. of Western Ont.; Tel. 455-5110.**
GALBRAITH, J. Douglas; Tor'35; IntMed(TB.); Staff, Dept. of National Health & Welfare, 12702-114th Ave., Edmonton, Alta.
GALBRAITH, Paul A.; Manitoba Clinic, 790 Sherbrook St., Winnipeg 2, Man.; Man' 56; M.Sc. (Med); FRCP(C), IntMed; Internist, Manitoba Clin., Dept. of Haem.; Att'd. Staff, Wpg. Gen. Hosp.; Clin. Instr. (Med.), U. of Manitoba; Tel. SP 4-6541.
GALBRAITH, Peter R.; Etherington Hall, Queen's University, Kingston, Ont.; 1108 Johnson St. (res); Qns '56; FRCP(C); IntMed; Att'd. Staff, Kingston Gen. Hosp.; Ass't. Prof., (Med.), Queen's U.; Tel. 546-1371, Loc. 508.
GALBRAITH, Ruth S.; 1108 Johnson St., Kingston, Ont.; Qns '57; Part-time Teach., Queen's Univ., Kingston.
GALE, Alan R.; Box 2135, Nipawin, Sask.; Box 297 (res); St. Andrew's (Scot.)'57; Tel. 2626.
GALE, Godfrey L.; 179 King St., Weston, Ont. **(res); Birmingham (Eng.) '35; FRCS(Edin.); Ass't. Surg., Toronto Hosp., for T.B., Weston;** Clin. Teach., U. of Toronto; Tel. RO 9-1162.
GALE, Herbert V. B.; Ste 801-802, 750 W. Broadway, Vancouver 9, B.C.; 1638-W. 20th Ave. (res); Alb '38; Tel. TR 6-2145
GALE, Robert A.; Ste. 450, Medical Arts Bldg., 1105 Pandora Ave., Victoria, B.C.; 3250 Weald Rd. (res); McG '47; M.C.G.P.; Active Staff, **Royal Jubilee Hosp. Tel. EV 3-3342.**
GALEA, Mario J.; Royal U. (Malta)'49; B.Sc (Oxon); Path(P.Q.); Staff, Lakeshore Gen. Hosp., Pointe Claire, P.Q.; Tel. 695-1310, Ext. 241.
GALIBOIS, Paul E.; 355-22eme rue, Quebec, P.Q.; Lav '43; Anaes; Staff (Anaes), Hop-de-l'Enfant **Jesus & Laval U.; Tel. 525-5846.**
GALIPEAU, Vianney; 12238 Notre Dame E., Pointe-aux-Trembles, Montreal, P.Q.; Mon '55; Tel. 635-3054.
GALIZIA, Edward J.; Box 10, Terrace, B.C.; London (Eng.)'61; Abroad.
GALL, D. Grant; Alb'65; Jr. Int., Vancouver Gen. Hosp., Vancouver 9, B.C.; Abroad.
GALL, Robert J.; McG'63; Res., Women's College Hosp., Toronto 5, Ont.
GALLAGHER, Donald J. P.; Haney, B.C.; Wes '48; M.C.G.P.
GALLAI, Zoltan; 643 Stuart Ave., Outremont, P.Q.; Geneva (Switz.) '38; Med. Adviser, Poulenc Ltd.; Tel. 271-6570.
GALLANT, Gilbert J.; Water St., Summerside, P.E.I.; 281 Schurman Ave. (res); Mon '44; **Anaes-in-Chief, Prince County Hosp.; Tel. 2-246.**
GALLANT, Joseph A.; 50 Dover St., Campbellton, N.B. (res); Dal '41; Supt. Prov. Hosp., Campbellton; Cons. Staff, Soldiers' Mem. & Hotel-**Dieu Hosp's; Tel. PL 3-4461.**
GALLANT, Omer J.; 2 St. Anne St., Shediac, N.B.; 25 Sackville St. (res); Lav '50.
GALLEGO, Miguel; 54 Brant Ave; Brantford Ont.; Valladolid (Spain)'53; Tel. 756-6333.
GALLET, Joseph P.; Box 220, Assiniboia, Sask.; Durham (Eng.)'54; FRCS(Eng.).
GALLIE, Hugh R.; 63 Academy Medical Bldg., 1812-14th St. W., Calgary, Alta.; 2918 Champlain St., (res); Tor '44; A.B.S., F.A.C.S., GenSurg; Att. Surg, Holy Cross, Calgary Gen., Alberta Children's & Col. Belcher Hosp's; Tel. 263-4495.
GALLIE, J. Gordon; 113 Buckingham Ave., Toronto, Ont.; Tor '10; Retired.
GALLIEN, Roger; Lav'65; Res., Hop. du St. Sacrement, Quebec 6, P.Q.
GALLIFORD, Brian W.; 816-103rd Ave., Dawson Creek, B.C.; UBC '64; Staff, St. Joseph's Gen. Hosp.; Tel. 782-4848.
GALLINGER, Angela A.; Man '46; Staff, Manitoba School, Box 1190, Portage-La-Prairie, Man.
GALLOWAY, Charles A.; 43 Dalton Cres. S., Orillia, Ont. (res); Qns '36; M.C.G.P.; Staff, **Ont. Hosp. School; Tel. 325-2175.**
GALLOWAY, G. D.; Main St., Oxbow, Sask.; Park St. (res); Man '45; M.C.G.P.
GALLOWAY, James D.; Wes'40; DHA; Med. Dir., St. Joseph's Hosp., Hamilton, Ont.; Field Surveyor, Cdn. Council on Hosp. Accreditation; Tel. 522-4941, Ext. 418.
GALLOWAY, Robert J. M.; 200 St. Clair Ave. W., Suite 220, Toronto, Ont.; 119 St. Leonard's Ave. (res); Tor '33; F.R.C.S.(E) & (C), GenSurg, OrthSurg; Surg., St. Joseph's Hosp.; Tel. WA 1-7100.
GALLOWAY, William R.; Assoc. Clinic, Box 669, Innisfail, Alta.; Edinburgh (Scot.) '46; Chief of Staff, Innisfail Municipal Hosp.; Tel. 227-3301.

GALSZECHY, **Julius C.; 310 Bloor St. W., Toronto 5, Ont.; Budapest (Hung.) '43; Tel. WA 3-2173.**
GALUTIRA, **Justo B.;** Santo Tomas (Philipp.)'57; Staff, Central Hosp., Grand Falls, Nfld.
GALWAY, **H. Paul; 1907 Baseline Rd., Ste. 2., Ottawa 3, Ont.; 1242 Stanton Rd. (res); Wes '59;** Paed; Tel. 725-2210.
GAMACHE, **Andre;** Lav'61; Psy; Staff, Hop Hotel Dieu, Levis, P.Q.
GAMACHE, **Andre;** Mon'65; Res., Hop du Christ Roi, Montreal 19, P.Q.
GAMACHE, **J. Paul, S/L;** Lav'55; Psy; 1 Cdn. Base Med. Unit, CFPO 5050, Cdn. Armed Forces, North-West Europe; Abroad.
GAMACHE, **Martin;** 32 Notre Dame est, Trois Pistoles, P.Q.; Lav'65.
GAMBLE, Charles S.; Calder Rd., Nanaimo, B.C. (res); McG '33; Staff, Nanaimo Indian Hosp. Tel. SK 3-4321.
GAMBLE, **Donald E.;** 2285 Carling Ave., Ottawa 14, Ont.; Tor '53; MCGP; Staff, Ottawa Civic Hosp.; Tel. 722-5351.
GAMBLE, **J. Errol;** 2285 Carling Ave., Ottawa 14, P.Q.; Tor'23; MCGP; Staff, Ottawa Civic & Grace Hosp's.; Tel. 722-5351.
GAMBLE, **Willard S.;** McG '59; Jr. Int'n., Montreal, Gen. Hosp., Montreal, P.Q.
GAMBLE, **W. J. Warren;** 291 Charlotte St., Peterborough, Ont.; 685 Walkerfield Ave. (res); Wes '49; M.C.G.P.: Staff, St. Joseph's & Civic Hosp's.: Tel. 742-8866.
GAMBOA, **Jose J.;** Neuvo Leon (Monterrey, Mexico) '57; Staff, Riverview Hosp., Essondale, B.C.; Tel. 521-1911.
GAMBRILL, R. Barry, Ste. 102, 396 Queen's Ave., London, Ont.; Wes '62; AMCGP; Tel. 433-3154.
GAMEZ-RUIZ, **David;** Box 308, Ste Pierre, Man.; Granada (Spain)'61.
GAMMIE, **Robert B.;** 46 Adam St., Hespeler, Ont.; Wes '44; MCGP; Staff, South Waterloo Mem. Hosp.; Med. Staff, Galt Mem. Hosp.
GAMULA, Stephan; Med. Arts Bldg., 420 East St. N., Sarnia, Ont.; Giessen (Germ.)'45; Tel. ED 7-5352.
GANDER, **T. A.;** 10004—105th St., Edmonton, Alta.; 9205—95th St. (res); Alb '40; F.A.A.P., Paed.; Attend. Staff, University of Alberta & **Royal Alexander Hosp's.; Assoc. Clin. Prof., U. of Alberta; Tel. GA 4-2121.**
GANDKIN, **Jacob;** Prague (Czech.)'25; Staff, Inst. Albert Prevost, 6555 boul. Gouin ouest, Montreal 9, P.Q.
GANGULI, **Adwaita K.;** Porters Lake, Hàlifax Co., N.S.; Calcutta (India)'49; GenSurg.
GANS, **Leo J.;** 407 Professional Bldg., 10830 Jasper Ave., Edmonton, Alta.; 9620-143rd St. (res); Alb '53; **ObstGyn;** Att'd. Staff, Misericordia & Gen. Hosp's.; Court. Staff, Royal Alexandra Hosp.; Sess. Instr., U. of Alberta; Tel. 422-6775.
GANS, **M. H.;** Tor'63; Res., Toronto Gen. Hosp., Toronto 2, Ont.
GANS, **Maurits;** 460 Main St., Exeter, Ont. (res)· Utrecht (Holl.) '50.
GANSHORN, **John A.;** 806 Fairmont Med. Bldg., 750 W. Broadway, Vancouver 9, B.C.; 5662 Laburnum St. (res); Man '32; M.S. (Surg.) (Minn.); GenSurg; Staff, Vancouver Gen. Hosp.; Clin. Ass't., U. of British Columbia; Tel. 875-5313.
GARAND, **Albert;** Mon '60; Anaes; Staff, Hop. Santa Cabrini, Montreal 36, P.Q.; Tel. CL 4-8311.
GARANT, L. Dollard; 225 Grande Allee E., Quebec 4, P.Q.; St. Anselme **(res); Lav '38; M.O. WCB (P.Q.); Tel. 522-4751.**
GARANT, **Oscar,** 32 Cote de la Fabrique, Quebec, P.Q.; 194 Ave. Brown (res); Lav '29; ObstGyn; Chief of Obst. & Gyn., Hotel Dieu; Prof. Gyn., Laval U.; **Tel. 529-9151.**
GARBE, William; 99 Avenue Rd., Toronto 5, Ont.; 11 Brownside Ave. (res); Tor '32; ABD; DermSyph; Sr. Att'd. Staff, New Mount Sinai Hosp.; Lect., School of Hygiene; Tel. WA 3-9809.
GARBER, Hyman; 4249 Ave. Esplanade, Montreal, P.Q.; McG '20; Otol.; Tel. VI 4-1257.
GARBUTT, **C. T. Percival;** 702 Coxwell Ave., Toronto 13, Ont.; 15 Douglas Dr. (res); Tor'18; **Tel. HO 6-9553.**
GARCEAU, **Eugene;** 406 Pine Ave. W., Montreal **18, P.Q.; Mon '27; DermSyph; Tel. VI 5-1398.**
GARCIA, **Eusebio;** Links Assoc. Clinic, 10951-124th St., Edmonton, Alta.; Madrid (Spain)'54; Staff, Royal Alexandra Hosp.; Tel. 454-4551.
GARCIA, **Liborio C.;** Res., Notre-Dame Mem. Hosp., Twillingate, Nfld.
GARCIA-MARTIN, **Alberto;** Queensway Medical Centre, 880 Queensway, Toronto 18, Ont.; Madrid (Spain) '51; GenSurg; Staff, Hamilton Gen. **Hosp., Hamilton, Ont.; Tel. CL 5-1161.**
GARD, Myrle A.; 581 Roberta, Winnipeg 15, Man.; Man '55; Anaes; Staff, Assoc. of Anaes; Dem. (Anaes.), U. of Manitoba; Tel. 943-7682.
GARDI, **Vito A.;** 162 Gore St., Sault Ste. Marie, Ont.; 124 Lake St. (res); Tor '29; Retired.
GARDINER, Douglas M.; 6039 Buckingham Ave., Burnaby, B.C.; Birmingham (Eng.)'56; Anaes; Staff, St. Mary's Hosp., New Westminster.
GARDINER, Harold M.; Minto, N.B.; Qns '27; M.C.G.P.; Dist. Coroner.
GARDINER, John H.; 25 Leonard Ave., Toronto 2B, Ont.; 3 Glenwood Terr. (res); Tor '43; DMRD; DiagRad; Paed; Act. Att'd. Staff, Toronto Western Hosp.; Clin. Instr., (Rad.), U. of Toronto; Tel. EM 3-1197.
GARDINER, Patricia A. (See Radcliffe).
GARDINER, Robert J.; Wes'61; Res., Montreal Gen. Hosp., Montreal, P.Q.
GARDINER, William A.; 320 Painted Post Dr., **Scarborough Ont.; 23 Burnview Cr., (res); Dal** '52; Staff, Scarborough Gen. Hosp.; Tel. AT 2-3471.
GARDINER, William J.; Tor '26; M.R.C.P. (Eng.), F.R.C.P.(C), PhysMed; Dir., Dept. of Phys. Med., Toronto Gen. Hosp.; Ass't. Prof. **(Therapeutics); U. of Toronto; Tel. EM 6-8211.**
GARDNER, Alexander J.; 213 Augustus St., Cornwall, Ont.; Liverpool (Eng.) '22; M.B., B.Ch.
GARDNER, Carstairs C.; 213 Medical Arts Bldg., 300 King St. W., Oshawa, Ont.; 981 Colborne St. E. (res); Edinburgh (Scot.) '40; F.R.C.S.(Edin.), F.A.C.S., F.R.C.S.(C), GenSurg; Surg., Oshawa Gen. Hosp.; Tel. 725-5844.
GARDNER, Elizabeth K. (Baker); R.C.P.S. (Lond.) '40; M.R.C.S., L.R.C.P.; M.O., Westminster DVA Hosp., London, Ont.; Tel. 432-6711, Loc. 331.
GARDNER, Harvey A.; Tor '61; Jr. Intn., New Mount Sinai Hosp., Toronto 2, Ont.
GARDNER, John S.; 3209 - 6th St. S.W., Calgary, Alta.; Alb'34; FACS, FRCS(C), GenSurg; Chief of Serv. (Surg), Col. Belcher Hosp. (DVA); Tel. AM 6-6760.
GARDNER, Lawrence G.; Box 80, Elkhorn, Man.; Edinburgh (Scot.)'62.
GARDNER, Patrick S.; 24 Archibald Ave., North Sydney, N.S.; 15 Queen St. (res); London U. (Eng.) '42; MRCS, LRCP; MRCOG; ObstGyn; Sr. Staff, St Elizabeth's Hosp.; Tel. 794-2264.
GARDNER, William; 1940 Lonsdale Ave., North Vancouver, B.C.; Glasgow (Scot.)'51; M.B., Ch.B.; DPM; Psy; Med. Spec., Provincial Mental Health Serv.; Staff, Riverview Hosp., Essondale; Tel. 987-0433.
GARDNER, William A.; 1158 Grosvenor, Winnipeg, Man. (res); McG '02; FACS; Retired.
GARDNER, W. P.; 250 Lawrence Ave. W., Ste 314, Toronto, Ont.; Tor '64; Staff, St. Joseph's Hosp.; Tel. 787-3771.
GARE, Douglas J.; 62 Glengarry Ave., Toronto 12, Ont.; Tor'60; FRCS(C), ObstGyn; Staff, Toronto Gen. Hosp.; Clin. Instr., U. of Torónto; Tel. EM 6-8211.
GAREAU, Emile P.; 830 Pierre Maufay, Ste. Foy, Quebec 10, P.Q.; Lav '50; Pulm. Dis. & TB (P.Q.); Cardiol. (P.Q.); Staff, Hop. Laval; Tel. 527-4162.
GAREAU, Jacques Y.; 350 rue Selby, Westmount, Montreal, P.Q.; Mon'57; AMCGP; Med. Dir., Charles E. Frosst & Co.; Staff, O.P.D., Queen Mary Vet's. Hosp.; Tel. 932-7111.

GAREAU, Robert; 960 boul Ste-Croix, Montreal 9, P.Q.; Mon '51; Tel. RI 7-6890.
GAREAU, Roger J.; 5535 Place d'Aiguillon, Montreal 9, P.Q. (res); Mon '48; Path (PQ); Staff, Hop.-Hotel-Dieu; Ass't. Prof., U. of Montreal; Tel. FE 4-0490.
GAREAU, Roland; 4167 Blvd. Lasalle, Verdun, P.Q.; 1112 Beatty (res); Mon '38; IntMed (P.Q.), Gastroent, (P.Q.); Gastroent. & Proct., Verdun Gen. Hosp.; Tel. 769-0202.
GAREAU, Serge; 106 Dussault, Laval-des-Rapides, Montreal 40, P.Q.; Mon '57. DiagRad.; Tel. 681-2832.
GAREAU, Urban J.; Medical Arts Clinic, 2125—11th Ave., Regina, Sask.; 55 Turgeon St. (res); McG '19; Paed; Head of Paed. Dept., Regina Gen. Hosp.; Cons. (Paed.), U. of Saskatchewan; Retired; Tel. LA 2-1811.
GAREAU, U. Paul; 316 Cook Medical Bldg., 1175 Cook St., Victoria, B.C.; McG'53; FRCS(C), PlasSurg; Active Staff, Royal Jubilee & St. Joseph's Hosp's. & Nanaimo Reg. Gen. Hosp., Nanaimo; Tel. 388-5222.
GARFIELD, Harry D.; The Doctors' Bldg., 394 Graham Ave., Winnipeg 1, Man.; Man '55; FICS; DiagRad.; Tel. 943-5144.
GARIEPY, Claude; Mon'65; Res., Hop. Maisonneuve, 5415 Boul. L'Assomption, Montreal, P.Q.
GARIEPY, Gilles; Mon'65; Res., Hop. Notre-Dame, Montreal 24, P.Q.
GARIEPY, J. Jacques; 145 Champlain, Hull, P.Q.; Lav '46.
GARIEPY, J. Jacques; Mon '64; Int., Hop. Notre-Dame, Montreal 18, P.Q.
GARIEPY, L. Henri; 520 rue Cherrier, Montreal, P.Q.; 70 Ave. Goodson, Dorval (res); Mon '21; F.R.C.P.(C), IntMed; Cons. Phys., Notre Dame Hosp.; Tel. VI 4-8411.
GARIEPY, Roger; Ste. 409, 3875 St. Urbain, Montreal 18, P.Q.; 3855 Maplewood (res); Mon '38; F.R.C.S.(C), Orth Surg; Chief, Dept. of Orth. Surg., Hotel Dieu de Montreal; Ass't., Orth., Hop. Sacre-Coeur, Cartierville; Ass't. Prof. Orth. Surg., U. of Montreal; Tel. LA 4-1119.
GARLAND, J. M. Boyd; Box 631, Brantford, Ont.; Glasgow (Scot.) '51; Anaes; Active Cons. Staff (Anaes.), Brantford Gen. Hosp., St. Joseph's Gen. Hosp. & Willet Hosp. Paris; Tel. 753-4492.
GARNEAU, Georges; 300 St. Louis Sq., Montreal, P.Q., & 5 Blvd. Taschereau, Pont-Viau; 6 Corbeil Terrace, Laval-des-Rapides (res); Lav '34; IntMed (P.Q.), Cardiol (P.Q.); Cardiol., Ste. Jeanne d'Arc Hosp., Montreal; Tel. VI 5-7309.
GARNEAU, Jean F.; 5430 des Sapins, Montreal 36; P.Q. (res); Lav '54; Anaes (P.Q.); Staff, Hop.-Maisonneuve; Tel. 254-8341.
GARNEAU, Jean-Jacques; 3781 Boulv. Laviolette, Trois Rivieres, P.Q. (res); Lav '41; MACR; D&T Rad; DiagRad (P.Q.); Chief, Dept. of Rad. & Cancer Clinic, St. Joseph's Hosp. & Hop. Cooke; Cons. Hop. Ste Marie & Hop. Clouthier; Tel. FR 4-6211.
GARNEAU, Noel; Mon'62; Psy; Staff, Ste-Justine Hosp., Montreal 26, P.Q.
GARNEAU, Robert P.; 2770 Blvd. Liégeois, Ste. Foy, Quebec 6, P.Q. (res); Lav '50; F.R.C.P.(C), Path; Chief Pathol., Hop. St. Sacrement; Assoc. Prof. Med., Laval U.; Tel. LA 7-3461.
GARNER, F. O. Roswell; c/o TB Control, 2647 Willow St., Vancouver 9, B.C.; 1705 W. 58 Ave., Vancouver 14 (res); Tor '34; D.P.H., P.H.; Dir., Travelling Clinics, Div. of TB Control, Dept. of Health, B.C.; Clin. Instr. (Med.), U. of British Columbia; Tel. TR 4-2331.
GARNER, Henry L. C.; Moose Jaw Clinic, 200 Scott Block, Moose Jaw, Sask.; 1116-2nd Ave. N.W. (res); Tor'43; IntMed; Tel. 692-2373.
GARNER, Mary K.; 925 W. Georgia, Vancouver B.C.; 1865 Quilchena Cres. (res); Man'41; MCGP; Tel. MU 5-0932.
GARNER, Richard W.; 100B-S. 3rd Ave., Port Alberni, B.C.; 311 Redford St. (res); Northwestern U. (USA) '32; GenSurg; Tel. 723-6211.
GARNHUM, Daniel G.; Stanley, York Co., N.B.; Dal'62; MCGP.

GARON, Jean; 298 Labelle, St.-Jerome, P.Q.; 594 Parent Ave. (res); Mon '45; Med. Bd. Hop.- Hotel-Dieu-de-St.-Jerome; Tel. 432-4301.
GARON, Nantel; 1762 St. Joseph, Lachine, P.Q.; Mon '39; Obst (P.Q.); Obst., Hop. St. Joseph de Lachine; Prof., Nursing Schl.; Tel. 637-6201.
GARRETSON, Henry D.; Neurological Inst., 3801 University Ave., Montreal 2, P.Q.; Harvard (U.S.A.)'54.
GARRETT, Douglas A.; Acton, Ont.; Tor '39; Staff, Guelph Gen. & St. Joseph's Hosp., Guelph; Tel. 853-0341.
GARRETT, D. Royden; 59 John St., Weston, Toronto 15, Ont. (res); Tor '29; FACCP, IntMed (T.B.); Phys., Toronto Hosp., Weston; Tel. CH 1-2053.
GARRIOCH, Henry G.; 626 Main St., Penticton, **B.C.; 445 Scott (res); McG '23; GenSurg.; Tel.** 492-3823.
GARRIOCK, James; 72 Pine St., Woodbridge, Ont.; Tor'51; MCGP; Vice-Pres. Med. Staff, Peel Mem. Hosp.; Vol. Ass't. (Med.), OPD, Toronto Gen. Hosp.; Tel. AT 8-0451.
GARRISON, T. W.; Fairview, Alta.; **Alb '41.**
GARRITY, James, S/L; National U. (Ire.) '57; Sr. Med. Officer, RCAF Station, Downsview, Ont.
GARROW, Barbara M. (Allan); 515 Fairmont Med. Bldg., 750 W. Broadway, Vancouver 9, B.C.; UBC '58; FRCP(C); Neur; Staff, Vancouver Gen. Hosp. & Shaughnessy Mil. Hosp.; Clin. Instr. Med., U. of British Columbia; Tel. TR 4-3334.
GARROW, David G.; 3590 Hudson St., Vancouver, B.C. (res); St. Andrews (Scot.) '49; D.M.-R.D., D.T.M.&H.; DiagRad; Rad. Staff, Vancouver Gen. Hosp.; Clin. Inst. (Rad.), U. of British Columbia; Tel. TR 9-4177.
GARSON, James E.; Box 1272, Saskatoon, **Sask.; 1922 Cairns Ave. (res); Madras (India) '35; LRCP: MRCS; Tel. 242-6166.**
GARSON, John Z.; Community Health Service Med. Clinic, 214 Avenue Bldg., 220-3rd Ave. S., Saskatoon, Sask.; 1028 University Dr. (res); London (Eng.)'46; DCH; MCGP; Assoc. Staff Saskatoon City & St. Paul's Hosp's.; Tel. 652-**0300.**
GARSON, Ronald D.; 161 Autumnwood Dr., Port Arthur, Ont. (res); Aberdeen (Scot.)'53; MCGP; Tel. DI 4-7271.
GARTHA, Ivan V.; Ste. 114, 400 Walmer Rd., Toronto 10, Ont.; Budapest (Hung.)'40; Med. Dir., Providence Hosp.; Court. Staff, St. Michael's Hosp.; Tel. 925-7313.
GARTHA, Susan (Vamos); 288 St. Claire Ave. W., Toronto 7, Ont.; Budapest (Hung.) '50; Paed; Staff, Hospital for Sick Children; Tel. 925-0809.
GARVEY, Julius W.; McG '61; Jr. Int., Royal Victoria Hosp., Montreal 2, P.Q.
GARVEY, M. Bernadette; Ott '60; FRCP(C), IntMed; Staff, St. Michael's Hosp., Toronto, Ont.; Abroad.
GARVIN, Kenneth; Qns '61; Res., Ottawa Civic Hosp., Ottawa, Ont.
GARVOCK, William B.; 3094 Danforth Ave., **Scarborough, Ont.; Qns' 54; Tel. 691-7912.**
GARWOOD, Gordon; 57 Erie St. N., Leamington, Ont.; 22 Danforth Ave. (res); Wes '53; Tel. FA 6-4711.
GARWOOD, John S.; Westwood Clinic, 3220 Portage Ave., Winnipeg 22, Man.; 8 Main St., Headingley (res); Durham (Eng.) '55; M.O.H., Brooklands; Tel. 832-1363.
GASCON, Bernard; 30 est boul. St. Joseph, Montreal 14, P.Q.; 8313B St.-Denis, Mtl. 11 (res); Mon'60; AMCGP; Tel. 274-7644.
GASCON, Jacques; Ste. 1012, 30 est, boul. St. Joseph, Montreal 34, P.Q.; Mon'55; IntMed; Teach. Staff, Hop. Notre-Dame; Tel. 845-0282.
GASCON, L. Phillippe; 440 L'Ange-Gardien, L'Assomption, P.Q.; **Mon '39.**
GASCON, Pauline M.; 1558 Ouellette Ave., Windsor, Ont.; Ott '61.
GASCON, Rene; 791 Legendre Est., Montreal 11, P.Q.; Mon '63; Tel. 388-8411.
GASEWICZ, Stanley A.; 2880 King St. E., Stoney Creek, Ont.; Wes'61; MCGP; Tel. 662-2222.

GASKELL, Peter; 826 Campbell St., Winnipeg, Man. (res); Wes '50; Ph.D. (Physiol., London); Staff, Clin Invest Unit, Wpg. Gen. Hosp.; Assoc. Prof., Dept. Physiol. & Med. Research, U. of Manitoba; Tel. GR 4-9110.
GASMANN, Henry C.; Qns '56; Staff, Deep River River Hosp., Deep River, Ont.; Tel. JU 4-3333.
GASS, Charles L.; Sackville, N.B.; Dal '19; IntMed; MCGP; Retired.
GASS, David A.; Moose Jaw Clin., 200 Scott Bldg., Moose Jaw, Sask.; 743 Elizabeth (res); Dal '52; MCGP; Tel. 692-2373.
GASS, George D.; Sackville Med. Centre, Sackville, N.B. 128 York St. (res); Dal '44; FACP; IntMed; Head, Dept. of Med. Sackville Mem. Hosp.; Tel. 536-0210.
GASS, K. V.; Pugwash, N.S.; Dal '53.
GASTLE, Hugh E.; Smith St. Lakefield, Ont.; Qns '44; M.C.G.P.; Staff, Civic & St. Joseph's Hosp's., Peterborough, Lakefield Private Hosp. & Apsley Red Cross Hosp.; M.O.H., Lakefield;
GATES, R. T.; Brigden, Ont.; Tor '39; M.C.G.P.
GATFIELD, Paul D.; 69 Hunt Club Rd., London, Ont.; Qns '57; Psy; Staff, Children's Psych. Research Inst.
GATFIELD, William T.; 1522 Ouellette Ave., Windsor, Ont.; 3654 Bruce (res); Qns '53; Paed; Tel. CL 6-8652.
GATIEN, Louis H.; 650 - 16th St., Lachine, **P.Q.; Mon '37; Anaes; Med. Dir., Hop.-St. Joseph. Tel. 637-2351.**
GATIEN, Romuald; 2185 Est rue Sherbrooke, Montreal 24, P.Q.; 268 St. Louis Sq. (res); Mon '21; Staff, Hotel Dieu; Assoc. Prof., U. of Montreal; Tel. LA 4-7353.
GATTEREAU, Antoine; Lausanne (Switz.) '60; FRCP(C), IntMed; Staff, Hop. Hotel Dieu, Montreal, P.Q.; Abroad.
GAUDET, Albert; 240 rue Elm, St.-Lambert, Cite-Jacques-Cartier, P.Q.; Mon '49; OrthSurg.; Tel. 672-1212.
GAUDET, Leonard J.; 113 rue Alma, Moncton, N.B.; Lav '36; MCGP; Surg., Hotel-Dieu-d'Edmunston; Tel. EV 4-7146.
GAUDET, Louis; Little Brook, N.S.; Lav'65.
GAUDET, Oliver P.; 535 Lafleur, LaSalle, P.Q.; 8543 Terrasse Georges (res); Lav '55; Tel. DO 6-2480.
GAUDET, Paul E.; Tracadie, N.B.; Lav '49; M.C.G.P.
GAUDET, Richard; Edifice Continental, 111 King W., Sherbrooke, P.Q.; 1267 Ave. Portland (res); Lav '19; F.A.C.S., F.I.C.S., GenSurg; Surg., Hop. St. Vincent de Paul & Hotel-Dieu; Tel. 562-5330.
GAUDETTE, Claude-E.; 22 ave. Bussieres, Vercheres, P.Q.; Mon '59; Tel. LU 3-3982.
GAUDETTE, Jean P.; 222 Blvd. Henri Bourassa E. Montreal 12, P.Q.; Mon '54; PlasSurg (P.Q.); Tel. DU 8-3752
GAUDIN, Donald A.; 204 Cook Med. Bldg., 1175 Cook St., Victoria, B.C.; 509 Foul Bay Rd. (res); Alb '56; OrthSurg; Tel. EV 2-5613.
GAUDIN, Frank H.; 624-6th St. New Westminster, B.C.; 540 Webster Ave. (res); Tor '27; DABP; Paed; Staff, Royal Columbian & St. Mary's Hosp's.; Tel. LA 1-1213.
GAUDIN, Melvin L.; Ste. 301, 625-5th Ave., New Westminster, B.C.; Alb'34; MRCOG; FRCS(C), ObstGyn.
GAUDREAU, Claude; 69 St. Francois, Edmundston, N.B.; 45 rue Beaulieu (res); Lav '50; FACS; FRCS(C), GenSurg; Chief Surg., Hop.-Hotel-Dieu-d'Edmunston; Tel. RE 5-3361.
GAUDREAU, Jacques,; Lav '57; Res., Hotel-Dieu, St-Vallier, Chicoutimi, P.Q.
GAUDREAU, J. B.; 14 rue Emerson, Edmundston, N.B.; Lav '34.
GAUDREAU, Noel; St. Jean-de-Dieu, Riviere-du-Loup, P.Q.; Lav '60.
GAUDREAULT, Jean R.; 8 Fafard, Baie-St-Paul, P.Q.; Lav '53; MCGP.
GAUDREAULT, Leonce; 1087 D'Avaugour, Val-de-Grace, Chicoutimi, P.Q. (res); Lav '42; P.H. **(P.Q.); Staff, Dept. of Health; Tel. 549-1193.**
GAUDREAULT, Yvon; Cap-d'Espoir, P.Q.; Lav '59.
GAUK, Ehor W.; Baker Clinic, 10004-105th St., Edmonton, Alta.; Man'58; B.Sc.(Med.); FRCP-(C), Paed; Staff, Royal Alexandra Hosp.; Court. Staff, U. of Alberta Hosp.; Sess. Instr., U. of Alberta; Tel. 474-3431.
GAUKRODGER, William T.; 180 Metcalfe St., Ottawa, Ont.; Box 349, R.R. 2 (res); Qns '53; FACS; A.B.O.; Ophth; Ass't. Surg., Ottawa Civic Hosp.; Lect., Clin. Ophth., Ottawa U.; Tel. CE 3-9321.
GAULD, Dorothy M.; Tor '58; Psy; Staff, Ontario Hosp., Toronto 14, Ont.
GAULD, E. Norman; 193 James St. S., Hamilton, Ont.; 1474 Scenic Drive (res); Aberdeen (Scot.) '37; M.R.C.P. (Lond.); F.A.C.C.P.; IntMed; Chief of Med., Chedoke Gen. Hosp.; Phys., Hamilton Gen. Hosp.; Cons. Phys., Brow Infirm; Tel. JA 8-3168.
GAULD, Flora (See Little)
GAULIN, Pierre; 545 King Edward Ave., Ottawa 2, Ont.; 416 Meadow Dr. (res); Ott '51; Urol; Chief, Dept. of Urol., Ottawa Gen. Hosp. & U. of Ottawa; Tel. 234-2938.
GAULIN, Robert; Ste Famille, Ile d'Orleans, P.Q.; Lav **'34**
GAULT, Mathew H.; 492 Lansdowne Ave., Westmount, Montreal 6, P.Q.; McG'54; IntMed; Dir., Dept. of Med. Chem. & Renal Serv., Queen Mary Vet's. Hosp.; Ass't. Outdoor Clinics & Cons. Renal Serv., Royal Victoria Hosp.; Research Ass't., Royal Victoria Hosp. & McGill U.; Dir. of Lab., Rehab. Inst.; Tel. RE 8-9481.
GAUM, Abraham R.; 820 Victoria Rd., Sydney, N.S.; 18 Howe St. (res); Dal'34; FICS; GenSurg; Tel. 564-8361.
GAUM, David; 820 Victoria Rd., Sydney, N.S.; Dal'43; Tel. 564-8361.
GAUM, Winston E.; Dal'65; Res., Montreal Children's Hop., Montreal 25, P.Q.
GAUMONT, Yves; Lav'65; Intern. c/o App. 6, 370 des Bouleaux ouest, Quebec 3, P.Q.
GAURON, Jean G.; 98-5th Ave., Ville St. Pierre, **Lachine, P.Q.; McG '56; Tel. 489-3666.**
GAUTAMA, Ved. B.; Northgate Med. Centre, Albert St. & 9th Ave. N., Regina, Sask.; R.C.P. & S. (Dublin, Ire.)'54; LRCP; LRCS(I); Staff, Regina Gen. & Grey Nuns Hosp's.; Tel. 568-2257.
GAUTHIER, Andre; 5079 est, Ste-Catherine, **Montreal 4, P.Q.; Mon '63; Tel. 256-2017.**
GAUTHIER, Bernard; 32 W. Blvd. St. Joseph, Montreal 14, P.Q.; 2240 Sheridan Rd., Ville Mont-Royal (res); Mon '47; OrthSurg; Ass't. (Orth.), Hop. Ste-Justine; Med. Staff, Victor Dore School for Sick Children; Tel. VI 2-9418.
GAUTHIER, Cajetan; R.R. No. 1, Montmagny, P.Q. (res); Lav '41; F.R.C.S.(C) GenSurg; Chief, **Dept. of Surg., Hop. Hotel-Dieu, Montmagny; Tel. 636.**
GAUTHIER, Charles A.; 1630 Chemin Gomin, Quebec, P.Q. (res); Lav '26; NeurPsy; Med. Dir., Dir. NeurPsy Clin., & Chief, Dept. of NeurPsy., Hop. de l'Enfant Jesus; Prof. Deontology & Med. Economics, Laval U.; Tel. 529-8711.
GAUTHIER, Denis; 581, boul des Laurentides, Pont-Viau, Laval-des-Rapides, P.Q.; Mon '64; Tel. 669-7334.
GAUTHIER, Fernand; 836, des Ursulines, Trois-Rivieres, P.Q.; Lav '58; ObstGyn (P.Q.); Tel. 378-4788.
GAUTHIER, Gaetan; 6 St-Jean Baptiste, Valleyfield, P.Q. (res); Mon '48; D.P.H.; P.H. (P.Q.); Staff, Dept. of Health, Valleyfield.
GAUTHIER, Georges A.; 7820 Marquette, Montreal 35, P.Q.; Lav'52; AMCGP.
GAUTHIER, Georges E.; 3875 St.-Urbain, Ste. 215, Montreal, P.Q.; 1630 Norway Rd., Ville-Mt. Royal (res); Mon'50; Urol(P.Q.); Staff, Hop.-Hotel-Dieu; Cons. Hop. Notre-Dame de l'Esperance; Tel. VI 5-2409.
GAUTHIER, Georges-Thomas; 627 Jacques Cartier E., Chicoutimi, P.Q.; Lav '38; Ophth; Otol. (P.Q.); Staff, Hotel-Dieu-St.-Vallier & Laval U.; Tel. 549-1452.
GAUTHIER, Gerard; 4395 Verdun Ave., Verdun & 5003 rue St. Denis, Montreal, P.Q.; 447 Stuart, Outremont (res); Mon '36; Gyn (P.Q.); Staff, Hop. Gen. de Verdun; Tel. 769-4811.

GAUTHIER, Germain J. E.; 1100 Main St. W., Hamilton, Ont.; 2 Grant Blvd., Dundas (res); Ott'63; Tel. 529-0913.

GAUTHIER, Guy; Saint-Michel des Saints, Cte. Berthier, P.Q.; Mon '47.

GAUTHIER, Herman; Saint-Georges San., Mont-Joli, P.Q. (res); Mon '34; F.A.C.C.P., Pulm. Dis. & TB (P.Q.), IntMed (T.B.); Med. Dir. & Adm., Saint-Georges San.; Tel. PR 5-4355.

GAUTHIER, Isidore M.; C. P. 10, Delisle, P.Q., Lav '30; Tel. 347-3005.

GAUTHIER, Jacques; 3423 St.-Denis, Montreal 18, P.Q.; 10612 d'Auteuil (res); Mon '55; Gyn (P.Q.); Haem. (P.Q.);

GAUTHIER, Jacques; 1165 Maguire, Sillery, Quebec 6, P.Q. (res); Lav '34; D.P.H., PH (P.Q.); Staff, Dept. Health, Parliament Bldgs., Quebec; Tel. LA 4-8411.

GAUTHIER, J. Charles A.; 1105 de Montigny, Sillery, Quebec, P.Q.; Lav '26; D.P.H.; Tel. LA 4-8411.

GAUTHIER, J. Dominique; 217 Premier Ave., Shippegan, N.B.; Lav'38; Ph.D.; M.C.G.P.; Prof. of Biol., Shippegan J.M. College; Tel. 336-2222.

GAUTHIER, Jean; St. Ubald, Cte. Portneuf, P.Q.; Lav '59.

GAUTHIER, Jean I.; C. P. 100, Delisle, P.Q.; Lav '59.

GAUTHIER, Jean J.; Mon'65; Res., Hop. Notre Dame, 1560 Est Sherbrooke, Montreal, P.Q.

GAUTHIER, Jean P.; 200 Beaupre, l'Assomption, P.Q.; Mon '62.

GAUTHIER, Jean-Pierre; Maria, Co. Bonnaventure, P.Q.; DiagRad(P.Q.).

GAUTHIER, J. Leon; 1051 rue St. Andre, Actonvale, P.Q.; Lav '11; Retired.

GAUTHIER, Joseph E. R.; 1645 Ainsley Dr., Ottawa, Ont.; Lav'59; Ophth.

GAUTHIER-LEBLANC, Therese; 193 Rue Notre-Dame, Maniwaki, P.Q.; Ott'51; MCGP; Tel. 555.

GAUTHIER, Louis J.; 3095 Sherbrooke St. E., Montreal, P.Q.; Mon '42; Paed (P.Q.); Staff, Pasteur Hosp.; Ass't. Prof. (Paed.), U. of Montreal; Tel. LA 3-1173.

GAUTHIER, Louis-Z.; Apt. 9, 4100 Chemin Ste. Catherine, Montreal 26, P.Q.; Lav '17; Retired.

GAUTHIER, Michel; 64 ave Begin, Levis, P.Q.; 13 du Parc (res); Lav '56; FRCS(C), GenSurg; Tel. 837-4356.

GAUTHIER, Michel; 1038 St.-Louis, Joliette, P.Q.; Mon '35.

GAUTHIER, Michel; 40 ouest Racine, Chicoutimi, P.Q.; Lav '26; PhysMed (P.Q.).

GAUTHIER, Patrice; 214 rue King W., Sherbrooke, P.Q.; Lav '43; OphthOtol (P.Q.); Staff, Hop. St. Vincent de Paul; Head of Studies, Nurses Schl., St. Vincent de Paul; Tel. 567-7682.

GAUTHIER, Paul-Andre; Lav'64; Res., Inst. Albert Prevost, Montreal 9, P.Q.

GAUTHIER, Paul J.; 956 est rue Sherbrooke, Montreal, P.Q.; 122 Ave. Maplewood, Outremont (res); Mon '37; F.I.C.S., Gyn; Sr. Ass't. (Gyn.), Hop. Notre Dame; Ass't. Prof. (Gyn.), U. of Montreal; Tel. LA 3-7376.

GAUTHIER, Pierre; 2692 Blvd. Pie IX, Montreal 4, P.Q.; Lav '21; Tel. CL 9-7511.

GAUTHIER, Pierre; Mon '64; Res., Hop. Ste-Justine, Montreal 26, P.Q.

GAUTHIER, Pierre-E.; 412 Blvd. desPrairies, Laval des Rapides, P.Q. (res); Mon '49; Pulm. Dis. & TB (P.Q.); Phys.-in-Charge, Broncho.-Oesoph., Hop. Sacre-Coeur. & Hop. Ste-Justine; Tel. FE 4-1210.

GAUTHIER, Pierre G.; 3142 Parkville, Montreal 5, P.Q.; Mon'60.

GAUTHIER, Raymond; 7940 Notre Dame E., Montreal, P.Q.; Mon '41; Phys., Cdn. Arsenals Ltd.; Tel. MI 5-9283.

GAUTHIER, Rejean; Mon '63; Res., Hop. Maisonneuve, Montreal, P.Q.

GAUTHIER, Rene; 6879 St. Denis, Montreal 10, P.Q.; Mon '32; Otol. (P.Q.); Tel. 277-0509.

GAUTHIER, Roger; 1053 St.-Andre, Acton-Vale, P.Q.; 1154 Dubois (res); Mon '50.

GAUTHIER, Roland; C.P. 850, 287 St.-Jerome, Matane, P.Q.; 10 St.-Joseph (res); Lav'43.

GAUTHIER, Roland; 2331 ouest Galt, Sherbrooke, P.Q.; Mon'60; AMCGP.

GAUTHIER, Vincent; 5000 Blvd. Gouin E., Montreal, P.Q.; 12191 Ste. Gertrude (res); Mon '50; Pulm. Dis. & TB (P.Q.); Staff, Hop. du Sacre-Coeur, Cartierville & Pt.-time Med. Dir. Marie Claret; Tel. 322-6661.

GAUTHIER, Vincent; 1100 Bougainville, Quebec 6, P.Q.; Lav '37; GenSurg (PQ); Staff, Hop.-St.-Francois-d'Assise & Laval U.; Tel. 527-8502.

GAUTHIER, Yvan A.; Mon '63; Res., Dept. of Biochem., Laval U., Quebec, P.Q.

GAUTHIER, Yvon; 475 de Lanaudiere, Joliette, P.Q.; Lav'53; OrthSurg; Chief OrthSurg., Hop. St. Eusebe & Hop. St. Charles; Tel. 756-8097.

GAUTHIER, Yvon; 560 Rockland Ave., Montreal 8, P.Q. (res); Lav '55; Psy (PQ); I/C Child Psy. Clin., Hop.-Ste. Justine; Tel. 273-4533.

GAUTIER, Emile; Centre Medical Fleury, 2157 Fleury E., Montreal 12, P.Q.; Mon'47; Tel. 381-2581.

GAUTREAU, Blair; Medical Arts Bldg., 640 Mountain Rd., Moncton, N.B.; Lav'49; Otol (P.Q.).

GAUTREAU, Raymond M.; 454 Bordeleau, Joliette, P.Q.; 475 de Lanaudiere (res); Lav'54; OrthSurg (P.Q.); Staff (Orth.), Hop-St-Eusebe; Tel. PL 6-8096.

GAUVIN, Gerald E.; 19 Ave. Laporte, Edmundston, N.B. (res); Lav '32; IntMed (T.B.); Med. Supt., San St. Joseph, St. Basile, N.B.; Tel. 263-5561.

GAUVIN, Jacques; 2205 Dickson, Sillery, Quebec 6, P.Q.; Lav '51; Anaes (P.Q.); Ass't. (Dept. of Anaes), Hop.-St.-Sacrement & St. Michel-Archange; Tel. 681-5818.

GAUVIN, Paul H.; 7488 ave Trudel, Quebec 7, P.Q.; Lav'46; Anaes(P.Q.); Staff, Hop. Francois d'Assise.

GAUVIN, Pierre; 1538 Sherbrooke St. ouest, Ste. 600, Montreal, P.Q.; Mon'60; Ophth; Tel. 937-9296.

GAUVIN, Roger; 750 St. Vallier ouest, Quebec 8, P.Q.; 170 Eymard (res); Lav'45; ObstGyn (P.Q.); Tel. 524-9488.

GAUVREAU, Adrien; New Richmond Centre, Co. Bonaventure, P.Q.; Lav '49; Surg., Hop. Notre Dame-de-Chartres-Maria.

GAUVREAU, Leo; 19 Ave.-Ste.-Genevieve, Quebec 4, P.Q. (res); Lav'43; FRCP(C), Bact; Bact., Hop.-St.-Sacrement; Cons. (Bact.), Hop.de-la-Misericorde & Prof. (Microbiol.), Laval U.; Tel. LA. 7-3461.

GAUZE, Joseph; Sask '64; Res., Jewish Gen. Hosp., Montreal 26, P.Q.; Abroad.

GAVANSKI, Milan S.; 55 Royal Ave., Ste. 201, New Westminster B.C.; Zagreb (Yugo.)'52; Psy.

GAVELIN, Gerald E.; 1103-42nd St. S.W., Calgary, Alta.; Sask.'58; FRCS(C), PlasSurg.

GAVILLER, Edwin A.; 128-10th St. W., Owen Sound, Ont.; 767-2nd Ave. W. (res); Tor '54; M.C.G.P.; Staff, Owen Sound Gen. & Marine Hosp.; Tel. 376-4184.

GAVSIE, William H.; 5091 Victoria Ave., Montreal, P.Q.; 5087 Victoria Ave. (res); McG '27; Paed; Sr. Phys., (Paed), Jewish Gen. Hosp.; Clin. Ass't., Montreal Children's Hosp.; Tel. RE 3-9372.

GAWENDA, Adam W.; 1290 Ottawa St., Windsor, Ont.; Lwow (Poland) '28; MCGP; Tel. 253-4154.

GAWMAN, William G.; Tor'55; DiagRad; Assoc. Rad., Hamilton Gen. Hosp., Hamilton, Ont.; Tel. 527-0271.

GAWTHROP, Paul C.; 140 Wallace St., Nanaimo, B.C.; 2345 Departure Bay Rd. (res); Ott'55; Active Staff, Nanaimo Gen. Hosp.; Tel. 754-5545.

GAY, Brian C.; 180 Metcalfe St., Ste. 308, Ottawa 4, Ont.; 2377 Georgina Dr., Ott. 14 (res); Ott'51; FACS; DABS; FRCS(C); GenSurg; Surg. Active Staff, Ottawa Civic & Grace Hosp's.; Tel. CE 2-0658.

GAY, Gabriel; 31 Montcalm, Hull, P.Q.; 89 Emond (res); Ott '52; MCGP; Phys., Canada Packers.

GAY, Keith E.; 991 Oxford St., London, Ont.; 455 Regal Dr. (res); Ott '53; IntMed; MCGP; Med. Dir. J. Labatt Co. Ltd.; Tel. GL 1-1330.
GAYMAN, George R.; 710 Seymour St., Vancouver 2, B.C.; 3904 W. 38th Ave. (res); Tor '41; Paed; Paed., Health Centre for Children & Children's Hosp.; Ass't Prof., U. of British Columbia; Tel. MU 4-1511.
GAYTON, Joseph L.; 4806 Narvaez Dr., Vancouver, B.C. (res); Man '31; D.P.H., PH; Ass't. Sen. M.O.H., Vancouver; Tel. TR 6-1313.
GAZINSKY, Wm.; 2369 Wellington St., Montreal 22, P.Q. Mon '54; Tel. WE 5-2013.
GAZLEY, Lorne A.; Tor '52; GenSurg; No. 3 Fighter Wing H.Q., CAPO 5055 Canadian Armed Forces, Europe.
GEAR, Douglas H.; 205 Bagot, Cobourg, Ont.; 230 King St. W. (res); Tor '47; Staff, Cobourg Gen. Hosp.; Tel. 372-2148
GEAR, Emily J. (See Berkman).
GEAR, George L.; Qns '57; Staff, Crease Clinic, Essondale, B.C.
GEAR, John R.; Hopedale Plaza, Oakville, Ont.; Tor'54; Staff, Oakville-Trafalgar Mem. Hosp.; Tel. 827-4144.
GEBBIE, Douglas M.; 35 Briarfield Cr., St. Catharines, Ont.; Glasgow (Scot.)'51; Tel. MU 4-3471.
GEDDES, Aubrey K.; 4342 Sherbrooke St. W., Montreal, P.Q.; Paed (P.Q.); Paed-in-Chief, Royal Victoria Hosp.; Phys., Montreal Children's Hosp.; Ass't, Prof. (Paed.), McGill U.; Tel. 933-1414.
GEDDES-SMITH, Elizabeth M.; Aberdeen (Scot.) '44; M.O., Chas. Camsell Indian Hosp., Edmonton, Alta.; Tel. GL 5-7141.
GEDGAUDAS, Eugenijus; 116 Med. Arts Bldg., Winnipeg, Man.; 157 Academy Rd., Wpg. 9 (res); Munich (Germ.) '48; DABR, FICS; DiagRad; Chief, Dept. of Rad., Misericordia Gen. Hosp.; Dem. (Rad.), U. of Manitoba; Tel. GL 3-7089.
GEDZ, William; Wes '59; DiagRad; Staff, Toronto Gen. Hosp., Toronto 2, Ont.; Tel. EM 6-8211.
GEE, Edgar M.; Ste. 500, Chinook Prof. Bldg., Macleod Trail, Calgary, Alta.; Man'42; AMCGP.
GEE, Evelyn A.; 2647 Willow St., Vancouver 9, B.C. (res); Tor '30; PathBact; Staff, Div. T.B. Control Vancouver; Tel. RE 3-1479.
GEER, Pitamer; Pine Falls, Man.; Man '58.
GEGGIE, Conrad G.; 12809 Stony Plain Rd., Edmonton, Alta.; Lav '09; Retired.
GEGGIE, David C.; Wakefield, P.Q.; McG '50; Staff Gatineau Memorial Hosp.; Tel. 459-2363.
GEGGIE, James H. S.; Wakefield, P.Q.; McG '40; D.A.; M.C.G.P.
GEGGIE, N. Stuart; Wakefield, P.Q.; McG '51; M.C.G.P.; Staff, Gatineau Mem., Hosp., Wakefield.
GEIGER, Donald W.; 150 King St. S., Waterloo, Ont.; McG'52; MCGP; Tel. 742-8652.
GEIGER, Douglas W.; 240 Brock St., Kingston, Ont.; Qns'52; Paed; Att'd. Phys., Hotel-Dieu Hosp.; Clin. Ass't. Paed., Queen's U.; Tel. 542-3093.
GEIGER, Linda M.; 4151 Sheppard Ave. E., Agincourt, Ont.; Tor'64; Court. Staff, Scarborough Gen. Hosp.; Tel. 293-4189.
GEISLER, William O.; 274 Riverside Dr., Toronto 3, Ont.; Tor '48; F.R.C.P.(C), IntMed, PhysMed & Rehab; Staff, Lyndhurst Lodge; Tel. WA 3-0928.
GEISSINGER, Max E.; Med. Assoc. Clin., 405 Hendryx St., Nelson, B.C.; R.R. 1 (res); Alb'32; FACS; FRCS(C); GenSurg; Att'd. Staff, Kootenay Lake Gen. Hosp.; Tel. 352-6611.
GEIST, Susanna; 2838 Thornton Ave., Regina, **Sask. (res); Marburg (Germ.) '47; Ass't. Path., Grey Nun's Hosp.; Tel. JO 9-9621.**
GELB, Reynold H.; Ste 201, 77 Westmount Rd., Guelph, Ont.; 11 Cedar St. (res); Capetown (S. Africa)'48; MRCOG; FACOG; ObstGyn; Chief (ObstGyn), Guelph Gen. Hosp.; Tel. 822-7232.
GELBER, Herman; 1025 Pine Ave. W., Montreal 2, P.Q.; McG'60; Psy; Clin. Ass't. (Psy.), Royal Victoria Hosp.; Lect. (Psy.), McGill U.; Tel. VI 2-1251.
GELBER, Shiela P.; 6875 LaSalle Blvd. Verdun, Montreal 19, P.Q.; Man '58.
GELBLOOM, Abraham J.; 155 Chiltern Hill Rd., Toronto 10, Ont. (res); Tor '56; Path; Staff. Toronto Gen. Hosp.; Tel. EM 6-8211.
GELDERT, G. M.; 516 Kenwood, Ottawa, Ont.; (res); Anaes; McG '13; Retired.
GELEFF, Thomas; 2112 Avenue Rd., Toronto 12, Ont.; 146 Bombay Ave., Downsview (res); Tor '45; Court. Staff (Obst.), Toronto Gen. Hosp.; Tel. HU 8-4465.
GELFAND, A. Sidney; 201 Medical Centre, 906 8th Ave. W., Calgary, Alta.; Man'30; FICS; Staff, Calgary Gen., Holy Cross, Grace & Children's Hosp's.; Tel. AM 2-6061.
GELFAND, Elliot T.; Alb'65; Res., University Hosp., Edmonton, Alta.; Abroad.
GELFAND, Morrie M.; 300 Ellendale Med. Bldg., 5845 Cote-des-Neiges Rd., Montreal 26, P.Q.; 5757 Decelles Ave. (res); McG '50; F.R.C.S.(C), ObstGyn; Tel. RE 3-3733.
GELINAS, Andre; 217 Javeline, Dorval, Montreal, P.Q.; Lav '32; FACP; Pulm. Dis. & TB (P.Q.); IntMed (TB); Staff, Veterans' Hosp., Ste. Anne de Bellevue; Tel. 453-5395.
GELINAS, Camille; 15 ave Begin, Levis, P.Q.; 22 rue Henry (res); Lav '40; Ophth, Otol (P.Q.); **Chief. Ophth. Otol., Hop. Dieu de Levis; Coroner; Tel. 837-9341.**
GELINAS, Charles; 241 Fleury Ouest, Montreal, P.Q.; 2250 Laure-Conan (res); Lav '57; Otol; Staff, Hop.-Sacre-Coeur, Cartierville & Hop.-Notre-Dame-de-l'Esperance, St. Laurent; Tel. DU 1-7281.
GELINAS, Conrad L.; 1840 St. Marc, Shawinigan, P.Q.; Lav'65.
GELINAS-DESAULINERS, Andre; 1915 Royale, Trois-Rivieres, P.Q.; Lav'57; AMCGP; Tel. FR 5-6820.
GELINAS, Georgette P.; Lav '43; PH(P.Q.); Paed; Staff, Health Dept., 777 Laurentian Blvd., Montreal 9, P.Q.; Tel. 744-6411.
GELINAS, Guy; 60 des Casernes, Trois-Rivieres, P.Q.; 2980 rue Duvernay (res); Lav '43; ObstGyn; Chief, Staff (Obst.), St. Joseph, & Cons. (Gyn.), St. Marie Hosp's.; Tel. FR 4-1414.
GELINAS, Henri; 2150 Sherbrooke ouest, App. 18, Montreal, P.Q.; Mon'24; IntMed (P.Q.); Tel. VI 4-4584.
GELINAS, Jacques; Parliament Bldgs., Quebec City, P.Q.; Mon '43; IntMed (P.Q.); Deputy Minister of Health, Prov. of Quebec; Tel. 693-6462.
GELINAS, Jean-Jacques; 1643 Boul. St-Louis, Trois Rivieres, P.Q.; Lav'62; FRCP(C), IntMed.
GELINAS, Jean P.; 5809 Gouin Blvd. W., Montreal 9, P.Q.; 12382 Reed (res); Mon '52; Tel. FE 4-6732.
GELINAS, Martial; St. Barthelemy, Co. Berthier, P.Q.; Lav '62
GELINAS, Michel; Lav '60; Cardiol (P.Q.); Staff, Hop. Santa Cabrini, Montreal 36, P.Q.; Tel. 254-8311.
GELINAS, Michel; 5760 de Jumonville, Montreal 5, P.Q.; Mon'65.
GELINAS, Real; 478 rue Principale, Ste.-Flore, Co. St. Maurice, P.Q.; Lav '52; IntMed (PQ); Tel. LE 8-2105.
GELINAS, Real-A.; 5809 Blvd Gouin O., Cartierville, Montreal P.Q.; 12356 Chevalier St. (res); Mon '47; F.R.C.P.(C) IntMed; Staff, Hop. de l'Esperance, Ville St. Laurent, P.Q.; Tel. FE 4-6732.
GELINAS, Richard M.; C.P. 1448, 141 Lorraine, Schefferville, P.Q.; Mon '65.
GELINAS-MACKAY, (Claire Gelinas); 3840 Parc Lafontaine, Montreal 24, P.Q.; Mon '43; Path. (P.Q.); Path., Hop. Notre-Dame; Tel. 525-6363.
GELL, Gordon W.; 642 S. E. Marine Dr., Vancouver 15, B.C.; 1137 Balfour, Van. 9 (res); UBC '55; MCGP; Tel. FA 5-9221.
GELLATLY, Thomas A.; Oak River, Man.; Glasgow (Scot.) '53.
GELLING, Barry M.; 3490 Saanich Rd., Victoria, B.C.; UBC'65.

GELLMAN, David D.; Winnipeg Clinic, Winnipeg 1, Man.; London (Eng.) '49; MRCP, FRCP (C), IntMed; Ass't. Phys., Winnipeg Gen. & Grace Hosp's.; Lect. (Med.), U. of Manitoba; Tel. 942-0551.

GELLMAN, Vera (Armett); Cambridge (Eng.) '50; MA; Paed; Dir., Poison Control Centre, & Lect. Paed., Wpg. Children's Hosp., Winnipeg, Man.; Tel. SP 5-8311.

GELPKE, Norman H.; Ste. 108, 1940 Lonsdale, North Vancouver, B.C.; London (Eng.)'51; FRCS(C), OrthSurg; Tel. 985-2227.

GELSON, John; Turtleford, Sask.; Birmingham, (Eng) '56.

GEMMELL, David; 95 S. Waterloo St., Stratford, Ont.; 176 Elizabeth St. (res); Tor '34; MCGP; Coroner, Perth County; Tel. 271-8852.

GEMMELL, John Patmore; 100 Medical College, **Bannatyne & Emily Sts., Winnipeg, Man.; 141 Montrose St. (res); Man'41; MRCP (London); FRCP(C); IntMed; Chief Phys., Winnipeg Gen. Hosp.; Assoc. Prof. (Med.) & Special Inst.** (Therapeutics), U. of Manitoba; Tel. SU 6-3569.

GEMMILL, Donald L.; Brandon Clinic, Box 280, Brandon, Man.; McG '55; MCGP; Tel. PA 9-6444.

GENCHER, Moses; Ste. 110, 225 Lisgar St., Ottawa 4, Ont.; Ott'56; Psy.; Tel. 235-8719.

GENDREAU, Cecil; 3761, ave. Lacombe, Montreal 26, P.Q.; Mon '58.

GENDREAU, Louis P.; Room 624, Justic Bldg., Ottawa, Ont.; 205 Faraday St. (res); Psy.; Tel. PA 2-5713.

GENDREAU, Lucien L.; Luceville, Co. Rimouski, P.Q.; Lav '56; Tel. 739-4477.

GENDREAU, Rene L.; Man '30; Supt., Ste. Rose **Hosp., Ste. Rose du Lac, Man.; Dist. Coroner; Tel. 1.**

GENDRON, Aristide; 310 Marchand, Drummondville, P.Q.; Lav '38; Hd. (Obst.), Hop.-Ste-Croix; Tel. GR 8-1381.

GENDRON, Claude P.; 635 Ouest Dorchester, Montreal 2, P.Q.; 725 Stuart, Outremont (res); Lav '51; FISH; Haem (P.Q.); MCGP; Staff Phys., & I/C Health Bureau, Hop.-Maisonneuve; (Haematol.), St. Francis-Xavier & Cabrini Hosp's.; M.O., Shell Oil Co. of Canada, Mtl.; Med. Dir., Cyanamide of Canada; Pres.-elect. College of G.P. of Canada; Tel. 527-2474.

GENDRON, Denis; 1248 Chemin Ste Foy, Quebec, **P.Q.; Lav '42; D.S. (Penn); GenSurg (PQ); Cons. Bell Telephone Co.; Tel. 525-7856.**

GENDRON, James B.; Man '45; Res., Vancouver Gen. Hosp., Vancouver 9, B.C.

GENDRON, J. Edmond; Workmen's Comp. Bd., 90 Harbour St., Toronto 1, Ont.; Tor'50; FRCS(C), GenSurg.

GENDRON, J. L.; 3156 Belanger E., Montreal, P.Q.; 6855—8eme Ave., Rosemount (res); Mon '42.

GENDRON, Lionel; 7738 St. Hubert, Montreal, **P.Q.; Mon '51; Tel. 272-3401.**

GENDRON, Moise; Bourget, Ont.; Mon '25; Dist. Coroner.

GENDRON, Olivier M.; 253 Rue Montcalm, Berthierville, P.Q.; Mon '56.

GENDRON, Oscar; Unite Sanitaire, 46, rue St-Charles, Dorion, P.Q.; Lav '29;

GENDRON, Phillippe; 2968 Blvd. du Carmel, Trois Rivieres; Lav '45; Anaes; Anaes., Hop. St. Joseph; Tel. FR 6-6211.

GENDRON, Pierre D.; Mon'64; Res. (DiagRad.); Hop. Notre-Dame, Montreal, P.Q.

GENDRON, Roland; 11109 L'Archeveque, Montreal, P.Q.; 4719 est Boul. Henri-Bourassa (res); Mon '42; M.O., Dept. of Health, Mtl.; Tel. DA 1-5590.

GENEEN, Benjamin; 99 Avenue Rd., Ste. 611, Toronto 5, Ont.; 27 Glenelm Ave. (res); Glasgow (Scot.) '39; D. Psy; Psy; Tel. 925-5692.

GENENDER, Lawrence J.; 243 Hyman Dr., Dollard Des Ormeaux, P.Q.; McG'59; FRCS(C), GenSurg.

GENEREUX, Arthur G.; 408 Canada Bldg., **Saskatoon, Sask.; 315 Poplar Cres. (res); Alb '26;** Ophth, Otol; Dist. Coroner; Ass't. Clin. Prof. **(Ophth), U. of Saskatchewan; Tel. 244-7822.**

GENEREUX, George P.; 1421 Argyle Ave., Saskatoon, Sask.; McG'60; DiagRad.

GENESOVE, L. Jack; 30 Bloor St. W., Toronto 5, Ont.; Tor'46; AMCGP.

GENEST, Armand; Ste. 818, 30 est, Boul. St. Joseph, Montreal 14, P.Q.; 5176 Blvd. Pie IX (res); Mon'43; D.D.S., PlasSurg, Chief, Dept. of PlasSurg, Hotel-Dieu Hosp; Prof., PlasSurg, U. of Montreal; Tel. VI 4-5773.

GENEST, Benoit; 3330 Mgr. Gauthier, Quebec, P.Q. (res); Lav '29; D.P.H.; Med. Off., Health Unit, Ste-Anne-de-Beaupre.

GENEST, Jacques; 1171 Blvd. Mont-Royal, Outremont, P.Q. (res); Mon '42; FACP; FRSC; FRCP(C); IntMed; Active Staff Dir., Clin. Research & Chief in Med., Hotel-Dieu Hosp.; Prof. of Med., U. of Montreal; Tel. VI 4-0161, Ext. 295.

GENEST, Jean-Paul; 168 St. Georges, Levis, P.Q.; Lav '48; MCGP; Staff, Hotel-Dieu Hosp.; Tel. 837-7915.

GENEST J. Pierre; 2 rue de l'Eglise St. Romuald, P.Q.; Lav '59; AMCGP.

GENEST, Leopold E.; 1096 rue Notre-Dame, Chicoutimi, P.Q. (res); Lav '53; DABTR; FRCP (C), TherRad; D&TRAD; Staff, Hotel-Dieu-St.-Vallier; Tel. 549-1293.

GENEST, Pierre; 30 est, boul. St. Joseph, Montreal 14, P.Q.; Mon '58; IntMed; Ass't. Med. Staff, Hop. Ste-Jeanne d'Arc; Tel. 845-4241.

GENEST, Pierre A.; 56 rue Principale N., Maniwaki, P.Q.; Mon '56; Memb. Bd. of Dir. & Pres. Med. Staff, Hop.-St. Joseph; Tel. 14.

GENEST, Robert; 809 Cherrier, Montreal, P.Q.; Mon '43; **F.R.C.P.(C), NeurPsy.; Tel. LA 1-5301.**

GENSER, Avron; 318 Med. Arts Bldg., Edmonton, Alta.; Alb'57; ObstGyn; Tel. 422-2286.

GENYK-BEREZOWSKI, Daria O.; 770 Barton St. E., Hamilton, Ont.; 94 Burris St. (res); Krakow **(Pol.) '38; M.O.H.; Tel. LI 4-2009.**

GENYK-BEREZOWSKI, Jaroslaw; 770 Barton St. E., Hamilton, Ont.; **94 Burris St. (res); Krakow (Pol) '33; Tel. LI 4-2009.**

GEOFFRION, Louise; 271 McDougall, Outremont, Montreal 8, P.Q.; Mon '51. Temporarily Retired.

GEOFFROY, Albert; 95 St. Charles Borromee St. N., Joliette, P.Q.; Lav '12. Retired.

GEOFFROY, Marc; 3576 est, Ontario, Montreal 4, P.Q.; 5590 Canterbury (res); Mon'49; DMRT (Lond.); D&T Rad; Hd., Dept. of Rad., Hop-St-Joseph-de-Rosemont, Hop-de-la-Misericorde; Cons., Inst. Bruchesi; Tel. CL 6-2681 & VI 2-5141.

GEOFFROY, Y. Guy; Ste. 444, 5757 Ave. Decelles, Montreal 26, P.Q.; Mon'60; Neurol(P.Q.); Staff, Hop. Ste-Justine; Tel. 739-6944.

GEOGHEGAN, John J.; 110 Queen St. W., Guelph, Ont. (res); Glasgow (Scot.) '30; D.Psy., Psy; Psych., Homewood San., Guelph; Tel. TA 4-1010.

GEORGE, C. H.; Lucan, Ont.; Lucan, Ont. (second off. and res); Tor '32.

GEORGE, Edward A.; Dal '64; Int., Vancouver Gen. Hosp., Vancouver 9, B.C.

GEORGE, Frederick H.; 101 Carleton St., St. John N.B.; 60 Wentworth St. (res); Dal '42; IntMed; Phys., St. John Gen. & St. Joseph's **Hosp's.; Cons., Lancaster DVA Hosp.; Tel. 693-3548.**

GEORGE, George G.; 1052 Drouillard Rd., Windsor, Ont.; 2039 Richmond St. (res); Wes '33; MCGP; Tel. 256-4949.

GEORGE, Herbert C.; 812 Med. Dental Bldg., Regina, Sask.; 3060 Albert (res); Tor '10; Int-Med; Staff, Regina Gen. & Grey Nun's Hosp's.; Tel. LA 2-5629.

GEORGE, J. Alexander; McG '49; DiagRad; Staff, St. Martha's Hosp., Antigonish, N.S.; Tel. 863-2830.

GEORGE, James P.; 604 Boyd Bldg., 388 Portage Ave., Winnipeg 1, Man.; 227 Academy Rd. (res); **Man '11; Retired.**

GEORGE, Kalarickal P.; Travancore (S. India) '56; FRCS(C), GenSurg; Staff, Victoria Gen. Hosp., Halifax, N.S.; Tel. 422-7371.

GEORGE, Morton B.; 238 Forsyth Dr., Waterloo, Ont. (res); Qns '33; D&TRad; Dir. of Rad. & Cancer Therapy, Kitchener-Waterloo Gen. Hosp., Kitchener, Ont.; Tel. SH 5-9451.

GEORGE, Stevan W.; 115 Lower Union St., Kingston, Ont.; Glasgow (Scot.)'56; MRC; MRCOG; FRCS(C); ObstGyn; Staff, Kingston Gen. Hosp.; & Hotel-Dieu Hosp.; Lect. (ObstGyn.), Queen's U.; Tel. 542-4124.

GEORGESCO, Miron; 825 rue Belvedere sud, Sherbrooke, P.Q.; Bucharest (Roum.) '41; IntMed (P.Q.); Haem (P.Q.); Tel. 569-3933.

GEORGIEVSKI, Aleksandar; 612 Sherbourne St., Toronto 5, Ont.; 21 Abitibi Ave. (res); Tel. 921-6677.

GERARD, J. A.; Quarantine Immig. Med. & Sick **Mariners Services, Box 145, Station B. Quebec, P.Q.**

GERARD, Ovide; 1015 rue Notre Dame, Lachine, P.Q.; Apt. 10, 6201 Sherbrooke W., Montreal 28 (res); Mon '23; Staff, Public Health Dept.

GEREIN, Alfred N.; 531 Medical, Dental Bldg., **925 W. Georgia St., Vancouver 1, B.C.; UBC '54;** ThorSurg; FACS; Assoc. Staff, St. Paul's Hosp.; Tel. MU 1-3724.

GERELUK, Madeline; Esperanza, B.C.; Alb '62.

GERGELY, Nicholas F.; 450 Central Ave., Ste. 209, London, Ont.; Budapest (Hung.)'51; FACC; FRCS(C), Cardiovasc & ThorSurg; Staff, Victoria & St. Joseph's Hosp's.; Teach. Staff, Victoria Hosp.; Clin. Instr. (Surg.), U. of Western Ont.; Tel. 432-2024.

GERHARD, Bruce L.; 182 Eagle St. W., Delhi, Ont.; Wes '28; MCGP; M.O.H., Delhi & Twp. Middletown; Tel. 582-1650.

GERIN-LAJOIE Gustave; Unite Sanitaire, Farnham, P.Q.; Lav '43; DPH; Tel. 293-4388.

GERLACHE, Freddy; Ste. 16, 5336 Queen Mary Rd., Montreal 26, P.Q.; Belgium '62; Tel. 488-1225.

GERLACH, Hans J.; 2605 Eglinton Ave. E., Scarborough, Ont.; Berlin (Germ.) '45; Otol; Staff, Central & Scarborough Gen. Hosp's.; Tel. 261-4371.

GERLITZ, James H. Sg./Lcdr.; Cornwallis Hosp., C.F.B. Cornwallis, Cornwallis, N.S.; Man'57; Psy.; Tel. 638-8214.

GERMAIN, Charles E.; 68 Sulpiciens, L'Epiphanie,, Co. L'Assomption, P.Q.; Mon '27; D.P.H., P.H. (P.Q.); M.O., L'Assomption-Montcalm Health Unit.

GERMAIN, Clement; 847 ave du Coteau, Quebec 10, P.Q.; Lav'50; DiagRad; Staff, Hop. St. Francois d'Assise.

GERMAIN, Gilbert; 44 rue Wellington, Coaticook, P.Q.; Lav '53; Tel. VI 9-3735.

GERMAIN, Guy; Lav '58; Res., Hop. St-Sacrement, Quebec, P.Q.

GERMAIN, Guy; Ste. 1018, 30 est Boul. St. Joseph, Montreal 14, P.Q.; Mon'52; FRCP(C); IntMed; Staff, Notre Dame Hop.; Ass't. Prof. (Med.), U. of Montreal; Tel. 845-0287.

GERMAIN, L. Marcel; 200-1ere Ave., Noranda, P.Q.; Mon'55; Paed.

GERMAIN, Louis A.; 875 des Recollets, Trois-Rivieres, P.Q.; Lav'56; GenSurg (P.Q.); Active Staff, St. Marie Hosp.; Tel. 378-3474.

GERMAIN, Marc A.; Ott'65; Res., Ottawa Gen. Hosp., Ottawa 2, Ont.

GERMAIN, Paul E.; Lav'65; Res., Hop. de l'Enfant Jesus, Quebec 3 ,P.Q.

GERMAIN, Romeo; 790 Sacre-Coeur, St-Hyacinthe, P.Q.; Lav '39; Path(P.Q.); Staff (Path.), Hop. St. Charles; Tel. PR 4-5331 .

GERMAINE, Clement; 47 ave du Coteau, Ste-Foy, Quebec 10, P.Q.; Lav '50; MCGP.

GERRARD, Alexander B.; Box 117, Glencoe, Ont.; Wes'63.

GERRARD, John W.; University Hosp., Saskatoon, Sask.; 809 Colony St. (res); Oxford (Eng.) '41; M.R.C.P. (Lond.), D.M. (Oxford); F.R.C.-P.(C), Paed; Prof. of Paed., U. of Saskatchewan; Tel. 242-7641.

GERRED, Ralph F.; 379 O'Connor Dr., Toronto 6, Ont.; Tor '39; IntMed; Staff, OPD, Toronto Gen. Hosp.; Clin. Ass't. (Med.), U. of Toronto; Tel. GA 1-2161.

GERRIE, John W.; Ste. 901, 1414 Drummond St., Montreal 25, P.Q.; McG '31; DDS; DLO; DABPS; FACS; FICS; Otol; PlasSurg; Dir., Div. of PlasSurg., Montreal Gen & Queen Mary Vet's. Hosp's.; Surg., St. Mary's Hosp.; Assoc. Prof. (Surg.), McGill U.; Tel. VI 9-9522.

GERRIE, Robert G.; 1125 E. Hastings St., Vancouver 6, B.C.; Man '61.

GERRY, James A.; Man '56; MCGP; Res., Victoria Hosp., London, Ont.

GERSHAW, Frederick W.; Med. Arts Clinic, 51-6th St. S.E., Medicine Hat, Alta.; Riverview Apts., (res); Man '08; FACS; GenSurg; Staff, Medicine Hat Gen. Hosp.; Senator, Gov't. of Canada; Tel. JA 7-2281.

GERSTEIN, Marvin C.; 1543 Victoria Pk. Ave., Scarborough, Ont.; Tor '52; FRCP(C), Paed; Ass't. Phys., Hosp. for Sick Children; Toronto; Assoc. (Paed.), U of Toronto; Tel. PL 9-0861.

GERSTEIN, William; 270 Seaforth Med. Bldg., 3550 Cotes des Neiges Rd., Montreal 25, P.Q.; Baylor (Texas) '56; FRCP(C); Derm; Staff, Montreal Gen. Hosp.; Tel. 935-2559.

GERTEL, Morris; McG'63; Res., Jewish Gen. Hosp., Montreal 26, P.Q.

GERTLER, Menard M.; 3406 Northcliffe Ave., Montreal, P.Q. (res); McG '43; D.A.B.I.M.C.

GERULA, George R.; Qns'63; Res., St. Joseph's Hosp., London, Ont.

GERULATH, Horst A.; Tor'63; Res., Women's College Hosp., Toronto 2, Ont.

GERVAIS, Andre G.; 84 St. Jacques, St. Jean, P.Q. (res); Mon '62; Staff (Anat.), U. of Montreal; Tel. RE 3-9951. Abroad.

GERVAIS, G.; 251 Frontenac St., Berthierville, P.Q.; McG '34.

GERVAIS, Gabriel A.; Mon'56; MCGP; DiagRad (P.Q.); Staff, Hop. Hotel-Dieu, Montreal 18, P.Q.

GERVAIS, Georges; 1285-9eme Ave., Charny, P.Q.; Lav'48.

GERVAIS, Gerard; 201 de la Gare, Alma, Cte. Lac St-Jean, P.Q.; Lav '52.

GERVAIS, Henry; 4065 Cote des Neiges, Montreal 25, P.Q.; Haiti '56; DiagRad.

GERVAIS, Jean-Guy; 139 Notre-Dame est, Victoriaville, P.Q.; Lav'60; MCGP; Tel. 752-7322.

GERVAIS, Jean-Pierre F/L; RCAF Station, Camp Borden, Ont.; Mon '65.

GERVAIS, Joseph; 324 Boul.-des-Prairies, Laval-des-Rapides, Montreal 40, P.Q.; Mon '22.

GERVAIS, Laurent; 37 Chemin Bellingham, Montreal 8, P.Q.; Mon '57; Psy; Staff, Inst. Albert Prevost.

GERVAIS, L.S. Marcel; 850 de la Terriere, Trois Rivieres, P.Q.; 3960 Des Cypres (res); Lav '51; Psy (P.Q.); Chief-of-Psy., Hop. Ste. Marie; Tel. FR 5-4242.

GERVAIS, Lucien E. J.; St. Francois, Cte. Montmagny, P.Q.; Lav '45.

GERVAIS, Marc; (Intern) c/o 433 Place Deauville, Laval des Rapides, P.Q.; Mon'64.

GERVAIS, Maurice; 4395 Ave. Verdun, Montreal 18, P.Q.; 74 Holyrood, Outremont (res); Mon '41; FICS, FACA, FICA; GenSurg (P.Q.); Surg. Hop. Gen.-de-Verdun; Cons. (Surg.), Hop. St.-Joseph & St. Lambert Gen.; Tel. VI 5-2450.

GERVAIS, Paul; 143 Nord, St.-Barthelemy, Joliette, P.Q.; Lav '29.

GERVAIS, Pierre B.; 1010, Chemin St. Roch, Tracy, P.Q.; Lav '64.

GERVAIS, Rodolphe; 1880 Sheppard, Quebec 6, P.Q.; Lav '44. Staff, Dept. of Health.

GERVAIS, Roger; 26 Cr. d'Avaugour, Duvernay, Mtl., P.Q.; Haiti '49; Anaes; Tel. MO 9-0559.

GERVAIS, Roland; 7967 rue Marquette, Montreal 35, P.Q.; Mon '53; M.C.G.P.; Tel. RA 2-3376.

GERVAIS, Simon J. J. B.; P.O. Box 307, Roberval, P.Q.; Mon '53; Anaes (P.Q.); Staff, Hop. Hotel Dieu St. Michel; Tel. 275-0110.

GERVAIS, Suzanne; Mon '63; Intn., Hop. Ste.-Justine, Montreal, P.Q.

GETTAS, Peter G., 210 Medical Dental Bldg., 450 Central Ave., London, Ont.; 568 Wellington St. (res); Wes '38; D.A.B. Otol. Otol; Clin. Instr. (Otol), U. of Western Ontario; Tel. GE 2-1906.

GETZLER, Nathan A.; 5174 Cote des Neiges Rd., Montreal 26, P.Q.; 4875 Grosvenor (res); Vienna (Austria) '22; **DermSyph (P.Q.); Clin. Asst.,** Royal Victoria Hosp., Royal Edward and Mtl. Children's Hosp's.; Tel. 733-7853.

GHABRIAL, Sobhy L.; 75 West King Edward, Vancouver 10, B.C.; Cairo (Egypt)'53; Paed.

GHAED-SHARAFY, Mohamad-A.; Tehran (Iran) '59; Psy; Staff, Riverview Hosp., Essondale, B.C.

GHAMANDE, Anat R.; 4870 Queen Mary Rd., Apt. 4, Montreal, P.Q.; Bombay (India)'59; FRCP(C), IntMed.

GHANY, Farouk; 1386 Fordon Ave., Bay Ridges, Ont.; Tor'63.

GHATAN, Said; Box 9, Foam Lake, Sask.; Geneva (Switz.)'58.

GHENT, Robert D.; Sudbury Clin., 130 Elm St. E., Sudbury, Ont.; Tor '56; MCGP; Tel. 673-7181.

GHENT, William R.; 10 Montreal St., Ste. 201, Kingston, Ont.; 29 Lakeland Point Dr. (res); Qns '47; FRCS(C); FACS; FICS; FAGS; GenSurg; Chief-of-Surg, Hotel-Dieu Hosp.; Att'd. Surg., Ongwanada San.; Att'd. Surg., Kingston Gen. Hosp.; Assoc. Prof., Queen's U.; Tel. 548-8123.

GHITTER, Earl I.; Wetaskiwin, Alta.; Man '55; MCGP; Tel. 352-3765.

GHYS, Roger; Liege (Belgium) '54; B.Sc.; TherRad; Staff, Inst. of Microbiology, U. of Montreal, Laval-des-Rapides, P.Q.; Tel. 681-2521.

GIALLORETO, Osmond Philip; Villa Medical Bldg., 225 Sherbrooke St. E., Montreal 18, P.Q.; 2365 Lakeshore Dr., Dorval (res); Padua (Italy) '46; FACC; Cardiol (P.Q.); Phys-in-Chief & Dir., Cardiovascular Dept., Santa Cabrini Hosp.; Tel. 254-8341.

GIAMMICHELE, Peter; Ott'62; Res., Montreal Gen. Hosp., Montreal 25, P.Q.

GIANNOTTI, Roberto; 6809 St. Laurent Blvd., Montreal 10, P.Q.; Rome (Italy)'59; ObstGyn (P.Q.).

GIARD, Claude; C.P. 1418, Ste Agathe Des Monts, P.Q.; Mon'61; FRCS(C); GenSurg.

GIARD, J. J. Capt.; Mon'62; Staff, Hop. Militaire, Camp Valcartier, P.Q.

GIARD, Normand; 1681 Parc Lafontaine, Montreal 34, P.Q.; Mon'56; FRCP(C); Neur.; Tel. 527-0555.

GIARDINE, Frank P.; 2489 Bloor St. W., Toronto, Ont., & 23 Applewood Village, Port Credit, Ont.; 589 **Mississauga Cr., Port Credit (res); Tor '45; ObstGyn; Staff, St. Joseph's, Queensway & South Peel Gen. Hosp's; Tel. RO 6-6631.**

GIARDINE, Joseph R.; 65 Balsam St. S., Timmins, Ont.; 379 Toke St. (res); Qns'38; Tel. AM 4-5880.

GIASSON, Carl; 7227 rue St. Denis, Montreal 10, P.Q.; 467 Bellevue, St. Vincent de Paul (res); **Mon '43; M.C.G.P.; Tel. 277-4224.**

GIBB, R. B.; 765 King St. W., Kitchener, Ont.; Tor'65.

GIBB, Robert B.; 253 Queen St. S., Kitchener, Ont.; Tor '35; FACOG ObstGyn; Staff, Kitchener-Waterloo & St. Mary's Hosp's.; Tel. 742-8084.

GIBBARD, Bruce A.; Qns'61; Psy; Staff, Allan Mem. Inst., 1025 Pine Ave. W., Montreal, P.Q.

GIBBINGS, John S.; Box 999, Taber, Alta.; 5119-50th Ave. (res); **Man '48.**

GIBBINS, Reginald R.; St. Walburg, Sask.; Bristol (Eng.) '58.

GIBBON, A. Douglas; 56 Coburg St., Saint John, N.B.; Dal'33; Paed; Chief (Paed), Saint John Gen. & St. Joseph's Hosp's.; Ass't. Prof. (Paed.), Prof. (Paed.), (Hon.), Dalhousie U.; Oral Exam. (Paed.), Royal College P & S of Canada; Tel. 693-3484.

GIBBON, George W.; 3rd St., Englehart, Ont.; 11-7th Ave. (res); **Tor '37; M.C.G.P.;** Chief. Surg. Staff, Englehart & Dist. Hosp.; M.O.H. Dack Twsp.; Dist. Coroner Timiskaming Dist.; Tel. 544-2321.

GIBBON, John E.; Box 639, Ponoka, Alta.; Dublin (Ire.) '61.

GIBBONS, A. Kenneth; Ste. 5, 6325 Fraser St., Vancouver 15, B.C.; Alb '42; Anaes; Staff, Shaughnessy Hosp.; Tel. TR 6-6767.

GIBBONS, James E.; 2300 Tupper St., Montreal 25, P.Q.; Qns '50; Cardiol, (P.Q.); F.A.A.P.; Ass't. Dir. Dept. of Cardiol., Montreal Children's Hosp.; Ass't. Prof. (Paed.), McGill U.; Tel. WE 7-8511.

GIBBONS, T. Gregory; P.O. Box 238, Woodstock, N.B. (res); McG '49. DiagRad; Staff, Carlton Mem. Hosp.; Tel. 328-6477.

GIBBS, John T.; Cambridge (Eng.) '53; Psy; Staff, University Hosp. & Ass't. Prof. (Psy), U. of Alberta, Edmonton, Alta.; Tel. 439-5911, Ext. 441.

GIBBS, P. Laird, CD; 603 St. George St. S., Dresden, Ont.; Wes'52; Coroner, Lambton & Kent Counties; Med. Exam. (Avia.), DOT; Att'd. Staff, Chatham Gen. & St. Joseph's Hosp's.; Staff, Sydenham Dist. Hosp., Wallaceburg; M.O.H., Dawn Twnsp.; Tel. 683-2411.

GIBEAULT, Herve; 4135 Ave. Papineau, Montreal 24, P.Q.; 45 des Erables (res); Mon '30; Obst; Ass't. Prof. U. of Montreal; Tel. LA 3-2035.

GIBEAULT, Robert; 3105 Montée St-Hubert, St-Hubert, P.Q.; Mon'65; Assoc. Med. Charles Lemoyne Hosp.; Tel. 676-7786.

GIBERSON, Herbert R.; Arnprior Med. Centre, Arnprior, Ont.; 20 Daniel St. (res); McG'41; MCGP; Tel. 623-3131.

GIBLON, Barnett I.; 2622 Eglinton Ave. E., Scarborough, Ont.; Tor '57; MCGP; Court. Staff, Scarborough & Toronto E. Gen. Hosp's; Tel. AM 7-0011.

GIBSON, A. Gordon; 2528 Montrose Ave., Abbotsford, B.C.; Alb'52; Tel. 853-1622.

GIBSON, Ann R.; Dublin (Ire.) '59; Jr. Intn., Grace Hosp., Toronto, Ont.

GIBSON, Donald A.; Toronto Professional Bldg., 123 Edward St., Toronto 2, Ont.; 3 Whitney **Ave., Tor. 5. (res); Tor '46; FRCS(Eng); FRCS (C); OrthSurg; Ass't. Surg., Hospital for Sick Children; Cons. Staff, Ontario Crippled Children's Centre; Clin. Instr. (Surg.), U. of Toronto; Tel.** 368-0744.

GIBSON, Edward S.; 24 Hope St. W., Tavistock, Ont.; Tor '54; MCGP; Staff, Stratford Gen. & Woodstock Gen. Hosp's.; 2nd I/C 12th Med. Co., RCAMC(M), Kitchener; Tel. 655-2322.

GIBSON, Gary A.; 8 George St. N., Galt, Ont.; Wes'65; Staff, South Waterloo Mem. Hosp.; Tel. 621-3680.

GIBSON, George A.; Box 970 Courteney, B.C.; Edinburgh (Scot.)'40; D.P.H.; PH; Dir., Upper Island Health Unit.

GIBSON, George J.; 208 Mary St., Chilliwack, B.C.; **Alb '49; MCGP.**

GIBSON, Glen P.; 145 Wellington St., Sarnia, Ont.; 1170 Colborne Rd. (res); Man'49; D.Psy.; Psy; Active Staff, St. Joseph's & Sarnia Gen. Hosp's.; Tel. 344-3220.

GIBSON, H. A.; 121 Medical Arts Bldg., Calgary, Alta.; 201 **Scarboro Ave. (res); Qns '03; F.R.** C.S.(C), **F.R.C.S. (Edin.), ObstGyn; Staff, Calgary Gen., Holy Cross & Grace Maternity Hosp's;** Retired.

GIBSON, Harry E.; 22 Academy Med. Bldg., 1812—4th **St. W., Calgary, Alta.; 503-30th Ave. S.W. (res); Alb '35; GenSurg; Tel. 269-3355.**

GIBSON, James A.; 91 Mott Cr., New Westminster, B.C. (res); Dal'54; Anaes; Chief-of-Anaes., St. Mary's Hosp.; Tel. LA 1-1881.

GIBSON, James D.; 159 Montreal St., Kingston, Ont.; **209 University Ave. (res); Qns '42.**

GIBSON, James W.; 176 East St., Sault Ste. Marie, Ont.; 267 Pim St. (res); Tor '41; IntMed.; Tel. AL 4-2771.

GIBSON, Janet B. (Grant); Okotoks, Alta.; Glasgow (Scot.)'39; MCGP; Tel. 683-4011.

GIBSON, J. Edward; 240 Brock St., Kingston, Ont.; Qns '40; FACP, FAGS, FCCP; IntMed; Med. Chief of Staff, Hotel-Dieu, and Att'd. Staff, St. Mary's-of-the-Lake Hosp's.; Sr. Treatment M.O., DVA; Ass't. Prof. (Med.), Queen's U.; Tel. 542-2712.

GIBSON, J. Henry; 145 Wellington St., Sarnia, Ont.; 579 Cathcart Blvd. (res); Tor '37; GenSurg; Tel. DI 4-1191.

GIBSON, John D.; 24 Kenaston Ave., Town of Mount Royal P.Q.; (res); Tor '54; DiagRad; Jr. Ass't. Rad., Montreal Gen. Hosp.; Dem. (Rad.), McGill U.; Tel. WE 7-6011. Loc 723.
GIBSON, John J.; 383 Ellis St., Penticton, B.C.; 112 Eckhardt Ave. W. (res); Qns '38; Dist. Coroner; Tel. 492-3024.
GIBSON, John M.; 6222 St. Georges, West Vancouver, B.C. (res); Glasgow (Scot.) '38; DMRT; FFR; TherRad; Clin. Instr. (TherRad), U. of British Columbia; Assoc. Dir., B.C. Cancer Inst.; Tel. TR 4-9321.
GIBSON, L. Melbourne; 360 Queen's Ave., London, Ont.; 560 Wellington St. (res); Qns'38; GenSurg; Court. Staff St. Joseph's & Victoria Hosp's; Tel. GE 9-6591.
GIBSON, Malcolm J.; 43 Inglewood Dr., Hamilton, Ont.; Qns '11; Retired.
GIBSON, Michael A.; The Med. Centre, Daysland, Alta.; Oxford (Eng.)'59; Abroad.
GIBSON, Robert; Box 1190, Portage-la-Prairie, Man.; Glasgow (Scot.) '33; M.D. (Psy. Glas.); DPM (Lond.); Clin. Dir. & Ass't. Med. Supt., Manitoba Training Sch.; Psy., Manitoba Rehab. Serv.; Lect. Psy., U. of Man.; Tel. 7-3404.
GIBSON, Robert S.; 178 George St., Belleville, Ont.; Qns '26; Anaes; Phys., International Hardware; Tel. WO 2-3828.
GIBSON, Samuel W. N.; Ste. 309, 4900 Kingsway, South Burnaby, B.C.; Queen's U. (Belfast, N. Ire.) '43; FRCS(Eng.), D.Ophth; FRCS(C), Ophth; Tel. HE 3-1258.
GIBSON, Scott M.; Cambridge (Eng) '60; Staff, Pangman Union Hosp., Pangman, Sask.; Tel 77.
GIBSON, Thomas C.; 499 Main St. E., Hamilton, Ont.; Tor'30; MCGP; Hon. Staff, four Hamilton Hosp's.; Tel. 522-4494.
GIBSON, Thomas C.; 5655 Cambie St., Vancouver 15, B.C.; Tor'62; Tel. AM 1-8155.
GIBSON, William C.; 5516 N.W. Marine Dr., Vancouver 8, B.C. (res); McG '41; D.Phil. (Oxon.); FACP; DABN; NeurPsy; Prof of Psy. Science & History of Med., U. of British Columbia; Tel. CA 4-3320.
GIBSON, William J.; Qns'62; Res., Queen Elizabeth Hosp., Montreal 28, P.Q.
GIBSON, William M.; 40 Main St., Okotoks, Alta.; Glasgow (Scot.) '39; MCGP; Staff, High River & Turner Valley Hosp's.; Tel. 683-4011.
GIBSON, William M.; Health Centre for Children, 715 W. 12th Ave., Vancouver, B.C.; 6598 Albion Way, R.R. 1, North Surrey (res); McG '50; DCH; DABP; Paed; Att'd. Staff, Vancouver Gen & Sunny Hill Hosp's.; Paed. Cons. CARS; Ass't. Prof. (Paed), U. of British Columbia; Tel. TR 6-3211. Abroad.

GIDDENS, Seymour W.; 605 Bloor St. W., Toronto, Ont.; Tor'36; FAAP; Paed; Ass't. Paed. Staff, New Mt. Sinai Hosp.; Tel. LE 1-6393.
GIDDINGS, C. Raymond, Capt.; Wes'65; National Defence Med. Centre, Ottawa 8, Ont.
GIDDINGS, E. Stirling; 78 Kent St., Charlottetown, P.E.I.; 18 Greenfield Ave. (res); Dal '30; ObstGyn; Gyn, P.E.I., & Charlottetown Hosp's.
GIES, Albert H.; Box 301, Winona, Ont. (res); Tor '26; Retired.
GIESBRECHT, Dennis R.; Steinbach, Man.; Man. '64.
GIESBRECHT, Richard; Box No. 580, Beausejour, Man.; Man '49; M.C.G.P.; M.H.O.; Dist. Coroner Tel. 44.
GIESBRECHT, Wilbert R.; Abbotsford, B.C.; Man'56; MCGP; Tel. 853-2500.
GIFFEN, Alan B.; 289 Cedar St., Sudbury, Ont.; 90 Windsor Cr. (res); Man'54; FRCS(C); ObstGyn; Chief-of-Obst., Sudbury Gen. Hosp.; Tel. 674-3131.
GIFFIN, Audley A.; Kentville Med. Bldg., Masters Ave., Kentville, N.S.; 40 Park St. (res); Dal '31; MCGP; Tel. 678-3140.
GIFFIN, Carl C.; Suite 305, Bank of Montreal Bldg., Truro, N.S.; Dal'51; Psy; Exec. Dir., Cobequid Mental Health Centre.
GIFFEN, J. W.; Strathmore, Alta.; Alb '29; Tel. 382-3211.
GIGNAC, Andre; Deschambault, Co. Portneuf, P.Q. (res); Lav '43; D.P.H., P.H. (P.Q.); M.O.H., Portneuf, P.Q.
GIGNAC, Fernand; 190 boul. des Etudiants, Loretteville, P.Q.; Lav '42.
GIGNAC, Guy; 1820 est, boul. St-Joseph, Montreal 34, P.Q.; Mon '50.
GIGUERE, Alphonse; 1160 rue Turnbull, Quebec 4, P.Q.; Lav '31; GenSurg; Staff, Laval U.
GIGUERE, Bertrand; 238 Notre-Dame S., Thetford Mines, P.Q.; Lav '53; IntMed; Tel. FE 8-1444.
GIGUERE, Gabriel; 1578 St. Edouard, Plessisville, Co. Megantic, P.Q.; 1525 Des Erables (res); Lav '48; GenSurg; Tel. 362-7777.
GIGUERE, Gaston; St.-Michel, Cte-Bellechasse, P.Q. (res.); Lav '57; Anaes (P.Q.); Staff, Hop.-Hotel-Dieu, Quebec City; Tel. 884-2584.
GIGUERE, Jean-Marie; C.P. 753, 1076, 7eme rue, Val d'Or, P.Q.; Lav'60; Staff, Hop. St-Sauveur; District Coroner; Tel. 824-6823.
GIGUERE, Paul-H.; 3755 Blvd. St.-Martin. Ste. 5, Chomedey, P.Q.; Lav'56; Paed; Hon. Staff, Hop. Ste-Justine; Cons. Hop. Gen. de Rose & Hop. Gen. St. Eustache; Tel. 681-2633.
GIGUERE, Raymond; 1500 rue 18eme, Quebec 3, P.Q.; 2255 Masson, Sillery (res); Lav'57; FRCP(C); Neurol; Staff, Hop.-de-l'enfant-Jesus; Tel. 525-4643.

GILBART, Frank O.; 295 St. Charles St., Victoria, B.C.; (res); Tor '02; Semi-retired.

GILBERT, André; 1070, de la Tour, Quebec 4, P.Q.; Lav'59; OrthSurg.; Tel. 524-3488.
GILBERT, Anthony; 603 Place Fleury, Montreal 12, P.Q.; Haiti'56; GenSurg.
GILBERT, Charles-A.; 109 Saint-Jean-Baptiste, Asbestos (Richmond), P.O.; Lav '44.
GILBERT, Claude; C.P. 610, Richmond, P.Q.; Lav'63; Tel. 826-5251.
GILBERT, Ghislaine; 5000 est Belanger, Montreal, P.Q.; Mon'49; IntMed(P.Q.); Cardiol(P.Q.); Staff, Inst. of Cardiol.; Tel. 336-3330.
GILBERT, Herbert H.; 918 Lavoisier St., Arvida, P.Q.; Wes '25; DTM & H(Eng.); GenSurg(P.Q.); Active Staff, Saguenay Gen. Hosp.; Chief Med. Cons., Aluminum Co. of Canada Ltd.; Tel. 548-5763.
GILBERT, Herman; 44 rue St.-Jean-Baptiste, Baie-St.-Paul, Cte. de Charlevoix, P.Q.; Lav '62.
GILBERT, James A. L.; University Hosp., Edmonton, Alta.; 8742-117th St. (res); Edinburgh (Scot.) '41; M.D. (Edin.); MRCP (Lond.), FRCP(Edin.); FACP; FRCP(C), IntMed; Prof. of Med. U. of Alberta; Tel. 439-5911.
GILBERT, James R.; 2045 Dufferin St., Toronto 10, Ont.; Tor'63.
GILBERT, J. Barry; Tor'61; Res., St. Michael's Hosp., Toronto 2, Ont.
GILBERT, Joseph J.; McG'65; Res., Jewish Gen. Hosp., Montreal 26, P.Q.
GILBERT, Jules; 4144 Marlowe, Montreal, P.Q. (res); Lav '26; D.P.H.; PH; Secretary, Schl. of Hygiene, U. of Montreal; Tel. RE 3-9951.
GILBERT, Michael J.; Box 9, Grenfell, Sask.; Birmingham (Eng.) '59; M.B., Ch.B., DRCOG; Hon. Phys., Grenfell Union Hosp.; Tel. 697-2881.
GILBERT, Paul; 563—10 Rue-Charney, P.Q.; 400—9e Ave. Charney (res); Lav '30; GenSurg (P.Q.); Supt. & Chief Surg., Hop. Notre Dame de Charny; Tel. 832-2981.
GILBERT, Paul-Emile; 495 avenue du Palais, St-Jerome, P.Q. (res); Lav '41; Anaes; Anaes, Hotel-Dieu Hosp.; Tel. GE 2-9711.
GILBERT, Philippe; Lav'62; Res., Hop. du St-Sacrement, Quebec 3, P.Q.
GILBERT, Richard G. B.; 3801 University St., Montreal 2, P.Q.; London (Eng.) '33; LRCP, DABA, FACA, FFARCS, FRCP(C), Anaes; Anaes., Mtl. Neurol. Inst., Royal Edward Laurentian San. & Queen Mary Vet's. Hosp.; Prof. and Chm. Dept. of Anaes., McGill U.; Tel VI 9-4955.

GILCHRIST, David A.; 7825 Saskatchewan Dr., Edmonton, Alta.; Cambridge (England) '56; D.A. (London); Anaes; Staff, Royal Alexandra Hosp.; Tel. GR 4-3431.
GILCHRIST, F. Ian; Dal'61; M.O. Indian Hosp., Moose Factory, Ont.
GILCHRIST, Harry A.; The Med. Clinic, 3009-31st Ave., Vernon, B.C.; R.R. 2 (res); Alb '48; MCGP; Tel. 542-4321.

GILCHRIST, John W.; 90 Harbour St., Toronto 1, Ont.; Wes '31; M.Sc. (Med.), MIMA; FIMA; M.O., WCB; Tel. 362-3411.

GILCHRIST, Morag M.; 3 Baby Point Rd., Toronto 9, Ont.; Tor '48; Paed; Staff, St. Joseph's Hosp., Sunnyside O.P.D. & Hosp. for Sick Children; Tel. RO 9-5913.

GILCHRIST, Robert A.; 205-2355 W. 1st Ave., Vancouver, B.C. (res); Tor '24; Retired.

GILCHRIST, William L.; Oshawa Clinic, 117 King St. E., Oshawa, Ont.; Edinburgh (Scot.)'56; MB, B.Ch; Paed; Tel. 728-1661.

GILDAY, A. Lorne., D.S.O., V.D.; 478 Mountain Ave., Westmount, P.Q. (res); McG '00; Hon. Cons., Med. Economics, Montreal Gen. Hosp.; Retired.

GILES, Charles R.; Box 400, Rosetown, Sask.; Alb '43.

GILES, John P.; Box 940, Barrhead Clinic, Barrhead, Alta.; London (Eng.) '56; LRCP; DA; DRCOG; Tel. 674-2231.

GILES, Roy; Ste. 14, 344 Furby St., Winnipeg 2, Man. (res); University College Hosp. London (Eng.) '53; M.B., B.S., M.R.C.S., L.R.C.P., D.A.; Anaes; Staff, Grace Hosp.; Tel. SU 3-7271.

GILFILLAN, Ronald R.; 205 Church St., Pembroke, Ont.; Glasgow (Scot.) '45; FRCPS (Glas.); FRCS(Ed.); FICS; GenSurg; Surg., Pembroke Cottage & Gen. Hosp's.; Tel. 732-2571.

GILFILLAN, Veronica J.; 205 Church St., Pembroke, Ont.; St. Andrews (Scot.)'56; Active Staff, Pembroke Gen. & Cottage Hosp's.; Tel. 732-2571.

GILHAM, Raymond E.; Box 70, Langley, B.C.; 20721 Trans-Canada Highway (res); Alb '41; M.C.G.P.; Med. Staff, Langley Mem. Hosp.

GILHOOLY, Joseph P.; 150 Metcalfe St., Ottawa, Ont.; 30 Goulburn Ave. (res); **McG '20;** Ophth, Otol; **Hd. Dept. of Ophth, Ottawa Gen.** Hosp.; **Prof. Emer. (Ophth), U. of Ottawa;** Retired.

GILL, George A. T.; Aberdeen (Scot.)'58; Jr. Res., Royal Victoria Hosp., Montreal, P.Q.

GILL, Guillaume; 8625 Rte. Marie-Victorin, Tracy, P.Q.; Lav '27; FACR; D&TRad; Cons. Canadian Army (Quebec Command); Staff, Hotel-Dieu de Sorel; Tel. RI 3-5521.

GILL, Gurdev S.; 624-6th St., New Westminster, B.C.; UBC '57; MCGP; Tel. 526-5454.

GILL, James R. P.; 22 Cambridge St. North, Lindsay, Ont.; Tor '49; GenSurg; Tel. 324-5601.

GILL, John M.; Aberdeen (Scot.) '55; Staff, Princess Margaret Hosp., Toronto 5, Ont.; Tel. 924-0671.

GILL, Norma M. (Dean); 22 Cambridge St., Lindsay, Ont.; Tor '49.

GILL, Richard K.; Tor '61; Jr. Intn., Hotel Dieu Hosp., Windsor, Ont.

GILL, Russell A.; Med. Arts Bldg., 300 King St. W., Oshawa, Ont.; Tyrone (res); Guy's H. (London, Eng.) '40; FRCS(Eng.), GenSurg; Orth Surg., Oshawa Gen., Pickering, Ajax & Bowmanville Hosp's.; Tel. 723-7823.

GILLAN, James G.; 206 Sheppard Ave. W., Willowdale, Ont.; Glasgow (Scot.)'39; DOMS; FICS; Ophth; Hd. Dept. of Ophth., Northwestern Gen. Hosp.; Chief of Ophth., Bethesda Gen. Hosp.; Cons. Ophth., North York Branson & Queensway Gen. Hosp's.; Tel. 221-2422.

GILLANDERS, David A.; Med. Clinic, 4794A Joyce Ave., Powell River, B.C.; UBC '57.

GILLEN, Charles W.; 132 King St., St. Catharines, Ont.; 50 Marsdale Dr. (res); Wes '43; FCCP, DMR; DiagRad; Rad., Hotel-Dieu Hosp.; Cons. Rad., West Lincoln Mem. Hosp., Grimsby; Tel. MU 4-9201.

GILLEN, Donald H.; 179 King St., St. Catharines, Ont.; Wes'50.

GILLEN, George R.; 117 King St. E., Oshawa, Ont.; 397 Mary St., (res); Ott '60; Tel. 728-1661.

GILLESPIE, Andrew E.; Ste. 120, 645 Fort St., Victoria, B.C.; 1414 Monterey Ave. (res); McG '48; DABP; FAAP; Paed; Chief (Paed.), St. Joseph's Hosp.; Assoc. Staff (Paed.), Royal Jubilee Hosp.; Tel. 383-2411.

GILLESPIE, C. Terrence; Dal'57; Paed; Staff, Children's Hosp., University Ave., Halifax, N.S.

GILLESPIE, Duncan J.; Man '63; Sr. Int., Wpg. Gen. Hosp., Winnipeg 3, Man.

GILLESPIE, Francis A.; National U. (Ire.)'54; Res., Hosp. for Mental & Nervous Dis., St. John's, Nfld.

GILLESPIE, Hector S.; 750 W. Broadway, Vancouver 9, B.C.; 4891 Paton (res); Tor'42; FRCS (C); **OrthSurg; Att'd. Staff, Van.Gen. & Shaugh**nessy Hosp's.; Clin. Instr., U. of British Columbia; Tel. 874-9334.

GILLESPIE, James W.; 164 St. Clair Ave. E., **Toronto 7, Ont.; Tor '50; MCGP; Tel. HU 5-9016.**

GILLESPIE, John C.; City Hall, Edmonton, Alta.; 15813-94A Ave. (res); Glasgow (Scot.) '49; DPH; DCH; Deputy M.O.H., City of Edmonton; **Sess. Instr., U. of Alberta; Tel. GA 4-0211.**

GILLETT, Peter G.; McG'63; Jr. Ass't. Res., Montreal Gen. Hosp., Montreal, P.Q.

GILLICK, Roy H.; 419 Dundas St., London, Ont.; 760 North Mile Rd. (res); Wes '59; MCGP; Tel. GE 3-3946.

GILLIES, Deirdre M.; Apt. 801, 4998 Western Ave., Montreal 6, P.Q.; Edinburgh (Scot.)'50; DA; Anaes; Anaes., Queen Elizabeth Hosp.; **Dem. (Anaes), McGill U.; Tel. HU 8-2311.**

GILLIES, George E.; Ste. 1124 Medical Dental Bldg., Vancouver, B.C.; McG '06; GenSurg.

GILLIES, James M.; Cancer Research Fdn., 700 Bannatyne Ave., Winnipeg 3, Man.; Glasgow (Scot.)'47; TherRad.

GILLIES, James N.; P.O. Box 39, New Carlisle, P.Q.; McG'26; MCGP; Dist. M.O., CNR; Tel. 752-2144.

GILLIES, John D.; Ste. 108, 280 Bloor St. W., Toronto 5, Ont.; Tor'44; ObstGyn; Fell. (ObstGyn), U. of Toronto; Teach. Staff, Toronto Gen. Hosp.; Tel. WA 2-6761.

GILLIES, John Z.; 103 Med. Arts Bldg., 280 Bloor St. W., Toronto, Ont.; 201 Cortleigh Blvd. (res); Tor '13; MCGP; Staff, OPD Med. Clin., Toronto Western Hosp.; Tel. WA 3-8292.

GILLIES, Richard R.; 340 McLeod St., Ottawa, Ont.; Qns'55; FRCP(C), IntMed; Hd. Gastroent. Serv., Ottawa Civic Hosp.; Cons. Gastroent, N.D.M.C.; Lect. (Clin. Med.), U. of Ottawa; Tel. 235-9683.

GILLIS, D. Alexander; 5880 Spring Garden Rd., Halifax, N.S.; Dal'53; FRCS(C); M.S. (Surg.) (U. of Minn.); GenSurg; ABOS; DABS; Chief Surg., Children's Hosp.; Cons. Surg., Halifax Infirmary and Grace Maternity Hosp.; Assoc. Prof. (Surg.), Dalhousie U.; Tel. 423-8693.

GILLIS, Frank G., F/L; Dal'65; Staff, Base Hosp., RCAF Station, Trenton, Ont.; Tel. 382-3511, Loc. 560.

GILLIS, John G.; 425, 2184 W. Broadway, Vancouver 9, B.C.; 5290 Maple St., (res); McG '49; IntMed; Assoc. Staff, St. Paul's Hosp.; Court. Staff, St. Joseph's Hosp.; Staff, B.C. Cancer Inst.; Tel. RE 6-6441.

GILLIS, John M.; Eldon, P.E.I.; Dal '59; MCGP; Court. Staff, Charlottetown & P.E.I. Hosp's.; Tel. 1-2.

GILLIS, Wilfred R.; 537 Mountain Rd., Moncton, N.B.; Dal'61; AMCGP.

GILLISON, Norman B.; Ste. 10, 10172—119th St., Edmonton, Alta. (res); London (Eng.) '53; Staff, **Charles Camsell Indian Hosp.; Tel. GL 5-7141.**

GILLMAN, Ross G.; Wes '59; GenSurg; Staff, U. of Western Ontario, London, Ont.

GILLRIE, R. Bruce; 628 Lister Bl., 42 James St. N., Hamilton, Ont.; Tor'21; Tel. 522-6533.

GILMORE, William M.; 43 Guthrie Ave., Stratford, Ont. (res); Wes '27; DABR; D & T Rad; Radiol., Stratford Gen. Hosp. and Memorial Hosp., Listowel, Ont.; Tel. 271-2120.

GILMOUR, David M.; 816-103rd Ave., Dawson Creek, B.C.; Alb '58; Staff, St. Joseph's Gen. & Pouce Coupe Comm. Hosp., Pouce Coupe; Tel. 782-5271.

GILMOUR, Joan (Sutherland); Sheffield (Eng.) '60; Staff, Manitoba Rehabilitation Hosp., Winnipeg, Man.; Tel. SP 5-0181.

GILMOUR, Joseph L.; 1214 Fairmont Medical Bldg., 750 W. Broadway, Vancouver 9, B.C.; Tor '54; GenSurg; Active Staff, Vancouver Gen. Hosp., St. Paul's & St. Vincent's Hosp's.; Tel. 874-7716.

GIMBEL, Hervey W.; North Hill Shopping Centre, 2nd Floor Office Ses., 1632 14th Ave. N.W., Calgary, Alta.; 1233-20th St. N.W. (res); Coll. of Med. Evang., Los Angeles (Calif., U.S.A.) '55; **M.C.G.P.; Staff, Calgary Gen., Holy Cross,** Grace Maternity & Alberta Crippled Children's **Hosp's.; Tel. AV 9-5044.**

GIMBEL, Howard V.; 103 Rideau Medical-Dental Centre, 1711-4th St. S.W. Calgary, Alta.; Loma Linda, Cal '60; Ophth; Tel. 269-4650.

GIMBERT, Shanna B. (Wright); 125 Yonge Blvd., Toronto 12, Ont.; Glasgow (Scot.) '38; D.P.H.; M.C.G.P.; Staff, (G.P., Div.) Women's College **Hosp.; Tel. HU 9-4505.**

GINGRAS, Gilles; Pont Rouge, Co. Portneuf, P.Q.; Lav'54; Tel. 873-2545.

GINGRAS, Gustave; 290 Morrison Ave., Town of Mt. Royal, P.Q. (res); Mon '43; ABPMR; FAAPMR; FRCP(C), PhysMed & Rehab; Exec. Dir. Rehab. Inst., 6300 Darlington Ave., Mtl. 26; Dir. Schl. of Rehab. & Prof. (P.M.R.), U. of Montreal; Dir., School of Rehab., Laval U.; Dir. P.M.R. Serv. D.V.A., Mtl. Dist.; Cons. P.M.R., WHO & Cdn. Forces Med. Council; Tel. 735-3741.

GINGRAS, Jacques; 700 St. Julie, Trois Rivieres, P.Q.; Lav '49; MCGP; Tel. FR 6-3344.

GINGRAS, Michel; 3460 Limoges, Ville St-Laurent, P.Q.; Lav'63; Med. Admin., Woods Gordon & Co.

GINGRAS, Pierre; Ste. 105, 11072 Ouest, Boul. Gouin, Pierrefonds, P.Q.; Mon '56; Tel. 684-3511.

GINGRAS, Roland; 523 St. Vallier W., Quebec, P.Q.; Lav '37; Tel. 523-2914.

GINGRAS, Rosaire L.J.; 1030 des Gouvenerneurs, Sillery, Quebec 6, P.Q.; Lav'34; Biochem. (P.Q.); Dir., Dept. of Biochem. & Dean, Fact. of Med., U. of Laval; Tel. LA 9-4511.

GINGRICH, David E.; West'65; Jr. Int., St. Joseph's Hosp., Toronto, Ont.; Abroad.

GINSBERG, Robert J.; Tor '63; P.G., U. of Toronto, Toronto 5, Ont.

GINSBERG, Samuel; 3 Alberta Ave., Toronto, Ont.; 50 Lynnhaven Rd. (res); Tor '49; M.C.-G.P.; Staff, New Mount Sinai Hosp.; Tel. LE 5-1541.

GINSHERMAN, Abraham B.; 3597 Lasalle Blvd., Verdun, P.Q.; 4721 Circle Rd., Montreal (res); McG'26; Tel. 767-5303; Abroad.

GINZBERG, Leibisch; 71 Howard Park Ave., Toronto 3, Ont.; Sask '53.

GIOVANDO, Lorenzo; 350 Albert St., Nanaimo, B.C.; 523 Vancouver Ave. (res); McG '30.

GIOVANNETTI, Joseph L.; Newcastle, N.B.; Dal '31; M.C.G.P.

GIRARD, Albert; 1058 rue St. Denis, Montreal **18, P.Q.; Mon '43; OrthSurg.; Tel. 842-4816.**

GIRARD, Armand E. A.; 236 Longueuil, St. Jean, **P.Q. Mon '33; Paed (P.Q.); Head of Paed. Dept., St. John's Hosp.; Inst'r., Local Nurses' School. Tel. 66871.**

GIRARD, Claude; Mon'61; Res., Hop. Notre-Dame, Montreal, P.Q.; Abroad.

GIRARD, Denis; 1460 Cap. Eternite, Duvernay, Ville de Laval, P.Q.; Lav'58; Anaes (P.Q.).

GIRARD, Fernando; 11109 L'Archeveque, Montreal-Nord, P.Q.; **Mon'55; MCGP; Ass't. Dir.,** Dept. of Health, Montreal (North); Tel. DA 2-1640.

GIRARD, Georges H.; Lac-aux-Sables, Co. Port-neuf, P.Q.; Lav '57.

GIRARD, Gerard; 1230 de Callieres, Quebec 6, P.Q. (res); Lav '48; F.R.C.S.(C), GenSurg; **Prof., Laval U.; Tel. LA 9-4511.**

GIRARD, Jean-Marie; St-Nazaire, Co. Lapointe, P.Q.; Lav '60.

GIRARD, Leo J.; 945 Parent St., Windsor, Ont.; Wes '23; Dist. Coroner.

GIRARD, Marc; 8160 Place Vaujours, Ville D'Anjou, Montreal 5, P.Q. (res); Lav '51; Diag-Rad; Staff, Queen Mary Vets Hosp.; Tel. RE 8-9481.

GIRARD, Marcel; 1820 Blvd. St. Joseph, Montreal, P.Q.; 860 Riviera, Laval W. (res); Mon '47; AMCGP; Chief, Dept. of G.P., Hop. Belle Chasse; Tel. LA 3-3563.

GIRARD, Michel; Lav'61; ObstGyn(P.Q.); Staff, Hop.-de-l'Enfant Jesus, Quebec, P.Q.

GIRARD, Paul M.; 590 McIntyre St. W., North Bay, Ont.; Mon '50; Sr. Treatment M.O., D.V.A.

GIRARD, Roland; 415 Ste-Helene, Longueuil, Cite-Jacques-Cartier, P.Q.; 810 Ste. Elizabeth, La Prairie (res); Lav'56; Tel. OR 4-8217

GIRARD, Yvan M.; 55 rue de l'Eglise, Verdun, Montreal 19, P.Q.; Mon'58; FRCS(C), ObstGyn; FACOG; Staff, Hop. Gen. de Verdun; Tel. 768-1802.

GIRARDIN, Guy; 55 Church St., Verdun, Mtl. 19, P.Q.; 4052 Oxford St. (res); Mon '49; Paed (Penn. & PQ); Hd. Dept. of Paed., LaSalle Gen. Hosp.; Ass't. (Paed), Hop.-de-Verdun; Ass't. Clin. Prof. U. of Mtl.; Tel. 766-3593.

GIRAY, Saim; M.O., Provincial Mental Hosp., Campbellton, N.B.; Istanbul (Turkey) '54.

GIRDAUSKAS, Grazina M.; Tor'63; Res., Toronto Western Hosp., Toronto 2B, Ont.

GIROUARD, J. Edgar; 336 rue High, Moncton, N.B.; Lav '51; FICS; GenSurg; Staff, Hotel-Dieu l'Assomption & Moncton Hosp.; Tel. 382-3700.

GIROUX, Andre; 18 St. Paul, Oka, P.Q.; Mon'65.

GIROUX, J. Cartier; 822 Sherbrooke est, Montreal 24, P.Q.; 465 Oakdale Ave., Town of Mount Royal (res); Mon '52; M.Sc.; FACS; FRCS(C); NeurSurg; Staff (NeurSurg.), Hop. Notr-Dame; Cons. (NeurSurg.), Hop. St-Vincent-de-Paul, Sherbrooke; Cons. (NeurSurg.), Hop. St-Charles, **St. Hyacinthe; Ass't. Prof. (Surg.), U. of Mont-**real; Tel. 526-9487.

GIROUX, Jean M.; 3875, rue St. Urbain, Montreal 18, P.Q.; Mon '58; FRCP(C); Derm; Staff, Hop. Hotel-Dieu; Ass't. Prof., U. of Montreal; Tel. 849-3445.

GIROUX, Leo L.; 462 Professional Bldg., 10830 Jasper Ave., Edmonton, Alta.; Alb'40; Urol; Clin. Instr., U. of Alberta; Tel. GA 2-6271.

GIROUX, Maurice; 1014 Mont-St.-Denis, Quebec, P.Q.; Lav '31; Path, Bact; Dir. Labs., Hop.-Laval, Ste-Foy; Prof. (Embriol.), Laval U.; Tel. LA 9-4511.

GIRVAN, G. Ralph; 927 Richmond St., London, Ont.; McG '36; ObstGyn; Sr. Fell; Obst & Gyn., U. of Western Ontario; Tel. 439-1581.

GIRVIN, John P.; 4331 Melrose Ave., Montreal 28, P.Q. (res); Wes '58; Research (Physiol.), McGill U. Abroad.

GIULIANELLI, Leonardo S.; Ste. 44, 1390 Sherbrooke St. W., Montreal, P.Q.; 2852 Masson St., Rosemount; Apt. 23, 4800 Cote des Neiges Rd. (res); McG '32; IntMed; Phys., St. Mary's Hosp.; Tel. AV 8-1954.

GIVAN, Kathleen F.; 69 Baby Point Cr., Toronto, Ont.; Tor'56; Bact.; Research Fell. Banting Inst..

GIVELAS, T. C.; Tor'62; Res., Hosp. for Sick Children, Toronto 2, Ont.

GIVENS, William C.; 3 Hill Cres., Scarborough, Ont.; Tor '16; MCGP; Retired.

GLADMAN, Donald J., Capt.; 1 Field Ambulance, R.C.A.M.C., C.F.P.O. 5050, Europe; UBC '62. Abroad.

GLADDY, Percy V.; 539 Exmouth St., Sarnia, Ont.; 113 Admiral Ave. (res); Qns '50; Obst-Gyn; Tel. DI 4-3695.

GLADSTONE, Norman; 1530 Bloor St. W., Toronto, Ont.; 2550 Bathurst St. (res); Tor '55; Tel. LE 4-7667.

GLADSTONE, Richard M.; Tor'64; Res., St. Michael's Hosp., Toronto, Ont.

GLADU, L. Maurice; 166 King St. W., Sherbrooke, P.Q.; Mon '53; Anaes (P.Q.); Tel. 569-3993.

GLADWIN, Kenneth D.; 34 Pleasant St., Dartmouth, N.S.; 32 Limardo Dr. (res); Dal '59; AMCGP; Tel. 469-2445.

GLAISHER, Ivor L.; 700 Med. & Dental Bldg., Regina, Sask.; 2099 Cross Pl. (res); London (Eng.)'52; MRCS; LRCP; Staff, Regina Gen. and Grey Nuns Hosp's.; Tel. 527-3060.

GLAISTER, Deborah (Mrs. Hannay); 15 Weber St. E., Kitchener, Ont.; Tor '32; Tel. 742-0919.

GLAS, Arnold P.; Hythe, Alta.; Prague (Czech.) '27; Alb '46; Dist. Coroner.

GLASGOW, Robert M.; Radway, Alta.; Alb'64.

GLASGOW, Robert R.; Alb '34; M.C.G.P.; Admin. Deputy Chief M.O., Workmen's Compensation Board, 10048-101A Ave., Edmonton, Alta.; Tel. GA 2-7151.

GLASS, Bernard; 3205 Wyandotte Ave. E., Windsor, Ont.; Wes'63.

GLASS, Irving H.; 340 McLeod St., Ottawa, Ont.; Tor '55; FRCP(C); FAAP; FACCP; Paed; Staff, Ottawa Civic, Ottawa Gen., St. Louis Marie de Montfort & Grace Hosp's.; Lect., U. of Ottawa; Tel. 233-2488.

GLASS, Leslie S.; 1904 Lonsdale Ave., North Vancouver, B.C.; 4035 St. Albans, (res); Edinburgh (Scot.) '40; MRCOG; FRCS(C), ObstGyn; Active Cons., Lion's Gate Hosp.; Tel. YU 5-1301.

GLASSCO, William G.; 526 Medical Arts Bldg., 404 Graham Ave., Winnipeg 1, Man.; 329 Elm St., Winnipeg 9 (res); London (Eng.) '31; D.P.M.; Psy.; Staff, Winnipeg Gen. & Misericordia Hosp's.; Lect. (Psy.,) U. of Manitoba; Tel. WH 3-2160.

GLASSEY, David W.; 8779 Yonge St., Thornhill, Ont.; Tor'30.

GLASSMAN; Max M.; Queensway Med. Centre, 880 Queensway, Toronto 18, Ont.; 19 Hilltop Rd., Tor. 10 (res); Tor '52; MCGP; Assoc. Staff, Queensway Gen. & St. Joseph's Hosp's; Tel. CL 5-1161.

GLASSMAN, Morris; Parkdale Med. Centre, 1271 Dundas W., Toronto 3, Ont.; 35 Warwick Ave., Tor. 10 (res); **Tor '37; GenSurg; Assoc. Surg. Staff, Doctor's Hosp.; Court. Surg. Staff, Central Hosp.; Tel. LE 5-6300.**

GLASSOW, Frank; 30 Colborne St., Thornhill, Ont.; Cambridge (Eng.) '42; MRCS(Lond.), LRCP(Eng.), FRCS(Eng.), FRCS(C), GenSurg., Surg., Shouldice Clinic; Tel. 889-1255.

GLATT, Benjamin S.; 150 The East Mall, Islington, Ont.; Tor'54; DAB; Paed; Tel. 621-2220.

GLAWDAN, Helena P. (Gromov); 734 Spadina Ave., Toronto 4, Ont.; Kharkov (Ukraine) '40; MCGP; Active Staff, Women's College Hosp.; Hypnother., The Bell Clinic; Tel. WA 2-4312.

GLAY, A.; 1240 Lucerne Rd., Town of Mount Royal, Montreal 16, P.Q. (res); Geneva (Switz.) '34; F.R.C.S.(C), D & TRad; Staff, Hop. Hotel Dieu; Tel. VI 4-0161.

GLAZIER, Edward; 136 Simcoe St. N., Oshawa, Ont.; 279 Glenview Ave. (res); Tor '49; MCGP; Tel. 723-7731.

GLAZMAN, Bernard; 546 Palmerston Blvd., Toronto 4, Ont.; Tor '56; AMCGP; Staff, Doctor's Hosp.; Tel. 531-5673.

GLEDHILL, Robert B.; Wes'60; FRCS(C), O rthSurg; Staff, Montreal Gen. Hosp., Montreal, P.Q.

GLEN, Norman G.; 1 Church St., Amherst, N.S.; 183 Victoria St. E. (res); Bristol (Eng.) '47; M.B., B.Ch., DRCOG; MCGP; Staff, Highland View Hosp.; Staff, Sackville Mem. Hosp., Sackville; Tel. 667-3426.

GLEN, William F.; 60 Grand Ave., W., Chatham, Ont.; 354 Victoria Ave. (res); Qns '32; MCGP; Tel. EL 4-2611.

GLENISTER, Ernest I.; 1791 Barrington St., Halifax, N.S.; Dal'25; Ophth; Staff, Halifax Infirmary & Glaucoma Clinic Victoria Gen. Hosp.; Tel. 423-8703.

GLENNIE, Gordon D.; 287 Queens Ave., London, Ont.; London (Eng.) '51; M.B., B.S., MRCS (Eng.), LRCP(Lond.); Anaes; Cons. Anaes., St. Joseph's Hosp.; Instr. (Anaes), U. of Western Ont.; Tel. GE 8-5143.

GLENNON, John; Ire. '56; Jr. Int'n., Regina Grey Nuns' Hosp., Regina, Sask.

GLICK, Daniel; 1192 Queen St. E., Toronto, Ont.; 18 Elway Ct., Apt. 3, (res); Tor '57; MCGP.; Tel. 463-4878.

GLICK, Harry; McG '62; Jr. Intn., Jewish Gen. Hosp., Montreal 26, P.Q.

GLICK, Hyman; McG'65; Res., Jewish Gen. Hosp., Montreal 26, P.Q.

GLICKMAN, Irvin B.; 600 Ellendale Med. Bldg., 5845 Cote des Neiges Rd., Montreal 26, P.Q.; 641 Victoria Ave., Westmount (res); McG '48; ObstGyn; Ass't., Jewish Gen. Hosp.; Chief, Dept. of ObstGyn, Bellechasse Hosp.; Tel. RE 1-9261.

GLIDDON, Edward C.; 10 Hincks St., St. Thomas, Ont.; 98 Sunset Dr. (res); McG '27; GenSurg. Retired.

GLOOR, Pierre; 3801 University Ave., Montreal 2, P.Q.; Basel (Switz.)'48; Ph.D.; Chief Electroenceph. & Neurophysiol., Mtl. Neurol. Inst.; Phys-I/C Electroenceph., Royal Victoria Hosp.; Assoc. Prof. (Experiment. Neur.), McGill U.; Tel. VI 2-1251, Loc. 605.

GLOSTER, Michael E.; Box 311, Red Lake, Ont.; London (Eng.) '57; MRCS(Eng.); LRCP (Lond.); Coroner, District of Kenora; Tel. R.L. 200.

GLOSTER, Owen C. L.; 149 Kenneth St., Duncan, B.C.; Glasgow (Scot.)'48; Tel. 748-8151.

GLOVER, Thomas J.; 110 Bloor St. W., Toronto 5, Ont.; 494 Avenue Rd., (res); Tor '11; Tel. WA 3-3719.

GLUBE, Mildred R; Box 1270, North P.O., Halifax, NS.; 22 Inglewood Dr. (res); Anaes. Tel. 423-8693.

GLUCK, Manuel; 2286 Carling Ave., Ottawa 3, **Ont.; 688 Hillcrest Ave. (res); Ott '56; ObstGyn; Staff, Ottawa Civic & Grace Hosp's.; Tel. 729-6704.**

GLYNN, John J.; Sick Mariners Clinic, Box 129, Halifax, N.S.; 33 Canary Cres., Rockingham (res); Galway (Ire.) '49; M.B., B.ch, BAO; L.M.; CPH (Dublin); DPH (Tor); Phys., Dept. of Nat. Health & Welfare; Tel. 423-7197.

GLYNN, Michael F.; 86 Queen's Park Cres., Toronto 5, Ont.; Loyola (Chicago, U.S.A.) '58; FRCP(C), IntMed; Abroad.

GNASS, J. Ernst; Trail-Tadanac Hosp., Trail, B.C.; Hamburg (Germ.) '55; Path.; Tel. 368-3311.

GNUECHTEL, Wolfgang; 327 Medical Arts Bldg., 750 Spadina Cres. E., Saskatoon, Sask.; Heidelberg (Germany) '52; OrthSurg. Abroad.

GOAD, F. D.; Deep River, Ont.; Tor '47; Gen**Surg; Staff, Deep River Hosp.; Tel. JU 4-2791.**

GOBA, Herberts K.; Evansburg, Alta.; Hamburg (Germ.) **'47; Tel. 156.**

GOBEIL, Jacques; Petit Saguenay, Cte Saguenay, **P.Q.; Lav '61.**

GOBEIL, J. Gerald; Box 159, Ste Anne, Man.; Ott '64.

GOBEIL, Louis J.; Victoria St., Grande Baie, P.Q.; Lav '41; M.C.G.P.

GOBIUS, Risto J.; Allin Clinic, 10155-120th St., Edmonton, Alta.; 9542-91st St. (res); Leyden (Holl.) '53; Paed; Tel. HU 8-7271.

GODARD, Denise; Mon '63; Res., Hop. St. Luc, Montreal, P.Q.

GODARD, Raymond; 12, rue Principale, Amos, P.Q.; Mon '61.

GODBERSON, Charles V.; Box 409, Barrhead Clinic, Barrhead, Alta.; Alb'56; AMCGP; Tel. 674-2231.

GODBOUT, J. Richard, F/L; Dal'64; Sr. M.O., RCAF Station, Bagotville, P.Q.; Tel. 677-2040, Ext. 307.

GODBOUT, Y.; 500 Lafontaine, Riviere du Loup, P.Q.; Lav '50

GODDARD, Ernest S.; 291 Dundas St., London, Ont.; Wes '35; F.A.P.A., D.Psy., Psy; Dir., Community Psy. Clin.; Sr. Assoc. (Psy.) & Instr. **(Med.), U. of Western Ontario; Tel. 439-8491.**

GODDARD, J. C.; Hensall, Ont.; Alb '38; Dist. Coroner.

GODDEN, John O.; 150 St. George St., Toronto 5, Ont.; 293 Dawlish Ave., Toronto 12, Ont.; Dal'51; M.Sc.(Minn.); IntMed; Assoc. Ed., CMA Publications; Cons. in Med. Communications; Tel. 924-0751 & 481-7091.

GODEL, John C.; Alb'55; Res., University Hosp., Edmonton, Alta.

GODFREY, Charles M.; 484 Church St., Toronto 5, Ont.; 2 Legato Ct., Don Mills (res); Tor '53; PhysMed & Rehab; Dir. Dept. of PhysMed & Rehab., Wellesley & Toronto East Gen. Hosp's.; Clin. Instr., U. of Toronto; Tel. WA 3-7127.

GODFREY, J. Godfrey; 514 Jarvis St., Toronto, Ont.; 81 Bannockburn Ave., Tor. 12 (res); Tor '55; D.Psy; Psy; Staff Phys., Toronto Mental Health Clinic; Tel. 924-7349.

GODIN, Andre; 2181 Pere Lelievie, Quebec 8, P.Q.; Lav'65.
GODIN, Lucien; Rawdon, P.Q.; 414 Queen St. (res); Mon '41; Dep. Coroner.
GODIN, P .E. Antonio; 359 Mt. Royal W., Montreal 8, P.Q.; Mon '23; Ophth, Otol; Ass't. Hop's. Notre Dame & Ste. Justine; Tel. 277-6422.
GODIN, Paul Emile; 1060 Ave. Royale, Villeneuve, Quebec 5, P.Q.; Lav '60.
GODON, Alain; Mon'60; Res., Hop. Hotel-Dieu, Montreal, P.Q.
GODRON, Eleonore R.; 3412 Atwater, Montreal 25, P.Q.; 5816 Palmer Ave. (res); Munich (Germ.) '30; Staff, Verdun Prot. Hosp.; Tel. WE 2-4577.
GODWIN, Thomas F.; Tor'61; FRCP(C), IntMed; Staff, Toronto Gen. Hosp., Toronto, Ont.
GOEL, Devendra P.; 1655 Commercial Dr., Vancouver 6, B.C.; Lucknow (India)'50; GenSurg.
GOEL, Joe N.; 8 George St., Galt, Ont.; Lucknow (India) '52; DOMS; M.Sc.(Ophth.); Ophth; Cons., South Waterloo Mem. Hosp.; Tel. 621-5140.
GOEL, Shash B.; 22 Hillcrest Dr., Galt, Ont.; Delhi (India)'54; FRCP(C), Anaes.
GOERTZ, Edwin P.; Box 490, Milk River, Alta.; UBC '59; AMCGP.
GOERTZ, Otto P.; Herbert, Sask.; St. Andrew's (Scot.) '60.
GOERTZEN, George; 755 W. Broadway Vancouver 9, B.C.; 925 W. 33rd Ave., Vancouver 13 (res); UBC '57; MCGP; Tel. TR 2-2541.
GOFTON, John P.; Ste. 250, 5780 Cambie St., Vancouver 15, B.C.; 5875 Yew (res); McG '50; FRCP(C), IntMed; Research Dir., Cdn. Arthritis & Rheum. Soc. (BC) Div.; Att'd. Staff, Shaughnessy Hosp.; Clin. Instr., U. of British Columbia; Tel. FA 7-3711.
GOGAN, Irial; 605 Renfrew House, Rideau Towers, Calgary, Alta.; Nat. U. (Dublin, Ire.) '43; DPH; MRSH; Med. Dir., Holy Cross Hosp.; Tel. 262-9409.
GOH, E. G.; Tor'64; Res., Hosp. for Sick Children, Toronto 2, Ont.
GOKCEN, Mehmet I.; 7200 Gouin Boul. E., Montreal 38, P.Q.; Istanbul (Turk.) '54; Psy; Staff, Hop. Mont Providence; Tel. 665-4971.
GOKIERT, J. Guy; Whissell Clinic, Westlock, Alta.; Alb'65; Assoc. Staff, Immaculata Hosp.; Tel. 342-3366.
GOKULANATHAN, Karakat, S.; Kerala (India) '56; FRCP(C), Paed; Staff, St. Joseph's Hosp., Toronto, Ont.; Tel. 534-9531.
GOLAB, Alexander; Sask'62; Res., New Mt. Sinai Hosp., Toronto 2, Ont.
GOLAB, Samuel; 1852 Bloor W., Toronto 9, Ont.; Paris (Fr.) '31; MCGP; Tel. RO. 6-5773.
GOLD, Allen; 3766 Cote-des-Neiges Rd., Montreal 25, P.Q.; 1680 St.-Clare Rd., Mtl. 16 (res); McG '42; M.Sc., FACP; FRCP(C), IntMed; Cons. (Endocrin. & Metab.), Queen Mary Vet's Hosp.; Assoc. Phys., Mtl. Gen. Hosp.; Lect. (Med. & Dent.), McGill U.; Tel. WE 5-8161.
GOLD, A. C.; Tor '64; Res., Hosp. for Sick Children, Toronto 2, Ont.
GOLD, Charles C.; Tor '64; Res. (Dept. of Obst-Gyn.), U. of Toronto, Toronto 5, Ont.
GOLD, Gerald; 68 Howard Pk. Ave., Toronto 3, Ont.; Tor '59; AMCGP; Tel. LE 6-6122.
GOLD, Lawrence H. A.; Man '62; Jr. Intn., Winnipeg Gen. Hosp., Winnipeg, Man.
GOLD, Marjorie E.; Ste. 207, 10405 Saskatchewan Dr., Edmonton, Alta.; Alb'64; Tel. 433-7553.
GOLD, Michael M. A.; 5845 Cote des Neiges, Montreal 25, P.Q.; 4705 Circle Rd. (res); McG '43; M.Sc.(Path.), D.A.B.I.M., F.R.C.P.(C) IntMed; Cardiol (P.Q.); Act. Phys.-in-Chief, Jewish Gen. Hosp.; Lect., Dept. of Invest. Med., McGill U.; Tel. WE 7-4070.
GOLD, Phil; McG'61; FRCP(C), IntMed; Med. Research Fell., Montreal Gen. Hosp., Montreal 25, P.Q.
GOLD, Reynold J. M.; 22nd Floor Ave. Bldg., 3rd Ave., Saskatoon, Sask.; Cambridge (Eng.)'58; Staff, St. Paul's & City Hosp's.; Clin. Fell., University Hosp.; Tel. 652-0300.
GOLD, Simon; 5845 Cote des Neiges Rd., Ste. 505, Montreal 26, P.Q.; McG '40; M.Sc., FACS; FACOG; ObstGyn; ObstGyn-in-Charge, Hop. Jean Talon Lect., McGill U.; Tel. 735-3131.
GOLD, Solomon; 6000 Cote des Neiges Rd., Montreal, P.Q.; McG '23; MCGP; Hon. Gyn., Jewish Gen. Hosp.; Court.(Obst.), Royal Victoria Hosp.; Tel. RE 8-4616.
GOLD, S. Samuel; 194 Coldstream Ave., Toronto 12, Ont.; Tor'45; FAAP; Paed; Clin. Ass't., Hosp. for Sick Children; Court. Staff (Paed.), Mount Sinai Hosp.; Clin. Instr., U. of Toronto; Tel. 481-0408.
GOLDBERG, A. H.; 116 Hinchey Ave., New Waterford, N.S.; R.C.S. (Ireland) '60.
GOLDBERG, Benjamin; Children's Psych. Research Inst., London, Ont.; Dal'55; Psy; Supt. Children's Psy. Research Inst.; Instr. (Psy.), U. of Western Ontario; Tel. GE 8-4185.
GOLDBERG, Erwin H.; 4560 Lasalle Blvd., Montreal 19, P.Q.; Dal '60; AMCGP; Staff, Bellechasse Hosp.
GOLDBERG, Howard I.; 1355 Barrington St., Halifax, N.S.; 11 Tobin St. (res); Dal '40; Derm-Syph; Lect. (Derm.), Dalhousie U.; Tel. 423-7594.
GOLDBERG, Ian L.; 805 Boyd Bldg., 388 Portage Ave., Winnipeg 1, Man.; Man'60; Paed.; Dem. (Paed.), U. of Manitoba; Tel. WH 3-0641.
GOLDBERG, John; 68 Howard Pk. Ave., Toronto 3, Ont.; 3236 Weston Rd., Weston; Tor '49; MCGP; Staff, Doctor's Hosp., Toronto; Tel. LE 6-6122; 241-9129.
GOLDBERG, Joseph; 47 Cote-St.-Catherine Rd., Outremont, Montreal, P.Q.; McG '29; MCGP; Tel. 272-4671.
GOLDBERG, Karolina; 5630 Durocher Ave., Montreal 8, P.Q.; Italy '38; Tel. 276-6412.
GOLDBERG, Leonard; 272 Roncesvalles Ave., Toronto, Ont.; 209 Hillhurst Blvd. (res); Tor '42; D.R., D.A.B.R., DiagRad; Dir. (Dept. Rad.), Northwestern Gen. Hosp.; Tel. LE 6-6023.
GOLDBERG, Melville; Tor'65; Jr. Int., Toronto Gen. Hosp., Toronto 2, Ont.
GOLDBERG, Michael R.; Tor'65; Jr. Int., New Mount Sinai Hosp., Toronto 2, Ont.
GOLDBERG, Melvyn; Tor'65; Res., 5th Floor, Banting Inst., Toronto 2, Ont.
GOLDBERG, Norman J.; 6000 Cote des Neiges Rd., Ste. 240, Montreal 26, P.Q.; McG '59; FRCP-(C), IntMed; Gastroent.(P.Q.); Jr. Ass't. Phys., Jewish Gen. Hosp.; Research Fell. (Gastroent.), McGill U.; Pt.-time Phys., Steinberg's Ltd.; Tel. 733-2232.
GOLDBERG, William M.; 78 Bertram Dr., Dundas, Ont. (res); Wes'49; FACP; FRCP(C), IntMed; Hd., Dept. of Med., St. Joseph's Hosp.; Memb. of Council (R.C.P. and S.C.); Pres. Elect., Hamilton Acad. of Med.; Tel. JA 8-7929.
GOLDBLOOM, Alton; 508 Medical Arts Bldg., 1538 Sherbrooke St. W., Montreal, P.Q.; 3980 Côte des Neiges (res); McG '16; D.C.L. (Bish.) DABP; FAAP; FRCP; Paed; Emeritus Prof. Paed., McGill U.; Cons. Montreal Children's, Montreal Gen. & Jewish Gen. Hosp's. & Royal Edward Laurentian San; Tel. WE 5-9762.
GOLDBLOOM, Richard B.; 2300 Tupper St., Montreal, P.Q.; 108 Thurlow Rd., Hampstead (res); McG '49; FRCP(C), Paed; Ass't. Phys., Montreal Children's Hosp.; Cons. (Paed.), Physician's Hosp., Plattsburg, N.Y.; Ass't. Prof. (Paed.), McGill U.; Tel. WE 7-8511.
GOLDBLOOM, Victor C.; 307, 1538 Sherbrooke St. W., Montreal 25, P.Q.; 5 Grove Pk, Mtl. 6 (res); McG '45; Paed; Ass't. Phys., Mtl. Children's & Jewish Gen. Hosp's.; Cons. (Paed.), Baron-de-Hirsch Inst.; 3rd VP, College of P & S (PQ); Dem. (Paed.), McGill U.; Tel. WE 5-2616.
GOLDEN, Clifford; 6000 Cote des Neiges, Montreal 26, P.Q.; 603 Algonquin Ave., Mt. Royal (res); McG '50; Paed; Staff. Mtl. Childrens and Jewish Gen. Hosp's and Health Dept., Twn. of Mount Royal; Tel. RE 7-8471.
GOLDEN, Isaac M.; 662 Bathurst St., Toronto, Ont.; 26 Dewbourne Ave. (res); Tor '23; Tel. LE 1-7160.

GOLDENBERG, Henry; 158 St. George St., Toronto, Ont.; 4 Shelborne Ave. (res); Tor '43; F.R.C.P.(C), IntMed; Sr. Att. Phys., New Mt. Sinai Hosp.; Ass't., Outpatient Dept., Toronto Gen. Hosp., & Dem., Clin. Microscopy, U. of Toronto; Tel. WA 1-4223.
GOLDENBERG, Gerald J.; Man '57; IntMed; Staff Cancer Research Fdn., 700 Bannatyne Ave., Winnipeg 3, Man.; Ass't. Prof., U. of Manitoba.
GOLDENBERG, Leon; 1466 Bathurst St., Toronto, Ont.; 53 Burnside Dr. (res); Tor '43; Paed; **Staff (Paed.), New Mt. Sinai Hosp.; Tel. LE 4-5925.**
GOLDENBERG, Louis M.; 345 Bloor St. W., Toronto, Ont.; 1840 Bathurst St., Apt. 106 (res); Tor '36; DermSyph; Staff (Derm.), New Mt. Sinai Hosp.; Tel. WA 2-1045.
GOLDENBERG, Marvin H.; McG'61; FRCP(C), DiagRad; Staff, Royal Victoria Hosp., Montreal, P.Q.
GOLDENBERG, Solomon; 1428 Ouellette Ave., Windsor, Ont.; Tor '48; F.A.C.S., F.I.C.S.; F.R.C.S.(C), GenSurg; Active Staff, Hotel-Dieu, Grace, & Metropolitan Hosp's; Cons. Surg., Riverview Hosp.; Tel. 252-4011.
GOLDFARB, Harry W.; Birmingham (Eng.) '52; Res., Hosp. for Mental & Nervous Diseases, St John's, Nfld.
GOLDFARB, H. P.; Ste 350, 6000 Cote des Neiges, Montreal 26, P.Q.; McG'49; AMCGP; Tel. 737-8010.
GOLDHAR, Albert; 2221 Keele St., Toronto 15, Ont.; 262 Wilson Ave., Downsview; 126 Ava Rd., Tor. 10 (res); Tor '49; DABOG; FRCS(C); FACOG; DNBUS; ObstGyn; Chief-of-ObstGyn., Northwestern Gen. Hosp.; Court. Staff, Branson Hosp.; Voluntary Ass't., New Mount Sinai Hosp.; Tel. CH 1-9115 & MU 5-1011.
GOLDIE, James H.; Tor'61; FRCP(C), IntMed; Staff, Princess Margaret Hosp., Toronto 5, Ont.
GOLDIE, John S.; 707 W. 37th Ave., Vancouver, B.C.; Glasgow (Scot.) '42; M.O., Workmen's. Comp. Bd.
GOLDING, Dorien R.; Birmingham (Eng.) '41; M.B., Ch.B.; Staff, James Paton Mem. Hosp., Gander, Nfld.
GOLDMAN, Bernard S.; Tor'60; Res. (Cardiovasc. Surg.), Hosp. for Sick Children, Toronto, Ont.
GOLDMAN, Hyman; 6000 Cote des Neiges, Montreal 26, P.Q.; Basel (Switz.)'58; FRCP(C), Paed; Staff, Montreal Children's Hosp.; Tel. WE 7-8511.
GOLDMAN, Ivan; Ste. 403, 99 Avenue Rd., Toronto 5, Ont.; Witwatersrand (S. Africa) **'50; MRCOG; ObstGyn; Staff, York Central Hosp.; Tel. WA 3-9095.**
GOLDMAN, Sol. E.; 310 Medical Arts Bldg., 1538 Sherbrooke St. W., Montreal, P.Q.; 4810 **Roslyn Ave. (res); McG '22; F.A.C.S.; Orth-**Surg; Hon. Att. Staff, Montreal Gen. Hosp.; **Cons. (OrthSurg), Jewish Gen. Hosp.; Cons. OrthSurg., Reddy Mem. Hosp. & Hosp. of Hope; Tel. WE 5-9942.**
GOLDMAN, William P.; 750 W. Broadway, Vancouver, B.C.; 6446 Churchill St. (res); Alb '38; F.R.C.S.(C), GenSurg; Tel. TR 4-4611.
GOLDSAND, George; 10104-140th Ave., Edmonton, Alta.; Alb '59; FRCP(C); IntMed. Abroad.
GOLDSTEIN, Abraham; Inglewood Med. Centre, 1897 Portage Ave., Winnipeg 12, Man.; Man '60; MCGP; Tel. 888-7794.
GOLDSTEIN, Albert S. Edinburgh (Scot.) '58; FRCS(C), GenSurg; Staff, Winnipeg Gen. Hosp., Winnipeg, Man.; Tel. SP 4-6511. Abroad.
GOLDSTEIN, Allan V.; 1729 Portage Ave., St. James 12, Man.; Tor '44; MCGP; Tel. 888-5019.
GOLDSTEIN, Arnold; Ste. 203, 440 Hinton Ave., Ottawa 3, Ont.; 29 Crescent Hgts. (res); Qns '49; MCGP; Assoc. Att'd. Staff, Grace Hosp.; Tel. PA 8-4611; PA 9-5008.
GOLDSTEIN, Ernest; Ste 210, 6000 Cote des Neiges Rd., Montreal 26, P.Q.; 4819 Lacombe (res); McG '31; IntMed (P.Q.); Assoc. Phys., Jewish Gen. Hosp.; Tel. RE 3-4473.
GOLDSTEIN, Marc B.; McG '64; Res., Royal Victoria Hosp., Montreal 2, P.Q.
GOLDSTEIN, Philip; 400 Norlyn Blvd., 309 Hargrave St., Winnipeg 2, Man.; 444 Enniskillen Ave., W. Kildonan (res); Qns '41; FICS; FACS; FRCS (Eng., Edin. & C.), GenSurg; Active Staff St. Boniface Hosp.; Ass't. Prof., (Surg.), U. of Man.; Tel. WH 7-0216.
GOLDSTEIN, Samuel; Man '61; Jr. Intn., St. Boniface Hosp., St. Boniface, Man.
GOLDSTEIN, Stanley E.; Ste. 480, 6000 Cote Des Neiges, Montreal 26, P.Q.; McG'60; Psy; Staff, Jewish Gen. Hosp.
GOLDSTRAW, Mary G. see McINTOSH, Mary G.
GOLDTHORPE, Arnold M.; 614 Med. & Dental Bldg., Regina, Sask.; London (Eng.)'39; MCGP; Tel. 523-2213.
GOLDTHORPE, Wilfred G.; Ste 508, 35 Walmer Rd., Toronto 4, Ont.; Tor '61.
GOLESIC, Stephen; 955 Queen St. E., Sault Ste. Marie, Ont.; Ott'52; Ophth.
GOLFMAN, Myer; Ste. 360, 5465 Queen Mary Rd., Montreal 29, P.Q.; McG'36; MCGP; Clin. Ass't., Jewish Gen. Hosp.
GOLFMAN, Sidney; 139 Carman Ave., Winnipeg 5, Man.; Man '39; M.C.G.P.
GOLLISH, Irvin; 1250 Victoria Pk. Ave., Toronto 16, Ont.; 62 Laurentide Dr., Don Mills (res); Tor '57; AMCGP; Tel. PL 9-3041.
GOLLOM, Joseph; 732 Spadina Ave., Toronto 10, Ont.; 204 Vesta Dr. (res); Tor '30; FRCS(C), Otol; Chief (Otol.), St. Joseph's & New Mt. Sinai Hosp's.; Teach. Staff Toronto Gen. Hosp.; Tel. WA 3-2233.
GOLT, Moses; 4828 Isabella Ave., Montreal, P.Q.; MCGP; Tel. RE 1-9538.
GOLUBOFF, Louis; 106 Med. Bldg., 217-3rd Ave. N., Saskatoon, Sask.; Man '31; MCGP; Cons. (ObstGyn.), City Hosp.; Teach. Staff (ObstGyn.), University Hosp.; Dir., V.D. Clinic, Saskatoon; Tel. 652-2600.
GOLUBOFF, Nathan; 105 The Medical Bldg., 217-3rd Ave. N., Saskatoon, Sask.; 1225 Elliott St. (res); Man '36; Paed; Ass't. Clin. Prof. (Paed.) U. of Saskatchewan; Tel. 242-3433.
GOLUMBIA, Joseph E.; Box 1690, Melfort, Sask.; 405 Stovel Ave. E. (res); Tor '50; MCGP; Tel. 752-2876.
GOMBERG, Charles L.; 325 Ellendale Med. Bldg., **5845 Cote-des-Neiges Rd., Montreal 26, P.Q.; 825 Burnet St., Mtl. 9, (res); Tulane (New Orleans) '52; IntMed; Clin. Phys., Jewish Gen. Hosp.; Tel. RE 3-8072.**
GOMEL, Victor; Ste. 1016, 750 West Broadway, Vancouver 9, B.C.; Istanbul (Turk.) '58; FRCS (C); ObstGyn; Staff, Vancouver Gen. Hosp.; Teach. Fell. (ObstGyn.), U. of British Columbia; Tel. 876-7011.
GOMES, F. G.; Tor '58; Jr. Int'n., Montreal Gen. Hosp., Montreal 25, P.Q.
GOMM, Audrey M.; 40 Swallow Cres., St. Albert, Alta.; Sydney (Aust.) '52.
GOMPF, John E.; 44 Mountain St., Aylmer, P.Q.; Wes'40.
GONDA, Andrew; 5757 Decelles Ave., Ste. 317, Montreal, P.Q.; Budapest (Hung.)'51; FRCP(C); IntMed; Att'd. Staff, Reddy Mem. Hosp.; Clin. Fell., Royal Victoria Hosp.; Research Ass't. McGill U.; Tel. RE 1-5179.
GONDOR, Ladislav J.; 3150 Constitution Blvd., Cooksville, Ont.; Bratislava (Slovak)'44.
GONDOR, Leslie P.; 3945 Tecumseh Rd. E., Windsor, Ont. (res); Staff, Riverview Hosp.
GONOR, Allan B.; North Battleford Medical **Clinic. 1332-100th St., N. Battleford, Sask.; 1392-97th St. (res); Man '52; M.C.G.P.; Staff,** Battleford Union Hosp.; Tel. 445-4415.
GONSALVES, Charles G.; 8330 Fairmont Dr., Calgary, Alta.; Tor'59; MCGP; Staff, Holy Cross Hosp.; Tel. 252-1161.
GONSALVES, Clive T.; 602 Dental Arts Bldg., 225 Vaughan St., Winnipeg 1, Man.; 335 Elm St. (res); McG '48; D.Psy., Psy; Cons. Psy., Children's Aid Soc.; Lect. (Psy.), U. of Manitoba; **Dir. of Treatment Planning, Children's Home; Tel. WH 3-2655.**
GONSALVES, Ralph C.; 349 Herring Cove Road, Spryfield, N.S.; Dal'60; AMCGP.

GONSIK, Helena; 283 Roncesvalles Ave., Toronto 3, Ont.; French U. (Beirut, Lebanon) '49; MCGP; Tel. LE 4-8551.

GONTHIER, Christine; Mon'65; Res., Inst. Albert Prevost, Montreal, P.Q.

GONTY, Joseph J. G.; Stonewall Health Unit, Stonewall, Man.; Man '35; DPH; Tel. 103.

GONZALES, Diosdado B.; Philippines '55; Staff, St-Sauveur Hosp., Val d'Or, P.Q.

GONZALES, Jorge; Colombia (S. Am.) '61; Jr. Intn., University Hosp., Saskatoon, Sask.

GONZALEZ, Victor; 611 Bloor St. W., Toronto 4, Ont.; Valladolid (Spain)'54.

GOOD, Harold G.; 371 Brunswick St., Fredericton, N.B.; Dal '54; ObstGyn; Tel. 475-7091.

GOOD, Harry E.; Haliburton, Ont., Box 120; Tor '52; Tel. 400.

GOOD, J. D.; 611 Med. Dental Bldg., Regina, Sask.; '55.

GOOD, Paul H.; 802 Med. Dental Bldg., Rose St. & 11th Ave., Regina, Sask., Man '57; Urol.; Tel. 522-2413.

GOOD, William C.; 471 Wallace St., Nanaimo, B.C.; Trinity Coll. (Dublin, Ire.)'38; BAO; GenSurg.

GOODALL, Robert G. W.; Ste.. 460, 5025 Sherbrooke St. W., Montreal 6, P.Q.; McG '53; D.Surg; FACS; GenSurg; Surg., Queen Elizabeth Hosp.; Tel. 489-9324.

GOODALL, Roger G.; UBC'58; Res., Vancouver Gen. Hosp., Vancouver 9, B.C.

GOODBRAND, James S.; 155 Ingram St., Duncan, B.C.; Qns'60; Tel. 746-5115.

GOODERHAM, Melville E.; 126 Underhill Dr. E., Don Mills, Ont. (res); Tor '42; Dir., Addiction Research Foundation, 1468 Victoria Pk. Ave., Toronto 16; Tel. 751-0955.

GOODFELLOW, Alice M.; Medical Arts Clinic, 2125-11th Ave., Regina, Sask.; 139 Angus Cres. (res); Tor '46; Paed; Clin. Instr. (Paed), U. of Saskatchewan; Tel. LA 2-1651.

GOODFELLOW, Ford M.; P.O. Box 72, Westport, Ont.; Qns '27; MCGP; MOH, Twp. Bedford, Frontenac Co.; Tel. 43.

GOODHALL, Patricia O.; 77-5 The West Mall, Etobicoke, Ont.; Liverpool (Eng.)'54; Anaes.

GOODHAND, Thomas K.; Abbott Clinic, 274 Osborne N., Winnipeg 1, Man.; 1306 Wolseley Ave. (res); Man '53; FACS, FRCS(C), GenSurg; Att'd. Surg. Staff, St. Boniface, Grace & Children's Hosp's.; Cons., Deer Lodge Hosp.; Tel. SP 4-4567.

GOODINE, Frederick S.; Med. Clinic, Woodstock, N.B.; Dal '59; MCGP; Staff, Carleton Mem. Hosp.; Tel. 328-3154.

GOODING, John T.; Port Arthur Clinic, 194 North Court St., Port Arthur, Ont.; 161 Blanchard St. (res); McG '54; FRCS(C); GenSurg; Tel. DI 4-7271.

GOODISON, Thomas J.; The Willows, Brockville, Ont.; Qns '26.

GOODMAN, Arthur W.; 30-6 Granderavine Dr., Downsview, Ont.; Tor '56; DiagRad; Staff, Northwestern Hosp.; Tel. 762-3641; Abroad.

GOODMAN, Benjamin; Ste. 260, 5655 Cambie St., Vancouver 15, B.C.; 6836 Laurel St., Van 14 (res) Alb '40; GenSurg; MCGP; Tel. 266-5121.

GOODMAN, George B.; 2656 Heather St., Vancouver, B.C.; Edinburgh (Scot.) '48; M.B., Ch.B., DMRT; FRCP(C), TherRad; Radiother., B.C. Cancer Inst.; Att'd. Staff, Vancouver Gen. Hosp.; Clin. Instr., U. of British Columbia; Tel. TR 4-9321.

GOODMAN, Jack M.; 158 St. George St., Toronto 5, Ont.; 349 Hillhurst Blvd., Toronto 19 (res); Alb '43; DermSyph; Att. Derm. New Mt. Sinai Hosp.; Hd. (Derm.) Doctors Hosp.; Tel. WA 3-4361.

GOODMAN, Wilfred S.; 506 Med. Arts Bldg., 170 St. George St., Toronto 5, Ont.; 118 Strathallan Blvd., Tor. 12 (res); Man '45; FRCS(C), Otol; Ass't. Otol., Tor. Gen. Hosp.; Cons. Otol., Sunnybrook DVA & Women's College Hosp's.; Clin. Instr., U. of Toronto; Tel. WA 1-8582.

GOODMAN, William E.; Ste. 602, 99 Avenue Rd., Toronto 5, Ont.; 10 Burton Rd., Tor. 10 (res); McG '43; DABO, Otol; Active Staff (Otol.), N. York Branson; Jr. Att'd. Staff, (Otol.), New Mt. Sinai & Vol. Ass't. (Otol.), Tor. Gen. Hosp's.; Tel. WA 1-7834.

GOODRIDGE, L. A.; 83 Church St., Moncton, N.B.; McG '19; Otol.; Tel. EV 4-5193.

GOODWIN, Alexander M.; Man. Clinic, 790 Sherbrooke St., Winnipeg 2, Man.; 1260 Wolsely Ave. (res); Man '22; ObstGyn; Ass't. in Obst. Gyn., Winnipeg Gen. Hosp.; Lect. Obst. Gyn., U. of Manitoba; Tel. SP 4-6541.

GOODWIN, Anna (See Flint).

GOODWIN, David A.; Ste. 5, 570 Milton St., Montreal 18, P.Q.; Man'59; IntMed; Abroad.

GOODWIN, James G.; 260 Muskoka St., Gravenhurst, Ont.; Wes '57; AMCGP; Staff, South Muskoka Hosp.; Dist.M.O., C.N.R. & D.O.T.; Med. Dir., Rubberset Co. Canada Ltd.; Tel 687-2271.

GOODWIN, James W.; University of Alberta, Ste. C. 129, University Hospital, Edmonton, Alta.; Tor '55; FRCS(C), ObstGyn; Assoc. Prof., Dept. of ObstGyn., U. of Alberta; Tel. GE 9-5911, Ext. 410.

GOODWIN, John M.; Teulon, Man.; **Man '21**; Dist. Coroner.

GOODWIN, Kenneth M.; Qns '53; MCGP; Res., Queen Mary Vet's. Hosp., Montreal, P.Q.

GOODWIN, Norman L.; 182 Humbervale Blvd., Toronto 18, Ont.; McG'47; LLB; (Br.Col.); Dir., Toronto Rehab. Centre; Dir., Health League of Canada; Med. Staff, Queen Elizabeth Hosp.; Tel. 239-7826.

GOODWIN, Philip; Leeds (Eng.) '57; Staff, Hosp. for Mental Diseases, St. John's Nfld.

GOOR, John H. Van; Associate Clinic, 214-6th Ave., Calgary, Alta.; Alta'65.

GOPAUL, Harold; Queensway Med. Centre, 880 The Queensway, Toronto 18, Ont. Dal '63.

GORAYEB, Eugene J.; P.O. Box 230, Grand Falls, N.B.; Lav '52; GenSurg; Tel. 458.

GORCHYNSKI, Orest; 299 Main St., Chilliwack, B.C.; Man '57; MCGP.

GORDON, Aaron; 5250 Rosedale, Montreal 29, P.Q. (res); Tor'46; Paed; Clin. Ass't. (Paed), Jewish Gen. & Mtl. Children's Hosp's.; Tel. RE 7-0752.

GORDON, Alan C.; Ridgeway Clinic, 1001 Ridgeway St., Fort William, Ont.; Liverpool (Eng.)'57.

GORDON, Alan S.P.; 505 O'Connor St., Ottawa 1, Ont.; 1088 Castle Hill Cr. (res); Qns '43; FAAP; Paed; Staff, Ottawa Civic & Grace Hosp's.; Tel. CE 2-5761.

GORDON, Alec L.; 1610 Pine St. W., Montreal, P.Q.; 518 Rockland Rd., Town of Mt. Royal (res); McG '39; F.R.C.P.(C), IntMed.; Ass't. (Med.), Montreal Gen. Hosp.; Lect. (Med.), McGill U.; Tel. WE 5-9875.

GORDON, Alfred; 108 Ochterloney St., Dartmouth, N.S.; 74 Slayter St. (res); Dal '53; FA GS; MCGP; Court. Staff, Victoria Gen. Hosp., Halifax Infirmary, Halifax Children's & Grace Maternity Hosp's.; Tel. 469-3511.

GORDON, Arthur A.; 1744 West Broadway, Vancouver, B.C.; 1736W. 57th Ave. (res); McG '43; IntMed.

GORDON, Athol R.; 419 Medical Arts Bldg., Winnipeg, Man.; 986 Grosvenor Ave. (res); Man '25; M.C.G.P.; Staff, Misericordia Hosp.; Staff, Dept. of Geriatrics, Deer Lodge Hosp.; Provincial Coroner; Tel. WH 2-3293.

GORDON, Bruce A.; Children's Psy. Research Inst., Sanatorium Rd., London, Ont.; Qns'57.

GORDON, Charles A.; 5991 Spring Garden Rd., Halifax, N.S.; 5840 Gorsebrook Ave. (res); Dal'44; FCCP; IntMed; Att'd. Staff, Camp Hill DVA Hosp; Assoc. Phys., Halifax Infirm.; Ass't. Prof. (Med.), Dalhousie U.; Tel. 422-5822.

GORDON, Douglas F. P.; 418 Med-Dental Bldg., Rose St. & 11th Ave., Regina, Sask.; Edinburgh (Scot.)'41; FRCS(Edin.), MRCOG; ObstGyn; Sr. Cons. (ObstGyn), Regina Grey Nuns' & Regina Gen. Hosp's.; Vis. Cons., Prov. Geriatric & Rehab. Centres; Tel. LA 3-0404.

GORDON, Duncan A.; 130 PPP, Toronto Gen. Hosp., Toronto 2, Ont.; Tor '55; FRCP(C), Int Med; Ass't Phys., Toronto Gen. Hosp.; Clin Teach., U. of Toronto; Cons., U. of Toronto Rheumatic Dis. Unit; Research Assoc., Cdn. Arthritis Soc.; Tel. EM 6-8411, ext. 2397.
GORDON, Elizabeth A.; 169 Roxborough Dr., Toronto 5, Ont.; '57; Staff, South Peele Mem. Hosp., Cooksville, Ont.; Tel. 279-7330.
GORDON, Esmond; Ste. 3337, 1 Place Ville Marie, Montreal 2, P.Q.; Geneva (Switz.) '55; Ophth (P.Q.); Jr. Ass't. (Ophth. & Path.), Montreal Gen. Hosp.; Clin. Ass't. (Ophth.), Montreal Children's Hosp.; Dem. (Ophth.), McGill U.; Tel. 861-8519.
GORDON, George; Ste. 107, 2096-W. 41st Ave., Vancouver 13, B.C.; UBC'64.
GORDON, Gilbert; 4621 Cambie St., Vancouver, B.C. (res); Tor '24; Tel. TR 9-3284.
GORDON, Helen E. (Currie); 134 Iroquois Place, Waterloo, Ont.; Qns'53; Anaes; Staff, Kitchener-Waterloo & St. Mary's Hosp's.
GORDON, Howard H.; 289 Sherwood Dr., Ottawa, Ont. (res); Tor '11; Anaes; Retired.
GORDON, James A. E.; 628 Davis Dr., Newmarket, Ont.; Tor'57; FRCP(C), IntMed.
GORDON, Lionel; 6235A Lennox St., Montreal, P.Q.; 6237 Lennox Ave. (res); McG '41; M.C.-G.P.; Clin. Ass't. (Med.), Jewish Gen. Hosp.; Tel. RE 7-3114.
GORDON, M. A.; Tor'65; Jr. Int., Toronto Western Hosp., Toronto 2B, Ont.; Abroad.
GORDON, Mary E.; UBC'55; MPH; Staff, Coqualeetza Hosp., Sardis, B.C.
GORDON, Peter C.; 6464 Waegwoltic Ave., Halifax, N.S. (res); Dal'55; MCGP; DPH; PH; Ass't. MOH, City of Halifax; Ass't. Prof. (PrevMed), Dalhousie U.; Tel. 2-4406.
GORDON, Robert B.; Box 6900, Campbell River, B.C.; UBC'59; AMCGP.
GORDON, Robert Ivan; 17 Weber St., W. Kitchener, Ont.; 140 Aberdeen Rd. (res); Tor '22; OphthtOtol; Staff, Kitchener Waterloo & St. Mary's Hosp's.; Tel. 742-3372.**
GORDON, Roderick A.; Toronto Gen. Hosp., 101 College St., Toronto 2, Ont.; Tor '37; DA (Eng. & Am. Bd.); FACA; FFARCS; FRCP(C), Anaes; Anaes-in-Chief, Toronto Gen. Hosp.; Cons. Anaes., Wellesley, Hosp. for Sick Children, Women's College, Sunnybrook & Princess Margaret Hosp's.; Editor, Canadian Anaesthetist's Soc. Journal; Prof. & Hd., Dept. of Anaes., U. of Toronto; Tel. 366-8211.
GORDON, Roderick J.; 866 Wellington St., London, Ont. (res); Wes '09; D.P.H., F.A.C.P., IntMed; Retired.
GORDON, Roger; Ste. 109, 780 Bord-du-Lac, Dorval, P.Q.; Mon'54; Tel. 631-8861.
GORDON, Stuart D.; Ste. 807, 170 St. George St., Toronto 5, Ont.; Tor'26; MS; FACS; FRCS(C), GenSurg; PlasSurg; Chief PlasSurg., Sunnybrook Hosp.; Cons. Surg., Toronto Gen., Hosp. for Sick Children, Women's College & Wellesley Hosp's.; Graduate Lect. Surg., U. of Toronto; Tel. 922-6726.
GORDON, Sydney; 99 Avenue Rd., Toronto 5, Ont.; 61 Elderwood Dr. (res); Tor '47; Urol; Jr. Att. Staff (Surg.), New Mt. Sinai Hosp.; Att. Surg. (Urol.), Northwestern Hosp.; Cons. (Urol.), Branson North York Hosp.; Tel. WA 2-8569.
GORDON, William H. M.; Box 409, Fort McLeod, Alta.; Alb '36; Retired.
GORDON, William J.; 483 George St. S., Peterborough, Ont.; 566 Gilmour St. (res); Qns '32.
GORECKI, Irena A. (Warszewska); Gdansk (Poland)'57; DMR; DiagRad; Staff, Kingston Gen. Hosp., Kingston, Ont.
GORECKI, Zbigniew; Pozan (Poland) '37; Ph.D.; ThorSurg; Supt., St. Lawrence San., Cornwall, Ont.; Cons. ThorSurg., Cornwall Gen. & Hotel-Dieu Hosp's.; Tel. WE 3-4975.
GORE-HICKMAN, Francis G.; Campbell Clinic, 430 Magrath Dr., Lethbridge, Alta.; 1131-17th St. A. S. (res); Alb '50; Paed; Staff, Lethbridge Mem. & St. Michael's Gen. Hosp's; Tel. FA 7-5737.**
GORELICK, Max M.; Ste 10G, 1521 Le Marchant St., Halifax, N.S.; Dal '55; Teaching, Victoria Gen. Hosp.; Tel. 422-7371.
GORESKY, Carl A.; 34 Ballantyne N., Montreal West, P.Q.; McG '55; FRCP(C); IntMed; Ph.D., Ass't. Phys; Mtl. Gen. Hosp.; Cons. Med., Queen Mary Vet's Hosp.; Ass't. Prof. (Med.) McGill U.; Tel. WE 7-6011.
GORESKY, Dorothy M.; 6069 Blenheim, Vancouver 13, B.C. (res); Alb'50; Staff, Health Serv., U. of British Columbia; Tel. AM 1-7022.
GORESKY, Walter V.; Ste. 1215, 750 W. Broadway, Vancouver 9, B.C.; Alb '50; Psy; Clin. Inst. (Psy.), U. of British Columbia; Cons. Shaughnessy Hosp.; Tel. 872-2910.
GORKIN, Murray; 1175 Denman St., Vancouver, B.C.; 4288 Cambie St. (res); Dal '39; Vis. Staff, St. Paul's, Vancouver Gen., St. Vincent's & Grace Hosp.'s; Tel. MU 5-0161.**
GORMAN, Alfred A.; 550 Professional Bldg., 10830 Jasper Ave., Edmonton, Alta.; 9728-84th St. (res); Alb '48; M.C.G.P.; Staff, Royal Alexandra, Edmonton Gen. & Misericordia Hosp's.; Tel. 424-5569.
GORMAN, Brian J.; Bashaw Clinic, Bashaw, Alta.; Bristol (Eng.)'60; Staff, St. Mary's Hosp., Camrose & Bashaw Gen. Hosp.; Tel. 372-3721.
GORMAN, Charles K.; Queen's (Belfast, Ire.) '56; FRCP(C), IntMed; Staff, Toronto Gen. Hosp., Toronto, Ont.; Research Assoc. (Med.), U. of Toronto.
GORMAN, Franklin J. A.; 502 Medical-Dental Bldg., Regina, Sask.; 3507 Garner Ave. (res); Man '45; GenSurg.; Tel. LA 2-8541.
GORMAN, John E.; Apt. 415, 3801 Riverside Dr. E., Windsor, Ont.; Qns'34; Anaes; Staff, Grace Hosp.; Tel. 945-5561.
GORMAN, Morley E.; 6 Angeline St. S., Lindsay, Ont.; 301 Kent St. W. (res); Tor '15; GenSurg; Chief of Staff, Ross Mem. Hosp.; Dist. Coroner; Retired.
GORMAN, Thomas W.; 30 Bay St., Antigonish, N.S.; 50 Hillcrest St. (res); McG '44; M.Sc.; FRCS(C); GenSurg; Chief, Res. Surg., St. Martha's Hosp.; Tel. 863-4308.
GORMLEY, Michael A.; 1132-100th St., North Battleford, Sask.; 1451-103rd St. (res); National U. (Dublin, Ire.) '52; M.B., B.Ch.; D.A.; Staff, Notre Dame Hosp.; Tel. 445-3756.
GORRELL, Douglas S.; 110-111 Med. Arts Bldg., Calgary, Alta.; 535 Salem Ave. (res); McG '37; Ophth, Otol.; Tel. 262-2665.
GORRIE, William A.; 50 Athlone Dr., Winnipeg 12, Man.; Man'50; Staff, Deer Lodge Hosp.
GORSSLINE, Raymond M. (D.S.O.); K. of St. J.; 22 Downing St., Ottawa, Ont. (res); Tor '11; D.P.H.; Retired.
GORT, George H.; 150 Delhi St., Guelph, Ont.; Alb'58; Psy; Active Staff, Homewood San.; Cons. Staff, Guelph Gen. & St. Joseph's Hosp's.
GORT, John; 308 Med. Arts Bldg., 1110 Jasper Ave., Edmonton, Alta.; 13915-119th Ave. (res); Alb'55; OrthSurg; Staff, University Hosp.; Chief Orth Surg., Misericordia Hosp.; Instr. Surg., U. of Alberta; Tel. 429-1883.
GORWILL, John A.; Seaforth, Ont.; Wes '35; M.C.G.P.; Tel. 527-0034.
GORWILL, P. Hugh; Wes'62; Res., Kingston Gen. Hosp., Kingston, Ont.
GOSLING, Richard E. G.; Ste. 9, 495 Dunsmuir St., Nanaimo, B.C.; London (Eng.)'50; MRCS (Eng.); LRCP(Lond.); Otol; Active Staff, Nanaimo Reg. Gen. Hosp.; Cons. Staff, West Coast Gen. Hosp., Port Alberni, Cumberland Gen. Hosp., Ladysmith Gen., Chemainus Gen. & Indian Health Serv. Hosp's.; Tel. 753-2112.
GOSSAGE, Charles D.; 9 Hillholm Rd., Toronto 7, Ont. (res); Tor '24; FRCS (Ed.); Chief Med. Dir., Confederation Life Assur., 321 Bloor St. E., Toronto; Tel. 924-6868 — HU 1-0441.
GOSSAGE, William; 454 Beaconsfield Blvd., Beaurepaire, P.Q.; 533B eaconsfield Blvd. (res); McG '53; M.C.G.P.; Active Staff, Lachine Gen. Booth Hosp's., Montreal; Plant Phys., General Foods Co.; Exam., Pte. Claire Protestant School Commission; Tel. 366-3600.

GOSSE, Clarence L.; Med. Arts Bldg., 5880 Spring Garden Rd., Halifax, N.S.; 6635 Norwood St. (res); Dal '39; FACS; FICS; GenSurg; Urol; Hd., Dept. of Urol. Victoria Gen. Hosp.; Chief, Urol., Camp Hill Hosp.; Prof. (Urol.), Dalhousie U.; Tel. 423-6400.

GOSSE, Norman H.; 5880 Spring Garden Rd., Halifax, N.S.; 1488 Birchdale Ave. (res); Dal '22; DCL (Hon., Kings & Dal.); D.Sc. (Hon., Laval); FACS; FRCS(C), GenSurg; Cons. Surg., Victoria Gen. Hosp.; Dir., NS Tumour Clinic; Tel. 423-6911.

GOSSELIN, A. Alexandre; St. Damase, St. Hyacinthe, P.Q.; Lav '33; MCGP; Tel. 797-3385.

GOSSELIN, Adrien; St. Ambroise-de-Kildare, P.Q.; Lav '43.

GOSSELIN, Arthur J.; 1011 Ouellette Ave., Windsor, Ont.; Ott'58; IntMed; Abroad.

GOSSELIN, Blandine Y.; Apt. 303, 1000 Pratt Ave., Montreal 8, P.Q. (res); Mon '51; Haem (P.Q.); Staff, Hop. Notre Dame.; Tel. 525-6363.

GOSSELIN, Camille; 1210-lere Ave., Quebec 3, P.Q.; Lav'56; FACS; FRCS(C); GenSurg; Ass't. Surg., Hop. St-Francois d'Assise Research & Teach. Staff (Med. & Anat.), U. of Laval; Tel. LA 9-4511.

GOSSELIN, Denis; L'ille (France)'62; Res., Queen Mary Vets Hosp., Montreal 26, P.Q.

GOSSELIN, Francois D.; 256 Blvd. St. Joseph, Hull, P.Q.; 267 Blvd. Gamelin (res); Lav '44; DPH; P.H. (PQ); MO, Dist. Health Unit; Tel. 771-6661.

GOSSELIN, Gaston; 3443 St. Hubert St., Montreal 24, P.Q. (res); Mon '29; Biochem. (P.Q.). Tel. 525-5063.

GOSSELIN, Gilles; Ste. 219, 3875 St-Urbain, Montreal, P.Q.; Mon '50; IntMed (P.Q.); Haem (P.Q.); Staff, Hop. Hotel Dieu; Ass't. Prof. (Med.), U. of Montreal; Tel. 844-7020.

GOSSELIN, Gustave; C.P. 113, 595 Ave. Royale, Quebec 5, P.Q.; Lav'63; Tel. 663-3236.

GOSSELIN, Jean; 200 Ave. St-Jerome, Matane, P.Q.; 2 rue Lebel (res); Lav '45; FRCS(C); GenSurg; Surg., Hop. St. Redempteur; Tel. 562-0441.

GOSSELIN, Jean-Yves; 1050 Chemin Ste-Foy, Quebec, P.Q.; 67 Ave. Bellevue, Que. 10 (res); Lav '55; Psy; Ass't. Phys., Hop. St-Michel-Archange; Cons. Staff, Hop-St-Sacrement; Tel. 663-3571.

GOSSELIN, J. A. Leon; 382 Assomption, Chicoutimi, P.Q. (res); Lav '51; FRCP(C), IntMed; Hd. Dept. of Endocrin. & Metabolism, Hotel-Dieu-St.-Vallier; Tel. 549-1452.

GOSSELIN, Jules L.; 580 Bowen-Sud, Sherbrooke, P.Q.; Lav '51; Bact(P.Q.); Dir., Bact. Labs., Hotel-Dieu Hosp.; Tel. 569-2551.

GOSSELIN, Roger A.; 1071 Ave Beatty, Montreal 19, P.Q.; Mon '57. Temporarily Retired.

GOSSELIN, Wilfrid; 3203 Ontario St. E., Montreal, P.Q.; Mon '40; Tel. LA 1-7443.

GOSSEN, Charles M.; 168 Lake St., St. Catharines, Ont.; 18 Hallcrest Ave. (res); Tor '56; Tel. MU 2-3588.

GOTTSCHLING, Kurt N.; Old Orchard Shopping Centre, 4429 Kingsway, S. Burnaby, B.C.; UBC'60; Active Staff, Burnaby Gen. Hosp.; Tel. 433-8274.

GOUDA, Salah E.; Cairo (Egypt) '58; Jr. Intn., Kingston Gen. Hosp., Kingston, Ont.

GOUDIE, James H.; Qns '64; Res., Hotel-Dieu Hosp., Kingston, Ont.

GOUDIE, Margaret M.; 101 Osborne Med. Bldg., 190 Osborne St. N., Winnipeg 1, Man.; Ste. 133 Birchwood Terr., 2440 Portage (res); Glasgow (Scot.) '32; Tel. SU 3-6250.

GOUDREAU, Michel; Lav'65; Res., Hop. St-Michel-Archange, Quebec 5, P.Q.

GOUGES, d'AGINCOURT, Raymond L. A.; 243 Marion St., St. Boniface, Winnipeg, Man.; 232 Hertford Blvd., Tuxedo (res); Guy's, London (Eng.) '43; F.R.C.S.(Eng.); F.I.C.S.; F.A.C.S.; Lect. (Gen. Surg.), U. of Manitoba; Assoc. Staff (Surg.), St. Boniface Hosp., & Children's Hosp., Winnipeg, Man.; Staff (Surg), Misericordia Hosp., Winnipeg. Tel. SP 4-6581.

GOUGH, David W.; Cornwall Clinic, 325 Hamilton Ave., St. John's, Nfld.; Dal '63.

GOUGH, H. Martin; 1175 Cook St., Victoria, B.C.; Cambridge (Eng.)'52; MRCOG; FACS; ObstGyn; Active Staff, Royal Jubilee & Court. Staff, St. Joseph's Hosp's.; Cons., Resthaven Hosp., Sidney; Tel. 385-0513.

GOUGH, James; Dal'44; Staff, James Paton Mem. Hosp., Gander, Nfld.; Tel. 256-3961, Ext. 218.

GOUGH, J. C.; Department of National Health & Welfare, c/o Regional Superintendent, European Region. Abroad.

GOUGOUX, Andre; Mon'65; Res., Hop. Notre-Dame, Montreal 24, P.Q.

GOUGOUX, Jacques; 241 Fleury W., Montreal 12, P.Q.; Mon '48; Pulm. Dis. & T.B. (P.Q.), F.C.C.P.; Staff (Med), Hop. du Sacre Coeur, Cartierville; Clinician (T.B.), La Chute Public Health Unit; Tel. DU 1-7281.

GOUIN, Jacques A.; 60 des Casernes, Trois Rivieres, P.Q.; 523 Radisson (res); Lav '46; Obst Gyn (P.Q.); Tel. FR 4-1414.

GOUIN, Leonard; 194 rue Brosseau, La Prairie, P.Q.; Mon '36; Tel. 659-1011.

GOUIN, Marcel; 6 rue Grenon, Laval-des-Rapides, P.Q.; Mon'43.

GOUIN, R.; 59 St. George St., Windsor Mills, P.Q.; Lav '52.

GOULD, A. Pauline; (See Hughes).

GOULD, Charles E. G.; 3195 Granville St., Vancouver, B.C.; 6151 St. Georges Cres., W. Vancouver (res); South. Calif. (U.S.A.) '38; Neur; Sr. Staff, Vancouver Gen. Hosp., Dept. Med. (Neur.); Cons. (Neur.), Shaughnessy Hosp. D.V.A.; Assoc. Clin. Prof. (Neur.), U. of British Columbia; Chmn., Med. Adv. Bd., Multiple Sclerosis Soc. Can.; Tel. RE 3-4211.

GOULD, C. Gerard; Cornwall Clinic, 325 Hamilton Ave., St. John's, Nfld.; Qns '57.

GOULD, David H.; 240 McNabb St., Sault Ste. Marie, Ont.; McG'58; IntMed; Sr. Active Staff, Plummer Mem. & Gen. Hosp's.; Tel. 254-6421.

GOULD, Grant A.; Medical Dental Bldg., 925 Georgia, Vancouver 1, B.C.; Tor '42; Tel. MU 3-2481. Abroad.

GOULDEN, Leila; Alberta Cancer Clinic, 11250-84th Ave., Edmonton, Alberta; McG'39; DiagRad.

GOULDING, A. M.; 305 Dawes Rd., Toronto, Ont.; Retired.

GOULDING, Gordon L.; 1519 Chestnut St., Halifax, N.S.; Dal '54; Anaes; Staff, Halifax Infirmary.

GOULEM, Yves; Doyles, Nfld.; Louvain (Belgium)'57; Trop. Med. (Antwerp); Dist. M.O., Dept. of Health, Nfld.; Tel. 27.

GOULET, Claude; Mon '56; Cardiol (P.Q.); Staff, Inst.-de-Cardiologie, 5000 est Belanger, Montreal 36, P.Q.; Tel. 254-8341.

GOULET, Fernand; 7820 Rue Marquette, Montreal 35, P.Q.; Lav'45; MCGP.

GOULET, Gerard; 212 Lockhart, Montreal 16, P.Q.; Mon'59; DiagRad; Staff, LaSalle Gen. Hosp.; Tel. 637-1161.

GOULET, Gilles; 2775 Bourdages, St. Hyacinthe, P.Q.; Mon '51; OrthSurg (P.Q.); Chief (Orth-Surg), Hop. St. Charles; Cons. Orth Surg., Hotel-Dieu Hosp., Sorel; Tel. PR 4-6873.

GOULET, Guy; Lav'58; AMCGP; Res., Hop. Hotel Dieu, Quebec 4, P.Q.

GOULET, Jean P.; 52 rue Laurier, Magog, P.Q.; Lav'59; GenSurg(PQ).

GOULET, Leo; Ste. 300, 969 Rte. de l'Eglise, Ste. Foy, P.Q.; Lav'51; OrthSurg(P.Q.); Chief of OrthSurg. Serv., Hop. Laval; Tel. 656-9177.

GOULET, Marc; Mon'62; OrthSurg(P.Q.); Staff, Hop. Ste-Justine, Montreal, P.Q.

GOULET, Roland; 7810 d'Aubigny, Ville d'Anjou, Montreal 5, P.Q.; Mon '59; Paed (P.Q.).

GOULET, Romeo; Lav '52; Staff, Centre de Re-adaptation, boul. Hamel, Quebec, P.Q.

GOULET, Yvon; 1012 Est, Boul. St.-Joseph, Montreal 34, P.Q.; Mon '55; Cardiol (P.Q.); F.R.C.P. (C), IntMed; Staff (Cardiol.) Hop-Notre-Dame; Tel. 525-6363.

GOUPIL, Jean L.; Lav '54; Staff, Hop. Ste. Anne, Ste. Anne des Monts, P.Q.; Tel. 117.

GOURDEAU, Robert; 2300 Tupper St., Montreal, P.Q.; 3793 Maplewood Ave. (res); Lav '44; Haem (P.Q.); F.R.C.P.(C), Paed; Ass't. Haem., Montreal Children's Hosp.; Clin. Ass't. (Paed.), Montreal Children's & Royal Victoria Hosp's.; Dem. (Paed.), McGill U.; Tel. WE 7-8511.
GOURDEAU, Yves S.; 1500-18e Rue, Quebec, P.Q.; 2543 Place Monceau, Sillery (res); Lav '46; FRCS(C), Urol; Hd. Dept. of Urol., Hop.-de-l'Enfant-Jesus; Ass't. Prof., Laval U.; Tel. 529-8711.
GOURGUE, Rene; 7685 Est 3eme Ave., Charlesbourg, Quebec 7, P.Q.; Lav'58; Psy(P.Q.).
GOURLAY, Donald E.; 62 Jane St., Toronto 9, Ont.; Tor '30; M.C.G.P.; Non-Active Att. Staff, St. Joseph's Hosp.; Tel. RO 9-4097.
GOURLAY, Robert H.; 3195 Granville St., Vancouver, B.C.; 6224 Carnarvon St. (res); McG '42; M.Sc., F.R.C.S.(C), GenSurg, ThorSurg; Surg.-in-Chief, St. Paul's Hosp.; Clin. Assoc. Prof. (Surg.), U. of British Columbia; Tel. RE 8-1014.
GOURLEY, Ian M.; 217 Adolphus St., Cornwall, Ont.; Qns '31; Paed; Att. Paed., Hotel Dieu Hosp. & Head of Dept. (Paed.), Cornwall Gen. Hosp.; Tel. WE 2-4725.
GOUTHRO, Alex. C.; Little Bras d'Or, N.S.; Dal '25.
GOUTHRO, Patrick J.; Med. Arts Bldg., 336 Kings Rd., Sydney, N.S.; McG'47; Tel. 562-3276.
GOUWS, Francis B.; 1139 Yates St., Victoria, B.C.; Edinburgh (Scot.) '51; LRCP; FRFPS (Glas.); LRCS (Edin.); FRCS(C); GenSurg; FACS; Att'd. Staff (Surg.), Royal Jubilee & St. Joseph's Hosp.; Tel. EV 2-2313.
GOVAN, W. R.; 925 W. Georgia St., Vancouver, B.C.; Man '43 FACS, FRCS(C), GenSurg.; Tel. MU 4-3912.
GOVATSOS, Sotiria; Athens (Greece)'58; Res., Halifax Path. Inst., Halifax, N.S.
GOVE, David I.; 206 Harwood S., Ajax, Ont.; 72 Hills Rd. (res); Tor '50; Tel. 942-6310.
GOVONI, Antonio F.; Modena (Italy) '45; DiagRad; Staff, General Hosp., Sault Ste. Marie, Ont.; Tel. AL 4-5181.
GOVINDASWAMY, Pandurangappa; Mysore (India); Res., St. Boniface Hosp., St. Boniface, Man.
GOW, George A.; 805 Med. Arts Bldg., 170 St. George St., Toronto 5, Ont.; 28 Brookfield Rd. Willowdale (res); Tor '48; FRCP(C), IntMed; Att'd. Phys., Wellesley Hosp.; Cons. DVA; Clin Teach. U. of Toronto Tel. 924-7067.
GOW, John A.; 15 Sydenham St., Dundas, Ont.; Tor '35; Active Staff, St. Joseph's Hosp., Hamilton; Tel. 627-7741.
GOW, Walter S.; 327 Charlotte St., Peterborough, Ont.; 25 Cindy St., R.R. 3 (res); McG '49; IntMed; Active Staff, Peterborough Civic & St. Joseph's Hosp.; Tel. 743-2040.
GOWER, Grahame F.; Ste. 808, 1849 Yonge St., Toronto 7, Ont.; Qns '53; D.Psy; Psy; Staff, Toronto East Gen. & Sunnybrook Hosp's.; Tel. 481-5595.
GOWETTE, SG/LT John G.; Wes'63; Staff, Shearwater Hosp., CFB, Shearwater, N.S.
GOWLER, Douglas R.; Man '57; D.Psy. Staff, Hosp. for Mental Diseases, Brandon, Man.; Tel. PA 6-2321. Abroad.
GOWOR, Lidia M.; (See ADAMKIEWICZ, Lidia M.).
GOWRON, Anthony T.; River Ave. Med. Bldg., 385 River Ave., Winnipeg 13, Man.; Man. '33; FICS; MCGP; Cons. Staff, (Surg.), St. Boniface Hosp.; Dir., River Ave. Med. Group Clinic; Tel. GL 2-8142.
GOYEAU, Francis R.; 504 Med. Arts Bldg., 1011 Ouellette Ave., Windsor, Ont.; Ott'61; Tel. 256-0982.
GOYER, Marcel; 259 Moisan St., Drummondville, P.Q.; Mon '36; Anaes.
GOYER, Paul; Mon'47; Staff, Norman Wells Hosp., Norman Wells, N.W.T.; Tel. 2146.
GOYETTE, Marc; Lav '48; Res. Hop-Notre-Dame, Montreal, P.Q.
GOYETTE, Roger; Apt. 710, 261 Cooper St., Ottawa 2, Ont. (res); Mon '37; DPH; Staff Dept. of Nat. Health & Welfare; Tel. CE 2-8211.
GOYO, Guery C.; 2030 Dufferin St., Toronto, Ont.; Turin (Italy) '48; MCGP; Staff, Northwestern Gen. Hosp.; Tel. LE 4-4162.
GOYO, Mario; 2030 Dufferin St., Toronto 10, Ont.; Turin (Italy) '49; Tel. LE 7-4554.
GRACE, Brian W., S/L; Glasgow (Scot.) '57; SMO, RCAF, St. Jean, P.Q.
GRACE, Donald A.; Alb '60; Res., University Hosp., Edmonton, Alta.
GRACE, Hyman B.; 493 Adelaide St., London, Ont.; Wes '30; Tel. 439-7721.
GRACE, Michael K.; 311 Day St., Transcona 25, Man.; Man'52; Tel. 222-4259.
GRACIE, James P.; 1050 Avenue Rd., Toronto 12, Ont.; Tor '50; MCGP; Med. Dir., Union Carbide Canada Ltd. & Atkinson Sch. of Nursing, Toronto Western Hosp.; Tel. HU 9-8954.
GRADER, Joseph; Ste 2. 2221 Keele St., Toronto, Ont.; Apt. 206, 2121 Bathurst St. (res); Tor '59; Ophth; Court Staff, North Western Gen. Hosp. Tel. CH 9-4222.
GRAF, Elca; 616 Broadway, Winnipeg, Man.; Modena (Italy) '38; Tel. SP 4-1653.
GRAF, Joseph; 616 Broadway, Winnipeg, Man. 125 Eastgate (res); Modena (Italy) '37; Paed; Cons. Staff (Paed.), St. Bonifice Hosp.; Tel. SP 4-1653.
GRAFTON, Ian G. S.; 248 Locke St. S., Hamilton, Ont.; McG '53; MCGP; Staff (GP), St. Joseph's Hosp.; Tel. JA 2-5252.
GRAHAM, Alexander; 5-6th St., Chatham, Ontario; Wes '60; Tel. 354-1451.
GRAHAM, Allen F.; 805 Med. Arts Bldg., 170 St. George St., Toronto 5, Ont.; 9 Doncliffe Dr. (res); Tor '39; FRCP(C), IntMed; Vis. Staff (Med), Sunnybrook Hosp.; Cons. (Pt-time), Toronto Gen. Hosp.; Tel. WA 3-4422.
GRAHAM, Bernard F.; 3801 University St., Montreal, P.Q.; 393 Roslyn Ave. (res); Dal '43; Neurol; Staff, Montreal Neurol. Inst., Mtl. Gen., Royal Victoria & Reddy Mem. Hosp's.; Staff, McGill U.; Tel. AV. 8-1023.
GRAHAM-BROWN, William D.; 506 Chinook Prof. Bldg., 6100 Macleod Trail, Calgary, Alta.; Cambridge (Eng.)'61.
GRAHAM, Bruce D.; 715 W. 12th Ave., Vancouver 9, B.C.; 6011 Wiltshire, Van. 13 (res); Vanderbilt (Tenn.) '42; Paed; Paed-in-Chief, Health Centre for Children, Van. Gen. Hosp.; Chief of Paed., Children's Hosp.; Prof. & Hd., Dept. of Paed., U. of British Columbia; Tel. TR 6-3211.
GRAHAM, C. Alexander; 130 Ross St., St. Thomas, Ont.; 85 Stanley Pl. (res); Wes '50; MCGP; Staff, St. Thomas Gen. Hosp.; MO. Elgin Co. Home for Aged & NYC Rlwy.; Tel. ME 3-0030.
GRAHAM, Charles H.; 1954 Oxford St., Halifax, N.S.; Dal'54; FRCS(C); GenSurg; Assoc. Surg., Camp Hill Hosp.; Ass't. Surg., Victoria Gen. Hosp.; Cons. Cdn. Forces Hosp.; Court. Staff, Halifax Infirmary & Halifax Children's Hosp's.; Lect. (Surg.), Dalhousie U.; Tel. 422-4594.
GRAHAM-CUMMING, George; 1009 Champlain Towers, 200 Rideau Terrace, Ottawa 2, Ont. (res); Edinburgh (Scot.)'29; MB; B.Chem; DPH(Ed.); DTM(Liverpool); FRSH; Med. Liaison Officer, Med. Serv., Dept. of National Health & Welfare; Tel. 992-4489.
GRAHAM, Cyril B.; 342 Lytton Blvd., Toronto, Ont. (res); Tor'26; IntMed; Tel. WA 2-2862.
GRAHAM, Donald C.; Office of the Dean, Faculty of Med., U. of British Columbia, Vancouver 8, B.C.; Tor'38; FRCP(C), IntMed; Assoc. Dean, Fac. of Med., U. of British Columbia; Tel. 228-2421.
GRAHAM, Donald N., Capt.; CBU, UNEF, CFPO 5049, CAF, Europe; Alb'64; Abroad.
GRAHAM, Donald V.; 6562 Norwood St. Halifax, N.S.; Dal '43; Anaes; Instr., Dalhousie U.; Tel. 422-4594.
GRAHAM, Duncan A., CBE; 343 Lytton Blvd., Toronto 12 (res); Tor '05; LL.D. (Qns); D.Sc. (Hon. Wes.); FACP; FRCP, FRSC, FRCP(C), IntMed; Adv. Med. Educ. & Research DVA, Ottawa; Cons. Phys., Toronto Gen. & Hosp. for Sick Children; Prof. Emer. (Med), U. of Toronto; Retired; Tel. HU 3-6700.

GRAHAM, E. R.; Luseland, Sask.; Qns '10.

GRAHAM, G. H.; Cdn. Forces Hosp. Rockcliffe, R.C.A.F. Stn. Rockcliffe, Ottawa, Ont.; Qns '36; Ophth; Tel. RE 3-6600.

GRAHAM, Glenn A.; Box 1089 Stouffville, Ont.; Tor'64; Staff, York County Hosp., Newmarket; Tel. 640-2300.

GRAHAM, Gordon A.; Qns '31; Psy; Staff, Ontario Hosp. School, Palmerston, Ont.

GRAHAM, Harold G.; Man '54; P.G., Psychopathic Hosp.; Winnipeg, Man.

GRAHAM, Harold M.; 453 Cumberland Rd., Box 119, Courtenay, B.C.; Qns '28; OphthOtol; Staff, Cumberland Hosp.; District Coroner; Tel. 334-2461.

GRAHAM, Henry; Box 60, Paradise Hill, Sask.; Glasgow (Scot.)'51; Tel. 10.

GRAHAM, James D.; Tor '63; Staff, Botwood Cottage Hosp., Botwood, Nfld. Abroad.

GRAHAM, James H.; 267 O'Connor St., Ottawa, Ont.; 309 Clemow Ave. (res); McG '42; F.R.C.P. (C), IntMed; Sr. Phys., Ottawa Civic Hosp.; Sec., Royal Coll. of Phys. & Surg. of Can.; Tel. 232-2655.

GRAHAM, James S.; 35 West Valley Rd., Corner Brook, Nfld.; Glasgow (Scot.)'55; MCGP; Active Staff, Western Mem. Hosp.; Tel. 634-5241.

GRAHAM, John; Medical Centre, 232 Metcalfe, Ottawa 4. Ont.; 67 Cartier St. (res); Tor '31; Staff, Ottawa Gen. & Civic Hosp's.; Tel. CE 2-2150.

GRAHAM, John C.; Winnipeg Clinic, N.E. St. Mary's & Vaughan, Winnipeg 1, Man.; 171 Waverley St. (res); Man '50; DABS, Gen & ThorSurg; GenSurg; Cons., Deer Lodge Hosp. and Wpg. Gen. Hosp.; Dem. (Surg.), U. of Manitoba; Tel. WH 2-6441.

GRAHAM, John D.; Tor '61; Res., St. Joseph's Hosp., Toronto 3, Ont.

GRAHAM, John E.; 625-5th Ave., New Westminster, B.C.; Ste. 10, 321 Agnes St. (res); McG '48; IntMed; Staff, Royal Columbian Hosp.; Tel. LA 2-0550.

GRAHAM, John E.; Tor '62; Fell. (Ophth.), U. of Toronto, Toronto 5, Ont.

GRAHAM, John G.; Qns '53; Staff, Coqualeetza Indian Hosp., Sardis, B.C.

GRAHAM, John K.; Box 669, Innisfail, Alta.; Dublin (Ire.) '56.

GRAHAM, John M.; Box 340, Blenheim, Ont.; Wes '37.

GRAHAM, John M.; Box 1810, Campbell River Plaza, Campbell River, B.C.; UBC '54; M.C.-G.P.; Tel. 287-4313.

GRAHAM, John R.; Qns '58; Psy; Staff, Dept. of Psy., Queen's U., Kingston, Ont.

GRAHAM, John S.; Alb '55; Res., University Hosp., Edmonton, Alta.

GRAHAM, Kathleen S.; 2107 W. 16th Ave., Vancouver 9, B.C.; 532 W. 26th Ave. (res); Alb '43; Tel. RE 3-4105.

GRAHAM, John W.; Tor'65; Res., St. Joseph's Hosp., Toronto, Ont.

GRAHAM, Malcolm D.; 1106 Cook St., Victoria, B.C.; McG'57; MS; FACS; FRCS(C), Otol; Staff, Royal Jubilee, St. Joseph's & Veteran's Hosp's.; Tel. 386-8448.

GRAHAM-MARR, John H.; Med. Assoc., 815 Victoria St., Trail, B.C.; Glasgow (Scot.) '53; DRCOG; MRCOG; FRCS(C), ObstGyn; Cons. ObstGyn., Trail-Tadanac Hosp. & Mater Misericordia Hosp., Rossland; Tel. 364-1234.

GRAHAM, M. David; 251 Crichton St., Ottawa, Ont.; Qns'14; Court. Staff, Ottawa Civic Hosp.; Tel. 749-6283.

GRAHAM, M. Edward; 275 Trafalgar Rd., Oakville Ont.; 278 Reynolds St. (res); Tor '56; FAAP; Paed; Staff, Oakville-Trafalgar Hosp., Tel. 845-6021.

GRAHAM, Michael R.; Box 29, Rexton, N.B.; Dal'66.

GRAHAM, Robert K.; Box 30, Palmerston, Ont.; Tor '48; FRCS(C), GenSurg; Tel. 133.

GRAHAM, Robert T.; 176A Roxborough St. E., Toronto 5, Ont.; Tor '33; Adm., Canada Life Assc. Co., Toronto; Tel. 368-7432.

GRAHAM, Robert W.; 330 University Ave., Toronto 1, Ont.; 3 Moorehill Dr. (Res); Tor '33; F.A.C.P.; IntMed; Ass't. Med. Dir., Canada Life Assurance Co.; Tel. 368-7432, Loc. 577.

GRAHAM, Ronald E.; Box 939, Mission City, B.C.; Tor'62; Staff, Mission Mem. Hosp.; Tel. 826-7111.

GRAHAM, Samuel S.; Glasgow (Scot.)'53; Supp. Wilson Mem. Hosp., Gilbert St., Marathon, Ont.; Coroner, District of Thunder Bay; Tel. 229-1740.

GRAHAM, V. Carolyn (Lewis); Wes '60; Res. (Med.), Victoria Hosp., London, Ont.

GRAHAM, William; 207 Cook Med. Bldg., 1175 Cook St., Victoria, B.C.; 3405 Cadboro Bay Rd. (res); Wes '49; GenSurg; Tel. EV 8-5577.

GRAHAM, William C.; 625-5th Ave., New Westminster, B.C.; Alb'53; FRCS(C), PlasSurg.

GRAHAM, W. Hugh; 8824-141st St., Edmonton, Alta.; Belfast (Ireland) '52; B.A.O.; Anaes; Staff, Royal Alexandra Hosp.; Tel GR 4-3431.

GRAHAM, William M.; P.O. Box 40, Fenelon Falls, Ont.; Tor'46; Active Staff (G.P.), Ross Mem. Hosp., Lindsay; Court. Staff, Peterborough Civic Hosp.; Tel. 887-2110.

GRAHAME, Gordon R.; Manitoba Clinic, 790 Sherbrook St., Winnipeg 2, Man.; Man '57; FRCP(C), IntMed. Tel. 774-6541.

GRAHAME, Ruth E.; Man'49; Lect., Dept. of Anat., U. of Manitoba, Winnipeg, Man.

GRAHAME, J. Wilson; Belfast (Ire.)'63; Res., Winnipeg Gen. Hosp., Winnipeg 3, Man.

GRAHOVAC, Zvonimir; Graz (Hung.) '47; DiagRad; Staff, Ottawa Gen. Hosp., Ottawa 2, Ont.; Tel. CE 6-0333.

GRAINGER, Frank A.; 164 Simcoe, Montreal 16, P.Q. (res); McG '43; DABR; D & T Rad; Assoc. Rad., Royal Victoria Hosp.; Lectr. (Rad.), McGill U.; Tel. 842-1251.

GRAINGER, Ronald S.; 503 Med. Centre, 906 8th Ave. S.W., Calgary, Alta.; Alb'60; AMCGP.

GRAINGER, R. Wayne; Wes'62; Res., Victoria Hosp., London, Ont.

GRAINGER, T. Roger; 116 Coulston Ave., Asbestos, P.Q. (res); Tor. '42; F.C.C.P.; Chief M.O. Johns-Manville Co.

GRAMLICH, Edwin; Box 1746, Wetaskiwin, Alta.; Alb'61.

GRAMKAU, Elizabeth; (See Pollonetsky).

GRANDBOIS, Claude; Lav'61; Paed; Staff, Montreal Children's Hosp., Montreal 25, P.Q.

GRANDBOIS, Jean; 1000 Chemin Ste-Foy, Quebec 6, P.Q.; Lav'41; FRCP(C), DermSyph; Chief of Derm., Hotel-Dieu Hosp.; Cons. Hop. St. Sacrement; Assoc. Prof. (Derm.) Hop. Laval & Laval U.; Tel. 681-6983.

GRANDY, John D.; 12 College St., Chilliwack, B.C.; Man '32; MCGP; Active Staff, Chilliwack Gen. Hosp.; Tel. 795-5727.

GRANGER, Harry P.; R.R. 6, Woodstock, Ont. (res); Qns '31; FACCP; FAGS; IntMed (T.B.); Supt. (Chest Dis. Div.), Ont. Hosp.; Tel. LE 9-1251.

GRANGER, M. Peter; Maple Plaza, Maple, Ont.; Tor'62; Dist. M.O., C.N.R.; Tel. 832-2201.

GRANGER, Pierre; Mon'65; Res., Hotel Dieu De Montreal, 3840 St-Urbain, Montreal, P.Q.

GRANSDEN, Godfrey M.; 61 King St. E., Brockville, Ont.; Cambridge (Eng.) '54; M.B., B.Ch., M.A., Ophth; Cons. Ophth., Ontario Hosp., Brockville Gen. & St. Vincent de Paul Hosp's.; Tel. 342-3843.

GRANT, Alfred M.; Crescent Ave., Souris, Man.; The Drive (res); Man '38; M.O.H., Glenwood Municipality.

GRANT, Alan E.; UBC'60; Res., St. Paul's Hosp., Vancouver 9, B.C.

GRANT, A. Ray; Charlottetown Clinic, 1 Rochford St., Charlottetown, P.E.I.; Dal '63; AMCGP.

GRANT, C. Ross; 65 King St. W., Beamsville, Ont.; 200 Hillside Dr. (res); Wes '52; MCGP; Tel. LO 3-8221.

GRANT, D. M.; 26 Quinn, Halifax, N.S.; Dal '31.

GRANT, Donald J. Capt.; Fort Osborne Barracks, Winnipeg, Man.; Alb'65.

GRANT, Donald K.; M.B.E.; 620 University Ave., Toronto 2, Ont.; 41 Hartfield Rd., Islington (res); Man '39; F.I.M.A.; Dir. of Med. Servs., Hydro-electric Power Comm. of Ont.; Chm., CMA Committee on Occup. Med.; Tel. 368-6767.

GRANT, Douglas A.; UBC'65; Jr. Int., Vancouver Gen. Hosp., Vancouver 9, B.C.

GRANT, Douglas J.; 751 King St. W., Kitchener, Ont.; 86 Dover St., Waterloo (res); Wes '55; Derm; Tel. SH 4-1791.

GRANT, Gordon H.; 1105 Pandora Ave., Victoria, B.C.; 3470 Upper Terrace (res); Tor '29; B.Sc., FRCS(C), GenSurg; Former Chief of Staff, Royal Jubilee Hosp.; Cons. Surg., Cdn. Armed Forces; Tel. EV 4-7622.

GRANT, Harold G.; 605 Med. Arts Bldg., 404 Graham Ave., Winnipeg 1, Man.; 232 Cordova St., Wpg. 9 (res); Man'54; D. Psy; Psy; Assoc. Staff, St. Boniface Gen. Hosp.; Cons. (Psy.), St. Boniface San.; Lect. (Psy.), U. of Manitoba; Tel. 943-8986.

GRANT, Ian M.; 204 Professional Bldg., 407 Graham Ave., Winnipeg 1, Man.; 888 Grosvenor Ave., Apt. 4, Wpg. 9 (res); St. Andrews (Scot.) '44; FRCS(Eng.), DTM&H; FRCS (Edin.); Chief of Staff, Misericordia Hosp.; Active Staff, Grace Hosp.; Court. Staff, Wpg. Gen., Children's, St. Boniface & Concordia Hosp's; Tel. WH 2-2431.

GRANT, James A. C.; 3147 Kingsway, Vancouver, B.C.; 4085 Trinity, Burnaby (res); Wes '53; Tel. HE 4-1307.

GRANT, J. E.; Regional Dir., Dept. of National Health & Welfare, c/o Regional Supt., European Region. Abroad.

GRANT, James P.; 834 Med. Arts Bldg., 170 St. George St., Toronto 5, Ont.; 286 Dawlish Ave., Tor. 12 (res); Qns '46; D. Psy; Psy; Ass't. Phys., Tor. Gen. Hosp.; Chief, Psy. Unit (Neurosis), Wellesley Hosp.; Assoc. Psy. & Clin. Instr. (Med.), U. of Toronto; Tel. 924-1723.

GRANT, Janet; (see Gibson.

GRANT, John C.B.; 74 Arjay Cres., Bayview, Toronto 12, Ont.; Edinburgh (Scot.) '08; FRCS (Edin.); Curator, Anatomy Museum, U. of Toronto; Tel. WA 3-6611.

GRANT, Joseph H. B.; Ste. 818, 925 W. Georgia St., Vancouver 1, B.C.; McG'21; Paed; Hon. Att'd. Staff, Vancouver Gen. Hosp., Staff Paed., Children's Aid Soc.; Tel. MU 1-5952.

GRANT, Kenneth C.; 1 Rochford St., Charlottetown, P.E.I.; Dal'57; FRCS(C), GenSurg; Chief of Surg., Charlottetown Hosp.; Tel. 894-5521.

GRANT, K. G.; 4-860 Winnipeg Ave., Winnipeg, Man. (res); McG '17; Retired.

GRANT, Kenneth M.; 1585 South Park St., Halifax, N.S.; 1583 South Park St. (res); Dal '29; FACOG; ObstGyn; Staff ObstGyn., Victoria Gen. & Grace Maternity Hosp's; Staff, Halifax Infirmary; Assoc. Prof. (ObstGyn) Dalhousie U. Tel. 423-6640.

GRANT, Lorna J.; UBC'65; Res., Victoria Hosp., London, Ont.

GRANT, Norbert C.; 362 Main St., St. John, N.B.; 2 Duncraggan Ct. (res); Dal '42; M.C.G.P.; Tel. 692-2207.

GRANT, P. Donald; 3603 Beaubien E., Montreal, P.Q.; 583 Rockland, Outremont (res); Qns '28; MCGP; Court. Staff, Royal Victoria Maternity & Catherine Booth Hosp's.: Hon. Att'd Staff, Mtl. Gen.; Med. Adviser, Phillips Electrical Co.; Paint Div. CIL & Dept. of Health, Outremont; Tel. 272-2277.

GRANT, Peter M.G.; 25 Glenbarr Rd., St. Catharines, Ont. (res); Tor '58; D. Psy; Psy; Staff, Mental Health Clinic, St. Catharines Gen. Hosp.; Tel. MU 4-7271.

GRANT, R. Carroll; Stephenville, Nfld. Tor. '28.

GRANT, R. Neville; 701—1029 Douglas St., Victoria, B.C.; St. Bart's (London, Eng.) '39; F.R.C.S. (Eng.), F.I.C.S., OrthSurg; Staff, Royal Jubilee & St. Joseph's Hosp's.; Tel. EV 4-4121.

GRANT, Robert S.; 7211 Quinpool Rd., Halifax, N.S.; 3 St. Matthias St. (res); Dal '48; AMCAA; Paed; Ass't. Prof., Dalhousie U.; Tel. 455-2186.

GRANT, Ronald J.; 9 Clintwood Gate, Don Mills, Ont.; 29 Pitcairn Cr., Tor. 16 (res); Tor '59; AMCGP; Staff (G.P.), Toronto East Gen. Hosp.; M.O.; Borden Co.; Tel. HI 7-9541.

GRANT, Ross A.; 765 King St. W., Kitchener, Ont.; 323 Longfellow Dr. Waterloo (res); Wes '52; MCGP; Tel. 576-4410.

GRANT, Stanley M.; McG '53; DABPath; Path; Staff, Nanaimo Gen. Hosp., Nanaimo, B.C.; Tel. 754-2141.

GRANT, T. Earle; 100 Hazen St., St. John, N.B.; 28 Garden St. (res); Dal 36; FACS; GenSurg; PlasSurg; Surg., St. John Gen. & St. Joseph's Hosp's; Cons., DVA & Provincial Hosp's.; Tel. 693-2276.

GRANT, Thomas P.; 21-4th Ave. N.W., Dauphin, Man.; St. Andrew's (Scot.)'44; MRCOG; Staff, Dauphin Gen. Hosp.; Tel. 638-3911.

GRANT, Thomas V.; Montague, P.E.I.; C.P.S. '13; Senator of Canada; Retired.

GRANT-TYRELL, Janet P.; McG'63; Res., Children's Hosp., Montreal 25, P.Q.

GRANT, W. Guthrie Y.; Brooklin Med. Centre, Brooklin, Ont.; Tor '47; Tel. 655-3321.

GRANT, William G.; 300 King St. W., Oshawa. Ont.; 333 Northcliffe Ave. (res); Tor '50; IntMed; Hd. (Med.) & Active Cons. Staff, Oshawa Gen. Hosp.; Cons., Ontario Hosp., Whitby; Tel. 728-6111.

GRANT, William M.; 94 Lake Shore Rd. E., Port Credit, Ont.; Man'45; Active Staff, G.P., South Peel Hosp., Cooksville; Tel. 278-6832.

GRANT, W. Wallace; 749 S. Drive, Winnipeg 19, Man. (res); Man '44; Paed; Psy; Dir., Child Development Clinic, Children's Hosp.; Cons. Paed., Soc. for Crippled Children; Assoc. Prof. (Paed), U. of Man; Tel. SP 5-8311.

GRANTHAM, Harry; 411 Boul. des Chutes, Beaupont, Quebec 5, P.Q.; Lav'60; FRCP(C), Psy; Scientific Dir., Hop. St. Michel Archange; Sec., Dept. of Psy., Fac. of Med., Laval U.; Tel. 663-6484.

GRANTHAM, Peter R.; 2184 W. Broadway, Vancouver 9, B.C.; 402-2366 York Ave. (res); UBC '58; MCGP; Assoc. Staff, St. Paul's Hosp.; Tel. RE 8-0042.

GRANTMYRE, Edward B.; 11 Westgate Dr., Fleming Glen. Armdale, N.S. (res); Dal '56; DiagRad; Ass't. Rad., Children's Hosp., Halifax; Ass't. Prof. (Rad.), Dalhousie U.; Tel. 423-1371, 422-8441, Loc. 30.

GRANTON, Bernard W.; 4 Church St. S., Richmond Hill, Ont.; Wes'61; Coroner Co. of York; Tel. 884-4471.

GRANT-WHYTE, Ian; 307 Eldorado, Pointe Claire, Lachine, P.Q.; Cambridge (Eng.)'55; Tel. 697-0740.

GRANVILLE, Edward T.; 1 Fleming Dr., Armdale, P.O., Halifax Co., N.S.; Dal'22; Med. Advisor, Dept. of Welfare, Government of N.S.; Tel. 477-4343.

GRAPENTINE, William L.; Biggar Clinic, Biggar, Sask.; Man'65.

GRAPES, Berton G.; 40 George St. N. Galt, Ont.; 39 Newman Dr. (res); Tor '48; FRCS(C), GenSurg; Active Staff (Surg.), S. Waterloo Mem. Hosp.; Cons. Surg. Staff, St. Mary's & Kitchener-Waterloo Hosp's.; Tel. 621-1905.

GRASSET, Anthony V.; Hollyburn Med. Centre, 520-17th St. W., Vancouver, B.C.; 4753 Clovelly Walk (res); Middlesex Hosp. (London, Eng.) '54; MCGP; Staff, Shaughnessy DVA Hosp. & Lionsgate Hosp.; Tel. 922-0211.

GRATTON-AMYOT, Monique; 3737 Sherbrooke est, Montreal 36, P.Q.; Mon '58.

GRATTON, Armand; Ste. 922, 30 est Boul. St. Joseph, Montreal 14, P.Q.; Mon'29; IntMed; Active Staff, Hop.-Notre-Dame; Cons. (Nutr.), Hop. St.-Joseph-de-Rosemont; Assoc. Prof. (Med.), U. of Montreal; Tel. 272-4311.

GRATTON, Jean D.; Ste. 1006, 30 est Boul. St. Joseph, Montreal 14, P.Q.; Mon'48; Cardiol. (P.Q.); Staff (Cardiol.), Hop. Notre Dame; Cons. Staff (Cardiol.), Hop. Sacre Coeur & Inst. Albert Prevost; Ass't. Prof., U. of Montreal; Tel. 844-9313.

GRATTON, J. Paul; Ott '59; AMCGP; Res., Ottawa Gen. Hosp., Ottawa, Ont.

GRAUER, Frederick W.; 5450 Laburnum St., Vancouver 13, B.C.; McG '36; FRCS(Edin. & C), FACS, FICS; GenSurg; OrthSurg; Att'd. Staff, Vancouver Gen. Hosp.; Vis. Staff, St. Paul's, St. Vincent's & Mt. St. Joseph's Hosp's; Clin. Instr. (Surg.), U. of British Columbia; Tel. AM 6-2133.

GRAUER, Harry; Ste. 14, 900 Sherbrooke St. W., Montreal 2, P Q.; Wes '54; Psy; Ass't. (Psy.), Jewish Gen. Hosp.; Phys., Royal Edward Laurentian Hosp.; Dem. (Med.), McGill U.; Tel. 849-7884.

GRAVEL, B-Gaston; 4 place du Fort, Repentigny, P.Q.; Mon '52; Psy; Hd. (Psy), Hop. St.-Jean-de-Dieu; Tel. 581-0660.

GRAVEL, Hector; Centre Medical de Laval, 915 Suzanne, St-Vincent-de Paul, Laval-des-Rapides, P.Q.; Lav '62.

GRAVEL, Hubert; 55 rue Church, Montreal 19, P.Q.; Mon '56.

GRAVEL, Jean P.; Lav'65; Res., Hop. Hotel-Dieu, Quebec 4, P.Q.

GRAVEL, Joffre A.; 1221 Place-Georges V, Quebec, P.Q.; 172 ouest Grande-Allee (res); Lav '41; FCCP, FACS, FRCS(C), GenSurg, ThorSurg; Thor Surg., Hop.-Hotel-Dieu, Hop.-Laval & Inst.-de-Cardiol.; Ass't Prof., Laval U.; Tel. 524-4378.

GRAVEL, Robert; 5 Lorne Ave., St. Lambert, P.Q.; Mon'52.

GRAVEL, Roland J. A. E.; 288 Worthington W., North Bay, Ont.; 810 Main West, Apt. 501 (res); Tor '62; Tel. 474-4640.

GRAVEL, Yvon; Mon '61; Anaes; Staff, Hop. St-Luc, Montreal 18, P.Q.; Tel. 861-7321.

GRAVELINE, Claude; 76 ave. Lorne, Longueuil, Cite Jacques Cartier, P.Q.; Mon '57; TherRad (P.Q.); Staff, Hop.-Hotel-Dieu; Tel. VI 4-0161.

GRAVES, C. A.; 377 Moncton St., Steveston, B.C.; 377 Garry St. (res); McG '10; Cor. in & for Prov. of B.C.: Tel. BR 7-7616. Retired.

GRAVES, Horace B.; 829 W. Broadway, Vancouver, B.C.; 6016 Alma St. (res); McG '42; FRCP(C); Anaes; Dir. (Anaes), Vancouver Gen. Hosp.; Assoc. Prof. (Dept. of Surg.), U. of British Columbia; Tel. TR 6-3211.

GRAY, Alice E. (Whiteside); 76 Grenville St., Toronto 2B, Ont.; 1 Chestnut Pk.; 1539 Mt. Pleasant Rd. (res); Tor '41; PathBact; Dir. of Labs., Women's College Hosp.; Staff, Cytopathology Assoc.; Dem. (Path), U. of Toronto; Tel. WA 3-7381, Loc. 347.

GRAY, Allen D.; Ste. 201, 121 Wellington St. W., Barrie, Ont.; Tor'34; Tel. 728-2476.

GRAY, Archie G.; 250 Medical Arts Bldg., 1105 Pandora Ave., Victoria, B.C.; 3050 Uplands Rd. (res); Man '45; FRCS (Edin.), GenSurg.; Tel. EV 3-8421.

GRAY, Brian G.; Leeds (Eng.)'59; D.ObstRCOG; Staff, Ottawa Civic Hosp., Ottawa 3, Ont.

GRAY, Cameron C.; Medical Arts Bldg., 170 St. George St., Toronto 5, Ont.; 118 Cheltenham Ave. (res); Tor '39; FRCP(C), IntMed; Assoc., Prof. (Med.), U. of Toronto; Tel. WA 2-9606.

GRAY, David G.; Aberdeen (Scot.)'55; DiagRad; Staff, Ottawa Gen. Hosp., Ottawa, Ont.

GRAY, David W.; 689 E. 49th Ave., Vancouver 15, B.C.; Tor'64.

GRAY, Doris M.; (see KAVANAUGH-Gray, Doris M.).

GRAY, E. John; Ste. 1312, 925 West Georgia St., Vancouver 1, B.C.; 1638 West 49th Ave. (res); Ott '54; FACS; FRCS(C), DABOS; GenSurg; Att'd. Staff, St. Paul's Hosp.; Instr. Med. Sch., U. of British Columbia; Tel. MU 1-3724.

GRAY, Francis R.; 399 Dibble St. W., Prescott, Ont.; Cork (Ire.)'48; BAO.

GRAY, George R.; Dept. of Path., Vancouver Gen. Hosp., Vancouver, B.C.; Qns'57; FRCP(C), Path; Staff, Vancouver Gen. Hosp.; Clin. Instr. (Med.), U. of British Columbia; Tel. TR 6-3211.

GRAY, George S.; Haig Clinic, Lethbridge, Alta.; 1811-12th Ave S. (res); Durham (Eng.) '42; M.R.C.P., IntMed; Staff, St. Nichols Gen. & Lethbridge Mun. Hosp's.; Tel. FA 7-3171.

GRAY, Gordon; 10216-132nd St., Edmonton, Alta. (res); Tor '40; OrthSurg; Med. Supt. & Cons. (OrthSurg), Chas. Camsell Hosp.; Instr. (OrthSurg), U. of Alberta; Tel. GL 5-7141.

GRAY, Harris M.; 310 Runnymede Rd., Toronto 9, Ont.; Tor '25; IntMed; Med, Cons., Manufacturers Life Ins. Co.; Tel. RO 9-1577.

GRAY, James C.; Uranium City, Sask.; London (Eng.) '41; L.R.C.P.(Lond.), M.R.C.S.(Eng.); Dist. Coroner.

GRAY, James N.; Qns'65; Res., Sunnybrook Hosp., Toronto 2, Ont.

GRAY, Jessie C.; 507 Med. Arts Bldg., 170 St George St., Toronto 5, Ont.; 21 Dale Ave., Apt. 742 (res); Tor '34; M.S., FRCS(C), GenSurg; Surg.-in-Chief, Women's College Hosp.; Ass't. Prof. (Surg.), U. of Toronto; Retired.

GRAY, John M.; St. Bart's (London, Eng.) '53; DRCOG; MRCP; Assoc. M.O., International Grenfell Assoc., St. Anthony, Nfld.; Tel. 2400.

GRAY, Kenneth C.; 135 King St. W., Gananoque, Ont.; Qns '32; M.O.H., Howe Island; Dist. Coroner; Tel. 382-3996.

GRAY, Kenneth G., Q.C.; Clarke Inst. of Psy., 250 College St., Toronto 5, Ont.; Tor'28; Psy; Chief of Forensic Serv., Clarke Inst. of Psy.; Prof. (Forensic Psy.), U. of Toronto; Tel. 924-6811.

GRAY, Leslie M.; 120 Overbrook Place, Downsview Ont.; Howard U. (Wash., U.S.A.) '55; AMCGP; Tel. 633-4984.

GRAY, L. Norman; Preeceville, Sask.; Man '53; Tel. 547-2027.

GRAY, Marion G (See Powell)

GRAY, Owen V.; 211 Toronto Western Medical Bldg., 25 Leonard Ave., Toronto 2B, Ont.; 14 Elderwood Dr. (res); Tor '44; F.A.C.S.; F.R.-C.S.(C), GenSurg; Attend. Staff (Surg.), Toronto Western Hosp., Assoc. Prof. Surg., U. of Toronto; Tel. EM 6-2076.

GRAY, Ronald C. V.; 39 Fuller Ave., Ottawa 3, Ont. (res); Qns '38; Staff, D.V.A., Ottawa. Tel. CE 2-8211.

GRAY, T.; 2511 E. Hastings St., Vancouver, B.C.; 1004 Douglas Cres. (res); Bologna (Italy) '33; Tel. AL 3-2110.

GRAY, Thomas W. A.; 403-1029 Douglas St., Victoria, B.C.; 1745 Rockland Ave. (res); Tor '25: M.C.G.P.; Staff, St. Joseph's Hosp.; Tel. EV 3-4011.

GRAY, W. Alexander; 420 East St. N., Sarnia, Ont.; Wes '52; DABS; FACS; GenSurg; Active Surg. Staff, St. Joseph's & Sarnia Gen. Hosp's.; Tel. 344-8941.

GRAY, Walter A.; Haig Clinic, 601-6th Ave. S., Lethbridge, Alta.; Sask '58; MCGP; Staff, St. Michael's, Lethbridge Municipal & Auxillary Hosp's.; Tel. 328-6641.

GRAY, W. Goldwin; Markdale, Ont.; Tor '24; M.C.G.P.; ObstGyn.; Tel. 52.

GRAYSON, William R.; Atikokan Clinic, Atikokan, Ont.; 140 Willow Rd. (res); Man '55; MCGP; Tel. 2721.

GREAVEN, Walter F.; 825 Granville St., Vancouver 2, B.C.; Argentine (S.A.)'38; Staff, St. Paul's Hosp.; Tel. MU 5-7747.

GREAVES, Kevin W.; 622 Upper Ottawa St., Hamilton, Ont.; Qns '54; Tel. 383-0611.

GREAVES, Patrick C. W.; 397 Park Ave., Newmarket, Ont.; London (Eng.)'50; Anaes; Med. Staff, York County Hosp.; District Coroner; Tel. 895-9605.

GREBEN, Stanley E.; 250 St. Clair Ave. W., Toronto 7, Ont.; Tor'53; DABPN; FAPA; Psy; Dir. Sect. of Psy., New Mount Sinai Hosp.; Cons. Clarke Inst. of Psy.; Ass't. Prof. (Psy.) & Assoc. Dept. of Med., U. of Toronto; Tel. 921-3325.

GREBEZS, Janis P.; 587 Queens Ave., London, Ont.

GREBNEFF, George A.; 16425-89th Ave., Edmonton, Alta.; Durham (Eng.)'57; FRCP(C), IntMed.

GRECO, Ernest J. M.; 316 Wellington St. W., Sault Ste. Marie, Ont.; 165 Upton Rd. (res): Tor 41; Chief, G.P., Sault Ste. Marie Gen. Hosp.; Tel. 253-2571.

GRECO, Frank L.; 70 Cedar St., Sudbury, Ont.; 200 Kingsmount (res); Naples (Italy) '40; M.C.-G.P.; Sr. Staff Memb., St. Joseph's, Sudbury Gen. & Sudbury Mem. Hosp's.; Tel. 675-8386.

GREEN, Albert H.; 3544A Bathurst St., Toronto 19, Ont.; 12 York Valley Cr., Willowdale (res); Wes '57; MCGP; Staff, New Mt. Sinai & N. York Branson Hosp's.; Tel. RU 9-4543.

GREEN, Andrew C.; 28 Catharine St., Blenheim, Ont.; 114 McGregor St. (res); Tor '36; Staff, St. Joseph's & Chatham Gen. Hosp's.; Tel. 676-5592.

GREEN, B. Lawrence; 6000 Cote des Neiges, Montreal 26, P.Q.; Dal'59; FRCS(C), OrthSurg; Staff, Jewish Gen. Hosp. & Maimonides Home for the Aged; Tel. 342-2912.

GREEN, C. Ross; Box 9, Thorndale, Ont.; Qns '53; MOH, W. Nissouri; Tel. 461-1780.

GREEN, David; 99 Avenue Rd., Toronto, Ont.; 100 Wembley Rd. (res); Tor '35; M.Sc. (Med.). Otol; Att. Otol., New Mount Sinai Hosp.; Tel. WA 1-0575.

GREEN, Derryl H.; Manitoba Clinic, 790 Sherbrooke St., Winnipeg 2, Man.; 51 Cordova St. (res Man '58; Ophth; Tel. SP 4-6541.

GREEN, Edward A., Major; 332 Maurepas Cr., Winnipeg 9, Man. (res); Man'52; MCGP; C.O. Wpg. Military Hosp.; Army Advis., Reg. Surg. Prairie Med. Reg.

GREEN, Eldon T.; 77 Peter St. N., Orillia, Ont.; Qns '36.

GREEN, Eric; The Polyclinic, 170 Fitzroy St., Charlottetown, P.E.I.; Glasgow (Scot.) '46; M.B., Ch.B.; Otol.; Tel. 894-7325.

GREEN, Floyd A.; 454 Glenwood Dr., Ridgeway, Ont. (res); Tor '56; Teach. Staff, State U., Buffalo, N.Y., U.S.A.

GREEN, Garth H.; Community Clinic, 110-8th St. E., Prince Albert, Sask.; Sheffield (Eng.) '61; MRCS (Eng.), LRCP (Lond.); Staff, Holy Family & Victoria Union Hosp's.; Tel. 763-6466.

GREEN, G. Edward; Qns'62; Res., University Hosp., Edmonton, Alta.

GREEN, Gerald R.; 151 Holland Ave., Ottawa 3, Ont.; Qns'55; MCGP.

GREEN, Howard C.; 101 Burrows Ave. E., Melfort, Sask.; Man '48; Tel. 752-3127.

GREEN, John E.; 475 Picadilly Ave., Ottawa 3, Ont.; Qns '50; Anaes; Staff, Ottawa Civic Hosp. **& Royal Ottawa Sanitorium; Tel. PA 9-2511; PA 2-6521.**

GREEN, John W.; Ste. 619, 1207 Douglas St., Victoria, B.C.; Tor'36; Anaes; Assoc. Staff, Royal **Jubilee Hosp.; Court. Staff, St. Joseph's Hosp.; Tel. 386-3131.**

GREEN, Kenwood; Ste. 206, 625-5th Ave., New Westminster, B.C.; Alb'45.

GREEN, Leo; 3643 Dutch Village Rd., Halifax, N.S.; Dal '43; IntMed., Tel. 454-1379.

GREEN, Lloyd S.; Cancer Clinic, Henderson Hosp., Hamilton, Ont.; Tor'41; DMRT(Eng.), D & TRad; Dir., Cancer Treatment & Research Fdn., Hamilton Clinic, Hamilton, Ont.; & Chief (TherRad.), Hamilton Civic Hosp's.; Tel. 389-1271.

GREEN, Mildred (Chernovsky); 131 Kilbarry Rd., **Toronto 7, Ont. (res); Tor '43; Tel. HU 9-6042.**

GREEN, Norman; Brunswick Diagnostic Clinic, 25 Brunswick Ave., Toronto 4, Ont.; 3 Prince Charles Dr. (res); Tor '53; MRCP(Lond.), FRCP (C), IntMed; Sr. Att'd. Staff (Med.), New Mt. Sinai Hosp.; Hd. (Dept. of Med.), Doctor's Hosp.; Tel. 924-9741.

GREEN, Oliver; Med. Arts Bldg., Empire Ave., St. John's, Nfld.; 42 Empire Ave. (res); Oxford (Eng.)'38; MCGP; Active Staff, St. Clare's Mercy & Grace Hosp's.; Tel. 578-5679.

GREEN, Ormond R.; 526 North Shore Blvd. E., Burlington, Ont.; Qns '43; DiagRad; Rad., St. Joseph's Hospital, Hamilton; Tel. 522-4941.

GREEN, Paul T.; Mall Med. Bldg., Winnipeg, Man.; 209 Oxford St. (res); Tor '40; FACP, FRCP(C), IntMed; Ass't. Prof. (Med), U. of Manitoba; Tel SP. 4-2411.

GREEN, Philip D.; 6790 Churchill St., Vancouver 14, B.C. (res); UBC '60.

GREEN, R. Glen; 301 Medical Bldg., Prince Albert, Sask.; 701-20th St. W. (res); McG '47; MCGP; Active Staff, Holy Family Hosp. & Victoria Union Hosp.; Dist. Coroner; Tel. 763-6401.

GREEN, Robert N.; McG'58; Res., Toronto General Hosp., Toronto 2B, Ont.

GREEN, Samuel S.; 503 Boyd Bldg., Winnipeg, Man.; 85 St. Cross (res); Man '21.

GREEN, Saul; 3663 Dutch Village Rd., Halifax, N.S.; 1667 Beech St. (res); Dal '45; FACS; GenSurg; Active Staff, Halifax Infirmary; Court. **Staff, Victoria Gen. & Halifax Children's Hosp's.; Tel. 454-1379.**

GREEN, Solomon A.; 2 York St., Glace Bay, N.S.; Dal '21; GenSurg; Sr. Surg., Glace Bay Gen. & St. Joseph's Hosp's.

GREEN, William G.; 211 Med. Arts Bldg., Hamilton, Ont.; 25 Fairleigh Cr. (res); Qns '45; FRCS (C); ObstGyn; Active Staff, Hamilton Gen., St. Joseph's, Chedoke Gen., & Children's Hosp's.; Court. Staff, West Haldimand & Joseph Brant Hosp's.; Tel. JA 9-0246.

GREEN, William O.; 17-11th Ave. S., Cranbrook, B.C.; McG '35; Dist. Coroner.

GREENAWAY, A. Clayton; 1658 St. Clair Ave. W., Toronto 9, Ont.; 19 Pricefield Rd. (res); Alb '46; Tel. RO 2-3336.

GREENAWAY, John R.; Qns'65; Res., Montreal Gen. Hosp., Montreal 25, P.Q.

GREENBAUM, Gerald H.; 3575 Bathurst St., Toronto, Ont.; Qns '58; Psy; Staff, Thistletown Children's Hosp.; Tel. 741-1210.

GREENBERG, A. B.; 207 Hastings St. W., Vancouver, B.C.; **Man '29; MCGP; Tel. MU 1-8922.**

GREENBERG, Arnold H.; Man'65; Res., Children's Hosp., Winnipeg 3, Man.

GREENBERG, Claude; Dept. of Veterans' Affairs, **Edmonton, Alta.; 10223-135th St. (res); Tor '29; Tel. Hu 8-4453.**

GREENBERG, Hyman; 16 Tower Dr., Scarborough, **Ont.; Tor '52; MCGP; Tel. PL 7-5048.**

GREENBERG, H. Joseph; 619 Bathurst St., Toronto 4, Ont.; Tor '25; AMCGP; Tel. 924-4965.

GREENBERG, Leonard; 400-309 Hargrave St., Winnipeg 2, Man.; 405 Bower Blvd. (res); Man **'46; FRCS(C); FACS; FICS; GenSurg; Active Staff, St. Boniface Hosp.; Lect., U. of Manitoba; Tel. WH 7-0216.**

GREENBLATT, Joseph; 340 McLeod, Ottawa 4, Ont.; Qns'40; FRCP(C); IntMed; Phys., Ottawa Civic Hosp.; Cons. (Med.), National Defence Med. Centre; Lect. (Clin.Med.), U. of Ottawa; Tel. CE 6-1728.

GREENE, Carrol B.; 214 Broad St. E., Dunnville, Ont.; 162 Victoria Ave. (res); Dal'44; **Sec. Med. Staff, Haldimand Mem. Hosp.; Pres. Haldimand Med. Assoc.; Tel. 774-6445.**

GREENE, Jerry G.; Man '60; Jr. Int'n., St. Boniface Hosp., St. Boniface, Man.

GREENE, L. Mitchell; 121 W. 2nd Ave., Prince Rupert, B.C.; 945 Borden St. (res); Tor '37; F.R.C.S.(Ed.), F.I.C.S., GenSurg; Att. Staff, Prince Rupert Gen. Hosp.; Tel. 624-9121.

GREENE, Thomas E.; 1604 Lonsdale Ave., North Vancouver; 2052 Inglewood W. (res); McG '48; A.B.D.R.; DiagRad; Rad.; Cons. Staff, North **Vancouver Gen. Hosp.; YU 8-3178.**

GREENHILL, Brian J. G.; 336 Professional Bldg., 10830 Jasper Ave., Edmonton, Alta.; St. Mary's Hosp. (London, Eng.) '57; FRCS(C); OrthSurg; Assoc. Staff, Royal Alexandra Hosp.; Dem. (Anat.), U. of Alberta; Tel. 424-4352.

GREENHILL, G. E.; 103 Glenmore Blvd., Edmonton, Alta.; Dept. of Nat. Health & Welfare.

GREENHILL, Stanley; Ste. C133, University Hosp., Edmonton, Alta.; 10223-137th St. (res); Tor '44; DPH; FACP; FIMA; MRSH; IntMed; Cons. (Med), DVA Cons. (Indus. Med.); Head & Prof. (Soc. & Prev. Med.) & Lect. (Med.) U. of Alberta; Tel. GE 9-5911. Loc. 413.

GREENHORN, Stanley M. (See **GRANT, Stanley M.**)

GREENHOW, D. Eric F.; 77 Westmount Rd., **Guelph, Ont.; 24 Lemon St. (res); Tor '56;** MCGP; Staff, Guelph Gen. & St. Joseph's Hosp's.; Sec. Wellington County Med. Soc.; Tel. TA 2-2666.

GREENHOW, Paul; Tor'59; Res., Victoria **Hosp., London, Ont.**

GREENIDGE, Arthur H.; 4308-108th Ave., Edmonton, Alta.; McG'43.

GREENIDGE, Herbert W., A/Col; 5 Westview Rd., Kingston, Ont. (res); Qns '45; IntMed; Hd. of Med. Cdn. Forces Hosp., Kingston; Lect. (Med.), Queen's U.; Tel. 546-3811.

GREENING, John R.; Box 448, Antigonish Clinic Antigonish, N.S.; McG '57; ObstGyn; Tel. 863-3871.

GREENLAW, Robert K.; Dal'58; Staff, Dept. of Surg., Queen's U., Kingston, Ont.

GREENWAY, Robert E.; Medical Dental Bldg., 450 Central Ave., London, Ont.; Wes. '45; FAAOO; FRCS(C), Otol; Chief of ENT Dept., Victoria Hosp.; Hon. Cons. St. Joseph's Hosp.; Clin. Prof. & Hd. Dept. of Otol., U. of Western Ont.; Tel. 439-6041.

GREENWOOD, Frederick A.; 700 Seaforth Med. Bldg., 3550 Cote des Neiges Rd., Montreal 25, P.Q.; 725 Upper Roslyn Ave., Westmount (res); McG'54; FRCS(C); OrthSurg; Ass't. OrthSurg., Montreal Gen. Hosp.; Tel. 937-5050.

GREENWOOD, Kemble; 645 Fort St. Victoria, B.C.; 687 Mount Joy Ave. (res); London (Eng.) '42, M.R.C.P. (Edin.), M.R.C.S. (Lond.), L.R.-C.P.(E); Derm Syph; Cons. Derm., Victoria Veterans' Hosp. (D.V.A.); Active Staff, Royal Jubilee Hosp.; Tel. EV 4-6232.

GREENWOOD, William F.; 628 Med. Arts Bldg., 170 St. George St., Toronto 5, Ont.; 124 Blythwood Rd. (res); Tor '37; FRCP(C), IntMed; Sr. Phys., Tor. Gen. Hosp.; Assoc. Prof. (Med.), U. of Toronto; Tel. WA 3-3377.

GREENWOOD, William R.; Wes '63; Int., Ottawa Civic Hosp., Ottawa, Ont.

GREER, Kenneth C.; Tor'40; Psy; Staff, Ontario Hosp., 999 Queen St., Toronto 3, Ont.

GREER, R. G.; 406 Medical Arts Bldg., Winnipeg, Man.; 347 Oak (res); Man '35; M.C.G.P.

GREEY, Philip H.; 100 College St., Toronto 5, Ont.; 122 Inglewood Dr., Tor 7 (res); Tor '28; B.Sc. (Med.); FRCP(C), Bact; Cons. Bact., Tor. Gen., Wellesley & Hosp. for Sick Children; Prof. **Bact. & Hd. of Dept., Banting Inst., U. of Toronto; Tel. 928-2547.**

GREGG, Ronald C.; Alb'65; Res., Royal Alexandra Hosp., Edmonton, Alta.

GREGOIRE, Andre; Mon '63; Res., Hop. Hotel-Dieu, Montreal 18, P.Q.

GREGOIRE, Bernard; 31 rue Montcalm, Hull, P.Q.; Ott'57; Ophth.

GREGOIRE, Charles J. A.; 334 St. Joseph, La Tuque, Co. Laviolette, P.Q.; Lav '60; GenSurg; Tel. 523-9111.

GREGOIRE, Claude; 1000 Chemin-Ste-Foy, Quebec, **P.Q.; 2645 Chemin St.-Louis (res); Lav '53;** FRCP(C); IntMed; Allergy (P.Q.); Ass't (Med.), Hop.-du-St.-Sacrement & Hop.-St.-Michel-Archangel; Tel. 681-7211.

GREGOIRE, Fernand S.; Clinque Lavoisier Inc., 5136 rue Bellechasse, Montreal 36, P.Q.; Lav '43; Pulm Dis & TB (P.Q.); FACP; FCCP; FRCP(C), IntMed; Chief, Dept. of Physio-Resp. Path., Hop. St. Joseph de Rosemont; Ass't Prof. (Med.), U. of Montreal; Tel. 254-4583.

GREGOIRE, Gregoire; 7826 St-Denis, Montreal 10, P.Q.; Lav '45; MCGP; Staff, Queen Mary Vet's. Hosp.; Tel. 276-4235.

GREGOIRE, H. Andre; 1715 1ere Avenue, Quebec **3, P.Q.; Lav'57;** FRCS(C); OrthSurg; Staff, Hop. **St. Francois d'Assise; Tel. 529-7311.**

GREGOIRE, Hubert; C.P. 981, 31 Montsec, Lor**raine, P.Q.; Mon '58; DiagRad; Staff, Hop.-Ste-Justine, Montreal; Tel. RE 1-4931.**

GREGOIRE, Jacques C.; Lav'65; Res., Hop. Hotel-Dieu, Sherbrooke, P.Q.

GREGOIRE, Jean; 135 ouest Grande-Allee, Quebec, P.Q. (res); Mon '24; DPH; Dr. PH (Johns Hopkins); PH (PQ); Prof. (PH), Laval U.; Tel. LA 9-4511.

GREGOIRE, Louis; 50 St. Joseph O., Quebec 8, P.Q.; 1368 rue Marechal Foch (res); Lav '29; Pulmon. Dis. & TB (PQ); IntMed (TB); Hd. Dept. of IntMed., Hop.-Hotel-Dieu-du-Sacre-Coeur; Ass't. Med. Dir., Anti-TB League of P.Q., Limoilou; Tel. 525-9960.

GREGOIRE, Marcel; Lav '61; Res., Hop. Notre-Dame, Montreal, P.Q.

GREGOIRE, Romeo; 1297 Masse, Sherbrooke, P.Q.; Lav '26; Staff, Unite Sanitaire.

GREGOIRE, Yves A.; 977 Route de l'Eglise, Ste-Foy, Quebec 10, P.Q.; Lav '55; Paed.; Tel. 653-9833.

GREGOR, Ronald D.; Qns'65; Res., Montreal Gen. Hosp., Montreal 25, P.Q.

GREGOR, Theodore J.; Qns'62; Res., Toronto Western Hosp., Toronto 2B, Ont.

GREGOR, William M.; 157 Lockhart Dr., St. **Catharines, Ont. (res); Glasgow (Scot.) '41; MD (Glas); Chest Phys. & Bronchoscopist, Niagara Pen. San.; Tel. CA 7-3731.**

GREGORIOV, Gregoriou; 189 Devon Ave., Twn. of Mount Royal, P.Q.; Athens (Greece) '56; Psy; Staff, Mont. Providence Hosp.; Tel. 665-4971.

GREGORY, Alexander G.; 104 Daniel St., Arnprior, Ont.; Ott'59; IntMed.

GREGORY, Alfred J.; 476 Victoria Ave., West**mount, Montreal 6, P.Q.; Mon '59; Tel. 484-6153.**

GREGORY, Bernard P.; Ste. 205, 1640-16th. Ave., N.W., Calgary, Alta.; London (Eng.) '54; Assoc. Staff, Holy Cross Hosp.; Staff, Calgary Gen. & Grace Hosp's.; Tel. 282-6149.

GREGORY, Charles; 685 Beach Dr. Victoria, B.C. (res); Liverpool (Eng.) '52; Psy; Dir. Mental Health Centre; Research Cons. & Lect., Dept. of Psychol., U. of Victoria; Tel. 386-5511.

GREGORY, Ian L.; 7100 Bowman Ave., Regina, Sask. Manchester (Eng.) '43; FRCS (Edin.) FRCS (Eng.); MRCS; LRCP; GenSurg.

GREGORY, John; 1019 Maple Ave., Quebec 6, P.Q.; Lav '46; Cons., Cdn. Gen. Electric Co.; Tel. 522-2215.

GREGORY, John D.; 225 Grand River St. N., Paris, Ont.; Tor'39; Tel. 442-4432.

GREGORY, Laszlo J.; 6138-90th Ave., Edmonton, Alta.; Szeged (Hung.) '28; Tel. 466-2388.

GREGORY, Robert A.; Box 20, Provincial Hosp., Lancaster, N.B.; 384 Lancaster Ave. (res); McG '31; NeurPsy; Supt. Prov. Hosp. Lancaster (DVA), Sr. Cons. (NeurPsy), Lancaster DVA, St. John Gen., St. Joseph's & T.B. Hosp's.; Tel. 694-2651.

GREGORY, Stanley J.; Bigelow-Fowler Clinic, 1605-9th Ave. S., Lethbridge, Alta.; Alb '54; Staff, Lethbridge Mun. & St. Michael's Hosp's.; Tel. 327-3121.

GREGSON, William E.; 538A Ewen Ave., New Westminster, B.C.; 4076 W. 31st Ave., Vancouver (res); McG '27; MCGP; Tel. CA 4-9419.

GREHAN, Anthony J.; Box 1088, Mission City, B.C.; R.C.P.S.(Ire.)'53.

GREHAN, John F.; 274 Linwell Rd., St. Catharines, Ont.; 194 Glendale (res); National U. (Dublin, Ire) '44; D.Obst., RCOG (Lond.); Active Staff, St. Catharines Gen. & Hotel-Dieu Hosp's; Tel. WE 5-5131.

GREIG, Charles H.; 955 Queen St. E., Sault Ste. Marie, Ont.; Tor'29; FRCS(C), GenSurg; OrthSurg; Urol; Chief of Staff, Sault Ste. Marie Gen. Hosp.; Tel. AL 4-2911.

GREIG, David H.; Tor'61; Otol; Staff, Royal Victoria Hosp., Montreal, P.Q.

GREIG, James H.; 211 Medical Dental Bldg., 925 W. Georgia St., Vancouver 1, B.C.; 4677 Belmont Ave., Vancouver 8 (res); Edinburgh (Scot.) '49; M.R.C.P. (Edin.), D.M.R.D., DiagRad; Cons. Staff, Shaughnessy D.V.A. Hosp.; Tel. RE 8-3188.

GREIG, John D.; 160 Brant Ave., Brantford, Ont.; Tor'48; ObstGyn; Cons. Staff (ObstGyn), Brantford Gen. & St. Joseph's Hosp's.; Tel. PL 3-6521.

GREINER, Anthony; 101 Royal Ave., New Westminster, B.C.; Budapest (Hung.) '37; IntMed; Dir. Med. Serv., Riverview Hosp.; Tel. LA 1-1911.

GRENIER, Andre; 6618, rue St-Denis, Montreal 10, P.Q.; Mon '55.

GRENIER, Bernard; 170 Saunders, Quebec 6, P.Q.; Lav '27; ObstGyn; Tel. 522-8808.

GRENIER, Georges; 241, Georges, St-Barnabe Nord, St-Maurice, P.Q.; Lav '46; MCGP.

GRENIER, Eugene; Apt. 105, 6950 Ave. Fielding, Montreal 29, P.Q. (res); Lav '06; FRCP(C), Retired.

GRENIER, Jacques; 2218 Marie Victorin, Sillery, P.Q. (res); Lav '54; Psy; Ass't. Psy., Hop. Archange & Hotel-Dieu, Quebec; Tel. 529-9151.
GRENIER, Jean; C.P. 459, Causapscal, Co. Matapedia, P.Q.; Lav '63.
GRENIER, Jean P., Capt.; 2 R.C.R.MIR, Soest, Germany, Abroad.
GRENIER, J. P., A/S/L; R.C.A.F. Station, Bagotville, P.Q.
GRENIER, Jocelyn; 1536, boul. Labelle, Chomedey, P.Q.; Mon '64.
GRENIER, L. Rosaire; 1010 St. Catherine St. E., Montreal, P.Q.; Mon '26; Tel. VI 2-4530.
GRENIER, Laurent J.; 960-3eme St., Richelieu, P.Q.; Mon '53.
GRENIER, Lucien; 477 St. Joseph, Est. Broughton, Beauce, P.Q.; Lav'59.
GRENIER, Marien; 1505 ave. Francois ler, Quebec, P.Q.; Lav '62; Tel. 523-8288.
GRENIER, Montcalm; Lille (France)'55; Res., Hop. Notre-Dame, Montreal 24, P.Q.
GRENIER, P. Emilien; Lav. '43; D.H.P., F.C.-C.P., Pulm. Dis. & TB (P.Q.); Head. Sanatorium Ross, Gaspe, P.Q.; Tel. 215.
GRENIER, Raynald; 42 rue Frontenac, Lac Megantic, P.Q.; Lav'65.
GRENIER, Richard; 960 boul. Ste-Croix, Montreal 9, P.Q.; Mon '65.

GRENNELL, Herbert J.; Box 413, 10 Montreal St., Kingston, Ont.; National U. (Ire.)'54; FRCP(C), Anaes; Att'd. Staff, Hotel-Dieu Hosp.; Clin. Ass't. Anaes., Queen's U.; Tel. 542-5609.
GRENON, Romeo G.; Casselman, Ont. (res); Mon '36; D.P.H.; Dir. & M.O.H., Prescott & Russell Health Unit, Hawkesbury, Ont.
GRESZCZYSZYN, E. R.; Tor '63; Staff, Ontario Hosp., Whitby, Ont.
GRETTON, Allan H.; Bowness Med. Centre, 6319 Bowness Rd., N.W., Bowness, Calgary, Alta.; 6911 Bow Cres (res); St. Bart's (London, Eng.) '53; MRCS; LRCP; DRCOG; MCGP; Staff (GP), Calgary Gen. Children's and Grace Hosp's. and Bowcrest Nursing Home; Tel. 288-2898.
GREVE, Donald I.; Sask'60; Res. (Paed.) Halifax Children's Hosp., Halifax, N.S.

GREVE, Doreen M. (See Mitchinson)

GREWAR, David A. I.; 265 Bruce Ave., St. James, Winnipeg 12, (res); St. Andrews (Scot.) '45; DCH, MRCP (Edin.); Paed; Med. Cons., Soc. for Crippled Children, Manitoba; Teach. Staff, Children's Hosp. & St. Boniface Hosp.; Ass't. Prof. (Paed.), U. of Manitoba; Tel. SP 5-8311.
GRIESER, Frank, 245 Campbell Ave., Windsor, Ont.; Graz (Austria) '24; Tel. 254-0481.
GRIEVE, Harry G.; 3295 Upper Terrace Rd., Victoria, B.C. (res); Man. '24; D.O.M.S. (Eng.), D.L.O. (Eng.), F.A.C.S., F.R.C.S. (C), Ophth-Otol, Cons. Staff, Royal Jubilee, St. Joseph's, & Victoria Vets' Hosp's; Tel. EV 2-7332.
GRIEVES, John K.; Med. Centre, Maple Ave., New Glasgow, N.S.; Guy's H. (London, Eng.)'47; DO (Lond.); Cons. & Hd. (Ophth), Aberdeen Hosp.; Tel. 752-5164.

GRIFFIN, Bruce M.; Children's Homes, 380 Sherbourne St., Toronto 5, Ont.; Tor '24.
GRIFFIN, Francis J.; 340 McLeod, Ottawa, Ont.; National U. (Dublin, Ire.) '49; Court. Staff, Ottawa Civic Hosp.; O.P.D. Staff, National Defence Med. Centre; Tel. 236-3863.
GRIFFIN, Jean; 41 Ennis Ave., St. John's, Nfld.; Leeds (Eng.)'58; M.O.H.; Dept. of Health; Staff, St. John's Gen. Hosp.
GRIFFIN, Jean H.; 21 Division St., Welland, Ont.; Tor'54.
GRIFFIN, John D.; 52 St. Clair Ave. E., Toronto 7, Ont.; 18 Bracondale Hill Rd. (res); Tor '32; D.Psy; Psy; Gen. Dir., Canadian Mental Health Assoc.; Tel. WA 5-4264.
GRIFFIN, John E.; 366 McIntyre St. W., North Bay, Ont.; 959 Pinewood Rd. (res); McG '53; Plant Phys., Cdn. Johns-Manville; Dist. M.O., C.N.R.; Tel. 474-2840.
GRIFFIN, M. B.; 4059 Dorchester St. W., Montreal, P.Q. (res); Royal College of Surg. (Ire.) '52.
GRIFFIN, Robt. C.; Staff, St. Martha's Hosp., Antigonish, N.S.; Dal '42; Tel. 863-2830.

GRIFFITH, George S.; 440 Med. Dental Bldg., Regina, Sask;. 3701 Dewdney Ave. (res); Man '37; DOMS(Eng.); District Coroner; Staff, Regina Gen. & Grey Nuns Hosp's.; Tel. 522-1645.
GRIFFITH, Geraint T., MBE; 195 Wellington St. W., Chatham, Ont.; 154 McNaughton Ave. E. (res); London (Eng.) '51; MRCS, LRCP; FRCP(C), IntMed; Chief, Dept. of Med., St. Joseph's Hosp.; Tel. EL 2-7020.
GRIFFITH, Harold R.; 3445 Northcliffe Ave., Montreal 28, P.Q.; McG '22; D.A.B.A., F.R.C.P. (C), F.F.A.R.C.S.(Eng.), F.I.C.A., F.A.C.A., Anaes; Anaes, Emer. Queen Elizabeth Hosp.; Emeritus Prof. (Anaes.), McGill U.; Tel. 484-8382.
GRIFFITH, Idris M.; Box 100, Blenheim, Ont.; London (Eng.)'24; MRCS(Eng.); LRCP(Lond.); Dir. O.P. Cedar Springs Hosp. School; Assoc. Children's Psy. Research Inst., London; Tel. 676-3629.
GRIFFITH, James J.; Ste. 660, 5025 Sherbrooke St. W., Montreal 28, P.Q.; McG'24; FACS; GenSurg; Surg. Emer., Queen Elizabeth Hosp., Tel. 488-2612.
GRIFFITH, John O.; 196 Church St., Westgate Apartments, Waltham, Mass., U.S.A.; Sask '58; Paed; Abroad.
GRIFFITH, L. A.; Department of National Health & Welfare, c/o Regional Superintendent, European Region. Abroad.
GRIFFITH, Martin N.; 109 Coe Hill Dr., Toronto 3, Ont.; 121 Parkside Dr., Tor. 3 (res); London (Eng.) '55; Tel. RO 2-7982.

GRIFFITHS, Alan L.; Box 857, 4718-51st Ave., Leduc, Alta.; Queen's U. Belfast (Ire.) '45; D.C.H.; Tel. 466-3310.
GRIFFITHS, Anthony J. M.; Conquerall Bank, P.O. Box 1455, Bridgewater, N.S. (res); London (Eng.) '44; MRCS (Eng.); LRCP (Lond.); DMRD; DiagRad; Rad., Bridgewater & Lunenburg Hosp's.
GRIFFITHS, Dorothy E.; Arkona, Ont.; Durham (Eng.)'62.
GRIFFITHS, E. Anthony; 39 Charlton Ave. E., Hamilton, Ont.; London (Eng.)'52; Ophth.; Tel. 525-1656.
GRIFFITHS, Frederick E.; Minden, Ont.; Tor '54; M.C.G.P.; Staff, Red Cross Hosp.; Dist. Coroner Tel. 17 W.I.
GRIFFITHS, G. Audrey (Meigh); 4718-51st Ave., Leduc, Alta.; Cambridge (Eng.)'46; LRCP; MRCS; DCH (Eng.); Tel. 446-3310.
GRIFFITHS, Helen L. M. (Partridge); 5 Victoria Blvd., Clinton, Ont. (res); Guy's Hosp., (London, Eng.) '52; Part-time G.P. & P.H.
GRIFFITHS, Marion M.; 6325 Fraser, Vancouver, B.C.; 1909 Quilchena Cres. (res); Alb '44; Anaes; Tel. FA 5-4040.
GRIFFITHS, Peter A. Capt.; RCAF Station, Camp Borden, Ont.; Tor'65.
GRIFFITHS, Wilfred L.; 24 Catherine St., Trenton, Ont.; London (Eng.)'53; Staff, Trenton Mem. Hosp.; Tel. EX 2-4032.

GRIGGS, F. C.; c/o Chief Med. Off., Dept. Nat'l. Health & Welfare, 61 Green St., London W.1, England.
GRIGGS, Francis C.; 707 Fairmont Medical Bldg., 750 W. Broadway, Vancouver 9, B.C.; Man '34; Tel. 876-4930.
GRIGGS, Gordon B.; Morris, Man.; Man '58; Tel. 280.
GRIGGS, W. D. P.; Department of National Health & Welfare, c/o Regional Superintendent, European Region. Abroad.

GRIGNON, Charles E.; 524 Sherbrooke St. E., Montreal, P.Q.; 3840 Marcil St. (res); Mon '30; FRCP(C), IntMed; Staff, Hop.-Notre-Dame; Tel. AV 8-0088.

GRIGNON, Gilles; C.P. 1029, Ste. Agathe de Monts, P.Q.; Mon '45; Med. Dir., Hop. Ste. Agathe des Monts; Tel. 326-2303.

GRIGNON, Jean; 524 Sherbrooke E., Montreal, P.Q.; 450 Champagneur, Outremont (res); Mon '43; F.R.C.P.(C) IntMed; Ass't. (Med), Hop. Notre-Dame; Ass't. Prof., U. de Montreal; Tel. AV 8-0088.

GRIGNON, Rene; 4281 Delormier, Montreal, P.Q.; Mon '41; F.A.C.S., F.I.C.S., F.I.A.P., GenSurg (P.Q.); Surg., Hop. Notre Dame; Ass't. Prof. (Surg.), U. of Montreal; Tel. LA 3-7577.
GRIMARD, Michel; App. 1, 2229 Maplewood, Montreal 26, P.Q.; Mon '64.
GRIMES, Sylvester E.; Suite 404, The Medical Arts Bldg., Ottawa 4, Ont.; 315 Holmwood Ave., Apt. 1014, (res); Qns '28; DermSyph; Cons. Staff, Ottawa Civic Hosp.; Tel. 233-1515.
GRIMSHAW, Isobel; 70 Vaughan Rd., Toronto, Ont.; 288 St. Clair W. (res); Tor '40; Anaes.; Tel. LE 5-6311.
GRIMSHAW, William L.; 75 Eglinton Ave. E., Toronto 12, Ont.; 283 Glencairn Ave. (res); Qns '40; Tel. HU 9-5763.
GRIMSON, Julius C.; 925 W. Georgia St., Vancouver, B.C.; Alb'25; Staff, Vancouver Gen., St. Paul's & St. Vincent's Hosp's.; Dist. Coroner; Tel. MU 1-9844.
GRINNELL, Diana M. (Gibbons); Qns'64; RCAF Station, Moosonee, Ont.
GRINSTEIN, Maxwell; 2436 Kensington Rd., Calgary, Alta.; 2716 Parkdale Blvd. (res); Middlesex H. (London, Eng.) '47; MRCS(Eng.), LRCP-(Lond.); Tel. AT 3-5957.
GRIPPER, Nigel D.; 112 Victoria St. E., Alliston, Ont.; London (Eng.) '56; DA; DRCOG; MRCS; LRCP; Tel. 435-6225.
GRISDALE, Lloyd C.; University Hosp., Edmonton, Alta.; Alb'46; Paed; Prof. of Community Med., U. of Alberta; Tel. 439-5911.
GRISDALE, William R.; Alb'63; Assoc. Res., University Hosp., Edmonton, Alta.
GRISE, Edmund A.; 194 Hugel Ave. E., Midland, Ont.; 275 Fifth St. (res); Tor '37; Tel. 526-5712.
GROBIN, Wulf; Ste. 706, 99 Avenue Rd., Toronto 5, Ont.; 130 Old Forest Hill Rd. (res); Basel (Switz.) '34; L.R.C.P.(Edin.), L.R.C.S.(Edin.), LRFPS (Glasgow) IntMed.; Tel. 923-3232.
GROBMAN, Jerry S.; Lynwood Shopping Centre, 8764-149th St., Edmonton, Alta.; 15423-75th Ave., Jasper Pl. (res); Sask '57; Tel. 489-6305.
GROCOTT, Hubert C.; Med. Arts Bldg., 2125-11th Ave., Regina, Sask.; London U. (Eng.) '54; MRCS(E), LRCP(Lond.); DABP; Paed; Att'd. Phys., Regina Gen. & Grey Nuns' Hosp's; Cons. Phys., Restoration Centre; Tel. 523-0961.
GRODZINSKI, Josef; 18 Croydon Rd., Toronto 10, Ont. (res); Cracow (Poland) '39; D.Psy; Psy; Sr. Phys., Ontario Hosp.; Clin Instr. (Psy), U. of Toronto; Tel. 787-6644.
GROENENDYK, John; Amsterdam (Neth.) '55; Ass't. Prof. (Anat.), U. of Saskatchewan, Saskatoon, Sask.; Tel. CH 2-7671.
GROGAN, Dallas R.; 6 Glen Watford Dr., Agincourt, Ont.; 28 Buena Vista (res); Tor '57; AMCGP.
GROGONO, Basil J. S.; 532 Med. Arts Bldg., 404 Graham Ave., Wpg. Man.; 989 Dorchester, Wpg. 9 (res); St. Mary's H. (London, Eng.) '45; F.R.C.S.(Eng.), F.R.C.S.(C), OrthSurg; OrthSurg., Deer Lodge Vet's. Hosp.; Tutor (Orthopaedics), U. of Manitoba; Tel. 942-3559.
GROH, George J.; Budapest (Hung.) '45; Staff, Hop.-des-Laurentides, L'Annonciation, P.Q.; Tel. 275-2118.
GROLEAU, Fernand; Lav'50; Path(P.Q.); Staff, Hop. Hotel-Dieu, Jonquiere, P.Q.
GROLEAU, Valere E.; 656-10 Ave. S., East Broughton Station, P.Q.; Lav'25.
GROLEAU, Yves; C.P. 159, St-Come, Liniere, Cte Beauce, P.Q.; Lav '44.
GROMOV, Helena (See Glawdan).
GRONDIN, Carrol; Lav'58; Bact(P.Q.); Teach. Fell. (Microbiol.), Laval U., Quebec, P.Q.
GRONDIN, Claude; 1525 rue Fradet, Drummondville, P.Q. (res); Mon '56; Staff, Hop.-Ste-Croix; Tel. GR 8-1381.
GRONDIN, Claude; Lav. '61; Res., Hop. St-Sacrement, Quebec 6, P.Q.
GRONDIN, Gerald E.; 722 Bank St., Ottawa, Ont.; Qns '28, Staff, Ottawa Gen. Hosp.; Tel. 235-1212.
GRONDIN, J. Georges; 640 Mountain Rd., Moncton, N.B.; Lav '53; GenSurg.; Tel. 382-8169.
GRONDIN, J. J. A. Guy; 625-9eme Ave., Charny, P.Q.; Lav '48.
GRONDIN, Leon; 53 George, Sorel, P.Q.; 131 Ch. Ste. Anne (res); Lav '43; Tel. RI 3-4253.
GRONDIN, Pierre; 5000 est Belanger, Montreal 36, P.Q.; Lav'51; FRCS(C), GenSurg; ThorSurg (P.Q.); Staff, Inst. of Cardiol; Tel. 254-8341.
GRONDIN, Romeo; 2684 Ave. de Soissons, Montreal 26, P.Q.; Lav '27; D&TRad.
GROOM, Richard H.; 922 Decarie Blvd., Ville St. Laurent, P.Q., & 1583 Graham Blvd., Town of Mt. Royal; 349 Morrison Ave., Town of Mt. Royal (res); Dal '52; Tel. RI 4-2404.
GROPPE, Hildegarde A.; (See Stein, Hildegarde A.).
GROSE, Paul S.; 539 Cassels St., North Bay, Ont.; Tor'59; Tel. 472-3620.
GROSHAW, Ronald E.; 1826 ½ Weston Rd., Weston, Ont.; 31 Princess Margaret Blvd., Islington (res); Wes '55; Ophth; Staff, Humber Mem. Hosp.; Cons. Staff, Sunnybrook Hosp.; Tel. 247-2550.
GROSLOUIS, Leon; Courcelles, Co. Frontenac, P.Q.; Lav '52.
GROSS, Allan E.; Tor '62; Research, Banting Inst., U. of Toronto, Toronto 5, Ont.
GROSS, Harrison S.; Box 340, Port Hardy, B.C.; Qns'32.
GROSS, Richard C.; Ste. 1, 10028-102nd St., Edmonton, Alta.; 11625 Edinboro Rd. (res); Qns '32; Ophth.; Tel. GA 2-4784.
GROSSMAN, Arnold A.; 3744 Cote-des-Neiges, Montreal 25, P.Q.; 122 Lockhart Ave., Twn. Mt. Royal (res); McG '39; FAAOO; FICS; FRCS(C), Ophth. Otol; Assoc. Dir. Dept. of Otol., Mtl. Gen. Hosp.; Lect. (Otol.), McGill U.; Tel. WE 2-1732.
GROSSMAN, Bernard M.; 538 St. Catherine Rd., Montreal, P.Q.; McG'27; Staff, Royal Victoria, Doctors' & Jewish Hosp's.; Tel. 272-7087.
GROSSMAN, Harold J.; 25 Brunswick Ave., Toronto 4, Ont.: Tor'46; FACS; FICS; DABS; FRCS(C), GenSurg; Staff, Doctor's Hosp., New Mount Sinai & St. John's Convalescent Hosp's.; Tel. 927-3041.
GROSSMAN, Sheila (Salamon); 4835 Lacombe, Montreal 26, P.Q.; Munich (Germ.) '50; Clin. Ass't., Jewish Gen. Hosp.; M.O. City of Montreal; Tel. UN 1-3811.
GROSSO, Roberto; Rome (Italy) '55; Staff, Copper Cliff Hospital, Copper Cliff, Ontario.
GROSZMAN, Michael; 5845 Cote des Neiges Rd., Montreal, P.Q.; Munich(Germ.) '50; FCCP; FAAMA; Med. Dir., Mt. Sinai Hosp.; Staff, Jewish Gen., & Royal Edward Hosp's.; Tel. 735-2818.
GROTELL, David; 895 Bloor St. W., Toronto, Ont.; Tor '55; MCGP.; Tel. 537-2527.
GROULX, Adelard; 11400 James Morrice, Montreal 12, P.Q.; Mon'24; MPH(Johns Hopkins); PH; Admin. Expo 67, Pavillion de l'Administration, Cite du Havre, Montreal.
GROULX, Georges; 300 rue de Lavaltrie, Trois-Rivieres, P.Q. (res); Lav '49; D. Bact (Paris); PathAnat. (PQ); Path; Chief of Pathol. Labs., Hop. St.-Joseph; Staff, Hotel-Dieu; Tel. FR 4-6211.
GROULX, Raoul; 1150 Est, Boul. St-Joseph, Montreal 34, P.Q.; 5590 Woodbury (res); Mon '44; Gyn; Chief of Gyn; Hop. Maisonneuve; Tel. LA 7-1241.
GROUSTRA, Fritz N.; 138-10th St. W., Owen Sound. Ont.; Netherlands '54.
GROVE, Joseph H.; 2649 Flannery Dr., Ottawa 8, Ont.; Tor '24; Tel. 733-2109.
GROVE, Ned. M.; 641 Med. Arts Bldg., 750 Spadina Cres., Saskatoon, Sask.; 2511 Wiggins Ave. (res); Tor '57; FRCS(C), OrthSurg; Assoc Staff, Dept. of Surg. (Orth), University Hosp. & St. Paul's Hosp.; Clin Teach., U. of Sask.; Tel. 652-7272. Abroad.
GROVER, B. Downey; Dal'60; Res., Hosp. for Sick Children, Toronto 2, Ont.
GROVER, Sunder D.; Nagpur (India)'59; FRCS(C), GenSurg; Staff, Royal Alexandra Hosp., Edmonton, Alta .
GROVES, John S.; 2418 Beacon, Sidney, B.C.; Brentwood Bay (res); Alb '60; Tel. GR 5-1164.

GROVES, John T.; London (Eng.) '49; M.B., B.S.; Path; Staff, Hamilton Gen. Hosp., Hamilton, Ont.

GROVES, Kenneth P.; 1404-925 W. Georgia St., Vancouver 1, B.C.; 1426 W. 48th Ave., Van. 13 (res); Tor '32; GenSurg; Vis. Staff, Vancouver Gen., Mt. St. Joseph's, Burnaby Gen., Grace & St. Vincent's Hosp's; Tel. 681-3857.

GROVES, R. A.; Alb '61; Jr. Intn., St. Michael's Hosp., Toronto 2, Ont.

GROVES, Terence D. Capt.; Nat. Defence Med. Centre, Smyth Rd. & Alta Vista, Ottawa 8, Ont.; Alb'65.

GROWSE, John M.; 287 Queen's Ave., London, Ont.; 219 Wortley Rd. (res); Qns '32; Anaes; Chief (Anaes), St. Joseph's Hosp.; Ass't. Prof. (Anaes), U. of Western Ont.; Tel. GE 8-5143.

GRUFFY, Marcel E.; 3719 Boul. Levesque, Chomedy, P.Q.; 715 Cardinal, St. Martin (res); Mon 55; Tel. 681-8331.

GRUNBERG, Frederic; Provincial Health Bldg., Regina, Sask.; 140 McNabb Cr. (res); Montpelier (Fr.) '52; DPM (Lond.); Psy; Dir. of Hospital's Branch Dept. of Public Health Sask.; Tel. 523-0661, Ext. 258.

GRUNBLATT, Leon; 44 Rogers Rd., Toronto, Ont.; Brussels (Bel.) '49; Staff, New Mt. Sinai, **Northwestern Gen. & Doctors' Hosp's.; Tel. RU 1-4278.**

GRUNDY, Eric C.; 2333 Bloor St. W., Toronto 9, Ont.; 53 Pinehurst Cres., Islington (res); Tor '43; FACS, FCCP, FRCS(C), GenSurg; Staff Surg., St. Joseph's Hosp.; Cons. Surg. (Thor & **Cardiovasc.), Queensway Gen. & S. Peel Hosp's.;** Tel. 766-4454.

GRUNER, O. Cameron; 231 Lazard Ave., Montreal 16, P.Q. (res); London (Eng.) '01; Retired.

GRUNER, Peter H.; Ste. 10, 1179 Decarie Blvd., Montreal 9, P.Q.; McG'59; Tel. 747-7103.

GRYFE, Arthur; 2085 Caroline St. E., Burlington, Ont.; Tor'60; Path.

GRYFE, Cyril I.; Tor'57; MCGP; Res., Toronto Western Hosp., Toronto 2B, Ont.

GRYMALOSKI, Martha R.; Apt. 170, 3550 Cote des Neiges Rd., Montreal, P.Q.; Sask '59; FRCP (C), DiagRad; Jr. Ass't. Rad., Montreal Gen. Hosp.; Tel. 937-9334.

GRYNOCH, Robert L.; 208-24th St., Fort Macleod, Alberta; 433-18th St. (res); Strasbourg (Fr.) '39; F.R.C.S. (Eng.); M.R.C.S. (Eng.); L.R.C.P. (Eng.); GenSurg; Staff, Macleod Municipal Hosp; Tel. 234-3828

GRZEBILISZEWSKI-COMBS, George; Poznan (Poland)'57; Jr. Int., Queen Mary Vets Hosp., Montreal, P.Q.

GRZYBOWSKI, Stefan; 1856 Allison Rd., Vancouver 8, B.C.; Polish School of Med., Edinburgh (Scot.) '45; MRCP (Lond.); FRCP(C); IntMed; Assoc. Prof. of Med., U. of British Columbia.

GUANZON, Alfredo Z.; Santo Tomas (Philipp.) '56; Anaes; Staff, University Hosp., Saskatoon, Sask.; Tel. 242-7641.

GUARD, Michael C.; Ste. 102, 1590 Bellevue Ave., West Vancouver, B.C.; Cambridge (Eng.)'53; DOBstRCOG; Staff, Lions Gate Hosp.; Tel. WA 2-0155.

GUAY, Gerald; Lav '58; Res., Toronto Gen. Hosp., Toronto 2, Ont.

GUAY, John; 300 Carre St. Louis, Montreal, P.Q.; 7650 Pie IX Blvd. (res); Mon '44; Urol; Staff (Urol.), Hop. Ste. Jeanne d'Arc; Prof. of Anatomy, School of Prev. Med., Hop. Ste. Jeanne d'Arc; Tel. VI 9-5421.

GUAY, Joseph M.; 1346 ave de Montmorency, Quebec 6, P.Q.; Lav'60; Paed.

GUAY, Louis-P.; 339 rue St. Joseph, Lauzon, P.Q.; Lav '27; DiagRad (P.Q.); MCGP; Phys., Davie Shipbuilding Ltd.

GUAY, Marcel; 62 rue Ste.-Ursule, Quebec, P.Q.; Lav '41; FRCP(C), IntMed; Staff, Hotel-Dieu & Laval U.; Tel. 523-3095.

GUAY, Pierre A.; Mon'65; Res., Hop. Notre Dame, Montreal 24, P.Q.

GUAY, Raymond M.; 15 Ave. Begin, Levis, P.Q.; 9 Belair (res); Lav '54; Otol; Staff, Hop. Hotel-Dieu; Tel. 837-4483.

GUBBAY, Eric R.; Ste. 705, 1538 Sherbrooke St. W., Montreal 25, P.Q.; 59 Windsor Ave., Westmount (res); London (Eng.) '39; MRCP; MRCS; M.D. (Lond.); FACP; FRCP(C); IntMed; Cardiol (P.Q.) Assoc. Phys., Jewish Gen. & Reddy Mem. Hosp's.; Med. Cons. (Cardiol.), Jewish Hosp. of Hope; Medical Dir., Steinbergs Ltd.; Tel. 933-8541.

GUBUAN, Ramon C.; Box 430, Herbert, Sask.; Santo Tomas (Philipp.)'55.

GUDGEON, Alfred B.; Med. Arts Clinic, Regina, Sask.; London (Eng.)'61; Tel. 523-0651.

GUEVREMONT, Pierre; Mon'65; Res., Hop. Notre Dame, Montreal 24, P.Q.

GUENETTE, Eug.; 6970 Louis-Hemon, Montreal '35; P.Q.; 215 Outremont, Montreal 8 (res); Mon '35; Tel. RA 7-7430.

GUENETTE, Paul J.; Apt. 207, 4300 Ave Western, Montreal 26, P.Q. (res); Mon '35; Med. Dir., Continental Can., Co. of Can. Ltd., The Ogilvie Flour Mills Co. Ltd., Atlas Asbestos Co. Ltd., Bathurst Container Ltd. & George Weston Ltd., Longueil; Tel. RI 7-0621.

GUENTER, Clarence A.; 1034 Cobb Rd., Saint Paul, Minn., U.S.A.; Man'61; FRCP(C), IntMed.

GUENTHER, Henry; Man'46; Psy; Staff, Psychiatric Inst., 75 Emily St., Winnipeg, Man.

GUERETTE, Georges — E.; C.P. 740, Amqui, Co. Matapedia, P.Q.; Lav '43; Med. Dir., Hospice du Lac-Au-Saumon; Dist. Coroner.

GUERETTE, Oscar; East Angus, P.Q.; Lav '58.

GUERIN, Gaetan R.; 149 de Normandie, St.-Bruno, Cte. Chambly, P.Q. (res); Mon '57; Anaes, Staff, Hop. Hotel-Dieu; Tel. VI 4-0161.

GUERIN, Ronald; Lav'65; Res., Hop. Notre-Dame, Montreal 24, P.Q.

GUERRETTE, Roger; 19 rue Fraser Edmundston, N.B.; Lav'51; Anaes; Chief Anaes., Hotel-Dieu Hosp.; Tel. 735-3361.

GUERTIN Claude; 835 rte. Marie Victorin, Tracey, P.Q.; Lav '40; Staff, Hop. St-Luc, Montreal; Staff, Hop. Hotel-Dieu & Hop. St-Sacremont, Quebec.

GUERTIN, Claude; 4207 est Beaubien, Montreal 36, P.Q.; 7960 des Vendeens, Ville-d'Anjou (res); Mon '53; Tel. RA 2-7297.

GUERTIN, J. A. Jean; 98 Laval, Granby, P.Q.; Mon '52; Med. Dir., Hop. Notre-Dame de Granby; Vice. Pres., Fed. des Omni Praticiens de Quebec; Tel. 378-6161.

GUERTIN, Paul; 837 Cherrier, Montreal, P.Q.; Mon '43; Otol; Staff, Hop. Notre Dame; Tel. 525-6363.

GUERTIN, Roger; 441 St. Patrice St. W., Magog, P.Q.; Mon '33.

GUERTIN, Roger; Mon'65; Res., Hotel-Dieu de Sherbrooke, Sherbrooke, P.Q.

GUEST, A. Barrie; Elliott Lake Clinic, 46 Ontario St., Elliot Lake, Ont.; Birmingham (Eng.)'53; DRCOG; Cons. Anaes., St. Joseph's Hosp., Elliott Lake & Blind River; Tel. 848-7176.

GUEST, Douglas B.; 117 Raglan St., Renfrew, Ont.; 66 Lochiel St. (res); McG '49; Dist. Coroner; Tel. HE 2-4141.

GUEST, George F.; 348 Fraser St., North Bay, Ont.; 647 Baywood (res); Qns '19; OphthOtol; Staff, Civic Hosp. & St. Joseph's Gen. Hosp.; Tel. 472-7070.

GUEST, Howard A.; 2416 Portage Ave., Winnipeg 12, Man.; Qns '53; M.C.G.P.; Tel. VE 2-2458.

GUEST, Joan E.; 64 Brookside Ave., Toronto 9, Ont. (res); Tor '60.

GUEST, R. Gerald; Ste. 1, 1703 Victoria Park Ave., Scarborough, Ont.; Tor '59; Staff, Toronto East Gen. Hosp.; Tel. 751-6141.

GUEST, Sheena G.; 2416 Portage Ave., Winnipeg 12, Man.; 2416 Assiniboine Cres. (res); Glasgow (Scot.) '52; Tel. VE 2-2458.

GUEST, Wilbur C.; 309 Med. Arts Bldg., Winnipeg, Man.; 343 Yale Ave. (res); Man '41; DABO; Ophth; Ass't. Ophth., Wpg. Gen. & Deer Lodge Hosp's.; Ass't. Prof. (Ophth), U. of Manitoba; Tel. WH 3-0507.

GUEST, William A.; Ste. 4, 215 Cooper St., Ottawa, Ont.; 714 Echo Drive (res); Tor '28; FACP; IntMed; Emer. Clin. Prof. of Med., U. of Ottawa; Tel. 233-5155.

GUEST, William A.; Tor '60; Psy; Staff, Ontario Hosp., Hamilton, Ont.; Tel. 385-5361.
GUEVIN, Raymond M.; 1058 rue St. Denis, Montreal, P.Q.; Mon '58; FRCP(C), IntMed; Staff, Hop. St. Luc.; Tel. 861-7321.
GUILBAULT, Claude; 181 Notre Dame, Oka, P.Q.; Lav '26
GUILBAULT, Georges H.; 1155 Terrasse Trepanier, Chomedey, P.Q.; Mon '54.
GUILBEAULT, Albert J.; Ste 1506, 1010 Cherrier, Montreal 24, P.Q.; 28 Roskilde, Outremont (res); Mon '31; Paed; Chief of Paed., Hop. Notre Dame; Prof. Paed., U. of Montreal; Tel. 522-2971.
GUILBAULT, Normand; 8531, rue St-Gerard, Montreal 11, P.Q.; Mon '64; Abroad.
GUILBERT, Jacques; Mon'65; Res., Montreal Gen. Hosp., Montreal, P.Q.
GUILBERT, Paul W.; 270 Henri Bourassa Ouest, Montreal, P.Q.; 5445 Place d'Argenteuil (res); **Mon '50; DABP; Paed. (P.Q.); Tel. 331-3550.**
GUILD, Julius; Suite 1243, **Royal Alexandra** Hospital, Edmonton, Alta.; Alb '46; D.P.M. (Lond.), D.-Psy., Psy; Dir. (Psy), Royal Alexandra Hosp.; Ass't. Clin. Prof. (Psy.), U. of Alberta; Cons, Family Service Bureau, City Welfare Dept.; Tel. GR 4-3431, Ext. 312.
GUILLEM, Jean S. (See SALVI-GUILLEM, Jean).
GUILLEMETTE, Louis P.; 31 des Saules, Quebec 3, P.Q.; Lav '25; Tel. 623-1069.
GUILLEMETTE, Marcel E.; 164 Metcalfe St., Ottawa, Ont.; Ott'54; DABP; FRCP(C); Paed; Clin. Ass't., U. of Ottawa; Tel. 233-1166.
GUILLERMO, Remedios A.; Santo Tomas (Philipp) '53; FACA; Staff, Winnipeg Gen. Hosp., Winnipeg, Man.; Abroad.
GUILLET, Mario A.; Buenos Aires'54; IntMed; Staff, Hop. St. Jean-de-Dieu, Montreal 5, P.Q.
GUILMETE, Charles; 832 est Boul. St. Joseph, Montreal 34, P.Q.; 235 ave. McDougall, Outremont (res); Lav '43; FRCS(C), GenSurg; Staff, Hop. Maisonneuve Hop. de-la-Misericorde & Hop. St. Joseph de Rosemont. Surg., CPR; Tel. 279-1498.
GUIMOND, J. Jacques; 960 Ste-Croix, Montreal 9, P.Q.; Mon '55; Paed.; Tel. 387-1030.
GUIMOND, Jean C.; Mon '62; Res., Hop. Notre-Dame, Montreal, P.Q.
GUIMOND, J. Claude; 2420 Noury, Quebec 6, P.Q.; Lav'59; Anaes (P.Q.); Anaes., Hop. Christ-Roi.
GUIMOND, Pierre; Mon'65; Res., Hop. Maisonneuve, Montreal 36, P.Q.
GUIMOND, Remi; 766 Grandin, Chicoutimi, P.Q. (res); Lav '55; PhysMed; Staff, Hop. Hotel Dieu **St. Vallier; Tel. 549-1452.**
GUIMOND, Vincent; 148 rue Price W., Chicoutimi, P.Q.; Lav '42; ObstGyn; Chief (ObstGyn). **Hotel-Dieu-St.-Vallier; Assoc. Prof., Laval U.; Tel. 543-5562.**
GUIMONT, Andre; 469 est Jacques-Cartier, Chicoutimi, P.Q.; Lav'60; FRCS(C), OrthSurg.
GUIMONT-BRICOUT, Louise; Mon'65; Res., Hop. Douglas, Montreal 19, P.Q.
GUIMONT, Celestin; 1195 Ave. des Erables, Que**bec 6, P.Q.; Lav '33; Paed (P.Q.); Tel. 523-6614.**
GUIMONT, Francois; 610-12eme rue, St. Georges W., Co. Beauce, P.Q. (res); Lav'29; Phys., Dept. of Health, Beauceville E.
GUIMONT, Roger; 258 Dorchester, Quebec, P.Q.; **821 Ave. Cardinal Rouleau (res); Lav '42; Tel. 523-6358.**
GUINDON, Michel; 3220 Forest Hill, Apt. 1103, Montreal, P.Q.; OrthSurg(P.Q.).
GUINDON, Noemi; Windsor Tower, Ouellette Ave., Windsor, Ont.; Ott'58; Tel. 253-5232.
GUIOU, Norman M.; 380 Driveway Ottawa, Ont.; McG '16; GenSurg; Gyn; Cons. Gyn., Ottawa **Civic Hosp.; Tel. 234-4311.**
GULATI, Des Raj; Punjab (India) '45; Res., Montreal Neurological Inst., Royal Victoria Hosp., Montreal, P.Q.
GULENS, Voldemars; Tor'63; Res., Toronto Western Hosp., Toronto, Ont.
GULENS, Voldemars; P.O. Box 34, Dashwood, Ontario; **Riga(Latvia) '37.**
GULKA, Orest N.; 107-2nd Ave. E., Kindersley, Sask.; Sask '61; AMCGP; Active Med. Staff, Kindersley Union Hosp.; Tel. 463-2621.
GULLEY, John L.; 100 Medical Dental Bldg., Edmonton, Alta.; 9122-116th St. (res); Tor '45; **OrthSurg; Instr., U. of Alberta; Tel. 424-1617.**
GULLIFORD, Eve F. (Forrest); Box 789, Salmon Arm, B.C.; Qns '50; Tel. TE 2-2220.
GULYAS, Julia; 96 Stream Ave., Dorval, P.Q.; Budapest (Hung.) '55; Paed; Tel. 631-9733.
GUNDRY, C. Hegler; 437 Somerset St., North Vancouver, B.C.; (res); Tor '30; Psy; Dir., Div. of Mental Hygiene, Metropolitan Health Comm., **Vancouver; Tel. TR 6-1313.**
GUNER, Ali I.; '43; Staff, Provincial Hosp., Lancaster, N.B.
GUNG, Edward B.; 193 E. Hastings St., Vancouver 4, B.C.; 436 W. King Edward Ave. (res); Tor '26; Vsi. Staff, Mount St. Joseph & Van**couver Gen. Hosp's.; Tel. MU 1-8610.**
GUNN, Dacie; Box 368, Duncan, B.C. (res); McG '45; DiagRad; Radiol., King's Daughters **Hosp.; Tel. 746-4141.**
GUNN, Donald R.; 1570 Crestview Ave., Port Credit, Ont. (res); Tor '31; Psy; Dir. of Clin. **Research, Ontario Hosp., New Toronto; Tel. CL 9-8291.**
GUNN, Gordon G.; 42 Newcroft Close, Hillingdon, Middx., Eng.; Wes'60; GenSurg; Abroad.
GUNN, Ian M.; 200 Greyhound Bldg., 622-1st S.W., Calgary, Alta.; 1204 Frontenac Ave. (res); Alb'50; AMCGP; Staff, Calgary Gen. Hosp.; Court. Staff, Holy Cross Hosp.; Tel. AM 2-5030.
GUNN, J. Struthers; 750 W. Broadway Vancou**ver, B.C.; 568 W. 27th Ave. (res); Man '46; MC-**GP Att'd. Staff, Vancouver Gen. Hosp.; Vis. Staff, Grace & Mt. Saint Joseph's Hosp's.; Tel. **TR 6-2145.**
GUNN, Sisvan W. A.; 810 Fairmont Med. Bldg., 750 W. Broadway, Vancouver 9, B.C.; 4625 Cherbourg Dr., W. Van. (res); Geneva (Switz.) '51; FACA, M.S. (Surg.); GenSurg; Active Staff (Surg.), Van. Hosp's.; Lect. (History of Med.), U of British Columbia; Tel. TR 2-2445.
GUNSTON, Frank H.; Man '63; Res. Winnipeg Gen. Hosp., Winnipeg 3 Man.
GUNTON, Ramsay W.; 1008 Harrison Ave., London, Ont.; Wes'45; D.Phil. (Oxon); FACP; FRCP(C), IntMed (Cardiol.).
GUNTSCHEFF, Nikola; 126-736 Granville St., Vancouver 2, B.C.; **Sofia (Bulgaria) '30; Tel. MU 3-0411.**
GUPTILL, Gerald A.; Starlite Bldg., Bayers Rd., **Halifax, N.S.; Dal '58; Tel. 454-0612.**
GURAVICH, J. Lionel; 19 Rosedale Cres., Champlain Hgts., N.B. (res); Dal '44; F.A.C.P., IntMed; Clin. Dir Med., Lancaster Hosp.; Ass't. Med. Dir., St. John Arthritis Clin.
GURALNICK, Melvin S.; McG'65; Res., Montreal Gen. Hosp., Montreal, P.Q.
GURBIN, Gary M.; Kincardine, Ont.; Wes'65.
GURD, Fraser N.; 1650 Cedar Ave., Montreal, P.Q.; 3180 The Boulevard, Westmount, Mtl. 6 (res); McG '39; M.Sc. (Med.), D.Surg., DABS; FACS; FRCS(C), GenSurg; Surg.-in-Chief, Mtl. Gen. Hosp.; Prof. & Chm. Dept. of Surg., McGill U.; Tel. 935-6750.
GUREVITCH, Ralph; Calgary Assoc. Clinic, 214-6th Ave. S.W., Calgary, Alta.; Alb'60.
GURJAR, Manoo; 2615 E. 49th Ave., Vancouver **16, B.C.; 2726 Alder St., Vanc. 9 (res); Gurajat (India) '54; Tel. 433-3818.**
GURRIN, Peter M.; 59 High Park Blvd., Toronto 3, Ont.; London (Eng.)'54; FRCP(C), Anaes; Staff, St. Joseph's Hosp., Toronto, Ont.
GURRIN, Teresa M., (Cassin); 59 High Park Blvd., Toronto 3, Ont.; London(Eng.)'56; M.B., B.S., FRCP(C); Anaes.
GURSAHANI, Lachman; Bombay (India)'58; Staff, Bay Med. Clinic, Glace Bay, N.S.
GUSELLE, Robert D. W.; Oshawa Clinic, 117 King St. E., Oshawa, Ont.; 50 Connaught (res); Qns '50; Tel. 728-1661.
GUSLITS, Samuel S.; 264 Henderson H'way, **Winnipeg 5, Man.;** 491 Hartford Ave. (res); **Man '54; MCGP; Tel. 533-5792.**

GUSTAINIS, Ona D. (Grajauskaite); 179 Cassandra Blvd., Don Mills, Ont.; Innsbruck (Austria) '47; Anaes.
GUTELIUS, John R.; 687 Pine Ave W., Montreal, 2, P.Q.; 607 Clarke Ave., Mtl. 6 (res); McG '55; FACS; FRCS(C); GenSurg; ThorSurg; Ass't. Surg., Royal Victoria Hosp.; Ass't. Prof. (Surg.), McGill U.; Tel. VI 2-1251. Loc. 504.
GUTHRIE, David G.; McG '44; DMRD, DiagRad; Staff, D.V.A. Hosp., Quebec 10, P.Q.
GUTHRIE, Donald; 20 Knollside Dr., Richmond Hill, Ont. (res); Wes '54; Path; Staff, York Central Hosp.; Tel. 884-1171.
GUTHRIE, John S.; 151 Metcalfe St., Ottawa, Ont.; 69 Cameron Ave. (res); Qns '27; GenSurg; **Cons. Surg., Ottawa Civic Hosp.; Tel. CE 3-3373.**
GUTKOWSKI, Andrezej; Trinity Coll. (Dublin, Ire.)'57; Res., St. Boniface Gen. Hosp., Winnipeg, Man.
GUTOWSKI, Willie D.; Altona, Man.; Man'65.
GUTTER, Zoigniew; 11414-75th Ave. Edmonton, Alta (res); Louvain (Belg.) '46; DTM (Belg.), D & T Rad (Belg. & Canada); Chief Rad., Edmonton Cancer Clinic & Archer Mem. Hosp., Lamont; Tel. GE 3-5807.
GUTTMAN, Alexander P.; 100 Osborne Med. Bldg., 190 Osborne St. N., Winnipeg 1, Man.; 315 Laidlaw Blvd., Tuxedo 29 (res); Man '24; FR-CS(Edin.); FICS; OrthSurg; Cons. OrthSurg., **Victoria Gen. Hosp.; Att'd. OrthSurg. Misericordia Gen. Hosp.; Tel. SU 3-5524.**
GUTTMAN, Frank M.; 6000 Cote-des-Neiges, Montreal 26, P.Q.; Geneva (Switz.)'57; FRCS (C); GenSurg; Staff, Hop. Ste. Justine, Montreal, P.Q.; Tel. RE 1-4931.
GUTTORMSSON, Peter B.; Box 580, Maple Creek Clinic, Maple Creek, Sask.; Man '28; FICS, FRCS(C), GenSurg; Abroad.
GUTTORMSSON, Vilhjalmer J.; West Summerland, B.C.; Man '43; MCGP.
GUY, Augustine M.; 181 Le Marchant Rd., **St. John's, Nfld.; 44 Cornwall Ave. (res); Dal '42; Tel. 578-6334.**
GUY, Roland; 788 Hartland Ave., Outremont, Montreal 8, P.Q. (res); St. Thomas (Philippines) **'40; Path (P.Q.); Path., Hop. Sacre Coeur, Montreal; Tel. FE 4-1210.**
GUY, William D.; 106 Ninth St., Brandon, Man.; Glasgow (Scot.)'56; MCGP; Med. Staff, Assiniboine & Brandon Gen. Hosp's.; Tel. PA 6-4509.
GUYDA, Harvey J.; Man '62; Jr. Ass't. Res., Children's Hosp., Winnipeg 3, Man.; Abroad.
GUYATT, Benjamin F.; 190 King St. W., Dundas, Ont.; West Flamboro (res); **Tor '41.**
GUYATT, John M.; 826 Main St. E., Hamilton, Ont.; Wes '43; MCGP; Tel. LI 4-0136.
GUYATT, Laurie A.; Tor '41; Not in practice.
GUYATT, Richard E.; 826 Main St. E., Hamilton, Ont.; Tor '11.
GUYOT, Henri; 580 Aulneau St., St. Boniface, Man.; Man'29; F.I.C.S.: Cons., Dept. Obst-Gyn, St. Boniface Hosp.; Lect. (Obst. Gyn.), U. of Manitoba; Tel. 233-7696.
GUZDZIOL, Wladyslaw; Port Hawkesbury, N.S., Poznan (Pol.) '37; D. Obst. R.C.O.G.; Tel. 189.
GUZMAN, Carole A.; Tor '58; Res., Royal Victoria Hosp., Montreal, P.Q.
GUZMAN, D. Antonio; 1610 Pine Ave. W., Montreal 25, P.Q.; McG'60; FRCP(C) Neur; Staff, (Neuropath.), Montreal Neurological Inst., Montreal, P.Q.
GUZMAN, Irene (See Aligaga-Guzman).
GUZMAN, Rolando; Philippines '55; Res., St. Boniface Hosp., St. Boniface 6, Man.
GWASSALIA, Schotha; 5 Welland Ave., St. Catharines, Ont.
GWIZDAL, Mary; Wes'64; Res., St. Michael's Hosp., Toronto, Ont.
GWOZDECKY, George; 107 Medical Arts Bldg., Port Arthur, Ont.; 172 Ruper St., 9A (res); Charles U., Prague (Czech.) '45; M.C.G.P.
GYDE, Maurice C.; 245 Marion St., St. Boniface 6,. Man.; Man '45; M.Sc.(Otol., Minn.); Otol; Active Staff, St. Boniface Hosp.; Cons. (ENT), St. Boniface San.; **Dem., U. of Manitoba; Tel. CH 7-9961.**
GYORFI, Alexander W.; 62 Harborview Dr., Sydney, N.S. (res); Brussells (Belg.) '50; D.T.M. & H.; Path., St. Rita Hosp., Sydney & St. Elizabeth Hosp., N. Sydney; Tel. 564-5528; 564-5507.
GYORKE, **Zoltan—(See Yorke).**
HAAG, Ann L.; Tor'65; Res., Women's College Hosp., Toronto 5, Ont.
HAAYEN, Peter J.; Ste 303, 77 Westmount Rd., Guelph, Ont.; 7 Exhibition St. (res); Leyden (Neth.) '52; MCGP; Tel. TA 2-3450.
HABER, Aurel; 187 St. Clair Ave. W., Toronto 5, Ont.; Bucharest (Roum.) '40; DiagRad; Staff (Rad), Sunnybrook & St. Joseph's Hosp's.; Tel. WA 2-9221.
HABER, Harold N.; 1771 Victoria Park Ave., Scarborough, Ont.; 1 Sagebush Lane, Don Mills (res); Tor '56; Tel. PL 5-0722.
HABER, Julius; 396 Pacific Ave., Toronto 9, Ont.; Tor '45; MCGP; Staff, New Mount Sinai Hosp.
HABERFELLNER, Helga (Samitz); 20 High Park Gdns., Toronto 3, Ont.; Innsbruck (Austria) '53.
HABERMAN, Herbert F.; 399 Bathurst St., Toronto, Ont.; Tor '59; FRCP(C), DermSyph; Active Staff, Toronto Western Hosp.; Research Assoc., Dept. of Med., U. of Toronto; Tel. EM 9-5101.
HABGOOD, Mary E.; London (Eng.)'55; D.Obst RCOG; Staff ,Inuvik Gen. Hosp., Inuvik, N.W.T.
HABIB, George G.; Winnipeg Clinic, St. Mary's & Vaughan, Winnipeg 1, Man.; Edinburgh (Scot.) '53; MRCP(Scot.).
HABROS, Joseph S.; 1428 Ouellette Ave., Windsor, Ont.; Ott'60; Tel. 252-8387.
HABROS, Ronald E.; 674 Fennell Ave E., Hamilton, Ont.; Wes '64; Tel. 383-6890.
HACHE, Alban G.; 15 Alma St., Moncton, N.B.; Ott'65.
HACHE, Lorenzo; 520 Sauve Blvd., St. Eustache, P.Q.; 117 Les Erables, Laval sur-le-lac **(res); Ott '57; M.Sc. (Surg.); DABOS; FRCS(C);** Gen-Surg; DABS; FACS; Chief-of-Surg., St. Eustache Gen. Hosp.; Tel. 473-6933.
HACKADON, Robert G.; Wes '60; Jr. Int'n. Toronto Gen. Hosp., Toronto 2, Ont.
HACKEMANN, Manfred A.; Norman Wells, N.W.T.; London (Eng.)'62; M.B., B.S.
HACKER, Allan H.; 1551 Kipling Ave. N., Rexdale, Ont.; Tor '53; Staff, New Mt. Sinai Hosp.; Tel. CH 4-1440.
HACKETT, Arnold A.; 955 Queen St. E., Sault Ste. Marie, Ont.; 97 Pageant Dr. (res); Ott'55; Active Staff, Sault Ste. Marie & Plummer Mem. Hosp's.; Tel. AL 4-5041.
HACKETT, John D.; 4773 Sherbrooke St. W., Montreal 6, P.Q.; London (Eng.) '51; MRCS; LRCP; D.Psy; Psy; Clin. Ass't. Psy., St. Mary's Hosp.; Assoc. Psy., Mental Hygiene Inst.; Dem. (Psy.), McGill U.; Tel. 937-7522.
HACKETT Roger M.; 10951-124th. St., Edmonton, Alta.; Dublin (Ire.) '56; FRCS (Ed.); FRCS(C); GenSurg; Tel. 454-4551.
HACKETT, Thomas J., see KIRKWOOD-HACKETT, Thomas J.
HACKNEY, John W.; 42 rue Ste.-Anne, Ste.-Anne-de-Bellevue, P.Q.; McG '39; Tel. 697-3900.
HACKNEY, Joseph C.; St. Mary's Med. Clinic, P.O. Box 1120, St. Mary's, Ont.; Wes '57; MCGP.
HACON, William S.; Nat. Health & Welfare, Brooke Claxton Bldg., Ottawa, Ont.; Guy's, Chief, Emergency Health Serv., Dept. of Nat. Health & Welfare; 251 Bank St.; Lect. (Admin.), U. of Ottawa; Tel. 992-5889.
HADDAD, Henry; Ott '63; Res., Montreal Gen. Hosp., Montreal 25, P.Q.
HADDAD, John W.; 67 Elm St. E., Sudbury, Ont.: 167 College St. (res); Tor '36; MCGP; AICS; Staff, St. Joseph's, Sudbury Mem. & Sudbury Gen. Hosp's.; Tel. OS 4-4303.
HADDAD, Nicholas N.; 67 Elm St. E., Sudbury, Ont.; 134 Adie St. (res); Tor '36; Cons. (Int-Med), St. Joseph's Hosp.; Tel. 674-4383.
HADDEN, Robert A.; 39 Charlton Ave. E., Hamilton, Ont.; **Tor '51; Otol.; Tel. 528-5233.**
HADE, Bernard; Mon '63; Res., Hop. St. Justine, Montreal 26, P.Q.

HADEN, Phillip; 188 Union St., Kingston, Ont. (res); Cambridge & Guy's Hosp. (Eng.) '40; MRCP, DPM (Lond.); Psy; Chief, Female Serv., Ontario Hosp.; Lect. (Psy), Queen's U.; Tel. LI 6-1101.

HADER, Walter J.; Ott'58; Res., Dept. of Neuropath., University Hosp., Saskatoon, Sask.

HADLEY, Donald K.; 84 Brant Ave., Brantford, Ont.; Tor'56; FRCS(C), GenSurg; Tel. 759-3100.

HADLEY, Gerald L.; 2769 Lundy's Lane, Niagara Falls, Ont.; 3231 Rolling Acres Cr. (res); Tor'52; FRCP(C); IntMed; Chief (Med.), Greater Niagara Gen. Hosp.; Tel. EL 6-2123.

HAFEZI, Douglas M; 2 Doris Dr., Toronto 16, Ont.; London (Eng.) '32; FRCS(Edin.); FICS; Active Surg. Staff, Central Hosp.; Tel. PL 5-1262.

HAFFEY, M. Joseph; Apt. 407, 169 Jameson Ave., Toronto 3, Ont.; Tor'09; MRCS, LRCP, Otol; Otol., St. Michael's Hosp.; Tel. WA 3-3434.

HAFFKE, Siegfried; Apt. 403, 5501 Randall Ave., Montreal 29, P.Q. (res); Frankfurt (Germ.) '49; DiagRad. (P.Q.); Staff, Queen Mary Vet's Hosp.; Tel. 342-2320.

HAFSO, Alice K. (Kjos); 4716-106th Ave., Edmonton, Alta.; Alb'51; Retired.

HAGAN, John N.; Tor'33; D. Psy; Psy; Staff, Brantford Gen. Hosp., Brantford, Ont.

HAGEN, Barry A.; 1669 Victoria St., Prince George, B.C.; UBC'65.

HAGEN, E. Odette (Faulkner); 6508-127th St., Edmonton, Alta. (res); Manchester (Eng.) '51; D.C.H. (Eng.); Ass't. Prof. (Anat.), U. of Alberta; Tel. GE 9-8721.

HAGEN, J. Martin; 6508-127th St., Edmonton, Alta. (res); Edinburgh (Scot.) '47; Anaes; Staff, Anaes. & Clinic. Instr., University Hosp.; Tel. 439-5911.

HAGEN, Paul B.; Sydney (Australia) '45; Prof. & Hd., Dept. of Biochem., Queen's U., Kingston, Ont.; Tel. 546-3871.

HAGEN, Victor J.; River Med. Group, 385 River Ave., Winnipeg 13, Man.; 106 Lyndale Dr., St. Boniface 6 (res); Man'44; FCCP; Ass't. Med. Dir., St. Boniface San., St. Vital; Dem. (Med.), U. of Manitoba; Tel. GL 2-8142.

HAGERMAN, E. Stanley; 238 Elm St., St. Thomas, Ont.; 101 Metcalfe St. (res); Qns'53; FRCP(C); IntMed; Cons. Active Staff, St. Thomas Elgin Gen. Hosp.; Tel. 633-0352.

HAGERMAN, Gerald E.; 80 Connell Ave., Virginiatown, Ont.; Qns '45.

HAGGAR, Robert A. J.; 877 Kingsway Dr., Longacres, Burlington, Ont. (res); Wes '50; M.Sc., F.A.C.P., F.A.S.C.P., D.A.B.Path; Path; Dir. of Lab., St. Joseph's Hosp., Hamilton, Ont.; Tel. NE 4-3846.

HAGMEIER, John E.; 155 Frederick St., Kitchener, Ont.; 37 Maragaret Ave. (res); Tor '11; AMCGP; Tel. SH 5-4022.

HAHN, Charlotte E.; Ste. 908, 1849 Yonge Street, Toronto 7, Ont.; Tor'45; IntMed; Tel. 487-0347.

HAIDASZ, Stanley, MP; 514 Lansdowne Ave., Toronto 4, Ont.; 77 Sir William's Lane, Islington (res); Tor '51; Assoc. Staff, St. Joseph's Hosp.; Parliamentary Sec. to Minister of Nat. Health & Welfare; Tel. LE 6-6604.

HAIG, Arthur A.; Haig Clinic, Lethbridge, Alta.; 1115-8th Ave. S. (res); McG '26; F.R.C.S. (Ed.), F.A.C.S., F.I.C.S., GenSurg.; Surg-in-Chief, St. Michael's Gen. Hosp.; Staff, Lethbridge Mun. Hosp.; Tel. FA 7-1531.

HAIG, T. Brian; Haig Clinic, 601-6th Ave. S., Lethbridge, Alta.; Sask'58; FRCS(C), GenSurg.

HAIG, Willard R.; Haig Clinic, 601—6th Ave. S., Lethbridge, Alta.; 720—11th St. S. (res); McG '26; F.I.C.S.; GenSurg; Staff, St. Michael's Gen. & Lethbridge, Mun. Hosp's.; Tel. 327-3171; Semi Retired.

HAIGH, Geoffrey; Three Hills, Alta.; Sheffield (Eng.)'53; MCGP; Tel. 443-5292.

HAIGH, James B.; Alta Guidance Clinic, 4734 Ross St., Red Deer, Alta.; Leeds (Eng.) '54 DPM (Leeds); Psy.

HAIGHT, Kenneth R.; Sask'65; Staff, Meadow Lake Union Hosp., Meadow Lake, Sask.

HAIGHT, Rachel K.; 224 Cooper St., Ottawa, Ont.; Tor '28; D.P.H., IntMed; Att. Staff, Ottawa Civic & Gen. Hosp's.; Tel. CE 3-3673.

HAIMSON, Jean; 1578 Jean Talon E., Montreal 35, P.Q.; Pavia (Italy) '38; Ass't. (Neur. Psy.), Hop. Ste. Justine; Tel. RE 1-4931.

HAIN, Cecil W.; 16 Brule Terr., Toronto 3, Ont. (res); Tor '26; MCGP; MO, U.S. Pub. Health Serv. & CPR; Tel. 769-2736.

HAIN, Gordon R.; Linwood, Ont.; Tor '21.

HAIN, Irene C.; 749 King St. W., Kitchener, Ont.; Linwood (res); Tor '52; MRCOG; Active Staff (ObstGyn), Kitchener-Waterloo & St. Mary's Hosp's.; Tel. SH 5-3821.

HAINES, Milton; Wes'56; Ph.D.; Research Dir., Westminster Hosp., London, Ont.

HAIR, H. Charles MBE; 816 Med. Arts Bldg., 170 St. George St., Toronto 5, Ont.; 34 Rochester Ave. (res); Tor '36; FRCP(C), DermSyph; Att'd Phys. (Derm), Toronto Western Hosp.; Cons. (DermSyph), Sunnybrook Hosp.; Ass't. Phys. (Derm) Hosp. for Sick Children; Ass't. Prof. Med. (Derm) U. of Toronto. Tel. WA 2-0111.

HAIST, Reginald E.; 56 Cheltenham Ave., Toronto, Ont. (res); Tor'36; Ph.D.; FRSC; Hon. Prof., Dept. of Med. Research, Banting & Best Inst. & Prof. & Chmn., (Physiol.), U. of Toronto; Tel. WA 3-6611.

HAJDU, Andrew; Ayerst Research Labs., 1025 Laurentian Blvd., Montreal 9, P.Q.; Budapest (Hung.)'52; Sr. Path.-Toxicol.

HAKSTIAN, Arthur; 2589 McBain Ave., Vancouver, B.C. (res); Tor '25 IntMed (TB); Dir., New Westminster Chest Clinic, Div., T.B. Control, B.C.; Tel. RE 1-8573. Retired.

HAKSTIAN, Robert W.; Drummond Med. Bldg., Ste 1009, 1414 Drummond St., Montreal 25, P.Q.; UBC'57; FRCS(C), PlasSurg.; Surg., St. Luc Hosp.; Tel. 288-3935.

HALAK, Joseph; 3147 Kingsway, Vancouver 6, B.C.; UBC '58.

HALAM-ANDRES, Alfred S.; 348 Simcoe St. N. Oshawa, Ont.; London (Eng.) '54; Tel. 723-3392.

HALDANE, James H., M.C.; Glasgow (Scot.)'41; LRCP&S (Glas.); MRCP (Glas. & Ed.); LRFPS (Glas.); FRFPS; Staff, Victoria Gen. Hosp., Halifax, N.S.

HALDENBY, David A.; 201 Western Med. Bldg., 25 Leonard Ave., Toronto 2B, Ont.; Tor'59; FRCS(C), Otol; Active Staff, Toronto Western Hosp.; Tel. 363-2978.

HALE, Burt B.; Royal Victoria Hosp., Montreal, P.Q.; 70 Stratford Rd., Hampstead, Mtl. 29 (res); McG '49; D.Rad; D&T Rad; Assoc. Rad., Royal Victoria Hosp.; Cons. Rad., Grace Dart Hosp.; Ass't. Prof. McGill U.; Tel. VI 2-1251.

HALE, Claude L.G.; 86 Bloor St. W., Toronto 5, Ont.; 416 Moore Ave., Tor. 17; Bristol (Eng.)'56; M.B., Ch. B., MRCS; LRCP; Assoc. Staff, Wellesley & Grace Hosp's.; Tel. WA 5-5511 & 425-5722.

HALE, George C.; 20 Hayman Court, London, Ont.; 124 St. James St., Apt. 112 (res); McG '09; LI.D., F.A.C.P., F.R.C.P.(C) IntMed; Prof. Emeritus of Med., U. of Western Ont.

HALE, Helena B.; 202 Vancouver St., Victoria, B.C.; Prague (Czech.)'28; FAPA, Psy.; Pt-time Psy., Gtr. Victoria Bd. of Health; Tel. 382-0257.

HALE, Thomas R.; Sun Life Bldg., Montreal, P.Q.; 224 Maple Ave., St. Lambert (res); McG '49; FRCP(C), IntMed, Cardiol (PQ); Ass't. Phys., Mtl. Gen. Hosp.; Assoc. Med. Dir., Sun Life Assurance Co. of Canada; Tel. UN 6-6411.

HALEY, Frank C.; Dept. of Anaes., University Hosp., Edmonton, Alta.; Alb '53; M.Sc., FACA; FRCP(C), Anaes; Att'd. Staff, University Hosp.; Hon. Ass't. Prof., U. of Alberta; Tel. 439-5911.

HALEY, Frank W.; 396 Queen's Ave., London, Ont.; Tor '52; MCGP.

HALEY, John F., Major; Tor '54; DMR(D); Diag Rad; No. 1, C.B.M.U., CAPO 5050, Canadian Armed Forces, Europe. Abroad.

HALIBURTON, Robert A.; 402 Med. Arts Bldg., 1011 Ouellette Ave., Windsor, Ont.; 660 Champlain Dr. (res); Tor '51; M.S. (OrthSurg., Minn.); DABOS; FACS; OrthSurg; Cons., Hotel-Dieu, Metropolitan, Grace & IODE Hosp's.; Tel. CL 3-5900.

HALINA, Flora; (See SCOTT, Flora).

HALINEN, Maire M. (VIHURI); 10815-60th Ave., Edmonton, Alta.; Helsinki (Finland) '39; DCLM.

HALKIEWICZ, Tadeusz J.; 3000 Lawrence Ave. E., Scarborough, Ont.; 37 Duncombe Blvd. (res); Lwow (Poland) '38; Anaes; Staff (Anaes), Scarborough Gen. Hosp.; Tel. AX 3-8681.

HALL, Alan B.; 350 Albert St., Nanaimo, B.C.; 135 Newcastle Ave. (res); McG '28; Staff, Nanaimo Gen. Hosp.

HALL, Allan S.; 14607 MacKenzie Dr., Edmonton, Alta.; London (Eng.) '38; MRCS; LRCP; Anaes (Alta.); Tel. HU 8-1613.

HALL, Arnold A.; Campbell River, B.C.; Sask'65.

HALL, C. William; 810 South Dr., Winnipeg 19, Man. (res); Man '38; DABR; FICS; DiagRad; Dir. Dept. of DiagRad., St. Boniface Hosp.; Ass't. Prof. (Rad.), U. of Manitoba; Tel. WH 3-0311, GR 5-5846.

HALL, David H., Lt/Col.; RCAF Station, Trenton, Ont.; Qns '43.

HALL, Dorothy L.; 3-9 Middlegate, Winnipeg 1, Man.; London (Eng.)'57; MPH(Minn.); Med. Dir., Kildonan St. Paul Health Unit.

HALL, Edwin R.; 815 King Georges Way, West Vancouver, B.C.; Alb'46; Anaes; Clin. Instr., (Anaes.), U. of British Columbia.

HALL, Elizabeth; Apt. 1002, 201 McLeod St. Ottawa, Ont. (res); Tor '54; Ph.D. (Ott.); Assoc. **Prof. Research Dept. of Anatomy, U. of Ottawa; Tel. CE 5-6751.**

HALL, F. Murray; 20 Victoria St., Toronto, Ont.; Tor'49; IntMed; Med. Spec., Imperial Life Assurance Co.; Tel. 364-8211.

HALL, G. Edward; 1836 Richmond St., London, Ont. (res); Tor '35; Ph.D. (Tor.); D.Sc. (Laval); LLD; FRSC; Pres. & Vice Chancellor, U. of **Western Ontario; Tel. GE 9-1681.**

HALL, George C. R.; 23 King St. S., Little Britain, Ont.; Tor '23; Staff, Ross Mem. Hosp. Lindsay, Port Perry & Uxbridge Hosp's.; Court. Staff, Peterborough Civic Hosp.; M.O.H., Mariposa Twp.; Coroner, Victoria & Haliburton Counties; Tel. 2R3.

HALL, George W.; Coldwater, Ont.; Wes '27; M.C.G.P.

HALL, Gordon R.; 550 Ingersoll Ave., Woodstock, Ont.; 119 Light St. (res); Tor '36; MCGP; Active Staff, Woodstock Gen. Hosp.; Tel. 537-2451.

HALL, Hector C.; 118 Simcoe St. N., Oshawa, Ont.; 42 Connaught St. (res); Tor '31.

HALL, Henry D.; 249 Main St. N., Brampton, Ont.; 15 Armstrong St. (res); Queen's U. (Belfast, N. Ire.)'55; AMCGP; Active Staff, Peel Mem. Hosp.; Tel. GL 1-1937.

HALL, Henry Gibson; 1050 Avenue Rd. N., Toronto, Ont.; 21 Lauderdale Dr., (res); Tor '29; IntMed; M.C.G.P.; Tel. HU 9-2106.

HALL, Herbert B.; 136 Devonshire, Iroquois Falls, Ont. (res); Alb '48; Tel. 3349.

HALL, Henry J.; 40 Coldwater St. E., Orillia, Ont.; Tor'59; AMCGP; Staff, Orillia Soldiers Mem. Hosp.; Vice Pres., Med. Soc.; Tel. 326-3541.

HALL, H. Kenneth; 5770 South St., Halifax, N.S.; **Dal '44; Psy; Assoc. Psy., Victoria Gen. Hosp.; Cons. Psy., Camp Hill & Dartmouth Hosp's.; Assoc. Prof. (Psy), Dalhousie U.; Tel. 423-8794.**

HALL, Howard H.; 201 Bliss Blk., Prince Albert, Sask.; 60—12th St. E. (res); Man '46.

HALL, Ian M.; 123 Woodward Ave., London, Ont.; Glasgow (Scot.) '48.

HALL, Jas. S.; 176 Catherine St., Port Colborne, Ont.; 151 Tennessee Ave. (res); Tor '54; M.C.-G.P.; Tel. 834-3638.

HALL, J. Leo; 2489 Bloor St. W., Toronto, Ont.; 56 High Park Blvd. (res); Tor '24; ObstGyn; Chief of Obst. Gyn., St. Joseph's Hosp.; Tel. RO 6-1352.

HALL, John; 93 Drake St., Sault-Ste-Marie, Ont. (res); Wes '45; Plant Surg., The Algoma Steel Corp. Ltd.; Tel. 4-5111, Loc. 2241.

HALL, J. Campbell; Tor'61; Res., Toronto Gen. Hosp., Toronto, Ont.

HALL, John E.; 123 Edward St., Toronto, Ont.; 110 Roxborough Dr. (res); McG '52; FRCS(C); OrthSurg; FACS; Chief OrthSurg., Hosp. for Sick Children; Cons. Orth., Ontario Crippled Children's Centre; Assoc. (Surg.), U. of Toronto; Tel. 368-0766.

HALL, John G.; Ste 1020, 143 James St. S., Hamilton, Ont.; Tor '43; D.Psy.; Psy.; Active Staff, Hamilton Civic Hosp's.; Tel. 525-2260.

HALL, John V.; Box 729, Castlegar, B.C.; 1145-**5th Ave. (res); UBC '56; MCGP; Tel. 365-6611.**

HALL, Kenneth A.; Guysborough, N.S.; Bristol (Eng.)'40; Staff, Guysborough Mem. Hosp.; Tel. 107.

HALL, LeRoy W.; Qns'57; MCGP; Res., Kingston Gen. Hosp., Kingston, Ont.

HALL, Malcolm R.; x-Ray, Med. Arts Bldg., 170 St. George St., Toronto 5, Ont.; 58 Church St., Brampton (res); Tor '28; FFR (Lond.), D & T Rad; Rad.-in-Chief, Toronto Gen. Hosp.; Prof. & Hd. Dept. (Rad.), U. of Toronto; Tel. WA 1-3118.

HALL, Mary C. (Armstrong); 249 Main St. N., Brampton, Ont.; Queens U. (Belfast, Ire.) '55; DCH; Ass't. Pt-time M.O.H., Peel County Health Unit; Tel. 451-1937.

HALL, Michael C.; 607 Medical Arts Bldg., 170 St. George St., Toronto 5, Ont.; 109 Belsize Dr., Tor. 7 (res); St. Bart's (London, Eng.) '52; Ph.D., B.Sc. (Med.), M.R.C.S., L.R.C.P., F.R.C.S.(C), OrthSurg; Ass't. Surg., Wellesley Hosp.; Ass't. Prof., Dept. of Anatomy Clin. Instr., Dept. of Surg. U. of Toronto; Tel. WA 1-3462.

HALL, Morton E.; Workmen's Comp. Bd., 707 W. 37th Ave., Vancouver 13, B.C.; Tor'40; FRCS(Eng.); GenSurg; M.O., WCB.

HALL, Morton E.; 12729 Stony Plain Rd., Edmonton, Alta.; Retired.

HALL, Noe, B.; Box 6900, Campbell River, **B.C.; McG '27; M.C.G.P.; Staff (Med.), Campbell** River Gen. Hosp.; Dist. Coroner; Retired.

HALL, Robert G.; The Campbell Clinic, 430 Mayor Magrath Dr., Lethbridge, Alta.; 2602—6th Ave. S. (res); Charing Cross Hosp. (London, Eng.) '42; M.R.C.S. (Lond.), L.R.C.P. (Lond.), M.R.C.-O.G.; FACOG; FRCOG; ObstGyn; Chief ObstGyn., St. Michaels Gen. Hosp.; Tel. FA 7-5737.

HALL, Robert T.; Qns '63; Res., Kingston Gen. Hosp., Kingston, Ont.; Abroad.

HALL, Roger M.; 6425 MacKenzie Place, Vancouver, B.C. (res); Tor'41; DMR (Lond.); DiagRad; Assoc. Dir., (Rad.), St. Paul's Hosp.; Tel. MU 3-2211.

HALL, Russel M.; Main St. Norwich, Ont.; Wes '50; MCGP; Dist. Coroner; Tel. 863-2338.

HALL, William E.; One Medical Place, 20 Wynford Dr., Don Mills, Ont.; 3 Governor's Rd. (res); Tor'38; FRCP(C), IntMed; Staff Phys., St. Michael's Hosp.; Ass't. Prof. (Med.), U. of Toronto; Tel. 429-1258.

HALL, W. Francis; 8008-119th St., Edmonton, Alta.; Alb '42; FACS; FRCS(C); GenSurg; Att'd. Staff, Royal Alex. Hosp. Lect. U. **of Alberta; M.O., Workmen's Comp. Bd., Edmonton; Tel. GA 2-6525.**

HALL, Wm. Mack; 5511 Wallace St., Vancouver 13, B.C. (res); Alb '37; F.A.C.A.; Anaes; Chief Anaes., Shaughnessy Hosp., D.V.A.; Clin. Instr., (Anaes.), U. of British Columbia; Tel. TR 6-6767.

HALLAM, Beverley H. B.; Burks Falls, Ont.; Tor '40.

HALLAM, Hugh T.; 821 Coxwell Ave., Toronto 13, Ont.; McG'58; FRCS(C); GenSurg; Staff, Toronto East Gen. Hosp.; Tel. 466-0388.

HALLE, Jules; 75 rue St.-Louis, Quebec, P.Q.; 1080 ave.-des-Governeurs, Sillery (res); Lav '35; Ophth, Otol; Chief of Otol., Hop. St. Sacrement; Cons. (Otol.), Hop. Jeffrey Hale; Assoc. Prof. (Ophth, Otol), Laval U.; Tel. 523-5605.

HALLE, Marc; 22 Henry St., Levis, P.Q.; Lav'59; Gastroent(P.Q.); Staff, Hop. Hotel-Dieu de Levis; Tel. 837-9990.

HALLETT, Roy E.; Psychiatric Centre, Yorkton, Sask.; 207-5th Ave. S. (res); Tor'59; **D.Psy.; Abroad.**

HALLETT, William M.; 5150 Dundas St. W., Islington, Ont.; Tor'54; FRCP(C), IntMed; Active Staff, Queensway Hosp.; Tel. 233-0447.
HALLEY, Janet G.; Liverpool (Eng.) '59; M.B.; Ch.B.; D.A.; Res., Vancouver Gen Hosp., Vancouver 9, B.C.
HALLEY, Leonard J.; 2074 Robie St., Halifax, N.S.; Dublin (Ire.) '56.
HALLGREN, Robert A.; Allen Clinic, 10155-120th St., Edmonton, Alta.; Alta'64.

HALLIDAY, Bruce; Box 249, 24 Hope St. W., Tavistock, Ont.; Tor'51; MCGP; Active Staff (Anaes.), Stratford Gen. Hosp.; Court. Staff, Woodstock Gen. Hosp.; Tel. 655-2322.
HALLIDAY Frank; Edinburgh (Scot.) '47; Med. Supt., Midale Union Hosp., Midale, Sask.
HALLIDAY, John A.; 200 Brant Ave., Brantford, Ont.; Tor '50; Ophth; Staff, Brantford Gen. Hosp. & St. Joseph's Hosp., Brantford; Tel. 752-7978.
HALLIDAY, Robert; Ste. 304, 4900 Kingsway, South Burnaby, B.C.; 1009 W. 33rd, Vancouver (res); Queen's U. (Belfast, N. Ire.)'42; DPM; Psy; Cons., Vancouver Gen. & Burnaby Gen. Hosp's.; Cons., Narcotic Addiction Fdn. of B.C.; **Clin. Instr. (Psy), U. of British Columbia; Tel. HE 4-8040.**

HALLIWELL, David; Man'46; Res. (Ophth.), Winnipeg Gen. Hosp., Winnipeg, Man.

HALLOWELL, Mary; Ste. 128, 624-6th St., **New Westminster, B.C.; 225 Royal Ave. (res); Leeds (Eng.) '50; DCH(Lond.); LRCP(Edin.);** MRCP(Ed.); Paed; Active Staff, Royal Columbian & St. Mary's Hosp's.; Cons. Staff, Surrey Mem. Hosp., N. Surrey & Maple Ridge Hosp., Hanney; Tel. 522-6447.

HALMAGYI, Andrew F.; Qns'61; GenSurg; Staff, St. Michael's Hosp., Toronto, Ont.
HALMOS, Veronica (Bereny); Ste. 1204, 123 Edward St., Toronto 2, Ont.; Budapest(Hung.) '53; FRCP(C); IntMed; Pt-time Research Fell., U. of Toronto; Tel. 363-5719.
HALPENNY, Gerald W.; Ste. 480, 4141 Sherbrooke St. W., Montreal 6, P.Q.; McG'34; FRCP(C), FACP, IntMed; Lectr., McGill U.; Senior Phys., Montreal Gen. Hosp.; Chief of Serv. (Med.), Queen Mary Veterans' Hosp.; Tel. 932-4255.
HALPERIN, David; Ste 590, 6000 Cote-des-Neiges, Montreal, P.Q.; 5020 Circle Rd. (res); McG '39; **DABOt; Otol; Otol.-in-Chief, Jewish Gen. Hosp.;** Cons., Mt. Sinai San.; Tel. 342-9520.
HALPERN, George I. J.; 172 Kenilworth Ave. N., Hamilton, Ont.; Tor'52; MCGP; Phys., Macassa Home for Aged; Active Staff, Hamilton Civic Hosp's.; Tel. LI 5-8683.
HALPERN, Israel; 892 Bloor W., Toronto 4, Ont.; 715 Palmerston Ave. (res); '39; Tel. LE 5-7033.
HALPERN, Norman N.; 6000 Cote des Neiges Rd., Montreal 25, P.Q.; Qns '46; Urol.; Tel. 844-7904.
HAM, Arthur W.; Tor'26; FRCS; Dept. of Anat., U. of Toronto, Toronto, Ont.
HAM, Trevor J.; McG '63; Res., Hosp. for Sick Children, Toronto 2, Ont.
HAMANN, Christa; Westmount Med. Bldg., 5025 Sherbrooke St. W., Montreal 28, P.Q.; Germany '47; AMCGP.
HAMBLEY, E. John; Tor'60; Ass't. Res., Urol., Sunnybrook Hosp., Toronto, Ont.
HAMBLIN, Garnet P.; 2333 Bloor St. W., Toronto, Ont.; Tor '32; Paed; Clin. Instr. (Paed), U. of Toronto. Tel. RO. 9-1124.
HAMDI, Fouad A.; 310-1070 Douglas St., Victoria, B.C.; Alexandria (Egypt)'48; DOMS (Lond.); Ph.D. (Edin.); NeurSurg; NeurSurg., Royal Jubilee & St. Joseph's Hosp's.; Tel. 386-1613.
HAMEED, Khalid; Punjab (Pakistan)'53; DAB (Path); Path; Staff, Pathology Inst., 5800 University Ave., Halifax, N.S.; Ass't. Prof., Dalhousie U.; Tel. 422-9661.
HAMEL, A. Oscar; 4800 Chemin Cote-des-Neiges, Montreal, P.Q.; Mon '47; Psy (P.Q.).
HAMEL, Christian J. C.; 219 Springdale, Pointe Claire, P.Q.; Lille (France)'61; Paed.
HAMEL, Come; 219 Springdale, Pointe Claire, Lachine, P.Q.; Lav'27; Tel. 695-3615.
HAMEL, Elzear; 55 rue Church, Montreal 19, Mon'40; A.M.C.G.P.; Tel. 766-6434.
HAMEL, Gerard; 880 est, Boul. Henri-Bourassa, Montreal, P.Q.; Mon'51; Pres. & Dir., Fed. des Omnipracticiens du Quebec; Tel. 382-2171.
HAMEL, Jacques; 3871 Belanger E., Montreal 36, P.Q.; 7037 Verdier (res); Mon '62; Tel. RA 9-5231.

HAMEL, Jean B.; St. Flavien, P.Q.; Lav '35.

HAMEL, John F.; 168 Charlotte St., Ste. 207, **Ottawa, Ont.; 727 Eastbourne Ave. (res); Mon '49; FACP; FCCP; FRCP(C); IntMed; Cardiol.,** St.Louis-Marie-de-Montford Hosp; Dir., Med. Serv. (Pt.-time), Rehab. Inst. of Ottawa; Cons., DVA; Lect. (PrevMed.), U. of Ottawa; Tel. 234-0040.
HAMEL, Maurice; 151 Scott, St. Jerome, P.Q.; Mon '44; Staff, Hotel-Dieu de St. Jerome.
HAMEL, Maxime; 980 rue Cherrier, Montreal, P.Q.; Mon '53.
HAMEL, P. Claude; 7630 rue Centrale, Ville-LaSalle, Lachine, P.Q.; Mon '51; Gen. Surg. (P.Q.).

HAMELIN, Albert; 1925 de la Ronde, Quebec 3. P.Q.; Lav '51; Anaes (P.Q.); Staff, Hop. Enfant-Jesus; Tel. 529-8711.
HAMELIN, Luc; 4667 Beaconsfield, Notre Dame de Grace, Montreal 28, P.Q. (res); Lav '52; D&TRad; Rad., Verdun Gen. Hosp.; Tel. 766-8511.
HAMELIN, Marc; 7820 Marquette, Montreal 35, P.Q.; 240 Provence, Auteuil, Co. Laval (res); Mon'52; IntMed (P.Q.); Tel. RA 9-6371.
HAMELIN, Paul; 2825 Blvd. du Carmel, Trois-Rivieres, P.Q.; Mon '55; Anaes; Staff, Hop. St.-Joseph; Tel. FR 4-6211.
HAMELIN, Paul-E.; 941 Cherrier, Montreal 24, P.Q.; Mon '43; DPH (Tor.); P.H. (PQ); Chief MOH (Lorimier Dist.), City of Mtl.; Tel. 872-3360.

HAMER, Henry E.; 113 McKenzie Ave., Revelstoke, B.C.; 420-9th St. (res); Tor '40; Dist. Coroner.

HAMERSKI, Henryk W.; 67 Pine St. S., Timmins, Ont.; 510 Patricia Blvd. (res); Polish Schl. of Med. (Edinburgh, Scot.) '47; MCGP; Lect. (Obst), Schl. of Nursing, St. Mary's Hosp.; Staff, St. Mary's & Porcupine Gen. Hosp's.; Tel. AM 4-3611.

HAMES, Clarence F. W.; 922-113th St. North Battleford, Sask.; Tor '24; DPH; PH; Chm., Sask. Cancer Comm.; Tel. 445-2285. Temporarily retired.
HAMES, W. Keith; Kenton, Man.; Tor '45; M.C.-G.P.

HAMILL, Alan S.; 1075 Pape Ave., Toronto, **Ont.; Tor '29; IntMed; Att. Med. Staff, Toronto East Gen. Hosp.; Tel. HO 5-1318.**
HAMILL, Frank C.; 18 Lawton, Blind River, Ont.; Tor '22; M.C.G.P.; M.O.H.; Tel. 356-7881.
HAMILTON, Frederick C.; 705 Med. Arts Bldg., 170 St. George St., Toronto 5, Ont.; 78 Inglewood Dr., Tor 7 (res); Tor '25; FACP; IntMed; Hon. Cons. Staff, Tor. Western Hosp.; Tel. WA 2-9900.
HAMILTON, Fraser B.; Medical Arts Bldg., Hamilton, Ont.; 3 Bull's Lane (res); Tor '27; F.R.C.S.(C), F.I.C.S., GenSurg; Staff, St. Joseph's & Hamilton Gen. Hosp's.; Tel. 383-4491.
HAMILTON, Gavin; Wes'55; Res. (DiagRad.), Victoria Gen. Hosp., London, Ont.; AMCGP.
HAMILTON, Glen F.; 185 Henderson Hwy., Winnipeg 5, Man.; 123 Green Ave. (res); Man '34; MCGP; Court. Staff, St. Boniface, Winnipeg Gen., **Children's & Concordia Hosp's.; Tel.** JU 9-7386.
HAMILTON, Harold G.; Shopping Centre, Smith's Falls, Ont.; Qns'59; GenSurg.; Tel. 283-5050.

HAMILTON, Harvey S.; Ste. 260, 403-6th St., New Westminster, B.C.; 12587-15A Ave., Ocean Park (res); Tor'38; Ophth; Staff, Royal Columbian Hosp.; Tel. LA 2-8227.

HAMILTON, Ian S.; McKinnon Industries, St. Catharines, Ont.; U.K.'55.

HAMILTON, James A.V.; Caledonia Med. Clinic, 340 Campbell St., Nanaimo, B.C.; 2510 Lynburn Cres. (res); Glas. (Scot.) '41; FRCS (Edin.); FRFPS (Glas.); AICS; GenSurg; Chief Surg., Nanaimo Reg. Gen. Hosp.; Tel. SK 3-3202.
HAMILTON, James D.; Ste 360, 5025 Sherbrooke St. W., Montreal 28, P.Q.; Wes'57; Tel. 488-6404.
HAMILTON, J. Douglas; Professional Bldg., 67 Talbot St., Essex, Ont.; Wes '56; GenSurg, Tel. PR 6-7366.

HAMILTON, John B.; Doaktown, N.B.; Qns'24.

HAMILTON, John D.; 73 Donwoods Dr., Toronto 12, Ont. **(res); Tor '35; FRCP(C), Path-Bact; Dean of Medicine, U. of Toronto; Tel. 928-2710.**
HAMILTON, John D.; 3260 Edgemont Blvd., North Vancouver, B.C.; UBC '54; Tel. YU 7-3931.
HAMILTON, John R.; 62 Farnham Ave., Toronto, Ont.; Tor '58; **FRCP(C),** Paed; Fell., Research, Hosp. for Sick Children; Clin Teach., U. of Toronto; Tel. EM 6-7242.
HAMILTON, Kenneth A.; 3 Tweedsmuir Cres., Edmonton, Alta. (res); Oxford (Eng.)'26; MRCP (Lond.); FACP; FRCP(C), IntMed; Psy; Staff, W.C.B. Rehab. Clinic; Spec. D.V.A.; Tel. 439-5911.
HAMILTON, Kenneth G.; McG'60; Jr. Int'n., Montreal Gen. Hosp., Montreal, P.Q.
HAMILTON, Norman E.; Alb'60; Chief Res. (OrthSurg.), Toronto Western Hosp., Toronto, Ont.
HAMILTON, Robert R.; Kelvington, Sask.; Trinity College (Dublin)'45; MCGP.
HAMILTON, Ronald W.; 240 McNabb St., Sault Ste. Marie, Ont.; Cambridge (Eng.)'59; FRCS(C), GenSurg.
HAMILTON, Rosemary (Haydock); 15312-73rd Ave., Jasper Pl., Edmonton, Alta. (res); Durham (Eng.)'51.
HAMILTON, Thomas R.; Box 2356, 11140-109th St., Edmonton, Alta.; 15312 Rio Terrace Dr., (res); Durham (Eng.)'51; MRCS, LRCP; Cons. Staff, Royal Alexandra Hosp.; Court. Staff, Edmonton Gen. Hosp.; Instr. (Prev. Med.), U. of Alberta; Reg. Phys., Imperial Oil Ltd.; Tel. 474-6421.
HAMILTON-SMITH, Barry; 1 Roxborough St. E., Toronto 5, Ont.; 502 Blythwood Rd., Tor. 12 (res); London (Eng.)'54; MCGP; O.P.D. Staff, St. Michael's Hosp.; Tel. WA 3-5514.
HAMLIN, George H.; 41 Royal Rd. N., Portage La Prairie, Man.; 67 2nd S.W. (res); Man'31; Staff, Portage Gen. Hosp.; Tel. 857-3471.
HAMLIN, J. Howard; 408, 267 O'Connor St., Ottawa 4, Ont.; 160 Leopold Dr., Ott. 10 (res); Qns'35; MCGP; Cons. Staff, Ottawa Civic Hosp.; Tel. 235-5700.

HAMM, John F.; Foord St., Stellarton, N.S.; Dal '63; AMCGP; Staff, Aberdeen Hosp.; Tel. 752-7823.
HAMMAN, Harold A.; McG'23; Med. Off., Baker Mem. San., Calgary, Alta.; Hon. Coroner.
HAMMERLING, Anne F. (Linder); 6777 Quinpool Rd., Halifax, N.S.; Dal'34; Tel. 423-3774.
HAMMERLING, James S.; 6777 Quinpool Rd., Halifax, N.S.; New York Med. Coll. (New York, U.S.A.) '33; FACS; FABOt; Hd., Dept. of Otol., Victoria Gen. Hosp.; Prof. &Hd. (Otol.), Dalhousie U.; Tel. 423-7884.
HAMMERLING, Judith D.; Dal'65; Intern., c/o 6777 Quinpool Rd., Halifax, N.S.
HAMMOND, Arnold A.; 1746 Jane St., Weston, Ont.; Manchester (Eng.)'50; Assoc. Med. Staff, Humber Mem. Hosp.; Tel. 244-5545.
HAMMOND, Keith C.; 206 Med. Bldg., 20-14th St. W., Prince Albert, Sask.; 600-20th St. W. (res); London (Eng.) '58; DRCOG; DA; Staff Holy Family & Victoria Union Hosp's.; Tel. 763-6401.
HAMONIC, Marcel; Lav '51; D.A.B.Path.; Assoc. Path. & Cyt., St. Boniface Hosp., St. Boniface, Man.; Lect., (Path.), U. of Manitoba; Tel. WH 3-0311.
HAMPSON, Kenneth W. W/C; Wes '50; MPH (Harvard); Reg. Surg.; Prairie Med. Reg., RCAF Station, Westawin, Sask.

HAMPSON, Lawrence G.; 540 Seaforth Med. Bldg., 3550 Cote des Neiges Rd., Montreal 25, P.Q.; McG'49; D.Surg.; DABS; FRCS(C); FACS; GenSurg; Ass't. Surg., Montreal Gen. Hosp.; Ass't. Prof., McGill U.; Tel. 937-1445.
HAMPSON, Lloyd M.; 42 Hereford Place, Ottawa 3, Ont.; Tor'40; DA; Anaes; Chief, Dept. of Anaes., Ottawa Civic Hosp.; Lect., U. of Ottawa; Tel. 729-0453.

HAMWEE, Cyril M.; Redvers, Sask.; Manchester (Eng.) '39; MRCS, LRCP.
HANAWAY, Joseph; McG '60; Research, Dept. of Anatomy, McGill U., Montreal 2, P.Q. Abroad.
HANCHARYK, George; 357 Ferguson St., North Bay, Ont.; Ott'62; Tel. 472-2300.

HANCOCK, Alan K.; Sam Campbell Med. Bldg., 10th Ave. & Alder, Campbell River, B.C.; Guys Hosp. (London, Eng.)'49; MRCS(Eng.); LRCP (Lond.); Staff, Phys., Campbell River & Dist. Gen. Hosp.; Tel. 287-7441.
HANCOCK, George R.; Drawer 608, 4826 Ross St., Red Deer, Alta.; 5555-45th Ave. (res); McG '39; FICS; Staff, Red Deer Mun. Hosp.; Tel. 346-2042.
HANCOCK, Ronald J.; 717 Fairmont Med. Bldg., 750 W. Broadway, Vancouver 9, B.C.; UBC '57; FRCS(C); GenSurg; Staff, O.P.D., Vancouver Gen. Hosp.; Tel. 874-3921.

HAND, Robert F.; Med. Arts Bldg., 5880 Spring Garden Rd., Halifax, N.S.; Glasgow (Scot.) '37; DTM&H(Lond.); DABOphth; OphthOtol; Ass't. Surg. (EENT), Halifax Infirmary & Children's Hosp's.; Vis. Surg., Camp Hill DVA Hosp.; Cons. Ophth., Cdn. Forces Hosp.; Tel. 423-7595.

HANDCOCK, Kenneth A.; 2111 Marlowe Ave., Montreal 28, P.Q. (res); Otago (N. Zealand) '56; M.B., Ch.B.; Psy; Staff, Queen Elizabeth Hosp.; Tel. HU 8-2311.
HANDFIELD, Georges Y.; Centre-Medical Ville-Marie, 3423 rue St.-Denis, Montreal 18, P.Q.; 36 Courcelette (res); Mon '40; Hd. Nutr. & Diab. & Clin., Prof. Anat. & Physiol., Schl. of Nursing. Hop. Notre-Dame-de-la-Merci; Vis Staff Hop. Notre-Dame de l'Esperance; Memb., Admin Council Hop. Notre-Dame de la Merci; Tel. 842-4892.
HANDFIELD, Roland H.; 3423 Saint Denis, Montreal, P.Q.; 5515 Place d'Aiguillon (res); Mon '44; GenSurg & Gyn (P.Q.); Ass't. Surg. & Gyn., Hop. St. Luc; Ass't. Prof. (Surg.), U. of Montreal; Prof. (Surg.), School of Nursing; Tel. VI 2-4892.
HANDFIELD, Therese; Ste. 56, 445 Boul St.-Joseph W., Montreal 8, P.Q.; Mon'64.

HANDFORD, Edward Y.; 225 Raglan St. S., Renfrew, Ont.; 580 Raglan St. S. (res); Qns '29; Tel. HE 2-3627.
HANDFORD, Herbert L.; 225 Raglan St., Renfrew, Ont.; 560 Raglan St. S. (res); Qns '40; Tel. HE 2-3627.
HANDFORD, Robert G.; 295 Cambridge St., Winnipeg 9, Man. (res); Man'55; IntMed; Ass't. Phys., Winnipeg Gen. Hosp.; Dir., Wpg. Gen. Hosp. Home Care Program; Dem. (Med.), U. of Manitoba; Tel. WH 2-5303.
HANDFORD, Sydney L.; 350-14th St. W., Owen Sound Ont.; 705-2nd Ave. W. (res); Qns '52; M.C.G.P.; Tel. FR 6-8510.
HANDFORTH, C. Peter; 2 Landsdoon Place, Truro, N.S. (res); London (Eng.) '50; M.C. Path; Path; Chief of Labs., Colchester County Hosp.; Tel. 893-9425.
HANDFORTH, James R.; Lancaster Hosp., St. John, N.B.; Cambridge (Eng.) '43; M.R.C.S., L.R.C.P., Psy., Chief Psy., Lancaster D.V.A. Hosp.; Tel. 4-2651.

HANDLEY, Grace I. J. (Richardson); 10 Cliffcrest Dr., Toronto, Ont. (res); Tor '30; Retired.
HANDLEY, Thomas R.; P.G. (Anaes.), Hamilton Gen. Hosp., Hamilton, Ont.
HANDY, Blake H.; 11 Coldwater St. E., Orillia, Ont.; 57 Penetang St. (res); Tor '41; Tel. 325-2271.
HANDYSIDES, Allan R.; Edinburgh (Scot.) '63; Res., Kingston Gen. Hosp., Kingston, Ont.
HANEY, Lorne; Mon'65; Sr. Int., Hopital Ste-Justine, Montreal, P.Q.

HANHAM, Wm. J.; Carleton Place, Ont.

HANIFORD, Ellis; Ste. 510, 1849 Yonge St., Toronto 7, Ont.; Glasgow(Scot.) '53; MCGP; Active Staff, Grace Hosp.; Tel. 489-6532.
HANKIN, Myers; Thorsby, Alta.; Man '29; AMCGP; Dist. Coroner; Tel. 16.
HANKINS, Gerald W.; Medical Dental Centre, 402 Rideau, Calgary, Alta.; Alb '51; FRCS(Eng.); FRCS(C); GenSurg; Staff, Calgary Gen. Alberta Childrens' & Holy Cross Hosp's.; Tel. 269-1609.
HANKINSON, Hazen W.; 701 Standard Bldg., 510 W. Hastings St., Vancouver 2, B.C.; 3591 Oak St., Van. 9 (res); Alb '50; MCGP; Vis. Staff, St. Paul's, St. Vincent's, Grace, Burnaby Gen. & Vancouver Gen. Hosp's.; Tel. MU 1-4412.
HANKO, Francis J.; 149 Ochterloney St., Dartmouth, N.S.; 6 Richards Dr. (ree); Ott '52; MCGP; Court. Staff, Victoria Gen., Hlfx. Children's, Grace Maternity & Hlfx. Infirm.; Tel. 466-1591.
HANKS, George; Baldur, Man.; London (Eng.) '49; L.R.C.P. (Lond.), M.R.C.S. (Eng.); Staff, Baldur District Hosp.
HANKS, Gerald A.; 377 Graham Ave., Winnipeg 1, Man.; 578 Oak St., Wpg. 9 (res); Bristol (Eng.) '49; DRCOG; FRCS (Edin.); GenSurg; Tel. WH 3-1313.
HANLEY, Edward J.; Ste 313, 10830 Jasper Ave., Edmonton, Alta.; National U. (Ire.) '45.
HANLEY, E. Guy S.; 434 Medical Arts Bldg., Toronto, Ont.; 288 Oriole Pkwy. (res); Tor '23; Anaes; Tel. WA 2-2356.
HANLEY, F. William; 750 West Broadway, Ste. 913, Vancouver 9, B.C.; Tor'43; Psy; Vis. Staff, Vancouver Gen. Hosp. & Cons. Staff, Burnaby Mental Health Centre; Tel. 876-1125.
HANLEY, James B.; 5 DuMaurier, Toronto, Ont. (res); Tor '15; Otol; Retired.
HANLEY, J. Lloyd; Ste. 6, 140 Wallace St., Nanaimo, B.C.; Ott'55; Active Staff & Dir. of Rehab., Nanaimo Reg. Gen. Hosp.; Hd. Dept. of Paed., Nanaimo Reg. Gen. Hosp.; Tel. 754-5545.
HANLEY, Phillis E.; 291 Avenue Rd., Toronto 2, Ont. (res); Tor '58; Tel. WA 1-1056.
HANLEY, Thomas R.; 178 St. George St., Toronto 5, Ont.; 21 Dunloe Rd. Tor. 7 (res); Tor '51; FRCP(C), Anaes; Anaes., Tor. Gen. Hosp.; Clin. Instr., U. of Toronto; Tel. WA 3-1154.
HANLEY, William B.; Ste. 207, 250 Lawrence Ave. W., Toronto 12, Ont.; Tor'54; Paed; Clin. Ass't., Hosp. for Sick Children; Cons. (Paed), N. York Branson & St. Michael's Hosp's.; Clin. Instr. (Paed.), U. of Toronto; Tel. RU 1-1805.
HANNA, Abdalla M.; O'Mara Martin Bldg., St. John's, Nfld.; Cairo (Egypt)'50; FRCS(C), GenSurg; Tel. 726-1182.
HANNA, Charles E.; 19 Parkview Blvd., Brockville, Ont.; Qns '14; Retired.
HANNA, Florence M. see ENGELBRECHT, (Hanna), Florence M.
HANNA, Herbert E.; Suite 103, 150 Metcalfe St., Ottawa, Ont.; 8 Lakeview Ter. (res); Qns '28; A.M.C.A.A.; Hon. Cons. Med. Staff Ottawa Civic Hosp.; Tel. 235-8826.
HANNA, Lloyd M.; Civic Health Centre, 2338 Dewdney Ave., Regina, Sask.; 2929-20th Ave. (res); Qns '19; D.P.H., P.H.; Ass't. M.O.H., City of Regina, Sask.; Dist. Coroner; Tel. 569-3853.
HANNA, Robert J.; 3310 Boundary, South Burnaby, B.C.; Ott '52.
HANNA, Robert J. E.; 90 Harbour St., Toronto 1, Ont.; 480 Oriole Pkwy., Tor 7 (res); McG '27; Memb. Med. Review Board, WCB (Ont.); Tel. 362-3411.
HANNAH, Beverley; 15 South Dr., Toronto, Ont. (res); Tor '09; M.R.C.S., L.R.C.P.; F.R.C.P.(C); Supt. Riverdale Isolation Hosp.; Cons. Infect. Dis., Hosp. for Sick Children; Lect. Comm. Dis., Schl. of Nursing, U. of Toronto; Retired.
HANNAH, Jason A.; 615 Yonge St., Toronto, Ont.; 9 Nesbitt Dr. (res); Qns '28; Path; Med. Dir., Associated Med. Services Inc.; Tel. WA 1-4193.
HANNAH, Walter J.; 202 St. Clair Ave. W., Toronto 7, Ont.; Wes'53; FRCS(C), ObstGyn; Chief, Dept. of ObstGyn., Women's College Hosp.; Ass't. Prof. (ObstGyn.), U. of Toronto; Tel. 921-3531.
HANNIWELL, David B.; 2150 Med. Arts. Bldg., Valley Way, Niagara Falls, Ont.; Qns '59; FRCS (C), ObstGyn; Tel. 354-2669.
HANNON, Gary T.; 7544-20 Ave. N.E., Seattle, Wash. 98115, U.S.A.; Alb'57; Path; Abroad.
HANRAHAN, Gorman E.; 1538 Sherbrooke St. W., Montreal, P.Q.; 1499 Painter Circle, St. Laurent (res); McG '51; D. Psy., Psy; Dir. O.P.D. (Psy.), Queen Mary Vet's Hosp.; Lect, (Psy.), McGill U.; Tel. RE 8-9481.
HANSEBOUT, Robert R.; Wes'60; Neur(P.Q.); Staff, NeurSurg., Montreal Neurological Inst., 3801 University Ave., Montreal 2, P.Q.
HANSEN, Alden R.; Woodlawn Med. Clinic, 110 Woodlawn Rd., Dartmouth, N.S.; Refinery Phys., Imperial Oil Ltd.; Refinery Phys., Texaco Ltd., Eastern Passage, N.S.; Ott'52; Tel. 469-1590.
HANSEN, Carl A.; McG '61; Res., Montreal Gen. Hosp., Montreal 25, P.Q.
HANSEN, Neils H., Capt.; Dal'65; Staff, Cdn. Forces Hosp., HMCS Stadacona, Halifax, N.S.
HANSEN, W. Bryce, Sg/Lt.; Box 563, Cdn. Forces Base, Greenwood, N.S.; Alb'64.
HANSLIK, Albin F.; 46-11th Ave., Roxboro, P.Q. (res); Graz (Austria) '49; Staff, Queen Mary Vet's. Hosp.; Tel. RE 8-9481.
HANSLIP, Arthur R.; 5116 Elbow Dr. S.W., Calgary, Alta.; UBC '59; Tel. 255-6647.
HANSON-DUNSE, Sidney; Moose Jaw Clinic, 200 Scott Bldg., Moose Jaw, Sask.; London (Eng.)'51; MRCS; LRCP; Tel. 692-2373.
HANSON, Samuel; 203 Professional Bldg., 10830 Jasper Ave., Edmonton, Alta.; 13628 Ravine Dr. (res); Alb '38; D.A.B.P.; PathBact; Dir. of Labs. Edmonton Gen. Hosp.; Assoc. Prof. U. of Alberta; Tel. 424-0061.
HANSTEIN, Gisela W.; Frankfurt (Germany) '52; Res., Reddy Mem. Hosp., Montreal, P.Q.
HANTHO, John A.; 2940-17th Ave. S.W., Calgary, Alta.; 176 Cherovan Dr. (res); Alb '55; MCGP; Tel. CH 9-5566.
HAQ, Badi-Uz-Zaman M.; Lahore (W. Pakistan) '59; AB Path; Staff, Pathol., Glace Bay & St. Joseph's Hosp's., Glace Bay, N.S.
HAQUE, Abulkalam W.; 4630 Mariette Ave., Montreal 28, P.Q.; Dacca (Pakistan)'58; DiagRad.
HARA, Victor; Apt. 28, 4790 Bouchette, Montreal 26, P.Q.; Beyrouth (Lebanon) '30; Tel. RE 3-7768.
HARAMIA, Joseph; Hudson Hope, B.C.; Prague (Czechoslovakia) '22.
HARASZTHY, Dennis J.; 305, 344 Bloor W., Toronto 5, Ont.; 2810 Bayview Ave., Willowdale (res); Budapest (Hung.) '48; ObstGyn; Court. Staff, Grace Hosp.; Tel. WA 2-1232.
HARBECK, Michel; 5260 rue Cadillac, Montreal 5, P.Q.; Mon '57; Tel. 256-5136.
HARBERT, Richard G.; 205 Medical Arts Bldg., 1538 Sherbrooke St. W., Montreal 25, P.Q.; 671 Grosvenor Ave., Westmount (res); McG '39; Assoc. Phys., Montreal Gen. Hosp.; Cons. Phys., Dupont Ltd.; Lectr. (Med.), McGill U.; Tel. WE 3-3196.
HARBINSON, Desmond J.; 2522 Keele St., Toronto 15, Ont.; 4 Calais Ave., Downsview (res); Belfast (Ire.)'48; MCGP; Sr. Active Staff, Northwestern Gen. & North York Branson Hosp's.; Court. Staff, Humber Mem. Hosp.; Tel. CH 4-3721.
HARBOTTLE, B. Gail; Man'65; Res., Montreal Gen. Hosp., Montreal 25, P.Q.
HARCOURT, John A.; Apt. 1212, 44 Jackes Ave., Toronto 7, Ont.; Tor'22; Retired.
HARDEN, Alec; Omincea Clinic, Vanderhoof, B.C.; Dublin (Ire.)'63; Abroad.
HARDER, David H.; Ste. 2, 321 E. Columbia St., New Westminster, B.C.; UBC'59; MCGP; Tel. 524-3621.
HARDER, Fred A.; 321 E. Columbia St., New Westminster, B.C.; 919 Laurel St. (res); UBC '54; MCGP; Tel. 524-3621.
HARDIE, Colin D.; 393 University Ave., Toronto, Ont.; Glasgow (Scot.) '58; DPH; M.O., Toronto Area, Bell Telephone Co. of Canada; Tel. 929-2811.

HARDIE, M. Jean; 3227 W. 35th Ave., Vancouver, B.C.; Wes '51; D.P.H.; Phys. Metropolitan Health Comm., City Hall.
HARDIE, Margaret B.; 3227 W. 35th Ave., Vancouver, B.C.; Tor '24; TherRad; Retired.
HARDIN, Earl D.; 705 Fairmont Med. Bldg., 750 W. Broadway, Vancouver 9, B.C.; Alb'58; Psy; Staff, Vancouver Gen. Hosp.; Tel. 876-1133.
HARDIN, Isidore; 453 Professional Bldg., 10830 Jasper Ave., Edmonton, Alta.; 10616-134th St. (res); Alb '43; D.A.B.D.S.; DermSyph; Att'd. **Staff, Gen. Royal Alexandria & Misericordia Hosp's.; Tel. 422-1822.**
HARDIN, Thomas; Alb'51; MCGP; Jr. Ass't. (res.), Phys Med., University of Alberta Hosp., Edmonton, Alta.
HARDING, A. W.; 18 Simcoe St. N., Oshawa, Ont.; 733 Simcoe St. N. (res); Wes '21; Ophth, Otol; Staff, Oshawa Gen. Hosp.; Tel. 723-2211.
HARDING, Harry G.; Carnduff, Sask.; Liverpool (Eng.) '54; D.ObstRCOG; Staff, Gainsborough Union Hosp.; Tel. 482-3404.
HARDING, Paul G.; 1686 Louise Blvd., London, Ont.; Wes'58; FRCS(C), ObstGyn.; Active Teach. Staff, Victoria Hosp.; Ass't. Prof. Depts. of Physiol. & ObstGyn., U. of Western Ontario; Tel. 432-5261, Loc. 225.
HARDING, Walter G.; 456 Wellington St. N., Preston, Ont.; Wes '44; Active Staff, S. Waterloo Mem. Hosp., Galt; Tel. 653-6801.
HARDMAN, Arthur C.; Food & Drug Directorate, Dept. of National Health & Welfare, Tunney's Pasture, Ottawa 3, Ont.; Tor'49; DPH; Dir., Bureau of Scientific Advisory Serv.; Tel. 992-5746.
HARDMAN, Anna B.; R.R. No. 3, London, Ont.; Tor '31.
HARDMAN, Jack G.; 131 Ontario St., St. Catharines, Ont.; McG '43; Paed.; Tel. 684-6581.
HARDMAN, R. D.; Dir., Div. of Epidem., Ont. Dept. of Health, Toronto, Ont.; Tel. EM 3-1211.
HARDWICK, David F.; 741 W. 26th Ave., Vancouver 9, B.C. (res); UBC'57; Path; Ass't. Pathol. (Paed.), Vancouver Gen. Hosp.; Ass't. Prof. (Path.), U. of British Columbia; Tel. 228-2682.
HARDY, Albert W.; 203 Med. Arts Bldg., 11010 Jasper Ave., Edmonton, Alta.; 11013-50th St. (res); Alb '36; FACS; FRCS(C); GenSurg; Ass't. Clin. Prof. (Surg.), U. of Alberta; Tel. 424-7433.
HARDY, Alburne N.; 613 McCallum-Hill Bldg., Regina, Sask.; McG '06; F.A.C.S., OphthOtol; Retired.
HARDY, Bruce C.; Lawrence Ave. Med. Centre, 3000 Lawrence Ave. E., Scarborough, Ont.; 77 Balsam Ave., Tor. (res); Tor '35; F.R.C.S.(Eng.), F.R.S.C.(C), GenSurg; Cons. D.V.A., Sunnybrook Hosp.; Tel. 293-8247.
HARDY, E. A.; Fort San, Sask.
HARDY, Ethelbert B.; 1602 The Croydon Towers, 19 Lascelles Blvd., Toronto 7, Ont. (res); Tor '05; Tel. HU 5-8259.
HARDY, Florence S.; (See McConney)
HARDY, George; 230 Wavell Ave., Winnipeg 13, Man.; Man'52.
HARDY, George E.; 223 Med. Arts Bldg., 335-339 6th Ave. S.W., Calgary, Alta.; Alb '53; Memb., Med. Advisory Bd., Calgary Gen. Hosp.; Tel. 266-2331.
HARDY, Jules; 1386 Sherbrooke St. E., Montreal 24, P.Q.; Mon'56; FACS; FRCS(C), NeurSurg; NeurSurg., Notre-Dame Hosp.; Ass't. Prof. (NeurSurg.), U. of Montreal; Tel. 526-0419.
HARDY, Larry W.; 208 Clarence Ave. S., Saskatoon, Sask. (res); Tor'54; FRCP(C), Paed; Staff, University Hosp.; Ass't. Prof. (Paed.), U. of Saskatchewan; Tel. 242-7641, Loc. 491.
HARDY, Quentin A.; Box 370, 20 Doctors Lane, King City, Ont.; Tor'53; MCGP; Staff, York County Hosp., Newmarket; Staff, York Central Hosp., Richmond Hill; Tel. TE 3-5331.
HARDY, Richard D.; 497 Victoria St., Sherbrooke, P.Q.; McG '01; D&TRad.
HARDYMENT, Archibald F.; 704 Fairmont Med. Bldg., 750 W. Broadway, Vancouver 9, B.C.; 6388 Marguerite St. (res); Man '36; F.A.A.P.; Paed; Phys.-in-Charge of Nurseries & Sr. Health Centre for Children, Vancouver Gen. Hosp.; Clin. Ass't. Prof. (Paed), U. of British Columbia; Tel. TR 9-5191.
HARE, Arthur; Carmel Med. Clinic, 124-1st Ave. N.W., Swift Current, Sask.; Glasgow, (Scotland) '57; Tel. 773-8333.
HARE, Robert B.; 125 Norfolk St. S., Simcoe, Ont.; Tor '22; FRCS(Edin), FACS, FRCS(C), GenSurg; MCGP; Chief of Surg., Norfolk Gen. Hosp.; Tel. 426-2653.
HAREL, Claude; Mon'58; DiagRad(P.Q.); Staff, Hop. Notre-Dame, Montreal, P.Q.
HAREL, Clement; 400 Fountainbleau, Duvernay, Laval-des-Rapides, P.Q.; Mon '58; Anaes(P.Q.); Staff, Hop. du Sacre-Coeur; Tel. 669-0831.
HAREL, Pierre; Mon '54; Haem(P.Q.); Staff, Hop. Sacre-Coeur, Montreal 9, P.Q.; Tel. 334-1210.
HARGAN, W. Alan; 146 Winnipeg Ave., Port Arthur, Ont. (res); Wes '41; D.R., D&TRad; Dir., Dept.s of Radiol., Port Arthur Gen. & St. Joseph's Gen. Hosp's.; Dir. of Radiotherapy, Thunder Bay Clin., Ontario Cancer & Research Fdn., Gen. Hosp.; Tel. DI 4-6621.
HARGARTEN, Benedict W.; 103 Medical Bldg., 217 3rd Ave. N., Saskatoon, Sask.; 307-31st W. (res); Alb '31; M.C.G.P.; Staff, St. Paul's, Hosp.; Vis. Phys., Saskatoon City and University Hosp's.; Clin. Teach. (ObstGyn), U. of Saskatchewan; Dist. Coroner; Tel. 244-6888.
HARGRAVE, Ralph; 3000 Lawrence Ave. E., Scarborough, Ont.; R.R. 2, Markham (res); Tor '17; Anaes; Tel. AX 3-8681.
HARITON Nicolas; Ste. 309, 1538 Sherbrooke St. W., Montreal 25, P.Q.; Montpellier (France) '36.
HARKER, James R.; 253 Queensway W., Simcoe, Ont.; Qns '46; Tel. 426-2815.
HARKER, Lawrence; Alb '60; Res., Montreal Gen. Hosp., Montreal 25, P.Q.
HARKINS, Edward B.; 219 Glenayr Rd., Toronto 10, Ont. (res); Tor'23; FAAP; FCPS; Paed.; Active Cons., Hosp. for Sick Children, St. Joseph's & Queensway Gen. Hosp's.; Med. Dir., Catholic Children's Aid Soc.; Tel. 532-9326.
HARKINS, John L.; 537 Med. Arts. Bldg., 170 St. George St., Toronto 5, Ont.; 18 Montclair Ave., Tor. 7 (res); Tor'50; FRCS(C); ObstGyn; Staff Toronto Gen. Hosp. Assoc. Staff, (Dept. **ObstGyn.), U. of Toronto; Tel. WA 3-2171.**
HARKNESS, James J.; Ste. 36, 800 Lakeshore Rd., Dorval, P.Q.; McG'36; GenSurg; Surg., Lachine Gen. & St. Joseph's Hosp's.; M.O.H., Dominion Bridge Co. & Dominion Engineering Works Ltd.; Tel. 637-2361.
HARLAND, John H.; Underhill Clinic, 1635 Abbott St., Kelowna, B.C.; 444 Morrison Ave. (res); Queen's U. (Belfast, N. Ire.) '49; M.B., B.Ch.; FACA; Anaes; Staff, Kelowna Gen. Hosp., Tel. 762-2740.
HARLEY, Brian J. S.; Med. Centre, West St., Corner Brook, Nfld.; London (Eng.) '47; M.D. (Lond.); MRCP; IntMed; Chief of Med., Western Mem. Hosp.; Cons. Phys., Cottage Hosp. Serv., Western Nfld.; Tel. 4-7474.
HARLEY, Charles H.; Alb'65; Res., University Hosp., Edmonton, Alta.
HARLEY, Harry C. M.P.; 129 Sparling Court, Oakville, Ont.; Tor '51; MCGP; Memb., House of Commons; Chmn., Spec. Committee on Food & Drugs & Health & Welfare; Tel. VI 5-3828.
HARLOS, Roland E.; 4900 Kingsway, South Burnaby, B.C.; 4356 Portland St. (res); UBC '55; Tel. HE 1-6696.
HARLOW, Charles M. CD; 5724 Harbour View Dr., Halifax, N.S. (res); McG '41; Ph.D. (Endocrin.); D.Sc. (Acadia); Dir. of Labs., Camp Hill DVA Hosp.; Cons. Path., RCN; Ass't. Prof., Dept. of Path., Dalhousie U.; Serving Brother, St. John's Ambulance; Tel. 423-1371.
HARMON, Thomas P.; 650 Fairmile Rd., West Vancouver, B.C.; UBC'63.
HARMON, Thomas R.; 650 Fairmile Rd., West Vancouver, B.C.; Dal'37; PathBact; Staff, Lions Gate Hosp., North Vancouver; Clin. Inst., U. of **B.C.; Tel. YU 8-3131.**

HARNICK, Louis R.; 106 Toronto Western Med. Bldg., 25 Leonard Ave., Toronto 2B, Ont.; 71 Shallmar Blvd. (res); Tor '43; FACR; D & T Rad; Chief Rad., Toronto Western Hosp.; Rad., Queensway Gen. Hosp.; Ass't. Prof. (Rad), U. of Toronto; Tel. EM 3-1197.

HARNOIS, Gaston P.; 20, rue Pharand, Hull, P.Q.; Ott'59; Psy.; Med. Supt., Hop. Pierre Janet; Tel. 771-7761.

HARNOIS, Marcel; 584 Manseau, Joliette, P.Q.; Mon '57.

HAROLD, Robert L.; Port Arthur Clinic, 194 North Court St., Port Arthur, Ont.; 187 Winnipeg Ave. (res); Tor '23; Obst; Staff, Obst., Pt. Arthur & St. Joseph's Gen. Hosp's.; Tel. DI 4-7271.

HAROLD, Thomas C.; 4676 W. 13th Ave., Vancouver 8, B.C. (res); Dal '34; Staff, W.C.B. 657 W. - 37th Ave.; Retired.

HARPER, Bertram H.; Box 9, Portland, Ont.; Qns'22; Tel. Elgin 26 Ring 24.

HARPER, Douglas W.; 2451A Bloor St. W., Toronto, Ont.; 14 Appledale Rd., Islington (res); Wes '52; Ophth; Active Cons., Oakville-Trafalgar & Sunnybrook Hosp's.; Vol. Ass't. (Ophth. Clinic), Toronto Gen. Hosp.; Court. Staff, Queensway Gen. Hosp.; Tel. RO 6-9522.

HARPER, Harold E.; Provost Med. Centre, Provost, Alta.; Durham (Eng.)'52; MCGP; Tel. 753-2271.

HARPER, Ian; 268 Newton Dr., Willowdale, Ont. **(res); Glasgow (Scot.) '46; Anaes; Staff, Branson Gen. Hosp., Willowdale; Tel. 639-9420.**

HARPER, John A.; 200 St. Clair Ave. W., Toronto 7, Ont.; Tor '48; FRCS(C), ObstGyn; Staff (ObstGyn), St. Michael's Hosp.; Clin. Instr. (ObstGyn), U. of Toronto; Tel. WA 2-4464.

HARPER, John F.; 1093 Fennell Ave. E., Hamilton, Ont.; 23 Edgewood (res); Wes '46; Staff, Hamilton Gen. & St. Joseph's Hosp's.; Phys., Otis Elevator Co.; Tel. 389-2228.

HARPER, Patricia J.; Provost, Alta.; Durham (Eng.)'52; Temporarily Retired.

HARPER, Reginald R.; 10730 King George **Hwy., N. Surrey, B.C.; 13665-107A St. (res); Man '44; Tel. 581-3348.**

HARPIN, Denis; 2225, boul Lapiniere, Ville-Brossard, Cite Jacques-Cartier, P.Q.; Lav '64.

HARPUR, Eleanor R. (Mackenzie); See MACKENZIE-HARPUR, Eleanor R.

HARPUR, G. D., F/L; MIR, RCAF Station, Downsview, Ont.; Tor '64.

HARRIES, Charles G.; Provost St., New Glasgow, N.S.; 312 Forbes St. (res); Dal '36; M.C.G.P.; Med. Staff, Aberdeen Hosp. & Exec., N.S. Med. Soc.; Dist. Coroner; Tel. 752-8311.

HARRIES, John D.; McG'64; Res., St. Mary's Hosp., Montreal 26, P.Q.

HARRIES, Thomas O.; U.K. '49; Staff, Calgary Gen. Hosp., Calgary, Alta.

HARRIGAN, Edward R.; 263 Toke St., Timmins, Ont. (res); Dal '43; D.R., D&TRad; Rad., St. Mary's Hosp., Timmins, Porcupine Gen. Hosp., South Porcupine; Tel. AM 4-1211; Ext. 237.

HARRIGAN, J. A.; Tor'63; Res., New Mount Sinai Hosp., Toronto 2, Ont.

HARRIGAN, James F.; 2 Hill St., Edmundston, N.B.; Dal '54; Chief of Med., Hotel Dieu Hosp.; Tel. RE 5-3361.

HARRIGAN, John R.; C. S. Williams Clin., 901 Helena St., Trail, B.C.; Man '48; A.M.C.A.A., Cons. (Derm.), & Vice-Chief, Med. Staff, Trail-Tadanac Hosp.; Memb., Bd. of Dirs., B.C. Div., C.M.A.; Tel. 368-5211.

HARRIMAN, Paul M.; Dal '62; Res., Royal Victoria Hosp., Montreal 2, P.Q.

HARRINGTON, Ian J.; Wes'65; Res., Dept. of Path., Victoria Hosp., London, Ont.

HARRINGTON, Robert W.; Ste. 501, 625-5th Ave., New Westminster, B.C.; Alb'51; Psy; Chief, Dept. of Psy., Royal Columbian Hosp.; Clin. Instr. (Psy), U. of British Columbia; Tel. 526-6422.

HARRIS, Arthur L.; 106 Med. Bldg., 217-3rd Ave. N., Saskatoon, Sask; 302 Lake Cr. (res); Alb '53; MCGP; Staff (G.P.), University & Saskatoon City Hosp's.; Clin. Instr. (ObstGyn.), U. of Saskatchewan; Tel. 653-2828.

HARRIS, Brian P.; Cambridge (Eng.) '32; DTM **& H; DRCOG; DPH; AMCGP; M.O., Elgin St.-** Thomas Health Unit, Court House, St. Thomas, Ont.

HARRIS, Brian R.; 4282 Dorchester Blvd. W., Apt. 703, Montreal, P.Q. (res); Otago (N. Zealand) '56; D.Psy; Psy; Staff, Royal Victoria & Mtl. Children's Hosp's.; Cons. Psy., Hartene Schls. Inc.; Tel. VI 2-1251.

HARRIS, Cecil E.; 3830 Lacombe Ave., Montreal, P.Q.; Glasgow (Scot.) '43; M.D.(Glas.), M.R.C.P. (Edin.) FRCP(Ed.); Haem(P.Q.); Haem. & Clin. Ass't. Phys, St. Mary's Hosp; Cons (Haem), Queen Elizabeth Hosp.; Tel. 735-3511.

HARRIS, Charles W.; 223 Forest Hill Rd., Toronto, Ont.; Tor '21; FRCS(Eng.); FRCS(C), GenSurg; Dir., Geriatric Study Centre; P.G. Lect. (Surg.), U. of Toronto; Tel. 531-5771.

HARRIS, Chester; Marystown, Nfld.; Edinburgh (Scot.) '16; M.H.O. Retired.

HARRIS, C. Strachan; Kirkland Lake Med. Group, Box 847, Kirkland Lake, Ont.; Tor '23; MCGP.

HARRIS, Dennis; Ste. 606, 625-5th Ave., New Westminster, B.C.; 755 Rochester Rd. (res); Guys Hosp. (London, Eng.)'53; MB, BS; Ophth; Chief Ophth., St. Mary's Hosp. & Royal Columbian Hosp.; Cons. Ophth., Surrey Mem. & Mapleridge Hosp's.; Tel. 522-2323.

HARRIS, Donald P.; 2300 Tupper St., Montreal, P.Q.; McG'57; Psy; Sr. Ass't. Res., Child Psy., Mtl. Children's Hosp.; Dem. (Psy.), McGill U.; Tel. WE 7-8511.

HARRIS, Edgar R.; Ste. 205, Med. Arts Bldg., 180 Metcalfe St., Ottawa, Ont.; Edinburgh (Scot.) '49; DiagRad; Cons. Rad., National Defence Med. Centre; Ass't. Rad., Grace Hosp.; Tel. 232-4256.

HARRIS, Edwin C.; 204 Bathurst St., Amherstburg, Ont.; Tor '09; Dist. Coroner.

HARRIS, Edward R.; 91 Duncan Ave., Kirkland Lake, Ont.; 126 First St. (res); Tor '30; PH; Dir. & Med. Off. of Health, Timiskaming Health Unit.

HARRIS, Ferguson F. C., D.S.O., MC; 92 Asquith Ave., Toronto 5, Ont.; Qns '01; M.R.C.S.(Eng.), L.R.C.P.(Lond.) F.R.I.P.H.(Eng.) D.N.B.(USA); Semi-retired

HARRIS, Fred; 458 Ossington Ave, Toronto 4, Ont.; 111 Frontenac Ave. (res); Tor '52; MCGP; P.G., St. Joseph's Hosp.; Tel. LE 2-7044.

HARRIS, George E.; Med. Arts Bldg., 420 East St. N., Sarnia, Ont.; 1282 Hillcrest Dr. (res); Wes '43; FACS, FRCS(C), GenSurg; Tel. DI 4-8362.

HARRIS, George W.; 235 Queen St. S., Hamilton, Ont.; 195 Charlton Ave. W. (res); Tor '22; Court. Staff, Hamilton Gen. & Civic Hosp's., St. Joseph's & Chedoke Gen. & Children's Hosp's.; Tel. JA 7-0960.

HARRIS, Gordon S.; 507 Fairmont Med. Bldg., 750 W. Broadway, Vancouver 9, B.C.; 6037 **Chancellor Blvd. (res); Tor'52; FRCS(C); Ophth; Staff, Vancouver Gen. & Shaughnessy Hosp's.;** Clin. Instr. (Ophth.), U. of British Columbia; Tel. 874-5321.

HARRIS, Gordon S.; Box 153, Annapolis Royal, N.S.; Qns '22; Retired.

HARRIS, Jean G.; 915 Ave. Suzanne, St.-Vincent-de-Paul, Laval-des-Rapides, P.Q.; 5682 Blvd. Levesque (res); Mon'59; AMCGP.

HARRIS, Jules E.; 11 Markdale Ave., Toronto 10, Ont.; Tor'59; FRCP(C), IntMed; Staff, Princess Margaret Hosp.; Abroad.

HARRIS, Kenneth S.; Rideau Med. Bldg., 1711-4th St. S.W., Calgary, Alta.; Man'57; FRCP(C), DiagRad; Staff, Calgary Gen. Hosp.

HARRIS, L. Duncan; 2159A Weston Rd., Weston, Ont.; Victoria U. (Manchester, Eng.) '52; Tel. 244-4845.

HARRIS, Louis J.; 99 Avenue Rd., Toronto 5, Ont.; 16 Rosedale Hgts. (res); Tor '29; FACOG; DABOG; FRCS(C); ObstGyn; Chief (ObstGyn & Gyn), New Mt. Sinai Hosp.; Tel. 924-2553.

HARRIS, Marguerite R.; Apt. 3, 3650 Lorne Cres., Montreal, P.Q.; McG '56; Psy.; Tel. 935-5211.

HARRIS, M. Joyce; Cambria Med. Bldg., 386 Cambria St., Stratford, Ont.; Dal'61; Anaes.
HARRIS, Mortimer E.; 1538 Sherbrooke St. W., Montreal, PQ.; 547 Lazard (res); Qns '43; MCGP; Tel. WE 5-5211.
HARRIS, Paul W.; Ste. 203, 1640-16th Ave. N.W., Calgary, Alta.; UBC '55; MCGP; Memb., Hosp. Executive & Dir. Emergency, Calgary Gen. Hosp.
HARRIS, Russel S.; Box 730, Virden Clinic, Virden, Man.; Tor '40; M.C.G.P.; Dist. Coroner; Tel. 461.
HARRIS, Stanley R.; London (Eng.) '55; FGSA; Res. (TherRad), Ont. Cancer Fdn., Ottawa Civic Hosp., Ottawa, Canada.
HARRIS, Walter C.; 21 Warbonnet Dr., Ottawa 5, Ont.; London (Eng.)'53.
HARRIS, Wilbur H.; Professional Bldg., 123 Edward St., Toronto 2, Ont.; Tor '58; FRCS(C), ObstGyn; Staff, Toronto East Gen. Hosp., Toronto 6, Ont.; Tel. 461-8272.
HARRIS, W. Robert; Medical Arts Bldg., 170 St. George St., Toronto 5, Ont.; 6 Clarendon Ave. (res); Tor'45; FRCS(C), OrthSurg; Assoc. (Surg), Toronto Gen. Hosp.; Chief (OrthSurg), Sunnybrook Hosp.; Tel. 923-8318.

HARRISON, A. Geoffrey; 57 King St., Port Hope, Ont.; London (Eng.)'53; MRCS(Eng.); LRCP (Lond.); Tel. 885-6112.
HARRISON, Alan W.; 54 Ravenscroft Circle, Willowdale, Ont. (res); Tor '49; FRCS(C), GenSurg; Chief (GenSurg), Sunnybrook Hosp.; Assoc. (Surg.), U. of Toronto; Tel. 485-8651, Loc. 303.
HARRISON, Anis; 72 Shippigan Cr., Willowdale, Ont. (res); London (Eng.) '40; Staff Phys., Bell Telephone Co. of Canada; Tel. 255-1502.
HARRISON, Colin P.; 5740 Cambie St., Vancouver 15, B.C.; Sydney (Aust.)'41; MCRA; DABR; DiagRad.; Tel. 325-3244.
HARRISON, Donald C .; 174 St. George St., Toronto 5, Ont.; 28 Wychwood Pk., Tor. 4 (res); Tor'50; IntMed; Staff, O.P.D., Tor. Gen. Hosp.; Staff Phys., Bell Telephone Co. & Atomic Energy of Canada Ltd.; Tel. 921-8581.
HARRISON, Elizabeth E.; 901 O'Connor Dr., Toronto 16, Ont.; 43 Rose Pk. Dr., Tor 7 (res); Tor '43; Staff, Women's College Hosp.; Tel. PL 5-6882.
HARRISON, Elizabeth Q. (Mrs. Alexander); 366 Central Ave., London, Ont.; Wes '52; Ophth; Staff, St. Joseph's, St. Mary's and Court. Staff, Victoria Hosp's.; Tel. GE 4-3934.
HARRISON, Glen S.; 3379 Kingsway, Van**couver 16, B.C.; 4650 Irmin St., South Burnaby (res); Man '51; M.C.G.P.; Staff, Burnaby Gen. Hosp.; Tel. HE 1-3388.**
HARRISON, Harold M.; 16 Thorncrest Rd., Islington, Ont. (res); Qns '12; A. B. Prev.Med.; Ass't., Toronto Western Hosp. Retired.
HARRISON, Jack E.; Ste. 906, 750 W. Broadway, Vancouver 9, B.C.; **705 Fairmile Rd., West Vancouver (res); McG '23; ObstGyn; Sr. Cons. (Gyn.), Vancouver Gen. Hosp.; Tel. RE 3-1193.**
HARRISON, Jas. F.; RCN Hosp., HMCS Naden, Esquimalt, B.C.; Qns'53.
HARRISON, Joan E. (Fletcher); 28 Wychwood Pk., Toronto 4, Ont. (res); Tor '51; Research Assoc. (Med.), U. of Toronto; Tel. 928-2940.
HARRISON, John P.; 222 Broad St. E., Dunnville, Ont.; Tor '08; Ophth.
HARRISON, R. Cameron; Alb'43; MS; DABS; FACS; FRCS(C), GenSurg; Staff, Dept. of Surg., Vancouver Gen. Hosp., Vancouver 9, B.C.; Prof. & Hd., Dept. of Surg., University of British Columbia; Tel. 876-3211.
HARRISON, R. Michael; 2 Young St., Hamilton, Ont.; Tor '49; FRCS(C), OrthSurg; GenSurg; Active Staff, St. Joseph's Hosp.; Cons., Crippled Children's Cerebral Palsy Clinic; Tel. JA 8-8601.
HARRISON, Samuel R.; 829 Blundell Rd., Richmond, Vancouver 14, B.C.; London (Eng.) '08. Retired.
HARRISON, W. Elliot; Ste. 808, 750 W. Broadway, Vancouver 9, B.C.; Man '27; F.A.C.S., F.C.C.P., Founder Memb., A.B.T.S.; GenSurg. ThorSurg; Chief Surg., B.C. Div. of T.B. Control; Hon. Att'd. Staff, Van. Gen. Hosp. & B.C. Cancer Inst.; Emer. Prof. (Surg.), U. of British Columbia; Tel. TR 2-5035.

HARROLD, Alan J.; Windsor Med. Clinic, 4505 Sources Rd., Roxborough, P.Q.; 128 Sheraton Dr., Montreal West (res); McG'61; AMCGP; Staff, Queen Elizabeth Hosp.; Tel. 684-7440.

HARROP, Albert H.; 195 Cordova St., Winnipeg, Man. (res); Man '53; Ass't. Med. Dir., Great West Life Assurance Co.; Tel. HU 9-1508.
HARROP, James; Apt. 306 1147 Ramsay View Crt., Sudbury, Ont.; London (Eng.) '52; Path (P.Q.); Staff, Memorial Hosp. Sudbury; Tel. 673-8421.

HARRY, Benjamin H. O.; 718 Granville St., Vancouver, B.C.; 1949 Beach Ave. (res); Man '15; Vis. Staff, (Ophth), St. Paul's & Vancouver Gen. Hosp's; Tel. MU 1-2850.
HARRY, John E.; Box 70, Luseland, Sask.; Man '55; Dist. Coroner; Tel. 202.
HARSHMAN, Jordan P.; 2401 Bloor St. W., Toronto 9, Ont.; 24 Strath Ave. (res); Tor '43; Ophth; Ophth, Staff, St. Joseph's, Queensway Gen. & S. Peel Hosp's.; Tel. RO 2-4640.
HARSANYI, I.; Oakville, Man.; Edinburgh, (Scot.) '61.

HART, Alan G.; 401 Med. Arts Bldg., 1 Young St., Hamilton, Ont.; Qns '58; FRCP(C); Paed; Tel. 529-6163.
HART, Gerald D; 821 Coxwell Avenue, Toronto 13, Ont.; 5 Hatherton Cr., Don Mills (res); Tor '52; FACP; FRCP(C) IntMed; Cons. Princess Margaret Hosp.; Att'd. Phys. & Dir., Dept. of Haem., Toronto East Gen. Hosp.; Clin. Ass't. (Med.), U. of Toronto; Tel. HO 6-2941.
HART, Howard D.; 325-21st St. E., Saskatoon, Sask.; 125 Sask Cres. W. (res); Man '35; Tel. 242-1208.
HART, Hugh; Gadshill Station, R.R.1., Ont. (res); Tor '13; Retired.
HART, Ian R.; Glasgow (Scot.)'60; Research Fell. (Endocrin.), Royal Victoria Hosp., Montreal 2, P.Q.
HART, Joseph; 322 Silverthorn Ave., Toronto, Ont.; 89 Dunloe Rd. (res); Tor '38; M.C.G.P.; Staff, N.W. Gen. & New Mount Sinai Hosp's.; Pt. Time, Canada Packers; Tel. RO 2-7795.
HART, Peter F.; 200 St. Clair Ave. W., Toronto 7, Ont.; Qns'60; Tel. 445-0428.
HART, Reginald G.; Ste. 360, 5780 Cambie St., Vancouver 15, B.C.; McG '40; Tel. FA 5-4611.
HART, R. Allan; Apt. 2, 63 Mallory Cres., Toronto 17, Ont.; Tor'61; IntMed.
HART, Robert.; Radville, Sask.; Durham (Eng.) '57; DRCOG; Abroad.
HART, Susan E.; Community Clinic, 110 - 8th. St. E., Prince Albert, Sask.; Durham (Eng.) '54; FRCS (Edin.); D.Obst. (Eng.); FRCS(C), GenSurg.; Tel. 763-6466.
HART, S. W. D.; 332 Main St., Picton, Ont.; **11 Hill (res); Qns '40; Gaol Surg.; Tel. GR 6-6590.**
HART, Vincent; 58 Bridge St. E., Napanee, Ont. (res); Qns '38; Retired.
HART, W. James; 189 Henderson H'wy., Winnipeg, Man., 19 Oakview Ave., East Kildonan (res); Man '40; M.C.G.P.; Tel. LE 3-5488.

HARTERRE, Donald J.; Medical Centre, 707 Charlotte St., Peterborough, Ont.; UBC'64.
HARTFORD, James J.; 97 Frederick St., Kitchener, Ont.; 305 Lourdes Cres. (res); Tor '45; Psy; Cons., Kitchener-Waterloo Hosp.; Cons., E.C.C.M.H. Serv., Buffalo, N.Y.; Tel. 745-6641.

HARTH, Manfred; 1231 Richmond St., London, Ont.; Tor'60; FRCP(C), IntMed.

HARTLEY, Bruce M.; 11 Doris Dr., Toronto 16, Ont.; Tor'62.
HARTLEY, Edward L.; 10730 King George Hwy., North Surrey, B.C.; Dal'62; AMCGP; Tel. 581-3348.
HARTLEY, Frederick C.; Ste. 309, 3614-30th Ave., Vernon, B.C.; Wes'56; FRCS(C), GenSurg; Cons. Surg., Vernon Jubilee Hosp., Shuswar Lake Gen. Hosp., Salmon Arm., Queen Victoria Hosp., Revelstoke, Enderby & Dist. Hosp. & Armstrong Hosp.; Tel. 542-2749.
HARTLEY, James M.; 405 Hendryx St., Nelson. B.C.; U.K.'60.

HARTOG, John H.; Wes'61; ObstGyn; Staff, Victoria Hosp., London, Ont.

HARTROFT, W. Stanley; 41 Sunnypoint Cres., Scarboro, Ont. (res); Alb '41; B.Sc. (Med.Anat.); LL.D.; Ph.D. (Path), (Tor.); FRCP(C); Dir. The Research Inst., Hosp. for Sick Children, Toronto; Prof. (Physiol). U. of Toronto; Tel. EM 6-7242.
HARTSELL, Dorothy L.; Tor '62; Jr. Intn., Women's College Hosp., Toronto, Ont.
HARTT, John N.; **500 Bridge St. E., Belleville, Ont.; Stanley Park Dr. (res); Qns '51; M.C.G.P.;** Staff, Belleville Gen. Hosp.; Tel. WO 2-6030.
HARTWELL, Leagh W.; 5914 Larch St., Vancouver 13, B.C. (res); UBC '54; Staff, Metro Health, Vancouver.
HARVEY, Donald C.; Fort Frances Clinic, 301 Victoria St., Fort Frances, Ont.; Cambridge (Eng.)'59.
HARVEY, Eoin S.; Box 268, Carlyle, Sask.; Tor '56; Abroad.
HARVEY, Georges H.; 13-3eme rue, Gagnon, Cte. Saguenay, P.Q.; Lav'63.
HARVEY, G. Lile; 119 Ottawa St. N., Hamilton, Ont.; 50 Rothsay Ave. (res); Tor '41; Tel. LI 5-1376.
HARVEY, Henri N.; Lav'58; Res., Hop. Hotel-**Dieu, Quebec 4, P.Q.**
HARVEY, J. Hamilton; 3000 Lawrence Ave. E., Scarborough, Ont.; 40 Regency Sq. (res); McG '53; Derm; Att'd. Staff, Scarborough Gen Hosp.; Tel. 291-1131.
HARVEY, J. Miln; 40 George St. N. Galt, Ont.; Tor'57; FRCS(C), ObstGyn.; Active Cons. Staff (ObstGyn.), S. Waterloo Mem. Hosp.; Tel. 623-0865.
HARVEY, John E.; Ste. 603, 1029 Douglas St., Victoria, B.C.; Tor '43; Ph.D(Surg.); NeurSurg; Staff, St. Joseph's & Royal Jubilee Hosp's.; Cons., Victoria Vet's. Hosp. & Queen Alexandria Solarium; Tel. 382-8030.
HARVEY, John H.; Ott'65; Res., Hop. Sacre-Coeur, Montreal 9, P.Q.
HARVEY, John P.; Box 1495, Churchill, Man.; Qns '33.
HARVEY, Joseph M.; 2455 Beach Dr., Victoria, B.C.; Tor'29; GenSurg; Ass't. Supt., Veteran's Hosp.; Tel. EV 2-4221.
HARVEY, J. P.; Reg. Supt., Sask. Region, Dept. of Nat. Health & Welfare, 735 Motherwell Bldg., Victoria Ave., Regina, Sask.
HARVEY, Melbourne R.; 14 Dundana, Dundas, Ont. (res); Wes '52; Anaes; Staff, Hamilton Gen. Hosp., Hamilton, Ont.; Tel. 527-0271.
HARVEY, Michael L.; 184 Lincoln Rd., Grand Falls, Nfld.; Bristol (Eng.) '55; Psy.
HARVEY, Miln C.; 131 Frederick St., Kitchener, Ont.; 148 John St. W., Waterloo (res); Tor '22; F.R.C.S. (Edin.), F.R.C.S.(C), GenSurg; Chief, Dept. of Surg., Kitchener-Waterloo Hosp., Kitchener; Tel. SH 5-7964.
HARVEY, Roger F.; McLennan Clinic, McLennan, Alta.; Bristol (Eng.)'50; Tel. 13.
HARVEY, Sylvain, Capt.; Nat. Defence Med. Centre, London, Ont.; Lav '65.
HARVEY, T. Jerome; Box 250, Cor. of Bell & 5th St., Nipigon, Ont.; Tor '60 AMCGP; & Chief of Staff, Nipigon Dist. Hosp.; Tel. 20.
HARVEY, William; 463 Eleventh St. "B" W., Owen Sound, Ont.; Tor '52; Staff, Gen. & Marine Hosp.; Tel. FR 6-6752.
HARVEY, William F.; Tor'60; Urol; Staff, Sunnybrook Hosp., Toronto, Ont.
HARVEY, William H.; 171 Queen St. S., Kitchener, Ont.; 70 Rusholme Rd. (res); Tor '22; Derm. Staff, St. Mary's Hosp., Kitchener; Retired.
HARVIE, Charles, A.; 40 Coldwater St. E., Orillia, Ont.; '09: GenSurg.; Tel. 326-3541.
HARVIE, Douglas A.; 201 Hurontario St., Collingwood, Ont.; 227 Minnesota St. (res); Tor '26; M.C.G.P.; Chief of Staff, Collingwood Hosp.; Tel. 445-2431.
HARVIE, Horace H.; 10 Sheppard, Espanola, Ont.; Tor '11; GenSurg; Med. Staff, Espanola Gen. Hosp.
HARVIE, James N.; 484 Church St., Apt. 210, Toronto 5, Ont. (res); Tor '52; DABR; DMR; DiagRad; Chief Radiol., Sunnybrook Hosp.; Clin. Assoc., U. of Toronto; Tel. 485-8651, Loc. 384.
HARVIE, R. Morley; 149 Alexandra Blvd. (Res), Toronto 12, Ont.; Tor'16; Sr. Examiner, Prudential Life Assur. of England; Retired.
HARWOOD-NASH, Derek; Cape Town (South Africa)'60; Res., Toronto Gen. Hosp., Toronto 2, Ont.
HARWOOD, Robert A.; Wes'60; DiagRad; Staff, Victoria Hosp., London, Ont.
HARWOOD, William L.; 53 Manor Rd. E., Toronto 12, Ont.; McG '23; D & T Rad; Tel. 487-0073.
HARYETT, Lorne E.; 440 Clarence, London, Ont. Wes '48; Tel. 439-5791.
HASE, Shoji; Bigelow-Fowler Clinic, Lethbridge, Alta.; 1506-12th Ave. S. (res); Kyoto (Japan) '50.
HASHI, David A. O.; McG'61; Res., Montreal Gen. Hosp., Montreal 25, P.Q.
HASHI, Jack I. O.; 15 Dolphin Bay, Regina, Sask.; McG'64.
HASHIMOTO, Stanley A.; Alb '62; Res., Vancouver Gen. Hosp., Vancouver 9, B.C.
HASHMI, Saeed; Box 241, Oxford, N.S.; Punjab (India)'62.
HASINOFF, Daniel J.; Alb'65; Res., University Hosp., Edmonton, Alta.
HASINOFF, David; Mannville, Alta.; Man '35; MCGP; District Coroner; Memb., Economics Commiss., C.M.A., Alberta; Tel. 763-3630.
HASKINS, Charles D.; 147 Buckingham, Iroquois Falls, Ont.; Tor '51; Staff, Anson Gen. Hosp.
HASLAM, Lewis C.; 630 Dorchester St. W., Montreal, P.Q.; 6 Waverley Rd., Pointe Claire, P.Q. (res); McG'35; Chief Med. Officer, C.I.L.; Tel. 874-3686.
HASLETT, William R. T.; 463 Waterloo St., London, Ont.; Wes '32; F.A.C.S., F.I.C.S., Gen Surg; Att. Surg., Victoria Gen. & St. Joseph's Hosp's.; Tel. GE 4-6253.
HASNAIN, S. Abid; 1447 Tecumseh Rd. E., Windsor, Ont.; 3076 Walker Rd. (res); U. of The Punjab (Lahore, Pakistan) '43; Tel. 256-2131.
HASSAN, Mervyn L.; 1146 Marine Dr., North Vancouver, B.C.; UBC'63; Tel. YU 8-5291.
HASSAN, Rayes; Montpellier (France)'60; Jr. Int., Hop. Laval, Quebec 10, P.Q.
HASSARD, Clarence E. A.; 41 Roehampton Ave., Toronto 12, Ont.; Tor '26; MCGP; Tel. HU 3-2881.
HASSARD, Donald T.; 410 Phys. & Surg's. Bldg., 8409 112th. St., Edmonton, Alta.; Alb '57; FRCS(C); Ophth; Otol; Staff, University Hosp.; Cons. (Ophth.), Charles Camsell Hosp.; Att'd. Staff, U. of Alberta Hosp.; Tel. 433-0229.
HASSARD, F. R.; 199 Parkside Dr., Toronto, Ont.; Tor '12; Retired. Tel. LE. 4-4533.
HASSELBACH, I.; Gottingen (Germ.) '45; Staff, Riverview Hosp., Essondale, B.C.
HASSELBACK, Richard; 500 Sherbourne St., Toronto, Ont.; 26 Underhill Dr., Ste. 708, Don Mills (res); McG '53; FRCP(C), IntMed; Haem., Princess Margaret Hosp.; Clin. Instr., (Med.), U. of Toronto; Tel. 924-0671.
HASSETT, Noel; 318 South Railway St. S.E., Medicine Hat, Alta.; National U. (Ire.) '53; M.B., B.Ch., B.A.O.
HASTINGS, David E.; 272 Bloor St. W., Toronto 5, Ont.; UBC'58; FRCS(C), OrthSurg; Attend. Staff, Wellesley Hosp.; Clin. Teach., University of Toronto; Tel. 921-7413.
HASTINGS, Donald J.; 132 Med. Arts. Bldg., Winnipeg 1, Man.; 111 Chataway Blvd. (res); Man'41; MCGP; Staff, Grace Hosp., Dept. of G.P.; Vice. Pres., College of Phy's. & Surg's.; Tel. WH 2-8727.
HASTINGS-JAMES, Richard T.; 23 Fleming Dr., Halifax, N.S. (res); Cambridge (Eng.) '40; M.R.C.P. (Lond.), D.M.R.D.; DiagRad; Rad., Victoria Gen. Hosp.; Assoc. Prof., Dalhousie U.; **Tel. 422-7371.**
HASTINGS, John E. F.; 18 McKenzie Ave., Toronto, Ont. (res); Tor'51; DPH, PH; Prof., PH & Prev. Med., School of Hygiene, U. of Toronto; Tel. WA 3-6611.
HASZNOS, Agnes E.; See LAU (Hasznos) Agnes E.
HATCH, Lorne R.; 45 9th Ave. S., Cranbrook, B.C.; Alb'65.

HATCHER, Gordon H.; School of Public Health, U. of Montreal, P.O. Box 6128, Montreal, P.Q.; McG'44; FAPHA.; DPH; PH; Prof. of PH (Med. Care Admin.), U. of Montreal; Part-time Cons., Dept. of Health for N.S., N.S. Hosp. Ins. Commiss., P.A.H.O., WHO & Dept. of National Health & Welfare; Tel. RE 3-9951, Loc. 435.

HATCHER, J. Donald; R.R. No. 1, Kingston, Ont. (res); Wes '46; Ph.D.; Prof & Hd. Dept. of Physiology, Queen's U.; Tel. 546-1731.

HATFIELD, C. Bruce; 008 Rideau Med. Centre, 1711-4th St. S.W., Calgary, Alta.; Alb'53; MSc; MRCP(Lond.); FACP; DABIM; FRCP(C); IntMed; Staff, Calgary Gen., Foothills Gen., Holy Cross & Calgary Auxiliary Hosp's.; Tel. 263-1454.

HATFIELD, George G.; Dal'36; MPH; Psy; Ass't. Med. Supt., Lancaster Prov. Hosp., Lancaster, N.B.; Tel. 694-4481.

HATFIELD, Jack, Major; National Defence Med. Centre, Ottawa 8, Ont.; Dal '61.

HATFIELD, Robert E.; 008 Rideau Med. Centre, 1711-4th St. S.W., Calgary, Alta.; Alb'53; AACP; FRCP(C); IntMed; Active Staff, Calgary Gen., Holy Cross, Calgary Auxiliary & Foothills Hosp's.; Cons., Home Oil Co. Ltd.; Tel. 263-1454.

HATFIELD, William H.; Medical Clinic, 710 Seymour St., Vancouver, B.C.; 1707 W 41 (res); Tor '26; F.C.C.P., IntMed; Assoc. Clin. Prof. of Med., U. of British Columbia; Tel. MU 4-1511.

HATHWAY, Wilfred W.; 508 Medical Arts Bldg., 750 Spadina Cres. E., Saskatoon, Sask.; Sask'57; Tel. 242-1291.

HAUCH, Cuyler Y.; 843—5th Ave. E., Owen Sound, Ont.; **R.R. No. 1, East Linton (res); Wes '31; F.A.C.S., M.A.B.S., F.I.C.S. GenSurg; Chm.,** Surg. Section, General & Marine Hosp.; Tel. 376-5390.

HAUCH, J. T.; 226 Roncesvalles Ave., Toronto 3, Ont.; Chicago (U.S.)'34; Ph.D., IntMed; Phys-in-Chief, St. Joseph's Hosp.; Tel. LE 4-1568.

HAUCH, Paul P.; 508 Waterloo St., London, Ont.; Wes '32; DMRD (Lond.); DiagRad; Cons. Rad., DVA, Westminster Hosp.; Sr. Assoc. (Rad), U. of Western Ontario; Tel. GE 2-6711.

HAUFFE, Herbert W.; 35 Frank St., Strathroy, Ont.; Oxford (Eng.)'63.

HAUGEN, Obert D; Box 190, Fort St. John, B.C.; Alb'62; Tel. 785-6677.

HAUGEN, Ragnvald; Box 217, Armstrong, B.C.; **Man '34; M.C.G.P.; Tel. 546-2036.**

HAUGH, Carman H.; 135 Jane St., Toronto 9, Ont.; Tor '32; Tel. RO 2-9122.

HAUGHTON, Thomas J.; Medical Arts Clinic, 2125-11th Ave., Regina, Sask.; 2816 McCallum Ave. (res); McG '35; **F.A.A.Ot., Otol; Sr.** Staff, Regina Gen. and Grey Nun's Hosp's.; Teaching Staff, Regina Grey Nuns' Hosp.; Cons.(Otol.) D.V.A.; Tel LA 2-1651.

HAUSER, Wolfgang; Austria'59; Path; Staff, Royal Inland Hosp., Kamloops, B.C.

HAUSLER, H. Richard; 477 Parkside Dr. Toronto 3, Ont. (res); Graz U. (Austria) '47; F.R.C.S.(C), Ophth; Research Assoc., Banting & Best Dept. of Med. Research; Teach. Staff, Dept. of Ophth., U. of Toronto; Cons. (Ophth), Oshawa Clinic; Tel. RO 6-5974

HAUST, H. L.; Heidelberg (Germ.) '56; M.Sc. (Med.); Ph.D.; Lect. (Biochem.), Queen's U., Kingston, Ont.; Tel. LI 6-1731.

HAUST, Maria D.; 205 Stuart St., Kingston, Ont. (res); Heidelburg (Germ.) '51 Path; Ass't. Prof. Path. Queen's U.; Tel. LI 6-1731.

HAVELKOVA, Milada; 320 Riverside Dr., Toronto 3, Ontario. (res); Prague (Czechoslovakia); '46; Psy.; Staff, Hosp. for Sick Children; Tel. EM 6-7242.

HAVENS, John R.; Box 1329, Avery Clinic, Quesnel, B.C.; Wes'62; Tel. 992-2171.

HAVER, John V. B.; Box 680, Wynyard, Sask.; Sask. '60; MCGP; Tel. 4-2303.

HAVEY, Harry B.; Stewiacke, Colchester Co., N.S.; McG '11; M.O.H., & Coroner, Colchester Co.; Phys., D.I.A., Micmac Res. & Indian Schl., Shubenacadie. Retired.

HAW, Beverley G.; 1 Alvinston Rd., Scarborough, Ont.; Tor '53; MCGP; Tel. PL 5-1431.

HAWES, Erwin G.; 441 Med. Arts Bldg., Saskatoon, Sask., 56 Kirk Cr. (res); Tor'43; IntMed; **Staff, Saskatoon City Hosp.; Clin. Assoc. (Med.),** U. of Saskatchewan; **Tel. 652-5161.**

HAWIRKO, Leonora (Mrs. Yaremovich); 301 Med. Arts Bldg., Winnipeg, Man. 181 Campbell St., Wpg. 9 (res); Man '37; Schl. Phys., City Health Dept., Pt.-time; Tel. WH 2-8859.

HAWK, Hubert E.; Dal'65; Res., Victoria Gen. Hosp., Halifax, N.S.

HAWKE, William A.; 555 University Ave., Toronto 2, Ont.; 92 Garfield Ave. (res); Tor '30; FRCP(Lond.), **FRCP(C), NeurPsy; Dir., Clin.** Psy. Med., Hosp. for Sick Children; Prof. (Paed), U. of Toronto; Tel. EM 6-7242.

HAWKE, W. M.; Tor'65; Ass't. Res. (Otol.), St. Michael's Hosp., Toronto, Ont.

HAWKES, Victor S.; 6188 Churchill St., Vancouver 13, B.C. (res); Sheffield (Eng.) '43; MRCS, LRCP; DPH (Tor.); FAPHA; Late Zone Supt., Med. Serv., Dept. of Nat. Health & Welfare, Van. 1; Tel. AM 6-9339.

HAWKINGS-FINK, Elma; 28 Chaplin Cr., Toronto 7, Ont.; '31; Tel. 485-6123.

HAWKINS, Arnot R.; Port Arthur Clinic, 194 N. Court St., Port Arthur, Ont.; 123 Cottonwood **Cres. (res); Sask '60; Active Staff, St. Joseph's Gen. & Pt. Arthur Gen. Hosp's.; Tel. DI 4-7271.**

HAWKINS, A. Russell; 10 Perry St., Woodstock, Ont.; 105 Vansittart Ave. (res); Tor '29; M.C.-G.P.; Surg. Staff, Phys., School of Nursing, Woodstock Gen. Hosp.; Tel. 537-2071.

HAWKINS, David G.; Dal '60; FRCP(C); IntMed; Staff, Dalhousie Public Health Clinic, Halifax, N.S.; Abroad.

HAWKINS, Nigel V.; 500 Sherbourne St., Toronto 5, Ont.; Sydney (Australia) '53; DMRT; FFR; TherRad; Staff, Princess Margaret Hosp.; Clin. Teach., U. of Toronto; Tel. 924-0671, Ext. 260.

HAWKINS, S. Jackson; c/o Freeport San., Kitchener, Ont.; R.R. 3, Kitchener (res); Tor '33; F.C.C.P., IntMed (TB); Med. Supt., Freeport San., Kitchener, Ont.; Tel. SH 5-4797.

HAWKS, Gordon H.; 116 Ridge Dr., Toronto, Ont. (res); Tor '43; Bact; Bact., St. Michael's Hosp., Toronto; Lect. in Bact., U. of Toronto; Tel. 362-4461.

HAWLEY, Richard T.; Ste. 1124, 925 W. Georgia St., Vancouver 1, B.C.; London (Eng.)'58; MRCS; Tel. MU 5-0046; Abroad.

HAWORTH, Derek H.; Lorne St., Cupar, Sask.; Edinburgh (Scot.) '48; AICS; MCGP; District Coroner; Chief of Med. Staff, Cupar Union Hosp.; Tel. 723-4222.

HAWORTH, George C.; Lacombe, Alta.; 5033-52 **St. (res); Alb '27.**

HAWORTH, Gordon L. S/L; London (Eng.) '53; DPH(C); c/o Reg. Surgeon, HMC Dockyard, Esquimalt, B.C.; Tel. EV 2-2911.

HAWORTH, James C.; Children's Hosp., Winnipeg 3, Man.; Birmingham (Eng.) '45; MRCP (Lond.); DCH; Paed; Paed., Children's Hosp.; Ass't Paed., Wpg. Gen. Hosp.; Ass't Prof.(Paed.), U. of Manitoba; Tel. SP 5-8311.

HAWTHORNE, Allan B.; 316 Grosvenor Ave., Westmount, Montreal 6, P.Q. (res); McG'21; FACS, Urol; Urol., Royal Victoria Hosp.; Urol. in Charge, Children's Memorial Hosp.; Lect. in Surg. (Urol.), McGill U.; Tel. WE 5-4044.

HAWTHORNE, Kenneth O.; 14 Wellington St., St. Catharines, Ont.; Tor '40; Assoc. Staff, Gen. & Hotel-Dieu Hosp's.; Tel. MU 2-4332.

HAY, A. J. Stewart; P.O. Box 185, Trochu, Alta.; Alb '42; Dist. Coroner.

HAY, Arthur W.S.; Box 420 Brandon, Man.; Man'59; D.Psy.; Psy.; Phys., Brandon Mental Hosp.; Tel. PA 6-2321.

HAY, Fraser E. J.; Main St., Listowel, Ont.; Victoria St. (res); Wes '37.

HAY, Gwendolen O. (See JOHNSON Gwendolen O.)

HAY, Hugh B.; 400 Collishaw St., Moncton, N.B.; Wes'49; MPH(Harvard).

HAY, Jack A.; 3520 Quadra St., Victoria, B.C.; Qns '44.
HAY, John; 238 St. John's Rd., Pointe Claire, Montreal 33, P.Q.; McG '45; M.C.G.P.; Staff, Lachine Gen. Hosp., Lachine.
HAY, John M.D.; 749 King St. W., Kitchener, Ont.; 366 Holly St., Waterloo (res); Tor'46; FRCS(Ed.); FACS; GenSurg; Cons. Surg., St. Mary's Gen., Kitchener-Waterloo & South Waterloo Mem. Hosp., Galt; Tel. SH 2-9290.
HAY, Malcolm D.; 322 Wellington St., Sarnia, Ont.; Tor'60.
HAY, Murray C.; 3724 Clark Dr., Vancouver, B.C.; 5193 Kersland Dr., Van. 15 (res); Qns '45; MCGP; Tel. TR 4-0424.
HAY, Ralph L.; Box 189, Rocky Mountain House, Alta.; Alb '53; MCGP.
HAY, Rankin K.; The Winnipeg Clinic, St. Mary's & Vaughan, Winnipeg 1, Man.; 226 Yale Ave., Wpg. 9 (res); **Durham (Eng.) '40; FRCS(Eng.), FACS, FRCS(C), NeurSurg; Ass't. NeurSurg.,** Wpg. Gen. Hosp.; **Hd. Dept. of NeurSurg., Deer** Lodge DVA Hosp.; **Lectr. NeurSurg., U. of Manitoba; Tel.** 942-0551.
HAY, W. D.; 124 Beverley St., Kingston, Ont.; Qns '21; PathBact; Staff, Queen's U.; Retired.
HAY, W. Ian; 2057 Caroline St. E., Burlington, Ont.; Durham (Eng.) '53; M.B., B.S., MCGP; Coroner, County of Halton; Tel. 637-5251.
HAY, William B.; 273 Glenairlie Dr., Victoria, B.C.; Qns '58; Path.

HAYAKAWA, Joseph; 35 Tod Dr., Winnipeg 8, Man. (res); Man '55; Anaes; Staff, St. Boniface Hosp.; Tel. WH 3-0311.
HAYDEN, D. Peter; McG '60; Res., Royal Victoria Hosp., Montreal 2, P.Q.

HAYES, Aubrey C.; 3 Acad. Med. Bldg., 1812-4th St. S.W., Calgary, Alta.; National U. (Ire.)'52; Tel. 263-7120.
HAYES, David F.; Manchester (Eng.) '61; Staff, Delisle Clinic, Delisle, Sask.
HAYES, Ethel M.; 139 Airdrie Rd., Toronto 17, Ont. (res); Tor '12; Tel. 421-3974.
HAYES, Herbert N.; Qns '63; Sr. Int. Hotel Dieu Hosp., Kingston, Ont.
HAYES, J. Kempton; 7193 Quinpool Rd., Halifax, N.S.; 1571 Le Marchant St. (res); Dal '62; AMCGP; Tel. 454-1547.
HAYES, Kenneth P.; 6052 Quinpool Rd., Halifax, N.S.; 31 Cherry St. (res); Dal '25; Tel. 423-7775.
HAYES, R. Marcus; 7989 Cambie St., Vancouver 14, B.C. (res); **Edinburgh (Scot.) '34; M.O.** Workmen's Comp. Bd.
HAYES, R. T.; 42 Coburg St., Saint John, N.B.; 198 King E. (res); **McG '27; Ophth,Otol; Cons., St. John T.B. & V.A. Prov. Lancaster Hosp's.;** Tel. 693-2081.

HAYHURST Robert J.; Med. Surg. Clinic, 2nd Ave. Whitecourt, Alta.; Edinburgh (Scot.) '54; DPH; DIH; Staff, Whitecourt Gen. Hosp.; Tel. 778-2671.
HAYLEY, Margaret A.; 183 Forest Hill Rd., Toronto 7, Ont. (res); St. Andrew's (Scot.) '44; Staff, Workmen's Comp. Bd.
HAYMAN, W. Philip; Wes'65; Ass't. Res. (Surg.), U. of Western Ontario & Victoria Hosp., London, Ont.

HAYNES, Elizabeth; Ire. '55; Int'n., St. John's Gen. Hosp., St. John's, Nfld.
HAYNES, Ernest R.; 300 Med. Dental Bldg., 10603-100th Ave., Edmonton, Alta.; Trinity Coll. (Dublin, (Ire.) '47; B.Ch., BAO; MCGP; Active Staff, Royal Alexandra Hosp.; Instr. (Dept. of Social & Prev. Med.), U. of Alberta; Tel. 422-1669.
HAYNES, Harold G.; RCP & S (Ire.)'55; Anaes; Staff, University Hosp., Emdonton, Alta.
HAYNES, J. David; 331 Sheddon Ave., Oakville, Ont.; Qns '50; D.A.B.S., F.I.C.S., F.R.C.S.(C), GenSurg; Cons Surg., Oakville-Trafalgar Mem. Hosp.; Assoc. Surg., Queensway Hosp., Islington.; Tel. VI 5-1711.
HAYNES, Thora W. (Lee); Ste 8, 331 Sheddon Ave., Oakville, Ont.; 260 Poplar Dr. (res); Johns Hopkins (U.S.A.) '56; FRCP(C); IntMed; Cons. IntMed., Oakville-Trafalgar Mem. Hosp.; Tel. **845-8761.**
HAYNES, W. Sterling; Alb'58; MCGP; Res., Vancouver Gen. Hosp., Vancouver 9, B.C.
HAY-ROE, E. Archer; 11156-64th St., Edmonton, Alta. (res); CP & S (Calif., U.S.A.) '16; Retired.

HAYTER, Francis W.; 333 Carpathia Rd., Winnipeg, Man. (res); Man '33; DiagRad; Rad., Deer Lodge Hosp., Winnipeg 12; Tel. 837-1301.
HAYTER, Russell R. P.; 800 Sherbrook St., Winnipeg 2, Man.; London (Eng.) '49; D.PhysMed (Eng.); PhysMed & Rehab; Dir. & Active Staff, (PhysMed.), Man. Rehab. Hosp.; Active Med. Staff (PhysMed.), Children's Hosp.; Lect. (PhysMed), U. of Manitoba; Tel. SP 5-0181.

HAYTHORNTHWAITE, James, C.H.; Asa St., Kemptville, Ont.; Trinity Coll. (Dublin, Ire.) '52; M.B., B.Ch.; BAO; LM (Rotun.); MCGP; Obst-Gyn; Staff, Kemptville, Dist. & Smiths Falls Public & Winchester Mem. Hosp's.; Tel. 258-2376.
HAYTON, Robert C.; 106 Med. Arts Bldg., 750 Spadina Cr. E., Saskatoon, Sask.; Alb'57; FRCP(C), IntMed; Staff, University Hosp.

HAYWARD, Ralph; Manitowaning Clinic, Manitowaning, Ont.; Tor'32; M.O. I/C of Manitowaning Clinic; Dept. of National Health & Welfare, Medical Services.
HAYWARD, R. S.; Ste. 12, 331 Sheddon Ave., Oakville, Ont.; Tor'65.

HAYWOOD, Gary L. Capt.; Man '62; CAPO 5050, Cdn. Armed Forces, Europe. Abroad.
HAYWOOD, George S.; 116 Marshall Cr., Winnipeg 19, Man.; Man '54.

HAZEL, Bernard; 52 Boul De-Guire, Ville St.-Laurent, Montreal 9, P.Q.; Mon'61; IntMed(P.Q.).
HAZEL, Joseph J.; Dal '52; TherRad; Staff, Dept. of TherRad., Royal Victoria Hosp., Montreal, P.Q.; Tel. VI 2-1251.

HAZELL, Howard C.; 42 Albert St., Stratford, Ont.; 119 Mornington St. (res); Tor '44; MCGP; Tel. 271-3123.
HAZELL, Shirley G.; Ste 104, 1050 W. 10th Ave., Vancouver, B.C.; Tor'60; Paed.; Staff, Vancouver Gen. Hosp.; Abroad.

HAZEN, G. Medley T.; 208 Canada Bldg., Saskatoon, Sask.; Tor'23; OphthOtol.; Tel. 242-3997.
HAZEN, James S.; Qns '34; FACCP; Supt., Brant San., Brantford, Ont.

HAZLETT, Barbara E. McKinnon; 16 Eastbourne Ave., Toronto, Ont.; Tor '49; F.R.C.P.(C), Int-Med.; Sr. Fell. (Med.), Toronto Gen. Hosp. Tel. EM 6-8211.
HAZLETT, John M.; 300 Bloor St. E., Toronto, Ont.; 496 Roselawn Ave. (res); Qns '19.
HAZLETT, John W.; 228 Brock St., Kingston, Ont.; Tor '47; DABOS; FRCS(C); OrthSurg; Att'd. OrthSurg., Hotel-Dieu Hosp.; Assoc. Staff, Kingston Gen. Hosp.; Ass't Prof. (OrthSurg.), Queen's U.; Tel. 542-2688.
HAZLEWOOD, Brenton F.; 38 Granite St., Copper Cliff, Ont.; 25 Park St. W. (res); Tor'36; **GenSurg; Surg., Copper Cliff Hosp.; Cons. Staff, St. Joseph's, Sudbury Mem. & Sudbury Gen. Hosp's.; Chief Surg., Internat. Nickel Co. of** Canada Ltd.; Coroner, Dist. of Sudbury; MOH, Copper Cliff; Tel. 682-4421.

HEAD, Philip W.; Rossburn, Man.; Man'14; Tel. 145.
HEAGY, Fred C.; 391 South St., London, Ont.; 1037 Brough St. (res); Wes'43; M.Sc., Ph.D.; Biochem. Ont. Cancer Fdn., London Clin.; Staff, Victoria Hosp.; Cons. (Nuclear Med.), Westminster DVA Hosp.; Hon. Cons. (Nuclear Med.), St. Joseph's Hosp.; Ass't. Prof. (Biochem. & TherRad), U. of Western Ont.; Tel. 432-5261.
HEAL, Frederick C.; Moose Jaw Clinic, 200 Scott Bldg., Moose Jaw, Sask.; Tor'35; F.A.C.P., F.R.C.P.(C), IntMed; **Chief of Med., Providence** Hosp.; Tel. 692-2373.
HEALY, Clifford J. M.; 157 Ontario St., St. Catharines, Ont.; 52 Hillcrest Ave. (res); Tor '41; Staff, St. Catharines Gen. & Hotel Dieu Hosp's.; Tel. 684-4130.
HEALY, D. E. L.; 86 Bloor St. W., Toronto, Ont.; 125 Merrill Ave. E. (res); Tor '28; Otol; Staff, St. Joseph's Hosp.; Tel. WA 2-4226.

HEALY, Robert W.; Park Med. Bldg., 150 Park St., Kentville, N.S.; 27 Colonial Ave. (res); Dal '53, Staff, Blanchard-Fraser Mem. Hosp. & Eastern Kings Mem. Hosp. Wolfville; Tel. 678-3144.

HEALEY, Ruth (See RUSSELL)

HEANEY, Adair G.; Belfast (N. Ire.) '59; M.B., B.Ch., BAO, DRCOG; Res., Queen Mary Vet's. Hosp., Montreal, P.Q.

HEARD, Frederick S.; Ste. 270, 1070 Douglas St., Victoria, B.C.; Liverpool (Eng.)'59.

HEARD, H. Stanley; 334 Queens Ave., London, Ont.; Highland Rd., R.R. No. 4 (res); Wes '35; Staff, St. Joseph's Hosp.; Court. Staff, Victoria Hosp.; Tel. GE 4-5322.

HEASLIP, David S.; 3040 Don Mills Rd. E., Willowdale, Ont.; Tor'64.

HEASMAN, Gerald A.; 535 Med. Dental Bldg., Regina, Sask.; London (Eng.)'54; D.Psy; DPM; Psy; Assoc. Staff, Regina Gen. & Grey Nuns Hosp's.; Tel. 527-9323.

HEATH, E. Sheldon; Allan Mem. Inst., 1025 Pine Ave. W., Montreal ,2 P.Q.; McG'57; Psy; Ass't. Psy., Royal Victoria Hosp.; Lect., McGill U.; Tel. 842-1251, Ext. 325.

HEATH, John W.; Bonavista, Nfld.; Edinburgh (Scot.) '37; M.C.G.P.; Supt., Bonavista Hosp.; M.H.O.; Tel. 7581.

HEATHCOTE, Anthony G. S.; 276 McKee Ave., Willowdale, Ont. (res); London (Eng.) '45; M.R.C.S. (Eng.); L.R.C.P. (Lond.); D.P.H.; Dist. M.O., Dept. Public Health, Toronto; Tel. EM 3-1211.

HEATON, Peter B.; 151 Holland Ave., Ottawa, Ont.; Tor '50; M.C.G.P.; Staff (G.P.), Ottawa Civic Hosp.; Tel. PA 2-1711.

HEBB, Alan R.; Dal'59; AMCGP; IntMed; Teach. & Research Fell., Dept. of Ther., University of Toronto.

HEBB, Harvey D.; 219 Professional Bldg., 10830 Jasper Ave., Edmonton, Alta.; Dal '34; GenSurg; Staff, Edmonton Gen. Hosp.; Tel. 424-1517.

HEBERT, A. J. Barlow; Ste. 9, Professional Bldg., 304 Dundas St. W., Whitby, Ont.; 865 Dundas St. W. (res); McG '12; Staff, Ajax & Oshawa Gen. Hosp's.; Tel. 668-2292. Retired.

HEBERT, Antoine; 825 rue Belvedere S., Sherbrooke, P.Q.; 160 rue Bryant (res); Lav '41; Tel. 569-1840.

HEBERT, Auguste; 3440 Hutchison, Montreal 18, P.Q.; Mon'30; Urol.

HEBERT, Charles E.; 3411 rue St. Denis, Montreal 18, P.Q.; 5002 Roslyn (res); Mon '22; F.A.C.S., F.R.C.S.(C), GenSurg; Chief of Surg., Hop Notre Dame; Tel. RE 8-6112.

HEBERT, Claude D.; 930 Courchesne, Ste. Foy, Quebec 10, P.Q.; Lav'56; Anaes; Staff, Hop. Laval and Laval U; Tel. 653-5251.

HEBERT, Dores; Yamaska, Co. Yamaska, P.Q.; Mon '58.

HEBERT, Emile; 300 Carre St. Louis, Montreal, P.Q.; 51 Ave. Cornwall, Ville Mont Royal (res); Mon '25; Gyn. (P.Q.); Chief Surg. (Gyn.), Hop Misericordia; Tel. VI 5-9439.

HEBERT, Fernand; 5600 Blvd. Gouin ouest, Montreal 9, P.Q. (res); Mon '28; F.A.C.C.P., Pulm. Dis. & TB (P.Q.); Med. Dir. Hop. Sacre Coeur; Tel. FE 4-1210, Loc. 255.

HEBERT, Francois; 4000 Blvd. Lasalle, Verdun, P.Q.; 201 Metcalfe Ave., Montreal 6 (res); Lav'53; DiagRad; Head, Dept. of Rad., Hop. General Du-Christ-Roi; Tel. WE 2-6230.

HEBERT, Georges; Medical Arts Bldg., 1538 Sherbrooke W., Montreal, P.Q.; 430 ave. Roslyn, Westmount (res); Mon '33; IntMed; Assoc. Prof., U. of Montreal; Staff, Hop. Notre-Dame; Tel. WE 2-2891.

HEBERT, Gilles; 1150 Est, Boul. St-Joseph, Montreal 34, P.Q.; 39 Cornwall Ave., Ville Mt-Royal (res); Mon '50; Gyn (P.Q.); Gyn., Hop. Maisonneuve; Tel. 254-8341.

HEBERT, Gustave; 2003 Nicolet St., Montreal, P.Q.; Mon '34; Tel. LA 4-2242.

HEBERT, Guy; Lav'61; Res., Hop. Notre Dame, Montreal, P.Q.

HEBERT, Henri J.; P.Q.; 22 rue Baie, Valleyfield, P.Q. (res); Mon'49; OrthSurg.(P.Q.); OrthSurg., Hop. Hotel-Dieu; Tel. 373-5560.

HEBERT, H. J. Louis; 513-2nd St. E., Cornwall, Ont.; Man '45; Staff, Cornwall Gen. & Hotel-Dieu Hosp's.; Tel. WE 2-0621.

HEBERT, Jean-Guy; 2101 Maplewood Ave., Montreal, P.Q.; 2360 Maurice, Ville Brossard (res); Mon '59; FRCP(C), IntMed; Med. Dir. Health Services, University of Montreal; Tel. 739-3271.

HEBERT, J. Gerard; 1150 Blvd. St. Joseph E., Montreal 34, P.Q.; 49 Linwood Cres. (res); Mon '40; PlasSurg; Staff, Hop Maisonneuve; Tel. 521-1241.

HEBERT, J. Louis; 265B Blvd. du Havre, Valleyfield, P.Q.; Lav '13; Retired.

HEBERT, Jean P.; 8476 St. Denis St., Montreal, P.Q.; Mon '42; Tel. DU 8-1471.

HEBERT, Louis; Ste. 230, 4 Taschereau St., Hull, P.Q.; Lav'61; Paed(P.Q.).

HEBERT, Louis; 400 Guilbeault, Longueuil, Jacques Cartier, P.Q.; Mon'61; FRCS(C), GenSurg; Staff, Hop. Maisonneuve.

HEBERT, Luc; 7282 St.-Denis, Montreal 10, P.Q.; Mon '59; Tel. 273-2052.

treal, P.Q.; Mon '27; Tel. 272-6959.

HEBERT, Paulin; Maskinonge, Co. Maskinonge, P.Q.; Lav '60.

HEBERT, Paul E.; 1270 Beaubien St. E., Mon- Notre-Dame, Montreal.

HEBERT, Roch; 148A Blvd. Ste. Rose, Ste. Rose, Co. Laval, P.Q.; Lav '55.

HECKADON, Robert G.; 504 Med. Arts Bldg., 1011 Ouellette Ave., Windsor, Ont.; Wes'60; FRCS(C), PlasSurg.

HECKING, Stephan J. H.; Bradford, Ont.; Muenster (Germ.) '37; Sr. Surg., York Co. Hosp., Newmarket; Tel. TW 5-4521.

HECTOR, R. Ian; Toronto Gen. Hosp., 101 College St., Toronto, Ont.; Tor'57; MRCP(Lond.); FRCP(C), Psy; Jr. Phys., Toronto Gen. Hosp.; Clin. Teach. Dept. of Psy. & Med., U. of Toronto; Tel. EM 6-8211.

HEDDLE, M. S.; 86 King St. E., Stoney Creek, Ont.; Qns '29; M.C.G.P.; M.O.H., Stoney Creek & Saltfleet Twp.

HEDDLE, Rognvald W.; Box 429, Rivers, Man. (res); Glasgow (Scot.) '46; M.B., Ch.B., FRCS(Edin.); Staff, Riverdale & Hamiota Hosp's; Tel. 69. Abroad.

HEDGES, Francis H.; Box 650, Rimbey, Alta.; London (Eng.)'44; MRCS(Eng.); LRCP(Lond.).

HEESE, Heinz B.; Rosthern, Sask.; Sask. '62; Tel. 232-4244.

HEFFELFINGER, Robert M.; 2255 Elgin St., Port Coquitlam, B.C.; 2610 Shaftesbury Ave. (res); Man '49.

HEFFERMAN, Angela; Ste. 502, 225 Lisgar St., Ottawa 4, Ont.; 1059 Chelsea Dr., (res); London (Eng.)'42; D.Psy; Psy; Ass't. Prof. (Psy), U. of Ottawa; Tel. CE 4-2223.

HEFFERNAN, James L.; 1139 Yates St., **Victoria, B.C.; 2131 Newton St. (res); McG '51; M.C.G.P.; Tel. EV 6-4211.**

HEFFEZ, G. Andre; Ste 101, 6945 Christophe Colomb, Montreal 10, P.Q.; 2295 Lucerne Rd., Twn. of Mt-Royal (res); Paris (France) '41; F.I.C.S., GenSurg; Vis. Staff (GenSurg.), Hop. Jean Talon; & Att'd. Staff, Doctor's Hosp.; Tel. 276-7517.

HEGGIE, David C.; 7 Main St. N., Brampton, Ont.; 73 Main St. (res); Tor '25; M.C.G.P.

HEGGTVEIT, H. Alexander; Ott'57; DABP; FCAP; FAGS; Path., Ottawa Gen. Hosp.; Ass't. Prof. (Pathol.), U. of Ottawa; Tel. 236-0333, Ext. 367.

HEICHMAN, Walter J.; 2417 Cairns Ave., Saskatoon, Sask.; Man'57.

HEIDE, Archie R.; 131 Ontario St., St. Catharines, Ont.; Tor'59; GenSurg; Active Staff, St. Catharines Gen. & Hotel-Dieu Hosp's.; Tel. 684-7644.

HEIMBACH, Michael; 607 Chinook Prof. Bldg., 6100 Macleod Trail, Calgary, Alta.; Man'54; Paed.

HEIMBECKER, Raymond O.; 607 Med. Arts Bldg., 170 St. George St., Toronto 5, Ont.; 75 Hillholm Rd., Tor. 7 (res); Tor '47; MA (Physiol.), MS; FACS, FRCS(C), GenSurg; Staff Surg., Toronto Gen. Hosp.; Cons. (Cardiovasc.), Wellesley Hosp.; Clin. Instr. (Surg.), U. of Toronto; Research Assoc. Ont. Heart Fdn.; Tel. 923-1603.

HEIMLICH, Hans-Joachim; Med. Bldg., 1175 Cook St., Victoria, B.C.; UBC'65.

HEIN, Samuel; 5106-50th St., Rocky Mountain House, Alta.; Alb'48; MCGP; Tel. 845-3461.

HEINE, Cezar; Ste. 313, 1669 Victoria St., Prince George, B.C.; Sask'59.

HEINE, Henry X.; The Med. Centre, 707 Charlotte St., Peterborough, Ont.; 40 Weller Cr. (res); Dal'55; MCGP; Med. Dir., Fairhaven Home for the Aged; Staff, Civic & St. Joseph's Hosp's.; Tel. RI 2-9229.

HEINISCH, Gerhart; 537 Ellice Ave., Winnipeg 2, Man.; Vienna (Austria)'49; Tel. SP 2-5597.

HEINRICH, Ronald G; Biggar, Sask.; Sask '62.

HEINRICHS, Erwin; 201 Plaza Bldg., 1538 Foster St., White Rock, B.C.; UBC'59; MCGP; Tel. 531-5575.

HEINRICHS, Peter D.; 3967 Kingsway, South Burnaby, B.C.; 2673 Waverley (res); UBC '59; Tel. HE 4-8781.

HEITNER, Adolph P.; 175 Church St., St. Catharines, Ont.; 11 Rivercrest Dr. (res); Prague (Czech.) '28; Spec. Obst Gyn (Czech.); Staff, St. Catharines Gen.; Court. Staff, Hotel Dieu Hosp.; Tel. MU 4-7271.

HELDE, Michael D.; Wes'63; Res., Ottawa Gen. Hosp., Ottawa 2, Ont.

HELEM, Edward V.; 818-6th Ave. N., Port Alberni, B.C.; 712 Anderson Ave. S. (res); Man '44; Tel. 723-2111.

HELEM, George B.; Port Alberni Med. Bldg., 818-9th Ave. N., Port Alberni, B.C.; 815-4th N. (res); Man '34; Tel. 723-2111.

HELEM, J. P.; Port Physician, Dept. of Nat. Health & Welfare, Port Alberni, B.C.

HELGASON, Robert E.; Ste. 501, 625-5th Ave., New Westminster, B.C.; Man'45; Psy.; Tel. 526-6422.

HELIE, Gilles A.; 45 est, rue Elm, Sudbury, Ont.; Lav '52; FRCS(C); FACS; FASAS; GenSurg; Tel. 673-8391.

HELIE, Pierre; Mon'64; Res., Hop. Ste-Justine, Montreal 26, P.Q.

HELLAT, Alexander; 116 Elm St. E., Sudbury, Ont.; 373 Nepahwin (res); Tartu (Estonia) & Helsinki '39; Staff, Sudbury Gen., Mem. & St. Joseph's Hosp's.; Tel. 675-6401.

HELLE, Stephen J.; 12437 Bergerac, Pierrefonds, P.Q.; McG '56; IntMed; Chmn., Dept. of Med., Lachine Gen. Hosp.; Active Staff, Lakeshore Gen. Hosp., Pointe Claire; Cons. (IntMed.), Queen Mary Vet's. Hosp.; Med. Adviser, Bank of Montreal; Tel. MU 4-4819.

HELLER, Benjamin P.; Medical Arts Bldg., 1538 Sherbrooke St. W., Montreal, P.Q.; 32 Joyce Ave., Outremont (res); McG '32; DermSyph; Assoc. Phys. (Derm.), Reddy Memorial Hosp.; Ass't. Phys. (Derm.), Jewish Gen. Hosp.; Tel. WE 5-4208.

HELLER, E. Maurice; Ste., 610, 99 Avenue Rd., Toronto 5, Ont.; 9 Berkindale Dr., Willowdale (res) Tor '37; M.Sc. (Med.), FRCP(Edin.), FACP, **FACC, FCCP; IntMed (Cardiol.); Att'd. Phys. (Med.), New Mt. Sinai Hosp.; Assoc. Phys. (Med.), Doctors' Hosp.; Cons., I/C Cardiol.** Northwestern Gen. Hosp.; Cons. Cardiol., Jewish Home for the Aged & Baycrest Hosp.; Tel. WA 5-2189.

HELLER, Irving H.; Ste. 10, 900 Sherbrooke St. W., Montreal 2, P.Q.; McG'50; PhD; Neur; Att'd. Staff, Mtl. Neurol. Inst., Royal Victoria & Jewish Gen. Hosp's.; Tel. VI 5-3812.

HELLER, Jacob M.; 459 Bloor St. W., Toronto 4, Ont.; Tor '33; Tel. WA 2-8388.

HELLER, Leon; 525 Ellendale Med. Bldg., 5845 Cote-des-Neiges Rd., Montreal 26, P.Q.; 686 Roslyn Ave., Westmount 26 (res); McG '51; M.S., F.A.C.S., F.R.C.S.(C), OrthSurg; Att'd. Orth Surg., Jewish Gen. & Reddy Mem. Hosp's.; Cons. (OrthSurg), Mt. Sinai San. & Grace Dart **Hosp's. & Jewish Hosp. of Hope; Sessional Lect'r. (Anat.), McGill U.; Tel. RE 1-9331.**

HELLER, Nathan; 590 Ellendale Med. Bldg., 5845 Cote-des-Neiges Rd., Montreal 26, P.Q.; Wes'49; FRCP(C), IntMed; Chief Phys., Jewish Convalescent Hosp.; Assoc. Phys., Jewish Gen. Hosp.; Att'd. Phys. & Dir. (Sub. Dept. of Metabolism), Reddy Mem. Hosp.; Tel. 735-3331.

HELLER, Vera (See PRICE, Vera H.)

HELLINGS-EVANS, Bennett M.; 49 Westlake Ave., Toronto 13, Ont.; London (Eng.) '55.

HELLIWELL, Maurice; Kincardine, Ont.; Tor '15; Dist. Coroner.

HELLMAN, J. E.; Department of National Health & Welfare, c/o Regional Superintendent, European Region. Abroad.

HELLMANN, Kurt; Mt. Sinai Hosp., Toronto, Ont.; 25 Forest Ridge Dr., Toronto 19, (res); Tor '44; Staff (Anaes.), Mt. Sinai Hosp.; Tel. EM 6-7361.

HELLMICH, S.; Alberton, P.E.I.

HELLMUTH, Fritz-Heinz K.; 700 Bannatyne Ave., **Winnipeg 3, Man.; 128 Talon Bay, Wpg. 8 (res); Christian-Albrechts (Kiel, Germ.) '53; TherRad; Radiotherap., Man. Cancer Fdn., Wpg.** Gen. Hosp.; Ass't. Radiother., Wpg. Gen. Hosp.; Tel. 786-4731.

HELLON, Charles P.; Edinburgh (Scot.)'56; Psy; Staff, Dept. of Psy., University Hosp., Edmonton, Alta.

HELLSTROM, John G.; 274 Sun Life Bldg., Montreal, P.Q.; 475 Fenton Ave. (res); McG'54; FRCP(C); IntMed; Ass't. Med. Officer, Sun Life Assur. Co. of Canada; Att'd. Phys., Montreal Gen. Hosp. and Queen Elizabeth Hosp.; Dem., McGill U.; Tel. UN 6-6411, Loc. 359.

HELM, A. Rennie; Medical Clinic, Box 2058, Whitehorse, Y.T.; London (Eng.)'45; Att'd. Staff, Whitehorse Gen. Hosp.; Tel. 7-2508.

HELMAN-ZALEWSKA, Maria (Gewere); 3285 Van Horn Ave., Montreal 26, P.Q.; Vilnuv (Poland)'30.

HELSON, Kenneth G.; Wes '56; DiagRad; Staff, Oshawa Gen. Hosp., Oshawa, Ont.; Tel. 723-2211.

HELSTON, Raymond H.; Ste. 104, 1593 Ellesmere Rd., Scarborough, Ont.; 36 Oakridge Dr. (res); Tor'62; Court. Staff (G.P.), Scarborough Gen. Hosp.; Tel. 293-8181.

HELT, Andries C.; 336 Locke St. S., Hamilton, Ont.; Amsterdam (Neth.) '55; Court. Staff, Hamilton Gen. St. Joseph's Hosp's.; Tel. JA 8-5480.

HELT, Maria C.; 336 Locke St., S. Hamilton, Ont Amsterdam (Neth.) '55; Tel. JA 8-5480.

HEMMING, Fred O.; Box 188, Sicamous, B.C.; Glasgow (Scot.) '57; Tel. 836-2511.

HEMMING, John H.; Qns'52; Staff, Westminster Hosp., London, Ont.

HEMMING, Sarah L. (Armour); Box 188, Sicamous, B.C.; Glasgow (Scot.) '56; Tel. 836-2511.

HEMMINGS, Charles H.; 9190 Canora Rd., R.R. 2, Sidney, B.C.; Alb'38; Med. Dir., Gorge Road Hosp., Victoria, B.C.; Staff, O.P. Clinic, D.V.A. Hosp., Victoria, B.C.

HEMMINGS, Lyle M.; 156 Greenwood, Dollard des Ormeaux, P.Q. (res); McG '56; GenSurg (P.Q.); Att'd. Surg Staff, Lakeshore Gen. Hosp., Pointe Claire; Tel. 695-1310.

HEMOND, Benoit G.; Clinique Med. Physique, 3001 boul. Levesque, Chomedy, P.Q.; Mon'52.

HEMOND, Charles J.; 1205 Poisson St., Tecumseh, Ont.; Tor '26; M.O.H., St. Clair Beach; Dist. Coroner; Tel. 735-2672.

HEMSTOCK, James W.; 5018—47th St., Lloydminister, Sask.; Alb '44; M.C.G.P.

HEMSTOCK, John R.; 512 Herald Bldg., 206-7th Ave., S.W., Calgary, Alta; Alb '52; DA; Anaes; Staff, Holy Cross & Alberta Children's Hosp's.; Tel. 266-1531.

HENAULT, Gaetan; 7662A rue St. Denis, Montreal 10, P.Q.; Mon '55; Tel. 276-1760.

HENAULT, Paul E.; St. Felix-de-Valois, Co. Joliette, P.Q.; 536 Manseau (res); Mon '43.

HENDELMAN, Myer; 1374 Sherbrooke St. W., Montreal, P.Q.; 4300 Western Ave., Apt. 410, Westmount (res); McG'41; FACS; FRCS(C); ObstGyn; Assoc. (ObstGyn.), Royal Victoria Hosp.; Assoc. Prof. (ObstGyn.), McGill U.; Tel. VI 4-4887.

HENDERSON, Alfred G.; Winnipeg Clin., 205 Vaughan St., Winnipeg 1, Man.; 143 Harris Blvd. (res); Man '37; DTM; MCGP; Staff (GP), Grace Hosp.; Tel. WH 2-6441.

HENDERSON, Charles U.; Newfoundland Anaesthesia Associates, 95 LeMarchant Rd., St. John's Nfld; Waterford Bridge Rd. (res); Dal '45; F.A.C.A., Anaes; Anaes., St. John's Gen., St. Clare's Mercy & Grace Hosp's. & St. John's San.; Tel. 578-7909.

HENDERSON, Christopher B.; 3040 Shelburne St., Victoria, B.C.; UBC'65.

HENDERSON, Clifford B.; 1635 Abbott St., Kelowna, B.C.; Tor '52; Paed.; Tel. 762-2740.

HENDERSON, David A.; P.O. Box 102, Bala, Ont. (res); Tor '07; M.R.C.S. (Eng.), L.R.C.P. (Lond.); Retired.

HENDERSON, D. Nelson; 502 Med. Arts Bldg., 170 St. George St., Toronto 5, Ont.; 233 Dunvegan Rd. (res); Tor '25; FRCS(C), ObstGyn; Sr. ObstGyn., Toronto Gen. Hosp.; Cons. Gyn., Peel Mem. Hosp., Brampton & Tor. Hosp., Weston; Prof. (Emer.), Dept. of ObstGyn & Assoc. in Path., U. of Toronto; Tel. WA 3-8111.

HENDERSON, Donald J.; Wes'64; Res., Victoria Hosp., London, Ont.

HENDERSON, Donald R.; Tor'63; Res., Dept. of Rad., Toronto Gen. Hosp., Toronto 2, Ont.

HENDERSON, D. R.; c/o Chief Med. Off., Dept. of National Health and Welfare, 61 Green St., London W.1, England.

HENDERSON, Erland E.; 54 Bell St., New Glasgow, N.S.; Dal '55; DiagRad; Staff, Aberdeen Hosp., New Glasgow, N.S.; Tel. 752-8311.

HENDERSON, Gordon L.; 204 Medical Arts Bldg., Windsor, Ont.; 2524 Lincoln Rd. (res); Qns '53; F.R.C.S.(C), Urol; Tel. CL 2-7284.

HENDERSON, Hartley H.; 181 Queen St. N., Kitchener, Ont.; McG '52; Staff, Kitchener-Waterloo & St. Mary's Hosp's.; Tel. SH 3-7432.

HENDERSON, H. William; Parliament Bldgs., Toronto 5, Ont.; 9 Averdon Cres., Don Mills (res); Qns '47; D.Psy; Psy; Dir., Commun., Mental Health Serv., Dept. of Health (Ont.); Spec. Lect., U. of Toronto; Tel. EM 3-1211.

HENDERSON, I. Nigel; 207 Strathcona Med. Dental Bldg., 8225-105th St., Edmonton, Alta.; 10519-52nd St. (res); Middlesex Hosp. (U. of London, Eng.) '55; M.B., B.S.; MCGP; Tel. GE 3-5545.

HENDERSON, Ian W. D.; 1650 Cedar Ave., Montreal 25, P.Q.; 3925 University St. (res); Glasgow (Scot.) '50; FRCS(C), GenSurg; Assoc. Dir. University Surg. Clinic, Mtl. Gen. Hosp.; Tel. WE 7-6011, Ext. 691.

HENDERSON, James C.; 10 Montreal St., Kingston, Ont.; Qns'59; FRCP(C), Anaes.; Clin. Ass't., Dept. of Anaes., Queen's U.; Tel. 542-5609.

HENDERSON, James C.; Applewood Acres Plaza, 1077 Queen Elizabeth Way, Cooksville, Ont.; 354 Dixon Park Cr., (res); Glasgow (Scot.) '53; MB., Ch.B.; Staff, Queensway Gen. & South Peel Hosp's.; Tel. 277-4451.

HENDERSON, James W.D.; Sudbury Clinic, 130 Elm St. E., Sudbury, Ont.; 160 Wembley Dr. (res); Man'55; FRCP(C); IntMed; Chief-of-Med., Sudbury Mem. Hosp.; Tel. 673-7181.

HENDERSON, John A. M.; Royal Victoria Hosp., Montreal 2, P.Q.; Manchester (Eng.) '52; MRCP; FRCP(C), IntMed; Staff, Royal Victoria & Royal Edward Laurentian Hosp's.; Tel. VI 2-1251.

HENDERSON, John R.; Box 730, Salom Arm, B.C.; Tor'60; MCGP; Tel. 832-2191.

HENDERSON, J. Stanley; 1944 Abbott St., Kelowna, B.C. (res); McG '26; Retired.

HENDERSON, Marion M. (Whitelaw); 199 Havelock Ave., Winnipeg 8, Man.; Glasgow (Scot.) '51; Res. Phys., St. Boniface San., St. Vital; Tel. AL 3-1311.

HENDERSON, Milton H.; 8 Baby Point Terr., Toronto 9, Ont. (res); Tor '43; IntMed; Teach. Staff (OPD), Toronto Western Hosp.; Assoc. Med. Dir., Excelsior Life & The Cdn. Reassurance Co.; Tel. EM 6-9771.

HENDERSON, Murray C.; 68 Charlton Ave. W., Hamilton, Ont.; 397 North Shore W., Burlington (res); Wes '55; FRCS(C), OrthSurg; Tel. JA 8-8563.

HENDERSON, Reginald S.; Merigomish, N.S.; McG '24; Sr. Pens. Med. Exam., Camp Hill DVA Hosp.; Retired.

HENDERSON, Robert B.; P.O. Box 9, Queen Charlotte City B.C.; Dal '63; AMCGP; Admin., Queen Charlotte Islands Gen. Hosp.; Tel. 639-4437.

HENDERSON, Robert D.; Edinburgh (Scot.) '59; FRCS(C), GenSurg; Staff, Toronto Gen. Hosp., Toronto 2, Ont.

HENDERSON, Robert S.; 336 Professional Bldg., 10830 Jasper Ave., Edmonton, Alta.; London (Eng.) '41; MRCS(Eng.), LRCP(Lond.); FRCS (Eng.); FACS; FRCS(C), OrthSurg; Hd. Dept. of Orth Surg., Royal Alexandra Hosp.; Court. Staff, U. of Alta. & Gen. Hosp's.; Tel. 424-4352.

HENDERSON, Rowland E.; Ste. 500, 5300 Cote-des-Neiges Rd., Montreal 26, P.Q.; 5587 Queen Mary Rd. (res); McG'38; FAA Otol; Otol(P.Q.); Chief (Otol.), St. Mary's Hosp.; Tel. RE 3-3562.

HENDERSON, Roy H.; 143 Frederick St., Kitchener, Ont.; Tor '10; Ophth,Otol; Staff, Kit-chener-Waterloo & St. Mary's Hosp's.; Retired.

HENDERSON, Smilja (Markovie); Belgrade (Yugo.) '38; Psy; Staff, Ontario Hosp., St. Thomas, Ont.

HENDERSON, Stewart C.; Man'48; Res., Dept. of Rad., Ottawa Civic Hosp., Ottawa 3, Ont.

HENDERSON, W. Ewart; 35 E. Princess Ave., Chilliwack, B.C.; McG '20; Retired.

HENDERSON, Walter E.; 60 First St., Orangeville, Ont.; Wes '43; Surg. Staff, Lord Dufferin Hosp.

HENDIN, I. Donald; Ste 210, 8409-112th St., Edmonton, Alta.; 14103-75th Ave. (res); Man **'56; DABR; DiagRad; Staff, (Rad), University** of Alberta Hosp.; Instr., U. of Alberta; Tel. 439-0272.

HENDRICK E. Bruce; Ste. 1225, 123 Edward St., Toronto 2, Ont.; Tor '46; FRCS(C) NeurSurg; Chief NeurSurg., Hosp. for Sick Children; Cons. (NeurSurg.), Queensway Gen. Hosp. & Ont. Soc. for Crippled Children's Treatment Centre; Med. Dir., Bloorview Home Hosp. & School; Ass't. Prof. (Surg.), U. of Toronto; Tel. 364-7504.

HENDRIE, John; 3038 Dewdney Ave., Regina, Sask.; Glasgow (Scot.) '44; Staff Regina Gen. & Grey Nuns Hosp's.; Tel. 527-0166.

HENDRY, James; 103 Clark Dr., Brandon, Man. (res); Aberdeen (Scot.) '47; DPH; Path; Pathol., Brandon Gen. Hosp. & San. Bd. of Manitoba; Tel. PA 6-7421.

HENDRY, James H.; Tor'61; Res. (Anaes.), Vancouver Gen. Hosp., Vancouver 9, B.C.

HENEGHAN, Walter D.; National U. (Ire.) '47; D&TRad; Staff, Dept. of Rad., St. John's Gen. Hosp., St. John's, Nfld.; Tel. 8-0471.

HENGEL Lowell M.; 45 Ninth Ave., Cranbrook. B.C.; Alb '61; Att'd., Staff, St. Eugene Hosp.; Tel. 426-4231.

HENGEN, Herman A. P. J.; 614 Med. & Dental Bldg., Regina, Sask.; 269 Leopold Cres. (res); Tuebingen (Germ.) '35; GenSurg; Staff, Regina Gen. & Grey Nuns Hosp.; Tel. LA 3-2213; Abroad.

HENKEL, Gunther G.; 1506 Victoria Ave., Windsor, Ont.; Philipp U. (Marburg, Germ.) '50; Tel. 254-9956.

HENNEBERG, Carl C.; Manitoba Clinic 790 Sherbrook St., Winnipeg, Man.; 1176 Dorchester Ave. (res); Man '32; M.R.C.O.G.; Ass't (ObstGyn), Winnipeg Gen. Hosp.; Lect. (ObstGyn), U. of Manitoba; Tel. SP 4-6541.

HENNECKE, Thea-Auguste (Doepner); 1558 Ouellette Ave., Windsor, Ont.; Tuebigen (Germ.) '30; Otol.; Tel. 253-8057.

HENNEN, Brian K.; Qns'62; Ass't. Res. (Med.), Kingston Gen. Hosp., Kingston, Ont.

HENNESSY, David B.; Lafleche, Sask.; St. Bart's (London, Eng.) '54; MB., MRCS(Eng.); Tel. 472-5545.

HENNESSY, John P.; 295 Cedar St., Sudbury, Ont.; 32 Lakeview Dr. (res); Ott '55; Paed; Chief of Paed., & Chm. Poison Control Comm., Sudbury Gen. Hosp.; Chief, Dept. of Paed., Sudbury Mem. Hosp.; Tel. OS 4-7672.

HENNESSY, Robert D.; 365 St. Peter Ave., Bathurst, N.B.; Dal'59; MCGP; Tel. 546-2514.

HENNING Elwood T.; Box 220, Humboldt, Sask.; Sask '64.

HENNING, James N.; UBC'55; Path; Pathol., Henderson Gen. Hosp., Hamilton, Ont.; Tel. 389-4411, Ext. 261.

HENNINGER, James R.; UBC '54; Res., Vancouver Gen. Hosp., Vancouver, B.C.

HENRICH, Clarence A.; Courtright, Ont.; Wes '36; Dist. Coroner.

HENRY, Alexander F.; 151 Holland Ave., Ottawa 3, Ont.; 521 Westminster (res); Aberdeen (Scot.) '50; M.B., Ch.B.; MCGP; Active Staff, Ottawa Civic Hosp. & Ottawa Grace Hosp.; Tel. PA 8-3788.

HENRY, Anthony P.; Carmel Clinic, 124-1st Ave. N.W., Swift Current, Sask.; London (Eng.)'62; LRCP(Lond.).

HENRY, A. Taylor; 750 W. Broadway, Vancouver, B.C.; 1589 Mathews Ave. (res); Tor '24; GenSurg; Ass't. Clin. Prof. Surg., U. of British Columbia; Tel. TR 2-5288.

HENRY, Benjamin; 84 Brant Ave., Brantford, Ont.; 18 Riverview Dr. (res); Tor '43; MCGP; Tel. 752-0048.

HENRY, Edwin W.; Ste. 202, 1669 Victoria St., Prince George, B.C.; Qn's. U. (Belfast, Ire.) '48; FRCP(C), IntMed; Cons. (Med.), Prince George Reg. Hosp.; Tel. 564-7074.

HENRY, E. Ross; 1207 Douglas St., Victoria, B.C.; 2025 Lansdowne Rd. (res); Edinburgh (Scot.) '50; Anaes; Staff, Royal Jubilee Hosp.; Tel. EV 3-3261.

HENRY, E. W.; Tor'64; Res., Sunnybrook Hosp., Toronto, Ont.

HENRY, Francois; Centre Medical, St.-Urbain, 3875 rue St.-Urbain, Montreal 18, P.Q.; 696 Victoria Ave., Westmount (res); Lav '29; Ophth, Otol; Hd. Dept. Ophth, Hop. Hotel-Dieu; Assoc. Prof. (Ophth), U. of Mtl.; Tel. VI 5-9076.

HENRY, G. Arnold; 328 Medical Arts Bldg., 170 St. George St., Toronto, Ont.; Tor'31; FACS, Otol; Chief of Staff (Otol.), St. Michael's Hosp.; Ass't. Prof. (Otol.), Toronto U.; Tel. WA 3-1179.

HENRY, Goldwin G.; 853 Main St. E., Hamilton, Ont.; Tor'24; FICS; GenSurg; Surg., Hamilton Gen. Hosp.; Tel. LI 4-2294.

HENRY, Hugh G.; 700 Campbell Bldg., 1029 Douglas St., Victoria, B.C.; McG'58; DiagRad; Tel. 382-9104.

HENRY, John A.; Little Current, Ont.; Tor '43; Tel. 78.

HENRY, J. Stewart; 1414 Drummond St., Montreal, P.Q.; 3057 Cedar Ave. (res); McG '24; F.R.C.O.G., F.A.C.S., F.R.C.S.(C), ObstGyn; Hon. ObstGyn, Royal Victoria Hosp.; Hon. Att. Staff, Montreal Gen. Hosp.; Tel. VI 9-3383.

HENRY, John S. Jr.; 1414 Drummond St., Montreal, P.Q.; Apt. 5, 5570 Decelles Ave. (res); McG '49; F.A.C.S., F.R.C.S.(C), ObstGyn; Clin. Ass't. (ObstGyn.), Royal Victoria Hosp.; Dem. (ObstGyn.), McGill U.; Tel. AV 8-7911.

HENRY, Laurence; 30 Sheppard Ave. E.; Willowdale, Ont.; London(Eng.) '55; MRCS; LRCP; Tel. 222-5431.

HENRY, LeRoy William; 225 Maxome Ave., Bayview Uplands, Willowdale, Ont.; Tor'37; Tel. BA 1-2900.

HENRY, Reginald B.; Arundel, P.Q.; McG '25. Tel. 687-2971.

HENRY, Robert I.; Brantford Clin., 54 Brant Ave., Brantford, Ont.; London (Eng.)'55; MRCS; LRCP; D.ObstRCOG.

HENRY, Sebert G.; 720 Dundas St., London, Ont.; Wes '21.; M.C.G.P.; Tel. 439-6871.

HENRY Thos. R.; Box 1, Bracebridge, Ont.; Tor '04; Retired.

HENRY, Thos. W. E.; 10104-108th St., Fort Saskatchewan, Alta. (res); Dublin (Ire.) '10; Retired.

HENRY, Violet I. E.; 211 Belsize Dr., Toronto 7, Ont.; Tor '30; M.C.G.P.; Staff, Women's College Hosp.; Tel. HU 9-9141.

HENRY, William A.; Lacombe Medical Centre, Lacombe, Alta.; McG '24; Retired.

HENSCH, Clara; Prague (Czecho-Slovakia) '31; Res., Ontario Hosp., North Bay, Ont.

HENSHAW, J. Douglas; Commercial Street, Berwick, King's County, N.S.; Edinburgh (Scot.)'57; FRCS(Ed.); Surgeon, West Kings Memorial Hospital; Tel. Berwick 9227.

HENTELEFF, Paul D.; Osborne Medical Bldg., 190 Osborne St. N., Winnipeg 1, Man.; 172 Kingston Row, St. Vital (res); Man'56; MCGP; Staff, St. Boniface San. & Prov. V.D. Control; Tel. 774-9157.

HEON, Maurice H.; Ste. 520, 1500-18eme rue, Quebec 3, P.Q.; Lav'51; FACS; FRCS(C), NeurSurg; Staff (NeurSurg), Hop.-de-l'Enfant-Jesus & Laval U.; Tel. 525-4643.

HEPBURN, Allan L.; 33 Academy Med. Bldg., 1812-4th St. W., Calgary, Alta.; 903 Edinburgh Rd. S.W. (res); Alb '48; M.S., FACS, FRCS(C), NeurSurg; Chief of NeurSurg., Calgary Gen. & Cons. Holy Cross & Children's Hosp's.; Tel. 269-2008.

HEPBURN, Howard H., MC; McG '10; FACS, FRCS(Edin.), FRCS(C), GenSurg; NeurSurg; Admin. Workmen's Compen. Bd., Edmonton, Alta.; Retired.

HEPWORTH, R. Gordon; 5780 Cambie St., Ste. 200, Vancouver 15, B.C.; Leeds (Eng.)'50; **MRCS, LRCP; Urol; Urol., St. Vincent's Hosp.; Research Fell., Shaughnessy Hosp.; Tel. AM 1-2711.**

HEPWORTH, Sheina A. (MacLean); 1042-28th St. S., Lethbridge, Alta.; Leeds (Eng.) '51; M.B., Ch.B.; MRCS, LRCP.

HERBA, Milton J.; Ste. 70, 3550 Cote des Neiges, Montreal 25, P.Q.; Man'59; DiagRad; Staff, Montreal Gen. Hosp.; Tel. 937-9334.

HERBERT, Armand; Lav '62; Res., Hop. Hotel-Dieu, Sherbrooke, P.Q.

HERBERT; Frank A.; 202 Med. Arts Bldg., 11010 Jasper Ave., Edmonton, Alta.; 7624-153rd St. (res); Man'55; M.Sc.; FRCP(C); ABIM; IntMed; Staff Phys., U. of Alberta Hosp.; Chest Cons., Charles Camsell Hosp.; Instr., U. of Alberta; Tel. 424-2424.

HERBERTS, Edward D.; 1305 Fairmont Med. Bldg., 750 W. Broadway, Vancouver 9, B.C.; 3651 Osler St. (res); Man '48; Urol; Vis. Staff, Vancouver Gen., Mt. St. Joseph's, Burnaby Gen. & St. Vincent's Hosp's.; Tel. TR 6-4733; 874-0311.

HERBERTS, Lewis T.; Ste. 309, 713 Columbia St., New Westminster, B.C.; 831 Massey St. (res); McG '48; Urol; Chief Urol, Royal Columbian & St. Mary's Hosp's; Med. Legal, Path. to City of New Westminster; Tel. LA 1-3939.

HERBIN, Charles A.; Arichat, Richmond Co., N.S.; Dal '25.

HERBST, W. Lilli; (See SOLLBACH, W. Lilli).

HERDMAN, John P.; Med. Arts Bldg., East St., Sarnia, Ont.; Glen Douglas Dr. (res); Oxford (Eng.) '45; FRCS(Eng.); GenSurg; Tel. 344-7179.

HERENDA, Maria M.; Bonn (Germ.) '55; P.G., Women's College Hosp., Toronto, Ont.

HERGOTT, Clifford W.; Calwood Clinic, 11816-124th St., Edmonton, Alta.; 8404-139th St. (res); Alb '54; MCGP; Att'd. Staff, Edmonton Gen.; Court Staff, Royal Alexandra Hosp.; Tel. 454-6571.

HERGOTT, Jerome J. T.; Box 54, Ayton, Ont.; Qns'33; Tel. 665-7721.

HERINGER, Richard; 195 Laurier Ave. E., Ottawa 2, Ont.; 246 Range Rd. (res); Ott'52; DABS; FRCS(C); GenSurg; Active Staff, Ottawa Gen. Hosp.; Sr. Lect. (Surg.), Ottawa U.; Tel. 234-2602.

HERINGER, Thomas M.; 212 Medical Arts Bldg., Port Arthur, Ont.; Ott'55; MCGP.

HERJANIC, Barbara L. (Moss); Michigan (U.S.A.) '50; Staff, Saskatchewan Hosp., Weyburn, Sask.

HERJANIC, Marijan; Box 700, Saskatchewan Hosp., Weyburn, Sask.; Zagreb (Yugo.)'56; Psy.

HERLICH, Samuel; 770 Outremont Ave., Montreal, P.Q.; 6762 Legare (res); Geneva (Switz.) '55; M.C.G.P.; **Staff, Jewish Gen., Queen Elizabeth, Catherine Booth Jean Talon Hosp's.;** Tel. 277-1063.

HERMAN, Irving H.; 2404-29th Ave. S.W., Calgary, Alta. (res); Tor '35; FCCP (Pulm. Dis. & Bronchoesoph.); Staff, Baker Mem. San. and Div of T.B., Dept. of Health Alberta; Tel. BU 8-2311.

HERMAN, M. L.; 1573 Eglinton W., Toronto 10, Ont.; 59 York Downs Dr. (res); Tor '47; MCGP; Tel. RU 3-3314.

HERMAN, Morris; Box 784, Davidson, Sask.; McG '26; MCGP; Pres. Davidson-Union Hosp. Med. Staff; Tel. 567-2041.

HERMAN, Myer; 63 Alma St., Moncton, N.B.; 73 MacBeath Ave. (res); Dublin (Ire.) '39; BAO; DPH; Pt.-time, Ass't. Dir., Matern. & Child Health Div., Dept. of Health (NB); Tel. 389-9846.

HERMANN, J. Douglas; Qns '34; FACS; Gen-Surg.; ThorSurg.; Staff, Norway House Hosp., Norway House, Man.; Tel. 301.

HERMESH, Irmgard E.; (Kirschstein); Wilkie, Sask.; Hamburg (Germ.) '48; Staff, Wilkie Hosp.; Tel. 843-2678.

HERMITTE, Gordon L.; 350 MacKay St., Pembroke, Ont.; Sheffield (Eng.) '43; MCGP; **Active Staff, Pembroke Gen. & Cottage Hosp's.; Coroner, County of Renfrew & Dist. of Nipissing;** Tel. 732-3946.

HERNANDO, Honesto M.; Santo Tomas (Philipp.) '56; Staff, Manitoba San., Ninette, Man.

HERNANDO, Honrado M.; 566 College St., Toronto 4, Ont.; Manila (Philipp.) '52; Tel. 922-5419.

HEROLD, Walter; 611 Bloor St. W., Toronto 4, Ont.; Leipzig (Germ.) '31; Ophth; Tel. 533-0300.

HERON, John S.; 4 Spinney Ct., Don Mills, Ont. (res); Tor '43; F.A.C.A.; Anaes; Staff, Toronto East Gen. Hosp., Toronto; Tel. 465-7533.

HEROUX, J. Roger, F/L; Mon '64; RCAF Station Hosp., St. Jean, P.Q.

HERRERO, Jose-Mariano M.; Valladolio (Spain) '53; Res. (Rad.), Kingston Cancer Clinic, Kingston, Ont

HERRICK, Robert D. B.; Ste. 107, 422 Royal Ave., New Westminster, B.C. (res); Ire '08; Psy.

HERRING, S. Friend; Dal '53; MCGP; Staff, Coloner Belcher Hosp., Calgary, Alta.; Tel. AM 6-7001.

HERRIOT, Ethel (See McPhail).

HERRIOT, Ross A.; 3252 Lawrence Ave. E., Scarborough, Ont.; 42 Rossander Ct. (res); Tor '51; MCGP; Assoc. Staff, Toronto E. Gen. & Scar. Gen. Hosp's.; Tel. AX 3-7201.

HERSAK, Eduard; 2199 Bloor St. W., Toronto 9, Ont.; '50; Tel. 766-2182.

HERSCOVITCH, Oscar; 5757 Decelles Ave., Montreal, P.Q.; 385 Glengarry Ave., Mt. Royal (res); McG '43; MCGP; Clin. Ass't., Jewish Gen. Hosp.; RE 1-6916.

HERSEY, Lewis W.; 287 Queen's Ave., London, Ont.; 1563 McClure Dr. (res); Wes '56; DABA; FACS; Anaes; Staff, Victoria Hosp.; Court. Staff, St. Joseph's Hosp.; Dem. (Pharm.), & Anaes., U. of Western Ont.; Tel. GE 8-5143.

HERSEY, M. Lewis R.; 1522 Ouellette Ave., Windsor, Ont.; 2052 Lorraine Ave. (res); Edinburgh (Scot.) '38; Surg. Staff Grace, Metropolitan Gen. & Hotel Dieu Hosp's.; Tel. 253-4079.

HERSHFIELD, Charles S.; 612 Somerset Bldg., Winnipeg, Man.; 318 Matheson Ave. (res); Man. '29; M.C.G.P.; (ObstGyn), Victoria Hosp. Clin. Tel. WH 2-7012.

HERSHFIELD, Earl S.; 612-294 Portage Ave., Winnipeg 1 Man.; Man '58; FRCP(C), IntMed; Ass't. Phys., Central T.B. Clinic; Active Staff, Grace & Victoria Hosp's.; Tel. 943-5665.

HERSHFIELD, Harry; 612 Somerset Bldg., Winnipeg, Man.; 280 Atlantic Ave. (res); Man'22; MCGP; Tel. WH 2-7012.

HERSHFIELD, Louis S.; Ste. 202, 956 Main St., Winnipeg 4, Man.; 445 Henderson Hwy (res); London (Eng.) '29; M.R.C.S., L.R.C.P., M.C.G.P.; Staff, Victoria & Misericordia Hosp's.; Tel. 582-6163.

HERSHFIELD, Noel B.; Ire'59; FRCP(C), IntMed; Staff, Winnipeg Gen. Hosp., Winnipeg, Man.

HERST, Murray; Concord Med. Clinic, 895 Bloor W., Toronto 4, Ont.; 3255 Bathurst St. (res); Tor '55; MCGP; Tel. 537-2527.

HERST, Roslyn (Ezrin); Tor'58; Ass't. Haem., Dept. of Haem., Toronto Gen. Hosp., Toronto 2, Ont.; Clin. Teach. (Med.), U. of Toronto.

HERSTEIN, Archie; Ste. 517, 750 W. Broadway, Vancouver 9, B.C.; 5770 Cartier (res); Man'34; **DRCOG; MRCOG; ObstGyn; Staff, Grace Hosp.; Clin. Ass't. Prof., U. of British Columbia; Tel. RE 6-9855.**

HERTZBERG, Friedrich S., see SCHMITZ-HERTZBERG, Friedrich S.

HERTZMAN, Victor O.; Ste. 1310-750 W. Broadway, Vancouver 9, B.C.; 1075 W. 51st (res); Tor '42; FACP; FRCP(C), IntMed; Att'd. Staff, Vancouver Gen. Hosp.; Instr. (Med.), U. of British Columbia; Tel. TR 4-2511.

HERZOG, Melvin; Wes'65; Res., Sunnybrook Hosp., Toronto, Ont.

HESELTINE, Gilbert F. D.; 3744 Cote des Neiges Rd., Montreal 25, P.Q.; London (Eng.) '58; D.Psy; Psy; Staff Psy., Allan Mem. Inst., Montreal Gen. Hosp. & Lakeshore Gen. Hosp.; Tel. 933-7277.

HESELTINE, Jeanne M.; Watrous Medical Clinic, Box 160, Watrous, Sask.; St. Andrew's (Scot.)'44; Tel. 946-3388.

HESELTINE, John R.; Watrous Medical Clinic, **Box 160, Watrous, Sask.; Leeds (Eng.) '44; F.R.C.S. (Eng.); M.O.H., Watrous; Staff, Wat**rous Union Hosp.; Tel. 946-3388.

HESLAM, R. Murray; Ste. 415, 5025 Sherbrooke St. W., Montreal 28, P.Q.; McG '50; Assoc. Phys., Queen Elizabeth Hosp.; Tel. 484-8821.

HESLER, Richard F.; 334 Broad St. W., Dunnville, Ont.; Qns '47; MCGP; Tel. 774-5823.

HESLIN, D. James; 139 Colin Ave., Toronto, Ont.; Qns'59; DiagRad; Staff (Rad), Hosp. for Sick Children; Dem. (Anat.), U. of Toronto; Tel. 362-4461.

HESLIP, Patrick G.; Med. Arts Clinic, 51 Sixth St., S.E., Medicine Hat, Alta.; Alb '63; Staff, Medicine Hat Gen. Hosp.; Tel. 527-2281.

HESS, Charles D.; Medical Arts Bldg., 5 Young St., Hamilton, Ont.; 217 Roseland Cres., Pt. Nelson, Burlington (res); Tor '33; D & TRad; Tel. JA 7-1238.

HESS, Frederick W.; 3329 Bloor St. W., Toronto 18, Ont.; 1445 Larchview Trail, Pt. Credit (res); Tor '46; FRSOG(N), ObstGyn; Active Staff, Queensway Hosp.; Tel. BE 3-4413.

HESSION, Lloyd B.; 301 Med. Dental Bldg., **450 Central Ave., London, Ont.; 31 Foxbar Rd. (res); Wes'37; M.Sc.; FACP; FRCP(C); IntMed.; Chief-of-Med., St. Joseph's Hosp.; Clin.** Assoc. **Prof. (Med.), U. of Western Ont.; Tel.** GE 9-8181.

HETENYI, Caroline (Scossa); 516 Med. Arts Bldg., 170 St. George St., Toronto 5, Ont.; Budapest (Hung.) '47; Ph.D.; FRCP(C); IntMed; Cons., Women's College Hosp.; Clin. Teach. U. of Toronto; Tel. 923-7493.

HETENYI, Geza J.; Budapest (Hung.) '47; Ph.D. (Tor.); Assoc. Prof., Physiol., Best Inst., 100 College St., Toronto, Ont.

HETHERINGTON, Harold G.; Bayfield, Westmoreland Co., N.B.; Dal '52; Assoc. Staff, Sackville Mem. Hosp.; Memb. Westmoreland County Sub. Dist. Bd. of Health; Tel. 538-2476.

HETHERINGTON, Herbert H.; 22 John St., Brampton, Ont.; 10 Scott St. (res); Tor '31; MCGP; Staff, Peel Mem. Hosp.; GL 1-0429.

HETHERINGTON, Robert F.; 72 Johnson St., Kingston, Ont.; Tor '50; D.Phil (Oxon); FRCS (C), NeurSurg; Cons. (NeurSurg), Kingston Gen., Hotel Dieu, Can. Forces & Ont. Hosp's. & DVA (Eastern Ont.); Ass't. Prof. (Surg., I/C NeurSurg.), Queen's U.; Tel. LI 542-2208.

HETHERINGTON, Robert N.; 84 Broad St., Lunenburg, N.S.; Queens U. (Belfast, Ire.) '38; Anaes; Staff, Fishermen's Mem. & Dawson Mem. Hosp's; Bridgewater.

HETHRINGTON, Hagar; 262 St. Clair Ave. W., Toronto; 31 Yonge St. N., Richmond Hill; R.R. 1, Kleinburg (res); Tor '28; MRCP(Lond.); FRCP(C), IntMed; Chief, Med. Dept., Richmond Hill Hosp.; Hon. Cons., St. Michael's & Cons. Sunnybrook Hosp's., Toronto; Chief Med. Exam., Sun Life Assur. Co.; Tel. WA 2-1212; 884-5034.

HETU, Jean; Maniwaki, Co. Gatineau, P.Q.; Mon '33; D.P.H.; Staff, Health Unit.

HETU, Marc A.; St-Chrysostome, Cte. Chateauguay, P.Q.; Mon '65.

HEUCHERT, Carl H.; 204A Med. Arts Bldg., **335-339-6th Ave. S.W., Calgary, Alta.; 4331 Britania Dr. (res); Man'38; Tel. 262-4240.**

HEVENOR, Donald W.; 40 Harvey St., Tillsonburg, Ont.; 86 Lisgar Ave. (res); Wes'51; Tel. VI 2-3682.

HEVEY, George; 795 Ste. Anne, St. Hyacinthe, P.Q.; 2736 Girouard St. (res); Mon '41; Tel. PR 4-7505.

HEVEY, J. Guy.; 1400 Girouard, St-Hyacinthe, P.Q.; Mon '54; GenSurg; Tel. PR 4-6717.

HEWAT, Colin M.; Workmen's Comp. Bd., 1840 Lorne St., Regina, Sask.; London (Eng.)'50; Staff, Regina Gen. & Grey Nun's Hosp's.

HEWAT, William A.; 286 Pelham St., Lunenburg, N.S.; 284 Pelham St. (res); Dal '28; M.C.G.P.

HEWITSON, A. Gordon; 179 Lakeview Ave., Pointe Clair, P.Q. (res); Qns '51; Paed; Clin. Ass't., Montreal Children's Hosp.; Tel. 695-6345.

HEWITT, W. John; 30 Main St. W., Smith's Falls, Ont.; Qns '57; Tel. 283-3424.

HEWSON, John R.; McG'65; Res., Montreal Gen. Hosp., Montreal 25, P.Q.

HEWSON, Roy T.; Med. Clinic, Box 998, Merritt, B.C.; UBC '55; MCGP; Staff Merritt Valley Gen. Hosp.; Tel. 378-2286.

HEYDON, Gordon K.; 9909 Esplanade. Chemainus, B.C.; UBC'54; Staff, Chemainus Gen. Hosp.; Tel. 246-3141.

HEYLAND, Peter L.; Tor'55; Res., Hosp. for Sick Children, Toronto, Ont.

HEYNE, Michel; Mon '64; Int., Hop. Hotel-Dieu, Montreal.

HEYNEMAND, Robert; 2950 des Ormeaux, Montreal 5 P.Q.; Mon '52.

HEYWOOD, Peter M.; 92 Dunvegan Rd., Toronto 7, Ont. (res); Tor '48; IntMed.; Vol. Ass't. Toronto Gen. Hosp.; Tel. HU 5-9527.

HIBBERD, John C.; UBC'58; Res., Vancouver Gen. Hosp., Vancouver 9, B.C.

HICK, W. Bernard M.; 320 Second Ave. W., Prince Rupert, B.C.; Tor '51.

HICKERTY, John C.; Man'53; DiagRad; Staff, Dept. of Rad., St. Paul's Hosp., Saskatoon, Sask.

HICKEY, Malcolm A.; 3650 St. Urbain St., Montreal, P.Q.; McG '34; FACCP; Pulm.Dis & TB **(PQ); IntMed; Ass't. Med. Dir., Royal Edward Laurentian Hosp.; Dem., Dept's. of Med. & PH, McGill U.; Tel. VI 9-5201.**

HICKEY, F/L Michael; RCAF Station, Comox, B.C.; Wes'65.

HICKS, Elbert; Cumberland, B.C.; McG'10.

HICKS, A. R.; Princeton, B.C.; McG '43.

HICKS, David V.; Liverpool (Eng.)'60; FRCP(C), Psy; Staff, Hosp. for Mental & Nervous Dis., St. John's, Nfld.

HICKS, Denis O.; Heart's Content, Trinity Bay, Nfld.; Dublin (Ire.) '40.

HICKS, F. H.; Department of National Health & Welfare, c/o Regional Superintendant, European Region, Abroad.

HICKS, Floyd C.; Glencoe, Ont.; Wes '58; Court. Staff, Strathroy Gen., & St. Joseph's & Victoria Hosp's., London; Tel. 287-2616.

HICKS, Gerald F.; UBC'54; MCGP; Res., Shaughnessy Hosp., Vancouver, B.C.

HICKS, John P.; 126½ Penetang St., Barrie, Ont. 94 Johnson St. (res); London (Eng.)'54; MCGP; Active Staff, Royal Victoria Hosp.; Tel. 726-1301.

HICKS, Merlin W.; 337 Dufferin Ave., Sherbrooke, P.Q.; 400 Quebec St. (res); Tor '36; Urol; Tel. LO 9-2322.

HICKS, Roger B.; Box 1150, Terrace B.C.; Tor '50; D.O.T. Examiner; Tel. 613-5444.

HICKS, W. H.; 517-8th St. S., Saskatoon, Sask. (res); Qns '16; Retired.

HIDDLESTON, J. Mitchell; 306-1137 Bute St., Vancouver 5, B.C.; Glasgow (Scot.)'48; DRCOG; DA; Anaes; Staff (Anaes.), Lions Gate Hosp.; Vis. Staff, St. Paul's Hosp.; Tel. MU 5-8623.

HIDVEGI, Robert; 5211 Earnscliffe Ave., Montreal 29, P.Q.; Budapest (Hung.)'52; DiagRad; Att'd. Staff, Queen Elizabeth Hosp.

HIER, David; 5600 Randall, Cote-St.-Luc, Montreal, P.Q. (res); Dal'49; GenSurg; Chief Surg., Eastern Hosp., 3800 Radisson, Mtl. 5; Jrn. Clin. Assoc. Surg., Jewish Gen. Hosp.; Tel. 489-4553.

HIERZ, Otto; Vienna (Austria) '49; ObstGyn; Staff, Royal Victoria Hosp., Montreal, P.Q.; Tel. 842-1251.

HIGGIE, Clement B.; Vere Clinic, Herbert, Sask.; London (Eng.) '51.

HIGGIN, John R.; 21 Academy Med. Bldg., 1812-4th St. S.W., Calgary, Alta.; 1319 Craig Rd. S.W. (res); Alb'56; FRCS(C), ObstGyn; Tel. 266-2500.

HIGGINS, Donald J.; 107a Carmarthan St., Saint John, N.B.; Dal'62; Tel. 693-7482.

HIGGINS, Gerald L.; Box 1500, Sherwood Med. Clinic, Sherwood Park, Alta.; Bristol (Eng.)'52.

HIGGINS, Gordon K.; 300 Medical Arts Bldg., Calgary, Alta.; 6 Granville Cres. (res); Dal '51; FACP; IntMed.; Tel. 269-2561.

HIGGINS, H. Patrick; Ste 1204 Toronto Professional Bldg., 123 Edward St., Toronto Ont.; 10 Douglas Dr. (res); Tor '50; FRCP(C); IntMed; Dir., Radioisotope Lab. & Endocrin. Clinic, St. **Michael's Hosp.; Cons. (Endocrin.), Scarborough Gen. Hosp.; Clin. Instr., U. of Toronto; Tel. 364-1615.**

HIGGINS, J. Elton; 2432 Thorold Stone Rd., Niagara Falls, Ont.; Dal '51.

HIGGINS, John F.; 3040 Shelbourne, Victoria, B.C.; Cambridge (Eng.)'52; Active Staff, Royal Jubilee Hosp.; Tel. 604-2531.

HIGGINS, John I.; Third St., Englehart, Ont.; Wes '46; M.C.G.P.; Tel. LI 4-2321.

HIGGINS, Leonard M.; c/o Mr. G. H. Lelewin, 685 Indian Rd., Windsor, Ont.; McG'61; FRCS(C), ObstGyn.

HIGGINS, R. Brian; 96 Cobourg St., St. John, N.B.; Lav '53; GenSurg; Tel. 692-3526.

HIGGINS, William J.; P.O. Box E.5122. 24 Cochrane St., St. John's, Nfld. (res); Dal '43; D.R.; Ass't. (D. & TRad.), St. John's Gen. Hosp.; Vis Rad., St. Clare's Mercy, Grace San. & Hosp. for Mental Nervous Diseases; Tel. 8-0471.

HIGH, Joseph H.; Wes'64; Res., Ontario Hosp., 999 Queen St. W., Toronto, Ont.

HIGHMAN, Saul; 333 Wilson Ave. W.; Downsview, Ont.; Tor '46; DABS; GenSurg; Staff, North York Branson Hosp.; Tel. 636-3553.

HIGNELL, Bruce; 380-5655 Cambie St., Vancouver **15, B.C.; 1469 W. 39th (res); Man '51; MCGP; Vis. Staff, Vancouver Gen. & Grace Hosp's.; Tel. 261-8155.**

HILBORN, David J.; Newell Med. Clinic, Brooks, Alta.; Qns '60; Staff, Brooks Gen. Hosp.; Tel. 362-3301.

HILDEBRAND Alvin F., 4-6 Finch Ave. W., **Willowdale, Ont.; 27 Tollerton Ave., Willowdale (res); McG '49; Anaes; Staff, North York Branson Hosp.; Tel. 633-9420.**

HILDEBRAND, Eugene W.; 14 Freshwater Rd., St. John's, Nfld., 108 Freshwater Rd. (res); Coll. Med. Evangel. (Loma Linda, Calif.); '53; Tel. 578-3178. Abroad.

HILDEBRAND, Henry; Ste. 1417, 750 W. Broadway, Vancouver, B.C.; Man'56; FRCS(C), GenSurg; Staff, Crease Clinic, Essondale; Tel. 872-2312.

HILDERMAN, Frederick A.; 300 Med. Arts Bldg., 335-6th Ave. S.W., Calgary, Alta. Alb '62.; Tel. 269-2561.

HILDES, John A.; 204 Montrose St., Winnipeg 9, Man.; Tor '40; M.R. C.P. (Lond.) F.R.C.P.(C); IntMed; Assoc. Prof. & Dir. of Arctic Med. Research Unit, U. of Manitoba; Ass't. Phys., Winnipeg Gen. Hosp.; Tel. GR 4-9110.

HILDITCH, John R.; 807 O'Connor Dr., Toronto 16, Ont. Tor '62; AMCGP; Staff, Chest Clinic, Toronto East Gen. Hosp.; Tel. PL 7-1441.

HILIOPOULOS, D.; Fort Que'Appelle, Sask.

HILL, Albert G.; 110 Joicey Blvd., Toronto, Ont. (res); Edinburgh (Scot.) '30; Staff Dept. of Health, Parliament Bldgs.; Tel. EM 3-1211.

HILL, Alfred E.; McG '40; DTM&H; D.IntMed; FRCP(C), IntMed; Pension Med. Exam., Canadian Pension Comm., Shaughnessy Hosp., Vancouver 9, B.C.; Tel. 876-3211.

HILL, Arthur C.; 309 Dufferin Ave., Sherbrooke P.Q.; 305 Dufferin Ave. (res); Wes '32; M.C.-G.P.; Staff (Surg.), Sherbrooke & Hotel Dieu **Hosp's.; Chm., G.P. Dept., Sherbrooke Hosp.;** Tel. 562-4222.

HILL, Cameron G.; 5 Academy Med. Bldg., **1812-4th St. S.W., Calgary, Alta.; 2326 Longridge** Dr. (res); Tor'48; FACP; FRCP(C); IntMed; Active Staff, Calgary Gen. Hosp.; Dir., Dept. of Med., Rockyview Gen. Hosp.; Cons., Colonel Belcher Hosp.; Tel. AM 9-7455.

HILL, Carl E.; 22 Hillcrest Ave., Willowdale, Ont. (res); Tor '21; M.O.H., Twp. of North York. Retired.

HILL, Clarence E.; Ste. 110, 321 Bloor St. W., Toronto 5, Ont.; 112 Blythwood Rd. (res); Tor '08; F.A.C.S.; F.R.C.S.(C), Ophth; Cons. (Ophth), Toronto Gen. Hosp.; Surg., Tor. Eye Inst.; Tel. WA 2-1132.

HILL, Donald P.; 1543 Botsford St., Ott 8 (res); Ott '54; DABP; Pathol., Ottawa Gen. Hosp.; Assoc. Prof. (Path.), U. of Ottawa; Tel. CE 6-0333, Loc. 367.

HILL, Elizabeth (Troup); 11121-89th Ave., Edmonton, Alta. (res); Durham (Eng.) '44; DPH (Tor); MOH., Sturgeon Health Unit, St. Albert, Alta.; Tel. 599-7561.

HILL, F. Marguerite; 76 Grenville St., Toronto, **Ont.; 70 Weybourne Cres. (res); Tor '52; F.R.-** C.P.(C), IntMed; Chief (Med.), Women's College Hosp.; Assoc. Prof. (Med.), U. of Toronto; Tel. **WA 3-7381.**

HILL, Frederick W.; 3033 - 7th. St. S.W., Calgary, Alta.; Durham (Eng.) '44; DA; FARCS; Anaes; Anaes., Calgary Gen. Hosp.; Tel. AM 6-7541.

HILL, Georges B.; Box 70, Chilliwack, B.C.; UBC '51. Abroad.

HILL, George H.; 9919 Fairmont Dr. S.E., Calgary, Alta.; Guys Hosp. (London, Eng.)'58.

HILL, George R.; 9919 Fairmount Dr. S.E., Calgary, Alta.; London (Eng.)'58.

HILL, George U.; 33-1st St., Orangeville, Ont.; Dal '50.

HILL, G. V.; Port Elgin, N.B.; Dal '50; Staff, Sackville Hosp.

HILL, Ian R.; Med. Arts Clinic, 2125-11th Ave., Regina, Sask.; London (Eng.)'61; Tel. 523-0691.

HILL, James C.; 8 Peter St. S., Orillia, Ont.; 261 Mississaga St. W. (res; Tor '19; Staff, Orillia Soldiers' Memorial Hosp.

HILL, James R.; Sask '59; Path; Staff, Univer-sity Hosp., Edmonton, Alta.; Tel. 439-5911.

HILL, Jean M. (Macpherson); 131 Royal York Rd. N., Toronto 18, Ont. (res): Tor '48 Staff, Humber Mem. Hosp.; Tel. 249-8111.

HILL, J. Gilbert; Div. of Clinical Chemistry, Hosp. for Sick Children, Toronto 2, Ont.; McG'56; Ph.D.; Assoc. Biochem., Hosp. for Sick Children; Tel. 366-7242.

HILL, John W.; 3500 Eglinton Ave. W., Toronto 15, Ont.; 31 Abilene Dr. Islington (res); Tor '48; Ass't. Dir., Industrial Relations, Cdn. Kodak Ltd. Tel. BE 1-6154.

HILL, Joseph C.; 174 St. George St., Toronto, Ont.; 20 Bennington Heights Dr. (res); Tor '39; Ophth; Assoc., Dept. Ophth., U. of Toronto; Ophth. Staff, Sunnybrook & Sr. Ophth., Toronto Gen. Hosp's.; Tel. WA 2-4838.

HILL, Kenneth C.; 4900 Kingsway, Ste. 301, Burnaby, B.C.; 3326 W. 21st Ave. (res); Man '56; OrthSurg; Cons. (OrthSurg), Burnaby Gen. Hosp.; Tel. 434-1211.

HILL, Malcolm B.; 450 Central Ave., London, Ont.; R.R. No. 1, Hyde Pk. (res); Qns '40; DiagRad; Radiol., St. Joseph's Hosp.; Sr. Assoc. (DiagRad), U. of Western Ont.; Tel. GE 9-3271.

HILL, Marian E.; Neurolog. Unit, Toronto Gen. Hosp., Toronto 2, Ont.; Sask'58; FRCP(C), Neur; Ass't. Phys., Toronto Gen. Hosp.; Clin. Teach. (Med.), U. of Toronto; Tel. EM 6-8211, Loc. 2494.

HILL, Maurice G.; 102 Watson St., Sarnia, Ont.; 120 Norman (res); Wes '39; IntMed; Tel. 337-6773.

HILL, Mary M. (Gastle); 120 Watson St., Sarnia, Ont.; Wes '39; Chief Dept. of Anaes., St. Joseph's Hosp.; Med. Dir, North American Benefit Assoc.; Tel. ED 7-6773.

HILL, M. Quinn, Capt.; 2 Rialto Dr., Don Mills, Ont. (res); Birmingham (Eng.) '57; M.B., Ch.B.; MIL.

HILL, Muriel S.; 716 Medical Arts Bldg., 170 St. George St., Toronto 5, Ont.; 22 Nesbitt Dr. (res); Edingurgh (Scot.) '49; L.R.C.P., L.R.C.S., D.R.-C.O.G., M.R.C.O.G., F.R.C.S.(C), ObstGyn Assoc Chief of Staff (ObstGyn), Women's College Hosp.; Clin. Instr., U. of Toronto; Tel. WA 1-6341.

HILL, Nicholas P.; 73 Welland Ave., St. Catharines, Ont. (res); McG '25; Anaes; Staff (Anaes.), St. Catharines Gen. & Hotel Dieu Hosp's.; Court. Staff, Niagara Hosp., Niagara-on-the-Lake; Tel. 685-8311.

HILL, Norman C.; 421 Med. Arts Bldg., 404 Graham Ave., Winnipeg 1, Man.; Man'52; FRCS(C), NeurSurg; Active Staff, St. Boniface, Children's, Deer Lodge & Misericordia Hosp's.; Court. Staff, Wpg. Gen. Hosp.; Tel. WH 2-1019.

HILL, Robert H.; 5731 Granville St., Vancouver, B.C.; Oxford (Eng.)'50; FAAP; Paed; Att'd. Staff, Vancouver Gen. Hosp.; Med. Dir., Sunnyhill Hosp.; Instr. U. of British Columbia; Dir. Children's Arthritis Programme CARS; Tel. AM 1-4248.

HILL, Ronald; Ste. 103, 729 Bank St., Ottawa, Ont.; Ott'58; AMCGP; Court. Staff, Ottawa Civic Hosp.; Tel. 731-6247.

HILL, Ross O.; 342 Ballantyne Ave. N., Montreal W., P.Q.; McG '48; D & TRad; Rad., Lachine Gen.; Jr. Ass't. Rad., Mtl. Gen.; Cons. Rad., Northern Electric Co.; Tel. HU 9-2341.

HILL, W. H. Phillip; 549 Roslyn Ave., Westmont, Montreal, P.Q. (res); McG '34; F.R.C.P. (Lond.); F.A.C.P., F.R.C.P.(C), IntMed; Phys., Royal Victoria Hosp.; Cons. Phys. (IntMed), Queen Mary Vets' Hosp.; Assoc. Prof., Med., McGill U.; Tel. VI 2-1251. Loc. 525.

HILL, William H.; City Hall, Calgary, Alta.; McG '19; D.P.H. (Tor.); PH.

HILLIARD, Irwin M.; Ste. 342, 399 Bathurst **St., Toronto 2B, Ont.; 123 Sylvan Ave., Scarborough (res); Tor '36; FACP, FRCP(C), IntMed; Phys.-in-Chief, Toronto Western Hosp.;** Prof., U. of Toronto; Tel. 368-4016.

HILLIARD, Joseph R.; 92 College St., Toronto 5, Ont.; Tor'50; FRCP(C), IntMed.

HILLMAN, Donald A.; 2300 Tupper St., Ste. 1131, Montreal 25, P.Q.; McG '51; Ph.D.; Paed (P.Q.); Dir. (Endocrin.), Montreal Children's Hosp.; Ass't. Prof. (Paed.), McGill U.; Tel. WE 7-8511.

HILLMAN, Elizabeth (Sloman); 2300 Tupper St., Montreal, P.Q.; 130 Brock Ave. S., Montreal West (res); Wes '51; Paed; Dir., O.P.D., & Poison Con-trol Centre, Montreal Children's Hosp.; Lect. Fell. (Paed.), McGill U.; Tel. WE 7-8511; Loc 355.

HILLS, Wm. H.; 29 Thursfield Cres., Toronto 17, Ont.; Tor '29; Phys.. Don Jail & Mercer Reformatory.

HILLSMAN, John A. B.; 332 Medical Arts, **Winnipeg, Man.; 214 Waverley St. (res); Med. Coll. Virginia (U.S.) '25; GenSurg; Tel. WH 2-**1349.

HILLSON, Raymond F., Capt.; Station Hosp., CFB, Trenton, Ont.; UBC'65.

HILTON, Caleb T.; 1100 Bruce St., Port Alberni, B.C. (res); London (Eng.) '99; Retired.

HILTON, Donald R.; 3105-31st Ave., Vernon, B.C.; Qns'65.

HILTON, James H. B.; 1053 Carling Ave., Ottawa 3, Ont.; McG'38; FACP; FRCP(C), IntMed; Chief & Chmn., Dept. of Med., Ottawa Civic Hosp.; Prof. of Clin. Med., U. of Ottawa; Pres., Canadian Med. Protective Assoc.; Tel. 729-2511, Ext. 535.
HILTZ, Carl W.; 14 Martin St., Milton, Ont.; 403 Campbell Ave. (res); Tor'55; MCGP; **Phys., Ont. Schl. for Deaf; Plant Phys., Jas. H. Matthews Co.; Tel. TR 8-6793.**
HILTZ, J. Earle; Dal '34; D.P.H., F.C.C.P., Int Med (TB); Med. Sup., Nova Scotia San., Kentville; Cons. T.B., Nova Scotia Hosp. (Mental), Dartmouth, N.S.; Dir., Division T.B. Control Serv., Dept. of P.H., Prov. of Nova Scotia; Tel. 678-3251.
HILTZ, John W.; 120 Eglinton Ave. E., Toronto 12, Ont.; 234 Forest Hill Rd. (res); Qns '33; Ophth; Inpatients Staff, Hosp. for Sick Children; Cons., Sunnybrook Hosp.; Tel. 488-6987.
HIMAL, Harry; Ott'63; Int., Royal Victoria Hosp., Montreal 2, P.Q.
HIMEL, Calvin; 869 Jane St., Toronto 9, Ont.; Tor '58. Tel. 766-0934.
HIMEL, Henry A.; 2020 Bathurst St., Toronto, Ont.; 89 Lynnhaven Rd., North York (res); Tor '36; IntMed; Att. Phys., Sunnybrook & New Mt. Sinai Hosp's.; Assoc. Chief of Staff & Dir. Geriatric Studies, Baycrest Hosp. & Jewish Home for Aged; Tel. RU 2-3822.
HINCH, Robert O.; Minnedosa Med. Group, Minnedosa, Man.; Man'53; MCGP; Tel. 867-2722.
HINCHEY, E. John.; Montreal Gen Hosp., Montreal, P.Q.; Qns '59; M.Sc., FRCS(C), GenSurg; Assoc. Dir., McGill Univ. Surg. Clinic, Montreal Gen. Hosp.; Ass't. Prof. (Experim. Surg.), & Lect., Dept. of Physiol., McGill U.; Tel. 933-8934.
HIND, Duncan H.; 1116 Barton St. E., Hamilton, Ont.; Wes'54; Tel. 547-2544.
HINDMARSH, Arthur W.; 928B-8th St. E., Saskatoon, Sask.; 1219 Ewart Ave. (res); Sask '57; A.M.C.G.P.; Tel. 343-1619.
HINES, Arthur; Cheverie, N.S.; Dal '16.
HINES, Charles H.; Cheverie, N.S.; Dal '52.
HINES, J. Douglas; 14 Mabou Ave., Armdale, N.S.; Dal'56; Abroad.
HINES, Rodger M.; 226 Randal St., Oakville, Ont.; Tor '50; MCGP; Chief (GP), Oakville-Trafalgar Mem. Hosp.; Tel. VI 5-3828.
HINGSTON, Etheline E. H. (Brady); 4655 Bellevue Dr., Vancouver 8, B.C. (res); Dublin U. (Ire.) '45; D.C.H.; Part-time Med. Off., Metropolitan Health Committee; Tel. RE 8-2102.
HINGSTON, James; Ste. 106, 3195 Granville St., Vancouver 9, B.C.; 4655 Bellevue Dr., Van. 8 (res); Nat. U. (Cork, Ire.) '44; BAO (Rotunda); MRCP (Edin.); FRCP(I), DCH; FAAP; L.M. (Rotunda) Paed; Att'd. Staff & Phys. I/C Speech Disorder Clin., Van. Gen. Hosp.; Vis. Staff, St. Paul's, Grace and St. Vincent's Hosp's.; Clin. Instr. (Paed.), U. of British Columbia; Tel. RE 8-2102.
HINTON, George G.; 391 South St., London, Ont.; McG'55; DCH; FRCP(C), Paed; Ass't. Prof. (Paed.), U. of Western Ontario; Tel. 432-5261.
HINTON, Norman A.; 180 McMahon Ave., Kingston, Ont. (res); Qns'51; M.Sc.(Med.); D.Bact. (Lond.); Bact; Bact., Kingston Gen. Hosp.; Cons. Bact., Hotel-Dieu & Canadian Forces Hosp's; Prof. & Hd., Dept. of Microbiol. & Immunol., Queens. U.; Tel. 546-1731, Local 403.
HIPPOLYTE, Raoul; 45 Elm St. E., Sudbury, Ont.; 165 McNaughten (res); Haiti '44; A.I.C.S., GenSurg.; Tel. 673-5190.
HIPWELL, Robert E.; 40 Coldwater St., Orillia, Ont.; 111 Peter St. N. (res); Tor '23; ObstGyn; Staff, Orillia Soldiers' Memorial Hosp.; Instr.. Nurses Training School.
HIPWELL, William T.; 170 College St. W., Belleville, Ont.; Tor'54.
HIRAKI, George Y.; 505 Med. Arts Bldg., 170 St. George St., Toronto 5, Ont.; Tor'53; FACS; FRCS(C), GenSurg; Active Staff, Women's College Hosp.; Att'd. Staff, O.P.D., Toronto Western Hosp.; Active Staff Surg., Doctor's Hosp.; Clin. Teach. Surg., U. of Toronto; Tel. 922-3362.
HIRSCH, Doris L. B.; 5855 Inglewood Dr., Halifax, N.S.; Johns Hopkins (USA) '50; Psy; Lect- (Psy), Dalhousie U.; Tel. 2-4406.
HIRSCH, Solomon; Med. Arts Bldg., 5880 Spring Garden Rd., Halifax, N.S.; 5855 Inglewood Dr. (res); Dal '49; Psy; Assoc. Psy., Victoria Gen. Hosp.; Cons. Psy., Camphill Hosp.; Prof. (Psy), Dalhousie U.; Tel. 422-6394.
HIRSCH, Werner P.; Brandon Med. Clinic, Box 280, Brandon, Man.; London (Eng.)'40; MRCS, LRCP; FRCS(Ed.), MRCOG; FACS; ObstGyn; FACOG; Chief of ObstGyn., Brandon Gen. Hosp.; Staff, Assiniboine Hosp.; Tel. PA 9-6444.
HIRT, Norman B.; 720 W. Broadway, Vancouver 9, B.C.; 3778 Hudson St., Van. 9 (res); Qns '46; Psy; Att'd. Staff, Vancouver Gen. Hosp.; Clin. Instr. (Psy), U. of British Columbia; Tel. TR 4-4636.
HIRTE, Wolfgang E.; University Hosp., Saskatoon, Sask.; 29 Moxon Cr. (res); Hamburg (Germ.) '46; DTM; IntMed; Sr. Assoc., Cancer Clinic & Active Staff University Hosp.; Court. Staff, Saskatoon City & St. Paul's Hosp's.; Clin. Teach. (Med.), U. of Sask.; Tel. 652-3850.
HIRTLE, Lloyd R.; 834 Ralston Bldg., Hollis St., Halifax, N.S.; 7128 Bayers Rd. (res); Dal'49; Med. Supt., National Health & Welfare, Atlantic Zone; Tel. 454-7577.
HIRTLE, Waldo E.; 10 Lansdowne St., Sackville, **N.B.; 14 Park St. (res); Dal '41; M.C.G.P. Tel. 536-0326.**
HISCOCK, R. James; St. Mary's Med. Clinic, Church St., St. Mary's, Ont.; Wes '61; AMCGP; Active Staff, Dept. of G.P., St. Mary's Mem. Hosp.; Court, Staff, Stratford Gen. Hosp.; Tel. 284-3450.
HISCOX, James L.; Wes'65; Res., Hosp. for Sick Children, Toronto 2, Ont.
HISCOX, Paul E.; Tor'59; FRCS(C), Ophth; Staff, Sunnybrook Hosp., Toronto, Ont.
HISEY, Lloyd G.; 4500 Sherbrooke St. W., Westmount, Montreal 6, P.Q. 4855 Cote St. Luc Rd. (res); Tor'41; D.Psy.; Psy(P.Q.(; **Assoc. Psy., Royal Victoria Hosp.; Ass't. Prof. (Psy.),** McGill U.; Registrar, Allen Mem. Inst. of Psy.; Cons. (Psy.), Civil Aviation, Cdn. Dept. of Transport; Tel. 937-7044.
HITCH, Donald A.; McGregor Clinic, 250 Main St. E., Hamilton, Ont.; R.R. 1, Ancaster, Ont. (res); Wes '49; Otol; Staff (ENT), Hamilton Gen. Hosp.; Tel. JA 7-2711.
HITCHIN, Edward; 540 Phys. & Surg. Bldg., 8409-112th St., Edmonton, Alta.; Alb '34; GenSurg; Lect. (Surg.), U. of Alberta.
HITESMAN, Robert J.; 405 Norlyn Bldg., 309 Hargrave St., Winnipeg 2, Man.; 62 Niagara St. (res); Man '33; Tel. WH 2-3822.
HITSMAN, Elden H.; Strasbourg, Sask.; Man '35; Tel. 725-3200.
HITSMAN, J. S., Col.; 1 Cdn. Base Med. Units, CAPO 5050, CAF Europe; Qns'43; IntMed; Abroad.
HIVON, Jules; Upton, Co. Bagot, P.Q.; Lav '57; Tel. 64.
HIVON, Marcel; 3414 MGR Gauthier, Quebec 5, P.Q.; Lav'51.
HJERTAAS, Orville K.; Community Clinic, 110-8th St. E., Prince Albert, Sask.; 530-20th St. W. (res); Man'42; FRCS(Edin.); Tel. 763-6466.
HNATKO, Stephen I.; 203 Professional Bldg., 10830 Jasper Ave., Edmonton, Alta.; Alb'55; MA(Bact); FASCP(Clin.Path); Bact; Med. Dir., Med. Bact. & Hd. Bact., Misericordia Hosp.; Cons. Bact., Royal Alexandra Hosp.; Grande Prairie & High Prairie Hosp's.; Lect. Med. Bact., U. of Alberta; Lect. Med. Bact. NAIT(Radiol); Chmn. & Inf. Control Officer, Misericordia Hosp.; Tel. 424-0061.
HNATUIK, John N.; Provost Medical Centre, Provost, Alta.; Alb '56; M.C.G.P.
HO, Ching; 566 Osborne St., Winnipeg 13, Man.; Hong Kong'53; DABS; FRCS(C), GenSurg; Active Staff, Victoria Gen. Hosp.; Assoc. Staff, Misericordia Hosp.; Tel. 452-8600.
HO, Cosmas V.; 14 Freshwater Rd., St. John's, Nfld.; Taiwan (Formosa)'61; MCGP.

HO, Edmund; 116 Elm St. E., Sudbury, Ont.; Ott '60; DPH; Staff, Sudbury Gen., Sudbury Mem. & St. Joseph's Hosp's.; Tel. 675-6401.
HO, Francis C.; 3268 Main St., Vancouver B.C.; UBC '61; AMCGP.
HO, Helena H.; McG'65; Res., Hosp. for Sick Children, Toronto 2, Ont.
HO, Julia W.; 10 Cobham Cr., Toronto 16, Ont.; Canton (China)'53; DMR(Tor); DiagRad.
HO, Thomas J.; 102 Med. Bldg., Prince Albert, Sask.; 124—19th St. E. (res); Rush Med. Coll., Chicago (U.S.) '36; FICA; DiagRad; Rad., Victoria Hosp. & Holy Family Hosp.; Tel. 763-8595.
HO, Wan Cheun; 802 East Hastings St., Vancouver 4, B.C.; Hong Kong (China)'58; GenSurg.
HO, Yau-Cheung; 150 Yardley Ave., Toronto 16, Ont.; Lingnan (China) '51; MCGP; Tel. PL 9-3911.

HOAG, S. R. R.; 1812 Buchanan Ave., Niagara Falls, Ont.; 2002 Lundy's Lane (res); Qns '43.

HOAKEN, Paul C. S.; 1050 Johnson St., Kingston, Ont.; Tor'57; FRCP(C), Psy; Staff, Kingston Gen. Hosp.; Ass't. Prof. Psy., Queen's U.; Tel. 546-3841, Ext. 348.

HOAR, Zella E.; Box 401, Edmonton, Alta. (res); Alb'46; Anaes; Staff, University Hosp.; Tel. 439-5911.
HOARE, Delbert S.; 250 Lawrence Ave. W., Toronto 12, Ont.; 1253 Don Mills Rd., Don Mills (res); Tor '28; Paed; Paed. Staff, St. Michael's Hosp.; Staff (OPD), Hosp. or Sick Children; Clin. Instr., U. of Toronto; Tel. RU 1-1474.
HOBAN, John J.; Ire. '56; Jr. Intn., St. Joseph's Hosp., Toronto, Ont.

HOBBS, Carolynne A.; Wes'61; D.Psy; Psy; Staff, Toronto Psychiatric Hosp., Toronto, Ont.
HOBBS, Frederick S.; 925 W. Georgia St., Vancouver, B.C.; 5747 Newton Wynd (res); McG '32; FACS; ObstGyn.; Hon. Cons., Staff, Van. Gen. Hosp.; Att'd. Staff, Grace Hosp.; Gyn., Shaughnessy Hosp.; Clin. Instr., U. of British Columbia; **Tel. MU 5-9658.**
HOBBS, G. Edgar; Med. Science Bldg., U. of Western Ontario, London, Ont.; Tor '33; MPH (Mich.); FRCP(C); NeurPsy; Cons. Psy., Westminster DVA & Victoria Hosp's; Prof. & Hd., Dept. of Psy. & Prev. Med. U. of Western Ont.; Tel. GE 9-1681.
HOBBS, Kenneth C.; Whitby Plaza, 65 Brock St. S., Whitby, Ont.; 112 Centre N. (res); Wes'55; Tel. 668-5835.
HOBBS, M. E.; Millbrook, Ont.; Tor '32; M.C.-G.P.
HOBBS, William G. R.; Gainsborough, Sask.; Bristol (Eng.)'56; MRSH (Eng.); MCGP; FAGS; FRSH; Staff, Gainsborough Hosp.; Tel. 40.
HOBBS, William K.; Tor '50; MPH; ABPM; Res., Toronto East Gen. Hosp., Toronto, Ont.
HOBSON, Arthur C. S., MC; 314 S. Railway St., Medicine Hat, Alta.; 1541-11th Ave. N.E. (res); London (Eng.) '39; B.S. (Lond), M.D., MRCS (Eng.); MRCP (Lond.); IntMed; Active Staff, Medicine Hat Gen. Hosp.; Tel. 527-4461.
HOBSON, George C.; 5885 Arbutus St., Powell River, B.C.; Man'54; GenSurg.
HOBSON, Jim D.; Box 310, Sechelt, B.C.; UBC '55.
HOBSON, Kenneth W.; 170 Woolwich St., Guelph, Ont.; 42 Lyon Ave. (res); Tor '52; FRCS(C), GenSurg; Tel. TA 2-0030.
HOBSON, Walter J.; Calabogie, Ont.; Tor '21; M.O.H.; Tel. 19.

HOCHGLAUBE, Jacques; UBC '62; Jr. Intn., Vancouver Gen. Hosp., Vancouver 9, B.C.
HOCKLY, Garth; Vanderhoof, B.C.; Cape Town (S. Africa)'61; Tel. 567-2361.
HODD, Donald G.; Harrington Harbour, P.Q.; Tor '25; M.O., Harrington Hosp.
HODD, Ralph N.; Qns'61; Res., Kingston Gen. Hosp., Kingston, Ont.
HODES, Harold; 1530 Albion Rd., Rexdale, Ont.; Queen's U. (Belfast, Ire.)'62; Staff, Humber Mem. Hosp.; Tel. 741-1622.
HODGE, Kenneth E.; 943 Scenic Dr., Hamilton, Ont. (res); Guy's H. (London, Eng.) '47; FRCP (C), DiagRad; Radiol., Chedoke Gen. & Children's Hosp. Tel. 385-5341.

HODGINS, Burton A.; Tor '24; Staff, Shute Inst., 10 Grand Ave., London, Ont.; Tel. 432-1884.
HODGINS, Emerson L.; 1000 Richmond St., London, Ont.; Tor '03; M.R.C.S.(Eng.), F.R.C.S. (Ed.); Dist. Coroner.
HODGINS, Gladys W.; 930 Diamond Rd., Richmond, B.C.; UBC '61.
HODGINS, Kenneth W.; Hosp. Services Branch, Dept. of Public Health, Regina, Sask.; Man'61; DHA; Dir. Hosp., Programs & Standards; Tel. 523-0661.
HODGINS, Thomas E.; 211 George St., Sarnia, Ont.; 800 Lakeshore Rd. (res); Wes '51; M.Sc., DABS, FRCS(C), GenSurg; Tel. DI 4-1325.
HODGKINSON, John R., F/L; Tor'61; CFMS Clinic, Goose Bay, Labrador.
HODGKISS, William R.; 1250 Victoria Park Ave., Toronto 13, Ont.; 132 Parkview Hill Cres. (res); Tor '43; M.C.G.P.; Assoc. Staff, Toronto East Gen. Hosp.; Chief, G.P. Dept., Scarborough Gen. Hosp.; Tel. PL 5-0500.
HODGSON, Gordon H.; Durham (Eng.) '54; M.B., B.S., Res., Toronto Western Hosp., Toronto 2B, Ont.
HODGSON, Murray R.; Pincher Creek Assoc. Clinic, Box 549, Pincher Creek, Alta.; Man'42; MCGP; Tel. 627-3322.
HODGSON, Roy O.; 305 Canada Bldg., Saskatoon, Sask.; 1207 Elliott St. (res); Tor '11; Ophth, Otol; Chief of Ophth. Otol., Saskatoon City Hosp.; Tel. 244-6051.
HODGSON, W. Morley; Box 880, Claresholm, Alta.; Alb '34; Tel. 235-3434.

HODJERA, Branislava M. (See COP-HODJERA)

HODKINSON, E. Spencer; Dingwall Clinic, Box 3004 Dryden, Ont.; 172 Van Horne (res); Qns '61; AMCGP; **Att'd. Staff, Dryden Dist. Gen. Hosp.; Tel. 223-2258.**
HODSON, Douglas S.; 985 Kingsway Dr., Burlington, Ont.; Tor '61; Tel. NE 4-4849.
HODSON, W. Alan; Man '59; Res., Children's Hosp., Winnipeg 3, Man.
HOE, Grant K.; 541 Professional Bldg., Edmonton, Alta.; 10327-135th St. (res); Man '50; Anaes; Att'd. Staff, Misericordia Hosp.; Tel. HU 8-5779.
HOEBERECHTS, Paul M.; 74 Chestnut Park, Toronto 5, Ont.; Amsterdam (Neth.) '37; F.N.-N.S.; NeurSurg; Staff, Scarborough Gen. Hosp., Lockwood Clin. & Oshawa Clin.; Tel. WA 2-4526.
HOFFER, Abram; University Hosp., Saskatoon, Sask.; 1027 University Dr. (res); Tor '49; Ph.D. (Minn.); Psy; Dir. Psy Research Dept., Public Health; Assoc. Prof. (Research Psy), U. of Saskatchewan; Tel. 242-7641.
HOFFMAN, Cecil M.; Rm. 5510, East Blk., Parliament Bldgs., Toronto 5, Ont.; 319 Rumsey Rd. (res); Tor '31; DPH; Dir., Maternal & Child Health Br., Ont. Dept. of Health; Tel. EM 3-1211.
HOFFMAN, D. V.; Port Arthur Clinic, 194 Court St. N., Port Arthur, Ont.; Tor'65.

HOFFMAN, Elsie M.; (see Crawford).

HOFFMAN, Harold J.; Ste. 1225, 123 Edward St., Toronto 2, Ont.; Tor '56; B.Sc.(Med.); FRCS(C); NeurSurg; Ass't. Surg., Hosp. for Sick Children; Cons. NeurSurg., Sunnybrook Hosp.; Clin. Teach. (Surg.), U. of Toronto; Tel. EM 6-5546.
HOFFMAN, Jack; Tor '59; FRCS(C), GenSurg; Staff, Kingston Gen. Hosp., Kingston, Ont. Abroad.
HOFFMAN, Martin M.; Royal Victoria Hosp., Montreal, P.Q.; 608 Victoria Ave., Wesmount (res); McG '47; Ph.D. (Experim. Med.); Int Med (P.Q.); Assoc. Phys., Royel Victoria Hosp.; Assoc. Prof. (Med.), McGill U.; Tel VI 2-1251.
HOFFMAN, Oscar; Apt. 405, 99 Cartier St., Ottawa 4, Ont. (res); Tor '39; Chief, Med. Rehab. Div., Dept. of National Health & Welfare; Tel. CE 2-8211.
HOFFMAN, Shirley G.; 364 Woolwich St., Guelph, Ont.; Tor. '54; Tel. 822-3162.
HOFFMANN, Meinrad W.; Ile-a-la-Crosse, Sask. (res); Breslau (Germ.)'44.
HOFFMANN, Norbert L; 3249 Montague St., Regina, Sask. (res); Germ '34; Ass't. Path, Regina Gen. Hosp.; Tel. LA 2-1811, Ext. 346.

HOFMANN, William G.; 1124 Medical-Dental Bldg., 925 W. Georgia St., Vancouver 1, B.C.; 1168 Pendrell St. (res); Ott'51; Tel. MU 5-0046.
HOFMANN, Rudolph; 6319 Bowness Rd. N. W., Calgary, Alta.; 1342 Hamilton St. N.W., Calgary (res); Vienna (Austr.)'54; Staff, Calgary Gen., Grace, Children's & Auxiliary Hosp's; Tel. BU 8-6711.
HOFSTADER, Emeric L.; Ste 210, 3000 Lawrence Ave. E., Scarborough, Ont.; 39 Bendale Blvd. (res); Dal '53; IntMed; Med. Staff, Scarborough Gen. Hosp.; Tel. 291-1129.
HOFSTADER, Sophie L.; 1126 Warden Ave., Scarborough, Ont.; Dal.'56; MCGP; Active Staff, Scarborough Gen. Hosp.; Tel. PL 7-8171.
HOGAN, J. J.; 85 Brockville, Smith's Falls, Ont.; Qns '42; Anaes.; Tel. 283-1414.
HOGAN, John T.; 1005 Main St., Sweetsburg, P.Q.; McG'56; MCGP; Indust. Phys., Bruck Mills, RCA Victor & Tupperware Plastics; Tel. 263-2929.
HOGAN, Martin W.; Dal'65; Ass't. M.O., Cottage Hosp., Placentia, Nfld.; Tel. 226-2013.
HOGAN, T. Guy; Dublin (Ire.)'60; ObstGyn; Staff, Mtl. Gen. Hosp., Montreal 25, P.Q.
HOGARTH, Barbara E. (Hossie); 102 Med. Arts Bldg., 101 May St. S., Fort William, Ont.; 705 Linwood Cr. (res); UBC '57; Active Staff, McKellar Gen. Hosp. Court. Staff, Port Arthur Gen. & St. Joseph's Hosp's; Cons. Derm., Fort William San.; Tel. MA 2-1834. Retired.
HOGARTH, Frederick S.; Apt. 202, 55 Oakmount Rd., Toronto 9, Ont.; Tor'49; Pensions Med. Exam., W.C.B.; Tel. 767-0971.
HOGARTH, R. Walter; Med. Arts Bldg., Fort William, Ont.; 705 Linwood Cr. (res); Wes '54; Urol; Active Staff, McKellar Gen. Hosp.; Court. Staff, Port Arthur Gen. & St. Joseph's Hosp's.; Staff, Fort William San.; Tel. MA 2-1834.
HOGARTH, Walter P.; 102 Med. Arts Bldg., Fort William, Ont.; 327 Syndicate (res); Tor '20; FACS; Urol; Urol. McKellar Gen. Hosp.; Cons. Urol., Fort William San. & St. Joseph's Gen. Hosp., Pt. Arthur; Tel. MA 2-1834.
HOGARTH, W. Jean; 208 Toronto Western Med. Bldg., 25 Leonard Ave., Toronto 2B, Ont.; Apt. 1407, 500 Avenue Rd. (res.); Tor '51; FRCP(C); IntMed; O.P. Teach. Staff, Toronto Western Hosp.; Clin. Teach. (Med.), U. of Toronto; Tel. 368-2100.
HOGG, Frederick, R.; 2187 Harcourt Cres., Applewood Acres, Ont.; Tor '50; DiagRad; Staff, Toronto E. Gen. Hosp.; Tel. 461-8272.
HOGG, Georgina; 1021 Wellington Ave., Winnipeg, Man.; Man '45; Path; Ass't. Path., Wpg. Gen. Hosp.; Lect. Path., U. of Manitoba; Tel. SP. 5-1786.
HOGG, James C.; Man'62; Res. (Path.), McGill U., Montreal, P.Q.
HOGG, J. H. Scott; George St., Arthur, Ont.; Isabella St. (res); Tor '35; Tel. 848-2021.
HOGG, Robert J.; 15496 North Bluff Rd., White Rock, B.C.; 664 Buena Vista (res); Wes '42; MCGP; Tel. 531-5595.
HOGG, Silva (Kuhar); Ljubljana (Yugo.)'57; Res., Toronto Gen. Hosp., Toronto 2, Ont.
HOGG, William A.; 1192 Newell St., Sarnia, Ont. (res); St. Andrews (Scot.) '48; DAB PrevMed; Staff, Sarnia Gen. & St. Joseph's Hosp's.; Reg. Phys., Imperial Oil Ltd.; Tel. 337-8221.
HOGG, William F.; 74 Hughson St. S., Hamilton, Ont.; Wes'57; Psy.
HOGGARTH, W. Bruce; Acadian Apts., 153 Nepean St., Ottawa 4, Ont.; Wes '35, DPH; Staff, Dept. of Health, Ottawa.
HOGUE, Guy; Ste 406, 2950 Masson, Montreal 36, P.Q.; Mon '59; A.M.C.G.P.
HOHN, Emil O.; 11511-78th Ave., Edmonton, Alta. (res); Guy's Hosp. (London, Eng.) '42; M.R.C.S.(Eng.), L.R.C.P.(Lond.); Assoc., Prof. (Physiol.), U. of Alberta; Tel. GE 9-8721, Ext. 449.
HOHN-SARIC, Rudolph; Austria '54; Res., Verdun Protestant Hosp., Montreal, P.Q.
HOLBROOK, J. David; 674 Broadview Ave., Toronto 6, Ont.; 187 Cottingham St., Tor. 7 (res); Tor '62; Court. Staff, Wellesley & Grace Hosp's.; Tel. HO 3-1323.
HOLBROOK, Robert H.; 24 Undermount Ave., Hamilton, Ont.; Qns '40; Anaes; Staff, Hamilton Gen. Hosp.; Court. Staff, St. Joseph's Hosp.; Tel. JA 7-0271.
HOLDCROFT, Donald J.; Havelock, Ont.; Qns '24.
HOLDEN, Fred. A.; 1805 Morgan Ave., Saskatoon, Sask. (res); London (Eng.) '44; D. Bact. (Lond.); Ass't. Bact., University Hosp.; Lect. (Bact.), U. of Sask.; Tel. CH 2-7641.
HOLDEN, George P.; Russell Medical Clinic, Cabri, Sask.; Manchester (Eng.)'48; Tel. 584-2286.
HOLDEN, John P. N.; 33 Regent St., Ottawa, Ont.; 267 Second Ave. (res); Tor '39; M.C.-G.P.; Tel. 235-2725.
HOLDEN-QUINLAN, Helen M.; Tor '40; F.C.-C.P., IntMed; Ass't. Supt., Nova Scotia San, Kentville, N.S.; Tel. 678-3251.
HOLLAND, Clyde W.; Ste. 1007, 5959 Spring Garden Rd., Halifax, N.S.; Dal'23; FACP, FRCP(C), IntMed; Sr. Phys., Victoria Gen. Hosp.; Cons. Phys., N.S. Hosp., Dartmouth; Prof. Clin. Med., Dalhousie U.; Tel. 2-4406.
HOLLAND, Eleonore (Gruenwald); 751 King St. W., Kitchener, Ont.; 1155 Queens Blvd. (res) Wes '57; Staff, St. Mary's & Kitchener-Waterloo Hosp's.; Tel. SH 3-4222.
HOLLAND, George A.; 1610 Pine Ave. W., Montreal 25, P.Q.; 65 Allan Pt., Dorval & St. Sauveur-des-Monts (res); McG '31; FRCS(C), GenSurg; Assoc. Surg. & Cons. (Vasc. Surg.), Mtl. Gen.; Surg. Cons. U. Health Serv. & Ass't. Prof. (Surg.), McGill U.; Tel. 937-4781, Loc. 227.
HOLLAND, James G.; Dal'63; Res., Victoria Gen. Hosp., Halifax, N.S.
HOLLAND, John B.; Ayr. Ont; London (Eng.) '51; M.R.C.S., D. Obst., R.C.O.G.; Tel. 632-7292.
HOLLAND, Lieselotte (Brown); Dal'54; Psy; Sr. Psy., Nova Scotia Hosp., Dartmouth, N.S.
HOLLAND, L. Gilbert; 6905 Tupper Grove, Halifax, N.S. (res); Dal '35; Ophth, Otol; Staff, Camp Hill (DVA) Hosp.; Tel. 423-1371.
HOLLAND, T. Edward; ED. QHS; 632 Med. Arts Bldg., 404-406 Graham Ave., Winnipeg, Man.; 172 Oxford St. (res); Man'29; FICS, FRCS (Edin.), FRCS(C), GenSurg; Cons. Surg., Deer Lodge DVA Hosp.; Lect. (Surg.), U. of Manitoba; Distr. M.O. CPR; Med. Cons. Manitoba Hosp. Comm.; Tel. WH 3-8579.
HOLLAND, William G.; 305 King St. W., Kitchener, Ont.; 190 Lester St., Waterloo (res); London (Eng.) '50; MRCS; LRCP(Eng.); DRCOG(Eng.); DA(Eng.); Anaes; Tel. 744-6551. Abroad.
HOLLAND, William H.; 751 King St. W., Kitchener, Ont.; 1155 Queen's Blvd. (res); Utrecht (Neth.) '50; M.C.G.P.
HOLLANDS, Raymond H.; West'65; Res. (Obs. Gyn.), University Hosp., Edmonton, Alta.
HOLLANDS, Wilbert W.; 531 Woodrowe Ave., Sarnia, Ont. (res); Wes '33; Path. Bact; Path., St. Joseph's Hosp., Sarnia; Tel. ED 6-6121.
HOLLENBERG, Charles, MBE; Mall Med. Group, 280 Osborne St. North, Winnipeg 1, Man.; 742 South Dr., Ft. Garry (res); Man '32; M.Ch.(Orth), FRCS(E) & (C), OrthSurg; Cons. OrthSurg., Wpg. & St. Boniface Gen., Deer Lodge Mil., Wpg. Mun., Children's Hosp's.; Ass't. Prof. (Orth), U. of Manitoba; Tel. SP 4-2411.
HOLLENBERG, Charles H.; 1650 Cedar Ave., Montreal 25, P.Q.; Man '54; FRCP(C), IntMed; Assoc. Phys. & Ass't. Dir., McGill Univ. Med. Clinic, Montreal Gen. Hosp.; Assoc. Prof., McGill U.; Tel. WE 7-6011, Loc. 703.
HOLLENBERG, Dorothy M. O.; 394 Graham Ave., Winnipeg, Man.; 810 St. Mary's Rd., St. Vital (res); Man '28; M.C.G.P.; Tel. WH 2-5305.
HOLLENBERG, Jacob; 203 Edmonton St., Winnipeg 1, Man.; 150 Waverley St., Wpg. 9 (res); Man '37; FICS; GenSurg; MCGP; Surg. Staff, Misericordia & St. Boniface Gen. Hosp's.; Lect. (Surg.), U. of Manitoba; Tel WH 2-5381.
HOLLENBERG, Joseph; 394 Graham Ave., Winnipeg, Man.; 810 St. Mary's Rd., St. Vital (res); Man '26; Dem. (Anat.), U. of Manitoba; Tel. WH 2-5305.

HOLLENBERG, Michael S.; Hollenberg Clinic, 394 Graham Ave., Winnipeg, Man.; 170 Waverley St. (res); Man '24; IntMed; Lect. Med., U. of Manitoba; Tel. WH 2-5096.

HOLLENBERG, Murray W.; Man'60; Ophth; Staff, Winnipeg Gen. Hosp., Winnipeg 3, Man.

HOLLENBERG, Norman K.; Man '60; Res., Winnipeg Gen. Hosp., Winnipeg, Man.; Abroad.

HOLLEY, D. Alexander; Box 1930, Holley Clinic, 348 Front St., Quesnel, B.C.; Alb'51; M.Sc., GenSurg; Chief of Med. Staff & Chmn., Surg., G. R. Baker Mem. Hosp.; Tel. 992-2158.

HOLLIES, E. G.; Pouce Coupe, B.C.; Alb '27.

HOLLING, F. Stanley; McG '21; Act. Dir., TB Preven., Ontario Dept., Parliament Bldgs., Toronto 5, Ont.

HOLLINGER, Donald M.; Med. Arts Bldg., 420 East St. S., Sarnia, Ont.; 904 Hagle St. (res); Qns '46; FRCS(C), ObstGyn; Staff (ObstGyn). St. Joseph's Hosp.; Tel. ED 7-8812.

HOLLINGER, Harvey Z.; Ste. 750, 3550 Cote des Neiges, Montreal 25, P.Q.; 4755 Vezina St., Mtl. 26 (res); McG '52; M.Sc. (Exp. Med.); FRCP(C); DABIM; IntMed.; (Allerg.) (P.Q.); Att'd Staff, Reddy Mem. & Jewish Gen. Hosp's.; Plant Phys., Imperial Tobacco Co.; Tel. 935-1593.

HOLLINGSWORTH, W. John, Sg/Lt.; HMCS Provider, FMO, Halifax, N.S.; Alb'64.

HOLLO, George; Jerusalem'54; Res. (Anaes.), U. of Manitoba, Winnipeg, Man.

HOLLO, Jelisaveta B.; Belgrade (Yugo)'52; Staff, Selkirk Mental Hosp., Selkirk, Man.

HOLLOWAY, Sydney H.; 624 Sifton Blvd. S.W., Calgary, Alta.; McG'44; MCGP.

HOLLOWS, Reginald K.; 230 Kent St. W., Lindsay, Ont.; London (Eng.) '47; FRCS(Eng.), Urol; GenSurg; Chief of Surg., Ross Mem. Hosp. & Uxbridge & Port Perry Hosp's.; Tel 324-6392.

HOLLO-ZELINGER, Agnes M.; Heidelberg (Germ.) '59; Paed; Staff, Montreal Children's Hosp., Montreal 25, P.Q.; Tel. WE 7-8511.

HOLLYWOOD, Brian C.; P.O. Box 188, St. Lawrence, Nfld. (res); Dublin (Ire.) '57; M.B., B. Ch.; BAO; Sr. Med. Officer, Cottage, Hosp.; Tel. 56-R-2.

HOLM, Arnold W.; 1220 Wellington Cres., Winnipeg 9, Man.; Man '37; D.A., Anaes; M.C.G.P.; Anaes., Winnipeg Children's Hosp.; Lect., U. of Manitoba; Tel. HU 9-7028.

HOLMES, Arthur B.; R.R. No. 3, Amherstburg, Ont.; Tor '15; Retired.

HOLMES, C. Brian; 543 Lawrence Ave., Kelowna, B.C.; 332 Strathcona Ave. (res); M.R.C.S., L.R.C.P. (Eng.) '44; IntMed; Derm.; Tel. 762-2003.

HOLMES, Clarence E.; 11804-92nd Ave., Edmonton, Alta.; Alb'34; D&TRad; Staff, University Hosp.

HOLMES, Edwin; Lanark, Ont.; Qns '47; Dist. Coroner; Tel. 69.

HOLMES, Francis R.; 168 Main St. W., Welland, Ont.; 9 Ridgewood Dr. (res); Man '53; Staff, Welland Co. Gen. Hosp.; Tel. RE 4-4622.

HOLMES, Gordon R., Sg. Lt.Cdr., CD.; Tor '50; CMO, Atlantic Coast, FMO, Halifax, N.S.

HOLMES, Ian H.; Parsons Clinic, Red Deer, Alta.; 4436-34th St. (res); Man '53; FRCP(C), IntMed; Med Staff, Red Deer Gen. Hosp.; Tel. 346-2042.

HOLMES, James A.; Knox Clinic, 1605 Glenmore St., Kelowna, B.C.; Alb '59; FRCP(C), IntMed.

HOLMES, John R.; 510 Wellington St., Wallaceburg, Ont.; 16 Warwick Dr. (res); Wes '53; IntMed; Tel. 7-3306.

HOLMES, R. Brian; 101 College St., Toronto 2, Ont.; Wes'43; M.Sc., FACR; FRCP(C), D & T Rad; Chief Rad., Tor. Gen. Hosp.; Prof. & Chmn. (Radiol.), U. of Toronto; Tel. EM 6-8211.

HOLMES, Robert G.; 122 2nd Ave. W., Prince Rupert, B.C.; London'59; FRCS(Ed).

HOLMES, Samuel E.; Eston, Sask.; Man '24; M.C.G.P.

HOLMES, S. John; 99 Avenue Rd., Toronto, Ont.; 14 St. Margaret's Dr. (res); Tor '40; Dip. Psy. (Tor.), Psy.; Cons. Psy., Sunnybrook Hosp. (D.V.A.); Psy., Brookdale Clin., Alcoholism Research Found.; Cons. Psy., Dept. of Reform Inst's., Ont.; Clin. Teacher (Psy), U. of Toronto; Tel. 924-3071.

HOLMES, Shirley M.; 5 Sixth St., Chatham, Ont.; 296 Wellington W. (res); Tor '10; Ophth.

HOLMES, Stewart E.; Eston, Sask.; Man'55; Tel. 4159.

HOLMES, Thomas C.; 626 Elstree Pl., North Vancouver, B.C. (res); McG '24; Retired.

HOLMES, Thomas H.; Tor '62; Staff, Dept. of Pharmacology, U. of Toronto, Toronto 2, Ont.

HOLMES, Willard S.; 217 Birks Bldg., Saskatoon, Sask.; 919 University Dr. (res); Chicago (U.S.) '29; Obst; Assoc. Cl. Prof. (Obst.), U. of Saskatchewan; Tel. 244-4563.

HOLMGREN, M. Grant; Sask '62; Res., University Hosp., Saskatoon, Sask.; Abroad.

HOLOWSKI, F. B.; 3578 Park Ave., Montreal, P.Q.; 3210 Maple Ave. (res); Paris '25.

HOLT, Ann R. (Gibson); 48 Grenview Blvd. S., Toronto 18, Ont.; Dublin (Ire.) '59; Tel. 231-8782.

HOLT, Danica M. (Lekich); 2525 S.W. Marine Dr., Vancouver 14, B.C.; UBC '62; School M.O., Richmond; Tel. TR 6-1313.

HOLT, William H.; UBC'62; Res., Vancouver Gen. Hosp., Vancouver, B.C.

HOLTON, Sylvia; (See Bensley).

HOLTZMAN, Jack H.; 415 The Westway, Weston, Ont.; Tor'59; MCGP; Staff, Queensway Gen. Hosp.; Tel. CL 5-2831 & 249-1644.

HOLUBITSKY, Isadore B.; Dept. of Surg., Fac. of Med. Bldg., Vancouver Gen. Hosp., Vancouver 9, B.C.; Alb '55; FRCS(C); GenSurg; Staff, Vancouver Gen. Hosp. & Shaughnessy Hosp.; Ass't. Prof. (Surg.), U.B.C.; Tel. TR 6-3211.

HOLUBITSKY, Nicholas D.; 207 Union Bldg., Edmonton, Alta.; 10725-125th St. (res); Alb '28; M.C.G.P.; Tel. GA 2-4543.

HOLVEY, David; London, (Eng.) '57; Jr. Intn., Sunnybrook Hosp., Toronto 12, Ont.

HOMBURGER, Helen R.; 2160 Weston Rd., Weston, Ont.; Marburg (Germ.) '50; Tel. CH 4-5566.

HOMER, Geoffrey F.; 260 Medical Arts Bldg., 1105 Pandora Ave., Victoria, B.C.; 3710 Cadboro Bay Rd. (res); Man '35; F.R.C.S.(Eng.), GenSurg; Chief of Surg., Victoria Veterans' Hosp.; Memb. Bd. of Governors, U. of Victoria; Tel. EV 2-7641.

HOMIK, Alexander M.; 115 Mountbatten St., Winnipeg 29, Man.; Man '41; Tel. HU 9-4250.

HOMONYLO, Michael; 358 Reynolds St., Oakville, Ont.; Tor'53; GenSurg; Urol; Staff, South Peel & Oakville Trafalgar Mem. Hosp's.; Tel. 845-8888.

HOMONYLO, William; 264 Humberside Ave., Toronto 9 (res); Tor '48; D.P.H., Chief M.O., Metro Police, Police Med. Bureau, 92 King St. E., Toronto 1.; Tel. EM 2-1711, Loc. 397.

HONEY, John W.; Pearson T.B. Hosp., 700 W. 57th Ave., Vancouver, B.C.; Liverpool (Eng.) '43; MRCS (Eng.); LRCP (Lond.)

HONEYMAN, D. Grant W.; 54 Brant Ave., Brantford, Ont.; Glasgow (Scot.)'49; GenSurg; Surg., St. Joseph's Hosp.; Att'd. Surg., Brantford Gen. Hosp. & Willett Hosp., Paris; Tel. PL 6-6333.

HONG, Chul. Y.; Staff, Regional Lab., Moncton, N.B.

HONIG, John L.; Main St., Swan River, Man.; London (Eng.)'53; MRCS; LRCP; DRCOG; Tel. 734-3141.

HOOD, Alan B.; McG '56; FRCP(C), IntMed; Haem(P.Q.); Staff, Queen Elizabeth Hosp., Montreal 28, P.Q.

HOOD, Angus M.; 514 Jarvis St., Toronto 5, Ont.; 152 St. Leonard's Ave., Tor. 12 (res); Qns '43; D.Psy; Psy; Dir., Toronto Mental Health Clinic; Assoc. Dept. of Psy. & Lect., Schl. of Social Work, U. of Toronto; Tel. 924-7349.

HOOD, Douglas C.; 6 Glenwatford Dr., Agincourt Plaza, Agincourt, Ont.; London (Eng.) '51; AMCGP; Tel. AX 3-2404.

HOOD, Eric; Medical Arts Bldg., 2150 Valley Way, Niagara Falls, Ont.; Glasgow (Scot.)'64.
HOOEY, Lawrence; Medical Arts Bldg., 260 Cedar St., Sudbury, Ont.; 259 Elm St. W. (res); Tor '26; Tel. 673-3695.
HOOEY, Mary A.; 419 Balliol St., Toronto 7, Ont.; Tor'59; FRCP(C), IntMed; Ass't. Phys., Wellesley Hosp.; Clin. Teach., Dept. of Med., U. of Toronto.
HOOGE, A. A.; 407 Preston Ave., Saskatoon, Sask.; Man'36; MCGP.
HOOGE, Peter D.; 107-2nd Ave. E., Kindersley, Sask.; 206-7th Ave. W. (res); Man '41; MCGP; Chief of Staff, Kindersley Union Hosp.; MOH; Dist. Coroner; Tel. 463-2621.
HOOGENRAAD, Arie; 47 Crawford St., Brockville, Ont. (res); Utrecht (Holland) '37; D.Psy.; Staff, Ontario Hosp.; Tel. DI 5-1461.
HOOGEWERF, Peter E.; 9905-101st. Ave., Grande Prarie, Alta.; London (Eng.) '54; MRCS (Eng.); LRCP (Lond.); AMCGP.
HOOGSTRATEN, Jan; 56 Queenston St., Winnipeg 9, Man. (res); Man '41; Ph.D., (Cantab.), Dir Lab. Children's Hosp.; Ass't. Prof. (Path), U. of Manitoba; Tel. HU 9-7665.
HOOK, James H.; Alb '55; Res., University Hosp., Saskatoon, Sask.
HOOPER, Donald G.; 240 Brock St., Kingston, Ont.; Qns'55; FRCS(C), Otol; Att'd. Surg., Kingston Gen. Hosp. & Hotel-Dieu Hosp.; Lect. (Otol.), Queen's U.; Tel. 546-5213.
HOOPER, G. David; 180 Metcalfe St., Ottawa 4, Ont.; 39 Madawaska Dr. (res); McG '50; D.Surg.; F.C.C.P.; F.R.C.S.(C), GenSurg; ThorSurg; Chief Cardiothor. Surg., Ottawa Civic Hosp.; Cardiothor. Surg. Ottawa Gen. Hosp.; Cons. (Thor Surg), Royal Ottawa San.; Ass't. Prof., (Cardiothor. Surg.), U. of Ottawa; Cons., (Cardio. Surg.); NDMC; Tel. 233-4604.
HOOPER, Georges; Mon '59; FRCS(C); GenSurg; Staff, Royal Victoria Hosp., Montreal, P.Q.; Tel. 842-1251.
HOOPER, George V.; 255 Metcalfe St., No. 8, Ottawa, Ont.; 194 Lansdowne Ave., Rockcliffe Pk. (res); Qns '15; LL.D. (Qns); FACS, FRCS(C), GenSurg; Gyn; Pres. Gen. Med. Bd., Chm. Adv. Bd. & Cons. (Gyn), Ottawa Civic Hosp.; Tel. CE 2-2211.
HOOPER, Harold S.; 520-8th St., Grand'Mere, P.Q.; McG '21; FACS; FICS; FRCS(C), GenSurg; Admin., Grand'Mere Gen. Hosp.; Tel. 538-3660.
HOOPER, James B.; 9210-95th Ave., Edmonton, **Alta.; Dal '53; Tel. 466-1185.**
HOOPER, Joseph E.A.G.; 1472 E. Blvd. St.-Joseph, Apt. 6, Montreal, P.Q.; Mon '59; GenSurg.
HOOPER, Robert L.; 1420 Birchwood Dr., Clarkson, Ont.; Tor'57; Anaes; Staff, South Peel Hosp.; Tel. 822-2775.
HOOPER, William T.; 22 St. Claire Ave., Charlottetown, P.E.I. (res); McG '45; TherRad; Dir., Div. of Cancer Control, Dept. of Health, P.E.I.; Tel. 894-8316.
HOOVER, Murray P.; 1042 William St., London, Ont.; Tor '40; Clin. Dir., Addiction Research Fdn.; Tel. 439-1311.
HOPE, Bertram K.; 394 Graham Ave., Winnipeg 1, Man.; Sidney (Australia) '51; M.B., B.S., MCRA; FRCS(Eng.); DiagRad; Tel. 943-5144.
HOPE, John D.; 208 Third Ave., Timmins, Ont.; McG '25; Chief, Dept. of Med., St. Mary's Hosp., Tel. 264-5025.
HOPE-GILL, Donald; Medical Arts Bldg., 2150 Valley View, Niagara Falls, Ont.; R.R. No. 1, Niagara-on-the-Lake; Edinburgh (Scot.) '32; Otol; Staff, Greater Niagara Hosp., & Niagara Cottage Hosp., Niagara-on-the-Lake; Tel. EL 8-5022
HOPE-GILL, Herbert F.; Seymour Med. Clinic, 192 Wellington St., Barrie, Ont.; Tor'65.
HOPKINS, Bruce H.; 95 King St. E., Kingston, Ont.; Tor '09; IntMed (TB); Ass't. Prof. (Med.), Queen's U.; Med. Dir., Ongwanada San.; Cons. DVA, Kingston; Tel. LI 8-4417
HOPKINS, Denis H. G.; London (Eng.) '55; Staff Phys., Mountain San., Hamilton, Ont.
HOPKINS, Donald R.; 749 King St. W., Kitchener, Ont.; Tor'58; FRCP(C), IntMed.
HOPKINS, John A.; 1121 Yates St., Victoria, B.C.; 2296 Dunlevy St. (res); Man '48; FRCS (C), Urol; Chief of Urol. Surg. St. Joseph's Hosp.; Cons. Urol., Royal Jubilee & HMCS Naden Hosp's.; Tel. 386-6151.
HOPKINS, Peter D.; Apt. 9, 324 Prince Edward **Dr., Toronto 18, Ont.; 30 Renown Rd., Islington (res); Tor '56; AMCGP; Med. Staff, O.P.D., Toronto Western Hosp.; Att'd. Staff, Runnymede** Hosp.; Tel. 233-7373.
HOPKINSON, Mervyn A.; Lion's Head, Ont.; Qns '50; M.C.G.P.; Tel. 34.
HOPKINSON, Norma E. (Cook); Lion's Head, Ont.; Wes '46; M.C.G.P. Dist. Coroner; Tel. 34.
HOPKYNS, John C.; 640 Professional Bldg., 10830 Jasper Ave., Edmonton, Alta.; 11009-80th Ave. (res); Oxford & London (Eng.) '40; MA (Oxon); MRCP(Lond.); IntMed; Instr. (ClinMed.), U. of Alberta; Tel. 422-2597.
HOPMANS, C. Clifford; 672 Brant St., Burlington, Ont.; 503 North Shore Blvd., Burl. (res); Tor'50; DABS, FRCS(C), GenSurg; OrthSurg; Chief (OrthSurg), Joseph Brant Mem. Hosp.; Staff (OrthSurg) Hamilton Gen. Hosp.; Tel. 637-5227.
HOPPER, John M.H.; E. Kootenay Health Unit, 102 S-11th Ave., Cranbrook, B.C.; Durham (Eng.) '49; DRCOG; DPH; Dir., East Kootenay Health Unit; Tel. 426-3361.
HOPPER, Peter W.; 925 W. Georgia St., Vancouver 1, B.C.; Guys H. (London, Eng.)'42; MRCS(Eng.); LRCP(Lond.); DRCOG; FRCS(C), GenSurg; ObstGyn.
HOPPER, S. Allan; 71 Church St., Moncton, N.B.; 12 Athlone Ave. (res); Dal'42; IntMed; Staff (Med.), Moncton City Hosp.; Tel. EV 4-5516.
HOPWOOD, Gerald M.; 309 Codrington St., **Barrie, Ont. (res); London (Eng.) '47; Staff, Ontario Hosp. School, Orillia; Tel. FA 4-7361.**
HORAN, Francis T.; Carnduff, Sask.; London (Eng.)'59; MRCS(Eng.); LRCP(Eng.); Abroad.
HORAN, J. Desmond; 600 Fairmont Med. Bldg., 750 W. Broadway, Vancouver 9, B.C.; Tor '51; FRCP(C), IntMed; Att'd. Phys., Allergy Clin., Van. Gen. Hosp.; Clin. Instr. (Med.), U. of British Columbia; Tel. 876-4411.
HORAN, Patrick J.; 183 Le Marchant Rd., St. **John's, Nfld.; Dal '45; M.Sc. (Surg., McG); Assoc. Surg., St. John's Gen.; Surg., St. Clare's** Mercy & Grace Hosp's.; Tel. 579-4271.
HORBACZEWSKI, Joseph; Warsaw (Pol.) '29; IntMed; Sr. Spec. IntMed, Saskatchewan Hosp., Weyburn, Sask.; Tel. 842-5461.
HORECZKO, Natalka; Alb '62; Res., University Hosp., Edmonton, Alta.
HORII, Akira; 1376 E. 57th Ave., Vancouver, B.C.; UBC '60; Tel. 325-6936.
HORLICK, Louis; Dept. of Med., U. of Saskatchewan, Saskatoon, Sask.; McG'45; FRCP(C), IntMed; Prof. (Med.), U. of Saskatchewan; Tel. 242-7641, Loc. 461.
HORN, Andrew A.; Qns '57; Path; Staff, Dept. of Path., South Waterloo Mem. Hosp., Galt, Ont.; Tel. 621-2330.
HORN, Harold I.; 200 Danforth Ave., Toronto 6, Ont.; Wales (U.K.)'56; FRCP(C), IntMed.
HORNE, Gordon M.; Ste. 211, 3000 Lawrence **Ave. E., Scarborough, Ont.; Apt. 701, 1300 York Mills Rd., Don Mills (res); Tor '54; Anaes; Staff, (Anaes), Scarborough Gen. Hosp.; Tel. AX 3-8681.**
HORNE, G. Robert; 50 Gore St., Kingston, Ont. **(res); Qns '54; Anaes; Staff, Kingston Gen. Hosp. & Queen's U.; Tel. LI 2-2821.**
HORNE, John S.; 1718 Lakeshore Rd. W., Clarkson, Ont.; Qns'54; GenSurg; Active Staff, Oakville-Trafalgar Mem. Hosp.; Tel. 822-9421.
HORNE, Leslie E.; Ste. 250, Bentall Bldg., 1070 **Douglas St., Victoria, B.C.; 2785 Tudor Rd. (res); Tor '49; ObstGyn; Cons. Staff, St. Joseph's & Royal Jubliee Hosp's.; Tel. 383-2621.**
HORNE, Margaret M. (Atkinson); 2416-23rd St. N.W., Calgary, Alta.; Man '49; Psy; Staff, Alberta Guidance Clinic; Tel. AM 6-1021.
HORNE, Norman C.; 2416-23rd St. N.W., Calgary, Alta.; London (Eng.) '37; L.R.C.P., M.R.C.S., D.P.M.; Dir. & Psy., I/C, Guidance Clinic.

HORNE, Scharley M. (Miller); Apt. 701, 1300 York Mills Rd., Don Mills, Ont. (res); Tor '53; DMR, DABR, DiagRad; Staff, Scarborough Gen. Hosp.; Tel. AX. 3-8181.
HORNE, S. Douglas; 225 Bridge St. E., Belleville, Ont.; Wes '54; MCGP; Examiner, D.O.T.
HORNE, William I.; Aberdeen (Scot.) '50; Path; Staff, Hotel-Dieu Hosp., Windsor, Ont.; Tel. CL 2-3631.
HORNER, Bennett A.; Suite 5, 140 Wallace St., Nanaimo, B.C.; Sask'60; FRCP(C), IntMed.
HORNER, Charlotte M.; R.R. 6., Box 20, Cobourg, Ont. (res); Tor '39; DPH; Staff, Northumberland-Durham Health Unit.
HORNER, E. Bruce; Shawville, P.Q.; McG '44; GenSurg (PQ); Tel. 647-2800.
HORNER, Frances A.; 140 Wallace St., Nanaimo, B.C.; Sask'60; FRCP(C), Derm.
HORNER, George S. H.; RCS (Dublin, Ire.)'57; FRSH; Path; Dir., Path. Labs., James Paton Mem. Hosp., Gander, Nfld.; Tel. 3961, Ext. 227.
HORNER, George H.; Clarenville, Nfld.; Royal Coll. of Surgeons (Ire.) '54.
HORNER, H. M.; Barrhead, Alta.; M.C.G.P.
HORNER, Ronald H.; 311 Med. Arts Bldg., 11010 Jasper Ave., Edmonton, Alta.; 7715 Saskatchewan Dr. (res); Alb '37; MRCOG; FRCOG; DABOG; FACS; ObstGyn; Staff, University Hosp. Court. Staff, Royal Alexandra Hosp.; Clin. Prof. (ObstGyn.), U. of Alberta; Tel. 422-2217.
HORNIMAN, Euan A.; 14819-108th Ave., North Surrey, B.C.; London (Eng.)'56; MCGP; MRCS (Eng.), LRCP(Lond.); Tel. 581-7777.
HORNING, C. E. Maxwell; 1703 Victoria Park Ave., Scarborough, Ont.; Tor '63; Staff, Toronto East Gen. Hosp.; Tel. 755-1316.
HORNUNG, Alisa; 3272 W. 33rd. Ave., Vancouver 13, B.C.; London(Eng.)'61; Pt.-time School M.O.; Tel. 736-0788.
HORNUNG, Judith (Mrs. Kalla); 2775 W. Broadway, Vancouver, B.C.; 2606 McBain Ave. (res); St. Mary's H. (London, Eng.) '58; Tel. RE. 8-4334.
HORNUNG, Leo; Ste. 205, 1541 W. Broadway, Vancouver 1, B.C.; Prague (Czech.) & Cardiff (Wales)'27; MRCS; MRCP; DCH; Tel. RE 6-6121.
HOROUPIAN, D.; Res., Winnipeg Gen. Hosp., Winnipeg 12, Man.
HOROVITCH, Roy M.; 256 Elgin, Ottawa 4, Ont.; Tor'60; IntMed; Tel. CE 3-7777.
HOROWITZ, Ben; 262 Wilson Ave., Downsview, Ont.; 63 Wasdale Cres. (res); Tor '52; ObstGyn; Staff, New Mount Sinai & Branson Hosp's.; Tel. ME 5-1011.
HOROWITZ, Isadore; Dept. of Epidem. & Health, 3775 University St., Montreal 2, P.Q.; McG'62.
HORRELT, Otto H.; Dal'60; Res., Victoria Gen. Hosp., Halifax, N.S.
HORSEY, Mary E.; Qns'63; Staff, Alberta Hosp., Ponoka, Alta.
HORSEY, William J.; St. Michael's Hosp., Toronto, Ont.; Tor'44; FACS; FRCS(C), NeurSurg; Surg.-in-Chief & Chief of NeurSurg. Div., St. Michael's Hosp.; Active Staff, (NeurSurg.), St. Joseph's Hosp.; Cons. NeurSurg., Hosp. for Sick Children; Prof. Surg., U. of Toronto; Tel. 368-0721.
HORSLEY, James I.; 50 Sheppard Ave. E., Willowdale, Ont.; 27 Southwell (res); Coll. of Med. Evang. (Calif.) '45; GenSurg; Tel. 222-2491.
HORTON, Donald R.; 300 Medical Arts Bldg., 1105 Pandora Ave., Victoria, B.C.; 2633 Beach Dr. (res); Alb'51; Tel. 385-7791.
HORTON, Howard R.; Cottam, Ont.; Tulane (Louisiana, U.S.A.) '56.
HORTON, T. Bevan; 1669 Victoria St., Prince George, B.C.; UBC '63; Tel. 564-6211.
HORWITZ, Aaron N.; 2159A Weston Rd., Weston, Ont.; Cape Town (S. Africa) '49; DRCOG; MRCOG; ObstGyn; Court. Staff (ObstGyn.), Toronto Gen. Hosp.; Vol. Ass't., New Mount Sinai Hosp.; Tel. 244-3555.
HOSEIN, Andrew A.; Roslin, Ont.; McG '60; MCGP; M.O.H., Twnsps. of Thurlow & Tyendinega; Coroner, County of Hastings; Tel. 477-2345.
HOSEIN, Lena; 2120 Austin Rd., Coquitlam, New **Westminster, B.C.; 303-125 Agnes St. (res); UBC** '61; Tel. 939-9434.
HOSIE, Robert T.; 220 Med. Arts Bldg., 1105 Pandora Ave., Victoria, B.C. 3543 Redwood Ave. (res); Tor'49; FRCS(C), GenSurg; Staff, Royal Jubilee Hosp.; Tel. EV 5-1614.
HOSKING, David J.; 236 Med. Bldg., U. of Saskatchewan, Saskatoon, Sask.; Westminster H. (London, Eng.)'52; DPH; AB (PrevMed); Staff, University Hosp.; Assoc. Prof. (PrevMed.), U. of Saskatchewan; Tel. CH 2-7641.
HOSPES, Donald E.; Box 820, Oliver, B.C.; UBC '62.
HOSPODAREWSKA, Sophie; 4163 Hingston Ave., Montreal 28, P.Q.; Mon'44; Tel. 484-9196.
HOSSEINI, Eshagh B.; 155 Ingram, Duncan, B.C.; Meshed (Iran)'56; Tel. 746-5115.
HOSSIE, Barbara (See Hogarth)
HOSTETLER, Howard W.; 825 Richmond St., London, Ont. (res); Wes'48; MCGP; Staff, Anaes. Assoc. of London.
HOTTE, Rodolphe; 4135 Ave. Papineau, Montreal 24, P.Q.; Mon'55; Obst(P.Q.); Abroad.
HOTTI, Allan R.; 710 Seymour St., Vancouver 2, B.C.; 3218 W. 31st (res); Tor '58; Tel. MU 4-1511.
HOTZ, Harry; 839 Main St. E., Hamilton, Ont.; 274 Mountain Brow Blvd. (res); Tor '44; F.A.-A.P., Paed; Staff (Paed.), St. Joseph's & Civic **Hosp's.; Tel. LI 9-3344.**
HOUDE, Denis; Lav'65; Res., Hop. St.-Sacrement, Quebec 6, P.Q.
HOUDE, Jacques; 1302 Lemoine, Sillery, Quebec 6, P.Q. (res); Lav '50; M.Ch.; Anaes; Staff (Anaes), Hotel-Dieu de Quebec & Laval U.; Tel. 527-6789.
HOUDE, Joseph P. E. Andre; 541 rue de l'Hopital, Jonquiere, P.Q.; 476 rue St. Pierre (res); Lav '54; Cardiol (P.Q.); F.R.C.P.(C), IntMed; Staff, Hotel-Dieu-de l'Assomption; Tel. 547-3651.
HOUDE, Laurent; 759 Hartland Ave., Montreal 8, P.Q.; Mon '53; D.A.A.P.C.C., Psy; Ass't. Dir. (Child Psy.) Hop.-Ste-Justine; Psy Cons., Montreal Orientation Centre; Ass't. Prof., U. of Montreal; Tel. RE 1-4931.
HOUDE, Pierre J.; Clinique Ste-Foy; 802 Chanoine Scott, Ste-Foy, P.Q.; Lav '61; Tel. 653-4931.
HOUDE, Real; 435 Blvd. St. Joseph, Roberval, P.Q.; Lav '51.
HOUGH, Earl K.; Ste. 203, 625-5th St., New **Westminster, B.C.; 1511 Edinburgh (res); McG '35.**
HOUGH, H. Bruce; 304 Med. Arts Bldg., 1011 Ouellette Ave., Windsor, Ont.; 1043 Victoria Ave. (res); Tor '28; FRCS (Edin.); GenSurg; Cons. Surg., Grace, Hotel-Dieu & Metropolitan Gen. Hosp's.; Tel. 253-5006.
HOUGH, John D.; Ste 106, 1175 Cook St., Victoria, B.C.; Oregon (U.S.A.) '51; DABS; FRCS-(C), GenSurg; Chief of Staff, St. Joseph's Hosp.; Tel. EV 4-9111.
HOUGHTLING, Walter J.; 821 Douglas St., Apt. 506, North Bay, Ont.; Qns '32; IntMed; Staff, Ontario Hosp., North Bay; Tel. 474-1200.
HOULD, Fernand; 1500-18e Rue, Quebec 3, P.Q.; Lav '54; FRCP(C), Paed; Staff, Hop. de l'Enfant Jesus & Laval U.; Tel. LA 4-4040.
HOULD, Jean; Lav'55; Res., Hop. Hotel-Dieu, Quebec 4, P.Q.
HOULD, Roland; 1185 Hart, Trois-Rivieres, P.Q.; 3520 Ludger, Duvernay (res); Lav '48; Anaes; Anaes., Hop. Ste.-Marie; Tel. FR 5-7721.
HOULE, Gaston A.; C.P. 1759, 13, rue de l'Eglise, Windsor, P.Q.; Lav '60; GenSurg(P.Q.).
HOULE, Germain L.; Ott'59; FRCP(C), Anaes; Staff, Royal Victoria Hosp., Montreal 2, P.Q.
HOULE, J. Antonio; 6412 rue Louis-Hebert, Montreal 35, P.Q.; Mon'28.
HOULE, Jean G.; 4 rue Ste Helene, Levis, P.Q.; Mon'60; Urol(P.Q.).
HOULE, Joseph A.; 155 Stillview Rd., Pointe Claire, P.Q.; Lav'60; OrthSurg(P.Q.); Cons. OrthSurg., Queen Mary Vets. Hosp.; Staff OrthSurg., Lakeshore Gen. Hosp.
HOULE, Normand J.; C.P. 754, 383 Heriot, Drummondville, P.Q.; Lav '60; IntMed.; Tel. 472-2520.

HOULE, Pierre; 875 des Recollets, Trois Rivieres, P.Q.; 781 De-Tonnacourt (res); Lav '54; MCGP; Tel. FR 4-2953.
HOULE, Robert; Mon'65; Res., Hop. Maisonneuce, 5414 Boul. L'Assomption, Montreal, P.Q.
HOUPT, Joseph B.; 99 Avenue Rd., Toronto 5, Ont.; Tor '58; FRCP(C), IntMed; Staff, New Mount Sinai Hosp.; Clin. Teach., U. of Toronto; Research Ass't., Sunnybrook Hosp.; Cons., Arthritis DVA; Tel. 921-7804.
HOURIGAN, John M.; 214 Main St. N., Moose Jaw, Sask.; 548 Oxford W. (res); Qns '05; Dist. Coroner.
HOURIGAN, Thomas S.; Swift Current Clinic, 129 Central N., Swift Current, Sask.; 1308 North Hill Dr. (res); Sask.'59; AMCGP Tel. 773-4681; Abroad.
HOUSE, A. Maxwell; 215 LeMarchant Rd., St. John's, Nfld.; Dal'52; Neur; Chief, Dept. of Neurol., Grace Hosp.; Ass't. Dir., Children's Rehab. Centre; Electroenceph., St. John's Gen. Hosp.; Cons. Neurol., Hosp. for Mental & Nervous Diseases; Tel. 579-2772.
HOUSE, Walter K.; 1710 Oxford St., Halifax, N.S.; Man '31; FRCS (Edin.), FRCS(C), GenSurg; Surg., Victoria Gen. Hosp.; Ass't. Prof. (Surg.), Dalhousie U.; Tel. 2-4406.
HOUSTON, Alexander C.; 273 N. Mitton St., Sarnia, Ont.; Queen's U. (Belfast) '45; M.R.C.P. (Edin.); F.R.C.P.(C), Int Med; Active Staff, Sarnia Gen. & St. Joseph's Hosp's.; Tel. ED 7-8183.
HOUSTON, Arnold B.; Manitoba Clinic, 790 Sherbrook St., Winnipeg 2, Man.; 158 Queenston St., Wpg. 9 (res); Man '39; FACP, FRCP(C), IntMed; Assoc. Phys., Wpg. Gen Hosp.; Assoc. Prof. Med., U. of Manitoba; Assoc. Med. Dir. Gt. West Life Assur. Co.; Memb. Bd. of Examiners Med. Council of Canada; Tel. SP 4-6541.
HOUSTON, Clarence J.; 11 Dunlop Blk., Yorkton, Sask.; 82 Fourth Ave. (res); Man '26; FACS; GenSurg; MCGP (Hon.); Chief of Staff, Yorkton Union Hosp.; Memb. Health Serv. Planning Comm., (Sask.); Tel. 783-2279.
HOUSTON, C. Stuart; 863 University Avenue Saskatoon, Sask.; Man '51; FRCP(C), DiagRad; MCGP; Ass't. Dir. Dept. of Rad., University Hosp.; Ass't. Prof. (DiagRad.), U. of Saskatchewan; Tel. 244-0742.
HOUSTON, E. Patrick; Ott '57; D.Psy; Psy; Staff, Royal Ottawa San., Ottawa, Ont.; Lect. Psy., U. of Ottawa; Cons., Boys' Training School, Alfred, Ont. & Elizabeth Fry Soc., Ottawa; Tel. 722-6521.
HOUSTON, Frederick; 605 Med. Arts Bldg., Young St., Hamilton, Ont.; Leeds (Eng.)'42; DMP(R); Psy; Court. Staff, St. Joseph's, Hamilton Gen. & Henderson Gen. Hosp's.; Pt.-time Cons. Psy., Addiction Research Fdn.; Tel. 528-2720.
HOUSTON, George F.; 430 Medical Arts Bldg., 1105 Pandora Ave., Victoria, B.C.; 2570 Arbutus Rd. (res); London (Eng.) '40; D.T.M. & H. (Lond.), M.R.C.S., L.R.C.P.; MCGP; G.P. Staff, Royal Jubilee Hosp.; Tel. EV 6-1712.
HOUSTON, George G.; The Polyclinic, Fitzroy St., Charlottetown, P.E.I.; 10 West St. (res); Dal '34; Otol.
HOUSTON, James E.; 106 Talbot St., Leamington, Ont.; Man '61; Tel. 326-3281.
HOUSTON, John A.; 201, 1840 Robson St., Vancouver 5, B.C. (res); Qns '10; Retired; Tel. MU 5-8012.
HOUSTON, John F.; 250 James St. S., Hamilton, Ont. Qns '20.
HOUSTON, Sigga C. (Christianson); Box 278, 11 Dunlop Blk., Yorkton, Sask.; 82-4th Ave. (res); Man '25; Tel. 783-2279.
HOUSTON, Stuart W.; 74 Johnston St., Kingston, Ont.; Qns '24; FRCS (Edin.), FRCS(C), GenSurg.; Staff Kingston Gen. Hosp.; Tel. 548-7661.
HOUSTON, W. Bradley; 9 Med. Arts Bldg., 626 Main St., Penticton, B.C.; 808 Barrington Pl. (res); Man '52; MCGP; Med. Staff, Penticton Gen. Hosp.; Tel. 492-8903.
HOUSTON, William H.; Trinity Coll. (Ire.) '44; B.A.O.; Path. & Dir. of Lab., Notre Dame Hosp., North Battleford, Sask.; Tel. 445-2411.
HOUTMAN, Siert G.; Utrecht (Neth.) '52; Psy; Staff, Mental Health Clinic, Ontario Hosp., Kingston, Ont.; Tel. LI 6-1101.
HOUZE, Graham N.; Qns'65; Res., Sunnybrook Hosp., Toronto 12, Ont.
HOVAN, Norman A.; Roy Clinic, 715 2nd Ave. S., Lethbridge, Alta.; Alb '50.
HOW, Richard K.; Wes'65; M.O., Sunnybrook Hosp., Toronto, Ont.
HOWARD, David L.; 410 Greyhound Bldg., Calgary, Alta.; 2412-12th Ave. N.W. (res); Tor '48; FRCP(C), IntMed.; Tel. 266-6621.
HOWARD, Michael J.; 273 Stewart St., Ottawa, Ont. (res); Qns '31; Med. Supt., Rideau H. & O. Centre, Ottawa; Tel. 235-2403.
HOWARD, Neville J.; Adelaide (Australia)'63; Res., Toronto Hosp. for Sick Children, Toronto 5, Ont.
HOWARTH, Brian G.; Lakeview Med. & Dental Centre, 63rd Ave. & 24th St. S.W., Calgary, Alta.; 2864 Lionel Cres. S.W. (res); Manchester (Eng.) '53; DRCOG; Staff Holy Cross Hosp.; Tel. 242-1716.
HOWARTH, Roy B.; 40 George St., Galt, Ont.; 171 Concession St. (res); Tor '47; Paed; Staff, South Waterloo Memorial Hosp., Galt; Tel. 621-0215.
HOWATSON, Douglas G.; London (Eng.) '39; LRCP (Lond); MRCS (Eng); Path; Staff, Gtr. Niagara Gen. Hosp., Niagara Falls, Ont.
HOWATT, Burton D.; Box 3000 Charlottetown, PEI; Bunbury (res); Dal '51; DPH; Ass't. Depty. Minister of Health & Chief, Emergency Health Services (PEI); Tel. 892-1293.
HOWATT, Wilfred B.; Flett Apts., Newcastle, N.B. (res); Dal '30; DiagRad; Rad., Miramichi Hosp.; Tel. MA 2-1341.
HOWDEN, Gordon D. G.; 211 Bastion St., Nanaimo, B.C.; 2545 Lynburn Cr. (res); Wes'42; Ophth; Chief of Surg., Nanaimo Reg. Gen. Hosp.; Tel. SK 3-2031.
HOWDEN, Robert L.; 273 Tache Ave., Norwood, Man.; Man'37; Anaes; Cons. Staff (ObstGyn), St. Boniface Gen. Hosp., St. Boniface; Tel. CH 7-3667.
HOWE, James B.; 137 Second Ave., Ottawa 1, Ont.; 265 First Ave. (res); Qns '56; M.C.G.P.
HOWE, William A.; 476 Portage Rd. N., Niagara Falls, Ont.; Wes'62.
HOWE, William D., M.P.; 58 Larkspur Dr., Ottawa 6, Ont.; 29 Parker Ave., Ott. 5 (res); Tor '41; Member of Parliament; Tel 828-4773.
HOWELL, Denis R., DSC; Medical Arts Bldg., 5880 Spring Garden Rd., Halifax, N.S.; 6030 Fraser St. (res); London (Eng.) '39; MRCS (Eng.), L.R.C.P. (Lond.), DermSyph; Cons. (Derm.), Camp Hill, Halifax Children's & Queen's Gen. Hosp's; Derm. & Hd. of Serv., Victoria Gen. Hosp.; Assoc. Prof. (Med.), Dalhousie U.; Tel 423-7768.
HOWELL, H. Doris; 140 Balmoral Ave., Toronto, Ont. (res); Tor '26; Path; Pathol., Ontario Dept. of Health, 360 Christie St., Toronto. Retired.
HOWELL, J. H.; 58 Water St., S., Galt, Ont.; 140 Blair Rd (res); Tor '28; Anaes.
HOWES, Edwin W.; 324 Prince Edward Dr., Toronto 18; Tor '40; OrthSurg; Surg. Staff, Orth. & Arthritic Hosp's.; Court. Staff (OrthSurg.), Doctor's and Queensway Gen. Hosp's.; Tel. BE 3-4042.
HOWES, Jos. E.; Med. Centre, 707 Charlotte St., Peterborough, Ont.; 635 Weller St. (res); Tor '38; FACS; FRCS(C), GenSurg; Surg Staff, Peterborough Civic, Surg. Staff, Campbellford Mem. Hosp. & Staff, St. Joseph's Hosp.; Tel. RI 2-3871.
HOWES, John M.; Suite 304, 291-9th St. E., Owen Sound, Ont.; Wes'44; FRCS(C), GenSurg; AMCGP; Tel. 376-0890.
HOWES, Merle E.; 445 Arlington Ave., Niagara Falls, Ont. (res); Tor '51; Staff, Dept. Health.
HOWETT, D. A.; 3280 Ridgewood Ave., Apt. 10, Montreal, P.Q.; U.K. '42.

HOWEY, Gilbert E.; Tor'62; Res., Clarke Inst. of Psy., 250 College St., Toronto 2B, Ont.
HOWEY, James R.; Caledonia Med. Clinic, 340 Campbell St., Nanaimo, B.C.; R.R. 1 Wellington (res); McG '51; ObstGyn; Hd., Dept. of ObstGyn., Nanaimo Reg. Gen. Hosp.; Cons. Gyn., Cumberland Gen. Hosp. and St. Joseph's Gen., Comox; Tel. 753-3202.
HOWIE, James L.; Box 807, Kindersley, Sask.; Sask'65.
HOWIE, John; 2090 Wyandotte St. E., Windsor, Ont.; 3550 Dougall Ave. (res); McG '27; DTM (Bengal); DPH; PH; MOH & Dir., Metropolitan Windsor Health Unit; Memb. Research Advis. Comm., Dom. Council of Health; Tel. CL 6-3416.
HOWIE, Mabel F.; 5691 Hutchison St., Montreal, P.Q. (res); McG '36; P.H., City of Montreal; Tel. 277-6569.
HOWITT, C. William E.; Ste. 307, 77 Westmount Rd., Guelph, Ont.; 32 Central St. (res); Tor'41; **MCGP; Tel. TA 2-9821.**
HOWITT, John R.; Tor '15; Psy; Supt., Ontario Hosp., Port Arthur, Ont.; Retired.
HOWLETT, John G.; 476 Mountain Ave., Westmount, Montreal 6, P.Q. (res); McG'33; M.Sc., MRCP(Lond.), FACP, FRCP(C), IntMed; Att'd. Phys., Royal Victoria Hosp.; Phys-in-Chief, St. Mary's Hosp.; Prof. (Med.), McGill U.; Tel. WE 7-7179.
HOWLETT, Lyall N., S/L; 3 Wing C.A.P.O. 5055, Can. Armed Forces, Europe; Wes '57. Abroad.
HOWSE, Christine R. (See Mason).
HOWSON, F. Ross; 68 Water St. S., Galt, Ont.; 31 Barrie St. (res); Wes '43; MCGP; Chief (Obst), South Waterloo Mem. Hosp.; Tel. 621-5120.
HRAB, Stanley W.; Tor'64; Res., Clarke Inst. of Psy., 250 College St., Toronto, Ont.
HRABAR, Stephen; 11614-130th St., Edmonton, Alta.; Graz (Austria)'26; MCGP; Retired.
HRADECKY, Rene A.; 5098 W. Broadway Montreal 29, P.Q.; Charles U. (Prague, Czech.) '35; M.O., Dept. of National Health & Welfare, Sick Mariners Clinic; Tel. HU 9-4133.
HRENO, Andrew; Qns '59; FRCS(C), GenSurg; Staff, Montreal Gen. Hosp., Montreal 25, P.Q.; Tel. 937-6011.
HRNCHIAR, Andrew; 1105 Carling Ave., Ottawa 3, Ont.; McG'58; Psy; Staff, Dept. of Children's Psy., Royal Ottawa San.; Tel. 722-1449.
HRUSHOVETZ, Semeon Bohdan; Winnipeg Clinic Research Inst., 205 Vaughan St., Winnipeg 1, Man.; Man'60; MSc(Alta); PhD(Tor); Dir., Research Lab., Winnipeg Clinic; Hon. Ass't. Prof. (Anat.), U. of Manitoba; Tel. 942-0551, Loc. 324.
HRYCIUK, Nestor, S/L; Cdn. Forces Base, Goose Bay, Labrador; Man'57.
HRYNIUK, William M.; Flin Flon, Man.; Man '61. Abroad.
HSIEH, Yang S.; Ste. 410, 2184 W. Broadway, Vancouver 9, B.C. 319 W. 15th (res); Shanghai (China) '51; ObstGyn; Staff, Grace Hosp.; Tel. RE 8-9814.
HSU, Chien L.; Box 40, Cranbrook, B.C.; Peking (China)'32; D&TRad.
HSU, Lillian C.; Medical Arts Clinic, 2125-11th Ave., Regina, Sask.; Cheeloo'46; DiagRad.
HSU, Nora; Peking (China) '51; Staff, Community Clinic, 2363 McIntyre St., Regina, Sask.
HSU, Shou H.; 6848 Ash St., Vancouver 14, **B.C. (res); Shanghai (China) '50; Anaes; Staff, Vancouver Gen. Hosp.; Tel. TR 4-3454.**
HUA, Johnson T. S.; National Defence Med. Centre, (Taiwan, Formosa)'61; Res., Royal Victoria Hosp., Montreal, P.Q.
HUANG, Erwin P. S.; Shanghai(China) '48; D. P. (Paed., McGill); DR(McG.); DABP; FRCP (C); Paed; DiagRad; Staff, Dept. of Rad., St. Joseph's Hosp. and Port Arthur Gen. Hosp., Port Arthur, Ont; Tel. DI 4-2431.
HUANG, Samuel H. S.; Medical Arts Clinic, Swift Current, Sask.; National Kiangsu Med. Coll. (Chungking, China)'45; Tel. 773-4636.

HUANG, Shao-Nan; 223 Park St., Kingston, Ont. (res); National U. (Taiwan)'56; Path; Ass't. Prof. Path., Kingston Gen. Hosp.; Ass't. Prof. (Path.), Queen's U.; Tel. 542-2259.
HUAPAYA, Luis V.; Lima (Peru)'53; Staff, Hop. Des Laurentides, L'Annonciation, Labelle, P.Q.
HUARD, Gilles; Mon '45; Paed (P.Q.); Med. Supt., Hop.-Marie Enfant, 5200 est, rue Belanger, Montreal 36, P.Q.; Tel. RA 7-2844.
HUARD, Ildebert; Lav '57; Med. Supt., Hop.- Notre-Dame-de-la-Garde, Cap-aux-Meules, Iles-de la Madeleine, P.Q.; Tel. 6-2000.
HUARD, Jacques; 40 Frontenac St., Lac Megan-tic, P.Q.; Lav'49; GenSurg (P.Q.); Chief Surg. & Dir. Corp., St. Joseph's Hosp.; Tel. 583-2672.
HUARD, J. Arthur.; 800 W. Blvd. Gouin, Montreal, P.Q.; 2219 Maplewood Ave. (res); Lav '27; F.A.P.A., Psy; Med. Supt., Hop. Bordeaux, Montreal; Tel. DU 9-1321.
HUARD, Louis G.; 2995 Lacombe Ave., Montreal, P.Q. (res); Lav '35; D.P.H.; Public Health, Div. of Child Hyg., Montreal; Tel. RE 1-5805.
HUBAR, Maurice; 4217 Dewdney Ave., Regina, Sask.; 2343 Broad St. (res); Dal '45; M.C.G.P.; Assoc. Staff, Regina Gen. & Grey Nuns' Hosp's.; Tel. 523-4878.
HUBBARD, Adrian R.; 906 Chateau St. Louis, 135 Grande Allee W., Quebec 6, P.Q.; London (Eng.) '02; MRCS; LRCP; FRCS(C); FACS; Hon. Surg. Staff, Jeffrey Hale's Hosp.
HUBBARD, E. Derry; 132 Wellington St., Bow-manville, Ont.; Tor'50; MCGP; Active Staff, Bowmanville Mem. Hosp.; Tel. 623-5910.
HUBBS, Donald H.; 216 St. Clair Ave, W., Toronto, Ont.; 272 Oriole Pkwy., Toronto 7 (res); Qns'23; MRCS, LRCP (Lond.); IntMed; Civil Aviation Examiner, Dept. of Transport; Tel. WA 1-8565.
HUBER, Walter A.; 93 Main St. S., Brampton, Ont.; Munich (Germ.) '47; Staff, Peel Mem. Hosp; Tel. GL 1-3433.
HUBERT, R. Pierre; C.P. 68, 484 rue Notre-Dame, Cap-de-la-Madeleine, P.Q.; 240 rue Rocheleau (res); Lav '44; Surg. & Pres. Med. Staff, Hop.-Cloutier; Coroner, Three-Rivers Dist.; Tel. FR 5-4714.
HUCKELL, John R.; 220 Phys. & Surg. Bldg., 8409-112th St., Edmonton, Alta.; McG '52; FRCS(C); FAAOS; OrthSurg; Active & Teach. Staff, University Hosp.; Court. Staff, Royal Alexandra Hosp.; Cons. Staff, Edmonton Gen. Hosp.; Chmn., Med. Advisory Bd., Alta. Council for Crippled Children; Tel. 439-4945.
HUCKELL R. Graham; 220 Phys. & Surg. Bldg., 8409-112th St., Edmonton, Alta.; McG '24; DABO (OrthSurg.); FACS.; FAAOS; OrthSurg; Staff, University of Alberta Hosp.; Cons.(OrthSurg.), Edmonton Gen. Hosp.; Prof. (Emer.), (OrthSurg.), U. of Alberta; Tel. 439-4945.
HUCKVALE, William S.; 405-1541 W. Broadway, Vancouver 9, B.C.; Alb '35; DIH; MCGP; M.O., **Workmen's Comp. Bd.; Tel. AM 6-0211.**
HUDEC, Albert V.; 538 Med. Dental Bldg., Rose St. & 11th Ave., Regina, Sask.; 3003 Westgate Ave. (res); Qns '45; MCGP; Sr. Staff, Regina Gen. & Gray Nuns Hosp.; Tel. 522-5013.
HUDECKI, Stanley M.; King East Med. Bldg., 987 King St. E., Hamilton, Ont.; 290 Caroline St. S. (res); Tor'40; FRCS(C), GenSurg; OrthSurg; Chief Orth Serv., St. Joseph's Hosp.; Cons., DVA and Cerebral Palsy Centre; Tel. 549-3541.
HUDON, Fernando; 254 Aberdeen, Quebec 6, P.Q.; Lav'32; FFARCS; FRCP(C); Anaes; Hd. (Anaes.), Hotel-Dieu, Hop.-Ste.-Foy, Hop.-Laval; Prof. & Hd., Dept. of Anaes, Laval U.
HUDON, Jacques, Cap.; Camp Hosp., Gagetown, N.B.; Lav'65.
HUDON, Maurice; Portneuf, P.Q.; Lav '27. Retired.
HUDON, Raymond; Lav '55; Anaes; MCGP; Staff, Hop. Hotel-Dieu, Montreal, P.Q.; Tel. VI 4-0161.
HUDON, R. Robert; Lav'59; Res., Hop. Hotel-Dieu, Quebec 4, P.Q.

HUDSON, Arthur J.; 403-Med Dental Bldg., 450 Central Ave., London, Ont.; 8 Doncaster Ave. (res); Tor '50; FRCP(C); Neurol.; Neurol., St. Joseph's Hosp.; Cons. Neurol. Westminster DVA Hosp.; Clin. Lect. (Med.) & Hon. Lect., Biochem., U. of Western Ontario; Tel. GE 8-9520.
HUDSON, Arthur L.; 1 Roxborough St. E., Toronto 5, Ont.; 219 Glen Rd. Tor. 5 (res); Tor '40; DermSyph; Derm. I/C, St. Michael's Hosp.; Cons., Sunnybrook DVA Hosp.; Clin. Instr., U. of Toronto; Tel. 922-0104.
HUDSON, **Aubrey D.**; Dal '54; Path; Staff, Calgary Gen. Hosp., Calgary, Alta.; Tel. 266-7541.
HUDSON, Henry D.; Pickle Crow Mines, Pickle Crow, Ont.; Tor'26.
HUDSON, John E.; Hamiota, Man.; Man '41; MCGP; Dist. Coroner; Chief of Staff, Hamiota Hosp.; Chmn., Bd. of Health, Manitoba.
HUDSON, P. W.; 4094 W. 33rd, Vancouver, B.C.; Alb '43; Anaes; Staff, Vancouver Gen. Hosp.; Clin. Instr. (Anaes), U. of British Columbia; Tel. TR 6-3211.
HUDSON, **Robert M.**; P.O. Box 220, Quyon Co. Pontiac, P.Q.; Man '35; Member. Bd. Dir., Pontiac Community Hosp., Shawville; Tel. 4.
HUEBERT, Helmut T.; Winnipeg Clinic, St. Marys & Vaughan, Winnipeg 1, Man.; Man'58.
HUESTIS, W. Stuart; 5991 Spring Garden Rd., Halifax, N.S.; Dal'56; FRCS(C), NeurSurg; Cons., Grace Maternity, Cdn. Forces, Convalescent, Children's, & Camp Hill Hosp's; Active Staff, Victoria Gen. Hosp.; Court. Staff, Halifax Infirmary; Instr., Dalhousie U.; Tel. 423-7015.
HUFFMAN, A. S.; Blenheim, Ont.; Tor '33.
HUFFMAN, Janice L.; 29 Woodside Ave., Toronto, Ont.; Tor '57; DiagRad; Staff, Wellesley Hosp.; Tel. WA 1-4111. Abroad.
HUGENHOLTZ, H.; Tor'65; Res., St. Michael's Hosp., Toronto 2, Ont.
HUGGINS, Donalda M. H.; Dept. of Anaes., Wpg. Gen. Hosp., Winnipeg, Man.; 99 Niagara **St. (res); Man '35; DABA; FACA; Anaes; Chief Anaes., Wpg. Gen. & Shriners' Hosp.; Anaes.,** Man. Rehab. & Wpg. Mun. Hosp's.; Asssoc. Prof. Surg. (Anaes.), U. of Manitoba; Tel. SP 4-6511, Loc. 225.
HUGHES, A. Pauline (Gould); 9 East Columbia St., New Westminster, B.C. (res); Alb '48; Psy; **Deputy Med. Supt., Woodlands School; Tel. LA 1-2611.**
HUGHES, Donald W.; Tor'61; Res., Shaughnessy Hosp., Vancouver 9, B.C.
HUGHES, Edward N.; 841 Collinson St., Victoria, B.C.; 2175 Kendal Ave. (res); Tor '47; Anaes; Active Staff (Anaes), St. Joseph's Hosp.; Tel. EV 4-5622.
HUGHES, **Gary F.**; Man '60; Res., Mtl. Gen. Hosp., Montreal 25, P.Q.
HUGHES, Harley J.; Spence Clinic, 910 Ridgeway, Ft. William, Ont.; 413 S. Norah St. (res); Man '49; FACOG; ObstGyn; Staff (ObstGyn), McKellar Gen. Hosp.; Court. Staff (ObstGyn), Gen. & St. Joseph's Hosp's., Port Arthur; Tel. MA 2-5301.
HUGHES, Harold V.; 218-1940 Lonsdale Ave., North Vancouver, B.C.; 655 Holmbury Pl., W. Vanc. (res); Qns '39; Anaes; Otol; Chief E.N.T. Lionsgate Hosp.; Tel. 987-3536.
HUGHES, Jack F.; 186 Norfolk St., Guelph, Ont.; Wes'63; Tel. 824-4510.
HUGHES, **John F.**; 326 Med. Arts Bldg., Winnipeg 1, Man.; Man'49; MSc; FRCP(C), IntMed; Chief, Dept. of Med., St. Boniface Hosp.; Cardiol. Municipal Hosp's.; Assoc. Prof. Med., U. of Manitoba; Tel. 943-5895.
HUGHES, Patrick; Nat. U. (Ire.) '62; Staff, Burin Hosp., Burin, Nfld.
HUGHES, Paul S.; Tor'64; Res., Wellesley Hosp., Toronto 5, Ont.
HUGHES, Raymond A.; Ste. 2000, 5300 Cote des Neiges Rd., Montreal 26, P.Q.; McG '38; Int-Med. (P.Q.); Phys., St. Mary's Hosp.; Tel. 731-3249.
HUGHES, R. Frederick; 501 Med. Arts Bldg., 1 Young St., Hamilton, Ont.; 38 Charlton Ave. W., Apt. 103 (res); Man '31; MCAA; Tel. JA 2-0224.
HUGHES, Robert A.; 68 Charlton Ave. W., Hamilton, Ont.; 586 Deborah Cres., Burlington (res); Wes '48; FACS, FRCS(C), NeurSurg; Staff, Hamilton Gen. & St. Joseph's Hosp's.; Tel. 528-7661.
HUGHES, **Roger**; Ste. 241, 243 Brock St., Kingston, Ont.; Qns'63.
HUGHES, Simon J.; 110-10th St. W., Owen Sound, Ont.; Tor '46; Otol; Tel. 376-5680.
HUGHES, Walter W.; Box 434, Lemberg, Sask.; Wes'31; MCGP; Med. Staff, Balcarres Union Hosp.; Tel. 335-2455 or 335-2231.
HUGHES, William; 179 Millard Ave., Newmarket, **Ont.; Sheffield (Eng.) '54; M.B., Ch.B.; Psy;** Dir., Psy. Services, York County Hosp., Newmarket; Tel. TW 5-4521.
HUGILL, Jean T.; 3855 Puget Dr., Vancouver, **B.C.; Alb '46; D.A. (McGill), D.A.B.A.; Anaes; Att. Staff, Vancouver Gen. Hosp.;** Assoc. Staff **Children's Hosp.; Staff, Clin. Surg., U. of British Columbia; Tel. RE 3-2070.**
HUHN, Otto H.; Alb'63; Res. (Path.), Vancouver Gen. Hosp., Vancouver 9, B.C.
HUITEMA, Pieter A.; 1737 Pandosy St., Kelowna, B.C.; Utrecht (Neth.)'50; GenSurg; Chief, Dept. of Surg., Kelowna Gen. Hosp.; Staff, Summerland Gen. Hosp.; Tel. 762-4212.
HULKA, Leslie; 934 Ottawa St., Windsor, Ont.; Marseille (Fr.)'47; Active Staff, Metropolitan Gen. Hosp.; Court. Staff, Grace, I.O.D.E., Mem. & Hotel-Dieu Hosp's.; Tel. CL 6-2533.
HULKE, Frederick P.; 199 Merritt St. W., Welland, Ont. (res); **Middlesex H. (London, Eng.) '43; DABR; DiagRad; DiagRadiol., Welland Co. Hosp.**; Tel. RE 2-6111.
HULL, Ralph F.; Brooklin Medical Centre, Brooklin, Ont.; Tor '59; AMCGP. Abroad.
HULYK, Raymond M., F/L; Canadian Forces Base, Station Hosp., Cold Lake, Alta.; Alb'64.
HUME, William E.; Daley Park Rd., R.R. 3, St. Catharines, Ont.; McG'24; GenSurg; Retired.
HUMENIUK, Roman B.; Apt. 1815, 666 Ontario St., Toronto 5, Ont.; Tor'61.
HUMES, H. Gordon; P.O. Box 580, Mission City, B.C.; 831 Main St. (res); Alb '52.
HUMPHREY, Barbara M.; 214-6th Ave. S.W., Calgary, Alta.; 515-38th Ave. S.W. (res); Alb '41; Tel. 263-7120.
HUMPHREY, John G.; 101 College St., Toronto 2, Ont.; 112 Clifton Rd., Tor. 7 (res); Tor '54; FRCP(C), Neurol; Ass't. Phys., Tor. Gen. Hosp.; Assoc. (Path), & Clin. Instr. (Med.), U. of Toronto; Tel. EM 6-8211.
HUMPHREY, **John N.; 10 N Sherbourne St., Toronto, Ont.; Tor '14; Staff, Grace Salvation Army Hosp.; Tel. WA 2-6503.**
HUMPHREYS, **Garry R., Capt.**; Sick Bay, CFB Stadacona, Halifax, N.S.; Tor'65.
HUMPHREYS, J. Charles; Ste. 205, 1105 Carling Ave., Ottawa 1, Ont.; 12 Ascot Ave., Ott. 6 (res); McG '21; GenSurg; Cons. (Surg.), Ottawa Civic Hosp.; Tel. 729-5402.
HUMPHREYS, **Robin P.**; Tor'62; Res., St. Michael's Hosp., Toronto, Ont.
HUMPHRIES, Helen A. (See Preston)
HUMPHRY, Alaric; 16 Balding Ct., Willowdale, Ont. (res); Wes '43; DMR; DiagRad; Ass't. Rad., Hosp. for Sick Children; Clin. Instr. (Rad.), U. of Toronto; Tel. EM 6-7242.
HUMPHRYS, Martin H.; Church St., St. Mary's, Ont.; King St. (res); Wes '48; M.C.G.P.
HUNEAULT, **Gaetan**; Box 100, Marier St., Azilda, Ont.
HUNT, A. Leigh; Ste. 214, 3195 Granville St., Vancouver 9, B.C.; 1450 West King Edward (res); McG '31; ObstGyn.; Tel. RE 3-1193.
HUNT, Brian R.; 1538 Sherbrooke St. W., Rm. 622, Montreal, P.Q.; 704 Grosvenor Ave., Westmount (res); Oxford (Eng.) '47; DPM; D.Psy; Psy; Ass't. (Psy), Montreal Children's Hosp.; Assoc. Prof. Psy., McGill U.; Tel. 933-1868.
HUNT, Barbara J.; Aberdeen (Scot.) '56; Staff, Dept. of Med., Ottawa Gen. Hosp., Ottawa 2, Ont.; Tel. CE 6-0333.
HUNT, **Brian M.**; 136 E. 15th St., North Vancouver, B.C.; UBC'64.

HUNT, Charles L.; 520-17th St., West Vancouver, B.C.; 5375 The Terrace (res); St. Bart's (London, Eng.) '25; M.R.C.S. (Eng.), L.R.C.P. (Lond.); IntMed; Dir. Registry & Rehab. Services, B.C. Prov. Dept. of Health; Tel. 922-2531.

HUNT, D. Earl; 56 Yates St., St. Catharines, Ont.; Tor '46 MCGP; Pres. Elect, College of G.P. of Canada; Tel. 684-1138.

HUNT, Dominic A.; Marlbank, Ont.; Qns'46; Active Staff, Lennox & Addington County Hosp's.; Tel. 478-5575.

HUNT, Douglas W.; Man'45; MCGP; Res., Psy. Inst., Winnipeg 3, Man.

HUNT, Edward H.; 406 Guelph Line, Burlington, Ont.; Wes '58; MCGP; Tel. 634-0408.

HUNT, Ernest A.; 25 Queen St., Port Hope, Ont.; 16 Bedford St. (res); McG '40; M.C.G.P. Tel. 885-5511.

HUNT, George G.; Marlbank, Ont.; Qns'33; Staff, Lennox & Addington County Gen. Hosp's.; Tel. 478-5575.

HUNT, Harry B.; 501 Hunt Bldg., Lethbridge, Alta.; 904-13th St. S. (res); McG '29; GenSurg; Act. Staff, St. Michael's & Galt Hosp's.; Tel. 327-3184.

HUNT, John Allan; 104-1718 Marine Dr., West Vancouver, B.C.; 1030 Ottawa Ave. (res); London (Eng.) '50; LRCP (Lond.); MRCS (Eng.); MCGP; Active Staff, Lions Gate Hosp.; Staff, O.P.D., Diabetic Clinic, Vancouver Gen. Hosp.; Pres., Canadian Diabetic Assoc.; Tel. 922-3288.

HUNT, John D.; 46 Ontario Ave., Elliot Lake, Ont.; Tor'62; Active Staff, St. Joseph's Hosp.; Tel. 848-7176.

HUNT, John E.; UBC'58; Res., Vancouver Gen. Hosp., Vancouver, B.C.

HUNT, John W.; Hunt Bldg., Lethbridge, Alta.; 525-16th St. S. (res); Alb '41; Staff, St. Michael's & Galt Hosp's.; Tel. 327-3184.

HUNT, John W.; Ste. 107, 1175 Cook St., Victoria, B.C.; McG'51; Tel. 386-2161.

HUNT, Norris E.; Med. Arts Bldg., 358 Reynolds St. N., Oakville, Ont.; Qns '51; M.C.G.P.; Staff, Oakville Trafalgar Memorial Hosp.; Tel. VI 5-0825.

HUNT, Paul A. K.; Red Lake Medical Group, Red Lake, Ont.; Wales '57; Tel. 200.

HUNT, Talmage E.; Dept. Rehab. Med., University Hosp., Saskatoon, Sask.; 213 Lake Cres. (res); Tor '44; FRCP(C), IntMed; PhysMed & Rehab; Prof. & Hd., Dept. of Rehab. Med., University Hosp.; Prof. & Chmn., Rehab. Med., U. of Saskatchewan; Tel. 242-7641, Ext. 471.

HUNT, Thomas; Barrett Clinic, 641-3rd. St. S. E., Medicine Hat, Alta.; National U. (Ire.) '51; Tel. 527-4461.

HUNT, Trevor M.; Ste. G.8, 250 Lawrence Ave. W., Toronto 12, Ont.; Lav'60; Paed; Tel. 789-1523.

HUNTER, A. C.B.E.; 2 Sultan St., Toronto, Ont.; M.B. (Edin.); F.R.F.P. & S. (Glas.), F.R.S.C.; Prof. Emer. (PathChem.), U. of Toronto; Tel. WA. 3-3660.

HUNTER, Alexander; Smith Clinic, 144 Main St., Hawkesbury, Ont.; 496 Stanley St. (res); Aberdeen (Scot.)'39; **DRCOG; MRCOG; FRCOG;** Staff, Hop. St.-Coeur-de-Marie & Notre-Dame; Tel. ME 2-2711.

HUNTER, Andrew T.; Ste. 101, 396 Queens Ave., **London, Ont.; 69 Wychwood Pk. (res); Wes '53;** MCGP.

HUNTER, Cameron W.; Ste. 202, 1195 W. 13th Ave., Vancouver 9, B.C.; 819-1445 Marpole Ave. (res); Man '46. Staff, Valleyview Hosp., Essondale; Tel. LA 1-1911.

HUNTER, Douglas D.; Ste. 211, 3000 Lawrence Ave. E., Scarborough, Ont.; Tor'60; Anaes.

HUNTER, Douglas R.; Ste. 302, 153 Seymour St., Kamloops, B.C.; McG '47; Psy; Staff, Royal Inland Hosp.; Tel. 874-4088.

HUNTER, H. Bruce M.; Brandon Clinic, Brandon, Man.; 7 Cedar Bay (res); Man '40; Staff, **Brandon Gen. & Assiniboine Hosp's.; Tel. PA 9-6444.**

HUNTER, Helen M.; 5637 Spring Garden Rd., Halifax, N.S.; 1434 Henry St. (res); Dal '49; Paed; Active Staff, Children's & Grace Maternity Hosp's.; Cons. (Paed.), Hearing & Speech Clin; Court. Staff, Halifax Infirm & Victoria Gen. Hosp's.; Lect., Dalhousie U.; Tel. 422-6390.

HUNTER, Ivan A.; 277 Main St., Milton, Ont.; Wes'65.

HUNTER, James M.; 2970 Lake Shore Blvd. W., Toronto 14, Ont.; Aberdeen (Scot.)'61; Tel. 384-4421.

HUNTER, James O.: 102 Hedgewood Dr., Moncton, N.B.; Dublin (Ireland) '50; BAO; DiagRad; Staff, Moncton Hospital.

HUNTER, J. Gordon; C.N.R. Medical Clinic, 1150 Station St., Vancouver 4, B.C.; Man '42; IntMed; Tel. MU 4-0171.

HUNTER, John D.; London (Eng.)'58; Res., Winnipeg Gen. Hosp., Winnipeg 3, Man.

HUNTER, John M.; 606 Chinook Prof. Bldg., 6449 MacLeod Trail, Calgary, Alta.; Alb'58; OrthSurg, FRCS(C).

HUNTER, Kenneth, A.; O.B.E., C.D., 2.H.P. (Major-General); 121 Powell Ave., Ottawa, Ont. (res); Wes '30; Hon. Phys., H.M. Queen Elizabeth 11.; Retired.

HUNTER, Margaret I. (Mrs. I. D. Mair); 945 Caledonia Rd., Montreal 16: P.Q. (res); **Alb '49; D.C.H. (Lond.); Paed; Clin. Asst., Montreal Children's Hosp.; Att'd. Staff, Catherine Booth Hosp.; Tel. 737-5294.**

HUNTER, Margaret I. (Mrs. A. Normand); 176 Dawlish Ave., Toronto 12, Ont. (res); Tor '48; **D.C.H. (Eng.); Paed; Staff, Children's Aid Soc.; Tel. WA 4-4646.**

HUNTER, Mary E.; 178 St. George St., Toronto 5, Ont.; Dal '57; FRCP(C), Anaes; Staff, Toronto Gen. Hosp.; Clin. Ass't., U. of Toronto; Tel. WA 3-1154.

HUNTER, Nigel J.; London (Eng.)'62; Res., Hosp. for Sick Children, Toronto 2, Ont.

HUNTER, Robert A.; Ste. 230, Medical Arts Bldg., 1105 Pandora Ave., Victoria, B.C.; 550 Transit Rd. (res); Man '31; M.R.C.P. (Lond.), F.R.C.P.(C), IntMed; Cons, Staff, Royal Jubilee Hosp.; Tel. EV 3-4714.

HUNTER, Robert D.; 357 Ferguson St., North Bay, Ont.; 715 Durril St. (res); Tor '54; MCGP; Tel. 472-2300.

HUNTER, Robin C. A.; 164 Barrie St., Kingston, Ont.; 26 Centre St., Kingston, Ont. (res); McG '50; D.Psy; Psy; Psy-in-Chief, Kingston Gen. Hosp.; Prof. & Hd. of Psy., Queen's U.; Tel. 546-3871, Loc. 317/318.

HUNTER, William S.; 176 St. George St., Toronto 5, Ont.; Tor '56; FRCS(C), Ophth; Staff, St. Michael's Hosp. & Sunnybrook DVA; Clin. Teach. (Eye Path.), U. of Toronto; Tel. 921-9623.

HUNTLEY, Margaret; London (Eng.) '55; P.G., St. Michael's Hosp., Toronto 2, Ont.; Tel. 362-4461.

HUNTSMAN, Archibald G.; 217 Indian Rd., Toronto 3, Ont. (res); Tor '07; Retired.

HUNZINGER, Werner W.; Manitoba Clinic, 790 Sherbrooke St., Winnipeg 2, Man.; 914 Borebank St. (res); Heidelberg (Germ.) '51; Psy; Lect., U. of Manitoba; Tel. SP 4-6541.

HUOT, Aurele; 170 rue Cote, Donnacona, P.Q.; Lav '34; M.C.G.P.; Phys., Donnacona Paper Co.; Tel. 35.

HUOT, Jean; Mon'57; MCGP; Res., Hop. Notre Dame, Montreal 24, P.Q.

HUOT, Jean M.; 343 Tache, St. Boniface, Man.; 631 Langevin (res); Man '46; M.C.G.P.; Dist. Coroner.

HUOT, J. Marcel; 2005 Champfleury, Quebec 3, P.Q.; Lav '39.

HUOT, Laurent; 5462 Isabella St., Montreal, P.Q.; Mon '52; DiagRad.

HUOT, Lucien A.; 822 est, rue Sherbrooke, Montreal 24, P.Q., Montreal 24, P.Q.; 415 Ste-Helene (2nd Off.); 66A St.-Catherine, Longueuil (res); Lav '50; Otol; Ass't. Otol., Hop. Notre-Dame; Tel. (Longueuil) OR 4-6281.

HUOT, Pierre; Lav'65; Res., Hop. Enfant Jesus, Quebec 3, P.Q.

HUOT, Roch E.; 240 Elm St., St. Lambert, Montreal 23, P.Q.; 137 De Touraine, **Preville (res); Lav '51.; Tel. 671-9202.**

HUOT, Roger; Mon'65; Res., Hop. St-Luc, Montreal 18, P.Q.
HUOT, Yves; 8 St.-Charles, Ste-Therese-de-Blainville, P.Q.; Mon. '60.
HURLBURT, F. William B.; 218-3195 Granville St., Vancouver, B.C.; 1603 Matthews Ave. (res); Tor '40; M.R.C.P.(Lond.), F.R.C.P.(C) IntMed; Act. Staff (Med.), St. Paul's Hosp.; Cons. Staff, Shaughnessy Hosp.; Instr. (Med.), U. of British Columbia; Tel. RE 8-6511.
HURLBURT, William E.; Vineland, Ont.; Tor '24.; Tel. LO 2-5115.
HURLEY, Charles G.; 92 Binkley Cres., Hamilton, Ont.; Tor '42; DiagRad; Ass't. Dir. X.-Ray Dept., Hamilton Gen. Hosp.; Tel. JA 9-3732.
HURLEY, Gerard A.P.; 3869 Cote-des-Neiges, Montreal, P.Q.; Nat. U. (Dublin, Ire.) '34; FACS, DABTS; FRCS(C), GenSurg; ThorSurg; Surg., St. Mary's, Royal Edward Chest & **Grace Dart Hosp's.; Cons. (ThorSurg.), Queen Elizabeth Hosp.; Tel. 932-9344.**
HURLEY, James D.; 402 Island Park Dr., Ottawa 3, Ont. (res); National U. (Galway, Ire.) '44; DCH; LM(Rotunda); FFR; DABR; DiagRad; Dir., Dept. of Rad., Riverside Hosp.; Deputy Dir. (Rad.), Ottawa Gen. Hosp.; Cons. Rad., St. Vincents & Ottawa Cancer Fdn.; Ass't. Prof. (Rad.), Ottawa U.; Tel. 731-6710.
HURLEY, Noel; R.C.S. (Ire.) '50; Med. Dir., St. James Health Unit, 2000 Portage Ave., St. James, Winnipeg 12, Man.
HURLEY, Robert M.; Wes'65; Res., War Mem. Children's Hosp., London, Ont.
HURLEY, Ronald C.; Fredericton Med. Clinic, 206 Rookwood Ave., Fredericton, N.B.; Dal '57; MCGP; Tel. 475-7701.
HURST, David W.; 97 Charlotte St., Port Colborne, Ont.; Qns '56; FRCS(C), GenSurg; Cons. Staff, Port Colborne Gen. Hosp.; Court. Staff, Welland County Gen. Hosp.; Tel. 834-4546.
HURST, Harold G.; 616 Medical Arts Bldg., Winnipeg, Man.; 237 Oxford St., Winnipeg 9 (res); Man '41; M.Sc.; D.A.B.D., Derm Syph; Cons. Staff, Winnipeg Gen. Hosp.; Lect., (Med., U. of Manitoba; Tel. WH 2-4808.
HURST, Lawrence N.; Tor'65; Res., Hosp. for Sick Children, Toronto 2, Ont.
HURTEAU, C. A. David G.; 65 Bruyere St., Ottawa 2, Ont.; McG '55; F.R.C.S.(C), ObstGyn; Staff, Ottawa Gen. Hosp.; Tel. CE 6-4592.
HURTEAU, Gilles; 1054 Riviera Dr., Ottawa 7, Ont. (res); McG '55; Obst; Lect. U. of Ottawa; Tel. CE 6-0333.
HURTEAU, J. L. A.; 612 Cumberland St., Ottawa, Ont.; Lav '23; Staff, Cndn. Pens. Comm., Daly Bldg. Montreal, P.Q.; Tel. 233-9093.
HURTIG, Abraham; Ste. 202, 150 Metcalfe St., Ottawa 4, Ont.; 162 Stewart St. (res); Alb '37; FICS; FACOG; GenSurg; **Staff, Ottawa Gen.** Hosp.; Cons. Gyn., St. Vincents Hosp; Court. **Staff, Ottawa Civic & St. Louis de Montford Hosp's.**; Assoc. Prof. (Gyn.), U. of Ottawa; Tel. CE 3-1233.
HURTUBISE, Francis A.; Smooth Rock Falls, Ont.; Staff, Smooth Rock Falls Hosp.
HURTUBISE, Marc; Mon '61; DiagRad; Staff, Hop. Notre Dame, Montreal 24, P.Q.
HUSAIN, S. Ishrat; Community Health Clinic, 2363 MacIntyre St., Regina, Sask.; Karachi (Pakistan)'54; LRCP&S (Edin.); LRFPS (Glas.); DO (Lond.); DLO (Lond.); FRCS (Ed.); Ophth Otol; Assoc. Staff Memb. & Dept. of Surg., Regina Gen. Hosp.; Tel. 527-0641.
HUSAIN, Siraj; Med. Clin., Fort Churchill Hosp., Fort Churchill, Man.; Osmania (India)'53; M.S. (Surg.); M.O., Dept. of National Health & Welfare.
HUSCHILT, **Nicholaus P.**; Box 639, 14 Alma N., Hagersville, Ont.: Tor '57; GenSurg.
HUSEL, Don H.; 10155—120th Ave., Edmonton, Alta.; 10210—133 St. (res); Alb '46; ObstGyn., Hon. Instr., U. of Alberta; Tel. 488-7271.
HUSSAIN, Shamshad; Osmania (India) '62; Staff, Miller Bay Hosp., Prince Rupert, B.C.
HUSTON, Arthur F.; Phys. Rehab. Centre, Regina, Sask.; London (Eng.) '45; M.B., B.S., PhysMed & Rehab; Med. Dir., Phys. Restoration Centre.
HUTCHINGS, Harold R.; 390 Orenda Rd., Bramalee, Ont.; Wes'60; MCGP; Med. Dir.. G. D. Searle Co. of Canada Ltd.
HUTCHINS, Donald T. A.; Med. Arts Bldg., 628 Davis Dr. E., Newmarket, Ont.; Tor '43; IntMed.; Tel. 895-9613.
HUTCHINS, E. Keith; 2374 Eglinton Ave. E., Scarborough, Ont.; UBC '55; Tel. PL 7-3217.
HUTCHINS, J. Donald; 1199 Austin Rd., New Westminster, B.C.; UBC '56; MCGP; Tel. WE 9-7345.
HUTCHINSON, D. Barry; Man'57; Res., Toronto Western Hosp., Toronto 2B, Ont.
HUTCHINSON, Duayne T.; UBC '60; Assoc. Res., Vancouver Gen. Hosp., Vancouver, B.C.
HUTCHINSON, Edgar B.; Box 629, Amherstburg, Ont.; Tor'50; AMCGP; Staff, Grace & Hotel Dieu Hosp's., Windsor; Tel. 736-2118.
HUTCHINSON, Edgar D.; Cor. Sandwich & Rankin Aves., Amherstburg, Ont.; 204 Dalhousie St. (res); Tor '16; M.O.H., Amherstburg, Twps. Anderdon & LaSalle, & Essex County; Tel. 736-2118.
HUTCHINSON, Gordon M.; Westmount Med. Bldg., 77 Westmount Rd., Guelph, Ont.; Tor '60; FRCS(C), Otol.; Staff, Guelph Gen. & St. Joseph's Hosp's.; Tel. 824-9510.
HUTCHINSON, H. H.; Mountain Ave., Neepawa, Man.; 2nd Ave. (res); Man '28.
HUTCHINSON, William E.; 955 Queen St. E., **Sault-Ste-Marie, Ont.; 55 Riverside Dr. (res); Tor '41; FACS, FRCS(C), GenSurg; Surg.-in-Chief, Sault-Ste-Marie Gen. Hosp.; Tel. AL 3-3301.**
HUTCHISON, Alan D.; 165 Kingston Rd., Toronto 8, Ont.; Tor '52; Tel. OX 4-5622.
HUTCHISON, Douglas A.; 331 South St., London, Ont.; 1200 Ivanhill Rd. (res); Tor '47; DPH; MOH, City of London Clin.; Ass't. Prof. (PrevMed.), U. of Western Ont.; Tel. 438-7255.
HUTCHISON, George A.; Apt. 4., 6815 Sherbrooke St. W., Montreal 28, P.Q.; 6801 Monkland Ave. (res); McG '40; GenSurg; Staff, Queen Elizabeth San. & Reddy Mem. Hosp's.; Teach (Med.), O.P.D., Montreal Gen. Hosp.; Tel. HU 6-7835.
HUTCHISON, George W.; Southey, Sask.; McG '10; GenSurg; Dist. Coroner. Abroad.
HUTCHISON, Harold C.; 171 Yale Ave., Winnipeg, Man. (res.); Man'37; Anaes; Anaes., Grace Hosp.; Tel. SU 3-7271.
HUTCHISON, Henry; 228 Dundas St., Trenton, Ont.; Edinburgh (Scot.) '41; L.M., Rotunda, D.R.-C.O.G., ObstGyn; Cons., Trenton Mem. Hosp.; Tel. EX 2-4651.
HUTCHISON, Huert M.; 13732-101st Ave., Edmonton, Alta.; Alb'36.
HUTCHISON, Ian E.; 145 Chester Ave., Mount Royal, Montreal 16, P.Q.; McG '54; IntMed; Att'd. Staff, Queen Elizabeth Hosp.; Clin. Ass't., OPD, Royal Victoria Hosp.; Tel. RE 3-3936.
HUTCHISON, J. Craig; 9 Mill St. W., Acton, Ont.; Tor'61; AMCGP; Tel. 853-2180.
HUTCHISON, James H.; 7136—80th St., Edmonton, Alta. (res); Tor '22; Admin., Workmen's Comp. Bd., Edmonton, Alta.
HUTCHISON, J. Lawrence; 1650 Cedar Ave., Montreal, P.Q.; 432 Roslyn Ave., Westmount 6 (res); McG '53; D.I.M.; F.R.C.P.(C), IntMed; Haem (P.Q.); Assoc., Montreal Gen. Hosp.; Ass't. Prof. (Med.), McGill U.; Tel. WE 7-6011.
HUTCHISON, John A.; Ste. 619, 1207 Douglas St., Victoria, B.C.; 3293 Henderson Rd. (res); U. of Wales'53; Anaes; Staff, Royal Jubilee Hosp.; Tel. EV 3-3261.
HUTCHISON, Patricia A.; Walton Health Centre, 1910 McIntyre St., Regina, Sask.; 2925 Cameron **St. (res); Qns '54; Paed; Paed., Regina City Health Dept.; Court. Staff (Paed.), Regina Gen.** Hosp.; Tel. 522-1621, Loc. 278.
HUTCHISON, W. Glen; Ste. 305, 77 Westmount Rd., Guelph, Ont.; Man'58; Ophth; Tel. 822-5500.
HUTSON, Richard E.; 39 Wesley Ave., Port Credit, Ont.; Wes'55; Path.
HUTTON, A. Lyle; 15 Maple Ave., Brantford, Ont.; Wes '34; MCGP; Tel. 753-4151.

HUTTON, Charles F.; London (Eng.) '44; MRCS; LRCP; DMRD; Staff, Melfort Union Hosp., Melfort, Sask.
HUTTON, Charles J.; Dal '56; Res., Children's Hosp., Montreal 25, P.Q.
HUTTON, Douglas V.; 1590 Ouellete Ave., Windsor, Ont.; 1924 Devonshire Court (res); Tor '27; Paed; Att. Paed., Grace, Hotel Dieu, & Metropolitan Hosp's.; Tel. 254-9108.
HUTTON, Gordon H.; 4211 Marguerite, Vancouver 9, B.C. (res); Tor '30; DABPsy; DPH; Psy; Cons. & Hd. Psy., (OPD), Shaughnessy Hosp.; Ass't. Clin. Prof. (Psy), U. of British Columbia; Tel. TR 6-6767.
HUTTON, Margaret M.; 202-10856-82 Ave., Edmonton, Alta.; 11321-79 Ave. (res); Alb '42; F.A.C.O.G., F.A.C.S., F.R.C.S.(C) ObstGyn; Staff, U. of Alberta Hosp; Court. Staff, Royal Alexandra & Gen. Hosp's.; Cons. Gyn., U. of Alberta Student Health Serv.; Ass't. Clin. Prof. (ObstGyn), U. of Alberta; Chmn. Alberta Perinatal Mortality Committee; Tel. GE 9-3681.
HUTTON, William F.; 20 Doctor's Bldg., 955 Queen St. E., Sault Ste. Marie, Ont.; 1071 Queen; **Wes '51; FRCS(C), ObstGyn; Staff Plummer Mem. & Gen. Hosp's.; Tel. AL 3-7442.**
HUTTON, W. Keith; 7121-112th Ave., Edmonton, Alta.; 11324-64th St. (res); Dublin (Ire.) '53; Tel. 477-5355.
HWANG, Frances L.; Shanghai Teng-De (China) '48; Staff, W.C.B.Rehab. Clinic, 7123 119th Street, Edmonton, Alta.
HWANG, Walter H.; Seoul (Korea) '48; Jr. Intn., Grace Hosp., Winnipeg, Man.
HWOZDECKI, Roman M.; Carmangay, Alta.; Prague (Czech.) '36.
HYAMS, Brahm B.; 470 Ellendale Med. Bldg., 5845 Cote des Neiges Rd., Montreal 26, P.Q.; McG '56; FRCS(C); Urol; Clin. Ass't. Urol., Jewish Gen. Hosp.; Cons. Urol., Maimonides Hosp. & Home for the Aged; Court. Staff, Queen Elizabeth & Mount Sinai Hosp's.; Tel. 733-4941.
HYATT, Blake W.; R.R.2, Peterborough, Ont.; Tor '51; Path; Ass't. Path., Peterborough Civic Hosp.; Tel. RI 2-3831.
HYATT, John; Wes'64; Res., Hamilton Gen. Hosp., Hamilton, Ont.
HYDE, Alexander P.; Boston (Mass., U.S.A.) '52; Psy; Staff, Hosp. for Mental & Nervous Dis. St. John's, Nfld.; Abroad.
HYDE, D. Margaret; 35 Emerson St., Hamilton, Ont.; 255 Hess St. S. (res); Wales (U.K.) '43; M.R.C.S., L.R.C.P.; School M.O.; Tel. JA 2-1583.
HYDE, Harry A.; 10004-105th St., Edmonton, Alta.; 14624-78th Ave. (res); Tor '53; F.R.C.S. (C), GenSurg; Sessional Instr. (Surg.), U. of Alberta; Tel. GA 4-2121.
HYDE, Reed W.; 137 Beaconsfield Blvd., Beaconsfield, P.Q.; 5025 Sherbrooke St. W., Ste. 425, Montreal 28, McG '44; FRCS(C), Otol; Att'd. Staff, Queen Elizabeth Hosp. & Lakeshore Gen. Hosp.; Tel. 695-6018 & 488-9471.
HYLAND, Herbert H.; 604 Med. Arts Bldg., 170 St. George St., Toronto 5, Ont.; 52 Lawrence Cres., Tor 12 (res); Tor '26; FRCP(Lond.), FRCP(C), NeurPsy; Cons. Phys., Toronto Gen., Wellesley & Sunnybrook Hosp's.; Tel. 922-4624.
HYMOVITCH, I. Victor; 5744 Durocher, Montreal 8, P.Q.; Mon '45; Indust. Phys., Richstone Bakeries Inc., 4222 St. Lawrence Blvd., Mtl. 18.
HYNDMAN, Charles F.; 8930-120th St., Edmonton, Alta.; Qns '41; DiagRad; Dir., Dept. of Rad., Royal Alexandra Hosp.; Lect. (Rad.), U. of Alberta; Tel. GR 4-3431.
HYNDMAN, W. W. Burton; 274 Dorval Ave., **Dorval, P.Q.; 62 Handfield Circle (res); McG '52; GenSurg (P.Q.); Surg. Staff, Lachine Gen. Hosp.; Tel. 631-6471.**
HYNES, Allan M.; 206 Med. Bldg., Prince Albert, Sask.; 306-19th St. W. (res); Alb '39; Urol; Chief Urol., Victoria Hosp.; Vis. Urol. Holy Family Hosp.; Tel. 763-7481.
HYNES, John A.; Abbott Clinic, 274 Osborne St. N., Winnipeg, Man.; Glasgow (Scot.) '55; MRCP (Glas.); FRCP(C), IntMed; Tel. 774-4567.

HYNSCHT, Robert O.; 220 St. George St., Port Dover, Ont.; Ludwig-Maximilian U. (Munich, Germany) '56; Tel. 582-1241.
HYSLOP, William A.; 608 Maritime Bldg., New Glasgow, N.S.; London (Eng.) '33; DO; Surg. (Ophth), Aberdeen Hosp.; Tel. 752-6121.
IACHELLI, Carmelo L.; 26 Barton St. W., Hamilton, Ont.; Catinia (Italy) '56.; AMCGP; Tel. JA 9-8980.
IBBERSON, John R.; Charles E. Frosst & Co.; Box 247, Montreal 3, P.Q.; Qns'44; MCGP; Exec. Med. Dir., Charles E. Frosst & Co.; Tel. 932-7111, Ext. 314.
IBBERSON, Olive; 516 Med. Arts Bldg., 170 St. George St., Toronto 5, Ont.; 450 Walmer Rd., Apt 1412, (res); London (Eng.) '51; FACS, FRCS(C), GenSurg; Assoc. Chief of Surg., Women's College Hosp.; Clin. Instr. (Surg.), U. of Toronto; Tel. WA 3-7493.
IBBOTSON, Colin; 193 West Lane, Moncton, N.B. (res); Liverpool (Eng.) '40; D. & T Rad; Assoc. Rad., Moncton Hosp.; Tel. EV 4-4421.
IBBOTT, J. William; 1081 Burrard St., Vancouver 1, B.C.; McG'54; FRCP(C), IntMed; Haem., St. Paul's & Shaughnessy Hosp's.; Clin. Instr. (Med.), U. of British Columbia; Tel. 682-2344.
IBRAHIM, Ali; Box 541, 288 Murdoch Ave., Noranda, P.Q.; Istanbul (Turkey)'54; DABA; FACA; FICS; D.A.; Anaes; Staff, Youville Hosp.; Tel. 762-9255.
IDESON, Roderick S.; Medical Arts Bldg., 121 Wellington St. W., Barrie, Ont.; Dal '42; Staff, Royal Victoria Hosp.; Tel. 728-5536.
IFFY, Leslie; Med. Arts Clinic, 147 Central St., Swift Current, Sask.; Budapest (Hung.)'49; FACOG; ObstGyn; Cons. ObstGyn., Swift Current Union Hosp.; Tel. 773-4636.
IGEL, Wilfried; Stittsville, Ont.; Ludwig-Maximilian U. of Munich (Germ.) '31; M.O.H. Twp. of Goulburn; Tel. 836-2361.
IGOE, John M.; Carmanville, Nfld.; Dublin (Ire.) '52.
ILES, John D.; 618 Church St., Toronto, Ont.; 160 Glen Rd., Tor. 5 (res); Cambridge (Eng.) '40; M.R.C.S., L.R.C.P.; M.C.G.P.; Staff, Shouldice Surgery; Tel. WA 3-3507.
ILLIEVITZ, A. Bernard; Apt. 1, 2156 Sherbrooke St. W., Montreal 25, P.Q.; McG '14; FAGS (Germ.); Hon. Med. Dir., Herzl Health Serv. Centre; Royal Norwegian & Swedish Consulate General for Mtl.; Phys., Sun Alliance & London Ins. Group; Tel. 933-8220.
IMPRIE Elizabeth P.; 421 Garden St., Hawkesbury, Ont.; Sheffield (Eng.) '49; MRCS; LRCP; Temporarily retired.
IMRIE, George G.; The Smith Clinic, Hawkesbury, Ont.; 421 Garden St. (res); Sheffield (Eng.) '52; M.B., Ch. B.; Tel. ME 2-2711.
IMRIE, Robert J.; 5110 Dundas St., Islington, Ont.; 15 Orkney Cres. (res); Tor '50; AMCAA; Paed; Dir., Poison Control Centre, Hosp. for Sick Children, Toronto; Clin. Instr., Hosp. for Sick Children; Tel. 231-1917.
INANKUR, Yuksel A.; Mall Med. Group, 280 Memorial Blvd., Winnipeg 1, Man.; 826 Ebby St. Wpg. 9 (res); Ankara (Turkey) '56; Paed; Staff, U. of Manitoba; Tel. SP 4-2411; Abroad.
INCH, F. Arthur; 421 Med. Arts Bldg., 1 Young St., Hamilton, Ont.; Qns'56; Ophth; Court. Staff, Hamilton Gen. & St. Joseph's Hosp's.; Tel. JA 8-0718.
ING, Moeuy C.; 112A Dundas W., Toronto 2, Ont.; Tor '29; Staff, Women's College Hosp.; Part-time Staff, Dept. of Health, City of Toronto; Tel. 368-9997.
ING, Robert Yun Kwing; 1004 Lawrence Ave. E., Apt. 212, Don Mills, Ont.; Tulane'61; FRCP(C), Paed.
ING, Tom G.; 3711 Riverside Dr. E., Riverside, Ont.; Wes'61; Ophth.
ING, Vincent W.; Tor '60; FRCP(C), IntMed; MRC Fell. Haem.; Staff, Victoria Gen. Hosp., Halifax, N.S.
INGHAM, George H.; 113 William St., Stratford, Ont.; Wes '14; Ophth, Otol; Ophth., Stratford Gen. Hosp.; Cons. Ophth, Otol., D.V.A. & W.C.-B.; Tel. 271-3950.

INGHAM, George K.; McGregor Clinic, 250 Main St. E., Hamilton, Ont.; 78 Mansfield Dr., Ancaster (res); Wes '43; FRCP(C), IntMed; Hd. Radio-Isotopes Dept., St. Joseph's Hosp.; Med. Dir. Hamilton Red Cross Blood Trans. Serv.; Med. Cons., Nuclear Reactor Project & Research Assoc., McMaster U.; Tel. JA 7-2711.

INGLIS, Alan M.; 750 W. Broadway, Vancouver 9, B.C.; 3751 Selkirk St. (res); Man '44; D.A.-O.A., F.R.C.S.(C), OrthSurg; Att'd. Staff, Vancouver Gen. Hosp.; Clin. Instr. (Surg.), U. of British Columbia; Tel. TR. 2-5696.

INGLIS, Douglas S.; Box 640, 160 Main St., Shediac, N.B.; Dal'66.

INGLIS, Frederic G.; 410 Seaforth Med. Bldg., 3550 Cote Des Neiges Rd.; 60 Simcoe Ave., Town of Mount Royal (res); Dal '55; M. Sc.; DABS; FRCS(C); GenSurg; Clin. Ass't., Royal Victoria Hosp.; Dem (Surg.), McGill U.; Tel. WE 7-9800.

INGLIS, Hugh F.; Med. Clinic, 1561 Gower Pt. Rd., Gibson's, B.C.; Alb '34; AMCGP; Staff, St. Mary's Hosp., Sechelt; Tel. 886-2221; Abroad.

INGLIS, J. Gordon; 985 Kingsway Dr., Burlington, Ont.; Glasgow (Scot.)'47.

INGLIS, John E.; 73 Queen St. E., Brampton, Ont.; Tor '62; Tel. 451-1244.

INGLIS, Robert; Estevan Med. Assoc., 1314-3rd St., Estevan, Sask.; 1217 First St. (res); Man '37; ObstGyn.; Tel. 634-2676.

INGRAHAM, Donald R.; 115 Hazen Ave., Saint John, N.B.; 256 Rodney St. (res); Dal '53; GenSurg.; Tel. 693-7771.

INGRAM, David W.; 1 Campbell Ave., St. John's, Nfld. Queen's U. (Belfast, N. Ire.) '50; M.B., B.Ch., BAO, M.S. (Med.) (Minn.), FRCP(C), IntMed.; Tel. 579-1199.

INGRAM, Geoffrey D.; Ste. 303, 1541 W. Broadway, Vancouver 9, B.C.; Manchester (Eng.)'60; FRCS(C), ObstGyn.

INGRAM, Herbert G. 143 Menzies St., Victoria, B.C.; 71 Beach Dr. (res); UBC'61; AMCGP; Tel. 385-3042.

INGRAM, Robert F.; 2300 Tupper St., Montreal, P.Q.; 348 Kensington Ave., Westmount, **Mtl. 6 (res); Dal '43; Executive Dir., Mtl. Children's Hosp.; Tel. WE 7-8511.**

INGRAM, William E.; 300 Medical Arts Bldg., Calgary, Alta.; Man '27; F.A.C.S., GenSurg; Chief Surg. Staff, Holy Cross Hosp.; Tel. 269-2561.

INMAN, Fay R.; 1745 Cedar Ave., Apt. 104, Montreal 25, P.Q.; Wes '57; FRCP(C), IntMed.

INMAN, G. S.; Montague, P.E.I.; Dist. Coroner.

INNES, Duncan M.; Bristol (Eng.)'57; Path: Staff, Kelowna Gen. Hosp., Kelowna, B.C.; Assoc. Path., Okanagan Regional Laboratories.

INNES, Ian R.; 575 Elm St., Winnipeg 9, Man. (res); Aberdeen (Scot.) '37; M.B., Ch.B., M.D.; Assoc. Prof (Pharmacol & Therapeut.), U. of Manitoba; Tel. GR 5-0810.

INNES, Roy; UBC '64; Res., Vancouver Gen. Hosp., Vancouver 9, B.C.

INNOCENTI, Giuseppe; 66 Treelawn Parkway, Toronto 15, Ont. (res); Florence (Italy) '50; M.O., W.C.B. Rehab. Centre & Hosp.

INTINO, Carmen A. D.; 133 Bay St., Sydney, N.S.; Dal '45.

INVIDIATA, Frank P.; 396 Royal York Rd. S., Toronto 18, Ont.; Tor '55; Tel. CL 9-8182.

IRA, Felix S.; U. of the Philippines '54; Jr. Int'n., Doctors' Hosp., 45 Brunswick Ave., Toronto 4, Ont.

IRELAND, Desmond J.; 35 Clement Blk., Brandon, Man.; Ste. 9, 256—29th St. (res); Sydney (Australia) '53; Otol; Otol. Staff, Brandon Gen. Hosp.; Cons. Otol., Brandon Hosp. for Mental Diseases, Assiniboine Hosp. & Ninette San.; Tel. PA 9-2478.

IRELAND, Franklin A. J.; 170 Bloor St. W., Toronto, Ont.; 108 Park Rd. (res); Tor '22; Derm-Syph.; Tel. WA 3-2525. Retired.

IRELAND, J. Allan; 1726 West Broadway, Vancouver 9, B.C.; 2157—W. 57th Ave. (res); Tor '26; D.M.R.D., DiagRad; Staff, Mount St. Joseph's Grace & St. Vincent's Hosp's.; Tel. RE 8-5118; 266-2388.

IRELAND, James R.; 625-5th Ave., New Westminster, B.C.; 1819 Acadia Rd. (res); **Man '39; Urol; Chief Urol., Royal Columbian Hosp.; Tel. LA 1-7761-2.**

IRELAND, L. Charles H.; 1020 Mackenzie Ave., Victoria, B.C.; UBC'61; Tel. 479-2433.

IRELAND, Percy E.; 330 Med. Arts Bldg., 170 St. George St., Toronto 5, Ont.; 494 Avenue Rd., Tor. 7 (res); Tor '29; FACS, FRCS(C), Otol; Cons. (Otol.), Hosp. for Sick Children & Women's College Hosp.; Otol-in-Chief, Toronto Gen. & Sunnybrook Hosp's.; Prof. & Hd., Dept. of Otol., U. of Toronto; Tel. WA 2-7456.

IRETON, H. J. 76 Lonsdale Rd., Toronto 7, Ont. (res); Tor '62.; Tel. HU 9-3116.

IRISH, Robert H.; Pearson Hosp., 700 W. 57th **St., Vancouver, B.C.**; 3592 Quesnelle Dr. (res); **Tor '36; F.C.C.P.; Ass't. Supt., Pearson Hosp., Pearson San., Vancouver; Tel. FA 1-3231.**

IRISH, Ronald; UBC'65; Staff, Royal Jubilee Hosp., Victoria, B.C.

IRLAM, L. Peter; Edinburgh (Scot.) '62; AMCGP; Res., Victoria Gen. Hosp., Halifax, N.S.

IRONSIDE, James J.; 710 Seymour St., Vancouver, B.C.; 6926 Churchill (res); Edinburgh (Scot.) '49; FRCS(Ed.), FRCS(C), GenSurg; Tel. MU 4-1511.

IRONSIDE, Nancy K.; 11 Coldwater St. E., Orillia, Ont.; Tor '56; Anaes; Staff, Soldiers Mem. Hosp.; Tel. 325-2271.

IRONSTONE, Paul S.; 247 Queen St., Cooksville, Ont. (res); McG '22; Retired.

IRVINE, Alan H.; 1105 Carling Ave., Ottawa 3, Ont.; 64 Geneva St. (res); Tor'52; FACS; FRCS(C), Urol; Att'd. Staff, Ottawa Civic Hosp.; Chief Cons. (Urol.), Nat. Defence Med. Centre (Ottawa); Clin. Ass't. (Surg.), U. of Ottawa; Tel. 729-1612.

IRVINE, George T.; Student Health Centre, 1220 College Dr., U. of Saskatchewan, Saskatoon, Sask.; Dal '33; Tel. 653-2522.

IRVINE, Ian F.; 27 Third St., Collingwood, Ont.; Glasgow (Scot.)'61.

IRVINE, I. G.; Tor '64; Jr. Int., Montreal Gen. Hosp., Montreal 25, P.Q.; Abroad.

IRVINE, John W.; 816-103rd Ave., Dawson Creek, B.C.; Alb '51; GenSurg.; Tel. 782-4848.

IRVINE, William G.; 1401 W. Broadway, Vancouver 9, B.C.; UBC'60.

IRVING, David W.; Baker Clinic, 10004-105th St., Edmonton, Alta.; Alb '57; FCCP; AFACC; IntMed; Att'd. Staff, Royal Alexandra Hosp.; Clin. Instr., U. of Alberta; Tel. 424-2121.

IRVING, Donald G.; Crystal City, Man.; Man. '49; Dist. Coroner.; Tel. 105.

IRVING, John A.; 3195 Granville St., Vancouver, B.C.; 1957 S.W. Marine Dr. (res); Qns '39; D.A.B.O., Ophth; Sr., Dept. of Ophth., Vancouver Gen. Hosp.; Clin. Ass't., U. of British Columbia; Tel. RE 3-3320.

IRVING, Rodney T.; Ste 230, 809 W-41st Ave., Vancouver 13, B.C.; Ott '55; GenSurg; M.C.G.P.; Att'd. Staff, St. Vincent's Hosp.; Tel. 263-6333.

IRVING, Ronald W.; 430 Mount Stephen Ave., Westmount, Montreal 6, P.Q. (res); Edinburgh (Scot.) '36; Staff, Ste. Anne's Hosp., Ste. Anne de Bellevue, P.Q.; Tel. 453-5395.

IRWIN, Aden C.; Regional Health Centre Bldg., Box, 938, Prince Albert, Sask.; 9B Paramount Apts. (res); Tor '51; DPH; MRSH; FRSH; MOH, Northern Health Dist.; Tel. 763-7240.

IRWIN, D. June; McG'61; Res. (Derm.), Montreal Gen. Hosp., Montreal, P.Q.

IRWIN, George E.; 165 Laurier E., Ottawa, Ont.; 671 Island Park Dr. (res); Lav '44; F.R.C.S.(C) GenSurg; Surg. Staff, Ottawa Gen. Hosp.; Ass't. Prof. Surg., Ottawa U.; Tel. CE 4-1335.

IRWIN, Herbert J. F.; 334 Old Muskoka Rd. Orillia, Ont. (res); Tor '47; Phys—I/C Orillia Dist. Chest Clinic (Br. of Gage Inst., Nat. San. Assoc.); Tel. 325-1482.

IRWIN, J. Kent; The Polyclinic, 170 Fitzroy St., Charlottetown, PEI; 16 Crestwood Dr. (res); Dal '40; ObstGyn; Chief (ObstGyn), PEI Hosp.; Court. Staff, Charlottetown Hosp.; Tel. 894-7325.

IRWIN, John; 11603-48th Ave., Edmonton, Alta.; Alb '64; Tel. 434-2701.

IRWIN, K. Maxwell; 238 Augustus St., Cornwall, Ont.; Tor'55; FACOG; FRCS(C), ObstGyn; Cons. Staff, ObstGyn, Hotel Dieu & Chief of ObstGyn, Cornwall Gen. Hosp's.; Tel. WE 2-8052.
IRWIN, Michael E.; 1539 Erie St. E., Windsor, Ont.; Tor'63.
IRWIN, Noble T.; Swift Current Clinic, 129 Central N., Swift Current, Sask.; 568-3rd N.E. (res); Man '50; ObstGyn; Chief (ObstGyn), Swift Current Union Hosp.; Tel. 773-4681.
IRWIN, Oscar M.; Swift Current Clinic, 129 Central Ave., Swift Current, Sask.; 412—4th Ave. E. (res); Tor '13; F.R.C.S.(Edin.), F.R.C.S.(C) GenSurg; Staff, Swift Current Union Hosp.; Retired.
IRWIN, Patricia J. (Scully); 109 Westmoreland St., Cornwall, Ont. (res); Tor '55; Temp. Retired.
IRWIN, Paul; Cooksville Med. Bldg., 21 Upper Middle Rd., Cooksville, Ont.; Tor '57; Pres. Med. Staff, South Peel Mem. Hosp.; Tel. 279-7330.
IRWIN, Robert N.; 168 Old Orchard Grove, Toronto, Ont.; Qns '26; Tel. HU 8-2983.
IRWIN, Robert W.; Swift Current Clinic, 129 Central Ave., Swift Current, Sask.; 371-4th N.E. (res); Man '52; GenSurg; Staff, Swift Current Hosp.; Tel. 773-4641.
IRWIN, Ross B. Sg/Cdr.; C.O., Cdn. Forces Hosp., Halifax, N.S.
IRWIN, Roy S.; 178 Simcoe St. N., Oshawa, Ont.; 438 Simcoe St. N., (res); Tor '43; Staff, Oshawa Gen. Hosp.; Tel. 723-2745.
IRWIN, Thomas G.; 14 Victoria E., Alliston, Ont.; Tor'45; Staff, Stevenson Mem. Hosp.; **Coroner, County of Simcoe; Tel. 435-6231.**

ISAAC, Geoffrey H.; 2901 Lawrence Ave. E., Scarborough, Ont.; London (Eng.) '50; MRCS; LRCP; MCGP; Staff, Scarborough Gen. Hosp.; Tel. AX 3-7551.
ISAAC, Jacob E.; Winnipeg Clinic, St. Mary's & Vaughan St., Winnipeg 1, Man.; Man '40; FICS; FRCS(C), GenSurg; Chief of Surg., Concordia Hosp.; Active Staff, Wpg. Gen. & Misericordia **Gen. Hosp's.; Lect., U. of Manitoba; Tel. 942-0551.**

ISAAK, Verner H.; 443 Reynolds St., Oakville, Ont.; Tor'65.

ISAACSEN, Ruth; 10408-118th Ave., Edmonton, Alta.; 8007-149th St. (res); Tor '47; M.C.G.P.; Att'd. Staff, Misericordia Hosp.; Assoc. Staff, Royal Alexandra Hosp.; Court. Staff, Edmonton Gen. Hosp.; Tel. GR 7-7871.
ISABELLE, Gaston; 31 Montcalm St., Hull, P.Q.; Aylmer Rd., Hull South (res); Mon '48; M.C.-G.P.
ISABEY, Amedee P.; Norwood Med. Bldg., 245 Marion St., St. Boniface 6, Man.; Man'61; MCGP.
ISBISTER, Earl G.; 103 Med. Arts Bldg., Hamilton, Ont.; 3050 Briarwood Cr., Burlington (res); McG '58; Urol; Tel. JA 2-8114.
ISCOVE, Arnold; 136 Carlton St., Toronto 2, Ont.; 728 Briar Hill Ave. (res); Tor '29; Staff, New Mt. Sinai Hosp.; Tel. WA 3-4191.
ISELI, Henry; 6674 Fraser St., Vancouver 15, B.C.; 5970 Athlone St. (res); Man '51; Vis. Staff, Vancouver Gen., Grace, St. Paul's, St. Vincent's & Mt. St. Joseph's Hosp's.; Tel. FA 7-4411.
ISHII, Masatatsu; 1217-17A St. N.W., Calgary, Alta.; Keio-Gijuku (Tokio, Japan); '54; Anaes; Dir. Dept. of Inhalation Ther. & Staff, Calgary Gen. Hosp.; Tel. AM 6-7541.
ISITT, Cyril L.; Shoal Lake Health Unit, Birtle, Man.; Edinburgh (Scot.)'42; LRCP&S (Edin.); LRFP&S (Glas.); DPH (Tor.).
ISMAN, Garry B.; Wolseley, Sask.; Man '24; Dist. Coroner.
ISOMURA, Soichi; 577 Ash St., Point-St.-Charles, Montreal, P.Q.; McG '55; Tel. WE 2-2610.
ISRAEL, J. A.; Tor'65; Res., Toronto Western Hosp., Toronto 2B, Ont.
ISRAELS, Esther D. (Hornstein); 502 South Dr., Winnipeg 19, Man.; Man '50; Research Assoc. (Paed.), U. of Manitoba.
ISRAELS, Lyonel G.; 502 South Dr., Winnipeg, Man. **(res); Man '49; F.R.C.P.(C), Int** Med; Prof. (Med.), U. of Manitoba; Tel. 786-4731.

ISRAELS, Max G.; 710 Seymour St., Vancouver 2, B.C.; Man '29; FACP; DABIM; FRCP(C), IntMed.
ISRAELS, Sydney; Man '39; FACP; FAAP; FR CP(C); IntMed; Paed; Chief Paed., Vancouver Gen. & Children's Hosp's.; Prof., Dept. of Paediatrics, U. of B.C., Vancouver, B.C.; Tel. CA 4-1111.

ISTVAN, Edward J.; Tor'60; FRCS(C), ObstGyn; Staff, Wellesley Hosp., Toronto 5, Ont.
ITTKIN, Paul; 535 Ellendale Med. Bldg., 5845 Cote des Neiges Rd., Montreal 26, P.Q.; McG'33; DABO; FACS; Otol; Att'd. Staff, Reddy Mem. Hosp. & Jewish Gen. Hosp.; Cons. Jewish Hosp. of Hope; Otol., Montreal Fashion Indus. Health Centre; Tel. RE 1-8881.
IUTCOVICH, Eugenia; Bucharest (Roum.)'54; Staff, Douglas Hosp., Montreal 19, P.Q.
IVAN, Leslie P.; 521 Bate Cres., Saskatoon, Sask. (res); Debrecen (Hung.) '44; FHCS; FRCS(C), NeurSurg; Active Staff, University & City Hosp's.; Assoc. Staff, St. Paul's Hosp.; Clin. Assoc. (NeurSurg), U. of Saskatchewan; Tel. 652-6977.
IVANANS, Peter; 537 College St., Toronto 4, Ont.; London (Eng.) '63.
IVANIC, Vuk; Box 23; Belgrade (Yugoslavia) '39; M.O., Industrial Farm, Dept. of Reform Institutions, Burwash, Ont.
IVE, F. Adrian; Haig Clinic, 601-6th Ave. S., Lethbridge, Alta.; Durham (Eng.), M.B., B.S.
IVERSEN, Paul J.; 91 Tudhope St., Espanola, Ont.; McG'54; Sr. Active Staff, Espanola Gen. Hosp.; Coroner, Dist. of Sudbury; Tel. 869-2620.
IVES, Elizabeth J.; 800 Spadina Cres. E., Saskatoon, Sask. (res); Glasgow (Scot.) '56; FRCP(C), Paed; DPH; DCH; DRCOG; Staff, University Hosp.; Ass't. Prof. Paed. & Lect. (Soc. & Prev. Med.), U. of Saskatchewan.
IVES, George Anthony; 78 Gore St., Kingston, Ont.; Edinburgh (Scot.)'52; DPM; FRCP(C), Psy.
IVES, Raymond E.; Stayner, Ont.; Tor '22; Dist. Coroner.
IVES, William G.; Stayner, Ont.; Tor '52; MCGP.
IVIE, L. Grant; Chinook Shopping Centre, 6449 Macleod Trail, Calgary, Alta.; Alb '54; MCGP; Tel. AL 5-5566.
IWACHNIUK, Nadia (Ruzycka); 409 Dovercourt Rd., Toronto, Ont.; 83 Shannon St. (res); Zagreb (Yugoslavia) '34; Assoc. Staff, Womens College Hosp.; Tel. LE 3-9992.
IWAN, Stanley R.; 900 King St. W., Kitchener, Ont.; Wes '55; FRCS(C), NeurSurg; Active Staff, Kitchener-Waterloo Hosp. & St. Mary's Gen. Hosp.; Cons., St. Joseph's Hosp. & Gen. Hosp. Guelph & South Waterloo Hosp., Galt; Tel. 742-4342.
IWANEC, Wasyl; 12911-114th Ave., Edmonton, Alta. (res); Cracow (Poland) '35; M.O., Chas. Camsell Indian Hosp.; Tel GL 5-7141.
IZATT, Jean A. (Ure); 359 St. James Cres., Vancouver, B.C.; UBC '55; Tel. 922-0942.
JACIW, George A.; Whitby Plaza, Whitby, Ont.; Ott '55.
JACK, Kenneth D.; Box 420, Hudson Hope, B.C.; Wes'64.
JACK, Richard D.; McG'62; Res., Dept. of Pharm., U. of British Columbia, Vancouver 8, B.C.
JACK, William; Box 339, Birch Hills, Sask. (res); Glasgow (Scot.) '47; L.R.C.P., L.R.C.S. (Edin.); Staff, University Hosp.
JACKH, Henry; 3028 Cadboro Bay Rd., Victoria, B.C. (res); Munich (Germ.) '44; DiagRad; Radiol., St. Joseph's Hosp.; Tel. EV 4-1131.
JACKS, Nathan B.; 900 Giles Blvd. E., Windsor, Ont.; 1599 Victoria Ave. (res); Tor '39; FACC, MCGP; Tel. CL 6-2347.
JACKS, Quentin D.; Ste. 1304, 750 W. Broadway, Vancouver 9, B.C.; 1222 Nanton Ave. (res); Man '40; Otol.; Tel. TR 6-5213.
JACKS, W. Grant; Lockwood Clinic, 300 Bloor St. E., Toronto 5, Ont.; Universidad National Del Sterest '60; Tel. WA 1-2121.

JACKSON, Alan B.; 36 Peel St., Simcoe, Ont.; 135 Union St. (res); Tor '16; F.A.C.C.; Rad & Cardiol., Norfolk Gen. Hosp.; Dist. Coroner.

JACKSON, Barton A.; 416 Avenue Bldg., Saskatoon, Sask.; 201-108th St., Sutherland (res); Tor '34; F.R.C.S.(Edin.), F.A.C.S., F.R.C.S.(C) GenSurg; Chief of Surg., Saskatoon City Hosp.; Surg. Cons., D.V.A.; Assoc. Clin. Prof. (Surg.), University Hosp.; Tel. 244-8504.

JACKSON, C. Colin; 745 W. Broadway, Vancouver, B.C.; 4922 Marine Dr., W. Vanc. (res); Man'44; M.Sc. (Proct.); DAB (Proct.); FAPS; Staff, Vancouver Gen., St. Vincents, Mount St. Joseph & Burnaby Gen. Hosp's.; Assoc. Staff, Lions Gate Hosp.; Tel. TR 4-1310.

JACKSON, Donald C.; 108 Medical Arts Bldg., 404-406 Graham Ave., Winnipeg, Man.; Sheffield (Eng.)'54; MRCS; MRCP; DMRD; FFR; FRCP(C), DiagRad; Staff (Rad.), St. Boniface Gen. Hosp. & Deer Lodge Vet's Hosp.; Tel. 943-7301.

JACKSON, Edwin J.; 17 Viamede Cr., Willowdale, Ont.; Tor '33; Anaes; Staff, Toronto East Gen. & Orth. Hosp.; Tel. 461-8272.

JACKSON, Francis L.; 9006-120th St., Edmonton, Alta.; London (Eng.)'46; MRCS (Eng.); LRCP (Lond.).

JACKSON, Frank I.; 540 Tegler Bldg., Edmonton, Alta.; Cape Town (S. Africa)'47; DPH; PH; DiagRad; Staff, Dept. of Rad., Royal Alexandra Hosp., Edmonton, Alta.; Tel. 421-8261.

JACKSON, George A.; 181 McIntyre St. W., North Bay, Ont.; 617 Jane St. (res); Tor '34; Head, Dept. of Obst., North Bay Civic, & St. Joseph's Gen. Hosp's.; Tel. GR 2-3660.

JACKSON, Harold M.; Ste. 201, 628 Davis Dr., Newmarket, Ont.; 198 Millard Ave. (res); Wes' '55; ObstGyn; Chief of Obst., York County Hosp.; Tel. 895-5561.

JACKSON, Ivan M.; 599-2nd Ave. E., Owen sound, Ont.; Tor'61; AMCGP; Tel. 376-9561.

JACKSON, James W.; Ste. 204, 414 Graham Ave., Winnipeg 1, Man.; Edinburgh (Scot.)'45; FICS; FRCS (Edin.); Otol; Otol., Children's, Winnipeg Gen. & Misericordia Hosp's.; Cons. Otol., Wpg. Mun. Hosp.; Dem. (Otol.), U. of Man.; Tel. 947-1561 or 947-1562.

JACKSON, John E.; 331 Russell St., Woodstock, Ont. (res); Tor '25; M.C.G.P.; Staff, Ontario Hosp., Woodstock; Tel. LE 9-1251. Retired.

JACKSON, John M.; Essondale, B.C. (res); Man '27; Psy; Rad., Crease Clinic; Retired.

JACKSON, John R., G/C; 437 Meadow Dr., Ottawa 2, Ont. (res); Birmingham (Eng.) '41; MRCS, LRCP, DTM & H, M.Sc., DPH (Tor.); **Path; Dir. of Labs., National Defence Med. Centre, Ottawa; Ass't. Prof. (Path), U. of Ottawa; Tel. CE 2-8211.**

JACKSON, Leonard G.; 5569 Borden Ave., Cote St. Luc, Montreal, P.Q.; London (Eng.)'44; MRCS (Eng.); LRCP (Lond.); FCCP; Med. Dir., Grace Dart Hosp.; Tel. 484-3464.

JACKSON, Mary E. P.; Keg River, Alta.; Birmingham (Eng.) '27; M.R.C.S. (Eng.), L.R.C.P. (Lond.), M.C.GP.

JACKSON, Mary V.; Clarke Inst. of Psy., 250 College St., Toronto 2, Ont.; Tor'29; Psy; Ass't. Med. Dir., Clarke Inst.; Assoc. Prof. (Psy.), U. of Toronto; Tel. 924-6811.

JACKSON, Neville J.; Durham (Eng.)'53; FRCS(Eng.); FRCS(C), GenSurg; Staff, Foothills Hosp., Calgary, Alta.

JACKSON, Norman C.; 58 Church St. Goderich, Ont.; Man '26; GenSurg; Chief of Surg., Alexandra Marine & Gen. Hosp.; Tel. 524-8622.

JACKSON, Paul P.; 417 Medical Dental Bldg., 925 W. Georgia St., Vancouver 1, B.C.; 6405 Cedarhurst res; Oklahoma (U.S.A.) '42; F.A.C.S.; GenSurg; Clin. Instr. Surg.), U. of British Columbia; Active Staff, St. Paul's Hosp.; Tel. MU 5-7201.

JACKSON, Peter D.; Plaza Med. Centre, Sydney River, N.S.; Guys Hosp. (London, Eng.) '56; FRCS(Ed.); Tel. 562-3134.

JACKSON, Robert; 310 O'Connor St., Ottawa, Ont.; 2036 Knightsbridge Rd. (res); McG '50; F.R.C.P.(C), DermSyph; Derm. Ottawa Civic Hosp.; Cons. (Derm), D.V.A.; Tel. CE 6-3637.

JACKSON, Robert W.; Orthopaedic Service, Toronto Gen. Hosp., Toronto, Ont.; Tor '56; FRCS(C); OrthSurg; Staff, Orthopaedic Research Lab., Rm. 526, Banting Inst., Toronto 2, Ont.; Ass't. Surg., Toronto Gen. Hosp.; Assoc. Surg., U. of Toronto; Markdale Scholar, Acad. Med.; Tel. EM 6-8211, Loc. 2684.

JACKSON, Ronald M.; 240 Algonquin Ave., North Bay, Ont.; 833 Morin St. (res); Man'44; FRCS (Edin.), GenSurg; Staff, St. Joseph's & Civic Hosp's.; Surg., Can. Int. Paper Co.; Tel. GR 2-8400.

JACKSON, Rosemary (See Lindan)

JACKSON, Russell F., W/C; Trinity Coll. (Ireland)'49; DPH(Tor); Deputy Reg. Surg., RCAF Station, Trenton, Ont.

JACKSON, Sydney G.; 3533 Eglinton Ave. W., Toronto, Ont.; 5 Reigate Rd. (res); Tor '38; Tel. RO 9-2203.

JACKSON, Thomas E.; Dawson Creek Med. Clinic, Dawson Creek, B.C.; Sask '58, MCGP.

JACKSON, William O.; Med. Arts Bldg., Hamilton, Ont.; 105 Arkell St. (res); Qns '50; IntMed; Active Staff, Hamilton Gen. Hosp.; Tel. JA 9-5148.

JACO, Nicholas T.; Oxford (Eng.)'45; MRCP (Lond.); DCH (Eng.); Paed; Staff, St. Joseph's Hosp., London, Ont.

JACOB, Chandy Vattakattucherry; Kerala (India)'58; FRCS(C), GenSurg; Staff, St. Boniface Hosp., St. Boniface, Man.

JACOB, David; 299 5th St., Quebec 3, P.Q.; 851 Bellevue, Que. 10 (res); Lav '53; Paed; Staff, Hop. St. Francois d' Assise; Tel. 529-4911.

JACOB, Jean L.; Mon'65; Res., Hop. Hotel-Dieu, Montreal 18, P.Q.

JACOB, Marcel; 11876, des Meulles, Montreal 12, P.Q.; Lav '59; Anaes; Staff, Royal Victoria Hosp.; Tel. 842-1251.

JACOB, Richard; 438 rue Thibeau, Cap-de-la-Madeleine, P.Q.; Lav '58.

JAN, James E.; Alb '63; Res., Vancouver Gen.

JACOBS, Alan A.; 326a College St., Toronto 2B, Ont.; 165 Jamieson Ave., Apt. 510, Tor. 3 (res); Howard, Washington (U.S.A.) '59; Tel. 923-7209.

JACOBS, C. Gloria (Brenner); 124-1st Ave. W., Swift Current Sask.; Liverpool (Eng.) '53; Staff, Swift Current Union Hosp.; Tel. 773-8333.

JACOBS, Harold; 560 Phys. & Surgs. Bldg., 8409 - 112th St., Edmonton, Alta.; Cambridge (Eng.) '53; M.Med. (Capetown); MRCP (Ed.); FRCP(C), Neurol; Ass't. Clin. Prof. (Neurol.), U. of Alberta.

JACOBS, H. E.; Freiburg (Germ.) '42; Delta, Ont.; Clin. Ass't., (Med.), Queen's U., Kingston, Ont.

JACOBS, John A.; 123 Edward St., Toronto 2, Ont.; Cambridge (Eng.) '58; M.B., B.Ch.; FRCP (C); Anaes; Staff, St. Michael's Hosp.; Tel. 362-4461

JACOBS, Robert; 124-1st St. N.W., Swift Current, Sask.; 865-8th St. N.E. (res); Queen's U (Belfast, N. Ire.) '45; **FICS, FRCS (Eng.); Gen Surg; Surg.; Swift Current Union Hosp.; Tel. PR 3-8333.**

JACOBS, William F.; Ste. 607, 62 Richmond St. W., Toronto, Ont.; Tor '50; Barr. & Solicitor; Tel. EM 4-2207.

JACOBSEN, John R.; 144 Hilton Ave., Toronto, Ont.; Tor '34; Anaes; Tel. LE 1-8482.

JACOBSEN, Lloyd W.; 459 Kingston Cres. Winnipeg, Man.; Man '57, PlasSurg.

JACOBSEN, Paul A.; 6039 Kingston Rd., West Hill, Ont.; Tor'65.

JACOBSON, Alf K.; 8693-10th Ave., Burnaby 3, B.C.; College of Med. Evangelists (Los Angeles) '53; Tel. LA 6-5538.

JACOBSON, Stephen A.; Dal'63; Res., Camp Hill Hosp., Halifax, N.S.

JACQUES, Alexandre J.; 853 Wyandotte St. E., Windsor, Ont. (res); Mon '23; B.Sc.; Surg., Essex County Gaol; Bd. of Health, Windsor, & Cons., Med., Hotel Dieu Hosp.; Tel. 253-1311.

JACQUES, Andre; 2379 Marie Victorin, Sillery, Quebec 6, P.Q.; Lav '41; F.R.C.P.(C) Anaes; Anaes. Ass't., Dept of Anaes., Hotel Dieu & Hops. Laval & Ste-Foy (D.V.A.); Head of Pharm, Course, Laval U.; Tel. LA 9-4511.
JACQUES, Elphege; 416 Main St., Farnham, P.Q.; Lav '16.
JACQUES, Guy; 1500-18eme rue, Quebec 3, P.Q.; Lav'48; D&TRad; Staff, Hop. l'Enfant Jesus, DVA & Hotel-Dieu-de-Hauterive.
JACQUES, Lucien A.; 7 Ottawa St., Kapuskasing, Ont.; Ott '58; GenSurg.
JACQUES, Maurice; Lav '43; Res., Hop. St-Sacrement, Quebec 6, P.Q.
JACQUES, Paul E.; 3244 Beaubien E. Montreal, P.Q.; Apt. 34, 3330 Ridgewood (res); Mon '47; Tel. RA 9-1891.
JACQUES, R. A.; 343 Tache, St. Boniface, Man.; 29 Ruskin Rd., (res); Man '42; M.C.G.P.
JACQUES, Raymond; App. 808, 600 ave Laurier, Quebec 4, P.Q.; Lav '54; DiagRad; Rad., Hop. St. Joseph, La Tuque & Beauceville; Tel. 524-1744.
JACQUES, Robert; 1840 rue St. Marc, Shawinigan, P.Q.; 900 Lambert (res); Lav '54; Tel. LE 7-0321.
JACQUES, William M.; 19 Market St., Copper Cliff, Ont.; Qns '56; Staff, Copper Cliff Hosp.; Tel. 682-4421.
JACQUES, Yvan; Lav'65; Res., Hop. Hotel-Dieu, Quebec 4, P.Q.
JACYK, William R.; Man'64; Res., Deer Lodge Hosp., Winnipeg 12, Man.
JAFFE, Doris J.; Glasgow, Scot. '48; Research, Princess Margaret Hosp., Toronto, Ont. Retired.
JAFFE, Frederick A.; 1367 Goldthorpe Rd., Port Credit, Ont. (res); McG '44; D.A.B.PathAnat; Path.; Ass't. Pathol., Toronto Western Hosp.; **Co-Director of Labs., Queensway Gen. Hosp.; Dem. (Pathol.), U. of Toronto; Tel. 368-2581; CL 9-6671.**
JAFFEY, B. David, Lt/Col.; 11 Det RCAMC, 4050 W-4th Ave., Vancouver 8, B.C.; Tor '44.
JAGLALSINGH, L. Harry; Mayerthorpe, Alta.; Alb'65.
JAHNKE, Volker; '61; Staff, Inst. of Experimental Surg., U. of Montreal, Montreal 26, P.Q.; Abroad.
JAIN, Kewal K.; 146 W. 15th St., North Vancouver, B.C.; Punjab (India)'57; FICS; FRCS(C), NeurSurg; NeurSurg., Lionsgate Hosp.; Tel. 987-4822.
JAIN, Roshan; Medical Clinic, Fox Valley, Sask.; Dublin (Ire.)'61; DPH.
JAKAB, Louis; 1692 Jane St., Weston, Ont.; Pazmany Peter U. (Budapest, Hung.)'49; Gen. Surg. (Hungary); Tel. CH 7-6671.
JAKEMAN, W. Alan; 20 Abercrombie Rd., New Glasgow, N.S.; Dal '57.
JAKIWCZYK, Nick; St. Barbara's Clinic, 266 Bathurst St., Toronto 2B, Ont.; Graz (Austria) '27.
JAKOBSON, Bodvar B.; 418 Mountain, Neepawa, Man.; Man'54.
JAKOVAC, Ema; Zagreb (Yugoslavia) '45; Res., Ontario Hosp., Toronto, Ont.
JAKUBOVICZ, Abraham; 7071 Bayers Rd., Halifax, N.S.; Hadassah U. (Jerusalem)'53; AMCGP; Tel. 455-5141.
JALBERT, Jean M.; Lav '63; Res., Hop. Ste-Justine, Montreal, P.Q.; Abroad.
JALIL, Syed Mazhar; Agra (India)'57; Gen-Surg; Staff, St. Joseph's Hosp., Toronto 3, Ont.; Tel. 534-9531.
JALKOTZY, Hannes; 8 Hardy Hts. Onaping P.O., via Sudbury, Ont.; Vienna (Aust.)'48; AMCGP; Indus. Phys., Falconbridge Nickel Mines Ltd.; MOH, Dist. of Onaping; Staff, Onaping Hosp.; Tel. 966-3311.
JALKOTZY, Martha (Mohr); Onaping, Ont.; 8 Hardy Hgts. (res); Innsbruck (Austria) '44; Cert. Paed. (Vienna, Aust.).
JAMES, Albert W.; Paris (France) '57; Path; Staff, St. Paul's Hosp., Vancouver, B.C.; Tel. 682-2344.
JAMES, Celia A., see VIETS, Celia A.
JAMES, Clifford W.; 208 Scott St., Walkerton, Ont.; Tor'47; MCGP; Tel. 881-0730.
JAMES, Courtenay V.; Unity Med. Assoc., 2nd Ave. W., Unity, Sask.; London (Eng.)'54; M.B., B.S.; Staff, Unity Hosp.; Coroner; Tel. 228-2638.
JAMES, Donald E.; Alb'65; Res., University Hosp., Edmonton, Alta.
JAMES, Edward H.; 802 Med. & Dental Bldg., Regina, Sask.; Sask '57; FRCS(C), Neur Surg.; Tel. 527-2035.
JAMES, Elmer A.; Kingston, Ont., R.R. No. 1; Qns '24; Psy; Retired.
JAMES, Elmer S.; Manitoba Clinic, Med. Arts Bldg., Winnipeg, Man.; 336 Oxford St. (res); Man '35; LRCP, MRCS, FRCS (Eng.), FRCS(C), Orth Surg; Ass't. OrthSurg., Wpg. Gen. Hosp.; Ass't. Prof. (Surg.), U. of Manitoba; Tel. WH 2-6441.
JAMES, E. Stewart; 5731 Granville St., Vancouver, B.C.; 6141 Alma St. (res); Tor '31; Paed; Sr. in Paed., Vancouver Gen. Hosp.; Clin. Ass't. Prof. (Paed), U. of British Columbia; Tel. AM 1-4248.
JAMES, Frank G.; 514 Danforth Ave., Toronto 6, Ont.; Tor '59; Tel. HO 5-5221.
JAMES, Kenneth W.; 1468 Wyandotte St. E., **Windsor, Ont.; Wes '53; Derm.; Tel. 256-2301.**
JAMES, Maurice M.; 88 Sydenham, Kingston, Ont.; 317 University Ave. (res); Qns '39; Civilian Surg. Spec., Can. Army, East Ontario Area; Tel. 546-3104.
JAMES, Nesta B.; Med. Clinic, Fort Simpson, N.W.T.; Edinburgh (Scot.)'58; DPH.
JAMES, Rajkumar D.; Medical Clinic, 1332-100th St., North Battleford, Sask.; Madras (India)'55; GenSurg.
JAMES, R. Hastings; Victoria Gen. Hosp., Halifax, N.S.; Fleming Glen (res); Cambridge (Eng.) '40; M.A., M.D., MRCS, LRCP, MRCP (Eng.), DMRD (Eng.); Assoc. Rad., Victoria Gen. Hosp.; Assoc. Prof., Dalhousie U.; Tel. 422-7371.
JAMES, Richard N.; Box 70, Amherst View, Ont.; Qns'59; MCGP.
JAMES, Robert T.; 772 Lawrence Ave. E., Don Mills, Ont.; London (Eng.)'54.
JAMES, Roger A.; 139 Carmen Ave., Winnipeg 5, Man.; London. (Eng.) '53; MRCS; LRCP; FRCS (Eng.); FRCS(C), GenSurg; Staff, Misericordia Gen. Hosp.; Tel. 533-5736.
JAMES, William A.; Ste. 910, 225 Cassandra Blvd., Don Mills, Ont.; Qns'61; FRCP(C), Anaes.
JAMES, William G.; Tor'63; Res., St. Michael's Hosp., Toronto 2, Ont.
JAMHARIAN, Jan; 125 Pierre Bourgery, Boucherville, P.Q.; Istanbul (Turkey)'53; Anaes. (P.Q.).
JAMIESON, Alastair; Ste. 207, 814 Cook Rd., Richmond, B.C.; Edin.(Scot.) '55; FRCS(C); GenSurg; Tel. 278-0114.
JAMIESON, Agnes Larkin; Ontario Hospital School, Orillia, Ont.; Creighton St., Atherley (res); Tor '35; M.O., Dept. of Health; Tel. 326-7361, Loc. 205
JAMIESON, Claude V.; 10236 Connaught Dr., Edmonton, Alta.; Tor '07; F.R.C.S.(C), Otol; Retired.
JAMIESON, D.; c/o Reg. Supt. Sask. Reg. Dept. of National Health & Welfare, 735 Motherwell Bldg., Victoria Ave., Regina, Sask.
JAMIESON, Duncan M.; 5 George St. W., Durham, Ont.; Tor'56; MCGP; Coroner, Grey County; Chief of Staff, Durham Mem. Hosp.; Tel. 369-2510.
JAMIESON, Fred L.; 532 Medical Arts Bldg., Winnipeg, Man.; 131 Campbell (res); Man '12; Dist. Coroner; Tel. WH 2-6880.
JAMIESON, Geoffrey G., Capt.; 1210 Meadowlands Dr. E.; Apt. 16, Ottawa 5, Ont.; Sask'65; M.O., Canadian Forces Med. Centre.
JAMIESON, James S.; 347 Sherbrooke St., North Bay, Ont.; Dal '42; OphthOtol; Tel. 474-7030.
JAMIESON, John; Carlyle Clinic, Carlyle, Sask.; Glasgow (Scot.) '50; Tel. 453-2464; Abroad.
JAMIESON, Robert C.; 10048-101A Ave., Edmonton, Alta.; Alb'49; MCGP; Staff, W.C.B.; Tel. 422-7151.
JAMIESON, Robert E.; Coboconk, Ont.; Tor '45; M.C.G.P.

JAMIESON, Ross A.; 922 Medical Arts Bldg., 170 St. George St., Toronto, Ont.; 47 Wanless Cres. (res); Tor '10; F.R.C.P.(C), IntMed; Retired.
JAMIESON, Thomas A. B.; 2800 Lundy's Lane, Niagara Falls, Ont.; 1939 Corwin Ave. (res); Tor '42.
JAMIESON, W. Eric; 206 Rookwood Ave., Fredericton, N.B.; Dal'66.
JAMIESON, William D. S.; 29 Rothmere Dr., Toronto 12, Ont. (res); McG '21; F.A.C.C.P.; M.O., Ont. Dept. of Health; Tel. 365-4091.
JAMIESON, William G.; 16 Lyndhurst Ave., London, Ont.; Wes'60; FRCS(C), GenSurg; Staff, Westminster Hosp.

JAMISON, Clarence A.; 5740 Cambie St., Vancouver, B.C.; Alb '42 DiagRad; Staff St. Paul's Hosp.; Tel. MU 3-2211.

JAMPOLSKY, Noel A.; 417 Med. Arts Bldg., Edmonton, Alta.; 14011-101A Ave. (res); Alb '56; DABD; DermSyph; Att'd. Staff, Royal Alexandra Hosp., Vancouver, B.C.

JAN, Roman A. (JANUSZEWSKA) Szymanska); **1658 Victoria Pk. Ave., Scarborough, Ont.; 14 Sulkara Ct. Tor 16 (res); Liverpool (Eng.) '56; AMCGP; Active (GP) Staff, Scarborough Gen. Hosp.; Tel. 757-3359.**

JANACK, Edwin S.; 42 King St. W., Stoney Creek, Ont.; 8 James Ave. (res); Qns '51; MCGP; Active Staff, Hamilton Civic & St. Joseph's Hosp's.; Tel. 662-4911.
JANAUSKAS, Antanas; Admin., Westminster D.V.A. Hosp., London, Ont.; Teubingen (W. Germ.) '48.; Tel. 432-6711.
JANCZUR, Stan; Med. Arts Clinic, 2125-11th Ave., Regina, Sask.; Madrid (Spain)'52; IntMed; Staff, Regina Gen. & Grey Nun's Hosp's.; Tel. 523-0691.
JANELLE, Leo Paul; 50 est, Trudel, St. Boniface, Co. of St. Maurice, P.Q.; Lav '45; Tel. LE 6-3117.
JANEK, Anna; (See Sirek, Anna).
JANES, Alan W.; Janeway Health Centre, St. John's, Nfld.; Dal'57.
JANES, W. C. Baird; Box 426, Duncan, B.C.; Man '46; GenSurg; Tel. 746-4401.
JANETOS, P. J.; Department of National Health & Welfare, c/o Regional Superintendent, European Region; Abroad.
JANIGAN, David T.; Dal'57; Res., Dalhousie U., Halifax, N.S.
JANIK, John; 1883 Baseline Rd., Ottawa 5, Ont.; Germany '57.
JANS, Ronald G.; Alb'65; Res., University Hosp., Edmonton, Alta.
JANSCH, Marjorie E. (Dupont); Ganges, B.C.; UBC '54.
JANSCH, Theodore L.; Ganges, B.C.; UBC'54.
JANSEN, Jan H.; Ste. 205, 3000 Lawrence Ave. E., Scarborough, Ont.; Berlin (Germ.) '44; Otol Tel. 291-1531.
JANSEN, Margaret G.; 29 Edmund Ave., Toronto 7, Ont. (res); Tor '49; Pt. Time Staff, Ont. Hosp.
JANSEN, Marinus G. W.; Suite 206, Med. Arts Bldgd., Toronto, Ont.; 7 Clarendon Ave. (res); Amsterdam (Neth.) '46; Teach, Staff, Toronto Gen. Hosp.; Cons., D.V.A., Sunnybrook Hosp.; Tel. WA 1-9566.
JANSSEN, Gesina E.; Apt. 310, 3801 Riverside Dr. E., Windsor, Ont.; Marburg (Germ.)'47; Anaes.
JANTZ, John; 844B Princess St., Kingston, Ont.; Tor'53.

JANUSZEWSKA, Roman A. (Szymanska) (See JAN)

JANZ, Leslie B.; 2489 Bellevue Ave., West Vancouver, B.C.; UBC'58; MCGP; Tel. WA 2-9377.
JANZEN, Andrew; Knox Clinic, 1605 Glenmore St., Kelowna, B.C.; UBC'61; AMCGP; Tel. 762-2002.
JANZEN, Herbert W.; Rosthern Med. Clinic, Rosthern, Sask.; Alb'64; Tel. 232-4432.
JANZEN, Homer K.; Man '57; Res., University Hosp., Saskatoon, Sask.
JANZEN, Jacob F.; Box 447, Rosthern, Sask.; Alb '53; MCGP; Hd., Med. Staff, Rosthern Union Hosp.; Tel. 232-4432.
JANZEN, M. Harry; Winnipeg Clinic, St. Mary's & Vaughan, Winnipeg, Man.; Man'60; FRCS(C), ObstGyn.
JAQUES, Norman A. G.; Ste. 604, 625 - 5th Ave., New Westminster, B.C.; 835 York St. (res); London (Eng.)'56; Tel. 522-5432.
JAQUITH, L. Everett; Terra Cotta, Ont.; Tor '26; Tel. 877-3234.
JARDINE, Kenneth; 100 Simcoe St. W., Beaverton, Ont.; Tor'42; MCGP; MOH Thorah Twp.; Sr. Active Staff, Orillia Soldiers Mem. Hosp.; District Coroner; Tel. 426-7331.
JARDINE, Phillip B.; Musquodoboit Harbour, N.S.; Dal '56.; AMCGP.
JAREMA, Maciej; Box 150, Mansonville, Cte. Brome, P.Q.
JAREMKO, Lois M. (Hokanson); Carberry, Man.; Man '52.
JARMAN, Ernest A.; Rainbow Rd., Ganges, Saltspring Island, B.C.; Qns'50; Pres., Med. Staff, Lady Minto Gulf Islands Hosp., Ganges; Tel. 537-5321.
JARON, P. W.; Ste 212, 1705-3rd Ave., Prince George, B.C.; Man '39.
JARROTT, Gilbert C.; 42 Albert St., Stratford, Ont.;Wes'33; ObstGyn; Dist. Coroner; Tel. 271-2120.
JARROTT, Thomas R.; 32 Broadway W., Paris, Ont.; Man '36; Obst.; Staff, Willet Hosp., Paris, Brantford Gen. & St. Joseph's Hosp's., Brantford; Tel. 442-3321.
JARRY, Gaetan; M.B.E.; 2225 Rachel St. E., **Montreal, P.Q.; 2082 Sherbrooke St. W., (res); Mon '35; F.C.C.P. Pulm. Dis. & TB (P.Q.); Med. Dir., Bruchesi Institute of Montreal Inc.; Cons. Chest Diseases, Queen Mary Veteran's Hosp.; Tel. LA 4-6825.**
JARRY, Leo; 55 Ave. de l'Eglise, Verdun, Montreal 19, P.Q.; 8730 Blvd. Lasalle, Ville Lasalle (res); Mon '42; F.R.C.S.(C), OrthSurg; OrthSurg, Verdun Gen. Hosp. & Hop-St. Joseph, Lachine; Tel. PO 9-7322.
JARRY-LAPORTE, Jocelyn; 1540 rue Elizabeth, Montreal 9, P.Q.; Mon '61.
JARVIS, Anita (Fellegi); Ott'59; Staff, Sunnybrook Hosp., Toronto 12, Ont.
JARVIS, Gregory J.; 8 Kingsway Med. Ctr., 2917 Bloor St. W., Toronto 18, Ont.; 44 Mill St. N., Brampton; 262 Poplar Plains Rd., Tor. 7 (res); Ott '58; Ophth; Staff, Queensway Gen. & Peele Mem. Hosp., Brampton; Tel. 451-4560.
JARZYLO, Stanley V.; 28 Parkwood Pl., Kingston, Ont.; Qns'59; DiagRad., Staff, Kingston Gen. Hosp., Kingston, Ont.; Tel. 542-2821.
JASEVICIUTE, Emily; Kaunas (Lith.) '34; Staff, Fort William San., Fort William, Ont.
JASEY, Gordon; 1386 Ouellette Ave., Windsor, Ont.; Dal'56; FRCS(C) ObstGyn; Tel. 256-5416.
JASMIN, Alban; 7541 Blvd. LaSalle, LaSalle, P.Q.; Mon '41; M.C.G.P.; Tel. DO 6-1724.
JASMIN, Florent; 1230 Beaubien E., Montreal 10, P.Q.; 3260 Fendal, Cote des Neiges (res); Mon '44; Vis. Staff, Hop. Notre-Dame; Tel. 277-2433.
JASMIN, Gaetan; 189 Glengarry, Montreal 16, P.Q. (res); Mon '51; Ph.D.; Assoc., Inst. Experimental Med.; Ass't. Prof., Dept. of Path., U. of Montreal; Tel. RE 3-9951.
JASPER, Herbert H.; Dept. of Physiol., U. of Montreal, C.P. 6128, Montreal, P.Q.; McG '43; Ph.D.; Research Prof. (Neurol. Science), U. of Montreal; Tel. 733-9951, Loc. 235.
JASTRZEBSKI, Zygmunt M.; 620 Bathurst St., Toronto 4, Ont.; UBC'65.
JAUREGUI, John G.; McG '60; Jr. Int'n., Royal Victoria Hosp., Montreal, P.Q.
JAVICOLI, Antonello; 5325 est rue Jean Talon, Montreal Nord, P.Q.; 5626 Boul. Maurice Duplessis (res); Rome (Italy) '49; IntMed (Gastroen.) **(P.Q.); Chief, Dept. of Med., Hop. Santa** Cabrini; Active Staff, Hop. Jean Talon; Tel. RA 5-5281.
JAVORSKY, Vjaceslav; 999 Merivale Rd., Ottawa 3, Ont.
JAWOROWSKY, Irene (See Dawosyr)

JAWORSKI, Zdzislaw F.; 43 Bruyere St., Ottawa 2, Ont.; Brussels (Belg.) '49; FRCP(C), IntMed; **Assoc., Med. Research Council of Canada; Ass't. Prof.** (Med.), **U. of Ottawa; Tel. CE 6-0333.**

JAY, H. J. D.; Forest, Ont.; Wes '38.

JAY, Howard; 130 Ellesmere Rd., Scarborough, Ont.; London (Eng.)'61; B. Chir.; Tel. 447-5531.

JEAN, Andre; 6029 Blvd. Monk, Montreal, P.Q. (res); Mon '39; Path (P.Q.); Path; Queen Mary Veteran's Hosp.; Tel. RE 8-9481.

JEAN, Bernard; Lav '56; Psy; Supt., Hop. Ste Anne, Baie-St. Paul, P.Q.; Tel. 435-2005.

JEAN, Claude; rue St.-Etienne, La Malbaie, P.Q.; Rue St.-Philippe (res); Lav '51; DPH; PH(P.Q.); MOH; Tel. MO 5-3264.

JEAN, Clement; 2767 La Silencieuse, Quebec 10, P.Q. (res); Lav'49; FRCP(C); Path; Dir., PathAnat. Lab., Hop-St-Francois-d'Assise; Assoc. Prof. (PathAnat.), Laval U.; Tel. 527-4555.

JEAN, Gaston; 12, rue Morissette, Loretteville, P.Q.; Lav '46; Huron Indian Reserve Loretteville Co.

JEAN, Jean D.; 839 Pierre Bedard, Chicoutimi, P.Q.; Lav'58; Cardiovasc Surg. (P.Q.).

JEAN, Jean P.; 2963 Chemin Ste-Catherine, Montreal 26, P.Q.; Mon'43; DABR; D&TRad; Dir., Dept. of Rad., Reddy Mem. Hosp.

JEAN, Laureat; 213 est, Maltais, Alma, P.Q.; Lav '51; Anaes.; Tel. 662-6624.

JEAN, Lionel; 41 ave. Sanatorium, Mont Joli, P.Q.; Lav '51.

JEAN, Paul; Lav '49; Baie des Sables, Co. Matane, P.Q.

JEAN, Pierre; 4405 Isabella, Montreal 26, P.Q. (res); Lav '58; Ph.D.; Ass't. Prof. (Anat.), U. of Montreal; Tel. 739-6080.

JEAN, Roger; L'Isletville, Co. L'Islet, P.Q.; Lav '60; AMCGP.

JEANES, Charles W. L.; 343 O'Connor St., Ottawa 4, Ont.; Guy's Hosp. (Lond., Eng.) '43; Exec. Sec., Can. Tuberculosis Assoc.; Tel. 237-1208.

JEDLICKI, Stanislaw M.; Box 39, North Battleford, Sask.; Warsaw (Poland) '31; Staff, Prov. Sask. Hosp.; Tel. 445-4461.

JEDWAB, Samuel J.; 1849 Yonge St., Ste. 418, Toronto 7, Ont.; Warsaw (Poland)'53; Psy; Cons. Psy., Forensic Clinic, Clarke Inst.; Cons. Psy., Catholic Children's Aid Soc.; Clin. Teach. (Psy.), U. of Toronto; Tel. HU 5-1375.

JEFFERSON, John C., Capt.; Dal'65; M.I.R., 2nd Battalion, P.P.C.L.I., Edmonton, Alta.

JEFFERY, E. S.; 307 Medical Dental Bldg., 450 Central Ave., London, Ont.; 1 Gammage St. (res); Wes '41; M.C.G.P.; Tel. 432-3023.

JEFFREY, Frederick W.; 505 O'Connor St., Ottawa, Ont.; 41 Monkland Ave. (res); Qns '28; F.A.A.P., Paed.; Tel. 232-5761.

JEFFREY, George S.; 3435 Church St., Windsor, Ont.; Tor '20; F.A.C.C.P.; IntMed (TB).; Retired.

JEFFREY, J. Ian; 201 McLeod Med. Bldg., 340 McLeod St., Ottawa 4, Ont.; Qns'46; DABOS; **FACS; OrthSurg; Att'd. OrthSurg., Ottawa Civic** Hosp.; Cons. Orth Surg., Grace Hosp.; Clin. Ass't. (OrthSurg.), Ottawa U.; Tel. CE 2-8352.

JEFFREY, Wendell H.; Shelburne, N.S.; Dal '53; Staff, Roseway Hosp.; Tel. 116.

JEFFRIES, Roy C.; 1205 Fairmont Med. Bldg., 750 W. Broadway, Vancouver 9, B.C.; UBC'54; IntMed; Att'd. Staff, Vancouver Gen. Hosp. & Shaughnessy Hosp.; Tel. 874-1253.

JEFFS, G. Douglas; R.R. 1, Stroud, Ont.; Tor '17; Retired.

JEFFS, James I.; 331 South St., London, Ont.; 21 Wychwood Pk. (res); Tor '32; DPH; Ass't. MOH, City of London; Tel. GE 8-7255.

JEFFS, Robert D.; 200 St. Clair Ave. W., Ste. 312, Toronto 7, Ont.; 51 Douglas Dr. (res); Tor '49; F.R.C.S.(C), Urol; Staff, Hosp. for Sick Children & Toronto Western Hosp.; Ass't. Prof (Surg.), U. of Toronto; Tel. 924-6341.

JEGIER, Wanda J.; 318 Cote St-Catherine, Montreal 8, P.Q.; Frankfurt (Germ.) '50; Paed; Cardiol (P.Q.); Staff, Montreal Children's Hosp.; Tel. WE 7-8511.

JEYGUD, Adelbert T.; Budapest (Hung.)'43; DA(Copenhagen); Staff, Dept. of Respiratory Dis., Grace Dart Hosp., Montreal, P.Q.; Fell., G.D. Research Inst., Montreal.

JELIU, Gloria; 3175 Cote St. Catherine Rd., Montreal, P.Q.; 1000 Pratt Ave. (res); Paris (France) '52; FRCP(C); Paed; Tel. RE 1-3011.

JEMSON, John A.; Box 9, Glenboro, Man.; Guy's Hosp., London U. (Eng.)'53; M.R.C.S., L.R.C.P.; M.O.H., Glenboro, Strathcona & South Cypress; Tel. 14R2.

JEN, Ivan; Hart House, 325-21st St. E., Saskatoon, Sask.; Sask'60; Tel. 242-1208.

JENEY, Leslie; 999 Queen St. W., Toronto 3, Ont.; Budapest (Hung.)'53; D.Psy; Psy; Psy., Ontario Hosp.; Tel. 533-8501, Ext. 329.

JENEY, Piroska (Kirschner); Budapest (Hung.) '53; Staff, (G.P.), Lakeshore Psychiatric Hosp., Toronto, Ont.

JENKIN, James R.; 230 St. Clair St., Chatham, Ont.; Wes'51; Tel. 354-4660.

JENKIN, Richard D. T.; 191 Stibbard Ave., Toronto 12, Ont. (res); London (Eng.) '58; FRCP (C); FFR; TherRad; TherRad., Princess Margaret Hosp.; Tel. 924-0671, Loc. 442.

JENKINS, Elaine; 4731-52nd Ave., Taber, Alta.; Sydney (Australia)'56.

JENKINS, Eunice K.; 702 Greyhound Bldg., 622-1st St. S.W., Calgary, Alta.; Alb'52; Pt.-time (IntMed), Col. Belcher Hosp.; Tel. 263-8309.

JENKINS, George E.; Mental Health Clinic, Ontario Hosp., London, Ont.; Wes'38; D.Psy; Psy; Dir., Mental Health Clinic; Tel. 455-5110.

JENKINS, Jack G.; King St., Gananoque, Ont.; Qns '40; M.C.G.P.; Tel. 382-3667.

JENKINS, John C.; 5 Brook St., Simcoe, Ont.; Dal '58; AMCGP; Staff, Norfolk Gen. Hosp.; Tel. 426-2043.

JENKINS, John R.; Gladstone, Man.; London (Eng.)'39.

JENKINS, Leonard C.; 3932 Osler St., Vancouver 9, B.C.; McG '52; FRCP(C), Anaes; Clin Ass't Prof. (Anaes), U. of British Columbia; Tel. 874-1626.

JENKINS, Ronald E.; Mental Health Clinic, Ste. 5, 1410 Central Ave., Prince Albert, Sask.; 385-24th St. W. (res); London (Eng.) '46; D.P.M. RCP&S(I); Psy; Clin. Dir., Mental Health **Clinic; Cons. Psy., Victoria Hosp., Head, Dept. of Psy., Holy Family Hosp.; Tel. 763-8477.**

JENKINS, Roy B.; 512 Goldstream Ave., Victoria, B.C. (res); Man '16; DPH; Retired.

JENKINS, Valerie E. see St. JOHN, Valerie E. (Jenkins)

JENKINS, W. M.; Gagetown, N.B.; McG '08.

JENKNER, Sarah M. (Elliott); 3565 St. Georges Ave., North Vancouver, B.C. (res); Qns'47; Staff, **B.C. Cancer Inst., 2656 Heather St., Vancouver.**

JENNER, Leonard C.; 15 Division St., Kingsville, Ont.; 50 Division St. N. (res); Tor '39; MCGP; D.O.T. Examiner; Tel. 733-2200.

JENNER, Morris R.; Sask'63; P.G. Dept. of Biochemistry, University of Western Ontario, London, Ont.

JENNINGS, Donald B.; 17 Jorene Dr., Kingston, Ont.; Qns '57; M.Sc.(Med.); Ph.D. (Physiol.); Research Assoc., Cdn. Heart Fdn.; Ass't. Prof. (Physiol.), Queen's U.; Tel. 546-3871, Loc. 636.

JENNINGS, Frederick C.; 458 Windsor St., Lancaster, N.B. (res); **Dal '31; Anaes; Dir. Anaes., Lancaster DVA Hosp.; Anaes., St. John TB Hosp.; Cons. (Anaes), Saint John Gen. Hosp.; Tel. 4-2651.**

JENNINGS, George H.; 29 Seneca Cres., Brantford, Ont.; Wes '23; Anaes; Tel. PL 3-5485.

JENNINGS, Harry N.; 300 Medical Arts Bldg., Calgary, Alta.; Calwin P.Q. (res); Tor '24; F.A.C.P., IntMed; Chief of Med., Cross Hosp.; Cons., Col. Belcher Hosp.; Retired.

JENNINGS, Kenneth H.; 691 Main St., **Moncton, N.B.; McG '54; Anaes.**

JENNINGS, Michael M.; 200 Brock St. N., Whitby, Ont.; Dal'64.

JENSEN, John K.; Leduc, Alta.; Alb '57; Tel. 446-2212.

JENSEN, Sven E.; 285 Prideaul St., Nanaimo, B.C.; Copenhagen (Denmark) '54; Psy; Dir., Mental Health Clinic; Tel. 754-4441.

JENSEN, William, G.; Ste. 217, 1940 Lonsdale Ave., North Vancouver, B.C.; Alb'52; Active Staff, Lionsgate Hosp.; Tel. YU 8-8588.

JENTZ, Lyle A.; 11 Hawarden Ave., Brantford, Ont. (res); Wes '51; Path; Dir. of Labs., Brantford Gen. Hosp.; Tel. PL 2-7872.

JEPSON, Gordon L.; 195 Dufferin Ave., London, Ont.; Wes '10; D.A., Anaes.

JEPSON, Joanne H.; Apt. 602, 3620 Lorne Cres., Montreal 18, P.Q.; McG '59; M.A.; Clin. Fell. (Haem.), Royal Victoria Hosp.; Tel. VI 2-1251.

JEPSON, Thomas E.; 47 Wilson St., Ancaster, Ont.; Wes'63; MCGP; Active Staff, Hamilton Civic Hosp.; Court. Staff, Chedoke Gen., Children's & St. Joseph's Hosp's.; Tel. MI 8-2911.

JERACE, Joseph R.; 1011 Ouelette Ave., Windsor Ont.; McG '47; ObstGyn.

JEREMIAS, Gabriel; 700 Main St. E., Hamilton, Ont.; Qns'58; OrthSurg; Active Staff, Hamilton Civic Hosp's.; Court. Staff, St. Joseph's, Chedoke & Joseph Brant Hosp's.; Tel. 527-4221.

JEREMIAS, Martin T.; 452 Main St. E., Hamil**ton, Ont.; 27 Forsythe Ave. S. (res); Qns '49; Urol; Active Staff, Civic Hosp.; Court. Staff, St. Joseph's, Brant & Chedoke Hosp's.; Tel. JA 8-7463.**

JERRY, L. Martin; Tor'61; FRCP(C), IntMed; Staff, Toronto Gen. Hosp., Toronto 2, Ont.; Abroad.

JESPERSEN, Reuben E.; 10155-120th St., Edmonton, Alta.; 10316-133 St. (res); Alb '35; F.A.C.S.; GenSurg; Pres. of Staff, Royal Alexandra Hosp.; Inst. in Surgery, U. of Alberta; Tel. 488-7271.

JESSAMINE, A. Gordon; 1108 Agincourt Ave., Ottawa, Ont.; Aberdeen (Scot.) '48; Med. Supt., Royal Ottawa San.; Cons. (TB & Chest Dis.), Ottawa Civic Hosp.; Tel. PA 2-6521, Local 68.

JESSEL, Levic; 2874 Keele St., Downsview, Ont.; Tor '23; MCGP; Staff, New Mt. Sinai & Northwestern Gen. Hosp's; Tel. 635-0423.

JESSEL, Sam J.; 122 Elm St. S., Timmins, Ont. (res); Tor'33; Active Staff, St. Mary's Hosp. & Lect. (Gyn.), Nurses Training School; Tel. 264-7170.

JESSOP, Charles P.; Box 590, 12-2nd Ave., Levack, Ont.; Tor'37; MCGP.

JETTE, Jean; 4495 Rue Lafontaine, Montreal, P.Q.; 5097 Blvd. Rosemont (res); Mon '53.

JETTE, Jean J.; 154, St.-Louis, St.-Eustache, P.Q.; Mon '63; Tel. 473-2121.

JETTE, M. Claude; 3731 Dandurand, Montreal, P.Q.; Mon '61; Tel. RA 5-1870.

JETTE, Yves; 5967 Boul. l'Assomption, Montreal 36, P.Q.; Mon'65.

JEWELL, Marion C.; 2171 Queen St. E., Toronto 13, Ont.; Tor'63.

JEWELL, Thomas C.; 332 Toronto Western Hosp., Toronto, Ont.; 21 High Park Gdns. (res); Tor'39; FRCS(C) ObstGyn; Staff, Dept. ObstGyn., Toronto Western Hosp.; Ass't Prof., (ObstGyn), **U. of Toronto; EM 6-2423.**

JEWETT, Beverly L.; 96 Parliament Square, Fredericton, N.B.; McG '43 ; GenSurg; Surg. Staff, Victoria Public Hosp.; Tel. 454-4532.

JEWETT, Marie A. C.; 96 Parliament Square, Fredericton, N.B.; Wes '43; Assoc. Staff, Victoria Public Hosp.; Tel. 454-4532.

JILEK, Wolfgang G.; Austria'56; D.Psy; Psy; Staff, Inst. Recherches Psych., 1000 boul. St. Anne, Joliette, P.Q.; Tel. 756-1681.

JIMENEZ, Jose; University Hosp., Edmonton, Alta.; Madrid (Spain)'50; PhysMed & Rehab; Ass't. Dir. (PhysMed. & Rehab.), Ass't. Clin. Prof., U. of Alberta Hosp.; Lect. (Phys Med & Rehab.), U. of Alberta; Tel. GE 9-5911, Loc. 300.

JINCHEREAU, Yvan; 196 Ave. St. Michel, St. Raymond Co. Portneuf, P.Q.; 26 St. Pierre (res); Lav '49.

JOANNETTE, Albert; 1 Saint-Joseph, Sainte-Agathe des Monts, P.Q.; Mon '25; Bact. (Lyon, Fr.); Pulm. Dis & TB (P.Q.); Med. Dir., Hop. Sainte-Agathe.; Tel. 326-3211.

JOANNETTE, Jean P.; 4930 Mayfair, Montreal 29, P.Q.; Mon'42; Tel. 488-6906.

JOASSIN, Guy; Louvain (Belg.) '62; Jr. Intn., Winnipeg Gen. Hosp., Winnipeg 3, Man.

JOB, Carla; c/o L. Eldridge, 141 Farnham Ave., Toronto 7, Ont.; Bologna (Italy) '56; FRCP(C); Anaes; Staff, Hosp. for Sick Children; Tel. EM 6-7242.

JOBIDON, Alfred; 2350 Coquette, Quebec 3, P.Q.; Lav '51; Anaes; Anaes., St. Francois d' Assise & Hop. Ste. Foy; Tel. 529-7311.

JOBIN, Andre; Smooth Rock Falls, Ont.; Lav'60; AMCGP.

JOBIN, Denys G.; 3363 Perigny, Quebec 10, P.Q.; Lav'59; FRCP(C), PhysMed. & Rehab.

JOBIN, Francois; 573 rue St-Jean, Quebec 4, P.Q.; Lav'61; FRCP(C), IntMed.

JOBIN, Jean-Baptiste; 610 Chemin St-Louis, Apt. 3, Quebec, P.Q., Lav '25; F.A.C.P., F.R.C.P.-(C), IntMed; Dean, Faculty of Med. Laval U.; Tel. LA 9-4511.

JOBIN, Joachim; 573 rue St.-Jean, Quebec 4, P.Q.; Lav '31; IntMed; Chief OPD (Med), Hop.-Hotel-Dieu; Chief (Med.) Rheum. Clinic; Ass't. Prof., Laval U.; Tel. 529-9151.

JOBIN, Maurice; Ste. 330, 5465 Queen Mary, Montreal 29, P.Q.; 4974 Coolbrook (res); Mon'54; Tel. 488-7502.

JOBIN, Michel; Lav '60; Research, Laval Univ., Quebec, P.Q.

JOBIN, Pierre; 91 d'Auteuil St., Quebec, P.Q. (res); Lav'32; FRCS(C), GenSurg; Prof. Anat. & Librarian, Laval U.; Tel. LA 9-4511.

JODIN, Gilles; Mon'65; Res., Hop. St-Luc, 1058 Rue St. Denis, Montreal 18, P.Q.

JODOIN, Pierre; 51A ouest, St.-Charles, Lon**gueuil, Cite Jacques-Cartier, P.Q.; Mon '30; Tel. Long 674-6525.**

JODOIN, Roderick; 298 Labelle, St.-Jerome, P.Q.; Mon '49; MCGP.

JODREY, James F.; 293 Water St., Summerside, P.E.I.; Dal'62; Active Staff, Prince County & Tyne Valley Hosp's.; Tel. 436-3906.

JOE, Byung K.; '50; Staff, Assiniboine Hosp., Brandon, Man.

JOE, M.; UBC'63; Res., Shaughnessy Hosp., Vancouver, B.C.

JOHANNESSON, Thorberg; 46 Cuthbertson Ave., Winnipeg 29, Man. (res); Man '45; Anaes; Staff, Winnipeg Gen. Hosp.; Tel. SP 4-6511.

JOHNS, David R.; 1871 King St. E., Hamilton, Ont.; Wes'65.

JOHNS, E. Ralph; Gertrude St., Alberni, B.C.; London (Eng.) '52.

JOHNS, George J.; 100 Sheppard Ave., Ste. 202, Willowdale, Ont.; 42 Almond Ave. (res); Tor '62; D.Psy.; Psy; Dir., Mental Health Unit of North York Branson Hosp.; Tel. 222-7701.

JOHNS, Ralph P.; 5043 Yonge St., Willowdale P.O., Toronto, Ont.; Tor '33; Dist. Coroner; Tel. BA 1-8011.

JOHNS, Walter S.; Business Administrators (Alta.) Ltd., 512 Herald Bldg., Calgary, Alta.; 512 Rideau Rd. (res); Alb '38; FACA; Anaes; Chief, Dept. of Anaes., Holy Cross Hosp.; Tel. AM 6-1531.

JOHNS, William R.; Anaes. Assoc., 900 King St. W., Kitchener, Ont.; Qns'53; DA(McG); Anaes; Tel. 744-7361.

JOHNSEN, Holger V.; 139 Brooks Ave., Greenacres, Chilliwack, B.C.; Man '52.

JOHNSON, A. M.; 710 Seymour St., Vancouver, B.C.; Wes '40; FRCP(C), IntMed; Staff, University of British Columbia Health Serv.; Tel. 224-1111.

JOHNSON, Aubrey E.; Great Village, N.S.; Dal '50;

JOHNSON, Arnold L.; 2300 Tupper St., Montreal, P.Q.; 370 Geneva Cres., Mount Royal (res); McG '40; F.R.C.P.(C), IntMed; Cardiol, (P.-Q.); Dir., C-V Div., Joint Cardioresp. Serv. **Royal Victoria and Montreal Children's Hosp's.;** Assoc. Prof. (Paed. & Med.), McGill U.; Tel. WE 7-8511.

JOHNSON, Arthur D.; Box 729, Castlegar, B.C.; **Dal '47; MCGP; Court. Staff, Trail Tadanac &** Castlegar & Dist. Hosp's.

JOHNSON, C. C. R.; 412 Med. Arts Bldg., 170 St. George St., Toronto 4, Ont.; Tor'48; Paed; Clin. Ass't., Hosp. for Sick Children; Tel. LE 6-1516.
JOHNSON, Charles A. Cameron Ave., Hudson, P.Q.; McG '54; Staff, Lachine Gen. Hosp.; Phys., Protestant Schl Bd.; Tel. 236-4083.
JOHNSON, Charles H.; 73 Fraser Ave., Edmundston, N.B. (res); Dal '30; M.O., Fraser Co. Ltd.
JOHNSON, David A.; St. Georges, Nfld.; Edinburgh (Scot.)'49.
JOHNSON, David M.; 135 Dalewood Ave. S., Hamilton, Ont.; Qns'64.
JOHNSON, Diana M.; Wes '51; Psy; Staff, Ontario Hosp., Woodstock, Ont.; Tel. 539-1251.
JOHNSON, Diane W.; 11412-73rd Ave., Edmonton, Alta.; Tor '55.
JOHNSON, D. L.; 838 Rosser Ave., Brandon, Man.; 341—13th (res); Man. '26.
JOHNSON, D. Michael; Res., Kingston Gen. Hosp., Kingston, Ont.
JOHNSON, Donald G.; Wes'64; Res., Vancouver Gen. Hosp., Vancouver 9, B.C.
JOHNSON, Douglas H.; 788 Eglinton Ave. E., Toronto 17, Ont.; Tor '57; Assoc. Staff, Toronto East Gen. Hosp.; Cons. Staff Sunnybrook Hosp.; Tel. 488-8973.
JOHNSON, Douglas S.; 1031 Carling Ave., Ottawa, Ont. (res); Qns '46; DiagRad; Rad., Ottawa Civic Hosp.; Tel. PA 9-2511.
JOHNSON, Dwight L.; Gibson, B.C.; Man '26.
JOHNSON, Edward; 75 Emily St., Winnipeg 3, Man.; Man '28; Psy; Dir. Psy. Serv., Prov. of Man.; Ass't. Prof. (Psy), U. of Manitoba; Supt., Psy. Inst.; Tel. SP 4-6511, Loc. 611.
JOHNSON, Edward A.; Kenmar Bldg., 4570 W. 10th, Vancouver B.C.; 5589 University Blvd. (res); Alb '28; Tel. 224-4455.
JOHNSON, Elizabeth M.; 710 Seymour St., Vancouver 2, B.C.; 1820 Bayswater, Van. 8 (res); Liverpool (Eng.) '48; **DRCOG; DCH; Paed; Tel. MU 4-1511.**
JOHNSON, Elmer W.; Workmen's Comp. Board, 90 Harbour St., Toronto 4, Ont.; Alb'48.
JOHNSON, Ernest A.; Johnson Eye Clin., Main Floor, Med. Centre Bldg., 906-8th Ave. S.W., Calgary, Alta.; Qns'38; FACS; FICS; FAAOO; Ophth; MCGP; Ophth-in-Chief, Holy Cross Hosp.; Active Staff, Calgary Gen. & Alberta Children's Hosp's,; Tel. 266-4011.
JOHNSON, Ernest B.; 6291 Coburg Rd., Halifax, N.S.; 18 Sherbrooke Dr., Rockingham (res); Dal'61; MCGP; Jr. Phys., OPD, Victoria Gen. Hosp.; Tel. 423-7167.
JOHNSON, Evjolfur; 327 Eveline St., Selkirk, Man. (res); Man'26; FRCS (Edin.); GenSurg; Staff, Selkirk Mental Hosp.
JOHNSON, F. Gordon; 477 Waterloo St., London, Ont.; 445 Averill Cres. (res); London (Eng.) '50; MB., BS., MRCS; LRCP; Psy; Pt. time Cons., Westminster DVA Hosp. & Cons., Alcoholism & Drug Addiction Research Fdn.; Lect. (Psy.), U. of Western Ont.; Tel. 433-3171.
JOHNSON, Frank L.; Campbell Clinic, 430 Mayor Magrath Dr., Lethbridge, Alta.; 410-14th St., S. **(res); Alb '40; Anaes; Tel. FA 7-5737.**
JOHNSON, Fred L.; 710 Medical Arts Bldg., 1 Young St., Hamilton, Ont.; 27 Paisley Ave. N. (res); Tor '36; D.A.B.O.G., F.R.C.S.(C) ObstGyn; Chief Obst. Gyn., Hamilton Gen. Hosp.; Hon Ass't. Prof. ObstGyn, U. of Western Ontario; Tel. JA 7-6654.
JOHNSON, George; 357 Legislative Bldg., Winnipeg, Man.; 299 Waverley St. (res); Man '50; MCGP; Minister, Dept. of Health, Prov. of Manitoba; Tel. WH 6-7207.
JOHNSON, Gerard; 1295 Ave. Patenaude, Sillery, Quebec 6, P.Q. (res); Lav '55; Psy; Staff, Clinique Roy Rousseau; Tel. 661-7735.
JOHNSON, Gwendolyn O. (Hay); Ste. 25, 659 Clyde Ave. W., Vancouver, B.C.; 71 Laurie Cres. (res); Qns '57.
JOHNSON, H. Desmond; McG'60; Res., St. Joseph's Hosp., London, Ont.
JOHNSON, Herman M.; 1800 Logan Ave., Winnipeg 23, Man.; Man '63.
JOHNSON, Hjalmar W.; 718 Fairmount Med. Bldg., 750 W. Broadway, Vancouver 9, B.C.; Man'56; FRCS(C), Urol; Att'd. Staff, Vancouver Gen. & Shaughnessy Hosp's.; Clin. Instr., U. of British Columbia; Tel. 876-1820.
JOHNSON, Hugh S.; Hastings St. N., Bancroft, **Ont.; Tor '52; M.O.H., Cardiff Twp.; Tel. 75.**
JOHNSON, John E.; 2676 Bayview Ave., Willowdale, Ont.; UBC'58.
JOHNSON, John E.; 350 Albert St., Nanaimo, B.C.; 1931 Bayview Ave. (res); Durham U. (Newcastle, Eng.) '57; MB, BS; Active Staff, Nanaimo Reg. Gen. Hosp.; Tel. 754-9552.
JOHNSON, John M.; 143 James St. S., Ste. 525, Hamilton, Ont.; Tor '56; D.Psy; Psy; Staff, Ontario Hosp.; Tel. 522-5925.
JOHNSON, Jonas G.; 59-1st Ave., Gimli, Man.; Man'48; MCGP.
JOHNSON, Joseph C.; Medical Centre, Ormstown, P.Q.; Sheffield (Eng.) '49; MCGP; Staff, Barrie Mem. Hosp.; Tel. 829-2331.
JOHNSON, Joseph H.; 2 Johnson Block, 114 Main St., Kenora, Ont.; 540 First Ave. S. (res); Tor'22; Otol; Tel. HO 8-6512.
JOHNSON, Kjartan I.; Man '37; MCGP; Med. Dir., Neepawa Health Unit, Neepawa, Man.; Tel. 200.
JOHNSON, Leavert E.; 5013—51st St., Wetaskiwin, Alta.; 5310—47A Ave. (res); Alb '40; M.C.G.P.
JOHNSON, Louis G.; Royal Victoria Hosp., Montreal 2, P.Q.; 19530 Gouin Blvd. W., Ste.-Genevieve (res); McG '39; FRCP(C), IntMed; Assoc. Staff, Royal Victoria Hosp.; Ass't. Prof. (Med.), McGill U.; Cons. Phys., Henry Morgan Co.; Dist. Coroner; Tel. VI 2-1251.
JOHNSON, Lyle O.; Port Arthur Clinic, 194 N. Court St., Port Arthur, Ont.; Man'59; AMCGP.
JOHNSON, Michael D.; Ste. 607, 170 St. George St., Toronto 5, Ont.; UBC'60; IntMed.
JOHNSON, Percival; 82 Church St., Flin Flon, Man.; 78 Church St. (res); Man '34; F.A.C.S., GenSurg; Med. Supervisor, Hudson Bay Mining Employees Health Assoc.; Chief, Med. Staff, Flin Flon Gen. Hosp.; Tel. 687-7571.
JOHNSON, Ralph L.; Campbell Clinic, Lethbridge, Alta.; Alb '48; GenSurg.; Tel. FA 7-5737.
JOHNSON, Ray; Fort Frances Clinic, Fort Frances, Ont.; Man'53; GenSurg; Vice Pres. Med. Staff, Laverendrye Hosp.; Tel. 274-3287.
JOHNSON, Reginald; 1012 Boul. St. Joseph E., Montreal 34, P.Q.; 212 Willowdale, Outremont (res); Mon '47; IntMed; Cardiol (PQ); I/C Cardiovasc. Unit, Hop.-Notre-Dame; Ass't. Prof. (Med.), U. of Montreal; Tel. LA 5-6363.
JOHNSON, Richard J.; 700 Bannatyne Ave., Winnipeg, Man.; 317 North Drive, Fort Garry (res); St. Bart's (London, Eng.) '51; D.M.R.T. (Lond.); Staff, Manitoba Cancer Fdn.; Ass't. Rad., Winnipeg Gen. Hosp; Tel. SP 5-0466.
JOHNSON, Richard W.; 807 Kent Trust Bldg., 500 Ouellette Ave., Windsor, Ont.; Qns'55; FACA; FRCP(C); IntMed; **Chief, Dept. of Med., Grace** Hosp.; Active Cons., Hotel Dieu, Metropolitan & IODE Hosp's.; Tel. 256-7631.
JOHNSON, Robert H.; 2149 Primate Rd., Cooksville, Ont.; Tor'48; FRCP(C), Paed; Active Cons., Queensway & South Peel Hosp's; Ass't. Phys. (Paed), Hosp. for Sick Children; Paed., Paed. Inst. of Child Study; Clin. Instr. (Paed.), U. of Toronto; Tel. 277-4171.
JOHNSON, Thomas C.; Ste. 25, 659 Clyde Ave., West Vancouver, B.C.; Qns '51; MCGP; Tel. WA 2-8216.
JOHNSON, Thomas E.; 3445 Cote des Neiges Rd,. Apt. 25, Montreal P.Q.; Chicago (Ill., U.S.A.) '52; GenSurg.
JOHNSON, Vernon A.; Ste 213, 1320-5th Ave., Prince George, B.C.; Man '59.
JOHNSON, W. Harold; Ste. 305, 672 Brant St., Burlington, Ont.; Wes'55; Ophth; Staff, Oakville-Trafalgar & Joseph Brant Hosp's.; Tel. 637-5944.
JOHNSON, Walter L.; Qns '55; Med. Missionary, c/o Can. Baptist Mission Bd., 190 St. George St., Toronto 5, Ont.; Abroad.

JOHNSON, William L.; 243 Loch Lomond Rd., Saint John, N.B.; Dal'63; AMCGP.
JOHNSON-MACLEOD, G. Enid; 8 Glenwood Ave.. Dartmouth, N.S.; Dal '37; Anaes.
JOHNSRUDE, Richard L.; Macklin, Sask.; UBC'65.
JOHNSTON, Alan F.; London (Eng.)'59; Psy; Staff, Riverview Hosp., Essondale, B.C.
JOHNSTON, Albert C.; Ste. 270, 5780 Cambie St., Vancouver 15, B.C.; 6710 Churchill St. (res); McG'53; Ophth; Att'd. Staff, Eye Dept., Vancouver Gen. Hosp.; Cons. Staff, Eye Dept., Shaughnessy Hosp.; Clin. Instr., U. of British Columbia; Tel. FA 7-5422.
JOHNSTON, Albert E.; 555 University Avenue, Toronto 2, Ont.; 15 Carnwath Cr., Willowdale (res); Dal '56; FRCP(C); Anaes; Ass't. Anaes., Dept. of Anaes., Hosp. for Sick Children; Tel. EM 6-7242.
JOHNSTON, Basil W.; Tor. '62; Res., Kingston Gen. Hosp., Kingston, Ont.
JOHNSTON, Bruce; 2971 Kingston Rd., Scarborough, Ont.; Tor'52; MCGP; Active Staff, Scarborough Gen. Hosp.; Chief of Staff, Scarborough Centenary Hosp.; Assoc. Staff, Toronto East Gen. Hosp.; Tel. AM 1-4025.
JOHNSTON, Chas H.; 17—22nd Ave., Edmundston, N.B. (res); Dal '30; Phys. Fraser Mills Ltd.
JOHNSTON, Charles M.; Port Arthur Clinic, Port Arthur, Ont.; 94 Winnipeg Ave. (res); Man '42; ObstGyn; Chief (ObstGyn), St. Joseph's Hosp.; Staff, Port Arthur Gen. Hosp.; Tel. DI 4-7271.
JOHNSTON, David; 74 Golden, South Porcupine, Ont.; 50 Cecil Ave. (res); Tor '32.
JOHNSTON, David; Young Clinic, 111-1st Ave. N.E., Swift Current, Sask.; Glasgow (Scot.)'56; Tel. 773-9393.
JOHNSTON, David R.; Alb '55; Staff, J. F. Haszard Clinic, Box 1239, Kimberley, B.C.; Tel. 427-2277.
JOHNSTON, David W. B.; Ste 103, 396 Queens Ave., London, Ont.; Wes '35; F.A.C.S., F.R.C.S. (C), GenSurg; Cons. Surg. & Att'd. Staff, Victoria & St. Joseph's Hosp's.; Cons. Surg. & Chief of Dept. of ThorSurg., Westminster Hosp.; Cons Surg., Ontario Hosp.; Assoc. Prof. Dept. of Surg., U. of Western Ont.; Tel. GE 2-4353.
JOHNSTON, D. Cooper; 220 Phys. & Surg. Bldg., 8409 112th St., Edmonton, Alta.; Alb'44; DABOS; FRCS(C); OrthSurg; Lect., Dept. of OrthSurg., U. of Alberta; Tel. 439-4945.
JOHNSTON, Dennis W.; 184 Portland St., Dartmouth, N.S.; Dal '58; ObstGyn.
JOHNSTON, Donald R.; Med. Arts Bldg., 2150 Valley Way, Niagara Falls, Ont.; 2220 Corwin Ave. (res); Qns'42; FACOG; ObstGyn; Chief, Dept. of ObstGyn., Gtr. Niagara Gen. Hosp.; Tel. EL 6-1351.
JOHNSTON, Douglas B.; Box 116, Kelliher, Sask.; McG'24; Dist. Coroner; Tel. 52; Retired.
JOHNSTON, Edmund B.; Box 940, St. Stephen, N.B.; McG '43; M.C.G.P.
JOHNSTON, Edward E.; 8108-98th Ave., Edmonton, Alta.; Tor'60; FRCS(C), ObstGyn.
JOHNSTON, E. Greer; Shelburne, Ont.; Qns '35.
JOHNSTON, Eric E.; 103 Med. Dental Bldg., 450 Central Ave., London, Ont.; 1462 Corley Dr. (res); Qns '43; DMR; D & T Rad; Rad., St. Joseph's Hosp.; Instr. (Rad.), U. of Western Ont.; Tel. 433-0791.
JOHNSTON, Frank T.; Ste. 2., 4761 Yonge St., Willowdale, Ont.; 17 Audubon Crt. (res); Tor '49; GenSurg; Cons., North York Branson & Bethesda Hosp's.; Tel. BA 1-6801.
JOHNSTON, H. Alan; P.O. Box 540, 131 Grove St. Danville, P.Q.; Tor '63; Plant Phys., Canadian Johns-Manville Co., Asbestos; Tel. 839-2158.
JOHNSTON, Harold W. J.; 622 Med. Arts Bldg., 170 St. George St., Toronto 5, Ont.; 734 Avenue Rd. (res); Tor '21; FRCS (Edin.), FRCS(C), ObstGyn; Assoc. Prof. (ObstGyn), U. of Toronto. Tel. WA. 2-5678. Retired.
JOHNSTON, Hugh D.; 315 Brant Ave., Brantford, Ont.; 18 Belholme (res); Tor '55; Otol; Staff, Brantford Gen., St. Joseph's & Willet Hosp., Paris; Tel. PL 3-3661.
JOHNSTON, Hugh J.; Moose Jaw Clinic, 200 Scott Blk., Moose Jaw, Sask.; 310 Oak St. (res); Man '52; Anaes; Staff, Moose Jaw Union & Providence Hosp's.; Tel. 692-2373.
JOHNSTON, James G.; 702 Norfolk Ave. N., Simcoe, Ont.; Wes'65.
JOHNSTON, J. Blain; Box 757, The Thompson Clinic, Thompson, Man.; 32 Hillside Cres. (res); Man'53 MCGP; M.O., Man. Div., Internat'l. Nickel Co. of Canada; Chief of Med. Staff, Thompson Hosp.; Tel. 677-2386.
JOHNSTON, J. Crosby; 1214—20 A St. N.W., Calgary, Alta. (res); Alb '39; D.H.A., F.A.C.H.A., FRSH; Admin., Calgary Gen. Hosp.; Tel. AM 6-7541, Loc. 1310.
JOHNSTON, J. Gordon; 29 Marmora St., Trenton, Ont.; 2 Catherine St. (res); Tor '38; L.R.C.P. & S. (Eng.); Staff, Trenton Mem. Hosp.; Assoc. Staff, Belleville Gen. Hosp.; Tel. EX 2-4811.
JOHNSTON, John A.; Box 1681, Carleton Place, **Ont.; Tor '23; M.C.G.P.; Tel. 288.**
JOHNSTON, John F. A.; 176 St. George St., Toronto, Ont.; 8 Burton Rd. (res); Tor '29; Ophth.; Tel. WA 2-5494.
JOHNSTON, John J.; Humphries Clinic, New Med. Bldg., Prince Albert, Sask.; 313-19th St. W. (res); McG '51; Staff, Victoria Union & Holy Family Hosp's.; Tel. 763-2681.
JOHNSTON, John L.; 135 St. Clair Ave. W., Toronto 7, Ont.; Qns'39; DPH; FACS; GenSurg; Dir., Medical Branch, Ontario Med. Serv. Ins. Plan; Tel. 365-5550.
JOHNSTON, John L., A/Col; 24B Sicily Dr., Kingston, Ont. (res); Tor'43; Psy; Psy., Cdn. Forces Hosp.; Lect. Psy., Queen's U.; Tel. 546-3811, Loc. 525.
JOHNSTON, Keith A.; 308½ Boler Rd., London, Ont.; Wes'57; MCGP; Staff (GP), Victoria Hosp.; Court. Staff, St. Joseph Hosp.; Tel. 471-6440.
JOHNSTON, Kenneth B.; Box 40. Como, P.Q.; McG '22; DABOphth; DOMS (Eng.); FRCS(C), Ophth; Cons. Staff, Royal Victoria Hosp., Mtl.; Tel. Mtl. VI 2-1251.
JOHNSTON, Kenneth D.; 20 Lake Dr., Hunts**ville, Ont. (res); Tor '46.**
JOHNSTON, Kenneth M.; 138 Geneva St., St. Catharines, Ont.; Tor'44; MCGP; Tel. 685-8636.
JOHNSTON, Lalia A.; Dal '62; Staff, Nova Scotia Hosp.; Halifax, N.S.
JOHNSTON, Lloyd W.; Haig Clinic, 601-6th Ave. S., Lethbridge, Alta.; Alb '44; FACS; FACOG; ObstGyn; Chief of ObstGyn., Lethbridge Municipal Hosp.; Active Staff, St. Michael's Hosp.; Cons., Lethbridge Auxiliary Hosp.; Tel. 328-6641.
JOHNSTON, MacAllister W.; Ste. 618, 1849 Yonge St., Toronto 7, Ont.; Tor'42; FRCP(C), IntMed; Ass't. Prof. (Med.), U. of Toronto; Tel. 487-5851.
JOHNSTON, Margaret M. (Movat); Ste. 270, 5780 Cambie St., Vancouver 15, B.C.; 6710 Churchill St., Van. 14 (res); McG '52; Derm; Att'd. Staff, Van. Gen. Hosp.; Vis. Staff, St. Vincent's Hosp.; Clin. Instr., U. of British Columbia; Tel. FA 7-5422.
JOHNSTON, Michael A.; 190 King St. W., Dundas, Ont.; 4 Mayfair Ct. (res); Dublin (Ire.) '54; BAO; MCGP; Active Staff, St. Joseph's Hosp.; Tel. 628-6745.
JOHNSTON, Patricia K.; 410-1207 Douglas St., Victoria, B.C.; UBC '60; AMCGP; Med. Advisor, Cerebral Palsy Clinic; Tel. 382-8691.
JOHNSTON, Robert J.; 316 Med. Arts Bldg., 11010 Jasper Ave., Edmonton, Alta.; 14623 Mackenzie Dr. (res); Alb '46; DABS, FACS; FRCS (C), GenSurg; Att'd. Staff, University of Alta. Hosp. & Union Hosp.; Court. Staff, Royal Alexandra Hosp.; Assoc. Clin. Prof. (Surg.), U. of Alberta; Tel. GA 2-4246.
JOHNSTON, Robert K.; 101 Vista Towers, 1270 Beach Dr., Victoria, B.C.; Qns '16; GenSurg; Retired.
JOHNSTON, Robert K.; Humphries Clinic, Prince Albert, Sask.; 510-25th St. W. (res); UBC '56; MCGP; Tel. 763-2681.

JOHNSTON, Robert V.; Miller Bldg., King St., North Battleford, Sask.; 622 Main St. (res); Durham (Eng.)'42; MRCP (Lond.); Phys., Battleford Union Hosp.; Tel. 445-3541.

JOHNSTON, Ronald E.; 142 Queenston St., St. Catharines, Ont.; 46 Marsdale Dr. (res); Tor '51; Psy; Cons. Psy., St. Catharines Gen. Hosp.; Tel. MU 4-7271.

JOHNSTON, Ross E.; 688 Coxwell Ave., Toronto 13, Ont.; 15 Navarre Cres., Guildwood Village, Scarboro (res); Tor '52; MCGP; Active Staff (GP), Tor. E. Gen. Hosp.; Tel. OX 9-4082.

JOHNSTON, Stephen R.; 180 Portland St., Dartmouth, N.S.; Dal'09; D&TRad; Tel. 466-7471.

JOHNSTON, T. Alexander; Park Royal Medical-Dental Centre, 856 Park Royal, West Vancouver, B.C.; 659 Clyde Ave. (res); Alb '32; M.I.C.S., GenSurg; Chief of Gen. Surg., Children's Hosp.; Att. Surg., St. Paul's Hosp.; Tel. WA 2-2141.

JOHNSTON, Thomas C.; 149½ Mitton St., Sarnia, Ont.; Wes '50; Urol.; Tel. YU 4-4194.

JOHNSTON, W. H.; 61 Victoria Ave., Chatham, Ont.; Tor '29.

JOHNSTON, William G.; 183 St. Clair Ave. W., Toronto 7, Ont.; 3000 Lawrence Ave. E., Scar.; 355 Inglewood Dr., Tor. 7 (res); Tor '31; FRCS (Eng.); GenSurg; Chief of Surg., Scarborough Gen. Hosp.; Tel. 922-5106; 291-0811.

JOHNSTON, William H.; 250 Lawrence Ave. W., Toronto, Ont.; 76 Hazelton Ave., (res); Tor '51; F.R.C.P.(C), Paed; Clin. Ass't. Hosp for Sick Children; Staff, U. of Toronto; Tel. WA 3-5262.

JOHNSTON, William M.; 301 Brant Arts Bldg., 672 Brant St., Burlington, Ont.; Qns '56; ObstGyn; Tel. 637-3213.

JOHNSTON, William S.; 361 Dufferin Ave., London, Ont.; Wes'31; Anaes; Tel. 434-1772.

JOHNSTON, W. Victor; 1260 Bay St., Toronto 5, Ont.; 83 Baby Pt. Rd. (res); Tor'23; Exec. Dir., College of Gen. Practice of Can.; Tel. WA 1-4376.

JOHNSTONE, Audrey K.; Fort Frances Clinic, 301 Victoria St., Fort Frances, Ont.; London (Eng.)'51.

JOHNSTONE, Brian; Fort Frances Clinic, 301 Victoria St., Fort Frances, Ont.; London (Eng.) '57.

JOHNSTONE, Charles G.; 305 St. Germaine Ave., Toronto 12, Ont.; Qns '20.

JOHNSTONE, D. W.; 1196 Fulton Ave., West Vancouver, B.C. (res); Tor '32; Staff, Shaughnessy Hosp.; Hosp. Supt. & Sr. Treatment Med. Officer, Dept. of Veteran's Affairs; Tel. TR 6-6767.

JOHNSTONE, Frederick R.; 4862 Angus Dr., Vancouver, B.C. (res); Edinburgh (Scot.) '45; FRCS (Edin.), FACS; GenSurg; Staff, Vancouver Gen. Hosp.; Assoc. Prof. (Surg) & Lect. (Anat), U. of British Columbia; Tel. CA 4-1111.

JOHNSTONE, George C.; Fenelon Falls, Ont.; Tor '37.

JOLICOEUR, Amyot; 401 Grande-Allee, Quebec, P.Q.; Lav '39; PlasSurg. (P.Q.); GenSurg.; Ass't. (Surg.), Hop-St.-Sacrement, l'Enfant-Jesus & St. Michel-Archange; Chief Clin. Hop.-Ste-Foy; Ass't Prof., Laval U.; Tel. MU 3-4951.

JOLICOEUR, Germain; Ste. 3017, 801 est, rue Sherbrooke Montreal 24, P.Q.; Mon '59; FRCS-(C); Otol; Tel. 527-1344.

JOLICOEUR, Gilbert; 4 Taschereau, Hull, P.Q.; 24 Lacasse (res); Ott '54; IntMed; Dir. Dept. of Med. & Head of GastroEnt. Hop-Sacre-Coeur; Tel. PR 7-2721.

JOLIVET, Georges-Y.; 1150 Boul. St. Joseph E., Montreal 34, P.Q.; 475 Lockhart, Ville Mount Royal (res); Mon '49; Paed; Ass't. Prof., U. of Montreal; Tel. LA 7-1551.

JOLLIFFE, Roy F.; Warkworth, Ont.; Wes '42; Staff, Campbellford Mem. Hosp.

JOLLY, Elaine E.; Qns'64; Ass't. Res., Ottawa Civic Hosp., Ottawa 3, Ont.

JOLLY, Robert D.; 2705 Lakeshore Blvd. W., Toronto 14, Ont.; Tor '43; Phys., Chest Clinic & Assoc. Staff (G.P.), St. Joseph's Hosp.; Tel. 255-3461.

JOLLY, Terence G.; 509 London St., Winnipeg 15, Man.; 1168 Kildonan Dr., Wpg. 16 (res); Queen's U. (Belfast, N. Ire.) '51; MB, BCh; BAO· Tel. ED 9-2275.

JOLLYMORE, George C.; Box 250, Chester, N.S.; Dal '63.; Tel. 275-3715.

JOLY, Jean G.; Mon'65; Res., Hop. St-Luc. 1058 Rue St-Denis, Montreal 18, P.Q.

JOLY, Jean G.; 3377 Grande-Allee, Lafleche, Cite, Jacques-Cartier, P.Q.; 1910 St.-Pierre, Ville Lemoyne (res); Mon '58; Tel. 676-4321.

JOLY, J. Jacques; Clinique Med. St-Remi, St. Remi, Cte. Napierville, P.Q.; Mon'57.

JOLY, J. Pacifique; 6338 St. Denis, Montreal, P.Q.; 745 Dunlop Ave. (res); Mon '27; Obst.

JOLY, Jean Raymond; 342 rue Labelle, St. Jerome, P.Q.; Mon '42; Anaes (P.Q.); Anaes., Hotel Dieu de Montreal.; Tel. GE 2-9711.

JOLY, Robert; 24 Place Bourget S., Joliette, P.Q. (res); Mon '51; D.P.H.; Staff, Health Unit, Joliette.

JOMM, Enn; McG'65; Res., Montreal Gen. Hosp., Montreal 25, P.Q.

JONASSON, Harold D.; 2-245 Marion St., St. Boniface 6, Man.; Man'57; MCGP; Tel. CH 7-8456.

JONAT, Glen H.; Moose Factory Indian Hosp., Moose Factory, Ont.; Sask '63; M.O., Med. Serv., Dept. of National Health & Welfare; Tel. 4500.

JONAT, Lorne V.; Dauphin Health Unit, Dauphin, Man.; Man '51.

JONAT, Percy G.; Nipawin, Sask.; Man '56.

JONCAS, Fernand; 1699 Parc Lafontaine, Apt. 2, Montreal, P.Q.; 6027 Ave. de Lorimier, Mon '40; IntMed (P.Q.); Ass't. Med. Staff in charge of Nutrition, Hop. Maissoneuve; Ass't. Prof. of Med., U. of Montreal; Tel. 254-8341.

JONCAS, Gerard; 1910 Arvida, St-Bruno-Montarville, Cte Chambly, P.Q.; Mon'38; Paed(P.Q.).

JONCAS, Jean H.; 12375 Frechette, Montreal 9, P.Q.; Mon'55; Paed; Ass't. in (Med.), Montreal Children's Hosp.; Research Ass't., Microbiol. Inst. & Ass't. Prof., U. of Montreal; Tel. ON 7-4892.

JONCAS, Roland; Newport Centre, Co. Gaspe, P.Q.; Lav '57.

JONEJA, Rajindar P.; Punjab (India)'56; Psy; Staff, Riverview Hosp., Essondale, B.C.

JONES, A. Bancroft; Box 119, Nipawin, Sask.; Liverpool (Eng.)'47; GenSurg.

JONES, Adrian B.; Alb '64; Res., University Hosp., Edmonton, Alta.

JONES, Arnold F.; Drummond Med. Bldg., 1414 Drummond St., Montreal, P.Q.; 17 Willow Ave., Westmount (res); McG '40; D.Surg.; FACS; FRCS(C): GenSurg; Ass't. Surg., Montreal Gen. Hosp.; Cons. in Periph. Vasc. Dis., Queen Mary Vet's. Hosp.; Surg-in-Chief, Reddy Mem. Hosp.; Ass't. Prof. (Surg.), McGill U.; Tel. VI 4-8079.

JONES, Arnold R.; C. S. Williams Clinic, Box 610, Fruitvale, B.C.; McG '53; Staff, Trail-Tadanac Hosp.; Tel. 367-9211.

JONES, Arthur; 2275 Leigh Square, Port Coquitlam, B.C.; Queens U. (Belfast, Ire.) '50; DPH; MCGP; Tel. 942-7227.

JONES, Arthur L.; 250 College St., Toronto 5, Ont.; 7 Wells Hill Ave., Tor. 4 (res); Dublin (Ire) '48; BAO, MRCP(I), D.Psy; DABPN, FRCP(C), Psy; Chief of Psy Serv., Clarke Inst. of Psy.; Assoc. (Med.), U. of Toronto; Tel. 924-6811.

JONES, Betty; Nipawin, Sask.; Liverpool (Eng.) '51.

JONES, Charles M.; 199 Inglis St., Halifax, N.S.; Dal '30; DABR, FACS, D & T Rad; Hd. Dept. of Radiol., Halifax Infirmary; Cons. Rad., Camp Hill & TB Hosp's.; Assoc. Prof. (Rad.), Dalhousie U.; Tel. 2-4406.

JONES, David P.; 710 Fairmont Med. Bldg., 750 W. Broadway, Vancouver 9, B.C.; 3181 Point Grey Rd. (res); Liverpool (Eng.) '38; M.R.-C.P. (Lond.), F.R.C.P.(C), Neur; Att'd. Neurol., Vancouver Gen. & Shaughnessy D.V.A. Hosp's.; Clin. Ass't. Prof. U. of British Columbia; Tel. TR 4-1232.

JONES, David T.; Wes'64; Res., Victoria Hosp., London, Ont.

JONES, Denis H.; Kemptville, Ont.; Liverpool (Eng.) '50; Staff, Kemptville Dist. Hosp.; Tel. 258-2486.
JONES, Dennis M.; Bengough, Sask.; London (Eng.) '54; Med. Staff, Bengough Union Hosp.; Tel. 18.
JONES, Donald R.; 2 Gary Ave., Hamilton, Ont.; Tor '41; Staff, D.V.A.; Tel. JA 9-3312.
JONES, Dora R.; 2006 Lafayette Towers W., Detroit, Mich., U.S.A.; Tor'61; Paed; Abroad.
JONES, Edward A.; 317 Medical & Dental Bldg., Regina, Sask.; 3003 Hill Ave. (res); Man '40; M.Ch.(Orth.), OrthSurg; Staff, Orth. Serv., Regina Gen. & Regina Grey Nun's Hosp's.; Tel. LA 3-2634.
JONES, Edward D.; Brigus, Nfld.; Dublin (Ire) '39.
JONES, Elmer A.; 2435 MacDonald St., Vancouver 8, B.C.; 6658 Angus Dr. (res); McG '43; MCGP; Staff (GP), Van. Gen. Hosp.; Tel. RE 8-0331.
JONES, Eloise A. E.; McG'56; Res., Royal Victoria Hosp., Montreal 2, P.Q.
JONES, Eloise M.; 213 Med. Arts Bldg., 750 Spadina Cres. E., Saskatoon, Sask.; Tor '43; DPH; Psy; Tel. 925-6522.
JONES, Eric E.; 11 Appleby Court, Islington, Ont.; Tor '48; DiagRad; Radiol., Humber Mem. Hosp. & Tor. Hosp. for T.B.; Tel. 249-8111.
JONES, Ernest R.; 855 Kipling Ave. N., Weston, Ont.; Tor '52; Tel. 247-2401.
JONES, F. Crawford; 292 Bay St., Orillia, Ont. (res); Tor '43; D.Psy; Psy; Ass't. Supt. Ontario Hosp. School; Cons. Psy., Orillia Soldier's Mem. Hosp.; Tel. 326-7958.
JONES, Frank M.; 26 Westland Dr., Mtl. W. P.Q. (res); McG '27; A.B. PrevMed (Occ. Med.); FACPM; DPH; Chief M.O., Dupont of Canada; Lect. (Occ. Toxicol.), McGill U.; Tel. 861-3861.
JONES, Gerald C.; 161 Hughson St. S., Hamilton, Ont.; University Coll. (Dublin, Ire.) '54; Psy; Active Staff, Hamilton Gen. Hosp.; Tel. 522-4693.
JONES, Gerald E.; 12 Parkwood Centre, 1277 York Mills Rd., Don Mills, Ont.; Tor'56; Assoc. Staff, Toronto East Gen. Hosp.; Tel. 444-8211.
JONES, G. Glyn; Box 1500, Hudson Hope, B.C.; London (Eng.) '40; LRCP; MRCS; DCH; Paed; IntMed.
JONES, G. R.; 109 Cedar St., Sudbury, Ont.: 44 Kingsmount Blvd. (res); Tor '20; GenSurg; Dist. Coroner; Tel. 673-9524.
JONES, Grant H.; 230 Metcalfe St., Ottawa, Ont.; 216 Metcalfe St. (res); Tor '26; Ophth, Otol.; Tel. 232-0452.
JONES, Harold; 25 Main St., Drayton, Ont.; Qns '44.
JONES, Hywel T.; Main St., Schomberg, Ont.; Welsh Nat. U. (Cardiff, Wales) '47; B.Sc.; MCGP; Active Staff, York Co. Hosp., Newmarket; Tel. 939-2112.
JONES, J. Daniel; 16 Main St. W., Huntsville, Ont.: Tor '56: AMCGP; Tel. 789-5581.
JONES, John A.; 250 Lawrence Ave. W., Toronto 12, Ont.: London (Eng.) '49; FRCP(C); DiagRad.; Cons., Sunnybrook Hosp.; Rad., Huntsville Dist. Mem. Hosp., York County & Central Hosp's.; Tel. 787-0029.
JONES, John H.; Copper Cliff Hosp., Copper Cliff, Ont.; Oxford (Eng.)'47; Staff, Coppercliff, St. Joseph's, Sudbury Gen. & Sudbury Mem Hosp's.; Tel. 682-4421.
JONES, John T.; Box 305, Shubenacadie, N.S.; Wales (U.K.)'61; Tel. 14.
JONES, Joseph R.; 2090 Wyandotte St., Windsor, Ont.; Wales (U.K.)'55.
JONES, Kathleen E. (See Sansom, Kathleen E. J.)
JONES, Neville C.; 1900 Lonsdale Ave., North Vancouver, B.C.; Portland (Oregon, U.S.A.) '52; PlasSurg; Active Staff, Lionsgate Hosp.; Tel. 988-9414.
JONES, Norman H.; 216 Argyle St., Port Alberni, B.C.; 611 Argyle St. (res); McG '33; F.R.C.S.(C), GenSurg; Staff, West Coast Gen. Hosp.; Tel. 724-1215.
JONES, Norman S.; 2910 Kingston Rd., Toronto 13, Ont.; Qns '52; MCGP.; Tel. AM. 1-8041.
JONES, Reginald A.; 509 Broadview Ave., Toronto, Ont.; 1082 Eastern Ave. (res); Tor '06; GenSurg; Tel. HO 6-3545.
JONES, Richard H. T.; 62 Portland Cr., Regina, Sask.; Liverpool (Eng.)'58; FRCP(C), Paed.
JONES, Robert A.; 940 King George's Way, West Vancouver, B.C. (res); McG '45; Anaes; Staff, St. Vincent's Hosp.; Tel. 922-2658.
JONES, Robert C.; 4027 E. Hastings St., Burnaby 2, B.C.; McG '53; GenSurg.; Tel CY 9-2677.
JONES, Robert O.; 1362 Robie St., Halifax, N.S.; Dal '37; FAPA; FRCP(C); Psy; Hd., Dept. of Psy., Victoria Gen. & Camp Hill Hosp's,; Cons. Psy., Canadian Forces, Children's & Nova Scotia Hosp's.; Prof. & Hd., Dept. of Psy., Dalhousie U.; Pres., Cdn. Medical Assoc.; Past Pres., Halifax Med. Soc.; Tel. 423-7677.
JONES, Stewart F.; 4187 Lakeshore Rd., Burlington, Ont.; Wes'61; Tel. 637-2098.
JONES, Trevor K.; U.S.A.'56; MCGP; Res., St. Paul's Hosp., Vancouver 1, B.C.
JONES, Wentworth W.; 2171 Queen St. E., Toronto 13, Ont.; Tor '56; Tel. 699-9823.
JONES, William A., OBE, VD, CD; 251 University Ave., Kingston, Ont. (res); Wes'14; FFR; FACR; FRCP(C), D&TRad; Hon. Cons. Rad., Kingston Gen. & Cdn. Forces Hosp's.; Emeritus Prof. (Rad.), Queen's U.; Retired.
JONES, William F.; 2146 Bloor St. W., Toronto, Ont.; 44 Ridgevalley Cres. (res); Tor. '42; IntMed; Staff, Dept. of Med., St. Joseph's Hosp.; Tel. RO 9-2514.
JONES, William M.; 31 Tournament Dr., Willowdale, Ont. (res); McG '54; FACA; DABA; FRCP (C); Anaes; Att'd. Anaes. Staff, Toronto Western Hosp.; Clin. Teach., U. of Toronto; Tel. 222-7206.
JONSSON, Bjorn; 105-8th Ave. N., Swan River, Man.; Reykjavik (Iceland)'47; Dist. Coroner.
JORDAN, David A.; 2953 Bathurst St., Toronto 19, Ont.; 48 Elderwood Dr. (res); Tor '47, Paed; Staff, Hosp. for Sick Children, New Mt. Sinai & N. York Branson Hosp's.; Tel. RU 2-5863.
JORDAN, Francis B.; 109 Le Marchand Mansion, 116th St. & 100th Ave., Edmonton, Alta.; 8127-80th Ave. (res); Alb '37; Psy; Lect. (Psy), Schl. of Nurses, Edmonton Gen. Hosp.; Tel. 488-5704.
JORDAN, Graham B.; 26 Canboro Rd., Fonthill Ont.; Wes'57; MCGP; Active Staff, Welland County Gen. Hosp.; Court. Staff, Hotel-Dieu Hosp., St. Catharines; Tel. 892-2421.
JORDAN, Lawrence T.; Medical Clinic, 3009-31st Ave., Vernon, B.C.; McG '52; ObstGyn; Tel. 542-4321.
JORDAN, Robert H.; McG'58; Neurol P.Q.); Staff, St. Annes Hosp., Ste Anne de Bellevue, P.Q.
JORDAN, Zoena A.; Black's Harbour, N.B.; Dal '63.
JORDANA, Jaime; '53; Res., Sunnybrook Hosp., Toronto, Ont.
JORIZZO, Alberto A.; Naples (Italy)'56; DAB (Path); Path; Staff, Santa Cabrini Hosp., Montreal 36, P.Q.
JORON, Guy E.; Ste. 200, 3550 Cote des Neiges, Montreal 25, P.Q.; McG'42; FACP; IntMed; Clin. Ass't., Dept. of Metabolism & Toxicol., Montreal Gen. Hosp.; Clin. Ass't., St. Mary's Hosp.; Dem. (Med.), McGill U.; Tel. VI 4-7645.
JORY, Thomas A.; 484 William St., London, Ont.; Wes '55; FACS; FRCS(C), GenSurg; Cons., Parkwood Hosp.; Instr. (Anat.), U. of Western Ontario; Tel. 432-4101.
JOSENHANS, W. T.; 30 Boutiliers Lane, Dartmouth, N.S. (res); Tubingen (Germ.) '50; Assoc. Prof. (Physiol.), Dalhousie U.; Abroad.
JOSEPHSON, Joseph E.; Waterford Bridge Rd., St. John's Newfoundland (res); Qns '34; F.A.C.P.; IntMed; PathBact; Chief Path., St. John's Gen. Hosp.; Govn't. Path for Newfoundland; Chief Cons. Path., St. Clare's & Grace Hosp's.; Dir. Prov. Public Health Labs; Med. Dir., Red Cross Blood Trans. Serv.; Tel. 578-0471, Loc. 238.
JOSIPOWICZ, Anna; see Josy, Anna.
JOSIPIWICZ, Isaac; see Josy, Isaac.

JOSLYN, Marcel; 328 Bathurst St., Toronto, Ont.; 38 Southgate (res); Paris (Fr.) '35; Tel. EM 3-4831.

JOSS, Sidney S., Capt.; 2 RHC Base, Gagetown, N.B.; Qns'64.

JOST, Harold M.; 317 Wellington St., Sarnia, Ont.; 928 Lakeshore Rd. (res); McG '47; D.Urol., Urol.; Tel. 336-3572.

JOST, Harold T.; 220 Island Park Cres., Ottawa 3, Ont.; McG '16; Anaes; Cons. Anaes., Ottawa Civic Hosp.; Tel. PA 9-2511.

JOSY, Anna; Paris (France) '40; Staff, Doctors Hosp., 45 Brunswick Ave., Toronto 4, Ont.; Tel. WA 3-5411.

JOSY, Isaac; 250 Lawrence Ave. W., Toronto 12, Ont.; Apt. 504, 211 College St. (res); Paris (France) '39; Derm; Tel. RU 9-4016.

JOUBERT, Doreen O., (Papageorgiou); 111 9th St., Brandon, Man.; Man'53; MCGP; Tel. PA 9-5471.

JOUBERT, Geo. A.; Price, Co. Matane, P.Q.; Lav '24; Gen. & Indust. Med., Price Co.

JOUBERT, Jacques; 116 rue Church, Buckingham, P.Q.; 561 rue Principale (res); Mon '52; GenSurg (P.Q.); Surg Staff, Gen. Hosp.; Tel. YU 6-3402.

JOUBERT, Lucien; 300 boul. Laurentian, Montreal 9, P.Q.; Mon'58; MCGP; Indust Med; Visiting Staff, Hop. Notre-Dame; Med. Dir., Smith, Kline & French Pharm.

JOUBERT, Marie; 1900, boul Levesque, Duvernay, Laval-des-Rapides, P.Q.; Mon '64; Research, U. of Montreal.

JOUBERT, Noel Y.; Western Med. Clinic, 111-9th St., Brandon, Man.; Man '56; MCGP; Active Staff, Brandon Gen. & Assiniboine Hosp's.; Tel. PA 9-5471.

JOURDAIN, Camille; 475 Boul. Talbot, Chicoutimi, P.Q.; Lav'49; AMCAA; Derm Syph.; Ass't. I/C Derm. & Allergy (Med.), Hotel-Dieu St.-Vallier; Tel. 549-3330.

JOURNET, Leon; 2200 Sherbrooke E., Montreal, P.Q.; 85 Courcelette Outremont (res); Mon '39; Obst. (P.Q.); Staff, Hop. de la Misericorde.; Tel. LA 2-2483.

JOUSSE, Albin T.; 153 Lyndhurst Ave., Toronto 4, Ont.; Tor'42; FRCP(C), PhysMed; Med. Dir., Lyndhurst Lodge Hosp.; Cons. PhysMed & Rehab., Sunnybrook & Crippled Children's Hosp's.; Cons. Med. Advisory Bd., Toronto Rehab. Centre; Dir. & Assoc. Prof., Div. of Rehab., U. of Toronto; Tel. WA 3-0928.

JOW, Eleanor P.; Ste. 5, 2240 Robinson St., Regina, Sask.; UBC'56; IntMed; Cons., Rehab. Centre, Sask. Prov. Public Health, Dept., Regina.

JOWSEY, John W.; Med. Arts Clinic, 2125-11th Ave., Regina, Sask.; Man '55; FRCS(C), OrthSurg.; Tel. 523-0691.

JOY, Clifton J.; Med. Arts Bldg., Empire Ave., St. John's, Nfld.; 2 Bonaventure (res); Dal '48; Paed; Paed., St. Clare's Mercy, Grace & Gen. Hosp's.; Cons. (Paed.), Prov. Dept. of Health & Pepperell Air Force Base; Tel. 578-0395.

JOYAL, Andre C.; Mon '58; FRCP(C), Anaes; Staff, Royal Victoria Hosp., Montreal, P.Q.; Tel. 842-1251.

JOYAL, Jean F.; 12245 Grenet, Montreal 12, P.Q.; 5575 Place d'Aiguillon, Mtl. 9 (res); Mon'48; Urol (P.Q.); Hd. (Urol.), Hop. Sacre-Coeur & Cons., Hop. Deux-Montagnes, St. Eustache; Tel. DU 1-7281.

JOYAL, Joseph A.; 420 Ferguson, Haileybury, Ont.; Lav '12; Med. Staff, Misericordia Hosp.

JOYAL, Paul E.; 369 Main St., Haileybury, Ont.; Lakeshore Rd. (res); Mon '47; MCGP; Tel. OS 2-3400.

JOYCE, Cecil R.; 3435 Drummond St., Apt. 24, Montreal 25, P.Q.; McG '14; Emer. Assoc. (Med.), Royal Victoria Hosp.; Tel. 845-5097.

JOYNT, George H.; 102 Toronto Western Medical Bldg., 25 Leonard Ave., Toronto 2B, Ont.; 183 Roxborough Dr. (res); Tor '34; F.R.C.S.(C); F.A.C.S.; GenSurg; IntMed; Attend. Staff, Toronto Western Hosp.: Cons. Thor.Surg., Sunnybrook Hosp. (D.V.A.); Assoc. Prof. (Surg.) U. of Toronto; Tel. EM 6-1710.

JOYNT, Robert L.; 1307 Highway No. 8, Winona, Ont.; Tor'60; AMCGP; Staff, West Lincoln Mem. Hosp.; Tel. 643-1755.

JUBA, Emil; 293 Wallace St., Hope, B.C. U.B.C. '56

JUBB, E. Dawne; Ste. 709, 99 Avenue Rd., Toronto 5, Ont.; Apt. 907, 267 St. George St. (res); Tor '51 FRCS(C), ObstGyn; Clin. Instr. (ObstGyn), U. of Toronto; Staff, Women's College Hosp.; Tel. WA 1-6881.

JUCKES, Angus W.; Med. Arts Cinic, 2125-11th Ave., Regina Sask.; 22 Bolell (res); Man '57; FRCS(C); GenSurg; Staff, Dept. of Surg., Regina Gen. & Grey Nuns Hosp's.; Tel. 523-0691.

JUDA, Tibor; Qns'61; Res., Toronto Western Hosp., Toronto, Ont.

JUDAH, Joseph I.; 3429 Gottingen St., Halifax, N.S.; Bombay (India) '49; Court. Staff, Halifax Infirmary, Victoria Gen., Grace, Children's & Maternity Hosp's.; Tel. 455-2159.

JUDD, Albert B.; 424 Med. Dental Bldg., 925 W. Georgia St., Vancouver 1, B.C.; Wes '48; FRCP-(C); IntMed; Tel. 681-3738.

JUDGE, David L.; 10004-105th St., Edmonton, Alta.; 13432-117A Ave. (res); Alb '51; F.R.C.P. (C), IntMed.; Tel. 424-2121.

JUDGE, Gordon A.; 45 King St. E., Burford Ont.; Qns'50; MCGP; Staff, Brantford Gen. Hosp.; Tel. 449-2444.

JUDGE, Ray H.; 257 Bessborough Dr., Toronto, Ont. (res); Qns '23; Staff, Dept. of Health, Provincial Civil Service, Toronto.

JUDSON, Arthur H.; 25 Victoria Ave., Brockville, Ont.; McG '04; FICS; GenSurg; Active Staff, Brockville Gen. & St. Vincent-de-Paul Hosp's.; Tel. DI 2-3766.

JUDSON, Graham; Ferguson Ave., Haileybury, Ont.; 620 Brewster St. (res); McG '56; Staff, Misericordia Hosp., Haileybury, & New Liskeard & District Hosp., New Liskeard; Abroad.

JULES, D. Roy; 62 Blvd. Tache, Hull, P.Q.; Lav '53; Staff (IntMed.), Hop. du Sacre Coeur.

JULIEN, Fernand; 4373 rue St. Hubert, Montreal, P.Q.; 3207 Fendall, Montreal 26 (res); Mon '34; Psy (P.Q.); Staff, St. Jean de Dieu Hop., Gamelin. Tel. RE 7-6040.

JULIEN, J.-Marc; 802 Ch. Scott S., Ste.-Foy, Quebec 10, P.Q.; 813 ave. John W. (res); Lav '54; B.Ph; Pulm Dis & T.B. (P.Q.); FRCP(C), IntMed; Hd. (IntMed) & Dir. Intern Instruction, Hop. Laval; Tel. 653-4931.

JULIEN, Lucien; 30 est, boul. St.-Joseph, Montreal 14, P.Q.; Mon '37; FACS; FICS; GenSurg. (P.Q.); Ass't. Surg. & Vice-Pres., Exec., Hop. Ste-Jeanne d'Arc; Tel. 845-4241.

JULIEN, Lucile; Ste. 405, 150 rue Metcalfe, Ottawa, Ont.; Mon'47; Active Staff (IntMed); Ottawa Gen. Hosp.; Ass't. Clin., U. of Ottawa; Tel. 232-2721.

JULIEN, Paul E.; 794—5th St., Shawinigan Falls, P.Q.; Lav '32; Ophth, Otol; Tel. LE 6-4342.

JULIEN, Pierre G.; Mon'64; Res., Hop. Notre-Dame, Montreal, P.Q.

JULIEN, Pierre-Paul; 1150 Blvd. St. Joseph E., Montreal 34, P.Q.; Mon '48; F.R.C.P.(C), IntMed; Head Dept. of IntMed, Hop-Maisonneuve; Assoc. Prof. (IntMed), U. of Montreal; Tel. LA 7-1241.

JULSON, Kenneth I.; Box 560, Riverside Dr. E., Drumheller, Alta.; Alb'56; MCGP; Staff, Drumheller Gen., Mun. & Joe Cramer Aux. Hosp's.; Tel. VA 3-3345.

JUNEAU, Archille; 34 Gamble E.; Rouyn, P.Q.; Lav '57.

JUNEAU, Claude; C.P. 222, Rue Dube, Block 1, Apt. "A". P.M.O., Camp Valcartier, P.Q.; Lav '60.

JUNEK, D. Victor; 19 Dunlop Blk., Yorkton, Sask.; 162-4th Ave. N. (res); Man '45; MCGP; FASAS; Sr. Staff Surg., Yorkton Union Hosp.; Tel. 783-2294.

JUNG, Anthony; Front St., LaSalle, Ont.; Retired.

JUNGER, Paul W.; 5300 Cote-des-Neiges Rd., Ste. 610, Montreal, P.Q.; Dusseldorf (Germ.) '52; Paed; Clin. Ass't. Paed., St. Mary's and Montreal Children's Hosp's; Teach. Staff, McGill U.; Tel. RE 3-2522.

JUNK, Gerald J.; Humboldt Clinic, Humboldt, Sask.; Sask '57; MCGP; Active Staff, St. Elizabeth Hosp.; Tel. 682-2618.

JUNKIN, Edward R.; 42 Academy Med. Bldg., 1812-4th St. S.W., Calgary, Alta.; 74 Glenpatrick Dr. (res); Tor '49; GenSurg; Staff Health Phys., Calgary Gen. Hosp.; Tel. 263-8268.

JURCIC, Predrag; 1940 Lonsdale Ave., North Vancouver, B.C.; Zagreb (Yugo.)'58; Ophth; DABOphth; Tel. 988-4433.

JURETIC, Filip; State U. (Perugia, Italy)'54; Staff, Provincial Hosp., Campbellton, N.B.; Tel. 753-4461, Ext. 237.

JURJANS, Valdis; St. Joseph's Hosp., London, Ont.; 101 Regent St. (res); Tuebingen (Germ.) '48; Psy; Active Staff, St. Joseph's Hosp.; Teach. Staff, U. of Western Ontario; Tel. GE 9-3271, Loc. 255.

JURIANSZ, Allan R.; Sydney (Australia)'63; Res., Hosp. for Sick Children, Toronto 2, Ont.

JURK, Volker; 153 Lyndhurst Ave., Toronto, Ont.; Bonn (W.Germ.)'52; PhysMed. & Rehab.; Staff, Lyndhurst Lodge Hosp.; Cons. PhysMed., Toronto Rehab. Centre; Tel. WA 3-0928.

JUST, Robert; St. Andrew's U. (Scot.) '45; D.-Psy.; Psy; Staff, Ontario Hosp., Whitby, Ont.

JUSTIK, Joseph C.; Strathcona Medical Dental Bldg., 83rd Ave. & 105th St., Edmonton, Alta.; 10704-78th Ave. (res); Alb '43; MCGP; Tel. 433-5877.

JUSTUS, Duane W.; Box 458, Winchester, Ont.; Qns '61; M.Sc. (Med.); FRCS(C), GenSurg; Surg. in-Chief, Winchester & Dist. Mem. Hosp., Winchester; Cons. Surg., Kemptville Dist. Hosp., Kemptville; Tel. 774-2635.

JUSTUS, Howard W.; Box 148, Chesterville, Ont.; Qns'28; Pres. of Med. Staff, Mem. Hosp., Winchester; Tel. HI 8-2356.

JUTEAU, Yvan; 101A Principale, Rouyn, Cte. Temiscamingue, P.Q.; Mon'37; Anaes. (P.Q.); Tel. 762-3702.

JUTRAS, Albert; Dept. of Rad., Hotel-Dieu de Montreal, 3875 rue St-Urbain, Montreal, P.Q.; 3682 rue Ste. Famille (res); Mon '25; F.R.-C.P.(C), D & TRad; Dir. of Dept. Rad., Hotel Dieu; Prof. & Dir., Dept. Rad., U. of Montreal; Tel. VI 5-7520.

JUTRAS, Michel; Ste. 1404, 3601 rue Ste Famille, Montreal 18, P.Q.; Mon'64; I/C Project Med. Science & Biology for Expo '67; Tel. 397-8986.

JUTRAS, Rene; Polyclinique Gravel, C.P. 26, 66 St-Jean-Baptiste, Victoriaville, P.Q.; Lav '52-Paed (P.Q.); Chief Paed., Hotel-Dieu, Arthabaska; Tel. 357-2031.

JUTRAS, Therese (See Martel-Jutras).

JUVSHIK, Alex; 124 Frederica St. E., Fort William, Ont.; Franz U. (Austria)49; Tel. 622-1274.

KAAN, David C.; Man'60; Res., Dept. of Anaes., St. Boniface Hosp., Winnipeg 6, Man.

KAARSOO, Maie; Man '61; Research, Dept. of Pathol., Banting Inst., 100 College St., Toronto 2, Ont.; WA 3-6611.

KABIR, M. Ahmed; Dacca (Pakistan)'56; Staff, Riverview Hosp., Essondale, B.C.

KABOLI, Khosrow S.; 166 King Hiram St., Ingersoll, Ont.; Teheran (Iran)'57; ObstGyn.; Abroad.

KACHAN, Ramkarran; Willow Bunch, Sask.; Royal Coll. (Ire.) '53.

KACZANOWSKI, Godfryd; 904 Centre St. S., Whitby, Ont. (res); Warsaw (Poland) '29; Psy; Clin. Dir., Ont. Hosp.; Tel. 668-5881.

KACZANOWSKI, Maria B.; Tor '59; Psy; Staff, Ontario Hosp., Hamilton, Ont.; Tel. 385-5361.

KADDISH, Greta L. (See Livingstone)

KADISH, Joan A. (Karen); Qns '60; Res., Royal Victoria Hosp., Montreal, P.Q.

KADISH, Manuel E.; Geneva (Switz.)'55; DiagRad; Staff, Royal Victoria Hosp., Montreal, P.Q.

KADYSIEWICZ, Michel M.; 401 Vaughan Rd., Toronto 10, Ont.; 59 Elm Ridge Dr. (res); Paris (Fr.) '54; MCGP; Staff, Northwestern Gen. Hosp.; Tel. RU 3-6762.

KADZIORA, Max B.; 1105 Carling Ave., Ste. 202, Ottawa, Ont.; 121 Powell Ave. (res); Dusseldorf (W.Germ.) '48; ObstGyn; Clin. Ass't. (ObstGyn.), U. of Ottawa; Att'd. Staff, (ObstGyn.), Ottawa Civic & Grace Hosp's.; Tel. 729-1997.

KAFATO, Kirino; 526 Guelph Line, Burlington, Ont.; Istanbul (Turk.)'50; Psy.

KADER, Fred J.; McG '64; Res., Montreal Gen. Hosp., Montreal 25, P.Q.; Abroad.

KAGAN, Joseph M.; 318 Medical Arts Bldg., Winnipeg, Man.; 851 Manitoba Ave. (res); Lav '46; FRCS(C), GenSurg; Lect. (Surg.), U. of Manitoba; Tel. WH 3-6996.

KAHANA Leo M.; Man '51; Pulm Dis and TB (P.Q.); Ass't. Lab. Dir., Mt. Sinai San., Ste.-Agathe-des-Monts, P.Q.; Tel. 326-2303.

KAHANOVITCH, Moses E.; 201-309 Hargrave St., Winnipeg, Man.; Man '41; MCGP; FAGS; FASAS; Chmn., Nursing Education Committee, Victoria Gen. Hosp.: Tel. WH 3-7861.

KAHN, Amnon; 5845 Cote des Neiges Rd., Ste. 590, Montreal, P.Q.; Qns '58; FRCP(C), IntMed; Clin. Fell., McGill U. Clinic; Staff Phys., Jewish Gen. Hosp.; Tel. 738-6771.

KAHN, David S.; 1301 Caledonia Rd., Mount Royal, Montreal 16, P.Q. (res); Tor '42; Path; Dir. of Labs., St. Mary's Hosp.; Ass't. Prof. Pathol., McGill U.; Tel. 735-3511. Abroad.

KAHNE, Harold M.; 5140 Victoria Ave., Montreal, P.Q.; 4802 Dornal Ave. (res); Mon '41; Paed; Clin. Ass't. (Paed.), Jewish Gen. & Montreal Children's Hosp's.; Tel. 737-5476.

KAINE, Gerald; 1154 Maple Ave., Shawinigan, P.Q.; McG '35; M.O. Aluminum Co. of Canada Ltd.; Tel. LE 9-5421.

KAJANDER, Ruth E. (Koeppe); 242 Hodder Ave., Port Arthur, Ont.; Goettingen (Germ.) '48; D.Psy; Psy; Tel. 683-6631.

KAKOS, Angelo; 520 Cherrier, Montreal 24, P.Q.; 4279 St. Catherine (res); Mon '51; IntMed.; Tel. AV 8-6873.

KALABUS, Francois; Unite Sanitaire, Rouyn, P.Q.; 818 Tardif (res); Paris (France) '51; DPH; PH(P.Q.); M.O., Dept. of Public Health.

KALANT, Harold; 39 Farnham Ave., Toronto 7, Ont.; Tor '45; Ph. D.; Ass't. Research Dir. (Biol.), Alcoholism & Drug Addiction Research Fdn.; Assoc. Prof. (Pharmacol.), U. of Toronto; Tel. WA 3-6611.

KALANT, Norman; 318 Monmouth Ave., Town of Mount Royal, P.Q.; Tor '47; Ph.D. (Exp-Med.); IntMed; Ass't. Dir. of Research, Jewish Gen. Hosp.; Ass't. Prof. (Invest. Med.), McGill U.; Tel. 735-3711.

KALAYCI, Mehmet; Ankara (Turkey); Staff, Hop Des Laurentides, L'Annonciation, P.Q.

KALB, Sidney; 174 Thistle Down Blvd., Rexdale, Ont.; Man '52; D.Psy; Psy; Staff, Ontario Hosp., New Toronto; Tel. CL 9-8291.

KALEAL, I. S.; 2992 W. Broadway, Vancouver, B.C.; Qns '43; MCGP; Tel. RE 3-6622.

KALINOWSKI, Maurice R.; 194 Glen Cedar Rd., Toronto 10, Ont. (res); Warsaw (Poland) '25; Staff, T.B. Provision Unit, Dept. of Health, Toronto; Tel 782-3697.

KALINOWSKI, Richard; 194 Glen Cedar Rd., Toronto 10, Ont.; Tor '59; DMR; DABR; Memb. Am. Coll. of Rad; FRCP(C), DiagRad; Tel. 782-1241. Abroad.

KALKMAN, Johannes W.; Fort Frances Clinic, 301 Victoria, Fort Frances, Ont.; 851-3rd St. E. (res); Tor'59; Tel. 274-3287.

KALLA, Frank P.; 2775 W. Broadway, Vancouver, B.C.; 2606 McBain Ave. (res); Budapest (Hung.) '51; Tel. RE 8-4334.

KALLA, Gabriel; 1307-11th Ave., Regina, Sask.; Debrecen (Hung.) '48; Tel. 522-7210.

KALLIO, Jean E.; Lucky Lake, Sask.; McG '44; Retired.

KALMAN, George S.; 805 Giles Blvd. E., Windsor, Ont.; 2261 Kildare Rd. (res); Debrecen (Hung.) '38; ObstGyn.; Tel. 252-3181.

KALNINS, Dagnisa M.; Tor'65; Res., St. Michael's Hosp., Toronto 2, Ont.

KALOW, Brigitte D.; 361 Blythwood Rd., Toronto 12, Ont. (res); Rostock (Germ.)'44; Anaes; Staff, Women's College Hosp.; Tel. WA 3-7381.

KALOW, W.; 53 Douglas Cr., Toronto 5, Ont. (res); Konigsberg (Germ.) '41; Assoc. Prof. (Pharm.), U. of Toronto; Tel. WA 3-6611.

KALUDI, Murat; 3423 rue St. Denis, Montreal 18, P.Q.; Paris (Fr.) '40; IntMed.; Tel. VI 2-4892.

KALYANA-SUNDARAM, Krishnaswami; Porcupine Med. Clinic, Porcupine Plain, Sask.; Madras (India) '53.

KALZ, Frederick; 1414 Drummond St., Ste. 620, Montreal 25, P.Q.; 3766 Marlowe Ave., Mtl. 28 **(res); Prague (Czechoslov.) '30; DPH; DermSyph; Chief, Dept. of Derm., Montreal Children's Hosp.; Staff (Derm), Queen Elizabeth Hosp.; Ass't. Prof. (Derm.), McGill U.; Tel. VI** 9-5833.

KALZ, Gertrude G.; 3766 Marlowe Ave., Montreal, P.Q. (res); Prague (Czech.) '31; D.P.H., Bact; Assoc. Prof. of Bact., McGill U.; Tel. VI 4-6311.

KAMBUROFF, Tonka D. (Dobreva); 5865 Sperling Ave., Burnaby 1, B.C.; (res); Karl's Univ. **(Czech) '45; M.O., The Woodlands School, New Westminster.**

KAMENICEK, Eve; (See FISHELL)

KAMINER, Mendel; 4052 New St., Burlington, Ont.; Witwatersrand (S. Africa)'52; FFA; Anaes; Staff, Joseph Brant Mem. Hosp.; Tel. 637-9753.

KAMINKER, Arthur; Ste. 203, 1543 Victoria Pk. Ave., Scarborough, Ont.; Tor '54; F.R.C.P.(C), IntMtd; Staff, Doctor's Hosp.; Tel. 759-6581.

KANDEL, Patricia F.; Apt. 206, 1178 Adelaide St., London, Ont.; Ott'61.

KANDEL, Stephen P.; Box 300, Port Perry, Ont.; Bucharest (Rum) '44.

KANDT, Robert; Brentwood Shopping Plaza, 3551 Charleswood Dr., Calgary, Alta. Abroad.

KANE, Ernest W.; 736 Granville St., Vancouver 2, B.C.; U.B.C.'62; Tel. 684-2481.

KANE, Louis Allin; 304 St. Clair Ave. W., Toronto, Ont.; 126 Kilbarry Rd., (res); Tor '35; M.Sc. (Med.); DABOT; Otol; Chief (Otol.), Northwestern Gen. Hosp.; Sr. Att'd. (Otol.), Mount Sinai Hosp.; Cons. Otol., North York Branson Hosp. & Oshawa Gen. Hosp.; Tel. WA 8-0997.

KANE, Thomas J.; The Spence Clinic, 910 Ridge**way St., Fort William, Ont.; 1425 Cuthbertson Pl.** (res); Wes '50; IntMed.; Tel. 622-5301.

KANEE, Ben; 203 Hycroft Medical Bldg., 3195 Granville St., Vancouver, B.C.; 2991 S.W. Marine Dr. (res); Man '34; D.A.B.D.S., A.M.C.A.A, DermSyph; Hon. Staff, Van. Gen. Hosp. & **U. of British Columbia; Tel. RE 3-2666.**

KANEE, Louis; 5152 Trunk Rd., Ladner, B.C.; McG'48; Tel. 946-4181.

KANG, Sang S.; Taegu Med. School (Kyong, Korea)'50; Staff, Manitoba Training School, Box 1190, Portage-La-Prairie, Man.

KANJILAL, Nirmalendu, F/L; Assam (India) '55; Cdn. Forces Hosp., Kingston, Ont.

KANOVSKY, Frank H.; Mon'61; Res. (Orth-Surg.), Shriner's Hosp. for Crippled Children, Montreal, P.Q.

KANOVSKY, Samuel; 54 Ontario St., St. Catharines, Ont.; Man '37; FICS; GenSurg; Sr. Active Surg. Staff & Chm., Comm. Surg. Infection, St. Catharines Gen. Hosp.; Court. Staff, Hotel-Dieu Hosp.; Tel. MU 4-7713.

KANTER, Yale C.; McDiarmid Clinic, 330 Clement Block, Brandon, Man.; Dal'60; Ophth; Tel. PA 9-2428.

KANTOR, Sam; 609 Boyd Bldg., Winnipeg, Man.; 849 Oak St. (res); Anaes; Staff, Misericordia Hosp.; Tel. SP 4-6581.

KAO, Hua; Canton (China) '43; PhysMed & Rehab; Staff, Moose Jaw Union Hosp., Moose Jaw, Sask.; Tel. 629-1841.

KAPKIN, Ihsan A.; Istanbul (Turk.) '49; Staff, Provincial Hosp., Lancaster, N.B.

KAPLAN, Samuel R.; 140 Brown's Line, Toronto 14, Ont.; 415 The Westway, Weston; Wes '56; MCGP; Med. Staff, Queensway Gen. Hosp.; Tel. 255-2831 & 249-1644.

KAPLAN, Sidney; Ste. 1104-750 W. Broadway, Vancouver 9, B.C.; 6080 Cartier St. (res); Tor '43; MCGP; Staff, Shaughnessy Hosp.; Vis. Staff, Vancouver Gen., St. Paul's & Grace Hosp's.; Clin. Instr. (Psy), U. of British Columbia; Tel. TR 4-1222.

KAPSOS, Joseph E.; 695 Markham Rd., Scarborough, Ont.; Tor '57; FRCS(C), ObstGyn; Active Staff, Scarborough Gen. Hosp.; Court. Staff, Grace Hosp.; Tel. AT 2-6698.

KAPUR, Prem L.; Edinburgh (Scot.) '51; DCH; DMRD; DTM&H; DiagRad; Rad., Hamilton Gen. Hosp., Hamilton, Ont.; Tel. 527-0271.

KAPUSTA, Michael; 86 Third St., New Toronto, Ont.; 264 Keele St., Toronto 9 (res); Ott '53; DDS, DDPH; MCGP; Staff, Queensway Gen. Hosp. M.O.H. New Toronto; Tel. CL 1-8571.

KAPUSTA, Morten A.; 2935 Maplewood Ave., Montreal, P.Q.; McG'59; FRCP(C), IntMed.

KAPUSTA, Ronald; McG'60; Res., Jewish Gen. Hosp., Montreal 26, P.Q.

KARABANOW, Oscar; 187 St. Clair Ave. W., Toronto 7, Ont.; Geneva (Switz.) '50; CEM (Geneva); Psy; Ass't. Dir., Mental Health Clin., Humber Mem. Hosp., Weston, Ont.; Cons. Psy., Northwestern Gen. Hosp.; Tel. 921-9663.

KARAKUC, Raymond J.; 15020 Greenfield Rd., Apt. 16, Detroit, Mich. 48227; Man'58; DiagRad; Abroad.

KARAM, Daoud B.; Apt. 26, 2780 Kent Ave., Montreal 26, P.Q.; Beirut (Lebanon)'62.

KARAM, Norman A.; 193 Railway St., Cochrane, Ont.; 237 Railway St. (res); Qns '42; MCGP; Tel. 272-4075.

KARASEWICH, Eugene G.; Man '54; FRCS(C), GenSurg; Staff, Memorial Hosp., New York 21, N.Y., U.S.A. Abroad.

KARASICK, Howard D.; Winnipeg Clinic, N.E. St. Mary's & Vaughan, Winnipeg 1, Man.; Man '55; FRCS(C), ObstGyn; Ass't. ObstGyn., Wpg. Gen. Hosp.; Clin. Teach. (ObstGyn.), U. of Manitoba; Tel. 942-0551.

KARASU, Toksoz; Istanbul (Turk.) '59; Staff, Two Hills Hosp., Box 160, Two Hills, Alta.; Abroad.

KARASZTHY, Dennis J.; 394 Bloor St. W., Toronto 5, Ont.; 59 Spadina Rd. (res); Pazmany Peter (Budapest, Hung.) '48; ObstGyn.

KARATEEW, Edward B.; Alb'56; Res., St. Paul's Hosp., Vancouver, B.C.

KARDASH, Sidney; Ott '63; Int., Montreal Children's Hosp., Montreal, P.Q.

KARDERA, Edward P., Capt.; MIR, C.F.B., Westwin, Man.; UBC'65.

KARGAS, Aristomenis K.; Athens (Greece) '50; Staff, Saskatchewan Hosp., Weyburn, Sask.

KARGER, Paul J.; 780 Eglinton Ave. W., Toronto 10, Ont.; 790 Eglinton Ave. W. (res); Berlin (Germ.) '15; Paed.; Tel. RU 2-3479.

KARJALA, Roy J.; 1734 W. Broadway, Vancouver 9, B.C.; UBC '56; FRCP(C), IntMed; Vis. Phys., Vancouver Gen. Hosp. & St. Paul's Hosp.; Cons. IntMed., St. Vincent's & Burnaby Gen. Hosp's.; Tel. 733-1919.

KARKALAS, Yani; 412 boul du Havre, Valleyfield, P.Q.; Istanbul (Turk.)'53; Abroad.

KARLINSKY, William; Winnipeg Clinic, Winnipeg 1, Man.; 827 Campbell St., Wpg. 9 (res); Man '45; FRCP(C), IntMed; Hon. Att'd. Staff, & Jr. Endo., Wpg. Gen. Hosp.; Cons. (Med.); DVA Hosp.; Ass't Prof. (Med.), U. of **Manitoba; Tel. 942-0551.**

KARME, Alan B.; 2317 Turner St., Vancouver 6, B.C.; UBC '59; Psy.

KARN, Gordon M.; 1130, 2300 Tupper St., Montreal 25, P.Q.; 259 Strathern Ave. N. (res); McG '43; M.Sc.; D.S.; FRCS(C); GenSurg (Cardiovasc.); **Assoc. Surg. & Ass't., Dept. of Cardio**vasc. Surg., Montreal Children's Hosp.; Cons. Catherine Booth Hosp.; Surg. Registrar, Mtl. Children's Hosp.; Lect. (Surg.), McGill U.; Tel. 937-8511.

KARNAUCHOW, Paul N.; 1158 Glenwood Ave., North Bay, Ont. (res); Krasnodar (USSR)'41; Path; Cons. Clin. Path, Dir. of Labs., St. Joseph's Gen. & North Bay Civic Hosp's.; Tel. GR 2-6100, GR 2-2700.

KAROLS, Janis; 455 Palmerston Blvd., Toronto 4, Ont.; Riga (Latvia) '31; Tel. LE 4-1681.
KARPATI, George; 215 Le Merchant Rd., St. John's, Nfld.; Dal '60; FRCP(C); Neur. Abroad.
KARPATI, Laszlo; 415 Bloor St. W., Toronto 4, Ont '31; Tel. 923-3436.
KARPETZ, Edward, Major; Mon '39; O.C., Alberta Military Hosp., Currie Barracks, Calgary, Alta.
KARR, A. William; Apt. 910, 16 Tremont Dr., St. Catharines, Ont.; Tor'62; AMCGP.
KARREL, Ben D.; 916 Prince St., Truro, N.S.; 357 Prince St. (res); Dal '53; MCGP.
KARRELL, Israel A.; 61 Peter St., St. John's, N.B.; 143 Sydney St. (res); Dal '49; FACP; IntMed; Assoc. Phys., St. John's Gen. Hosp.; Cons. **(Gastroent.), Lancaster DVA Hosp.; Tel. 693-2361.**
KARSGAARD, Andrew T.; Winnipeg Clinic, N.E. St. Mary & Vaughan, Winnipeg, Man.; Man '43; Ophth.; Tel. 942-0551.
KARVELLAS, Penelope; Alb '64; Staff, Alberta Hosp., Ponoka, Alta.
KASARI, Leili (Marks); 602 Indian Rd., Toronto, Ont.; Tartu (Estonia) '36; Tel. LE 2-9863.
KASARI, Voldemar; 602 Indian Rd., Toronto, Ont.; Tartu (Estonia) '39; Tel. LE 2-9863.

KASCHUB, Robert W.; McG'65; Res., Royal Victoria Hosp., Montreal 2, P.Q.
KASDORF, William; Box 280, Brooks, Alta.; Sask '59; Tel. 362-3001.
KASIAN, Peter; 413 Selkirk Ave., Winnipeg, Man.; 35 Primrose Cres. (res); Man '42; Courtesy Staff, St. Boniface, Childrens' Hosp.; Staff, Victoria Hosp.; Med. Examiner, Manufacturer's Life.; Tel. JU 2-6855.
KASIRER, Paul; McG'65; Res., Royal Victoria Hosp., Montreal 2, P.Q.
KASLER, David; Ste 407, 99 Avenue Rd., Toronto, Ont.; 575 Avenue Rd. (res); Tor '34; FCCP; IntMed; Att., Staff (Med.), New Mount Sinai Hosp.; Dir., Chest Clinic, New Mount Sinai Hosp.; Member, Chest Clinic, Toronto Western Hosp.; Tel. WA 1-0584.
KASMAR, James J.; McG '51; MCGP; Res., (DiagRad.), University Hosp., Saskatoon, Sask.
KASNER, Martin; Dal '59; Res., Jewish Gen. Hosp., Montreal, P.Q.

KASPARDLOV, Melvin; Medical Arts Bldg., 11011 Ouellette St., Windsor, Ont.; Wes'56; DiagRad.

KASPER, Thaddeus A.; 203 Professional Bldg., 10830 Jasper Ave., Edmonton, Alta.; Alb'56; **Path; Ass't. Prof. (Path.), U. of Alberta Provincial Labs.;** Tel. 454-5707.
KASSAY, Guido I.; 727 Scarborough Golf Club Rd., Scarborough, Ont.; Ferenc-Jozsef-Kolozsvar (Hung.) '44; D.Psy.; Staff, Ontario Hosp., Whitby; Tel. 668-5881.
KASSERRA, Monika E. (v. Tappeiner); Freelton, Ont.; Cologne (Germ.) '54; MCGP; Staff, St. Joseph's Hosp., Hamilton & Guelph; Tel. 659-3302.
KASSERRA, Wolfgang; Freelton, Ont.; Cologne (Germ.)'52; MCGP; Staff, St. Joseph's Hosp., Hamilton & Joseph Brant Hosp., Burlington; Tel. 659-3302.
KASSNER, Edward; Souris, P.E.I.; Vienna (Austria) '37; M.C.G.P.; Staff, PEI Hosp.; Tel. 33.
KASTEN, Sydney L.; 316 St. Clair Ave. W., Toronto 7, Ont.; 552 Deloraine Ave. (res); Tor '57; D.Psy.; Psy; Tel. 923-7668.
KASTNER, Aaron; 2293 Carling Ave., Ottawa, Ont.; 1069 Chelsea Dr. (res); Man '50; MCGP; Tel. 725-2801.
KASYAPAN, Nelpakkam, D.; 4565 Queen Mary Rd., Montreal 26, P.Q.; Madras (India) '55; FRCS(C), Neur. Surg.; Tel. 342-2330.

KASZA, Leslie; Delaware, Ont.

KATO, Joichi G.; Matheson Bldg., 10410-81st Ave., Edmonton, Alta.; Alb '41; MCGP; Hosp. Advisory Bd. & Teach. Staff, General Hosp.; Tel. 488-8181.
KATO, Laszlo; 6 Kilburn Cr., Montreal 29, P.Q.; Budapest (Hung.) '39; Hd., Dept. of Physiopath., Inst. of Microbiology & Hygiene, U. of Montreal; Tel. MU 1-2521.

KATONA, Veronica (See Gal)

KATTY, Virupax S.; Bombay (India) '50; FACS; GenSurg; Staff, Cancer Clinic, University Hosp., Saskatoon, Sask.; Tel. 242-7641. Abroad.

KATZ, Abraham S.; McG'64; Res., Royal Victoria Hosp., Montreal 26, P.Q.
KATZ, Allan; 38 Whitehall Rd., Toronto 5, Ont.; Man'57; Path; Ass't. Path., St. Michael's Hosp.; Dem., U. of Toronto; Tel. 362-4461.
KATZ, Arnold H.; 565 Ellendale Med. Bldg., 5845 Cote-des-Neiges Rd., Montreal 26, P.Q.; 375 Revere Ave., Twn. of Mt. Royal (res); McG '40; DOMS (Eng.); FRCS(C), Ophth; Att'd. Staff, Jewish Gen., Mtl. Children's Hosp's. **& Queen Mary Vet's Hosp.; Tel. RE 3-2927.**
KATZ, Deborah; Ste. 1005, 123 Edward St., Toronto 2, Ont.; 209 Raglan Ave. (res); Paris (France)'42; PCN (France); MCAA, IntMed; Chief Allergy Clin. & O.P.D. IntMed., Women's College Hosp.; Tel. WA 3-3375.
KATZ, Eli; 5025 Sherbrooke St. W., Montreal 28, P.Q.; McG '38; Otol; Assoc. Otol; Queen Elizabeth Hosp.; Tel. 488-8011.
KATZ, Max; McG '64; Staff, Cottage Hosp., Come-by-Chance, Nfld.
KATZ, Morris; Ste. 645, 5845 Cote des Neiges Rd., Montreal 26, P.Q.; Alb'60; Psy.
KATZ, Mortimer; 2020 Alta. Vista Dr., Ottawa 8, Ont.; Tor '50; MCGP; Tel. 733-7202.
KATZ, Moises; 160 Foster St., Waterloo Co., Shefford, P.Q.; Mon'30; Staff, Brome-Missisquoi **Perkins Hosp., Sweetsburg; Tel. 539-1244.**
KATZ, Philip; 72 Hargrave St., Ste. 100, Winnipeg 1, Man.; 887 Ash St. (res); Man'55; Psy; Active Staff, St. Boniface Gen., Winnipeg Gen. & Children's Hosp's.; Cons. (Psy.) to Children's, Eastern Man. Family Bureau of Greater Winnipeg, Wpg. Child's Guidance Clin. & Jewish Child & Family Service; Ass't. Prof. (Psy.), U. of Man.; Tel. 943-6242.
KATZ, Sydney; Ste. 206, 280 Bloor St. W., Toronto 5, Ont.; Man '57; FRCS(C), Urol; Staff, Toronto Gen. Hosp.; Tel. 924-7666.

KAUFFMAN, Philip P.; 2090 Eglinton Ave. W., Toronto, Ont.; Tor '44; Tel. RU 2-5600.

KAUFMAN, Barry J.; 245 Wellington Cres., Winnipeg 9, Man.; Man '57; FRCP(C), IntMed; Staff, Wpg. Gen. & Deer Lodge Hosp's.; Dem. (Med.), U. of Manitoba; Tel. 284-3970.

KAUFMAN, John J.; 119 Forest Ave., St. Thomas, Ont. (res); Ott '52; Psy; Phys., Ontario Hosp., St. Thomas.; Tel. ME 1-2020.

KAUFMAN, Paul M.; 74 Stormont Ave., Toronto 12, Ont.; Tor '44; DMR; DiagRad; Staff, St. Michael's Hosp.; Clin. Instr., U. of Toronto; Tel. RU 3-1874.

KAUFMAN, Ruebin; 400 Norlyn Bldg., 309 Hargrave St., Winnipeg 2, Man.; Man '53; IntMed.; Active Staff, (IntMed.), Victoria Gen. Hosp.; Court. Staff, St. Boniface Gen. Hosp.; Tel. 943-7754.

KAUFMAN, V. S.; 11027-87th Ave., Edmonton, Alta. (res); Tor '08; Retired.

KAUFMANN, August F.; 23 Queen St., Campbellford, Ont.; 119 Oliver Rd. (res); Graz (Aust.) '50.
KAUFMANN, Mark; 4773 Sherbrooke St., Montreal, P.Q.; 771 Upper Belmont St., Westmount (res); McG '19; GenSurg; Hon. Att. Staff, Royal Victoria Hosp.; Tel. WE 5-1498; Abroad.
KAUFMANN, M. I. H.; 4773 Sherbrooke St. **W., Westmount, Montreal 6, P.Q.; 4687 Bonavista Ave. (res); McG '36; DOMS; DABOph;** FAAOO; Ophth (P.Q.); Assoc. Ophth., Jewish Gen. Hosp.; Ass't. Ophth., St. Mary's Hosp.; Cons. Ophth., Mt. Sinai San., Prefontaine; Tel. 935-1498.
KAUFMANN, Noel R.; 1055-64th Ave., Fabreville, P.Q.; Mon'61; MCGP; Ass't. Med. Dir., Hoffman Laroche Ltd.; Tel. 748-8751.

KAVANAGH, Aidan J.; 309 Med. Centre, 906-8th Ave. S., Calgary, Alta.; National U. (Ire.) '51; DABP; Paed; Dir. (Paed.), Calgary Gen. Hosp.; Tel. 266-4775.
KAVANAGH, Gerald J.; 2171 Queen St. E., Toronto 13, Ont.; Tor'63.

KAVANAGH-GRAY, Doris; 1638 W. 49th Ave., Vancouver 13, B.C.; Ott'54; FRCP(C), IntMed; Teach. Staff, St. Paul's Hosp.; Tel. MU 3-2211.

KAVANAGH, Norwood W.; 508 Medical Arts Bldg., 750 Spadina Cr., Saskatoon, Sask.; Sask'57.

KAVANAGH, Patrick J. Caledonia, Queens Co., N.S.; Dal'59; AMCGP; Tel. Caledonia 14.

KAVANAGH, Terence; 329 Bloor St. W., Toronto 5, Ont.; Manchester (Eng.) '53; DRCOG; Chief Pensions M.O., WCB (Ont.) 90 Harbour St.; Tel. PL 5-2393.

KAVECKAS, Anthony; 645 Hamilton Rd., London, Ont.; 571 Lambton St. (res); Kaunas (Lith.) '41; MCGP; Tel. 455-0480.

KAVELMAN, Douglas A.; 280 Belfield Rd., Rexdale, Ont.; Tor '56; IntMed; Vol. Ass't. Med., Toronto Gen. Hosp.; Med. Dir., Ames Co. of Canada; Tel. 677-1820.

KAWA, Krystyna M.; 92 Cedarbrae Blvd., Scarborough, Ont.; Polish Sch. Med. (Edinburgh, Scot.)'49; MB; ChB; D.ObstRCOG.

KAWA, Mieczyslaw Z.; 693 McCowan Rd., Scarborough, Ont.; Edinburgh (Scot.) '48; Otol; Att'd. Staff (Otol.), Scarborough Gen. Hosp.; Tel. 267-0263.

KAWULA, Leo; Nat. Health & Welfare, Brooke Claxton Bldg., Ottawa, Ont.; Ludwig (Germ.)'45; MPH(Calif.); FAPHA; FACOG; Obst.

KAY, Elspeth S. K. (Campbell); 2010 Bel-Air Dr., Ottawa 5, Ont.; Edinburgh (Scot.) '45; DRCOG; DCH; FAAP; Paed; Active Staff, Ottawa Gen. & Grace Hosp's.; Ass't. M.O., Public School Bd., Ottawa; Clin. Ass't. (Paed.), Ottawa U.; Tel. 729-3628.

KAY, George D.; Ste. 105, One Medical Place, 20 Wynford Dr., Don Mills, Ont.; Glasgow (Scot.)'47; FRCS(C), OrthSurg; Att'd. Staff, Scarborough Gen. & Bethesda Hosp's.; Assoc. Staff, Toronto East Gen. Hosp.; Tel. 429-1032.

KAY, Harold E.; 65 Shaughnessy Blvd., Willowdale, Ont. (res); Western Reserve (Cleveland, Ohio)'60; Court. Staff, Tor. E. Gen. & Grace Hosp's.; Tel. 447-6721.

KAY, Harold T.; 163 Laurier Ave. E., Ottawa 2, Ont.; London (Eng.)'45; FACA; Anaes; Staff, Ottawa Gen. Hosp.; Acting Hd. (Anaes.), U. of Ottawa; Tel. 235-5025.

KAY, K. K.; c/o Chief Occupational Health Div., Jackson Bldg., Ottawa, Ont.

KAY, Marvin S.; 12 Peveril Hill S., Toronto 10, Ont.; Tor '57; Tel. 781-6818.

KAY, Ronald B.; 11 Crescentwood Rd., Scarborough, Ont. (res); Tor '35; D.Psy; Psy; Staff, Ont. Hosp. Whitby; Tel. MO 8-5881.

KAY, Samuel; Mall Med. Bldg., Osborne St. & St. Mary's Blvd., Winnipeg, Man.; 834 Waterloo (res); Man '45; FRCS (Edin.), FRCS (C), GenSurg; Staff, St. Boniface Hosp.; Dem. (Surg.), U. of Manitoba; Tel. SP 4-2411.

KAYE, Christopher H.; 5798 Victoria Dr., Vancouver 16, B.C.; 1992 Trimble St., Van. 8 (res); Oxford (Eng.) '46; DRCOG; MCGP; Tel. FA 5-1288.

KAYE, Henry A.; Melita, Man.; Lav '45; Dist. Coroner.

KAYE, Michael; 7 Douglas Ave., Montreal 6, P.Q.; St. Bart's (London, Eng.) '50; MRCS; LRCP; FACP; FRCP(C); IntMed; Sr. Att'd. Staff, Montreal Gen. & Queen Mary Vet's Hosp's.; Ass't. Prof., McGill U.; Phys., Gen. Foods Ltd.: Tel. 482-7884.

KAYE, Peter P.; Castor, Alta.; Man '33.

KAYLER, Travis D.; 132 Weber St. N., Waterloo, Ont.; 100 Weber St. S. Kitchener (res); Wes '57.

KAZANDJIAN, Zareh; Beirut (Lebanon) '65; Res., Inst. de Cardiologie, 5000 est rue Belanger, Montreal 36, P.Q.

KAZDAN, Jerome J.; Tor'60; FRCS(C), Ophth; Staff, Toronto Gen. Hosp., Toronto 2, Ont.

KAZDAN, Louis; Ste. 308, 99 Avenue Rd., Toonto 5, Ont.; 406 Richview (res.); Tor '27; Ophth.; Tel. 927-1214.

KAZDAN, Martin S.; Ste. 308, 99 Avenue Rd., Toronto 5, 12A Finch Ave., Willowdale, Ont.; 33 Tollerton Ave., Willowdale (res); Tor '54; M.S. (Ophth, Minn.); DAB-Ophth; FRCS(C), Ophth; Court. Staff, North York Branson, New Mt. Sinai & Vol. Ass't., Toronto Gen. Hosp's.; Tel. 927-1214 and 221-0243.

KAZUN, Walter J.; Ste. 206, 1541 W. Broadway, Vancouver 9, B.C.; 5472 Manson St. (res); Ott '52; Tel. 738-9424.

KEALEY, Owen J.; 257 Lisgar St., Ottawa, **4, Ont.; 37 Monkland (res); Ott '55; IntMed; Active Staff, St. Vincent's Hosp.; Assoc. Staff, Ottawa Gen. Hosp.; Cons. (IntMed.), DVA; Lect. Med. U. of Ottawa; Tel. 233-1991.**

KEAN, Cecil D.; 17 Topsail Rd., St. John's, Nfld.; McG'15; M.C.G.P.; Anaes.; Staff, St. John's Gen., Grace Maternity & St. Clare's Hosp's.

KEAN, Gerald T.; 213 Lemarchand Rd., St. John's, Nfld.; National U. (Ire.)'55; ObstGyn.

KEARNEY, Derek D.; Box 508, Harbour Grace Clin., Harbour Grace, Nfld.; Dal'63; AMCGP.

KEARNEY, Garnet H.; Fort St. John, B.C.; McG '11; Dist. Coroner.

KEARNS, Hubert J.; 130 Bessborough Dr., Toronto 17, Ont. (res); McG '24; Retired.

KEARNS, Joseph A.; Kazabazua, P.Q.; Qns '30 GenSurg.

KEARNS, Joseph R.; Qns'60; FRCS(C), Otol; Staff, Henry Ford Hosp., Detroit, Mich., U.S.A.; Abroad.

KEATING, Douglas W.; 496 Parkside Dr., Bathurst, N.B. (res); Dal '49; DiagRad; Staff, Hotel-Dieu Hosp.; Tel. LI 6-4471.

KEATING, Walter J.; 2169 Gottingen St., Halifax, N.S.; **Dal '25.**

KEAY, Charles C.; 178 Riverview Blvd., St. Catharines, Ont.; Glasgow (Scot.)'53; FRCS(C), OrthSurg.

KEAYS, Claude F.; Med. Arts Bldg., 5880 Spring Garden Rd., Halifax, N.S.; 870 Greenwood Ave. (res); Dal '45; FACS; FAAOO, FICS, Ophth; Hd. Dept. (Ophth, Otol), Children's Hosp.; Ass't. Ophth, Otol., Victoria Gen. & Camp Hill DVA Hosp's; Assoc. Prof. (Ophth, Otol), Dalhousie U.; Tel. 423-8704.

KEAYS, James F.; Newcastle, N.B.; Dal '43.

KEDDIS, Erna; 311 Morton, Port Alberni, B.C.; Tartu (Estonia) '25; Tel. 723-7511.

KEDDY, David B.; Box 320, Mahone Bay, N.S.; Dal '62.

KEDDY, D. Bruce; 56 Victoria St., Lunenburg, N.S.; Dal '51; Staff, Fishermen's Mem. Hosp.; Tel. 634-8527.

KEDDY, George W.; 115 Hazen St., Saint John, N.B.; Sandy Pt. (res); Dal '35; FRCS(Ed.), FRCS(C), GenSurg; Orth. Spec. Saint John Gen. St. Joseph's Lancaster DVA & TB Hosp's.; Tel. 693-2890.

KEE, C. Graham; 126 Elm St., Wodstock, N.B. (res); **Qns '43.**

KEECH, William A.; Medical Arts Bldg., 539 Cassells St., North Bay, Ont.; 899 McLaren St. (res); Wes '50; Tel. 472-3620.

KEEGAN, David L.; Box 700, Estevan Med. Assoc., Estevan, Sask.; Sask '64.

KEELER, W. Raymond; 484 Avenue Rd., Ste. 102, Toronto 7, Ont.; Tor'44; BSc(Med.); D.Psy; Psy; Pt.-time Psy. Cons., Toronto Bd. of Education; Tel. WA 2-2921.

KEELEY, Charles D.; 274 King St. W., Chatham, Ont.; R.R. 3, Chatham (res); Wes '41; F.A.C.S., F.R.C.S.(C), GenSurg; Cons. Surg., St. Joseph Hosp.; Chief of Surg., Public Gen. Hosp.; Tel. 352-4140.

KEELING, Clifford J.; 347-9th St. E., Owen Sound, Ont.; Wes'61; IntMed.

KEELING, Patricia A.; Wes '64; Res., Kingston Gen. Hosp., Kingston, Ont.

KEEN, William H.; 3195 Granville St., Vancouver 9, B.C.; Alb'57; DiagRad; Tel. RE 1-5241.

KEENBERG, A. Alexander; 306 Boyd Bldg., 388 Portage Ave., Winnipeg 1, Man.; 310 Oxford St. (res); Man '34; M.C.G.P.; Tel. 943-2315.

KEENE, J. D.; 212 Burrows Bldg., Swift Current, Sask.; 378—2nd Ave. East (res); Man '39; Anaes; Staff, Swift Current Union Hosp.; Dist. Coroner; Tel. 773-7277.

KEENLEYSIDE, Donald W.; 574 Princess St., Kingston, Ont.; 180 Victoria (res); Qns '56 AMCGP; Clin. Ass't. Queen's University; Tel. 546-2434.

KEENLEYSIDE, Edward A.; 153 Forest Hill Rd., Toronto 7, Ont. (res); Tor'28; Bd. Life Ins. Med.; Tel. 485-7775.

KEENLEYSIDE, Hubert B.; 287 Queens Ave., London, Ont.; 104 Elworth Ave. (res); Tor '51; Anaes; Anaes. Staff, Victoria Hosp.; Instr. (Anaes), U. of Western Ont.; Tel. GE 8-5143.

KEENLEYSIDE, John G.; Sherway Dr., Etobicoke, Ont.; 1247 Cloverbrae Cres., Port Credit (res); Tor '54; DiagRad; Assoc. Radiol., Queensway Gen. Hosp.; Tel. 231-3369.

KEERI-SZANTO, Michael; 6, Russell, Montreal 16, P.Q.; Budapest (Hung.)'46; FACA; Anaes; Ass't. Prof., U. of Montreal; Tel. 733-6174.

KEET, Sylvia J.; 1667 Preston St., Halifax, N.S.; London (Eng.)'53; DCH(Eng.); DObst RCOG.

KEEVIL, Ralph F.; 15 Elwood, Chatham, Ont.; Tor '39; DiagRad, Staff, Chatham Public Gen. Hosp.; Tel EL 2-6400.

KEFFER, Glen W.; 38 Dorothy St., Welland, Ont.; Wes. '61; Tel. 734-9746.

KEIDAN, Herbert; Ste. 20, 306 Boler Rd., London, Ont.; Liverpool (Eng.)'47; DRCOG; MCGP; Tel. 471-4400.

KEIJZER, Johannes J.; 755 Brimley Rd., Scarborough, Ont.; Leiden (Neth.) '62.

KEIL, Alan M.; 2729 Lindstrom Dr. S.W., Calgary, Alta. (res); Cambridge (Eng.)'53; DA (Lond.); MRCS(Eng.); LRCP(Lond.); FFARCS; Anaes; Staff, Holy Cross & Alberta Children's Hosp's.; Tel. 266-1531.

KEIL, William; 17 Metamora Cres., London, Ont. (res); Wes '54; Psy; Staff, Victoria Hosp.; Tel. GE 2-5261.

KEILLOR, Clifford M.; Box 721, Kingsville, Ont. (res); Wes '14; Retired.

KEIR, William R.; Barrhead Clinic, Box 940, Barrhead, Alta.; Alb '44; FICS; FASAS; MCGP; Chief of Staff, St. Joseph's Hosp.; Tel. 674-2231.

KEIRSTEAD, Eric R., Sg/Lcdr; Institute Aviation Med., 1107 Avenue Rd., Toronto 12, Ont.; Qns'52.

KEITH, Douglas; 145 Wellington St., Sarnia, Ont.; Glasgow (Scot.) '47.

KEITH, John D.; 555 University Ave., Toronto, Ont.; 451 Blythewood (res); Tor '32; Paed; Phys. I/C Dept. of Card., Hosp. for Sick Children; Prof. (Paed), U. of Toronto; Tel. EM 6-7242.

KEITH, Roger G.; 300 Med. Arts Bldg., 335-339 6th. Ave. S.W., Calgary, Alta.; Alb '64; Staff, Holy Cross Hosp.; Tel. 269-2561.

KEITH, W. Elliott; 2450 Lincoln Rd., Windsor, Ont.; Tor '42; Anaes; Chief Anaes., Hotel Dieu Hosp.; Tel. 254-9393.

KEITH, Wm. S., MBE; 207 Toronto Western Med. Bldg., 25 Leonard Ave., Toronto 2B, Ont.; 55 St. Leonard's Cres. (res); Tor '27; NeurSurg; NeurSurg., Toronto Western Hosp. & Hosp. for Sick Children; Assoc. Prof. (Surg.) U. of Toronto; Tel. EM 6-3233.

KELEMEN, Andor; Allin Clinic, 10155-120th St., Edmonton, Alta.; Hung. '56; MCGP; Tel. 488-7271.

KELEN, Andrew; Ormstown Medical Centre, Ormstown, P.Q.; 17 Church St. (res); McG '43; M. Sc. (Neurol.); IntMed(P.Q.); M.C.G.P.; Chief of Staff, Barrie Mem. Hosp.; Cons., Hotel-Dieu, Valleyfield; Tel. 829-2331.

KELEN, Leslie; 2567 Bedford Rd., Montreal 26, P.Q.; Pazmany Peter U. (Budapest, Hung.) '38; FAGS; Tel. 735-1062.

KELEN, Marian (Francis); 17 Church St., Ormstown, P.Q.; McG '45.

KELLAM, Hewson I. J.; 406 Med. Arts Bldg., 180 Metcalfe St., Ottawa, Ont.; 1281 Parkhill Cir. (res); Tor '35; F.A.C.S., ABOS, FICS, FRCS(E) & (C), GenSurg; OrthSurg; Sr. OrthSurg., Ottawa Civic Hosp.; Cons. OrthSurg., DVA; Assoc. Prof. (Orth), U. of Ottawa; Tel. CE 3-1139.

KELLAM, Shirley Y.; 24 Nanwood Dr., Brampton, Ont.; Tor '62; Active Staff, Peel Mem. Hosp.; Tel. 451-8563.

KELLER, Edward S.; McG'55; Path; Staff, Dawson Mem. Hosp., Bridgewater, N.S.

KELLER, Harry W.; 184 Finch Ave. W., Willowdale, Ont.; 7 Bunty Lane (res); Tor '50; MCGP; Staff, North York Branson Hosp.; Tel. BA 5-3441.

KELLER, Jules; 4074 LaSalle Blvd., Verdun, Montreal 19, P.Q.; 421 Mount Pleasant Ave., Westmount (res); Geneva (Switz.) '39; FICS, Obst (P.Q.), D.Bact (Fr.); Assoc. Staff, Queen Elizabeth & Catherine Booth Hosp's.; Tel. 767-4930.

KELLER, Rhona J.; Apt. 201, 3500 Linton Ave., Montreal 26, P.Q.; McG'61.

KELLEY, Cecil W.; 180 Metcalfe St., Ottawa, On.; 105 Kenilworth Ave. (res); Qns '28; F.A.-C.S., F.I.C.S., GenSurg; Sr. Surg., Ottawa Civic Hosp.; Ass't. Prof. Surg., Queen's U.; Tel. CE 2-9507.

KELLEY, Edward G.; 48 Havelock St., Amherst, N.S.; Dal '53; Staff, Highland View Hosp.; Tel. 667-3680.

KELLEY, Francis J.; Med. Arts Bldg., 336 Kings Rd., Sydney, N.S.; McG'52; FACS; GenSurg.; Tel. 562-1102.

KELLEY, Hugh Edgar; 71 Commercial St., Middleton, N.S.; 58 Connaught Ave. (res); Dal '26; Sec., Med. Staff, Soldiers' Mem. Hosp.; Tel. 825-2693.

KELLINGTON, William T.; Freelton, Ont.; Qns'53; Active Staff, St. Joseph's Hosp., Hamilton; Court. Staff, Joseph Brant Hosp., Burlington; Tel. 659-3301.

KELLNER, Joseph; 105 Duke St., Ingersoll, Ont.; St. Charles St. (res); Naples (Itzly) '31; Tel. 485-0770.

KELLOCK, Marie G.; Apt. 438, 261 Goulet St., Winnipeg 6, Man.; St. Andrew's (Scot.)'59.

KELLS, George W.; 206 Richmond St., London, Ont.; Tor '11; Retired.

KELLY, Allan; 707 Charlotte St., Peterborough, Ont.; 1443 Sherwood Cres. (res); Glasgow (Scot.) '45; F.R.S.C. (Eng.), GenSurg; Surg. Staff, St. Joseph & Civic Hosp's.; Tel. RI 2-3871.

KELLY, Allison C.; 1745 Manawagonish Rd., Lancaster, N.B.; Dal'56; Anaes; Staff Anaes., St. Joseph's, Lancaster DVA, & Gen. Hosp's., Saint John; Tel. 672-2013.

KELLY, Arthur D.; 150 St. George St., Toronto, Ont.; 5 Edmund Gate (res); Tor '25; Managing Editor, C.M.A. Publications, 150 St. George St., Toronto; Tel. 924-0751.

KELLY, Beverley A.; 2917 Bloor St. W., Toronto 18, Ont.; Ott'54; Psy; Dir., Mental Health Clinic, Queensway Gen. Hosp.

KELLY, Charles B.; 76 John St., Port Hope, Ont.; Tor. '10.; Tel. 885-2113.

KELLY, Charles W.; Box 760, Fredericton, N.B.; 781 MacLaren Ave. (res); Qns '43; Admin., Public Health; Tel. 475-7711, Ext. 257.

KELLY, Colin L.; Box 280, Brandon Clinic, Brandon, Man.; London (Eng.)'57; Tel. PA 9-6441.

KELLY, Daniel; 7244-101st Ave., Edmonton, Alta.; Ire '52; MCGP; Tel. 466-0263.

KELLY, Douglas B.; Medical Centre, Charlotte St., Peterborough, Ont.; 479 Thompson Ave. (res); Tor '39; F.R.C.P.(C) IntMed.; Tel. RI 2-3871.

KELLY, Francis O.; Ste. 104, 3000 Lawrence Ave. E., Scarborough, Ont.; '54; Urol.

KELLY, Francis P.; The Leamington Clinic, 9 Talbot St. E., Leamington, Ont.; R.R. 1 (res); McG '48; GenSurg; Pres. Med. Staff, Leamington Hosp.; Tel. 326-6765.

KELLY, Gordon C.; 700 Med. Arts Bldg., Young St., Hamilton, Ont.; 167 Aberdeen Ave. (res); Tor'26; GenSurg; OrthSurg; Hon. Cons. (OrthSurg.), Hamilton Civic Hosp.; Tel. JA 9-2561.

KELLY, H. Garfield; Etherington Hall, Stuart St., Kingston, Ont.; 77 Alwington Ave. (res); Qns '40; F.A.C.P., F.R.C.P.(C), IntMed; Prof. of Med. & Continuing Educ., Queen's U.; Tel. 542-3542.

KELLY, Jerome J.; 423 Roslyn Ave., Westmount, Montreal 6, P.Q. (res); McG '31; Anaes; Assoc. Anaes., Montreal Gen. Hosp.; Dem. Anaes., McGill U.; Tel. WE 7-6011.
KELLY, John M.; 269 Lesperance Rd., Tecumseh, Ont.; Wes '45; Active Staff, ObstGyn., Metropolitan Gen. Hosp., Windsor; Tel. 969-4080.
KELLY, John W. M.; Ste. 202, 1248 St. Foy Rd., Quebec 6, P.Q.; Lav'55; FRCS(C), GenSurg; Active Med. Staff, Jeffery Hale Hosp.; Tel. 681-0529.
KELLY, J. Ross; 300 Medical Dental Bldg., 106th & 100th Ave., Edmonton, Alta.; 10518—134th St. (res); Alb '38; M.C.G.P.; Tel. 422-1704.
KELLY, Maurice J.; 284 David St., Sudbury, Ont.; Tor '30; Anaes; Staff, Sudbury Gen., Sudbury Mem. & St. Joseph's Hosp's.; Tel. 673-0788.
KELLY, Michael A.; Med. Arts Bldg., 2150 Valley Way, Niagara Falls, Ont.; Glasgow (Scot.)'58; FRCS(Glas.); Otol.
KELLY, Michael A.; 121 York St., Cornwall, Ont.; McG '27; M.C.G.P.; Staff, Hotel-Dieu & Cornwall Gen. Hosp's.
KELLY, Michael J. A.; 115 Doctor's Bldg., 995 Queen St. E., Sault Ste. Marie, Ont.; Oxford (Eng.)'55; M.A., B.M., B.Ch., MRCOG; FACOG; FRCOG; FRCS(C), ObstGyn; Cons. (ObstGyn.), Plummer Mem. Hosp. & Gen. Hosp.; Tel. AL 3-4845.
KELLY, Norman H.; 4208 Bathurst St., Downsview, Ont.; Tor '59; Tel. ME 3-9090.
KELLY, Patrick A.; National U (Dublin, Ire.) '50; M.C.G.P.; Staff, Marine Hosp., Sydney, N.S.
KELLY, Peter; 1192 Weston Rd., Toronto 15, Ont.; 7 Anglesey Blvd.., Islington (res); Sheffield (Eng.) '49; M.R.C.S., L.R.C.P.; Staff, Mem. Hosp., Weston; Tel. RO 6-7611.
KELLY, Peter F.; London (Eng.)'60; Res., Dept. of Psy., Hotel-Dieu Hosp., Kingston, Ont.
KELLY, R. Arnold; 93 King St. W., Kingston, Ont.; Qns '38; DPH; M.O.H., City of Kingston; Ass't. Prof. Public Health, Queen's U.
KELLY, Robert; Univ. Coll. (Dublin, Ire.) '63; Ass't. M.O.; Staff, Cottage Hosp., Brookfield, Nfld.; Tel. 2181.
KELLY, Robert G.; Tor'64; Res., Montreal Gen. Hosp., Montreal 25, P.Q.
KELLY, Robert G. C.; Ste. 902, 1849 Yonge St., Toronto 7, Ont.; Tor '32; Ophth; Chief of Ophth., St. Michael's Hosp.; Ass't. Prof. (Ophth.), U. of Toronto; Tel. 485-3636.
KELLY, William J.; 325 Doctor's Bldg., 955 Queen St. E., Sault Ste. Marie, Ont.; 12 Sisson Ave. (res); Ott'53; FACS, FRCS(C), GenSurg; Cons., Gen. & Plummer Mem. Hosp's.; Tel. AL 3-7352.

KELSEY, Henry A.; 403-6th St., New Westminister, B.C.; 538A Ewen Ave.; 410-3rd St. (res); London (Eng.) '38; MRCOG; ObstGyn; Tel. LA 6-8313.

KELTZ, Irwin; 5927 Yonge St., Willowdale, Ont.; Tor'59; AMCGP; Staff, North York Branson Hosp.; Court. Staff, Bethesda Hosp.; Tel. 221-5588.

KELTZ, Maurice; 572 Eglinton Ave. W., Toronto 12, Ont.; 582 St. Clements Ave. (res); Tor '57; Tel. HU 1-0661.

KEMKARAN, Samuel K.; Man'58; Res., Deer Lodge Hosp., Winnipeg 6, Man.
KEMP, Allen E.; Tor'60; Staff, Toronto Western Hosp., Toronto 2B, Ont.
KEMP, C. Robert; 23 King St. W., Stoney Creek, Ont.; 1 Wardrope Ave. S. (res); Wes '38; MCGP; Coroner, Co. of Wentworth; Treas., Ont. Chapt., College of GP; Memb. Educ. Comm., Ham. Assoc. for Retarded Children; Tel. 662-8535.
KEMP, William N.; 2414 Main St., Vancouver 10, B.C.; 4743 Belmont Ave. (res); McG '22; Anaes; Tel. TR 6-2627.
KEMPER, F. Dean; Imperial Oil Ltd., Don Mills at Eglinton, Don Mills, Ont.; 40 Almond Ave., Willowdale (res); McG '47; AACP; IntMed; Vol. Ass't. Phys. (OPD), Tor. Gen. Hosp.; Regional Phys., Imperiol Oil Co.; Tel. 429-2000, Loc. 410.

KEMPFF, Johan G.; Groningen (Neth.) '50; DiagRad; Head, X-Ray Dept., Peterborough Civic Hosp., Peterborough, Ont.; Tel. 743-2121, Ext. 243.
KEMPTON, A. Russell; Box 458, Leduc, Alta.; Dal '52; M.C.G.P.; Staff, Misericordia & Court. Staff, Royal Alexandra Hosp's., Edmonton; Tel. 446-2212.
KENDALL, Alan G.; Ste. 81, 3465 Cote des Neiges Rd., Montreal 25, P.Q.; McG '54; M.A. (Oxon.); FACP; FRCP(C), IntMed; Haem(P.Q.); Ass't. Phys., Royal Victoria Hosp.; Lect. (Med.), McGill U.; Tel. WE 5-3535.
KENDALL, David; 5880 Spring Garden Rd., Halifax, N.S.; Oxford (Eng.)'36.
KENDALL, John M.; 672 Brant Arts Bldg., Brant St., Burlington, Ont.; Durham (Eng.) '57; MRCP (Lond.); FRCP(C), IntMed; Tel. 637-3500.
KENDALL, W. Thomas; 1286 Wellington St., Ottawa, Ont.; Qns '41; Dist. Coroner.
KENDRICK, G. Bryce; 206 Riverside Dr., Toronto 3, Ont.; Qns '11; M.R.C.S., L.R.C.P., E.E.N. & T (Poly Clinic, Chicago), OphthOtol; Coroner, Essex County.
KENDRICK, William W.; 310-1070 Douglas St., Victoria, B.C.; 2002 Ferndale Ave. (res); Tor '49; FRCS(C), Urol.; Tel. 383-8911.
KENMUIR-EVANS, Anthony; 407 Rideau Med. Centre, 1711 - 4th. St. S.W., Calgary, Alta.; Cambridge (Eng.) '53; Tel. 266-7496.
KENNARD, Antony B.; 340 The Westway, Weston, Ont. (res); London (Eng.) '53; Staff, Workmen's Comp. Bd., 115 Torbarrie Rd., Downsview; Tel. 244-1761, Loc. 309.
KENNEDY, Alexander; Georgetown, P.E.I.; McG '19.
KENNEDY, Alexander J.; Qns'61; Res., Toronto East Gen. Hosp., Toronto 13, Ont.
KENNEDY, Arthur M.; Deer Lake Clinic, Nfld.; National U. (Cork, Ire.) '54; Tel. NE 5-2358.
KENNEDY, Bernard J.; 45 Queen's Rd., St. John's, Nfld.; UK '39.; Capt., R.C.A.(Militia).
KENNEDY, Cormac; Imperial, Sask.; National U. (Ireland) '57.
KENNEDY, Douglas W.; 420 N. East St., Sarnia, Ont.; Tor '56; Paed; Staff, Sarnia Gen. & St. Joseph's Hosp's.; Tel. 336-6562.
KENNEDY, Edmund J.; 402 Boyd Bldg., 388 Portage Ave., Winnipeg 1, Man.; Prague (Czechoslovakia) '39.
KENNEDY, Garfield G.; 5010-106th Ave., Edmonton, Alta.; Alb '49; GenSurg; Tel. HO 6-9063.
KENNEDY, George E.; Carbonear, Nfld.; McG '45.
KENNEDY, Henry K.; 828 W. 10th Ave., Vancouver, B.C.; Man '49; DPH; PH; Dir., Div. of Venereal Dis. Control; Tel. TR 4-2321.
KENNEDY, Irving F.; Cumberland, Ont.; Tor '50; MCGP; Staff, St.-Louis-Marie-de-Montfort, Ottawa Civic & Grace Hosp's., Ottawa; Tel. 762-4720.
KENNEDY-JACKSON, Irlma; Box 240, Station D., Hamilton, Ont.; Tor'19; DABPN; D.Psy; Psy; Court. Staff, Hamilton Gen. Hosp., St. Joseph's, Chedoke Gen. & Children's Hosp's.; Tel. 389-3229.
KENNEDY, James C.; 144 Church St., Weston, Ont. (res); Tor '61; Research Fell., Ntl. Cancer Inst. of Canada.
KENNEDY, J. C.; 212 Med. Dental Bldg., 450 Central Ave., London, Ont.; 191 Cheapside St. (res); Wes '42; FRCS(C), GenSurg; OrthSurg; Staff, Victoria & Westminster D.V.A. Hosp's.; Ass't. Prof. (Surg.), U. of Western Ont.; Tel. GE 9-5551.
KENNEDY, James E.; 4765 St. Catherine E., Montreal, P.Q.; 1637 Aird Ave. (res); Lav '42; Staff, St. Mary's & Royal Edward Laurentian Hosp's.; Cons. Phys., Union Carbide Ltd.; Tel. CL 5-7510.
KENNEDY, John S.; Ste. 202, 625-5th Ave., New Westminster, B.C.; 6925 Granville St., Vancouver 14 (res); Wes'49; FRCS(C), Urol; Tel. 526-0011.
KENNEDY, Margaret (See Campbell)
KENNEDY, Ralph D.; 245 Queen St., Charlottetown, P.E.I.; Dal'64; Tel. 892-2932.
KENNEDY, Raymond J.; 9123-143rd St., Parkview, Edmonton, Alta.; London (Eng.)'52; P.G., Dept. of Anaes., University Hosp.

KENNEDY, Richard; 15 Le Marchant Rd., St. John's, Nfld.; McG '51; F.R.C.S.(C), GenSurg.; Tel. 579-4808.
KENNEDY, Richard J.; Qns '63; Res., Montreal Gen. Hosp., Montreal, P.Q.
KENNEDY, Roger A.; Dept. of Health, 495 Richmond Rd., Ottawa 13, Ont.; Cambridge (Eng.) '28; DPH; MRCS; M.O.H., City of Ottawa; Tel. 725-1171.
KENNEDY, Ruth L. (Clements); Ste. 202, 625-5th Ave., New Westminster, B.C.; Wes'49; Psy; Cons., St. Mary's Hosp. & Surrey Mem. Hosp., Surrey; Teach. Staff, Student Nurses, Royal Columbian Hosp.; Tel. LA 6-0011.
KENNEDY, Sylvia; 324 Prince Edward Dr., Toronto 18, Ont.; Tor '61; Staff, St. Joseph's & Our Lady of Mercy Hosp's.; Tel. BE 9-4644.
KENNEDY, Walter W.; 422 Birks Bldg., 718 Granville, Vancouver, B.C.; 206 W. 35th (res); Qns '13; Tel. MU 1-1617.
KENNEDY, W. Roland; Ste. 320, 1538 Sherbrooke St. W., Montreal 25, P.Q.; 3456 Harvard Ave., Mtl. 28 (res); McG '25; IntMed; Hon. Att'd. Phys., Mtl. Gen. Hosp.; Tel. WE 5-3201.
KENNER, H. B.; 117 Waterloo S., Stratford, **Ont.; 325 St. David St. (res); Qns '20; F.A.C.S., GenSurg; Surg.; Chief of Staff, Stratford Gen. Hosp.; Tel. 271-2120.**
KENNEY, Athol S.; 14 Kippewa Dr., Ottawa 1, Ont. (res); Qns '33; Paed; Anaes; Sr. Paed., Ottawa Civic Hosp.; Paed., Grace Hosp.; Cons. Paed., Royal Ottawa San.; Ass't. Prof. (Clin. Paed.) U. of Ottawa; Retired.
KENNEY, Francis W.; Rexton, N.B.; Dal '41.
KENNEY, William G. C.; 43A Mill St. E., Acton, Ont.; Tor. '26. Retired.
KENNING, Ian S.; Ste. 312, 1175 Cook St., **Victoria, B.C.; McG '49; D.Psy.; Psy; Instructor, Dept. of Psy., Univ. of B.C.; Tel. CA 4-1111.**
KENNING, Stuart G.; 645 Fort St., Victoria, B.C.; 806 Dereen Place (res); McG '21; IntMed; Chief of Med., Victoria Veteran's Hosp.; Cons. Staff, St. Joseph's Hosp.; Tel. EV 4-7106.
KENNING, Stuart P.; 645 Fort St., Victoria, B.C.; 2642 Dalhousie St. (res); McG '56; FRCP (C), IntMed; Chest Cons., DVA Hosp.; Tel. 384-7106.
KENNY, George E.; Hantsport, N.S.; Dal '53; MCGP; Tel. 684-3325.
KENNY, John G.; National U. (Ire.) '48; Res., Mtl. Gen. Hosp., Montreal, P.Q.
KENNY, Kevin J.; Broadview, Sask.; National U. (Galway, Ire.) '56; M.B., B.Ch., BAO; Staff, St. Michael's Hosp.; Tel. 696-2255.
KENNY, Michael M.; 306 Medical-Dental Bldg., Ross St. & 11th Ave., Regina, Sask.; Nat. U. (Ire.) '44; DiagRad; Tel. 523-7653.
KENNY, Patricia I.; Qns'60; D.Psy; Res., Ont. Hosp., Toronto, Ont.
KENNY, Patrick, N. J.; 1492 W. 45th St., Vancouver, B.C. (res); Wes'43; Anaes; Staff, Dept. of Anaes., St. Paul's Hosp.; Tel. MU 3-2311.
KENNY, Randal Y.; 163 King St., Peterborough, Ont.; 319 Pearl Ave. (res); Tor '07; L.R.C.P. (Lond.), M.R.C.S. (Eng.); OphthOtol; Retired.
KENSHOLE, Anne B.; London (Eng.)'61; DRCOG; MRCS; LRCP; Res., Women's College Hosp., Toronto 5, Ont.
KENT, Elspeth M.; 74 Westgate, Winnipeg 1, Man.; Man '48.
KENT, Eric T.; Westwood Clinic, 3220 Portage **Ave., Winnipeg 22, Man.; Durham (Eng.) '55;** Tel. VE 2-6881.
KENT, Geraldine (Hall); 475 Gordon Pl., West Vancouver, B.C.; UBC '55; Anaes; Tel. 922-8271.
KENT, Heino A.; Dental-Med. Bldg., 59 N. Court St., Port Arthur, Ont.; Tartu (Estonia)'40; MCGP.
KENT, Henry Peter; 18 Rutta Cr., Saskatoon, Sask. (res); Cambridge (Eng.) '42; DMRD; DiagRad; Prof. & Head, Dept. of DiagRad, University Hosp. and U. of Saskatchewan; Tel. CH 2-7641, Ext. 427.
KENT, Ian; 1203 Med-Dental Bldg., 925 W. Georgia St., Vancouver 1, B.C.; London (Eng.)'49; MRCS; LRCP; Psy.
KENT, Lois E., see **TWEEDLE, Lois E. (Kent).**
KENT, Trevor; Bank of Commerce Bldg., 1 Saskatchewan Ave., Portage La Prairie, Man; Durham (Eng.) '55.
KENT, Wallace R.; 43 Floradale Dr., Cooksville, Ont.; Wes '53; GenSurg; Cons. Staff, South Peel Hosp.; Tel. 277-8923.
KENYON, Anthony; Box 594, Fort Nelson Med. Clinic, Fort Nelson, B.C.; Cambridge (Eng.)'58; FRCS(Ed.); LRCP; MRCS; Tel. 774-2355.
KEOGH, John H.; Westminster Med. Bldg., 625-5th Ave., New Westminster, B.C.; McG'48; ABDR; DiagRad; Staff, Surrey Mem. Hosp.; Tel. 522-6818.
KEOGH, Richard K.; 105 Northgate Bldg., 10049 Jasper Ave., Edmonton, **Alta.; 9007-141st St.,** (res); McG'56; DABR; DiagRad; Alternate Chief, Dept. of Rad., Royal Alexandra Hosp.; Tel. 429-2508.
KEOHANE, John T. F.; 703 Professional Bldg., 10830 Jasper Ave., Edmonton, Alta.; Dublin (Ire.) '51; M.Ch. (ROL); DLO (Eng.); Otol; Att'd, Staff, Royal Alexandra Hosp.; Tel. 422-0191, 439-2126.
KEON, Harold C.; Chapeau, P.Q.; Ott'52; District Coroner; Tel. 689-2565.
KEON, Thomas P.; 619 Brock St. S., Whitby, Ont.; Ott'65.
KEON, Wilbert J.; Ott'61; FRCS(C), GenSurg; Staff, Toronto Gen. Hosp., Toronto 2, Ont.
KEPKAY, Paul H., 2184 W. Broadway, Vancouver 9, B.C.; 1371 Oakwood, North Vancouver (res); Wes '47; IntMed; Tel. RE 1-3171.
KERBEL, Gordon A.; 1849 Yonge St., Ste. 512, Toronto 7, Ont.; Tor '59; FRCP(C), Derm; Clin. Teach., U. of Toronto; Tel. HU 7-3453.
KERBEL, Norman C.; 2221 Keele St., Toronto 15, Ont.; Tor '51; FRCP(C), IntMed; Staff, O.P.D. (Endocrin.), Toronto Western Hosp.; Att'd. Phys., Northwestern Gen. Hosp.; Tel. CH 7-1122.
KERBEL, Norman J.; Ste. 210, 305 Finch Ave. W., Willowdale, Ont.; Apt. 1, 2 Meadowbrook Ave. (res); Tor '59; AMCGP; Tel. BA 1-5544.
KERENYI, Albert B.; 475 Ellendale Med. Bldg., 5845 Cote-des-Neiges Rd., Montreal 26, P.Q.; Apt. 16, 3201 Forest Hill, Mtl. 26 (res); Munich (Germ.) '50; Psy; Staff, Jewish Gen. Hosp.; Tel. 733-7001.
KERENYI, Norbert A.; 5800 University Ave., Halifax, N.S.; Med. U. (Budapest, Hung.) '52; M.C. (Path.); Path; Dir., Div. of Anatomical Path., Pathology Inst.; Assoc. Prof. (Path.), Dalhousie U.; Tel. 422-9661.
KERESTECI, Ara G.; 408 Med. Dental Bldg., 1849 Yonge St., Toronto 7, Ont.; Istanbul (Turk.)'54; B.Sc.(Med.); FRCS(C), Urol; Surg. (Urol.), Wellesley Hosp.; Cons. Urol., Princess Margaret Hosp.; Research Fell., Ontario Cancer Fdn.; Clin. Instr. (Surg.), U. of Toronto; Tel. 487-1243.
KERESZTES, Sylvia (Gruenwald); 202 Queen St. S., Kitchener, Ont.; 261 Belmont Ave. W. (res); Utrecht (Neth.) '53; MCGP; Active Staff, Kitchener-Waterloo & St. Mary's Hosp's.; Tel. SH 5-5914.
KERESZTURI, Joseph; 215 Greyhound Bldg., 622-1st St. S.W., Calgary, Alta.; Cluj (Roumania)'48; DiagRad.
KERFOOT, David A.; Pincher Creek, Alta.; St. Andrew's (Scot.) '55; MRCP (Edin.).
KERFOOT, H. Wilfred; 26 Maple Ave. N., Smiths Falls, Ont.; McG '06; L.R.C.P., M.R.C.S.; M.O.H., Town of Smith Falls; Retired.
KERGIN, Alan J.; Ste. 703, 625-5th Ave., New Westminster, B.C.; Ste. 3, 13665-96th Ave., N. Surrey; Tor '46; DABS; FACS; FRCS(C), GenSurg; Active Staff, Royal Columbian & St. Mary's Hosp's.; Active Staff, Surrey Mem. Hosp., N. Surrey; Cons. Staff, Maple Ridge & Chilliwack Gen. Hosp's.; Tel. 521-2025 & 581-3232.
KERGIN, Frederick G.; Sunnybrook Hosp., 2075 Bayview Ave., Toronto 12, Ont.; Tor'30; MS (Tor.); MA (Oxon.); FACS; FRCS (Eng.); FRCS(C), GenSurg; Assoc. Dean & Prof. of Surg., U. of Toronto; Trustee, R. Samuel McLaughlin Fdn., 174 St. George St.; Tel. 921-6966 & 485-8651.

KERGIN, William S.; 153—3rd Ave. W., Prince Rupert, B.C.; Tor '30; F.I.C.S., GenSurg.; Tel. 3331.

KERI, Jolan; Raxlen Clin., 500 Parliament St., **Toronto 5, Ont.; Sask '59; Tel. WA 5-4381.**

KERINS, Timothy A.; Med. Centre, Corner Brook, Nfld.; Nat. U. (Ire.) '62.

KERNAHAN, Desmond A.; Manitoba Clinic, 790 Sherbrook St., Winnipeg 2, Man.; 232 Oak St., Wpg. 9 (res); Otago New Zealand) '46; FRCS (Edin.); FRCS(C), PlasSurg; Hd. PlasSurg., Children's Hosp.; Cons. PlasSurg., Man. Rehab. Hosp.; Assoc. Prof. & Hd., Dept. of PlasSurg., (Surg.), U. of Manitoba; Tel. SP 4-6541.

KERNER, Ilona; Apt. 603, 3665 Ridgewood, Montreal 26, P.Q.; Budapest (Hung.) '48; Path; Pathol., Medico-Legal Inst. of Mtl.; Pt-time Lect. McGill U.; Tel. 873-3300.

KERNOHAN, David; Box 326, Parrsboro, N.S.; Queens, Belfast (N. Ire.) '46.; Tel. 181-X2.

KERNOHAN, Henry R.; Box 100, Lashburn, Sask.; Queen's U. (Belfast, N. Ire.) '54; MCGP. Staff, Lashburn Hosp.; Tel. 58.

KEROACK, Real; 207 Richelieu, St. Jean, P.Q.; 190 Latour (res); Mon '49; Staff (Med.), St. Jean Hosp.; M.O., Singer Manufacturing Co.

KERPEL, Martha; 9017-16th Ave., North Battleford, Sask.; Budapest (Hung.)'52; Radiol., Union Hosp., North Battleford; Tel. 445-2411.

KERR, Archibald L.; 6 Maple N., Smiths Falls, Ont.; **McG'49.**

KERR, Ashton L., Col.; McG'40; Dir., Med. Plans & Requirements, Cdn. Forces HDQS, D. Med. P.R., Ottawa 4, Ont.; Tel. 992-2401.

KERR, Douglas L.; 321 Med. Arts Bldg., 404-406 Graham Ave., Winnipeg 1, Man.; 177 Brock St. (res); McG '43; Paed; Att'd. Staff, Wpg. Children's Hosp.; Instr. (Paed), U. of Manitoba; Tel. WH. 2-0949.

KERR, Hugh T.; 218 Jane St., Toronto, Ont.; Tor '24; Phys., Aluminum Goods Ltd., Toronto; Can. General Electric Co. Ltd.; **Alcoholism Research Fndn.;** Tel. RO 7-3381.

KERR, James H.; Anaes. Assoc., 178 St. George St., Toronto 5, Ont.; Cambridge (Eng.)'52; MA; DA; LMSSA (Lond.) Eng.; FRCP(C) Anaes; Sr. Anaes., Tor. Gen. Hosp.; Clin. Instr. (Anaes.), U. of Toronto; Tel. WA 3-1154.

KERR, J. Ian; Ste. 21, 31 Yonge St. N., Richmond Hill, Ont.; Tor '55; FRCS(C), GenSurg; Chief of Surg., York Central Hosp.; Tel. 884-5034.

KERR, John R.; Annapolis Royal, N.S.; Dal '42; Surg. Cons., H.M.C.S. Cornwallis.

KERR, John W.; 574 Princess St., Kingston, Ont.; 119 Queen's Cres. (res); Qns '53; FACS; FRCS(C), GenSurg; Att'd. Staff, Kingston Gen. Hosp.; Lect. (Surg.), Queen's U.; Tel. Area 613; 546-2511.

KERR, Norman D.; 31 Centre St., Brampton, Ont.; Tor'58; FRCS(C), ObstGyn; Tel. 451-4411.

KERR, Norman W.; Elgin, Ont.; Qns '32; Dist. Coroner.

KERR, Robert B., O.B.E.; 1549 Western Cres., Vancouver, B.C. (res); Tor '33; F.R.C.P. (Lond.), **F.A.C.P., F.R.C.P.(C), IntMed; Prof. & Head, Dept. of Med., U. of British Columbia; Head,** Dept. of Med., Vancouver Gen. Hosp.; Cons., DVA Shaughnessy Hosp.; Tel. TR 6-3211, Loc. 2541.

KERR, William H.; Ste. 1103, 123 Edward St., Toronto 2, Ont.; Tor'56; FRCS(C), GenSurg; Staff, Toronto Gen. Hosp.; Tel. EM 6-8211.

KERR, William K.; 516 Medical Arts Bldg., 170 St. George St., Toronto, Ont.; 134 Inglewood Dr. (res); Tor'40; FRCS(C); Urol; Surg., Toronto Gen. Hosp.; Cons. Urol., Toronto Hosp. for T.B.; Sr. Cons. (Cancer of the G.U. Tract), Ontario Cancer Inst.; Cons., Women's College Hosp.; **Cons. Urol., R.C.A.F.; Assoc. (Dept. of Surg.),** U. of Toronto.; WA 2-5555.

KERRIDGE, John H.; 1740 Davie St., Vancouver 5, B.C.; London (Eng.)'54; IntMed; Staff, Shaughnessy Hosp., & Pt.-time Staff, B.C. Hydro & Power Authority; Assoc. Staff, St. Paul's Hosp.; Tel. 681-3619.

KERRIGAN, Aiden J.; National U. (Ire.) '49; Staff. West Coast San., Corner Brook, Nfld.

KERRIN, Hugh F.; 5300 Cote-des-Neiges Rd., Montreal 26, P.Q.; Mon '53; IntMed; Staff Phys., Health Serv., St. Mary's Hosp.; Tel. RE 7-9091.

KERSHAW, Thomas G.; Box 190, Esterhazy, Sask.; Sheffield (Eng.)'53; Tel. 745-3971.

KERSTER, George G.; Med. Arts Clinic, 2125-11th Ave.. Regina, Sask.; 29 Culliton Cr. (res); Man '41; MRCOG; ObstGyn; Tel. 523-0691.

KERTESZ, Andrew; Qns'60; FRCP(C), IntMed; Neur; Staff, Hosp. for Sick Children, Toronto 2, Ont.; Abroad.

KERWIN, Alfred J.; Ste. 210, Toronto Western Med. Bldg., 25 Leonard Ave., Toronto 2B, Ont.; 21 Dale Ave. (res); Tor '33; MRCP(Lond.) FRCP **(C); IntMed(Cardiol.); Att'd. Phys., Toronto Western Hosp.; Assoc. Prof. (Med.), U. of Toronto; Tel. EM 3-2565.**

KERWOOD, Lionel A.; Dublin (Ire.) '45; DPM; Psy; Staff, Verdun Protestant Hosp., Montreal 19, P.Q.; Tel. 766-8511.

KESSLER, Jacques I.; Jewish Gen. Hosp., 3755 St. Catherine Rd., Montreal 26, P.Q.; Jerusalem (Israel)'55; Gastroent. (P.Q.); **FRCP(C), IntMed;** Dir Lab. for Metabolic Research; **Tel. 735-3771.**

KESTER, Harold A.; 6476 Granville St., Vancouver 13, B.C.; Wes'40; Anaes; Staff (Anaes), **Vancouver Gen. Hosp.; Clin. Instr. (Anaes), U. of British Columbia.; Tel. TR 6-3211.**

KESTER, Norman M.; 242 Kenaston Blvd., Winnipeg 9, Man.; Tor'51.

KETCHESON, Ross B.; 203 Medical Arts Bldg., 335-339, 6th Ave. S.W., Calgary, Alta.; Man '46; ObstGyn; Tel. 262-9326.

KETCHUM, Jesse; 2483 Chilver Rd., Windsor, Ont.; Tor '43; F.A.C.O.G., ObstGyn; Court. Staff, ObstGyn Wm. Beaumont Hosp., Woman's Hosp., Receiving Hosp., Detroit; Ass't. Instr., Gyn. Wayne U.

KETCHUM, Katherine D.; 181 Rosedale Heights Dr., Toronto 7, Ont. (res); McG'31; Clin. Ass't., **Women's College Hosp.; Tel. WA 3-7381.**

KETENE, Vahdettin; Istanbul (Turk.)'52; Staff, Camp Hill Hosp., Halifax, N.S.

KETTLE, William W.; 194 Hugel Ave., Midland, Ont.; Qns '61.

KETTLES, John S.; 160 Balmoral Ave., Toronto 7, Ont. (res); McG'43; Sr. Cons., Hospital Programmes, Ontario Hosp. Services Commission, 2195 Yonge St., Toronto 7; Tel. 487-1711.

KETTLEWELL, John W.; 1190 King St. W., Toronto 3, Ont.; Tor'39.

KETTNER, Joseph; Mall Med. Group, 280 Memorial Blvd., Winnipeg 1, Man., 434 Forrest Ave. (res); Man '53; MCGP; Tel. SP. 4-2411.

KETTYLS, G. Donald; Provincial Labs., 828 W. 10th Ave., Vancouver 9, B.C.; Alb '52; B.Sc. (Med); DPH; PH; Dip. Bact; Virol., Div. of Labs., B.C. Health Branch; Staff, Vancouver Gen. Hosp.; Clin. Instr. (PrevMed.), U. of British Columbia.

KEY, James A.; 628 Med. Arts Bldg., 170 St. George St., Toronto 5, Ont.; 534 Blythwood Rd., Tor. 12 (res); Edinburgh (Scot.) '39; FRCS (Eng.); GenSurg; Assoc. Surg., Toronto Gen. Hosp.; Sr. CardioVasc Surg., Sunnybrook Hosp.; Cons. Surg., Women's College & Tor. E. Gen. Hosp's.; Ass't. Prof. (Surg.), U. of Toronto; Tel. WA 2-9843.

KEYES, Sean A.; 131 Main St., Lancaster, N.B.; Dal '60; AMCGP.

KEYL, Anne; Ste. 614, 86 Bloor St. W., Toronto 5, Ont.; Tor'37; Dir., Special Clinic, Women's College Hosp.; **Tel. WA 2-8855.**

KEYS, David N.; 2202-3rd St. N.E., Calgary, Alta.; 4540 Chapel Rd. N.W. (res); Durham (Eng.) '34; DPH; M.O.H., Mountview Health Unit.

KEYS, James H.; Box 210, Boyle, Alta.; Dublin (Ire.) '46; L.R.C.P.(I), L.R.C.S.(I).

KHAIRAT, Omar; 911 W-64th Ave., Vancouver, B.C.; Cairo (Egypt)'33; PhD; DTM&H (Lond.); FRPS.

KHAKEE, Abdulaziz G.; 301 Montreal Ave., Lancaster, N.B.; Bombay (India) '54; Staff, Lancaster Prov. Hosp.

KHALIFA, A. Momin; Bay Med. Group, Glace Bay, N.S.; Punjab (Pakistan)'58.

KHALIL, Elhamy F.; 2315-7th St. E., Ste. 9, Saskatoon, Sask.; Cairo (Egypt); Paed.
KHALIQ, Abdul; Karachi (Pakistan)'59; IntMed; Staff, Royal Alexander Hosp., Edmonton, Alta.; Abroad.
KHAN, Abdullah Y.; Ste. 108, 688 Coxwell Ave., Toronto 13, Ont.; McG'64; Tel. 465-1230.
KHAN, Airudin S.; Man'65; Res., St. Boniface Hosp., Winnipeg 6, Man.
KHAN, Anthony C.; 1691 Tecumseh Rd. W., Windsor, Ont.; Ott '62.
KHAN, Durr-i-Kamil; Punjab (India) '55; Derm; Staff, Toronto General Hospital, Toronto 2, Ont.
KHAN, Feroze; Winkler Clinic, Winkler, Man.; Man'63; Staff, Bethel Hosp.; Tel. 325-8934.
KHAN, Habib U.; 720 McDermit Ave., Winnipeg 3, Man.; West Pakistan'52; Paed.
KHAN, Imran; McG'61; Anaes; Staff, Royal Victoria Hosp., Montreal 2, P.Q.
KHAN, Mohamed I.; Sask '63; Res., University Hosp., Saskatoon, Sask.
KHAN, Naeem A.; Osmania (India)'60; Staff, Ontario Hosp., Whitby, Ont.
KHAN, Nazir A.; Strathclair, Man.; Man '62.
KHAN, Otto; Tor '61; Res., St. Michael's Hosp., Toronto 2, Ont.
KHANNA, Ranbir 50 Queen St. E., Brampton, Ont.; Bombay (India)'49; FRCS (Edin.); GenSurg; Active Staff, Peel Mem. Hosp.; Tel. 459-4121.
KHARE, Umesh; 215 Professional Centre, 1705-3rd Ave., Prince George, B.C.; Lucknow (India) '60.
KHAZEN, Roch S.; Maternal & Child Health, Dept. of Health, Fredericton, N.B.; Beirut (Lebanon)'57; MPH; Paed. Maternal & Child Health Div.
KHERA, Shamsher, A.K.; Punjab (India) '56; FRCP(C), Paed; Staff, Royal Victoria Hosp., Montreal, P.Q.; Tel. 842-1251.
KHOBREH, Mohamed; 3777 St. Urbain St., Montreal, P.Q.; Switzerland '57; GenSurg; Tel. 849-8917.
KHODADADEH, Manuchehr; Box 640, Steinbach, Man.; Tehran (Iran) 54.
KHOO, EE C.; 11044-132nd St., Edmonton, Alta. (res); Indiana (USA) '55; IntMed; Staff, Cancer Clin., Dept. of Health, Edmonton. Abroad.
KHOO, Priscilla S. H.; (See Suffel).
KHOSLA, Santosh V.; 107-1st Ave. W., Kindersley, Sask.; Edinburgh (Scot.)'53; Tel. 463-2532.
KIDD, Andre; Lav'62; Res., Hop. St. Michel Archange, Quebec 5, P.Q.
KIDD, B. S. Langford; 555 University Ave., Toronto 2, Ont.; 511, 23 Underhill Dr., Don Mills (res); Queen's (N. Ire.) '54; M.B., B.Ch., BAO, M.D., MRCP(E); Clin. Cardiovas. Physiologist., Hosp. for Sick Children; Tel. EM 6-7242.
KIDD, Derek J. S/G CDR; DSC, CD, RCN; Inst. of Aviation Med., 1107 Avenue Rd., Toronto 12, Ont.; London (Eng.) '52; M.B., B.S., MRCS; LRCP; Officer-in-Charge, Royal Canadian Navy Personnel Research Unit; Tel. 633-4240.
KIDD, Edward G.; 202 Med. Arts Bldg., 11010 Jasper Ave., Edmonton, Alta.; Alb '45; IntMed; Staff, University Hosp.; Clin. Instr. (Med.), U. of Alberta; Med. Dir., Cdn. Arthritis & Rheum. Soc., Edmonton Div.; Tel. GE 9-5911.
KIDD, Honor M.; 4874 Fannin Ave. Vancouver 8, B.C. (res); McG'47; Hon. Att'd. Staff, B.C. Cancer Inst., Research Assoc. (Med.) & Hon. Lect., History of Med. & Sc., U. of British Columbia; Tel. TR 4-9321.
KIDD, J. A.; Foster St., Perth, Ont.; Qns '35; M.C.G.P.
KIDD, Langford; 555 University Ave., Toronto 2 Ont; Queen's U. (Belfast, N. Ire.) '54; Cardiovas. Physiol. Research Inst., Hosp. for Sick Children; Clin. Instr., U. of Toronto; Tel. EM 6-7242.
KIDD, Richard L.; Qns'63; Jr. Int., Montreal Gen. Hosp., Montreal, P.Q.; Abroad.
KIDD, Thomas W.; 15 Maple Ave., Brantford, Ont.; London (Eng.) '51; L.R.C.P. (Lond.), M.R.C.S.(Eng.), D.Obst R.C.O.G.; Tel. PL 3-4151.
KIEFER, Heinz G. R.; 330 King St., Midland, Ont.: Hamburg (Germ.) '53; Tel. 526-5641.
KIELMANN, Arnfried A.; McG'65; Jr. Int., Hop. Hotel-Dieu, Montreal 18, P.Q.
KIERLUK, Edward W.; 140 Wellington St., St. Thomas, Ont.; Wes '43; GenSurg; Staff, Memb. & Surg. Cons., St. Thomas-Elgin Gen. Hosp.; Tel. 631-9465.
KIERNAN, Anald S.; (Mooradian); 51 Cordova St., Winnipeg 9, Man. (res); Man '42; Retired.
KIERNAN, Matthew K.; 25 Medical Arts Bldg., Winnipeg, Man.; Man '42; D.A.B.R. (Roent), F.A.C.R.; D&TRad; Ass't. Rad., Winnipeg Gen. & Children's Hosp's. Ass't. Prof. (Rad.), U. of Manitoba; Tel. WH 2-6453.
KIFF, Raymond D.; Med. Arts Bldg., 17 Dunedin St., Orillia, Ont.; Wes '61; Ophth; Active Staff, Soldiers Mem. Hosp.; Tel. 325-1982.
KIHM, Ruth S.; McG '59; Res., Rehab. Inst., Montreal 26, P.Q.
KIKINDAY, Ladislaus; York Hotel, 13th St. N., Lethbridge, Alta.; Hungary '21.; Tel. 327-7070.
KILBANE, Michael; St. George's, Nfld.; U. Galway (Ire.) '51.
KILBORN, Jean E.; Park Terrace, Apt. 113, 125 Raymond St., Guelph, Ont.; Wes '31; Anaes; Retired.
KILBORN, Leslie G.; Park Terrace Apt. 113, 125 Raymond St., Guelph, Ont.; Tor '21; MA; Ph.D. Physiol; Retired.
KILBORN, Robert M.; 305 King St. W., Ste. 1101, Kitchener, Ont.; 174 Lydia St. (res); Tor '50; Anaes; Tel. 744-6511.
KILBY, Thomas H.; Box 160, Flin Flon, Man.; Man'38; Tel. 687-7571.
KILDUFF, Christopher J.; 602 Med. Arts Bldg., Spadina Cr., Saskatoon, Sask.; Nat. U. (Dublin, Ire.) '49; FACA; Anaes; Chief Anaes., Saskatoon City Hosp.; Ass't. Prof. (Anaes.), U. of Saskatchewan; Tel. 434-1930.
KILGOUR, Charles S.; Victoria Medical Bldg., 215 Victoria St., Toronto 1, Ont.; 108 Glen Rd., Toronto 5 (res); Tor '43; PlasSurg; Cons, Northwestern Hosp. & Branston Hosp., Willowdale; Tel. 364-5325.
KILGOUR, John A.; 180 Wellington St., Ottawa 4, Ont.; 33 Lyall St., Ott. 5 (res); Tor '49; IntMed; Assoc. Med. Dir., Metropolitan Life Ins. Co.; Court. Staff, Med. Clin., Ottawa Civic Hosp.; Tel. 232-2631.
KILGOUR, John M.; Wpg. Clinic, Winnipeg, Man.; 275 Harvard Ave. (res); Man '36; MRCP (Lond.), FACP, FRCP(C), IntMed; Phys., Wpg. Clinic; Assoc. Prof. (Med), U. of Manitoba; Tel. WH 2-6441.
KILLETT, J. R.; 4824 Fraser St., Vancouver, B.C.; Staff, Dept. Nat. Health & Welfare, Vancouver.
KILLIKELLY, Eva T.; Ireland '49; Part-Time M.O., Immigration Medical Services, Toronto International Airport, Malton Ont.
KILLIKELLY, Harry; 8 Hillavon Dr., Islington, Ont. (res); Dublin (Ire.) '49; Staff, Dept. of Immigration, Malton Airport; Tel. 233-0373.
KILLINGBECK, Robert N.; 7th St., Matheson, Ont.; Qns '43; FICS.
KILLINGER, Donald W.; Wes'57; Res., Wellesley Hosp., Toronto 5, Ont.
KILLOH, J. Allan; Ste. 311, 1669 Victoria St., Prince George, B.C.; Man'53; Ophth; DAB Ophth; Staff, Prince George Regional Hosp.; Tel. 564-2108.
KILLORN, Leo H.; 129 Kent St., Charlottetown, P.E.I.; McG '49; MCGP; Phys., Beach Grove Home for the Aged; Tel. 4-3015.
KILPATRICK, Carman D.; 150 Delhi St., Guelph, Ont.; Wes'29; Phys., Homewood Sanitarium; Tel. TA 4-1010.
KILPATRICK, Elizabeth; 948 Greenwood Ave., Halifax, N.S.; Dal '15: C.H., Dip. Psy (USA), DAIP; Lect. (Psy), Dalhousie U.; Tel. 423-7905.
KILSHAW, Miles F.; 550 Trafford Cr., Oakville, Ont.; Manchester (Eng.)'60.
KILTY, Harold C.; 3094 Danforth Ave., Scarborough, Ont.; Tor'54; Tel. 691-7710.
KILTZ, Herbert; Box 1015, Athabasca, Alta.; Alb'57.

KIM, Chang H.; Kyungpook (Korea) '58; DiagRad; ABDR; Dir. Dept. of Rad., Holy Family Hosp., Prince Albert, Sask.; Tel. 763-2605.
KIM, Dook T.; Seoul (Korea)'54; Res., St. John's Sanatorium, St. John's, Nfld.
KIM, Hyeong S.; Ste. 32, 50-20th St. S.W., Portage La Prairie, Man.; Seoul (Korea)'56.
KIM, James H. K.; 3026 Parliament Ave., Regina, Sask.; Yonsei (Korea)'59; Anaes.
KIM, John P.; Med. Arts Clinic, 2125-11th Ave., Regina, Sask.; Kwangju (Korea) '52; OrthSurg; Staff, Regina Gen. & Grey Nuns Hosp's.; Tel. 523-0691
KIM, Pung W.; 396 Francis Rd., Richmond, B.C.; Kyungpook (Korea)'54.
KIM, Yang G.; '56; Res., St. Paul's Hosp., Vancouver 1, B.C.
KIMBER, Ronald W.; 417 Lawson Rd., London, Ont.; Wes '59; FRCP(C), IntMed; Staff, Victoria Hosp.; Ass't. Prof., Dept. of PathChem., U. of Western Ontario; Tel. 432-5261.
KIMLER, Ronald D.; Sask '60; Res., Dept. of Anaes., University Hosp., Saskatoon Sask.
KIMM, George E.; Dept. of Nat. Health & Welfare. Laboratory of Hygiene, Ottawa, Ont.; 425 Richardson Ave. (res); Ott '53.; Tel. CE 2-8211.
KIMMERLY, Ralph J.; 152 Simcoe N., Oshawa, **Ont.; 920 Mohawk St. (res); McG '50; MCGP; Tel. 723-2973.**
KIMMITT, Patrick J.; 215 Le Marchand Mansions, Edmonton, Alta.; 7331-118A St. (res); Alb'46; Paed; Chief, Dept. of Paed., Gen. Hosp.; Clin. Instr. (Paed), U. of Alberta; Tel. 488-5784.
KIMOFF, Richard; 309 Dufferin, Sherbrooke, P.Q.; 579 Bois Joli (res); Tor '53; MCGP; Tel. 567-6207.
KIMPTON, Albert J.; St. George San. Mont-Joli, P.Q., Mon '41; F.A.C.C.P., Pulm. Dis & TB (P.Q.); Ass't. Med. Dir. & Chief of Serv. San. St. Georges; Tel. PR 5-4355.
KINAHAN, Patrick J.; 1669 Victoria, Prince George, B.C.; UBC'55; Tel. 563-3024.
KINASH, Barney R.; 1593 Wilson Ave., Downsview, Ont.; 10 Elmwood Ave., Willowdale (res); Tor '57; Tel. CH 1-3017.
KINASH, Thomas E.; Gilbert Plains, Man.; Man '48; Prov. Coroner; Tel. 150.
KINCADE, Gordon F.; 2647 Willow St., Vancouver 9, B.C.; 4706 W. 4th Ave., Van 8 (res); McG '31; IntMed. (TB); Dir. of TB Control; Clin. Assoc. Prof. (Med.), U. of British Columbia; Tel. CA 4-1622.
KINCAIDE, Cyril M.; Ste. 322, 200 St. Clair W., Toronto 7, Ont.; 57 Glenrose Ave., Tor. 7 (res); Dal '45; Anaes; Staff, Wellesley Hosp.; Tel. WA 2-4348.
KINCH, Kenneth E.; 442 Maxwell St., Sarnia, Ont. (res); Tor'48; IntMed; Chief of Med., St. Joseph's Hosp.; Tel. DI 4-5162.
KINCH, Robert A.H.; 375 South St., London, Ont.; 264 St. James St. (res); London (Eng.)'43; MRCS; MRCP; FRCOG; FRCS(C); ObstGyn; **Hd. & Chief of Staff (ObstGyn.), Victoria Hosp.; Prof. (ObstGyn.), U. of Western Ont.; Tel. 432-5261.**
KINDRACHUK, John; Fort St. John, B.C.; Alb '64.
KINDRACHUK, Walter; 137 Wellington St., Sarnia, Ont.; Tor '53.
KINDRACHUK, William H.; 602 Medical Centre, 906-8th Ave. S.W., Calgary, Alta.; Qns'42; DABOS; FACS; FICS; OrthSurg.
KINDREE, LaVerne C.; Squamish, B.C.; Tor '47.
KINDREE, William A.; Ste. 2., 986-3rd Ave. E., Owen Sound, Ont.; Wes '59.
KINDY, Alexander; 209 St. Joseph St. W., Montreal, P.Q.; Lav '57; Psy. (PQ); Psy., St. Vincent de Paul, Sherbrooke, P.Q.
KINDY, Dagmar; 209 Boul. St. Joseph W., Montreal, P.Q.; McG '60; DiagRad.
KING, A. Ben; 4939-50th St., Vermilion, Alta.; Alb'43; MCGP.
KING, Alexander; 2201 Como Lake Ave., Coquitlam, B.C.; Glasgow (Scot.)'59.
KING, Archie E.; 243 King St. E., Oshawa, **Ont.**; 1141 Hortop Ave. (res); Med. Evangelists (Cal., U.S.A.) '53.
KING, Brian M.; Biggar, Sask.; Cambridge (Eng.) '56.
KING, David L.; Med. Clinic, Jeffrey's, Nfld.; Dal'64; AMCGP.
KING, Dolores; Eatonia Clinic, Eatonia, Sask.; Trinity Coll. (Dublin, Ireland)'58.
KING, Donald M.; 350, 5780 Cambie St., Vancouver 15, B.C.; 1855 W. 43rd Ave. (res); Tor '31; MCGP; Clin. Instr., U. of British **Columbia; Tel. FA 5-3511.**
KING, Donald W. Capt.; Qns '64; Canadian Forces Hosp., Kingston, Ont..
KING, Douglas; Trinity Coll. (Ire.) '54; DMRT (Eng.); TherRad; Staff, Hamilton Cancer Clinic, Henderson Gen. Hosp., Hamilton, Ont.
KING, E. Garner; Alb'63; Res., University Hosp., Edmonton, Alta.
KING, E. Peter; 8 Eastwood Avenue, Scarborough, Ont.; 25 Hill Cr. (res); Tor'48; MCGP; Staff (G.P.), Toronto East Gen. & Scarborough Gen. Hosp's; **Tel. OX 8-1684.**
KING, Frank; Tor'64; Res., St. Michael's Hosp., Toronto 2, Ont.
KING, Franklin G. E.; 1886 Weston Rd., Weston, Ont. North Dr., Islington (res); Tor '43; MRCOG, ObstGyn.; Tel. CH 1-0872.
KING, Gordon; c/o Imperial Oil Ltd., Norman Wells, **N.W.T.; Dublin (Ire) '52.**
KING, Hollister F.; Box 540, Bella Coola, B.C.; Tor'57; MCGP; Staff, Burns Lake & Dist. Hosp.; Tel. 9.
KING, Howard F.; Box 309, 101 Chipman St., Kenora, Ont.; Man'46; MCGP.
KING, Jacob H.; Medical Arts Bldg., Corner Brook, Nfld.; 12 West St. (res); McG '38; Otol.
KING, James A.; Tor'64; Res., Hosp. for Sick Children, Toronto 2, Ont.
KING, J. Barry; Box 310, Rothesay, N.B.; McG '54; MCGP; Assoc. Staff, Saint John Gen. and St. Joseph's Hosp's.; Tel. 847-7542.
KING, John K.; 22 Main St. W., Grimsby, Ont.; Tor'54; FRCS(C), GenSurg; Tel. 945-8513.
KING, John K.; 118 Water St., Almonte, Ont.; 189 Spring St. (res); McG '54; Pres., Med. Staff, Almonte Gen. Hosp.; Staff, Carleton Place Dist. Mem. Hosp.; Tel. 299.
KING, John L.; 21 Wellington St., Galt, Ont.; 9 Brant Rd. S. (res); Tor '17; F.A.C.S., GenSurg; Staff, South Waterloo Memorial Hosp., Galt, St. Mary's & Kitchener-Waterloo Hosp's., Kitchener; Retired.
KING, Kenneth C.; 766 Queen St., Preston, Ont.; Tor '41; GenSurg; Surg. Staff, South Waterloo Mem. Hosp.; Tel. 653-4141.
KING, Michael F.; 599 Cheapside St., London, Ont.; McG '60; AMCGP; Staff, Victoria Gen., St. Joseph's & St. Mary's Hosp's.; Tel. 438-4611.
KING, Michael H.; Tor'65; Res., Banting Inst., Toronto 2, Ont.
KING, Michael R.; Third St., Englehart, Ont.; Edinburgh (Scot.) '50; Chief of Staff, Englehart & Dist. Mem. Hosp.; Tel. 544-2321.
KING, Paul A.; 8 Cassandra Blvd., Don Mills, Ont.; London (Eng.)'53; M.B., B.S., FRCP(C), IntMed; Cons., Sunnybrook Hosp., Toronto; Clin. Teach., U. of Toronto; Tel. 485-8651.
KING, Ruth A.; Ste. 404, University Hosp., Edmonton, Alta.; Alb'64.
KING, William E.; Oakview Cr., R.R. 1, Union, Ont.; Ott'55; Psy; Staff, Ontario Hosp., St. Thomas; Tel. 631-8510.
KING, William L.; Tor'65; Res., St. Michael's Hosp., Toronto 2, Ont.
KING, W. L. MacKenzie; 7 Moira St., Dartmouth, N.S. (res); Dal '60; Phys., Nova Scotia Hosp. Abroad.
KING-BROWN, Richard; Campbell Clinic, 480 Mayor Magrath Dr., Lethbridge, Alta.; 636—19th St. S., (res); London (Eng.) '42; M.D. (Lond.), M.R.C.P.(Lond.), IntMed; Staff, Mun. Hosp. & St. Michael's Hosp.
KINGHORN, Malcolm G. C., F/L; M.O., Station Hosp., RCAF, Portage La Prairie, Man.; Glasgow (Scot.)'60.
KINGMA, Herre; 168 Charlotte, Ottawa, Ont.; 20 Stewart (res); Groningen (Neth.)'42; DermSyph; **Staff, Ottawa Gen. Hosp.; Assoc. Prof. (Derm.), U. of Ottawa; Tel. 234-6090.**

KINGSLEY, Dudley J.; 121 Cameron St., Sarnia, Ont.; 1694 Lakeshore Rd. (res); McG'37; FACS; FICS; FACOG; DABOG; ObstGyn; Hon. Cons., Staff, St. Joseph's & Sarnia Gen. Hosp's.; Tel. ED 7-5331.

KINGSMILL, Diana P.; Box 867, 136 Lasalle, Baie-Comeau, P.Q. (res); McG '57; Retired.

KINGSMILL, Sheila de N.; (See, LEITCH, Sheila de N.).

KINGSTON, Mark B.; 35 Edward Laurie Dr., Rockingham, N.S.; Dal'53; ObstGyn.

KINGSTON, Paul T.; 768-3rd Ave., Val-d'Or, P.Q.; Bourlamaque (res); McG '30; GenSurg; Surg. Staff, Hop.-St.-Sauveur; Tel. 824-2524.

KINGSTON, William B.; Dal'63; AMCGP; Staff, Student Health Clinic, Dalhousie University, Halifax, N.S.

KINGSTONE, Eddie; 1025 Pine Ave. W., Montreal 2, P.Q.; McG '56; D.Psy; Psy; Ass't. Psy., Royal Victoria Hosp.; Att'd. Psy., Queen Elizabeth Hosp.; Lect. (Psy.), McGill U.; Tel. VI 2-1251, Ext. 267.

KINGSTONE, Henry; 1862 Eglinton W., Toronto, Ont., 45 Park Hill Rd. (res); Tor '33; M.C.G.P.; Staff, Northwestern Gen. Hosp.; Court. Staff. North York Branson Hosp.; Tel. RU 2-6111.

KINGSTONE, Robert A.; 1862 Eglinton Ave. W., Toronto 10, Ont.; Tor '63; Tel. RU 2-6111.

KINGSTONE, Sheldon I.; 1862 Englinton Ave. W., Toronto 10, Ont.; Apt. 10, 80 Neptune Dr., Tor. 19 (res); Tor '57; MCGP; Tel. RU 2-6111.

KINLEY, C. Edwin; 5849 University Ave., Halifax, N.S.; Dal '56; M.Sc.(Surg.); FRCS(C); GenSurg; Ass't. Surg., Victoria Gen. & Halifax Children's Hosp's.; Ass't. Prof. (Surg.), Dalhousie U.; Tel. 423-7458.

KINLEY, Richard H.; Dal'65; Res., Deer Lodge Hosp., Winnipeg 12, Man.

KINLOCH, David R.; P.O. Box 87, Whitehorse, Y.T.; Alb '58; DPH (Lond.); Zone Supt., Yukon Northern Health Serv.

KINMAN, Humphrey L.; Regional Health Office 11, Tisdale, Sask.; Edinburgh (Scot.)'50.

KINNAIRD, Francis A.; Box 40, Russell, Ont.; Qns '33; M.C.G.P.

KINNEAR, Douglas G.; 1650 Cedar Ave., Montreal, P.Q.; 461 Mt. Pleasant, Westmount (res); McG '52; FACP; FRCP(C), IntMed. (Gastroent.); Ass't. Phys., Mtl. Gen. Hosp.; Lect. (Med.), McGill U.; Tel. WE 7-6011, Loc. 722.

KINNEAR, William S.; 213 Canada Bldg., Saskatoon, Sask.; 702 Queen St. (res); Tor '33; Paed; Chief, Paed. Serv., Saskatoon City Hosp.; Staff (Paed.) St. Paul's & University Hosp's.; Ass't. Clin. Prof. (Paed.) U. of Saskatchewan; Tel. 242-4323.

KINSELLA, T. Douglas; 1 Fourth Ave. S., Roxboro, P.Q.; McG '57; FRCP(C), IntMed; Att'd. Staff, Royal Victoria & Lakeshore Gen. Hosp's.; Cons. (Med.), Queen Mary Vet's. Hosp.; Lect. (Med.), McGill U.; Phys., Bank of Montreal Hd. Office; Tel. 684-3764; Abroad.

KINSEY, Francis E.; Ste. 408, 625-Fifth Ave., New Westminster, B.C.; Qns'40; ObstGyn; Tel. 521-3622.

KINSMAN, Glen W.; 742 King St. W., Kitchener, Ont.; 156 Ripplewood Cr. (res); Qns'45; Anaes; Active Staff, Kitchener-Waterloo & St. Mary's Gen. Hosp's.; Tel. 742-7337.

KINSMAN, John L.; 53 Carruthers St. Kingston, Ont. (res); Tor '40.

KINSMAN, Paul E.; Aylesford, Kings Co., N.S.; Dal '57; Tel. 427-3446.

KINSMAN, R. P.; 925 W. Georgia St., Vancouver, B.C.; Paed; McG '22; Retired.

KINTZEN, Charlotte M. (Mambourg); 181 Argyle, Sherbrooke, P.Q. (res); Berne (Switz.) '49.

KINTZEN, Walter; 181 Argyle St., Sherbrooke, P.Q. (res); Berne (Switz.) '50; Path; Dir., Path. Lab., Sherbrooke Hosp.; Tel. LO 9-3661.

KIORS, Antons; 481½ William Ave., Winnipeg 2, Man.; Riga (Latvia) '28.

KIPKIE, George F.; 41 Dickens Dr., Kingston, Ont. (res); Qns '39; M.Sc. (Path); D.A.B. Path., PathBact; Dir. of Labs. Kingston Gen. Hosp.; Assoc. Prof. of Path., Queen's U.; Tel. 542-2822, Loc. 277

KIPPEN, Duncan L.; Winnipeg Clinic, Winnipeg, Man.; 269 Oxford St. (res); Man '42; FACP; IntMed; Hon. Att'd. Staff, Wpg. Gen. Hosp.; Ass't. Prof. (Med.), U. of Manitoba; Tel. 942-0051.

KIRBY, Alan R.; 208 Garrison Cr., Saskatoon, Sask.; Durham (Eng.) '47; FRCS(Eng.); Lect. (NeurSurg), University Hosp.; Tel. 242-7641, Ext. 448.

KIRBY, John W.; Ste 301, 77 Westmount Rd., Guelph, Ont.; Tor '42; GenSurg.; Tel. 822-3111.

KIRBY, Orville E.; 925 W. Georgia St., Vancouver 1, B.C.; McG '33; Ophth; Otol.; Tel. MU 4-6488.

KIRBY, Royal C.; Smith Clinic, Hawkesbury, Ont.; 47 Main St. E. (res); McG '52; MCGP; Tel. ME 2-2711.

KIRK, Bryan; Man '60; FRCP(C), IntMed; Staff, Winnipeg Gen. Hosp., Winnipeg 3, Man.; Tel. SP 4-6511.

KIRK, Carman J.; 478 Victoria St., London, Ont. (res); Tor '32; M.Sc.; FACHA; Supt., Victoria Hosp.; Retired.

KIRK, David K.; 689 E. 49th Ave., Vancouver 15, B.C.; 4176 Cartier St. (res); Alb '43; Tel. FA 7-3837.

KIRK, Donald E.; Box 2511, Campbell River, B.C.; Alb'57.

KIRK, J. Lawrence; 422 Ash St., Sudbury, Ont.; Wes '23; Med. Exam., Metropolitan Life Ins.; Tel. 674-5159.

KIRK, Mary E.; Wes'64; Res., Montreal Gen. Hosp., Montreal 25, P.Q.

KIRK, T. Edwin; McG'27; M.A.C.H.A.; FACHA; MRSC; Med. Supt., Camp Hill Hosp., Halifax, N.S.; Sr. Treatment M.O., D.V.A., Prov. of N.S.; Assoc. Prof. (Hosp. Admin.), Dalhousie U.; Tel. 423-1371.

KIRKALDY-WILLIS, William H.; University Hosp., Saskatoon, Sask.; Cambridge (Eng.)'39; FRCS(Ed.); FACS; FRCS(C), OrthSurg; Ass't. Prof. Rehab. Med., University Hosp.; Ass't. Prof. Surg., U. of Saskatchewan; Tel. CH 2-7641.

KIRKBRIDE, John; Durham (Eng.) '57; DPH (Tor.); M.O., Indian Hosp., Sioux Lookout, Ont.; Tel. 463.

KIRKBRIDE, R. A.; 3862 Valdez Rd., Vancouver, B.C.; 3849 W. 19th Ave. (res); McG '42; IntMed; Tel. MU 2-1228.

KIRKBY, Robert W.; 836-20th St. W., Prince Albert, Sask. (res); Qns '19; FACCP; IntMed (T.B.); Staff Prince Albert Chest Clinic; Staff, Anti-T.B. League & Holy Family Hosp's.; Lect. (T.B.), Victoria Union Hosp.; Tel. 763-3266.

KIRKEBECK, Ebba; 509-15th Ave. N.E., Calgary, Alta.; Tor '52; Anaes; Staff (Anaes.), Calgary Gen. Hosp.; Tel. AM 6-7541.

KIRKER, Gilbert E.; UBC'63; Res., Shaughnessy Hosp., Vancouver 9, B.C.

KIRKHAM, Frederick R.; 12 Lawton Blvd., Toronto, Ont.; Tor '15; Tel. 924-4775.

KIRKLAND, A. Stanley; Rothesay, N.B. (res); McG '13; D.A.B.R., F.R.C.P.(C), D. & TRad; Rad., Ass't. Dir., St. John Gen.; Cons., St. John T.B., & Lancaster D.V.A. Hosp's.; Tel. 693-3351.

KIRKPATRICK, Crosby; New Hamburg, Ont.; Tor '29.; MCGP;

KIRKPATRICK, Donald H.; Park Med. Bldg., 150 Park St., Kentville, N.S.; Layton Ave. (res); Dal '50; Med. Staff, Blanchard-Fraser Mem. Hosp.; Exam. Dept. of Transport.

KIRKPATRICK, Fenwick; Ste. 21, 810-820 McBride Blvd., New Westminster, B.C.; Dublin (Ire.) '47; Tel. LA 2-3656.

KIRKPATRICK, Garnet J.; 3195 Granville St., Vancouver 9, B.C.; 5342 Angus Dr., Van. 13 (res); Man'34; FRCS (Ed.); GenSurg; Tel. RE 8-4342.

KIRKPATRICK, Gordon M.; Mental Health Centre, 4400 W. Grandview-Douglas Hwy., Burnaby 2, B.C.; 2049 W. 45th Ave. (res); Tor '28; Psy.

KIRKPATRICK, Hartley W.; P.O. Drawer 461, Wolfville, N.S.; Dal '16; Ophth, Otol.

KIRKPATRICK, P. Hugh; 8 Peppett Street, North Sydney, N.S.; Dal'54; Staff, St. Elizabeth Hosp., & Harbour View Hosp., Sydney Mines; Tel. 794-2712.

KIRKPATRICK, T. C.; New Hamburg, Ont.; Tor '29; M.C.G.P.
KIRKWOOD-HACKETT, Thomas J.; Campbellford Clinic, 49 Doxsee Ave. S., Campbellford, Ont.; RCS(Ireland)'53; LRCP; LRCS; LMRCSI; LM(Rotunda); Chief of Staff, Campbellford Mem. Hosp.; Staff, Peterborough Civic & Trenton Mem. Hosp's.; Tel. 653-3550.
KIRKWOOD, William K.; 4027 E. Hastings St., North Burnaby, B.C.; 6083 Buchanan St. (res); Edinburgh (Scot.) '47; Tel. CY 9-2677.
KIRSCH, Archie; 1538 Sherbrooke St. W., Montreal, P.Q.; 5533 Fyon (res); McG '40; Clin. Ass't. Med., Jewish Gen. Hosp.; Tel. WE 5-7230.
KIRSCHBERG, Leo S. S.; Ste. 25, 1390 Sherbrooke St. W., Montreal 25, P.Q.; 3429 Grey Ave. (res); McG '39; Ophth; Assoc. Ophth., Royal Victoria Hosp., Lect. in Ophth., McGill U.; Cons. (Ophth.), Dept. of Transport; Tel. VI 2-6407.
KIRSCHNER, Piroska (See Jeney)
KIRSH, Erving L.; 1495 Kipling Ave. N., Rexdale, Ont.; 24 Kilburn Pl., Weston (res); Wes '55; MCGP; Tel. CH 1-5264.
KIRSH, Jerry J.; 976A Bloor St. W., Toronto 4, Ont.; Tor '57; MCGP; Tel. LE 1-7779.
KIRSHNER, Abe W.; Ste. 209, 688 Coxwell Ave., Toronto 6, Ont.; Cape Town (S. Africa)31; DTM; Staff, Toronto East Gen. Hosp.; Tel. 461-8272.
KIRVAN, Frank J.; 177 Norfolk St., Guelph, Ont.; 82 Oxford St. (res); Wes '32; MCGP; Staff, St. Joseph's & Guelph Gen. Hosp's.; Tel. 2-2530.
KISS, Alexander; 73 Hellems Ave., Welland, Ont.; Qns '56.
KISS, Andrew; 322 College St., Toronto 2B, Ont.; Budapest (Hun.); '51; FAGS; FHCS; MCGP; Adjunct (GP), New Mt. Sinai & Grace Hosp's.; Tel. 921-7192.
KISS, Jozsef; Pecs (Hung.) '56; DiagRad; Staff, Mtl. Gen. Hosp., Montreal, P.Q.; Tel. WE 7-6011.
KISS, Zenon; 604 Medical Arts Bldg., 1 Young St., Hamilton, Ont.; Qns'58; Gen. Surg.; Assoc. Staff, Hamilton Gen. & Henderson Gen. Hosp's.; Court. Staff, Chedoke Gen. & St. Joseph's Hosp's.
KISTER, Earle; 27 Academy St., St. Catharines, Ont.; Tor '11; Ophth.
KITCHEN, Borden; 502 Med. Dental Bldg., Rose St. & 11th Ave., Regina, Sask.; 1008 College Ave. (res); Qns '56; Tel. LA 2-8541.
KITCHEN, George H.; 402 Medical Arts Bldg., Toronto, Ont.; 150 Wimbleton Rd. Islington, Ont. (res); Tor '32; F.I.C.S., F.R.C.S.(Eng.), F.R.C.S.(C) GenSurg; Surg Staff, St. Joseph's Hosp; Cons. Staff, Queensway Gen. Hosp.; Tel. WA 2-1737.
KITCHEN, H. D.; Manitoba Clinic, 790 Sherbrooke St., Winnipeg, Man.; 364 Montrose St. (res); Man '21; FACP, FRCP(C), IntMed.; Tel. SP 4-6541.
KITCHEN, S. F.; Lab. of Hygiene, 45 Spencer St., Ottawa, Ont.; Wes '26.
KITCHING, Donald C.; 185 Britannia Ave., Hamilton, Ont.; Tor '55.; Tel. 544-2760.
KITCHING, John S.; 74 Hughson St. S., Hamilton, Ont.; 4 North Oval, No. 2. (res); Tor '31; DPH; PH; M.O.H., Hamilton; Tel. 528-1441.
KITEALA, John; McG'61; Paed; Staff, Montreal Children's Hosp., Montreal 25, P.Q.
KITELY, Elizabeth L.; 15 Charles St. E., Toronto, Ont. (res; Tor '19; Div. of Maternal & Child Hygiene, Dept. of Health, Parliament Buildings, Toronto, Ont.; Retired.
KITELEY, John E.; Riverhurst, Sask.; Man '13; Dist. Coroner; Retired.
KITZ, Alice D.; 1110 Rockcliffe St., Halifax, N.S.; Aberdeen (Scot.)'39; Instr. (Anat.), Dalhousie U.
KLAASSEN, David J.; Sask'61; FRCP(C), IntMed; Staff, Cancer Clinic, University Hosp., Saskatoon, Sask.
KLADY, Alvin M.; 750 W. Broadway, Ste. 1410, Vancouver 9, B.C.; Man'61; MCGP; Active Staff, Vancouver Gen., Grace, Children's & St. Vincent's Hosp's.; Tel. TR 2-5601.
KLAHSEN, Abraham W.; 253 Josephine St., Wingham, Ont.; Wes '54; MCGP; Active Staff, Wingham Dist. Hosp.; Tel. 357-2500.
KLAJN, Roman P.; 9832-71st St., Edmonton, Alta. (res); National U. (Dublin, Ire.) '55; Staff, Edmonton Mental Inst.
KLASS, Alan A.; Mall Med. Bldg., Winnipeg, Man.; 594 Oak St., Wpg. 9 (res); Man '32; FICS, FRCS (Edin.), FRCS(C), GenSurg; Assoc. Surg., Winnipeg Gen. & Misericordia Hosp's.; Ass't. Prof. (Anat.) & (Surg.), U. of Manitoba; Tel. SP. 4-2411.
KLASS, William A.; Box 998 Med. Clinic, Merritt, B.C.; Sask'57; MCGP; Tel. 378-2286.
KLASSEN, Bernhard G.; 3 Gore Ave., Chilliwack, B.C.; Alb '61.
KLASSEN, David; Ste. 103, 299 Main St., Chilliwack, B.C.; Alb'49; FRCS(C), Otol; MCGP; Staff, Chilliwack Gen. Hosp.; Tel. 792-6921.
KLASSEN, Gerald A.; UBC'57; FRCP(C); Int. Med.; Cardiol (P.Q.); Attend. Staff, Cardio-Respiratory Div., Royal Victoria Hosp.; Staff, McGill University Clinic; Ass't. Prof. (Experimental Med.), McGill University; Tel. VI 2-1251-1759.
KLASSEN, John; Man '62; Res., Royal Victoria Hosp., Montreal 2, P.Q.; Abroad.
KLASSEN, Leonard; Box 267, Milk River, Alta.; Alb. '59; MCGP.
KLASSEN, Peter W.; 303 Fairmont Med. Bldg., 750 W. Broadway, Vancouver 9, B.C.; Tor'54; Anaes.
KLASSEN, William; Med. Arts Bldg., 2125-11th Ave., Regina, Sask.; 2 Langley St. (res); Tor '54; MCGP; Sr. Staff, Regina Grey Nuns' & Regina Gen. Hosp's.; Tel. LA 3-0691.
KLEIDER, Victor N.; 1489 Prince Rd., Windsor, Ont.; 1941 Richmond St. (res); Vienna (Aust.) '41; NeurSurg; Chief of NeurSurg., IODE Mem. Hosp., Sr. Cons. (NeurSurg), Metropolitan Gen., Salvation Army & Hotel-Dieu of St. Joseph Hosp's.; Dir. of Electroenceph., Metropolitan Hosp.; Tel. CL 4-1350.
KLEIMAN, Harry J.; 25 Brunswick Ave., Toronto, Ont.; Tor'58; DiagRad; Assoc. Radiol., Doctor's Hosp.; Tel. WA 7-3202.
KLEIN, Agnes V.; Tor'64; Staff, New Mount Sinai Hosp., Toronto 2, Ont.
KLEIN, Allan; Viking, Alta.; Man '52.
KLEIN, David; 5845 Cote-des-Neiges Rd., Montreal 26, P.Q.; 6280 Northcrest Pl., Apt. 616 (res); McG '22; DPH; FAAP; Paed; Sr. Phys. (Paed), Jewish Gen. Hosp.; Ass't. Phys., Montreal Children's Hosp.; Dem. (Paed), McGill U.; Tel. RE 9-1291.
KLEMCHUCK, Stephen E.; 3423, St. Denis, Montreal 18, P.Q.; 6827 Molson St. (res); Mon '42; Otol; Staff, E.N.T. Serv., St. Luke's Hosp.; Tel. 842-4892.
KLIFFER, Earl; 8431 Granville St., Vancouver 14, B.C.; Man'44; MCGP; Att'd. Staff (G.P.), St. Vincent's Hosp.; Tel. 261-3135.
KLIMAN, Murray R.; 510 Fairmont Med. Bldg., 750 W. Broadway, Vancouver 9, B.C.; 4215 Cambie St., Van. 9 (res); Tor '46; FRCS (Eng.), FRCS(C), FACS; GenSurg; Att'd. Surg., Children's Hosp. & Vancouver Gen. Hosp.; Clin. Tutor, U. of British Columbia; Tel. TR 9-5791.
KLIMCZYNSKI, Jerzy; Ste. 221, 1940 Lonsdale Ave., North Vancouver, B.C.; Edinburgh (Scot.)'46; M.D. (Neur); Psy.; Chief Psy. Div., Lionsgate Hosp; Tel. YU 5-2452.
KLIMKOWSKI, Edmund J.; 1110 Ouellette Ave., Windsor, Ont.; Ott '58; Tel. 252-6524.
KLIMUK, Thomas F.; Alb '62; Res., Shaughnessy Hosp., Vancouver 9, B.C.; Abroad.
KLINCK, William J.; 22 Church St., Lennoxville, P.Q.; Wes '37; GenSurg; Staff, Sherbrooke Hosp.
KLINE, Harvey; c/o Albany Medical Clinic, 200 Danforth Ave., Toronto 6, Ont.; Tor'58; MCGP; Tel. 461-0761.
KLINE, Hubert J.; 200 Danforth Ave., Toronto, Ont.; 607 Briar Hill Ave. (res); Tor '40; M.C.-G.P.; Tel. HO 5-1171.
KLING, Samuel; 302 Medical Arts Bldg., Edmonton, Alta.; 13818—101 Ave. (res); Tor '43; MCGP; FACS, FRCS(C) GenSurg; Ass't. Clin. Prof., Surg. & Dir. Dept. of Central Med. Educ., U. of Alberta; Tel. GA 2-4715.
KLISOWSKY, Anthony; 137 Catherine St., Fort Erie, Ont.; 25 Emerich Ave. (res); Tor '51.

KLOSS, Gerd A.; Berlin (Germ.) '36; DPH; FACCP; Staff Phys., Nova Scotia Sanatorium, Kentville, N.S.; Tel. 678-3251.

KLOTZ, Max O.; Ottawa Civic Hosp; 181 Carleton, Rockliffe, Ottawa, Ont. (res); Tor '35; PathBact; Dir. of Labs. Ottawa Civic Hosp.; **Prof. (Clin. Path.), U. of Ottawa; Tel. 729-2511,** Ext. 243.

KLOTZ, Philip G.; 158 St. George St., Toronto, Ont.; 99 Old Colony Rd. (res); Tor '48; F.A.C.S., F.R.C.S.(C), Urol; Att. Urol., New Mt. Sinai & Scarboro Gen. Hosp's.; Vol. Ass't. (Urol.). Toronto Gen. Hosp.; Tel. WA 3-5551.

KLOTZEK, Jerzy S.; Reston, Man.; National U. (Ire.) '55; MB, B.Ch.; BAO; Tel. 3794.

KNAPP, Bruce E.; 1013 Vancouver St., Victoria, B.C.; Qns '22; Staff, Royal Jubilee & St. Joseph's Hosp's.; Tel. EV 2-4796.

KNAPP, John E.; 460 Eglinton Ave. E., Toronto 12, Ont.; 8 Red Oaks Cres. (res); Tor '52; Staff, Wellesley & Grace Hosp's.; Tel. HU 3-5134.

KNAPP, Noel S.; 516 Evered Ave., Ottawa 3, Ont. (res); Qns '24; Med. Adviser, Canadian Pensions Commission.; Tel. 722-4381.

KNEALE, Hugh A.; 720 Professional Arts Bldg., 155 James St. S., Hamilton, Ont.; 16 Inverness Ave. W. (res); Tor '39; Psy; Psy. Staff, St. Joseph's & Hamilton Gen. Hosp's.; Tel. JA 7-8281.

KNEESHAW, R. Selby; 5 Hilldowntree Rd., Islington, Ont.; Tor '45; Anaes; Staff, St. Joseph's Hosp.; Tel. 534-9531.

KNICKERBOCKER, W. James; Fairmont Med. Bldg., 750 W. Broadway, Vancouver 9, B.C.; Man '57; DiagRad; Ass't. Rad., Vancouver Gen. Hosp.; Tel. TR 9-4177.

KNIEWASSER, Andrew V.; 226 Argyle Ave., Ottawa, Ont.; Qns '21; Hons. Cons. Surg., Ottawa Civic Hosp.; Assoc. Obst., Grace Hosp.; Tel. 722-4381.

KNIGHT, Allan; 900 Sherbrooke St. W., Montreal, P.Q.; 421 Argyle Ave., Westmount (res); McG '50; AMCAA; FRCP(C), IntMed. (Allerg.); Clin. Ass't. McGill U. Clinic, Dept. of Med., McGill U.; Tel AV 8-1645.

KNIGHT, Charles, Sg/Lcdr; Inst. of Aviation Med., 1107 Avenue Rd., Toronto 12, Ont.; Wes'57.

KNIGHT, Charles P.; Consort, Alta.; Alb '52.; MCGP; Tel. 101.

KNIGHT, Charles R.; 606 Med. Arts Bldg., 770 **Spadina Cres. E., Saskatoon, Sask.; Wes '55;** FRCS(C), PlasSurg; Instr. PlasSurg., U. of Saskatchewan; Tel. 242-8082.

KNIGHT, Leslie W.; Crescent Ave., Souris, Man.; Man '46; Staff, Souris Dist. Hosp. & Hartney Hosp.; M.O., Reserve Army, 12th Man. Dragoons; Coroner, Souris Dist., Chm., Souris School Bd.; Tel. 527.

KNIGHT, M. Ross; Tor'60; DiagRad; Active Cons., South Peel Hosp., Cooksville, Ont.; Tel. 279-7330.

KNIGHT, Russell W.; 54 Brant Ave., Brantford, Ont.; Wes'22; DABR; DiagRad; GenSurg; Tel. 756-6333.

KNILL, James R.; 989 Colborne St., **London, Ont.; Wes '58; Research, U. of Western** Ont.; Tel. GE 9-1681. Abroad.

KNIPF, Joseph; 136 Eagle St., Delhi, Ont.; 217 Orchard Ave. (res); Tor '48; M.C.G.P.; Staff, Norfolk Gen. Hosp.; Tel. 582-0310.

KNIRSCH, Anthony K.; Health Group Assoc., 240 McNabb St., Sault Ste. Marie, Ont.; Wes'62; Staff, Sault Ste. Marie Gen. Hosp. & Plummer Mem. Hosp.; Tel. AL 4-6421, Ext. 74.

KNISTER, Charles E.; Comber, Ont.; Tor '03.

KNODELL, Herbert L.; 6450 Quinpool Rd., Halifax, N.S.; Dal'37; MCGP; Courtesy Staff, Victoria Gen., Halifax Infirmary, Children's & Grace Maternity Hosp's.; Tel. 422-5992.

KNOLL, F. Graham; Torryburn, N.B.; Qns '41; Obst; Ass't. ObstGyn., St. John Gen. Hosp.; Chm., Obst. Serv., St. Joseph's Hosp.

KNOTT, Nairn D.; 1309 Fairmont Med. Bldg., **750 W. Broadway, Vancouver 9, B.C.; 7007 Churchill St., Van. 14 (res); New York U. (USA) '43; IntMed.; Staff, Vancouver Gen.;** Tel. 872-7788.

KNOWLES, Betty P.; 32 Wellington St. E., Aurora, Ont.; London (Eng.)'48; Tel. 727-9481.

KNOWLES, James; 32 Wellington St. E. **Aurora,** Ont.; 100 Wells St. (res); Aberdeen **(Scot.)** '49; Tel. 727-9481.

KNOWLES, James A.; Kirkfield, Ont.; Tor '52; MOH, Eldon & Carden Twp.; Tel. 438-3122.

KNOWLES, Ronald J., S/L; Dal'57; DiagRad; Staff, Canadian Forces Hosp., Halifax, N.S.

KNOWLES, Vernon R.; 312 Medical Arts Bldg., Saskatoon, Sask.; 1304 Main St. E. (res); Man '51; Ophth.; Tel. 652-4800.

KNOWLING, Eithne (MacLaughlin); 13 Glenridge Cres., St. John's, Nfld. (res); Dublin (Ire.) '45; Phys., TB Dispensary.

KNOWLING, Thomas A.; 13 Glenridge Cres., St. John's, Nfld. (res); Edinburgh (Scot.) '35; IntMed (T.B.); Ass't. Dep. Minister, Dept. of Health, Nfld.; Tel. 9-5011.

KNOWLTON, Charles E.; Knight Commander, Order of St. Gregory the Great; 530 St. Clair Ave. W., Toronto, Ont.; 201 Vesta Dr. (res); Tor '25; GenSurg; Chief of Staff, St. Joseph's Hosp.; Tel. LE 2-9100.

KNOWLTON, Robert J.; 408 Med. Arts Bldg., 170 St. George St., Toronto 5, Ont.; Tor'59; FRCS(C), PlasSurg.

KNOWLTON, Thomas G.; 262 St. Clair Ave. W., **Toronto 7, Ont.; Tor '31; ObstGyn; Tel. WA 1-2261.**

KNOX, Frederick W.; 2nd Ave., Hanna, Alta.; London (Eng.) '59; LRCP; MRCS; Staff, Hanna Gen. Hosp.; Tel. 854-3342.

KNOX, J. Edward; 699 Coxwell Ave., Toronto 6, Ont.; Tor '14; Tel. HO 5-1113.

KNOX, Stanley H.; 1090 Marlatt, Montreal 9, P.Q.; McG'48; MCGP; Med. Dir., Montreal Gen. Hosp., 1650 Cedar Ave., Montreal 25, P.Q.; Tel. 937-6011.

KNOX, William J., OBE; Knox Clinic, 1605 Glenmore St., Kelowna, B.C.; 1855 Pandossy St. (res); Qns '03; FACS, LL.D.; Tel. 762-2002. Retired.

KNUDSEN, Albert M.; Ste. 117, 3195 Granville St., Vancouver 9, B.C.; UBC'54; MCGP.

KNUTSON, Gordon H.; Western Med. Bldg., 25 Leonard St., Toronto 2B, Ont.; McG'58; DDS; FRCS(C), PlasSurg; Clin. Teach., U. of Toronto; Tel. 363-2793.

KNUPP, Graydon C.; Box 59, Sutton West, Ont.; Tor '54; Tel. 722-5161.

KO, H. Y.; Gull Lake, Sask.; Taiwan (Formosa) '57.

KOBACS, Michael C.; Mon '57; Res., Hosp. for Mental Diseases, Selkirk, Man.

KOBER, Dorothy S.; 152 Caulder Dr., Oakville, Ont. (res); Tor'41; MCGP; Staff, Oakville-Trafalgar Mem. Hosp.; Tel. VI 5-1281.

KOBER, Werner R.; 5050 de Sorel, Montreal 9, P.Q.; 15 Gables Court, Beaconsfield (res); Wuerzurg (Germ.) '51; Staff, Lakeshore Gen. Hosp.; Med. Dir., FBA Pharmaceuticals, Cdn. Subsidiary Farben Fabriken Bayer, Germany; Tel. 739-3197.

KOBERNICK, David; Ste. 4, 1452 **Bishop St., Montreal 25, P.Q.; McG '43.; MCGP.**

KOBRINSKY, Louis; 208 Edmonton St., Winnipeg, Man.; Man '33; FRCS(Edin.); FICS; Court. Staff, St. Boniface, Winnipeg Gen., Grace & Misericordia Hosp's.; Tel. WH 2-6391.

KOBRINSKY, Sidney; 208 Edmonton St., Winnipeg 1, Man.; 379 Kingston Cres. (res); Man '34.

KOBRYNSKI, Borys; 83 Trugeon Cr., Regina, Sask.; Stefan Batory U. (Wilno, Poland) '38; FCCP; IntMed: Med. Dir., Provincial Geriatric Centres, Dept. of Social Welfare and Rehab., Saskatchewan; Cons. (Ger.) Phys. Rehab. Centre; Tel. 536-4114.

KOCH, Bernd R.; Hamburg (Germ.) '56; FRCP (C), IntMed; Hd., Renal Lab., Ottawa Civic Hosp., Ottawa 3, Ont.

KOCH, Carl A.; 16011 TransCanada Hwy., R.R. 5, North Surrey, B.C.; P.O. Box 119, Cloverdale (res); Utrecht (Neth.) '54; MCGP; Tel. 596-5215.

KOCH, Eduard A.; Municipal Bldg., 550 Burnhamthorpe Rd., Etobicoke, Ont.; McG '57; DPH; Tel. BE 1-4161, Ext. 278.

KOCH, Katharina; 15 John St., Leamington, Ont.; 66 John St. (res); Qns '52; Tel. FA 6-6621.
KOCSIS, Lorant F.; Room 212, 394 Graham Ave., Winnipeg 1, Man.; Pecs (Hung.)'44; MCGP.
KOEGLER, Siegfried J.; Mental Retardation Centre, 2 Surrey Place, Toronto 5, Ont.; Wes'44; DCH; Paed; Supt., Mental Retardation Centre; Tel. 365-5000.
KOEHLER, B. E.; Port Arthur Clinic; Port Arthur, Ont.; Tor'65.
KOEN, Leon; '56; Staff, Cottage Hosp., Brookfield, Nfld. Abroad.
KOENIG, Lucile; App 406, 1060 Raymond Casgrain, Quebec 6, P.Q.; Lav'58; DPH.
KOEPPE, Ruth E.; See KAJANDER.
KOFMAN, Oscar S.; 99 Avenue Rd., Ste. 608, Toronto 5, Ont.; 233 Douglas Dr., (res); Tor '46; FRCP(C), Neurol.; Sr. Att'd. Phys. I/C Neurol., New Mt. Sinai Hosp.; Clin. Ass't. (Neurol.), Tor. Gen. Hosp.; Cons. (Neurol.), Scarborough Gen. Hosp.; Assoc. Dept. of Med., U. of Toronto; Tel. WA 2-7008.
KOHARI, Joseph; 86 Bloor St. W., Toronto 5, Ont.; Budapest (Hung.) '37; MRCS (Eng.); LRCP (Lond.); FRCS (Edin.); GenSurg; Pt-time Research Fell., St. Michael's Hosp.; Tel. WA 1-8882.
KOHLHEPP, Helmut; 6870 Chester Ave., Montreal 29, P.Q.; Munich (Germ.)'47; Corps. St. John's Ambulance Brigade; Tel. 482-1393.
KOHLI, Jai D.; Food & Drug Directorate, Tunney's Pasture, Ottawa, Ont.; Punjab (India)'40; Ph.D.; Tel. 992-4334.
KOHLMEIER, Amandus C.; 291 Wellington St., Sarnia, Ont.; 152 Watson St. (res); Man '49; ObstGyn; Staff, Sarnia Gen. & St. Joseph's Hosp's.; Tel. ED 7-3771.
KOHLMEYER, Werner A.; Goettingen (Germ.) '45; Res. (Psy), Allan Memorial Inst., 1025 Pine Ave. W., Montreal, P.Q.
KOHUT, Camille D.; 3509—17th Ave. S.E., Calgary, Alta.; Alb '55; Tel. BR 2-4149.
KOHUT, Donald R.; 4820 MacLeod Trail, Calgary, Alta.; 2204 Kelwood Dr. (res); Alb '53; Tel. CH 3-7229.
KOKAN, Peter; Selkirk Health Unit; 502 Front, Nelson, B.C.; Zagreb (Yugo.) '56.
KOKNEL, Yusuf Edip; Istanbul (Turkey)'48; DiagRad; Staff, Hop. Sacre-Coeur, 5400 Boul Gouin O., Montreal 9, P.Q.; Abroad.
KOLADICH, Carol J.; Tor '63; Staff, Psy. Hosp., 3131 Lakeshore Blvd., Toronto 14, Ont.
KOLADICH, Stephen; 77 Upper Middle Rd., Ste. 100, Cooksville, Ont.; Tor'58; D.Psy.; Psy.; Cons., Psy., South Peel Hosp.; Cons., New Toronto Mental Health Clinic; Cons., Dept. of Reform Inst.; Tel. 277-9744.
KOLAROMI, Gabor; Budapest (Hung.) '49; Res., St. Mary's Hosp., Montreal, P.Q.
KOLBER, Benjamin; 5610 Durocher Ave., Montreal, P.Q.; McG '26; M.C.G.P.; Med. Staff, Jewish Gen. Hosp.; Tel. 735-3711.
KOLBER, Stanley L.; McG '64; res., Jewish Gen. Hosp., Montreal, P.Q.; Abroad.
KOLCHE, Eugene; '42; Staff, Ontario Hosp., Brockville, Ont.
KOLESNICHENKO, Elizabeth; 407 Boyd Bldg., 388 Portage Ave., Winnipeg 1, Man.; Kharkow (USSR)'41; MCGP; Tel. 943-9653.
KOLIA, Ahmed; 453 Lakeshore Rd., Port Credit, Ont.; Bombay (India) '42; MCGP; Staff, Doctor's & South Peel Hosp's.; Tel. PA 2-6521
KOLKE, Richard H.; Box 1690, Associate Med. Clinic, Melfort, Sask.; Sask'61; AMCGP; Tel. 752-2876.
KOLKIND, Thomas K.; Alb. '57; MCGP; Staff, Burris Clinic, Kamloops, B.C.
KOLLER, Lloyd A.; Alb '56; Res., University Hosp., Edmonton, Alta.
KOLOTYLUK, Kenneth; 5682 Victoria Dr., Vancouver 16, B.C.; Alb'65; Tel. FA 5-1717.
KOLOTYLUK, Wm.; 5682 Victoria Dr., Vancouver, B.C.; 554 W. 21st St. (res); Alb '54; MCGP; Tel. FA 5-1717.
KOMAR, Leon; 8431 Granville St., Vancouver 14, B.C.; 4850 Hudson St., Vancouver 9 (res); St. Mungo's Coll. (Glasgow, Scot.) '44; M.C.-G.P.; Phys., Eburne Saw Mills & Pacific Meat Co.; Tel. AM 6-8044.
KOMAROMI, Gabor; 5845 Cote-des-Neiges Rd, Montreal, P.Q.; 5195 Earnscliffe Ave. (res); Peter Pazmany U. (Budapest, Hung.) '49; FRCP (C), IntMed; Tel. 739-1522.
KOMJATHY, C. Adalbert; 414 Medical & Dental Bldg., Rose St. & 11th Ave., Regina, Sask.; Budapest (Hung.) '48; ObstGyn (Budapest); Assoc. Staff, Regina Gen. & Grey Nuns Hosp's.; Tel. 522-4330.
KONRAD, Daniel B.; 1669 Victoria St., Prince George, B.C.; UBC'58; MCGP; Tel. 564-5531.
KONDZIELEWSKI, Zygmont; Cudworth, Sask.; Sask '58. Staff St. Michael's Hosp.
KONG, Glen P.; 750 W. Broadway, Vancouver 9, B.C.; UBC '58; Otol; Att'd. Staff, Dept. of Surg. (Otol.), Vancouver Gen. Hosp.; Clin. Instr., U. of British Columbia; Tel. 874-5816.
KONIK, Walter; Zenon Park, Sask.; Sask '63; Tel. 767-2212.
KONKAL, Peter J.; Man'64; Res., Winnipeg Gen. Hosp., Winnipeg 3, Man.
KONKIN, Fred; Box 1329, Quesnel, B.C.; UBC'64.
KONOK, George P.; Tor'64; Res., Montreal Gen. Hosp., Montreal 25, P.Q.
KONTAXOPOULOS, George; Aristotelion (Greece) '54; Staff, Riverview Hosp., Essondale, B.C.
KONYER, Charles; 221 Kent St. W., Lindsay, Ont.; Tor '50; Chief of Med., Ross Mem. Hosp.; Staff, Peterborough Civic Hosp.; Tel. 324-6061.
KOOP, Walter H.; 1645 Commercial St., Vancouver, B.C.; UBC '55; Tel. AL 4-1355.
KOPE, Jacob H.; Enderby, B.C.; Man '40; M.C.-G.P.; Tel. 838-2244.
KOPP, Clemens M.; Ott '59; Path; Pathol., Pembroke Cottage Hosp., Pembroke, Ont.; Tel. RE 2-3663; Abroad.
KOPPLIN, Peter A.; Tor'63; Res., St. Michael's Hosp., Toronto 2, Ont.
KOPSTEIN, Jerome B.; 1579 Ouellette Ave., Windsor, Ont.; Tor'53; Derm.
KOPYTEK, Stefan; 180 Berry Rd., Toronto 18, Ont.; 8 Breezewood Dr. (res); Tor '56; AMCGP; Active Staff, Queensway Gen. & Court. Staff, Toronto Western Hosp.; Tel. BE 3-6601.
KORANYI, Erwin K.; Ste 470, 6000 Cote des Neiges Rd., Montreal 26, P.Q.; Innsbruck (Austria) '50; D.Psy.; Psy; Staff, Jewish Gen. Hosp.; Tel. RE 1-8351.
KOREC, Vladimir; 3147 Kingsway, Vancouver 16, B.C. 406-1050 Chilco St., (res); Prague (Czechos.) '15; Retired.
KORECKY, Borivoj V.; Ass't. Prof., Dept. of Physiol., U. of Ottawa, Ottawa, Ont.
KORENBERG, Lyon J.; Ste. 228, 5757 Decelles Ave., Montreal 26, P.Q.; McG '31; IntMed (P.Q.), Cardiol. (P.Q.). Assoc. Phys., Jewish Gen. Hosp.; Ass't. Phys. (O.P.D.), Montreal Gen. Hosp.; Dem. (Med.), McGill U.; Tel. RE 1-0400.
KORENBERG, Morton; 1538 Sherbrooke St. W., Montreal, P.Q.; 626 Algonquin, Mount Royal (res); McG '39; IntMed (P.Q.); Ass't. Phys., Jewish Gen. Hosp.; Tel. WE 5-9202.
KORENTAGER, Harold; Box 422, Malton Medical Group, Malton, Ont.; Queen's (Belfast, N. Ire.) '50; Pres. Med. Staff, Peel Mem. Hosp.; Tel. 677-4200.
KORHONEN, Annie E.; Tor '64; Staff, Grenfell Med. Mission, St. Anthony, Nfld.
KORHONEN, Paul A.; Ste. 303, Brant Arts Bldg., 672 Brant St., Burlington, Ont.; 2134 Harris Cr. (res); Tor'62; Tel. 634-0434.
KORMAN, David; 5585 Clanranald Ave., Montreal 29, P.Q.; Montpellier (Fr.) '55; Anaes.; Tel. 486-0622.
KORMAN, Henry; 6000 Cote des Neiges Rd., Montreal 26, P.Q.; McG'48; GenSurg.
KORMAN, Irvine A.; 200 Bloor St. E., Toronto 5, Ont.; Tor '55; FRCP(C), IntMed; Ass't. Med. Dir., Manufacturers Life Ins. Co.; Tel. 928-4250.
KORMOLSKA, Lillian T. (See Lome)

KORN, Gerald W.; 414 Medical Arts Bldg., Saskatoon, Sask.; 2106-14th St. E., (res); London **(Eng.) '46; M.R.C.S., L.R.C.P., D.R.C.O.G., M.R.COG.; ObstGyn; Staff (ObstGyn), University Hosp.; Assoc. Staff, City & St. Paul's** Hosp's.; Ass't. Clin. Prof., U. of Saskatchewan; Tel. 244-6144.

KORNDER, Lee D.; Box 310, Boundary Health Unit, Cloverdale, B.C.; UBC'56; MCGP; DPH; Dir., Boundary Health Unit; Tel. 594-0441.

KORNELL, Simon; 560 Professional Bldg., 10830 **Jasper Ave., Edmonton, Alta.; 9423-145th St. (res); Witwatersrand (Jo'burg, S. Africa) '51;** FCPSA; FRCP(C), IntMed; Teach., Misericordia Hosp.; Lect. U. of Alberta; Tel. 429-3351.

KOROL, Paul; LeRoy, Sask.; Sask '59; Tel. 286-3272.

KORSAK, Christina M.; 416 Moore Ave., Toronto 17, Ont.; Tor'62; Staff, Women's College Hosp.; Tel. 425-1272.

KORT, Kees; 13 Garden St., Brockville, Ont.; 1 Granite St (res); Utrecht (Neth.) '51; MCGP.

KORTH, Virgil H.; 23 Springvale Ave., Armdale, N.S.; Alb '53; Anaes; Staff, Cdn. Forces Hosp., Halifax.

KORTHALS, Theodore H.; 8030 Guelph Rd., Montreal, P.Q. (res); State U., Leiden (Neth.) '50; Pulm Dis & TB (P.Q.); Med. Dir., Grace Dart Hosp.; Tel. CL 5-2831. Abroad.

KORVIN, Christopher; Community Clinic, 110-8th. St. E., Prince Albert, **Sask.; London (Eng.)** '60; MRCP (Lond.); **MRCS (Eng.); LRCP** (Lond.); Staff, Holy Family & Victoria Union Hosp's.; Tel. 763-6466.

KORWAN, George J.W.; 2547 Danforth Ave., Toronto, Ont.; Wurzburg (Germ.)'53; DiagRad; Cons. Rad., Dufferin Area Hosp., Orangeville & Gen. Hosp., Ajax; Tel. OX 4-4434.

KORYAK, Ozker T.; Ankara (Turk.)'54; Staff, Hop. des Laurentides, L'Announciation, Cte Labelle, P.Q.

KOSAR, Eugene W.; 45 First Ave., Coniston, Ont.; Tor '61.

KOSAR, Stephen J.; 161 Larch St., Sudbury, Ont.; 109 Windsor Cr. (res); Tor '57; Tel. 674-1013.

KOSLOWSKI, Walter; 22 Livingston Ave., Grimsby, Ont.; Wes'65.

KOSMAL, Richard J.; 131 Dundas St., Thamesford, Ont.; Frankfurt (Germ.)'51; Att'd. Staff, Alexandra & Victoria Hosp's., Ingersoll; Court. Staff, St. Joseph's Hosp., London; Tel. 264.

KOSOWSKI, Mikolay; 611 Bloor W., Toronto 3, Ont.; Prague (Czech.) '24.

KOSOY, Martin; 100 Sheppard Ave. W., Willowdale, Ont.; Tor'59; FRCP(C); Paed; Staff, Hosp. for Sick Children, Toronto 2, Ont.; Tel. EM 6-7242.

KOST, Walter F.; 341 Med. Arts Bldg., Saskatoon, Sask.; 1032 University Dr., (res); Man '52; Staff, St. Paul's Hosp.; Tel. 652-5414.

KOSTA, Sofia (Konstantinidi); Ste. 203, 99 Avenue Rd., Toronto 5, Ont.; Istanbul (Turkey) '46; Tel. WA 3-6524.

KOSTER, Basil M.; 7 Union St. W., Kingston, Ont.; 162 Barrie St. (res); McG '22; GenSurg; Surg. Staff, Hop. Hotel Dieu; Lect. in Surg., Queen's U.; Tel. 546-6222.

KOSTICK, Evan L.; 414 Main St., Saskatoon, Sask. (res); Ass't. Prof. (Anat.), U. of Saskatchewan; Tel. CH 2-7671.

KOSTUIK, John P.; Qns '61; Res., Toronto General Hosp., Toronto, Ont.

KOSTIUK, Joseph A.; Alb'62; Res., University Hosp., Edmonton, Alta.

KOSTUK, William J.; Wes'65; Res., Victoria Hosp., London, Ont.

KOTKAS, Lawrence J.; 1279 3rd Ave. S., Lethbridge, Alta.; Alb'56; Psy.

KOSZEGI, Bela S.; 401 Johnston Rd., Alberni, B.C.; Zagreb (Yugo.) '55; Tel. 723-3581.

KOTLOWSKI, Kazimiers; 831 Cherry Tree Lane, Lancaster, N.B.; Warsaw (Poland) '36; Psy; Cons. Psy., Lancaster D.V.A. Hosp.; Tel. 694-4481.

KOTWALL, Aspi N.; Meadow Lake Med. Centre, Meadow Lake, Sask.; Karachi (India)'53; LRCP (Ed.); LRCS(Ed.); LRFPS(Glas.); Staff, Meadow Lake Union Hosp.; Tel. 236-5636.

KOUDOURIS, Spyros D.; Apt. 607, 1185 Fennell Ave. E., Hamilton, Ont.; Athens (Greece)'52.

KOVACH, John C.; 20 Spence St., Regina, Sask. (res); Tor'38; GenSurg; Staff, Dept. of Health, Regina.

KOVACS, Alexander J.; 166 Lake St., Sault Ste. Marie, Ont.; Debrecen (Hung.)'47.

KOVACS, Edith; Dal '62; Staff, Nova Scotia Hosp., Dartmouth, N.S.

KOVACS, Eleonora I. — see **PAPP-KOVACS, Eleonora I.**

KOVACS, Ernest E.; 2 Spadina Rd., Toronto 4, Ont.; 70 Hillcrest Dr. (res); Budapest (Hung.) '35.

KOVACS, Eva M.; Szeged (Hung.) '52; Staff, Dept. of Pharm., McGill U., Montreal 2, P.Q.

KOVACS, George; Budapest (Hung.)'52; Psy; Staff, Riverview Hosp., Essondale, B.C.

KOVACS, Ida (Diosi); 398 Bloor St. W., Toronto, Ont.; 583 Dundas W. (res); Vienna (Austria) '32; Tel. 922-0901.

KOVACS, Lajos; 408½ Selkirk Ave., Winnipeg, **Man.;** 917 Palmerston Ave. (res); **Budapest (Hung.) '31; Tel. JU 6-1069.**

KOVACS, Laszlo L.; Budapest (Hung.)'52; Psy; Staff, Nova Scotia Hosp., Dartmouth, N.S.

KOVACS, Leslie; Ste. 51, 3465 Cote-des-Neiges Rd., Montreal 25, P.Q.; 5784 Westminster, Mtl. 29 (res); Brussels (Belg.) '51; FACP; FRCP(C), IntMed; Clin. Ass't. Royal Victoria Hosp.; Lect., McGill U.; Cons. Aluminium Co. of Canada; Tel. WE 3-7189.

KOVACS, Michael C.; Hosp. for Mental Diseases, P.O. Box 9600, Selkirk, Man.; Man '57; Psy; Tel. 482-3810.

KOVACS, Simon J.; 363 Markham Rd., Richmond Hill, Ont.; Qns '62; Active Staff, York Central Hosp.; Tel. 884-1008.

KOVACS, Stephen F.; 869 Palmerston Ave., Winnipeg 10, Man. (res); Budapest (Hung.) '32; Staff, Princess Elizabeth Hosp.; Tel. SU 3-5228.

KOVACS-BIMBI, Agnes E.; 3465 Cote-des-Neiges Rd., No. 51, Montreal, P.Q.; 5784 Westminster Ave., Cote-St-Luc (res); Brussels (Belgium) '52; Paed; Clin. Ass't., Montreal Children's Hosp.; Phys. Prot. Schl. Bd., Gtr. Mtl.; Tel. WE 3-7189.

KOVAL, Andrew; R.R. No. 1, Kingston, Ont. (res); Wes '53; FRCP(C), IntMed; Assoc. Staff (Med.), Hotel-Dieu Hosp.; Ass't. Prof. (Med), Queen's U.; Tel. 546-1451.

KOVAL, Robert J.; Box 60, Minden, Ont.; Ott'65.

KOVALIK, Michael; 5160 Pie IX Blvd., Montreal 36, P.Q.; McG '48; IntMed (P.Q.); Staff, Dept. of Med., St. Mary's & Montreal Gen. Hosp's.; Tel. RA 7-7610.

KOVEN, Irving H.; Ste. 302, 99 Avenue Rd., Toronto 5, Ont.; 63 Rollscourt Dr., Willowdale (res); Dal'54; FACS; FRCS(C), GenSurg; Att'd. Surg., New Mt. Sinai Hosp.; Clin. Teach. Dept. of Surg., U. of Toronto; Tel. WA 4-9005.

KOWALEWSKI, Jan E.A.; 48 Joicey Blvd., Toronto 12, Ont.; Warsaw (Poland)'33; Dir. Corp. Med. Serv., Dept. of Public Health, City of Toronto; Tel. HU 1-8164.

KOWALEWSKI, Konstanty P.; 11650-74th Ave., Edmonton, Alta. (res); Brussels (Belg.) '47; Ph. D; DTM; IntMed; Cons. Endocrinol., Alberta Cancer Clinic; Assoc. Prof. Experim. Surg.; Dir. Surg. Research & Admin. Surg-Med. Research Inst., U. of Alberta; Tel. GE 9-8721.

KOWALISHIN, Paul; 8 Albert St., Sault Ste. Marie, Ont.; Qns'47; Urol; Tel. 947-0439.

KOWALL, Monte H.; 912 Boyd Bldg., 388 Portage Ave., Winnipeg 1, Man.; Man '54; Paed.

KOWALSKY, Nestor B., F/L; McG'65; Rivers Station Hosp., Rivers, Man.

KOWALSKY, Nicholas; 211 Simcoe St. S., Oshawa, Ont.; Innsbruck (Aust.) '47; MCGP.

KOWALSON, Bella; 208 Edmonton St., Winnipeg, Man.; 1226 Wellington Cres. (res); Man'35; Tel. 942-6391.

KOYL, Leon F.; 250 Lawrence Ave. W., Toronto 12, Ont.; Tor'40; DTM & H, FRCP(C), IntMed; Dir. A & R Unit, Sunnybrook DVA Hosp.; Chief of Med., Bethesda Hosp.; Med. Cons., DeHaviland Aircraft; Tel. RU 7-2577.

KOZAK, Peter; 1250 Ste. Foye Rd., Quebec 6, P.Q.; Apt. 601, 135 Grande Allee W. (res); Alb '45; F.R.C.S.(C), Urol.; Tel. 681-5692.

KOZAKIEWICZ, Mieczyslaw; Room 1410, Brooke Claxton Bldg., Ottawa, Ont.; Warsaw (Poland) '36; DPH.

KOZIAK, Peter H.; 709 Tegler Bldg., Edmonton, Alta.; 12407-65th Ave. (res); Alb '42; Ophth; Att'd. Staff, Edmonton Gen. Hosp.; Court Staff, Royal Alexandra & Misericordia Hosp's.; Tel. 422-8815.

KOZIN, Frank; 311 Day St., Winnipeg 25, Man.; Graz (Austria) '34; Tel. 222-9892.

KOZIOL, Jan K.; 82 Sherman Ave. S., Hamilton, Ont.; Edinburgh (Scot.) '46; Tel. LI 5-9596.

KOZIOL, Miecyzslaw E. F.; P.O. Box 86, Vulcan, Alta.; Warsaw (Poland) '46; L.R.C.P., M.R.C.S.; Staff, Vulcan Clin.

KOZLIK, Theodore J.; Box 847, Kirkland Medical Group, Kirkland Lake, Ont.; Nat. U. (Galway, Ire.) '56; M.B., Ch.B.; BAO.

KOZLOWSKI, F. Bratek; 3610 Durocher, Montreal 18, P.Q.; 3210 Maplewood Ave., Outremont (res); Paris (Fr.) '21; MCGP; Tel. VI 9-3101.

KOZNER, Alice S. (Mrs. Breglia); 31 Edenbrook Hill, Islington, Ont.; Tor'55; Paed; Active Staff, St. Joseph's Hosp.; Tel. BE 9-7824.

KOZUB, Paul; Assoc. Med. Clinic, P.O. Box 790, Peace River, Alta.; Alb '53; MCGP.

KRAFT, Barbara N. (PEAD); McG '47; FACA; Anaes; Staff, Kitimat Hosp., Kitimat, B.C.; Tel. 789.

KRAFT-GODDARD, David G.; Associate Clinic, Pincher Creek, Alta.; London (Eng.)'59; MRCS; LRCP; D.Obst. RCOG; Staff, St. Vincent's Hosp.; Tel. 627-3321.

KRAHN, Abram; 28 Cheadle St. E., Swift Current, Sask.; Tor '50; DPH; Reg. Med. Officer, Swift Current Health Reg.; Cons. (PH), Swift Current Union Hosp.; Tel. 773-8391.

KRAHN, Henry P.; 115 Medical Arts Bldg., 404-406 Graham Ave., Winnipeg 1, Man.; Man '58; FRCS(C); Urol; Tel. 942-2607.

KRAHN, John J.; Box 640, Clearbrook, B.C.; UBC '55.

KRAICER, Jacob; Dept. of Physiol., Queen's University, Kingston, Ont.; Tor'58; Ph.D. (Physiol.); Ass't. Prof. (Physiol.), Queen's U.; Tel. 6-1731.

KRAJBICH, George P.; 1727 Dufferin St., Toronto 10, Ont.; Prague (Czech.) '49; Tel. LE 1-4560.

KRAJICEK, Josef (see Craig, Joseph)

KRAL, Katherine (Neumark); Ste. 560, 5300 Cote-des-Neiges Rd., Montreal 26, P.Q.; Apt. 30, 4145 Blueridge Cres., Montreal 25 (res); German U. (Prague, Czech.) '34; Ophth.; Tel. RE 9-3503.

KRAL, Vojtech A.; 1025 Pine Ave. W., Montreal 25, P.Q.; Prague (Czech.) '27; Psy; Neur; Staff, Royal Victoria Hosp.; Cons. Psy., Maimonides, Queen Mary Vet's., & Douglas Hosp's.; Assoc. Prof. (Psy.), McGill U.; Tel. VI 2-1251.

KRAMER, Simon; 61 Denley Apts., 253 River Ave., Winnipeg 13, Man. (res); London (Eng.) '43; D.M.R.T., F.F.R.; Dir. Rad. Dept., St. Boniface Hosp., St. Boniface, Man.; Tel. WH 3-0311.

KRAMOLC, Nicholas; 939 Lawrence E., Don Mills, Ont.; 53 Banbury Rd., Don Mills (res); Tor '57; MCGP; Court. Staff, Tor. E. Gen. Hosp.; Court Staff, Wellesley & Scar. Gen Hosp's.; Tel. HI 4-6221.

KRAR, Frank; 301 Med. Arts Bldg., 1 Young St., Hamilton, Ont.; 717 Highcliffe Ave. (res); Ott '53; ObstGyn; Active Staff, St. Joseph's Hosp.; Tel. JA 8-4710.

KRASINS, Berta; Apt. 304, 575 Avenue Rd., Toronto 7, Ont. (res); Riga (Latvia) '33; Staff, Gage Inst.; Tel. 924-2191.

KRATZ, Hanna M.; 500-10th St., Fairview, Alta.; Frankfurt (Germ.) '32; FAGS; MRSH; Chm. Med. Staff, Fairview Mun. Hosp. & Hotel-Dieu, Whitelaw; Tel. 835-2360; 835-2126.

KRATZ, Julius C.; Medical Bldg., Fairview, Alta.; Basel (Switz.) '34; FAGS; MRSH; Staff Fairview Mun. Hosp. & Hotel-Dieu-St.-Joseph, Whitelaw; Dist. Coroner; Tel. 835-2360.

KRAUSE, Calvin C; Med. Arts Clinic, Regina, Sask.; 3455 Portnall Ave. (res); McG '51; FRCS (C); Urol; Tel. 522-1651.

KRAUSE, Donald A.; 4012A E. Hastings St., North Burnaby, B.C.; Alb '60; Tel. 299-2422.

KRAUSE, Michael E.; Apt. 802, 2121-W 44th Ave., Vancouver 13, B.C.; Alb'26.

KRAUSE, Robert G.; 1288 Pembina Highway, Winnipeg 19, Man.; Edinburgh (Scot.)'47; D.ObstRCOG; AMCGP; Tel. 474-1351.

KRAUSE. Vernon W.; 5880 Balmoral Rd., Halifax, N.S. (res); Alb '48; Path; Dir. of Labs., Children's Hosp.; Ass't. Prof. (Pathol), Dalhousie U.; Tel. 422-8441.

KRAVITZ, Henry; 1745 Cedar Ave., Ste. 211, Montreal 25, P.Q.; 4994 Circle Rd. (res); McG '49; D. Psy; Psy; Clin. Dir. (Psy), Jewish Gen. Hosp.; Ass't. Prof. (Psy.), McGill U.; Sec., Cdn. Psychoanalytic Soc.; Tel. WE 2-4039.

KRAWETZ, Michael; Bala, Ont.; Wes'57; Tel. 762-3210.

KRAYENHOFF, John J.; 300 Med. Arts Bldg., 1105 Pandora Ave., Victoria, B.C.; 1540 Montgomery Ave. (res); Utrecht (Neth.) '50; AMCGP; Tel. 385-7791.

KREBES, Andrew J.; Box 10, Coleman, Alta.; Alb'59.

KREDENSTER, Bernard; Strathcona Medical Bldg., 83rd Ave. & 105th St., Edmonton, Alta.; 6720-112th St. (res); Mon '51; Obst-Gyn.; Tel. 439-7772.

KREIM, Alice—See Csoka.

KREINDLER, Simon; McG'65; Jr. Int., Jewish Gen. Hosp., Montreal 26, P.Q.; Abroad.

KREINER, Harold O.; Ste. 3, 65 Balsam St., Timmins, Ont.; 300 Toke St. (res); Wes '44. Tel. 264-6118.

KREKORIAN, George D.; 103 Riverview, St. Catharines, Ont.; Tor '52.

KRESTOW, Michael; Heidelberg (Germ.)'60; Anaes; Staff, Hosp. for Sick Children, Toronto 2, Ont.

KREUTZ, D. Melvin, Major; Alb'50; IntMed; Staff, Canadian Forces Hosp., Kingston, Ont.

KREYES, Wilhelm; Cologne (Germ.) '49; D.-Psy; Psy; Clin, Dir., Hosp. for Mental Diseases, Box 9600, Selkirk, Man.; Cons. Psy., Selkirk Gen. Hosp.; Dem. Psy., U. of Manitoba; Tel. 482-3810.

KRIEGER Earl.; 6014 Yonge St., Willowdale, Ont.; Tor '47; Paed; Staff, Hosp. for Sick Children & North York Branson Hosp's.; Cons., Mount Sinai Hosp.; Clin. Teach., U. of Toronto; Tel. BA 1-8255.

KRINGHAUG, Olaf; 210 E. 50th Ave., Vancouver 15, B.C.; 1646 E. 56th Ave. (res); UBC '54; Tel. FA 1-3474.

KRISHNAYYA, Kummarapurugu V.; Madras (India) '57; Staff, Dept. of Path., Saskatoon City Hosp., Saskatoon, Sask.; Tel. 242-6681.

KRISMAN, Ashley M.; 755 W. Broadway, Vancouver 9, B.C.; 812 Cook Rd., Richmond, B.C.; Man'54; M.Sc.; FRCS(C); ObstGyn.; Tel. 876-6933 & 278-1636.

KRISTAL, Louis; 62 Avondale Blvd., Bramalea, Ont.; Dal'43.

KRISTJANSON, Grettir V.; Atikokan Clinic, Marks St., Atikokan, Ont.; Qns '49; Tel. 2721.

KRISTJANSON, Kristjan R.; Osoyoos, B.C.; Tor '61.

KRISTJANSSON, Gestur; Westbrook Med. Centre, S.W. Keewatin & Logan Ave., Brooklands, Winnipeg 23, Man.; Man '53; M.C.G.P.; Tel. SP 2-9453.

KRISTOF, Alexander C.; 343 Tache Ave., St. Boniface, Man.; 465 Kingston Cres., Winnipeg 8 (res); Budapest (Hung.)'43; MCGP.

KRISTOF, Francis E.; 1538 Sherbrooke St. W., Montreal, P.Q.; Budapest (Hung.) '55; D.Psy; Psy; Admitt. Staff, St. Mary's & Lakeshore Gen. Hosp's.; Ass't., O.P.D. (Psy.), Royal Victoria Hosp.; Tel. WE 7-8886.

KRITZINGER, Viljoen; The Medical Centre, Stony Plain, Alta.; Edinburgh (Scot.) '52; LRCP; LRCS; LRFPS(Glas.); MCGP; Staff, Stony Plain Municipal Hosp.; Tel. 777-2226.
KRIVEL, Harold; 1734 W. Broadway, Vancouver 9, B.C.; Alb'44; Paed; Clin. Ass't. Prof. (Paed.), U. of British Columbia.
KROCH, M. N.; Tor'65; Res., Toronto Gen. Hosp., Toronto 2, Ont.
KROCHAK, Michael B.; 1513-20th St. W., Saskatoon, Sask.; 2713 Jarvis Dr. (res); Sask '57; A.M.C.G.P.; Assoc. Staff, St. Paul's & Saskatoon City Hosp's.; Tel. 382-1144.
KROFT, Frederick E.; Qns'65; Res., Clarke Inst., 250 College St., Toronto 2B, Ont.
KROHN, Hans S.; 37 Cote St. Antoine Rd., Westmount, P.Q.; Heidelberg (Germ.) '40.

KROLMAN, Gordon M.; 200 Power Bldg., 428 Portage Ave., Winnipeg 1, Man.; 4495 Roblin Blvd., Charleswood (res); Man '55; DO(Lond.), FRCS(Ed.), FRCS(C), Ophth; Hd. (Ophth), Wpg. Gen. Hosp.; Staff, Deer Lodge DVA. St. Boniface & Man. Rehab. Hosp's.; Prof. (Ophth), U. of Manitoba; Tel. WH 3-1654.
KROMAR, Leon; 8431 Granville St., Vancouver, B.C.; 4850 Hudson St. (res); London (Eng.) '44; Indust. Phys., Pacific Pine Co. & Pacific Meat Co.
KRONICK, Sydney; 340 McLeod St., Ottawa 4, Ont.; Qns'47; FACOG; ObstGyn; Active Staff, Ottawa Civic Hosp. and Grace Hosp.; Clin. Ass't. (Med.), U. of Ottawa; Tel. CE 5-6442.

KRUEGER, Karl H.; 333 Reimer Ave., Box 640, Steinbach, Man.; 375 Elmdale Dr. (res); Danzig **(Germ.) '41; Surg. (Germ.); Tel. DA 6-3463.**
KRUGER, George W.; Med. Arts Bldg., 550 Ingersoll Ave., Woodstock, Ont.; 755 Wilton Cres. (res); Tor'42; DiagRad; Radiol., Alexandra Hosp., Ingersoll; Tel. 537-5552.
KRUMINS, Janis; Riga (Latvia) '38; Staff, Freeport San., Kitchener, Ont.; Tel. 742-5891.
KRUPA, S. Alison M.; 14 Putnam, Ottawa 2, Ont.; 76 Springfield Rd., Ott. 2 (res); Leeds (Eng.)'52; M.B., B.Ch., DCH (Lond.); Active Staff, Grace Hosp.; Court. Staff, Ottawa Gen. Hosp.; Tel. SH 9-9868.
KRUSPE, Robert C.; 136 Market St., Brantford, Ont.; 75 Golfdale Rd. (res); Tor '50; Staff, Brantford Gen. & St. Joseph's Hosp; Tel. 752-1441.
KRUYFF, Elizabeth; 22 Brucedale Cr., Willowdale, Ont.; Amsterdam (Neth.)'49; FRCP(C), IntMed; DiagRad; Tel. 223-4358.
KRUYFF, Everet; Amsterdam (Neth.) '47; Diag Rad; Staff, Dept. of Rad., Hosp. for Sick Children, Toronto, Ont.; Tel. EM 6-7242.
KRYGIER, Jechiel; 6235 Wilderton Ave., Montreal **26, P.Q.; Poland '30.; Tel. 737-5629.**
KRYN, Stanislas; 441 Huron Street, Woodstock, Ontario; '21.
KRYNSKI, Zdzislaw; Warsaw (Poland)'45; Res., Ottawa Civic Hosp., Ottawa, Ont.
KRYSZEK, Stanley H.; Box 612, Windsor, N.S.; Edinburgh (Scot.) '42; Dir., Emergency Health Serv., Dept. of Public Health.
KRYT, Maria (Lecewicz); Women's College Hosp., 78 Grenville St., Toronto, Ont.; 355 Castlefield Ave., Tor 12 (res); Brussels (Belgium) '52; Anaes.; Staff Anaes., Women's College Hosp.; Tel. WA 3-7381.
KRYWULAK, Wolodymyr; 1055 Atlantic Ave., Winnipeg 14, Man.; Lvov (Ukraine)'44; AMCGP.
KRZYSKI, Tadeusz K.; Box 608, Point Edward Hosp., Sydney, N.S.; Polish Med. School (Edinburgh, Scot.)'49; Ch.B.; Staff Phys., Point Edward Hosp.
KRZYSKI, Thomas; Kracow (Poland) '17; Staff, **Bayview Hosp., Advocate Harbour, N.S.; Tel. 15.**
KUAN, Peter W.; 114 Langley, Regina, Sask. (res); Hsia Ya Med. Coll. (China)'46; TherRad; Clin. Assoc., Allan Blair Mem. Clinic; Tel. 527-9651.
KUBIKOVA, Eva; Mon'65; Res., Hop. Notre-Dame, Montreal 24, P.Q.
KUBILIUS, Vincas; 1410 Woodward Ave., Ottawa, Ont. (res); Kaunas (Lithuania) '33; Staff Phys., Royal Ottawa San.; Tel. PA 2-6521.

KUBINSKI, Halina M. (Drzewicka); 210 Hammond Bldg., 310 Main N., Moose Jaw, Sask.; 1113 Grafton Ave. (res); Brussels (Belgium) '49; Active Staff, Moose Jaw Union & Providence Hosp's.; Tel. 692-1858.
KUBINSKI, Zbigniew T.; Moose Jaw Clin.. 200 Scott Bldg., Moose Jaw, Sask.; 1113 Grafton Ave. (res); Warsaw (Poland)'37; Anaes; Staff Anaes., Moose Jaw Hosp.; Tel. 692-2373.
KUBRYK, David; 1257 Checkers Rd., Ottawa 3, Ont.; Bologna (Italy) '36; DPH; PH Cons., Emergency Health Serv., Dept. of Natl. Health & Welfare, 1346 Brooke-Claxton Bldg., Ottawa 3; Tel. 992-5893.
KUCHARSKA, Wanda M. (Wojciechowska); **652 Brimley Rd., Scarborough, Ont.; Edinburgh** (Scot.) '49 .
KUCHARSKI, Jerzy W.; 652 Brimley Rd., Scarborough, Ont.; Edinborough (Scot.) '47; M.C.-G.P.; Staff (G.P.), Scarborough Gen. Hosp.; Tel. AM 1-9436.
KUCHARYSZEN, Mykola; 4579 Park Ave., Montreal 8, P.Q.; McG '29; MCGP; Tel. VI 5-5306.
KUCHEREPA, John W.; 29 Edenbridge Dr., Islington, Ont.; Tor'45; AMCGP; Ass't. Registrar, College of Physicians & Surgeons of Ont., **Tel. WA 4-2577.**
KUCKERTZ, Berta E. (Frank); Meadow Lake Medical Centre, Meadow Lake, Sask.; Bonn (Germ.)'53; Retired.
KUCKERTZ, Harald W.; Meadow Lake Med. Centre, Meadow Lake, Sask.; Bonn (Germ.) '52; Retired.
KUCZMENDA, Stephan; 2199 Boor St. W., Toronto 9, Ont.; Tel. 766-3311.
KUDER, Gerald; Alb'59; Res., Dept. of Radiology, Kingston Gen. Hosp., Kingston, Ont.
KUDER, Gordon G.; Alb '59; Res., Montreal Gen. Hosp., Montreal, P.Q.
KUDO, Catherine F.; McG '62; Res., Royal Victoria Hosp., Montreal 2, P.Q.
KUGLER, Michael; 204-200 St. Clair Ave. W., Toronto 7, Ont.; Guy's (London, Eng.)'46; FRCS (Eng.), OrthSurg; Surg. Staff (Orth), North Western Gen. Hosp.; Tel. WA 2-9011.

KUHAR, Sylvia; (See HOGG, Silvia).

KUHARIK, Laszlo; 294 Hellems Ave., Welland, Ont.
KUHBACHER, Ferenc G.; Szeged (Hung.) '21; F.R.C.O.&G. (Szeged & Kolozsvar, Hungary); Staff Phys., Saskatchewan Hosp., Cottage No. 3, Box 7000, Weyburn, Sask. Retired.

KULA, Edward D.; 433 Jarvis St., Toronto 5, Ont.; Sorbonne U. (Paris, France)'36; Cert. T.B. Hop. Laeunec (Paris); Tel. 921-7694.

KULASALU, Heino A; (see KENT)

KULCSAR, Desider D.; 511 Med. Arts Bldg., 1538 Sherbrooke St. W., Montreal 25, P.Q.; 5628 MacDonald Ave., Hampstead (res); Hungary '35; ObstGyn; Sec.-Treas., Cdn. Cytology Council (Div. Cdn. Assoc. of Pathol.); Tel. 932-7287.
KULCZYCKI, Ihor G.; Ott'64; Res., Royal Victoria Hosp., Montreal 2, P.Q.
KULIS, Dorothea F. (Liedtke); Tor'57; D.Psy; Psy; Staff, Psy. Serv., Kitchener-Waterloo Hosp., Kitchener, Ont.

KUMAR, Ganraj; McG'61; FRCP(C), IntMed; Staff, Kingston Gen. Hosp., Kingston, Ont.
KUMAR, Kamla; 1605 MacPherson, Regina, Sask.; Delhi (India)'53; FRCP(C), Paed.
KUMAR, Krishna; 535 Med. Dental Bldg., Rose St. & 11th Ave., Regina, Sask.; Agra (India) '53; FRCS(C), NeurSurg; Cons., Regina Gen. Hosp.; Hd. Dept. of NeurSurg., Regina Grey Nuns Hosp.; Tel. 527-9323.
KUMAR, Stanley E.; Res. (Surg.), Royal Alexandra Hosp., Edmonton, Alta.
KUMAR, Sukh D.; 612 Med-Dental Bldg., Rose St. & 11th Ave., Regina, Sask.; Lucknow (India) '54; FRCP(C), IntMed.

KUMMEL, George E.; Med. Arts Bldg., 31 Centre St. S., Brampton, Ont.; Kiel (Germ.)'50; FACS; GenSurg; Sr. Surg. Cons., Peel Mem. Hosp.; Hon. Surg. Cons., Georgetown & Dist. Mem. Hosp.; Tel. 451-2551.

KUNICA, Richard D.; 443 Reynolds St., Oakville, Ont.; 145 Dornie Rd. (res); Tor'62; AMCGP; Active Staff, Oakville-Trafalgar Mem. Hosp.; Tel. 844-3281.

KUNKEL, Melvin G.; 641 Medical Arts Bldg., Saskatoon, Sask.; 507 Garrison Cres. (res); Tor '45; M.Sc.(Orth); D.A.B.O.S., F.A.C.S., F.R.C.S. (C), OrthSurg; Chief of OrthSurg., University Hosp.; Cons. (Scoliosis), Saskatoon Phys. Restoration Centre; Clin. Ass't. Prof. (Surg), U. of Saskatchewan; Tel. 652-7272.

KUNKEL, Rudolph G.; Box 66, Rouyn, P.Q.; 30-7th St., Noranda (res); Tor '34; Tel. 762-1155.

KUNSTLER, Walter E.; 408 Medical Arts Bldg., 1538 Sherbrooke W., Montreal 25, P.Q.; 30 Thurlow Rd., Hampstead (res); Frankfort (Germ.) '30; Ch.D., Dip. Surg., F.R.C.S.(C), F.C.C.P., ThorSurg, GenSurg; Surg., Royal Edward Chest Hosp.; Cons. Surg., & Lieut.-Col., Canadian Army, Quebec Command; ThorSurg (in charge), Reddy Memorial Hosp.; Surg.-in-Chief, Santa Cabrini Hosp.; Tel. WE 5-1658.

KUNSTLER-MEYER, Margaret S.; 408 Medical Arts Bldg., 1538 Sherbrooke St. W., Montreal 25, P.Q.; 30 Thurlow Rd., Hampstead (res); Leipzig (Germ.) '33; Dip.Paed.; Pulm Dis. & TB (P.Q.; Paed; Phys., Royal Edward Chest Hosp., M.O., YWCA & Marianapolis College; Dem., McGill U.; Tel. WE 5-1658.

KUNTZ, J. David; Tor'65; Res., Shaughnessy Hosp., Vancouver 9, B.C.

KUNYK, Miroslaw B. J.; 121 Church St., St. Catharines, Ont.; Johannes Casimir '31.

KUNYCKYJ, Theofan G.; Berlin (Germ.) '45; **Staff, Hosp. for Mental Diseases, Box 420, Bran**don, Man.; Tel. PA 6- 2321, Ext. 123.

KUOLAS, L. R.; 1364 Islington Ave. N., Rexdale, Ont.; Tor '64.

KUPFERSZMIDT, Irena; (Korn); 5757 Descelles Ave., Montreal 26, P.Q.; 27 Maplewood (res); Moscow (Russia) '44.

KURDYAK, Ruth O.; 27 First Ave., Coniston, Ont.; Tor '60; Retired.

KURDYAK, Victor B.; Tor'60; FRCP(C), ObstGyn; Staff, Women's College Hosp., Toronto 5, Ont.

KURESHI, Aziz H.; Box 1570, Comer Clinic, Williams Lake, B.C.; Panjab (Pakistan)'57; FAAP; Paed; Vice Chmn. & Att'd. Staff, Cariboo Mem. Hosp.; Tel. 392-4465.

KURKJI, Henry S.; 149 Cartier Ave., Pointe Claire, Montreal, P.Q.; American U. (Beirut, Lebanon)'46; FACS; FACCP; FICA; FRCS(C), GenSurg; Thor. Surg. to the Lakeshore Gen., Queen Elizabeth, Lachine Gen. & Santa Cabrini Hosp's.; Tel. 697-6612.

KURSELL, Peter O.; 205 Norfolk N., Simcoe, Ont.; Wes '60.

KURTZ, J. Aube; 57 Clansman Blvd., Willowdale, Ont.; Qns '63; Med. Staff, North York Branson Hosp.; Tel. ME 3-6560.

KURTZE, William L.; 502 Broder Bldg., Regina, Sask.; 2839 Victoria Ave. (res); Man '38; GenSurg.

KUSHEVICH, Zvonimir A.; 412 College St., Toronto 4, Ont.; 821 Palmerston Ave. (res); Zagreb (Yugoslavia) '41; Tel. 922-9140).

KUSHNER, Arnold G.; Ellendale Med. Bldg., 5845 Cote-des-Neiges Rd., St. 235, Montreal 26, P.Q.; 6525 Wilderton Ave., Apt. 408 (res); McG '54; DABOPh; Ophth; Clin. Ass't. (Ophth), Jewish Gen. & Reddy Mem. Hosp's.; Tel. 739-3191.

KUSHNIRUK, Mackim; Northgate Prof. Bldg., 12946-97th St., Edmonton, Alta.; Alb'56; MCGP; Tel. GR 4-8036.

KUSHNIRUK, William; 333 Medical Arts Bldg., Saskatoon, Sask.; 614 Leslie Ave. (res); McG '50; M.Sc.; Derm.; Staff, University, St. Paul's & City Hosp's.; Tel. CH 4-7971.

KUSNIERCZYK, Reginald G.; Sudbury Clinic, 130 Elm St. E., Sudbury, Ont.; Ott '62; Tel. 673-7181.

KUSSIN, Larry; Man '61; Jr. Intn., Winnipeg Gen. Hosp., Winnipeg 3, Man.

KUSSNER, Jacob; 90 Harbour St., Toronto 1, Ont.; 575 Avenue Rd., Apt. 601 (res); Qns '38; MO, WCB; Tel. 362-3411.

KUSSNER, Norman; Queensway Med. Centre, 880 Queensway, Toronto 18, Ont.; 121 Dewbourne Ave., Tor. 10 (res); Ott '52; MCGP; Active Staff, Queensway Gen. Hosp.; Tel. CL 5-1161.

KUTASY, William; 1430 King St. W., Toronto 3, Ont.; Sask '50; Tel. 536-1678.

KUTSCHERA, Joe N.; 3980-3rd St., Chomedy, Cte Laval, P.Q.; Karl Franzens (Graz, Austria) '30.

KUTZNER, Waldemar; 109 King St. E., Oshawa, Ont.; Loma Linda (California, U.S.A.) '64.

KUWABARA, Edward H.; Ste. 201, 344 Bloor St. W., Toronto 5, Ont.; 81 Poplar Plains Cres. (res); Alb '34; Tel. WA 1-2612.

KUWAYTI, Kamal; Ste. 305, 1105 Carling Ave., Ottawa 3, Ont.; 1899 Highland Terr. Ott. 8 (res); Beirut (Lebanon) '51 M.S. (Minn.); IntMed; Staff, (Metab. Serv.), Ottawa Civic Hosp.; Phys., Riverside Hosp.; Cons. (Med.), DVA & (Endocrin.), Ont. Cancer Fdn.; Tel. 728-4893.

KUZMINSKI, Donald J.; 58 Thorncliffe Park Rd., Toronto 17, Ont.; Tor'61.

KUZYK, Nicholas J.; Vegreville Clinic, 5006-51 Ave., Vegreville, Alta.; 4539-54 Ave. (res); Qns '45; Chief of Surg. & Teaching Staff, St. Joseph's Gen. Hosp.; M.O.H., Innistree; Coroner, Vegreville; Tel. 2121.

KWAK, John; 211 Simcoe St. S., Oshawa, Ont.; Ott '55; GenSurg; Tel. 728-3941.

KWAN, James Chung-Y.; Oshawa Clinic, 117 King St. E., Oshawa, Ont.; Sun Yat-Sen (Canton, China)'52; Tel. 728-1661.

KWAN, Yin-Ching (Yeung); Sun Yat Sen U. (Canton, China) '52; Res. (Anaes.), Hotel Dieu Hosp., Montreal, P.Q.

KWITKO, Marvin L.; 400 Linton Med. Bldg., 6000 Cote-des-Neiges Rd., Montreal 26, P.Q.; **5731 Lockwood Ave., Mtl. 29 (res); Wes '56;** DABO; FAAO; FICA; **Ophth; Ophthal., Jewish Gen. Hosp.; Tel. 735-1133.**

KWO, Chin; Taiwan (Formosa)'52; Jr. Int., Jewish Gen. Hosp., Montreal 26, P.Q.

KWONG, Min Kun; 334 Alberta Corner Bldg., 804-1st St. S.W., Calgary, Alta.; Paris (France) '31; Tel. 263-4409.

KYAW, Myo; St. Louis (U.S.A.)'63; Ass't. Res. (Rad.), St. Boniface Gen. Hosp., Winnipeg 6, Man.

KYLE, Clarence A.; Med. Arts Bldg., 2150 Valley Way, Niagara Falls, Ont.; 104 Rolling Acres Dr. (res); Tor'39; FRCS(C); GenSurg; Staff, Greater Niagara Gen. Hosp.; Tel. EL 4-6535.

KYLE, Joseph L.; Med. Arts Bldg., 2150 Valley Way, Niagara Falls, Ont.; 2077 Corwin Ave. (res); Tor '44; D. Ophth (Eng.); Ophth; Staff, Dept. of Ophth., Gtr. Niagara Gen. Hosp.; Tel. EL 4-4812.

KYLE, M. Joan; 740 Brimley Rd., Scarborough, Ont.; Tor '57; Tel. OX 4-4641.

KYLE, Paul R.; Med. Arts Bldg., 260 Cedar St., Sudbury, Ont.; 283 David St. (res); Tor '35; FACOG; FICS; ObstGyn; Chief of Gyn., Sudbury Gen. & Mem. Hosp's.; Tel. 673-3695.

KYLE, Victor N.; Port Arthur Clinic, 194 N. Court St., Port Arthur, Ont.; Tor'57; FRCS(C); Urol.; Tel. 344-7271.

KYLE, William D.; 7618-119th St., Edmonton, Alta. (res); Alb '51; Anaes; Staff, University Hosp.; Tel. 439-5911.

KYLES, John N.; 212 James St. S., Hamilton, Ont., Tor '33; Anaes; Staff (Anaes.), St. Joseph's Hosp.; Tel. 528-8437.

KYNE, William P.; 200 St. Clair Ave. W., Toronto 7, Ont.; 221 Riverside Dr., (res); National U. (Galway, Ire.) '51; B.A.O., D.Psy; Psy; Active Staff & Admin. Psy. Unit, St. Joseph's Hosp.; Tel. WA 5-6282.

LABARRE, Gillies; 75 St. Jean Baptiste, Chateauguay, P.Q.; Mon '60.

LABBE, Paul; 1500-18e rue, Quebec 3, P.Q.; Lav'49; FACS; FRCS(C); GenSurg; Ass't. Surg., Laval U.

LABBE, Pierre; 5612 Ave. Canterbury, Montreal, P.Q.; Mon '53; Psy (P.Q.).

L'ABBE, Robert; 11799 de Tracy, Montreal 9, P.Q. (res); Mon '51; D & T Rad; Hd. (Rad.), Hop.-Gen. Fleury & Hop. Notre-Dame-de-la-Merci; Ass't. Prof. (Rad.), U. of Mtl.; Tel. DU 1-6235; 331-2320.

LABELLE, Andre; App. 2, 4575 St. Kevin, Montreal 26, P.Q.; Mon'51; Tel. 342-9277.

LABELLE, Arthur R.; 964 Cherrier, Montreal 24, P.Q.; McG '51; OphthOtol (P.Q.).; Tel. 525-0215.

LABELLE, Avila; 92 St. Andre, St. Remi, Napierville, P.Q.; Lav '18.

LABELLE, Bernard; 222 Eramosa Rd., Guelph, Ont.; Tor'37; MCGP; Staff, St. Joseph's & Guelph Gen. Hosp's.

LABELLE, Claude; Mont-Laurier, Cte. Labelle, P.Q.; Lav '58.

LABELLE, Emilien; 45 Kelvin Ave., Outremont, Montreal 8, P.Q.; Mon'48; Med. Dir., Hop. Gen. Fleury; Tel. 381-9311.

LABELLE, Jacquelin; Clinique Lachapelle rue Madone, Mont Laurier, P.Q.; Lav'65.

LABELLE, M. H. Suzanne; Ott'64; Res., Hop. du Sacre-Coeur, Hull, P.Q.; Abroad.

LABELLE, Paul E.; 24 Blvd. Montclair, Hull, P.Q.; Mon '41.

LABELLE, Pierre F.; Mon'65; Res., Hop. Maisonneuve, Montreal 36, P.Q.

LABELLE, Pierre H.; 32 ouest Blvd. St. Joseph, Montreal 14, P.Q.; 850 Lapointe, Ville, Ville St. Laurent (res); Mon' 47; F.R.C.S.(C) OrthSurg; Staff, Orth. Surg., & Cerebral Paralysis Clinic, Hop. Ste. Justine; Memb. Med. Staff. Victor Doré Children's Infirmary; Memb., Med. Comm., Cerebral Paralysis, Prov. of Quebec; Tel. VI 2-9418.

LABERGE, Claude; Lav'62; Res., Hop. Hotel-Dieu, Quebec 4, P.Q.

LABERGE, Denis; 175 Doody, Chambly, P.Q.; Mon'65.

LABERGE, Edouard; 4104 rue St. Jacques W., Montreal 30, P.Q.; 7150 rue Hurteau (res); Mon '43; Paed (P.Q.).; Tel. 935-4330.

LABERGE, Ivan; 1656 est Sherbrooke, Montreal 24, P.Q.; 3500 Ridgewood, Mtl. 26 (res); Mon '49; FRCS(C), Urol; Ass't. Urol., Hop. Notre-Dame & Hop. Ste. Justine; Tel. 526-3783.

LABERGE, J. Roger; 7 Bell, Chateauguay Centre, P.Q.; Mon '63; Tel. 691-1353.

LABERGE, Jules; 91 Ave. Brittany, Montreal 16, P.Q.; (res); Mon '47; D&T Rad; Dir. (Rad.), Hop. Maisonneuve; Chief, Dept. of Rad., Inst. de Cardiol; Tel. 254-8341.

LABERGE, Lassale; 635 Quebec, Sherbrooke, P.Q. (res); Mon '24; F.C.C.P., Pulm. Dis. & TB (P.Q.); Med. Dir., San. St. Francois, Sherbrooke; Tel. LO 9-2551. Retired.

LABERGE, L. Philippe; Ott'59; Res. (Anaes.), Montreal Neurological Inst., Montreal, P.Q.

LABERGE, Marie-Jean; 5757 Blvd. Rosemont, Montreal 36, P.Q.; 2 Plateau Belmont Ave., Repentigny, Co. L'Assomption (res); Mon '51; Pulm. Dis. & TB (P.Q.); Staff, Institut Lavoisier, Hop. Maisonneuve, Verdun Gen. Hosp., Montreal, & Sacred Heart Hosp., Cartierville; Tel. 256-7885.

LABERGE, Martin; 65 Grande Allee E., Quebec 6, P.Q.; 820 Ave. des Erables (res); Lav '51; GenSurg (P.Q.); Staff (Surg.), Hop. Hotel-Dieu & Laval U.; Tel. 529-9691.

LABERGE, Pierre; Lav'60; Psy(P Q.); Staff, Albert Prevost Inst., Cartierville, Montreal, P.Q.

LABERGE, Raymond; Centre Medicale, 750 St. Vallier Ouest, Quebec, P.Q.; 756 St. Vallier Ouest (res); Lav'44; Tel. 527-3748.

LABERGE-NADEAU, Claire; 43 Springrove Cres., Montreal 8, P.Q.; Mon '54; Asst. Med. Dir., Hop. Ste-Justine; Tel. RE 1-4931.

LABOSSIERE, Marcel; 222 Henri Bourassa E., Montreal 12, P.Q.; Mon '49; Pulm. Dis. & TB (P.Q.); Tel. DU 7-4551.

LABOSSIERE, Sylvio D.; 64 rue Wilfrid, Valleyfield, P.Q.; '48; M.C.G.P.; Med. Staff, Hop. Hotel-Dieu de Valleyfield; Tel. 373-4622.

LABRANCHE, Dorian A.; 15 rue Gill, Granby, P.Q.; 23 Chapleau (res); Mon '63; Tel. FR 2-2133.

LABRECQUE, Andre; Lav '59; Anaes; Staff, Hop. St.-Francois-d'Assise, Quebec, P.Q.; Tel. 529-7311.

LABRECQUE, Benoit; 3015 Chemin St. Louis, Quebec 10, P.Q. (res); Mon '44; Staff, Dept. of Health, Prov. of P.Q.; Tel. VI 9-9371.

LABRECQUE, Benoit; Mon'55; FRCP(C), Anaes; Staff, Hop. Hotel-Dieu, Montreal 18, P.Q.

LABRECQUE, Claude; 5575 Notre-Dame-de-Grace, Montreal 28, P.Q.; Mon'51; Staff, Dept. of Health, City of Montreal.

LABRECQUE, Francois; 892 St. Cyrille, Quebec, P.Q. (res); Lav '24; D.Hyg.; Retired.

LABRECQUE, Jean P.; 3840 St. Urbain, Montreal, P.Q.; Mon'48; Psy(P.Q.); Tel. VI 4-0161.

LABRECQUE, J. Emile; 2159 Bois-Joli, Sillery, P.Q. (res); Lav '44; F.C.C.P.; Pulm. Dis. & TB (P.Q.); Supt. Quebec Immigration Hosp.; Staff, Laval U.

LABRECQUE, Martin; 2980 Ave. Royale, Giffard, **Quebec 5, P.Q.; Lav '58; Tel. 661-4543.**

LABRECQUE, Paul; 3423, St.-Denis, Montreal 18, P.Q.; Lav '35; GenSurg; Tel. VI 2-4892.

LABRECQUE, Raymond; 383 Blvd. St. Joseph E., Montreal 14, P.Q.; Mon '38; Paed; Med. Dir., Hop-Ste-Justine; Tel. RE 1-4931.

LABRIE, Eudore; Grindstone, Iles-de-la-Madeleine, P.Q.; Lav '48; M.C.G.P.

LABRIE, Gerard; 870 rue Holland, Quebec, P.Q.; **Lav '28; Tel. 527-3815.**

LABRIE, Henri; Clinique Medico-Chirurgical, 2775 rue Bourdages, St-Hyacinthe, P.Q.; 2755 rue Bourdages (res); Lav '46; GenSurg (P.Q.); Tel. PR 4-4818.

LABRIE, Jacques M.; Lav'60; Psy; Staff, Hop. St.-Michel-Archange, Quebec, P.Q.

LABROSSE, Claude; Lav'57; Res., Hop. St-Luc, Montreal 18, P.Q.

LABUN, Clarence H.; Man '60; Res., University Hosp., Edmonton, Alta.

LACASSE, Fernand; Batiscan, P.Q.; Lav '48.

LACASSE, Jean; 228 rue Longueil, Iberville, P.Q.; Lav'54; Anaes.; Tel. 347-3677.

LACASSE, Paul H., Major; 1 Field Ambulance, RCAMC, CFPO 5050, CAF, Europe; Lav'60; Abroad.

LACASSE, Yves P.; Mon'65; Res., Hop. St-Luc, Montreal 18, P.Q.;

LACERTE, Jean; 34 Fabrique, Quebec, P.Q.; 1130 Ave. du Parc (res); Lav '29; F.R.C.S.(C) Ophth Otol; Chief, Dept. of Ophth., Hop. Hotel **Dieu; Prof. (Ophth.), Laval U.; Tel. 524-1786.**

LACERTE, Jean-Francois; Lav'64; Res., Montreal Gen. Hosp., Montreal 25, P.Q.

LACERTE, Marc; 275 Racine, Arvida, P.Q.; Lav '51; Industrial Phys., Aluminum Co. of Can.

LACERTE, Marcel; Centre Med. St. Vallier, 750 ouest St. Vallier, P.Q.; Lav'57; IntMed (Gastroent.) (P.Q.); Staff, Hop. Christ-Roi; Tel. 681-8220.

LACHAINE, Georges A.; 55 Ave de l'Eglise, Verdun, Montreal 19, P.Q.; 277 Beatty, Verdun (res); Mon'41; IntMed(P.Q.); Cardiol(P.Q.); Cardiol., Hop. Gen de Verdun; Tel. 768-5532.

LACHANCE, Claude R.; 26 rue Metcalfe, Sherbrooke, P.Q.; Mon'60.

LACHANCE, Jean C.; Centre Medica de Chicoutimi, **1508 ouest rue Price, Chicoutimi, P.Q.;** Lav '58; A.M.C.G.P.

LACHANCE, Jean Y.; 1384 Jean-Talon E., Montreal 10, P.Q.; 10788 Berri (res); Lav '57; M.C.-G.P.; Tel. 274-5583.

LACHANCE, J. Willie; 2 Eglise, St-Romuald, Cte Levis, P.Q.; Lav'44; MCGP.

LACHANCE, Marc; 1375 Notre Dame, Lachine, P.Q.; 3740 St. Joseph (res); Lav '40; GenSurg **(P.Q.); Pres., Med. Bureau, St. Joseph's Hosp.; Tel. 637-3088.**

LACHANCE, Paul; 3525 Aylmer, Montreal 18, P.Q.; Lav '55; D&TRad; Radiol., Royal Victoria Hosp.; Tel. VI 2-1251.

LACHANCE, Paul A.; 77 Charles Martin, Quebec, P.Q.; Lav '55; F.R.C.P.(C), PhysMed. & Rehab.; Staff, Hop.-St-Sacrement; Tel. LA 7-3461.

LACHANCE, Pierre A.; 31 ouest King, Sherbrooke, P.Q.; Lav '61.

LACHANCE, Pierre M.; Ste. 306, 825 Belvedere Sud, Sherbrooke, P.Q.; Lav'61; FRCP(C), Derm.

LACHANCE, Robert; 50 ave. de-l'Eglise, Verdun, Montreal 19, P.Q.; 3782 ave. Vendome, Mtl. 28 (res); Mon '34; FACP; FAGS; IntMed; Staff, Hop. Gen.-du-Christ-Roi; Tel. 769-3331.

LACHANCE, Robert R.; 5000 Boul. Perras, Montreal 39, P.Q.; Mon '60; A.M.C.G.P.; Tel. 323-1535.

LACHANCE, Roch; St. Damien, Co. Bellechasse, P.Q.; Lav '52.

LACHANCE, Roger; 440 sud Notre-Dame, Champlain, P.Q.; Lav'48; Staff, Hop. Cloutier, Cap. de la Madeleine; Tel. 295-3411.

LACHANCE, Roger; Lav '41; FACCP; Pulm. Dis. & TB (P.Q.); Med. Dir., Hop. du Sacre-Coeur, 230 boul. Gamelin, Hull, P.Q.; Tel. PR 7-2721.

LACHANCE, Roger; Lav '63; Res., Montreal Children's Hosp., Montreal 25, P.Q.; Abroad.

LACHANCE, Valere L.; 916 rue Hebert, Desbiens, Lac-St-Jean, P.Q.; Lav '64; Tel. 346-5443.

LACHANCE, Wilfrid; Chemin Sydenham, Chicoutimi, P.Q. (res); Lav '36; Haem (P.Q.); Path-Bact; Dir. of Labs., Hop. Hotel-Dieu St. Vallier, Chicoutimi; Staff, Laval U.; Tel. 549-1452.

LACHAPELLE, Georges; Mont Laurier, P.Q.; Ott '45.

LACHAPELLE, Pauline; Mont Laurier, P.Q.; Lav '44.

LACHARITE, Herve; 205 Centre-Medical St.-Urbain, 3875 rue St.-Urbain, Montreal 18, P.Q.; 47 Granville Rd., Hampstead (res); Mon '23; DMRI (Paris & Cambridge); PhysMed (P.Q.); D & TRad; Dir. (Rad.), Hop. St.-Michel, Mtl. & Hop. St.-Charles, St.-Hyacinthe; Assoc. Rad., Jewish Gen. Hosp. Mtl.; Tel. RA 2-2571.

LACKEY, Allison W.; McG'62; Res., New Mount Sinai Hosp., Toronto, Ont.

LACKNER, H. Allister; 86 Queen St. N., Kitchener, Ont.; Tor'34; FACS; GenSurg; Surg.-in-Chief, St. Mary's Hosp.; Tel. 743-1451.

LACKNER, H. John; Tor'63; Res., Sunnybrook Hosp., Toronto 12, Ont.

LACKEY, Arthur A.; 592 Victoria Ave., St. Lambert, Cite Jacques Cartier, P.Q.; 429 Wickham St. (res); McG '55; Tel. OR 1-1661.

LACNY, Jan; Edin. (Scot.) '48; Phys., Saskatchewan Training School, Moose Jaw, Sask.; Tel. 692-6491.

LACOMBE, Henry; Taschereau, P.Q.; Lav '49; Dist. Coroner; Tel. 796-3333.

LACOMBE, Michel; 1150 E. Boul. St-Joseph, Montreal 34, P.Q.; Mon '55; Haem (P.Q.); F.R.C.P.(C), IntMed; Tel. LA 7-1241.

LACOURCIERE, Helen; Ott'64; Staff, Frobisher Gen. Hosp., Frobisher Bay, N.W.T.

LACOURCIERE, Victor; La Malbaie, Charlevoix, P.Q.; Lav '34.

LACOURCIERE, Yves; Rue Baril, Warwick Cte., Arthabaska, P.Q.; Lav'65.

LACOURSE, Marcel; 12 rue Champagne, Landraie, Cté Berthier, P.Q.; Lav'65.

LACOURSIERE, A.; 142 Champlain, Hull P.Q.; Mon '40.

LACOURSIERE, Jean-Pierre; Lav '64; Res., Hop. Sacre-Coeur, Montreal 9,P.Q.

La CROIX, E. Bertin; Lameque, Gloucester Co., N.B.; Lav '56; Med. Supt. & Chief of Med., Hotel-Dieu St-Joseph; Tel. 344-2250.

LACROIX, Jean P.; 12470 Notre Dame E., Pointe -aux-Trembles, Montreal 5, P.Q.; Mon '54; M.C.-G.P.; Tel. 645-3635.

LACROIX, John R.; Medical Centre, Kapuskasing, Ont.; Man'38; GenSurg; Staff, Sensenbrenner Hosp.

LACROIX, J. Rheal; 274 Friel, Ottawa 2, Ont.; Ott '59; MCGP.

LACROIX, Paul; 2934 de la Promenade, Quebec 10, P.Q.; Lav '35; MCGP; Phys., St. Lawrence Co-op.

LACROIX, Raymond; 309 Renaud, St. Eustache, P.Q.; Mon '60.

LACROIX, Real; 152 St. Louis St., Terrebonne, **P.Q.; Mon '51; Tel. 666-3007.**

LACROIX, William R.; 250 Lawrence Ave. W., Toronto 12, Ont.; 9 Steele Valley Rd., Thornhill (res); Man '44; DiagRad; Radiol., York Co. Hosp., Newmarket; Tel. RU 7-0229.

LACY, Edward; 2489 Bloor St. W., Toronto 9, Ont.; 351 Dickson Park Cr., Cooksville (res); National U. (Ire.) '47; MRCOG; FRCS(C); MAO; ObstGyn; Cons. ObstGyn., St. Joseph's Hosp.; Tel. 766-1030.

LADOUCEUR-DUPUIS, Paule — see **DUPUIS, Paule.**

LADOUCEUR, Ernest C.; 10 Elm Ave., Amherstburg, Ont.; 502 Sandwich St. (res); Wes '35; Tel. 736-4241.

LADOUCEUR, Frederic; Casselman, Ont.; McG '19.; Tel. 38.

LADOUCEUR, Jacques; 175 Doody, Chambly, P.Q.; Mon'65.

LADOUCEUR, Joseph H. C.; 559 King Edward Ave., Ottawa 2, Ont.; 351 Summit (res); **Lav '48; ObstGyn.; Tel. 235-5956.**

LADOUCEUR, Leo; 574 McEachran, Montreal, **P.Q.; 305 est Mt. Royal (res); Mon '23.; Tel. 274-3204.**

LAEVENS, Leslie V.; 216-3rd Ave., Kamsack, Sask.; 1000 Boulevard (res); Man '48; MCGP; Tel. 542-2251.

LAFARGA, Angel M.; Zaragoza (Spain) '53; Path; Staff, Trenton Mem. Hosp., Trenton, Ont.; Tel. 392-3526.

LAFAVE, Hugh G.; Box 1056, Weyburn, Sask.; McG '53; DABPN; Sup., Saskatchewan Hosp.; Tel. 842-5461; Abroad.

LAFAVE, Wallace John; Suite 230, 5300 Cote des Neiges Rd., Montreal 26, P.Q.; 1705 Caledonia Rd., Town of Mt. Royal (res); McG'35; FICS, ObstGyn (P.Q.); **Staff (ObstGyn.), St. Mary's Hosp.; Tel. RE 3-1851.**

LAFERRIERE, Jacques; Mon'65; Res., Hop Hotel-Dieu, Montreal 18, P.Q.

LAFERRIERE, Real; Staff, Hop. Sacre Coeur, Hull, P.Q.; Lav '51; D&TRad.; Tel. 777-2721.

LAFERRIERE, Ronald; 11900 ave Salk, Montreal Nord, P.Q.; Mon '59.

LAFERRIERE, Ulysse; Unite Sanitaire, 181 Champlaine & 1121 Frontenac, Berthierville, P.Q.; 269 Montcalm (res); Mon'35; D.P.H., PH (P.Q.); M.O.H., Co. of Berthier; Tel. 836-4422 & 836-4356.

LAFLAMME, A. Maurice; Lav '57; Res., Hop. St. Sacrement, Quebec 6, P.Q.

LAFLAMME, Charles; 505 Grande Allee E., Quebec, P.Q.; 1130 ave de la Tour (res); Lav '30; IntMed; Med. Dir., Inst. St. Joseph de la Deliverance; Phys. to Local Ins. & Indust. Co's.; Tel. 522-8069.

LAFLAMME, Denis; Lav'61; OrthSurg(P.Q.); Staff, Hop. Sacre-Coeur, Montreal 9, P.Q.

LAFLAMME, Henri; 556 Iere rue, Iberville, P.Q.; Mon'29; IntMed; Med. Cons., Hop. St. Jean, St. Jean, P.Q.; Tel. 346-3633.

LAFLAMME, Jacques; 505 Grande-Allee Est., Quebec 4, P.Q.; Lav'62.

LAFLAMME, Jean; Mon '63; Res., Hop. Notre-Dame, Montreal, P.Q.

LAFLAMME, Louis-Emile K.; 700, ave. Laurier, Sept-Iles, P.Q.; Lav '53; Quarantine Officer & Phys. to Sick Mariners; M.O.H., Sept-Iles.

LAFLAMME, Pierre; Mon'65; Res., Hop. Hotel-Dieu, Montreal 18, P.Q.

LAFLAMME, Michel; Mon'65; Staff, Hop. Manic 5, Manicouagan, P.Q.

LAFLAMME, Raymond; 505 Grande-Allee E., Quebec 4, P.Q.; 1334 de-Repentigny, (res); Lav '56; DIH; FRCP(C), IntMed; Tel. 522-8069.

LAFLECHE, Francois, Lt/Col.; McG'53; OrthSurg(P.Q.); Staff, Cdn. Forces Hosp., Kingston, Ont.

LAFLECHE, J. Georges M.; 720 Sherbrook, Winnipeg, Man; Lav '21; MCGP; Tel. SP 4-2170.

LA FLECHE, Leo R.; 625 Rockland Rd., Montreal 16, P.Q.; McG'50; ThorSurg; GenSurg (P.Q.); Att'd. Surg., Hop. Notre-Dame & Cons. Surg., Inst. Bruchesi; Cons. (Thor. & Cardiovasc.), Hotel-Dieu, St. Jerome.

LAFLECHE, Magloire; Box 548, Senneterre, Co. Abitibi E., P.Q.; Lav '51.

LAFLEUR, Francois; 1560 est Sherbrooke, Montreal, P.Q.; 440 Curzon, St. Lambert (res); Mon '50; Anaes; Staff, Hop. Notre-Dame; Tel. LA 5-6363.

LAFLEUR, Henri; 20 Brebeuf Sorel, P.Q. (res) Mon'40; Anaes. (P.Q.); Med. Dir., Marine Industries, Sorel, P.Q.; Tel. RI 3-3586.
LAFLEUR, Jean; 150 Boul. Salaberry, Chateauguay, P.Q.; Mon '54.
LAFLEUR, J. Claude; St.-Apollinaire, Cte. Lotbiniere, P.Q.; Lav '62.; Tel. 269-4333.
LAFLEUR, Lionel; 1420 Redpath Cres., Montreal 25, P.Q. (res); Mon '41; D&TRad (P.Q.); Staff, St. Joseph's Hosp.; Tel. 637-2351.
LAFLEUR, Lucette; Mon '60; FRCP(C), Bact; Hop. Ste.-Justine, Montreal 26, P.Q. Tel. RE 1-4931.
LAFLEUR, Richard; Ott'64; Res., Royal Victoria Hosp., Montreal 2, P.Q.
LAFOND, Andre; 1259 Hart St., Trois Rivieres, P.Q.; Lav '54; F.R.C.P.(C), IntMed.; Tel. FR 5-5769.
LAFOND-LETARTE, C. Therese; 2753 Valcourt, Ste. Foy, Quebec 10, P.Q.; Lav '57.
LAFOND, Guy; 12245 Grenet, Montreal, P.Q.; 5475 Place D'Aiguillon (res); Lav'46; FRCS(C) OrthSurg; Ass't. Staff (Orth.), Hop. du Sacre-Coeur; Tel. WE 2-3113.
LAFOND, Jean J.; Mon'54; Res., Hop. Notre-Dame, Montreal 24, P.Q.
LAFOND, Jean R.; 535 Mondor Ave., St. Hyacinthe, P.Q.; Par. Douville (res); Lav '38; Tel. PR 4-7844.
LAFOND, Jean Y.; 529 Notre Dame Ave., Sudbury, Ont.; Lav '58; Tel. 674-7361.
LAFOND, Real; 138 Brooks S., Sherbrooke, P.Q.; 1499 Desjardins (res); Lav '41; ObstGyn (P.Q.); Tel. 562-1101.
LAFONTAINE, Guy; 400, Boul. Ste.-Madeleine, Cap-de-la-Madeleine, P.Q.; Lav '63; Tel. FR 5-2788.
LAFONTAINE, Raymond; Ste. 233, 5757 Decelles Ave., Montreal 26, P.Q.; Mon'54 Neur(P.Q; Neurol., Hop. Ste-Justine; Staff, Faculty of Med. & Fac. of Science Education, U. of Montreal & U. of Sherbrooke; Tel. 739-5633.
LAFOREST, Berchmans; 12245 Grenet, Montreal 9, P.Q.; 2325 Nicholas Perrot (res); Mon'48; FRCS(C); ObstGyn; Chief-of-Service (Gyn.), Hop. Sacre-Coeur, Cartierville; Tel. 381-2421.
LAFOREST, Marc G.; 20 Ave. Du Quai, Montmagny, P Q.; Lav'60; IntMed(P.Q.).
LAFOREST, Raymond A.; Ste. G05, 3000 Lawrence Ave. E., Scarborough, Ont.; 5 Burnview Cres. (res); Ott'53; Paed; Chief, Dept. of Paed., Scarborough Gen. Hosp.; Tel. 291-1117.
LAFORTUNE, Claude; 489 rue Ste.-Anne, Joliette, P.Q.; 422 Manseau (res); Mon '55; FRCS(C), GenSurg; Surg., Hop. St.-Eusebe & St. Charles; Tel. PL 6-8073.
LAFORTUNE, Gerard O.; 7312 Papineau Ave., Montreal, P.Q. (res); Mon '49; Anaes; Anaes., Hop. St. Luc; Tel. UN 1-7261.
LAFORTUNE, Jean G.; Mon '59; Res., Hop. Sacre-Coeur, Montreal 24, P.Q.
LAFORTUNE, Joseph A.; 422 Manseau St., Joliette, P.Q.; Mon '25; Anaes (P.Q.).
LAFORTUNE, J. Omer; 5505 Cote St. Antoine, Montreal, P.Q.; Mon '29; M.C.G.P.
LAFORTUNE, Luc L.; 1150 St. Joseph Blvd. E., Montreal, P.Q.; 153 Pagnuelo Ave., Outremont (res); Mon '47; F.R.C.S.(C) GenSurg; Gen. Surg., Hop. Maisonneuve, Montreal; Tel. LA 7-1241.
LAFORTUNE, Marcel; 12 rue Beaudry, St-Jacques, Co. Montcalm, P.Q.; Mon '50; Tel. 839-2626.
LAFORTUNE, Paul E.; 2057 Dezery, Montreal, P.Q.; Mon '52.
LAFRAMBOISE, Georges E.; 95 Rideau St., Ottawa, Ont.; 16 Lakeview Ter. (res); Mon '23; Ophth, Otol; Act. Staff, Ottawa Gen. Hosp.; Cons., Hop. St. Louis-Marie de Montfort; Clin. Instr., Ottawa U.; Tel. CE 3-6517.
LAFRAMBOISE, G. Guy; 225 Metcalfe St., Ottawa 4, Ont.; Ott '54; FRCS(C), Otol; Acting Chief, Dept. of Otol., Ottawa Gen. Hosp.; Cons., Tri Service Hosp. & Sacred Heart Hosp., Hull; Hon. Cons., Ottawa Civic Hosp.; Memb. Cdn. Otol. Soc.; Lect. (Otol.), U. of Ottawa; Memb., American Rhinol. Soc.; Ass't. Sec., Ottawa Academy of Med.; Tel. 237-0971 & 237-0972.
LAFRAMBOISE, Jean B. E.; 692 St. Patrice St., Ottawa, Ont.; 249 River Rd., Eastview (res); Lav '49; F.R.C.S.(C), GenSurg; Surg., Hop. St. Louis-Marie-de-Montfort; Clin. Ass't (Surg.), U. of Ottawa; Tel. CE 4-2636.
LAFRANCE, Charles E.; 247 est rue Main, Hawkesbury, Ont.; Mon '30; MCGP.
LAFRANCE, J. Romeo; 3817 Boul. Decarrie, Montreal 18. P.Q.; Lav'57; FRCS(C), Gen-Surg; Staff, Hop. St. Luc; Ass't. Prof., U. of Montreal; Tel. 521-8585.
LAFRANCE, W. Andre; 5124 Cadillac, Montreal 5, P.Q.; Ott'61; Derm.
LAFRENIERE, Jean; 875 des-Recollets, Trois Rivieres, P.Q.; Lav '54; ObstGyn.; Tel. FR 6-6690.
LAFRENIERE, Rene; Thurso, P.Q.; Lav '49; Phys., Pulp & Paper Co. & Singer Mfg. Co.
LAFRENTIERE, Robert E.; Ste.-Anne, Man.; Lav'56; MCGP; Tel. GA 2-5377.
LAGACE, Gilles; 513 Ste-Cecile, Trois Rivieres, P.Q.; Lav'65.
LAGACE, Rene; 4399 ave. Bannantyne, Montreal 19, P.Q.; Mon '50; MCGP; Inspect. Hygiene, Catholic Schls. of Verdun.
LAGACE, Vincent; 18 O'Leary, Campbellton, N.B.; Lav'55; OrthSurg(P.Q.).
LAGARDE, Jean P.; 7229 St. Denis, Montreal, P.Q. (res); Mon '49; Pulm. Dis. & TB (P.Q.); Staff, Med., Hop. Sacre Coeur, Cartierville, & Hop. Ste. Jeanne d'Arc, Montreal.; Tel. VI 2-5201.
LAGASSE, Philippe; 150 King W., Sherbrooke, P.Q.; 434 rue Quebec (res); Mon '43; Urol; Chief, Dept. Urol., St. Vincent de Paul Gen. Hosp.; Tel. LO 9-6381.
LAGER, Louis H.; 188 Giles Blvd. E., Windsor, Ont.; 1529 Victoria Ave. (res); Wes '42; FACA; Tel. 254-4501.
LAGUE, Paul A.; Ste. Madeleine, Co. St. Hyacinthe, P.Q.; Mon '45; M.C.G.P.; Med. Dir., Foyer Dieppe, St. Hilaire; Tel. 795-3313.
LAHAI, E. Maurice; 4391 St.-Hubert, Montreal 34, P.Q.; Lav '28; Phys., Cdn. Celanese Ltee.
LAHAISE-LEVESQUE, Francois D.; App. 1, 3270 E. rue Sherbrooke, Montreal 4, P.Q.; Lav'57; Psy; Staff, Hop. Ste Justine.
LAHAY, W. Douglas; UBC'57; Res., Shaughnessy Hosp., Vancouver, B.C.
LAI, Suke-Yen; 108 Lagauchetiere W., Montreal, P.Q.; Canton (China) '52; GenSurg.
LAIDLAW, Campbell; 608 Parkview Rd., Ottawa, Ont.; Qns '07; F.R.C.P.(C); Retired.
LAIDLAW, James H.; 60 Stanley Ave., Ottawa 2, Ont.; Qns '03; F.R.C.P.(C), PathBact; Retired.
LAIDLAW, John C.; 101 College St., Toronto, Ont.; 36 Hudson Dr. (res); Tor '44; Ph.D. (Lond.); F.R.C.P.(C), IntMed; Assoc. Prof. of Med., U. of Toronto; Sr. Phys., and Dir. Clin. Invest Unit, Toronto Gen. Hosp.; Tel. EM 6-8211.
LAIDLAW, Robert A.; Rm. 428, Vancouver Bld., 736 Granville, Vancouver 2, B.C.; 2049 W-59th. Ave. (res); Man '49; Vis. Staff, St. Paul's, Vancouver Gen., St. Vincent's, Grace, & Burnaby Gen. Hosp's.; Tel. MU 3-2221.
LAIDLAW, Robert G.; Manotick, P.O., Ont. (res); Qns '37; Psy., Civil Service Health Div., Dept. of Natl. Health & Welfare, Ottawa, Ont.
LAIDLAW, Thomas A.; 170 Fitzroy St., Charlottetown, P.E.I.; 48 Summer St. (res); Dal '41; F.R.C.S.(C), GenSurg; Att. Surg., Prince Edward Island San.; Chief of Staff, P.E.I. Hosp.; Tel. 894-7325.
LAIDLAW, William R.; 703 Danforth Ave., Toronto, Ont.; 13 Burnham Rd., Tor 17 (res); Tor '50; Psy; Psy., Mental Health Clinic for Leaside & East York; Tel 466-5544.
LAILEY, Whitney W.; 324 Spadina Rd., Toronto 4, Ont.; Tor '08; FACS; Tel. WA 3-3488.
LAIMON, Harold; 510 Fairmont Med. Bldg., 750 W. Broadway, Vancouver 9, B.C.; 6968 Ash, Van. 14 (res); McG '53; FRCS(C); GenSurg; Vis. Staff, Vancouver Gen., St. Paul's, St. Vincent's & Children's Hosp's.; Tel. TR 9-5791.

LAINE, C. Antoine; Ste. Rose du Degelis, Temiscouata, P.Q.; Lav '32; Sec., Med. Staff & Staff, Hop. Notre Dame du Detour, Notre Dame du Lac.
LAING, Charles A.; 589 Pelissier St., Windsor, Ont.; 826 Argyle Rd. (res); McG '52; M.Sc., D.S., FACS; FRCS(C), GenSurg; Chief Surg., IODE Mem. Hosp.; Tel. CL 6-2158.
LAING, Iain M.; 513 Med. Arts Bldg., 404-406 Graham Ave., Winnipeg 1, Man.; Aberdeen (Scot.)'51; GenSurg.; Tel. 837-4323.
LAING, Lorne P.; 179 Courtleigh Blvd., Toronto 12, Ont. (Res.); Tor'51; MCGP; Active Staff, O.P.D., Wellesley Hosp., Toronto, Ont.; Teach. Staff, U. of Toronto.
LAING, Ronald R.; Ottawa St. W., South River, Ont.; Loma Linda U. (Calif., U.S.A.) '54; Hon. Cons., Branson Hosp., Willowdale; Active Staff, Red Cross Hosp., Burk's Falls; Tel. 386-2331.
LAING, Richard; 1414 Drummond St., Montreal 25, P.Q.; 456 Strathcona Ave. (res); McG'42; DIM; FCCP; IntMed; Att'd. Staff, Mtl. Gen. Hosp.; Dem. Med., McGill U.; Tel. AV 8-3900.
LAING, W. Bruce; 818-9th Ave. N., Port Alberni, B.C.; St. Andrew's (Scot.) '43; D.P.H.; Tel. 723-2111.
LAING, W. Vardy; 3344 36th Ave. S.W., Calgary, Alta. (Res.); McG'40; MCGP; Staff, Colonel Belcher Hosp., Calgary, Alta.; Sr. Pension Med. Examiner.
LAIR, Remi H.; 167 St. Joseph, Hull, P.Q.; Lav '64.
LAIRD, Reginald R.; 4383 Erwin Dr., West Vancouver, B.C.; Qns'37; Retired.
LAIRD, Robert C.; 405 Toronto Western Medical Bldg., 25 Leonard Ave., Toronto 2B, Ont.; R.R.2, Woodbridge, Ont. (res); Tor '28; F.A.C.S.; F.R.-C.S. (Eng.); F.R.C.S.(C), GenSurg; OrthSurg; ThorSurg; Surg-in-Chief, Toronto Western Hosp.; Prof. of Surg., U. of Toronto; Tel. EM 6-1227.
LAJEUNESSE, Andre; Lav'60; FRCS(C), ObstGyn; Staff, Hop. Misericorde, Quebec 6, P.Q.
LAJEUNESSE, Claude; 116 Morissette, Loretteville, P.Q.; Lav '65.
LAJOIE, Gustave (See Gerin-Lajoie, Gustave).
LAJOIE, Jean L.; 1064 rue Michel-Moreau, Boucherville, P.Q. (res); Lav '57; Anaes; Staff, Hop. Ste.-Jeanne-d'Arc; Tel. 2-5201.
LAJOIE, Real, Capt.; Camp Shilo, Shilo, Man.; Lav'65; Staff, Shilo Military Hosp.; Tel. 765-2102.
LAJOS, Thomas Z.; 91 King St. E., Kingston, Ont.; Pecs (Hung.)'56; FRCS(C), GenSurg.
LAKE, John R.; 4349 E. Hastings, Burnaby 2, B.C.; Qns'65.
LAKEY, William H.; Ste. 241, University Hospital, Edmonton, Alta.; Alb'53; FACS; FRCS(C), Urol; Assoc. Prof. of Surg., U. of Alberta; Tel. 439-5911, Ext. 462.
LAKINS, Jill E.; Vulcan, Alta.; Leeds (Eng.)'59; D.ObstRCOG.
LAKINS, John P.; Vulcan, Alta.; Leeds (Eng.) '60.
LAL, Lakhan; Patna (India) FRCS(C), Otol; Staff, Montreal Gen. Hosp.; Tel. WE 7-6011.
LAL, Samarthji; London (Eng.) '62; Res., Queen Mary Vet's Hosp., Montreal 26, P.Q.
LALANCETTE, Ange M.; Lav '63; Sr. Int., Hop. Notre-Dame, Montreal 24, P.Q.
LALANDE, Emile; 6830 St. Denis St., Montreal, P.Q.; Mon '28.; Tel. 271-5863.
LALANDE, Eugene; Ville Marie, Co. Temiscamingue, P.Q., Mon '45; GenSurg.
LALANDE, Roger; 805 Henri Bourassa, Montreal, P.Q.; Mon '48.; Tel. DU 8-0737.
LALIBERTE, Albert; Lav '61; Res., Hop. Notre-Dame, Montreal 24, P.Q.
LALIBERTE, Benoit; 93 Belanger, Quebec, P.Q.; Lav '26.
LALIBERTE, Bruno; St. Celestin, P.Q.; Lav '47.
LALIBERTE, Chas.; 335 Ste. Foye Rd., Quebec 6, P.Q.; Cap Rouge (res.); Lav '51; IntMed.(P.Q.); Med. Staff, Hop. de l'Enfant Jesus; Prof. Pt.-time, Laval U.; Tel. 527-2444.
LALIBERTE, Jean; Fortierville, P.Q.; Lav '48.
LALIBERTE, Jean M.; St. Bernard, Cte. Dorchester, P.Q.; Lav'63; Tel. 253-4255.
LALIBERTE, J. Henri; 335 Chemin Ste-Foye, Quebec, P.Q.; Lav '19; IntMed (Cardiol.) (PQ); Vis. Phys. all Quebec Hosp's.; Semi-retired; Tel. 527-2444.
LALIBERTE, L. A.; 160 Ste.-Famille, Kenogami, P.Q.; Lav '52.
LALIBERTE, Lionel; Acton-Vale, Co. Bagot, P.Q.; Lav '42.
LALL, Hugh D.; Staff, Alberta Hosp., Ponoka, Alta.
L'ALLIER, P. Andre; St. Andre Est., Co. d'Argenteuil, P.Q.; Ott '57.
L'ALLIER, Pierre; Labelle P.Q.; Lav '57; A.M.-C.G.P.
L'ALLIER, Raymond A.; 8230 Champagneur, Montreal 15, P.Q.; Mon '53; Anaes; Staff, Hop. Hotel-Dieu.; Tel. VI 4-0161.
LALONDE, Alban J. G. H.; 360 Wellington St. W., Sault Ste. Marie, Ont.; Ott'49; GenSurg; Active Cons. Surg., Plummer Mem. & Gen. Hosp's.; Tel. AL 4-6421.
LALONDE, Charles E.; 1554 Ave. de L'Eglise, Montreal 20, P.Q.; Mon '33.; Tel. 768-6549.
LALONDE, Charles F.; 200 Adolphus St., Cornwall, Ont.; Ott'55; ObstGyn.
LALONDE, Jean-B.; 8415 rue St. Denis, **Montreal 11, P.Q.; 575 Ave. Davaar, Outremont (res); Lav '49; Cardiol (P.Q.); Tel. 381-5311.**
LALONDE, Jean L.; 12245 Grenet, Montreal 9, P.Q.; Mon'56; NeurSurg(P.Q.).
LALONDE, J. Leo; 169 Notre Dame, Hull, P.Q.; Mon. 22. Retired.
LALONDE, Real P.; 744 Avenue Royale, Beauport, P.Q. (res); Lav '45; Phys., Quarantine & Immigration Dept.; Tel. 522-7209.
LALONDE, Wilfrid; 33 Kindersley Ave., Montreal, P.Q.
LALOR, Terence P.; 2202 Dixie Rd., Port Credit, Ont. (res); Man '50; DiagRad; Chief, X-Ray Dept., South Peel Hosp., Cooksville; Tel. 277-2761.
LALOUETTE, Jacques M.; 240 McNabb St., Sault Ste. Marie, Ont.; London (Eng.)'59; MRCOG; ObstGyn.
LAM, Anthony K.; 122A-16th Ave. N.E., Calgary, Alta.; McG'62; MCGP; Pt.-time Quarantine M.O., Calgary International Airport; Tel. 277-6333.
LAM, Kwok C.; Box 760, Lake Cowichan, B.C.; UBC '61.; Tel. 749-6621. Abroad.
LAM, Sing P.; Whissell Clinic, Westlock, Alta.; Taiwan (Formosa)'60; IntMed.
LAMARCHE, Andre; 12450 Notre Dame E., Pointe-Aux-Trembles, Montreal 5, P.Q.; Mon '57; A.M.C.G.P.
LAMARCHE, Claude; Ste. Therese de Blainville, P.Q.; Lav '09.
LAMARCHE, Guy; 2943 Summerside, Ste-Foy, Quebec 10, P.Q. (res); Lav '52; Research, Laval U.
LAMARCHE, Jean; Mon '53; Res., Hop. Maisonneuve, Montreal 36, P.Q.
LAMARCHE, Louis; 2606 St. Jacques St. W., Montreal, P.Q.; Mon '25; Tel. WE 2-0566.
LAMARCHE, Yves; 2855 Gigault, Quebec 10, P.Q.; Lav '54; Anaes; Staff, Hop. Christ-Roi; Tel. MU 3-3607.
LAMARRE, Andre; Mon'65; Res., Hop. St-Justine, Montreal 26, P.Q.
LAMARRE, Charles J.; Lav'56; Psy; Teach. Staff, Dept. of Psy., University of Sherbrooke, Sherbrooke, P.Q.
LAMARRE, C. Jules; Lav '56; Res., Saskatchewan Hosp., North Battleford, Sask.
LAMARRE, Claude; 347 rue St. George, St-Jerome, P.Q.; Lav'58; FRCS(C); OrthSurg; Staff, Hotel-Dieu; Tel. GE 8-1792.
LAMARRE, Francois; 170 Guilbeault, Longueuil, Montreal 23, P.Q.; 150 St.-Laurent (res); Mon '48; Phys., Scott Clothing Co.; Tel. OR 4-9386.
LAMARRE, Gerard; 2521 Ste. Catherine Rd., Montreal, P.Q.; Mon '37; IntMed (P.Q.); Tel. RE 3-0986.
LAMARRE, Jean P.; C.P. 1025, 518 Wilson, Chibougamau, P.Q.; Lav '63.
LAMARRE, Leo; 423 Glengarry, Mont Royal, Montreal 16, P.Q.; Mon '47; Pulm. Dis. & TB (P.Q.); Phys., Hop. St. Joseph de Rosemont; Tel. 256-2681.

LAMARRE, Pierre; 80 Francois-Gauthier, Boucherville, P.Q.; Mon '62; Tel. OR 7-8880.
LAMARRE, Roger; 415 Ste-Helene, Longueuil, P.Q.; Mon '51; Tel. 674-8215.
LAMARRE, Suzanne; Lav'65; Res., Montreal Gen. Hosp., Montreal 25, P.Q.
LAMARRE, Yves; Mon '60; Research, U. of Montreal, Montreal, P.Q.
LAMB, Ewart R.; 5 Empress Ave., Hamilton, Ont.; 60 Inverness Ave. W. (res); Wes '43; MCGP; Staff G.P. Div., Chedoke Gen. & Hamilton Gen. Hosp's.; Tel. 383-8431.
LAMBERD, William G.; 2549 Pinewood Dr., Winnipeg 12, Man.; Liverpool (Eng.)'52; M.Sc. (Med.); Psy; Chief Psy. Serv., Deer Lodge Hosp.; Ass't. Prof. (Psy.), U. of Manitoba; Tel. 832-0270.
LAMBERT, Benoit; 29 Montcalm St., Hull, P.Q.; Lav '45; OphthOtol (P.Q.); Staff, Hop. du Sacre Coeur.; Tel. 777-2721.
LAMBERT, Bernard; 3875 St. Urbain, Ste. 501, Montreal 18, P.Q.; Mon '55; FRCS(C), ObstGyn; Ass't. Serv. (Gyn.), Hotel-Dieu Hosp.; Staff (ObstGyn.), U. of Montreal; Tel. 849-7260.
LAMBERT, Calvin S.; Box 129, Leoville, Sask.; London (Eng.)'43; LRCP; MRCS; Staff, Leoville Hosp.; District Coroner; Tel. 35.
LAMBERT, C. Andre, Capt.; Y Wing Infirmary, CFPO 5056, Belleville, Ont.; Lav'65.
LAMBERT, Dominique; 8750 Marjolaine, Montreal Nord, P.Q.; Lav'48; Ass't. Med. Dir., Hop. Notre-Dame; Tel. 525-6363.
LAMBERT, Edward H. N.; 48 Lakeshore Dr., Morrisburg, Ont.; Qns'50; Tel. KI 3-3124.
LAMBERT, Fernand; New Richmond, Cte. Bonaventure, P.Q.; Lav'65; Tel. 392-5351.
LAMBERT, Georges A.; 1027 Commerciale St. Romuald, P.Q.; Lav '45; Anaes (P.Q.).
LAMBERT, Harold F.; Med. Centre, 292 Oakdale Ave., St. Catharines, Ont.; Tor '35.
LAMBERT, Jacques; 239 boul. Deguire, App. 623, Ville St. Laurent, P.Q.; Mon'60; GenSurg.
LAMBERT, J. Adrien; 418 Sherbrooke E., Montreal, P. Q.; 465 Ave. Champagneur, Outremont (res); Mon '23; DermSyph; Derm., Hop. Notre-Dame; Ass't. Prof. Derm., U. of Montreal; Tel. VI 4-7661.
LAMBERT, Jean J., F/L; RCAF Station, St. Jean, P.Q.; Lille (France)'55.
LAMBERT, J. Jacques; 475 Wiseman Ave., Outre Montreal 8, P.Q.; Mon '45; Anaes.; Tel. 271-3162.
LAMBERT, Julien; Ste. 4, 1395 est, rue Fleury, Montreal 12, P.Q.; Mon'49; Pulm. Dis. (TB), (P.Q.); Staff, Hop.-du-Sacre-Coeur; Tel. FE 4-1210.
LAMBERT, Joseph; Rue St. Etienne, La Malbaie, Co. Charlevoix, P.Q.; Lav '46; M.C.G.P.; T.B. Clin.; Tel. MO 5-2366.
LAMBERT, J. Jules; 1643 de Bruyere, Quebec 10, P.Q.; Lav '52; Psy; Med. Sup., Hop. St. Michel Archange; Sec. Treas., Social Med. Centre for Children: Prof. (Psy.), Laval U.; Tel. 663-6373.
LAMBERT, Kenton G.; 85 South St., Goderich, Ont.; 53 North St. (res); McG '55; GenSurg; Staff, Alexandra Marine & Gen. Hosp.; Staff, Clinton Gen. Hosp., Clinton; Tel. 524-9183.
LAMBERT, Michel J.; 204 Blvd. Ste. Rose, Ste. Rose, Laval, P.Q.; Lav '28.
LAMBERT, Paul E.; 875 des Recollets, Trois Rivieres P.Q.; 898 rue Ste. Julie (res); Lav'46; Otol(P.Q.); Tel. FR 5-7323.
LAMBERT, Ralph C.; Birmingham (Eng.) '52; IntMed; Staff, Assiniboine Hosp., Brandon, Man.
LAMBERT, Richard; Medical Center, 238 S. Notre-Dame, Thetford Mines, P.Q.; 648 Alphonse (res); Lav '54; F.R.C.S.(C), GenSurg; Surg., Hop.-St.-Joseph; Tel. FE 8-1277.
LAMBERT, Suzanne; 2060 rue Mont-Thabor, Quebec 3, P.Q.; Bact(P.Q.).
LAMBERT, Yvan; 459 St. Dominique, Jonquiere, Co. Chicoutimi, P.Q.; Lav '45.
LAMBERTI, Armand J. D.; Ste. 206, 2211 Riverside Dr., Ottawa, Ont.; 151 Bayswater Ave. (res); Tor'45; DPH; Psy; Dir., In-Patient (Psy) & Staff Psy., (Child Psy. Div.), Ottawa Gen. Hosp.; Clin. Ass't. (Psy), U. of Ottawa; Tel. CE 4-5057.
LAMBERTI, Joseph W.; 1600 Wolseley Ave., Winnipeg, Man. (res); Ott '54; Psy; Staff, Psychopathic Hosp.; Lect., U. of Manitoba; Tel. SP 4-6511. Abroad.
LAMBERTSEN, Gudmundur; 1800 Logan Ave., Winnipeg, Man.; Man '48; Tel. SP 2-9453.
LAMBIE, Ronald S.; 416 Med. Arts Bldg., 404-406 Graham Ave., Winnipeg, Man.; Birmingham (Eng.)'52; D.A.(Eng.), M.R.C.S.(Eng.), L.R.C.P. (Lond.); D.A.B.M.H., F.A.C.A., F.I.C.S.; Anaes; Active Staff, St. Boniface Hosp.; Lect. (Dept. of Surg.), U. of Manitoba; Tel. GR 5-6377.
LAMBIN, Jacques; Lav'61; Res., Hop. Maisonneuve, Montreal, P.Q.
LAMBIN, Louise C.; Lav'65; Res., Hop. St. Sacrement, Quebec 6, P.Q.
LAMENSA, Francesco A.; '52; Res., Wellesley Hosp., Toronto 5, Ont.
LAMER, Laurent; Suite 510, 801 est rue Sherbrooke, Montreal 24, P.Q.; Mon '59; FRCS(C); Ophth.; Ass't. Ophth., Hop. Notre-Dame; Tel. 524-3049.
LAMON, Charles B.; 50 Franklin St., Brantford, Ont. (res); Tor '53; D.M.R.D.; DiagRad; Staff, Brantford Gen. Hosp.; Tel. 752-7871.
LAMOND, Donald E.; Abbott Clinic Bldg., Winnipeg, Man.; 531—2265 Portage Ave., St. James (res); Man '53.
LAMOND, William J.; Main St., Sydney Mines, N.S.; Shore Rd. (res); Dal '37; Sr. Staff, Harbour View Hosp., & Hamilton Mem. Hosp.
LAMONDE, Jean L.; 190 rue Wolfe, Levis, P.Q.; Mon'58; ObstGyn.
LAMONDE, Robert; 127A du Prince, Sorel, P.Q.; Lav '41; Tel. RI 3-6569.
LAMONDE, Robert; 94 rue Frontenac, Lac Megantic, P.Q.; Lav'65.
LAMONICA, Jean; 1230 McGregor, app. 402, Montreal 25, P.Q.; GenSurg(P.Q.).
LAMONT, Campbell T.; Elizabeth St., Thamesville, Ont.; Wes '46; M.C.G.P.; Active Staff, Public Gen. Hosp., Chatham.; Tel. 181.
LAMONT, David A.; Wes'63; Res., Victoria Hosp., London, Ont.
LAMONT, J. Archibald; 893 Main St. E., Hamilton, Ont.; 140 Sherman Ave. S. (res); Wes '24; M.C.G.P.; Staff, Convalescent Serv., Hamilton Gen. Hosp.; Tel. 527-0271.
LAMONT, Jean E.; Ste. 230, 4 Tachereau, Hull, P.Q.; 8 Cayer (res); Ott '55; Paed; Tel. 771-6867.
LAMONT, Keith A.; 1227 Johnston Rd., White Rock, B.C.; Man'56; DABS; FRCS(C), GenSurg.; Tel. 536-7121.
LAMONT, Kenneth G.; Wes'61; FRCS(C), ObstGyn; Staff, St. Joseph's Hosp., London, Ont.
LAMONT, Robert W.; Tor '63; Int., Sunnybrook Hosp., Toronto, Ont.
LAMONT, Thomas W. H.; 305 Nelson St., Wallaceburg, Ont.; 126 Margaret Ave. (res); Man '45; FRCS(Ed.); FRCS(C); GenSurg; Chief of Staff, Sydenham District Hosp.; Tel. 627-5932.
LAMONT, William E.; 893 Main St. E., Hamilton, Ont.; 222 Concession St., Apt. 401 (res); Wes '34; Obst; Hon. Cons. Staff, Henderson Gen. Hosp.; Tel. 544-3010 or 383-5655.
LAMONTAGNE, Armand; 394 La Canardiere, Quebec, P.Q.; Lav '46; Anaes (P.Q.).
LAMONTAGNE, Charles E.; Apt. 1, 1883 St. Marc, Shawinigan, P.Q.; 2233 Blvd. Royal, Apt. 2 (res); Lav'58; Tel. LE 6-2782.
LAMONTAGNE, Charles H.; 10610 rue Papineau, Montreal 12, P.Q.; Lav'46; Psy (P.Q.); Psy., Hop. Mont Providence; Tel. 387-9144.
LAMONTAGNE, Claude; 1000 Chemin Ste-Foy, Quebec 6, P.Q.; Lav '64; Tel. 681-0659.
LAMONTAGNE, Gerard; 750 St. Vallier ouest, Quebec 8, P.Q.; Lav'59.
LAMONTAGNE, Guy; 271 ouest, St.-Vallier, Quebec 8, P.Q.; Lav '62; Tel. 523-9217.
LAMONTAGNE, Horace; 517 Medical Arts Bldg., Winnipeg, Man.; McG '37.; Tel. WH 2-7339.
LAMONTAGNE, Jean M.; Lav '60; Otol; Staff, Clinque Pasteur, 770-lere Ave., Quebec 3, P.Q.; Tel. 529-0042.
LAMONTAGNE, Joseph; St. Apollinaire, P.Q.; Lav '32.

LAMONTAGNE, Joseph; St. Ferdinand d'Halifax, P.Q.; Lav '25; Med. Sup't., Hop. St. Julien.
LAMONTAGNE, J. Paul; 111 Eveche, Rimouski, P.Q.; Lav '52; Tel. 723-2777.
LAMONTAGNE, Langis; 298 rue St-Germain, Rimouski, P.Q.; Lav '50; GenSurg.; Tel. 723-2274.
LAMONTAGNE, Leon F/L.; Lav '64; Staff, Hop. Ste-Foy, Quebec 10, P.Q.
LAMONTAGNE, Raymond; Inst. de Cardiologie, 5000 est rue Belanger, Montreal 36, P.Q.; Mon'61; Cardiol(P.Q.).
LAMOS, Steven; 896 Erie St. E., Windsor, Ont.; Qns '62.
LAMOTHE, Armand; 25 St.-Jacques, Longueuil, Cite Jacques-Cartier, P.Q.; Lav '17; Obst(P.Q.); Obst. Clin., Ste-Jeanne-d'Arc Hosp.; Ass't. Prof. (Obst.), Montreal U.; Retired.
LAMOTHE, Francois; 1820 Blvd. St. Joseph, Apt. 10, Montreal, P.Q.; 270 Labonte, Longueuil (res); Mon '47; Staff, **Med. Clin. d'Urgence.**
LAMOTHE, Laurent; 31 Montcalm St., Hull, P.Q.; Qns '56; MCGP; Phys., Canada Packers.
LAMOTHE, Marcel; 580 rue Provost, Lachine, Montreal 32, P.Q.; **642-25th Ave. (res);** Mon '58; **AMCGP; Tel. 634-1691.**
LAMOUREUX, Andre; 351 rue Labelle, St-Jerome, P.Q. (res); Mon '56; DPH; Staff, Dept. of Health.
LAMOUREUX, Charles E.; 1005 St.-Prosper, Trois-Rivieres, P.Q.; 2995 Blvd.-du-Carmel (res); **Mon '38; D.A.B.O.S., F.R.C.S.(C), OrthSurg; Staff, Hop.-St. Joseph; Tel. 378-1272.**
LAMOUREUX, Christian; Mon'60; FRCP(C), Path; Staff, Hop.-Maisonneuve, Montreal, P.Q.
LAMOUREUX, Etienne; 3897 Ontario St. E., Montreal, P.Q.; Lav '07; Tel. 522-7722.
LAMOUREUX, Gilles; Lav'63; Res., Hosp. for Sick Children, Toronto 2, Ont.
LAMOUREUX, Jacques; Lav'61; PhD (Physiol); Staff, Hop. Notre-Dame, Montreal 24, P.Q.
LAMOUREUX, Joseph; 907 Royale St., Three Rivers, P.Q.; **1543 Blvd. des Forges (res);** Mon '22; Ophth, Otol.
LAMOUREUX, Julien; 565 Lindsay, Drummondville, P.Q.; Grantham W., Co. Drummond (res); Lav '42; P.H. (P.Q.); M.O.H., Dept. of Health, Quebec.
LAMOUREUX, Louis; 12150 James Morrice, Montreal 12, P.Q.; Mon '40; Anaes; Chief Anaes., **Hop.-Notre-Dame; Tel. LA 5-6363.**
LAMOUREUX, Marcel; 1150 St. Joseph Blvd. E., Montreal 34, P.Q.; 5 Springrove Cresc., Outremont (res); Mon '40; F.R.C.S.(C) GenSurg; Chief **Surg., Hop. Maisonneuve; Prof. & Hd., Dept. of** Surg., Montreal U.; Tel. LA 7-1241.
LAMPLUGH, Anthony N.; 180 Portland St., Dartmouth, N.S.; 289 Portland St. (res); London (Eng.) '52; A.M.C.G.P.
LAMPLUGH, Charles M.; 619 Brock St. S., Whitby, Ont.; St. Andrew's (Scot.)'61.
LAMQUIN, Roland; 5647 ave Canterbury, Mont**real, P.Q. (res); Mon '44.; Tel. 271-4834.**
LAMY, Fernand; 44 St-Andre, Metabetchouan, Cte Lac St-Jean, P.Q.; Lav '38; Dist. Coroner.
LAMY, Jean-Louis; 1150 est Blvd. St-Joseph, Montreal 34, P.Q.; Mon'51; FRCS(C), GenSurg; OrthSurg(P.Q.); Surg., Hop. Maisonneuve; Tel. LA 7-1241.
LAMY, J. Lionel; 278 Carre St. Louis, Montreal **18, P.Q.; 36 Ave. Beloeil, Outremont (res); Lav '16; Phys., Hotel-Dieu Hosp., Montreal.; Tel. VI 4-0161.**
LAMY, L. P. Rouville; 191 Brooks Sud, Sherbrooke, P.Q.; 217 Brooks Sud (res); Lav '35; Anaes; Anaes., Hop. St. Vincent de Paul.; Tel. LO 9-6381.
LAMY, Paul; Yamachiche, P.Q.; St. Anne (res); Lav '41.
LAMY, Romeo L.; Lav '29; Travelling Med. Off., C.N.R. Medical Clinic, **Montreal, P.Q.**
LANCTOT, Claude; McG '57; ObstGyn; Staff, Harvard School of Public Health, 55 Shattuck St., Boston, Mass., U.S.A. Abroad.
LANCTOT, Jean; 415 Ste Helene, Longueuil, P.Q.; Mon'65.

LAND, Harry D.; 390 Charlotte St., Sydney, N.S.; 65 Whitney Ave. (res); McG '26; Ophth, Otol; Staff, Sydney City & St. Rita Hosp's.; Tel. 564-8438.
LAND, Jacob; 736 Water St. W.; Box 479, St. John's, Nfld.; McG '30; Ophth Otol.; Tel. 578-5574.
LAND, Vita J.; McG'65; Res., Montreal Children's Hosp., Montreal 25, P.Q.
LANDA, S.; 212—1st Ave. S., Saskatoon, Sask.; 930 Saskatchewan Cresc. E. (res); Man '38.
LANDE, Joseph; 1117 St. Catherine St. W., Montreal, P.Q.; 2219 Maplewood (res); McG '21; **Staff, Royal Edward Laurentian Hosp.; Tel. VI 9-5201.**
LANDELLS, David G.; LeMarchant Rd. & Campbell Ave., St. John's, Nfld.; 107 Rennie's Mill Rd. (res); Glasgow (Scot.) '48; M.B.Ch.B.; OrthSurg; Active Staff, St. Clare's Mercy, St. John's Gen., Children's & Grace Hosp's.; Cons. (Orth), TB San; Tel. 579-6920 or 579-7087.
LANDER, David; Black Diamond, Alta.; Alb '36; MCGP.; Tel. 625-3052.
LANDER, Harold A.; Man'42; MCGP; Res., Children's Hosp., Winnipeg 3, Man.
LANDER, Jacob J.; 410 Norlyn Bldg., 309 Hargrave St., Winnipeg 2, Man.; 1368 Mathers Bay East (res); Man '33; MCGP; Tel. WH 3-6521.
LANDIS, Noah; 391 Dundas St. W., Toronto, Ont.; Tor'25; MCGP; Tel. 368-6555.
LANDREVILLE, J. Auguste; 1462 Blvd St. Joseph E., Apt. 2, Montreal 34, P.Q. (res); Mon '28; PH (P.Q.); Ass't. Chief, Dept. of Health, Montreal.; Tel. LA 3-1200.
LANDRIAULT, Guy; 5088 Bellechasse, Montreal, P.Q.; Lille (Fr.) '54.
LANDRIAULT, Raoul; 6387 St. Denis, Montreal, P.Q.; **Mon '23;** Industrial Phys., Montreal Transport Comm; Tel. 877-6300.
LANDRIGAN, Paul L.; 5880 Spring Garden Rd., Halifax, N.S.; Dal '54; FRCP(C), IntMed; Ass't. Phys., Victoria Gen. Hosp.; Lect. (Med.) Dalhousie U.; Tel. 423-7052.
LANDRY, Alfred; 2245 boul. Connaught, Montreal 9, P.Q.; Mon'20; AMCGP; Retired.
LANDRY, Conrad; 60 Iberville, Riviere-du-Loup, P.Q.; Lav'60; Tel. 862-5823.
LANDRY, Edmond L.; 470 Victoria St., Dalhousie, N.B.; Lav'54; Tel. 684-4142.
LANDRY, Henry J.; 5170 Ave. Verdun, Verdun, Mtl. 19, P.Q.; Paris (Fr.) '55; IntMed (P.Q.); Jr. Clin. Ass't. **St. Mary's Hosp., Mtl.; M.O., TCA; Tel. PO 7-7452.**
LANDRY, Jacques; RCAF Station, Mont Apica, P.Q.; Mon'65.
LANDRY, J. Jacques; 80-17eme Ave., Lachine, P.Q.; Lav '57; Tel. 634-1570.
LANDRY, J. Gerard; 228 rue Longueuil, St. Jean, P.Q.; Mon '55.
LANDRY, Jean P.; 2200 Blvd. O'Brien, St. Laurent, Montreal 9, P.Q.; Lav '49; OrthSurg; Staff, Hop.-du-Sacre-Coeur; Tel. RI 4-1622.
LANDRY, Paul; Mon'62; Res., Hop. Ste-Justine, Montreal 26, P.Q.
LANDRY, Philippe; 2395 Beaubien E., Montreal 36, P.Q.; 327 de l'Epee (res); Lav '40; F.C.C.P., Pulm. Dis. & TB (P.Q.); M.C.G.P.; Staff, Bruchesi Institute and Hop. St. Joseph de Rosemont; Tel. CR 2-2345.
LANDRY, Real; Metagami Clinic, 10 Petite Allee, Matagami, P.Q.; Mon'65.
LANDRY, Real; Lav'64; Res., Hop. St. Michel Archange, Quebec 5, P.Q.
LANDRY, Raoul D.; Department of Health, 400 Collishaw St., Moncton, N.B.; Lav '36; Tel. EV. 2-6056.
LANDRY, Robert B.; Lav'63; Res., Montreal Gen. Hosp., Montreal 25, P.Q.
LANE, G. Alan; 720 Professional Arts Bldg., **Hamilton, Ont.; 8 Auchmar Rd. (res); Tor '40;** M.S., F.R.C.S.(C), GenSurg; **Chief of Surg., St. Joseph's Hosp.; Tel. JA 7-3821.**
LANE, Graham B.; 70 Balsam St. S., Timmins, Ont.; 270 Preston St. S. (res); Tor '32; FCCP; IntMed (TB); MOH & Dir., Porcupine Health Unit; Clin., Ont. Dept. of Health (TB); Tel. AM 4-2377.

LANE, John S.; 303 Goldstream Ave., Victoria, B.C.; Dublin (Ireland)'48; DObstRCOG.

LANE, Oliver G.; 585-25th St. W., Prince Albert, Sask.; Guys Hosp. (London, Eng.) '39; M.B., B.S., LRCP(Lond.); MRCS(Eng.); M.D.(Lond.); F.C.(Path.); Path; Chief Pathol., Victoria Union Hosp. & Holy Family Hosp.; Tel. 763-7481.

LANE, Richard A.; Ste. 608, 1055 Lucknow St., Halifax, N.S.; Tor '39; Cons. (Derm.), Cdn. Forces Hosp.; Tel. 422-2179.

LANE, Robert F.; 299 Main St., Chilliwack, B.C.; Tor'53; MCGP; Active Staff, Chilliwack Gen. Hosp.; Cons. Staff, Coqualeetza Indian Hosp., Sardis; Tel. 792-9071.

LANE, Robert M.; 500 Beach Dr., Victoria, B.C. (res); McG '44; DPH; IntMed; Staff, Victoria Island Health Centre; Tel. EV 3-8761.

LANG, Alexander P.; 220 Greenwood Avenue, Toronto 8, Ont.; Freiburg (Germ.)'54; MCGP; Staff, Dept. of Gen. Practice, Toronto East Gen. & Central Hosp's.; Tel. HO 3-6642.

LANG, **Donald W.;** 155 Howard St., Kimberley, B.C.; Alb'55; MCGP; Tel. 427-2277.

LANG, **Herbert B.; Innsbruck (Aust.) '45; Path;** Assoc. Pathol., Halifax Infirmary, 1335 Queen St., Halifax, N.S.; Ass't. Prof. (Path.), Dalhousie U.; Tel. 422-1511, Loc. 282.

LANG, **Janet K. (See Ross)**

LANG, **Louis V.; 74 Weber St. W., Kitchener, Ont.; 137 Stirling N. (res); Tor '26; M.C.G.P.;** Chief (Med), St. Mary's Hosp., Kitchener: Dist. Coroner; Tel. SH 5-9101.

LANG, **Stanley R.;** 42 Cheritan Ave., Toronto 12, Ont.; Qns '51.

LANGDALE-GREGORY, Ian — see GREGORY, Ian L.

LANGDON, Rex L.; 6044 Quinpool Rd., Halifax, N.S.; 12 Fleming Dr., Armdale (res); Dal '57; AMCGP; Tel. 422-4534.

LANGDON, William A.; 362 Queens Ave., London, Ont.; Wes'54; Paed; Research Fell., Ontario Heart Fdn.; Instr. (Paed.), U. of Western Ontario; Tel. 439-9872.

LANGE, **Hugo N.;** Russell Clinic, Russell, Man.; Man'56; MCGP; Tel. 310.

LANGE, John A.; 9720—106th St., Edmonton, Alta. (res); Jr. Int'n., Royal Alexandra Hosp., Edmonton.

LANGELIER, Leon P.; Lav '43; D&TRad; Staff, Hop. Hotel-Dieu, Arthabaska, P.Q.; Tel. 357-2031.

LANGELIER, Reginald; Lav'63; Staff, Hop. Notre-Dame, Montreal 24, P.Q.

LANGER, Bernard; Room 138, Private Patients' Pavillion, Toronto Gen. Hosp., Toronto, Ont.; **180 Gordon Rd., Willowdale (res); Tor '56; FRCS(C); GenSurg; Ass't. Surg., Toronto Gen. Hosp.; Clin. Teach. (Surg.), U. of Toronto; Tel.** EM 6-8211, Loc. 2684.

LANGER, **Frederick;** Tor '64; Res., Dept of Surg., U. of Toronto, Toronto 5, Ont.

LANGER, Joseph; 1428 Ouellette Ave., Windsor, Ont.; Wes '56; OrthSurg; Tel. 256-1833. Abroad.

LANGER, Melvin H.; 214 Avenue Blgd., 220-3rd Ave. S., Saskatoon, Sask.; 105 Poplar Cr. (res); Tor '46; GenSurg; Tel. 652-0300.

LANGEVIN, **Benoit;** St-Hubert, Cte. Temiscouata, P.Q.; Lav '65.

LANGEVIN, Ernest; 30 E. Blvd. St. Joseph, Montreal, P.Q.; 5430 Blvd. Pie IX (res); Mon '43; Ophth, Otol (P.Q.); Staff (Ophth., Otol.), Hotel Dieu; Clin. (Ophth.), U. of Montreal, & Hotel Dieu; Tel. AV 8-2088.

LANGEVIN, Georges E.; Paspebiac, Co. Bonaventure, P.Q.; Mon '27.

LANGEVIN, Hebert; 484 Chemin Ste-Catherine, Montreal 8, P.Q.; Mon '56; Psy; Staff, Hop. Notre-Dame; Tel. 274-3242.

LANGEVIN, Jean; 404 Woodlea, Ville Mont-Royal, Montreal, P.Q.; Mon '41; Tel. RE 1-4640.

LANGEVIN, **Pierre;** Lav'65; Res., Hop. Ste-Justine, Montreal 26, P.Q.

LANGEVIN, Pierre; Hop. Notre Dame, Montreal 24, P.Q.; 4260 Chemin St. Michel, St. Leonard de Port-Maurice (res); Mon'49; Paed; Vol. Ass't. (Paed); Hop. Notre Dame; Tel. 523-1137.

LANGEVIN, Raymond; 241 rue Fleury W., Montreal 12, P.Q.; Mon '47; OrthSurg; Active Staff (OrthSurg), Hop. Sacre-Coeur; Tel. DU 1-7281.

LANGEVIN, Stephen; 330 Sherbrooke St. E., Montreal, P.Q.; Mon '10; FRCM (Lond.); FACS; FRCOG; FRCS(C); Tel. AV 8-5589.

LANGEVIN, **Suzanne;** 245 Beverley Ave., Ville Mont Royal, Montreal 16, P.Q. (res); Mon'59; Staff, Dept. of Health, Mtl.; Tel. 872-3360.

LANGFORD, Arthur; 500 Lafontaine, Riviere-du-Loup, P.Q.; Lav '58; FRCS(C); GenSurg.; Tel. UN 2-3563.

LANGFORD, E. Robert; School of Hygiene, U. of Toronto, Toronto 5, Ont.; Qns '58; DPH; Ass't. Sec., School of Hygiene & Assoc. Prof. (PH), U. of Toronto; Tel. 928-2751.

LANGFORD, Joan F.; Health Unit, 38 Augustus St., Cornwall, Ont.; U.K. '51; D.P.H.; Ass't. M.O.H., Cornwall, Ont. Abroad.

LANGFORD, **Walton W.,** 623 Brant St., Burlington, Ont.; **Qns '51; M.C.G.P.**

LANGILLE, David C.; Mahone Bay, N.S.; Dal '62.

LANGILLE, James A.; Medical Arts Bldg., 107 Church St., Amherst, N.S.; 213 E. Victoria St. (res); Dal '32; D.O.M.S., D.L.O., Ophth, Otol; F.A.C.S.; Med. Staff, Highland View Hosp.; Dist. Coroner; Tel. 667-8600.

LANGIS, Antonio; 10 Picard, Ste. Martine, Chateauguay C., P.Q.; Lav '31; PH (P.Q.); M.O.H., Unite Sanitaire.

LANGIS, Camille; 1005 rue St. Prosper, Trois Rivieres, P.Q.; Lav'54; Gastroent. (P.Q.).

LANGIS, **J. Claude;** Maria, Cte Bonaventure, P.Q.; Lav'53; Otol(P.Q.).

LANGIS, **Jules G.;** 380 Princess, Bathurst, N.B.; Lav'17; Tel. LI 6-2326.

LANGIS, L. Jacques; Disraeli, P.Q. Lav '49; A.M.C.G.P.

LANGIS, Napoleon; 293 St. Germain, Rimouski, P.Q.; Lav '41; Anaes (P.Q.); Chief Anaes., St. Joseph's Hosp., Rimouski.; Tel. 723-7851.

LANGIS, **Pierre Eustache; 38 Ave. d'Amours, Matane, P.Q.; Lav '19; Phys., Matane Prison.**

LANGIS, Rodolphe L.; 177 rue Gillespie, Sherbrooke, P.Q.; 38 Peel St. (res); Mon '39; Paed (P.Q.); Chief Paed., Hop. St. Vincent de Paul; Tel. 562-0525.

LANGLAIS, Jean C.; C.P. 1177, Mont Joli, P.Q.; Lav'46; PH(P.Q.); Staff, Dept. of Health, Mont Joli.

LANGLAIS, Jean P.; C.P. 39, Trois Pistoles, Co. Riviere du Loup, P.Q.; Lav '51.

LANGLAIS, L. Dominique; 790—18eme rue, Quebec, P.Q.; Lac St. Charles (res); Lav '28; Tel. 524-8120.

LANGLAIS, **Louis M., Major;** Lav '53; IntMed; Chief of Med., Quebec Military Hosp., Ste. Foy, P.Q.; Tel. 653-7201.

LANGLEY, George E.; 718 Granville, Vancouver, B.C.; 1141 W. 43rd (res); Man '34; F.R.C.S. (Ed.); GenSurg; Att. Surg., St. Paul's & Children's Hosp's; Tel. MU 1-9451.

LANGLEY, **George R.;** Dalhousie Public Health Clinic, University Ave., Halifax, N.S.; Dal'57; FACP; FRCP(C), IntMed; Ass't. Phys., Victoria Gen. Hosp.; Ass't. Prof., Dalhousie U.; Tel. 429-1420, Loc. 489.

LANGLEY, Hugh G.; 168 Ontario St., St. Catharines, Ont.; 96 Glenwood Ave. (res); Qns '56; AMCGP; Tel. MU 2-0073.

LANGLEY, Robert K.; 241 Brant Ave., Brantford, Ont.; 43 Franklin St. (res); Tor '54; Ophth; Staff, Brantford Gen. & St. Joseph's Hosp's.; Tel. 756-5532.

LANGLOIS, **Charles A.;** 3860 St. Urbain, Montreal, P.Q.; **Lav '17; D&TRad (P.Q.); Ass't. Med. Dir., Hotel Dieu, Montreal; VI 4-0161.**

LANGLOIS, **Claude;** 3766, Chemin Reine-Marie, Montreal 26, P.Q.; Mon'55; IntMed; Allergy (P.Q.).

LANGLOIS, Claude H.; 5270 Ave. Beaconsfield, Montreal 29, P.Q.; Mon'58; FRCP(C), IntMed.; Tel. 731-3211.

LANGLOIS, Jean-L.; 3 Ave. Kelvin, Outremont, Montreal 8, P.Q.; 660 ave Hartland (res); Mon '48; DABPN; Dip. Boston Psychoanal. Soc.; Psy. (P.Q.); Cons. (Psy.), Inst-Albert-Prevost, U. of Mtl.; I/C Course Dept. of Psy., U. of Montreal; Tel. 737-2881.

LANGLOIS, J. Denis; 832 St. Joseph Blvd. E., Montreal 34, P.Q.; Mon '42; Pulm. Dis. & TB (P.Q.).; Tel. 525-1335.

LANGLOIS, Leonard E.; 31 King St. W., Sherbrooke, P.Q.; 441 rue Labarre (res); Mon '57; F.R.C.P.(C), Paed; Staff, Hop.-St.-Vincent-de-**Paul; Tel. LO 9-5931.**

LANGLOIS, Marcel; 1345 rue Patenaude, Sillery, P.Q.; Lav '56; Psy; Staff, Hop.-St.-Michel Archange; Tel. 661-7781.

LANGLOIS, Maurice; 31 King ouest, Sherbrooke, P.Q.; Mon '57; FRCP(C); IntMed; Tel. 567-8844.

LANGLOIS, Peter L.; 1274 Kingston Rd., Scarborough, Ont.; Tor'63; Abroad.

LANGLOIS, Pierre R.; 190 Bonaventure, Trois-Rivieres, P.Q.; Lav'54; Otol; Tel. FR 6-2549.

LANGLOIS, Yves; 1005 rue Principale, Cowansville, P.Q.; Mon'59.

LANGMUIR, Robin M.; Ste. 5, 331 Sheddon Ave., Oakville, Ont.; Glasgow (Scot.)'51; Tel. 845-3415.

LANGS, Edwin R.; Lynden, Ontario; Tor '32; MCGP; Staff, Brantford Gen. & St. Joseph's Hosp's. & Willett Hosp., Paris; District Coroner; Tel. 647-3422.

LANGSTAFF, James R.; 50 Yonge St. N., Richmond Hill, Ont.; 106 Yonge St. N. (res); Tor **'35; M.C.G.P.; Tel. 884-1154.**

LANGSTAFF, Lillian C. (Carroll); 27 Church St. N., Richmond Hill, Ont. (res): Tor '05; Retired.

LANGSTAFF, Rolph L.; 27 Church St. N., Richmond Hill, Ont. (res); Tor '91; L.R.C.P.(Ed.); Retired.

LANGSTON, M. Kathleen W.; 3280 Mathers Ave., West Vancouver, B.C. (res); Alb '28; D.A., **Anaes.; Anaes., Shaughnessy Hosp., Vancouver; Tel. TR 6-6767.**

LANGSTON, Robert G.; 925 W. Georgia St., Vancouver 1, B.C.; **3280 Mathers Ave., West Vancouver (res); Alb '29; F.A.C.S., PlasSurg, GenSurg; Chief of Plas. Surg., Shaughnessy & Vancouver Gen. Hosp's.; Att. Staff, St. Paul's Hosp.; Cons. Plas. Surg., Children's Hosp., B.C. Cancer Control; Clinic. Ass't. Prof. Plas. Surg., U. of British Columbia; Tel. MU 2-5696.**

LANNON, Stanislaus G.; 73 Fernhill, Outremont, Montreal, P.Q.; Dal'57; FRCS(C), Urol.; Research Fell., Royal Victoria Hosp.

LANOIE, Jean M.; 699 rue St.-Louis, Joliette. P.Q.; Lav'46; IntMed, Cardiol, (P.Q.); Tel. 756-8921.

LANSDALL, Frederick C.; 212 Victoria St., Kamloops, B.C.; Dal '52; Urol.; Tel. 372-3211.

LANSDOWN, Edward L.; Apt. 609, 26 Underhill Dr., Don Mills, Ont.; Man '57; DMR; FRCP(C), DiagRad; Ass't. Rad., Toronto Gen. Hosp.; Cons., Lakeshore Psy. Hosp., New Toronto; Principal Med. Off., HMCS "York"; Clin. Teach., U. of Toronto; Tel. EM 6-8211, Loc. 2054.

LANSDOWN, Leslie P.; 1204 Wolseley Ave., Winnipeg 10, Man.; Man '25; DPH; Bact; Dir. of Lab. Serv., Prov. of Man.; Ass't. Prof. (Bact.) & Lect. (Soc. & Prev. Med.), U. of Man.

LANSKAIL, James C.; **215 Victoria St., Ste. 503,** Toronto 2, Ont.; Tor '46; FRCS(C), GenSurg; Active Staff, St. Michael's Hosp.; Cons. Staff, Stevenson Mem. Hosp., Alliston; Court. Staff, Scarborough Gen. & Queensway Gen. Hosp's.; Clin. Teach., U. of Toronto; Tel. 366- 1780.

LANSKY, Gerald; Ste. 3, 749 King St. W., Kitchener, Ont.; Tor'59; FRCS(C), GenSurg.; Tel. 576-1830.

LANSPEARY, William D.; 75 Giles Blvd. W., Windsor, Ont.; Tor '20; Tel. 253-4751. Retired.

LANTHIER, Andre; 1880 de la Duchesse, St-Bruno, Cte Chambly, P.Q.; Mon '53; FRCP(C); IntMed; Dir. (Endocrine Lab.), Hop. Notre Dame; Ass't. Prof. (Med.), U. of Montreal; Tel. RE 3-9951.

LANTHIER, Henri J.; 3244 Beaubien, Rosemont, **Montreal, P.Q.; 4735 St. Zotique (res); Mon '52; M.C.G.P.; Tel. RA 9-1891.**

LANTHIER, John C.; McG '34; DiagRad; Staff, St. Vincent-de-Paul Hosp., Brockville, Ont.; Tel. DI 2-4461.

LANTHIER, Suzanne; Centre Medical, 520 Notre-Dame, Repentigny, P.Q.; Mon'65.

LANTIER, Robert; 1395 Guertin, Ville-St-Laurent Montreal 8, P.Q. (res); Mon '52; PhysMed & Rehab; Staff, Rehab. Inst.

LANTZ, J. Brodie; 170-72 Fitzroy St., Charlottetown, P.E.I.; Dal '65; Tel. 894-7325.

LANTZ, J. P.; 170-172 Fitzroy St., Charlottetown, P.E.I.; 98 Brighton Rd. (res); McG '25; Ophth, Otol.; Tel. 4-7325.

LAO, Han L.; Santo Tomas (Philippines) '59; Jr. Intn., Winnipeg Gen. Hosp., Winnipeg 3, Man.

LAPALME, Roger; Apt. 17, 4395 Ave. Verdun, Montreal 19, P.Q.; Mon'57; FRCS(C); Urol; Staff, Hop. Hotel-Dieu; Tel. PO 9-5222.

LAPCHINSKI, Ernest S.; 289 Cedar St., Sudbury, Ont.; Tor'63; Tel. 674-3131.

LAPERRIERE, Aubert; 184 rue Brassard, Nicolet, P.Q.; 448 St. Jean Baptiste (res); Mon '42; DPH (Tor.); PH(P.Q.); Med. Dir., Nicolet Health Unit & Hop. Nicolet; Tel. 293-4412.

LAPERRIERE, Jean; 11675 Claude Legault, Montreal-Nord, P.Q.; Lav '58; MCGP; Tel. 321-2790.

LAPERRIERE, Vincent; 469 rue Cartier E., Chicoutimi, P.Q.; 476 de Sales (res); Mon '43; F.R.-C.S.(C) OrthSurg; Chief of Orth. Surg., Hotel-**Dieu St. Vallier, Chicoutimi; Ass't. Prof., Laval U.; Tel. 549-1452.**

LAPIERRE, Andre; 2122 Jean-Talon E., Montreal 35, P.Q.; Mon '55; M.C.G.P.; Tel. RA 2-9017.

LAPIERRE, Aquilla A.; 847 Dunlop Ave., Omt., Montreal, P.Q. (res); Lav '12.

LAPIERRE, Armand P.; Ste. 104, Medical Arts Bldg., 131 Ontario St., St. Catharines, Ont.; 15 Wood-Dale Dr. (res); Tor'44; Paed; Chief of Paed., St. Catharines Gen. Hosp.; Tel. 684-6581.

LAPIERRE, Bernard; 1352 Ontario E., Montreal, P.Q.; 1956 est, rue Sherbrooke (res); Mon '48.

LAPIERRE, Camille; 3575 Sherbrooke St. E., **Montreal 4, P.Q.; Mon '24.; Tel. LA 4-4578.**

LAPIERRE, Claude; 175 rue Doody, Chambly, P.Q.; Mon'65

LAPIERRE, Guy; 35 Main St., Beebe, P.Q.; McG'46; MCGP; Active Staff, Broadview Gen. Hosp. & Court. Staff, Orleans Mem. Hosp., Newport, Vermont; Tel. 876-2316.

LAPIERRE, Irene; 1213 rue Commerciale, St. Romuald d'Etchemin, P.Q. (res); Lav '33; Anaes; Anaes.-in-Chief, Hotel-Dieu, Levis; Tel. 837-9341.

LAPIERRE, Jean Jr.; Mon'64; Res. (Psy.), Jewish Gen. Hosp., Montreal, P.Q.

LAPIERRE, Jean; 11810 est Notre-Dame, Pointe-aux-Trembles, Montreal E. 5, P.Q.; 12286 est **Notre Dame (res); Mon '36; MCGP. M.O., Pointe-Aux-Trembles.**

LAPIERRE, Jean L.; 249 rue St.-Pierre, St.-Constant, Cte. Laprairie, P.Q.; Mon '45; Vist. Staff, Gen. Hosp., Verdun, St. Joseph & Lachine.

LAPIERRE, Jeanne; 350 18e rue, Quebec 3, P.Q.; Mon '50.

LAPIERRE, Louis; 1560 rue Sherbrooke E., Montreal, 24, P.Q.; Mon '56; FRCP(C), IntMed (PQ); Staff, Hop. Notre-Dame; Tel. 525-6363.

LAPIERRE, Rene; 3 St. Jean Baptiste, Vercheres, P.Q.; Mon '22.

LAPIERRE, Robert; Mon'64; Res., Hop. Hotel-Dieu, Montreal 18, P.Q.

LAPIERRE, Romeo; 8880 Lajeunesse, Montreal, P.Q.; Lav '19.

LAPIERRE, Yvon D.; Ott'61; Res., Hop. Notre Dame, Montreal 24, P.Q.

LAPIN, Albert W.; 4119 Sherbrooke St. W., Montreal, P.Q.; 3785 Vendome Ave. (res); McG '35; M.R.C.P., F.A.C.P., D.A.B.I.M., F.R.C.-P.(C), IntMed, Cardiol. (P.Q.); Dir. of Cardiol, Jewish Gen. & Queen Mary Vet's. Hosp.; Ass't. **Phys., Montreal Gen. Hosp.; Lect. (Med.), McGill U.; Tel. WE 2-1906.**

LAPIN, Irving; Ste. 208, 5757 Decelles Ave., Montreal 26, P.Q.; 189 Dufferin Rd., Hampstead (res); McG '49; Staff, Jewish Gen. & Royal Edward Laurentian Hosp's.; Dem. (Med.), McGill U.; Tel. RE 3-6588.

LAPIN, Lyon; Ste. 580, 6000 Cote des Neiges Rd., Montreal 26, P.Q.; McG'41; FACP; IntMed; Assoc. Phys., Jewish Gen. Hosp.; Chief Arthritis Clinic, Jewish Gen. Hosp.; M.O.H., City Cote St. Luc; Tel. 733-4687.

LAPKO, Alexander P.; Box 420, Brandon, Man.; Stalino (Ukraine) '41; D.A.B.P.; FCAP; Path; Staff. Provincial Labs., Dept. of Health.; Tel. PA 6-3230.

LAPLANTE, Aime-E.; 30 Blvd. St. Joseph E., App. 714, Montreal 14, P.Q.; Mon '28; GenSurg; Chief of Surg., Hop. Ste-Jeanne-d'Arc; Tel. 845-4241.

LAPLANTE, Albert; 281 St. Georges, St. Jerome, P.Q.; 378 Rolland **(res); Mon '39; Chief Paed., Hop. Hotel Dieu; Indust. Phys., Dominion Rubber Co. & Rolland Co.**

LAPLANTE, J. Paul; 1058 St. Denis St., Montreal 18, P.Q.; McG '30; Dir. Gen., Hop. Sainte-Luc; Tel. 861-7321.

LAPLANTE, Marcel; 800 est Blvd. St. Joseph, Montreal, P.Q.; 225 rue Fleury est (res): Mon **'44; Gyn; Gyn. Staff, Hop. Ste. Jeanne d'Arc.; Tel. VI 2-5201.**

LAPLANTE, Michael P.; McG '62(Hons.); Prize in Paed.; Res., Royal Victoria Hosp., Montreal 2, P.Q.

LAPLANTE, Pierre; Mon '63; Res., Hop. Notre-Dame, Montreal 24, P.Q.

LAPOINTE, Andre; 809 ave. Paradis, Quebec 10, **P.Q. (res); Lav '48; D & TRad; Staff (DiagRad), Hop. Hotel-Dieu & Laval U.; Tel. 529-9151.**

LAPOINTE, Andre; 138 rue Angers, Jonquiere, P.Q.; Lav'62; FRCP(C), Anaes.

LAPOINTE, Antoine; 335 St.-Dominque, Jonquiere, P.Q.; Lav '31; Paed (P.Q.).

LAPOINTE, Carol; 7820 Marquette, Montreal 35, P.Q.; Mon '62.

LAPOINTE, Constance K.; 1387 Athlone Rd., Montreal 16, P.Q.; Women's Med. Coll. (Pa., U.S.A.)'59.

LAPOINTE, Donat; 570 Grande Allee E., Quebec 4, P.Q.; Lav '31; FRCP(C), Paed; Chief of Newborn Infant Serv., St. Vincent-de-Paul Hosp.; Prof. & Hd., Dept. of Paed., Laval U.; Tel. **656-2827.**

LAPOINTE, Fernand; 15 ave Begin, Levis, P.Q.; Lav '50; Tel. 837-9990.

LAPOINTE, Gaston; 475 Boul. Talbot, Chicoutimi, P.Q.; Lav '37; IntMed; Clin. Instr. (Med.), Hotel-Dieu-St.-Vallier; Assoc. Prof. Laval U. Tel. 549-1542.

LAPOINTE, Gaston A.; Clinique St. Georges, 627 Jacques Cartier E., Chicoutimi, P.Q.; Lav 54; DABOphth; Ophth; Staff, Hotel-Dieu St. Valier; Tel. 549-0292.

LAPOINTE, Gerald; C.P. 88, Val d'Or, P.Q.; Lav'61; Tel. 824-6853.

LAPOINTE, Gilles; Lav'65; Res., Hop. Maisonneuve, Montreal 36, P.Q.

LAPOINTE, Henri; 169 Cadillac, Bourlamaque, P.Q.; Lav'25; FACR; PhysMed(P.Q.); D & T Rad.

LAPOINTE, J. Audet — (See Audet-Lapointe, J.)

LAPOINTE, Jean A.; 300 St. Louis Sq., Montreal 18, P.Q.; **Mon '25; Ophth,Otol.**

LAPOINTE, Jean J.; Box 600, The Med. Clinic, Valleyview, Alta.; Ott '60.

LAPOINTE, Jean L.; 518, 5757 Ave. Decelles, Montreal 26, P.Q.; Mon '55; D. Psy; Psy; Dir. OPClin. Child Psy., Hop. Ste.-Justine; Med. Supt., Hop. Mont-Providence; Cons. Mental Hyg. Inst., McGill U.; Ass't. Prof., U. of Mtl.; Tel. RE 9-4055.

LAPOINTE, Leon R.; Man'65; Res., Winnipeg Gen. Hosp., Winnipeg 3, Man.

LAPOINTE, Leonard; 2157, Fleury est, Montreal 12, P.Q.; Lav'57; IntMed; Cardiol (P.Q.); Tel. 381-2581.

LAPOINTE, Marcel L.; 2539 Belanger, Montreal 37, P.Q.; **Mon '63.**

LAPOINTE, Marcel; 1146 rue Melancon, Chicoutimi, P.Q. (res); Lav'43; M.Sc., (Hosp. Adm.); Med. Dir., Hotel Dieu St. Vallier; Tel 549-2195 Loc. 214.

LAPOINTE, Marielle R. (Pharand); 292 Donald St., Ottawa 7, Ont.; Ott '61; Pt.-time PH.; Tel. 745-5924.

LAPOINTE, Michel A.; 3248 rue Ste.-Lucie, Cite-de-St.-Michel, Montreal N., P.Q.; Mon '63.

LAPOINTE, Normand; Mon '63; Res., Hop. Ste-Justine, Montreal 26, P.Q.

LAPOINTE, Pierre A.; Mon '60; Res., Hop. Maisonneuve, Montreal, P.Q.

LAPOINTE, Roger; 822 E. Sherbrooke, Montreal, P.Q.; 6264 MacDonald, Hampstead (res); Mon '49; F.R.C.S.(C), ObstGyn; Ass't., (Gyn.), Hop. Notre-Dame; **Tel. LA 5-6363.**

LAPOINTE, Roland; 7612 Christophe Colomb, **Montreal 10, P.Q.; Mon '34; Ophth, Otol; Active Staff, Hotel-Dieu; Ass't. Prof. (Ophth.), U. of Montreal; Tel. CR 7-9380.**

LAPOINTE, Vincent; 1144 de l'Acadie, Chicoutimi, P.Q.; Lav'50; D&TRad; Staff, Hotel-Dieu Hosp.

LAPORTE, Andre F.; 6635 Christophe-Colomb, Montreal 10, P.Q.; Mon '59.; Tel. DU 8-1219.

LAPORTE, Guy; 30 est Blvd. St. Joseph, Montreal 34, P.Q.; 1681 Winton, V.M.R. (res); Mon '52; M.C.G.P.; Tel. VI 5-4241.

LAPORTE, Jacques; 596 Blvd. Manseau, Joliette, P.Q.; Mon '56.

LAPORTE, Jean; 415 Dobie, Mont Royal, Montreal 16, P.Q. (res); Mon '51; Anaes; Chief Anaes., Hop. Hotel-Dieu, Montreal; Tel. VI 4-0161. Loc. 281.

LAPORTE, Jean; 162 Hepworth, Ville Lasalle, P.Q.; Mon'61; Psy (P.Q.).

LAPORTE, Jean M.; Ste. 802, 30 est, boul. St-Joseph, Montreal 14, P.Q.; Mon '53; Cardiol (France); Active Staff, Hop. Gen. Fleury; Tel. 845-4241.

LAPORTE, J. Marius; 30 est Boul. St. Joseph, Montreal 14, P.Q.; Mon'43; MCGP; Med. Dir., Hop-Notre-Dame-de-Rosaire; Tel. 845-4241, Loc. 51.

LAPORTE, Joseph N.; 1410 Chemin Lucerne, Mont-Royal, Montreal 16, P.Q. (res); Mon '21; D.P.H., PH (P.Q.); Ass't. Dir., Health Serv., Montreal Hotel de Ville, Annexe Viger.; Tel. RE 9-8848.

LAPORTE, L. Maurice; 12245 Grenet, Montreal 9, P.Q.; 10020 Laverdure (res); Mon'53; GenSurg (P.Q.); Surg., Hop. Sacre-Coeur; Tel. FE 4-1210.

LAPORTE, Louis J.; 835 Blvd. St. Joseph E., Montreal 34, P.Q.; Mon '50; F.R.C.S.(C), GenSurg; Tel. VI 5-1134.

LAPORTE, Louis P.; 489 Boul. Ste-Anne, Joliette, P.Q.; Mon '34; F.I.C.S., Urol (P.Q.); Urol. Hop.-St-Eusebe.; Tel. 756-8073.

LAPORTE, Marcellin; 1204 est, Fleury, Montreal **12, P.Q.; Bordeaux (Fr.) '57.; Tel. 389-5888.**

LAPORTE, Paul C.; Box 365, 95 rue St. Francois, Edmundston, N.B.; Lav'09; MRSH; GenSurg; Ll.D. (St. Louis U.); Dist. M.O.H., Madawaska Co.

LAPORTE, Raymond; 416 Jarry St. E., Montreal, P.Q.; Mon. '48.; Tel. DU 7-1858.

LAPORTE, Sylvain; 598 Manseau, Joliette, P.Q.; Mon '51.

LAPP, Carl A.; Qns '59; Staff, Ontario Hosp., London, Ont.; Tel. 455-5110.

LAPP, E. Gordon; Alb'51; Res., St. Paul's Hosp., Vancouver 1, B.C.

LAPP, Frederick H.; 130 North Shore E., Burlington, Ont.; Qns'47; Anaes; Staff, Brant Mem. Hosp.; Tel. 634-3308.

LAPP, Paul W.; McGregor Clinic, 250 Main St. E., Hamilton, Ont.; 73 Cloverhill Cres. (res); Tor '50; Otol; Chief (Otol.), & Med. Advisory Bd., Hamilton Gen. Hosp.; Cons. (ENT), DVA & RCAF; Tel. JA 7-2711.

LARAMEE, Andre; 1700 Sherbrooke St. E., Apt. 20, Montreal, P.Q.; 325 Ste. Catherine St., Outremont (res); Mon'43; Psy (P.Q.); Tel. LA 4-1972.

LARAMEE, Bernard; 1150 est Boul. St. Joseph, Montreal 34, P.Q.; Mon'48; Obst (P.Q.); Head (Dept. of Obst.), Santa Cabrini Hosp.; Vol. Ass't. (Obst), Hop-Maisonneuve; Tel. AV 8-5341.

LARAMEE, Francois; 76 rue Willowdale, Montreal 8, P.Q. (res); Mon '44; Pulm Dis. & TB (P.Q.); IntMed (P.Q.); Ass't. Prof. (Med.), U. of Mtl.; Med. Dir., Hotel-Dieu-de-Mtl.; Tel. VI 4-0161, Loc. 300.

L'ARCHEVEQUE, Andre; 222 est Henri-Bourassa, **Montreal 12, P.Q.; 10570 Vianney, Mtl. 12 (res); Mon '57; DABP; Paed; Staff, Pasteur, Sacre-Coeur & Ste.-Justine Hosp's.; Tel. 381-4555.**

L'ARCHEVEQUE, Marcel A.; 207 Blvd. St. Joseph E., Montreal 14, P.Q.; Mon '48; Obst. **(P.Q.); Tel. VI 4-2591.**

LARETEI, Aksel; 10 Foster St., Kentville, N.S.; Tartu (Estonia)'41; Staff, Nova Scotia Sanatorium.

LARGE, Alfred W.; Tor'39; Ass't. Res., Vancouver Gen. Hosp., Vancouver, B.C.

LARGE, George E.; 3450 Enniskillen Circle, Erindale Ont. (res); Qns '39; D.P.H.; Dir., Epi**demiology, Dept. of Health, Ontario; Tel. EM 3-**1211.

LARGE, Gordon C.; 5780 Cambie St., Vancouver 15, B.C.; 1420 W. 46th Ave. Van. 13 (res); Tor '28; F.A.C.S., D.A.B.Ot;Otol; Att'd. Staff, St. Vincent's, & Children's Hosp's.; Vis. Staff, Richmond, St. Paul's & Vancouver Gen. Hosp's.; Clin. Instr., U. of British Columbia; Tel. FA 1-1111.

LARGE, R. Geddes; P.O. Box 487, 219-2nd Ave. W., Prince Rupert, B.C.; Tor'23; FACS, FICS, GenSurg; Chief of Med. Staff, Prince Rupert Gen. Hosp.; Cons. Staff (Surg.), Miller Bay Hosp.; Tel. 624-5143.

LARGE, William A. Winnipeg Psychiatric Inst. Emily & Bannatyne, Winnipeg, Man. Man '46; Psy; AMCGP.

LARICHELLIERE, Raymond; 80 Blvd. St. Joseph W., Montreal 41, P.Q.; Mon'33; OrthSurg (P.Q.); Tel. 845-6201.

LARINI, Gian Paolo; 3033 Sherbrooke W., Westmount, Montreal, P.Q. (res); Parma (Italy) '46; D & TRad; FICS; Rad-in-Chief, Reddy Mem. Hosp.; Tel. WE 5-9641.

LARIOSA, Augustus P.; Santo Tomas (Philipp.) '60; Jr. Int., Regina Gen. Hosp., Regina, Sask.

LARIVEE, Luc; 3577 Ste-Catherine E., Montreal 4, P.Q.; Mon '54; M.C.G.P.; Phys., Dominion **Rubber Co.; Tel. LA 2-2111.**

LARIVIERE, Paul; 3484 Laval Ave., Montreal, P.Q.; 1532 Pine Ave. (res); Mon '27; NeurPsy; Assoc. Prof. (Psy.), U. of Montreal.; Tel. VI 5-7666.

LARIVIERE, Paul M.; 433 Blvd. St. Joseph E., Montreal 34, P.Q.; 4880 Cavendish (res); Mon '38; Paed; Dir. Med. Soc. Serv., Hop.-Ste-Justine; Tel. AV 8-8826.

LARKE, R. Bryce; Qns '60; Res., Hosp. for Sick Children, Toronto, Ont.

LARKING, Eric W.; 770 Seaforth Med. Bldg., 3550 **Cote des Neiges Rd., Montreal 25, P.Q.; 161 Monterrey, Pointe Claire, Lachine (res); McG '49; Anaes; Ass't. Anaes., Montreal Gen. Hosp.; Tel. WE 7-6011.**

LAROCHE, Albert G.; 1197 Transit Rd., Victoria, B.C.; Lav '16; Urol; Retired.

LAROCHE, Andree; Apt. 1, 1955 rue Genest, Cartierville, **Montreal, P.Q.; Mon '56.**

LAROCHE, Francois; Lav'60; FRCP(C), DiagRad; Staff, Hop. St-Sacrement, Quebec 6, P.Q.

LAROCHE, Gaston; 13350 Notre Dame E., Pointe-aux-Trembles, Montreal 5, P.Q.; Mon '59.; Tel. 642-2631.

LAROCHE, Guy; 314 Principale Farnham, P.Q.; 4 rue St. Paul (res); Mon '50; Coroner, Bedford Dist.

LAROCHE, Luc; 349 Boul. Alexandre-Tache, Hull, P.Q.; Ott'58; Tel. 771-6412.

LAROCHE, Noel; Ste. 5, 4395 rue Verdun, Verdun, Montreal 19, P.Q.; 74 Kelvin Ave., Outremont (res); Mon '42; Urol (P.Q.); Urol., Verdun **Gen. Hosp.; Tel. PO 6-3551.**

LaROCHELLE, Guy; 1016 Medical Arts Bldg., 1538 Ouest, rue Sherbrooke, Montreal 25, P.Q.; 35 rue Beloeil, Outremont Mtl. 8 (res); Mon '50; Psy.

LAROCHELLE, Jean; 475 boul. Talbot, Chicoutimi, P.Q.; Lav'60; Paed; Tel. 549-1034.

LAROCHELLE, Jean L.; 34 de la Fabrique, Quebec, P.Q.; 1403 Parc Champoux (res); Lav '40; OrthSurg; Ass't. Orth., Hotel Dieu; Cons. Orth., Veterans' Hosp.; Assoc. Prof. Anatomy, Laval U.; Med. Adv., C.N.R. & T.C.A.; Tel. 525-9817.

LAROCHELLE, Jean Y., Ste., Justine, Cte. Dorchester P.Q.; Lav '63.

LAROCHELLE, Louis A.; Lav'65; Res., Hop. Hotel-Dieu, Quebec 4, P.Q.

LAROCHELLE, L. N.; 80 rue St. Louis, Quebec, P.Q.; Lav '32; IntMed; Chief, Clin. Med., Hotel Dieu, Quebec; Prof. Therapeutics, Laval U; Tel. 529-9151.

LAROCHELLE, Leopold; 116 Morissette, Loretteville, P.Q.; Lav '37; Tel. 842-7474.

LAROCHELLE, Paul R.; 1500, de la Canardiere, Quebec 3, P.Q.; Lav '26; OphthOtol; Hd., Ophth-Otol., Hop.-de-l'Enfant-Jesus & Hop.-St-Michel-Archange; Assoc. Prof., Laval U.

LAROCHELLE, Remi; 3253 rue Beaubien E., Montreal 36, P.Q.; 7257 rue Lisieux, Ville St.-Leonard (res); Lav '54; ObstGyn; Tel. 721-4191.

LAROCHELLE, Yvette B. (See Brissette)

LAROCQUE, Andre; App. 402, 4335 Ave. Broadway, Lachine, P.Q. (res); Ott '53; GenSurg (P.Q.); Admin., Immigration Med. Serv., Dorval Airport; Tel. 631-1861.

LAROCQUE, Antonio; 161-4e Ave., Ville-St.-Pierre, P.Q.; Mon '47; F.A.S.A.S.; Ass't. Surg., Hop-St-Joseph-de-Lachine; Tel. HU 1-6768.

LAROQUE, Edmond; Plantagenet, Ont.; Qns '14.

LAROCQUE, Henri; 1415 Boul. d'Auteuil, Duvernay, P.Q.; Mon'55.

LA ROCQUE, J. Alfred; 418 Rideau St., Ottawa, Ont.; Mon '33; Gyn; F.I.C.S.; Surg. Staff, Ottawa Gen. Hosp.; Lect. Surg. & Clin. Surg., Ottawa U.; Tel. CE 3-9454.

LAROCQUE, Jean J.; 3423 St. Denis, Montreal 18, P.Q.; Mon '51; Obst(P.Q.).; Tel. VI 2-4829.

LAROCQUE, Gilles J.; 53 rue William, Sturgeon Falls, Ont.; Highway 17 E. (res); Lille (Fr.) '55; MCGP; Tel. 753-2650.

LAROCQUE, Raymond D. J.; 1539 Erie St. E., Windsor, Ont.; Wes '53; F.R.C.S.(C), GenSurg; Tel. CL 2-2733.

LAROSE, Claude L.; 4 Tashereau St., Hull, P.Q.; Ott '56; IntMed(P.Q.); Allergy(P.Q.); M.Sc (ExperimMed.); Cons. (Med&Allergy), Hop. Sacre-Coeur.; Cons.(Allergy), Nat. Med. Defence Centre; Tel. 771-5491.

LAROSE, Gilles; C.P. 7, 547 rue Notre-Dame, **Notre-Dame-des-Laurentide, P.Q.; Lav '60.**

LAROSE, Henri; 260 St. Anne, Varennes, Co. Vercheres, P.Q.; Mon '54.

LAROSE, J. Avila; 10 rue St. Charles, Ste. Therese de Blainville, Co. Terrebonne, P.Q.; Mon '21.

LAROSE, J. Claude; Mon '59; Res., Hop. St. Luc, Montreal 18, P.Q.

LAROSE, J. Guy; 693 St-Pierre, Terrebonne, P.Q.; Mon'59; Tel. 666-4421.

LAROSE, Leopold; C.P. 200, 260 rue Foster, Waterloo Co., Shefford, P.Q.; Lav'31.

LAROSE, Marcel; 68 St.-Jean, East Angus, Co. Compton, P.Q.; Lav '43; Phys., St. Lawrence Corp.

LAROSE, Michel; 4169 Papineau, Montreal 24, P.Q.; Mon'65.

LAROSE, Raoul; 2083 de la Canardiere, Quebec 8, P.Q.; Lav '51; A.M.C.G.P.; Tel. 661-5892.

LAROUCHE, Dollard; 158 ouest rue Price, Chicoutimi, P.Q.; Lav '50 MCGP.

LAROUCHE, Gerard; 14 Laurier, Arthabaska, P.Q.; Lav '52; IntMed(P.Q.).

LAROUCHE, Gerard-L.; 825 sud, rue Belvedere, Sherbrooke, P.Q.; Lav '44; FRCP(C), IntMed; Cardiol(P.Q.); Tel. 567-8575.

LAROUCHE, Jacques; Mon'59; DiagRad; Staff, Hop. Ste Jeanne d'Arc, Montreal 18, P.Q.

LAROUCHE, Norman; rue La Falaise, C.P. 700, Hauterive, (Saguenay), P.Q.; Lav '58; A.M.C.-G.P.

LAROUCHE, Raymond; 177 rue Collard, Alma, P.Q.; 230 Blvd. Auger (res); Lav '51; IntMed; Cardiol (P.Q.); Hd. Dept. of Med., Hop.-Hotel-Dieu; Tel. VI 4-0161.

LAROUCHE, Roland; Lav'59; Res., Hop. l'Enfant-Jesus, Quebec 3, P.Q.
LARRIVEE, Roger; Lav'65; Res., Hop. Hotel-Dieu, Quebec 4, P.Q.
LARSEN, Anthony A.; Alb '46; DPH; MPH; PH; Dir., Div. of Epidemiology & Dir. Emergency Health Services, Dept. of Health, B.C., Parliament Bldgs., Victoria, B.C.; Clin. Instr. U. of British Columbia; Tel. EV 2-6111.
LARSEN, Trygve E.; Sask '61; Res., University Hosp., Saskatoon, Sask.
LARSEN-LUNG, Violet A. (Larsen); Box 34, Regina, Sask.; 2845 Athol St. (res); Alb '40; Anaes; Anaes., Regina Gen. & Grey Nuns' **Hosp's.; Tel. LA 2-1811; JO 9-9621; Retired.**
LARSON, Burns J.; Cardston Clinic, Cardston, Alta.; Alb '50; GenSurg; Chief of Med. Staff, Cardston Municipal Hosp.; Tel. 653-3546.
LARUE, Antoine; 1193 des Erables, Quebec, P.Q.; 124 Preston **(res); Lav '44;** F.A.A.P.; Paed (PQ); Paed., Med. Soc. Centre; Clin. Ass't., Creche-St.-Vincent-de-Paul; Staff, Laval **U.; Tel. 524-9529.**
LARUE, Georges H.; rue de la Canardiere, Quebec 5, P.Q.; 512 ave Royale (res); Lav '30; NeurPsy; Hd. Male Serv., Hop. St.-Michel-Archange; Tel. 661-7781.
LARUE, Lucien; 964 rue Casot, Quebec, P.Q. (res); Lav '24; F.R.C.P.(C), NeurPsy; Med. Supt., Hop.-St.-Michel-Archange; Prof. (Psy), **Laval U.; Tel. 663-3571.**
LARUE, P. Antoine; Lav'35; Staff, San. Begin, Ste Germaine, Cte Dorchester, P.Q.
LARUE, Pierre; Ste 260, 3440 est Ontario Montreal 4, P.Q.; 5450 des Sapins (res); Lav '46; F.C.C.P. Pulm Dis. & TB (P.Q.), IntMed; Chief of Serv. Hop-San St. Joseph, 5689 Blvd., Rosemont, Montreal; Tel. CL 6-2681.
LARUE, Robert; App. 1, 3471 boul. Neilson, Quebec 10, P.Q.; Lav'45; DPH; PH (P.Q.); Tel. 653-5621.
LARUE, Vianney; 5 Laurier, Magog, P.Q.; Lav '55; Cardiol (P.Q.); Tel. 843-9233.
LARYEA, E. A.; Tor'65; Res., Shaughnessy Hosp., Vancouver 9, B.C.
LaSALLE, Gerald; Dean, Faculte de Medecine, Universite de Sherbrooke, Sherbrooke, P.Q.; Lav'40; DHA; Tel. 567-3901.
LaSALLE, M. J. M.; Department of National Health & Welfare, c/o Regional Superintendent, European Region; PH. Abroad.
LASALLE, Roger; Hop. Ste-Justine, 3175, chemin Ste-Catherine, Montreal 26, P.Q.; Mon'57; FAAP; Paed; Ass't. Prof. (Paed.), U. of Montreal; Tel. 731-4931.
LASCHIAZZA, Dominic; Box 160, Flin Flon Clinic, Flin Flon, Man.; McG '60.
LASKARIS, Michael A.; 697 St-Roch St., Park Extension, Montreal 15, P.Q.; Athens (Greece) '52.
LASKI, Bernard; 99 Avenue Rd., Toronto 5, Ont.; Tor '39; FAAP; FRCP(C), Paed; Chief (Paed.), New Mt. Sinai Hosp.; Phys., Hosp. for Sick Children; Ass't. Prof. (Paed.), U. of Toronto; Tel. WA 3-1768.
LASKIN, Manual M.; 10022-103rd St., Edmonton, Alta.; Tor '48; FRCS(C), GenSurg; Instr., U. of Alberta; Tel. GA 4-8076.
LASNIER, Raymond; 328 Cartier, Laval-des-Rapides, P.Q.; Mon '60.
LASSONDE, Michel; Mon'65; Res., Hop. Notre-Dame, Montreal 24, P.Q.
LASZLO, Clara E.; Apt. 211, 5725 Cote St. Luc, Montreal 29, P.Q.; Debrecen (Hungary)'55.
LASZLO, Theodore A.; 1428 Ouellette Ave., Windsor, Ont.; Ott'60; Paed.
LATHAM, Curtis F.; 465 N. Dollarton Hwy., North Vancouver, B.C.; 110 W. 14th St., North Vancouver; UBC'62; Tel. 987-2810 & 929-2422.
LATHAM, Harold D.; 65 King St., Beamsville, Ont.; 255 King St. (res); Qns '38; Med. Dir., Bethesda Home, Vineland; MCGP; Tel. LO 3-8221.
LATHAM, Harry O.; 340 Campbell St., Nanaimo, B.C.; Sheffield (Eng.)'57; Tel. 753-3202.
LATHE, Frank E.; Box 70, 4528A Kingston Rd., West Hill, Ont.; 96 Danforth Rd., Scarborough (res.); Tor '55; Tel. AT 2-1573.
LATHI, Dewayani S.; Poona (India); Res., Victoria Gen. Hosp., Halifax, N.S.
LATHI, Subhashchandra; Bombay (India); Jr. Int., Victoria Gen. Hosp., Halifax, N.S.
LATHOURAS, Nicolas G.; 123 Erie Ave., Brant**ford, Ont.; Athens (Greece) '51; Tel. 752-3791.**
LATHOURIS, George; Bell Island, Nfld.; Athens (Greece)'57.
LATIMER, John W.; Kapuskasing Med. Centre, **Kapuskasing, Ont.; 70 Dominion St. (res); Qns** '41; M.C.G.P.; Staff, Sensenbrenner Hosp.; Dist. **coroner; Tel 335-4115.**
LATIMER, Robert H.; Queen St., St. Mary's, Ont.; Widder St. (res); Tor '24; M.C.G.P.; M.O.H., Town of St. Mary's; Med. Rep., D.V.A. Tel. 284-2797.
LATOUR, Gerard; 3570 St.-Urbain, Montreal 18, P.Q.; 7598 Pl. Ornains, Ville d'Anjou, Mtl. 5 (res); Lav '43; D & TRad; Rad., Hop. Ste.-Jeanne-d'Arc; Tel. VI 2-5201.
LATOUR, Jean P.; 31 Menard, Roberval, P.Q. (res); Mon '59; DiagRad; Staff, Hop. Hotel-Dieu; Tel. 275-0110.
LATOUR, J. P. A.; 4820 Western Ave., Westmount, P.Q. (res); McG '40; F.A.C.S., F.R.C.S. (C), ObstGyn; Ass't. ObstGyn., Royal Victoria & Montreal Gen. Hosp's.; **Ass't. Prof., McGill U.;** Tel. VI 4-3122.
LATOUR, Paul; 501—6th Ave., Pointe aux Trembles, P.Q.; 14344 Notre Dame E. (res); Mon '25.
LATOUR, Yves; Mon'64; Res., Hop. Saint-Luc, Montreal 18, P.Q.
LATOURELLE, Rodrigue; 7 St. Laurent, Louiseville, P.Q. (res); Mon '30; PH (P.Q.); M.O.H., Health Unit, Cte. Maskinonge, Dept. of Health, P.Q.
LATRAVERSE, Valmore; 287 St. Louis Sq., Montreal, P.Q.; Mon '35; Otol; Staff, Hop. Notre **Dame; Tel. LA 5-6363.**
LATTEY, R. Michael; The Med. Clinic, 3009-31st Ave., Vernon, B.C.; 2500-28th St. (res); Oxford (Eng.) '39; Tel. 542-4321.
LATULIPPE, Lucien; 113 Commerciale, Cabano, Cte Temiscouata, P.Q.; Lav'65.
LAU, Agnes E.; Tor'61; Res., Shaughnessy Hosp., Vancouver 9, B.C.
LAU, George Y.; 20 Hewitt Ave., Toronto 3, Ont.; UBC'58; GenSurg; Abroad.
LAUBER, R. W.; 608 Elgin St., Wallaceburg, Ont.; 1234 Wallace (res); Tor '38; Staff, Sydenham Dist. Hosp.; Tel. 627-3611.
LAUCHLAN, Stuart C.; 1954 Henderson H'way, N. Kildonan, Winnipeg 16, Man. (res); Edinburgh (Scot.) '54; FRCP(C); Path; Staff, Winnipeg Gen. Hosp.; Dem. Dept. of Path., U. of Manitoba; Tel. SP 4-6511.
LAUDAN, John C.; 323 E. Columbia St., New Westminster, B.C.; DiagRad; Staff, X-Ray Dept., Royal Columbian Hosp.
LAUENER, Roland W.; 755 W. Broadway, Vancouver 9, B.C.; 6112 Wiltshire St. (res); UBC '56; FRCP(C), IntMed; Att'd. Staff, Van. Gen. Hosp.; Clin. Instr. (Med.), U. of British Columbia; Tel. TR 2-2115.
LAUERMAN, Joseph M.; Calwood Clinic, 11816-124th St., Edmonton, Alta.; Alb '48; MCGP; Active Staff, Edmonton Gen. Hosp.; Tel. 454-6571.
LAUFER, Frederick; 6380 Joseph Renaud Blvd., Ville d'Anjou, Montreal 5, P.Q.; Paris (France) '51; Staff, Hop. Jean Talon & Hop. Bellechasse; Tel. 352-2230.
LAUFER, Otto; 611 Bloor St. W., Toronto, Ont.; 36 Peveril Hill, N. (res); Vienna (Austria) '21; Tel. LE 4-1211.
LAUFER, Srul T.; 1788 Oxford St., Halifax, N.S. '30; F.A.C.P.; F.A.C.C; IntMed; **Head Dept. of Med., Halifax Infirmary; Assoc. Prof. (Med.), Dalhousie U.; Tel. 422-7153.**
LAUGHLAND, William W.; Liverpool MB., B.-Ch., Psy. (Ed); (Eng) '31; Depty. Med. Supt., Woodlands Schol., New Westminster, B.C.; Tel. LA 1-2611.
LAUGHREA, Patrick R.; P.O. Box 264 ,515 Fecteau St., Thetford Mines, P.Q. (res); Lav '48; Anaes; Chief (Anaes.), St. Joseph's Hosp.

LAUGHTON, John S.; Ste. 203, 3000 Lawrence Ave. E., Scarborough, Ont.; Tor '48; F.R.C.S. **(C), GenSurg; Tel. 291-0931.**
LAUKS, Anna (Bersins); 86 Bloor St. W., Toronto, Ont.; 241 Evelyn Ave. (res); Riga (Latvia) '28; Gyn. & Obst. (Latvia); M.C.G.P.; Staff, **Women's College Hosp.; Tel. 924-7002.**
LAUNAY, Marc P.; Mon '61; Res. Royal Victoria Hosp., Montreal 2, P.Q.
LAUNDY, Patrick W.; Sheffield (Eng.) '56; Dir. Med. Serv. Div., Prov. Welfare Dept., 800 Cassiar St., Vancouver 6, B.C.; Tel. CY 9-9131.
LAURENCE, Gabriel C.; 30 est boul St-Joseph, Montreal 14, P.Q.; 3402 Sherbrooke St. E. (res); Mon'54; FRCP(C); IntMed; I/C Gastroent. Serv., Ste Jeanne d'Arc; Tel. 845-4241.
LAURENCE, Marcel; 259 St-Georges, St-Jerome, P.Q.; Mon '48; ObstGyn; Staff, Hop. Hotel-Dieu-de-St.-Jerome.; Tel. GE 2-9711.
LAURENDEAU, Edmond; 1117 Est Blvd. St. Joseph, Montreal, P.Q.; Lav '32; **IntMed (P.Q.),** Cardiol (P.Q.); **Phys.-in-Chief, Hop. Notre Dame de la Merci; Tel. 331-2320.**
LAURENDEAU, Fernand; 1150 est Boul. St. Joseph, Montreal 35, P.Q.; Mon'60; FRCS(C), GenSurg; Surg., Hop. Maisonneuve.
LAURENDEAU, Pierre; 1229 Notre Dame St., Lachine, P.Q.; Mon '51; Otol(P.Q.); Sec., Med. Office, St. Joseph's Hosp. Tel. 637-9488 .
LAURENSON, R. Duncan; Aberdeen (Scot.) '53; Ass't. Prof. (Anat.), Queen's U., Kingston, Ont.
LAURENT, Eugene C.; Man'64; Res., St. Boniface Hosp., St. Boniface 6, Man.; Abroad.
LAURENT, Guy; 201-9eme ave., Dieux Montagnes, P.Q.; Mon'62.
LAURIAULT, Claude D.; 132 Principale, Maniwaki, P.Q.; Ott'62.
LAURIAULT, Louise; B.P. 337, Unite-Sanitaire, Thetford Mines, P.Q.; Lav. 61.
LAURIE, Neil M.; 35 Owen St., Barrie, Ont.; 40 Lettitia (res); Wes '28; Tel. PA 8-2552.
LAURIER, Claude; C.P. 329, 1221 Islemere, Ste-Dorothee, P.Q.; Mon '60.
LAURIER, Jean-Jacques; Ottawa Gen. Hosp., 43 Bruyere St., Ottawa 2, Ont.; 1881 Rideau Garden Dr. (res); **Mon '43; F.A.C.C.P., F.A.C.H.A.; Pulm. Dis. & TB (P.Q.); Med. Dir., Ottawa Gen.** Hosp.; Tel. 236-0333, Loc. 211.
LAURIER, Ruben; 10550 Papineau Ave., Montreal, P.Q.; **Mon '41; Pulm. Dis. & TB (P.Q.), IntMed. (P.Q.); Tel. DU 7-3355.**
LAURIMAA, Ivar; 23 King St. W., Stoney Creek, Ont.; Durham (Eng.)'60; AMCGP.
LAURIN, Andre; Mon'59; DiagRad(P.Q.); Staff, Hop. Maisonneuve, Montreal 36, P.Q.
LAURIN, Camille; 66 Pagnuelo Ave., Outremont, Montreal 8, P.Q. (res); Mon'50; Psy (P.Q.); Scien. Dir., Albert Prevost Inst.; Prof. (Psy.), U. of Mtl.; Tel. FE 4-2440.
LAURIN, Carroll A.; Ste 209, 3875 St-Urbain, Montreal 18, P.Q.; McG '52; FRCS(C); Orth-Surg.; GenSurg., Hotel-Dieu Hosp ; Tel. 849-8391.
LAURIN, Gilles; 14 rue Green, St. Lambert, P.Q.; 26 rue Macaulay (res); Mon'54; GenSurg (P.Q.); Staff Surg., Hop. Charles Lemoine; Tel. 671-9693.
LAURIN, Jean G.; 55, ave de l'Eglise, Montreal 19, P.Q.; Mon '50; Haem (P.Q.) Staff, Verdun Protestant Hosp.; Tel. 766-8511.
LAURIN-JOLY, Marjolaine; Mon'65; Res., Dept. De Physiologie, Universite De Montreal, Montreal 26, P.Q.
LAURIN, Paul E.; 4599 Jeanne d'Arc, Montreal, P.Q. (res); Mon '35; PathBact; Chief, Path.-Anat. Labs., Hop. Ste. Jeanne d'Arc; Telephone CL 5-5475.
LAURIN Robert; 5095 ouest Boul. Gouin, Montreal, P.Q.; Mon '57; MCGP; Vis. Phys., Hop. Sacre-Coeur-de-Cartierville; Tel. 334-6220.
LAURIN, Suzanne T.; Mon '56; Haem (P.Q.); Staff, Hop. Notre-Dame, Montreal 24, P.Q.; Tel. 525-6363.
LAUZE, Simon; 6773-32ieme Ave., Rosemont, P.Q. (res); Lav '41; Path (P.Q.); Ass't. Path., Anat. Lab., Hop. Notre Dame, Montreal, Ass't. Prof., (Path.), U. of Montreal; Tel. LA 5-6363.
LAUZER, Rosaire; 364 est, rue Sherbrooke, Montreal, P.Q.; Lav '26; GenSurg; Surg., Hop. Pasteur & Hon. Surg., Hop. St. Luc; Tel. 845-0853.
LAUZIER, J. Maurice; 2550 rue Holt, Montreal 36, P.Q.; Lav'60.
LAUZIER, Leo; 769 Boul. Walberg, Dolbeau, Co. Lac St. Jean, P.Q.; Lav '49; GenSurg; Chief **Surg., Hotel Dieu Sacre Coeur; Tel. 31.**
LAUZON, Gilles; Apt. 3, 5591 Cote des Neiges Rd., Montreal 26, P.Q.; Mon '59; FRCS(C); GenSurg; PlasSurg(P.Q.); Staff, Hop. Notre-Dame; Tel. LA 5-6363.
LAUZON, Maurice; 4044 est, Jean Talon, Cite St-Michel, Montreal-Nord, P.Q.; 7112-22eme Ave. (res); Mon '51; MCGP.
LAUZON, Rene; 2250 Bon-Air, Montreal, P.Q.; Mon '51.; Tel. 728-1142.
LAUZON, Roland; 1 Fox St., Penetanguishene, Ont.; 25 Robert E. (res); Lav '52; MCGP; Staff, Penetang Gen. & St. Andrews, Midland; Tel. 549-7092.
LAVALLE, Alfred B.; Ott'65; Res., Ottawa Gen. Hosp., Ottawa, Ont.
LAVALLEE, Alfred; Ste 704, 30 est, boul St-Joseph, Montreal 14, P.Q.; Mon '47; FICS; Urol; Active Staff (Urol.), Hop. Ste. Jeanne d'Arc; **Cons. (Urol.), Hop. St. Michel, Rosemont, Misericordia & Hop. Le-Gardeur, Repentigny; Tel. LA 4-9881.**
LAVALLEE, Bernard W.; 25 Belton Rd., Pointe Claire, P.Q.; Tor '56; MCGP.
LAVALLEE, Gerard; 981 Notre-Dame, Lavaltrie, Co. Berthier, P.Q.; Lav '58.
LAVALLEE, Guy; 52 Grande-Ile, Valleyfield, P.Q.; Mon '57; Tel. 373-6242.
LAVALLEE, Hugues; 875, boul des Recollets, Trois-Rivieres, P.Q.; Lav '55; Paed; Staff, Hop. St. Joseph; Tel. FR 4-6211.
LAVALLEE, Jean C.; Lav'65; Res., Hop. St. Michel Archange, Quebec 5, P.Q.
LAVALLEE, Jean-L.; Lav '61; Ophth; Staff, Hop.-Notre-Dame, Montreal, P.Q.; Tel. 525-6363.
LAVALLEE, Jean G.; 490 - 17eme rue, Grand' Mere, P.Q.; Lav '56; FRCP(C); ObstGyn.; Tel. LE 8-8935.
LAVALLEE, Joseph; Ott'65; Jr. Int., Ottawa Gen. Hosp., Ottawa 2, Ont.
LAVALLEE, J. Paul; 465 Lockhart, Montreal 16, P.Q.; Mon '52; Anaes; Staff, Hop. Notre-Dame; Tel. 525-6363.
LAVALLEE, Marc; 1582 ave des Pins, Montreal 25, P.Q.; Mon '58; Prof., U. of Montreal.
LAVALLEE, Marguerite O.; 9537—108th Ave., Edmonton, Alta. (res); Alb '51; Staff, Alberta Hosp.
LAVALLEE, Rene; Mon'61; Haem(P.Q.); Int-Med; Staff, Hop Maisonneuve, Montreal, P.Q.
LAVENTURE, Arthur R.; Spirit River, Alta.; Sask. '59.
LAVERGNE, J. Neree; 155 rue St-Jean, Quebec 4, P.Q.; Lav '24; Urol (PQ); Hd. & Clin. Instr. (Urol.), Hop. du-St.-Sacrement; Tel. 523-3500.
LAVERGNE, Paul H.; 10 Holyrood, Outremont, P.Q. (res); Lav '42; Pulm. Dis. & TB (PQ); Ass't. Dir. Hosp. Stat., Quebec Hosp. Serv.; Tel. 844-3781.
LAVERS, Harlan D.; 36 Logan St., Truro, N.S.; 96 Queen St. (res); Dal '43; D.P.H.; M.C.G.P.; **Med Staff, Colchester County Hosp.; Tel 893-9161.**
LAVERTY, S. George; 114 Barrie St., Kingston, Ont.; 75 L'Union St. (res); **Edinburgh (Scot.)** '46; MRCP (Lond); DPM (Lond.); Psy; Assoc. Prof. (Psy), Queen's U.; Tel. 546-1731, Loc. 318.
LAVIGNE, Arthur; 74 Principale, Granby, P.Q.; 37 rue Principale (res); Lav '54; ObstGyn(P..Q); Tel. FR 2-6270.
LAVIGNE, Jean; 2403 Principale, Farnham, P.Q.; Lav '59.
LAVIGNE, Louis R.; 1976 Rachel St. E., Mont**real 24, P.Q.; Mon '41; Tel. LA 1-5392.**
LAVIGNE, Pierre; McG'58; OrthPaed(P.Q.); Staff, Hop. Gen.-de-Verdun, Montreal 19, P.Q.
LAVIGNE, Robert; 1010 rue Tasse, Ville-St.-Laurent, Montreal 9, P.Q.; Mon '54; Active Staff, Hop.-Notre-Dame-de-l'Esperance; Vis. Staff **(Obst), Hop.-Sacre-Coeur; Tel.** RI 7-6892.

LAVIGNE, Rodolphe; 171 Montreal Rd., Cornwall, Ont.; 709 McConnell Ave. (res); Lav '45; Tel. WE 2-3177.
LAVIGNE, Roger; 65 rue Hamelin, Lachute, Co. Argenteuil, P.Q.; Mon '47; M.C.G.P.
LAVIOLETTE, Roland; L'Original, Ont.; Mon '33.
LAVOIE, Aurele; 260 rue Principale, Ste. Rose du Degeles, Cte Temiscouata, P.Q.; Lav'65.
LAVOIE, Bertrand; Lav'63; Res., Hop. Ste.-Justine, Montreal 26, P.Q.
LAVOIE, Bertrand; Lav '63; Res., Hop. Sacre-Coeur, Montreal 9, P.Q.
LAVOIE, Clarice M. see McKIERNAN-LAVOIE, Clarice M.
LAVOIE, Clement; 400 rue Tache, St.-Boniface, Man.; 641 rue Langevin (res); Lav '50; Tel. CE 3-6762.
LAVOIE, Daniel; Ste. 2, 6770 Boul. Pie IX, Montreal 36, P.Q.; Lav '54; FRCS(C), GenSurg; Staff, Hop. Bellechasse; Tel. 722-1808.
LAVOIE, G. Pierre; 1150 est Boul. St. Joseph, Montreal 34, P.Q.; Mon'58; FACS; FICA; FRCS(C), GenSurg; Sr. Surg., Hop. St. Luc; Ass't. Prof., U. of Montreal; Tel. 527-1241.
LAVOIE, Henri; 1051 rue St. Hubert, Montreal 24, P.Q.; Lav'56; ObstGyn(P.Q.); Staff, Misericorde Hosp.; Tel. 842-7181.
LAVOIE, J. Charles; Clinique St. Georges, 627 Jacques-Cartier E., Chicoutimi, P.Q.; Lav '49; Otol.
LAVOIE, J. Gerard; Lav '55; Anaes; Staff, Dept. of Anaes., Hop. Maisonneauve, Montreal 36, P.Q.; Tel. 254-8341.
LAVOIE, Jules A.; C.P. 1330, 335-1ere Ave., St.-Georges-de-Beauce Est, P.Q.; 133 Blvd. Lacroix (res); Lav'42; FICS; GenSurg; Chief Surg., Hotel-Dieu-Notre-Dame-de-Beauce; Tel. 228-3912.
LAVOIE, J. Victor; 1961 ouest, St-Cyrille, Quebec, P.Q.; Lav '18; OphthOtol; Retired.
LAVOIE, Lionel A.; Box 1690, Assoc. Medical Clinic, Melfort, Sask.; Ott'64; AMCGP; Staff, Melfort Union Hosp. & Melfort Geriatric Centre; Tel. 752-2876.
LAVOIE, Lucie; 112 boul. St-Joseph ouest, Montreal 14, P.Q.; McG '51; Tel. 272-3335.
LAVOIE, M. B.; 8415 St. Denis, Montreal, P.Q.; 460 Blvd. des Prairies, Laval-des-Rapides (res); Mon '50.; Tel. 681-4341.
LAVOIE, Pierre; 6650 - 25 ieme Ave., Rosemont, Mtl., P.Q.; Mon. '58; FRCS(C), GenSurg.
LAVOIE, Raynald; Clinique St-Georges, 627 Jacques-Cartier, Chicoutimi, P.Q.; Lav '58; Otol.; Tel. 549-0292.
LAVOIE, Real; 1606 rue Boucher, Rimouski, P.Q.; Lav'59.
LAVOIE, Rejane Josette; 1970 St-Just, Montreal, P.Q.; Mon'62; Paed.
LAVOIE, Rene G.; Ste. 201, 915 ouest, Boul. St.-Cyrille, Quebec 6, P.Q.; 1346 Pere-Jamay, Ste.-Foy (res); Lav '51; Ophth; Ass't Ophth, St-Francois-d'Assise; Tel. 681-6081.
LAVOIE, Roland; 915 Ste-Cyrille ouest, Quebec 6, P.Q.; 610 Chemin St.-Louis (res); Lav '45; D.A.B.Ot; Otol; Ass't. Staff, Hop.-de-l'Enfant **Jesus & Ste.-Foy Hosp's.; Ass't. Prof., Laval U.; Tel. 681-6081.**
LAVOIE, Vial; 208 St-Jacques, St-Jean, P.Q.; 230 Blvd. Montcalm (res); Mon '42; Phys. (O.P.D.), Hop. de St-Jean.
LAW, Choon L.; China '41; Staff, Coqualeetza Hosp., Sardis, B.C.
LAW, Douglas T.; 163 Laurier Ave. E., Ottawa 2, Ont.; Qns'42; Anaes.
LAW, Fong M.; Spirit River, Alta.; McG '37; Dist. Coroner; Tel. 9.
LAW, Frank F.; 211 Birks Bldg., Edmonton, **Alta.; Alb '25; Tel. GA 2-2072.**
LAW, George A.; 108 Regent Ave. E., Transconna 25, Man.; Man '33; MCGP; Active Staff, Concordia Hosp.; Court. Staff, St. Boniface Hosp.; Tel. CA 2-4422.
LAW, John T.; 11186—84th Ave., North Surrey, B.C.; Alb '62; Tel. 596-3384.
LAW, Maureen M.; Carleton Co. Health Unit, 1683 Merivale Rd., Ottawa, Ont.; Qns '64; Tel. 729-1438.
LAW, William B.; 190 Laurier Ave. E., Ottawa, Ont.; Qns '42; Med. Staff, Ottawa Gen. Hosp.; **U. of Ottawa Med Journal; Tel. CE 6-4592.**
LAWDER, John O.; UBC'65; Res., Vancouver Gen. Hosp., Vancouver 9, B.C.
LAWEE, Da'oud; 2045 Dufferin St., Toronto **10, Ont.; 525 Chaplin Cres., Apt. 507, Tor. 12 (res); Paris (Fr.) '53; L.Sc. (Paris); Tel. LE 6-2128.**
LAWLER, Arthur W.; Workmen's Comp. Bd., 657 W. 37th Ave., Vancouver 13, B.C..; 302-1111 Jervis St., Vancouver 5 (res); Man '32; M.R.C.-**O.G.; IntMed.; Phys., Physiother, Dept., W.C.B.;** Tel. AM 6-0211.
LAWLER, Robert H.; 2433 Assiniboine Cr. Winnipeg 12, Man. (res); Man '48; Psy; Dir., Dept. of Psy., Children's Hosp.; Ass't. Prof. (Psy), U. of Manitoba; Tel. SP 5-8311.
LAWLER, William R.; 289 Cedar St., Sudbury, **Ont.; 276 Wilson St., Lockerby (res)); Tor '47 D.A.B.S., F.R.C.S.(C), GenSurg; Tel. OS 4-3131.**
LAWLEY, Alan M.; James St., Inverness, N.S.; Dal '52.
LAWRASON, Douglas M.; Med. Arts Clinic, 51-6th St. S.E., Medicine Hat, Alta.; 403-5th St. S.W. (res); Wes '30; M.Sc., DABR; DiagRad; Staff, Medicine Hat Gen. Hosp.; Tel. 527-2281.
LAWRENCE, D. D'Arcy; Tor'65; Res., Vancouver Gen. Hosp., Vancouver 9, B.C.
LAWRENCE, George A.; Amherst, N.S.; London (Eng.)'50; FRCS(Eng.); FRCS(Ed.); MRCS (Eng.); LRCP(Lond.); GenSurg.
LAWRENCE, Hugh J.; 106 Talbot St. W., Leamington, Ont. Elizabeth Village Apts. Rob**son Rd.; (res); Tor '56; FRCS(C), GenSurg;** Tel. 326-3281.
LAWRENCE, James A.; St. George St., Annapolis Royal, N.S.; Dal'58; Staff, Annapolis Gen. Hosp.; Tel. 532-2144.
LAWRENCE, John H.; 1404-70th Ave. S.W., Calgary, Alta. (res); McG'50; Anaes.; Dir. Dept. of Anaes., Rockyview Gen. Hosp.; Tel. 266-1531.
LAWRIE, S. Wallace; Associate Med. Clinic, P.O. Box 790, Peace River, Alta.; Alb '57; MCGP.
LAWRIE, Thomas R., SG/LCDR; Aberdeen (Scot.)'51; M.B., Ch.B.; DiagRad; Chief of Radiol., Cdn. Forces Hosp., Kingston, Ont.
LAWS, H. Wyatt; 1509 Sherbrooke St. W., Apt. 17, Montreal, P.Q.; McG'40; D.Ophth, Ophth; Ophth-in-Chief, Queen Elizabeth Hosp., Ophth. Ass't. Surg., Montreal Children's Hosp.; Tel. WE 5-6936.
LAWS, James E.; Ott'55; DiagRad; Staff (Rad.), Ottawa Civic Hosp., Ottawa, Ont.
LAWSON, Alan K.; Dal'61; Res., Royal Alexandra Hosp., Edmonton, Alta.
LAWSON, David A.; 200 King St. S., Waterloo, **Ont.; Wes '57; AMCGP; Tel. SH 3-6328.**
LAWSON, Frank L.; Med. Centre, 68 King St. E., Cobourg, Ont.; 265 D'Arcy St. (res); Tor '40; DNB; FACS; FRCS(C), GenSurg; Surg. Cons., Ontario Hosp., Cobourg; Tel. 372-5494.
LAWSON, F. Samuel; Apt. 807, 121 Allan St., Oakville, Ont.; Tor'28; D.Psy; Psy; Retired.
LAWSON, Gordon A.; 58 Lawrence Ave. E., Toronto, Ont. (res); Man '26; PhysMed; Head **Phys. Med., Sunnybrook Hosp., Toronto; Tel. 485-8651.**
LAWSON, Gordon E.; Minto, N.B.; Dal '51; FAGS.
LAWSON, James T.; 35-6th St., New Westminster, B.C.; 301-5th Ave. (res); Man '31; Tel. LA 1-5757. Retired.
LAWSON, Jean (MacDonald); Box 32, Southampton, Ont.; Dal'44; ObstGyn.
LAWSON, John; 60 King St. W., Ingersoll, Ont.; Edinburgh (Scot.) '41; Tel. 485-1100.
LAWSON, John B.; 1291 Ouellette Ave., Windsor, Ont.; Oakleigh, Matchette Rd., River Canard (res); Wes '45; Tel. 252-8591.
LAWSON, Ray N.; 4459 Sherbrooke St. W., Montreal, P.Q.; 37 Church Hill (res); Wes '37; D.-Surg., F.A.C.S., F.R.C.S.(C), GenSurg; Lect. Surg. McGill U.; **Ass't. Surg., Royal Victoria Hosp.; Tel. WE 5-1265.**

LAWSON, Victor G.; Tor'60; Ass't. Res., Wellesley Hosp., Toronto, Ont.
LAWTON-GREGORY, Michelle V.; 476 Victoria Ave., Montreal 6, P.Q.; Mon '59; Part-Time Practice; Tel. 484-6153.
LAWTON, Louis E.; 41 Queens Rd., St. John's, Nfld.; 155 Elizabeth Ave. (res); Dal '43; Pt.-time MO, WCB; Assoc. Surg. Staff, St. John's Gen. Hosp.; Tel. 8-4373.
LAWTON, Robert D.; O'Mara Martin Bldg., 135 Military Rd., St. John's, Nfld.; Dal '50; Ophth; Active Staff, St. John's Gen., St. Clare's Mercy & Grace Hosp's.; Tel. 578-2770.
LAXDAL, Arni T.; Indian Head Sask.; Man '60.
LAXDAL, Oliver E.; Medical Arts Clinic, Regina, Sask.; 26 Langley St. (res); Tor '47; F.R.-C.P.(C), Paed; Chief, Paed. Serv. Regina Gen. Hosp.; Sr. Staff Member, Regina Grey Nuns' Hosp.; Vis. Cons. U. Hosp., Saskatoon; Paed. Cons. Dept. of Public Health & Dept. Indian **Affairs, Regina; Tel. LA 2-1811.**
LAY, Richard A. Q.; 3313 Roblin Blvd., Charleswood, Man.; London (Eng.) '33; MRCS; LRCP; MCGP; Court. Staff, Grace, Misericordia, Rehab. & Children's Hosp's.; Tel. VE 2-1613.
LAYCOCK, Harold E.; Fort Coulonge, P.Q.; Qns '52; Coroner, Pontiac Co.; Tel. 68.
LAYCRAFT, George H.; 1010 McCallum Hill Bldg., 1874 Scarth St., Regina, Sask.; Alb '53; Anaes.; Tel. 522-8400.
LAYDEN, J. Murray; Mulgrave, N.S.; Dal '58. Tel. 52-2.
LAYNG, James L.; Roblin, Man.; Royal Coll. of Surg. (Dublin, Ire.)'54; D.Anaes. (Lond.); Tel. 22.
LAYNG, John M.; 1541 West Broadway, Ste. No. 403, Vancouver 9, B.C.; 4702 W., 7th Ave. (res); **Ott '53; MCGP; Tel. RE 6-0107.**
LAYTNER, Bernard D.; 262 Wilson Ave., Downsview, Ont.; 46 Himount, Willowdale (res); Tor '43; Paed; Jr. Att'd. Staff, New Mount Sinai Hosp.; Tel. ME 6-2200.
LAYTON, Basil D. B.; 211 Sunnyside Ave., Ottawa, Ont. (res); Tor '31; M.P.H. (Harvard), PH; Principal M.O., Research Development & International Health, Dept. of Nat'l Health & Welfare, **503 Copeland Bldg., Ottawa; Tel. CE 2-**8211.
LAZAR, Gregory; Apt. 18, 4935 Queen Mary Rd., Montreal 29, P.Q.; Ferencz-Joseph, Szeged **(Hungary) '35; Tel. RE 9-7042.**
LAZARCHUK, Myron; 476 Tranquille Rd., North Kamloops, B.C.; Vienna (Austria) '47; GenSurg; Tel. 376-5811.
LAZARCHUK, Olga; 476 Tranquille Rd., North Kamloops, B.C.; Tel. 376-5811.
LAZAROU, Lazaros P.; 514 Danforth Ave., Toronto, Ont.; Salonica(Greece) '52; DiagRad; Staff, St. Michael's Hosp.; Tel. 362-4461.
LAZAROVITS, Stephen; 1147 Dundas St. W., Toronto 3, Ont.; 79 Collegeview Ave. (res); Pazmany U. (Budapest, Hung.) '45; M.C.G.P.; Staff, Doctor's & Grace Hosp's.; Tel. LE 1-5441.
LAZARUK, William G.; Willingdon, Alta.; Alb **'41; Dist. Coroner; Tel. 24 R 2.**
LAZARUS, Sarill S.; 909 Sherritt Ave., Lynn Lake, Man.; London (Eng.)'50; MRCS(Eng.); LRCP(Lond.).
LAZENBY, Frederick S.; 170 St. George St., Toronto 5, Ont.; 200 Forest Hill Rd. (res); Tor '18; DermSyph; Derm. Staff, Toronto Western Hosp. & St. Joseph's Hosp.; Tel. WA 1-4840.
LAZORKO, Wolodymyr; **2596 E.—18th Ave., Vancouver, B.C.; Lviv (Ukraine) '35; Staff, Prov.** Mental Hosp., Essondale.
LAZURE, Denis; 3100 Ellendale, Montreal 26, P.Q.; Mon'52; Psy; AAPCC (Paed.Psy.); Assoc. Prof. Psy., U. of Montreal; Cons. Ministry of Health P.Q.; Tel. 731-4931.
LEA, R. Gordon; The Polyclinic, 170 Fitzroy St., Charlottetown, PEI; 1 Green St. (res); Dal '38; Chief of Med. PEI Hosp.; Registrar, Med. Council of PEI: Tel. 894-7325.
LEA, Robert H.; Simmons Med. Clinic, 243 Loch Lomond Rd. East, Saint John, N.B.; Dal'65; Staff, Saint John Gen. & St. Joseph's Hosp's.; Tel. 657-3920.

LEACH, Clifton E.; 182 Winnipeg Ave., Port Arthur, Ont. (res); Tor'50; D.Psy; Psy; Clin. Dir., Ont. Hosp.; Tel. DI 4-3571.
LEACH, Clifford G.; Man'65; Jr. Int., Winnipeg Gen. Hosp., Winnipeg 3, Man.; Abroad.
LEACH, J. E. K.; 340 McLeod, Ottawa 4, Ont.; Qns'43; DermSyph; Derm., Ottawa Civic & Cons. Derm., Grace Hosp's.; Cons. Derm., Kemptville Dist. Hosp.; Tel. CE 5-2567.
LEACH, N. Gary; Ott '60; Assoc. Res. (Surg.), **Harper Hosp., Detroit 1, Mich., U.S.A.; Abroad.**
LEACH, W. G., W/C; 1107 Avenue Rd., Toronto 12, Ont.; 8A William Baker Pk., Downsview (res); Wes '52; W/C & O/C, Flying Personnel Med. Estab. Inst. of Aviation Med., R.C.A.F.; Tel. ME 3-7985.
LEACH, William J.; Manotick, Ont.; Tor '11.
LEACH, Wilson G., G/C; Surgeon General's Hdqs., Ottawa, Ont.; Wes'52.
LEACOCK, Arthur M.; 11219-57th Ave., Edmonton, Alta.; McG'52; Anaes; AMCGP.
LEACY, J. William; 253 Ontario St., Kingston, Ont.; Qns'60; Tel. 546-1474.
LEADMAN, Thomas P.; 190 MacLaren St., Ottawa, Ont.; 90 Sunnyside Ave. (res); Qns '43; **F.R.C.S. (Eng.), GenSurg.; Tel. 235-2613.**
LEAHY, Carl F.; Ott '64; Res., Ottawa Civic Hosp., Ottawa 3, Ont.
LEAHY, Denis W.; Grandview, Man.; Ireland'49; Phys. & Surg., Grandview Dist. Hosp.; Tel. 53.
LEAHY, Philip J.; Box 189, Teeswater, Ont.; Tor '52; MCGP; Active Staff, Wingham Dist. Hosp. & County of Bruce Gen. Hosp.; Tel. 392-6813.
LEAHY, W. Harry; 141 Tancred St., Sault-Ste-Marie, Ont.; Qns '19; Tel. AL 6-9790.
LEAKOS, James; **556 Medical Arts** Bldg., 750 Spadina Cres., Saskatoon, Sask.; 34 McDermid Cres. (res); Alb '54; Otol; Att'd. Staff, Uni**versity, Saskatoon City & St. Paul's Hosp's.; Tel. 652-5585.**
LEAMY, Peter J.; 3310 Boundary Rd., Vancouver 12, B.C.; McG'51; Active Staff, Burnaby Hosp.; Vis. Staff, Vancouver Gen., Mt. St. Joseph's & Grace Hosp's.; Tel. 434-3131.
LEATH, Nathan; 72 Burnaby Blvd., Toronto 12, Ont. (res); Alb '46; D.M.R.; TherRad; Staff, Princess Margaret Hosp.; Clin. Instr. (Rad.), U. of Toronto; Tel. 924-0671.
LEATHERBARROW, Albert T.; Hampton Station, King's Co., N.B.; Qns '16; F.A.C.P., F.R.-I.P.H. & H. (Lond.); Dist. Coroner; Tel. 832-5522.
LEATHERDALE, Charles L.; Port Burwell, Ont.; Wes '60.
LEAVINE, Desta F.; 667 King St. W., Kitchener, Ont.; Qns '54; Derm; Active Staff, St. Mary's Gen. & Kitchener-Waterloo Hosp's.; Tel. SH 5-5353.
LEAVITT, Clark T.; 32 Academy Medical Bldg., 1812-4th St. W., Calgary, Alta.; 1440 Richland Rd. (res); Alb '54; IntMed.; Tel. 263-7272. Abroad.
LEAVITT, Joseph; 4489 Maplewood Ave., Mont**real P.Q.; McG '16; Anaes.; Tel. RE 8-6300.**
LEAVITT, Preston M.; 115 Hazen St., Saint John, N.B.; Dal'65.
LEBBETTER, Thomas A.; Winnipeg Clinic, Winnipeg, Man.; 614 Park Towers, 2300 Portage Ave. (res); Dal '14; F.A.C.P., IntMed; Memb. Div. Med., Winnipeg Clinic; Retired.
LEBBETTER, Thomas A.; Winnipeg Clinic, N.E. St. Mary's & Vaughan, Winnipeg 1, Man.; Man '56; Urol; Tel. WH 2-6441.
LEBEAU, Rene; 3725 Maplewood St., Montreal, **P. Q.; Mon '37; Anaes.; Tel. RE 8-7046.**
LEBEL, Etiennette; Mon'57; FRCP(C), Anaes; Staff, Hop. Hotel-Dieu, Montreal 18, P.Q.; Tel. VI 4-0161.
LEBEL, Georges; 4565 Queen Mary Rd., Montreal 9, P.Q.; Lav '41; Paed (P.Q.); Staff, Queen Mary Vet's. Hosp.; Tel. FE 4-9232.
LEBEL, Georges A.; 137 Hotel de Ville, 67 Albert St., Aylmer, P.Q.; Lav '45; Staff, Hop. Prive.
LEBEL, Jacques; 3875 St. Urbain, Montreal 18, P.Q.; 316 Willowdale, Outremont (res); Mon'48; Obst (P.Q.); **Hd. (Med. Dept.), Hop. de la Misericorde; Staff Ophth., Hop. Ste-Justine; Tel.** VI 2-5141.

LEBEL, J. Etienne; 34 ave. Maplewood, Montreal 8, P.Q. (res); Mon '54; TherRad (P.Q.); **Staff, (Radio-isotope), Hop.-Hotel-Dieu; Tel. VI 4-0161.**
LEBEL, L. Leon; 3875 St. Urbain, Ste. 215, Montreal 18, P.Q.; Mon'43; IntMed; Cardiol (P.Q.); Staff, Hotel-Dieu Hosp.; Tel. 843-5681.
LEBEL, Rejean; 132 est Notre-Dame, Trois Pistoles, P Q.; Lav'65.
LeBER, S. Marshall; Tor'50; Staff, Royal Alexandra Hosp., Edmonton, Alta.
LEBEUF, Jacques, 2815 Willowdale, Montreal 26, P.Q.; Lav '58; Psy (P.Q.); Psy., Hop. des Laurentides, L'Annonciation; Cons. & Research Dept. of Psy., Hop. Notre-Dame; Teach. Staff, Albert-Prevost Inst.; Tel. 733-1663.
LEBLANC, Alphonse E.; Ste. 406, 302 Ouellette, Windsor, Ont.; **417 Askin Blvd. (res); Lav '51; M.C.G.P.; Tel. 252-2185.**
LEBLANC, Claude; 55 Church Ave., Montreal 19, P.Q.; Mon'57; FRCS(C), GenSurg; Ass't. Surg., Verdun Gen. Hosp.; Tel. PO 8-8531.
LEBLANC, Francis E.; Ott'59; Ph.D. (Physiol.); Sr. Fell. (Neurosurgery), Neurological Inst., 3801 University St., Montreal 2, P.Q.; Dem. (Neurology & Neurosurg.), McGill University.
LEBLANC, Gerard; 681 Blvd. Talbot, Chicoutimi, **P.Q. (res); Lav '55; FRCS(C), NeurSurg; Staff, Hop. Hotel-Dieu St.-Vallier, Chicoutimi; Tel. 549-1452.**
LEBLANC, Guy; Mon'56; Res., Hop. St. Charles, Joliette, P.Q.
LEBLANC, Guy; Lav'63; Res., Hop. Ste-Justine, Montreal, P.Q.
LEBLANC, Henri C.; 97 Alma St., Moncton, N.B.; Lav'32; Tel. 855-8547.
LEBLANC, Irenee; 225 Grande Allee E., Quebec 6, P.Q.; 1055 Chemin St.-Louis (res); Lav '40; M.O., WCB (P.Q.); Tel. 522-4751.
LEBLANC, J. A. Roland; 3692 Chemin St-Louis, Quebec 10, P.Q.; Lav'54.
LEBLANC, Jean J.; 27 rue Gendron, Hull, P.Q.; Lav '44; Anaes.
LEBLANC, Jean L.; Lav '60; AMCGP; Res., Albert-Prevost Inst., Montreal, P.Q.
LEBLANC, Jean L.; Ste. 531, 465 Victoria, St. Lambert, P.Q. (res); Mon'52; MCAA; Paed; Clin. **Ass't., Montreal Chilren's Hosp., Montreal; Tel. WE 7-8511.**
LEBLANC, J. Marc; Carleton-sur-Mer, Cte Bonnaventure, P.Q.; Lav'51; Anaes., Hop. Notre-Dame de Chartres-Maria; Tel. 59.
LEBLANC, Joseph A.; 80 Mgr. Tessier, Rouyn, P.Q.; 575 Perreault E. (res); Lav '36; PH (P.Q.); Staff, Health Unit, Rouyn-Noranda.
Le BLANC, L. Claude; Elbow Drive Medical Dental Centre, 5116 Elbow Dr., Calgary, Alta.; **Ott '60; AMCGP; Tel. AL 5-6647.**
LEBLANC, Lionel G.; Mon '43; IntMed (P.Q.); Med. Sup., Hop. de Ste-Anne, Ste-Anne de Bellevue, P.Q.; Tel. 453-3440.
LEBLANC, Lomar; 986 Brant St., Ottawa 7, Ont.; Ott '55; MCGP; Tel. SH. 9-9492.
LEBLANC, Loyola E.; 55 Rue Emmerson, Edmundston, N.B.; 30 Rue Fraser (res); Mon '49; **Paed; Dir. Paed. Serv., Hotel Dieu & St Joseph's Hosp's.; Edmundston; Tel. RE 5-3361.**
LeBLANC, L. Philippe; 77 Westmount Rd., Guelph, Ont.; Ott'53; GenSurg; DABS; Chief of Surg., St. Joseph's Hosp.; Tel. TA 4-8810.
LEBLANC, Marcel; Mon'52; D&T Rad.; Staff, Hop. Ste. Croix, Drummondville, P.Q.
LEBLANC, Marien; 227 Notre Dame E., Victoriaville, P.Q.; Lav '55.
LEBLANC, N. Adelard; St. Gabriel, Co. Rimouski, P.Q.; Lav '19.
LEBLANC, Paul; Matapedia, Cte Bonaventure, P.Q.; Lav'65.
LEBLANC, Paul E.; Buctouche, N.B.; Lav '53; Tel. 743-2496.
LEBLANC, Paul-E.; Lyster, Co. Megantic, P.Q.; Lav '56.
LeBLANC, Phillip H.; Little Brook, Digby Co., N.S.; Lav '43; M.C.G.P.
LeBLANC, Pierre; Clinique Metropolitaine, 1150 est, boul. St-Joseph, Montreal 34, P.Q.; Mon'57; FRCS(C); GenSurg; NeurSurg (P.Q.); Staff, Hop. Maisonneuve; Cons., Dept. of NeurSurg., Hop. St. Joseph de Rosemont & Hop. Ste-Justine; Tel. LA 7-1241.
LEBLANC, Pierre; Mon'63; Res., Hop. Hotel-**Dieu, Montreal 18, P.Q.**
LEBLANC, Rene; 700 Route Marie-Victorin, Tracy, P.Q.; Lav'52; Tel. RI 3-5944.
LeBLANC, Richard; C.P. 2657, Outardes 4, Cte Saguenay, P.Q.; Lav '62.
LEBLANC, Rodolphe F.; C.P. 1297, 355 rue Oxford, Fredericton, N.B.; Lav'53; AFACCP.
LEBLANC, Roland P.; Gravelbourg, Sask.; Lav '51; Tel. 648-2277.
LEBLANC, Roland; 1010 Chemin St-Roch, Tracy, P.Q.; Mon'59; Paed; Tel. 742-2253.
LEBLANC, Victor; Tracadie, N.B.; Lav '46. est, Montreal 11, P.Q.; Mon'65.
LEBLANC, Wilfrid; Clinique Jarry, 150 Jarry est, Montreal 11, P.Q.; Mon'65.
LEBLANC, W. L.; Maniwaki, P.Q.; Hotel de Ville (res); Ott '51.
LEBLOND, Andre; 198 Notre-Dame Sud, Thetford Mines, Cte Megantic, P.Q.; Lav'57; ObstGyn. (P.Q.); Tel. 335-2505.
LEBLOND, Charles P.; 68 Chesterfield Ave., Westmount, P.Q. (res); Paris (Fr.) '34; D.Sc. (Sorbonne); Ph.D. (Montreal); Cons. Staff (Anat.), Montreal Gen. Hosp.; Prof. (Anat.), McGill U.; Tel. VI 9-3057.
LEBLOND, Jean M.; 49 Government Rd. W., Kirkland Lake Ont.; 56 McCamus (res); Lav '36; MCGP; Coroner for Temiskamingue.
LEBLOND, Joseph; 317 Pere Marquette, Quebec, P.Q.; Lav '07; Staff, Workmen's Comp. Bd., 225 Grande Allee, Quebec.
LeBLOND, J. W. Rupert; 310 Medical Dental Bldg., Rose St. & 11th Ave., Regina, Sask; 2800 McCallum Ave. (res); Tor'51; Sr. Staff, Regina General & Grey Nuns Hosp's.; M.O., **Carling Breweries; Tel. LA. 3-7681.**
LEBLOND, Pierre; Lav'65; Res., Hop. St. Sacrement, Quebec 6, P.Q.
LEBLOND, Sylvio; 475 Boul. Talbot, Chicoutimi, P.Q.; Lav '28; IntMed; Chief of Med. Hotel-Dieu-St.-Vallier; Prof. (ClinMed), Laval U.; Tel. 549-1621.
LeBLOND, Wilfrid; 3060 Petit Village, Quebec 5, P.Q.; Lav '26; DPH(France); Haematol.(Paris); Microbiol.(France); ClinPath(P.Q.); PathBact; IntMed; Dir., Health Serv., Hop. de l'Enfant Jesus; ClinPath., Hop. Notre-Dame de l'Esperance; Dir. of Labs., San. Begin; Hon. Prof., Industrial Hygiene, Laval U.; Dir. of Health Serv., Goodyear Factory; Phys., Joseph Morneau Inc., Charlesbourgh; Tel. MO 3-0653.
LEBOEUF, Bernard; 1560 Est Sherbrooke, Montreal 24, P.Q.; Mon'55; FRCP(C); IntMed.; Ass't., Dept. of Biochemistry, Hop. Notre-Dame; Ass't. Prof., Dept. of Med., University of Montreal; Tel. 525-6363, Local 216.
LEBOEUF, Gilles S. R.; Mon '56; Int'n., Hosp. for Sick Children, Toronto, Ont.
LEBOEUF, Jean Louis; 349 boul. Tache, Hull, P.Q.; Lav '64.
LEBOEUF, Yves; 1125 Blvd. D'Auteuil, Duvernay, P.Q.; Mon '58; Research (Hosp. Admin.), University of Montreal.
LeBOLDUS, Gordon M.; 396 Queens Ave., London, Ont.; Wes'60; FRCS(C); Otol; Instr. in Otology, Rhinology & Laryngology, St. Joseph's Hosp. & University of Western Ontario; Tel. 434-9151.
Le BOLDUS, J. Martin; 1820 Victoria Ave., Regina, Sask.; **2503 Winnipeg St. (res); Wes '32;** M.C.G.P.; Sr. Att'd. Staff, Regina Gen. & Regina **Grey Nuns Hosp's.; Tel. LA 2-6117.**
LEBOURDAIS, Paul E.; Aurigny, Iles-de-la **Madeleine, P.Q.; Lav '42.**
LEBOUTHILLIER, Perley; Caraquet, N.B.; Lav '57.
LEBRUN, Andrew; Mon'64; Res., Hop. Maisonneuve, Montreal 36, P.Q.
LEBRUN, Claudette; Mon'65; Res., Hop. Hotel-Dieu, Montreal 18, P.Q.

LEBRUN, Conrad J.; 440 Hinton Ave., Ottawa 3, Ont.; Ott '55; FRCS(C); Otol; Staff, Ottawa Civic Hosp.; Tel. 729-2312.
LEBRUN, Gerald J.; Bedford, N.S.; Dal '37; GenSurg; Lect. (Surg.), Dalhousie U.; Tel. 2-4406.
LEBRUN, J. Adrien; 7464 rue St. Denis, Montreal 10, P.Q. (res); Mon'24; Staff, Hop. Ste-Justine; Tel. RE 1-4931.
LECHOW, Bohdan; Ste. 205, 59 N. Court St., Port Arthur, Ont.; 500 Red River Rd. (res); Man '53; Tel. DI 4-2122.
LECHTER, Mortimer; Qns '62; Intn., Jewish Gen. Hosp., Montreal, P.Q.
LECKEY, Robert G.; 915 King St. W., Toronto 3, Ont.; 47 Willingdon Blvd., Tor. 18 (res); Tor '50; GenSurg; Plant Phys., Massey-Ferguson Ltd.; Tel. EM 6-6911.
LECKIE, Garnet B.; Lake of the Woods Clinic, 112 Matheson St. S., Kenora, Ont.; Man '58; MCGP; Tel. HO 8-6423.
LECKIE, George G.; 810 Canada Bldg., Saskatoon, Sask.; 501—7th St. E. (res); Man '25; Dist. Coroner.
LECLAIR, Claude Capt.; Mon '65; 3 RCHA, Fort Osborne Barracks, Winnipeg, Man.
LECLAIR, J. Edgar; C.P. 430, 147 Notre Dame St., Azilda, Ont.; Lav'57.
LECLAIR, J. Maurice; McG'51; Haem(P.Q.); FRCP(C), IntMed; Dir., Faculté Medecine, Universite Sherbrooke, Sherbrooke, P.Q.
LECLAIR, Paul E.; 3871 est Belanger, Montreal, P.Q.; 7050 rue Verdier, St-Leonard-de-Port-Maurice, Montreal-Nord (res); Mon '58; Cardiol (P.Q.); Staff, Hop. Belle-Chasse, Hop. Gen. Fleury & Hop. Belanger; Tel. 729-5231.
LECLAIR, Rene B.; 3827 Ave. Lacombe, Montreal, P.Q.; **3823 Ave. Lacombe (res); Mon '30; M.C.G.P.; Tel. RE 7-5004.**
LECLAIRE, Yves, Lt-Col.; Cdn. Forces Base, Borden, Ont.; 4050 Grey, N.-D.-G., Montreal (res); Mon'43; DPH; Army M.O.
LECLERC, Claude; App. 4, 19 Arnaud, Baie-Comeau, P.Q.; Lav'63.
LECLERC, Georges; 418 Sherbrooke St. E., Montreal 24, P.Q.; 521 Sherbrooke E. (res); Mon '38; D.A.B.D.; FRCP(C), DermSyph; Hd. Dept. of Derm. Hop.-Notre-Dame; Cons. (Derm.), Queen Mary Vet's. Hosp; Prof. of Derm., U. of Montreal; Tel. VI 4-7647.
LECLERC, Georges E.; Mon'65; Res., Hop. Notre-Dame, Montreal 24, P.Q.
LECLERC, Gilles; Lav'59; Res.(Anaes.), Hop. St. Joseph, Trois-Rivieres, P.Q.
LECLERC, J. Arthur; C.P. 305, Pointe-au-Pic, Cte Charlevoix, P.Q.; Lav'28; GenSurg(P.Q.); AMCGP.
LECLERC, Jean; 34 Fabrique, Quebec, P.Q.; Lav '48; FRCS(C), OrthSurg; Staff (OrthSurg), Hotel-Dieu & Laval U.; Tel. 523-2410.
LECLERC, Jean L.; 1014 ave des Erables, Quebec 6, P.Q.; Lav '55; FRCS(C), GenSurg.; Tel. 681-5592.
LECLERC, Jean P.; C.P. 42, Ste. Claire, Co. Dorchester, P.Q.; Lav **'53.**
LECLERC, J. Flavius; Health Unit, Count. of Terrebonne, 351 rue Labelle, St. Jerome, P.Q.; Lac Guindon, Cte. Terrebonne, P.Q. (res); Lav '29; D.P.H.; Staff, Phys., Dept. of Health (P.Q.).
LECLERC, Jules E.; 1000 Chemin-Ste.-Foy, Quebec 6, P.Q.; 2405 Noury, Sillery (res); Lav '54; FRCS(C), ObstGyn; Ass't. (ObstGyn), Hop. St.-Sacrement; Tel. 527-9944.
LECLERC, Laval; Lav'62; FRCS(C), OrthSurg; Staff, Hop. de l'Enfant-Jesus, Quebec, P.Q.
LECLERC, Leon; C.P. 7, Imperial Tobacco Co., Granby, P.Q.; Mon'44; Staff(Anaes.), Hop. St. Joseph De Granby; Indus. Phys., Imperial Tobacco Co., Miner Rubber Co., Cdn. Westinghouse, Simonds Canada Saw, Thor Mills, Stedfast Rubber & Laiterie Leclerc.
LECLERC, Leonidas; St. Phillipe de Neri, Co. Kamouraska, P.Q.; Lav '50; Dist. Coroner.
LECLERC, Louis; 10375 rue Papineau, Montreal, P.Q.; 2117 Sauveur (res); Mon '56; A.M.C.G.P.; Tel. DU 1-0061.
LECLERC, Louis P.; L'Islet, P.Q.; Lav '19.
LECLERC, Louis-P.; 1193 ave. des Erables, Que**bec 6, P.Q.; 2071 Chemin-Ste.-Foy, Quebec 10 (res); Lav '26; GenSurg; Surg. Staff, Hop. St.-**Sacrement; Ass't. Prof., Laval U.; Tel. 523-2601.
LECLERC, Marc Y.; 7911 Wilfrid-Pelletier, Ville d'Anjou, Montreal 5, P.Q.; Lav '55. Anaes.
LECLERC, Michel; 218 Ave. St. Jerome, Matane, P.Q.; Lav '46; GenSurg.
LECLERC, Roger; Box 1300, C.C.C.S. John Cabot, St. John's, Nfld.; Lav '62.
LECLERC, Roland; 1500-18eme rue, Quebec 3, P.Q.; Lav'61; Paed.
LECLERC, Therese M.; 6371 rue St. Hubert, Apt. 1, Montreal 10, P.Q.; Mon '55.; Tel. 277-1010.
LECOQ, Henri; 5654 Laurendeau, Cote St. Paul, Montreal 20, P.Q.; Mon '59.; Tel. 766-5114.
LECOQ, J. Pierre; 118 Denison Ave. W., Granby, P.Q.; McG '52; Tel. 372-3456.
LECOT, Albert; Man '45; Staff, East General Hosp., Toronto 6, Ont.; Tel. 461-8272.
LECOURS, Antonio; 445 Ouest Boul. St-Joseph, Montreal 8, P.Q.; Lav'34; FACS; FRCS(C), GenSurg.
LECOURS, Henri; C.P. 278, 198a rue Notre-**Dame, Black Lake, P.Q.; Lille (France) '60.**
LECOURS, J. Raymond; 900 Boul. Decarie, St. Laurent, Montreal 9, P.Q.; 1655 de-l'Eglise (res); Mon '31; IntMed (PQ); Staff, Notre-Dame-de-l'Esperance; Tel. 747-1329.
LECOURS, Roch H.; 49 Charles, Aylmer, P.Q.; Ott '54; **M.C.G.P.**
L'ECUYER, Jean T.; Maniwaki, P.Q.; Mon **'29; Dist. Coroner.**
L'ECUYER, Maurice; 912 est Sherbrooke, Montreal 24, P.Q.; 11995 Boul. Fredmir, Mtl. N. (res); Mon'58; OrthSurg (P.Q.); Tel. 524-4133.
LEDDY, John E.; 605 Canada Bldg., Saskatoon, Sask.; McG '37; F.A.C.S., F.R.C.S.(Edin.), F.R.C.S.(C) GenSurg; Surg. Staff, St. Paul's & City **Hosp's.; Surg. Staff, & Ass't Clin. Prof., U. of Saskatchewan; Tel. 244-5355.**
LEDERER, Ludwig; 1538 Sherbrooke St. W., Montreal, P.Q.; 434 Dufferin Rd. (res); Prague **(Czech.) '20; Tel. WE 3-4820.**
LEDERMAN, John J.; 606 Fairmont Med. Bldg., 750 W. Broadway, Vancouver 9, B.C.; UBC '60; LI.B; AMCGP; Tel. TR 4-9236.
LEDGER, John L.; Wpg. Gen. Hosp., 700 William Ave., Wpg. 3, Man.; Man'59; Psy.; Admin.(Psy.), Wpg. Gen. Hosp.; Ass't. Prof., Dept. of Psy., University of Manitoba; Tel. 774-6511.
LEDGERWOOD, Ernest F.; 5798 Victoria Dr., Vancouver 16, B.C.; 2056 W. 58th Ave., Van. 14, (res); UBC '60; MCGP; Tel. FA 5-1288.
LEDINGHAM, Margaret E.; 64 Academy Medical Bldg., 1812 - 4th St. W., Calgary, Alta.; 416 Roxboro Rd. (res); Man '48; ObstGyn.; Tel. 269-2238; Abroad.
LEDOUX, Armand; 126 Brooks S., Sherbrooke, P.Q.; Deauville (res); Mon '38; GenSurg (P.Q.); **Staff, Hotel-Dieu; Tel. 562-8100.**
LEDOUX, Leon; 1251 St. Denis, Montreal, P.Q.; Mon '43; OrthSurg; Orth., Hop. St. Luc; Tel. UN 1-7261.
LEDOUX, Roger; 6452 Guillaume Couture, Montreal 5, P.Q.; Mon'60; DiagRad; Staff, Hop. Notre-Dame.
LEDUC, Aime; 79 Ste. Cecile, Valleyfield, P.Q.; Mon '31; Gyn; M.C.G.P.; Tel. 373-3663.
LEDUC, A. Michel; 7630 Centrale, Ville Lasalle, P.Q.; Mon'65.
LEDUC, Andre; 1560 Sherbrooke St. E., Montreal, P.Q.; 5635 Canterbury, Mtl. 26 (res); Mon '42; Bact (P.Q.); Chief, Dept. of Bact., Hop.-Notre-Dame; Ass't. Prof. (Bact.), U. of Montreal; Assoc. Exec. Dir. Assoc.-des-Medecins-de-Langue-Francaise-du-Canada, 5064 ave-du-Parc, Mtl. 8; Tel. LA 5-6363, Loc. 562.
LEDUC, Bernard; Mon '63; Sr. Int., Hop. Notre-Dame, Montreal, P.Q.
LEDUC, Claude; 5751 ave Northmount, Montreal 26, P.Q.; Mon'53; Anaes; Staff, Hop-Ste-Justine, Montreal, P.Q.; Tel. RE 1-4931.
LEDUC, Gaston; Mon '42; F.C.C.P., Pulm. Dis. & TB (P.Q.), Ass't. Med. Dir., Hop. San St. Joseph 5689 Rosemont Blvd., Montreal, P.Q.; Tel. CL 6-2681.

LEDUC, G. Gilles; Centre-Medical St.-Urbain, 3875 St.-Urbain, Montreal 18, P.Q.; 2582 Blvd. Pius IX (res); Mon '50; IntMed (P.Q.); Cardiol (P.Q.); Staff Phys., Hop. Hoteu-Dieu; Cons. Hop. Ste.-Justine; Tel. 842-6933.
LEDUC, Guy; 361 est, St-Joseph, Montreal 14, P.Q.; Mon'55; Psy; Staff, Hop. Maisonneuve; Tel. 255-8301.
LEDUC, Ishbel; N.A. Inst. of Technol., 11762-106th St., Edmonton, Alta.; Ott'54.
LEDUC, Jacques R.; 30 est Boul. St. Joseph, Ste. 718, Montreal 14, P.Q.; 4653 Ave. Lacombe (res); Mon'47; Ph.D.; Staff, Hop. Maisonneuve; Tel. 845-4241.
LEDUC; Jean H., Major; Camp Hosp., Gagetown, N.B.; Ott'54.
LEDUC, Jean M.; 960, boul Ste-Croix, Montreal 9, P.Q.; McG'55; Tel. RI 8-8133.
LEDUC, L. Jacques; 2160 Capitaine Bernier, Montreal 12, P.Q. (res); Mon '44; Anaes; Staff, Hop-St-Luc; Tel. 861-7321.
LEDUC, Paul Emile; 4395 Ave. Verdun, Verdun, P.Q.; 775 Beatty (res); Mon '42; IntMed (P.Q.).
LEDUC, Pierre; Ste. 2, 260 rue Ball, Sherbrooke, P.Q.; Lav'64; Tel. 567-3854.
LEDUC, Pierre; 62 ouest Blainville, Ste Therese, P.Q.; Mon'65.
LEE, Albert; Rangoon (Burma)'59; Paed; Staff, Shaughnessy Hosp., Vancouver, B.C.
LEE, Anathalie W. (Heath); 212 Yarrow Bldg., Victoria, B.C.; Alb '40; DiagRad; Part-time Staff, Royal Jubilee Hosp.; Tel. 386-7538.
LEE, Anthony, J.; 295 Cedar St., Sudbury, Ont.; Bristol (Eng.) '48; M.R.C.S., L.R.C.P.; Path., **St. Joseph's Hosp.; Tel. 674-8411.**
LEE, Arthur H.; 1199 Austin Rd., New West-minster, B.C.; Sask '61; AMCGP; Tel. LA 2-2557.
LEE, Charles C.; 40 London St., Tillsonburg, Ont.; 22 Bidwell St. (res); Wes '34; M.C.G.P.; Tel. VI 2-3636.
LEE (Wong), Clara; 30 Newbold Dr., Burlington, Ont. (res); Wes '37; Not practising.
LEE, Clemens; Chiba (Japan)'62; Res., Halifax Infirmary, Halifax, N.S.
LEE, David B.; 338 Mission, B.C.; 7592 Stave Lake Rd. (res); McG'52; Tel. 826-7211.
LEE, D. H. Taylor; 1605 York Pl., Victoria, B.C. (res); Tor '51; D.M.R.; DiagRad; Assoc. Rad, Royal Jubilee Hosp.; Tel. EV 6-3131.
LEE, Ding-Tsai; 1257 Henry St., Halifax, N.S.; Taiwan (Formosa)'54; ECFMG; FRCS(C), ObstGyn; Staff, Grace Maternity Hosp.; Research Fell. (ObstGyn.), Dalhousie U.; Tel. 422-2616.
LEE, Dou H.; Soeul (Korea) '48; Path; Staff, Provincial Hosp., Campbellton, N.B.; Tel. 753-4461.
LEE, Earl R.; 23 George St., St. Stephen, N.B.; Dal '48; DiagRad; Staff, Charlotte County Hos-pital; Tel. 466-1140.
LEE, Eldon E.; 1669 Victoria St., Prince George, B.C.; Washington (U.S.A.) '55; ObstGyn.; Tel. 564-8070.
LEE, Eric H.; 1880 Rideau Gdn. Dr., Ottawa 1, Ont. (res); Man '34 Adm., Can. Pension Comm; Tel. CE 2-8211.
LEE, Flaviana S.; 3105 Oak St., Vancouver 9, B.C.; Santo Tomas (Philipp.) '59.
LEE, Garth G.; Ste. 102, 1940 Lonsdale Ave., North Vancouver, B.C.; Man'57; GenSurg; Tel. YU 5-1939.
LEE, George H.; Medical Centre, 5 Central St., Summerside, P.E.I.; Edinburgh (Scot.) '48.
LEE, G. G.; 168 Dundas St. W., Toronto, Ont.; 441 Glengarry (res); Tor '32; Tel. 368-9592.
LEE, Han C.; Box 490, Williams Lake, B.C.; Seoul(Korea)'48; GenSurg; Med. Staff, Cariboo Mem. Hosp., Williams Lake, B.C.; Tel. 392-7221.
LEE, Henry H.; 196 George St., Hamilton, Ont.; Colquhoun Cres., (res); M.C.G.P.; Wes '43; Obst Gyn; Staff, Hamilton Gen., & Obst. Staff, St. Joseph's Hosp.; Tel. JA 7-1545.
LEE, Henry J.; 405 No. 5 Rd., Richmond, B.C.; Seoul(Korea)'48; Staff, Richmond Gen., Vancouver Gen., & St. Paul's Hosps.; Public Health Officer, Richmond School Board; Tel. 278-8638.
LEE, Ian N.; 142 Simcoe St. N., Oshawa, Ont.; 954 Mowhawk St. (res); London (Eng.) '55; FRCS(Endin.); DLO; Otol; Active Staff, Oshawa Gen. Hosp.; Active Cons., Ajax & Pickering Gen., Port Perry Mem., Bowmanville & Uxbridge Hosp's.; Tel. 728-4646.
LEE, Jae R.; 181 Lincoln Rd., Grand Falls Nfld.; Seoul (Korea) '54; FRCP(C), IntMed; Chief of Med., Central Newfoundland Hosp.; Tel. 2802.
LEE, Jane; 150 Yardley Ave., Toronto 16, Ont.; 189 Ferris Rd. (res); Lingnan (China) '51; MCGP; Tel. PL 9-3911.
LEE, John Y.; 2161 Danforth Ave., Toronto 13, Ont.; McG'65.
LEE, Kyoo H.; Seoul (Korea) '50; Jr. Intn., Queen Elizabeth Hosp., Montreal, P.Q.
LEE, Randolph; 200 Danforth Ave., Toronto 6, Ont.; Tor'63; Staff (G.P.), Toronto East Gen. & Doctors Hosp.; Court. Staff, Wellesley Hosp.; Tel. 461-0761.
LEE, Richard B.; 1 Hopecrest Cres., Scarborough, Ont.; 9 Foxwarren Dr., Willowdale (res); Tor '57; MCGP; Staff, (G.P.), Scarborough Gen. Hosp.; Tel. AM 1-9360.
LEE, Richard W.; 115 Hazen St., Saint John, N.B.; Dal '55; IntMed.; Tel. 692-9674.
LEE, Richmond J.; Box 800, 41 Broadway Ave., Wawa, Ont.; Man'63; Active Staff, Lady Dunn Gen. Hosp.; Tel. 856-2379.
LEE, Robert E.M.; 4609 Lazelle Ave., Terrace, B.C.; 4820 Davis Rd. (res); Man'52; FRCS(C); FACS; GenSurg; Staff, Mills Mem. Hosp., Terrace & Kitimat Gen. Hosp., Kitamat; Tel. VI 3-2242.
LEE, Robert G.; Tor '60; Res., Toronto Gen. Hosp., Toronto 2, Ont.; Abroad.
LEE, Robert H.; Qns'52; Staff, Parry Sound Gen. Hosp., Parry Sound, Ont; Abroad.
LEE, Simon J.; Soeul (Korea) '57; FRCP(C), IntMed; Staff, University Hosp., Edmonton, Alta.; Clin. Instr., U. of Alberta; Tel. 439-5911, Loc. 277.
LEE-SING, Mamin S.; 123 1st Ave. E., Canora, Sask.; Sask '64; Tel. 563-5672.
LEE-SING, Swithin; 123 1st Ave. W., Canora, Sask.; Sask '64; Tel. 563-5672.
LEE, Siu-Pik; (See LEE, Jane).
LEE, Stuart B.; Tor'59; FRCS(C), GenSurg; Staff, Ottawa Civic Hosp., Ottawa, Ont.
LEE, Thomas; Avon Med. Bldg., 2715 Avonhurst Dr., Regina, Sask.; London(Eng.) '43.
LEE, Thora W. (See HAYNES)
LEE, William A.; Man '64; Res., Winnipeg Gen. Hosp., Winnipeg 3, Man.
LEE, Wilson J.; 175 Llydican Ave., Ext. Chatham, Ont. (res); McG '43; Paed; Chief of Paed., Public Gen., & St. Joseph's Hosp's.; Chm., Med. Staff, Public Gen. Hosp.; Tel. EL 2-6400.
LEEDER, James R.; 101 Le Marchand Mansion, 116th St. & 100th Ave., Edmonton, Alta; 14115-96th Ave. (res); Alb '48; FACOG; ObstGyn; Instr,. ObstGyn., U. of Alberta; Tel. HU 8-3333.
LEEDS, John H.; Mount Hope, Ont.; Qns '15.
LEERS, Wolf D.; 49 Renault Cres., Weston, Ont.; Wuerzburg (Germ.) '55; D. Bact. (Tor.); Bact; Fitzgerald Mem. Fell., (Microbiol.), Schl. of Hygiene, U. of Toronto; Tel. WA 3-6611.
LEES, Brian; 35 West Valley Rd., Corner Brook, Nfld.; London (Eng.) '41; M.R.C.S., L.R.C.P., M.R.C.P.; Vis. Anaes., West Coast San., Corner Brook; Tel. 634-5232.
LEES, C. D.; 401 Medical Arts Bldg., Winnipeg, Man.; 62 Riverside Dr., Wpg. 19, (res); Man '50; Adm., W.C.B.; Tel. GL 2-8809.
LEES, H. Hislop; 1150 Chilver Rd. Windsor, Ont. (res); Qns '19; Anaes; Chief of Anaes, Metropolitan Hosp.; Cons. (Anaes.), Hotel Dieu & Grace Hosp's.; Tel. 254-4016.
LEES, Joan see McCausland, Joan.
LEES, M. Anne; 5370 Larch St., Powell River, B.C.; Liverpool (Eng.)'49; DCH; Tel. 486-7515.
LEESON, C. Roland; 395 Days Rd., Kingston, Ont.; Cambridge (Eng.) '50; M.B., B.Ch., M.A., M.D. (Cantab.); Assoc. Prof. (Anat.), Queen's U.; Tel. LI 6-1731.
LEESON, Helen J.; 939 Lawrence Ave. E., Don Mills, Ont.; Tor'39; DPH; Paed; Staff, Hosp. for Sick Children.

LEESON, James I.; Box 88, Wiarton, Ont.; Wes '51; MCGP; Staff, Mem. Hosp., Wiarton; Tel. 534-1160.

LEESON, John F.; 68 King St. E., Cobourg, Ont.; 257 Walton St. (res); Tor '48; Staff, Cobourg Gen. Hosp.; Tel. FR 2-5494.

LEESON, Paul F.; 92 Mary St., Orillia, Ont.; 34 Maple Dr. (res); Tor '48; Staff, Orillia Soldiers' Mem. Hosp.; Tel. 325-5061.

LEESON, Thomas S.; Cambridge (Eng.) '50; M.D. (Cantab.); Prof. & Hd. Dept. of (Anat.), U. of Alberta, Edmonton, Alta.; Tel. GE 9-8721.

LeFAVE, Lawrence R.; 1466 Ouellette Ave., Windsor, Ont.; Qns '32; Tel. 253-9446.

LEFCOE, Neville M.; Victoria Hosp., 375 South St., London, Ont.; R.R. 3, Komoka (res); Vanderbilt (Nashville, Tenn.)'50; FRCP(C), IntMed; Staff, Victoria Hosp.; Assoc. Prof. (Med.), U. of Western Ont.; Tel. 432-5261.

LEFEBVRE, Adrien; 46 Towzin St., Dorval, P.Q. (res); Mon '33; Staff, Can Pensions Comm.

LEFEBVRE, Albert; 1910 de l'Eglise, Ville St. Laurent, Montreal, P.Q.; Mon '52.; Tel. RI 4-2518.

LEFEBVRE, Andre; Roxton Falls, Cte. Shefford, P.Q. (res); Lav '34.

LEFEBVRE, B. Arthur; 3977 Hochelaga St., Montreal, P.Q.; Mon '57.; Tel. CL 6-3931.

LEFEBVRE, Bernard M.; 43 rue Bruyere, Ottawa, Ont.; 1575 Balena, Ott 8 (res); Lav '54; FRCS(C), GenSurg; Staff, Ottawa Gen. Hosp. & Geographical Lect. (Surg.), U. of Ottawa; Tel. 233-7377.

LEFEBVRE, Charles E.; 106 Le Marchand Mansions, 116th St. & 100th Ave., Edmonton, Alta.; 9845-110th St. (res); Alb '35; IntMed (Alb); Lect., U. of Alberta; Tel. 488-5932.

LEFEBVRE, Eugene; 847 Sherbrooke St. E., Montreal, P.Q.; Mon '23.

LEFEBVRE-GAGNON, Louise; Lav'65; Res., Hop. St-Sacrement, Quebec 6, P.Q.

LEFEBVRE, G. T. G.; 29 Bouchette St., Huntingdon, P.Q.; McG '44; Dist. Coroner; Tel. 264-5416.

LEFEBVRE, Guy; 825 Belvedere S., Sherbrooke, P.Q.; Lav '48.

LEFEBVRE, Guy A.; Mon'58; Anaes; Staff, Hop. St. Luc, Montreal 18, P.Q.

LEFEBVRE, Jacques; 1252 est Belanger, Montreal, P.Q.; Mon'52.

LEFEBVRE, J. Andre; 832 Blvd. St. Joseph E., Montreal 14, P.Q.; Mon '56.; Tel. LA 4-9772.

LEFEBVRE, J. F. A.; 46 Touzin, Dorval, P.Q. (res); Mon '33; Staff, D.V.A., Federal Govt., Montreal; Dist. Coroner.

LEFEBVRE, J. Lucien; 595 Blvd. Charest E., Quebec, P.Q.; 884 Eymard Ave.) Res); Lav '39; Ophth. Otol; Part-time Staff, Mun. Clin., Dept. of Ophth. Otol., Quebec; Tel. 529-9721.

LEFEBVRE, Josephat; 17 St. Gabriel, St-Gabriel-de-Brandon, Co. Berthier P.Q.; Lav '22.

LEFEBVRE, Matthieu C., Capt.; Military Hosp., Kingston, Ont; Mon'65.

LEFEBVRE, Paul; 3412 Atwater, Montreal, P.Q.; 715-45th Ave., Lachine (res); Mon '52; Psy; Staff Psy., Notre Dame Hosp., Mtl.; Tel. WE 7-2669.

LEFEBVRE, Pierre; 2930 Maplewood, Apt. 405, Montreal 26, P.Q.; Mon '50; Psy (P.Q.).

LEFEBVRE, Rene R.; 850 - 38eme Ave., Lachine, P.Q. (res); Mon '50; D.Sc. (Med.); Path (P.Q.); Staff (Path.), Hotel-Dieu, Montreal; Assoc. Prof., U. of Montreal; Tel. 637-5907.

LEFEBVRE, Rodrigue; 1300 est rue Sherbrooke, Montreal, P.Q.; 1302 est rue Sherbrooke (res); Mon '29; IntMed (P.Q.), Cardiol (P.Q.); Chief, Dept. of Cardiol., Hop. Hotel-Dieu; Assoc. Prof., Med. Path., U. of Montreal; Tel. VI 4-0161.

LEFEBVRE, Roger; 600-12th Ave., St.-Louis De Terrebonne, Cte. Terrebonne, P.Q.; Mon '51; Anaes.; Staff, Hop. Ste. Jeanne D'Arc, Montreal, P.Q.

LEFEBVRE, Rosaire; Mon'63; Res., Hop. Maisonneuve, Montreal 18, P.Q.

LEFEBVRE, Yves; Hop. Notre-Dame, 1560 Sherbrooke Est., Montreal 24, P.Q.; 7643 Ave. Defougeray, Ville D'Anjou; Mon'58; FRCS(C); ObstGyn; Staff, Dept. of ObstGyn, Hop. Notre-Dame; Teach. Staff, University of Montreal; Tel. 525-6363, Ext. 216, or 352-1411.

LEFRANCOIS, Jacques; 825 sud, rue Belvedere, Sherbrooke, P.Q.; Lav '58; OrthSurg.; Tel. 567-3611.

LEFRANCOIS, Robert; Mon '62; Res., Hop. Notre-Dame, Montreal 24, P.Q.

LEGARE, Adolphe M.; 382 Grosvenor Ave., Westmount, P.Q. & 367 Place Des Fleurs, Dollard Des Ormeaux, P.Q.; Ott'55; PlasSurg; Staff, Lakeshore Gen. Hosp., Pointe Claire, P.Q.; Tel. HUI-5869 & 626-1805.

LEGARE, Andre; 4506, Boul. Pie IX, Rosemont, Montreal 36, P.Q. (res); Mon '57; DiagRad; Staff, Hop. St. Luc.; Tel. VI 2-5201.

LEGARE, Benoit J.M.; 770 lere Ave., Quebec 3, P.Q.; 18-1/2-10th E., St. Rodrique (res); Lav'52; ObstGyn; Tel. 523-7253.

LEGARE, Jean P.; 7155 Ave., Charlesbourg, Quebec 7, P.Q.; 265 Blvd. Henri-Bourassa (res); Lav '58; Tel. 623-3713.

LEGARE, Laurier; 644 Rideau St., Ottawa 2, Ont.; McG'42; AMCGP; Tel. 235-2767.

LEGARE, Luc; C.P. 279, St. Joseph, Co. Beauce, P.Q.; Lav '58.

LEGARE, Marguerite; 11820 Notre Dame E., Pointe-Aux-Trembles, Montreal 5, P.Q.; Mon'49; Tel. 645-8267.

LEGARE, Maurice; 2171 Sherbrooke est, Montreal, P.Q.; Mon '27; Anaes; Anaes., Hotel Dieu de Montreal; Tel. VI 4-0161.

LEGATE, W. Stephen; 181 Main St., Milton, Ont.; Tor'35; GenSurg; Tel. 878-3352.

LEGAULT, Gaston; 1896 ouest Dorchester, Montreal, P.Q.; Lav'51; MAH; ISAH(Mtl.); Dir. Med. Serv., Quebec Coll. of Medicine & Surgery.

LEGAULT, Gerard; 1553 Viel, Montreal 12, P.Q.; 12087 Bois-de-Boulogne (res); Mon '60.; Tel. 4-3470.

LEGAULT, Jean-Paul; CH 507, 3875 St-Urbain, Montreal 18, P.Q.; Mon '34; FACS; FICS; Urol; Chief, Dept. of Urol., Hop. Hotel-Dieu; Assoc. Prof., U. of Montreal; Tel. 845-3159.

LEGAULT, Leonard; 300 Carre St. Louis, Montreal 18, P.Q.; 1120 Bernard (res); Mon'35; FICS; Anaes; Hd., Dept. of Anaes., Hop. de la Misericorde; Ass't. Prof., U. of Montreal; Tel. VI 4-9700.

LEGAULT, Maurice; 261 Hubert, Greenfield Pk., Cite Jacques-Cartier, P.Q.; Mon '63.

LEGAULT, Pierre; 240 Elm, St-Lambert, Cite Jacques-Cartier, P.Q.; Mon'51; Cardiol (P.Q.); Tel. 671-5637.

LEGAULT, Raymond; Mon'52; Psy; Staff, Hop. St. Jean-de-Dieu, Montreal 5, P.Q.

LEGAULT, Robert; 6565, Christophe-Colomb, Montreal 10, P.Q.; Mon'64; Staff, Dept. of Med., Hop. Santa Cabrini; Tel. 272-8012.

LEGENDRE, J. Alfred; 1077 Ave. Fournier, Ste.-Foy, P.Q.; Lav '54; MCGP; Tel. 653-9413.

LEGENDRE, Jeanne; 1035 Boul. Bellerive, Longueuil, Cite Jacques-Cartier, P.Q. (res); Mon '59; Staff, Dept. of Health, Mlt.; Tel. VI 9-9371.

LEGENDRE, J. H.; 967 Blvd. St. Joseph E., Montreal, P.Q.; Mon '20; F.R.C.P.(C), IntMed.; Cons., Hotel Dieu Hosp., Phys., Hop. St. Jean de Dieu; Tel. VI 5-0322.

LEGER, Anthony F.; Apt. 7, 3410 Rosedale Ave., Montreal 28, P.Q. (res); Lav '53.

LEGER, Aurele; 8 Maple St., Ste-Anne-de-Bellevue, P.Q.; Mon '56; Tel. 453-5692.

LEGER, Eugene; 640 Mountain Rd., Moncton, N.B.; Lav '50; Tel. 384-5257.

LEGER, F. Emery; 186 Archibald St., Moncton, N.B.; 184 Archibald St. (res); Lav '42; M.C.G.P.; Tel. EV 4-8711.

LEGER, Francois; 3766 Queen Mary Rd., Montreal 26, P.Q.; 760 Pratt, Outremont (res); Mon '52; A.M.C.A.A., F.R.C.P.(C), IntMed; Cons. (Med.), Queen Mary Vet's. Hosp.; Tel. RE 1-3211.

LEGER, Gerard C.; 260 Westmount Blvd., Moncton, N.B.; Lav'28; D.P.H., M.C.G.P.; Med. Dir., La Societe L'Assomption (Assur.), & Hop.-Hotel Dieu-de-L'Assomption.
LEGER, Hugette; Lav'60; FRCP(C), IntMed; Staff, Hop. Hotel-Dieu, Montreal, P.Q.
LEGER, Jacques; 1681 Parc Lafontaine, Montreal, P.Q.; Mon '42; Ph.D., F.A.A.A., M.C.A.A., All. (P.Q.), IntMed (P.Q.); Vice-Pres., Cdn. Acad. of All.; Pres., Soc. of All. of P.Q.
LEGER, Jean L.; 1560 Sherbrooke St. E., Montreal, P.Q.; 365 Leacross, Ville Mont Royal (res); Mon '43; D.& T. Rad.; Chief Radiol., Hop. Notre Dame; Assoc. Prof. Rad., U. of Montreal; Tel. 527-2164.
LEGER, J. Euclide; 28 rue Alma, Moncton, N.B.; Lav '22; GenSurg; Cons. Staff, Hotel-Dieu & Moncton Hosp's.; Tel. 855-3201.
LEGER, L. Paul; Box 260, Tracadie, Cte. Gloucester, N.B.; Lav'51; DiagRad.
LEGER, Yvan; 1037 Est, Boul. St-Joseph, Montreal 34, P.Q.; 2551 Beauclerk (res); Mon '52; **Psy; Psy., Hop. St.-Jean-de-Dieu; Tel. VI 5-7804.**
LEGERE, Hermel; Lav'62; DiagRad(P.Q.); Staff, Hop. Hotel-Dieu, Sorel, P.Q.
LEGERSKI, Roger; 106 Northgate Bldg., Edmonton, Alta.; Cologne (Germ.) '54; Tel. GA 2-1184.
LEGGETT, Laurence H.; 319 Speedvale Ave. E., Guelph, Ont.; Qns '24; F.R.C.S.(Ed.), F.R.C.S.(C), F.I.C.S., GenSurg; Tel. TA 4-8550. Abroad.
LEGRAND, Herve; 916 rue Cherrier, Montreal, P.Q.; Mon'20; Ophth, Otol; Cons.(Med.), Hotel Dieu Hosp.; Prof., University of Montreal; Tel. LA 3-1611.
LeGRESLEY, Louis P.; App. T.6, Pavilion A., Havres des Iles, Chomedy, P.Q.; Mon'45; DABP; FRCP(C), Path; Pathol., Hop. Maisonneuve; Ass't. Prof. (Pathol.), U. of Mtl.; Tel. 254-8341.
LEGRIS, A. J.; Ridgeway, Ont.; Crystal Beach (res); Qns '38; Dist. Coroner.
LEGROS, J. Guy; Mon '63; Res., Hop. Maisonneuve, Montreal 36, P.Q.
LEGROW, Charles L.; Port-aux-Basques, Nfld.; McG '34; M.C.G.P.; M.O., Channel., Hosp., Channel, Nfld.; Tel. 695-2151.
LEGZDINS, Alexandra; 60 Marlowe Cres, Ottawa, Ont.; Latvia '35.
LEHINANT, Volker W. A.; Bancroft, Ont.; Prague (Czech.) '39.
LEHMAN, Geoffrey W.; Ste. 25 1390 Sherbrooke St. W., Montreal 25, P.Q.; McG'53; D.Surg. (McG); DABS, FACS, FRCS(C), GenSurg; Clin. Ass't. (Surg.), Royal Victoria Hosp.; Court. Staff, Queen Elizabeth Hosp.; Lect., McGill U.; Tel. 842-4971.
LEHMANN, Elsa; 396 Francis Rd., Richmond, B.C.; McG'45.
LEHMANN, Eric C. H.; 925 W. Georgia, Vancouver, B.C.; Tor '45; F.R.C.S.(C), OrthSurg; Active Staff, St. Paul's Hosp. & Children's Hosp.; Clin. Ass't., U. of British Columbia; Tel. MU 1-9464
LEHMANN, Heinz E.; 6875 LaSalle Blvd., Montreal 19, P.Q.; 6603 LaSalle Blvd. (res); Berlin (Germ.)'35; Psy; Clin. Dir., Douglas Hosp.; Prof. (Psy), McGill U.; Vis. Prof. Psy., U. of Cincinnati; Tel. 766-8511., Ext. 218.
LEHMANN, Maurice J.; 302 Boyd Bldg., Winnipeg 1, Man.; 550 Queenston St., Wpg. 9 (res); Man '45; FACS, FICS; FRCS(C), GenSurg; Active Staff (Surg.), St. Boniface Hosp.; Cons. Surg., Man. Rehab. Hosp.; Court. Staff, Wpg. Hosp's.; Ass't. Prof. (Surg.), U. of Manitoba; Tel. WH 3-6437.
LEHMANN, Peter O.; 750 W. Broadway, Vancouver 9, B.C.; 3304 Radcliff (res); Man '37; D.A.B.N., NeurSurg; Assoc. in Neur. Surg., Vancouver Gen. Hosp.; Cons. in Neur. Surg., Shaughnessy Hosp.; Clin. Instr., U. of British Columbia; Tel. TR 4-1211.
LEHOCZKY, Leslie; 499 Main St. E., Hamilton, Ont.; Budapest (Hung.)'53.
LEHOUX, Armand; Lav'63; Ass't. Res., Hop.-Notre-Dame, Montreal, P.Q.
LEHOUX, Louis M.; 299-5th rue, Quebec 3, P.Q.; 1330 rue Patenaude, Sillery, Quebec 6 (res); Lav '53; Otol; Tel. 524-8924.
LEHUQUET, J. Raymond; Ste. 201, 1625 Oak Bay Ave., Victoria, B.C.; **1398 Oliver St. (res); U.B.C. '55; M.C.G.P.; Staff, O.P.D., Victoria Vet's. Hosp.; Assoc. Staff, Royal Jubilee Hosp.; Tel. EV 6-1523.**
LEIBEL, Bernard S.; 200 St. Clair Ave. W., Toronto 7, Ont.; London (Eng.) '38; Cons. (Diab.), Sunnybrook Hosp.; Dir. Dept. of Med. Research & Cons. (Metabol.), Mount Sinai Hosp.; Tel. 924-9275.
LEICESTER, Joseph; Man'46; Res., General Hosp., Winnipeg, Man.
LEIGHTON, Claude M.; 195 Bonaccord, Moncton, N.B.; 20 Athlone Ave. (res); Dal '43; Paed; Active Staff, Moncton & Hotel-Dieu Hosp's.; Tel. EV 4-8630.
LEIGHTON, K. Macrae; 3227-W. 28th Ave., Vancouver, B.C.; Aberdeen(Scot.)'47.
LEISHMAN, John D.; 635 Glenmaroon, Vancouver, B.C. (Res.); Man'35; Urol.
LEITCH, Douglas B.; 210 McLeod Bldg., Edmonton, Alta.; 6220—111 Ave. (res); Tor '13; F.A.A.P., F.R.C.P.(C), **Paed**; Emeritus Phys., University & Royal Alexandra Hosp's.; Staff (P.H.) Child Welfare Clinics; Tel. 422-7412.
LEITCH, Gary T.; Alb '64; Res., U. of Alberta Hosp., Edmonton, Alta.
LEITCH, Jack R.; 85 South St., Goderich, Ont.; 27 Nelson St. E. (res); Wes'52; MCGP; Tel. 524-9511.
LEITCH, Sheila de N. (Kingsmill); Mental Health Clinic, Ontario Hosp., London, Ont.; Wes'55; D.Psy; Psy; Staff Psy., Mental Health Clinic, Ontario Hosp.; Tel. 455-5110.
LEITH, Arthur B.; 3550 Cote des Neiges Rd., Montreal 25, P.Q.; McG '55; Ophth; Staff, Montreal Gen., Children, & Catherine Booth Hosp's.; Staff, McGill U.; Tel. 935-6020.
LEITH, John D. F.; 50 Place Cremazie, Montreal 11, P.Q.; Queen's U. (Belfast, Ire.) '45; M.B., B.Ch., BAO(Hon.); MCGP; Vice. Pres. & Dir. of Med. Affairs, Pfizer Co. Ltd.; Tel. 381-9331.
LEITH, Mary P.; 645 Fort St., Victoria, B.C.; 2423 Currie Rd. (res); Wes'51; Tel. 385-3632.
LEITH, Wilfred; 4119 Sherbrooke St. W., Montreal, P.Q.; 20 Highfield (res); Dal '42; M.C.A.A., All. (P.Q.), IntMed; Clin. Ass't., Royal Victoria Hosp.; Assoc. Res., McGill U. Clin.; Dem., McGill U.; Tel. WE 7-1805.
LEITMAN, H. Reuben Robert; 6501 Fielding Ave., Montreal, P.Q.; 5619 Westluke Ave., Cote St. Luc (res); Lausanne '51; D.Psy; Ass't. Psy., Verdun Protestant Hosp.; Tel. 766-8511.
LEIZNER, Harry; 10 Regina Ave., Toronto 19, Ont.; Tor'30; Staff Phys., Ontario Hosp., Whitby, Ont.
LEJEUNE, Louis P.; 31 King St. W., Sherbrooke, P.Q.; 2360 Verdun (res); Mon '55; F.R.C.S.(C), GenSurg.; Tel. 569-7822.
LEKICH, Denise M. — see — HOLT, Danica M.
LEKIE, Rene; Montpelier (France)'63; Staff, Ecole d'Hygiene, U. of Montreal, Montreal 26, P.Q.
LEKISCH, Edmund; 10808-129th Ave., Edmonton Alta.; 10325 Villa Ave. (res); Graz (Austria) '13; Tel GR 7-6682.
LELIEVRE, Michel L.; Lav'65; Res., Hop. Enfant-Jesus, Quebec 3, P.Q.
LEMAIRE, Charles; 3362, rue Houde, Trois Rivieres, P.Q.; Lav '37.
LEMAIRE, J. Charles; 122 rue St. Jean, Drummondville, P.Q.; Lav'52; GenSurg (P.Q.); Tel. 478-5152.
LEMAIRE, Marcellin; 27 Desbraves, Terrebonne, P.Q.; Lav'61.
LEMAIRE, Raymond; 241 Quest, Fleury, Montreal 12, P.Q.; Lav '56; F.R.C.S.(C), OrthSurg; Staff, Hop. Sacre Coeur, Cartierville; Tel. FE 4-1210.
Le MASTERS, George S.; 476 Portage Rd. N., Niagara Falls, Ont.; Wes '62; MCGP; Active Staff (G.P.), Greater Niagara Gen. Hosp.; Bd. of Dir., Welland County Mental Health Unit; Tel. 356-0434.
LEMAY, Andre; Lav'65; Res., Hop. Hotel-Dieu, Quebec 4, P.Q.
LEMAY, Charles A.; 3367 Masson, Montreal 36, P.Q.; Mon'58; Tel. 721-7178.

LEMAY, Conrad; 1965 Belanger Ave., Montreal 35, P.Q.; 267 Dauphin Pont Viau (res); Man '50; Tel. RA 7-4627.

LEMAY, Guy; 1 rue Champlain, Pointe Gatineau, P.Q.; Lav'63.

LEMAY, Jacques; 6985 Christophe-Colomb, Montreal 10, P.Q.; Mon'65; Tel. 276-3466.

LEMAY, Jean D.; 165 King St. E., Sherbrooke, P.Q.; Lav'51; Anaes(P.Q.); Tel. 569-2961.

LEMAY, J. Fernand; 34 Gamble E., Rouyn, P.Q.; Lav '43; GenSurg (PQ); Hd. Surg., Hop. You-ville-de-Noranda; Tel. 762-6511.

LEMAY, Jean; 274 rue Friel, Ottawa 2, Ont.; 139 Granville, Eastview (res); Lav '53; ObstGyn; Staff, Ottawa Gen. & St. Louis-Marie-de-Montfort Hosp's.; Tel. CE 3-7407.

LEMAY, J. Robert; Mon'65; Res., Hop. St-Luc, Montreal 18, P.Q.

LEMAY, Marcel; Lav'58; Res., Hop. St-Luc, Montreal 18, P.Q.

LEMAY, Pierre M.; 428 Rideau St., Ottawa 2, Ont.; McG '56; **ObstGyn; Staff, Ottawa Gen. Hosp.; Clin. Asst. ObstGyn U. of Ottawa; Tel. CE 6-4592.**

LEMAY, Raymond; Deschaillons, P.Q.; Lav '31.

LEMAY, Richard; 183 St.-Georges, Levis, P.Q.; Lav'53; Paed (P.Q.); Tel. 478-5152.

LEMAY, Rodrigue; Manic 2, C. P. 12000, Baie Comeau, P.Q.; Lav '60.

LEMAY, Yves; 541 rue de l'Hopital, Jonquiere, P.Q.; 509 rue Pasteur (res); Lav '51; FICS; GenSurg; Chief (Surg.), Hotel-Dieu; Active Staff (Surg.), Saguenay Gen. Hosp.; Tel. 547-9341.

LEMELIN, Fernand; 750 St. Vallier Ouest, Quebec 8, P.Q.; Lav'42; Psy.(P.Q.); Chief Cons, Dept. of Psy., Hop. Christ Roi, Quebec, P.Q.; Tel. 683-3116.

LEMESURIER, Arthur B.; 606 Medical Arts Bldg., 170 St. George St., Toronto, Ont.; 22 St. Thomas St. (res); Tor '10; F.R.C.S.(C) OrthSurg, GenSurg; **Cons. Surg., Hosp. for Sick Children; Tel. WA 1-3007.**

LEMIEUX, Andre; Le Centre Medico-Social, 898 rue Richelieu, Quebec 4, P.Q.; Lav'55; Psy; Cons. Child Psy., Hop. Hotel-Dieu; Ass't. Prof. (Psy.), School of Social Sciences, Laval U.; Ass't. Dir., Le Centre Medico-Social; Tel. 529-9211.

LEMIEUX, Bernard G.; 15 Arthur Ave. S.E., Minneapolis, Minn., U.S.A.; Lav'61; FRCP(C), Neur.; Abroad.

LEMIEUX, Gerard; 3010, La Promenade, Ste-Foy, Quebec 10, P.Q.; Lav '33.

LEMIEUX, Gerard; C.P. 515, Gagnon, Cte. Saguenay, P.Q.; Lav'58; GenSurg.

LEMIEUX, Germain; St-Charles, Cte Bellechasse, P.Q.; Lav'62.

LEMIEUX, Guy; 146 rue Notre Dame, St. Jean, P.Q. (res); Mon '53; Int Med (P.Q.); Res. (Clin. Research), Hosp. Hotel-Dieu, Montreal, P.Q.; Tel. VI 4-0161.

LEMIEUX, Hector H. L.; 311 ave. Ste-Famille, Chicoutimi, P.Q.; Lav '44; Gastroent. (P.Q.), Gastroenterol. & Endoscop., Hotel-Dieu-St.- Vallier; Staff, Laval U.

LEMIEUX, Jean; 1050 Chemin St. Foy, Quebec, P.Q.; 2164 Dickson, Sillery (res); Lav '46; OrthSurg (P.Q.); Ass't Orth. Surg. Serv., Hop's du St. Sacrement & Laval; Cons. Orth. Surg., Hop. St. Michel Archange; Tel. 523-4752.

LEMIEUX, Jean M.; 246 St. Jean St., Quebec, P.Q.; 1175 Park Ave. (res); Lav '37; GenSurg, ThorSurg; Staff, Laval, & St. Sacrement Hosp's.; Assoc. Prof., Laval U.; Tel. 523-4752.

LEMIEUX, J. Edouard; Mont Laurier, P.Q.; Mon '37; GenSurg (P.Q.).

LEMIEUX, J. Rejean; C.P. 34, Grand'Mere, P.Q.; Lav '64.

LEMIEUX, J. Renaud; 1401 Parc Champoux, Quebec, P.Q.; (res); Lav '26; D.Sc. (Hon.), F.A.C.P., F.R.C.P.(C), IntMed; Med. Dir., Hop.-St.-Sacrement; Cons. Hop.-Ste-Foy; Prof. (Med), Laval U.; Tel. 681-7211.

LEMIEUX, Laurier, 88 Jacques-Cartier, Mont-Joli, P.Q.; Lav '64.

LEMIEUX, Lionel H.; Clinique Roy-Rousseau, Quebec, P.Q.; 2064 Dixon St., Sillery (res); Lav '46; F.R.C.P.(C), Neur; Staff, Clinique Roy-Rous**seau & Laval U.; Tel. 663-7856.**

LEMIEUX, Marcel; 480 Filion, St. Jovite, Cte Terrebonne, P.Q.; Lav'55; Psy(P.Q.).

LEMIEUX, Real; Mon '60; Res., Hop. Notre-Dame, Montreal 24, P.Q.

LEMIEUX, Richard; Main St., Buckingham, P.Q.; Lav '49; M.C.G.P.; Anaes., Hop. St. Michel de Buckingham; Tel. 986-3341.

LEMIEUX, Rock (Claude); C.P. 848, 81 Notre-Dame S., Ste. 102, Thetford Mines, P.Q.; 707-8th Ave. (res); Lav'55.

LEMIEUX, Roger; 910 est boul St-Joseph, Montreal 34, P.Q.; 86 Willowdale, Outremont (res); Mon'43; Tel. 524-0493.

LEMIEUX, Roger R.; 6555 Boul. Gouin Ouest, Montreal 9, P.Q.; 710 Chemin-Ste.-Catherine, Mtl. 8 (res); Mon '44; DABPN; Psy (PQ); FAPA; Educ. Dir., Inst., Albert-Prevost; Prof. (Med., Psy & Rehab), U. of Mtl.; Tel. RE 3-9951.

LEMIRE, Alphonse; Baieville, Cte. Yamaska, P.Q.; Mon '24.

LEMIRE, Andre; 5628 Leopold Pouliot, Montreal Nord, P.Q. (res); Mon '54; Ass't. Prof. (Histol.), U. of Montreal.

LEMIRE, Claire; App 1, 258 Willowdale, Montreal 8, P.Q.; Lav'59; Anaes.; Staff Anaes., Hop. Jean Talon.

LEMIRE, Claude; 1811 des Cascades St. Hyacinthe, P.Q.; Lav '57; Tel. PR 3-2066.

LEMIRE, Fernand; 700, rue Ste-Julie, Trois-Rivieres, P.Q.; 3810 Pie X (res); Lav '52; F.R.C.S. (C), GenSurg.; Tel. FR 5-6381.

LEMIRE, Gaetan; Ste. Anne des Monts, Co. Gaspe, P.Q.; Mon '49; F.R.C.S.(C), GenSurg; Surg., Hop. Ste. Anne.; Tel. 498.

LEMIRE, Jacques; 192 Iberville, Repentigny, P.Q.; Mon'58; FRCS(C), Ophth.

LEMIRE, Paul G.; App 2, 184 boul. Thomson, Montreal 9, P.Q.; Mon'61; DiagRad.

LEMIRE, Joseph J.; 127 Laflamme, St-Jerome, P.Q.; Mon'57; GenSurg.; Tel. GE 8-4549.

LEMIRE, Jean; Mon'51; Res., Hop, Maisonneuve, Montreal 36, P.Q.

LEMIRE, Robert; Mon'63; Int., Hop. Maisonneuve, Montreal, P.Q.

LEMIRE, Suzanne; Ste. 302, 1248 Chemin Ste-Foy, Quebec 6, P.Q.; Lav '55; FRCS(C); ObstGyn.; Tel. 681-1816.

LEMIRE, Suzanne; Lav '62; Res., Hop. de l'Enfant Jesus, Quebec, P.Q.

LEMIRE, Yvette; 258 Willowdale, Outremount (res); Lav '53; Cardiol (P.Q.); Staff, Inst. de Cardiologie, 5000 est, rue Belanger, Montreal 36, **P.Q.; Tel. 254-8341.**

LEMISZKA, John.; Vonda, Sask.; Prague (Czech.) '29; M.H.O., Municipalities 372 & 373; Dist. Coroner.

LEMKE, Dieter W.; Alb '64; Res., Royal Alexandra Hosp., Edmonton, Alta.

LeMOINE, Menna (Jones); R.R. 5, Woodstock, Ont. (res); Aberdeen (Scot.) '40; FACCP; Phys., Ont. Hosp.; Tel. LE 9-1251.

LEMYRE, Georges E.; rue St. Georges, St. Cesaire, P.Q.; Mon'40.

LEMYRE, Germain; Lav'62; Res., Hop. Notre-Dame, Montreal 24, P.Q.

LEMYRE, Robert; 5531 Verdun Ave., Verdun, P.Q.; 470-90th Ave., LaSalle; Lav '55; MCGP; Indust. Phys., Ralston Purina; Med. Exam., Sun Life, Prevoyants, & Union of Canada; Ass't. Dir., Desjardins, Dominion Life, & Prudential; Med. Staff, Hop. Archambault; Tel. 768-4702 & 366-6582.

LENCZNER, Michael M.; 2 Forest Hill Rd., Toronto 7, Ont.; Bologna (Italy) '32; IntMed; O.P.D. Med. Clin., & Teach. Staff, Toronto Gen. & Western Hosp's.; Tel. WA 3-9191.

LENECK, Charles M.; 3042 Keele St., Downsview, Ont.; Tor'65; Tel. ME 3-6560.

LENGYEL, George; 1509 Ottawa St., Windsor, Ont.; 4545 Pleasant Pl. (res); Munich (Germ.) '50; Tel. 253-6762.

LENIS, George J.; Room 2076, DVA Bldg., Wellington St., Ottawa, Ont.; Warsaw (Poland) '33; F.C.C.P.; Med. Adv., Can. Pension Comm., Ottawa.
LENK, Czeslaw; Hastings Health Unit, Belleville, Ont.; Cracow (Poland)'39; DPH; PH.
LENKEI, Susan C.; Cardiovascular Unit, Toronto Western Hosp., 399 Bathurst St., Toronto 2B, Ont.; Zurich (Switz.)'51; FCCP; FRCP(C); IntMed (Card.); Staff, Toronto Western Hosp.; Research Assoc.; Ont. Heart Fdn.; Clin. Teach., U. of Toronto; Tel. 369-5713.
LENNOX, Bruce M.; 425 Davis Dr., Newmarket, Ont.; Tor'63.
LENNOX, Thomas E.; Uxbridge, Ont.; Tor '50; Coroner, Uxbridge Town & Twp.
LENOIR, Ernest; Cheneville, Co. Papineau, P.Q.; Mon '22.
LENSON, Frank W.; Mall Med. Bldg., 280 Osborne St. N., Winnipeg 1, Man.; 877 Sherburn St. (res); Man'58.
LEON, Eva (See Powell)
LEON, Joseph M.J.; 165 Plymouth Rd., Welland, Ont.; 70 Parkway Dr. (res); Ott'56; IntMed; Tel. 735-5015.
LEON, Wolf H.; Dublin (Ire.) '48; Staff, Riverside Hosp., Charlottetown, P.E.I.
LEONARD, C. E.; Centre-Medicale, St.-Jerome, P.Q.; Mon '48; MCGP; Staff Phys., Rolland Paper Co.
LEONARD, Claude; 1150 Blvd. St. Joseph E., Montreal 34, P.Q.; 6012 Wilderton Ave. (res); Mon '39; F.A.A.P., Paed (P.Q.); Chief Paed., Hop. Maisonneuve; Paed., Creche d'Youville; **Ass't. Prof. Paed., U. of Montreal; Tel. LA 7-1551.**
LEONARD, Fernand; 1020 est, rue Sherbrooke, Montreal 24, P.Q.; Mon '55; Psy; Jr. Ass't. Psy., Hop. Notre-Dame; Cons. Psy., Psychio-Social, St. Jerome; Tel. 525-1616.
LEONARD, Gerard; 1951 Blvd. St. Joseph E., Montreal, P.Q.; 826 Blvd. St. Joseph E. (res); Mon '40; Obst (P.Q.); Chief of Obst. Serv., Misericordia Hosp.; **Ass't Prof., Obst., U. of** Montreal; Tel. LA 3-1441.
LEONARD, Gerard J.; 30 est boul St.-Joseph, Montreal 14, P.Q.; 3050 de Versailles, Durvenay (res); Mon'54; Tel. 845-4241.
LEONARD, John G.; Murray & George Sts., Amherstburg, Ont.; Tor '46; Tel. 736-4114.
LEONG, Saw T.; Schwartz Bldg., 415-3rd Ave. S., Lethbridge, Alta.; 517-15th St. S. (res); Punjab (India) '44; DOMS (Eng.); DO (Oxon); FRCS (Eng.); Ophth; Staff, St. Michael's Gen. Hosp.; Tel. 327-4166.
LEONG, Wing; 212 James St. S., Hamilton, Ont; Tor'53; Tel. 528-8437.
LEPAGE, Antoine J.; 3485 ave. Atwater, Montreal 25, P.Q.; 3181 Glencoe, Mtl. 16 (res); Mon '54; D.Psy (McG); Psy; Hd. Dept. of Psy., Hop St. Luc; Hd. Dept. of Psy., Inst., Albert Prevost, 6555 Boul. Gouin W.; Teach. Staff, U. of Montreal; Tel. 932-6510.
Le PAGE, Blois C.; 64 Bayview Ave., Newmarket, Ont.; Dal '43; DPH; Ass't. M.O.H., York County Health Unit.
LEPAGE, Claude; Lav '56; Anaes; Staff, Hop. Notre-Dame, Montreal, P.Q.; Tel. 525-6363.
LEPAGE, Gilles; 5000 est Belanger, Montreal 36, P.Q.; 455 Lockhart, Mtl. 16 (res.); Mon'51; FRCS(C); ThorSurg; Staff, Inst. of Cardiology; Cons. ThorSurg., Hop. Jean Talon; Tel. 376-3330.
LEPAGE, Jean M.; Mon'65; Staff, Clinique Med. Candiac, Candiac, P.Q.
LEPAGE, Paul M.; 8415 St. Denis, Montreal 11, P.Q.; Lille (Fr.) '55; IntMed (P.Q.); Tel. 381-1801.
LEPAGE, Rene A.; 46 Blvd. Jacques-Cartier, Mo Joli, P.Q.; Lav '28; MCGP; First-Aid Instr., St. John's Ambulance; Tel. 775-3339.
LEPAGE, Victor; 242 St-Germain, Rimouski, P.Q.; Lav'35; Ophth.
LEPARD, Sidney F., 31 James St., Parry Sound, Ont.; Tor '52; MCGP; Chief of Staff, Parry Sound & St. Joseph's Hosp's.; Indust. Phys., Dept. of Indian Affairs & Canadian Motorlamp; Tel. 746-9382.
LEPINE, Aurele M.; rue Principale, Cookshire, P.Q.; Mon '43.
LEPINE, Charles; 10107 Fabre St., Montreal 12, P.Q.; 861 Wilder Ave. (res); Mon '49; Pulm. Dis. & TB (P.Q.); **Chief (Cardio-Pulm.), Inst. Lavoisier; Tel. CL 6-1686.**
LEPINE, Edgar; 1150 Blvd. St. Joseph E., Montreal 34, P.Q.; Man '43; F.R.C.S.(C), OrthSurg; Chief, OrthSurg., Hop. Maisonneuve; Tel. LA 7-1421.
LEPINE, Ernest F.; 570 Queens, London, Ont.; Wes '36; MCGP; Active Staff, St. Joseph's & St. Mary's Hosp's.; Hon. Phys., Marian Villas; Tel. 432-7603.
LEPINE, Henri; Mon'56; AMCGP; Anaes(P.Q.); Staff, Hop. Ste-Jeanne-d'Arc, Montreal, P.Q
LEPINE, Ivan; 259 rue St. George, St. Jerome, Cte. Terrebonne, P.Q.; 489 du Palais (res); Lav '59; Paed; Ass't. (Paed.), Hotel-Dieu Hosp.; Tel. 438-8519.
LEPINE, Raymond; 6899-14eme Ave., Montreal 36, P.Q.; Lille (Fr.) '55; Tel. RA 8-1901.
LEPINSKIE, Fredrick F.; 212 James St. S., Hamilton, Ont.; 913 Gorton, Burlington (res); Qns '55; Anaes; Tel. 528-8437.
LE RICHE, Jean (Macdonald); 11823 87th Ave., Edmonton, Alta.; Liverpool(Eng.)'57; MRCS, LRCP.
LERICHE, Leroy H.; College of Physicians & Surgeons, 9905-108th St., Edmonton, Alta.; Liverpool (Eng.)'53.
le RICHE, W. Harding; 150 College St., Toronto 5, Ont.; **30 Golfdale Rd., Tor. 12 (res); Witwatersrand (S. Africa) '43; Hon. Vis. Phys., Queen Elizabeth Hosp.; Cons. Med. Stat., Hosp. for Sick Children; Cons. Physicians' Services** Inc.; Prof. & Hd. Dept. of Epidem. & Biometrics, Schl. of Hygiene, U. of Toronto; Tel. 928-2020.
LERNER, Arthur I.; 100 Osborne Medical Bldg., Winnipeg, Man.; 357 Scotia St. (res); Man '38; F.I.C.S., F.R.C.S.(C) GenSurg; Surg. Staff, Misericordia Hosp.; Tel. SU 3-4513.
LERNER, Maxwell; 512 Boyd Bldg., Winnipeg 1, Man.; 466 Inkster Blvd., Wpg. 4 (res); Man '34; DOMS; Staff, St. Boniface Gen. Hosp.; Tel. WH 2-7162.
LEROUX, George W.; Box 250, 120 Victoria Ave., Fernie, B.C.; 11 Howland Ave. (res); Man'34; Staff, Fernie Gen. Hosp.; Tel. 739.
LEROUX, Hector; 8618 rue Chaumont, Ville d'Anjou, P.Q.; GenSurg(P.Q.).
LEROUX, Henri; 14 ouest Victor, St-Janvier, Co. Terrebonne, P.Q.; Lav'51; Tel. 435-3357.
LEROUX, John A.; 501 Fairmont Med. Bldg., 750 W. Broadway, Vancouver 9, B.C.; 2425 W. 33rd Ave. (res); Man'37; DPH; FRCP(C); IntMed; Att'd. Staff, Vancouver Gen. Hosp.; Cons. Staff, Shaughnessy DVA Hosp.; Clin. Instr. (Med.), U. of British Columbia; Tel. 879-4312.
LEROUX, Olivier; University of Montreal, Montreal, P.Q.; 4137 Jean Brilliant (res); Mon '33; Pub. Health Admin.; Ass't. to Dean, Schl. of Hygiene; Tel. RE 3-9951.
LEROUX, Paul; Ott'62; Res., Jewish Gen. Hosp., Montreal 26, P.Q.
LEROY, Alfred; 175 Sherbrooke E., Montreal, P.Q.; Mon '25; Obst; Chief. Serv. of Obst., Hop St. Luc; Assoc. Prof. Obst., U. of Montreal; Tel. UN 1-7261.
LEROY, Maurice J.; 1384 Jean-Talon est, Montreal 35, P.Q.; 8545 boul-de-l'Acadie, App 5 (res); Louvain (Belgium) '52; AMCGP; Vis, Staff, Jean Talon & Santa Cabrini Hosp's.; Tel. **274-5583.**
LERTZMAN, Morley; 46 Wildwood Pk., Winnipeg 19, Man (res); Man '55; IntMed; Dir., Respiratory Lab., Children's Hosp.; Phys., Rehab. Hosp.; Instr. (Paed.), U. of Manitoba; Tel. SP 5-8311.
LESACK, Bohdan J.; 624-6th St., New Westminster, B.C.; Man'53; FRCS(C), GenSurg; Tel. LA 1-6021.
LESAGE, Earl E.; 5657 Park Ave., Apt. 2, Montreal, P.Q.; McG'30; IntMed (P.Q.); Staff Phys. & Phys.-in-charge (All.), St. Mary's Hosp.; Med. Dir., Mtl. Catholic School Comm.; Tel. 277-4516

LESAGE, Gilles; Mon'52; Res., Hop. Notre-Dame, Montreal 24, P.Q.
Le SAGE, J. Bernard; 1639 Chemin Norway, Montreal 9, P.Q.; 4647 ave. Verdun, Mtl. 19; Mon '45; GenSurg; Chief Surg., Hop. Ste-Rose de Laval & Med. Dir., Hop. Archambault; Tel. 733-0251.
LESAGE, Marcel; 3525 Masson, Montreal, P.Q.; 5043 Jeanne-d'Arc (res); Mon '47; Tel. RA 7-1919.
LESAGE, Michel; Lav'62; Res., Hop. Notre-Dame, Montreal 24, P.Q.
LESAGE, Robert; Mon'63; Res., Montreal Gen. Hosp., Montreal, P.Q.
LeSAGE, Roger; App. 304, 1000 Ste.-Foy, Quebec, P.Q., 911 Brown (res); Lav B.L.L.'39; M.D.'44; Gastroent (P.Q.); I/C, Ther. Gastroent., **Laval U.**; Ass't. (Med.), Hop. du St.-Sacrement; Tel. 681-6241.

LESCHE, Konrad M.; Box 1241, Saskatoon Sanatorium, Saskatoon, Sask; Leipzig (Germ.) '33; Tel. 652-8877.

LESK, David M.; Alb '63; Res., Westminster Hosp., London, Ont.
LESK, Louis; 713 Columbia St., New Westminster, B.C.; 1525 Dublin St. (res); Alb '31; M.C.-G.P.; **Tel. LA 2-5152.**

LESLIE, B. Scott; Department of National Health & Welfare, c/o Regional Superintendent, European Region; Dal '56; PH. Abroad.
LESLIE, Douglas; 1312 Rebecca St., Oakville, Ont.; Aberdeen (Scott.) '53; Chief, Dept. of G.P., Oakville Trafalgar Hosp.; Tel. 827-3301.
LESLIE, Samuel W.; 386 Bloor St. W., Toronto, Ont.; 157 Lytton Blvd. (res); Tor '30; D.D.S.; M.C.G.P.; Tel. WA 2-9700.
LESLIE-SPINKS, Arthur J.; 12730—102nd Ave., Edmonton, Alta. (res); Oxford (Eng.) '28; MOH & Dir. Vegreville Health Unit, Box 99, Vegreville, Alta.; Tel. 632-2744.
LESLIE, William L.; 283 Metcalfe St., Ottawa, Ont.; 275 MacLaren St. (res); Qns '43; Staff, **Ottawa Civic Hosp.; Tel. PA 9-2511.**

L'ESPERANCE, Alphonse; 520 Chemin St. Louis, Quebec, P.Q. (res); Lav '24; F.A.C.C.P., Pulm. Dis. & TB (P.Q.), IntMed (TB); Med. Dir., Hop. **Laval, Ste-Foy, P.Q.; Tel. 653-5251.**
LESPERANCE, Jacques; 12 Algonquin, Fabreville, P.Q.; Mon '56; D & TRad; Staff, Hop. Maisonneuve, Montreal; Ass't. Prof. (Radiol.), U. of Montreal; Tel. 254-8341.
L'ESPERANCE, Paul; 65 est Grande-Allee, Quebec 4, P.Q.; Lav '50; F.R.C.S.(C), GenSurg; Ass't. Surg., Hotel-Dieu-de-Quebec; Staff, Laval **U.; Tel. 529-9691.**
LESPERANCE, Richard R.; McG'62; Res., Royal Victoria Hosp., Montreal, P.Q.; MCGP.

LESSARD, Alphee; Box 817, Chicoutimi, P.Q.; Lav '50; IntMed (P.Q.).

LESSARD, Andre; 1626 Cascades, St. Hyacinthe, P.Q.; 855 Bernard (res); **Lav '56; M.C.G.P.**

LESSARD, Andree; 1135 ave. Ploermel, Quebec 6, P.Q.; Lav '62, Staff, Dept. of Health.

LESSARD, Camille; 189 Notre Dame S., Thetford Mines, P.Q.; 1269 d'Youville (res); Lav '61; Tel. FE 5-7373.
LESSARD, Camille; 8250 rue Chatillon, Ville-Anjou, Montreal 5, P.Q.; Mon'59; MCGP; Tel. 352-1820.
LESSARD, Camille; 2596 Lapointe, Ste. Foy, Quebec, P.Q. (res); Lav '46; Pulm Dis. & TB (P.Q.); Med. Staff, Hop. Laval; Med. Ass't., Anti-T.B. Disp., Quebec; Tel. 653-5251.

LESSARD, Francoise; 44 Fraser, Levis, P.Q.; Apt. 15, 1195 Brown Ave., Quebec 6 (res); Lav'48; PH(P.Q.); Staff, Dept of Health; Tel. 837-8808.
LESSARD, Guy; Centre Med St. Vallier, 750 St. Vallier Quest, Quebec 8, P.Q.; Lav'60; PhysMed & Rehab (P.Q.).

LESSARD, Henri P.; St. Jean de Matha, Co. Joliette, P.Q.; Lav '46.

LESSARD, Ivan; 2 rue de la Cour, Riviere-du-Loup, P.Q.; Mon '48 IntMed; (Cardiol.); (P.Q.); Tel. 862-6066.

LESSARD, Jean M.; 240 rue St. Jean, Quebec, P.Q.; 818 Ave. Cardinal Rouleau (res); Lav '42; F.A.C.S., F.R.C.S.(C), OrthSurg; Chief, Serv. of Orth. Surg., **Hop. de l'Enfant-Jesus**; Clin. Ass't., **Orth Surg., Laval U.; Tel. 523-2610.**
LESSARD, Jean-M.; 3840 St. Urbain, Montreal, P.Q.; Lav '35; PhysMed (P.Q.); Chief, Dept. of Phys. Med., Hotel Dieu; Ass't. Prof. Med., Montreal U.; Tel. VI 4-0161.
LESSARD, Jean-N.; 754 3rd Ave., Val d'Or, P.Q.; Lav'46; Gen Surg.(P.Q.); Tel. 824-6807.
LESSARD, Louis; 225 Grande-Allee, Quebec, P.Q.; 1595 Chemin St. Louis (res); Lav '32; **GenSurg (P.Q.); Indust. Phys., W.C.B., P.Q.; Tel. 522-4751.**
LESSARD, Pierre; Lav'64; Res., Hop Notre-Dame, Montreal 24, P.Q.
LESSARD, Pierre; 167 St. Joseph, Hull, P.Q.; Mon'56; Tel. PR 1-8186.
LESSARD, Pierre A.; 10965 Joseph-Casavant, Montreal 12, P.Q.; Mon'57; Anaes (P.Q.); Tel. 334-3172.
LESSARD, Raymond; 960 chemin Ste-Foy, Quebec 6, P.Q.; Lav '60; FRCP(C), Derm.
LESSARD, Richard; 115 est, Grande-Allee, Quebec 4, P.Q.; 870 Ave. des Braves (res); Lav '29; Paris (France) '33; F.A.C.P., F.R.C.P.(C), IntMed; Cardiol. (P.Q.); Chief of Med., Hop. Hotel **Dieu; Prof. of Med. Path., Laval U.; Tel. 523-1003.**

LESSARD, Robert; 71-rue Latour, St.-Jean, P.Q.; Mon '49; DPH; PH (P.Q.).
LESSARD, Robert; 1214 Luxembourg Ave., Sillery, P.Q. (res); Lav '40; D&TRad; Chief, Diag-Rad., Hotel-Dieu-de-Quebec; Ass't. Prof., Laval **U.; Tel. 529-9151.**
LESSARD, Robert; Montmagny, Co. Montmagny, P.Q.; Lav '62
LESSARD, Roger; 294 rue Notre Dame, Ste Marie, Cte Beauce, P.Q.; Lav '65.

LESSER, Arthur L.; 221 Brant Ave., Brantford, Ont.; 18 Springfield Dr., (res); **Dal '56; Psy**; Dir. Psy Unit, Brantford Gen. Hosp.; Tel. 752-8900.

LESTER, Evangelie (Papamatheaki); 1025 Pine Ave. W., Montreal 2, P.Q.; 509 Pine Ave. W. (res); Athens (Gr.) '48; Psy; Hd. Children's Psy. Clin., Allan Mem. Inst.; Lect. (Psy), McGill U.; Tel. VI 2-1251.
LESTER, Marvin G.; 505, 99 Avenue Rd., Toronto 5, Ont.; 101 Wembley Rd. (res); Tor '55; Derm; Cons. Derm; W.C.B.; Tel. WA 2-5445.
LESTER, Michael L.; Tor '64; Res., Hosp. for Sick Children, Toronto 2, Ont.
LESTER, Robert S.; Tor'62; Res., Sunnybrook Hosp., Toronto 12, Ont.

LESZCZYNSKI, Janusz; The Clinic, Melville, **Sask.; 213-7th Ave. E. (res); Nat. U. (Ire.) '53; Tel. 728-5411.**

LETAIN, Fernand A.; Somerset, Man.; Man'65.

LeTARTE, Andre; Ste. 230, 4 Taschereau, Hull, P.Q.; R.R. 2, Aylmer E. (res); Lav'57; Paed (P.Q.); Dir. Poison Control, Hop. du Sacre-Coeur; Tel. 771-0027.
LETARTE, Francois; 84 rue St.-Louis, Quebec, P.Q.; Lav '35; Ophth, Otol; Chief, Ophth, Otol., Hop.-St.-Francois-d'Assise; Cons. Veterans' Hospital; Prof. (ORL), Laval U.; Tel. 523-2138.
LETARTE, Paulette; 2155 ave. Maplewood, Montreal 26, P.Q.; Mon '62. Abroad.

LETELLIER, Edouard H.; 149 St. Laurent, **Longueuil, P.Q.; Mon '43.**

LETENDRE, Georges A.; 2976 de la Promenade, Quebec 10, P.Q.; Lav'38.
LETENDRE, Gerard; 106 Principale, Danville, Co. Richmond, P.Q.; Lav '50.
LETENDRE, Joseph; 2-2eme Ave ouest, Amos, cte Abitibi, P.Q.; Lav'60; **Orth Surg (P.Q.).**

LETENDRE, Paul; Ste. 319, 3875 St-Urbain, Montreal 18, P.Q.; Mon '37; FRCP(C); Gastroent P.Q.); Int. Med; Chief of Med., Hotel-Dieu; Prof. of Clin. Med., U. of Montreal; Tel. 288-1289.
LETENDRE, Samuel P. J.; 418 Sherbrooke St. E., Montreal, P.Q.; 1721 Lajoie (res); Mon '29; Gyn (P.Q.); Ass't. Etrang. U. of Paris (Fr.), F.I.C.S.; Gyn.; Tel. VI 2-1078

LETIENNE, Gerrard J. E.; 604 Med. Arts Bldg., Winnipeg, Man.; 597 Lyndale Dr., Norwood (res); Lav '45; DPH; Ophth; Att'd. Staff, St. Boniface Hosp.; Dem. (Ophth.), U. of Manitoba; Tel. WH 3-4369.

LETIENNE, Louis; 1005 St. Prosper, Trois Rivieres, P.Q.; Lav '41; F.R.C.S.(C), OrthSurg; OrthSurg; Hop. St.- Joseph; Tel. FR 4-6611.

L'ETOILE, Marcel; 2289 rue Viel, Montreal 12, P.Q.; Lav '54; Anaes; Anaes., Private Hosp's.

LETONDAL, Paul; 97 rue St-Jude, St-Eustache-sur-le-Lac, P.Q.; Mon '22; Paris (Fr.) '22; F.R.-C.P.(C), Paed. Dir., L'Union Medicale.

LETOURNEAU, A. Guy; 1522 Ouellette Ave., Windsor, Ont.; Lav '58; Psy; Ass't. Dir. Dept. of Psy., Metropolitan Gen. Hosp.; Tel. 254-2451.

LETOURNEAU, Georges, Major; Lav'55; 3516 Herman St., Fabreville, P.Q. (res); C.M.O. Headquarters, Quebec Command, 3530 Atwater Ave., Montreal 25.

LETOURNEAU, Jacques; 5800 Beaumont, Quebec 7, P.Q.; Lav'54; PH(P.Q.).

LETOURNEAU, Jacques; Lav '59; TherRad; Staff, Hop. Notre-Dame, Montreal 24, P.Q.; Tel. 525-6363.

LETOURNEAU, J. L.; 479 St. Vallier W., Quebec, P.Q.; Lav '37; GenSurg (P.Q.); Tel. 522-6115.

LETOURNEAU, Paul E.; 512 rue School, Arvida, P.Q.; Lav '48; M.C.G.P.; Tel. 548-4663.

LETOURNEAU, Richard; Box 485, 12 MacMillan, Campbellton, N.B.; Mon '60; Paed; Chief Paed., Hop. Hotel-Dieu; Tel. 753-4294.

LETOURNNEAU, Jean L.; 875 des Recollets, Trois-Rivieres, P.Q.; Lav'53; GenSurg. (P.Q.); Tel. 375-8696.

LETT, Georges; 352 boul des Laurentides, Pont-Viau, Laval-des-Rapides, P.Q.; Mon'55.

LETTAU, H. Frances; Dept. of Nat. Health & Welfare, Tunney's Pasture, Ottawa 4, Ont.; Tor '60; M.A. (Pharm.).

LETTS, Albert E., Apt. 803, 1265 Richmond St., London, Ont.; Wes '32; Staff, Veteran's Affairs, Westminster Hosp.; Tel. 434-1511.

LETTS, G.D. James; 405 Rideau Medical Centre, 1711-4th St. S.W., Calgary, Alta.; Alb '53; Psy; Tel. 262-6672.

LETTS, Harry W.V.; 6512-109B Ave., Edmonton, Alta. (res); Ott'57; FRCP(C) Path; DNBME; DABPA; Assoc. Path., Royal Alexandra Hosp.; Lect. U. of Alberta; Tel. GR 4-3431.

LETTS, Robert M., F/L; Camp Marina, El Erish, Egypt; Man'64. Abroad.

LETTS, T. Blake; 205 Med. Dental Bldg., 8225-105th St., Edmonton, Alta.; 11715-83rd Ave. (res); Alb '40; MCGP; Tel. GE 3-1598.

LETWIN, Ervin; Alb'60; FRCS(C), GenSurg; Staff, Charles Camsell Hosp., Edmonton, Alta.

LEUNG, Fung; Taiwan (Formosa); Staff, Cottage Hosp., Come-By-Chance, Nfld.

LEUNG, Jock; Ste. 500, 1541 W. Broadway, Vancouver, B.C.; UBC'60; MCGP; Assoc. Staff, St. Paul's Hosp.; Tel. RE 1-6011.

LEUNG, So Won; Ste. 3—426 Main St., Vancouver, B.C.; 4612 Pine Cres. (res); Tor '43; Tel. MU 4-4934.

LEVAC, Armand; 4395 Verdun Ave., Verdun, Montreal 19, P.Q.; Mon'47; Anaes(P.Q.); Staff, Hop. Verdun; Tel. 679-4071.

LEVAC, Therese; 1033 Blvd. St. Joseph E., Montreal 34, P.Q.; Mon '47; Neur (P.Q.).

le VANN, Leonard J.; Box 580, Red Deer, Alta.; Edinburgh (Scot.) '43; Supt., Alberta School Hosp.; Dir. Linden House Unit for Emotionally Disturbed Children; Cons. Psy., Red Deer Gen. Hosp.; Lect. (Psy.), U. of Alberta; Tel. 346-2760.

LEVANT, Marvin N.; Man '63; Int., Royal Victoria Hosp., Montreal, P.Q.

LEVASSEUR, C. Auguste; Ste. Angele de Laval, Co. Nicolet, P.Q.; Lav '44.

LEVASSEUR, Louis J.; 1605 lere Ave., Quebec 3, P.Q.; Lav '50; FACS; FRCS(C), GenSurg; Staff, Hop. St. Francois d'Assise; Prof. (Geog.), U. of Laval; Tel. 529-7311.

LEVASSEUR, Marc; 362 St. Cyrille St., Normandin, P.Q.; Lav '59; Tel. 274-2014.

LEVEILLE, Antonio; 200 est Blvd. Gouin, Montreal, P.Q.; Mon '33; Paed (P.Q.); Staff, Hop. Ste.-Justine; Tel. DU 8-4751.

LEVEILLE, Bernard; 5664 Laurendeau, Montreal 20, P.Q.; Mon '43; Tel. 768-6931.

LEVEILLE, Jean; Mon'65; Res., Hop. Maisonneuve, Montreal 36, P.Q.

LEVEILLE, Michel; Mon'63; Res., Hop. Maisonneuve, Montreal, P.Q.

LEVELL, Gerald W.; 8 Madrona Bldg., 140 Wallace St., Nanaimo, B.C.; Tor'53; DiagRad; Staff, Nanaimo Gen. Hosp.; Tel. SK 3-4351.

LEVENE, Donald L.; 496 W. 40th Ave., Vancouver 15, B.C.; Man '62.

LEVENTHAL, Abraham; Ste. 303, 333 Wilson Ave., Downsview, Ont.; 773 Spadina Rd. (res); Tor'36; Paed; Sr. Att'd. Phy. (Paed.), New Mount Sinai Hosp.; Med. Dir., Children's Div., Jewish Family & Child Services; Staff Phys., Dept. of Paed., Doctor's Hosp.; Tel. 635-1281.

LEVENTHAL, Joseph I.; 1340 Wilson Ave., Downsview, Ont.; Tor '50; MCGP; Active Staff, North York Branson & North Western Gen. Hosp's.; Rep. of Bd., Coll. of G.P. (Ont. Div.); Memb., Committee Child Welfare O.M.A.; Tel. CH 1-6651.

LEVEQUE, Cedric P.; 5341 Duquette Montreal, P.Q. (res); McG '29; Staff, United States Consulate, 1558 McGregor Ave.; Tel. 484-4283.

LEVER, Malcolm A.; 705 Med. Arts Bldg., 1011 Ouellette Ave., Windsor, Ont.; R.R. 1., Tecumseh (res); Wes'42; DABR; DiagRad; Rad., Metropolitan Gen. & Leamington Dist. Hosp's.; Tel. 254-7551.

LEVERS, Peter E.; Ste. 207, Med. Arts Bldg., 628 Davis Dr., Newmarket, Ont.; 191 Yonge St. S., Richmond Hill, Ont.; 111 Lewis Dr., Newmarket (res); London (Eng.) '55; FRCS(C); Urol; (Active) Staff, York County Hosp.; Court. Staff York Central Hosp.; Tel. 895-9411 & 884-3811.

LEVERT, Guy; C.P. 6, Clinique Sainte-Foy, Quebec 10, P.Q.; Lav'65.

LEVESQUE, Andre J.; Lav'65; Res., Hop. St. Francis d'Assise, Quebec 3, P.Q.

LEVESQUE, Benoit, Lav '63; Res., Hop. Notre-Dame, Montreal, 24, P.Q.

LEVESQUE, Etienne; Ste. Marie, Co. Beauce, P.Q.; Lav '51.

LEVESQUE, Fernand H.; 19 Durham N., Sudbury, Ont.; 509 Willard (res); Ott '53; GenSurg.; Staff, St. Joseph's Hosp.; Tel. 673-9623.

LEVESQUE, Georges H.; 6801 Ave., Royale, L'Ange-Gardien E., Co. Montmorency, P.Q.; Lav '50; MCGP; Tel. 822-1588.

LEVESQUE, Georges H.; 69 St - Francois, Edmunston, N.B.; Mon'61; FRCP(C), IntMed.; Tel. 735-7515.

LEVESQUE, Henri P.; Centre Med. St. Urbain, 3875 St-Urbain, Montreal 18, P.Q.; Mon '53; DiagRad; Staff, Hop. Hotel-Dieu; Tel. VI 4-0161.

LEVESQUE, Jean-M.; Lav'60; FRCS(C); OrthSurg; Ass't., Dept. of OrthSurg, Hop. St-Sacrement, Quebec 6, P.Q.

LEVESQUE, Louis M.; 520 Montcalm St., Chicoutimi, P.Q.; 407 Cote-St.-Ange (res); Lav '53; M.C.G.P.

LEVESQUE, Lucien; 105 Angus, East-Angus Cté Compton, P.Q.; Lav'63; Tel. 832-2929.

LEVESQUE, Paul A.; 100B Jacques Cartier Blvd., Mont Joli, P.Q.; Lav '36.

LEVESQUE, Roch; Bonaventure, P.Q.; Lav '62.

LEVICZKY, Bela E.; 1741 East Broadway, Vancouver 12, B.C.; Budapest (Hung.)'40; Tel. TR 9-3320.

LEVIN, Douglas C.; Ste. 108, 3545 Cote-des-Neiges, Montreal 25, P.Q.; London (Eng.)'51; M.B., B.S.; Psy.; Tel. 932-5932.

LEVIN, Herman; 1538 Sherbrooke St. W., Montreal, P.Q.; 5043 Grosvenor Ave. (res); McG '38; Clin. Ass't. (Surg.), Reddy Memorial Hosp.; Tel. WE 3-2828.

LEVIN, Manly B.; 801 Boyd Bldg., 388 Portage Ave., Winnipeg 1, Man.; Man'52; DABS; FRCS(C), GenSurg; Tel. 947-0481.

LEVIN, Raymond C.; Ste. 210, 305 Finch Ave. W., Willowdale, Ont.; Tor '59; AMCGP; Tel. BA 1-5544.
LEVIN, Richard L.; USA '61; Res., Hosp. for Sick Children, Toronto 2, Ont.
LEVIN, Sam R.; 641 St. Mary's Rd., Winnipeg Man.; 110 Elm Park Rd. (res); Man '41; Anaes.; **Staff (Anaes), Deer Lodge (D.V.A.) Hosp.; Tel. TU 8-4861.**

LEVINE, Arthur H.; 6770 Pius IX, Montreal, P.Q.; 2480 Decelles St., St. Laurent (res); McG '48; DABS, GenSurg (P.Q.); Chief Surg., Bellechasse Hosp.; Att'd. Staff, Jewish Gen. Hosp.; Tel. 725-9317.
LEVINE, Benjamin P.; 523 Outremont Ave., Montreal 8, P.Q.; McG '27; IntMed; **Ass't. Phys.**, Jewish Gen. Hosp.; Tel. 277-3777.
LEVINE, E. Calderwood; Box 250, Lillooet, B.C. Glasgow (Scot.)'46; Staff Psy., Lillooet & Dist. Hosp.; Tel. 62.
LEVINE, Harry H.; 5 Watercliffe Rd., Rexdale, Ont.; Tor '49; F.R.C.S.(C), GenSurg.
LEVINE, Jon H.; Tor'65; Res, Room 316, Banting Int., Toronto 2, Ont.
LEVINE, Joseph D.; 4949 Bathurst St., Willowdale, Ont.; Lausanne (Switz.)'58; DMR; DiagRad; Staff, North York Branson Hosp.; Tel. 223-5460.
LEVINE, Morris; Ste. 212-213, 175 East Broadway, Vancouver 10, B.C.; Manchester (Eng.)'28; Tel. 874-0624.
LEVINE, Morris H.; 452 Main St. E., Hamilton, Ont.; 44 Proctor (res); Tor '35; OphthOtol.; Tel. JA 2-5407.
LEVINE, Robert M.; Linton Clin., 6000 Cote des Neiges Rd., Montreal 26, P.Q.; McG'42; FACS; FRCS(C); GenSurg; Assoc. Surg. & Dir. of Tumour Clinic, Jewish Gen. Hosp.; Court. Staff, Queen Elizabeth Hosp.; **Chief M.O., RCA Victor** Co.; Tel. 342-2912.

LEVINNE, Nathan N.; 1353 Dundas St. W., Toronto 3, Ont.; Tor '41; MCGP; Chief Dept. of GP, New Mt. Sinai Sosp.; Tel. 533-5365.

LEVINSKAS, Leo; 570 King St. E., Hamilton, Ont. (res); Albertus U. (Koenigsberg, Germ.) '45; D.Psy (Tor); AMCGP; Staff, Ontario Hosp.; Tel. 385-5361.
LEVINSON, Edward D.; 620 Ellendale Med. Bldg., 5845 Cote-des-Neiges Rd., Montreal 26, **P.Q.; McG '53; Psy.; Tel. 737-7301.**
LEVIS, William H., Major; 28 Fairhill Cres., Don Mills, Ont. (res); UBC'54; DiagRad; DMR(D); M.O., CAFMS, Sunnybrook Hosp.; Tel. 485-8651.
LEVISON, Henry; Ireland'53; Res., Hosp. for Sick Children, Toronto 2, Ont.
LEVITAN, Benjamin A.; Ste. 114, 3545 Cote des Neiges, Montreal 25, P.Q.; McG '44; FRCP(C); IntMed; Cardiol (P.Q.); Ass't. Phys., Royal Victoria Hosp.; Cons. (Med.), Queen Mary Vet's. Hosp.; Lect. (Med.), McGill U.
LEVITSKY, Philip; 290 Ellendale Med. Bldg., 5845 Cotes des Neiges Rd., Montreal 26, P.Q.; 5930 Dolbeau (res); McG'34; IntMed (Gastroent.) (P.Q.); Staff, Jewish Gen. Hosp.; Tel. 735-0401.
LEVITT, Martin; Alb'63; Jr. Int., Winnipeg. Gen. Hosp., Winnipeg, Man.
LEVITT, Michael N.; 620 Seaforth Med. Bldg., 3550 Cote des Neiges Rd., Montreal 25, P.Q.; McG '58; Otol (P.Q.) Clin. Ass't (Otol.), Royal Victoria Hosp.; Tel. 933-3700.
LEVITTAN, Edwin D.; 787 Main St., Moncton, N.B.; Shediac Rd., Lewisville (res); Dal '40; MRCP; Tel. EV 4-4307.
LEVITZ, Abraham; 11 Harland Place, Hampstead, Montreal 29, P.Q.; Dal'49; F.A.C.A.; **Anaes; Staff Anaes., Jewish Gen. Hosp.**; Tel. 484-1003.
LEVSON, Harry; Ste. 402, 1040 Barclay St., Vancouver 5, B.C.; 3191 Crown St. (res); Man '38; MCGP.
LEVY, Alan H.; 163 Hunter St. W., Peterborough, Ont.; Bristol (Eng.) '48; FRCS (Eng.); GenSurg; Active Surg Staff, St. Joseph's & Civic Hosp's; Tel. 745-2455.
LEVY, Daniel; 810 King St. E., Hamilton, Ont.; **812 King St. E. (res); Tor '38; Neur; Cons. Neur., Hamilton Gen., St. Joseph's & Ontario Hosp's.; Dir. E.E.G. Lab. St. Joseph's; Tel. LI 4-8605.**

LEVY, Edith P.; 818 Upper Belmont Ave., Westmount 6, P.Q.; McG '42; Staff, Quebec Heart Assoc.

LEVY, Frances (Gula); 810 King St. E., Hamilton, Ont.; 812 King St. E. (res); Tor '40; MCGP; Tel. LI 4-8605.

LEVY, H. Roland; 1656 est rue Sherbrooke, Montreal 24, P.Q.; Paris (France) '58; FRCS(C); ThorSurg (Cardiovasc.); Staff, Hop. Notre-Dame; Tel. LA 5-6363.

LEVY, Irving; 1390 Main St. E., Hamilton, Ont.; 505 Maple Ave. (res); Tor '41; MCGP; Tel. LI 9-1244.

LEVY, Jacob; Granada (Spain); Staff, Hop. St-Vincent-de-Paul, Sherbrooke, P.Q.

LEVY, Leonard; 1025 Pine Ave. W., Montreal, **P.Q.; 52 Summit Circle (res); Dublin (Ire.) '52; Psy; Ass't. Psy., Royal Victoria Hosp.; Clin. Ass't., Jewish Gen. Hosp.; Tel. VI 2-1251.**

LEVY, Lyall A.; 1025 W. 67th St., Vancouver, B.C.; UBC'61; Tel. AM 6-5131.

LEVY, Mortimer; Ste. 3, 3800 St. Kevin, Montreal 26, P.Q. (Res.); Clin. Fell., Renal Diseases, Royal Victoria Hosp., Montreal; McG'61; FRCP(C), IntMed; Abroad.

LEVY, Ronald A.; 929 Liverpool Rd., Bay Ridges, Ont.; Tor'58; Staff(G.P.), Ajax & Bethesda Hosps.; Tel. 839-5851.

LEWCHUK, Wm.; 402 1541 W. Broadway, Vancouver, B.C.; UBC '55; Tel. RE 3-7525.

LEWIN, Oscar; 2428 Kingston Rd., Toronto 13, **Ont.; Tor '34; Tel. AM 1-1441.**

LEWIN, Peter K.; Room 113, Banting Inst., Toronto 2, Ont.; London (Eng.)'59; MRCS; LRCP; Research Fell., Dept. of Path., Banting Inst.

LEWIS, Archdale S.; 323 Hamilton Ave., Cornwall Drug Bldg., St. John's, Nfld.; Nagles Hill (res); Dal '43; F.I.C.S., F.R.C.S.(Edin.), GenSurg; Surg. Cons., D.V.A., D.A.D.M.S., Nfld. Area; Surg. Staff, St. Clare's, Grace & Gen. Hosp's.; Tel. 578-6870.
LEWIS, Anthony J.; 1075 Wellington St., Halifax, N.S.; London (Eng.) '49; D.Path. (Eng.); DTM&H (Eng.); Path; Neuropathol., Dalhousie U.
LEWIS, A. Franklin; 8 Sussex Ave., Toronto 5, Ont. (res); Tor '62; P.G., U. of Toronto.
LEWIS, Beverley A.; 53 St. Nicholas St., Toronto 5, Ont. (res); Tor '57; Path; Dir. of Labs., Queen Elizabeth Hosp., 130 Dunn Ave., Toronto 3; Tel. 534-7513.
LEWIS, Clarence H.; 2 Sultan St., Apt. 503, Toronto 5, Ont. (res); Qns '29; Psy; Ass't. Dir., Ontario Hosp's., Mental Health Div., Ontario **Dept. of Health; Tel. 365-2446.**
LEWIS, David J.; 1025 Pine Ave. W., Montreal, P.Q.; Tor'50; FAPA; FRCP(C); Psy; Assoc. Psy., Royal Victoria Hosp.; Co-ordinator P.G. Educ., Dept. of Psy. & Assoc. Prof. (Psy.), McGill U.; Tel. VI 2-1251, Loc. 695.
LEWIS, David J.; Box 480, Drayton Valley, Alta.; London (Eng.) '56; Tel. 542-3301.
LEWIS, Donald F.; Medical Arts Clinic, 51—6th **St. S.E., Medicine Hat, Alta.; 286 Prospect Dr. (res); Tor '45; IntMed; Staff, Medicine Hat Mun. Hosp.; Tel. 527-2281.**
LEWIS, Douglas E.; Water St., Digby, N.S.; Warwick St. (res); Dal '51; MCGP; Tel. 245-**2112.**
LEWIS, D. Sclater; 1390 Sherbrooke St. W., Ste. 35, Montreal 25, P.Q.; 31 Ramezay Rd., Westmount Montreal 6 (res); McG '12; D.A.B.I.M., F.A.C.P., LL.D.(Dal.), F.R.C.P.(C), IntMed; Hon. Att. Staff, Royal Victoria Hosp.; Tel. WE 5-4110.
LEWIS, Frederick I.; 430 Medical Arts Bldg., 170 St. George St., Toronto 5, Ont.; 48 Arjay Cres., Willowdale (res); Tor '23; F.R.C.S. (Edin.), F.R.C.S.(C), GenSurg; Cons. Surg., Toronto Gen. Hosp.; Ass't. Prof., U. of Toronto.; Tel. WA 5-8432.
LEWIS, Frederick N.; 542 Middlewoods, London, Ont.; Wes '52; Path; Assoc. Pathol., Victoria Hosp.; Clin. Ass't. Prof. (Path.), U. of Western Ontario; Tel. 432-5261.

LEWIS, George A.; 308 Charlotte St., Peterborough, Ont.; 942 Weller St. (res); Tor '45; ObstGyn; D.Obst (RCOG), MRCOG; Staff, Peterborough Civic, St. Joseph's, Port Hope, Cobourg, Campbellford & Lindsay Hosp's.; Tel. RI 2-0414.
LEWIS, George A.; 12 Bord du Lac, Beaconsfield, Ste. Anne de Bellevue, P.Q.; Mon'42; Anaes.(P.Q.).
LEWIS, George F.; 131 Park St. W., Windsor, Ont.; 1141 Kildare Rd. (res); Tor '16; Staff, Grace Hosp.; Tel. 253-5711.
LEWIS, George H.; Med. Arts Bldg., 2150 Valley Way, Niagara Falls, Ont.; 2361 Orchard Ave. (res); Qns'35; Ophth; Staff, Grt. Niagara Gen. Hosp.; Tel. EL 8-3911.
LEWIS, Henry John; 302-625 Fort St., Victoria, B.C.; Apt. 6, 1337 Rockland (res); M.R.C.S., L.R.C.P. (England) '44; Derm.; Tel. EV 2-6232.
LEWIS, Henry S.; Tor'61; Res., Vancouver Gen. Hosp., Vancouver 9, B.C.
LEWIS, Irwin; 5985 Souart Ave., Apt. 11, Montreal, P.Q.; McG '58; FRCP(C), Neurol. Abroad.
LEWIS, Ivor H.; Aberdeen (Scot.) '49; DPH (Leeds); M.O., Edson Health Unit, Edson, Alta.
LEWIS, James W.; River John, Pictou Co., N.S.; Dublin (Ire.)'50; BAO; Vis. Staff, Sutherland Mem. Hosp., Pictou & Lillian Frazer Mem. Hosp., Tatamagouche; Tel. 12.
LEWIS, John; Bennett St., Bell Island, Nfld.; Oxford (Eng.) '61.
LEWIS, John A.; Ste. 207, Medical Dental Bldg., 450 Central Ave., London, Ont.; 385 Wortley Rd. S. (res); Wes '35; F.A.C.P., F.C.C.P., F.R.C.P.-(C), IntMed; Chief of Med. Serv., Westminster D.V.A. Hosp.; Clin Assoc. Prof. (Med.), U. of Western Ontario; Tel. GE 2-9202.
LEWIS, John A.; 194½ Ontario St., St. Catharines, Ont.; 4 Rivercrest Dr. (res); Tor '43; Pres. Med. Staff, St. Catharines Gen. Hosp.; Telephone MU 4-4222.
LEWIS, John E.; 24 Pine St. S., Timmins, Ont.; 275 Hemlock St. (res); Qns '33; F.A.A.O.O., Ophth; Memb., Can. Ophth. Soc.; Tel. 264-5140.
LEWIS, J. William; 795 Carson Ave., Dorval, Lachine, P.Q.; 50 St. Joseph Blvd., Apt. 2 (res); Tor '51.
LEWIS, Leopold; Med. Arts Clinic, 51-6th St. S.E., Medicine Hat, Alta.; 125-2nd St. S.W. (res); Tor'36; MCGP; Staff, Medicine Hat Gen. Hosp.; Dist. Coroner; Tel. 527-2281.
LEWIS, Mervyn J.; 10547-52nd Ave., Edmonton, Alta.; London (Eng.)'59; Anaes.
LEWIS, Ralph S.; 299 Brock St., Kingston, Ont.; Qns '58; Tel. 546-7506.
LEWIS, Ronald D. M.; Box 449, High Prairie, Alta.; Birmingham (Eng.)'51; MCGP; Active Staff, Providence Hosp.; Chmn. of Health Unit; Dist. Coroner; Tel. 3-3354.
LEWIS, Ross A.; 877 Riverside Dr. London, Ont. (res); McG '42; M.C.G.P.; Vis. Staff, St. Joseph's & Victoria Hosp's.; Tel. 438-2464.
LEWIS, T. H. Christopher; 1665 W. Broadway, Vancouver 9, B.C.; 1351 Laurier Ave., Van. 9 (res); Oxford (Eng.) '49; IntMed; Att'd. Staff, Van. Gen. & Shaughnessy DVA Hosp's.; Tel. RE 1-4144.
LEWIS, V. D.; UBC '63; Res., Shaughnessy Hosp., Vancouver 9, B.C.
LEWIS, William S.; Glendon, Alta.; London (Eng.)'41; MRCS; LRCP.
LEWISON, Edward; 1414 Medical Dental Bldg., 925 W. Georgia St., Vancouver 1, B.C.; 801 Anderson Cres. West Van. (res); Tor '37; Otol.; Cons. (Otol.), Oakalla Prov. Gaol; Tel. MU 3-1755.
LEWITSKY, George; 375 Dorchester Rd. N., Niagara Falls, Ont.; Innsbruck (Austria)'48; Tel. 354-8211.
LEWKE, Hans S.; 632-16th Ave. N.W., Calgary, Alta.; Vienna (Aust.)'42; MCGP; FAGS; Tel. 289-2501.
LEWKIN, Dij; The Port Arthur Clinic, 194 N. Court St., Port Arthur, Ont.; 44 Winnipeg Ave. (res); Vienna (Aus.) '49; Psy; Tel. 344-7271.
LEWKOWITZ, Iveranda; 127 Ontario St., St. Catharines, Ont.; U. of Brazil (S.Am.)'56; Tel. 684-6774.
LEWONUK, Victor G.; Tor'60; Res., Hosp. for Sick Children, Toronto, Ont.
LEY, Dorothy C. H.; Room 384, 399 Bathurst St., Toronto, Ont.; Tor '48; B.Sc. (Med.); FACP; FRCP(C), IntMed; Dir. of Haem. & Att'd. Phys., Toronto Western Hosp.; Cons. Haem., Oakville-Trafalgar Mem. Hosp. & Queensway Gen. Hosp.; Assoc. Med., U. of Toronto; Tel. 366-1778.
LEYLAND, Eric E.; 714 Fairmont Med. Bldg., 750 W. Broadway, Vancouver 9, B.C.; 367 St. James Cres., West Van. (res); London (Eng.) '44; M.B., B.S. (Lond.), F.A.P.A.; D.R.C.O.G.; Psy; Tel. TR 4-7913.
LEZNOFF, Arthur; 610 Dawson Ave., Mont Royal, Montreal 16, P.Q. (res); McG '55; M.Sc. (Experimen. Med.); Allergy (P.Q.) F.R.C.P.(C), IntMed; Nat. Research Council, Fell. (All.), Royal Victoria Hosp.; Staff, Jewish Gen. Hosp.; Tel. RE 9-8384.
L'HEUREUX, J. A.; 532 rue St. Antoine, La Tuque, P.Q.; McG '56.
L'HEUREUX, Jean; 8415 rue St. Denis, Montreal 10, P.Q ; Mon'58; MCGP; Tel. Du 8-8195.
L'HEUREUX, Philippe L.; Man'61; Ass't. Res., St. Boniface Hosp., St. Boniface, Man.
L'HEUREUX, P. J. Paul; 22 Cherokee, St. Boniface, Man. (res); Man '33; D.P.H., PH.; Med. Dir., St. Boniface Hosp.; Tel. WA 3-0311.
LI, Kai T.; '62; Res., Children's Hosp., Winnipeg 3, Man.
LI, Mok-Dock; Taiwan (Formosa)'58; ABP; Res., St. Joseph's Hosp., London, Ont.
LI, Teng T.; St. Lawrence, Nfld.; Taiwan (Formosa)'63.
LIANG, David Y.; 309 Lancaster St. W., Kitchener, Ont.; Witwatersrand (S. Africa)'54; MRCOG; FRCS(C), ObstGyn; Staff (ObstGyn.), at St. Mary's Gen. Hosp. & Kitchener-Waterloo Hosp's.; Tel. 744-4552.
LIARD, Jean; 12774 Gouin Blvd. W., Pierrefonds, P.Q.; Mon '51; Psy (P.Q.); Ass't. (Dept. of Psy.), Jewish Gen. Hosp.; Cons., Federal Training Centre (Penit.).
LIAW, Yih-Chen; 224 East Broadway, Vancouver 10, B.C.; National Taiwan (Formosa)'62.
LIBERTY, Gordon L.; Suite 409, 340 McLeod St., Ottawa 4, Ont.; 33 Millbrook Cr., Ott. 5 (res); Qns'53; GenSurg; Att'd. Surg., Ottawa Civic, Riverside & Grace Hosp's.; Tel. 233-1252.
LIBMAN, David; Tor '53; Sr. Ass't. Res. (Clin. Lab), University Hosp., Edmonton, Alta.
LIBMAN, Israel; Linton Clin., 6000 Cote-des-Neiges Rd., Montreal 26, P.Q.; 493 Mitchell Ave., Twn. of Mt. Royal (res); McG'56; FRCP(C), Neur; Cons. Neurol. & Dir. (EEG) Lab., Jewish Gen. Hosp.; Tel. 735-1993.
LIBOIRON, Gilles; 378 Cartier, Laval-des-Rapides, P.Q.; Mon '63.
LIBRACH, Morris M.; 330 Oakwood Ave., Toronto 10, Ont.; Tor '56; Assoc. Staff, Doctor's & Northwestern Gen. Hosp., Tel. 781-4111.
LIBRACH, Samuel; 25 Brunswick Ave., Ste. 302, Toronto 4, Ont.; Tor '52; FRCS(C), ObstGyn; Ass't. Chief (ObstGyn.), Doctor's Hosp.; Tel. 923-7311.
LI CHONG, Pook C.; National U. (Ire); FRCS (Ed.); Res., Hamilton General Hosp., Hamilton, Ont.
LICHTBLAU, Steven I.; 35 Sherman Ave. S., Hamilton, Ont.; 108 Dufferin St. (res); Munich (Germ.)50; AMCGP; Active Staff, St. Joseph's & Hamilton Gen. Hosp's.; Tel. LI 9-6951.
LICHTENHELDT, John E.; Box 310, 19 Boullee St., New Hamburg, Ont.; Leipzig (Germ.) '44; M.C.G.P.
LICKLEY, H. Lavina; Tor'62; Res., Women's College Hosp., Toronto, Ont.
LIDDLE, Clive A. W.; 2322 St. Marc St., Shawinigan Falls, P.Q.; McG '54; M.C.G.P.; Staff, **Joyce Mem. & Ste.lTherese Hosp.; Tel. LE 9-3661.**
LIDDY, Bryan; Dublin (Ire.) '52; Ophth; Staff, Sunnybrook Hosp., Toronto 12, Ont.; Tel. 485-8651.

LIDDY, Edith B.; 473 Baker St., Apt. 4, London, Ont. (res); Tor '05; Retired.

LIDINGTON, Edgar W.; 151 Holmwood Ave., Ottawa, Ont.; 30 Woodlawn Ave. (res); Qns '42; M.C.G.P.; Staff, Ottawa Civic, & Grace Hosp's.; Courtesy Staff, Ottawa Gen. Hosp.; Tel. 235-4036.

LIDSTER, Donald K.; Rivers Med. Clin., Rivers, Man.; Sask '58.

LIEBE, Herman K.; 2441 Lake Shore Blvd. W., Toronto 14, Ont.; 47 Reid Manor Dr. Tor. 18 (res); Ernst-Moritz-Arndt U. (Greifswald, Germ.) '43; OrthSurg (Hamburg); Staff, St. Joseph's & Queensway Gen. Hosp's.; MOH, Mimico; CNR, Dist. M.O.; Tel. 259-6243.

LIEBLICH, Bruno A.; 3696 Dandurand, Montreal 36, P.Q.; Cluj (Roumania)'45.

LIEDTKE, Dorothea (See Kulis).

LIEFMANN Robert; 3283 Cedar Ave., Montreal 6, P.Q.; McG '45; Tel. WE 2-4281.

LIEPA, Egils V.; 250 Fairmont Ave., Ottawa 3, Ont. (res); Tuebingen (Germ.) '49; Path; Path., Ottawa Civic Hosp.; Vis. Lect. (Path), U. of Ottawa; Tel. PA 9-2511.

LIEPINA, Gerda (See MENETREZ, Gerda).

LIESEMER, Eldon J.; 13324-106th Ave., Edmonton, Alta. (res); Alb '25; Adm., Workmen's Comp. Bd., Edmonton.

LIGHT, A. Wolfe; 4565 Queen Mary Rd., Montreal, P.Q.; 4725 Fulton Ave. (res); McG '42; D&T Rad; Ass't. Rad., Queen Mary Veterans' Hosp.; Tel. RE 8-9481.

LIGHT, Irwin J.; McG '59; Res., Montreal Children's Hosp., Montreal, P.Q.

LIKAR, Ivan; Carmel Med. Clinic, 124—1st Ave. N.W., Swift Current, Sask.; London (Eng.)'62; MRCS(Eng.); LRCP(Lond.).

LIKELY, John C.; Fredericton Med. Clinic, 206 Rookwood Ave., Fredericton, N.B.; 86 Alexandra St. (res); McG '43; Otol; Tel. 475-7701.

LIKWORNIK, Herman; '33; Staff, Ontario Hosp., Whitby, Ont.

LILL, Frank J.; Ott '59; Jr. Int'n., Montreal Gen. Hosp., Montreal 25, P.Q.

LILLEY, Kenneth, S/L; Cdn. Forces Base, Chatham, N.B.; Liverpool (Eng.)'58; Sr. M.O., Cdn. Forces Base, Chatham.

LILLIE, John B.; Windsor Medical Clinic, 4505 Sources Road, Roxboro, P.Q.; McG'61.

LIM, Chong W.; Soeul (Korea) '57; DiagRad; Staff, Prince George Regional Hosp., Prince George, B.C.; Tel. 564-4411.

LIM, Dick S.; Manitoba Clinic, 790 Sherbrooke St., Winnipeg, Man.; Santo Tomas (Phillipp.) '55; IntMed; Staff, Misericordia Gen. Hosp.; Tel. 774-6541.

LIM, Don W.; 543 Lawrence Ave., Kelowna, B.C.; 1120 Hillcrest Rd. (res); Qns '47; Ophth.; Tel. 762-2003.

LIM, Eusebio G.; Westminster Hosp., London, Ont.; Santo Tomas (Philipp.)'52.

LIM, Jonathan S.; 805 Boyd Bldg., 388 Portage Ave., Winnipeg 1, Man.; Santo Tomas (Philip) '58.

LIM, Robert; Medical Clinic, 49-13th St. W., Prince Albert, Sask.; Santo Tomas (Philipp.) '55; Tel. 764-4241.

LIM, Richard A.; St. Boniface Clinic, 343 Tache Ave., St. Boniface, Man.; 963 Autumnwood Dr., Windsor Park (res); Santa Tomas (Manila, Philipp.) '52; M.S.; DABS; DABTS; FACS; FRCS(C), ThorSurg; Staff, St. Boniface Gen., Children's Misericordia, Winnipeg Gen. & Victoria Hosp's., Winnipeg; Dem. Surg., U. of Manitoba; Tel. 947-1581; Abroad.

LIM-LU, Margaret; Russell Clinic, Russell, Man., Santo Tomas (Philippines) '58.

LIM, Toh B.; North West. Univ. (Chicago Ill., U.S.A.)'62; Ass't Res., Toronto Gen. Hosp., Toronto 2, Ont.

LIM, William; Ste. 706, 1101 Pacific St., Vancouver 5, B.C.; Santo Tomas (Phillipp.)'56.

LIMOGES, Andre; 51 Blainville W., Ste. Therese de Blainville, Co., Terrebonne, P.Q.; Mon '56.

LIMOGES, Guy; 184 Blvd-Ste-Anne, Ste-Anne-des-Plaines, P.Q.; Mon '58.

LIMOGES, Joseph E.; 3977 Hochelaga, Montreal 4, P.Q.; Mon. '34; Tel. CL 5-3722.

LIMOGES, Philippe; 1336 Lemoine, Sillery, Quebec 6, P.Q.; Lav '59; MAH; Med. Dir., Hop. Hotel-Dieu; Tel. 529-9151, Loc. 227.

LIMOGES, Richard; Mon'65; Res., Verdun Gen. Hosp., Montreal 19, P.Q.

LIMONGELLI, Fulvio M.; 5325 Jean Talon E., Ville St. Leonard, Montreal N. P.Q.; Genoa (Italy)'55; FRCS(C), GenSurg.

LIN, David T. W.; 1531 Place-Ville-Marie, Montreal 3, P.Q.; 406 Beverley Ave., Twn. of Mt. Royal (res); McG'40; FACA; GenSurg (P.Q.); Ass't. Surg., Royal Victoria Hosp.; Lect. (Surg.), McGill U.; Pres., Mtl. Chinese Hosp.; Tel. 866-7127.

LIN, Sylvia J.; McG'61; Paed; Staff, Children's Hosp., Montreal 25, P.Q.

LIND, Jack R.; 630 St. Clair Ave. W., Toronto, Ont; 24 Austin Cres. (res); Tor '30; MCGP; Tel. LE 2-7773.

LIND, James F.; 1422 Mathers Bay East., Winnipeg 9. Man. (Res.); Qn's'51; FRCS(C); GenSurg.; Surg-in-Chief, Winnipeg Gen. Hosp.; Prof. (Surg.), University of Manitoba.

LIND, John A.; 112 Market St., Brantford, Ont.; Glenwood Rd. (res); Wes '36; Tel. 752-5712.

LINDENFELD, Bela; 736 Granville St., Vancouver, B.C.; 1370 W. 59 Ave. (res); Vienna (Austria) '10; Tel. MU 1-6640. Retired.

LINDENFELD, Elda; Ste. 909, 750 W. Broadway, Vancouver 9, B.C.; 1807 Knox Rd. (res); Vienna (Aust.) '22; Psy; Cons Children's Aid Soc.; Tel. TR 2-2913.

LINDENFIELD, Charles E.; 198 Muskoka St. N., Gravenhurst, Ont.; Tor '32; FCCP; Surg. Staff, Muskoka Hosp.

LINDSAY, Alexander; 4581/2 Main St., Kentville, N.S.; Glasgow (Scot.)'43; DOMS; Ophth; Staff (Ophth.Surg.), Blanchard-Fraser Mem. Hosp., Kentville; Soldiers Mem. Hosp., Middleton; Digby Gen. Hosp., Digby; West King's Mem. Hosp., Berwick; Tel. 678-3358.

LINDSAY, C. Crawford; 360 Seaforth Med. Bldg., 3550 Cote des Neiges Rd., Montreal 25, P.Q.; 11 Northcote Rd. (res); McG '50; FACOG; FRCS(C); ObstGyn; Ass't. (ObstGyn.), Montreal Gen., St. Mary's Mem., Herbert Reddy Mem. & Verdun Protestant Hosp's.; Jr. Ass't. & Sec. Med. Bd., Catherine Booth Maternity Hosp.; Tel. 935-6592.

LINDSAY, Donald S.; 401 Medical Centre, 906 8th Ave. W., Calgary, Alta.; 1245-19th Ave. W. (res); Dal '47; D.Psy., Psy.; Psy., Calgary Gen. Hosp.; Cons. in Psy., Colonel Belcher Hosp.; Tel. AM 3-6323.

LINDSAY, George C.; 20 Elizabeth St., Kingston, Ont.; Qns '23; Clin. Ass't., Dept. of Surg., Queen's U.; Tel. LI 6-1731; Retired.

LINDSAY, George E.; 221 Brant Ave., Brantford, Ont.; 1849 Yonge St., Toronto; Tor '56; DiagRad; Dir. of Rad., Norfolk Gen. Hosp., Simcoe; Tel. PL 3-8666 & 485-9154.

LINDSAY, Ian; Cambria Med. Bldg., 386 Cambria St., Stratford, Ont.; 62 John St. N. (res); Edinburgh (Scot.)'45; FRCS (Ed.), FRCS (Eng.); FRCS(C) GenSurg; Tel. 271-4051.

LINDSAY, James H.; 318 Gilmore Ave. S., Burnaby 2, B.C.; Qns'47.

LINDSAY, J. Gordon; 87 Adelaide St. N., Lindsay, Ont.; Sask '61; Tel. 324-2561.

LINDSAY, John H.; Manitoba Clinic, 790 Sherbrook St., Winnipeg 2, Man.; 225 Dromore Ave. (res); Wes '43; Psy; Hon. Att. Staff, Winnipeg Gen. Hosp., Lect., Psy. U. of Manitoba; Tel. SP 4-6541.

LINDSAY, Peter B.; 550 Ingersoll Ave., Woodstock, Ont.; 578 Devonshire Ave (res); Tor '40; Anaes; MCGP; Anaes. Staff, Woodstock Gen. Hosp.; Tel. 539-1526.

LINDSAY, Robert W.; Box 177, Dundalk, Ont.; Tor '33; M.C.G.P.

LINDSAY, William G.; Man '64; Res., Minneapolis U. Med. Centre, Minneapolis, Minn., U.S.A.; Abroad.

LINDSAY, William K.; 619 Med. Arts Bldg., 170 St. George St., Toronto 5, Ont.; 222 Balmoral **Ave. (res); Tor '45; F.A.C.S., M.S., F.R.C.S.-**(C), PlasSurg; Assoc. Surg., Hosp. for Sick Children; Assoc. Prof. (Dept. of Surg.), U. of Toronto; Chm., Med. Advis. Comm. & Treatment Centre, Ont. Soc. Crippled Children; Tel. WA 2-5246.

LINDSAY, William R.N.; Ste. 505, Med. Dental Bldg., 1849 Yonge St., Toronto, Ont.; 2374 **Eglinton Ave. E., Scarboro; 22 Rochester Ave.** (res); Alb'49; M.S. (Tor.); FRCS(C); GenSurg; PlasSurg; Att'd. Staff, Toronto East & Scarboro Gen. Hosp's.; Tel. 485-0465.

LINDSAY, W. Stewart; 812A Spadina Cres. E., Saskatoon, Sask.; Edinburgh (Scot.) '12; Path-Bact; Sec. University Hosp. Bd.; Tel. CH 2-7641. Retired.

LINDSEY, George W.; 200 Brock St. N., Whitby, **Ont.; 306 John St. W. (res); Tor '40; Tel. 668-3378.**

LINDZON, Martin; 305 Brunswick Diagnostic Clinic, 25 Brunswick Ave., Toronto 4 Ont.; 15 West Grove Cres. (res); Tor '53; FAAP; FR-CP(C), Paed; Chief of Paed., Doctors' Hosp.; Tel. 921-5322.

LINEGAR, Kevin L.; 222 Le Marchant Rd., St. **John's, Nfld., Dal '52; Paed.; Tel. 578-7074.**

LINELL, Eric A.; 253 Blythwood Rd., Toronto 12, Ont. (res); Manchester (Eng.) '14; M.B., Ch.B., M.D., Path; **Cons. (NeurPath), Hosp. for** Sick Children & Toronto East Gen. Hosp.; **Emer. Prof. (NeurPath), U. of Toronto; Tel. HU 9-3469.**

LING, Chin H.; 8th Floor, Confederate Bldg., Winnipeg, Man.; 20 Glengarry Dr., Wpg. 19 (res); Peking Union Med. College (China) '26; OphthOtol; Med.Spec. OphthOtol, Indian & North**ern Health Service, Dept. Nat. Health & Welfare; Tel. WH 3-1414.**

LING, Grace; Ste. 100, 77 Upper Middle Rd., Cooksville, Ont.; Tor '61.

LINGARD, William F.; Ste 660, 5025 Sherbrooke St. W., Montreal 28, P.Q.; Qns '47; Urol; Ass't. Urol. Montreal Gen. Hosp.; Cons. Urol., Queen Mary Vet's Hosp.; Staff (Urol.), Queen Elizabeth & Reddy Mem. Hosp's; Dem. (Surg.), McGill U.

LINKLATER, E. W.; Imperial Bank Bldg., Nor**anda, P.Q.; 17 Murdoch Ave. (res); GenSurg.** Retired.

LINKLETTER, Alfred M.; 317 Eldorado Ave., Pointe-Claire, P.Q.; 23 Claremont Ave. (res); McG '48; ObstGyn; Att'd. Staff, Catherine Booth, Lakeshore Gen. & Lachine Gen. Hosp's.; Tel. OX 7-2317.

LINKS, Harold; 10951-124th St., Edmonton, Alta.; 11827-91st Ave. (res); Dublin (Ire.) '43; Gen-Surg.; Tel. GL 4-4551.

LINSDELL, Francis J.; 450 Central Ave., London, Ont.; 125 Wychwood Park (res); Wes '52; Diag Rad; Staff, St. Joseph's Hosp.; Lect. (Diag-Rad.), U. of Western Ontario; Tel. 433-2841.

LINTON, F. Douglas; 1206 Wyandotte St., River**side, Ont.; Tor '27; Tel. 945-3921.**

LINTON, Harold; 305 Finch Ave. W., Willowdale, Ont.; 48 Ridelle Ave. (res); Tor'39; Gen**Surg; Court. Staff, Bethseda North York Branson Hosp's.; Tel. BA 1-5544.**

LINTON, Robert C.; Wes '59; Res., Victoria Hosp., London, Ont.

LINTON, William T.; 1 Roxborough St. E., Toronto 5, Ont.; 59 Bellgrave Ave. (res); Tor '55; **FRCP(C); Derm; Staff, St. Michael's Hosp.** & Hosp. for Sick Children; Cons. Derm., York Central Hosp.; Clin. Ass't. (Med.), U. of Toronto; Tel. 922-0105.

LIONANAG, Emilia M.; Santo Tomas (Phillipp.) **'52; Staff, Union Hosp., Moose Jaw, Sask.; Tel.** 692-1841.

LIPA, Michael; Qns'61; FRCP(C), Path; Staff, Toronto Western Hosp., Toronto 2B, Ont.

LIPCSEI, Joseph; 44 Ellesmere Rd., Scarborough, Ont.; Budapest (Hung) '56; Staff, Doctors' & Tor. E. Gen. Hosp's.; Tel. 447-9452.

LIPINSKI, Edwin; 4400 W. Grandview, Douglas Highway, Burnaby 2, B.C.; UBC'60; Psy.

LIPINSKI, John J.; 8505-118th Ave., Edmonton, Alta.; 11042-108th St. (res); Alb '48; MCGP; Tel. 477-6111.

LIPITCH, Henry S.; Hodgerille, Sask.; Edinburgh (Scot.)'62.

LIPMAN, May; (See Cohen, May).

LIPOWSKA, Barbara (Przygodzka); 3478 Grey **Ave., Montreal, P.Q. (res); Dublin (Ire.) '53;** Clin. Ass't. OPD, Mtl. Gen. Hosp.; Tel. WE 7-6011, Loc. 691.

LIPOWSKI, Zbigniew; 1025 Pine Ave. W., Mont**treal 2, P.Q.; University Coll. (Dublin, Ire.) '54;** D.Psy.; Psy(P.Q.); Ass't. Psy., Royal Victoria Hosp.; Ass't. Prof. (Psy.), McGill U.; Tel. VI 2-1251.

LIPP, James A.; Sect. of Physiol., Suffield Experimental Station, Ralston, Alta.; U.S.A. '60.

LIPPERT, Frederick G.; USA '65; Jr. Int., Royal Victoria Hosp., Montreal 2, P.Q. Abroad.

LIPPERT, Gerard G.; 80 Queen St. N., Kitchener, Ont.; 211 Stanley Dr., Waterloo (res); McG '42; F.A.C.S., F.R.C.S.(C), GenSurg; Staff, Kitchener-Waterloo & St. Mary's Hosp's.; Cons. Staff, S. Waterloo Mem. Galt, St. Joseph's & **Guelph Gen. Hosp's. & Freeport San., Kitchener; Tel. 742-8421.**

LIPPMANN, H. Hugo; 410 Norlyn Med. Bldg., 309 Hargrave St., Winnipeg 2, Man.; Man '44.; **Urol; Tel. 943-8943.**

LIPSETT, W. Barry; Salmon Arm, B.C.; Man '53; AMCGP; Tel. 832-2191.

LIPSON, Martin H.; 1271 Dundas St. W., Toronto, Ont.; Tor '62; AMCGP; Staff, Dept. of G.P., New Mt. Sinai & Doctor's Hosp's.; Tel. LE 5-3164.

LIPTON, Irving H.; Tor '62; Res., Toronto Gen. Hosp., Toronto, Ont.

LIQUORNIK, Clara (Rudich); 690 Eglinton Ave. E., Toronto 17, Ont.; Bucharest (Roum.)'34; Tel. HU 3-5044.

LIRENMAN, David S.; 715 W. 12th Ave., Vancouver 9, B C.; Man'60; FRCP(C), Int.Med.

LISBONA, Andre; Mon'64; Res., Montreal Gen. Hosp., Montreal 25, P.Q.

LISTER, J. Godfrey; Mental Health Clinic, 514 Jarvis St., Toronto 5, Ont.; 19 St. Andrews Gdns., Tor 5 (res); Tor'55; D. Psy; Psy; MCGP; Clin. Dir., Toronto Mental Health Clinic; Clin. Teach. Psy., U. of Toronto; Tel. 924-7349.

LISTGARTEN, C.; Tor'64; Res., Royal Victoria Hosp., Montreal 2, P.Q.

LISTON, Ambrose J.; 595 King St. W., Hamilton, Ont.; Qns '31; M.C.G.P.; Chief, G.P. Section, St. Joseph's Hosp.; Tel. JA 2-6616.

LISTON, William P.; 360 Professional Bldg., Edmonton, Alta.; Dublin (Ire.)'47; DMRD; Diag-Rad; Assoc. Radiol., Edmonton Gen. Hosp.; Tel. 424-0496.

LITCH, S. W.; Tor '64; Res., Vancouver Gen. Hosp., Vancouver, **B.C.; Abroad.**

LITHE, Wolfgang; 5300 Cote-des-Neiges Rd., Montreal 26, P.Q.; Hamburg (Germ.) '47.

LITHERLAND, Henry K.; Ste. 1417, 750 W. Broadway, Vancouver 9, B.C.; Cambridge (Eng.) '57; M.B., B.Ch.; DRCOG; FRCS(C), GenSurg; Staff, Vancouver Gen. & Shaughnessy DVA Hosp's.; Tel. 872-2312.

LITHERLAND, Oswald K.; 1940 Lonsdale Ave., North Vancouver, B.C.; 2709 Mathers Ave., West Van. (res); Cambridge (Eng.) '51; FRCP(C), IntMed; Active Staff, Lion's Gate & Cons. Staff, Shaughnessy DVA Hosp's.; Tel. YU 8-3242.

LITHGOW, Alexander D; 933 Ottawa St., Windsor, Ont.; 935 Ottawa (res); Tor '39; Tel. 253-4171.

LITTLE, Adam S.; Edmonton Cancer Clinic, 85th Ave., Edmonton, Alta.; Man '42; F.R.C.P. (C), IntMed; Dir. O.P.D., University Hosp.; Assoc. Prof. (Med.), U. of Alberta; Tel. 439-5911.

LITTLE, A. Hugh; Tor'59; IntMed; Staff, Sunnybrook Hosp., Toronto, Ont.

LITTLE, Andrew W.; Nanton, Alta.; London (Eng.) '38; M.R.C.S., L.R.C.P.; Tel. 486-2131.

LITTLE, Barry J.; 1 Strathearn Rd., Toronto 10, Ont.; Tor'59; FRCP(C); Neur; Staff, St. Michael's Hosp.; Tel. 362-4461.

LITTLE, Desmond C.; 250 Main St. E., Hamilton, Ont.; 131 Chedoke Ave. (res); Manchester (Eng.) '41; DCH; MRCP (Lond.); IntMed; Tel. JA 7-2711.
LITTLE, Flora G. (Gauld); 264 Woolwich St., Guelph, Ont.; Tor '23; Tel. TA 2-5221.
LITTLE, G. A.; 1152 Downing, Winnipeg, Man. (res); Man '30; Psy; Staff, U. of Manitoba; Tel. GR 4-9110.
LITTLE, George E.; 3310 Boundary Rd., Vancouver 12, B.C.; Man '41; Tel HE 1-7424.
LITTLE, George D.; 722 Medical Arts Bldg., Montreal, P.Q.; 3245 Cedar (res); McG '21; F.A.C.S.; GenSurg; Hon. Att'd. Staff, Montreal Gen. Hosp.; Tel. WE 5-6864.
LITTLE, G. Meldrum; 770 City Hall, Edmonton, Alta.; 12203 Jasper Ave. (res); Man '21; D.A.B., P.M.P.H., D.P.H., PH; M.O.H., City of Edmonton; Tel. 424-0211.
LITTLE, Hanna B. (Brinkop); 127 Elgin Cres., Waterloo, Ont.; Munich (Germ.) '41; TherRad; Staff, Kitchener-Waterloo & St. Mary's Hosp's. Guest. Lect., Waterloo Lutheran U.; Tel. 742-1996.
LITTLE, Harry; 18-3rd Ave. N.W., Dauphin, Man.: Man '51; Dist. Coroner.
LITTLE, James A.; 30 Bond St., Toronto 2, Ont.; 361 Glengrove W., Tor. 12 (res); Tor '46; MA; FRCP(C), IntMed; Dir. Clin. Invest. Unit & Hemodialysis Unit, & Diabetic Clin; St. Michael's Hosp.; Research Assoc., Sunnybrook DVA Hosp.; Assoc. (Med.), U. of Toronto; Tel. EM 2-4461.
LITTLE, J. Graham; Ste. 150, 3550 Cote des Neiges, Montreal 25, P.Q.; 5791 Melling St., Mtl. 29 (res); McG'54; DABO, FAAOO; FRCS(C), Ophth; Staff, Jr. OphthPath. & Ass't. Dir. Glaucoma Clinic, Montreal Gen. Hosp.; Att'd. Staff, Montreal Children's Hosp.; Tel. VI 9-8551.
LITTLE, John M.; McG'61; Ophth; Staff, Montreal Gen. Hosp., Montreal, P Q.; Abroad.
LITTLE, Kenneth J., S/L; Dal '57; Staff, Can. Forces Hosp., Kingston, Ont.
LITTLE, Lewis N.; Ste. 402, 267 O'Connor St., Ottawa, Ont.; 139 Ruskin Ave. (res); Tor '44; Otol; Cons., D.V.A.; Cons., Dept. of Natl. Defence; Att. Staff, Otol., Ottawa Civic Hosp.; Tel. CE 3-9447.
LITTLE, Lloyd G.; 1250 Victoria Park Ave., Toronto 16, Ont.; Tor '49; MCGP: Tel. PL 5-2541.
LITTLE, Meldrum W.; Box 1418, Weyburn Med. Clinic, Weyburn, Sask.; Alb '50; FRCS(C); GenSurg; Staff, Union Hosp.; Tel. 842-5404.
LITTLE, M. Harvey; Apt. 842, 21 Dale Ave., Toronto 5, Ont.; Tor'41; Anaes.
LITTLE, Perley R.; 893 Prince St., Truro, N.S.; Dal'26.
LITTLE, Robert B.; 475-3rd Ave. N.E., Swift Current, Sask. (res); McG'53; DiagRad; Staff, Union Hosp.; Tel. 773-4641.
LITTLE, Robert D.; Assoc. Med. Clinic, Westlock, Alta.; Aberdeen (Scot.) '53; GenSurg; Tel. 342-3341.
LITTLE, Robert M.; 27 Cedar St. N., Timmins, Ont.; Ott '60; Staff, St. Mary's Hosp. & Porcupine Gen. Hosp., South Porcupine; Tel. 264-1234.
LITTLE, Shauna G.; 4529 W. 10th Ave., Vancouver 8, B.C.; Alb '48; Psy; Staff, Child Guidance Clinic; Tel. CA 4-7824.
LITTLE, Walter M.; 343 Markland Dr., Markland Wood, Etobicoke, Ont. (res); Tor '48; DABR; DiagRad; Staff, Dept. of Rad., St. Joseph's Hosp., Toronto 3; Tel. 534-9531.
LITTLE, William C.; Simcoe Medical Group, Ste. 201, 121 Wellington St. W., Barrie, Ont.; Tor'20; Tel. 728-2476.
LITTLE, William F.; Tor'54; Staff, Nanaimo Indian Hosp., Nanaimo, B.C.; Indian Health Serv., Dept. of National Health & Welfare; Tel. SK 3-4322.
LITWIN, Jaroslaw; Punnichy, Sask. (res); Cracow (Poland) '38; M.O., Dept. of Nat. Health & Welfare, Fort Smith, N.W.T.
LITZENBERGER, Don; Raxlen Clinic, 500 Parliament St., Toronto 5, Ont.
LIU, Lillian W. M.; 3225 Wyandotte St., Riverside, Windsor, Ont.; 237 Belle Isle View Blvd. (res); National Central U. (Nanking, China) '49; Paed.; Tel. 948-3961.
LIU, Sim F.; 219 St. Clair Ave. W., Toronto 7, Ont.; 58 Moore Ave. (res); Shanghai (China) '44; DTM&H (Eng.), FCCP; FACP; FAGS; IntMed; Staff (OPD), Toronto Western Hosp.; Cons. Phys., Lambert Lodge & Geriatric Centre; Tel. 923-6201.
LIVELY, Frank M.; 2753 Bathurst St., Toronto 19, Ont.; Tor'26; MCGP; Assoc. Staff, OPD, St. Joseph's Hosp.; Tel. RU 2-4232.
LIVER, John A.; 1933 Fairmeadow Cr., Ottawa 8, Ont.; Edinburgh (Scot.)'49; DiagRad; Staff, Ottawa Gen. Hosp.; Clin. Ass't., U. of Ottawa; Tel. 236-0333.
LIVERMORE, Marilyn L.; Tor '59; D.Psy.; Psy; Staff, Ont. Hosp., St. Thomas, Ont.; Tel. 631-8510.
LIVERPOOL, J. Alban; 326A College St., Toronto 2B, Ont.; McG '55; MCGP; Chief, Dept. G.P. Doctor's Hosp.; Tel. WA 5-4396.
LIVESEY, Robert J.; 39 Earl St., Kingston, Ont.; Qns '40; Tel. 548-8068.
LIVINGSTON, John M.; 98 Queen St. N., Kitchener, Ont. (res); Tor '11; Retired.
LIVINGSTON, Michael C.; 1083B No. 4 Rd., Richmond, Vancouver 14, B.C.; Alb '53; Tel. BR 7-8922.
LIVINGSTON, Sir Philip C.; KBE., C.B., A.F.C.; Box 220, Qualicum Beach, Vancouver Island, B.C.; Cambridge (Eng.) '19; L.R.C.P. (Lond.); F.R.-C.S. (Eng.); F.R.C.S. (Edin.); D.O.M.S.; DPH; Ophth; Tel. SK 2-6012.
LIVINGSTONE, Arthur G.; Ste. 2, Metcalfe Bldg., Lethbridge, Alta.; 310—28th St. (res); Alb'46; Urol; Tel. 327-7666.
LIVINGSTONE, Cecil S.; 303-720 W. Broadway, Vancouver, B.C.; 6652 Granville (res); National U. (Wales) '48; M.D. (Lond.); DCH (Eng.), M.R.C.P. (Eng.); Paed; Teach. Fell. (Paed.), U. of British Columbia; Tel. TR 9-2133.
LIVINGSTONE, Donn A., F/L; Station Infirmary CFB, North Bay, Ont.; UBC'65.
LIVINGSTONE, Edward S.; 462-25th Ave. N.W., Calgary, Alta.; Glasgow (Scot.) '54; Tel. CR 7-3887.
LIVINGSTONE, Frank; 76 Wellington St., St. Thomas, Ont. '20.
LIVIU, Andreiu, 238 S. Notre-Dame, Thetford Mines, P.Q.; Roumania '42.
LIZEWSKI, Waldemar J.; 2917 Bloor St. W., Toronto 18, Ont.; 456 Crawford St., Tor 4 (res); Tor '60; Tel. 534-6379.
LIZOTTE, Fernand; MPP; Lav '33; MCGP; Supt. Hop. St.-Jean-de-Port-Joli, St. Jean-de-Port Joli, Cte. L'Islet, P.Q.; Tel. 303.
LIZOTTE, Joseph A.; Notre Dame du Lac, Co. Temiscouata, P.Q.; Lav '28.
LIZOTTE, J. Adrien.; 2172 Desormeaux, Montreal, P.Q.; Lav '22; Tel. CL 5-6039.
LIZOTTE, Laurent; 924 Cardinal Rouleau, Quebec 6, P.Q. (res); Lav '46; MCGP; Staff Dept. of Health, PQ; Tel. LA 4-8411.
LIZOTTE, Paul; 10858 rue St-Vital, Montreal-Nord, P.Q.; Lav'43; MCGP; Tel. DA 1-1520.
LIZOTTE, Real; Unite Sanitaire, St. Jean, Port Joli, Cte. l'Islet, P.Q.; Lav '54; DPH; Tel. 175.
LLEWELLYN, Anne; Dublin (Ire.)'58; Staff, Wpg. Municipal Hosp., Winnipeg, Man.
LLEWELLYN-THOMAS, Edward R.; Inst. of Bio-Medical Electronics, U. of Toronto, Toronto 5, Ont.; McG '55; Assoc. Dir., Inst. of Bio-Med Electronics; Clin. Ass't., Dept. of Anaes., Toronto Gen. Hosp.; Prof. (Pharm.), U. of Toronto; Tel. 928-3114.
LLOYD Ann; London (Eng.) '57; Jr. Intn., Vancouver Gen. Hosp., Vancouver, B.C.
LLOYD, Gary R.; Qns'65; Res., Hosp. for Sick Children, Toronto 2, Ont.
LLOYD, H. Alan; 300 Medical Dental Bldg., Edmonton, Alta.; 9235-118th St. (res); Alb '43; M.C.G.P.; Tel. 422-2232.
LLOYD, Hubert H.; 34 Beckwith St. S., Smith's Falls, Ont.; Qns '43; Staff, St. Francis Gen. & Smiths Falls Public Hosp's.; Coroner, Co. of Lanark; Tel. 283-3345.

LLOYD, J. Ewart; Box 220, Claresholm, Alta.; Wales'40.

LLOYD Lois A.; 507 Med. Arts Bldg., 170 St. George St., Toronto 5, Ont.; 148 Strathallan Blvd., Tor. 12 (res); Tor '49; FRCS(C), Ophth; Staff (Ophth.), Tor. Gen. & Assoc. Staff, Hosp for Sick Children; Assoc. (Ophth.), U. of Toronto; Tel. WA 1-9342.

LLOYD, Merrick H.; 1093 Fennel St. E., Hamilton, Ont.; Birmingham (Eng.)'36; D.ObstRCOG.

LLOYD-SMITH, Donald L.; 3801 University St., Montreal, P.Q.; 637 Belmont Ave., Westmount (res); McG '41; MRCP (Lond.); FRCP(C), Neurol; Neurol., Mtl. Neurol. Inst. & Royal Victoria Hosp.; Cons. (Electroencephal.), Queen Mary Vet's. Hosp.; Assoc. Prof. (Neurol), McGill U.; Tel. VI 5-3838 & 484-4914.

LLOYD-SMITH, Walter C.; Box 640, 5025 Sherbrooke St. W., Montreal 28, P.Q.; 530 Argyle Ave., Westmount (res); McG '43; F.A.C.S.; F.R.-C.S. (Edin.), F.R.C.S.(C), GenSurg; Assoc. Surg., Queen Elizabeth & Herbert Reddy Mem. Hosp's.; Tel. 489-9324.

LO, Louis Y.; Man '61; Res., Wpg. Gen. Hosp., Winnipeg 3, Man.

LO, Mei C.; 10 Argyle St., Campbellton, N.B.; Taiwan (Formosa)'48; Urol; Active Staff, Soldiers' Mem. Hosp.; Assoc. Staff, Hotel Dieu Hosp.; Cons., Provincial Hosp.; Cons., St. Joseph Hosp., Dalhousie, N.B.; Tel. 753-4329.

LOACH, Lynn F.; Room 132, Private Patients' Pavillion, Toronto Gen. Hosp., Toronto 2, Ont.; Tor'59; FRCP(C); IntMed; Clin. Ass't., Toronto Gen. Hosp.; Sr. Teach. Fell., University of Toronto; Tel. EM 6-8211, Loc. 2398.

LOADMAN, A. Evelyn; 137 Montrose St., Winnipeg 9, Man.; Man '41; Paed; Part-Time Staff, City Health Dept. & Children's Hosp.

LOADMAN, Bruce E.; Winnipeg Clinic, Winnipeg, Mon.; 137 Montrose St. (res); Man '41; Orth Surg; Staff (Orth.), Winnipeg Gen., Children's **& Misericordia Hosp's.; Lect., (Surg.), U. of** Manitoba; Tel. WH 2-6441.

LOANE, Anna L. (Miller); 608 Queen St., Fredericton, N.B.; 384 Parkhurst Dr. (res); McG '44; ObstGyn; Chief Dept. of ObstGyn, Victoria Public Hosp.; Tel. GR 5-3201. Abroad.

LOBAN, Louis; 2193 Portage Ave., Winnipeg, Man.; Man '28; Anaes; Chief of Anaes., Deer Lodge Vet's. Hosp.; Lect. (Anaes), U. of Manitoba; Tel. TU 8-4861.

LOBAY, Fred; Smoky Lake, Alta.; Alb '55.

LOBB, Ross A.; X-Ray Dept., Med. Arts Bldg., 170 St. George St., Toronto 5, Ont.; 296 Oriole Parkway, Tor. 7 (res); Tor '43; DMR; D&TRad; Ass't. Rad., Toronto Gen. Hosp.; Clin. Teach. (Rad.), U. of Toronto; Tel. EM 6-8211.

LOBLEY, Percy G.; 1415 Lawrence Ave. W., Toronto, Ont.; 28 North Park Dr. (res); Tor '45; Staff, St. Joseph's & Humber Memorial, & North**western Gen. Hosp's.; Tel. 247-3991.**

LOBSINGER, Allan J.; 242 Birks Bldg., Edmonton, Alta; 26 Riverside Cres. (res); Man '29; GenSurg.; Tel. GA 2-2563.

LOBSINGER, William J.; Wes'51; Res., Victoria Hosp., London, Ont.

LOCAT, Wilfrid; St. Roch de L'Achigan, P.Q.; Mon '41.

LOCHEAD, John A.; McG'63; Res., St. Paul's Hosp., Vancouver 1, B.C.

LOCHHEAD, William E.; Ste. 14, 222 Blvd. Henri Bourassa E., Montreal, P.Q.; 241 rue Fleury W.; 10520 rue Hoque (res); Mon'50; GenSurg (P.Q.); GenSurg , Hop. du Sacre Coeur, Cartierville; Tel. DV 7-3454.

LOCKE, Arthur C.; 52 Bridge St. E., Belleville, Ont.; Qns '21; OphthOtol; Tel WO 8-6560.

LOCKE, Clair J.; 878 Armoury St., Niagara Falls, Ont.; Qns '35.

LOCKE, F. Dean; Lacombe, Alta. (res); Tor '19; Retired.

LOCKE, Howard A.; 176 Provost St., New Glasgow, N.S.; 665 East River Rd. (res); Dal'45; **MCGP; Staff, Aberdeen Hosp.; Tel. 752-6266.**

LOCKE, H. W. Beecher; John St., Thornhill, Ont. (res); Tor '18; Urol.; Cons. Surg. (Urol.), Toronto Western Hosp.

LOCKE, John C.; Ste. 1012, 1414 Drummond St., Montreal, P.Q.; 1 Cressy Rd., Hampstead (res); McG '42; Med. Sc.D.(Columbia), D.A.B.O., F.A.-C.S., F.R.C.S.(C), Ophth; Ophth.-in-Chief, Royal Victoria Hosp.; Cons. Ophth., Catherine Booth Maternity Hosp.; Prof. & Chairman, Dept. of Ophth., McGill U.; Cons. (Ophth), Physician's **Hosp., Plattsburgh, N.Y.; Tel. VI 2-4024.**

LOCKHART, Earle A.; Tor'65; Res., Hosp. for Sick Children, Toronto 2, Ont.

LOCKHART, Henry B.; Ste. 450, 2184 W. Broadway, Vancouver 9, B.C.; 5795 Churchill St. (res); Tor '44; D.A.B. Ot., F.A.A.O.O.; F.R.C.S.(C); **F.A.C.S.; Otol; Hd. (Otol.) St. Paul's & Staff Children's Hosp.; Vis. Staff Vancouver Gen.** Hosp.; Clin. Instr. Dept. Surg., U. of British **Columbia; Tel. RE 3-0327.**

LOCKHART, John A.; Bath Hosp. Ltd., Bath, N.B.; McG '45; Pres. & Chm., Bath Hosp. Ltd.

LOCKHART, J. Osler; 632 King St. E., Hamilton, Ont.; 976 Concession (res); Wes '39; MCGP; Tel. JA 8-5926.

LOCKIE, John G.; 5798 Victoria Dr., Vancouver 16, B.C.; Qns'65; Tel. FA 5-1288.

LOCKIE, John M.; Brandon Health Unit, Brandon, Man.; 2736 Princess Ave. (res); Edinburgh (Scot.) '34; D.M.R.(D) (Lond.); Cons. Rad., Dept. Health & Welfare, Prov. of Man. Gov't.

LOCKINGTON, W. A.; Wes'43; Res., Clarke Inst. of Psy., 250 College St., Toronto 2B, Ont.

LOCKNER, Patricia A.; McG'65; Jr. Int., Royal Victoria Hosp., Montreal 2, P.Q.; Abroad.

LOCKWOOD, Ambrose L.; 300 Bloor St. E., Toronto, Ont.; McG '10; F.A.C.S., F.R.C.S.(C), GenSurg; Dir. & Sr. Surg., Lockwood Clinic Hosp.

LOCKWOOD, Charles A.; Glencoe, Ont.; Wes '24; Dist. Coroner.

LOCKWOOD, Charles; Wes '53; FRCP(C), Int-Med; Staff, Ont. Hosp., Box 155, Woodstock, Ont.; Tel. LE 9-1251.

LOCKWOOD, Peter; 288 Duckworth St., St. **John's, Nfld.; "Wessenden", Nagles Hill (res);** Leeds (Eng.)'51; Hd., Ophth. Div., Grace Hosp.; Assoc. Staff, St. Clare's Hosp.; Tel. 8-0237.

LOCKWOOD, Thomas M.; 21 Upper Middle Rd., Ste 211, Cooksville, Ont.; McG '42; F.A.C.S., F.C.C.P., F.R.C.S.(C), GenSurg; Cons., (Active Staff), South Peel Hosp.; Cons. (Court. Staff), Queensway & Oakville-Trafalgar Gen. Hosp's.; Tel. 279-6113.

LOCKYER, Norman S.; 2470 Lansdowne Rd., Victoria, B.C.; London (Eng.)'39; MRCS; DMRT, TherRad; Med. Dir., Victoria Cancer Clin., Royal **Jubilee Hosp.; Rad., Royal Jubilee Hosp.; Rad. Ther., St. Joseph's Hosp.; Tel. EV 6-3131.**

L'ODDO, Giovanni; 7039 St. Denis, Montreal 10. P.Q.; Palermo (Italy) '24; Tel. 271-6322.

LODER, Peter G.; 225 McDonald Ave., Belleville, Ont.; Dal '47; DiagRad; Dir. Dept. of Rad., Belleville Gen. Hosp.; Tel. WO 8-5511.

LOEB, Jacques A.; 331 Sheddon Ave., Oakville, Ont.; 272 Pinehurst Dr. (res); London (Eng.) '49; FRCS (Eng.); FRCS(C), FACS; GenSurg; Cons. (Surg.), Oakville-Trafalgar Mem. Hosp.; Surg. Staff, St. Joseph's & Queensway Hosp's., Toronto; Tel. 845-7092.

LOEB, Lazarus J.; 256 Elgin St., Ottawa 4, Ont.; M.Sc., DIM, FAAA, FRCP(C), Int-Med; (Allergy); Staff & Dir. Allergy Clin. & Lab., Ottawa Civic Hosp.; Chief, Allergy Clinic, Nat. Defence Med. Centre; Cons. Allergy, Royal Ottawa San; Pres., Cdn. Acad. of Allergy (1965-66); Lect. (Bact. & Immunol.), U. of Ottawa; Tel. CE 3-7777.

LOEWEN, George; 16 Capilano Mall, Edmonton, Alta.; Alb'64; Tel. 699-5671.

LOEWEN, Lowell M.; 356 Medical Arts Bldg., Saskatoon, Sask.; **322 Ash St. E. (res); Sask '57.**

LOEWEN, Margaret; 125 Willowdale Pl., Winnipeg 16, Man. (res); Odessa (Ukraine) '39; D.A.; Anaes; Staff, St. Boniface Hosp.; Tel. WH 3-0311.

LOEWEN, William; Box 908, Altona, Man., Man '58; MCGP; Med. Staff, Altona Hosp.; Dist. Rep., Manitoba Med. Assoc.; Tel. 324-5575.

LOFCHY, A. Norman; 200 Danforth Ave., Toronto 6, Ont.; Tor '54; MCGP; Active Staff, Doctors' Hosp.; Assoc. Staff, Tor. E. Gen. Hosp.; Tel. 461-0761.

LOFFT, Thomas F.; 155 College St., Toronto 2B, Ont.; Wes'59; Psy; School Psy., Toronto Board of Education, Child Adjustment Service; Tel. 362-4931, Ext. 410.

LOFTHOUSE, Robert N.; McGregor Clinic, 250 Main St. E., Hamilton, Ont.; 60 St. Clair Ave. (res); Tor '43; FRCS(C), GenSurg; OrthSurg; Chief, OrthSurg., & Chm., Med. Staff Advisory Committee, Hamilton Gen. Hosp.; Staff, Chedoke Gen. & Children's Hosp's.; Sec.-Treas., Cdn. Orth. Assoc.; Tel. JA 7-2711.

LOFTUS, Louis J.; Wes '29; Admin. Staff, Med. Serv., Dept. of National Health & Welfare, 816 Government St., Victoria, B.C.; Tel. EV 6-2488.

LOGAN, Herbert L. (Mons Medal); 28 Crescent Dr., Sussex, N.B. (res); McG '23; D.P.H. (Tor.), F.A.P.H.; Retired.

LOGAN, Jane E.; (See SCHUNK, Jane E.).

LOGAN, Lawther; Ste. 201, Med. Arts Bldg., 6th Ave. & 3rd St. W., Calgary, Alta.; 4716 Britania Dr. (res); McG'46; MRCP(Ed.); FCCP; FACC; FICA; FACP; FRCP(C); IntMed; Dir., Alberta Heart Fdn.; Cons. Staff, Alberta Children's Gen. & Holy Cross Hosp's.; Tel. 266-1313.

LOGAN, R. I.; 713 Columbia St., New Westminster, B.C.; 725 Royal Ave. (res); Man '45; Anaes; Tel. LA 2-4241.

LOGEL, Robert; 99 Tyndal Ave., Toronto 3, Ont. (res); Munich (Germ.) '38; M.O., Workmen's Comp. Bd., Rehab. Centre, Downsview.

LOGIE, Frank A.; Avenue Bldg., 220-3rd Ave. S., Saskatoon, Sask.; Birmingham (Eng.) '49; M.B., Ch.R.; MRCS (Eng.); LRCP (Lond.); Tel. 652-0300.

LOGIER, Paul E.; 134 Mayrand, St. Jean, P.Q.; 132 Mayrand (res); Mon '52; Staff, Hop. de St. Jean.

LOGOTHETOPOULOS, J.; Ass't. Prof., Banting & Best Dept. of Med. Research, U. of Toronto, Toronto, Ont.

LOGUINOFF, Gerry B.; Rosemont Med. Centre, 5062-4th Ave., Regina, Sask.; 100 Donahue Ave. (res); Aurora U. of (Shanghai, China) '44; Tel. JO 9-6097.

LOH, George; 802 E. Hastings St., Vancouver 4, B.C.; Dal '58; Tel. 254-2622.

LOHRENZ, John G.; 517 Pine Ave. W., Montreal 2, P.Q.; Man'49; D.Psy(McG); Psy; Assoc. Psy., Royal Victoria Hosp.; Dir., University Health Service & Ass't. Prof., Dept. of Psy., McGill University; Tel. V-4-6311, Ext. 585.

LOIGNON, Gaston; 370 Lethbridge, Ville Mt. Royal, P.Q. (res); Mon '23; Psy; Med. Supt., Hop. St.Jean de Dieu, Gamelin & Hop. Mt. Providence, Montreal; Tel. CL 4-5361.

LOISEL, Rejean; Lav'64; Res., Hop. Hotel-Dieu, Montreal 18, P.Q.

LOISELLE, Guy; 565 Commerciale, La Tuque, P.Q.; 19 Laviolette (res); Mon '56; FRCP(C), IntMed (Cardiol.) (P.Q.); Chief, Dept. of Med., Hop. St. Joseph; Tel. 523-5300.

LOISELLE, Jean M.; 3028 William Stuart St., Ste. Foy, Quebec 10, P.Q. (res); Lav'51; Med. BioChem (P.Q.); Ph.D. (Sc., McG); Cons. (Biochem.), Hop.-Hotel-Dieu; Ass't. Prof. (Biochem.), U. of Laval.

LOKEN, John D.; Med. Arts Clinic, 2125-11th Ave., Regina, Sask.; Sask'65.

LOMAX, Walter W.; Carruthers Clinic, 137 Wellington St., Sarnia, Ont.; 889 Hollands Ave. (res); Qns'51; ObstGyn; Active Cons. Staff, Sarnia Gen. & St. Joseph's Hosp's.; Tel. DI 4-5261.

LOME, Lillian T. (Kormolska); 901 O'Connor Dr., Toronto 16, Ont.; Tor'41; MCGP; O.P.D. Staff, Women's College Hosp.; Tel. PL 5-8281.

LOMMERSE, Peter G.; Box 89, Dunrea, Man.; Guy's Hosp. (London, Eng.) '49; LRCP, LRCS, DPH; DIH; Med. Dir. Northern Health Serv.; Tel. Minto 301-11.

LONE, Frank J.; 35 South High St., Port Arthur, Ont. (res); Man '45; F.R.C.P.(C), Path; Dir. of Labs, St. Joseph's Gen. & Port Arthur Gen. Hosp's.; Cons. (Path.), Geraldton Mem Hosp. & Port Arthur Clinic; Tel. DI 4-2431 & 344-6621.

LONEY, Elgin M.; Box 99, Langton, Ont.; Tor '48; Med. Staff, Tillsonburg Dist. Mem. Hosp.; Tel. 875-4484.

LONEY, E. E. Milton; 2969 Kingston Rd., Scarborough, Ont.; Apt. 3, 29 Cliffside Dr. (res); Tor '57; MCGP; Tel. 261-1961.

LONG, George S., Workmen's Comp. Bd., Prov. Bd., Edmonton, Alta.; 11822-91stAve. (res); Alb '33.

LONG, J. Edwin; 2276 Queen St. E., Toronto 13, Ont.; 87 Silverbirch Ave. (res); Tor '31; Tel. OX 1-7128.

LONG, Leopold A.; 3742 Ave. Lacombe, Montreal 26, P.Q. (res); Mon '45; L.Sc., M.Sc., IntMed (P.Q.); Clin. Path. (P.Q.); Chief (Haematol.), Hop. Hotel Dieu; Ass't. Prof. (Med.), U. of Montreal; Tel. VI 4-0161.

LONG, Richard; 23—21e Ave., Edmunston, N.B.; Lav '60; Urol; Abroad.

LONG, Richard C.; 1374 Sherbrooke St. W., Montreal, P.Q.; 120 Strathcona Dr., Mount Royal (res); McG '40; F.R.C.S.(C), F.A.C.S., D.A.-B.S., GenSurg.; Ass't. Surg., Royal Victoria Hosp.; Cons. Surg., Queen Mary's Veteran Hosp.; Assoc. Prof., McGill U.; Tel. AV 8-0586.

LONGDEN, Douglas E.; Cambridge (Eng.) '55; M.R.C.S. (Eng.), L.R.C.P. (Lond.), D.P.M. (Eng.); Exec. Dir., South Shore Mental Health Centre, Box 1173, Bridgewater, N.S.; Tel. 543-4411.

LONGFIELD, G. Maxwell; 4 Alderway Ave., Brampton, Ont. (res); Wes '45; D.A.B.P.; FACP; Pathol., Peel Mem. Hosp., Dufferin Area Hosp., Orangeville; Reg. Pathol., Peel & Dufferin Co's., Attn'y-Gen. Dept.; Tel. GL 1-1710 & 941-2410.

LONGFORD, U. Dazell; McBirnie-Cleland Clinic, 218 Catherine St., Port Colborne, Ont.; Dublin (Ire.)'53.

LONGINOTTO, Michael B.; 210 Rideau Medical Bldg., 1711-4th St. S.W.,, Calgary, Alta.; London (Eng.) '40; MRCS; LRCP; DOMS (London); Ophth; Otol; Staff, Calgary Gen. & Holy Cross Hosp's.; Tel. AM 2-9243.

LONGLEY, J. Donald; Fairmont Med. Bldg., 750 W. Broadway, Vancouver 9, B.C.; McG '52; DiagRad; Ass't. Rad., Vancouver Gen. Hosp.; Clin. Instr., U. of British Columbia; Tel. TR 9-4177.

LONGLEY, Joy C.; Fairmont Med. Bldg., 750 W. Broadway, Vancouver 9, B.C.; UBC '60; Fell. Paed.; U. of British Columbia; M.O.H., Burnaby; Tel. TR 9-4177.

LONGMORE, Allan J.; 648 King St. W., Kitchener, Ont.; 784 Dunbar Rd. (res); Tor'41; FRCP(C); IntMed; Chief, Dept. of Med. & Staff, Kitchener-Waterloo Hosp.; Staff, St. Mary's Gen. Hosp.; Tel. 744-8911.

LONGMORE, Robert D.; 260 Cedar St., Sudbury, Ont.; 1925 Miller Cres. (res); Tor '53; Chief (GP), Sudbury Gen. Hosp.; Tel. 673-3695.

LONGO, Anthony J.; 1762 Danforth Ave., Toronto, Ont.; 1762 Danforth Ave. (res); Tor '45; Tel HO 1-3221.

LONGO, Thomas N.; 26 Queen St. S., Thorold, Ont.; Tor'55; Staff, Hotel-Dieu Hosp., St. Catharines Gen. Hosp.; Tel. CA 7-4117.

LONGPRE, Bernard; Ediface Central, 31 King St. W., Sherbrooke, P.Q.; Mon '55; Haem (P.Q.); IntMed; Tel. 569-6266.

LONGPRE, Daniel; 5592 Queen Mary Rd., Hampstead, Montreal 29, P.Q. (res); Lav '19; FRCP (C); Paed; Hon. Cons. (Paed.), Hop. St-Luc; Tel. 272-9016.

LONGPRE, Leo F., 718-750 W. Broadway, Vancouver 9, B.C.; Man '46; Urol.

LONGRIDGE, David M. N.; 1029 Douglas St., Victoria, B.C.; 1220 Transit Rd. (res); Cambridge (Eng.) '40; M.R.C.S. (Eng.), L.R.C.P. (Lond.), F.R.C.S.(Ed.), GenSurg; Active Staff (Surg.), Royal Jubilee Hosp.; Assoc. Staff (Surg.), St. Joseph's Hosp.; Tel. EV 2-3456.

LONGTIN, Jean; 3440 est, Ontario, Montreal 4, P.Q.; Mon '44; Pulm. Dis & T.B. (P.Q.); Cardiol (P.Q.); IntMed; Staff, St. Joseph's Hosp.; Tel. 534-9531.

LONGTIN, Leon; 45 Hazelwood, Outremont, P.Q. (res); Mon '35; F.R.C.P.(C) **Anaes; Ass't Anaes.,** Hotel Dieu, Montreal; **Dir. (Anaes.), Hop. San., Rosemont; Assoc. Prof. (Anaes.), U. of Montreal; Tel. VI 4-0161.**

LONGTIN, Marcel; Ste. 205, 3875, rue St. Urbain, Montreal 18, P.Q.; Mon '41; **D&TRad; Hd., Dept.** of DiagRad., Hop. Hotel-Dieu; Assoc. Prof. (Rad.), U. of Montreal; Tel. 844-3418.

LONGTIN, Pierre; Mon '64; Res., Hop. Ste-Justine, Montreal, P.Q.

LONTOK, Rodolfo M.; Manila (Philipp.)'48; Staff, Dept. of Rad., Swift Current Union Hosp., Swift Current, Sask.

LOO, Laine (Mathiesen); 2398 W. 34th Ave., Vancouver 13, B.C.; **Tartu (Estonia) '44; Tel.** AM 6-0800.

LOOMIS, Gordon B.; 444 Dufferin Ave., Sherbrooke, P.Q.; McG '34; GenSurg; Staff, Sherbrooke Gen. Hosp.; Tel. LO 9-3661.

LOOS, A. J. Ruddy; Oshawa Clinic, 117 King St. E., Oshawa, Ont.; Tor'36; DABR; DiagRad; Radiol., Oshawa Clinic, Oshawa Gen. Hosp. & Mem. Hosp., Bowmanville; Rad., General Motors of Canada; Tel. 723-2211.

LOPEZ, Basilio; 138 Prowse Ave., St. John's, Nfld. (res); Madrid (Spain) '52; Cons. PhysMed., Dept. of Public Health.

LOPEZ, Jeronimo; Brandon Clinic, 620 Dennis St., Brandon, Man.; Madrid (Spain)'49.

LOPEZ, Jose F.; University Hosp., Saskatoon, Sask.; Seville (Spain)'55; IntMed; Assoc. Dir., CardioPulm. Lab., University Hosp.; Assoc., Med. Research Council of Canada; Ass't. Prof. of Med., University of Saskatchewan; Tel. 652-8821, Ext. 233.

LOPEZ-PEREZ, Jeronimo; Box 1078, The Pas, Man.; Madrid (Spain) '49.

LORANGE, Gilles C.; 1681 est Rachel, Montreal 34, P.Q.; 5125 Charlemagne (res); Mon '51; FCCP; Pulm Dis. & T.B. (P.Q.); IntMed (P.Q.); Ass't. (Med.) & I/C Resp. Physiol. Lab., Hop.-Notre-Dame; Ass't. Prof. (Med.), U. of Montreal; Tel. LA 6-5909.

LORANT, Denis; 97 Manuel Dr., Dollard Des Ormeaux, P.Q.; Budapest (Hung.)'51; Paed (P.Q.); Med. Staff (Paed), Lachine Gen. Hosp., Lachine, P.Q.; Tel. 684-2863.

LORD, Julien; Lav'63; Res., Hop. Notre-Dame, Montreal, P.Q.

LOREE, Luke A.; 360 Woolwich St., Guelph, Ont.; Tor '31; M.C.G.P.

LOREN, Philip; 454 Midland Ave., Scarboro, Ont.; Tor'46; MCGP; Staff, Doctor's Hosp.; **Tel. 267-2181.**

LORENZ, Mervin A.; 8330 Fairmont Dr., Calgary, Alta.; Alb '60; MCGP; Tel. 252-1161.

LORENZEN, David I.; Ste. 6, Pen Centre, Glendale W., St. Catharines, Ont.; Tor'62; Active Staff, Hotel Dieu Hosp.; Assoc. Staff, St. Catharines Gen. Hosp.; Tel. 682-4271.

LORENZETTI, Dario; McG'60; FRCS(C), Ophth; Staff, Montreal Gen. Hosp., Montreal, P.Q.; Abroad.

LORIMER, Alan; Provincial Labs., Castle St., Saint John, N.B.; Aberdeen (Scot.) '49; M.B., Ch. B.; M.C. (Path); Path; Pathol., Prov. Labs., Saint John; Tel. 692-2644.

LORIMER, Donald G.; 64 Queen St., St. Catharines, Ont.; Tor '63.

LORIMER, William R.; Ste. 322, 200 St. Clair Ave. W., Toronto 7, Ont.; Tor'57; FRCP(C); D.A.(Tor.); Anaes; Staff, Wellesley Hosp.

LORINC, Janos; 118 St. Leonard's Ave., Toronto 12, Ont.; Budapest (Hung.) '50; Path; Ass't. Path., Central Labs.; Tel. EM 3-1211.

LORRAIN, Jacques; 12,190 Poutrincourt, Montreal, P.Q.; Mon '59; FRCS(C), Obst-Gyn; Staff, Hop. Sacre-Coeur; Tel. FE 4-1210.

LORRAIN, Jean; Ste. Rose de Lima, P.Q.; Lav '40; Dist. Coroner.

LORTIE, Bruno C.; 364 Joseph, St. Raymond, Co. Portneuf, P.Q.; Lav '34.

LORTIE, Edouard; 6531 rue Molson, Montreal, P.Q.; Mon '43; Anaes; Staff (Anaes.), Hop. Ste. **Justine; Tel. RE 1-4931.**

LORTIE, Gilles; 4207 Jean Brillant, Montreal 26, P.Q.; Mon '54; Psy(P.Q.); Dir., O.P.D., Inst. Albert Prevost; Ass't. Prof. (Psy.), U. of Montreal; Tel. 731-4013.

LORTIE, Marcel; 2157 est rue Fleury, Montreal 12, P.Q.; **Lav'65.**

LOSIER, E. Barry; 173 Wellington St., Chatham, N.B.; Ott'51.

LOSIER, Percy J.; Lobban Ave., Chatham, New Brunswick; Tor'35; D.P.H.; PH; MCGP; Tel. 3-3456.

LOSSING, Edward H.; 3203 Riverside Dr., Billings Bridge, Ottawa, Ont.; Qns'30; MPH; Dir.-General, Health Ins. & Resources, Dept. of National Health & Welfare; Tel. CE 2-8211.

LOTIMER, Leonard E.; 613 Med. Arts Bldg., 1 Young St., Hamilton, Ont.; Tor '37; DRCOG; MRCOG; FRCOG; FRCS(C); ObstGyn; Staff, Dept. of ObstGyn., Hamilton Civic Hosp.; Tel. JA 9-3511.

LOTT, Gordon G.; Ste. 106, 1175 Cook St., Victoria, B.C.; McG'53; FRCS(C), GenSurg.

LOTTO, Wallace N.; 101 Toronto Western Med. Bldg., 25 Leonard Ave., Toronto 2B, Ont.; 62 St. Andrews Gdns., Tor. 5 (res); Tor'47; FRCS (C); FACS; GenSurg; OrthSurg; Staff & Hd. (Orth-Surg.), Toronto Western Hosp.; Ass't. Prof. (Surg.), U. of Toronto; Tel. EM 6-1381.

LOU, Peter; Aurora (Shanghai, China) '41; GenSurg; Staff, Hop. Hotel Dieu, Dolbeau, P.Q.; Tel. 276-1420.

LOU WU; 802 Chanoine Scott S, Quebec 10, PQ.; Aurora U. (Shanghai, China) '41; FACS, FRCS(C), GenSurg; Surg., Hop. Laval & Inst.-de-Cardiol-de-Quebec; Ass't. Prof. Laval U., Tel. 653-4931.

LOUCH, Robert E.; Wes'62; Res., Toronto Western Hosp., Toronto 2B, Ont.

LOUDEN, C. Gordon; 2286 Carling Ave., Ottawa 14, Ont.; Qns '49; Tel. 722-3511.

LOUDON, Esther D. H.; 254 Sherbourne St., Toronto 2, Ont.; Tor '21; Gyn; Hon. Staff, **Women's College Hosp.; Tel. 921-4870.**

LOUDON, James L.; Victoria Hosp., London, Ont.; Tor'55; FRCP(C); IntMed; Ass't. Dir. (Med.), Victoria Hosp.; Med. Cons., Westminster Hosp.; Clin. Instr. (Med.), University of Western Ontario; Tel. 432-5261.

LOUDOUN, James R.; 185A Woolwich St., Guelph, Ont.; Qns '42; MCGP; Med. Staff, Guelph Gen. & St. Joseph's Hosp's.; Med. Advisory, Fed. Wire Div. of H. K. Porter Co. & Armco Drainage Co.; Tel. TA 2-0570.

LOUGH, John O.; 4678 Hingston Ave., Montreal 28, P.Q.; McG'57; **FRCP(C), Path; Lect., Dept. of Path., McGill University.**

LOUGHEED, Gladstone W., MC, ED; 289 Forest Hill Rd., Toronto 7, Ont. (res); Tor '13; F.R.-C.P.(C), IntMed; Path,Bact; Med. Dir., Confederation Life Assoc., Toronto; Tel. 924-6868.

LOUGHEED, Jeva U. R. (Rogers); 561 Broadview Ave., Toronto 6, Ont.; Tor '45; Anaes; Staff, Dept. of Anaes., Women's College Hosp.; Tel. HO 5-7194.

LOUGHEED, Lawrence E.; Ste. 508, 625-5th Ave., **New Westminster, B.C.; 6588 Lambert Cres., R.R. 1, N. Surrey (res); Man '51; FRCS(C); NeurSurg; Chief of NeurSurg., Royal Columbian Hosp.; Tel. LA 2-9808.**

LOUGHEED, Marvin N.; 3550 Cote des Neiges Rd., Ste. 170, Montreal P.Q.; McG'47; FRCP(C); D&TRad; Rad., Montreal Gen. & Children's Hosp's.; Ass't. Prof. (Rad.), McGill U.; Tel. 937-9334.

LOUGHEED, Morley S.; City Hall, Winnipeg, Man.; 169 Lanark St. (res); Man '17; D.P.H.; M.H.O., Winnipeg; Retired.

LOUGHEED, William M.; 430 Med. Arts Bldg., 170 St. George St., Toronto 5, Ont.; 67 Ridge Dr. (res); Tor '47; FRCS(C); NeurSurg; Chief NeurSurg., Sunnybrook Hosp.; Surg. (Div. of NeurSurg.), Toronto Gen. Hosp.; Cons. Staff, Toronto East Gen. Hosp. & Wellesley Hosp.; Assoc. Surg., U. of Toronto; Tel. 925-7081.

LOUGHLIN, Edward I.; 446 Queen's Ave., London, Ont.; Wes '20; ObstGyn; Instr. (Obst. Gyn.), U. of Western Ontario; Staff, St. Joseph's & Victoria Hosp's.; Tel. 439-3271.

LOUGHLIN, Hubert J.; 289 Dufferin Ave., London, Ont.; 340 St. James (res); Wes '30; Paed; Lect. (Paed.), U. of Western Ontario; Staff, (Paed.), **Victoria, Children's & St. Joseph's** Hosp's.; Tel. 434-4142.

LOUGHREY, Robert S.; 13 Garden St., Brockville, Ont.; 123 James St. E. (res); Queen's U. (Belfast, N. Ire.) '53; MCGP; Active Staff, Brockville Gen. & St.- Vincent-de-Paul Hosp's.; Tel. DI 2-7666.

LOUGHREY, Theohane; 201 Med. Centre, 8th Ave & 8th St. S.W., Calgary, Alta.; '61.

LOUIE, Norman V., F/L; R.C.S.M.E., Chilliwack Stn. Hosp., Veddar Crossing, B.C.; Alb '63.

LOUIE, Richard A.; Burris Clinic, 242 Victoria St., Kamloops, B.C.; Alta'64; Tel. 372-6303.

LOUIE, William L.; 12918-127th St., Edmonton, Alta.; Alb '59; Tel. 455-1616.

LOUKRAS, Chris; 2374 Eglinton Ave. E., Toronto, Ont.; 25 Wigmore Dr. (res); Tor '56; Staff, Scarboro Gen. & Toronto E. Gen. Hosp.; Tel. PL 7-3217.

LOUNDER, James H., Major; 1 CBMU, Cdn. Forces, Europe; Dal'54; FRCP(C), Anaes; Staff, British Mil. Hosp., Iserlohn, W. Germany; Abroad.

LOUNGNARATH, Vilaysoun; Mon'62; FRCS(C), GenSurg; Staff, Hop. Jean Talon, Montreal 36, P.Q.

LOUTTIT, Ronald T.; Box 460, Kinistino, Sask.; Edinburgh (Scot.)'42; FRCS(Ed.).

LOVATT, George E.; 289 Dufferin Ave., London, Ont.; 329 Victoria St. (res); London (Eng.) '54; B.Sc. (Physiol., Lond.); MRCS; LRCP; DRCOG; IntMed; Cons., Westminster DVA Hosp. & Ont. Hosp.; Active Staff, St. Joseph's Hosp.; Lect., University of Western Ont.; Tel. GE 8-8831.

LOVE, Edgar J.; 319 Westminster Ave., Apt. 2, London, Ont.; Wes '56; ObstGyn; Staff, Victoria Hosp.; Tel. 434-3588.

LOVE, James W.; 108 Medical Arts Bldg., Calgary, Alta.; 4516 Britannia Dr. (res); Alb '42; Active Memb. Calgary Gen. & Holy Cross Hosp's.; Tel. 262-9270.

LOVE, Robert A.; C. S. Williams Clinic, 901 Helena St., Trail, B.C.; McG '50; DNBME; DABIM; IntMed; Staff, Trail-Tadenac Hosp.; Tel. 368-5211.

LOVE, William R.; 39 Charlton Ave. E., Hamilton, Ont.; 624 Edgewater Cres. Burlington (res); Qns '44; D.A.B.Ot.; Otol; Chief of ENT Serv. St. Joseph's Hosp., Hamilton & Joseph Brant Mem. Hosp., Burlington; **Staff, Hamilton Gen. Hosp.;** Tel. JA 8-5763.

LOVE, William R.; 240 Broadway St., Orangeville, Ont.; Wes'54; Staff, Dufferin Area Hosp.; Tel. 941-3950.

LOVEGROVE, Thomas D.; Westminster Hosp., London, Ont.; Wes '53; M.O., Dept. of Vet's. Affairs; Instr. (Pharm.), U. of Western Ont.

LOVEGROVE, William M.; 4027 E. Hastings St., **North Burnaby, B.C.; Wes '42; Tel. CY 9-2677.**

LOVELL, Barry A.; London (Eng.) '55; DRCOG; Staff, Riverdale Hosp., Rivers, Man.; Tel. 328-5305.

LOVELL, Dorcas M. (Beaton); 104 Celina St., Oshawa, Ont.; **55 Connaught St. (res); Tor '46.**

LOVERING, John H. D.; 2009 Danforth Ave., Toronto 6, Ont.; 14 Fleming Cres. (res); Tor '44; **Dist. Coroner; Tel. OX 8-5565.**

LOVETT-DOUST, John W.; Clarke Inst. of Psy., 250 College St., Toronto, Ont.; 338 Steeles Ave. E., R.R. 1, Thornhill (res); London (Eng.)'42; LRCP (Lond.); MRCS (Eng.); MRCP (Lond); AKC; FRCP(C); Psy; Sr. Psy. & Hd., Dept. of Physiol., Clarke Inst. of Psy.; Hon. Cons., & Dir., Research Unit, Ontario Hosp.; Hon. Cons., North York Branson Hosp.; Prof. (Psy.), U. of Toronto; Cons. Psy. Research, Ontario Dept. of Health; Vis. Lect. (Psy.), U. of South Carolina; Tel. 924-6811, Ext. 462.

LOVEYS, N. Craig; 207 Le Marchant Rd., St. John's, Nfld.; Tor'50; Tel. 579-2213.

LOW, Donald M.; Medical Arts Bldg., Toronto, Ont.; 97 Hudson Dr. (res); Tor '18; F.R.C.O.G., F.R.C.S.(C), ObstGyn; Cons. (ObstGyn.), Toronto Gen. Hosp.; Grad. Lect., U. of Toronto; Tel. WA 2-6007; Retired.

LOW, Eugene W.; Edinburgh (Scot.)'31; DPH; Staff, Saskatoon Sanatorium, Saskatoon, Sask.

LOW, George A.; 3000 Lawrence Ave. E., Scarborough, Ont.; 8 Landfair Cres. (res); Tor '46; IntMed; FRCP(C); Sr. Att'd. Phys., Scarborough Gen. Hosp.; Tel. 291-0241.

LOW, James A.; Tor '49; FRCS(C), ObstGyn; Staff, Dept. of ObstGyn., Kingston Gen. Hosp., Kingston, Ont.; Tel. 542-8642.

LOW, John S.; 20 Church Ave., Raymond, Alta.; Alta'59; Tel. 752-3067.

LOW, Ronald W., S/L; R.C.A.F. Station, Gimli, Man.; St. Andrews (Scot.) '52.

LOWDEN, Arnold G.; 383 Ellis St., Penticton, B.C.; Tor'51; DPH; MCGP.

LOWDEN, J. Alexander; Tor '57 Ph.D. (Biochem.) Res.; Hosp. for Sick Children, Toronto, Ont.

LOWE, Anne C.; George St., Durham, Ont.; Queen's U. (Belfast, Ire.)'56; Staff, Durham Mem. Hosp.; Tel. 369-2510.

LOWE, Frank C.; 1241-100th St. N. Battleford, Sask.; 1432-98th St. (res); Shanghai (China) '43; MCGP; Tel. 445-2714.

LOWE, Thomas; 210 Hammond Bldg., Moose Jaw, Sask.; 1304 Grace St. (res.); Dublin (Ire) '52; Staff, Moose Jaw Union and Providence Hosp's.; Tel. 692-1814.

LOWENSTEIN, Louis; Royal Victoria Hosp., Montreal, P.Q.; 631 Victoria Ave., Westmount (res); Vanderbilt U. (Nashville, Tenn.) '33; Haem (P.Q.); A.B.I.M., F.A.C.P., F.S.I.H., F.I.S.A., IntMed; Haematologist-in-Chief & Assoc. Phys. Dept. of Med., Royal Victoria Hosp.; Assoc. Prof. (Med.), McGill U.; Tel. VI 2-1251.

LOWER, Alfred H.; 1408 Brown St., Fort William, Ont.; Qns'54; Tel. 623-7378.

LOWES, John N.; 73 Centre St., Oshawa, Ont.; Tor'61.

LOWI, R. Naomi (Paltiel); Food & Drug Directorate, Dept. of National Health & Welfare, Ottawa, Ont.; McG'51; M.Sc. (Exp. Med.).

LOWINGS, Keith L.; Roy Clinic 715 2nd Ave. S., Lethbridge, Alta.; 1402-20th St. (res); **Guy's (London, Eng.) '54; M.R.C.S., L.R.C.P., M.B.-B.S.; Staff, Lethbridge Mun. & St. Michael's** Hosp's.; Tel. 327-3134.

LOWREY, Arthur V.; St. Davids, Ont.; Tor '36.

LOWREY, H. Evans D.; 357 Ferguson St., North Bay, Ont.; 630 Jane St. (res); Tor '26; FACS; GenSurg; Active & Cons. Staff (Surg.), St.- Joseph's & Civic Hosp's.; Retired.

LOWREY, Stanley R.; 914 Medical Arts Bldg., 170 St. George St., Toronto, Ont.; 212 Hillhurst Blvd.; Tor '32; Urol.; **Assoc. (Surg.), U. of Toronto.; Tel. WA 3-9861.**

LOWRIE, Howard A.; 4 Humewood Dr., Toronto 10, Ont.; Tor '20; Tel. LE 3-1220.

LOWRY, Curtis H.; Sawyerville, P.Q.; Lav '48; M.C.G.P.

LOWRY, R. Brian; 715 W. 12th Ave., Vancouver 9, B.C.; Queens U. (Belfast, Ire.) '56; DCH; FRCP(C), Paed; Attend. Staff, Vancouver Gen. Hosp.; Med. Cons., Provincial Health Branch; Registry for Handicapped Children; Instr. (Paed.), U. of British Columbia; Tel. TR 6-3211.

LOWSON, Colin; Estevan Med. Associates, 1314 3rd St., Estevan, Sask.; London (Eng.)'54; MRCS; LRCP; Tel. 634-2676.

LOWTHER, Glen H; Box 1190, Portage la Prairie, Man. (res); Glasgow (Scot.)'49; Med. Supt., Manitoba School for Retardates, Portage La Prairie, Man.

LOWY, Frederic H.; McG'59; Psy; Clin. Ass't., Allan Mem. Inst., 1025 Pine Ave. W., Montreal, P.Q.; Tel. 842-1251.

LOYNES, James S.; 274 Charles St. Belleville, Ont.; 219 Foster Ave. (res); Qns '44—M.Sc. (Pharm.); Staff, Belleville Gen., Trenton, Campbellford & Picton Hosp's.; Lect. (Med.), Queen's U., Kingston; Tel. WO 8-8888.

LOZINSKI, Ezra; 255 Ellendale Med. Bldg., 5845 Cote-des-Neiges Rd., Montreal 26, P.Q.; 4300 Western Ave. Apt. 610, Mtl. 6 (res); McG '20; M.Sc.; IntMed; Hon. Att'd. Phys., Jewish Gen. Hosp.; Med. Dir., Charles E. Frosst & Co.; Tel. 731-6978.

LU, Frank C.; 76 Leopold Dr., Ottawa 10, Ont. (res); Cheeloo U. (China) '39; Hd., Pharm. & Toxicol. Sect., Food & Drug Directorate, Dept. of National Health & Welfare; Tel. 992-4334.

LU, Kui L.; Russell Clinic, Russell, Man.; Santo Tomas (Manilla, Phillipines) '57.

LU, Lawrence C-T; 2820 W. 39th Ave., Vancouver 1, B.C.; Taiwan (Formosa)'56; Path.

LUBINSKI, G. A.; M.B., B.S., M.Sc. (Kiev, U.S.S.R.); Ph.D. (McGill); Ass't. Prof. (Zoology), U. of Manitoba, Winnipeg, Man.; Tel. GR 4-9110.

LUBINSKI, Herbert H.; 560 Glengarry St., Town of Mt. Royal, P.Q. (res); Breslau (Germ.) '17; Bact; Prof. Emer.; Bact. & Chief of Transfusion Serv., Jewish Gen. Hosp., Montreal; Tel. RE 8-3019.

LUBORSKY, Benjamin; 1980 Ottawa St., Windsor, Ont.; 3408 Church St. (res); Tor '36; M.C.-G.P.; **Chief, Dept. of ObstGyn., Grace Hosp.; Tel. 254-2288.**

LUCAS, Gordon R.; 326 S. Syndicate Ave., Fort William, Ont.; 611 Hyde Pk. (res); Man '44; Tel. 24272.

LUCAS, Jan P.; 11 Laxton Ave., Toronto 3, Ont.; '60.

LUCAS, Oscar C.; Medical Arts Bldg., 1105 Pandora Ave., Victoria, B.C.; 5024 Echo Dr. (res); **Pennsylvania '33; Tel. EV 2-3322.**

LUCAS, Sydney I.; 114 West St., Waterford, Ont.; Wes '51; MCGP; Staff, Norfolk Gen. Hosp.; Tel. 443-5333.

LUCCIOLI, Giuliano M.; Italy '55; Res., Royal Victoria Hosp., Montreal 2, P.Q.

LUCE, Anna L.; 249 Halls Mill Rd., London, Ont.; Wes'63.

LUCIANI, Donato; Tor '49; Psy; Staff, Childrens Psych Inst., London, Ont.

LUCIS, Ojars J.; Pathology Inst., Halifax, N.S.; McG'61; M.Sc. (Invest. Med.); Ph.D.; Ass't. Pathol., Dept. of Public Health, Province of N.S.; Ass't. Prof. (Path.), Dalhousie University; Tel. 422-9661.

LUCK, Donald E. R.; Skeena Health Unit, 333-5th St., Prince Rupert, B.C.; West Indies '50; DPH; PH; Dir., Skeena Health Unit; Tel. 624-6735.

LUCKE, Hans H.; Frankfurt (Germ.) '36; Path; Staff, Mountain Sanatorium, Hamilton, Ont.

LUCY, John D.; Manitoba Clinic, 790 Sherbrook St., Winnipeg 2, Man.; 671 Waterloo St., Wpg. 9 (res); London (Eng.) '45; MRCS(Eng.), DPM (Lond.); Psy; Staff, Misericordia Gen. & Wpg. Gen. Hosp's.; Lect. (Psy), U. of Manitoba; Tel. SP 4-6541.

LUDWIG, Bernard L.; 99 Avenue Rd., Toronto 5, Ont.; 25 Gardiner Rd., Forest Hill (res); Tor '45; ObstGyn; Staff, New Mt. Sinai Hosp.; Tel. WA 4-2553.

LUDWIG, Joseph A.; 313 Boyd Bldg., 384 Portage Ave., Winnipeg, Man.; 125 Scotia St. (res); London (Eng.) '48; DDS; M.S., FICS; Staff, St.- Boniface & Victoria Hosp's.; Tel. WH 3-1746.

LUGSDIN, Gordon H.; 106 Paris Rd., Brantford, Ont.; Tor '36; D.Psy (Tor); Psy; Dir. of Psy., Brantford Gen. Hosp.; Tel. 752-6878.

LUGSDIN, James G.; 1590 Bellevue Ave., West Vancouver, B.C.; Qns'65.

LUHOVYJ, Ihor R.; Mon'64; Sr. Asst. Res., Royal Victoria Hosp., Montreal, P.Q.

LUKAS, Martha (Kerpel); 9017-16th Ave., North Battleford, Sask.; Budapest (Hung.) '52; **Radiol. (Hung.); Tel. 445-2411.**

LUKAS, William J.; 9017-16th Ave., North Battleford, Sask. (res); Budapest (Hung.) '52; D&T Rad; Hd. Dept. of Radiol., Notre Dame Hosp.; Tel. 445-2411.

LUKE, Josephus C.; Lakeshore Gen. Hosp., Pointe Claire, P.Q.; McG '31; FRCS (Eng.); FRCS(C); FACS; GenSurg; Surg-in-Chief & Chmn., Med. Bd., Lakeshore Gen. Hosp.; Surg., Royal Victoria Hosp.; Assoc. Prof. (Surg.), McGill U.; Tel. 695-1310.

LUKE, William R. F.; 316 Medical Arts Bldg., 170 St. George St., Toronto 5, Ont.; 31 Errington Ave. (res); Tor '23; Ophth; Sr. Ophth., Toronto Gen. Hosp.; Inst., U. of Toronto; Tel. WA 3-2114.

LUKEMAN, Richard; Box 430, Noranda, P Q.; Man'56; GenSurg; Staff, Youville Hosp.; Tel. RO 2-0711.

LUKENCHUK, John J.; Medical Centre, Box 279, Vegreville, Alta.; UBC '55; MCGP; Tel. 632-2822.

LUKOWSKI, Maria; 90 Castleknock Rd., Toronto 12, Ont.; Lwow (Poland) '41; Anaes; Staff, Doctor's Hosp.; Tel. WA 3-5411.

LUKSS, Linard; 277 Scarboro Cres., Scarborough, Ont.; Tor'65; Staff, New Mt. Sinai Hosp.; Tel. 261-7211.

LUMB, S. S.; Bancroft, Ont.; Qns '20.

LUMSDEN, Walter F.; 66 Broadway, Toronto 12, Ont.; Tor'42; FACS; FRCS(C), GenSurg; Tel. 485-7896.

LUNA, Salvador P.; Philippines'59; FRCP(C), IntMed; Staff, Dept. of Card., Ottawa Civic Hosp., Ottawa, Ont.

LUNAM, J. B.; Box 1419, Courtenay, B.C.; **McG '40; M.C.G.P.**

LUNAN, Maxwell D.; 2401 Bloor St. W., Toronto 9, Ont.; 19 Riverside Trail, Swansea (res); Tor '41; Otol; Active Staff, St. Joseph's, Queensway & Northwestern Gen. Hosp's.; Tel. RO 7-3171.

LUND, George E.; 105½ Carmarthen St., Saint John, N.B.; 66 Coburg St. (res); Dal '56; MCGP; Tel. 693-7482.

LUNDE, Finn; Norway '52; Res., Montreal Gen. Hosp., Montreal, P.Q.

LUNDELL, Frederick W.; Ste. 1019, Med. Arts Bldg., 1538 Sherbrooke St. W., Montreal 25, P.Q.; 389 Devon Ave., Twn. of Mt. Royal (res); McG'51; D. Psy; Psy; Dir. Psy. Research & Cons., DVA, St. Annes Hosp. & Assoc. Psy., Queen Mary Vet's Hosp.; Dir. Mental Assess. & Guidance Clin. Mtl. Children's Hosp.; Ass't. Psy., Mtl. Gen Hosp.; Ass't. Prof. (Psy), McGill U.; Tel. WE 5-5939.

LUNDERVILLE, C. William P.; 178 St. George St., Toronto 5, Ont.; 27 Ruden Cres., Don Mills (res); McG '49; Anaes; Staff (Anaes), Tor. Gen. Hosp.; Clin. Instr. (Anaes), U. of Toronto; Tel. WA 3-1154.

LUNDGREN, Frederick M.; Alb '59; Res., Shaughnessy Hosp., Vancouver 9, B.C.

LUNDON, John R.; Tor'60; Research Fell., St. Michael's Hosp., Toronto 2, Ont.

LUNDQUIST, Ahti S. M.; 452 Charlotte St., Peterborough, Ont.; 878 Kawartha Dr. (res); Tor'53; Anaes.; Chief, Dept. of Anaes., Civic Hosp.; Tel. 745-2491.

LUNDY, Frank E.; Ste. 405, 209—8th Ave. S.W., Calgary Alta.; Man '37; D.A., Anaes; Cons. Anaes., Holy Cross Hosp.; Tel. 266-1531.

LUNEY, F. W.; 223 Base Line Rd., London, Ont. (res); Wes '14; DPH; PathBact; Staff, St. Joseph's Hosp.; Tel. 439-3271.

LUNN, Douglas F.; 541 Professional Bldg., 10830 Jasper Ave., Edmonton, Alta.; 14604-99th Ave. (res); London (Eng.) '53; DA (Eng.); Anaes. Active staff, Misericordia Hosp.; Tel. 422-6552.

LUNN, James, T.; 731 Renfrew St., Winnipeg 9, Man. (res); Edinburgh & Belfast (Gr. Brit.) '51; B.A.O., L.R.C.P., L.R.C.S., L.R.F.P. & S., D.M. R.D.; **Rad., Dept. of Health, Manitoba; Tel.** WH 6-7207.

LUNNEY, E. W.; 70 Elliott Row, Saint John, N.B. (res); McG '17; **Anaes; Staff, Assoc. Anaes.,** Saint John.

LUNNEY, Thomas E.; 43 Mount Pleasant, Saint John, N.B.; McG'43; DA (McGill); DABA; **Anaes; Staff & Med. Admin., Lancaster DVA** Hosp.; Tel. 694-2651.

LUPIEN, Jules E.; 11111 Frigon, Montreal 12, P.Q.; Mon '58; Anaes; Staff, Hop. Hotel-Dieu; Tel. VI 4-0161.
LUPIEN, Louis C.; 2015 Blvd., St. Paul, Trois-Rivieres, P.Q.; 60 St. Louis (res); Lav'58; Tel. 374-1247.
LUPIEN, Martial; 401 de la Salle, Grand'Mere Est, P.Q.; 455 Champlain (res); Lav '51; M.C.-G.P.
LUPIN, Alan J.; Tusket, Yarmouth Co., N.S.; London (Eng.) '59; LRCP; MRCS; Tel. 25.
LUPU, G. Harvey; Ste. 570, 6000 Cote des Neiges Rd., Montreal, P.Q.; McG '59; FRCP(C), Paed; Jr. Ass't. (Paed.), Jewish Gen. Hosp.; Clin. Ass't. (Med.), Montreal Children's Hosp.; Tel. RE 1-6366.
LUSH, Norman; 62 Cornwall Cr., St. John's, Nfld.; Dal'59; FRCP(C), Neur.
LUSK, John B. H.; 11787-8½ Ave., Haney, B.C.; 11957 Acadia Cres. (res); Trinity Coll. (Dublin, Ire.)'46; CPH(I); MCGP; Chief of Med. Staff, Maple Ridge Hosp.; Tel. 463-4162.
LUSSIER, Andre; 55 de l'Eglise, Verdun, P.Q.; Mon'59; IntMed; Tel. 766-8588.
LUSSIER, Claude; 45-48e Ave, Lachine, P.Q.; Apt. 3, 3555 Linton (res); Mon '55; GenSurg (P.Q.); Tel. 637-8681.
LUSSIER, Gisele; 1810 rue Ducharme, Mon 8, P.Q.; Mon '56; DiagRad; Staff, Hop. Notre-Dame de l'Esperance; Tel. RI 7-4771.
LUSSIER, J. Jacques; 596, Driveway, Ottawa 1, Ont.; Mon '45; Ph.D. (Camb.); FICS (Hon.); Dean, U. of Ottawa; Tel. CE 5-6751.
LUSSIER, Jules; 6428 Boul. Monk, Montreal 20, P.Q.; Mon '24; IntMed (P.Q.).
LUSSIER, Leo; 2789 1eme Ave., Quebec 3, P.Q.; Lav'40; MCGP; Tel. 524-3165.
LUSSIER, Marcel; 30 Blvd. St. Joseph E., Montreal 14, P.Q.; 5935-26th Ave., Rosemont (res); Mon '52; DABOph; FAAO; Ophth.; Tel. VI 2-3072.
LUSSIER, Robert; 522 Notre-Dame, Repentigny, P.Q.; Mon '53; M.C.G.P.
LUSSIER, Roger; 176 Church Ave., Verdun, Montreal 19, P.Q.; Mon '40; Anaes (P.Q.); Head, Dept. of Anaes., Verdun Gen. Hosp.; Tel. PO 6-3551.
LUTHE, Wolfgang; Medical Centre, 5300 Cote-des-Neiges Rd., Montreal, P.Q.; 4933 Piedmont St. (res); Hamburg (Germ.) '47; Tel. RE 1-3100.
LUTTOR, Charles; Ste. 305, 344 Bloor St. W., Toronto 5, Ont.; 533 Briar Hill Ave. (res); St. Elizabeth U. (Hung.)'42; ObstGyn; Staff (Obst-Gyn.), St. Michael's Hosp.; Clin. Instr., U. of Toronto; Tel. WA 2-4620.
LUUS, George J.; Sault Ste.- Marie & Dist. Group Health Assoc., 240 McNabb St., Sault Ste.-Marie, Ont.; Tor '62; Tel. 254-6421.
LUZOD, Ernest R.; Michel, B.C.; Manila (Philipp.)'55; Staff, Michel-Natal Dist. Hosp. & Fernie Mem. Hosp., Fernie; Tel. 425-6212.
LWAI, San; Bay Medical Clinic, Glace Bay, N.S.; Rangoon (Burma) '62. Abroad.
LYALL, W. Alan; Wes'61; Res., Clarke Inst. of Psy., 250 College St., Toronto 2B, Ont.
LYDON, M. J.; 41 Harvard Ave., Ottawa, Ont.; Nat. U. (Ire.) '49; IntMed.
LYMBURNER, Ross M.; Medical Arts Bldg., Hamilton, Ont.; 56 Chedoke Ave. (res); Tor '29; M.Sc. (Med.), F.A.C.P., IntMed; Chief of Serv., Med. Div., Hamilton Gen. Hosp.; Tel. JA 7-0271.
LYNCH, D.O.'G.; Springarden Terr. Apts., 5885 Spring Garden Rd., Halifax, N.S.; Qns'22; FAPA; Psy; Cons. Psy., Halifax County Hosp., Cole Harbour; Sr. Instr. (Psy.), Dalhousie U.; Tel. 422-2744.
LYNCH, John; National U. (Ire.) '51; DiagRad; Staff, St. Joseph's Hosp., Sarnia, Ont.; Tel. ED 6-6162.
LYNCH, John B.; 1875 Bay St., Nanaimo, B.C.; McG '38; Anaes; Staff, Nanaimo Reg. Hosp.; Tel. 758-6113.
LYNCH, John F.; R.R. 1, Dundas, Ont. (res); Liverpool (Eng.) '48; FRCP(C); Path; Dir. of Path., Henderson Gen. Hosp., Hamilton; Tel. 389-4411.
LYNCH, John G.; 109 Charlotte St., Sydney, N.S. (res); McG '08; Chief M.O., Dominion Steel & Coal Co. Ltd.; Tel. 564-5991.
LYNCH, John G.; 317 Duckworth St., St. John's, Nfld.; "Richmond," Topsail Rd. (res); McG '32; Optth. Otol; Tel. 578-2269.
LYNCH, Leo; 1570 rue St.- Hubert, Montreal, P.Q.; 11845 ave. Norwood (res); Lav '38; DPH; FCCP; MRSH; Pulm Dis. & TB (PQ); Registrar, Anti-TB League of Mtl.; Staff, Dept. of Health, Mtl.; Tel. 331-5937.
LYNCH, Matthew J.; Nat. U. (Ire.) '42; MRCP (Lond.); FCAP; FRCP(C), Path; Staff, Hosp. for Sick Children, Toronto 2, Ont.; Tel. EM 6-7242.
LYNCH, M. G.; Department of National Health & Welfare, c/o Regional Superintendent, European Region. Abroad.
LYNCH, Roland F.; 209 Rideau Med. Centre, 1711-4th St. S.W., Calgary, Alta.; Dublin (Ire.) '43; DPH; Psy; Tel. 266-3789.
LYNCH, Stephen H.; 2915B - 97th St., Edmonton, Alta.; Ott '55; Att'd. Staff, Misericordia Hosp.; Tel. GA 4-4959.
LYNCH, Theodore J.; 51 King St. E., Brockville, Ont.; 43 King St. W. (res); Tor '36; M.C.G.P.
LYNE, P. E. (See HILLOCK, Phyllis E.).
LYNES, Frank S.; 301 Medical Arts Bldg., 1 Young St., Hamilton, Ont.; Wes '58; FRCS(C), ObstGyn; Staff, St. Joseph's Hosp., Hamilton; Tel. 527-0331.
LYNES, Patrick G.; Tor'52; D.Psy; Psy; Supt., Ontario Hosp., Whitby, Ont.; Tel. 668-5881.
LYNN, R. Beverley; Etherington Hall, Queen's U., Kingston, Ont.; R.R. 1, Westbrook (res); Qns '45; F.R.S.C. (Eng.), F.R.C.S. (Edin.), F.A.C.S.; ThorSurg; Thor. & Cardiovasc, Surg., Kingston Gen. Hosp.; Cons. ThorSurg., Hotel Dieu & Kingston Mil. Hosp's.; Chief of Surg., Ongwanada San.; Prof. of Surg., Queen's U.; Hon. Cons. (Thor. & Cardiovasc. Surg.), Ont. Cancer Fdn., Kingston Clin; Tel. 546-3871.
LYNNE-DAVIES, Gerald; 9 Pleasant Ave., Kitchener, Ont.; Oxford (Eng.) '55.
LYNNE-DAVIES, Patricia; London (Eng.) '61; IntMed; Staff, U. of Alberta Hosp., Edmonton, Alta.; Dem. (Physiol), U. of Albert; Tel. 439-3911.
LYNNES, Howard M.; Box 310, Ashcroft, B.C.; Alb '54; M.C.G.P.
LYON, Harry T.; Ste. 809, 1414 Drummond St., Montreal 25, P.Q.; McG '39; Tel. 844-7309.
LYON, E. Kirk; 106 Talbot St. W., Leamington, Ont.; Seacliffe Dr. (res); Tor '23; FACS; Gen-Surg; Chief of Surg., Leamington Dist. Mem. Hosp.; Dist. Coroner; Deputy Pres., CMA for HRH, Prince Philip, The Duke of Edinburgh; Tel. FA 6-3281.
LYON, R. Kirk; 1755 Steeles Ave., Willowdale, Ont. (Res.); Wes'52; GenSurg; Clin. Assoc., Connaught Research Lab., Toronto 4, Ont.; Tel. 635-2645.
LYON, Sheila M.; 3535 Lakeshore Blvd., Toronto 14, Ont.; U.K.'65.
LYON, William R.; 117 S. John St., Fort William, Ont.; 328 Catherine St. (res); Tor '51; Staff (Med.), McKellar Gen. Hosp.
LYONS, Anthony A.; Davis St., Jarvis, Ont.; Ott'65.
LYONS, Benjamin H.; 407 Norlyn Med. Bldg., 309 Hargrave St., Winnipeg, Man.; 677 Waverley (res); Alb '31; F.R.C.P.(C), F.A.C.P., IntMed; Lect., U. of Manitoba; Active Att. Staff, St. Boniface & Victoria Hosp's.; Ass't. Phys., General Hosp.; Cardiol., Victoria Hosp.; Tel. WH 2-8950 & WH 2-7713.
LYONS, George; 32 Alma St., Moncton, N.B.; McG 16; GenSurg; Tel. EV 4-3275.
LYONS, Gerald M.; 305 Victoria St., Kingston, Ont. (res); Qns '59; Ass't. Prof. (Anat.), Queen's U.; Tel. 546-3871.
LYONS, Peter; 32 Alma St., Moncton, N.B.; 81 Donald Ave. (res); McG '47; GenSurg.; Tel. EV 2-2198.

LYONS, Ruvin; Mall Medical Bldg., Winnipeg, Man.; 420 Niagara St. (res); St. Batholomew's (London, Eng.) '34; F.R.C.O.G., F.A.C.S., F.A.-C.O.G., F.I.C.S., ObstGyn; Assoc. ObstGyn.. Winnipeg Gen. Hosp.; Assoc. Prof., ObstGyn., U. of Manitoba; Tel. SP 4-2411.

LYSACK, Allan; 18-3rd Ave. N.W., Dauphin, Man.; Man '60; FRCS(C), GenSurg.

LYTHGOE, Colin; 206 Rookwood Ave., Fredericton, N.B.; Oxford (Eng.)'57; Tel. 475-7701.

LYTHGOE, Leyda S. (Sestrap); 1207 Douglas St., Victoria, B.C.; 901 Ellery (res); Alb '34; D.A.B. Psy.; Tel. EV 5-2212.

MAALOUF, Hanna; 7437 rue Fabre, Montreal, P.Q.; Beiruth (Leb.) '60; GenSurg.

MA, Alex; South Peel Med. Arts Bldg., 77 Upper Middle Rd., Cooksville, Ont.; Tor '58; FRCS(C), GenSurg.; Staff, South Peel Hosp.; Tel. 279-1871.

MA, G. L.; Tor '61; Jr. Intn., University Hosp., Saskatoon, Sask.

MA, Grace L. (Ling.); Tor '61; Int., University Hosp., Saskatoon, Sask.

MA, Hung F.; 214 Avenue Bldg., 220-3rd Ave. S., Saskatoon, Sask.; Taiwan (China)'61; MCGP.

MABBOTT, James D.; Alb'63; Res., University Hosp., Edmonton, Alta.

MABEE, Horace C.; 79 William St., Kingston, Ont.; Qns '10. Retired.

MABEE, Keith W.; 247 Pine St E., Gananoque, Ont.; 249 Pine St. E. (res); Qns '60; MCGP; Court. Staff Kingston Gen. & Hotel-Dieu Hosp's. Tel. 382-3974.

MABERLEY, Al L., SG/LT; Nat. Defence Med. Centre, Ottawa, Ont.; Alb '64.

MABON, George; Somerset, Man.; Lav '57.

MACALLUM, A. Bruce; R.R. 3, Lunenburg, N.S. (res); Tor '09; Retired.

MacARTHUR, Angus; 604 Brant St., Burlington, Ont.; Edinburgh (Scot.) '61; Active Staff, Joseph Brant Hosp.; Tel. 637-3931.

MACARTHUR,Edward D.; Commercial St., Berwick, N.S.; Dal '52.

MacARTHUR, Frederic C.; Ste. 230, 955 Queen St. E., Sault Ste. Marie, Ont.; 118 Leo Ave. (res); Dal'42.

MACARTHUR, J. Lorne; Seaforth Med. Bldg., 3550 Cote des Neiges Rd., Montreal 25, P.Q.; 654 Roslyn (res); Wes '37; DABOG; FACS; FRCOG; FRCS(C); ObstGyn; Chief Obst. Catherin Booth Hosp.; Ass't., Royal Victoria Hosp.; Assoc. (Obst. & Gyn.), Montreal Gen. Hosp.; Ass't. Prof., McGill U.; Tel. 932-8275.

MacARTHUR, W. J. Campbell; 358 Reynolds St. N., Oakville, Ont.; R.R. 1, Hornby (res); McG '38; FACS; FICS; GenSurg; Chief of Staff, Oakville-Trafalgar Mem. Hosp.; Surg. (OPD), Tor. Western Hosp.; Tel. 844-3201.

MACARTNEY, Hugh H.; Queen's U. (Belfast, N. Ire.) '49; FRCP(C), Anaes; Staff, Dept. of Anaes., St. Joseph's Hosp., Victoria, B.C.; Ass't. Prof. (Anaes.), U. of British Columbia; Chm., B.C. Div., Cdn. Anaes. Soc. & Sec. (B.C. Div., CMA); Tel. 384-1131.

MacASKILL, Alexander D.; Ste. 7, 13656-102nd. Ave., North Surrey, B.C.; Man '55; Ophth; Cons. Staff, St. Mary's Hosp.; Active Staff, Royal Columbian & Surrey Mem. Hosp's.; Tel. 581-7710.

MACAULAY, A. F.; 252 Buena Vista Rd., Ottawa. Ont.; South March Rd. (res).

MACAULAY, Charles J.; 4021A East Hastings **St., North Burnaby, B.C.; 8146 Government Rd. (res); Glasgow (Scot.) '56; DRCOG; MRCOG;** ObstGyn; Staff, Burnaby Gen.; Vis. Staff, Vancouver Gen. & St. Paul's Hosp's.; Tel. 298-8444.

MACAULAY, Donald N.; 1 Roxborough St. E., Toronto 5, Ont.; Wes '62.

MACAULAY, John D.; Marydale Ave., R.R. 1, Long Sault, Ont.; Oxford (Eng.)'55; B.Ch.; Path.

MACAULAY, Malcolm A.; Dal '58; Path; Staff, Magee-Women's Hospital, Pittsburgh, Penn. U.S.A.; Abroad.

MACAULAY, Malcolm J.; Dal '31; Staff, Sydney City Hosp., Sydney, N.S.

MACAULAY, Margaret H.; R.R. 1, Long Sault, Ont.; Liverpool (Eng.)'55.

MACAULAY, M. Grant; 527 Professional Bldg., 10830 Jasper Ave., Edmonton, Alta.; 10039-108th St. (res); Alb '32; Ophth; Ophth., Dept. of Veterans' Affairs; Tel. 422-1245.

MACAULAY, W. Donald; 206 Rookwood Ave., Fredericton, N.B.; McG'57; ABIM; IntMed; Phys., Victoria Public Hosp.; Tel. 475-7701, Loc. 222.

MACBEAN Eric; London (Eng.) '48; DPH; MRCS; LRCP; M.O.H., York Township Health Dept., 2700 Eglinton Ave. W., Toronto 15, Ont.; Tel. RO 6-3481.

MACBETH, Robert A.; Ste. C 148 University Hosp., Edmonton, Alta.; 14120-96th Ave. (res); Alb '44; M.Sc., D.Surg., F.A.C.S., F.R.C.S.(C), GenSurg; Dir. of Surg. Serv., U. of Alberta Hosp.; Surg. Cons., DVA; Prof. & Hd. of Dept. of Surg., U. of Alberta; Tel. GE 9-5911, Loc. 415.

MacCALLUM, A. P.; 4249 Petrolia St., Petrolia, Ont.; Tor'23; MCGP; Dist. Coroner; Tel. 882-0150.

MacCALLUM Evan A.; 510 Seaforth Med. Bldg., 3550 Cote des Neiges Rd., Montreal 25, P.Q.; 9 Ellerdale Rd. (res); McG '45; FRCS(C); Obst-Gyn; Assoc. (ObstGyn.), Montreal Gen. Hosp.; **ObstGyn-in-Chief, Reddy Mem. Hosp.; Cons., Verdun Protestant & Lachine Gen. Hosp's.; Clin. Ass't., Royal Victoria & Catherine Booth Hosp's.;** Lect. (ObstGyn.), McGill U.; Tel. 932-2511.

MACCALLUM, Jean M.; Tor '51; Phys., The Ontario Hosp., London, Ont.

MacCANNELL, Keith L.; Man '58; FRCP(C), IntMed; School of Med., Emory Univ., Atlanta, Ga., U.S.A. Abroad.

MacCHARLES, Clarence W.; Apt. 1115, Faircrest Apts. 1833 Riverside Dr., Ottawa, Ont. (res); Man '23; D.Ph.; Science Staff Officer (Med.), Defence Research Bd. Headquarters, Dept. of National Defence; Retired.

MacCHARLES, Ernest D.; Medical Arts Clinic, 51—6th St. S.E., Medicine Hat, Alta.; 540—7th S.W. (res); Man '40; GenSurg; Staff, Medicine Hat. Gen. Hosp.; Tel. 527-2281.

MACCHARLES, M. R.; Manitoba Clinic, 790 Sherbrooke St., Winnipeg, Man.; 128 Grenfell Blvd. (res); Man '20; F.R.C.S. (Edin. & Can.), **F.A.C.S.; Emer. Prof (Surg.), U. of Manitoba; Tel. SP 4-6541.**

MacCONNACHIE, Hugh F.; 52 Daleside Cres., Toronto 16, Ont. (res); Edinburgh (Scot.) '52; Path; Staff, Sunnybrook Hosp.; Tel. 485-8651.

MacCORMICK, John A.; Box 663, Antigonish Clinic, Antignonish, N.S.; Dal'43; MCGP.

MacCORMICK, L. D.; 108 Howe St., Sydney, N.S.; Dal '57; MCGP.

MACCROSTIE, M. Watson; 3062 S.W. Marine Dr., Vancouver 13, B.C. (res); Alb '45; Anaes; Att. Staff Dept. of Anaes., St. Vincent's Hosp.; Tel. TR 6-7171.

MacDERMOT, H. Ernest; 138 Dunrae Ave., Twn. of Mt. Royal, Montreal, P.Q. (res); McG '13; F.R.C.P.(C), Affil. Memb. C.A.A.; Retired.

MacDERMOT, John H.; 1807 W. 10th St., Vancouver, B.C.; 1835 Morton Ave. Ste. 904, Van. 5 (res.); McG '05; M.C.G.P.; Hon. Editor, BC Med. Jrl.; Hon. Instr. (Hist. Med.), U. of British **Columbia; Tel. MU 2-1066.**

MacDERMOT, Pembroke N.; 1620 Pine Ave. W., Montreal 25, P.Q.; 629 Belmont St. (res); McG '27; Paed; Pulm. Dis. & TB (P.Q.); Staff, Royal Edward Laurentian & Catharine Booth Hosp's.; Tel. WE 3-6806.

MACDONALD, Alan A.; Ste. 160, 5780 Cambie St., Vancouver 15, B.C.; Ott'55; MCGP; Att'd. Staff, Mount St. Joseph's Hosp.; Assoc. Staff, St. Vincent's Hosp.; Tel. 325-3348.

MacDONALD, A. Craig; 74 Normandy Gdns., London, Ont.; Wes'55; Path; FRCP(C), Diag-Rad; Tel. 471-4431.

MacDONALD, A. Edward; 1940 Lonsdale Ave., North Vancouver, B.C.; No. 203, 461 W. 16th St. (res); UBC' 57; Tel. YU 5-4177.

MacDONALD, Alexander E.; MC; ED; 421 Med. Arts Bldg., 170 St. George St., Toronto 5, Ont.; 74 Spadina Rd., Apt. 900 (res); Tor '16; DOMS (Eng.); FRCS(C), Ophth; Cons. (Ophth), Tor. Gen. Hosp. & Cdn. Nat. Inst. for the Blind; Memb. Int'l. Council of Ophth; Vice-Pres. Intern'l. Assoc., Prevention of Blindness; Tel. WA 2-4244.

MACDONALD, Alexander G.; 206 Rookwood Ave., Fredericton, N.B.; Dal'66.

MacDONALD, Allan S.; Dal'63; Res., Camp Hill Hosp., Halifax, N.S.

MacDONALD, Allison D.; Ste. 1721, Place Ville-Marie, Montreal, P.Q.; 380 Simcoe Ave., Twn. of Mt. Royal (res); McG '44; MRCP (Edin.); FACP; FRCP(C), IntMed (Cardiol); Assoc. Phys., **Royal Victoria Hosp.; Cons., Queen Mary Vet's.** Hosp.; Ass't. Prof. McGill U.; M.O., Steel Co. of **Canada; Tel. 861-8103.**

MACDONALD, Allison R.; Edson Med. Centre, 502-50th St., Edson, Alta.; Alta'43; Tel. 723-3366.

MacDONALD, Allister J.; 29 Erb St. E., Waterloo, Ont.; McG'49; Tel. SH 5-7129.

MacDONALD, Angus C.; Dal'63; Res., Victoria Gen. Hosp., Halifax, N.S.

MACDONALD, Angus J.; 141 Simcoe St. S., Oshawa, Ont.; 836 Masson St. (res); Dal '33; **GenSurg; Tel. 723-3262.**

MACDONALD, Archibald J.; 17 Brunswick St., Stratford, Ont.; 69 William St. (res); Bristol (Eng.)'53; Tel. 271-1731.

MACDONALD, Arthur G.; Box 340. Qualicum Beach, B.C.; Qns '39.

MacDONALD, Augustine A.; Souris, P.E.I.; McG '02.

MACDONALD, Austin; 232 St. Clair St., Chatham, Ont.; 35 Gregory Dr. (res); McG '43; MCGP; Active Staff, St. Joseph's & Public Gen. Hosp's; Tel. EL 4-3515.

MacDONALD, Austin A.; Med. Arts Bldg., 336 Kings Rd., Sydney, N.S.; Dal'42; IntMed.; Chief of Staff, City of Sydney Hosp.; Tel. 562-1202.

MacDONALD, Catherine (see Thomas)

MacDONALD, C. Alexander; 278 George St., Sydney, N.S.; Tor '34; Tel. 564-6252.

MACDONALD, Charles C.; Apt. 102, 6950 Fielding Ave., Montreal 29 P.Q.; 195 Welseley Ave. N. (res); McG '41; IntMed; Dem. (Med.), McGill U. & Montreal Gen. Hosp.; Tel. WE 7-6011.

MACDONALD, Charles J.; 6337 Cornwall St., Halifax, N.S.; Dal '37; Ass't. Med. Supt., Camp **Hill DVA Hosp.; Tel. 423-1371.**

MACDONALD, Charles J.; 1980 Oxford St., Halifax, N.S.; Dal'53; GenSurg; Vis. Staff, Victoria Gen. & Halifax Gen. Hosp's. & Halifax Infirmary; Tel. 422-4554.

MACDONALD, Clive S.; Baddeck, N.S.; Dal'60.

MacDONALD, C. Nolan; Tor'58; Res., Victoria Hosp., London, Ont.

MacDONALD, Colin E.; 215 Hammond Bldg., 310 Main St. N., Moose Jaw, Sask.; St. Andrews (Scot.) '46.; M.B., Ch.B., Dip. Ophth; Assoc. Med. Staff, Union & Providence Hosp's.; Tel. 692-2227.

MACDONALD, D'Arcy K.; Suite 911, 1849 Yonge, Toronto 7, Ont.; 93 Glengowan Rd. (res); DOMS, DABOphth; F.R.C.S.(C), Ophth; Ophth-in-Chief, Toronto Western Hosp.; Ass't. Prof. (Ophth), U. of Toronto; Tel. 485-5276.

MACDONALD, D. Chisholm; 3 Craig Bldg., 1092-101st St., North Battleford, Sask.; Dal'25; Ophth-Otol; Attend. Staff, Battleford's Union Hosp.; Tel. 445-3782.

MacDONALD, Dennis A.; Man'65; Jr. Int., St. Boniface Hosp., Winnipeg 6, Man.

MACDONALD, D. James; 9 Kenridge Ave., Toronto 18, Ont.; Tor'59; D. Psy; Psy; Abroad.

MACDONALD, D. Keith; 3579 W. 41st Ave., Vancouver 13, B.C.; 3205 W. 24th Ave. (res); UBC '60; MPH; MCGP; Tel. AM 1-6361.

MacDONALD, Donald; 615 Fraser, Quebec 6, P.Q.; Lav '40; P.Q., Veterans' Hosp.

MacDONALD, Donald A.; 915 Fairmont Med. Bldg., 750 W. Broadway, Vancouver 9, B.C.; 5311 Cypress St. Van. 13 (res); McG '52; FRCS (C), Urol; Att'd. Staff, Vancouver Gen. Hosp.; ClinInstr., U. of British Columbia; Tel. 874-7010.

MACDONALD, Donald C.; Ste. 502, 1541 Broadway W., Vancouver 9, B.C.; 2248 Wenonah (res); Qns'39; Psy; Cons., Hollywood Hosp., New Westminster; Cons. B.C. Penitentiary, New Westminster; Tel. RE 3-8219.

MacDONALD, Donald G.; 3220 Portage Ave., Winnipeg 22, Man.; Glasgow (Scot.)'49; MB; Ch.B.

MacDONALD, Donald G.; 172 Queen St. W., Brampton, Ont.; 58 Main St. (res); Tor '37; DPH; PH; MOH Peel Co. Health Unit; Staff, Peel Mem. Hosp.; Tel. 451-1262.

MACDONALD, Doreen I. (Mathers); 1449 Chrisenden Dr., Port Credit, Ont.; Tor '50; DiagRad; **Staff, Oakville-Trafalgar Hosp.; Abroad**

MacDONALD, Douglas A.; P.O. Box 852, Charlottetown, P.E.I.; Dal '51; Anaes; Staff, Charlottetown Hosp.; Tel. 894-5561.

MACDONALD, Douglas F.; 305 Main St., Yarmouth, N.S.; 35 Brunswick St. (res): Dal '29; **IntMed; Chief of Med., Yarmouth Hosp.; Tel.** 742-2041.

MACDONALD, Douglas O.; 10 Rosemount Ave., Montreal 6, P.Q.; McG '22; Tel. 488-7153.

MacDONALD, Duncan D.; Deer Lake Clinic, Deer Lake, Nfld.; Dublin (Ire.) '50. M.B., B.Ch., BAO; L.M. (Rotunda); Hon. M.P.S.; Tel. 5-2925.

MacDONALD, Earle M.; 197 Charles St., **Belleville, Ont.; Qns '37; Tel. WO 8-7670.**

MACDONALD, E. Fraser; Dal'62; Res., Pathological Inst., 5808 University Ave., Halifax, N.S.

MACDONALD, Eric W.; Reserve Mines, N.S. (res); Dal '22; F.A.C.S., F.R.C.S.(C), GenSurg; Retired.

MACDONALD E. Stuart; 170 St. George St., Ste. 216, Toronto, Ont.; Tor '40; F.R.C.S.(C) ObstGyn; Att. Staff, Obst. Gyn St. Michael's Hosp.; Ass't. Prof., Dept. of Obst. Gyn., U. of Toronto; Tel. 924-1787.

MACDONALD, Eva; (Mader); 58 Glengowan Rd., Toronto 12, Ont. (res.); Dal '27; DPH; Bact; Dir. PH Women's College Hosp.; Tel. WA 3-7381.

MacDONALD, Floyd D.; Box 430, 328 Main St., Liverpool, N.S.; 70 Bristol Ave (res); Dal'62; Staff, Queen's Gen. Hosp; Tel. 354-4312.

MacDONALD, Francis B.; 224 Charlotte St., Sydney, N.S.; 587 Kings Rd. (res); Dal '44; M.Sc. (Med.); MCGP; Active Staff, Sydney City & St. Rita's Hosp's.; Tel. 564-6110.

MACDONALD, Frederick R.; 276 Morrison Ave., Mont Royal, Montreal 26, P.Q. (res); Dal '50; **DiagRad; Staff, Royal Victoria Hosp.; Tel. VI 2-1251.**

MacDONALD, George; Woodlawn Med. Clinic, 110 Woodlawn Rd., Dartmouth, N.S.; Dal'62.

MacDONALD, Gerard F.; Yater Clin., 1780 Massachusetts Ave. N.W., Washington 6, D.C.; McG'42; FRCS(C), GenSurg; DABS. Abroad.

MacDONALD, Giles F.; 11816-124th St., Edmonton, Alta.; Alb '61. Abroad.

MacDONALD, Gordon C.; Box 454, Sydney, N.S.; 17 Auberville St. (res); Dal '36; Staff, Sydney City & St. Rita Hosp's.; Tel. 564-4577.

MACDONALD, Gordon M.; 305 Main St., Yarmouth, N.S.; 24 Chestnut St. (res); Dal '44; Att. Phys., Yarmouth Gen. Hosp.; Tel. 742-2041.

MacDONALD, Harold S.; Med. Arts Bldg. Sydney, N.S.; 455 Kings Rd. (res); Ott'51.; Tel. 562-1119.

MACDONALD, Hugh; 1088 Pembina Highway, **Winnipeg, Man.; Qns '52.**

MacDONALD, Hugh Neil A.; 5880 Spring Garden Rd., Halifax, N.S.; 2908 Doug Smith Dr. (res); Dal'53; FRCP(C); Neurol; Neurologist-in-Chief, Victoria Gen. Hosp.; Cons. Neurol. & Electroenceph., Children's Nova Scotia & Camp Hill DVA Hosp's.; Assoc. Prof. (Neurol.), Dalhousie U.; Tel. 423-8862.

MacDONALD, Innis M.; 144 Main St. N., Markham, Ont.; Tor'27; DO (Oxon); FRCS (Edin.); Ophth.; Tel. 294-2300.

MACDONALD, J. A.; Bay Med. Group, Glace Bay, N.S.; MCGP.

MACDONALD, James D.; 1505 Victoria Ave., Windsor, Ont.; Tor '18; Staff, Hotel Dieu Hosp.; **Dist. Coroner; Tel. 254-4401.**

MacDONALD, James H.; 14463 Malabar Cr., White Rock, B.C.; 14462 Blackburn Cr. (res); Tor '35; DAB; Ophth; Ophth. Staff, White Rock Hosp.; Tel. 531-4727.

MACDONALD, J. Cameron; 1428 Ouellette Ave., Windsor, Ont.; 840 Argyle Rd. (res); Dal '51; DiagRad; Hon. Cons. (Rad.), IODE Mem. Hosp.; Tel. CL 2-2789.

MACDONALD, J. Claude; 204-3000 Lawrence Ave. E., Scarborough, Ont.; Tor '51; F.R.C.S.(C), GenSurg; Intn. Dir., Scarborough Gen. Hosp.; Tel. 293-5533.

MACDONALD, J. D. C.; 620 Berkshire Rd., Sarnia, Ont. (res.); Wes '38; F.A.C.A., Anaes; Supervisor Med. Dept., Polymer Corporation Ltd.; Tel. ED 7-8251.

MACDONALD, J. Fyfe; 3535 New Metropolitan Blvd., Pointe Claire, Lachine, P.Q.; McG '49; Assoc. Med. Dir., Schering Corp. Ltd.

MacDONALD, John A.; 1000 Toronto Prof. Bldg., 123 Edward St., Toronto 2, Ont.; Tor'53; FRCS (C), GenSurg; Active Staff (Surg.), St. Michael's Hosp.; Clin. Teach. (Surg.), U. of Toronto; Memb., Editorial Bd., "Applied Therapeutics"; Tel. WA 2-4981.

MacDONALD, John A.; Qualicum Beach, B.C.; Qns '38; MCGP; Tel. 752-6731.

MACDONALD, John A.; 4349 Hastings St. E., North Burnaby, B.C.; 3814 Oxford St. (res); Alb **'44; Tel. CY 9-4388.**

MACDONALD, Joseph B.; Foord St., Stellarton, N.S.; Park St. (res); McG '37; M.C.G.P.; Staff, **Aberdeen Hosp., New Glasgow; Tel. 2-6131.**

MACDONALD, Keith G.; Streetsville Medical Clinic, Streetsville, Ont.; Wes '60

MacDONALD, Keith M.; Sask '62; Res., University Hosp., Saskatoon, Sask.

MACDONALD, L. Vance; 211 Le Marchand Mansions, Edmonton, Alta.; Alb '35; NeurSurg; Chief of NeurSurg., Royal Alexandra Hosp.; Tel. 488-6567.

MacDONALD, Malcolm H.; 61 Academy Med. Bldg., 4th & 19th Ave. S.W., Calgary, Alta.; McG '51; FRCS(C); GenSurg; ThorSurg; Surg. Staff, Calgary Gen. & Holy Cross Hosp's.; Tel. 262-9061.

MacDONALD, Malcolm M.; Allen St., Thedford, Ont.; Wes'50.

MacDONALD, Martin P.; Fitch St. Plaza, Welland, Ont.; Ott '53; FACS; DABS; FRCS(C), GenSurg; Active & Cons. Staff, Welland County Gen. Hosp.; Cons. Staff, Port Colborne Gen. Hosp.; Tel. 732-7511.

MacDONALD, Martin S.; 149 Octerloney St., Dartmouth, N.S.; 181 Crichton Ave. (res); Dal '45; MCGP; Tel. 466-7530.

MACDONALD, Mary J. (Murray); Dal'53; Res., Halifax Infirmary, Halifax, N.S.

MACDONALD, Michael R.; 30 Armshore Dr., Armdale, Halifax, N.S. (res); McG '38; D.P.H., F.A.P.H.A., PH; Ass't. Admin., Victoria Gen. Hosp., Halifax; Registrar, Prov. Med. Bd. of N.S.; Hd. of Dept. of Prev. Med., Victoria Gen. Hosp.; Ass't. Prof., Dalhousie U.; Tel. 422-7371.

MacDONALD, Neil; Med. Arts Bldg., 1011 Ouellette Ave., Windsor, Ont.; 2228 Victoria Ave. (res); Tor '24; FATS, FACS; FRCS(C), GenSurg; Cons. Surg., Hotel-Dieu, Grace, Metropolitan Gen. & I.O.D.E. Mem. Hosp's.; Tel. 256-7162.

MACDONALD, Peter M.; 285 Mansfield Place, Lancaster, N.B.; Dal'53.

MACDONALD, Phillip; Harshman Blk., Sydney, N.S.; 19 Union St. (res); Dal '45; Staff, Sydney City & St. Rita Hosp's.; Tel. 564-4557.

MACDONALD, R. Glen; 115 Hazen St., Saint **John, N.B.; 23 Seely St. (res); Dal '45; Paed; Paed., Saint John Gen. & St. Joseph's Hosp's.;** Cons. East Saint John TB Hosp., Tel. 693-3466.

MacDONALD R. Ian.; 312Med. Arts Bldg., 170 St. George St., Toronto 5, Ont.; 39 Chestnut Park Rd. (res); Dal '30; FRCP (Lond.); FRCP(C); IntMed; FACP; Sr., Phys., Toronto Gen. **Hosp.; Dir., Div. of P.G. Med. Educ.; Prof. & Assoc. Dean, Dept. of Med. U. of Toronto; Tel. WA 3-8974.**

MacDONALD, Richard; Elbow Drive Medical Centre, 51st Ave. & Elbow Drive, Calgary, Alta.; 27 Hallbrook (res.); Alb '52; Tel. AL 5-6647. Abroad.

MACDONALD, R. J.; 1030 Medical-Dental Bldg., Vancouver 1, B.C.; 2578 Ottawa Ave., West Van**couver (res); Man '35; D.P.H.; Tel. MU 1-4828.**

MACDONALD, R. Keith; 421 Medical Arts Bldg., 170 St. George St., Toronto, Ont.; 15 Walmsley Blvd. (res); Tor '45; Ophth; Res. Fell., U. of Toronto; Tel. WA 3-6711.

MacDONAL, R. Neil; McG'59; Haem(P.Q.); FRCP(C), IntMed; Clin. Ass't., Royal Victoria Hosp., Montreal 2, P Q.; Dem., McGill U.; Tel. AV 8-8848.

MacDONALD, Robert; Nfld. Anaes. Associates, 95 LeMarchant Rd., St. John's, Nfld.; 3 Roche St. (res); Edinburgh (Scot.) '52; FACA; Anaes; Staff, St. John's, Grace, St. Clare's Mercy Hosp's.; Tel. 578-7909.

MacDONALD, Robert E.; 308 Med. Arts Bldg., 170 St. George St., Toronto 5, Ont.; Tor'58; FRCS(C), Otol; Teach. Staff, Hosp. for Sick Children; Assoc. Staff, Toronto Gen. Hosp.; Cons. Staff, Oakville Trafalgar Hosp.; Tel. 923-1030.

MacDONALD, Robert G.; Man'57; Res., Winnipeg Gen. Hosp., Winnipeg 3, Man.

MacDONALD, Robert G.; 8 George St. S., Galt, **Ont.; Wes '59; A.M.C.G.P.; Tel. 621-3880.**

MacDONALD, Robert M.; Med. Arts Bldg., 5880 Spring Garden Rd., Halifax, N.S.; 1820 Armview Terr. (res); Edinburgh (Scot.) '39; FRCP(C); IntMed; Chief of Med. Services, Camphill DVA Hosp.; Assoc. Phys., Victoria Gen. Hosp.; Prof. of Med. & Dean, Faculty of Health Professions, Dalhousie U.; Tel. 423-7984.

MacDONALD, Robert L.; 7184 King George VI Hwy., Newton, B.C.; Sask '59.

MacDONALD, Samuel A.; 570 Seaforth Med. Bldg., 3550 Cote des Neiges Rd., Montreal 25, P.Q.; 697 Aberdeen Ave., Westmount (res); Edinburgh (Scot.) '30; FICS; FRCS(C); Urol; Assoc. Urol., Montreal Gen. Hosp.; Ass't. Prof. (Surg.); McGill U.; Tel. 933-9933.

MacDONALD, Stewart; 206 Spring Park Rd., Charlottetown, P.E.I. (res); Dal '53; Pension Med. Exam. & Sr. Treatment M.O. (D.V.A.), Dominion Bldg. (D.V.A.) Charlottetown, P.E.I.; Tel. 894-5316.

MacDONALD, Stewart A.; 385 Wellington St. W., Chatham, Ont.; St. Thomas's (London, Eng.) '42; Otol; Staff (ENT), Chatham Public Gen. & St. Joseph's Hosp's.; Tel. EL 4-4552.

MACDONALD, Thomas S.; Community Clinic, 110-8th St. E., Prince Albert, Sask.; Nat. U. (Ire.)'49; MB; BCh; BAO; MRCOG; Staff (Obst-Gyn), Community Clinic, Holy Family Hosp. & Victoria Union Hosp.; Tel. 763-6466.

MacDONALD, Walter C.; 2656 Heather St., Vancouver 9, B.C.; UBC '55; FRCP(C), IntMed; Ass't. Cytol., Vancouver Gen. Hosp.; Instr., U. of British Columbia; Tel. TR 4-9321.

MACDONALD, W. Dean; 14 King St., St. Catharines, Ont.; Tor '32; F.A.C.S., GenSurg; Surg. Staff, St. Catharines Gen. & Hotel Dieu Hosp's.; Tel. 682-4730.

MACDONALD, Wendell L.; 94 Brighton Rd., Charlottetown, P.E.I. (res); Edinburgh (Scot.) '37; D.R.; D&TRad, Prince Edward Island & **Charlottetown Hosp's.; Tel. 8352; 894-5561.**

MacDONALD, William A.; 1119-71st Ave., Edmonton, Alta. (res); Alb'27; DPH; MRSH.; Tel. 434-5202.

MacDONALD, William B.; Dept. of Anaes., University Hosp., Saskatoon, Sask.; Sask'59; FACA; DABA; FRCP(C), Anaes; Active Staff, University Hosp.; Ass't. Prof., U. of Saskatchewan; Tel. 652-8221, Loc. 413.

MACDONALD, William D.; 166 Victoria St., Moncton, N.B.; Dal '44; Otol; Staff (E.N.T.), Moncton Hosp.; Cons. Staff, Hotel-Dieu Hosp.; Tel. 855-4218.

MACDONALD, William G.; 254 Queen St. S., Kitchener, Ont.; Tor '22; M.C.G.P.; Industrial (Med).

MACDONALD, William J.; 300 Medical Arts Bldg., Calgary, Alta.; 330 Scarboro Ave. (res); Alb '45; ThorSurg; Tel. 269-2561.

MACDONALD, William J.; 124 Victoria St., Truro, N.S.; Wes'56; GenSurg.

MacDONALD, William J.; 297 Main St., Yarmouth, N.S.; Dal '56.

MacDONALD, William J.; Box 144, Truro, N.S.; Wes '57.

MacDONALD, William K.; 3535 Metropolitan Blvd., Pte.- Claire, P.Q.; 54 Winston Circle (res); McG '43; MCGP; Research Staff, Mtl. Gen. Hosp.; Vice-Pres. (Clin. Research), Schering Corp. Ltd.; Tel. 695-1320.

MACDONELL, A. Bruce; 227 Medical Arts Bldg. & 102 Canada Bldg., Saskatoon, Sask.; 1066 Spadina Cr. E. (res); Qns '29; D&T Rad; Dept. Head, Rad., Saskatoon City Hosp.; Vis. Cons. (Rad.), St. Paul's & University Hosp. & Saskatoon Cancer Clin.; Clin. Ass't. Prof. (Rad.), U. of Saskatchewan; Tel. 244-1169.

MACDONELL, J. Kennedy; Ott'54; DiagRad; Staff, X-Ray Dept., Royal Inland Hosp., Kamloops, B.C.; Tel. 372-3131, Local 252.

MACDONELL, John A.; 256 Winchester St., St. James, Winnipeg 12, Man. (Res.); Man'43; AMCAA; IntMed; Con. in Geriatrics & Chest Diseases, Deer Lodge Hosp., Winnipeg 12, Man.; Ass't. Prof., Dept. of Med., U. of Man.; Tel. 837-1301.

MacDONELL, John A.; 212 Yarrow Bldg., 645 Fort St., Victoria, B.C.; McG'49; D&TRad.; Tel. 386-7538.

MacDONELL, John E.; 33 Hawthorne St., Antigonish, N.S. (res); McG '48; IntMed; Staff, St. Martha's Hosp.; Tel. 863-3871.

MacDONELL, Josefina A. (Kristjansson); 256 Winchester St., Winnipeg 12, Man. (res); Man '43; Ass't Dir., Deer Lodge Veteran's Hosp.; **Tel. TU 8-4861.**

MACDOUGAL, J. Raymond; 20030 Lakeshore Rd., Baie d'Urfe, Ste-Anne-de-Bellevue, P.Q. (res); Tor '53; MCGP; Med. Dir., Burroughs Wellcome & Co. Can., Ville-La-Salle; Tel. DO 6-9211.

MacDOUGALL, Charles H.; 390 Burnham St., Peterborough Ont.; Tor'55; Staff, St. Joseph's & Peterborough Civic Hosp's.; Tel. RI 2-9234.

MacDOUGALL, Charles S.; 200 Med. Arts Bldg.. 170 St. George St., Toronto 5 Ont.; 12 Silverwood Ave. (res); Tor '17; DLO; FRCS(Ed.); FRCS(C); Otol; Cons. Staff, St. Michaels Hosp.; Tel. 921-3689.

MacDOUGALL, Daniel A.; Dal '55; Staff, St. Martha's Hosp., Antigonish, N.S.; Tel. 863-2830.

MacDOUGALL, James I.; Tor'60; FRCP(C), IntMed; Staff, Montreal Gen. Hosp., Montreal 25, P.Q.

MACDOUGALL, John A., OBE; 750 W. Broadway, Vancouver, B.C.; 4130 Burkehill Rd. (res); Man '34; FACS; F.R.C.S. (Eng.), F.R.C.S.(C), GenSurg; Att'd Surg., Van. Gen. Hosp., & B.C. Cancer Inst.; Ass't Clin. Prof., (Dept. of Surg.), U. of British Columbia; Tel. TR 2-5288.

MACDOUGALL, John A.; Tor '63; M.O., RCAF Station, Gimli, Man.

MACDOUGALL, John T., DSO; Abbott Clinic, 274 Osborne St. N., Winnipeg, Man.; 613 South Drive (res); McG '37; F.R.C.S.(Edin.), F.A.C.S., F.I.C.S., F.R.C.S(C), GenSurg; Ass't Surg., Wpg. Gen. Hosp.; **Chief Surg. Deer Lodge Hosp.; Surg., Grace Hosp., Assoc. Prof. (Surg.) U. of Manitoba; Tel. SP 4-4567.**

MACDOUGALL, Joseph A.; 20 Queen Squ., Saint John, N.B.; (res); Dal '42; Anaes.; Tel. 693-4447.

MACDOUGALL, Walter G.; 812 Medical & Dental Bldg., Regina, Sask.; 2926 Rae St. (res); **Edinburgh (Scot.) '36; M.R.C.P.(Edin.), IntMed.; Tel. LA 2-5629.**

MACDOWALL, C. Ross; 153 Bridge St., Carleton Place, Ont.; Qns'32. Retired

MACE, William E.; 99 Ridout St. S., London, Ont.; 775 Riverside Dr. (res); Wes '22; MCGP; Court. Staff, Victoria Hosp.; Tel. 471-5636.

MacEACHEN, Donald A. G.; 322 Wellington St., Sarnia, Ont.; Dal'52; GenSurg.; Tel. 337-5414.

MacEACHERN, William N.; 307½ Lancaster St. W., Kitchener, Ont.; Tor'58; DABD; FRCP(C), Derm; Active Staff, Kitchener-Waterloo & St. Mary's Hosp's.; Court. Staff, South Waterloo Mem. Hosp.; Tel. 742-0591.

MACEWAN, Douglas W.; 30 Aldershot Blvd., Winnipeg 9, Man.; McG'52; FRCP(C); D&TRad; Prof. of Rad., University of Manitoba; Dir., Rad. Dept., Winnipeg Gen. Hosp.

MACEWAN, William R.; 925 W. Georgia St., Vancouver, B.C.; 5969 Cartier St. (res); Alb '45; D. Obst. R.C.O.G.; ObstGyn; Attend. Staff, Grace Hosp.; Clin. Instr., U. of British Columbia **Med. School; Tel. MU 1-7716.**

MacEWEN, H. Bruce; Box 389, Squamish, B.C.; McG '60; Anaes.

MacEWEN, Kenneth F.; 170 St. George St., **Toronto 5, Ont.; 10 Green Valley Rd., Willow-**dale (res); Tor'39; DR; FACS; DiagRad; Rad.-in-**Chief, Wellesley Hosp.; Sr. Cons. (DiagRad), Princess Margaret Hosp.; Ass't. Prof. (Rad),** U. of Toronto; Tel. WA 1-3118.

MACEY, Henry P.; 343 Ridge St., Ridgeway, Ont.: McG '32; Staff, Port Colborne Gen. Hosp.; **M.O.H. Twnsp. of Bertie; Tel. 869-3661.**

MacFADYEN, Donald A.; 683 Prince St., Truro, N.S.; Dal '59; Active Staff, Colchester Hosp.; Tel. 893-3738.

MacFADYEN, D. John; Dept. of Med., Vancouver Gen. Hosp., Vancouver, B.C.; Tor '53; FRCP(C), Neurol. Hd. Sub-Dept. of Neurol., Vancouver Gen. Hosp.; Assoc. Prof. (Neurol.) U. of British Columbia; Tel. TR 6-3211, Loc. 2544.

MACFADYEN, Lennis R.; Scarborough Radiologists, Ste. GO 1, 3000 Lawrence Ave., Scarborough, Ont.; Dal'54; DiagRad; Member, X-Ray Dept., Scarborough Gen. Hosp.

MACFARLAND, H. N.; Occupational Health Laboratory, 200 Kent St., Ottawa, Ont.

MACFARLAND, Maxwell T.; Second Floor, 201 Kennedy St., Winnipeg 1, Man.; 104-333 Welling-ton Cres., Wpg. 9 (res); Qns '30; Registrar, Coll. of Phys & Surg. of Manitoba; Tel. 947-0424.

MacFARLANE, A. L.; 304 Med. Arts Bldg., 1 Young St., Hamilton, Ont.; Tor'65.

MACFARLANE, E. Blakely; 610 Medical **Arts** Bldg., Hamilton, Ont.; 25 Glenfern (res); **Tor** '47; D.A.B.Op., Ophth; Staff, Ophth., Hamilton Gen. Hosp.; Tel. 528-2629.

MACFARLANE, Edward J.; 2911 Bayview Ave., Ste. 115, F., Willowdale, Ont.; Glasgow (Scot.) '55; MB, ChB; OrthSurg; MO, WCB, Downsview; Tel. 483-9837.

MacFARLANE, Gordon N.; 407 Brant Arts Bldg., 672 Brant St., Burlington, Ont.; 40 Auchmar Rd. (res); Trinity Coll. (Dublin, Ire.) '37; FICS; FRCS (Edin.); FRCS(C); GenSurg; Chief-of-Surg, Joseph Brant Mem. Hosp.; Surg. Staff, Hamilton Gen. & St. Joseph's Hosps.; Tel. 637-2121.

MacFARLANE, James; 105 The Stratford House, 3477 Drummond St. Montreal 25, P.Q.; Edinburgh (Scot.) '32; FRS; M.B., Ch.B. (Ed.); B.Comm.; DPH; Post-Grad, McGill U.; Tel. VI 4-6311.

MacFARLANE, John K.; McG '63; Jr. Ass't. Res. Montreal Gen. Hosp., Montreal, P.Q.

MacFARLANE, J. Wallace; 492 Locust St., Burlington, Ont.; Tor '43; MCGP; Tel. NE 4-2133.

MacFARLANE, Kenneth T.; 500 Seaforth Med. Bldg., 3550 Cote des Neiges Rd., Montreal 25, P.Q.; 64 Forden Cr., Westmount (res); Wes '29; FRCOG; FACS; FACOG; FRCS(C); ObstGyn; ObstGyn-in-Chief & Memb., Med. Bd., Montreal Gen. Hosp.; Cons., St. Mary's Hosp. Mtl., Barrie Mem. Hosp., Ormstown, Douglas Mem. Hosp. & Lake Placid Mem. Hosp.; Prof. (ObstGyn.), McGill U.; Tel. 932-6058.

MACFIE, Donald D. W/C; Unit 20, 670 Sir J. A. MacDonald Blvd., Kingston, Ont. (res); Glasgow (Scot.) '50; Otol; Cons. Otol., Canadian Forces Hosp.; Clin. Ass't Otol., Queen's U.

MacGILL, Robert D.; Turtleford Clin., Turtleford, Sask.; Glasgow (Scot.)'56.

MacGILLIVRAY, Leo F.; 114 Queen St., St. Catharines, On.; 14 Cliff Rd. (res); McG '49; Paed.; Tel. 682-7778.

MacGILLIVRAY, Patrick C.; Spence Clinic, 910 Ridgeway St., Fort William, Ont.; Edinburgh (Scot.) '46; M.R.C.P. (Edin.), D.C.H.; Paed; Med. Staff, McKellar Gen. Hosp.; Tel. 622-5301.

MacGILLIVRAY, Roderick A.; 1940 Lonsdale Ave., North Vancouver, B.C.; UBC'63; Staff, Lionsgate Hosp.; Tel. YU 8-8770.

MacGOUGAN, Melrose K.; 121 Medical Arts Bldg., 335-339-6th Ave. S.W., Calgary, Alta.; 3409 **Elbow Dr. (res); McG '35; Ophth, Otol.; Tel. 262-2663.**

MACGOWAN, George A.; 71 Yonge Blvd., Toronto 12, Ont.; 21 Don Ridge Dr., Willowdale (res); Tor '25; Tel. HU 8-5017.

MACGREGOR, Alexander H.; 1605-9th Ave. S., Lethbridge, Alta.; 1050-18th St. S. (res); Edinburg (Scot.) '56; LRCP (Edin. & Glas.); LAH (Ire.); ObstGyn; Tel. 327-3121. Abroad.

MacGREGOR, Arthur J.; 1026 Cook St., Victoria, B.C.; 3021 Phyllis St. (res); UBC '58; MCGP; **Active Staff, St. Joseph's Hosp.; Court. Staff,** Royal Jubilee & Gorge Rd. Hosp's.; Tel. 388-4341.

MacGREGOR David C.; Tor '62; Ass't. Res., Toronto Gen. Hosp., Toronto Ont.

MacGREGOR, Donald J.; 408 Rideau Medical-Dental Centre, 1711-4th St. S.W., Calgary, Alta.; 1211 Beverly Blvd. (res); Dal '52; ObstGyn; **Staff, Calgary Gen., Holy Cross & Grace Hosp's.;** Tel. AM 2-5282.

MACGREGOR, H. Ian; 5691 Duffus St., Halifax, N.S.; Dal '43; M.C.G.P.; Ass't., Clin. Med. (OPD), Victoria Gen. Hosp.; Lect. (Urol.) (VD), Dalhousie U.; Tel. 422-7371.

MACGREGOR, John W.; 11139-86th Ave., Edmonton, Alta (res); Alb '30; F.R.C.P.(C), PathBact.; Prof. & Chm., Dept. of Path., U. of Alberta; Tel. GE 3-3589.

MACGREGOR Marguerite A.; Alb '63; Res., University Hosp., Edmonton, Alta.

MacGREGOR, Peter A.; Dal '58; FRCP(C), IntMed; Staff, Victoria Gen. Hosp., Halifax, N.S.; Tel. 422-7371.

MACGREGOR, R. Roy; 148 Earl St., Kingston, Ont.; Qns '16: F.R.C.P.(C), Paed; Staff, Kingston Gen. Hosp. Tel. 542-2821.

MacGUIRE, Gerald F.; 62 Charlotte St., Sydney, N.S.; Ott '52.

MACHABBIE, Nicole; Mon'65; Res., Hop. Notre-Dame, Montreal 24, P.Q.

MACHABEE, Gilles; 3871 est Belanger, Montreal 46, P.Q.; Mon'65.

MacHABEE, Yvan; Belanger Med. Clinic, 3871 Belanger Ave., Montreal 36, P.Q.; 8120 Place Dalkeith, Ville-d'Anjou (res); Mon '58; Tel. 729-5231.

MACHAFFIE, Lloyd P.; 155 Gilmour St., Ottawa, Ont. (res); McG '12; Paed; Chief Paed., Ottawa Pub Sch. Health Serv.; Retired.

MACHAN, James R.; 1001 Ridgeway St., Fort William, Ont.; 1303 Ridgeway (res); Wes '48; F.A.C.P., F.R.C.P.(C), IntMed.; Tel. MA 2-0601.

MACHATTIE, Frederick G. W., Sg.Capt.; c/o National Defence Med. Council, Smyth Rd. & Alta Vista Dr., Ottawa 8, Ont.; Tor '39; DPH; DHA; C.O., N.D.M.C.; Reg, Surg., Ottawa Valley Med. Region.

MACINNES, Angus; Med. Arts Clinic, 51-6th St. S.E., Medicine Hat, Alta.; Aberdeen (Scot.) '51; DTM&H; D.ObstRCOG; Staff, Medicine Hat Gen. Hosp.; Tel. 527-2281.

MacINNES, Frederic C.; Box 460, Summerland, B.C.; Dal '58; Tel. HY 4-4356.

MACINNES, Ian; Broadway Med. Clinic, 1319 Broadway Ave., Regina, Sask.; Manchester (Eng.) '60; M.B.; CHB; DRCOG; Tel. 527-3355.

MacINNIS, Daniel F.; Shubenacadie, N.S.; Dal '18; Court Staff, Colchester County Hosp., Truro; Tel. 14.

MACINNIS, Donald R.; Shubenacadie, Hants Co., **N.S.; Dal '49; Tel. 14.**

MACINNIS, Frank H.; Smith Clinic, Camrose, Alta.; Qns '41; F.A.C.P.; IntMed; Chief, Med. Staff, St. Mary's Hosp.; Tel. 672-2424.

MACINNIS, James A.; Bath, N.B.; Dal '50.

MACINTOSH, Alistair E.; 116 Mountainview Rd. S., Georgetown, Ont.; Aberdeen (Scot.)'43; MCGP; MRCP(Lond); Coroner, Halton County; Tel. 877-2639.

MacINTOSH, Allan S.; 5871 Spring Garden Rd., Halifax, N.S.; 599 Tower Rd. (res); Dal '41; FACA; Anaes; Ass't. Anaes., Victoria Gen. **Hosp.; Ass't. Prof. (Anaes) Dalhousie U.; Tel. 423-8484.**

MACINTOSH, Carmen N.; Antigonish, N.S.; Dal '45; M.C.G.P.; Gen. Staff, St. Martha's Hosp., Antigonish; Tel. 863-2830.

MACINTOSH, David L.; 812 Med. Arts Bldg., 170 St. George St., Toronto 5, Ont.; 10 Moorehill Dr., Tor. 12 (res); Dal '39; F.R.C.S.(C), OrthSurg; Surg., Toronto Gen. Hosp.; Cons. OrthSurg., Princess Margaret Hosp.; Staff Surg., Hart House, U. of Toronto. Ass't Prof. (Surg.), U. of Toronto; Tel. WA 3-7823.

MacINTOSH, Donald J.; 1610 Pine Ave. W., Montreal 25, P.Q.; 356 Kensington Ave., Mtl. 6 (res); McG '47; DIM; FCCP; FRCP(C); IntMed; Assoc. Phys. & Dir., Cardio Resp. Sub-Dept., Montreal **Gen. Hosp.; Phys.-in-Chief, Royal Edward Chest** Hosp.; Ass't. Prof. McGill U.; Tel. WE 7-3653.

MACINTOSH, James H. M.; Med. Arts Clinic, Regina, Sask.; Man '52; Tel. LA 2-1651.

MacINTOSH, James F.; 911 Wellington St. E., Sault Ste. Marie, Ont. (res); Tor '52; Anaes; Anaes., Plummer & Gen. Hosp's.; Tel. 254-5161.

MACINTOSH, John W.; 6076 Coburg Rd., Halifax, N.S.; Dal '22; F.A.C.P.; IntMed; Telephone 423-7928.

MACINTOSH, John W., Jr.; 6076 Coburg Rd., Halifax, N.S.; Dal '51; Ass't. Phy. (OPD), Victoria Gen. Hosp.; Court Staff, Halifax Infirmary, Children's & Convalescent Hosp's.; Instr. Med., Dalhousie U.; Tel. 423-7928.

MACINTOSH, Mary L.; Tor'63; Res., Dept. of Psy., U. of Toronto, Toronto 5, Ont.

MacINTOSH, Nadine; 356 Kensington Ave., Montreal 6, P.Q.; '45.

MacINTOSH, O. Carvell; Dal'40; MC Path; Path; Dir. of Labs., Halifax Infirmary, Halifax, N.S.

MacINTOSH, Robert A.; Fredericton Med. Clinic, 206 Rookwood Ave., Fredericton, N.B.; 134 Parkhurst Dr. (res); McG '42; F.A.C.S., F.R.C.S.(C), GenSurg; Staff, Victoria Public Hosp.; Telephone 475-7701.

MacINTYRE, George D.; High St., Vankleek Hill, Ont.; McG '13; Tel. 678-2010.

MACINTYRE, H. I.; Belmont, R.R. 1, Ont.; Wes '53; M.C.G.P.

MacINTYRE, Iain D.; 327 N. Christina St., Sarnia, Ont.; 1292 Lakeshore Rd. (res); Glasgow **(Scot.) '40; M.R.C.O.G., F.A.S.E.A.; ObstGyn;** Staff (ObstGyn.), Sarnia Gen. & St. Joseph's **Hosp's.; Tel. DI 4-0851.**

MacINTYRE, John A.; Ste. 4, Carnduff B'dg., Yorkton, Sask.; Man '53; Active Staff, Yorkton Union Hosp.; Tel. 783-2755.

MacINTYRE, Kenneth R.; Lunenburg, N.S.; Dal '64; Staff, Fishermen's Mem. Hosp.; Tel. 634-4454.

MACINTYRE, Mary W.; 104 St. Clair Ave., Ham**ilton, Ont.; 24 Rosedene Ave. (res); Dal '39; Tel. LI 5-2433.**

MacISAAC, Cyril A.; 409 Braidwood Ave., Peterborough, Ont.; Ott '56; Tel. RI 5-1341.

MacISAAC, Cyril J.; McG '60; Res., Hosp. for Sick Children, Toronto, Ont.

MacISAAC, Stephen G.; Dal'61; Urol; Staff, Queen Mary Vet's Hosp., Montreal 26, P.Q.

MACISAAC, Wilfred; Margaree Forks, N.S.; Dal '38; Otol; Bronchoscopist, Point Edward Hosp., Sydney; Tel. 564-5531.

MACIVER, Donald A., Surg. Capt.; National Defence Med. Centre, Ottawa 8, Ont.; Edinburgh (Scot.) '42; GenSurg; Chief of Surg., NDMC; Assoc. Prof. (Surg.), U. of Ottawa; Tel. 733-6600.

MACIVOR, John; 986 Third Ave. E., Owen Sound, Ont.; 764 Second Ave. W. (res); Tor '45; **Ophth.; Staff, Owen Sound Gen. & Marine Hosp.; Tel. FR. 6-6936.**

MACK, B. H. Raymond; 23 Baldwin St., Port Hope, Ont.; Qns'46; Tel. 885-4341.

MACK, F. Gordon; Med. Arts Bldg., 5880 Spring Garden Rd., Halifax, N.S.; 5660 Ogilvie St. (res); Dal '44; FRCS(C); Urol; Hd., Dept. of Urol., Halifax Infirmary & Chidren's Hosp's.; Assoc. Urol. Victoria Gen. Hosp.; Assoc. Prof. (Urol.), Dalhousie U.; Tel. 423-7924.

MACK, Gordon J.; Box 820 Kitimat, B.C.; 1457 **Albatross (res); Qns '49; FACS; FRCS(C); GenSurg; Chief of Staff, Kitimat Gen. Hosp.; Chief MO, Aluminum Co. of Canada; Kitimat Works; Tel. 982.**

MACKAY, Alward M.; Albert, Albert Co., N.B.; Dal'64.

MACKAY, Andre; 1681 Rachel, Montreal 34, P.Q.; 3840 Parc Lafontaine (res); Mon '43; F.C.C.P.; Pulm. Dis. & TB (PQ); F.R.C.P.(C), IntMed; **Ass't. Dept. of Med.**, Hop.-Notre-Dame; Ass't. Prof. (Clin.Med.), U. of Mtl., & Med. Dir. Alliance Assur. Co.; Tel. LA 6-5909.

MACKAY, Bruce K.; Irving Clinic, 74 W. Seymour, Kamloops, B.C.; 299 St. Paul St. W. (res); Tor'41; FACP; FICA (Ang.); FCCP; IntMed; Chief, Dept. of Med., Royal Inland Hosp.; Tel. 372-5251.

MACKAY, C. MacKenzie; 43 Vansittart, Woodstock, Ont. (res); Tor '03; Retired.

MACKAY, Donald; Rosedale Ave., Stettler, Alta.; Edinburgh (Scot.) '39; L.R.C.P. & S. (Edin.), L.R.F.P.S.(Glas.), D.P.H.; M.O H., Alberta East Central Health Unit No. 10; Tel. 742-2636.

MACKAY, Donald G.; 4458 Sherbrooke St. W., Westmount 6, Montreal, P.Q.; Edinburgh (Scot.) '45; M.O.H., City of Westmount; Att'd. Staff, Montreal Gen. Hosp.; Med. Adviser, Provincial Transport Co.; Tel. WE 7-2907.

MacKAY, Donald H.; X-Ray Dept., Chatham Gen. Hosp., Chatham, Ont.; Dal'53; DABR; DiagRad; Court. Staff, St. Joseph's Hosp. & Sydenham Dist. Hosp., Wallaceburg.

MACKAY, Doris E. (Watson); Ste. 150, 5780 Cambie St., Vancouver, B.C.; Alb '48; Anaes; PhysMed. & Rehab; Dir., Dept. of PhysMed., St. Paul's Hosp.; Med. Dir., Soc. for Rehab. Adult Cerebral Palsied; Tel. FA 1-3713.

MacKAY, Duncan W.; Box 188, Victoria Harbour, Ont.

MacKAY, Elizabeth N.; 415 Walmer Rd., Apt. 21, Toronto 4, Ont. (res); McG '40; DPH; PH; M.O. I/c Cancer Sect., Med. Statistics, Ont. Dept. of Health; Tel. EM 3-1211.

MACKAY, George; 801-2 Fairmont Med. Bldg., 750 West Broadway, Vancouver 9, B.C.; 1757 W. 40th Ave. (res); Man '36; F.R.C.S. (Edin.); GenSurg; Tel. TR 6-2145.

MACKAY, Harold V.; Peterborough Clinic, 327 Charlotte St., Peterborough, Ont.; 798 Norwood Terr. (res); Dal '51; Active Med. Staff, Peterborough Civic & St. Joseph's Hosp's.; Tel. 743-2040.

MACKAY, Harriet A.; (see CAWTHORPE).

MACKAY, H. F.; Mar Bldg., New Glasgow, N.S.; 89 High St. (res); Dal '25; GenSurg; Med. Staff, Aberdeen Hosp.; Tel. 752-6838.

MACKAY, Hugh J.; 113 McKenzie Ave., Revelstoke. B.C.; 202—6th St. E. (res); Edinburgh (Scot.) '43.

MACKAY, Ian D.; 215 College St., Apt. 241, Toronto 2B, Ont.; Wes'60; GenSurg.

MACKAY, Ian E.; 12 Acadia Ave., Stellarton, N.S.; McG '37; MCGP; Staff, Aberdeen Hosp. New Glasgow; Tel. 752-1565.

MACKAY, Iain M.; 230 Rosedale Heights Dr., Toronto 7, Ont.; Tor'43; DABA, FACA; Anaes; Sr. Anaes., Toronto Gen Hosp.; Cons., Princess Margaret & Wellesley Hosp's; Assoc. (Anaes.), U. of Toronto; Tel. 489-0535.

MACKAY, Jacques R.; Ste C824, 3100 Ave, Ellendale, Montreal 26, P.Q.; Mon '55; Psy; Staff, Mtl. Children's Hosp.; Dem. Queen Mary Vets'. Hosp.; Tel. 737-8346.

MACKAY, James; 440 Brown's Line, Toronto 14, Ont.; Tor'49; D.Psy; Psy; Dir. of Psy. Unit, Queensway Gen. Hosp.; Tel. 251-7291.

MACKAY, J. Alastair; 541 Professional Bldg., Edmonton, Alta.; Alb '48; Anaes; Chief, Dept. of Anaes., Misericordia Hosp.; Tel. GA 2-6552.

MACKAY, Jean C.; St.-Roch-des-Anulnaies, P.Q.; Mon '16; Med. Bd., Notre-Dame-de-Fatima, Ste-**Anne-de-la-Pocatiere & Hop.-St-Jean, Port-Joli; Tel. 353.**

MACKAY, John A.; Box 610, C. S. Williams Clinic, Fruitvale, B.C.; 355-3rd St. (res); McG '53; IntMed; Staff, Trail-Tadanac Hosp., Trail; Tel. 367-9211.

MacKAY, John A.; Sask '64; Res., University Hosp., Saskatoon, Sask.

MACKAY, John E.; Fredericton Med. Clinic, 206 Rookwood Ave., Fredericton, N.B.; McG '54; ObstGyn.; Tel. 475-7701.

MacKAY, John P.; 57 James St., Parry Sound, Ont.; Tor'45; MCGP; Dist. Coroner; Staff, Parry Sound Gen. & St. Joseph's Hosp's.; Tel. RI 6-2181.

MACKAY, John S.; 150 College St., Toronto, Ont.; Dal'61; FRMS; AOA; LAMCUK; FASCP; Path; MRC Fell., Dept. of Microbiol., School of Hygiene, U. of Toronto; Tel. 278-6517.

MacKAY, Kenneth H.; Ste. 107, 3000 Lawrence Ave. E., Scarborough, Ont.; 31 Pineridge Dr. Tor. 13 (res); Tor '50; ObstGyn.; Tel. 291-1361.

MACKAY, Kenneth J.; Staff, Ontario Hosp., Owen Sound, Ont.; Aberdeen (Scot.) '54. Abroad.

MACKAY, Malcolm I.; 1105 Pandora Ave., Victoria, B.C.; 1287 Rockland Ave. (res); Tor '47; DABS; FRCS(C); GenSurg; Tel. EV 5-1614.

MacKAY, Mary C.; 435 Oxford St., Halifax, N.S.; Dal '60.

MacKAY, Ritchie J.; Ste. G. 02, 3000 Lawrence Ave. E., Scarborough, Ont.; 104 Cedarbrae Blvd. (res); Path; Staff, Scarborough Gen. Hosp.; Dem. (Path), U. of Toronto; Tel. AX 3-8181.

MACKAY, Ronald A.; 146 Main St., **Milton,** Ont.; Charles St. (res); Tor '50; Staff, Milton Gen. Hosp.; Tel. TR 8-2383.

MacKAY, Ronald D.; Ste. 310, 5780 Cambie St., Vancouver 15, B.C.; 1164 W. 40th Ave. (res); **Dal '50; M.C.G.P.; Tel. FA 5-1712.**

MacKAY, Ross C.; 301 Russell Hill Rd., Toronto 7, Ont. (res); Tor '51; IntMed; O.P. Teach. Staff (Med.), Toronto Western Hosp.; Assoc. Med. Dir., Crown Life Insce. Co.; Tel. 924-6811.

MACKAY, R. W. Murray; Dal '28; F.A.P.A., M.R.C.P.S., Psy; Supt., Nova Scotia Hosp., Dartmouth, N.S.; Ass't. Prof. of Psy., Dalhousie U., **Halifax, N.S.; Tel. 466-7411.**

MACKAY, W. Allan; Med. Centre, 5 Central St., Summerside, P.E.I.; Dal'66.

MacKAY, Willard W.; Newcastle Medical Clinic, Box 1360, 246 Delano Ave., Newcastle N.B.; Dal '56.

MacKECHNIE, Graeme S.; Golden Manor, 481 Melrose, Timmins, Ont.; Tor '28; GenSurg.

MACKECHNIE, Hugh A.; 718 Granville St., Vancouver, B.C.; 1541—29th Ave. W. (res); Tor '28; DermSyph; Att. Staff, Vancouver Gen. Hosp.; **Sub., Dept. of Derm., U. of British Columbia; Tel. MU 4-7012.**

MacKEEN, Albro D.; 6150 Oakland Rd., Halifax, N.S.; Dal'59; DiagRad. Ass't Radiol. Victoria Gen. Hosp.

MacKEIGAN, Donald S.; 40 Crichton Pk. Rd., Dartmouth, N.S. (res); Dal '44; GenSurg; **M.C.-G.P.; Staff, Camp Hill Hosp., Halifax; Tel. 423-1371.**

MACKENZIE, Adrian; Pathology Inst., 5800 University, Halifax, N.S.; Dal'54.

MacKENZIE, Alexander D.; 21 Water St., Penetanguishene, Ont.; 13 Fox St. (res); Tor '48; Dist. Coroner; Tel. 549-2516.

MACKENZIE, A. Lewen; 417 Islington Ave. N., Islington, Ont.; Tor '32; AMCGP; FRCS(Edin.); GenSurg; Assoc. Staff, Toronto Western Hosp.; Tel. 233-7115.

MACKENZIE, Allan D., F/L; McG'64; Ass't. Res. (Surg.), Canadian Forces Hosp., Kingston, Ont.; Tel. 546-0981.

MACKENZIE, C. Grant.; 309 Lancaster St. W., Kitchener, Ont.; Qns'52; Psy; Tel. 744-6673.

MacKENZIE, Charles R. S.; 131 Ontario St., St. Catharines Ont.; 40 Marsdale Dr. (res); McG '49; ObstGyn; Staff. Hotel Dieu & Gen. Hosp's.; Tel. MU 4-9201

MACKENZIE, Cortland J. G.; Dept. of PrevMed., Fac. of Med., U. of British Columbia, Vancouver 8, B.C.; Qns'51; DPH; PH; Ass't. Prof. (Prev-Med.), UBC; Tel. 228-2772.

MACKENZIE, C. R.; 2 Southwick St., St. Thomas, Ont.; Tor '08.

MacKENZIE, David J.; 208 St. Clair Ave. W., Toronto 7, Ont.; Tor '41; FRCP(C), IntMed; Staff Phys. & Dir., Special Treatment Clin., St. Michael's Hosp.; Ass't. Prof. (Med.), U. of Toronto; Tel. 924-4748.

MACKENZIE, David W. Jr.; Eldon, P.E.I.; McG '36, M.A. (Cantab.); D.Sc. (Columbia); GenSurg.

MacKENZIE, Donald A.; Ste. 204, 450 Central Ave. London, Ont.; 1067 The Parkway (res); Wes '46; M.Sc.; FACS; FRCS(C); GenSurg; Teach. Staff, St. Joseph's Hosp.; Court. Staff Victoria Hosp.; Surg. Cons., Ontario Cancer Fdn., London Clinic; Instr. (Surg.), U. of Western Ont.; Tel. GE 9-1161.

MacKENZIE, Donald E.; 336 Kings Rd., Sydney, N.S.; Dal '58; IntMed; Assoc. Staff, Sydney City & St. Rita's Hosp's.; Tel. 562-3194.

MACKENZIE, Donald H.; Apt. 1705, 111 Raglan Ave., Toronto 10, Ont.; Tor'54; IntMed; Phys., New Toronto Health Serv.

MACKENZIE, Donald J.; R.R. No. 2, Marion Bridge, Cape Breton Co., N.S.; Dal '18; F.A.-P.H.A., F.R.C.P.(C), Bact; Dir. of Labs (PH), Prov. of N.S.; Retired.

MacKENZIE, Douglas H.; 588 Charlotte St., Sydney, N.S.; 380 Cottage Rd. (res); Dal '47; F.A.-C.S.; GenSurg; Staff, Sydney City & St. Rita Hosp's.; Tel. 564-8301.

MacKENZIE, Elmer A.; Musquodoboit Harbour, N.S.; Dal '56; AMCGP.

MACKENZIE, F. Douglas; Willow Chest Centre, 2647 Willow St., Vancouver, B.C.; 6030 Blenheim (res); McG '40; F.R.C.S. (Edin.); GenSurg; Surg., Willow Chest Centre; Att. Staff, Vancouver Gen. Hosp.; Tel. TR 2-1733.

MACKENZIE-HARPUR, Eleanor R.; 51 Cedar Ave., Pte. Claire, P.Q. (Res.); McG'39; Path-Bact; Dir. (Biochem. & Metabolism), Montreal Children's Hosp.; Dem. (Paed.), McGill U.; Tel. WE 7-8511.

MacKENZIE, Henry H.; 511 Ash St., New Westminster, B.C. (res); McG '14; Coroner for Province of B.C. in New Westminster.

MACKENZIE, Hugh N.; Medical Centre, Nipawin, Sask; Aberdeen (Scot.) '57; Tel. 2626.

MacKENZIE, Ian D.; 194 E. King Edward St., Vancouver 10, B.C.; Tor'64.

MACKENZIE, James R.; 5915 McLynn Ave., Montreal 29, P.Q.; McG '59; FRCS(C), GenSurg.

MACKENZIE, J. Conrad; Ste. 140, 5780 Cambie St., Vancouver 14, B.C.; 4561 Angus Dr. (res); McG '49; M.C.G.P.; Tel. FA 7-6318.

MACKENZIE, J. E. Gordon; Strathclair, Man.; Man '30.

MacKENZIE, John K.; 811 St. Charles St., Toronto 5, Ont. (res); **Qns '51; Staff, Workmen's** Compensation **Hosp., 115** Torbarrie **Rd.,** Downsview; **Tel. 244-1761.**

MACKENZIE, J. Robert; Mitton-Essex Med. Bldg., 168 Essex St., Sarnia, Ont.; 1375 Robin Lane (res); Tor '54; M.C.G.P.; FAGS; Hd. Dept. of G.P. Sarnia Gen. Hosp.; Active Staff, St. Joseph's Hosp.; Bd. of Governors Physicians Serv. Inc., Toronto; Tel. 337-3245.

MacKENZIE, J. Ross; 257 Springbank Ave., Woodstock, Ont. (res); Aberdeen (Scot.) '46; **FACP; FRCP(C), Path; Pathol., Woodstock Gen. Hosp.; Cons. (Path), Stratford Gen.; Pathol., Att'y. Gen. Dept.; Tel. LE 7-5511; Abroad.**

MACKENZIE, John W. S.; Elmvale, Ont.; Tor '58; Staff, Penetanguishene Gen. Hosp.; Tel. 130.

MACKENZIE, John W.; 427 Med. Arts Bldg., Saskatoon, Sask.; 856 University Dr. (Res.); **Glasgow (Scot.) '37; MD; Paed; Att. Paed., University, St. Paul's & Saskatoon City Hosp's.; Clin. Assoc. (Paed.), U. of Saskatchewan; Tel. 242-0991.**

MACKENZIE, J. Wendell; 170 Fitzroy St., Charlottetown, P.E.I.; McG'12; IntMed.; Tel. 894-7325.

MACKENZIE, K. B.; 21 Wellington St. N., Woodstock, Ont.; 187 Vansittart (res); Tor '31; Dist. Coroner; Tel. 537-5241.

MACKENZIE, Kenneth R.; 687 Pine Ave. W., Montreal 2, P.Q.; 3655 Ridgewood Ave., Apt. 602 (res); St. Barts (Eng.) 38; MRCS; LRCP; Ph.D. (Exper. Med.); IntMed (PQ); Ass't. Phys. & Dir. Clin. Labs., Royal Victoria Hosp.; Att'd. Phys., Mtl. Prot. Hosp.; Cons. (Rheum.), Queen Mary Vet's. Hosp.; Ass't. Prof. (Med.), McGill U.; Tel. VI 2-1251.

MACKENZIE, Kenneth S.; Dal '65; Staff, Queen Charlotte Hosp., Queen Charlotte City, B.C.; Tel. 629-4437.

MACKENZIE, Kenneth W.; 125 Botsford St., Moncton, N.B.; Dal '35; F.A.C.S., GenSurg; Surg. Staff, Moncton Hosp.; Tel. EV 4-4217.

MACKENZIE, Malcolm B.; 206 Cote St. Antoine Rd., Westmount, Montreal, P.Q. (res); McG '42; Path. (P.Q.); Path., Reddy Memorial Hosp., 4039 Tupper St., Montreal; Dem. (Path.) McGill U.; Tel. WE 5-9641, Loc. 25.

MacKENZIE, R. Gordon; 440 Hinton Ave., Ottawa, Ont.; 193 Island Park Dr., Ott. 3 (res); Dal '43; Anaes; Staff Anaes., Ottawa Civic Hosp.; Tel. PA 9-2511.

MACKENZIE, Robert A.; 1 Field Ambulance, SOEST CFPO 5050, CAF, Europe; Sask'63; Abroad.

MACKENZIE, Robert N.; 1401 Ridgeway St., Fort William, Ont. (res); Tor '52; DMR; DABR; DiagRad; Dir., Dept. of Rad., McKellar Gen. Hosp.; Tel. 622-7140.

MACKENZIE, Ross G.; 3000 Yonge St., Toronto, Ont.; 127 Sandringham Dr. (res); Tor '31; Ass't. Prof. (Anat.), U. of Toronto; Telephone HU 3-8967.

MACKENZIE, Seymour G.; 36 Logan St., Truro, N.S.; 187 Queen St. (res); Dal '40; F.R.C.S.(C) GenSurg; Staff, Colchester County Hosp.; Tel. 893-9161.

MacKENZIE, Thomas C.; 3256 Cambie, Vancouver 9, B.C.; Tor '57; Tel. TR 4-0261.

MacKENZIE, Veronica (Willis); 257 Springbank Ave., Woodstock, Ont. (res); Liverpool (Eng.) '51; Temp. Retired.

MACKENZIE, Walter C.; 504 Med. Arts Bldg., Edmonton, Alta.; 10131 Clifton Pl. (res); Dal '33; F.A.C.S., F.R.C.S.(C), GenSurg; Sr. Surg. Cons. DVA, Nr. Alta.; Dean, Fac. of Med. & Prof. of Surg., U. of Alberta; Tel. GA 2-6956.

MACKENZIE, Walter F.; 22 Livingston Ave., Grimsby, Ont.; 16 Cherryhill Dr. (res); Tor '52; MCGP; Tel. 945-4811.

MacKENZIE, Wilfred F.; 901 O'Connor Dr., Ste. 6, Toronto 16, Ont.; 216 Parkview Hill Crt. (res); Tor '41; Tel. PL 5-8281.

MACKENZIE, William J.; 5309 W. Blvd., Vancouver 13, B.C.; Tor '11.

MACKERCHER, Donald A.; Cobden, Ont.; McG **'28; Dist. Coroner; Tel. 464-2073.**

MACKEY, Arthur G.; 340 McLeod St., Ottawa Ont.; McG '52; MCGP; Staff, Ottawa Civic & Grace Hosp's.; Tel. 235-7553.

MACKEY, Lawrence R.; C.N.R. Med. Division, C.N.R. Depot, Winnipeg 9, Man.; Man'31; Urol; D.P.H. (Tor.).

MACKEY, Leslie W.; Guy's Hosp. (London, Eng.)'49; Staff, Athabasca Health Unit, Athabasca, Alta.

MACKICHAN, H. Gerald; 42 Wharncliffe Rd. N., London, Ont.; 822 Clearview Ave. (res); Wes '50; MCGP; Tel. 432-6786.

MACKID, L. Stewart; 220-6th Ave. E., Calgary, Alta.; McG '04; F.A.C.S., GenSurg; **Retired.**

MACKIE, Andrew T.; 270 Lochiel St., Renfrew, **Ont.; Qns '41; Tel. HE 2-4334.**

MACKIE, Kenneth W.; 74 Johnson St., Kingston, Ont.; Tor '56; DiagRad; Radiol., Kingston Gen. Hosp.; Lect. (Rad.), Queen's U.; Tel. 542-2821.

MacKIMMIE, John C.; 595 Main St., Lachute, P.Q.; McG'52; MCGP; Tel. 562-2919.

MacKIMMIE, Suzanne S.; Box 142, 593 Main St., Lachute, P.Q.; Mon '52; Tel. 562-2919.

MACKINLAY, Archie K.; 350 Wellington St., Sarnia, Ont.; 146 S. Mitton St. (res); Tor '47. Tel. 337-3221.

MACKINLAY, Robert; 350 Wellington St., Sarnia, Ont.; Coilavoulin, Camlachie, Ont. (res); Tor '16; GenSurg; Dist. Coroner.
MacKINLEY, R. Douglas; 350 Wellington St., Sarnia, Ont.; 930 Lakeshore Rd. (res) Wes '50; Dist. Coroner; Tel. ED 7-3221.

MACKINNON, Alpin G.; 9 Kinnear St., Ottawa 3, Ont.; Tor'38; Admin. Cdn. Pension Comm.; Tel. CE 2-8211.
MACKINNON, A. M.; Ste. 204, 77 Westmount Rd., Guelph, Ont.; Tor'45.
MacKINNON, Archibald L.; 86 Callander Dr., Guelph, Ont. (res); Tor '24; Psy; Part-time Staff, Dept. of Reform Inst., Prov. of Ont.; Tel. TA 2-0020.
MACKINNON, Arthur H.; 405 Medical Centre, 906-8th Ave. Calgary, Alta.; 505 Somioa Ave. (res); Edin. (Scot.) '43; Tel. 263-0676.
MacKINNON, Bernard L.; 200 Douglas Ave., Saint John, N.B.; Dal '60; AMCGP; Staff, Lancaster DVA Hosp.; Tel. 694-2651.
MACKINNON, C. Gordon; 23 Balmoral Road, Halifax, N.S.; Dal '31; Anaes; Chief, Dept. of Anaes., Camp Hill DVA Hosp.; Ass't. Prof. (Anaes.), Dalhousie U.; Tel. 423-1371.
MACKINNON, George E. L.; 405-12th Ave. S., Cranbrook, B.C. (res); McG '02; Retired.
MacKINNON, George L.; 1010 Fairmont Med. Bldg., 750 W. Broadway, Vancouver 9, B.C.; 5887 Highbury St. Van. 13 (res); McG '48; ObstGyn; Att'd. Staff, St. Vincent's Hosp.; Telephone TR 2-5467.
MacKINNON, Hector H.; Tor'41; DTM; FACP; FRCP(C), IntMed; Staff, Inst. of Path., Dalhousie U., Halifax, N.S.
MACKINNON, Kenneth J.; 4500 Sherbrooke St. W., Westmount, Montreal 6, P.Q.; 465 Argyle Ave., Westmount (res); Dal '45; F.R.C.S.(C), Urol; Urol.-in-Chief, Royal Victoria Hosp.; Cons. (Urol.), Montreal Children's Hosp.; Assoc. Prof. (Surg.) (Urol.), McGill U.; Tel. 845-5376.
MACKINNON, Malcolm H.; 135 Main St., Woodstock, N.B.; Qns '34.
MACKINNON, Michael A.; 199 Westminster Blvd., La Salle, Ont.; Dal '62; AMCGP.
MacKINNON, Neil D.; Tor '37; D.P.H.; Zone Supt., Indian & Northern Health Services, 304 Customs Bldg., Calgary, Alta.
MACKINNON, Stuart J.; 300 Med. Centre, 906-8th Ave. S.W., Calgary, Alta.; 505 Sonora Ave. (res); Edinburgh (Scot.) '45; L.R.C.P. & S. Edin.), L.R.F.P.S.(Glas.); Staff, Calgary Gen., Holy Cross & Grace Hosp's.; Tel. 269-1593.
MacKINNON, William B.; 532 Med. Arts Bldg., Winnipeg 1, Man.; 182 Montrose St., Wpg. 9 (res); Man '37; Ch.M. (Man.); F.I.C.S., F.R.C.S. (C), OrthSurg; Chief (Orth Dept.), St. Boniface Gen. Hosp.; Chief Surg., Shriner's Hosp.; Orth. Cons., Sanitorium Bd. of Manitoba, Ninette & St. Boniface San. & Dept. of Indian Affairs; Ass't. Prof. (OrthSurg.), U. of Manitoba; Tel. WH 2-3559.

MACKLEM, Peter T.; 20150 Lakeshore Rd., Baie d'Urfe, Ste-Anne-de-Bellevue, P.Q. (res); McG '56; FRCP(C), IntMed; Staff, Royal Victoria Hosp., Montreal; Tel. VI 2-1251.

MACKRELL, Estelle V.; (Peters); 2057 Caroline St. E., Burlington, Ont.; 790 Partridge Dr. (res); London (England) '51; MRCS; LRCP; AMCGP; Active Staff, Joseph Brant Mem. Hosp.; Tel. 634-5073.

MACLACHLAN, Peter N.; 115 LaMennais, Buckingham, P.Q.; Qns '32; GenSurg (PQ); M.C.-G.P.; Chief Surg., St. Michael's Hosp.; Indus. Phys., Electric Reduction Co.; Tel. YU 6-3447.

MacLACHLAN, Robert G.; 814 Cook Rd., Richmond, B.C.; Wes '57; FRCS(C), OrthSurg; Cons. Staff, Shaughnessy DVA Hosp.; Assoc. Staff, St. Paul's Hosp.; Tel. 278-9333.

MACLACHLAN, Thomas B.; Tor'52; FRCS(C), ObstGyn; Staff, University Hosp., Saskatoon, Sask.; Ass't. Prof., U. of Saskatchewan; Tel. 242-7641.

MacLAREN, Douglas B.; 204 Jeffcoat Dr., Toronto, Ont.; Tor '37; FRCS(C), GenSurg; Tel. 244-1928.

MACLAREN, Lloyd B.; Alert Bay, B.C.; Woss Camp, Englewood (res); Alb '44; Staff, St. George's Hosp.; Tel. 974-5215.
MACLAREN, Mary C. (Chisholm); 746 Eastbourne Ave., Ottawa 7, Ont.; Dal'58; Retired.
MACLAREN, R. Douglas; 925 W. Georgia St., Vancouver, B.C.; 5909 Cartier St. (res); Tor '37; M.C.A.A.; Cons., Allergy Clin. Shaughnessy (D.V.A.) Hosp.; Tel. MU 1-7188.
MacLAREN, Robert G. C.; Ontario Cancer Fdn., Henderson Gen. Hosp., Hamilton, Ont.; Kings Coll. (London, Eng.) '46; DMRT; FRCS(Eng.); DMRT; TherRad; Active Staff, Hamilton Civic Hosp.; Staff, St. Joseph's Hosp.; Tel. 389-1371.

MacLAUGHLIN, James P.; 811 Boyd Bldg., Portage Ave., Winnipeg 1, Man.; 500 Laidlaw Blvd. (res); Dublin (Ire.) '39; M.Rad. (Liverpool); DMRD (Lond.); DiagRad; Cons. Rad., Winnipeg Municipal & Victoria Gen. Hosp's.; Tel. WH 2-1836.

MacLEAN, Alastair D.; Fort MacLeod, Alta.; Qns '44; Dist. Coroner; Tel. 262.
MACLEAN, Alexander C.; Box 100, New Richmond, Bon Co., P.Q.; Dal '33.
MacLEAN, Arnold E.; Dal '63; Res., Montreal Gen. Hosp., Montreal 25, P.Q.
MacLEAN, Bruce L.; 128-10th St. W., Owen Sound, Ont.; 548-4th St. W. (res); Tor '49; MCGP; Staff, Owen Sound Gen. & Marine Hosp's; Tel. 376-3895.
MacLEAN, Catriona D.; 734 Blueridge Ave., North Vancouver, B.C. (res); McG '54; Paed; Ass't. Dir., HCC, O.P.D., Vancouver Gen. Hosp.; Tel. YU 5-5455.
MACLEAN, Charles A.; 1407-750 W. Broadway, Vancouver, B.C.; 3890 Osler St., Van. 9 (res); McG '47; F.R.C.P.(C), IntMed; Att'd. Staff, Shaughnessy & St. Vincent's Hosp's.; Vis. Staff, Van. Gen. Hosp.; Clin. Instr. (Med.), U. of British Columbia; Tel. TR 4-2211.
MacLEAN, Christina R.; Advocate Harbour, Cumberland Co., N.S.; Glasgow (Scot.) '41.

MACLEAN, Charles B.; Maple St., Inverness, N.S.; Church St. (res); Dal '61; AMCGP; Tel. 299.

MACLEAN, C. Peter; 171 King St., St. Catharines, Ont.; 2 Pine Hill (res); McG '23.

MacLEAN, Donald; Box 490, Williams Lake, B.C.; Edinbugh (Scot.) '60; Tel. 392-7221.

MACLEAN, Donald J. G.; 159 Marion, Winnipeg, Man.; Man '24.

MACLEAN, Donald L., OBE; 94 Chatsworth Dr., Toronto 12, Ont. (res); Tor'25; DABPH & PrevMed; DPH; PH; Assoc. Dir., Connaught Med. Research Labs., U. of Toronto; Prof. Epid. & Sec. Schl. of Hygiene; Tel. 928-2741.

MacLEAN, Douglas R.; 28 Weber St. W. Kitchener, Ont.; 327 Longfellow Dr., Waterloo (res); Tor'60; AMCGP; Sec. Med. Staff, Kitchener-Waterloo Hosp.; Tel. 745-5617.

MacLEAN, Hugh M.; 97 Botsford St., Moncton, N.B.; Dal '28; F.A.C.S., GenSurg; Surg., Moncton Hosp.; Tel. EV 4-3939.

MACLEAN, Ian S.; 111 Medical Arts Bldg., 404 Graham Ave., Winnipeg 1, Man.; 73 Harvard Ave. (res); Man '39; D.I.H. (Lond.); Med. Dir., Bristol Aero Indus. (Wpg.) Ltd. & Paulin Chambers Ltd.; Tel. WH 3-9640.

MACLEAN, James G.; 115 Hazen St., Saint John, N.B.; Dal'42; DermSyph; Attend. Staff, Gen. Hosp., St. Joseph's & DVA Hosps., Lancaster, N.B.; Tel. 692-3604.

MACLEAN, John; 54 Third St., Collingwood, Ont.; 255 Minnesota St. (res); McG '37; GenSurg.; Tel. 445-2030.

MacLEAN, John A.; 1849 Yonge St., Toronto 7, Ont.; 177 Inglewood Dr. (res); Tor '43; Paed; Clin. Ass't., Hosp. for Sick Children; Chief of Paed., Northwestern Gen. Hosp.; Clin. Teach. U. of Toronto; Tel. HU 8-8876.

MACLEAN, John P.; 194 Kingsway, Winnipeg 9, Man.; Man '50; IntMed; Dir. Research, St. Boniface Hosp.; Ass't. Prof. (Med.), U. of Manitoba; Tel. GL 3-4243.

MACLEAN, John T.; 1538 Sherbrooke St. W.; Ste 202, Montreal, P.Q.; 599 Victoria Ave., Westmount (res); Man '34; D.A.B.U., F.A.C.S., F.R.C.S.(C), Urol.; Urol., Royal Victoria Hosp.; Dir(Urol.), Queen Mary Vets. Hosp.; Cons. (Urol.), Grace Dart. Hosp.; Ass't. Prof. (Surg.) McGill U.; Tel. WE 5-2352.

MACLEAN, J. Robert; St. 3; 1306-750 W. Broadway, Vancouver 9, B.C.; 982 W. 18th Ave. (res); Tor '50; Paed; Clin. Ass't. Prof. U. of British Columbia; Tel. TR 9-4564.

MacLEAN, J. Ross; 7020 Adera St., Vancouver, B.C. (res); Man '49; MCGP; Med. Dir., Hollywood Hosp., Ltd., 515 Fifth Ave., New Westminster; Tel. LA 2-8621.

MacLEAN, Kenneth; Wellandport, Ont.; Wes '09.

MacLEAN, Lloyd D.; 687 Pine Ave. W., Montreal 2, P.Q.; 5 Renfrew, Westmount (res); Alb '49; **Ph.D. (Minn.); DABTS; DABS; FRCS(C); Surg-in-Chief, Royal Victoria Hosp.; Prof of Surg., McGill U.; Tel. VI 2-1251, Loc. 1559.**

MacLEAN, Lloyd R.; 816 Woodbine Blvd., Jackson, Mich., U.S.A.; Qns'59; Urol; Abroad.

MACLEAN, Mairi M. (See Narod).

MACLEAN, Margaret J.; 177 Inglewood Dr., Toronto 12, Ont. (res); Tor '43; Not practising.

MACLEAN, N. Bruce; 625-5th Ave., New Westminster, B.C.; 1910 Dublin St. (res); Man '45; Urol; Tel. LA 1-7761.

MACLEAN, Norman J.; Maple St., Inverness, N.S.; Dal '41; Tel. 36.

MACLEAN, Randall R.; Box 1000, Ponoka, Alta.; **Alb '27; F.A.P.A., NeurPsy; Hon. Staff, U. of** Alberta; Dir., Mental Health Div., Alberta; Retired.

MACLEAN, R. Bruce; Brickyard Rd., R.R.1., Wellington B.C.; UBC '56; Anaes; Active Staff, Nanaimo Reg., Ladysmith Gen. & Nanaimo Indian Hosp's.; Tel. SK 3-8998.

MacLEAN, Sheina (See Hepworth).

MacLEAN, S. Keith; 30 George St. N., Galt, Ont.; 180 Salisbury Ave. (res); Qns '52; GenSurg; Staff, South Waterloo Mem. Hosp., Galt & St. Mary's Hosp. & Freeport San., Kitchener; Tel. 621-4600.

MACLEAN, T. Ray; 5750 South St., Halifax, N.S.; 518 Young St. (res); Dal '30; MCGP; Tel. 423-7093.

MacLEAN, Walter D.; 20 Abercrombie Rd., New Glasgow, N.S.; 60 Herbert St. (res); Dal'53; Clin. Ass't. Surg., Aberdeen Hosp.; Tel. 2-5261.

MACLEAN, William A.; 1004-105th St., Edmonton, Alta.; 14408-95th Ave. (res); Man '49; FACS; DABS; FRCS(C), GenSurg; Active Staff, Royal Alexandra Hosp.; Court. Staff, University Hosp.; Lect. (Surg.), U. of Alberta; Chmn. Comm. on Cancer, Alta Div. C.M.A.; Tel. GA 4-2121.

MacLEAN, W. Robert; 327 Charlotte St., Peterborough, Ont.; 739 Wellet St. (res); McG '49; Paed; **Paed., Peterborough Clinic & Peter-**borough Civic & St. Joseph's Hosp's.; Tel. 743-2040.

MacLELLAN, C. Lorway; Charlotte St., Sydney, N.S.; McG '42; Staff, St. Rita's & Sydney City Hosp's.; Tel. 564-8408.

MACLELLAN, Donald I.; 114 Highfield St., Moncton, N.B.; Dal'54; FRCS(C), OrthSurg.

MacLELLAN, John A.; Dal '57; DiagRad; Staff, Charlottetown Hosp., 17 Haviland St., Charlottetown, P.E.I., Tel. 894-5561.

MacLELLAN, Robert A.; Upper Rawdon, R.R. No. 1, Hants Co.; N.S.; Dal '08; Tel. 1-12.

MACLENNAN, David A.; 78 Roseberry St., Campbellton, N.B.; 154 Roseberry St. (res); McG '29; F.R.C.S. (Edin.), F.R.C.S. (C) GenSurg; Gyn; Tel. PL 3-3156.

MacLENNAN, D. Stirling; Doulton Dr., R.R. No. 2, Port Credit, Ont. (res), Tor '16; Plant Phys., Anaconda American Brass Co.; M.O.H. New Toronto; Retired.

MacLENNAN Ian A.; Provincial Labs., Castle St. Saint John, N.B.; East Riverside, Kings Co. (res); McG '37; FCAP; DTM; PathBact; Path.-in-Chief, St. John's Gen. & St. Joseph's Hosp's.; Dir. of Labs., Dept. of Health, N.B.; Tel. 692-2644.

MacLENNAN, Jean M.; 206-5600 Dalhousie Rd., Vancouver 8 B.C. (res); Edinburgh (Scot.) '30; DPH; Paed; Hon. Vis. Staff, Vancouver Gen. Hosp. & Children's Hosp.; Med. Staff, Children's Aid Soc. & City Health Dept.; Clin. Instr. (Paed.), U. of British Columbia; Tel. CA 4-3826.

MACLENNAN, John A.; 13130 Riverside Dr., Tecumseh, Ont. (res); Wes '29; Med. Dir., Chrysler Corp. of Canada Ltd., Windsor; Tel. 252-3651.

MACLENNAN, John A.;12 Grant Cres., Saint John, N.B. (res); Dal'62; Tel. 693-3943.

MACLENNAN, John G.; 206 James S., Hamilton, Ont.; R.R. 1, Dundas (res); Alb '40; F.A.-C.A.; **Staff, Allergy Clin, Hamilton Gen. Hosp.; Tel. JA 9-0460.**

MacLENNAN, Myles R.; 3 Chippewa Dr., Chatham, Ont. (res); Man'57; DMR; DiagRad; Staff **St. Joseph's Hosp.; Te. EL 2-2500.**

MACLENNAN, N. Kenneth; Med. Arts Bldg., 336 Kings Rd., Sydney, N.S.; Dal '48; Obst-Gyn; Hd. (Obst.), St. Rita & Sydney City Hosp's.; Tel. 564-6185.

MACLEOD, A. G.; 53 King St., Dartmouth, N.S.; Dal '32; MO, WCB.

MACLEOD, Alan J.; 5880 Spring Garden Rd., Halifax, N.S.; Dal'50; IntMed; Ass't. Phys., Victoria Gen. Hosp.; Ass't. Prof. (Med.), Dalhousie University; Tel. 423-8968.

MacLEOD, Alastair W.; 3690 Peel St., Montreal, P.Q.; Glasgow (Scot.) '41; DPH; DPM; MRCP (Lond.); Psy; Assoc. Dir., Mental Hygiene Inst.; Att'd. Psy., Royal Victoria Hosp.; Assoc. Prof. Dept. of Psy., & Spec. Lect., School of Social Work, McGill U.; Training Analyst, Cdn. Inst. of Psychoanalysis; Tel. 844-3971.

MACLEOD, Angus A.; Bonshaw, P.E.I.; Dal '49.

MACLEOD, Ben M.; Brooks, Alta.; McG '48; Dist. Coroner.

MACLEOD, Bruce A.; 117 St. John St., Fort William, Ont.; Vickers Heights P.O. (res); Tor '35; FICS; ObstGyn; Chief-of-staff, McKellar Gen. Hosp.; Cons. ObstGyn., Fort William San.; Court. **Staff, Port Arthur Gen. & St. Joseph's Gen. Hosp's.; Tel. 622-5363.**

MacLEOD, David E.; 153 Pinnacle St., Belleville, Ont.; Dal'54; Ophth.; Active Staff, Belleville Gen. Hosp.; Tel. 962-1296.

MacLEOD, C.; Sunnybrook Hosp., Bayview Ave., Toronto 12, Ont.; Dal '23; Sr. Treatment Off., **D.V.A.; Tel. 485-8651; Retired.**

MACLEOD, Donald R. E.; 22 Austin Cr., Toronto, Ont. (res); Tor '35; D.P.H., Bact; Assoc. Prof., Dept. of Epidemiology & Biometrics, School of Hygiene & Research Assoc., Connaught **Med. Research Labs., U. of Toronto; Tel. RO 7-3807.**

MACLEOD, Enid (Johnson); 8 Glenwood Ave., Dartmouth, N.S. (res); Dal '37; Anaes; Retired.

MacLEOD, Eric C.; 231 Boland Ave., Sudbury, Ont. (res); Aberdeen (Scot.) '54; DPM; Psy; Dir., Psy. Unit, Sudbury Gen. Hosp., Tel. 674-1941.

MacLEOD, Frederick H.; 13 Garden St., Brock-ville, Ont.; 3 Hardy Cres. (res); Dal'40; FACS; **GenSurg; Chief of Surg., St.-Vincent-de-Paul Hosp.; Active Staff, Brockville Gen. & Cons. Surg., Ont. Hosp.; Tel. 345-5196.**

MACLEOD, Iain C.; Botwood, Nfld.; Glasgow (Scot.) '61.

MacLEOD, Ian D.; 611 Medical Arts Bldg., 404-406 Graham Ave., Winnipeg 1 Man.; Man '53; FRCS(C); GenSurg; Urol; Hd., Dept. of Urol., Deer Lodge & St. Boniface Hosp's.; Lect. Dept. of Surg., U. of Manitoba; Tel. 942-5879.

MacLEOD, Ian M.; Halifax Infirm. Queen St., Halifax, N.S.; 15 Lawnsdale Dr., Dartmouth (res); Dal '43; D.M.R., F.C.C.P.; D&T Rad; Assoc. Radiol., Halifax Infirmary; Cons. Rad., Nova Scotia Hosp., Dartmouth; Tel. 422-1511.

MACLEOD, James H.; 23 Court St., Liverpool, N.S.; Dal '52; GenSurg; Staff, Queens Gen. Hosp.; Tel. 354-3530. Abroad.

MacLEOD, James L.; Med. Clinic, 4794A Joyce Ave., Powell River, B.C.; 800 Maple (res); Alb '45; MCGP; Tel. HU5-6261.

MACLEOD, John A.; 265 Heneker St., Sherbrooke, P.Q.; McG '41; F.R.C.S. (Edin.); FACS; GenSurg (P.Q.), Att. Staff (Surg.), Sherbrooke Hosp.; Courtesy Staff, Hotel Dieu & St. Vincent de Paul Hosp's.; Tel. LO 2-0434.

MACLEOD, John G.; Finch, Ont.; Qns '20; Tel. 984-2316.

MACLEOD, J. Peter; McG'64; Res., Kingston Gen. Hosp., Kingston, Ont.

MACLEOD, J. Wendell, OBE; 75 Albert St., Ottawa 4, Ont.; 17 Avenue Rd. (res); McG '30; F.A.C.P., F.R.C.P.(C), IntMed; Exec. Sec., Assoc. of Cdn. Med. Colleges, Cdn. Universities Fdn.; Tel. 233-8431.

MacLEOD, Lloyd A.; 135 Main St., Liverpool, N.S.; Dal '43; Staff, Queen's Gen. Hosp.; Tel. 354-423.

MACLEOD, R. Keith; 1466 Ouellette Ave., Windsor, Ont.; Qns '59; ObstGyn; Active Staff (ObstGyn.), Grace, Metropolitan & Hotel-Dieu Hosp's.; Tel. 254-3261.

MACLEOD, Roderick J.; Sask'64; Res., Dept. of Psy., Montreal Gen. Hosp., Montreal 25, P.Q.

MACLEOD, S. Clair; 5880 Spring Garden Rd., Halifax, N.S.; Dal'59; FRCS(C); ObstGyn; Ass't. Gyn., Victoria Gen. Hosp.; Ass't. Prof. (ObstGyn), Dalhousie University; Tel. 423-7073.

MacLEOD, Ronald B.; 208 Mary St., Chilliwack, B.C.; Glasgow (Scot.) '58; Tel. 795-7228.

MACLURE, Hugh L.; Drayton Valley, Alta.; London (Eng.) '40; MRCS; LRCP; DTM & H (Lond.); MCGP; Chm., Med. Staff, Drayton Valley Mun. Hosp.; Tel. 542-3301.

MacMASTER, Duncan R; New Waterford, N.S.; Dal '60.

MACMASTER, John C.; 599 Empress St., Winnipeg 10, Man.; 353 Brock St., Wpg. 9 (res); Glasgow (Scot.) '29; M.B., Ch.B.; Ex. Dir., Manitoba Med. Serv.; Tel. SP 5-8371.

MACMILLAN, Albert C.; 2876 Rae St., Regina, Sask. (res); Qns '19; GenSurg.; Retired.

MACMILLAN, Angus B.; 302 Medical Arts Bldg., 1 Young St., Hamilton, Ont.; 120 W. 19th St., (res); Qns '55; F.R.C.P.(C), Paed; Chief of Paed., Chedoke Gen. & Children's Hosp.; City Staff, St. Joseph's & Hamilton Gen. Hosp's., Hamilton & Joseph Brant Mem. Hosp., Burlington; Tel. JA 2-9207.

MACMILLAN, Angus H.; 68 Charlton W., Hamilton, Ont.; Qns'50; DAAOS; FAAOS; OrthSurg; Chief (OrthSurg), Chedoke Gen. & Children's Hosp.; Attend. Staff, Hamilton Civic Hosp.; Cons., DVA, Hamilton; Tel. JA 8-8563.

MACMILLAN, Carleton L.; Chebucto St., Baddeck, N.S.; Dal '28; Public Health Off.; Dist. Coroner.

MacMILLAN, Charles C.; 42 Wellington Row, Saint John, N.B.; McG '54; Ophth; Staff, Saint John Gen., St. Joseph's & Lancaster DVA Hosp's.; Tel. 657-1084.

MacMILLAN, Charles W.; 359 Melville Ave., Westmount, Montreal 6, P.Q. (res); Dal '24; DPH; PH; Prof. & Hd. Dept. of Health & Social Medicine, McGill U.; Retired.

MACMILLAN, C. Lamont; '62; Res., Victoria Gen. Hosp., Halifax, N.S.

MacMILLAN, Clarence; 260 Islington Ave. N., Islington, Ont.; Tor '31.

MACMILLAN, Donald W.; 1165 Maple Ave., Quebec, P.Q.; Lav '40; Anaes (P.Q.); Chief of Anaes., Jeffrey Hale's Hosp.; Tel. 683-4471.

MacMILLAN, Francis A.; Charlottetown Clinic, 1 Rochford St., Charlottetown, P.E.I.; 76 McGill Ave. (res); McG '42; Staff, Charlottetown Hosp.; Tel. 4-5521.

MacMILLAN, H. Allan; Box 604, Charlottetown Clinic, 1 Rochford St., Charlottetown, PEI; 126 N. River Rd. (res); Ott '52; MCGP; Staff, Charlottetown & City Hosp's.; Att'd Phys., Beech Grove Chronic Care Unit; Dir. VD Control, P.E.I.: Tel. 894-5521.

MacMILLAN, Ian C.; 129 Kent St., Charlottetown, P.E.I.; Dal '55; Tel. 894-4297.

MACMILLAN, James A.; Newcastle, N.B.; McG '48.

MacMILLAN, James H.; 325 Main St. W., Grimsby, Ont.; Qns '24; MCGP; Retired.

MACMILLAN, John A.; 768 Seymour St., Vancouver, B.C.; McG'33; Att'd. Staff (Med.), Vancouver Gen. Hosp.; Dir., Indust. Med. Assoc.; Med. Dir., B.C. Tel. Co. Tel. 662-8144.

MacMILLAN, Joseph C.; 1499 Pharmacy Ave., Scarborough, Ont.; Tor '56; MCGP; Active Staff, Toronto East Gen., Scarborough Gen. & St. Michael's Hosp's.; Tel. HI 4-4466.

MacMILLAN, Ralph V.; Woodland Plaza, Cooksville, Ont.; 2095 Grange Dr. (res); Tor '60; AMCGP; Tel. 277-2842.

MacMILLAN, Robert L.; Room 136, Private Patient's Pavilion, Toronto Gen. Hosp., Toronto, Ont.; Tor'41; MRCP (Lond.); FACP; FRCP(C), IntMed; Phys., Toronto Gen. Hosp.; Ass't. Prof., U. of Toronto; Tel. 928-2720.

MacMILLAN, Robert M.; Apsley, Ont.; Qns '64.

MACMILLAN, Vernon H.; Sask'61; Res., New Mount Sinai Hosp., Toronto 2, Ont.

MacMURDO-MacMILLAN, Margaret; Box 172, Bedford, N.S.; Dal'57; MCGP.

MACNAB, Ian; Ste. 516, 1849 Yonge St., Toronto 7, Ont.; 230 Lytton Blvd. (res); Birmingham (Eng.) '43; Ch.B., M.B., FRCS (Eng.); FRCS (C); OrthSurg; Ass't. Surg. (Orth.Serv.), Toronto Gen. Hosp.; Assoc. (Surg.), U. of Toronto; Tel. 481-7295.

MACNAMARA, Harold O.; 109 Humberside Ave., Toronto, Ont.; Tor '22; Tel. Ro 9-5419.

MacNAUGHTON, Donald B.; 574 Princess St., Kingston, Ont.; 90 Collingwood St. (res); Qns '54; MCGP; Tel. 546-1714.

MacNAUGHTON, Eric A.; Ste. 330, Seaforth Med. Bldg., 3550 Cote des Neiges Rd., Montreal 25, P.Q.; 34 Thurlow Rd., Hamstead (res); McG'26; FRCS(C); GenSurg; ThorSurg (P.Q.); Cons. Surg., Montreal Gen. Hosp.; Sr. Cons. Surg., **Queen Mary Vet's Hosp.; Ass't. Prof. (Surg.), McGill U.; Tel. 935-7787.**

MacNAY, Kenneth R.; Wes '63; Staff, Inuvik Hosp., Inuvik, N.W.T.

MACNEIL, Frank A.; 529 Medical Arts Bldg., Winnipeg, Man.; 255 Dromore Ave. (res); Man **'16; F.A.A. Op.Ot.; Ophth; Tel. WH 2-6707.**

MacNIEL, Hugh C.; 1316 Fairmount Med. Bldg., 750 W. Broadway, Vancouver 9, B.C.; Tor'57; FRCS(C), OrthSurg; Teach. Fell., University of British Columbia.

MACNEIL, John D.; The Manitoba School, 3rd St. N.E., Portage La Prairie, Man.; Man'56; Psy. Med. Officer; Tel. 857-3403.

MacNEIL, John J.; Beech Clinic 350 Beech Ave., Toronto 13, Ont.; London (Eng.) '42; MRCS (Eng.); LRCP (Lond.); PlasSurg.

MACNEIL, John R.; Bay Medical Group, Glace Bay, N.S.; 133 Main St. (res); Dal '30; M.C.G.P.; **Staff St. Joseph's & Glace Bay Gen. Hosp.; Tel. 849-5521.**

MACNEIL, Robert W.; 2333 Portage Ave., Winnipeg, Man.; 113 Parkside Dr. (res); Man '43; Paed; Lect., (Paed.), U. of Manitoba; Hon. Att. Staff, Children's, Misericordia & Grace Hosp's.; Ass't. Paed., Winnipeg Gen. Hosp.; Tel. SP 2-9777.

MACNEILL, Donald D.; 22 Peachtree Park, Fonthill, Ont. (res); Tor '43; DiagRad; Dir., Dept. of Rad., Welland County Gen. Hosp.; Tel. RE 2-6111.

MACNEILL, Neil F.; Provincial Bldg., Prince St., Sydney, N.S.; Dal '43; DPH; Tel. 564-4447.

MacNEILL, Roy D.; Ste. 402, 625-5th Ave., New Westminster, B.C.; McG'48; FRCS(C), GenSurg; ThorSurg.

MacNICOLL, Wilfred T.; 576 Willard Ave., Toronto 9, Ont. (res); Tor '28.

MACNIVEN, F. M.; Tor '64; Res., Toronto Gen. Hosp., Toronto 2, Ont.

MACNUTT, Louis W.; 3195 Granville St., Vancouver 9, B.C.; 5946 Angus Dr. (res); McG '12; Tel. RE 3-8711.

MACOOMB, Richard K.; Winnipeg Clinic, St. Mary & Vaughan St., Winnipeg 1, Man.; Man '57; M.Sc., Dip. Surg; OrthSurg; Tel. 942-0551.

MacPHAIL, A. Sinclair; Capitol Bldg., Larder Lake, Ont.; Glasgow (Scot.) '52; MB; Ch.B; Tel. 26.

MACPHAIL, Franklin L.; Ste. 200, 5300 Cote-des-Neiges Rd., Montreal 26, P.Q.; 4835 Lacombe (res); Dal '38; ObstGyn (P.Q.); Staff, Catherine Booth Hosp. Tel. HU 1-0431.
MACPHAIL, Hugh R.; 7227-114 A St., Edmonton, Alta. (res); Man '48; F.A.S.A.; Anaes; Staff, Misericordia Hosp.; Dist. Coroner; Tel. GE 9-1280.
MacPHAIL, Ian A.; 600 Norfolk St., Windsor, Ont.; Tor'56; MCGP; Sec. Med. Advisory, Metropolitan Gen. Hosp.; Tel. 969-0580.
MACPHEE, Archibald E. R.; 314 York St., Cornwall, Ont.; Tor '36; F.C.C.P.; IntMed; Chief of Med., Hotel Dieu Hosp.; Staff, Cornwall Gen. & MacDonell Mem. Hosp's.; Tel. WE 2-3730.
MacPHEE, Douglas M.; 560 Professional Bldg., **10830 Jasper Ave., Edmonton, Alta.; 10406 Park** Rd. (res); Edinburgh (Scot.) '49; MCGP; Active Staff, Misericordia Hosp.; Hon. Instr. (Prev. **Med.), U. of Alberta; Tel. 429-3351.**
MACPHERSON, Alexander D.; Alb '29; Psy; Med. Supt., Albert Hosp., Box 307, Edmonton, Alta.; Ass't. Clin. Prof., U. of Alberta; Tel. GR 7-0221.
MACPHERSON, Alexander S.; Tor'56; Psy; Chief, Psy. Service, Ste. Anne's Hosp., Ste. Anne De Bellevue, P.Q.; Ass't. Prof., Dept. of Psy., McGill University; Tel. 453-3440.
MacPHERSON, Archibald M.; 360 Professional Bldg., 10830 Jasper Ave., Edmonton, Alta.; Dal '50; DiagRad.
MacPHERSON, Bruce; 15 John St., Weston, Ont.; 20 Blair Athol Cres., Islington (res); Tor '50; Staff, (IntMed), Humber Mem. Hosp. & Orenda Engines; Tel. 247-6066.
MACPHERSON, Donald M.; 8 Canal St. E., Tilbury, Ont.; **Wes '26; Dist. Coroner.**
MACPHERSON, Enid; 6178 Quinpool Rd., Halifax, N.S.; Glasgow (Scot.)'52.
MacPHERSON, George W.; 1075 Bayview Ave., Toronto 12, Ont.; 323 Ridgewood Rd., West Hill (res); Qns '37; MO (Admin.), Sunnybrook Hosp.; Tel. 485-8651.
MACPHERSON, Gordon B.; 221 King St. E., Kingston, Ont.; 629 Earl St. (res); Qns '30; Ophth, Otol; Cons. (ENT), Kingston Gen & Hotel-Dieu Hosp's.; Ass't. Prof. Ophth & Act. Hd. (ENT), Queen's U.; Tel. 548-3915.
MACPHERSON, Iain G.; 6178 Quinpool Rd., Halifax, N.S.; Edinburgh (Scot.)'54; MCGP.
MACPHERSON, J. Archibald; Duart, Ontario; Wes'51; MCGP; Chmn., Kent County Health Unit; Tel. 678-3301.
MACPHERSON, J. Campbell; 11608-78th Ave., Edmonton, Alta.; Alb. '34; Ass't. Med. Supt., Aberhart Mem. San.; Tel. GE 9-0051.
MACPHERSON, John R.; Highgate, Ont.; Wes '14; MCGP; Tel. 678-3911.
MACPHERSON, Kenneth D.; 950 Oxford St., London, Ont.; 192 Taylor St. (res); **Wes '48.**
MACPHERSON, Lauchlan; Hampton, N.B.; Dal '49; F.A.C.S.
MACPHERSON, Malcolm M.; 750 West Broadway, Vancouver, B.C.; 6288 Wiltshire St. (res); **Man '35; GenSurg; Vis. Staff, Vancouver Gen., St. Paul's & Children's Hosp's.; Med. Dir., B.C. Sugar Refinery; Tel. 874-1613.**
MACPHERSON, Robert A.; 25 Medical Arts Bldg., Winnipeg, Man.; **150 Oak St. (res); Qns** '29; F.A.C.R., D. & TRad; **Prof. of Rad., & Chairman, Dept. of Rad., U. of Manitoba; Tel.** WH 2-6453.
MACPHERSON, Robert N.; 58 Collier St., Barrie, Ont.; Wes '33.
MACPHERSON, Roderick I.; Ste. 211, 925 W. Georgia St., Vancouver 1, B.C.; Man'58; FRCP(C), DiagRad; Clin. Dem. (DiagRad), University of British Columbia; Tel. MU 4-4177.
MACPHERSON, Ronald H.; 304 Medical Arts Bldg., Saskatoon, **Sask.; 301 Lake Cres. (res);** McGill'43; FACS; FACOG, FRCS(C), Obst-**Gyn; Chief ObstGyn., St. Paul's Hosp.; Vis. Cons., City Hosp.; Assoc. Clin., Prof., ObstGyn, U. of Saskatchewan; Tel. 242-7188.**
MACPHERSON, Ronald T.; Prov. Lab., Castle St., St. John, N.B.; Aberdeen (Scot.) '50; DABPA; FCAP; MC Path; Path; Pathol., Prov. Lab.; Tel. 692-2644.
MACPHERSON, William C.; South Plant Med. Centre, General Motors Canada Ltd., Oshawa, Ont.; Glasgow (Scot.)'47; DPH; Plant Phys., General Motors of Canada; Tel. 725-7311.
MACPHERSON, William J.; 10 Subway St., Campbellton, N.B.; McG'58; IntMed.
MacQUARRIE, Alastair W.; Box 1138, Weller Fdn. Bldg., Banff, Alta.; 500 Banff Ave. (res); Edinburgh (Scot.)'27; FRCS (Edin.); LM (Rotunda, Dublin); MCGP; Phys. & Surg., Mineral Springs Hosp.; Tel. 762-2925.
MacQUARRIE, Kenneth T.; Smith Clinic, Camrose, Alta.; Oxford (Eng.)'55; MA; MCGP.
MACQUARRIE, M. Jeanette (Morrison); Camrose, Alta.; Alb'54; MCGP.
MACQUARRIE, William A.; Ste. 411, Maritime Bldg., New Glasgow, N.S.; Dal'48; MCGP; Staff, Aberdeen Hosp., New Glasgow, N.S.; M.O., Hawker-Siddeley (Dom. Steel & Coal Corp.), Trenton, N.S.; Tel. 752-4177 & 752-4176.
MACQUEEN, Donald G.; 526 Lougheed Bldg., 604-1st St. S.W., Calgary, Alta.; 811-48th Ave. S.W. (res); Man '20 FACS; GenSurg; Staff, Workmen's Comp. Board; Tel. 242-5323; Retired.
MACRAE, Alexander I.; 222 Eramosa Rd., Guelph, Ont.; **18 Gladstone Ave. (res); Tor '49; IntMed; Staff, Guelph Gen. & St. Joseph's Hosp's.; Tel. TA 4-5091.**
MacRAE, Alvin E.; 34 Queen St., Dartmouth, N.S.; Dal'51; Tel. 466-7561.
McRAE, C. G.; Department of National Health & Welfare, c/o Regional Superintendent, European Region. Abroad.
MacRAE, Donald; Apt. 909, 416 The Westway, Weston, Ont. (res); Glasgow (Scot.) '44; M.B., Ch.B.; M.D. (High Commend.); Staff, Quarantine Immigration Med. Serv., Toronto International Airport, Malton; Tel. BU 6-3661.
MACRAE, Donald M.; Med. Arts Bldg., 5880 Spring Garden Rd., Halifax, N.S.; 247 Jubilee Rd. (res); Dal '34; Ophth, Otol; Assoc. Surg., Ophth, Otol., Victoria Gen. & Children's Hosp's.; Bronchoscopist, Nova Scotia San.; Cons., Halifax TB Hosp.; Prof. Hd. (Ophth, Otol), Dalhousie U.; Tel. 423-6309.
MacRAE, Duncan R.; 27 Leinster St., St. John, N.B.; 849 Anderson Dr. (res); Dal '42; Ophth-Otol; Staff, (Ophth) St. John Gen. & St. Joseph's Hosp's.; Tel. 692-3676.
MacRAE, Emerson E.; Oromocto, N.B.; Dal '60.
MACRAE, Frank R.; Ste. 303, 1248 St. Foy Rd., Quebec 6, P.Q.; McG '42; D.I.M. (McG.), FRCP (C); IntMed; Chief of Med. Serv. & Med. Staff, Jeffery Hale's Hosp.; Tel. 681-0228.
MACRAE, Harry M.; Ste. 226, Medical Arts Bldg., 170 St. George St., Toronto, Ont.; 290 Oriole Parkway (res); Tor '28; Ophth; Sr. Surg., Toronto Gen. Hosp.; Assoc. Prof. of Ophth., U. of Toronto; Tel. WA 1-8527.
MACRAE, William D.; 611 Med & Dental Bldg., Rose St. & 11th Ave., Regina, Sask.; Sask '59; FRCS(C), GenSurg; Staff, Regina Gen. & Grey Nun's Hosp's; Tel. 522-7671.
MACRAE, William G.; Tor'65; Res., Shaughnessy Hosp., Vancouver 9, B.C.
MacRAE, William M.; 6301 Quinpool Rd., Halifax, N.S.; 1784 Cambridge St. (res); Dal '55; Staff, Victoria Gen., Hfx. Infirm., Grace & Children's Hosp's.; Tel. 422-4555, 422-9374.
MACRANDER, Hans; 15272 Fraser Highway, New Westminster, B.C.; Amsterdam (Neth.) '57. Tel. 581-7722.
MacSEARRAIGH, Eamonn S.; Nat. U. (Galway, Ire.) '23; M.B., B.Ch.; BAO; DPH; LM (Rotunda); Staff, Walwyn Hosp., Come-by-Chance, Nfld.
MacSWEEN, George B.; 64 Queen St., St. Catharines, Ont.; **Simpson Road (res); McG '49; Staff, St. Catharines Gen. Hosp.**
MacSWEEN, H. Miller; 206 Rookwood Ave., Fredericton, N.B.; Dal'66.
MACSWEEN, Michael; Victoria Gen. Hosp., Halifax, N.S.; Dal'57; MCGP; Tel. 422-7454.
MacTAVISH, John N.; Qns'61; Psy; Staff, Thistletown Hosp., Rexdale, Ont.
Mac VICAR, Alexander S.; Glasgow (Scot.) '46; Ass't. Res. (Psy), Montreal Gen. Hosp., Montreal, P.Q.

MacVICAR, Archibald A.; 1030 Ouellette Ave., Windsor, Ont.; Dal '42; Psy; Dir., Psy. Unit, Hotel-Dieu Hosp.; Active Cons., Psy., Hotel-Dieu Hosp. & Cons. Psy., Maryvale Vocat. Girl's School; Tel. 252-3631.
MacVITTIE, Jerrold A.; 64 Robert St. E., Penetanguishene, Ont.; Qns '54; Staff, Ontario Hosp., Penetanguishene.
MacWATT, David J. L.; 38 Thornton Ave., Montreal 16, P.Q.; Edinburgh (Scot.) '43; Anaes; Anaes-in-Chief, Lakeshore Gen. Hosp.; Staff Anaes., St. Mary's & Catherine Booth Hosp's.; Tel. 735-3511.
MacWHIRTER, Robert B.; 471 Herring Cove Rd., Spryfield, N.S.; Dal '62; Tel. 477-4660.
MacWILLIAM, Herbert D.; Ste. 220, 1175 Cook St., Victoria, B.C.; Dal '50; Otol; Tel. EV 5-8931.
MacWILLIAM, John C.; 44—3rd St., Chatham, Ont.; 243 Wellington St. W. (res); Wes '39; M.A.R.S., M.A.I.S., M.C.G.P.; Surg., C.N.R., Pere Marquette & C & O Rwy's., & Kent Co. Jail; Indust. Surg., Campbell Soup Co. Ltd., & Canada Packers, Ltd.; Surg. Staff, St. Joseph's & Public Gen. Hosp's.; Dist. Exam., Prudential Insce. Co., Bank of Montreal, & Metropolitan Life Insce. Co. Ltd.; Tel. 352-2420.
MacWILLIAM, John U.; South Ohio, Yarmouth Co., N.S.; Lond. (Eng.) '52; Staff, Yarmouth Reg. Hosp.; Tel. 742-4412.
MADDEFORD, William R.; 599 Cheapside St., London, Ont.; Wes '60; AMCGP; Staff, St. Mary's Hosp.; Phys., C.P.R.; Tel. 438-4611.
MADDIN, W. Stuart; 745 W. Broadway, Vancouver 9, B.C.; 242 Onslow Pl., West Van. (res); Dal '47; DABDS; DermSyph, Staff Van. Gen. Hosp.; Dir. VD Control, Dept. of Health (BC); Tel. TR 4-8138.
MADDISON, G. Edward; 260 Germain St., Saint John, N.B.; Rothesay (res); Dal '37; D.P.H., PH; Dir., T.B. Control, N.B. Dept. of Health; Tel. GR 5-7711.
MADDISON, George D.; Dal'64; Ass't. Res., Winnipeg Gen. Hosp., Winnipeg 3, Man.
MADELY, Patricia M. (Mrs. R. S. Chaikoff); Apt. 2, 419 Lawrence Ave. W., Toronto 12, Ont.; Retired.
MADGWICK, Keith S.; 243 King St. E., Oshawa, Ont.; London (Eng.)'59; MRCS (Eng.); LRCP (Lond.); DObstRCOG; DA (Eng.).
MADIGAN, Joseph L.; 2571 Lakeshore Blvd. W., Toronto 14, Ont.; Tor '63; Tel. 259-4219.
MADILL, John S.; 1081 Burrard St., Vancouver 1, B.C.; Ste. 501, 6060 Balsam St., Van. 13 (res); Alb '31; D & TRad; Dir. Dept. of Rad., St. Paul's Hosp.; Tel. MU 2-2344, Loc. 300.
MADILL, Mervyn F.; Ste. 109, Medical Dental Centre, Chilliwack, B.C.; Tor '61; Tel. 792-2513.
MADILL, N. Stewart; 136 E. 15th St., North Vancouver, B.C.; UBC'59; MCGP; Tel. YU 7-1455.
MADOR, Manning L.; Med. Arts Bldg., 260 Cedar St., Sudbury, Ont.; 470 Lakepoint Ct., R.R. 2, **Site 9 (res); Tor '42; FICS; Urol; Chief (Urol.),** St. Joseph's, Sudbury Gen. & Mem. Hosp's.; Cons. Urol., Sudbury Algoma San.; Tel. 673-3695.
MADORE, Fernand; 1063 d'Avaugour, Chicoutimi, P.Q. (res); Lav '51; ObstGyn (P.Q.); Staff, Hop. Hotel-Dieu-St.-Vallier; Tel. 549-0214.
MADORE, Patrick; Ste. 615, Medical Arts Bldg., 1538 Sherbrooke St., Montreal 25, P.Q.; Dal '43; ThorSurg (P.Q.); F.R.C.S.; GenSurg; Hosp. Appt's.; Tel. WA 2-4980.
MADORE, Paul R.; Mon'52; TherRad; Staff, Notre Dame Hosp., Montreal, P.Q.
MADRAS, Nathan P.; McG'65; Res., Jewish Gen. Hosp., Montreal 26, P.Q.; Abroad.
MADRONICH, John S.; 311 Med. Arts Bldg., 1 Young St., Hamilton, Ont.; Wes'60; Ophth.; Tel. 525-0545.
MAE, August; 11 Alderbrook Dr., Don Mills, Ont.; Stockholm (Sweden) '47; Tel. 444-8425.
MAEHLE, Waldemar, M.; Raxlen Clinic, 500 Parliament St., Toronto 5, Ont.; Tor '62.
MAEND, Alexander; 144 Ontario St., St. Catharines, Ont.; Kharkov (Russia) '40; Staff, St. Catharines Gen. & Hotel-Dieu Hosp's.; Tel. 684-4995.

MAGAT, Exequiel; Manila Central (Philippines) '59; Staff, West Coast San., Corner Brook, Nfld.
MAGDER, David M.; McG'65; Jr. Int., Jewish General Hosp., Montreal 26, P.Q.
MAGDER, Harry; 6000 Cote des Neiges Rd., Montreal 26, P.Q.; Tor '34; Ophth; Chief (Ophth.), Jewish Gen. Hosp.; Cons., Reddy Mem. Hosp.; Tel. RE 9-1092.
MAGDER, John H.; 3094 Danforth Ave., Scarborough, Ont.; 7 Love Cresc. (res); Tor '56; Tel. 267-5111.
MAGEAU, Guy; 4327 Delorimier, Montreal 34, P.Q.
MAGEE, Douglas E.; Ste. 1, 1703 Victoria Pk. **Ave., Scarborough, Ont.; Tel. PL 5-1316.**
MAGEE, Donald R.; 309 Medical Arts Bldg., Winnipeg, Man.; 149 Brock St. (res); Man. '49; D.A.B. Ophth; Ophth; Ass't. (Ophth.), Winnipeg GenHosp.; Cons., Municipal Hosp's.; Lect., Ophth., U. of Manitoba; Tel. WH 3-0507.
MAGEE, Edward L.; 452 Charlotte St., Peterborough, **Ont.; Middleton Dr. (res); London (Eng.) '48; Anaes; Chief-of-Anaes., St. Jo**seph's Hosp.; Staff, Anaes., Peterborough Civic Hosp.; Tel. RI 5-2491.
MAGEE, Gary L.; Willowdale Clinic, 30 Sheppard Ave. E., Willowdale, Ont.; Tor'65.
MAGEE, Mrs. Russell K.; (see MOFFAT, Agnes K.).
MAGEE, Russell K.; The Peterborough Clinic Ltd., 327 Charlotte St., Peterborough, Ont.; 597 Weller St. (res); Tor '30; F.A.C.S., F.R.C.S. (Eng.), F.R.C.S.(C), GenSurg, OrthSurg, Urol; Sr. Surg., Peterborough Clin.; Tel. 743-2040.
MAGIAN, Victor de C.; Winnipeg Clinic, St. Mary's & Vaughan, Winnipeg, Man.; 127 Chataway Blvd., Tuxedo (res); Edinburgh (Scot.) '45; DLO; Otol; Staff, Winnipeg Gen. Children's & Misericordia Hosp's.; Tel. WH 2-0551
MAGILL, Frank; Apt. 607, 5353 Sherbrooke St. W., Montreal 28, P.Q.; McG'60; IntMed(P.Q); Staff, Royal Victoria Hosp., Montreal 2, P.Q.
MAGNAN, J. Antonio; Lav '56; Psy (P.Q.); Staff, Hop. St.-Michael-Archange, Mastai, Quebec 5, P.Q.; Tel. 663-3571.
MAGNAN, L. Arthur; 822 est rue Sherbrooke, Montreal, P.Q.; 1469 Drummond St. (res); Mon '22; M.D. (Paris), F.A.C.S., F.R.C.S.(C), ObstGyn.; VI 5-5058.
MAGNAN, Roland; 405 Manseau, Joliette, P.Q.; Mon '32.
MAGNER, Desmond E. O.; 231 Clemow Ave., Ottawa, Ont. (res); Tor '36; F.R.C.P.(C), PathBact.; Prof. & Hd. Dept. of Path., U. of Ottawa; Tel. 235-7594.
MAGNER, Raymond G.; 005 Rideau Med. Centre, 1711-4th St. S.W., Calgary, Alta.; 1314 Riverdale Ave. (res); Dublin (Ire.) '42; M.B., B.Ch.; BAO; DCH; Tel. 269-6697.
MAGNUSON, Dale W. S.; 1284-56th St., R.R.2. Ladner, B.C.; 855 Bayview Dr. (res); Sask '60; Tel. 943-2241.
MAGTIBAY, Luis Z.; Regional Lab., 71 Brunswick St., Fredericton, N.B.; Santo Tomas (Phillip.) '55; DABPath; Pathol., Regional Lab., & Victoria Public Hosp., Fredericton, N.B.
MAGUIRE, Frederick P.; 266 Oxford St. E., London, Ont.; Man'48; D.Psy.
MAGUIRE, Gerard H.; 3550 Cote des Neiges Rd., Montreal, P.Q.; 306 Strathearn N., Montreal West (res); McG '54; D&TRad; Ass't. Rad., Montreal Gen. Hosp.; Tel. 937-9334.
MAGUIRE, J. Eudes; Nouvelle, Bonaventure Co., P.Q.; Lav '40; M.C.G.P.
MAGUIRE, John Gordon, 1538 Sherbrooke St. W., Ste. 324, Montreal, P.Q. McG '59; Psy.; Cons. Queen Mary Vet's. Hosp.; Clin. Ass't. (O.P.D.), Mtl. Gen. Hosp.; Lect. Dept. of Psy., McGill U.; Tel. 933-7932.
MAGUIRE, Nancy S. (Marsden); 3603 7th St. S.W., Calgary, Alta. (res); London (Eng.) '52; M.B., B.S.; LRCP; MRCS; Pt.-time School M.O., Dept. of Health; Tel. CH 9-0738.
MAGUIRE, Webster T.; 2696 W. Broadway, Vancouver 8, B.C.; 5907 Chancellor Blvd., Van. 8 (res); Tor '36; FASAS; Staff, Van. Gen., St. Paul's & Grace Hosp's.; Tel. RE 8-0824.

MAGUIRE, Wilfrid L.; 95 Main St., St. Catharines, Ont.; Wes '25; Court. Staff, Hotel-Dieu & St. Catharines Gen. Hosp's.; Dist. Coroner, Tel. WE 4-3711.

MAGWOOD, Kathleen; 233 N. Syndicate Ave., Fort William, Ont.; Ott'62; Tel. 622-6033.

MAGWOOD. S. J. Newton; 86 Braeside Rd., Toronto, Ont. (res.); Tor'06; FRCS(C), Obst.; Retired.

MAGYAR, Sandor; 1081 St. Clair Ave. W., Toronto 10, Ont.; Budapest (Hung.) '53; MCGP; Staff, St. Michael's Hosp.; Tel. LE 5-5510.

MAHABIR, Ramkhelawan N.; Dal '60; FRCP(C), IntMed; Staff, Halifax Infirmary, Halifax, N.S.; Tel. 422-1511.

MAHABIR, Winston J.; McG'48; Res., Riverview Hosp., Essondale, B.C.

MAHAFFY, Charlotte E.; Box 513, Sylvan Lake, Alta.; Alb '30; MPH & PH.

MAHANEY, Gordon R.; Bridgetown, Annapolis Co., N.S.; Dal '34; M.C.G.P.; Dist. Coroner.

MAHARAJ, Deodath T.; Neil's Harbour, N.S.; Dal'65; Tel. 762.

MAHARAJ, Charles; Benito, Man.; Paris (France) '62; District Coroner; Tel. 119.

MAHARAJ, Gunness R.; 112-6th Ave. S., Swan River, Man.; Dal'65.

MAHBOOB, Shahnaz; 30 Beaton Ave., New Waterford, N.S.; Panjab (West Pakistan)'56.

MAHER, Leonard A.; Ste 304, 153 Seymour St., Kamloops, B.C.; Alb '49; Otol.

MAHEU, J. Odilon; 1135 Provost, Lachine, P.Q.; 535-38th Ave. (res); Lav '33; PH (P.Q.).

MAHEU, Pierre; Mon '62; Res., Hop.-Notre-Dame, Montreal, P.Q.

MAHEUX, Carol E.; 1618 ouest, rue King, Sherbrooke, P.Q.; Lav '64; Tel. 562-4409.

MAHEUX, Paul; C.P. 233, Outremont, Montreal 8, P.Q. (res); Lav'48; Path (P.Q.); Staff, Hop.-Maisonneuve; Tel. 254-8341.

MAHEUX, Rodolphe; Ville St. Georges Est, Beauce Co., P.Q.; Lav '35; M.C.G.P.; Med. Staff, Hop. Notre Dame de Beauce; Dist. Coroner.

MAHON, John D.; 912 Greyhound Bldg., Calgary, Alta.; 313—38th Ave. S.W. (res); McG '44; **GenSurg.; Tel. 262-5633.**

MAHON, Michael A.; Ste. 103, 460 Eglinton Ave., E., Toronto 12, Ont.; Tor '63; Tel. HU 3-5134.

MAHON, William A.; Dept. of Pharmacology, Toronto Gen. Hosp., Toronto 2, Ont.; Edinburgh (Scot) '52; S.M. (Hygiene, Harvard); FRCP(C); IntMed; Assoc. Prof. (Pharm.) & Ass't. Prof. (Ther.), U. of Toronto.

MAHON, William K., Capt.; Qns '63; Staff, Can. Forces Hosp., Kingston, Ont.

MAHON, Winston S.; 32 The Queensway N., Keswick, Ont.; Tor'36; MCGP; Staff, York County Hosp., Newmarket, Ont.; Tel. Area 416-476-4133.

MAHONEY, James L.; 1014 Victoria Ave., Niagara Falls, Ont.; Tor '13; Staff, Greater Niagara Falls Gen. Hosp.; Tel. 354-6622.

MAHONEY, Leo J.; Ste. 120, 200 St. Clair Ave. W., Toronto 7, Ont.; 95 Inglewood Dr. (res); Tor'44; M.S.; FACS; FRCS(C); GenSurg; Staff Surg., St. Michael's Hosp.; Cons. Surg., Princess Margaret Hosp.; Ass't. Prof. Dept. of Surg., U. of Toronto; Tel. WA 1-1052.

MAHONEY, Paul R., SG/LT; H.M.C.S. Stadacona, Halifax, N.S.; Tor '64.

MAHONY, John B.O.; 327 Christina St., Sarnia, Ont.; Wes'39.

MAHOOD, James H. S.; 29 Hillcroft Dr., Kingston, Ont. (res); Qns '48; Anaes; Att. Staff, Anaes., Kingston Gen. Hosp.; Lect., Dept. of (Anaes), Queen's U.; Tel. 542-2821.

MAHOOD, Margaret C. (Fisher); 214 Avenue Bldg., Saskatoon, Sask.; 327 Lake Cres. (res); McG'55; Psy; Active Staff, University Hosp.; Med. Cons. Rehab. Branch Dept. of Social Welfare; Tel. 652-0300.

MAIDENBERG, Robert O.; 659 Hamilton Rd., London, Ont.; Wes'61; AMCGP; Tel. 455-2850.

MAIER, Margaret M. (See Guest)

MAILE, John K.; Box 1930, Quesnel, B.C.; London (Eng.) '61; M.B., B.S.; MRCS (Eng.); LRCP (Lond.); Tel. 992-2158.

MAILHOT, Maurice; 4074 Boul. LaSalle, Verdun, Montreal 19, P.Q.; Mon '51; Vis. Staff, Verdun & Lachine Hosp's.

MAILHOT, Paul; 347 rue St-Georges, St. Jerome, Cte. Terrebonne, P.Q.; Mon'54; FRCS(C), OrthSurg; Tel. GE 8-1792.

MAILHOT, Roger; 825 Belvedere S., Sherbrooke, P.Q.; Mon'55; DABS; FACS; FASAS; GenSurg (P.Q); Active Staff, Hotel-Dieu Hosp.; Tel. LO 2-8126.

MAILLE, Gilles; 912 est Sherbrooke, Montreal 24, P.Q.; 6965-20th Ave., Rosemont (res); Mon'50; FRCS(C), OrthSurg; Orth. Surg., Hop. Ste. Jeanne d'Arc; Tel. VI 2-5201.

MAILLE, Jean-Guy; 11239 Drouart, Montreal, P.Q.; Mon '55; Anaes; Staff Anaes., Ste-Jeanne d'Arc & St-Michel Hosp's.; Tel. VI 2-5201.

MAILLE, Rene; 3205 Viel St., Montreal 12, P.Q. (res); Mon '41; DPH; P.H. (PQ); D. Vit Stat. (Johns Hopkins); Supt. Vit. Statistics, Mtl. Dept. of Health; Tel. 872-1111.

MAILLOUX, G.; Department of National Health & Welfare, c/o Regional Superintendent, European Region. Abroad.

MAILLOUX, Jean; 245 Victoria Ave., Westmount, Montreal 6, P.Q.; Mon'53; BSc; MCGP; Staff, Hop. Gen. de Verdun; Dir. of Med. Services, Merck, Sharp & Dohme Ltd.; Tel. 933-7371.

MAILLOUX, Laurent; 2902 Ave. Lacombe, Montreal, P.Q.; **2900 Ave. Lacombe (res); Mon '28;** M.C.G.P.; (Hon.); Retired.

MAILLOUX, Luc; 525 Cherrier St., Montreal, **P.Q.; Mon '37; Ophth,Otol; Tel. AV 8-4792.**

MAILLY, Georges A.; Nominingue, Co. Labelle, P.Q.; Lav '35.

MAINMAN, Edwin R.; Longlac Infirmary, Birchcrest Rd., Longlac, Ont.; Leeds (Eng.) '51.

MAINPRIZE, George J.; Prudential Ins. Co. of America, 4 King St. W., Toronto, Ont.; Tor'50; Staff, O.P.D., Toronto Gen. Hosp.; Tel. 366-6971, Loc. 284.

MAINPRIZE, Graham W.; Central Butte, Sask.; Tor '53; M.C.G.P.; Dist. Coroner.

MAINPRIZE, William G.; Midale, Sask.; Tor '11; Dist. Coroner.

MAINVILLE, Jean C.; Mon'64; Res., Hop. Ste-Justine, Montreal 26, P.Q.

MAINVILLE, Lodois L.; Lancaster DVA Hosp., Lancaster, N.B.; Mon'43; C. (Gross Anat.) (Sorbonne, Paris, Fr.); CHOM; MACHA; Dir., District Admissions Services For N.B. Province; Tel. 694-2651, Loc. 306.

MAINVILLE, Maurice; 163 est, rue Laurier, Ottawa 2, Ont.; Lav '46; Staff (Anaes.), Ottawa Gen. Hosp.; Lect. (Anaes.), U. of Ottawa.

MAIR, C. Mellis; Med. Arts Bldg., 1105 Pandora Ave., Victoria, B.C.; 2533 Killarney Pl. (res); Alb '43; MRCOG; FRCOG; FACS; FACOG; ObstGyn; Active Staff, Royal Jubilee Hosp.; Cons. Queen Alexandra Solarium; Tel. 382-3741.

MAIR, George T.; 1576 Weston Rd., Weston, **Ont.; 6 Limerick Ave. (res); Glasgow (Scot.)** '49; F.R.C.S. (Edin.) GenSurg; Gen. Surg **Humber Mem. Hosp.; Tel. CH 1-2441.**

MAISONNEUVE, Jacques; 2630-30th rue, Laval Ouest, P.Q.; Mon '52.

MAISONVILLE, Philippe S.; Hycroft Medical Bldg., 3195 Granville St., Vancouver 9, B.C.; 4310 Curle Ave. S. Burnaby (res); Tor '46; D.A.B.O., F.A.B.O., M.R.C.S., Ophth; Assoc. **Staff, St. Paul's & Children's Hosp's.; Tel. RE 8-2826.**

MAJEAU, Guy; Ste. 208, 2120 est rue Sherbrooke, Montreal 34, P.Q.; Mon'60; MCGP.

MAJKA, Mieczyslaw; Austria '51; Staff, Regional Lab., Moncton, N.B.

MAJOR, Emile J.; 119½ Charlotte, Ottawa 2, Ont.; McG '24; M.C.G.P.; Staff, St. Louis Marie de Montford Hosp., Ottawa; Vist. Staff, Ottawa Gen. Hosp.; Coroner Carleton Co.; M.O.H. Gloucester Twp.; Tel. 233-2326.

MAJOR, Real; Apt. 1, 5797 Beaubien E., Rose**mont, Montreal 36, P.Q.; Mon '57; Tel. 721-9885.**

MAJOR, Willie; Mon'29; Paed. (P.Q.); Staff, Hop. Ste.-Jean-De-Dieu, Montreal 5, P.Q.

MAJURY, Arthur S.; Winnipeg Clinic, Winnipeg **1, Man.; 148 Elm St., Wpg. 9 (res.); Queen's U.** (N. Ire.) '41; BAO; FACOG; FRCOG; ObstGyn; Ass't. ObstGyn., Wpg. Gen. Hosp.; Ass't. Prof. ObstGyn., U. of Manitoba; Tel. 942-0551.
MAKAROFF, Robert P.; 4529-W. 10th Ave., Vancouver 8, B.C.; 3896 W-13 Ave. (res); Alb '48; Tel. 224-4142.
MAKHAN, Bernard A.; 350 Beech Ave., Toronto 13, Ont.; Dal '63.
MAKINS, David J. B.; 14920 Stony Plain Rd., **Edmonton, Alta.; 10939-60th Ave. (res), Edin**burgh (Scot.) '52; Court. Staff, Misericordia & Gen. Hosp's.; Tel. 489-4820.
MAKKAY, Zoltan; Dal'63; Res., Toronto Gen. Hosp., Toronto 2, Ont.
MAKSYMIUK, Lore (See Burkhardt)
MALAVIYA, Devesh; Heidelberg (Germ.)'61; Res., Gen. Hosp., St. Boniface, Man.
MALCHO, Thomas J.; 2530 Jane St., Downsview, Ont.; Tor'64; AMCGP; Active Staff, Northwestern Gen. Hosp.; Tel. 633-6633.
MALCHY, David; Man '62; Jr. Intn., St. Boniface Hosp., St. Boniface, Man.
MALCOLM, Andrew I.; Ste. 1003, 123 Edward St., Toronto 2, Ont.; Tor '51; DABP; Psy; Acting Hd., Narcotic Addiction Unit, Alcohol & Drug Addiction Research Fdn.; Tel. 366-1083.
MALCOLM, Arthur H. H.; Geraldton Dist. Clinic, Box 610, Geraldton, Ont.; Tor'47; MCGP; MOH, Geraldton & Nakina; M.O., MacLeod-Cockshutt Gold Mines Ltd., Consolidated Mosher Mines Ltd., Kimberley-Clark of Canada Ltd. & The Algoma Steel Corp. Ltd.; Memb. Bd. of Governors, Geraldton Dist. Hosp.; Tel. 854-0800.
MALCOLM, D. Ian; 98 Sherman S., Hamilton, Ont.; 2 Desjardins Ave., Dundas (res); Wes '57; MCGP; Active Staff, St. Joseph's & Hamilton Civic Hosp's.; Tel. LI 4-1067.
MALCOLM, Donald A.; Dal '51; DiagRad; Staff, Saint John Gen. Hosp., Saint John, N.B.; Tel. 693-3351.
MALCOLM, Findlay Lt. Col.; 6 Hall's Rd., Boul**derwood, Halifax Co., N.S. (res); Edinburgh** (Scot.) '49; DMR; DiagRad; Rad-in-Chief, Cdn. Forces Hosp., Halifax, N.S.; Lect. (Radiol. Anat.), Dalhousie U.
MALCOLM, Frank F.; 184 Portland St., Dart**mouth N.S. (res); Dal '20; Chief M.O., Halifax** Co. Hosp.; Tel. 466-7411.
MALCOLM, John M.; Box 1210, Med. Centre, Stettler, Alta.; Man'43; Tel. 742-2194.
MALCOLM, Thomas F.; Box 1028, Swan River, Man.; Man'30; MRCS; MRCP; Med. Dir., Swan Valley Health Unit; Tel. 734-3495.
MALCOLMSON, Alexander S.; 228 King, St. Catherines, Ont.; 12 Rodman Hall Dr. (res); Tor '21; Cons. Serv., St. Catherines Gen. Hosp., Ind. Phys., Foster Wheeler Co.; Dist. M.O., C.N.R.; Retired.
MALCOLMSON, Charles H.; 672 Brant St., Burlington, Ont.; Qns '58; FRCP(C); Paed; Staff, Joseph Brant Hosp.; Tel. 637-0352.
MALCOLMSON, Samuel A.; Medical Clinic, 60 Albert St. W., Thorold, Ont.; Tor'64; Tel. 227-5255.
MALE, Brian M.; 117 Rennie's Mill Rd., St. John's Nfld. (res); London (Eng.) '60; Staff, Dept. of Health, St. John's; Tel. 578-7091.
MALE, Thomas W.; Tor'65; Res., Clarke Inst., Toronto 2B, Ont.
MALEK, David L.; 2091 Alta Vista Dr., Ottawa 8, Ont.; Ott '63; Staff, Ottawa Civic Hosp.; Tel. 731-6296.
MALEY, Stephen C.; 168 Charlotte St., Ottawa 2, Ont.; Man '38; MCGP; Court. Staff, Ottawa Civic, Grace & St. Louis Marie de Montfort Hosp's.; Tel. 233-8489.
MALEZIEUX, Jacques P. (see Paget, Jacques)
MALHOMME, Bernard E.; Birch Hills, Sask.; Man '55.
MALHOTRA, Jagadish C.; Bombay (India) '40; Staff, Riverview Hosp., Essondale, B.C.; Abroad.
MALKIN, Aaron; Sunnybrook Hosp., Toronto 12, **Ont.; 163 York Mills Rd., Willowdale (res); Man** '49; Ph.D. (Biochem.); IntMed; Dir. (Biochem.), **Sunnybrook Hosp.; Tel. 485-8651.**
MALKIN, Dina (Gordon); Tor '48; M.Sc. (Path.); Bact. Staff, Sunnybrook Hosp., Toronto 12, Ont.; Tel. 485-8651.
MALKIN, Edwin; 15 James St., Parry Sound, Ont.; Qns'31; Tel. 746-9382.
MALKIN, Solomon; 857 Sargent Ave., Winnipeg 3, Man.; 776 Queenston St. (res); Man '40; **M.C.G.P.; Tel. SP 2-0401.**
MALKUS, Edmund; Seaforth Med. Clinic, 42 Goderich St. W., Seaforth, Ont.; Dusseldorf (Germ.)'48; MCGP; Active Staff, Seaforth Community Hosp.; Court. Staff, Stratford Gen. Hosp.; Tel. 527-1770.
MALLAM, William W.; Bay Robert Med. Group, Bay Roberts, Nfld.; Dal '63.
MALLEK, Howard; 736 Granville St., Vancouver 2, B.C.; 1588 Wesbrook Cres. (res); McG '37; D.O.M.S., Ophth; Staff, Ophth., St. Paul's & **Children's Hosp's.; Ophth., Burnaby Schl. Bd.; Tel. MU 4-4388.**
MALLEK, Josephine; 736 Granville St., Vancouver 2, B.C.; 1588 Wesbrook Cres. (res); McG '36; IntMed; Staff, Int. Med., St. Paul's & Children's **Hosp's.; Tel. MU 4-4388.**
MALLEN, Richard W.; Ste. 240, 8409-112th St., Edmonton, Alta.; Alb'59; FRCS(C), Otol.
MALLETT, James J.; West Pubnico, Yarmouth Co., N.S.; Dal'56; MCGP; Tel. 117-1.
MALLETT, Lawrence L.; 540 Tegler Bldg., Edmonton, Alta.; 14116-97th Ave. (res); Alb '52; D.M.R., DiagRad; Staff, Misericordia Hosp.; Tel. **424-8261.**
MALLETT, Marshall; 540 Tegler Bldg., Edmonton, Alta.; 10946-82 Ave. (res); McG '24; Diag**Rad; Rad., Misericordia Hosp.; Lect. (Rad.), U. of Alberta; Tel. HU 8-0921.**
MALLICK, Sushil; Glasgow (Scot.) '49; LRCP, LRCS, LRFPS; Staff, Indian Hospital, Sioux Lookout, Ont.
MALLOUH, George E.; 200 Avenue Bldg., 200-3rd Ave. S., Saskatoon, Sask.; Cairo (Egypt) '54; FACOG; FRCS(C), ObstGyn; Tel. 652-0300.
MALLOW, W. E.; 3rd Ave., Kamsack, Sask.; 721 Boulevard **(res); Man '32;** Dist. Coroner.
MALLOY, John J.; Ridgeway Clinic, 1001 Ridgeway St., Fort William, Ont.; Ott '57; FRCS(C) ObstGyn; Tel. 622-0601.
MALLOY, L.; Ridgetown, Ont.; Qns '51.
MALLOY, Leon P.; 8330 Fairmount Dr., Calgary, Alta.; 9428 Fairmount Dr. (res); Ott '56; **ObstGyn; Staff, (Obst), Holy Cross Hosp.; Tel.** 252-1161.
MALLY ,Martha C.; Apt. 1503, 1101 Lafontaine Park, Montreal 34, P.Q.; Rome (Italy)'41.
MALMSTROM, Eric; Buenos Aires (Argentine) '62; Res., Montreal Gen. Hosp., Montreal, P.Q.
MALO, Gilles; Mon '59; Res. Hop. Notre-Dame, Montreal 24, P.Q.
MALO, Jean-M; 4495 Lafontaine, Montreal, P.Q.; Mon '53; Tel. CL 5-3649.
MALO, Muriel; 2266 rue Hochelaga, Montreal 24, P.Q.; Mon'60; PH(P.Q.).
MALO, Robert A.; 3645 Beausejour, St-Laurent, P.Q.; Ott '51; Med. Dir. Hoechrt Pharmaceuticals of Canada.
MALO, Robert F.; 144 Irving Ave., Ottawa, Ont.; **McG '21; Med. Supt., St. Vincent's Hosp.; Tel. CE 3-4041.**
MALONE, Edward W.; Dept. of Health, 278 Le Marchand Rd., St. John's, Nfld.; 344A Hamilton Ave. (res); Dublin (Ire.) '50; DiagRad; Staff, St. John's Gen. Hosp.; Tel. 8-0471.
MALONE, George M.; Box 158, Fort Vermilion, Alta.; Qns '36; GenSurg.
MALONE, James M. F.; 669 Laviolette Ave., Three Rivers, P.Q. (res); McG'15; GenSurg; Surg. in Charge, A. Serv., St. Joseph's Hosp.; Surg., Can. Internat. Paper Co. & St. Lawrence Corp.; Tel. FR 4-8824.
MALONE, Maurice C.; Lacombe, Alta.; Man'42; Tel. 782-3351.
MALONEY, Geraldine C.; 321 Med. Arts Bldg., 170 St. George St., Toronto 5, Ont.; 5 Glen Edyth Pl. Tor. 7 **(res);** Tor '37; F.A.C.S., F.R.C.S.(C), ObstGyn; Tel. **WA 1-6843.**
MALONEY, John; Lav'61; Res., Hop. St-Jeande-Dieu, Montreal 5, P.Q.

MALONEY, John A.; 184 Cedar St., Sudbury, Ont.; 76 Cranbrook Cres. (res); Wes '55; ObstGyn; Staff, St. Joseph's, Sudbury Gen. & Mem. Hosp's.; Tel. OS 3-2121.

MALONEY, John H.; Charlottetown Clinic, 1 Rochford St., Charlottetown, P.E.I.; 11 Churchill Ave. (res); McG '42; M.R.C.O.G., ObstGyn; Staff, Charlottetown & P.E.I. Hosp's., Charlottetown; Tel. 894-5561.

MALONEY, Patrick J.; 267 O'Connor St., Ottawa, Ont.; 250 Island Park Dr. (res); Qns '31; Paed; Active Staff, Ottawa Gen. Hosp.; Court. Staff, Ottawa Civic, Grace & St. Louis Marie de Montford Hosp's.; Teaching Staff, U. of Ottawa; Tel. CE 3-5645.

MALOUF, Hanna; Beyrouth (Leb.) '60; GenSurg; Staff, Hop. Jean-Talon, Montreal 35, P.Q.

MALOWANY, Allan J.; Alb'64; Res., Shaughnessy Hosp., Vancouver 9, B.C.

MALOWNEY, Vernon C.; 2221 Keele St., Ste. 26, Toronto 15, Ont.; 19 Greenbrook Dr. (res); Qns '33; MCGP; Chief-of-Staff, Northwestern Gen. Hosp.; Tel. RU 2-5888.

MALPASS, Alfred J.; 132 Parkdale Ave. S., Hamilton, Ont.; Qns'60; MCGP; Active G.P. Staff, Hamilton Gen. Hosp.; Tel. LI 4-3309.

MALTAIS, Benoit; 769 Boul. Wallberg, Dolbeau, P.Q.; Lav '54.

MALTAIS, Roger; 3 rue St.-Jean, Longueuil, P.Q.; Mon '56; F.R.C.P.(C), DiagRad; Staff, Hop.-Notre Dame, Montreal; Tel. 525-6363.

MALTBY, E. J.; 310 Medical Arts Bldg., 170 St. George St., Toronto, Ont.; Tor '24; F.R.C.P.(C), IntMed.; Tel. WA 1-1413.

MALTBY, J. Roger; Okotoks, Alta.; Cambridge (Eng.) '62; D(Obst.) RCOG; Tel. 683-4011.

MALTBY, Lila F. (Coates); 2701 Eglinton Ave. W., Apt. B1, Toronto 9, Ont.; 54 Heath E. (res)· Tor '26; D. Psy; Psy; Dir. York Twp. Child and Adolescent Guidance Clinic; Tel. RO 9-0894.

MALYON, Morley H.; Ste. 208, 688 Coxwell Ave., Toronto 6, Ont.; 23 Lionel Hts. Cres., Don Mills (res); Tor '55; F.R.C.P.(C), IntMed; Staff, Toronto East Gen. Hosp.; Tel. 463-2852.

MALYON, Roy H.; 794 Coxwell Ave., Toronto, Ont.; Tor '18; M.C.G.P.; Cons., Toronto East Gen. Hosp.; Retired.

MALYSKA, Elizabeth (Mrs. Shelton); 773 Selkirk Ave., Winnipeg 4, Man.; 43 Forest Park Dr. (res); Man '50; Tel. 582-5509.

MALYSKA, William; Deloraine, Man.; Man '39; MCGP; MRSH; MOH, Deloraine, Man.; Tel. 277.

MANACE, Bernard A.; 106 Park Towers W., 400 Walmer Rd., Toronto 10, Ont.; 768 Spadina Rd. (res); Tor '26; M.C.A.A., F.A.A.A., F.A.C.A., IntMed; Cons. (Allergy Dept.), New Mt. Sinai Hosp.; Tel. WA 1-1432.

MANACE, Gordon; Apt. 103, 300 St. Clair Ave. W., Toronto 7, Ont.; Tor '26; F.A.A.P., Paed; Cons. Paed. Div., New Mount Sinai Hosp.; Tel. 922-8214.

MANACKI, J. Alexander; 33 Edgemore Dr., Toronto 18, Ont. (res); Lwow (Poland) '41; D.P.H.; Staff, P.H., Forest Hill Health Unit; Tel. HU 1-5918.

MANAX, Stanley J.; Wes '64; Jr. Int., Victoria Hosp., London, Ont.

MANCER, James F.; Man'65; Jr. Int., St. Boniface Hosp., Winnipeg 6, Man; Abroad.

MANCHESTER; G. H.; 2797 Douglas Rd., South Burnaby, B.C. (res); McG '94; Retired; Part-time Police Work.

MANCHESTER, J. Stewart; 5885 Spring Garden Rd., Halifax, N.S. (res); Dal '41; D&TRad; Prof. (Rad.), Dalhousie U., Head, Dept. DiagRad., Victoria Gen. Hosp.; Cons. (Rad.) R.C. N.H.; Tel. 422-7371.

MANCUSO, Ferdinand; Medico-Dental Bldg., 1396 St. Catherine St. W., Montreal, P.Q.; 1905 Tupper St. (res); McG '26; Tel. 866-1628.

MANCUSO, Salvatore; 6864 St. Denis St., Montreal, P.Q.; McG '38; M.O.H., City of Montreal; Tel. 272-6666.

MANDAVIA, Mansukhlal G.; Bombay (India) '49; Staff, Dept. of Anat., McGill U., Montreal 2, P.Q.

MANDEL, Bernard; 5835 Verdun Ave., Verdun Montreal 19, P.Q.; 3645 Northcliffe Ave. (res); Mon '38; Paed (P.Q.); Tel. 481-6677 & 761 5363.

MANDELL, Howard; Ott '62; Research, Toronto Western Hosp., Toronto, Ont.

MANDELSTAM, Jocelyn P.; Associated Anaesthetists, Winnipeg Gen. Hosp., Winnipeg 3, Man.; Ste. 4, 54 Donald St. (res); London (Eng.) '47; M.R.C.S. (Lond.), L.R.C.P. (Eng.) D.A.; Anaes.; Tel. WH 3-7682.

MANDERSON, Henry J. B.; Royal Victoria Hosp., Montreal, P.Q.; Glasgow (Scot.) '51; ObstGyn.; Tel. 842-1251.

MANDERVILLE, Eugene A.; 500 Bridge St. E., Belleville, Ont.; Dal '62.

MANDEVILLE, Alexander F.; 11967 Bailey Rd., R.R. 9, New Westminster, B.C.; 13307—96th Ave., R.R. 13 (res); UBC '55; Tel. 596-3391.

MANDEVILLE, Audrey M. (Underwood); 11967 Bailey Rd., R.R. 9, New Westminster, B.C.; 13307 — 96th Ave., R.R. 13 (res); UBC '55; Tel. 596-3391.

MANDEVILLE, H. Paul; Mon '50; AMCGP; DiagRad; Staff, Hop. Notre-Dame, Montreal, P.Q.

MANDIN, Henry; Alb '63; Res., University Hosp., Edmonton, Alta.

MANDIN, Joseph A.; Box 160, Carrot River, Sask.; Lav '51; Tel. 768-2711.

MANDRYK, Eugene W.; Tor'63; Res., Clarke Inst. of Psy., 250 College St., Toronto 2B, Ont.

MANES, John D.; McG'51; MCGP; Med. Dir., Holy Cross Hosp., Calgary, Alta.; Exec. Dir., Cdn. Assoc. of Med. Clinics; Tel. 266-7231.

MANGAN, Michael A.; Nat. U. (Ire.) '54; Staff, Dept. of Health, 278 Le Marchant Rd., St. John's Nfld.

MANGEL, Roman; McG'63; Res., Montreal Gen. Hosp., Montreal, P. Q.

MANIAR, Atish; Bombay (India); Staff, Dept. of Bact., Winnipeg Gen. Hosp., Winnipeg 3, Man.; Tel. SP 4-6511.

MANINGAS, Carlos S.; Medical Arts Bldg., 1255-100th. St., North Battleford, Sask.; Santo Tomas (Phillipp.)'55; Paed; Staff, North Battleford Union & Indian Hosp's.; Tel. 445-8146.

MANION, Robert A.; Norway House, Man.; Ott '64.

MANITIUS, Danuta; 211 Simcoe St. S., Oshawa, Ont.; 46 Thickson Rd., R.R. 3 (res); Polish School of Med. (Edinburgh, Scotland) '48; Tel. 725-8502.

MANKIEWICZ, Edith M. (Meyer); 760 Wilder Ave., Outremont, Montreal 8, P.Q.; Lyon (Fr.) '38; Dir. Labs., Royal Edward Laurentian San.; Lect. McGill U.; Tel. VI 9-5201.

MANKIEWICZ, Stanley; Oshawa Clinic, 117 King St. E., Oshawa, Ont.; 308A Park Lane Apts., 15 Adelaide St. E. (res); Man '56; Urol; Active Staff (Urol.) Oshawa Gen. Hosp.; Tel. 728-1661.

MANKTELOW, Ralph T.; 44 Kimberley, Bracebridge, Ont.; Tor'64; Tel. 645-2281.

MANN, A. Douglas; Box 359, Burns Lake, B.C.; Tor '60; Tel. 288.

MANN, Alan M.; 324 Medical Arts Bldg., Montreal, P.Q.; 170 Simcoe Ave., Mount Royal (res); McG '49; D.Psy, Psy; Ass't. Psy., Montreal Gen. Hosp.; Cons. (Psy.), Queen Mary Veterans' Hosp.; Dem. (Psy.), McGill U.; Tel. WE 2-2792.

MANN, Dorothy M. K.; 220 Med. Arts Bldg., 1 Young St., Hamilton, Ont.; 5314 Lakeshore H'way E., Burlington (res); Tor '47 MRCOG (Eng.); ObstGyn; Staff, St. Joseph's Hosp.; Tel. JA 9-0393.

MANN, Harry B.; 5179 Park Ave., Montreal, P.Q.; 746 Wilder, Outremont (res); Mon '47; M.C.G.P.; Staff, Jewish Gen. Hosp; Tel. GI 3-3452.

MANN, I. Walter; 442 North Christina St., Sarnia, Ont.; Wes '37; Anaes; Chief Anaes., Sarnia Gen. Hosp.; Staff Anaes., St. Joseph's Hosp.; Tel. 344-1451.

MANN, John A.; 612 Medical Arts Bldg., 750 Spadina Cr. E., Saskatoon, Sask.; Sask '59; Tel. 653-0112.

MANN, John J.; 2558 Lakeshore Blvd. W., Toronto 14, Ont.; Tor '43; M.C.G.P.; Tel. 251-9471.

MANN, Margaret B.; Man '57; Staff, Hosp. for Mental Diseases, Selkirk, Man.
MANN, Robert W.; '37 Roxborough St. E., Toronto, Ont.; Tor '06; Tel. WA 1-3070.
MANN, Wm. H.; 10 Hincks St., St. Thomas, Ont.; 363 Wellington St. (res); Frankfurt (Germany) '51; OphthOtol; FAAOO; Active Cons. Staff, St. Thomas Elgin Gen. Hosp.; Tel. 631-0298.
MANNERS, Douglas O.; 450 Central Ave., London, Ont.; 1055 Patricia Ave. (res); Wes '56; FRCS(C); ObstGyn; Instr., (ObstGyn), U. of Western Ont.; Tel. 432-7891.
MANNING, Clinton E.; 157 Dufferin St., Richmond, P.Q. (res); McG '21; Adm., The Wales Home; Tel. 826-3060.
MANNING, George W.; 9 Harrison Cr., London, Ont. (res); Tor '40; Ph.D., FRCP(C), IntMed; Dir., Cardiovasc. Unit, Victoria Hosp.; Cons. (Cardiac.), D.V.A.; Prof. of Med., U. of Western Ontario; Tel. GE 2-5261.
MANNING, Glen; Box 490, Williams Lake, B.C.; UBC'64.
MANNING, H. Kent; 280 Bloor W., Toronto 5, Ont.; 118 Montgomery Ave. Apt. 211E; Tor '11; ObstGyn; Retired.
MANNING, R. Elizabeth; 3931 Sunnycrest Blvd., North Vancouver, B.C. (res); Tor '56; Staff, Woodlands School, New Westminster.
MANNING, Walter L.; 8584 Granville St., Vancouver, B.C.; 6126 Olympic (res); UBC '54; MCGP; Tel. AM 6-8010.
MANOUVRIER, Frans P.; C.P. 280, rue Principale, Van Kleek Hill, Ont.; Mon '61; Tel. 678-2011.
MANSEAU, J. Arthur; 960 Blvd. St. Joseph E., Montreal 34, P.Q. Mon '21; Obst (P.Q.).
MANSEAU, Philippe; 5689 Boul. Rosemount, Montreal 36, P.Q. (res); Mon '47; Pulm. Dis. & TB (P.Q.); Staff, Hop. St. Joseph de Rosemount, Montreal; Tel. CL 6-2681.
MANSFIELD, Gordon R.; Kootenay Mental Health Centre, 1325 McQuarrie St., Trail, B.C.; Tor'52; D.Psy; Psy; Dir., Kootenay Mental Health Centre; Cons. Staff, Trail-Tadanac, Kootenay Lake Gen., Castlegar & District Hosps.
MANSON, Arthur B.; 925 W. Georgia St., Vancouver 1, B.C.; 5976 Tisdall St. (res); McG '26; GenSurg; Att'd. Staff Surg., Vancouver Gen. Hosp.; Tel. MU 1-9655.
MANSON, Arthur D. C.; 935C Homestead Village Lane S.E., Rochester, Minn., U.S.A.; UBC'61; GenSurg; Abroad.
MAN-SON-HING, Clyde T.; Calgary Assoc. Clinic, 214 Sixth Ave. S.W., Calgary, Alta.; Cambridge (Eng.)'59; FRCP(C), Neur.
MANTHA, Leopold; 333 rue Besserer, Ottawa 2, Ont.; Mon '23; IntMed; Cons., Hop. St. Vincent; Tel. 234-0411.
MANUEL, F. Russell; 1076 Roper Ave., Port Credit, Ont.; Tor'57; DPH; DTM&H (Eng.).
MANZ, Herbert J.; Wes'63; Res., Montreal Gen. Hosp., Montreal 25, P.Q.
MANZI, Jean; Mon '63; Res., Hop. Hotel-Dieu, Montreal 18, P.Q.
MAQUERA, Andres G.; 318 Alberta Corner Bldg., 804-1st St. S.W., Calgary, Alta.; Santo Tomas '52; Tel. 262-5003.
MAR, Peter G.; 2464 Huntley Ave., Ottawa 8, Ont.; Man '34; Chemist I/C, Biol. Lab., Radiation Protection Div., Dept. of National Health & Welfare; Tel. CE 2-8211.
MAR, P. S.; c/o Chief Med. Off., Dept. Nat. Health & Welfare, 61 Green St., London W.1, England.
MAR, Rhoda; UBC'64; Res., Shaughnessy Hosp., Vancouver 9, B.C.
MARANDA, Emilien; 216 St.-Vallier, ouest, Quebec 8, P.Q.; 1047 Chaumont, Sillery (res); Lav '34; Ophth,Otol; Ass't. Dept. of Ophth,Otol., Hop.-de-l'Enfant-Jesus; Ass't. Prof. Laval U.; Tel. 522-5832.
MARC-AURELE, Julien; 3840 rue St.-Urbain, Montreal 18, P.Q.; 27 Nelson, Outremont (res); Mon'55; IntMed(P.Q.); Assoc. Dir., Clin. Research, Hotel-Dieu; Tel. VI 4-0161.
MARCEAU, Gilles; 1573 Chemin Gomin, Sillery, Quebec, P.Q. (res); Lav '45; F.R.C.S.(C), F.A.C.S., GenSurg; Surg., D.V.A. Hosp., St. Foy; Ass't. Prof., Anat. Dept., Laval U.; Tel. MU 3-4951.
MARCEAU, Helene; Lav'65; Res., Allan Mem. Inst., 1025 Pine Ave. W., Montreal 2, P.Q.
MARCEAU, Laurent M.; Lav'59; Res., Hop. Hotel-Dieu, Montreal 18, P.Q.
MARCEAU, Michel; Lav'62; Otol; Staff, Queen Mary Vet's Hosp., Montreal, P.Q.
MARCEAU, Picard; Lav '58; FRCS(C), GenSurg; Staff, Hop. Laval, Quebec 10, P.Q.; Tel. 653-5251.
MARCEAU, Rene H.; Lav'61; Res., Queen Elizabeth Hosp., Montreal 28, P.Q.
MARCELIN, Andre; Lav'63; Staff, Hop. St. Louis, C.P. 580, Terrebonne, P.Q.
MARCELLUS, C.R.; Iroquois, Ont.; Qns '37; Dist. Coroner.
MARCELLUS, Donald F.; Health & Welfare Bldg., Albert & Hills St., Regina, Sask.; Tor '40; Dir., Med. Branch, Med. Care Ins. Comm.; Tel. 527-9681.
MARCELLUS, Edward E.; Qns. '65; Res., Kingston General Hosp., Kingston, Ont.
MARCELLUS, James A.; Goodchild Bldg., Mission City, B.C.; 963 Main St. (res); Qns '46; M.C.G.P.; Tel. 826-2523.
MARCH, Bernard W.; Dublin (Ire.) '57; DABPN; Psy; Deputy Sup., Saskatchewan Hosp., Box 7000, Weyburn, Sask.
MARCH, Raymond J.; 625-5th Ave., Ste. 607, New Westminster, B.C.; 317-4th Ave. (res); Ott'55; DABS; GenSurg; Active Staff, Royal Columbian Hosp.; Cons. Staff, St. Mary's & Surrey Mem. Hosp's.; Tel. 526-4606.
MARCHAND, Andre; 391 Blvd. Ste-Madeleine, Cap-de-la-Madeleine, P.Q.; 67 Guillet (res); Lav '58; Cardiol (P.Q.); Tel. FR 5-4776.
MARCHAND, Ernest; 11 Ste. Famille, Kenogami, P.Q.; Man '23; F.I.M., M.C.G.P.; Ind. Phys., Aluminum; Price Bros. & Co., (Jong & Kenog. Mills); Dist. M.O.H.
MARCHAND, Jacques; 3817 Boul. Decarie, Montreal 28, P.Q.; Mon'63; Tel. 488-5424.
MARCHAND, Jean C.; 161 Notre Dame, Ste. Thecle, Co. Laviolette, P.Q.
MARCHAND, Jean R.; 370 St. Jacques, Ste. Thecle, Co. Laviolette, P.Q.; Lav '58.
MARCHAND, Joseph A.; Mon'49; Res., Hop. St.-Jean-De-Dieu, Montreal 5, P.Q.
MARCHAND, Leopold; 12245 Grenet, Montreal 9, P.Q.; 5595 Place D'Aiguillon, Cartierville (res); Mon'50; DABOt., FAAOO, Otol (P.Q.); Chief of Otol., Hop.-du-Sacre-Coeur, Cartierville; Tel. DU 7-1413.
MARCHAND, Louis-J.; 55 St. Louis, Beauharnois, P.Q.; Mon '43; Staff, Hotel-Dieu Hosp., Valleyfield; Tel. 268-3434.
MARCHAND, Marc A.; 1005 rue St. Prosper, Trois Rivieres, P.Q.; 575 des Volontaires (res); Mon '49; M.C.G.P.; Ass't., Med. Staff, Hop. St. Joseph; Phys., K. of C.; Phys., Bell Telephone Co., a/M.O., RCAF., 6 GOBC Unit; Tel. 274-1944.
MARCHAND, Marcel; C.P. 490, 321 rue St. Laurent, Louiseville, P.Q.; Lav'50.
MARCHAND, Pierre; 50 rue du Couvent, St.-Tite, Cte. Champlain, P.Q.; Lav '45.
MARCHAND, Pierre; 451 de l'Hopital, Jonquiere, P.Q.; Lav'58; Paed; Tel. 547-9341.
MARCHAND, Rene; 1010, ouest, StCyrille, Quebec 6, P.Q.; Lav'46; Obst (P.Q.); Tel. 681-3242.
MARCHAND, Roger; Lav'59; Anaes(P.Q.); Staff, Hotel-Dieu Hosp., Sherbrooke, P.Q.
MARCHAND, Roger; Lav'63; Res., Hop. Ste. Justine, Montreal, P.Q.
MARCHANT, Peter; 178 St. George St., Toronto 5, Ont.; 56 Pine Cres., Tor. 13 (res); Tor '41; Anaes; Anaes., Toronto Gen. Hosp.; Cons. Anaes., Princess Margaret Hosp.; Clin. Instr. (Anaes.), U. of Toronto; Tel. WA 3-1154.
MARCHESSAULT, Victor J. H.; 14 rue Green, St. Lambert, P.Q.; Mon'55; FRCP(C), Paed; Clin. Ass't. Med., Mtl. Children's Hosp.; Lect. McGill U.; Tel. 671-0555.

MARCHILDON, Andre; 30 est, boul St.-Joseph, Montreal 14, P.Q.; Mon '56; IntMed (P.Q.); FRCS(C), Ophth; Teach. Staff Hop. Notre-Dame; Cons. Hop. Charles Lemoine, St. Lambert; Tel. 845-4241.

MARCHILDON, Paul A.; 519 Cherrier St., Montreal, P.Q.; 7 Querbes (res); Mon '25; GenSurg.

MARCHILDON, Roland B.; 145 Hampshire Rd., Beaconsfield, P.Q.; GenSurg(P.Q.).

MARCHUK, Peter; Box 70, Belmont, Ont.; R.R. No. 7, London (res); Wes '53; Tel. 644-1260.

MARCIL, **Gilles;** Mon'65; Res., Hop. Notre-Dame, Montreal 24, P.Q.

MARCIL, Pierre-Paul; 34 est Gamble, Rouyn, P.Q.; Mon'58; GenSurg; Staff, Hop. Youville; Tel. 762-6511.

MARCIL, Roland; 415 Ste. Helene, Longueuil, **Montreal P.Q.; Mon '43; Tel. OR 4-6281.**

MARCINIAK, Joseph L.; 20 Porteous Cres., Saskatoon, Sask. (res); Ott '53; IntMed; Active Staff, University Hosp.; Sr. Assoc., Sask. Cancer Clinic; Vis. Staff, St. Paul's & City Hosp's.; Clin. Instr., U. of Saskatchewan; Tel. CH 2-7641.

MARCINKOVSKY, Emilian; Box 600, Guelph, Ont.; R.R. 6, (res); Zagreb (Yugoslav.) '45 (Microbiol); M.O., Guelph Reformatory; Tel. TA 2-8403.

MARCOLIN, Lorenzo; 162 Gore St., Sault-Ste-Marie, Ont.; 126 Promenade Dr. (res); Tor '58; M.O.H.; Tel. 3-9142.

MARCOLONGO, Vincenzo, 1268 St. Clair Ave. W., Toronto, Ont.; '48.

MARCON, Norman E.; Qns'62; Res., St. Michael's Hosp., Toronto 2, Ont.

MARCOTTE, Emile; 12774 ouest Boul. Gouin, Pierrefonds, P.Q.; Lav'58; Cardiol (P.Q.); FRCP(C), IntMed; Part-time Teach. Staff, Hop. Hotel-Dieu; Cardiol. & Internist, Lakeshore Gen. Hosp.; Tel. 684-8460.

MARCOTTE, Gaston, C.P. 457, Cap-de-la-Madeleine, P.Q.; Mon '47; Surg., Hop. Cloutier.

MARCOTTE, J. E. Alexandre; 2165 Mount Royal E., Montreal, P.Q.; 20 Beloeil, Outremont **(res); Mon '25; Psy; Chief Psy., Montreal Health Serv.; Assoc. Prof. (Psy.) U. of Montreal; Tel. 872-5599.**

MARCOTTE, Michel; Coteau du Lac, Co. Soulanges, P.Q.; Mon '59.

MARCOTTE, Yvan; Mont-Laurier, P.Q.; Lav **'55; Med. Dir., Hop. Mont-Laurier; Tel. 440.**

MARCOUX, Agathe; Lav'64; Res., Hop. St-Jean-de-Dieu, Montreal 5, P.Q.

MARCOUX, Andre; Valcourt, Cte Shefford, P.Q.; Lav'62.

MARCOUX, Camille; Lourdes-du-Blanc-Sablon, Cte. Duplesis, P.Q.; Lav '57.

MARCOUX, Gendron; 1500-18eme rue, Quebec 3, P.Q.; Lav'46; FACS; FRCS(C), GenSurg; Chief of Surg., Hop. de l'Enfant Jesus; Ass't Prof. Laval U.; Tel. 525-5505.

MARCOUX, Gonzague; 5809-11eme Ave., Montreal 36, P.Q.; Mon '53; Tel. 721-7144.

MARCOUX, Guy P.; 540 Ave. Royale, Beauport, Quebec 5, P.Q.; Mon '52; P.C.B.; Phys., Canadian Cancer Soc.; Reg. Surg., St. John's Ambulance; Memb., Infect. Comm., Hop. de l'Enfant-Jesus; M.P.; Tel. 663-3832.

MARCOUX, Henri; 1050 Ploermel Ave., Quebec, P.Q. (res); Lav '29; PathBact; Chief, Clin. Lab's. (Bact. & Clin. Chem.), Hop. Hotel Dieu; **Prof. (Clin. Chem.), Laval U.; Tel. 529-9151.**

MARCOUX, Jean; Lav'65; Res., Hop. Ste-Justine, Montreal 26, P.Q.

MARCOUX, Jean R.; 1010 Chemin St. Roch, **Tracy, P.Q.; 2500 Bvd. Courvoyer (res); Mon '44; Cardiol (P.Q.); Chief-ofMed. & Cardiol., Hotel-Dieu Hosp., Sorel; Tel. RI 3-3725.**

MARCOUX, Paul; 298 rue Labelle, St.-Jerome, P.Q.; Lav '37; Anaes; Staff, Hop. Hotel-Dieu; Tel. GE 2-9711.

MARCOUX, Raymond; Lav '62; Res., Hotel-Dieu-St-Vallier Chicoutimi, P.Q.

MARCOUX, Rene; 1908 est Rachel, Montreal, P.Q.; Mon'42; 6591 Blvd. Pie IX (res); Mon'42; Tel. 521-1873.

MARCOUX, Robert; 10303 Ave. Sacré-Coeur, Montreal, P.Q.; **10830 Blvd. Olympia (res); Lav** '38.

MARCOUX, Romeo; 96 St. Charles St., St. Jean, P.Q.; Mon'40; Tel. 347-2560.

MARCUS, Anthony M.; Dept. of Psy., Vancouver Gen. Hosp., Vancouver, B.C.; Cambridge & Guy's H. (Eng.) '56; MA (Cantab.); **DPM (McG); Psy; Dir. Psy., OPD, Van. Gen. Hosp.; Ass't. Prof. (Psy), U. of British Columbia;** Tel. 876-3211.

MARCUS, David M.; 590 Seaforth Med. Bldg., 3550 Cote des Neiges Rd., Montreal 25, P.Q.; 5792 Wolseley Ave., Cote-St-Luke (res); Qns '50; FRCP(C); IntMed; Att'd. Phys., O.P.D., Montreal Gen. Hosp.; Dem. (Med.), McGill U.; Cons., Aviation Electric Ltd.; Tel. 933-4801.

MARCUS, Samuel; 37 Pleasant St., Bridgewater, N.S.; Dal'25; GenSurg (N.S.); Sr. Surg. & Chmn. Surg. Committ. & Med. Staff, Dawson Mem. Hosp.; Surg. Staff, Queen's Gen. Hosp., Liverpool; Tel. 543-3922.

MARECHAUX, E. W.; 1590 LaSalle Blvd. E., Sudbury, Ont.; 732 Falconbridge Hwy. (res).

MARECHAUX, Susanne, 1590 LaSalle Blvd. E., **Sudbury, Ont.; Freiburg U. (Germ.) '43; Staff,** Sudbury-Algoma San.

MARENGERE, Oliviere G.; 234 Levesque St., Sturgeon Falls, Ont.; Ott '61; AMCGP; Tel. 753-0830.

MARET, Eric P.; Eastport, Bonavista South, Nfld.; Bonn (Germ) '36.

MARFLEET, Teddy L.; Box 399, Maidstone, Sask.; **Alb '46; Dist. Coroner.; Tel. 893-2362.**

MARGETS, Philip G.; Box 880, Campbell River, B.C.; McG'44; GenSurg.

MARGETTS, Edward L.; McG '44; F.A.P.A.; D.Psy; Psy; Prof., Dept. of Psy., U. of British Columbia, Vancouver, B.C.; Tel. TR 6-3211, Loc. 2560.

MARGISON, Malcolm E.; Woodstock, N.B.; Dal '59; MCGP.

MARGOLESE, Richard G.; McG'60; FRCS(C), GenSurg; Staff, Jewish Gen. Hosp., Montreal, P.Q.; Abroad.

MARGOLIAN, Joseph; 1989 Queen St. E.; Toronto 8, Ont.; Tor '51; GenSurg; Tel. OX 9-7216.

MARGOLIS, Jack; 312 Boyd Bldg., Winnipeg 1, **Man.; 33 Scotia St. (res); Man '43; Ophth.; Tel. WH 3-3856.**

MARGOLIS, Neil; 423 Med. Arts Bldg., 404-406 Graham Ave., Winnipeg 1, Man.; Man'60; Paed; Active Paed. Staff, Winnipeg Children's & Misericordia Hosp's.; Dem. Paed., U. of Manitoba; Tel. 942-6405.

MARGOLUS, Benjamin D.; 560 Professional **Bldg., 10830 Jasper Ave., Edmonton, Alta.;** 1003-140th St. (res); Alb '37; FRCS(C), Gen Surg; Sess. Lect. (Med.), U. of Alberta; Tel. 422-6311.

MARGULIES, Alfred I.; 99 Avenue Rd., Ste. 809, Toronto, Ont.; 52 Beechwood Ave., Willowdale; Tor'59; D.Psy; Psy; Vol. Ass't., New Mount Sinai Hosp.; Staff, Baycrest Hosp. & Jewish Home for the Aged; Tel. CL 9-8291.

MARI, Paul; 800 Sherbrook St., Winnipeg 2, Man.; 28 Armour Cres. (res); Aurora (Shanghai, China) '46; Staff, Man. Rehab. H., Central TB Clinic; Instr., U. of Manitoba; Tel. SP 5-0181.

MARIAN, John J.; 617 Med. Arts Bldg., Saskatoon, Sask.; St. Bartholomew's Hosp. (London, Eng.) '41; MRCS (Eng.); LRCP (Lond.); FACS; FICS; FRCS(C), GenSurg; Cardiovasc & ThorSurg; Urol; Att'd. Surg., University, Saskatoon City & St. Paul's Hosp's.; Clin. Assoc. (Surg.), U. of Saskatchewan; Tel. 242-3525.

MARIE, E.; Ott '64; Res., Hop. Sacre-Coeur, Hull, P.Q.

MARIEN, Breen; 660 Westmount Med. Bldg., 5025 Sherbrooke St. W., Montreal 28, P.Q.; McG '49; FRCS(C); GenSurg; Ass't. Surg., Queen Elizabeth Hosp.; Tel. 488-2612.

MARIER, Louis P.; 191 Granville, Ottawa 7, Ont.; Ott'54; Anaes; Chief, Dept. of Anaes., St. Louis de Monfort Hosp.

MARIN, Charles E.; 367 est, boul St-Joseph, Montreal 14, P.Q.; Mon'56; Psy (P.Q.); Dem., U. of Montreal; Tel. 844-5554.

MARIN, Gerald A.; 221 Brant Ave., Brantford, Ont.; Guy's Hosp., London (Eng.) '52; FRCS (Ed.); FRCS (Eng.); FICS; OrthSurg; Active Staff, Brantford Gen. Hosp., St. Joseph's Hosp., Brantford & Willett Hosp., Paris; Tel. 753-4831.
MARIN, Reginald L.; 127 Conseil St., Sherbrooke, P.Q.; Lav '34 Anaes; Tel. 562-0225.
MARINEAU, Jean M.; 3424 rue St-Denis, Montreal 18, P.Q.; Mon'64; Tel. 842-4892.
MARINIER, Maurice; 207 Blvd. St. Joseph E., Montreal 14, P.Q.; Mon '54; Obst (P.Q.); Tel. VI 4-2591.
MARINKER, Simon; 240 McNabb St., Sault Ste. Marie, Ont.; London (Eng.) '36; MRCS; LRCP (Eng.); FRCS (Eng.); FRCS(C); GenSurg; Tel. 254-6421.
MARION, Donatien; 326 E. Blvd. St. Joseph, Montreal, P.Q.; 801 Riverside Dr., St. Lambert (res); Mon '20; F.R.C.S.(C), Obst (P.Q.); Professor Emer. Obst., & Memb. Board of Governors, U. of Montreal; Tel. 844-2991.
MARION, Gilles; Ste. 201, 168 Charlotte St., Ottawa 2, Ont.; 761 Hemlock Rd., Ott. 7 (res); Qns '47; FAAP; Paed; Chief (Paed), St.-Louis-Marie-de-Montfort Hosp.; Lect. (Paed.), U. of Ottawa; Tel. 236-3234.
MARION, Gilles; Mon'65; Res., Hop. Gen. Verdun, Montreal 19, P.Q.
MARION, J. Eustache; 538 Beaubieu E., Montreal, P.Q.; Lav '12; Tel. 277-6300.
MARION, Jean; 7525 Louis Hemon, Montreal 35, P.Q.; Mon '41; Tel. RA 5-4232.
MARION, Pierre G.; 326 E. Blvd. St. Joseph, Montreal 14, P.Q.; 528 Bloomfield Ave., Outremont (res); Mon '43; F.A.C.C., IntMed (P.Q.), Cardiol. (P.Q.), Head Dept. of Cardiol., Hop. Ste. Justine; Cardiol., Hotel Dieu, Montreal & Sorel; Ass't. Prof. (Med.), U. of Montreal; Member of the Board of the American College of Cardiology; Sec.-Treas., Cardiol, Assoc. (P.Q.); Tel. RE 1-4931.
MARIONI, Peter; Aberdeen (Scot.) '47; FRCS-(Ed.); FRCS (Eng.); GenSurg; Chief Res. (Gen-Surg.), Royal Alexandra Hosp., Edmonton, Alta. Abroad
MARITS, Maldus; Box 730, Salmon Arm, B. C.; 3577 W. 35th Ave. (res); UBC '58.
MARIZ-FERNANDEZ, Segundo; 1591 Jalna Ave., Clarkson, Ont.; Madrid (Spain) '51; Path.
MARJANOVICH, Katarina; (See ADLER, Kay).
MARJERRISON, Gordon L.; Box 39, North Battleford, Sask.; McG '55; FRCP(C), Psy; Staff, Saskatchewan Hosp.; Vis. Cons., University Hosp., Saskatoon; Clin. Teach. (Psy.), U. of Saskatchewan; Sr. Spec. Psy. Research, Dept. of Public Health; Tel. 445-2421, Ext. 334.
MARK, Alexander L.; Qns '63; Jr. Ass't. Res. (Path.), Kingston Gen. Hosp., Kingston, Ont. Abroad.
MARK, Frederick G. F.; 1101 Victoria Park Ave., Toronto 16, Ont.; 28 Beechwood Dr. (res); Tor '52; Tel. PL 5-0626.
MARK, Ivan G. C.; 2806 Danforth Ave., Toronto 13, Ont.; 87 Sylvan Ave., Scarboro (res); Tor '47; O.P.D., Toronto Western Hosp.; Plant Phys., American Motors of Canada & Perfect Circle Ltd.; Tel. OX 9-8105.
MARK, Mary (See WONG-MARK)
MARK, Richard J.; Nipawin, Sask.; Man'65.
MARKARIAN-DEMERS, Angik; 11758 l'Acadie, Montreal 12, P.Q.; Ophth(P.Q.).
MARKENS, Isaac J.; 1271 Dundas St. W., Toronto, Ont.; Tor '48; MCGP; Att'd. Staff, Mount Sinai & Doctor's Hosp's.; Tel. LE 5-3164.
MARKHAM, James D.; Fort William Clinic, Fort William, Ont.; 427 S. Marks St. (res); Tor '37; IntMed.; Internist, McKellar Gen. Hosp; Tel. 622-5363.
MARKHAM, William G.; UBC '55; Anaes; Staff, Hosp. for Sick Children, Toronto 2, Ont.; Tel. EM 6-7242.
MARKKANEN, V. William; 3225 Wyandotte E., Riverside, Ont.; 1104 Riverside Dr., Riverside (res); Tor '36; FRCS(Edin); Tel. 945-7365.
MARKO, Arthur M.; 419 Albert Ave., Saskatoon, Sask. (res); Tor '49; Ph.D.; Ass't. Prof. (Biochem.) & Research Assoc. (Paed.), Saskatchewan U.; Tel. CH 2-7671.
MARKO, John; 11131-85th Ave., Edmonton, Alta.; Alb'58; FRCS(C), ObstGyn; MacLaughlin Travelling Fell. 1967-68.
MARKOV, Bozidar H.; Stoughton, Sask.; Sofia (Bulgaria); '61.
MARKOVA, Fodorka; Box 37, Stoughton, Sask.; Sofia (Bulgaria)'54.
MARKOVIC, Smilja (See Henderson)
MARKOVITS, Molly H.; 207 Bond St., Winnipeg 25, Man.; Man'39; Tel. CA 2-1345.
MARKOVITS, Samuel L.; 207 Bond St., Transcona, Man.; 78 St. Mary's Rd., Norwood (res); Man'29; Tel. CA 2-1345.
MARKOWITZ, Jacob, M.B.E.; 46 Forest Hill Rd., Toronto, 7, Ont.; Tor '23; Ph.D. (Physiol.), M.S. (Experi.Surg.), M.C.G.P.; Prof. (Physiol.), U. of Toronto; Vis. Prof. (Physiol.), Ont. Veterinary Coll., Guelph; Tel. WA 3-8606.
MARKOWSKI, Edwin G.; Box 70, 5761 Pacific Highway, Cloverdale, B.C.; McG '47. Tel. 574-4423.
MARKS, Cyril P.; Ste. 201, 1200 Lawrence Ave. E., Don Mills, Ont.; 18 Donway E., Apt. 301 (res); Tor'58; AMCGP; Adj. Ass't., New Mt. Sinai Hosp.; Court. Staff, Tor. E. Gen. & Grace Hosp's.; Tel. 444-4497.
MARKS, Leili (See Kasari)
MARKS, Lionel; 605 Bloor St. W., Toronto 4, Ont.; 15 Shallmar Blvd., Apt. 704 (res); Tor '31; FACG; IntMed; Att'd. Staff, New Mt. Sinai & Doctors' Hosp's.; Memb. Bd. of Trustees, Am. Coll. Gastro-enterology; Tel. LE 1-2181.
MARKS, Malcolm M.; 359 Fraser St., North Bay, Ont.; Dublin (Ire.) '57; Active Staff, North Bay Civic & St. Joseph's Hosp's.; Tel. 474-4780.
MARKS, Melvin L.; McG'65; Res., Children's Hosp., Montreal 25, P.Q.
MARKSFIELD, Wm. C.; 308-40th Ave., Lachine, Montreal 32, P.Q.; 4566 Hampton Ave. (res); McG '43; F.I.C.S., F.R.C.S.(C), GenSurg; Surg. Staff, Lachine Gen. Hosp.; Tel. 637-7262.
MARKSON, Chas. A.; Ste. 612, 99 Avenue Rd., Toronto 5, Ont.; 1603 Bathurst St. (res); Tor'22; IntMed; Cons., Baycrest Hosp.; Tel. 924-2444.
MARKSON, Elliott R.; 288 St. Clair Ave. W., Toronto 7, Ont.; Tor '48; Psy; Vol. Ass't. New Mt. Sinai Hosp.; Cons. Forensic Clinic; Clin. Inst. (Psy), U. of Toronto; Tel. WA 1-5282.
MARKSON, Moses; 5A Main St., Alexandria, Ont.; Kenyon St. (res); McG '20; Dist. Coroner.
MARKSON, Sari S. (Hockman); 288 St. Clair Ave. W., Toronto 7, Ont.; Tor '48; Psy; Staff (OPD), Tor. Psychiatric Hosp.; Tel. WA 1-5282.
MARKUS, Arthur J.; 5041 Park Ave., Montreal, P.Q.; 431 Lethbridge Ave., Twn. of Mt. Royal (res); McG '52; Paed; Staff, Montreal Children's & Jewish Gen. Hosp's.; Chief of Paed., Santa Cabrini Hosp.; Teach Fell., McGill U.; Tel. 277-7700.
MARKUS, Frank; King St., Shelburne, N.S.; Budapest (Hung.) '50; MCGP; Active Staff, Roseway Hosp.; Tel. 519.
MARKUS, Newton; 25 Brunswick Ave., Toronto 4, Ont.; 84 Chiltern Hill Rd., Tor 10 (res); Tor '56; DABR; DiagRad; Assoc. Rad., Doctor's Hosp.; Tel. WA 3-5411.
MARLATT, Donald C.; Ste. 2, Boyd Bldg., 3 Gore St., Chilliwack, B.C.; 516 Maple Ave. (res); Man'35; IntMed (TB); Tel. 792-1735.
MARLATT, Helen M.; 401 Medical Arts Bldg., Winnipeg, Man.; 550 Campbell St. (res); Man '26; Paed; Staff, Winnipeg Children's Hosp.; Lect. (Paed.), U. of Manitoba; Retired.
MARLBOROUGH, Marcus; Jewish Gen. Hosp., Montreal 26; P.Q.; Glasgow (Scot.) '43; D.M.R. (T), TherRad.; Tel. 735-3771.
MARLEAU, Denis; Mon'65; Res., Hop. St Luc, Montreal 18, P.Q.
MARLISS, Errol B.; Alb '64; Res., Royal Victoria Hosp., Montreal 2, P.Q.
MARLOW, John N.; 615A Main St., Lively, Ont.; 186—6th Ave.; Tor '52.
MARMAR, M.; 135 Osborne, Winnipeg, Man.; 442 Montrose St. (res); Man '32; M.C.G.P.; Tel. GR 5-6854.
MARMINA, Joseph V.; 1417 Danforth Ave., Toronto 6, Ont.; 149 Valley Dr., Don Mills (res); Tor '62; Tel. 444-5359.

MAROIS, Andre; 234 rue St. Jean, Quebec 4, P.Q.; 828 ave Bellevue, Quebec 10 (res); Lav '46; Cardiol. (P.Q.); Hd. Cardiol., Hop. de l'Enfant Jesus; Tel. 525-9128.
MAROIS, Martial; Ott '58; Phys Med. & Rehab; Staff, Hop. St. Vincent, Ottawa 4, Ont; Tel. 233-4041.
MAROIS, Michel; Lav '60; Path (P.Q.); Staff, Hop. St. Francois d'Assise, Quebec 3, P.Q.
MAROIS, Michel; Lav'60; Path (P.Q.); Staff, Hop. St. Francois d'Assise, Quebec 3, P.Q.
MAROOSIS, John P. G.; 195 Simcoe St. N., Oshawa, Ont.; 494 King St. E. (res); Tor '43; Chief of Med. Div., Oshawa Gen. Hosp.; Tel. 725-6811.
MAROTTA, Joseph T.; Ste. 203, 215 Victoria St., Toronto 1, Ont.; Tor '49; F.R.C.P.(C), Neur; Staff, St. Michael's Hosp.; Clin. Instr. (Med), U. of Toronto; Tel. 364-1072.
MAROTTE, Germain; Mon'60; Res., Hop. Maisonneuve, Montreal 36, P.Q.
MAROUN, Falah B.; Beirut (Lebanon) '60; FRCS(C), NeurSug;r Staff, Hop. Hotel-Dieu, Montreal 18, P.Q.
MARQUETTE, Claude; Mon'65; Sr. Int., Institute Albert Prevost, Montreal 9, P.Q.
MARQUIS, Andre B.; 299 - 5th Ave., Quebec 3, P.Q.; 324 - 21st St. (res); Lav '52; F.R.C.S.(C), ObstGyn.; Staff. Hop-l'Enfant - Jesus & Laval U.; Tel. 524-4972.
MARQUIS, Jacques; 1660 Parc Chesnaye, Quebec 6, P.Q.; Lav '57; Anaes; Staff, Hop. Hotel-Dieu; Tel. 529-9151.
MARQUIS, John A. D.; 138 Market St., Brantford, Ont.; 136 Market St. (res); Tor '33; IntMed; Staff, Brantford Gen. & St. Joseph's Hosp's; Tel. 752-1441.
MARQUIS, Michel; Lav'58; Anaes (P.Q.); Staff, Hop. St. Vincent-de-Paul, Sherbrooke, P.Q.
MARQUIS, Paul A.; Lav'54; Psy; Staff, Hop. St.-Michel-Archange, Quebec, P.Q.
MARQUIS, Yves; Lav '61; Res., Cardiovasc. Unit, Toronto Gen. Hosp., Toronto 2, Ont.
MARR, Peter F.; 4900 Kingsway, Burnaby 1, B.C.; 6226 Gilpin St. (res); Wes '50; FRCS(C), Urol; Tel. HE 3-0545.
MARRACK, Alexander; 194 N. Court St., Port Arthur, Ont.; London (Eng.) '55; FRCP(C), Anaes.
MARRIOTT, Frank G.; 144 Geneva St., St. Catharines, Ont.; Glasgow (Scot.)'53; Ophth; Tel. MU 5-7739.
MARRIOTT, Ian A., W/C; CFMS Training Centre, Camp Borden, Ont.; Cambridge & St. Thomas's. H. (Eng.) '42; MIH (Harvard).
MARRIOTT, R. Douglas; Parsons Clinic, 4826 Ross St., Red Deer, Alta.; Wes '53; FRCS(C), GenSurg; Chief of Surg., Red Deer Municipal Hosp.; Tel. 346-2042.
MARSAN, Richard G.; 3737 est rue Sherbrooke, Montreal 36, P.Q.; 1135 ouest Laurier, Outremont (res); Mon '56; Med. Dir., Catholic School Comm.; Tel. 525-6311, Loc. 379.
MARSDEN, John; 2184 W. Broadway, Vancouver 9, B.C.; Cambridge (Eng.) '55; Tel. RE 1-3171.
MARSH, David W.; Transcona Med. Group, 311 Day St., Transcona 25, Man.; Durham (Eng.) '61; Tel. 222-4259.
MARSH, G. Stewart; Sydney Med. Arts Bldg., 336 Kings Rd., Sydney, N.S.; Ott '59; Staff, St. Rita's & Sydney City Hosp's.; Tel. 562-1282.
MARSH, Joan E.; Aberdeen (Scot.) '49; Res., Jewish Gen. Hosp., Montreal 26, P.Q.
MARSH, John K. McK.; 277 Scarboro Cres., Scarborough, Ont.; Tor '49; Tel. AM 1-7211.
MARSH, Margaret L. (Peddie); 2529 Estevan Ave., Victoria, B.C.; 954 Newport Ave. (res); Qns '53; Tel. EV 5-1717.
MARSH, Peter E.; 350 Albert St., Nanaimo, B.C.; Liverpool (Eng.)'64.
MARSHALL, A. Cleland; R.R.4, Middle Musquodoboit, Halifax Co, N.S.; Dal'63; Sec. Eastern Shore Med. Soc.; Sec., Standards Committ., Musquodoboit Valley Mem. Hosp.; Memb. & Nominating Committ., N.S. Med. Soc.; Tel. Upper Musquodoboit 3.
MARSHALL, Albert H.; Box 138, Dunnville, Ont.; Tor '32; Dist. Coroner; Tel. 774-6445.
MARSHALL, Ann T. (Bowden); 66 Oxford St., Strathroy, Ont. (res); Qns'52; Tel. 245-0333.
MARSHALL, Arthur M.; 6086 Quinpool Rd., Halifax, N.S.; 7020 Armview Ave. (res); Dal '22; F.R.C.S.(Edin.); Assoc. Surg., Children's Hosp.; Tel. 423-6555.
MARSHALL, Brian M.; 178 St. George St. Toronto 5, Ont.; **25 Eastbourne Ave. (res); Tor '50; FRCP(C); Anaes; Staff (Anaes.) Toronto Gen. Hosp.; Clin. Instr., U. of Toronto; Tel. WA 3-1154.**
MARSHALL, Clyde; Dept. of PH., Prov. Bldg., Hollis St., Halifax, N.S.; 1779 Beech St. (res); Dal '24; NeurPsy; Admin. Mental Health Serv. Dept. of PH; Assoc. Prof. (Med., (Neurol.)), Dalhousie U.; Tel. 422-7341, Loc. 485.
MARSHALL, Donald G.; 532 Waterloo St., London, Ont.; 376 Ridout St. S. (res); Wes '49; FAAP; FRCS(C); GenSurg; Paed. Surg; St. Joseph's Hosp.; Instr. (Surg.), U. of Western Ontario; Tel. GE 9-7381.
MARSHALL, Donald G.; 73 Queen St. E., Brampton, Ont.; 193 Elizabeth St. S., Tor '56; Active Staff, Peel Mem. Hosp.; Tel. GL 1-1244.
MARSHALL, Ernest B.; 1554A Bloor St. W., Toronto 9, Ont.; Dal '65; MCGP; Tel. LE 3-1731.
MARSHALL, Frederick C.; 518 Med. Arts Bldg., 11010 Jasper Ave., Edmonton, Alta.; Alb. '54; FRCS(C), Urol; Active Staff, Royal Alexandra Hosp.; Cons. Urol. Mult. Handicapped Children's Unit, Glenrose Prov. Gen. Hosp.; Instr. (Surg.), U. of Alberta; Tel 488-9357.
MARSHALL, George; 502 Chinook Prof. Bldg., 6449 Macleod Trail, Calgary, Alta.; St. Andrews (Scot.) '58.
MARSHALL, George M.; 230 Norfolk S., Simcoe, Ont.; 249 Dean St. (res); Wes '43; Med. Staff, Norfolk Gen. Hosp.; Tel. 426-3530.
MARSHALL, Gladys D.; 560 Professional Bldg., 10830 Jasper Ave., Edmonton, Alta.; Alb'64.
MARSHALL, Judith A.; (see Meade).
MARSHALL, Kelvin H. A.; 277 Duckworth St., St. John's, Nfld.; 7 Glenridge Cres. (res); Oxford & London (Eng.) '36; M.R.C.S. (Eng.), L.R.C.P. (Lond.); Ass't. Orth. Surg., St. John's Gen. Hosp.; Sr. Dist. MOH, CNR; Tel. 722-2120.
MARSHALL, Kenneth G.; McG '58; FRCP(C); Path; Staff, Dept. of Path., Kingston Gen. Hosp., Kingston, Ont.; Tel. 546-3842.
MARSHALL, Mark R.; University of Alberta Hosp., Edmonton, Alta.; 11125 Saskatchewan Dr. (res); McG'26; DLO (Eng.), FRCS(C), FACS, Ophth; Prof. of Ophth., U. of Alberta; Tel. GE 3-3531.
MARSHALL, Mary E. (Mrs. A. A. Bailey); 243 Med. Arts Bldg., Saskatoon, Sask.; Tor'35; Psy; Part-time Teach. Staff, University Hosp.; Tel. 242-2290.
MARSHALL, Maurice M.; Lethbridge Mun. Hosp., Lethbridge, Alta.; 2113-20th Ave. S. (res); **Alb '46; M.A.C.R., D.A.B.R., DiagRad;. Tel. FA 7-8591.**
MARSHALL Norman L.; 103 Med. Arts Bldg., Windsor, Ont.; Wes'52; FACS; FCCP; GenSurg; Chief, Dept. of Surg., IODE Hosp.; Surg. Cons., Metropolitan, Hotel-Dieu, Grace & Riverview Hosp's.; Tel. 256-3871.
MARSHALL, Robert E.; Box 1088, Mission, B.C.; McG '52; M.C.G.P.
MARSHALL, Russell H.; 750 W. Broadway, Vancouver, B.C.; 6176 Alma Rd. (res); Tor '46; F.R.C.S.(C), GenSurg.; Tel. TR 2-2595.
MARSHALL, S. Alison; (See Krupa).
MARSHALL, T. David; Cayuga, Ontario.; Tor '63.
MARSHALL, W. Douglas; Medical Arts Bldg., 1105 Pandora St., Victoria, B.C.; 615 Foul Bay Rd. (res); Wes'37; FRCOG, FRCS(C), FACS, ObstGyn; Staff, Royal Jubilee Hosp.; Cons. Staff, St. Joseph's Hosp.; Tel. EV 4-5931.
MARSHALL, William L.; Southwest Health Unit, Killarney, Man.; Edinburgh (Scot.) '50; DPH.
MARSOLAIS, Almanzor; 447 Querbes, Montreal 8, P.Q.; Mon '30; Anaes; Ass't. Anaes., Hop. Hotel-Dieu; Ass't. Prof. (Anaes.), U. of Montreal; Tel. 279-6036.

MARSON, F. Graham; 220 Med. Arts Bldg., 1 Young St., Hamilton, Ont.; 86 **Mansfield** Dr., Ancaster (res); Birmingham (Eng.) '44; M.R.-C.S.(Eng.), M.R.C.P.(Lond.), L.R.C.P.(Lond.), FRCP(C), IntMed; Active Cons. Staff, Hamilton Civic & Chedoke Gen. & Children's Hosp's; Tel. JA 9-6161.

MARSTON, John G., F/L; Canadian Forces Hosp., Halifax, N.S.; Dal'64.

MARTEINSSON, Brandur T. H.; 1410 Med. Dental Bldg., 925 W. Georgia St., Vancouver, B.C.; 5911 Wiltshire St. (res); Man '31; F.R.-C.S.(Eng.); GenSurg; Surg. Staff, St. Paul's Hosp.; Clin. Instr. (Surg.), U. of British Columbia; Tel. MU 1-4161.

MARTEL, Andre; 875 boul. des Recollets, Trois-Rivieres, P.Q.; 680 des Metezes (res); Lav '52; FACS, FRCS(C), GenSurg; Active Staff (Surg.), Hop. Ste.-Marie; Vis. Staff, Hop. St.-Joseph & Hop. Comtois, Louisville; Tel. FR 5-5531.

MARTEL, Antonio; 590 St-Cyrille, ouest, Quebec 6, P.Q.; 620 Chemin St. Louis, Apt. 6 (res); Lav '32; IntMed; Lect. (Med.), Laval U.; Tel. 681-9433.

MARTEL, Claude R.; 298 rue St. Germain, Rimouski, P.Q.; Lav'60; Cardiol(P.Q.).

MARTEL, F.; 3800 Dandurand St., Montreal, 48, P.Q.; 2513 Fullum (res); Mon '48.; Tel. 721-6618.

MARTEL, Gilles; Mon'64; Res., Hop. Ste-Justine, Montreal 26, P.Q.

MARTEL, J. Alcide; 2207 Fullum St., Montreal, P.Q.; Mon '33; Paed. Tel. LA 3-3647.

MARTEL, Jean C.; 300 Carre-St.-Louis, Montreal 18, P.Q.; 947 Macnaughton Rd., Ville-Mt. Royal (res); Mon '49; DAB (Proct.); Vol. Surg., Hop. Jeanne-d'Arc; Tel. VI 9-6485.

MARTEL, Jean-Guy; Lav '61; Res., Hop. Hotel-Dieu, Quebec 4, P.Q.

MARTEL, M. C. Roland; 4 Blvd. Joliet, Hauterive, Co. Saguenay, P.Q. (res); Mon. '43; Gen Surg; Med. Dir. & Surg., Hotel-Dieu de Hauterive; Tel. 589-3701.

MARTEL, Pierre G.; 1000 Boul. Ste.-Anne, Joliette, P.Q.; 879 St.-Louis (res); Lav '55; Psy; Med. Supt., Hop. St.-Charles; Tel. PL 6-8021.

MARTEL-JUTRAS, Therese; Polyclinique Gravel, **66 St.-Jean-Baptiste, Victoriaville, P.Q.; 42 St.** Paul (res); Lav '52; Staff, Hotel-Dieu-d'Arthabaska; Tel. 752-7292.

MARTEL, Serge B.; 170 Saunders, Quebec, P.Q.; Paed(P.Q.).

MARTENS, Robert G., F/L; Station Infirmary, CFB Edmonton, Lancaster Park, Alta.; Man'64.

MARTENSTYN, Henry R. L.; 46 Roosevelt Ave., Truro, N.S.; Ceylon '55; DiagRad; Radiol., Colchester County Hosp.; Tel. 895-5421.

MARTH, Edmund A.; 308 Boler Rd., Byron, Ont.

MARTIMBEAU, Emile; 3165 Tremblay, Montreal 26, P.Q.; Mon '34; Anaes. (P.Q.).

MARTIN, Alberto G.; 600 Caledonia Rd., Toronto 10, Ont.; 345 Lonsdale Rd. (res); Madrid (Spain) '51; GenSurg; Court. Staff, Doctors' Hosp.; Tel. RU 1-7511.

MARTIN, Alice M. (Mrs. F. G. Dance); 166 Langton St., Peterborough, Ont. (res); Tor '49; A.M.-C.G.P.; M.H.O., Smith Township.

MARTIN, Antoine; Lav '54; Res., Montreal Gen. Hosp., Montreal 25, P.Q.

MARTIN, Benoit; Maria, Co. Bonaventure, P.Q.; Lav '35; GenSurg (P.Q.); Med. Supt., Hop. Notre Dame de Chartres, Maria; Tel. 443.

MARTIN, Charles A.; Clinique Roy-Rousseau, Mastai, P.Q.; Lav '38; FRCP(C), Psy; NeurPsy (P.Q.); Chief of Serv., Clinique Roy-Rousseau; **Dir., Dept. of Psy., Laval U.; Tel. 661-7735.**

MARTIN, David J.; 10730 Trans Canada Hwy., North Surrey, B.C.; Sask '57; Tel. 581-3348. Abroad.

MARTIN, Dennis; 2917 Bloor St. W., Toronto 9, Ont.; Ireland '54; D.Psy; Psy; Staff, Toronto Psychiatric Hosp.; Tel. WA 5-6371.

MARTIN, Donald C.; UBC '57; Int'n., Shaughnessy Hosp., Vancouver, B.C.

MARTIN, Douglas T.; 440 Medical-Dental Bldg., Regina, Sask.; 2900 College Ave. **(res); Man '37; D.A.O.(Eng.), Otol.; Tel. 522-1645.**

MARTIN, Elizabeth C. (Stockdale); 6 Delhi St., Guelph, Ont. (res); Tor '33; Part-time P.H. Med. Exam.

MARTIN, Francois; Mon '64; Res., Hop. St-Luc, Montreal 18, P.Q.; Abroad.

MARTIN, Gabriel; 10690 d'Auteuil, Montreal 12, P.Q.; Lav'51; PhysMed. & Rehab.; Tel. 381-6291.

MARTIN, Gerard; 9050 Blvd. St. Michel, Ville St. Michel, Montreal 38, P.Q.; Mon '52; A.M.C.G.P. Tel. DU 7-0397.

MARTIN, Gerard; 770-lere Ave., Quebec 3, P.Q.; Mon '59.

MARTIN, Glen M.; 650 Tunstall Cres., Kamloops, B.C. (res); Qns '49; FCAP; Path; Pathol., Royal Inland Hosp.; Dir. Reg. Pathol. Serv.; Tel. 372-8113.

MARTIN, Gordon K.; Parliament Bldgs., Toronto 5, Ont.; 40 Foursome Cr., Willowdale (res); Tor '48; DPH; Dir., PH Admin. Br., Ont. Dept. of Health; Tel. 365-2426.

MARTIN, Harold S.; 11 Sherwood Rise, Hamilton, Ont. (res); Tor '14; Tel. 385-2174.

MARTIN, Hugh J.; Sydney Mines, N.S.; Dal'31.

MARTIN, Jacques; 8020 Papineau Ave., Montreal 35, P.Q.; 11920 Zotique (res); Mon '59; Tel. 728-4508.

MARTIN, James; Queen's U. (Belfast, Ire.)'57; BAO; Res., Dept. of DiagRad., Toronto Gen. Hosp., Toronto 2, Ont.

MARTIN, J. David; Fort Rae, N.W.T.; Tor'64; M.O., Fort Rae Med. Serv., Dept. of National Health & Welfare.

MARTIN, Jean; 1229 Notre Dame St., Lachine, P.Q.; Mon '43; GenSurg (P.Q.); Surg., Hop. St. **Joseph, Lachine; Tel. 637-8681.**

MARTIN, Jean C.; 836, des Ursulines, Trois-Rivieres, P.Q.; Lav '61.

MARTIN, Jeffrey L.; London (Eng.) '59; MRCS; LRCP; Staff, Doctor's Hosp., Toronto, Ont.

MARTIN, John H.; 415 Medical Arts Bldg., Winnipeg, Man.; 200 Ash St. (res); Man '43; Int-Med; Cons. Gastroent. Deer Lodge (DVA) Hosp.; Med. Staff, St. Boniface & Misericordia Hosp's.; **Lect. (Med.), U. of Manitoba; Tel. TU 8-4861.**

MARTIN, J. Campbell; Apt. 406, 110 Park Rd. N., Oshawa, Ont. (res); Tor '54; Staff, Oshawa Gen. Hosp.; Tel. 723-2211, Loc. 294.

MARTIN, J. Henri; Edifice Medical de Hull, 31 Montcalm, Hull, P.Q.; Ott '57; M.C.G.P.

MARTIN, J. Kenneth; Dept. of Paed., University Hosp., Edmonton, Alta.; 10224 Churchill Cr. (res); London (Eng.) '41; MRCP; DCH; DRCOG; FRCP(C); Paed; Staff. University Hosp.; Prof. & Hd., Dept. of Paed., U. of Alberta; Tel. 439-5911.

MARTIN, John M.; Med. Clinic, Invermere, B.C.; UBC'56; MCGP; Med. Staff, Windemere Dist. Hosp.; Tel. 342-9221.

MARTIN, John P.; 3 Maple Ave. W., Georgetown, Ont.; Dal '59; AMCGP; Tel. 877-6541.

MARTIN, John R.; 1414 Drummond St., Ste. 706, Montreal 23, P.Q.; McG'45; MRCP (London), FACP; FRCP(C), IntMed; Att'd. Staff, Montreal Gen. Hosp.; Cons. (Arthritis), Queen Mary Vet's. Hosp.; Phys. Cdn. Industries Ltd.; Tel. VI 9-8804.

MARTIN, J. Walter; 524 Brant St., Burlington, Ont.; Wes '54; GenSurg.; Tel. 637-2915.

MARTIN, Jules; Mon '62; Ass't. Res., Hop. Notre -Dame, Montreal, P.Q.

MARTIN, Laura; (Levine); 902 King St. E., **Hamilton, Ont.; 2 St. Clair Ave. (res); Tor '38; A.M.C.A.A., DermSyph; Med. Staff, Hamilton Gen. Hosp.; O.P.D. (Derm.), Toronto Western Hosp., Toronto; Tel. LI 9-9796.**

MARTIN, Morgan G.; Box 639, Almonte, Ont. (res); Qns '44; M.Sc., Admin. Med.; MHA; Psy; Chief, Mental Health Div., Dept. Natl. Health & Welfare, Ottawa; Lect. Civil Defence College, Arnprior; Tel. 992-6937; Abroad.

MARTIN, Paul; 55 Bellingham Rd., Montreal, P.Q. (res); Mon '34; PathBact; Ass't Dir. Medico Legal Lab. of P.Q.; Chief Path & Dir. Lab's., Hop. St. Luc; Cons. Path. Queen Mary D.V.A. Hosp.; Prof. Path., U. of Montreal; Tel. 861-7321.

MARTIN, Pierre; C.P. 160, Gracefield, Cte Gatineau, P.Q.; Lav'63; Tel. 463-2818.
MARTIN, Pierre R.; Mon'63; Res., Hop. Hotel-Dieu, Montreal, P.Q.
MARTIN, Richard R.; Mon'65; Res., Hop. Maisonneuve, Montreal 36, P.Q.
MARTIN, Robert F.; Ontario Crippled Children's Centre, 350 Rumsey Rd., Toronto, Ont.; Tor'57; FRCS(C), OrthSurg.
MARTIN, Robert G.; 240 McNabb St., Sault Ste. Marie, Ont.; Wes'56; FACOG; FRCS(C), ObstGyn; Cons. Staff, local Hosp's.; Tel. 254-4653.
MARTIN, Robert H.; 98 Sherman Ave. S., Hamilton, Ont.; Wes '46; Phys., Dominion Foundry & Steel Co.; Tel. LI 9-5211.
MARTIN, Roch; C.P. 320, Amqui, Cte. Matapedia, P.Q.; Lav '54; Tel. 677.
MARTIN, Ross L.; Grand Falls, Nfld.; Dal '60.
MARTIN, Saul A.; Ste. 440, 5845 Cote des Neiges Rd., Montreal 26, P.Q.; Sask'58; Psy; Ass't., Jewish Gen. Hosp.; Tel. 739-8002.
MARTIN, S. Jameson; Ste. 480, 4141 Sherbrooke St. W., Westmount 6, P.Q.; McG'28; FRCS (Ed. & Eng.); FRCS(C), GenSurg; Sr. Surg., Montreal Gen. Hosp.; Assoc. Prof. (Surg.), McGill U.; Tel. 931-1081.
MARTIN-SMITH, Bernard; Martin-Smith Assoc. Clinic, Lakeview Med. Dental Bldg., Lethbridge, Alta.; London (Eng.) '54; Active Staff, Lethbridge Mun. & St. Michael's Gen. Hosp's.; Tel. 328-5538.
MARTIN, Thomas H.; Wes'64; Res., Westminster Hosp., London, Ont.
MARTIN, Thomas R.; Durham (Eng.) '59; Res., Victoria Gen. Hosp., Halifax, N.S.
MARTIN, William E.; 528—12th Ave. N., Port Alberni, B.C. (res); UBC'60; FRCP(C), IntMed.
MARTIN, William E.; Torrance, Ont.; Tor'16; Anaes.; Retired.
MARTIN, William J.; Box 240, Cyanamid of Canada, Ltd., Niagara Falls, Ont.; Tor'49; Dir. of Med. Serv., Cyanamid of Canada Ltd.; Tel. EL 8-3681.
MARTIN, William R.; Ste. 309, 4900 Kingway, South Burnaby, B.C.; UBC '54; Ophth; Tel. HE 3-1258.
MARTIN, William S.; 666 Victoria Dr., Baie d'Urfe, P.Q.; McG '50; M.Eng. (Electrical); Phys., Ste. Anne's Hosp., Ste. Anne de Bellevue; Biophysicist, Queen Mary Vet's. Hosp., Montreal.
MARTIN, William W.; 1125 Moncton Ave., Quebec 6, P.Q.; Lav '33; Anaes; Techn. Adviser, Hosp. Construction (PQ).; Tel. 683-9664.
MARTINE, Paul; Stettler, Alberta; Lav '55; Abroad.
MARTINE, R.; Meadow Lake, Sask.
MARTINEAU, Bernard; 2525 Cote Ste. Catherine, Montreal 26, P.Q.; Mon'49; Bact. (P.Q.); Assoc. Prof. Montreal U.; Bact. & Chief Labs., Hop. Ste. Justine; Tel. RE 1-4931, Loc. 460.
MARTINEAU, Gerard A.; 1300 Ave. Green, Ste.-Foy, P.Q. (res); Lav'49; DPH; PH (P.Q.); MPH (Johns Hopkins); Staff, Dept. of Health, Quebec, P.Q.
MARTINEAU, Guy; C.P. 117, Rimouski; P.Q.; Mon'55; FRCS(C), OrthSurg; Tel. 723-8680.
MARTINEAU, Jean E.; 5240 Wellington, Verdun, Montreal 19, P.Q.; Mon '32; Retired.
MARTINEAU, Joseph A. G.; Lav'62; FRCS(C), GenSurg; Staff, Hop. St. Sacrement, Quebec 6, P.Q.
MARTINEAU, Maurice; 5105 Delorimier Ave., Montreal, P.Q.; Mon '43; Tel. LA 1-5737.
MARTINEAU, Real; Apt. 11, 2525 Sherbrooke E., Montreal 24, P.Q.; McG '50; GenSurg; Tel. LA 6-5144.
MARTINEAU, Roger; Natashquan, Saguenay, P.Q., Mon '47.
MARTINEAU, Yves; 1150 Blvd. St. Joseph E., Montreal 34, P.Q.; 728 Ave. Davaar, Outremont (res); Mon '49; F.R.C.S.(C), GenSurg; Staff Surg., Hop. Maisonneuve; Tel. 254-8341.
MARTINEZ, S. Napoleon; 1392 est rue Sherbrooke, Montreal 24, P.Q.; St. Dominique '53; FRCS(C), NeurSurg; Staff, Hop. Notre-Dame; Ass't. Surg. Research, U. of Montreal; Tel. LA 6-0491.
MARTINEZ, Victor; Box 10, Coleman, Alta; Valladolid (Spain) '55.
MARTINOFF, Ivan; Ste. 320, 5780 Cambie St., Vancouver 15, B.C.; 144 W. 26th Ave. (res); Ott '51; MCGP; Att'd. Staff, St. Vincent's Hosp.; Tel. FA 1-8822. Abroad.
MARTINS, Anna W.; 120 Herkimer St., Hamilton, Ont.; Crimean '23; D.Psych., Psy; Staff, St. Joseph's & Hamilton Gen. Hosp's.; Tel. JA 7-3821.
MARTINSON, Herbert A.; 110-8th St. E., Prince Albert, Sask.; Nat. U. (Ireland) '51; MB; BCH; DCH (Eng.).; Assoc. Staff, Victoria Union & Holy Family Hosp's. Tel. 763-6466.
MARTIN-VILLAR, Jose; 266 Barclay Rd., Ottawa 7, Ont.; Valencia (Spain) '45; Staff, Ottawa Gen. Hosp.; Clin. Ass't., Ottawa U.; Tel. CE 6-4592.
MARTON, Dominique; Mon'64; Res., Hop. Notre-Dame, Montreal 24, P.Q.
MARTOSH, Andrew E.; Ste. 203, 344 Bloor St. W., Toronto 5, Ont.; Szeged (Hung.) '49; Tel. WA 1-7426.
MARTYN, Donald M.; 200 St. Clair Ave. W., Toronto 7, Ont.; 7 Vernham Ave. (res); Tor '52; ObstGyn; Staff, St. Michael's Hosp.; Tel. WA 1-8252.
MARTYN, Gordon E.; McGregor Clinic, 250 Main St. E., Hamilton, Ont.; Wes'59; Urol.; Tel. 527-2771.
MARTYN, John W.; 294 Aylmer St., Peterborough, Ont.; Tor'54; FRCS(C); GenSurg; FICA; FACS; Surg. Staff, Peterborough Civic & St. Joseph's Hosp.; Tel. 742-3811.
MARTYNIUK, Anthony; Graz (Austria) '40; Staff, Alberta Hosp., Box 307, Edmonton, Alta.; Tel. 7-0221.
MARTYNIUK, Frank J.; 770 Barton St. E., Hamilton, Ont.; 100 Melrose Ave. S. (res); Wes '42; M.C.G.P.; Tel. LI 4-5708.
MARWOOD, Leonard R.; 378 Fairlawn Ave., Toronto, Ont.; Tor '29; M.C.G.P.; Staff, Grace Hosp.; Tel. RU 3-2300.
MARX, Richard; 123 Victoria St. W., Alliston, Ont.; Dublin (Ire.) '43; BAO; ObstGyn; Staff, Stevenson Mem. Hosp.; Tel. HE 5-6720.
MARYANKA, Eva; 41 Covington Rd., Toronto 10, Ont. (res); M.C.G.P.; Staff, Women's College Hosp.; Tel. RU 1-0015.
MARYNIAK, Oleh Capt.; Ott '64; Petawawa Mil. Hosp.; Camp Petawawa, Ont.
MARYNOWSKI, Bohdan; Weinlos Clinic, 10022-103rd St., Edmonton, Alta.; Alb'65.
MASCARIN, Telesforo A.; 3945 Tecumseh Rd., Windsor, Ont.; Ott'59; Abroad.
MASHAL, Jamil; 520-17th St. W. Vancouver, B.C.; 1940 Lonsdale, N. Van.; 870 Fairmile Rd., W. Van. (res); Beirut (Lebanon) '47; Paed; Instr., U. of British Columbia; Tel. WA 2-2912; YU 7-9911.
MASON, Bernard L.; 113-3rd Ave. E., Biggar, Sask.; Man'65.
MASON, Christine R. (Howse); 4224 LeBow Dr., Calgary, Alta. (res); Tor '49; Temp. Retirement.
MASON, David R.; Harshman Block, Sydney, N.S.; London (Eng.) '42; MRCS (Eng.); LRCP (Lond.).
MASON, Donald M.; 142 Queenston St., St. Catharines, Ont.; 30 Briarfield Cr. (res); Wes '48; Path; Ass't. Pathol., St. Catharines Gen. Hosp.; Tel. MU 4-7271.
MASON, Edward H.; 3465 Cote des Neiges Rd., Montreal, P.Q.; McG '14; D.A.B.I.M.; F.A.C.P., F.R.C.P.(C) IntMed.; Hon. Att. Staff, Royal Victoria Hosp.; Tel. WE 5-3535.
MASON, John L.; Box 189, Killam Med. Centre, Killam, Alta.; Liverpool (Eng.) '58; MCGP; Staff, Killam Gen. & Beaver Auxillary Hosp's. Abroad.
MASON, John T.; 540 Tegler Bldg., Edmonton. Alta.; 6608-124th St. (res); Alb '52; DiagRad; Rad., Misericordia Hosp.; Tel. 424-8261.
MASON, Lawrence H.; Bassano, Alta; Man '46; Dist. Coroner.
MASON, L. V.; 4012A East Hastings, Vancouver, B.C.; 4315 Grandview Hwy. (res); Tor '45; Tel. 298-3717.

MASON, Robert J.; 1453 Prince Rd., Windsor, Ont.; Wes'59; Psy; Dir. Psy., Ontario Mental Health Clinic.

MASON, Vaughan T.; Calgary Assoc. Clinic, 214-6th Ave. W., Calgary, Alta.; Victoria U. (Manchester, Eng.) '47; DRCOG; ObstGyn; Chief (ObstGyn), Holy Cross Hosp.; Tel. 263-7120.

MASON, William E.; 3465 Cote-des-Neiges Rd., Montreal 25, P.Q.; McG '51; F.R.C.P.(C), Int-Med.; Clin. Ass't., Royal Victoria Hosp.; Jr. Clin. Ass't., St. Mary's Hosp.; Dem. (Med.), McGill U.; Tel. WE 5-3525.

MASON, William F.; Dal '61; Res., Victoria Gen. Hosp., Halifax, N.S.

MASON-BROWNE L. (See Browne)

MASOTTI, Ronald E.; 857 Princess St., Kingston, Ont.; 85 College St. (res); Qns '58 Paed; Att'd. Staff (Paed.), Kingston Gen. Hosp. & Queen's U.; Tel. 546-7575.

MASSE, Jean; Hop. Notre Dame, Montreal 24, P.Q.

MASSE, J. E. Rosaire; 489 Blvd. Ste-Anne, Joliette, P.Q.; 1090 Notre Dame (res); Mon '30; F.I.C.S.; GenSurg (P.Q.); Clin. Prof. Hop -St-Eusebe; Tel. PL 6-8093.

MASSE, Jules, 367 St. Louis Sq., Montreal, P.Q.; McG'34; Tel. 845-8852.

MASSE, Laurent; 122 St. Jean, Drummondville, P.Q.; Lav '43; GenSurg (P.Q.); 1st Ass't. (Surg.), Hop. Ste. Croix; Tel. GR 8-5152.

MASSE, Louise R.; St. Nicolas, Levis, P.Q.; Lav '33; Phys., Hop., St. Joseph de Bellevue, Quebec; Vis. Phys., Hop. St. Francois d'Assise, Quebec.

MASSE, Maurice A.; 8541 Hochelaga St., Montreal, P.Q.; Mon '51; M.C.G.P.; Tel. CL 5-5444.

MASSE, Regis; Lav'65; Res., Hop. Notre-Dame, Montreal 24, P.Q.

MASSE, Rosaire; 489 Blvd. Ste-Anne, Joliette, P.Q.; 1090 Notre-Dame (res); Mon '30; GenSurg P.Q.); FICS; Staff, Hop. St. Eusebe & Hop. St. Charles; Tel. 756-8073.

MASSEY, Douglas G.; Tor'51; DNB; MRCP(E); MSc (McGill); FCCP; Pulm Dis & TB (P.Q.); FRCP(C), IntMed; Staff, University Hosp., Sherbrooke, P.Q.; Ass't. Prof. U. of Sherbrooke.

MASSEY, Luebert W. C.; London (Eng.)'41; LRCP Lond.), MRCS (Eng.); M.B., B.S., FACCP; Int-Med; Med. Spec. (Chest Dis. Div.), Ontario Hosp., Woodstock, Ont.; Tel. LE 9-1251.

MASSEY, William K.; 405 Hendryx St., Nelson, B.C.; 608-3rd St. (res); Man '38; DiagRad; Chief of Staff, Kootenay Lake Gen. Hosp.; Tel. 352-6611.

MASSICOTTE, Clement; 6015 boul. du Jardin, Orsainville, P.Q.; Lav'58.

MASSICOTTE, Gilles A.; 825 sud, rue Belvedere, Sherbrooke P.Q.; Mon '59; PlasSurg; Tel. 569-6945.

MASSICOTTE, J. P. Henri; Victoriaville, P.Q.; 40 Notre Dame W. (res); Lav '02.

MASSICOTTE, Paul; Mon '58; A.M.C.G.P.; Paed; Staff, Hop.-Ste.-Justine, Montreal, P.Q.; Tel. RE 1-4931.

MASSIE, R. A.; 4 Bayside Dr., Saint John, N.B. (res); McG '24; Anaes; Staff M.O., Lancaster Hosp. D.V.A.; Tel. 694-2651.

MASSIG, Eric; Tor'32; Path; Dir. of Labs., St. Joseph's Hosp., Sarnia, Ont.; Tel. ED 6-6121.

MASSON, Anne M.; 5740 Plantagenet Ave., Montreal 26, P.Q. (res); Paris (Fr.) '42; Ass't. Prof. (Bact), McGill U.; Tel. 738-1548.

MASSON, Edward L.; 16 Regency Sq., Scarborough, Ont. (res); Tor '51; M.C.G.P.; Med. Dir., Upjohn Co. of Canada, 865 York Mills Rd., Don Mills, Ont.; Tel. HI 4-4433.

MASSON, Gaston; 31 ouest, rue King, Sherbrooke, P.Q.; 230 rue Heneker (res); Lav '48; IntMed (P.Q.); Head Dept. (IntMed) & Adm. (Electrocardiol.), Hop-St-Vincent-de-Paul; Tel. LO 9-6381.

MASSON, J.A. Richard; 447 Du Domaine, St. Jerome, Cte Terrebonne, P.Q.; Ott'54; DiagRad.

MASSON, Pierre; 83 de l'Eveche, Rimouski, P.Q.; 39 rue Ste-Marie (res); Lav '58; Paed; Staff (Paed.), Hop. St-Joseph de Rimouski; Tel. 723-7851.

MASSON, Rene N.; 11245-60 eme Ave., Riviere des Prairies, P.Q.; Mon '52.

MASSON, Victoria; 738 Jacques Berthiaume, Ste.-Foy, P.Q. (res); Lav '53; Anaes; Staff, Hop. St. Sacrement; Tel. 681-7211.

MASTER, W. McKee; 1011 Ouellette Ave., Windsor, Ont.; 2089 Willistead Cres. (res); Tor '28; M.C.G.P.; Tel. 256-8351

MASTERSON, Thomas L.; Okanagan St., Salmon Arm, B.C.; Lakeshore Rd. (res); St. Andrews (Scot.) '24; FRCS(Ed.); FRCS(C); GenSurg; Cons. Surg., Shuswab Lake Gen. Hosp.; Tel. 832-3949.

MASTROMATTEO, Ernest; 5402 Parliament Bldgs., Toronto 2, Ont.; 19 Carey Rd., Tor 7 (res); Tor '47; DIH; DPH; DABPM (Occup. Med.); FACPM; Staff (OPD), St. Michael's Hosp.; Ass't. Dir. Indus. Hygiene Br., Ont. Dept. of Health; Ass't. Prof., Schl. of Hygiene, U. of Toronto; Tel. 365-2493.

MASTROPASQUA, Corrado A.; Naples (Italy) '53; Anaes; Staff, Santa Cabrini Hosp., Montreal 36, P.Q.

MATAS, Harry; 857 Notre Dame Ave., Winnipeg, Man.; 560 Waterloo St. (res); Man '36; M.C.G.-P.; Tel. SP 4-7047.

MATAS, John; 314 Boyd Bldg., Winnipeg, Man.; 525 Cordova (res); Man '34; Psy; Dir., Psy. Serv's, St. Boniface Hosp.; Assoc. Prof. (Psy.), U. of Manitoba; Tel. 943-3554.

MATAS, Matthew; 11344-128th St., Edmonton, Alta.; 9022-120th St. (res); Alb '26; FCCP; Reg. Supt., Foothills Reg. Med. Services, Dept. of National Health & Welfare; Lect. Med. (T.B.), U. of Alberta; Tel. GL 5-6622.

MATE, Maria J.; 4371 Greta St., South Burnaby, B.C.; Qns '50; Anaes; Active Staff (Anaes), St. Paul's Hosp.; Staff, (Anaes), U. of British Columbia; Tel. MU 5-8623.

MATHE, Charles J. W.; 3038 A Bloor St. W., Toronto 18, Ont.; Tor '43; Tel. BE 1-6721.

MATHENS, Marvin S.; 2767 Maplewood, Montreal, P.Q. (res); Sask. '60.

MATHER, Cecil E.; 20th Floor C.N. Tower, 10139-103rd St., Edmonton, Alta.; Man'34; DPH.

MATHER, James M.; 4036 W. 8th Ave., Vancouver 8, B.C. (res); Tor '36; D.A.B.P.M. & P.H., F.A.C.-Prev. Med.; D.P.H., PH; Ass't. Dean, Prof. & Head, Dept. of Prev. Med., U. of British Columbia; Retired.

MATHER, J. Hartley; 209 Medical Arts Bldg., Winnipeg, Man.; 450 Waterloo St. (res); Man '26; M.C.G.P.; Tel. WH 2-3896.

MATHERS, Doreen I.; (see MacDonald, Doreen I.).

MATHES, Edward J.; Medical Centre, 106 Talbot St. W., Leamington, Ont.; Tor'64.

MATHESON, Donald; 2885 W. 34th Ave., Vancouver, B.C. (res); Aberdeen (Scot.)'38; F.F.A., D.A., (R.S.C., Eng.); Anaes; Att'd. Staff, Van. Gen. Hosp.; Clin. Instr. (Anaes.), U. of British Columbia; Tel. 874-5291.

MATHESON, Donald C.; 48 Sydenham Street, Kingston, Ont. (res); Qns '15; Emer. Prof. (Anat.), Queen's U.; Retired.

MATHESON, Donald C.; 4900 Kingsway Ave., South Burnaby, B.C.; UBC'57; FRCS(C), Ophth; Vis. Staff, Vancouver Gen. Hosp.

MATHESON, D. I.; Qns '54; Intn., Toronto Gen. Hosp.; Toronto, Ont.

MATHESON, Donald I.; Brockville Medical Clinic, 224 King St. E., Brockville, Ont.; 67 North Augusta Rd. (res); Qns '34; M.C.G.P.; Staff, Brockville Gen. & St. Vincent de Paul Hosp's.; Tel. DI 2-4477.

MATHESON, Donald I.; 50 Fallingbrook Dr., Scarborough, Ont.; Tor '55; FRCP(C); Anaes; MCGP; Staff, Toronto East Gen. Hosp.; Tel. 461-8272.

MATHESON, D. Torquhil; Dobson Assoc. Med. Clinic, 10102-101st St., Grande-Prairie, Alta.; 9313-102nd St. (res); London (Eng.) '51; L.R.-C.P. (Lond.), M.R.C.S.(Eng.), A.M.C.G.P.; Tel. 532-4444

MATHESON, Grant M., F/L; Dal '64; M.O., RCAF Station, Trenton, Ont.

MATHESON, John A.; 1156-3rd. Ave. N. W., Moose Jaw, Sask.; Tor '26; GenSurg; Med. Dir., Moose Jaw Union Hosp.; Tel. 692-1841.

MATHESON, J. Murray; Box 280, Brandon Clinic, Brandon, Man.; Man '34; FICS; GenSurg.; Tel. PA 9-6444.
MATHESON, W. Allan; Fonthill, Ont.; U.K. '52
MATHEU, Heracleo; Box 39, North Battleford, Sask.; Santo Tomas (Manila, Philippines) '42; DABPN; Clin. Dir., Saskatchewan Hosp.; Vis. Cons. (Psy.), University Hosp., Saskatoon; Tel. 445-2421.
MATHEWS, Frederick A. J.; Bonn (Germ.) '62; Res., Ottawa Gen. Hosp., Ottawa, Ont.
MATHEWS, Raymond E.; Tor '60; FRCS(C), GenSurg; Toronto Gen. Hosp., Toronto 2, Ont.; Tel. EM 6-8211.
MATHEWS, William H.; 1002 McNaughton Rd., Mount Royal, Montreal 16, P.Q. (res) McG '36; FRCP(C), PathBact; Chief Pathol., Montreal Gen. Hosp.; Cons. Path., Reddy Mem. Hosp.; Assoc. Prof., McGill U.; Tel. 937-6011, Loc. 291-292.
MATHEWSON, Francis A. L.; 326 Medical Arts Bldg., 404-406 Graham Ave., Winnipeg, Man.; 283 Yale Ave. (res); Man'31; F.A.C.P., IntMed; Assoc. Prof. (Med.), U. of Manitoba; Assoc. Phys. & Dir. Dept. of Electro-Cardiography, Winnipeg Gen. Hosp.; Med. Dir., Great West Life Assur. Co.; Tel. WH 2-8684.
MATHIES, Helmut D.; 69 Margaret Ave. N., Waterloo, Ont.; 215 Lincoln Rd. (res); Wes '55; AMCGP; Staff, Kitchener-Waterloo & St. Mary's Hosp's.; Tel. 744-3397.
MATHIESON, David W.; 1940 Lonsdale Ave., North Vancouver, B.C.; 1500 Grand Blvd. (res); Aberdeen (Scot.)'43; Att'd. Staff, Lionsgate Hosp.; Tel. YU 7-2522.
MATHIESON, Gordon; Mtl. Neurol. Inst., 3801 University St., Montreal 2, P.Q.; 6275 Northcrest Pl., Mtl. 8 (res); Aberdeen (Scot.) '49; M.Sc. (McGill); Neuropath., Mtl. Neurol. Inst. & Ass't. Prof. (Neurol & NeurSurg.), McGill U.; Tel. VI 2-1251, Loc. 242.
MATHIESON, Laine; (see Loo, Laine).
MATHIESON, M. Joan L. (Hall); 1940 Lonsdale Ave., North Vancouver, B.C.; 1500 Grand Blvd. (res); London (Eng.)'49; D. Ophth. (Eng.); Tel. YU 7-2522.
MATHIESON, Robert; 84 Union St., Sydney, N.S.; Glasgow (Scot.) '48; Path. & Dir. of Labs., City Hosp.; Tel. 564-6234.
MATHIESON, William A.; Ste. 9, Medical Arts Bldg., 335-339-6th. Ave. S.W., Calgary, Alta.; Man '55; DiagRad; Staff, Holy Cross Hosp.; Tel. 262-9183.
MATHIEU, Charles L.; 349 Cote St. Catharine, Montreal, P.Q.; Mon 27; Ophth,Otol.
MATHIEU, Claude; 8390 Ave. Royale, Chateau Richer, Cte. Montmorency, P.Q.; Lav '60.
MATHIEU, Emile; 2553 Gascon Ave., Montreal, P.Q.; Mon'21; Retired.
MATHIEU, Guy; 30 est Boul. St. Joseph, Montreal 14, P.Q.; 6559 Pie IX (res); Mon '48; Psy; Ass't. NeurPsy., Hop. Ste. Jeanne d'Arc; Tel. VI 2-5201.
MATHIEU, Jean; 1150 Boul. St. Joseph est, Montreal, P.Q.; Mon'50; FRCP(C), IntMed; Cardiol. (P.Q.); Internist, Hop. Maisonneuve; Tel. LA 7-1241.
MATHIEU, Jean-Pierre; Lav'65; Res., Hop. Notre-Dame, Montreal 24, P.Q.
MATHIEU, J. Euclide; 169 St. Laurent St. W., Longueuil, P.Q.; Mon '23; GenSurg.
MATHIEU, Michel; 30 est boul. St-Joseph, Ste. 220, Montreal 14, P.Q.; Mon'43; Ophth; Chief, Dept. of Ophth., Hop. Maisonneuve; I/C Basic Science Courses (Ophth.) affil., U. of Montreal; Cons., W.C.B.; Tel. 845-0274.
MATHIEU, Michel P.; Mon'65; Res., Hop. Notre-Dame, Montreal 24, P.Q.
MATHIEU, Raymond; 2495 ave. Vitre, Quebec 3, P.Q.; Lav '55; Tel. 529-2468.
MATHIEU, Yves; 5 rue Legault, St.-Jerome, P.Q.; Mon '58.
MATHISEN, Arne K.; 1027 Med. Dental Bldg., 925W. Georgia St., Vancouver 1, B.C.; 3989 Angus Dr. (res); McG '41; FRCP(C); FACP; FCCP; IntMed; Att'd. Staff, Vancouver Gen. Hosp.; Clin. Instr. Med., U. of British Columbia; Tel. 683-1444.
MATHUR, Kailash C.; 45 Aberdeen Ave., New Glasgow, N.S.; Lucknow (India) '57; Anaes.
MATHUR, Parshottam S.; 110 Woodlawn Rd., Dartmouth, N.S.; Agra (India) '52; FRCS(Ed.); FRCS(Eng.); FRCS(C), GenSurg; Court. Staff, Halifax Infirmary, Victoria Gen. & Children's Hosp's.; Tel. 463-3370.
MATIKO, Reuben; 3520 Quadra, Victoria, B.C.; 3140 Humber Rd. (res); Coll. of Medical Evangelists (U.S.)'45; Tel. EV 6-6161.
MATRICK, Lawrence E.; 7263 Inlet Dr., North Burnaby, B.C.; Man'57; Psy.; Tel. 298-9144.
MATSALLA, Florian S.; Tor'60; AMCGP; Res., Toronto Western Hosp., Toronto, Ont.
MATSUSAKI, Hishashi; 106 Wellington St. N., Hamilton, Ont.; Tor '57; A.M.C.G.P.; Tel. JA 9-4224.
MATTE, Gerard; 369 rue St.-Jean, Quebec 4, P.Q.; Lav'30; Tel. 438-2381.
MATTE, Gerard; St. Louis de l'Isle aux Coudres, P.Q.; Lav'50; Tel. 526-2816.
MATTE, Joseph A. R.; 5219 Acadia Ave., Bethseda, Maryland, 20014, U.S.A.; Lav '60; Anaes; Abroad.
MATTE, Roger; Lav'60; Anaes (P.Q.); Staff, Hop. St. Sacrement, Quebec 6, P.Q.
MATTEAU, Jean C.; 444 Laviolette, Trois Rivieres, P.Q.; 2010 rue Lajoie (res); Lav '48; Gastroent. (P.Q.); Chief, Dept. Gast., Hop. Sainte-Marie; Tel. FR 5-1196.
MATTEAU, Philippe; 561 Beaumont St., St. Bruno, Co. Chambly, P.Q.; Lav '51.
MATTEAU, Pierre; Lav '54; Res., Hop. St-Francois d'Assise, Quebec 3, P.Q.
MATTEAU, Rene; 975 St. Prosper, Trois Rivieres, P.Q.; Lav '50; FACS; Urol(P.Q.); Chief of Urol. Serv., Hop. St. Joseph; Cons. Urol., Hop. Cooke & Hop. Ste-Marie; Tel. FR 5-4914.
MATTHEWS, Alan R.; Box 637, Fort Qu'Appelle, Sask.; London (Eng.) '54.
MATTHEWS, Aubrey M.; Regina Med. Centre, 1847 Rose St., Regina, Sask.; Glasgow (Scot.)'55.
MATTHEWS, Charles A.; 3147 The Kingsway, Vancouver 16, B.C.; 6270 Domen St. (res); Man '48; Active Staff, Mt. St. Joseph & Burnaby Gen. Hosp's.; Tel. HE 1-4441.
MATTHEWS, John A.; Hamilton Cancer Clinic, Henderson Gen. Hosp., Hamilton, Ont.; Witwatersrand (South Africa) '53.
MATTHEWS, Raymond L.; 178 St. George St., Toronto 5, Ont.; Apt. 1006, 19 Lascelles Blvd. Tor. 7 (res); Wes '52; F.R.C.P.(C), Anaes; Anaes., Toronto Gen. Hosp.; Clin. Instr., U. of Toronto; Tel. WA 3-1154.
MATTHEWS, Ross M.; 327 Charlotte St., Peterborough, Ont.; R.R.3. Greenhill (res); Tor '33; Paed.; Tel. 743-2040.
MATTHEWS, Vincent L.; 236 Med. Bldg., U. of Saskatchewan, Saskatoon, Sask.; Tor'45; DPH; PH; Prof. & Hd., Dept. of Social & PrevMed., U. of Saskatchewan; Tel. 242-7641.
MATTHEWS, Vivian M.; C.N.R. Med. Clinic, Moncton, N.B.; London (Eng.) '22.
MATTHEWS, William H.; 762A Commissioners Rd., London, Ont.; Tor'51; Staff Phys., DVA, Westminster Hosp., London, Ont.
MATTHEWS, William R.; Ste. 219, Medical Arts Bldg., Hamilton, Ont.; Tor'56; FRCS(C), GenSurg; Tel. 525-0702.
MATTIMOE, Peter F.; 98 Guestville Ave., Toronto 9, Ont.; National U. (Ire.) '65.
MATTIS, Martha; 2631 Columbia Court, Windsor, Ont.; Marburg (Germ.) '49.
MATUK, Naeema; 189 Harris Blvd., Winnipeg 12, Man.; Karashi (Pakistan) '58.
MATTON, Jean; 407 Blvd. St. Joseph Est., Montreal, P.Q.; 5500 Legare, Cote des Neiges (res); Lav '30; Tel. AV 8-8056.
MATUKAS, Antanas; Ontario Hosp., Woodstock, Ont.
MATVENKO, Jack; Tor '54; Res., Dept. of Ophth., U. of Saskatchewan, Saskatoon, Sask.
MATWICHUK, Zenon; McGregor Medical Centre, 561 Machray Ave., Winnipeg 4, Man.; Erlangen (W. Germ.)'60; Tel. 586-5076.

MATZINGER, Karl E.; 255 Broadview Dr., Pembroke, Ont. (res); Bratislava (Czech.) '44; D&T Rad; Rad., Pembroke Cottage, Pembroke Gen. & Deep River Hosp's. & Plant Hosp. of Atomic Energy of Canada Ltd., Chalk River; Tel. 732-4785.

MATZINGER, Lucy M.; (Dylownan); 251 Broadview Dr., Pembroke, Ont. (res); Edinburgh (Scot.) '47; Retired.

MATZKO, Alexander; 1650 Cedar Ave., Montreal 25, P.Q.; McG '51; FACA; FRCP(C), IntMed; Anaes; Staff, Montreal Gen. Hosp.; Lect. McGill U.; Tel. WE 7-6011.

MATZKO, Peter; 43 Ridgemoor Ave., Scarborough, Ont.; McG '58; Tel. AM 1-4159.

MAUDSLEY, Robert F.; Qns '62; Res., Kingston Gen. Hosp., Kingston, Ont.

MAUFFETTE, Andre; Mon'65; Res., Inst. Albert Prevost, Montreal 9, P.Q.

MAUFFETTE, Jean; 7433 St. Denis, Montreal, P.Q.; 5765 Deom (res); Mon'37; MCGP; Full-time Phys., Town of Outremont; Tel. 272-7338.

MAUGER, Jacques; Mon'65; Res., Institute Albert Prevost, Montreal 9, P.Q.

MAUGHAN, George B.; 619 Sydenham Ave., Westmount, Montreal, P.Q. (res); McG '34; F.A.C.S., F.R.C.O.G., F.R.C.S.(C), ObstGyn; Obst & Gyn.-in-Chief, Royal Victoria Hosp.; Cons., St. Mary's, Montreal Gen., Queen Elizabeth & Reddy Mem. Hosp's.; Prof. & Chm. (ObstGyn), McGill U.; Tel. 849-4870.

MAUGILE, Dumas; 4265 rue Isabella, Montreal, P.Q.; Haiti '56; Psy.

MAURICE, Rolland R.; Suite 220, 236 St. George St., Moncton, N.B.; Mon'55; Otol; MCGP; Active Staff, Moncton City & Hotel-Dieu de l'Assomption Hosp's.; Tel. 382-2794.

MAURIELLO, Antoine H.; 1384 est, Jean-Talon, Montreal, P.Q.; 2 ave. Derome, Laval-des-Rapides (res); Mon '51; M.C.G.P.; Tel. 274-5583.

MAURIELLO, Ginette; 9 Venise Croissant, Duvernay, Laval-des-Rapides, P.Q. (res); Lav '58; Staff, Dept. of Health, Laval U.; Tel. 669-2496.

MAURIELLO, Vincent; 71 Ave. Duchastel, Montreal 8, P.Q.; Man '53; Psy.

MAURINS, Janis; 4961 Queen Mary Rd., Montreal, P.Q.; 513 Saraguay Blvd., Pierrefonds (res); Riga (Latvia) '32; GenSurg (Latvia); Court. Staff, Queen Elizabeth Hosp.; Tel. 731-2827.

MAUS, John H.; 1995 Lens Ave., Windsor, Ont.; 73 Reedmere Rd., Riverside (res); Tor '42; TherRad; Dir. Windsor Clinic, Ont. Cancer Treatment & Research Fdn.; Tel. CL 3-9587.

MAUTNER, Lawrence S.; 203 Oakmount Rd., Toronto, Ont.; Vienna (Aust.) '38; PathBact; Path., St. Joseph's Hosp.; Dem. (Pathol.), U. of Toronto; Tel. LE 4-9531.

MAX, Paul; 1003 Harrison Ave., London, Ont.; Wes'57; Psy; Ass't. Prof. (Psy.), Victoria Hosp. & U. of Western Ontario; Tel. 432-5261.

MAXFIELD, Frederick B.; Box 130, Nakusp, B.C.; Man '40; Med. Advisor, Calgar Ltd., Woods Div.; Tel. 265-3232.

MAXMEN, Marvin D.; 4 Parmbelle Cr., Don Mills, Ont.; Wes'51; GenSurg; Med. Dir., Campbell Soups Canada, Anaconda American Brass & Employees Health Unit, Hosp. for Sick Children; Tel. HI 4-4165.

MAXWELL, Benjamin R.; Glace Bay Gen. Hosp., Glace Bay, N.S.; 178 South St. (res); McG '38; DiagRad.; Tel. 849-8515.

MAXWELL, Brian E. S/L; Inst. of Aviation Med., 1107 Avenue Rd., Toronto 12, Ont.; Sask'65.

MAXWELL, Gordon A.; 7742 Elbow Dr. S.W., Calgary, Alta.; 643B-69th Ave. S.W. (res); Alb **'57; Staff, Holy Cross & Calgary Gen. Hosp's.; Tel. AL 5-5225.**

MAXWELL, Ian; Winnipeg Clinic, N.E. St. Mary's & Vaughan Winnipeg 1, Man.; Glasgow (Scot.) '57; MRCP(Edin.); MRCP(Lond.); FRCP (C), IntMed.; Tel. 942-0551.

MAXWELL, Ian D.; 1175 Studley Ave., Halifax, N.S.; Edinburgh (Scot.) '42; Path; Assoc. Dir. **(Pathol.), Halifax Infirm.; Assoc. Prof. (Pathol.), Dalhousie U.; Tel. 2-4406.**

MAXWELL, John A.; Alb '43; Staff, Colonel Belcher Hosp., Calgary, Alta.; Tel. AM 6-7001.

MAXWELL, John B. W.; 513 Med. Arts Bldg., Winnipeg, Man.; Dublin (Ire.) '55; MCGP; Tel. WH 2-8063.

MAXWELL, Lenwood T.; Ste 210, 1320-5th Ave., Prince George, B.C.; 2425 Laurier Cres. (res); Man '44; GenSurg; Tel. 564-8262.

MAXWELL, Marthta R. (See Grymaloski)

MAXWELL, Maureen P. (Briscoe); Qns '59; Paed; Staff, Kingston Gen. Hosp., Kingston, Ont.

MAXWELL, W. John B.; 412 Danforth Ave., Toronto, Ont.; 20 Rivercourt Blvd. (res); Tor '31; Urol; Staff (Urol.), Toronto East Gen. Hosp.; Tel. HO 3-1413.

MAXWELL, W. Keith; McG '60; Anaes; Staff, Vancouver Gen. Hosp., Vancouver, B.C. Abroad.

MAY, Gerald A.; 645 Fort St., Victoria, B.C.; Dal'50; MCGP; Tel. 388-5032.

MAY, Jack R.; 548 King St. W., Port Colborne, Ont.; Dal'55; MCGP; Tel. 834-3684.

MAY, Malcolm J.; M.B.E.; 306 Medical Bldg., Prince Albert, Sask.; 317-20th St. W., (res); Guy's Hosp. (London, Eng.) '42; **F.R.C.S. (Eng.);** Tel. 763-6401.

MAY, William; Winnipeg Clinic, St. Mary's & Vaughan, Winnipeg 1, Man.; 1345 Wellington Cres., Wpg. 9 (res); London (Eng.) '51; DO (Eng.); Ophth; Hon. Staff, Wpg. Gen. & Children's Hosp's.; Dir. Contact Lens Clinic, U. of Manitoba; Dem. (Ophth), U. of Manitoba; Tel. 942-0551.

MAY, William L.; Box 1090, Murdochville, P.Q.; 517-8th St. (res); McG'52; MCGP; Admin. Murdochville Hosp.; Phys., Gaspe Copper Mines Ltd., Med. Sup. GCML Employees Med. Serv. Ass'n.; Tel. 2561.

MAYBA, Ihor; 790 Sherbrook St., Winnipeg 2, Man.; Man'57; FRCS(C), GenSurg; Tel. SP 4-6541.

MAYBEE, T. Keir; Alb'59; FRCP(C), IntMed; Staff, Vancouver Gen. Hosp., Vancouver, B.C.

MAYER-CARRE, M. Aline; 616 Cote Ste. Catherine, Montreal 8, P.Q.; Mon'61.

MAYER, George A.; 847 Princess St., Kingston, Ont.; Budapest (Hung.) '37; MSc (Med.); Att'd. Staff & Dir. Anti-Coag. Serv., Kingston Gen. Hosp.; Lect. (Med.), Queen's U.

MAYER, George P.; 1274 Kingston Rd., Scarborough, Ont.; 16 Briar Dale Blvd. (res); Tor '50; M.C.G.P.; Vis. Staff, St. Michael's, Toronto East Gen. & Scarborough Gen. Hosp's.; Tel. OX 4-4944.

MAYER, Harold; Alb '57; Res., Sunnybrook Hosp., Toronto 12, Ont.

MAYER, Jack A.; 605 Bloor St. W., Toronto, Ont.; 490 Wilson Ave. (res); Tor '49; F.R.C.S.-(C), NeurSurg.; Tel. LE 3-4893.

MAYER, Joseph M.; 2045 Dufferin St., Toronto 10, Ont.; 1 Ealing Dr., Willowdale (res); Baghdad (Iraq) '44; L.R.C.P.(Lond.), MRCS(Eng.), FRCS(Ed.), FRCS(C), GenSurg; FACS; Tel. 651-1210.

MAYER, M. Aline; Mon '62; Intn., Hop. Hotel-Dieu, Montreal, P.Q.

MAYERS, James R.; 2405 Lake Shore Blvd. W., Toronto 14, Ont.; London (Eng.) '44; M.B., B.S., M.D., MRCS(Eng.), LRCP(Lond.)* DPH; Tel. 259-1231.

MAYMAN, Abe B.; 690 Ellendale Med. Bldg., 5845 Cote-des-Neiges Rd., Montreal 26, P.Q.; 139 Finchley Rd., Hampstead (res); McG '47; M.C.G.P.; Staff, Jewish Gen. Hosp.; Mem. Med. Bd., Herzl Health Clin. & Jewish Hosp. of Hope; Tel. RE 1-9636.

MAYMAN, Chaim I.; 11 Turner Terrace, Newtonville, Mass., U.S.A. 02160; Man '54; FRCP(C), Neur. Abroad.

MAYMAN, David; Man '63; Int., Winnipeg Children's Hosp., Winnipeg, Man.

MAYNARD, Harrison C.; 307 Grosvenor Ave. N., Hamilton, Ont.; Alb '53.

MAYNARD, Jean J.; 282 est rue Principale, Hawkesbury, Ont.; Mon'61.

MAYNARD, M. Douglas; Wes'62; Res., Victoria Hosp., London, Ont.

MAYNES, Earl A.; 277 Scarboro Cr., Scarborough, Ont.; Tor'51; MCGP; Med. Dir., Litton Systems (Canada) Ltd.; Staff, Scarborough Gen. Hosp.; Tel. 267-5851.

MAYR, Heinz O.; 1864 Dundas, London, Ont.; Vienna (Austria) '42; Facharzt Int. Med. (Vienna); Tel. 451-4000.

MAYRAND, Gerald; Ste. 209, 550 Bonaventure, Trois-Rivieres, P.Q.; Mon'43; Tel. 374-7636.

MAYRAND, Leonce; Lachevrotiere, Cte. Portneuf, P.Q.; Lav'46.

MAYRAND, Martin; 272 Principale, St.-Felix-de-Valois, Cte. Joliette, P.Q.; Lav '53.

MAYRAND, Placide; 10390 Royale, Ste-Anne-de-Beaupre, P.Q.; Lav '48; Tel. 263-2901.

MAYRAND, Yves; 991 rue Riel, St-Vincent-de-Paul, Laval-des-Rapides, P.Q.; Mon'56; DiagRad (P.Q.); MCGP; Staff, Hop. Notre-Dame; Tel. LA 5-6363.

MAZEROLLE, Antoine; C.P. 296, 4th St., Shippegan, N.B.; Lav'61.

MAZER, Irwin H.; 205 Doctors' Bldg., 394 Graham Ave., Winnipeg 1, Man.; 874 Elm St., Wpg. 9 (res); Man '42; DLO (Eng.); FICS; Otol; Active Staff (ENT), St.-Boniface & Misericordia Hosp's.; Tel. 943-5230.

MAZEROLLE, Denis; St. Leonard, N.B.; Lav '58. Abroad.

MAZEWSKI, Stanislaw M., Major; National U. (Ire.) '51; Otol; c/o RCN Hosp., HMCS "Naden", Victoria, B.C.

MAZIADE, Pierre I.; Centre Medical Fleury, 2157 est, Fleury, Montreal 12, P.Q.; Mon '63; Tel. 381-2581.

MAZIEC, Konstanty; 989 Bronson Ave., Ottawa, Ont.; 257-4th Ave (res); Edinburgh (Scot.) '42; **Lect. & Slin. Instr. (Med.), U. of Ottawa; Tel. 235-2281.**

MAZUGI, Ali; Tehran (Iran.); Jr. Int., Children's Hosp., Halifax, N.S.

MAZUR, Jan; Mon'61; DiagRad(P.Q.); Staff, Hop. Ste-Jeanne d'Arc, Montreal 18, P.Q.

MAZUREK, Leon, Major; Sask'59; Canadian Base Unit, UN Emergency Forces, CFPO 5049 Europe.

MAZZOLANI, Luciano; 824-3rd St. N.E., Calgary, Alta.; 2531-11th Ave. N.W. (res); Milan (Italy) '53; Tel. 283-7066.

McADAM, Ronald; 133 E. 14th St., North Vancouver, B.C.; 1950 Orchard Way, West Van. (res); Edinburgh (Scot.) '50; MRCP (Edin.); IntMed; Chief of Med., Lion's Gate Hosp.; Tel. YU 5-2424.

McADAM, W. Murray.; 437 Highland Rd. E., Kitchener, Ont.; Tor '59; Active Staff, St. Mary's Gen. & Kitchener-Waterloo Hosp's.; Tel. 744-7922.

McALEER, Joseph; RCS (Ire.) '58; Staff, Alberta Hosp., Box 1000, Ponoka, Alta.

McALISTER, Harold R.; 406 Med. Arts Bldg., Hamilton, Ont.; Tor '24; IntMed; Hon. Cons., Hamilton Civic Hosp.; Cons., St. Joseph's Hosp.; Active Staff, St. Peter's Infirmary; District Coroner; Tel. JA 7-3962.

McALISTER, Stanley L.; 631 Med. Arts Bldg., 750 Spadina Cr. E., Saskatoon, Sask.; Sask'65.

McALLISTER, Arthur; 50 Main St. N., Georgetown, Ont.; Tor '10.

McALLISTER, John E.; 216 Med. Arts Bldg., Calgary, Alta.; 339-6th Ave. W.; Alb '39; FACS; FACOG; ObstGyn; Cons. Holy Cross & Calgary Gen. Hosp's.; Tel. 262-4321.

McALLISTER, Neal J.; 7510-101st Ave., Edmonton, Alta.; Royal Coll. of Surg. (Dublin, Ire.) '38; Court. Staff, Royal Alexandra Hosp.; Att'd. Staff, Misericordia Hosp.; M.O., Premier Steel; Tel. HO 9-7717 & HO 9-7676.

McALPINE, Donald G.; 9123-139th St., Edmonton, Alta. (res); Alb '43; MCGP; Pres., Med. Staff, Royal Alexandra Hosp.; Dist. Coroner; Tel. 474-3431.

McALPINE, Douglas F.; 1010 McCallum Hill Bldg., Regina, Sask.; 2876 Rae St. (res); Glasgow (Scot.) '42; D.A., F.A.C.A., F.F.A.R.C.S., Anaes; Dir., Dept. of Anaes, Grey Nuns' Hosp.; Staff, Sr. Member (Anaes.), Regina Gen. Hosp.; Vis. Cons. (Anaes) University Hosp.; Clin Teach (Anaes), U. of Saskatchewan; Tel. 522-0704.

McALPINE, Hugh T.; 887 Richmond St., London, Ont.; Wes'39; Dip. IntMed (McG); Clinical Lect. (Med.), U. of Western Ont.; Tel. 439-8051.

McALPINE, Kenneth L.; 332 Queens Ave., London, Ont.; 255 Grosvenor St. (res); Wes '31; Paed; Staff, St. Joseph's & War Mem. Children's Hosp.; Tel. 432-8282.

McAMMOND, Ernest N. C.; Ste. 817, 925 W. Georgia St., Vancouver, B.C.; Tor '36; D.T.M. & H(Eng.), F.I.C.S., GenSurg; Proctology; Staff, St. Paul's Hosp. & Sick Children's Hosps.; Vis. Staff, St. Vincent's, Vancouver Gen. & Mount St. Joseph's Hosp's.; Sec., Int'nl. College of Surgeons (Can. Sect.); Tel. MU 4-6477.

McANDREW, Irene; (See Cassells).

MCANINCH, Lloyd M.; 301 Victoria Bldg., 111 Waterloo St., London, Ont.; Wes'45; FACS; FRCS(C) Urol; Chief of Urol. Serv., Victoria Gen. Hosp.; Att'd. Urol., St. Joseph's Hosp.; Cons. (Urol.), Westminster Hosp. & Beck Mem. San.; Assoc. Prof. (Surg.), U. of Western Ont.; Tel. GE 8-8835.

McANULTY, James; Box 50, Oyama, B.C.; Edinburgh (Scot.)'57; DPH; Tel. 548-3818.

McARDLE, Edward J.; Nat. U. (Ire.) '50; DPH; DIH; Staff, Health Unit, 442-1st St. S.E., Medicine Hat, Alta.

McARTHUR, E. C.; 705 Brock S., Whitby, Ont. (res); Tor '10; Staff, Ontario Hosp.

McARTHUR, James E.; 165 Murdoch Ave., Noranda, P.Q.; 136 3rd Ave. (res); McG '29; F.A.-C.S., F.I.C.S., GenSurg; Chief of Staff, Youville Hosp.; Tel. 762-1711, 1712.

McARTHUR, Mervin I.; 310 Med. Centre, 906-8th **Ave. S.W., Calgary, Alta.; Alb '61; AMCGP; Tel. 263-4685.**

McASKILE, Kenneth; One Medical Place, 20 Wynford Dr., Don Mills, Ont.; 11 Wimpole Dr., Willowdale (res); Tor '39; **Otol**; Sr. Otol., St. Michael's Hosp.; Cons. Otol., Sunnybrook Hosp.; Assoc., Dept. Otol., U. of Toronto; Tel. 429-1580.

McATEER, D. K.; 46 Hillcrest, Willowdale, Ont.; Tor '30; Ass't. Coroner, York County; Tel. BA 1-4262.

McATEER, F. Michael; Maple Medical Clinic, Maple Plaza, Maple, Ont.; Tor '62; Staff, York Central Hosp., Richmond Hill; Tel. 832-2201.

McAULEY, Robert D. J.; King St., P.O. Box 603, Kingston, Ont.; 56 Hill St. (res); Qns '54; D.Psy; Psy; Ass't. Supt., Ont. Hosp.; Clin. Ass't. (Psy), Queen's U.; Tel. 546-1101.

McAULEY, Ronald G.; 132 Parkdale S., Hamilton, Ont.; 171 Sherwood Rise (res); Qns '54; MCGP; Active Staff, Hamilton Civic & St. Joseph's Hosp's Court. Staff, Chedoke & Joseph Brant Hosp's.; Tel. LI 4-8945.

McAVOY, Allen V.; 247 Main St., Port Colborne, Ont.; Tor '50; GenSurg.; DABS; Tel. TE 5-8322.

McAVOY, James R.; 35 Buell St., Brockville, Ont.; Qns '21; F.A.C.S., GenSurg; Tel. 345-5913.

McBAIN, Robert W.; 18 Sunnylea Cres., Grimsby, Ont.; Tor '24; DiagRad.

McBEATH, John H.; Manitoba Clinic, 790 Sherbrook St., Winnipeg 2, Man.; 50 Guelph St., Wpg. 9 (res); Glasgow (Scot.) '40; FRCS(Edin.), FRCS(C), Urol; Chief (Urol.), Children's Hosp.; and Wpg. Gen. Hosp's.; Hd. Dept. of Urol., U. of Manitoba; Tel. SP 4-6541.

McBIRNIE, John E.; McBirnie-Cleland Clinic, 218 Catharine St., Port Colborne; 2 Steele St. (res); Toronto '47; FRCS(C); GenSurg; Chief of Surg., Port Colborne Gen. Hosp.; Tel. 834-3656.

McBRIDE, C. D.; 407 McLeod Bldg., Edmonton, Alta.; 10713—11th Ave. (res); McG '21; Retired.

McBRIDE, George A.; Medical Clinic, Outlook, Sask.; 403 Semple St. S. (res); Sask'63; Tel. 867-8626.

McBRIDE, Richard L.; Alb'61; FRCS(C), ObstGyn; Staff, Toronto Gen. Hosp., Toronto, Ont.

McBRIEN, G. Ernest; 2078 Lawrence Ave. E., Scarborough, Ont.; Tor '51; MCGP; Assoc. Staff, Tor. E. Gen. & Scarborough Gen. Hosp's.; Tel. PL 5-3528.

McBROOM, George L.; 77 Upper Middle Rd., Cooksville, Ont.; Tor '44; FRCP(C); IntMed; Chief of Med., South Peel Hosp.; Assoc. Med. Staff, St. Joseph's Hosp.; **Cons. (IntMed.),** Queensway Gen.; Tel. 277-8301.

McBROOM, J. Gilbert; 275 Ontario St., Kingston, **Ont.; 165 University Ave. (res); Qns '34; OphthOtol; Hd. (OphthOtol.), Hotel-Dieu Hosp.; Active Staff, Kingston Gen. Hosp.; Ass't. Prof. (OphthOtol.), Queens U.; Tel. 548-4811.**

McBROOM, Wilbert T.; 217 St. Clair Ave. W., Toronto 7, Ont.; Wes '07.

McBURNEY, Donald A.; Box 300, Oak Ridges, Ont.; Man '34; Tel. 773-5327.

McBURNEY, R. James; 20 Faulkner St., Orangeville, Ont.; Wes '51; MCGP; Active Med. Staff, Dufferin Hosp.; Tel. 941-0642.

McCABE, John; 321 Tecumseh Blvd. E., Windsor, Ont.; 1316 Riverside, Riverside (res); Tor '38; **FRCS(1); GenSurg.; Tel. 252-2867.**

McCABE, John P.; 561 Middlewoods Dr., London, Ont. (res); Qns '39; DHA; Admin. Victoria Hosp.; Retired.

McCABE, Philip C.; 233 Coronado Dr., Tecumseh, Ont.; Tor '45.

McCAFFERTY, William J.; 359 Wellington St., Preston, Ont.; 347 King St. (res); Qns '53; AMCGP; Tel. 653-4791.

McCAFFREY, Francis W.; 1219 Harwood St., Apt. 1202, Vancouver 5, B.C.; Lav'41; Anaes; Staff, Dept. of Anaes., St. Paul's Hosp.; Tel. MU 3-2211.

McCAFFREY, Robert P.; Ste. 380, 5780 Cambie St., Vancouver 15, B.C.; Tor'40; Att'd. Staff, Dept. of Surg., St. Vincent's Hosp.

McCALDON, Robert J.; 837 Princess St., Kingston, Ont.; Tor'60; D.Psy; Psy; Psy., Penitentiary Service; Court. Staff, Kingston Gen. & Hotel Dieu Hosp's.; Staff, Inst. of Psychotherapy; Tel. 548-8209.

McCALL, William J.; Ste. 102, 1718 Marine Dr., West Vancouver, B.C.; St. Mary's(London) '52; Tel. 926-1510.

McCALLA, Robert I.; Alb '51; Anaes; Staff, University Hosp., Edmonton, Alta.; Tel. 439-5911.

McCALLUM, A. B.; 616 Talbot St., St. Thomas, Ont.; 122 Myrtle St. (res); London (Eng.) '30; Phys. & Surg., Timken Roller Bearing Co.

McCALLUM, Alan G.; 940 King St. W., Kitchener, Ont.; London (Eng.) '48; DLO; Otol; Staff, Kitchener-Waterloo, St. Mary's & South Waterloo Mem. Hosp's.; Tel. 744-3526.

McCALLUM, Archie; 430 Armadale Ave., Toronto, Ont. (res); Tor '16; Retired.

McCALLUM, Barbara J.; (See Blake).

McCALLUM, J. Lester; Room 647, Montreal Gen. Hosp., Montreal 25, P.Q.; 3466 Grey Ave. (res); McG'43; DIM; FACP; FRCP(C), IntMed; Ass't. Phys., Montreal Gen. Hosp.; Phys-in-Chief, Reddy Mem. Hosp.; Assoc. Prof. (Med.), McGill U.; Tel. WE 7-3458.

McCALLUM, John A.; Ormstown Med. Centre, Ormstown, P.Q.; McG '56; GenSurg; Tel. 829-2331.

McCALLUM, Malcolm G.; Alb '31; D.P.H., PH; Deputy Minister, Department of Health, Alberta, Administration Bldg., Edmonton, Alta.; Tel. CA 9-3208.

McCALLUM, Ronald F.; 124 Eagle St., Delhi, Ont.: Wes '39; MCGP; Tel. 582-2370.

McCALLUM, W. M.; 2525 Pine St., Vancouver 9, B.C.; Alb'39.

McCAMMON, Joseph; Assoc. Anaes. of Wpg., 805 Power Bldg., 428 Portage Ave. Winnipeg 1, Man.; 176 Old Mill Rd., Wpg. 12 (res); Man '36; FACA; FRCP(C), Anaes; GenSurg; Ass't. Anaes., Wpg. Gen.; Dem. (Anaes), U. of Manitoba; Tel. 943-7682. Abroad.

McCANN, Gerard J.; 50 Dart Shopping Centre, Dartmouth, N.S.; Glasgow (Scot.) '49.

McCANN, Harold D.; Stinson St., Rodney, Ont.; Wes '45; M.C.G.P.

McCANN, J. Alan; Box 1419, Courtenay, B.C.; Man '55.

McCANN, Kevin; Lourdes Clinic, Lourdes, Port au Port, Nfld.; Dublin (Ire.)'41; DPH; M.O., Lourdes Med. District; Tel. 642-5371.

McCANN, Maureen; Queensway Med. Centre, 880 The Queensway, Toronto 18, Ont.; Glasgow (Scot.)'60; DObstRCOG.

McCANN, Nessan; Nat. U. (Ire.) '49; Staff, Queen Elizabeth Hosp., Toronto, Ont.; Abroad.

McCANNEL, John A.; McG'53; DiagRad; Staff, Dept. of Rad., Royal Columbian Hosp., New Westminster, B.C.

McCANNEL, John S.; 357 Montgomery St., Fredericton, N.B.; McG'37.

McCANNEL, N. Bruce; 402 Medical-Dental Bldg., Regina, Sask.; 152 Connaught Cres. (res); Qns '50; D.A.B., FACOG; ObstGyn. Staff, Regina Gen. & Regina Grey Nuns Hosp's; Tel. LA 3-9653.

McCARLEY, John S.; Wes'44; Staff, Ontario Hosp., Smiths Falls, Ont.

McCARNEY, J. Robert; 275 Trafalgar Rd., **Oakville, Ont.; 1312 Hillhurst Rd. (res); Ott** '53; GenSurg; Active Cons. Staff, Oakville-Trafalgar Hosp.; Tel. VI 5-1455.

McCARRON, Edward; Dal '61; Res., Sunnybrook Hosp., Toronto 12, Ont.; Abroad.

McCARTEN, Alan B.; Ste 340, 3429-112th St., Edmonton, Alta.; 8007 Saskatchewan Dr. (res); Man '42; F.R.C.S.(Eng.), F.A.C.S., F.R.C.S.(C), GenSurg; Ass't. Clin. Prof., U. of Alberta; Tel. 433-0904.

McCARTHY, D. Dale; 41 Ridley Blvd., Toronto 12, Ont.; Tor'55.

McCARTNEY, Eric D.; McG'65; Res., Montreal General Hosp., Montreal 25, P.Q.

McCARTHY, Dermot; 250 Lawrence Ave. W., Toronto 12, Ont.; 10 Hammok Cres., R.R. 1, Thornhill (res); Tor '44; D.R.; DABR; D&TRad Radiol., York Co. Hosp., Newmarket; Cons. Rad., York Central Hosp., Richmond Hill; Tel. 787-0229.

McCARTHY, Patrick J.; R.C.A.F., Cold Lake, Alta.; Wales '58; M.B., B.Ch.

McCARTHY, Thomas F.; 47 Southern Dr., Ottawa 1, Ont.; Qns '53; Staff, Health Serv. Dir., Dept. of Natl. Health & Welfare; Tel. CE 2-8211.

MCCARTNEY, Harold J.; Medical Centre, 707 Charlotte St., Peterborough, Ont.; Qns'60; Ophth; Tel. 742-3871.

McCAUGHEY, Thomas J.; 70 Kingsway, Winni**peg 9, Man. (res); Dublin (Ire.) '50; D.A.; Anaes; Chief Anaes., Children's Hosp.; Ass't.** Prof. (Anaes), U. of Manitoba; Tel. SP 5-8311.

McCAUL, Evelyn K. (Johnston); Cambria Med. Bldg., 386 Cambria St., Stratford, Ont.; Tor'40; Staff, Stratford Gen. Hosp.

McCAUL, Herman C.; Princeton, Ont.; London **(Eng.) '09; Dist. Coroner; Tel. 458-4615.**

McCAULEY, Martin M.; Perth Med. Clinic, Perth, N.B.; Queens (Belfast, N. Ire.) '60; M.B., B.Ch., B.A.O., D.A. (Eng.); Tel. 491.

McCAULEY, W. Douglas; 149 Kenneth St., Duncan, B.C.; 2897 Phillips St. (res); Alb'49; Tel. 748-8151.

McCAUSLAND, Archibald; Qns '12; NeurPsy; Med. Supt., Ontario Hosp., London, Ont.; Retired.

McCAUSLAND, D. J. M.; c/o Long Lac Pulp & Paper Co., Terrace Bay, Ont.; Dist. Coroner.

McCAUSLAND, Joan (Lees); 23 Lascelles Blvd., Apt. 301, Toronto, Ont.; Aberdeen (Scot.) '60; DCH.

McCAW, Iain F.; Dept. of Nat. Health & Welfare, Terminal Rd., Halifax, N.S.; Glasgow (Scot.)'42; DPH; Port M.O.; Tel. 423-6636.

McCAW, J. W.; Craik, Sask; Dublin (Ire.) '48.

McCAWLEY, J. Comrie; 227 Medical Arts Bldg., Winnipeg, Man.; 233 Niagara St. (res); Man '46; M.R.C.O.G., F.R.C.S.(C), ObstGyn; Ass't ObstGyn, Winnipeg Gen. & Misericordia Hosp's; Ass't. Prof., (ObstGyn), U. of Manitoba; Tel. WH 3-0633.

McCENDIE, Ross G.; Blind River, Ont.; Tor '47; **Staff, St. Joseph's Hosp.; Tel. EL 6-9852.**

MCLEAN, Charles M.; Glasgow (Scot.) '39; DOMS (Eng.); Ophth; Staff, Eastern Reg. Med. Serv., Dept. of Ntl. Health & Welfare, Ottawa, Canada; Tel. 235-3932.

McLEAN, Janette S.; Box 158, Cold Lake, Alta.; McG '60; Staff, John Neil Hosp.; Tel. 20.

McCLEARY, Paul H.; Wes '62; Jr. Intn., Victoria Hosp., London, Ont.

McCLEAVE, J. Graham; 166 Main St., Nashwaaksis, N.B.; Dal '63; AMCGP.

McCLEAVE, John R.; Digby, N.S.; Dal '30; Gen Surg; Staff, Digby Gen. Hosp.; Tel. 245-2434.
McCLELLAND, James C.; Apt. 510, 25 Lascelles Blvd., Toronto 7, Ont. (res); Tor '16; FRCS(C), Urol; Retired.
McCLELLAND, J. Harold C.; 153 Royal York Rd. N. Toronto 18, Ont.; Tor '18; Retired.
McCLEMENTS, Sheila M.; (See Rotgans, Sheila M.).
McCLENAHAN, Claude A.; 1053 Mohawk, Burlington, Ont.; Tor '13; Med. Spec., Ontario Hosp., Hamilton, Ont.; Tel. 385-5361.
McCLINTOCK, Hugh T.; 84 Strath Ave., Toronto 18, Ont. (res); Tor '40; Dir., Gage Institute Chest Clin., 223 College St., Toronto; Tel. 924-2191.
McCLINTOCK, William B.; 206 Med. Arts Bldg., 628 Davis Dr., Newmarket, Ont.; 6 Church St., Mimico (res); Tor '45; GenSurg; Act. Staff, York County Hosp.
McCLINTON, James B.; 46 Pine St. S., Timmins, Ont.; 144 Hemlock St. (res); Tor '24; GenSurg; Staff, St. Mary's Hosp.; Dist. Coroner.
McCLISH, Andre; Apt. 4, 756 Place Philippe, Quebec 10, P.Q. (res); Lav '55; FRCP(C), Anaes; Staff, Laval Hosp.; Tel. 653-5251.
McCLURE, David; Medical Clinic, Eatonia, Sask.; UBC '57; Staff, Eatonia Union Hosp.; Tel. 967-2501.
McCLURE, J. David; 73 Queen St. E., Brampton, Ont.; R.R. 1, Caledon (res); Qns '54; Tel. 451-1244.
McCLURE, Joseph A., F/L; Canadian Forces Base, Trenton, Ont.; Qns'63.
McCLURE, Peter D.; 73 Wicklow Dr., Agincourt, Ont. (res); Qns '56; FRCP(C), Paed; Ass't. Path. (Haem.), Hosp. for Sick Children; Clin. Teach. Paed., U. of Toronto; Tel. EM 6-7242.
McCLURE, Raymond; St. Guillaume d'Upton, Cte. Yamaska, P.Q.; Mon '59.
McCLURE, William G.; College of Phys. & Surg., 1807-W. 10th Ave., Vancouver 9, B.C.; Tor '41; MCGP; Registrar, Coll. of Phys. & Surg.; Tel. 736-5551.
McCLUSKEY, Kenneth A.; 161 Larch St., Sudbury, Ont.; 142 McNaughton St. (res); London (Eng.) '46; M.B., B.S., F.R.C.S. (Ed.), F.R.C.S. (Eng.), F.R.C.S.(C), Orth Surg; OrthSurg., St. Joseph's Hosp's.; Tel. OS 3-7131.
McCLUSKEY, Lawrence U.; 610 Pembroke St. W., Pembroke, Ont.; Ott'52; GenSurg; Chief of Surg., Pembroke Gen. Hosp.; Staff Surg., Pembroke Cottage Hosp.; Tel. 732-3101.
McCOLGAN, James W.; 39 Arjay Cres., Willowdale, Ont.; Man '19; Retired.
McCOLL, Duncan T. R.; 4850 MacKenzie St., Vancouver 8, B.C.; 5469 Manson St., Van. 13 (res); Qns '33; Vis. Staff, St. Paul's, Vancouver Gen., St. Vincent's, Grace & Mount St. Joseph's Hosp's.; Tel. AM 6-4250.
McCOLL, J. D., Box 959, Frank W. Horner Co. Montreal, P.Q.; 722 Church, Dorval (res); Tel. RI 7-6575; 631-3261.
McCOLLUM, James L.; 930 Medical Arts Bldg., 170 St. George St., Toronto, Ont.; Tor '28; Urol.; Tel. WA 2-5747.
McCOMB, C. Renwick; 208 Medical Arts Bldg., Port Arthur, Ont.; 74 Winnipeg Ave. (res); Tor '46; F.R.C.S.(C), GenSurg, Urol.; Tel. 344-1813.
McCONACHIE, Donald B.; 350-14th St. W., Owen Sound, Ont.; 700-2nd Ave. W. (res); Tor '50; Staff, Owen Sound Gen. & Marine Hosp's.; Tel. 376-8510.
McCONKEY, Arthur S.; 925 W. Georgia St., Vancouver 1, B.C.; 1658 W. 28th Ave. (res); Alb'35; FICS, OrthSurg; Chief, Dept. of Orth. Surg., St. Paul's Hosp.; Staff, Children's Hosp.; Clin. Ass't. Prof. (OrthSurg), U. of British Columbia; Tel. MU 1-9464.
McCONN, Sheila; Staff, Dept. of Health, 278 Le Marchant Rd., St. John's, Nfld.
McCONNACHIE, Charles C.; Box 279, Redvers, Sask.; London (Eng.) '61; M.B., B.S.; MRCS (Eng.); LRCP (Lond.); DObstRCOG.
McCONNACHIE, Thomas; 38 Highcliffe Ave., Hamilton, Ont.; Tor '40; Anaes; Anaes. Staff, Hamilton Gen. Hosp.; Tel. 383-9104.
McCONNEL, Lorne H.; 414 Avenue Bldg., Saskatoon, Sask.; Man '12; NeurSurg.
McCONNELL, Aileen P.; Ste. 1402, 11025-82nd Ave., Edmonton, Alta.; Qns'55; IntMed.
McCONNELL, Doreen E.; 340 Campbell St., Nanaimo, B.C.; 22 Rosehill (res); Bristol (Eng.) '53; DRCOG; Paed; Retired.
McCONNELL, Fleming; Suite 1402, 11025-82nd Ave., Edmonton, Alta.; Tor'52; FRCP(C), Diag-Rad; Dir., Dept. of Rad., University of Alberta Hosp.; Prof. of Rad., U. of Alberta.
McCONNELL, John A.; 7187 Beechwood St., Vancouver 14, B.C.; Wes'53; Anaes; AMCGP; Att'd. Staff, Vancouver Gen. & Children's Hosp's.; Tel. 874-1626.
MCCONNEY, Florence S. (Hardy); 275 Glencairn Ave., Toronto 12, Ont.; Tor '20; F.A.C.P.; IntMed; Hon. Staff, Women's College Hosp.; Tel. HU 8-3379.
McCONVILLE, Brian J.; Otago (N. Zealand) '57; Psy; Staff, Kingston Gen. Hosp., Kingston, Ont.; Lect. Child Psy. & Paed., Queen's U.; Tel. 546-3841.
McCORD, Walter J.; Abbott Clinic, Winnipeg, Man.; 1184 Wolseley Ave. (res); Man '34; F.R.C.-O.G., F.A.C.O.G., F.A.C.S., F.R.C.S. (C), ObstGyn; Assoc. Prof. (ObstGyn), U. of Manitoba; Tel. SP 4-4567.
McCORKELL, Wilfred J.; 304 Birks Bldg., Saskatoon, Sask.; Alb'53; MCGP; Chmn. Dept. of G.P., University Hosp.; Clin. Teach., U. of Saskatchewan; Tel. 242-0056.
McCORMACK, C. W.; M.O., Charles Camsell Indian Hospital, Edmonton, Alta.
McCORMACK, Francis; Invermay Clinic, Invermay, Sask.; Glasgow (Scot.)'52.
McCORMACK, James T.; 168 Ontario St., St. Catharines, Ont.; Tor'36; ObstGyn.; Staff, St. Catharines Gen. & Hotel-Dieu Hosp's.; Tel. 685-0481.
McCORMACK, Mary A.; Invermay Clinic, Invermay, Sask.; Glasgow (Scot.)'47.
McCORMACK, Oliver Y.; 1938 Gerrard St. E., Toronto, Ont.; 82 Normandy Blvd. (res); Tor '23; Tel. OX 4-6263.
McCORMACK, Philip C.; C. S. Williams Clinic, 2105 Columbia, Rossland, B.C.; London (Eng.)'62; DObstRCOG (Eng.).
McCORMICK, Andrew Q.; 2775 Heather St., Vancouver 9, B.C.; McG'60; FRCS(C), Ophth; Staff, Vancouver Gen. Hosp., Vancouver 9, B.C.
McCORMICK, A. M.; 150 Driveway, Ottawa 4, Ont.; Qns '07; Retired.
McCORMICK, C. Palmer; 303 Med. Arts Bldg., 170 St. George St., Toronto 5, Ont.; 189 Old Yonge St., Willowdale (res); Wes '35; GenSurg; NeurSurg; Vis. NeurSurg., Wellesley Hosp.; Tel. 922-5777.
McCORMICK, G. Ralph; 406 Medical Arts Bldg., 1011 Ouellette Ave., Windsor, Ont.; Ott '56; GenSurg.; ThorSurg.; Tel. 256-1990.
McCORMICK, Myra J.; McG '62; Res., Ottawa Civic Hosp., Ottawa 3, Ont.
McCORMICK, Norman A.; 1687 Wyandotte St. E., Windsor, Ont.; Tor '26; D.A.B.R., F.R.C.S. (Edin.), F.A.C.R., Gen Surg, TherRad; Dir., Ontario Cancer Foundation, Windsor Clin., Chief Neoplastic Serv., Metropolitan Hosp.; Tel. 256-3461.
McCORMICK, Robert W.; Box 351, Harrow, Ont.; Tor'43; MCGP; Court. Staff, local Hosp's., Windsor; Dist. Coroner, Tel. RE 8-2912.
McCORMICK, William J.; 16 Gothic Ave., Toronto 9, Ont.; Med. Missionary Coll. (U.S.A.) '05; Tel. RO 9-4460.
McCORMICK, William K.; 1440 Tecumseh Rd. E., Windsor, Ont.; Riverdale Manor, Riverside (res); Tor '23; Tel. 253-5767.
McCORRISTON, James R.; Etherington Hall, Stuart St., Kingston, Ont.; Qns '43; M.Sc., FACS; DABS; FRCS(C), GenSurg; Surg-in-Chief, Kingston Gen. Hosp.; Cons.Surg., Hotel-Dieu Hosp; Sr. Cons. Surg., Cdn. Forces Hosp.; Hon. Cons. Staff, Royal Victoria Hosp., Montreal; Prof. & Hd., Dept. of Surg., Queen's U.; Tel. 542-2188.
McCORRISTON, Lila (See REDMOND, Lila).

McCOSH, Robert A.; 187 Widder St., Goderich, Ont.; Tor '24.
McCOURT, John F.; Box 160, Ituna, Sask.; Nat. U. (Ire.) '48.; DPH; Tel. 795-2632.
McCOURTIE, David R.; Wes'62; Res., Wellesley Hosp., Toronto 5, Ont.
McCOWAN, Conrad W.; Ste. 203, 1640-16th Ave. N.W., Calgary, Alta.; Alb'59; Tel. 289-4431.
McCOY, Edwin C.; 1807 W. 10th, Vancouver, **B.C.; 5358 Angus Dr. (res); McG '39; M.C.G.P.;** Exec. Dir., CMA (BC), (Dept. of Prev. Med.), Hon. Lect., U. of British Columbia; Tel. 736-5551.
McCOY, Hugh D.; 8 Sydenham, Dundas, Ont.; R.R. No. 3 (res); Qns '52; Tel. MA 8-8251.
McCOY, R. Hall; 600 Seaforth Med. Bldg., 3550 Cote des Neiges Rd., Montreal 25, P.Q.; 601 Kenilworth Rd., Town of Mount Royal (res); McG '36; Otol Tel. 932-8409.
McCRACKEN, Eric C.; 1364 Islington Ave. N., Rexdale, Ont.; 32 Blair Athol Cr., Islington, (res); Glasgow (Scot.) '53; Tel. 741-2020.
McCRACKEN, George; 346 Guildwood Pkwy. West Hill, Ont. (res); Royal Coll. (Edin. & Glasgow) '25; FRFPS (Glasgow), FCCP; MRCP (Glas.); Med. Dir., Riverdale Hosp., Toronto; Tel. 461-8251.
McCRACKEN, James A.; Oyen, Alta.; Alb '50; Dist. Coroner.
McCRACKEN, William J.; 64 Charlton Ave. W., Hamilton, Ont.; Tor'45; MS; FRCS(C), GenSurg; Active Surg. Staff, St. Joseph's & Chedoke Hosp's.; Court. Staff, Hamilton Gen., Henderson & Joseph Brant Hosp's.; Tel. 529-1795.
McCRANK, Ernest W.; Qns'64; Res., Kingston Gen. Hosp., Kingston, Ont.
McCRAE, William H.; 672 Brant St., Burlington, Ont.; Tor '55; B.Sc (Med.); FRCS(C), Urol; Chief of Urol., Joseph Brant Mem. Hosp.; Hon. Cons. Urol., Oakville-Trafalgar Hosp. & Milton Hosp., Milton, Ont.; Tel. 637-7404.
McCREA, James C.; 149 Highfield St., Moncton, N.B.; McG '43; Staff, Moncton Hosp.; Court. **Staff, Hotel-Dieu Hosp.; Tel. EV 2-6647.**
McCREARY, Bruce D.; Qns '62; Res., Psych. Research Inst., London, Ont.; Abroad.
McCREARY, John F.; 4762 W. 2nd Ave., Vancouver, B.C. (res); Tor '34; DABP; FRCP(C), Paed; Dean, Fac. of Med., U. of British Columbia; Tel. CA 4-4725.
McCREARY, Robert H.; Arnprior Med. Centre, 104 Daniel St., Arnprior, Ont.; 115 John St. (res); Qns '29; FAAP; Paed; Pres. of Staff, Arnprior & Dist. Mem. Hosp.; Tel. 623-3131.
McCREATH, Norman D.; Grace Gen. Hosp., Winnipeg 10, Man.; New Zealand'39; MRCP (Lond.); MRACP; Med. Dir., Grace Gen. Hosp.; Tel. SU 3-7271.
McCREDIE, John A.; 469 Waterloo St., London, Ont.; 485 Windamere Rd. (res); Queen's U. (Belfast, N. Ire.) '46; M.Ch., F.A.C.S., F.R.C.S. (Eng. & Ed.), F.R.C.S.(C), GenSurg; Surg. Staff, St. Joseph's Hosp.; Research Fell., Ont. Cancer Fdn.; Hon. Lect. (Surg.), U. of Western Ont.; Tel. GE 8-6751.
McCREERY, Robin G.; Ste. 130, 5780 Cambie St., Vancouver 15, B.C.; Wes '54; Ophth; Att'd. Staff, Vancouver Gen. Hosp.; Tel. FA 1-1818.
McCRIMMON, Donald R.; 510 Medical Arts Bldg., 1538 Sherbrooke St. W., Montreal, P.Q.; 511 Clarke Ave., Westmount (res); McG '34; Paed; **Assoc. Phys., Mtl. Children's, Chief Paed., St. Mary's Hosp's; Dem. (Paed), McGill U.; Tel. WE 3-1234.**
McCRIMMON, F. Gordon; 15 King St., Huntingdon, P.Q.; 32 Prince St. (res); McG '31; GenSurg; Tel. 264-5344.
McCRIMMON, John R.; Pincher Creek, Alta.; Man '27.
McCRORY, Thomas P.; 1538 Sherbrooke St. W., **Montreal 25, P.Q.; McG '59; Tel. WE 3-3327.**
McCRUM, John R.; Sexsmith, Alta.; Alb '45; Dist. Coroner.
McCRYSTAL, Frank; 309 Lancaster W., Kitchener, Ont.; Ireland'52; Am. Bd. Psy. & Neurol; Cons. Psy., St. Mary's & Kitchener-Waterloo Hosp's.; Tel. 743-7521.
McCUAIG, C. Homer; Ontario Hosp., Kingston, Ont.; 117 College St. (res); Qns '21; Psy.
McCUAIG, Kenneth O.; Tor '57; Assoc. Prof., Dept. of Anatomy, U. of Toronto, Toronto 5, Ont.; Tel. 928-2620.
McCUE, Daniel; 1217 Oxford St. W., London, Ont.; Glasgow (Scot.) '50; MCGP; Tel. 471-6570.
McCUE, Francis J.; Tweed, Ont.; Tor '37; **M.O.H.; Tel. 478-3240.**
McCULLAGH, Malachy S.; 604 Brant St., Burlington, Ont.; Wes'64; Tel. 634-7255.
McCULLOCH, A. Ernest; 165 St. Clair Ave. W., Toronto 7, Ont.; 60 Warren Rd. (res); Tor '13; MCGP; Retired.
McCULLOCH, Allan W.; 108 Medical Arts Bldg., 404-406 Graham Ave., Winnipeg, Man.; Man '38; DiagRad; Cons. & Chief of Rad. Serv., Deer Lodge & Grace Hosp's.; Staff, St. Boniface Hosp.; Court. Staff, Concordia Hosp.; Chief Cons. in Radiol., Dept. of Health Manitoba Gov't.; Tel. 943-7301.
McCULLOCH, Charles F.; 813 Greyhound Bldg., **Calgary Alta.; 2424 Sovereign Cr., (res); Qns** '45; GenSurg; FACS; Clinician, Calgary Cancer Clin.; Tel. 269-7512.
McCULLOCH, Donald J.; 71 Grangemill Cresc., Don Mills, Ont. (res); Tor '48; F.R.C.S.(C), Psy; Dip. Psy.; Assoc. Staff (Psy), & Special Lect., Psy., School of Social Work, U. of Toronto; Dir., Community Mental Health Clinic, Ont. Hosp., **999 Queen W., Toronto, Ont.; Tel. LE 3-8501.**
McCULLOCH, Ernest A.; Ontario Cancer Inst., 500 Sherbourne St., Toronto, Ont.; 58 Binscarth Rd. (res); Tor '48; F.R.C.P.(C), IntMed; Ass't. Phys., Toronto Gen. Hosp.; Research Haematol., Princess Margaret Hosp.; Ass't. Prof. (Med. Bio**physics), U. of Toronto; Tel. 924-0671.**
McCULLOCH, J. Clement; 830 Medical Arts Bldg., 170 St. George St., Toronto, Ont.; 165 Teddington Park Ave. (res); Tor '39; FRCS(C); Ophth; Hd., Ophth. Dept., Toronto Gen. Hosp.; Prof., U. of Toronto; Tel. WA 2-4131.
McCULLOCH, John; 2678 Yonge St., Toronto 12, Ont.; Tor'42.
McCULLOCH, J. A.; Tor'63; Res., Toronto Western Hosp., Toronto 2B, Ont.
McCULLOCH, Keith G.; 430 Edgewood Rd., Beaconsfield, P.Q.; Man'57; FRCS(C), GenSurg.; Tel. 695-9299.
McCULLOCH, Michael A.; 229 Church St., Oakville, Ont.; Dal'59; Assoc. Staff, Oakville Mem. Hosp.; Tel. 845-8771.
McCULLOCH, Peter B.; Tor '64; Res., Montreal Gen. Hosp., Montreal 25, P.Q.
McCULLOCH, Thomas A., Sg./Lcdr; Tor'55; Psy; Chief of Psy., Cdn. Forces Hosp., Halifax, N.S.
McCULLOUGH, Crawford C.; 225 N. Syndicate Ave., Fort William, Ont. (res); Qns '04; F.A.-**C.S., F.R.C.S. (C), Ophth; Otol; Retired.**
McCULLOUGH, David W.; Ste. 206, 96 Larch St., Sudbury, Ont.; Tor'39; Ophth; Staff, Sudbury Gen. & Sudbury Mem. Hosp's.; Tel. 675-7015.
McCULLOUGH, D. Louis; 4742-55th St., Red Deer, Alta. (res); Dublin (Ire.) '14; D.P.H.; D.P.M.; B.A.O.; L.M., Rotunda; Psy; Retired.
McCULLOUGH, James T.; 2 Park Rd., Elmira, Ont.; R.R. 4 (res); Wes '30; MCGP; Active Staff, Kitchener-Waterloo & St. Mary's Gen. Hosp's.; Tel. 669-5471.
McCULLOUGH, John A.; Box 160, Carrot River, Sask.; Lav'40; Dist. Coroner; Tel. 768-2711.
McCULLOUGH, John F.; Sudbury Med. Arts Ltd., 260 Cedar St., Sudbury, Ont.; 894 Roderick Ave., Site 7, R.R. No. 2, Box 5 (res); Tor **'30; F.I.C.S.; GenSurg; Tel. 673-3695.**
McCULLOUGH, Mary G. C.; 4742-55th St., Red Deer, Alta. (res); Dublin (Ire.) '11; B.A.O., D.P.H.; Retired.
McCULLOUGH, Robert S.; 3935 Bloor St. W., Toronto 18, Ont.; Tor '51; M.C.G.P.; Staff, **Queensway Gen. & Runnymede Hosp's.; Tel. BE 1-0239.**
McCULLY, J. Alden; 134 Victoria St., Amherst, N.S.; Dal'60; MCGP; Tel. 667-8555.
McCUNN, P. Donald; 340 McLeod, Ottawa 4, Ont.; Ott'55; Ophth; Assoc Staff, Ottawa Gen. Hosp.; Clin. Ass't. (Ophth), Ottawa U.; Tel. 233-4904.

McCURDY, David G.; 1 Burns Dr., Fleming Glen, Halifax, N.S.; Dal '41; D.P.H.; Administrator, Cons. Serv., Dept. of Health, Nova Scotia, Hollis St.; Tel. 5-8271.
McCURDY, Margaret J.; 300 Islington Ave. N., Toronto, Ont.; 44 Kingsway Ave. (res); Tor '54; M.C.G.P.; Assoc. Staff, Women's College Hosp.; Court. Staff, Humber Mem. Hosp.; Tel. WA 3-7381.
McCURLIE, John M.; 2 St. Margaret's Rd., Ancaster, Ont.; Wes '50.
McCURRACH, Allan C.; 2058 Commercial Dr., Vancouver 12, B.C.; 4661 Drummond St. (res); Alb '38; D & T Rad.; Tel. 253-7505.
McCUSKER, Emmet A.; Medical Arts Clinic, Regina, Sask.; McG '21; Ophth; Retired.
McCUTCHEON, Caswell W. V.; 168 Essex St., Sarnia, Ont.; 206 MacKenzie N. (res); Tor '35; F.R.C.S.(C), GenSurg; Surg. Staff, Sarnia Gen. & St. Joseph's Hosp's.; Dist. M.O., C.N.R.; Memb. Occupational Health Assoc., Canada; Tel. DI 4-1873.
McCUTCHEON, Elgin; Tor'61; Res., Kingston Gen. Hosp., Kingston, Ont.
McCUTCHEON, John D.; 1605-9th Ave. S., Lethbridge, Alta.; 2716 South Parkside Dr. (res); Alb '46; Staff, Lethbridge Mun. & St. Michael's Hosp's.; Tel. 7-3121.
McCUTCHEON, John E.; Tor '35; Anaes; Staff, Ontario Hosp., Port Arthur, Ont.; Tel. D14-3571.
McCUTCHEON, J. W.; 157 Main St., Milton, Ont.; 57 Victoria St. (res); Tor'31; Home Phys., Halton Manor; Tel. TR 8-9223.
McCUTCHEON, Richard M.; Qns'61; Anaes; Staff, Hosp. for Sick Children, Toronto, Ont.
McDADE, Frederick D.; Medical Centre, Golden Mile Plaza, Regina, Sask.; Qns'38; Tel. 536-1169.
McDANIEL, Bernard M.; Box 490, Ocean Falls, B.C.; McG '51; MCGP.
McDERMENT, Robert; 136 Walton St., Port Hope, Ont. '27.
McDERMID, James M.; 159 Bidwell St., Tillsonburg, Ont.; Wes '61; AMCGP; Tel. VI 2-8172.
McDERMOT, Rebecca S. R. (MacLean); 1911 Wembley Ave., Ottawa 13, Ont.; Tor '54; TherRad; Staff, Ont. Cancer Fdn., Ottawa.
McDERMOTT, Aod; National U. (Cork, Ire.) '44; DPH (Tor.); DMRD (Liverpool); Chief (Rad.), Central Nfld. Hosp., Grand Falls, Nfld.; Tel. 2123.
McDERMOTT, James G.; 236 Ontario St., Stratford, Ont.; 44 Haig St., Wes '33; F.I.C.S.; GenSurg; Chief of Staff, Stratford Gen. Hosp.; Tel. 271-2558.
McDIARMID, Howard R.; Tofino, B.C.; Man '54; MCGP; Tel. 725-3282.
McDIARMID, Roper O.; 35 Clement Block, Brandon, Man.; 1605 Victoria Ave. (res); Man '36; Ophth, Otol; E.E.N.T. Dept., Brandon Gen. & Ninette Hosp's.; Cons., Brandon, & Ninette Sans., Brandon Mental Hosp., DVA; Tel. PA 9-2478.
McDONAGH, E. Christina; Cape Breton Mental Health Centre, 337 Prince St., Sydney, N.S.; National U. (Dublin, Ire.) '45; BAO; Psy; Tel. 562-3202.
McDONAGH, John E.; 414-925 W. Georgia St., Vancouver 1, B.C.; 1716 West King Edward (res); Man '46; ObstGyn; Att'd. Staff, Van. Gen. Hosp.; Sec.-Treasur., Pacific Northwest ObstGyn Assoc.; Lect., U. of British Columbia; Tel. MU 3-2737.
McDONALD, A. Donald; 15010-75th Ave., Edmonton, Alta.; Guy's H. (London, Eng.) '37; Staff, Chas. Camsell Hosp., Dept. of Indian & North Health Serv.; Tel. GL 5-7141.
McDONALD, Alexander W.; 4665 Prince of Wales Ave., Montreal, P.Q. (res); McG '50; Anaes; Staff Anaes, Montreal Children's & Reddy Mem. Hosp's.; Staff, McGill U.; Tel. WE 7-8511.
McDONALD, Alice; Harrison Springs Hotel, Harrison Hot Springs, B.C.; Alb '33.
McDONALD, Donald J.; 2917 Bloor St. W., Toronto 18, Ont.; Tor'56; FRCS(C); Ophth; Active Staff, St. Joseph's Hosp.; Court. Staff, South Peel Hosp., Cooksville; Tel. 239-3843.
McDONALD, Donald J.; Tor'61; ObstGyn; Staff, Toronto Western Hosp., Toronto 2B, Ont.
McDONALD, Donald M.; 319-E Columbia St., New Westminster, B.C.; Deer Lake Dr., Burnaby 2 (res); Alb '48; OrthSurg; Chief of Surg., Royal Columbian Hosp.; Cons., St. Mary's & Surrey Mem. Hosp's.; Tel. LA 2-9312.
McDONALD, Glen A.; 272 Bloor St. W., Toronto 5, Ont.; 99 Tyndale Ave. (res); Tor '49; F.R.C.S.(C), GenSurg, OrthSurg; Staff, St. Joseph's & Queensway Hosp's.; Clin. Instr. (Surg.), U. of Toronto; Tel. WA 2-4511.
McDONALD, G. V.; Apple Hill, Ont.; Qns '28.
McDONALD, Harriet E.; 308½ Boler Rd., London, Ont.; Wes '62.
McDONALD, Hector A.; 2481 Kingston Rd., Scarboro, Ont.; 4369 Lawrence Ave. E. (res); Tor '51; Staff Scarborough Gen. Hosp., Tel. 261-6767.
McDONALD, Hugh D.; Man '48; Med. Dir., St. Paul's Hosp., Vancouver, B.C.; Tel. MU 2-2334.
McDONALD, Hugh R.; Kilbride, Ont.; McG '22.
McDONALD, Ian M.; 19 Weir Cres., Saskatoon, Sask. (res); Man '53; Psy; Staff, University Hosp.; Assoc. Prof. (Psy), U. of Saskatchewan; Tel. 242-7641, Ext. 481.
McDONALD, Ida M.; Tor '39; D. Psy; Staff, Ontario Hosp., London, Ont.; Tel. 455-5110.
McDONALD, J. Corbett; London (Eng.) '49; DPH; MRCP; MRCS; LRCP; DIH; MSc (Harvard); Prof. & Chmn., Dept. of Epidem. & Health, McGill U., Montreal 2, P.Q.
McDONALD, John; 80—50th Ave., Lachine, P.Q. (res); McG 17; GenSurg; Retired.
McDONALD, John L.; 532 Med. Arts Bldg., 170 St. George St., Toronto 5, Ont.; 8 Silverwood Ave. (res); Tor '16; FRCS(C), GenSurg; OrthSurg; Cons. (Surg.), Wellesley Hosp.; Hon. Cons. (Surg.), Hosp. for Sick Children; Grad. Lect. (Surg.), U. of Toronto; Tel. WA 3-7834.
McDONALD, John O.; 1287 N. Shore Dr., Sudbury, Ont.; 197 Nicholas (res); McG'22; GenSurg; M.O.H., McKim, & Phys., Pioneer Manor; Tel. 675-7565.
McDONALD, John W.; 120 Grand Ave., Apt. 601, London, Ont. (res); Wes '61; MRC Fell., Dept. of Biochem., Univ. of Western Ont.
McDONALD, Joseph A.; Bay Medical Group, Glace Bay, N.S.; 174½ Main St. (res); Dal '33; M.C.G.P.; Sr. Med. Staff, St. Joseph's & Glace Bay Gen. Hosp's.; Tel. 849-5521.
McDONALD, Lyle T.; 423 Med. Arts Bldg., Winnipeg, Man.; 354 Campbell St. (res); Man '51; Paed; Dem. (Paed), U. of Manitoba; Telephone WH 2-6405.
McDONALD, Malcoln E.; Aberdeen (Scot.) '51; M.O. Brookfield Cottage Hosp., Brookfield, Nfld.; Tel. 2151.
McDONALD, Millard H.; No. 239, Star City, Sask.; Qns '11.
McDONALD, Robert C.; Ste. 1803, 625 Milton St., Montreal, P.Q.; Sydney (Australia)'58; D.Psy; Clin. Fell. Psy., Royal Victoria Hosp.; Ass't. Psy., McGill Student Health Serv.; Dem. Psy., McGill U.; Tel. 844-6311.
McDONALD, W. Leslie; Ste. 3, 21 Quinte St., Trenton, Ont.; 72 Byron St. (res); Qns'41; FACS, FRCS(C), GenSurg; Cons. (Surg.), Belleville Gen. Hosp.; Hd., Dept. of Surg., Trenton Mem. Hosp.; Tel. EX 2-3945.
McDONNELL, Charles E.; Ste. 480, 2184 W. Broadway, Vancouver 9, B.C.; McG '51; FRCP (C), IntMed; Chief of Staff, Holy Family Hosp.; Clin. Instr., UBC; Tel. RE 1-3171.
McDOUGALL, Allan N.; Chatsworth, Ont.; Wes '62; AMCGP.
McDOUGALL, Alexander D.; Irving Clinic, 74 W. Seymour, Kamloops, B.C.; 674 Tunstall Cres. (res); Tor '51; MCGP; Staff, Royal Inland Hosp.; Tel. 372-5251
McDOUGALL, E. Peter; 1849 Yonge St., Ste. 505, Toronto 7, Ont.; Tor '56; FRCS(C), PlasSurg; GenSurg; Att'd. Staff, Toronto East Gen. Hosp.; Tel. HU 1-5531.
McDOUGALL, Gerald M.; 380-2184 West Broadway, Vancouver 9, B.C.; Alb'60; Psy; Tel. 731-9636.
McDOUGALL, Hector A.; 143 Longmore Ave., Pointe Claire, P.Q.; McG '42; GenSurg; DABS; FACS; Staff, Lakeshore Hosp.; Tel. 697-5268.

McDOUGALL, James A.; 223 Doris Ave., Willowdale, Ont.; 52 Hillcrest Ave. (res); Qns '44; M.C.G.P.; G.P. Staff, Grace Maternity Hosp., Toronto & Branson & St. John's Convalescent **Hosp's., Willowdale; Tel. BA 1-8333.**

McDOUGALL, John W.; 35 Garden St., Brockville, Ont.; Qns '37; M.C.G.P.; Med. Staff, Brockville Gen. & St. Vincent de Paul Hosp's.; Vis. Staff, Ontario Hosp.

McDOUGALL, Ruth; Dept. of Health, 5970 University Ave., Halifax, N.S.; McG '45; DPH; PH; Dir. of Maternal & Child Health, City of Halifax; Tel. 422-8571.

McDOWELL, H. Trevor; 300 Bloor St. E., Toronto 5, Ont.; Apt. 1403, 450 Walmer Rd. (res); **Qns** '27; Staff, Lockwood Clinic.

MCDOWELL, James D.; Winnipeg Clinic, Winnipeg, Man.; 255 Thurso St. (res); Belfast (Ire.) '48; F.R.C.P.(C), IntMed; Lect. (Med.), U. of Manitoba; Tel. WH 2-6441.

McDOWELL, Martin F.; 442 Christina St. N., Sarnia, Ont.; 750 London Rd. (res); Tor '56; IntMed; Active Staff (IntMed.), St. Joseph's & Sarnia Gen. Hosp's.; Tel. 336-3046.

McDOWELL, S. Earl; Shawville, P.Q.; Ont '22; Tel. 647-2511.

McDOWELL, Walter; 1535 Notre-Dame, Lachine, P.Q.; McG'46.

McDUFF, R. E.; 478 Notre Dame, St. Paul l'Ermite, P.Q.; 350 Notre Dame (res); Mon '49; M.C.G.P.

McEACHERN, Kenneth D.; 631 Med. Arts Bldg., 170 St. George St., Toronto 5, Ont.; 66 Roxboro St. E. (res); Tor '32; IntMed; Ass't. Phys., Toronto Gen. Hosp.; Clin. Ass't., U. of Toronto; Tel. WA 2-9491.

McEACHERN, Margaret A.; 66 Roxborough St. E., Apt. 402, Toronto, Ont.; Tor'32; Otol; Retired.

McEACHERN, Robert A.; 5224 Kingsway, South Burnaby, B.C.; 2036 Stride Ave., New Westminster (res); Coll. of Med. Evangelists (Calif., U.S.A.) '53; Tel. HE 3-1268.

McELLIGOTT, Joseph C.; Ott '59; Res., Ottawa Civic Hosp., Ottawa, Ont.

McELLIGOTT, Timothy F.; Box 157, Cartwright Point, Kingston, Ont.; National U. (Ire.)'52; BAO; DPH; MC Path.

McELMAN, George W.; 221 Gibson St., Fredericton, N.B.; Dal '41; Med. Advisor, N.B. Mother's Allowance Comm.; Federal Memb., N.B. Total Disability Pensions Bd.; Anaes. Staff, Victoria Public Hosp.

McELMOYLE, William A.; 110 Med. Arts Bldg., 1105 Pandora Ave., Victoria, B.C.; 1509 Rockland Ave. (res); Man '29; F.R.C.S.(Edin.), F.R.C.S. (C) GenSurg.; Tel. EV 4-8631.

McEVOY, John V.; 482 Cote-St.-Catherine Rd., Montreal, P.Q.; McG '27; MCGP; Cons. Phys., Toilet Laundries; Tel. WE 2-5121.

McEWAN, Mary C. (Fee); Glasgow (Scot.)'42; D. Psy; MCGP; Res., Clarke Inst. of Psy., 250 College St., Toronto 5, Ont.

McEWEN, Bennett B.; 664 Hillcrest Ave., Ottawa 3, Ont. (res); McG '32; Clin., Dept. Nat. Health & Welfare.

McEWEN, Donald C.; 34 Academy Med. Bldg., 1814-4th St. W., Calgary, Alta.; 5711 Elbow Dr. (res); Man '45; MRCOG; FRCOG; FACOG; FRCS(C), ObstGyn; Staff, Calgary. Gen. & Holy **Cross Hosp's.; Tel. 262-3956.**

McEWEN, D. Sanger; 630 Med. Arts Bldg., 404 Graham Ave., Winnipeg, Man.; 275 Dromore Ave. (res); Man'31; MCAA; IntMed; Cons., St. Boniface Gen. & Municipal Hosp's.; Assoc. Prof. (Med.), U. of Manitoba; Tel. WH 2 7706.

McEWEN, Howard; 402 E. Rideau Medical Centre, 1711-4th St. S.W., Calgary, Alta.; 1427-24th St. S.W. (res); Man '43; FACP; IntMed; Cons. Staff, Calgary Gen. Hosp.; Court. Staff, Holy Cross & Alberta Crippled Children's Hosp's.; Tel. 262-9807.

McEWEN, John A.; 154 Bridge St., Carleton Place, Ont.; Tor'08; District Coroner.

McEWEN, Robert B.; 237 William St., Pembroke, Ont.; **McG '53; GenSurg; Tel. 735-5722.**

McEWEN, Sydney F.; 550 Belfast St., Medicine Hat, Alta. (res); Tor '09; Retired.

McFADDEN, Danny; 656 Med. Arts Bldg., 750 Spadina Cr. E., Saskatoon, Sask.; Dublin (Ire.) '50; BAO; FRCS(C), GenSurg; Clin. Assoc., University Hosp.; Active Staff, St. Paul's Hosp.; Lect. (Surg.), U. of Saskatchewan; Tel. 242-5519.

McFADDEN, David G.; 940 King St. W., Kitchener, Ont.; Wes '46; DABOS; OrthSurg; Surg. Staff, Kitchener-Waterloo & St. Mary's Hosp's.; Tel. 743-4541.

McFADDEN. G. F.; Strathroy, Ont.; Qns '18.

McFADDEN, Kieran A.; 108—16th Ave. N.E. Calgary, Alta.; 2216 Capital Hill Cres. (res); Dublin (Ire.) '45; Tel. CR 7-0397.

McFADYEN, E. Hector; Box 161, Jasper, Alta.; Alb '40; DABOG, FAAOG, FACS; ObstGyn.

McFADZEAN, Wilfrid T.; 947 Colborne St., Brantford, Ont.; Wes '35; Tel. PL 3-2951.

McFARLAND, Donald W.; Box 20, Cookstown, Ont.; Tor '54; FAGS; Active Staff, Stevenson Mem. Hosp., Alliston; Coroner, Simcoe Co.; Tel. Area 705; 458-4321.

McFARLAND, H. Melville, C/O; Shilo Military Camp, Camp Shilo, Man.; McG '55.

McFARLAND, Ian W.; McFarland-Lewis Clin., High Prairie, Alta.; St. Andrew's (Scot.) '51; **F.R.C.S.(Ed.); GenSurg; Abroad.**

McFARLAND, Joseph D.; Ste. 9, 2730 Main St., Saskatoon, Sask.; Glasgow (Scot.)'59; FRCP(C), Anaes.

McFARLANE, Allan H.; 304 Med Arts Bldg. Hamilton, Ont.; 89 Inverness Ct. (res); Qns **'57; MCGP; Tel. JA 2-9767.**

McFARLANE, Clara J.; 205 Med. Arts Bldg., **Winnipeg, 1, Man.; 156 Winston Rd., Wpg. 12 (res); Man '51; MRCOG; FRCS(C), ObstGyn; Clin. Tutor (ObstGyn), U. of Manitoba; Tel. WH 3-3913.**

McFARLANE, Donald C.; 382 Queen's Ave., London, Ont.; 1674 Greenacres Dr. (res); Wes '51; D.A.B.Ophth; Ophth; Court. Staff, St. Joseph's Hosp.; Teach. Staff, Victoria Hosp.; Ophth. Cons., Children's Psych. Research Inst.; Clin. Lect., (Ophth), U. of Western Ontario; Tel. GE 9-4161.

McFARLANE, Douglas V.; 71 Buckingham Ave., Toronto 12, Ont.; McG '51; DMR; FRCP(C), DiagRad; Staff, Toronto Western Hosp.; Tel. 369-5871.

McFARLANE, G. M.; Sackville, N.B.; Tor '27.

McFARLANE, Gordon L.; Carbon, Alta.; Tor '11; Retired.

McFARLANE, Robert M.; 382 Queens Ave., London, Ont.; Wes'51; FACS, FRCS(C), GenSurg; PlasSurg; Victoria Hosp.; Cons. (PlasSurg), Westminster DVA Hosp.; Assoc. Prof. (PlasSurg); U. of Western Ont.; Tel. GE 8-8984.

McFARLANE, Ronald H.; Manitoba Clin., 790 Sherbrooke St., Winnipeg 2, Man.; 414 Campbell St., Winnipeg 9 (res); Man '41; F.A.C.P., IntMed; Ass't. Phys., Winnipeg Gen. Hosp.; Cons. (Med.), Deer Lodge & Winnipeg Mun. Hosp's.; Lect. (Med.), U. of Manitoba; Tel. SP 4-6541.

McFARLANE, William J. G.; 517 St. James Rd. W., North Vancouver, B.C. (res); UBC '55; D.-Psy; Psy; Unit. Dir., Crease Clinic, Riverview Hosp., Essondale; Clin. Instr. (Hon.) (Psy.), U. of British Columbia; Tel. LA 1-1911.

McFETRIDGE, James D.; Lacombe, Alta.; Dal '43.

McFETRIDGE, James G.; Medical Arts Clin., Regina, Sask.; Man '37; F.R.C.S.(Edin.); GenSurg.

McFETRIDGE J. Grant; Med. Arts Clinic, 2125-11th Ave., Regina, Sask.; 30 Davis Pl. (res); Man '44; IntMed; Chief of Med., Regina Grey Nuns Hosp.; Cons Med., DVA Hosp.; Tel. LA 2-1651.

McFETRIDGE, Samuel A.; 520 Birks Bldg., Vancouver, B.C.; **3937 Osler St. (res); Man '25; F.R.C.S. (Edin.), F.I.C.S., GenSurg; Assoc. Surg., Vancouver Gen. Hosp., Surg. Clin. Instr., U. of British Columbia; Tel. MU 1-9451.**

McGARRITY, Philip B.; Sarnia Med. Arts Bldg., 420 East St. N., Sarnia, Ont.; Ott'52; FACS, GenSurg; Chief of Surg., St. Joseph's Hosp.; Tel. ED 7-3431.

McGARRY, Garrett G.; 613 Meadow View Place, Calgary S.W., Alta.: Nat. U. (Ire.)'51; DPH; DRCOG.
McGARRY, George C.; 997 St. Paul St., Niagara Falls, Ont.; Tor '31; IntMed; Staff, Grt. Niagara Gen. Hosp.; Phys., Cdn. Carborundum Co.; Tel. EL 4-1418.
McGARRY, Howard H.; 219 Huron St., Niagara Falls, Ont.; 819 Portage Rd. (res); Tor '30; Paed; Staff, Niagara Falls Gen. Hosp.; Tel. 354-2707.
McGARRY, James R.; 1827 Main St., Niagara Falls, Ont.; 2150 Lundy's Lane (res); Tor '22; ObstGyn; Tel. EL 6-0721.
McGARRY, Patrick M. F.; c/o Grace Hosp., Winnipeg, Man.; National U. (Ire.) '46; D.A. (Ire. & Eng.); F.F.A.R.C.S.I., F.A.C.A., Anaes; Active Staff, Deer Lodge Hosp. & Chief Anaes. Grace Hosp.; Lect. (Surg.), U. of Manitoba; Tel. SU 3-6732.
McGARRY, Peter D.; Ste. 109, 3000 Lawrence Ave. E., Scarborough, Ont.; 693 McGowan Ave. **(res); Ire. '48; ObstGyn; Tel. 291-1861.**
McGAUGHEY, Hugh R.; Ireland '56; Paed; Staff, Soldier's Mem. Hosp., Campbellton, N.B.; Tel. 753-3897.
McGAVIN, Kenneth R.; 61 Colborne St. S., Simcoe, Ont.; 6 Summit Circle (res); Man '51; Chief of Paed., Norfolk Gen. Hosp.; Tel. 426-1037.
McGAVIN, Merritt F.; Ford Motor Co., Windsor, Ont.; 12602 Riverside Dr., Tecumseh (res); Tor '37; DPH(Tor); DAB(OccMed); Surg. Staff, Me-tropolitan Gen. Hosp.; Med. Dir., Ford Motor Co. of Canada Ltd.; Tel. 256-5555.
MCGEACHY, William G.; 600 Chinook Prof. Bldg., Chinook Centre, Calgary, Alta.; Sask'58; MCGP; Tel. AL 5-5566.
McGECHEN, John A.; Wainwright Clinic, 401-10th St., Wainwright, Alta.; Edinburgh (Scot.) '54; FRCS(Edin.); GenSurg.
MCGEE, Andrew R.; 261 Glenmanor Dr., Toronto, Ont. (res); Tor '26; F.A.C.R., D & T Rad; Chief of Rad. Dept., Toronto East Gen. Hosp.; Tel. HO 1-8272.
McGEE, Donald A.; Suite 2, 825 Coxwell Ave., Toronto 13, Ont.; Wes'57; FRCP(C), Neurol; Staff, Neur., Toronto East Gen. Hosp.; Research Assoc., Dept. of Path., Div. of Neuropath., U. of Toronto; Tel. 463-0830.
McGEE, G. Paul; 444 Beaconsfield Blvd., Beaconsfield, Ste.-Anne-de-Bellevue, P.Q.; McG '51; Paed; Tel. 453-8701.
McGEE, R. B.; 239 Broadway, Orangeville, Ont.; Tor '34; M.C.G.P.; Dist. Coroner.
McGEE, Robert J.; Tor'65; Res., St. Joseph's Hosp., Victoria, B.C.
McGEER, Patrick L.; 4727 W. 2nd Ave., Vancouver 8, B.C. (res); UBC '58; Ph.D.; Ass't. Dir. Kinsman Lab. & Neur. Research & Assoc. Prof. Med., U. of B.C.; MPP; Tel. CA 4-1111.
McGETTIGAN, James; National U. (Ireland)'59; Staff, Kelvington Union Hosp., Kelvington, Sask.
McGEOUGH, Vincent L.; 85 South St., Goderich, Ont.; 98 Britannia Rd. W. (res); Ott '55; Staff, Alexandra, Marine & Gen. Hosp.; Tel. JA 4-8441.
MCGHEE, John J.; Ste. 307, 1669 Victoria St., Prince George, B.C.; UBC'56; FRCS(C) GenSurg; FRCS (Ed.); FRCS (Eng.); Tel. 564-2634.
McGHIE, Ambrose G.; 250 Main St. E., Hamilton, Ont.; 17 Thorndale Ave. N. (res); Qns '16; MRCP (Edin.); FACP; FAIM; FRCP(C); IntMed; Tel. 527-2711.
McGIBBON, Dianne L. (Boyd); Tor '61; Res., Princess Margaret Hosp., Toronto, Ont.
McGIBBON, D. P.; Tor'63; Res., Hosp. for Sick Children, Toronto 2, Ont.
McGIBBON, Kenneth C.; 532 Med. Arts Bldg., 404 Graham Ave., Winnipeg 1, Man.; 25 Ruskin Row, Wpg. 9 (res); Tor '27; FICS; OrthSurg; Hon. Chief Cons., Shriners' Hosp., St. Boniface & Crippled Children's Hosp's; Tel. WH 2-2493.
McGILL, Alan F.; Ste. 603, Campbell Bldg., 1029 Douglas St., Victoria, B.C.; McG'36; GenSurg; Active Staff, St. Joseph's Hosp.; Court. Staff, Royal Jubilee Hosp.; Tel. EV 2-2811.
McGILL, Kenneth J.; 4900 Kingsway, South Burnaby, B.C.; 4373 Hurst Ave. (res); Loma Linda U. (Calif.) '51; ABOG; DNB; ObstGyn; Cons. ObstGyn., Burnaby Gen. Hosp.; Tel. 433-1281.
McGILL, William L. C.; 200 Brant Ave., Brantford, Ont.; 29 Westmount Blvd. (res); Tor '40; FACS, FRCS(C), GenSurg; Cons. Surg., Brantford Gen. & St. Joseph's Hosp's; Tel. 752-5000.
McGILL, Yuoell K.; 411-6th St., Saskatoon, Sask. (res); UBC '60.
McGILLIVRAY, Alexander M.; 526 Sydney St., Cornwall, Ont. (res); McG '21; DiagRad; Rad., Cornwall Gen. Hosp.; Cons. (Rad.), St. Lawrence San.
McGILLIVRAY, Donald C.; Tor'62; Res., Sunnybrook Hosp., Toronto 12, Ont.
McGILLIVRAY, D. Wray; 88 Wentworth St. S., Hamilton, Ont.; Wes '54; Ophth; Chief of Ophth., Joseph Brant Hosp.; Staff, St. Joseph's Hosp., Hamilton; Tel. 522-3563.
McGILLIVRAY, James; 402 Boyd Bldg., Winnipeg, Man.; 77 Niagara St. (res); Man '05; Ophth; Retired; Tel. HU 9-1083.
McGILLIVRAY, James W.; 144 Hurontario St., Collingwood, Ont.; 189 Minnesota St. (res); Tor '53; FRCS(C), GenSurg; Chief Surg., Collingwood Gen. & Marine Hosp's.; Cons. Surg., Meaford Gen. Hosp., Meaford.
McGILLIVRAY, John S., ED; 502 Med. & Dental Bldg., Regina, Sask.; London (Eng.) '39; MCGP; Staff, Regina Gen. & Ger. Centre; Grey Nuns' Hosp's.; Surg. Regina Prov. Correctional Inst.; STMO, DVA; Lt.-Col., RCAMC; Tel. LA 2-8541.
McGILLIVARY, Joseph I.; 302 Baldwin Ave., Cornwall, Ont., Dal '58; Anaes.
McGIRR, Robert E.; 106 Talbot St. W., Leamington, Ont.; Qns '54; MCGP; Chief of Paed., Leamington Dist. Mem. Hosp.; Tel. 326-3281.
McGIVERN, Bernadette P.; Ire. '50; P.G. Anaes., Winnipeg Gen. Hosp., Winnipeg 3, Man.
McGIVERN, Edward A.; 7575 Cambie St., Vancouver, B.C.; 5756 Angus Dr. (res); Nat. U. (Ire.) '44; FRCS(Dublin); MCGP; Vis. Staff, Vancouver Gen. Hosp.; Tel. FA 1-9161.
McGOEY, James S.; 306 Med. Arts Bldg., Winnipeg 1, Man.; 226 Handsart (res); Tor '43; DABS; DABTh.S; GenSurg; ThorSurg; Lect. **(Surg.), U. of Manitoba; Tel. WA 3-2918.**
McGOEY, Janet M. (Waugh; 1400 Sheppard Ave. E., Don Mills, Ont. (res); Glasgow (Scot.) '41.
McGOEY, John E.; Manitoba Clinic, 790 Sherbrook St., Winnipeg, Man.; Man '48; Otol; Lect. (Otol.), U. of Manitoba; Tel. SP 4-6541.
McGOEY, Paul F.; One Medical Place, 20 Wynford Dr., Don Mills, Ont.; Tor '40; FRCS(C); OrthSurg; Orth. Surg., Scarborough Gen. Hosp.; Chief Surg., Centennary Hosp.; Tel. 429-1502.
McGOVERN, John E.; 5300 Cote des Neiges Rd., Montreal 26, P.Q.; McG'38; GenSurg; Clin. Ass't., St. Mary's Hosp.; Cons. Phys., Labatt's Brewery Ltd.
McGOVERN, Murray G.; 275 Trafalgar Rd., Oakville, Ont.; **289 Dundas St. (res); Ott '53; Paed; Hd., Dept. of Paed., Oakville-Trafalgar Mem. Hosp.; Tel. VI 4-6046.**
McGOWAN, Angus; 204 Professional Bldg., 407 Graham Ave., Winnipeg 1, Man.; 85 Triton Bay, St. Vital, Wpg. 8 (res); Glasgow (Scot.) '53; M.B., Ch.B.; Tel. WH 2-2431.
McGOWAN, David G.; Glasgow (Scot.)'61; Staff, Cancer Clinic, University Hosp., Saskatoon, Sask.
McGOWAN, Donald A.; 38 Young St., Capreol, Ont.; Tor '51; M.O.H., Town of Capreol & Capreol Twp.; Dist. M.O., C.N.R.; Tel. 969-2233.
McGRAIL, J. Simon; 160 Wellesley St. E., Toronto, Ont.; Manchester (Eng.)'55; FRCS(C), Otol; Chief of E.N.T., Wellesley Hosp.; Assoc. E.N.T., U. of Toronto; Ass't. Prof. Anat., U. of Toronto; Tel. 966-6943.
McGRAND, Frederic A.; Fredericton Junction, N.B. (res); McG '23; **Dist. Coroner; Retired; Senator, Gov't. of Canada.**
McGRATH, Brian H.; Tor'64; Res., Sunnybrook Hosp., Toronto, Ont.

McGRATH, James M. F., Hon., M.P.P.; 119 Rennies Mill Rd., St. John's, Nfld. (res); National U. (Dublin, Ireland) '27; PH; Minister of Health, Newfoundland; Tel. 9-5011.

McGRATH, John J.; 95 Le Marchand Rd., Harbour Grace, Nfld.; Queen's U. (N. Ire.) '54; M.B., B.Ch., BAO, Anaes.

McGRATH, J. Percy; 20 Cornwallis St., Kentville, N.S.; 14 Canaan Ave. (res); Dal '17; Ophth,Otol; Staff, Blanchard-Fraser Memorial Hosp., Kentville; Eastern Kings Memorial Hosp., Wolfville; Cons., Nova Scotia San.

McGRATH, William P.; 1310 Ouellette Ave., Windsor, Ont.; Wes '48; D.A.B.O.; Ophth; Chief, Dept. of Ophth., Hotel-Dieu Hosp.; Tel. 254-8060.

McGRAW, Jean Y.; 3840 St-Urbain St., Montreal 18, P.Q.; 3011 Cedar Ave. (res); Lav '54; M.B., M.Sc., D.Sc., Ph.D., M.Chir; Gen-Surg (P.Q.); Surg. Staff, Hotel-Dieu Hosp.; Cons., St. Johns Hosp., St. Johns; Cons Surg., CFMS; Ass't Prof. (Surg.), U. of Montreal; Tel. VI 4-0161, Local 224.

McGRAW, Robert; UBC'60; FRCS(C), OrthSurg; Staff, Vancouver Gen. Hosp., Vancouver 9, B.C.

McGREAL, Douglas A.; 213 Med. Arts Bldg., **170 St. George St., Toronto 5, Ont.; 131 Glenrose Ave., Tor. 7. (res); St. Andrews (Scot.) '46; MRCP(Lond.); DCH(Eng.); Neur; Ass't. Neurol., Hosp. for Sick Children; Neurol., Crippled Childrens' Centre; Clin. Instr., U. of Toronto; Tel. 922-8229.**

McGREERY, Robin G.; 619 Medical Dental Bldg., Vancouver 1, B.C.

McGREGOR, Donald F.; 363 Markham Rd., Richmond Hill, Ont.; 18 Bridgeford St. (res); Wes '56; Staff, York Central Hosp.; Tel. TU 4-1008.

McGREGOR, Frank R.; 5441 Bannantyne Ave., Verdun, Montreal 19, P.Q.; 5923 Lasalle Blvd. (res); McG '31; Tel. 767-4242.

McGREGOR, Herbert B.; 125 Nanaimo Ave. W., Penticton, B.C.; McG '37; MCGP; Tel. 492-4066.

McGREGOR, James S.; Delaware, Ont.; Wes '35; Staff, Beck Mem. San., London.

McGREGOR, J. Kenneth; 35 Emerick St., Fort Erie, Ont.; McG '55.

McGREGOR, John A.; 1010 McCallum Bldg., 1830 Hamilton St., Regina, Sask.; Alb'52; Anaes.

McGREGOR, John C.; 13665-96th Ave., North Surrey, B.C.; 13032-104th Ave., Ste. 3 (res); UBC '56; MCGP; Tel. 581-2040.

McGREGOR, Keith M.; Wes '35; Psy; Ass't. Supt. Ontario Hosp., St. Thomas, Ont.; Tel. 631-8510.

McGREGOR, Maurice; 687 Pine Ave. W., Montreal, P.Q.; 7430 rue Bayard, Mtl. 16 (res); Witwatersrand (Jo'burg, S. Africa) '42; MRCP (Lond.); FRCP(C); IntMed (Cardiol)(P.Q.); Assoc. Phys., Royal Victoria Hosp.; Prof. (Experim. Med.), McGill U.; Tel. VI 2-1251, Loc. 738.

McGREGOR, Norval R.; 1548 Lonsdale Ave., North Vancouver, B.C.; Wes'50; Tel. 985-5381.

McGRUTHER, William J. B.; Creighton Mine, Ont.; Tor '41; AMCGP; Tel. 692-3517.

McGUGAN, Angus C.; 8324-111th St., Edmonton, Alta.; Alb '29; D.P.H.; F.A.C.H.A.; Supt. University of Alberta Hosp., Edmonton; Tel. GE 9-7057.

McGUGAN, R. Gibb; 191 Highland Rd., London, Ont.; Wes '39; Admin., Victoria Hosp. Retired.

McGUIGAN, John P.; 151 Front St. W., Toronto 1, Ont.; 130 Glenrose Ave., Tor 7 (res); Alb '39; DABPrevMed (OccMed); Reg. M.O., CNRlwys & Air Canada; Tel. 365-3328.

McGUINESS, Frederick G.; 18 Roslyn Cres., Winnipeg, Man. (res); Man '17; F.A.C.S., F.R.C.O.G., F.R.C.S.(C), ObstGyn; Emer. Prof. (ObstGyn), U. of Manitoba; Hon. Cons. (ObstGyn), Wpg. Gen Hosp.; Retired; Tel. VE 2-5977.

McGUIRE, Clyde T.; 175 Church St., St. Catharines, Ont.; Lakeshore Rd., R.R. No. 3 (res); Tor '26; Tel. 682-5511.

McGUIRE, Gerald F.; 275 Trafalgar Rd., Oakville, Ont.; '52; Tel. VI 5-5661.

McGUIRE, J. Hugh; 37 Dundas St. W., Cooksville, Ont.; Qns '63.

McGUIRE, John A.; 215 Sydney St., Cornwall, Ont.; McG '25; Chief of Surg., Cornwall Gen. Hosp.

McGUIRE, John J.; 42 William St. E., Smiths Falls, Ont.; Qns '33; Tel. 283-3060.

McGUIRE, John J.; Qns'65; Res., St. Michael's Hosp., Toronto 2, Ont.

McGUIRE, M. G.; 12 Victoria Ave., Brockville, Ont.; Qns '37.

McGUIRE, W. Bruce; 132 Norfolk St. S., Simcoe, Ont.; 7 Summit Circle (res); Tor '48; Tel. 426-4462.

McHAFFIE, David S.; Quarantine Service, 816 Government St., Victoria, B.C.; 1725 Beach Dr. (res); Wes '29; M.C.G.P.; Retired.

McHARG, Robert G.; 154 Wilson St. Ancaster, **Ont.; Wes '48; Med. Staff, St. Joseph's Hosp., Hamilton; Tel. MI 8-3052.**

McHUGH, Brian; Box 42, Moosomin, Sask.; Dublin (Ire.) '49.

McHUGH, Hollie E.; St. 475, 2055 Peel St., Montreal 2, P.Q.; 564 Kenaston Ave., Twn. of Mt. Royal (res); McG '36; D.L.O. (R.C.P. & S. Lond.); A.B.O.; Otol; Otol-in Chief, Royal Victoria Hosp.; Cons. Civil Aviation Med., Dept of National Health & Welfare; Lect. (Otol.) Northwestern U., Chicago.; Prof & Chmn., Dept. of Otol, & Dir. Otol. Inst., McGill U.; Tel. 844-7653.

McHUGH, John J.; 275 Trafalgar Rd., Oakville, **Ont.; 323 Division St. (res); Ott '53; IntMed; Hd., Dept. of Med., Oakville-Trafalgar Mem. Hosp.; Tel. VI 4-9320.**

McILQUHAM, Morven C.; McG '62; Staff, Neurological Inst., Montreal 2, P.Q.

McILRAITH, John B.; 1631 Islington Ave. N., Rexdale, Ont.; Tor '51; Tel. 741-0410.

McILROY, William J.; Ste. 401, 25 Leonard Ave., Toronto 2B, Ont.; 3 St. Andrews Gdns., Tor 5 (res); Tor '56; FRCP(C); Neurol; Neurol. Staff, Toronto Western Hosp.; Cons. Neurol. Sunnybrook & Queensway Hosp's.; Clin. Teach. (Med.), U. of Toronto; Tel. EM 6-2483.

McILVEEN, Charles E.; 152 Simcoe St. N., Oshawa, Ont.; 21 Aberdeen (res); Qns '46; Staff, Oshawa Gen. Hosp.

McILVEEN, Gilbert Norman; Professional Bldg., 228 Harwood Ave. S., Ajax, Ont.; 45 Forest Rd. (res); Qns'50; Chief Surgery Ajax & Pickering Gen. Hosp's.; Tel. 942-0201.

McILVEEN, Jean E.; Apt. 304, 850 Cook St., Victoria, B.C.; Qns '60; Retired.

McILWRAITH. William; Scott St. Plaza, St. Catharines, Ont.; Glasgow (Scot.)'48; Tel. 684-8061.

McINERNEY, Arthur J.; 651 Loyalist Ct., Fredericton, N.B. (res); McG '45; MPA (Cornell); Cons. Hosp. Admin., N.B., Dept. of Health; Tel. 475-7711, Loc. 348.

McINERNEY, John F. MPP; Fredericton Med. Clinic, 206 Rookwood Ave., Fredericton, N.B.; 101 Alexandra St. (res); McG '39; Anaes; M.O.H., & Soc. Serv.. Gov't. of N.B., 680 King St.; Tel. 475-7701.

McINERNEY, James P.; 36 Mecklenberg St., St. John, N.B.; 29 Douglas Ave. (res); McG '29; GenSurg.

McINNES, John D.; 70 Cedar St., Sudbury, Ont.; 262 McNaughton St. (res); Wes '40; F.I.C.S., F.R.C.S.(C), GenSurg; Active Surg. Staff, Sudbury Gen. & Sudbury Mem. Hosp.; Cons. Sudbury & Algoma San.; Tel. OS 5-8386.

McINNES, Malcolm F.; 790 Sherbrook St., Winnipeg 2, Man.; 282 Kingsway Wpg. 9 (res); Man '51; FRCP(C), IntMed; Active Staff, Winnipeg **Gen. & Children's Hosp's; Tel. SP 4-6541.**

McINNIS, A. Campbell; 523 Med. Arts Bldg., Winnipeg 1, Man. 466 Montrose St. Wpg. 9 (res); Man '49; M.R.C.O.G.(Lond.), F.R.C.S.(C), ObstGyn; Staff (ObstGyn), Wpg. Gen., St. Boniface & Misericordia Hosp's.; Lect. (ObstGyn), U. of Manitoba; Tel. WH 3-5416.

McINNIS, David B.; 420 Lock St. W., Dunnville, Ont.; 105 Lock St. (res); Wes'54; MCGP; Tel. **774-7541.**

McINNIS, Elmore L.; 420 Lock St. W., Dunnville, Ont.; 629 Lock St. (res); Wes '21; M.C.G.P.; Coroner, Co. of Haldimand; M.O.H., Dunnville; **Surg., CNR & TH & B. Rlwy.; Tel. 774-7541.**

McINNIS, Frank P.; 280 Bloor St. W., Ste. 106, Toronto 5, Ont.; Tor '36; FACOG; ObstGyn; Staff, St. Michael's & Grace Hosp's.; Court. Staff, Toronto Gen. & Wellesley Hosp's; Pres. Society of ObstGyn. of Canada; Tel. WA 2-6566.
McINNIS, Thomas J.; 44 Church St., St. Mary's, Ont.; Tor '23; M.O.H. Blanchard Twp.; Coroner, Perth County; Tel. 284-1170.
McINNIS, William P.; 367 Princess Ave., London, Ont.; 25 Doncaster Ave. (res); Wes '52; Neurol., Victoria Gen. & St. Joseph's Hosp's.; Cons. (Neurol.), Westminster DVA & RCAF; Electro-enceph. Ont. Hosp., St. Thomas; Sr. Fell. (Neurol.), U. of Western Ont.; Tel. GE 2-5511.
McINTOSH, Alan D.; 1635 Abbott St., Kelowna, B.C.; 859 Saucier Ave. (res); Tor '53; MCGP; Tel. 762-2740.
McINTOSH, Anna M. H.; 469 Roselawn Ave., Toronto 12, Ont. (res); Tor '32; Public Health (part-time).
McINTOSH, Clarence A.; 900 Sherbrooke St. W., Montreal 2, P.Q.; McG '24; FRCS(C); GenSurg; ThorSurg (P.Q.); Tel. 845-7726.
McINTOSH, Gavin J.; Box 730, Med. Centre, Barrhead, Alta.; Oxford (Eng.) '62; Tel. 674-2246.
McINTOSH, Hamish W.; Van. Gen. Hosp., Vancouver, B.C.; 1402 Ottawa, W. Van. (res); McG '43; M.Sc., D.I.M.(McG); F.R.C.P.(C), IntMed; Dir. of Research, Shaughnessy Hosp.; Ass't. Med., Van. Gen. Hosp.; Assoc. Prof. (Med.), U. of British Columbia; Tel. TR 6-3211.
McINTOSH, Harold A.; Humphreys Clinic, 201 Med. Bldg., Prince Albert, Sask.; 563-25th W. (res); Man '46; M.Sc. (IntMed.); FCCP; IntMed; Chief (Med.), Victoria Union Hosp.; Tel. 763-2681.
McINTOSH, H. David; Man '58; Psy; Staff, Burnaby Mental Health Centre, 4400 W. Grandview-Douglas Hwy., Burnaby 9, B.C.; Tel. 434-4247.
McINTOSH, James D.; 36 Peel St., Simcoe, Ont.; 301 South Dr. (res); Wes '61; Staff, Norfolk Gen. Hosp.; Tel. 426-2290.
McINTOSH, John D.; 302 S. Syndicate Ave., Fort William, Ont.; Tor'36; Vice Pres., Med. Staff, Mackellar Gen. Hosp.; Assoc. Staff, St. Joseph's & Gen. Hosp's.; Port Arthur; Tel. MA 2-4733.
McINTOSH, Keith M.; 36 Peel St., Simcoe, Ont.; 39 Gibson Dr. (res); Tor '33; Phys., Home for the Aged; Gaol Surg., Co. of Norfolk; Post Chairman & Memb. of Med. Staff, Norfolk Gen. Hosp.; Dist. Coroner; Tel. 426-2290.
McINTOSH, Mary G. (Goldstraw); Medical Centre Box 730, Barrhead, Alta.; London (Eng.) '63; M.B., B.S.
McINTOSH, Ronald W.; Ste. 603, 237 Cassandra Blvd., Don Mills, Ont.; Tor'61; FRCP(C), Anaes.
McINTOSH, William C.; 139 Gloucester St., Ottawa, Ont.; 6 Lakeview Terr. (res); Qns '36; Staff, Ottawa Civic & Grace Hosp's.; Tel. CE 2-2580.
McINTYRE, Archibald J.; 302 Oxford St., Apt. 2, London, Ont. (res); Qns '19; Retired.
McINTYRE, D. Ian; 672 Brant St., Burlington, Ont.; Qns '56; FRCS(C), OrthSurg; Surg. Staff, Toronto Gen. Hosp., Toronto; Tel. 637-5227.
McINTYRE, Donald F.; 332 Medical Arts Bldg., Winnipeg, Man.; 258 Dromore Ave. (res); Man '09; F.A.C.S.; Tel. WH 2-2519.
McINTYRE, Donald H.; 123 Welland Ave., Toronto 7, Ont. (res); Alb '41; D.A.B.A., D.A. (McGill); Anaes; Staff, Lockwood Clinic & Grace Hosp's.
McINTYRE, Donald N. C.; 332 Med. Arts Bldg., Winnipeg, Man.; 4321 Roblin Blvd., Charleswood (res); Man '38; MCGP; Tel. WH 2-2159.
McINTYRE, Dougald; 112 Bartlett Ave., Winnipeg, Man. (res); Man '11; Med. Ref., Manitoba Hosp. Service Assoc.; Retired.
McINTYRE, Grant J.; 366 McIntyre W., North Bay, Ont.; Wes '52; Tel. 474-2840.
McINTYRE, Helen I. D. (Doan); Harrietsville, Ont.; Wes '33; M.C.G.P.
McINTYRE, Hugh M.; Man '52; DiagRad; Staff, McKellar Gen. Hosp., Fort William, Ont.; Tel. 623-6471.
McINTYRE, Hugh R.; 108 Scott Blk., Moose Jaw, Sask.; 1159 Redland Ave. (res); Alb '39; GenSurg; Chief, Med. Staff, Moose Jaw Union Hosp.; Tel. 692-1827.
McINTYRE, J. Alexander; 183 St. Clair Ave. W., Toronto 7, Ont.; 61 Highland Ave. Tor. 5 (res); Tor '46; F.A.C.S., F.R.C.S.(C), GenSurg; Chief of Surg., St. Joseph's Hosp.; Cons. Surg., South Peel Hosp.; Tel. WA 2-1466.
McINTYRE, James L.; St. Andrew's (Scot.)'57; DMR; FRCP(C), DiagRad; Staff, Rad., St. Michael's Hosp., Toronto 2, Ont.
McINTYRE, John A.; 450 Central Ave., London, Ont. 147 Highland Rd. (res); Qns '38; F.C.C.P.; DiagRad; Staff, Beck Mem. Hosp.
McINTYRE, John A.; 94 Dominion St., Uxbridge, Ont.; Tor '51; FRCS(C), GenSurg; Surg. Cons., Cottage Hosp.; Tel. UL 2-3822.
McINTYRE, John W. R.; 11110-86th Ave., Edmonton, Alta. (res); **London (Eng.) '48; M.R.-C.P.(Eng.), L.R.C.P.(Lond.), D.A., F.F.A.R.C.S (Eng.); Anaes; Staff, University Hosp.; Ass't. Prof (Anaes.) U. of Alberta; Tel. GE 3-1444.**
McINTYRE, J. Murray; Room 536, 2300 Tupper St., Montreal 25, P.Q.; McG '37; FRCS(C), OrthSurg; Dir. (Orth.), Montreal Children's Hosp.; Cons. (Orth.), Queen Mary Vet's. & Alexandra Hosp's.; Ass't. Surg., Reddy Mem. Hosp.; Assoc. Surg., St. Mary's Hosp.; Dem. (Orth.), McGill U.; Tel. 937-8511.
McINTYRE, Marjorie; 202 Med. Arts Bldg., 170 St. George St., Toronto 5, Ont.; 46 Wells Hill Ave. (res); Man '29; Hon. Staff, Women's College Hosp.; Tel. 922-7136.
McINTYRE, Norman R.; 2 Maple Ave. N., Burford, Ont.; 86 Brant Ave. (res); Tor '46; Tel. 449-2421.
McINTYRE, Preston; Montague, P.E.I.; McG '21; GenSurg; Chief, Med. Staff, King's Co. Mem. Hosp.; Tel. 838-2471.
McINTYRE, Richard W.; 102 Medical Arts Bldg., 750 Spadina Cres. E., Saskatoon, Sask.; Alb '55.
McINTYRE, Robert W.; 104 Johnson St., Ste. 3, Kingston, Ont.; 204 Churchill Cres. (res); Qns '42; MCGP; Tel. 542-9363.
McINTYRE, Ruaraidh W.; Aberdeen (Scot.)'57; Res., Dept. of Anaes., Sunnybrook Hosp., Toronto, Ont.; DRCOG; D.A.
McINTYRE, William J.; Box 1930, Holley Clinic, Quesnel, B.C.; UBC '63.
McISAAC, Elmer R.; 224 Queen St., Streetsville, Ont.; Dal '57; Tel. TA 6-1761.
McIVER, John R.; 1243 Amesbrook Dr., Ottawa 3, Ont.; Glasgow (Scot.) '52; M.B., Ch.B.; DiagRad; Staff, Ottawa Civic Hosp.; Tel. 729-2511, Loc. 525.
McJANNETT, William A.; Wes'53; Anaes; Staff, Hosp. for Sick Children, Toronto 2, Ont.
McKAY, Alexander L.; 465 Bay St., Toronto, Ont.; 111 Lawton Blvd. (res); Tor '20; D.P.H.; PH; Director, Community Health Serv., City of Toronto; Retired.
McKAY, A. Robert; 1428 Ouellette Ave., Windsor, Ont.; Wes'59; GenSurg.
McKAY, Berta E.; 1428 Ouellette Ave., Windsor, Ont.; Wes'59.
McKAY, David E.; 147 McLeod St., Ottawa 4, Ont.; Qns'59; FRCS(C), Urol.
McKAY, Donald H.; 27 Third St., Collingwood, Ont.; 242 Third St. (res); Tor '37; GenSurg; Staff, Gen. & Marine Hosp.; Tel. 445-4111.
McKAY, Frances L. (Mulligan); 242-3rd St., Collingwood, Ont. (res); Tor'37.; Tel. 445-4111.
McKAY, Joseph B.; Laboratory, Dept. of PH of Ont., 360 Christie St., Toronto 4, Ont.; Wes'34; PathBact; Sr. Med. Spec. (Prov.Pathol.), Sect. on Pathol. Lab., Dept. of Health, Ontario; Tel. LE 4-3511.
McKAY, Joseph W.; 1700 McGregor St., Montreal, P.Q. (res); Dal '18; F.R.C.P.(C) D & TRad; Dir., Dept. of Rad., Montreal Gen. Hosp.; Assoc. Prof., McGill U.; Tel. WE 7-6011.
McKAY, Malcolm H.; 44 Third St., Chatham, Ont.; 312 Wellington St. W. (res); Tor '54; MCGP.

McKAY, Wilson G.; 340 Simcoe St. N., Oshawa, Ont.; 845 King St. E. (res); Tor '34; ObstGyn; ObstGyn. Staff, Oshawa Gen. Hosp.; Chmn., Bd. of Health, Oshawa; Tel. 728-8443.

McKAY, W. W.; R.R. No. 1, Aylmer, Ont. (res); Qns '16; Staff, Dept. Nat'l. Health & Welfare, **Jackson Bldg., Ottawa, Ont.;** Special Court. **Lect., Prev. Med. on Alcoholism, Ottawa U.; Tel. 455-2328.**

McKAY, Yves; Mon'55; Path. (P.Q.); Staff, Hop. Hotel-Dieu, Montreal, P.Q.; Tel. VI 4-0161.

McKEAN, H. R.; 600 Prince, Truro, N.S.; 127 Park (res); Dal '34; Staff, Dept EENT, Colchester Co. Hosp.; Tel. 893-8081.

McKEAN, J. Douglas; 3915 E. Hastings St., North Burnaby, B.C.; Glasgow (Scot.)'56; Tel. CY 8-7252.

McKECHNIE, Robert E.; Ste. 302, 1030 W. Georgia St., Vancouver, B.C.; McG'31; MS (Surg); FACS; FICS; GenSurg; Sr. Surg., Vancouver Gen. Hosp.; Hon. Cons. Surg., St. Paul's Hosp. & B.C. Cancer Inst.; Instr. Surg., U. of British Columbia; Woodward Lect., Dept. History of Med.; Med. Dir., Seabord Life Insur. Co. & Mr. & Mrs. P. A. Woodward Fdn.; Tel. MU 3-8494.

McKEE, Beverley W.; AMCGP; Res., Montreal Gen. Hosp., Montreal 25, P.Q.

McKEE, David C.; 366 Vaughan Rd., Toronto 10, Ont.; Tor'64; Staff, Northwestern Gen. Hosp.; Tel. 651-0211.

McKEE, **Elisabeth F.;** 132 Woodbridge Cr., Ottawa 14, Ont.; Tor'51; Abroad.

McKEE, Geo. H.; 3967 Kingsway, S. Burnaby, B.C.; 4209 Maywood St. (res); Man '42; Tel. HE 4-8781.

McKEE, James A.; Ottawa Civic Hosp., Ottawa, Ont.; Tor '51; FRCP(C), Paed; Paed-in-Chief, Ottawa Civic Hosp.; Assoc. Prof. (Paed.), U. of Ottawa; Tel. 729-2511.

McKEE, M. Elizabeth; 206 Med. Arts Bldg., 170 St. George St., Toronto 5, Ont.; Tor '54; FRCS-(C), Otol; Staff, St. Michael's & Women's College Hosp's.; Clin. Instr., U. of Toronto; Tel. 923-9665.

MCKEE, Thomas D.; Tor'54; Res. (Otol.), U. of Toronto, Toronto 5, Ont.

McKEE, William N.; Quarantine Immigration Burrard Bldg., Vancouver, B.C.; Qns '34.

McKEEN, Albro D.; Dal '59; Res., Victoria Gen. Hosp., Halifax, N.S.

McKEEN, James L.; 242 Victoria St., Kamloops, B.C.; 171 Connaught Rd. (res); Alb'51; Tel. 372-3303.

McKEEVER, Robert W.; Dublin (Ire.)'54; Anaes; Staff, St. John's Gen. Hosp., St. John's, Nfld.

McKELLAR, James C.; 301 Toronto Western Med. Bldg., 25 Leonard Ave., Toronto 2B, Ont.; 7 Ansley St. (res); **Tor '35; F.R.C.S.(C), ObstGyn; Tel. EM 4-7914.**

McKELLAR, John M.; 202 Professional Centre, 1705-3rd Ave., **Prince George, B.C.; 690** Ewert St. (res); Man'53; Tel. 564-7612.

McKELVEY, Alexander D.; 628 Medical Arts **Bldg., 170 St. George St., Toronto 5, Ont.; 109 Douglas Dr. (res); Tor '43; FRCP(C), IntMed.; Phys., Toronto Gen. Hosp.; Assoc. (Med.), U. of Toronto; Tel. WA 3-3175.**

MCKENDRICK, Alistair J.; Glasgow (Scot.)'42; DPH; DMRD (Ed.); Staff, Highland View Hosp., Amherst, N.S.

McKENDRICK, William H.; Box 449, High Prairie Med Clinic, High Prairie, Alta: London (Eng.) '51; Active Staff, Providence Hosp.; Tel. 2-3354.

McKENDRY, **James B. J.; 3 Jackson Ave., Toronto, Ont.; Tor '46; F.A.A.P.; Paed; Clin. Ass't., Hosp. for Sick Children & Staff (Paed), U. of Toronto; Tel. EM 6-7242.**

McKENDRY, J.B. Ralph; 267 O'Connor St., Ottawa, Ont.; 50 Lynwood Ave. (res); Qns '43; M.Sc., FACP; FRCP(C), IntMed; Chief, Metabol. Serv., Ottawa Civic Hosp.; Tel. CE 2-6355.

McKENNA, A. Carmel; T.B. Div. Dept. of Health, 875 Bay St., Toronto 5, Ont.; Dublin (Ire.) '40; DPH; FCCP; Tel. 365-2302.

McKENNA, Brian; 121 Med. Arts Bldg., 750 Spadina Cr. E., Saskatoon, Sask.; National U. (Ire.)'52; FRCS(C), OrthSurg.

McKENNA, Frank E.; Windsor Med. Serv. Inc., 1427 Ouellette Ave., Windsor, Ont.; Tor'44; MPH; Med. Dir., Windsor Med. Serv. Inc.; Tel. 256-7861.

McKENNA, Joseph P.; Alb. '63; Res., St. Michael's Hosp., Toronto 2, Ont.

McKENNA, Leo B.; 1226 West 49th Ave., Vancouver 13, B.C. (res); McG '27; Pension Med. Examiner, Can. Pension Comm. Retired.

McKENNA, **Peter B.;** Lower Floor, Med. Arts Bldg., Calgary, Alta.; Ireland'53; LRCP&S(I); DiagRad.

McKENNA, Reginald L.; 105 Alma St., Moncton, N.B.; Dal '42; Tel. 389-9348.

McKENNA, Richard D.; 1390 Sherbrooke St. W., Montreal 25, P.Q.; 19 Grenville Ave., Westmount (res); McG '38; D.A.B.I.M., F.A.C.P., Gastroent. (P.Q.) F.R.C.P.(C), IntMed; Chief Gastroent. Assoc. Phys., Royal Victoria Hosp.; Cons. (Med.) **Queen Mary Vet's Hosp.; Ass't Prof. (Med. & Clin. Med.), McGill U.; Tel. VI 2-7391.**

McKENTY, John Stewart; 604 Med. Arts Bldg., 404 Graham Ave., Winnipeg 1, Man.; 74 Westgate (res); Man'38; DO (Oxon.); DOMS (Lond.); Ophth; Active Staff, St. Boniface Hosp.; Dem. **(Ophth.), U. of Manitoba; Tel. WH 3-1688.**

McKENTY, Mary R.; 301 Med. Arts Bldg., 404-406 Graham Ave., Winnipeg Man.; Man '41; Pt.-time Staff, Children's Hosp.; Tel. GR 5-6463.

McKENTY, Vincent J.; 385 Montrose St., Winnipeg, Man. (res); Man '32; Sr. Med. Exam., Cndn. Pension Comm., Winnipeg; Tel. TU 8-4861.

McKENZIE, Alan F.; Orono, Ont.; Tor '36; Tel 186.

McKENZIE, **Allan D.;** Ste 1200, 750 W. Broadway, Vancouver 9, B.C.; Alb '42; DABS; FRCS-(C), GenSurg; Prof. & Hd., Dept. of Surg., U. of British Columbia; Sr. Surg., Vancouver Gen. Hosp.; Cons. Surg. Shaughnessy Hosp.; Tel. 876-5828.

McKENZIE, Alvin H.; 222 Medical Arts Bldg., 11010 Jasper Ave., Edmonton, Alta.; Alb '52; M.Ch.Orth.; FRCS(C); OrthSurg; Staff, Royal Alexandra Hosp.; Clin. Instr. (OrthSurg.), U. of Alberta; Tel. 482-3666.

McKENZIE, Andrew W.; 42 Albert St., Stratford, Ont.; Cambridge (Eng.) '61; MB; B.Chir.; MRCS; LRCP; D.O.; Tel. 271-5600.

McKENZIE, Frederick A.; 635 Santa Monica Rd., London, Ont.; Wes '56; Psy; Staff, Children's Psy. Research Inst.

McKENZIE, George J.; 50 Med. Arts Bldg., 1105 Pandora Ave., Victoria, B.C.; McG '45; Paed; Active Med. Staff (Paed), Royal Jubilee Hosp.; Tel. EV 2-3612.

McKENZIE, Hector; 4-3885 Cambie St., Vancouver, B.C.; Qns '15; Retired.

McKENZIE, Herbert F.; Medical Arts Clinic, 51—6th St. E., Medicine Hat, Alta.; Man '40; TherRad; MCGP; Staff, Medicine Hat Mun. Hosp.; Cons. Cancer Clinic; Tel. 527-2281.

McKENZIE, **J. Maxwell;** 567 Walpole Ave., **Town of Mount Royal, Montreal 16, P.Q.; St. Andrews (Scot.) '58; IntMed; MRCP (Eng.); Clin. Ass't., Royal Victoria Hosp.; Ass't. Prof. (Med.), McGill U.; Tel. VI 2-1251, Loc. 729.**

McKENZIE, John G.; Ste. 211, 1320-5th Ave., Prince George, B.C.; Man'45; MCGP; Tel. 564-8018.

McKENZIE, Kenneth D.; 2333 Portage Ave., Winnipeg 12, Man.; 2507 Assiniboine Cr. (res); Man '55; MCGP; Hon. Sectary Man. Med. Assoc.; Tel. VE 7-1327.

McKENZIE, Lloyd A.; Bay Medical Group, Glace Bay, N.S.; 19 Park St. (res); Dal '55.

McKENZIE, Lloyd D.; Archibald Ave., North Sydney, N.S.; Prince St. (res); Dal '55.

McKENZIE, **Lloyd E.;** 2045 Dufferin St., Toronto 10, Ont.; Tor'65; Tel. 651-1210.

McKENZIE, Robert B.; Newcastle Med. Clinic, 246 Delano Ave., Newcastle, N.B.; 165 King George H'way (res); McG '40; MCGP; Staff, Miramichi Hosp., Newcastle & Hotel Dieu Hosp., Chatham; Tel. 622-3344.

McKENZIE, Roderick E.; Okotoks, Alta.; Aberdeen (Scot.) '38. Retired.

McKENZIE, Sheila M.; Alb '53; Res., Royal Alexandra Hosp., Edmonton, Alta. Retired.

McKENZIE, Thomas R.; 1428 Ouellette Ave., Windsor, Ont.; 1542 Bruce (res); Wes '54; Ophth; Active Staff, Grace, Hotel-Dieu & Metropolitan Gen. Hosp's.; Cons., Riverview Hosp.; Instr. (Ophth.), Wayne State Med. Schl. & Lect'r. (Histol & Ophth Path), Kresge Eye Inst., Detroit, U.S.A.; Tel. 256-3251.

McKENZIE, W. G.; Esterhazy, Sask.; Man '21; Dist. Coroner.

McKEOUGH, Liam L.; Commercial St., North Sydney, N.S.; 54 King St. (res); Dal '49; GenSurg; Sr. Surg. Staff, St. Elizabeth Hosp. & Harbour View Hosp., Sydney Mines; Tel. 794-2753.

McKEOUGH, Thomas J.; Main St., Sydney Mines, N.S.; Shore Rd. (res); Ott '51; Staff, Harbour View Hosp., Sydney Mines & St. Elizabeth Hosp's. North Sydney; M.P.P. (N.S.).

McKEOWN, John; 221 Adolphus St., Cornwall, **Ont.; 219 Adolphus St. (res); Tor '38; GenSurg; Tel. WE 2-3722.**

McKEOWN, Robert A.; Ste. 565, 5025 Sherbrooke St. W., Montreal 28, P.Q.; 3581 Marlowe Ave., **Mtl. 28 (res); Queen's (Belfast, N. Ire.) '53; FACOG; MAH; ObstGyn; Att'd. Staff, St. Mary's, Queen Elizabeth & Catherine Booth Maternity Hosp's.; Tel. RE 1-1944.**

McKEOWN, Thomas J.; 1077 Queen Elizabeth Way, Cooksville, Ont.; Tor '61;

McKEOWN, William; McG'43; Staff, c/o Regional Dir., European Reg., Dept. of National Health & Welfare, 38 Grosvenor St., London W.1, England; Abroad.

McKERCHER, Alexander E.; 255 Briscoe St., London, Ont. (res); Qns '30; Psy; Psy., Westminster Hosp., DVA, London; Tel. 432-6711.

McKERCHER, D. Douglas; 501 Med. Arts Bldg., 180 Metcalfe St., Ottawa 4, Ont.; Qns '43; Otol; Chief Otol., Ottawa Civic Hosp.; Tel. 233-8034.

McKERCHER, Lawrence A.; 31 Academy Medical Bldg., 1812-4th St. W., Calgary, Alta.; 8203-5th St. S.W. (res); Tor '52; MCGP; Tel. 263-8219.

McKERRACHER, Donald G.; 103 Poplar Cres., Saskatoon, Sask. (res); Tor'35; FRCP(C); Psy; Prof. of Psy. & Chairman, Dept. of Psy., U. of Saskatchewan; Chief (Psy.), University Hosp.; Tel. CH 2-7671.

McKERRACHER, Finlay; Carling Ave., Ottawa 3, Ont.; 5 Lipstan Ave., Ott. 5 (res); St. Andrew's (Scot.) '46; MACHA; Ass't. Dir. (Serv.), Ottawa Civic Hosp.; Tel. 729-2511.

McKERRELL, D. Manus; Swift Current Clinic, 129 Central Ave. N., Swift Current, Sask.; St. Andrew's (Scot.)'52; Staff, Swift Current Union Hosp.; Tel. 773-4681.

McKERRICHER, Donald E.; 211 Bastion St., Nanaimo, B.C.; McG'50; DABOph; Ophth; Staff, Nanaimo Reg. Gen. Hosp.; Tel. 753-2031.

McKIBBIN, Gilles T.; 55 Ave. de l'Eglise, Verdun,, Montreal 19, P.Q.; Mon '51; GenSurg (P.Q.); Tel. 766-4897.

McKIBBIN, John; Box 551, Lacombe, Alta.; Coll. of Med. Evangelists (U.S.A.) '28; M.C.G.P.; Dist. Coroner; Tel. 782-6101.

McKIBBON, Walton A.; Wingham, Ont.; Wes '35; MCGP; Tel. 357-1911.

McKIE, Joseph G.; **Morrison Rd., Oakville, Ont.; Wes '13; Tel. VI 5-1388.**

McKIERNAN-LAVOIE, Clarice M.; Dublin (Ire.) '52; BAO; Anaes; Staff Anaes., Hop. Maisonneuve, Montreal 36, P.Q.; Tel. 254-8341.

McKIGGAN, John J.; Ste. 302, 5880 Spring Garden Rd., Halifax, N.S.; Dal'60; FRCP(C), IntMed.

McKILLIGIN, Helen R.; 222 LeMarchant Rd., St. John's, Nfld.; Aberdeen (Scot.) '58; Paed.; Tel. 579-8149.

McKILLIP, T. H.; Nakina, Ont.; Tor '13.

McKILLOP, Angus N.; 3050 Lakeshore Blvd. W., Toronto 14, Ont.; 1549 Lochlin Trail, Pt. Credit (res); Wes '26; FACPrevMed; GenSurg; Vol. Ass't. OPD, (Surg.), Tor. Gen. Hosp.; Med. Dir., Goodyear Tire & Rubber Co. of Canada Ltd.; Tel. CL 1-4111.

McKIM, Anson; 6412 Bay St., West Vancouver, B.C.; 136-27th St. (res); McG '44; IntMed; Staff Phys. (Part-Time), Pearson TB Hosp.; Telephone **921-7120.**

McKIM, J. C.; Lucknow, Ont.; Wes '58; MCGP; Tel. 528-2907.

McKIM, John S.; Psy. Research Inst., Sanatarium Rd., London, Ont.; Wes'46; DCH; Paed; Phys., Children's Psy. Research Inst.; Research Instr. (Paed.), U. of Western Ont.; Tel. 438-1111.

McKIM, Laurie H., ED; 1002 McGregor Ave., **Apt. 203, Montreal 2, P.Q.; McG '12; FACS;** FRCS(C), GenSurg; Tel. VI 9-1092.

McKIM, Mary E.; Tor'49; Res., St. Joseph's Hosp., London, Ont.

McKINLAY, **William D.;** 730 Birks Bldg., Vancouver, B.C.; 4075 W. 15th (res); McG '48; Ophth; Vis. Staff, Van. Gen.; Clin. Instr. (Ophth), **U. of British Columbia; Tel. MU 4-4949.**

McKINLEY, A. Colin; Wabush Mines, Wabush Lake, Lab.; Qns '58. Abroad.

McKINLEY, Helen I.; 715 Danforth Ave. & 244 **Bloor St. W., Toronto; 107 Hudson Dr. (res); Tor '33; Paed; Staff Women's College & Hosp. for Sick Children; Tel. HO 1-3006.**

McKINLEY, John N.; 94 Inglewood Dr., Toronto, Ont.; Qns '08; Retired.

McKINLEY, William H.; Richmond Shopping Centre, 3224-28th St. S.W., Calgary, Alta.; **Queen's U. (Belfast, N. Ire) '55; Tel. 242-3330.**

McKINNA, Alfred J.; 814 Med. Arts Bldg., 1538 Sherbrooke St. W., Montreal 25, P.Q.; 770 Haude Blvd., St. Lambert (res); McG '52; DABOphth; Ophth; Att'd. Staff, & Ass't. Glaucoma Clinic, Mtl. Gen. & Dir. Dept. of Ophth., Mtl. Children's Hosp's.; Dem., McGill U.; Tel. WE 5-0866.

McKINNA, Colin; St. James Med. Group., 633 Lodge Ave., Winnipeg 12, Man.; London (Eng.) '51; MCGP; Tel. 832-1644.

McKINNEY, J. H.; Brooklin, Ont.; Tor '30; MCGP.

McKINNEY, John A.; 224 Centre St., Napanee, Ont.; Qns'63.

McKINNON, Carl R.; 657 W. 37th Ave., Vancouver 13, B.C.; Man '39; PhysMed & Rehab; Ass't. Med. Dir., Rehab. Centre, WCB (BC); Tel. AM 6-0211, Loc. 102.

McKINNON, Francis A.; 347 Sherbrooke St., North Bay, Ont.; Qns '52; GenSurg; Surg. Staff, St. Joseph's & North Bay Civic Hosp's.; Tel. 472-2220.

McKINNON, J-Albert; 65 Grande-Allee est, Quebec 4, P.Q.; 1274 Fitzpatrick, Sillery (res); Lav '52; Tel. 529-9691.

McKINNON, Jean-P.; Lav '57; IntMed (PQ); Hd. Dept. of Med., Hotel-Dieu-St.-Michel, Roberval, P.Q.; Tel. 275-0110, Loc. 40.

McKINNON, J. Roy; 199 Westminster, La Salle, Ont.; Dal '55; GenSurg.; Tel. 734-7561.

McKINNON, M. H.; Woodstock, N.B.; Qns '34.

McKINNON, Neil E.; 16 Eastbourne Avenue, Toronto, Ont.; Tor '21; Bact., PH; Staff, School of Hygiene **U. of Toronto; Tel. HU 9-7248.**

McKISHNIE, Eunice (Oestreicher); West Lorne, Ont.; Wes '49; AMCGP.

McKISHNIE, John; Box 190, West Lorne, Ont.; Wes '54; AMCGP.

McKNIGHT, Claude K.; Clarke Inst. of Psy., 250 College St., Toronto 2B, Ont.; Wes'55; D.Psy; Psy; Dir., Inpatient Forensic Serv.; Clin. Teach., U. of Toronto; Tel. 924-6811.

McKNIGHT, Russel D.; Qns'60; Acting Dir., Continuing Care Prog., Ontario Hosp., Kingston, Ont.

McKONE, Barclay; 483 George St. S., Peterborough, Ont.; Tor'40; MCGP; Tel. 742-0461.

McLACHLIN, Angus D.; Victoria Hosp., London, Ont.; 437 Commissioners Rd. E. (res); Wes '32; M.Sc., D. Phil. (Oxon.); M.S. (Tor.); FRCS (Eng.); FACS; FRCS(C); GenSurg & OrthSurg; Chief Surg., Victoria Hosp.; Prof & Hd., Dept. of Surg., U. of Western Ont.; Tel. 432-5261.

McLACHLIN, J. A.; 236 Elm St., St. Thomas, Ont.; Wes '40; F.A.C.S., F.R.C.S.(C), GenSurg; Cons., Westminster DVA Hosp., London; Instr. (Surg.) U. of Western Ont.; Tel. 631-0567.

McLACHLIN, Sheilah; 287 Queens Ave., London, Ont.; Wes '36; Anaes; Tel. GE 8-5143.

McLAGAN, A. D. Campbell; 552 King St., Preston, Ont.; Wes'43; MCGP; Staff, S. Waterloo Mem. Hosp., Galt & St. Mary's & Kitchener-Waterloo Hosp's., Kitchener; Tel. 653-6524.

McLAINE, Peter N.; Qns '62; Res., Montreal Children's Hosp., Montreal, P.Q.

McLANDRESS, Murray; Ste. 102, 225 Vaughan St., Winnipeg 1, Man.; Man'41; Paed; Att'd. Staff, Winnipeg Children's & Gen. Hosp's.; Cons. Staff, Municipal Hosp.; Ass't. Prof. Paed., U. of Manitoba; Tel. 943-9822.

McLAREN, Alexander G., Col.; Alb '42; DPH Reg. Surg., Alberta Med. Reg., CAFMS, Griesbach Barracks, Edmonton, Alta.

McLAREN, David K.; South Shore Rd., Pointe-Au-Baril Station, Ont.; Ste. 109D, 321 Bloor St. W., Toronto; McG '41; Med. Staff, Parry Sound Gen. Hosp. & St. Joseph's Hosp.; Court. Staff, Grace Hosp., Toronto; Tel. 366-2308.

McLAREN, Kenneth A.; 321 Bloor St. W., Toronto, Ont.; 504 Dovecourt Rd. (res); Tor '10; WA 2-8700.

McLAREN, Wm. J.; Burris Clinic, Kamloops, B.C.; 705 Fraser St. (res); St. Andrew's (Scot.) '44; F.R.C.S.(Eng.); GenSurg; Att'd. Staff, Royal Inland Hosp.; Tel. 372-3303.

McLARTY, Thomas D.; 450 Central Ave., London, Ont.; 10 Grosvenor St. (res); Wes '52; FRCS(C); GenSurg; Staff, Victoria Hosp.; Surg. Cons., Ontario Cancer Fdn.; Cons. Westminster DVA; Clin. Lect. (Surg.), U. of Western Ont.; Tel. 438-5405

McLATCHIE, Lola D.; 738 Rideau Rd., Calgary, Alta. (res.); Tor'22; MCAA, DABPA & CA; PathBact; Path. & Dir., Dept. of Path, Calgary Gen. Hosp.; Path., Alb. Red Cross Hosp. for Children; Legal Path., Calgary & Prov. of Alberta; Tel. 262-9016.

McLAUGHLIN, Graydon A.; 136-E. 15th St., North Vancouver, B.C.; 4120 Delbrooke Ave. (res); Man'37; FICS, GenSurg; MCGP; Chief, Dept. Gen. Surg., North Vancouver Gen. Hosp.; Tel. YU 8-3747.

McLAUGHLIN, John A.; Westfield, King's Co., N.B.; McG '35; Chief M.O., N.B. Workmen's Comp. Bd., Saint John; Dist. Coroner.

McLAUGHLIN, John H.; 20 Emerald Park Rd., Regina, Sask. (res); Glasgow (Scot.) '37; DPH; DTM & H; Dir. Med. Standards Hosp. Branch & **Dir., Emergency Health Serv. Br., Dept. of Health, Prov. of Saskatchewan; Health & Welfare Bldg.; Tel. LA 3-0661 Ext. 223.**

McLAUGHLIN, Patrick G.; 7045 St. Denis St., Montreal, P.Q.; **41 Ave. Vivian (res); Lav '32; Anaes; Tel. 272-8060.**

McLAUGHLIN, Victor D.; 104 Alma St., Moncton, N.B.; McG '52; F.R.C.S.(C), ObstGyn; Att. Staff, Moncton Hosp.; Cons. Staff, Hotel-Dieu Hosp.; Tel. 384-5079.

McLEAN, A. Joseph; 309-2nd St. W., Cornwall, Ont.; Qns. '52; GenSurg; Chief of Surg., Hotel-Dieu Hosp.; Chief of Surg., Glengarry Mem. Hosp., Alexandria; Tel. WE 2-0879.

McLEAN, Alan R., Capt.; 7 Med. Det. RCAMC, Wolseley Barracks, London, Ont.; UBC'65.

McLEAN, Alexander P.; McG'57; FRCS(C), GenSurg; Staff, Dept. of Exp. Surg., Royal Victoria Hosp., Montreal 2, P.Q.

McLEAN, Charles D.; Pine St., Woodbridge, Ont.; Qns '45; Staff, Peel Memorial Hosp., Dist. Coroner; Tel. AT 8-0701.

McLEAN, Charles M.; 183 Metcalfe St., Ottawa, Ont.; 85 Range Rd. (res); Glasgow (Scot.) '39; M.D. (Glas); DOMS (Lond.); Ophth; Reg. Ophth., Eastern Reg. Med. Serv., Dept. of Nat. Health & Welfare; Tel. 235-3932.

McLEAN, Charles S.; 502 Med. Dental Bldg., Regina, Sask.; 2275 Montague St. (res); Man '29; Chmn. Med. Assessment Bd.; Business Mgr., Medical & Surgical Associates; Retired.

McLEAN, Chester R.; 399 Bathurst St., Toronto 2B, Ont.; 1343 Nocturne Ct., Port Credit (res); Queen's (N. Ire.) '42; M.Sc. (McG); DABP; FRCP(C), Path; Pathol-in-Chief, Tor. Western Hosp.; Path., Queensway Gen. Hosp.; Assoc. Prof. (Path.), U. of Toronto; Tel. EM 8-2581, Loc. 303.

McLEAN, Clifford C.; Isleview Place, Lions Bay, West Vancouver, B.C.; Tor '36; FACCP; Staff, Pearson T.B. Hosp., Vancouver; Div. T.B. Control, B.C.

McLEAN, D. Bruce; 453 O'Connor Dr., Toronto, Ont.; Tor '43; MCGP; Tel. HO 3-0107.

McLEAN, Donald J.; 201 Medical Arts Bldg., 300 King St. W., Oshawa, Ont.; 107 Connaught St. (res); Tor '50; M.C.G.P.; Tel. 725-3512.

McLEAN, Donald M.; 555 University Ave., Toronto 2, Ont.; 22 Oriole Gdns., Tor. 7 (res); Melbourne (Australia) '50; Virol., Hosp. for Sick Children; Assoc. Prof. (Virol.), Schl. of Hygiene & Assoc. (Paed), U. of Toronto; Tel. EM 6-7242.

McLEAN, Donald W.; 422 Med. Arts Bldg., 1 Young St., Hamilton, Ont.; Qns '55; MCGP; Active Staff, Hamilton Gen. & St. Joseph's Hosp's.; Tel. JA 7-1413.

McLEAN, Edwin M.; 52 Erie St. N., Wheatley, Ont.; Qns'40; Tel. 825-4302.

McLEAN, Frederick J.; 724-13th St. N. Lethbridge, Alta.; **646-15th St. S. (res); Man '41; D. Phil. (Oxon) (Pathol); MCGP; Tel. FA 8-4451.**

McLEAN, Herman A.; Man '28; Supt. Esperanza Gen. Hosp., Esperanza, B.C.

McLEAN, I. Ross; 214-6th Ave. S.W., Calgary, Alta.; Qns 51; FRCP(C), IntMed; Cons. Staff, Holy Cross, Calgary Gen., Alberta Children's & Colonel Belcher Hosp's; Tel. 263-7120.

McLEAN, James William; Apt 209, 2 Milepost Place, Toronto 17, Ont.; Wes '60; FRCS(C), Otol; Staff, Sunnybrook Hosp.

McLEAN, J. Douglas; 42 Coburg St., Saint John, N.B.; Dal'60; Psy.

McLEAN, J. Leo; 183 James St. S., Hamilton, Ont.; Ott '54; Tel. 528-1252.

McLEAN, John A.; Merlin, Ont.; Wes'28. MCGP.

McLEAN, John A.; 1211-750 W. Broadway, Vancouver, B.C.; 1644 W. 40th Ave. (res): Tor '31; Ophth; Chief, Dept. of Ophth, Vancouver Gen. Hosp.; Assoc. Prof. Ophth., U. of British Columbia; Tel. TR 6-2121.

McLEAN, John D.; 2200 Dixie Rd., Cooksville, Ont.; Tor'64; Staff, South Peel & Queensway Hosp's.; Tel. 279-1700.

McLEAN, J. William; Ste. 1038, 751 King St. W., Kitchener, Ont.; Wes'60; FRCS(C), Otol; Tel. 576-2200.

McLEAN, Malcolm J.; UBC'65; Res., Vancouver Gen. Hosp., Vancouver, B.C.

McLEAN, Palmer M.; Ste. 607, 625-5th Ave., New Westminster, B.C.; Man '39; MCH (Orth.); OrthSurg; Staff, Royal Columbian & St. Mary's Hosp's.; Tel. 526-4606.

McLEAN, T. B., Sg. Rear Adm., C.D., QHS.; Dept. of National Defence, Ottawa 4, Ont.; 12 Birch Ave., Ott. 7 (res); Alb '39; Surg. Gen., CAFMS; Tel. 992-0431.

McLEAN, William S.; 308 Main St., Stayner, Ont.; Wes'55; Staff, Collingwood Gen. & Marine **Hosp's.; Tel. 428-2544.**

McLEAN, Winston G.; Tor'65; Res., New Mount Sinai Hosp., Toronto 2, Ont.

McLEAN, W. Neil; Ste. 600, Chinook Prof. Bldg., Calgary, Alta.; 2410 Longridge Dr. (res); Alb'54; MCGP; Tel. AL 5-5566.

McLEESE, Ruth V.; Dal'59; Diag Rad; Staff, Dept. of Rad., Saint John Gen. Hosp., Saint John, N.B.

McLEISH, John C.; St. Joseph's Hosp., London, Ont.; Wes'53; Psy; Lect. Paed. & Clin. Psy., U. of Western Ont.; Tel. 439-3271.

McLEISH, William A.; Wes '62; Intn., Kingston Gen. Hosp., Kingston, Ont.

McLELLAN, Allister M.; McG '60; Res., Montreal Gen. Hosp., Montreal 25, P.Q.
McLELLAN, Charles L.; Bishop Blk., Charlotte St., Sydney, N.S.; McG'42; Tel. 564-8408.
McLELLAN, James R.; Box 712, 164 Charlotte St., Sydney, N.S.; 16 Whitney Ave. (res); Dal '37; Ophth; Staff, Sydney City & St. Rita's Hosp's.; Tel. 564-6300.
McLELLAN, Norman W.; Westfield, King's Co., N.B. (res); McG '29; IntMed, Bact; Med. Spec., Lancaster Hosp., D.V.A., St. John, N.B.
McLELLAN, Robert A.; 138 East St.Napanee, Ont.; 58 Ridge St. E. (res); McG '52; Court. Staff, Hotel-Dieu & Kingston Gen. Hosp's.; Tel. 354-3524.
McLELLAN, T. Allan; 221 Queensdale Ave. E., Hamilton, Ont.; 27 Millen Ave. (res); Qns '43; M.C.G.P.; Indoor Staff, Hamilton Gen. Hosp.; Tel. TA 7-0271.
McLELLAN, Wilfrid G.; 710 Hartland, Montreal 8, P.Q.; McG '20; FRCP; MCAA; Allerg (PQ); IntMed; Hon. Att'd. Staff, Royal Victoria Hosp.
McLELLAN, William; The Cancer Clinic, 11250-84th Ave., Edmonton, Alta.; Glasgow (Scot.)'41; DMRT.
McLEMAN, Daniel; Smith Clinic, 144 Main St. E., Hawkesbury, Ont.; Aberdeen (Scot.) '55; DRC-OG; DCH; Staff, Smith Clinic; Tel. ME 2-2711.
McLENNAN, D. William; 68 Main St. E., Grimsby, Ont.; Qns'54; MCGP; Tel. 945-5424.
McLENNAN, James A.; Ste. 2, 604 Royal Ave., New Westminster, B.C.; Ste. 5, 43 Elliot St. (res); Ott '57; Tel. LA 6-5747.
McLENNAN, John D.; 108 Otter Cres., Toronto, Ont. (res); Tor '34; F.C.C.P., IntMed, T.B.; Prov. Dept of Health, Ontario; Tel. RU 3-4458.
McLENNAN, Thomas A.; 17 Hatherton Cr., Don Mills, Ont. (res); Tor '50; DABS; FACS; FRCS-(C) Cardiovasc Surg; Chief Res., (Cardiovasc Surg.), Toronto Gen. Hosp.; Research Cardiovasc., Banting Inst.; Tel. EM 6-8211.
McLENNAN, Trevor M.; 242 Lawrence Ave., Orillia, Ont. (res); Qns'32; DiagRad; Dir., Dept. of Radiol., Orillia Soldiers Mem. Hosp.; Tel. 325-2201.

McLEOD, Allan; 202 Marlborough St., Cornwall, Ont.; Ott '51; Tel. WE 2-3464.
McLEOD, Angus M.; 1003 Medical Arts Bldg., 170 St. George St., Toronto, Ont.; 29 Bayview Ridge, York Mills, Willowdale P.O. (res); Tor '24; Otol; Sr. Surg., Dept. of Otol., Toronto Gen. Hosp.; Assoc., Dept. of Otol., U. of Toronto; Tel. WA 3-7169.
McLEOD, Clarke K.; 5292 Queen Mary Rd., Montreal, P.Q.; McG '27; F.A.C.S.; GenSurg; Hon. Att'd. Staff, Mtl. Gen. Hosp.; Cons. Phys., Electrolux Ltd.; Tel. WE 7-6011.
McLEOD, David A.; 106 Alma St., Moncton, N.B.; Aberdeen (Scot.)'56; FRCS(C), Urol.
McLEOD, David L.; 5 Kirkdale Cr., Don Mills, Ont. (res); Tor'52; Paed; Assoc. Prof. (Histol.), U. of Toronto; Tel. 928-2714.
McLEOD, Ewen C.; 1587 W 41st Ave., Vancouver 13, B.C.; McG'22.
McLEOD, James Gordon; 3137 Athol St., Regina, Sask. (res); McG '38; Sr. Med. Exam., Canadian Pensions Commission; Tel. LA 2-0189.
McLEOD, Janey M.; 291 Christina St. N., Sarnia, Ont.; Tor '43; Derm.; Tel. 337-3517.
McLEOD, Lionel E.; 12904-65th Ave., Edmonton, Alta.; Alb '51; M.Sc. (Med.); FRCP(C); IntMed. (Endocrin); Hd., Div. of Endocrin., University Hosp.; Assoc. Prof., Alberta U.; Tel. GE 9-5911.
McLEOD, Neil S.; Fort William Clinic, 117 John St. S., Fort William, Ont.; Man'65.
McLEOD, Norman D.; 47 Lisgar Ave, Tillsonburg, Ont. (res); Tor'19; Dist. Coroner; Tel. VI 2-4231.
McLEOD, Peter J.; Man'65; Res., Montreal Gen. Hosp., Montreal 25, P.Q.
McLEOD, Presley A.; 221 King St. E., Kingston, Ont.; 96 Queen's Cres. (res); Qns' '26; F.R.C.-O.G., F.R.C.S.(C) ObstGyn; Att. Obst. Gyn., Kingston Gen. Hosp.; Cons. Obst. Gyn., Ontario Hosp. & Cdn. Forces Hosp.; Assoc. Prof. Obst. Gyn., Queen's U.; Dist. Coroner; Tel. 542-5851.
McLEOD, Roderick A.; 1629 London St., New Westminster, B.C.; Ste. 201, 410—8th Ave. (res); McG '20.
McLEOD, Scott H.; 615 Greyhound Bldg., Calgary, Alta.; 206 Roxboro Rd. (res); McG '23; Retired.
McLEOD, William A.; 925 W. Georgia St., Ste. 318, Vancouver 1, B.C.; Alb'58; FRCP(C), Derm.
McLISTER, John C.; 482 Pelissier St., Windsor, Ont.; 1422 Ouellette Ave. (res); Tor '44; A.M.-C.G.P.; Vice-Pres. Gen. Med. Staff & Exec. Comm. & Sec., Dept. of Surg., Grace Hosp.; Tel. 252-9511.
McLOUGHLIN, Diarmuid P.; 83 Ottaway Ave., Barrie, Ont.; Dublin (Ire.)'58; DMRD; DiagRad.
McLUHAN, William J.; Associate Clinic, Ross St., Red Deer, Alta.; 4 Savoy Cr., (res); Alb 57; Staff. Red Deer Mun. Hosp.; Pres., Central Alta. Med. Soc.; Tel. 346-2057.
McLURG, John J. A.; Medical Arts Clinic, Regina, Sask.; Alb '34; Psy; Dist. Coroner; Tel. LA 2-1651.
McLURG, Robert J.; 812 Med. Dental Bldg., Rose St. & 11th Ave., Regina, Sask.; Sask '61; AMCGP; Tel. 527-2234.
McMAHAN, Jay S.; 574 Princess St., Kingston, Ont.; 46 Toronto St. (res); Qns '60; Tel. 548-4352.
McMAHEN, Willard J.; 120 Med. Arts Bldg., Victoria, B.C.; Alb'42; Urol; Staff, Veteran's Hosp.; Tel. EV 2-4221.
McMAHON, Alexander J.; Tor'62; Res., Toronto Gen. Hosp., Toronto 2, Ont.
McMAHON, James M.; 100 Church Ave., Chilliwack, B.C.; Man'52; AMCGP.
McMAHON, L. Paul; 166 King St. W., Sherbrooke, P.Q.; 275 Bryant St. (res); Lav '42; Anaes; Chm. Anaes. Dept., Hotel-Dieu & Sherbrooke Hosp's.; Phys. Cdn. Ingersoll-Rand; Tel. LO 9-2551.
McMAIN, Peter B.; 168 Ontario St., St. Catharines, Ont.; Glasgow (Scot.)'53; Paed; Chief of Paed., Hotel-Dieu Hosp.; Tel. 682-8072.
McMANUS, Francis R.; 600 Herald Bldg., 206-7th Ave. W., Calgary, Alta.; 4012 Crestview Rd. (res); Man'39; GenSurg; Staff, Calgary Gen. & Col. Belcher Hosp's.; Tel. 262-1200.
McMANUS, John J.; 550 Talbot St., St. Thomas, Ont.; Wes '29.
McMANUS, John P.; Northern Trans Co. Ltd., 10040-105th St., Edmonton, Alta.; Qns'37; MCGP.
McMARTIN, John W.; 5025 Sherbrooke St. W., Ste. 425, Montreal, P.Q.; McG '42; Staff, Phys., Queen Elizabeth Hosp.; Tel. 488-4849.
McMARTIN, W. Finlay; Ste. 340, 5025 Sherbrooke St. W., Montreal 28, P.Q.; McG '35; IntMed; Tel. 488-0394.
McMASTER, Ervin A.; Lake Rd., Grand Bend, Ont.; Tor '23; FACCP (Cardiol.); MCGP; Tel. 238-2315.
McMASTER, E. Susan; Ste. 602, W. 44th Ave., Vancouver 13, B.C.; Berlin (Germ.)'34; DPH; PH.
McMICHAEL, Lawrence A.; Regent Park Clinic, Sherwood Dr., Regina, Sask.; Birmingham (Eng.) '55.
McMILLAN, Donald A.; Thorold Medical Clinic, 60 Albert St. W., Thorold, Ont.; 33 Claremont St. (res); Qns'49; Tel. CA 7-5255.
McMILLAN, Donald B.; 28 Weber St. W., Kitchener, Ont.; Ott '54; M.C.G.P.; Staff. St. Mary's & Kitchener-Waterloo Hosp's.; Tel. SH 5-'617.
McMILLAN, Donald W.; 305 Northgate Bldg., Edmonton, Alta.; Ste. 3, 11414-132nd St. (res); Alb '48; Ophth; Staff, Edmonton Gen Hosp.; Tel. GA 4-2942.
McMILLAN, Douglas G.; Crysler, Ont.; McG '50; M.C.G.P.; Att'd. Staff, Winchester Mem. Hosp.; Tel. WU 4-2780.
McMILLAN, Gardner C.; 370-41st Ave., Lachine, P.Q. (res); McG '44; Ph.D.; FRCP(C), Path; Cons. Path., Montreal Gen. Hosp.; Strathcona Prof. of Path., McGill U., Montreal; Tel. WE 7-6011.
McMILLAN, Jack D.; Silver Heights Medical-Dental Bldg., 2333 Portage Ave., St. James 12, Wpg., Man.; Man '55; M.C.G.P.; Coroner, Prov. of Manitoba; Tel. VE 7-1327.

McMILLAN, Joseph A.; Charlottetown Clinic, 1 Rochford St., Charlottetown, P.E.I.; 45 Greenfield Ave. (res); McG '38; M.C.G.P.; Staff, Charlottetown Hosp.; Assoc. Staff, P.E.I. Hosp. & Med. Dir., Maritime Health Serv. Assoc.; Tel. 894-5521.

McMILLAN, Mark L.; 10951-124th St., Edmonton, Alta.; 14346 Park Dr. (res); Glasgow (Scot.) '51; DRCOG; MCGP; Att'd. Staff, Royal Alexandra Hosp.; Tel. GL 4-4551.

McMILLAN, Neil L.; Elliot Lake Clinic, 46 Ontario St., Elliot Lake, Ont.; Edinburgh (Scot.) '53; Tel. 848-7176.

McMILLAN, Robert M.; 140 Seaforth Med. Bldg., 3550 Cote des Neiges Rd., Montreal 25, P.Q.; Alb '52; Otol; Staff, Montreal Gen. & St. Mary's Hosps'; Tel. 935-1363.

McMILLAN, William H.; 28 Claremont, Thorold, Ont.; Qns'16; Hon. Staff, St. Catharines Gen. & Hotel-Dieu Hosp's.; Tel. 227-5255; Retired.

McMILLAN, William J. P.; 205 Kent St., Charlottetown, P.E.I.; McG '08; F.A.C.S., F.I.C.S., F.R.C.S.(C), GenSurg; Chief Med. Staff, Charlottetown Hosp.; Staff, Prince Edward Island Hosp.; Tel. 894-5561.

McMILLAN, W. Robert; 132 Parkdale S., Hamilton, Ont.; 80 Irene Ave., Stoney Creek (res); Qns '54; MCGP; Tel. 219-6611.

McMILLEN, Gordon R.; 546 Pharmacy Ave., Scarborough, Ont.; 57 Florens Ave. (res); Tor '53; Tel. PL 7-3237.

McMILLEN, Norman R. J.; 1961 Allison Rd., Vancouver, B.C. (res); Tor '40; D.A.B.A., F.A.C.A., Anaes; staff, St. Paul's Hosp.; Tel. MU 3-2211.

McMILLIN, Robert S.; 2160 Weston Rd., Weston, Ont.; Tor '54; M.C.G.P.; Chief, Dept. of G.P., Humber Mem. Hosp.; Tel. CH 4-5566.

McMORLAND, Graham H.; 589 Scenic Dr., Hamilton, Ont.; Cape Town (S. Africa) '51; DA (Eng.); Anaes; Staff, Hamilton Civic Hosp's.; Tel. 389-7595.

McMORRIS, Lawrence S.; Pathology Dept., Winnipeg Gen. Hosp., Winnipeg, Man.; Man'46; Path; Lect. (Path.), U. of Manitoba; Tel. SP 4-6511.

McMULLEN, David; 11 Trent St., Frankford, Ont.; Tor'15; MOH, Village of Frankford & Twp. of Sydney; Dist. Coroner! Tel. EX 8-6021.

McMULLEN, Monica (See Murdoch)

McMURCHY, A. Donald; 288 Worthington St. W., North Bay, Ont.; 41 Campbell Ave. (res); Ott '52; MCGP; Tel. 474-2630.

McMURCHY, John G. M.; Medical Assoc. Clin., 405 Hendryx St., Nelson, B.C.; 808 Kokanee St. (res); Man '34; M.C.G.P.

McMURCHY, N. Ray; 215 Frederick St., Kitchener, Ont.; Tor '42; M.C.G.P.; Staff, Kitchener-Waterloo & St. Mary's Hosp's.; Tel. SH 5-5551.

McMURRAY, Leith E.; Tor '61; Jr. Intn., Toronto East Gen. Hosp., Toronto 6, Ont.

McMURRAY, Mary B.; Ste. 306, 825 Granville St., Vancouver 2, B.C.; Glasgow (Scot.)'62; Tel. RE 8-1343.

McMURTRY, Shirley O.; 1224 St. Catherine St. W., Montreal, P.Q.; 1710 Dorchester W. (res); McG '05; Ophth., Moorfield (London); Cons. Ophth., Montreal Gen. Hosp.; Tel. UN 6-6177. Semi-Retired.

McMURTRY, Thomas S. G.; 3009-31st Ave., Vernon, B.C.; "Kal-View" (res); Man '41; FRCP (C), IntMed; Tel. 542-4321.

McNAB, James, S/L; Sick Bay, Canadian Forces Base, Halifax, N.S.; Aberdeen (Scot.)'53.

McNAB, John A.; 6325 Fraser St., Vancouver 15, B.C.; 2474 W. 36th (res); Man '37; DA (Lond.); Anaes; Anaes. Staff, Burnaby Gen. Hosp.; Tel. FA 5-4040.

McNABB, Alan R.; Henderson Gen. Hosp., Hamilton, Ont.; Wes'46; PhD; FRCP(C), IntMed; Chief, Dept. of Med., Hamilton Civic Hosp.; Tel. 389-4933.

McNABB, Malcolm W.; 672 Brant St., Burlington, Ont.; Wes'50; ObstGyn; MCGP; Active Staff, Joseph Brant Mem. Hosp.; Tel. 634-1560.

McNAIR, Alan Y.; 420 Med. Dental Bldg., 925 W. Georgia St., Vancouver 1, B.C.; 5874 Marguerite St., Van. 13 (res); Tor '16; IntMed; PathBact; Cons. IntMed., St. Paul's Hosp.; Tel. 682-3232.

McNAIR, Francis E.; 1737 Pandosy St., Kelowna, B.C.; 822 Saucier (res); McG '43; Psy; Dir., Okanagan Mental Health Centre; Clin. Instr., U. of British Columbia; Tel. PO 2-5354.

McNALLY, James A.; Alb '50; Staff, Lethbridge Mun. Hosp., Lethbridge, Alta.; Tel. 327-8591.

McNALLY, Lawrence B.; 12774 Gouin Blvd. W., Pierrefonds, P.Q.; McG '63; Staff, Lakeshore Gen. & Lachine Gen. Hosp's.; Tel. 684-8960.

McNALLY, Norman H., Col.; 123 Talbot Dr., Oakville, Ont. (res); Wes '42; Anaes; Hon. Med. Staff, Oakville-Trafalgar Hosp.; Reg. Surg., CFMS (Ont.), Ortona Barracks, Oakville, Ont.

McNALLY, William J.; 1509 Sherbrooke St. W., Montreal 25, P.Q.; 25 Redpath Place (res); Dal '22; M.Sc., D.Sc., LL.D., F.R.C.S.(C), Otol; Hon. Cons. Otol., Royal Victoria Hosp.; Tel. 935-2500.

McNAMARA, J. Arch; 182 Patrick St., St. John's Nfld.; National U. (Ire.) '39; M.C.G.P.; Staff, St. John's Gen., St. Clare's Mercy & Grace Maternity Hosp's.; Tel. 8-2558.

McNAUGHT, David R.; 86 St. Georges Cr., Edmonton, Alta.; Alb'60; FRCS(C), OrthSurg.

McNAUGHTON, Francis L.; 3801 University St., Montreal 2, P.Q.; 618 Victoria Ave., Westmount (res); McG '31; F.R.C.P.(C), NeurPsy; Cons. Neur., Montreal Gen. Hosp.; Neur., Royal Victoria Hosp. & Montreal Neurological Inst.; Prof. Neur., McGill U.; Tel. VI 2-1251, Ext. 349; 845-6781.

McNAUGHTON, Robt. H.; 503—1541 W. Broadway, Vancouver 9, B.C.; McG '49; ObstGyn.; Tel. RE 3-9514.

McNEEL, Burdett H.; Dept. of Health, Parliament Bldgs., Toronto 5, Ont.; 125 Sylvan Ave., Scarborough (res); Tor '36; D.Psy; FAPA; Psy; Assoc. Prof. (Psy), U. of Toronto; Dir. Prof. Serv. Branch, Mental Health Div., Parliament Bldgs.; Tel. 365-2446.

McNEEL, Robert W.; 2069 Gore St., Burlington, Ont.; 3037 South Dr. (res); McG '50; Paed; Prin. MO, HMCS "Star", RCN(R); Tel. 634-1302.

McNEELY, Donald T.; Med. Arts Bldg., 358 Reynolds St., Oakville, Ont.; Tor '56; IntMed; Active Cons. Staff, Oakville-Trafalgar Mem. Hosp.; Assoc. Med. Dir., Rheumatic Dis. Unit, Chedoke Hosp., Hamilton. Tel. 845-5942.

McNEELY, Ross G. D.; 939 Foul Bay Rd., Victoria, B.C. (res); Man '41; Path; Dir. of Labs. Royal Jubilee Hosp.; Chief of Serv. (Path.) Victoria Veterans' Hosp.; Hon. Pathol., Queen Alexandra Solarium; Dir. Branch Public Health Lab.; Tel. EV 6-3131.

McNEIL, Donald L.; Calgary Assoc. Clinic, 214-6th Ave. W., Calgary, Alta.; Man'39; FACP; FRCP(C), IntMed; Cons., Holy Cross Hosp.; Hon. Cons., Foothills Gen. Hosp.; Dir. Student Health Serv., U. of Calgary; Past Pres. CMA (Alta. Div.); Tel. 263-7120.

McNEIL, John K.; 103 Deer Park Circle, London, Ont.; Wes'56.

McNEIL, John O.; 5 Commercial St., Glace Bay, N.S.; Dal '45; GenSurg.; Tel. 849-7733.

McNEIL, M. Ross; 260 Wharncliffe Rd. S., London, Ont.; 207 Windsor Ave. (res); Wes '52.

McNEILL, Alexandre; 222 est Henri-Bourassa, Montreal 12, P.Q.; 115 Lockhart (res); Mon '44; Obst; Tel. 387-7607.

McNEILL, Clarence G.; 1548 Lonsdale Ave., North Vancouver, B.C.; 1617 Grand Blvd. (res); Alb '41; MCGP; Tel. 985-5381. Abroad.

McNEILL, George T.; Box 10, Virden Health Unit, Virden, Man.; Man '39.

McNEILL, Hubert B.; 5 Central St., Summerside, P.E.I.; 260 Green St. (res); Dal '53; A.M.C.G.P.

McNEILL, J. A.; 1319 Monaghan Rd., Peterborough, Ont.; Tor '43.

McNEILL, John F.; 253 Church St., Summerside, P.E.I.; McG '02; Retired.

McNEILL, Laurie K.; Dal'65; Res., Children's Hosp., Halifax, N.S.

McNEILL, O. Redmond; Tor'59; Res., General Hosp., St. John's, Nfld.
McNEILL, Stuart R. Sg/Lt; Tor '64; RCN Air Station, Shearwater, N.S.
McNEILLY, Kenneth A.; Box 422, Malton, Ont.; Belfast (Ire.)'63; Tel. 677-4200.
McNEILLY, Walter E., 2045 Dufferin St., Toronto 10, Ont.; Tor '63; Tel. LE 6-2128.
McNICHOL, John F.; 58 Ainslie St. S., Galt, Ont.; 27 Barrie St. (res). Qns '36; Tel. 621-7210.
McNICHOL, J. Wallace; 700 Medical Arts Bldg., Hamilton, Ont.; 403 Queen St. S. (res); Tor '37; F.A.C.S.; F.I.C.S.; F.R.C.S.(C), PlasSurg; GenSurg; Chief, **Plas. Surg. Serv., Hamilton Gen., & St. Joseph's Hosp's.; Tel. JA 8-6789.**
McNICHOLAS, Patrick J.; 288 Duckworth St. John's, Nfld. Dublin (Ire.) '41; DOMS; DLO; Ophth.; Tel. 578-3109.
McNICOLL, Andre; 54 rue Lapointe, Clermont Co., Charlebois, P.Q. (res); Lav '45; MCGP; Staff, Hop. St. Joseph, LaMalbaie.; Tel. MO 5-3711.
McNICOL, Harvey L.; 159 Oak St., Winnipeg 9, Man.; Man '35; FACS; GenSurg; MCGP.
McNIVEN, Errol L.; Bank of Toronto Bldg., 1405 Douglas, Victoria, B.C.; 520 Falkland Rd., Oak Bay (res); Tor '28; Staff, Royal Jubilee Hosp.
McNULTY, P. H.; 264 Edmonton St., McNulty Clinic Bldg., Winnipeg, Man.; 138 Harrow St. (res); Man '17; F.R.C.S.; F.A.C.S.; F.I.C.S., GenSurg; Tel. WH 3-0735.
McPHAIL, Donald M.; 367 N. Railway, Boissevain, **Man.; Man '45; M.C.G.P.; Tel. 534-2425.**
McPHAIL, Ethel M. (Herriot); Box 400, Boissevain. Man.; **678 Johnson St. (res); Man '45; Tel. 534-2425.**
McPHAIL, John A.; 336 Kings Rd., Sydney, N.S.; Dal'61; AMCGP; Assoc. Staff Memb., Sydney City & St. Rita Hosp's.; Tel. 562-1143.
McPHAIL, Mary (Kujawa); 500-11th Ave., North Battleford, Sask.; Man '45; Tel. 445-8646.
McPHAIL, Neil V.; Tor'61; Res. (Surg.), Ottawa Civic Hosp., Ottawa 3, Ont.
McPHAIL, W. Grant; 10169 - 104 St., Edmonton, Alta.; **6002—111 Ave. (res); Man '46; M.C.G.P.; Hon. Sess. Instr., U. of Alta.; Dir. of Med.** Servs., Med. Servs. (Alberta) Inc.; Tel. 429-1731.
McPHEDRAN, N. Tait; 138, Private Patients Pavilion, 101 College St., Toronto 2, Ont.; Tor'50; FACS; FRCS(C), GenSurg; Ass't. Surg., Tor. Gen. Hosp.; Assoc. (Surg.), U, of Toronto; Tel. 364-2046.
McPHEDRAN, Robert S.; Wellesley Hosp., Toronto 5, Ont.; Wes'56; FRCP(C), NeurPsy; Phys., Wellesley Hosp.; Research Assoc. (Path.) & Clin. Teach., Dept. of Med., U. of Toronto; Tel. 925-7742.
McPHEE, James A.; 20 Doctors' Lane, King City, Ont.; Tor '53; MCGP; Chief (GP), York Central Hosp., Richmond Hill; Sr. Active Staff, York Co. Hosp., Newmarket; Tel. TE 3-5331.
McPHEE, James G.; 323 E. Columbia St., New Westminster, B.C.; 865 Highland Dr., W. Van. (res); Man '44; D.A.B.R.; D&T Rad; Att'd. Staff, Royal Columbian Hosp., New Westminster. Tel. LA 2-2771.
McPHEE, Malcolm S.; Qns'65; Res., University Hosp., Edmonton, Alta.
McPHERSON, Archie; 1331 Elliott St., Saskatoon (res): Sask '60.
McPHERSON, A. Russell; 1320 Ave. K. S. Saskatoon, Sask.; Man '28; FCCP; IntMed (TB); Med. Supt., Sask. San.; Retired.
McPHERSON, C. F. S.; Centre St., Prescott, Ont.; Qns '96; Dist. Coroner; Retired.
McPHERSON, Colin A.; 15 Riddell St., Woodstock, Ont.; Wes'29; FIAP, FICS, GenSurg; Surg. Staff, Woodstock Gen. Hosp.; Cons. Surg., Alex**andra Hosp.; Cons. Surg., Ont. Hosp.; Tel. 537-7101.**
McPHERSON, Douglas F.; 1605-9th Ave. S., Lethbridge, Alta.; 612-11th St. S. (res); McG '44; Paed; Chief Paed., St. Michael's Hosp.; Tel. 327-3121.
McPHERSON, G. Duncan; Ste. 706, 750 W. Broadway, Vancouver 9, B.C.; Wes'56; M.Sc. (UBC); FRCS(C), OrthSurg; Cons. Staff, Shaughnessy Hosp.; Vis. Staff, Vancouver Gen. Hosp.; Staff, U. of British Columbia; Tel. 874-4717.
McPHERSON, Gordon R.; Med. Centre, Sandwich St., Amherstburg, Ont.; Wes '60; Tel. 736-2118.
McPHERSON, Merle (MacRae); 1331 Elliott St., Saskatoon, **Sask. (res); Sask '60.**
McPHERSON, R. H.; Mount Forest, Ont.; Tor '36; M.C.G.P.
McPHERSON, Victor A.; National Defence Med. Centre, Alta Vista Dr., Ottawa 8, Ont.; UBC '54; FRCS(C); GenSurg; Tel. 733-6600.
McPHILLIPS, Alexander St. G.; 1051 Denman St., Vancouver 5, B.C.; 6387 Cambie St. (res); St. George's (London, Eng.) '40; LMSSA; Vis. Staff, St. Paul's, St. Vincent's & Kelowna Gen. Hosp's.; Tel. MU 5-7039.
McPHILLIPS, Brian; R.C.P.S. (Ire.) '43; L.M. (Rotunda), D.A.B.R., D & TRad; Rad., St. Catharines Gen. Hosp., St. Catharines, Ont. Tel. MU 4-7271.
McQUADE, G. D.; Ass't. Reg. Dir. & Chief Cons., Department of National Health & Welfare, c/o Regional Supt., European Region; Abroad.
McQUADE, G. William; 1110 Townsend St., Sydney, N.S.; Dal '63.
McQUADE, M. Margaret; 514 Jarvis St., Toronto 5, Ont.; 51 Alexander St., Apt. 917 (res); Wes '48; Ph.D.; D.P.M. (Lond.); Psy; Clin. Instr. Psy., U. of Toronto; Special Lect'r., School of Social Work, U. of Toronto; Staff Psy., Toronto Mental Health Clinic; Tel. 924-7349.
McQUAIG, Keith D., 346 Carpathia Rd., Winnipeg, Man. (res); McG '43; D.P.H.
McQUAY, John B.; Mindemoya, Ont.; Qns '44; MCGP; Tel. 2R22.
McQUAY, Norman W.; 742 King St. W., Kitchener, Ont.; 166 Norman St., Waterloo (res); Qns '45; DABIM; IntMed; Active Staff, Kitchener-Waterloo & St. Mary's Hosp's.; Cons. Staff, South Waterloo Mem. Hosp.; Ass't. Med. Dir., Dominion Life Assurance Co.; Tel. 743-2573.
McQUEEN, Beryl M. (Gee); Stonewall & Rockwood Health Area, Stonewall, Man.; London U. **(Eng.) '40; M.R.C.S., L.R.C.P., M.B., B.S.** (Lond.); Mun. Phys, Stonewall & Rockwood Health Area.
McQUEEN, David; 221 Medical Arts Bldg., 404 Graham Ave., Winnipeg 1, Man.; Stonewall (res); London (Eng.) '52; L.R.C.P., M.R.C.S.; D.Surg., OrthSurg; Clin. Ass't. Wpg. Children's & Gen. Hosp's.; Cons. Brandon Gen. Hosp's.; Dem. (Surg). U. of Manitoba; Tel. WH 3-1153.
McQUEEN, Kenneth E.; Box 290, 44 Main St., Picton, Ont.; Qns'30; MCGP.
McQUEEN, Roberta J. (Mrs. R. W. Keyes); 456 W. Broadway, Vancouver 10, B.C.; 765 Southborough Dr. W. Van. (res); Man '45; D. Psy (Tor); Psy; Ass't. Psy., Mental Hyg. Div., Metro. Health Serv., City of Van.; Tutor Pre-Clin. Year, U. of British Columbia; Tel. TR 6-**1313, Loc. 375.**
McQUEEN, Ross C.; 111-9th St., Brandon, Man.; Glasgow (Scot.) '59; D.ObstRCOG; MCGP; Surg. Lt., Royal Cdn. Sea Cadet Corps; Tel. PA 9-5471.
McQUEEN, Thomas A.; Qns'65; Res., Dept. of Surg., U. of British Columbia, Vancouver, B.C.
McQUIBBAN, George A.; 172 Queen St. W., Brampton, Ont.; Rideau Towers (res); Tor '63; Active Staff, Peel Mem. Hosp.
McQUITTY, George D.; 225-226 Med. Arts Bldg., 335-339 6th Ave S.W., Calgary, Alta.; St. Andrews (Scot.) '40; Tel. 262-4244.
McQUITTY, Melvyn; 5977 Marceau Ave., Ste. Genevieve, P.Q. (res); Tor '21; F.C.C.P., IntMed (TB); Head (T.B.), Queen Mary Veterans' Hosp.; Dem., McGill U.; Clin Phys., Royal Edward Laurentian Hosp.
McRAE, Colin A.; 230 Russell Hill Rd., Toronto, Ont.; Tor '33; MCGP; Phys., Royal York Hotel; Tel. 924-4567.

McRAE, Donald L.; 3801 University St., Montreal 2, P.Q.; Wes'38; FACR; D&TRad; Rad.-in-Chief, Montreal Neurol. Inst.; Ass't. Radiol., Royal Victoria Hosp.; Assoc. Prof. (Radiol. & Neurol. & NeuroSurg.), McGill U.; Tel. VI 2-1251.

McRAE, Donald S.; 1075 Bayview Ave., Toronto 12, Ont.; 141 Highland Cres., Willowdale (res); Tor'50; FCCP; Clin. Staff, Sunnybrook Hosp.; Tel. 485-8651, Loc. 260.

McRAE, Joseph R.; 20 Widdecombe Hill, Weston, Ont.; Tor '30; PhysMed & Rehab; Staff, St. Michael's, St. Joseph's & St. Bernard's Hosp's.

McRAE, Kenneth N.; 358 Elm St., Winnipeg, Man.; Man '55; Paed; Dir., O.P.D., Children's Hosp.; Ass't. Dir., Child Guidance Clinic; Lect. (Paed.), U. of Man.; Tel. 775-8311, Local. 220.

McRAE, William D.; 502 Medical Dental Bldg., Regina, Sask.; Sask '59.

McRITCHIE, Murdo; Box 820, Fernie, B.C.; Man '39; MCGP; Staff, Fernie Mem. Hosp.; Tel. 13.

McROBERTS, A. T.; Okanagan Agency, c/o Reg. Sup., Pacific Region, Dept. Nat. Health & Welfare, 4824 Fraser St., Vancouver, B.C.

McROBERTS, Allan F.; 3105-31st St., Vernon, B.C.; 2403-26th (res); Qns '39; Tel. 542-2830.

MCRUER, Enid E.; Box 1136, Morden, Man.; Man'49; Retired.

McSHEFFREY, J. Brian; 710 Canada Bldg., 21st E. & 1st Ave. S., Saskatoon, Sask.; Sask'60; Paed; Assoc. Med. Staff, University Hosp.; Clin. Teach., U. of Saskatchewan; Tel. 244-1116.

McSHERRY, J. Brendan; 249 William St., Belleville, Ont.; Queens (Belfast) '50; MCGP; Staff, Belleville Gen. Hosp.; Tel. 968-7888.

McSWEENEY, E. Douglas; Ott '58; Res. Royal Victoria Hosp., Montreal, P.Q.; Nat. Research Council Fell. (Exper.Surg) McGill U.

McSWEYN, Norman F. A.; 267 O'Connor St., Ottawa, Ont.; Aylmer Rd. (res); Man '43; ThorSurg; **Sr. Lect. (ThorSurg), U. of Ottawa;** Tel. 236-1722.

McTAGGART, Andrew N.; Dept. of Psy., University of British Columbia, Vancouver, B.C.; McG'55; Psy.

McTAGUE, Gerald A.; 1539 Erie St. E., Windsor, Ont.; 743 Devonshire Rd. (res); **Wes '29; Chief of Staff, Hotel Dieu Hosp; Tel. CL 2-2733.**

McTAVISH, D. Ross; Wes'60; Res., Toronto Western Hosp., Toronto 2, Ont.

McTAVISH, J. Edward; 1512-9th Ave. S., Lethbridge, Alta.; **1107-16th St. S. (res); Man '45;** MCGP; Dist. Coroner; Tel. 7-1123.

McTAVISH, John N.; Qns '61; Res., Toronto Psy. Hosp., Toronto 5, Ont.

McTAVISH, Stanley; Kapuskasing Med. Centre, Kapuskasing, Ont.; **Tor '30; M.C.G.P.**

McTAVISH, Willson A.; 424 Medical Arts Bldg., 170 St. George St., Toronto, Ont.; **162 Forest Hill Rd. (res); Tor '29: M.R.C.P. (Lond.); IntMed; Phys., Upper Canada College; Tel. WA 2-8311.**

McTAVISH, William B.; 189 Henderson Hwy., Winnipeg 5, Man.; Man'56; AMCGP; Tel. 533-7631.

McVICKER, Daniel D. C.; 85 Centre St., Deseronto, Ont.; **Wes '39; Staff, Belleville Gen. Hosp., Belleville; M.O.H. & Coroner, Hastings Co.; Tel. 396-2443.**

McVICKER, Maurice A.; 2 Exploits Street, Lewisporte, Nfld.; Trinity Coll. (Dublin, Ire.)'52; MCGP; Ass't. MHO, Lewisporte; Tel. 6701.

McWILLIAM, Ranald S.; 17 Brunswick St., Stratford, Ont.; 110 John St. N. (res); **Edinburgh (Scot.) '45; DCH (Lond.); Staff (Paed), Stratford Gen. Hosp.; Tel. 271-0430.**

McWILLIAM, Maureen H.; (See Roberts, Maureen M.).

McWILLIAM, Margaret B.; Student Health Serv., U. of Alberta, Edmonton, Alta.; Alb'43; IntMed.

MEADE, Frederick C.; Tor '60; Res., Sunnybrook Hosp., Toronto 12, Ont.

MEADE, Judith A. (Marshall); 67 Magpie Rd., Wawa, Ont.: Tor '60.

MEADS, G. E.; Wes'61; FRCS(C), GenSurg; Staff, Westminster Hosp., London, Ont.

MEAGHER, Pierre Y.; Lav'66; Staff, Hop. Temiscaming, **Temiscaming, P.Q.**

MEAKIN, J. William; 500 Sherbourne St., Toronto 5, Ont.; Qns '53; M.A., F.R.C.P.(C), IntMed; Phys. Ont. Cancer Inst.; Cons. Wellesley Hosp.; Assoc. (Med.). U. of Toronto; Tel. 924-0671.

MEAKINS, Jonathan F.; 687 Pine Ave. W., Montreal 2, P.Q.; McG '36; M.A., FACP; FCCP; Pulm. Dis. & T.B. (P.Q.); FRCP(C), IntMed; Phys., Royal Victoria Hosp.; Phys-in-Chief, Lakeshore Gen. Hosp.; Cons., Queen Mary Vet's. & Royal Edward Chest Hosp's.; Memb., Silicosis Bd. Prov. of Que.; Hon. Cons., Bruchesi Inst. & Grace Dart Hosp.; Ass't. Prof. (Med.), McGill U.; Tel. 849-3249.

MEARS, Trevor S.; Box 114, Barrington Passage, Shelburne Co., N.S.; London (Eng.)'62; M.B., BS, D.ObstRCOG; Staff, Roseway Hosp.; Tel. 43.

MEASHAM, Anthony R.; 180 Portland St., Dartmouth, N.S.; Dal'65; Tel. 466-7471.

MECH, Z. Romuald; 31 Centre St. W., Brampton, Ont.; Tor '56; D. Psy.; Psy; Dir.. Psy. Unit., Peel Mem. Hosp.; Tel. 451-2470.

MEDD, Dallas; Winnipeg Clinic, Winnipeg, Man.; 736 Oak St. (res); Man '45; Tel. 942-0551.

MEDHURST, John D.; 29 Hatherton Cr., Don Mills, Ont.; Bristol (Eng.)'45; MRCS; LRCP; DPH; DHA.

MEDINA, Carlos A.; McG'64; Res., Royal Victoria Hosp., Montreal 2, P.Q.

MEDINA, Ernest S.; Santo Tomas (Philippines) '54; Res., St. Boniface Hosp., St. Boniface 6, **Man.**

MEDINA, Gideon; Manila Central (Philipp.)'61; Staff, Fogo Cottage Hosp., Fogo, Nfld.

MEDINE, Sidney M.; Family Med. Centre, 269 Lesperance Rd., Tecumseh, Ont.; 1715 Riverside Dr., Riverside (res); McG '40; MRCOG; ObstGyn; Sr. ObstGyn Staff, Grace, Hotel-Dieu & Metropolitan Hosp's., Windsor; Tel. 735-2128.

MEDLEY, Archie J.; R.R. No. 1., Glenburnie, **Ont. Qns '39.**

MEDLICOTT, Henry G.; Box 483, Pincher Creek, **Alta.; Trinity C. (Ire.) '53; B.A.O.**

MEDLINE, Alan; Wes'63; Res., Toronto Gen. Hosp., Toronto, Ont.

MEDLINE, Norton; Tor'60; Path; Staff, Kingston Gen. Hosp., Kingston, Ont.

MEDOVY, Harry; Rm. 12, Children's Hospital, Winnipeg 3, Man.; 133 Elm St. (res); Man '28; B.A.; FRCP(C); Paed; Paed-in-Chief, Children's Hosp.; Prof. & Hd., Dept. of Paed, U. of Man.; Cons., Child Health, City of Winnipeg; Tel. SP 5-8311.

MEDWAY, John G.; Box 728, Brooks, Alta.; Man '41.

MEECH, Lloyd R.; Peppem St., North Sydney, N.S.; Dal '15; GenSurg.

MEEHAN, Joseph E.; 540 Mount Pleasant Rd., Toronto, Ont.; Wes'50; Tel. HU 8-9528.

MEEKISON, William G.; UBC'62; Res., School of Hygiene, U. of Toronto, Toronto, Ont.

MEEMA, H. Erik; 106 Toronto Western Med. Bldg., **25 Leonard Ave., Toronto 2B, Ont.; 38 Princess Margaret Blvd., Islington (res); Karolinska Inst., (Stockholm, Sweden) '50;** DMR: DiagRad; Staff, Tor. Western Hosp.; Assoc. (Rad.), U. of Toronto; Tel. EM 3-1197.

MEEMA, Silvia (Veerus); 38 Princess Margaret Blvd., Islington, Ont. (res); Stockholm (Sweden) '51; Temp. Retired.

MEEN, Richard; Wes'63; Res., Ontario Hosp., Toronto 3, Ont.

MEERAFEL, Otto; Bienfait Coalfields Union Hosp., Bienfait, Sask.; Tel. 25; London (Eng) '58.

MEGILL, A. H.; 151 Holland Ave., Ottawa, Ont.; Qns '41; GenSurg.; Tel. 728-3788.

MEHL, Joseph F.; 340 McLeod, Ottawa 4, Ont.; Tubingen (Germany)'49; Otol.; Tel. 235-0469.

MEIHUIZEN, Sytse H.; 1940 Lonsdale Ave. N., Vancouver, B.C.; Amsterdam (Neth.) '52; Tel. YU 8-0414.

MEIKLE, Alexander L.; 88 River Rd., Winnipeg 8, Man. (res); Edinburgh (Scot.) '42; D.T.M. & H. (Eng.), D.M.R.(T), (Edin.); TherRad; Staff TherRad), St. Boniface Hosp.; Lect. (Rad.), U. of Manitoba; Tel. AL 3-1311.

MEIKLEJOHN, Robert B.; Ste. 329, Toronto-Western Hosp., Toronto, Ont.; Tor '32; F.R.C.-O.G., ObstGyn; Chief, Obst. Gyn., Toronto Western Hosp.; Prof. (Obst. Gyn), U. of Toronto; Tel. EM 6-3161.
MEILLEUR, Paul A.; Ste. 330, 4 Taschereau, Hull, P.Q.; Ott '55; IntMed. (P.Q.); Tel. PR 1-4975.
MEILLEUR, Rene; 1987 Boul. Rosemont, Montreal, P.Q.; Mon '46; M.C.G.P.; Tel. 272-1960.
MEILLEUR, Robert; 65 est, Grande-Allee, Quebec 4, P.Q.; Lav '62.
MEINDL, Alexander G.; 315 Medical Arts Bldg., Winnipeg, Man.; 924 Dorchester Ave. (res); McG '03; Hon. Staff, Misericordia Hosp., Winnipeg, Man.; Tel. WH 2-6174.
MEINDOK, Harry; London (Eng) '58; M.B., B.S., FRCP(C), IntMed; Staff, Toronto Western Hosp., Toronto, Ont.; Research Ass't., U. of Toronto; Tel. 368-2581.
MEINERS, Jean M.; (See Davey).
MEISELS, Alexandre K.; 2949 Gentilly, Quebec 10, P.Q. (res); Mexico '51; Dir. Dept. of Cytol., Dept. of Path., U. of Laval; Tel. 656-2702.
MEJIA, Manuel S.; Manila (Philipp.)'56; Sr. Psy., Saskatchewan Hosp., North Battleford, Sask.
MEKDECI, Anthony; Flemingdon Pk. Med. Centre, 747 Don Mills Rd., Don Mills, Ont.; West Indies'62; Tel. 429-1755.
MEKLER, Bernard S.; 262 Wilson Ave., Ste. 202, Downsview, Ont.; Tor '50; M.C.G.P.; Court. Staff, Northwestern Gen. Hosp., Toronto; Tel. ME 5-6611.
MELANCON, Denis; Mon'60; DiagRad(P.Q.); Staff, Hop. Ste-Justine, Montreal 18, P.Q.
MELANCON, Henri; Apt. 25, 1840 St. St. Marc, Shawinigan Falls, P.Q.; 1832 Georges (res); Lav '38; Otol (P.Q.); Tel. LE 6-5520.
MELANCON, Jacques J.; 3871 est, Belanger, Montreal 36, P.Q.; Mon '58; FRCP(C), IntMed; Staff, Hop. Hotel-Dieu; Tel. VI 4-0161.
MELANCON, Serge B.; Mon'65; Res., Hop. Notre-Dame, Montreal, P.Q.
MELANCON, Wilfrid; 955 Jean de Brebeuf, Drummondville, P.Q.; 643 Lindsay (res); Lav'19; GenSurg; Surg., Hop. Ste. Croix.
MELANSON, Emile R.; Grand-Vallee, Cte. Gaspe Nord, P.Q.; Lav'42.
MELANSON, Flavien J.; 305 Main St., Yarmouth, N.S.; Ste. Anne du Ruisseau (res); Lav '39; GenSurg; Staff, Regional Hosp.; Tel. 742-3242.
MELANSON, H. Paul; 1111 Main Et., Moncton, N.B.; McG '29; GenSurg; MCGP; Retired.
MELANSON, J. Arthur, Box 760, Dept. of Health, Fredericton, N.B.; 895 Charlotte St. **(res); Edinburgh (Scot.) '28; DPH; PH; Deputy** Minister of Health, Prov. of N.B.; Retired.
MELANSON, Jean L.; Memracook, N.B.; Ott '61. Abroad.
MELE, Victor L.; 846 Danforth Ave., Toronto 6, Ont.; Wes '62; Staff, St. Michael's & Toronto East Gen. Hosp's.; Tel. HO 1-0785.
MELGRAVE, Anthony P.; 2020 Glasgow Dr., Calgary, Alta. (res); London (Eng.) '54; M.B., B.S., M.R.C.S., L.R.C.P.; Anaes; Staff, Gen. Hosp.; Tel. CH 9-3801.
MELHADO, Gerald C.; 900 Sherbrooke W., Montreal, P.Q.; 900 Sherbrooke St. W. (res); McG '14; F.A.C.S., F.R.C.O.G., F.R.C.S.(C) ObstGyn; Hon. Att. Staff, Royal Victoria & Montreal Gen. Hosp's.; Tel. VI 5-5609.
MELINGRANA, Francesco: Ste 1128, 123 Edward St., Toronto, Ont.; Naples (Italy) '53; FRCP(C), IntMed; Staff, Cardiovasc. Unit, Toronto Gen. Hosp.; Tel. 366-0841.
MELILLO, Carlo; 112 St. Joseph's Blvd. W., Montreal 18, P.Q.; Naples (Italy) '29; Staff, Santa Cabrini Hosp.; Tel. 272-3335.
MELILLO, Ennio; 247 King St. Welland, Ont.; Naples (Italy) '47; Tel. 734-6410.
MELLING, John; Mulhurst, Alta.; Alb '57.
MELLING, M. Thomas; Hunt Clinic, 501 Hunt Bldg., Lethbridge, Alta.; Glasgow (Scot.)'57.
MELLING, Peter; 12920-103 Ave., Edmonton, **Alta.; Tor '23; Tel. HU 8-6327.**
MELLING, Thomas; Cancer Clin., Holy Cross Hosp., Calgary, Alta.; 2606-10th St. S.W. (res); Alb '31.
MELLISH, H. L.; Petitcodiac, N.B.; Dal '33.
MELLOR, Edmund; Manchester (Eng.) '45; Staff, Riverview Hosp., Essondale, B.C.
MELLOR-FRICKER, Mary D.; 619 Belmont Ave., Westmount 6, P.Q. (res); McG'30; IntMed; Ass't. Phys., Royal Victoria Hosp.; Tel. VI 2-1251.
MELLOR, Keith V.; Durham, Ont.; London (Eng.) '58; LRCP (Lond.), MRCS (Eng.); MCGP; Tel. 369-2510.
MELLOR, Norman; 2325 Central Ave., Victoria, B.C.; Leeds (Eng.) '46; Pt-time Phys., B.C. Alcoholism Fdn.; Tel. 386-2833.
MELLOW, Gordon A.; 51 Cambridge St., Guelph, Ont. (res); Qns '29; M.O., Ont. Reformatory, Guelph.
MELLOW, Ross C.; 42 King St. W., Stoney Creek, Ont.; 103 Grosvenor Ave. S., Hamilton (res); Tor '38; Tel. NO 2-7935.
MELLOWS, Frank S.; Cambridge (Eng.)'48; Paed; Staff, Hosp. for Sick Children, Toronto 2, Ont.
MELNYK, Demitro; 216 Northgate Bldg., Edmonton, Alta.; 10986-129th St. (res); Alb '43; MCGP; Sec. Med. Staff, Edmonton Gen. Hosp.; Tel. GA 4-2323.
MELNYK, Ferdinand; 2199 Bloor St. W., Toronto 9, Ont.; Heidelberg (Germ.) '49; MCGP; Tel. 762-2212.
MELOCHE, Bernard R.; 1150 est Boul. St.-Joseph, Montreal 34, P.Q.; 406 Ellerton, Ville Mt.-Royal (res); Mon '49; DABNS; FRCS(C), NeurSurg; Hd. (NeurSurg), Hop. Maisonneuve; Cons. Surg, Hop. Ste.-Justine, St.-Joseph-de-Rosemont & Misericordia Hosp.; Cons. Inst. Radium; Tel. LA 7-1241.
MELOCHE, Lorenzo; 4286 W. 8th Ave., Vancouver 8, B.C.; Mon '38; Anaes; Tel. CA 4-7585.
MELOCHE, Roger A.; Mon '60; Sr. Int., Hop. Notre-Dame, Montreal 24, P.Q.
MELOCHE, Rolland; Centre Medical de l'Est, 5965 Sherbrooke E., Montreal, P.Q.; Mon'65; Tel. 254-5394.
MELTZER, David B.; 1054 Brough St., London, Ont. (res); Wes '50; F.R.C.P.(C), IntMed; Haematol. & Cons. Med., St. Joseph's Hosp.; Cons., Med., Westminster Hosp.; Ass't. Prof. (Med. & PathChem) & Lect. Pharmacol., U. of Western Ontario; Tel. GE 9-3271.
MELTZER, Herbert; 505 Med. Arts Bldg., Edmonton, Alta.; 14127-98th Ave. (res); Man '29; D.A.B.T.S., F.A.C.S.; ThorSurg; Chief Surg. Serv. & ThorSurg., Chas. Camsell Hosp.; Att'd. Surg., Alberta University & Gen. Hosp's.; Lect. (Surg.), U. of Alberta; Tel. GA 4-1441.
MELVIE, Olaf A.; Ste. 213, 1632-14th Ave. N.W., Calgary, Alta.; Alb'62.
MELVILLE, Kenneth I.; 4937 Circle Rd., Montreal, P.Q. (res); McG '26; Hon. Cons. Staff, Royal Victoria Hosp.; Prof. of Pharm., & Chairman, Dept. of Pharm., McGill U.; Tel. VI 4-6311.
MELVILLE, Philip H.; Clarke Inst. of Psy., 250 College St., Toronto, Ont.; Tor'51; D.Psy; FRCP(C), Psy; Staff, Clarke Inst. & Wellesley Hosp.; Tel. 924-6811.
MELVIN, Roy; 200 Danforth Ave., Toronto, Ont.; 568 Castlefield Ave. (res); Tor '44; M.C.-G.P.; Tel. HO 5-1171.
MELVIN, W. James; 76 Johnston St., Kingston, Ont.; Qns '43; FRCS (Eng.); OrthSurg; Cons. OrthSurg., DVA, Brockville Gen. Hosp., Smiths Falls Public Hosp., Belleville Gen. Hosp. & Prince Edward County Hosp.; Assoc. Prof. (Surg.), Queen's U., Tel. 546-5775.
MEMON, Yacob M.; Sind (W. Pakistan) '62; Res., Victoria Gen. Hosp., Halifax, N.S.
MENARD, Albani; 226 St. Francois St., Southby Stn., Co. Wolfe, P.Q.; Lav '33.
MENARD, A. Eugene; 261 rue Hubert, Greenfield Pk., Cite-Jacques-Cartier, P.Q.; Mon '63.
MENARD, Bernard S.; 241 ouest rue Fleury, Montreal 12, P.Q.; 5560 ave. Stirling, Outremont (res); Mon '56; Psy; Staff, Hop. Notre-Dame; Tel. DU 1-7281.

MENARD, Claude; C.P. 2140, 346 Blvd. Gilman, Chibougamau, P.Q.; Lav'58; GenSurg(P.Q.); Med. Dir., Hop. Chibougamau; Tel. 276-3344.
MENARD, Claude-E.; Lav'64; Res., Hop. St-Sacrement, Quebec 6, P.Q.
MENARD, Emile; 1327 Blvd. St. Joseph E., Ste. 3, Montreal 34, P.Q.; 4090-Olivar-Asselin (res); Mon '25; IntMed; Sr. Ass't. (Med.), & Dir., Med. Library, Hop. Notre Dame; Tel. LA 5-6363.
MENARD, Jean; 2205 Place Richard, Shawinigan-Sud, Cte Maurice, P.Q.; Lav'59; Anaes; Staff, Hop. Ste-Therese; Tel. Le 6-4446.
MENARD, Jean C.; 912 est rue Sherbrooke, Montreal 24, P.Q.; McG'54; GenSurg (P.Q.); Staff, Hop.-Ste-Jeanne-d'Arc.
MENARD, Jules A.; 3094 Edgar, Fabreville, P.Q.; Mon '65.
MENARD, J. Victor; App 2, 899 Obrien St., North Bay, Ont.; Mon'29.
MENARD, Marcel; C.P. 217, Montebello, Co. Papineau, P.Q.; Mon'50; Staff, Hop. St. Michel, Buckingham; Tel. 423-6930.
MENARD, Yvon; Mon '64; Res., Hop. Hotel-Dieu; Sherbrooke, P.Q.
MENDELSOHN, Melvin; McG '61; Jr. Ass't. Res. (Otol.), Royal Victoria Hosp., Montreal, P.Q.; Abroad.
MENDELSON, Hyman I.; 1538 Sherbrooke St. W., Montreal, P.Q.; 5418 Victoria Ave. (res); McG '40; Staff, Jewish Gen. Hosp.; Tel. 735-3771.
MENDELSON, Jack; 203 Boyd Bldg., Winnipeg, Man.; 711 Borebank St. (res); Tor '44; D.A.B. Ophth., Ophth; Staff, Children's & Misericordia Hosp's.; Tel. WH 3-4859.
MENDELSON, Jack; 5789 Melling Ave., Montreal 29, P.Q.; McG'60; Bact(P.Q.).
MENDELSON, Murray; Anaesthesia Associates, 178 St. George St., Toronto, Ont.; 173 Old Forest Hill Rd. (res); Anaes; Staff, Toronto Gen. Hosp.; Tel. WA 3-1154.
MENDES, Peter C.; Baker Clinic, 10004-105th St., Edmonton, Alta.; Mon'59; Int.Med.; Tel. 424-2121.
MENETREZ, Gerda; Germany '49; Anaes; Staff, Queensway Gen. Hosp., Etobicoke, Ont.
MENG, Maurice; M.O., C.N.R. Clinic, 935 Lagauchetiere St. W., P.O. Box 8100, Montreal 3, P.Q.; McG '51; Tel. 877-5430.
MENGEBIER, Robert A.; 116 Indiana Dr., Sault-Ste.-Marie, Ont. (res); Wes '62; Staff, Sault-Ste.-Marie & Dist. Group Health Assoc.; Tel. AL 4-6634.
MENKES, Harold A.; 4326, W. 10th Ave., Vancouver 8, B.C.; UBC '63. Abroad.
MENTICOGLOU, Kyriacos; 227 Blvd. St. Joseph E., Montreal 14, P.Q.; Greece '49; Tel. VI 2-4582.
MENYASZ, Leslie; 208 Hammond Bldg., 310 Main St. N., Moose Jaw, Sask.; Pecs (Hung.) '37; Otol; Staff, Union & Providence Hosp's:; Tel. 692-1333.

MENZIES, Alexander M.; 2226 W. 40th Ave., Vancouver, B.C. (res); Man '21; D.P.H.; Retired.
MENZIES, Ernest C.; Fairville, N.B.; McG '24; Psy; Staff, Saint John Gen. Hosp., Saint John; Retired.
MENZIES, F. H.; 733 Pape Ave., Toronto, Ont.; 83 Airdrie Rd. (res); Tor '25; Tel. 421-3564.
MENZIES, James C.; Morden, Man.; Man '49; M.C.G.P.
MENZIES, M. Albert; 317 Royal Bank of Canada Bldg., 1489 W. Broadway, Vancouver 9, B.C.; 1476 W. 26th Ave. (res); Qns '45; D.Psy; Psy; Active Staff, Children's Hosp.; Pt.-time Psy., Mental Health Centre, Burnaby; Cons. Psy., Elizabeth Fry Group Living Home; Tel. RE 3-2042.
MENZIES, Nanette; 1476 W. 26th Ave., Vancouver 9, B.C. (res); U.K. '45; Part-time, Metro Health Comm.
MENZIN, A. W.; M.S., M.D. (Geneva, Switz.); Med. Staff, Ciba Co., Dorval, P.Q.
MEPHAM, Thomas E.; 451 King St. W., Hamilton, Ont.; Wes '31; Tel. JA 2-2088.
MERA, Zoltan; 2nd Ave., Bowladrome, Wilkie, Sask.; U. of Kolozsvar '37; FHCS (Hung.); LRCP&S (Edin.); LRCPS (Glasgow); Tel. 843-2235.

MERCANTINI, Edward S.; 280 Metcalfe St., Ottawa 4, Ont.; Ott'55; DABD; Derm; Active Staff & Pres. Advisory Council, School of Nursing, Ottawa Gen. Hosp.; Cons. (Derm.), St.-Louis-Marie-de-Montford, Ott. & Sacred Heart Hosp., Hull; Ass't. Prof. (Derm.), Ottawa U.; Tel. CE 5-7935.

MERCER, Alvin R.; Med. Arts Bldg., Empire Ave., St. John's, Nfld.; 157 Patrick St. (res); Dal'49; Urol; Staff, Gen. Hosp.; Tel. 578-0387.

MERCER, Donald D.; Box 150, Southampton, Ont.; Wes '58.
MERCER, Edward N.; 4077 W. 32nd Ave., Vancouver 8, B.C.; UBC'60; FRCP(C), IntMed.
MERCER, John E.; 8330 Fairmont Dr., Calgary, Alta.; Belfast (Ire.) '50; GenSurg; Staff, Holy Cross, Children's & Calgary Gen. Hosp's.; Tel. 252-1161.
MERCER, Mona C.; 14 Brock Ave. N., Montreal West, P.Q.; McG '50; Tel. 488-6179.
MERCER, Stanley; Central Med. Bldg., 1105 Carling Ave., Ottawa 3, Ont.; 542 Hillcrest (res); Queen's U. (Belfast, N. Ire.) '47; D.Obst; R.C.O.G.; F.A.A.P.; F.R.C.S.(C), GenSurg; Paed; Surg., Ottawa Civic Hosp.; Lect., Clin. Surg., U. of Ottawa; Tel. PA 9-2741.

MERCIER, Alcide; 908-6eme Ave., La Pocatiere, P.Q.; Lav'65.
MERCIER, Arthur; Lav '42; Urol (PQ.); Staff, Hop.-St.-Sacrement, Quebec, P.Q.; Ass't. Prof., Laval U.
MERCIER, Cecilius; 117 Notre Dame S., Thetford Mines, P.Q.; 512 rue Dute (res); Lav '36.
MERCIER, Gaston; Ste 640, 1500 18eme rue, Quebec 3, P.Q.; Lav'55; IntMed & Cardiol. (P.Q.); Teach Staff, Hop. Enfant Jesus; Tel. 525-8118.
MERCIER, Jean; 8415 St.-Denis, Montreal 11, P.Q.; Mon '53; Urol (PQ); Tel. 381-1801.
MERCIER, Jean J.; 313 Laurier Ave. E., Ottawa 2, Ont.; 511 Blair (res); Lav '49; F.R.C.P.(C); IntMed; Staff, (Med.), U. of Ottawa; Tel. CE 6-2055.
MERCIER, Jean P.; Lav'65; Res., Hop. Hotel-Dieu, Quebec 4, P.Q.
MERCIER, Lucien; 912 E. rue Sherbrooke, Montreal 24, P.Q.; Lav'51; ObstGyn.
MERCIER, Marc; 760-3rd Ave., C.P. 537, Val-d'Or, P.Q.; 900-6th Ave. (res); Lav '48; MCGP.
MERCIER, Marcel; 15 Ave Begin, Levis, P.Q.; Lav '55; Ophth; Tel. 837-4483.
MERCIER, Raymond; 1308 de la Visitation, Quebec 10, P.Q.; Lav '45; MCGP. Retired.
MERCIER, Roger J.; Ste. 208, 2120 est rue Sherbrooke, Montreal 24, P.Q.; Mon'60.

MERCURE, Justin; 62 Sacre-Coeur, Charlemagne, P.Q.; Lav '55; Tel. 581-1900.
MERCURE, L. Claude; Mon '61; Paed; Staff, Hop.-Ste.-Justine, Montreal, P.Q.; Tel. RE 1-4931.

MEREDITH, Allan R.; Ilderton, Ont.; Wes '58; MCGP.
MEREDITH, John T.; 11 Coldwater St., Orillia, Ont.; 331 Colborne St. W. (res); Tor '39; M.C.G.P.
MEREDITH, Rice H.; 82 Old Mill Rd., Toronto 18, Ont.; Tor '28; F.I.C.A.; Anaes; Cons. Toronto Western Hosp.; Ass't. Prof. (Anaes), U. of Toronto; Tel. BE 3-9611.

MEREI, Leslie; 742 King St. W., Kitchener, Ont.; 100 Foresthill Dr. (res); Pecs (Hung.) '39; D.L.O.; Otol; Staff, Kitchener-Waterloo, St. Mary's & S. Waterloo Mem. Hosp's.; Tel. 744-5219.

MERGELAS, James E.; Tor'61; Res., Dept. of Rad., St. Michael's Hosp., Toronto, Ont.

MERGLER, Leo; 530 Seaforth Med. Bldg., 3550 Cote des Neiges Rd., Montreal 25, P.Q.; McG '50; Psy; Clin. Ass't. (Psy.), Allan Mem. Inst.; Cons. (Psy.), Rehab. Inst.; Dem. (Psy.), McGill U.; Tel. 932-5057.

MERKELEY, Norman P.; 325 Med. Arts Bldg., Winnipeg, Man.; 230 Queenston St. (res.); Man '40; Ch.M., F.A.C.S., F.R.C.S.(C), GenSurg; PlasSurg; Staff, Wpg. Gen. & Children's Hosp's.; Chief of Surg, Grace Hosp.; Ass't. Prof. Surg.; U. of Man.; Tel. WH 3-0073.

MERLER, Claudio; 2661 E. Hastings St., Vancouver 6, B.C.; Lav '55; Gen Surg.
MERLER, Thomas; 2661 E. Hastings St., Vancouver 6, B.C.; Innsbruck (Aust.) '18; Tel. 255-2120.
MERRIAM, Richard K.; Drawer 608, Red Deer, Alta.; 3423 Spruce Dr. (res); Dal'52; DMR (McG); D & TRad; Cons. Staff, Red Deer Mun. & Dist. Hosp's.; Tel. 346-2042.
MERRICK, Bruce W.; 2160 Weston Rd., Toronto 15, Ont.; Tor '61; Tel. CH 4-5566.
MERRICK, Harold K., F/L; Man '64; Staff, Can. Forces Med. Service, Camp Borden, Ont.
MERRICK, William G.; Man '58; Jr. Int'n., St. Boniface Hosp., St. Boniface, Man.
MERRIMAN, John E.; Qns '47; F.R.C.P.(C), IntMed(Cardiol.); Dir. Cardiopulm. Lab., University Hosp., Saskatoon, Sask.; Att'd. Phys., University Hosp.; Cons. Phys. City & St. Paul Hosp's.; Assoc. Prof. (Med.), U. of Saskatchewan; Tel. CH 2-7641.
MERRITT, John O.; 49 Main St., Lambeth, Ont.; Wes '43; M.C.G.P.; Dist. Coroner; Tel. 652-3255.
MERRITT, Lorne E.; 121 Oakdale, St. Catharines, Ont.; Tor '46; M.C.G.P.; Staff (Paed.), St. Catharines Gen. Hosp.; Staff (Paed.), Hotel-Dieu Hosp.; Tel. MU 5-8700.
MERRITT, Robert L.; Ste. 2, 168 Ontario St., St. Catharines, Ont.; Qns'50; FRCS(C); ObstGyn.
MERRY, Colin C.; 25 Turgeon Cr., Regina, Sask. (res); London (Eng.) '59; LRCP; MRCS; Assoc. Path., Regina Grey Nuns Hosp.; Tel. 527-9641.
MERRY, George M.; 253 Ontario St., Kingston, Ont.; Ott'65; Tel. 548-7819.
MERTENS, Donald J.; 89 Ambridge Dr., Ansonville, Ont.; Durham (Eng.) '63; Staff Phys., Anson Gen. Hosp., Iroquois Falls; Tel. 1043.
MERTENS, Gustaaf A.; R.R.1. Hespeler, Ont. (res); Leiden (Neth.) '50; Path; Dir. of Labs., South Waterloo Mem. Hosp., Galt, Ont.; Tel. 621-2330
MESBUR, J. Boris; Regina Med. Centre, 1847 Rose St., Regina, Sask.; 3230 Retallack St. (res); Man '36; M.C.G.P.; Sr. Staff, Regina Gen. & Regina Grey Nuns' Hosp's.; Teaching Staff, Nurses Training School, Regina Grey Nun's Hosp.; Tel. 522-6661.
MESBUR, Kenneth H.; Box 99, Arkona, Ont.; Ireland'57; Tel. 822-3563.
MESAGLIO, N. R.; Tor'65; Res., St. Michael's Hosp., Toronto 2, Ont.
MESSECAR, Clyde R.; Apt. 910, 265 Markland Dr., Etobicoke, Ont.; Tor'37; FCCP; FAGS; Temporarily Retired.
MESSENGER, Donald B.; Kirkland Med. Group, **42-2nd St., Kirkland Lake, Ont.; 95 Government** Rd. E. (res); Tor '28; M.C.G.P.
MESSER, Vernon R.; 2222 Alexis Rd., Windsor, Ont.; 5 Vernon Court, Riverside (res); Wes '47; Tel. 945-1149.
MESSIER, Alain; Clinique Medicale de Bedford, Place d'Estrie, Bedford, P.Q.; Mon'63; Tel. 248-3336.
MESSIER, Charles A.; 3600 Ave. Barclay, Ste. 360, Montreal 26, P.Q.; Mon '44; F.C.C.P.; Head (Broncho-Oesoph.) & Teach. Staff, Hop. Ste. Justine; Member, Civil Defense of Canada; Tel. RE 1-4931.
MESSIER, Michel; Mon '64; Res., Inst. Albert Prevost, Montreal, P.Q.; Abroad.
MESSIER, Myrto; 228 Longueuil, St. Jean, P.Q.; Mon'58; IntMed(P.Q.); Cardiol(P.Q.).
MESSINGER, Moses J.; 271 Cote-St.-Catherine Rd., Montreal 8, P.Q.; McG '22; FAAA; MCAA (All. PQ); IntMed; Hon. Att'd. Staff, Jewish Gen. Hosp.; Tel. 274-6655.
MESTER, Zoltan; 262 St. Clair Ave. W., Toronto 7, Ont.; 5889 Bathurst St., Willowdale, Ont.; Cluj (Hung.)'37; GenSurg; Staff, Central Hosp., & North York Branson Hosp., Willowdale; Tel. 222-6761.
MESZAROS, Anthony F.; 604 cote St-Antoine, Montreal 6, P.Q.; Budapest (Hung.) '39; Psy; Psy., D.V.A., St. Anne's & Queen Mary Hosp's.; **Tel. 483-4340.**
MESZAROS, George; Mall Med. Bldg., 280 Osborne St. N., Winnipeg, Man.; Man'52.
METCALFE, Earl V.; 24 Renwick Ave., London, Ont.; Wes '33; D.Psy; Psy; Chief of Serv. (Psy), Westminster Hosp.; Ass't. Prof. (Psy. & Prev.Med.), U. of Western Ont.; Telephone GE 4-7630.
METCALFE, Herbert G.; 340 McLeod St., Ottawa 4, Ont.; Qns'51; Urol; Staff (Urol.), Ottawa Civic & Grace Hosp's. & DND Med. Centre; Tel. 233-5953.
METCALFE, James O.; 421 Medical Arts Bldg., 11010 Jasper Ave., Edmonton, Alta.; Alb'46; FACS, FRCS(C), Urol.; Dir. Div. of Urol., University Hosp.; Clin. Prof. (Urol.), Div. of Urol. (Surg.), U. of Alberta; Tel. 422-2174.
METCALFE, McColl; 87 Bessborough Dr., Toronto, Ont.; McG '16. Tel. 421-9587.
METELSKY, Natalie J.; (See Romanick).
METH, Bernard; 407 North Rd., New Westminster, B.C.; Wes'39; MCGP; Chmn., Educ. Committ., Royal Columbian Hosp.; Indust. Phys., Imperial Oil Co. & Crane of Canada Ltd.; Exec., College of G.P., B.C. Chapter; Tel. 939-9232.
METHOT, Andre L.; Lav'61; Res., Hop. St. Sacrement, Quebec 6, P.Q.
METHOT, J. Paul; 12260 Taylor, Bordeaux, Montreal, P.Q.; Mon '49; Anaes (P.Q.); Staff, Hop. St. Joseph de Rosemont; Tel. CL 6-2681.
METHOT, Yvan; 1656 est, rue Sherbrooke, Montreal 24, P.Q.; 5558 Blvd. Pie (res); Lav '49; D&T Rad; Staff, Hop. Notre-Dame; Tel. LA 5-6363.
METIVIER, Pierre; St. Isidore, Cte. Dorchester, P.Q.; Lav'65; Tel. 646-5690.
METRAKOS, Katherine; 3757 Marlowe, Montreal, P.Q.; McG'49; Dir. of Electroenceph., Montreal Children's Hosp.; Chief Phys., Convulsive Disorders Clin.; Ass't. Neurol., O.P.D.; Tel. WE 7-8511, Loc. 320, 371.
METTEN, Damian; Box 594, Fort Nelson, B.C.; London (Eng.)'61; Staff (G.P.), Fort Nelson Gen. Hosp.; Tel. 774-6555.
METZLER, William S.; 1516 Bathurst St., Toronto 10, Ont.; 362 Glencairn Ave., Toronto 12 (res); Tor '39; F.R.C.P.(C), IntMed; Staff, St. Joseph's Hosp.; Tel. LE 5-3424.
MEUNIER, Andre; 3005, Viel, Montreal 12, P.Q. (res); Mon '57; Diag Rad; Staff, Hop. Sacre Coeur; **Tel. FE 4-1210.**
MEUNIER, Pierre E.; Ste. 309, 3875 rue St-Urbain, Montreal 18, P.Q.; Mon '36; FRCS(C); Gyn; Chief, Dept. of Gyn., Hop. Hotel-Dieu; Assoc. Prof. (Gyn.), U. of Montreal; Tel. 288-9465.
MEUNIER, Robert C.; Apt. 1, 1402 Blvd. Pius **IX, Montreal 4, P.Q.; Min '45; M.C.G.P.; Tel. LA 7-2419.**
MEUWISSEN, Hilaire; Holland '57; Res., Vancouver Gen. Hosp., Vancouver 9, B.C.
MEWBURN, Robert H.; 1070 W. 53rd Ave., Vancouver 14, B.C.; McG '50; Research Fell., Dept. **of Neurological Research, U. of British Columbia; Tel. AM 1-1762.**
MEWHORT, Cuthbert W.; Box 760, Lake Cowichan, B.C.; Park Rd. (res); Tor '41; MCGP; Tel. 749-6621.
MEYER, Clifford R.; Qns'65; Res. (ObstGyn.), Kingston Gen. Hosp., Kingston, Ont.
MEYER, Dietmar, F/L; R.C.A.F., Baden Soellinger, Germany; Man '64. Abroad.
MEYER, Edith (See Mankiewicz)
MEYER, Ernest G.; Tor'38; FRCS(C), Urol; GenSurg; Staff, W.C.B. Rehab. Hosp., Torbarrie Rd., Downsview, Ont.
MEYER, Ivan H.; Climax, Sask.; St. Bart's (London, Eng.) '40; MRCS(Eng.), LRCP(Lond.); FRCS; FAGS; Ph.D., Med. Supt., Climax-Bracken Union Hosp. MOH, Lone Tree Mun.; Dist. Coroner; Tel. 17.
MEYER, J. P. O.; Hamburg (Germ.) '57; Fell., Nat. Research Council (Path), Queen's U., Kingston, Ont.
MEYER, Maurice J. M.; 8 Albert St. E., Sault Ste. Marie, Ont.; 99 Pine St. (res); Qns '58; Active Staff, Plummer & Gen. Hosp's.; Tel. AL 4-3141. Abroad.
MEYERS, John F.; Mon'61; GenSurg(P.Q.); Staff, Hop.-Hotel-Dieu, Montreal, P.Q.

M'GONIGLE, Arthur C.; 776 Westcot Place, West Vancouver, B.C.; Tor'34; FRCS(C), GenSurg.
M'GONIGLE, Rowland H.; Saint Andrews, N.B.; Tor '26; M.A.; Retired.
MHEIR-EL-SAADI, Abdul-Halim; 2965 rue de Louisbourg, Montreal 12, P.Q.; Paris (France) '56; DiagRad.
MIAN, Maqbul A.; Mental Health Centre, Cape Breton Plaza, Sydney River, N.S.; Punjab (India) '56; Tel. 562-3202.
MICHAELS, Leon; Manitoba Clinic, 790 Sherbrook St., Winnipeg 2, Man.; 154 Queenston St. (res); London (Eng.) '46; MRCP(Lond.); Ph.D. (Lond.); FRCP(C), IntMed; Phys., Wpg. Gen. Hosp.; Cons. (Cardiol.), Man. Rehab. Hosp.; Dem. (Med.), U. of Manitoba; Tel. SP 4-6541.
MICHAELS, Leslie; Sudbury Gen. Hosp., Sudbury, Ont.; London (Eng.) '49; M.D. (Lond.); MC (Path); DABP; D.Path; FCAP; Path; Dir. of Labs., Sudbury Gen. Hosp.; Tel. 673-3601.
MICHALKOFF, Michael W.; 260 St. Patrick St., Ottawa 2, Ont.; Innsbruck (Austria) '49; Staff, (Anaes), St.- Louis-Marie-de-Montfort; Tel. SH 6-4621.
MICHALOVSKY, Leo; 495 Bathurst St., Toronto 2B, Ont.; 238 Lonsmount Dr. (res); **Prague (Czech) '29; MCGP; Court. Staff, New Mt. Sinai Hosp.; Tel. WA 1-8843.**
MICHALSKI, Adam; 20 Sherman Ave. N., Hamilton, Ont.; 45 London S. (res); Man '30; Active Staff, Hamilton Civic Hosp.; Court Staff, St. Joseph's Hosp.; Dist. Coroner; Tel. LI 4-2565.
MICHALYSHYN, Bohdan; 403 Medical Arts. Bldg., Edmonton, Alta.; 7505—1118 St. (res); Alb '42; F.A.C.S.; F.R.C.S.(C) GenSurg; Clin. Prof. **(Surg.), U. of Alberta; Tel. 422-2767.**
MICHAUD, Alphee; Lav'65; Res., Hop. St. Sacrement, Quebec 6, P.Q.
MICHAUD, Andre; 395 rue Collard, Alma, P.Q.; Lav'49; FRCS(C); GenSurg; Joint Head, Surg. Staff, Hop. Hotel-Dieu d'Alma; Tel. 662-9642.
MICHAUD, Andre J.; 1120 Ouellette Ave., Windsor, Ont.; Ott'58; Tel. 252-6525.
MICHAUD, Camille; St-Paulin, P.Q.; Dist. Coroner; Lav '32.
MICHAUD, Charles E.; 794-5th St., Shawinigan, P.Q.; McG '51; Active Staff, Joyce Mem. & Grand 'Mere Gen. Hosp's.; Med. Dir., City of Shawinigan; Plant Phys., Consolidated Paper Corp.; Med. Exam., Hydro Quebec, Shawinigan Area; Tel. 537-6411.
MICHAUD, Claude; Suite 510, 801 est rue Sherbrooke, Montreal 24, P.Q.; Mon'55; Ophth; Tel. 524-3049.
MICHAUD, Gilbert; 1500 18eme rue, Quebec 3, P.Q.; 11 Ave. Beaumont (res); Lav '56; ObstGyn (P.Q.); Tel. 661-6692.
MICHAUD, J. Baptiste; 98 Longueuil St., Longueuil, Montreal, **P.Q.;** Mon '27.
MICHAUD, Jean G.; Lav '58; Res., Hop. Notre-Dame, Montreal, P.Q.
MICHAUD, J. Raymond; Spiritwood, **Sask.;** Lav '55; Tel. 68.
MICHAUD, J. Rheal; 45 Elm St. E., Sudbury, Ont.; Ott'53; FRCS(C), GenSurg; Pres., Sudbury Cardio-Thoracic Research Fdn.; Tel. 674-5951.
MICHAUD, Laurent J.; 565 rue Commerciale, La Tuque, P.Q.; 21 rue Corbeil (res); Lav '44; FICS; GenSurg; Staff, Hop. St.-Joseph; Tel. 523-4581.
MICHAUD, Laurent-V.; 391 Blvd. Ste. Madeleine, Cap de la Madeleine, P.Q.; Lav '43.
MICHAUD, Marc R.; 700 Ste-Julie, Trois Rivieres, P.Q.; Lav'60; OrthSurg(P.Q.).
MICHAUD, Paul; 554 King est, Sherbrooke, P.Q.; Mon'65.
MICHAUD, Richard; 800 ouest boul. Gouin, Montreal 12, P.Q.; Mon'60; Psy.
MICHAUD, R. J.; 195 Laurier Ave. E., Ottawa, **Ont.; Att. Cons. (Rad.), Ottawa Gen. Hosp.; Tel. CE 6-4592.**
MICHAUD, Robert; 241 ouest Fleury, Montreal 12, P.Q.; Lav'54; FCCP; FACCP; FAGS; IntMed; Cardiol. (P.Q.); Chief of Med. Serv., Hop. Gen. Fleury, Montreal; Cons. (Med.), St. Charles Hop.; Tel. PR3-1362.
MICHAUD, Rodolphe; 195 Ave. Laurier E., Ottawa, Ont.; 150 Driveway **(res); Mon '16; D & TRad.; Tel. 232-1490.**
MICHAUD, Roger; 8415 rue St. Denis, Montreal 11, P.Q.; 11965 **Bois** de Boulogne, Bordeaux; Lav '51; **Tel. 334-7871.**
MICHAUD, Roger C.; 34 rue Frontenac, Lac Megantic, P.Q.; '62.
MICHAUD, Thomas W.; St. Pacome, P.Q.; Lav '01.
MICHAUD, Yvan; Mon'64; Res., Hop. Notre-Dame, Montreal 24, P.Q.
MICHAUD, Yvan C.; Lav'62; Res., Neurological Inst., 3801 University, Montreal 2, P.Q.
MICHEL, Ernest R.; Tor'65; Res., Dept. of Anaes., Toronto Western Hosp., Toronto 2B, Ont.
MICHEL, Philippe; 103-1111 Bldg., Main St., Moncton, N. B.; Haiti '42; Psy.; Tel. 382-5081.
MICHELL, W. A. Rupert; 312 Fairmont Ave., Ottawa, Ont. (res); Tor '02; D.P.H.; Retired.
MICHIE, Thomas C.; 302 Admin Bldg., 109th St. & 98th Ave., Edmonton, Alta.; Alb'26; Psy.; Clin. Prof. Psy., U. of Alberta.
MICHON, J. Bertrand; Ste. 208, 30 est Boul. St. Joseph, Montreal 14, P.Q.; Mon'58; FRCS(C); ObstGyn; Staff, Hop. Notre-Dame; Tel. LA 5-6363.
MICKELSON, Cecil H.; 742 King St. W., Kitchener, Ont.; Alb'48; D.Psy.; Psy; Dir., Mental Health Clinic, Kitchener-Waterloo Hosp.; Tel. 745-0711.
MICKELSON, W. Phillip; 195 Woodruffe Ave., Ottawa 13, Ont.; Alb'60; **Staff,** Dept. of National Health & Welfare.
MICKEVICIUS, V. Alexander; Box 425, Renfrew, Ont.; Tor'63.
MICROYS, Gisele I. (Michael); Albany Clinic, 200 Danforth Ave., Toronto, Ont.; Tor '63.
MIDDLEBRO, Arthur S.; 138—10th St. W., **Owen Sound, Ont.; 1114—4th Ave. W. (res); Tor '36;** Anaes.; Tel. 376-0108.
MIDDLEBRO, J. Geldard; 3052-3rd Ave. W., Owen Sound, Ont.; Tor '36; Staff, Phys., Ontario Hosp.
MIDDLEBRO, John P.; 3052-3rd Ave. W., Owen Sound, Ont.; Tor '25; FRCS (Edin.); FACS; FRCS(C), GenSurg; Sr. Surg. Staff, Owen Sound Gen. & Marine Hosp.; Tel. 376-0385.
MIDDLEMASS, Ian B.; 254 Robina Rd., Ancaster, Ont. (res); Edinburgh (Scot.) '47; MB., Ch. B., M.D.; DMRD; DiagRad; Rad., Chedoke & Children's Hosp's.; Rad., West Haldimand Gen. Hosp., Hagersville; Tel. 385-4341.
MIDDLEMASS, Joseph G.; 1202-4th Ave., Wainwright, Alta.; Tor '06; Dist. Coroner.
MIDDLEMISS, Kenneth C. H.; 122 First St., Kirkland Lake, Ont. (res); Tor '51; DMR; D&T-Rad; Cons. Rad., Kirkland & Dist. Hosp., New Liskeard & Dist. Hosp., Englehart Dist. Hosp. & Misericordia Hosp., Haileybury; Tel. 567-5251.
MIDDLETON, Donald G.; Qns'65; Res., Sunnybrook Hosp., Toronto 12, Ont.
MIDDLETON, Frederick C., M.B.E.; 2322 Robinson St., Regina, Sask. (res); Tor '07; D.P.H.; Retired.
MIDDLETON, Kenneth R.; Ste. 101, 15496 North Bluff Rd., White Rock, B.C.; 14472 Malabar Cr. (res); Edinburgh (Scot.) '51; Staff, Peace Arch Dist. Hosp.; Tel. 531-5595.
MIDDLETON, Lyall A.; 658 Grace St., Lachute, P.Q.; McG '25.
MIDDLETON, Peter M.; London (Eng.)51; DPM; Psy; Clin. Dir., Riverview Hosp., Essondale, B.C.; Clin. Instr., U. of British Columbia; Tel. LA 1-1911.
MIDDLETON, Raymond J.; 14 King St., Hespeler, Ont.; Qns'57; Tel. 658-4361.
MIDDLETON, William L. C.; Murrayville, B.C.; Urol; Retired.
MIDDLETON, William W.; Beck Mem. San., London, Ont.; 570 Wellington St. (res); **Wes '31;** F.C.C.P.; IntMed(TB); Ass't. Med. Dir., Beck Mem. San.; Cons. DVA Westminster Hosp.; Clin. Lect., U. of Western Ontario; Tel. 471-1440
MIDGLEY, G. Harold; 14 George St. N., Galt, Ont.; Tor '39; M.C.G.P.

MIDGLEY, Robert D.; McG'60; FRCS(C), PlasSurg; Staff, Montreal Gen. Hosp., Montreal, P.Q.

MIELKE, Bruce W.; 11044-80th Ave., Edmonton, Alta.; Alb '59; FRCP(C), Path; Instr. (Path.), U. of Alberta; Tel. GE 9-8721.

MIERAU, Peter H.; 200 Glenwood Cres., Winnipeg 9, Man. (res); Odessa (U.S.S.R.) '39; Ass't. Path., Misericordia Gen. Hosp.; Tel. SP 4-6581.

MIGHTON, Albert K., M.B.E.; 206 Medical Arts Bldg., Hamilton, Ont.; 126 Aberdeen Ave. (res); Tor '41; F.R.C.S.(C), GenSurg; Surg., Staff, Hamilton Gen. & St. Joseph's Hosp's.; Tel. JA 7-8773.

MIGNAULT, Alexander A.; 146 Sanborn St., Sherbrooke, P.Q.; 1381 Ontario St. (res); Lav '26; ObstGyn (P.Q.); Tel. 562-1233.

MIGNAULT, Gerard; 12485 St. Castin Pl., Montreal 12, P.Q. (res); Mon '49; Anaes; Ass't. Hd. Dept. of Anaes., Hop.-Hotel-Dieu; Tel. 331-5272.

MIGNAULT, Jean de L.; 3840 St. Urbain, Montreal, P.Q.; 7660 des Vendeens, Mtl. 5 (res); Mon '51; FACC; FCCP, Cardiol (PQ); Dir. Hemodynam. Lab., Hotel-Dieu; Ass't. Prof. (Med.), U. of Montreal; Tel. VI 4-0161, Loc. 371.

MIGNEAULT, Pierre; Inst., Albert-Provost, 6555 ouest, boul Gouin, Montreal 9, P.Q.; Mon '63; Tel. 372-2148; Abroad.

MIGUELINO, Oliver M.; Santo Tomas (Philipp.) '57; Staff, Botwood Cottage Hosp., Botwood, Nfld.

MIKEL, Donald E.; 205 Bagot St., Cobourg, Ont.; Front Rd. E. (res); Tor'47; Tel. 372-2148.

MIKELSONS, Velta K. (Slesers); Riga (Latvia) '42; Anaes (P.Q.); Staff, Montreal Children's Hosp., Montreal 25, P.Q.; Tel. 937-8511.

MIKI, Patrick Y.; 127 Church Ave., Chilliwack, B.C.; 2441 McCallum Rd., Abbotsford; Box 760, Langley, B.C.; Man'55; DiagRad; Cons. Rad., Chilliwack Gen. Hosp., MSA Hosp., Abbotsford, Mission Mem. Hosp., Mission, Langley Mem. Hosp., Langley; Tel. 795-7205, 859-4888, 534-4114.

MIKLOS, Laszlo S.; P.O. Box 39, Newcastle Ont.; Budapest (Hungary) '43; M.C.G.P.; Staff, Bowmanville Mem. Hosp.; Tel. 987-4220.

MIKLOSIK, Stephen; Tor '60; Res., Queen Mary Vet's. Hosp., Montreal, P.Q.

MIKOLAJEWSKI, Jerzy; 410 Boyd Bldg., 388 Portage Ave., Winnipeg 1, Man.; London (Eng.) '56; Psy; Psy., Child Guidance Clinic of Greater Wpg., Psychiatric Inst., Care Services; University of Manitoba Counselling Service; Lect., (Dept. of Psy.), University of Manitoba; Tel. 947-1820.

MILANESE, Charles A.; 203 Halter Bldg., 419 Graham Ave., Winnipeg 1, Man.; Man '48; Ophth; Staff, St. Boniface, Misericordia, Children's, & DVA Hosp's & St. Boniface San.; Tel. WH 3-8102.

MILAWSKI, William; 604 Brant St., Burlington, Ont.; Wes '61; AMCGP.

MILBANK, Reginald J.; Workmen's Comp. Bd., 7123-119th St., Edmonton, Alta.; Guys H. (London, Eng.)'26; Tel. 433-4231.

MILBRANDT, W. E.; Heather & 37 Ave., Vancouver, B.C.; 6925 Cypress (res); Man '38; Med. Dir., Rehab. Dept., Workmen's Comp. Board of B.C.; Tel. AM 6-0211.

MILBURN, Charles W.; 210 Dixon Rd., R.R. No. 1. Weston, Ont.; Tor '53; Assoc. Staff, Humber Mem. Hosp.; Tel. 249-8111.

MILBURN, Helen Y. B.; 376 Willard Ave., Toronto, Ont. (res); Tor '19; D & TRad; Retired.

MILBURN, Lewis H.; Wes'57; (Intern), c/o 1396 Goyeau, Windsor, Ont.

MILBURN, T. Henry H.; 2435 MacDonald St., Vancouver, B.C.; 1915 Haro St. (res); Qns '08; Cons. in Med., St. Paul's Hosp.; Ind. Phys., American Can. Co.; Tel. RE 3-9214.

MILEIKO, William; 537 College St., Toronto, Ont.; 159 Sorauren Ave. (res); Ott'63; MCGP; Court. Staff (G.P.), St. Joseph's Hosp.; Tel. 921-2052.

MILES, Albert E.; 126 Dufferin St., Belleville, Ont.; Qns'42; MCGP; Active Staff, Dept. of G.P. & Surg., Belleville Gen. Hosp.; Tel. WO 2-0666.

MILES, James E.; McG '53; MCGP; Res., Vancouver Gen. Hosp., Vancouver 9, B.C.; Abroad.

MILETTE, Rosaire; 200 St. Damase, Ste. Jean Baptiste, Drummondville, P.Q.; Lav '50; Anaes (P.Q.); Tel. GR 2-5055.

MILFORD, Donald M.; 111 Queen St. E., Toronto 1, Ont.; Dal '60.

MILIAN, Edmund Z.; 501 Dundas St. E., Whitby, Ont.; Lwow (Poland) '34.

MILICEVIC, Jure; Federal Electric Corp., International Airport, Winnipeg, Man.; Zagreb (Yugo.)'55; MCGP; Tel. SU 6-1441.

MILLAN, Victor G.; 598 Selkirk Avenue, Winnipeg 4, Man.; Ste. 217-571 Wardlaw Ave. (res); Man '58; MCGP; Tel. JU 9-4897.

MILLAR, Herbert A.; 1960A Eglinton Ave. W., Toronto 10, Ont.; 77 Greenbrook Dr., Tor 15 (res); Queen's U. (Belfast, N. Ire.) '50; M.C.-G.P.; Tel. RU 3-4901.

MILLAR, Irene E.; Box 816, New Westminster, B.C.; 15469-86th Ave., N. Surrey (res); Qns '54; M.Sc. (Med.); Anaes; Tel. LA 1-5197.

MILLAR, J. Charles; 495 Annette St., Toronto 9, Ont.; 207 Riverside Dr. (res); Qns '41; Staff, Toronto Western Hosp.; Tel. RO 7-2525.

MILLAR, John; The Clinic, Sioux Lookout, Ont.; Glasgow (Scot.) '44.

MILLAR, John W.; Ste. 340, 5780 Cambie St., Vancouver 15, B.C.; Man '38; ObstGyn; Chief of Staff, Grace Hosp.; Ass't. Clin. Prof., U. of British Columbia; Tel. FA 5-6113.

MILLAR, Kenneth G.; 69 King St., Picton, Ont.; St. Andrew's (Scot.)'59.

MILLAR, Leslie P.; P.O. Box 610, 9 Saskatchewan Ave., Portage-la-Prairie, Man.; 635 Queen Ave. E. (res); Glasgow (Scot.) '54; Pres. Med. Staff, Portage Dist. Hosp.; Med. Adviser, Public Health Unit; Tel. 857-4398; Abroad.

MILLAR, Owen B.; Ste. G. 01, 3000 Lawrence Ave. E., Scarborough, Ont.; 37 Hill Cres. (res); Tor '41; D.R., F.F.R. (Eng.), D.A.B.R., F.R.-C.P.(C), D & T Rad; Rad., Scarborough Gen. Hosp.; Cons. (Rad.), Sunnybrook & Women's College Hosp's.; Tel. 291-1121.

MILLAR, Robert D.; 2175 W. 49th Ave., Vancouver 13, B.C.; Alb '37; Anaes; Anaes., St. Vincent's Hosp., Vancouver; Tel. TR 6-7171.

MILLAR, Teresa A.; Box 610, Portage La Prairie, Man.; Man'52; Abroad.

MILLAR, Thomas P.; 913 Fairmont Medical Bldg., 750 W. Broadway, Vancouver 9, B.C.; McG '51; Psy.; Tel. 874-5936. Abroad.

MILLARD, Oliver H.; 5880 Spring Garden Road, Halifax, N.S.; Dal '55; FRCS(C); Urol; Ass't. Urol., Victoria Gen. Hosp.; Tel. 429-3224.

MILLARD, William E.; 57 Mack St., Kingston. Ont.; Qns '36; Tel. 546-6112.

MILLEN, Donald B.; 1206 Ouellette Ave., Windsor, Ont.; Wes '34; Gen Surg; Surg. Staff, Grace, Hotel-Dieu & Metropolitan Hosp's.; Tel. 254-9977.

MILLER, Abraham; 27 Highbourne Rd., Toronto 12, Ont. (res); Tor '34; D.Psy., Psy; Clin. Dir., Ontario Hosp., Toronto; Ass't. Prof. (Psy.). U. of Toronto; Tel. LE 3-8501.

MILLER, A. Bruce; 207 LeMarchand Rd., St. John's, Nfld.; 26 Baird Pl. (res); Glasgow (Scot.)'50; MRCOG; ObstGyn; Active Staff, Grace, St. Clare's Mercy & St. John's Gen. Hosp's.; Tel. 579-2213-14.

MILLER, Alexander, Ste 706, 1414 Drummond St., Montreal, P.Q.; 577 Grosvenor Ave., Westmount (res); McG '47; FRCP(C); IntMed; Cons. Med. Queen Mary Vet's Hosp.; Ass't. Phys., Montreal Gen. Hosp.; Lect., McGill U.; Tel. 842-4555.

MILLER, Allan P.; 216 Argyle St., Port Alberni, B.C.; 607 Cres. 3. (res); Man '31; Tel. 723-3211.

MILLER, Andrew P.; 350 Albert St., Nanaimo, B.C.; Glasgow (Scot.)'49; Staff, Nanaimo Reg. Gen. Hosp.; Tel. 753-3431.

MILLER, Bernard F., MBE; 401 Med. Arts Bldg., 5880 Spring Garden Rd., Halifax, N.S.; 1526 Lilac St. (res); Dal '31; M.Ch. (Orth, L'pool); FRCS(Ed); FRCS(C), OrthSurg; OrthSurg., Victoria Gen.; Assoc. OrthSurg., Childrens' & Camp Hill DVA Hosp's.; Cons. (Orth), NS Polio Clinic & NS San; Assoc. Prof. (OrthSurg), Dalhousie U.; Tel. 423-8868.

MILLER, Borden C.; 60 Stone St., Gananoque, Ont.; Qns '37; 382-4123.

MILLER, Carol J.; McGill Health Service, 555 Sherbrooke W., Montreal, P.Q.; 520 Abercorn Ave., Montreal 16, P.Q. (Res.); Ott'64; M.O. of Health, McGill U.; Tel. VI 4-6311, Ext. 420.

MILLER, Charles; Box 190, McCreary, Man.; M.B., Ch.B., Aberdeen (Scot.)'49; GenSurg.

MILLER, Charles P.; New Waterford Medical Clinic, New Waterford, N.S.; 213 Plummer Ave. (res); Dal '47; Staff, New Waterford Gen. Hosp.; M.O.H., New Waterford; Tel. 862-6570.

MILLER, Chauncey A.; Sundre, Alta.; McG '29; Coroner.

MILLER, C. Hugh O.; P.O. Box 450, Knowlton, P.Q.; Tor '56; Staff, Brome Missisquoi Perkins Hosp., Sweetsburg, P.Q.

MILLER, David; Med. Dir., American Motors Canada, Kennedy S., Brampton, Ont.; Dublin (Ire.)'50.

MILLER, Donald M.; Courtenay, B.C.; Alb '51; M.C.G.P.

MILLER, Eleanor W.; (See Sutherland, Eleanor W.).

MILLER, Frank; Ste. 415, 3875 rue St-Urbain, Montreal 18, P.Q.; Mon '42.

MILLER, Fred G.; Elk Point, Alta.; **McG '19;** Dist. Coroner.

MILLER, Frederick R.; 280 Carlton St., Toronto 2, Ont.; Munich (Germ.) '11; F.R.S., F.R.C.P.-(C), IntMed.

MILLER, Geoffrey M.; Apt. 711, 10 Beechwood Pl., London, Ont. (res); Wes'50; TherRad; Research, Victoria Hosp.; Tel. GE 2-5261.

MILLER G. Cumming; Box 21, Sundre, Alta.; Glasgow (Scot) '57.

MILLER, George E.; 214-6th Ave. W., Calgary, Alta.; 2316 Sunset Ave. (res); Alb '46; M.S. (Minn.); ThorSurg; Chief (ThorSurg.), Holy Cross Hosp.; Tel. AM 3-7120.

MILLER, George E.; Tor'65; Ass't. Res., St. Joseph's Hosp., Toronto 3, Ont.

MILLER, George W.; 95 Wellesley St., Toronto, Ont.; Tor '30; D.P.H.; PH; Nat. Dir., Red Cross Blood Transfusion Service; Tel. WA 3-6692.

MILLER, Georges; 791 ave, Dalquier, Quebec 10, P.Q.; Lav '55; Path; Staff, Hop. Hotel-Dieu.; Tel. 529-9151.

MILLER, G. Thomas; 110 Stone St., Gananoque, Ont.; Qns '62.

MILLER, Harold W.; Alb '52; Res., University Hosp., Edmonton, Alta.

MILLER, Henry G.; 238 Wellington St., Preston, Ont.; 102 Highland Crest (res); Tor '29; M.C.-G.P.; M.O.H.

MILLER, Hugh S.; 816 Fairmont Med., Bldg., 750 W. Broadway, Vancouver 9, B.C.; 6200 MacDonald St. W., Van. 13 (res); McG '52; F.R.-C.S.(C), Orth Surg; Dir., Emergency Serv., Van. Gen. Hosp.; Clin. Instr. Dept. of Surg., U. of British Columbia; Tel. TR 2-7181.

MILLER, Ian H.; Box 519, Disbury, Alta.; London (Eng.) '40; MRCS; LRCP; MCGP; Staff, Didsbury Gen. Hosp.; Tel. 335-3141.

MILLER, I. E.; 182 Jarvis St., Toronto 2, Ont.; 12 Hillholme Rd. (res); **Tor '37; Tel. EM 8-8564.**

MILLER, Jack D. R.; Witwatersrand (S.Africa) '56; DABR; DiagRad; Staff, Dept. of Rad., University Hosp., Edmonton, Alta.; Instr., U. of Alberta; Tel. 439-0709, Ext. 308.

MILLER, James A.; 400 Norlyn Med. Bldg., 309 Hargrave St., Winnipeg, Man.; 5 Mohawk Bay, St. Boniface (res); **Wes '46; F.I.C.S., F.R.C.S.-(C), Gen Surg.; Staff Surg., St.-Boniface Hosp.** & Victoria Gen. Hosp.; Tel. WH 7-0216.

MILLER, James; 6411 Quinpool Rd., Halifax, N.S.; Dal '52; MCGP; Tel. 422-5843.

MILLER, James E.; 3394 Grank Forks Rd., Cooksville, Ont.; Tor'64; Tel. 625-1241.

MILLER, James H.; 270 Runnymede Rd., Toronto, Ont.; 32 Kingslynn Rd. (res); Tor '31; Assoc. Staff, Toronto Western Hosp.; Exam., Dept. of Transport, Canada; Tel. RO 6-5451.

MILLER, James M.; 301-6455 W. Blvd., Vancouver 13, B.C.; Tor '26; Retired.

MILLER, James R.; Alb'62; Res., Toronto Western Hosp., Toronto 2B, Ont.

MILLER, J. E. Harris; 6411 Quinpool Rd., Halifax, N.S.; 596 Young Ave. (res); Dal '52; MCGP; Chief, Dept. of G.P., Halifax Infirmary; Staff Faculty, Dalhousie Med. School; Faculty, Mount St. Vincent College, Rockingham; Pres., Defence Med. Assoc. of Canada; Tel. 422-5843.

MILLER, J. Lance; Oromocto Med. Clinic, 101 Hersey St., **Oromocto, N.B.; Dal'66.**

MILLER, John D.; Alb'61; Anaes; Staff, University Hosp., Edmonton, Alta.

MILLER, John E.; 714 Carbon Ave., Bienfait, Sask.; Durham (Eng.)'56; Active Staff, St. Joseph's & Union Hosp's.

MILLER, John R.; Corner Dundas & Davis Dr., **Iroquois, Ont.; 151 Dundas St. (res); Tor '19; Staff, Brockville Gen. Hosp., St. Vincent de Paul Hosp., Brockville & Winchester Dist. Mem. Hosp.; Tel. 652-4484.**

MILLER, John S.; P.O. Box 270, Canyon St., Creston, B.C.; Alice Mine Rd. (res); Dal '39.

MILLER, Joseph E.; Alb'55; OrthSurg; Staff, Montreal Gen. Hosp., Montreal 25, P.Q.

MILLER, Josephino W.; Child Guidance Clinic, 700 Elgin Ave., Winnipeg 3, Man.; Man'54; D. Psy.; Tel. SP 5-7101.

MILLER, Kenelm C.; Elk Point, Alta.; Alb '51; Dist. Coroner.

MILLER, Kenneth R.; Medical Arts Clinic, Bradbrooke Block, Swift Current, Sask.; Alb'57; FAAP; FRCP(C); Paed; Hd., Dept. of Paed., Swift Current Union Hosp.; Tel. 773-4636.

MILLER, Leonard A.; 5 Forest Ave., St. John's, Nfld. (res); Dal '30; PH; Dep. Minister of **Health, Prov. of Nfld.; Tel. 9-5011.**

MILLER, Lloyd L.; 5224 Kingsway, South Burnaby, B.C.; 5445 Buckingham Ave. (res); Loma Linda (Calif., U.S.A.) '56; Tel. HE 1-5585.

MILLER, Louis A.; 309 Tegler Bldg., Edmonton, Alta.; 8 Riverside Cres. (res); McG '20; GenSurg; Att'd. Staff (Surg.), Misericordia Hosp.; Retired.

MILLER, Marvin E.; Ste. 511, 99 Avenue Rd., **Toronto 5, Ont.; 29 Charnwood Rd., Don Mills (res); Tor '55; D.Psy; Psy; Cons. Psy., Baycrest Hosp. & Jewish Home for the Aged; Vol. Ass't; New Mount Sinai Hosp.; Tel. WA 3-9293.**

MILLER, Mary L.; 6200 Macdonald St., Vancouver 13, B.C.; McG'53; Anaes; Staff, Vancouver Gen. Hosp.

MILLER, Max J.; Ste. 220, 3550 Cote des Neiges Rd., Montreal 25, P.Q.; **Qns'43; Cons., Mtl. Gen.** & Lakeshore Gen' Hosp's.; Memb. Expert Committ. on Parasitic Diseases W.H.O.; Research Prof., School of Hygiene, U. of Montreal; Tel. 932-9415.

MILLER, Melvin J.; 7325-101st Ave., Edmonton, Alta.; Alb '42; MCGP; Tel. HO 6-9133.

MILLER, Meyer S.; 404 Med. Centre, 906-8th Ave. S.W., Calgary, Alta.; 1114 Premier Way (res); Man '37; D.A.B.O.L., F.A.A.Ophth, Otol, F.A.C.S. F.I.C.S.; Ophth,Otol; Chief, **EENT, Holy Cross Hosp.; Tel. AM 2-9854; AM 2-5972.**

MILLER, M. Keith; Castor, Alta.; Alb'65.

MILLER, M. M.; Aylmer, Ont.; Wes '33; M.C.-G.P.

MILLER, Morris; 700 Bathurst St., Toronto, Ont.; 201 Richview Ave. (res); Tor '35; M.C.-G.P.; **Staff, Mount Sinai Hosp.; Tel. LE 1-9875.**

MILLER, Morris C.; 1625 Sherbrooke St. W., Montreal, P.Q.; 4515 Dupuis Ave. (res); McG '48; Gastroent. (P.Q.), IntMed: **Staff, Jewish Gen. & Victoria Hosp's.; Tel. 735-3771.**

MILLER, M. Sue; Alb'65; Res., Victoria Hosp., London, Ont.

MILLER, Norman E.; 955 Queen St. E., Sault Ste. Marie, Ont.; 59 Palace Dr. (res); Qns '53; M.Sc., FACOG; ObstGyn; Pres. Med. Staff, Sault-Ste.-Marie Gen. Hosp.; Cons. Plummer Mem. Hosp.; Tel. PH 4-2821.

MILLER, Patrick J.; Humboldt Med. Clin., Humboldt, Sask.; Man '54; A.M.C.G.P.

MILLER, Ralph G.; 200 Medical Arts Bldg., 73 N. Cumberland, Port Arthur, Ont.; 109 Rupert St. (res); Qns '37; M.C.G.P.

MILLER, Ralph P.; 174 Hartley St., Brockville, Ont. (res.); McG'53; D.Psy; Psy; Ass't. Supt., Ontario Hosp.; Tel. 345-3461.

MILLER, Raymond; 1077 Clifton Ave., Moose Jaw, Sask. (res); Ire. '43; DPH; Regional Med. Health Officer.

MILLER, R. Bruce; 88 Pineview Cres., New Glasgow, N.S. (res); Dal '49; DiagRad; Hd. Dept. of Rad., Aberdeen Hosp.; Tel. 752-8311.

MILLER, Robert E.; 405 Hendryx, Nelson, B.C.; Dal '58; Staff, Kootenay Lake Gen. Hosp., Nelson; Tel. 357-9313.

MILLER, Robert H.; Qns'64; Staff, Mem. Hosp., Labrador City, Nfld.

MILLER, Robert K.; 14 Alexandra St., Oshawa, Ont.; 105 Alexandra St. (res); Tor '52; FRCS(C); ObstGyn; Tel. 728-5931.

MILLER, Robert L.; 423—1445 Marpole Ave., Vancouver, B.C. (res); McG '09; Retired.

MILLER, Ronald J.; 514 Agnes St., New Westminster, B.C.; 227-3rd Ave., New Westminster (res); Liverpool (Eng.)'39; MCGP; Staff, Royal Columbia Hosp.; Assoc. Staff, St. Mary's Hosp.; Tel. LA 2-7818.

MILLER, Saul; Ste. 412, 750 W. Broadway, Vancouver 9, B.C.; 7088 Marguerite St., Van. 14 (res); McG '39; DR; DABR; D & TRad; Cons. Rad., Health Serv. & Clin. Assoc. Prof. (Anat.), U. of British Columbia; Tel. TR 2-7595.

MILLER, Scharley-May; (See—Horne).

MILLER-TAIT, Robert; 1669 Victoria St., Prince George, B.C.; 1921-3rd Ave. (res); McG '24; DiagRad.

MILLER, Telford W.; Box 190, Fort St. John, B.C.; Man'50; GenSurg.

MILLER, W. Douglas; 115 Hazen St., Saint John, N.B.; Sandy Pt. (res); Dal '45; M.Sc., D.S. (McG); FACS; FRCS(C), GenSurg; Chief of Surg., Saint John Gen. & Lancaster DVA Hosp's.; Surg., Saint John TB & St. Joseph's Hosp's.; Tel. 693-2449.

MILLER, W. R. A.; 114 Lankin Blvd., Toronto, 6, Ont.; Tor '43; Tel. HO 5-3401.

MILLET, Rene; 112 Lindsay, C. P. 336, Drummondville, P.Q.; Mon '22; Dist. Coroner.

MILLETTE, Honorius; 930 Boul. Saraguay, Pierrefonds, P.Q.; Lav'57.

MILLETTE, Lucien J. N.; Western Med. Clinic, Brandon, Man.; Lav'60; FRCS(C), GenSurg; Am. Bd. Surg; Tel. PA 9-5471.

MILLETTE, Ovila J.; 221 Main, Melville, Sask.; Lav '50; Dist. Coroner.

MILLIGAN, Francis D.; 1105 Pandora Ave., Victoria, B.C.; John Hopkins U. (U.S.A.) '57; FRCP(C), IntMed; Active Staff, St. Joseph's Hosp.; Court. Staff, Royal Jubilee Hosp.; Dir. Med. Educ., St. Joseph's Hosp.; Tel. 382-8742.

MILLIGAN, John E.; 167 Rusholme Rd., Toronto 4, Ont.; Tor '59; FRCS(C), ObstGyn; Staff, Women's College Hosp. Abroad.

MILLIGAN, William A.; 330-2nd Ave. E., Cornwall, Ont.; McG '27; Staff, Cornwall Hosp.; Tel. WE 2-0332.

MILLIKEN, John A.; 106 Alwington Place, Kingston, Ont.; Qns '46; FACP; FRCP(C), IntMed; Head (Med.), Hotel-Dieu Hosp.; Assoc. Prof. (Med.), Queens U.; Tel. 546-1451.

MILLINGTON, Malcolm; 131 Balsam, Snow Lake, Man.; London (Eng.)'61; MB, B.S.; D.A.; D.(Obst.)RCOG; Ass't. Med. Supervisor, Hudson Bay Mining & Smelting Employees Health Association, Snow Lake; Tel. 358-2241.

MILLIONS, James V.; Eastend, Sask.; Man '29.

MILLMAN, William L.; Wes'65; Res., Victoria Hosp., London, Ont.

MILLS, Cecil V.; 408 Canada Bldg., Windsor, Ont.; Tor'16; MCGP; Coroner, Essex Co.; Local Insp. of Anat.; Tel. 254-1781.

MILLS, Donald W.; 225 Queens Ave., London, Ont.; Wes '57; FRCS(C); Ophth; Staff, Victoria Hosp.; Tel. GE 2-5261.

MILLS, Douglas G.; 348 Simcoe St. N., Oshawa, Ont.; Tor'55; FRCS(C); FACS; GenSurg; Staff, Oshawa Gen. Hosp.; Tel. 728-2961.

MILLS, D. Keith; Ste. 401, 267 O'Connor St., Ottawa 4, Ont.; Wes'56; Psy; Att'd. Staff (Psy.), Ottawa Civic Hosp.; Lect. (Psy.), U. of Ottawa; Tel. 237-2492.

MILLS, Douglas V. M.; Dept. of Path., St. Joseph's Hosp., London, Ont.; Wes'48; Path; Chief of Path., St. Joseph's Hosp.; Cons. Path., St. Mary's Hosp.; District Path., Attorney General's Dept., Ontario; Clin. Assoc. Prof. of Path., U. of Western Ontario; Tel. 439-3271, Local 323.

MILLS, Edgar J.; Shouldice Surgery, 618 Church Street, Toronto 5, Ont.; '48; Tel. WA 3-3507.

MILLS, Edward S.; 567 Grosvenor Ave., Westmount, P.Q. (res); McG '22; F.A.C.P., F.R.C.P. (C) IntMed; Phys.-in-Chief, & Dir., McGill U. Clin., Montreal Gen. Hosp.; Hon. Treas., Canadian Med. Assoc.; Prof. of Med., McGill U.; (Retired; After Sept./57, Address—Foxboro Rd., Essex, Conn., U.S.A.).

MILLS, F. Graham; Ste. 105, 520-17th St., West Vancouver, B.C.; Man '45; Psy.; Tel. 922-0333.

MILLS, Fred C.; 422 London St., Sherbrooke, P.Q.; McG '56; M.Sc. (Exp.Med.); IntMed (P.Q.); Staff, Sherbrooke Hosp.; Tel. 562-8901.

MILLS, G. Franklin; 1 Nelson Ave. E., Goderich, Ont.; Wes'51; MCGP.

MILLS, J. Grant; 218 Medical Arts Bldg., Calgary, Alta.; 3336-39th St. S.W. (res); Wes '54; MCGP; Tel. 266-2139.

MILLS, J. R. Frank; 1015 Medical Arts Bldg., Toronto, Ont.; 207 Dawlish Ave. (res); Tor '33; F.R.C.S. (Edin.), F.A.C.S., F.R.C.S.(C), GenSurg, OrthSurg, ThorSurg; Sr. Surg., Toronto Gen. Hosp.; Cons. Surg., Sunnybrook D.V.A. Hosp.; Assoc. Prof. (Surg.), U. of Toronto; Tel. WA 2-2565.

MILLS, Oscar G.; 117 King St. E., Oshawa, Ont.; 743 Simcoe St. N. (res); Tor '21; IntMed; Med. Staff, Oshawa Gen. Hosp; Tel. 728-1661.

MILLS, Thomas J.; 201 Med. Arts Bldg., Winnipeg 1, Man.; 5011 Roblin Blvd., Wpg. 20 (res); Trinity College (Dublin, Ire.) '47; M.Ch. (Orth)(Liverpool); F.R.C.S.(I), F.R.C.S.(C), OrthSurg; OrthSurg., Children's, Grace, St. Boniface Gen. Hosp's.; Lect. (Orth.Surg.), U. of Manitoba; Tel. WH 3-1153.

MILLS, Wilfrid C.; Med. Centre, 420 Lock St. W., Dunnville, Ont.; Wes '41; M.C.G.P.; Med. Staff, Haldimand War Mem. Hosp.; Dist. MOH; Tel. 774-7541.

MILLSON, Jerry W.; Ste. 304, 25 Leonard Ave., Toronto 2B, Ont.; Tor '50; FRCS(C); ObstGyn; Clin. Instr., Toronto Western Hosp. & U. of Toronto; Tel. 364-3013.

MILNE, Donald A. D.; Durham St., Kincardine, Ont.; Tor '51; M.C.G.P.; Staff, Kincardine Gen. Hosp.; Tel. 440.

MILNE, Donald H.; Paisley, Ont.; Tor '32.

MILNE, Douglas R. S.; Suite 225, 925 W. Georgia St., Vancouver, B.C.; 5876 Angus Dr. (res); Edinburgh (Scot.)'38; Tel. MU 4-4646.

MILNE, Eric N. C.; Victoria Hosp., London, Ont.; Edinburgh (Scot.) '56; DMRD (Edin.); FFR; DiagRad; Ass't. Rad., Victoria Hosp.; Instr. (DiagRad.), U. of Western Ontario; Tel. 432-5261; Abroad.

MILNE, G. Craig; McG'65; Res., Royal Victoria Hosp., Montreal 2, P.Q.

MILNE, Glenn D.; 1541 W. Broadway, Vancouver 9, B.C.; 1813-W.36th (res); UBC '59; MCGP; Tel. 736-5661.

MILNE, Ian G.; 385 Seaforth Med. Bldg., 3550 Cote des Neiges Rd., Montreal 25, P.Q.; McG'49; FRCP(C); IntMed; Cardiol (P.Q.); Assoc. Phys., Montreal Gen. Hosp.; Ass't. Prof. Med., McGill U.; Cardiol., Montreal Gen. Hosp.; Cons., British Petroleum; Tel. 932-6601.

MILNE, J. Kenneth; Wes'65; Res., Victoria Hosp., London, Ont.

MILNE, John D.; 912 Greyhound Bldg., 622-1st Ave., S.W., Calgary, Alta.; 2205-22nd St. S.W. (res); Alb '59; Tel. 262-4345.
MILNE, John E.; Flesherton, Ont.; Tor '25; Temp. Retired.
MILNE, Kenneth W.; Med. Clinic, 327 Charlotte St., Peterborough, Ont.; Tor '39; D.M.R., Diag-Rad; Dir. of Rad., St. Joseph's Hosp., & Peterborough Clin.

MILNE, Lorna; (See Boag).

MILNE, M. Norman; 3519 Lake Shore Blvd. W., Toronto 14, Ont.; 8 Kenridge Ave., Tor 18 (res); Tor '45; M.C.G.P.; Imm. M.O. & U.S. PH Serv., Malton Airport; Retired.
MILNE, Peter L.; 357 Ferguson St., North Bay, Ont.; 458 McIntyre St. E. (res); Dal '58; Tel. 472-2300.
MILNE, Richard T. G.; 240 Brock St., Kingston, Ont.; Qns '58; MCGP; Preceptor (PrevMed.), Queen's U.; Indust. Phys., Dupont of Canada; Tel. 546-4318.

MILNER, Frederick J.; 270 Victoria St., London, Ont.; Wes '34.
MILNER, Macey; 4622 Bowness Rd. N.W., Calgary, Alta.; 539-34A St. N.W. (res); Qns '43; Tel. 266-6990.
MILNER, Robert W.; 169 St. Vital Rd., Wpg. 8, Man. (res); Aberdeen (Scot.) '49; DA (Ire.); FRCP & FFARCS (Lond.); Staff (Anaes), St.-Boniface & Victoria Hosp's.; Lect., U. of Manitoba; Tel. WH 3-0311.

MILOBAR, Tony; Alb '58; MCGP; Res., University Hosp., Edmonton, Alta.

MILOS, Paul; 1011 Ouellette Ave., Windsor, Ont.; Qns'59; FRCP(C), IntMed; Tel. 256-1226.

MILOT, Claude; Centre Commercial, Ste. Adele en Bas, Cte. Terrebonne, P.Q.; Lav'65.
MILOT, Jean; Mon '62; Res., Hop. Maisonneuve, Montreal, P.Q.
MILOT, Jean P.; 450 Monmouth Rd., Montreal, P.Q.; Mon '48; Pulm. Dis. & TB (P.Q.); Staff, Hop. Mont Providence.
MILOT, J. Jacques; 2 St. Stanislas, St. Therese, P.Q.; Mon '64.
MILOT, Leonard, 5 rue St. Nicholas, St. Eustache, Co. Deux Montagnes, P.Q. (res); Mon '37; DPH; PH(P.Q.); Health Officer, Deux Montagnes Co.
MILOT, Paul E.; 7690 Querbes Ave., Montreal 15, P.Q.; 139 Glengarry Ave. (res); Ott '56; Tel. 272-1300.

MILROD, Samuel; 44 Coburg St., Saint John, N.B.; 45 Seely St. (res); Tor '43; F.A.C.S., F.I.C.S.; GenSurg; Att'd. (Surg.), Saint John Gen., St. Joseph's & Lancaster DVA Hosp's.; Tel. 693-3601.
MILTINS, Alfred; Canmore, Alta.; Latvia '35; Staff, Conmore Hosp.; Dist Coroer; Tel. 678-5001.
MILTON, Gordon L.; Port Williams, N.S.; Dal '48.
MILTON, Margaret E. (Russell); 115 North Toronto Med. Bldg., 250 Lawrence Ave. W., Toronto 12, Ont.; Tor'62; Ph.D. (Edin.); AMCGP; Med. Dir., St. John's Convalescent Hosp.; Court. Staff, Toronto Gen. Hosp.; Tel. 782-4552.
MINC, Paul H.; Doctor's Bldg., 955 Queen St., Sault Ste. Marie, Ont.; London (Eng.)'56; M.B., B.S.; MCGP; Med. Staff, Plummer Mem. & Gen. Hosp's.
MINDE, Klaus K.; Munich (Germany)'57; Psy; Staff, Children's Hosp., Montreal 25, P.Q.

MINDEN, Joseph H.; 452 Main St. E., Hamilton, Ont.; 34 Chedoke Ave. (res); Tor '38; D.A.B.S., F.A.C.S., F.R.C.S.(C) GenSurg; Staff, Hamilton Gen & St. Joseph's Hosp's.; Tel. JA 9-6267.
MINEAU, Michelle; Mon'64; Res. (ObstGyn.), Hop. Notre-Dame, Montreal, P.Q.
MINGIE, Peter G.; Park Towers, 400 Walmer Rd., Ste. 1ll, Toronto, Ont.; McG '59; D. Psy; Psy; Cons. Psy., U. of Toronto Health Serv.; Tel. 921-7158.
MINGIE, Walter J.; 22 Linwood Cr., Montreal 16, P.Q.; McG'15; FIAMA; Med. Dir., Macdonald Tobacco Inc.; Tel. 844-2501.

MINICH, John; 908½ Garth St., Hamilton, Ont.; Qns '56; MCGP; Active Staff, Hamilton Civic, St. Joseph's, Chedoke & Children's Hosp's.; Tel. 385-2841.
MINIELLY, Herbert A.; 771 Alexander St., Woodstock, Ont. (res); Wes '32; FACCP; Phys., Ontario Hosp., Woodstock.

MINISH, Nathaniel J.; 11222-123rd St., Edmonton, Alta. (res); Man '20; Hon. Ass't. Prof. of Anat.; Retired.

MINK, L. Murray; 2043 Courtland Dr., Burlington, Ont. (res); Tor '50; Path; Assoc. Path., St. Joseph's Hosp., Hamilton; Tel. 522-4941.
MINK, Morris M.; 853 Bathurst St., Toronto, Ont.; 7 Elderwood Dr. (res); Tor '33; M.C.G.P.; Sr. Att. Staff (O.P.D.), New Mt. Sinai Hosp.; Night Phys., Dept. of Public Health, City of Toronto; Tel. LE 6-1871.

MINNES, Allen G.; 1134 Victoria Ave., Niagara Falls, Ont.; Qns '35.
MINNES, H. E.; 232 Metcalfe St., Ottawa, Ont.; 456 Lansdowne Rd. (res); McG '31; GenSurg; A/Staff (Traum. Surg.), Ottawa Civic Hosp.; Lect'r. (Traum. Surg.), Queen's U.; Surg.; C.N.R.; Tel. 235-6141.
MINNES, James F.; 3195 Granville St., Vancouver, B.C.; 3065 Capilano Rd. (res); McG '34; D.A.B.Op., D.Op., Ophth; Att. Staff, Vancouver Gen. Hosp.; Vist. Staff, St. Paul's & Children's Hosp's.; Clin. Instr., U. of British Columbia; Tel. RE 3-5220.

MINO, Roland; 43 des Frenes E., Quebec 3, P.Q.; 2005 Chemin-Ste.-Foy (res); Ott '59; Tel. 623-0525.

MINORGAN, George A.; 1069 W. 26th Ave., Vancouver, B.C.; 969 Montroyal, N.V. (res); Edinburgh (Scot.) '47; M.R.C.P., M.B., Ch.B. IntMed.; Tel. RE 8-3546.
MINOVITZ, Osher; 175 West Broadway, Vancouver 10, B.C.; McG'47; IntMed; Ass't. Clin. Dir., The Alcoholism Fdn. of B.C.; Tel. 879-5755.

MINSHULL, Fred A.; Dal '30; Staff Phys., Med. Dept. Can. Nat. Rlwys., Moncton, N.B.

MINUCK, Max; 799 Waterloo St., Winnipeg 1, Man.; Man'46; Anaes; Dir., Dept. of Anaes., St. Boniface Hosp.; Ass't. Prof. Surg. (Anaes.), U. of Manitoba; Tel. WH 3-9565.
MIRABEL, Ludovic; Ste. 406, 625 - 5th Ave., New Westminster, B.C.; Edinburgh (Scot.)'47; MRCP(Ed.); IntMed.; Tel. VA 6-6543.
MIRANDA, Rosman F.; Hamburg (Germ.)'58; Res., Victoria Gen. Hosp., Halifax, N.S.
MIRCHANDANI, Gopi R.; 98 Old Sambro Rd., Spryfield, Halifax, N.S.; Bombay (India)'48; DGO (Bombay); Cytologist, Pathology Inst., Halifax; Tel. 422-9661.
MIREAULT, Jean P.; 339 rue Papineau, Joliette, P.Q.; Mon '45; M.C.G.P.
MIREHOUSE, Orville J.; 68 Charlton Ave. W., Hamilton, Ont.; 79 Irma Ct., Ancaster (res); Wes '48; PlasSurg; Staff, Hamilton Gen. & St. Joseph's Hosp's.; Tel. JA 8-3914.
MIRHADY, Fereidoun; 7947 Granville St., Vancouver, B.C.; 1679 W. 65th (res); Vienna (Aust.) '45; Paed; Clin. Instr., U. of British Columbia; Tel. AM 1-2022.
MIRHADY, Katharine E. (Stouffer); 1679 W. 65th St., Vancouver 14, B.C.; Tor '48; Pt. Time P.H., M.O.H.
MIRLIN, Walter; Med. Centre, 25 St. Michael St., St. Albert, Alta.; Witwatersrand (S. Africa) '39; Staff, Edmonton Gen. & Royal Alexandra Hosp's.; Tel. 599-7705.
MIRON, Donat; 991 Girouard, Montreal 28, P.Q.; Mon '25.
MIRON, Rose D.; Ott '57; Anaes; Staff, Hamilton Gen. Hosp., Hamilton, Ont. Tel. 527-0271.
MIRONOWICZ, Halina K.; 99 Burris St., Hamilton, Ont.; Warsaw (Poland) '40; D.P.H.
MIRSKY, Samuel; 306 Med. Arts Bldg., 180 Metcalfe St., Ottawa 4, Ont.; 122 Argylle Ave. (res); McG'24; FACP; DIM; IntMed; Phys., Emer. Civic Hosp.; Cons., DVA; Assoc. Prof. (Med.), Ottawa U.; Tel. 232-5970.
MIRZAI, Mahmood; 16 Clement Block, Brandon, Man.; Tehran (Iran) '55.

MISENER, Clair C.; 423 Crestview Rd., Ottawa 8, Ont. (res); Tor'30; Dir., Admission Serv., D.V.A.
MISENER, F. J.; 28 Fairview St., Kentville, N.S. (res); Dal '48; Rad., Nova Scotia San., Kentville.
MISHKIN, Seymour; McG'65; Jr. Int., Royal Victoria Hosp., Montreal 2, P.Q.; Abroad.
MISHRA, Raghunandan; Rajasthan (India)'60; Res., Pathol. Inst., Halifax, N.S.
MISIK, Charles; Hampden, Nfld.
MISIR, Hari; Dal'59; Res. (GenSurg.), Providence Hosp., Detroit, Michigan; Tel. 969-6667.
MISKELLY, Lorna M. (Sansom); Box 113, R.R. 1, Hull, P.Q. (res); Tor'43; NDMC, Ottawa; Tel. 733-6600.
MISKEW, John W.; 406 Medical Arts Bldg., 1011 Ouellette Ave., Windsor, Ont.; Alb'32.
MISUMI, Yoshiyuki D.; Royal York Plaza, 1500 Royal York Rd., Weston, Ont.; 41 Fernalroy Blvd. Tor. 18 (res); Tor '55; MCGP; Tel. CH 9-4641.
MITAREWSKI, Walter W.; 253 E. 14th St., North Vancouver, B.C.; UBC'58.
MITCHELL-BANKS, William H.; Greene Clinic, 122-2nd Ave. W., Prince Rupert, B.C.; Oxford (Eng.) '54; B.M., B.Ch.; Tel. 624-9121.
MITCHELL, David P.; 3116 Geneva St., Los Angeles, Calif. 90005, U.S.A.; Tor'59; FRCS(C), Otol; Abroad.
MITCHELL, David R.; 407 Medical Arts Bldg., 170 St. George St., Toronto, Ont.; 57 Garfield (res); Tor '27; M.S.(Tor.), F.R.C.S.(Eng.), F.R.C.S.(C) Urol; Chief Urol., Toronto Gen. **Hosp.; Assoc. Prof. Surg., U. of Toronto; Tel. WA 3-4345.**
MITCHELL, Donald M.; 106 Med. Arts Bldg., Saskatoon, Sask.; 1020 Victoria Ave. (res); Man '46; DABIM; IntMed; Active Staff (Med.), University Hosp.; Med. Dir., Sask. Div. CARS; Ass't. Clin. Prof. (Med.), & Dir. Rheumatic Dis. Unit, U. of Saskatchewan; Tel. 653-3737.
MITCHELL, Donald S.; 1414 Drummond St., Montreal 25, P.Q.; 497 Mt. Pleasant Ave., Westmount, Montreal 6, (res); Northwestern U. **(U.S.A.) '31 DermSyph; Tel. 845-1040.**
MITCHELL, Douglas G.; 50 Church St., St. Catharines, Ont.; 456 Queen St., Niagara-on-the-Lake (res); Alb'52; Ophth.; Tel. 682-3832.
MITCHELL, Elizabeth (See Richards)
MITCHELL, Elmer W.; 7 Rosemary Lane, Toronto 10, Ont.; GenSurg; Tel. RU 2-8774.
MITCHELL, H. Douglas; Apt. 1005, 9 Deer Park Cres., Toronto 7, Ont.; Tor '25; Psy.
MITCHELL, Helen C. (Craw); 293 Glen Rd., Toronto, Ont.; Tor '30; D. Psy; Psy; Child Adjustment Serv., Bd. of Education, Toronto.
MITCHELL, Howard S.; 1414 Drummond, Montreal, P.Q.; 3787 Cote des Neiges (res); Qns '27; F.A.C.P.; F.A.A.A.; M.C.A.A., IntMed; **Assoc. Prof. Med. McGill U.; Phys., Montreal Gen. Hosp.; Cons., Queen Mary Veterans', Children's Memorial, & Alexandra Hosp's.; Tel. VI 4-3210.**
MITCHELL, Hugh A.; 707 Charlotte St., **Peterborough, Ont.; Bridge North, Ont. (res); Man** '27; F.R.C.P.(C), IntMed (Cardiol).
MITCHELL, Ian A.; 105 Bernard Ave., Toronto, Ont (res); Tor '51; Fellow (Haem), Dept. of **Path., Toronto Sick Children's Hosp.; Tel. EM 6-7242.**
MITCHELL, Jack; 200 Danforth Ave., Toronto, Ont.; Man '39; GenSurg; Active Staff, Doctor's Hosp.; Assoc. Staff, Toronto East Gen. Hosp.; Tel. 461-0761.
MITCHELL, James R.; 523 Medical Arts Bldg., Winnipeg, Man.; 760 Dowker, Winnipeg 9, (res); Man '43; F.R.C.S.(C), ObstGyn; Staff (ObstGyn), Winnipeg Gen., St. Boniface & Grace **Hosp's.; Lect., (ObstGyn.), U. of Manitoba; Tel. WH 3-5416.**
MITCHELL, John; Box 1520, Med. Centre, Lloydminster, Sask.; Glasgow (Scot.)'52.
MITCHELL, John C.; 614 Fairmont Med. Bldg., 750 W. Broadway, Vancouver 9, B.C.; 766 Grand Blvd., N. Van. (res); London (Eng.) '48; MRCP (Lond.); FRCP(C), DermSyph; Hd. Div. of Derm., Shaughnessy Hosp.; Ass't. Prof. Derm., U. of British Columbia; Tel. TR 2-2814.
MITCHELL, John E.; 602 Professional Bldg., Red Deer, Alta.; Man '42; FACS; FRCS(C); GenSurg; Staff, Red Deer Mun. Hosp.; Tel. 347-2911.
MITCHELL, Lorne I.; Rideau Med Centre, 1711-4th St. S.W., Calgary, Alta.; 4007-5th St. (res); Qns '42; Urol; Chief (Urol); Calgary Gen. & Pres. Med Staff, Children's Hosp.; Court. Staff, Holy Cross Hosp.; Instr. Schl. of Nursing, Calgary Gen. Hosp.; Tel. 263-6464.
MITCHELL, Marvin, 10022-103rd St., Edmonton, Alta.; Alb '57; FAAP; Paed; Court. Staff, Royal Alexandra Hosp.; Active Staff, Misericordia & Glenrose Hosp's. & Cerebral Palsy Clinic; Tel. 429-3781.
MITCHELL, Mary E.; Addiction Research Fdn., **221 Elizabeth St., Toronto 2,; Tor '58.**
MITCHELL, Michael D.; 115-116 Medical Arts Bldg., Calgary, Alta.; 2112-10th St. W. (res); Man'27; AMCGP; Tel. 262-9379.
MITCHELL, Nelson S.; McG'59; FRCS(C), Orth Surg; Staff, Shriner's Hosp., Montreal 25, P.Q.
MITCHELL, Norman H.; 1020 North Shore E., Burlington, Ont.; Tor '21; Dist. Coroner; Tel. NE 4-3885.
MITCHELL, Peter J.; Box 700, Ladysmith, B.-C.; UBC'59; MCGP.
MITCHELL, Ralph E.; 112 Royal Ave., New Westminster, B.C. (res); Dal '33; (DiagRad); **Staff, Royal Columbian Hosp., New Westminster; Tel. LA 2-2771.**
MITCHELL, R. Blair; Box 1089, 154 Main St. W., Stouffville, Ont.; Tor'52; MCGP; Sr. Staff, York County Hosp., Newmarket.
MITCHELL, R. Gordon; Windsor Park Med. Centre, 844 Autumnwood Dr., Winnipeg 6, Man.; Glasgow (Scot.)'56; Tel. 253-1324.
MITCHELL, R. Morrison; 289 Cedar St., Sudbury, Ont.; 295 Riverside Dr. (res); Tor '29; F.R.C.S.(C), F.A.C.S., GenSurg; Pres. Med. Staff & Chief of Surg., Sudbury Mem. Hosp.; Memb. of Council & Exec., Coll. of Phys. & **Surg. of Ont.; Tel. OS 4-3131.**
MITCHELL, Robert I.; Ste. 234, 200 St. Clair Ave. W., Toronto 7, Ont.; 82 Forest Grove Dr., Willowdale (res); Sydney (Australia) '50; FRCS (Eng); FRACS; FACS; FRCS(C); GenSurg; ThorSurg; Surg., Wellesley Hosp.; Cons. Surg., **Princess Margaret Hosp.; Tel. WA 1-2742.**
MITCHELL, Rosslyn B.; 506-1650 Pembina Highway, Winnipeg 19, Man.; Man '06; FACS; FRCP(C), ObstGyn; Hon. Cons. Staff, Winnipeg Gen. Hosp.; Retired.
MITCHELL, Sara; (See Alexander).
MITCHELL, Sheila C.; 105 Bernard Ave., Toronto 5, Ont. (res); Tor '51; Temp. Retired.
MITCHELL, Thomas M.; UBC'54; Res., Vancouver Gen. Hosp., Vancouver 9, B.C.
MITCHELL, William; 19 Parklane Cr., St. Catharines, Ont. (res); Glasgow (Scot.) '54; M.B., B.Ch.; DiagRad; Staff, Dept. of Rad., St. Catharines Gen. Hosp.; Tel. MU 4-7271.
MITCHELL, William B.; 22 Second St., Collingwood, Ont.; 224 Minnisota St. (res); Tor '38; Staff, Collingwood Gen. & Marine Hosp's.; Tel. 445-3711.
MITCHELL, William E. M., MC; Med. Arts Bldg., 1105 Pandora Ave., Victoria, B.C.; 2171 Granite St. (res); London (Eng.) '24; L.R.C.P. (Lond.), M.R.C.S.(England), M.R.C.P.(London), F.R.C.S.(Eng. & C), GenSurg; Urol; **Cons. Surg., Royal Jubilee & DVA Hosp's.; Tel. EV 2-2313.**
MITCHELL, William J.; 3256 Cambie St., Vancouver 9, B.C.; 6892 Laurel St. (res); UBC '55; MCGP; **Med. Dir., British Pacific Life Ins. Co.; Tel. TR 4-0261.**
MITCHELL, Winston M.; Qns'65; Res., Kingston General Hosp., Kingston, Ont.
MITCHINSON, Doreen M. (Greve); 612 Med. Arts Bldg., 750 Spadina Cr. E., Saskatoon, Sask.; 306 Whitney Ave. N. (res); Sask'58; Semi-retired; Tel. 343-1619.
MITIS, Livia H.; 901 Medical Arts Bldg., 170 St. George St., Toronto 5, Ont.; 284 Spadina Rd. (res); Edinburgh (Scot.) '46; Neur; Neurol., **Women's College Hosp.; Clin. Ass't., Dept. (Neur.), Toronto Gen. Hosp.; Tel. WA 3-2002.**

MITMAKER, Benjamin; Linton Clinic, 6000 Cote des Neiges Rd., Montreal 26, P.Q.; 4943 Lacombe Ave. (res); Geneva (Switz.) '57; M.Sc.; FRCS(C), GenSurg; Staff, Jewish Gen. Hosp.; Tel. 733-5691.

MITRA, Atin K.; 3643 Dutch Village Rd., Halifax, N.S.; Calcutta (India)'57.

MITSUI, Ken K.; Ste. 2058, 1920 Weston Rd., Weston, Ont.; 11 Foxmeadow Rd. (res); Tor'53; IntMed; Cons. (IntMed), Humber Mem. Hosp.; Att'd. Staff (Allerg. Clin.), Tor. Western Hosp., Toronto; Tel. 247-5891.

MITTLER, Nicholas L.; Ste. 403, 1849 Yonge St., Toronto 7, Ont.; Paris (France)'40.

MITTON, Claude C.; 304 Tournelle, Pont-Viau, P.Q.; Haiti'56; Anaes.

MIVILLE, Jacques; St-Anne-des-Monts, P.Q.; Lav '50.

MIVILLE-DECHENE, Gaston; 214 ouest, rue King, Sherbrooke, P.Q.; Lav '43; Derm.

MIYA, Robert T.; 83 Smith Ave., Hamilton, Ont.; 103 Wiseman Cr. (res); Tor '52; Tel. 528-5666.

MIYAGISHIMA, Robert T.; UBC'60; FRCS(C), GenSurg; Staff, Toronto Western Hosp., Toronto 2B, Ont.

MIYAUCHI, David K.; 11120-102nd St., Edmonton, Alta.; Alb'60; Psy.

MIZBAH, Geoffrey; Box 250 Smooth Rock Falls, Ont.; Liverpool (Eng.) '45; LRCP; FRSM; FRCS (Eng.); FICS; GenSurg; Surg., Smooth Rock Falls Hosp. & Abitibi Power & Paper Co.; Tel. 370.

MIZGALA, Henry F.; 3550 Cote des Neiges Rd., Ste. 350, Montreal 25, P.Q.; McG '57; FRCP(C), IntMed; Cardiol (P.Q.); Staff, St. Mary's, Montreal Gen. & Lakeshore Gen. Hosp's.; Tel. WE 2-6881.

MIZRAHI, Aslan M.; Mental Health Clinic, 140-1st St. N.W., Swift Current, Sask.; Alexandria (Egypt)'55; Psy; Clin. Dir., Swift Current Mental Health Clin.; Tel. 773-7263.

MLYNARYK, Peter; 1390 Sherbrooke St. W., Ste. 25, Montreal 25, P.Q.; Mc '56; Gastroent (P.Q.); Dip. IntMed; FRCP(C); IntMed; Clin. Ass't., Dept. of Med., Royal Victoria Hosp.; Dem., McGill U.; Tel. VI 2-1396.

MOAR, James D.; 424 Water St., Chatham, N.B.; Ott '52.

MOCKLER, Gordon R.; 33 Beaverbrook Ave., Saint John, N.B.; Dal '65.

MODE, G. Stuart; 5890 Monkland Ave., Montreal, P.Q.; 14 Glenmore Rd., Hampstead (res); McG '35; Assoc. Surg., Queen Elizabeth Hosp.; Tel. 486-8565.

MODI, Suman; Bombay (India) '35; MRCS (Eng.); Staff, Alberta Hosp., Edmonton, Alta.; Tel. 7-0221.

MOES, C. A. Frederic; 27 Glenrose Ave., Toronto 7, Ont. (res); Tor'46; D.R., D&TRad; Ass't. Rad., Hosp. for Sick Children; Clin. Teach., U. of Toronto; Tel. EM 6-7242, Loc. 2138.

MOFFAT, Agnes K. (Mrs. Russell K. Magee); 327 Charlotte St., Peterborough, Ont.; 597 Weller St. (res); McG'31; M.A.; Anaes; Paed; Chief of Anaes., Peterborough Civic & St. Joseph's Hosp's.; Tel. 743-2040.

MOFFAT, David J.; 14511 Mackenzie Dr., Edmonton, Alta.; Alb '41; Anaes.; Tel. HU 8-3133.

MOFFAT, Frederick K.; 1884 Weston Rd., Weston, Ont.; Tor'51; FRCS(C), GenSurg; Tel. 244-6111.

MOFFAT, James F.; 692A Coxwell Ave., Toronto, Ont.; 40 Barbara Cres. (res); Tor '50; F.R.C.S.(C), ObstGyn; Att. Staff (ObstGyn), Toronto East Gen. Hosp.; Tel. HO 1-6356.

MOFFAT, John G.; Tor'60; FRCS(C), GenSurg; Staff, Toronto Gen. Hosp., Toronto 2, Ont.

MOFFAT, John H.; 30A George St. N. Galt, Ont.; Tor'54; FRCS(C), GenSurg; Staff, South Waterloo Hosp.; Tel. 621-2860.

MOFFAT, Robert G.; 250 Main St. E., Hamilton, Ont.; Man'34; DMRE (Cambridge); D&TRad.; Rad. McGregor Clinic; Active Cons., Oakville-Trafalgar Mem. Hosp., Oakville.

MOFFAT, William W.; 1884 Weston Rd., Weston, Ont.; McG '53; FRCS(C); GenSurg; Staff, Toronto Western Hosp.; Tel. 244-6111.

MOFFATT, Alexander J.; 277 Scarborough Cr., Scarborough, Ont.; Tor'62; AMCGP.

MOFFATT, Clarence D.; 1647 Angus Dr., Vancouver 9, B.C. (res); U.S.'24; Staff, Workmen's Comp. Bd.; Tel. AM 6-0211.

MOFFATT, Donald W.; 1127 Medical-Dental Bldg., 925 W. Georgia St., Vancouver 1, B.C.; 1550 W. 26th Ave. (res); S. California (U.S.) '35; MCGP; Staff, St. Paul's Hosp.; Tel. MU 5-0046.

MOFFATT, Garfield M.; Fredericton Med. Clinic, 206 Rockwood Ave., Fredericton, N.B.; 838 Regent St. (res); Dal '47; IntMed; Chief-of-Med., Victoria Public Hosp.; Cons. Med., Hotel-Dieu & St. Joseph's Hosp's., Perth; Tel. GR 5-7701.

MOFFATT, Thomas I.; 215 Cooper St., Ottawa, Ont.; 732 Parkdale Ave. (res); Tor '29; Obst; Active Staff, Ottawa Civic Hosp.; Courtesy Staff, Ottawa Gen. Hosp.; Tel. PA 9-2511.

MOFFATT, Wm.; 333 Willard Ave., Toronto, Ont. (res); McG '27; Staff, Public Health Dept.; Tel. EM 3-1211.

MOFFITT, John A.; R.C.S. (Ire.) '52; Sr. Int'n. (Psy.), Ontario Hosp., Toronto, Ont.

MOFFITT, Kathleen J.; Med. Arts Clinic, 2125-11th Ave., Regina, Sask.; Alb'54; Paed; Staff, Regina Gen. & Grey Nun's Hosp's.; Tel. 523-0691.

MOFFOOT, Alexander G.; Box 370, Sidney, B.C.; Edinburgh (Scot.) '45; F.R.C.S. (Eng.); GenSurg.; Staff, Resthaven Hosp.; Tel. 656-1164.

MOGA, Traian J.; 116 Elm St. E., Sudbury, Ont.; 213 Bowland Ave. (res); Bucharest (Roumania) '48; MCGP; Staff, Psy. Unit, Sudbury Gen. Hosp.; Tel. 674-0166.

MOGAN, John J.; 4 Church St. S., Richmond Hill, Ont.; Tor '61; M.A.; Staff, York Central Hosp.; Tel. 884-4471.

MOGHADAM-KAZVINI, Hossein K.; 1815 W. 37th Ave., Vancouver 13, B.C.; Zurich (Switz.) '53; MPH; PH; Paed; Dir. of Med. Serv., Vancouver City Health Dept.; Tel. AM 1-6700.

MOGHAL, Ali N.; Karachi (Pakistan)'56; Am. Bd. Surg.; GenSurg; Staff, Ottawa Civic Hosp., Ottawa 3, Ont.

MOHACSY, Jeno; 344 Bloor St. W., Ste. 203, Toronto 5, Ont.; 35 Dunlace Dr., Willowdale; Debrecen (Hung.) '50; Tel. 927-3521.

MOHAJERIN, Amir H.; Med. Arts Bldg., 2125-11th Ave., Regina, Sask.; Tehran (Iran)'52.

MOHAN, Lajja M.; 36 Collingwood St., Kingston, Ont.; Punjab (India) '40; Tel. 546-2846.

MOHAMED, Gerald E.; Man '64; Staff, Birtle District Hosp., Birtle, Man.

MOHAMED, J. Kenneth; Mall Med. Bldg., 280 Osborne St. N., Winnipeg 1, Man.; Man'57; Urol.

MOHANNA, Mohamed; Montpellier (France)'55; Staff, L'Ecole de Hygiene, U. of Montreal, Montreal 26, P.Q.; Abroad.

MOHER, Herbert J.; 1229 The Queensway, Toronto 18, Ont.; Tel. CL 9-5961.

MOHER, Murray J.; 2 Aberdeen St., Peterborough, Ont.; Qns '16; Ophth; Retired.

MOHIDEEN, Koraishia (See Robinson).

MOHR, Armin A., Sg/Lt; HMCS Yukon, F.M.O., Victoria, B.C.; Alb'62; Abroad.

MOINEAU, Andre; 69 Beaver Ridge, Ottawa, Ont.; Mon '55; DPH; M.O., Dept. National Health & Welfare, Health Services Directorate.

MOIR, Donald M.; 151 Holland Ave., Ottawa 3, Ont.; 22 Fairfax Ave. (res); Aberdeen (Scot.) '50; M.C.G.P.; Att'd. Staff. Ottawa Civic & Grace Hosp's.; Tel. PA 9-2511.

MOIR, James H.; Knox Clinic, 1605 Glenmore St., Kelowna, B.C.; 3152 Watt Rd. (res); Man '36; FRCS(C), GenSurg; Tel. 762-2002.

MOIR, J. Bruce; Knox Clinic, 1605 Glenmore St., Kelowna, B.C.; Okanagan Mission (res); Man '44; MCGP; Staff, Kelowna Gen. Hosp.; Tel. 762-2002.

MOIR, J. David; 362 Main St., Saint John, N.B.; Dal '57; MCGP; Tel. 693-4855.

MOIR, Robert S.; Ste. 5, 6325 Fraser St., Vancouver 15, B.C.; Glasgow (Scot.) '54; M.B., B.Ch.; Anaes; Tel. FA 5-4040.

MOISAN, Andre; Hop. Laval, Ste. Foy, Quebec 10, P.Q.; Lav'59; MSc; Cardiol(P.Q.); FRCP(C), IntMed; Tel. 653-5251.

MOISAN, Fernand; 65 rue des Chenes E., Quebec, P.Q. (res); Lav '51; Pulm. Dis. & TB (P.Q.); Staff, Hop. Laval, Ste. Foy; Cons., Anti-T.B. League (P.Q.); Tel. 653-5251.

MOISAN, Octave; 360 St-Joseph, St-Raymond, Cte Portneuf, P.Q.; Lav '24.

MOISE, Andre L.; 2747 Maplewood, App. 5, Montreal 26, P.Q.; Haiti'44; Anaes.

MOK, George C. K.; Ontario Cancer Fdn., Windsor Clinic, Windsor, Ont.; 237 Belle Isle View Blvd., Riverside (res); Lingnan U. (Canton, China) '50; TherRad; Radiotherap. Ontario Cancer Fdn.; Active Staff, Metropolitan Gen. Hosp.; Tel. CL 3-7455.

MOK, Lillian W. (See Liu)

MOK-DOCK, Li; '58; Res., Victoria Hosp., London, Ont.

MOKKHAVESA, Suprija; McG'64; Res., Shaughnessy Hosp., Vancouver 9, B.C.

MOKUENA, John M.; Staff, Glendon Hosp., Glendon, Alta.; Tel. 16. Abroad.

MOLARO, Alphonso L.; 3195 Granville St., Vancouver 9, B.C.; Man'57; IntMed; M.O. in charge of Admission Serv., Shaughnessy Hosp.; Instr. (Med.), U. of British Columbia; Tel. RE 1-1282.

MOLBERG, Carey R.; Box 399, Fort Churchill, Man.; Sask'63; Tel. 336.

MOLDOFSKY, Harvey; Clarke Institute of Psychiatry, 250 College Street, Toronto, Ont.; Tor'59; D. Psy.; FRCP(C), Psy; Assoc. Psy., Clarke Institute of Psychiatry; Tel. 924-6811.

MOLDOFSKY, Jack; 158 St. George St., Toronto 5, Ont.; 148 Dalemount Ave., Tor. 19 (res); Tor '48; Psy; Cons. Psy., North York Branson Hosp.; Tel. WA 2-0785.

MOLGAT, Andre; 617 Med. Arts Bldg., Winnipeg 1, Man.; 209 Kingston Row, St. Vital 8 (res); Lav '48; M.Sc. (Chir.); FRCS(C), FACS; FICS; GenSurg; Active Staff (Surg.), St.-Boniface Hosp.; Ass't Prof. (Med.), U. of Manitoba; Tel. 943-5265

MOLINEUX, Robin R.; Belleoram, Nfld.; London (Eng.) '61; M.B., B.S.; Dist. Med. Officer & M.O.H.

MOLL, Albert E.; 570 Seaforth Med. Bldg., 3550 Cote des Neiges Rd., Montreal 25, P.Q.; 4342 Westmount Ave., Westmount (res); McG '37; FAPA; Psy; Psy-In-Chief, Mtl. Gen. Hosp.; Cons. Psy., Queen Elizabeth, Reddy Mem. & Queen Mary Vet's. Hosp's.; Prof (Psy.), McGill U.; Tel. 933-4552.

MOLLE, Alfred; 29 Nairn Ave., Kenora, Ont. (res); Tartu (Estonia) '35; D&TRad; Staff, Kenora Gen. & St. Joseph's Hosp's.

MOLLER, Evert S.; 49 W. Lake Ave., Toronto 13, Ont.; 5 Anewen Dr. (res); Tor '49; Ass't. Med. Dir., Crown Life Ins. Co.; Tel. OX 1-4669.

MOLLERUP, Victor; Alb'62; Res., Shaughnessy Hosp., Vancouver 9, B.C.

MOLLOY, J. Hubert; 6387 Coburg Rd., Halifax, N.S.; 5851 Inglis St. (res); Dal '43; Ophth; Ass't. Ophth., Victoria Gen. & Children's Hosp's.; Tel. 423-7822.

MOLONEY, Patrick J.; 4041 W. 40th Ave., Vancouver 13, B.C.; Seattle (U.S.A.)'52; FRCS(C), Urol.

MOLONY, Ronald J.; Otaga (N. Zealand)'60; Res., Kingston Gen. Hosp., Kingston, Ont.

MOLONY, Terence J.; 170 St. George St., Toronto, Ont.; Royal Coll. (Ire.) '46; F.R.C.S.(C), Otol; Staff, St. Michael's Cons., Scarborough Gen. & Oakville Mem. Hosp's.; Clin. Inst. U. of Toronto; Tel. WA 2-8651.

MOLOT, Michael J.; Ott'63; Res., Montreal Gen. Hosp., Montreal 25, P.Q.

MOMOSE, K. Jack; 350 Mayfield Ave., Eastview Ont. (res); McG '48; D.M.R., F.F.R.(Eng.), DABR (D&T), FCCP (USA); FRCP(C), D&T-Rad; Rad., Ottawa Gen. Hosp.; Lect'r., U. of Ottawa; Tel. 749-1866; Abroad.

MONAGHAN, Edmond D.; 267 Glengarry Ave., Town of Mount Royal, P.Q. (res); Lav '57; M.Sc. (Exper. Surg.); FRCS(C), GenSurg; Clin. Ass't. Surg., Royal Victoria Hosp.; Dem., McGill U.; Tel. VI 2-1251, Loc. 1567.

MONAGHAN, Theodore T.; Medical Arts Bldg., Corner Brook, Nfld., 16 Cobb Lane (res); Dal '32; Zeugnis (Vienna); GenSurg; Head, Dept. of ObstGyn., & GenSurg., Dept. of Surg., Western Mem. Hosp.; Tel. 4-5232.

MONAGHAN, Thomas G.; Iroquois, Ont.; Ott '59.

MONAGLE, J. Edgar; 5 Crystal Beach Dr., Ottawa 14, Ont. (res); Alb '51; Chief, Nutrition Div., Dept. of Nat. Health & Welfare; Tel. CE 2-8211.

MONAHAN, Gordon J., Major; National Defence Med. Centre, Smyth Rd. & Alta Vista Dr., Ottawa, Ont.; Ott'54; FRCP(C); IntMed.; Deputy Chief Med. NDMC; Clin. Ass't. Med., U. of Ottawa.

MONAST, N. Etienne; 107 rue Davignon, Cowansville, P.Q.; Mon '55; Phys., Albany Felt Co.

MONCKTON, George; University Hosp., Edmonton, Alta.; St. Bart's (London, Eng.) '44; M.D. (Lond.), M.R.C.P.(Lond.), F.R.C.P.(C), Neurol; Assoc. Prof. (Neur.), U of Alberta; Telephone GE 9-5911, Ext. 345.

MONDAY, Louise; Mon'65; Res., Hop. Hotel-Dieu Montreal 18, P.Q.

MONDOR, Albert; 4902 Verdun Ave., Verdun, P.Q.; Mon '25; Anaes (P.Q.).

MONDOR, Eugene; 3719 Blvd. Levesque, Chomedey, P.Q.; Mon'25; DPH.

MONDOR, La Salle; 630-6e rue, Grand'Mere, P.Q.; Mon '40; Anaes (P.Q.).

MONDOUX, Gaetan; 8415 St.-Denis, Montreal 11, P.Q.; Mon '61.

MONESTINE, S. Firmin; Box 520, Mattawa, Ont.; Haiti'36.

MONETTE, Lucie; 945 Didace, Magog, P.Q.; Mon '54; Paed. (P.Q.); Tel. 843-5571.

MONFETTE, Claude B.; 364 est Sherbrooke, Montreal, P.Q.; 789 Dunlop (res); Mon '43; Ophth, **Otol (P.Q.); Ass't. Ophth., Hotel Dieu; Tel. VI 4-0161.**

MONGEAU, Bernard; Ste. 203, 825 sud, rue Belvedere, Sherbrooke, P.Q.; Mon '53; Staff (Med.) & Chief, Radio-isotopes Clin., Hotel-Dieu de Sherbrooke; Tel. 567-5088.

MONGEAU, J. Andre; 305 Grande Cote, Rosemere, Cte. Terrebonne, P.Q.; Mon '62.

MONGEAU, Jean-Guy; 302 Varry Ville St. Laurent, Montreal 9, P.Q.; Mon'58; FRCP(C), Paed.

MONGEAU, Maurice; 6300 Darlington Ave., Montreal, P.Q.; 2330 Seneca St. (res); Mon '48; DABPhysMed & Rehab; PhysMed & Rehab; Hd. Dept. (PhysMed & Rehab), Inst. de Rehab.-de-Mtl.; Cons., Hop. Pasteur; Ass't. Dir., Schl. of Rehab & Assoc. Prof. (PhysMed & Rehab), U. of Mtl.; Tel. 735-3741.

MONGEAU, Serge; 5285 Aurele, St.-Hubert 1, P.Q.; Mon '63; Tel. 676-2321.

MONGEON, Roland; Mon'63; Res., St. Mary's Hosp., Montreal 25, P.Q.

MONK, William S. M.; Bracebridge, Ont.; Tor 51; FACS, FRCS(C), GenSurg.; Tel. 645-2541.

MONKMAN, Evan J.; 1050 Avenue Rd., Toronto 12, Ont.; Tor'64; Assoc. Staff, Toronto Western Hosp.; Tel. 489-9374.

MONKS, H. Thomas J.; 5327 Queen Mary Rd., Montreal, P.Q.; 8 Merton Cres., Hampstead (res); McG '39; Derm. Syph; Derm., St. Mary's & Montreal Children's Hosp's.; Cons., Derm., Catherine Booth Maternity Hosp.; Clin Med. McGill U.; HU 1-8800.

MONKS, James G.; 227 Med. Arts Bldg., Saskatoon, Sask.; 225 Saskatchewan Cres. W. (res); Nat. U. (Dublin, Ire.) '47; BAO; DMRD; DiagRad; Radiol., St. Paul's Hosp.; Lect. (Rad.Anat.), U. of Saskatchewan; Tel. 242-1169.

MONTEITH, D. A.; Shedden, Ont.; Wes '37.

MONTEITH, John S.; 710 Seymour St., Vancouver 2, B.C.; 5230 Marguerite, Van. 13 (res); Man '43; MCGP; Tel. MU 4-1511.

MONTEL, Georges B.; 127 du Prince, Sorel, P.Q.; Lyon (Fr.) '28; GenSurg (P.Q.); Tel. RI 3-8153.

MONTEMURO, Thomas J.; 207-208 Med. Arts Bldg., Port Arthur, Ont.; 54 Summit Ave. (res); Tor '43; FRCP(C); IntMed; Chief of Med., St. Joseph's Hosp.; Tel. 4-2692.

MONTEMURRO, G. A.; Streetsville, Ont.; Tor **'31; Dist. Coroner; Tel. TA 6-1616.**
MONTFORT, Frank G.; 1192 The Queensway, Toronto 18, Ont.; 2 Amattice Rd., Islington (res); London (Eng.)'49; MRCS; LRCP; MCGP; Pres., Queensway Gen. Hosp Med. Staff; Tel. 259-0956.
MONTGOMERY, A. Eugene; 802 Medical Arts Bldg., 170 St. George St., Toronto, Ont.; Tor '23; Tel. WA 2-1545.
MONTGOMERY, Cecil B.; Box 130, Cumberland, B.C.; Man '53.
MONTGOMERY, Donald B.; 3240 Bloor St. W., Toronto 18, Ont.; Tor '54; FRCP(C), IntMed; Cons. & Hd., Dept. of Med., Queensway Gen. Hosp.; Hon. Cons., South Peel Hosp.; Tel. 239-7621.
MONTGOMERY, Donald C.; 310 O'Connor St., Ottawa, Ont.; 89 Seneca St. (res); **Qns '44; D.A.B.D.S., F.A.A.D., DermSyph; Sr. Derm., Ottawa Civic Hosp.; Cons. (Derm.), Winchester Hosp.; Lect. (Derm.) U. of Ottawa; Tel. 236-3637.**
MONTGOMERY, Harold; 15 Oakridge Park Terr., London, Ont. (res); London (Eng.) '52; Path; MRCP (Ed.); Path., Victoria Hosp.; Ass't. Prof., U. of Western Ontario; Tel. 432-5261.
MONTGOMERY, Lorne C., O.B.E., M.C., V.D., Legion of Merit; 1414 Drummond St., Montreal, P.Q.; 556 Grosvenor Ave., Westmount (res); McG '20; F.R.C.P. (Lond.), F.R.S.M. (Hon.), F.R.C.P.(C), IntMed; Cons. Med., Montreal Gen. **Hosp.; Emeritus Prof. (Med.), McGill U.; Tel. AV 8-2284.**
MONTGOMERY, Richard C.; 116 Stratford Cres., Toronto 12, Ont. (res); Tor '21; M.O., Manufacturers Life Ins. Co., 200 Bloor St. E.; Tel. 924-4111.
MONTGOMERY, Robert C.; 72 Highbourne Rd., Toronto, Ont. (res); Tor '24; Psy; Retired.
MONTGOMERY, Thomas E.; Philipsburg, P.Q. (res); Bishops (U.S.) '94; Retired.
MONTGOMERY, Wesley G.; Somerset Bldg., **Winnipeg, Man.; 17 Purcell Ave. (res); Tor '10; Tel. SU 3-3022.**
MONTGRAIN, Noel-Henri; 352 rue Dolbeau, Quebec 6, P.Q.; Lav'59; FRCP(C), Psy.
MONTGRAIN, Pierre; 1975 rue Henri Bourassa est, Apt. 6, Montreal 12, P.Q.; Lav'60; IntMed. (P.Q.); Gastroent (P.Q.).
MONTMINY, Lionel; 802 Chanoine Scott, **Quebec 10, P.Q.; 941 ave Fournier, Ste.-Foy (res); Lav '49; Pulm. Dis. & TB (PQ); Staff, Hop. Laval; Memb. Anti-TB League (PQ); Staff, Laval U.; Tel. 653-4931.**
MONTMINY, Roger; Lav '59; Res., Hop. Notre-Dame, Montreal 24 P.Q.
MONTOUR, Jean; 7494 St. Denis, Montreal, **P.Q.; Mon '45; Staff, Hop. Ste. Justine; Tel. RE 1-4931.**
MONTPETIT, Jean; Mon'59; Psy(P.Q.); c/o 9 Rue Burton, Montreal 6, P.Q.
MONTPETIT, Pierre; Mon '62; Res., Hop. Hotel-Dieu, Montreal 18, P.Q.
MONTPETIT, Vital J.A.; Montreal Neurological Inst., 3801 University St., Montreal, P.Q.; Ott'61; Path(P.Q.).
MONTREUIL, Fernand; 801 est Sherbrooke, Mon**treal 24, P.Q.;** 310 Cote St-Antoine, Westmount **(res); Lav '39; DABO; FAAOO; FALA; FABES; FACS; FRCS(C); Otol; Chief, Dept. of Otol. & Dir., Speech & Hearing Clin., Hop. Notre Dame Dir., Otol. Serv., Queen Mary Vet's. Hosp.; Prof. & Hd., Dept. of Otol., U. of** Montreal; Tel. 527-1344.
MONTY, Lomar A.; Adm., Immigration Serv., Dept. of National Health & Welfare, 150 St. **Paul W., Montreal 1, P.Q.; Mon '50; Tel. VI 9-4165.**
MONTY, Pierre; Clinique Med. Belanger, 3871 Est Belanger, Montreal 36, P.Q.; Mon '61.
MONYPENNY, A. Doris; 99 Wanless Cres., Toronto 12, Ont. (res); Tor '23; Paed; Cons., Child Health Centre for Dept. of P.H., Toronto; Retired.
MOODIE, C. Alastair; 157 Ontario St., Ste. 3, St. Catharines, Ont.; St. Andrews (Scot.) '48; MC(Path.); Path; Dir. of Labs., Hotel-Dieu Hosp.; Tel. 682-8316.
MOODIE, George E.; Bayview Towers, 15 Vancouver St., Barrie, Ont.; McG '23; DPH; M.O.H., Simcoe County Health Unit; Tel. 728-5967.
MOODY, Arthur D., SG Lt; RCAF Station, Comox, B.C.; Qns '63.
MOODY, Dwight L.; 1669 Victoria St., Prince George, B.C.; '47; Psy.; **Tel. 563-0800.**
MOODY, Frederick J.; 71 Westlake Ave., Toronto 13, Ont.; Tor '55; Assoc. Staff, Toronto East Gen. Hosp.; Tel. OX 1-1441.
MOODY, Joseph P.; 46 Ontario St., Elliot Lake, **Ont.; 47 Axmith (res); Wes '46; MCGP; M.NYASc; Chief of Staff, Elliot Lake Hosp.;** Dist. Coroner (Algoma); Tel. VI 8-7176.
MOOGK, Donald H.; Ste. 204, 824 King St. W., Kitchener, Ont.; Tor'50; Psy.; Tel. 576-2270.
MOON, Chang S.; 7601 Côte St. Luc Rd., Apt. 403, Montreal, P.Q.; Taegu (Korea)'48; DiagRad.
MOON, Isobel D.; Winnipeg Clinic, St. Mary's & Vaughan, Winnipeg, Man.; 333 Wellington Cres., Apt. 607 (res); Tor '45; IntMed; Tel. 942-0551.
MOONEY, Alvin W.; Drawer 890, Vanderhoff, B.C.; Alb '46; F.R.C.S.(C), GenSurg; FACS; Chief of Staff, St. John Hosp.; Tel. 567-2361.
MOONEY, Bernard R.; 2716 Dominion Blvd., Windsor, Ont. (res); **Wes '10;** D&TRad; Retired.
MOONEY, Harold A. L.; Box 68, Comox, B.C.; Man '34; MCGP.
MOONEY, John K.; Ste. 455, 5025 Sherbrooke St. W., Montreal 28, P.Q.; Qns '46; IntMed P.Q.); Tel. 488-3304.
MOONEY, Malcolm C.; 151 Main St., Cowansville, P.Q.; McG'36; GenSurg; Surg., Brome-Missisquoi-Perkins Hosp.; Tel. 263-2777.
MOONIE, George T.; 11515-77th Ave., Edmonton, Alta. (res); Alb '48; D.A.B.A., F.A.C.A.; Anaes; Att. Staff, Dept. of Anaes., U. of Alberta **Hosp.; Tel. 439-5911.**
MOONJE, Vijay B.; Nagpur (India) '59; Res., Ottawa Gen. Hosp., Ottawa, Ont.
MOORADIAN, Anaid S.; 244 Waverley St., Winnipeg 9, Man. (res); Man'42; Retired.
MOORE, Allin H.; 710 Seymour St., Vancouver 2, B.C.; 1550 W. 29th (res); Man '44; F.R.C.S. **(Ed.); F.R.C.S. (Eng.); F.R.C.S.(C), GenSurg; Tel. MU 4-1511.**
MOORE, Amer H.; Box 540, North Bay, Ont.; Qns '35; Adm., Cdn. Pension Comm.; Tel. 472-2000.
MOORE, Brian P. L.; 95 Wellesley St. E., Toronto 5, Ont.; Queen's U. (Belfast, N. Ire.) '42; M.B., B.Ch., BAO; MC Path; Dir., Nat. Blood Group Ref. Lab., Cdn. Red Cross Blood Transfusion Serv.; Tel. WA 3-6692.
MOORE, Carl A.; 1507 Main W., Hamilton, Ont.; Wes'59; MCGP; Active Staff, Hamilton Gen. & St. Joseph's Hosp's.; Court. Staff, Chedoke Gen. & Children's Hosp's.; Tel. JA 9-6870.
MOORE, Charles E.; Hermitage, Hermitage Bay, Nfld.; Missouri (U.S.A.) '64.
MOORE, Claude A.; 1414 Drummond St., Montreal **25, P.Q.; 420 Clarke Ave., Westmount (res); Wes '42; FRCS(C);** Urol; Assoc. Urol., **Montreal Gen. Hosp.; Cons. Urol., Lachine Gen. Hosp's.; Lect. (Surg.), McGill U.; Tel. VI 2-4370.**
MOORE, Christopher H.; 340 Med. Arts Bldg., 1105 Pandora Ave., Victoria, B.C.; 3450 Upper Terr. (res); Man '41; M.S. (Minn.); Ophth; Chief (Ophth), Royal Jubilee Hosp.; Tel. EV 3-3282.
MOORE, David S.; 681 Prince St., Truro, N.S.; Ott '55.
MOORE, Denis; Box 2347, Smithers, B.C.; Edinburgh (Scot.) '54; MCGP.
MOORE, Donald C.; 321 Med. Arts Bldg., 170 St. George St., **Toronto 5, Ont.; Dal '53; F.R.-C.S.(C), ObstGyn; Active Staff (Indoor), Women's College Hosp.; Clin. Instr., U. of Toronto; Tel. WA 2-1902.**
MOORE, Donald F.; 217 Saskatchewan Cres., W., Saskatoon, Sask.; Tor '34; B.Sc. (Med.), F.R.C.P.(C), Path,Bact; Dir. of Labs., University Hosp.; Prof. & Hd. (Path), U. of Saskatchewan; Tel. CH 2-7641, Loc. 321.

MOORE, Duncan J. McB.; London (Eng.) '52; Sr. Intn. (Med.), St. Joseph's Hosp., Toronto 3, Ont.

MOORE, Eamonn A.; 6252 Quinpool Rd., Halifax, N.S.; RCS (Ireland) '53; Psy; Staff, Nova Scotia Hosp.; Dir., Alcoholism Unit; Tel. 423-0604.

MOORE, Fred C.; 241 Lakeview Ave., Pointe-Claire, P.Q.; McG '50; IntMed; Att'd. Phys., Queen Elizabeth & Lachine Gen. Hosp's.; Tel. 695-6471.

MOORE, Gerald F. W.; Perth, N.B.; McG '48; **Gen Surg; M.C.G.P.; Surg., Hotel Dieu Hosp.;** Tel. 430.

MOORE, J. B.; Mitchell, Ont.; Nelson St. (res); Wes '43; M.C.G.P.; Dist. Coroner.

MOORE, Jean E.; 67 College St., Toronto 2, Ont.; London (Eng.)'50; MRCS; LRCP; DPH (Tor); Ass't. Dir., Maternal & Child Health Branch, Ont. Dept. of Health; Tel. 365-4066.

MOORE, J. Albert; 139-6th Ave., Box 790, Cochrane, Ont.; 87-7th St. (res); Qns '45; MCGP; G.P., & Regional Pathol., Att'y. Gen. Dept.; Tel. 272-5227.

MOORE, John B.; 42 Albert St., Stratford, Ont.; Wes'43; MCGP; Tel. 271-4280.

MOORE, John D.; McGregor Clinic, 250 Main St. E., Hamilton, Ont.; London (Eng.) '52; IntMed; Court. Staff, St. Joseph's & Hamilton Civic Hosp's.; & Hamilton Health Assoc.; Tel. 527-2711.

MOORE, John H.; 1405 Douglas St., Victoria, B.C.; 2941 Sea View Rd. (res); Qns '12; F.A.-C.S., GenSurg.; Tel. EV 3-6331.

MOORE, John H.; 722—12th St., Saskatoon, Sask. (res); Mon '20; Exam. Can. Pension Comm.; Tel. 653-1186.

MOORE, John R.; 4500 Sherbrooke St. W., Montreal 6, P.Q.; 3655 Ridgewood Ave. (res); McG '41; DABS; FACS; FRCS(C); GenSurg; Clin. Ass't., Royal Victoria Hosp.; Cons. Surg., Queen Mary Vet's. Hosp.; Dem. Surg. McGill U.; Tel. WE 2-2723.

MOORE, Joseph D.; 17 Gore Ave., Chilliwack, B.C.; McG '17; Tel. SY 2-2241.

MOORE, Laurence H.; 752 Commissioner's Rd. E., London, Ont.; Alb'64.

MOORE, Marjorie B. (Bremner); 288 St. Clair Ave. W., Toronto 7, Ont.; 32 Cornish Rd. (res); Tor '48; MRCOG; ObstGyn; Staff, Women's College Hosp.; Tel. WA 3-2757.

MOORE, Maurice B.; 406 Med. Centre, Calgary, Alta.; 4223 Brisebois Dr. N.W. (res); Durham (Eng.) '46; Psy; Psy., Calgary Gen. Hosp.; Assoc. (Psy), Holy Cross Hosp.; Tel. 262-2538.

MOORE, Mayhew G.; 118 John Blvd., Waterloo, Ont.; Lond. (Eng.) '45.

MOORE, M. John; 306 King St., Midland, Ont.; London (Eng.)'57; DRCOG; Ass. Member Medical Staff, St. Andrew's Hosp. & Penetang General Hosp., Penetang; Tel. 526-5326.

MOORE, Percy E.; 65 Sunnyside Ave., Ottawa, Ont.; Man '31; DPH; PH; Dir., Med. Services Directorate, Dept. of National Health & Welfare; Tel. CE 2-8211.

MOORE, Peter C. F.; 262 St. Clair Avenue W., Toronto 7, Ont.; Tor'49; Psy; Assoc. Clarke Inst. for Psychiatry; Staff, Psy., Univ. of Toronto; Tel. 927-5499.

MOORE, Peter S.; Ste. 40, 3195 Granville St., Vancouver 9, B.C.; 733-1050th St., Van. 9 (res); Oxford (Eng.) '47; Paed; Att'd. Staff, St. Vincent's Hosp.; Clin. Instr. (Paed.), U. of British Columbia; Tel. 731-2155.

MOORE, Robert F.; 300 Islington Ave. N., Islington, Ont.; 6 Hampshire Hgts. (res); Tor '53; Active Staff, Queensway Gen. Hosp.; Court. Staff, St. Michael's Hosp.; Pt-time Dept. of Health, City of Toronto; Tel. BE 1-3511.

MOORE, Sean; 498 Lansdowne Ave., Westmount, P.Q. (res); Queen's U. (Belfast, N. Ire.) '50; Path; Assoc. Pathol., Mtl. Gen. Hosp.; Cons. Path., Queen Mary Vet's & Catherine Booth Hosp's.; Ass't. Prof. (Path.), McGill U.; Tel. WE 7-6011.

MOORE, T. Brian; 2 Main St. N., Acton, Ont.; Tor '61.

MOORE, Terrence L.; Wes'65; Res., Shaughnessy Hosp., Vancouver 9, B.C.

MOORE, Thomas; Med. Centre, 5 Central St., Summerside, P.E.I.; 223 Commerce Ave. (res); Sheffield (Eng.) '54; DRCOG; FACS; FACOG; **ObstGyn; Chief, Dept. of ObstGyn., Prince Co. Hosp.; Tel. 436-2277.**

MOORES, Arthur A.; 19 Virginia Ave., Dartmouth, N.S.; College of Med. Evangelists (Loma Linda, Calif., U.S.A.)'53; GenSurg; Staff, Victoria Gen. Hosp., Halifax.

MOORES, Edwin F.; 29 Cornwall Heights, St. John's, Nfld.; Qns '19; FACS; FRCS(C); GenSurg; Tel. 578-3631.

MOORES, William G.; Dal '60; Res., Grace Maternity Hosp., Halifax, N.S.

MOORHEAD, Peter B.; St. George St., Dresden, Ont.; London U. (Eng.) '53; A.M.C.G.P.

MOORHOUSE, David J.; Sackville Med. Centre, 10 Lansdowne St., Sackville, N.B.; Cambridge (Eng.)'55; MRCS(Eng.); LRCP(Lond.); D.Obst RCOG; DCH(Eng.).

MOORHOUSE, H. Clayton; Wes '31; Psy; Supt. Ontario Hosp., 3131 Lake Shore Blvd. W., Toronto 14, Ont.; Tel. CL 9-8291.

MOORHOUSE, John A.; 148 Seven Oaks, Winnipeg 17, Man.; Man '50; Ass't. Prof. (Physiol.), U. of Man.; Tel. GR 4-9110.

MOORHOUSE, Victor H. K.; 32 Amanda St., Orangeville, Ont. (res); Tor '10; F.R.C.S.; Prof. Emeritus (Physiol.), U. of Manitoba; Retired.

MOORS, David E.; Ste. 207, 1105 Carling Ave., Ottawa 3, Ont.; Qns'52; FRCS(C), Urol.

MORA, Julio; 537 College St., Toronto 4, Ont.; Madrid (Spain) '51.

MORAIS-ROCHON, Therese; Mon'63; Res., Hop. Ste-Justine, Montreal 26, P.Q.

MORALEJO, Richard V.; 400-5300 Cote-des-Neiges Rd., Montreal 26, P.Q.; 5604 Notre-Dame-de-Grace Ave. (res); McG '49; F.R.C.S.-(C), GenSurg; Assoc. Surg., St. Mary's Hosp.; Cons. Sperry-Gyroscope Co.; Tel. RE 7-3722.

MORAN, D. J. Lyall; 239 Broadway, Orangeville, Ont.; 79 McCarthy St. (res); Tor '57; Staff, Dufferin Area Hosp.; Tel. 941-1551.

MORAN, Donald B.; One Medical Place, 20 Wynford Dr., Don Mills, Ont.; 25 Governor's Rd. (res); Tor'39; FRCP(C), IntMed; Assoc. Prof. (Med.), U. of Toronto; Cardiol., St. Michael's Hosp.; Tel. 429-1560.

MORAN, Edward J.; 4151 Sheppard Ave. E., Agincourt, Ont.; Tor'57; AMCGP; Tel. 293-4189.

MORAN, Francis J.; Bolton St., Bobcaygeon, Ont.; Tor'53; MOH, Bobcaygeon; Tel. 738-2441.

MORAN, John H.; Anaesthesia Associates, 178 St. George St., Toronto, Ont.; Tor'54; DA; FRCP(C), Anaes; Staff, Toronto Gen. Hosp.; Cons., Princess Margaret Hosp.; Clin. Ass't., U. of Toronto; Tel. WA 3-1154.

MORAND, Claude; Mon'65; Res., Institute Albert Prevost, Montreal 9, P.Q.

MORAND, J. Charles; 1691 Tecumseh Rd. W., Windsor, Ont.; Tor '58; Tel. 252-6022. Abroad.

MORCH, John E.; McG '56; FRCP(C), IntMed; Ass't. Dir., Cardiovascular Unit, Toronto Gen. Hosp., Toronto 2, Ont.; Tel. EM 6-8211.

MORDRET, Claude; Lav'63; Res., Hop. Ste-Justine, Montreal 26, P.Q.

MORE, Charles G. R.; 4758 - 32nd St., Red Deer, Alta.; 3657-41st Ave. (res); Aberdeen (Scot.) '43; DPH; MRSH; FRSH; FAPHA; M.O.H., No. 9 Red Deer Health Unit; Tel. 347-1166.

MORE, John H.; Box 138, Rimbey, Alta.; Man'51.

MORE, Robert H.; R.R.3., Collins Bay, Ont. (res); Tor '39; M.Sc.(Path.) (McGill); FRC-P(C); Path; Path-in-Chief, Kingston Gen. Hosp.; Prof. (Path.), & Hd. of Dept. Queen's U.; Tel. 546-3871.

MOREASH, Roy A.; Commercial St., Berwick, N.S.; Dal '31; F.I.C.S., GenSurg; Staff, Western King's Mem. Hosp; Surg., Cambridge Stn., Indian Reserve.

MOREAU, Alphonse; 1193 des Erables, Quebec, P.Q.; 1054 Chaumont, Sillery (res); Lav '46; Ophth,Otol (P.Q.); Clin. Ass't. & Dem. Hop.-St.-Sacrement; Staff, Laval U.; Tel. 524-2642.

MOREAU, Antonio; App 18, 10140 Place Meilleur, Montreal 12, P.Q.; Mon '56; FRCS(C); GenSurg; Staff, Gen. Hosp., St. Eustache; Tel. 627-2848.

MOREAU, Francois A.; 3801 Barclay, Montreal, P.Q.; Mon '47.

MOREAU, Joseph P.; 104 Lemarchand Bldg., Edmonton, Alta.; 9728-111 Ave. (res); Alb '44; DABOS; FACS; FRCS(C); OrthSurg; Chief of OrthSurg., Edmonton Gen. Hosp.; Instr. (OrthSurg.), U. of Alberta; Tel. HU 8-5235.

MOREAU, Marcel; R.R. 1, St. Jean, P.Q.; Mon '61; GenSurg(P.Q.).

MOREAULT, Philippe; Suite 21, 5757 ave Decelles, Montreal 26, P.Q.; Lav '54; Psy; Staff, Rehabilitation Inst.; Tel. 733-8881.

MOREHOUSE, Charles N.; Bayers Rd. Shopping Centre, Halifax, N.S.; Dal'43.

MOREHOUSE, Douglas D.; Dept. of Urol., Royal Victoria Hosp., Montreal 2, P.Q.; McG'58; FRCS(C), Urol; Staff, Royal Victoria & Queen Mary Vet's Hosp's.; Staff, McGill U.; Tel. 844-1881.

MOREHOUSE, Oscar E.; Burtt's Corner, N.B.; McG '33; Tel. Keswick 110.

MOREL, Robert A.; 590-5th Ave., Chibougamau, P.Q.; Ott'53; Tel. 276-2111.

MORELAND, Stewart W.; Qns'65; Res., Montreal General Hosp., Montreal 25, P.Q.

MORENCY, Pierre; Lav'65; Res., Hop. du Christ-Roi, Quebec 8, P.Q.

MORES, George P.; 440 Scarborough Ave., Calgary, Alta.; Alb '40 F.A.C.A.; Anaes; Tel. CH 4-1532.

MORESIDE, J. William; 170 Fitzroy St., Charlottetown, P.E.I.; 45 York Lane (res); Dal '49; Ophth; Tel. 894-7325.

MORF, Gustave; 2983 Soissons, Montreal 26, P.Q.; Berne U. (Switz.)'38; Psy(P.Q.); Cons. Psy., Rehab Inst.

MORGAN, A. Lloyd; Ste. 1116, 123 Edward St., Toronto 2, Ont.; Tor '27; Ophth; Active Cons. Ophth., Hosp. for Sick Children; Ass't. Prof. Ophth. (Emer.), U. of Toronto; Tel. 368-2661.

MORGAN, Bruce E., Lt/Col.; Qns'51; FACS; FRCS(C), GenSurg; Chief of Surg., Toronto Military Hosp.; Tel. 485-8561, Loc. 319.

MORGAN, Charles A.; 109 King St. E., Oshawa, Ont.; 718 Glengrove (res); Loma Linda (Los Angeles) '60; AMCGP; Tel. 728-9361.

MORGAN, Deane K.; 183 James St. S., Hamilton, Ont.; 148 Buckingham (Dr.), (res); London (Eng.) '48; L.R.C.P., M.R.C.S., F.F.A.-R.C.S., D.A.R.C.S.; Anaes; Head of Anaes; Chedoke Gen. & Children's Hosp's.; Staff, Hamilton Gen. & West Lincoln Mem. Hosp.; Tel. JA 9-8875.

MORGAN, Edward A.; 416 Medical Arts Bldg., 170 St. George St., Toronto, Ont.; Tor'09; FRCP(C) Paed.; Cons. Hosp. for Sick Children; Tel. WA 2-9754.

MORGAN, E. Laurie D.; 109 Coe Hill Dr., Toronto 3, Ont.; 15 Grenadier Hgts. (res); Tor '45; AMCGP; Tel. RO 2-6776.

MORGAN, Ethel A. M.; (Matt); 27 Douglas Cres., Toronto 5, Ont. (res); Columbia (N.Y.) '28; Path Bact; Dem. (Path.), U. of Toronto; Tel. WA 3-6611. Retired.

MORGAN, Henry V.; Calgary Assoc. Clinic, 214-6 Ave. W., Calgary, Alta.; Man. '28; F.R.C.S.-(Ed.), F.A.C.S., GenSurg.; Cons. (Gen Surg.), Holy Cross Hosp. & Calgary Assoc., Clinic; Tel. AM 3-7120.

MORGAN, H. Robert; 307 Medical Arts Bldg., Hamilton, Ont.; 1097 Scenic Dr. (res); Wes '43; ObstGyn; Active Staff, Hamilton Civic Hosps.; Chief Gyn., Chedoke Hosp.; Tel. JA 8-6369.

MORGAN, J. Edwin; 157 Roxborough St. E., Toronto 5, Ont.; Tor'58; FRCS(C), ObstGyn; Staff, Toronto Gen. Hosp.; Tel. EM 6-8211.

MORGAN, John C.; 62 Academy Med. Bldg., 1812-4th St. W., Calgary, Alta.; 1219 Bel Air Dr. (res); Qns '50; FRCP(C), IntMed (Cardiol.); Cardiol., Col. Belcher Hosp.; Staff, Holy Cross Hosp.; Tel. AM 3-2251.

MORGAN, John E.; Metcalfe Bldg., 5th St. S., Lethbridge, Alta.; 1522-11th Ave. S. (res); London (Eng.) '41; L.R.C.P., M.R.C.S., D.Obst., R.C.O.G.; MR.C.O.G.; ObstGyn; Staff (ObstGyn), St. Michael's Gen. & Lethbridge Mun. Hosp's.; Dist. Coroner; Tel. FA 8-2831.

MORGAN, John F.; 74 Sunset Blvd., Kingston, Ont.; Tor '56; FRCS(C), Ophth; Chief, Dept. of Ophth., Cdn. Forces Hosp.; Clin. Ass't. (Ophth.), Queen's U.; Tel. 8-3060.

MORGAN, J. Russell; 707 Charlotte St., Peterborough, Ont.; 900 Armour Rd. N. (res); Tor '31; B.Sc. (Med.), F.A.C.P., M.C.A.A.; IntMed; Staff, Peterborough Civic & St. Joseph's Hosp's.; Tel. RI 2-3871.

MORGAN, Leonard I.; 115 Hazen St., Saint John, N.B.; 58 Quinton Dr. (res); McG '53; MCGP; Att'd. Staff, St. John Gen. & St. Joseph's Hosp's.; Tel. 693-1618.

MORGAN, Marion (Webster); 307 Med. Arts Bldg., 1 Young St., Hamilton, Ont.; 1097 Scenic Dr. (res); Wes '43; Anaes; Staff (Anaes), Chedoke Gen. Hosp.; Tel. JA 8-6369.

MORGAN, Philip J.; 335 Matthew Brady Blvd., Windsor, Ont.; Ott'55; Tel. 948-0896.

MORGAN, Robert W.; 2946 Tillicum, Victoria, B.C.; 55 Tovey Cr. (res); UBC '61; AMCGP; Tel. 385-6112.

MORGAN, Roderick A.; Alb '61; Res., University Hosp., Edmonton, Alta.

MORGAN, Roger E.; 260 Cedar St., Sudbury, Ont.; 62 Cranbrook Cr. (res); Tor '56; MCGP; Tel. 673-3695.

MORGAN, Waldo B.; Wilson-Hall Clinic, 176 Catharine St., Port Colborne, Ont.; Cardiff (Wales)'50; Active Medical Staff, Port Colborne General Hospital; Tel. 834-3638.

MORGENSTERN, Gert F.; 4633 Sherbrooke St. W., Montreal 6, P.Q. (res); McG '58; Staff, Jewish Gen. Hosp.; Tel. 735-3771.

MORGENTALER, Henry; 2990 Beaugrand St., Montreal 5, P.Q.; Mon '53; Tel. 351-0290.

MORIARITY, Andrew; 300 Laurentian Blvd., Montreal 9, P.Q.; 395 Northcote, Rosemere (res); Wes '49; Dir. of Research, Smith Kline & French (Senneville); Tel. RI 7-6565.

MORIARTY, Joseph E., 117 Medical Arts Bldg., Calgary, Alta.; 1320 Quebec Ave. (res); Qns '43; MCGP; Tel. 262-4474.

MORIN, Benoit; Trahan Bldg., 490-17th Ave., Grand'Mere, P.Q.; Lav '51; Otol (P.Q.).

MORIN, Claude, Capt.; RCAF Station, Cold Lake, Alta.; Lav'66.

MORIN, Claude; 3817 boul. Decarie, Montreal 28, P.Q.; Mon '58; FRCP(C), IntMed; Staff, St. Luc. Hosp.; Tel. 488-5424.

MORIN, Claude L.; Mon'62; Paed(P.Q.); Staff, Hosp. for Sick Children, Toronto 2, Ont.

MORIN, Gaspard; 1475 Ave Desjardins, Montreal, P.Q.; Mon '33; Paed; Prof. of Paed., U. of Montreal; Ass't. Chief (Paed.), Hop. Ste. Justine; Tel. RE 1-4931.

MORIN, Gaston D.; 232 Metcalfe, Ste. 22, Ottawa 4, Ont.; Mon'51; Psy; Chief Psy., Royal Ottawa San.; Ass't. Prof. Psy., Ottawa U.

MORIN, Gerard; 6452 Delorimier, Montreal '35, P.Q.; 6450 Delorimier, Apt. 1 (res); Mon '34; IntMed; Phys., Hotel Dieu Hosp.; Ass't. Clin. Prof., U. of Montreal; Tel. RA 9-1201.

MORIN-GONTHIER, Mariette; 221 Ave Outremont, Montreal 8, P.Q.; Mon '61.

MORIN, Guy M.; Lav'58; Bact; Staff, Hop. du Sacre-Coeur, 5400 ouest Blvd. Gouin, Montreal, P.Q.; Tel. 334-1210.

MORIN, Jacques; Lav'59; Res., Hop. Maisonneuve, Montreal 36, P.Q.

MORIN, J. Donald; 1050 Avenue Road, Toronto 12, Ont.; Tor'59; FRCS(C); Ophth; Staff, St. Michael's Hospital; Tel. 485-3888.

MORIN, Jeanine; Lav'62; Path(P.Q.); Staff, Hop. Hotel-Dieu, Quebec 4, P.Q.

MORIN, Jean-Marc; 28 rue Berard, Drummondville, P.Q.; Lav '40; DPH; OphthOtol (P.Q.); Tel. 472-5474.

MORIN, Jean M.; 238, Bellevue Dr., Pincourt, P.Q.; Lav '53; Tel. 453-6561.

MORIN, Jean R.; 310 Maple N., Brownsburg, P.Q.; Mon'65.

MORIN, J. Eustace; 1140 de-la-Tour, Quebec, P.Q.; Paris (Fr.) '34; IntMed; Hd. Dept. of Clin.Med., Hop.-Ste-Foy; Prof. (Med.), Laval U.; Tel. 522-5448.
MORIN, Laurier; Lav'64; Res., Montreal Gen. Hosp., Montreal 25, P.Q.
MORIN, Leonard H.; 221 est rue Laurie, Ottawa 2, Ont.; Mon'51; Paed; Chief of Paed Serv. & Newborn Infants & Prematures, Hop. St. Louis Marie de Montfort; Tel. 236-7244.
MORIN, Leo P.; Ville-Marie, P.Q.; Lav '45; M.C.G.P.
MORIN, Lorenzo; 1061, boul. Mont Royal, Montreal 8, P.Q.; Mon'50; Psy.; Tel. 272-1483.
MORIN, Luc; Lav'65; Res., Douglas Hospital de Verdun, Montreal 19, P.Q.
MORIN, Noel; 550 Blvd. Walberg, Dolbeau, Co. Roberval, P.Q.; 760 Blvd. Walberg (res); Lav '46; Anaes; Anaes., Hotel-Dieu-de-Dolbeau; Tel. 276-0778.
MORIN, Paul; 680 St. Denis, St. Hyacinthe, **P.Q.; 2385 Laframboise (res); Mon '24; GenSurg ; Tel. PR 4-7163.**
MORIN, Paul G.; Paspebiac, Co. Bonaventure, P.Q.; Qns '39.
MORIN, Paul J. F.; 306 Blvd. St. Joseph E., Montreal, P.Q.; 215 Kindersley, Ville Mont Royal (res); Mon '29; Cardiol. (P.Q.), IntMed; Cardiol., Hop. Notre-Dame de l'Esperance; Tel. 842-1910.
MORIN, Philippe A.; 807C Harve-des-Iles, Chomedy, P.Q.; Lav'42.
MORIN, Philippe A.; 69 rue St. Levis, P.Q. (res); Mon'48; Instr., Neuro Psy., Hop. Ste. Croix de Drummondville, P.Q.
MORIN, Raymond M.; 229 rue St.-Joseph, Lauzon, P.Q.; Lav'60; AMCGP; Tel. 837-2454.
MORIN, Rosario E.; Rue Principale, Gravel**bourg, Sask.; Lav '45; Tel. PA 9-2511.**
MORIN, T. J.; 381 Churchill, Ottawa, Ont. (res); Qns '33; Dir. of Diseases Div., Ottawa Civic Hosp.
MORIN, Wilfred; St-Camille, Cte Bellechasse, P.Q.; Lav '33.
MORIN, Yves L.; 1290 Pelletier, Quebec 6, P.Q.; Lav '53; FRCP(C); IntMed; Cardiol (P.Q.); Staff, Hotel-Dieu Hosp.; Tel. 529-9151.
MORIN, Yvon; 298 St-Germain, Rimouski, P.Q.; Lav '54; OrthSurg; Staff, Hop. St. Joseph; Tel. 723-8680.
MORINVILLE, Yvon; boul Comtois, Louiseville, P.Q.; Lav '50.
MORISON, Elsie; (See Ritch, Elsie).
MORISON, Aileen (See Calder).
MORISON, James B.; 654 Riverwood Ave., Winnipeg 1, Man.; 665 Oakenwald Ave., Wpg. 19 (res); Man'50; DPH; Dir. Health Serv., Wpg.; Lect. Soc. & Prev. Med., U. of Manitoba; Tel. WH 6-7763.
MORISSET, Jacques; Lav '61; Anaes; Staff, Hotel Dieu de Levis, Levis, P.Q.; Tel. 837-9341.
MORISSET, Jean; 313 St.-Germain, Rimouski, P.Q.; Lav '35; Paed (P.Q.).
MORISSET, Pierre; 217-1ere Ave., Ville St. Georges, Cte. Beauce, P.Q.; Lav'32; IntMed(P.Q.); Med. Staff, Hop. Notre-Dame de Beauce.
MORISSET, Richard; Mon '64; Ass't. Res., Hop. Hotel-Dieu, Montreal, P.Q.
MORISSETTE, Amaury; 1494 Laurier Ave. E., Montreal, P.Q.; 1492 Laurier Ave. E. (res); Mon **'28; Obst. (Paris); Tel. LA 2-9333.**
MORISSETTE, Andre L.; Mon '63; Res., Hop. Maisonneuve, Montreal, P.Q.
MORISSETTE-DELAGE, Jacqueline; Lav '63; Staff, Hop. St. Sacrement, Quebec, P.Q.
MORISSETTE, Gaston; 7956 Place des Jesuites, Charlesbourg, Quebec 7, P.Q.; 44 Colombiere ouest (res); Lav. '50; OrthSurg; Orth., Hop. St.-Francois-d'Assise; Tel. 524-3488.
MORISSETTE, Gilles; 20 rue St. Georges, Giffard, Quebec 5, P.Q.; Lav '51.
MORISSETTE, Guy; 145 St. Laurent, Longueuil, **Cite, Jacques-Cartier, P.Q.; 181 Victoria (res); Mon '53; Paed; Ass't. (Paed), Hop.-Ste-Justine;** Tel. OR 4-1222.
MORISSETTE, Jean; 6241 Boul. Monk, Montreal 20, P.Q.; Mon '61; Tel. 769-2783.
MORISSETTE, Jean J., Capt.; H.M.C.S. Naden Hosp., Victoria, B.C.; Lav'64.
MORISSETTE, J. Guy; 4 Taschereau, Hull, P.Q.; Ott '55; OrthSurg (P.Q.).
MORISSETTE, Leopold; 3766 Queen Mary Rd., Montreal 26, P.Q.; Mon '36; M.S. Med. (Minnesota), F.I.S.H., IntMed (P.Q.); Haem (P.Q.); Staff Hop. Notre Dame; Assoc. Prof. (Med.), U. of Montreal; Tel. RE 1-3211.
MORISSETTE, Raymond; Lav'63; Res., Hop. Notre-Dame, Montreal 24, P.Q.
MORISSETTE, Yves; Mon '63; Res., Hop. Maisonneuve, Montreal 36, P.Q.
MORRISSETTE, Yvon; Lav '59; Res., Hop. Notre-Dame, Montreal, P.Q.
MORISSETTE, Yvon C.; Edifice Lavoie, Hauterive, P.Q.; Lav'63.
MORITZ, Denis V.; 232 Metcalfe St., Ottawa, Ont.; 360 Driveway (res); Budapest (Hung.) '28; Paed; Active Med. Staff, Ottawa Gen. Hosp.; Court. Med. Staff, Hop. St. Louis-Marie-de-Montfort, Ottawa Civic & Grace Hosp's.; Lect. **(Paed), U. of Ottawa; Tel. CE 6-4461.**
MORLEY, Helen M. (Briggs); 111 Ridge Dr., Toronto 7, Ont. (res); Oxford (Eng.) '43; DCH; Pt.-time M.O., East York-Leaside Health Unit & Catholic Children's Aid Soc.; Tel. HU 5-9779.
MORLEY, Thomas P.; 906 Med. Arts Bldg., 170 St. George St., Toronto 5, Ont.; 111 Ridge Dr., Tor. 7 (res); Oxford (Eng.) '43; F.R.C.S. (Eng.), F.R.C.S.(C), NeurSurg; Sr. Surg., Toronto Gen. Hosp.; Assoc. Prof. (Surg.), U. of Toronto; Tel. WA 2-3386.
MORLOCK, Frederick J.; 197 Ashcroft Place, Waterloo, Ont. (res); Wes '51; DiagRad; Staff, Rad. Dept., Kitchener-Waterloo Hosp., Kitchener; Tel. 742-2244.
MOROS, George P.; 23 Blvd. St. Joseph W., Montreal 14, P.Q.; Tel. 272-1413.
MOROZ, Leonard A.; The Rockfeller Inst., New York, N.Y. 10021, U.S.A.; Man '59; FRCP(C), IntMed; Abroad.
MORPHET, John A.; Tor'57; Res., Dept. of Med., University of Toronto, Toronto 5, Ont.
MORPHY, Geo. P.; 652 Kingston Rd., Toronto, Ont.; Wes '30; Tel. OX 9-2311.
MORPHY, R. Stevenson; 216 McDonald Ave., Belleville, Ont.; Wes'48; Urol; Cons. & Surg. Staff, Belleville Gen. & Trenton Mem. Hosp's.; Cons. Staff, Prince Edward Co. Hosp.; Tel. WO 8-9994.
MORRICE, Peter; Paediatric Centre, 505 O'Connor St., Ottawa 1, Ont.; Qns '59; Paed.
MORRILL, Stanley F.; 1146 Marine Dr., North Vancouver, B.C.; Qns '49; MCGP.
MORRIN, Peter A.; 2 Gibson Ave., Kingston, Ont. (res); National U. (Ire.) '54; M.B., B.Ch., B.A.O., F.R.C.P.(C), IntMed; Staff, Kingston Gen. Hosp.; Ass't. Prof. (Med.), Queen's U.; Tel. Area 613; 546-1731, Loc. 517.
MORRIS, Alexander G.; 64 Elmwood Ave., London, Ont.; Wes '31; Anaes.
MORRIS, Betty; (See Steiner, Betty).
MORRIS, C. Arthur; O'Mara-Martin Bldg., 135 Military Rd., St. John's, Nfld.; Ireland '54; AMCGP.
MORRIS, Cecil W.; 70 Binswood Rd., Toronto 6, Ont. (res); Wes '32; D.P.H.; Chm., Med. Adv. Bd., Dept. of Welfare of Ontario, Parliament Bldgs., Toronto; Tel. 365-5395.
MORRIS, Charles J.; Edinburgh (Scot.) '60; Jr. Intn., Victoria Hosp., London, Ont.
MORRIS, Darryl; 4326 W. 10th Ave., Vancouver 8, B.C.; UBC'64; AMCGP; Tel. CA 4-1355.
MORRIS, Donald E.; 60 Old Ferry Rd., Dartmouth, N.S.; Dal'56; FRCS(C), GenSurg; Staff, Victoria Gen. & Camp Hill Hosp's.
MORRIS, Donald J.; 84 Grey St., Windsor, N.S.; Dal'61; AMCGP; Staff, Payzant Mem. Hosp.; Tel. 798-2324.
MORRIS, Everton J.; 405 Wyandotte St. W., Windsor, Ont.; 416 Rosedale Blvd. (res); Wes '52; MCGP; Tel. 256-4908.
MORRIS, Fred R.; Moose Jaw Clinic, 200 Scott Bldg., Moose Jaw, Sask.; Man'57; FRCS(C), GenSurg; Tel. 692-2373.
MORRIS, George D.; Algoma Mills, Ont.; McG '24; GenSurg; **Retired.**

MORRIS, Harry V.; 3120 Highland Blvd., North Vancouver, B.C.; Qns '37; Tel. 988-2444.
MORRIS, James; 765 Upper Gage Ave., Hamilton, Ont.; 7 Bertram Dr., Dundas (res); Tor '56; Active Staff, Hamilton Civic & St. Joseph's Hosp's.; Tel. 385-7002.
MORRIS, James M.; 34 Amherst Hgts., St. John's, Nfld. (res); National U. (Galway, Ire.) '56; M.B., B.Ch., BAO; Psy; Chief of Serv. (Female Div.), Hosp. for Mental & Nervous Diseases; Tel. 9-5061.
MORRIS, Jeffrey E.; Wpg. Clinic, St. Mary's Ave., Winnipeg, Man.; 1582 Wellington Cres. (res); Rochester (NY) & Manchester (Eng.) '45; MRCP (Eng.); FACP; IntMed; Ass't. Phys. Wpg. Gen. Hosp.; Ass't. Prof. (Med.), U. of Manitoba; Tel. 942-0551.
MORRIS, Leo C.; 162 Sedgefield Ave., Pointe Claire, Lachine P.Q.; McG '58; IntMed.; Tel. 695-5503.
MORRIS, Mary E.; Apt. 3, 2177 Lincoln Ave., Montreal 25, P.Q.; Qns'55; Anaes.
MORRIS, Maurice L.; 118 Simcoe N., Oshawa, Ont.; 112 Kingsdale Dr. (res); Tor '38.
MORRIS, Neil; Tor '64; Res., Hosp. for Sick Children, Toronto, Ont.
MORRIS-OAKLEY, Margery U.; 22 Ochterloney St., Dartmouth, N.S.; 5 Limardo Dr. (res); Dal '54; M.O.H.; Pt.-time, City of Dartmouth; Tel. 466-7680.
MORRIS, Robert N.; Grace Anaes. Clinic, 200 Arlington St., Winnipeg 10, Man.; London (Eng.) '54; M.S., B.S.
MORRIS, Starling O.; 395 College St., Cobourg, Ont. (res); Qns '23; Retired.
MORRIS, Sylvia (Kliman); 2221 Keele St., Ste. 1, Toronto 15, Ont.; 474 Oriole Parkway (res); Glasgow (Scot.) '49.
MORRIS, Walter G.; 8 Eastwood Ave., Scarborough, Ont.; Tor'63; Tel. OX 8-1684-5.

MORRISH, Hugh F.; Alb'58; D&TRad; Staff, Foothills Hosp., 29th St. & 16th Ave. N.W., Calgary, Alta.
MORRISH, Walter; McLeod Bldg., Edmonton, Alta.; 8925—112 St. **(res); McG '18; D.M.R.E.** (Cantab), DiagRad; **Assoc. Dir. Cancer Clinics, Prov. of Alberta; Tel. GA 2-4511.**

MORRISON, A. Lindsay; 120 Lakeshore Rd., Port Credit, Ont.; Tor '64; Tel. CR 8-1551.
MORRISON, Angus E.; 200 Greyhound Bldg., 622 1st St. S.W., Calgary, Alta.; Alb'51; AMCGP; Att. Staff, Calgary Gen. & Holy Cross Hosp's.; Tel. 263-5030.
MORRISON, Charles G. R.; Ste. 8, 1940 Lonsdale Ave., North Vancouver, B.C.; 1480 Nelson Ave., West Vancouver (res); Man '40; Ophth; Chief of Staff (Ophth.), **North Vancouver** Gen. Hosp.; **Cons. (Ophth), Shaughnessy Hosp.; Tel. YU 7-**1733.
MORRISON, Gary C.; UBC '62; Res., Royal Victoria Hosp., Montreal 2, P.Q.
MORRISON, George E.; 2096 W. 41st Ave., Vancouver 13, B.C.; UBC'56; MCGP; Tel. 261-9626.
MORRISON, George H.; 117 S. John St., Fort William, Ont.; 2720 Sillscourt (res); Tor '52; FRCP(C), IntMed; Active Staff, McKellar Hosp.; Court. Staff, Port Arthur Gen. & St. Joseph's Hosp's.; Tel. MA 2-5363.
MORRISON, Hugh G.; 942 Oshawa Blvd. N., Oshawa, Ont.; Qns '54; BAO; Indust. Phys., General Motors of Canada Ltd.
MORRISON, Ian; Glasgow (Scot.) '59; Res., Winnipeg Gen. Hosp., Winnipeg 3, Man.
MORRISON, Irene S.; 12 Sherwood Rd. W., Pickering, Ont. (res); Queens U. (N. Ire.) '47; Part-time South. Ont. Co. Health Unit.
MORRISON, Jack H.; Ste. 308, 1175 Cook St., Victoria, B.C.; UBC '59; MCGP; Tel. 386-1446.
MORRISON, James E.; 1687 W. Broadway, Vancouver 9, B.C.; Alb'35; FACA; Retired.
MORRISON, J. Kemp; 1075 Bayview Ave., Toronto 12, Ont.; 16 Larkfield Dr., Don Mills (res); Dal '43; DHA (Tor); Supt., Sunnybrook Hosp.; Tel. 485-8651.
MORRISON, Joseph S.; 375 Main St. E., Hamilton, Ont.; Wes '55; Tel. 522-7944.
MORRISON, Mackenzie; Ste. 1410, 750 W. Broadway, Vancouver 9, B.C.; 5962 Adera St. (res); Alb '35; MCGP; Tel. TR 2-5601.
MORRISON, M. Jeannette; (see MacQuarrie).
MORRISON, Murray G.; Ste. 318, 1175 Cook St., Victoria, B.C.; Alb '59; ObstGyn; Tel. 385-6771.
MORRISON, N. Alastair; 20 Golf St. N., Truro, N.S. (res); **Dal '43; D.P.H.; Staff, Dept. of** Health, Truro.
MORRISON, N. Alister; 262 Queen St. S., Kitchener, Ont.; Tor '10; M.C.G.P.
MORRISON, Neil E.; Medical Assoc. Clin., 405 Hendryx St., Nelson, B.C.; 422 Maple St. (res); Qns '34; MCGP; Tel. 352-6611.
MORRISON, Peter V.; Eastend, Sask.; London (Eng.)'62; Abroad.
MORRISON, Robert D.; Box 1088, Hope, B.C.; Man' 41; Tel. 869-5637.
MORRISON, Roy E.; 2 Paisley Ave. S., Hamilton, Ont.; Tor '36; Tel. JA 7-7481.
MORRISON, Thomas; Medical Clinic, Carberry, Man.; Glasgow (Scot.) '61; M.B., Ch.B.
MORRISON, W. Ross; 163 E. Victoria St. Amherst, N.S. (res); Dal '45; Staff, Highland View Hosp.; Phys. (V.D.), Dept of Public Health.

MORRISSETTE, Yvon; Lav '59; Res., Hop. Notre-Dame, Montreal 24, P.Q.

MORRISSY, R. Herbert; Pleasant St., Newcastle, N.B.; McG '24.

MORROW, A. Meyer; 130 Ellesmere Rd., Scarborough, Ont.; Tor '56; Assoc. Staff, Toronto East Gen. Hosp.; Court. Staff, Scarborough Gen. Hosp.; Tel. 447-5531.
MORROW, B. M.; 73 Erie St. S., Leamington, Ont.; 16 Morgan St. (res); Tor '40.
MORROW, Carl E. L.; 50 Monk St., Ottawa, Ont.; Metcalfe (res); McG '28; M.C.G.P.; Staff, Memorial **Hosp., Winchester & Grace Hosp's., Ottawa; Tel. PA 8-4611.**
MORROW, Desmond F.; Kelowna Gen. Hosp., Kelowna, B.C.; Qns '51; Path.; Tel. 762-4000.
MORROW, Donald R.; Sask '62; Int., Montreal Gen. Hosp., Montreal 25, P.Q.
MORROW, Ian M.; Man '57; DiagRad; Staff, Winnipeg Gen. Hosp., Winnipeg, Man.; Tel. SP 4-6511.
MORROW, James J.; Box 760, Lake Cowichan, B.C.; 841 Stevens Cres. (res); Man '52; MCGP; Tel. 749-6621.
MORROW, John D.; 201 Medical Arts Bldg., 170 St. George St., Toronto 5, Ont.; Wes '46; F.R.C.P.(C), IntMed; Cons. (Cardiol.), D.V.A., Sunnybrook Hosp.; Clin. Teach. (Med.), Toronto Gen. Hosp., & U. of Toronto; Tel. WA 1-2593.
MORROW, Mary M.; Apt. 406, 3325 Decelles Ave., Montreal 26, P.Q.; McG '51; Neur (P.Q.).
MORROW, Nathan; 4208 Bathurst St., Downsview, Ont.; Tor '60.

MORSE, Frank W.; Lawrencetown, N.S.; Dal '38; GenSurg; Att. Surg., Soldier's Mem. Hosp., Middleton.
MORSE, Lewis R.; 151 King St. E., Saint John, N.B.; East Riverside (res); Tor '36; Urol; Chief (Urol.), Saint John Gen. Hosp.; Urol., St. Joseph's & Lancaster (DVA) Hosp's.; Tel. 693-3150.
MORSE, Peter G.; 18 Centre St., Thornhill, Ont.; Tor '55; MCGP; Staff, North York Branson & York Central Hosp's.; Tel. AV 5-3634.
MORSE, Philip W.; 808 Fairmont Med. Bldg., **750 W. Broadway, Vancouver 9, B.C.; 6037 Wiltshire St. (res); Oxford (Eng.) '36; M.R.C.P.** (Lond.), **IntMed; Cons., Willow Chest Centre, Shaughnessy D.V.A. Hosp.; Silicosis Cons.,** W.C.B.; Staff, Coqualeeza & Miller Bay Indian Hosp's.; Tel. 872-5330.
MORSE, William I.; 33 Vancouver St., Yarmouth, N.S.; Dal'45; D.IntMed (McG); FRCP(C), IntMed.

MORTELLARO, Antonino; Balcarres, Sask.; Italy'54; MCGP; Tel. 334-5260.

MORTIMER, Clive B.; 1001 Med. Arts Bldg., 170 St. George St., Toronto 5, Ont.; Cambridge (Eng.)'54; M.B., B.Ch. (Cantab.), M.D. (Cantab.), FRCS(C), Ophth; Ophth., Toronto Gen. Hosp.; Tel. 922-9832.

MORTIMER, Donald C.; 219 St. Clair Ave. W., Toronto 7, Ont.; 3 Gleneverest Rd. (res); Tor'55; Gastroent., O.P.D., Toronto General Hosp.; Ass't. Med. Dir., Excelsior Life Ins. Co.; Tel. 921-5674.
MORTIMER, H. F.; Department of National Health & Welfare, c/o Regional Superintendent, European Region; Ott '51. Abroad.
MORTIMER-LAMB, Charles; 1324 W. 57th Ave., Vancouver, B.C.; UBC'65.
MORTIMER, Norman W.; 200 Med. Arts Bldg., 628 Davis Dr., Newmarket, Ont.; 191 Park Ave. (res); Tor '54; B.A.; FACS; FRCS(C); GenSurg; Sr. Staff Surg., York County Hosp.; Tel. TW 5-5461.
MORTIS, Eric A.; Elbow Dr. Med. Centre, 51st Ave. & Elbow Dr., Calgary, Alta.; 1123 Beverley Blvd. (res); Oxford (Eng.) '56; Tel. AL 5-6647.
MORTON, Alexander E.; Med. Centre, 707 Charlotte St., Peterborough, Ont.; 27 Benson Ave. (res); Glasgow (Scot.) '50; DMR; DiagRad; Staff, Civic & St. Joseph's Hosp's.; Tel. RI 2-3871.
MORTON, Allan; 915-1538 Sherbrooke St. W., Montreal, P.Q.; McG '43; M.Sc. (Neur); Dip. Neur (McG); Neurol (P.Q.); Lect. (NeurAnat.), McGill U.; Tel. WE 2-8282.
MORTON, Allan R.; 6950 Armview Ave., Halifax, N.S. (res); Dal '25; MPH(Johns Hopkins); FAPHA; PH; Prof. Emer. (P.H.), Dalhousie U.; Research Med. Soc. Retired.
MORTON, Bruce S.; Bayer's Rd., Shopping Centre, Halifax, N.S.; **26 Rowe Ave. (res); Dal** '50; **Paed; Instr., Hlfx. Children's Hosp.; Lectr. Dalhousie U.; Tel. 422-8441.**
MORTON, Guy K.; 440 Phys. & Surg. Bldg., 8409-112th St., Edmonton, Alta.; Alb '39; NeurSurg; Clin. Prof. (NeurSurg.), Alberta University Hosp.
MORTON, G. M.; Med. Arts Bldg., Windsor, Ont.; Wes '41; F.A.C.S.; F.R.C.S.(C), GenSurg; Tel. CL 3-8958.
MORTON, Harry S., OBE, CD; 4500 Sherbrooke St. W., Westmount, Montreal 6, P.Q.; London (Eng.) '32; MB BS; M.Sc.; ObstGyn (PQ); FACS, FRCS (Eng.), FRCOG; FRCS(C), GenSurg; Surg.-in-Chief, Queen Mary Vet's. Hosp.; Surg., Royal Victoria Hosp.; Assoc. Prof. (Surg.), McGill U.; Tel. WE 7-6761.
MORTON, James W.; 2330 Queens Ave., West Vancouver, B.C. (res); McG '48; IntMed; Staff, Central TB Clinic, Vancouver & Clin. Instr., U. of British Columbia; **Tel. WA 2-6266.**
MORTON, Kenneth S.; 617 Fairmont Medical Bldg., 750 W. Broadway, Vancouver 9, B.C.; 7909 Laburnum St. (res); McG '50; F.R.C.S.(C), OrthSurg; Ass't. Prof (Orth) & Asst. Dir., Trauma Research Unit, Dept. of Surg., U. of British Columbia; Tel. TR 2-5665.
MORTON, L. M.; Main St., Yarmouth, N.S.; Cliff St. (res); Dal '14; GenSurg.
MORTON, M. Vivyan (Mrs. J. A. Forrester); 440 Hinton Ave., Ottawa 3, Ont.; Tor '46; Anaes.
MORTON, Philip L.; 2077 Danforth Ave., Toronto 6, Ont.; 64 Leacrest Rd. (res); Tor '54; F.R.C.S.(C), Ophth; Tel. OX 4-3741.
MORTON, William A.; 903 Fairmont Med. Bldg., 750 W. Broadway, Vancouver 9, B.C.; 1712 Acadia Rd. (res); Edinburgh (Scot.) '33; FRCS (Edin.); GenSurg; Clin. Ass't. (Surg.), U. of British Columbia; Tel. 876-3934.
MORTON, W. Ross; Suite 202, 2525 Pine Street, Vancouver 9, B.C.; Qns'59; DABO; Ophth; Tel. RE 1-3108.
MOSBAUGH, Marjorie M.; Tor '40; Staff, Beck Mem. San., London, Ont.
MOSCARELLO, Mario A.; 202 Rusholme Rd., Toronto, Ont. (res); Tor '55; Research Inst., Hosp. for Sick Children.
MOSCARELLO, Rebeka (Sheinin); 1849 Yonge St., Ste. 907, Toronto 7, Ont.; Tor '59; D.Psy; Psy; Staff, Women's College Hosp. & Addiction Research Fdn.; Tel. 488-8393.
MOSCOVICH, Bernard B.; 720 W. Broadway, Vancouver, B.C.; 4725 Chancellor Blvd. (res); Alb '34; IntMed; Clin. Instr., U. of British Columbia; Clin. Dir., Alcoholism Fdn., B.C.; Tel. TR 4-4202.
MOSCOVICH, Jacob C.; 720 West Broadway, Vancouver, B.C.; 3190 Travers Ave. (res); McG '28; F.A.C.P., IntMed; Med. Staff, Vancouver Gen. Hosp.; Dir. Med. Serv., Provincial Welfare Dept.; Med. Teaching Staff, U. of British Columbia; Tel. TR 4-4202.
MOSCOVITCH, Michael D.; UBC'63; Res., Montreal Gen. Hosp., Montreal 25, P.Q.
MOSELEY, H. Frederick; Ste. 1106-1414 Drummond St., Montreal, P.Q.; 3781 Westmount Blvd. (res); Oxford (Eng.) '33; MA, M.Ch. (Oxon), D.M., MRCS(Eng.), LRCP(Lond.), FACS, FR-C.S.(Eng. & C), GenSurg, OrthSurg; Dir. Accident Serv. & Surg., Royal Victoria Hosp.; Assoc. Prof. Surg., McGill U.; Tel. 845-4882.
MOSES, Rosalind; Res., Winnipeg Gen. Hosp., Winnipeg, Man.
MOSHER, D. Thornton; Box 69, Louisburg, N.S.; Dal '55.
MOSHER, Garth E.; St. James Med. Dental Group, 633 Lodge Ave., Winnipeg, Man.; McG '58; MCGP; Active Staff, Grace Hosp.; Tel. 837-1363.
MOSKALUK, Raymond; Ott'62; Res., Montreal Gen. Hosp., Montreal 25, P.Q.
MOSLEY, William; East York Municipal Bldg., Coxwell & Mortimer, Toronto 6, Ont.; 20 Lankin Blvd. (res); McG '28; D.P.H., PH; M.O.H., East York-Leaside Health Unit; Teach. Staff, School of Hygiene, U. of Toronto; Tel. HO 5-1192.
MOSS, Barbara A.; Box 839, Summerland, B.C.; London (Eng.)'56; DCH; DRCOG(Lond.) Paed; Tel. 494-3431.
MOSS, Clive B.; 234 Lawrence Ave., Kelowna, B.C.; Manchester (Eng.)'54; DMRD(Liverpool); DMRD(Eng.); DiagRad.
MOSS, George W. O.; 67 Rose Park Dr., Toronto, Ont. (res); Tor '45; D.P.H.; Dep. M.O.H., City of Toronto; Vis. Staff, School of Hygiene, U. of Toronto; Tel. 367-7403.
MOSS, Michael S.; London (Eng.)'64; MRCS; LRCP; Staff, University Hosp., Saskatoon, Sask.
MOSSER, Herbert A.; Carruthers Clinic, 137 Wellington St., Sarnia, Ont.; 139 Cecil St. (res); Wes '33; Path; Tel. DI 4-5261.
MOSSING, Doris S.; (See Richardson, Doris S.).
MOTKE, A. William; 902 King St. E. Hamilton, Ont.; 11 Sherman St. (res); Utrecht (Neth.) '48; ObstGyn; Court. Staff, Hamilton Civic Hosp's & Joseph Brant Mem. Hosp., Burlington; Tel. 544-2458; Abroad.
MOTT, Frederick D.; Apt. 602, 1 Clarendon Avenue, Toronto 7, Ont.; McG'32; PH; Prof. of Medical Care, School of Hygiene (Full time), Univ. of Toronto; Tel. 928-2758.
MOTT, George A.; 456 W. Broadway, Vancouver, B.C. (res): Cambridge (Eng.) '41; M.R.C.S. (Eng.), L.R.C.P. (Lond.) A.B.P.M., D.P.H., PH; Deputy Sr Med Health Officer, Greater Vancouver Metropolitan Health Dept.; Tel. TR 6-1313.
MOTTA, James A.; 602 Chinook Prof. Bldg., 6100 MacLeod Trail S.W., Calgary, Alta.; Man'59; FRCS(C), ObstGyn.; Staff, Calgary Gen. Hosp.
MOTTRAM, Leslie E.; 20 Millburn Dr., Islington, Ont.; Tor'43.
MOULDEY, R. Gordon; Qns'58; Psy; Staff, Royal Ottawa San., Ottawa 3, Ont.; Tel. 722-6521.
MOULDS, Godfrey G. S.; 340 McLeod St., Ottawa 4, **Ont.; 157 Ruskin Ave. (res); Qns '42; Tel. 236-7183.**
MOULE, John W.; 751 King St. W., Kitchener, Ont.; McG '62; Tel. 744-7041.
MOULSON, Robert A. L.; Fort William Clinic, 117 S. John St., Fort William, Ont.; Tor '61; AMCGP; Active Staff, McKellar Gen. & Westmount Chronic Hosp's.; Court. Staff, Port Arthur Gen. & St. Joseph's Hosp's., Port Arthur; Med. Staff, Alcoholic Research Fdn., Fort William; Tel. MA 2-5363.
MOULTON, Richard; Fort Frances Clinic, Fort Frances, Ont.; Cambridge (Eng.)'56; Active Staff, La Verendrye Hospital; Tel. 274-3287.
MOUNCE, Aubrey R.; Napanee, Ont.; Tor'22.
MOUNT, Harry T. R.; 276 Elgin St., Ottawa 4, Ont.; Tor'24; GenSurg; NeurSurg; Staff, Ottawa Civic Hosp.; Cons., Ottawa Gen. & St. Louis Marie de Montfort Hosp's.; Tel. 232-5719.

MOUNT, H. T. James; 340 McLeod St., Ottawa, Ont.; Qns'57; Ophth; Clin. Ass't., Ottawa U.; Tel. 235-1792.

MOUNTAIN, Harold E.; Chatsworth, Ont.; Wes '32; Anaes; Dist. Coroner.

MOUNTAIN, Harold E. Jr.; 532 Waterloo St., London, Ont.; 26 Hunt Village Cr. (res); Wes '58; Psy; Active Staff, St. Joseph's Hosp.; Instr. (Psy.), U. of Western Ont.; Tel. 439-5442.

MOUNTAIN, Thomas C.; Ponoka, Alta.; Wes'62.

MOUSSEAU, Jean M.; 7227 St. Denis, Montreal 10, P.Q.; Mon '41; MCGP.

MOUSSEAU, Paul; 150 est Jarry, Montreal 11, P.Q.; Mon'30.

MOUT, Robert; P.O. Box 23, Aldergrove, B.C.; Leiden (Neth) '51; Tel. 856-2717.

MOVAFAGH, Parviz; Manitoba Clinic, 790 Sherbrook St., Winnipeg 2, Man.; 844 Winnipeg Ave. (res); Tehran (Iran) '57; Paed; Tel. SP 4-6541.

MOVAT, Henry Z.; 17 Truxford Rd., Parkway Woods, Don Mills, Ont. (res); Innsbruck (Austria) '48; PhD. (Qns); Path; Assoc. Prof. (Path.), U. of Toronto; Tel. 928-2550.

MOWAT, Charles D.; St. Walburg, Sask.; Aberdeen (Scot.) '57.

MOWAT, David; 750 W. Broadway, Ste. 201, Vancouver 9, B.C.; Man '45; F.R.C.P.(C) IntMed; Clin. Dir., Willow Chest Centre; Clin. Instr. (Med.), U. of British Columbia; Tel. TR 4-4828.

MOWAT, Harold F.; 906 Whittier Cres., Port Credit, Ont.; Tor '23; M.S. (Tor.); FACS; FRCS (Eng.), FRCS(C), GenSurg; Retired; Tel. 278-4131.

MOWAT, Margaret A. (Riddell); 15 Park St. W., Copper Cliff, Ont. (res); Tor '51; IntMed; Temp. Retired.

MOWBRAY, John H.; University Hosp., Saskatoon, Sask.; Tor'48; FRCP(C), IntMed; Ass't. Prof. (Med.), U. of Saskatchewan; Tel. 242-7641.

MOWCZAN, Ivan; Aborg., Man.; Dnepropetrovsk (U.S.S.R.) '38.

MOWRY, Albert E.; 534 Waterloo St., London, Ont.; 1651 Gloucester Rd. (res); Wes '28; Obst-Gyn; Cons., Victoria, St. Joseph's, Westminster, Woodstock Gen. & St. Thomas Elgin Gen. Hosp's.; Cons., Beck Mem. San.; Assoc. Prof. (Clin.), U. of Western Ont.; Tel. 432-6033.

MOYER, Arthur A.; 208 Ridout St. S., London, Ont.; Wes '50; IntMed; Staff, Westminster DVA Hosp. & U. of Western Ont.; Tel. GE 2-6711.

MOYER, Donald J.; 10155—120th St., Edmonton, Alta.; 13224—102nd Ave. (res); Wes '51; ObstGyn. Hon. Instr., U. of Alberta; Tel. 488-7271.

MOYER, Ernest L.; 3302—19th St., Vernon, B.C. (res); Man '25; Ophth,Otol; Retired.

MOYES, Alexander; 99 Victoria Dr., Vancouver, B.C.; UBC '61; Tel. AL 5-5253.

MOYES, Andrew H.; St. Andrew's (Scot.) '49; DPM Leeds (Eng.); Med. Supt., Hosp. for Mental Dis., Box 420, Brandon, Man.; Dem. (Psy.), U. of Manitoba; Tel. PA 6-2321.

MOYES, Peter D.; 903 Fairmont Med. Bldg., 750 W. Broadway, Vancouver 9, B.C.; Ste. 302, 2726 Alder St. (res); London (Eng.) '50; FRCS(C), NeurSurg; Clin. Instr. (NeurSurg), U. of British Columbia; Tel. 876-2325.

MOYLE, Allan H.; Room 320, Du Pont of Canada Ltd., Box 660, Montreal 3, P.Q.; McG'42; Medical Director, Du Pont of Canada Ltd.

MOYO, Charles T.; Ott '59; Res., Ottawa Civic Hosp., Ottawa 3, Ont.

MOYSE, Henry W.; 5 Central St., Summerside, P.E.I.; 186 Belmont St. (res); Dal '33; MCGP; Tel. 2277.

MUCZIJ, Theodor; 154 Machray Ave., Winnipeg, Man.; Carl's U. Prague (Czech) '28; Tel. JU 2-9253.

MUDGE, Peter B.; London (Eng.) '60; Res., Vancouver Gen. Hosp., Vancouver, B.C. Abroad.

MUDIE, Ian S.; Box 10, Lee Nicholson Clinic, Terrace, B.C.; St. Andrews (Scot.)'45; DTM&H (Lond.); Active Staff, Mills Mem. Hosp.; Tel. VI 3-2242.

MUDIE, Lawrence H.; 2 Citation Dr., Willowdale, Ont.; Tor '57; MCGP; Active Staff, N. York Branson Hosp.; Staff (OPD), Tor. Western Hosp.; Sec. Metro-Tor. Chapt., Coll. GP of Canada; Tel. BA 5-8351.

MUDRY, Walter J.; 1815 Cayuga Cr., Calgary, Alta.; Alb '51; Anaes; Tel. 289-4431.

MUEHLENBECK, Erich C.; 1812 Broad St., Regina, Sask.; 241 Durham Dr. (res); Frankfurt-am-Main (Germ.)'49; Tel. LA 2-1276; Abroad.

MUELLER, Lebrech H.; 71 Howard Park Ave., Toronto 3, Ont.; 11 Radford (res); Krakow (Poland) '28; M.C.G.P.; Tel. LE 6-3750.

MUELLER-WILM, Ingrid; 43 Quinan Dr., Toronto 15, Ont.; Heidelberg (Germ.) '51; Tel. 244-7391.

MUGAN, John F. M.; 17-11th Ave. S., Cranbrook, B.C.; 232-14th Ave. S. (res); Man '42; **MCGP; Staff, St. Eugene Hosp.**

MUIR, Andrew P.; 518 Brant St., Burlington, Ont.; Glasgow (Scot.) '30; MCGP; Active Staff, Joseph Brant Mem. Hosp.; Tel. NE 4-3372.

MUIR, David, 412 Danforth Ave., Toronto 6, Ont.; Tor '19; MCGP; Tel. HO 3-2835.

MUIR, Donald M.; Dal '45; Staff Phys., Point Edward Hosp., Sydney, N.S.

MUIR, Douglas M. K.; London (Eng.) '48; DMRD (Lond.); DiagRad; Rad., Royal Jubilee Hosp., Victoria, B.C.; Tel. 386-3131.

MUIR, John Maxwell; 602 Med. Arts Bldg., 750 Spadina Cr., Saskatoon, Sask.; Glasgow (Scot.) '59; FRCP(C), Anaes; Inst. (Anaes.), U. of Saskatchewan.

MUIR, J. Ronald; Woodside Shopping Centre, 205 Pleasant St., Dartmouth, N.S.; Dal '63; Court. Staff, Oceanview Mun. Home, Eastern Passage & Pleasantview Foster Villa; Tel. 463-2055.

MUIR, Robert K.; 90 Harbour St., Toronto 1, Ont.; 4 Alvarado Pl., Don Mills (res); Dal '31; PathBact; M.O., WCB; Lt-Col. RCAMA & IMS (Ret'd.); Tel. 362-3411.

MUIRHEAD, William; 23 West 33rd St., Hamilton, Ont.; Edinburgh (Scot.) '51; D.M.R.T. (Ed.); TherRad; Radiother., Ontario Cancer Fdn., Henderson Gen. Hosp.; Tel. 389-1371.

MUIRHEAD, William R.; 2055 W. 30th Ave., Vancouver 9, B.C.; Qns '33; Staff, Dept. of National Health & Welfare, Med. Services Clinic, Immigration Bldg., Vancouver.

MULARCHYK, Edward J.; Wes'62; Ophth; Staff, Victoria Hosp., London, Ont.

MULCAIR, John G.; Ste. 330, 5300 Cote-des-Neiges Rd., Montreal 26, P.Q.; McG'48; FACOG, ObstGyn; Att. Staff, St. Mary's Mem. & Catherine Booth Maternity Hosp's.; Tel. RE 1-3357.

MULDER, David S.; Sask '62; Intn., Mtl. Gen. Hosp., Montreal 25, P.Q.

MULDOON, Alfred D.; Associate Clin., 214-6th Ave. S.W., Calgary, Alta.; Ste. 9, Windsor Apts., 206-26th Ave. S.W. (res); University Coll., Dublin (Ire.)'43; MRCP (Edinburgh), FRCP(C), IntMed; Active Staff, Holy Cross Hosp. & Calgary Gen. Hosp.; Tel. AM 3-7120.

MULHOLLAND, Alastair B.; Aberdeen (Scot.) '56; DA; FFARCS; Anaes; Staff, Dept. of Anaes., St. Joseph's Hosp., Victoria, B.C.

MULL, John D.; Tor'57; Path; Dir. of Labs, Norfolk Gen. Hosp.; Simcoe & Tillsonburg District Mem. Hosp., Tillsonburg; Regional Path. for Norfolk, Oxford & Haldimand Counties; Tel. 426-5570.

MULLEN, Leslie M.; 2260 Capitol Hill Cres., Calgary, Alta. (res); Tor'29; FACP; IntMed; Staff, Calgary Gen. Hosp. & Colonel Belcher Hosp.; Tel. 282-3592.

MULLEN, Lorne H.; Tor'49; MCGP; Res., St. Joseph's Hosp., London, Ont.

MULLENS, J. Edward; 914 Med. Arts Bldg., 170 St. George St., Toronto 5, Ont.; 34 Ridge Dr. (res); Wes '49; FACS; FRCS(C), GenSurg; Surg., Wellesley Hosp.; Ass't Prof., U. of Toronto; Tel. WA 3-9432.

MULLER, A. Karola; Allan Mem. Inst., 1025 Pine Ave. W., Montreal, P.Q.; Cologne (Germany)'52; Phys-in-charge, Dept. of Electroenceph., Allan Mem. Inst.; Lect., McGill U.; Tel. 842-1251, Loc. 637.

MULLER, Herbert F.; 118 Arlington, Montreal 6, P.Q. (res); Cologne (Germ.) '51; Psy; Staff, Verdun Protestant Hosp.; Lect. (Psy.), McGill U.; Tel. 935-6893.
MULLIGAN, G. William; 4145 Blueridge Cr., Apt. 24, Montreal 25, P.Q.; GenSurg(P.Q.).
MULLIGAN, Mona D.; 91 King St. E., Kingston, Ont. (res); Manchester (Eng.) '54; DPH; Ass't. M.O.H., City of Kingston; Lect. (PrevMed.), Queen's U.
MULLIN, George L.; 29 St. Lawrence St. E., Madoc, Ont.; Qns '49; MCGP; Active Staff (G.P. & IntMed.), Belleville Gen. Hosp., Belleville; Tel. 473-4252.
MULLIN, Gower M.; Omineca Clinic, Vanderhoof, B.C.; Dal'55.
MULLINGER, Margaret A.; (see BOGOCH, Margaret A.).
MULLOY, John K.; 1417 Prospect Ave., Calgary, Alta.; McG '21; Retired.
MULLOY, William H.; 2940-17th Ave. S. W., Calgary, Alta.; McG '52; MCGP; Tel. CH 9-5566.
MULVIHILL, Julia; Ott'65; Res., St. Michael's Hosp., Toronto 2, Ont.
MULVIHILL, Louis J.; Box 272, 196 Argyle St. S., Renfrew, Ont.; Qns' 42; Dist. Coroner; Tel. HE 2-2375.
MULYK, Iwan; Med. Arts Bldg., 420 East St. N., Sarnia, Ont.; (Germ.) '49; Active Staff, Sarnia Gen. & St. Joseph's Hosp's.; Tel. DI 4-2208.
MUNCEY, Nancy D. (Robinson); Qns '64; Res., Hotel-Dieu Hosp., Kingston, Ont.
MUNDAY, Albert D.; Sask'63; Res., St. Paul's Hosp., Saskatoon, Sask.
MUNDLE, Robert M.; McG'59; Res., Victoria Gen. Hosp., Halifax, N.S.
MUNDY, Harcourt B.; Wes'65; Res., Victoria Hosp., London, Ont.
MUNGALL, Andrew N.; McG '45; Anaes; Anaes., Rooyal Victoria Hosp., Montreal, P.Q.; Tel. VI 2-1251.

MUNGER, Louis P.; 142 St. Dominique, Jonquiere, P.Q.; Lav '26; Clin. Anaes., St. Joseph's Hosp.; Tel. 542-6881.

MUNHOLLAND, Ralph J.; 2975 Longfellow Ave., Windsor, Ont.; 3210 Bruce Ave. (res); McG '52; MCGP; Tel. 969-4300.
MUNHOLLAND, Walter L.; 2115 Gladstone Ave., Windsor, Ont.; Sask '57; Staff, Grace & Metropolitan Hosp's.; Tel. 252-5883.

MUNIO, Natalie; 1179 Decarie Blvd., St. Laurent, Montreal 9, P.Q.; 2175 Scott (res); Liban '35; Tel. RI 4-0602.

MUNKITTRICK, Ronald C.; 2037 Alton St., Ottawa, Ont. (res); **Wes '51;** D.A.B.Path.Anat. D.A.B.C.P.; Path; Path., Ottawa Civic Hosp.; Med. Dir., Eastern Ont. Red Cross Blood Transfusion Serv.; Vis. Lect. (Path), U. of Ottawa; Tel. PA 9-2511.

MUNKLEY, Franklyn H.; 300 Lawrence Ave. E., Scarborough Ont.; 10 Landfair Cr. (res); Tor '44; FRCS(C); ObstGyn; Cons., Scarborough Gen. Hosp.; Tel. 291-1361.

MUNN, Donald J.; Professional Bldg., 360 Wallace St. N., Listowel, Ont.; Wes'52; Tel. 291-2290.
MUNN, John D.; 61 Fleming Cres., Leaside, Toronto, Ont. (res); **Wes '38; Dip. Rad., D & TRad; Dir. Dept. of Rad., Hosp. for Sick Children; Assoc. Prof. Rad., U. of Toronto; Tel.** EM 6-7242.
MUNN, W. H. Blanchard; Medical Clinic, West Summerland, B.C.; Hospital Hill (res); McG '27; Tel. HY 4-4356. Abroad.
MUNN, William D.; 360 Wallace N., Listowel, Ont.; Wes'55.

MUNNICH, Matthew; 355½ Dutch Village Rd., Halifax, N.S.; 25 Fairmount Rd. (res); McG '55.

MUNNOCH, Norman M.; Medical Dental Bldg., 111 Huron St., Woodstock, Ont.; 169 Graham St. (res); Edinburgh (Scot.) '52; M.B., Ch.B.; M.C.G.P.; Staff, Woodstock Gen. Hosp.; M.O., Standard Tube & T.I.; Tel. LE 9-1111.
MUNRO, Allan T.; Box 369, Nepawa, Man.; 290 Hospital St. (res); Dal '59; DPH; Med. Dir., Nepawa Health Unit; Tel. 200.
MUNRO, Carman B.; 237 Pembroke St. W., Pembroke, Ont.; 253 Broadview Dr. (res); Qns '40; MCGP; Chief of Med., Cottage Hosp.; Interpreter, Cardiographs Pembroke Gen. & Cottage Hosp's.; Tel. RE 2-2451.
MUNRO, Darrell D.; Dept. of Surg., Royal Victoria Hosp., 687 Pine Ave. W., Montreal, P.Q.; McG'44; M.Sc (Exp. Surg.); FACS; ThorSurg (P.Q.); Surg.-in-Chief, Royal Edward Chest Hosp.; Sr. Att'd. Surg., Royal Victoria Hosp.; Ass't. Prof. Surg., McGill U.; Tel. 849-9716.
MUNRO, Don C.; St. Marys Med. Clinic, P.O. Box 1120, St. Marys, Ont.; James St. N. (res); Wes '55; MCGP; Chief of Staff, St. Mary's Hosp.; Tel. 284-3450.
MUNRO, Elizabeth A.; McG '57; Res. (Rad.), Toronto Gen. Hosp., Toronto 2, Ont.
MUNRO, Jeptha S.; 18 Archibald Ave., North Sydney, N.S.; 92 Pierce St. (res); Dal '19; M.C. G.P.; Staff, St. Elizabeth & Harbour View Hosp's.; Tel. 794-2695.
MUNRO, Raymond M.; 64 Cameron St., Moncton, N.B.; 614 Wedgwood Ave., Riverview Hgts. (res); Dal '54; Staff, Moncton Hosp.; Court. Staff, Hotel Dieu Hosp.

MUNRO, R. E.; Middleton, N.S.

MUNROE, Alexander T.; Dalkeith, Ont.; Qns '04; L.R.C.P.(Edin.), L.R.C.S.(Edin.), L.R.C.P. & S. (Glasgow).
MUNROE, Donald H.; 250 Main St. E., Hamilton, Ont.; Jerseyville Rd., Ancaster (res); Qns '45; Urol; Staff, St. Joseph's, Hamilton Gen., Chedoke & Henderson Gen. Hosp's.; Tel. JA 7-2711.
MUNROE, Donald S.; 2765 Heather St., Vancouver 9, B.C.; Man'36; MRCP(Eng.), FACP, FRCP(C), IntMed; Sr. in Med. & Dir. Heart Stn., Vancouver Gen. Hosp.; Pt.-time Assoc. Prof. (Med.), U. of British Columbia; Tel. 872-1251.
MUNROE, Gladys A.; 33 Galt St., Oakville, Ont., Tor '36; Anaes.
MUNROE, James D.; 1638 W. 52nd Ave., Vancouver 14, B.C. (res); Man '33; DPH; DTM&H; Indust. Med., Sick Mariners Clinic.

MUNROE, James P.; Ste. 4, 1155 W. 13th Ave., Vancouver 9, B.C.; McG '60; FRCP(C), Anaes; McLaughlin Travelling Fell. (1 year).

MUNROE, Roy G.; Maritime Bldg., New Glasgow, N.S.; Birch St., Stellarton (res); Dal '52; GenSurg; Tel. 752-5291.

MUNT, Peter W.; Oshawa Clinic, 117 King St. E., Oshawa, Ont.; Tor '64; Assoc. Clin., Oshawa Gen. Hosp.; Tel. RA 8-1661.

MURAKAMI, Ernest K.; 360 Wallace St., Hope, B.C.; 566-3rd Ave. (res); UBC '58, Nomin. Comm., BC Div. CMA; Tel. 869-5637.

MURAFSKY, Meyer; (see Morrow, A. Meyer).

MURBY, William H.; 221 Med. Arts Bldg., 170 St. George St., Toronto 5, Ont.; 38 Hillholm Rd. (res); Tor '33; ObstGyn; Chm. (ObstGyn), St. Michael's Hosp.; Ass't. Prof. (ObstGyn), U. of Toronto; Tel. WA 3-7459.

MURCHLAND, Charles A.; Box 80, Oromocto Med. Clinic, Oromocto, N.B.; Dal'64.

MURCHISON, Alexander J.; Dal'63; Res., Victoria General Hosp., Halifax, N.S.

MURDOCH, Douglas A.; 628 Davis Dr., Newmarket, Ont.; Tor '59.
MURDOCH, Frank T.; 658 W. 32nd Ave., Vancouver 9, B.C.; Wes'59.
MURDOCH, George W.; 903 Fairmont Med. Bldg., 750 W. Broadway, Vancouver 9, B.C.; Tel. 876-3612.
MURDOCH, John H.; 240, 5655 Cambie St., Vancouver 15, B.C.; 806 W. 19th Ave., Van. 9 (res); Aberdeen (Scot.) '44; MCGP; Att'd. Staff, St. Vincent Hosp.; Tel. 261-6944.
MURDOCH, Monica E.; Ste. 905, 750 W. Broadway, Vancouver 9, B.C.; Qns'52; Psy.

MURDOCK, Alan I.; McG'63; Res., Children's Hosp., Montreal 25, P.Q.

MURENBEELD, William H.; 560 Professional **Bldg., 10830 Jasper Ave., Edmonton, Alta.;** Amsterdam (Neth.)'42; MCGP; Tel. 429-3351.
MURIE, John J.; Box 309, Sardis, B.C.; Qns'53.

MURNAGHAN, Donal P.; 333 Med. Arts Bldg., 170 St. George St., Toronto 5, Ont.; 2 Beaumont Rd., Tor. 5 (res); Nat. U. (Dublin, Ire.) '37; FRCP(C), IntMed (Cardiol.); Att'd. Staff, Wellesley Hosp.; Hon. Cons. (Cardiol.), Princess Margaret Hosp.; Ass't. Prof. (Med.), U. of Toronto; Tel. WA 2-9320.

MURNAGHAN, Maurice F.; Dept. of Pharmacology, University of Ottawa, Ottawa 2, Ont.; 600 Parkdale Ave. Ott. 3 (res); National U. Dublin (Ire.), '42; M.B. B.Ch., M.Sc.(Med.), M.D.; Prof. & Hd. Dept of Pharm., U. of Ottawa; Tel. CE 5-6751. Abroad.

MURPHY, A. Patrick; 153 St. George St., Moncton, N.B.; Tor '44; Tel. EV 4-3566.

MURPHY, Arthur B.; 49 Main St. E., Smiths Falls, Ont.; 39 Russel St. E. (res); Qns '37; MCGP; Tel. 283-2400.

MURPHY, Arthur L.; 1488 Carleton St., Halifax, N.S.; 6009 Inglis St. (res); Dal '30; FACS, FAAST; GenSurg; Sr. Surg., Victoria Gen. Hosp.; Cons., Hlfx. Infirm.; Assoc. Prof. Surg., Dalhousie U.; Tel. Area 902; 423-6620.

MURPHY, Beverley E. (Pearson); Queen Mary Vet's Hosp., Montreal, P.Q.; Tor'56; M.Sc., Ph.D.; Research Assoc., Queen Mary Vet's Hosp.; Lect., McGill U.; Tel. 342-2320, Loc. 295.

MURPHY, Brian J.; 924 Crescent Blvd. S. W., Calgary, Alta.; (res); Man '38; DiagRad; Assoc. Rad., Calgary Gen. & Alberta Children's Hosp's.; Tel. 262-2912.

MURPHY, Claude H.; Ste. 100, 219 Kennedy St., Winnipeg 1, Man.; Man '53; M.C.G.P.; Tel. WH 2-8648.

MURPHY, C. Walter; 200 Montreal-Toronto Blvd., Dorval, Lachine, P.Q.; McG '50; Med. Adviser, Ciba Co. Ltd.; Tel. ME 1-4211.

MURPHY, David A.; McG'60; FRCS(C), GenSurg; Staff, Royal Victoria Hosp., Montreal 2, P.Q.; Abroad.

MURPHY, David R.; The Montreal Children's Hosp., 2300 Tupper St., Montreal, P.Q.; 31 Forden Ave., Westmount (res); McG '42; F.A.C.S., F.R.C.S.(C), GenSurg; Surg-in-Chief & Dir., Sub-Dept. of Cardiovasc. Surg., Montreal Children's Hosp.; Surg., Alexandra Hosp.; Prof. (Surg.), McGill U.; Tel. WE 7-8511.

MURPHY, Dermot P.; Stephenville Crossing, St. George's Bay, Nfld.; National U. (Ire.) '44; MCGP; Med. Sup't., Stephenville Crossing Hosp.; Tel. 6-2233.

MURPHY, D. Kent; Med. Arts Bldg., 2150 Valley Way, Niagara Falls, Ont.; 260 Rolling Acres Dr. (res); Tor '43; GenSurg; Surg. Staff, Gtr. Niagara Gen. Hosp.; Tel. 358-8711.

MURPHY, Donald E.; 31 Yonge St. N., Richmond Hill, Ont.; 126A Lucas St., Richmond Hill (res); Wes '58; FRCS(C); ObstGyn; Staff, York Central Hosp.; Tel. 884-7007.

MURPHY, Donald M.; Ste 214-1320-5th Ave., Prince George, B.C.; 1765-5th Ave. (res); Qns '41.

MURPHY, D. Raymond; Queen's U. (Belfast, N. Ire.) '49; M.B., B.Ch.; BAO; FRCP(C); Path; Staff, St. Mary's Hosp., 3830 Lacombe Ave., Montreal 26, P.Q.

MURPHY, E. Gordon; Cooksville Med. Centre, 21 Upper Middle Rd., Cooksville, Ont.; London (Eng.) '45; DCH; Paed; Ass't. Phys., Hosp. for Sick Children; Chief Paed., South Peel Hosp.; Cons. Neurol., Crippled Children's Centre; Clin. Instr., U. of Toronto; Tel. 277-4455.

MURPHY, Fergus A.; 2525 Albert Ave., Saskatoon, Sask.; Man '52; Path; Ass't. Path., University Hosp.; Lect. (Path.), U. of Saskatchewan; Tel. 242-7671, Ext. 234.

MURPHY, Frederick G.; 5 John St., Moncton, N.B.; McG '54; GenSurg.; Staff, Moncton City & Hotel-Dieu Hosp's.; Tel. 382-8331.

MURPHY, Frederick W.; 333 Main St., Picton, Ont.; 46 Queen St. (res); Qns '52; MCGP; Staff, Prince Edward County Hosp.; Court. Staff, Kingston Gen. & Hotel-Dieu Hosp's.; Tel. GR 6-5621.

MURPHY, Gerard F.; McG'64; Res., St. Mary's Hosp., Montreal 26, P.Q.

MURPHY, Gerald M.; 217 LeMarchant Rd., St. John's Nfld.; Nat. U. (Ire.) '53; IntMed; Tel. 587-4347.

MURPHY, Giles B.; 707 W. 37th Ave., Vancouver, B.C.; 813—W. 69th Ave. (res); McG '08; Retired.

MURPHY, G. Ross; Ste. 460, 3550 Cote des Neiges Rd., Montreal 25, P.Q.; McG'57; FRCS(C), OrthSurg; Jr. Ass't. OrthSurg., Montreal Gen. Hosp.; Clin. Ass't., Reddy Mem. Hosp.; Cons. OrthSurg., The Douglas Hosp.; Dem. (OrthSurg), McGill U.; Tel. 932-8234.

MURPHY, Harold R.; 1001 Ridgeway, Fort William, Ont.; '31.

MURPHY, Harry B.; 72 Mullock St., St. John's, Nfld. (res); Dal '41; D & TRad; Dir. Rad., St. John's Gen. Hosp.; Cons. Rad., St. Clare's Mercy, Grace, D.V.A., W.C.B. & U.S. Air Comm.; Tel. 8-0471.

MURPHY, Hazel (Jones); 64 Cameron St., Moncton, N.B.; 614 Wedgwood Ave., Riverview Hgts. (res); Dal '54; MCGP; Tel. 382-3385.

MURPHY, Herbert H.; 3230 Ripon Rd., The Uplands, Victoria, B.C. (res); McG '04; F.A.C.S., D & TRad; Retired.

MURPHY, H. Ormond; 755 W. Broadway, Vancouver 9, B.C.; 4770 W. Second Ave. (res); Qns '51 IntMed; Att'd. Staff, Shaughnessy & Vancouver Gen. Hosp's.; Clin. Instr. (Med.), U. of British Columbia; Tel. TR 2-2115.

MURPHY, James E.; Gambo, Nfld.; Dublin (Ire.) '57; MCGP; Tel. 651-4496.

MURPHY, J. Kevin; 108 Med. Dental Bldg., Regina, Sask.; 2629 Grant Rd. (res); Trinity C. (Dublin, Ire.) '54; M.B., B.Ch., BAO; ObstGyn; Staff, Regina Gen., Regina Grey Nuns Hosp's. & Sask. Cancer Comm.; Tel. LA 3-7631.

MURPHY, John; 1061 Simcoe St., Moose Jaw, Sask. (res); Glasgow (Scot.) '41; DPM; Sr. Psy., Moose Jaw Union Hosp.; Tel. 692-1841.

MURPHY, John B.; Dept. of Nat. Health & Welfare, Tunney's Pasture, Ottawa, Ont.; 2543 Regina St., Ott. 14 (res); Tor '56; MA (Pharmacol.); Chief MO, Food & Drug Directorate; Tel. 992-5746.

MURPHY, John P.; 950 Ennislaire Ave., Sarnia, Ont.; Ott'59; IntMed.

MURPHY, J. P.; Wawota, Sask.; Durham (Eng.) '44.

MURPHY, Marie L. B.; 37½ Western Ave., Ottawa, Ont. (res); McG '44; Not practising.

MURPHY, Mary A.; Box 70, 5761 Pacific Highway, Cloverdale, B.C.; Wes '47; Tel. 574-4423.

MURPHY, Michael; Port Hood, N.S.

MURPHY, Noel F., MPP; 22 Cobb Lane, Corner Brook, Nfld.; London H. (Eng.) '42; Staff, Western Mem. Hosp.; Tel. 4-5202.

MURPHY, Patrick G.; 545 King Edward Ave., Ottawa 2, Ont.; Ott '55; FACS; FRCS(C), Urol; Urol., Ottawa Gen. Hosp.; Cons. Urol., Tri-Service, N.D.M.C. & St. Vincents Hosp.; Lect. (Surg.), U. of Ottawa; Tel. CE 4-2938.

MURPHY, Patrick J.; Mankota, Sask.; Durham (Eng.)'44.

MURPHY, Patrick V.; Medical Centre, West St., Cornerbrook, Nfld.; National U. (Cork, Ire.)'54; DAnaes(Lond.).

MURPHY, P. Noel; 32 Fairview S., Antigonish, N.S. (res); Nat. U. (Ire) '39; Psy; Exec. Dir., Eastern Co. Mental Health Centre; Assoc. Prof. (Psy), St.- Francois-Xavier U.; Tel. 863-4511.

MURPHY, Raymond M.; 64 Cameron St., Moncton, N.B.; 614 Wedgewood Ave. (res); Dal '54; MCGP; Tel. 382-3385.

MURPHY, Richard; 991 Alder St., Campbell River, B.C.; Murphy St. (res); University Coll. (Cork, Ire.) '43; Active Staff, Campbell River Dist. Hosp.; Tel. 287-7441.

MURPHY, Robert S.; Med Arts Bldg., 5880 Spring Garden Rd., Halifax, N.S.; Dal '57; Otol.

MURPHY, Sean B.; 322, 1414 Drummond St., Montreal 25, P.Q.; 578 Claremont Ave., Mtl. 6 (res); McG '47; DABOph; FRCS(C), Ophth; Assoc. Ophthalmologist, Royal Victoria Hosp.; Lect., McGill U.; Tel. VI 5-0987.

MURPHY, Thomas B.; 86 Church St., Antigonish, N.S. (res); Dal '34; MCGP; Staff, St. Martha's Hosp.

MURPHY, Vincent J.; 214-6th Ave. W., Calgary, Alta.; Alb '51; OrthSurg.; Tel. 263-7120.

MURPHY, Wm. J.; 2630 Eglinton Ave. E., Scarborough, Ont.; Queen's (Belfast, N. Ire.) '53; Tel. 261-3500.

MURPHY, William O.; 49 Main St. E., Smith Falls, Ont.; Qns '45; MCGP; Tel. 283-2400.

MURPHY, W. J.; 376 Main St., St. John, N.B.; Dal '31; IntMed.

MURRAY, Alastair A.; 1109, 750 W. Broadway, Vancouver 9, B.C.; 1226 Laurier (res); Edinburgh (Scot.) '36; FRCS(E); GenSurg; Tel. 879-2520.

MURRAY, Alastair M.; Wes'64; Res., Vancouver Gen. Hosp., Vancouver, B.C.

MURRAY, Alistair S., S/L; Glasgow (Scot.)'60; Senior Medical Officer, R.C.A.F. Station, North Bay, Ontario; Tel. 474-6600, Loc. 266.

MURRAY, Andrew B.; 601 Fairmont Med. Bldg., 750 W. Broadway, Vancouver 9, B.C.; Capetown (S. Africa) '51; MRCP (Edin.); DCH; Paed; Vis. Staff, Van. Gen. Hosp.; Clin. Instr., (Paed), U. of British Columbia; Tel. TR 6-0424.

MURRAY, A. Edward; 6461 Quinpool Rd., Halifax, N.S.; 6933 Armview Ave. (res); Dal '30; GenSurg; Lect. (Med. Juris.), Dalhousie U.; Tel. 423-7947.

MURRAY, Arnold R.; 10102-101st St., Grande Prairie, Alta.; 8801-102nd St. (res); Alb '54; MCGP; Tel. 532-4444.

MURRAY, Bernard; 94 Main St., Curling, Nfld.; National (Ire.) '49; M.O.H., Lourdes.

MURRAY, Cyril V.; Ste. 930, 123 Edward St., Toronto 2, Ont.; Nat. U. (Ire.) '42; DPH; D.-Psy; Psy; Staff, St. Michael's Hosp.; Clin. Teach. (Psy.), U. of Toronto; Tel. 366-5382.

MURRAY, Daniel; Tatamagouche, N.S.; Dal '03; Retired.

MURRAY, David C.; Dal '63; Res., Sunnybrook Hosp., Toronto 12, Ont.

MURRAY, Donald J.; Smith Clinic, 4825-51st Street, Camrose, Alta.; Alb'54; ObstGyn; Tel. 672-2424.

MURRAY, Donald R.; 4567 Sunset St., South Burnaby, B.C.

MURRAY, Douglas G.; 1783 Mountain Highway, North Vancouver, B.C.; UBC '54; Path; Staff, Royal Columbian Hosp., Vancouver; Tel. LA 2-2771.

MURRAY, Douglas K.; 6038 Quinpool Rd., Halifax, N.S.; Dal'35; FACS; FICS; Ophth; Staff, Victoria Gen., Halifax, Children's & Grace Maternity Hosp's.; Tel. 423-7482.

MURRAY, Duncan; Hinton Med. Clinic, Box 2327, Hinton, Alta.; 120 Dorin Dr. (res); Aberdeen (Scot.) '54; Tel. 865-2695.

MURRAY, Eric J.; 2374 Eglinton Ave. E., Scarborough, P.Q., Ont.; 52 Doonaree Dr. (res); Wes '49; M.C.G.P.; Plant Phys., John Inglis Scarborough Works; Tel. PL 7-3217.

MURRAY, Ernest J.; 6014 Yonge St., Willowdale, Ont.; National U. (Ire.)'35.

MURRAY, Florence J.; Canadian Mission, 190-102 Ka, Choong Chung Ro, Su Tae Moon Ku, Seoul, Korea; Dal '19; Staff, Severance Union Med. College Hosp. & Lect'r. in Gyn.

MURRAY, Foster S.; Veterans' Home, 312 Albert Ave., Saskatoon, Sask.; Dal '23; Psy; M.O., D.V.A.; Tel. 652-8876.

MURRAY, Gordon D. W.; 500 Medical Arts Bldg., Toronto 5, Ont.; 56 Sandringham St. (res); Tor '21; F.A.C.C., F.I.C.S., F.R.C.S. (Eng.), F.R.C.S.(C) GenSurg; Cons. Surg., Toronto Gen. Hosp.; Graduate Lect. (Surg.), U. of Toronto; Med. Dir., Gairdner Med. Research Fdn.; Tel. WA 2-4981.

MURRAY, Haakon O.; Irving Clinic 74 W. Seymour, Kamloops, B.C.; 166 W. St. Paul St. (res); McG '47; DTM&H; FACS; FRCS(C); GenSurg; Staff, Royal Inland Hosp.; Tel. 372-5251.

MURRAY, Hugh M.; Community Health Clin., 2363 McIntyre St., Regina, Sask.; Edinburgh (Scot.)'58; DRCOG.

MURRAY, Ian H.; 1428 Ouellette Ave., Windsor, Ont.; Edinburgh (Scot.) '57.

MURRAY, Jacques; Mon'65; Res., Montreal Gen. Hosp., Montreal 25, P.Q.

MURRAY, James F.; 534 Medical Arts Bldg., 170 St. George St., Toronto 5, Ont.; 209 Cortleigh Blvd. (res); Tor '43; F.R.C.S.(C), GenSurg, Plas Surg; Att. Plas. Surg., Toronto East Gen. Hosp.; Tel. WA 1-2933.

MURRAY, James F.; 117 King Street E., Oshawa, Ont.; Tor'64; Staff, Oshawa Gen. Hosp.; Tel. 728-1661.

MURRAY, James G.; 21 Alpaca Dr., Scarborough, Ont.; McG '51; Anaes; Staff, Sunnybrook **Hosp., Court Staff, Toronto Gen. Hosp.; Tel. 485-8651.**

MURRAY, James H., W/C; Inst. of Aviation Med., 1124 Avenue Rd., Toronto 12, Ont.; Wes'50; MPH (Harvard); DAB (PrevMed.).

MURRAY, James K.; 420 Med. Arts Bldg., 1 Young St., Hamilton, Ont.; 3089 Woodward Ave., Burlington (res); Tor '53; FRCS(C), NeurSurg; Active Staff, Hamilton Civic, St. Joseph's & Joseph Brant Mem. Hosp's.; Tel. 527-2753.

MURRAY, James N.; Wes'50; MPH(Harvard); FACPM; C.O., Cdn. Forces Inst. of Aviation Med., Toronto, Ont.

MURRAY, J. Bryson; Springfield Hgts. Shopping Centre, 1161 Rothesay, Winnipeg 16, Man.; 193 Larchdale Cres., Wpg. 16 (res); Man'57; MCGP; Tel. 338-9323.

MURRAY, J. Carson; Springhill Medical Centre, Springhill, N.S.; 131 Main St. (res); Dal'32; Tel. 597-3613.

MURRAY, J. Leo; 4 King Cres., Weston, Ont.; 10 Riverstone (res); Tor '41; M.C.G.P.

MURRAY, John C.; 170 Queen St., P.O. Box 1090, P.Q.; McG '58; MCGP.

MURRAY, John D.; 50 Sheppard Ave. E., Willowdale, Ont.; Tor'60; Paed; Staff, Hosp. for Sick Children; Tel. BA 1-6200.

MURRAY, John R.; 812 Cook Rd., Richmond, B.C.; UBC '61; **AMCGP; Tel. 278-5191.**

MURRAY, Joseph J.; Tor'62; Res., Children's Hosp., Montreal, P.Q.

MURRAY, J. Vernon; The Med. Clinic, Box 670, Creston, B.C.; Tor '34; MCGP; Coroner; Tel. 356-2224.

MURRAY, Kenneth W.; 10104-124th St. Edmonton, Alta.; 11915-119th Ave. (res); Alb '52; Tel. HU 8-4336.

MURRAY, Leslie L.; Medical Centre, 140 Brown's Line, Toronto 14, Ont.; Tor'26; AMCGP; Tel. CL 1-8831.

MURRAY, Malcolm M. E.; 452 Main St. E., Hamilton, Ont.; Qns '56; MRCOG; D.ObstRCOG; FRCS(C), ObstGyn; Active Staff (ObstGyn.), St. Joseph's Hosp.; Court. Staff, Chedoke & Hamilton Civic Hosp's.; Tel. 522-9400.

MURRAY, Mary P.; 206 Rookwood Ave., Fredericton, N.B.; Ireland'55; LRCP & LRCS(I); LM; DA(Eng.).

MURRAY, Peter C.; Res., Winnipeg Children's Hosp., 685 Bannatyne Ave., Winnipeg 3, Man.

MURRAY, Peter J. B.; Rowell Clinic, Carbonear, Nfld.; Edinburgh (Scot.) '52; FRCS(Ed.); Surg., Carbonear Hosp.; Tel. 5018.

MURRAY, Robert G.; 739 Taylor St., Saskatoon, Sask. (res); Tor '41; F.A.C.S., F.A.A.O.O., F.R.-C.S.(C), Ophth; Hd., Dept. of Ophth., University Hosp.; Prof. of Ophth., U. of Saskatchewan; Tel. CH 2-7641.

MURRAY, Robert G. E.; Dept. of Bact. & Immunol., U. of Western Ontario, London, Ont.; McG'43; FRSC; Hon. Cons. Microbiol., Victoria Hosp., & St. Joseph's Hosp.; Prof. & Hd., Dept. of Bact. & Immunol., U. of Western Ontario; Tel. 679-3751.

MURRAY, Shirley B.; McG'61; Res., Toronto Gen. Hosp., Toronto 2, Ont.

MURRAY, Timothy M. F/L; Qns '62; M.O., RCAF Station North Bay, North Bay, Ont.

MURRAY, T. John; Dal'63; AMCGP; Res., Victoria Gen. Hosp., Halifax, N.S.

MURRAY, William A.; 5880 Spring Garden Rd., Halifax, N.S.; 6113 Oakland Rd. (res); Dal '43; IntMed; Assoc. Phys., Victoria Gen. Hosp.; Cons. (Med.), DVA, RCAF, Hlfx. Conval. Hosp.; Dir. Student Health Serv. & Lect. (Med.), Dalhousie U.; Tel. 423-6666. Retired.

MURRAY, William A.; 3811 Royal Ave., Montreal 28, P.Q.; McG '23; Hon. Att. Staff, Montreal Gen. Hosp.; Dir., Med. Serv. Molson's Brewery Ltd.; Tel. 484-7621.
MURTAGH, Andrew P.; Beachburg, Ont.; McG '17; Staff, Pembroke Gen. Hosp.; MOH, Beachburg; Tel. 582-3580.
MURUVE, Gabriel; Manitoba Clinic, 790 Sherbrook St., Winnipeg 2, Man.; Turkey '55; Paed; Tel. SP 4-6541.
MUSCH, Ludwig; Strathcona Med. Dental Bldg., 8225-105th St., Edmonton, Alta.; Prague (Czecho-Slov.)'43; Tel. 433-5877.
MUSGRAVE-McCONNELL, Aileen P.; 3625 Ridgewood Ave., Montreal 26, P.Q.; Queen's U. (Belfast, N. Ire.) '55; DRCOG; IntMed. Staff, Mtl. Gen. Hosp.
MUSGROVE, James E.; 925 W. Georgia St., Vancouver, B.C.; 461 Southborough Dr., West Vanc. (res); Man '39; M.S.(Surg.); FACS; FRCS(C); DABOS; GenSurg; Instr. (Surg.), U. of British Columbia Tel. MU 1-4161.
MUSGROVE, Wilfred M.; 1578 Wellington Cres., Winnipeg, Man. (res); Man '22; Psy; Head of Psy., Deer Lodge Hosp.; Ass't. Prof. (Psy.), U. of Manitoba; Tel. TU 8-4861.
MUSKOVITCH, Zol F.; 322 Wellington St., Sarnia, Ont.; 620 Berkshire St. (res); Sask '58; Staff, Sarnia Gen. & St. Joseph's Hosp's.
MUST, Christopher J.; 327 Charlotte St., Peterborough, Ont.; Aberdeen (Scot.)'57.
MUSTARD, H. Arthur; Box 370, Cardinal, Ont.; Tor'55; GenSurg.
MUSTARD, H. Jean; (See Shepley, H. Jean).
MUSTARD, James F.; Dept. of Path., McMaster University, Hamilton, Ont.; Tor'53; Cambridge (Eng.)'56; Ph.D.(Cantab); FRCP(C), Path; Tel. 522-4971.
MUSTARD, Kenneth I.; 420 Lock St. W., Dunnville, Ont.; 155 Elizabeth Cr. (res); Tor'53; DABS; FACS; GenSurg; Active Surg. Staff, Haldiman Mem. & West Haldiman Hosp's.; Tel. 774-7541.
MUSTARD, Robert A., MBE; Ste. 1007, Med. Arts Bldg., 170 St. George St., Toronto 5, Ont.; Tor '38; FACS; FRCS(C), GenSurg; Surg., Tor. Gen. Hosp.; Cons. Surg., Princess Margaret & Women's College Hosp's.; Assoc. Prof. (Surg.), U. of Toronto; Tel. WA 1-0215.
MUSTARD, William T.; M.B.E.; Ste. 1225, 123 Edward St, Tor. 2, Ont.; 482 Russell Hill Rd. res); Tor'37; FACS; FRCS(C), Orth Surg; Chief, Cardiovas. Surg., Hosp. for Sick Children; Assoc. Prof. (Surg.), U. of Toronoto; Tel. 364-2564.
MUTCH, John; Box 788, Fort Qu'Appelle, Sask.; London (Eng.)'43; M.B., B.S. (Lond.); FRCS (Eng.).
MUTCH, John F.; Box 392, Maxville, Ont.; Tor '42; Staff, Cornwall Gen. Hosp.
MUTCHNIK, Alfred; 377 Graham Ave., Winnipeg 1, Man.; R.C. of Surg., Dublin (Ire.) '53; M.C.G.P.; Staff, St. Boniface & Misericordia Hosp's.; Tel. WH 2-5915.
MUTH, Harvey A.; 901 Helena St., Trail, B.C.; **Man '48; IntMed; MCGP.**
MUTH, H. John; C. S. William Clinic, Rossland, B.C.; Park St. (res); Man '32; Coroner.
MUTHANNA, K. C.; Staff, Riverview Hosp., Essondale, B.C.
MUTRIE, Eric T.; 111 Norfolk St., Guelph, Ont.; Qns'37; MCGP; Active Staff, Guelph Gen. & St. Joseph's Hosp's.; Tel. 822-7831.
MUTRIE, Robert R.; Ontario Soc. for Crippled Children, 350 Rumsey Rd., Toronto 17, Ont.; Qns '34; FRCS(Ed.); FACS; FRCS(C), GenSurg; OrthSurg; Med. Dir., Ontario Soc. for Crippled Children; Tel. 487-5311.
MUTTITT, Eldon L. C.; Baker Clinic, 221 Medical Arts Bldg., 11010 Jasper Ave., Edmonton, Alta.; Man'49; IntMed. (Allerg.); Lect. Med., U. of Alberta; Tel. 488-0141.
MUZYCHKA, Julita; Madrid (Spain)'56; Res., **St. John's Fever Hosp., St. John's, Nfld.**
MYATT, Donald G.; 260 Cedar St., Sudbury, Ont.; 370 Laura Ave. (res); Tor '32; F.R.C.S.(Edin.), F.R.C.S.(C), GenSurg.; Tel. OS 3-3695.
MYCYK, Modest D.; 2 Grenview Blvd. N., Toronto 18, Ont.; Ott'57; AMCGP.

MYDLAND, Wallace E.; 214-6th Ave. S.W., Calgary, Alta.; 924 Kerfoot Cres. (res); Alb '52; DABS; FACS; FRCS(C), GenSurg; Ass't. Chief of Surg., Holy Cross Hosp.; Tel. AM 3-7120.
MYER, Donald S.; 60 Albert St., Thorold, Ont.; 35 Lawrence Dr. (res); Wes '54; Tel. 227-5525.
MYERS, Beverly A.; McG'61; Paed; Staff, Montreal Children's Hosp., Montreal, P.Q.; Abroad.
MYERS, Charles A.; 507 Federal Bldg., Saskatoon, Sask.; Tor '37; Med. Exam., Canadian Pension Comm.
MYERS, Earl D.; Ste. 202, 158 St. George St., Toronto 5, Ont.; Tor'45; FACS; FRCS(C), GenSurg; Att'd Surg., Mt. Sinai & Cons. Proct., Baycrest Hosp.; Assoc. Surg., Doctor's Hosp.; Tel. 923-3892.
MYERS, Gerald R.; 1516 Merivale Rd., Ottawa 5, Ont.; Tor '64.
MYERS, Henry A.; 102 Church St., Amherst, N.S.; Edin. (Scot.) '43; L.R.C.P., L.R.C.S. (Edin.), L.R.F.P.&S. (Glasgow); M.C.G.P.; Staff, Highland View Hosp., Amherst; Med. Examiner, County of Cumberland; Tel. 667-8432.
MYERS, Herman A.; 405 Northgate Bldg., 10049 **Jasper Ave., Edmonton, Alta.; Alb '45; GenSurg; Tel. 422-1184.**
MYERS, Lois M.; 81 Georgia Rd., London, Ont.; Wes '51; Ph.D. (Leeds) (Path); DMRT (Eng.) TherRad; Radiotherapist, Ont. Cancer Fdn., London Clin; Lect. (TherRad), U. of Western Ont.
MYERS, Louis; Ste. 303, 25 Brunswick Ave., Toronto 4, Ont.; 363 Glencairn Ave. (res); Tor '43; DOMS (Eng.); Ophth; Staff, Doctor's Hosp.; Tel. 924-2686.
MYERS, Ralph P.; 15 Alma, Moncton, N.B.; Edinburgh (Scot.) '38; LRCP & S (Edin.), LRCP & S (Glas.), AICS, MCGP; Surg. Serv., Moncton City Hosp.; Sr. Surg., Hotel-Dieu-l'Assomption; Dist. Coroner; Tel. EV 4-4624.
MYERS, Robert F. M.; Box 280, Brandon Clinic, Brandon, Man.; Man'41; Paed; **Tel. PA 9-6444.**
MYERS, Violet (Morrow); Alb '45; Staff, Alberta Hosp., Box 307, Edmonton, Alta.; Tel. 799-8383.
MYERS, William N.; Alb '61; Res., Royal Alexandra Hosp., Edmonton, Alta.
MYHAL, Bohdan; 603 Simpson St., Fort William, Ont.; Lemberg (Pol.) '40; Staff, McKellar Hosp.; Tel. 622-8322.
MYHAL, Daniel R.: Mon '63; Res., Hop. Notre-Dame, Montreal, P.Q.
MYLECHREEST, Peter H.; The Medical Clinic, Gibsons, B.C.; Cambridge (Eng.)'62; MRCS; LRCP(conjoint); Tel. 886-2221.
MYLES, John M.; 10040-87th Ave., Edmonton, Alta.; Edinburgh (Scot.) '51; M.B., Ch.B., DA (Lond.); Anaes; Staff, Edmonton Gen. Hosp.; Tel. MU 8-8181.
MYLES, Joyce M.; Galahad, Alta.; Manchester (Eng.)'57.
MYLES, Patrick J.; Galahad, Alta.; Dublin (Ire.)'50.
MYLES, S. Terence; Alb'65; Res., Children's Hosp., Montreal 25, P.Q.
MYLKS, Gordon R. W.; 122 Wellington St., Kingston, Ont.; 77 Kensington Ave. (res); Qns '29; DABOG; FACOG; FACS, ObstGyn; Att. Staff, ObstGyn., Kingston Gen. Hosp.; Sr. Chief, Att. Staff Hotel Dieu Hosp.; **Assoc. Prof., Obst** Gyn., Queen's U.; Tel. 546-0901.
MYMIN, David; Witwatersrand (S.Africa) '52; MRCP (Lond.); St. Boniface Hosp., St. Boniface, Man.; Ass't. Prof. (Med.), U. of Manitoba; Tel. WH 3-0311.
MYRDEN, J. Allen; 5880 Spring Garden Rd., Halifax, N.S.; 1777 Bloomingdale Terr. (res); Dal '50; FRCS(C); GenSurg; Assoc. Surg., Victoria Gen. Hosp.; Dir., Nova Scotia Tumour Clinic; Ass't. Prof. (Surg.), Dalhousie U.; Tel. 423-8773.
MYRHOLM, Gunnar S.; Box 126, Hay River, N.W.T.; Alb'64.
MYSAK, Joseph; 1083 Bloor St. W., Toronto 4, Ont.; 17 Riverside Cres., Tor. 3 (res); Zagreb (Yugoslavia) '39; **MCGP; Tel. 536-1712.**
NABETA, Saeko S.; Apt. 43, 16 St. Joseph St., Toronto 5, Ont.; Tor '57; FRCP(C); Anaes; Staff Hosp. for Sick Children; Tel. EM 6-7242; Abroad.

NADASDI, Miklos; Apt. 3, 444 Lawrence Ave. W., Toronto 12, Ont.; Budapest (Hung.) '56; Ph.D. (Mtl.); Med. Dir., British Drug Houses (Canada) Ltd.
NADEAU, Alexander R.; St. Charles de Bellechase, P.Q.; Lav'26; MCGP; Coroner.
NADEAU, Andre; St-Michel, Cte. Bellechasse, P.Q.; Lav '60; AMCGP.
NADEAU, Claude; 700 rue Ste-Julie, Trois Rivieres, P.Q.; Lav'61; Otol (P.Q.).
NADEAU, Conrad; 15 rue St. Jean, P.Q.; 1277 rue des Calliers (res); Lav '43; Cardiol, (P.Q.); Cons. (Cardiol.), Notre-Dame de l'Esperance & Immigration Hop's.; Tel. 523-1563.
NADEAU, Denis; 633 rue Dequen, Chicoutimi, P.Q.; Lav '53; M.C.G.P.; Staff (Med, Obst & Anaes), Hotel-Dieu-St.-Vallier, Chicoutimi.
NADEAU, Germain; St. Francois du Lac, Co. Yamashaka, P.Q.; Lav '52; Tel. 568-2248.
NADEAU, Guy; 180 Boul. Laval, Ste Rose, P.Q.; Lav'62; Paed(P.Q.).
NADEAU, Jacques; 1000 Chemin Ste-Foy, Quebec 6, P.Q.; Lav '45; Tel. 683-9463.
NADEAU, Marc; Lav'63; Res., Hop. Sacre Coeur, Montreal 9, P.Q.
NADEAU-JODOIN, Marie; App. 3, 4375 Jeanne d'Arc, Montreal 36, P.Q.; Mon '64.
NADEAU, Nelson; Lav'65; Res., Hop. Enfant Jesus, Quebec 3, P.Q.
NADEAU, Nidgar; 4 Prince William St., Campbellton, N.B.; Lav'44; Ophth, Otol; Chief (Ophth., Otol.), Hotel-Dieu Hosp.; Cons., Soldier's Mem. & Provincial Hosp's.; Tel. 753-4427.
NADEAU, Norbet; St. Alexandre, Co. Kamouraska, P.Q.; Lav '53; Tel. 495-2022.
NADEAU, Pierre; 43 Springrove Cres., Montreal 8, P.Q.; Mon '54; PulmDis & TB (P.Q.); FRCP-(C); IntMed; Teaching Staff, Hop. Hotel Dieu; Ass't. to Dean, Fac. of Med., U. of Montreal; Tel. 279-0752.
NADEAU, Reginald A.; 745 rue St-Aubin, Ville St. Laurent, P.Q. (res); Mon '57; FRCP(C), IntMed; Cardiol (P.Q.); Staff, Dept. of Cardiol., Hotel-Dieu Hosp.; Staff, Dept. of Physiol., U. of Montreal; Tel. VI 4-0161.
NADEAU, Roger; Lav '63; Staff, Clinique d'Urgence, 1820 est St. Joseph, Montreal 34, P.Q.
NADEN, John R.; W.C.B. 707 W. 37th Ave., Vancouver 13, B.C.; Ste. 302, 5616 Yew St. (res); Tor '25; OrthSurg; Hon. Cons. (OrthSurg), Vancouver Gen. Hosp.; Chief M.O., B.C. Workmen's Compensation Bd.; Retired.
NADIAK, Olga S.; Innsbruck (Austria)'48; Anaes(P.Q.); Clin. Fell., Dept. of Anaes., Santa Cabrini Hosp., Montreal 36, P.Q.; Tel. 254-8311.
NADLER, Norman J.; 5845 Cote-des-Neiges Rd., Montreal, P.Q.; 4929 Fulton St. (res); McG '51; Ph.D.; IntMed (PQ); Ass't. Phys., Jewish Gen. Hosp.; Assoc. Prof., McGill U.; Tel. 738-5555.
NADON, Alban; 234 Chemin Montreal, Ottawa 7, Ont.; Mon '54; MCGP; Tel. 746-8634.
NADON, Andre; 210 de Martigny, St-Jerome, P.Q.; Mon'65; Tel. 438-1800.
NADON, Grant W.; Tor '61; Res., Sunnybrook Hosp., Toronto 12, Ont.
NAFTOLIN, Leigh Z.; Ste. 408, 450 Central Ave., London, Ont.; Wes'63; AMCGP; Staff (G.P.) Victoria & St. Joseph's Hosp's.; Tel. 438-8339.
NAGLER, Frederick P. O.; Lab. of Hygiene, Tunney's Pasture, Ottawa 4, Ont.; 45 Barrie Ave. (res); Frankfurt (Germ.) '34; Chief, Virus Labs., Dept. of National Health & Welfare; Cons. Virol., Ottawa Civic Hosp.; Tel. 992-8140.
NAGY, Ferenc; 110-3rd St. N.E., Weyburn, Sask.; Budapest (Hung.) '56; Staff, Saskatchewan Hosp., Weyburn, Sask.; Tel. VI 2-3812.
NAGY, Katrina P.; Med. Bldg., Bannatyne & Emily, Winnipeg 3, Man.; 150 Lockwood St., Wpg. 9 (res); Man '59; Ass't. Prof. Anat., U. of Manitoba; Tel. GR 4-9110.
NAGY, Zoltan; Physicians & Surgeons Bldg., 86 Bloor St. W., Toronto, Ont.; Cluj (Roumania) '39; GenSurg; Court. Staff (Surg.), Toronto Gen. Hosp. & Toronto Central Hosp.; Tel. WA 2-7726.
NAHORNICK, Boris A.; Box 560, Drumheller, Alta.; Alb '56; Active Staff, Drumheller Mun. Hosp.; Tel. VA 3-3345.
NAIBERG, Murray B.; Concord Med. Clinic, 895 Bloor W., Toronto 4, Ont.; 340 Lonsdale (res); Tor '55; MCGP; Tel. 537-2527.
NAIDOO, Dayanand; London (Eng.) '43; M.B., B.S., MRCP (Edin.), LRFPS (Glas.); DCH (Eng.); DPM (Glas., Lond., Boston & Stockholm); Ph.D. (Lond.); Psy; Staff, Clin. Research Dept., Ontario Hosp., Toronto 3, Ont.; Tel. LE 3-8501; Abroad.
NAIDU, Paul; Davis St., Chesley, Ont.; Ireland '58; DCH; LAH (Dublin).
NAIDU, Rangaswamy L.; Calcutta (India) '49; M.O., Dept. of Nat. Health & Welfare, Moose Factory Indian Hosp., Moose Factory, Ont.
NAIHOUSE, David M.; 464 Villeneuve W., Montreal, P.Q.; McG '19; Tel. CR 1-7433.
NAIKEN, Veerasamy; Leeds (Eng.)'55; Staff, St. Joseph's Hosp., Brantford, Ont.
NAIMAN, James; 3555 Atwater Ave., Apt. 102, Montreal 25, P.Q.; McG '49; D.Psy; Psy; Assoc. Psy., Jewish Gen. Hosp.; Ass't. Prof. (Psy.), McGill U.; Tel. 935-9860.
NAIMAN, Sheldon C.; Tor '62; Res., Vancouver Gen. Hosp., Vancouver 9, B.C.
NAIMARK, Allan P.; 6000 Cote des Neiges Rd., Montreal 26, P.Q.; McG'60; Diag Rad (P.Q.).
NAIMARK, Arnold; 205 Girton Blvd., Winnipeg 29, Man.; Man '57; FRCP(C); IntMed; Staff, Winnipeg, Gen. Hosp.
NAIRNSEY, Colman; 410 Hammond Bldg., 310 Main St. N.; Moose Jaw, Sask.; Trinity Coll. (Dublin, Ire.) '23; BAO; Tel. 693-3661.
NAISMITH, Archibald G.; Mahood Falls, B.C. (res); Tor '08; D.P.H.; Retired.
NAISMITH, James T.; 103 Dundas St., Kingston, Ont. (res); Glasgow (Scot.) '45; FCCP; Dir. Chest Clin., Ongwanada San.; Clin. Instr. (Prev-Med & IntMed)., Queen's U.; Tel. 548-4417.
NAKIELNY, Wladyslaw; Berne (Switz.) '51; D. Psy; Staff Psy., Selkirk Mental Hosp., Selkirk, Man.; Tel. 482-3810, Loc. 378.
NALBANTOGLU, Henri; Sanatorium Notre-Dame, De-Lourdes, Vallee Lourdes, N.B.; Istambul (Turkey)'48.
NANCEKIEVILL, Ivan W.; Cameron St., Cannington, Ont.; Wes '61; Staff, Ross Mem. Hosp., Lindsay; M.O.H., Cannington; Tel. 432-2569.
NANCEKIVELL, Arthur F.; McG '42; FRCP(C); IntMed; Staff, Queen Elizabeth Hosp., Montreal 28, P.Q.; Tel. 488-2311.
NANCEKIVELL, Eric W.; 569 Concession St., Hamilton, Ont.; 43 Knyvett Ave. (res); Tor '43; M.C.G.P.; Tel. 383-3351.
NANCEKIVELL, Harold K.; 117 S. John St., Fort William, Ont.; 447 Heather Cres. (res); Tor '44; F.A.C.S., F.C.C.P., GenSurg; Cons. (Chest Surg.), Fort William San.; Chief of Surg., Mc-Kellar Hosp.; Tel. MA 2-5363.
NANSON, Eric M.; 802 Idylwyld Cres., Saskatoon, Sask.; Otago (New Zealand) '39; FRCS (Eng.), FACS, FRCS(C), GenSurg; Prof. & Hd. Dept. of Surg., U. of Saskatchewan; Huntarian Prof. RCS (Eng.), 1959; Tel. CH 2-7671.
NANSON, Geoffrey L.; 3256 Cambie St., Vancouver 9, B.C.; 6111 Mackenzie St. (res); Wes'50; MCGP; Att'd. Staff, Vancouver Gen. Hosp.; Tel. TR 4-0261.
NANTEL, Albert; Mon '64; Research, U. of Montreal, Montreal, P.Q.; Abroad.
NANTEL, Jacques; C.P. 244, Salaberry-de-Valleyfield, P.Q.; Mon '56.
NANTEL, Marcel; 4515 Ouest Notre Dame, Montreal 30, P.Q.; Mon '43; M.C.G.P.; Tel. 935-7747.
NAPIER, Robert; 6044 Quinpool Rd., Halifax, N.S.; Dal'62; AMCGP; Tel. 423-7973.
NAPKE, Edward; Food & Drug Directorate, Tunney's Pasture, Ottawa 5, Ont.; Tor '51; M.O. in-Charge, Drug Adverse Reaction Prog. & Poison Control Centres; Tel. 992-1877.
NAPRAWA, Thaddeus S.; Tor '57; FRCS(C), ObstGyn; Staff, St. Michael's Hosp., Toronto, Ont. Abroad.
NAQUI, S. Mahmood; New Waterford Med. Clinic, New Waterford, N.S.; Karachi (Pakistan) '58. Abroad.
NARINE, Toolsie; 36 Wilson St., Hamilton, Ont.; Dal '64.

NAROD, Mairi M. (MacLean); 15496 North Bluff, White Rock, B.C.; 12581 North Bluff (res); McG '64; Tel. 531-5541.
NAROD, Phillip; 15496 North Bluff Rd., White Rock, B.C.; 12581 North Bluff (res); UBC '55; Active Staff, Peace Arch Dist. Hosp.; Tel. 531-5541.
NARWANI, Kishore; McG '62; Int., Montreal Gen. Hosp., Montreal, P.Q.
NASH, Arthur B.; 322 Cook Medical Bldg., 1175 Cook St., Victoria, B.C.; 9502 Ardmore Dr., R.R. 2., Sidney (res); McG '26; DABOG; FACOG; FACS; FRCOG; FRCS(C); ObstGyn; Cons. Obst-Gyn., Royal Jubilee Hosp., Med. Att'd. Staff, Victoria Cancer Clinic; Retired.
NASH, Everard T.; 1139 Yates St., Victoria, B.C.; 3019 Quadra St. (res); Tor '32; M.C.G.P.; Staff, St. Joseph's Hosp.; Tel. EV 4-1131.
NASH, Frederick C.; Wes'65; Res., Victoria Hosp., London, Ont.
NASH, M.; Tor '61; Jr. Intn., New Mount Sinai Hosp., Toronto 2, Ont.
NASH, Martin; Bloor Med. Clinic, 609 Bloor W., Toronto 4, Ont.; Tor '61; AMCGP; Tel. LE 4-4214.
NASH, Peter H.; 5400 Cote-de-Liesse Rd., Montreal 9, **P.Q.; 228 Portland Ave. Mtl. 16 (res); Cambridge (Eng.) '41; DPH, DIH, MCGP; Clin. Med. Assoc., Royal Victoria Hosp.; Cons. (Pharm.), Dept. of Experim. Surg., McGill U.; Med. Dir., Abbott Laboratories; Tel. 735-2411.**
NASH, Richard M.; 1288 Pembina Hwy., Fort Garry, Winnipeg 9, Man.; 695 Queenston St. (res); Ire. '39.
NASH, Samuel S.; 123 Edward St., Toronto 2, **Ont.; 1 Briancliffe Dr., Don Mills (res); Tor '45; F.R.C.S.(C), ObstGyn; Staff, (ObstGyn), New Mount Sinai Hosp.; Tel. 924-7960.**
NASH, T. W.; 1320 King St. E., Hamilton, Ont.; Wes '31; Tel. LI 4-1346.
NASON, Harold O.; Dal '59; Res., Victoria Gen. Hosp., Halifax, N.S.
NASSR, Donald G.; Ste. 409, 362 Dundas St., London, Ont.; Wes'60; DPM; Psy; Staff Psy., Ontario Hosp., St. Thomas, Ontario; Tel. 433-3571.
NATAROS, Harry S.; Box 717, Langley, B.C.; Qns '54; Tel. 534-3717.
NATESAN, Ramasamy; Madras (India) '60; Res., Allan Memorial Inst., Montreal 2, P.Q.
NATHAN, Max T.; 452 Main St. E., Hamilton, Ont.; 173 Cline Ave. S. (res); Wes '55; DABP, FAAP; Paed; Tel. JA 7-2092.
NATHAN, Sidney N.; 1746 Jane St., Weston, Ont.; 323 Hillhurst Blvd. Tor. 19 (res); Leeds (Eng.) '43; MCGP; Sr. Active Staff, Humber Mem. Hosp.; Tel. CH 4-5545.
NATHANSON, Daniel S.; New Waterford Med. Clinic, New Waterford, N.S.; Dal '53; GenSurg; Tel. 862-6495.
NATHANSON, Martin M.; McG'65; Jr. Int., Jewish Gen. Hosp., Montreal 26, P.Q.; Abroad.
NATHENS, Marvin S.; Sask '60; DiagRad; Staff, St. Mary's Hosp., 3830 Lacombe Ave., Montreal 26, P.Q.; Tel. 735-3511.
NATION, Eric W.; Cambridge (Eng.) '45; MR-CP (Lond.); IntMed; Med. Spec., Colonel Belcher **Hosp.; Med. Dir. Calgary Dept., Cdn. Red Cross Blood Transfusion Serv., Calgary, Alta.; Tel.** 266-4820.
NATSUK, Antony W.; 609 Boyd Bldg., 388 Portage Ave., Winnipeg 1, Man.; 301 Carpathia Rd. (res); Man '42; Anaes; Staff, Misericordia Gen. Hosp.; Tel. SP 4-6581.
NATTA, Clayton L.; Tor '61; Res., Ottawa Civic Hosp., Ottawa 3, Ont.; Abroad.
NATTRESS, J. Ronald; Box 440, Lloydminister, **Sask.; Alb '49; M.C.G.P.**
NAUD, Robert; 100 Carre Youville, Quebec, P.Q.; Lav'38; GenSurg.; Tel. 523-8937.
NAULT, Albert; St.-Philippe, Co. Laprairie, **P.Q. (res); Mon '63; Research, U. of Mtl.**
NAUMOFF, Peters; 345 Bloor St. W., Toronto 5, Ont.; Munich (Germ.) '41; Tel. WA 1-1277.
NAVIN, Stephen J.; Cassiar, B.C.; London (Eng.) '35; MCGP.
NAVRATIL, Frantisek; 66 Joyce Parkway, Tor**onto 19, Ont. (res); Carolinensis (Prague, & Lausanne (Switz.) '18; Retired.**
NAYLOR, Gerald A.; 41 Chelsea St., Calgary, **Alta., 2316 Cherokee Dr. (res); Bristol (Eng.) '55;** MRCS; LRCP; Staff, Calgary Gen., Grace & Children's Hosp's.; Tel. AV 9-1901.
NAZARENO, Sesinando; Manila (Philippines) '56; Jr. Intn., St. Joseph's Hosp., Toronto 3, Ont.
NAZIF, Aziz; Ste. 501, 625-5th Ave., New Westminster, B.C.; Cairo (Egypt)'57; Psy.; Tel. 526-6422.
NAZURUK, Eileen; Ott'65; Jr. Int., Ottawa Gen. Hosp., Ottawa 2, Ont.
NEAGA, Arcadie; 455 Ave. Oakdale, Montreal 16, P.Q. (res); Jassy (Roumania) '44; Path; Path., Hop.-Jean-Talon; Tel. CR 3-5151.
NEAL, William S.; 975 Waterford Ave., Fort Garry, Man.; 122 Ruttan Bay (res); Man '53; MCGP; Tel. GR 5-0574.
NEALE, William F.; 240 Yonge St., Midland, Ont.; Tor '56; Act. Staff, St. Andrew's Hosp.; Court. Staff, Penetang Gen. Hosp., Penetang.; Tel. 526-7266.
NEAMAN, Montague P.; 105 Northgate Bldg., 10049 Jasper Ave., Edmonton, Alta.; 8911-146th St. (res); Man '55; DABDR; DiagRad; Tel 424-5735.
NEARING, Thomas N.; 500, 5300 Cote-des-Neiges **Rd., Montreal 26, P.Q.; 27 Stratford Rd., Hampstead (res); McG '49; FRCS(C), Urol; Urol., St. Mary's Hosp.; Ass't. Urol., Mtl. Children's Hosp.; Dem. (Surg.), McGill U.; Tel. RE 1-3131.**
NEARY, Angus J.; 10 Ordnance St., St. John's, Nfld.; 26 Campbell Ave. (res); Dal '48; D.A.B.S., F.R.C.S.(C), GenSurg; Surg. Staff, Gen., St. Clare's & Grace Hosps.; Tel. 578-3760.
NEAVE, Margaret (Taylor); Man '35; D.C.H.; Med. Dir., Tranquille School, Tranquille, B.C.
NEDILSKI, Morris M.; Ste. 925, 123 Edward St., Toronto 2, Ont.; Tor'54; IntMed; I/C Allergy, St. Michael's Hosp.; Clin. Ass't. Dept. of Med., U. of Toronto; Tel. 366-2451.
NEEDHAM, William L.; 3816 Seminole St., Windsor, Ont.; 2567 Buckingham Dr. (res); Wes '40; DRCOG; MCGP; Staff, Metropolitan Gen. Hotel-Dieu I.O.D.E. Mem. & Grace Hosp's.; Tel. 945-4261.
NEELANDS, Lucy (See Marritt)
NEELANDS, Peter J.; 1119 Victoria Ave., Fort William, Ont.; 110 Med. Arts Bldg., Port Arthur, Ont.; Tor'55; Paed; Active Staff, McKellar Hosp., Fort William; Court. Staff, Port Arthur Gen. & St. Joseph's Hosp's.; Cons. Staff, Children's Diagnostic Centre, Ontario Hosp., Port Arthur, & Fort William San.; Tel. 344-1813 & 623-0414.
NEELIN, W. Eric E.; 604 Besserer St., Ottawa 2, **Ont.; Tor '24; Tel. 233-5452.**
NEESON, George B.; 55 Avondale Blvd., Bramalea, Ont.; Tor '62; Tel. 451-7575.
NEGRETTE, Juan C.; Tucuman (Argentine)'61; Psy; Staff, Mont Providence Hosp., Montreal 39, P.Q.
NEGRYCH, Sylvia; Man'62; Res., Wellesley Hosp., Toronto 5, Ont.
NEHRA, Narendra N.; 4 King Cr., Weston, Ont.; Liverpool (Eng.) '53.
NEIL, Andrew J.; Box 550, Carlyle, Sask.; Glasgow (Scot.) '55; Tel. 453-2464.
NEIL, S. Christella (Gardiner); Box 550, Carlyle, Sask.; Glasgow (Scot.) '55; Tel. 453-2464.
NEIL, Duncan; 2030 Larch St., Vancouver, B.C. (res); UBC '60.
NEIL, Rhonda B.; (See Robertson, Rhonda B.).
NEILL, Raymond; Tor '54; FRCP(C); Anaes; Staff, Kingston Gen. Hosp., Kingston, Ont.; Lect. Med., Queen's U.; Tel. 546-3841.
NEILMEYER, Cuncliffe L.; Langenburg, Sask.; (Ireland) '59; Staff, Langenburg Union Hosp.; Tel. 6.
NEIL-SERS, Phyllis M.; Goldboro, Guys Co., N.S. (res); St. Andrews (Scot.) '44; D.C.H.; Retired.
NEILSON, David B.; R.R. 1, Boutiliers Point, Halifax Co., N.S. (res); Glasgow (Scot.) '47; M.C.; Path; Ass't. Path., Path. Inst., Halifax; Lect., Dalhousie U.

NEILSON, George; Box 99, Fort Langley, B.C.; 21734 Telegraph Trail (res); Glasgow (Scot.) '52; Tel. 534-3415.
NEILSON, H. Kenneth; Med. Arts Bldg., 180 Metcalfe St., Ottawa, Ont.; 252 Metcalfe St. (res); McG '15; Ophth, Otol; Hon. Cons., Ottawa Civic Hosp.; Retired.
NEILSON, James M.; Box 99, Fort Langley, B.C. Glasgow, Scotland '53; Tel. 534-3415.
NEILSON, John B.; 304 Rossmore Blvd., Burlington, Ont. (res); Tor '37; Chm., Ont. Hosp. Services Commission, 2195 Yonge St., Toronto 7, Ont.; Tel. EM 3-1211.
NEILSON, Thomas H.; 455 E. Columbia St., New Westminster, B.C.; Glasgow (Scot.) '52; MCGP; Tel. LA 6-4655.
NEILSON, Walter I.; Qns '51; Anaes (P.Q.); Staff, Montreal Gen. Hosp., Rm. 839, Montreal 25, P.Q.; Tel. We 7-6011.
NEILY, Harold H., S/L; 3 Wing RCAF, CFPO 5055, Canadian Armed Forces, Overseas; Dal'53; Anaes.
NEIMAN, Gregory M.A.; Ste. 320, 6000 Cote des Neiges Rd., Montreal, P.Q.; 4840 Cote St. Luc. (res); Dal '48; M.Sc. (Med.), D.I.M.; IntMed; Clin. Ass't., Jewish Gen. Hosp.; Tel. RE 3-0239.
NEKUS, Valentinas A.; Box 413, 10 Montreal St., **Kingston, Ont.; 34 Hillcroft Dr. (res); Kaunas (Lithuania) '44; F.A.C.A.; Anaes; Chief, Dept. of Anaes, Hotel-Dieu Hosp.; Staff, Kingston Gen.** Hosp.; Ass't. Prof., Queen's U.; Tel. 542-5609.
NELEMS, Beverley G. (See Barron)
NELKO, Sidney L.; 1757 Main St., West Kildonan, Winnipeg 17, Man.; Man '57; FACG; MCGP; Pt-time Civilian M.O., Winnipeg Military Hosp.; Tel. ED 4-4945.
NELLES, Jas. E.; 100 Victoria Ave., Belleville, Ont.; 24 Rosewood Ave. (res); Qns '50; Paed; Chief of Paed & Dir. Poison Control Centre, Belleville Gen. Hosp.; Cons. (Paed), Trenton Mem. Hosp.; Tel. 968-8156.
NELLES, J.V.; Port Elgin, Ont.; Qns '35; IntMed (TB).
NELLES, Thomas R. B.; 925 W. Georgia St., Vancouver, B.C.; 1500 W. 16th Ave. (res); McG 05; Tel. MU 5-9412.
NELLIGAN, Patrick L.; 4958 St. Catherine St. E., Montreal, P.Q.; 241 McDougall (res); McG '26; GenSurg; Indus. Phys., BA & Shell Oil Co's; Tel. CL 5-7347.
NELSON, A. John; 970 Burrard St., Vancouver 1, B.C.; 1075 Groveland Rd., West Van. (res); Glasgow (Scot.) '45; DPH; MD; PH; Dir. Health Serv., BC Hydro & Power Authority; Clin. Assoc. Prof. (PrevMed), U. of British Columbia; Tel. 683-8711.
NELSON, Clifton L.; 7525-110th Ave., Edmonton, Alta. (res); Alb '54; M.Sc., (Physiol.); Med. Missionary, Africa Inland Mission, Tanganyika, East Africa; Abroad.
NELSON, Donald G.M. A/C; 48 Rideau St., Ottawa 4, Ont.; Tor '39; DPH; DAB (Prev.Med.) (Avia.Med.); FACPM; Deputy Surg. General, Cdn. Forces; Tel. 992-2564.
NELSON, George F.; 576—20th St. W.; Prince Albert, Sask. (res); Wes '12; Psy; Cons. Psy., Saskatchewan Penit.
NELSON, James D.; 5740 Cambie St., Vancouver, B.C.; 1555 W. 58th Ave. (res); Glasgow (Scot.) '46; M.B., Ch.B., DMRD (Lond.); DiagRad; Active Staff, Royal Columbian Hosp.; Cons. Staff, Maple Ridge Hosp.; Clin. Instr., U. of British Columbia; Tel. FA 5-3244; Abroad.
NELSON, Jean C. (Taylor); 11603-89th Ave., Edmonton, Alta. (res); Aberdeen (Scot.) '45; M.B., Ch.B., D.C.H. (Lond.), M.R.C.P. (Edin.); Paed; Cons. Paed. Dept. of Public Health, Edmonton; Instr. (Paed.), U. of Alberta; M.O., Detention Home for Girls & Alberta Inst. for Girls; Dir., Well Child Prog., U. of Albetra; Tel. 433-0050.
NELSON, John W.; Box 670, Creston, B.C.; London (Eng.)'41; MRCP(Ed.); MRCS(Eng.); LRCP(Lond.); Tel. 356-2224.
NELSON, Robert F.; Dal '59; Res., Montreal Neurological Inst., Montreal 2, P.Q.
NELSON, Robert J.; 88 Blake St., Barrie, Ont.; McG'32; GenSurg; Tel. 726-0173.
NELSON, Rodger A.C.; 605-5th Ave., New Westminster, B.C.; 1912-7th Ave. (res); UBC '56; Tel. LA 2-5445.
NELSON, Thomas R.; 330 Phys. & Surg. Bldg., 8409-112th. St., Edmonton, Alta.; Edinburgh (Scot.)'44; MRCOG(Lond.); FRCOG; FRCS(C); ObstGyn; Staff, University Hosp.; Clin. Assoc. Prof. (ObstGyn), U. of Alta.; Tel. 439-1672.
NEMETHY, Nicholas I.; 5853 Spring Garden Rd., Halifax, N.S.; 2121 Newton Ave. (res); Debrecen (Hung.) '39; Derm; Assoc. Prof. (Anat.), Dalhousie U.; Tel. 422-5801.
NENADKEVICH, Antonina; USSR '19; M.O., Fisher River Indian Hosp., Hodgson, Man.
NEPVEU, Theodule; Ste. Ursule, P.Q.; Lav '13.
NERI, Luciano C.; 423 Bronson Ave., Ottawa, Ont.; Italy '47; MCGP; Tel. CE 4-3914.
NERMAN, Yale; Ste. 310, 5845 Cote-des-Neiges Rd., Montreal 26, P.Q.; 2957 Soissons Ave. (res); Dublin (Ire.)'57; D.Psy(McG); Psy; Ass't. (Dept. of Psy), Jewish Gen. Hosp.; Lect. (Psy.), McGill U.; Tel. 737-2211.
NERO, Richard P.; 77 Upper Middle Rd., Cooksville, Ont.; Tor'56; ObstGyn; Active Staff, South Peel Hosp.; Court. Staff, St. Joseph's Hosp., Toronto; Tel. 277-2252.
NESSETH, Merrill E.; 580 Mill St., Windsor, Ont.; 3350 Bruce (res); McG '47; M.C.G.P. Active Med. Staff. Windsor Hosp's.; Tel. 254-9279.
NESSIM, Raymond; Ste. 205, 77 Upper Middle Rd., Cooksville, Ont.; Paris (France)'56; Pres. of Med. Staff, South Peel Hosp.; Coroner, County of Peel; Tel. 279-1340.
NESTEL, Maurice B.; 4810 Queen Mary Rd., Montreal, 26, P.Q.; 5835 Decelles Rd. (res); Prague (Czecho-slov.) '34; MCGP; Tel. RE. 1-1522.
NESTLER, H. Adelbert; 1271 Portage Rd. S., Niagara Falls, Ont.; Prague (Czech.) '43; GenSurg; Tel. EL 6-2475.
NESTMAN, Jerry M.; 1933 W. Broadway, Vancouver 9, B.C.; **3155 W. 13th Ave. (res); UBC '56; Tel. RE 8-3414.**
NETT, Alvina E.; Ste. 18, 10445-57th Ave., Edmonton, Alta.; Alb'61.
NETTLETON, John M.; Apt. 103, 100 Oriole Pkwy., Toronto 7, Ont.; Tor '10; Retired.
NEUBAUER, Edward; Bratislava (Czech.) '35; Staff, Montreal Gen. Hosp., Montreal, P.Q.; Tel. 937-6011.
NEUBAUER, Ernest; 183 James St. S., Hamilton, Ont.; Vienna (Austria) '24; O.P.D., Gen. Hosp.; Tel. JA 2-8887.
NEUFELD, Abram H.; Dept. of PathChem., U. of Western Ontario, London, Ont.; 1071 Colborne St. (res); McG '50 M.Sc., Ph.D. Biochem. (P.Q.); Dir. ClinPath, Victoria Hosp., Head & Prof., Dept. of PathChem., U. of Western Ont.; Tel. GE 2-5261.
NEUFELD, Bernard; Box 399, Outlook, Sask.; Alb '53; AMCGP; Tel. 867-8626.
NEUFELD, Nicholas J.; Ste. 201, 171 Donald St., Winnipeg 1, Man.; Crimea (Russia) '23; Man '26; Tel. WH 3-7519.
NEUFELD, Wilhelm P.; 4927 Kingsway, South Burnaby, B.C.; 1335 Nanton Ave. (res); **Man '29; Tel. MU 4-4174.**
NEULANDER, Arthur; King Ferdinand U. (Klausenburg) '40; Jr. Intn., Regina Grey Nun's Hosp., Regina, Sask.
NEUMAN, Alan A.; 5845 Cote des Neiges, Montreal 26, P.Q.; Chicago (U.S.A.)'60; FRCS(C), ObstGyn.
NEUMAN, Alice; 1820 est-Joseph, Montreal 34, P.Q.; Mon'62.
NEUMAN, Harold W.; 240 Brock St., Kingston, Ont.; 1 Marley St. (res); Qns '46; M.Sc., D.N.B., D.A.B.S., F.R.C.S.(C), GenSurg; ThorSurg; FACS; Ass't. Prof. (Surg.), Queen's U.; Tel. 542-9290.
NEUMANN, Alfred L.; 714 Boyd Bldg., 388 Portage Ave., Winnipeg 1, Man.; 1200 Henderson Hwy., East Kildonan (res); Vienna (Austria)'49; Tel. WH 2-1212.
NEUMANN, Peter Z.; 12 Belcourt Rd., Dollard des Ormeaux, Montreal 26, P.Q.; Szeged (Hung.) '56; Paed; Research Assoc., Montreal Children's Hosp.; Tel. 684-1248.

NEVE, Clement R.; J. F. Haszard Clinic, Howard St., Kimberley, B.C.; Guys's Hosp. (London, Eng.) '45; FRCS (Eng.); FACS; GenSurg; Chief of Surg., Kimberley & Dist. Hosp.; Surg., St. Eugene Hosp., Cranbrook; Tel. 427-2277.

NEVEU, Michel; 875 des Recollets, Trois Rivieres. P.Q.; 2879 Place Harper (res); Lav'54; Ophth, **Chief of Ophth. Serv., Hop. Ste-Marie; Tel. TR 5-0366.**

NEVILLE, John J.; 397 Reid St., Peterborough, Ont.; 550 Homewood (res); Qns'49; Tel. 742-2291.

NEVILLE, John W.; Box 699, High St., Ladysmith, B.C.; Walker Ave. (res); Man'44; MCGP; Chief Med. Staff, Ladysmith Gen. Hosp.; Tel. 245-3413.

NEWALL, John R.; Tor'64; Res., St. Michael's Hosp., Toronto, Ont.

NEWBERRY, Peter D., S/L; Inst. of Aviation Med., 1107 Avenue Rd., Toronto 12, Ont.; Witwatersrand (S. Africa)'53.

NEWBIGGING, Donald K.; 505 Albert St., Sault Ste. Marie, Ont.; 407 McDonald Ave. (res); Tor '32; Otol; Staff, Plummer Memorial & Gen. Hosp's. Retired.

NEWBIGGING, P. D.; Tor'64; Res., Toronto Western Hosp., Toronto, Ont.

NEWBIGIN, Brian; Cambridge (Eng.)'58; Ass't. Res., Sunnybrook Hosp., Toronto, Ont.

NEWBY, R. C.; 1207 Douglas St., Victoria, B.C.; 1161 Camrose Cres. (res); Alb '35; M.C.G.P.; Temp. Retired.

NEWBY-GOOD, Frederick W.; 2 Prairie Lane, Beaconsfield, Ste-Anne-de-Bellevue, P.Q.; St. Mary's Hosp. (London, Eng.) '40; D.I.H.; Tel. 695-9181.

NEWCASTLE, Neill B.; U. of St. Andrews (Scot) '55; Sr. Int'n. (Path.), Shaughnessy Hosp., Vancouver, B.C.

NEWCOMBE, Edward H.; McG '61; Res., Montreal Children's Hosp., Montreal 25, P.Q.; Abroad.

NEWEDUK, Michael W.; 1364 Islington Ave. N., Rexdale, Ont.; 16 Sage Ave., Tor. 19 (res); Wes '58; Tel. 741-2020.

NEWELL, Alan N.; 221 Brant Ave., Brantford, Ont.; Tor '49; IntMed; Tel. 753-5683.

NEWELL, Edith C.; 109 Cedar, Sudbury, Ont.; Lockerby P.O. (res); Tor '50; Tel. 673-9524.

NEWELL, Jack E.; Man '45; M.Sc.; Path; Dir. of Labs., Foothills Hosp., Calgary, Alta.; Tel. 283-0751.

NEWELL, Philip G.; Liverpool (Eng.)'52; Staff, Barrhead Clinic, Barrhead, Alta.

NEWHOUSE, Alan L.; Merritt, B.C.; UBC '55; AMCGP; Tel. 378-2262.

NEWHOUSE, Michael; 217 James St. S., Hamilton, Ont.; Qns '59; IntMed; Staff, St. Joseph's Hosp., Hamilton, Ont.

NEWLAND, Frank M.; Huron St., Clinton, Ont.; Tor '46; M.C.G.P.

NEWLANDS, William J.; Brown Clinic, 700-8th St. S.W., Calgary, Alta.; Edinburgh (Scot.)'52.

NEWMAN, Donald E.; Qns '62; Staff, Winnipeg Gen. Hosp., Winnipeg, Man.

NEWMAN, Harvey E.; Box 298, Leamington, Ont.; Man '52; DPH.

NEWMAN, John D.; Qns'60; Res., Toronto Western Hosp., Toronto 2B, Ont.

NEWMAN, Michael J.; 632 Med. Arts Bldg., Winnipeg 1, Man.; 1286 Wolseley Ave., Wpg. 10 (res); Cambridge (Eng.) '50; MD; MRCP (Lond.); FRCP(C), IntMed; Neur; Active Staff, St.-Boniface Hosp.; Ass't. Phys., Wpg. Gen. Hosp.; Cons. Neurol., Man. Rehab. & Brandon Gen. Hosp's.; Tel. 943-8579.

NEWMAN, M. Jean; 1040 Gilles Blvd. E., **Windsor, Ont.; Tor '31; Staff, Grace Hosp.; Tel. 254-1907.**

NEWMAN, Richard L.; 714 Fairmont Med. Bldg., 750 W. Broadway, Vancouver 9, B.C.; 725 W. 41st Ave., Van. 13 (res); Leiden (Neth) '56; Psy; Teach. Fell. (Psy), U. of British Columbia; Tel. TR 6-8226.

NEWMAN, William G.; 101 Medical Arts Bldg., Winnipeg, Man.; 456 Ash St. (res); Man '42; M.C.G.P.; Med. Staff (ObstGyn), Grace Hosp.; Dem. (ObstGyn), Manitoba U.; Tel. WH 2-5962.

NEWSON, Dora A.; 121 Med. Arts Bldg., 11010 Jasper Ave., Edmonton, Alta.; 14307 Mackenzie Dr. (res); Alb'31; FACP; Tel. 488-0974.

NEWSTONE, John M.; 310-311, 718 Granville St., Vancouver 2, B.C.; 4887 Cambie St. (res); Man'32; AMCGP; Tel. MU 5-8058.

NEWTON, John B.; 10426-81st Ave., Edmonton, Alta.; Liverpool (Eng.)'51; DPH; M.O. of Health; Tel. 439-7348.

NEWTON, Orville R.; Box 446, Strathroy, Ont.; Wes '44.

NEWTON, Robert A.; 330 Med. Arts Bldg., 170 St. George St., Toronto 5, Ont.; McG '58; DDS; FRCS(C); PlasSurg; Surg., Toronto Gen. Hosp.; Clin. Teach. (Surg.), U. of Toronto; Tel. 924-4851.

NEWTON, William E.; 1175 Cook St., Victoria, B.C.; McG'51; GenSurg.

NEY, Philip G.; Ste. 1103, 750 W. Broadway, Vancouver 9, B.C.; UBC'60; Psy.

NG, Anastacio C.; Santo Tomas (Manilla) '58; DiagRad; Staff, Dept. of Rad., Regina Gen. Hosp., Regina, Sask.

NG, Edward H.; 1466 Ouellette Ave., Windsor, Ont.; Ott'60; AMCGP; Tel. 252-8466.

NG, Robert Y.; Tulane '61; Res., Dept. of Haem., Hosp. for Sick Children, Toronto 2, Ont.

NG, Ronnie Y.; Man '60; Res., Toronto Gen. Hosp., Toronto 2, Ont.; Abroad.

NGAI, Shihk; 221 St. Clair Ave. W., Toronto, Ont.; Hunan-Yale Med. Coll. '29; Tel. WA 3-8262.

NGUYEN, Dong; 233 rue Beauchesne, Arthabasca, P.Q.; Paris (France)'56; Diag Rad; Staff, Hop-Hotel-Dieu.

NIBLETT, Douglas H.; National Health & Welfare, Brooke Claxton Bldg., Ottawa, Ont.; Calcutta (India)'43; DPH; Med. Cons., Hospital & Med. Services, Emergency Health Services Div., Dept. of National Health & Welfare, Ottawa.

NICAS, James A.; 105 Med. Dental Bldg., Lethbridge, Alta.; Alb'56; Active Staff, Dept. of Orth-Surg., Lethbridge Municipal & St. Michael's Hosp's.; Tel. 327-3121.

NICHINI, Antonio; 1811 Delaney Dr., Clarkson, Ont.; London (Eng.)'56; MRCS, LRCP.

NICHINI, Franco M.; London (Eng.) '56; TherRad; Staff, Princess Margaret Hosp., Toronto 5, Ont.; Abroad.

NICHKA, Bohdan A.; 408-1541 W. Broadway, Vancouver 9, B.C.; 3767 Edgemont Blvd., N. Van. (res); Alb '56; FRCS(C), Otol; Vis. Staff, St. Paul's, Mt. St. Joseph, Van. Gen. & Shaughnessy DVA Hosp's.; Tel. RE 6-4123.

NICHOL, Hamish; Dept. of Psy., Fac. of Med., 717 W. 10th & Heather, Vancouver 9, B.C.; Cambridge (Eng.)'52; MRCS (Eng.); LRCP (Lond.); DPM; Psy; Ass't. Prof. & Hd., Child Psy., U. of British Columbia; Memb. Sub-Committee on Children's Serv. and Mental Retardation of the Nat. Committee on Mental Health; Tel. 876-3211, Loc. 3302.

NICHOL, James T.; Carling Ave., Ottawa 3, Ont.; 2458 Rosewood Ave., Ott 14 (res); Wes '53; M.Sc.; Ph.D. (Biophysics); TherRad; Radiotherapist, Ont. Cancer Fdn. & Research Fell. (Radioisotope Lab.), Ottawa Civic Hosp.; Tel. 728-3745.

NICHOL, Walter W.; 1569 Dixie Rd., Port Credit, Ont.; McG'51; MCGP; Courtesy Staff, Peel Memorial Hosp., Brampton; Tel. CR 8-1049.

NICHOLAS, Godfrey J.; Calcutta (India)'35; LRCP; MRCS; DPH; Staff, Lady Willingdon Hosp., Ohsweken, Ont.

NICOLAS, Tomas D.; Santo Tomas (Philipp.) '57; Staff, Saskatchewan Hosp., Weyburn, Sask.

NICHOLAS, William C.; 6097 Roxton Rd., Halifax, N.S.; Dal '58; FRCP(C), IntMed; Active Staff, Victoria Gen., Camphill DVA & Halifax Infirmary; Tel. 429-2323.

NICHOLL, Joan O.; 2723 Retallack St., Regina, Sask. (res); Liverpool (Eng.) '43; Bact; Bacteriolist, Regina Gen. Hosp.; Tel. LA 2-1811.

NICHOLLS, Doris (McEwan); 9 Pinevale Rd., Willowdale, Ont.; Wes '59; B.Sc., M.Sc., Ph.D. (Bio-Chem.); Assoc. Prof. (Biochem.), York U.

NICHOLLS, George W.; 111 Queen St. E., Toronto 1, Ont.; 33 Farmcote Rd., Don Mills (res); Tor '46; Tel. 368-1828.

NICHOLLS, John H.; Box 89, Linden Bldg., Wolfville, N.S.; Sheffield (Eng.)'51; DA(Eng.).

NICHOLLS, John V. V.; 1414 Drummond St. Montreal 25, P.Q.; 5690 Queen Mary Rd., Mtl. 29 (res); McG '34; D.A.B.Ophth, F.A.C.S., F.R.C.S. (C), Ophth; Ophth., Royal Victoria Hosp.; Cons. Ophth., Catherine Booth Hosp. Mtl. & Physician's Hosp., Plattsburg, N.Y.; Assoc. Prof (Ophth), McGill U.; Tel. VI 9-9916.

NICHOLS, Erwin B.; 385 Miller Ave., Eastview, Ont.; 1885 Rideau Garden Dr. (res); Ott'57; MCGP; Court. Staff, Ottawa Gen. Hosp.; Cons., Dept. of National Defence; Tel. 749-2477.

NICHOLS, Florence L.; 200 Fairview Ave., Toronto 9, Ont.; Tor '37; D.P.M. (Tor.); Ph.D.; D.A.B.P.; Psy; Pt.-time, Day-Care Centre, Lakeshore Psy. Hosp., New Toronto; Pt.-time Instr. Clergy & private practice; Tel. RO 7-5757.

NICHOLS, Gerald B.; 98 Guestville Ave., Toronto 9, Ont.; 4 Astoria Ave. (res); Dal '42; Tel. RO 3-1171.

NICHOLS, Jack S.; 742 King St. W., Kitchener, Ont.; Wes '45; ObstGyn; Tel. 742-4001.

NICHOLS, **Peter R.;** Box 29, North Sydney, N.S.; Dal'66.

NICHOLS, **Roberta;** see BOND-Nichols, Roberta.

NICHOLS, **Thomas M.;** McG'59; Res. (Path.), Vancouver Gen. Hosp., Vancouver 9, B.C.

NICHOLSON, Clyde G.; Box 420, Stony Plain, Alta.; London U. (Eng.) '39; M.R.C.S., L.R.C.P.; MCGP; Chief of Staff, Stony Plain Municipal Hosp.; Tel. 777-2226.

NICHOLSON, **Allan J.;** Box 388, Fort McMurray, Alta.; Alb'62.

NICHOLSON, **Donald M.;** 5750 South St., Halifax, N.S.: Dal'60; FRCS(C), GenSurg.

NICHOLSON, G. M.; 128 Kenilworth St. S., Hamilton, Ont.; 130 Kenilworth St. (res); Tor '43; M.C.G.P.; Tel. JA 2-8887.

NICHOLSON, James K.; 305 Main St., Toronto 13, Ont.; Tor '60; Tel. OX 1-0972.

NICHOLSON, J. Fraser; Medical Arts Bldg., 5880 Spring Garden Rd., Halifax, N.S.; Boulderwood (res); Dal '37; Psy; Ass't. Psy., Victoria Gen. Hosp.; Cons. Psy., Camp Hill Hosp., & Nova Scotia Hosp., Dartmouth; Assoc. Prof. (Psy.), Dalhousie U.; Tel. 422-6310.

NICHOLSON, John R.; Box 10, Terrace, B.C.; UBC'55; ObstGyn; Med. Staff, Mills Mem. Hosp.; Tel. VI 3-2242.

NICHOLSON, **J. Robert;** 284 Central Ave., London, Ont.; Wes'53; FAAP; Paed; Teach. Staff, Victoria Hosp. Tel. GE 8-5500.

NICHOLSON, Mary A.; (Mrs. Wright); 416-111th St., Saskatoon, Sask.; Tor '25; FACA; Anaes; Cons. Anaes., City Hosp.; Staff, St. Paul's Hosp.; Retired.

NICHOLSON, Murdoch A.; 1401 W. Broadway, Vancouver, B.C.; 6042 N.W. Marine Dr. (res); **Tor '32; Med. Exam., Imperial Oil Co.; Tel. 736-5661.**

NICHOLSON, **Robert E.;** Steel Company of Canada, Wilcox St., Hamilton, Ont.; Tor '29; GenSurg; Med. Dir., Steel Co. of Canada; Surg. Staff, Hamilton Gen. Hosp.

NICHOLSON, William M.; Bay Medical Group, Glace Bay, N.S.; Dal '42.

NICKERSON, Granville H.; 350 Kenaston Ave., Mont Royal, Montreal 16, P.Q. (res); McG '45; D.Paed; FRCP(C), Paed; Paed., I/C, Royal Victoria Hosp.; Staff Paed., Montreal Children's Hosp.; Ass't. Prof. (Paed.), McGill U.; Tel. VI 5-3405.

NICKERSON, John A.; 385 Hebert St., Port Arthur, Ont.; 121 Pine St. (res); Qns '54; MCGP; Tel. 344-8475.

NICKERSON, **Kenneth G.;** Ste 1013 750 W. Broadway, Vancouver 9, B.C.; 1331 West 46th (res); McG '48; F.R.C.S.(C), ObstGyn; Assoc. (ObstGyn.), Van. Gen. Hosp.; Clin. Ass't. Prof. (ObstGyn), U. of British Columbia; Tel. TR 2-5484.

NICKERSON, Mark; 256 Kingsway Ave., Winnipeg, Man. (res); Utah (U.S.A.) '50; Ph.D. (Johns Hopkins U.); Cons. Staff, Winnipeg Gen., Winnipeg Children's, Winnipeg Municipal & Deer Lodge D.V.A. Hosp's; Prof. & Head of Pharmacol & Therapeutics, U. of Manitoba; Tel. 786-3514.

NICKEL, **Arnold J.;** Rosthern, Sask.; Sask'60.

NICKLIN, H. R.; 73 Erie St. S., Leamington, Ont.; 88 Erie St. S. (res); Qns'16; MCGP; Tel. 326-6441.

NICOLAS, Monica T.; Santo Tomas (Philipp.)'57; Staff, Saskatchewan Hosp., Box 700, Weyburn, Sask.

NICOLAS, Tomas O.; Santo Tomas (Philipp.)'57; Staff, Saskatchewan Hosp., Box 700, Weyburn, Sask.

NICKOLOFF, Boris J.; Qns '55; Anaes; Staff, Kingston Gen. Hosp., Kingston, Ont.; Clin. Ass't. Anaes., Queen's U.; Tel. 542-9385.

NICKORICK, **Elsie;** Wakaw, Sask.; Sask. '63; Tel. 233-4411.

NICOL, Douglas A.; 103 Med. Dental Bldg., 450 Central Ave., London, Ont.; Tor '44; DABR, D.R., D & T Rad; Assoc. Rad., St. Joseph's Hosp.; Instr. (DiagRad), U. of Western Ont.; Tel. GE 3-2841.

NICOL, John F/L; Glasgow (Scot.) '61; RCAF Station Infirmary, North Bay, Ont.

NICOL, Thomas; Flin Flon Clinic, Flin Flon, Man.; Glasgow (Scot.)'61; Staff, Flin Flon Gen. Hosp.; Tel. 687-5216.

NICOL, William G.; C. S. Williams Clinic, **Trail, B.C.; 3270 Laburnum Dr.** (res); Alb '57; **Ophth; Tel. 368-3255.**

NICOLAIDES, Telemachus; 5006 Park Ave., **Montreal 8, P.Q.; Tel. 277-7862.**

NICOLLE, Frederick V.; Ste. 430, Seaforth Med. Bldg., 3550 Cote des Neiges Rd., Montreal 25, P.Q 589 Lansdowne Ave. (res); Cambridge (Eng.) '56; M.B., B.Chir.; FRCS(C); PlasSurg; Ass't. Surg., Montreal Gen. & Children's Hosp's.; Tel. 933-5667

NICOLSON, Donald N.; 47 Sheppard Sq., Willowdale, Ont.; Edinburgh (Scot.) '53; Tel. BA 1-6072.

NICOLSON, **George A.;** Tor '43; Path; Staff, Riverview Hosp., Essondale, B.C.

NIEBOER, L. P.; Phys., Imperial Oil Ltd., Norman Wells, N.W.T.

NIELSEN, John S.; 287 Queens Ave., London, Ont.; London (Eng.) '51; Anaes; Teach. Staff, Victoria Hosp. & U. of Western Ontario; Tel. GE 8-5143.

NIELSEN, Sigurd; 2057 Caroline St. E., Burlington, Ont.; 223 Poplar Dr. (res); Wes '50; Assoc. Staff, St. Joseph's Hosp., Hamilton & Hamilton Gen. Hosp.; Tel. 634-5336.

NIESEN, William C.; 2150 Valley Way, Niagara Falls, Ont.; 5273 Hewitt Pky., Lewiston, N.Y. **(res); Buffala (NY) '43; DABS (Urol); Urol; Att'd. Urol., Mem. Hosp., NF (Ont.) & Mt. St. Mary's Hosp., NF(USA); Clin. Ass't., U. of Buffalo; Tel. EL 6-2030.**

NIETO, **Alvaro;** Apt. 1807, 55 Maitland St., Toronto 5, Ont.; '57; Tel. 924-2697.

NIEUWENHUIZEN, Maarten; 136 Logan Cres. W., Yorkton, Sask.; Utrecht (Neth) '53; Psy; Clin. Dir., Yorkton Psy. Centre, Dept. of PH (Sask.); Tel. 783-2401, Loc. 200. Abroad.

NIEWCHAS, W. S.; 541 Tegler Bldg., Edmonton, Alta.; Alb '31; Staff, Royal Alexandra Hosp.; Tel. GA 2-2132.

NIGAM, **Krishna K.;** Mall Med. Group, 280 Osborne St. N., Winnipeg 1, Man.; Agra (India) '58; FRCP(C), Paed.; Tel. 774-2411.

NIGAM, **Prabba S.;** 2169 Gottingen St., Halifax, N.S.; Agra (India)'58; AMCGP; Tel. 454-7834.

NIGAM, Sneh; 414 Kilbride Ave., Winnipeg 17, Man.; Delhi (India)'58; Paed.; Tel. 339-8002.

NIGAM. **Sneh;** 412 Kilbride Ave., Winnipeg 17, Man.; Delhi (India) '58; Paed.

NIKAIDO, H.; Bow Island, Alta.; Tor '47.

NIKIFORUK, William J.; Suite T, Craig Block, North Battleford, Sask.; 1501 Queen St. (res); Alb '34; M.C.G.P.; Dist. Coroner.

NIKOLAJEVICH, Vladimir; 2045 Dufferin St., Toronto 10, Ont.; Belgrade (Yugo.) '41; Tel. 651-1210.

NIKSIC, Vera; Zagreb (Yugo.)'40; Staff, Lakeshore Psy. Hosp., 3131 Lakeshore Blvd. W., Toronto 14, Ont.; Tel. 259-8291.
NILOFF, Paul H.; Linton Clinic, 6000 Cote-des-Neiges Rd., Montreal 26, P.Q.; McG '43; F.A.C.S., F.R.C.S.(C), GenSurg; Ass't. Surg., Jewish Gen. Hosp.; Tel. RE 1-9961.
NIP, Ho C.; Man'60; Res., Royal Victoria Hosp., Montreal 2, P.Q.
NIP, Yuen-C.; 1723-18th Ave., N.W., Calgary, Alta.; Hong Kong (China) '54; M.B., B.S.; Anaes; Staff, Calgary Gen. Hosp.; Tel. AM 6-7541.
NIRENBERSKI, Jerry; Allencourt Plaza, 423 Markham Rd., Richmond Hill, Ont.; Poland '55.
NIRENBERSKI, Susan Z.; Allencourt Plaza, 423 **Markham Rd., Richmond Hill, Ont.; Tor '62.**
NISHIKAWA, Frederick S.; Ste. 130, 400 Walmer Rd., Toronto 4, Ont.; Tor'31; Tel. 924-2694.
NISHIKAWA, Ryoichi; 152 Carlton St., Toronto, Ont.; Tor'54; MCGP; Tel. YA 1-2882.
NISHIOKA, Hiro; Dept. of Surg., University Hosp., State University of Iowa, Iowa City, Iowa, U.S.A.; Man '54; DABNS; NeurSurg; Abroad.
NITIKMAN, Gladys (See Ellison).
NIX, Harold L.; 541 Professional Bldg., 10830 Jasper Ave., Edmonton, Alta.; Alb. '27; Tel. GE 9-2494.
NIX, Nelson W.; 14016 Valleyview Dr. Edmonton, Alta. (res); Alb '41; FACA Anaes; Hd. Dept. of Anaes. Royal Alexandra Hosp.; Ass't. Clin. Prof. (Anaes), U. of Alberta; Tel. GR 4-3431.
NIXON, Arthur; Leduc, Alta.; Liverpool (Eng.) '52; FRCS(Ed.); GenSurg; Tel. 446-3432.
NIXON, Helen M.; R.R. No. 5, Simcoe, Ont. (res); Wes '34; Not practising.
NIXON, James R.; 815 Greyhound Bldg., Calgary, Alta.; 504 Crescent Rd. (res); McG '35; GenSurg; Part-time Surg., Col. Belcher Hosp. (D.V.A.); City Coroner; Tel. AM 2-3218.
NIXON, John C.; 1283 Wesmar Dr., Ottawa 8, Ont.; Qns'53; M.Sc; Ph.D. (Biochem.); Biochem., NDFM; Lect. (Biochem.), U. of Ottawa.
NIXON, John E.; 5515 Laburnum St., Vancouver, 13, B.C. (res); Wes'50; Anaes; Att. Staff, Dept. of Anaes., Vancouver Gen. Hosp.; Clin. Instr. (Anaes.), U. of British Columbia; Tel. TR 6-3211.
NIXON, Lloyd H.; 231 Victoria St., Kamloops, B.C.; Alb'55; MCGP; Tel. 372-5522.
NIXON, Murray D.; 115 Hazen St., Saint John, N.B.; McG'60; AMCGP; Tel. 657-1871.
NIXON, Ronald D.; Mountain Health Unit, 755 Upper Wentworth, Hamilton, Ont.; McG '50; Psy; Dir. of Mental Health Serv., City of Hamilton; Tel. 389-2203.
NKANSAH, John; Tor'64; Res. (Psy.), U. of Toronto, Toronto 5, Ont.
NOAKES, John A.; 106 Med Centre, 1711-4th St., S.W., Calgary, Alta.; 3910-3rd St. S.W., Qns '45; Urol; Tel. 263-6464.
NOBERT, Andre; 125 St. Charles, Joliette, P.Q.; Mon'54.
NOBLE, Alan B.; 316 Lethbridge Ave., Town of Mount Royal, Montreal, P.Q. (res); Tor '34; FACA; FRCP(C); Anaes; Chief Anaes., Royal Victoria Hosp.; Assoc. Prof., Dept. of Anaes., **McGill U.; Tel. VI 2-1251.**
NOBLE, Allan J.; 8 Kilkenny Dr., Agincourt, Ont.; Tor '54; Path; Ass't. Pathol., Toronto East Gen. Hosp.; Tel. 461-8272.
NOBLE, Alison E.; 26-35th St., Long Branch, Ont.; Tor '37; Staff, Queensway Gen. Hosp.; M.O.H., Village of Long Branch; District Coroner, County of York; Tel. CL 1-9381.
NOBLE, Charles S.; High St., Sutton West, Ont.; Tor '48.
NOBLE, Donald M.; Ajax Shopping Centre, Ajax, Ont.; Wes'60.
NOBLE, E. Clark; OBE, ED; 216 St. Clair Ave. W., Toronto 7, Ont.; Tor'25; MA (Tor); MRCP (Lond.); Med. Dir., Global Life Ins. Co. & Zurich Life Ins. Co.; Med. Examiner, D.O.T.; Tel. WA 2-0022.
NOBLE, Edward J.; 216 St. Clair Ave. W., Toronto 7, Ont.; 139 Imperial St., Tor. 7 (res); Tor '55; FRCP(C); IntMed (Cardiol.); Staff, Toronto Gen. & Wellesley Hosp's.; Clin. Teach., U. of Toronto; Tel. 923-4446.
NOBLE, J. Arnold, OBE, ED; Glen Margaret, Halifax, N.S. (res); Edinburgh (Scot.) '30; FRCS (Edin.); FRCS(C); GenSurg; Chief-of-Surg., Camp Hill DVA Hosp.; Assoc. Prof. (Surg.), Dalhousie U.; Tel. 423-1371.
NOBLE, James H.; Haig Clinic, Lethbridge, Alta.; 2222—9th Ave. S. (Res); Glasgow (Scot.) '43; GenSurg; Staff, Lethbridge Mun. & St. Michael's Gen. Hosp's.; Cons. Picture Butte Hosp.; Tel. 328-6641.
NOBLE, John G.; 121 Med. Arts Bldg., 750 Spadina Cr. E., Saskatoon, Sask.; Durham (Eng.) '48; MRCS; LRCP; FICS; FRCS(C), OrthSurg; Staff, University, City & St. Paul's Hosp's.; Clin. Instr. (OrthSurg.), U. of Saskatchewan; Tel. 244-0994.
NOBLE, John G.; Smith Clinic, 144 Main St. E., Hawkesbury, Ont.; Aberdeen (Scot.) '56; M.B., Ch. B.; DObstRCOG; Psy., Smith Clinic; Tel. 632-2711.
NOBLE, Robert L.; 4746 W. 2nd Ave., Vancouver 8, B.C.; Tor '34; Ph.D., D.Sc., FRSC; Dir., Cancer Research Centre & Prof. (Physiol.), U. of British Columbia; Tel. CA 4-1111.
NOBLE, Samuel; 266 Oxford St., London, Ont.; Tor '40; M.C.G.P.; Tel. 439-5841.
NOBLE, William H.; Tor'64; Res., Toronto Gen. Hosp., Toronto 2, Ont.
NODWELL, G. Ross; 714 Highland Ave., Ottawa, Ont.; Tor '22; Chief, Heart & Chest Div., Med. Adv. Staff, Can. Pension Comm.
NODWELL, Robert J.; 399 Bathurst St., Toronto **2B, Ont.; 3 Alexandra Wood, Tor. 12 (res); Tor '32; Hosp. Org. & Mgt., Med. Dir., The Toronto** Western Hosp.; Tel. EM 8-2581.
NOEL, Clement; Mon'65; Res., Hop. Hotel Dieu, Montreal 18, P.Q.
NOEL, Frank; 385—121st St., Shawinigan Sud, P.Q.; Mon '26; Dist. Coroner.
NOEL, Gaston; 177 Collard E., Alma, Co. Lac St. Jean, P.Q.; 94 rue Bergeron (res); Lav '51; IntMed (Gastro) (P.Q.); Staff, Hop.-Hotel-Dieu-d'Alma.
NOEL, Gerard; C.P. 728, 8 Blvd. des Veterans, Lac Megantic, P.Q.; Lav '38.
NOEL, J.-Ovila; 301 Conseil, Sherbrooke, P.Q.; Lav '21; F.A.S.A., Anaes; Staff Anaes., Hotel-Dieu Hosp.; Tel. LO 9-2551.
NOEL, J. Maurice; Centre Medical St.-Urbain, 3875 rue St.-Urbain, Montreal 18, P.Q.; 6900 Blvd. Pius IX, Apt. 4 (res); Mon '49; ObstGyn (P.Q.); Ass't. ObstGyn, Hop. Ste.-Justine; Tel. RE 1-4931.
NOEL, Maurice; 274 Friel St., Ottawa, Ont.; Mon '45; Clin. Ass't. (ObstGyn), U. of Ottawa; Tel. CE 5-6751.
NOEL-de-TILLY, Bernard; 184 Cedar St., Sudbury, Ont.; Ott'61.
NOEL, Henri P.; Lav'65; Res., Hop. St-Sacrement, Quebec 6, P.Q.
NOEL, Jacques F.; Mon'65; Res., Hop. Hotel-Dieu, Montreal 18, P.Q.
NOEL, Louis; Lav'65; Res., Hop. Hotel-Dieu, Quebec, P.Q.
NOGRADY, Bernadette; Pecs (Hungary) '54; DiagRad; Staff, Dept. of Rad., Children's Hosp., Montreal 25, P.Q.; Tel. WE 7-8511.
NOGRADY, George L.; 4378 Draper, Montreal 28, P.Q.; Kolozsvar (Hung.)'44; Bact.; Tel. RE 1-4462.
NOGRADY, Marie B.; 2767 Maplewood Ave., Apt. 404, Montreal 26, P.Q.; Pecs (Hung.) '54; DiagRad; Tel. RE 1-4462.
NOGUCHI, Ayao; 2221 Keele St., Toronto 15, Ont.; 8 Paulson Rd., Tor. 15 (res); Tor '54; Anaes; Active Staff (Anaes); Northwestern Gen. Hosp.; Tel. 762-6452.
NOISEUX, Jacques; 485 Ellendale Med. Bldg., 5845 Cote-des-Neiges, Montreal 26, P.Q.; 27 Blvd. Chambord, Cillege Lorraine (res); Mon '50; Ophth; Hd. Ophth, Hop. Sacre-Coeur; Tel. 731-3696.
NOISEUX, Maurice; 9 rue Dufferin, Granby, P.Q.; Mon'47; M.C.G.P.; Tel. 372-5844.
NOLAN, W. J.; 532 St. Clair Ave. W., Toronto, Ont.; 43 Sandringham Dr. (res); Tor '39; Tel. LE 3-1007.

NOLIN, G. Henri; Unite Sanitaire, Matane, P.Q.; Lav '23.

NOLIN, Jacques; Lav'65; Res., Hop. St. Francois d'Assise, Quebec 3, P.Q.

NOLIN, P. Gaetan; 960 boul Ste-Croix, Montreal 9, P.Q.; Mon '51; Paed; Staff, Hop-Ste-Justine; Tel. 747-3501.

NONAMAKER, E. Paul; 5991 Spring Garden Rd., Halifax, N.S.; Dal '42; FRCS(C), GenSurg; ThorSurg; Chief of Surg., Victoria Gen. Hosp.; Cons. (ThorSurg.), Cdn. Forces Hosp., Camp Hill DVA & Children's Hosp's.; Assoc. Prof., Dalhousie U.; Tel. 423-7578.

NOON, William E.; Sandalwood Apts. 3, 7 Osler Court, Dundas, Ont. (res); Tor '53; Staff (Med. Admin.) Hamilton Gen. Hosp.; Tel. JA 7-0271.

NOONAN, John F.; 22 Foster St., Perth, Ont.; Qns '24.

NOONAN, James S.; 317 St. George St., Moncton, N.B.; Dal'62; MCGP.

NOONAN, William E.; 2125 Gary Cres., Burlington, Ont. (res); Tor '53; Staff, Nora Frances Henderson Hosp., Hamilton.

NOONAN, William T.; 244 St. George St., Toronto 5, Ont.; Tor '21; DGO; FRCS(I), ObstGyn; Sec., Maternal Welfare Committee, Ont. Med. Assoc.; Ex-Chief ObstGyn., St. Michael's Hosp.; Ex-Assoc. Prof. (ObstGyn.), U. of Toronto; Tel. 489-7383.

NORELL, Merle V.; 149 Ingram St., Duncan, B.C.; Sask'59.

NORHEIM, N. George; Box 549, 8779 Yonge St., Thornhill, Ont.; Ott'56; Tel. 889-2621.

NORMAN, Hugh R. C.; 104 Toronto Western Med. Bldg., 25 Leonard Ave., Toronto 2B, Ont.; 251 Dunvegan Rd. (res); Tor '32; FRCS(Eng.),; FACS; FRCS(C); GenSurg; Sr. Surg., Toronto **Western Hosp.; Cons Surg., Sunnybrook DVA &** Princess Margaret Hosp's.; Assoc. Prof. (Surg.), **U. of Toronto; Tel. EM 6-2177.**

NORMAN, James; 1045 Bloor St. W., Toronto 4, Ont.; 11 Woodland Hts. Swansea (res); Qns '13; Retired.

NORMAN, Margaret G.; Tor'58; Path; Ass't. Path., Toronto Gen. Hosp., Toronto, Ont.

NORMAN, Nils; 3505 Linton Ave., Apt. 14, Montreal 26, P.Q. (res); Olso (Norway) '50; IntMed; Staff, McGill U.; Tel VI 4-6311.

NORMAND, Denis; 310-6eme Ave., Grand'Mere, P.Q.; Lav '58; Gen. Surg (P.Q.); Tel. LE 8-9833.

NORMAND, Georges; 975 St. Prosper, Trois Rivieres, P.Q.; Lav'50; GenSurg (P.Q.); Tel. 375-4913.

NORMAND, Hudon; 1241 Blvd. St.-Louis, Trois-Rivieres, P.Q.; Lav '24; Indus. Phys., Cd. Iron Foundries Ltd., Cdn. Westinghouse Ltd. & Wabasso Cotton Co.; Tel. FR 5-1331.

NORMAND, Joseph M.; 1027 Blvd. Laviolette, Trois-Rivieres, P.Q.; Lav '27; Fell. Indus. Med. (P.Q.); Indus. Phys., Consolidated Paper Corp., Divisions Wayagamack; Tel. FR 4-5429.

NORMAND, Michel; Lav'65; Res., Hop L'Enfant Jesus, Quebec 3, P.Q.

NORMAND, Yves; 700 rue Ste-Julie, Trois Rivieres, P.Q.; Lav'54; FRCS(C); OrthSurg; Active Staff, Hop. Ste-Marie; Tel. 378-3465.

NORMANDEAU, Fernand W.; 610 Calixa-Lavallee, Quebec 6, P.Q.; Lav '50.

NORMANDEAU, Gerard; 155 Provencher Ave., St. Boniface, Man.; 108 Harvard Ave., Winnipeg 9 (res); Lav '38; Tel. 233-7927.

NORMANDIN, Antonio; 615 rue Notre Dame, Cap-de-la-Madeleine, P.Q.; 223 rue St. Paul (res); Lav '49; DPH (Hyg.); PulmDis. & TB (P.Q.); Cons. Hyg. & Pneum., Hop. Cloutier & Hop. Ste-Marie; Med. Dir., Unite San.; Tel. FR 5-4849 & FR 5-4840.

NORMANDIN, Jean; Mon'48; Anaes(P.Q.); Staff, Hop. Maisonneuve, Montreal, P.Q.

NORONHA, Aloysius; One Med. Place, 20 Wynford Dr., Don Mills, Ont.; Bombay (India)'51; FRCS(C), GenSurg; PlasSurg; Cons. Staff, S. Waterloo Hosp., Galt, St. Joseph's & Guelph Gen. Hosp's.; Cons. Staff, Peel Mem. Hosp., Brampton & Scarborough Gen. Hosp.; Tel. 429-1028.

NORRIS, Albert S.; 113 Lower Union St., Kingston, Ont.; Wes '51; Psy.

NORRIS, Charles K.; Box 170, 767 Foster, Waterloo, P.Q.; McG'40; Att'd. Staff, Brome-Missisquoi-Perkins Hosp., Cowansville, P.Q., & St. Joseph's Hosp., Granby, P.Q.; Tel. 539-2373.

NORRIS, James R.; 419 Med. Arts Bldg., 170 St. George St., Toronto 5, Ont.; 106 Highland Ave., Tor. 5 (res); Otago (New Zealand) '42; MRCOG (Lond.), FRCS(C), ObstGyn; Chief (ObstGyn), Wellesley Hosp.; Ass't. Prof. (ObstGyn), U. of Toronto; Tel. WA 3-7661.

NORRIS, Philip L.; Box 362, Salmo, B.C.; London (Eng.)'58.

NORRIS, Robert L.; Wyoming, Ont.; Tor '33; M.C.G.P.; Tel. 845-3432.

NORRIS, Samuel; 158 St. George St., Toronto, Ont.; 56 Strathearn Rd. (res); Tor '28; D.A.-B.O.G., F.A.C.S., F.I.C.S., A.B.O.G., A.A.O.G., FACOG; ObstGyn; Sr. Att. Obst. Gyn., New Mount Sinai Hosp.; Act. Cons., ObstGyn., Northwestern Gen. Hosp.; Tel. WA 1-3000.

NORRY, Harry T.; 3 Mountsfield Dr., Sub. 14, London, Ont. (res); Wes '38; D.A.B.A., Anaes; Instr. Dept. of Anaes., U. of Western Ont.; Tel. GE 9-1681.

NORTH, Donald P.; 160 Medical Arts Bldg., 1105 Pandora Ave., Victoria, B.C.; The Orchard 4585 Sumner Pl. (res); London (Eng.) '46; M.R.C.S., L.R.C.P., D.O.M.S.; Ophth; Staff, Royal Jubilee Hosp.; Court. Staff, St. Joseph's Hosp.; Vis. Staff, Victoria Vet's Hosp.; Tel. EV 4-8512.

NORTH, H. W. Clinton; Carman, Man.; Man '41; Dist. Coroner.

NORTH, Robert H.; Wes'63; Res., Toronto Gen. Hosp., Toronto 2, Ont.

NORTHOVER, Robert J.; 23 Mory St., Gloucester, Ont. (res); Tor '40; DPH; PH; Staff, Dept. Nat. Health & Welfare, Ottawa; Tel. CE 2-8211.

NORTON, Clair H.; Box 60, Raymond, Alta.; Alb'60.

NORTON, George I.; 925 W. Georgia St., Vancouver, B.C.; 4634 W. 2nd Ave. (res); Alb '36; D.A.B.R., D. & TRad; Staff, Shaughnessy Hosp.; Tel. MU 4-4177; RE 8-3188.

NORVELL, Stevens T. Jr.; 208 O.P.D. Bldg., Victoria Gen. Hosp., Halifax, N.S.; Chicago (U.S.A.) '47; FRCS(C); GenSurg; Staff, Victoria Gen. & Camp Hill DVA Hosp's.; Ass't. Prof. (Surg.), Dalhousie U.; Tel. 422-7371, Ext. 755.

NORWELL, David M.; Glasgow (Scot.)'51; Res., Vancouver Gen. Hosp., Vancouver 9, B.C.

NORWICH, Kenneth H.; 100 Raglan Ave., Apt. 404, Toronto 10, Ont.; Tor '63; Tel. 536-0695.

NORYS, Walter J.; 605 Chinook Professional Bldg., 6449 Macleod Trail, Calgary, Alta.; Alb'55; Psy.

NOTKIN, Louis J.; Ste. 1008, 6800 Cote St. Luc Rd., Montreal 29, P.Q.; McG'20; IntMed; Gastroent(P.Q.); Retired.

NOTKIN, Myron; 502 Med. Arts Bldg., Montreal, P.Q.; 18 Grenville Ave. (res); McG '20; F.C.C.P.; IntMed; Pulm. Dis. & TB (P.Q.); Phys. & Med. Bd., Royal Edward Laurentian Hosp.; Hon. Att'd Phys., Montreal Gen. & Jewish Gen. Hosp's.; Lect. (Med.), McGill U.; Tel. WE 5-7500.

NOTT, Robert F.; 707 Charlotte St., Peterborough, Ont.; **696 Stannor Dr. (res); Tor '32; Obst; Staff, Peterborough Civic & St. Joseph's Hosp's.; Tel. 742-3871.**

NOVAK, Michael C.; Ste. 1, Dunlop Blk., Yorkton, Sask.; 81—3rd Ave. (res); Man '32; Supt., Yorkton Gen. Hosp.; Retired.

NOVAK, Sylvia J.; 4388 W. 15th Ave., Vancouver 8, B.C.; Sask '59.

NOVEK, Arnold M.; Tor '61; Res., New Mount Sinai Hosp., Toronto 2, Ont.

NOVELLA, Carman, Spain '49; Psy; Staff, Douglas Hosp., Montreal 19, P.Q.

NOVICK, William H.; DFC; 1538 Sherbrooke St. W., Montreal 25, P.Q.; 2445 Nantal, St. Laurent (res); Qns '54; FRCS(C); Otol; Ass't. Otol., **Royal Victoria Hosp.;** Dem., Montreal **Children's Hosp.; Cons., Alexandra Hosp.;** Lect., **McGill U.; Tel. WE 5-3211.**

NOVOTNY, George M.; Tor '58; P.G. (Otol.), McGill U., Montreal, P.Q.

NOVOTNY, Milan E.; Kipling, Sask.; Prague (Czech.) '48.

NOWELL, Albert L.; Main St., Kipling, Sask. Edinburgh (Scot.) '46; LRCP; LRCS; LRFP; Tel. 736-2575.
NOWLAN, Bernard E.; Main St., Grand Falls, N.B.; Lav '55.
NOWOSELECKI, Pawel; Virgil Med. Centre, Stone Rd., Virgil, Ont.; Wilno (Poland) '39.
NOWOSIELSKI, Joseph; Poznan (Poland)'53; Staff, Physical Rehab. Centre, Regina, Sask.
NOYEK, Arnold M.; Ste. 602, 99 Avenue Rd., Toronto 5, Ont.; Tor'61; FRCS(C), Otol.
NUCCI, Constant; Ste. 430, 5300 Cote-des-Neiges Rd., Montreal, P.Q., 4269 Isabella (res); Ott'56; FACOG; FRCS(C), ObstGyn; Ass't. ObstGyn., St. Mary's Hosp.; Tel. RE 9-0676.
NUGENT, Brock O.; 24 Catherine St., Trenton, Ont.; Ott'54; Chief Med. Staff, Trenton Mem. Hosp.; Tel. 392-4633.
NUGENT, Edward A.; Box 449, Peterborough, Ont.; Tor'52; FRCS(C), GenSurg; Med. Dir., Ethicon Sutures Ltd.; Tel. 743-2220.
NUGENT, James M.; 3643 Dutch Village Rd., Halifax, N.S.; Dal '64; Tel. 454-1379.
NUGENT, John R.; 122 Carleton St., Saint John, N.B.; McG '17; FACS, GenSurg; Registrar, Med. Council of New Brunswick; Tel. OX 3-2266.
NUGENT, Thomas E.; Bath, N.B.; Qns '34; M.C.G.P.
NUMBERS, Alex A.; 216 Medical Arts Bldg., Hamilton, Ont.; 543 Scenic Dr. (res); Tor '30; IntMed; Tel. JA 7-8311.
NUNAN, Thomas; Box 10, Nokomis, Sask.; National U. (Ire.)'57.
NUNEZ, Juan; 539 College St., Toronto 4, Ont.; Madrid (Spain) '59.
NUNEZ, Matias; 153 Delhi St., Guelph, Ont.; Madrid (Spain) '51; Psy; Staff, Homewood San.; Tel. TA 4-1010.
NUSSBAUM, Marvin A.; Tor'65; Res., Hosp. for Sick Children, Toronto 2, Ont.
NUTIK, Harry L.; Linton Clinic, 6000 Cote des Neiges, Montreal, P.Q.; 4888 Victoria Ave. (res); **McG '38; GenSurg; Sr. Surg., Jewish Gen. Hosp.;** Att'd. Surg., Reddy Mem. Hosp.; Tel. WE 5-1362.
NUTIK, Oscar; 409 Clarke Ave., Montreal 6, P.Q.; McG '31; FACS, FACOG; ObstGyn; Att. Staff, Reddy Memorial Hosp.; Tel. WE 5-2800.
NUTIK, Stephen L.; McG'64; Res., Neurological Inst., 3801 University, Montreal 2, P.Q.
NUTTAL-SMITH, John; 350 Albert St., Nanaimo, B.C.; R.R. 1, Wellington (res); Cambridge (Eng.) '39; MRCP; DCH; Paed; Staff (Paed), Nanaimo Reg. Gen. Hosp.; Tel. SK 3-3431.
NUTTYCOMBE, Hugh; University Hosp., Edmonton, Alta.; Alb '58.
NUYENS, Andreas J. J.; 313 Laurier Ave. E., Ottawa 2, Ont.; 35 Marlborough Ave. (res); Utrecht U. (Neth.) '46; ObstGyn; Assoc. Prof. (ObstGyn), U. of Ottawa; Tel. CE 5-8107.
NYHOF, Andre; Executive House, 730 Humboldt, Victoria, B.C.; Leiden (Neth.)'51; AMCGP; Active Staff, Royal Jubilee, Veteran's & St. Joseph's Hosp's.; Tel. 383-3473.
NYHUS, Tron P.; Ste. 100, 477 Martin St., Penticton, B.C.; 1414 Wilton Cres (res); Alb '52; Staff, Penticton Gen. Hosp.; Tel. 492-8802.
NYKIFORUK, Edward; Box 100 Hafford, Sask.; Sask '58.
OAKE, Chesley M.; P.O. Box 93, Saint John, N.B.; 13 Germain St. (res); Dal '28; D.P.H., D.I.H.; M.C.G.P.; M.O., Dept. of Health, Saint John.
OAKES, Richard G.; Moose Jaw Clinic, 200 Scott Block, Moose Jaw, Sask.; Sask '63. Abroad.
OAKES, Walter A.; 69 Victoria St., Clinton, Ont.; Tor '26; GenSurg; Tel. 482-9443.
OAKES, W. Harris; Tor'60; FRCS(C), GenSurg; Staff, Sunnybrook Hosp., Toronto, Ont.

OAKEY, Roy J.; 710 Seymour St., Vancouver 2, B.C.; Birmingham (Eng.) '60; MB, Ch.B.; Tel. MU 4-1511.

OAKLEY, Anthony R. H.; 12725 Fort Rd., Edmonton, Alta.; 11322-58 St. (res); London (Eng.) '36; M.R.C.S. (Eng.), L.R.C.P. (Lond.); Hon. Coroner; Tel. GR 9-2466.
OAKLEY, Donald; 319 Third Ave., Prince Rupert, B.C.; 127 Hays Cove Circles (res); Qns'49; Tel. 624-6242.

OATWAY, R. Douglas; 1705 Corydon Ave., Winnipeg 9, Man.; Man '42; FRCS (Edin.); FRCS-(C); GenSurg; Tel. 489-8228.
OATWAY, W. Arthur; Moncton Anaesthetic Serv., 691 Main St., Moncton, N.B.; 136 Bromley Ave. (res); Qns '43; Anaes; Ass't. Admin. Moncton Hosp. & Active Staff (Anaes); Cons. Staff (Anaes.), Hotel-Dieu-Hosp.; Tel. 389-9467.
OBERDIECK, Karl E.; Munich (Germ.)'54; Psy; Staff, University Hosp., Saskatoon, Sask.
OBNEY, Nicholas; 618 Church St., Toronto, Ont.; 24 Longbridge Rd., Thornhill (res); Tor '43; Chief Surg., Shouldice Hosp.; Tel. WA 3-3507.

OBORNE, Harry G.; Department of National Health & Welfare, c/o Regional Superintendent, European Region; Tor '38; DIFA; Abroad.

OBRENOVITCH, Milena; Ste. 36, 4145 Blueridge Cres., Montreal 25, P.Q.; Paris (France) '51; Psy.; Tel. 935-0850.
O'BRIEN, Allan; 134 Spruce St., Elliott Lake, Ont.; Tor '55.
O'BRIEN, Brian; 15 Kilbarry Cres., Ottawa 7, Ont.; Dublin (Ire.) '31; Psy; Tel. 749-3646.
O'BRIEN, Brian J.; 83 East Valley Rd., Corner Brook, Nfld.; Nat. U. (Ire.) '43; DPH; Staff, West Coast San., Corner Brook, Nfld.
O'BRIEN, David E.; Res., Vancouver Gen. Hosp., Vancouver 9, B.C.; UBC'65.
O'BRIEN, D. Brian; Medical Arts Bldg., 5880 Spring Garden Rd., Halifax, N.S.; Dal '57; Ophth; Active Staff, Victoria Gen.; Teach. Staff, Dalhousie U.; Tel. 429-2760.
O'BRIEN, Dennis F.; 67 College St., Toronto 2, Ont.; Tor'61.
O'BRIEN, Edward G.; The Med. Clinic, 3009-31st Ave., Vernon, B.C.; McG'52; DABS, FACS; FRCS(C), GenSurg; Chief Surg. Staff, Vernon Jubilee Hosp.
O'BRIEN, Frederick F.; 410 S. Vickers St., Fort William, Ont. (res); Ott '55; DABPA; DABCP; MC Path; FCAP; FRCP(C), Path; Dir. of Labs., McKellar Gen. Hosp.; Tel. 623-0346.
O'BRIEN, Gerald J.; 64 Cochrane St., St. John's, Nfld.; National (Ire.) '42; Psy; Cons. in Psy., St. John's Gen. Hosp.; Staff, St. Clare's Hosp.; Tel. 578-2279.
O'BRIEN, Herbert L.; Alb'65; Jr. Int., Holy Cross Hosp., Calgary, Alta.; Abroad.
O'BRIEN, Hugh J.; Ste. 100, 1136-103rd Ave., Dawson Creek, B.C.; McG'41.
O'BRIEN, James V.; Baddeck, N.S.; Dublin (Ire.)'61.
O'BRIEN, John C.; Coronation, Alta.; '37; District Coroner.
O'BRIEN, John H.; Geddes St., Elora, Ont.; Wes '30.
O'BRIEN, John M., W/C; National Defence Med. Centre, Smyth & Alta Vista Dr., Ottawa 8, Ont.; Glasgow (Scot.)'46; PhysMed. & Rehab.
O'BRIEN, John R.; 680 Seaforth Med. Bldg., 3550 Cote des Neiges Rd., Montreal 25, P.Q.; McG '58; FRCS(C); ObstGyn; Staff, Royal Victoria Hosp.; Jr. Admin & Teach. Staff McGill U.; Tel. 937-2376.
O'BRIEN, Joseph A.; 403 Northgate Bldg., Edmonton, Alta.; 11603-78 Ave. (res); Alb '48; M.C.G.P.; Staff, Edmonton Gen. Hosp.; Courtesy Staff. Misericordia & Royal Alexandra Hosp's.; Tel. GA 2-1748.
O'BRIEN, Kennedy J.; O'Mara Martin Bldg., Rawlins Cross, St. John's, Nfld.; Dublin (Ire.)'49.
O'BRIEN, Mary S.; Nat. Defence Med. Centre, Smyth Rd. & Alta Vista Dr., Ottawa 8, Ont.; Edinburgh (Scot.) '47.
O'BRIEN, Michael J.; 262 St. Clair Ave. W., Toronto, Ont.; 32 Bennington Heights Dr. (res); Tor '42; F.R.C.P.(C), Paed; Ass't. Prof. (Paed.), U. of Toronto; Tel. WA 1-5542.
O'BRIEN, Michael M.; UBC'63; Res., Vancouver Gen. Hosp., Vancouver 9, B.C.
O'BRIEN, Milton W.; 253 Main St., Yarmouth, N.S.; Dal '55; Tel. 742-2215.
O'BRIEN-MORAN, Seamus M.M.; 160-14th St., Brandon, Man.; National U. (Dublin, Ire.) '49; DA; Anaes; Chief, Dept. of Anaes., Brandon Gen. Hosp.; Cons. Anaes., Assiniboine Hosp & Man. Sanitorium, Ninette; Cons. (Anaes.), Brandon Hosp. for Mental Dis.; Tel. PA 6-2086

O'BRIEN, Sabina J.; Ire. '47; Int'n., West Coast San., Corner Brook, Nfld.

O'BRIEN, Stephen E.; Ste. 208, Medical Arts Bldg., 1 Young St., Hamilton, Ont.; 150 Chedoke Ave. (res); Tor'47; FACS, FRCS(C), GenSurg; Chief of Serv. (GenSurg), St. Joseph's Hosp.; Tel. JA 8-5403.

O'BRIEN, Stephen H.; 86 Sherman Ave. S., Hamilton, Ont.; 20 Auchman Rd. (res); McG '18; MCGP; Tel. HI 4-0038.

O'BRIEN, Willard C.; Wedgeport, N.S.; Dal '19.

O'CALLAGHAN, John J.; Foam Lake, Sask.; Nat. U. (Ire.)'53; M.B., B.Ch.; BAO; MCGP; Staff, Foam Lake Union Hosp.; Tel. 272-3533.

O'CALLAGHAN, William J.; Alb'61; Res., St. Michael's Hosp., Toronto 2, Ont.

O'CANA, Antonia; 539 College St., Toronto 4, Ont.; Granada (Spain)'52; Tel. 924-5871.

OCKENDEN, Kenneth A.; 15 Lakeview Ave., Onaping, Ont.; Tor'65.

O'CONNEL, Charles L.; Ste. 4., 824 King St. W., Kitchener, Ont.; R.C.P.S., Dublin (Ire.) '53. L.M. (Rotunda); GenSurg; Staff, Kitchener-Waterloo & St. Mary's Hosp's.; Tel. 742-6111.

O'CONNELL, John J.; 84 Sevenoaks, Brockville, Ont.; Qns '32; D.S.B.P.N., Psy; Ass't. Supt. & Act. Clin. Dir., Ontario Hosp.; Assoc. Prof. (Psy.), U. of Ottawa; Tel. CE 5-6751.

O'CONNOR, Denis A.; Main St., Curling, Nfld.; Galway (Ire.) '50.

O'CONNOR, Fergus J. Jr.; 145 William St., Kingston, Ont.; 73 Sydenham St. (res); Qns '36; FAAP; Paed; Chief of Paed., Hotel-Dieu Hosp.; Lect. (Paed); Queens U.; Tel. 546-0511.

O'CONNOR, Fergus J., Sr.; 193 Earl St., Kingston, Ont.; Qns '06; Obst; Tel. 548-4055.

O'CONNOR, Francis B.; Nat. U. (Dublin, Ire.)'55; Res., Pathological Inst., McGill U., Montreal 2, P.Q.

O'CONNOR, Francis X.; 263½ King St. E., Kingston, Ont.; Qns '15; Ophth, Otol.; Tel. 548-8677.

O'CONNOR, James A.; Ste. 3, Medical Bldg., 188 Prince St., Pembroke, Ont.; 173 Maple Ave. (res); Glasgow (Scot.) '38; F.A.A.P., D.C.H., R.C.P. (Lond.), R.C.S. (Eng.); Chief, Dept. Paed., Pembroke Gen. & Cottage Hosp's.; Med. Examiner, Civil Aviation Med Div.. Dept. Transport, Ottawa.; Tel. 732-2811.

O'CONNOR, James P.; Erin, Ont.; Tor '58; Active Staff, Guelph Gen. & St. Joseph's Hosp's., Guelph; Tel. 833-2277.

O'CONNOR, Laurence N.; Ste. 1, 104 Johnson St., Kingston, Ont.; 437 Frontenac St. (res); Qns'43; F.A.C.O.G.; ObstGyn; Co-Chief, ObstGyn., Hotel-Dieu Hosp.; Cons. (Gyn), Canadian Forces & St. Mary's Hosp's.; Lect. (ObstGyn), Queen's U.; Tel. 546-5873.

O'CONNOR, Maurice J.; 45 Richmond St. W., Toronto, Ont.; 1426 Bayview Ave., Willowdale (res); McG'24; Phys., Simpson's Ltd.; Retired.

O'DEA, Francis L.; 281 Duckworth St., St. John's, Nfld.; 8 Winter Pl. (res); National U. (Ire.) '44; Chief Obst., Ste. Clare's Mercy Hosp.; Tel. 726-9315.

O'DEA, John J.; Shaunavon, Sask.; National U. (Ire.)'47; Coombe H. (Dublin'48); MCGP; Tel. 297-2625.

O'DEA, Mary M.; 102 Osborne Med. Clinic, 190 Osborne St. N., Winnipeg 1, Man.; Glasgow (Scot.) '54; Tel. 774-3835.

O'DELL, John H.; 191 Bay St., Gravenhurst, Ont.; Michigan (U.S.A.) '44; AMCGP; Tel. 687-2411. Abroad.

O'DONNELL, Joseph P.; 4116 W.8th Ave., Vancouver 8, B.C.; Alb '39; FACA; DABA; Anaes; Tel. CA 4-7474.

O'DONNELL, Manus; Main St., Palmerston, Ont.; Dublin (Ire.) '51.

O'DONNELL, Walter J.; 1635 Abbott St., Kelowna, B.C.; 379 Park Ave. (res); Dal '45; GenSurg; Surg. Staff, Kelowna Gen. Hosp.; Tel. 762-2740.

O'DONOGHUE, Pearse; Box 70, Yellowknife, N.W.T.; National U. (Ire.) '46; M.B., B.Ch.; FRCS(Eng.); Gen Surg; Staff, Stanton Yellow Knife Hosp.; Tel. 4456.

O'DONOUGHUE, Robert; Med. Centre, 401 South St., Cowansville, P.Q.; R.R. 1, Sweetsburg (res); Mon '54; Tel. 263-0774.

O'DRISCOLL, Robert F.; 170 Lincoln Rd., Grand Falls, Nfld.; 45 Carmelite Rd. (res); Dal '50; GenSurg; Surg., Central Nfld. Hosp.; Tel. 4848.

O'DWYER, M. Gerald; 170 Queen St. W., Brampton, Ont.; Tor'56; DABS; FACS; FRCS(C), GenSurg; Active Cons. Surg., Peel Hosp.; Cons. Surg., Georgetown Hosp. & Milton Dist. Hosp.

O'DWYER, Michael P., SG/LT; Wes '64; Staff, Royal Can. Navy Hosp., HMCS Naden, Esquimalt B.C.

OESTREICHER, Donald L.; 38 Tecumseh Rd., Chatham, Ont.; Wes '43; F.A.C.P., F.R.C.P.(C), IntMed; Cons. in Med., St. Joseph's Hosp.; Chief, Dept. of Med., Public Gen. Hosp.; Tel. 352-4144.

OESTRICHER, Eunice; (See McKishnie).

OFFORD, David R.; Qns '57; Psy; Dept. of Psy., U. of Florida, Gainesville, Fla., U.S.A. Abroad.

O'FLAHERTY, William J.; Roberts Med. Group, 95 LeMarchant Rd., St. John's, Nfld.; Wickham Pl. (res); McG '60; Staff, Grace & St. Clare's Mercy Hosp's.; Tel. 8-2230; 8-4487.

OGDEN, Erskine; 320 St. Clair Ave. E., Toronto, Ont. (res); London (Eng.) '27; M.R.C.S. (Eng.), L.R.C.P. (Lond.); Phys., City Hall; Tel. 366-8411.

OGG, Marie; Manning, Alta.; Sheffield (Eng.) '56. Retired.

OGILVIE, G. M.; c/o Chief M.O., Dept. Nat. Health & Welfare, 61 Green St., London W.1, England.

OGILVIE, Richard I.; Tor'60; FRCP(C), IntMed; Staff, Montreal Gen. Hosp., Montreal 25, P.Q., & Teach. Fell., McGill U.

OGILVY, W. Lindsay; Ste. 230, 3550 Cote Des Neiges, Montreal, P.Q.; 4524 King Edward Ave. (Res); St. Andrew's (Scot.)'50; M.Sc. (Exper. Surg.)(McG.); D.S.; FRCS(C); GenSurg; Ass't. Surg., Montreal Gen. Hosp.; Cons. Surg., Queen Mary Vets Hosp.; Ass't. Prof., Dept. of Surg., McGill U.; Tel. 932-2255.

OGRYZLO, Metro A.; Wellesley Hosp., Toronto, Ont.; Man'38; FRCP(C), IntMed; Staff Phys., Wellesley Hosp.; Cons., Sunnybrook Hosp.; Dir., U. of Toronto Rheumatic Dis. Unit; Assoc. Prof. Med., U. of Toronto; Tel. 966-6600.

OGULNIK, F. Victor; Ste. 301, 1396 St. Catherine St. W., Montreal 25, P.Q.; 5 Belfrage Rd., Westmount 6 (res); McG '36; MCGP; Staff, Jewish & Reddy Mem. Hosp's.; Tel. UN 6-9037.

O'HALLORAN, Peter B.; 64 Queen St., St. Catherines, Ont.; Glasgow (Scot.) '55; Staff, St. Catharines & Hotel-Dieu Hosp's; Tel. 685-4851.

O'HANLEY, J. Hubert; Charlottetown Clinic, 1 Rochford St., Charlottetown, P.E.I.; 60 Green St. (res); McG '50; Paed.; Tel. 894-5521.

O'HARA, John G.; 88 Rosedale Heights Dr., Toronto 7, Ont.; Tor '47; MCGP; Staff (Med.), O.P.D., St. Michael's Hosp.

O'HARA, Peter J.; Ste. 102, 3000 Lawrence Ave. E., Scarborough, Ont.; 88 Rosedale Hgts. Dr., (res); Tor '44; ObstGyn; Chief (ObstGyn), Scarborough Gen. Hosp.; Tel. 291-1751.

O'HARA, William J., F/L; Tor '63; RCAF Station, Winnipeg, Man.

O'HASHI, David A.; McG '61; Res., Montreal Gen. Hosp., Montreal, P.Q.

O'HASHI, Jack I.; McG '64; Res., Regina Gen. Hosp., Regina, Sask.

O'HEA, Thomas P.; Box 534, Carstairs, Alta.; Glasgow (Scot.) '49.

O'HEANY, Jean M. (Mrs. E. C. Dowd); 636 Pharmacy Ave., Scarborough, Ont.; 134 Balsam Ave., Tor. 13 (res); Tor'56; Assoc. Staff, Scarborough Gen. & Toronto East Gen. Hosp's.; Tel. PL 5-2393.

O'HEANY, Terence M.; One Medical Place, 20 Wynford Dr., Don Mills, Ont.; Tor'56; DNBME; FACS; FRCS(C); ObstGyn.

O'HIGGINS, John W.; Med. Centre, Sackville, N.B.; London (Eng.) '59; D.Obst. R.C.O.G.; DA(Eng.); Staff Anaes., Sackville Mem. Hosp.; Tel. 536-0567.

OHLKE, Rudolph F.; Qns '39; F.A.C.A., Anaes; Chief, Dept. of Anaes., Queensway Gen. Hosp., Toronto, Ont.; Tel. CL 9-6671.

OHRI, Haquiqat Rai; Allan Memorial Inst., Montreal, P.Q.; D.Psy; Psy.; Fellow (Psy.), Colombo Plan; Tel. VI 2-1251.

OHRT, Harry A.; 408 Medical Arts Bldg., 404-406 Graham Ave., Winnipeg 1, Man.; Man '49; DiagRad. Abroad.

OILLE, William A.; 1010 Medical Arts Bldg., 170 St. George St., Toronto, Ont.; 106 Glen Rd. (res); Tor '36; F.A.C.P., F.R.C.P.(C); Int Med.; Phys., Toronto Gen. Hosp.; Assoc. Prof. (Med.), U. of Toronto; Tel. WA 2-3835.

OKAMURA, Yoshiyuki; N. Lethbridge Med. Centre, 718-13th St. N., Lethbridge, Alta.; Man '49; FRCS(C), ObstGyn.; Tel. 328-5445.

O'KEEFE, John F.; 456 Medical Arts Bldg., Saskatoon, Sask.; 2106 Cairns Ave. (res); National U. (Ire.) '51; D.Obst., R.C.O.G., M.A.O. (Ire.), F.R.C.S.(C), ObstGyn; Staff, University City & St. Paul's Hosp's.; Clin.Asst., U. of Saskatchewan; Tel. 242-2429.

O'KEEFE, John M.; Ste. 8, 1211-7th St. S.W., Calgary, Alta.; Man '45; DPH.

O'KELLY, Francis; Ste. 104, 3000 Lawrence Ave. E., Scarborough, Ont.; National U. (Ire.)'54; BAO; FACS; FRCS(C); Urol; Cons. Urol., Toronto East Gen. Hosp. & Scarborough Gen. Hosp.; Tel. 293-8030.

OKO, Jan K.; Vilna (Poland) '30; Phys., Baker Mem. San., Calgary, Alta.

OKTEM, Milagros R.; Ste. 6, 1538 Alexandria St., Regina, Sask. (res); Philippines '54; Staff, Regina Gen. Hosp.; Tel. LA 2-1811.

OKUMURA, Richard T.; 910 Ridgeway St., Fort William, Ont.; Man. '55; FRCS(C), OrthSurg; Staff, McKellar Hosp.; Staff, Westmount & Port Arthur Gen. Hosp's.; Staff, St. Joseph's Gen., Port Arthur & Cons. Orth., Atikokan Gen. Hosp.; Tel. MA 2-5301.

OLACKE, Frank A.; 505 Fairmont Med. Bldg., 750 W. Broadway, Vancouver 9, B.C.; 1903 Cedar Cr. (res); Man '40; DiagRad; Clin. Instr., U. of British Columbia; Tel. RE 3-9379.

OLARIU, Jean; 522 George St., Sarnia, Ont.

OLDFIELD, Frederick S. J.; 3405 Cote Ste-Catherine, Apt. 72, Montreal, P.Q.; Belfast (Ire.)'59; Path.

OLDROYD, Kenneth; Big River, Sask.; Leeds (Eng.) '59; Staff, Union Hosp.; Tel. 52.

OLDS, John M.; Twillingate, Nfld.; John Hopkins (Baltimore, U.S.A.) '31; GenSurg; Med. Div., Notre Dame Bay Mem. Hosp.

O'LEARY, Donal A.; 693 McCowan Rd., Scarborough, Ont.; 26 Underhill Dr., No. 1014, Don Mills (res); Dublin (Ire.) '54; Paed; Att'd. Staff, Scarborough Gen. Hosp.; Tel. 267-6104.

OLEKSIUK, Stanley; 944 Ottawa St., Windsor, Ont.; Ott'56; Otol; Chief (Otol.), Metropolitan Gen. Hosp.; Med. Dir., Remedial Speech Assoc. of Essex County; Tel. 254-0191.

OLENSKI, Stanley; 8 Henrietta St., Brantford, Ont.; Lwow (Poland) '38; Tel. 752-9029.

OLESKER, Norman H.; 5835 Verdun Ave., Verdun, Montreal 19, P.Q.; 323 Melville Ave., Westmount (res); McG '37; Ass't., Obst., Reddy Mem. Hosp.; Tel. PO 7-5363.

OLIN, Jack S.; Ste. 402, 1849 Yonge St., Toronto 7, Ont.; 14 Croydon Rd. (res); Man '54; FACP; FRCP(C); IntMed; Staff, Wellesley Hosp.; Cons., Sunnybrook Hosp.; Cons. Orthopaed. & Arthritic Hosp.; Dir. Detoxification Assess. Unit, Alcoholic & Drug Addiction Fdn.; Teach. Fell. (Path-Chem.), U. of Toronto; Tel. 489-7544.

OLIVA, Filippo G.; 558 College St., Toronto 4, Ont.; 149 Christie St. (res); Padua (Italy) '54; Tel. 925-0889.

OLIVER, Elizabeth A.; 178 St. George St., Toronto, Ont.; Tor '57; FRCP(C); Anaes; Ass't. Anaes., Toronto Gen. Hosp.; Clin. Teach. (Anaes.), U. of Toronto; Tel. WA 3-1154.

OLIVER, Glen L.; Wes'60; Ophth; Staff, Victoria Hosp., London, Ont.; Abroad.

OLIVER, H. D., Sg.Cdr.; 1107 Avenue Rd., Toronto 12, Ont.; 62 Upwood Ave., Tor. 15 (res); London (Eng.) '49; FACPM; DABAv.Med; Surg/Cdr., RCN; O/C, Central Air Med. Bd., Inst. of Aviation Med.; Abroad.

OLIVER, Bernard R.; Tor'61; Res., Toronto Gen. Hosp., Toronto 2, Ont.

OLIVIER, Guy; Lav'65; Res., Hop. St-Sacrement, Quebec 6, P.Q.

OLIVER, Jacques; App. 401, 3445 Drummond, Montreal 25, P.Q.; Mon'42; PathBact.; Tel. 844-4536.

OLIVER, John A.; 4500 Sherbrooke St. W., Montreal 6, P.Q.; McG '56; FRCS(C); Urol; Urol., Royal Victoria Hosp.; Cons. Staff, Queen Mary Vet's Hosp.; Dem. (Surg.), McGill U.; Tel. 937-7508.

OLIVIER, Andre; Mon '64; Res., Dept. of Physiology, Laval U., Quebec, P.Q.

OLIVIER, Michel; Mon '64; Res., Hop. Notre-Dame, Montreal 24, P.Q.; Abroad.

OLIVIERI, Fernando A.; 658 Barton St. East, Hamilton, Ont.; 33 Edgemont Ave. S. (res); Tor '48; Paed.; Staff (Paed.), Hamilton Gen. & St. Joseph's Hosp's.; Tel. JA 7-0271.

OLLERHEAD, William W.; 241 Queen's Ave., London, Ont.; Wes'29; M.Ch.Orth.(Eng.), Orth-Surg; Staff, Dept. of Orth.Surg., St. Joseph's Hosp.; Tel. GE 4-7443.

OLMSTEAD, G. Allison; Upper Main St., Woodstock, N.B. (res); Edinburgh (Scot.) '40; Surg. Staff, Carleton Memorial Hosp.; Tel. 328-6485.

OLMSTED, Alexander I.; McGregor Clinic, 250 Main St. E., Hamilton, Ont.; 85 Chedoke Ave. (res); McG '29; F.I.M.A.; Surg. Staff, Hamilton Gen. Hosp.; Tel. JA 7-2711.

OLNEY, Gerald P.; 5924 McLynn Ave., Montreal 29, P.Q.; McG '59; GenSurg (P.Q.); Staff, Jewish Gen. Hosp.; Tel. 731-0481.

OLSEN, Gordon B.; Alb '62; Res., University Hosp., Edmonton, Alta.

OLSEN, Philip P.; UBC'62; Res., Vancouver Gen. Hosp., Vancouver 9, B.C.

OLSON, Clifford J.; 550 Clarke Rd., New Westminster, B.C.; Wes '53; Tel. WE 9-1212; 939-5220.

OLSON, G. Paul; Box 25, Streetsville, Ont.; 266 Hillside Dr. (res); Tor '55; M.C.G.P. Abroad.

OLSON, R. Marvin; 358 Reynolds St. N., Oakville, Ont.; 80 Ennisclare Dr. E. (res); Qns '56; Tel. 845-4221.

OMABOE, Narh; Geneva (Switz.)'60; DTM; Res. Fell., New Mount Sinai Hosp., Toronto 1, Ont.

O'MAHONY, J. B.; 327 Christina St., Sarnia, Ont.; 124 Pearl St. (res); Wes '39; R.C.S.(Eng.); D.L.O.; Staff, Sarnia Gen. Hosp.; Chief of Staff, (E.N.T.), St. Joseph's Hosp.; Tel. ED 6-6121.

O'MALLEY, Brian P.; Nat. U. (Galway, Ire.) '54; M.B., B.Ch.; BAO; DiagRad; Staff, Henderson Gen. Hosp., Hamilton, Ont.

O'MALLEY, Thomas A.; 3217 Hill Ave., Regina, **Sask. (res); Liverpool (Eng.) '56; Staff, Allen** Blair Mem. Clinic. Abroad.

OMARALI, Unus; 2372 Lake Shore Blvd., Toronto 14, Ont.; RCS (Dublin, Ire.)'55; MCGP; DPA; DLO.

O'MEARA, Bernard B.; 1374 Baseline Rd., Ottawa 5, Ont.; Ott'56; MCGP; Staff, Ottawa Civic Hosp.; Tel. 728-4862.

OMELCHUK, Alex; 6414-118 Ave., Edmonton, Alberta; Alb'62; AMCGP; Active Staff, Royal Alexandra Hosp.; Tel. 474-6487.

O'MULVENNY, Thoreau W., Box 126, Fort Erie, Ont.; Wes '28.

O'NASON, Harold; Dal '59; MCGP; Res., Victoria Gen. Hosp., Halifax, N.S.

ONEL, Joseph; Istanbul (Turkey) '54; Staff, Saskatchewan Hosp., Box 39, North Battleford, Sask.; Tel. 445-2421, Loc. 335.

O'NEIL, Agnes J. E. (Eagles); 426 Superior Ave., Calgary, Alta. **(res)**; Tor '43; DPH; DAB-PreMed; FAPA; MRSH; PH; Deputy M.O., City of Calgary; Tel. 269-0110.

O'NEIL, Albert A.; 426 Superior Ave., Calgary, Alta.; Man '43; FACA; Anaes; Staff (Anaes.), Calgary Gen. Hosp. & Holy Cross Hosp. Dir. (Anaes.), Alberta Red Cross & Crippled Children's Hosp's.; Tel. 244-2920. Abroad.

O'NEIL, Frank B.; Perth, N.B.; McG '48; Tel. Andover 118J.
O'NEIL, James J.; 389 est Boul. St. Joseph, Montreal, P.Q.; Lav '43; NeurPsy. (P.Q.).
O'NEIL, Jean M. (McCallum); 100 Arnold St., Richmond Hill, Ont. (res); Tor '51; Staff, York Co. Health Unit.
O'NEIL, Murray R.; Wes '51; (Intern.) c/o 350 Talbot St., Essex, Ont.
O'NEIL, T. J.; 1635 Abbott St., Kelowna, B.C.; 2185 Abbott St. (res); Dal '50; Tel. 762-2740.
O'NEILL, Anna (Biechl); Box 570, Bridgewater, N.S.; Innsbruck (Austria)'52; MCGP; Tel. 543-2242.
O'NEILL, Dermot A. J.; Come-by-Chance, Nfld.; Dublin (Ire.)'60; LRCP(I); LRCS(I); DMO; Sr. M.O., Cottage Hosp.; Tel. 2121.
O'NEILL, Eric P.; 157 Ontario St., St. Catharines, Ont.; 30 Rockcliffe (res); Madras (India) '40; L.M. (Rotunda); D.Obst, R.C.O.G.; M.R.C.O.G.; ObstGyn; Tel. 684-6133.
O'NEILL, Hugh P.; St. Andrew's, N.B.; Columbia (U.S.A.) '02; Retired.
O'NEILL, James H.; Ste. 630, 5300 Cote-des-Neiges Rd., Montreal 26, P.Q.; 8 Kilburn Cres., Hampstead (res); McG '37; Paed; Paed. in Charge, Catherine Booth Hosp.; Assoc. Phys., Montreal Children's Hosp.; Phys., St. Mary's Hosp.; Lect. (Paed.), McGill U.; Tel. RE 3-2451.
O'NEILL, John D.; 385 Wellington St. W., Chatham, Ont.; 42 Robertson (res); Wes '46; ObstGyn, Staff, Chatham Gen. & St. Joseph's Hosp's.; Tel. 352-1340.
O'NEILL, John J.; 440 Victoria St., Kamloops, B.C.; McG'49; Tel. 372-7321.
O'NEILL, J. Patrick; Ste. 210, 955 Queen St. E., Sault Ste. Marie, Ont.; Tor'56; FRCS(C), Otol.
O'NEILL, Matthew J.; Box 250 Clarks Harbour, Shelburne Co., N.S.; Sheffield (Eng.) '54; M.R.C.S.(Eng.), L.R.C.P.(Lond.).
O'NEILL, Tim; Qns'56; Staff, Ontario Hosp., Kingston, Ont.
ONERHEIM, William O.; 4728 Ross St., Red Deer, Alta.; Wes'53; FRCS(C), GenSurg; Staff, Red Deer Gen. Hosp.; Tel. 346-2057.
ONHAUSER, Claire M.; 811-17th. St., West Vancouver, B.C.; Man'25; Tel. 922-1120.
ONHAUSER, Joseph B.; 1424 Main St. E., Hamilton, Ont.; 279 Graham Ave. S. (res); Man '25; Cons. Staff, St. Joseph's Hosp.; Dist. Coroner; Tel. 545-2465.
OOSTERHUIS, Jan; 678 Hale St., London, Ont.; 472 Blake St., Byron (res); Groningen (Neth.) '51; MCGP; Tel. 451-0720.
OPIE, Clarence H.; Lac du Bonnet, Man.; London (Eng.) '52.
OPIE, J. Anthony; 1871 King Street East, Hamilton, Ont.; Wes'62; AMCGP; Tel. 545-3003.
OPSETH, Melvin O.; Sask'59; Staff, Cudworth Clinic, Cudworth, Sask.
O'RAFFERTY, Edward F.; 149 Church Ave., Sussex, N.B.; Dublin (Ire.) '49; LM (Rotunda); DPH; Dist. M.O.H., King's, Queen's & Sunbury Co's; Tel. 1168.
ORAL, Orhan; Istanbul (Turk.)'56; Res., Toronto Western Hosp., Toronto, Ont.
ORANGE, Robert; 205 Wembley Dr., Sudbury, Ont.; Qns '32; F.A.C.A., F.I.C.S., Anaes; Chief Dept. of Anaes., Sudbury Gen. Hosp.; Cons. Anaes., St. Joseph's, Sudbury Memorial & Algoma San.; Tel. OS 3-3601.
ORBECK, Kenneth W., F/L; RCAF Station, Uplands, Ottawa, Ont.; Alb. '64.
ORCHARD, Basil C.; Tor'61; Psy; Staff, Ontario Hosp., Penetanguishene, Ont.
ORCHARD, C. Bryce; 327 Med. Arts Bldg., 750 Spadina Cres. E., Saskatoon, Sask.; 1038 University Dr. (res); Man '35; FRCS(C), GenSurg; Surg. Staff (Orth), University, City & St. Paul's Hosp's.; OrthCons., DVA & Sask. Physical Restoration Centre; Clin. Assoc. (Surg.), U. of Saskatchewan; Tel. 242-0264.
ORCHARD, Donald B.; 710 Seymour St., Vancouver 2, B.C.; Sask '62; Tel. MU 4-1511.
ORCHARD, John W.; 934 Oxford St. W., London, Ont.; Wes'58; MCGP; Tel. GE 9-9082.
ORCHARD, Stewart A.; 102 Medical Bldg., 217-3rd Ave. N., Saskatoon, Sask.; 670 Sask Cres. (res); Man '43; M.C.G.P.; Clin. Instr. (Surg.), Saskatchewan U.; Tel. 652-1020.
ORD, John V. R.; Ste. 636, Medical Arts Bldg., 170 St. George St., Toronto, Ont.; 334 Inglewood Dr. (res); Tor '38; F.R.C.S.(C), PlasSurg, GenSurg; Plas & Paed Surg., St. Joseph's Hosp.; Cons. (PlasSurg), Queensway Gen. & South Peel Hosp's.; Tel. WA 2-1383.
ORD, John W.; 102 Riverview Blvd., St. Catharines, Ont. (res); McG '16; Staff, Hotel-Dieu & St. Catharines Gen. Hosp's.
ORDMAN, Jack A.; 703 Quinn House, 9940-112th St., Edmonton, Alta.; Witwatersrand (S. Africa) '57; FRCS(C); OrthSurg.
O'REGAN, John B.; 113 Palisades, 23rd. St., Saskatoon, Sask.; Dublin (Ire.) '57; BAO; Psy; Staff, Dept. of Psy., University Hosp.; Staff, Med. Serv., City Hosp. & St. Paul Hosp.; Clin. Teach., U. of Saskatchewan; Tel. 244-1529.
O'REGAN, Kenneth R.; 175 Norwood Ave., Pte-Claire, Lachine, P.Q. (res); Dal '52; DPH; Staff, Dept. of National Health & Welfare, Internat. Airport, Dorval.
O'REILLY, F. Joan; Fort San, Sask.; Ireland '45.
O'REILLY, Frank L., Capt.; Nat. Defence Med. Centre, Ottawa 8, Ont.; Ott '64.
O'REILLY, Hugh; Fort San, Sask.; Ireland '40.
O'REILLY, James J.; 818 Douglas St., Victoria, B.C.; 1015 Gillespie Place (res); Qns '24; **Ophth Otol; Staff, St. Joseph's Hosp.; Court. Staff, Royal** Jubilee Hosp.; Retired.
O'REILLY, John A.; 3240 Bloor St. W., Toronto 18, Ont.; 63 Sir William's Lane, Islington (res); Tor '49; PhysMed & Rehab; Dir. PhysMed. & Rehab., Dept., Queensway Gen. Hosp.; Cons. (PhysMed) WCB Rehab. Centre, Downsview & to Ont. Crippled Children's Centre; Tel. 239-4942.
O'REILLY, Julia; 1010 Tower Gardens, 1100 Broadway Ave., Regina, Sask.; RCS (Ire.) '49; L.M. (Rotunda).
O'REILLY, K. Shirley (Ashmore); 63 Sir William's Lane, Islington, Ont.; Tor '49; Anaes; Staff (Anaes.), Queensway Gen. Hosp.; Tel. BE. 3-8374.
O'REILLY, P. O.; 1123 Connaught St., Moose Jaw, Sask. (res); Dublin (Ire.) '48; Psy; Dir. Dept. of Psy., Moose Jaw Union Hosp.; Cons. Psy., University Hosp.; Clin. Teach. (Psy.), U. of Saskatchewan; Tel. 692-1841.
ORFORD, Thomas J.; 500 Derrick Bldg., Regina, Sask.; Qns '32; F.C.C.P.; Reg. Sup. Saskatchewan Med. Serv. Directorate, Dept. of National Health & Welfare; Tel. 523-7615.
ORGAN, Leslie W.; Tor '57; Research, Banting Inst., U. of Toronto, Toronto 5, Ont.
ORIZAGA, Manuel; Dept. of Path., U. of Ottawa,, Ottawa, Ont.; Mexico'50; Path; Pathol., Ottawa Gen. Hosp.; Lect. (Path.), U. of Ottawa; Tel. CE 5-6751.
ORLANDO, Mario P.; 5300 Cote des Neiges Rd., Ste. 220, Montreal 26, P.Q.; 59 Thurlow Rd., **Hampstead (res); McG '35; F.I.C.S., GenSurg;** Surg., St. Mary's Hosp.; Chief Surg. & Dir. of Dept., Santa Cabrini Hosp.; Tel. RE 8-7900.
ORLAW, Richard G.; UBC'65; Res., Vancouver Gen. Hosp., Vancouver 9, B.C.
ORLICK, Eric G.; 169 Ontario St., St. Catharines, Ont.; Prague (Czech.)'38; IntMed; Chief, Dept. of Med., Hotel-Dieu Hosp.; Tel. MU 5-9512.
ORLICKI, Joseph; Warsaw (Germ.) '42; Jr. Int'n., Miller Bay Hosp., Prince Rupert, B.C.
ORMEROD, Brian; Medical Dental Clinic, Biggar, Sask.; Liverpool (Eng.)'62.
ORMEROD, Melville J.; 60 Russell St. W., Lindsay, Ont.; Tor '26; Retired.
ORMEROD, Richard O.; 302 Med. Bldg., 20-14th St. W., Prince Albert, Sask.; London (Eng.) '54; M.B., B.C.; MRCS (Eng.); LRCP (Lond.); Tel. 763-7435.
ORMISTON, A. W.; 309 Charlotte St., Sydney, N.S.; 61 Tain St. (res); Dal '42.
ORMSBY, Hugh L.; 51 Glenview Ave., Toronto 12, Ont.; Alb '37; FRCS(C); Ophth; Tel. HU 5-5243.

O'ROONEY, Patrick; 10075-156th St., Edmonton, Alta.; Liverpool (Eng.)'37; Tel. 484-2550.

OROSDY, Bela E.; '40; Jr. Int., St. Joseph's Hosp., Toronto 3, Ont.

O'ROURKE, Sharon O.; UBC'64; Res., Hamilton Gen. Hosp., Hamilton, Ont.

O'ROURKE, Stephen J.; Ste. 507, 215 Victoria St., Toronto 1, Ont.; 27 Denewood Cres., Don Mills (res); Ire '49; Anaes; Staff, St. Michael's Hosp.; Tel. HI 7-4556.

ORR, Alfred M.; Burris Clinic, Kamloops, B.C.; 633 Tunstall Cres. (res); Glasgow (Scot.) '57; MCGP; Staff, Royal Inland Hosp.; Tel. 372-3303.

ORR, Findlay R.; 250 Main St. E., Hamilton, Ont.; Edinburgh (Scot.) '56; MRCP (Edin.); FRCP(C); IntMed; Tel. 527-2711.

ORR, John; Fort San., Sask.; Man '16; IntMed (TB); Dir. of Med. Serv. & Gen. Supt., Fort San.; Retired.

ORR, Kenneth F.; 170 Main St., Sturgeon Falls, Ont. (res); Tor '51; Staff, St.-Jean-de-Brebeuf Hosp.; Tel. 753-2300.

ORR, Ross K.; 46 Ontario St., Thorold, Ont.; Wes '47; Staff, G.P. Dept., St. Catharines Gen. Hosp.; Assoc. Staff, Hotel Dieu Hosp.

ORR, Wilbert H.; Main & Erie St., Ridgetown, Ont.; 2 Church St. (res); Wes '37; M.C.G.P.; Dist. Coroner; Tel. 674-3381.

ORR, William J.; 196 King St., St. Catharines, Ont.; Tor '43; FRCS(C), GenSurg; Active Staff, St. Catharines Gen. Hosp.; Chief of Surg., Hotel-Dieu Hosp.; Cons. Staff, Niagara Pen. San.; Tel. 684-2521.

ORR, W. Leonard, G/C; Canadian Forces Base, St. Hubert, P.Q.; McG'40; DiagRad.

ORSER, W. Blair; 508 King Ave., Bathurst, N.B.; 370 Allison Cr. (res); Dal'54; MCGP; Active Staff, **Hotel-Dieu Hosp.; Tel. LI 6-4725.**

ORT, Reginald R.; 17 Bear St., Tillsonburg, Ont.; 19 Broadway (res); Wes'57; FRCS(C); GenSurg.; Tel. 842-2101.

ORTEZA, Josefina M.; '45; Staff, Regina Grey Nuns Hosp., Regina, Sask.; Retired.

ORTENBERG, Samuel L.; 1538 Sherbrooke St. W., Montreal, P.Q.; 166 Willowdale (res); McG '08; IntMed; Hon. Att. Phys., Montreal Gen., Jewish Gen. & Reddy Mem. Hosp's.; Med. Bd., Mt. Sinai San., Ste.- Agathe; Tel. 932-7414.

ORTIZ, Armando; 1466 Ouellette Ave., Windsor, Ont.; '50; Tel. 253-9884; Abroad.

ORTON, Thomas H.; 153 Simcoe St. N., Oshawa, **Ont.; 39 Grandview St. N. (res); Tor '43; Active** Staff, Oshawa Gen. Hosp.; Tel. 725-2312.

ORTVED, William E.; Ste. 7, 825 Coxwell Ave., Toronto 13, Ont.; Tor'41; FACS, FRCS(C), Urol; Att. Surg. (Urol.) & Chief Dept. of Urol., Toronto East Gen. Hosp.; Tel. HO 1-2722.

OSBALDESTON, George J.; 884 Concession St., Hamilton, Ont.; Tor '51; Tel. 383-1921.

OSBALDESTON, James B.; 2182 King St. E., Hamilton, Ont.; 682 North Shore E., Burlington (res); Tor '50; Chief of Staff, St. Joseph's Hosp.; M.O., Canadian Westinghouse Co.; Field Rep., Cdn. Council on Hosp. Accreditation; Tel. 544-8269.

OSBERG, Edwin A.; Ste. 20, 3195 Granville St., Vancouver 9, B.C.; Man'52; DiagRad.

OSBORN, N. J.; 17 Chesley Ave., Toronto 4, Ont. (res); Tor '54; Tel. CE 5-9903.

OSBORNE, Darrell F.; Irving Clinic, 74 W. Seymour St., Kamloops, B.C.; Man '45; FACS; ObstGyn; Chmn., Dept. of ObstGyn., Royal Inland Hosp & Chmn., Dept. of Continuous Educ., Royal Inland Hosp.; Tel. 372-5251.

OSBORNE, James C.; Ste 101, 1940 Lonsdale, North Vancouver, B.C.; 502 St. Andrews Rd., W. Vanc. (res); Man '46; FACS; FRCS(C); GenSurg; Cons. Staff & Chief Div. of Surg., Lionsgate Hosp.; Tel. YU 7-6940.

OSBORNE, John A.; 3340 Westmount Rd., West Vancouver, B.C. (res); Alb '48; FACC; IntMed; Dir. Dept. of Cardiol., Van. Gen. Hosp.; Clin. Instr. (Med.), U. of British Columbia; Tel. TR 6-3211.

OSBORNE, Ronald J.; RCS (Ire.) '58; FRCS (Eng.); GenSurg; Staff, Children's Hosp. & Wpg. Gen. Hosp., Winnipeg, Man.

O'SHAUGHNESSY, Brian D.; 65 Balsam St. S., Timmins, Ont.; 536 Eyre Blvd. (res); Sask'61; Tel. 264-1357.

OSHIRO, James H.; Coaldale, Alta.; Man '52.

OSITIS, Aleksandrs; Box 400 Medical Clinic, Rosetown, Sask.; Riga (Latvia)'37; MCGP; Med. Staff, Rosetown Union Hosp.

OSLER, Thomas R.; 607 Fairmont Med. Bldg., 750 W. Broadway, Vancouver 9, B.C.; McG '45; FRCS(C); GenSurg; Staff, Shaughnessy Hosp.; Vis. Staff, Vancouver Gen. Hosp.; Clin. Instr. (Surg.), U. of British Columbia; Tel. 872-5033.

OSMOLSKI, Edward; 11055 Pasteur, Montreal 12, P.Q.; '51; Anaes.; Tel. 331-2075.

OSOBA, David; Princess Margaret Hosp., 500 Sherbourne St., Toronto 5, Ont.; Alb'56; FRCP(C), IntMed.

OSTAFICHUK, Nicholas; 17 John St., Oshawa, Ont.; Innsbruck (Austria) '48; M.C.G.P.; Tel. 725-9921.

OSTAFICHUK, Robert N.; Tor '52; P.G. (Rad.), Port Arthur Gen. Hosp., Port Arthur, Ont.

OSTAPOVITCH, John J.; 3482 Park Ave., Montreal, P.Q.; 3425 Ridgewood Ave., Apt. 301 (res); Man '36; Gen. Surg (P.Q.); Sr. Surg., Queen Elizabeth Hosp.; Tel. AV 8-7302.

OSTAPOVITCH, William H.; Holland, Man.; Man '44; Health Officer, R.M. Victoria; Tel. 4.

OSTERREICHER, Marianne; 3261 Forest Hill, Montreal, P.Q. (res); Prague (Czech.) '34; F.A.C.C.P., Spec. (Chest Dis.), St. Anne's Hosp., **Ste. Anne de Bellevue; Tel. 453-5395.**

OSTIGUY, Gaston; 6525 Henri-Miro, Montreal 5, P.Q.; Mon'61; FRCP(C), IntMed; Pul. Dis. & TB (P.Q.); Staff, Hotel-Dieu Hosp.

OSTIGUY, Gerard; Clinique Medicale-de-Montreal, 8415 rue St.-Denis, Montreal 11, P.Q.; 7412 Baudelaire, St.-Leonard-de-Pt. Maurice (res); Mon '54; ObstGyn; ObstGyn & Cytol., Exfoliat., Hop.-Jean-Talon; Tel. DU 1-5311.

OSTIGUY, Jean P.; App. 1402, 135 est rue Sherbrooke, Montreal 18, P.Q.; Mon'54.

OSTIGUY, Lucien; 222 Melville, Westmount, P.Q. (res); Mon '29; Anaes (P.Q.); Ass't. Anaes., Hop du Sacre Coeur, Montreal; Tel. FE 4-1210.

OSTIGUY, Marcel; 3707 St. Hubert, Montreal, P.Q.; 515 Kenaston, Mont Royal (res); Mon '30; OphthOtol; Chief, Dept. of Ophth & O.R.L., Hop. St. Luc; Tel. UN 1-7261.

OSTIME, Maurice J.; Pine St., Woodbridge, Ont.; Cheltenham Ave. (res); London (Eng.) '54; MCGP; Tel. 288-0451.

OSTOLOSKY, Raymond J.; Baker Clinic, 10004-105th St., Edmonton, Alta.; Alb'53; MRCOG; FRCS(C); ObstGyn; Active Staff, Royal Alexandria Hosp.; Court. Staff, University Hosp.; Instr. (ObstGyn.), U. of Alberta; Tel. 424-2121.

OSTRANDER, Albert B.; Box 127, Invermere B.C.; Man '44; GenSurg.

OSTRO, Solomon; 611—1538 Sherbrooke St. W., Montreal, P.Q.; 5940 Decelles, Apt. 1 (res); Mon '40; Tel. WE 7-1959.

OSTRY, Edward I.; 304 Med. Centre, Calgary, Alta.; London (Eng.) '40; MRCS(Eng.), DPH. MRCOG, FACOG; ObstGyn; Cons., (ObstGyn), Calgary Gen. Hosp.; Tel. AM 3-8391.

OSTRY, Harry; 471 Wallace St., Nanaimo, B.C.; McG '30; Urol.; Tel. SK 4-2012.

O'SULLIVAN, Alvin B.; 69 Mohawk Rd. E., Hamilton, Ont.; Wes'64; Tel. 389-1525.

O'SULLIVAN, Jeremiah G.; 604 Med. Centre, 906 - 8th Ave. S.W., Calgary, Alta.; No. 6, National U. (Cork, Ire.)'47; M.A.O. (Ire.), M.R.C.O.G. (Lond); ObstGyn; Staff, Holy Cross, Calgary Gen. & Grace Hosp's.; Tel. AM 2-1395.

O'SULLIVAN, John; Macklin, Sask.; Nat. U. (Dublin, Ire.) '55.

O'SULLIVAN, John L.; Emo, Ont.; Cambridge (Eng.) '55; M.B., B.Chr.; Tel. 157.

O'SULLIVAN, Michael A.; Med. Arts Bldg., 5104-51st Ave., Ponoka, Alta.; National U. (Cork, Ire.) '45; M.B., B.Ch., LM (Rotunda); M.Ch., FRCS(I.); FRCS (Edin.); FICS; FRAMI; FRSM; GenSurg; Tel. 783-3306.

O'SULLIVAN, Patrick; Moose Jaw Clinic, 200 Scott Bldg., Moose Jaw, Sask.; Cork (Ire.) '55; Tel. 692-2373. Abroad.

O'SULLIVAN, Paul M.; One Medical Place, 20 Wynford Dr., Don Mills, Ont.; Tor '44; FRCP-(C), IntMed; Hd. Dir. of Gastroenterology, Sunnybrook Hosp.; Ass't. Prof. (Med.), U. of Toronto; Tel. 429-1146.

OSWALD, John M.; 1101 Avenue Rd., Toronto, Ont.; 340 St. Clements Ave. (res); Tor '34; Tel. HU 8-4976.

OSYANY, Bela G.; Med. Arts Bldg., 336 Kings Rd., Sydney, N.S.; Pecs. (Hung.) '32; Derm. (Budapest); Staff, City & St. Rita's Hosp's.; Tel. 562-6125.

OSZADSZKY, Sandor; Ste. 600, 5300 Cote des Neiges Rd., Montreal 26, P.Q. (res); Budapest (Hung.) '51; DiagRad; Staff, St. Mary's Hosp., Montreal; Tel. 735-3511.

OTKE, Edward; Medical Service, 83 Maple St., Winnipeg 4, Man.; Man'51.

O'TOOLE, George W.; 208 Scott St., Walkerton, Ont.; McG '30; Pres. Med. Staff, Bruce County Hosp.; Tel. 881-0970.

O'TOOLE, James W.; 633 Lodge Ave., Winnipeg, Man.; 284 Guilford St., St. James (res); Man '52; M.C.G.P.; Staff, Children's, Grace & Misericordia Hosp's.; Tel. SP 5-8311.

OTTON, Paul E.; 687 Pine Ave. W., Montreal 2, P.Q.; 72 Strathcona Dr., Twm Mt. Royal (res); Wes '54; FRCP(C), Anaes; Ass't. Anaes., Royal Victoria Hosp.; Lect. (Anaes), McGill U.; Tel. VI 2-1251, Loc. 530.

OUELLET, Bertrand; Sixth Ave., La Pocatiere, P.Q.; Lav '61; Tel. 856-2391.

OUELLET, Camille; 171 Hickson, St.-Lambert, P.Q. (Res.); Mon'56; Anaes; Staff, Hop. General Du Christ-Roi; Tel. 766-8511.

OUELLET, Gilles; 70 rue Ste.-Marie, Rimouski, P.Q.; Lav '50; MCGP; Med. Staff, Hop.-St.-Joseph; Tel. 723-7777.

OUELLET, Guy; C.P. 130, Forestville, P.Q.; Lav '51; Dist. Coroner.

OUELLET, J. R. Albert; 165-80th St. E., Charlesbourg, Quebec 8, P.Q.; 155-80th St. E. (res); Lav '35; Tel. 623-1621.

OUELLET, Laurent; 32 St. Philippe, Clermont, P.Q.; 35 Ave. Cartier (res); Lav '56; MCGP; Tel. GE 9-3947.

OUELLET, Paul G.; 2007-1st Ave., Quebec 3, P.Q.; Lav '51; Tel. 524-8318.

OUELLET, Treffle; Riviere Bleue, Cte Temiscouata, P.Q.; Lav '46.

OUELLET, Yvon; Lav'63; Res. Fell., Royal Victoria Hosp., Montreal, P.Q.

OUELLETTE, Andre; 264 rue de la Madore, Mont Laurier, P.Q.; Lav '55.

OUELLETTE, Edmond; Unite Sanitaire, St. Gervais, Co. Bellechasse, P.Q.; Lav '11; PH (P.Q.).

OUELETTE, Gilles G. O.; 3253 Beaubien Rosemont, P.Q.; Mon'62; Staff, Eastern Hosp. & Bellechasse Hosp.; Tel. 728-1549.

OUELLETTE, Nicol; Lav'63; Res., Hop. Hotel Dieu, Quebec 4, P.Q.

OUIMET, Arthur; Napierville, P.Q.; Mon '49.

OUIMET, Charles; Chambre 409, 3875 rue St-Urbain, Montreal, P.Q.; 15 Glencoe Westmt. (res); Mon'45; FICS; Gyn; Prof. (Gyn.), Hotel Dieu Hosp. & U. of Montreal; Tel. 844-7932.

OUIMET, Denise; Hop.-Notre-Dame, 1560 Sherbrooke E., Montreal, P.Q.; Mon '56; D&T Rad; Tel. LA 5-6363.

OUIMET, Marc; St. Jovite, P.Q.; Mon '47; Staff, St. Paul's Hosp. & Hotel Dieu, St. Jerome; Tel. 425-2741.

OULTON, John L.; 485 Southborough Dr., West Vancouver, B.C. (res); McG'50; Anaes.; Att. Staff, Vancouver Gen. & Children's Hosp's.; Lect. (Anaes.), U. of British Columbia; Tel. TR 6-3211.

OUTERBRIDGE, Eugene W.; McG '63; Res., Children's Hosp., Montreal 25, P.Q.

OUTERBRIDGE, Ralph E.; Ste. 500, 713 Columbia St., New Westminster, B.C.; Tor'36; FACS; FRCS(C); GenSurg, OrthSurg; Active Staff, Royal Columbian, St. Mary's, Chilliwack Gen., M.S.A., Abbotsford, Surrey Mem., Langley Mem., Maple Ridge Gen., Mission Mem. & Riverview Hosp's.; Teach. Staff, Royal Columbian & Riverview Hosp's.; Tel. LA 2-2332.

OUTRED, James T.; Markham Shopping Plaza, Markham, Ont.; 116 Lincoln Green Dr. (res); Guy's H. (London, Eng.) '59; DRCOG; Tel. 294-0531.

OVEREND, F. B.; 1514 Main St. E., Hamilton, Ont.; Tor '38; Tel. LI 4-5442.

OVERHOLT, Bluett M.; 221 Brant Ave., Brantford, Ont.; Tor '62; Staff, Brantford Gen. & St. Joseph's Hosp's.; Tel. 752-4752.

OWEN, Herbert F.; 2300 Tupper St., Montreal 25, P.Q.; 43 Brock Ave. N. (res); McG '42; D. Surg.; F.R.C.S.(C), GenSurg; Ass't. Surg., Montreal Children's Hosp.; Ass't. Prof. McGill U.; Tel. WE 7-8511.

OWEN, J. Grahame; 305 Sherin Dr., Oakville, Ont.; London (Eng.) '55; Staff, Oakville Trafalgar Mem. Hosp.; Tel. 827-1562.

OWEN-FLOOD, Joseph H.; 411 Tegler Bldg., Edmonton, Alta.; 10832—75th St. (res); R.C.P. & S. (Dublin, Ire.) '24; D.P.H., D.O.M.S.; Tel. GA 2-5411.

OWENS, Audrey L.; 321 Med. Arts Bldg., Winnipeg 1, Man.; Liverpool (Eng.) '49; Paed; Lect. (Paed.), U. of Manitoba; Tel. WH 2-0949.

OWENS, Margaret; 625 Medical Arts Bldg., Winnipeg, Man.; 291 Scotia St., West Kildonan (res); Tor '25; Tel. 942-4719.

OWERHEIM, William O.; Kroshus Bldgd., 4th Ave. W., Assiniboia, Sask.; 300-4th Ave. E. (res); Wes '53.

OXENHAM, Lawrence W.; London (Eng.)'46; MRCS; LRCP; Anaes., Oshawa Gen., Port Perry & Uxbridge Hosp's.; Tel. 3-2211.

OXLEY, P. L.; Hillsborough, N.B.; Dal '29.

OXORN, Harry; 680 Seaforth Medical Bldg., 3550 Cote des Neiges Rd., Montreal 25, P.Q.; Dal '45; FACS; FRCS(C); ObstGyn; Assoc. ObstGyn., Royal Victoria Hosp.; Jr. Ass't. ObstGyn., Montreal Gen. Hosp.; Lect., McGill U.; Tel. 937-2376.

OZCAN, Erdogan; 432 Water St., Chatham, N.B.; Istanbul (Turk.)'58.

OZERE, Rudolph L.; 11 Scarlet Rd., Rockingham, N.S., Ott '53; Paed; Teaching, Children's Hosp., Halifax; Tel. 422-8441.

OZKAN, Adnan; 437 Jarvis St., Apt. 405, Toronto, Ont.; Ankara (Turk.)'57; Path.

OZMAN Ihsan M.; Istanbul (Turk.) '46; Staff (Psy.), Brandon Mental Hosp., Brandon, Man. Abroad.

OZVEGY, Frank L.; Szeged (Hung.) '44; DiagRad; TB (Budapest); Staff, Yarmouth Hosp., P.O. Box 255, Yarmouth, N.S.; Tel. 742-3541.

PAAS, Pritt; Tartu-Dorpat U. (Estonia) '29; Res., Ontario Hosp., Penetanguishene, Ont.

PAASUKE, Rein T.; Box 910, Olds, Alta.; McG'65.

PABST, Henry F.; Alb '62; Res., Children's Hosp., Montreal 26, P.Q.

PACE, A. Murray; Medical Arts Bldg., 539 Cassells St., North Bay, Ont.; 639 Reynolds St. (res); Tor '55; ObstGyn; Ass't. Chief (Obst Gyn), North Bay Civic & St. Joseph's Hosp's.; Tel. 472-7038.

PACE, F. Cecil; Apt. 1, 412 Sparks St., Ottawa 4, Ont.; Man '28; Med. Cons., Spec. Weapons Sec., Emerg. Health Serv., Dept. of Natl. Health & Welfare; Tel. CE 2-8211.

PACE-FLORIDA, Albert; Malta '58; FRCP(C), Anaes; Staff, Neurol. Inst., Montreal 2, P.Q.

PACE, Graham C.; Woodland Med. Clinic, 110 Woodlawn Rd., Dartmouth, N.S.; Dal '57; AMCGP; Tel. 469-1590.

PACE, William E.; 205 Medical-Dental Bldg, 450 Central Ave., London, Ont.; 321 Victoria St. (res); Wes '41; M.Sc. (Biochem.), F.R.C.P.(C), DermSyph; Staff (Derm. Syph.), Victoria & Westminster Hosp's.; & Beck Mem. San.; Clin. Lect., U. of Western Ont.; Tel. 432-4241.

PACEVICIUS, Anthony; 280 Roncesvalles Ave., Toronto 3, Ont.; Kaunas (Lith.) '42; Bonn (Germ.) '47; MCGP; Tel. LE 4-4778.

PACEVICIUS, Stanislovas; 25 Cedarcrest Dr., Islington, Ont.; Kaunas (Lithuania) '41; F.C.-C.P.; Staff, Workmen's Comp Bd.

PACIS, Andresito B.; Manila Central (Philipp.) '62; Jr. Int., Hotel-Dieu-St-Joseph, Bathurst, N.B.

PACKHAM, John S.; 325 Victoria Ave., Chatham, Ont.; Qns '49.

PADDELL, Harry W.; 309 Princess Ave., Apt. 208, London, Ont. (res); Wayne (U.S.A.) '08; Retired.

PADDON, William A.; Grenfell Mission, Northwest River, Labrador, Nfld.; New York State (Brooklyn, U.S.A.) '40; DPH; MCGP; M.O. I/C Grenfell Mission & Supt. North West River Hosp.; Tel. 946-0241.

PADWICK, Peter H.; 1940 Lonsdale Ave., North Vancouver, B.C.; 4344 Quinton Pl. (res); London U. (Eng.) '51; MRCS, LRCP; Paed; Att'd. Staff, Van. Gen. & Cons. Staff, Lion's Gate Hosp's.; Lect., U. of British Columbia; Tel. YU 7-4613.

PAETKAU, Eric J.; Box 10 Sechelt B.C.; Sask '57; Tel. 885-2257.

PAEZ, Pedro N.; Fitness Research Unit, University of Alta., Edmonton, Alta.; Cordoba Nat. U. (Argentina)'51.

PAGACZ, Alexis; Mon '64; Res., Hop. Notre-Dame, Montreal, P.Q.

PAGAN, Robert T.; 113-05 104th St., Grande Prairie, Alta.; St. Bartholomew's Hosp. (London, Eng.) '54; M.B., B.S., MRCS; LRCP; DPH; M.O.H., Grande Prairie Health Unit; Tel. 532-4441.

PAGE, Arthur A.; 12245 Grenet, Montreal 9, P.Q.; Mon'55; FRCS(C), GenSurg; DABS; FACS; Staff, Hop. du Sacre-Coeur.

PAGE, Denis; Ott'65; Res., Ottawa General Hosp., Ottawa 2, Ont.

PAGE, E. Lawrence; 85 Blake St., Hamilton, Ont.; Qns '18; IntMed; Med. Dir., St. Peter's Infirmatory; Tel. LI 4-1229.

PAGE, G. Benson, Sg. Lcdr; No. 1 CBMU, CFPO 5050, Cdn. Armed Forces, Overseas; Tor '52; Otol. Abroad.

PAGE, Graham C.; 114 Tacoma Dr., Westphal, Halifax Co., N.S.; Dal '57.

PAGE, Guy; Thurso, Co. Papineau, P.Q.; Mon '52; AMCGP.

PAGE, John; Med. Clinic, 224 King St. E., Brockville, Ont.; 14 Weston Cr. (res); Qns '50; FACP; IntMed; Cons. IntMed., Ontario Hosp.; Staff. Brockville Gen. & St. Vincent de Paul Hosp's.; Clin. Ass't., Queen's U.; Tel. DI 2-4477.

PAGE, J. Ulric; 500 Blvd. St. Joseph E., Montreal, P.Q.; Mon '30; Cons. (Medico-Legal), W.C.B.; Tel. LA 1-4457.

PAGE, L. Adrien; 170 King E., Sherbrooke, P.Q.; 267 Blvd. Queen N. (res); Mon '43; Paed (P.Q.); Tel. 569-1737.

PAGE, Leopold; 7227 St. Denis, Montreal, P.Q.; Mon '43; Paed (P.Q.), Staff (Paed.), Hop. Ste. Justine; Tel. RE 1-4931.

PAGE, Michael A.; Mount Denis Med. Group 98 Guestville Ave., Toronto 7, Ont.; Leeds (Eng.) '56; AMCGP; Sr. Active Staff, Humber Mem. Hosp., Weston; Tel. RO 3-1171.

PAGE, P. Renauld; Mon '64; Res., Hop. Maisonneuve, Montreal, P.Q.; Abroad.

PAGE, Robert; 1500 18e rue, Quebec 3, P.Q.; Lav '48; FACS; FRCS (C), OrthSurg; MCH (Orth.) (Liverpool); OrthSurg., Hop. Enfant Jesus; Chief of Serv., Hop. Christ Roi; Ass't. Surg., Hop. Ste-Foy.

PAGE, Roger H.; UBC '59; Staff, R. W. Large Mem. Hosp., Campbell Island P.O., Bella Bella, B.C.; Tel. 287-6221.

PAGE, William E.; Med. Centre, Cobourg, Ont.; 49 Abbott Blvd. (res); Tor '53; MCGP; Tel. FR 2-5494.

PAGER, Antonio; St. Hermas, P.Q.; Mon '22; IntMed.

PAGER, Robert; Ste. 220, 30 est boul. St-Joseph, Montreal 14, P.Q.; Mon'47; Ophth; Dir. Glaucoma Clin., Hop. Maisonneuve; Prof. Ophth., I/C Basic Science Courses (Ophth) affil., U. of Montreal; Tel. 845-0274.

PAGET, Jacques P.; 153 Bellevue St., Edmundston, N.B. (res); Lille (Fr.) '49; Path; Dir. of Edmundston Reg. Lab., N.B. Dept. of Health; Tel. 735-8484.

PAHAPILL, Raimund; Ste. 202, 1849 Yonge St., Toronto 7, Ont.; 336 Glen Park Ave., Tor 19 (res); Tor '60; Tel. 924-7455.

PAIDRE, Juhan; Newburgh, Ont.; Heidelberg (Germ.)'47; Active Staff, Lennox & Addington County Gen. Hosp.; Courtesy Staff, Kingston Gen. & Hotel Dieu Hosp's., Kingston; Belleville Gen. Hosp., Belleville; Tel. 378-2613.

PAIEMENT, Bernard; 73 Manuel Dr., Dollard-des-Ormeaux, St-Genevieve, P.Q.; Lav '54; Anaes; Staff, Hop. Maisonneuve, Montreal; Tel. 254-8341.

PAIEMENT, Jacqueline M.; Ott'57; Res., Jewish Gen. Hosp., Montreal 26, P.Q.

PAIEMENT, J. Germain; 330 Montreal Rd., Cornwall, Ont.; Mon '35.

PAIEMENT, Lionel; 101A Main, Rouyn, P.Q.; 71 Richelieu, Noranda (res); Mon '47; Orth (P.Q.); Staff, Orth.; Hop. Youville, Noranda; Con. Orth, Hop. St. Francois, La Sarre, Hop. St. Sauveur, Val d'Or, San. St. Jeann, Macamic; Tel. 762-1945.

PAIEMENT, Lucien; 1919 Ave. Paradis, Vimont, Ville De Laval, P.Q.; Mon'58.

PAIEMENT, P. A.; 4234 Adam St., Montreal, P.Q.; Lav '06; Tel. CL 4-1571.

PAIEMENT, Raymond; 287 Montreal Rd., Ottawa, Ont.; 630 Malartic (res); Ott '52; Orth-Surg.; Tel. 746-6745.

PAIGE, Bruce F.; 708 Fairmont Med. Bldg., 750 W. Broadway, Vancouver 9, B.C.; 5726 Angus Dr., Van. 13 (res); Sydney (Aust.) '45; IntMed; Att'd. Staff, Van. Gen. Hosp.; Clin. Instr. (Med.), U. of British Columbia; Tel. 872-1207.

PAIKEN, Harry; 250 Hughson St. N.; Hamilton, Ont.; Tor '30; Chm., Bd. of Health, Hamilton; Tel. JA 2-6212.

PAILLE, George A.; 3993 W. 10th Ave., Vancouver, B.C. (res); Man '16; Retired.

PAILLE, J. B. J. Guy.; 308 rue Celanese, Drummondville, P.Q.; Lav '56; F.R.C.S.(C), GenSurg; Staff, Hop.-Ste.-Croix; Tel. GR 8-3700.

PAIN, Albert M.; 706 Med. Arts Bldg., Hamilton, Ont.; Wes'37; ObstGyn; Court. Staff, Joseph Brant Hosp., Burlington; Court. Staff, Chedoke Gen. Hosp., Hamilton & West Lincoln Mem. Hosp., Grimsby; Court. Staff, St. Joseph's & Henderson Gen. Hosp's.

PAINCHAUD, Charles A.; 1211 Delaune, Sillery, P.Q. (res); Lav '28; Haem (P.Q.); Dip. Serol. (Paris); Bact; Hd. of Lab., Hop.-St.-Michel-Archange; Clin., Roy-Rousseau; Assoc. Prof., Laval U.; Tel. 663-3571.

PAINCHAUD, Lionel A.; Box 98, Montmartre, Sask.; Sask '61.

PAINCHAUD-MARCOUX, Claude; Le Centre-Medico-Social Pour Enfants, Inc., 898 rue Richelieu, Quebec 4, P.Q.; Lav '61; Psy.

PAINCHAUD, Paul; 902 Rue St. Jean, Quebec, P.Q.; 124 Murray (res); Lav '26; F.R.C.S.(C) Otol; Chief, Otol. Serv., Hotel-Dieu Hosp.; Prof. Clin. Otol., Laval U.; Tel. 522-1675.

PAINE, Alfred L.; Ninette, Man. (res); Man '29; ThorSurg; Med. Supt., Manitoba Sanatorium; Tel. 3322.

PAINE, David L.; Ste. 204, 1121 Yates St., Victoria, B.C.; 1164 St. Patrick St. (res); London (Eng.) '49; FRCS (Edin.); DO (Eng.); Ophth; Active Staff, Royal Jubilee & Court. Staff, St. Joseph's Hosp's.; Tel. 383-4425.

PAINE, Donald; Med. Arts Bldg., 539 Cassells St., North Bay, Ont.; R.R. No. 3 (res); Guy's H. (London, Eng.) '44; FRCS(Eng.), FACS, FRCS(C), GenSurg; Urol; Chief of Urol., St. Joseph's Gen. Hosp.; Cons. Urol., Mattawa Gen., New Liskeard Hosp. & St.-Jean-de-Breboeuf, Sturgeon Falls; Tel. 472-6950.

PAINE, George C.; Stillwater, B.C.; McG '16.

PAINE, Kenneth W.; 1703 Grosvenor Ave., Saskatoon, Sask. (res); London (Eng.) '44; LRCP; MRCS; FRCS (Eng.), FRCS(C), NeurSurg; Chief (NeurSurg), University Hosp.; Neur Surg., Yorkton, City & St. Paul Hosp's.; Prof. of Surg., U. of Saskatchewan; Tel. 242-7641.

PAINE, R. Joseph; 925 W. Georgia St., Vancouver 1, B.C., 1930 Leyland St. (res); McG '40; M.S.; Ophth; Clin. Instr., Vancouver Gen. Hosp.; Tel. MU 5-9436.

PAINE, William A.; Falher, Alta.; Dublin (Ire.) '43; Staff, Sacred Heart Hospital, MacLennan, Alta.; Tel. 29.

PAJE, Alfredo O.; Manilla (Philipp.)'39; GenSurg; Staff, Murdochville Hosp., Murdochville, P.Q.
PAJKOVICH, A. P.; Tor'65; Jr. Int., St. Michael's Hosp., Toronto 2, Ont.
PAKES, Eddy H.; Alb'61; Psy; Staff, Montreal Children's Hosp., Montreal, P.Q.; Staff, Jewish Gen. Hosp. & Teach. Staff, McGill U.; Tel. 733-9141.
PAKIAM, Anthony; Cambridge (Eng.)'63; Staff, Dept. of Surg., U. of Manitoba, Winnipeg 3, Man.
PAKOZDY, Stephen P.; 57 Division St., Welland, Ont.; 15 Elgin st. E. (res); Qns '39; M.C.G.P.; Tel. 732-5233.
PALACIO, Angelo; Manilla (Philipp.)'57; Res., **Laurentian Chest Hosp., Ste Agathe des Monts, P.Q.**
PALACIOS, Edward; Raxlen Clinic, 500 Parliament St., Toronto 5, Ont.; Madrid (Spain) '54; Tel. WA 5-4381.
PALANEK, Frank G.; 147 Thames St., Chatham, Ont.; 321 Victoria Ave. (res); Qns '43; Staff, St. Joseph, & Public Gen. Hosp's. Coroner Kent County; Tel. 352-3435.
PALARDY, Jacques; St. Michel, Cte. Napierreville, P.Q.; Mon'65.
PALARDY, Roland; 2767 rue Rouen, Motreal 24, P.Q.; Mon '61; Tel. LA 3-3621.
PALAYEW, Max J.; 6000 Cote des Neiges Rd., Montreal, P.Q.; Montpellier (France)'56; FRCP(C), DiagRad; Assoc. Rad., Jewish Gen. Hosp.; Tel. 735-3771.
PALERME, Gaston R.; 91 ouest Beaumont, St Bruno Montarville, P.Q.; Mon'58; FRCS(C), Obst-Gyn.
PALETZ, Solly G.; 7505-118th St., Edmonton, Alta.; Edinburgh (Scot.) '39; FACA; Anaes; Staff, Leduc, Stony Plain, Devon Municipal, Aberhart San., Oliver Mental Inst. & University Hosp's.; Tel. 439-5911.
PALIJ, Boris; 288 St. Clair Ave. W., Toronto 7, Ont.; 92 Arlington Ave. (res); **Helsinki (Finland) '47; Staff (OPD), St. Michael's Hosp.; Tel. 925-9052.**
PALKO, P. Dale; 335 Medical Arts Bldg., 750 Spadina Cres. E., Saskatoon, Sask.; Sask'60; Staff, St. Paul's & City Hosp's.; Tel. 242-1208.
PALMER, Bernard K.; Ste. 103, 77 Upper Middle Rd., Cooksville, Ont.; Bristol (Eng.)'55; D.Obst RCOG.
PALMER, Cecil F.; 306 Medical Bldg., Prince Albert, Sask.; London (Eng.)'58.
PALMER, Geoffrey R. C.; 439 Mayor Magrath Dr., Lethbridge, Alta.; London (Eng.)'34; MRCS; DA; MFARCS; **Staff, St. Michael's & Municipal** Hosp's.; Dir., **Barons-Eureka Health Unit**, Coaldale; Tel. 327-3230.
PALMER, James D. K.; 243 Highway 53, Ancaster, Ont.; London (Eng.)'48; M.B., B.S., M.D. (London.); D. PhysMed; PhysMed & Rehab; Cons. Physiatrist, Hamilton Civic Hosp.; Abroad.
PALMER, J. Eric; Box 548, 496 Adelaide St., Woodstock, Ont.; 813 Bayswater St. (res); Wes '57; Tel. 539-1152.
PALMER, J. Gordon; 53 Reidmount, Agincourt, Ont. (res); Tor '39; Admin. Med. Officer, Phys, Serv. Inc.; Tel. 487-3311.
PALMER, John A.; 530 Med. Arts Bldg., 170 St. George St., Toronto 5, Ont.; **105 Strathhallan Blvd. (res); Tor '48; FACS, FRCS(C), GenSurg; Surg. Staff, Toronto Gen. Hosp.; Cons. Surg., Princess Margaret Hosp.; Clin. Teach. (Surg.),** U. of Toronto; Tel. WA 1-6765.
PALMER, John D.; 1414 Drummond St., Montreal, P.Q.; 295 Vivian Ave. (res); McG '41; D.A.B.S., F.A.C.S., F.R.C.S.(C), GenSurg; Assoc. Surg., Montreal Gen. & Reddy Mem. Hosp's.; Cons. Surg., Queen Mary Vet's. Hosp.; Ass't. Prof. (Surg.), McGill U.; Tel. AV 8-8744.
PALMER, L. L.; Department of National Health & Welfare, c/o Regional Superintendent, European Region. Abroad.
PALMER, Luben (Panojotov); 1369 Barton St. E., Hamilton, Ont.; Tel. LI 5-9961.
PALMER, Marven F.; Fredericton Med. Clinic, 206 Rookwood Ave., Fredericton, N.B.; 161 Winslow St. (res); McG '54; FACS; GenSurg; Surg., Victoria Public Hosp.; Tel. 475-7701.
PALMER, Mary; '34; Staff, Ontario Hosp., Brockville, Ont.: Tel. DI 5-1461.
PALMER, R. Bruce; Wes'41; Psy; MCGP; Staff, Ontario Hosp., London, Ont.; Tel. 455-5110.
PALMER, Russell A.; 925 W. Georgia St., Vancouver, B.C.; 1826 King Edward Ave. W. (res); McG '31; MRCP(Edin.) FACP, FRCP) (Edin.), FRCP(C), IntMed; Phys., Van. Gen. Hosp.; Cons. (Med.) BC Cancer Inst.; Hon. Cons., Shaughnessy DVA Hosp.; Ass't. Clin. Prof. (Med.), U. of British Columbia; MU 4-1720.
PALMER, Wilfred H.; 337 Roslyn Ave., Westmount, Montreal 6, P.Q. (res); McG '54; FR-CP(C), IntMed (Cardiol.); Ass't. Phys., Royal Victoria Hosp.; Ass't. Prof. Med., McGill U.; Tel. VI 2-1251.
PALOC, S. Geza; Ste 303, 76 Avenue Rd., Toronto 5, Ont.; Queen Elizabeth U. (Hung.) '35; Derm.; Tel. 921-3701.
PALOSCHI, Gian B.; Ste. 201, 10 Montreal St., Kingston, Ont.; Italy'55; FRCS(C); Gen.Surg.
PALTER, Harry; Tor '61; Res., Toronto Western Hosp., Toronto 2B, Ont.
PALTIEL, R. Naomi; (see Lowi, R. Naomi).
PAMENTER, Edward J.; 18 Centre St., Thornhill, Ont.; Tor '62; AMCGP; Tel. 889-3634.
PAMIR, Tolon A.; Ankara (Turkey) '55; Staff, Provincial Hosp., Campbellton, N.B.
PAMUKOFF, Maria; 62 Cartier, Roxboro, P.Q.; Innsbruck (Austria) '50; Paed (P.Q.); Tel. 684-2759.
PAMUKOFF, Nicola; 669 Barton St. E., Hamilton, Ont.; Innsbruck Austria) '50; Tel. 549-0423.
PAN, Alexander; 243 Marion St., Winnipeg 6, Man.; Man'58; FRCP(C); IntMed; Assoc. Staff, St. Boniface Gen. Hosp.; Clin. Instr. (Med), Univ. of Man.; Tel. 947-1581.
PAN, Peter; 1312 Valley Dr., Kenora, Ont.; Man'58; Path; Dir. of Labs., Kenora Gen. Hosp., St. Joseph's Hosp. & La Verendrye Hosp., Fort Frances; Tel. HO 8-9861.
PAN, Wen M.; National U. (Taiwan)'59; Staff, Indian Hospital, Hodgson, Man.
PANABAKER, J. Paul; 116 Mountain View Rd. S., Georgetown, Ont.; Tor'60; Tel. 877-3661.
PANACCIO, Lucien; 249 Chemin Ste Catherine, Montreal 8, P.Q.; Mon'39; Psy (P.Q.).
PANACCIO, Nicolas; Mon'65; Sr. Int., Hop Hotel-Dieu, Montreal 18, P.Q.; Abroad.
PANACCIO, Victor; 100 St. Joseph St. W., Montreal, P.Q.; Mon '43; DermSyph; Hd. (Dept. of Derm.), Hop.-Hotel-Dieu; Ass't. Prof., U. of Montreal; Tel. CR 9-7495.
PANCARO, Luigi; 96 Larch, Sudbury, Ont.; Rome **(Italy) '25; FAGS; FICA; GenSurg; Cons., St. Joseph's Hosp.; Tel. OS 3-7623.**
PANCHAM, S. R.; Tor '64; Res., Humber Mem. Hosp., 200 Church St., Weston, Ont.
PANCARO, Luigia M.; Jr.; 96 Larch St., Sudbury, Ont.; 296 Morris St. (res); Rome (Italy) '60; Tel. OS 3-7623.
PANEGOS, Ezio R.; Bologna (Italy) '60; Jr. Intn., Princess Margaret Hosp., Toronto 5, Ont.
PANET-RAYMOND, Jean A.; 64 ave. Nelson, **Montreal 8, P.Q.; Mon '30; NeurPsy;** NeurSurg; **Chief of Neur. & Electroen., St.-Jean-de-Dieu Hosp.**
PANGALOS, Constantine; Nat. U. (Greece) '53; DiagRad; Staff, Toronto East Gen. Hosp., Toronto, Ont.; Tel. 461-8272.
PANIKKAR, Mohan K.; Northern Health Unit, **Flin-Flon, Man.; London (Eng.) '51; MRCS(Eng.); LRCP(Lond.); DTM&H;** DPH(Tor.); **Tel. 687-3459.**
PANISSET, Alain; Mon'65; Sr. Int., Hop Notre-Dame, Montreal 24, P.Q.
PANKHURST, Ruth D.; 4128-126th St., Edmonton, Alta. (res); McG '60; Pt-time U. of Alberta Infirmary.
PANNEL, Raymond W.; 402 Main St., Melfort, **Sask.; 613 Crawford Ave. E. (res); MCGP**; Man '55; Tel. 752-2303.
PANNETON, Andre; 825 Belvedere, Sherbrooke, P.Q.; 444 Vimy (res); Mon '50; Paed; Staff, Hotel-Dieu, Sherbrooke, **P.Q.; Tel. LO 9-2551.**
PANNETON, Lucie —see— **PETROVITCH-PANNETON, Leposova.**

PANNETON, Michel; 43 Gendron St., Hull, P.Q. (res); Mon'57; AMCGP; Med. Cons., Employee Health Serv., Ottawa Gen. Hosp.; Med. Dir., Metropolitan Life Ins. Co., Ottawa 4, Ont.; Tel. 232-2631.

PANOJOTOV, Luben; (See Palmer)

PANTALONY, Dominic; Wes'58; Path; Staff, Dept. of Hematology, Toronto Gen. Hosp., Toronto 2, Ont.

PANTON, Frances I.; 340 Christina St. N., Sarnia, Ont.; 1607 Lakeshore Rd., R.R. 3 (res); King's College (Durham, Eng.) '45; MCGP; Active Staff, Sarnia Gen. & St. Joseph's Hosp's.; MOH Plympton Twp.; Tel. DI 4-1743.

PANTON, William D.; 1394 Kingsway, Vancouver, B.C.; 4375 Locarno Cres. (res); McG '47; MCGP; Gaol Phys., Van. City Police; Tel. TR 6-6121.

PANWAR, Krishnasingh M.; 400 Maria St., Sarnia, Ont.; **Bombay (India) '55; DA; FACA; Anaes;** Chief, Dept. of Anaes., St. Joseph's Hosp.; Tel. 344-9806.

PAPADOPOULOS, Dennis; Brooks, Alta.; Athens (Greece) '53; IntMed.

PAPAGEORGES, Constant J. S.; 599 rue Malouin, Sherbrooke, P.Q.; Mon'53; Phys Med & Rehab.

PAPAGEORGIOU, Doreen O.; (see Joubert, Doreen O.).

PAPALAZARDU, Lazarus; see Lazarou, U. C.; Lazaros, P.

PAPAMATHEAKI-LESTER, Evangelie; (see LESTER, Evangelie P.)

PAPICH, Dragutin F.; Ste 1015, Medical Arts **Bldg., 1538 Sherbrooke St. W., Montreal 25, P.Q.; McG '54; GenSurg; Tel. WE 2-8898.**

PAPILLION, Robert; 1966 Sherbrooke St. E., Montreal, P.Q.; Mon '49; Tel. LA 1-3967.

PAPINEAU, Louis; 30 est Boul. St. Joseph, Montreal 14, P.Q.; Mon'52; FRCS(C), GenSurg; OrthSurg; Staff, Hop.-Notre-Dame, Tel. 526-3783.

PAPINEAU, Marc; 456 rue Principale, Lachute, P.Q.; 452 rue Principale (res); Lav '41; M.C.G.P.; Phys. Pres. Med. Staff, Hop., Province; Med. Dir., Hop.-Notre-Dame-du-Sourire; Tel. LO 2-2266.

PAPP-KOVACS, Eleonora I.; Group Health Centre, 240 McNabb St., Sault Ste. Marie, Ont.; Debrecen (Hung.)'49; Paed.

PAPP, Gabor; 1751 Parent Ave., Windsor, Ont.; Debrecen (Hung.) '26; MCGP; Tel. 256-4477.

PAPP, Otto A.; 444 Beaconsfield, Beaupaire, Ste-Anne-de-Bellevue, P.Q.; Debrecen (Hung.)'52; D.IntMed(McG); Cardiol (P.Q.); Tel. 453-1481.

PAPPALARDO, Carlos; 5366 Cumberland, Montreal, P.Q.; Argentina (S.A.) '53; FRCS(C), PlasSurg; Tel. VI 5-1650.

PAPPELBAUM, Stanley J.; UBC'63; Res., Children's Hosp., Montreal 25, P.Q.

PAPRICA, Gordon M.; Qns '63; Res., Kingston Gen. Hosp., Kingston, Ont.

PAPROSKI, Kenneth R.; 10022-103rd St., Edmonton. Alta.; 42 Valleyview Cr. (res); Alb '56; MCGP; Teach. Preceptor (Dept. of Social & Prev-Med.), U. of Alberta; Alternate Chief (G.P.) Misericordia Hosp.; Tel. 429-3781.

PAPSIN, Frederick R.; Suite 353, East Wing, Toronto Western Hospital, Toronto 2B, Ont.; Tor'58; FRCS(C); ObstGyn; Attending Staff, Toronto Western Hospital; Clin. Teacher, Univ. of Toronto; Tel. 366-3218.

PAQUET, Alphonse E.; 890 Decarie Blvd., St-Laurent, Montreal 9, P.Q.; Mon '48; Paed; Dir., O.P.D., Hop. Ste-Justine; Tel. 744-4747.

PAQUET, Andre; 750 Ouest St. Vallier, Quebec 8, P.Q.; Lav'65.

PAQUET, Berchmans; 1069 Boul. du Jardin, Orsainville, P.Q.; Lav'31; P.H.(P.Q.); IntMed (P.Q.); Hd. Dept. of Contg. Dis., Civic Hosp.; Prof., Laval U.; Tel. 527-6242.

PAQUET, Bernard; 960 boul. Ste-Croix, Ville St. Laurent, Montreal 9, P.Q.; Mon '59; Staff, Hop. Notre-Dame-de l'Esperance; Vis. Staff (ObstGyn.), Hop. du Sacre-Coeur; Tel. 747-3501.

PAQUET, Edmond; Lav '50; FCCP, FRCP(C), IntMed; Hd. (Dept. of Med.), Hop.-St.-Ambroise, Loretteville, P.Q.; Tel. 842-3651.

PAQUET, Eleonore; Lav'63; Res., Hop. Hotel-Dieu, Quebec 4, P.Q.

PAQUET, J. Aime; 16-23 eme rue St. Georges, Cte Beauce, P.Q.; Lav '57.

PAQUET, Jean; 1666 Montcalm, Montreal 24, P.Q.; Mon '56; Tel. 525-4257.

PAQUET, Jean-Pierre, 1500-18eme rue, Quebec 3, P.Q.; Lav'59; Urol.; Tel. 653-4734.

PAQUET, Joseph E.; 6986 Louis Hemon, Montreal, P.Q.; Mon '31; Cons., Hop. Hotel-Dieu; Tel. VI 4-0161.

PAQUET, Leo P.; Lav '60; Res., Hop. Hotel-Dieu, Montreal 18, P.Q.

PAQUET, Pierre P.; 341A St. Dominique, Jonquiere, P.Q.; Lav'54; Anaes.

PAQUET, Romuald; 1216-6th St., Val-d'Or, P.Q.; 847 ave. Chapais (res); Lav '46; Tel. 824-3219.

PAQUET, Ronald; Ott'65; Res., Ottawa Gen. Hosp., Ottawa 2, Ont.

PAQUETTE, Cyrille; 3871 Belanger E., Montreal, P.Q.; Lav'53; FRCS(C), GenSurg; Staff Surg., Hop.-Jean-Talon; Tel. 729-5231.

PAQUETTE, Guy; 5078 rue Ste. Catherine E., Montreal 4, P.Q.; Mon '60; Tel. CL 6-9851.

PAQUETTE, J. A.; Mont Laurier, P.Q.; Lav '19; Prov. Dept. Health.

PAQUETTE, Jean C.; Ferme Neuve, P.Q.; Lav '53; Dist. Coroner.

PAQUIN, Antoine; App. 56, 445 ouest boul. St. Joseph, Montreal 8, P.Q.; Mon'54; DPH; Staff, Mtl. Dept. of Health.

PAQUIN, Charles A.; 2909 rue Masson, Montreal 36, P.Q.; Mon'37; MCGP; Tel. RA 7-5006.

PAQUIN, Francois; 278 St. Joseph, Terrebonne, **P.Q.; 132 St. Louis (res); Mon '39; Tel. 666-3762.**

PAQUIN, Gilles; 8333 Blvd. Gouin E., Riviere-des-Prairies, P.Q.; Mon '56.

PAQUIN, Hector; 25 du Chalet, Ville-de-St. Pierre, Lachine, P.Q.; Lav '40; GenSurg (P.Q.).

PAQUIN, J. Gilles; Mon'62; Sr. Int., Hop. Hotel-Dieu, Montreal 18, P.Q.

PAQUIN, Jean Louis; St. Anne de Bellevue, P.Q.; Mon '45; Tel. 453-4428.

PAQUIN, J. Jacques; 933 Royale, Trois Rivieres, P.Q.; 2141 Blvd. St. Louis (res); Lav '37; GenSurg (P.Q.). Tel. FR 4-9141.

PAQUIN, Michel, F/L; Box 60, RCAF Station, Chatham, N.B.; Mon'65.

PAQUIN, Pierre; Centre d'Achats, St. Hilaire, P.Q.; Lav'60.

PAQUIN, Pierre Paul; Les Cedres, Co. Soulanges, P.Q.; Lav '58.

PAQUIN, Rene; 1005 St. Prosper St., Trois Rivieres, P.Q.; Lav '58; M.C.G.P.; Tel. FR 5-7865.

PARADIS, Adrien; CP 725, 622-4e rue, Shawinigan Falls, P.Q.; 702 Blvd. St. Maurice (res); Mon '41; Int-Med (P.Q.); Tel. LE 7-8955.

PARADIS, Antonio; 56 Amyot St., Riviere du Loup, P.Q.; 54 Amyot St. (res); Lav '18; GenSurg; Dist. Coroner.

PARADIS, Bernard; 2110 Bourbonniere, Quebec, P.Q.; 2110 Bourbonniere (res); Lav '43; Anaes; **Staff, Anaes., Hop. St. Francois d'Assise, & Veteran's Hosp. & Laval U.; Tel. 527-3110.**

PARADIS, Claude; 1248 Chemin Ste-Foy, Quebec 6, P.Q.; Lav '55; IntMed (P.Q.); Staff, Jeffrey Hale's Hosp.; Tel. 681-0529.

PARADIS, Denis; Lav'65; Res., Hop. Hotel-Dieu St. Vallier, Chicoutimi, P.Q.

PARADIS, Gerard; 745 ave. Eymard, Quebec 6, P.Q. (res); Lav '50; Pulm. Dis., TB (P.Q.); Staff, Hop. Laval; Tel. 653-5251.

PARADIS, Guy; 1260 Fitzpatrick, Sillery, Quebec, **P.Q. (res); Lav '46; Psy; Ass't., Hop.-St.-Michel-Archange, Mastai; Cons. Hop.-St.-Francois-d'Assise, Que.: Staff, Laval U.; Tel. 663-3571.**

PARADIS, Hubert; Lav'58; Res., Inst. Albert Prevost, Montreal 9, P.Q.

PARADIS, Jacques; 117 Principale, LaSarre, P.Q. (res); Lav '50; GenSurg; Staff, Hop. St. Francois, LaSarre; Tel. 333-2311.

PARADIS, Jacques D.; 193 Hyman Dr., Dollard-des-Ormeaux, P.Q.; Lav'61; FRCS(C), ObstGyn.

PARADIS, Joseph L.; Ste. Scholastique, P.Q.; Lav '46.

PARADIS, Lavergne; 54 rue Amyot, Riviere-du-Loup, P.Q.; Lav '49; GenSurg.; Tel. UN 2-3538.

PARADIS, Maurice; 628 Caribou Cres., Labrador City, Nfld. (res); Lille (Fr.) '57; Staff, Capt. William Jackman Hosp.; Tel. 944-2632.
PARADIS, Roger Capt.; 891 Ave. Laurier, Quebec 4, P.Q.; Lav '63; M.O., Cdn. Army; Tel. 529-3311, Ext. 309; Abroad.
PARADIS, Viateur; 63 Principale, Vercheres, P.Q.; Mon '35; Dist. Coroner.
PARADIS, Yvon; 24 Henry, Levis, P.Q.; 6 rue St. Jean (res); Lav '42; F.C.C.P., Pulm. Dis. & TB (P.Q.), Cardiol (P.Q.); Ass't. Dept. of Med., Hotel-Dieu de Levis; Tel. 837-4227.
PARAMONOFF, Alexander; 520-17th St., West Vancouver, B.C.; 4867 Skyline Dr. (res); Marburg (Germ.) '41; DiagRad; Rad., North Vancouver Gen. Hosp.; Tel. WA 2-5144.
PARANT, Francois; 6875 Place du Roi, Quebec 7 **P.Q.; Lav '56; Anaes; Phys Med. & Rehab; Staff, Hop. St. Sacrement; Tel. LA 7-3461.**
PARASKEVAS, Frixos; 700 Bannatyne, Winnipeg 3, Man.; Thessaloniki (Greece).
PARASKEVOPOULOS, George; 115 Hazen St., Saint John, N.B.; Istanbul (Turk.)'51; Paed.
PARCHMENT, Alwin; 6070 Yonge St., Willowdale, Ont.; U.S.A.'50; Tel. 221-3431.
PARDY, W. V. V.; Mount Brydges, Ont.; Wes '19; Dist. Coroner.
PARE, Claude; 55 ave de l'Eglise, Verdun, Montreal 19, P.Q.; 340 Beatty (res); Mon '56; Paed (P.Q.); Tel. PO 6-3593.
PARE, Gilles; Lav'64; Res., Hop. Ste. Justine, Montreal 26. P.Q.
PARE, Hubert; 45 Ave. Goyette, Iberville, P.Q.; Mon '45; Staff (Med.), Hop-St.-Jean, St.-Jean; Lect., Pharm., Nurses School, Hop-St.-Jean; Tel. 6-6871.
PARE, J. Peter; 4500 Sherbrooke St. W., Westmount, P.Q.; McG'43; D.IntMed; IntMed; Dir. Diag. Serv., Resp. Div., Cardioresp. Unit, Royal Victoria Hosp.; Tel. VI 2-1251, Loc. 1727.
PARENT, Bernard; C.P. 5., Hull, P.Q.; Lav '51; D&TRad; Staff, Hop. Sacre-Coeur; Tel. 777-2721.
PARENT, Charles E.; Sedley, Sask; Lav '11, Dist. Coroner.
PARENT, Jacques-F.; 10232 rue Waverley, Montreal 12, P.Q.; Mon '49; Otol (P.Q.); M.O., Prov. Dept. of Health; Tel. 849-9371.
PARENT, Jacques H.; 4662 ave Patricia, Montreal 28, P.Q. (res); Mon '48; OrthSurg (P.Q.); Staff, Hop.-St. Luc; Tel. 484-7518.
PARENT, Jean-Guy; 8606 Centrale, App 205, LaSalle, P.Q.; 595-45th Ave. (res); Mon '62; Active Staff. LaSalle Gen. Hosp.; Vis. Staff, Verdun Gen. Hosp.; Tel. DO 6-8411.
PARENT, Jean M.; 874 St. Pierre, Terrebonne, P.Q.; Mon'47.
PARENT, Jean P.; 1210-1ere Ave., Quebec 3, P.Q.; Lav'55; IntMed (Gastro)(P.Q.); Tel. 529-9981.
PARENT, J. Fabien; 570 Bord-du-Lac, Dorval, **P.Q.; Mon '48; Staff, Hop. St. Joseph de Lachine & Lachine Gen. Hosp's.; Tel. ME 1-3131.**
PARENT, J. Maurice; Ste. 201, 1656 est rue Sherbrooke, Monteal 24, P.Q.; 6240 Bois de Coulonge, Anjou (res); Mon'53; FRCS(C); GenSurg.
PARENT, Joseph P.; 940 Pillette Rd., Windsor, Ont.; Mon '19; M.O.H., Sandwich East, Ont.; Dist. Coroner; Tel. 945-1602.
PARENT, Julien; Ste 210, 4 Taschereau, Hull, P.Q.; R.R. 1, Mountain Rd. (res); Lav '53; Orth-Surg (P.Q.); Tel. 771-2119.
PARENT, Marcel; Service de Sante, Hotel-de-Ville, Montreal 19, P.Q.; Mon '56.
PARENT, Paul E.; 175 Branson Ave., Ottawa, Ont.; 742 Cooper St. (res); Ott '52; Staff, Ottawa **Gen. Hosp.; Ass't. Med. Dir., St. Vincent's Hosp.; Clin. Ass't. (Med.), U. of Ottawa; Tel. 236-3950.**
PARENT, Roger; 1295 Leblanc, Sillery, P.Q. (res); **Lav '54; Psy; Dir., Psy. Serv., Hotel-Dieu, Levis;** Tel. 837-9341.
PARENT, Yves; Ste.-Gertrude, P.Q. Lav '56.
PARENTEAU, Andre; Ste. 403, 3875 St-Urbain, Montreal 18, P.Q.; Mon '43; DABNS; NeurSurg (P.Q.); Chief, Dept. of NeurSurg., Hotel-Dieu & St. Justine Hosp's.; Ass't. Prof. (Surg.), U. of Montreal; Tel. 842-1382.

PARENTEAU-CARREAU, Suzanne; **App. 11, 2219 rue Maplewood, Montreal 26, P.Q.; Mon '62; Tel.** 342-9614.
PARENTEAU, Gilles R.; 84 Gordon, Sherbrooke, P.Q.; 574 Newton (res); Mon '48; D.A.B.O.S., Orth Surg (P.Q.); Chief Orth., Hotel Dieu Hosp.; Cons. (Orth.), Sherbrooke & St. Vincent's Hosp.; Con. Prov. Hosp.; Magog; Tel. 567-5475.
PARENTEAU, Jean M.; Mon'61; Res., Hop. Notre-Dame, Montreal 24, P.Q.
PARENTEAU, Rosaire; Lav'65; Res., Hop St-Michel-Archange, Quebec 5, P.Q.; Abroad.
PARFITT, Kathleen P.; 6 Mons Ave., Calgary, Alta.; London (Eng) '59.
PARFITT, Hugh L.; London (Eng.)'59; MRCS; LRCP; Res., University Hosp., Edmonton, Alta.
PARIS, Jean P.; 321 Woodward, Sherbrooke, **P.Q. (res); Lav '37; Chief of Serv., San Saint-Francois, Sub. 8, Sherbrooke, P.Q.; Tel. LO 9-2551.**
PARIS, Robert P.; Fairmont Med. Bldg., 750 W. Broadway, Vancouver 9, B.C.; Lav '58; Paed; Tel. TR 2-7111.
PARISER, Marcel; 301 Mitchell St., Port Col**borne, Ont.; Paris (France) '39; Tel. 834-6253.**
PARISH, J. Gordon; Ste. 12, 9819-111th St., Edmonton, Alta. (res); Edinburgh (Scot.) '47; M.D., D.PhysMed; PhysMed & Rehab.; Ass't. Dir. Rehab. Centre, University Hosp.; Tel. 424-7888.
PARISI, Alfonso; 66 Charlton W., Hamilton, Ont.; Ott'55; GenSurg.
PARISIEN, Richard S.; 439-2nd St. E., Cornwall, Ont.; Ott '52; MCGP; Tel. WE 2-4582.
PARISIEN, Victor; Ott '62; Res. Royal Victoria Hosp., Montreal 2, P.Q.
PARIZEAU, Polina, (Zdanowicz); 1686 Pear St., Victoria, B.C. (res); Leningrad (Russia) '40; Assoc. Staff, St. Joseph's Hosp., Victoria.
PARK, Andrew M.; 209 Toronto Western Medical Bldg., 25 Leonard Ave., Toronto 2B Ont.; 234 Rosedale Hghts. Dr. (res); Tor '43; F.R.C.P.(C); Neur; Att. Staff, Toronto Western Hosp. Assoc. Med.; U. of Toronto; Tel. EM 4-6962.
PARK, Donald Capt., Petawawa Military Hosp., Petawawa, Ont.; Man '63.
PARK, In H.; MacNeill Clinic, 514 Queen Street, Saskatoon, Sask.; Soeul (Korea)'52; Dir. Adult Service, MacNeill Clinic, Dept. of Public Health; Tel. 652-4640.
PARK, James N.; 151 Hillcrest Ave., New Glasgow, N.S.; Edinburgh (Scot.) '52; MA; MRCP (Edin.); Pathol., Aberdeen Hosp.; Tel. 752-8311.
PARK, J. Malcolm; 2286 Carling Ave., Ottawa 13, Ont.; 8 Kitimat Cres., Bells Corners (res); Birmingham (Eng.) '50; FAAP; Paed; Staff, Ottawa Civic & Grace Hosp's.; Clin. Ass't., U. of Ottawa; Tel. 728-9288.
PARK, Norman S.; 282 Bessborough Dr., Toronto 17, Ont.; Tor '39; Anaes; Anaes. Staff, Hosp. for Sick Children; Clin. Teach. (Anaes.), U. of Toronto; Tel. EM 6-7242.
PARK, R. J. Grierson; Ridgeway Clinic, 1001 Ridgeway St., Fort William, Ont.; 1810 Isabella St. (res); Tor '36; ObstGyn; Staff, McKellar Gen. Hosp.; **Tel. MA 2-0601.**
PARKER, Charles B.; 149 South Dr., Toronto, Ont.; Tor '09; F.R.C.S.(C), GenSurg; Retired.
PARKER, C. William; 164 Norfolk St., Guelph, Ont.; Tor '43; GenSurg; Staff, St. Joseph's & Guelph Gen. Hosp.; Tel. TA 4-2640.
PARKER, Donald; Brown Clinic, 700-8th. St. S.W., Calgary, Alta.; Liverpool (Eng.) '56: D. Ophth. (Lond.); Ophth; Staff, Calgary Gen., Holy Cross Children's & Auxiliary Hosp's.; Tel. 263-1340.
PARKER, George H.; Glasgow (Scot.)'54; FRCS (Edin); Asst. Res. Urology, Winnipeg General Hospital, Winnipeg, Manitoba.
PARKER, George M.; 80 Charles St. W., Toronto, Ont.; Tor'60; DiagRad.
PARKER, Gilbert P.; 228 Medical Arts Bldg., 170 St. George St., Toronto 5, Ont.; 45 Rose Park Dr. (res); Tor '10; IntMed.; Tel. WA 1-7101.
PARKER, G. M.; 3509 Church, Windsor, Ont.; Tor '36; Staff, Ford Motor Co.

PARKER, James E.; Ste. 220, 1940 Lonsdale Ave., N. Vancouver, B.C.; Dublin (Ire.) '54; ABPaed; Paed; Active Staff, Lions Gate Hosp.; Vis. Staff, Vancouver Gen. Hosp.; Cons. Phys., P.K.U., Dept. of Paed; Tel. 988-3738.
PARKER, John A.; Tor'61; Ophth; McLaughlin Fell., Dept. of Ophth., U. of Toronto, Toronto, Ont.
PARKER, John M.; Box 2005, Canada Duphar Ltd., London, Ont.; Man '41; DPH; Ph.D. (Pharm.).
PARKER, John O.; Etherington Hall, Kingston, Ont.; 54 Kensington Ave. (res); Qns '54; M.Sc. (Meds.); F.R.C.P.(C), IntMed.; Att'd. Phys., Kingston Gen. Hosp.; Ass't Prof. (Med.), Queen's U.; Tel. 546-1731, Loc. 519.
PARKER, K. Ross; Polyclinic 170 Fitzroy St., Charlottetown, P.E.I.; 255 North River Rd. (res); Dal '56; D.C.H. (Lond.); Paed; Head, Paed. Dept. P.E.I. Hosp.; Tel. 8532.
PARKER, Richard H.; P. O. Box 420, Hospital for Mental Diseases, Brandon, Man.; Man '48; Dir., Adult O.P.D. & Child Guidance Clinic; Tel. PA 9-5496.
PARKER, Ross G.; 132 Norfolk St. S., Simcoe, Ont.; Wes '43; FACS; FICS; FRCS (Edin.); FRCS (C); GenSurg; Chief Surg., Norfolk Gen. Hosp.; Tel. 426-3031.
PARKER, Shirley E. (Swail); 51 Eastgate, Winnipeg 1, Man. (res); Man '55; Bact; Ass't. Bact., Wpg. Gen. Hosp.; Lect. (Bact.), U. of Manitoba; Tel. SP 4-6511, Loc. 273.
PARKER-SUTTON, Geoffrey A.; 10216-128th St., North Surrey, B.C.; 12733-100th Ave. (res); Durham (Eng.) '56; M.B., B.S.; Tel. 581-8033.
PARKER, Vernon H. T.; Stellarton, N.S.; Pleasant Ave. (res); McG '17; M.C.G.P.; Staff, Aberdeen Hosp.
PARKER, William L.; Dept. of Bact. & Immunol., U. of Manitoba Winnipeg, Man.; Edinburgh (Scot.) '51; M.Sc., MC(Path); Path; Cons. Virol., Wpg. Gen. Hosp.; Path., Concordia Gen. Hosp.; Ass't. Prof., U. of Manitoba; Tel. SU 6-3522.
PARKER, William R.; 10028-142nd St., Edmonton, Alta.; Glasgow (Scot.) '31; LRCP & S (E); LRFPS(G); DMRD (Eng.); DiagRad; Staff, University & Leduc Municipal Hosp's.; Ass't. Lect., U. of Alberta; Tel. 439-5911.

PARKIN, Alan C.; 276 St. Clair Ave. W., Toronto 7, Ont.; Tor'49; Training Analyst Cdn. Inst. of Psychoanalysis.; Ass't. Prof. (Psy), U. of Toronto; Tel. WA 1-7225.
PARKIN, Herbert G.; 7 Forsyth St. Marmora, Ont.; Qns '49; M.O.H.; District Coroner; Tel. 472-2747.
PARKIN, Robert P.; 25 Summit St., Dartmouth, N.S.; Dal'56; Psy; Staff, Halifax Children's & Victoria Gen. Hosp's.; Cons., Nova Scotia Hosp. & Halifax School for the Blind; Cons., Halifax Mental Health Clin. for Children; Staff, Dalhousie U.; Tel. 469-1589 & 463-3840.
PARKINS, Gerald A.; 200 Scott Bldg., Moose Jaw, Sask.; River Drive (res); McG '21; Urol; Dir., Moose Jaw Clin.; Retired.

PARKINSON, Dwight; 418 Medical Arts Bldg., Winnipeg 1, Man.; McG'41; DABNS, FACS, FRCS(C), NeurSurg; Chief (NeurSurg), Winnipeg Gen. & Children's Hosp's; Assoc. Prof. (Head Dept. of NeuroSurg.), U. of Manitoba; Tel. WH 3-1627.
PARKINSON, Raymond; 714-750 West Broadway, Vancouver 9, B.C.; 3065 Capilano Rd., N. Van. (res); UBC'54; Psy; Att'd. Staff, Vancouver Gen. Hosp.; Cons., Narcotic Addiction Fdn.; Clin. Instr. (Med.), & Staff, Dept. of Contin. Educ., U. of British Columbia; Tel. 874-8636.
PARKINSON, Thomas J.; 4822-51st St., Red Deer, Alta.; 4001-37th Ave. (res); St. Andrew's (Scot.) '46; DCH, MRCP (Lond.); Paed.; Tel. 346-5276.
PARKS, Arthur E.; 330 University Ave., Toronto 1, Ont.; 70 Highland Cres., Willowdale (res); Tor '30; MRCP (Lond), FACP, FRCP(C), IntMed; Vol. Clin. Ass't., OPD, Toronto Gen. Hosp.; Med. Dir., The Canada Life Assurance Co.; Tel. 368-7432.
PARKS, John; 3379 Kingsway, Vancouver 16, B.C.; 4339 Southwood St., S. Burnaby (res); McG '44; Staff, Burnaby Gen. Hosp.; Tel. HE 1-3388.
PARKS, Wilfred R.; 27 Manor Rd. E., Toronto, Ont.; Tor '18; M.C.G.P.; Tel. HU 9-4195.
PARLA, Nusret; 4710 Wyandotte St. E., Windsor, Ont.; Istanbul (Turk.) '47; Staff Phys., Riverview Hosp.; Tel. 945-1621.
PARLEE, H. Bruce G.; 142 Charlotte St., Saint John, N.B.; 19 Seely St. (res); McG '43; MCGP; Chief Dept. of G.P., St. John Gen. Hosp.; A.A. Surg., U.S. Public Health, Consular Dist.; District M.O., C.P.R.; Tel. 693-3754.
PARLEE, Stephen S.; 1004—105th St., Edmonton, Alta.; 13916 Valley View Dr. (res); Alb '38; D.A.B.O.G., F.A.C.S., M.R.C.O.G.; Att. Staff, Royal Alexandra & U. of Alberta Hosp's.; Lect. (ObstGyn.), U. of Alberta; Tel. GA 4-2121.
PARLIAMENT, David R.; 311 Annex, 67 College St., Toronto 2, Ont.; Man'57; DPH; Medical Officer, Industrial Hygiene Branch, Ont. Dept. of Health; Tel. 365-4601.
PARLIAMENT, Wallace J.; 176 Yonge St., Toronto; 2 Boldmere Cr., Willowdale (res); Tor '46; Sr. M.O., Robert Simpson Co.; Tel. UN 1-9111, Loc. 2767.

PARMENTER, Ellice A., see DRYER, Ellice A.

PARMLEY, J. Robert; 4843 Paton St., Vancouver, B.C. (res); McG '30; Staff, Workmen's Compensation Board, 707-37th Ave. W., Vancouver, B.C.; Tel. AM 6-0211.
PARNELL, John L.; 1735 W. Broadway, Vancouver, B.C.; 410 Rabbit Lane, Pk. Royal (res); Edinburgh (Scot.) '39; F.A.C.P., F.R.C.P.(C), IntMed; Phys., Schl. of Nursing & Att'd. Staff, Vancouver Gen. Hosp.; Cons. (Med.), Shaughnessy (DVA) Hosp.; Clin. Instr. (Med.), U. of British Columbia; Tel. RE 3-2327.
PARNEY, Frederick L.; Alb'58; FFARCS; FRCP(C), Anaes; Dir., Dept. of Anaes., Foothills Hosp., Calgary, Alta.
PARNEY, Fred S.; 655 Rideau St., Ottawa, Ont. (res); Tor '17; Retired.
PARRAGA, Ricardo; 116 Elm St. E., Sudbury, Ont.; Madrid (Spain)'54.

PARRISH, Robert M.; 26 Underhill Dr., Apt. 505, Don Mills, Ont. (res); Tor '53; FRCP(C), DiagRad; Ass't. Radiol., Tor. Gen. Hosp.; Clin. Instr. (Rad.), U. of Toronto; Tel. EM 6-8211.

PARROT, J. J. Clement; C.P. 280, Normetal, Abitibi, P.Q.; Lav'46.
PARROT, Paul; 1328 Ave.-des-Pins, Sillery, Quebec 6, P.Q. (res); Lav '22; D.P.H., M.O.H., F.A.P.H.A.; Chief Demographer, Dept. of Health, Province of P.Q.; Staff, Laval U.; Tel. LA 4-8411.

PARROTT, Fraser C.; 215 West River Rd., Galt, Ont. (res); Tor'44; DMR; DiagRad; Active Cons., South Waterloo Mem. Hosp., Georgetown District Mem. Hosp. & Milton Dist. Hosp.; Tel. 621-2330, Ext. 69.
PARROTT, Kenneth B.; 74 Johnson St., Kingston, Ont.; McG '55; Dip.Rad. (McG.); DiagRad; Clin. Ass't., Queen's U.; Tel. 546-1151.
PARROTT, Ross; 2969 Kingston Rd., Scarborough, Ont.; 216 Scarborough Golf Club Rd. (res); Tor '43; Dir., OMA; Tel. AM 1-4141.

PARRY, John C.; 574 King St. W., Chatham, Ont.; Wes'50; Anaes.; Tel. 352-5220.
PARRY, John D.; Port Arthur Clinic, 194 Court St. N., Port Arthur, Ont.; London (Eng.)'60.

PARSON, Joseph V.; 1249 Ross Rd., North Vancouver, B.C.; London (Eng.) '53; M.B., B.S.; M.C.G.P.; Active Staff, Lion's Gate Hosp.; Tel. YU 5-4545.

PARSONS, Christopher J.; Arnprior Med. Clinic, 107 Damiel St., Arnprior, Ont.; Tor'64.
PARSONS, Daphne W.; 133 LeMarchant Rd., St. John's Nfld. (res); Dal. '50; Staff TB. Dispensary.
PARSONS, George V.; 691 Main St., Moncton, N.B.; 78 Henry St. (res); Dal '40; F.A.C.A., F.R.C.P.(C), Anaes; Anaes., Moncton & Hotel-Dieu Hosp's.; Tel. 9-9467.
PARSONS, Kenneth W.; P.O. Box 395, 15 W. Valley Rd., Corner Brook, Nfld.; Dal '34; Staff, Western Mem. Hosp. Semi-retired.
PARSONS, Melvin L. W.; Glovertown South, Bonavista Bay, Nfld.; Dal '55; M.C.G.P.; Local M.O.H.; Tel. 5581.

PARSONS, R. MacGregor; The Parsons Clinic, Drawer 608, Red Deer, Alta.; 5140-43 Ave. (res); Tor '30; F.A.C.S., F.R.C.S.(C), GenSurg; M.C.G.P.; Chief of Staff, Red Deer Mun. Hosp.; Cons. Surg, Provincial Hosp's.; Tel. 346-2042.

PARSONS, R. Milton; 740 Seaforth Med. Bldg., 3550 Cote des Neiges Rd., Montreal 25, P.Q.; 4596 Mont Clair Ave. (res); McG '43; FACOG; FRCS(C); ObstGyn; Staff (ObstGyn.), Montreal Gen., Royal Victoria & Catherine Booth Hosp's.; Cons. ObstGyn., Douglas, & Champlain Valley Hosp's.; Staff, McGill U.; Tel. WE 2-4552.

PARSONS, William B.; Parsons Clinic, Red Deer, Alta.; 5045 - 45th Ave. (res); Tor '34; DiagRad; Rad., Red Deer Gen. Hosp.; Tel. 346-2042.

PARSONS, W. David; 215 LeMarchant Rd., St. John's, Nfld.; McG '51; IntMed; Cons. St. John's Gen. & Grace Hosp's.; Cons. (IntMed), DVA; Tel. 579-9642.

PARTHENIS, Alexander; Shute Inst., 10 Grand Ave., London, Ont.; Wes '61; Tel. 432-1884.

PARTINGTON, Cyril N.; 1878 Lakeshore Rd., Sarnia, Ont. (res); Liverpool & London (Eng.) '41; MRCS; LRCP; FC(Path.); DCP(Lond.); Path; Dir. of Path., Sarnia Gen. Hosp., Sydenham & Dist. Hosp., Wallaceburg & Strathroy Middlesex Hosp.; Tel. DI 4-3661.

PARTINGTON, Michael W.; 31 Garrett Ave, Kingston, Ont. (res); London U. (Eng.) '48; MRCP (Edin.), DCH (Lond.), Ph.D. Lond.); Assoc. Prof. (Paed), & Lect. (Physiol.), Queen's U.; Tel. 546-3871.

PARVARESH, Goudarz A.; Teheran U. (Iran); Staff, Mental Health Clin., Union Hosp., Moose Jaw, Sask.

PARVIN, Mohamed; Tehran (Iran)'60; ObstGyn; Staff, Queen Mary Vet's Hosp. & McGill U., Montreal, P.Q.

PASCAL, Oscar; 2002 Bathurst St., Toronto 10, Ont.; Tor '43; DiagRad.; Tel. RU 9-2929.

PASCOE, Herbert; 523 Med. Arts Bldg., 11010 Jasper Ave., Edmonton, Alta.; 9115-139th St. (res); Tor '53; D.Psy; FRCP(C), Psy; Att'd. Staff, Royal Alexandra Hosp.; Clin. Instr. (Psy), U. of Alberta; Tel. 424-6542.

PASCOE, M. Gilbert; 194 Dufferin Ave., Brantford, Ont.; 95 Parkside Dr. (res); Tor. '49; D.A.-B.P., F.A.A.P.; DNBME; Cons. (Paed), Brantford Gen. & St. Joseph's Hosp's.; Tel. 753-3586.

PASCOE, William W.; 1706 Danforth Ave., Toronto, Ont.; 608 Vesta Dr. (res); Tor '40; M.C.-G.P.; Assoc. Staff, Toronto East Gen. Hosp.; Tel. HO 3-2600.

PASE, Peter R. P.; 21 Kenilworth Ave. S. Hamilton, Ont.; Wes'54; FAGS; Active Staff, O.P.D., Allergy Clin., Hamilton Gen. Hosp.; Tel. LI 5-0913.

PASHAYAN, Hermine; Cairo (Egypt)'61; Res., Montreal Gen. Hosp., Montreal 25, P.Q.

PASHBY, Thomas J.; 1050 Avenue Rd., Toronto, Ont.; 24 Donlea Dr. (res); Tor '40; Ophth; Staff, Toronto Western & Sick Children's Hosp's.; Tel. HU 3-3975.

PASKEVICIUS, Lydia; Qns'65; Jr. Int., Kingston General Hospital, Kingston, Ont.

PASLEY, Francis C.; Ott '57; Staff, Ontario Hosp. Schl., Smith Falls, Ont.

PASQUALE, Mario; Ste. 214, 5325 est, Jean Talon, Montreal-Nord, P.Q.; 333 Wiseman Ave., Outremont (res); Mon '53; GenSurg (P.Q.); Staff, Hop. Ste. Justine; Tel. 725-5281.

PASQUET, Andre F.; 6010 Inglis St., Halifax, N.S. (res); Qns '43; Anaes; Chief Anaes., Grace Maternity Hosp.; Anaes., Victoria Gen. Hosp.; Assoc. Prof. (Anaes), Dalhousie U.; Tel. 422-6501; 422-7371.

PASSI, Ronald B.; Wes '60; FRCS(C), GenSurg; Staff, Westminster Hosp., London, Ont.; Tel. 432-6711.

PASTERSHANK, Stephen P.; Sask '62; Int., Royal Victoria Hosp., Montreal 2, P.Q.

PATAKI, John I.; 225 Lisgar St., Ottawa, Ont.; Budapest (Hung.) '55; IntMed; Assoc. Staff Med., Ottawa Civic Hosp.; Tel. 234-4200.

PATCHEL, Robert D.; Tor '44; FRCS(C), ObstGyn; Staff, Harlem Hosp. Centre, New York, U.S.A.; Abroad.

PATCHELL, Douglas J.; Box 189, Elmvale, Ont.; Tor '46; Staff, Penetang Gen. Hosp.

PATEL, Dinubhai; Box 189, Killam, Alta.; Dublin (Ire)'58; DGO; D.Obst. RCOG; Chief of Staff, Killam Gen. Hosp.; Tel. 388-3721.

PATEL, Dorab, Fl/Lt.; Bombay (India)'52; RCAF Hosp., Greenwood, N.S.

PATEL, Hawa; 4000 Yonge St., Apt. 321, Toronto 12, Ont.; Cape Town (S. Africa)'48; Paed.

PATEL, Manubhai P.; Box 788, Eston, Sask.; Bristol (Eng.) '58; Tel. 962-3607.

PATENAUDE, Edgar S.; 1131 est Rachel, Montreal, P.Q.; Mon '24; Clin. Ass't., Queen Mary's Vet's Hosp.; Tel. 521-9332.

PATENAUDE, Etienne-L.; 1125 Ontario est, Montreal, P.Q.; Mon'41; DPH; PH; Supt., Dept. of National Health, Montreal.

PATENAUDE, Nicol H.; Field, Ont.; Mon '48; M.C.G.P.; Staff, Hop. St. Joseph de Brebeut, Sturgeon Falls; M.O.H.; Tel. 758-6671.

PATERAS, Vincent R.; 445 Westmount Med. Bldg., 5025 Sherbrooke St. W., Montreal 28, P.Q.; McG '57; IntMed (P.Q.; Chief & Cons. Nephrol., Sub. Dept.. St. Mary's Hosp.; Cons. Nephrol., Santa Cabrini Hosp.; Tel. 489-2326.

PATERSHANK, Stephen P.; Sask '62; Res. (Rad.), Royal Victoria Hosp., Montreal, P.Q.

PATERSON, Donald H.; 1707 Angus Dr., Vancouver 9, B.C.; Edinburgh (Scot.) '16; FRCP-(Lond.), FAAP (Hon.), FRCP(C), Paed; Cons. Paed., Vancouver Gen. Hosp.; Chm. Med. Advisory Comm. of Handicapped Children's Registry of B.C.; Tel. RE 3-2401.

PATERSON, Hugh H., F/L; Tor '63; National Defence Med. Centre, Ottawa, Ont.

PATERSON, Ian S.; 1995 Sasamat Pl., Van. 8, B.C. (res); St. Bart's (London, Eng.) '53; FFARCS; Anaes; Att'd. Staff (Anaes), Van. Gen. Active Staff, Children's Hosp's.; Clin. Instr. (Anaes.), U. of British Columbia; Tel. TR 4-5291.

PATERSON, James C.; The Medical Centre, Box 420 Stony Plain, Alta.; Edinburgh (Scot.) '50; MCGP; Tel. 198.

PATERSON, James C., OBE; 14 Mayfair Dr., London, Ont. (res); Tor '25; Path, Bact; Chief, Lab. Serv., Westminster Hosp.; Prof. in Path., & Prof. (Med. Research), U. of Western Ont.; Path., Byron San., Byron; Tel. GE 9-1681. Abroad.

PATERSON, James E.; 34 Drury St., Kapuskasing, Ont.; Glasgow (Scot.)'40; DMRD(Eng.); DiagRad; Staff, Notre Dame Hosp., Hearst, Lady Minto Hosp., Cochrane, Anson Gen. Hosp., Ansonville & Sensenbrenner Hosp., Kapuskasing.

PATERSON, James L.; Alb '48; Psy; Clin. Dir., Alberta Hosp., Box 307, Edmonton, Alta.; Tel. 7-0221.

PATERSON, John F.; 403 Toronto Western Med. Bldg., 25 Leonard Ave., Toronto 2B, Ont.; 37 Whitney Ave. (res); Cambridge (Eng.) '36; MD (Cantab); MRCP (Lond.), FRCP(C), IntMed; Hd. Dept. of Med., Sunnybrook Hosp.; Prof. (Med.), U. of Toronto; Tel. 368-6676.

PATERSON, William P., Jr.; 506, Med. Arts Bldg., 180 Metcalfe St., Ottawa 4, Ont.; Qns '56; ObstGyn; Staff, Ottawa Civic & Grace Hosp's.; Tel. CE 2-5487.

PATIENCE, C. R.; 179 Huron St., Woodstock, Ont.; 179 Huron St. (res); Qns '28; Ophth,Otol; Staff, Woodstock Gen. Hosp.; Tel. LE 7-5511.

PATODIA, Girdhari L.; 1½ Prince St., Glace Bay, N.S.; Calcutta (India)'59; Staff, Glace Bay Gen. & St. Joseph's Hosp's.

PATOINE, Jean G.; 176 Ave. Royale, St.-Laurent d'Orleans, Cte. Montmorency, P.Q. (res); Lav '52; Anaes; Staff, Hop.-de-l'Enfant-Jesus; Tel. 529-8711.

PATOINE, Lionel; 6635 Christophe-Colomb, Montreal 10, P.Q.; Mon '35; Phys-in-Chief, Artisans Soc., 333 Craig E.; Tel. 271-9811.

PATOINE-LAPORTE, Mireille; 6635 Christophe-Colomb, Montreal 10, P.Q.; Mon '59, Retired.

PATON, James P.; 305 Matheson St. S., Kenora, Ont.; Tor '10.

PATRIARCHE, M. Elizabeth; 1377 Rockland, Victoria, B.C.; Man'36; Part-time Phys., Gtr. Victoria Met. Bd. of Health; Teach. Family Life Educ., Gtr. Victoria School Bd.; Tel. EV 5-0404.

PATRICK, Andrew; 837 Professional Bldg., Edmonton, Alta.; 9728-64th Ave. (res); Glasgow (Scot) '54; FRCS(C); Ophth; Tel. 422-0461.

PATRICK, Daphne (Mrs. P. W. Yaremko); 41 Tollerton Ave., Willowdale, Ont.; Queen's U. (Belfast, N. Ire.) '48; MCGP; Active OPD Staff, Women's College Hosp.; Tel. BA 5-9671.

PATRICK, Doreen; 9728-64th. Ave., Edmonton, Alta. (res); Glasgow (Scot.) '54; Part-time School M.O., Edmonton, Retired.

PATRICK, Evan; Port Arthur Clinic, 194 N. Court St., Port Arthur, Ont.; Liverpool (Eng.)'51; MRCP (Lond.); Assoc. IntMed., Port Arthur Gen. & St. Joseph's Hosp's.; Tel. 344-7271.

PATRICK, John W.; 5025 Sherbrooke St. W., Ste. 440, Westmount, 28, P.Q.; McG '43; FACOG; ObstGyn; Staff, Catherine Booth, Queen Elizabeth & Reddy Mem. Hosp's.; Med. Dir., Catherine Booth Hosp.; Tel. 488-3151.

PATRICK, Murray C.; Fredericton Med. Clinic, 206 Rookwood Ave., Fredericton, N.B.; 31 Woodfield Cres. (res); McG '53; AMCGP; Att'd. Staff, Victoria Public Hosp.; Treas. N.B. Chapter, College of G.P.; Tel. 475-7701.

PATRICK, Terry R., Sg/Lt.; RCN Hosp., HMCS "Naden", Esquimalt, B.C.; Alb'63.

PATRICK, W. H. Laurence; 3195 Granville St., Vancouver 9, B.C.; Glasgow (Scot.) '36; MCGP; Staff, St. Vincent's Hosp.; Vis. Staff, Vancouver Gen., St. Paul's & Grace Hosp's.; Tel. RE 3-1224.

PATRIQUIN, Heidi B. (Rumscheidt); McG'64; Res., Princess Margaret Hosp., Toronto 5, Ont.

PATRY, Bernard; 12774 ouest boul. Gouin, Pierrefonds, P.Q.; Mon'65.

PATRY, Georges; Lav'65; Res., Hop L'Enfant Jesus, Quebec 3, P.Q.

PATRY, Jean C.; Polyclinique Gravel, 66 St.-Jean-Baptiste, Victoriaville, P.Q.; Lav '54; OrthSurg; Staff, Hop.-Hotel-Dieu-d'Arthabaska; Tel. 752-7511.

PATRY, J. Maurice M.; 258 Crowland Ave., Welland, Ont.; Ott '55; MCGP; Tel. RE 2-5912.

PATRY, Laurent; 30 ave-des-Berniers, Quebec, P.Q. (res); Lav '32; Psy; Chief of Serv., (Men's Dept.), Clin. Roy-Rousseau, Mastai; Cons. Psy., Military & Jeffrey Hale's Hosp's.; Ass't., San., Mastai & Hop.-Hotel-Dieu-de-Sacre-Coeur; Staff, Laval U.; Tel. 663-7856.

PATRY, Paul-E.; 63 ouest Notre-Dame, Victoriaville, P.Q.; Lav'54; FACS; FRCS(C); GenSurg; Assoc. Surg., Hotel-Dieu D'Arthabaska; Tel. 752-2254.

PATRY, Raymond; 1205 rue La Promenade, Douville, St-Hyacinthe, P.Q. (res); Lav'59; Anaes; Staff, Hop. Generale St. Hyacinthe, P.Q.; Tel. 773-3453.

PATRY, Sauveur; St. Alban, P.Q.; Lav '37; Obst (P.Q.).

PATT, Norman L.; One Medical Place, 20 Wynford Dr., Don Mills, Ont.; X-Ray Dept., St. Michael's Hosp., Toronto; Tor'55; DMR; FRCP(C); DiagRad; Clin. Instr., Rad., Faculty of Med.; Dem. Anat., U. of Toronto; Tel. 429-0757.

PATTEE, Chauncey J.; 1390 Sherbrooke St. W., Apt. 25, Montreal, P.Q.; 636 Murray Hill, Westmount (res); McG '36; FACP; IntMed (PQ); Assoc. Phys., Royal Victoria Hosp., Dir., Clin. Investigation Unit, Queen Mary Veteran's Hosp., Ass't., Dept. of Obst. Gyn., Montreal Gen. Hosp.; Hon. Cons. Endocrin., Herbert Reddy Memorial Hosp.; Ass't. Prof. of Med. McGill U.; Tel. VI 2-9604.

PATTEN, Donald E.; Wes'65; Res., Ottawa Civic Hosp., Ottawa 3, Ont.

PATTEN, John F.; Suite 408, Med. Dental Bldg., 450 Central Ave., London, Ont.; 704 Huron St. (res); Wes '57; MCGP; Tel. 438-7771.

PATTEN, Robert L.; McG '62; Jr. Intn., Montreal Gen. Hosp., Montreal 25, P.Q.

PATTERSON, Bryson C.; 436 Hinton Ave., Ottawa 3, Ont.; Qns '11; Ophth; Hon. Cons., Ottawa Civic Hosp.; Retired.

PATTERSON, Donald M.; 286 King St. W., Chatham, Ont.; 112 Lydican Ext. (res); Wes '54; GenSurg.; Tel. 352-0501.

PATTERSON, Earl R.; Box 136 Lucan, Ont.; Wes'38; M.O.H.; Tel. 227-4752.

PATTERSON, Frank P.; Room 1015, 750 West Broadway, Vancouver 9, B.C.; McG '40; FACS; FRCS(C), OrthSurg; DABOS; Chief OrthSurg., Vancouver Gen. Hosp.; Cons., Shaughnessy DVA, Children's & St. Paul's Hosp's.; Assoc. Prof. (Surg.), U. of British Columbia; Tel. TR 2-5665.

PATTERSON, Ian S.; Apt. 3, 321 Stradbrook Ave., Winnipeg 13, Man.; London (Eng.) '53.

PATTERSON, John A. MC; Oshawa Clinic, 117 King St. E., Oshawa, Ont.; R.R. 2, Port Perry (res); Tor '42; FCCP; IntMed; Dist. Coroner; Tel. 728-1661.

PATTERSON, John G.; Ste. 214, 895 Fort St., Victoria, B.C.; McG '47; MAAGP; MCGP; Tel. 388-5481.

PATTERSON, L. A.; Ste. 724, Vancouver Block 736 Granville St., Vancouver, B.C.; Coll. of Med. Evangelists (Los Angeles, Calif.) '43; M.C.G.P.; Tel. MU 4-2481.

PATTERSON, Leonard J.; 4826 Ross St., Red Deer, Alta.; 5829-45th Ave. (res); Qns '42; MCGP; Tel. 346-2042.

PATTERSON, Leslie D.; Box 70, Hastings, Ont.; Tor'52; Chief of Staff, Campbellford Mem. Hosp.; Tel. 696-2231.

PATTERSON, Maxwell C.; 1276 Tyondoya Park Dr., Burlington, Ont. (res); McG'55; FRCP(C), Path; Pathol., Henderson Gen. Hosp., Hamilton.

PATTERSON, Randolph J.; 199 Clemow Ave., Ottawa, Ont. (res); Qns '43; DiagRad; Staff, Dept. of Rad., Otaawa Civic Hosp.; Tel. PA 9-2511.

PATTERSON, Russell K.; 100B Victoria Ave., Belleville, Ont.; Qns '60; MCGP; Active Staff (GP), Belleville Gen. Hosp.; Tel. 962-8711.

PATTERSON, Thomas A.; Ste 609, 1849 Yonge St., Toronto 7, Ont.; Tor'56; Staff Phys., U. of Toronto Health Serv.; Tel. 485-1789.

PATTERSON, Thomas D.; Wes '53; Path; Pathol., St. Joseph's Hosp., Chatham, Ont.; Tel. EL 2-2500.

PATTERSON, Thomas H.; Occupational Health Div., Environmental Health Centre, Dept. of National Health & Welfare, Ottawa 3, Ont.; Dal'45; DPH; MPH; Tel. 992-5601.

PATTERSON, Wm. J.; Ste. 450, 2184 W. Broadway, Vancouver 9, B.C.; 1250 Netley Pl. (res); Ott '53; Otol.; Hd. Dept. of Otol., Children's Hosp.; Staff, St. Paul's Hosp.; Clin. Instr. (Otol.) Hosp.; Staff, St. Paul's Hosp.; Clin. Instr. (Otol.), U. of British Columbia; Tel. RE 8-2511.

PATTERSON, W. Stuart; 221 King St. E., Kingston, Ont.; 337 Union St. W. (res); Qns '44; ObstGyn; Assoc. Staff, Kingston Gen. & Hotel-Dieu Hosp's.; Prin. MO, HMCS Cataraqui & RMC; Surg. Cdr., RCN (R); Clin. Ass't., ObstGyn, Queen's U.; Tel. 548-8962.

PATTON, Donna; Manitoba Clinic, 790 Sherbrooke St., Winnipeg 2, Man.; Man'50; Tel. SP 4-6541, Ext. 260.

PATTON, D. Robert; 200 Beacon Hill Rd., Beaconsfield, P.Q.; Dal '60; Court. Staff, Lachine Gen. & Lakeshore Gen. Hosp's.; Schl. Phys., West Island Comm. (Pte. Claire & Beaconsfield); Tel. 697-1080.

PATTON, Gordon O.; 671 Westchester Dr., Baie d'Urfee, P.Q.; Alb '37; Psy; M.O. (Psy), D.V.A., Montreal Dist.; Med. Spec. (Psy.) Ste-Anne Hosp.; Dem. (Psy.), McGill U.; Tel. 453-2342.

PATTON, I. Jocelyn; 1501 Shell Tower Bldg., 1255 University, Montreal 2, P.Q.; 2171 St. Catherine W., Mtl. 25 (res); State U. (Iowa, U.S.A.) '33; Med. Dir., Paul, Phelan & Perry, Public Relations; Tel. VI 9-8061; Retired.

PATTON, John O.; 647 Sherbourne Rd., Ottawa 3, Ont. (res); Qns '40; Path; Assoc. Path., Ottawa Civic Hosp.; Ass't. Prof. (ClinPath), Ottawa U.; Tel. PA 9-2511, Loc. 245.

PATTON, Weldon W.; Glace Bay, N.S.; 14 Yorke (res); Dal '08.

PATTON, William D.; 1637 Cedar Cres., Vancouver, B.C. (res); McG '09; Retired.

PATZAUER-VOTSCH, Anna; Ste. 208, 77 Upper Middle Rd., Cooksville, Ont.; Vienna (Aust.) '51; FRCP(C), IntMed; Active Staff, Queensway Gen. & South Peel Hosp's.; Tel. 277-4432.

PAUL, Donald J.; 27 Third Street, Collingwood, Ont.; Tor'59; Staff Phys., Collingwood Gen. & Marine Hosp.; Tel. 445-4111.

PAUL, Edward B.; Box 1220, 224 Centre St., Napanee, Ont.; Qns'43; Tel. 354-4215.
PAUL, Godfrey M.; 314 Cook Medical Bldg., 1175 Cook St., Victoria, B.C.; 1895 Landsdowne Ave. (res); Qns '43; Staff, St. Joseph's Hosp.; Tel. EV 3-1732.
PAUL-HUS, Gilles; 1037 est Boul. St. Joseph, Montreal 34, P.Q.; Mon'52; FRCP(C); Psy; Chief of Geriatric Serv., Hop. St. Jean de Dieu; Ass't. Prof., U. of Montreal; Tel. VI 5-7804.
PAUL, John A. D.; Qns '42; Staff, Dept. of Vet's Affairs, University Hosp., Saskatoon, Sask.
PAUL, M. Marvin; 403-158 St. George St., Toronto 5, Ont.; 3455 Bathurst St., Tor. 10 (res); Tor '57; MCGP; Tel. LE 4-4214.
PAUL, William M.; Room 134, Private Patients Pavilion, Toronto Gen. Hosp., College St., Toronto 2, Ont.; Tor'47; FRCS(C); ObstGyn; Obst & Gyn-in-Chief, Toronto Gen. Hosp.; Prof. & Hd. Dept. of ObstGyn., U. of Toronto; Tel. EM 6-8211, Loc. 2375.
PAUL, William R.; 149 Jeffery St., Asbestos, P.Q.; Tor '48; GenSurg; MCGP; M.O., Cdn. Johns-Manville Co.; Tel. 879-5471.
PAULETTE, Robert E.; 420 Montreal St., Sherbrooke, P.Q.; McG '54; ThorSurg(P.Q.); FACS; **FCCP; DABS; DABTS; FRCS(C), GenSurg; Att'd. Surg., Sherbrooke Hosp.,** Tel. 569-8626.
PAULIN, Claude; 912 est Sherbrooke, Montreal 24, P.Q.; Lav'51; IntMed; Staff, Hop. Ste. Jeanne d'Arc; Con., Hop. de la Misericorde; Tel. LA 7-2521.
PAULIN, J. Ernest; Tracadie, N.B.; Lav '18; D.P.H.
PAULIN, J. Roger; Tracadie, N.B.; Dal '48.
PAULIN, Roger; Ste. 22, 2115 Drummond St., Montreal 25, P.Q.; Lav'45; ThorSurg(P.Q.); GenSurg(P.Q.); Dir., Dept. of Surg., Hop. St. Joseph de Rosemont & Hop. Misericorde; Provincial Surg., St. John's Ambulance Assoc.; Tel. 842-9497.
PAULS, Henry; 101-299 Main St., Chilliwack B.C.; 45405 Bernard Ave. (res); UBC '54; FACS; DABS; GenSurg; Cons., Matsqui-Sumas-Abbotsford, Misson & Chilliwack Gen. Hosp's.; Tel. 795-7944.
PAULS, Leon A.; 907 Boyd Bldg., Winnipeg, Man.; 418 Brock St. (res); **Man '33; Ophth, Staff, St. Boniface Hosp.; Tel. WH 3-0311.**
PAULSE, Douglas T.; Witwatersrand (S. Africa) '49; Psy; Dir., Day Care Centre, Hosp. for Mental Dis., **St. John's, Nfld.; Tel. 9-5061.**
PAULSON, Gudmundur; Lundar, Man; Man '28; M.C.G.P.; Dist. Coroner.
PAUPST, James C.; 215 Victoria Street, Toronto, Ont.; Tor'62; Staff, Diagnostic Clinic, St. Michael's Hosp.; Tel. 364-5325.
PAVELEY, George E.; 2905-13th Ave., Regina, Sask.; Edinburgh (Scot.)'56; Tel. 527-4104.
PAVILANIS, Vytautas; C.P. 100, Laval des Rapides, P.Q.; Kaunas (Lith.) '42; Bact (P.Q.); Chief, Virus Lab., Inst. of Microbiology & Hyg., **& Assoc. Prof., Schl. of Hyg., U. of Montreal.;** Tel. 681-2521.
PAWLOVITCH, John; Spirit River, Alta.; Sask '59.
PAWLOWSKI, Gerald J.; 902 Davenport Rd., Toronto 4, Ont.; Tor '61; Assoc. Staff (Med.), Toronto Gen. Hosp.; Tel. 533-5581.
PAWLOWSKI, Joseph; 155 Ingram, Duncan, B.C.; Alb'51; Tel. 746-5115, 746-5116.
PAWLUK, William; Suite 203, 8225-105th St., Edmonton, Alta.; Alb'54; FRCS(C); GenSurg; Clin. Inst., Dept. of Surg., Univ. of Alberta; Tel. 439-4321.
PAYETTE, Hector; 4545 Queen Mary Rd., Montreal, P.Q.; Mon '29; Sr. Pen. Med. Exam., Cdn. Pen. Comm.; Tel. 738-9451.
PAYETTE, Lorenzo; 201 Blvd. L'Ange Gardien, L'Assomption, P.Q.; Lav '30.
PAYETTE, Yvon; 3437 Sherbrooke E., Montreal, P.Q.; 8211 rue de la Seine, Ville d'Anjou (res); Mon '55; A.M.C.G.P.; Tel. 525-8112.
PAYEUR, Leo; 7 d'Auteuil, Quebec, P.Q. (res); **Lav '28; D & T Rad; PhysMed (PQ); Staff, Hotel-Dieu; Assoc. Prof. Laval U. Tel. 529-9151.**
PAYNE, Donald E.; Baie Verte, Nfld.; Tor '63.
PAYNE, Eric N.; 12th St. N.E., Grand Forks, B.C.; Cambridge (Eng.)'58.
PAYNE, Hubert; 10690 Verville St., Montreal 12, P.Q.; Mon '57; Tel. 331-5451.
PAYNE, Lloyd G.; Box 110, Dresden, Ont.; Wes '35; M.C.G.P.; Tel. 683-4522.
PAYNE, Peter F.; 423 Medical Arts Bldg., 11010 Jasper Ave., Edmonton, Alta.; Sheffield (Eng.)'55; Psy.
PAYNE, Walter J.; Nat. U. (Dublin, Ire.) '50; Staff, General Hosp., St. John's Nfld.
PAZARATZ, Bozidar; 686½ Main St. E., Hamilton, Ont.; Belgrade (Yugoslav.) '40; Tel. JA 2-0021.
PAZDER, Lawrence H.; Alb'61; Res., University Hosp., Edmonton, Alta.
PEACHEY, Arthur B.; 14 McKay Ave., Cornwall, Ont.; Tor'46; DPH; Dist. Coroner; Tel. 932-0825.
PEACHEY, John E.; Qns'61; Res., Mental Health Clinic, 514 Jarvis St., Toronto 5 ,Ont.
PEACOCK, Elaine G. S.; 520-17th St., West Vancouver, B.C.; 504 Eastcot Rd. (res); Man '33; Tel. WA 2-4188.
PEACOCK, George W.; 932 Spadina Cres. E., Saskatoon, Sask.; 802—8th Ave. N. (res); Tor '32; D.H.A.; Sec. Sask. Div., C.M.A.; Registrar, Coll. of Physicians & Surgeons of Saskatchewan, 932 Spadina Cres. E., Saskatoon; Tel. CH 4-7355.
PEACOCK, Henry A.; McGregor Clinic, 250 Main St. E., Hamilton, Ont.; 260 Aberdeen Ave. (res); McG '26; IntMed; Hon. Cons., D.V.A.; Tel. JA 7-2711.
PEACOCK, John J.; Ste. 204, 280 Bloor St. W., Toronto 5, Ont.; Tor'59; FRCP(C); Neur; Staff, St. Joseph's Hosp.
PEACOCK, Kenneth A.; 520—17th St., West Vancouver, B.C.; Man '38; Tel. WA 2-4188.
PEACOCK, Peter N. B.; 516-2nd Ave. N., Saskatoon, Sask.; 1416 Main St. (res); Cape Town (S. Africa) '45; DPH; DIH; DTM&H; Reg. M.O.H., Dept. of Public Health; Ass't. Prof. (Dept. of Soc. & Prev. Med.), U. of Saskatchewan; Tel. 244-0191. Abroad.
PEACOCK, P. Michael; Glasgow (Scot.)'53; Staff, General Hosp., Port Colborne, Ont.
PEAD, Barbara (See Kraft)
PEARCE, Charles F.; 407 Canada Bldg., Windsor, Ont.; Tor'61; Urol.
PEARCE, George A.; 210 Church St., Belleville, Ont.; 592 Bridge St. E. (res); Wes '55; MCGP; WO 8-9211.
PEARCE, James W.; 10303—121st St., Edmonton, Alta. (res); Qns '47; D. Phil (Oxon); Hon. Cons. (Med.) U. Hosp.; Prof. & Head, Dept. of Physiology & Pharmacology, U. of Alberta; Tel. GE 9-8721. Abroad.
PEARCE, Jocelyn C.; 2 Scholfield Ave., Toronto 5, Ont. (res); Wes '56; DMR; DiagRad; Ass't. Radiol., Toronto E. Gen. Hosp.; Tel. 461-8272.
PEARCE, J. P.; 352 Main St. E., Picton, Ont.; Qns '40; Tel. GR 6-2724.
PEARCE, Keith I.; MRCS(Eng.); LRCP(Lond.); Psy; Dir., Dept. of Psy., Foothills Hosp., Calgary, Alta.; Tel. 283-0751.
PEARCE, Lois C. (Craig); 249 Victoria Ave., Chatham, Ont.; Tor '45; Tel. EL 4-3220.
PEARL, Hyman; 35 St. Joseph St., Granby, P.Q.; McG'53; Tel. 372-4216.
PEARL, Gerald J.; 4565 Michel-Bibaud, Montreal, P.Q.; UBC'60; FRCS(C); GenSurg.
PEARL, Manuel J.; Qns '56; Staff, Jewish Gen. Hosp., Montreal, P.Q.; Tel. 735-3771.
PEARLMAN, David; 377 Graham Ave., Winnipeg 1, Man.; 6 McCurdy St. (res); Alb'53; MCGP; Court. Staff, all Winnipeg Hosp's.; Staff (G.P.), St. Boniface Hosp.; Tel. 942-7241.
PEARLMAN, Lyon N.; 505 O'Connor St., Ottawa, Ont.; 759 Manitou Dr., Ott. 13 (res); Tor '34; FAAP; Paed; Paed., Ottawa Civic & Grace Hosp's.; Court. Staff, Ottawa Gen. Hosp.; Lect. (Paed), U. of Ottawa; Tel. CE 2-5761.
PEARMAN, Robert W.; 600 Seaforth Med. Bldg., 3550 Cote des Neiges Rd., Montreal 25, P.Q.; 140 Easton Ave. (res); McG '45; Ophth; Assoc. Ophth., Queen Elizabeth Hosp.; Clin. Ass't. Montreal Gen. Hosp.; Lect., McGill U.; Tel. 932-6948.

PEARSALL, Howard E.; 260 Cedar St., Sudbury, Ont.; 139 Bowland Ave. (res); Tor '44; FACS; Otol; Chief, Dept. of Otol, Sudbury Gen. Hosp.; Cons. (Otol.), Sudbury-Algoma San.; Surg. Staff, Sudbury Mem. & St. Joseph's Hosp's.; Tel. 675-1346.

PEARSON, Beverley (See Murphy)

PEARSON, Cecil L.; 228 Administration Bldg., 98th Ave. & 109th St., Edmonton, Alta.; Alb'38; DPH; Ass't. Dir., Med. Serv., Dept. of Public Health, Prov. of Alta.; Exec. Sec., Special Legislative & Lay Committ., Prev. Health Serv.; M.O.H., Northern Alberta Health Serv.; Tel. 229-3550.

PEARSON, Frank B.; 104 Norlyn Med. Bldg., 309 Hargrave St., Winnipeg 2, Man.; 457 Kingston Cres., St. Vital (res); Man '50; MCGP; Court. Staff, all Winnipeg Hosp's.; M.O. Militia, Tel. WH 3-7596.

PEARSON, Frederick G.; 134 Lawton Blvd., Toronto 7, Ont.; Tor '49; FRCS(C), GenSurg; Staff, Toronto Gen. Hosp.; Clin. Instr. (Surg.), U. of Toronto; Tel. 364-4802.

PEARSON, Georges; App. 1, 5715 ave. Darlington, Montreal 26, P.Q.; Mon '23; Bact (P.Q.); Bact., Research Dept., Ste. Jeanne d'Arc Hosp.; Tel. VI 2-5201

PEARSON, Gertrude E.; 125 Vimy St., Sherbrooke, P.Q. (res); McG '33; Not practising.

PEARSON, J. Campbell; Port Arthur Clinic, Port Arthur, Ont.; 22 Summit Ave. (res); Tor '47; FACS, FRCS(C), GenSurg; Chief of Surg., Port Arthur Gen. Hosp.; Tel. DI 4-7271.

PEARSON, Lawson J.; Med. Centre, 106 Talbot St. W., Leamington, Ont.; Bayshore Dr. (res); Birmingham (Eng.) '54; DRCOG; Anaes., Leamington Dist. Hosp.; Tel. FA 6-3281.

PEARSON, Margaret; 305 Medical Centre, 8th Ave. S.W., Calgary, Alta.; Alb'52; Paed; Dir., Southern Alberta Poison Information Centre; Tel. 266-4494.

PEART, Arthur F. W.; M.B.E. (Mil.); 150 St. George St., Toronto, Ont.; 70 York Mills Rd., Willowdale (res); Qns '40; M.R.S.H., D.P.H., PH; Ass't. Sec., Cdn. Med. Assoc.; Memb. Council, School of Hygiene, U. of Toronto; Tel. 924-0751.

PEART, Harry E.; Tor '26; F.A.C.C.P. F.C.C.P; IntMed (T.B.); Staff, Mountain San., Hamilton, Ont.; Tel. 385-5341.

PEART, J. Arthur; 33 White St., St. Thomas, Ont.; 217 Gravel Rd. (res); Tor '38; D.A. (Eng.), Anaes.; Tel. 631-5090.

PEAT, Gilbert B.; Hampton Rd., Rothesay, N.B. ObstGyn.; Mcg. '06.

PEAT, Robert S.; 144 Bombay Ave., Downsview, Ont.; Tor '36; D.P.H., PH; Staff, Ontario Hosp. Servs. Comm., Toronto; Tel. 487-1711.

PECK, Jack G.; Alb'49; Res., Vancouver Gen. Hosp., Vancouver 9, B.C.

PECKHAM, Gerald B.; 11 Alderdice Pl., St. John's, Nfld.; Dal'60; FRCP(C), IntMed.; Dir. Cardiac Unit & Cardiovasc Research, St. John's Gen. Hosp.; Tel. 726-5967.

PECO, Henry C.; 148 Llydican Ave., Extension, Chatham, Ont.; Wes '30; Tel. 352-4233.

PEDDLE, David B.; Dal'64; Staff, St. John's Gen. Hosp., St. John's, Nfld.

PEDDLE, Leo J.; Dal '62; Res., Winnipeg Gen. Hosp., Winnipeg 3, Man.

PEDERSEN, B. A. T.; 55 Avondale Blvd., Bramalea, Ont.; Tor '64.

PEDLER, John A.; 28 Chatsworth Dr., Toronto 12, Ont.; London (Eng.) '50; LRCP(Lond.); MRCS(Eng.); MDS(Lond.); FDS(Eng.); Dental Surg-in-Chief, Toronto Gen. Hosp.; Prof. & Hd., **Dept. of Oral Diag., Fac. of Dentistry, U. of Toronto; Tel. EM 6-8211.**

PEDLEY, Ernest W.; 97 Charlotte St., Port Colborne, Ont.; Qns'56; MCGP; Staff, Port Colborne Gen. Hosp.; Tel. 834-4216.

PEDLEY, Frank G.; Hudson, P.Q.; McG '16; M.P.H. (Johns Hopkins), P.H. (Harvard); Retired.

PEDLEY, W. H.; 53 Lincoln Sq., Brantford, Ont. (res); Tor '21; Retired.

PEDLOW, Alan L.; Man'48; DiagRad; Staff, Dept. of Rad., Royal Columbia Hosp., New Westminster, B.C.; Tel. LA 2-2771.

PEDNAULT, Jean R.; Ste-Catherine, Cte Pontneuf, P.Q.; Lav '62.

PEDVIS, Sydney; Ste. 420, 5300 Cote-des-Neiges Rd., Montreal 26, P.Q.; 430 Kindersley, Twn. of Mt. Royal (res); McG '43; M.C.A.A.; All. (P.Q.); Paed; Paed-in-Chief, Jewish Gen. Hosp.; Ass't. Phys., Montreal Children's Hosp.; Dem. (Paed). McGill U.; Tel. RE 9-8451.

PEEL, Hugh R.; 801 Prince St., Truro, N.S.; 46 Highland Dr. (res); Edinburgh (Scot.) '31.

PEER, Edgar T.; 24 Church St., St. Catharines, Ont; Tor '46; F.C.C.P.

PEERLESS, S. John; UBC'61; Res., Hosp. for Sick Children, Toronto 2, Ont.

PEERS, Anthony L.; 515 Med. Arts Bldg., 11010 Jasper Ave., Edmonton, Alta.; 10025-143rd St. (res); Cambridge (Eng.) '36; MRCS (Eng.), LRCP (Lond.); Part-time Phys. Edmonton Public School Bd.; Tel. 422-5656.

PEET, Robert M.; 401 Campbell Bldg., 1029 Douglas St., Victoria, B.C.; 3460 Upper Terr. (res); Dublin (Ire.) '47; MRCP(I), FRCP(I); M.S. (Neurol., Minn.); FRCP(C), Neur; Active Staff, (NeurPsy), Royal Jubilee & St. Joseph's Hosp's.; Dir. EEG Dept., Royal Jubilee Hosp.; Research Assoc. U. of Victoria; Tel. EV 2-1911.

PEET, Thomas A. M.; 1105 Pandora Ave., Victoria, B.C.; 516 Dallas (res); St. Andrew's (Scot.) '54; M.B., Ch.B.; MCGP; Active Staff, Royal **Jubilee Hosp.; Lect. (Pt. time), Vic. College; Tel. 383-3342.**

PEEVER, George M.; 161 Church St., Newmarket, Ont.; Qns '35.

PEEVER, Irvin C.; Manitoba Clinic, 790 Sherbrook St., Winnipeg 2, Man.; Man'54; FACOG; FRCOG; FRCS(C); ObstGyn; Clin. Tutor, ObstGyn, Univ. of Manitoba; Tel. SP 4-6541.

PEIKOFF, Samuel S.; 400 Norlyn Bldg., 309 Hargrave St., Winnipeg, Man.; 99 Wellington Cr (res); Man '25; F.A.C.S., F.I.C.S., F.R.C.S. (Edin.), FRCS(C), GenSurg; Active Surg, Staff, St. Boniface & Victoria Hosp's.; Ass't. Prof. (Surg.), U. of Manitoba; Tel. 947-0216.

PEINTNER, Inge; 50 Harrow Cres., Haysboro, Calgary, Alta. (res); Vienna (Austria) '50; Staff, Dept. of Health, Calgary.

PEIRCE, Carleton B.; 472 Strathcona Ave., Westmount, Montreal 6, P.Q.; U. of Michigan (USA) '24; M.Sc; DABR; FACR; FACP; FRCP(C), D&TRad; Hon. Cons., Royal Victoria & Royal Edward Chest Hosp's.; Hon. Cons., Cdn. Armed Forces, Med. Council; Cons. Med. & Life Sciences, Cdn. Corp. for 1967 World Exposition; Cons. to Fac. of Med., U. of British Columbia, Vancouver.

PEISLEY, Hazel N.; Newfoundland Anaesthesia Associates, 95 Le Marchant Rd., St. John's Nfld.; Sydney (Australia) '50; Anaes.

PEKELSKY, Karel; 297 Sunnyside Ave., Ottawa 3, Ont.; Charles U. (Prague)'45; AMCGP; Civilian M.O., R.C.A.F. Stn. Hosp., Rockcliffe; Tel. 235-4961.

PELCHAT, Conrad; 3423 St. Denis St., Montreal 18, P.Q.; 2080 Jeanne-Mance St. (res); Lav '55; Part-time Staff, St Luke's Hosp.; Tel. VI 2-4892.

PELISSIER, Roch; St. Cyrille de Wendover, Co. Drummond, P.Q.; Lav '46; M.C.G.P.

PELLAND, A. Marthe; 1475 Boul. Sir Wilfred Laurier, Quebec 6, P.Q.; Mon'30; Neur; Retired.

PELLER, Joseph A.; 302 Medical Arts Bldg. Hamilton, Ont.; Box 122, Ancaster (res); Tor '48; MRCP(Eng.); FRCP(C), IntMed.; PhysMed. Staff & Dir. Radio-Isotope Lab., Hamilton Gen. Hosp.; Staff, Hamilton Civic Hosp; Med. Dir., Western Life Assur. Co., Hamilton; Tel. JA 8-7253.

PELLERIN, Camille G.; 875 des Recollets, Trois Rivieres, P.Q.; Lav'55; Urol.; Tel. 375-8220.

PELLERIN, J. Richard; Lav'60; Res., Dept. of Health, U. of Montreal, Montreal, P.Q.

PELLERIN, Roland; 1800 Blvd. Pie IX, Montreal, P.Q.; 5160 des Sorbiers (res); Mon '31; Otol (P.Q.)., Ophth; Ass't. Clin. Instr. (Ophth.), Hotel Dieu de Montreal; Phys., Workmen's Comp. Bd., P.Q.; Tel. 522-1044.

PELLERIN, Wilfrid; 176 rue Sherbrooke, Magog, P.Q.; Lav'45; Anaes (P.Q.); Tel. 843-3440.

PELLETIER, Clement; St-Anselme, Cte Dorchester, P.Q.; Lav '61.

PELLETIER, Emile; Cap Chat, Cte. Gaspe, P.Q.; Lav '36; Otol (P.Q.); FAGS; M.C.G.P.; Dir., S. Shore St. Lawrence Med. Assoc.; Vice-Pres., Med. Staff, Hop. Ste. Anne des Monts; Tel. 786-5767.

PELLETIER, Fernand E.; 10 Lindsley, Chapais, Cte Abitibi, P.Q.; 30 Dufresne (res); Lav '53; Tel. 5516.

PELLETIER, Georges; Lav'65; Res., Dept. of Pharmacologie, University Laval, Quebec, P.Q.

PELLETIER, Georges E.; 298 Blvd. Labelle, St. Jerome, P.Q.; 608 Grande Allee (res); Lav '43; OphthOtol (P.Q.); Head, Dept. Otorhino & Ophth., Hotel Dieu, St. Jerome; Tel. 432-4301.

PELLETIER, Gerard, 114 Principale, St.-Guillaume-d'Upton, P.Q.; Lav '63.

PELLETIER, Gerard J.; 2 Rexgate, Rexdale, Ont.; Lav'45; Tel. CH 4-0431.

PELLETIER, Gilles; Mon'65; Res., Hop. des Laurentides, L'Annonciation, P.Q.

PELLETIER, Guy; App. 4, 768 Place Philippe, Quebec 10, P.Q.; Lav'59; Ph.D. (Experim. Med.).

PELLETIER, Helene E.; 5812 Pascale, Montreal-Nord, P.Q.; Mon '54; Staff, U. of Montreal.

PELLETIER, J. Alphonse; 1030 ave du-Parc, Quebec, P.Q. (res); Lav '28; NeurPsy; Psy-in-Chief, Women's Div., Hop.-St.Michel-Archange, Mastai; Staff, Laval U.; Tel. 663-3571.

PELLETIER, Jean; Lav '63; Int., Hop. St. Justine, Montreal, P.Q.

PELLETIER, Jean P.; 3958 Belanger est, Montreal, P.Q.; Lav '53; ObstGyn.; Tel. RA 5-3333.

PELLETIER, J. Emile; 34 de-la-Fabrique, Quebec 4, P.Q.; Lav '34; Opth, Otol; Staff (Ophth), Hotel-Dieu; Assoc. Prof., Laval U.; Tel. 523-0033.

PELLETIER, J. Jacques; 1229 de-la-Vigerie, Quebec 10, P.Q. (res); Lav '54; Anaes; Ass't., Hop.-Hotel-Dieu; Tel. MU 1-1264.

PELLETIER, J. O. Aime; 4395 Verdun, Verdun, P.Q.; Mon '40.

PELLETIER, J. Roger; 27 Henderson, Ottawa 2, Ont.; Ott'59; Psy; Staff, Ottawa Gen. Hosp.; Clin. Instr. Psy., U. of Ottawa; Tel. CE 3-5242.

PELLETIER, Leon; Gaspe, P.Q.; Lav '28; Gen. Surg.

PELLETIER, Leonard; 1577 Notre-Dame, Ancienne-Lorette, P.Q.; Lav '65.

PELLETIER, Louis A.; 1564-5eme Ave. Shawinigan-Sud, P.Q.; Lav '61.

PELLETIER, Louis C.; Mon'64; Res., Hop. Ste Justine, Montreal 26, P.Q.

PELLETIER, Louis P.; Pied de-la-Montagne, Ste-Melanie, P.Q.; Lav '31; IntMed (Cardiol.) (P.Q.).

PELLETIER, Micheline; Mon'65; Res., Hop. Notre-Dame, Montreal 25, P.Q.

PELLETIER, Noel; 122 St. Jean, Drummondville, P.Q.; 137 Blvd. Garon (res); Lav '57.

PELLETIER, Normand; 3145 Chemin Ste.-Foy, Quebec 10, P.Q.; Lav '58; Paed; Tel. 653-0235.

PELLETIER, Robert M.; 171 Mary St., Orillia, Ont.; Tor '52; Tel. 325-1394.

PELLETIER, Roger; R.R. No. 1, Edmundston, N.B.; Lav'60; Otol.; Tel. 735-7309.

PELLETIER Roger; 55 Emmerson, Edmundston, N.B.; Lav '64.

PELLETIER, T.; St. Leon Le Grand, Co. Matapedia, P.Q.; Lav '48.

PELLETIER, Urgel; 700 Edifice Laure, Sept-Iles, P.Q.; Lav '60.

PELOQUIN, Andre; 2730 Beaubien E., Apt. 5, Montreal, P.Q.; Mon '50; MCGP; Tel. RA 7-3232.

PELOQUIN, Antonin; 84 Ramesay, Sorel, P.Q.; Mon '50; Tel. RI 3-5869.

PELOQUIN, Andre B.; 1656 est, rue Sherbrooke, Ste. 201 Montreal 24, P.Q.; 7530 Boischatel (res); Mon '58; FRCS(C); GenSurg; Staff Hop. Notre-Dame; Tel. 521-2116.

PELOQUIN, Louis P.; 260 Main Ouest, Magog, P.Q.; 314 des Pins (res); Lav '36; D.P.H.

PELOQUIN, Lucien; 770 Hotel de Ville, St. Hyacinthe, P.Q.; Lav '30; Tel. PR 4-8148.

PELOQUIN, Robert; Mon'63; Res., Royal Victoria Hosp., Montreal 2, P.Q.

PELOQUIN, Ronald; 3576 Ontario St. E., Montreal 4, P.Q.; Mon '56; Tel. 525-6022.

PELTIER J. Andre; 240 rue Elm, St. Lambert, Cite Jacques-Cartier, P.Q.; Mon '51; FAGS; FASAS; NeurSurg; Chief of NeurSurg., St. Lambert Gen. Hosp.; Cons. NeurSurg., Hop. du Christ Roi & Hop. St. Jean; Tel. 671-1762.

PELTON, David A.; 31 Foursome Cres., Willowdale, Ont. (res); Tor '54; FRCP(C), Anaes; Staff, Hosp. for Sick Children; Clin. Teach. U. of Toronto; Tel. EM 6-7242.

PEMBER, Frank R.; Box 340, Division St., Colborne, Ont.; Tor'26; MCGP; Active Med. Staff, Cobourg Gen. Hosp.; Tel. 355-2101.

PENDER, Charles B.; 119 Sydney St., Cornwall, Ont.; 7 McKay Ave. (res); Qns '47; FAAP; Paed; Hd. Dept. of Paed., Hotel-Dieu Hosp.; Att'd. Staff (Paed), Cornwall Gen. Hosp.; Tel. WE 3-2123.

PENDELTON, Ralph L.; 100B-3rd Ave. S., Port Alberni, B.C.; 609-17th St. N. (res); Sask '57; MCGP; Tel. 723-6211.

PENDRIGH, R. M.; 219 Guilford St. W., St. John, N.B.; McG '21; GenSurg; Chief. Dept. of Surg., St. John Gen. Hosp.; Dist. Coroner; Tel. 693-3351.

PENDRY, Margaret A.; Box 382, Salmo, B.C.; London (Eng.)'62.

PENFIELD, Wilder G.; O.M., C.M.G., Legion of Hon. (Fr.); 4302 Montrose Ave., Montreal, P.Q. (res); Johns Hopkins (U.S.) '18; D.Sc. (McGill, Oxon, Princeton, UBC, Toronto, Leeds, Yale, N.Y.U., Man., Delhi, Wisconsin, Dartmouth); D.M. (U. of Montreal, Laval), D.C.L. (Bishop's, Oxon, Queen's); F.R.S.C., Hon. F.R.C.S. (Eng.), Hon. F.R.C.P. (Eng.), F.R.S. (Lond.), Ll.D. (U. Wales, Qns, Dal., St. Lawrence, Sask., Edin.), Litt.B. (Princeton) D. de l'U. (Paris), Med. Freedom (U.S.A.), F.R.S.M. (Lond.), F.R.C.S.(C), NeurSurg; Emer. Dir., Montreal Neurol. Inst., McGill U.; Mem. Bd. of Governors, McGill U.; Tel. AV 8-7320.

PENGELLY, G. Allan; 20 McKee Ave., Willowdale, Ont.; 810 Doris Ave. (res); Tor '51; A.M.-C.A.A., M.C.G.P.; Diabetic O.P.D., Toronto Western & Branson Hosp's.; Tel. 221-6383.

PENIKETT, Eric J.; Victoria Hosp., London, Ont.; London (Eng.) '53; MRCS; LRCP; M.C. (Path.); Ph.D.(Bact.); Dir., Dept. of Microbiol., Victoria Hosp.; Clin. Prof. (Bact.), U. of Western Ontario; Tel. 432-5261.

PENISTAN, John L.; 109 Mornington St., Stratford, Ont. (res); London (Eng.) '39; MD(Lond.); MRCP; LRCS; M.C.(Path.); Path; Chief, Dept. of Path., Stratford Gen. Hosp.; Cons. Path., St. Mary's Mem. Hosp.; Listowel Mem. Hosp. & Bruce County Gen. Hosp., Walkerton; Reg. Path., Dept. of Attorney Gen.; Tel. 271-2120, Ext. 255.

PENMAN, David; 53 Haultain Cr., Regina, Sask.; Edinburgh (Scot.) '50; M.B., Ch.B.; DPH; DTM&H.

PENMAN, Lillias E. (See Beale)

PENN, Israel; 109 Med. College, Emily & Bannatyne Sts., Winnipeg, Man.; Witwatersrand (S. Africa) '52; FRCS(Eng.); FRCS(C), Gen. Surg; Sr. Research Assoc., U. of Manitoba; Tel. 786-3575; Abroad.

PENN, Michael J. W.; 4474 W. Saanich Rd., Royal Oak, Vancouver Island, B.C.; 4045 Rainbow Rd., Victoria (res); Cambridge (Eng.) '53; M.R.C.S. (Lond.). Tel. GR 9-2593.

PENNAL, George F.; 272 Bloor St. W., Toronto 5, Ont.; 433 Kingsway (res); Tor '37; M.Ch. (Orth). D.A.B.O.S., F.R.C.S. (Edin.), F.R.C.S.(C), OrthSurg; Chief Surg. St. Joseph's Hosp.; Chief Orth Serv., Sunnybrook Hosp.; Clin. Instr., U. of Toronto; Tel. 924-2109.

PENNECOTT, Clifton W.; 49 Carfrae Cres., London, Ont.; Park Towers Apt., 808, 10 Beechwood Pl. (res); Wes '18; MCGP; Active Staff Victoria & St. Joseph's Hosp's.; Sec. & Memb. Advisory Comm. Parkwood Hosp.; Tel. CE 4-3441.

PENNER, Donald W.; 700 William Ave., Winnipeg 3, Man.; 56 River Rd., St. Vital (res); Man '42; FCAP; DABP; Path; Dir. & Chm. (Path), Wpg. Gen. Hosp.; Chief Path. & Chief of Staff, Victoria Gen. Hosp.; Path., Shriner's Hosp.; Cons. (Medico-legal), Prov. of Man.; Ass't. Prof. (Path), U. of Manitoba; Sec.-Treas., Cdn. Assoc. of Pathol.; Tel. SP 2-7487.

PENNER, Edgar; Man '61; Res., Deer Lodge Hosp., Winnipeg, Man.

PENNER, Ernest P.; Haig Clinic, 601-6th Ave. S., Lethbridge, Alta.; Alb'62; AMCGP.

PENNER, Erwin H.; 310 Nairn Ave., Winnipeg 5, Man.; Man'55; Tel. 533-2604.

PENNER, Harold U.; Man'51; MCGP; Res., Hosp. for Mental Diseases, Selkirk, Man.

PENNER, Leonard U.; 107-2nd Ave. E., Kindersley, Sask.; 200-7th Ave. E. (res); Man '51; MCGP; Active Staff, Union Hosp.; Assoc. Staff, Eston Union Hosp., Eston; District Coroner; Tel. 463-2621.

PENNER, Lorne; Box 640, Steinbach, Man.; Man'58.

PENNER, Raymond C.; 1940 Lonsdale Ave, North Vancouver, B.C.; Man'62; Tel. YU 5-4177.

PENNEY, Robert H.; Ste. 14, East Gen. Hosp., 825 Coxwell Ave., Toronto 13, Ont.; 1 Alder Rd. (res); Tor'42; FRCP(C), IntMed; Att'd. Staff, Toronto East Gen. Hosp.; Tel. HO 6-8123.

PENNINGTON, P. W.; 396 Queens Ave., London, Ont.; Tor '63; AMCGP; Tel. 433-3154.

PENNOCK, George M.; 7 Clarendon Ave., Ottawa, Ont.; 557 Dovercourt Ave. (res); Tor '21; Hon Cons. Staff, Civic & Grace Hosp's.; Tel. 728-9548.

PENNY, Cherer G.; 10155-120th St., Edmonton, Alta.; Witwatersrand (S. Africa)'47; DTM&H; Plant Phys., Chemcell (Canada) Ltd.; Preceptor, Dept. of Commun. Med., U. of Alberta; Tel. 488-7271.

PENNY, S/L John A.; Sask'59; Staff, Canadian Forces Hosp., Kingston, Ont.

PENNY, Stuart F.; 526 Fourth Ave. W., Owen Sound, Ont.; Tor'34; PathBact; Pathol., General & Marine Hosp.

PENROSE, George S.; Medical Arts Clinic, 51-6th St. S.E., Medicine Hat, Alta.; McG'52; Anaes.; Staff, Medicine Hat Gen. Hosp.; Tel. 527-2281.

PENTLAND, Ernest S.; Middlesex County Bldg., Ridout St. N. & King, London, Ont.; Tor'40; DPH; MCGP.

PENTON, R. Bruce; 141 Church St., St. Catharines, Ont.; Tor '50; MCGP; Active Staff, St. Catharines Gen. & Hotel-Dieu Hosp's.; Coroner & Inspector of Anatomy; Tel. MU 4-9477.

PEPIN, Andre; 31 Montcalm, Hull, P.Q.; Mon '60; AMCGP; Tel. 776-1273.

PEPIN, Gerard; 73 rue Laval, Hull, P.Q.; Mon '50; ObstGyn (PQ); AMCGP; Staff, (ObstGyn), Hop.-Sacre-Coeur; Tel. PR 7-5582.

PEPIN, Jean M.; 31 King St. W., Sherbrooke, P.Q.; 590 Villeneuve (res); **Mon '55; F.R.C.P.(C), IntMed; Tel. 569-5838.**

PEPPER, Verne W.; Ste. 305, 625-5th Ave., New Westminster, B.C.; Tor'38; B.Sc.; FRCS(C); ObstGyn; Staff, Royal Columbian & St. Mary's Hosp's.

PEQUEGNAT, Homer M.; 193 Frederick St., Kitchener, Ont.; Tor'32; Tel. SH 5-7742.

PEQUEGNAT, Leon A.; 390 Christie St., Toronto, Ont.; Tor'19; D.A.B. Prev. M. & P.H.; PH; Med. Admin., Pilot Home Care Programme, Dept. of Public Health, Toronto; Tel. LE 3-2601.

PERALES, Alberto; San Marcos (Lima, Peru)'59; B.Sc.; Staff, Hop. St. Charles, Joliette, P.Q.

PERAMAKI, Raymond T.; Wes'62; Res., Ottawa Civic Hosp., Ottawa 3, Ont.

PERCHANOK, Morris R.; Med. Arts Bldg., 420 East St. N., Sarnia, Ont.; Dal '50; IntMed.; Chief of Med., Sarnia Gen. Hosp.; Tel. ED 6-6381.

PERCHESON, Anne C.; 573 Mountain Ave., Winnipeg 4, Man.; Tor'61; Tel. 586-1058.

PERCHESON, John A.; 262 St. Clair Ave. W., Toronto.; 835 Bayview (res); Qns '33.

PERCHESON, Paul T.; 573 Mountain Ave., Win-nipeg 4, Man.; Tor'56; D.P.H.; Tel. 586-1058.

PERCHESON, Peter B.; 6325 Fraser St., Vancouver 15, B.C.; 3837 Cypress St., Van. 9, (res); Qns '43; DA (Eng.); FACA; FRCP(C), Anaes; Active Staff, Grace & Burnaby Gen. Hosp's.; Clin. Instr., (Anaes), U. of British Columbia; Tel. FA 5-4040.

PERCIVAL, Eleanor S.; 280 Seaforth Med. Bldg., 3550 Cote des Neiges Rd., Montreal 25, P.Q.; McG '22; FRCS(C); ObstGyn; Assoc. Obst-Gyn., Montreal Gen. Hosp.; ObstGyn., Royal Victoria Hosp.; **Obst., Catherine Booth Hosp.; Cons. Gyn.,** Reddy Memorial Hosp.; Ass't. Prof. (ObstGyn.), McGill U.; Tel. 935-9344.

PERCIVAL, John A.; 262 St. Clair Ave. W., Tor-onto 7, Ont.; 9 Valleyanna Dr. (res); Qns '33; **Tel. WA 3-9645.**

PERCIVAL, Ralph; 85 Clyde St., Lachute, P.Q.; Dal '31; Tel. LO 2-5151.

PERCIVAL-SMITH, Robin K.; 814 Cook Rd., Richmond, B.C.; 830 Granville Ave. (res); Cambridge (Eng.) '56; Tel. 278-2191.

PERCIVAL, Walter L.; 1598 Ouellette, Windsor, Ont.; 889 Kildare Rd. (res); McG '43; D.S., F.A.C.S., F.I.C.S.; GenSurg; Att. Staff, Grace, Hotel Dieu & Metropolitan Gen. Hosp's.; Tel. CL 3-2282.

PERCY, Edward C.; 700 Seaforth Med. Bldg., **3550 Cote des Neiges Rd., Montreal 25, P.Q.; 15 Grenville Ave., Westmount (res); McG '51;** M.Sc., FACS; FRCS(C); OrthSurg; Staff, Montreal Gen. & Children's Hosp's.; Lect. McGill U.; Tel. 932-0683.

PEREIRA, Cecil J.; Sedgewick, Alta.; Welsh Nat. School of Med. (Cardiff, Wales) '50; DMS (Madras, India); LRCP (Lond.); MRCS (Eng.); Staff, Killam Gen. Hosp.; Tel. 384-3805.

PEREIRA, Ethel E.; 5991 Spring Garden Rd., Halifax, N.S.; Madras(India) '53; MRCOG; FRCS(C), ObstGyn; Active Staff, Halifax Infirmary; Court. Staff, Grace Maternity & Victoria **Gen. Hosp's.; Lect., Dalhousie U.; Tel. 423-8647.**

PEREIRA, Valdemar L.; Coimbra (Portugal)'59; FRCP(C), Paed; Staff, Hop. de l'Enfant Jesus, Quebec 3, P.Q.

PERERA, Frank A.; 5903 Arbutus Ave., Powell River, B.C.; Cambridge (Eng.) '55; FRCP(C), IntMed; Tel. 483-9355.

PERESZLENYI, Akos; 964 Albion Rd., Rex-dale, Ont.; Pecs. (Hungary)'49; Tel. 741-1421.

PERETZ, Arthur W.; Hollyburn Med. Centre, **520-17th St., West Vancouver, B.C.; 890 Anderson Cres. (res); Vienna (Aust.) '36 FAGS, FIGA;** Att'd. Staff, Lionsgate Hosp.; Vis. Staff, St. Paul's Hosp.; Tel. WA 2-4720.

PERETZ, Dwight I.; 1081 Burrard St., Vancouver 1, B.C.; UBC '56; M.Sc. (Exper.Med.); FRCP-(C), IntMed; Dir. Intensive Care, (Cardiores.) Unit, St. Paul's Hosp.; Clin. Instr. Med., U. of B.C.; Tel. 685-3131.

PEREY, Bernard J.; 687 Pine Ave. W., Montreal 2, P.Q.; 54 Roxton Cres., Montreal West (res); McG '56; M.Sc.; Dip Surg. (McGill); FRCS(C); GenSurg; Ass't. Surg. & Dir. of Clinics & Emergency, Royal Victoria Hosp.; Ass't. Prof. Surg., McGill U.; Tel. VI 2-3080.

PERFECT, Kenneth E.; 201 Annette St., Toronto, Ont. Tor '29; Tel. RO 9-0628.

PERIGNY, Yvon; 1259 Hart, Trois Rivieres, P.Q.; 280 de Lavaltrie (res); Lav '53; FRCS(C); GenSurg; Surg., Hop. St. Joseph; Tel. FR 5-6679.

PERITI, G. C.; Workmen's Comp. Bldg., 90 Harbour St., Toronto 1, Ont.; Tel. 362-3411.

PERKIN, Reginald L.; 2200 Dixie Rd., Cooksville, Ont.; Tor '54; M.C.G.P.; Active Staff, Queensway Gen. & South Peel Hosp's.; Tel. 277-2761.

PERKINS, James R.; 460 Eglinton Ave. E., Toronto 12, Ont; 48 Wanless Cres. (res); Tor. '56; Tel. HU 3-5134.

PERKINS, Stanley H.; 901 Barton St. E., Hamilton, Ont.; 42 Rothsay Gdns. (res); Qns '19; Psy., Indust. Surg., Wallace Barnes Co. Ltd.; Staff, Hamilton Gen. Hosp.; Ont. Athletic Comm. Doctor, Hamilton; Tel. LI 4-3682.

PERL, Anthony F.; 137 Wellington St., Sarnia, Ont.; (res); Vienna (Aust.) '36; FACP, FCCP; IntMed; Cons. Staff, St. Joseph's & Sarnia Gen. Hosp's.; Tel. 344-5261.

PERLER, Zelick; 40 Elm St., Tenafly, N.J., U.S.A.; Alb'59; Urol; Abroad.

PERLEY, Donald A.; Box 400, Grand Forks, B.C. Alb '39; M.C.G.P.; Dist. Coroner.

PERLIN, Irving A.; 5750 South St., Halifax, N.S.; 966 Greenwood Ave. (res); Dal '43; FACS, FICS, FACOG; ObstGyn; Assoc. Gyn., Victoria Gen. Hosp.; Assoc. Obst., Grace Matern. Hosp.; Assoc. Prof. (ObstGyn), Dalhousie U.; Tel. 423-8864.

PERLMAN, Isaac; Ste. 606, 750 W. Broadway, Vancouver 9, B.C.; Sask'62; AMCGP; Tel. 874-4433.

PEROT, Phanor L.; 3801, University St., Montreal, P.Q.; Tulane (New Orleans, U.S.A.) '52; Ph.D., FACS; Ass't. Neurosurg., Montreal Neurological Inst.; Clin. Ass't. (Neurol.), Royal Victoria Hosp.; Ass't. Prof. (NeurSurg.), McGill U.; Tel. AV 8-0764.

PERRAS, Colette; 3737 ave Lacombe, Montreal 26, P.Q.; 6255 North Crest Pl., Apt. 502 (res); Mon '48; PlasSurg (P.Q.); Instr. (Surg.), Hotel-Dieu-de-Montreal; Tel. 737-3105.

PERRAS, J. Rene; 267 O'Connor St., Ottawa, Ont.; 60 Onslaw Cres. (res); Tor '32; Obst (P.Q.); Tel. 232-1383.

PERRAS, Loyola; 1153 rue Sussex, Montreal, P.Q.; 530 ave. Grosvenor, Westmount (res); Mon '26; FICA; Anaes.; Dir. Anaes., Hop. Ste. Justine; Tel. RE 1-4931.

PERRAS, Pierre; Lav '55; DiagRad; Staff, Hop. Jean-Talon, Montreal 35, P.Q.

PERRAULT, Antonio; 535 St.-Anne, St. Hyacinthe, P.Q.; 2655 Girouard (res); Mon '29; GenSurg.; Surg., St. Hyacinthe Gen. Hosp.; Tel. PR 4-6811.

PERRAULT, Marcel; 805 Ste. Anne St., St. Hyacinthe, P.Q.; Lav '51; Staff, St. Charles Hosp.; Tel. PR 4-5419.

PERRAULT, Rene; Clinique Medico-Chirurgicale, 2775 rue Bourdages, St. Hyacinthe, P.Q.; Mon '57; FRCS(C), GenSurg; Tel. PR 3-0461.

PERRAULT, Roger A.; Apt. 108, 344 Dundas St., Ottawa, Ont.; Ott '63; Research Ass't. Dept. of Path, NDMC.

PERREAULT, Gaston; 4582 boul. Ste-Rose, Fabreville, P.Q.; Mon '58.

PERREAULT, Gerard A.; Lav'65; Res., Hop. St. Sacrement, Quebec 6, P.Q.

PERREAULT, Gilles; Mon'63; Res., Hop. Notre-Dame, Montreal 24, P.Q.

PERREAULT, Gilles P.; 8415 St. Denis, Montreal, P.Q.; Mon '58; IntMed(P.Q.); Gastroent (P.Q.); Staff, Hop. Jean Talon; Tel. 381-5311.

PERREAULT, Henri; 407 ave-de-Lorraine, Longueuil, Cite-Jacques-Cartier, P.Q. (res); Mon '57; Anaes; Staff, Hop. Gen., St. Lambert; Tel. 677-7288.

PERREAULT, J. Daniel; Mon'65; Res., Hop. Maisonneuve, Montreal 36, P.Q.

PERREAULT, Jean-Guy; 1740 du Bocage, St-Bruno, P.Q.; Mon'55; DiagRad.

PERRAULT, Jean L.; Mon'65; Res., Hop. Notre-Dame, Montreal 24, P.Q.

PERREAULT, Joseph C.; 15105 Stony Plain Rd., Edmonton, Alta.; **McG '23; Tel. 489-6222.**

PERREAULT, J. Philibert; 4402 St. Hubert St., Montreal, P.Q.; 4400 St. Hubert St. (res); Mon '27; Obst (P.Q.); Tel. LA 1-6100.

PERREAULT, Luc; 11300 Frigon, Montreal 12, P.Q.; Lav '52; Anaes (P.Q.); Staff, Hop. Ste-Jeanne-d'Arc; Tel. VI 2-5201.

PERRAULT, Raymond; Lav'65; Res., Hop. Ste-Justine, Montreal 26, P.Q.

PERREAULT, Robert; 585 Villeray, Montreal 10, P.Q.; Mon '65.

PERRAULT, Roger Sg/Lt.; Nat. Defence Med. Centre, Smyth Rd. & Alta Vista, Ottawa 8, Ont.; Ott'63.

PERREAULT, Wilfrid J. E.; 3482 est Ste Catherine, Montreal, P.Q.; 5175 des Sorbiers (res); Mon '36; GenSurg; Surg., Hop. Ste. Jeanne d'Arc; Tel. LA 3-1665.

PERRETT, Thomas S.; 707 W. 37th Ave., Vancouver 13, B.C.; 5761 Marguerite St. (res); Tor '32; FRCS(C), GenSurg; Att'd. Staff, Vancouver Gen. Hosp.; Staff, WCB; Ass't. (Surg.), U. of British Columbia; Tel. MU 4-1511.

PERRIER, Arcade; 282 Principale est, Hawkesbury, Ont.; **Mon '40; Dist. Coroner.**

PERRIER, Romeo; 5591 Cote-des-Neiges, Montreal 26, P.Q.; Mon '60; Tel. RE 1-7291.

PERRIGARD, Gordon Eric; Ste. 1009, Med. Arts Bldg., 1538 Sherbrooke St. W., Montreal, P.Q.; McG '41; AICS; GenSurg; M.O., Dept. of Public Health, City of Montreal; Vis. Staff, Hop. Jean Talon; Tel. WE 2-2844.

PERRIN, Donald R.; 15 Court House Ave., Brockville, Ont.; 16 Church St. (res); Qns '57; DNBME; FABAS; GenSurg; Cons. Surg., Ontario Hosp.; Active Surg. Staff, Brockville Gen. & St. Vincent de Paul Hosp's.; Tel. 345-1068.

PERRIN, Jyneen G.; 6 Court Terrace, Brockville, Ont.; Qns'61; Ophth.

PERRIN, W. Harper; 6 Court House Ave., Brockville, Ont.; Qns'24.

PERRON, Jacques; 1000 Chemin-Ste-Foy, Quebec 10, P.Q.; Lav'57; Ophth; Tel. 681-7977; Abroad.

PERRON, Jean M.; Mon '62; Res., Vancouver Gen. Hosp., Vancouver 9, B.C.

PERRON, Jean-Luc, Major; CFPO 5050, IFA RCAMC, via Belleville, Ont., MRS Cdn. Forces Europe; Lav'61; Abroad.

PERRON, Joseph; 589 Bennett, Montreal 4, P.Q.; **Mon '51; Tel. 255-9894.**

PERRON, Joseph M.; 12 ave. Mercier, Shawinigan Falls, P.Q.; Mon '20; DiagRad (P.Q.), Anaes; Retired.

PERRON, Louis; 9023 boul. Lasalle, Lasalle, P.Q.; Mon'61; FRCP(C); IntMed.

PERRON, Lucien; 964 rue Cherrier, Montreal 24, P.Q.; 61 Riverside Dr. (res); Mon '36; Ophth-Otol.; Tel. LA 6-3339.

PERRON, Marcel; Mon'62; Staff, Hop. Hotel-Dieu, Alma, P.Q.

PERRON, Marcel; 389 Boul. St.-Jude, Alma, P.Q.; Mon '62.

PERRON, Paul; 2915 Maplewood, Apt. 505, Montreal 26, P.Q.; Lav '53; Anaes; Staff, Hop.-Hotel-Dieu; Tel. 733-7337.

PERRON, Stanislas; 5160 Notre Dame Ouest, Montreal 30, P.Q.; 2930 Maplewood, Apt. 209 (res); Mon '21; Tel. WE 3-4738.

PERRY, Albert E. B.; 306 Medical & Dental Bldg., Regina, Sask.; 2187 Montague St. (res); Tor '30; D&TRad; Dir., Dept. Rad., Grey Nuns' Hosp.; Cons., Cancer Clin., Regina; Tel. JO 9-9621.

PERRY, Albert W.; 316 Yarrow Bldg., 645 Fort St., Victoria, B.C.; 804 Foul Bay Rd. (res); Qns '45; FRCP(C), IntMed; Active Staff, Royal Jubilee & D.V.A. Hosp's.; Assoc. Staff, St. Joseph's Hosp.; Tel. EV 6-1812.

PERRY, Barbara E.; 19 Totteridge Rd., Islington, Ont.; Tor '39.

PERRY, John R.; 909 Sherritt Ave., Lynn Lake, Man.; Sheffield (Eng.)'58; Med. Supt., Sherritt Gordon Mines Hosp.; District Coroner; D.O.T. Examiner; M.O., C.N.R.; Deputy M.O.H., Lynn Lake; Surg. Lieut., RCSCC; Tel. FL 6-2288.

PERRY, John W.; Medical Clinic, Innisfail, Alta.; Wales'62; Medical Staff of local Hospitals; Tel. 227-3419.

PERRY, Kathleen V.; Box 640, Innisfail, Alta.; Cardiff (Wales)'64.

PERRY, Paul E.; Tor '58; D.Psy; Psy; Dir. O.P.D., York County Hosp., Newmarket, Ont.; Tel. 895-4521.

PERRY, Robert J.; Qns'64; Res., Kingston Gen. Hosp., Kingston, Ont.

PERRY, Roland A.; 2-251 Bedford Highway, Rockingham, N.S.; Dal'61; AMCGP; Medical Examiner, Halifax County; Tel. 455-3121.

PERRY, Victor R., M.B.E.; 19 Totteridge Rd., Islington, Ont.; Tor '39; Phys., Indust., Steel Co. of Canada, Swansea, Toronto 3 & Continental Can Co. of Can.

PERRY-WHITTINGHAM, B. D.; Box 138, Sooke, B.C.; UBC '63.

PERRY, William F.; 145 McLaughlin Ave., St. James, Man. (res); **Qns '46; FACS; Dir., Clin. Chem., Winnipeg Gen. Hosp.; Assoc. Prof. (Physiol), U. of Manitoba; Tel. SP 4-6511.**

PERSYKO, Lucien; Wes '64; Res., Victoria Gen. Hosp., Halifax, N.S.

PERVERSEFF, John I.; Box 9, Hardisty, Alta.; Man '31; MCGP; Dist. Coroner.

PESANT, Laurent; Mon'41; FRCS(C); GenSurg; Staff, Hop. St. Luc, Montreal 18, P.Q.

PESANT, Pierre, J. A.; Clinique Metropolitaine, 1150 est, Boul. St.-Joseph, Montreal 34, P.Q.; 77 Le-moyne Repentigny (res); Mon '52; IntMed; Tel. LA 7-1241.

PESTRI, Tatiana; 7 Raymond St., St. Catharines, Ont.

PETERFY, George; Allan Mem. Inst., 1025 Pine Ave. W., Montreal 2, P.Q.; 6 Simcoe Ave., Mtl. 16; Budapest (Hung.)'54; Psy; Ass't. & Research Psy., Allan Mem. Inst.; Ass't. Psy., Royal Victoria Hosp.; Lect., McGill U.; Tel. VI 2-1251, Loc. 742.

PETERKIN, Edith K.; 216 McDonald Ave., Belleville, Ont.; Man '46; Paed; Active Cons. Staff, Belleville Gen. Hosp., Tel. 968-7400.

PETERKIN, F. David; 887A Corydon Ave., Winnipeg 9, Man.; Man '52; Tel. 475-0876.

PETERS, Ago; 1192 Weston Rd., Weston, Ont.; Wes '58; Tel. RO 6-7611.

PETERS, Alexander; 6 Glen Watford Dr., Agincourt, Ont.; Tor'65.

PETERS, Charles A.; D.S.O.; 1414 Drummond St., Montreal, P.Q.; 17 Decasson Rd., Westmount (res); McG '01; L.L.D., D.C.L. (Bishop's), M.R.C.S. (Eng.), L.R.C.P. (Lond.), F.R.C.P.(C), Cons. Staff, Montreal Gen. Hosp.; Tel. WE 7-6011.

PETERS, Ella L.; 401 Boreham Blvd., Tuxedo. Winnipeg, Man. (res); Man '35; M.P.H. (Harvard); Dir., Bureau of Maternal & Child Hygiene, Dept. of Health & Public Welfare, Prov. of Man.; Tel. WH 6-7207.

PETERS, Estelle **(See Mackrell)**

PETERS, E. S.; McG '33; IntMed; West Coast San., Corner Brook, Nfld.; Tel. 634-5232.

PETERS, James A.; 132 Norfolk St. S., Simcoe, Ont.; Wes'56; FRCS(C), GenSurg.; Tel. 426-3031.

PETERS, John C.; Manitoba Clinic, 790 Sherbrook St., Winnipeg 2, Man.; Man'60; Paed; Active Staff, Children's & Grace Hosp's.; Lect., U. of Manitoba; Tel. SP 4-6541.

PETERS, M. Vera (Lobb); 15 Blyth Hill Rd., Toronto 12 (res); Tor '34; TherRad; Sr. TherRad., Princess Margaret Hosp. & Dept. of TherRad., Toronto Gen. Hosp.; Assoc. Prof. (TherRad. & Biophysics), U. of Toronto; Tel. 924-0671.

PETERS, Olivier R.; Rothesay, N.B.; McG '02; Dist. Coroner.

PETERS, Paul F.; Box 489, Steinbach, Man.; Man. '59; Tel. DA 6-3404.

PETERS, Rudolph V.; 169 William St., Pembroke, Ont.; Cambridge (Eng.) '43; DPH; Dir. & M.O., Renfrew County Health Unit; Tel. 735-5784.

PETERS, William G.; 399 Dibble St. W., Prescott, Ont.; Qns'53; MCGP; Chief of Staff, St. Vincent de Paul Hosp., Brockville; Tel. 925-2839.

PETERSEN, John E.; 3490 Saanich Rd., Victoria, B.C.; 1200 Judge Pl. (res); Alb '58; AMCGP; Tel. 388-5321.

PETERSON, Arnold D.; Smith Clinic, Camrose, Alta.; Alb '58.

PETERSON, Clinton P.; Apt. 412, 200 Ridley Blvd., Toronto 12, Ont.; Qns '23; Staff Phys., Health Centre, Parliament Bldg's.

PETERSON, Constantine L.; Med. Centre, 1428 Ouellette Ave., Windsor, Ont.; 863 Kildare Rd. (res); Tor'45; FRCS(N), FICS; FACA; FRCS(C), GenSurg; Sr. Surg., Hotel-Dieu & Metropolitan Gen. Hosp's.; Chief (Cardiovas. & Thor. Surg.), Grace Hosp.; Cons., ThorSurg., Neoplas Clin., Cdn. Cancer Fdn.; Tel. 256-0440.

PETERSON, David M.; Box 279, Parksville, B.C.; Man '55.

PETERSON Edward R.; 241 Canada Bldg., Saskatoon, Sask.; 931 University Dr. (res); McG '38; FACS, FICS, GenSurg; Att. Surg., St. Paul's, University & City Hosp's.; Clin. Teacher, Saskatchewan U. Med School; Tel. 244-4937.

PETERSON, Eric W.; 300 Cooper St., Ottawa 4, Ont.; 2 DeLong Dr., Rothwell Hgts. (res); McG '42; DABNS; FRCS(C), NeurSurg; Sr. NeurSurg., Ottawa Gen. & NeurSurg., Ottawa Civic Hosp's.; Cons. (NeurSurg), St. Louis-Marie-de-Montfort, St. Vincent's & Sacred Heart Hosp's. & NDMC; Assoc. Prof. (NeurSurg), U. of Ottawa; Tel. 233-3851.

PETERSON, John; 94 Guestville, Toronto, Ont.; Tor '53; MCGP; Tel. RO 3-1171.

PETERSON, Natalie; St. Barbara's Clinic, 226 Bathurst St., Toronto 2B, Ont.; Latvia'35; Tel. 366-3134.

PETITCLERC, C.; 3038 De La Forest, app. 2, Ste-Foy, P.Q.; '61; Haem(P.Q.).

PETITCLERC, Lucien; St. Augustin, Co. Portneuf, P.Q.; Lav '30.

PETITCLERC, Robert; Lav'65; Res., Hop. Notre-Dame, Montreal 24, P.Q.

PETITCLERC, Roland; Lav '55; Psy; Staff, Clinique Roy-Rousseau, Chemin de la Canardiere, Quebec 5, P.Q.; Tel. 661-7735.

PETKAU, Abram; Whiteshell Nuclear Research, Atomic Energy of Canada Ltd., Pinawa, Man.; **Man '60; Hd. of Med. Research; Tel. 753-2311.**

PETKOVICH, Narcis J.; 1303 Elliot St., Saskatoon, Sask.; Zagreb (Yugo.)'57; IntMed.

PETRASEK, Anthony; 38 Surrey Dr., Montreal 16, P.Q.; Tor '53; FRCP(C); Anaes; Anaes., St. Mary's Hosp.; Dem. (Anaes.), McGill U.; Tel. 735-2511.

PETRELLA, Nick J.; 30 St. Joseph Blvd. E., Montreal 14, P.Q.; Ott'65.

PETREMAN, Melvin C.; 401 Johnston Rd., Alberni, B.C.; Sask'65.

PETRIE, Charles B.; 215 Cooper St., Ottawa, Ont.; 124 Springfield (res); McG '35; GenSurg; Chief of Staff, Ottawa Civic Hosp.; Sr. Lect. (ClinSurg.), U. of Ottawa; Tel. CE 4-4080.

PETRIE, David P.; McG'64; Res., St. Michael's Hosp., Toronto 2, Ont.

PETRIE, Donald J.; Stouffville Med. Centre, 200 Main St. W., Stouffville, Ont.; 115 Lloyd St. (res); Tor '57; MCGP; Staff, Tor. E. Gen., Scarboro Gen. & Uxbridge Cottage Hosp's.; Tel. 640-3100.

PETRIE, Edward A.; Rothesay, N.B. (res); **McG '24; FACR, DABR, D&TRad; Rad., St. Joseph's Hosp.; Cons. Rad., Lancaster & Provincial Hosp's., Lancaster; Kings County Hosp., Sussex; Tel. 4-2651.**

PETRIE, Edward A.; 206 Rookwood Ave., Fredericton, N.B.; McG'59; Anaes; Active Staff, Victoria Public Hosp.; Tel. 475-7701.

PETRIE, Ian B.; 55 Avondale Blvd., Bramalea, Ont.; Edinburgh (Scot.)'62; D.ObstRCOG.

PETRIE, James G.; 1374 Sherbrooke St. W., Montreal, P.Q.; 3230 Westmount Blvd. (res); McG '36; FRCS(C), OrthSurg; Surg.-in-Charge (Orth.). Royal Victoria Hosp.; Chief Surg., Shriner's Hosp. for Special Surg.; Tel. VI 9-5164.

PETRIE, Richard A.; McG'63; Res., Royal Victoria Hosp., Montreal 2, P.Q.

PETRIN, Philippe; 333 Marie Victorin, Vercheres, P.Q.; Mon'61; Tel. 583-3755.

PETRINACK, Nicholas F.; Box 360, Birtle, Man.; Man'58; MCGP; Chief of Staff, Birtle District Hosp.; Tel. 842-5250.

PETRIW, Joseph; Ste 202, 1541 West Broadway, Vancouver 9, B.C.; 1520 Harwood (res); Vienna (Austria) '47; Tel. RE 1-5388.

PETROPOULAKIS, Ares; 329 St. George St., Toronto 5, Ont.; Athens (Greece) '38; M.S. (Tor.); Court. Obst. Staff, Toronto Gen. Hosp.; Active Surg. Staff, Central Hosp.; Tel. WA 5-1291.

PETROVITCH-PANNETON, Leposova; Mon '57; Staff, Sanatorium St-Laurent, 20 rue Pharand, Hull, P.Q.

PETROWSKI, Igor; 239 Niagara St., St. Catharines, Ont.; Rostov (Russia)'41; Tel. 684-5363.

PETRYK-POTOSKI, Stephanie (Petryk); See Potoski, Stephanie).

PETT, L. Bradley; 270 Harmer Ave., Ottawa 3 Ont.; Alb'41; MA; PhD; CPH; PH; Deputy Dir General, Health Serv., Dept. of National Health & Welfare; Tel. 992-5394.

PETTIGREW, Antoine; App. 6, 610 Chemin St-Louis, Quebec 6, P.Q.; Lav'33; GenSurg; Assoc. Prof., Laval U.

PETTIGREW, Jacques; Ayer's Cliff, Co. Stanstead, P.Q.; Lav '49; GenSurg (P.Q.).

PETTIGREW, Michael; 533 Taylor St., Saskatoon, Sask.; Sheffield (Eng.) '47.

PETTIGREW, Reginald W.; 18 Pinecrest, Fonthill, Ont.; Edinburgh (Scot.)'43; FCCP; DMR; DiagRad; Radiol., Port Colborne Gen. Hosp., Douglas Mem. Hosp., Fort Erie & Haldimand Dist. Hosp., Dunnville.

PETTIMAN, Frank E.; 3504-20th St., Vernon, B.C.; (res); Tor '10; Retired; Staff (Med.), I.O.D.E. Hosp.

PETTY, Ross E.; Sask'65; Res., University Hosp., Saskatoon, Sask.

PFEIFER, John R.; Peterborough Clinic, 327 Charlotte St., Peterborough, Ont.; Sask'58; DABS; Tel. 743-2040.

PFEIFFER, Walter M.; 555 Casgrain, St. Lambert P.Q. (res); Lav '30; MCGP; M.O., Dept. of Nat. Health & Welfare; Tel. 845-1300. Retired.

PFLUG, Michael; 43 Woodlawn Ave. W., Toronto 7, Ont.; Paris (France)'60; FRCP(C); Int Med; Senior Fellow, Research Assoc., Toronto General Hospital.

PHAIR, William B.; 98 Guestville Ave., Toronto 9, Ont.; R.R. 3, King (res); Tor '40; IntMed; Staff, Humber Mem. Hosp., Weston; Tel. 763-1171.

PHANEUF, Gabriel; 2775 Bourdages, St-Hyacinthe, P.Q.; Mon '60; IntMed (P.Q.), Cardiol (P.Q.); Tel. 774-5050.

PHANEUF, Georges .; 6544 St. Denis St., Montreal, P.Q.· Mon '38; Tel. 279-3898.

PHANEUF-FILION, Gisele; Apt. 5, 4343 Jeanne d'Arc, Montreal 36, P.Q. (res); Mon '48; Staff, Health Serv., Montreal; Tel. 872-3360.

PHANEUF, Irene A.; 5655 St. Zotique St. E., Montreal 36, P.Q.; Man'45; Anaes; Dir., Dept. of Anaes., Santa Cabrini Hosp.; Tel. CL 4-8311, Ext. 238.

PHANEUF, Jacques; 230 rue Longueuil, St.-Jean, P.Q.; 320 St.-Hubert (res); Mon '47; F.A.C.S., F.R.C.S.(C), GenSurg; Surg., Hop.-St.-Jean; Tel. 6-6871.

PHANEUF, Jean; 24 des Erables, Co. Rouville, St. Hilaire, P.Q. (res); Mon '47; Anaes; Staff, (Anaes), Hop. St. Charles; Tel. PR 4-5331.

PHANEUF, Jean G.; 228 Longueuil, St. Jean, P.Q.; 230 Longueuil (res); Mon'52; Anaes.; Tel. 843-6856.

PHANEUF, Marcel; 12774 ouest Gouin, Pierrefonds, P.Q.; Mon'56; GenSurg.

PHANEUF, Paul; 230 Longueuil, St. Jean, P.Q.; **99 Bouthillier (res); Mon '52; FRCS(C); FACS; GenSurg; Tel. FI 7-3210.**

PHARAND, Marielle (See Lapointe).

PHELPS, Albert H.; 299 Main St., Chilliwack, B.C.; 30 - 1st Ave. (res); Tor '47; **F.A.C.S., GenSurg; Att. Staff, Chilliwack Gen. Hosp.; Cons.** Staff, Coqualeetza Indian Hosp.; Tel. 792-1556.

PHELPS, Eric L.; Ste 440, 5025 Sherbrooke St. W., Montreal, P.Q., 5761 Cote-St.-Luc (res); McG '44; ObstGyn; Staff, Queen Elizabeth, Catherine Booth, & Herbert Reddy Mem. Hosp's; Cons., Verdun Prot. Hosp.; Tel. 482-5158.

PHELPS, F. Learn; 32 Albert St., Ste. Agathe des Monts, P.Q. (res); McG '16; F.C.C.P., IntMed (TB); Med. Dir., Royal Edward Laurentian Hosp., Laurentian Div., Ste. Agathe des Monts; Retired.

PHELPS, Roy C.; 176 Oakdale Ave., Merritton, Ont.; Tor '13; Retired.

PHENIX, Georges A. F.; 83 St. Jacques St., St. Jean, P.Q.; 81 St. Jacques St. (res); Lav '12. Retired.

PHILCOX, Herbert A.; 350 Albert St., Nanaimo B.C.; R.R. No. 2 (res); Guy's Hosp. (London, Eng.) '44; OrthSurg; Tel. 753-3431.

PHILIBERT, R. Paul; Lav '54; Path; Dir. of Labs. & Pathol., Hop. Ste-Marie, Trois-Rivieres, P.Q.; Tel. FR 5-7721.

PHILIP, William F.; Tor '61; Jr. Intn., Toronto East Gen. Hosp., Toronto 6, Ont.

PHILIPPIDJIS, Paris J.; Ste. 32B, 31 Yonge St. N., Richmond Hill, Ont.; Athens (Greece)'54; Urol.

PHILIPPON, Fernand; Lav '61; FRCP(C), IntMed; Staff, Hop.-Hotel-Dieu-de-Quebec, Quebec 4, P.Q.; Abroad.

PHILIPPON, Pontien; 2012, Chapdelaine, Quebec 10, P.Q.; Lav'54; GenSurg (P.Q.); Tel. 683-3260.

PHILIPS, T. Bruce; 340 McLeod, Ottawa 4, Ont.; McG'50; FRCP(C), D&TRad; Tel. 232-2493.

PHILLIPS, Barrie L.; Qns'64; Res., St. Paul's Hosp., Vancouver 1, B.C.

PHILLIPS, Bertram A. A.; Cape Town (S. Africa)'52; MB; Ch.B.; Res., School of Hygiene, Toronto 5, Ont.

PHILLIPS, David L. C.; Alb '44; D.Psy., Psy; Clin. Dir., Alberta Hosp., Ponoka, Alta.; Lect. (Psy.), U. of Alberta; Tel. 3-3301.

PHILLIPS, Eileen M.; Box 89, Kincaid, Sask.; Sask'59.

PHILLIPS, Gerald C.; 1161 Royal York Rd. N., Islington, Ont.; Lond. (Eng.) '48; Tel. 239-5604.

PHILLIPS, G. Keith; Medical Arts Bldg., 358 Reynolds N., Oakville, Ont.; 441 Chamberlain Lane, (res); Wes '50; M.C.G.P.; Staff, Oakville Trafalgar Memorial Hosp.; Dist. Coroner; Tel. VI 5-4221.

PHILLIPS, Gordon K.; McG '62; Jr. Intn., Royal Victoria Hosp., Montreal 2, P.Q.

PHILLIPS, H. Ralph; 6178 Quinpool Rd., Halifax, N.S.; 11 Aikens Ave. (res); Dal '50; MCGP; Teach. Staff, Dalhousie U.; Tel. 422-4489.

PHILLIPS, Hubert H.; 306 Med. Dental Bldg., **Regina, Sask.; Sask '58; DiagRad; Staff, Regina** Grey Nuns Hosp.; Tel. 523-7653.

PHILLIPS, James N.; Suite 205, 77 Westmount Rd., Guelph, Ont.; Qns'57; Urol; Staff Urol., Guelph Gen. & St. Joseph's Hosp's.; Tel. TA 4-7272.

PHILLIPS, John E.; Mental Health Clinic, 1904 Fort St., Victoria, B.C.; Cardiff (Wales)'59; DPM; Psy., Mental Health Service, Mental Health Centre.

PHILLIPS, John K.; Box 89, Kincaid, Sask.; Edinburgh (Scot.)'57; MB, ChB; MRCOG.

PHILLIPS, John R.; Medical Arts Bldg., 121 Wellington St. W., Barrie, Ont.; Qns'49; MCGP; Staff, Ross Mem. Hosp.; Tel. 728-4242.

PHILLIPS, Kenneth G.; 2917 Bloor St. W., Toronto 18, Ont.; Tor '44; Paed; Clin. Ass't., Hosp. for Sick Children; Chief Paed., St. Joseph's Hosp.; Tel. 239-3165.

PHILLIPS, Leslie J.; Medical Arts Clin., 51-6th St. S.E., Medicine Hat Alta.; 202-1st S.W., (res); London (Eng.) '52; M.B., B.S., F.R.C.S. (Edin.); D.Otol. (Lond.); Otol; Staff, Medicine Hat Gen. Hosp.; Tel. JA 7-2281.

PHILLIPS, Melville J.; Banting Inst., Dept. of Path., U. of Toronto; Paperbirch Drive, Don Mills, Ont. (res); McG'56; M.C. (Path.); FCAP; FRCP(C); Path; Pathol., Toronto Gen. Hosp.; Staff, Banting Inst., Ass't. Prof. (Path.), U. of Toronto; Tel. 928-2555.

PHILLIPS, Morley F.; UBC'65; Res., Royal Alexandra Hosp., Edmonton, Alta.

PHILLIPS, W. Carlyle; 5750 South St., Halifax N.S.; Dal '61; AMCGP.

PHILLIPS-WOLLEY, Clive J. F.; 520—17th St., West Vancouver, B.C.; 1885-15th St. (res); McG '40; M.C.G.P.; Tel. WA 2-7858.

PHILLIPSON, Eliot A.; Alb '63; Res. University Hosp., Edmonton, Alta.

PHILLIPSON, Gerald J.; Chemainus, B.C.; UBC '56.

PHILLS, James A.; 5056 Cote des Neiges Rd., Montreal, P.Q.; 5320 Bessborough Ave. (res); Dal '51; M.C.G.P.; Staff, Queen Elizabeth and Royal Edward Laurentian Hosp's.; Tel. HU 8-2311.

PHILP, Ian J.; 3009 31st. Ave., Vernon, B.C.; Sask '64; Staff, Vernon Jubilee Hosp.

PHILPOTT, Newell W.; 3465 Cote-des-Neiges Rd., Montreal, P.Q.; McG '26; D.Sc. (Laval); Hon. FRCS(Ed.); FACOG; FRCOG, FACS, FRCS(C), ObstGyn; Staff, Royal Victoria Hosp.; Cons. (ObstGyn), Montreal Gen. Hosp.; Tel. WE 5-5366.

PHIN, John M.; 282 Wildwood Dr., Calgary, Alta. (res); Tor '55; MHA. (MINN.); Ass't. Admin. Foothills Prov. Hosp.; Surveyor, Cdn. Council on Hosp. Accreditation; Tel. 283-0751.

PHIN, Kenneth G.; 711 Kent Trust Bldg., 500 Ouellette Ave., Windsor, Ont.; Qns'49; Staff, I.O.D.E. Comm., Psy. Hosp.; Staff Psy. Sect., Metropolitan Gen. Hosp.; Staff, Hotel-Dieu Hosp.; Member New York Academy of Sciences; Tel. 252-7759.

PHINNEY, Willoughby M.; Kenney Bldg., Yarmouth, N.S.; 615 Main St. (res); Edinburgh (Scot.) '30; D.O.; Staff & Lect. (E.E.N.T.), Nurses' Training School, Yarmouth Hosp.; Tel. 2-3646.

PHOENIX, Paul E.; 4720 le boulevard, Westmount, Montreal 6, P.Q.; Mon '51; Psy; Chief of O.P.D. (Psy.), Hop. Notre-Dame; Tel. 489-9458.

PIASECKI, Anthony J.; 137 Cedar St., Sudbury, Ont.; Ott '55; Active Staff, St. Joseph's & Sudbury Mem. Hosp's.; Assoc. Staff, Sudbury Gen. Hosp.; Tel. 674-2433; Abroad.

PIASECKI, George; 4500 Sherbrooke St. W., Montreal 6, P.Q.; McG'58; FRCP(C), IntMed.; Tel. 933-3420.

PICARD, Carrol; St-Gervais, Cte Bellechasse, P.Q.; Lav '63; Tel. 116.

PICARD, Henri; 74 Principle St., Granby, P.Q.; Lav '45.

PICARD, J. Louis; 822 Sherbrooke St. E., Montreal 24, P.Q.; Mon '49; Paed.; Tel. 523-1137.

PICARD, Joseph; 429 Medical Arts Bldg., Winnipeg, Man.; 349 Elm St. (res); Man'14; Retired.

PICHE, Arthur J. A.; 10 Le Marchand Apts., Edmonton, Alta.; 11646-111A Ave. (res); Lav '29; Hon. Coroner; Tel. 488-0497.

PICHE, Bernard; 1290 est Belanger, Montreal, P.Q.; Mon '47; Psy (P.Q.).; Tel. 272-1516.

PICHE, Claude; 2325 rue Benjamin-Sulte, Montreal 12, P.Q. (res); Mon '56; FRCP(C), Path; Staff, Hop. Ste-Jeanne-d'Arc; Tel. VI 2-5201.

PICHE, Gilles; 53 Ave. des Erables, Arthabaska, P.Q.; Lav '48; Anaes; Anaes.-in-Chief, Hotel-Dieu d'Arthabaska; Tel. 357-2031.

PICHE, G. D. M.; Department of National Health & Welfare, c/o Regional Superintendent, European Region. Abroad.

PICHE, Joseph A.; 110A Le Marchand Mansion, Edmonton, Alta.; 11646-111A Ave. (res); Lav'29; Tel. HU 8-0497.

PICHE, Lucien G.; 6664 St. Denis St., Montreal, P.Q.; 801 Rockland Rd. (res); Mon '31; Tel. 277-7647.

PICHE, Paul; Nicolet, P.Q.; Mon '57. GenSurg (P.Q.); Tel. 293-5210.

PICHETTE, Joseph L.; 177 Principale, Hull, P.Q.; Lav '27; GenSurg (P.Q.); Surg., Hop. Sacre Coeur.

PICHETTE, Louis P.; 87 Church St., Edmundston, N.B.; Lav'36; Ophth, Otol.; Tel. 735-6373.

PICHETTE, L. Paul; Centre Medical St. Urbain, 3875 rue St.-Urbain, Montreal 18, P.Q.; Lav '52; Gastroent. (P.Q.); FRCP(C), IntMed; Staff, Hop. Hotel-Dieu; Tel. VI 4-0161.

PICHETTE, Roland; 3395 Guimont, Giffard, P.Q.; Lav '49; Phys., Hop.-Ste-Foy (DVA), Hop.-St.-Augustin, Ancienne-Lorette & Hop.-du-Mont, St.-Aubert, St.-Pierre, Charlesbourg; Staff, Laval U.; Tel. 663-9152.

PICK, Charles A.; 2162 Sherbrooke St. W., Ste. 1, Montreal 25, P.Q.; 149 Cote St. Antoine Rd., Westmount (res); McG '42; Haem (P.Q.); D. IntMed. (McGill); FAAAS; F.R.C.P.(C), IntMed; Cons., Queen Mary Veterans Hosp.; Phys. St. Mary's Hosp.; Tel. WE 7-1856.

PICKARD, Edgar W.; 428 Medical Arts Bldg., Winnipeg, Man.; 892 Lyon St., Fort Garry (res); Man '34; PlasSurg; Staff, Deer Lodge Hosp. D.V.A.; Winnipeg Gen., Children's & St. Boniface Gen. Hosp's; Lect., Dept. Med., U. of Manitoba; Tel. GL 3-0143.

PICKARD, Harold A.; 304 Med. Dental Bldg., 450 Central Ave., London, Ont.; Wes '47; FRCP(C), IntMed; Staff, Victoria Hosp.; Instr. (Med.), U. of Western Ont.; Tel. 432-5261.

PICKARD, Harry T.; 5A Fountain House, 300 Roslyn Rd., Winnipeg 13, Man.; Man'25.

PICKARD, Patricia A.— see **WIGHTMAN, Patricia A.**

PICKERING, John W.; Ste. 210, Med. Arts Bldg., 300 King St. W., Oshawa, Ont.; 220 Winona Ave. (res); Qns '41; Otol; Chief ENT, Oshawa Gen. Hosp.; Tel. 723-2302.

PICKERING, Nigel A.; 6555 Fraser St., Vancouver 15, B.C.; 187 W. 47 (res); Man '45.

PICKERING, Richard J.; Sask '61; Jr. Intn., University Hosp., Saskatoon, Sask.

PICKETT, Charles H.; St. George, Ont.; Tor '57; MCGP.

PICKETT, George E.; McG '61; Jr. Intn., Royal Victoria Hosp., Montreal 2, P.Q.

PICKLES, Archibald C.; Glasgow (Scot.) '45; Med. Dir., Regina Gen. Hosp., Regina, Sask.; Tel. LA 2-1811.

PICKUP, H. Jackson; Alert Bay, B.C.; Qns '42; M.C.G.P.; M.O.H., Alert Bay District; Chief of Staff, St. George's Hosp.; Tel. 974-5215.

PIDDE, William J.; Man '53; AMCGP; Res., Wpg. Gen. Hosp., Winnipeg, Man.

PIDERMAN, John P.; 801 W. 41st Ave., Vancouver 13, B.C.; Qns'47; MCGP; Vis. Staff, St. Paul's, Vancouver Gen. & Burnaby Gen. Hosp's.

PIDGEON, Thomas V.; 765 King St. W., Kitchener, Ont.; 225 Bruce St. (res); Tor '53; MCGP; Tel. 745-8465.

PIDUTTI, Joseph A.; 70 Cedar St., Sudbury, Ont.; 140 Roxborough Dr. (res); Qns '43; Phys., Home for the Aged; Dist. Coroner; Tel. 673-2613.

PIE, Lionel; 22 rue Cusson, Delson, P.Q.; Mon '61.

PIELORZ, Hildegard (See Schmidt-Malo)

PIERCE, Anne; 77 Lord Seaton Rd., Willowdale, Ont.; Tor '47; M.C.G.P.; O.P. Staff, Women's College Hosp.; Tel. BA 5-3001.

PIERCE, Harry H.; Box 563, 179 Queen St., Charlottetown, P.E.I.; Dal '26; Obst; Staff, PEI Hosp.; Tel. 894-4212.

PIERCE, Maurice M.; 627 Med. Arts Bldg., 404 Graham Ave., Winnipeg 1, Man.; 153 Ash St., Wpg. 9 (res); Man '35; Otol; Hd., Dept. of Otol., St.-Boniface, Misericordia, Grace & Deer Lodge DVA Hosp's.; Dem. U. of Manitoba; Tel. 943-0629.

PIERCY, Dorothy I.; 4143 Virginia Cres., N. Vancouver, B.C. (res); McG '55; Pt-time Med. Health Officer, North Shore Union Bd. of Health.

PIERCY, George I.; 2006 - 8th Ave., New Westminster, B.C.; 1808 Edinburgh St. (res); McG '49; M.C.G.P.; Staff, Royal Columbian & St. Mary's Hosp's.; Tel. LA 2-1742.

PIERCEY, W. Douglas; Can. Hosp. Assc., 25 Imperial St., Toronto 7, Ont.; Dal '34; Tel. HU 1-2244.

PIERON, A. Paul; Amsterdam (Holland)'62; Res., Winnipeg Gen. Hosp., Winnipeg 3, Man.

PIERSON, D. G.; Tor'64; Res., Sunnybrook Hosp., Toronto 12, Ont.

PIERSON, Roger V.; 430 King St. W., Chatham, Ont.; London (Eng.)'52; Dir. Mental Health Clinic & Chief Psy., Public Gen. Hosp.; Cons Psy., St. Joseph's Hosp.; Tel. 354-4507.

PIETAK, Tanya F.; Qns '63; Int., Toronto East Gen. Hosp., Toronto, Ont. Abroad.

PIETILAINEN, Esko K.; 208 Med. Arts Bldg., 73 Cumberland St. N., Port Arthur, Ont.; Helsinki (Finland) '46; GenSurg; Tel. 344-1813.

PIETTE, Edmond; 35 St. Charles Borromee St. S. Joliette, P.Q.; 37 St. Charles Borromee St. S (res); Lav '15; GenSurg; Surg., Hop. St Eusebe; Tel. PL 6-4000.

PIETTE, Jean; 5200 est Boulanger, Montreal P.Q.; Mon '44; Paed (P.Q.); Staff, Hop. Notre Dame; Tel. 525-6363.

PIETTE, Yves; 3766 Queen Mary Rd., Montreal 26, P.Q.; 11839 De Meulles (res); Mon '50; F.R.C.P.(C), IntMed.; Ass't. (Med.), Hop. Notre Dame; Cons., D.V.A.; Ass't. Prof. (Med.), U. of Montreal; Tel. RE 1-3211.

PIETZ, Carl O.; Ste. 105, 1516 Bathurst St., Toronto 10, Ont.; 59 Heathdale Rd. (res); Giessen (Germ.) '34; ObstGyn (Berlin); M.C.G.P.; Staff Northwestern Gen. Hosp.; Tel. LE 4-9681.

PIGEON, Gilles; 55 rue de l'Eglise, Verdun, P.Q. Mon '56; IntMed (P.Q.); Staff, Verdun Gen. Hosp. Ass't. Prof. Med., U. of Montreal; Tel. PO 7-9785.

PIGEON, Jean; 43a Woodward Ave., Blind River, Ont.; Lav'37; FRSH; Chief of Staff, St. Joseph's Gen. Hosp.; MOH & District Coroner; Tel. 356-2621.

PIKE, Eric; Tor '54; D.A.B.P.; Ass't. Dir. Labs., St. John's Gen. Hosp, St. John's, Nfld.; Tel. 8-0471.

PIKE, Roy D.; 33 Beaverbrook Ave., Saint John, N.B.; Dal'63; Tel. 657-3920.

PILKEY, Ray M.; 692 Coxwell Ave., Toronto 6, Ont.; 50 Glenwood Cres., Toronto 16 (res); Tor '41; F.R.C.S.(C), ObstGyn; Staff (ObstGyn.), Toronto East Gen. Hosp.; Tel. 461-6356.

PILLAR, Paul P.; '55; Staff, Dept. of Health, St. John's, Nfld.; Tel. 578-7091.

PILLET, Jean V.; Buenos Aires (Argent.)'55; Staff, Ecole d'Hygiene, Universite de Montreal, Montreal, P.Q.

PILLOW, William M.; 3507-34th Ave. S.W., Calgary, Alta.; Queen's U. (Belfast, N. Ire.)'55; DA; Anaes; Staff, Calgary Gen. & Alberta Children's Hosp's.; Tel. 242-3330.

PILO, Leo; 855 Kipling Ave. N., Weston, Ont.; 66 Waterford Dr. (res); Tor '58; Tel. CH 9-3441.

PILON, Alcide; App. 41, 445 ouest St-Joseph, Montreal 8, P.Q.; Mon '29; NeurPsy; Chief of Serv., Hop. St. Jean de Dieu; Tel. CL 4-5361.

PILON, Bernad; 8415 Rue St-Denis, Montreal, P.Q.; Apt. 207, 350 Graham Blvd. (res); Mon'49; FRCS(C); GenSurg; Ass't. (Surg.), Hop. Notre-Dame-de-l'Esperance; Tel. VI 9-1540.

PILON, Henri; 251 Blvd. St. Joseph, Hull, P.Q.; Mon '25; Anaes.

PILON, J. Louis; 389 Blvd. St. Joseph E., Montreal, P.Q.; 5701 Northmount (res); Mon '38; **Pulm. Dis&TB (P.Q.); Tel. VI 2-1662.**

PILON, Louis D.; 1970 Blvd. Rosemont, Montreal, P.Q. (res); Mon '44; M.C.G.P.; Staff, Rosemont Hosp.; Tel. CR 4-2511.

PILON, Louis J.; 5 Linden Terrace, Ottawa, Ont.; Mon '44; MCGP; Med. Advisor, Cdn. Pension Commission.

PILOTE, Lomer; 6770 Blvd. Pie IX, Montreal, P.Q.; Lav '55; FRCS(C), GenSurg; Staff, Hop. Bellechasse; Tel. 722-1808.

PIMBLETT, Thomas; 88 Lindsay Dr., Saskatoon, Sask. (res); London (Eng.) '49; DA (Eng.); FACA; Anaes; Anaes., University Hosp.; Ass't. Prof. (Anaes.), U. of Saskatchewan; Tel. 242-7641.

PINARD, Gilbert D.; Mon'65; Res., Hop. St. Jean de-Dieu, Montreal 5, P.Q.

PINARD, Herve E.; Alfred, Ont.; Lav '44; Tel. 679-2882.

PINARD, Roger; 622 Blvd. du-Domaine, St. Jerome, P.Q.; Mon '50; D & T Rad; Rad.-in-Chief, Hop.-Hotel-Dieu; Tel. GE 2-9711.

PINAULT, Andree; 843 Riverside Dr., St-Lambert, Cte. Chambly, P.Q.; Mon'55; Anaes.; Tel. 671-7638.

PINAULT, Paul; 315 ouest Peupliers, Quebec 3, P.Q.; Lav'58.

PINCHIN, Arthur H.; 208 King St., Midland, Ont.; 270 Fifth St. (res); Tor '24; F.I.A.P., M.C.G.P.; Staff, St. Andrew's Hosp.; Tel. 526-6311.

PINCOCK, James G.; 501 Churchill Dr., Winnipeg 13, Man. (res); Man'43; FACP; IntMed; Dir., Assessment & Rehab. Unit, & Hd. PhysMed., Deer Lodge Hosp.; Cons. Neurol., Deer Lodge & Grace Hosp's.; Fed. Med. Rep. (Man.), Disallowance Bd.; Lect., U. of Manitoba; Tel. 837-1301.

PINCOCK, Thomas A. 75 Emily St., Winnipeg, Man.; 247 Duffield St. (res); Man '21; Psy; Clin. Dir., Alcoholism Foundation of Man.; Ass't. Prof. (Psy.), U. of Manitoba; Tel. SP 4-6511.

PINCOTT, Robert S.; 1005 Main St., Cowansville, P.Q.; McG'60; Tel. 263-2955.

PINE, Enid; London (Eng.) '46; Res., Vancouver Gen. Hosp., Vancouver 9, B.C.

PINEAU, Alcime J.; Coin Ash & Erie, Kapuskasing, Ont.; 10 rue Erie (res); Mon'50; Tel. 335-2620.

PINEAULT, J. E. H.; c/o Regional Superintendent, Department of National Health & Welfare, Eastern Region, Booth Bldg., Ottawa, Ont.

PINEAULT, Raynald; Lav'65; Res., Hop. St. Michel Archange, Quebec 5, P.Q.

PINEO, Graham F.; Dal'62; FRCP(C), IntMed; Staff, Victoria Hosp., Halifax, N.S.

PINILLA, J. Vicente; Apt. 602, 200 Jameson Ave., Toronto 3, Ont.: Colombia (S. America)'60.

PINKERTON, Alexander C.; 900 W. 27 Ave., Vancouver 9, B.C.; 1195 Renton Pl. (res); Glasgow (Scot.) '45; DPM (Eng.); PhysMed & Rehab; Med. Dir., G. F. Strong Rehab. Centre & Cerebral Palsy Assoc. of Greater Vancouver; Hon. Cons. (PhyscMed), Pearson Polio Pavilion, Dept. of Health & Welfare, B.C.; Clin. Instr., U. of British Columbia; Tel. RE 1-3111.

PINKERTON, Edwin K.; 925 W. Georgia St., Vancouver, B.C.; **McG '32; Tel. MU 5-6660.**

PINKERTON, Ronald M. H.; Etherington Hall, Stuart St., Kingston, Ont.; Queen's U. (Belfast, N. Ireland)'55; FRCS (Lond.); FRCS(C); Ophth; Att'd. Staff, Kingston Gen. & Hotel-Dieu Hosp's.; Ass't. Prof. (Ophth.), Queen's U.; Tel. 546-1040.

PINSONNAULT, Jean P.; 1840 St.-Marc, Shawinigan Falls, P.Q.; Lav'49; GenSurg.; Tel. LE 6-3403.

PINSONNEAULT, Germain; Apt. 401, 2505 Maplewood Ave., Montreal 26, P.Q. (res); Lille (France) '28; D&TRad, PhysMed (P.Q.); Chief Rad., Hop. Hotel Dieu; Assoc. Prof. (Rad.), U. of Montreal; Tel. VI 4-0161.

PINTAR, Karl; 475 Cardinal St., Montreal 9, P.Q.; Vienna (Austria) '54; Path. (P.Q.); Ass't. Path., Jewish Gen. Hosp.; Tel. 735-3771. Abroad.

PINTO, Bernardo; Madrid (Spain)'59; Staff, Dept. of Biochem., Queen's U., Kingston, Ont.

PINTO, Ricardo; Madrid (Spain)'58; Psy; Staff, **Ontario Hosp., 999 Queen St. W., Toronto 3, Ont.**

PION, Pierre P.; 115 Heriot St., Drummondville, **P.Q.; Mon '35; D.P.H.; DermSyph** (Paris); Staff, Hop. Ste. Croix; Phys., Can. Celanese; Tel. GR 8-1381.

PION, Rene; Clin. Roy-Rousseau, Mastai, P.Q.; 1576 du Ruisseau (res); Lav '51; Psy; Ass't. (Fem. Serv.), Clin. Roy-Rousseau & NeurPsy., Hop.-de-l'Enfant-Jesus; Staff, Laval U.; Tel. 661-7735.

PIOTROWSKI, Adolph; 396 Royal York Rd., **Toronto 18, Ont.: Tor '55; Tel. CL 9-8182.**

PIPER, Athol V.; 3663 Shelbourne St., Victoria, B.C.; 4451 Narvaez Cr. (res); Loma Linda (Calif., USA) '58; MCGP; Tel. 477-3323.

PIPER, Gary A.; Ste. 306, 77 Westmount Rd., Guelph, Ont.; Tor'60; MCGP; Phys., Imperial Tobacco Co. Ltd.; Tel. 824-6200.

PIPER, George W.; 516-2nd Ave. N., Saskatoon, Sask.; London (Eng.)'48; M.B., B.S., MRCS (Eng.); LRCP (Lond.); DPH; Regional Med. Health Officer, Saskatoon Rural Health Region; Ass't. Clin. Prof., Dept. of Social & Prev. Med., University of Saskatchewan; Tel. 244-0191.

PIPER, Sherman A.; 106 Toronto Western Medical Bldg., 25 Leonard Ave., Toronto 2B, Ont.; 1458 Skyline Dr., Orchard Hghts., Port Credit, Ont. (res); Tor '43; DiagRad; Staff (Rad.), Toronto Western & Queensway Gen. Hosp.; Tel. EM 3-1197.

PIPER, W. Archibald; 36 Wilson St., Hamilton, Ont.; Dal'66.

PIRIE, Gordon E.; 5187 Pine Cr., Vancouver 13, B.C. (res); McG '54; Paed; Research, Vancouver Gen. Hosp.; Instr., U. of British Columbia; Tel. TR 6-3211, Loc. 2597.

PIRNAZAR, Rahmatollah; Teheran (Iran); Staff, Dept. of Anat., U. of Man., Winnipeg, Man.

PIROZYNSKI, Witold J.; 3775 University St., Montreal 2, P.Q.; 4804 Cote des Neiges Rd., Apt. 25 (res); Zurich (Switzerland)'45; DABP; Path; Assoc. Prof. (Path.), McGill U.; Tel. 842-1251, Ext. 416.

PIRQUET, Anton S.; Ste 213, 1669 Victoria St., Prince George, B.C.; Vienna (Austria)'41; Tel. 564-4645.

PISESKY, Walter; 305 Professional Bldg., 10830 Jasper Ave., Edmonton, Alta.; 13943-107th Ave. (res); Alb '55; DABS; FACS; FRCS(C), GenSurg; Att'd Staff, Edmonton Gen. Hosp.; Clin. Instr., (Surg.), U. of Alta.; Tel. 422-8207.

PITERS, John; 4014 Cambie St., Vancouver, B.C.; 3338 Radcliffe Ave. W., Van. (res); Tor '34; A.M.C.A.A.; Paed; Sr. Staff (Paed) & Chief, Children's Allergy Clin., Vancouver Gen. Hosp.; Clin. Ass't. Prof. (Paed.), U. of British Columbia; Tel. 876-1616.

PITMAN, Richard G.; London (Eng.)'44; MRCP; MRCS; LRCP; FFR; DMRD; FRCP(C), IntMed; Diag Rad; Staff, St. Paul's Hosp., Vancouver 1, B.C.

PITT, Dennis C.; 80 Bond St., Lindsay, Ont. (res); Dal '52; DiagRad; Rad., Ross Mem. Hosp.; Tel. 324-6111.

PITT, Paul L.; Ste. 104, 1593 Ellesmere Rd., Scarborough, Ont.; Tor'64; Court. Staff, Scarborough Gen. Hosp.; Tel. 293-6660.

PITT-PAYNE, Bruce; Dobson Clinic, 10102-101st. St., Grande Prairie, Alta.; London (Eng.) '58; MRCS (Eng.), LRCP (Lond.); Tel. 532-4444.

PITTS, Harry H., Sr.; 1550 W. 11th Ave., Vancouver 9, B.C. (res); McG '18; PathBact; Retired.

PITTS, Harry H. Jr.; 2184 W. Broadway, Vancouver 9, B.C.; 1691 Somerset Cres. (res); McG '49; FACS; FRCS(C), Urol; Staff, St. Paul's Hosp., Children's Hosp. & B.C. Cancer Clinic; Assoc. Prof., U. of British Columbia; Tel. RE 6-4451.

PITTS, William C.; 213 Victoria Quay, Alberni, B.C.; 390 Elizabeth (res); Qns '29; Tel. 723-8141.

PIUZE, J. Maurice; 432 St. Jerome, Matane, P.Q.; Lav '35.

PIUZE, Yves E.; 970 Clement, St. Laurent, Montreal 9, P.Q.; Mon '44; Anaes (P.Q.); Ass't. (Anaes), Hop. Sacre Coeur; Tel. RI 8-7683.

PIVNICK, Bernard; 488 Victoria St., London, Ont. (res); Tor '51; Psy., Staff, St. Joseph's Hosp.; Cons. Staff, St. Mary's Hosp., London; Instr. (Psy), U. of Western Ontario; Tel. GE 9-3271, Ext. 279.

PIVNICKI, Dimitrije; Allan Mem. Inst., 1025 Pine Ave. W., Montreal, P.Q.; 2460 Montclair Ave. (res); Belgrade (Yugoslavia) '49; D.Psy; Psy; Ass't. Psy., Royal Victoria Hosp. & Allen Mem. Inst.; Ass't. Prof. Psy., McGill U.; Tel. VI 2-1251, Ext. 634.

PIYAPONGSE, Metta; Thailand'58; FRCP(C), Anaes; Staff, Toronto Western Hosp., Toronto, Ont.

PIZANS, Antons; 627 King St. E., Kitchener, Ont.; 94 Weber St. E. (res); Tel. SH 5-9862.

PIZER, T. H.; Tor'65; Jr. Int., Vancouver Gen. Hosp., Vancouver 9, B.C.

PLACE, Ronald E. G.; 595 Victoria Ave., Westmount 6, P.Q.; McG '39; D.I.M., D.A.B.I.M., Pulm Dis. & TB (P.Q.), F.R.C.P.(C), IntMed; Ass't. Phys., Royal Victoria Hosp.; Phys. (Respir. Physiol.), Royal Edward Laurentian Hosp.; Dir., Respir. Function Lab., Queen Mary Vet's. Hosp.; Lect., McGill U.; Phys., McGill Health Serv., Tel. HU 9-6641.

PLAMONDON, Charles A.; Ste. 400, 922 Pl. d'Aiguillon, Quebec 4, P.Q.; 1095 Bougainville (res); Lav '49; FRCP(C), IntMed; Hd. Dept. of Med., Hop. de-l'Enfant-Jesus; Assoc. Prof., Laval U.; Tel. 522-8905.

PLAMONDON, Gabriel; 92 St. Denis Jonquiere P. Q.; Lav '42.

PLAMONDON, Guy; 8052, St-Michel, Cite St-Michel, Montreal Nord, P.Q.; Mon '49; Tel. RA 7-4853.

PLAMONDON, Marc; 35 Cote-du-Palais, Quebec, P.Q.; 1325 ave des Gouveneurs, Sillery (res); Lav '48; Ophth; Staff, Hotel-Dieu & Laval U.; Tel. 523-7442.

PLAMONDON, Marcel; ave Patenaude, Sillery, P.Q.; Lav '40; Anaes; Staff, Hop.-de-l'Enfant-Jesus & Hotel-Dieu; Tel. 529-8711.

PLAMONDON, Romain R.; 240 rue Elm, St. Lambert Co., Chambly, P.Q.; Lav'55; MCGP.

PLANT, J. Stewart; 140 Fairview Cres., Woodstock, Ont. (res); Tor '45; FACCP, DMR; DiagRad.; Staff, Woodstock Gen. Hosp.; Tel. LE 7-5511.

PLANTE, Adrien; Hotel Dieu St. Michel, Roberval, P.Q.; 18 rue Lizzotte (res); Lav '40; Ophth, Otol (P.Q.); Tel. 275-0683.

PLANTE, Albert; Mon'65; Res., Inst. Albert Prevost, Montreal 9, P.Q.

PLANTE, Anatole; 12408 Cousineau, Montreal, P.Q. (res); Lav '18; Phys.-in-Chief, La Commission des Ecoles Catholiques de Montreal, 117 Ste. Catherine Ouest, Montreal; Retired; Tel. FE 4-6754.

PLANTE, Charles U.; Ste. Angele de Merci, Co. Rimouski, P.Q.; Lav '59; Tel. 775-5151.

PLANTE, Claude; 3422 rue St. Hubert, Montreal 24, P.Q.; Lav'58; Psy(P.Q.); Staff, Hop. St-Jean-de-Dieu; Tel. 845-3605.

PLANTE, Claude A.; 55 Church, Montreal 19, P.Q.; Mon '59; FRCS(C), OrthSurg.

PLANTE, Fernand; 66 St-Jean-Baptist, Victoriaville, P.Q.; Lav'51; Tel. 752-6404.

PLANTE, Gabriel; 252 Lemoyne, Longueil, Cite Jacques Cartier, P.Q.; Mon '59.

PLANTE, Gabriel; 698 Gamache, Sept-Iles, P.Q.; Lav '57; Anaes (P.Q.); Staff, Hop. des Sept-Iles.

PLANTE, Gerard; Mon '64; Res., Hop. Hotel-Dieu, Montreal, P.Q.

PLANTE, Gilles C.; Ott '59; Psy; Staff, Dept. of Psy., Hop. Notre-Dame, Montreal 24, P.Q.; Tel. 525-6363.

PLANTE, Gustave; 60 de la Gare, Montmagny, P.Q.; Lav'56; MCGP.

PLANTE, Henri J. J.; Mon'56; Res. (Psy.), Hop. des Laurentides, L'Annonciation, P.Q.

PLANTE, Jean L.; 16 Levac, Rigaud, Cte.-Vaudreuil, P.Q.; Mon '60; Tel. 238-4321.

PLANTE, Jean M.; Lav '58; Res., Hop. St-Sacrement, Quebec, P.Q.

PLANTE, J. N.; Disraeli, P.Q.; Lav '19.

PLANTE, Louis J.; C.P. 38, Bic, Co. Rimouski, P.Q.; Lav '28.

PLANTE, Lucien; 58 Notre Dame, Louiseville, P.Q.; Lav '08.

PLANTE, Normand; 2537 rue Biencourt, Quebec 10, P.Q.; Lav '56; Psy; Staff, Hop. St-Michel-Archange; Tel. 663-3571.

PLANTE, Robert; 1210-1ere Ave., Quebec 3, P.Q.; Lav'52; Urol (P.Q.); Tel. 529-9981.

PLANTE, Roger; 201, 1656 est, Sherbrooke, Montreal 24, P.Q.; 379 de Lorraine, Longueuil (res); Mon '57; FRCS(C), GenSurg; Surg., Hop. Notre-Dame; Tel. 521-2116; LA 5-6363.

PLASTER, Ernest L.; Arcola, Sask.; Man '51; Weyburn Estevan Reg. Bd. of Public Health.

PLATT, John C.; 286 Donnelly Dr., Port Credit, Ont. (res); Wes '57; Med. Dir. South Peel Hosp., Cooksville, Ont.; Tel. 277-2761.

PLATT, Shirley (see Deneka)

PLATTS, Marjorie E.; Apt. 1117, 484 Church St., Toronto 5, Ont. (res); Tor '55; Path; Pathol., Wellesley & Princess Margaret Hosp's.; Pt-time Dem., U. of Toronto; Tel. WA 1-4111.

PLAYFAIR, F. David; 168 Ontario St., St. Catharines, Ont.; 36 Woodruff Dr. (res); McG '42; IntMed; Chief of Med., Hotel Dieu; Active Cons. Staff, St. Catharines Gen. Hosp.; Cons. (Med.), D.V.A.; Tel. MU 4-9201.

PLAYFAIR, John A. F.; 4071 Kingsway, South Burnaby, B.C.; 5058 Carson St. (res); Qns '53; MCGP; Tel. HE 3-4411.

PLAYFAIR, Lawrence L.; 41 Duke St., Hamilton, Ont. (res); Qns '06; F.R.C.S. (Edin.), GenSurg; Retired.

PLAYFAIR, Peter F.; 221-2nd St. N., Kenora, Ont. (res); Qns '43; DPH; MCGP; MOH Exec Dir., Northwestern Health Unit; Tel. HO 8-7072.

PLECASH, Myles; 477 Martin St., Penticton, B.C.; 620 Winnipeg St. (res); McG '45; Urol; Tel. 492-4232.

PLEDGER, Robert G.; Barrington Passage, N.S. London (Eng.) '53. Abroad.

PLENDERLEITH, Ian H.; 9 Ruskin St., Ottawa 3, Ont.; George Washington U. (Washington U.S.A.)'58; FRCP(C), IntMed; Med. Cons., Ottawa Clinic & Ontario Cancer Foundation.

PLEWES, Burns; 825 Coxwell Ave., Ste. 9, Toronto 13, Ont.; 40 Taylor Dr. (res); Tor'32; MA M.S., FACS, FRCS(Edin.), FRCS(C), GenSurg; Cons. (Surg.), Toronto East Gen. Hosp.; Cons (Surg.), Ont. Hosp.; Clin. Instr., U. of Toronto Pres. Tor. Academy of Med.; Tel. 465-5971.

PLEWES, William F.; 40 Taylor Dr., Toronto 13, Ont.; Tor'08; Retired.
PLIMBLEY, W. Roger; Box 999, Taber, Alta.; Box 2078, Taber (Res); Birmingham (Eng.)'59; D.A. (Eng.); Assoc. Med. Staff, Taber Gen. Hosp.; Tel. 223-3525.
PLOUFFE, Adrien; C.P. 590, 73 rue Ouimet, Terrebonne, P.Q. (res); Mon '12; D.P.H.; Ass't. Dir., Health Services. Hotel de Ville, Montreal. Retired.
PLOUFFE, Donald; 349 boul. Tache, Hull, P.Q.; Lav '64.
PLOUFFE, Gabriel; 4601 Chambord, Montreal, P.Q.; 8415 St. Denis, Montreal 11, P.Q.; Mon '51; Obst (P.Q.).; Tel. LA 1-0905.
PLOUFFE, Maurice; St. Constant de Laprairie, P.Q.; Mon '57.
PLOUGHMAN, Robert; Water St., Bay Roberts, Nfld.; Dal'64; AMCGP.
PLOURDE, Andre; Metabetchouan, P.Q.; Lav'62.
PLOURDE, Camille; 1124 Chopin, Chicoutimi-Nord, P.Q.; Lav '59; Psy; Staff, Hotel-Dieu St-Vallier; Tel. 549-2195.
PLOURDE, Jacques; C.P. 159, Barraute, Cte. Abitibi-est, P.Q.; Lav '51; Tel. 734-2565.
PLOURDE, Jean L.; Isle-Verte, Cte Riviere-du-Loup, P.Q.; Lav '51.
PLOURDE, Paul; R.R. No. 1, Montmagny, P.Q. (res); Lav '40; **Anaes; Anaes., Hotel Dieu de Montmagny.**
PLOURDE, Sabin; 81 Eveche, Rimouski, P.Q.; Lav'55; FACS; FRCS(C), GenSurg; **Staff, Hop.** de-Rimouski; Tel. 723-7851.
PLUMB, Louis M.; 77 St. Edmunds Dr., Toronto 12, Ont; **Wes '46; D.Psy.; Psy; Psy-in-Charge.** Psych. **Ward, Women's College Hosp.; Tel. HU** 7-2231.
PLUMMER, Paul; 1669 Victoria St., Prince George, B.C.; UBC '64
PLUNKETT, Earl R.; Colborne Bldg., Victoria Hosp., London, Ont.; 34 Kingspark Cres. (res); Wes'46; Ph.D.; FACOG; Cons. (Endocrin.), Victoria Hosp.; Assoc. Prof. (Endocrine) (ObstGyn & Med. Research) & Ass't. Prof. (Med.), U. of Western Ont.; Tel. 432-5261, Loc. 613.
POCHEREVA, William; 444 Beaconsfield Blvd., Beaconsfield, P.Q.; 689 Victoria Dr., Baie-d'Urfe **(res); McG '54; GenSurg; Court. Staff, Lachine Gen. Hosp.; Tel. Area 514; 695-6302.**
POCOCK, Wilfred T.; Emsdale, Ont.; Qns '18; **Staff, Huntsville Hosp.; Coroner Parry Sound & Nipissing; Tel. 50.**
PODEDWORNY, Walter M.; 225 James St. S., Hamilton, Ont.; 95 Arcade Cr. (res); Qns '59; Ophth; M.Sc. (Med. Sc.), (Ohio State U.); Staff, Hamilton Gen. & St. Joseph's Hosp's.; Tel. JA 7-0442.
PODILSKY, Myroslau; Box 39, North Battleford, Sask.
PODKOMORSKA, Danuta M.T.; 1800 Logan **Ave., Winnipeg 23, Man.; 1467 Wellington Cr. (res); Poznan (Poland) '47; Otol; Tel. 783-0840.**
POGONOWSKI, Stanislaw J. B.; 146 David St., Sudbury, Ont. (res); Edinburgh (Scot.)'47; FACCP; Dir., Miners' Chest Clinic, WCB; Tel. 675-7181.
POHLMAN. E. Ralph; 45 Birgitta Cr., Toronto, Ont. (res); Qns '58; Path; Staff, St. Joseph's Hosp.; Tel. 534-9531, Ext. 407.
POHRAN, Nicholas; Med. Arts Bldg., 2150 Valley Way, Niagara Falls, Ont.; McG'53; MCGP; Tel. 358-9668.
POHU, Andre; Mon '64; Res., Hop. Notre Dame, Montreal, P.Q.
POIRIER, Fernand; 1150 est, boul. St. Joseph, **Montreal 34, P.Q.; Ott '53;** FRCP(C), Neur; Staff, Hop. Maisonneuve; Tel. LA 7-1241.
POIRIER, Florian; 341A St. Dominic, Jonquire, P.Q.; **Lav '51; Anaes; Staff, Hop. Notre-Dame-de-l'Assomption;** Tel. 547-3651.
POIRIER, Gaston; Lav'65; Res., Hop St-Sacrement, Quebec 6, P.Q.
POIRIER, Gerard; Lav'51; Staff, Hop. Christ Roi, Quebec 8, P.Q.
POIRIER, Gilles; 395 Bois-des-Filion, Cte. Terrebonne, P.Q.; Mon '59; Med. Dir. **Abbott Labs.,** Montreal, P.Q.; **Tel. 735-2411.**
POIRIER, Henri W.; 124 Claude-Ramsay nord, **Marieville, Cte. Rouville, P.Q.; Mon '65.**
POIRIER, J. Alphee; Lav '38; Staff, San. Begin, Lac Etchemin, Cte. Dorchester, P.Q.
POIRIER, Jean R.; 971 boul. Ste-Croix, Montreal **9, P. Q.; Mon '43; Ophth; Ophth.,** Notre Dame de l'Esperance Hosp.; Cons., Sacre-Coeur Hosp.; Tel. 747-1323.
POIRIER, Jean P.; 174 Westcliffe, Pointe-Claire, Lachine, P.Q.; Mon '51; Paed; Tel. 697-3975.
POIRIER, John L.; 180 King St., St. Catharines, Ont. (res); Tor '10; Cons. Phys., St. Catharines **Gen. & Hotel Dieu Hosp's.; Tel. MU 5-5811.**
POIRIER, Louis; 1310 Dolan, Quebec 10, P.Q.; Mon '47; Ph.D. (Mich.).
POIRIER, Normand; Mon'65; Res., Royal Victoria Hosp., Montreal 2, P.Q.
POIRIER, Paul; 1386 est, rue Sherbrooke, Montreal 24, P.Q.; Lav '26; Derm; FAAD; Cons., Hop. Hotel-Dieu; Prof. (Emer.), U. of Montreal; Tel. LA 3-9055.
POIRIER, Paul E.; Maria, Co. Bonaventure, P.Q.; Lav '48; IntMed (P.Q.); Internist, Hop. Notre Dame de Chartres; Tel. 443.
POIRIER, Rene; 30 est, boul St-Joseph, Montreal 14, P.Q.; Mon '49; Tel. 845-4241.
POIRIER, Richard A.; Ste. 105 Le Marchand Mans., Edmonton, Alta.; 10205-137 St. (res); Mon '36; Paed., Chief of Staff, Paed. Dept., Edmonton Gen. Hosp.; Instr., Paed., U. of Alberta; **Tel. 488-2134.**
POIRIER, Roger; 3423 Notre-Dame St. W., Montreal, P.Q.; **3766 Harvard Ave.** (res); Mon '34; MCGP; Staff, Verdun Gen. Hosp.; Med. Dir., Foyer St. Henri; Tel. WE 2-1950.
POIRIER, Roger; 3175 Cote-Ste.-Catherine Rd., Montreal 26, P.Q.; Mon '51; Paed; Staff, Hop.-Ste.-Justine; Tel. RE 1-3011.
POIRIER, Roger; 227, Longueuil, St-Jean, P.Q.; Mon '43.
POISSANT, Alain; 127A rue du Prince, Sorel, P.Q.; Mon'65.
POISSON, Andre; C.P. 427, Grand'Mere, **Cte. Lav-iolette, P.Q.; Lav '33; Dist. Coroner.**
POISSON, Emile; 1300 Galt St. W., Sherbrooke, P.Q.; Lav '33; **D.P.H.; M.O., Health Serv., Sherbrooke, P.Q.; Tel. LO 9-5464.**
POISSON, Jacques; Lav'59; Res. (Rad.), Hop. St. Sacrement, Quebec 6, P.Q.
POISSON, Paul; 120 Ste Rose Ave., Windsor, Ont.; Wes'09.
POISSON, Roger; 30 Boul. St. Joseph est; Montreal 14, P.Q.; Ott '56; FRCS(C), GenSurg; Research Fell. (Experimental Surg.), Royal Victoria Hosp. & McGill U.; Tel. VI 2-1251.
POISSON, Thomas C.; 548 Notre Dame, Belle River, Ont.; Wes '58; MCGP.
POITEVIN, Normand; 960, boul Ste-Croix, Montreal 9, P.Q.; 2040 Depatre (res); Mon '54.
POITRAS, Benoit; 513 Ste Cecile, Trois Rivieres, P.Q.; Lav'65.
POITRAS, Jean P.; 496 Ave. St. Jerome, Matane, P.Q.; Lav '57.
POITRAS, Vincent S.; 24 Beaconsfield Blvd., Beaconsfield, P.Q.; Mon'53; Active Staff, Dept. of G.P., Lakeshore Gen. Hosp., Pointe Claire; Tel. 695-5751.
POKOLY, Thomas B.; Tor'65; Intern, rotating various Toronto Hosp's.
POLAK, Danuta; Box 118, Gravenhurst, Ont.; Dublin (Ire.) '57; DA.
POLAK, Jaroslav M. J.; 229 St. Clair Ave. W., Toronto 7, Ont.; Tor '64; Tel. WA 3-6537.
POLACK, Stanley S.; 130 Elm St. E., Sudbury, Ont.; 416 Ramsay Lake Rd. (res); Tor '23; FACS, FICS, GenSurg; Gyn; Cons., Sudbury Gen. & St. Joseph's Hosp's.; Tel. OS 3-7181. Retired.
POLAN, W. Desmond; Ste. 565, 5025 Sherbrooke **St. W., Montreal 28, P.Q.; McG '47; ObstGyn; Staff, St. Mary's, Queen Elizabeth & Catherine** Booth Hosp's.; Tel. 482-0838.
POLAND. Betty J.; 1856 Allison Rd., Vancouver 8, B.C.; London (Eng.) '43; MRCOG (Eng.); ObstGyn.
POLEC, Edward M.; Greer St., Wynyard, Sask.; Man '33; Dist. Coroner.

POLIQUIN, Jacques; 1010 rue Jacques, Terrasse Bon Air, Quebec 7, P.Q.; Lav'57; Anaes (P.Q.); Staff, Hop. de l'Enfant Jesus; Tel. 529-8711.
POLIQUIN, Jacques; Mon'65; Res., Verdun Gen. Hosp., Verdun, P.Q.
POLIQUIN, L. Philippe; Maniwaki, Co. Gatineau, P.Q.; Lav '30; D.P.H. Med. Dir. St. Joseph's Hosp.; Tel. 449-1333.
POLIQUIN, Paul A.; 71 Ste. Anne, Quebec, P.Q.; 508 St. Cyrille Ouest (res); Lav '18; F.A.C.S., GenSurg; Cons., Hop. St. Francis d'Assisi & Hop. de l'Enfant Jesus; Vis. Staff, Hop. St. Sacrement & Jeffery Hale's Hosp.; Prof. of Clin. Surg., Laval U.; Tel. 522-1501.
POLIQUIN, Robert W.; 90 Salaberry, Valleyfield, P.Q.; Lav'59; GenSurg.
POLISIUK, Adolf; 107 Medical Bldg., 217-3rd Ave. N., Saskatoon, Sask.; 402 Queen St. (res); Vienna (Aust.) '32; M.C.G.P.; Staff, City & St. Paul's Hosp's.; Tel. 242-6681.
POLITI, Vincent L.; 192 Sherwood Rise, Hamilton, Ont.; Qns '50; Anaes; Staff, Hamilton Gen. Hosp.; Tel. JA 7-0271.
POLLACK, Hymie; 8218—104th St., Edmonton, Alta.; 10030—83rd Ave. (res); Alb '48; Att. Staff, Misericordia Hosp.; Court. Staff, Edmonton Gen. Hosp.; Tel. GE 3-3501.
POLLACK, Jacob; 1709 Bathurst St., Toronto, Ont.; 55 Ava Rd. (res); Tor '22; Med. Dir., New Annex Hosp.; Retired.
POLLACK, Samuel L.; 1070 des-Braves Quebec, P.Q. (res); McG '37; DABR, ObstGyn (PQ); Chief of Staff, (ObstGyn), Jeffery Hale's Hosp.; Tel. 683-4441.
POLLAK, Bernard; 3650 St. Urbain St., Montreal 18, P.Q.; 4116 Melrose Ave. (res); Prague (Czech.) '37; FCCP; Pulm.Dis. & T.B. (P.Q.); Med. Dir., Royal Edward Chest Hosp.; Lect. (Med.), McGill U.; Tel. VI 9-5201. Ext. 212.
POLLAK, John E.; 1604 Lonsdale Ave., North Vancouver, B.C.; 4374 Skyline Dr. (res); Qns '42; DiagRad; Staff (Rad.), St. Paul's Hosp. & Lions Gate Hosp.; Tel. YU 5-5352.
POLLALIS, S.; 6565-44th Ave., Montreal, P.Q.; Athens (Greece) '55; Ophth; Tel. 725-3503.
POLLETT, Harry F.; 340 Campbell St., Nanaimo, B.C.; Dal'66.
POLLETT, William E.; 2005 Kline St., Halifax, N.S.; 1140 Rockcliffe (res); Dal '34; FRCS (Edin.), FRCS(C), GenSurg; Assoc. Surg., Children's Hosp.; Lect'r. (Surg.), Dalhousie U.; Tel. 423-8770.
POLLOCK, Alexander; 335 Med. Arts Bldg., Saskatoon, Sask.; 870 University Dr. (res); Qns '54; FRCS(C), GenSurg; Active Staff, University, St. Paul's & Saskatoon City Hosp's.; Clin. Assoc. (Surg.) & Sess. Lect. (Anat.), U. of Saskatchewan; Tel. 652-4481.
POLLOCK, Allan D.; 117-10th St. W., Owen Sound, Ont.; 1000—1st Ave. W. (res); Tor '31; F.A.C.S., GenSurg; Sr. Cons. (GenSurg), General & Marine Hosp.; Tel. FR 6-4508.
POLLOCK, A. Walter L.; Lewisporte, Notre Dame Bay, Nfld.; Dublin (Ire.)'51; MCGP; M.O.H.; Tel. 6791.
POLLOCK, Francis D.; The Underhill Clinic, 1635 Abbott St., Kelowna, B.C.; Qns'62; AMCGP; Tel. 762-2740.
POLLOCK, Frederick H.; 636 Pharmacy Ave., Scarborough, Ont.; 21 Fallingbrook Road (res); Tor '50; Tel. 755-2393.
POLLOCK, Ilse E. S.; Community Clinic, 108-8th St. E., Prince Albert, Sask.; Edinburgh & Glasgow (Scot.)'59 & '64; DCH; Paed; Tel. 763-6466.
POLLOCK, Ira J.; 417 Bloor St. W., Toronto 4, Ont.; 34 Alexandra Wood (res); Tor '44; M.C.-G.P.; Sr. Clin. Phys., New Mount Sinai Hosp.; Tel. WA 1-1141.
POLLOCK, John M.; Avonmore, Ont.; McG '14; Dist. Coroner.
POLLOCK, Maurice A.; 417 Bloor St. W., Toronto, Ont.; Tor, '11; IntMed.; Tel. WA 1-1141.
POLLOCK, Oscar; 417 Bloor St. W., Toronto, Ont.; 416 Lytton Blvd. (res); Tor '39; M.C.G.P.; Staff, Chest Clinics, New Mt. Sinai Hosp.; Tel. WA 1-1143.
POLLOCK, Piney; Ste. 402, 340 McLeod, Ottawa 4, Ont.; Ott'51; DIM (McG); IntMed; Assoc. in Med., Ottawa Civic Hosp.; Tel. CE 4-4807.
POLLONETSKY, Elizabeth; 2080 DVA Bldg., Wellington St., Ottawa, Ont.; Shanghai (China) '45; Med. Adviser, Cdn. Pensions Commission, Ottawa.
POLNICKY, Thaddee; Box 667, 817A George St., Hearst, Ont.; Ott '55.
POLO, Rafael F.; 160-14th St., Brandon, Man.; 40 Almond Cr. (res); Cartagena (Columbia, S. America) '55; Staff, Brandon Gen. Hosp.; Tel. PA 6-2086.
POLOWIN, Moses I.; 38 Coburg St., St. John, N.B.; 647 Manawagonish Rd., Lancaster (res); Qns '47; GenSurg; Att'd. Staff, St. John's Gen., & St. Joseph's Hosp.; Cons., Dept. of OrthSurg & Dir. Physio & Occup. Therapy, Lancaster DVA Hosp.; Tel. 692-6290.
POLSON, J. Stewart; Ste. 200, 3550 Cote de Neiges, Montreal 25, P.Q.; McG'45; FRCP(C); IntMed; Ass't. Phys., Montreal Gen. Hosp.; Chief of Med., Ste-Anne's DVA Hosp.; Ass't. Prof. (Med.), McGill U.; Chief M.O., Dominion Steel & Coal Corp.; Tel. 931-1061.
POLSON, Robert A.; Wpg. Clinic, N.E. St. Mary's & Vaughan, Winnipeg, Man.; 377 Oxford St., Wpg. 1 (res); Man '45; FACP; FRCP(C), IntMed; Ass't. Phys., Wpg. Gen. Hosp.; Lect. (Med.), U. of Manitoba; Tel. 942-0551.
POLYMENAKOS, L. G.; 57 Bloor St. W., Toronto, Ont.; 133 Braemar (res); Athens (Greece) '31; Tel. 924-2000.
POLYNCHUK, Dora (See CULLIMORE, Dora).
POMAHAC, Anthony; Campbell Clinic, 430 Mayor Magrath Dr., Lethbridge, Alta.; Alb '61; Tel. FA 7-5737.
POMERANTZ, Daniel; Apt. 8, 4850 Walkley Ave., Montreal 29, P.Q.; Montpellier (France)'59.
POMERANTZ, Harold Z.; Ste 340, 6000 Cote des Neiges Rd., Montreal 26, P.Q.; 18 Lazard Ave., Twn. of Mt. Royal (res); McG '47; FACP; FACC; FICA; IntMed; Cardiol (PQ); Ass't. Phys., Jewish Gen. Hosp.; Assoc. Phys., Reddy Mem. Hosp.; Tel. WE 3-6071.
POMERLEAU, Albany; C.P. 26, Beauceville Ouest, Co. Beauce, P.Q.; Lav'54; Tel. 390.
POMERLEAU, C.; 175 St. Cyrille, Quebec, P.Q.; Lav '33; D.P.H.; Dept. of Health, Quebec.
POMERLEAU, Damien; Mon '63; Res., Hop. Ste-Justine, Montreal 26, P.Q.
POMERLEAU, Guy; Lav'65; Sr. Int., Hop St. Michel-Archange, Quebec 5, P.Q.
POMERLEAU, Pierre A.; 1210-lere Ave., Quebec 3, P.Q.; Lav '50; GenSurg (PQ).; Tel. 522-1712.
POMEROY, James K.; 72 Donahue Ave., Regina, Sask.; Qns '22; 900 Garnet St., Regina (res); Tel. 568-1000.
POMPA, Carmelo; 784 est, rue Jean-Talon, Montreal, P.Q.; Mon '58; AMCGP; Tel. 277-4397.
PON, Franklin W.; Wes'65; Res., Victoria Hosp., London, Ontario.
POND, John C.; 115 Hazen St., Saint John, N.B.; Renforth, King's Co. (res); London (Eng.) '51; IntMed; Path; MRCP; MRCP(Ed.); MC (Path); Cons. Haem., DVA Hosp., Lancaster; Haematol., Prov. Lab.; Internist, St. John's Gen & St. Joseph's Hosp's.; Tel. OX 3-2449.
POND, Ronald A.; Mackenzie Clinic, 97 Charlotte St., Port Colborne, Ont.; 199 Rosemount (res); Qns '56; MCGP; Tel. 834-4216.
PONESSE, David J.; 3040 Don Mills Rd. E. Willowdale, Ont.; Tor'64.
PONTBRIAND, Roger; 72 boul Cure Labelle, L'Abord-a-Plouffe, P.Q.; 258 Cure Labelle, Chomedey, Laval-des-Rapides (res); Mon '49.
PONTIFEX, Alexander H.; UBC '54; Staff, Dept. of Pathol., Royal Columbian Hosp., New Westminster, B.C.; Tel. LA 2-2771.
POOLE, James B.; 550 Ingersoll Ave., Woodstock, Ont.; 336 Light St. (res); Wes '32; Staff, Woodstock Gen. Hosp. & Alexander Hosp., Ingersoll; Tel. 537-2951.
POOLE, John C.; 1049 Devonshire Cres., Vancouver, B.C. (res); Man '36; DABA; Anaes; Staff, Vancouver Gen. Hosp.; Clin. Instr. (Anaes), U. of British Columbia; Tel. RE 3-9086.

POOLE, John K.; 4900 Kingsway, South Burnaby, B.C.; McG '53; Paed.; Clin. Instr., U. of British Columbia; Tel. HE 4-6681.
POOLE, Norman L.; 45 de Rouville, Baie Comeau, P.Q. (res); McG '54; FACS; GenSurg; Chief Surg., Boisvert Mem. Hosp.; Att'd. Surg., & Dir. of Labs., Hotel-Dieu, Hauterive; Tel. 584-2261.
POOLE, Robert W.; 130 Drinkwater St., Sudbury, Ont.; Dublin (Ire.)'46; FRCS(I); GenSurg; Chief of Surg., Sudbury Gen. Hosp.; Tel. OS 4-0936.
POOTS, A. Vaughan; 194 Talbot St. E., Aylmer, Ont.; 52 Harvey St. (res); Trinity Coll. (Dublin, Ire.) '42; MCGP; Staff, St. Thomas-Elgin Hosp.; Tel. 68.
POPHAM, Harold; 121 Chataway Blvd., Winnipeg 29, Man. (res); Man '23; Paed; Hon. Cons., Winnipeg Children's Hosp.; Retired.
POPOV, Cyril; Burwash, Ont.; Kiel (Germ.) '31; M.O., Dept. of Reform Inst'ns.
POPOV, Theodore; 30 est, boul. St-Joseph, Montreal 14, P.Q.; Sofia (Bulgaria) '42.
POPOWICH, John W.; Weinlos Clinic, 10022-103rd St., Edmonton, Alta.; Alb '61; Tel. GA 4-8076.
PORLIER, Jean P.; Lav'65; Res., Hop St-Sacrement, Quebec 6, P.Q.
POROVNE, Franc; 2406A Dufferin St., Toronto 10, Ont.; Spain '52; Tel. RU 1-8162.
PORRITT, Peter N.; Manitoba Clinic, 790 Sherbrook St., Winnipeg 2, Man.; 4829 Roblin Blvd., Wpg. 20 (res); London (Eng.) '46; LRCP (Lond.); MRCS (Eng.); FRCS (Eng.); FRCS(C); OrthSurg; Active Staff, Grace, Wpg. Gen. & Children's & Manitoba Rehabilitation Hosp's.; Lect. (Orth.), U. of Manitoba; Tel. 774-6541.
PORT, Muriel E.; Manitoba Clinic, 790 Sherbrook St., Winnipeg 2, Man.; 211 Brock St., Wpg. 9 (res); Cape Town (S. Africa) '39; MRCP (Lond.); LMSSA (Eng.); Active Staff, Grace Hosp.; Tel. SP 4-6541.
PORTELANCE, Herbert J.; 303 Goldstream Ave., Victoria, B.C.; U.S.A. '58; Tel. GR 8-1744.
PORTER, Allan S.; Port Arthur Clinic, 194 N. Court St., Port Arthur, Ont.; 169 Blanchard St. (res); Qns'51; Abroad.
PORTER, F. Thomas; 244 St. George St., Toronto, Ont.; 5 Pinevale Rd. (res); Tor '52; Ass't. Sec., O.M.A.; Tel. WA 5-3264.
PORTER, Harry; St. Leonard, Nicolet, P.Q.; Lav '49.
PORTER, James S.; 11 Dumont St., Willowdale, Ont.; Tor '51; Tel. BA 5-2676.
PORTER, J. Gordon McM.; P.O. Box 97, St. Thomas, Ont.; Qns '21; F.I.C.S.; GenSurg; Staff, St. Thomas Elgin Mem. Hosp.; Tel. ME 1-3843.
PORTER, John J.; 501 Chinook Prof. Bldg., 6449 Macleod Trail, Calgary, Alta.; Alb'40; DABR; MACR; D&TRad; Cons., Colonel Belcher Hosp. & Mineral Springs Hosp., Banff; Tel. 262-9184.
PORTER, John M.; Ste. 606, 1849 Yonge St., Toronto 7, Ont.; Tor'44; Coroner, County of York; Tel. 489-8500.
PORTER, Robert H.; 393 University Ave., Toronto 2, Ont.; 854 Caldwell Ave., Port Credit (res); Wes '55; MCGP; Med. Dir., West Area, Bell Telephone Co.; Tel. 929-2811.
PORTH, Frank J.; Box 815, Fort Qu'Appelle, Sask.; Man '31; DPH.
PORTIGAL, Evelyn P.; (See ASHLEY, Evelyn P.).
PORTIGAL, Sheila; Man '58; Res., Queen Mary Vet's. Hosp., Montreal 26, P.Q.
PORTNUFF, Harry A. L.; 19 Dunlop Block, Yorkton, Sask.; 49 Darlington E. (res); Man '26; A.I.C.S.; FICS; FASAS; M.C.G.P.; Sr. Staff (Surg) & Chief of Staff, Yorkton Union Hosp.; Tel. 783-2294.
PORTNUFF, Joseph C., MC; 5845 Cote-des-Neiges, Ste. 600, Montreal 26, P.Q.; Man '40; DABOS; FACS; FRCS(C), ObstGyn; Assoc. ObstGyn., Jewish Gen. Hosp.; Cons., Jean-Talon & Bellechasse Hosp's.; Dem., McGill U.; Tel. 735-3122. Abroad.
POS, Robert; Toronto Gen. Hosp., Toronto 2, Ont.; 18 Denewood Cres., Don Mills (res); Amsterdam (Holl.) '51; D. Psy (Tor.); Ph.D. (Utrecht); FRCP(C), Psy; Ass't. Phys., Tor. Gen. Hosp.; Clin. Instr. (Med. & Psy), U. of Toronto; Tel. EM 6-8211.
POSEN, David; 4208 Bathurst St., Downsview, Ont.; Tor'65.
POSENER, Louis J.; 2184 W. Broadway, Vancouver 9, B.C.; 1392 West 45th Ave., (res); London (Eng.) '52; LRCP, MRCS; Paed; Att'd. Staff, Van. Gen. Hosp.; Active Staff, St. Paul's & Children's Hosp's; Dem. (Paed.) U. of British Columbia; Tel. RE 6-0921.
POSNER, Barry I.; Man '61; Res. (IntMed), Winnipeg Gen. Hosp., Winnipeg, Man.
POSNER, Hertha F.; Wes '39; D.P.H. Staff Saskatoon Sanatorium, Box 1241, Saskatoon, Sask.
POSNER, Kenneth S.; Man'61; FRCP(C), Neur; Staff, Winnipeg Gen. Hosp., Winnipeg 3, Man.; Abroad.
POST, Arthur R.; Central Medical Bldg., 33 White St., St. Thomas, Ont.; 321 Sunset Dr. (res); Wes '23; GenSurg; MCGP; Surg Staff, St. Thomas-Elgin Gen. Hosp.; Vice Pres., Staff of Hosp. & Member Bd. of Governors, St.-Thomas-Elgin Gen. Hosp.; Tel. ME 1-5090.
POSTMA, Klaas J.; 321 Med. Arts Bldg., Saskatoon, Sask.; 1025-10th St. (res); Groningen (Neth.) '55; Clin Fell., (Med.), University Hosp.; Tel. 244-1137.
POSTNIKOFF, John; Medical Arts Bldg., 121 Wellington St. W., Barrie, Ont.; Tor '44.
POSTUK, Peter; 160 Jubilee St., P.O. Box 1180, Duncan, B.C.; Gibbons Rd. (res); UBC '55; M.C.G.P.; Tel. 746-4102.
POTHIER, Andre; 700 Ste. Julie, Trois Rivieres, P.Q.; 2565 Marie-Le Neuf (res); Lav '46; Pulm. Dis. & TB (P.Q.). Chief of T.B., Cooke & Ste. Marie Hosp's.; Tel. FR 6-3721.
POTHIER, Benedict E.; 497 Victoria St., Dalhousie, N.B.; Lav '40; GenSurg; Dist. Coroner. Tel. 684-3107.
POTHIER, Guy; 9 Hazlewood, Montreal 8, P.Q.; Mon '37; GenSurg; Tel. 735-0211.
POTHIER, H. J.; Lower Saulnierville, Digby Co., N.S.; Dal '19.
POTHIER, Paul; 1009 de Grenoble, Quebec 10, P.Q.; Lav'51; Psy(P.Q.); Staff(Psy.), Hop. St.-Michel Archange, Quebec.
POTHIER, Yves; 1230 Dessaulles, St. Hyacinthe, P.Q.; Mon'43; Anaes (P.Q.); Tel. 774-6717.
POTOSKI, Michael; Potoski Bldg., 190-3rd Ave., N.E., Dauphin, Man.; 328 River (res); Man '26; M.C.G.P.; Staff, Dauphin Gen. Hosp.
POTOSKI, Peter; 4 Dunlop Blk., Yorkton, Sask.; 18 Logan Cres. W. (res); Man '26; M.C.G.P.; Active Staff, Yorkton Union Hosp.; Lect. (Orthopaed.), Nursing Schl.; Tel. 783-2401.
POTOSKI, Stephanie (Petryk); 4 Dunlop Block, Yorkton, Sask.; 18 Logan Cres. W. (res); Man '46; MCGP; Tel. 783-2233.
POTTER, John M.; 435 Adelaide St., Dalhousie, N.B.; McG '48; MCGP; Dist. Coroner; Staff, St. Joseph's Hosp. & Soldier's Mem. Hosp., Campbellton; Pt.-time Phys., C.I.L.; Tel. 684-3108.
POTTER, Richard T.; 276 Charles St., Belleville, Ont.; Qns '39; MCGP; Dist Coroner; Tel. WO 2-1818.
POTTER, Stanley W.; Sheet Harbour, N.S.; Dal '54; Staff, Eastern Shore Mem. Hosp.; Tel. 200.
POTTLE, Clarence H.; 4 Bonnycastle Cr., St. John's. Nfld. (res); Dal '44; Psy; Hosp. Admin.; Dir., Mental Health Serv., Dept. of Health; Ass't. Prof. (Psy), Dalhousie U.; Tel. 579-5061.
POTTS, David W.; 2615 E. 49th Ave., Vancouver 16, B.C.; Cambridge (Eng.)'57; Visiting Active Staff, Vancouver Gen. Hosp., Grace Hosp., St. Paul's Hosp., Children's Hosp., St. Vincent's Hosp. & Mount St. Joseph's Hosp.; Tel. 433-3818.
POTTS, Donald A.; Cambrian Med. Dental Clinic, 41 Chelsea St., Calgary, Alta.; London (Eng.)'53; MRCS(Eng.), LRCP(London); Tel. AV 9-1901.
POTTS, John L.; Dingwall Med. Clinic, 56 King St., Dryden, Ont.; 181 Whyte Ave. (res); Dal '58; MCGP; Staff, Dryden Dist. Hosp.; Tel. 223-2258.

POTVIN Andre; 1225 rue Ernest Lavigne. Sillery, Quebec 6, P.Q.; Lav '49; Bact; Staff (Path.). Hotel Dieu; Staff (Microbiol.), Laval U.; Tel. 529-9151.
POTVIN, D. A. Rosario; 47 ave.-Ste-Genevieve, Quebec, P.Q. (res); Lav '17; DiagRad; Chief Rad., Hotel-Dieu Hosp.; Emer. Prof. (Histol.), Laval U.; Tel. 529-9151.
POTVIN, Earl J.; Ott '64; Res., Ottawa Civic
POTVIN, Jacques; Lav'64; Res., Hop. Hotel-Dieu, Quebec 4, P.Q.
POTVIN, Jacques J.; Lav'54; Res., Hop. Ste. Justine, Montreal 26, P.Q.
POTVIN, Jean G.; 210 de Martigny, St-Jerome Cte. Terrebonne, P.Q.; Mon '65.
POTVIN, J. Y. Laurent; 623 Noranda, Ottawa 2, Ont. (res); Lav '46; F.R.C.P.(C), IntMed, Gastroent (P.Q.); Head of Dept. of Med., Hop. St. Louis-Marie de Montfort; Ass't. Prof. (Clin-Med.), U. of Ottawa; Tel. SH 6-4621.
POTVIN, Leonce; Hebertville, P.Q.; Lav '50; Staff, Notre Dame d'Hebertville Hosp.
POTVIN, Paul; 5750 boul. Gouin ouest, Montreal 9, P.Q.; Mon '39; OrthSurg.
POTVIN, Real; 143 Wolfe, Levis, P.Q.; Lav '59; Psy (P.Q.).
POTVIN, Pierre; 1915 rue Bourbonniere, Quebec 6, P.Q.; Lav'55; Ph.D. (Tor.); Prof. (Physiol.), Laval U.; Tel. LA 9-4511.
POTVIN, Robert; 770-lere ave., Quebec 3, P.Q.; **Lav '53; FRCP(C), IntMed; Cardiol (P.Q.); Teach. Staff, Hop-St-Francois-d'Assise & Laval U.; Tel. 529-0042.**
POTVIN, Victor; 313 rue St. Joseph, La Tuque, P.Q.; Lav '31; GenSurg; Med. & Surg. Supt., Hop, St. Joseph; Tel. 3-2161.
POUDRIER, Claude; 1401-18e rue, Quebec 3, **P.Q.; Lav '59; PhysMed & Rehab; Staff, Hop-de-l'Enfant-Jesus; Tel. 529-8711.**
POULAKAKIS, George M.; Athens (Gr.) '48; Deputy Dir., Munroe Wing & Clinic, Regina Gen. Hosp., Regina, Sask.
POULIN, Gerald; Lav '61; Res., Hop. St-Sacrement, Quebec 6, P.Q.
POULIN, Fabien; 1555 rue Latour St. Hubert Co. Chambly, P.Q.; Lav '55.
POULIN, Gilles; 802 Chanoine-Scott, Quebec 10, P.Q.; 1950 Raymond Casgran (res); Lav '56; Otol (P.Q.); Ass't. (Oral), Hop Laval; Tel. 653-9833.
POULIN, G. R.; c/o Chief Medical Officer, Dept. Nat. Health & Welfare, 61 Green St., London W.1, England.
POULIN, Jacques; St-Ephrem, Cte Beauce, P.Q.; Lav'65.
POULIN, Jacques G.; MIR, RCAF Station, Winnipeg, Man.; Mon '65.
POULIN, Jean C.; Lav '60; Anaes; Staff, Hop. St-Joseph, Rimouski, P.Q.; Tel. 723-7851.
POULIN, Marc; Lav '49; Path (P.Q.); Haem (P.Q.); Path & Med. Dir., Hop. St-Joseph, Thetford Mines, P.Q.; Tel. FE 5-2971.
POULIN, Michel; 26, 20eme rue, St-Georges-de-Beauce, P.Q.; Lav '65.
POULIN, Nil; 490-17eme rue, Grand'Mere, P.Q.; Lav'65.
POULIN, Omer.; Lauvaine (Belg.) '63; Res., Hop. Notre-Dame, Montreal 24, P.Q.
POULIN, Raoul; St. Martin, Co. Beauce, P.Q.; Lav '26.
POULIN, Rheo; 198B Notre Dame, Thetford Mines, P.Q.; Lav'65.
POULIN, Roch; Lav'53; Res., Hop. Notre-Dame, Montreal 24, P.Q.
POULIN, Yvan; Ste-Agathe, Cte Lotbiniere, P.Q.; Lav '64.
POULIOT, Claude; 4, rue Taillenbourg, Courville, P.Q.; Lav '59.
POULIOT, C. Eugene; 52 Murray, Sherbrooke, P.Q. Mon '24.
POULIOT, Gerard E.; 176A, Ave. de l'Eglise Verdun 19, P.Q.; 4052 Ave. Marlowe, N.D.G. (res); Lav '30; Ophth (P.Q.); Chief, Dept. of OphthOtol., Verdun Gen. Hosp.; Tel. PO 6-3551.
POULIOT, J. Claude; 2979 rue Matapedia, Quebec 10, P.Q. (res); Lav '57; Anaes; Staff, Hop. Enfant-Jesus; Tel. 529-8711.
POULIOT, Jean P.; St. Agapit, P.Q.; Lav '39; Dist. Coroner.
POULIOT, Louis; 1186 Ave. des Erables, Quebec, P.Q.; 1318 des Gouverneurs, Sillery (res); Lav '48; AMCAA, FRCP(C), IntMed; Ass't. Dept. of Med.. Hop. St. Francois d'Assisi; Assoc. Prof., Laval U.; Tel. 683-8013.
POULIOT, Louis; St.-Pierre-les-Becquets, Cte. Nicolet, P.Q.; Lav '62.
POULIOT, Marc A.; Gaspe, P.Q.; Lav '56. Paed (P.Q.); Tel. 699.
POULIOT, Marcel J.; 3058 Rue Laforest, Quebec 10, P.Q.; Lav'60; Biochem.(P.Q.).
POULIOT, P.; c/o Regional Dir., European Reg., Dept. of National Health & Welfare, 38 Grosvenor St., London W.1., England; Abroad.
POULIOT, Paul E.; 897-3eme Ave., Quebec, P.Q.; 368-15rue (res); Lav '37; FR.C.S.(C), GenSurg.; Tel. 524-2659.
POULIOT, Paul E.; Lav'61; Path(P.Q.); Staff, Hotel Dieu St. Vallier, Chicoutimi, P.Q.
POULOS, Harry P.; 90 Crichton Ave., Dartmouth, N.S.; Dal'51; Psy; Clin. Dir., Nova Scotia Hosp.; Tel. 466-7727.
POULSEN, Ernest R.; 1605 - 9th Ave. S., Lethbridge, Alta.: Alb '43.
POULSEN, James B.; Irving Clinic, 74 W. Seymour St., Kamloops, B.C.; Alb '64; Tel. 372-5251.
POUPART, Gerard; 825 est boul. St. Joseph, Montreal, P.Q.; Mon '37; Pulm. Dis. & TB (P.Q.).; Tel. VI 5-5955.
POURBAIX, William E.; 107 Le Marchand Mansions, 116th St. & 100th Ave., Edmonton, Alta.; Alb '42; IntMed; Active Staff, Edmonton Gen. Hosp.; Tel. 482-1737.
POVAH, Arthur H.; 115 Clement Block, Brandon, **Man.; 241-29th St. (res); Man '45; Staff, Assini**boine Hosp.; Tel. 9-8488.
POW, Cyrus G.; 203-1541 W. Broadway, Vancouver, B.C.; 1750 Allison Rd., Van. 8 (res); McG '45; FICS; PlasSurg; Att'd, Staff, Children's Hosp.; Vis. Staff, Van. Gen. & St. Paul's Hosp's.; Cons. Staff, St. Mary's Hosp.; Tel. RE 3-5725.
POW, Robert E.; Ste. 35, Academy Med. Bldg., 1812-4th St. S.W., Calgary, Alta; 3611-7th St. S.W. (res); Alb '43; FRCS(Ed.); FRCS(C); GenSurg; Cons. Staff, Colonel Belcher Hosp.; Att'd. Staff, Calgary Gen., Holy Cross & Children's Hosp's.; **Tel. 269-4258.**
POWELL, A. Bailey C.; 12 Feldbar Crt., Willowdale, Ont. (res); Tel. 221-6696; Tor'38; GenSurg; Dir. Med. Serv., W.C.B., 90 Harbour St., Toronto; Tel. 362-3411.
POWELL, Alan H.; 5300 Cote des Neiges Rd., Montreal 26, P.Q.; McG'59; IntMed.
POWELL, Anne M.; Apt. 912, 124 Springfield Rd., Ottawa 2, Ont.; McG'64.
POWELL, Elinor D. U.; 567 Montery Ave., Victoria, B.C.; FRCP(C), IntMed.
POWELL, Eva G. (Mrs. Leon); 7 Smallwood Cr., Charlottetown, P.E.I. (res); Dal'54; Psy; Staff, Riverside Hosp.; Tel. 4-5581.
POWELL, Evan; Medical Arts Bldg., 73 Cumberland N., Port Arthur, Ont.; 126 Winnipeg Ave. (res); Tor '42; Ophth; Med. Staff, McKellar Gen. Hosp.; Tel. DI 4-6681.
POWELL, Gordon W.; 350 Portage Rd. N., Niagara Falls, Ont.; **Tor '51; Coroner, Welland Co.; Tel. EL 8-3244.**
POWELL, Henry C.; Ste. 506, 1906 Barclay St., Vancouver 5, B.C. (res); Charing Cross H. (Lon.) '20; M.R.C.S., L.R.C.P.; Adm., Workmen's Comp. Bd., Vancouver; Tel. AM 6-0211.
POWELL, Lloyd G.; Box 70, Yellowknife, N.W. T.; McG '59; AMCGP; Pres., Med. Staff, Stanton Hosp.; M.O.H.; Coroner; Tel. 4456.
POWELL, Marion G. (Gray); 2001 Eglinton Ave. E., Scarborough, Ont.; Tor '46; DPH; Ass't. M.O.H., Scarborough Dept. of Health; Tel. 759-4747.
POWELL-SMITH, Cyril J.; 5295 Westmore Ave., Montreal 28, P.Q.; London (Eng.)'56; FRCP(C), TherRad; Staff, Montreal Gen. Hosp., Montreal, P.Q.
POWELL, Thomas J., G/C; Tor '39; DABAviaMed; FACPrevMed; Ottawa Valley Reg. Surg., Air Materiel HQ., Ottawa, Ont.

POWELL, Tom E.; Ste. 2103, 2055 Pendrell St., Vancouver 5, B.C.; Oxon & London (Eng.)'51; Anaes; Staff, Assoc. Anaes.

POWELL, William C.; 16 King St. W., Hagersville, Ont.; Qns'37; Dist. Coroner, County of Haldimand; M.O.H., Hagersville & Oneida; Tel. 768-3387.

POWELL, W. Gayner; 2115 Victoria Ave., Windsor, Ont. (res); Tor'20; GenSurg; Surg. Staff, Grace Hosp.; Tel. 253-1622.

POWER, David J.; 3830 Lacombe Ave., Montreal 26, P.Q.; 49 Franklin Ave., Mtl. 16 (res); Nat. U. (Ire) '47; FFARCSI, FFARCS; DA; DABA; FRCP(C), Anaes; Anaes-in-Chief, St. Mary's Hosp.; Ass't. Prof. (Anaes), McGill U. Tel. 735-3511.

POWER, Frank L.; 130 Elm St. E., Sudbury, Ont.; 376 Laura (res); Ott '51; FACS; FRCS(C); GenSurg; Sr. Surg., Sudbury Gen., Sudbury Mem. & St. Joseph's Hosp's.; Tel. 673-7181.

POWER, George R. I., S/L; 6 Woodfield Cres., Westbrook, Ont. (res); Dal '53; DMR (Tor.); DiagRad; Chief, Dept. of Rad., Cdn. Forces Hosp., Kingston; Lect., (Rad), Queen's U.; RCAF; Tel. 8-3060.

POWER, Phillip G.; 209 Church St., Comox, B.C.; Box 400; Wes '51; MCGP; Active Staff, St. Joseph Gen. Hosp.; Tel. 339-2266.

POWER, Richard M. H.; Sr.; 1610 Sherbrooke St. W., Ste. 11, Montreal, P.Q.; 57 Forden Ave., Westmount (res); McG '20; M.Sc. (McG), D.Sc. (Lav), F.A.C.S., F.I.C.S., D.A.B.O.G., F.A.C.O.G., ObstGyn; Sr. Att. Obst. & Gyn., St. Mary's Hosp., Montreal; Cons. Gyn., Hop. Notre Dame de l'Esperance, Ville St. Laurent; Tel. WE 5-7722.

POWER, R. M. Hugh; 1610 Sherbrooke St. W., Montreal 25, P.Q.; Ott'55; MRCOG; FRCS(C), ObstGyn; Clin. Ass't. (ObstGyn), Royal Victoria Hosp., St. Mary's & McGill U.; Tel. WE 5-7722.

POWERS, Annie; Rockland, Ont.; Ott '45; M.C.G.P.

POWERS, Arthur; 135 Gloucester, Ottawa 4, Ont.; 11 Front St., Hull, P.Q. (res); Lav '32; F.C.C.P., Cardiol, (P.Q.), Pulm. Dis. TB (P.Q.); IntMed; Lect. (Med.), U. of Ottawa; Tel. 233-3614.

POWERS, Charles G.; 541 William St., Preston, Ont.; 452 Duke St. (res); McG '37; Staff, S. Waterloo Mem., St. Mary's, Kitchener-Waterloo & Freeport San.; Tel. 653-3031.

POWERS, Neil; 2363 McIntyre St., Regina, Sask.; Cambridge (Eng.)'58; Tel. 527-0641.

POWERS, Oscar C.; Woodstock, Ont.; Thamesford, R.R. No. 4 (res); Wes '27; D.P.H.; Dir., Oxford Health Unit; M.O.H., Oxford Co.; Retired.

POWERS, Robert; 73 Ave. Begin, Levis, P.Q.; Lav '46; GenSurg (P.Q.).

POWLES, G.P.S.; 201 Med. Bldg., Prince Albert, Sask.; Man '40; MCGP; Tel. 763-2681.

POWLES, William E.; McG'43; Psy; Staff, Dept. of Psy., Queen's U., Kingston, Ont.

POY, Neville G.; McG '60; Res., Montreal Gen. Hosp., Montreal, P.Q.

POZNANSKI, Wojciech J.; Metabolism Serv., Dept. of Med., Ottawa Civic Hosp., Ottawa, Ont.; Brussels (Belgium) '49; IntMed; Tel. 729-2511, Ext. 420.

POZNER, Samuel N.; 1884 Eglinton Ave. E., Scarborough, Ont.; Tor '52; ObstGyn.; Tel. PL 9-2331.

POZNAN, Zoltan; Ste. 101, 3311 Bayview Ave., Willowdale, Ont.; '56; Tel. 223-2089.

POZSONYI, Joseph; 10 Beechwood Pl., London, Ont. (res); Staff Psych., Research Inst. for Children.

PRADOS, Miguel; Apt. 48, 1390 Sherbrooke St. W., Montreal, P.Q.; 432 Metcalfe Ave. (Westmount (res); Madrid (Spain) '19; F.A.P.A., Psy; Cons. Psy., Montreal Neurological Inst.; Spec. Lect., Allan Mem. Inst. of Psych.; Tel. VI 2-1804. Retired.

PRAG, Joe J.; Johannesburg (S. Africa)'38; MB; B.Ch; BSc(Hons.); DPH; Pathol. (S. Africa); Staff, Gen. Hosp., Sault Ste. Marie, Ont.

PRASAD, Lakshman; Patna (India)'58; Staff, Saskatchewan Hosp., North Battleford, Sask.

PRASLOSKI, Peter F.; Ste. 204, Westminster Med. Bldg., 625 Fifth Ave., New Westminster, B.C.; UBC'56; ABOph; Ophth; Staff, Royal Columbian & St. Mary's Hosp's.; Tel. 521-3232.

PRAT, Alain; 1150 est, boul. St. Joseph, Montreal 34, P.Q.; Mon'59; FRCP(C), IntMed; Tel. 527-1241.

PRATT, Charles H.; 150 Gurnett St., Aurora, Ont. (res); Tor '24; NeurPsy; Med. Supt., Ontario Hosp., Aurora; Retired.

PRATT, Charles M.; 1 Chipman Hill, Saint John, N.B.; McG '02; Retired.

PRATT, Glenn E.; 40 Alexander St., London, Ont.; Wes '52; MCGP; Fell. (Med.), U. of Western Ont.; Tel. 439-2281.

PRATT, Henry H.; 9 Chartwell Rd., Toronto 18, Ont. (res); Dal '61; AMCGP; Staff, Ontario Hosp.; Tel. LE 3-8501.

PRATT-JOHNSON, John A.; 507 Fairmont Med. Bldg., 750 W. Broadway, Vancouver 9, B.C.; 1715 W. 16th St. (res); Witwatersrand (Jo'burg, S. Africa) '51; FRCS (Edin); DO (Lond.); FRCS(C), Ophth; Cons. Ophth, Shaughnessy DVA Hosp.; Att'd. Staff, Van. Gen. Hosp.; Instr. (Ophth), U. of British Columbia; Tel. 874-0644.

PRATT, Kenneth E.; 235A Danforth Ave., Toronto, Ont.; Tor '31; Tel. HO 6-8811.

PRATT, Roy F.; UBC'63; Res., Vancouver Gen. Hosp., Vancouver 9, B.C.

PRATTEN, John S.; 213 Mowat Ave., Kingston, Ont. (res); Qns '43; D.Psy; Psy; Supt., Ontario Hosp.; Assoc. Prof. (Psy.), Queen's U.; Tel. 546-1101.

PREECE, Clifford G.; 111 St. Clair Ave. W., Toronto 7, Ont.; 47 Citation Dr., Willowdale (res); Tor '42; IntMed; Vol. Ass't. (Med.) O.P.D., Toronto Gen. Hosp.; Regional Phys., Imperial Oil Co. Ltd.; Tel. 924-9111.

PREFONTAINE, Georges; 5689 Boul. Rosemont, Montreal 36, P.Q. (res); Mon '23; Bact. (P.Q.); Dir. of Labs., Hop. St. Joseph, de Rosemont, Montreal 36, P.Q.; Hon. Prof. & Memb. Admin. Council, Inst. of Microbiol. & Hygiene, U. of Montreal: Tel. CL 6-2681.

PREFONTAINE, Lionel L.; Montmartre, Sask.; Lav '52; Tel. 72.

PREFONTAINE, Real G.; 150 St. George St., Toronto 5, Ont.; 15 Esterbrooke Ave., Ste. 26, Willowdale (res); Lav '61; Ass't. Sec., Canadian Med. Assoc.; Tel. 924-0751.

PREGELJ, Srecko; Madrid (Spain)'54; Res., Royal Ottawa San., Ottawa 3, Ont.

PRELIPP, Joan B.; 658 Sequin Cres., Port Credit, Ont.; Tor '51; Anaes; Anaes. Staff, South Peel Hosp.; Tel. 279-7330.

PREMACHUK, Peter G.; Flin Flon Clin., Flin Flon, Man.; 384 Parkway Blvd. (res); Ott '54; M.C.G.P.; Staff, Flin Flon Gen. & Company Hosp's.; Tel. 687-5211.

PREMI, John; 310 Med. Arts Bldg., 1 Young St., Hamilton, Ont.; 819 Garth St. (res); Tor '55; MCGP; Tel. JA 9-6762.

PRENDERGAST, D'Arcy; Ste. 63A, 2 Bloor St. E., Toronto 5, Ont.; 124 Crescent Rd. (res); Tor '22; M.R.C.P. (Eng.); IntMed; Tel. 921-3385.

PRENDERGAST, Walter F.; 306 Glenayr Rd., Toronto 10, Ont. (res); Tor '50; Cons. (Indust. Med.), Scarborough Gen. Hosp.; Staff O.P.D., St. Michael's Hosp.; Med. Dir., T. Eaton Co. of Canada; Tel. UN 1-5111.

PRENOVEAU, Yolande; Mon'65; Res., Inst. Albert Prevost, Montreal 9, P.Q.

PRENTICE, Alexander W.; Malton Med. Centre, Malton, Ont.; 18 Tampa Terr. (res); Cambridge (Eng.)'55; Tel. 677-4200.

PRENTICE, Robert S.; Camp Hill Hosp., Halifax, N.S.; Qns'60; Path; Pathol., Camp Hill Hosp.; Ass't. Path., Inst. of Path., Dalhousie University; Lect. (Path.), Dalhousie University; Tel. 423-1371, Ext. 282.

PRESTAGE, Patrick T.; Esterhazy Med. Clinic, Esterhazy, Sask.; National U. (Ire.)'47; DPH; Tel. 745-3971.

PRESTON, Alan J.; 25 Leonard Ave., Ste. 303, Toronto 2B, Ont.; 216 Cortleigh Blvd., Tor. 12 (res); Tor'53; D.Psy; FRCP(C), Psy; Chief, Dept. of Psy., Tor. Western Hosp.; Ass't. Prof., Dept. of Med. & Psy., U. of Toronto; Tel. 368-1355.

PRESTON, A. Mary; 272 Glasgow St., Kitchener, Ont.; Dal'57.

PRESTON, David N.; Tor'60; FRCP(C), IntMed; Staff, Hosp. for Sick Children, Toronto 2, Ont.

PRESTON, David R.; Lamont Clinic, Lamont, Alta.; Tor '55; Tel. 55-15.

PRESTON, Frederick C.; Ste. 816, 750 W. Broadway, Vancouver 9, B.C.; 1307 W. 33 (res); Tor'34; **F.R.C.S.(C), GenSurg, OrthSurg; Att. Staff, Vancouver Gen. Hosp. & B.C. Cancer Inst; Clin.** Assoc. Prof., Dept. of OrthSurg., U. of British Columbia; Tel. TR 2-7181.

PRESTON, Fred T.; Med. Dental Bldg., Lethbridge, Alta.; Man '39; MCGP; Tel. 327-6737.

PRESTON, H. E.; 62 King St. E., Brockville, Ont.; Qns '16; F.I.C.S.; ObstGyn.; Dist. Coroner.

PRESTON, Helen A. (Humphries); 25 Leonard Ave., Ste. 303, Toronto 2B, Ont. 216 Cortleigh Blvd., Tor. 12 (res); Tor '56; D.Psy; Psy; Psy., Ont. Hosp., New Toronto; Tel. 368-1355.

PRESTON, Joseph H.; 1 Sunset Blvd., Brockville, Ont. (res); Qns '35; DPH (Tor); Staff, Ont. Hosp.; Tel. DI 5-1451.

PRESTON, Kenneth S.; Allan Blair Mem. Clinic, Regina, Sask.; Edinburgh (Scot.) '44; DMRT (Edin.); Sr. Assoc. (TherRad), Sask. Cancer Clinic; Tel. 527-9651.

PRESTON, Margaret T.; 3831 Albert St., Regina, Sask.; Glasgow (Scot.)'46; Staff, Sask. T.B. League.

PRESTON, William H. B.; Ste. 5, 498A Brant St., Burlington, Ont.; Tor'51; MCGP; Tel. NE 4-5316.

PRESUTTI, Henry J.; Box 458, Brighton Clinic, Main St., Brighton, Ont.; Dal '56; MCGP; Tel. 475-2100.

PRETO, Hannibal; UBC '64; Res., Vancouver Gen. Hosp., Vancouver 9, B.C.

PRETTY, Geoffrey C.; 3331 Bloor W., Toronto 18, Ont.; 1591 Wembury Rd., Clarkson (res); London (Eng.) '52; Staff, C.N.R. Clinic, Toronto & Dept. G.P., Queensway Gen. Hosp.; Tel. BE 1-8430.

PRETTY, H. Gurth; 906-1414 Drummond St., Montreal, P.Q.; 600 Rockland Ave., Outremont (res); McG '25; F.A.C.S., D.A.B.S., F.A.C.A.; GenSurg; Hon. Att'd. Surg., Montreal Gen. Hosp.; Cons. Surg., Verdun Protestant & Cornwall Gen. Hosp'.; Tel. AV 8-2912.

PRETTY, Harry M.; Mon'61; Haem(P.Q.); Staff, Hotel-Dieu Hosp., Montreal, P.Q.; Abroad.

PREVILLE, Guy; 94 Deguire, Chateauguay Centre, P.Q.; Mon'51; Anaes (P.Q.).

PREVILLE, Rene; 21 St. Charles, Joliette, P.Q.; Mon '49.

PREVOST, Edward C.; 318 Cook Medical Bldg., 1175 Cook St., Victoria, B.C.; 4491 Shore Way (res); Seattle (Washington, U.S.A.) '51; ObstGyn; Tel. EV 5-7033.

PREVOST, J. A. Remi; 86-88 St. Thomas, Montmagny, P.Q.; Lav '60; AMCGP; Tel. 248-0942.

PREVOST, Jules; 1681 Parc Lafontaine, Montreal 34, P.Q.; Mon '29; F.C.C.P., Pulm. Dis. & TB (P.Q.); IntMed; Dir., Thor. Clin. & Phys., Hop. Notre Dame; Prof. of Med., U. of Montreal; Tel. LA 6-5903.

PREVOST, Marcel J.; 115 Cedar St., Sudbury, Ont.; Lav'53; FRCS(C), GenSurg.; Tel. 674-7812.

PREVOST, Maurice; Lav'59; Otol; Staff, Hop. Maisonneuve, Montreal 36, P.Q.

PREVOST, Paul; 450 rue Principale, Lachute, P.Q.; Mon '63.

PREVOST, Yves; Ste 200, 1656 est rue Sherbrooke, Montreal 24, P.Q.; 6229 Deacon Rd., Mtl. 8 (res); Mon '48; FRCS(C), PlasSurg; GenSurg; Tel. 527-1528.

PRICE, Carmen S.; Dal '65; Staff, Grand Bank Cottage Hosp., Fortune Bay, Nfld.

PRICE, David C.; Tor '58; FRCP(C), IntMed; Staff, Toronto Gen. Hosp., Toronto, Ont. Abroad.

PRICE, Derek L.; Oakville, Man.; Sheffield (Eng.) '51; Deputy MOH, Portage-la-Prairie; Tel. 7.

PRICE, D. King; Ste. 103, 688 Coxwell Ave., Toronto 6, Ont.; Guys Hosp. (London, Eng.)'56; FRCP(C), Anaes; Ass't. Anaes., Toronto East Gen. Hosp.

PRICE, F. E.; Norwich, Ont.; Qns '19.

PRICE, George E.; UBC '59; FRCP(C); IntMed; Staff, Vancouver Gen. Hosp., Vancouver 9, B.C.; Tel. 876-3211.

PRICE, George M.; Tofield, Alta.; Loma Linda (Calif., U.S.A.)'52; Tel. Riley 58.

PRICE, Gerald F.; 84 Rogers Rd., Toronto 10, Ont.; Tor '28; Sr. Att'd. Staff, Northwestern Gen. Hosp.; Tel. 651-1431.

PRICE, Harold W.; 214-6th Ave. S.W., Calgary, Alta.; 2917-10th St. S.W. (res); Johns Hopkins (U.S.A.) **'24; A.B.P.; F.A.A.P.; Paed; Chief of Paed., Holy Cross Hosp.; Tel. AM 6-7231; Retired.**

PRICE, Ivan; 334 Queen's Ave, London, Ont.; R.R. No. 7 (res); Dal'42; FAAD; DermSypth., Sr. Cons. (Derm.) DVA, Western Ont; Instr. (Med.), U. of Western Ont.; Tel. 439-9211.

PRICE, John; Fredericton Med. Clinic, 206 Rookwood Ave., Fredericton, N.B.; 121 Winslow St. (res); Queen's U. (Belfast, N. Ire.) '55; DA (McG); **Anaes; Staff, Victoria Public Hosp.; Tel. 475-7701.**

PRICE, John D.; Dept. of Med., Vancouver Gen. Hosp., Vancouver 9, B.C.; McG'54; FRCP (C); IntMed; Assoc. Phys., Vancouver Gen. Hosp.; Cons. (Med.) Shaughnessy Veterans Hosp.; Assoc. Prof. (Med.), U. of British Columbia; Tel. TR 6-3211.

PRICE, Norman E.; Medical Arts Bldg., Hamilton, Ont.; 227 Queensdale Ave. E. (res); **Wes '50;** M.C.G.P.; Tel. JA 2-6207.

PRICE, R. M.; Medical Centre, Brooklin, Ont.; Tor'65.

PRICE, Vera H. (Heller); 314 St. Clair Ave. W., Toronto 10, Ont.; Tor '58; FRCP(C); Derm; Staff, Toronto Gen. & Women's College Hosp's.; Clin. Teach. (Med.), U. of Toronto; Tel. EM 6-8211.

PRICHARD, John S., MC; 555 University Ave., Toronto 2, Ont.; 25 St. Leonard's Ave. Tor. 12 (res); Cambridge (Eng.)'38; MRCP; FRCP (Lond.); Neur; Cons. Paed. Neurol., Hosp. for Sick Children; Assoc. Prof. (Paed.), U. of Toronto; Tel. EM 6-7242, Loc. 345.

PRIDDLE, William W.; 618 Medical Arts Bldg., Toronto, Ont.; 4272 Dufferin St., Downsview (res); Wes'26; F.A.C.P.; IntMed; Att'd. O.P.D., Toronto Western Hosp., Cons., Geriatrics, Prov. of Ont.; Tel. WA 3-3824.

PRIDHAM, Guy R.; 150 Jarry St. E., Montreal 11, P.Q.; Mon '59; Tel. DU 1-2313.

PRIDHAM, W. E.; Mitchell, Ont.; St. David's St. (res); Wes '30.

PRIEBE, Victor H.; 1574 Ouellette Ave., Windsor, Ont.; Wes'57; DiagRad; Staff, Hotel-Dieu of St. Joseph Hosp.; Tel. 256-4914.

PRIETZ, Hans; 59 Park St. W., Port Credit, Ont. (res); Rorloik (Germ.) '35; Phys., Mimico Reformatory.

PRIEUR, George O.; 214-6th Ave. W., Calgary, Alta.; 3635-9th St. S.W. (res); Alb '35 FAAP; Paed.; Tel. 263-7120.

PRIME, F. Michael; Tor '57; D. Psy; Staff, Riverview Hosp., Essondale, B.C.

PRIME, Ralph L.; 3220 Cambridge St., Niagara Falls, Ont.; Dal'53; Anaes.

PRIMEAU, Bertrand; 4470 Lacombe, Montreal 26, P.Q. (res); Mon '33; MPH; Med. Dir., Institut de Rehabilitation de Montreal, 6300 ave. **Darlington, Mtl. 26; Tel. 735-3741.**

PRIMEAU, Robert; 8415 St. Denis, Montreal, P.Q.; Mon'54; IntMed(P.Q.); Tel. DU 1-1801.

PRIMEAU, Robert; Mon'61; Cardiol(P.Q.); FRCP(C), IntMed; Staff, Hop.-Hotel-Dieu, Montreal 18, P.Q.; Abroad.

PRIMROSE, Thomas; 2332 Fulton Rd., Town of Mount Royal, Montreal, P.Q. (res); Edinburgh (Scot.) '40; F.A.C.S., F.R.C.S.(C), ObstGyn; Obst. & Gyn., Royal Victoria Hosp. & Ass't. ObstGyn., Montreal Gen. Hosp.; Assoc. Prof., McGill U.; Tel. AV 8-5307.

PRINCE, Douglas A.; 116 Elm St. E., Sudbury, Ont.; 22 Cranbrook Cr. (res); Qns '62; Active Staff, Sudbury Gen. & Mem. Hosp's.; Tel. 682-4421.

PRINCE, Frederick W.; Hillcrest Clinic, Bridgewater, N.S.; 78 Dufferin St. (res); Dal '56; AMCGP; Staff, Dawson Mem. Hosp.; Tel. 543-4314.

PRINCE, Garry E.; Tor'63; Res., Ontario Hosp., Toronto 3, Ont.

PRINCE, Gilles; 222 rue Longueuil, St.-Jean, P.Q.; Mon'57; Paed.; Chief, Dept. of Paed., Hop. St. Jean; Tel. 346-4348.

PRINCE, Jack E.; 1310 Ouellette Ave., Windsor Ont.; Wes '49; IntMed.; Dir. of Radioisotope Lab., Met. Gen. Hosp.; Chief of Med., Grace Hosp.; Tel. CL 3-2495.

PRINCE, Jacques; 55 de l'Eglise, Verdun, Montreal 19, P.Q.; 181 Blvd. St. Joseph E. (res); Mon '47; GenSurg (P.Q.).; Tel. 769-6181.

PRINCE, J. B.; 181 Blvd. St. Joseph E., Montreal, P.Q.; Lav '06; GenSurg (P.Q.).; Tel. VI 9-5877

PRINCE, M. C.; Tor'65; Res., Sunnybrook Hosp., Toronto 12, Ont.

PRINCE, Raymond H.; 1266 Pine Ave. W., Montreal 25, P.Q.; Wes'50; Psy; Research Dir., Urban Social Redevelopment Project; Tel. VI 4-6311, Local 631.

PRINCE, W. Ross; Ste 4, 331 Sheddon, Oakville, Ont.; Tor'59; Urol.; Staff, Oakville-Trafalgar Mem. & Joseph Brant Hosp's.; Tel. 845-3272.

PRINGLE, Donald F.; 1535 Notre-Dame, Lachine, P.Q.; Qns '63; Staff, Lachine Gen. Hosp.; Tel. 637-1161.

PRINS, Vincent Winkler; Hermitage, Nfld.; Groningen (Neth) '48.

PRIOR, Burton C.; Queensway Gen. Hosp., X-Ray Dept., Sherway Dr., Toronto 18, Ont.; 5150 Dundas St., Islington; 501 Temagami Cres., Port Credit (res); Tor'43; DABR, DiagRad; Dir., Dept. of Rad., Queensway Gen. Hosp.; Tel. CL 9-6671, Loc. 491.

PRIOR, John D.; Coldwater, Ont.; Tor '28.

PRIORESCHI, Plinio; Pavia (Italy)'54; Staff, Dept. of Pharm., Queen's U., Kingston, Ont.

PRISSICK, Frances H.; 27 Bellevue Ave., Westmount, Montreal, P.Q. (res); McG '39; Bact; Staff, Montreal Children's Hosp.; Tel. WE 7-8511.

PRITCHARD, Elizabeth J.; Ott'62; Staff, Children's Hosp., Montreal 25, P.Q.

PRITCHARD, Joseph E.; 239 Lazard Ave., Mount Royal, Montreal 16, P.Q. (res); Man '17; Path, Bact; Cons. Path., Mtl. Gen. Hosp.; Hon. Cons. (Path), Mtl. Children's & St. Mary's Hosp's.: Tel. RE 8-4082.

PRITCHARD, Raymond E.; 641 Med. Arts Bldg., 750 Spadina Cr. E., Saskatoon, Sask.; Alb '56; Staff, University, St. Paul's & City Hosp's.; Tel. 652-7272.

PRITCHARD, Robert W.; 539 Exmouth St., Sarnia, Ont.; 606 Cathcart Blvd. (res); Tor '41; FC-CP; Active Staff I/C Inhalation Therapy & Chest Clin., St. Joseph's Hosp.; Head Anaes., Sarnia Gen. Hosp.; Tel. DI 4-3695.

PRITCHARD, Ruggles B.; Box 178, George St., Havelock, Ont.; Dal '54; Staff, Campbellford Mem., St. Joseph's & Peterborough Civic Hosp's., M.O.H. Havelock; Tel. 778-3361.

PRITCHETT, Edwin A.; Bellingham Med. Center, Bellingham, Wash., U.S.A.; Wes '51; D.A.B.O.G.; ObstGyn.

PRITCHETT, Leonard W.; 54 Ainslie St. N., Galt, Ont.; 445 Dover St. N., Preston (res); Wes '19; Surg. Staff, South Waterloo Memorial Hosp.; Schl. M.O., City of Galt.

PRIVE, Lucien; 736 rue Murdock, Chicoutimi, P.Q.; Lav '54; Path (P.Q.); DAB (Path); Staff, Hop.-Hotel-Dieu-St. Vallier; Tel. 549-2195.

PROBERT, Lloyd A.; 510 Scott Bldg., Moose Jaw, Sask.; Tor '45; Ophth; Staff, Moose Jaw Union & Providence Hosp's.; Tel. 692-3095.

PROBERT, Ralph I.; 17 Mount Royal Ave., Hamilton, Ont.; Tor '40; D.A. (R.C.P. & S.E.), Anaes; Anaes. Staff, Hamilton Gen. Hosp.; Tel. JA 7-0271.

PROCTER, Henry A., DSO; Apt. 909, 200 Rideau Terr., Ottawa 2, Ont. (res); Tor '38; Ph. D.; Dir., Med. Serv., Dept. of Nat. Health & Welfare; Tel. CE 2-8211.

PROCTER, William C.; 480 Guelph Line, Burlington, Ont.; 239 Elmhurst (res); Tor '59; Active Staff, Joseph Brant Mem. Hosp.; Tel. 637-2349.

PROCTOR, Anthony P.; Tor'65; Res., Hosp. for Sick Children, Toronto 2, Ont.

PROCUNIER, Cecil W.; Wes '28; Staff, Dept. of Can. Pension Commiss., Sunnybrook Hosp., Toronto 12, Ont.; Tel. 485-8651.

PROCUNIER, Frederick A.; 44 Alice St., Waterford, Ont.; Tor '38; MCGP; Active Staff, Norfolk Gen. Hosp.; Tel. 443-8223.

PROHASKA, Gertrude; '53; (Intern); c/o Apt. 3, 8011 Champagneur, Montreal 15, P.Q.

PROKIPCHUK, Edward J.; 87 Grenview Blvd. S., Toronto, Ont. (res); Wes '54; FRCP(C); IntMed (Gastroent.); Staff, St. Michael's Hosp.; Clin. Teach., U. of Toronto; Tel. 362-4461, Loc. 552.

PROKOPETZ, George V.; 3000-30th St., Vernon, B.C.; Innsbruck (Austria) '60.

PROKOPETZ, Vadim; 263 Niagara St., St. Catharines, Ont.; Innsbruck (Aust.) '50; ObstGyn; Active Staff, St. Catharines Gen., Hotel-Dieu & Niagara-on-the-Lake Hosp's.; Tel. MU 4-6141.

PROKOPISHYN, Harold; Haig Clinic, Lethbridge, Alta.; Sask'59; GenSurg.

PRONGER, Ralph C.; 645 Fort St., Victoria, B.C.; 2780 Dover Rd. (res); McG '47; Otol; Staff, St. Joseph's & Victoria Veteran's Hosp's.; Tel. EV 4-1131.

PRONOVOST, Adrien; Lav'48; DermSyph(P.Q.); Staff, Hop. Notre-Dame, Montreal 24, P.Q.

PRONOVOST, Roch; C.P. 160, 112 Racine, Loretteville, P.Q.; Tel. 842-7655.

PROPP, Albert G.; Steinbach Med. Clinic, Steinbach, Man.; Man '59.

PROSEN, Harry; 1362 Mathers Bay E., Winnipeg 9, Man. (res); Man '55; M.Sc.(Med.); DABPN; Psy; Dir., Psy. O.P.D., Wpg. Gen. Hosp.; Cons. Psy., Deer Lodge Veteran's Hosp.; Co. Dir., Residency Training Program (Psy.) & Assoc. Prof. (Psy.), U. of Manitoba; Tel. SP 4-6511, Ext. 333.

PROSSER, Robert G., Capt.; Dal'64; Staff, Gagetown Station Hosp., Oromocto, N.B.

PROSSER, Robert R.; 218 Bonaccord St., Moncton, N.B.; Edinburgh (Scot.) '31; D.Psy; Psy; Dir. Mental Health Serv., Prov. of N.B.; Ass't. Prof. (Psy), Dalhousie U.; Tel. GR 5-7711.

PROSSIN, Albert J.; Westmount North, Co. Cape Breton, N.S.; Dal '55; M.C.G.P.; Co. Health Off., Cape Breton Co.

PROSTERMAN, D. Barnett; Ste. 202, 720 W. Broadway, Vancouver 9, B.C.; Qns '46; OrthSurg.; Tel. TR 2-7568.

PROUD, John D.; 150 Norfolk St., Guelph, Ont.; Wes '53; ObstGyn; Tel. TA 2-2602.

PROUDFOOT, William A.; 2940 - 17th Ave. S.W., Calgary, Alta.; Alb '54; MCGP; Tel. CH 9-5566.

PROULX, Andre; Manseau, P.Q.; Lav '46; A.M.-C.G.P.; Tel. 30.

PROULX, Andre; 12245 rue Grenet, Montreal 9, P.Q.; Mon '51; F.R.C.P.(C), IntMed.; Tel. VI 2-4892.

PROULX, George H.; 1315 Chemin Ste-Foy, Sillery, Quebec 6, P.Q.; Lav '45; Tel. 681-4846.

PROULX, Jacques; Lav'60; Path(P.Q.); Staff, Hotel-Dieu de Sorel, Sorel, P.Q.

PROULX, Jacques; 1150 est St-Joseph, Montreal 34, P.Q.; Mon'61; Cardiol (P.Q.).

PROULX, Joseph L. C.; 1075 rue Godin, Verdun, P.Q.; Mon'62; Paed.

PROULX, Leo; 14 Prince Albert, Danville, P.Q.; Lav '49.

PROULX, Maurice; St. Jovite, P.Q.; Mon '56.

PROULX Pierre; 3073-1st Ave., Quebec 3, P.Q.; 3077-1st Ave. (res); Lav '54; Tel. 623-3209.

PROULX, Pierre-Y.; 66 St. Jean Baptiste, Victoriaville, P.Q.; Lav'60; IntMed; Tel. 758-8338.

PROUSE, F. Hewetson; 21 Upper Middle Rd., Cooksville, Ont.; Tor'46; OrthSurg; Hd. (OrthSurg.), South Peel Hosp.; Tel. 279-7621.

PROVENCHER, Bruno; 475 boul. Talbot, Chicoutimi, P.Q.; Lav'53; Allerg (P.Q.); Tel. 549-3330.

PROVENCHER, Jean; Centre d'Achats, Baie-Comeau Nord, P.Q.; 23 de Ramezay (res); Mon '54; AMCGP; Indus. Phys., Cdn. British Aluminum Co. Ltd.; Tel. 584-3347.
PROVENCHER, Jean-P.; 42 Blvd. Carignan, Victoriaville, P.Q.; Lav'56; MCGP; Tel. 752-2194.
PROVIS, Hugh S.; 3313 Roblin Blvd., Charleswood, Winnipeg 20, Man.; 4727 Roblin Blvd. (res); Edinburgh (Scot.) '38; M.B., Ch.B(Edin.); D.C.H. (Eng.); Court. Staff (G.P.), Winnipeg Gen., Children's, Grace & Misericordia Hosp's.; Tel. VE 2-1613.
PROVONOST, Roch; 126 St. Jean Jonquiere, Co. Chicoutimi, P.Q.; Lav '48.
PROVOST, Andre; 4453 Beaubien E., Montreal 36, P.Q.; Mon '48; Obst (PQ); Ass't. (Obst), Hop de-la-Misericorde; Ass't. Prof., U. of Montreal; Tel. 721-0730.
PROVOST, A. Remi; 38 du Depot, Montmagny, P.Q.; Lav '60.
PROVOST, Guy; 4074 LaSalle Blvd., Montreal 19, P.Q.; Mon'48; Pulm. Dis & TB (P.Q.); IntMed; Ass't. (Med.), Hop. Gen.-de-Verdun; Ass't. Prof. (Med.), U. of Montreal; Sr. Exam., Sun Life & Canada Life Assur. Co.; Tel. 766-8511.
PROVOST, Jean G.; 4256 Delorimier, Montreal 34, P.Q.; Mon '47; Tel. LA 4-1805.
PROVOST, Leon; 4256 Delormier Ave., Montreal, P.Q.; 5784 Deom (res); Lav'11; Retired.
PROVOST, Maurice; 222 Henri Bourassa E., Montreal 12, P.Q.; Mon '48; Gyn (P.Q.); Tel. DU 7-6629.
PROVOST, Yves; 1656 Sherbrooke St. E., Montreal 24, P.Q.; 6229 Deacon Rd. Mtl. 8 (res); Mon '48; FRCS(C), PlasSurg, GenSurg; Ass't. Dept. (PlasSurg.), Hop.-Notre-Dame; Tel. 525-6363.
PROWSE, Gordon G.; 6 Glenwatford Dr., Agincourt, Ont.; 32 Marydon Cr. (res); Tor '58; Tel. 293-2404.
PROWSE, Lemuel E.; 29 Greenfield Ave., Charlottetown, P.E.I.; Tor '40; Anaes; Dir. of Anaes., Prince Edward Island Hosp.; Dir. V.D. Control, Dept. of Health & Welfare, P.E.I.; Dist. Coroner; Tel. 8932.
PROWSE, William A.; 56 Avenue Rd., Ottawa, Ont. (res); Qns'43; DPH(Tor.); DIH(Tor.); DABPM; Cons. (Aerospace Med.), Dept. of National Health & Welfare; Tel. 992-5250.
PROWSE, William C.; Box 459, Carstairs, Alta.; Alb '43.
PRUCHA, Zdenek S.; 3481 Danforth Ave., Toronto 13, Ont.; 51 Beech Ave. Tor. 13 (res); Tor '52; MCGP; Assoc. Staff, Tor. E. Gen. & Scarborough Gen. Hosp's.; Tel. OX 4-6488.
PRUD'HOMME, Claude; 1252 est, Belanger, Montreal, P.Q.; Mon '62.
PRUD'HOMME, Gilles; 11067, rue Tanguay, Montreal 12, P.Q.; '61; Anaes.
PRUD'HOMME, Gustave L.; 3551 Park Ave., Montreal, P.Q.; Ste. St. Adele en Haut, B.P.107, Co. Terrebonne (res); Lav '11; Retired.
PRUD'HOMME, Hector; 428 Beaubien St. E., Montreal, P.Q.; Lav '18; Tel. 277-5070.
PRUD'HOMME, Hortense; 131 Graham Blvd., Ville Mt. Royal, Montreal 16, P.Q. (res); Mon '55; Anaes (P.Q.); Staff, Hop.-Sacre-Coeur; Tel. FE 4-1210.
PRUD'HOMME, Jean A.; 1150 est Blvd. St. Joseph, Montreal 34, P.Q.; 2084 de la Regence, St.-Bruno (res); Mon '47; FRCP(C), IntMed; Ass't. (Med.), Hop. Maisonneuve; Cons. (IntMed), Queen Mary Vet's. (DVA) Hosp.; Ass't. Prof., U. of Montreal; Tel. LA 7-1241.
PRUETER, Gordon W.; 284 Central Ave., London, Ont.; Tor'44; MRCOG; FRCS(C); ObstGyn.
PRUETER, R. Douglas; 274 Wright Ave., Toronto 3, Ont. (res); Tor '48; F.R.C.P.(C), IntMed., Med. Spec., Ontario Hosp., 999 Queen St. W., Toronto; Tel. LE 3-8501.
PRUNEAU, Charles; rue de Puyjalon, Hauterive, Cte. Saguenay, P.Q. Lav '62.
PRUS, R. D.; Shoal Lake, Man.; Man '52; MCGP; Staff, Shoal Lake Hosp.; Tel. 27.
PRYCE, Harold A.; 569 Concession St., Hamilton, Ont.; Wes '62; Tel. 383-3351.
PRYMAK, Vladimir; 4250 Wyandotte St. E., Riverside, Ont.; Ott '60.
PRYTULAK, Walter; 61 Northland Cres., Woodstock, Ont. (res); Innsbruck (Austria) '47; D.Psy; Psy; Dir. Mental Health Clinic, Ontario Hosp., Woodstock; Tel. LE 9-1251.
PRZIBISLAWSKY, Laszlo; Budapest (Hung.) '50; Staff, Stonewall Hosp., Stonewall, Man.; Tel. 383-5680.
PSUTKA, Dennis A.; 16 Ontario St., Grimsby, Ont.; Tor'63; AMCGP; Tel. 945-2144.
PTAK, Lumir L.; 400 Med. Arts Bldg., 1105 Pandora Ave., Victoria, B.C.; 2875 Beach Dr. (res); Nebraska (Omaha, Neb.) '38; FRCS (Edin.); Chief of Surg., Royal Jubilee Hosp.; Past Pres., Coll. of Phys. & Surg., B.C.; Tel. 383-6533.
PTAK, Theadore W.; Ott'63; Ass't. Res. (Med.), Toronto Gen. Hosp., Toronto 2, Ont.
PUBLOW, Charles A.; 73 King St., Picton, Ont.; Qns '06; OphthOtol; Member, Prince Edward County Health Unit; Tel. GR 6-3611; Retired.
PUDDEN, A. J.; Tor'64; Res., Toronto Gen. Hosp., Toronto 2, Ont.
PUDDEN, Beverley E.; Tor'64; Res., Toronto Gen. Hosp., Toronto 2, Ont.
PUDDICOMBE, Paul G.; 180 Metcalfe St., Ottawa 4, Ont.; Qns'61.
PUDDICOMBE, Robert T.; Box 300, Rossland, B.C. (Res.); MRCS; LRCP; FCCP; FICP; DiagRad; Radiol., Castlegar & District Hosp. & Grand Fork's Hosp.; Ass't. Radiol., Trail Hosp.
PUDDINGTON, B. A.; Grand Falls, N.B.; McG '03; GenSurg; Retired.
PUDYMAITIS, Oscar J.; Munich (Germ.) '27; Staff, Nova Scotia Hospital, Dartmouth, N.S.
PUETZ, Irene M.; Ste. 7, 1108 Williams Rd., Richmond, B.C.; Sask'63; Tel. 277-3181.
PUFFER, A. D.; Ste 302, 262 Wilson Ave., Downsview P.Q., Ont.; 2125 Avenue Rd., Toronto (res); Tor '50; Assoc., Staff, Northwestern Gen. & St. Joseph's Hosp's.; Tel. ME 5-6502.
PUFFER, DeWillett S.; 118 Hillhurst Blvd., Toronto 12, Ont. (res); Tor '20; D.P.H., PH. Retired.
PUGH, Duncan S.; 1206, 51 Alexander St., Toronto 5, Ont.; Qns '33; D.P.H.; Staff, Dept. of Ont.; 125 Snalford Cr. (res); Tor '15; Staff, Toronto East Gen. & Grace Hosp's.; Tel. 466-0065.
PUGH, Edgar C.; 7 Caithness Ave., Toronto 6, Health; Tel. EM 3-1211.
PUGH, Paul A.; 230 Highfield St., Moncton, N.B.; Dal '53; ObstGyn; Staff, Moncton Hosp.; Tel. 382-2162.
PUGH, Rodger F.; 2505 Taylor St. E., Saskatoon, Sask.; Man'56; Anaes.
PUGSLEY, E., Bliss M. (MacQuarrie); 390 First Ave., Ottawa 1, Ont.; Tor '35; Phys., Children's Aid Soc. of Ottawa & Carleton Co.; Tel. CE 5-4619.
PUGSLEY, Herbert E.; R.R. 1, Willowdale, Ont (res); Tor '27 F.R.C.P.(C), IntMed; Cons. (Med.), Toronto Hosp. for TB, Weston; Assoc. Med. Dir., Confederation Life Assurance Co. 321 Bloor E., Toronto; Tel. 924-6868.
PULLIN, Lloyd B.; 8 East Ave., Corner Brook W., Nfld.; McG '50; M.C.G.P.; Staff, Western Mem. Hosp.
PULLIN, William A.; 32 Bessborough Ave., Moncton, N.B.; Dal '22; Ophth; Staff, Moncton City Hosp.; Tel. 855-4140.
PUMP, Karl K.; 508 Fairmont Med. Bldg., 750 W. Broadway, Vancouver 9, B.C.; 5550 Kingston Rd. (res); Alb '42; FCCP; F.R.C.P.(C). IntMed; Att'd. Staff, Vancouver Gen. Hosp.; Clin. Instr. (Med.) U. of British Columbia; Tel. 874-4422.
PUN, Ronald; Dal '61; Res., Royal Victoria Hosp., Montreal 2, P.Q.
PURCELL, W. Barry; Ste. 105, 815 Park Rd., Richmond, B.C.; McG'60; Ophth; Tel. 278-8515.
PURCHASE, Emerson C.; 256 Elgin St., Ottawa 4, Ont.; 707 Sherbourne Rd. (res); Tor '46; IntMed.; Staff, Ottawa Civic Hosp.; Cons. (Allergy), Ottawa Gen. Hosp. & N.D.M.C.; Lect. (Med.), U. of Ottawa; Tel. CE 3-7777.
PURDELL-LEWIS, J. Geoffrey; London (Eng.) '63; MRCS (Eng.); LRCP (Lond.); Staff, Grenfell Assoc. Hosp., St. Anthony, Nfld.
PURDIE, Francis J.; Brandon Clinic, Brandon, Man.; Man'44; GenSurg; Staff, Brandon Gen. & Assiniboine Hosp's.; Tel. PA 9-6444.

PURKIN, Noel; 201 Med. Centre, 906 - 8th Ave. S.W., Calgary, Alta.; Sask.'60.

PURDON, Arnold L.; 165 Plymouth Rd., Welland, Ont.; 153 Aqueduct St. (res); Tor '40; Anaes; Dist. Coroner; Tel. 734-6431.

PURDON, Derek H.; 303 Goldstream, Victoria, B.C.; McG '64.

PURDY, Arthur D. T.; 353 East Wing, Toronto Western Hosp., Toronto, Ont.; Tor'24; ObstGyn; Cons. Obst. Gyn., Toronto Western Hosp.; Chief Cons. (ObstGyn), Humber Mem. Hosp.; Ass't. Prof. (ObstGyn), U. of Toronto; Tel. EM. 6-6000.

PURDY, Mary E.; 102 Med. Arts Bldg., Hamilton, Ont.; Wes '48; IntMed; Br. Dir., Ont. Alcoholism Drug Addiction Research Fdn.; Tel. 529-3567.

PURKIS, Ian E.; 5871 Spring Garden Rd., Halifax, N.S.; 5865 Balmoral Rd. (res); London U. (Eng.) '53; FFARCS; Anaes; Att'd. Staff, Victoria Gen. Hosp.; Ass't. Prof. (Anaes), Dalhousie U.; Tel. 423-8484.

PURKIS, Raymond S. A.; 330 University Ave., Toronto, Ont.; 157 Wimbleton Rd. (res); Tor '43; Int Med; Ass't. Med. Dir. Canada Life Assurance Co.; Tel. 368-7432, Ext. 238.

PURKIS, Robert S.; 1401 W. Broadway, Vancouver 9, B.C.; UBC'54.

PURRES, Jaak; Ott'65; Res., St. Joseph's Hosp., Toronto 3, Ont.

PURSER, Margaret J.; Federal Hosp., Moose Factory, Ont.; London (Eng.) '53; M.B., B.S., LRCP; MRCS; DRCOG; M.O., Dept. of Health & Welfare.

PURVES, Jas. K.B., DFC; 5991 Spring Garden Rd., Halifax, N.S.; 6435 Cobourg Rd. (res); Dal '51 F.R.C.S.(C), GenSurg; Ass't Surg., Victoria Gen. Hosp.; Cons. (Surg.), Camp Hill DVA Hosp.; Instr. (Surg.), Dalhousie U.; Tel. 422-5808.

PURVIS, James H.; Wes '64; Res., Montreal Gen. Hosp., Montreal 25, P.Q.

PURVIS, James R.; Brock Medical Bldg., 240 Brock St., Kingston Ont.; 266 Albert St. (res); Qns '52; D.L.O.; Otol; Clin. Ass't (Otol.), Queen's U.; Tel. 542-8818.

PURVIS, William M.; 955 Woodbine Ave., Toronto 13, Ont.; 23 Southlea Ave., Leaside (res); Qns '33; Tel. 699-4924.

PUSEY, John H.; Mayerthorpe, Alta; London Eng.)'63; LRCP (Lond.) MRCS (Eng.); Abroad.

PUSEY, Valdine A.; Man '64; Res., Wpg. Children's Hosp., Winnipeg 3, Man.

PUSHMAN, Donald R.; 340 Macleod, Ottawa 4, Ont.; Tor'50; Psy; Dir. Inpatient Serv., Ottawa Civic Hosp.; Cons., DVA; Ass't. Prof. (Clin. Psy.), U. of Ottawa; Tel. CE 4-3042.

PUTNAM, Malcolm J. M.; 170 Fitzroy St., Charlottetown, P.E.I.; 80 Greenfield Ave. (res); McG '40; FRCS(C); GenSurg; Staff, Prince Edward Island Hosp.; Tel. 894-7325.

PUTTEE, M. Eleanor; Man'63; Res., St. Boniface Hosp., Winnipeg 6, Man.; Abroad.

PUVREZ, Marie-Genevieve P.; (see Stegen, Marie-Genevieve P.).

PYE, Eduard C.; Morton St., Cobden, Ont.; Leeds (Eng.) '59; M.O.H., Cobden; Tel. 646-2200.

PYESMANY, Allan F.; Alb '61; Res., Mtl. Children's Hosp., Montreal 25, P.Q.; Abroad.

PYLE, I. Roger; 108 Med. Arts Bldg., 404-406 Graham Ave., Winnipeg 1, Man; Durham (Eng) '51; FRCP(C), DiagRad; Tel. 452-8402.

PYLE, Walter; 1539 Parkside Crt., Sandwich West Twp., Windsor, Ont.; Tor '32; FACCP; IntMed. (T.B.); Staff, Essex County San.; Tel. 252-2771.

PYLYPUK, Eugene S.; 80 King St., Welland, Ont.; Alb '48; GenSurg; Tel. 735-1121.

PYLYPIUK, John A.; 770 Barton St. E., Hamilton, Ont.; 1338 Cumberland Ave. (res); Alb '35. Tel. LI 4-5708.

PYPER, Joanna F.; Northern Health Unit, 1461-6th Ave., Prince George, B.C.; Melbourne (Aust.) '54; DPH.

PYPER, John E.; Cambria Med. Bldg., 386 Cambria St., Stratford, Ont.; 29 Jaffre St. (res); Queen's (Belfast)'45; DOMS(Eng.); Ophth; Ophthalmologist, Stratford Gen. Hosp.; Tel. 271-0417.

PYUN, Kwang W.; Korea'50; Staff, Hosp. Mental Diseases, Box 420, Brandon, Man.

QUACKENBUSH, H. Arnley; 5 Owen St., Barrie, Ont. McG '27.

QUAN, Paul; 2300 Tupper St., Montreal 25, P.Q.; Tor '53; DABA; Anaes; Ass't. Anaes., Mtl. Children's & Reddy Mem. Hosp's.; Dem. (Anaes), McGill U.; Tel. WE 7-8511; Loc. 463.

QUANTZ, Marie C.; Tor'65; Res., Montreal General Hosp., Montreal 25, P.Q.

QUARRINGTON, Albert J.; 2286 Carling Ave., Ottawa 14, Ont.; Qns'62; Tel. 725-1316.

QUARRY, John G.; 490 Brant St., Burlington, Ont.; 3095 Woodward Ave. (res); Wes '54; MCGP; Active Staff, Joseph Brant Hosp.; Court. Staff, Hamilton Gen. & St. Joseph's Hosp's.; Tel. NE 4-2307.

QUARTZ, Bradley F.; Tor'61; Res., Wellesley Hosp., Toronto 5, Ont.

QUASTEL, Michael R.; McG '57; Staff, Radiation Prot. Div., N.H.W. Brookfield Rd., Ottawa 8, Ont.; Tel. 997-4621.

QUASTEL, J. H.; D.Sc., Ph.D., F.R.I.C., F.C.I.C., F.R.S., F.R.S.C., Dir. Research Inst., Memb. Med. Bd., Montreal Gen. Hosp.; Hon. Cons., Children's Mem., Jewish Gen. & Verdun Protestant Hosp's.; Prof. Biochem., McGill U.; Tel. VI 4-6311.

QUAYLE, James T. B.; Ste. 210, 624-6th St., New Westminster, B.C.; 13128 Coulthard Rd., R.R. 1., Cloverdale (res); McG '50; PlasSurg; Chief Plas. Surg., Royal Columbian Hosp.; Tel. LA 1-6021.

QUE, Mariano; Santo Tomas (Phillip.) '57; Staff, Douglas Hosp., Montreal, P.Q.

QUEHL, Eby; 208 Medical Arts Bldg., 11010 Jasper Ave., Edmonton, Alta.; 9119-117 St. (res); Alb'35; DRCOG, MRCOG; ObstGyn; Lect'r., ObstGyn., Alberta University; Tel. 424-1273.

QUEMUEL, Ruperto S.; Santo Tomas (Phillipp.) '55; Staff, Wawanesa Dist. Hosp., Wawanesa, Man.; Abroad.

QUENNEVILLE, Emile; 210 rue Principale, Granby, P.Q.; 778 Principale (res); Mon '33.

QUENNEVILLE, Jean M.; Clinique Medicale Jarry, 150 Jarry E., Montreal 11, P.Q.; Mon '59.

QUENNEVILLE, J. Guy; 3567 Lagarde, St. Vincent-de-Paul, P.Q. (res); Mon'54; FRCP(C), IntMed; Staff, Hop. Notre-Dame; Ass't. Prof., U. of Montreal; Tel. LA 4-0986.

QUENNEVILLE, Paul; 12061 Tecumseh St. W., Tecumseh, Ont.; Lav '51; MCGP; Tel. 735-2164.

QUENNEVILLE, Robert; 365 Blvd. Manseau, Joliette, P.Q.; Mon '47.

QUENTIN, Margaret R.; 26 Eglinton Ave. W., Toronto 12, Ont.; 63 Glengrove Ave. W. (res); Tor '39; Paed; Clin. Ass't., Dept. Med., Hosp. for Sick Children; Paed., Women's College Hosp.; Tel. HU 9-1774.

QUENVILLE, Noel F., Box 1239, Kimberley, B.C.; UBC '56; Tel. 427-2277.

QUERENGESSER, Earl I.; 473 Queen St. S., Kitchener, Ont.; 50 Forest Hill Dr. (res); Wes '47; Ophth; Staff, Kitchener-Waterloo & St. Mary's Hosp's; Tel. SH 3-8131.

QUESADA, Honorio; Wes'59; Res., Wellesley Hosp., Toronto 5, Ont.

QUESNEL, Albert E., Port Daniel Station, Co. Bonaventure, P.Q.; Mon '37.

QUESNEL, Bernard; 4395 Ave. Verdun, Montreal 19, P.Q.; 423 Senecal, Ville LaSalle (res); Mon '56; Paed; Clin. Staff, Mtl. Children's Hosp.; Tel. PO 8-9719.

QUESNEL, Georges; Mon'65; Res., Hop. Hotel-Dieu, Montreal 18, P.Q.

QUESNEL, Louis A.; 109 York St., Cornwall, Ont.; Ott'61.

QUIGGIN, F. H. Stewart; Fillmore, Sask.; London (Eng.) '56; Staff, Fillmore Union Hosp.

QUIGLEY, Gerard J.; 208 Med. Arts Bldg., 1 Young St., Hamilton, Ont.; 15 Forsythe Pl. (res); Tor '43; FACS, MRCOG, FRCS(C), ObstGyn; Staff (ObstGyn), St. Joseph's Hosp.; Court. Staff, Hamilton Gen. Hosp.; Tel. JA 7-3821.

QUIGLEY, Hadsel G.; 6389 Coburg Rd., Halifax, N.S.; Dal'42.

QUIGLEY, John H.; 1674 Oxford St., Halifax, N.S.; Dal '51; **DNBME (US); DABOph; Ophth; Active Staff, (Ophth.), Victoria Gen. Hosp.; Chief of Ophth., Halifax Infirmary; Lect., Dalhousie U.;** Tel. 423-7650.
QUIGLEY, John P.; 245 Johnson St., Kingston, Ont.; Qns '03; MRCS(Eng.), LRCP(Lond.), FRCP(C).
QUIGLEY, Michael P.; Sg/Lt; Dal '64; M.O., Gagetown Station Hosp., Oromocto, N.B.
QUIMPER, Alfred; C.P. 489, 494 rue St.-Pierre, Rimouski, P.Q.; Lav '45; PH (P.Q.); Staff, Dept. of Health, Rimouski; Tel. 723-7631.
QUINLAN, Edmund J.; Cornwall Clinic, 325 Hamilton Ave., St. John's, Nfld.; 7 Curtis Pl. (res); Dal '58; MCGP; Tel. 578-0257.
QUINLAN, Harry F.; 181 King St., St. Catharines, Ont.; McG'28; MCGP; Staff, Obst. Gyn., St. Catharines Gen. & Hotel Dieu Hosp's.; Tel. MU 2-3881.
QUINLAN, John J.; Nova Scotia Sanatorium, Kentville, N.S.; Dal '41; FCCP; ThorSurg; ThorSurg., Nova Scotia San. & Cons. ThorSurg., Blanchard-Fraser Mem. Hosp.; Tel. 678-3251.
QUINLAN, John J.; 54 Brant Ave., Brantford, Ont.; 7 Parkside Dr. (res); Tor '43; M.C.G.P.; Active Staff, Brantford Gen. & St. Joseph's Hosp's.; Tel. 756-6333.
QUINLAN, Peter T.; Ste. 250, 8409-112th St., Edmonton, Alta.; Manchester (Eng.) '43; M.B., Ch B., FRCS (Edin.); Otol; Chief of Otol., Misericordia Hosp.; Att'd. Staff (Otol.), University Hosp.; Lect. (Otol.), U. of Alberta; Tel. 439-3803.
QUINLAN, Vincent P.; 1 Erie St., Stratford, Ont.; Wes '57; FRCP(C); IntMed; Staff, Stratford Gen., St. Mary's & Listowel Hosp's.; Tel. 273-0770.
QUINN, Louis J.; Ste. 230, 5300 Cote des Neiges Rd., Montreal, P.Q.; 357 Portland Ave., Mount Royal (res); McG '36; F.R.C.O.G., F.A.C.O.G., F.R.C.S.(C), ObstGyn; **ObstGyn I/C. St. Mary's Hosp.; Cons. Gyn., Queen Mary Veterans' Hosp.; Cons., Catherine Booth Hosp.; Tel. RE 3-1861.**
QUINN, Michael H.; 1390 Grand Marais Rd. W., Windsor, Ont.; Ott'55; GenSurg; ThorSurg; Tel. 969-2272.
QUINN, William R.; 496 Waterloo St., London, Ont.; Wes '22; M.C.G.P.; Court. Staff, Victoria & St. Joseph's Hosp's.; Tel. GE 4-6616.
QUINTAL, David; 5025 A, Delorimier, Montreal, P.Q.; 200 ave-des-Champs, Repentigny, Verdun (res); Mon '49; AMCGP.; Tel. LA 4-1882.
QUINTAL, Jean F.; 77 rue Brock, Drummondville, P.Q.; Mon '53; Anaes (P.Q.); Staff, Hop. Ste. Croix; Tel. GR 8-3353.
QUINTIN, Thomas James; 422 London St., Sherbrooke, P.Q.; 1550 White St. (res); McG'30; FACP, IntMed; Staff, Sherbrooke, Hotel Dieu & St. Vincent de Paul Hosp's.; Lect., McGill U.; Tel. LO 9-3444.
QUINTO, Manrique G.; 108 Medical-Dental Bldg, Rose St. & 11th Ave, Regina, Sask.; Santo Tomas (Philipp.)57; Paed; Medical Staff, Regina Gen. & Regina Grey Nuns Hosps.; Tel. 523-7633.
QUINTYN, Elmer A.; 17 Bear St., Tillsonburg, Ont.; 274 Broadway St. (res); Wes '51; FICS; GenSurg; Chief of Surg., Tillsonburg Mem. Hosp.; Tel. VI 2-2101.
QUIRION, Renaud, Capt.; Mon'65; St. Jean Armee Base, St. Jean, P.Q.
QUIRK, John; 172 Queen W., Brampton, Ont.; Cardiff (Wales)'52; Urol.
QUIRK, Keith C.; 350-14th St. W., Owen Sound, Ont.; 75-5th St. E. (res); McG '52; M.C.G.P.; Staff, Owen Sound Gen. & Marine Hosp's.; Tel. 376-8510.
QUIRK, Louis A.; Ste. 23, 4429 Kingsway, South Burnaby, B.C.; 102-1025 Wolfe Ave., Vanc. 9, **(res); Alb '38; LM (Dublin); DNB; Tel. HE 1-0717.**
QUIRKEBECK, Ebba; Tor '52; P.G. Anaes., Hosp. for Sick Children, Toronto 2, Ont.; Tel. EM 6-7242.
QUIRON, Renauld Capt.; Lav'66; St. Jean Armee Base, St. Jean, P.Q.
RABATICH, Steven; Plaster Rock, N.B.; McG '45; Dist. Coroner.
RABB, Haddon R.; Fort Coulonge, P.Q. (res); Qns'31; D.P.H.; M.O., Pontiac Health Unit, **Dept. of Health, P.Q.; Tel. 62.**
RABBAT, Antoine G.; Alexandria (Egypt) '63; Jr. Int., Royal Victoria Hosp., Montreal 2, P.Q.
RABIN, Elijah Z.; Qns'61; FRCP(C), IntMed; Staff, Montreal Gen. Hosp., Montreal, P.Q.
RABIN, Harvey R.; Wes'65; Res., Montreal General Hosp., Montreal 25, P.Q.
RABINOVICH, Solomon; Tor '57; Path; Staff, Toronto Western Hosp., 399 Bathurst St., Toronto 2B, Ont.; Dem. Path., U. of Toronto; Tel. 369-5722.
RABINOVITCH, Alexander; McG'65; Res., Royal Victoria Hosp., Montreal 2, P.Q.
RABINOVITCH, Boaz; 373 St. Catherine Rd., Montreal 8, P.Q. (res); McG'28; Tel. AV 8-3927.
RABINOVITCH, Edward M.; Tor '63; Res., Mtl., Children's Hosp., Montreal 25, P.Q.
RABINOVITCH, Irving I.; 35 Nelson Ave., Montreal 8 ,P.Q.; Mon'37; Tel. 279-2570.
RABINOVITCH, Phineas; 4351 Esplanade Ave., **Montreal, P.Q.; McG '25; Tel. VI 4-2200.**
RABINOVITCH, Sam; 3 Bellingham Rd., Montreal, P.Q.; **Mon '34; IntMed.; Tel. RE 8-1711.**
RABINOWITCH, Israel., O.B.E.; Box 9, Val David, P.Q.; McG'30; D.Sc., FACP, FI, Biol., FRCP(C), IntMed; Cons. Staff, (Metab & Toxicology), Montreal Gen. Hosp.; Tel. 937-6011.
RABINOWITZ, Mabel; Mountain Sanatorium, Hamilton, Ont.; Tor '18.
RABINOWITZ, Paul; Mountain Sanatorium, Hamilton, Ont.; Berlin (Germ.) '25; F.A.C.C.P., **Otol.; Tel. 385-5341.**
RABKIN, Fred B.; 979 McPhillips St., Winnipeg 14, Man.; Qns'46; MCGP.
RABSON, Lawrence R.; 280 Memorial Blvd., Winnipeg 1, Man.; 545 Queenston St., Winnipeg 9 (res); Man '36; F.R.C.S. (Edin.), F.R.C.S.(C), GenSurg; Surg., St. Boniface Hosp.; Ass't. Prof. (Surg.) U. of Manitoba; Tel. SP 4-2411.
RABY, Paul, F/L; RCAF Station, Val d'Or, P.Q.; Lav '65.
RACETTE, Lois J.; Med. Arts Clinic, Medicine Hat, Alta.; Alb'54; Tel. 527-2281.
RACETTE, Paul C.; Alb '52; Path; Staff, Diagnostic Lab., 709-1st Ave. S.E., Medicine Hat, Alta.; Staff, Medicine Hat Gen. Hosp.; Tel. 527-3989.
RACHMEL, Israel; 224 Queen St., Charlottetown, P.E.I.; North River Rd. (res); Strasbourg (France) '36; M.C.G.P.; Active Staff, P.E.I. Hosp.; Tel. 894-4844.
RACICOT, Gilles; 50 rue Jacques Cartier, Valleyfield, P.Q.; 149 Edouard (res); Mon '55; Paed; Tel. 373-9393.
RACICOT, Georges N.; 1252 rue Royale, Trois Rivieres, P.Q.; 1284 rue Royale (res); Lav '28; **Pulm Dis & TB (P.Q.); IntMed (T.B.); T.B. Clin., Dept. of Health; Phys. & Ass't. Med. Dir., San.** Cooke; Tel. FR 6-3721.
RACICOT, Jules; 64 Begin, Levis, P.Q.; Lav '55; FRCS(C); GenSurg; Tel. 837-1177.
RACICOT, Maurice; 213 rue Principale, La Sarre, Cte. Abitibi, P.Q.; Lav '65.
RACICOT, Paul; 62 rue Begin, Levis, P.Q.; Lav '28; GenSurg; Chief of Serv. "B" Surg., Hotel-Dieu; Tel. 837-4356.
RACINE, Eva C. (Arendt); 1650 Cedar Ave., Montreal 25, P.Q.; McG'49; FRCP(C) Int Med; Ass't. Phys. & Dir., Nursing Health Service, Montreal Gen. Hosp.; Lect. (Med.), McGill U.; Tel. WE 7-6011.
RACINE, Gerard; 965 Ave. Eymard, Quebec, P.Q.; 1495 de Repentigny (res); Lav '48; Tel. 681-1002.
RACINE, Jacques; 816 Dunlop Ave., Montreal, P.Q.; Lav '50; DiagRad; Staff, Verdun Gen. Hosp.; Tel. 766-8511.
RACINE, Luc; 1150 est, boul. St-Joseph, Montreal 34, P.Q.; Mon'59; FRCS(C); OrthSurg; Staff, (Orth. Surg.), Hop. Maisonneuve; Tel. LA 7-1241.
RACINE, Paul A.; 8 rue McQuaig E., Rouyn, P.Q.; 359 E. Perreault St. (res); Lav '48.
RACINE, Pierre Y.; Mon '64; Int., Hop. Hotel-Dieu, Montreal 18, P.Q.

RACINE, Roger; 3549 boul Levesque, Chomedey, Laval-des-Rapides, P.Q.; Mon '44; Psy (P.Q.); Tel. MU 1-1110.

RACZ, Ferenc; Debrecen (Hung.)'47; Staff, Central Hosp., Toronto 2, Ont.; Tel. 925-8991.

RAD, Manzar J.; Tehran (Iran)'56; Staff, Grey Nun's Hosp., Regina, Sask.

RAD, Shamsedin F.; Medical Arts Clinic, 2125-11th Ave., Regina, Sask.; Tehran (Iran)'56; GenSurg.

RADACOVICI, C. Eugene; 12245 Grenet, Montreal 9, P.Q.; (Bucharest, Roumania'44; GenSurg; (P.Q.); Tel. DU 8-0528.

RADCLIFFE, Patricia A. (Gardiner); Ste. 3, Madrona Bldg., 140 Wallace St., Nanaimo, B.C.; 2905 Haliday Cres. (res); Qns '53; ObstGyn.; FACOG; Cons. Staff (ObstGyn.), Nanaimo Reg. Gen. Hosp.; Tel. 754-6323.

RADCLIFFE, Roland W.; Ste. 3., 140 Wallace St., Nanaimo, B.C.; Qns '53; DABOG; FACS; FACOG; ObstGyn; Cons. ObstGyn., Nanaimo Reg. Gen., Ladysmith Gen., Chemainus Gen., West Coast Gen. & Nanaimo Indian Hosp's.; Ass't. Clin. Prof. (Anat.), U. of British Columbia; Tel. 754-6323.

RADDE, Ingeborg C.; 555 University Ave., Toronto 2, Ont.; 70 Delisle Ave., Tor 7 (res); Frankfurt (Germ.) '49; Ph.D. (Tor); FRCP(C); IntMed; Research Assoc., Hosp. for Sick Children & Dept. of Pharm., U. of Toronto; Tel. EM 6-7242.

RADFORD, Charles J.; 644 Willowburn Cr. S.E., Calgary, Alta.; Tor'59; Ophth.

RADFORD, Hugh W.; Ste. 7, 825 McBride Blvd., New Westminster, B.C.; 2777 Noel Dr. (res); UBC'55; Tel. LA 6-3013.

RADHAKRISHNAN, Mothalampet; Madras (India)'58; Anaes; Staff, Montreal Children's Hosp., Montreal 25, P.Q.

RADIN, Steve; 1011 Ouellette Ave., Windsor, Ont.; Wes'59; FRCS(C), GenSurg.

RADO, Eva (Mrs. Balazs); 4 MacRae Ave., Dartmouth, N.S. (res); Man '56; Psy; Staff, **Nova Scotia Hosp.; Tel. 466-7411. Abroad.**

RADO, Ivan P.; 44 Inglewood Dr., Hamilton, Ont.; Munich (Germ.) '51; Anaes; Staff, St. Joseph's Hosp.; Tel. 528-4990.

RADO, Karoly; 394 Bloor St. W., Toronto 4, Ont.; 5 Berkindale Cres. (res); Szeged (Hung.) '34; Tel. 924-7963.

RADO, Peter P.; 1452 Bathurst St., Toronto 10, Ont.; Budapest (Hungary) '40; Tel. 535-8717.

RADOMSKI, Tadeusz; Humboldt Clinic, 637-9th St., Humboldt, Sask.; National U. (Ire.) '55; M.B., B.Ch., BAO; D(Obst.) R.C.G.O.; Hd., Dept. of ObstGyn., St. Elizabeth Hosp.; Tel. 682-2618.

RADOUX, Victor H.; App 6, 902, Mgr. Grandin, Quebec 10, P..Q(res); Lav '43; Adm. Hop. Ste.-Foy; Tel. MU 3-4951.

RAE, Donald W.; Prairie Med. Assoc., 156-6th St. S.E., Portage-la-Prairie, Man.; 115 Dufferin Ave. (res); Man '57; MCGP; Staff, Portage Gen. Hosp.; Tel. 857-6873.

RAE, Edgar; 412 Danforth Ave., Toronto, Ont.; **670 Broadview (res); Tor '09; Anaes; Retired.**

RAE, James M.; 402 Toronto Western Medical Bldg., 25 Leonard Ave., Toronto 2B, Ont; **Qns '43; D.Psy; F.R.C.P.(C), Psy; Psy.I/C Psy; Ward, Toronto Western Hosp.; Con.Psy., Sunnybrook** Hosp., Assoc. Psy., U. of Toronto; Tel. EM 6-1453.

RAE, M. Viola; Shaughnessy Hosp., Vancouver, B.C.; 4175 Cartier St. (res); Alb '29; PathBact; Path., Shaughnessy Hosp.; Curator, Path. Museum, U. of British Columbia; Retired.

RAE, Peter L.; Box 398, Wiarton, Ont.; Wes'62; Tel. 534-1093.

RAEDER, Henry A.; 61 Elliott St. E., Windsor, Ont.; Poznan (Poland) '33; Tel. 256-6778.

RAFAAT, Massoud; 108 Med. Dental Bldg., Rose St. & 11th Ave., Regina, Sask.; Geneva (Switz.) '53; DTM; DCH(Lond.); Paed; Tel. 523-7633.

RAFF, David; 540 Ellendale Med. Bldg., 5845 Cote-des-Neiges Rd., Montreal 26, P.Q.; 622 Murray Hill, Westmount (res); McG '27; IntMed (P.Q.); Med. & Cardiol. Staffs, Jewish Gen. Hosp.; Tel. RE 1-9931.

RAFF, Moe J.; 5757 Decelles, Montreal 38, P.Q.; McG '24; Otol (P.Q.). Tel. RE 3-3796.

RAFFAN, Hamish M.; 75 Woolwich St., Guelph, Ont.; 153 Riverview Dr. (res); Aberdeen (Scot.) '43; M.B., Ch.B., M.D.(Commend.), MRCP (Lond.); IntMed; Active Staff, Guelph Gen. & St. Joseph's Hosp's.; Tel. TA 4-8400.

RAFI-ZADEH, Ebrahim; 110 The Palisades, Saskatoon, Sask.; Tehran (Iran) '56; IntMed; Staff, University Hosp., Saskatoon, Sask.; Tel. 242-7641.

RAFUSE, Edward V.; Dal'61; Res., Toronto Gen. Hosp., Toronto 2, Ont.

RAFUSE, Elwood R.; 302 Linwood St., St. James, Man.; U.S.A. '30; Dir., Bureau of Hosp., Dept. of Health & Public Welfare, Prov. of Man.

RAGAN, Edward J.; Wes'65; Jr. Int., Toronto Western Hosp., Toronto 2B, Ont.; Abroad.

RAGAN, John D.; 1215-736 Granville St., Vancouver 2, B.C.; Alb'49; FACS; FAAOO; DABO, Ophth; Assoc. Staff, St. Paul's & Children's Hosp's.; Tel. MU 4-2825.

RAGAN, Terrence M.; 331 Birks Bldg., 718 Granville St., Vancouver 2, B.C.; 6475 Wiltshire St. Van. 13 (res); Alb '43; M.Sc., Active Vis. Staff, Vancouver Gen. & Children's Hosp's.; Assoc. Staff, St. Paul's Hosp.; Tel. MU 1-0935.

RAGINSKY, Bernard B.; 376 Redfern, Apt. 2, Montreal 6, P.Q.; 220 Chester Ave., Mtl. 16 (res); McG '29; FICA; FAAAS; FACC; FAMWA; FAPM; FISCEH; IntMed; Psy; Hon. Staff, Jewish Gen. Hosp.; Tel. WE 5-5084.

RAGONA, Paolo; 421 Birks Bldg., 718 Granville St., Vancouver, B.C.; 2601 Pt. Grey Rd. (res); Palermo (Italy) '28; Tel. MU 1-7643.

RAGULA, Boris D.; 756 Adelaide St., London, Ont.; Louvain (Belgium) '51; M.C.G.P.; Tel. 438-1709.

RAHAMAN, Abdul R.; Box 379, Gladstone, Man.; Dublin (Ire.)'58; BAO.

RAHMAN, Fazal U.; Punjab (Pakistan)'53; Staff, Pathol. Inst., 5800 University Ave., Halifax, N.S.

RAI, Jyotsna; Apt. 502, 232 Oakland Ave., London, Ont.; Calcutta (India)'48; Staff, Ontario Hosp.

RAIBECK, William A.; Qns '64; Res., Kingston Gen. Hosp., Kingston, Ont.

RAIL, J. Romeo, Major; Lav'55; Res., National Defence Med. Centre, Smyth Road & Alta Vista Dr., Ottawa 8, Ont.

RAILTON, Richard H.; 165 Plymouth Rd., Welland, Ont.; Tor'55; FACS; FRCS(C); GenSurg; Tel. 732-6181.

RAILTON, S. Victor; Med. Arts Bldg., 165 Plymouth Rd., Welland, Ont.; Tor'29; FRCS(C); Gen. Surg.; Chief of Surg., Welland County Gen. Hosp.; Cons. (Surg.), Douglas Mem. Hosp., Fort Erie, Port Colborne Gen. Hosp., Haldimand War Mem. Hosp., Dunnville; Tel. 732-6181.

RAINDA, Hilda (Scheffler); 26 Church Ave., Willowdale, Ont.; 17 Purbrock Crt. (res); Loma Linda (Calif., U.S.A.)'57; Tel. 222-2331; Abroad.

RAINE, Robert J., Sg/Lt.; Alb'62; Res. (GenSurg.), National Defence Med. Centre, Ottawa 8, Ont.

RAINVILLE, Bernard; Lav'60; Res., Montreal Gen. Hosp., Montreal, P.Q.

RAINVILLE, Normand; 6986, boulv. l'Assamption, Montreal, P.Q.; Apt. 14, 3940 Belanger **E. (res); Mon '58; MCGP; Tel. RA 9-5231.**

RAINVILLE, P. H.; 1039 ave. des Erables, Quebec, P.Q.; Lav '19; Retired.

RAISBECK, William A.; 12 Ipswich Cr., Agincourt, Ont.; Qns'64.

RAJA, Khaliq D.; Punjab'57; FRCS(C), GenSurg; Staff, Emergency Dept., Henderson Gen. Hosp., Hamilton, Ont.; Tel. 389-4411, Ext. 227.

RAJAN, P. V.; India '57; Jr. Int'n., Ottawa Gen. Hosp., Ottawa, Ont.

RAJANI, Manohar R.; Bay Medical Clinic, Glace Bay, N.S.; Bombay (India)'57; FRCS (Eng.); FRCS(C), GenSurg.

RAJIC, Dimitrije S.; 1588 Stoney Brook Cres., N., London, Ont. (res); Graz (Austria) '49; D.A.B.R., DiagRad; Rad., I/C., War Mem. Children's Hosp.; Clin. Lect. (Rad), U. of Western Ontario; Tel. GE 2-5261, Ext. 651.

RAJNOVICH, Edward; 598 Upper Sherman, Hamilton, Ont.; 54 Garside St. S. (res); Tor '55; DAAP; Tel. 544-4278.

RAJOTTE, Paul; Mon'57; Psy; Dir., Inst. of Psy. Research of Joliette, Hop. Saint-Charles, Joliette, P.Q.; Tel. 756-1681.

RAJPUT, Ali H.; Sind (W. Pakistan)'58; FRCP(C), Neur; Staff, Kingston Gen. Hosp., Kingston, Ont.

RAKOFF, Vivian M.; 3755 Cote St. Catherine Rd., Montreal, P.Q.; London (Eng.) '57; MRCS; LRCP; FRCP(C), Psy; Ass't. Phys. & Assoc. Dir. of Research, Dept. of Psy., Jewish Gen. Hosp.; Lect., McGill U.; Tel. 735-3771.

RALLEY, Dintcho L.; 23 Castleview Ave., Toronto 4, Ont:; Tor '56; Psy.; Tel. 922-5339.

RALLEY, D. Lenin.; Upper Duplex, 23 Castleview Ave., Toronto 4, Ont. (res); Tor '56; Psy; Staff, Ontario Hosp., New Toronto; Tel. CL 9-8291.

RALLING, Antony; 206 Wellington St., Wallaceburg, Ont.; McG'48; FRCS(C); GenSurg; Chief of Med. Staff, Sydenham Dist. Hosp.; Tel. 627-2462.

RALLY, Charles R.; 408-750 W. Broadway, Vancouver 9, B.C.; McG'52; FRCP(C), IntMed; Att'd. Staff, Vancouver Gen. Hosp.; Clin. Inst'r., U. of British Columbia; Ass't. Med. Dir., Fidelity Life Ins.; Tel. 872-2211.

RALPH-EDWARDS, E. S.; 795 Warden Ave., Scarborough, Ont.; Beirut (Lebanon) '42; MRCS (Eng.), LRCP (Lond.); FRCS (Edin.), FRCS(C), GenSurg; MCGP; Assoc. Staff, Toronto E. Gen. Hosp.; Tel. 461-8272.

RALPH, Gordon L.; 60 Albert St. W., Thorold, Ont.; 31 Clairmont St. (res); Tor '50; M.C.G.P.; Staff, St. Catharine's Gen. & Hotel Dieu Hosp's.; Part-Time Indust., McKinnon Industries; Tel. CA 7-5255.

RALPH, Robert E.; 1057 Avenue Rd., Toronto 12, Ont.; Qns'34; DIH, MCGP, FRSH; Assoc. Staff, Toronto East Gen. Hosp.; M.O., Toronto Fire Dept.; Tel. HU 3-8600.

RAM, Anantha A.; Mysore (India) '56; FRCS (C), Otol; Staff, Queen Mary Vets Hosp., Montreal, P.Q.; Tel. 342-2320.

RAMAGE, Howard C.; 462 Professional Bldg., Edmonton, Alta.; Alb'54; FRCS(C); Urol; Attend. Staff, Misericordia, Edmonton Gen., Glenrose Provincial Gen., & Good Samaritan Auxiliary Hosp's.; Tel. 422-6271.

RAMANOWSKI, Edward; Poznan (Poland); Staff, Charles Camsell Hosp., Edmonton, Alta.

RAMCKE, Elsbeth; (see FISCHER, Elsbeth).

RAMESAR, Simon; 196 Alwington Place, Kingston, Ont.; Sheffield (Eng.)'49; DPM; Psy.

RAMEY, F. F.; Department of National Health & Welfare, c/o Regional Superintendent, European Region. Abroad.

RAMON-MOLINER, Ouida; 2961 Longfellow, Ste-Foy, Quebec 10, P.Q.; Trinity Coll. (Dublin, Ire.) '53; Pt time Res., Laval Hosp.

RAMOS, Angeles; Santo Tomas (Philipp.)'56; Staff, Children's Hosp., Montreal 25, P.Q.

RAMOS, Fernando B.; Manila Central (Philipp.) '50; Staff, Riverview Hosp., Essondale, B.C.

RAMOS, Virginia G.; Santo Tomas'54; Staff, Riverview Hosp., Essondale, B.C.

RAMPHAL, Premdath J.; 3544A Bathurst St., Toronto 19, Ont.; Jamaica (West Indies) '62; M.B., B.S. (Lond.)

RAMSAY, Allan G.; 375 South St., London, Ont.; Wes '48; FRCP(C), IntMed (Nephrology); Phys., Victoria Hosp.; Ass't. Prof. (PathChem), Clin. Lect. (Med), & Hon. Lect. (Pharmacol.), U. of Western Ont. Tel. 432-5261. Abroad.

RAMSAY, Donald W.; Calgary Assoc. Clinic, 214-6th Ave. W., Calgary, Alta.; 929 Ridge Rd. (res); Dal '38; FACS; GenSurg; Chief of Gen. Surg., Holy Cross Hosp.; Tel. AM 3-7120.

RAMSAY, Elbern L.; 160 Highfield St., Moncton, N.B.; 351 Lutz St. (res); Dal '42; D.A.B.Ophth., Ophth Otol; Staff, Moncton City & Hotel Dieu Hosp's.; Tel. EV 2-8694.

RAMSAY, Francis G.; 11719 Edinboro, Edmonton, Alta.; Man '24; S.T. M.O., DVA, Edmonton; Retired.

RAMSAY, Francis W.; Academy Med. Bldg., 1812-4th St. S.W., Calgary Alta. 1801 Cayuga Dr. (res); Alb '54; F.R.C.P.(C), Neurol; Staff, Calgary Gen. & Holy Cross Hosp's.; Cons. Col. Belcher (DVA) Hosp.; Tel. 262-3505.

RAMSAY, James D.; 1718 Parker Ave., Regina, Sask. (res); St. Andrews (Scot.) '42; DPH; Dir. Pub. Health Research & Planning, Prov. Health Dept.; Tel. LA 3-0661.

RAMSAY, R. Alec.; McG'62; Res., Hop. Notre-Dame, Montreal 24, P.Q.

RAMSAY, R. M.; 125 Medical Arts Bldg., Winnipeg, Man.; 111 Handsart Blvd., Tuxedo (res); Man '37; M.Sc. (Ophth-Minn.), Ophth; Ophth., St. Boniface, Grace & Winnipeg Gen. Hosp's.; Ass't. Prof. (Ophth.), U. of Manitoba; Tel. WH 2-3383.

RAMSAY, T. Osborne; 550 Ingersoll Ave., Woodstock, Ont.; 72 Vansittart Ave. (res); Glasgow (Scot.)'51; Pres., Med. Staff, Woodstock Gen. Hosp.; Tel. 539-1112.

RAMSEY, Colin G.; 640 Professional Bldg., 10830 Jasper Ave., Edmonton, Alta.; 8428-109th St. (res); McG '48; IntMed; Pt.-time Indust. Phys., Imperial Oil Ltd.; Pt.-time PH Quarant. M.O., Dept. of Nat. Health & Welfare; Inst'r. (Med.), U. of Alta.; Tel. 422-8218.

RAMSEY, G. A. Stuart, VD; 1414 Drummond St., Montreal, P.Q.; 1469 Drummond St. (res); McG '12; FACS, FAAOO, FRCS(C), Ophth; Cons. (Ophth), Mtl. Gen. & Reddy Mem. Hosp's.; Tel. VI 2-2982.

RAMSEY, Michael S.; Belfast (Ire.)'61; Res., Winnipeg Gen. Hosp., Winnipeg 3, Man.

RAMSEY, Ronald K.; 519 Med. Arts Bldg., 11010 Jasper Ave., Edmonton, Alta.; Sask'59; MCGP; Tel. 488-0670.

RAMSEY, R. Bruce; Ste. 222, 1414 Drummond St., Montreal, P.Q.; McG'49; DAB; Ophth; Att'd. Staff, Children's Mem. Hosp. & Montreal Gen. Hosp.; Lect., McGill U.; Tel. VI 2-2982.

RANALLI, Joseph P.; 78 Barton St. W., Hamilton, Ont.; 31 Auchmar Rd. (res); Tor '52; MCGP; Active Staff, Hamilton Gen. & St. Joseph's Hosp's. Tel. JA 2-4633.

RANCE, C. Phillips; Hosp. for Sick Children, 555 University Ave., Toronto 2, Ont.; 181 Cortleigh Blvd., Toronto (Res.); Tor'42; FRCP(C); Paed; Assoc. Phys., Hosp. for Sick Children; Ass't. Prof., Dept. of Paed., U. of Toronto; Tel. 366-7242.

RANCOURT, Denis; 1500-18eme rue, Quebec 3, P.Q.; Lav'60.

RAND, Charles G.; Dept. of Nat. Health & Welfare, Brooke Claxton Bldg., Ottawa, Ont.; McG '42; MPH; IntMed; Cons. in Chronic Dis. & Ageing.

RANDALL, Herbert S.; 4786 W. 2nd Ave., Vancouver, B.C.; McG '43; Anaes; Staff, Vancouver Gen. Hosp.; Instr. (Anaes), U. of British Columbia; Tel. CA 4-0222.

RANDALL, John D.; 657 W. 37th Ave., Vancouver 13, B.C.; London (Eng.) '39; F.R.C.S. (Eng.); Sr. M.O.; W.C.B.; Tel. AM 6-0211.

RANDALL, M. T. Clare; London (Eng.)'51; MRCS; LRCP; Paed; Staff, Douglas Hosp., Montreal, P.Q.

RANDELL, Owen T.; Box 1329-1359, Med. Assoc., Parry Sound, Ont.; London (Eng.) '46; LRCP; MRCS; GenSurg; Staff, Parry Sound Gen. & St. Joseph's Hosp's.; Tel. 746-9382.

RANDLETT, Ralph P.; 227 York St., Cornwall, Ont.; McG '49; FRCS(C); FACS; GenSurg; Staff, (Surg.) Hotel Dieu & Cornwall Gen. Hosp's.; Tel. WE 2-3113.

RANGACHARI, Samavedam; Andhra '53; FRCS-(C), Cardiovasc & ThorSurg; Staff, University Hosp., Edmonton, Alta.

RANGER, Claude J.; Ott '57; Psy; Staff, Ontario Hosp., North Bay, Ont.; Tel. 474-1200.

RANGER, Hubert; 234 Lakeshore, Point-Claire, P.Q.; Mon '23; Anaes.; Tel. 695-4405.
RANGER, Louis; Mon'65; Res., Hop. Maisonneuve, Montreal 36, P.Q.

RANGNO, Robert E.; Man'63; Res., Montreal Gen. Hosp., Montreal 25, P.Q.

RANKIN, Allan C.; 9005-112th St., Edmonton, Alta. (res); McG '04; D.P.H., F.R.C.P.(C); Retired.

RANKIN, Roy W.; 24 Ridout St. E., Tillsonburg, Ont.; Tor '18; Tel. VI 2-2331.

RANKINE, James A.; 1635 Abbott St., Kelowna, B.C.; Dal '39; F.A.C.S., F.I.C.S., F.R.C.S.(C), GenSurg; Att'd. Staff, Kelowna Gen. Hosp.; Tel. 762-2740.

RANKING, Gerald N.; Ste. D, 403A Toronto Western Medical Bldg., 25 Leonard Ave., Toronto, Ont.; 354 Russell Hill Rd. (res.); Witwatersrand (S. Africa) '41; FRCS (Eng.), FRCS(C), Urol; Surg. Staff (Urol.), Toronto Western Hosp.; Clin. Instr., U. of Toronto; Tel. 368-7227.

RANNEY, E. Kenneth; Tor'53; Res., New Mount Sinai Hosp., Toronto 2, Ont.

RANOSKY, Michael J.; River Ave. Medical Bldg., 385 River Ave., Winnipeg, Man.; 234 Glenwood Cres.(res); Man '42; M.C.G.P.; Dem. (Obst.), U. of Manitoba; Tel. GL 2-8142.

RANSFORD, Peter M.; 216 Cook Medical Bldg., 1175 Cook St., Victoria, B.C.; 3422 Mayfair Dr. (res); Middlesex Hosp. (London, Eng.) '42; MRCS; LRCP; DCH; Paed; Chief of Paed, Royal Jubilee Hosp.; Tel. 383-5022.

RANTA, Lawrence E.; 4182 W. 8th Ave., Vancouver 8, B.C. (res); Tor '36; DPH; PH; Bact; Dir. (Med.), Vancouver Gen. Hosp.; Hon. Lect. (Med. Ed.), U. of British Columbia; Tel. TR 6-3211.

RAO, Sirivaram V. K.; 102 Canada Bldg., 21st St. E. & 1st Ave. S., Saskatoon, Sask.; Madras (India) '57; DiagRad.

RAPHAEL, Stanley S.; Hotel Dieu Hosp., 1030 Ouellette Ave., Windsor, Ont.; London (Eng.)'46; Path; Staff (Path.), Hotel Dieu & Riverview Hosp's., Windsor; Tel. 252-3631.

RAPIER, Dunbar O. C.; 11454-50th Ave., Malmo Plains, Edmonton, Alta. (res); Edinburgh (Scot.) '57; Psy; Psy., Unit for Emotionally Disturbed Children, U. of Alberta Hosp.; Lect. (Psy.), U. of Alberta; Tel. GE 9-5911, Loc. 409.

RAPOPORT, Abraham; Tor. Western Hosp., 399 Bathurst St., Toronto 2B, Ont.; 10 Heathdale Rd., Tor. 10 (res); Tor '49; FACP; FRCP(C), IntMed; Dir. (Biochem. Dept.), Tor. Western Hosp.; Assoc. (Med.) & Research Assoc. (PathChem.), U. of Toronto; Tel. 369-5133.

RAPP, Clarence R.; Ste. 3, Tor. East Gen. Hosp., 825 Coxwell Ave., Toronto 6, Ont.; 49 Garfield Ave. (res); Tor '31; B.Sc. (Med.), MA (Cantab.), FRCS(Eng.), FRCS(C), GenSurg; Tel. HO 1-8834.

RAPP, Morton S.; Tor'61; Psy; Staff, Toronto Western Hosp., Toronto 2B, Ont.

RAPPAPORT, Aron M.; 134 St. Clements Ave., Toronto 12, Ont. (res); Prague (Czech.) '29; Ph.D. (Physiol.); Prof. (Physiol.), U. of Toronto; Tel. 928-2594.

RAPPAPORT, Rosa K.; (Koslowsky); 1 Roxborough St. E., Toronto 5, Ont.; 134 St. Clements Ave. Tor. 12 (res); Tashkent (U.S.S.R.) '41; Derm; Staff, Hosp. for Sick Children & O.P.D. Women's College & Toronto Gen. Hosp's.; Tel. 924-6433.

RAPSON, Linda M.; 350 Beech Ave., Toronto 13, Ont.; Tor'65; Tel. OX 4-1126.

RARAGOSKY, Terrence M. (See Ragan, Terence M.).

RASCHKA, Leslie; Budapest (Hung.) '49; D.Psy; Staff, Ontario Hosp., Toronto, Toronto 3, Ont.

RASHEED, Abdur; Punjab (India)'51; Staff, Provincial Hosp., Lancaster, N.B.

RASHID, Abdur; 161 Augusta St., Ottawa, Ont.; Dacca (India)'57; FRCP(C), IntMed.

RASHID, Syed A.; Staff, Provincial Mental Hosp., Lancaster, N.B.; Bihar U. (India) '55; D. Psy.; Tel. 694-4481.

RASKIN, Norman; 300 King St. W., Oshawa, Ont.; 324 Northcliffe Ave. (res); Tor '46; D.Psy; Psy; Staff, Oshawa Gen. & Ajax & Pickering Gen. Hosp's.; Tel. 728-1241.

RASMINSKY, Bernard J.; Tor'65; Res., Toronto Western Hosp., Toronto 2B, Ont.

RASMUSSEN, George; 2946 Tillicum Rd., Victoria, B.C.; UBC'64; Staff, Royal Jubilee, St. Joseph's, & Gorge Road Hosp's.; Tel. EV 5-8761.

RASMUSSEN, Theodore B.; 3801 University St., Montreal 2, P.Q.; 29 Surrey Dr., Mtl. 16 (res); U. of Minnesota (Minn., USA) '34; M.S., ABNS; FRCS(C), NeurSurg; Dir. & NeurSurg., Mtl. Neurol. Inst.; Neurol. & NeuroSurg.-in-Chief, Royal Victoria Hosp.; Cons. (NeurSurg.), Queen Mary Vet's., DVA, Montreal Children's & Jewish Gen. Hosp's.; Prof. of Neurol. & NeurSurg., McGill U.; Tel. AV 8-7320.

RASSELL, John A., W/C; 2218 Circle Place, Ottawa 8, Ont.; London (Eng.)'51; DPH; D.Psy.; Hd., Dept. of Psy., National Defence Med. Centre, Ottawa; Lect., Dept. of Psy., U. of Ottawa; Tel. 733-3859.

RASTOGI, Pratap N.; Lucknow (India)'52; FRCP(C), Paed; Staff, Women's College Hosp., Toronto, Ont.; Tel. WA 3-7381.

RATAS, Iivi—see CAMPBELL, Iivi

RATCHFORD, Harold A.; Cheticamp, N.S.; Dal '25; GenSurg; Surg.-in-Chief, Sacred Heart Hosp.

RATELLE-CHARTIER, Germaine; 5105 des Melezes, Montreal, P.Q. (res); Mon '52; D&T Rad; Jr. Ass't. Dept. of Rad., Hop. Maisonneuve; Tel. 254-8341.

RATH, Otto J.; 705 Commercial Bldg., 169 Pioneer Ave., Winnipeg 1, Man.; 45 Galinee Bay, Wpg. 22 (res); Alb '48; MPH (Mich.); Reg. Dir., (Med. Serv.), Dept. of Nat. Health & Welfare; Tel. WH 3-1414.

RATHANA - NAKINTARA, Thaworn; Bangkok, Thailand'57; Sr. Psy., Munroe Wing (Mental Health Clinic), Regina Gen. Hosp., Regina, Sask.

RATHBONE, Eric D.; 100 Medical Arts Bldg., Fort William, Ont.; 429 Norah (res); Qns '39; Active Staff, McKellar Gen. Hosp.; Courtesy Staff, St. Joseph's Port Arthur Gen. Hosp's.; Tel. MA 3-9242.

RATHBUN, John C.; War. Mem. Children's Hosp., London, Ont.; R.R. No. 6 (res); Tor'39; FAAP, FRCP(C), Paed; Phys-in-Chief, War Mem. Children's Hosp.; Cons., Byron San. & Children's Psy. Inst.; Prof. & Hd. Dept. of Paed., U. of Western Ontario; Tel. GE 2-5261.

RATHJEN, Beryl (See Bishop).

RATNER, Jack T.; 5845 Cote des Neiges Rd., Montreal 26, P.Q.; McG '54; FRCP(C), IntMed; Gastroent (P.Q.); Staff, Jewish Gen., Reddy Mem. & Lakeshore Gen. Hosp's.; Staff Phys., Bell Telephone Co.; Tel. 731-8071.

RATTE, Viateur; 4 Durocher, Riviere du Loup, P.Q.; Lav'51; DHP; PH(P.Q.); Reg. M.O., Dist. No. 3; Tel. 862-4287.

RATZLAFF, Elmer H.; UBC'65; Res., Kingston Gen. Hosp., Kingston, Ont.

RATZLAFF, Victor J.; Alb'62; Res., University Hosp., Edmonton, Alta.

RAUF, M. Naseem; 3218 Yonge St., Toronto 12, Ont.; McG '59; Tel. 485-5381.

RAVARY, Pierre; 3239 Maplewood Ave., Montreal 26, P.Q.; Mon '23; Tel. RE 9-1552.

RAVENSCROFT, Alan K.; 121 Wellington St. W., Barrie, Ont.; Edinburgh (Scot.)'59; Staff, Royal Victoria Hosp. of Barrie; Tel. 728-5536.

RAVINSKY, Ely; Ste. 401, 99 Avenue Rd., Toronto 5, Ont.; 28 Farrington Dr., Willowdale (res); Qns '54; FRCS(C), ObstGyn; Active Staff (ObstGyn), New Mt. Sinai Hosp. Court Staff, Grace Hosp.; Tel. WA 5-6280.

RAWLING, Edward G.; 2254 Gordon Dr., Cooksville, Ont.; 358 Reynolds St., Oakville; Wes '57; FRCS(C), GenSurg; Staff, South Peel & Oakville Trafalgar Mem. Hosp's.; Tel. 277-0618;

RAWLINSON, Herbert E.; Alb '27; Ph.D. (McGill Physiol.); Emer. Prof. of Anat., U. of Alberta, Edmonton, Alta.

RAWLINSON, M. P .C.; Department of National Health & Welfare, c/o Regional Superintendent, European Region. Abroad.

RAXLEN, Alexander; Brunswick Diagnostic Group, 25 Brunswick Ave., Toronto 4, Ont.; 68 Wembley Rd. (res); Tor '34; M.A., FRCS (Edin.), FRCS(C), GenSurg; Chief, Dept. of Surg., & Dir. of Med. Affairs, Doctor's Hosp.; Tel. 927-3641.

RAXLEN, Benjamin; Brunswick Diagnostic Group, 25 Brunswick Ave., Toronto 4, Ont.; 26 Burnside Dr. (res); Tor '37; Anaes; Staff, Doctor's Hosp.; Tel. 924-9741.

RAYES, Hassan; 715 Myrand Nord, app. 4, Quebec 10, P.Q.; GenSurg(P.Q.).

RAYMAN, M. Raza; Citizens' Clinic, Main St., Biggar, Sask.; Sixth Ave. E. (res); Liverpool (Eng.)'54; FRCS(Ed); Tel. 948-3378.

RAYMAN, Paul; 727 Jane St., Toronto, Ont.; 66 Bywood Dr. (res); Warsaw (Poland) '23; Court. Staff, Toronto Gen. Hosp.; Tel. 767-0849.

RAYMERS, Milton P.; 15 Saguenay, Toronto 12, Ont. (res); Tor'29; M.Sc. (Penn.); FACOG; ObstGyn; Sr. Att. ObstGyn.; New Mount Sinai Hosp.; Tel. 922-7111.

RAYMOND, Cyril; App. 4, 2135 Bellechasse, Montreal 35, P.Q.; Mon'61; FRCS(C), GenSurg; Staff, Hop. St. Joseph de Rosemont; Abroad.

RAYMOND, George H.; Brockville Medical Clinic, 224 King St. E., Brockville, Ont.; 13 N. Augusta Rd., Brockville, Ont. (res); McG'35; FACS, FRCS(C), GenSurg; Active Staff Surg., Brockville Gen. & St.-Vincent-de-Paul Hosp's.; Tel. DI 2-4477.

RAYMOND, Georges; 512 School, Arvida, P.Q. McG '50; Tel. 548-4663.

RAYMOND, Gerard; Mon '56; Res., Hop. Notre-Dame, Montreal 24, P.Q.

RAYMOND, Laurent; St. Jean Port Joli, Co. L'Islet, P.Q.; Lav '59.

RAYMOND, Odilon; 241 Fleury W., Montreal, P.Q.; 5605 Place d'Aiguillon (res); **Lav '49; FACA; D & T Rad; Head, Dept. of Rad., Hop. du** Sacre-Coeur; Tel. DU 1-7281.

RAYMOND, Paul E.; C.P. 58, St-Eleuthere, Cte Kamouraska, P.Q.; Lav'65.

RAYMOND, Raymond M.; 800-1eme, Ville La Pocatiere, Co. Kamouraska, P.Q.; Med. Dir. & Anaes., Hop. de Notre-Dame de Fatima; Tel. 789.

RAYMOND, Rene; St. Esprit, Co. Montcalm, P.Q.; Mon '43; M.C.G.P.; Dep. Coroner.

RAYMOND, Richard; 3175 Chemin Ste-Catherine, Montreal, P.Q.; 324 Thomas-Pepin, Boucherville (res); Mon '52; Paed (PQ); Haem. (PQ); I/C (Haem.) Lab., Hop. Ste-Justine; Tel. RE 1-4931, Loc. 462.

RAYMOND, Willie J. A.; 520-4eme ave., Quebec 3, P.Q.; Lac Beauport (res); Lav '45; Tel 849-8145.

RAYNAULD, Pierre; 4135 ave. Papineau, Montreal 24, P.Q.; 5880 Bld. Roi-Rene, Ville d'Agou (res); Mon '59; Obst; Staff Hop. Notre-Dame; Tel. LA 4-4451.

RAYNER, Douglas C.; 233 N. Franklin St., Fort William, Ont. (res); Capetown (S. Africa) '56; Path; Assoc. Pathol., McKellar Gen. Hosp.; Tel. MA 3-6471.

RAYNHAM, Frederick; 8941-82nd Ave., Edmonton, Alta.; 8531-88th Ave. (res); London (Eng.) '49; Tel. HO 6-2735.

RAYNOR, Everett F.; Ste 277, 5655 Cambie St., Vancouver 15, B.C.; 1611-W. 45th Ave., Van. 13 (res); Qns '35, Ophth; Cons. (Ophth), Shaughnessy & Van. Gen. Hosp's. & Health Centre for Children; Clin. Instr. (Ophth), U. of British Columbia; Tel. 263-3939.

RAYPORT, Mark; McG '48; Ph. D., D.N.S.; Research Fell. of U.S. P.H. Serv., Montreal Neurol. Inst., Montreal, P.Q.

RAYSON, John H.; Mission City, B.C.; Man'65.

RAZ, Victor M.; Cher Radio Bldg., 56 Inglis St., Sydney, N.S.; Calcutta (India)'53; FRCS(C), OrthSurg.

RAZA, Lorne N.; 10-5th Ave., Pointe-Claire, Montreal, P.Q.; Geneva (Switz.) '54; GenSurg, Staff, Lakeshore Gen. & Lachine Gen. Hosp's.; Tel. 697-1263.

RAZACK, Abdool; Main St., Palmerston, Ont.; Dal'65.

REA, D. Homer; 428 Rideau St., Ottawa 2, Ont.; London (Eng.)'44; MRCS; LRCP; MRCOG; FACS; FRCS(C), ObstGyn.

REA, George W.; 215 Saskatchewan Cres. W., Saskatoon, Sask. (res); Queen's (N. Ire.) '14; D.P.H., D.Bact.(Lond.), Bact.; Retired.

READ, Anthony M.; 1541 W. Broadway, Vancouver 9, B.C.; UBC '60; AMCGP; Tel. RE 6-0611.

READ, Harold C.; 5808 University Ave., Halifax, N.S.; 151 Inglis St. (res); Dal '43; IntMed; Att'd. Phys., Victoria Gen. Hosp.; Cons. (Haem. & Med.), Camp Hill DVA Hosp.; Assoc. Prof. Dalhousie U.; Staff, Path. Inst. Prov. Dept. of PH; Tel. 423-6493.

READ, John G.; Wes'61; Staff, University Hosp., Edmonton, Alta.

READ, John H.; 7 Lakeland Pt. Dr., Kingston, Ont. (res); McG '50; DPH; Paed; Staff Kingston Gen. Hosp.; Prof. & Hd. Dept. of PrevMed. & Ass't. Prof. (Paed), Queen's U.; Tel. 546-1731.

READ, Paul A.; Box 429, Didsbury, Alta.; London (Eng.) '48; MRCS; LRCP.

READ, Robert M.; Dal '56; Res., Victoria Hosp., London, Ont.

READ, R. Wallace; 286 Main St., Exeter, Ont.; Wes '52; MCGP; Tel. 235-2290.

READ, Stanley E.; Alb'65; Res., University Hosp., Saskatoon, Sask.

READ, Walter W.; 6 Kingsway Blvd., General Delivery, Grimsby, Ont.; **McG '19.**

READ, Wesley R.; 401 Oakridge Towers, 6026 Tisdall St., Vancouver 13, B.C.; Tor'39; D.Psy; Psy; MCGP.

READER, Norman; Lav '62; Res., Hop. St-Sacrement, Quebec, P.Q.

READY, Morris H.; 809 Dunlevie Ave., Ottawa 13 Ont. (res); Qns '55; Anaes; Staff, Ottawa Civic Hosp.; Tel. PA 9-2511.

REARDON, C. Henry; 6389 Coburg Rd., Halifax, N.S.; 1036 Ridgewood Dr. (res); Dal '45; MCGP; Assoc. Staff Memb. of all Halifax Hosp's.; Instr., Dalhousie U.; Tel. 422-7454.

REARDON, F. L.; Canadian Pension Comm., D.V.A., Ottawa, Ont. (Med. Exam.).

REASON, H. T. Ward; 538 Dundas St., London, Ont.; 1084 The Parkway (res); Wes '42; MCGP; Att'd. Staff, Victoria & St. Joseph's Hosp's.; Tel. 439-7311.

REBBECK, Patricia M.; Edinburgh (Scot.)'59; FRCS(C), GenSurg; Staff, Riverview Hosp., Essondale, B.C.

REBHAN, Auguste W.; 32 Rowanwood Ave., Toronto 5, Ont.; J. W. Goethe (Frankfurt, Germ.) '50; Paed; Chief of Paed., Women's College Hosp.; Med. Dir., Children's Aid, Metropolitan Toronto; Tel. WA 4-5982.

RECESTER, Tamara; 804 Jean Talon W., Montreal 15, P.Q.; Italy'39; AMCGP; Tel. 274-4064.

RECHNITZER, Peter A.; 304-450 Central Ave., London, Ont.; 1000 Wellington St. (res); **Wes '48; MRCP (Edin.), FRCP(C), IntMed; Cons.** Med., St. Joseph's Hosp.; Cons., Norfolk Gen. Hosp.; Clin. Instr., U. of Western Ont.; Tel. GE 9-9851.

REDDING, Ralph A.; Alb'60; FRCP(C), IntMed; Staff, Toronto Western Hosp.; Abroad.

REDDY, S. R.; 1741 Portage Ave., Winnipeg 12, **Man. Mysore (India) '53.**

REDFEARN, Donald S.; 4052 New St., Burlington, Ont.; 4133 Lorraine Cr. (res); Qns '56; MCGP: Active Staff, Hamilton Gen. & Joseph Brant Hosp's.; Phys., Shell Oil Co.; Tel. 637-2323.

REDFEARN, R. Graham; 4052 New St., Burlington, Ont.; 552 Bridgman (res); Qns '57; MCGP; Tel. NE 7-2323.

REDFORD, Hamish; 818-9th Ave N., Port Alberni, B.C.; UBC'64; Abroad.

REDINGER, Richard N.; Wes '62; Res., Victoria Hosp., London, Ont.; Abroad.

REDMAN, John A.; 2390 Eglinton Ave. E., Scarborough, Ont.; Edinburgh (Scot.)'59.

REDMOND, Lila; Ste 520, 1538 Sherbrooke St. W., Montreal, P.Q.; 3600 Ridgewood, (res); McG '43; Derm; Clin. Staff, Mtl. Children's & Reddy Mem. Hosp's.; Teach. Staff, McGill U.; Tel. WE 7-2269.

REDPATH, Edward L.; Man '43; P.G. (Path.), Vancouver Gen. Hosp., Vancouver, B.C.
REE, Rhoda; UBC'64; Res., Shaughnessy Hosp., Vancouver 9, B.C.
REED, Carol A.; Wes'63; Res., 526 Banting Inst., 100 College St., Toronto 2, Ont.
REED, Charles E.; 176 Woolwich St., Guelph, Ont.; Tor'51.
REED-DAOUST, Lise; 222 Henri Bourassa est, Montreal, P.Q.; 11355 Drouart (res); Mon '56; IntMed; Ass't., Dept. of Med., Hop. Sacre-Coeur; Tel. VI 2-4892.
REED-DAVIS, Royston; Med. Arts Bldg., Hamilton, Ont.; Westminster H. (London, Eng.) '46; MRCS, LRCP, FRCS (Eng. & Ed.); OrthSurg; Staff, Chedoke Hosp.; Tel. 529-9061.
REED, George E.: Baysville P.O., Ont.; Tor '26; NeurPsy.; Retired.
REED, Howard N.; Winnipeg Clinic, Winnipeg 1, Man.; 210 Oak St., Winnipeg 9 (res); London (Eng.) '41; M.R.C.S. (Eng.), L.R.C.P. (Lond.), D.O. (Oxon.), D.O.M.S. (Eng.), F.R.C.S. (Eng.), M.S. Ophth (Lond.), F.A.C.S., F.R.C.S.(C), Ophth; Ophth. Winnipeg Gen. Children's & Misericordia Hosp's.; Ass't. Prof., U. of Manitoba; Tel. WH 2-0551.
REED, R.H.B.; Ste. 420, 2184 W. Broadway, Vancouver 9, B.C.; 4750 Angus Dr. (res); Tor '37; F.I.C.S., OrthSurg; Chief of Staff & Chmn. Orth. Serv., Children's Hosp.; Cons. Orth., Shaughnessy Hosp.; Orth. Staff, St. Paul's Hosp.; Tel. RE 1-3722.
REED, Roger W.; 3775 University St., Montreal 2, P.Q.; 79 Ballantyne Ave. N., Westmount (res); McG '49; FRCP(C), Bact; Bact., Royal Victoria Hosp.; Prof. & Chm. Dept. of Bact. & Immunol., McGill U.; Tel. VI 2-1251. Loc 595.
REED, William, Col.; H.Q. Mobile Command, Longueuil, P.Q.; McG'40; DPH; Command Surgeon, H.Q. Mobile Command; Tel. 671-3711, Local 394.
REEDS, W. Robert; Beaverton, Ont. (res); Tor '14; Retired.
REES, Donald L.; 303 Med. Arts Bldg., Edmonton, Alta.; 9106-120th St. (res); Alb '48; DAB-Ophth; Staff, University Hosp.; Instr. (Ophth), U. of Alberta; Tel. 424-7417.
REES-DAVIES, Eudora M., 6079 Grandview, Douglas Hwy. E., S. Burnaby, B.C. (res); Bristol (Eng.) '47; M.R.C.S. (Eng.), L.R.C.P. (Lond.), M.O., Columbia Hosp. Ship (Minstrel Island).
REES-DAVIES, Peter E.; Ste 303, 1541 W. Broadway, Vancouver 9, B.C.; 376 Keith Rd. West Van. (res); London H. (Eng.) '39; LRCP(Lond), MRCS (Eng.), FACS, F.R.C.S. (Eng.), FRCS(C), GenSurg; Att'd. Staff, St. Paul's Hosp.; Cons. Surg., Cancer Inst. & Dept of Indian Affairs; Clin. Ass't., U. of British Columbia; Tel. RE 1-7616.
REES, Elihu; McG'63; Res., Royal Victoria Hosp., Montreal 2, P.Q.
REES, Howard J.; Box 219, Blenheim, Ont.; Tor 51; Staff, St. Joseph's & Gen. Hosp's., Chatham; Tel. 676-3394.
REESAL, Michael R.: 851 Prieur, Apt. 3, Cite Jacques Cartier, P.Q.; Belfast (N. Ire.)'55; FRCP(C), Path; Ass't. Path., Reddy Mem. Hosp., Montreal.
REESE, Lawrence W.; 271 Lucas St., Richmond Hill, Ont. (res); Loma Linda (Calif, USA) '51; DABPath; Hd., Dept. of Path., North York Branson Hosp., Willowdale; Tel. 633-9420, Loc. 229. Abroad.
REESE, Lionel; 450 Central Ave., London, Ont.; 22 Linksgate Rd. (res); Qns '47; FACS; FRCS(C); Urol; Chief Urol., St. Joseph's Hosp.; Cons. Urol., Ontario Cancer Fdn., London Clinic, St. Mary's Hosp., & Ontario Hosp.; Dir. of Nuclear Med., St. Joseph's Hosp.; Instr. (Surg.), Lect. (Physiol.), U. of Western Ontario; Tel. 438-0611.
REES-JONES, Thomas Glyn, Sg.Lt.; London (Eng.)'52; MRC; LRCP; D.(Obst.) RCOG; Med. Centre, Verden, BFPO 32, Germany; Abroad.
REESOR, Helen L. (Eydt); 323 Batavia Place, Waterloo, Ont.; Tor'51: Campus Phys., U. of Waterloo; Tel. SH 3-4286.
REEVE, Charles E.; McG'62; Res., Vancouver Gen. Hosp., Vancouver 9, B C.
REEVES, Andre; 3575 rue la Garde, Duvernay, Ville de Laval, P.Q.; Mon'55; Haem (P.Q.); Staff, Hop. Jean Talon; Tel. CR 3-5151.
REEVES, R. L.; Eganville, Ont.; Qns '40; Dist. Coroner.
REGAN, K. J.; 163 Brock St., Kingston, Ont.; 301 Barrie St. (res); Qns '32; Tel. 548-8288.
REGAUDIE, Bernard; 70 Place Bourget S., Joliette, P.Q.; Lav '59; Paed; Chief Paed., Hop. St. Eusebe; Tel. 756-1811.
REGEHR, John I.; Man'65; Staff, Morris Gen. Hosp., Morris, Man.; Tel. 280.
REGIMBALD, Andre; 110 boul Laurentides, Pont-Viau, Laval-des-Rapides, P.Q.; Mon '63.
REGNAULT, Paul C.; 30 est, boul. St-Joseph, **Montreal 34, P.Q.; Paris (France) '45; FRCS(C);** GenSurg; PlasSurg; Surg., St. Luc Hosp.; Tel. 861-7321.
REICH, Carl J.; 300 Calgary Med. Centre, 906-8th Ave. S.W., Calgary, Alta.; Qns'43; IntMed; Tel. 262-5696.
REICH, Samuel; 1538 Sherbrooke W., Montreal, P.Q.; 1001 Mount Royal Blvd. (res); Vienna (Austria) '31; DiagRad; Cons. Rad., Mt. Sinai San., St. Agathe; Tel. WE 5-6288.
REICHENFELD, Hans; Box 590, Hamilton Health Assoc., Hamilton, Ont.; London (Eng.)'52; DObst-RCOG.
REICHER, Agnes E.; Tor'62; Res., Sunnybrook Hosp., Toronto 12, Ont.
REICHERT, John N.; 530 Eglinton Ave. E., Toronto 12, Ont.; 18 Valley View, Tor. 7 (res); Tor '60; Med. Dir., St. Michael's Hosp. Employees Health Clinic; Tel. 483-3996.
REID, Andrew N.; 213 Scollard Bldg., 1207 Douglas St., Victoria, B.C.; 3311 Richmond Ave. (res); Edinburgh (Scot.)'35; FRCS(Ed.), FACS, FRCS(C), GenSurg, OrthSurg; Surg. Staff, St. Joseph's & Royal Jubilee Hosp's.; Tel. EV 4-6931.
REID, Anne M. (Mitchell); Box 2327 Hinton Alta.; Aberdeen (Scot.) '54.
REID, Antoine; Ste. 50, 1610 Sherbrooke St. W., Montreal 25, P.Q.; Lav '54.
REID, Byron L.; 5750 South St., Halifax, N.S.; Dal '61; AMCGP; Court. Staff, Victoria Gen., Grace Maternity, Halifax Infirmary, Halifax Clinic & Children's Hosp's.; Tel. 423-9239.
REID, Charles D.; 866 3eme ave., Val d'Or, Cte. Abitibi, P.Q.; Lav '60; AMCGP.
REID, David W. J.; 311 Med. Arts Bldg., 11010 Jasper Ave., Edmonton, Alta.; Alb'56; FRCS(C); ObstGyn; Staff, University Hosp.; Instr. (Obst-Gyn), U. of Alberta; Tel. GA 2-2217.
REID, Earle L.; Dal '57; MCGP; Res., Dept. of Med., Victoria Gen. Hosp., Halifax, N.S.
REID, E. A. Stewart; 650 Seaforth Med. Bldg., 3550 Cote des Neiges Rd., Montreal 25, P.Q.; 485 Strathcona Ave. Westmount (res); McG '42; FACC; FACP; FACCP; Cardiol (P.Q.); FRCP (C); IntMed; Dir. Div. of Cardiol & Sr. Phys., Mtl. Gen. Hosp.; Assoc. Prof. (Med.), McGill U.; Tel. 932-7857.
REID, Eric M. W.; 6745 Hastings St. E., North Burnaby, B.C.; Glasgow (Scot.) '45; Active Staff, Burnaby Gen. Hosp.; Vis. Staff, Vancouver Gen. Hosp.; Tel. CY 8-5747.
REID, E. Paul; Tor'62; Res., Kingston Gen. Hosp., Kingston, Ont.
REID, Everett C.; Ste 550, 3550 Cote des Neiges Rd., Montreal 25, P.Q.; McG '48; FRCS(C), Urol; Staff, Montreal Gen. Hosp., Montreal 25, P.Q.
REID, George R.; 24 Wellesley St. E., Toronto, Ont.; Qns '05; DiagRad; Tel. WA 2-5343.
REID, Grainger W., O.B.E.; 20 Cheltenham Ave., Toronto 12, Ont.; Edinburgh (Scot.)'39; MB; Ch.B; MRCS(Edin.).
REID, Henri; Mon '41; PulmDis & TB (P.Q.) Chief of Surg., San. St. George, Mount Joli, P.Q.; Tel. PR 5-4355.
REID, Ian L.; Box 4000, Selkirk, Man.; Man'56; GenSurg; Tel. 482-3321.
REID Ian W. C.; 5 Utilities Bldg., P.O. Box 2327, Valley Rd., Hinton, Alta.; Lodge Pole Dr. (res); Aberdeen (Scot.) '54; M.O., North Western Pulp & Power Ltd.; Dist. Coroner.

REID, James D.; 77 Upper Middle Rd., Cooksville, Ont.; Tor '47; ObstGyn; Staff, Dept. of ObstGyn, South Peel Hosp., Cooksville; Tel. 279-6383.
REID, James F.; Medical Centre, 4902-50th St., Vegreville, Alta.; 5102-51st St. (res); Alb '41; GenSurg; M.C.G.P.; Staff, St. Joseph's Gen. Hosp.; Instr. Schl. of Nursing; Tel. 632-2822.
REID, James W.; 6033 Cobourg Rd., Halifax, N.S.; Dal '26; M.R.C.G.P. (Lond.), F.R.C.P.(C), IntMed; Assoc. Prof. Dalhousie U.; Tel. 423-6874.
REID, John A. G., MBE; 710 Seymour St., Vancouver, B.C.; Tor '38; FCCP, FRCP(C), IntMed; Att'd. Staff, Van. Gen. Hosp.; Clin. Instr., U. of British Columbia; Tel. MU 4-1511.
REID, John B.; 600 Prince St., Truro, N.S.; 90 King St. (res); Dal '42; FACAS; Chief (Urol.), Colchester Co. Hosp.; Tel. 893-8603.
REID, John C.; 42 King St. W., Stoney Creek, Ont.; Qns'52; MCGP; Active Staff, Hamilton Civic Hosp's.; Tel. 662-4911.
REID, Joseph D.; Hotel-Dieu Hosp., Kingston, Ont.; Qns'53; MRCP(Eng.); FRCP(C), Paed; Hd., Dept. of Paed., Hotel-Dieu Hosp.; Ass't. Prof. Paed., Queen's U.; Tel. 546-2446.
REID, J. Yvan, Major; Base Hosp., Cdn. Forces Base, St. Hubert, P.Q.; Lav'51.
REID, Leonide; 425 est Blvd. Charest, Quebec, P.Q.; Moulin des Meres, Loretteville (res); Lav '21; ObstGyn; Assoc. Prof. (Gyn.), Laval U.; Chief of Gyn., Hop. Enfant Jesus, Quebec; Tel. 524-0611.
REID, Leslie T.; Box 428, Lakefield, Ont.; Tor '54; MCGP; Active Staff (GP), Peterboro Civic & St. Joseph's Hosp's., Peterboro; Tel. OL 2-3151.
REID, Lloyd G.; 205 Church St., Pembroke, Ont. 485 Irving St. (res); Qns '39; Tel. RE 2-2611.
REID, Raymond A.; Wellington, P.E.I.; Mon '33; M.C.G.P.; Staff, Prince Co. Hosp.; Summerside; Tel. 2246.
REID, Robert F.; Medical Arts Bldg., 121 Wellington St. W., Barrie, Ont.; Edinburgh (Scot.) '48.
REID, Robert G.; 1414 Drummond St., Montreal, P.Q.; McG '28; Urol.
REID, Robert L.; 257 Highland Ave., Fort Erie, Ont.; Tor'63.
REID, Samuel I.; 215 Laurier Ave. E., Ottawa 2, Ont.; 894 Eastbourne Ave. (res); Ott '53; ObstGyn; Clin. Instr., Ottawa U.; Tel. CE 3-6457.
REID-SMITH, Edward A. M.; Dublin (Ire.) '59; M.B., B.Ch.; BAO; DMRD (Eng.); DiagRad; Staff, Woodstock Gen. Hosp., Woodstock, Ont.; Tel. 537-5511.
REID, Wilfrid; Mon'65; Res., Institute Albert-Provost, Montreal 9, P.Q.
REID, William D.; Wes '64; Jr. Int., Montreal Gen. Hosp., Montreal, P.Q.
REID, William H.; Main St., Port Rowan, Ont.; Tor '06.
REID, William J.; 274 King St. W., Chatham, Ont.; 48 Robertson (res); Tor '38; Tel. 352-3320.
REID, William S.; 353 Eveline St., Selkirk, Man.; Man '39; Staff, Selkirk Gen. Hosp.; Dist. Coroner.
REIHER, Jean; Mon '59; Int'n., Hop. Hotel Dieu, Montreal, P.Q.
REIKIE, Robert D.; Smith Clinic, Camrose, Alta.; Alb '48.
REILLY, Bernard J.; 10 Whitehall Rd., Toronto 5, Ont. (res); Glasgow (Scot.) '49; DiagRad; Ass't. Rad., Hosp. for Sick Children; Clin. Instr. (Rad.), U. of Toronto; Tel. EM 6-7242.
REILLY, Douglass H.; 73 Westminster Ave., Montreal West, P.Q.; 85 Easton (res); McG '43; M.R.C.P.(Lond.), M.R.C.P.(Ed.), IntMed; Att'd. Phys., Queen Elizabeth Hosp.; Tel. 484-0480.
REILLY, Gordon L.; Ste. 210, 1175 Cook St., Victoria, B.C.; 3413 Henderson Rd. (res); Glasgow (Scot.)'58; AMCGP; Tel. 384-9621.
REILLY, Guy O.; Qns'65; Jr. Int., University Hosp., Saskatoon, Sask.; Abroad.
REILLY, Mary M.; 10 Whitehall Rd., Toronto 5, Ont.; Glasgow (Scot.)'49; Pt.-time Ass't. O.P.D., Princess Margaret Hosp.; Tel. 924-0671; Ext. 221.
REILLY, Nelson B.; 302 Cook Medical Bldg., 1175 Cook St., Victoria, B.C.; 2357 Pacific Ave. (res); McG '43; MCGP; Tel. 382-7462.
REILLY, Ruth A.; Manitoba Sanatorium, Ninette, Man.; Dublin (Ire.)'52; BAO; Sr. Staff Phys., Manitoba Sanatorium; Tel. Ninette 3322.
REIMER, Donald H.; Thompson Clinic, Thompson, Man.; Man '61.
REIMER, Jacob; Medical Clinic, 5102-48th St., Lloydminster, Alta.; Man'65.
REIN, Allan; 30 Sheppard Ave E., Willowdale, Ont.; Tor'55; MCGP; Tel. 221-6760.
REINGOLD, Albert A.; 217 Bathurst St., Toronto, Ont.; 20 Fernwood Rd. (res); Tor '47; M.C.G.P.; Staff, New Mt. Sinai Hosp.; Tel. EM. 4-1934.
REINGOLD, Maurice M.; 99 Avenue Rd., Toronto 5, Ont.; Tor '43; FACS; FCCP; FRCS(C), GenSurg; ThorSurg; Att'd. Surg., New Mount Sinai Hosp.; Clin. Teach. Surg., U. of Toronto; Tel. WA 1-7552.
REINGORF, Carl A.; London (Eng.) '57; Intn., Hosp. for Sick Children, Toronto 2, Ont.
REINE, Jacob W.; 68 Strathearn Rd., Toronto 10, Ont.; Tor '54; Anaes; Staff, Doctor's Hospital; Tel. WA 3-5411.
REINHARDT, Georges H.; 616 St.-Cyrille, ouest, Quebec 6, P.Q.; Lav '49; NeurSurg; Staff, Hop.-de-l'Enfant-Jesus; Cons. Hop.-St.-Francois-d'Assise, St. Sacrement, St.-Ambroise-delorette-ville & Hop. Ste.-Foy DVA; Staff, Laval U.; Tel. 683-9875.
REININGER, Siegfried M. M. T.; Ste: 1101, 123 Edward St., Toronto 2, Ont.; Munich (Germ.) '41; MCGP; Staff, St. Michael's, Wellesley & Central Hosp's.; Tel. 364-8882.
REINKE, Ernst E.; 103 Renrew St., Pembroke, Ont.; Qns '31; M.C.G.P.; Staff, Pembroke Gen. & Cottage Hosp's.; Tel. RE 2-3091.
REISLER, Hyman; 3550 Cote des Neiges Rd., Ste. 350, Montreal 25, P.Q.; Melbourne (Austral.) '56; Cardiol (P.Q.); FRCP(C), IntMed; Att'd. Phys., Jewish Gen. Hosp. & Dir., Cardiovasc. Lab.; Tel. 937-3442.
REIST, Harvey A.; Daysland, Alta.; Alb '53.
REIVE, Wilfred G.; 178 Claremont Ave., Kitchener, Ont.; Tor'41; DABA, FACA, Anaes.; Tel. 774-6551.
REJNOVICH, Edward; 527 Brant St., Burlington, Ont.; Tor '55.
REJSKIND, Mojzesz D.; 21 Lamont Cres., Regina, Sask. (res); Paris (Fr.) '39; Psy; Dir., Munroe Wing & Regina Mental Health Clinic, Regina Gen. Hosp.; Tel. LA 2-1811.
REKAI, John; 331 Sherbourne St., Toronto 2, Ont.; Peter Pazmany U. (Budapest, Hung.)'36; Admin., Central Private Hosp.; Tel. WA 3-2395.
REKAI, Paul; 331 Sherbourne St., Toronto 2, Ont. 323 Walmer Rd., Tor 4, (res); Budapest (Hung.) '36; Admin., Central Hosp.; Tel. WA 3-2395.
RELLE, Alexander; 30 Knightswood Rd., Toronto 12, Ont. (res; Munich (Germ.) '50; Anaes; Staff, New Mount Sinai Hosp.; Tel. EM 6-7361.
RELTON, John E. S.; Hosp. for Sick Children, Toronto, Ont.; London (Eng.) '54; M.B.; B.S., LRCP; MRCS; FFARCS; DA(Lond.); Anaes; Staff, Hosp. for Sick Children; Clin. Teach. (Anaes.), U. of Toronto; Tel. EM 6-7242.
REMARTINEZ, Felix C.; Madrid (Spain) '57; M.O., Dept. of Health, Mary's Town, Nfld.; Tel. 440.
REMILLARD, Benoit; 8415 rue St.-Denis, Montreal 11, P.Q.; Mon '51; M.C.G.P.
REMILLARD, Francis; 234 rue Longueuil, St-Jean, P.Q.; Mon'58; GenSurg(P.Q.); Surg., Hop. Gen. de St-Jean; Tel. 347-1252.
REMILLARD, Paul E.; 4515 ouest, Notre Dame, Montreal 30, P.Q.; 497-38th St. (res); Mon '52; Gen. Surg (P.Q.); Tel. WE 7-1880.
REMINGTON, James H.; 5906 Boul. Gouin ouest, Montreal 9, P.Q.; 10804 rue Verville, Mtl. 12 (res); Mon '23; Med. Adviser, Catholic Schl. Comm. of Mtl., 3737 est rue Sherbrooke, Mtl. 36; Tel. FE 4-5130.
REMUS, Leonard A.; 1001 Ridgeway St., Fort William, Ont.; 1800 McGregor St. (res); Qns '34; MIMA; FACS; GenSurg; Staff Surg. Div., McKellar Gen. Hosp.; Court. Staff, St. Joseph's & Port Arthur Gen. Hosp's.; Tel. MA 2-0601.

REMY, Huguette; Mon'65; Res., Hop. Notre-Dame, Montreal 24, P.Q.
REMY, Marcel; 30 est, boul St-Joseph, Montreal 14, P.Q.; Mon '49; ObstGyn; Tel. 845-4241.
RENAUD, Georges; 11178 Royale, Beaupre, Co. Montmorency, P.Q.; Lav '52; Tel. 263-3131.
RENAUD, Leo P.; Ott'65; Res., Montreal General Hosp., Montreal 25, P.Q.
RENAUD, Michael A.; 132 Hellems Ave. Welland, Ont.; Mon '18; M.C.G.P., Med. Staff, Welland Co. Hosp.; Tel. RE 2-6111.
RENAUD, Paul E.; 7637, Fontanelle, Cite-de-St-Leonard, Montreal-Nord, P.Q.; Mon '57; GenSurg.; OrthSurg(P.Q.); Tel. 259-8932; Abroad.
RENAUD, Reginald E.; 399 Bathurst St., Toronto 2B, London (Eng.) '41; M.R.C.S., L.R.C.P., M.C.G.P.; PhysMed & Rehab.; Tel. 368-2581.
RENAULT, Benoit; C.P. 220, Shediac, N.B.; Lav '57.
RENAULT, C. Guy; Lav '57; Staff, Hop. Provincial, C.P. 10, Campbellton, N.B.; Tel. PL 3-4461.
RENDELL, Wallace B.; Ste. 5, 539 Cassells St., North Bay, Ont.; Dal '54; FRCP(C); IntMed; Tel. 472-1140.
RENECKER, Glenn T.; 400 Walmer Rd., Toronto 4, Ont.; Wes'60; D.Psy; Psy.; Staff Psy., University of Toronto.
RENNER, Willi W.; 11 McKay Ave., Cornwall, Ont.; (res); Hamburg (Germ.) '45; D & T Rad; Chief, X-Ray Dept., Hotel-Dieu Hosp., Tel. WE 2-4630.
RENNERT, Charles; 7375 Papineau, Montreal 35, P.Q.; 6624 Parkview, Cote St. Luc (res); Bolgna (Italy) '38; MCGP; Tel. RA 8-5451.
RENNIE, Charles S.; Ste. 1212, 750 W. Broadway, Vancouver 9, B.C.; 5011 Collingwood St., Vanc. 13 (res); Man'40; MRCP(Lond.); FACP; IntMed. Att'd. Staff, Vancouver Gen. Hosp.; Clin. Instr., U. of British Columbia; Tel. TR 2-2111.
RENNIE, George M.; Port Perry, Ont.; Qns '23; Staff, Oshawa Gen. Hosp.; Dist. Coroner.
RENNIE, James W. R.; Manitoba Clinic 790 Sherbrooke St., Winnipeg, Man; 386 Brock St. (res); Man '34; DABS; FACS; F.R.C.S. (Ed), F.R.C.S. (C), GenSurg; Ass't Prof. of Surg., U. of Manitoba; Assoc. Surg., Winnipeg Gen. Hosp.; Tel. SP 4-6541.
RENNIE, John A.; Crestview Plaza, Port Credit, Ont.; Tor '62.
RENNIE, John C.; Portage Medical Services Clinic, Portage La Prairie, Man.; 227 Dufferin Ave. W. (res); Man '37.
RENNIE, Richard T.; Box 119, Bienfait, Sask.; London (Eng.) '47; MRCS; LRCP; Staff, Bienfait Hosp.; Tel. 388-2466.
RENOUF, John H.; Tor'63; Res., Toronto Gen. Hosp., Toronto 2, Ont.
RENPENNING, Hans J.; 112 The Palisades, 514 23rd. St. E., Saskatoon, Sask.; Sask '60; Tel. 244-1534.
RENSAA, Margaret A.; Apt. 1607, 8510-111th St., Edmonton, Alta.; Alb'55; FRCP(C), Anaes.
RENSHAW, H. Vaughn; 419 Medical Arts Bldg., Hamilton, Ont.; 50 Arkledun Ave. (res); Tor '32; F.I.C.S., PlasSurg; PlasSurg., St. Joseph's & Hamilton Gen. Hosp's.; Tel. JA 8-0077.
RENTIERS, Paul L.; 210 Medical Arts Bldg., 11010 Jasper Ave., Edmonton, Alta.; 13626—100 Ave. (res); Alb '41; M.Sc. (Minn., Derm. Syph.), D.A.B.D.S., DermSyph; Dir., Div. of Soc. Hygiene, Prov. of Alberta; Cons. Derm., D.V.A.; Prof. (Derm. Syph.), U. of Alberta; Tel. GA 2-4589.
RENTON, Alexander J.; 526 Guelph Line, Burlington, Ont.; McG'55; Psy.
RENTON, George E.; Med. Arts Bldg., 121 Wellington St. W., Barrie, Ont.; Tor'61; Tel. 726-0331.
RENWICK, Cynthia (Ward); 356 Woodroffe Ave., Ottawa 13, Ont.; Oxford (Eng.) '52; DRCOG (Eng.); Court. Staff, Ottawa Civic & Grace Hosp's.; Tel. 722-8505.
RENWICK, Gordon J.; 356 Woodroffe Ave., Ottawa 13, Ont.; Oxford (Eng.) '51; Staff, Ottawa Civic & Grace Hosp's.; Tel. 722-8505.
RENWICK, Wells A.; 38 Fallingbrook Dr., Scarborough, Ont.; Tor'54; FRCP(C), Anaes; Chief Anaes., Toronto East Gen. Hosp.; Clin. Instr., U. of Toronto; Tel. OX 5-6033.
RENY, Pierre; 1618 ouest King, Sherbrooke, P.Q.; Lav'65.
RENY, Raymond; St. Prosper de Dorchester, P.Q.; Lav '35.
RENZI, Gildo; 1681 Rachel est, Montreal, P.Q.; 875 Boissy, St. Lambert (res); Mon '58; Pulm Dis & TB (P.Q.); FRCP(C) IntMed; Clin. Ass't., Hop. Notre-Dame & Santa Cabrini Hosp.; Tel. 526-5909.
RENZI, Nelio; 240 Elm St., St.-Lambert, Cite-Jacques-Cartier, P.Q.; Mon '53; IntMed (P.Q.). Tel. 671-1255.
REPO, R. U.; Tor'64; Staff, Wabush Lake Clinic, Wabush, Labrador.
REQUENA, Calixto; 1129 est, Mont-Royal, Montreal 34, P.Q.; Tel. 523-0704.
RESNICK, Morris; 150 Metcalfe St., Ottawa, Ont.; 85 Avenue Rd. (res); Tor '52; MCGP; Dir., Nurses Health Serv. & Dir., Communicable Diseases, Ottawa Civic Hosp.; Tel. CE 5-3492.
RESNIK, Max M.; 510 W. Hastings St., Vancouver, B.C.; 1370 W. King Edward (res); Man '26.
RETFALVI, Andor A.; St. Basile, N.B.; Royal Hungarian Elizabeth U. (Pecs, Hung.) '39; F.C.C.P., F.A.G.S.; Ass't. Med. Supt., St. Joseph San.; Tel. 263-5561.
RETY, Nicholas A.; London (Eng.)'58; MB; BS; MRCS(Eng.); LRCP(Lond.); MSc(Surg.); Res., University Hosp., Edmonton, Alta.
RETZER, Oskar O.; Med. Arts Clinic, Bradbrooke Bldg., Swift Current, Sask.; Alb'56; FRCS(C), GenSurg; Att'd. Staff, Swift Current Union Hosp.; Tel. 773-4636.
REVELL, Daniel G.; 4441 Shore Way, Victoria, B.C. (res); Alb '32; Anaes; Sr. Anaes., St. Joseph's Hosp.; Tel. EV 4-1131.
REVELLE, Ian E.; 67 Pine St. S., Timmins, Ont.; 551 Elm S. (res); Qns '27; Tel. AM 4-7811.
REVICH, Stanley J.; 53 Forest Grove Dr., Willowdale, Ont.; Tor '56; Med. OPD, Sunnybrook Hosp.; Staff, (GP), North York Branson Hosp.; Tel. 221-4503.
REVIE, Maureen; Ste. 401, 428 Portage Ave., Winnipeg 1, Man.; Man '55.
REWA, Tetiana; 568 Dovercourt Rd., Toronto 4, Ont.; Austria '48; Tel. LE 4-6933.
REYES, Cesar N.; Santo Tomas (Philipp.)'55; ABPath; Path; Assoc. Path., St. Boniface Hosp., Winnipeg 6, Man.; Tel. WH 3-0311, Ext. 252.
REYNAR, John A.; Brooks, Alta.; Alb '51.
REYNOLDS, Edward N.; 490 Main St., Sussex, N.B.; Dal'52; AMCGP.
REYNOLDS, F. Barry; Sask'62; Res., University Hosp., Saskatoon, Sask.
REYNOLDS, Harold A.; 309-3rd Ave. N.E., Calgary, Alta.; Dublin (Ire.) '55; Path; Staff, Calgary Gen. Hosp.; Tel. AM 6-7541.
REYNOLDS, Margaret (See Beaumont).
REYNOLDS, Peter J.; 5861 Arbutus Ave., Powell River, B.C.; Leeds (Eng.)'48; DPH(Eng.).
REYNOLDS, W. John; 1209 Avenue Rd., Toronto 12, Ont.; Tor '58; FRCP(C), IntMed; Staff, Toronto Gen. Hosp.; Fell., Rheumatic Dis. Unit, U. of Toronto; Tel. EM 6-8211.
REZNOWSKI, L. W.; 346 Selkirk Ave., Winnipeg, Man.; Man '27; M.C.G.P.; Tel. JU 2-6804.
RHAMEY, Lorne E.; Ste. 505, 143 James St. S., Hamilton, Ont.; Wes '50; D.Psy; Psy; Active Staff (Psy.), Hamilton Gen. Hosp's.; Court. Staff (Psy.), St. Joseph's Hosp.; Tel. 529-1518.
RHEA, L. David; 260 Seaforth Med. Bldg., 3550 Cote des Neiges Rd., Montreal 25, P.Q.; McG '56; FRCS(C); ObstGyn; Staff, Montreal Gen. Hosp.; Tel. 932-8397.
RHEAULT, Florian; 1564 est Blvd. St.-Joseph, Montreal 34, P.Q.; 5215 Garnier, Mtl. 34 (res); Mon '53; MCGP; Tel. 527-1433.
RHEAULT, Gustav; 250 rue Principale, LaSarre, P.O.; 5-2ieme Ave. (res); Lav '30; M.C.G.P.
RHEAULT, Jean; 3615 Ave. Ridgewood, Apt. 402, Montreal, P.Q.; Lav '50; Anaes; Staff, Hop. Notre-Dame; Tel. 525-6363.

RHEAULT, Marcel J.; 3875 St-Urbain, Ste. 215, Montreal 18, P.Q.; Mon'58; MS; FRCS(C); GenSurg; McLaughlin Travelling Fell.; Surg., Hotel-Dieu Hosp.; Staff, U. of Montreal; Tel. 843-5681.
RHEAUME, Denis; Clinique Medicale, Forestville, P.Q.; Lav'65.
RHEAUME, Roland; Mon '64; Res., Hop. Maisonneuve, Montreal 36, P.Q.
RHEAUME, Serge; Lav'65; Res., Hop. Notre-Dame, Montreal 24, P.Q.
RHO, Yong M.; Soeul (Korea) '55 Staff, St. John's Gen. Hosp., St. John's Nfld.; Tel. 578-0471.
RHODES, Andrew J.; 79 Rochester Ave., Toronto 12, Ont. (res); Edinburgh (Scot.) '34; **FRCP (Ed.); FRSC; Bact; Prof. & Hd. Dept. of Microbiol. & Dir. Schl. of Hygiene, U. of Toronto; Cons. (Virol.), Hosp. for Sick Children; Tel.** 928-2748.
RHODES, John R.; 940 King St. W., Kitchener, Ont.; Wes '55; DiagRad; Staff, Kitchener-Waterloo Hosp.; Tel. SH 5-9451.
RHODES, Robert C.; 12051 Haney Plaza, Haney, B.C.; Tor '53; MCGP; Staff, Maple Ridge, Hosp.; Tel. 463-6636.
RHYS-JONES, Wyn; Trinity Coll. (Dublin, Ire.) '59; Res., School of Hygiene, U. of Toronto, Toronto 5, Ont.
RICARD, Alcidas; 427 St. Joseph Blvd. E., Montreal, P.Q.; Mon '22; Obst.; Tel. VI 4-2286.
RICARD, Gilles; App 302, 4101 est, Jarry, Montreal-Nord, P.Q.; Mon '61; Tel. 722-5714.
RICARD, Hector; 350 est Blvd. St.-Joseph, Montreal 14, P.Q.; 1455 Blvd. Morgan (res); Mon '33; Obst; Hd. Dept. of Obst., Hop.-de-la-Misericorde; Assoc. Prof., U. of Montreal; Tel. VI 2-6520.
RICARD, Jean; 2438 Jolicoeur St., Montreal, P.Q.; 475 Riverside Dr., St. Lambert (res); Mon '35; Obst. (P.Q.); Staff, Hop. Gen. de Verdun; Tel. 768-4913
RICARD, J. Marc; 17 Ave. des Sources, Strathmore, P.Q.; Mon '48.
RICARD, J. Paul; Ste. 919, 30 est Boul. St. Joseph, Montreal 14, P.Q.; Mon'29; FACCP; GenSurg & Thor Surg(P.Q.); Surg., Hop. Notre-Dame; Cons., Mtl. Chinese Hosp.; Assoc. Prof. Surg., U. of Montreal.
RICARD, Pierre; Mon'64; Res., Hop. Notre-Dame, Montreal 24, P.Q.
RICARD, Raymond; Ste. 502, 30 est Boul. St. Joseph, Montreal 14, P.Q.; Mon'54; PlasSurg; Cons., Hop. Notre Dame de L'Esperance, Ville St. Laurent, Hop. St. Eusebe, Joliette, & Clinique Medico-Esthetique.
RICCI, Elio E.; 666 Barton St. E., Hamilton, Ont.; 284 Mountain Brow (res); Tor '51; Staff, St. Joseph's Hosp.; Tel. LI 9-1580.
RICE, Alan D.; 123 W. Main St., Welland, Ont.; Tor'37; Staff, Welland Gen. Hosp.; Tel. 732-1234.
RICE, Arthur L.; 166 Elizabeth Grove, King City, Ont. (res); Tor '32; FCCP; Supt., Ont. Hosp., Aurora, Ont.; Tel. WA 1-4795.
RICE, Donald A.; Roy Clinic, 715—2nd Ave. S., Lethbridge, Alta.; 2515—5th Ave. S. (res); **Alb '45; Staff, Lethbridge Mun. & St. Michael's Hosp's.; Assoc. Dir., Lethbridge Cancer Clinic; Tel. FA 7-8591.**
RICE, Donald I.; Dal '51; MCGP; Exec. Dir., College of General Practice, 1260 Bay St., Toronto 5, Ont.; Tel. 923-7367.
RICE, Duncan M.; Site 6, Box 31, St. John's, Nfld. (res); London (Eng.) '55; MCGP; Ass't. Supt., St. John's San.; Tel. 9-0072.
RICE, Harold V.; 455 Burhill Rd., West Vancouver, B.C.; Tor '36; **Ph.D.; Dir. of Research, Clin. Physiol., St. Paul's Hosp.; Tel. 682-2344.**
RICE, J. H. Melville; 78 Roseberry St., Campbellton, N.B.; 37 Arran St. (res); McG '33; F.A.C.S.; GenSurg; M.C.G.P.; Staff, Soldiers' Memorial & Hotel Dieu Hosp's; Cons. Surg., Prov. Mental Hosp.; Coroner, Restigouche Co.; Tel. 753-2350.
RICE, Murray C.; Woodview Park Med. Centre, 3236 Weston Rd., Weston, Ont.; 10 Fullwell Cr., Downsview (res); Ott '59; MCGP; Assoc. Staff, Humber Mem. Hosp.; Court. Staff, Doctor's Hosp.; Tel. CH 1-9129.
RICE, William C.; 12 King St., Wolfville, N.S.; **McG '42; GenSurg.**
RICH, Charles B.; Ste. 103B, 1175 Cook St., Victoria, B.C.; Charing Cross H. (London, Eng.) '24; FACP; FRCP(C); IntMed.; Active Staff, Royal Jubilee Hosp.; Cons. Staff, St. Joseph's Hosp.; Tel. EV 4-5912.
RICH, E. John; 175 Collier St., Toronto 5, Ont.; London (Eng.) '46; DPM; Ph.D; Cons. Psy., Big Sisters Counselling Serv., St. John's Training School & Powell-Brown Nursery School; Assoc. Dept. of Psy, U. of Toronto; Vis. Lect., Queen's U., Kingston; Tel. 921-6863.
RICH, J. Harry; 128 Cameron St., Moncton, N.B.; 79 Allison Dr. (res); **Dal '56; GenSurg, Active Staff, Moncton & Hotel Dieu Hosp.; Tel. 382-**5274.
RICH, Park J.; 49-13th St. W., Prince Albert, Sask.; Man '44; GenSurg; AMCGP; Tel. 764-4241.
RICH, W. T.; 45 Cambridge St. N., Lindsay, Ont.; Tor '06; Retired.
RICHARD, Arthur; 112 rue St.-Thomas, Montmagny, P.Q.; Lav'49; Staff, Hotel-Dieu.
RICHARD, Arthur L.; 117 Stewart St., Ottawa, Ont.; 211 River Rd., Kingsview Park, Eastview **(res); Lav '28; GenSurg, Gyn; Staff, Ottawa Gen. Hosp.; Prof. & Hd., ObstGyn, Fac. of Med., U. of Ottawa; Tel. CE 5-6751.**
RICHARD, Ferdinand; 4377 Blvd. Rosemont, Apt. 19, Montreal, P.Q.; Haiti '58; FRCS(C), GenSurg; Staff, Hop. Notre-Dame; Tel. LA 5-6363.
RICHARD, Harol L.; Allin Clinic, 10155-120th St., Edmonton, Alta.; Alb '37; FACS; FRCS(C); GenSurg; Court. Staff, University Hosp.; Surg., Att'd. Staff, Royal Alexandra Hosp.; Ass't. Clin. Prof. (Surg. & Surg. Anat.), U. of Alberta; Tel. HU 8-7271.
RICHARD, J. B. Liguori; 1213 Ave. St. Viateur, Outremont, Montreal 8, P.Q.; Lav '45; D.P.H.
RICHARD, Jean P.; 855 rue St.-Louis-Ville-St.-Joseph, St.-Hyacinthe, P.Q.; Mon '58; Tel. PR 3-1120.
RICHARD, Jean P.; Lav '63; Res., Hop. St-Sacrement, Quebec, P.Q.
RICHARD, J. Edouard; 75 St-Louis, Quebec 4, P.Q.; Lav'59; Otol; Tel. 523-5605.
RICHARD, Joseph P.; Petit Rocher North, N.B. (res); Lav '07; Retired.
RICHARD, Leon; 166 Victoria St., Moncton, N.B.; Lav'51; Ophth.; Tel. 382-5524.
RICHARD, Maurice; 1215 des Pins, Quebec 6, P.Q.; Lav '46; Paed; Chief of Paed. Serv., Hotel-Dieu Hosp.; Tel. 683-7011.
RICHARD, Maurice; 165 est, rue King, Sherbrooke, P.Q.; Mon'45; Tel. 562-2755.
RICHARD, R.; 1477 Parc Lafontaine, Montreal, P.Q.; Mon '23; Psy; Retired.
RICHARD, R. Vital; 366 St. Vallier W., Quebec, P.Q.; 397 Ch. St. Foy (res); Lav '45; Tel. 525-5502.
RICHARDS, A. Gerald; Ste. 105, 605 Princess St., New Westminster, B.C.; Alb '50; F.R.C.P.(C), IntMed; Att. Staff, Royal Columbian & Shaughnessy Hosp's.; Tel. LA 4-3133.
RICHARDS, A. Guyon; 1328 Elliott St., Saskatoon, Sask.; Cambridge (Eng.) '42; Active Staff (Med.), Saskatoon City Hosp.; Tel. 653-0922.
RICHARDS, Alan J.; 1190 Danforth Ave., Toronto 6, Ont.; 250 Lawrence Ave. E. (res); Tor '43; D.Rad; D. & T Rad; Ass't Rad., Toronto East Gen. Hosp.; Tel. 461-0945.
RICHARDS, Burke A.; Box 366, Ste. 308, 672 Brant St., Burlington, Ont.; Wes'53; FRCP(C), IntMed; Staff, Joseph Brant & Hamilton Gen. & St. Joseph's Hosp's.; Tel. 637-5713.
RICHARDS, C. Alvin; Box 187, 102 Bidwell St., Tillsonburg, Ont.; Tor '24; MCGP; Chief, Med. Staff, Tillsonburg Dist. Mem. Hosp.; Tel. VI 2-2451.
RICHARDS, D. A. Rankin; 401 Pitt St. W., Whitby, Ont.; Qns '23; FRCS(Ed.); FRCS(C); GenSurg; Staff Surg., Ontario Hosp.; Tel. 668-5881.
RICHARDS, Elizabeth M. (Mitchell); 1328 Elliott St., Saskatoon, Sask.; London (Eng.) '39; Active Staff (ObstGyn), University Hosp.; Tel. 653-0922.

RICHARDS, Frank; 350-14th St. W., Owen Sound, Ont.; Liverpool (Eng.)'56.

RICHARDS, Frances M. (Forrest); Alb '51; Psy; Staff, Riverview Hosp., Essondale, B.C.

RICHARDS, Jo-Anne; 375 Strathallan Ave., & Burlington, Ont. (res); Wes '53; Part-time Dept. of Health, Hamilton.

RICHARDS, John M.; Turtleford Clinic, Turtleford, Sask.; Cardiff (Wales)'48; AMCGP; Tel. 58.

RICHARDS, John S. F.; 301-1125 Jarvis St., Vancouver, B.C.; UBC'60; Ophth.

RICHARDS, Michael T.; 14213 Stony Plain Rd., Edmonton, Alta.; 10108—144 St. (res); London (Eng.) '53; Tel. HU 8-5019.

RICHARDS, Robert N.; 324 Vesta Dr., Toronto 10, Ont.; Tor '62; P.G., Toronto East Gen. Hosp.

RICHARDS, Robert T.; Wes'62; Res., Henderson Gen. Hosp., Hamilton, Ont.

RICHARDS, Terence A.; 220 Med. Arts Bldg., 1 Young St., Hamilton, Ont.; 375 Strathallan, Burlington (res); Wes '53; M.Sc.; FACS; FRCS(C), GenSurg; Active Cons. Staff, Hamilton Gen. & Joseph Brant Mem. Hosp's., Burlington; Tel. JA 7-7810.

RICHARDS, Terence J.; Bigelow Fowler Clinic, 1605-9th Ave. S., Lethbridge, Alta.; Durham (Eng.)'59; DObstRCOG; MCGP; Active Staff, St. Michael's & Lethbridge Mun. Hosp's.

RICHARDS, William H.; 391 Lakeshore Dr., Cobourg, Ont. (res); Dal '54; DiagRad; Rad., Cobourg & Port Hope Gen. Hosp's.; Cons. Rad., Ontario Hosp., Cobourg; Tel. FR 2-5451.

RICHARDS, William L.; 207 Lakeshore Rd. E., Port Credit, Ont.; 1581 Birchwood Dr., Clarkson (res); Temple U. (Philadelphia) '51; F.R.C.P.(C), IntMed; Active Cons., South Peel Hosp., Cooksville; Tel. CR 8-0051.

RICHARDSON, Andrew L.; Petitcodiac, N.B.; Dal '26; Cons. Staff, & Member Hosp. Board, Moncton City Hosp.; Tel. EV 4-4421.

RICHARDSON, Anne B.; Dal '52; Anaes; Staff, (Anaes), Royal Victoria Hosp., Pine Ave., Montreal P.Q.; Tel. VI 2-1251.

RICHARDSON, Charles D.; 145 Wellington St. Sarnia, Ont.; 1256 Glen Douglas (res); Wes '50; Active Staff, Sarnia Gen. Hosp.; Vice Pres. Med. Staff, St. Joseph's Hosp.; Tel. DI 4-1191.

RICHARDSON, Clifton A.; Qns '43; DiagRad; Staff, St. Joseph's Hosp., Toronto 3, Ont.; Tel. 534-9531.

RICHARDSON, C. Douglas; 145 Wellington St., Sarnia, Ont.; Wes '50; Act. Staff (G.P. & Anaes.), St. Joseph's & Sarnia Gen. Hosp's.; Tel. 344-1191.

RICHARDSON, Donald A.; 40 Coldwater St. E., Orillia, Ont.; Tor'59; Staff, Soldier's Mem. Hosp.; Tel. 326-3541.

RICHARDSON, Derek S.; Elrose, Sask.; St. Mary's H. (London, Eng.) '49; Tel. 378-2223.

RICHARDSON, D. Shirley; 3515-17th Ave. S.W., Calgary, Alta.; Wes'55.

RICHARDSON, Ernest A.; 544 Windermere Ave., Toronto, Ont. (res); Tor '11; Retired.

RICHARDSON, Harold F.; 11 Kingsbury Cres., Scarborough, Ont. (res); Tor'34; GenSurg; Chief Med. Dept., WCB, Toronto; Tel. 362-3411.

RICHARDSON, Horace J.; 696 Golden Ave., Ottawa, Ont. (res); Tor '33; Med. Adviser, Cndn. Pensions Comm.; Tel. 992-3056.

RICHARDSON, J. F.; 14 Queen N., Tilbury, Ont.; 4 Canal W. (res); Wes '35.

RICHARDSON, James W.; 220 Medical Arts Bldg., 335-339 6th Ave. S.W., Calgary, Alta.; 815 Prospect Ave. (res); McG'10; MRCS(Eng.), LRCP(Lond.), FACS, FRCS(Edin.), FRCS(C) GenSurg; Att. Surg., Holy Cross & Calgary Gen. Hosp's.; Tel. AM 9-2673.

RICHARDSON, J. Clifford; M.B.E.; 170 St. George St., Ste. 305, Toronto 5, Ont.; Tor '32; FRCP (Eng.); FRCP(C); Neur; Sr. Phys. (Neur.), Toronto Gen. Hosp.; Cons. (Neur.), Sunnybrook D.V.A. Hosp. & W.C.B.; Assoc. Prof. I/C Neur., U. of Toronto; Tel. WA 2-4520.

RICHARDSON, John; 149 Ochterloney St., Dartmouth, N.S.; London (Eng.)'64; Temporar Court. Staff, Halifax Infirmary; Tel. 466-1591.

RICHARDSON, Kenneth R.; 239 Ridout St. S., London, Ont.; Wes '31; Anaes; Sr. Assoc. Anaes., Victoria Hosp., & U. of Western Ontario; Tel. GE 2-5261.

RICHARDSON, Noel L.; Ste. 3, 133 E. 14th St., North Vancouver, B.C.; 1111 Crestline, W. Vanc. (res); McG '43; Psy; Lect. (Psy.), U. of British Columbia; Tel. 987-4845.

RICHARDSON, Oscar B.; 1314 Clonsilla Ave., Peterborough, Ont.; Tor '42; D.A.B. Ophth; Ophth., Staff, Civic & St. Joseph's Hosp's; Tel. RI 2-8342.

RICHARDSON, Peter; Box 210, 135 6th Ave., Cochrane, Ont.; Durham (Eng.)'54; DABS; FRCS(C); GenSurg; Staff, Lady Minto Hosp.; Tel. 272-3276.

RICHARDSON, Peter M.; Tor '62; Res., Toronto General Hosp., Toronto 2B, Ont.

RICHARDSON, R. Norman C.; 5162 Dundas St. W., Islington, Ont.; Tor '21.

RICHARDSON, Robert L.; 1179 Decarie Blvd., Ville-St.-Laurent, Mtl., P.Q.; Tor '51; Cons. Phys., Internat.; Tel. & Telegraph (Canada) Ltd; Tel. 389-8221.

RICHARDSON, Roy B.; 64 Wellesley St. E., Toronto 5, Ont.; Qns '13; NeurPsy.; Tel. WA 2-0662.

RICHARDSON, Roy W., OBE; 432 Med. Arts Bldg., Winnipeg, Man.; 191 Brock St. (res); Man '26; GenSurg; Ass't. Prof. (Surg.), U. of Manitoba; Tel. WH 2-6389.

RICHARDSON, Seton-Leslie; 1414 Drummond St., Montreal 25, P.Q.; 34 Finchley Rd., Hampstead (res); McG '32; IntMed. (Cardiol.) (P.Q.); Staff, Montreal Gen. Hosp.; Tel. 288-9555.

RICHARDSON, Stanley J.; 510 Wellington St., Wallaceburg, Ont.; Wes'53; Tel. 627-3306.

RICHARDSON, Stephen R.; 3515-17th Ave. S.W., Calgary, Alta.; Wes'56.

RICHARDSON, Thomas A.; 220 Medical Arts Bldg., Calgary, Alta.; 1318 Crestview Rd. (res); McG '43; M.S. (Orth), D.A.B.O.S., F.A.C.S., FRCS(C), OrthSurg.; Tel. AM 9-3311.

RICHARDSON, William F.; 14 George St. N., Galt, Ont.; Wes '50; Staff, South Waterloo Mem. Hosp.; Dist. Coroner; Tel. 621-3131.

RICHER, Bernard; Mon '64; Res., Hop. Maisonneuve, Montreal, P.Q.

RICHER, Claude L.; 3770 Cote Ste-Catherine, App. 14, Montreal 26, P.Q.; Mon'54; M.Sc. (Exper. Med.); Ass't. Prof., Dept. of Anat., U. of Montreal; Tel. RE 3-9951.

RICHER, Clement; 5920A Viau, Montreal 36, P.Q.; 6575 LeMay (res); Mon '59; AMCGP; Tel. CL 9-2001.

RICHER, Gilles; C.P. 910; 933 St. Louis, Terrebonne, P.Q.; Mon'59.

RICHER, P. Arthur; 7052 St.-Denis St., Montreal, P.Q.; 797 Hartland (res); Mon '36; M.C.G.P.; Tel. CR 7-5175.

RICHER, P. Fernando; 5870 Park Ave., Montreal 8, P.Q.; Mon '25

RICHER, Simon; 3100 Ellendale Ave., Montreal 26, P.Q. (res); Mon '57; Psy; Staff, Montreal Children's Hosp. & Ass't. Dir. Mental Assessment Clinic; Cons. Richmond Schl., Soc. for Mentally Disturbed Adolescents.

RICHER, Yves; Mon'65; Res., Hop Notre-Dame, Montreal 24, P.Q.

RICHES, John V.; The Port Arthur Clinic, 194 North Court St., Port Arthur, Ont.; McG '32; FACS; GenSurg; Chmn., Cons. Staff, Thunder Bay Clinic & Ont. Cancer Treatment & Research Fdn.; Memb. of Council, Coll. of Phys. & Surg. of Ontario; Tel. DI 4-7271.

RICHMAN, Alex; Faculty of Med., 10th & Heather Sts., Vancouver 9, B.C.; Man '53; M.P.H. (Johns Hopkins); Psy; Assoc. Prof (Psy), U. of British Columbia & Hd. Sect. of Social Psy.; Tel. TR 6-3211, Loc. 2599; Abroad.

RICHMAN, Norman A.; 2 South Dr., St. Catharines, Ont.; Wes'35; GenSurg; Memb. S.A.A.S.; Chief of Surg., Hotel-Dieu Hosp.; Tel. MU 4-7271.

RICHMOND, Clifford R.; 315 Main St., Picton, Ont.; Paul St. (res); Qns '37; Dist. Coroner; Tel. GR 6-6225.

RICHMOND, Hugh A.; Ste 208, 300 King St. W., Oshawa, Ont.; 120 Connaught St. (res); Tor '53; FRCS(C); Urol; GenSurg; Staff, Oshawa Gen. & Ajax-Pickering Hosp's.; Cons., Ontario Hosp., Whitby; Tel. 728-4861.
RICHMOND, Richard G.; 1773 Eastern Dr., Port Coquitlam, B.C. (res); U.K. '28; M.R.C.S. (Eng.), L.R.C.P. (Lond.); Phys., Oakalla Prison Farm, S. Burnaby.
RICHMOND, William; Goldboro, N.S.; Glasgow (Scot.)'35; Tel. 11; Abroad.
RICHTER, Maxwell; McG'64; Staff, Royal Victoria Hosp., Montreal 2, P.Q.
RICHTER, Helmut; McG'47; Anaes; DABA; Staff, Lachine Gen. Hosp., Lachine, P.Q.; Tel. 637-1161.
RICHTER, Katherine E.; 11 Grace Ave., Brantford, Ont.; Berlin (Germ.)'47; I/C Chest Clinic, Brant Sanatorium; Tel. PL 3-2658.
RICHTER, Robert R.; Med. Arts Bldg., 1 Young St., Hamilton, Ont.; 15 Ravenscliffe (res); Tor '47; FRCS(C); OrthSurg; Staff, St. Joseph's Hosp's; Tel. JA 8-8355.
RICKARD, John H.; 304 Danforth Ave., Toronto 6, Ont.; Tor'36; IntMed; Vis. Phys., St. Michael's & Tor. E. Gen. Hosp's.; Tel. HO 6-4545.
RICKETTS, Thomas G.; 184 Lincoln Road, Grand Falls, Nfld.; Dal '58; Tel. 4243.
RIDDELL, Alan D.; 221 Brant Ave., Brantford, Ont.; 26 Kingsway Cres. (res); Wes '33; Tel. 752-8213.
RIDDELL, Andrew R.; 38 Kingsley Cr., Waterloo, Ont.; Tor '45; Anaes; Staff, Dept of Anaes., Kitchener-Waterloo Hosp.; Staff, Dept of Surg., Anaes, Serv., St. Mary's Hosp.; Courtesy Staff, South Waterloo Memorial Hosp.; Tel. SH 5-9451.
RIDDELL, Denis M.; 790 Sherbrook St., Winnipeg, Man.; London (Eng.) '50; FRCS(C), OrthSurg.; Tel. 774-6541.
RIDDELL, John R.; Box 249, Palmerston, Ont.; Tor '23; GenSurg; Sr. Surg., Palmerston Gen. Hosp.; Coroner, Perth & Wellington Counties. Abroad.
RIDDELL, Margaret A. (see MOWAT, Margaret A.)
RIDDLE, William J.; 10155—120th St., Edmonton, Alta.; 10832-77 Ave. (res); Alb '51; M.C.G.P.; Staff, Royal Alexandra Hosp.; Tel. 488-7271.
RIDDOLLS, Wilfrid E.; 19 Broadway E., Paris, Ont.; Wes '33; Tel. 442-4151.
RIDEOUT, Chester F.; 3967 Kingsway, S. Burnaby, B.C.; McG'52; Tel. HE 4-8781.
RIDEOUT, David A.; 508 Main St., Sussex, N.B.; Stewart Ave. (res); Dal'63; AMCGP; Tel. 28W.
RIDEOUT, Vernon K.; 10 Starrs Rd., Yarmouth, N.S.; Dal'53; DPH.
RIDER, Robert C.; 1574 Ouellette Ave., Windsor, Ont.; 1989 Ontario St. (res); Wes '35; F.A.C.S., F.R.C.S.(Edin.), F.R.C.S.(C), OrthSurg.; GenSurg; Chief of Orth Surg., Hotel-Dieu Hosp.; Tel. CL 6-4594.
RIDER, Walter D.; Ont. Cancer Inst., 500 Sherbourne St., Toronto, Ont.; Edinburgh (Scot.)'45; M.B., Ch.B., FFR, DMRT; TherRad; Sr. Radiotherap., Princess Margaret Hosp.; Ass't. Prof. (Rad.), & Assoc. Med. Bio-Phys., U. of Toronto; Tel. 924-0671.
RIDGE, John M.; Man'41; Path; Staff, Dept. of Path., Rockyview Gen. Hosp., Calgary, Alta.
RIDGE, John W.; Box 209, Mount Hope, Ont.; Tor '49; M.C.G.P.; Staff, O.P.D., Hamilton Gen. Hosp.; Tel. 527-0271.
RIDGE, Priscilla (See Barnes)
RIDGE, Robert W.; Box 189, Mount Hope, Ont.; Tor '56.
RIDGE, William W.; Mount Hope, Ont.; Tor '24; Coroner, Co. of Wentworth; M.O.H., Tsp. of Seneca; Tel. 679-4241.
RIDGWAY, Clayton R.; 430 Tegler Bldg., 10189 101st St., Edmonton, Alta.; Man'55; Ophth.
RIDLEY, Charles M.; 711 Brown's Line, Toronto 14, Ont.; Tor '51; Tel. CL 1-1331.
RIDSDEL, Wm. B.; Clinic Blk., 3rd Ave., Yorkton, Sask. London (Eng.) '35.
RIEDEL, Otto; Warsaw (Poland) '23; Res., Phys. (Med), Nova Scotia Hosp., Dartmouth N.S.
RIEDL, Frank W.; Wes'65; Res., University Hosp., Edmonton, Alta.
RIEDWEG, Edward A.; Alb'65; Jr. Int., Holy Cross Hospital, Calgary, Alta.
RIESBERRY, Annjane; (See Carter, Annjane).
RIESE, Karl T.; 605 Med. Arts Bldg., 404 Graham Ave., Winnipeg 1, Man.; 894 Borebank St. (res); Man '54; DABS; FACS; FRCS(C), GenSurg; Att'd. Surg., St-Boniface & Deer Lodge Hosp's.; Dem. & Pt-time Tutor, (Surg.), U. of Manitoba; Tel. 943-8845.
RIFAAT, Mostapha R.; Freelton, Ont.; Edinburgh (Scot.)'41.
RIGBY, Frederick N.; 2255 Elgin Ave., Port Coquitlam, B.C.; Guy's H. (London, Eng.) '55; MRCS, LRCP; Staff, Royal Columbian Hosp.; Tel. WH 2-7292.
RIGBY, John E.; Carleton St., St. Andrews, N.B.; Dal '49.
RIGG, Charles B.; Box 51, 287 Davy St., Niagara-on-the-Lake, Ont.; Tor '40; MAA (Allerg.); MCGP; Tel. HO 8-3251.
RIGG, Frederick D.; 443 Broad St. W., Dunnville, Ont.; Tor '39; Tel. 774-5934.
RIGG, F. J.; 287 Davy St., Niagara-on-the-Lake, Ont.; 80 Front St. (res); Tor '43; M.C.G.P.; Tel. HO 8-3251.
RIGG, J. Michael; Hycroft Med. Bldg., 3195 Granville St., Vancouver 9, B.C.; 3350 W. 43rd Ave. (res); Cambridge (Eng.) '52; MA, MB; B.Ch.; DCH (Lond.); FAAP; Paed; Att'd. Staff, Van. Gen. & Van. Children's Hosp's.; Tel. RE 8-2102.
RIGGS-WOOD, A. Eleanor C.; 4 Dunloe Rd., Toronto 7, Ont. (res); Tor '35; D.P.H.; not practising.
RIIVES, Johannes; 554 Lewin Park, Lancaster, N.B. (res); Tartu/Dorpat (Estonia) '27; Neur: Sr. Med. Off., Provincial Hosp., Lancaster; Tel. 694-2331.
RILEY, C.; P.O. Box 608, Sydney, N.S.; Edwardsville St., (res); Edinburgh (Scot.) '43.
RILEY, G. Terence; Box 1720, Campbell River, B.C.; Tor '60; AMCGP; Tel. 287-7166.
RILEY, John M.; 217 Laurier Ave. E., Ottawa 2, Ont.; 63 Birch Ave. (res); Ott '51; Clin. Ass't. Ottawa Gen. Hosp. & U. of Ottawa; Med. Dir., Island Lodge & Geriatric Centre; Tel. 234-5711.
RIML, Otto G.; Graz (Austria) '30; Staff, King George Hosp., Winnipeg, Man.; Sr. Phys., Winnipeg Municipal Hosp.; Tel. GL 2-3411.
RIMMER, Hugh; Box 830, Squamish, B.C.; London (Eng.)'53; Tel. 892-3313.
RINFRET, Charles; 885 E., rue St. Joseph, Quebec, P.Q.; 2064 rue Brulart (res); Lav '26; Tel. 524-0461.
RINFRET, Gilbert G. F.; 1063, St. Denis, Montreal 18, P.Q.; Mon '43; FRCS(C); NeurSurg; Chief of Serv., Verdun Gen. Hosp.; Cons., Hop. St-Luc & Gen. Hop. de St-Lambert; Tel. 842-4816.
RINFRET, Leonard; 2320 Ontario St. E., Montreal, P.Q.; Lav '08.
RINFRET, Lucien; 1045 ave Begin, Quebec 6, P.Q.; Lav '39; Anaes; Staff, Hop.-St.-Sacrement & Laval U.; Tel. LA 7-3461.
RINFRET, Paul C. E.; Med. Serv. Clinic, Dept. of National Health & Welfare, Foot Burrard St., Vancouver 3, B.C.; Ott'51; Tel. 682-1377.
RING, Edward D.; 2125 - 11th Ave., Regina, Sask.; 3312 - 15th Ave. (res); Man '46; IntMed; Staff, Regina Gen. & Grey Nun's Hosp's.: Cons., D.V.A. & Cons. Arthritis, Yorkton Gen. Hosp.; Tel. 523-0691.
RINGHAM, Malcolm C.; Stony Plain Med. Centre, Stony Plain, Alta.; Sheffield (Eng.) '60; M.B., Ch.B., MCGP; Tel. 777-2226.
RINGROSE, C. Douglas; 836 Professional Bldg., 10830 Jasper Ave., Edmonton Alta.; Alb. '54 F.R.C.S.(C) ObstGyn; Assoc Staff, Royal Alexandra & Misericordia Hosp's Court. Staff, Edmonton Gen. Hosp.; Tel. 422-3802.
RINGUET-GAGNON, Madeline; 2421, boul du Carmel, Trois-Rivieres, P.Q.; Mon '57; Staff, Hop. Ste. Marie; Tel. FR 5-7721.
RINGUET, J. Jacques; 68 Ave de la Cathedrale, Rimouski, P.Q.; Lav '38; F.R.C.S.(C) GenSurg; Chief, Dept. of Surg. Hop. St. Joseph; Tel. 723-2459.

RINGWOOD, John B.; Williams Lake, B.C. Alb '39 GenSurg; Tel. 392-4451.
RINNE, Herman H. F.; 184 Cedar St., Sudbury, Ont.; 466 Yale St. (res); Hamburg (Germ.) '41; Derm; Tel. 674-1243.
RIOPELLE, Joseph L.; 3130 Fendall St., Montreal, P.Q.; Mon '31; F.R.C.P.(C), Path Bact; Path., Hotel-Dieu Hosp.; Prof. (Path) Fac. of Med., U. of Montreal; Tel. VI 4-0161.
RIOPELLE, Philippe; 271 ouest St.-Laurent, Longueuil, Cite-Jacques-Cartier, P.Q.; Mon '43.
RIOUX, Andre; 5531 Verdun Ave., Montreal 19, P.Q.; Lav '55; Anaes.; Tel. 768-4702.
RIOUX, Armand; 1175, Ave. des Erables, Quebec 6, P.Q.; Lav '28; ObstGyn; MCGP; Gov., Coll. of Phys. and Surg. of Quebec; Tel. 523-1154.
RIOUX, Ernest; Lav'60; Haem(P.Q.); IntMed (P.Q.); Staff, Hop. L'Enfant-Jesus, Quebec 3, P.Q.
RIOUX, Henri; Cacouna, Cte. Riviere Loup, P.Q.; Lav '65.
RIOUX, Jacques; Lav'60; ObstGyn(P.Q.); Staff, Hop.-de-l'Enfant-Jesus, Quebec 3, P.Q.; Abroad.
RIOUX, Euclide; Clair, N.B.; Lav '50.
RIOUX, Lionel; Riviere-au-Renard, Co. Gaspe, P.Q.; Lav'46; Prof., St. Martin Clin.; Tel. 145.
RIOUX, Marcel; Mon'59; Res., Hop. Notre-Dame, Montreal 24, P.Q.
RIOUX, Marcel; Oromocto, N.B.; Lav '62.
RIOUX, Monique; 496 D'Aguillon, Quebec 4, P.Q.; Lav'63.
RIOUX, Paul L.; Main St., Sutton, P.Q.; Lav '49; Coroner, Brome; Chm., Records Committee; Tel. 538-2401.
RIOUX, Pierre; App. 2, 146 rue Roy, Ville Lemoyne, P.Q.; Lav'60; Anaes(P.Q.).
RIPLEY, Howard R.; 14 Arlington Dr., Moncton, N.B. (res); Dal 40 F.A.C.R., D & T Rad; Dir., Dept. of Rad., Moncton Hosp., Moncton, N.B.; Cons. (Rad.), CNR (Atlantic Div.); Tel. EV 4-4421.
RIPSTEIN-SOICHER, Riva B. (Ripstein); 445 Greenwood Dr., Beaconsfield, P.Q.; McG'44; Med. Dir., Employees Health Serv., Lakeshore Gen. Hosp., Pointe Claire; M.O., West Island School Commiss., Pte. Claire.
RISDON, Ernest Fulton; 60 Chestnut Park, Toronto 5, Ont. (res); Tor '14; DDS; FRCS(C), PlasSurg; Cons. (PlasSurg), Toronto Western Hosp.; Tel. WA 2-3750.
RISHIKOF, Jack R.; 520 Seaforth Med. Bldg., 3550 Cote des Neiges Rd., Montreal 25, P.Q.; Qns'58; Teach. Fell., Mtl. Gen. Hosp. & McGill U.; Staff Phys., Bell Tel. of Canada; Tel. 932-2197.
RITCEY, Edgar L.; 312 Med. Arts Bldg., 170 St. George St., Toronto 5, Ont.; Tor'60; FRCP(C), IntMed.; Tel. 923-9457.
RITCH, Elsie (Morison); 6325 Fraser St., Vancouver 15, B.C.; 3779 Blenheim St., Van. 8 (res); St. Andrews U. (Scotland) '46; FACS; FACA; Anaes; Att'd. Staff, Grace & St. Paul's Hosp's.; Tel. FA 5-4040.
RITCHIE, Alexander C.; 100 College St., Toronto 2, Ont.; New Zealand '44; M.B., Ch.B.; D.Phil. (Oxon.); M.C. (Path.); FCAP; FRCP(C), Path; Hd., Div. of Path. Dept. of Lab's., Toronto Gen. Hosp.; Cons., Dept. of Clin. Path., Wellesley Hosp.; Cons. (Path.), Hosp. for Sick Children & Ont. Dept. of Health; Cons., Cdn. Tumour Registry on Tumours of Soft Tissues; Cons. (Path.), Women's College Hosp. & Ont. Cancer Inst.; Prof. & Hd.; Dept. of Path., U. of Toronto; Tel. 928-2557.
RITCHIE, Douglas C.; 10011-103rd St., Edmonton, Alta.; 11843 Saskatchewan Dr. (res); Alb '41; F.A.C.S., D.A.B.O.G., ObstGyn; Staff, University Hosp.; Ass't. Clin. Prof., U. of Alberta; Tel. 422-7221.
RITCHIE, Gordon W.; 108 Med. Arts Bldg., 404-406 Graham Ave., Winnipeg 1, Man.; Man'48; DMRD; DiagRad; Dir., Dept. of Rad., St. Boniface Gen. Hosp.; Rad., Shriner's Hosp.; Cons. Rad., Deer Lodge Hosp.; Tel. 943-7301.
RITCHIE, J. Graham; 1664 W. Broadway, Vancouver 9, B.C.; Cambridge (Eng.) '51; Anaes.
RITCHIE, John A.; 122 Main St., Newmarket, Ont.; 120 Arden Ave. (res); Dal '42; GenSurg; Tel. 895-2661.
RITCHIE, Kenneth C.; 107 Medical Arts Bldg., 73 N. Cumberland St., Port Arthur Ont.; 31 Marlboro Rd. (res); Wes '50; M.O.H., Dorion Twp. Sec., St. Joseph's Hosp., Med. Staff; Tel. 344-3021.
RITCHIE, Kenneth S.; Room 5028, Veteran's Affair's Bldg., Ottawa, Ont.; 3860 Revelstoke Dr. (res); McG'36; Dir., General Treatment Serv., Dept. of Vet's Affairs; Tel. 992-5679.
RITCHIE, Railton G.; Dal'47; Staff, Nova Scotia Hosp., Dartmouth, N.S.
RITCHIE, Robert C.; The Old Manse, R.R. 2, King City, Ont. (res); Tor '45; Path; Path. & Dir. of Labs., North York Branson Hosp.; Regional Path., Attorney-General's Dept., Ontario; Supervisor, Committee on Exper. Research & Research Assoc. (Part-time), Dept. of Path., U. of Toronto; Tel. 762-3641.
RITCHIE, Robert E. C.; Main St., Brock, Sask.; Box No. 93 (res); Man '46; M.C.G.P.; Dist. Coroner; Tel. 43.
RITCHIE, Robert S.; 927 Liverpool Rd., Bay Ridges, Ont.; Aberdeen (Scot.)'48; DA(Eng.).
RITCHIE, Ronald M.; 1584 Robie St., Halifax, N.S.; 2251 Armcrest E. (res); Dal '43; FAAP; Paed; Assoc. Phys., Children's Hosp. & O.P.D., Nova Scotia Tumour Clinic; Assoc. Prof. (Paed.), Dalhousie U.; Tel. 423-6831.
RITCHIE, William G.; 31-3rd Ave. N.E., Dauphin, Man.; 37 River Ave. (res); Mon '45; Tel. 638-3723.
RITZ, Irwin; 99 Avenue Rd., Toronto 5, Ont.; Tor'46; Urol; Jr. Att. Urol., New Mount Sinai Hosp.; Tel. WA 2-9877.
RITZEN, Alex A.; Alb '57; Staff, Provincial Training School, Red Deer, Alta.
RIVARD, Fernand; Lav '61; Res., Hop. Notre-Dame, Montreal 24, P.Q.
RIVARD, Gerard; 3482 est, rue Ste. Catherine, Montreal 4, P.Q.; 1477 Nicolet (res); Mon'41; Tel. 523-1665.
RIVARD, Guy; 262 Cooper Place, New Haven, Conn., U.S.A.; Paed(P.Q.); Abroad.
RIVARD, Jules; 75 Racine, Loretteville, P.Q.; Lav '58; Tel. 842-2998.
RIVARD, Paul-L.; 6 Dollard, La Tuque, P.Q.; Mon'28; GenSurg; Phys. & Surg., Hop.-St.-Joseph; M.O., Cdn. Internat. Paper Co.; Tel. 523-5222.
RIVARD, Roland; Lav'62; OrthSurg(P.Q.); Staff, Hop. de l'Enfant Jesus, Quebec, P.Q.
RIVEN, David J.; 296 St. Joseph Blvd., Montreal 8, Westmount, P.Q.; 598 Kindersley Ave., Twn. of Mt. Royal (res); McG '41; M.C.G.P.; Clin. Ass't. Jewish Gen. Hosp.; Ass't. Med. Dir., Montreal Fashion Industries Health Centre & M.O., Fina & B.P. Oil Refineries; Tel. 279-0576.
RIVERIN, Leopold; C.P. 99, Unite Sanitaire, Sept-Iles, P.Q.; Lav '60.
RIVERS, E. Paul, F/L; C.J.A.T.C., Rivers, Man.; Tor '62.
RIVERS, Ian; 321 E. Columbia St., New Westminster, B.C.; UBC'64.
RIVERS, Norman; UBC'65; Res., Shaughnessy Hosp., Vancouver 9, B.C.
RIVERS, William A.; 6668 Fraser St., Vancouver 15, B.C.; 6161 Wiltshire St., Van 13. (res); McG '55; AMCGP; Att'd. Staff, St. Vincent's Hosp.; Tel. FA 7-4252.
RIVEST, Pierre; Mon'65; Res., Dept. of Physiologie, Universite de Montreal, Montreal, P.Q.
RIVEST, Raymond; 8415 St. Denis, Montreal 11, P.Q.; Mon'61.
RIVEST, Simon P.; 960 Boulv. Ste-Croix, Montreal 9, P.Q.; 345 Ave. Barton, Ville Mont-Royal (res); Mon '53; D&TRad; Radiol., Hop. Notre-Dame-de-l'Esperance; Tel. RI 7-3501.
RIVEST, Yvon; 10949 St.-Vital, Montreal North 39, P.Q.; Mon '57; Tel. DA 1-5910.
RIVET, Marc G.; 225 McIntyre W., North Bay, Ont.; 130 Worthington E. (res); McG '51; MCGP; Tel. 472-8445.
RIVET, Roland; 3905 Est, Ste-Catherine, Montreal 4, P.Q.; Mon '41; Tel. LA 3-4264.
RIVIERE, Leon; Lav '54; Path; Staff, Hop. St-Joseph, Rimouski, P.Q.; Tel. 723-7851.

RIX, Don B.; Wes'57; MCGP; Res. (Path.), Vancouver Gen. Hosp., Vancouver, B.C.
RIX, Edwin J.; 284 Lakeshore Rd. E., Port Credit, Ont.; Birmingham (Eng.)'52; MCGP; Court. Staff, South Peel Hosp.
RIZZA, Marta; Staff, Hop. des Laurentides, L'Annonciation, P.Q.
RIZZO, Nicholas A.; Qns'58; Res., Clarke Inst. of Psy., 250 College St., Toronto 4, Ont.
ROA, Sylvia; Philippines'57; Staff, Riverview Hosp., Essondale, B.C.
ROACH, Cecil J.; 2612 Waterloo St., Vancouver, B.C.; Tor '25; Anaes; Staff, Dept. of Anaes., St. Paul's Hosp.; Tel. MU 3-2311.
ROACH, Kenneth E.; Ste. 208, 3000 Lawrence Ave. E., Scarborough, Ont.; 97 Sylvan Ave. (res); Tor'51; IntMed; Indoor Staff, Scarborough Gen. Hosp.; Tel. 291-1331.
ROACH, Joseph A.; Plummer Avenue, New Waterford, N.S.; Dal'47; Tel. 862-6495.
ROACH, Margot R.; 400 Princess Ave., London, Ont.; McG '59; **FRCP(C)**, IntMed; Ph.D. (Biophysics); Ass't Prof., Dept. of Biophysics & Med., U. of Western Ontario, London, Ont.; Tel. 438-8694.
ROAD, David A.; 2363 McIntyre St., Regina, Sask.; London (Eng.)'47; DRCOG; MCGP; Tel. LA 7-0641.
ROADHOUSE, Robert C.; 4 King St. W., Toronto 7, Ont.; 16 Ormsby Cres., Tor. 7 (res); Tor '50; Vol. Ass't. (Med.), Tor. Gen. Hosp.; Assoc. Med. Dir., Prudential Ins. Co.; Tel. EM 6-6971.
ROBB, Diana S.; 7 Manitou Rd., Manitouwadge, **Ont.; Tor '60; Staff, Manitouwadge Hosp.; Tel. TA 6-4161.**
ROBB, Donald S.; Dal '42; Med. Supt., Point Edward Hosp., Sydney, N.S.; Tel. 564-5531.
ROBB, Douglas M.; P.O. Box 87, **Hampton Stn., King's Co., N.B.; Dal '56; AMCGP; Active Staff, Saint John Gen. & St. Joseph's Hosp's.; Assoc. Staff, King's Co. Mem. Hosp., Sussex; Tel. 330.**
ROBB, George M.; 4017 E. Hastings St., North Burnaby, B.C.; Aberdeen (Scot.)'53; FRCS(C), GenSurg; Staff, St. Paul's Hosp., Vancouver; Tel. 298-5833.
ROBB, J. Preston; 1610 Pine Ave. W., Montreal 25, P.Q.; 419 Roslyn, Westmount (res); McG '39; Neur; Neurol., Mtl. Children's Hosp.; Dir. Cerebral Palsy Clin.; Assoc. Neur., Royal Victoria Hosp.; Cons. Neur., Mtl. Gen. Hosp.; Dir. (Hosp.) & Assoc. Neur., Mtl. Neurol. Inst.; Assoc. Phys. (Neur.), St. Mary's Hosp.; Cons. Neur., Douglas & Reddy Mem. Hosp's.; Tel. WE 3-9317.
ROBB, K. Ian, Capt.; M.I.R.B.C. Area Hq.; 4050 W. 4th. Ave., Vancouver 8, B.C.; Dal '65.
ROBB, William A.; Ste. 106, 1711-45th St. S. W., Calgary, Alta.; 627-61st Ave. S. W. (res); Wes '43; FRCS(C); GenSurg; Urol; Tel. 263-6464.
ROBB, W. McConnell; 233 Ridley Blvd., Toronto, Ont. (res); Qns '05; D.P.H., P.H; Res. Phys. Lambert Lodge, Toronto; Retired.
ROBBIE, Stanley J.; Beausejour, Man.; Ott'55; Tel. 70.
ROBBINS, Evelyn Edwin; 5827 Clanranald Ave., Montreal 29, P.Q. (res); McG '06; IntMed; Hon. Cons. (Med.), Montreal Gen. Hosp.; Tel. 735-3867.
ROBBINS, Frederick C.; 56 Bessborough Ave., Leaside, Ont. (res); Tor '20; Assoc. Staff, Toronto East Gen. Hosp.; Tel. 425-2338.
ROBBINS, George E.; 1926—11th St. W., Calgary, Alta.; Berne U. (Switz.) '25; Ophth.; Retired.
ROBBINS, James H.; Dal '50; Staff, Camp Hill Hosp., Halifax, N.S.; Tel. 433-1371, Ext. 479.
ROBBINS, Sterling; Box 220, Lockport, N.S.; Dal '56.
ROBERGE, Andre; Lav '61; Res., Neurological Inst., 3801 University, Montreal 2, P.Q.
ROBERGE, Claude; Lav'65; Res., Hop. St. Frances d'Assise, Quebec 3, P.Q.
ROBERGE, Gerard; St. Ephrem de Beauce, P.Q.; Lav '34.
ROBERGE, Jacques G.; Lav'58; Res., Hop. Maisonneuve, Montreal 36, P.Q.
ROBERGE, Jean J.; 805 Rue Royale, Malartic, P.Q.; Mon'59; Abroad.
ROBERGE, Jean P.; 805 rue Royale, Malartic, P.Q.; Mon'59; Tel. 100.
ROBERGE, Marie-Louise; Lav '61., Res., Hop. St-Michel-Archange, Quebec 5, P.Q.; Abroad.
ROBERGE, Pierre A.; Lav '63., Montreal Gen. Hosp., Montreal 25, P.Q.
ROBERGE, Raoul; 1000 Chemin Ste-Foy, Quebec 6, P.Q.; 1180 Belvedere (res); Lav '50; Cardiol (PQ); FRCP(C), IntMed; Ass't. Staff, Hop. du-St.-Sacrement & Laval U.; Tel. 681-2783.
ROBERGE, Rene; Lav'65; Res., Hop. Christ Roi, Quebec 3, P.Q.
ROBERGE, Roger; Notre Dame des Laurentides, P.Q.; Lav '50; Tel. 849-4106.
ROBERGE, Roger; Lav'65; Res., Hotel-Dieu St-Vallier, Chicoutimi, P.Q.
ROBERGE, Roger T.; St. Henry, Co. Levis, P.Q.; Lav '49.
ROBERGE, Yvan; 201-9eme Ave., Deux-Montagnes, P.Q.; Mon '57.
ROBERT, Adrien; 1317 Parc Lafontaine, Montreal, P.Q.; Mon '33; Tel. LA 3-5000.
ROBERT, A. Hermenegilde; 5119 St. Denis, Apt. 1, Montreal, P.Q.; 769 Algonquin, Mount Royal (res); Lav '09; IntMed.
ROBERT, Andre; 2917 Haskell, Kalamazoo, Mich. (res); Mon '50; Ph.D (Exp. Med. & Surg.), (Mon); Research Assoc., Upjohn Co.
ROBERT, Andre; 480 ave Bloomfield, Outremont, Montreal, P.Q.; Mon '58; Bact.
ROBERT, Antonio; 119 Cremazie, Quebec 6, P.Q.; Mon '30; AMCGP; Tel. 523-1202.
ROBERT, Arthur; 969 Blvd. St. Joseph E., Montreal, P.Q.; Lav '12; Tel. VI 5-6651.
ROBERT, Francoise; 726 McEachran, Outremont, Montreal 8, P.Q. (res); Mon '53; Path (P.Q.); Staff, Hop. Notre-Dame; Tel. LA 5-6363.
ROBERT, Gerard; Lav'59; Res., Hop. St. Michel Archange, Quebec 5, P.Q.
ROBERT, Gisele; 483 est, Boul. St.-Joseph, Montreal 34, P.Q.; 478 Ave. Bloomfield, Outremont (res); Mon '59; Psy.; Staff Hop. Maisonneuve; Tel. VI 2-2672.
ROBERT, Jean; Mon '63; Res., Hop. St. Luc., Montreal, P.Q.
ROBERT, J. M. Paul Emile; Clinique Metropolitaine, 1150 est Boul. St.-Joseph, Montreal 34, **P.Q.; Lav '39; M.D. (Paris), F.R.C.P.(C), IntMed.; Staff, Hop. St-Jean-de-Dieu; Tel. LA 7-1241.**
ROBERT, Leo; 969 Ave. des Erables, Quebec 6, P.Q.; Lav '28; Tel. 522-1003.
ROBERT, Lionel; 1275 De Salaberry, Co. Chambly, (res); Mon '17; Retired.
ROBERT, Louis P.; 17 rue Mauranlt, Pierreville, Cte. Yamaska, P.Q. Mon '30; MPH (Johns Hopkins); Tel. 568-2717.
ROBERT, Maurice J. A.; 242 Montreal Rd., Eastview, Ont.; Lav '48; M.C.G.P.
ROBERT, Rene; Case Postal 426, 490-17e rue, Grand-Mere, P.Q.; Lav'58; IntMed(P.Q.); Tel. 538-1088.
ROBERT, Telesphore; 232 Longueuil St., St. Jean, P.Q.; Lav '51; Tel. FI 6-4681.
ROBERTO, Sarah; Santiago (Chile)'49; Staff, Hop. St. Charles, Joliette, P.Q.
ROBERTS, Alexander; 997 Mt. Pleasant Rd., Toronto, Ont.; Tor '54; Tel. HU 9-6024.
ROBERTS, Athol L.; Polyclinic, Charlottetown, P.E.I.; Dal '54. MCGP.
ROBERTS, Charles A.; 250 College St., Toronto 2B, Ont.; Dal '43; FAPA; Psy; Exec. Dir., Clarke Inst. of Psy.; Assoc. Prof. (Psy. & Hygiene), U. of Toronto; Tel. 365-1511.
ROBERTS, Douglas G., SG/LT; HMCS Naden, Esquimalt, B.C.; Sask '64.
ROBERTS, F. Barry; 331 Sheddon Ave., Oakville, Ont.; Tor'56; FRCP(C), Paed; Hd., Dept. of Paed., Oakville-Trafalgar Mem. Hosp. & Joseph Brant Mem. Hosp., Burlington; Tel. 845-8271.
ROBERTS, Frederick J.; Sask'60; Path; Ass't. Path., Vancouver Gen. Hosp.; Clin. Inst. Path., Univ. of B.C.; Tel. 876-3211.
ROBERTS, George A. C.; 299 Main St., Chilliwack, B.C.; 38 E. Princess (res); McG '24.

ROBERTS, Harry D.; Roberts Prof. Bldg., 95 LeMarchant Rd., **St. John's, Nfld.**; **5 Pringle Pl. (res)**; **Dal '36**; **GenSurg**; **Staff Surg., St. John's** Gen. Hosp.; Sr. Cons. Surg., Grace Hosp.; Tel. 726-4560.

ROBERTS, H. Elgin; 1645 Commercial Dr., Vancouver 6, B.C.; Wes'50.

ROBERTS, James B.; **c/o Med. Consultants Group, 1 Campbell Ave., St. John's, Nfld.**; **14 Pine Bud Ave. (res)**; **Tor '42**; **IntMed**; **Chief Phys., Grace Hosp.**; **Sr. Phys., General Hosp.**; **Cons. Phys., St. Clare's Hosp.**; **Chief of Med., DVA Gen. Hosp.**; **Tel. 579-1199.**

ROBERTS, James B.; 1029 **Douglas St., Victoria, B.C.**; **2745 Beach Dr. (res)**; **Qns '36**; **D & TRad EV 2-9104.**

ROBERTS, James F.; 450 Charlesworth Lane, Sarnia, Ont.; Tor'32; MS(Tor); FICS; MASA; MSWSA; GenSurg; Cons. Surg., Sarnia Gen. & St. Joseph's Hosp's.; Tel. DI 4-2232.

ROBERTS, James V.; 1514 Stonybrook Cr., London, Ont.; Wes'50; DiagRad.; Tel. 433-4153.

ROBERTS, John A. G.; 1022 **Waterdown Rd., Burlington, Ont.**; **916 Condor Dr. (res)**; **Qns '54. MCGP**; Tel. NE 4-3568.

ROBERTS, Kenneth A.; **Ste. 906, 11 Adelaide St. W., Toronto 1, Ont.**; **R.R. No. 2, Pickering, Ont. (res)**; **Qns '32**; **Tel. EM 4-3397.**

ROBERTS, Lawrence H.; **695 Station St., Shawinigan Falls, P.Q.**; **1156 Maple Ave. (res)**; **McG '14**; **F.I.M.A. (U.S. & P.Q.)**; **Staff, Joyce Mem. Hosp. & Can. Resin & Chemicals Ltd.**; **Retired.**

ROBERTS, Llewellyn N.; **Ste. 240, 1105 Pandora Ave., Victoria, B.C.**; **Tor '44**; **DPH**; **M.Sc. (Clin. Research)**; FACP, FRCP(C); IntMed.; Tel. 383-5023.

ROBERTS, Maureen H. (McWilliam); 351 Mountbatten **Ave., Ottawa 8, Ont.**; **Edinburgh (Scot.) '37**; DCH(Eng.); Paed.; Sr. Lect. Paed., U. of Ottawa.

ROBERTS, Melville G.; Wes'65; Res., University Hospital, Edmonton, Alta.

ROBERTS, Michael T.S.; 110-8th St. E., Prince Albert, Sask.; Cambridge (Eng.)'61; LMSSA; FFARCS; Assoc. Staff, Victoria Union & Holy Family Hosp's.; Tel. 763-6466.

ROBERTS, Paul W.; **120 Bloor St. E., Toronto 5, Ont.**; **112 Chatsworth Dr., Tor. 12 (res)**; **Tor '47**; **M.D. (Quito, S. America)**; **MCGP**; **Assoc. Med. Dir., Crown Life Ins. Co.**; **Tel. 928-4656.**

ROBERTS, Percy H.; **625 Westmount Med. Bldg.,** 5025 Sherbrooke **St. W., Montreal 28, P.Q.**; **McG '31**; FICS; **FACOG**; **ObstGyn**; **Staff, Queen Elizabeth Hosp.**; Tel. 482-8523.

ROBERTS, Peter C.; 42 Albert St., Stratford, **Ont.**; **170 Douglas St. (res)**; **Wes '50**; **MCGP**; Tel. 271-4461.

ROBERTS, Richard, Sg/Capt.; Nat. Defence Med. **Centre, Ottawa 8, Ont.**; Liverpool (Eng.) '38; MRCS (Eng.); **LRCP (Lond.)**; FACP; IntMed; Hd., Dept. of Med., N.D.M.C.; Assoc. Prof. (Med.), U. of Ottawa.

ROBERTS, Richard W.; 183 James St. S., Hamilton, Ont.; Wes '55; Anaes; Tel. JA 9-8875.

ROBERTS, T. Michael F.; 5880 Spring Garden Road, Halifax, N.S.; London (Eng.)'53; D(Obst) RCOG; FRCS(C); PlasSurg; Ass't. Surgeon, Victoria Gen. & Halifax Children's Hosp.; Tel. 423-6994.

ROBERTSEN, John R.; Witwatersrand (S. Africa)'51; Res., University Hosp., Edmonton, Alta.

ROBERTSHAW, Arthur M.; **7311 Kingsway, Burnaby 1, B.C.**; **Tor '52**; **Tel. LA 4-3422.**

ROBERTSON, Alan R.; New Prov. Bldgs., 110 Charlotte St., Saint John, N.B.; 322 Balmoral Cr., Lancaster (res); Glasgow (Scot.)'56; DPM (Eng.); Dir. of Mental Health Clinic; Tel. 692-0181.

ROBERTSON, Alexander D.; **924A Saskatchewan Cres., Saskatoon, Sask. (res)**; **Edinburgh (Scot.) '49**; **DPH**; **Vis. Cons., University Hosp.**; **Tel. 242-7641.**

ROBERTSON, Alexander L.; **Old Orchard Shopping Centre**, 4429 Kingsway, South Burnaby, B.C.; Wes '52; Act. Staff, Burnaby Gen., Vancouver Gen. & Grace Hosp's.; Memb. of Med. Bd., Burnaby Gen. Hosp.; Tel. HE 3-8274.

ROBERTSON, A. St. Clair; **810 Greyhound Bldg., Calgary, Alta.**; **3032—1st St. W. (res)**; **Edinburgh (Scot.) '36**; **F.R.C.S. (Edin.), F.A.C.S., F.I.C.S., GenSurg**; **Surg. Cons., Calgary Gen., Holy Cross & Alberta Children's Hosp's.**; **Tel. 263-7399**; **Abroad.**

ROBERTSON, Basil D.; **1490 Sherbrooke W., Montreal, P.Q.**; **1575 Summerhill Ave. (res)**; McG '28.

ROBERTSON, C. Eric; **Lions Gate Hosp., North Vancouver, B.C.**; **2207 W. 35th Ave., Van. 13 (res)**; **Tor '43**; **Path**; **Ass't. Pathol., Lions Gate Hosp.**; **Tel. YU 8-3131.**

ROBERTSON, Charles A.; 34 High Street, Pictou, N.S.; Glasgow (Scot.)'58; Senior Staff, Sutherland-Harris Memorial Hosp.; Tel. 485-4171.

ROBERTSON, Charles T.; **825 Coxwell Ave., Toronto 6, Ont.**; **3 Fallingbrook Woods (res)**; **Tor '39**; **F.R.C.S.(C), GenSurg**; **Surg-in-Chief, Toronto** East Gen. Hosp.; **Tel. HO 3-3521.**

ROBERTSON, Clyde H.; **1 Wood Glen Rd., Scarborough, Ont. Tor '10**; **Tel. OX 1-6122**; **Retired.**

ROBERTSON, Cyril M.; **24 Ferrand Dr., Don Mills,** Ont.; Alb'40; Dir., Medical Records Inst.; Tel. 429-0464.

ROBERTSON, David; **812 Cook Rd., Richmond,** B.C.; 786 Afton Dr. (res); Man'52; MCGP; Memb. Med. Advisory Bd. & Chmn. Paed. Sec., Richmond Gen. Hosp.; Tel. 278-5191.

ROBERTSON, David A.; **Aberdeen (Scot.) '59**; **M.B., Ch.B.**; **Sr. Intn., (Anaes), Sunnybrook** Hosp., **Toronto 12, Ont.**

ROBERTSON, David E.; **233 Med. Arts Bldg.,** Saskatoon, Sask.; 206 Garrison Cres.(res); **St. Andrew's (Scot.) '42**; **FRCS(Edin.)**; **OrthSurg**; **Active Staff, University, City & St. Paul's Hosp's.**; Tel. 242-9992.

ROBERTSON, David M.; **56 Ellerbeck St., Kingston, Ont. (res)**; **Qns '55**; **M.Sc. (Med.)**; **Path**; **Ass't. Pathol. & Neuropathol., Kingston Gen.** Hosp.; Cons. Neuropath.; Ottawa Civic Hosp., Ottawa; Ass't. Prof. (Path) (Neuropathol.), **Queen's U.**; **Tel. 546-1731.**

ROBERTSON, Donald C.; 330 **Medical Arts Bldg.,** 170 **St. George St., Toronto, Ont.**; **232 Cortleigh Blvd. (res)**; **Tor '43**; F.R.C.S.(C), GenSurg, PlasSurg; Sr. Surg. & Chief PlasSurg., Toronto Gen. Hosp.; Cons. Surg., Princess Margaret Hosp.; Ass't. Prof., Dept. of Surg., U. of Toronto; Tel. 924-4868.

ROBERTSON, Donald M.; Box 488, Morrisburg, Ont.; Ott '53; F.A.G.S., M.C.G.P.; Chief of Med., Winchester & Dist. Mem. Hosp.; Court Staff, Hotel Dieu Hosp.; Tel. KI 3-3153.

ROBERTSON, Donald P.; 7 Maytree Rd., Willowdale, Ont.; Man'38; FRCS(Eng.); FACS; GenSurg.; Tel. 483-9595.

ROBERTSON, Donald S.; **Deep River Hosp., Ste. 3, Deep River, Ont.**; **35½ Faraday (res)**; **Tor '59**; **MOH, Twps. Rolph, Wylie, Buchanan &** McKay; Dist. Coroner; Tel. 584-4744.

ROBERTSON, Edwin M.; **Etherington Hall, Stuart St., Kingston, Ont.**; **Edinburgh (Scot.) '26**; FRCS (Edin.), FACOG, FRCOG, MRCOG, FRCS(C), ObstGyn.; ObstGyn., Kingston Gen. Hosp.; Prof. of ObstGyn., Queen's U.; Tel. 542-4340.

ROBERTSON, Elizabeth (Chant); **503 Davenport Rd., Toronto, Ont. (res)**; **Tor '24**; **Ph.D.**; **Paed**; Clin. Cons. & Research Assoc., Hosp. for Sick Children; Tel. EM 6-7242.

ROBERTSON, Fred G.; **Cobourg Clinic, 188 King St. W., Cobourg, Ont.**; **180 King St. W. (res)**; **Tor '33**; **Staff, Cobourg Gen. Hosp.**; **Tel.** 372-3323.

ROBERTSON, Gordon D.; 925 W. Georgia St., Vancouver, B.C.; Tor '60; MCGP; Tel. MU 1-9454.

ROBERTSON, Gordon L.; 10 Treadgold Cr., Don Mills, Ont.; Alb'53; IntMed; Staff, Princess Margaret Hosp.

ROBERTSON, H. A.; Chest Cons., Dept. of Nat. **Health & Welfare, c/o Regional Superintendent,** European Region. Abroad.

ROBERTSON, Harold F.; 802 Med. Arts Bldg., 170 St. George St., Toronto 5, Ont.; 82 Rosedale Hgts. Dr. (res); Tor '28; FRCS(C), GenSurg; Staff (Surg.), U. of Toronto; Tel. WA 2-1545.
ROBERTSON, H. Rocke; 604 Clarke Ave., Westmount, Montreal, P.Q. (res); McG '36; F.R.C.S. (Edin.), F.A.C.S., F.R.C.S.(C), GenSurg; Principal, & Vice-Chancellor, McGill U.; Tel. WE 7-6011.
ROBERTSON, Hugh E.; 353 Dalhousie St., Ottawa 2, Ont.; 2063 Thorne Ave. (res); Qns '24; F.C.C.P.; IntMed; Dir., Eastern Ontario Chest Clinic; Tel. 234-1361.
ROBERTSON, Hugh J. F.; 225 Lisgar St., Apt. 908, Ottawa 4, Ont.; Ott'59; DiagRad.
ROBERTSON, J. Douglas; 250 Lawrence Ave. W., Toronto 12, Ont.; 387 Greer Rd., Tor 12 (res); Tor '57; MCGP; Court Staff, Wellesley Hosp.; Tel. RU 1-8737.
ROBERTSON, Joan S.; R.R. No. 2, King City, Ont. (res); McG '41; DiagRad; Tel. 833-6809.
ROBERTSON, John G.; 713 Columbia St., New Westminster, B.C.; 210 First St. (res); Man '29; Ophth, Otol; Tel. LA 1-0630.
ROBERTSON, J. Sinclair; Prov. Bldg., Hollis St., Halifax, N.S.; Dal '34; DPH; PH; Deputy Minister, Dept. of Public Health (N.S.); Assoc. Prof. (PrevMed.), Dalhousie U.; Tel. 5-8271.
ROBERTSON, Joseph A.; 3 Orchard St., Port Hope, Ont.; Qns '40.
ROBERTSON, Kenneth; Assiniboia, Sask.; Dublin (Ire.) '57; Tel. 642-3364.
ROBERTSON, Kenneth K.; 4 Main St. N., Waterdown, Ont.; Glasgow (Scot.) '56.
ROBERTSON, Mary E.; 280 Bloor St. W., Toronto 5, Ont.; Tor'57; FRCP(C); IntMed.
ROBERTSON, Maryon S.; 302 Med. Centre, 906-8th Ave. S.W., Calgary, Alta.; 1702-32nd Ave. S.W. (res); Alb'62; AMCGP; Att'd. Staff, Calgary Gen., Holy Cross & Grace Hosp's.; Tel. 263-0140.
ROBERTSON, Patrick A. M.; Box 1056, Weyburn, Sask. (res); Edinburgh (Scot.) '39; L.R.C.P.&S., L.R.F.P.S.; Psy., Saskatchewan Hosp., Weyburn; Retired.
ROBERTSON, Ralph O.; Box 4000, 353 Eveline St., Selkirk, Man.; Qns'55; ObstGyn.; Tel. 482-3121.
ROBERTSON, Rhoda B. (Neil); Box 88, Mindapore, Alta. (res); Alb'44; Anaes; Staff, Holy Cross & Children's Hosp's., Calgary; Tel. AM 6-7231.
ROBERTSON, Ritter W.; 51 Orrin Ave., Ottawa 3. Ont. (res); Tor '44; M.O., Dept. of Nat. Health & Welfare; Tel. 992-0818.
ROBERTSON, Robert F.; 10951-124th St., Edmonton, Alta.; 7808-143A St. (res); Liverpool (Eng.) '58; MCGP; Assoc. Staff, Royal Alexandra Hosp.; Tel. 454-4551.
ROBERTSON, Robina (Herd); Glasgow (Scot.) '56; M.B., Ch.B.; Staff, Children's Hosp. School, Lancaster, N.B.
ROBERTSON, Ross; 410 Fairmont Med. Bldg., 750 W. Broadway, Vancouver 9, B.C.; 6076 Blink Bonnie Rd. (res); Tor '26; F.R.C.S.(C), F.A.C.S.; GenSurg; OrthSurg; ThorSurg; Cons. (ThorSurg), Shaughnessy Vet's. Hosp.; Hon. Att'd. Staff, Vancouver Gen. Hosp.; Surg. Cons., Civil Aviation Med. Cons. Bd.; Clin. Ass't. Prof. (Surg.) U. of British Columbia; Tel. TR 9-5355.
ROBERTSON, Struan F.; 2842 Bloor St. W., Toronto 18, Ont.; Tor'35; MCGP; Tel. 233-9721.
ROBERTSON, William J.; 955 Queen St. E., Sault Ste. Marie, Ont.; 94 Lansdowne (res); Tor '44; Paed; Chief, Paed Dep't., Plummer Memorial & Sault Ste. Marie Gen. Hosp's.; Tel. AL 4-5166.
ROBERTSON, W. M. D., Shad Bay, Halifax Co., N.S.; Glasgow (Scot.) '28, MCGP; Tel. 130.
ROBICHAUD, A.; Box 20, Tracadie, N.B.; Mon '33; GenSurg; Chief Surg., Hotel-Dieu Hosp.; Chief M.O., Dominion Govern't Hosp.; Tel. 46.
ROBICHAUD, Ephrem; 7159 des Erables, Montreal 35, P.Q.; Mon'43; Staff, Mtl. Gen. Hosp.; Tel. RA 7-5830.
ROBICHAUD, Philippe A.; 7350 St. Denis St., Montreal, P.Q.; Mon '07; All (P.Q.).
ROBICHON, Jacques R.; 178 Laurier E., Ottawa, Ont.; 789 Lonsdale St. (res); Lav '43; F.A.C.S., F.R.C.S.(C), OrthSurg; Head (Dept. of OrthSurg) Ottawa Gen. Hosp.; Assoc. Prof (OrthSurg) U. of Ottawa; Tel. CE 6-0586.
ROBILLARD, Eugene; 524 Cote Ste-Catherine, Montreal 8, P.Q. (res); Mon '36; M.Sc.; Vice Dean, Faculty of Med., U. of Montreal; Tel. RE 3-9951.
ROBILLARD, Francis A.; 1650 Cedar Ave., Montreal 25, P.Q.; 4039 Marlowe Ave. (res); McG '51; Anaes; Ass't. (Anaes), Mtl. Gen. Hosp.; Dem. (Anaes), McGill U.; Tel. WE 7-6011.
ROBILLARD, Gaston; 358 Beverley Ave., Mount Royal, Montreal 16, P.Q. (res); Mon '47; DiagRad.; Staff (Rad.), Hop. Ste Justine.; Tel. RE 1-4931.
ROBILLARD, John O.; 272 Bronson Ave., Ottawa 4, Ont.; McG '21.
ROBILLARD, J. Maurice; 4000 Ave. Marlowe, Montreal, P.Q.; Mon '40; Anaes. (P.Q.); Anaes., Hop. St. Joseph, Lachine; Tel. 527-7348.
ROBILLARD, Pierre; 525 rue Leonard, St. Jovite, P.Q.; Mon'65.
ROBILLARD, Raymond; Ste. 1001, 801 Est Rue Sherbrooke, Montreal 24, P.Q.; Mon'53; FRCP(C), Neurol.; Chief of Neurol. Serv., Hop. Maisonneuve; Tel. 254-8341, Loc. 249.
ROBILLARD, Rene; 116 Willowdale, Montreal 8, P.Q.; Mon'47; MCGP; TherRad; Staff, Inst. du Radium, Montreal; Tel. LA 3-3151.
ROBILLARD, Rosario; 8423 rue Saint-Denis, Montreal, P.Q.; 2574 Blvd. Pie IX (res); Mon '40; IntMed; Assoc. Phys., Hop. St. Luc; Assoc. Prof. (IntMed.), U. of Montreal; Tel. VI 2-4892.
ROBIN, E. Peter; 201 Plaza Bldg., 1538 Foster St., White Rock, B.C.; UBC'54; MCGP; Tel. 531-5575.
ROBIN, Jean P., Capt.; Lav'65; 4th Detachment, Canadian Armed Forces, Longueuil, P.Q.
ROBINOW, Carl F.; Hamburg (Germ.) '34; F.R.S.C., Prof. Act. Hd., Dept. of Immunol. U. of Western Ont., London, Ont.; Tel. GE 9-1681.
ROBINS, R. Edward; 750 W. Broadway, Vancouver, B.C.; 2081 S.W. Marine Dr. (res); Wes '48; F.R.C.S.(C), GenSurg; Attend. Staff, Vancouver Gen. & Shaughnessy Hosp's; Clin. Instr. (Surg.) U. of British Columbia; Tel. TR 2-5461.
ROBINSON, Barbara J. (Mrs. R. A. Watson); Fredericton Med. Clin., 206 Rockwood Ave., Fredericton, N.B.; Dal'47; Paed; Att'd. Staff, Victoria Public Hosp.; Tel. 475-7701.
ROBINSON, Barbara L.; Alb'65; Staff, Respir. Unit, Vancouver Gen. Hosp., Vancouver 9, B.C.
ROBINSON, Cecil E.; 3195 Granville St., Ste. 221, Vancouver 9, B.C.; 5988 Adera St. (res); Qns '43; FRCP(C), IntMed; Ass't. Chief Med., Shaughnessy DVA Hosp.; Staff St. Vincent's & Vancouver Gen. Hosp's.; Clin. Instr., U. of British Columbia; Tel. RE 1-1282.
ROBINSON, Clarence E.; 46 Westleigh Cres., Toronto 14, Ont. (res); Qns '42; D.P.H. D.Psy; Psy; Staff, Lakeshore Psy. Hosp.; Spec. Lect. (Schl. of Hyg.) U. of Toronto; Tel. 367-7416.
ROBINSON, Clayton L.; Ste. 814, 750 W. Broadway, Vancouver 9, B.C.; Qns'43; FRCS(Eng.); FRCS(C), GenSurg.
ROBINSON, D. Alexander; Box 70, Langley, B.C.; 2521—200th St. (res); McG '41; M.C.G.P.; Med. Staff, Langley Memorial Hosp.; Tel. 534-4413.
ROBINSON, David C.; Meaford, Ont.; Wes '58; AMCGP; Tel. 103.
ROBINSON, Donald C.; McGregor Clinic, 250 Main St. E., Hamilton, Ont.; Wes'57; FRCS(C), ObstGyn; Active Staff, Hamilton Civic Hosp's.; Court. Staff, St. Joseph's & Chedoke Gen. Hosp's.; Tel. JA 7-2711.
ROBINSON, D. Roberta (Noble); 46 Westleigh Cres., Toronto 14, Ont.; Tor '44; D.P.H.; Tel. CL 9-4525.
ROBINSON, Edward G.; 710 Seymour St. Vancouver, B.C.; Alb '63; Tel. MU 4-1511.
ROBINSON, Edward S.; 1838 W. 57th Ave., Vancouver, B.C.; 3876 S.W. Marine Dr. (res); Oxford (Eng.) '55; B.M., B.Ch., M.A.; Tel. AM 6-1557.

ROBINSON, Eleanor M.; 2401 Bloor St. W., Toronto 9, Ont.; 60 Runnymede Rd. (res); Tor '34; M.C.A.A., IntMed; Staff, Diabetic Dept., Women's College Hosp.; Tel. RO 9-2445.

ROBINSON, F. T.; 17 King St. W., Stoney Creek, Ont.; Wes '47.

ROBINSON, G. C. F.; 715 W. 12th Ave., Vancouver, B.C.; Qns '45; F.R.C.P.(C), Paed; Med. O.P.D., Health Centre for Children; Ass't. Prof. (Paed.), U. of British Columbia.

ROBINSON, Gaston L.; 3725 W.29, Vancouver, B.C. (res); Lav '42; Anaes; Anaes. Staff, St. Paul's Hosp.; Tel. MU 3-2211.

ROBINSON, Geoffrey E.; Montague, P.E.I.; London (Eng.)'51; MRCS; LRCP.

ROBINSON, Gordon E.; 21 Upper Middle Rd., Cooksville, Ont.; Tor'45; FRCS(C), GenSurg.; Tel. 277-9434.

ROBINSON, Hadley V.; 4480 Sherbrooke St. W., Westmount, Montreal 6, P.Q.; Retired.

ROBINSON, Harold C., G/C; 3 F. Wing RCAF, C.F.P.O. 5055, Can. Armed Forces, Europe; Wes '50; Otol.; Abroad.

ROBINSON, H. Campbell; 308-1/2 Boler Rd., London, Ont.; Wes'59; MCGP; Active Staff, Victoria Hosp.; Teach. Fell., U. of Western Ontario; Tel. 471-6440.

ROBINSON, Harold S.; 900 W. 27th Ave., Vancouver 9, B.C.; 4335 W. 3rd Ave., Van. 8 (res); McG '42; IntMed; Att'd. Staff, Van. Gen. Hosp.; Med. Dir., Cdn. Arthritis & Rheum. Soc. (BC) Div.; Clin. Instr., U. of British Columbia; Tel. RE 3-1128.

ROBINSON, Harry C.; 908 King St. E., Hamilton, Ont.; Qns '30; MCGP; Tel. LI 4-2974.

ROBINSON, Henri; 44 Champlain, Pointe Gatineau, P.Q.; Mon'34; Paed.

ROBINSON, James B.; Beck Mem. San., London, Ont.; Tor'28; IntMed(T.B.); Med. Dir., Beck Mem. San.; Clin. Ass't. Prof. of Med. (T.B.), Med. School & Lect. (T.B.) Public Health Nurses, U. of Western Ontario; Tel. 471-1440.

ROBINSON, James M.; 1461-6th Ave., Prince George, B.C.; Belfast (Ire.) '59; DPH; Dir., & M.O. of Health, Northern Interior Health Unit; Tel. 563-1631.

ROBINSON, J. Dean; 1130 Fulton Ave. W., Vancouver, B.C. (res); McG '17; Retired.

ROBINSON, J. Graham; 2221 Keele St., Toronto 15, Ont.; 42 Greenbrook Dr. (res); Tor '52; FAC-A; Anaes; Anaes. Staff, Northwestern Gen. Hosp.; Tel. 249-1555.

ROBINSON, John; 70 Melville St., Dundas, Ont.; Queens (N. Ire.)'57; Staff, Hamilton Civic Hospitals & St. Joseph's Hospital; Tel. 672-0342.

ROBINSON, John B. C.; 420 Oxford St., London, Ont.; 973 Waterloo St. (res); Wes '31; M.Sc.; MCGP; Lect. (Med. Ethics), U. of Western Ont.; Coroner, Middlesex Co.; Tel. GE 2-0112.

ROBINSON, John D.; Box 100, Durham St., Flesherton, Ont.; Tor '52; M.C.G.P.; M.O.H., Flesherton; Coroner, Grey County; Tel. 150.

ROBINSON, John D.; 81 Bruce Ave., South Porcupine, Ont.; Durham (Eng.)'61; DA.

ROBINSON, John E.; Man '60; Jr. Int'n., St. Boniface Hosp., St. Boniface, Man.

ROBINSON, John G.; 308 Med. Arts Bldg., 1 Young St., Hamilton, Ont.; Tor '49; M.Sc., MRCP (E); FACC; FRCP(C), IntMed; Phys., Hamilton Gen. Hosp.; & Dir., Heart Invest. Unit; Cardiologist, Cardiac Work Eval. Unit, Hamilton Health Assoc.; Tel. 528-2635.

ROBINSON, J. T. Harold; Walkerton, Ont.; Tor '24; MCGP; Dist. Coroner; Tel. 881-0564.

ROBINSON, Koraishia (Mohideen); 250 Lawrence Ave. W., Toronto 12, Ont.; Hong Kong (China) '52; ObstGyn; Tel. 782-7351.

ROBINSON, Lorne K.; 2055 Carling Ave., Ottawa, Ont.; Britannia Heights (res); Tor '43; Tel. 722-4121.

ROBINSON, Louis; Ste. 210, North Toronto Med. Bldg., 250 Lawrence Ave. W., Toronto 12, Ont.; St. Mungo's (Glasgow, Scot.)'50; LRCP & S (Edin.); IntMed; Staff (Med.), OPD, Toronto Western Hosp.; Phys. ADARF; Tel. RU 2-7351.

ROBINSON, Lyn (Ashworth); Brant Arts Lab., Brant Arts Bldg., Burlington, Ont.; London U. (Charing Cross Hosp., Eng.)'56; M.B., B.S., D.Obst., RCOG; MCGP; Tel. 637-1976.

ROBINSON, Marc; Ottawa Gen. Hosp., Bruyere St., Ottawa, Ont.; Ott'59; IntMed; Teach. Staff, U. of Ottawa; Tel. CE 6-0333.

ROBINSON, Margaret J. L.; 340 N. Christina St., Sarnia, Ont.; 1607 Lakeshore Rd. (res); Durham (Eng.) '51; DRCOG; MCGP; Tel. DI 4-1743.

ROBINSON, Martin L.; 367 Princess Ave., London, Ont.; Wes '53; MRCOG; FACS; FACOG; FRCS(C); ObstGyn; Staff, Victoria & St. Joseph's Hosp's.; Lect. (ObstGyn.), U. of Western Ont.; Tel. 434-4711.

ROBINSON, Ralph B.; 156 Ontario St., St. Catharines, Ont.; 23 Yates St. (res); Tor '31; F.A.C.S., GenSurg; Chief Surg., Hotel Dieu Hosp.; Sr. Surg. Staff, St. Catharines Gen. Hosp.; Surg. Cons., Niagara Peninsular San.; Court. Staff, Niagara-on-the-Lake Cottage Hosp.; Tel. MU 4-9201.

ROBINSON, Ralph T.; 606 Boyd Bldg., 388 Portage Ave., Winnipeg 1, Man.; 125 Elm St., Wpg. 9 (res); Man '28; MCGP; Tel. WH 2-8728.

ROBINSON, Robert E.; 14 Donalda Cr., Agincourt, Ont.; Tor '47; MCGP; Tel. AX 3-4189.

ROBINSON, Samuel S.; 301 Brock St., Kingston, Ont.; Qns '33; Staff, Kingston Gen. Hosp.; Lect. (Med.), Queen's U.; Tel. 546-0335.

ROBINSON, Shaun M.; Alb '64; Res., University Hosp., Edmonton, Alta.

ROBINSON, Stuart C.; 5880 Spring Garden Rd., Halifax, N.S.; 4 Hall's St., Armdale (res); Tor'44; FACOG; ObstGyn; Assoc. Prof., Dalhousie U.; Dir., Uterine Cancer Detect. Programme, Prov. of N.S.; Tel. 423-8441.

ROBINSON, Theodore J.; Man '63; Res., Shaughnessy Hosp., Vancouver 9, B.C.; Abroad.

ROBINSON, Wilfred G.; 53 Whyte St., Dryden, Ont.; Tor '33; M.C.G.P.; Dist. Coroner.

ROBINSON, Wilfrid R.; McG '57; Jr. Int'n., Montreal Gen. Hosp., Montreal, P.Q.

ROBINSON, William E.; Sir John A. MacDonald Blvd., 670, No. 14, Unit 6, Kingston, Ont.; Qns'60; Psy.

ROBISON, Donald L.; 2200 Dixie Rd., Cooksville, Ont.; Tor '61; Tel. 277-2271.

ROBITAILLE, Jean C.; 1605—1st Ave., Quebec 3, P.Q.; Lav '40; D&TRad; Head, Dept. of Radiol., Hop. St. Francois d'Assise & Hop. Ste Anne de Beaupre; Tel. 529-7311.

ROBITAILLE, J. Noel; Box 800, Espanola, Ont.; Lav '59; AMCGP.

ROBITAILLE, Lucien; 1805 Maufils, Quebec, P.Q.; Lav '39; Tel. 661-1821.

ROBITAILLE, Marcel; St. Zacharie, Dorchester, P.Q.; Lav '50; Tel. 2-2341.

ROBITAILLE, Pierre; Mon'65; Res., Hop. Hotel-Dieu, Montreal 18, P.Q.

ROBITAILLE, Robert, Colonel; Canadian Forces Base, St. Hubert, P.Q.; Mon'43.

ROBSON, B. E.; Tor'65; Res., The Clarke Inst., 250 College St., Toronto 2B, Ont.

ROBSON, Charles C.; 3252 Lawrence Ave. E., Scarborough, Ont.; Glasgow (Scot.)'52; Tel. 293-7551.

ROBSON, Charles H.; 96 Chatsworth Dr., Toronto, Ont.; McG '13; F.I.C.A., Anaes; Cons, in Anaes., Hosp. for Sick Children; Anaes-in-Chief, Toronto Hosp. for Tuberculosis; Tel. 769-1161.

ROBSON, Charles J.; 1017 Med. Arts Bldg., 170 St. George St., Toronto 5, Ont.; 185 Roxborough Rd. (res); Tor '42; FACS, FRCS(C), Urol; Staff Surg. (Urol.), Toronto Gen. Hosp.; Cons. (Urol.), Sunnybrook DVA., Women's College Hosp. & Hosp. for Sick Children; Ass't Prof Surg (Urol.), U. of Toronto; Tel. 924-3614.

ROBSON, David B.; 191 Yonge St. S., Richmond Hill, Ont.; 27 Thornbank Rd., Thornhill (res); Tor 50; GenSurg; Surg. Cons., North York Branson & York Central Hosp's.; Tel. TU 4-5981.

ROBSON, George W.; 270 Medical Arts Bldg., 1105 Pandora Ave., Victoria, B.C.; 2855 Lansdowne Rd. (res); Tor '33; F.R.C.O.G., ObstGyn; Head, Dept. ObstGyn., Royal Jubilee Hosp.; Cons. Staff, St. Joseph's Hosp.; Tel. EV 3-3834.

ROBSON, Hugh G.; 4855 Cote-St-Luc Rd., Montreal 29, P.Q.; McG'60; FRCP(C), IntMed.

ROBSON, James G.; 301 Victoria Dr., Baie d'Urfee, P.Q. (res); Glasgow (Scot.) '44; D.A., F.F.A.R.C.S.(Eng.); Research Prof., McGill U.; Cons. (Anaes.) Royal Victoria, Montreal Gen. Queen Elizabeth, Montreal Children's, St. Mary's, Notre Dame de l'Esperance Hosp's. & Montreal Neurol. Inst.; Tel. VI 4-6311.
ROBSON, Peter A.; Box 1088, Mission City, B.C.; Horne Ave. (res); London (Eng.) '58; MRCS (Eng.) LRCP(Lond.); Tel. 826-6231.
ROBSON, Thomas B.; 1504 Ouellette Ave., Windsor, Ont.; 907 Chilver Rd. (res); Tor '49; FRCS(C), ObstGyn; Chief of ObstGyn., Metropolitan Gen. Hosp.; Tel. CL 6-5851.
ROBURN, Michael; London (Eng.)'57; FRCP(C), Psy; Staff, Vancouver Gen. Hosp., Vancouver, B.C.
ROBUTKA, Leo P.; 609A Medical Centre, 8th Ave. & 8th St. S.W., Calgary, Alta.; Tor'45.
ROBY, Harold R.; 2 Clifton Ave., Windsor, N.S.; Dal '45; DiagRad.; Tel. 798-2749.
ROCHE, Albert J.; McG'63; Res., Montreal Gen. Hosp., Montreal 25, P.Q.
ROCHE, James W.; 2209 Arch St., Ottawa 8, Ont.; Dublin (Ire.)'44.
ROCHEFORT, Jean M.; 288 Worthington St. W., North Bay, Ont.; Lav'55; MCGP; Tel. 472-8220.
ROCHEFORT, Julien; Lav '50; DiagRad(P.Q.); Staff, Hop. La Providence, Magog, P.Q.; Tel. 843-3381.
ROCHELEAU, J. Ferdinand; 3431 Ave. Laval, Montreal 18, P.Q.; 4174 St.-Denis (res); Lav '18; Tel. 288-2424.
ROCHETTE, Emilien; C.P. 83, 14 Place Orleans, App. 1, Beauport, Quebec 5, P.Q.; Lav'59; Med. Dir., Centre Hop. St. Francois; Tel. 661-5943.
ROCHETTE, Lucien; 417 ave. Jacques-Cartier, Disraeli, P.Q.; Lav '62; Tel. 437.
ROCHETTE, Madeleine; Lav'61; Paed(P.Q.); Staff, Hop. Hotel Dieu, Montreal 18, P.Q.
ROCHETTE, Marcel; 225 Grande Allee E., Quebec 4, P.Q.; 421 ouest 67e rue, Charlesbourg (res); Lav '56; M.O., W.C.B. (P.Q.); Tel. 522-4751.
ROCHETTE, Marcellin; Rue St. Etienne, La Malbaie, Charlevoix, P.Q.; Pointe au Pic (res); Lav '41; Ophth, Otol (P.Q.); Ophth. Otol., St. Joseph's Hosp.; Tel. MO 5-3711.
ROCHMAN, Harvey; 307 Huron St., London, Ont.; Tor'49; Psy; Med. Spec. Psy., Westminster DVA Hosp.; Clin. Lect., (Psy), U. of Western Ont.; Tel. GE 2-6711.
ROCHMAN, Saul; 7655 Querbes Ave., Montreal, P.Q.; 366 Kindersley Ave. (res); McG '40; Paed; Clinical Ass't., Montreal Children's Hosp., & Jewish Gen. Hosp's.; Tel. 272-3901.
ROCHON, Bruno; 644 Parent, St-Jerome, P.Q.; Mon '25.
ROCHON, Guy; 9 rue Dufferin, Granby, P.Q.; 10 Ottawa (res); Mon'44; Ophth, Otol (P.Q.); Tel. 372-5844.
ROCHON, Jean; 2643 Beaubien E., Montreal, P.Q.; Mon '56; Staff, Hop. Bellechasse, Jean-Talon, & de-la-Misericorde; Tel. RA 2-3807.
ROCHON, Jean L.; 201 rue Charron, Ville-Le Moyne, Cite-Jacques-Cartier, P.Q.; Mon '63.
ROCHON, Jean L.; 7630 Centrale, Lasalle, P.Q.; Mon'65.
ROCK, W. Kenneth; 705 Glengarry Ave., Windsor, Ont.; 1221 Louis Ave. (res); Tor '51,; Tel. 252-2785.
ROCKEL, Albert C.; 68 Queen St. N., Kitchener, Ont.; Tor '37; M.C.G.P.; Tel. SH 5-9596.
ROCKMAN, J. B.; 436 Palmerston Blvd., Toronto 4, Ont.; Tor '31; M.C.G.P.; Tel. LE 1-4721.
RODDICK, John E.; 248 Dalhousie St., Brantford, Ont.; 480 Chatham St. (res); Qns '38; Tel. 752-2512.
RODEN, Rudolph G.; 4330 Sherbrooke St., Montreal 6, P.Q. 3295 Cedar Ave, Westmount (res); Qns '55; Ph.D., MCGP; Court. Staff, Reddy Memorial, Catherine Booth & Jean Talon Hosp's.; Tel. 932-6191.
RODENBURG, Martin; Leiden (Neth.) '55; Res., Kingston Gen. Hosp., Kingston, Ont.
RODERIQUE, Eastmond M.; UBC '62; Res., Montreal Gen. Hosp., Montreal, P.Q.
RODERICK, J. Homfray; 372 Wilson St., Ancaster, Ont.; Tor'27; Sr. Treatment M.O., DVA Hamilton Dist.; Tel. JA 2-3522.
RODGER, David E.; 2125 - 11th Ave., Regina, Sask.; 3131 Angus St. (res); McG '35; F.A.C.P., M.R.C.P. (Lond.), F.R.C.P.(C), IntMed; Dir. of Med., R.A. Dist D.V.A.; Head of Med., Regina Gen. Hosp.; Fed. Rep., Dept of Nat. Health & Welfare, Disability & Rehab. Com'ttee; Tel. 522-1651.
RODGER, Kenneth C.; 19 Wellington Row, Saint John, N.B.; 270 King St. E. (res); Dal '47; IntMed; Attend. Staff, Saint John Gen., St. Joseph's, Lancaster D.V.A. & East Saint John T.B. Hosp's.; Tel. 693-3138.
RODGER, N. Wilson; Man '60; FRCP(C), IntMed; Staff, Royal Victoria Hosp., Montreal 2, P.Q.; Tel. 842-1251.
RODGER, William A.; 21 Wellington St., Galt, Ont.; 35 Lansdowne Rd. N. (res); Tor'60; Tel. 623-0400.
RODGERS, Christine A.; 232 King St., Bathurst, N.B.; '57.
RODGERS, C. Lawrence; 198 Brant Ave., Brantford, Ont.; Tor '47; Paed; Staff, Brantford Gen. Hosp.; Tel. PL 3-8631.
RODGERS, Donald D.; 73 Agassiz Dr., Winnipeg 19, Man.; Man '57; Psy.
RODGERSON, James S.; 4 King Cres., Weston, Ont.; 38 Yorkleigh Ave. (res); Tor '59; Staff, Humber Mem. Hosp.; Tel. 248-1741.
RODIN, Alvin E.; 15001 - 86th Ave., Edmonton, Alta. (res); Man '50; M.Sc. (Med.); D.A.B.P.A. & C.P., F.R.C.S.(C), Path; Pathol., Miscericordia Hosp.; Inst., U. of Alta.; Tel. HU 8-9021.
RODKO, Eugene A.; 34 Munro Pl., Regina Sask.; Man '53; DiagRad; Dir. Dept. of Rad., Regina Gen. Hosp.; Tel. LA 2-1811.
RODMAN, Floyd B.; Ste. 450, 8409-112th St., Edmonton, Alta.; Alb '48; M.Sc., Ph.D., IntMed; Staff, U. of Alberta Hosp.; Ass't. Clin. Prof., U. of Alberta; Tel. 439-3019.
RODRIGUE, Berchmans; Lac Etchemin, Cte Dorchester, P.Q.; Lav '63.
RODRIGUE, Denis; Lav'65; Res., Hop. St. Francois d'Assise, Quebec, P.Q.
RODRIQUE, Eastmond M.; Box 69, Princeton, B.C.; UBC '62; Tel. 23.
RODRIGUE, Florian; Case Postale 159, Station Outremont, Montreal 8, P.Q.; Mon'54.
RODRIGUE, Gaston; 66, boul Gall, Drummond-ville, ouest, P.Q. (res); Lav '43; D&TRad; Med. Dir. & Dir. of Rad. Serv., Hop. Ste. Croix; Tel. GR 8-1381.
RODRIGUE, Lionel J.; Lav '56; Res. University Hosp., Saskatoon, Sask.
RODRIGUE, Marcel; 389 boul. Leclerc, Granby, P.Q.; Mon '61; Staff, Hop. St. Joseph; Tel. FR 8-7411.
RODRIGUE, Venant; St-Samuel, Cte. Frontenac, P.Q.; Lav '54.
RODRIGUEZ, Carlos; St. Albans, Bay d'Espoir, Nfld.; Kyoto Imperial (Japan) '54.
ROE, Alan A.; 809 Kipling Ave. N., Weston, Ont.; Guy's (London, Eng.) '53; M.B., B.S. (Lond.), M.R.C.S. (Eng.), L.R.C.P. (Lond.); Tel. CH 4-3662.
ROE, Bernadine V.; 347 Salter St., Winnipeg 4, Man. (res); Man '45; Anaes.; Tel. 586-7428.
ROE, John A.; 306 Royal Trust Bldg., 612 View St., Victoria, B.C.; 1870 Cochrane St. (res); McG '50; M.C.G.P.; Staff, Royal Jubilee Hosp.; Tel. EV 2-5129.
ROE, John A.; 249 Victoria Ave., Chatham, Ont.; Wes '58; FRCS(C), ObstGyn; Chief of ObstGyn., Chatham Public Gen. Hosp.; Tel. 354-3220.
ROE, Richard H.; Man'56; Res., Toronto Gen. Hosp., Toronto 2, Ont.
ROE, Robert D.; 215 E. 31st St., New York, N.Y. 10016., U.S.A.; Tor '57; FRCP(C), Neur; Abroad.
ROEBUCK, Marvin J.; 5 Fraserwood Ave., Toronto 19, Ont.; Tor '57; Anaes.; Tel. 782-5583.
ROEMMELE, Edward A.; 1590 Ouellette Ave., Ste. 203, Windsor, Ont.; 433 Askin Blvd. (res); Wes '50; M.C.G.P.; Staff, Grace & Hotel Dieu Hosp's; Tel. 252-6464.

ROFFMAN, Ruth; 11075 Trans Canada Hwy., North Surrey, B.C.; Breslau (Germ.) '41; Tel. 581-4242.

ROGER, J. David; 205 Medical Arts Bldg., 180 Metcalfe St., Ottawa 4, Ont.; 21 Withrow Ave., Ott. (res); Tor'39; MRCP(Lond.); FACP, FACC, MRCP(Lond.); FCCP; FRCP(C), IntMed; DiagRad; Phys., & Electrocard., Ottawa Civic Hosp.; Phys. & Chief of Rad., Grace Hosp.; Cons. Phys. & Cardiol., Dept. Nat. Health & Welfare; Tel. 232-4256.

ROGER, Jean P.; 1050 Ste.-Foy Rd., Quebec 6, P.Q.; 480 Pere-Marquette St. (res); Lav '26; OrthSurg; ThorSurg; Staff, Hop.-St.-Sacrement, Laval & DVA; Assoc. Prof., Laval U.; Tel. 681-7211.

ROGERS, Alicja J. (Strzalkowska); 66 Broadway Ave., Toronto 12, Ont. (res); National U. (Dublin, Ire.) '54; M.B., B.Ch., BAO; Anaes; Staff, Lockwood Clinic, 300 Bloor St. E., Toronto 5.; Tel. WA 1-2121.

ROGERS, Arnold G.; Doctor's Bldg., 394 Graham Ave., Winnipeg 1, Man.; 780 Elm St., Wpg. 9 (res); Man '50; M.Sc. (Minn.); FRCP (C), IntMed; Dir. Interne Education, Misericordia Gen. Hosp.; Lect. (Med.), U. of Manitoba; Tel. 943-9108.

ROGERS, Benson T.; Med. Dir., Northern Electric Co., 1600 Dorchester Blvd. W., Box 6123, Montreal 25, P.Q.; Tor '37; FRCP(C), IntMed; Clin. Ass't. (Indus.), Montreal Gen. Hosp.; Chmn. CMA Committ. on Occ. Med.; Dir. Counsellor, Quebec & Maritimes & Am. Indust. Med. Assoc.; Tel. 937-8541, Ext. 8415.

ROGERS, D. Daniel; Ste. 101, Med. Arts Bldg., 300 King St. W., Oshawa, Ont.; 984 Mowhawk St. (res); Tor '53; MIMA; MCGP; Tel. 728-6041.

ROGERS, Donald B.; 775 Cranston Crt., Burlington, Ont.; Tor '50; DiagRad; Staff, X-Ray Dept., St. Joseph's Hosp., Hamilton; Tel. 522-4941.

ROGERS, Francis J.; 168 Ontario St., St. Catharines, Ont.; 30 Ridgewood Dr. (res); Tor '48; DermSyph.; Tel. MU 2-8404.

ROGERS, George W.; Essex, Ont.; Tor '08.

ROGERS, Harold P.; 207 Oakwood Ave., Toronto, Ont.; Tor '13; Tel. RU 2-5102.

ROGERS, H. Derrick; 3834 Cadboro Bay Rd., Victoria, B.C.; Leeds (Eng.)'57; Tel. 477-3311.

ROGERS, Jeva U. R.; (see Lougheed, Jeva U. R.)

ROGERS, John R.; Gage Institute Chest Clinic, 223 College St., Toronto, Ont.; 4 Moccasin Terr. Don Mills (res); Tor '30; F.A.C.S., F.C.C.P., F.R.C.S.(C). GenSurg.: Tel. 924-2191.

ROGERS, J. W., Sg. Capt.; Qns '41; DPH; PH; Cdn. Forces Med. Serv., 48 Rideau St., Ottawa 2, Ont.

ROGERS, Joseph E.; 4380 Washtenaw Ave., Ann Arbor, Mich., U.S.A.; Tor'60; Psy; Abroad.

ROGERS, Joslyn W.; 419 Medical Arts Bldg., 170 St. George St., Toronto, Ont.; 161 Roxborough Dr. (res); Tor '42; F.R.C.S.(C), ObstGyn; Clin. Teacher (Obst. Gyn.), U. of Toronto, Ass't. Att. Obst. Gyn., Toronto Gen. Hosp.; Tel. WA 3-7924.

ROGERS, K. Eric; St. Catharines Med. Centre, 292 Oakdale Ave., St. Catharines, Ont.; Wes '44; FRCS(C), GenSurg.; Active Staff, St. Catharines Gen. Hosp.; Tel. MU 2-9302.

ROGERS, L. M.; 11114—87th Ave., Edmonton, Alta.; Man '19; Retired.

ROGERS, R. Hayward; Room 221, 175 E. Broadway, Vancouver, B.C.; UBC'59; Tel. 879-4551.

ROGERS, Stewart; Med. Arts Bldg., 170 St. George St., Toronto 5, Ont.; Tor '34; DermSyph; Ass't. Phys. (Derm.), Toronto Gen. Hosp.; Cons. Ontario Cancer Inst.; Ass't. Phys. I/C Derm., Princess Margaret & Hosp. for Sick Children; Assoc. (Med.), U. of Toronto; Tel. WA 1-2227.

ROGERS, Syd; Man '64; Staff, Little Long Hosp., Little Long Rapids, Ont.

ROGERS, Victor A.; 3173 Douglas St., Victoria, B.C.; 1777 Hollywood Cr. (res); Liverpool (Eng.) '39; FACA; DMRD; Anaes; Tel. 385-8332.

ROGOMAN, Edith P.; Room 15, 501 Yonge St., Toronto 5, Ont.; Sask'57; FRCP(C), Anaes; Staff, Women's College Hosp.; Tel. WA 3-7381.

ROGSTAD, Vernon J.; Watson, Sask.; UBC'56; Staff, Watson Union Hospital; Tel. 287-3344.

ROHM, Walter; Vienna (Aust.) '52; DABPN; Psy; Staff, Hosp. for Mental Diseases, Brandon, Man.; Tel. PA 6-2321. Abroad.

ROHR, Ernest A.; 104 Dental Medical Bldg., 59 Court St. N., Port Arthur, Ont.; 29 Strathcona Ave. (res); Greifswald (Germ.) '40; F.C.C.P.; A.M.C.G.P.; Tel. 345-9981.

ROJKO, Andrew; Tor'60; Anaes; Staff, Branson Hosp., Willowdale, Ont.

ROLAND, Charles G.; American Med. Assoc., 535 North Dearborn St., Chicago, Ill., U.S.A.; Man'58; MCGP; Abroad.

ROLFE, Hedley C.; The Pas Assoc. Med. Clinic, The Pas, Man.; Birmingham (Eng.)'55; DPH (Tor); MRCS(Eng.); LRCP(Lond.); Staff, St. Anthony's Hosp.; Tel. 3-3477.

ROLLAND, Gaston; 29 rue Picard, Ste.-Martine, Co. Chateauguay, P.Q.; Mon '60; AMCGP; Tel. 457-2219.

ROLLAND, Gerard; Clinique Jeanne Mance, 7820 rue Marquette, Montreal 35, P.Q.; Mon '31; F.I.C.S., GenSurg; ThorSurg (P.Q.); Tel. 729-6371.

ROLLAND, Paul E.; 165 Victoria, Longueuil, Montreal, P.Q.; Lav'42; Tel. 674-8048.

ROLLAND, Romeo; 5523 Wellington, Verdun, Montreal 19, P.Q.; Mon '44; Vis. Staff, Hop.-Gen.-de-Verdun; Tel. 767-4882.

ROLLAND, Walter; 221 Brant Ave., Brantford, Ont.; 34 Kingsway Cres. (res); Tor '49; F.A.C.S., F.R.C.S.(C), GenSurg; Active Cons. Staff, Dept. of Surg., Brantford Gen. & St. Joseph's Hosp's.; Tel. PL 3-6322.

ROLLINS, Nelles; Box 111, Wadena, Sask.; Man '14.

ROMAGNOLI, Alexander; 44 Highfield Ave., Montreal 16, P.Q. (res); Florence (Italy) '49; **D.A. (McGill); Anaes., Jewish Gen. Hosp.; Tel. 735-3771.**

ROMAN, Leslie; St. George St., Alexandria, Ont.; Ott'62.

ROMANICK, Natalia; 376 The Kingsway N., Islington, Ont.; Tel. BE 3-0144.

ROMANO, Walter L.; 705 Medical Arts Bldg., 1011 Ouellette Ave., Windsor, Ont.; Tor '57; Diag-Rad.; Tel. 254-7551.

ROMANOWSKI, Edward; 10316-132nd Street, Edmonton, Alta.; Poznan (Poland)'37; Chief, Internal Medicine, Charles Camsell Hospital.

ROMBOUGH, William G.; 749 King St. W., Kitchener, Ont.; Tor'56; **Ophth; Staff, St. Mary's** Gen. & Kitchener-Waterloo Gen. Hospitals; Tel. 576-4450.

ROMEO, Michael A.; Tor'61; Res., Toronto Gen. Hosp., Toronto 2, Ont.

ROMERA-SIERRA, Cesar; Zaragoza (Spain); Staff, Dept. of Anat., U. of Ottawa, Ottawa, Ont.

ROMEYN, James A.; Dept. of Bact. & Immun., Manitoba Med. Schl., Emily and Bannatyne Sts., Winnipeg, Man.; 320 Waverley St., Wpg. 9 (res); Tor '39; D.Phil. (Oxon), Dip. Bact. (Tor.); Bact; Assoc. Prof. Bact., U. of Manitoba; Tel. 786-3522.

ROMNEY, David; Ste. G04, 3000 Lawrence Ave. E., Scarborough, Ont.; 41 Bendale Blvd. (res); **Trinity College (Dublin, Ire.) '50; IntMed; Att'd. Staff, Scarborough Gen. Hosp.; Tel. 291-1481.**

RONA, Agnes (Szilas); Budapest (Hung.) '52; Staff, Path. Inst., McGill U., Montreal 2, P.Q.

RONA, George; 80 Henley Ave., Twn. of Mount Royal, Montreal 16, P.Q.; Budapest (Hung.) '49; Ph.D., FCAP; DABP; M.C.Path; FRCP(C), Path; Path. & Dir. of Labs., Lakeshore Gen. Hosp.; Ass't. Prof. (Path.), McGill U.; Tel. 695-1311.

RONA-REVESZ, Clara; 4474 Circle Rd., Montreal, P.Q.; Budapest (Hung.) '36; Paed; Sr. Endocrin., Ayerst, McKenna & Harrison; Tel. 739-7517.

RONA, Steven; 615 Westmount Med. Bldg., 5025 Sherbrooke St. W., Montreal, P.Q.; Budapest (Hung.) '34; DIM (McG.); MCGP; M.O., Health Serv., Queen Elizabeth Hosp.; Tel. 488-5782.

RONALD, Alfred C.; 2917 Bloor St. W., Toronto; Ste. 3, Humbertown Centre, Islington, Ont.; 9 Hartfield Ct. (res); Capetown (S. Africa) '47; M.B., Ch.B., M.R.C.P. (Lon.); IntMed; Staff Phys., Toronto Hosp., Weston; Assoc. Staff, St. Joseph's Hosp., Toronto; Tel. BE 3-4511.

RONAN, Alice K.; 4742 Drummond Dr., Vancouver 8, B.C.; McG'47; FACA; Anaes.; Tel. 224-7181.

RONCAIOLI, Joseph S.; Tor'60; Res., Wellesley Hosp., Toronto 5, Ont.

RONCARI, Daniel A.; Qns '61; Jr. Intn., Montreal Gen. Hosp., Montreal 25, P.Q.

RONDEAU, Guy; Huberdeau, Co. Argenteuil, P.Q.; Mon '60; Instr., Soc.-Peda. Centre, Mtl.; Tel. Area-819; 687-3233.

RONDEAU, Jacques; St-Denis-sur-Richelieu, P.Q.; Mon. '61; Tel. 787-2112.

RONDEAU, Rene; 2279 Blvd. des Chutes, St. Louis de Courville, P.Q. (res); Lav '50; Retired.

RONDEAU-RIVARD, Lucie; 415 rue Lemesurier, Quebec 6, P.Q.; Lav '61.

RONDEAU, Yvon; 757 Thibault, Ste-Therese-en-Haut, Cte Terrebonne, P.Q.; Mon'56; Anaes.; Staff, Hop. Gen. St-Eustache.

ROOK, Lionel A.; Box 998 Vernon, B.C.; 2403 - 23rd Ave. (res); Cambridge (Eng.) '42; M.R.C.S., L.R.C.P., D.O.M.S.; Ophth.; Tel. 542-5800.

ROOKS, John H.; Wes '52; Staff, Inuvik General Hosp., Inuvik, N.W.T.

ROOS, Jaan O.; 3252 Lawrence Ave. E., Scarborough, Ont.; Tor '63; Court. Staff, Scarborough Gen. Hosp.; Tel. 293-7201.

ROOT, Howard S.; 4858 Westmount Ave., Westmount, P.Q. (res); McG'40; Retired.

ROPER, Peter D. L.; 1025 Pine Ave. W., Montreal 2, **P.Q.; 43 Mont Savage Rd., Ste-Adele** (res); **Glasgow (Scot.) '51; D.P.M. (Lond.); Psy; Cons. Staff, Royal Victoria & Queen Mary Vet's Hosp's.; Teach Staff. McGill U.; Tel. VI 2-1251.**

ROQUE, Nabor G.; 340 Campbell St., Nanaimo, B.C.; Philipp.'55; OrthSurg.; Tel. 753-3202.

RORABECK, Cecil H.; Dept. of Health, Parliament Bldgs., Queen's Park, Toronto 5, Ont.; Tor '40; Dir., T.B. Prev. Branch, Dept. of Health; Spec. Lect. (T.B.), U. of Toronto; Memb. Silicosis Referee Bd.: Tel. 365-2528.

ROSALES, Jose K.; 2300 Tupper St., Montreal 25, P.Q.; 64 Banstead Rd., Mtl. W. (res); Santo Tomas (Manila, Philippines) '49; DABA; FACA; FRCP(C), Anaes; Staff (Anaes). Mtl. Children's & Reddy Mem. Hosp's.; Lect. Anaes), McGill U.; Tel. WE 7-8511.

ROSE, Arnold; 90 Erie Ave., Brantford, Ont.; Tor '39; M.C.G.P.; Staff, Brantford Gen. & St. Joseph's Hosp.; Tel. 753-6904.

ROSE-BERNSTEIN, Vera; 201 Coldstream Ave., Toronto 12, Ont.; London (Eng.) '52; Paed; Clin. Ass't. & Research Assoc., Dept. of Cardiol., Hosp. for Sick Children; Tel. EM 3-1211.

ROSE, Bram; 636 Victoria Ave., Westmount, Montreal, P.Q. (res); McG '33; Ph.D.; FACP; FRSC; MCAA; Allerg (P.Q.); IntMed Phys., & Dir., Div of Immunochem., Royal Victoria Hosp.; Assoc. Prof., McGill U.; Tel. VI 2-1251, Loc. 455/439.

ROSE, Clayton C.; 37 Wellington St. E., Aurora, Ont.; Tor '52; MCGP; Vice Pres., York County Hosp.; Tel. 727-9447.

ROSE, Crawford; 37 Wellington St. E., Aurora, Ont.; Man '26; M.C.G.P.

ROSE, Frederick L.; 848 Dundas St., London, Ont.; 1128 Sunset Ave. (res); Wes '30; M.C.G.P.; 1st Vice-Pres., London Acad. of Med. & Mem. Exec. Comm. Victoria Hosp.; Tel. 439-5141.

ROSE, Hugh A.; Tor '56; Res., Vancouver Gen. Hosp., Vancouver, B.C.

ROSE, Ian R.; Irving Clinic, 74 W. Seymour, Kamloops, B.C.; 325 McGill Rd. (res); London (Eng.) '48; M.B. B.S., MRCS; LRCP; Active Staff, Royal Inland Hosp.; Tel. 372-5251.

ROSE, John E.; 306 Medical Arts Bldg., Winnipeg, Man.; 222 Harvard Ave. (res); Man '40; D.A.B.O., Ophth; Ass't. Ophth., Winnipeg Gen. & Children's Hosp's.; Ass't. Prof., Ophth., U. of Manitoba; Tel. WH 3-4839.

ROSE, John W.; Cobourg Clinic, 188 King St. W., Cobourg, Ont.; Durham (Eng.) '51; Staff, Cobourg Dist. Gen. Hosp.; Tel. 372-3323.

ROSE, Lewis C.; 111—9th St., Brandon, Man.; 97 Clark Dr. (res); London (Eng.)'54; MCGP; D.Obst. RCOG; Staff (Med.), Brandon Gen. Hosp **& Assiniboine Hosp.; Tel. PA 9-5471.**

ROSE, Mervyn; 147 Northover Street, Downsview, Ont.; Dublin (Ire.)'57; LRCS; MCGP; Tel. 636-6677.

ROSE, Patrick B.; 8311-120th St., Edmonton, Alta (res); Alb '42; M.C.G.P.; Dir., Div. of Medical Services, Dept. of Health, Alberta; Sess. Instr., U. of Alta; Tel. GE 3-5545.

ROSE, Ralph; 1383 Davenport Rd., Toronto, Ont.; Tor '37; M.C.G.P.; Tel. LE 5-8000.

ROSE, Roger C.; 60 Albert St. W., Thorold, Ont.; Birmingham (Eng.)'64; MRCS; LRCP.

ROSE, R. Viola (Vail); 137 Park Ave., Brantford, Ont.; R.R. No. 1, St. George (res); Wes '36; MCGP; D.Psy; Psy Staff St. Joseph & Brantford Gen. Hosp's.; Tel. 753-0432.

ROSE, Theodore F.; 645 Fort St., Victoria, B.C.; 905 Pemberton Rd. (res); McG '43; IntMed. Tel. EV 2-3641.

ROSE, Vera (Bernstein); London (Eng.) '53; Paed; Research Assoc., Cardiol Dept., Hosp. for Sick Children, Toronto, Ont.; Tel. 366-7242.

ROSEBOROUGH, George F.; Ste. 307, 723 Fort St., Victoria, B.C.; Qns '55; Ophth; Tel. 383-7833.

ROSEBOROUGH, Jane F.; Ste 603, 1849 Yonge St., Toronto 7, Ont.; Tor'63; O.P.D. Staff, St. Michael's Hosp.; Tel. 485-8117.

ROSEN, David A.; Etherington Hall, Stuart St., Kingston, Ont.; 45 Hillcroft Dr. (res); McG '49; FACS, FRCS(C), Ophth; Hd. Dept. of Ophth, Kingston Gen. Hosp.; Cons. (Ophth), DVA, Cdn. Forces Hosp.; Prof. Ophth, Queen's U.; Tel. 546-2974.

ROSEN, Edward J.; Clarke Inst. of Psy., 250 College St., Toronto 2, Ont.; McG'42; D.Psy; Psy; Ass't. Prof. Psy., U. of Toronto; Tel. 924-6811.

ROSEN, Fred; Tor '62; Res., Toronto Gen. Hosp., Toronto 2, Ont.

ROSEN, Gerald P.; 732 Spadina Ave., Toronto 4, Ont.; Tor '59; FRCS(C), Otol; Active Staff, St. Joseph's & New Mount Sinai Hosp's.; Clin. Teach (ENT), U. of Toronto; Tel. WA 3-2233.

ROSEN, Harold J.; Med. Arts Bldg., 115 Hazen St., Saint John, N.B.; 38-5th St. (res); McG '44; M.Sc., Dip., NeurSurg; FACS; FRCS(C), NeurSurg; Dir. (NeurSurg), St. John Gen. Hosp.; Cons. (NeurSurg.), St. Joseph's Lancaster DVA, St. John's TB & Prov. Mental Hosp's.; Tel. 693-2837.

ROSEN, Irving B.; 99 Avenue Rd., Ste. 606, Toronto 5, Ont.; 82 Heathcote Ave. (res); Tor '54; FRCS(C), GenSurg; Att'd. Surg., New **Mt. Sinai Hosp.; Clin. Teach. U. of Toronto;** Tel. WA 4-9824.

ROSEN, Irving E.; Tor'60; FRCP(C), DiagRad; Staff, Hosp. for Sick Children, Toronto, Ont.

ROSEN, Ivor; 620 Jane St., Toronto 9, Ont.; 2 Brentwood Rd. N. (res); St. Bart's (London, Eng.) '44; M.B., B.S. (Lond.), M.R.C.S. (Eng.), L.R.C.P. (Lon.); Tel. RO 6-8833.

ROSEN, Lawrence J.; 333 Wilson Ave., Ste. 201, Downsview, Ont.; 235 Betty Ann Dr., Willowdale (res); Tor '54; Paed; Allergy; Staff Toronto Western Hosp., Allergy Clin.; Staff, Mount Sinai & North York Branson Hosp's.; Tel. ME 5-5581.

ROSEN, Martin S.; Woodview Park Med. Centre, 3236 Weston Rd., Weston, Ont.; 8 Alonzo Rd., Willowdale (res); Tor '50; M.C.G.P.; O.P.D. Staff, New Mt. Sinai & Doctor's Hosp's., Toronto; Tel. Tel. CH 1-9129.

ROSEN, Norman J.; Man '59; Jr. Int'n., Winnipeg Gen. Hosp., Winnipeg, Man.

ROSEN, Phillip S.; Ste. 402, 99 Avenue Rd., Toronto 5, Ont.; Tor'52; FRCP(C), IntMed; Cons., D.V.A. Sunnybrook Hosp.; Clin. Teach. Med., U. of Toronto; Tel. 921-4912.

ROSEN, Sydney I.; 333 Wilson Ave., Downsview, Ont.; 7 St. Margaret's Dr., Tor 12 (res); Tor '46; DABP; Paed; Staff, New Mt. Sinai, Hosp. & Hosp. for Sick Children; Tel. ME 5-5581.

ROSENBAUM, Peter; 1414 Drummond St., Montreal, P.Q.; McG '54; Ophth; Ass't. Ophth., Royal Victoria Hosp.; Cons. Ophth., Royal Edward Hosp.; Dem. Ophth., McGill U.; Tel. VI 5-8021.

ROSENBERG, Albert; 1868 Portage Ave., St. James, Man.; 45 Fidler Ave., Silver Heights (res); Man '52; M.C.G.P.; Tel. TU 8-2309.

ROSENBERG, Arthur; Qns '61; Jr. Intn., Hotel Dieu Hosp., Kingston, Ont.

ROSENBERG, Edwin M.; Dal'65; Res., Victoria General Hosp., Halifax, N.S.

ROSENBERG, Gilbert, 5845 Cote-des-Neiges Rd., Ste. 350, Montreal 26, P.Q.; 5015 Hingston Ave., Mtl. 29 (res); McG '49; DIM; M.Sc., (Exper. Med.); IntMed; Ass't. Phys., Jewish Gen. Hosp.; Phys.-in-Chief, Maimonides Hosp. & Home for the Aged; Clin. Ass't. (Med.), Reddy Mem. Hosp.; Tel. 735-0001.

ROSENBERG, Horace D.; 2333 Tampa Ave., Ottawa 1, Ont. (res); Edinburgh (Scot.) '37; M.C.G.P.; M.O., Can. Pension Comm. Tel. CE 2-8211.

ROSENBLATT, Adam; 159 Vaughan Rd., Toronto 10, Ont.

ROSENBLATT, Jacob; Qns'58; Staff, Div. of TB Control, Vancouver Gen. Hosp., Vancouver 9, B.C.

ROSENFELD, Hirsh; 4575 Park Ave., Montreal, P.Q.; 31 Maplewood, Outremont (res); Strassbourg (Fr.) '36; MCGP; Med. Dir., Doctor's Hosp. Inc.; Tel. RE 9-7771.

ROSENFELD, Jacques; 3945 Tecumseh Rd. E., Windsor, Ont.; Jerusalem (Israel)'58.

ROSENFELD, Michael W.; 2660 E. Hastings St., Vancouver 6, B.C.; 2190 W. 43rd Ave. (res); UBC '60; AMCGP; Vis. Staff, Vancouver Gen., Grace & St. Paul's Hosp's.; Active Staff, Holy Family Hosp.; Tel. AM 6-4334.

ROSENFELD, Robert; Geneva (Switz.)'64; Res., Children's Hosp., Montreal 25, P.Q.

ROSENFIELD, Morley; 530 Broadway Ave., Winnipeg, Man.; 175 Academy Rd. (res); Man '52; F.R.C.S.(C), GenSurg.; Tel. SU 3-7214.

ROSENFIELD, Victor L.; Rosenfield Med. Bldg., 530 Broadway Ave., Winnipeg, Man.; 766 Wellington (res); Man '35; M.C.G.P.; Pres. Med. Staff, Victoria Hosp.; Tel. SU 3-7214.

ROSENHEK, Clarence; 1248 Chemin Ste-Foy, Quebec 6, P.Q.; McG '40; Staff, Jeffrey Hale's Hosp.; Tel. 683-4878.

ROSENQUIST, G. E. (see SWENSSON-ROSENQUIST)

ROSENRAUCH, Salomon; 710 College St., Toronto 4, Ont.; Rome (Italy)'37.

ROSENSWEIG, Jacob; 3755 Cote-St.-Catherine Rd., Montreal 26, P.Q.; McG'55; FACS; FRCS(C), GenSurg; ThorSurg; Assoc. Surg., Jewish Gen. Hosp.; Cons. (ThorSurg), Mt. Sinai Hosp., Prefontaine; Tel. 735-3771, Loc. 550.

ROSENTHAL, Donald; Ste 520, 143 James St. S., Hamilton, Ont.; Tor '58; FRCP(C), Derm; Acting Chief Derm. Serv., St. Joseph's Hosp.; Tel. 525-1450.

ROSENTHALL, Leonard; 5719 Sunrise Ave., Cote-St.-Luc, Montreal 29, P.Q. (res); McG '56; DABR; D & T Rad; Staff, Mtl. Gen. Hosp.; Teach. Staff, McGill U.; Tel. WE 7-6011.

ROSERE, L. A.; 152 Ochterloney St., Dartmouth, N.S.; Dal '32.

ROSHER, Frank W.; 412 Canada Bldg., 101-21st St. E., Saskatoon, Sask.; 201-6th St. E. (res); Alb '31; M.C.G.P.; Staff, St. Paul's Saskatoon City & University Hosp's.; Teach (Surg.), University Hosp.; Tel. 244-7477.

ROSMAN, Michael A.; Ott'65; Res., Montreal General Hosp., Montreal 25, P.Q.

ROSMAN, Norman P.; McG '59; FRCP(C), Neur; Staff, Massachusetts Gen. Hosp., Boston 14, Mass. U.S.A.; Abroad.

ROSMUS, Horst; Hamburg (Germ.) '44; Res., Royal Victoria Hosp., Montreal 2, P.Q.

ROSOL, Tadeusz; 312 Roncesvalles Ave., Toronto, Ont.; Poznan (Poland) '33; Tel. LE 3-1558.

ROSS, Alan S.; 2300 Tupper St., Montreal 25, P.Q.; 653 Belmont Ave., Westmount (res); McG '27; F.R.C.P.(C), Paed; Phys-in-Chief Montreal Children's Hosp.; Chm. Dept. of Paed., McGill U.; Tel. WE 7-8511.

ROSS, Alexander G.; Elk Point, Alta.; McG '22.

ROSS, Anthony L.; 358 Reynolds St. N., Oakville, Ont.; Birmingham (Eng.)'50; MRCS(Eng.); LRCP(Lond).

ROSS, Arthur E.; 331 Sheddon Ave., Oakville, Ont.; Qns '49; MCGP; Tel. 845-3415.

ROSS, Arthur W.; 272 St. George, Moncton, N.B.; Dal '31; OphthOtol; Sr. Ophth. Otol., Moncton Hosp.; Tel. 855-7262.

ROSS, Cecil C., OBE; 291 Dundas St., London, Ont.; 406 Regent St. (res); Man '24; FRCS (Edin.), FRCS(C), GenSurg; OrthSurg; Surg., Victoria Gen. & St. Joseph's Hosp's.; Asst't. Prof. (Surg.), U. of Western Ont.; Retired.

ROSS, Charles B.; 320 Muskoka St., Gravenhurst, Ont.; McG '21; IntMed (TB); Tel. 687-2586.

ROSS, Colin A.; 508 Med. Arts Bldg., Edmonton, Alta.; Alb '43; FICS, FCCP, FACS, FRCS(C), GenSurg; ThorSurg; Lect. (ThorSurg), U. of Alberta; Tel. GA 4-6242.

ROSS, Colin S.; North Toronto Med. Bldg., 250 Lawrence Ave. W., Toronto 12, Ont.; 189 Dunvegan Rd., Tor. 7 (res); Tor '50; MCGP; Att'd. Staff (OPD) Tor. Western Hosp.; Med. Dir. Munich Reinsurance Co. (Canada); Tel. 789-4981.

ROSS, Donald A.; 3310 Boundary, Vancouver 12, B.C.; Tor'51; Tel. 434-3131.

ROSS, Douglas R.; Box 370, Sidney, B.C.; McG '33; GenSurg; Chief of Staff, Resthaven Hosp.; Tel. 656-1164.

ROSS, Dudley E., ED; St.-Adolphe d'Howard, P.Q.; McG '21; F.A.C.S., F.R.C.S.(C).

ROSS, Edward L.; 800 Sherbrook, Winnipeg 2, Man.; 418 Kingston Cres., St. Vital (res); Man '25; IntMed (TB); Lect. (Med.), U. of Manitoba; Admin., Sanatorium Bd. of Manitoba; Tel. 755-0181.

ROSS, Edwin F.; 5880 Spring Garden Rd., Halifax, N.S.; Dal '31; FACS; FRCS(C), GenSurg; Att'd. Surg., Victoria Gen. & Halifax Children's Hosp's.; Cons. Surg., Camp Hill DVA Hosp.; Assoc. Prof. Surg., Dal. Med. School; Tel. 423-8540.

ROSS, Elizabeth (Douglas); 1929 Rosebank Ave., Halifax, N.S. (res); Dal '52; Paed; Active Staff, Children's Hosp.; Lect. Dalhousie U.; Tel. 423-0394.

ROSS, Francis R.; 15 E. Moira St., Belleville, Ont.; Qns '36; Tel. WO 8-8511.

ROSS, Gordon T.; 166 Main St. W., North Bay, Ont.; 925 Beattie St. (res); Wes '45; M.C.G.P.; Tel. 472-3770.

ROSS, Helen E.; Wes '64; Res., Montreal Gen. Hosp., Montreal 25, P.Q.

ROSS, Henry B.; 6252 Quinpool Rd., Halifax, N.S.; 10 Connaught Ave (res); Dal '42; FAAP; Paed; Assoc. Phys., Halifax Children's Hosp.; Staff (Paed), Grace Matern. Hosp.; Assoc. Prof. (Paed), Dalhousie U.; Tel. 423-9147.

ROSS, Henry G.; 519 Med. Arts Bldg., 11010 Jasper Ave., Edmonton, Alta.; Capetown (S. Africa)'52; ObstGyn.

ROSS, H. Graham; 657 Lansdowne Ave., Montreal 6, P.Q. (res); McG'24; Phys., Bathurst Containers Ltd., & Rolls-Royce Co.; Tel. HU 6-0807.

ROSS, H. Raymond; 69 Townsend St., Sydney, N.S.; Dal '21; F.A.C.S.; GenSurg.

ROSS, Hugh M.; 211 Oxford St., Winnipeg 9, Man. (res); Tor '42; Path; Assoc. Path., Winnipeg Gen. Hosp; Lect. (Path.), U. of Manitoba; Tel. SP 4-6511; Loc. 657.

ROSS, Hugh M.; 5929 Athlone St., Vancouver, B.C. (res); Tor '26; M.O., W.C.B. of B.C.; Tel. AM 6-0211.

ROSS, Hugo F.; Weyburn, Sask.; Man'49; Psy; Ass't Supt., Saskatchewan Hosp.; Tel. 842-5461, Ext. 290.

ROSS, James B.; 122A-16th Ave. N.E., Calgary, Alta.; Man'59.

ROSS, James F.; Ste 406, Med. Arts Bldg., 5880 Spring Garden Rd., Halifax, N.S.; 1929 Rosebank Ave. (res); Dal '51; FRCS(C), PlasSurg; GenSurg; Cons. (PlasSurg), Victoria Gen., Hlfx. Infirm., Children's, Camp Hill & Cdn. Forces Hosp., HMCS Stadacona; Tel. 423-7008.

ROSS, James L.; 422 London, Sherbrooke, P.Q.; McG'54; FRCS(C); GenSurg; AMCGP; Staff, Sherbrooke & St. Vincent De Paul Hospitals; Tel. 569-2715.

ROSS, James W.; 2A Glengrove Ave. W., Toronto 12, Ont.; 14 Glenrush Blvd (res); Tor '15; FACS; GenSurg.

ROSS, Janet K. (Lang); 461 Eglinton Ave. E., Toronto 12, Ont.; 1 Orchard Green, Tor. 17 (res); Tor'38; MCGP; Assoc. Staff, Women's College Hosp.; Tel. 425-1272.

ROSS, J. Barrie; 8 Campbell Ave., St. John's Nfld.; Durham (Eng.) '54; D.ObstRCOG; FRCP (C), Derm; Chief of Derm., Grace Hosp.; Active Staff, St. Clare's Hosp.; Assoc. Staff, Gen. Hosp.; Tel. 579-9672.

ROSS, J. Donovan; 8211 - 107th St., Edmonton, Alta.; 10604 83rd Ave. (res); Alb '37; M.C.G.P.; Minister of Health (Alta.); Tel. CA 9-3443.

ROSS, John A.; 170 Ripplewood Cres., Kitchener, Ont.; Tor '38; MCGP; Staff, Kitchener-Waterloo & St. Mary's Hosp's.; Tel. 742-2435.

ROSS, John C.; 96 West St., Goderich, Ont.; Tor '24; M.C.G.P.; Retired.

ROSS, John E.; 1010 Fairmont Med. Bldg., 750 W. Broadway, Vancouver 9, B.C.; Qns '44; Clin. Instr. U. of British Columbia; Tel. TR 2-5467.

ROSS, John G.; 290 Sheldon Ave. N., Kitchener, Ont. (res); Tor '44; Cert. Life Ins. Med.; Assoc. Medical Dir., Mutual Life Assurance Co. of Canada., 227 King St. S., Waterloo; Tel. 744-6171.

ROSS, John M.; Aberdeen (Scot.) '53; MCGP; Staff, Placentia Hosp., Placentia, Nfld.

ROSS, John R.; Box 880, Campbell River, B.C.; UBC '56.

ROSS, John R.; 216 St. Clair Ave. W., Toronto, Ont.; 3 Bluejay Pl. (res); Tor '26; A.A.A., M.C.A.A., Paed; Assoc. Phys., Hosp. for Sick Children; Tel. WA 3-9119.

ROSS, John T.; 34 Paget St., New Liskeard, Ont.; 30 Paget St. (res); Tor '50.

ROSS, Lorne E.; Box 310, Ashcroft, B.C.; Qns '52; Tel. 453-2525.

ROSS, Louis H.; 403 Dundas St. West, Toronto, Ont.; Tor'31; MCGP; Court. Med. Staff, New Mt. Sinai Hosp.; Tel. 368-9780.

ROSS, Malcolm M.; Apt. 207, 5820 Decarie Blvd., Montreal 9, P.Q.; McG '29.

ROSS, Marion; 58 Forest Heights Blvd., Willowdale, Ont.; (res); Tor '34; Dip. Bact. (London), Bact; Dir. of Bact., Sunnybrook Hosp.; Lect., (Bact.), U. of Toronto; Tel. 485-8651.

ROSS, Michael A.; Ste. 270, 1070 Douglas St., Victoria, B.C.; 2197 Lafayette (res); Liverpool (Eng.) '59; Tel. 282-8895.

ROSS, M. B.; Tor '59; Jr. Int'n., New Mount Sinai Hosp., Toronto, Ont.

ROSS, Peggy L. (Andreen); 18 Denver Cres., Willowdale, Ont.; UBC'58; Anaes; Tel. 368-2581.

ROSS, R. Alexander; Dal'65; Med. Officer in charge, Padden Memorial Hospital, Happy Valley, Labrador.

ROSS, Robert T.; 317-404 Graham Ave., Winnipeg 1, Man.; Man '48; MRCP (Lond.), FRCP(C), Neur; Neurol., Wpg. Gen. Hosp.; Assoc. Prof. (Med.), U. of Manitoba; Tel. WH 2-3341.

ROSS, Roderick C.; Dept. of Path., St. Michael's Hosp., Toronto 2, Ont.; Tor'40; MSc(Path); FRCP (C), Path; Path-in-Chief, St. Michael's Hosp.; Assoc. Prof. Path., U. of Toronto; Tel. 362-4461, Loc. 580.

ROSS, Roderick C.; 117 King St. E., Oshawa, Ont.; 24 Rossland Rd. E. (res); Tor '48; ObstGyn. Tel. 728-1661.

ROSS, S. Graham; DSO; 1390 Sherbrooke St. W., Montreal, P.Q.; 65 Rosemount Cres., Westmount (res); McG '13; FRCP(Lond.), FRCP(C), Paed; Hon. Att'd Staff, Royal Victoria Hosp.; Retired.

ROSS, Stephen R.; Medical Centre, 707 Charlotte St., Peterborough, Ont.; Tor'60; FRCS(C), GenSurg.

ROSS, Thomas H.; Proctor St., Hanover, Ont.; Wes'44; Tel. 364-1990.

ROSS, William C.; 1625 Oak Bay Ave., Victoria, B.C.; 601-240 Douglas (res); UBC'54; Tel. EV 5-8513.

ROSS, William R.; Box 878, Steinbach, Man.; Man. '56; Tel. DA 6-2522.

ROSS, W. Jack; 273 Tache Ave., Winnipeg 4, Man.; 385 Dubue St., St. Boniface (res); Man '57; A.M.C.G.P.

ROSS, Winifred M.; Apt. 604, 3620 Ridgewood Ave., Montreal 26, P.Q.; McG '52; ObstGyn; TherRad; Dip. Radiotherapy (McGill); Clin. Ass't. Dept. of TherRad, Royal Victoria Hosp.; Dem. Rad., McGill U.; Tel. VI 2-1251.

ROSS, W. J.; Man '57; P.G., St. Boniface Hosp., St. Boniface, Man.

ROSSALL, Richard E.; 8831 Saskatchewan Dr., Edmonton, Alta.; Leeds (Eng.) '50; M.B., Ch.B., MRCP(Lond.); FRCP(C), IntMed; Active Staff, University Hosp.; Cons. Cardiol., DVA & Student Health Serv., U. of Alberta; Ass't. Prof. (Med.), U. of Alberta; Tel. 439-5911, Loc. 348.

ROSSET, Mark; 314 St. Clair Ave. W. Toronto 10, Ont.; Paris (Fr.)'40; FRCP(C), DermSyph; Staff (Derm.), St. Joseph's Hosp.; Cons. (Derm.), Queensway Gen. & Hon. Cons. (Derm.), South Peel Hosp's.; Tel. WA 2-0061.

ROSSI, Servio; 6809 Lawrence Blvd., Montreal 10, P.Q.; Rome (Italy)'50; ObstGyn (P.Q.); Tel. CR 1-6667.

ROSSIGNOL, Jean P.; 374 Besserer, Ottawa 2, Ont.; Mon '52; Anaes; Anaes., Hop. St. Louis-Marie-deMonfort; Lect. (Anaes.), U. of Ottawa; Tel. SH 6-4621.

ROSSITER, Helen M. (Randell); 287 Queens Ave., London, Ont.; 504 Colborne St. (res); Edinburgh (Scot.) '40; DA; FFARCS; Active Staff St. Joseph's Hosp.; Tel. GE 8-5143.

ROSSISTER, Roger J.; 504 Colborne St., London, Ont. (res); Oxford (Eng.) '41; D.Phil.; DM; FRIC (Eng.); FRCS; Cons. Med., Westminster, St. Joseph's & Victoria Hosp's.; Dean, Fac. of Graduate Studies & Prof. of Biochem., U. of Western Ontario; Tel. GE 9-1681.

ROSSITTER, Fergus P.; Suite 507, 215 Victoria St., Toronto 2, Ont.; 4 Hi Mount Dr., Willowdale (res); Tor '36; Anaes; Staff Anaes., St. Michael's Hosp.; Tel. 362-4461.

ROSTANT, John; McG'52; Res., Montreal Gen. Hosp., Montreal 2, P.Q.

ROSTANT, Leonard A.; R.R. No. 1, Monastery, N.S.; London (England) '26; Surg., Hydrographic Ship, Baffin; Staff, Dept. of National Health & Welfare.

ROSTOCKA, Maria; Louvain (Belgium) '51; Staff, Nova Scotia San., Kentville, N.S.

ROSTOCKY, Winona M.; (See Copping, Winona).

ROSTRON, Barbara J.; Manchester (Eng.) '57; DObstRCOG; Res., Colonel Belcher Hosp., Calgary, Alta.

ROSTRUP, Olav; 108 Med. Arts Bldg., Edmonton, Alta.; 8926 Windsor Rd. (res); Alb '37; FACS, DABOS, FAAOS, FRCS(C), OrthSurg; Cons. OrthSurg., DVA & Chas. Camsell Hosp.; Cons. Royal Alexandra Hosp.; Chief OrthSurg., University Hosp.; Prof. & Dir. (OrthSurg). U. of Alberta; Tel. 422-6216.

ROTA, Alexander N.; 35 Rosewood Ave., Belleville, Ont.; Tor'49; M.Sc.; Path; Chm. Dept. of Lab. Med., Belleville Gen. Hosp.; Dir. Clin. Lab., Prince Edward County Mem. Hosp.; Instr. (Path), Queen's U., Kingston; Reg. Path., Attorney Gen. Dept.; Tel. WO 8-5511.

ROTENBERG, Cyril; 5 Glen Rush Blvd., Toronto, Ont. (res); Tor '43; D&TRad; Ass't. Att. Rad., Toronto East Gen. Hosp.; Staff, Doctors' Hosp.; Tel. 927-3202.

ROTENBERG, Hertzel; Albany Clinic, 200 Danforth Ave., Toronto 6, Ont.; Tor'45; Otol; Tel. 461-0761.

ROTENBERG, Manie; 732 Spadina Ave., Toronto, Ont.; 26 Farrington Dr., Willowdale (res); Tor '52; Anaes; Staff, New Mt. Sinai Hosp.; Tel. HU 7-7405.

ROTGANS, Sheila M. (McClements); Box 248 Sooke, B.C.; Bristol (Eng.) '56; MB, Ch.B; Tel 472-3114.

ROTH, Edward; Jewish Hosp. of Hope, 7745 Sherbrooke St. E., Montreal 5, P.Q.; Tor'53; Med Dir., Jewish Hosp. of Hope; Tel. RI 8-8127.

ROTH, F. Burns; 95 The Kingsway, Toronto 18, Ont. (res); Wes '36; Prof. & Hd., Dept. of Hosp. Admin., School of Hygiene. U. of Toronto; Tel. 928-2736.

ROTHBART-FOX, Zelda R.; 5037 Ponsard Ave., Montreal 29, P.Q.; Tor'47; AMCAA; Paed; Allergy (P.Q.); Att'd. Staff, Paed. & Allergy, Montreal Children's Hosp.; Tel. 484-5683.

ROTHER, Irving; 316 St. Clair Ave. W., Toronto 7, Ont.; Tor'43; FRCP(C) Int Med; Clin. Ass't. (Med.), Toronto Gen. Hosp.; Sr. Att. Staff, New Mt. Sinai Hosp.; Dem. (Clin. Microscopy), U. of Toronto; Tel. 924-3123.

ROTHSTEIN, Bernard; Ste. 435, 6000 Cote des Neiges Rd., Montreal 26, P.Q.; McG'51; FRCS (C), GenSurg; Staff, Jean Talon & Jewish Gen. Hosps.; Tel. 733-1461.

ROTHWELL, Alfred; 2104-14th St., Calgary, Alta.; 2411-9th Ave. N.W. (res); Cambridge (Eng.) '32; DCH; Tel. AV 9-3182.

ROTHWELL, G. Sheldon; 605-5th Ave., New Westminster, B.C.; 125-4th (res); McG '37; Staff, Royal Columbian Hosp.; Tel. LA 2-5445.

ROTHWELL, William O.; 200 Greyhound Bldg., 622-1st St. S.W., Calgary, Alta.; McG'37; FACS; GenSurg.

ROTMAN, Harold H.; Tor '58; FRCP(C), IntMed; Staff, Toronto Gen. Hosp., Toronto, Ont.; Abroad.

ROTMAN, Louis; 368-8th Ave., Lachine, Montreal, P.Q.; McG '49; GenSurg.; Tel. 637-6841.

ROTSTEIN, Matthew I.; 929 Liverpool Rd., Bay Ridges, Ont.; Tor'45; MCGP; FACS; Tel. 839-5851.

ROTSTEIN, Morris L.; 99 Avenue Rd., Toronto 5, Ont.; 35 Old Park Rd. (res); Tor '40; D.A.B.-O.G., ObstGyn; Sr. Att. Obst. Gyn., New Mt. Sinai Hosp.; Tel. WA 3-5862.

ROTSTEIN, Murray; 676 Old Weston Rd., Toronto 9, Ont.; 283 Grace (res); Tor '48; MCGP; Dist. Coroner; Tel. RO 9-4878.

ROUILLARD, J. Michel; Lav '60; Res., Hop. Enfant-Jesus, Quebec 3, P.Q.

ROUKEMA, Joe; Box 160, 18 Springside Dr., Ryckmans Corners, Ont.; Amsterdam (Holland) '53.

ROULEAU, Andre; 4395 Ave. Verdun, Montreal 19, P.Q.; Mon'55; Otol (P.Q.); Tel. 768-6751.

ROULEAU, Claude; Lav '62; Res., Hop. St. Francois d'Assise, Quebec, P.Q.

ROULEAU, Claude; Mon'63; Res. Royal Victoria Hosp., Montreal 2, P.Q.

ROULEAU, Georges A.; Mon'48; Med. Dir., Comission hydroelectrique du Quebec, 75 ouest Dorchester, Montreal 1, P.Q.; Tel. 334-9677.

ROULEAU, J. M.; St. Gregoire, P.Q.; Mon '23; Dist. Coroner.

ROULEAU, Paul; 6632 Christopher Columbus St., Montreal, P.Q.; 268 Glengarry (res); Mon '32; Tel. 272-5053.

ROULEAU, Roger L. L. J.; 294 Chemin Montreal, Ottawa 7, Ont.; 342 Frontenac (res); Lav '46; M.C.G.P.; M.O.H., Eastview; Coroner, Carleton Co.; Active Staff, Ottawa Gen. Hosp.; Clin. Ass't. (Obst.), U. of Ottawa; Tel. 749-4542.

ROULEAU, Yvan; 1681 Parc Lafontaine, Montreal 34, P.Q.; 12335 Place-de-la-Capricieuse (res); Mon '50; IntMed, Cardiol (PQ); Teach. Staff, Hop. Notre-Dame; Tel. LA 6-6061.

ROULEAU, Yves; 1227 William, Sillery, Quebec 6, P.Q.; Lav '48; Psy; Dir. Dept. of Psy., Hop.-St.-Sacrement; Assoc. Prof., Laval U.; Tel. 681-7211.

ROULIOT, Marcel R.; Lav '60; Res., Hospital Hotel-Dieu, Quebec 4, P.Q.

ROULSTON, Thomas M.; Dept. of ObstGyn., The Chown Bldg., McDermot & Emily Sts., Winnipeg, Man.; Queens (Belfast, Ire.) '43; M.B., B.Ch., BAO; DRCOG; FRCOG; FACOG; ObstGyn; ObstGyn-in-Chief, Wpg. Gen. Hosp.; Prof. of ObstGyn., U. of Manitoba; Tel. 786-3596.

ROUNDHILL, Ashleigh; Wright Clinic, 57 James St., Parry Sound, Ont.; Laird Ave. (res); Queen's (Belfast, N. Ire.)'54; DRCOG; Active Staff, Parry Sound Gen. & St. Joseph's Hosp's.; Tel. 746-2181.

ROUNTHWAITE, F. John; Medical-Dental Bldg., 450 Central Ave., London, Ont.; 276 Regent St. (res); McG '49; DABOt; FRCS(C), Otol; Chief of Otol., St. Joseph's Hosp.; Cons., Westminster Hosp., Ontario Hosp. & Children's Psy. Research Inst.; Clin. Assoc. Prof. (Otol.) & Sess. Lect. Physiol., U. of Western Ont.; Tel. 439-3931.

ROUNTHWAITE, Harry L.; 137 Wellington St., Sarnia, Ont.; 1271 Ridgewood Dr. (res); McG '49; DABS; FACS; FRCS(C) GenSurg; Surg. Carruthers Clinic; Tel. DI 4-5261.

ROUSE, Frank V.; Ste. 310, 345 Lake Shore Rd. E., Oakville, Ont.; Qns '57; Tel. 845-4511.

ROUSSE, Georges; 6539 St. Denis St., Montreal, P.Q.; 6537 St. Denis St. (res); Mon '37; Tel. 277-5060.

ROUSSEAU, Agnes; 6162 Laurendeau, Montreal 20, P.Q.; Mon '57; Retired.

ROUSSEAU, Alain P.; 1010 St-Cyrille ouest, Apt. 1, Quebec 6, P.Q.; Lav '56; FRCS(C); Ophth; Ass't. Ophth., Hop. de-l'Enfant-Jesus; Tel. 527-0522.

ROUSSEAU, Bernard; Mon '64; Int., Hop. Notre-Dame, Montreal, P.Q.

ROUSSEAU, Conrad; 56 rue Lamontagne, Quebec 3, P.Q.; 1041 Mont St. Denis (res); Lav '46; Tel. 522-2901.

ROUSSEAU, Jean; 1193 ave.-des-Erables, Quebec 6, P.Q.; 1180 de Salaberry (res); Lav '41; IntMed (P.Q.); Chief Med., Hop. Ste.-Foy; Hd., Arthritis Hosp. & Jeffrey Hale's Hosp.; Staff, Laval U.; Tel. 522-2140.

ROUSSEAU, Jean M.; 112A Rue St. Louis, Warwick, P.Q.; Lav'63.

ROUSSEAU, J. M.; Vallee Jct., P.Q.; Lav '07.

ROUSSEAU, Leon; Lav'63; Res., Hop. Notre Dame, Montreal, P.Q.

ROUSSEAU, Louis; Lav '26; IntMed (TB); Med. Dir., San-du-Lac-Edouard, Lac-Edouard, P.Q.; Prof., Laval U.

ROUSSEAU, Marie; 155 Chemin Ste. Foy, Quebec, P.Q.; Lav '45; Paed; Staff, Hop. du St. Sacrement & Laval U.; Tel. 522-7564.

ROUSSEAU, M. Suzanne; Mon'65; Res. Hop. Maisonneuve, Montreal 36, P.Q.

ROUSSEAU, Paul W.; Box 520, Oliver, B.C.; McG '55; MCGP.

ROUSSEAU, Pierre; Mon'62; Anaes; Staff, Hop. Maisonneuve, Montreal, P.Q.

ROUSSEAU, Therese M.; Ste 809, 30 Blvd. St.-Joseph E., Montreal 34, P.Q.; 3885 Lacombe (res); Mon '48; Paed; Tel. 845-4241.

ROUSSEL, Jacques; 1780 ave Champfleury, Quebec 3, P.Q.; 312 de-la-Ronde (res) Lav '51; Dir. Dept. of Health; Tel. 661-3863.

ROUSSEL, Jean M.; 443 rue St. Vincent, Montreal 1, P.Q.; 70 ave. Cornwall, Ville-Mt-Royal (res); Mon '31; Med. Legis. (U. de-Paris); Dir. de-l'Inst.-de-Medecine legale et de police scientifique (PQ); Prof. (Med. Légale), U. of Montreal; Tel. 873-3300.

ROUSSEL, Leonard; 222 Daly, Ottawa, Ont.; Mon '43; Staff, Ottawa Gen. Hosp.; Ass't Prof. (Med.) Ottawa U. Medical School; Tel. CE 6-2365.

ROUSSIN, Camille; 131 St. Charles Borommee St. N., Joliette, P.Q.; Mon '37; Tel. 756-4770.

ROUTLEDGE, James H.; 740 Seaforth Med. Bldg., 3550 Cote des Neiges Rd., Montreal 25, P.Q.; 54 Winston Circle, Pointe Claire (res); McG '41; MRCOG; FRCOG; FRCS(C); ObstGyn; Ass't. ObstGyn., Montreal Gen. & Royal Victoria Hosp's.; Lect. (ObstGyn.), McGill U.; Tel. 937-3595.

ROUTLEY, John V.; Caledonia Medical Bldg., 340 Campbell St., Nanaimo, B.C.; UBC '54; MCGP.

ROUX, Augustin; 32 Madeline, St-Benoit, Cte Deux Montagnes, P.Q.; Mon '53; MCGP; Tel. 258-3477.

ROUX, Francois C.; Mon'61; Urol(P.Q.); Staff, Hop. Hotel-Dieu, Montreal, P.Q.

ROUX, J. Rene; 417 Centre-Medical-St.-Urbain, 3875 rue St.-Urbain, Montreal 18, P.Q.; 3182 ave. Kent (res); Mon '40; FICS; GenSurg (P.Q.); Surg., Hop. Hotel-Dieu; Ass't. Prof. (Med.), U. of Mtl.; Tel. VI 9-4184.

ROUX, Louis; 585 Ave. Champagneur, Montreal 8, P.Q.; Lav '09; Medico-Legal Expert, City of Montreal; Retired; Tel. 272-3273.
ROUX, Roland; Clinique Medicale-LeMoyne, 201 Charron, Ville-LeMoyne, Cite-Jacques-Cartier, P.Q.; 55 Rene Philippe No. 4 (res); Mon '63; Tel. OR 1-5585.
ROVINESCU, Ionel A.; 2195 St. Louis, Montreal 9, P.Q.; Bucharest (Roum.)'48; Urol.
ROW, Robert K.; 751 King St. W., Kitchener, Ont.; McG'55.
ROWAN, Arthur A.; 130 St. John St., Fredericton, N.B.; McG '24; Otol; Active Staff, Victoria Public Hosp.; Tel. GR 5-3351.
ROWAN, Jack; 2638 Eglinton Ave. W., Toronto, Ont.; Tor '37; Tel. RO 2-1756.
ROWAN-LEGG, C. Kingsley; 215 Cooper St., Ottawa, Ont.; 320 Cloverdale Rd., Rockcliffe (res); McG '32; D.C.H.(Eng.) Paed; Paed., Ottawa Civic Hosp.; Lect. (Paed.), U. of Ottawa; Tel. CE 2-4424.
ROWAT, Floyd L.; 303 Medical Centre, 906-8th Ave. S.W., Calgary, Alta.; Alb'62; Tel. 263-4686.
ROWE, Arthur R.; Cambria Med. Bldg., 386 Cambria St., Stratford, Ont.; Bristol (Eng.)'42; D.L.O. (Eng.); Otol; Staff, Stratford Gen. Hosp.; Tel. 271-1420.
ROWE, Augustus T.; Water St., Carbonear, Nfld.; St. Mary's H. (London, Eng.) '53; Med. Supt., Carbonear Comm. Hosp.; Tel. 5018.
ROWE, William D.; Medical Arts Bldg., Corner Brook, Nfld.; 93 Reid St. (res); St. Mary's Hosp., London (Eng.) '43; M.R.C.S., L.R.C.P.; Staff, Western Memorial Hosp.; Vis. Staff, West Coast San.; Tel. 634-2268.
ROWE, William J.; 128 Westminster Ave., Penticton, B.C.; Okanagan Falls, (res); Wes '51; Ophth.; Staff, Penticton Gen. Hosp.; Tel. 492-5900.
ROWED, Robert B.; Manitouwadge, Ont.; Man '41; GenSurg; Staff Phys., Manitouwadge Gen. Hosp.; Tel. 826-4161.
ROWELL, Peter F.; Box 421, Sylvan Lake, Alta.; Durham (Eng.)'54; M.B., B.S.; DObstRCOG; Tel. 887-2565.
ROWLAND, E. Murray; 32 Valentine Dr., Don Mills, Ont. (res); London (Eng.) '36; MRCS (Eng.); LRCP (Lond.); DPH (Lond.); Examiner, Can. Pension Comm.; Tel. 485-8651.
ROWLAND, William A.; 807 Med. Arts Bldg., 170 St. George St., Toronto 5, Ont.; R.R. 1, York Mills (res); Tor '40; FACCP, FRCP(C), IntMed; Staff, Wellesley Hosp.; Assoc. (Med.), U. of Toronto; Tel. WA 1-1758.
ROWLANDS, John E.; 27 Clement Blk., Brandon, Man.; 331—7th St. (res); Guy's Hosp., London (Eng.) '33; M.R.C.S., L.R.C.P., F.R.C.S. (Edin.); GenSurg; Staff Surg., Brandon Gen. Hosp.; Tel. PA 9-5461.
ROWLEY, John C.; Tor'58; DiagRad; Staff, Dept. of Rad., Wellesley Hosp., Toronto, Ont.
ROWSELL, H. Roy; 300 King St. W., Oshawa, Ont.; 736 Jasmine Cres. (res); Tor '50; F.R.C.P. (C), IntMed; Cons. (IntMed), Ontario Hosp., Whitby; Tel. 725-8632.
ROWSELL, Peter W.; 235 Church St., Oakville, Ont.; Cambridge (Eng.)'46; MRCP(Lond.); DPM (RCPI); D.Psy (McG); Psy; Phys., O.P. D. Toronto Western Hosp.; Active Cons., Oakville-Trafalgar Mem. Hosp.; Tel. 845-7652.
ROWSOM, John W.; 71 King St. W., Ingersoll, Ont.; Tor '32; Staff, Alexandra Hosp.; Indust. Phys., C.I.L.; Tel. 485-2460.
ROWSWELL, Arthur C.; 1554 Merivale Rd., Ottawa 5, Ont. (res); Tor '13; Med. Adviser, Cdn. Pension Comm. Veteran's Mem. Bldg., Ottawa; Retired.
ROWTER, Robert M.; King St., Bridgewater, N.S.; Aberdeen Rd. (res); Dal '43; Staff, Dawson Mem. Hosp.; Tel. 543-2411.
ROXBURGH, Douglas B.; 291 King George Terrace, Victoria, B.C. (res); Alb '32; PathBact; Dir., Dept. of Path., St. Joseph's Hosp., Victoria; Tel. EV 4-1131.
ROY, Alexander K.; Medical Arts Clinic; 2125-11th Ave., Regina, Sask.; 2 Calder Cres. (res); Dal'44; Derm; Staff, Regina Gen. & Grey Nun's Hosp's.; Tel. 523-0691.
ROY, Alfred M.; 34 ave. Begin. Levis, P.Q.; 30 ave. Begin (res); Lav '32; Surg., Hotel Dieu de Levis; Tel. 837-9341.
ROY, Almanzors; 635 Gilbert St., Magog, P.Q. (res); Lav '18; D.P.H.; Phys., Dept. of Pub. Health.
ROY, Andre; St-Raphael, Cte. Bellechasse, P.Q.; Lav '64.
ROY, Antoine; Riviere-au-Renard, P.Q.; Lav '30; M.C.G.P.
ROY, Arsese, C.P.; C.P. 550, Beauceville E., P.Q.; Lav '56.
ROY, Augustin; 1896 ouest Dorchester, Montreal, P.Q.; Lav '54; DPH; MAH; PH(P.Q.); Registrar, College of Phys. & Surg. of Quebec; Tel. 935-2591.
ROY, B.; 60 St. Patrice, Quebec 10, P.Q.; Lav '30.
ROY, Bernard; 780 St. Patrice, Quebec, P.Q.; Lav '30.
ROY, Brien R.; 2784 Kingsway, Vancouver 16, B.C.; Durham (Eng.) '56; Tel. 433-2461.
ROY, Bruno J. P. E.; 82 Frontenac, Lac Megantic, P.Q.; 16 rue Agnes (res); Lav '38; DPH; Staff, Frontenac Health Unit; Tel. 583-0151.
ROY, C. Gustave; 313 Rue La Madone, Mont Laurier, P.Q.; 375 Carre Laurier (res); Lav '34.
ROY, Charles E.; Suite 53, 445 ouest boul. St. Joseph, Montreal 8, P.Q.; Mon'29; Anaes; Anaes., Hop. St. Luc; Tel. 861-7321.
ROY, Claude; 1250 Chemin Ste-Foy, Quebec 6, P.Q.; 2885 Valmont (res); Lav '56; TherRad; Staff, Jeffery Hale Hosp.; Tel. 683-4471.
ROY, Claude; St. Jean Port Joli, Co. L'Islet, P.Q.; Lav '59.
ROY, Claude C.; 539 Grande-Allee E., Quebec 4, P.Q.; 61 Laurier Ave. (res); Lav '54; FRCP(C), Paed; Ass't. (Dept. of Paed.), Hotel-Dieu Hosp.; Clin. Instr., U. of Laval; Tel. 524-7914. Abroad.
ROY, Claudette; Mon'65; Res., Hop. Hotel-Dieu, Montreal 18, P.Q.
ROY, Clovis; C.N.R. Medical Clinic, 935 Lagauchetiere St. W.; P.O. Box 8100, Montreal 3, P.Q.; 7415 Blvd. Lasalle, Verdun (res); Lav '34; Dip., Gen. Surg.; OrthSurg., U. of Paris (Fr.); C.N.R. Med. Off. in Montreal; Tel. 877-5430.
ROY, Donald E.; 267 O'Connor Ave., Ottawa 4, Ont.; Qns'58; IntMed; Staff, Ottawa Civic Hosp.; Tel. 235-6507.
ROY, Douglas G.; Roy Clinic, 715 - 2nd Ave. S., Lethbridge, Alta.; 1307-13 Ave. S .(res); Alb'45; Tel. 327-3134.
ROY, Douglas L.; The Children's Hosp., Halifax, N.S.; Dal'48; IntMed; Assoc. Prof. Paed. (Cardiol.), Dalhousie U. & The Children's Hosp.; Tel. 422-8441, Loc. 34.
ROY, Edgar; App. 1, 3045 Hochelaga, Quebec 10, P.Q.; Lav'50; Admin. Hop. Ste-Foy.
ROY, Fernand; 4765 - 1st Ave., Charlesbourg, Quebec 7, P.Q.; Lav '58; MCGP; Tel. 623-9172.
ROY, Francois; 59 Grande Allee E., Quebec 4, P.Q.; 1140 Vauquelin, Sillery (res); Lav '29; F.A.C.S., F.R.C.S.(C), GenSurg; PlasSurg (P.Q.); Chief Surg., Hop. Hotel Dieu; Cons (Surg), Hop. Ste. Foy; Prof. (Cin. Surg.), Laval U.; Tel. 524-3784.
ROY, Gaston; Lav '62; R.C.A.M.C.
ROY, Gaston M.; St. Placide, Co. Deux Montagnes, P.Q.; Mon. '30.
ROY, George E.; 244 Notre-Dame Est., Victoriaville, P.Q.; Lav '26; Tel. 752-5000.
ROY, Georges E.; 270 Brassard, Nicolet, P.Q.; Laval'27; GenSurg; Hop. du Christ-Roi.
ROY, Gerard; 2200 ouest Boulv. Dionne, St-Georges ouest, Cte Beauce, P.Q.; Lav '60.
ROY, Germain J.; Man '61; (Intern) c/o 224 Prado Place, Windsor, Ont.; Abroad.
ROY, Gustave; 7113 Christophe-Colomb, Montreal 10, P.Q.; Mon '52; MCGP; Cons. American Can.; Tel. 272-4488.
ROY, Hughes; 127 rue du Prince, Sorel, P.Q.; Lav '49; Tel. RI 3-6654.
ROY, Jacques; 1811 boul. Laurentide, Vimont, P.Q.; Mon'63.
ROY, J. Claude; Lav '58; Int'n., Hop. Hotel Dieu, Quebec, P.Q.

ROY, Jean, 1550 est Boul. St. Joseph, Montreal 34, P.Q.; 7820 St.-Denis (res); Lav '43; M.C.A.A., All. (P.Q.), IntMed (P.Q.); Head, (Dept. of Allerg.), Hop.-Maisonneuve & Hop.-Sacre-Coeur. Tel. LA 6-7729.
ROY, Jean P.; 1248 Chemin Ste-Foy, Quebec 6, P.Q.; McG '51; ObstGyn (P.Q.); Staff (ObstGyn.), Jeffery Hale's Hosp.; Tel. 683-4441.
ROY, Joseph C.; 1405 Ave. Fitzpatrick, Sillery, Quebec 6, P.Q.; Lav'50; Staff, Hop. Laval; Tel. 653-5251.
ROY, Jules D.; 62A Blvd. Tache, Hull, P.Q.; Lav '53; IntMed; Staff (IntMed), Hop.-du-Sacre-Coeur; Tel. 777-9752.
ROY, J. Lionel; Lille (France) '56; GenSurg (P.Q.); Staff, Hop. Ste-Jeanne-d'Arc, Montreal, 18, P.Q.; Tel. VI 2-5201.
ROY, Leon; 755 rue Ste. Anne, St. Hyacinthe, P.Q.; Lav '18; Tel. PR 4-7979.
ROY, Louis; Mon'65; Res., Hop. Maisonneuve, Montreal 36, P.Q.
ROY, Louis; 64 Ave. Begin, Levis, P.Q.; 13 rue-de-l'Esplanade (res); Lav '46; GenSurg (PQ); Surg., Hotel-Dieu-de-Levis; Tel. 837-1177.
ROY, Louis; 1337 ave Lemoine, Quebec 6, P.Q.; Lav'55; Psy(P.Q.).
ROY, Louis; Lav '63; Res., Hop. Hotel-Dieu, Quebec, P.Q.
ROY, Louis E.; Port-au-Prince (Haiti) '37; Res., Hop. St.-Joseph, Montreal, P.Q.
ROY, Louis F.; Richibucto, N.B.; Lav '53.
ROY, Louis J.; Suite 22, Edifice Laure, Sept-Iles, P.Q.; Lav'55; GenSurg (P.Q.); Tel. 942-6160.
ROY, Lucien; 750 ouest St-Vallier, Quebec 8, P.Q.; Lav'50.
ROY, Madeleine; Lav '64; Res., Hotel-Dieu de Quebec, Quebec 4, P.Q.
ROY, Marcel; 1500-18eme rue, Quebec 3, P.Q.; Lav '54; DABD; FRCP(C), DermSyph; Staff, Hop. Enfant Jesus, Hop. St-Francoise d'Assise, Hotel Dieu, Levis, & U. of Laval; Tel. 529-3553.
ROY, Marcel; 144 DeQuoy, St-Gabriel-de-Brandon, P.Q.; Lav '62.
ROY, Maurice; 34 Ave. Begin, Levis, P.Q.; 30 Ave. Begin (res); Lav'32; GenSurg (P.Q.); Tel. 837-7482.
ROY, Maurice; St. Placide, P.Q.; Mon '30.
ROY, Paul; 3875 St-Urbain, Ste. 205, Montreal, P.Q.; Mon '54; DiagRad; Staff, Hop. Hotel-Dieu; Tel. 844-3418.
ROY, Paul B.; 1717 Ducharme, Outremont, Montreal 8, P.Q.; (res); Lav '54; Psy (P.Q.); Staff Psy., Hop. Bordeaux; Tel. DU 1-2581.
ROY, Paul-E.; Lav '62; Res. (Ophth.), Hotel-Dieu-de-Quebec, Quebec, P.Q.; Abroad.
ROY, Paul E.; 401 Sud, Cowansville, P.Q.; Lav '39; Dist. Coroner.
ROY, Paul E.; 655 Boul. Bastien, Neufchatel, P.Q.; Lav'50.
ROY, Paul Emile; Paspebiac, P.Q.; Mon '45.
ROY, Paul E.; Lav'58; Path(P.Q.); Staff, Hop. Hotel-Dieu, Quebec, P.Q.
ROY, Paul M.; 307 Ave. Arnaud, Sept. Iles, P.Q.; Lav '40.
ROY, Philippe A.; Lav '55; Path (P.Q.); Chief of Labs., Hop.-Hotel-Dieu de Gaspe, Gaspe, P.Q.; Tel. 400.
ROY, Pierre; 3275 Ave. Royale, Giffard, Quebec 5, P.Q.; Lev '21; Tel. 663-9386.
ROY, Pierre; Lav'64; Res., Hop. Notre-Dame, Montreal 24, P.Q.
ROY, Regent; 69 rue Principale, Danville, P.Q.; Lav '65.
ROY, Richard; Dunrea, Man.; Man '16; Dist. Coroner; Retired.
ROY, Robert; 52 ave. Grand-Ile, Valleyfield, P.Q.; Mon '60; Tel. 373-4647.
ROY, Robert L.; Arnprior Med. Centre, 104 John St., Arnprior, Ont.; Lav '58; MCGP; Tel. 623-3131.
ROY, Roger; 1619 Stanley Ave., Ste-Foy, Quebec 10, P.Q.; Lav '49; Path; Anat; (P.Q.) Dir. of Path., Hotel-Dieu Hosp.; Lect. (Path.), Laval U; Tel. 837-9341.
ROY, Roger; 270 Brassard, Nicolet, P.Q.; Lav '56; OrthSurg.
ROY, Roland; Wolfe's Cove Clinic, Champlain Harbour Station, Quebec 2, P.Q.; Lav'51; DNB (USA); Staff, Quarantine & Sick Mariners Serv., Dept. of National Health & Welfare; Tel. 522-7029.
ROY, Theodore E.; 4 Wendigo Way, Toronto, Ont. (res); McG '31; PathBact; Dir., Dept. of Bact., Hosp. for Sick Children; Ass't. Prof. (Bact.), U. of Toronto; Spec. Lect., School of Hygiene; Tel. EM 6-7242.
ROY, Viateur; St.-Ulric, Cte. Matane, P.Q.; Lav '54.
ROY, Wallace M.; 30 The Queensway, Toronto 18, Ont.; 7 Edenbrook Hill (res); Dal '38; M.A.C.R., D & T Rad; Head, Dept. of Rad., St. Joseph's Hosp.; Tel. LE 4-9351.
ROY, Wilfred A.; 89 Beckwith St., Carelton Place, Ont.; Qns '49; M.C.G.P.; Med. Staff Mem. Hosp.; Tel. 4.
ROY, Yvon; Lav'65; Res., Dept. of Biophysics, U. of Toronto, Toronto 5, Ont.
ROYAL, Harold O.; Debert, N.S.; Brandeis U. (Waltham, Mass.)'22.
ROYER, Albert; St. Pacome, Co. Kamouraska, P.Q.; Lav '34.
ROYER, Albert; 3175 Chemin Ste-Catherine, Montreal, P.Q.; 258 Outremont (res); Mon '43; F.I.S.H., F.R.C.P.(C), Paed; Haem, (P.Q.); Paed. & Chief of Dept. of Haem., Hop.-Ste-Justine; Prof. (Paed), U. of Montreal; Tel. RE 1-4931.
ROYER, Jean L.; 18 rue Bellevue, Arthabaska, P.Q.; Lav'61; Ophth.
ROYER, Louis; 370 Ste.-Cyrille ouest, Quebec 6, P.Q.; Lav '42; Otol; Staff (Otol.), Hotel-Dieu & Laval U.; Tel. 683-8281.
ROYER, Maurice; Apt. 220, est Grande Allee, Quebec, P.Q.; 140 ave, des-Berniers (res); Lav'35; OrthSurg; Chief of Orth. & Traum. Surg., Hop-St. Francois-d'Assise & Staff, Laval U.; Tel. 524-3488.
ROYER, Paul-H.; Lav'56; Diag. Rad. (P.Q.); Staff, Hop. Gen. Fleury, Montreal 12, P.Q.
ROYLE, N. Derek; 901 Helena St., Trail, B.C.; 305 Ritchie Ave. (res); Manchester (Eng.) '55; FRCS(C), ObstGyn; Tel. 368-5211.
ROZDILSKY, Bohdan; Dept. of Path., U. of Saskatchewan, Saskatoon, Sask.; Lwow (Ukraine) '41; M.Sc., Ph.D.; Path; Neuropathol., University Hosp.; Cons., Weyburn & North Battleford Hosp's.; Assoc. Prof. (Neurpath), U. of Saskatchewan; Tel. 242-7671, Loc. 373.
ROZECKI, William A.; Box 430, Selkirk, Man.; Man '60.
RUBENSTEIN, Alfred I.; Medical Centre, 1428 Ouellette Ave., Windsor, Ont.; 2352 Hall Ave. (res); Tor '46; Tel. 256-3403.
RUBENSTEIN, Wanda (See Schiffmann).
RUBENZAHL, Sam; 3042 Keele St., Downsview, Ont.; 2910 Keele St. (res); Tor '54; MCGP; Tel. ME 3-6560.
RUBIN, I. C.; 1437 MacKay St., Montreal 25, P.Q.; Mon '33; MCGP; Clin. Ass't. (Med.), Jewish Gen. Hosp.; Tel. 842-9789.
RUBIN, Jack A.; 603 Boyd Bldg., Winnipeg, Man.; 816 Elm St. (res); Man '50; DABOtol; M.Sc. (Otol); FACS; Otol; Chief E.N.T. Dept., Children's Hosp.; Cons. Otol., Deer Lodge Hosp. & Pre School Deaf Programme; Otol. Winnipeg Gen. Hosp.; Ass't. Prof., Dept. of Otol., U. of Manitoba; Tel. WH 3-4668.
RUBIN, Jack H.; Ste. 23, 5757 Decelles St., Montreal, P.Q.; 6607 Nice Rd. (res); McG '36 F.C.C.P., Pulm. Dis. & T.B. (P.Q.); Clin. Ass't., Jewish Gen. Hosp.; Phys., Royal Edward Laurentian Hosp.; Dem. (Med.), McGill U.; Tel. RE 9-1590.
RUBIN, Joseph W.; McG'65; Jr. Int., Royal Victoria Hosp., Montreal 2, P.Q. Abroad.
RUBIN, Leon; Mall Med. Bldg., Winnipeg, Man.; Man '45; MRCOG; ObstGyn; Active Staff, Wpg. Gen. & Misericordia Hosp's.; Ass't. Prof. (ObstGyn.), U. of Manitoba; Hon. Sec., Manitoba Med. Assoc.; Tel. SP 4-2411.
RUBIN, Mitchell; Ste 110, 809 West 41st Ave, Vancouver 13, B.C.; Man'36; MCGP; Att'd. Staff, St. Vincent's Hosp., Tel. 261-3135.

RUBIN, Samuel S.; 615 Ellendale Med. Bldg., 5845 Cote des Neiges Rd., Montreal 26, P.Q.; 536 Bloomfield (res); Geneva (Switz.) '51; FCCP; IntMed (P.Q.); Tel. 738-3792.

RUBINYI, Lea; 183 Trenton Ave., Montreal 16, P.Q.; Budapest (Hung.) '50; Anaes.

RUBLACK, Alexander E.; 240 Med. & Dental Bldg., Regina, Sask.; 3619 Hill Ave. (res); Qns '45; FICS, FRCS (Edin.), FRCS(C), GenSurg; Tel. LA 2-8328.

RUBLEE, Jack D.; 2 Waubeek St., Parry Sound, Ont.; McG '43; M.Sc.(Path); Path; Dir. of Labs., Parry Sound Gen. & St. Joseph's Hosp's.; Regional Pathologist; Tel. 746-2161.

RUBY, Ralph A.; 12 Fort St., Tilbury, Ont.; Tor '26; Tel. 682-2412.

RUBY, Ralph R.; Wes '63; Res., Westminster Hosp., London, Ont.

RUDD, Douglas R.; Moose Jaw Clinic, 200 Scott Bldg., Moose Jaw, Sask.; 707 Elizabeth St. (res); Tor '51; Tel. 692-2373.

RUDD, Elias J. K.; 130 Lytton Blvd., Toronto 12, Ont.; Qns '19; Ophth; Retired.

RUDD, Michael S. K.; 99 St. Clair Ave. W., Toronto, Ont.; Tor '25; F.R.C.S.(Eng.); Retired.

RUDD, William W.; 215 Dunvegan Rd., Toronto 7, Ont.; Tor'59; GenSurg.

RUDDELL, J. Shegog; 2402-5th Ave. S., Lethbridge, Alta.; Dublin (Ire.) '33; MB, MD; DA; FFARCS; FFARCS(I); Anaes; Vis. Anaes., St. Michael's Hosp.; Tel. 238-2124.

RUDDICK, Donald W.; 2015 Crescent St., Montreal 25, P.Q.; 271 Glengarry Ave., Twn. of Mount Royal (res); McG '42; FRCS(Eng.); FRCS(C); GenSurg; FACS; Ass't. Surg., Montreal Gen. Hosp.; Ass't. Prof. (Surg.), McGill U.; Tel. 288-5002.

RUDDICK, William W., VD; 2015 Crescent St., Montreal 25, P.Q.; McG '14; GenSurg; Cons. (Surg.) Mtl. Gen. Hosp.; Cons. Phys., T. Eaton Co. Ltd.; Tel. 842-4587.

RUDDY, J. O.; 200 Brock N., Whitby, Ont.; (res); Tor '26; Dist. Coroner.

RUDERMAN, Robert L.; Ste. 702, 99 Avenue Rd., Toronto 5, Ont.; Tor'53; DABS, FACS; FRCS(C), GenSurg; Assoc., Dept. of Surg., The Doctors Hosp.; Vol. Ass't. (Surg.), New Mount Sinai Hosp.; Clin. Teach. Surg., U. of Toronto; Tel. WA 5-5421.

RUDIS, Leonids A.; 27 Nanwood Dr., Brampton, Ont.; Riga (Latvia) '40; GenSurg.; Tel. GL 1-2310.

RUDNICK, Alexander; 211 Simcoe St., Oshawa, Ont.; Dublin (Ire.)'50; Tel. 728-9459.

RUDNICK, K. Vincent; 1507 Main St. W., Hamilton, Ont.; 99 Dalewood Ave. S. (res); Qns '51; MCGP; Active Staff, St. Joseph's Hosp.; Court. Staff, Hamilton Gen., Henderson & Chedoke Gen. Hosp's.; Tel. 528-8517.

RUDNICK, Leon R.; 671 Sheppard Ave. W., Downsview, Ont.; Tor'55; Staff, Branson Hosp.; Tel. 633-9566.

RUDOLPH, Cecil R.; Apt. 404, 437 St. Paul Ave., Brantford, Ont.; Tor '27; M.C.G.P.; Tel. 752-5221.

RUEBEN, Erich F.; Heidelberg (Germ.) '51; Res., Vancouver Gen. Hosp., Vancouver 9, B.C.

RUEBSAAT, Helmut J.; Ste 504, 1541 W. Broadway, Vancouver 9, B.C.; Friedrich Wilhelm (Bonn, Germ.) '46; Tel. RE 1-5514.

RUEDY, John; Qns'56; FRCP(C), IntMed; Staff, Montreal Gen. Hosp., Montreal 25, P.Q.

RUEL, Adrien H.; 222 Henri-Bourassa E., Montreal, P.Q.; 10922 Tanguay (res); Lav '50; Gastroent (P.Q.); Staff, Hop. Sacre-Coeur, Cartierville, Mtl.; Tel. DU 8-7608.

RUEL, Jean M. Capt.; Lav'64; Staff, Valcartier Stn. Hosp., Camp Valcartier, P.Q.

RUELLAND, Raymond; 1305 Ave. Patenaude, Sillery, Quebec 6, P.Q. (res); Lav '55; Psy.; Tel. 683-8416.

RUELLAND, Yves; 4072 Blvd. Ste. Anne, Montmorency, P.Q.; Lav '53; Tel. 663-0450.

RUETHER, Bernard A.; Alb'61; FRCP(C), IntMed; Staff, University Hosp., Edmonton, Alta.

RUFF, Helen L. (Fill); 840 Upper Wellington, Hamilton, Ont.; Budapest (Hung.) '50; Tel. 389-5144.

RUFF, Peter; 840 Upper Wellington, Hamilton, Ont.; Apt. 9, 143 Stinson St. (res); Budapest (Hung.) '45; Tel. 389-1319.

RUGGERI, Ferdinand A.; 350 Selby St., Montreal, P.Q.; Bristol (Eng.) '48; Med. Dir., International Div., Charles E. Frosst & Co.; Tel. 932-7111.

RUHMAN, Walter; 4549 Sherbrooke St. W., Montreal, P.Q.; Berlin (Germ.) '24.

RUIZ, Carlos; Dal'63; Res. (Paed.), U. of British Columbia, Vancouver 9, B.C.

RULAND, Notrid W.; 311 Wilson St., Ancaster, Ont.; Heidelberg (Germ.) '53; Tel. 648-4620.

RUMBALL, N. H.; 997 Gerrard St. E., Toronto 8, Ont.; Tor '43; IntMed.; Tel. HO 3-9911.

RUMBALL, Wilbur C.; Kirkland Med. Group, 42-2nd St., Kirkland Lake, Ont.; 90 First St. (res); Tor '25; M.C.G.P.

RUMBALL, William G.; Medical Centre, 707 Charlotte St., Peterborough, Ont.; Tor'58; Otol; Staff, Peterborough Civic & St. Joseph's Hosp's.; Cons., Ross Mem. Hosp., Lindsay; Tel. 742-3871.

RUMBALL, W. James S.; 42 Second St., Kirkland Lake, Ont.; Tor '59; GenSurg.; Tel. 567-5331.

RUNDLE, F. William; 117 King St. E., Oshawa, Ont.; 839 Glenbrae St. (res); Tor '55; M.Sc. (Otol.); FRCS(C). Otol; FACS; Active Surg. Staff, **Oshawa Gen. Hosp.; O.P.D. Staff, (Otol.), St.** Michael's Hosp., Toronto; Cons. Staff, Bowmanville Mem. Hosp.; Tel. 728-1661.

RUNDLE, George A.; 44 Colborne St. E., Oshawa, Ont.; 728 Jasmine Cr. (res); Wes '55; FAAP; Paed; Tel. 725-8453.

RUNDLE, James E.; 300 King St. W., Oshawa, Ont.; 364 Simcoe St. N. (res); Tor '45; A'ttd. Phys., Hillsdale Manor, Home for the Aged; Tel. 725-3523.

RUNDLE, L. Gordon; 955 Queen St. E., Sault Ste. Marie, Ont.; Dal '49; IntMed; Tel. 253-1852.

RUNDLE, L. Howard B.; 79 Queen St., Bowmanville, Ont.; Tor '36; Tel. 623-5488.

RUNIONS, J. Ernest; Ponoka, Alta.; Alb'63.

RUNNALLS, Kenneth W.; Wes '44; Psy; Supt., **Ontario Hosp., North Bay, Ontario; Tel. 474-1200.**

RUNNELLS, George W.; 10 Selkirk Ave., Hudson, P.Q.; McG '21.

RUSE, James L.; 129 Eastborne Ave., Toronto 7, Ont.; Tor '54; Research Staff, Banting Inst.

RUSEN, Samuel D.; 190 Osborne St. N., Winnipeg, Man.; 541 Queenston St. (res); Man '41; IntMed; Act. Staff, IntMed., Deer Lodge, Grace, St. Boniface & Municipal Hosp's.; Lect. Dept. IntMed., U. of Manitoba; Tel. SU 3-5533.

RUSH, Raymond D.; 175 E. Broadway, Vancouver, B.C.: 275-W. 21st Ave. (res); Alb. '29; Tel. TR 4-1023.

RUSHFORTH, John N., MC; 217 Laurier Ave. E., **Ottawa 2, Ont.; 782 Eastbourne Ave. (res); St. Andrew's (Scot.) '49; Court. Staff, Ottawa Gen., Ottawa Civic & St. Vincent's Hosp's.; Tel. CE 6-7263.**

RUSHTON, Shirley J.; Ste. 260, 2184 W. Broadway, Vancouver 9, B.C.; King's College (Durham, Eng.) '57; MCGP; Tel. RE 6-4341.

RUSIEWICZ, E.; Tor'63; Res., Toronto Gen. Hosp., Toronto 2, Ont.

RUSKIN, Samuel G.; 1015 Hillside Ave., Victoria, B.C.; 1182 Old Esquimalt Rd. (res); Man '44; Tel. EV 2-7321.

RUSNAK, Conrad H.; 502 Med. Dental Bldg., Rose St. & 11th Ave., Regina, Sask.; Sask'61; GenSurg.

RUSSELL, Alexander; Edinburgh (Scot.) '54; Res., Toronto East Gen. Hosp., Toronto 2, Ont.

RUSSELL, Axel; 296 St. Joseph Blvd. W., Montreal 8, P.Q.; Graz (Aust.) '51; D.Psy; Psy; **Staff, Jewish Gen. Hosp.; Teach. Staff, McGill U.; Tel. CR 2-7145.**

RUSSELL, Bernice O. (See WYLIE, Bernice).

RUSSELL, Brian; North York Health Dept., 5000 Yonge St., Willowdale, Ont.; Belfast (Ire.)'46; MOH, Twp. of North York.

RUSSELL, Charles D.; 110 Green St., Whitby, Ont.; Wes'34; Tel. 668-8991.

RUSSELL, C .Scott; 25 Leonard Ave., Toronto 2B, Ont.; Tor'55; FRCS(C), ObstGyn; Clin. Teach. (ObstGyn.), U. of Toronto; Tel. EM 4-2549.
RUSSELL, Donald B., Capt.; 1 Field Ambulance, CAPO 5050, Germany; Alb'64; Abroad.
RUSSELL, Earl S.; 86 MacDonnell St., Kingston, Ont. (res); Wes '50; Anaes.; Clin. Ass't., Queens U.; Att. Staff, Kingston Gen. Hosp.; Tel. 542-2821.
RUSSELL, Edgar A.; 214 Med. Arts Bldg., 750 Spadina Cres. E., **Saskatoon, Sask.; Man '46;** ObstGyn.; Tel. 652-4967.
RUSSELL, Eric N.; 13665-96th Ave., North Surrey, B.C.; Belfast (N. Ire.) '55; Tel. 581-3230.
RUSSELL, Gregory F.; Cornwall Clinic, 325 Hamilton Ave., St. John's, Nfld.; Dal'59; MCGP; Assoc. Staff, St. Clare's Mercy & Grace Maternity Hosp's.; Tel. 579-0055.
RUSSELL, James E., F/L; P.M.Q. 188, 14015-101st St., Edmonton, Alta.
RUSSELL, J. L. Thomas; 627 Medical Arts Bldg., 170 St. George St., **Toronto, Ont.; 214 Strathallan Wood (res); Tor '41; F.R.C.S.(C), GenSurg, Urol; Chief, Dept. of Urol., St. Michael's Hosp.; Cons., Urol., Sunnybrook Hosp., & Princess Margaret Hosp.; Ass't. Prof., Surg.,** U. of Toronto; Tel. 924-2022.
RUSSELL, John; UBC '64; Res., Grenfell Hosp., St. Anthony, Nfld.
RUSSELL, Joseph R.; 1088 Pembina Hwy., Winnipeg 19, Man.; Man'62; Tel. 453-3303.
RUSSELL, Kelvin J.; 327 Charlotte St., Peterborough, Ont.; Wales (U.K.) '61; D.ObstRCOG.
RUSSELL, Mary G.; Abbott Clinic, 274 Osborne St. N., Winnipeg 1, Man.; London (Eng.) '56.
RUSSELL, Neville; Dal'64., Toronto Gen. Hosp., Toronto 2, Ont.
RUSSELL, Nicholas C.; London (Eng.) '58; Res., Kingston Gen. Hosp., Kingston, Ont.
RUSSELL, Robert W.; Alb '56; Res., Vancouver Gen. Hosp., Vancouver 9, B.C.
RUSSELL, Ruth; Ste. IIA, 6 Vendome Place, Don Mills, Ont.; St. Andrews (Scot.) '56.
RUSSELL, Thomas F.; 175 Provost Lane, Fergus, Ont.; 240 St. David St. (res); Wes '31; Tel. 843-3210.
RUSSELL, Wayne H.; 2333 Portage Ave., Winnipeg 12, Man.; Man'63; Tel. 837-1327.
RUSSELL, W. Andrew M.; 65 King St. W., Beamsville, Ont.; 194 King St. W. (res); Wes '42; M.C.G.P.; Staff, West Lincoln Mem. Hosp., Grimsby; Tel. LO 3-8221.
RUSSELL, Welford H.; Lockwood Clinic, 300 Bloor St. E., Toronto, Ont.; 49 Dalewood Rd. (res); Tor '25; F.I.C.S., GenSurg; Surg-in-Chief, Lockwood Clinic; Surg. Cons., Sunnybrook D.V.A. Hosp.; Tel. WA 1-2121.
RUSSELL, William F.; Blairmore, Alta.; Alb '43; Dist. Coroner. Retired.
RUSSELL, William G.; 70 Roncesvalles Ave., Toronto, Ont.; Wes '07; Dist. Coroner.
RUSSON, Gordon W.; Med. Arts Clinic, 2125 11th Ave., Regina, Sask. (res); Tor'48; Psy; Cons. Psy., Corrections Branch, Dept. Soc. Welfare & Rehabilitation, Regina, Sask.
RUSTED, Ian E. L. H.; 1 Campbell Ave., St. John's, Nfld.; 17 Exeter Ave. (res); Dal'48; M.Sc (McG); FACP; FRCP(C), IntMed; MCGP (Hon); Cons. (Internist), Dept. of Health, St. John's; Phys. & Dir. of Interne Educ., St. John's Gen. Hosp.; Dir. P.G. Med. Educ., Memorial U. of Nfld.; Tel. 579-1199.
RUSTED, Nigel F. S.; 28 Monkstown Rd., St. John's, Newfoundland; Dal '33; F.A.C.S., F.I.C.S., GenSurg; Chief of 3rd Surg. Serv., St. **John's Gen. Hosp.; Chief Surg., Grace Hosp.;** Cons. Surg., St. Clare's Mercy Hosp.; Tel. 726-8834.
RUSTIGE, Louis R.; 51 William, Brantford, Ont.; Leiden (Neth.) '52; Staff, Brantford Gen. Hosp.; Tel. 753-6111.
RUSTON, Francis G.; 44 Beulah Ave., Hamilton, Ont.; Wes '40; Anaes; Active Staff, Hamilton Gen. Hosp.; Court. Staff, Chedoke Gen. Hosp.; Tel. JA 9-2661.
RUTHERDALE, John A.; 2403 Redfern Rd., Burlington, Ont. (res); Tor '50; IntMed.; Tel. 637-6781.
RUTHERFORD, Allan P.; Qns '64; Jr. Int., Kingston Gen. Hosp., Kingston, Ont.
RUTHERFORD, Donald D.; 261 Riverside Drive W., Windsor, Ont.; Tor'46; Active Staff (Anaes.), Grace, Hotel Dieu & Metropolitan Hosp's.; Tel. 253-1590.
RUTHERFORD, Isobel; 158 S. Front St., Sarnia, Ont. (res); Qns '57; Path; Ass't. Path., Sarnia Gen. Hosp.; Tel. DI 4-3661.
RUTHERFORD, Reginald W.; 821 Coxwell Ave., Toronto 6, Ont.; 18 Rochester Ave. (res); Tor '48; F.R.C.P.(C), IntMed; Med. Staff, Toronto East Gen. Hosp; Tel. HO 3-4121.
RUTHERFORD, Samuel N.; 4 Highland Ave., Ridgeway, Ont.; Nye Rd. (res); Dublin (Ire.) '44; M.B., B.Ch., BAO; MCGP; FRCS (Ire.); Tel. 869-1311.
RUTHERFORD, Scott E.; 345 Victoria Ave., Windsor, Ont.; 2559 Riverside Dr. W. (res); Qns'21; Hon. Cons. Surg., Grace Hosp.; Tel. CL 3-7091.
RUTHERFORD, Terence F.; UBC'56; Path; Staff, St. Paul's Hosp., Vancouver 1, B.C.
RUTHERFORD, Thomas F.; 277 King St. E., Kingston, Ont.; 251 Mack St. (res); Qns '29; Ophth. Otol; Tel. 548-8522.
RUTHERFORD, Wilfrid B.; 183 S. Christina St., **Sarnia, Ont.; 158 S. Front St. (res); Tor '16; Gaol. Surg., County of Lambton; Staff, Cons. (IntMed), Sarnia Gen. Hosp.; Dist. Coroner.**
RUTLEDGE, Earl J.; 200 Helmsdale Ave., East Kildonan, Man.; 683 Clifton St., Winnipeg (res); Qns '19; D.P.H; Med. Dir., Kildonan-St. Paul Health Unit.
RUTLEDGE, George; Mall Med. Group, 280 Osborne St. N., **Winnipeg 1, Man.; Belfast (N. Ire.)** '49.
RUTLEDGE, Stuart L.; The Peterborough Clinic, 327 Charlotte St. W., Peterborough, Ont.; Roper Dr., R.R. No. 3 (res); McG '45; F.R.C.S.(C), GenSurg; Surg. Staff, Peterborough Civic & St. Joseph's Hosp's; Tel. 743-2040.
RUTT, John M.; Slave Lake, Alta.; Philadelphia (U.S.A.) '64; Tel. 849-3806.
RUTTER, Philip E. H.; Box 449, High Prairie, Alta.; London (Eng.) '51; MRCS; LRCP; D.ObstRCOG; MCGP; Tel. 3-3354.
RUTTAN, Henry R., O.B.E., C.D.; Ste. 108, North Toronto Med. Bldg., 250 Lawrence Ave. W., Toronto 12, Ont.; Qns'35; Derm; Staff, Sunnybrook Hosp.; Tel. 787-3575.
RUTTLE, John A.; Dresden, Ont.; Wes '33.
RUTZ, Harold; Box 907, Langley, B.C.; Man'48; Staff, Langley Mem. Hosp.; Tel. 534-6711.
RYALL, David B.; McBride, B.C.; Tor **'27;** M.C.G.P.
RYALL, Patrick P.; The Humboldt Clinic, Humboldt, Sask.; 903 Main St. (res); Cork (Ire.) '54; MCGP; Tel. 682-2618.
RYAN, Catherine C.; 718 Water St., St. John's, Nfld.; **National U. (Ireland) '52; M.B.; B.Ch., Staff, St. Clare's Mercy & Grace Hosp's.; Tel.** 9-8078.
RYAN, Clarence A.; 4660 W. 2nd Ave., Vancouver 8, B.C.; McG'20; FICS; OrthSurg; Semi-Retired; Tel. 224-3892.
RYAN, Doreen B.; Box 2387, **Smithers, B.C.;** Qns'55; Tel. 847-9411.
RYAN, Edmond; McQueen Res., Highland View Hosp., Amherst, N.S.; 17 Rupert St. (res); Nat. **U. (Ire) '52; Psy; Exec. Dir., Cumberland Mental Health Centre; Tel. 667-3879.**
RYAN, Ernest A.; Ste 202, 3000 Lawrence Ave. E., Scarborough, Ont.; 160 Rosedale Hgts. Dr., Tor 7 (res); Tor '42; M.A. (Biochem.), Ph.D. (Physiol.), M.S. (Tor.), F.R.C.S.(C), GenSurg; Att'd. Surg. Staff, Scarborough Gen. Hosp.; Tel. 291-1104.
RYAN, Gabriel V.; Marshall Clinic, Cayuga, Ont.; National U. (Ireland) '40; Tel. 772-3370.
RYAN, G. Clifford; 1010 McCallum Hill Bldg., Regina, Sask.; 50 Langley St. (res); London, (Eng.) '47; Anaes; Tel. 527-4922.

RYAN, George H.; Winnipeg Clinic, Winnipeg, Man.; 141 Yale Ave. (res); Man '29; M.S. (Minn.), FACS; OrthSurg; Cons., Wpg. Gen. & Grace Hosp's.; Tel. 942-0551.
RYAN, Ivan G.; 27 Foster St., Perth, Ont.; 10 Drummond St. E. (res); National U. (Dublin, Ire.) '54; MB, B.Ch., BAO; Tel. 267-1771.
RYAN, James G.; 569 Concession St., Hamilton, Ont.; Qns '59.
RYAN, James V.; 718 Water St. W., St. John's, Nfld. National U. (Ire.) '52; B.A.O., L.M.; Tel. 9-7009; Abroad.
RYAN, J. Martin; 10022-103rd St., Edmonton, Alta.; Dal'50; FACP; IntMed; Chief of Med., Misericordia Hosp.; Lect. Med., U. of Alberta; Tel. 429-3781.
RYAN, Joseph J.; Apt. 501, 3380 Ridgewood Ave., Montreal, P.Q.; McG'24; GenSurg (P.Q.); Att'd. Cons. GenSurg., St. Mary's Hosp.; Semi-retired; Tel. 737-7729.
RYAN, Michael; 843 Princess St., Kingston, Ont.; 148 Indian Rd. (res); U. Coll. (Dublin, Ire.) '50; MCGP; Assoc. Staff, Kingston Gen. & Hotel-Dieu Hosp's.; Preceptor, Queen's U.; Med. Staff, Aluminum Co. of Canada; Tel. 542-7366.
RYAN, Patrick J.; Islay, Alta.; Dublin (Ire.) '63; MRCS (Lond.); LRCP.
RYAN, Philip A.; 229 St. Clair Ave. W., Toronto 7, Ont.; 103 Heath St. E., Tor 7 (res); Tor '39; FRCP(C), IntMed; Phys.-I/C, OPD, St. Michael's Hosp.; Clin Ass't. Med. U. of Toronto; Tel. WA 2-0721.
RYAN, Valerie P.; 843 Princess St., Kingston, Ont.; 148 Indian Rd. (res); Edinburgh (Scot.) '52; Tel. 542-7366.
RYBAK, Francis A.; 359 Selkirk Ave., Winnipeg 4, Man.; McG '26; Tel. 586-1903.
RYBAK, Stanley E.; Sydenham, Ont.; Lav '48; M.R.S.H., M.C.G.P.; M.O., Portland & Hinchinbrooke Townships; Tel. 376-3447.
RYCKEBOSCH, James L., Surg/Lt.; Man '61; M.O., RCAF Station, Comox, B.C. Abroad.
RYCKMAN, Maxwell B.; 542 Talbot St., St. Thomas, Ont.; 177 Wellington St. (res); Wes '35; Indus. Phys; Phys., C.P.R. & L.& PS Rlwys.
RYDER, Donald E.; 53 Dinnick Cr., Toronto 12, Ont. (res.); Edinburgh (Scot.) '49; DPH; Path; Ass't. Dir. of Labs., Women's College Hosp., Toronto; Reg. Pathol., Metro Toronto & Ont.; Tel. WA 3-7381.
RYDER, John; Glasgow (Scot.) '33; F.C.C.P., Med. Supt., Baker Memorial Sanatorium, Calgary, Alta.; Cons. (Disease of Chest), D.V.A., Col. Belcher Hosp.; Tel. BU 8-2311.
RYDER, Joseph B.; Dublin (Ire.) '44; M.R.C.P. (I); M.R.C.P. (Lond.); IntMed; Staff, Mountain San., Hamilton, Ont.; Tel. 385-5341.
RYERSON, E. S.; 14 Delisle St., Toronto 12, Ont. (res); Dublin (Ire.) '00; F.A.C.S.; Retired.
RYLEY, Thomas G.; 1849 Yonge St., Toronto 7, Ont.; Tor'51; FRCS(C), ObstGyn; Clin. Ass't. Wellesley Hosp. & U. of Toronto; Tel. 489-6555.
RYLL, Hertha; Vienna (Aust.) '39; P.G., Holy Cross Hosp., Calgary, Alta.
RYMAL, Lloyd C.; 506 York St., Hamilton, Ont.; Tor '18.
RYNARD, P. Bernard, M.P.; 11 Coldwater St., Orillia, Ont.; Qns '26; FIAP; FAGS; M.O.H., Twp's. of Carden, Dalton & Rama; M.P. Simcoe East; Tel. 325-2271.
RZADKI, Edward J.; Tor'60; D.Psy.; Psy; Staff Psy., Toronto Gen. Hosp., Toronto, Ont.
SAAR, Hilja (Ostra); 43 Clarendon Ave., Ottawa 3, Ont. (res); Tartu (Estonia) '28. Bact., Ottawa Civic Hosp.; Tel. 729-1976.
SAASK, Linda; Tuebingen (Germ.) '46; D.Psy (Tor.); Psy; Staff, Ontario Hosp., 999 Queen St. W., Toronto 3, Ont.; Tel. LE 3-8501.
SABEAN, H. Burgess; 2940 Dublin St., Halifax, N.S. (res); Dal '56; DiagRad; Staff, Hlfx. Infirm; Teach. Fell., Dalhousie U.; Tel. 422-1511.
SABEL, Barbara; New York (U.S.A.) '64; Staff, Placentia Cottage Hosp., Placentia, Nfld.
SABETTA, Vittorio; 150 Metcalfe St., Ottawa 4, Ont.; Tel. 235-3832.
SABIA, Michael J.; 94 Church St., St. Catharines, Ont.; 29 Edgedale Rd. (res); McG '38; F.I.C.S., GenSurg; Chief Dept. of Surg., St. Catharines Gen. Hosp.; Tel. MU 4-7271.
SABIN, Morris; 255 Ellendale Med. Bldg., 5845 Cote-des-Neiges Rd., Montreal 26, P.Q.; 5502 Rosedale (res); McG '50; FRCS(C), FACOG; ObstGyn; Tel. RE 1-9971.
SABO, Gabriel; Maple Med. Centre, Maple, Ont.; Ott'62; Staff, York Central Hosp.; Tel. 832-2201.
SABOURIN, Georges A.; St. Boniface Clinic, 343 Tache Ave., St. Boniface, Man.; Lav '43; M.C.G.P.; Tel. 233-3486.
SABRY, Elsayeed; Med. Dental Clinic, 321 Central Ave., Swift Current, Sask.; Alexandria (Egypt) '55.
SACHAROFF, Mortimer; 2161 Wyandotte St. W., Windsor, Ont.; 2405 Lincoln Rd. (res); Qns '45; Att'd. Med. Staff, Grace Hosp.; Tel. 252-1590.
SACHIS, Jacob H.; 1429 Bathurst St., Toronto, Ont.; 53 Melgund Rd. (res); Tor '37; Staff, New Mt. Sinai & Doctors' Hosp's.; Tel. LE 1-2326.
SACHS, Harold J.; 200 Rideau Terrace, Apt 1016, Ottawa, Ont.; Ott '54; FRCS(C) Cardiovasc & Thor Surg; GenSurg.; Tel. 233-8688.
SACKVILLE, George A.; Ste. 304, 625-5th Ave., New Westminster, B.C.; Alb'50.
SADA, Mitsuko; Apt. 7, 1254 Princess St., Kingston, Ont.; Tor'53; IntMed; Medical Specialist, Ontario Hosp.; Tel. 546-1101.
SADLER, Bruce G.; 294 Labelle St.-Jerome, P.Q.; Qns '53; F.R.C.S.(C), OrthSurg; Staff, Hosp. Hotel-Dieu-de-St. Jerome; Tel. GE 2-9711.
SADLER, Olive M.; 330 East Columbia St., New Westminster, B.C.; McG '40; TherRad; Staff, TherRad. Dept., Royal Columbian Hosp.; Tel. LA 1-7556.
SADOWSKI, Paul D.; Apt. 205, 2525 Bathurst St., Toronto 19, Ont.; Tor '63; Research, Banting Inst.
SADOWSKI, S.; 1347 Ouellette Ave., Windsor, Ont.
SADRO, Teimur; Ste. 2, 2021-7th St. E., Saskatoon, Sask.; Berlin (Germ.)
SAEZ, Antonio J.; 558 College St., Toronto 4, Ont.; Seville (Spain) '55; Tel. 923-6941.
SAGER, Henry S.; 600 University Ave., Toronto, Ont.; 503 Russell Hill Rd. (res); Tor '39; D.A.B.N.S., Psy; Att. Staff, (Psy.), New Mount Sinai Hosp.; Tel. 368-5592.
SAGLE, Lloyd A.; 955 Queen St. E., Sault Ste. Marie Ont.; 445 Lake St. (res); Qns '55; MCGP; Tel. AL 6-6904.
SAGRITALO, Guillermo C.; Manilla (Phillip.) '56; Staff, F. Horner Research Lab., 5485 Ferrier, Montreal 9, P.Q.
SAHAY, P. Ajoy S.; 45 Overlea Blvd., Ste. 4, Toronto 17, Ont.; Patna (India) '51; Staff, Toronto East Gen. & Scarborough Gen. Hosp's.; Tel. 421-4415.
SAHAY, Usha; Ste. 4, 976 Brimorton Dr., Scarborough, Ont.; '51.
SAHIN, A. Fuat; 445 Varsity Ave., Niagara Falls, Ont.; Istanbul (Turk.) '50; Urol.
SAIBIL, David; Ste 370, 6000 Cote des Neiges Rd., Montreal 26, P.Q.; McG'36; IntMed (P.Q.); MCGP; Assoc. Phys., Jewish Gen. Hosp.; Tel. RE 7-7271.
SAIBIL, Maurice; 430 Bloomfield Ave., Montreal, P.Q.; 1201 St. Viateur W. (res); McG '32; IntMed; AMCGP; Att. Phys., Jewish Gen. & Royal Edward Laurentian Hosp's.; Tel. 277-0464.
SAIKEWICH, Peter; 1633 University Ave. W., Windsor, Ont.; Graz (Austria) '34; Tel. 253-7858.
SAIKI, John H.; McG '61; Jr. Intn., Royal Victoria Hosp., Montreal 2, P.Q.
SAINDON, Denis; Henryville, Co. Iberville, P.Q.; Mon '50.
SAINDON, Dominique; 405 Lafontaine, Riviere du Loup, P.Q.; B.P. 116 (res); Mon '21; Anaes.
SAINDON, Zoel; P.O. Box 158, Professional Center of Lachute, Regd., 446 Main St., Lachute, P.Q.); 176 St-Jacques (res); Lav '46; F.A.B.-A.S.; Assoc. Fell., A.B.Gastroent; Surg. Staff, D'Argenteuil Hosp.; Tel. LO 2-2127.
SAINE, George; 184 Aberdeen St., Sherbrooke. P.Q.; Lav '39.

SAINE, Joseph; 7063 rue St. Denis, Montreal 10, P.Q.; Lav '39.; Tel. 279-2368.

ST-AMAND, Jacques; Lav'62; Anaes(P.Q.); Staff, Hop. St-Joseph, Trois-Rivieres, P.Q.

ST. AMAND, Maurice; 594 Theberge, Terrebonne, P.Q.; Haiti '40.

ST-ARNAUD, Gregoire; Ste. 430-450, 34 Cote de la Fabrique, Quebec 4, P.Q.; Lav '44; Gyn; Tel. 523-1641.

ST.-ARNAUD, Louis; Lav '51; Res., Queen Mary Vet's. Hosp., Montreal, P.Q.

ST-ARNEAULT, Guy; Lav'65; Res., Hop. Enfant Jesus, Quebec, P.Q.

ST. CLAIR, John D.; 14204-75th Ave., Edmonton, Alta. (res); Edinburgh (Scot.) '50; FFARCS; DA (Eng.); Anaes. Att'd Staff Edmonton Gen. Hosp.; Tel. 488-8924.

ST. CLAIR, W. Roy; 536 Professional Bldg., 10830 Jasper Ave., Edmonton, Alta.; 10717-108th St. (res); Edinburgh (Scot.) '46; M.R.C.P. (Edin.); IntMed.; Instr. (Clin. Med.), U. of Alta; Tel. 424-6703.

ST-CYR, Bernard; Lav '62; Res., Hop. du St.-Sacrement, Quebec, P.Q.

ST-CYR, Jacques; 1012 Pierre-Bedard, Chicoutimi, P.Q.; Lav '54; PhysMed & Rehab; Tel. 549-0116.

ST. CYR, Laval; 660-2 Ave., Quebec, P.Q.; Lav '35; Tel. 523-5786.

ST. CYR, Rene; C.P. 100, Albanel, Cte. Roberval, P.Q.; Lav '64.

ST. DENIS, Joseph A. M.; 259 St. Georges, St. Jerome, P.Q.; Lav'62; Paed.

ST. DENIS, Joseph A. P.; 2344 rue Martin, Ville de Brossard, P.Q.; Mon'62; Paed.

ST-DENIS, Raymond A.; 51 Elgin St. N., Sudbury, Ont.; Lav '54; MCGP.

ST.-GEORGES, Fernand; 541 De L'Hopital, Jonquiere, P.Q.; Lav'65.

ST. GEORGES, Pierre; 3300 Tracy, Durvernay, P.Q.; Mon '57; Med. Dir., Hop. Jean Talon; Tel. 273-5151.

ST GERMAIN, Jacques, Capt.; Camp Gagetown, N.B.; Lav'65.

ST. GERMAIN, J. Prud'homme; 300 Carre St. Louis, Montreal, P.Q.; Mon '34; Staff, Hop. Ste. Jeanne d'Arc.; Phys., Cdn. National Bank; Tel. VI 5-3787.

ST.-HILAIRE, Gerard SG/LT; Nat. Defence Med. Centre, Ottawa 8, Ont.; Lav'63.

ST-HILAIRE, Gilles; Lav'65; Res., St. Michael Archange, Quebec 5, P.Q. Abroad.

ST. HILAIRE, Jacques; Mon'65; Res., Hop. St. Jean de Dieu, Montreal 5, P.Q.

ST. HILAIRE, Jean L.; Princeville, Co. Arthabaska, P.Q.; Lav '46.

ST-HILAIRE, J. Marc.; 1681 Parc Lafontaine, Montreal, P.Q.; Lav'60; FRCP(C), Neur.; Ass't. Neur., Hop. Notre-Dame; Cons. Hop. Maisonneuve & Inst. of Cardiol & Hop. St. Luc.; Teach. Staff, U. of Montreal; Tel. 527-0555.

ST. JACQUES, Andre; 3117 rue Jean Brillant, Montreal 26, P.Q.; Mon '55; DiagRad.

SAINT-JACQUES, J. Antoine; C.P. 66, Ste. Marie, Co. Beauce, P.Q.; Lav '33.

ST. JACQUES, Marie (See Bastarache).

ST-JEAN, Andre; 906 ave Wilder, Montreal 8, P.Q.; Mon '57; Psy (P.Q.); Tel. RE 7-3292.

ST. JEAN, Conrad; 9 Dufferin, Granby, P.Q.; 201 Dufferin (res); Lav '44; GenSurg.; Tel. 372-5844.

ST.-JEAN, Marc; 1055 Bruxelles, Montreal 5, P.Q.; Mon '52; M.C.G.P.; Tel. CL 5-7151.

ST. JOHN, J. Russell; 107 Toronto St. S., Uxbridge, Ont.; 55 Dominion St. (res); Tor '44 M.O.H., Uxbridge; Tel. 852-3311.

ST. JOHN, Valerie E. (Jenkins); Box 810; Minnedosa, Man.; Man '63; Tel. 867-2722.

SAINT LAURENT, Claude; 700 McEachran, Montreal 8, P.Q.; Lav '55; Psy.

ST. LAURENT, Francois-X.; 25½ Prince William St., Campbellton, N.B. (res); Lav '49; DiagRad; Rad., Hotel Dieu & Soldier's Mem. Hosp's., Campbellton & Hop. St. Joseph, Dalhousie; Tel. PL 3-3301.

ST-LAURENT, Jacques J-C.; 1025 ave des Pins, Montreal 2, P.Q.; Lav'59; Psy; Clin. Ass't., Royal Victoria Hosp.; Lect. (Psy.), McGill U.; Tel. VI 2-1251, Loc. 1618.

ST. LAURENT, Joseph, 2205 des Ormeaux, Montreal, P.Q.; Lav '43.

ST.-LAURENT, P. Guy; 822 Sherbrooke St. E., Montreal, P.Q.; 1230 la Tour, Cite-St.-Laurent (res); Mon '52; F.A.A.P.; Haem (P.Q.); Paed; Tel. LA 3-1137.

ST. LAURENT, Romulus; 50 est, boul. Cremazie, Montreal 11, P.Q.; Lav '51; FRCS(C); GenSurg.

ST. LOUIS, Fernand; Pont Rouge, P.Q.; Lav '41.

St. LOUIS, Gregorie; Mon '64; Res., Hop. Maisonneuve, Montreal, P.Q.

ST. LOUIS, Henri E.; 1541 W. Broadway, Vancouver, B.C.; 3330 W. 44th Ave. (res); Mon '45; M.C.G.P.; Staff, St. Vincent's Hosp.; Vis. Staff, Vancouver Gen. & St. Paul's Hosp's; Tel. RE 8-2611.

ST. LOUIS, Hubert; CP 70, St. Andre Avellin, P.Q.; Lav'55; AMCGP.

STE. MARIE, Sr.; Ott '64; Int., St. Mary's Hosp., Montreal, P.Q.

SAINT-MARTIN, Jean; Quarantine Office, Immigration Bldg., Quebec, P.Q.; 176 Grando Allee (res); Mon '42.

SAINT-MARTIN, Maurice; 277 Blvd. Gouin E., Montreal, P.Q. (res); Mon '42; Bact; Bact., Hotel-Dieu Hosp.; Cons. Bact., St. Luc & Pasteur Hosp's.; Tel. VI 4-0161.

ST-MARTIN, Robert; 1315 Provost, Lachine, P.Q.; Mon '48; DPH; Paed (P.Q.).

St.-ONGE, Armand; 370 rue Brassard, Nicolet, P.Q.; Lav '56; A.M.C.G.P.

ST. ONGE, Claude; 117 Dufferin Rd., Valleyfield, P.Q.; Mon '30; Med. Dir., The Montreal Cottons Ltd. & The Nichols Chemical Co. Ltd.; Tel. WE 7-5711.

ST.-ONGE, Francoise; 7 rue Bell, Chateauguay Centre, P.Q.; Mon '63; Tel. 691-1353.

ST.-ONGE, Gerard; Centre-Medical-St.-Urbain, 3875 rue St.-Urbain, Montreal 18, P.Q.; 460 Wiseman, Outremont (res); Mon '36; FACS; FICS; GenSurg; Surg., Ass't. Prof. Surg & Pres. Med. Bdg., Hop. Hotel-Dieu; Tel. VI 4-0161.

ST. ONGE, L. F. Gilles; 171 Blvd. Garon, Drummondville, P.Q.; Mon '41; Ass't Etranger (Paed.), Paris (Fr.); Paed (P.Q.;); Head of Paed., Hop. Ste-Croix; Dist. Coroner; Tel. GR 8-1381.

ST. ONGE, Marie G.; Mon'65; Res., Royal Victoria Hosp., Montreal 2, P.Q.;

ST-ONGE, Paul; 2130 Bourgogne, Chambly, P.Q.; Mon'30.

ST. ONGE, Real; St. Etienne des Gres, Co. St. Maurice, P.Q.; Lav '50; Tel. LE 7-0664.

ST. PIERRE, Antonotien; St. Dominique, Co. Bagot, P.Q.; Lav '30.

ST-PIERRE, Charles E.; 116 rue Martin, Edmundston, N.B.; Lav'56; DiagRad; Staff, Hop. Hotel-Dieu.

SAINT-PIERRE, Claire; 475 boul. Talbot, Chicoutimi, P.Q.; Lav '61; DPH; Ass't. Dir., Dept. of Health.

ST. PIERRE, Francois; 66 St. Jean Baptiste, Victoriaville, P.Q.; Lav'59; FRCS(C); ObstGyn.

ST.-PIERRE, Gerald L.; 2095 Wyandotte St. W., Windsor, Ont.; 712 Devonshire (res); Wes '50; Tel. 252-2585.

ST. PIERRE, Guy; 690 Concord St., Hyacinthe, P.Q.; 1175 rue Tellier (res); Mon '49; Tel. PR 3-3656.

ST-PIERRE, Guy J.; 354 Inglewood Dr., Fredericton, N.B.; Lav '60.; DPH; AMCGP; Co-ord., Public Health Serv.

SAINT-PIERRE, Hubert L.; C.P. 754, 383 rue Heriot, Drummondville, P.Q.; 1355 Boulv. Fradet **(res); Mon '50; FRCP(C); IntMed; Chief of Med. Serv., Hop. Ste-Croix; Tel. GR 2-2520.**

ST-PIERRE, J.-Paul E.; 2890 De Courcelles, Quebec 10, P.Q.; Lav'54; FRCS(C), GenSurg.

ST. PIERRE, L. Jacques; 658 Fleury E., Montreal, P.Q.; 680 Fleury E. (res); Mon '45; Pulm. Dis. & TB (P.Q.); Staff, Hop. Sacre-Coeur; Cons., T.B., Hop. St. Jean de Dieu.; Tel. DU 8-2138.

ST.-PIERRE, Marc; Mon '63; Res., Hop. Notre-Dame, Montreal, P.Q.; Abroad.
ST.PIERRE, Maurice G.; 130 Water St., Campbellton, N.B.; Lav'65.
ST.-PIERRE, Paul; 36, Puyjalon, Hauterive, P.Q.; Lav '63.
ST. PIERRE, Paul M.; 514 du Palais, St. Jerome, P.Q.; Mon '31; GenSurg (P.Q.).
ST.-PIERRE, Raymond; Mon '62; Res., Hop. Maisonneuve, Montreal, P.Q.
ST. PIERRE, Rosaire; 1005 St.-Prosper, Trois-Rivieres, P.Q.; 2337 Place de Vaudreuil (res); Lav '43; F.R.C.P.(C), IntMed, Cardiol(P.Q.); Hd. Dept. of Med. & Cardiol., Hop.-St. Joseph; Teach Staff, Hop. Ste Marie & Cons. Inst. of Cardiol, Montreal.; Tel. 378-1331.
ST-PIERRE, Yves; Weedon, P.Q.; Lav'62; Tel. 194.

ST-ROME, Gabriel; Paris (Fr.) '57; Paed; Staff, Hop. Ste-Justine, Montreal 26, P.Q.; Tel. RE 1-4231.

SAINT-VICTOR, Jean; (See de Saint-Victor, Jean).

SAIPHOO, Carl S.; Dal'62; FRCP(C), IntMed; Staff, Toronto Western Hosp., Toronto 2B, Ont.
SAIPHOO, Moses M.; Dal'57; Res., St. Joseph's Hosp., Toronto 3, Ont.

SAKAMOTO, Kenneth K.; Glen Agar Plaza, 50 Firwood Cres., Islington, Ont.; 350 Beresford **Ave. (res); Tor '54; M.C.G.P.; Tel. BE 3-7951.**
SAKKAL, Kanal A.; 36 rue Ste-Famille, Montreal, P.Q.; Paris (Fr.) '54; FRCS(C), GenSurg.
SAKRAN, Bishara F.; Ste. 212, One Medical Place, 20 Wynford Dr., Don Mills, Ont.; Tor'65; Tel. 429-2925.
SALAMA, Youssef A.; 192 Moore Ave, Toronto, Ont.; Cairo (Egypt.) '54; Ch.B., Paed; Staff, Hosp. for Sick Children.
SALARUDDIN, A.; Kettle Valley Clinic, Grand Forks, B.C.; Patna (India) '55.
SALCEDO, German; Santo Domingo (Dominican Republic) '55; Int'n., Ottawa Gen. Hosp., Ottawa 2, Ont.
SALDIVAR, Ezequiel; Mexico '52; Staff, Saskatchewan Hosp., North Battleford, Sask.; Tel. 5-2421.
SALEH, W. S.; Cairo (Egypt)'57; FRCS(C), GenSurg; Staff, Ottawa Civic Hosp., Ottawa, Ont.
SALEM, Isaiah; Hagersville, Ont.; Qns '64; Abroad.
SALES, Jack L.; 450 Central Ave., London, Ont.; Wes'55; FRCS(C), GenSurg; Urol; Staff, Victoria Hosp.; Instr. (Surg.), U. of Western Ont.; Tel. 433-3801.
SALGADO, Isidro; 58 Water St., Campbellton, **N.B.; Madrid (Spain) '51; GenSurg; Tel. 3-5533.**
SALISBURY, Gladys M.; 2525 Albert Ave., Saskatoon, Sask.; Man '54; MO, Cairns Schl. Temporarily Retired.
SALKUS, Anthony; 1125 Dundas H'way, Cooksville, Ont.; Munich (Germ.) '55; Active Staff, South Peel Hosp.; Tel. 277-3812.
SALMON, Harold A.; Rosetown, Sask.; Birmingham (Eng.) '54; Ass't. Prof. U. of Saskatchewan. Abroad.
SALMON, J. Douglas; 559 O'Connor Dr., Toronto 6, Ont.; Tor '55; FRCS(C); GenSurg; Tel. 421-4972.
SALMON, Peter A.; 84 Quesnel Cr., Edmonton, Alta.; Washington (U.S.A.) '55.
SALMON, Robert W.; 72 Main St., Huntsville, Ont.; 19 Church St. (res); Tor '39; Dist. Coroner.
SALNA, Marta-E.; 547 Hillsdale Ave. E., Toronto, Ont. (res); Riga (Latvia) '37; Retired.
SALONEN, Otto; 208 Med. Arts Bldg., Port Arthur, Ont.; Wes'59; MCGP; Sec. Treas., Port Arthur Gen. Hosp.; Tel. 345-9722.
SALSBURY, C. Russell; D.C.M., E.D.; 707 W. 37th Ave., Vancouver 13, B.C.; 4784 W. 7th Ave. (res); Qns '24; F.R.C.S.(Eng.), F.R.C.S. (C) GenSurg; Chief Clin. M.O., W.C.B.; Retired.
SALTER, Elizabeth; Alb'61; Paed; Staff, Children's Hosp., Montreal 25, P.Q.
SALTER, Robert B.; 5 Edgar Ave., Toronto 5, Ont. (res); Tor'47; M.S., F.A.C.S., F.R.C.S.(C), OrthSurg; Chief of OrthSurg., Hosp. for Sick Children; Ass't. Prof. (Surg.), U. of Toronto; Tel. WA 3-1704.

SALTIEL, Jacques J.; 14 Ave. Courcelette, Montreal 8, P.Q. (res); Athens (Greece) '47; Diag Rad; Staff, Hop. Maisonneuve; Tel. 254-8341.
SALTMAN, Kenneth; Water St., Harbour Grace, Nfld.; Harvey St. (res); Edinburgh (Scot.) '47; Staff Anaes., Carbornear Hosp.; M.O.H.; Tel. 6153, 6604.
SALTON, William; 54 Ontario St., St. Catharines, Ont.; Buffalo (N.Y., U.S.A) '64
SALVADOR, Herminia S.; Ste. 10, 865 W. 10th Ave., Vancouver 9, B.C.; Far Eastern (Manila, Philipp.)'61; ObstGyn.
SALVI-GUILLEM, Jean; 4934 St.-Denis, Montreal, P.Q.; 5582 des Marguerites (res); Vienna (Aust.) '53; Psy (PQ); Tel. VI 9-8753.
SAMIS, J. Clifford; 267 O'Connor St., Ottawa, Ont.; 68 Reid Ave. (res); Qns '32; FRCS (Edin.), FRCS(C), GenSurg; Sr. Surg., Ottawa Civic Hosp.; Assoc. Prof. (Surg.), Ottawa U.; Tel. 236-5341.
SAMAD, Abdus; Karachi (Pakistan) '55; Staff, Nova Scotia Hosp., Dartmouth, N.S.
SAMAD, Iqbal Abdus; 666 Ontario St., Apt. 802, Toronto 5, Ont.; Osmania (India)'60; IntMed.
SAMAROO, Leslie L.; 1204 10th Ave., New Westminster, B.C.; UBC'65.
SAMIS, T. Tweed; 92 Warren Rd., Toronto 7, Ont.; 25 Strathallan Blvd. (res); Qns '24; Ophth. Tel. 923-1203.
SAMIS, William D.; Ste. 904, 1849 Yonge St., Toronto 7, Ont.; Tor'56; Ophth; Staff, Toronto Western Hosp.; Tel. HU 5-7044.

SAMITZ, Helga (See Haberfellner).

SAMS, Norman H.; General Delivery, Peterborough, Ont.; North Palmerston (N. Zealand)'65.
SAMSON, Andre; Clinique Samson & Dechene, Coaticook, P.Q.; Wellington St. (res); Lav '46.
SAMSON, Andre; 596 E. St. Francois, Quebec, P.Q.; 34 Begin (res); Lav '36; C.P.R., City Med. Officer & Phys., Quebec Power Co.; Tel. 522-7041.
SAMSON, Eucharistе; 60 St. Ursule, Quebec, **P.Q.; Lav '37; DABS; F.A.C.S., GenSurg; Chief Clin. Surg., Hotel Dieu; Assoc. Prof. U. of Laval;** Tel. 529-9151, Loc. 498.
SAMSON, George A.; Coaticook, Co. Stanstead, P.Q.; Lav '43; GenSurg (P.Q.).
SAMSON, G. Henri; 2174 Sherbrooke St. W., Montreal 25, P.Q.; **Lav '32; Ph.D.(Psy.), Psy; Prof. of Psychopath, & Dir., Psychotherapy (Que. & Montreal Inst.), Laval U.; Tel. WE 2-**0486.
SAMSON, Herman A.; Cheticamp, N.S.; Ott '61; Tel. 74.
SAMSON, Hugh R.; 2215 Sheridan St., Montreal 16, P.Q.; Wes'45; Abroad.
SAMSON, Jacques; 4280 rue Adam, Montreal 4, P.Q.; Mon '53; Vis. Phys. (Med. & Obst.), Hop. Maisonneuve; Tel. CL 9-5228.
SAMSON, J. Wilfrid; 1210—lere Ave., Quebec, **P.Q.; Lav '25; M.C.G.P.; Tel. 524-0633.**
SAMSON, Laurent M.; 8415 St. Denis, Montreal, P.Q.; 1001 Waverly (res); Mon '50.; Tel. DU 1-1801.
SAMSON, **Louis;** 2181 Pere Lelievre, Quebec 8, P.Q.; Lav'65.
SAMSON, **Louis-Marie;** 826 Alexandra St., Hearst, Ont.; Tel. 362-4565.
SAMSON, Mathieu; 1060 ave. Parc, Quebec 6, P.Q. (res); Lav '26; DiagRad; Radiol., Hop. St.-Michel-Archange, & Sacre-Coeur; Cons. (Rad.), WCB; Prof. (Rad.), U. of Laval; Tel. 663-3571.
SAMSON, Maurice; 585 est, Boul. Charest, Quebec 2, P.Q.; Lav '42; GenSurg (P.Q.); Staff, Hop. l'Enfant—Jesus & Laval U.; Tel. 523-9728.
SAMSON, Michel; 970 Ave. Cartier, Quebec 6, P.Q.; Lav'49; Cardiol (P.Q.); IntMed; Staff, Inst. de Cardiologie; Tel. 525-9986.
SAMSON, Roger P.; 12245 rue Grenet, Montreal 25, P.Q.; Lav '51; OrthSurg.; Tel. WE 2-3113.

SAMU, Desiderius C.; 316 St. Clair Ave. W., Toronto 10, Ont.; Wurzburg (Germ.) '30; Derm.; Tel. WA 2-5161.
SAMUELL, C. Neville; 560 Professional Bldg., 10830 Jasper Ave., Edmonton, Alta.; Liverpool (Eng.)'41; MCGP; Tel. 429-3351.
SAMUELS, Norman; Med. Arts Clinic, Estevan, Sask.; Cape Town (S. Africa) '51; LRCP; MRCS; FRCS (Eng.); Active Med. Staff, St. Joseph's Hosp. & Bienfait Coalfields Union Hosp.; Tel. 634-3646.
SANBORN, C. Shannon; 1466 Ouellette Ave., Windsor, Ont.; 2088 Willistead Cres. (res); Wes '53; Otol; Hd. Dept. of EENT, Hotel-Dieu; Tel. CL 2-6505.
SANBORN, Clare S.; 1011 Ouellette Ave., Windsor, Ont.; 2033 Niagara St. (res); Wes '24; IntMed; Tel. 253-2024.
SANBORN, D. Kathleen; Medical Arts Bldg., 1011 Ouellette, Windsor, Ont.; 2033 Niagara St. (res); Wes '24.
SANCHE, Hector; 3707 St. Hubert, Montreal, P.Q.; 437 Brookfield, Mont Royal (res); Mon '19; Obst; Hon. Phys., Hop. Misericordia; Prof., Emer., U. of Montreal.; Tel. LA 1-8542.
SANCHE, Pierre; 3707 St. Hubert, Montreal 24, P.Q.; 5485 Beaubien (res); Man '54; Obst. (P.Q.).; Tel. LA 1-8542.
SANCHEZ, Adolfo; Ste 19, 4328 Sherbrooke St. W., Montreal 6, P.Q.; Valladolid (Spain) '57; D.Psy(McGill); Psy(P.Q.); Tel. 935-2846.
SANCHEZ-ARROYO, Emilio; '55; DiagRad (P.Q.); Staff, Lakeshore Gen. Hosp., Pointe Claire, P.Q.
SANCHEZ, Arturo; 2917 Bloor St. W., Ste. 10, Toronto 18, Ont.; National U. of Colombia (S. America) '58; Paed; Assoc. Staff, St. Joseph's Hosp.; Tel. 239-3165.
SANCHEZ, Yolanda E.; Santo Tomas (Philip.) '54; Intn., Ottawa Civic Hosp., Ottawa, Ont.
SAND, Nicholas; Ste. 716, 1849 Yonge St., Toronto 7, Ont.; Prague (Czech.)'33; MCGP; Staff, New Mount Sinai & Central Hosp's.; Tel. HU 3-1008.
SANDBORN, B. Edmund; 85 avenue Woodland, Beaconsfield, P.Q. (res); Man '45; Ass't. Prof., Dept. d'Anatomie, U. of Montreal; Tel. 733-9951, Loc. 320.
SANDBORN, Lillian S. (Floyd); R.R. 1, Kingston, Ont. (res); Man '45.
SANDERS, Britain M.; 280 Bloor St. W., Toronto, Ont.; 84 Heathcote Ave. (res); Wes '48; DermSyph; Staff, Toronto Gen. & Sick Children's Hosp's.; Teach., U. of Toronto; Tel. 924-5105.
SANDERS, C. Borden; 23 Division St., Welland, Ont.; 62 Pine St. (res); Wes '44; F.R.C.P.(C) IntMed; Chief, Med. Dept., Welland Co. Gen. Hosp.; Tel. RE 4-6605.
SANDERS, David H.; 180 Portland St., Dartmouth, N.S.; Dal'66.
SANDERS, Douglas E.; Med. Arts Bldg., 170 St. George St., Toronto, Ont.; Tor'49; DMR; FRCP(C), DiagRad; Sr. Rad., Toronto Gen. Hosp.; Assoc. in Rad., U. of Toronto; Tel. WA 1-3118.
SANDERS, Maurice R.; Glencoe, Ont.; Wes'63; M.O.H.. Cafrid Twnsp.; Phys., C.N.R.; Tel. 287-2616.
SANDERS, Michael G.; Qns'65; Res., Shaughnessy Hosp., Vancouver 9, B.C.
SANDERSON, Harry M.; 117 King St. East. Oshawa, Ont.; Tor'59; MCGP; Active Staff, Oshawa Gen. Hosp.; Tel. 728-1661.
SANDERSON, Moira; Cancer Clinic, University Hosp., Edmonton, Alta.; Qns'60; IntMed.
SANDFORD, John R.; 213 Church St., Oakville, Ont.; Cambridge (Eng.) '56; MA; MB; B.Chir; MRCS; LRCP; FRCS(C), Otol; Staff, Oakville-Trafalgar Mem. Hosp., Oakville, Ont.
SANDHU, Manmohan S.; Raxlan Clinic, 500 Parliament St., Toronto 5, Ont.; London (Eng.) '62; D.ObstRCOG (Eng.); ECFMG; Tel. 925-4381.
SANDILANDS, James; 3195 Granville St., Vancouver 9, B.C.; 4816 Selkirk St. (res); Edinburgh (Scot.) '34; M.R.C.P.(Edin.), IntMed; Att. Staff, (Med.), Vancouver Gen. Hosp., Cons. Staff, Shaughnessy (DVA) Hosp.; Pt-time Phys., Spec. Div. TB Control (B.C.); Tel. RE 3-4214.
SANDLER, Allan; 120 Overbrook Place, Downsview, Ont.; Tor '63.
SANDOMIRSKY, Stanley K.; Qns '64; Res., Kingston Gen. Hosp., Kingston, Ont.
SANDOR, Kathleen (See Stavraky).
SANDS, Colin A.; 4705 Chancellor Blvd., Vancouver 8, B.C.; Tor'43; Anaes; Att'd. Staff, Vancouver Gen. Hosp.; Clin. Instr., U. of British Columbia; Tel.
SANDY, J. Trevor; 708 Fairmont Med. Bldg., 750 W. Broadway, Vancouver 9, B.C.; Wes '51; FRCS (C), GenSurg; Vis. Staff, Vancouver Gen., St. Paul's, St. Vincent's & Burnaby Gen. Hosp's; Clin. Instr., U. of British Columbia; Tel. 874-3921.
SANESI, Lorenzo; Bologha, Italy '58 Jr. Intn., University Hosp., Edmonton, Alta.
SANGHI, Jodh K.; Kentville Med. Arts Bldg., Masters Ave., Kentville, N.S.; Agra (India) '49; FAGS; OrthSurg; Hd., Dept. of OrthSurg., B.F.M. Hosp.; Tel. 678-2062.
SANGOWICZ, Jadwiga; 509 Pine Ave. W., Montreal 18, .PQ.; '50.
SANSOM, Kathleen E. J. (Parry).; 22 Dalton Cres. S., Orillia, Ont.; Cardiff (Wales) '43; MRCS; LRCP; DPH; M.O., Ontario Hosp. School; Tel. 326-7361.
SANSOM, Lorna (See Miskelly).
SANSONE, Anthony J.; 750 King St. W., Hamilton, Ont.; Tor '23.
SANSONE, D.; 360 Spadina Rd., Toronto, Ont.; Naples (Italy) '24; Tel WA 2-0266.
SANSOUCY, Jacques; 51 rue Gault, Valleyfield, P.Q.; Mon'61; DiagRad; Radiol., Hop. Hotel-Dieu & Barrie Mem. Hosp., Ormstown; Tel. 373-3162.
SANSREGRET, Andre; Ste. 71, 445 ouest St. Joseph, Montreal 18, P.Q.; Lav'55; DiagRad; D. & T. Rad (P.Q.); Staff, Hop. Maisonneuve; Tel. 254-8341.
SANSREGRET, Dollard; 6876 Delorimier, Montreal, P.Q.; 6874 Delorimier (res); Mon '45; M.C.G.P.
SANSREGRET, Edmond; 1277 Blvd. St. Joseph E., Montreal, P.Q.; Mon '31; Obst; Obst., Hop.-Notre-Dame; Teach., Staff, U. of Montreal; Tel. 522-0981.
SANSREGRET, Jean; 3707 St. Hubert, Montreal 24, P.Q.; Obst(P.Q.); Tel. LA 3-8211.
SANSREGRET, Victor; 832 Blvd. St. Joseph E., Montreal 34, P.Q.; 6546 Louis Hebert (res); Lav '39; Staff, Hop. Notre Dame.; Tel. LA 6-0001.
SANTOS, Amado; Santo Tomas (Philipp.) '58; Staff, Hotel Dieu Hosp., Kingston, Ont.
SAPIRSTEIN, Wolf; Ste 926, 123 Edward St., Toronto Ont.; 4 Campbell Cres., Willowdale (res); Capetown (S. Africa) '49; FACS; FRCS(C); GenSurg, FRCS(C), Cardiovasc & ThorSurg; Staff (Thor. & Cardiovas. Surg.) St. Michael's Hosp.; Clin. Instr. (Surg.), U. of Toronto; Tel. 922-0701; Abroad.
SARABIA, Luis G.; 10 Errington St., Chelmsford, Ont.; Valladolid (Spain) '55.
SARDA, Pierre; Ste. 11, 161 Augusta St., Ottawa 2, Ont.; Paris (France) '46; DTM; MCGP; Staff, St. Louis-de-Montfort Hop; Tel. 234-9090.
SARGEANT, Everett J.; 425 Roselawn Dr., Windsor, Ont.; Qns '62; Staff, Hotel-Dieu, Grace, Metropolitan & I.O.D.E. Hosp's.; Tel. 969-4160.
SARGEANT, H. Lynn; 16 Main St. W., Huntsville, Ont.; 25 Lake Dr. (res); Qns '54; Tel. 789-5581.
SARGENT, Austin U.; 570 Milton St., Montreal 18, P.Q.; McG '57; Research, Royal Victoria Hosp.; Tel. VI 2-1251.
SARGENT, Raymond D.; Wes'51; Res., Vancouver Gen. Hosp., Vancouver 9, B.C.
SARJEANT, Donald A.; 674 Broadview Ave., Toronto 6, Ont.; Tor '53; M.C.G.P.; Tel. HO 3-1323.
SARJEANT, Pamela E.; (See Cooper, Pamela E.).
SARJEANT, Thomas R.; 925 W. Georgia St., Vancouver, B.C.; 1784 Drummond Dr. (res); Tor '31; F.R.C.S.(Eng.), F.A.C.S., F.R.C.S.(C), GenSurg; Sr. Surg., Van. Gen. Hosp.; Clin. Prof. (Surg.), U. of British Columbia; Tel. MU 5-5940.
SARJEANT, W. Ross; Tor'55; Res., Wellesley Unit, Sunnybrook Hosp., Toronto 12, Ont.

SARKAR, Nellie N.; Far Eastern U. (Philipp.) '57; Staff, Path Inst., 5800 University Ave., Halifax, N.S.

SARKAR, Sushil; 60 Queen St., Dartmouth, N.S.; Bihar (India)'53; Am.Bd. (Paed.); Paed.; Active Staff, Halifax Children's Hosp.; Cons., Nova Scotia Hosp.; Court. Staff, Halifax Infirmary & Grace Maternity Hosp.; Lect., Dalhousie U.; Tel. 466-1507.

SARLES, Sally A.; 109 Main St., Picton, Ont.; Tor '54; 35 King Street, (res).; Tel. GR 6-5536.

SARNE, Andrew J.; Ste. 1, 23 Applewood Village, Cooksville, Ont.; London (Eng.) '61.

SARRASIN, Paul; 287 Ave. St. Jerome, Matane, P.Q.; 10 Rue Thibault (res); Mon '48; OrthSurg (P.Q.); Staff, Hop. St. Redemption.

SARTOR, Victor E.; 1687B Marina Court, San Mateo, California, U.S.A.; Alb'61; IntMed; Abroad.

SARTORELLI, Anthony; Suite 904, Greyhound Bldg., 622-1st St. S.W., Calgary, Alta.; Tor'49.

SARWER-FONER, Gerald J.; 613 Cote-Saint-Antoine Rd., Montreal 6, P.Q.; Mon'51; DNB; D.Psy(McG); FAPA; FAAA, Sc.; DABNP (Psy); FACON; Psy; Memb. Cdn. Psychoanalytic Soc. & Int. Psychoanalytic Assoc.; Assoc. Psy. & Dir. of Psy. Research, Jewish Gen. Hosp.; Cons. Psy., Notre Dame Hosp.; Vis. Prof. (Psychother.), Laval U.; Ass't. Prof., McGill U.; Tel. HU 6-9996.

SASSEVILLE, J. Hubert; Mon '63; Res., Hop. Ste-Justine, Montreal 26, P.Q.

SASSEVILLE, Real; Lav'60; Otol(P.Q.); Staff, Hop. Hotel-Dieu-St-Michel, Roberval, P.Q.

SASS-KORTSAK, Andrew; 555 University Ave., Toronto 2B, Ont.; 1347 Mt. Pleasant Rd. (res); Peter Pazmany U. (Budapest, Hung.) '40; Paed; Phys. & Research Memb., Hosp. for Sick Children; Assoc. Prof. (Paed). & Research Assoc. (Pathol.), U. of Toronto; Tel. EM 6-7242., Ext. 463.

SASYNUIK, Michael E.; Birtle, Man.; Man '55; M.C.G.P. Abroad.

SATANOVE, Abraham; Ste. 201, 625-5th Ave., New Westminster, B.C.; Alb'48; DermSyph.

SAUCIER, Cosette; 11, Marguerite de 'Youville, Levis, P.Q. (res); Lav '54; M.O., Levis Health Unit, Quebec.

SAUCIER, Guy; 2531 Place de Monceaux, Quebec 6, P.Q. (res); Lav '55; B.Ph.; F.R.C.P.(C), IntMed; Ass't. (Med.), Hop.-St.-Sacrement; Ass't. Prof. (Physiol.), U. of Laval; Tel. LA 7-3461.

SAUCIER, Jean; 1414 Drummond St., Montreal 25, P.Q.; Mon '22; Paris (France) '27; FRCP(C), NeurPsy; FANA; FAPA; Chief of NeurPsy., Hop. Hotel-Dieu; Prof. of Neur., U. of Montreal; Tel. 842-3633.

SAUCIER, J. Francois; 1266 ouest, ave. des Pins, Montreal 25, P.Q.; Lav '58; Psy; Research Assoc., Allan Mem. Inst.; Cons. Research, Hop. Notre-Dame; Tel. VI 4-6311, Ext. 631.

SAUCIER, J. Tancrede O.; 823-12th St., Saskatoon, Sask. (res); Lav '96; Retired.

SAUCIER, Roland; 475 Boul. Talbot, Chicoutimi, P.Q.; Lav '48; (For. Hosp. Ass't. Paris, Fr.); Psy (PQ); Dir. Dept. of Neurpsy.; Prof. of Psy., Nurses' Schl. & Ass't. (Med.) Hotel-Dieu-St.-Vallier; Prof. (Psy), Laval U.; Tel. 549-1452.

SAUER, Emil K.; Medical Arts Clinic, Regina, Sask.; 2705 McCallum (res); Qns '26; GenSurg; Tel. 522-1651.

SAUER, Jean F. (COVERT); 2210 Navaho Dr., Ottawa 3, Ont. (res); U. of Minnesota (U.S.A.) '56; Research, Ottawa Civic Hosp.

SAUKS, Arvo A.; Heidelberg (Germany) '50; Staff, Ontario Hosp., North Bay, Ont.; Tel. 474-1200.

SAULNIER, Andre; 52 Grand-Ile, Valleyfield, P.Q.; Mon '47; GenSurg (P.Q.); Tel. 373-6464.

SAULNIER, Georges; 115 est Grande-Allee, Quebec 4, P.Q.; 12 rue Couvent, Beauport (res); Lav '44; F.R.C.P.(C), IntMed; (Cardiol) (P.Q.); Med. Ass't., Hop.-Hotel-Dieu; Ass't. Prof., Laval U.; Tel. 523-1003.

SAUNDERS, Allison L.; 98 Prince St., Charlottetown, P.E.I.; 36 Brighton Rd. (res); Dal '48; Staff, P.E.I. Hosp.; Tel. 894-5642.

SAUNDERS, David R.; Dept. of Med., Royal Victoria Hosp., Montreal 2, P.Q., McG '57, FRCP(C), IntMed; Tel. VI 2-1251.

SAUNDERS, Frederick E.; 925 W. Georgia, Vancouver, B.C.; 5450 Cypress (res); McG '35; F.A.C.S., F.A.C.O.G.; ObstGyn; Cons. (ObstGyn), Vancouver Gen. Hosp.; Assoc. Staff, ObstGyn., Grace Hosp.; Att. Staff, ObstGyn., St. Vincent's Hosp.; Tel. MU 1-7716.

SAUNDERS, George M.; 2 Church St., Amherst, N.S.; 175 Victoria St. E. (res); Dal '47; FACS; F.R.C.S.(C), GenSurg; Chief of Surg., Highland View Hosp.; Tel. 667-8740.

SAUNDERS, Jack A.; 20 Doctors Lane, King City, Ont.; R.R. No. 1, King City, Ont. (res); Tor '60; MCGP; Active Staff, York Co. & York Central Hosp's.; Tel. TE 3-5331.

SAUNDERS, James L.; 5 Central St., Summerside, PEI; Dal '60; AMCGP.

SAUNDERS, Maurice H.; The Rocanville Clinic, Rocanville, Sask.; Bristol (Eng.) '58; Staff, Moosomin Union Hosp.; Tel. 237.

SAUNDERS, Michael G.; E.E.G. Dept., Winnipeg Gen. Hosp., Winnipeg, Man.; Manchester (Eng.) '44; Dir. E.E.G. Wpg. Gen. Hosp.; Cons. E.E.G., Children's Hosp., St. Boniface, & Prov. of Man.; Assoc. Prof. (Med.), U. of Manitoba; Tel. SP 4-6511, ext. 385.

SAUNDERS, Reginald M.; Lunenberg, N.S.; Dal '11; M.C.G.P.; Dist. Coroner.

SAUNDERS, Reginald O.; Black's Harbour, Charlotte Co., N.B.; Dal '57; Staff, Fundy Hosp.; Tel. 456-3344.

SAUNDERS, Richard L. deCH.; 1401 Embassy Towers, Spring Garden Rd., Halifax, N.S.; Edinburgh (Scot.) '32; F.R.S.E., F.R.S.A.; Prof. & Hd. (Anat.), Dalhousie U.; Tel. 2-4406.

SAUNDERS, Sarah C. (MacIntyre); 1401 Embassy Towers, Spring Garden Rd., Halifax, N.S.; Edinburgh (Scot.) '38; Staff, Dept. of Anat., Dalhousie U.

SAUNDERS, Thomas C.; 48 Academy Bldg., 1812-4th St. W., Calgary, Alta.; McG'51; MCGP; Staff, Holy Cross & Calgary Gen. Hosp's.; Tel. 266-4467.

SAUNDERS, Walter G.; 710 Seymour St., Vancouver, B.C.; 3931 Sunnycrest Dr. (res); Alb '26; D.P.H.; Tel. MU 4-1511. Retired.

SAURET, Pedro; 539 College St., Toronto 4, Ont. '54.

SAUVE, Andre; 556 Blvd. Bedard, Lachute, P.Q.; Mon '56; MCGP; Tel. LO 2-2666.

SAUVE, Clement; 186 boul. Harwood, Dorion, P.Q.; Mon '62.

SAUVE, Gaston; 663 Echo Dr., Ottawa 2, Ont. (res); Mon '50; Staff, Ottawa Gen. Hosp. Lect. (Med.), U. of Ottawa.

SAUVE, Jean M.; C.P. 60, Chateauguay Village, P.Q.; Mon '55; Tel. 692-8731.

SAUVE, Noel; 217 Laurier Ave. E., Ottawa, Ont.; 54 Wayling Eastview Rd. (res); Mon '23; Anaes; Active Staff, Ottawa Civic Hosp.; Tel. CE 3-7342.

SAVAGE, Donald C.; 115 Woolwich St., Guelph, Ont.; 28 Crestwood Pl. (res); Tor '33; Ophth.; Staff (Ophth.), Guelph Gen. & St. Joseph's Hosp's.; Tel. TA 2-9381.

SAVAGE, E. Margaret; Cold Lake, Alta.; Wes '29; M.O.H., Cold Lake.

SAVAGE, Howard G.; 250 Lawrence Ave. W., Toronto 12, Ont.; 97 Glenview Ave. (res); Tor '37; A.M.C.A.A., Paed.; Clin. Ass't., Hosp. for Sick Children; Tel. RU 1-4040.

SAVAGE, John P.; 180 Portland St., Dartmouth, N.S.; Belfast (N. Ire.)'56; BAO.

SAVARD, Germain; 3840 Monselet, Montreal N., P.Q. (res); Mon '52; Staff, Hop. Notre Dame.

SAVARD, Guy; Lav'54; Res., Hop. St. Michel-Archange, Quebec 5, P.Q.

SAVARD, Lucien; 309 Montcalm, Chicoutimi, P.Q.; Lav '46; M.C.G.P.; Staff, Hop.-Hotel-Dieu-St.-Vallier.

SAVARD, Martial; 34 rue de l'Hopital, Lorettville, P.Q.; Lav '51; Pres. Med. Council, St-Ambroise Hosp.; Tel. 842-3246.

SAVARD, R. Marc.; 1150 est Boulv. St. Joseph, Montreal 34, P.Q.; 310 Lockhart, Mtl. 16 (res); Mon '52; M.Sc. (Minn.); Cardiol. (P.Q.); Staff, Hop. Maisonneuve; Dem. (Clin.Med.), U. of Montreal; Tel. LA 7-1241.

SAVARD, Yves; 102 rue Principale, St. Victor, Cte. Beauce, P.Q.; Lav'64.

SAVARY, Paul; 1010 ouest St. Cyrille, Quebec 6, P.Q.; 3196 Neuville (res); Lav '58; Otol; Ass't. (Oral Serv.), Hotel-Dieu; Tel. 527-3252.

SAVIGNAC, Bernard; 55 du Roi, Sorel, P.Q.; 34 rue Georges (res); Lav '45; M.C.G.P.; Tel. RI 3-4292.

SAVISKY, Michael F.; Ste. 102, 299 Main St., Chilliwack, B.C.; Man '38; Ophth; Tel. SY 4-8891.

SAVOIE, A. M.; c/o Chief Medical Officer, Dept. National Health & Welfare, 61 Green St. London W.1, England.

SAVOIE, Andre; Lav. '61; Res., Hop. Notre-Dame, Montreal., P.Q.

SAVOIE, Bernard; St. Quentin, N.B. (res); Mon '54.

SAVOIE, C. Bertrand; 1570 rue St.-Louis, Plessisville, P.Q.; 1384 rue du-College (res); Lav '55; Med. Dir., Hop. Notre-Dame-du-Champs; Tel. 362-7517.

SAVOIE, Eudore; Ste. 217, 3875 rue St.-Urbain, Montreal 18, P.Q.; Mon'47; FRCS(C), GenSurg; Tel. 288-3320.

SAVOIE, Guy; 109 rue Rice, Edmunston, N.B.; Lav'58; Tel. 735-3181.

SAVOIE, Isabelle; Caraquet, N.B.; Lav'50; Tel. 727-3030.

SAVOIE, Jean M.; Lav'65; Res., Hop Enfant Jesus, Quebec, P.Q. Abroad.

SAVOIE, J. Romeo; Lav '32; GenSurg (P.Q.); Staff, Hotel-Dieu-du-Sacre-Coeur, Quebec 8, P.Q.; Tel. 523-5049.

SAVOIE, Laval; St. Ferdinand d'Halifax, Cte. Megantic, P.Q.; Lav '46.

SAVOIE, L. Philippe; 230 Longueuil, St.-Jean, P.Q.; Mon '40; GenSurg (P.Q.).

SAVOIE, Monique; 685 Cathcart St., Montreal, P.Q.; 3124 Fendall Ave. (res); Lav '53; Supt., Med. Serv., Dept. of National Health & Welfare; Tel. 866-7314.

SAVOIE, Pierre; Ste. 101, 68 boul. Cartier, Laval-des-Rapides, P.Q.; Mon '64.

SAVOIE, Raymond; Caraquet, N.B.; Lav '51; M.C.G.P.; Vice Pres. Staff, Hop. Infant Jesus; Staff, Hop. Hotel Dieu St. Joseph, Tracadie; Port Phys., Caraquet; Coroner, Gloucester Co.; Tel. 727-3030.

SAVOIE-BOURGEOIS, Isabelle Y.; Caraquet, N.B. (res); '50; Not practising.

SAVRAN, Nebahat; '46; Staff, Riverview Hosp., Essondale, B.C.

SAWADA, Kamio; Box 999, Taber, Alta.; 5003-48th (res); Alb '55; Tel. 223-3525.

SAWATZKY, Harvey J.; Box 490, Enderby, B.C.; Sask'64.

SAWCHUK, Victor N.; Wainwright, Alta.; Alb '60; MCGP; Tel. 842-3341.

SAWREY, Kendall R.; Qns '55; Res., Kingston Gen. Hosp., Kingston, Ont.

SAWYER, Glenn; 244 St. George St., Toronto 5, Ont.; 408 Fairview Dr., Whitby (res); Wes '36; Gen. Sec., Ont. Med. Assoc.; Editor, Ont. Med. Review; Tel. 925-3264.

SAXON, Roland D.; Dal'63; Res., Victoria Gen. Hosp., Halifax, N.S.

SAXTON, Dorothy E. (Pound); 1607—W. 28th Ave., Vancouver, B.C. (res); Man '34; Retired.

SAXTON, George D.; Ste 1205, 750 W. Broadway, Vancouver, B.C.; 1607 W. 28th Ave. (res); Man '32; F.R.C.S. (Edin.); GenSurg; Assoc. Surg., Vancouver Gen. Hosp.; Cons. Surg, B.C. Cancer Inst.; Thor Surg., Indian Health Dept., Sardis; Cons. T.B. Dir. Dept. of Health. Prov of B.C.; Ass't. Prof., Dept. of Surg., U. of British Columbia; Tel. TR 2-1510.

SAYEGH, Victor; 5469 Trans-Highland Ave., Montreal, P.Q.; Bagdad (Iraq) '48; DiagRad.

SAYLES, Una J.; Richards Landing, Ont.; College of Med. Evangelists (Calif.) '57.

SAZANT, Marvin; Raxlen Clinic, 500 Parliament St., Toronto, Ont.; Tor'61; Staff, Doctors Hosp.; Tel. WA 5-4381.

SCALA, Salvatore; 2032 Gerrard St. E., Toronto 13, Ont.; 177 Sweeney Dr. (res); Tor '58; Assoc. Staff, Tor. E. Gen. Hosp.; Tel. OX 8-5311.

SCALES, E. John; Box 90, Mayerthorpe, Alta.; Trinity Coll. (Dublin, Ire.) '53.

SCALES, J. J.; 10970—124th St., Edmonton, Alta.; Tor '46; Anaes.; Anaes, Edmonton Gen. Hosp.

SCAMMELL, Harold L.; 5736 Atlantic St., Halifax, N.S.; Dal '27; Exec. Dir., Nova Scotia Alcoholism Research Fdn.; Lect., Dalhousie U.; Tel. 423-7002.

SCANDIFFIO, Michael A.; 86 Bloor St. W., Toronto, Ont.; 10 Hillcrest Dr. (res); Tor 31; M.C.G.P.; O.P.D. Spec. Clinic, V.D.S.; St. Michael's Hosp., Tel. 924-1700.

SCANTLEBURY, Thomas H.; Bridgewater, N.S.; Dal'66.

SCAPPATURA, Anthony R.; 110 Main W., North Bay, Ont.; Ott '52; Tel. 472-3240.

SCARFF, Michael A.; 1112 Riverside Dr. E., Riverside, Ont.; Wes'61; Path.

SCARFO, John R.; 13656-102nd Ave., North Surrey, B.C.; 13790-101A Ave. (res); UBC '55; Staff, Dept. of Nat. Health & Welfare; Tel. 581-1515, 581-4314.

SCARFONE, Francis P.; 1310 Ouellette Ave., Windsor, Ont.; 2093 Ypres Blvd. (res); Wes '48; M.C.G.P.; Staff, Hotel-Dieu, Metropolitan & Grace Hosp's; Tel. 254-7712.

SCARLATESCO, Alexander J.; North End Med. Center; 663 Jarry St. W., Montreal, P.Q.; 3445 Ridgewood Ave., Apt. 408 (res); Bucharest (Roumania) '42; Staff, Dept. of Anat., U. of Montreal; Tel. 274-4949.

SCARLETT, Earle P.; 214-6th Ave. W., Calgary, Alta.; 409 Roxboro Rd., (res); Tor '24; LL.D., F.A.C.P., F.R.C.P.(C) IntMed; Chancellor, U. of Alberta; Retired.

SCARROW, Gordon R; 159 Watson St., Sarnia, Ont. (res); Wes '36; DiagRad; Rad., Sarnia Gen. & Petrolia Gen. Hosp's.; Tel. DI 4-3361.

SCARROW, Hartford G.; 3009—31st Ave., Vernon, B.C.; R.R. 4 (res); Man '36; GenSurg; Tel. 542-4321.

SCARTH, Alastair G.; McG'51; Res., Princess Margaret Hosp., Toronto 5, Ont.

SCATLIFF, John R.; 21 Sandra Bay, Winnipeg 9, Man.; London (Eng.) '41; DPH; MCGP (Hon.); Med. Dir., Misericordia Gen. Hosp.; Tel. SP 4-6581.

SCHACHER, Nathan; 159 Sherbrooke St. E., Montreal, P.Q.; Bishops (U.S.A.) '05; Retired.

SCHACHERL, Ugo; Delisle, Sask.; Dal '62.

SCHACTER, Brent A.; Manitoba Cancer Fdn., 700 Bannatyne Ave., Winnipeg 3, Man.; Man'65.

SCHACHTER, Harry; 5 Menin Rd., Toronto 10, Ont.; Tor '59; Ph.D.; Assoc. Prof. Biochemistry, U. of Toronto; Tel. WA 3-6611; Abroad.

SCHACTER, Irving B.; 99 Avenue Rd., Toronto 5, Ont.; 411 Richview Ave. (res); Tor '49; FRCS(C), NeurSurg; Att'd. Staff, Mt. Sinai Hosp.; Assoc. Staff, Doctor's Hosp.; Clin. Teach. (Surg.), U. of Toronto; Tel. WA 2-8773.

SCHACTER, Melville; 8719 Saskatchewan Dr., Edmonton, Alta.; McG'46.

SCHACHTER, Ricky (Kanee); 314 St. Clair Ave. W., Toronto 10, Ont.; Tor'43; DermSyph; Teaching Staff, Women's College Hosp.; Clin. Teach. (Med.). U. of Toronto; Tel. WA 2-9620.

SCHAEFER, John P.; Dal'64; Res., Victoria Gen. Hosp., Halifax, N.S.

SCHAEFER, Otto; 12815-116th Ave., Edmonton, Alta. (res); Heidelberg (Germ.) '45; IntMed; M.O. Chas. Camsell Indian Hosp., Dept. of Indian Affairs, Natl. Health & Welfare; Clin. Inst. Med., U. of Alberta; Tel. GL 5-7141.

SCHAFFER, Henri; 605 Erie St. E., Windsor Ont.; 1987 Ypres Blvd. (res); Naples (Italy) '33; MCGP; Tel. 256-0379.

SCHAFFER, Louis; The Pilot, 604 E. Cordova St., Vancouver 4, B.C.; Glasgow (Scot.) '37.

SCHAFFNER, Vernon D.; 12 Cornwallis St., Kentville, N.S.; McG '30; DABTS; FACS; GenSurg; ThorSurg; Chief of Staff, Blanchard-Fraser Mem. Hosp., & Hd. Dept. of Surg.; Surg., Nova Scotia San.; Cons. Surg., Western Kings Mem. Hosp., Berwick; Dist. M.O., Cnd. Pacific Railways; Tel. 678-4626.

SCHAFFRIN, Miriam; Sask '63; Staff, Woodlands School, New Westminster, B.C.; Tel. LA 1-2611.

SCHAFFRIN, Roger M.; Sask '63; Res., Dept. of Chem., U. of British Columbia, Vancouver, B.C.

SCHARF, Arthur A.; 206 Canada Bldg., Saskatoon, Sask.; 1137 Elliott St. (res); Wes '28; Ophth.Otol; Teaching & on Medical Board, City Hospital; Tel. 242-2570.

SCHARF, Forrest L.; McG '56; Staff, Dept. of Pathol., Trenton Mem. Hosp., Trenton, Ont. Abroad.

SCHARF, Robert F., Major; McG '48; FRCS(C); GenSurg; OrthSurg; Staff, Canadian Forces Hosp., Halifax, N.S. & Lect. Surg., Dal. University.

SCHARFE, Ernest E.; 1414 Drummond St., Montreal, P.Q.; 620 Victoria Ave., Westmount (res); McG '23; D.L.O.(Eng.), D.A.B.Ot., Otol; Chairman, Dept. of Otol, Montreal Gen. Hosp.; Ass't. Prof., Dept. of Otol., McGill U.; Tel. VI 9-3149.

SCHATZ, Douglas L.; Suite 301, Tor. Western Hosp., Toronto 2B, Ont.; Tor'56; FRCP(C); IntMed; Staff, Toronto Western Hosp.; Clin. Teach. (Med.), U. of Toronto; Tel. 364-4694.

SCHATZ, J. I.; c/o Chief Medical Officer, Dept. Nat. Health & Welfare, 61 Green St., London W.1, England.

SCHATZ, Stanley W.; 123 Edward St., Ste. 1025, Toronto 2, Ont.; Tor '53; FRCS(C), NeurSurg; Active Staff, St. Michael's & St. Joseph's Hosp's.; Cons. Staff, Sunnybrook Hosp.; Assoc. Surg., U. of Toronto; Tel. 368-1264.

SCHATZKER, Joseph; Tor'60; FRCS(C), OrthSurg; Staff, Dept. of OrthSurg., Toronto Gen. Hosp., Toronto, Ont.

SCHECTER, Nathan; 297 Laurier Ave. E., Ottawa, Ont; 434 Daly Ave. (res); McG '36; FACP; A.M.A.P.; IntMed; Att. Phys., Ottawa Civic Hosp. & Chmn., Pharm & Ther. Committee; Tel. 233-5075.

SCHEFFER, Yvon; Ott'61; Res., Hop. Ste. Justine, Montreal 26, P.Q.

SCHEFFLER, Hilda (Rainda); 5193 Yonge St., Willowdale, Ont.; College of Med. Evangelists (Loma Linda, Calif.) '57; Staff, North York Branson Hosp.; Tel. 633-9420.

SCHENKER, Marianne; 1911 Baseline Rd., Ottawa 4, Ont.; Ott '62.

SCHERER, Guy; 7707 Edouard, Ville LaSalle, Lachine, P.Q.; 325-80th Ave. (res); Mon '59; AMCGP; Staff, Hop. Gen. Lasalle; Tel. DO 6-9661.

SCHERRER, H. F.; 4762 W. 6th Ave., Vancouver 8, B.C.; Graz (Aust.) '51; Assoc. Prof. (Anatomy), U. of British Columbia; Tel. CA 4-1111.

SCHERRER, Roland; 1500-18eme rue, Quebec 3, P.Q.; 1900—4th Ave. (res); Lav '46; ObstGyn (P.Q.); Ass't. ObstGyn., Hop. de l'Enfant-Jesus; Tel. 523-5446.

SCHERZ, Markus; Box 35, Oak Lake, Man.; Brussels (Belg.) '41; Med. Staff, Brandon Gen. & Assiniboine Hosp's.; Tel. 110.

SCHEURLEN, Martin W.; 51 Ahrens St. W., Kitchener, Ont.; Tuebingen (West Germ.) '45; Gen Surg; Active Staff, Kitchener-Waterloo & St. Mary's Hosp.; Hon. Cons., South Waterloo Mem. Hosp.; Tel. SH 3-9222.

SCHICK, Raphael J.; Parkdale Med. Clinic, 1271 Dundas St. W., Toronto 3, Ont.; London (Eng.) '61; Tel. 535-3164.

SCHICKLER, Oskar; 5596 Park Ave., Montreal, P.Q.; 610 Champagneur Ave. (res); Hamburg (Germ.)'36; MCGP; Staff (G.P.), Clin., Queen Mary Vet's Hosp.; Tel. 276-8809.

SCHIETTEKATTE, Fernand; Mon'62; Res., Hop. Hotel-Dieu, Montreal 18, P.Q.

SCHIEWE, Sigmund N.; Port Arthur Clinic, 194 North Court St., Port Arthur, Ont.; Man '39; Tel. DI 4-7271.

SCHIFFER, Irvine; 300 St. Clair Ave. W., Toronto 7, Ont.; Tor '41; DABNP (Psychoanal.); Psy., Toronto Psychiatric Hosp.; Ass't. Prof. (Psy.), U. of Toronto; Tel. WA 5-1781.

SCHIFFMAN, Stella; 4 Chester, Valois, P.Q.; Vienna (Aust.) '37; Staff, Lachine Gen. Hosp.; Tel. 697-1701.

SCHIFFMANN, Wanda (Rubenstein); 109 Finchley Rd., Montreal 29, P.Q. (res); Aurora (Shanghai, China)'48; Neurol; Staff, Hop. Ste. Justine; Tel. HU 1-4363.

SCHILDER, Gustav; 1955 W. Broadway, Vancouver 9, B.C.; 5612 Chancellor Blvd. (res); Graz (Austria) '25; D.P.H.; IntMed.; Tel. RE 1-4414.

SCHILLER, Honore A.; 4400 Wyandotte St. E., Windsor, Ont.; 301 Belleperche Pl., Riverside, Ont. (res); Wes '53; M.C.G.P.; Tel. 945-9671.

SCHILLER, M. G.; Tor '64; Jr. Int., New Mount Sinai Hosp., Toronto 2, Ont.

SCHIMANEK, Tadeusz A.; 300 Bloor St. E., Toronto 5, Ont.; 87 Ascolda Blvd., Scarborough (res); Budapest (Hun.) '42; F.I.C.S.; Staff Surg., Lockwood Clinic; Tel. WA 1-2121. Abroad.

SCHINBEIN, John E.; 153 Third Ave. W., Prince Rupert, B.C.; Tor '51; FACS; GenSurg.

SCHINCARIOL, Elfio A.; 1428 Ouellette, Windsor, Ont.; '56; Tel. 253-7220.

SCHINDLER, Quentin R.; 1401-17th St. S., Lethbridge, Alta.; 1702-14th Ave. S. (res); Man '35; Ophth, Otol; Staff, St. Michael's & Mun. Hosp.; Tel. 327-8643.

SCHIPPER, Hirsh L.; 4505 Sources Rd., Roxboro, P.Q.; Paris (Fr.) '54; FRCS(C), GenSurg; Staff, Jewish Gen. Hosp., Montreal 26, P.Q.; Tel. 735-3771.

SCHIRMER, Kurt E.; 5300 Cote des Neiges Rd., Montreal, P.Q.; 327 Dorval Ave., Montreal; Vienna (Austria) '51; Ophth; Staff, Phys., St. Mary's & Queen Mary Vet's Hosp's; Tel. 631-0452.

SCHISLER, Joseph E.; Box 70, Emeryville, Ont.; Wes '57; MCGP.; Indust. Phys., Chrysler Corp. of Canada Ltd., Windsor; Tel. 252-1956.

SCHLAGINTWEIT, Hugo E. O.; 11968-8th Ave., Haney, B.C.; Heidelberg (W. Germ.)'47; Staff, Maple Ridge Hosp.; Tel. 463-4102.

SCHLAPPNER, Otto L.; 805 Giles Blvd., Windsor, Ont.; Qns'65.

SCHLESINGER, I. Arthur; 5757 Decelles Rd., Ste. 327-8, Montreal, P.Q.; 2920 Graham Blvd., Mt. Royal (res); McG '28; M.C.G.P.; Ass't. Phys., Jewish Gen. Hosp.; Tel. RE 8-2829.

SCHLICHTHER, Wolfgang; Innsbruck (Aust.) '48; Psy; Staff, Riverview Hosp., Essondale, B.C.; Tel. LA 1-1911.

SCHLOSS, Eric; Alb '63; Res., University Hosp., Edmonton, Alta.

SCHLOSS, S. Morton; 552 Columbia St., New Westminster, B.C.; UBC '62; Active Staff, Royal Columbian Hosp.; Assoc. Staff, St. Mary's Hosp.; Tel. LA 2-7530.

SCHLUDERMANN, Eduard; 730 Somerset Bldg., 294 Portage Ave., Winnipeg 1, Man.; 41 Kingsway (res); Vienna (Austria) '32; Tel. WH. 3-3942.

SCHMALTZ, Stephen M.; 9107-118th St., Edmonton, Alta. (res); Alb '32; Exec. Dir., Med. Servs. (Alta.) Inc.; Tel. 429-1731.

SCHMELKA, Daniel; Ott '63; Res., Montreal Gen. Hosp., Montreal 25, P.Q.; Abroad.

SCHMIDEK, Henry H.; Wes '63; Jr. Res., Royal Victoria Hosp., Montreal, P.Q.

SCHMIDT, C. Henri; 2850 Marcel Ave., St.-Laurent, Montreal 9, P.Q. (res); Lav'50; M.O. Hydro Quebec; Tel. 875-4311.

SCHMIDT, Donald J.; Sask '57; Res., University Hosp., Saskatoon, Sask.

SCHMIDT, Ernest W.; 2409 Cairns Ave., Saskatoon, Sask. (res); McG '51; Staff, Cancer Clinic, University Hosp.; Tel. 652-3850.

SCHMIDT, Ingeborg; 220 Bloor W., Toronto 5, Ont.

SCHMIDT, Kenneth E.; 402 Med. Arts Bldg., Edmonton, Alta.; 10201-83rd St. (res); Man '57; GenSurg; Staff, Cancer Clinic; Tel. 422-6525.

SCHMIDT-MALO, Hildegard (Pielorz); 2235 Harcourt Cres., Cooksville, Ont.; Breslau (Germ.) '41; D.Psy.; Psy; Staff, Ontario Hosp.; Tel. LE 3-8501.
SCHMIDT, Nis; Alb '61; Int; c/o 9131-117th St., Edmonton, Alta.
SCHMIDT, Otto A.; 227 Med. Arts Bldg., Winnipeg 1, Man. 200 Waverley St. (res); Man '41; F.A.C.S., F.A.C.O.G., F.R.C.O.G., F.R.C.S. (C), ObstGyn; Ass't. ObstGyn., Wpg. Gen. Hosp.; Assoc. Prof. (ObstGyn), U. of Manitoba; Tel. WH 3-0633.
SCHMIDT, Peter P.; Med. Arts Bldg., 73 N. Cumberland St., Port Arthur, Ont.; 136 Winnipeg Ave., (res); Oxford (Eng.) '44; FRCS(Edin.); GenSurg; Staff, Pt. Arthur Gen. & St. Joseph's Hosp's.; Tel. DI 4-2327.
SCHMIDT, P. Wesley; Sask '58; Res., Winnipeg Gen. Hosp., Winnipeg 3, Man.
SCHMIDT, R. Brenda; 10516-52nd St., Edmonton, Alta.; Man'54; Paed.
SCHMITT, Nikolaus; West Kootenay Health Unit, Trail, B.C.; Heidelberg (Germ.) '45; DPH; PH; FACCP.
SCHMITZ-HERTZBERG, Friedrich S.; Dunbarton, Ont.; Munich (Germ.) '39; M.D. (Goettingen); MCGP; Hd., Medical Dept. & Various Committees, Ajax-Pickering Gen. Hosp.; Tel. 839-2471.
SCHMOK, Arthur C.; Newton Plaza, 7184 King George Hwy., North Surrey, B.C.; 13794 Burkhart Rd. (res); UBC '54; Tel 596-6201.
SCHNEIDER, Ralph J.; Qns '58; FRCS(C); Ophth; Staff, University Hospital, Saskatoon, Sask.; Tel. CH 2-7641.
SCHNEIDER, Robert; 415 Bloor St. W., Toronto, Ont.; 300 St. Clair Ave. W. (res); Peter Pazamy U. (Budapest, Hung.) '51; MCGP; Tel. 921-5736.
SCHNEIDERMAN, Clarence; 435 Ellendale Med. Bldg., 5845 Cote-des-Neiges Rd., Montreal 26, P.Q.; 115 Stratford Rd. Hampstead (res); McG '41; F.A.C.S., Urol; Chief Urol., Jewish Hosp.; Cons. (Urol), Queen Mary Vet's. & Queen Elizabeth Hosp's.; Tel. RE 1-8921.
SCHNEIDERMAN, Gerald; 6000 Cote des Neiges Rd., Ste 395, Montreal, P.Q.; Wes '58; Psy; Jr. Ass't. Psy., Jewish Gen. Hosp.; Cons. Mt. Sinai San.; Dem. (Psy.), McGill U.; Tel. 733-1255.
SCHNEIDERMAN, John L.; Ott' 63; Res., Hotel Dieu Hosp., Kingston, Ont.
SCHNURR, Ilona; Budapest (Hung.) '34; Staff, Hop. St. Charles, Joliette, P.Q.
SCHOBER, Alfred; UBC '64; Res., Shaughnessy Hosp., Vancouver B.C.
SCHOEMPERLEN, C. Benjamin; Manitoba Clinic, 790 Sherbrook St., Winnipeg 2, Man.; 351 Yale Ave., Wpg. 9 (res); Man '37; FACP; FCCP; IntMed; Ass't. Phys. & Endoscopist, Wpg. Gen.; Endoscopist, Children's & Deer Lodge DVA Hosp's.; Chest Phys. & Endoscop., Man. Rehab. Hosp.; Assoc. Prof. (Med.), U. of Manitoba; Tel. SP 4-6541, Loc. 206.
SCHOFER, Roy C.; 829 W. Broadway, Vancouver 9, B.C.; UBC '56; Anaes; Staff, Vancouver Gen. Hosp.
SCHOFIELD, C. Campbell; 102 Med. Arts Bldg., 628 Davis Dr., Newmarket, Ont.; 379 Botsford St. (res); McG'48; Coroner, County of York; Tel. 895-6421.
SCHOFIELD, Robert; London (Eng.) '24; Staff, Alberta Hosp., Ponoka, Alta.
SCHOFIELD, Thomas E.; 703 Danforth Ave., Toronto, Ont.; 833 Coxwell Ave., Toronto, Ont.; Tor'49; D.Psy; Psy; Dir. East-York Leaside Mental Health Clinic; Tel. 466-5544 & 421-9900.
SCHOLTZ, Martin K.; Box 100, Norquay, Sask.; Berlin & Breslau (Germ.) '29; LRCP, LRCS, LRFPS (Edin. & Glas.); Staff, Canora Union & Norquay Hos'p.; Tel. 49.
SCHOM, Charles; 736 Granville St., Vancouver 2, B.C.; 1058-W.41st (res); Man '32; MCGP; Tel. 681-8458.
SCHOPFLOCHER, Paula H.; 789 Upper Belmont Ave., Westmount, P.Q. (res); Heidelberg (Germ.) '28; DermSyph; Clin. Ass't., Royal Victoria Hosp.; Dem., McGill U.; Tel. VI 2-1251.
SCHRAG, A. Ralph; 9259 Strathearn Dr., Edmonton, Alta. (res); Alb '37; Psy; Ass't. Dir. Div. of Mental Health, Alberta; Assoc. Clin. Prof. Psy., U. of Alberta; Tel. CA 9-3443.
SCHRAM, E. Russell; 30 Hayman Ct., 274 Queen's Ave., London, Ont.; 1568 Richmond St. (res); Wes '37; DABOG; FACS, FRCS(C), ObstGyn; Sr. Assoc. (ObstGyn), U. of Western Ont.; Tel. 432-1441.
SCHRAMM, William D.; 619 Brock St. S., Whitby, Ont.; Sask '61; Tel. 668-5835.
SCHROEDER, Warren W. E.; 68 Main St. E., Grimsby, Ont.; 31 Orchard Pkwy. (res); Wes '54; MCGP; Active Staff, West Lincoln Mem. Hosp.; Tel. 945-4922.
SCHROPP, Jerome H.; Box 246, Peace River, Alta.; Tuebingen (Germ.) '37; M.C.G.P.
SCHRYER, Kenneth R.; Ste. 2, 2286 Carling Ave., Ottawa 14, Ont.; Ott '51; MCGP; Staff, Ottawa Civic & Grace Hosp's.; Tel. 728-1454.
SCHRYER, Maurice J.P.; 440 Greenwood Ave., North Bay, Ont.; Ott'58; Path; Staff, Civic Hosp.; Tel. 472-2700.
SCHUBERT, de Schwertenau, Joseph F.; 1870 Bloor St. W., Toronto 9, Ont.; Budapest (Hungary) '37; Tel. RO 7-9369.
SCHUH, Elfriede K. (Zimmermann); 386 Cambria, Stratford, Ont.; Muenster (Germ.) '46; MCGP; Active Staff, Stratford Gen. Hosp.
SCHUH, Otto W.; 386 Cambria St., Stratford Ont.; Erlangen (Germ.) '46; FACA; Anaes; Active Staff, Stratford Gen. Hosp.; Tel. 271-7855.
SCHULDE, Joseph M.; 2085 Tecumseh Rd. E., Windsor, Ont.; 1981 Arras (res); Wes '43; GenSurg; Tel. CL 3-6620.
SCHULER, Graham T.; Room 180, Bldg M50, National Research Council, Ottawa, Ont.; Qns '60.
SCHULMAN, Irvin; 701 Canada Bldg., Saskatoon, Sask.; 1126 Spadina Cres. E.; Man '45; Active Staff, St. Paul's & Saskatoon City Hosp's. 244-4356.
SCHULMAN, Louis; 701 Canada Bldg., Saskatoon, Sask.; 1126 Spadina Cres. E. (res); Man '26; M.C.G.P.
SCHULTE-STEINBERG, Ottheinz; Goettingen (Germ.) '46; Staff, Dept. of Anaes., Scarborough Gen. Hosp., Scarborough, Ont. Abroad.
SCHULTHIES, Lloyd G.; 17 Brunswick Street, Stratford, Ont.; Wes '54.
SCHULTZ, Arthur G.; 322 Wellington St., Sarnia, Ont.; Germany '32.
SCHULTZ, Edward B.; 2271 King St. E., Kitchener, Ont.; Wes '61; AMCGP; Tel. 745-0401.
SCHULTZ, Maxwell H.; 162 Stevens Dr., West Vancouver, B.C.; Qns'46; Anaes; Clin. Instr., (Anaes.), U. of British Columbia; Tel.
SCHULTZ, Stuart D.; Man '27; M.R.C.S.(Eng.), L.R.C.P.(Lond.), Psy; Med. Supt. & Dir., Research, Brandon Mental Hosp.; Brandon, Man.; Cons. in Psy., Brandon Gen. Hosp.; Retired.
SCHULZE, Werner B.; 318 Med. Arts Bldg., Edmonton, Alta.; 8225-112th St. (res); Philipps U., Marburg (Germ.) '54; ObstGyn; Att'd. Staff, Misericordia Hosp.; Court. Staff, Royal Alexandra & Edmonton Gen. Hosps.; Tel. 422-3274.
SCHULZER, Geza; 3029 W. 3rd Ave., Vancouver 8, B.C.; Vienna (Austria) '34; Tel. RE 8-8131.
SCHULZER, Michael; 3029 W. 3rd Ave., Vancouver 8, B.C. (res); UBC '63; Research, U. of British Columbia.
SCHUMACHER, Julius M.; 1120 Ouellette Ave., **Windsor, Ont.; 2799 Avondale St. (res); Innsbruck** (Austria)'53; ObstGyn; Tel. 253-3439.
SCHUMM, B. J.; 16 Laurel W., Waterloo, Ont.; Wes '40.
SCHUNK, H. K. G.; 6039 Kingston Rd., West Hill, Ont.; Heidelberg (Germ.) '48; M.C.G.P. Staff, Ajax-Pickering & Scarborough Gen. Hosp's.; Tel. AT 2-2242.
SCHUNK, Jane E.; (Logan); 6039 Kingston Rd., West Hill, Ont.; Qns '53; Staff, Ajax-Pickering & Scarborough Gen. Hosp's; Tel. AT 2-2242.
SCHUTT, Charles C.; Broadview Ave., W., Smith's Falls, Ont.; Tor '46; D.Psy; Psy; Ass't. Supt., Ont. Hosp. Schl., Tel. 283-2990.
SCHUTZ, Hart; Tor'63; Res., Sunnybrook Hosp., Toronto, Ont.

SCHWAB, Elizabeth M. (Collett); 447 Professional Bldg., 10830 Jasper Ave., Edmonton, Alta.; Alb'57; Psy; Cons. Staff, Royal Alexandra Hosp.; Tel. 424-9328.
SCHWAB, Joseph A.; 1069 Avenue Rd., Toronto 12, Ont.; Tor. '25; Tel. HU 1-6746.
SCHWAB, Wilfred; 1573 Dupont St., Toronto 9, Ont.; 53 Wembley Rd. (res); Tor '34; Tel. LE 5-6191.
SCHWAGER, Paul G.; 742 King St. W., Kitchener, Ont.; 152 Norman St. (res); McG '39; IntMed; Tel. 742-6062.
SCHWANN, Paul G.; 502 Medical Dental Bldg., Regina, Sask.; Alb'58; MCGP; Tel. LA 2-8541.
SCHWARTZ, Arthur M.; Ste. 245, 6000 Cote des Neiges Rd., Montreal, P.Q.; Qns'59; FRCP(C), Neur.
SCHWARTZ, Benjamin; 1868 Portage Ave., Winnipeg 12, Man.; 134 Oakdean Blvd. (res); Man '45.; Tel. TU 8-2309.
SCHWARTZ, Jack P.; 2110 Nantel, Montreal 9, P.Q.; Lausanne (Switz.) '57; Haem. (P.Q.); Staff, Jewish Gen. Hosp.
SCHWARTZ, Maurice H.; 6525 Somerled Ave., Ste. 6, Montreal 29, P.Q.; Paris (France) '56; F.A.G.S.; M.C.G.P.; **Ass't.,** Jewish Gen. Hosp.; Court. Staff, Catherine Booth Hosp.; Tel. HU 8-6262.
SCHWARTZKOPFF, Othild M.; 59 White Oak Dr., Sault Ste.-Marie, Ont. (res); Goettingen (W. Germ.) '46; Staff, Sault Ste. Marie & Dist. Health Clin.
SCHWARTZMAN, Jacob C.; Ste. 7, 1390 Sherbrooke St. W., Montreal 25, P.Q.; 4572 Michel **Bibaud (res); McG '27; F.A.C.S.; Staff, Reddy, Mem. Hosp.; Chief Surg. Doctor's Hosp.; Tel. 844-1331.**
SCHWARZ, Conrad J.; Dept. of Psy., Faculty of Med., U. of British Columbia, Vancouver, B.C.; Glasgow (Scot.) '57; Psy; Instr. (Psy.) & Cons. Psy., Student Health Serv., U. of British Columbia; Tel. TR 6-3211.
SCHWARZ, Harald A.; 405 Northgate Bldg., Edmonton, Alta.; 9712 Riverside Dr. (res); Alb '48; M.C.G.P.; Att. Staff, Misericordia Hosp.; Court. Staff, Edmonton Gen. & Royal Alexandra Hosp's.; Tel. 429-2895.
SCHWARZ, Herbert T.; 6940 Fielding Ave. Montreal 29, P.Q.; 492 Ballantyne N., Montreal West (res); Sheffield (Eng.) '44; M.R.C.S. (E), L.R.C.P. (Lond.), IntMed (P.Q.); Cons. Nordic Biochemicals Ltd.; Tel. HU 8-4513.
SCHWARZL, Johann F.; 955 Queen St. E., Sault Ste. Marie, Ont.; Graz (Aust.)'48; Psy; Staff, Gen. Hosp.; Tel. AL 4-5181.
SCHWEDA, Norbert; 7912-157A St., Edmonton, Alta. (res); Munich (Germ.) '56; M.O., Charles Camsell Hosp.; Tel. GL 5-7141.
SCHWEIGEL, Joseph F.; UBC'62; Res., Victoria Hosp., London, Ont.
SCHWENGER, Cope W.; 39 Tranby Ave., Toronto 5, Ont. (res); Tor '48; DPH; Assoc. Prof. (PH), Schl. of Hygiene, U. of Toronto; Tel. 928-2740.
SCIME, Carmelo; 666 Barton St. E., Hamilton, Ont.; Tor'58; MCGP; Active Staff, St. Joseph's, Hamilton Gen., Henderson & Chedoke & Children's Hosp's.; Tel. LI 9-1679.
SCIME, Ignatius; 250 Main St. E., Hamilton, Ont.; 339 E. 34th St. (res); Ott '56; FRCP(C), IntMed; Active Staff, St. Joseph's & Hamilton Hosp's.; Tel. JA 7-2711.
SCOBIE, Donald H.; McLeod Med. Centre, 340 McLeod St., Ottawa 4, Ont.; 730 Dovercourt Ave. (res); McG '50; FRCS(C), GenSurg; Att'd. Surg., Ottawa Civic Hosp.; Lect. (Surg.), U. of Ottawa; Tel. CE 5-3481.
SCOBIE, T. Keith; McLeod Med. Centre, 340 McLeod St., Ottawa, Ont.; 243 Harmer (res); McG '49; M.Sc., D.A.B.S., F.A.C.S., F.R.C.S.(C), GenSurg; Ass't. Prof. (Surg), U. of Ottawa; Tel. CE 5-1975.
SCOFFIELD, Mary E.; 379 Wortley Rd., London, Ont.; Tor '33; DermSyph; Staff, Dept. of Health, City Hall; Lect. (PrevMed), U. of Western Ont.; Tel. 438-7530. Retired.
SCOSSA, Caroline (See Hetenyi).

SCOTT, Alan C.; Ste. 207, 1105 Carling Ave., Ottawa 3, Ont.; 2244 Alta Vista Dr. (res); Tor '46; FRCS(C), Urol; Staff, Ottawa Civic Hosp.; Tel. CE 3-1903.
SCOTT, Alice (Kakushavish); Cochenour, Ont.; McG '50.
SCOTT, Anthony F. C.; Glazier Med. Centre, 136 Simcoe St. N., Oshawa, Ont.; Dublin (Ire.) '52; G.P. Staff, Oshawa Gen. Hosp.; Tel. 728-7571.
SCOTT, Arthur A.; Tor'53; Res., St. Michael's Hosp., Toronto 2, Ont.
SCOTT, B. H.; 5148 Westbury, Montreal, P.Q.; Qns '43; M.C.G.P.; Tel. 486-2963.
SCOTT, Caroline P.; 1988 Killarney Dr., Ottawa 13, Ont. (res); Dal'51; M.O. Food & Drug Directorate, Dept. of Nat. Health & Welfare; Tel. CE 2-8211.
SCOTT, Charles M.; 343 Stewart St., Peterborough, Ont.; Qns '14; F.A.C.S.; Ass't. M.O.H., Peterborough; **Hon. Staff Member, Civic & St. Joseph's Hosp's.; Tel. 745-5213.**
SCOTT, Christopher R.; Spalding, Sask.; London (Eng.) '61.
SCOTT, David I.; Qns'64; Res., Ottawa Civic Hosp., Ottawa 3, Ont.
SCOTT, David J.; 33 First St., Orangeville, Ont.; Tor'56; FRCS(C), GenSurg; Cons. Staff, Dufferin Area Hosp.; Tel. 941-0700.
SCOTT, Donald J., SG/LT; M.I.R., R.C.A.F. Station, Winnipeg, Man.; Man '61.
SCOTT, Donald L.; Ste. 40q, 811 Grosvenor Ave., Winnipeg 9, Man. (res); Man '26; IntMed (TB); Med. Supt. Ward C 3, Wpg. Gen. Hosp.; Lect. (Med.), U. of Manitoba; Ass't. Med. Div., San. Bd. of Manitoba; Tel. SP 4-6511.
SCOTT, Elizabeth (See Everard).
SCOTT, Flora H. (Halina); 10119-84th St., Edmonton, Alta (res); Alb '54; Psy; Staff, Alberta Hosp.
SCOTT, Florence A. G. (Griffiths); 3 Harvard **Ave., Toronto 3, Ont. (res); Tor '38; D.Psy., Psy;** Psy., Child Adjustment Centre, Board of Edu., **Toronto; Tel. 362-4931.**
SCOTT, Francis G. E.; St. Mary's Med. Clinic, St. Mary's, Ont.; Wes '64; Tel. 284-3450.
SCOTT, Frank; Box 190, Loon Lake, Sask.; Durham (Eng.) '56; Med. Staff, Loon Lake Union Hosp.; Tel. 20.
SCOTT, G. Allan; Fort William San., 300 N. Lillie St., Fort William, Ont.; Edinburgh (Scot.) '34; FCCP; FRCP (Ed.); Cons. Chest. Dis., McKellar Gen., St. Joseph's Gen. & Port Arthur Gen. Hosp's.; Tel. 623-7493.
SCOTT, Geoffrey F.; McG '50; Staff, Ste. Anne's **Hosp., Ste. Anne de Bellevue, P.Q.; Tel. 453-5395.**
SCOTT, George B.; Cochenour, Ont.; McG '49; GenSurg.
SCOTT, George D.; 113 Lower Union St., Kingston, Ont.; R.R. 3, Collins Bay (res); Qns '39; D.Psy (Tor.); Psy; Att'd. Staff, Kingston Gen. & Hotel Dieu Hosp's.; Med. Dir., Inst. of Psychotherapy; Cons. Psy., DVA & Chief Psy., Dept. of Justice (Kingston Pen., Collins Bay & Prison for Women); Lect., Queen's Theolog. College & Queen's U.; Tel. 546-3116.
SCOTT, Gerald W.; 404 Rideau Med. Centre, 1711-4th St. S.W., Calgary, Alta.; London (Eng.) '55; M.S.; DABS; FRCS(C), GenSurg; Surg., Foothills, Holy Cross, Calgary Gen. & Alberta Children's Hosp.; Tel. 263-7120.
SCOTT, Gordon M.; 33 White St., St. Thomas, Ont.; Queens U. (Belfast, N. Ire.) '52; BAO; **Staff, St. Thomas Elgin Hosp.; Tel. 633-0458.**
SCOTT, Grace E.; Qns '61; Staff, Ontario Hosp. School, Cedar Springs, Ont.; Tel. 676-5431.
SCOTT, G. Raymore; Scott Clinic, 483 George St. S., Peterborough, Ont.; 33 Manning Ave. (res); Tor '16; ObstGyn; Pres., Cdn. Army Med. Bd.; Tel. RI 2-0461.
SCOTT, Henry; 925 W. Georgia St., Vancouver, B.C.; 3906 Quesnel Dr. (res); McG '32; IntMed; Cons. (IntMed), D.V.A.; Instr., Dept. of Med., U. of British Columbia; Tel. MU 1-7188.
SCOTT, Henry J.; 540 Seaforth Med. Bldg., 3550 Cote des Neiges Rd., Montreal 25, P.Q.; 611 Sydenham Ave., Westmount (res); McG '42; FRC-S(C); GenSurg; **ThorSurg (P.Q.) Chief Surg., Div. of Thor & Cardiovasc. Surg., Mtl. Gen. Hosp.;** Assoc. Prof. (Surg.) McGill U.; Tel. 932-9112.

SCOTT, Herbert W.; 193 Appleby Line, Burlington, Ont.; Man '28; M.C.G.P.
SCOTT, **Hugh MacKay;** 5905 Trans Island Ave., Montreal 29, P.Q.; Qns'61; FRCP(C), IntMed.
SCOTT, **Ian S.;** Ste. 601, 4700-55th St., Red Deer, Alta.; Glasgow (Scot.)'52; MCGP; Staff, Red Deer Mun. Hosp. & Alberta School Hosp.; Tel. 347-2340.
SCOTT, J. Alan; 22 Laurier St., Magog, P.Q.; 551 Merry St. S. (res); McG '40; Tel. 843-3543.
SCOTT, James; Ire. ('62); Staff, Placentia Cottage Hosp., Placentia, Nfld.
SCOTT, James H.; 117-10th St., Brandon, Man.; Edinburgh (Scot.) '44; M.B., Ch.B., DO; Ophth; Ophth., Brandon Gen. Hosp.; Tel. PA 9-8119.
SCOTT, James R.; 254 Main St., Markham, Ont.; 468 Church St. (res); Qns '50; M.C.G.P.; Med. Staff, Scarborough Gen. Hosp.; Tel. 293-8181.
SCOTT, John A. L.; 191 Woolwich St., Guelph, Ont.; 45 Mont St. (res); Tor '32; FRCS(Ed.); GenSurg; Chief of Surg., Guelph Gen. Hosp.; Surg. Staff, St. Joseph's Hosp. Tel.; Tel. TA 4-3361.
SCOTT, **John G.;** Qns'58; FRCP(C), IntMed; Staff, Dept. of Haem., Toronto Gen. Hosp., Toronto 2, Ont.
SCOTT, John W.; 101 College St., Toronto 2, Ont.; 36 Cheritan Ave., Tor. 12 (res); Tor '41; Dir. EEG Lab., Toronto Gen. Hosp.; Prof. (Physiol.), U. of Toronto; Tel. EM 6-8211, Loc. 2742.
SCOTT, John W.; 420 Physicians & Surgeons Bldg., 8409 - 112th St., Edmonton, Alta.; McG '21; FACP; FRCP(C); IntMed; Phys., University Hosp.; Tel. 433-5896.
SCOTT, Josef; 92 Le Marchant Rd., St. John's, Nfld.; '62.
SCOTT, J. Russell; 91 Bridge St. E., Belleville, **Ont.; 200 John St. (res); Qns '41; M.C.G.P. Staff, O.P.D. Toronto Western Hosp.; Plant Phys., Mead Johnson of Canada Ltd., Stephens-Adamson Mfg. Co. Ltd. & Stewart-Warner Corp. of Canada; Tel. WO 2-2345.**
SCOTT, Kenneth E.; McG '55; Paed; Staff, Children's Hosp., Halifax, N.S.; Tel. 422-8441.
SCOTT-KERR, Michael T.; 350 Albert St., Nanaimo, B.C.; London (Eng.) '60; M.B., B.Chir.; MRCS; LRCP; Staff, Nanaimo Reg. Gen. Hosp.; Tel. 753-3431.
SCOTT, Michael A.; 19 Third St., Chatham, Ont.; Qns'61.
SCOTT, Michael B.; 40 Coldwater St. E., Orillia, Ont.; London (Eng.) '51; D.ObstRCOG; Assoc. Staff, Orillia Soldier's Mem. Hosp.
SCOTT, Moira A.; 9035 Saskatchewan Dr., Edmonton, Alta.; Alb '57; Ass't. Path., Misericordia Hosp.
SCOTT, Norman A.; 452 Charlotte St., Peterborough, Ont.; 478 Albertus Ave. (res); Qns '49; Anaes.; Tel. 745-2491.
SCOTT, Paul A.; 354 Codrington St., Barrie, Ont. (res); Qns '24; D.P.H.; Dir., & M.O.H., Simcoe County Health Unit, Barrie.
SCOTT, Peter A.; 249 William St., Belleville, Ont.; Qns'57; GenSurg; Cons. Surg., Belleville Gen., Trenton Mem., Prince Edward County & Campbellford Mem. Hosp.; Tel. 962-9312.
SCOTT, Peter F.; Med. Assoc. Bldg., 31 James St., Parry Sound, Ont.; Edinburgh (Scot.) '45; M.B., Ch.B., MCGP; Staff, Parry Sound & St. Joseph's Hosp's.; Memb., Planning & Dev. Committee, Parry Sound Gen. Hosp.; Phys., C.P.R. & Lowphos Ore Ltd.; Tel. 746-9382.
SCOTT, Robert M.; 704 Sask. Cres. E., Saskatoon, Sask. (res); Edinburgh (Scot.) '33; Sr. Treatment Off., D.V.A., Federal Bldg., Saskatoon, Sask.
SCOTT, Robert S.; 68 King St. E., Cobourg, Ont.; Edinburgh (Scot.)'57.
SCOTT, Stuart M.; 11121-82nd Ave., Edmonton, Alta.; Man '20; Treatment Staff, D.V.A., Colonel Mewburn Pavilion, U. of Alberta Hosp.; Retired.
SCOTT, Thomas B.; Ste. 302, 688 Coxwell, Toronto 6, Ont.; Cambridge (Eng.)'50; MRCS, LRCP, DermSyph; Att. Ass't. Phys., O.P.D., Toronto East Gen. & Toronto Gen. Hosp's.; Tel. 466-4098.
SCOTT, Walter A.; 115 Woolwich St., Guelph, Ont.; 40 Stuart St. (res); Tor '36; FACS; FRCS (C), GenSurg; Chief of Staff, Guelph Gen. Hosp.; Tel. TA 4-2831.
SCOTT, W. Clifford; 1516 Pine Ave. W., Montreal 25, P.Q.; Tor '27; DPM; Psy(P.Q.); Cons. Montreal Children's Hosp.; Assoc. Dir., Canadian Inst. of Psychoanalysis; Tel. 932-1333.
SCOTT, **William;** Breton Med. Clinic, Breton, Alta.; Glasgow (Scot.) '52; LRCP, LRCS (Ed.); LRFPS (Glas.).
SCOTTI, Raymond; 784 Jean Talon E., Montreal 10, P.Q.; Mon '60; AMCGP; Tel. 273-7421.
SCOTT-MONCRIEFF, Ronald; 315 Medical Arts Bldg., 1105 Pandora Ave., Victoria, B.C.; 663 Radcliffe Lane (res); McG '31; D.A.B.Ot., Otol; Chief E.N.T., Victoria Veterans' Hosp's.; Staff (E.N.T.), Royal Jubilee & St. Joseph's Hosp's.; Memb., Council of Coll. of Phys. & Surg., B.C.; Tel. EV 3-3615.
SCOUGALL, **Keith H.;** 1530 Albion Rd., Rexdale, Ont.; Cambridge (Eng.) '43; MRCS (Eng.); LRCP (Lond.); MCGP.
SCRAGG, Richard D.; 12209-101st St., Edmonton, Alta.; Alb '51; Anaes; Instr. (Pharmacol.), U. of Alberta.
SCRATCH, John A.; Maymont, Sask.; Tor '05.
SCRATCH, John R.; Cutknife, Sask.; Man '37.
SCRATCH, Norvel W.; 386 Cambria, Stratford, **Ont.; 12 Denison St. (res); Wes '43; IntMed; Tel. 271-4151.**
SCREECH, Guy; Ste. 1101, 2060 Comox St., Vancouver 5, B.C.; Cambridge (Eng.) '52; Anaes; Att'd. Staff, Vancouver Gen. Hosp.; Clin. Instr., U. of British Columbia.
SCRIBNER, Charles R.; Gimli Medical Centre, Gimli, Man.; 66—5th Ave. (res); Man '38; Dist. Coroner.
SCRIBNER, Franklin E.; Gimli, Man.; Man '36; Chief of Staff, Johnson Mem. Hosp.; Dist. Coroner.
SCRIMGEOUR, John W. F.; Spence Clinic, Fort William, Ont.; 441 S. Norah St. (res); St. Andrew's (Scot.) '43; M.R.C.O.G., F.R.C.S.(C), ObstGyn; Staff (ObstGyn.), McKellar Hosp.; Tel. MA 2-5301.
SCRIMGEOUR, William G.; Parkhill, Ont.; Tor '50; M.C.G.P.; M.O.H., W. Williams Twp., Middlesex County; Tel. 294-6881.
SCRIVER, Charles R.; 232 Strathearn Ave., Montreal West 28, P.Q. (res); McG '55; F.R.C.P. (C), Paed; Staff, Montreal Children's Hosp.; Tel. HU. 6-9929.
SCRIVER, Jessie B.; 4500 Sherbrooke St. W., Montreal 6, P.Q.; 510 Roslyn Ave., Westmount **(res); McG '22; F.A.A.P., F.R.C.P.(C) Paed; Hon. Att. Staff, Royal Victoria & Montreal Children's Hosp.; Tel. VI 2-6446.**
SCRIVER, Walter de M.; 4500 Sherbrooke St. W., Montreal 6, P.Q.; 510 Roslyn Westmount (res); **McG '21; FACP; FRCP(C); IntMed; Registrar-in-Chief, Royal Victoria Hosp.; Prof. (Emer.) Med.,** McGill U.; Tel. 935-4426.
SCROGGIE, D. G.; Box 2058, Medical Clinic, Whitehorse, Yukon; Tor '64.
SCUDAMORE, M. June; London (Eng.) '49; MRCOG; Hd. Dept. of Exfoliative Cytology, Henderson Gen. Hosp., Hamilton, Ont.
SCULLY, Hugh E.; Qns'65; Res., Queen's U., Kingston, Ont.
SCULLY, L. Terence; 104 Med. Arts Bldg., 638 Davis Dr., Newmarket, Ont.; Tel. 895-6551.
SCULLY, **Peter D.;** McG'61; Res., Douglas Hosp., Verdun, P.Q.
SEAGRAM, C. Geoffrey; Mc'G '63; Res., Hosp. for Sick Children, Toronto, Ont.
SEAH, Stanley K.; Thorold Med. Clinic, 60 Albert St. W., Thorold, Ont.; Man '61; Tel. CA 7-5255. Abroad.
SEALE, C. M. (See Onhauser, C.M.).
SEALE, Carl W. E.; 1734 W. Broadway, Vancouver, B.C.; Man '19.
SEAMAN, Donald M.; Med. Arts Bldg., Masters Ave., Kentville, N.S.; Dal'57; Tel. 618-2830.
SEAMAN, Killem; 115 Hazen St., Saint John, N.B.; 66 Rocky Terr. (res); Dal '42; OrthSurg; Staff, Saint John Gen. & St. Joseph's Hosp's.; Tel. 693-3647.

SEAMANS, Keith B.; Dal'59; FRCP(C), Neur; Staff, Mtl. Neurol. Inst., 3801 University, Montreal 2, P.Q.
SEARBY, Brian; Haig Clinic, 601-6th Ave. S., Lethbridge, Alta.; London (Eng.) '62; M.B., B.S., D.ObstRCOG; MRCS; DA; Assoc. Staff, Lethbridge Municipal & St. Michael's Hosp's.; Tel. 328-6641.
SEARBY, Mary, (Shipp); London (Eng.) '62; LRCP; MRCS; Ass't. Res., Royal Alexandria Hosp., Edmonton, Alta.
SEARLE, Howard G.; 2347 Edgewood Blvd., Berkley, Mich., U.S.A.; Wes '49; GenSurg; Abroad.
SEARLES, Gerald K.; Schreiber, Ont.; Tor '63.
SEARS, Charles F.; Box 998, Merritt, B.C.; **Tor '43; Staff, Nicola Valley Gen. Hosp.;** Tel. 378-2286.
SEARS, Gerald A.; 727 Westmount Hill, London, **Ont.; Wes '52;** FACC; FRCP(C), IntMed; Active **Teach. Staff, Victoria Hosp.; Ass't. Prof. (Med.),** U. of Western Ontario; Tel. 471-4476.
SEARY, John M.; 92 Lemarchant Rd., St. John's, Nfld.; London (Eng.) '63; MRCS (Eng.); LRCP (Lond.); Tel. 579-0102.
SEAVER, Robert; 113 Main St., Markham, Ont.; Tor'56; AMCGP.
SEBASTIEN, Guy; 1384 est Jean Talon, Montreal 10, P.Q.; Mon'58; FRCS(C), GenSurg; PlasSurg; Cons. Hop. Gen. Fleury; Tel. 274-5583.
SEBGHATI, Mahmoud; 23-725 McGee St., Winnipeg 3, Man. (res); Tehran (Iran) '57; FACA; Anaes; Staff, Wpg. Gen. Hosp.; Abroad.
SECORD, Geoffrey; 75 Park Ave., Guelph, Ont.; **80 London Rd., (res); Tor '52; M.C.G.P.; Tel. TA 2-3061.**
SECTER, John J.; 2232 W. 41st Ave., Vancouver 13, B.C.; 3844 S.W. Marine Dr. (res); Man. '52; Tel. AM 1-1734.
SECTER, Max B.; 340 Superior Ave., Calgary, Alta. (res); Man '30; IntMed; Staff Cons. Int. Med., Colonel Belcher Hosp. D.V.A., Calgary; Tel. AM 6-7001.
SEDDON, Thomas T.; 623 Bedford Rd., Saskatoon, Sask.; Alb '41; Tel. 244-5089.
SEDGWICK, William S.; 550 Ingersoll Ave., Woodstock, Ont.; Tor '43; MCGP; Tel. 537-3791.
SEDLEZKY, Isadore; 3755 Cote-St.-Catherine Rd., Montreal 26, P.Q.; 1460 McGregor, Apt. 501, Mtl. 25 (res); McG '38; MACR; DABR; D & TRad (PQ); Radiol.-in-Chief, Jewish Gen. Hosp.; Tel. 738-1164.
SEDLMEIR, Marcus J.; 755 Brimley Rd., Scarborough, Ont.; **3 Fraserton Cres. (res); Tor '50; Tel. 261-6131. Abroad.**
SEELIG, Gustav M. F.; Ste. 2, 901 O'Connor Dr., Toronto 16, Ont.; Qns'44; D.Obst.RCOG, ObstGyn; Clin. Ass't. (ObstGyn), Toronto East Gen. Hosp.; Tel. PL 9-7541.
SEELY, John F.; McG'62; Res., Royal Victoria Hosp., Montreal 2, P.Q.
SEEMAN, Jacob; 1279 St. Clair Ave. W., Toronto, Ont.; 16 Steven Ave. (res); Heidelberg (Germ.) '48; Tel. LE 1-2277.
SEGAL, Perry M.; Ste. 395, 6000 Cote des Neiges Rd., Montreal 26, P.Q.; McG'59; Psy; Clin. Ass't. O.P.D., Jewish Gen. Hosp.; Dem. (Psy.), McGill U.; Tel. 737-5809.
SEGAL, Sydney; 715-W. 12th Ave., Vancouver 9, B.C.; 4338 Quinton Pl., North Van. (res); Qns '50; M.A. (Physiol.); Paed; Research Dir. & Att'd. Phys., Health Centre for Children; Att'd. Staff, Vancouver Gen. Hosp.; Assoc. Prof. (Paed), U. of British Columbia; Tel. TR 6-3211.
SEGALL, Harold N.; 390 Ellendale Med. Bldg., 5845 Cote-des-Neiges Rd., Montreal 26, P.Q.; 4100 Cote-des-Neiges Rd. (res); McG '20; F.A.C.P.; **F.R.S.A.; IntMed; Cardiol (P.Q.); Staff,** Montreal Gen. Hosp., Cons. (Med.), Jewish Gen. Hosp.; **Cons. (Cardiol.), Queen Elizabeth Hosp.;** Tel. RE 1-8181.
SEGALL, M. L. Joseph; 10951-124th St., Edmonton, Alta.: 8204-149th St. (res); London (Eng.) '48; MCGP; Med. Exam., Independent Order of Foresters; Staff, Royal Alexandra Hosp.; Staff, Norwood & Good Samaritan Aux. Hosp's.; Tel. 454-4551.
SEGALL, Sydney; 670 Ellendale Med. Bldg., **5845 Cote-des-Neiges Rd., Montreal 26, P.Q.;** 179 **Dufferin Rd. (res); McG '42;** D.I.M., D.A.B.I.M., F.A.C.P.; **IntMed; Cardiol. (P.Q.); Assoc. Phys.,** Jewish Gen. & Reddy Mem. Hosp's.; Cons. (Cardiol), Mt. Sinai Hosp., St. Agathe; Cons. (Cardiol.), Montreal Fashion Industry Health Centre; Tel. RE 1-9011.
SEGOVIA, C. G.; Staff, Saskatchewan Hosp., Weyburn, Sask.; Tel. 842-3812.
SEGUIN, Fernand; 417 Centre-Medical-St.-Urbain, 3875 rue St.-Urbain, Montreal 18, P.Q.; 2927 Fendall (res); Mon '34; IntMed, Cardiol. (PQ); Ass't. Prof. (Med.), U. of Mtl.; Tel. VI 4-1862.
SEGUIN, Gerard A.; Ott'65; Res., St. Joseph's Hosp., Hamilton, Ont.
SEGUIN, Gerard; 50, Jacques-Cartier, Valleyfield, P.Q.; Mon '55. Anaes (P.Q.).
SEGUIN, Hermas; 30 Est Boul St. Joseph, Montreal 14, P.Q.; Mon'56; ObstGyn. (P.Q.)..
SEGUIN, Herve L.; Penhold, Alta.; Ott '55.
SEGUIN, Julien; 6385 est Sherbrooke, Montreal 5, P.Q.; Mon '60.
SEGUIN, Real; 5399 Place Grovehill, Montreal 28, P.Q.; Mon'57; DiagRad.
SEGUIN, Roger; 287 Montreal Rd., Eastview, Ottawa. Ont.; Lav'50; MCGP; Tel. 749-1274.
SEGUIN, W. Gerard; Mon '55; Res., St. Mary's Hosp., Montreal 26, P.Q.
SEHDEV, Harcharan S.; 3252 Lawrence Ave. E., Scarborough, Ont.; Apt. 533, 10 St. Dennis Dr., Don Mills (res); UBC '63; AMCGP; Tel. AX 3-7551.
SEHL, John R.; 742 King St. W., Kitchener, Ont.; 20 Juniper Cres. (res); Wes '54; FRCS(C), ObstGyn; Tel. 744-8561.
SEHL, Willard A.; 111 Westmount S., Waterloo, Ont.; Tor '35; Obst; Med. Dir., Dominion Life Assurance Co.; Tel. 744-4471.
SEIDE, James; St. Joseph's, Nfld.; Rigia Pavia (Italy) '37.
SEIFER, Roman; 615 Princess St., Brandon, Man.; National U. (Dublin, Ire.) '57.; Staff, Brandon Hosp. for Mental Diseases; Tel. PA 9-1280.
SEITZ, Helmut H.; Bigelow-Fowler Clinic, 1605-9th Ave. S., Lethbridge, Alta.; 1017-20th **St. S. (res); Muenster (Germ.) '46; IntMed;** Staff, Lethbridge Mun., St. Michael's & Lethbridge Aux. Hosp's; Tel. 327-3121.
SEKIGUCHI, Susumu; Tokyo (Japan)'57; Staff, Toronto Western Hosp., Toronto 2B, Ont.; Fell. in Med., U. of Toronto; Tel. 369-5148.
SELAND, T. Peter Sg. Lt.; R.C.A.F. Hosp., Comox, B.C.; Alb '64.
SELBY, David A.; Tor'56; FRCP(C), IntMed; Staff, Toronto Western Hosp., Toronto, Ont.
SELBY, Gordon W.; Allin Clinic, 10155-120th St., Edmonton, Alta.; Man '51; D.A.B.P.; FRCP (C), Paed.; Instr., U. of Alta.; Tel. 488-7271.
SELBY, Raymond C.; 43 Academy Medical Bldg., 1812-4th St. W., Calgary, Alta.; 711 Crescent Blvd. (res.); Man. '52; Tel. 266-5029.
SELDON, George E.; 1354 Matthews Ave., Vancouver 9, B.C. (res); Tor '05; LRCP(Lond.), M.R.C.S.(Eng.), F.A.C.S., F.R.C.S.(C), GenSurg; Cons. Surg., Van. Gen. Hosp.: Retired.
SELENY, Frank L.; Apt. 8, 319 Westminster Ave., London, Ont.; Budapest (Hung.) '50; Anaes; Staff, Victoria Hosp.; Tel. GE 2-5261; Abroad.
SELIGMAN, Gerald M.; Tor'64; Res., Toronto Gen. Hosp., Toronto, Ont.
SELINGER, Zelig; 9929-108th St., Edmonton, Alta.; Mon '41; Psy; Cons. Royal Alexandra Hosp. & Misericordia Hosp.; Psy., Dept. of Public Health, City of Edmonton; Lect. (Psy.), U. of Alberta; Tel. GA 4-5724.
SELLERS, A. Hardisty; 35 Oriole Pkwy., Toronto, Ont. (res); Tor '32; D.P.H., PH; Dir. Med. Stat., Dept. of Health for Ontario; Cons. Stat., Workmen's Compensation Board; Med. Stat., Ontario Cancer Treatment & Research Foundation; Cons. Stat., R.C.A.F., Mem. Cons. Bd., Can. Ins. Med. Council; Lect. P.H. Admin., Epidem. & Biometrics, School of Hygiene, U. of Toronto; Tel. EM 3-1211.

SELLERS, Clayton S.; Wellesley, Ont.; Wes '51; A.M.C.G.P.
SELLERS, Edward A.; 21 Valleyview, Toronto, Ont. (res); Man. '39; Ph.D.; Prof., Banting & Best Inst's., Dept. of Med. Research; Head, Dept. of Pharmacol., U. of Toronto; Tel. WA 3-6111, Loc. 381.
SELLERS, E. M.; Tor'65; Res., Toronto Western Hosp., Toronto 2B, Ontario.
SELLERS, Frank J.; 1227 Osler St., Saskatoon, Sask.; Qns '55; Paed; Staff, (Paed), University Hosp., Saskatoon, Sask.; Ass't. Prof. (Paed.) U. of Saskatchewan; Tel. 242-7641, Loc. 491.
SELLERY, Gordon R.; Tor'60; Res., Sunnybrook Hosp., Toronto 12, Ont.
SELMECI, T. George; Budapest (Hung.) '52; Staff, Memorial Hosp., Oakville, Ont.
SELWOOD, Michael; 477 Martin, Penticton, B.C.; Man. '54; Tel. 492-5716.
SELYE, Hans; 659 Milton St., Montreal, P.Q. (res); Prague (Czech.) '29; Ph.D. (Prague), D.Sc. (McG); FRS(C); Prof. & Dir., Int. of Exper. (Med. & Surg.), U. of Montreal; Tel. RE 3-9951.
SELZNICK, Maurice W.; 99 Avenue Rd. Ste. 605, Toronto 5, Ont.; 145 Old Forest Hill Rd. (res); Tor '32; D.A.O. (Trinity), L.M. (Rotunda), F.A.C.O.G., ObstGyn; Sr. Att. ObstGyn., I/C Gyn., New Mount Sinai Hosp.; Att'd. Staff, Tor. Gen. & Western Hosp's.; Tel. WA 2-3930.
SEMCHISEN, Orest M.; 6220-128th St., Edmonton, Alta.; Alb'56; DiagRad; Med. Staff, Edmonton Gen. Hosp.; Tel. 424-0496.
SEMELKA, Donna L.; Man'53; DiagRad; Staff, Wpg. Gen. Hosp., Winnipeg, Man.
SEMELKA, Gunther; 416 Med. Arts Bldg., Winnipeg, Man.; 412 Kelvin Blvd. (res); Innsbruck (Austria) '47; Anaes; Active Staff, St. Boniface & Victoria Gen. Hosp's.; Lect. Surg. (Anaes.), U. of Manitoba; Tel. WH 3-9565.
SEMENCHUK, Peter W.; 645 Fort St., Victoria, B.C.; Man '40; FRCP(C), IntMed; Tel. 383-4953.
SEMENIUK, Konstantin H.; Alb'59; Res., Neurol. Inst., 3801 University Ave., Montreal 2, P.Q.
SEMKULEY, Myron; Cowichan Lake, B.C.; Alb '64.
SEMOGAS, Jonas; 5441 Bannatyne Ave., Verdun, Montreal 19, P.Q.; 7491 LaSalle Blvd., Mtl. 32 (res); Kaunas (Lith.) '35; GenSurg; Att'd. Staff, Lachine Gen. Hosp.; Court. Staff, Verdun Gen. Hosp.; Tel. PO 7-3175.
SEN, Susanta; Sen Clinic, Battleford, Sask.; Cambridge (Eng.) '33; M.D.(Cantab.); MRCP (Lond.); FRCS (Edin.); Med. Staff, Notre Dame Hosp.; Tel. 937-2636.
SENAY, R. Gerald; Apt. 1, 8097 St.-Hubert, Montreal, P.Q.; Mon '56; A.M.C.G.P.
SENAY-BELIVEAU, Pierrette; Mon '60; Res., Inst. Albert Prevost, Montreal 9, P.Q.
SENDBUEHLER, Joseph M.; Queen Elizabeth Hosp., Montreal, P.Q.; McG '57; D.Psy; Psy; Staff, Queen Elizabeth Hosp. & McGill U.; Tel. 489-5422.
SENECAL, Chomedey; 485 est, boul. St. Joseph, Montreal 34, P.Q.; 5087 Cote Ste Antoine (res); Mon '31; Chief of DermSyph., Hop. Ste-Jeanne-d'Arc; Tel. VI 2-5201.
SENECAL, Joseph G.; Rougemont, P.Q.; McG '25.
SENECAL, Leo; Mon'52; Path.(P.Q.); Staff, Hop. Hotel-Dieu, Montreal, P.Q.
SENECAL, Pierre M.; 5300 Cote-des-Neiges, Ste. 310, Montreal, P.Q.; 3485 Vendome (res); McG '43; D.P.H., Paed; **Ass't. Paed., St. Mary's Hosp.**; Clin. Ass't. Montreal Children's Hosp.; Ass't. M.O.H., City of Westmount; Dem. (Paed.), McGill U.; Tel. RE 1-7281.
SENENSKY, Errol R.; 341 Med. Arts Bldg., Saskatoon, Sask.; Man'65; Staff, St. Paul's Hosp.
SENG, Magnus I.; 615 Medical Arts Bldg., Montreal, P.Q.; 4466 Western (res); F.R.C.S.(C); Staff, Royal Victoria Hosp.; Tel. WE 5-2936.
SENIKAS. Joseph; 226 Longueuil St., St. Jean, P.Q.; 14 Mercier (res); Leipzig (Germ.) '45; Munich '56.
SENIOR, Margaret T.; (see Campaigne, Margaret T.).
SENN, Dilip K.; 216 Highfield St., Moncton, N.B.; U. of Calcutta (India) '45; D.T.M. & H. (Liverpool), D.A. (Eng.); Anaes (P.Q.); Active Med. Staff, Moncton City & Hotel Dieu **Hosp's; Tel. EV 2-1546.**
SENN, John M.; Tor '25; Psy; Staff, Dept. of Health, Mohawk & Upper Wentworth, Hamilton, Ont.
SENN, John S.; 728 Medical Arts Bldg., 170 St. George St., Toronto, Ont.; Tor'53; FRCP(C), IntMed; Cons. IntMed., Sunnybrook Hosp.; Fellow IntMed., Toronto Gen. Hosp. & Associate IntMed., U. of Toronto; Tel. WA 3-9774.
SENNEWALD, George; 110 Columbia St., Kamloops, B.C.; Wes'59.
SENNEWALD, Lothar F.; 1958 Crescent Rd., Victoria, B.C.; Leipzig (Germ.) '33; Ph.D.; MHD; Tel. 385-8565.
SEPP, Hans; 55 Duggan Ave., Toronto 7, Ont. (res); Bonn (Germ.)'51; PathBact; Bacteriol. & Ass't. Pathol., Toronto Western Hosp., Dem. (Path), U. of Toronto; Tel. 369-5158.
SEQUEIRA, Hamilton; '62; Staff, Psychiatric Centre, Yorkton, Sask.
SERAGLIA, Mario L.; Ste. 505, 1541 W. Broadway, **Vancouver 9, B.C.; Padua (Italy) '52; IntMed; Cons. (IntMed.), Shaughnessy DVA Hosp.; Active Staff, Pearson Hosp. for TB; Tel. RE 1-6911.**
SERBU, John; 902 Lariat Dr., Eugene, Oregon, U.S.A.; Alb '57; FRCS(C), NeurSurg; Abroad.
SEREDA, Lawrence E.; 1680 Albany Ave., Hartford, Conn., U.S.A.; Tor '53; Psy; Med. Dir., Hartley-Salmon Child Guidance Clinic; Abroad.
SEREDA, Mitro M.; 403 Northgate Blvd., Edmonton, Alta.; 10603 Saskatchewan Dr. (res); Alb '36; MCGP; Ass't Prof. (Path), & Lect. (Clin.Med.), U. of Alta; Tel. 422-1748.
SERENO, Luciano R.; 2661 E. Hastings, Vancouver 6, B.C.; 1148 Commercial Dr.; 5662 McMaster Rd., Van. 8 (res); Rome (Italy) '55; MCGP; Tel. RE 8-1343.
SERENY, George; Ste. 4., 459 Bloor St. W., Toronto 4, Ont.; Munich (Germ.) '50; IntMed (Cardiol.); O.P.D. Staff, St. Michael's Hosp.; Research Phys., Alcoholism Research Fdn.; Tel. 924-2933.
SERGERIE, Claude; 2678 Lacordaire, Montreal 5, P.Q.; 8780 Bourgjoly, St. Leonard de Port Maurice (res); Mon '61; Ass't. Dir. Health Serv., Hop. Notre-Dame; Dir. Health Serv., Hop. Marie; Tel. 254-6363.
SERPELL, Barry W.; Malton Med. Centre, Malton, Ont.; Edinburgh (Scot.) '59.
SERRES, Robt.; 3800 St. Catherine E., Montreal, P.Q.; Mon '36.; Tel. LA 3-1551.
SERS, Phyllis M. (Neil); Box 778, Antigonish, N.S.; St. Andrew's U. (Scot.)'44; DCH(Eng.); Physician, Mount St. Bernard College.
SERS, Rolf; P.O. Box 778, Main St., Antigonish, N.S.; 49 Archie St. (res); Riga (Latvia)'40; MCGP; Tel. 863-3871.
SERVICE, C. William McD.; 11 Adelaide St. N., Lindsay, Ont.; 64 Albert St. N. (res); Tor '39; FACS; FRCS(C); GenSurg; Chief of Med. Staff, Ross Mem. Hosp.; Tel. 324-6159, 324-6150.
SERVICE, Gwendolyn F. (Barber); 830 McLean St., Apt. 32, Halifax, N.S. (res); London (Eng.) '40; Research, Dept. of Med., Dalhousie U.; Tel. 2-4406.
SESTRAP, Leyda S.; (see Lythgoe, Leyda S.).
SETTERINGTON, Eleanor M. (See Davies).
SETTERINGTON, Melvin J.; 106 Talbot St. W., Leamington, Ont.; 44 Marlboro St. W. (res); Tor '34; IntMed; Tel. 326-3281.
SETTLE John R.; 1161 C Northmount Dr., Calgary, Alta.; 1012 Northmount Dr. (res); Alb '52; MCGP; Tel. 282-3168.
SEVENSMA, Jaap; 1000 McCaw St., Sarnia, Ont.; Amsterdam (Neth.)'53; Tel. KI 2-9571.
SEVERS, David; Oxford (Eng.) '55; D.P.H.; Ass't. Chief M.O., Dept. of Health, St. John's Nfld.
SEVIGNY, Andre; 5901 Boul. Pie IX, Montreal 36, P..Q; Lav '57; Tel. 727-1274.
SEVIGNY, Jacques; 214 Bonaventure, Trois Rivieres, P.Q.; Lav '50.
SEVIOUR, George R.; Qns '63; Staff, Cornwall Clinic, 325 Hamilton St., St. John's Nfld.

SEVIOUR, James F.; 238 Lemarchant Rd., St. John's, Nfld.; National U. (Ire.) '55; FRCS(C), ObstGyn; Chief, Dept. of Gyn., St. John's Gen. Hosp.; Tel. 579-8852.

SEWARD, Francis W.; 194 Concession Rd., Galt, Ont.; Guy's (London)'46; MRCS (Eng.); LRCP (Lond.); Dist. Coroner; Tel. 623-1400.

SEWELL, Ian M.; Spence Clinic, 910 Ridgeway, Fort William, Ont.; 1312 Ridgeway (res); Tor '50; GenSurg.; Tel. MA 2-5301.

SEXSMITH, Edgar L.; 33 Sheldrake Blvd., Toronto, Ont.; Tor '24; Tel. HU 3-4600.

SEXTON, George B.; 455 Waterloo St., London, Ont.; 890 Riverside Dr. (res); Qns '30; DABDS; DermSyph; Dir. London Venereal Dis. Clinic; Staff, Victoria, St. Joseph's & Westminster DVA Hosp's.; Assoc. Clin. Prof. (Med.), U. of Western Ont.; Tel. GE 4-1108.

SEYMOUR, Bruce A.; 9 Lytton Blvd., Toronto, Ont.; Tor '43; Anaes; Anaes., Sunnybrook Hosp.; Tel. HU 9-5917.

SEYMOUR, Burwell; 3801 Karen St., Windsor, Ont.; 1924 Devonshire Ct. (res); Wes '33; Tel. 269-2670.

SEYMOUR, George C.; Ste. 303, Medical Arts Bldg., 121 Wellington St. W., Barrie, Ont.; Tor '33; Active Staff, Royal Victoria Hosp.; Tel. 728-5536.

SGRO, Giuseppe; Box 51, Peace River, Alta.; Rome (Italy) '56.

SHABANAH, E. H. (See ABOU-SHABANAH).

SHABSOVE, Harold B.; 402 Greenfield St., Petrolia, Ont.; Apt 4., Wellington Crt. (res); Wes '63; Tel. 882-2110.

SHACK, Leo; 235 Dixon Rd., Weston, Ont.; 40 Hallsport Cres. (res); Tor '51; Paed; Staff, New Mount Sinai Hosp., St. Joseph's & Queensway Gen. Hosp's.; Tel. CH 7-2131.

SHACKLETON, Harry O.; 2090 Wyandotte St. E., Windsor, Ont.; Tor '63; Dip. Bact; Dir. Regional Lab., Ontario Dept. of Health; Tel. 254-5565.

SHACKLETON, Monica; 32 Hortie Ave., Pierrefonds, P.Q.; Sheffield (Eng.) '56; DPH (Lond.); Staff, Dept. of Public Health, City of Westmount.

SHACKLOCK, Herbert T.; 11186-84th Ave., North Surrey, B.C.; U.K.'56; MCGP; Tel. 596-3385.

SHAFFER, Eldon A.; Qns'65; Res., Montreal General Hosp., Montreal 25, P.Q.

SHAFFER, Henry E.; 337 Brock St., Kingston, Ont.; 40 Hillcroft Dr. (res); Edinburgh (Scotland) '31; M.C.G.P.; D.P.M. (Leeds); Staff, Ontario Hosp., Kingston; Tel. 542-4406.

SHAFRAN, Murray; 2221 Keele St., Toronto, Ont.; 182 Hillhurst Blvd., Tor. 12 (res); Tor '49; IntMed; Chief, Dept. of Med., Northwestern Gen. Hosp.; Tel. 241-4694.

SHAFTO, C. Maxwell; 315 Greyhound Bldg., Calgary, Alta.; London (Eng.)'41; MRCS(Eng.), LRCP(Lond.), DOMS; Ophth.; Dir. Glaucoma Clin., Foothills Hosp.; Tel. 269-1319.

SHAH, Chandulal M.; '61; Res., Vancouver Gen. Hosp., Vancouver 9, B.C.

SHAHARIW, William; 929 Rosser Ave., Brandon, Man.; Ukraine '41.

SHAIKH, Mohammed A.; Main St., Sydney Mines, N.S.; '54.

SHAKER, Galal T.; 2493 Commercial Dr., Vancouver 12, B.C.; Beirut (Lebanon) '45; Tel. TR 4-8333. Abroad.

SHALLARD, Bruce T.; 1744 W. Broadway, Vancouver 9, B.C.; Sydney (Austr.) '26; MRACP; IntMed; Staff, Dept. of Med., St. Paul's Hosp.; Cons. (Med.), Burnaby Gen. Hosp.; Clin. Instr. (Med.), U. of British Columbia; Tel. RE 3-5511.

SHALOM, Maurice S.; Haysboro Shopping Centre, 903C—82nd Ave. S.W., Calgary, Alta.; London (Eng.) '54; D.Obst. R.C.O.G.; Tel. AL 5-5868.

SHAMEHORN, Garnet; 115 Lower Union St., Kingston, Ont.; Qns '52.

SHAMESS, Samuel A.; 955 Queen St. E., Sault Ste. Marie, Ont.; Tor'40; Ophth.

SHAMSIE, S. Jalal; 8417 George Terrace, Ville **La Salle, P.Q.; Punjah (India) '53; Psy; Dir.** Adolescent Unit, Douglas Hosp.; Clin. Ass't. (Psy.), Montreal Children's Hosp.; Lect. (Psy.), McGill U.; Tel. 766-8511.

SHANDLING, Barry; Ste. 1120, 123 Edward St., Toronto 2, Ont.; Capetown (S. Africa)'50; FRCS(Eng.), FRCS(C), GenSurg; Staff Surg., Hosp. for Sick Children; Clin. Instr., U. of Toronto; Tel. 364-3695.

SHANDRO, William A.; 214 LeMarchand Bldg., Edmonton, Alta.; 8614 W. Saskatchewan Dr. (res); McG '33; FICS, FRCS(C), GenSurg; Urol; Teach. Co-ordinator, Gen. Hosp.; Lect. (Surg.), U. of Alberta; Tel. 488-9797.

SHANE, Arthur G.; 6156 Quinpool Rd., Halifax, N.S.; 22 Bellvue Ave. (res); Dal '42; DOMS; Otol; Ass't. Otol. Surg., Halifax Children's Hosp.; **Lect., Dalhousie U.; Tel. 423-9326.**

SHANE, Aubrey M.; 5770 South St., Halifax, N.S.; 5830 Inglewood Dr. (res); Dal '55; Psy; Assoc. Chief (Psy), Hlfx. Infirm. Pt-time Psy. Hlfx. Mental Health Clinic for Children; Civilian Cons. Camp Hill DVA Hosp.; Staff (Psy), Victoria Gen. & Hlfx. Children's Hosp's.; Ass't. Prof., Dalhousie U.; Tel. 422-4579.

SHANE, Frederick H.; Man'65; Res., Children's Hosp., Winnipeg 3, Man.

SHANE, Rita; 565 Ellendale Med. Bldg., 5845 Cote-des-Neiges, Montreal 26, P.Q.; 375 Revere Ave. Twn. of Mt. Royal (res); McG '42; Paed (P.Q.); Att'd. Staff, Jewish Gen. Hosp.; Tel. RE 3-2927.

SHANE, Samuel J.; 5849 University Ave., Halifax, N.S.; 7141 Morningside Dr. (res); Dal '40; DIM; FACP; FCCP; FACC; FRCP(C); IntMed; Dir., Cardiac Unit, Victoria Gen. Hosp.; Assoc. Cardiol., Halifax Children's Hosp.; Cons. Cardiol. & Pulm. Dis., N.S., Rehab. Centre; Cons. Cardiol., Halifax Infirmary; Cons. Cardiol., Cdn. Forces Hosp.; Assoc. Prof. (Med.) Dalhousie U.; Tel. 429-1420, Loc. 366.

SHANFIELD, Isidore; McG '64; Res., Royal Victoria Hosp., Montreal 2, P.Q.

SHANKS, George; 1184 Clovelly Terrace, Victoria, B.C.; McG '08; PathBact; Cons. (Path.), Victoria Veterans' Hosp., Victoria; Retired.

SHANKS, John; Ste. 1, 2162 Sherbrooke St. W., Montreal, P.Q.; 3445 Ridgewood Ave. (res); McG '50; F.R.C.P.(C), IntMed; Clin. Ass't. Royal Victoria Hosp.; Lect., McGill U.; Tel. WE 5-1626.

SHANKS, John A.; Ste. 207, Glenwood Med. Centre, Brockville, Ont.; Aberdeen (Scot.)'48; MRCOG; FRCS(C); ObstGyn; Tel. 342-1313.

SHANNETTE, Archie T.; Morrisburg, Ont.; Qns '29.

SHANNON, Eugene H.; 323 Bloor St. W., Toronto, Ont.; 215 Cortleigh Blvd. (res); Tor '20; F.F.R.(Lond.); D.R.; D&TRad; Dir. of Rad., St. Michael's Hosp.; **Ass't. Prof. of Rad., U. of Toronto; Tel. WA 1-7700.**

SHANNON, Francis; Box 333, Barrie, Ont.; Tor'33; MCGP; Staff, Royal Victoria Hosp.; District Coroner; Tel. 728-4242.

SHANNON, Jane C. S. (MacLachlan); 9 Old Orchard Ave., Cornwall, Ont.; Liverpool (Eng.) **'42; Part-time M.O., St. Lawrence San. Retired.**

SHANNON, James G.; 1019 Drummond Med. Bldg., 1414 Drummond St., Montreal, P.Q.; 784 Upper Belmont Ave., Westmount (res.); Tor '28; FACS, DABOS, FRCS(C), OrthSurg.; Orth. Surg-in-Chief, Montreal Gen. Hosp.; Dir. of OrthSurg., Queen Mary Vet's Hosp. Cons. Orth. Surg., Montreal Children's Hosp.; Assoc. Prof. of Surg., McGill U.; Tel. VI 5-3856.

SHANNON, Malcolm P.; 22 Milson St., Armdale, Halifax, N.S.(res); Edinburgh (Scot.) '51; D.M.-R.D.; DiagRad; Staff, Halifax Infirmary; Lect. Rad., Dal. U.; Tel. 422-1511.

SHANNON, William J.; 1407 Peter St., Cornwall, Ont.; London (Eng.) '38; M.R.C.S., L.R.C.P., F.R.C.P.(C), Path; Path., Cornwall Gen. & Hotel Dieu Hosp's; Cons. (Path.), Alice Hyde Hosp., Malone, N.Y.; Assoc. Path., Prov. of Ont.; Tel. WE 2-4577.

SHANOFF, Henry M.; Brunswick Diagnostic Clinic, 25 Brunswick Ave., Toronto 4, Ont.; Tor'48; B.Sc.; FACC; FACP; FRCP(C), IntMed; Chief of Cardiol., Doctor's Hosp.; Research Assoc., Sunnybrook Hosp.; Ass't. Cardiovasc. Clinic, Toronto Gen. & New Mt. Sinai Hosp's.; Tel. 924-9741.

SHANTZ, William L.; 200 King St. S., Waterloo, Ont.; Tor '49; MCGP; Active Staff, St. Mary's Gen. & Kitchener-Waterloo Hosp's.; Tel. 743-6328.

SHAPERA, George H.; 805 Boyd Bldg., 388 Portage Ave., Winnipeg 1, Man.; 20 Colish Dr. (res); Man'20; FRCP(Eng.); FAAP; FRCP & S(Eng.); Paed; Hon. Staff, Children's & St. Boniface Hosp's.; Tel. WH 2-4259.

SHAPERO, Gerald D.; Semans, Sask.; Durham (Eng.) '59; M.B., B.S.

SHAPIRO, Bernard J.; 550 University Ave., Toronto, Ont.; 79 Munro Blvd., Willowdale (res); McG '43; M.A.C.R., F.R.C.P.(C), DiagRad; Chief, Dept. of Rad., New Mt. Sinai & Baycrest Hosp's.; Tel. EM 6-7361.

SHAPIRO, Charles E.; Ste. 2, 800 Cooper, Ottawa 4, Ont.; McG '22; Staff, Ottawa Gen. Hosp.; Dist. Coroner.

SHAPIRO, Edward I.; 150 Metcalfe St., Ottawa, Ont.; 1879 Highland Terrace (res); Tor '43; **GenSurg.; Surg., Ottawa Civic Hosp.; Tel. 236-0533.**

SHAPIRO, Ernest K.; Ste. 118, 3545 Cote des Neiges, Montreal 25, P.Q.; Lav '45; Ophth.

SHAPIRO, Franklyn; 36 Wilson St., Hamilton, Ont.; 80 Bertram Dr. (res); Wes '44; M.C.G.P.; Tel. JA 7-2325.

SHAPIRO, Israel; 158 St. George St., Toronto, Ont.; 214 Strathearn Rd. (res); Tor '30; OrthSurg; Sr. Surg., (OrthSurg) New Mt. Sinai Hosp.; Cons. (OrthSurg) N. Western Hosp.; Tel. WA 1-6585.

SHAPIRO, Lorne; 4119 Sherbrooke St. W., Westmount, P.Q.; 345 Lansdowne Ave. (res); McG '39; F.A.C.P., F.R.C.P.(C) IntMed; Haem (P.Q.); Assoc. Phys., Royal Victoria Hosp.; Cons. (Haem.), Queen Mary Vets' Hosp.; Ass't. Prof. (Md.), McGill U.; Tel. WE 3-6464.

SHAPIRO, Maynard; UBC '60; Research. McGill U., Montreal, P.Q.

SHAPIRO, Samuel J.; 1218 Islington Ave. N., Rexdale, Ont.; Tel. 244-5111.

SHAPIRO, Simon B.; 4740 Maplewood Ave., Montreal, P.Q.; McG '35; A.M.C.A.A.; Paed; Staff, Montreal Children & Jewish Gen. Hosp's.; Tel. RE 3-3335.

SHAPLEY, James M.; 8 St. Margaret's Dr., Toronto 12, Ont. (res); Qns '39; Anaes., Chief of Anaes., Sunnybrook Hosp.; Tel. 485-8651.

SHAPTER, A. Edward; Med. Arts Bldg., Empire & Mayor Ave., St. John's, Nfld.; 36 Shea St. (res); Dal '51; OrthSurg; Chief (OrthSurg), St. John's Gen. Hosp.; Chief Cons. (OrthSurg.), St. John's TB San. & Hosp. for Ment. & Nervous Dis.; Med. Dir., Children's Rehab. Centre; Tel. 579-2146.

SHAPTER, Robert K.; Dal '58; Res. (Path.), St. John's Gen. Hosp., St. John's, Nfld.

SHARDT, Antony; 2045 Dufferin St., Toronto 10, Ont.; Zagreb (Yugo.) '47; MCGP; Tel. 651-1210.

SHARIFF, Fariduddin K.; Dacca (Pakistan) '59; Res., Winnipeg Gen. Hosp., Winnipeg, Man.

SHARKEY, Patrick J.; 751 King St. W., Kitchener, Ont.; McG '48; MCGP; Staff, St. Mary's & Kitchener-Waterloo Hosp's.

SHARMA, Shiv R.; Box 579, Port Hawkesbury, N.S.; Agra (India) '62.

SHARMAN, William J.; Box 31, Clanwilliam, Man. (res); Man '13; Retired.

SHARP, Allan S.; 316 St. Clair Ave. W., Toronto 10, Ont.; 150 Sandringham Dr., Wilson Hgts. (res); Tor '47; F.R.C.P.(C), IntMed; Att'd. Staff, New Mt. Sinai Hosp.; Clin. Instr. (Med.), U. of Toronto; Tel. 922-6104.

SHARP, Fletcher B.; 86 Bloor St. W., Toronto, Ont.; 4 Hawthorne Gardens (res); Qns '18; Tel. WA 2-2920.

SHARP, J. Douglas; 3505 Broadway Ave., Lachine, P.Q.; Man '49; Paed; Tel. 637-8342.

SHARP, W. Lindsay; Clyde Ave. Med. Centre, 660 Clyde Ave., West Vancouver, B.C.; 761 Burley Pl. (res); Dublin (Ire.) '39; L.R.C.P.(Lond.), L.R.C.S.(Lond.), M.R.C.P.(Edin.), F.R.C.P.(C), IntMed; Assoc. Staff, St. Paul's & Lions Gate Hosp's.; Tel. WA 2-7234.

SHARPE, Anna E. (Wilson); Ste. 208, 267 O'Connor, Ottawa 4, Ont.; Alb '30; FAAP; Paed; School M.O., Ottawa Public School Bd.; Clin. Lect., U. of Ottawa.

SHARPE, D. M.; Strathroy, Ont.; Wes '38; Pres. Med. Staff, Strathroy Gen. Hosp.

SHARPE, H. H.; Sussex, N.B.; McG '22; Ophth.

SHARPE, Herbert S.; The Bigelow Clinic, Clement Blk., Brandon, Man.; 1414 Victoria Ave. (res); Man '05; F.A.C.S., OrthSurg; Staff, Brandon Gen. Hosp.; Tel. PA9-1469.

SHARPE, J. E., O.B.E.; 213 Hillhurst Blvd., Toronto 12, Ont. (res); Wes '30; F.A.C.H.A.; Psy; Supt., Toronto Gen. Hosp.; Tel. EM 6-8211.

SHARPE, John R.; Wes '63; Res., Sunnybrook Hosp., Toronto 12, Ont.

SHARPE, Noble C.; 8 Jarvis St., Toronto 1, Ont.; Brooklin, Ont. (res); Tor '11; Path, Bact; Med. Dir., Attorney-Gen.'s Lab., Prov. of Ont.; Tel. 365-2561.

SHARPE, Sydney S.; 384 Bloor St. W., Toronto, Ont.; 1644 Bathurst St. (res); Tor '35; Derm Syph; Att. Derm., New Mount Sinai, & Northwestern Hosp's.; Cons. Derm., Jewish Home for Aged; Tel. WA 1-2800.

SHARPE, Victor J. H.; Bigelow Clinic, Brandon, Man.; 1635 Lorne Ave. (res); Man '44; IntMed; Staff, Brandon Gen. Hosp.; Tel. PA 9-1469.

SHARPE, William C.; Beck Mem. Sanatorium, London, Ont.; Tor '24; F.A.C.C.P., IntMed(T.B.), Supt. Beck Mem. San.; Ass't. Prof. (Med.), U. of Western Ont.; Retired.

SHATFORD, Robert C.; 65 Ruskin St., Ottawa, Ont. (res); Dal '52; Med. Adviser, Can. Pension Comm.; Tel. CE 2-8211.

SHATZ, Richard M.; Sask'63; Res., Royal Victoria Hosp., Montreal 2, P.Q.

SHATZKO, Paul; UBC'60; Res., Vancouver Gen. Hosp., Vancouver 9, B.C.

SHAUL, David L.; Ste. 1112, 123 Edward St., Toronto 2, Ont.; Tor'47; FACOG; FRCS(C) ObstGyn; Jr. Att. Staff (ObstGyn), New Mt. Sinai Hosp.; Tel. LE 4-7021.

SHAVER, Cecil G.; 356 Martindale Rd., St. Catharines, Ont. (res); Tor '26; FACCP; IntMed (T.B.); Supt., Niagara Peninsula San.; Tel. CA 7-3731.

SHAVER, Charles H.; 955 Queens St. E., Sault Ste Marie, Ont.; 122 Leo Ave. (res); Qns '36; Staff, Plummer Memorial & Gen. Hosp's.

SHAVER, Eloise M.; (see Jones, Eloise M.).

SHAVER, Elspie R. E. (Halnan); 133 Heddington Ave., Toronto 12, Ont.; Tor '38; Pt.-time PH; Tel. HU 8-9533.

SHAVER, Frank W.; 600 Seaforth Med. Bldg., 3550 Cote des Neiges Rd., Montreal 25, P.Q.; 105 Radcliffe Rd. (res); McG '23; Otol (P.Q.); Assoc. Otol., Montreal Gen. Hosp.; Lect. (Otol.), McGill U.; Tel. 932-3050.

SHAVER, Jack E.; Scotland, Ont.; Wes '55; MCGP; Tel. 446-2231.

SHAW, Albert J.; 9 Shaw Cres., Armdale, Halifax, N.S. (res); Dal '52; DiagRad; Staff, Victoria Gen. Hosp.; Instr. (Rad.), Dalhousie U.; Tel. 422-7311.

SHAW, Alexander G.; 513 Medical Arts Bldg., Toronto 5, Ont.; 3 Garland Ave. (res); Tor '31; F.R.C.S.(C) GenSurg; Clin. Teach. (Surg.), U. of Toronto; Tel. WA 1-7956.

SHAW, Arthur E.; 705A Pape Ave., Toronto, Ont.; Apt. 407, 45 Glen Rd. (res); Tor '23; MCGP; Staff, Grace & Toronto East Gen. Hosp's.; Tel. HO 6-6266.

SHAW, David T.; Alb'59; MCGP; Res., University Hosp., Edmonton, Alta.

SHAW, D. Barry; McG '57; Staff, Victoria Hosp., London, Ont.

SHAW, Edward C.; 1705 Corydon Ave., Winnipeg 9, Man.; 440 Lanark St., (res); Man '55; M.C.G.P.; Exec. Memb., Coll. of Gen. Practice, Man. Chapter.; Tel. HU 9-8228.

SHAW, George B.; 69 Arlington Ave., Armdale, Halifax, N.S. (res); Dal '45; Med. Dir., Maritime Medical Care Inc.; Tel. 422-7461.

SHAW, Harry; 2255 Elgin St., Port Coquitlam, B.C.; Alb '49.
SHAW, Ian M.; 198 Bagot St., Cobourg, Ont.; 214 King St. E. (res); Qns '45; M.C.G.P.
SHAW, James M.; Man '48; Staff, Workmen's Comp. Bd., 707 W. 37th. Ave., Vancouver 9, B.C.; Tel. 266-0211.
SHAW, J. P.; Box 1056, Weyburn, Sask.; Oxford (Eng.) '23; Staff, Saskatchewan Hosp.
SHAW, Leonard B.; 222 Third Ave., Ottawa 1, Ont.; Ott '60; Tel. CE 4-3284.
SHAW, Melville H.; 1203 Fairmont Med. Bldg., 750 W. Broadway, Vancouver 9, B.C.; 1630 Western Pkwy. (res); Qns '49; FRCP(C), IntMed; Att'd. Staff, Van. Gen. Hosp.; Vis. Staff, St. Paul's, St. Vincent's & Mt. St. Joseph's Hosp's.; Clin. Instr., U. of British Columbia; Tel. 874-3722.
SHAW, Mervin G. Capt.; Dal '65; RCAMC, Camp Gagetown, N.B.
SHAW, Ralph W.; Tor'64; Res., Toronto Gen. Hosp., Toronto 2, Ont.
SHAW, R. Bruce; 577 Baker St., Nelson, B.C.; 422 Vernon St. (res); **McG '27; Dist. M.O., C.P.R.; Tel. 352-2121.**
SHAW, Reginald E.; 27 Cedar St. N., Timmins, Ont.; Oxford (Eng.) '43; FRCS (Eng.); D.Obst-RCOG.
SHAW, Robert M.; 11050-89th Ave., Edmonton, Alta. (res); McG '06; **D.P.H., F.R.C.P.(C); Retired.**
SHAW, Robert S.; 194 Elm St. W., Sudbury, Ont.; Apt. 3, 372 Wellington Heights (res); **Wes '53; Paed.; Tel. 674-5472.**
SHAW, Ross A.; 599-2nd Ave. E., Owen Sound, Ont.; Tor '62; AMCGP; Tel. 376-3581.
SHAW, Thomas W.; Deer Lake Clinic, Deer Lake, Nfld.; Oxford (Eng.) '62; B.M., B.Ch., MRCS (Eng.), LRCP (Lond.); D.Obst RCOG; Tel. 635-2925.
SHAW, Walter M.; 117 King St. E., Oshawa, Ont.; 773 Glencairn (res); Dal '48; M.Sc.; IntMed; Staff, Oshawa Gen. Hosp.; Tel. RA 8-1661.
SHAW, William H.; 250 Lawrence Ave. W., Toronto 12, Ont.; Tor'55; DCH (Lond.); Paed; Psy; Child Psy., North York Gen. Hosp.; Tel. 782-6200.
SHAW, Williamson F.; 825 Granville St., Vancouver, B.C.; 1406 Anderly St., Beach Grove, **B.C. (res); Man '14; Tel. MU 3-4618.**
SHAY, G. Douglas; Box 369, Main St., Winnipegosis, Man.; Tor'55; MCGP; Staff, Crerer Gen. & Dauphin Gen. Hosp's.; M.O.H.; Tel. OL 6-4677.
SHEA, D. Robert; 314 Med. Arts Bldg., 11010 Jasper Ave., Edmonton, Alta.; Alb '55; Paed; Staff, University Hosp.; Tel. 422-3213.
SHEA, John B.; Toronto Professional Bldg., 123 Edward St., Toronto, Ont.; 11 Donmac Dr., Don Mills (res); National U. (Ire.) '50; BAO; FRCP(C); DiagRad; Radiol., St. Michael's Hosp.; Dir., X-Ray Dept., Scarborough Centenary Hosp.; Tel. 362-8651.
SHEA, Marguerite B.; 1530 W. 37th Ave., Vancouver 13, B.C.; Tor '33; Anaes.; Tel. AM 1-6055.
SHEA, Michael; Rm. 828 Medical Arts Bldg., 170 St. George St., Toronto 5, Ont.; Nat. U. of Ire.'51; FRCS(C), Ophth; Ophth., St. Michael's Hosp.; Assoc. (Ophth.), U. of Toronto; Tel. 923-6554.
SHEARER, Robin S., F/L; R.C.A.F. Station, Armstrong, Ont.; Wes'64; Tel. 62.
SHEARS, Arthur H.; 5950 University Ave., Halifax, N.S.; 1775 Roseland Ave. (res); Dal '50; PhysMed & Rehab; Med. Dir., N.S. Rehab. Centre; Ass't Phys., Victoria Gen. & Hlfx. Children's Hosp's.; Ass't. Phys. & Co-Dir., PhysMed., Hlfx. Infirm.; Ass't. Prof. Med. & Dir. Schl. of **Physiotherapy, Dalhousie U.; Tel. 422-6367.**
SHEDDEN, Douglas A.; Central Newfoundland Hosp., Grand Falls, Nfld.; Edinburgh (Scot.) '60; M.B., Ch.B., DPH; Infection Control Officer & Memb. of Active Staff, Central Nfld. Hosp.; Reg. M.O., Dept. of Public Health; Tel. 2123, Ext. 375.
SHEEDY, Francis T.; 258 Tache Ave., St. Boniface, Man.; 371 Kingston Cres., St. Vital (res); Man '51; MCGP; Tel. CE 3-2156.
SHEEHAN, Donal B.; Clarks Harbour, Shelburne Co., N.S.; Cork (Ire.) '42; MB; BCh; BAO.
SHEEHAN, Margaret M.; 11 Rainham Pl., Don Mills P.O., Ont.; Tor '47; Anaes; Staff, Hosp. for Sick Children, Toronto; Clin. Ass't. (Anaes), U. of Toronto; Tel. EM 6-7242.
SHEER, William T.; Main St. N.W., Gravelbourg, Sask.; 2nd Ave. W. (res); Man '45; Dist. Coroner; Pres. of Med. Staff, St. Joseph's Hosp.; Tel. 648-2277.
SHEFFMAN, Edward J.; 182 Fenn Ave., Willowdale, Ont.; Qns '53; DA; FACA; Anaes; Adjunct. (Anaes.), New Mount Sinai Hosp.; Tel. BA 2-4343.
SHEINER, Nathan M.; 659 Alexis Nihon, Montreal 9, P.Q. (res), Mc'G '57; FRCS(C); Thor-Surg (Cardiovasc.); FRCS(C), GenSurg; Staff, Jewish Gen. Hosp.; Tel. 735-3771.
SHEKTER, Jack J.; 1100 Main St. W., Hamilton, Ont.; Qns '57; MCGP; Tel. JA 8-0136.
SHELDON, Huntingdon; 3775 University, Montreal 2, P.Q.; Johns Hopkins (Baltimore, Md., U.S.A.) '56; Prof., Pathological Inst.
SHELL, Ben; 811 Lanark St., Winnipeg 9, Man. (res); Man '50; Anaes; Staff Winnipeg Gen. Hosp.; Tel. SP 4-6511.
SHELLEY, Robert P.; Med. Centre, Amherstburg, Ont.; Wes '56; Tel. 736-2118.
SHELTINGA, Douglas J.; 2904 Wascana St., Regina, Sask.; McG'48.
SHELTON, Elizabeth; (see Malyska, Elizabeth).
SHELTON, Peter J.; 773 Selkirk Ave., Winnipeg 4, Man.; 43 Forest Park Dr., Wpg. 17 (res); Man '50; GenSurg; Chief of Staff, Victoria **Hosp.; Tel. JA 2-5509.**
SHENKEN, Ellis; Ste. 603, 2 St. Clair Ave. W., Toronto 7, Ont.; Edinburgh (Scot.) '44; DOMS; Ophth.; Sr. Att'd. Eye Surg., Scarborough Gen. Hosp.; Tel. 927-2023.
SHENOUDA, Gamal-Zaki; 110-8th St. E., Prince Albert, Sask.; Cairo (Egypt) '53; FRCS (Eng.); FRCS (Ed.); GenSurg; Surg., Community Clinic, Victoria Union & Holy Family Hosp's.; Tel. 763-6466.
SHENSTONE, Norman; 904 Med. Arts Bldg., 170 St. George St., Toronto 5, Ont.; 65 Hillholm (res); Columbia (U.S.A.) '05; F.R.C.S.(Eng.) (Hon.), F.R.C.S.(C), GenSurg; Hon. Surg., Toronto Gen. Hosp.; Retired; Tel. WA 1-2189.
SHEPHARD, David A.; London (Eng.) '55; DA; Anaes; Staff, Dept. of Anaes., Halifax Infirmary, Halifax, N.S.; Lect. (Anaes.) Dalhousie U.; Tel. 422-1511.
SHEPHARD, Kenneth B.; 545 Prince St., Truro, N.S.; Dal '59; Active Staff, Colchester Co. Hosp.; Tel. 893-7344.
SHEPHARD, Roy J.; 150 College St., Toronto 5, Ont.; London (Eng.)'52; Prof. Applied Physiology, U. of T.
SHEPHERD, E. Dale; 216 Argyle St., Simcoe, Ont.; Sask. '60; Tel. 426-2014.
SHEPHERD, Gordon H.; Box 330, Osoyoos, B.C.; Alb '51; MCGP; Tel. HY 5-4311.
SHEPHERD, Grosvenor H.; 805 Lawrence Rd., Windsor, Ont.; 60 Jefferson Blvd., Riverside (res.); McG '34; Tel. 945-2509.
SHEPHERD, Ian L.; 198 Walkers Line, Burlington, Ont.; Aberdeen (Scot.) '44.
SHEPHERD, James K.; Main St., Neudorf, Sask.; Leeds (Eng.) '60; M.B., Ch.B., MRCP; Tel. 748-2566.
SHEPHERD, John T.; Tor'59; Res., Toronto East Gen. Hosp., Toronto 13, Ont.
SHEPHERD, Robert R.; Wes'63; Res., Westminster Hosp., London. Ont.
SHEPHERD, Robert W.; 64 Gables Ct., Beaconsfield, P.Q. (res); Tor '53; MCGP; Att'd. Phys. (O.P.D.), Royal Victoria Hosp.; Med. Advisor, CIBA Co. Ltd.; Tel. 631-4211.
SHEPHERD, W. Earl; 3994 - W 35th Ave., Vancouver 8, B.C. (res); Man'53; Path; Path. & Bact., Shaughnessy Hosp.; Clin. Assoc. Prof. Path., U. of British Columbia; Tel. CA 4-1111.
SHEPLEY, Donald J.; I.B.M., 36 King St. E., Toronto 1, Ont.; Tor'65; Systems Engineer I.B.M. Med. Team; Assoc. of Inst. of Bio-Medical Electronics, U. of Toronto; Tel. 362-6051.

SHEPLEY, Jean M. (Mustard); Res. & Mailing Address—601 Victoria Ave., Chatham, Ont.; Office —219 Wellington St. W.; Tor '33; MCGP; Tel. 354-2240.
SHEPLEY, Ledson J.; Res. & Mailing Address—601 Victoria Ave., Chatham, Ont.; Office—219 Wellington St. W.; Tor '34; MCGP; Tel. 354-2240.
SHEPPARD, Dorothy A. (Mrs. R. B. Babyn); 576 Christie St., Toronto 4, Ont.; Tor '49; ObstGyn; Active O.P.D. Staff, Women's College Hosp.; Tel. LE 2-4000.
SHEPPARD, Edward J.; 17-11th Ave. S., Cranbrook, B.C.; Tor'51; DRCOG; Med. Staff, St. Eugene Hosp.; Tel. 426-2201.
SHEPPARD, Elizabeth (See Barr.).
SHEPPARD, George G.; Mount Stewart, P.E.I.; Dal '47.
SHEPPARD, Lawrence D.; Ste. 10, Capital Apts., Fort Saskatchewan, Alta. (res.); Alb. '56; Tel. 453-2180.
SHEPPARD, Mabel L. (Mrs. Halliday); 755 Kingston Rd., Toronto 8, Ont.; Tor '49; Staff (G.P.), Toronto East Gen. Hosp.; Tel. OX 1-1405.
SHEPPARD, Richard J.; 35 Church St., St. Catharines, Ont.; Tor '21; Ophth. Otol.; Tel. MU 2-1344.
SHEPPARD, Robert D.; 35 Church St., St. Catharines, Ont.; Wes'60; Otol.; Tel. 682-1344.
SHEPPARD, Robert H.; 308 Toronto Western Medical Bldg., 25 Leonard Ave., Toronto 2B, Ont.; 122 Laurentide Dr., Don Mills, Ont. (res); Tor '48; F.R.C.P.(C), IntMed; Staff Phys., Toronto Western Hosp.; Cons.(Endocrine), Ontario Cancer Inst.; Clin. Instrt., U. of Toronto; Tel. EM 4-3852.
SHEPPARD, Thomas J.; 327 Charlotte St., Peterborough, Ont.; Tor'53; FRCS(C), ObstGyn; Active Staff (ObstGyn), Peterborough Civic & St. Joseph's Hosp's.; Tel. 743-2040.
SHER, Nathan; 170 The Donway W., Don Mills; 21 Briancliffe Dr. (res); Glasgow (Scot.) '41; M.D. (Glas); MRCP (Edin.); FRFPS (Glas); DCH (Lond.); Paed; Staff, Tor. E. Gen. Hosp.; Tel. 444-5881.
SHERBANIUK, Richard W.; 202 Medical Arts Bldg., 11010 Jasper Ave., Edmonton, Alta.; Alb '52; M.Sc., F.R.C.P.(C), IntMed; Staff, University Hosp.; Chief Phys., Student Health Serv. & Instr., U. of Alberta; Tel. 424-2424.
SHEREMATA, William A., Capt.; Canadian Forces Hosp., Kingston, Ont.; Alb'59.
SHERIDAN, Bernard B.; 4 Taschereau Ave., Hull, P.Q.; 691 Highland Ave., Ottawa 3 (res); Qns '44; Ophth; Chief Eye Serv. & Dir., Glaucoma Clinic, Sacred Heart Hosp., Hull; Cons. Ophth, St.-Louis-Marie-de-Montfort Hosp., Ottawa; Tel. PR 7-2721.
SHERIDAN, C. Arthur; 687 Pine Ave. W., Montreal 2, PQ; 1960 Laird Blvd., Mtl. 16 (res); Qns '46; Anaes; Anaes., Royal Victoria Hosp.; Tel. VI 2-1251, Loc. 530.
SHERIDAN, Philip A.; Ave. Q & 29th. St., Saskatoon, Sask.; Sask '64; Staff, Saskatoon City & St. Paul's Hosp's.; Tel. 652-6968.
SHERIN, John P.; Queen St., Lakefield, Ont.; Regent St. (res); Tor '55; MCGP; Staff, Civic & St. Joseph's Hosp's.; MOH; Tel. OL 2-3441.
SHERITON, Jack E.; Ste. 105, 170 Donway W., Don Mills, Ont.; Queen's U. (Belfast, N. Ire.) '56; ObstGyn.
SHERK, Boyce E.; St. Catharines Med. Centre, 292 Oakdale Ave., St. Catharines, Ont.; 49 Carleton St., S., Thorold (res); Wes '38; F.I.C.S., F.R.C.S.(C), GenSurg.; Active Staff, St. Catharines Gen. & Hotel-Dieu Hosp's.; Instr. (PG), St. Michael's Hosp., Toronto; Tel. MU 2-8344.
SHERK, Iva R.; (see Taves, Iva R.).
SHERKAT, Abolhassan; Teheran (Iran) '56; DiagRad; Staff, Dept. of Rad., St. Paul's Hosp., Vancouver 1, B.C.; Tel. 682-2344.
SHERMAN, E. David; 4330 Hampton Ave., Montreal 28, P.Q.; McG '32; F.A.C.P., D.I.M.; IntMed; Co.-Phys-in-Chief. Maimonides Hosp. & Home for the Aged; Dir. Research, Rehab. Inst.; Staff, Jewish Gen. Hosp.; Lect. (Geriat.) Schl. of Rehab., U. of Montreal; Tel. HU 6-6448.
SHERMAN, Ludwik; Ste. 405, 11010 Jasper Ave., monton, Alta.; 10803-138th St. (res); Poznan (Poland) '46; FACP; IntMed; Alternate Chief of Med., Royal Alexandra Hosp.; Cons. Staff, Edmonton Gen. Hosp.; Instr. (Med.), U. of Alberta; Tel. GA 2-8987.
SHERRIN, Adrienne; 1635 Abbott St., Kelowna, B.C.; UBC '59.
SHERRIN, Darrell A.; The Underhill Clinic, 1635 Abbott St., Kelowna, B.C.; UBC '58; FRCS(C), GenSurg.; Staff, Kelowna Gen. Hosp.; Tel. 762-2740.
SHERSTAN, James H.; Lloydminster Clinic, Lloydminster, Alta.; Alb'60; FRCS(C), GenSurg.
SHERWIN, Allan L.; 3801 University St., Montreal 2, P.Q.; McG '57; Ph.D., FRCP(C), Neurol; Ass't. Neurol., Mtl. Neurological Hosp.; Staff, Royal Victoria Hosp.; Ass't. Prof. (Neurol.), McGill U.; Markle Scholar, Academic Med., McGill U.; Tel. 845-6781 & VI 2-1251, Loc. 349.
SHETISKY, Gerald M.; Tor '62; Res. (Ophth.), Henry Ford Hosp., Detroit, Mich., U.S.A. Abroad.
SHEWCHUK, Alan B.; Tor'60; Res., Women's College Hosp., Toronto 2, Ont.
SHEWCHUK, Henry W.; Calgary Associate Clinic, 214-6th Ave. S.W., Calgary, Alta.; Alb '55; IntMed; Tel. AM 3-7120.
SHIAU, Edwin L.; McG '63; Res., Vancouver Gen. Hosp., Vancouver 9, B.C.
SHEWCIW, Zenon; St. Paul Med. Clinic, St. Paul, Alta.; Alb '60.
SHIBATA, Henry R.; Hiroshima '55; GenSurg; Teach Fell., Royal Victoria Hosp., Montreal 2, P.Q.; Tel. 842-1251.
SHIELDS, Garwood; Box 320, Young St., Capreol, Ont.; Tor'55; Med. & G.P. Staff, Sudbury Gen. & Mem. Hosp's.; Tel. 969-2233.
SHIELDS, Harry J.; 744 Duplex Ave., Toronto 12, Ont. (res); Tor '11; D.A., F.F.A.R.C.S.9 (Eng.), F.A.C.A., F.R.C.P.(C), Anaes; Hon. Cons. (Anaes), Toronto Gen., Sick Children's & Women's College Hosp's; Retired.
SHIELDS, Yehudi P.; 1271 Dundas St. W., Toronto 3, Ont.; Tor '62; AMCGP; Tel. LE 5-6300.
SHIER, Arthur A.; 2435 MacDonald St., Vancouver 8, B.C.; Man. '58; Tel. RE 8-0134.
SHIER, Crawford B.; 1020 Med. Arts Bldg., 170 St. George St., Toronto 5, Ont.; 289 Inglewood Dr. (res); Tor '40; F.R.C.S.(C), ObstGyn; Sr. ObstGyn., Toronto Gen. Hosp.; Sr. Cons. (ObstGyn), Ont. Cancer Inst.; Ass't. Prof., U. of Toronto; Tel. WA 1-5926.
SHIER, Donald J.; 2971 Kingston Rd., Scarborough, Ont.; 77 Deerfield Rd. (res); Tor '57; MCGP; Tel. AM 1-4025.
SHIER, John W.; 1314 Fairmont Med. Bldg., 750 W. Broadway, Vancouver 9, B.C.; Tor '28; MCGP.
SHIER, Karl J.; 2862 Riviera Dr., Windsor, Ont. (res); Vienna (Aust.) '47; Path; Staff, IODE Mem. Hosp.; Tel. CL 2-2771.
SHIER, Leonard V.; 215 Kent St. W., Lindsay, Ont.; Tor '22; Chief of Staff, & Chief Obst., Ross Memorial Hosp.; Dist. Coroner; Tel. 324-6111.
SHIER, Stanley G., O.B.E., C.D., Q.H.P. (Retired); Box 25, Hornings Mills, Ont.; Tor '30.
SHIERS, J. Anthony; 4593 Lakeside Rd., Penticton, B.C.; Cambridge (Eng.) '44; DMRD; DiagRad; Radiol., Penticton Hosp.; Tel. HY 2-4000.
SHIFF, Theodore; McG '64; Res., Jewish Gen. Hosp., Montreal 26, P.Q.; Abroad.
SHILETTO, Maurice D.; 249 Beta St., Toronto 14, Ont.; Univ. Coll. of West Indies '58; Dip. Anaes; Staff, Doctor's Hosp.; Tel. 251-9604.
SHIM, Sunshik S.; Dept. of Surg., U. of British Columbia, Vancouver Gen. Hosp., Vancouver, B.C.; M.Sc.; PhD; OrthSurg; Ass't. Prof. of Surg., U. of British Columbia; Cdn. Med. Research Council Scholar; Tel. TR 6-2565.
SHIME, J.; 275 Keewatin Ave., Toronto 12, Ont.; Tor '64.
SHIMIZU, Arthur G. S.; 1603 Bryn Mawr, Apt. 5, Cleveland, Ohio 44112, U.S.A.; Ott'59; IntMed; Abroad.

SHIMIZU, Henry J.; Ste. 430, 8409-112th St., Edmonton, Alta.; Alb '54; FRCS(C); PlasSurg; Staff, University Hosp.; Cons., Royal Alexandra Hosp.; Teach. Staff, U. of Alberta; Tel. 433-7642.

SHIMIZU, Keiji; Osaka (Japan) '49; Staff, Kitimat Gen. Hosp., Kitimat, B.C.

SHIMIZU, Raymond M.; Ott '59; Res., Montreal Gen. Hosp., Montreal 18, P.Q.

SHIMOKURA, Harold M.; 872E Hastings St., Vancouver, B.C.; 2797 William St. (res); Tor '32; Tel. MU 4-7917.

SHIMO-TAKAHARA, George; 2055 Peel St., Ste. 476, Montreal, P.Q.; 138 Brock Ave. N., Mtl. W. (res); McG '44; D.A.B.O.T., F.R.C.S.(C), Otol; Assoc. Otol., Royal Victoria & Mtl. Children's Hosp's.; Cons., Royal Edward Laurentian Hosp.; Lect. (Otol.), McGill U.; Tel. 288-8701.

SHINOBU, Roy R.; One Medical Place, 20 Wynford Dr., Don Mills, Ont.; Tor'49; D.Psy; Psy; Staff, Mental Health Clinic, North York Gen. Hosp., (Part-time); Tel. 429-1736.

SHIPPAM, Frederick; 146 Jasper Ave., Twn. of Mt. Royal, P.Q. (res); McG '26; M.R.C.P. (Edin.) Paed; Dem., Montreal Children's Hosp.; Hon. Staff, Montreal Gen. Hosp.; Dem. (Paed.), McGill U.; Retired.

SHIRLEY, Samuel Y.; Ste. 301, 180 Metcalfe St., Ottawa, Ont.; 458 Piccadilly Ave. (res); Dal '42; FACS, FRCS(C), Ophth; Chief, Dept. of Ophth., Ottawa Civic Hosp.; Assoc. Prof. (Ophth.), U. of Ottawa, Tel. 232-9321.

SHISTER, Hyman E.; 216 Medical Arts Bldg., 1538 Sherbrooke St. W., Montreal, P.Q.; 4630 Stanley Weir St. (res); McG '32; M.C.A.A., Cardiol. (P.Q.), IntMed; Att. Phys. & Card., Reddy Memorial Hosp.; Lect. in Pharmacol., McGill U.; Tel. WE 5-1454.

SHIZGAL, Harry M.; McG '63; Clin. Fell., Royal Victoria Hosp., Montreal 2, P.Q.

SHLESER, Isaac H.; 703 Spadina Ave., Toronto, Ont.; 203 Hillhurst Blvd. (res); Tor '37; D.A.B.I.M., IntMed; Att. Phys., Mount Sinai Hosp.; Ass't., Cardiac Clin., Toronto Gen. Hosp.; Clin. Teach., U. of Toronto; Tel. WA 2-6838.

SHLOSSBERG, Allan H.; Dal '64; Res., Montreal Gen. Hosp., Montreal 25, P.Q.

SHLOSSBERG, Reuben S.; 6432 Quinpool Rd., Halifax, N.S.; Dal '28; Ophth, Otol; Tel. 423-8956.

SHNEIDMAN, Nina; Ste. 1, 605 Bloor St. W., Toronto 4, Ont.; Vilnius State (Lith.) '53; Tel. 534-7205.

SHNIDER, Maurice; 1151 Pembina Hway, Winnipeg 19, Man.; 1007 Queenston Bay (res); Man '51; Tel. GL 3-6479.

SHNIDER, Mervyn; 400 Norlyn Med. Bldg., Hargrave St., Winnipeg 2, Man.; Man '57.

SHNITKA, Theodor K.; Dept. of Path., Prov. Lab., U. of Alberta, Edmonton, Alta.; 9823-106th St. (res); Alb '53; M.Sc., Path; Assoc. Prof. (Pathol.), U. of Alberta; Att. Staff, U. of Alberta Hosp.; Tel. 433-5811, Loc. 216.

SHOJANIA, A. Majid; Dept. of Haem., St. Boniface Gen. Hosp., Winnipeg 6, Man.; Tehran (Iran) '57; Paed; Dir. of Haem., St. Boniface Gen. Hosp.; Lect. in Paed., U. of Manitoba; Tel. 943-0311, Ext. 255.

SHOLDRA, E. P.; Tor'65; Res., Ottawa Gen. Hosp., Ottawa 2, Ont.

SHOMODY, Stephen H.; 276 Elgin St., Ottawa 4, Ont.; 158 Ruskin St., Ott. 3 (res); Peter Pazmany (Budapest, Hung.) '44; Jr. Staff, Ottawa Civic Hospital; Tel. 236-1583.

SHONE, John D.; London (Eng.) '53; Paed; Staff, Hosp. for Sick Children, Toronto 2, Ont.; Tel. EM 6-7242.

SHONIKER, Thomas J.; 12 Russet Place, Kitchener, Ont.; Wes'57; Path; Assoc. Pathol., St. Mary's Hosp.; Tel. 744-3311, Loc. 324.

SHOONER, Fernand; 815 Queen, St.-Lambert, Cite Jacques Cartier, P.Q. (res); Lav '55; Anaes; Staff, Hop.-General-de-Lambert.

SHORE, Alfred E.; 135 Greyhound Bldg., Calgary, Alta.; 815 Durham Ave. (res); Wes'10; Ophth, Otol.; Tel. 269-4838.

SHORE, Ben; McG'65; Res., Montreal General Hosp., Montreal 25, P.Q.

SHOREY, Kenneth M.; Apt. 707, 137 Isabella St., Toronto 5, Ont. (res); Qns '16; Adm., Dept. of Health, Toronto; Tel. EM 3-1211.

SHORT, Edwin J.; Box 910, 1 Evergreen Rd., Bridgewater, N.S.; McG '28; M.H.O.; Phys., Western Union Telegraphs. Retired.

SHORT, Hugh A.; 1403 Terminal Towers, 105 Main St. E., Hamilton, Ont.; Wes' 59; FRCS(C), ObstGyn; Tel. 525-2283.

SHORTING, Donald M. L.; Ste. 119, 645 Fort St., Victoria, B.C.; 2651 Queenswood Dr. (res); UBC '60; AMCGP; Active Staff, St. Joseph's Hosp.; M.O., Vancouver Island Unit of Oakalla Prison Farm; Tel. 384-7223.

SHORTREED, Robert D.; 189 N. Mitton St., Sarnia, Ont.; Tor'58; FRCS(C), Otol; Active Staff, Sarnia Gen. Hosp.; Assoc. Staff, St. Joseph's Hosp.; Tel. 337-6661.

SHORTT, Charles D.; 935 Lagauchetiere W., Montreal, P.Q.; 120-48th Ave., Lachine (res); Tor '31; DAB; PrevMed; (Occup. Med.); Sr. M.O., Cdn. National Railways, Box 8100, Montreal; Tel. 877-5635.

SHORTT, James D.; Dal'65; Res., Toronto Gen. Hosp., Toronto 2, Ont.

SHOSTACK, Bernard; 150 The East Mall, Islington, Ont.; Tor '54; MCGP; Assoc. Staff, Queensway Gen. Hosp.; Tel. BE 9-4315.

SHOTTON, John A.; 34 Talbot St. W., Leamington, Ont.; 62 Mill St. W. (res); McG '28; M.C.-G.P.; Tel. FA 6-4421.

SHOULDICE, Earle B.; Shouldice Surgery, 618 Church St., Toronto 5, Ont.; Wes. '61; Tel. WA 3-3507.

SHRAGOVITCH, Israel; 3755 Cote St. Catherine Rd., Montreal 26, P.Q.; 328 Redfern Ave., Westmount (res); McG '39; FRCS(C); GenSurg; Surg.-in-Chief, Jewish Gen. Hosp.; Assoc. Surg., Montreal Children's Hosp.; Cons. Reddy Mem. Hosp.; Lect. Surg., McGill U.; Tel. 735-3771, Loc. 525.

SHUBERT, Sydney; Taylor Clinic, 1746 Jane St., Weston, Ont.; Manchester (Eng.)'50; Active Staff, Humber Mem. Hosp.; Tel. CH 4-5545.

SHUGAR, Gerald; Clarke Inst., 250 College St., Toronto, Ont.; Tor'60; Psy.

SHUGAR, Joseph L.; Linton Clinic, 6000 Cote des Neiges Rd., Montreal 25, P.Q.; 4530 Madison Ave. (res); McG '43; DABOS; FACS; FRCS(C); OrthSurg Sr. Orthopaed. I/C Orth. Serv., Jewish Gen. Hosp.; Assoc. Surg., Mtl. Children's & Reddy Mem. Hosp's.; Lect. (OrthSurg.), McGill U.; Tel. 342-2912.

SHUKYN, David; 575 Euclid Ave., Toronto, Ont.; Tor '34; Tel. LE 1-6291.

SHULMAN, Abraham; 5195 Victoria Ave., Montreal, P.Q.; 4750 Fulton Ave. (res); McG '31; FAGS; FACP; IntMed; Assoc. Phys., Outdoor, Montreal Gen. Hosp.; Ass't. Phys., Jewish Gen. Hosp. Assoc. (Neur.), Hosp. of Hope; Tel. RE 8-5225 .

SHULMAN, Morton P.; 378 Roncesvalles Ave., Toronto 3, Ont.; 66 Russell Hill Rd., Tor. 7 (res); Tor '48; Chief Coroner, Metro Toronto; Tel. LE 6-8942.

SHULMAN, Philip N.; 99 Avenue Rd., Toronto 5, Ont.; 28 Glentworth Rd., Willowdale (res); Tor '55; Tel. 921-7472.

SHULMAN, Robert; Ste. 509, 1538 Sherbrooke St. W., Montreal, P.Q.; 2127 Noel St., St. Laurent (res); Geneva (Switzerland)'59; FRCP(C), IntMed; Clin. Ass't. O.P.D., Mtl. Gen. Hosp.; Jr. Phys., Reddy Mem. Hosp.; Dem. Med., McGill U.; Tel. 937-4300.

SHUM, T. W.; Box 490, Ocean Falls, B.C.; '55.

SHUMAK, K. H.; Tor '65; Res., Toronto General Hosp., Toronto 2, Ont.

SHUMAK, Rene S.; Tor'65; Res., Toronto Western Hosp., Toronto 2B, Ont.

SHUMAN, Ben; 1734 W. Broadway, Vancouver 9, B.C.; 825 W. 52nd (res); Tor '42; Paed; Att'd. Staff, Van. Gen. & Children's Hosp's.; Clin. Ass't. Prof. (Paed), U. of British Columbia; Tel. RE 1-2184.

SHUREN, Alex; 944 Ottawa St., Windsor, Ont.; Qns'60; Otol; Tel 254-8664.

SHUSTER, Samuel; 3521 Girouard Ave., Montreal, P.Q.; McG '36; F.C.C.P., IntMed (P.Q.); Clin. Ass't., Jewish Gen. Hosp.; Ass't. Phys., Royal Edward Inst; Cons. Phys., Steinberge Ltd.; Tel. 484-5225.

SHUSTERMAN, Morris; 72 St. Clair Ave W., Toronto, Ont.; 399 Brock Ave. (res); Tor '45; D.A.B.O., F.R.C.S.(C), Ophth; Active Staff, St. Joseph's & Mt. Sinai Hosp's.; Clin. Ass't. (Ophth), Hosp. for Sick Children; Telephone WA 2-6235.

SHUTE, Dennis; Provincial Lab., Southern Br., U. of Alberta, Calgary, Alta.; 7028 Bow Cres., Bowness (res); Manchester (Eng.) '35; M.B., Ch.B., M.D., DTM (Liverpool); Dir., Prov. Lab., Calgary; Tel. BU 8-2965.

SHUTE, Evan V.; Heronspool, Arva, Ont. (res); Tor '27; D.A.B.O.G., F.R.C.S.(C) ObstGyn, GenSurg; Med. Dir., Shute Inst., 10 Grande, London, Ont.; Editor, The Summary; Tel. GE 2-1884.

SHUTE, Wallace B.; 276 Elgin St., Ottawa, Ont.; 300 Island Pk. Dr. (res); Wes '36; D.A.B.O.G., M.R.C.O.G., F.A.C.S., F.R.C.S.(C), ObstGyn; Staff, Ottawa Civic & Grace Hosp's.; Tel. CE 2-7677.

SHUTE, Wilfrid E.; 299 Lakeshore Rd. E., Port Credit, Ont.; 1549 Trimble Ct. (res); Tor '33; Tel. CR 8-2711.

SHUTT, Ken; Alb '63; Res., University Hosp., Edmonton, Alta.

SHWARTZ, Issie; 606 Boyd Bldg., Winnipeg, Man.; 803 Elm St. (res); Man '50; MCGP; Court. Staff, Wpg. Gen., Children's & Grace Hosp's.; Tel. 942-3920.

SHYDLOWSKI, Walter; Bassano, Alta; Alb '55; Tel. 187.

SHYKOFF, Henry J.; Ste 103, 688 Coxwell Ave., Toronto 6, Ont.; Tor'49; Anaes; Staff, Toronto East Gen. Hosp.; Tel. 461-8272.

SIAHAAN, Corry; Staff, Children's Hosp., Montreal 25, P.Q.

SIBLEY, John C.; Rose Valley, Sask.; London (Eng.)'48; Tel. 85.

SIBLEY, John C. A.; 407 Brant Arts Bldg., 672 Brant St., Burlington, Ont.; Qns'47; MRCP (Lond.); FACP; FACC; FRCP(C), IntMed; Hd. Dept. of Med., Joseph Brant Mem. Hosp.; Hon. Cons. Dept. of Med., Hamilton Civic & St. Joseph's Hosp's.; Tel. 637-0302.

SICARD, Andre; 30 St. Joseph Blvd. E., Montreal 14, P.Q.; Mon '53; Derm; Tel. 845-5970.

SICARD, Julien; 959 St. Maurice, Trois Rivieres, P.Q.; Mon '27.

SICOTTE, Jules; Churchill Blk., Mountain Ave., Neepawa; Man.; **Ste. 1, Keer Blk. (res); Lav '57.**

SIDDALL, Alvin M.; Yarmouth, N.S.; 20 Baker St., (res); Dal '25; MCGP; Tel. 2-3233.

SIDDALL, Edward R.; 28 Maple St., Pine Falls, Man.; Man '49.

SIDDALL, Jack R.; Ste. 309, 4900 Kingsway, South Burnaby, B.C.; Wes '44; Ophth; F.A.C.S., D.A.B. Ophth., F.R.C.S.(C), Ophth.; Clin. Instr. (Physiol.), U. of British Columbia; Tel. HE 3-1258.

SIDDALL, Wilson R; Port Hawkesbury, N.S.; Dal '57.

SIDDHARTH, Padmanabhan; Madras (India) '58; Res., Victoria Gen. Hosp., Halifax, N.S.

SIDDOO, Jagdis K.; Tor '49; Staff, Vancouver Gen. Hosp., Vancouver, B.C.; Tel. 876-3211.

SIDEBOTHAM, Richard E.; Lynwood Med. Office, 6622-20A St. S.E., Calgary, Alta.; 6644-18th St. S.E. (res); London (Eng.)'46; LRCP, MRCS; Tel. BR 9-4581.

SIDENBERG, Roy E.; 320 Davis St., Sarnia, Ont.; Tor '41; M.C.G.P.

SIDENBERG, Sidney H.; 320 Davis St., Sarnia, Ont.; 1338 Kim St. (res); Tor '46; D.A.B.S.; Chief of Surg., St. Joseph's Hosp.; Surg. Staff, Sarnia Gen. Hosp.; Tel. ED 6-6121.

SIDGWICK, A. Mary (Sibly); 1277 Sheppard Ave. E., Willowdale, Ont.; 26 Chipping Rd. (res); Cambridge (Eng.) '46; M.R.C.S. (Eng.), L.R.-C.P. (Lond); AMCGP Assoc. Staff North York Branson Hosp.; Tel. 225-0213.

SIDLOFSKY, Saul; Ste. 302, 99 Avenue Rd., Toronto 5, Ont.; Tor'58; Am. Bd. Surg; FRCS (C), GenSurg; Adjunct, Dept. of Surg., Mount Sinai Hosp.; Clin. Teach. Surg., U. of Toronto; Tel. WA 4-9005.

SIDOROV, J. J.; Suite 201, 5880 Spring Garden Rd., Halifax, N.S.; Zagreb (Yugo.) '51; FRCP (C); IntMed; Ass't. Phys., Victoria Gen. Hosp.; Cons. (Med. Gastroen.), DVA Camphill Hosp., Cdn. Forces Hosp. "Stadacona". & Halifax Infirm.; Ass't. Prof. (Med.) Dalhousie U.; Tel. 454-7836.

SIEGEL, Elliott J.; Ste. 302, 151 Eglinton Ave. W., Toronto 12, Ont.; 97 Old Colony Rd., Willowdale, (res); Tor '44; DMD (Harvard); Tel. 487-5264.

SIEGEL, Theodore; 546 Barton St. E., Hamilton, Ont.; 30 Colquhoun Cres. (res); Wes '45; MCGP; Staff, Hamilton Gen. & St. Joseph's Hosp's.; Tel. JA 9-1221.

SIEGENBERG, Joe; 406 Med. Arts Bldg., 11010 Jasper Ave., Edmonton, Alta.; Witwatersrand (S. Africa) '53; FRCS(C); GenSurg; Instr. (Surg. & Anat.), U. of Alberta.

SIEGMUND, Konstantin; 214 Church St., Pembroke, Ont.; 301 Dominion St. (res); Zagreb (Yugoslavia)'39; GenSurg; Chief Surg., Pembroke Cottage Hosp.; Tel. RE 2-7231.

SIEMENS, Herman; 328 Administration Bldg., Edmonton, Alta.; Alb'37; Dr.PH; DIH; Spec. Am.Bd., PM & PH; PH; Dir. of Div. of Industrial Health Serv., Dept. of Public Health, Govn't. of the Province of Alta.; Tel. 229-3033.

SIEMENS, Peter; Box 489, Outlook, Sask.; Sask '57.

SIENIEWICZ, James D.; Montreal Gen. Hosp., Montreal, P.Q.; 715 Grosvenor Ave., Westmount, Montreal 6 (res); Dal '50; DABR; D & TRad; Rad.-in-Chief, Montreal Gen. Hosp.; Assoc. Prof. (Rad.), McGill U.; Tel. WE 7-6011.

SIENIEWICZ, Thaddeus M.; 1803 Armview Terr., Halifax, N.S. Dal '17; M.C.A.A., F.C.C.P., F.R.C.P.(C) IntMed; Cons. in Dis. of Chest & All. Victoria Gen. Hosp.; Cons. in All., D.V.A. Camp Hill Hosp.; Cons. in Med., Halifax T.B. Hosp.; Assoc. Prof. of Med., Dalhousie U.; Tel. 423-6655.

SIEVENPIPER, Stanley H.; 3310 Boundary Rd., South Burnaby, B.C.; Tor'22.

SIFRER, Asuncion G.; 1658 Victoria Park Ave., Scarborough, Ont.; Madrid (Spain) '52.

SIFTON, John A.; 6th Floor, 151 Bloor St. W., Toronto 5, Ont.; Wes '26.

SIGAL, Cecil; Ste. 403; 750 W. Broadway, Vancouver 9, B.C.; UBC'59; FRCP(C), Derm.

SIGMAN, Gerald; McG '62; Intn., Jewish Gen. Hosp., Montreal 26, P.Q.

SIGMAN, Harvey H.; 6000 Cote des Neiges Rd., Montreal 25, P.Q.; McG '57; M.Sc. (Exper. Surg.); FRCS(C), GenSurg; Surg., Jewish Gen. Hosp. & Queen Mary Vet's Hosp.; Dem. (Surg.) McGill U.; Tel. 342-2912.

SIGSWORTH, Pius M.; 7140 Bayers Rd., Halifax, N.S.; Dal '48; Paed; Staff, Children's, Grace Maternity & Hlfx. Infirmary; Lect. (Paed), Dalhousie U.; Tel. 454-0682.

SIGURDSON, Frank T.; 3091 W. Broadway, Vancouver 8, B.C.; 4689 Haggart St. (res); Alb '59; Tel. RE 8-3848.

SIGURDSON, Jon F.; Man '59; FRCS(C), OrthSurg; Staff, Winnipeg Gen. Hosp., Winnipeg, Man.; Abroad.

SIGURDSON, Larus A.; 528 Medical Arts Bldg., Winnipeg, Man.; 1246 Wolseley Ave. (res); Man '27; M.A. (Stand.); M.C.G.P.; Assoc. Prof. Anat., U. of Manitoba.

SIHLER, James C. T.; 61 Colborne St. S., Simcoe, Ont.; **Tor '32.**

SIKORA, Stanislaus; 201 Main W., Welland, Ont.; Warsaw (Pol.) '22; Tel. 732-3010.

SIKSAY, Nicholas E.; 111 St. Clair Ave., Hamilton, Ont.; Tor '62.

SILBERMAN, Max; 316 St. Clair Ave. W., Toronto 7, Ont.; Tor'30; FAAP, Paed; Att. Paed., New Mt. Sinai Hosp.; Tel. 924-2433.

SILBERMANN, Olaf H.; Dodsland, Sask.; Alb '56.

SILDVEE, Oivo; 71 Westlake Ave., Toronto 13, Ont.; Man '63; Tel. OX 1-1441.
SILIVASK, Helvi; Tartu (Estonia) '42; Staff, Saint John T.B. San., East Saint John, N.B.; Tel. 693-6551.
SILLAPERE, Ann; (see Barrett, Ann).
SILLER, Theodore N.; Wes '59; FRCS(C), OrthSurg; Staff, Montreal Children's Hosp., Montreal 25, P.Q. Abroad.
SILLERS, Donald E.; 1707 Weston Rd., Weston, Ont.; Tor'58; Ophth; Staff, Humber Mem. & Sunnybrook Hosp's.; Tel. 249-1174.
SILLS, H. L.; 751 Hamilton Rd., London, Ont.; **176 Sherwood (res); Tor '40**; Tel. 451-6160.
SILNY, John; 569 Newton St., Sherbrooke, P.Q. (res); McG '48; D&TRad; Chief of Rad., Sherbrooke Hosp.; Tel. 569-3661.
SILUCH, Kazie A.; Alb'54; Urol; Staff, University Hosp., Edmonton, Alta.
SILUCH, Malcolm D.; Adelaide (S. Australia) '56; Jr. Ass't. Res. (Path.), Royal Victoria Hosp., Montreal, P.Q.; Dem. (Path.), McGill U.
SILVA-AZAUSTRE, Jesus; Madrid (Spain) '53; PhysMed & Rehab; Staff, Montreal Gen. Hosp., Montreal 25, P.Q.; Staff Physiatrist, Occupational Therapy & Rehab. Center.
SILVA, Yvan J.; Bombay (India)'61; FRCS(C), GenSurg; Staff, Royal Victoria Hosp., Montreal 2, P.Q.
SILVEIRA, C. John; 201-1543 Victoria Pk. Ave., Scarborough, Ont.; **Durham (Eng.) '44; M.C.-G.P.; F.A.G.S.; Staff, Scarborough Gen. & Toronto E. Gen. Hosp's.; Tel. 759-2671.**
SILVER, Archie; 6000 Cote Des Neiges Rd., Montreal, P.Q.; McG'45; DABNP, Psy; Clin. **Ass't.,** Jewish Gen. Hosp. & O.P.D., Royal Victoria Hosp.; Tel. VI 2-1251.
SILVER, Daniel; McG'64; Res., Douglas Hosp., Montreal 19, P.Q.
SILVER, Gordon L.; Sherbrooke, N.S.; Dal '35.
SILVER, Harold L.; 314 St. Clair Ave. W., **Toronto 7, Ont.; 33 Scarth Rd. Rosedale (res); London (Eng.) '52; PlasSurg; Staff, Women's** College Hosp.; Tel. WA 7-3015.
SILVER, Jack B.; Hudson Bay, Sask.; Man '33; Dist. Coroner.; Tel. 865-2641.
SILVER, Meredith M.; 118 South Dr., Toronto 5, Ont.; '57.
SILVER, Samuel; 38 Coburg St., Saint John, N.B.; 26 Highwood Dr. (res); **McG '38; Ophth,** Otol.; Chief, Dept. of Oph.Otol., Saint John Gen. Hosp.; Tel. 693-3646.
SILVER, William A.; McG'56; AMCGP; Res., **University Hosp., Saskatoon, Sask.**
SILVERBERG, L. R.; 25 Brunswick Ave., Toronto 4, Ont.; Tor'65.
SILVERBERG, Mervin; 5300 Cote-des-Neiges Rd., Montreal 26, P.Q.; 2255 Benjamin Sulte, Mtl. 12 (res); McG '54; FRCP(C), Paed; Ass't. (Metab.) & Dir., Liver Function Lab., Mtl. Children's Hosp.; Clin. Ass't., Jewish Gen. Hosp.; Dem. (Paed), McGill U.; Hosmer Teach. Fell; Tel. 937-8511, & RE 1-5048.
SILVERBERG, S. A.; Tor'65; Jr. Int., Toronto Western Hosp., Toronto 2B, Ont. Abroad.
SILVERMAN, Baruch; 3690 Peel St., Montreal 2, P.Q.; McG '21; FAAMD; FAPA; Psy; Dir., Mental Hygiene Inst.; Sess. Lect. (Psy), McGill U.; Tel. 844-3971.
SILVERMAN, Bernie; Ste. 121. 400 Walmer Rd., Toronto 10, Ont.; Tor'55; D.Psy; Psy.; Clin. Teach. (Psy.) U. of Toronto; Tel. 923-8533.
SILVERMAN, Marvin; 1105 Carling Ave., Ste. 304, Ottawa 3, Ont.; 465 Island Park Dr. (res); Ott '56; Psy; Staff, Ottawa Gen. & Civic Hosp's.; Tel. 729-2933.
SILVERSIDES, John L.; 211 Toronto Western Medical Bldg., 25 Leonard Ave., Toronto 2B, Ont.; 19 Dunbar Rd., Tor. 5 (res); Man '40; F.R.C.P.(C), IntMed; Neurol; Neurologist, Toronto Western Hosp.; Cons.Neurol., W.C.B. Hosp., Downsview; Assoc. Prof. (Med.), U. of Toronto; Tel. EM 6-2606.
SILVERSTEIN, Ezra A.; 99 Avenue Rd., Ste. 405A, Toronto 5, Ont.; Tor '54; FRCS(C), OrthSurg; Staff Surg., Mount Sinai Hosp.; Clin. Teach. Surg., U. of Toronto; Tel. 925-6416.
SILVERSTEIN, Henry; 550 University Ave., Toronto, Ont.; 28 Yorkdowns Dr., Downsview, (res); Tor '40; D.A.B.P.M., PhysMed & Rehab; Chief. Dept. of Phys. Med. & Rehab., New Mount Sinai Hosp. & Baycrest Hosp. & Jewish Home for Aged; Tel. EM 6-7361.
SILVERTHORNE, L. Nelles; 204 Med. Arts Bldg., 170 George St., Toronto 5, Ont.; 8 Brendan Rd. (res); Tor '26; Paed; Staff, Connaught Labs.; Sr. Phys., Hosp. for Sick Children; Assoc. Prof. (Paed), U. of Toronto; Tel. WA 2-5986.
SIM, David G.; Ste 505, 143 James St. S., Hamilton, Ont.; 216 Chesley St. (res); Wes '49; D.Psy; Psy; Active Staff (Psy), Hamilton Civic Hosp's.; Court. Staff (Psy), St. Joseph's & Chedoke Gen. Hosp's.; Tel. JA 9-1518.
SIMAO, Antonio; Coimbre (Portugal) '55; DiagRad; Staff, St. Joseph's Hosp., Saint John, N.B.
SIMARD, Arthur; 10030 rue Royale, Ste. Anne de Beaupre, P.Q.; 279 rue Royale (res); Lav '33; M.C.G.P.; Dir., Hop. Notre Dame du Sacre-Coeur, Dist. Coroner; Tel. 263-4003.
SIMARD, Camille; Box 1500, Sioux Lookout, Ont.; Lav '60.
SIMARD, Charles E.; 24B Victoria, Bagotville, P.Q.; 2A Notre Dame (res); McG '53.
SIMARD, Denis; Lav'65; Res., Hop Enfant Jesus, Quebec, P.Q.
SIMARD, Dollard; 81 rue de-l'Eveche, Rimouski, **P.Q.; 65 ave. Rouleau (res); Lav '43; M.C.G.P.**
SIMARD, Dominique; 1248 Chemin Ste Foy, Quebec 6, P.Q.; Lav'65.
SIMARD, F.; Tor'65; Jr. Int., Toronto General Hosp., Toronto 2, Ont.
SIMARD, Francois X.; 865 rue d'Iberville, Chicoutimi, P.Q.; Lav '44; Anaes; Staff, Hop.-Hotel-Dieu-St. Vallier; Tel. 549-1452.
SIMARD, Gaston; Baie Comeau, Co. Saguenay, P.Q.; Lav '48.
SIMARD, Herve, Capt.; Camp Gagetown, N.B.; Lav '65.
SIMARD, Jacques G.; 1150 Blvd. St. Joseph E., Montreal 34, P.Q.; 345 Strathcona Dr., Mont Royal (res); Mon '50; F.R.C.S.(C), GenSurg; Surg., Hop. Maisonneuve; Tel. LA 7-1241.
SIMARD, J. A. Rene; 540 rue St. Jean, Quebec, P.Q.; 2595 des Quatre Bourgeois (res); **Lav '37; FRCS(C); ObstGyn; Prof. of Clin. Obst., & Chief, Dept. of Obst., Laval U.; Tel. LA 9-4511.**
SIMARD, J. Conrad; 209 Blvd. St. Joseph, Hull, P.Q.; Lav '38; Tel. PR 7-1388.
SIMARD, J. Emile; 42 Blvd. Riviere du Moulin, Chicoutimi, P.Q. (res); Lav '39; F.A.C.S., F.R.-C.S.(C) GenSurg; Surg., Hotel-Dieu St. Vallier Hosp., Chicoutimi; Assoc. Prof., Laval U.; Tel. 549-1452.
SIMARD, Louis C.; 624 Dunlop Ave., Montreal, P.Q. (res); Mon '23; F.R.C.S.(C) PathBact; Chief Path., & Dir. & Pres., Cancer Inst., Notre-Dame Hosp.; Assoc. Prof., U. of Montreal; Tel. LA 5-6363.
SIMARD, Louis P.; 505 de Sales, Chicoutimi, P.Q. (res); **Lav '43; F.R.C.S.(C).** Urol; Staff, Hop. Hotel-Dieu & Laval U.; Tel. 549-2212.
SIMARD, Michel; Mon. '62; Res., Hop. Notre-**Dame, Montreal, P.Q.**
SIMARD, Michelle; Lav'65; Res., Royal Victoria Hosp., Montreal 2, P.Q.
SIMARD, Normand; Lav'64; Res., Hop. Enfant Jesus, Quebec 3, P.Q.
SIMARD, Padoue; Notre Dame du Nord, Co. Temiscaminque, P.Q.; Lav '45; Hop. de Paris (Fr.).; Tel. 3261.
SIMARD, Paul; Lav '41; D&TRad; Staff, Hop. St-Jean, St-Jean, P.Q.
SIMARD, Paul R.; 4515 ouest, Notre-Dame, Montreal 30, P.Q.; **Mon '57.**; Tel. 932-2248.
SIMARD, Philippe; 945 Joffre, Quebec 6, P.Q.; 8 Terrasse Dufferin (res); Lav '30; OphthOtol; **Staff, O.R.L., Hop. Ste-Foy; Tel. 523-9384.**
SIMARD, Pierre; Apt. 301, 1000 ave Pratt, Outremont, P.Q.; Mon'58; Path(P.Q.); Staff, Hop. Jean-Talon; Teach. Staff, U. of Montreal.
SIMARD, Pierre-Paul; Lav'62; Res., Hop. Maisonneuve, Montreal, P.Q.

SIMARD, Raymond; 1656 est rue Sherbrooke, Montreal 24, P.Q.; 6540 Pie IX Blvd. (res); Mon '35; F.I.C.S., F.R.C.S.(C), Gyn; Clin. Instr. (Gyn), Notre Dame Hosp.; Ass't. Prof. (Gyn), Montreal U.; Tel. 526-3783.
SIMARD, Raymond-M.; 1500 - 18e rue, Quebec 4, P.Q.; Lav'54; ObstGyn(P.Q.); Tel. 529-3083.
SIMARD, Raymond M.; Lav '58; Res., Hop. Hotel-Dieu, Montreal 25, P.Q.
SIMARD, Real; rue St.-Edmond, Normandin, Cte. Roberval, P.Q.; Lav '58.
SIMARD, Renald; 2 Rouville, Baie Comeau, P.Q.; Ott'62; Tel. 584-3347.
SIMARD, Rene; 246 rue St. Jean, Quebec 4, P.Q.; 2595 des Quartre-Bourgeois (res); Lav '37; **FRCS(C); ObstGyn; Head Dept. of Obst., Hop.** Misericorde; **Chm. & Prof. (Dept. of ObstGyn), Laval U.; Tel. 522-4415.**
SIMARD, Roch; 541 rue de l'Hopital, Jonquiere, P.Q.; Lav '56; Paed (P.Q.).
SIMARD, Roger P.; 1384 est, Jean Talon, Montreal, 35, P.Q.; Mon '51; GenSurg (P.Q.).
SIMARD, Roland; 1260 est Boul. St.-Joseph, Montreal 34, P.Q.; Mon '42; F.R.C.S.(C), Gyn.; Tel. LA 6-6608.
SIMARD, Sylvain; Lav '64; Res., Hop. Hotel-Dieu, Montreal 18, P.Q.
SIMARD, Victorien; Ste. 209, 2120 est rue Sherbrooke, Montreal 24, P.Q.; Lav'55; GenSurg (P.Q.); Tel. 526-8521.
SIMARD, Yvan; Lav'59; Res., Hop. Hotel Dieu, Montreal 18, P.Q.

SIMINOVITCH, Jack; Ste. 300, 5300 Cote des Neiges Rd., Montreal 26, P.Q.: 766 McEachran Ave., Outremont (res); McG '35; IntMed (P.Q.); Ass't. Phys., Jewish Gen. Hosp.; Tel. RE 1-4590.
SIMINOVITCH, Moses; Linton Clinic, 6000 Cote-des-Neiges Rd., Montreal 26, P.Q.; 4990 Glencairn Ave. (res); McG'40; FACS, D.Urol., FRCS(C) Urol; Ass't. Urol., Jewish Gen. Hosp.; Urol.-in-Charge, St. Mary's Hosp.; Tel. RE 3-1542.

SIMMONS, Edward H.; 272 Bloor St. W., Toronto 5, Ont.; One Med. Place, 20 Wynford Dr., Don Mills; Tor '48; B.Sc. (Med), M.S. (Tor); FACS; FRCS(C), OrthSurg; GenSurg; Att'd. OrthSurg., Tor. E. Gen. & Sunnybrook DVA Hosp's.; Memb. Med. Advisory Bd., Cnd. Rehab Fdn. for Disabled & Tor. Rehab. Centre; Memb. Council, Tor. Med-Legal Assoc.; Clin. Instr., U. of Toronto; Tel. 923-3565.
SIMMONS, Robert J.; Ott '62; Res., c/o 80 Brookdale Ave., Toronto 12, Ont.; Abroad.

SIMMS, David C.; Tor '59; Res., St. Michael's Hosp., Toronto 2, Ont.
SIMMS, Douglas C.; 31 Queen's Rd., St. John's Nfld.; 27 Long Pond Rd. (res); Dal '43; Paed; Staff, St. John's Gen., & Grace Hosp's.; Chief Paed., St. Clare's Hosp.; Tel. 578-7837.
SIMMS, G. Graham G.; 2260 Connaught Ave., Halifax, N.S. (res); Dal '38; DPH; PH; Vice-Chm. & Exec. Dir., N.S. Hosp. Ins., Comm.; Assoc. Prof. (Hosp. Ins.), Dept. of Prev. Med., Dalhousie U.; Tel. 423-7341.
SIMMS, Hugh M.; Wolfville, N.E.; Dal '53; Phys., Acadia U.
SIMMS, John G.; 168 Charlotte St., Ottawa, Ont.; 798 Dunloe (res); McG '50; M.C.G.P.; Tel. 234-1135.
SIMMS, Robert J.; 31 Queens Rd., St. John's, Nfld.; 23 Cornwall Hgts. (res); Guy's H. (Lond.) '37; IntMed; Chief (Dept. of Med.), St. John's Gen. & St. Clare's Hosp's.; Tel. 726-8366.

SIMO, Jose; 505 O'Connor St., Ottawa 1. Ont.; **Santo Thomas (Philippines) '46.; Tel. 232-5761.**

SIMON, Albert V.; 4865 Queen Mary Rd., Montreal, P.Q.; **4075 Maplewood (res); Tor '41;** Anaes.
SIMON, F.; Albany Med. Clinic, 200 Danforth Ave., Toronto 6, Ont.; Tor'65; Tel. 461-0761.
SIMON, Jean C.; 3871 Belanger E., Rosemont, Montreal 36, P.Q.; No. 2, 6435 Pie IX Blvd. (res); Mon '58.
SIMON, Jerome B.; Qns '62; Jr. Ass't. Res. (Med.), Mtl. Gen. Hosp., Montreal, P.Q.; Abroad.
SIMON, John B.; 4304-17th Ave. S.E., Calgary, Alta.; Szeged (Hung.)'52; Tel. BR 2-0510.
SIMON, Leslie; 288 St. Clair W., Toronto, Ont.; 34 Poplar Plains Cres. (res); Budapest (Hung.) '29; Tel. WA 1-6614.
SIMON, Louis M.; 114 Carleton St., St. John, N.B.; Dal'64; AMCGP; Staff, St. John's & St. Joseph's Hosp's.; Tel. 692-1432.
SIMON, Morris A.; 279 Kenaston Ave., Mount Royal, Montreal, P.Q. (res); Cleveland (U.S.A.) '31; FASCP, FCAP, PathBact; Dir. of Lab., Jewish Gen. Hosp.; Ass't. Prof. in Path., McGill U.; Tel. 737-6464.
SIMON, Solomon A.; 1831 Rose St., Regina, Sask.; Tor '42; Assoc. Med. Staff, Regina Gen. & Regina Grey Nuns Hosp's.; Tel. 522-7886.
SIMONDS, Patricia E.; Alb'57; Res., Vancouver Gen. Hosp., Vancouver 9, B.C.
SIMONEAU, Roger; 32 ouest Blvd. St. Joseph, Montreal 14, P.Q.; Mon'53; OrthSurg; Ass't. OrthSurg., Hop-SteJustine; Tel. VI 2-9418.
SIMONEAU, Roger; 367 St. Joseph est, Montreal, P.Q.; Mon'60; Psy(P.Q.); Staff, Hop. St. Jean-de-Dieu; Tel. 254-8381.
SIMONEAU, Roland J. H.; 6697 Christophe Colomb St., Montreal, P.Q.; Lav '33; M.O.H., Child Health, Town of Montreal.
SIMONETTA, Luigi R.; C.S. Williams Clinic, 901 Helena St., Trail, B.C.; UBC'56; Tel. 368-5211.

SIMONS, Siebert P.; 3597 Papineau Ave., Montreal 24, P.Q.; Amsterdam (Neth.)'51; Psy(P.Q.); Research, Beatty Hall, Montreal.

SIMONSEN, Leif E.; 110 Med. Arts Bldg., Port Arthur, Ont.; Qns '53; Anaes; Chief, Dept. of Anaes., Port Arthur Gen. Hosp.; Active Staff, St. Joseph's Gen. Hosp.; Court. Staff, McKellar Gen. Hosp., Fort William; Cons. Staff, Fort Wm. San. & Nipigon Mem. Hosp.; Tel. 344-1813.

SIMOR, Imre S.; 550 University Ave., Toronto 2, Ont.; 16 Farrington Dr., Willowdale (res); Munich (Germ.) '50; FRCP(C), DiagRad; Sr. Att'd. Radiol., New Mt. Sinai Hosp.; **Tel. EM 6-7361,** Loc. 321.
SIMOR, Laszlo; 4085 Maplewood Ave., Montreal 26, P.Q.; Budapest (Hung.)'50; Staff, Johnson & Johnson; Tel. RE 1-1607.

SIMPSON, Albert A.; 3 Gloria Ave., Beaverbank, Lower Sackville, N.S.; Aberdeen (Scot.) '25; Court. Staff, Halifax Hosp's.; Tel. 865-2960.
SIMPSON, Alan W.; Anaesthesia Assoc., 900 King St. W., Kitchener, Ont.; Aberdeen (Scot.) **'53; DObstRCOG; Anaes; Staff, Kitchener-Water**loo & St. Mary's Hosp.; Tel. 744-7361.
SIMPSON, Carl; 3256 Cambie St., Vancouver, B.C., 3777 Cambie (res); Wes '51; Tel. TR 4-0261.
SIMPSON, Charles A.; 790 Sherbrook St., Winnipeg 2, Man.; Edinburgh (Scot.)'59; MRCP(Ed.); FRCP(C), Neur; Neurol., Grace Hosp.; Neurol. & Electroen., Manitoba Rehab. Hosp.; Tel. 774-6541.
SIMPSON, Derek G.; Ste. 1402, 750 W. Broadway, Vancouver 9, B.C.; U. of New Zealand'40; FRCS(Edin.), FRCS(Eng.); DOMS, Ophth; Sr. Surg., Vancouver Gen. Hosp.; Ass't. Prof. (Clin. Ophth.), U. of British Columbia; Tel. 876-2236.
SIMPSON, Errol R.; Prov. Bldg., North Battleford, Sask.; U. of London (Eng.) '46; DPH (Lond.); DIH; Reg. M.H.O., North Battleford Health Reg. No. 13, Sask. Dept. of Health; Tel. 445-2492.
SIMPSON, Ernest R.; Tor'63; Res., Montreal Gen. Hosp., Montreal 25, P.Q.
SIMPSON, George A.; 1374 Sherbrooke St. W., Ste. 19, Montreal, P.Q.; 462 Wood Ave., Westmount (res); McG '30; F.R.C.O.G., F.A.C.S., F.R.C.S.(C) **ObstGyn; ObstGyn., Royal Victoria** Hosp.; Assoc. ObstGyn., Montreal Gen. Hosp.; Cons. (ObstGyn), **Royal Edward Laurentian Hosp.; Assoc. Prof. (ObstGyn), McGill U.;** Tel. AV 8-2596.
SIMPSON, Glenn; 60 Medical Arts Bldg., 1105 Pandora Ave., Victoria, B.C.; 2858 Seaview Rd. **(res); Man '27; DABP; FAAP, Paed; Cons. Staff, Royal Jubilee Hosp.; Tel. 383-7615.**
SIMPSON, H. Murray; 292 Queen's Ave., London, Ont.; Wes'22; FRCS(Edin.), GenSurg; Tel. 434-3363.

SIMPSON, Ian McD.; Medical Centre, Cornerbrook, Nfld.; Cambridge (Eng.) '60.
SIMPSON, Jack C.; Avery Clinic, Quesnel, B.C.; Alb '55; FRCS(C), GenSurg; Tel. 992-2171.
SIMPSON, Jack F.; 200 St. Clair Ave. W., Toronto, Ont.; 1201 Avenue Rd. (res); Wes '30; Tel. WA 1-9051.
SIMPSON, James S.; 730 Med. Arts Bldg., 170 St. George St., Toronto 5, Ont.; 226 Inglewood Dr. (res); Tor '44; FAAP; FACS, FRCS(C), GenSurg; Assoc. Surg., Hosp. for Sick Children; Assoc. (Dept. of Med.), U. of Toronto; Tel. 923-8361.
SIMPSON, J. Claude; Summerside, P.E.I.; Gen. Surg.; Tel. 436-2277.
SIMPSON, James W.; 108 Med. Arts Bldg., 404 Graham Ave., Winnipeg 1, Man.; 9 Glengarry Dr., Wpg. 19 (res); Man '21; DiagRad; Dept. of Rad., Grace Hosp.; Tel. WH. 2-3521.
SIMPSON, John S., Sg. Cdr; Tor'43; OrthSurg; RCAF Station, Cold Lake, Alta.
SIMPSON, R. Gordon; 26 Rigby Rd., Sydney, N.S.; Dal '50; Tel. 562-1200.
SIMPSON, Robert E.; 1281 W. 32nd Ave., Vancouver, B.C.; Qns '45; Anaes; Staff, Shaughnessy DVA Hosp., S. Burnaby; Clin. Instr. (Anaes), U. of British Columbia; Tel. RE 3-1230.
SIMPSON, Robert N.; Tor '23; Staff, Nanaimo Indian Hosp., Nanaimo, B.C.; Retired.
SIMPSON, Richard T.; 2773 Lake Shore Blvd. W., Toronto 14, Ont.; Tor '46; AMCGP; Tel. 251-8941.
SIMPSON, Walter; 201 Ming Bldg., 4909 Gaetz Ave., Red Deer, Alta.; 4586 Waskasoo Cr. (res); St. Mary's Hosp. (London, Eng.) '37; Dip.Ophth (Oxon); Active Staff, Municipal & Richard Parsons Auxiliary Hosp's.; Tel. 924-0671.
SIMPSON, William; Med. Arts Bldg., 550 Ingersoll Ave., Woodstock, Ont.; 285 Light St. (res); Edinburgh (Scot.) '35; FRCS(Edin.), FRCS(C), GenSurg; Surg. Staff & Chief of Urol., Woodstock Gen. Hosp.; Cons. Ont. Hosp. & Alexandra Hosp., Ingersoll; Tel. LE 7-2401.
SIMPSON, William John K.; 500 Sherbourne St., Toronto 5, Ont.; 31 Alexander St. Apt. 1117 (res); Tor '51; DMRT; FRCP(C); IntMed; TherRad; Radiother., Princess Margaret Hosp.; Assoc. (Rad.), U. of Toronto Tel. WA 4-0671.
SIMPSON, W. Wesley; 925 W. Georgia St., Vancouver, B.C.; 5511 Chancellor Blvd., University Hill (res); Tor '33; Ph.D., F.A.C.P., IntMed; Cons. in Med., Shaughnessy Hosp. D.V.A.; Sr. in Med., Vancouver Gen. Hosp.; Clin. Instr. in Med., U. of British Columbia; Tel. MU 3-1503.
SIMS-COCHEN, Sandra J.; Box 162, Cooksville, Ont.; Qns'57; FRCP(C), Anaes.; Staff, Queensway Hosp.; Tel. CL 9-6671.
SIMS, Henry A.; 267 O'Connor St., Ottawa, Ont.; 268 Second Ave. (res); Tor '40; F.R.C.P. (C) IntMed; Sr. Phys., Ottawa Civic Hosp.; Sr. Lect. (Clin. Med.), U. of Ottawa; Tel. CE 2-1650.
SIMS, Stuart D.; 206 Medical Arts Bldg., 280 Bloor St. W., Toronto 5, Ont.; 1576 Weston Rd., Weston, Ont.; Tor '54; FRCS(C); ObstGyn; Tel. WA 5-8631.
SIMPSON, Stanley E.; Wes'58; Res., Toronto Gen. Hosp., Toronto 2, Ont.
SIMURDA, John; 165 Maloney Blvd. W., Gatineau, P.Q.; Ott '51; GenSurg; Tel. MO 3-4426.
SIMURDA, Michael A.; 344 Johnson St., Kingston, Ont.; 211 Stuart St. (res); Tor '53; F.R.C.S.(C), OrthSurg; Att'd. Staff (Orth), Kingston Gen. Hosp.; Clin. Ass't., Queen's U.; Tel. 546-7887.
SINAISKY, Martin J.; Man '61; Jr. Intn., Winnipeg Gen. Hosp., Winnipeg 3, Man. Abroad.
SINANAN, Eddison G.; Ste. 107, 3195 Granville St., Vancouver 9, B.C.; Belfast (Ire.)'53; Otol.
SINANAN, Kenneth; Souris, Man.; Dublin (Ire.) '65; BAO.
SINANAN, Ranvir H.; '60; Res., Vancouver Gen. Hosp., Vancouver 9, B.C.
SINCERBOX, Gary A.; 346A Upper Ottawa St., Hamilton, Ont.; Tor'62; AMCGP; Tel. 389-0023.
SINCLAIR, Abraham S.; 1831 Rose St., Regina, Sask.; Man'27; MCGP; Coroner; Phys., Sask. Gov't. School for Boys; Tel. 522-1147.
SINCLAIR, Albert M.; 5750 South St., Halifax, N.S.; Dal'52; FRCS(C), OrthSurg; Hd. Dept. of OrthSurg., Children's Hosp.; Cons. OrthSurg., Grace Maternity & Nova Scotia Soc. for Care of Crippled Children; Assoc. ProfSurg., Dalhousie U.; Tel. 422-5895.
SINCLAIR, Alexander; Sebringville, Ont.; Wes '32; M.O.H., Ellice & Downie Twps.; Tel. 393-6143.
SINCLAIR, Alexander B.; 955 Queen St. E., Sault Ste. Marie, Ont.; 1033 Queen St. E. (res); Tor'44; FRCS(C) GenSurg; Chief of Staff, Plummer Memorial & Gen. Hosp's.; Tel. AL 3-2431.
SINCLAIR, Alexander B.; 120 Medical Arts Bldg., 1105 Pandora Ave., Victoria, B.C.; 1860 Bowker Pl. (res); Tor '37; F.R.C.S.(C), Urol.; Tel. EV 4-3936.
SINCLAIR, Alexander C.; St. Boniface Sanatorium, Winnipeg 8, Man.; 245 Wellington Cres., Wpg. 9 (res); Man '30; F.C.C.P.; ThorSurg; Med. Dir., & ThorSurg., St. Boniface San.; Cons. (ThorSurg), St. Boniface Hosp.; Lect. (Med), U. of Manitoba; Tel. AL 3-1311.
SINCLAIR, Duncan W.; 155 Talbot St., Aylmer, Ont.; Wes'63; AMCGP; Tel. 773-9234.
SINCLAIR, Gerald E.; 612 Medical Dental Bldg., Regina, Sask.; Man. '53; IntMed; Staff (Med.), Regina Gen. & Regina Grey Nuns' Hosp's.; Tel. LA 3-6522.
SINCLAIR, Gerald M.; Ste. 590, 6000 Cote des Neiges Rd., Montreal 26, P.Q.; McG '59; FRCS-(C), Otol.; Staff Otol., Jewish Gen. Hosp.; Tel. 342-9520.
SINCLAIR, Gordon; 111 St. Clair Ave. W., Toronto 7, Ont.; 9 Rothmere Dr., Tor. 12 (res); Tor '26; DABPrev Med. & Occ. Med; IntMed; Med. Dir., Imperial Oil Ltd.; Tel. 924-9111, Ext. 2100.
SINCLAIR, Harry A.; Ste. 510, 6000 Cote des Neiges Rd., Montreal 26, P.Q.; McG'28; IntMed (P.Q.).
SINCLAIR, James D.; 1051 Capri St., Sarnia, Ont.; Wes '48; DMR; DiagRad; TherRad; Rad., Sarnia Gen. Hosp. Tel. DI 4-3661.
SINCLAIR, James M.; Ste. 130, Med. Arts Bldg., 1105 Pandora Ave., Victoria, B.C.; 555 Monterey Ave. (res); Alb'42; FACP; FRCP(C), IntMed.; Active Staff, St. Joseph's Hosp.; Med. Cons., Veterans' Hosp.; Tel. EV 3-3443.
SINCLAIR, John A.; 306 Braid St., New Westminster, B.C.; 431-3rd St. (res); Alb '44; M.C.-G.P.; Tel. LA 6-8631.
SINCLAIR, John D.; 14 Emery Circle, Weston, Ont.; Tor'34; M.O., Liquor Control Bd., Aluminum Goods & Chrysler Castings; Staff, O.P.D., Toronto Western Hosp.
SINCLAIR, John D.; Tor'62; Jr. Intn., Toronto East Gen. Hosp., Toronto, Ont.
SINCLAIR, John N.; 11 Coldwater St. E., Orillia, Ont.; 70 Brant St. (res); Ott '53; GenSurg.; Tel. 325-2271.
SINCLAIR, Jonathan C.; 83 Lascelles Blvd., Toronto 7, Ont.(Res.); Tor'43; MRCP(Lond.); FRCP(C); IntMed.; Research, Banting Inst., U. of Toronto; Tel. 483-4812.
SINCLAIR, Kenneth Y.; Tor '22; Staff, Ont. Hosp., North Bay, Ont.; Tel. 474-1200.
SINCLAIR, Olive M.; Queen's, (Belfast, Ire.) '49; Staff, Riverview Hosp., Essondale, B.C.; Tel. LA 1-1911.
SINCLAIR, Robert A.; 288 Worthington St. W., North Bay, Ont.; Tor '56; M.C.G.P.; Tel. 474-2430.
SINCLAIR, Ronald M.; Apt. 40, Churchill Sq. Apts., St. John's, Nfld.; Aberdeen (Scot.) '49; DPH; M.O., Dept. of National Health & Welfare.
SINCLAIR, Wilfred; Leigh Sq. Med. Centre, Port Coquitlam, B.C.; 1863 Windermere Ave. (res); Belfast (N. Ire.) '49; DPH (Lond.) '57; Active Med. Staff, Royal Columbian Hosp. Court. Staff, St. Mary's Hosp., New Westminster; Tel. WH 2-7227.
SINCLARE, Ross G.; 1139 Yates St., Victoria, B.C.; Alb '58; MCGP; Tel. EV 6-4211.
SINDER, Slema; 1247 Jean-Talon E., Montreal 10, P.Q.; Palermo (Sicily) '56; M .C.G.P.; Tel. 279-9103.

SINDON, Andre; Mon'62; FRCP(C), Anaes; Staff, Hop. Maisonneuve, Montreal 36, P.Q.

SINGER, Edgar B.; 3489 Kingston Rd., Scarborough, Ont.; Tor. '54; MCGP; Tel. AM 1-0261.

SINGER, George E.; Ste. 803, 1550 W. 10th Ave., Vancouver 9, B.C.; McG'48.

SINGER, Henry N.; Tor'61; FRCS(C), Urol; Staff, Sunnybrook Hosp., Toronto 12, Ont.

SINGER, Hyman O.; 597 King St., Welland, Ont.; 99 Fitch St. (res); Tor'37; Chief of Med. Staff, Welland County Gen. Hosp.; Tel. 735-5627.

SINGER, Oscar P.; Ste. 635, 5845 Cote des Neiges Rd., Montreal 26, P.Q.; RCP&S (Dublin, Ire.) '55; FAAP; Paed; Staff, Jewish Gen. & Reddy Mem. Hosp's.; Research Ass't., U. of Montreal.

SINGER, William; 1258 Pembina Hgwy., Winnipeg 19, Man.; Innsbruck (Austria) '47; MCGP; Tel. 475-4015.

SINGH, Chanan; 5050 Cavendish Blvd, N.D.G., Montreal 29, P.Q.; Paris (France) '59; Anaes.

SINGH, Chandra P.; 415 Med. Arts Bldg., 1105 Pandora Ave., Victoria, B.C.; Lucknow (India) '50; Urol.; Tel. 386-3733.

SINGH, Dilmohan C.; Melita, Man.; Man'64; Tel. 522-3987.

SINGH, Gur S.; 310 Bentall Bldg., 1070 Douglas St., Victoria, B.C.; Punjab (India)'58; FRCS(C), NeurSurg.; Staff, Royal Jubilee & St. Joseph's Hosp's.; Tel. 386-1613.

SINGH, Gurdeep; Edinburgh (Scot.) '42; Staff, Fort Qu'Appelle San., Fort Qu'Appelle, Sask.; Tel. 332-5785.

SINGH, Harbhajan; 340 McLeod, Ottawa 4, Ont.; Nagpur (India)'54; DABP; Psy; Staff, Ottawa Gen. Hosp.; Clin. Instr., U. of Ottawa; Tel. 729-4426.

SINGH, Indarjit; 1100 Main St. W., Hamilton, Ont.; Sheffield (Eng.)'64.

SINGH, Neeranjan; Man '57; Anaes; Staff, Humber Mem. Hosp., Weston, Ont.; Tel. 249-8111.

SINGH, Santokh; 11412-128th St., Edmonton, Alta. (res); Punjab (India) '50; FRCS(C), Orth Surg; Staff, Chas. Camsell Hosp.; Tel. GL 5-7141.

SINGH, Sinanan; P.O. Box 310, Hartney, Man.; Man'62; Tel. 183.

SINGH, Virick; 63 Charlotte St., Sydney, N.S.; Christian Med. Coll. (India) '61.

SINGH, Walter S. A.; Dal '54; FRCP(C), Paed; Staff, Hosp. for Sick Children, Toronto, Ont.

SINGLETON, Alfred C. B.; Ste. 260, 2184 W. Broadway, Vancouver 9, B.C.; Aberdeen (Scot.) '39; DPH; DTM&H; MCGP; Vis. Staff, Vancouver Hosp's.; Med. Dir., North West Life Assur. Co.; Tel. RE 6-4341.

SINGLETON, Arthur C., M.B.E., E.D.; Med. Arts Bldg., 170 St. George St., Toronto 5, Ont.; Tor '23; F.F.R. (Hon.), F.A.C.R., F.R.C.P.(C), D & T Rad; Cons. (Rad.), Toronto Gen. Hosp.; Emer. Prof. & Hd. of Dept. of Rad., U. of Toronto; Tel. WA 1-3118.

SINGLETON, Frederic Brian; Box 413, Kingston, Ont.; 325 Kingscourt Ave. (res); London H. (Eng.) '52; MB, BS; DA (Eng.); Anaes; Att'd. Staff, Hotel-Dieu Hosp.; Clin. Ass't. (Anaes.), Queen's U.; Tel. 542-5609.

SINGLETON, Jean A. (Robertson); 1530 West 8th Ave., Vancouver, B.C.; Ste. 227, 4875 Valley Dr. (res); McG'45; DPH; DTM&H; M.O., City of Vancouver Health Dept.; Tel. RE 1-5727.

SINKINS, James M.; 132 S. Victoria St., Sarnia, Ont.; R.R. 1, Camlachie (res); Qns '44; ObstGyn; Chief of ObstGyn., & Pres. of Med. Staff, St. Joseph's Hosp.; Tel. DI 4-1181.

SINNOTT, J. Cyrill; Charlottetown Clinic, 1 Rochford St., Charlottetown, P.E.I.; 135 Nassau St. (res); McG '53; M.Sc., D.I.M., F.R.C.P.(C), IntMed; Att. Staff, Charlottetown Hosp.; Telephone 894-5521.

SINOTTE, Lorenzo; 2888 Masson, Montreal, P.Q.; Lav '28.

SINTON, Eric J.; 608 Professional Bldg., 4808 Ross St., Red Deer, Alta.; Aberdeen (Scot.) '51; M.B., Ch.B., D.O. (Lond.); Ophth; Staff, Red Deer Gen., Dr. Richard Parsons Aux. & Innisfail Mun. Hosp's.; Tel. 346-2244.

SIPOS, John K.; 4530 Cote des Neiges Rd., Montreal 26, P.Q.; '60.

SIPOS, Louis; 107 Guildwood Pkwy., Scarborough, Ont.; Qns '60; Tel. 261-1471.

SIREK, Anna (Janek); C. H. Best Inst., 112 College St., Toronto, Ont.; 93 Farnham Ave., Tor. 7 (res); Bratislava (Czech.) '46; MA; Ph.D.; Ass't. Prof. (Physiol.), U. of Toronto; Tel. 928-2593.

SIRETT, Morley A.; 214 Robindale Rd., Winnipeg 20, Man. (res); Man '52; MCGP; Dir. Manitoba Hosp. Serv. & Comm.; Tel. 837-5360.

SIRETT, Nancy K. (GREEN); 214 Robindale Rd., Winnipeg 20, Man.; Man '52; Tel. 837-5360.

SIRKIS, Hymie; 1750 Main St., Winnipeg 17, Man.; 167 Scotia St. (res); Man '52; Tel. ED 4-4339, WH 3-5683.

SIROIS, Emilien; 38 boul. Valcartier, Loretteville, P.Q.; Lav '57.

SIROIS, Georges; Mon'60; Res., Rop. Hotel-Dieu, Quebec 4, P.Q.

SIROIS, Jean; 580 Grande-Allee E., Apt. 100, Quebec, P.Q.; 2025 Brulart, Sillery (res); Lav '35; Neur; NeurSurg; Chief (NeurSurg.), Hop.-de-l'Enfant-Jesus; Cons. (NeurSurg), Hop's. DVA, Hotel-Dieu; Jeffrey Hales & St. Sacrement; Prof. (NeurSurg.), Laval U.; Tel. 525-4643.

SIROIS, Jean; 145 Chemin Cameron, Hull, P.Q. (res); Lav '52; M.C. Path; FASCP; FRCP(C), Path; Dir. of Labs., Hop. du-Sacre-Coeur; Dir. (Path.), U. of Ottawa; Tel. PR 7-2721.

SIROIS, J. Sarto; 725 ave. Chouinard, Quebec 6, P.Q. (res); Lav '31; D.P.H., M.O.H.; Ass't. Chief, Hosp. Insur. (P.Q.), Quebec Area.

SIROIS, L. G.; c/o Chief Med. Officer, Dept. National Health & Welfare, 61 Green St., London W.1, England.

SIROIS, Paul E.; 16 Lacasse, Hull, P.Q.; Lav '51; Anaes; Tel. 771-8713.

SIROIS, Rodolphe, J. G. (Reeves); 1009-2nd E., Cornwall, Ont.; Mon '54; Staff, Cornwall Gen. & Hotel-Dieu Hosp's.

SISLER, George C; Med. College Bldg., Bannatyne & Emily Sts., Winnipeg, Man.; 714 Ash St. (res); Man '46; D.A.B.N.P.; F.R.C.P.(C), Psy; Prof. & Hd. Dept. of Psy., U. of Manitoba; Tel. GR 4-9110.

SISON, Alfredo; Medical Centre, West St., Cornerbrook, Nfld.; Santo Tomas (Philipp.) '56.

SISSON, Barry V.; Ste. 116, 2135 Avenue Rd., Toronto 12, Ont.; 148 Tamworth Rd., Willowdale (res); Tor '53; Phys., Brookside Clinic; O.P.D., St. Michael's Hosp.; Tel. 485-1214.

SITTLINGER, George; 11 White Blvd., Red Rock, Ont.; Graz (Austria) '51; M.O.H. Improvement Dist. of Red Rock.

SIVASANKAR, Ramachandran; Madras (India) '63; Jr. Int., Shaughnessy Hosp., Vancouver 9, B.C.

SIVILOTTI, Enzo U.; 787 Richmond St., London, Ont.; Wes'62.

SIWAK, Theodore H.; Alb '56; MCGP; Res., University Hosp., Edmonton, Alta.

SIWAK, Walter J.; Smith Clinic, 4815 - 51st St., Camrose, Alta.; Alb '51; DABS; FRCS(C), GenSurg; Chief, Med. Staff, St. Mary's Hosp.; Tel. 672-2424.

SKAFEL, Einar J.; 11 Clement Blk., Brandon, Man.; 525-14th St. (res); Man '27; Staff, Brandon Gen. Hosp.; Tel. PA 6-2968.

SKAIN, Frank J.; 250 Lawrence Ave. W., Toronto 12, Ont.; 2110 Keele St., Apt. 607 (res); Tor '54; F.R.C.S.(C), ObstGyn; Active Staff, Northwestern Gen. Hosp.; Assoc. Cons. Staff, North York Branson Hosp.; Tel. RU 9-3102.

SKALA, Gustav K.; 2676 Lake Shore Blvd. W., Toronto 14, Ont.; Tor '48; M.C.G.P.; O.P.D., St. Joseph's Hosp.; Tel. 251-2791.

SKALING, James H.; 21538 Nelson Rd., Haney, B.C. (res); Man '21; M.C.G.P.; Retired.

SKEET, Brian J.; Moose Jaw Clinic, 200 Scott Bldg., Moose Jaw, Sask.; London (Eng.) '59; MRCS; LRCP.

SKEET, Harold J.; Knowlton, P.Q.; McG '24. Retired.

SKELHORNE, Gordon P.; 399 Dibble St. W., Prescott, Ont.; Wes'50; Tel. 925-4766.

SKELLY, William R.; Ste. 1, Deep River Hosp., Deep River, Ont.; Tor'37; Med. Supt., Deep River Hosp.; MOH; Tel. JU 4-2201.

SKENE, John S.; Drawer 890, Lloydminster, Alta.; Alb '49; MCGP; Med. Staff, Lloydminster Mun. Hosp.

SKIADAS, George D.; 75 Fernhill Ave., Outremont, P.Q.; Athens (Gr.) '52; AMCGP; Tel. CR 6-9812.

SKINNER, Basil S.; London (Eng.)'43; MRCS (Eng.), LRCP (Eng.), FACA; DA (McG.); Anaes; Staff, Foothills Hosp., Calgary, Alta.

SKINNER, Edison B.; Maple St., New Glasgow, N.S.; Dal'59; MCGP.

SKINNER, Edward G. F.; Medical Arts Clinic, 51—6th St. S.E., Medicine Hat, Alta.; 19—8th St. N.E. (res); Sheffield (Eng.) '38; Staff, Medicine Hat Gen. Hosp.; Coroner.; Tel. 527-2281.

SKINNER, F. Leslie; 923 Birks Bldg., Vancouver 2, B.C.; 3463 S.W. Marine Dr. (res); McG '36; M.R.C.P., IntMed; Staff, St. Paul's, St. Joseph's, & Children's Hosp's.; Cons., Chest Unit, Shaughnessy D.V.A. Hosp.; Electrocardiol., St. Vincent's Hosp.; Tel. MU 3-1828.

SKINNER, G. Bernard; 3551 Vendome Ave., Montreal 28, P.Q. (res); McG '54; F.R.C.P (C), DiagRad; Clin. Ass't., (Rad), Royal Victoria Hosp.; Dem. (Rad.), McGill U.; Tel. VI 2-1251, Loc. 771.

SKINNER, George F.; 36 Coburg St., Saint John, N.B.; McG '23; F.A.C.S., F.R.C.S.(Edin.), F.R.C.S.(C), GenSurg; ThorSurg; Surg., Saint John Gen. & Saint John TB Hosp's.; Tel. 693-3351.

SKINNER, H. Alan; 846 Richmond St., London, Ont. (res); Tor '22; F.R.C.S.(C), Prof. of Anat., U. of Western Ontario. Retired.

SKINNER, James H.; Fort Frances Clinic, 301 Victoria St., Fort Frances, Ont., Man '52; MCGP.

SKINNER, John H. B.; 80-Fourth Ave., Hornepayne, Ont.; Tor '50; D.A.B.S.; M.O.H., Twnp. of Wickstead; Tel. 465.

SKINNER, Leslie C.; 2701 Regina Ave., Regina, Sask. (res); Aberdeen (Scot.)'50; Anaes; Anaes., Regina Gen. & Regina Grey Nuns' Hosp's.; Tel. 522-0704.

SKINNER, Lyle A.; Commercial St., North Sydney, N.S.; Queen St. (res); Dal '52; M.C.G.P.

SKINNER, Norman S.; 89 Hawthorne Ave., Saint John, N.B.; McG '34; FACP; Cons. Rad, St. John T.B. Hosp.; Dir. Dept. DiagRad., Saint John Gen. Hosp.; Ass't. Prof. (Rad), Dalhousie U.; Tel. 693-3351.

SKINNIDER, Leo F.; Glasgow (Scot.) '51; Int., Ottawa Civic Hosp., Ottawa, Ont.

SKITCH, Clifford H.; 6875 Lasalle Blvd., Montreal 19, P.Q.; Alb'30; Psy; Med. Supt., Douglas Hosp.; Lect. Psy., McGill U.; Tel. 766-8511.

SKOLL, Louis S.; Capetown (S. Africa) '48; M.B., Ch.B.; Staff, Public Health & Welfare, Albert & Hill, Regina, Sask.; Tel. LA 3-0661.

SKOLNICK, Marvin; 221 Brant Ave., Brantford, Ont.; Tor '59; FRCP(C), Derm; Staff, St. Joseph's & Brantford Gen. Hosp's.

SKORBINSKI, Abraham W.; 1334 King St. W., Toronto 3, Ont.; Cape Town (S. Africa) '52; GenSurg; Staff, Queen Elizabeth Hosp.

SKORYNA, Stanley C.; 4427 Sherbrooke W., Westmount, Montreal, P.Q.; 14 Forden Ave. (res); Vienna (Aust.) '43; M.Sc., Ph.D.; FACS; GenSurg (P.Q.); Ass't. Surg., St. Mary's Hosp.; Vis. Surg., Royal Victoria Hosp.; Ass't. Prof. of Surg. Research & Div. Gastrointest Research Lab., McGill U.; Tel. WE 5-3088.

SKORUPSKI, Lois J.; (See RACETTE, Lois J.).

SKOULAS, Achilles; Athens (Greece) '51; Jr. Intn., University Hosp., Saskatoon, Sask.

SKREPNEK, Stan V.; Box 1117, Peace River, Alta.; Alb '57; AMCGP; Staff, Peace River Municipal Hosp.; Tel. 624-2581.

SKROBOT, Walter M.; 25 St. Michael St. St. Albert, Alta.; 10 Greshan Blvd. (res); Alb '58; Tel. 599-6066.

SKRYPUCH, John; 266 Park Ave., Brantford, Ont.; Heidelberg (Germany) '48; Tel. PL 3-1454.

SKULLY, Hyman J.; 504-6th Ave., New Westminster, B.C.; 7554 Burris St., S. Burnaby (res); Man. '33; Tel. LA 1-8801.

SKWAROK, Eugene W.; 2184 W. Broadway, Vancouver 9, B.C.; 675 Parkside Rd. W. Vanc. (res); Alb '44; DABNS; NeurSurg; Active Staff, St. Paul's & Hd. Dept. of NeuroSurg; Children's Hosp's.; Clin. Instr., U. of British Columbia; Tel. RE 1-1810.

SKWAROK, Romeo L.; 325-2184 W. Broadway, Vancouver 9, B.C.; 1675-19th St., West Van. (res); Alb '50; Psy; Staff, St. Euphrasia Schl. for Girls; Tel. RE 1-1810.

SKY, Kenneth; Tor'63; Res., Montreal Gen. Hosp., Montreal 25, P.Q.

SKY, Ruth (Mrs. H. J. Shykoff); Tor '49; MCGP; Staff, Riverdale Hosp., Toronto 8, Ont.; Tel. 461-8251.

SLADE, H. Clyde; Vancouver Gen. Hosp., Vancouver, B.C.; Dal'41; FRCP(C), IntMed; Psy; Att'd. Staff, Vancouver Gen. Hosp.; Ass't. Prof. (Med.), U. of British Columbia; Tel. 876-3211, Loc. 3128.

SLADE, Reginald H.; 4012 New St., Burlington, Ont.; Qns '64

SLADE, Samuel E.; Box 559. Cleveland Ave., Squamish, B.C.; London U. (Eng.) '49; Chief of Staff, Squamish Gen. Hosp.; Court Staff, Lions Gate Hosp., N. Vancouver; Tel. 892-3313.

SLADEN, Joseph G.; Ste. 320, 2184 W. Broadway, Vancouver 9, B.C.; Tor'54; FRCS(C), GenSurg; Assoc. Staff, St. Paul's Hosp.; Pt-time Staff, Shaughnessy Hosp.; Tel. RE 6-4451.

SLAKOV, Roy I.; 301, 720 W. Broadway, Vancouver 9, B.C.; 6550 Marine Cres. (res); U. of Oregon (Portland) '53; Psy; Clin. Instr., (Psy), U. of British Columbia; Tel. TR 4-4722.

SLAPAK, Maurice; Cambridge (Eng.)'56; FRCS(C), GenSurg; Staff, Royal Victoria Hosp., Montreal 2, P.Q.

SLATER, Gerald; Ste. Clotilde de Horton, Co. Arthabaska, P.Q.; Lav '51.

SLATER, Harry M.; Ste. 30, 5810 Cote St. Luc Rd., Montreal 29, P.Q.; Tor'43; DA; FACA; FAAP; Anaes; Dir. Montreal Anaes. Centre; Dir. Inhalation Therapy, Cons. & Co-Dir., Dept. of Anaes., Jewish Gen. Hosp.; Cons Alexandria Hosp.; Tel. HU 6-2386.

SLATER, John G.; Box 210, 135-6th Ave., Cochrane, Ont.; McG'55; Active Staff, Lady Minto Hosp.; Tel. 272-3276.

SLATER, Jules; 204-452 Main St. E., Hamilton, Ont.; 829 Forest Glen Ave., Burlington (res); Tor '47; FAAO; D.A.B.Oph; Ophth; Staff, Hamilton Gen. Hosp.; Tel. JA 7-0402.

SLATER, Paul E.; 119 Highland Rd., London, Ont.; Wes '47; Anaes; Research Ass't., Dept. of Pharm., U. of Western Ont.; Tel. GE 9-1681.

SLATER, Stuart; 192 Principale, Hull, P.Q.; Lav '51; Urol.; Tel. 777-6831.

SLATKOFF, William R.; Jewish Gen. Hosp., 3755 Cote St. Catherine Rd., Montreal, P.Q.; McG '34; Hosp. Adm., Med. Dir., Jewish Gen. Hospital; Tel. 735-3771.

SLATT, Bernard; 1849 Yonge St., Ste. 918, Toronto 7, Ont.; Tor'59; FRCS(C), Ophth; Staff, Toronto Gen. Hosp.; Clin. Instr., U. of Toronto; Tel. 487-4697.

SLAVENS, John J.; Ste. 201, 151 Eglinton Ave. W., Toronto 12, Ont.; Tor'30; DABP; Paed; Ass't. Phys., Hosp. for Sick Children; Sr. Att'd. Paed., New Mount Sinai Hosp.; Clin. Instr. (Paed), U. of Toronto; Phys., Forest Hill Schools; Tel. 483-2500.

SLAVIK, R. J., Major; Greisbach Barracks, Edmonton, Alta.; Alb'59.

SLAYTER, John H.; Boscobel, Armdale, N.S.; London (Eng.) '39; Staff, Victoria Gen., Halifax Infirmary, Grace Maternity & Children's Hosp's.; Med. Cons., N.S. Hosp. Insurance Comm. Tel. 477-4635.

SLEATH, G. Edward; 6007 Blenheim St., Vancouver 13, B.C. (res); Alb'46; DABA, Anaes; Att. Staff, Vancouver Gen. Hosp.; Lect. (Anaes.), Dept. of Surgery, U. of British Columbia; Tel. TR 6-3211.

SLEATH, G. William; 2850 Willoughby Ave., Burnaby 3, B.C.; UBC '56; FRCP(C), Anaes; Staff, Assoc. Anaes., Vancouver; Research, U. of British Columbia; Tel. WE 9-5200.

SLEEVA, A. Nicholas; 150 Steeles Ave. E., Willowdale, Ont.; Ott. '56; Tel. 285-1311.

SLEEVA, Gertrude F. (Wagner); 150 Steeles Ave. W., Willowdale, Ont.; Ott '61; Staff, North York Branson Hosp.; Tel. AV 5-1311.

SLEIGH, Alfred D.; 1030 Wildwood Lane, West Vancouver, B.C. (res); UBC '55; Psy; Staff, Prov. Mental Health Services.

SLEMON, Harold V.; 103 Toronto Western Medical Bldg., 25 Leonard Ave., Toronto 2B, Ont.; 40 Austin Terr. (res); Tor '37; F.R.C.S.(C), GenSurg; Att. Surg., Toronto Western Hosp.; Clin-Instr.(Surg), U. of Toronto; Tel. EM 6-3343.

SLEMON, Keith W.; 38 Centre St., Bowmanville, Ont.; Tor '46.

SLESAR, Stephan J.; 163 Queenston, St. Catharines, Ont.; McG '59; FRCP(C), IntMed; Tel. 684-1412.

SLESS, Phillip; 50 Sheppard Ave. E., Willowdale, Ont.; 29 Bayview Court (res); Edinburgh (Scot.) '50; Tel. BA 1-4424.

SLINGER, Robert P.; Victoria Hosp., London, Ont.; Tor '55; Path; Staff, Victoria Hosp.; Clin. Ass't. Prof. (Path.), U. of Western Ontario.

SLINGERLAND, J. Owen; Box 40, Mount Albert, Ont.; West London H. (Eng.) '57; MRCS; LRCP; MCGP; Sr. Staff, York Co. & Uxbridge Hosp's.; MOH, Scott Twp.; Tel. 473-2443.

SLIPP, Leslie B.; Hubbards, N.S.; Dal '60.

SLOAN, Ian A.; 555 University Ave., Toronto 2, Ont.; 10 Campbell Cres., Willowdale (res); Capetown (S. Africa) '53; F.F.A.R.C.S.(Eng.), F.R.C.P.(C), Anaes; Staff, (Anaes), Hosp. for Sick Children; Clin. Instr. (Anaes), U. of Toronto; Tel. EM 6-7242.

SLOAN, Sophia E. (Murray); 477 Martin St., Penticton, B.C.; Okanagan Falls (res); Glasgow (Scot.) '40; Tel. 492-4274.

SLOAN, William L.; 216 Medical Dental Bldg., 925 W. Georgia, Vancouver 1, B.C.; 1291 Devonshire Cres. (res); Tor '38; D.R., D&TRad; Att. Staff, Shaughnessy Hosp., Vancouver; Powell River Gen. Hosp., Powell River, B.C.; Tel. RE 8-3188.

SLOANE, R. Bruce; 26 Centre St., Kingston, Ont.; London (Eng.) '45; M.R.C.P.(Lond.), D.P.M.; Psy; Prof. (Psy) & Hd. of Dept., Queen's U. & Kingston Gen. Hosp.; Cons. DVA & Dept. of Nat. Defence Hosp.; Tel. 546-1630. Abroad.

SLOBODZIAN, Michael S.; Cavalier Plaza, Saskatoon, Sask.; Man'52.

SLOMAN, Leon; Montreal Children's Hosp., Montreal 25, P.Q.; Royal Free Hosp. (Lon., Eng.)'56; M.R.C.S., L.R.C.P.; D.Psy(McG); Psy; Clin. Fell., Allan Mem. Inst.; Staff, Mtl. Children's Hosp; Tel. WE 7-8511.

SLONIM, Rodney O.; Man'64; Res., Hosp. For Mental Diseases, Selkirk, Man.

SLOWIK, Danuta M.; Apt. 3, 171 Elizabeth Ave., St. John's, Nfld. (res); Polish School of Med. (Edinburgh, Scot.) '49; Staff. Hosp. for Mental Diseases.

SLOWIK, Oskar J.; 500 Medical Centre, 906-8th Ave. S.W., Calgary, Alta.; Edinburgh (Scot.)'48; MB., Ch.B., DPM; Psy.; Staff, Calgary Gen. & Holy Cross Hosp's.; Tel. 262-6051.

SLUZAR, Roman L.; 3302 Credit Heights, Erindale Woodlands, Cooksville, Ont.; Ott '53; Anaes; Chief Anaes., South Peel Mem. Hosp.; Tel. 277-9065.

SMAILES, Colin L.; 13620 Grosvenor Rd., North Surrey, B.C.; Cambridge (Eng.) '59; Tel. 584-0141.

SMAILL, W. Donald; Ste. 207, 1541 W. Broadway, Vancouver, B.C.; 5790 Cartier St. (res); McG'35; GenSurg; Vis. Staff, Vancouver Gen. Hosp., St. Paul's & Mount St. Joseph's Hosp's.; Tel. RE 3-4011.

SMALL, Allen A.; 345 Bloor St. W., Toronto, Ont.; 11 Starmont Ave. (res); Tor '44; D.A.-B.D., DermSyph; Adjunct, New Mount Sinai Hosp.; Derm., Med. Staff, Scarborough Gen. Hosp.; Tel. WA 3-1774.

SMALL, James; 306 King St., Midland, Ont.; Qns '41; Tel. 526-5291.

SMALL, James H.; Qns'62; Res., Hotel-Dieu Hosp., Kingston, Ont.

SMART, Hugh T.; Qns.'65; Res.. University Hosp., Edmonton, Alta.

SMART, Iain H. M.; Edinburgh (Scot.) '51; Staff, Dept. of Anat., McGill U., Montreal, P.Q.

SMART, John B.; Box 234, Waterdown, Ont. (res); Tor '23; Retired.

SMART, John E.; Box 440, Waterdown, Ont.; Wes '60; AMCGP; Active Staff, Joseph Brant Hosp., Burlington; Tel. 689-1242.

SMART, John M.; Box 787, Langley, B.C.; UBC '57.

SMART, Margaret C. (Lee); 561 London St., Sherbrooke, P.Q.; Edinburgh (Scot.) '51; MCGP; Active Staff, Sherbrooke Hosp.; Tel. 562-0055.

SMART, Maxwell R.; North Okanagan Health Unit, Vernon, B.C.; Sask'57; DPH; PH; Cons. PrevMed., Vernon Jubilee Hosp., Shuswap Lake Gen. Hosp. & Queen Victoria Hosp., Revelstoke; Tel. 542-2742.

SMART, Michael J.; 140 Wallace St., Nanaimo, B.C.; 2555 Holyrood Dr. (res); London (Eng.) '54; DiagRad; Tel. SK 3-4351.

SMART, Robert E.; 180 Metcalfe St., Ottawa 4, Ont.; 243 McLeod St. (res); Tor '30; DOMS; DABOphth; FACS; FICS; Ophth; Sr. Ophth., Ottawa Civic Hosp.; Tel. 353-9321.

SMART, Ronald W.; 1050 Queens Blvd., Kitchener, Ont.; Glasgow (Scot.)'55.

SMEETON, F. Rance; 1309 Windermere Rd., Windsor, Ont.; Wes '59.

SMELLIE, Thomas H.; 399 Dibble St. W., Prescott, Ont.; Qns'32; Court. Staff, Brockville Gen. & Hon. Active Staff, St. Vincent de Paul Hosp's., Brockville; Plant Phys., RCA Victor Co. Ltd., & Parke Davis Co., Brockville; Tel. 925-2467.

SMILEY, R. Kennedy; Ottawa Gen. Hosp., Ottawa, Ont.; Qns '46; FRCP(C), IntMed; Prof. & Ass't. Dean (Med.), U. of Ottawa; Tel. 236-0333.

SMILLIE, Alex. B.; 837 Valleyway, Niagara Falls, Ont.; 2226 Clare Cres. (res); Tor '05; M.R.C.S. (Eng.), L.R.C.P. (Lond.). Retired.

SMILLIE, Ivan G.; Burris Clinic, 242 Victoria St., Kamloops, B.C.; 57 Clarke St. (res); Tor '30; Dist. Coroner; Tel. 372-3303.

SMILLIE, R. A., Lt./Col.; 3 Field Ambulance, Camp Sarcee, Calgary, Alta.; Tor'41; Retired.

SMITH, Alasdair J.; Oxford (Eng.) '57, Staff, St. Anthony's Hosp., St. Anthony, Nfld.; Tel. 2211.

SMITH, Alexander R.; St. Andrews (Scot.)'42; Staff, Bonne Bay Hosp., Norris Point, Nfld.

SMITH, Allen J.; 50 Yonge St. N., Richmond Hill, Ont.; 370 Sugar Maple Lane (res); Tor '52; M.C.G.P. Staff York Central Hosp.; Tel. 884-1171.

SMITH, Ann R. (Whyte); 37 Dundas St. W., Box 40, Cooksville, Ont., or 2106 Truscott Dr., Clarkson; George Washington U. (U.S.A.)'49; Tel. 277-2933.

SMITH, Alan G.; Alb'61; FRCS(C), GenSurg; Staff, University Hosp., Edmonton, Alta.

SMITH, A. O. Code; 58 Fyfeshire Rd., Willowdale, Ont. (res); Tor'45; FACA; FRCP(C); Anaes; Ass't. Anaes., Hosp. for Sick Children; Clin. Teach., Dept. Anaes., U. of Toronto; Tel. EM 6-7242.

SMITH, Arthur G.; 26 Dunvegan Rd., Toronto, Ont.; Tor '26; O.P.D. Staff, Toronto Western Hosp.; Staff, Health Service, U. of Toronto; Tel. WA 2-2842.

SMITH, Carl H.; 681 Prince, Truro, N.S.; 31 Smith Ave. (res); Dal '30; Staff (OphthOtol.), Colchester County Hosp.

SMITH, Carlton G.; 2141 Bloor St. W., Apt. 10, Toronto, Ont. (res); Tor '35; M.Sc., Ph.D.; Prof. of Anat., U. of Toronto; Tel. RO 7-7194.

SMITH, C. Conway; Ste. 921 Medical Arts Bldg., 1538 Sherbrooke St. W., Montreal, P.Q.; 637 Cote St. Catherine Rd., Outremont (res); McG '49; D.Psy; Psy; Clin. Ass't., Montreal Gen. Hosp.; Cons. (Psy), D.V.A., Queen Mary Vet's. Hosp.; Lect. (Psy) McGill U.; Tel. WE 5-5751.

SMITH, C. Hampton; Smith Clinic, Camrose, Alta.; Alb'41; Tel. 672-2424.

SMITH, Charles B.; 34 High St., Pictou, N.S.; Dal'31; MCGP; Staff, Sutherland Mem. Hosp.; Tel. 485-5377.

SMITH, Clare Neville; Cambridge (Eng.) '45; Paed; DPH(Tor); Schl. M.O., Province of Nfld, St. John's, Nfld.; Tel. 9-5011.

SMITH, Clarence B.; 3220 Mayfield Ave., Halifax, N.S.; Dal '55; Staff, Nova Scotia Hosp., Dartmouth; Tel. 466-7411.

SMITH, Clifford B.; 3421 Draper Ave., Montreal, P.Q.; McG '26; Hon. Att. Staff, Montreal Gen. Hosp.; Tel. 484-7112.

SMITH, Colin M.; University Hosp., Saskatoon, Sask.; 9 Weir Cres., Saskatoon, Sask. (res); Glasgow (Scot.) '49; M.B., Ch.B., M.D., D.P.M., F.R.C.P.(C), Psy; Deputy Dir., Psy. Research, Sask. Dept. of Public Health; Assoc. Prof. (Psy), U. of Saskatchewan; Tel. 242-7641, Loc. 481.

SMITH, D. A.; Department of National Health & Welfare, c/o Regional Superintendent, European Region. Abroad.

SMITH, David F.; Qns'65; Res., Hosp. for Sick Children, Toronto 2, Ont.

SMITH, David M.; Wes '62; Res., Westminster Hosp., London, Ont.

SMITH, David M.; Box 1180, Duncan, B.C.; Briar St. (res); UBC '55; MCGP; Tel. 746-4102.

SMITH, David P.; Tor '62; Jr. Intn., Toronto Gen. Hosp., Toronto, Ont.

SMITH, David R.; 26 Dunvegan Rd., Toronto 7, Ont.; 88 Roxborough (res); Tor '54; M.C.G.P.; Ass't. Dir., Men's Health Serv., U. of Toronto; Indust. Phys., O.H.S.C.; Tel. 922-2842.

SMITH, David R.; McG'64; Res., Dept. of Ophth., U. of Toronto, Toronto 5, Ont.

SMITH, Donald E. MC; Oshawa Clinic, 117 King St. E., Oshawa, Ont.; McG'50; DIM; IntMed; Tel. 728-1661.

SMITH, Donald F.; 6086 Quinpool Rd., Halifax, N.S.; 995 Beaufort Ave. (res); Dal '45; FICS; FACOG; ObstGyn; Vist. Staff, Hlfx. Infirmary, Victoria Gen., Grace Maternity & Children's Hosp's.; Inst. (ObstGyn), Dalhousie U.; Tel. 423-7460.

SMITH, Donald H.; Box 1089, Stouffville, Ont.; Tor'52; Staff, York County Hosp., Newmarket; Tel. 640-2300.

SMITH, Donald R.; 450 Central Ave., London, Ont.; Wes'51; FRCP(C), IntMed; Teach. Staff, Victoria Hosp.; Ass't. Med. Dir., London Life Ins. Co.; Tel. 434-6318.

SMITH, Donald W.; Tor'59; Res., New Mount Sinai Hosp., Toronto 2, Ont.

SMITH, Donne W.; 93 Frederick St., St. Andrews, N.B.; Dal'47; MCGP; Staff, Charlotte County Hosp., St. Stephen; Tel. 529-3255.

SMITH, Douglas M.; 213 Marsh St., Maple Creek, Ont. (res); Cambridge (Eng.) '56; MA; DRCOG; Staff, Maple Creek Union Hosp.; Tel. 667-2611.

SMITH, Edward W.; 408 Canada Bldg., 21st St. E. & 1st Ave. S., Saskatoon, Sask.; Alb '55; Ophth; AMCGP.

SMITH, Edwin R.; Provincial Cancer Clinic, 2104—2nd St. S.W., Calgary, Alta.; 116 Westminster Dr. (res); Durham (Eng.) '45; D.M.-R.T. (Eng.), TherRad; Staff, Holy Cross Hosp.; Tel. AM 6-7231.

SMITH, E. John; 570 Seaforth Med. Bldg., 3550 Cote des Neiges Rd., Montreal 25, P.Q.; Dal '38; FAAOC; FRCS(C); Otol; Sr. Otol., Montreal Gen. Hosp.; Assoc. Surg. (Otol.), St. Mary's Hosp.; Cons. (Otol.), Catherine Booth Hosp.; Ass't. Prof. (Otol.), McGill U.; Tel. WE 3-3663.

SMITH, Elizabeth A.; 59 Victoria St., London, Ont.; Wes '62.

SMITH, Elizabeth M.; Ste. 111, 10830 Kingsway Ave., Edmonton, Alta. (res); Aberdeen (Scot.) '44; Ass't. Pathol., Edmonton Gen. Hosp.; Tel. HU 8-8181.

SMITH, Elmer L.; 5402-48th Ave., Lloydminster, Sask.; Alb'48; MCGP; Tel. 875-2221.

SMITH, Eric L.; 750 W. Broadway, Vancouver 9, B.C.; 1650 Acadia Rd., Vancouver 8 (res); McG '49; Ophth; Att. Staff, Vancouver Gen. Hosp.; Part-time Att. Staff, Shaughnessy Mil. Hosp.; Lect. (Ophth), U. of British Columbia; Tel. TR 2-5533.

SMITH, E. H. Newel; 1120 Ouellette Ave., Windsor, Ont.; Wes '57; M.Sc. (Ophth); Ophth; Active Staff, Hotel-Dieu & Grace Hosp's.; Court. Staff, I.O.D.E. Hosp.; Cons. Ophth., Riverview Hosp.; Tel. 253-5112.

SMITH, E. Stuart O.; 190 Glendowynne Rd., Toronto 9, Ont.; Cambridge (Eng.)'47; LRCP; MRCS; DIH; DPH; PH.

SMITH, Everett A.; Dal'56; Staff, Nova Scotia Hosp., Dartmouth, N.S.

SMITH, F. Hartley; 60 Osborne St. N., Winnipeg 1, Man.; 214 Handsart Blvd. Wpg. 29 (res); Man '29; IntMed; Assoc. Med. Dir., Gt. West Life Assur. Co.; Tel. 946-9316.

SMITH, Florence M.; 414 Med. Arts Bldg., 5 Young St., Hamilton, Ont.; 4 Mountain Brow Blvd. (res); Tor '26; Tel. JA 7-3213.

SMITH, Foster; Ste. 322, 200 St. Clair Ave. W., Toronto 7. Ont.; Tor'36; DA(Lond.); Anaes; Chief, Dept. of Anaes., Wellesley Hosp.; Cons. Anaes., Princess Margaret Hosp.; Assoc. (Anaes.), U. of Toronto; Tel. 966-6900.

SMITH, Frank A.; St. Barbaras Clinic, 226 Bathurst St., Toronto 2B, Ont.; McG'64.

SMITH, Frank M.; Smith Clinic, Camrose, Alta.; 4712-51st St. (res); Alb '35; F.R.C.S. (Ed.), F.I.C.S.; M.C.G.P.; Tel. 672-2424.

SMITH, Frank R.; 195 Main St. E., Welland, Ont.; 40 Glen View (res); Tor '17.

SMITH, Frederick B.; St. Barbaras Clinic, 226 Bathurst St., Toronto 2B, Ont.; McG'65.

SMITH, Gaetan; Lav'65; Res., Hop. St. Sacrement, Quebec 6, P.Q.

SMITH, Garnet H.; Box 100, Jordan Stn., Ont.; Wes '45; Staff, St. Catharines Gen. Hosp.; Court. Staff, Hotel Dieu Hosp., St. Catharines; Tel. 562-5221.

SMITH, G. Douglas; 59 Forest Hill Dr., Lancaster, N.B. (res); Glasgow (Scot.) '48; D.M.-R.T. (Eng.), TherRad; Ass't. Dir., Dept. of Rad., Saint John Gen. Hosp.; Tel. 693-3351

SMITH, George M.; P.O. Box 1210, Windsor, N.S.; Dal '43; D.P.H.; Div. M.H.O., Dept. of P.H., Prov. of Nova Scotia.

SMITH, George W.; 807 Medical Arts Bldg., 170 St. George St., Toronto, Ont.; 26 Greenvalley Rd., Willowdale (res); Tor '44; F.R.C.P.(C), IntMed; Att. Phys., Tor. Wellesley Hosp.; Sr. Cons. IntMed., Orthopaed. Hosp.; Assoc. Staff (Med.), U. of Toronto; Tel. WA 1-3851.

SMITH, Gerald L.; 4027 Hastings St., North Burnaby, B.C.; 1650 Fell Ave. (res); Man '38; GenSurg; Tel. CY 9-2677.

SMITH, G. L.; Hillside Rd., Creston, B.C.; Alb '46; M.C.G.P.

SMITH, Glen G.; 1309 Fairmount Med. Bldg., 750 W. Broadway, Vancouver, B.C.; 6112 Adera St., Van. 13 (res); Tor '43; FRCS(C), ObstGyn; Clin. Instr. (ObstGyn), U. of British Columbia; Tel. 879-3422.

SMITH, G. L. Morgan, Brig.; CBE, CD, QHP; Tor '34; Eblana, Bayfield, Ont.; Tor '34.

SMITH, G. Murray; Box 908, Windsor, N.S.; Dal '43; DPH; Dir. of Fundy Health Unit; Teach. Staff, N.S. San. Kentville & Payzant Mem. Hosp.

SMITH, Gordon J.; Man'48; Psy; Staff, Psy. Inst., 75 Emily St., Winnipeg 3, Man.

SMITH, Gordon K.; Prince St., Hantsport, N.S.; Dal '22; M.C.G.P.; Pres. Med. Staff, Payzant Mem. Hosp., Windsor; M.O.H.; Hantsport; Tel. 684-3321.

SMITH, Harry C.; Elliott Lake, Ont.; Qns '54.

SMITH, H. Austin; 1857 Bayview Ave., Toronto 17, Ont. (res); Tor '43; IntMed (Cardiol.); Staff, O.P.D. Cardiol. Clin., Toronto Western Hosp.; Assoc. Med. Dir. Confederation Life Assoc.; Tel. 924-6868.

SMITH, Hazel M. (Thompson); 4309 Dufferin St., Downsview, Ont. (res); Wes '52.

SMITH, H. Dorothy (Snell); 107 Windsor Ave., London, Ont. (res); Wes '30; Part-time Phys., Victoria Hosp.

SMITH H. Drummond; 144 Main St. E., Hawkesbury, Ont.; 31 McGill St. (res); McG '39; GenSurg; Surg., Smith Clin.; Tel. ME 2-6912.

SMITH, Henri G.; 745-5th St., Shawinigan Falls, P.Q.; 645-118e St. (res.); Lav '34; D.H.P.; Att. Staff Hop.-Ste-Therese; Tel. LE 6-4510.

SMITH, Henri H.; 3423 rue St.-Denis, Montreal 18, P.Q.; Lav '29; DermSyph; Chief of Derm. Serv., Hop. Gen. de Verdun; Tel. PO 6-3551.
SMITH, Herbert B.; 209 Canada Bldg., Windsor, Ont.; 810 Riverside Dr., Riverside, Ont. (res); **McG '21; GenSurg.; Cons. (Surg), Staff, Grace Hosp.; Tel. 253-6242.**
SMITH, H. Goldwin; 340 McLeod, Ottawa 4, Ont.; Qns'37; FACOG; FICSI ObstGyn; Sr. ObstGyn. & Pres. of Med. Staff, Ottawa Civic & Riverside Hosp's.; Sr. Lect., Ottawa U.; Tel. 233-9965.
SMITH, H. Gordon; Maple Creek Clinic, H'way 21, Maple Creek. Sask.; Alb'50; MCGP; Tel. 667-2681.
SMITH, H. Hedley; Box 39, Shelburne, Ont.; Qns'66; FAGS; Chief of Staff, Shelburne Dist. Hosp.; Home Phys., Dufferin Oaks Home for the Aged; Tel. 925-3110.
SMITH, H. James; Port Arthur Clinic, 194 Court St. N., Port Arthur, Ont.; Qns'59; FRCP(C), IntMed.
SMITH, Howard A.; Ste. 103, 1940 Lonsdale Ave., North Vancouver, B.C.; Belfast (Ire.)'41; FRCS(Ed.); FRCS(C), GenSurg; Urol; Clin. Instr. (Urol.), U. of British Columbia.
SMITH, Hubert H.; Shelburne, Ont.; Qns '56.
SMITH, Hugh C.; Man '65; Res., Winnipeg General Hosp., Winnipeg, Man.
SMITH, Ian McD.; Edam, Sask.; Edinburgh (Scot.) '55; MCGP; Med. Staff, Lady Minto Union Hosp.; Court. Staff, Battleford Union Hosp., North Battleford; Tel. 397-2233.
SMITH, I. Ruebert; 124 St. George St., Toronto, Ont. (res); Tor '12; L.R.C.P., M.R.C.S.; Retired.
SMITH, Irwin; Apt. 1411, 120 Shelborne Ave., Toronto 19, Ont.; Tor '31.
SMITH, Irwin T.; The Smith Clinic, 144 Main St., Hawkesbury, Ont.; 67 Main St. (res); McG '40; Co-Partner, The Smith Clinic.
SMITH, Isidor J.; 1771 Victoria Pk. Ave., Scarborough, Ont.; 774 Lawrence Ave. E., Don Mills (res); Tor '48; DNB; Staff, Tor. E. Gen. Hosp.; Tel. PL 5-0722.
SMITH, Ivor S.; Inglewood Med. Centre, 1897 Portage Ave., Winnipeg 12, Man.; Cambridge (Eng.) '58; Tel. TU 8-6076.
SMITH, Jacqueline A.; London (Eng.)'56; Res., Shaughnessy Hosp., Vancouver 9, B.C.
SMITH, James; 7215 Main St., Vancouver 15, B.C.; 1204-10th Ave., New Westminster; 632-W. 50th Ave., Van. 14 (res); Glasgow (Scot.) '51; DRCOG; Vis. Staff, Vancouver Gen. & St. Vincent's Hosp's.; Tel. FA 5-0616; LA 6-6121.
SMITH, James A.; Mount Forest, Ont.; Tor '49; MCGP; Tel. 14.
SMITH, James A.; Woodlawn Clinic, 110 Woodlawn Rd., Dartmouth, N.S.; Dal'64; AMCGP; Tel. 469-1563.
SMITH, J. Donald; 37 Dundas St. W., Cooksville, Ont.; 2364 Hurontario S. (res); Tor '45; GenSurg; Active Staff Surg., South Peel & Doctor's Hosp's.; Court. Staff, Queensway Gen. Hosp.; Tel. 277-2933.
SMITH, J. Dwight; 496-½ Adelaide St., Woodstock, Ont.; R.R. 6. (res); Wes '47; FRCS(C); GenSurg; **DABS; Surg. Staff, Woodstock Gen. Hosp.; Court Staff, Alexandra Hosp., Ingersoll; Tel. 539-2811.**
SMITH, J. Harold N.; Med. Arts Bldg., 121 Wellington St. W., Barrie, Ont.; Tor '30; Chief of Staff, Royal Victoria Hosp.; Tel. 728-5951.
SMITH, J. Hartley; 828 W. 10th Ave., Vancouver 9, B.C.; Queen's U. (Belfast, Ire.) '49; DPH (Tor); DIH (Lond.); PH; AB.PrevMed; Dir. Div. of Occupational Health, B.C. Health Dept.; Ass't. Prof. (PrevMed.), U. of British Columbia; Tel. TR 4-2331.
SMITH, J. K. Brydon; One Medical Place, 20 Wynford Dr., Don Mills, Ont.; Tor'43; FACS; FICS; FRCS(C), Otol; Staff, St. Michael's Hosp.; Cons., Defence Research Lab., (Downsview), Sunnybrook Hosp., RCAF & Ont. Cancer Inst.; Clin. Ass't. U. of Toronto; Tel. 429-1580.
SMITH, John A.; Box 968, College Rd., Windsor, N.S.; Dal '55; Anaes; Staff, Payzant Mem. Hosp. & Eastern Kings Mem. Hosp., Wolfville; Tel. 798-2966.
SMITH, John D.; Qns '62; Res., Kingston Gen. Hosp., Kingston, Ont.
SMITH, John R.; 2900—31st Ave., Vernon, B.C.; **Kalamalka Lake (res.); McG '39; GenSurg.; Tel. 542-5634.**
SMITH, J. Tolson; 37a Forest Rd., St. John's, Nfld.; Dal '32; GenSurg; Chief of B. Surg. Serv., St. John's Gen. Hosp.; Cons. Staff, Grace Hosp.; Vis. Staff, St. Clare's Mercy Hosp.; Tel. 578-3343.
SMITH, Kevin P.; 349 Herring Cove Rd., Spryfield, N.S.; Dal '54; M.C.G.P.
SMITH, Laurence A. E.; 64 Third St., Collingwood, Ont.; 91 Third St. (res); Man '25.
SMITH, Leighton; 132 Surrey Dr., Town of Mt. Royal, P.Q. (res); **McG '43; Ass't. Med., O.P.D., Royal Victoria Hosp.; Vice-Pres. & Med. Dir.,** Ayerst Laboratories; P.O. Box 6115; Tel. RI 4-6771.
SMITH, Leonard; One Medical Place, 20 Wynford Dr., Don Mills, Ont.; Tor '52; DABOG; FACOG; FRCS(C); ObstGyn; Att'd. Staff (ObstGyn.), Toronto East Gen. Hosp.; Tel. 429-1188.
SMITH, Leslie W.; Westbrook Med. Centre, 157 Westbrook Mall, Calgary, Alta.; Birmingham (England) '55; Tel. 249-0738.
SMITH, Malcolm B.; Edinburgh (Scot.)'58; Staff, Dept. of Path., Wellesley Hosp., Toronto 5, Ont.
SMITH, M. Anne; Ste. 204, 407 Graham Ave., Winnipeg, Man.; St. Andrew's (Scot.)'47; Tel. 942-2431.
SMITH, Marcia; 327 Charlotte St., Peterborough, Ont.; Wes '57; Paed; Staff, Civic Hosp. & St. Joseph's Hosp's.; Tel. 743-2040.
SMITH, Marjorie L.; Herring Cove Rd., Spryfield, N.S.; Dal '54; M.C.G.P.
SMITH, Mary L.; One Hundred Mile House, B.C.; USA'46; Abroad.
SMITH, Maurice W. J.; 2009 Danforth Ave., Toronto 6, Ont.; Glasgow (Scot.)'57; D.Obst RCOG; Tel. OX 8-5565.
SMITH, McIver; 640 Seaforth Med. Bldg., 3550 Cote des Neiges Rd., Montreal 25, P.Q.; 631 Roslyn Ave. (res); McG '30; FACP; IntMed; Assoc (Med.) Montreal Gen. Hosp.; Ass't. Prof. (Med.), McGill U.; Tel. 932-3868.
SMITH, Michael J.; 210 Avenue Bldg., 220-3rd Ave. S., Saskatoon, Sask.; Birmingham, (Eng.); Tel. 652-0300.
SMITH, Michael S.; Box 679, Radville, Sask.; Birmingham (Eng.)'62.
SMITH, M. S.; 22 William St., Smith's Falls, Ont.; Tor'63; AMCGP; Tel. 283-0711.
SMITH, Neville S. H.; 3044 Retallack St., Regina, Sask. (res); Tor'41; MCGP; Med. Dir., Cooperative Life Ins. Co.; Med. Dir., Kaliam Chemicals Co.; Tel. 522-1651.
SMITH, Norman E.; 402 Metropolitan Blvd., Pointe Claire, P.Q.; McG '57; FRCS(C), ObstGyn; Tel. 697-3413.
SMITH, Norman K.; Ste. 204, 407 Graham Ave., Winnipeg 1, Man.; St. Andrews (Scot.) '44; M.B., Ch.B.; MRCP (Ed.)
SMITH, Peter C.; Box 429, Barry's Bay, Ont.; Ott '61; Tel. 486.
SMITH, Peter M.; 221 King St. E., Kingston, Ont.; Leeds (Eng.)'47; D.ObstRCOG; Tel. 542-5517.
SMITH, Philip E.; Ste. 433, Med. Arts Bldg., 170 St. George St., Toronto, Ont.; Wes '52; FRCS(C), Otol.; Staff, St. Michael's Hosp.; Clin. Teach. (Otol.), U. of Toronto; Tel. 922-8651.
SMITH, Pierre; 300 St. Louis Sq., Montreal, P.Q.; Mon '22; GenSurg; Staff, St. Luc Hosp.
SMITH, Raleigh D.; Belledune, Gloucester Co., N.B.; Qns'40.
SMITH, Ralph C.; 212 Cook Medical Bldg., 1175 Cook St., Victoria, B.C.; 3446 Plymouth Rd. (res); Wes '49; D.S. (McGill); DABS; DABTS; ThorSurg; Cardiovasc & ThorSurg; Staff, Royal Jubilee & St. Joseph's Hosp's. Cons. (ThorSurg.), Veteran's Hosp.; Tel. EV 5-5151.
SMITH, Robert B.; 3490 Saanich Rd., Victoria, B.C.; UBC'55; Tel. 382-8011.

SMITH, Robert L.; 555 University Ave., Toronto 2, Ont.; 4 Superior Ave., Tor. 14 (res); Tor '51; Psy; Clin. Ass't. (Psy), Hosp. for Sick Children; Cons. (Psy), Bloorview Hosp. & Boys Village; Clin. Instr. (Psy), U. of Toronto; Tel. EM 6-7242.

SMITH, Robert L.; 452 Charlotte Street, Peterborough, Ont.; Tor'56; FRCS(ED); FRCS (ENG); FACS; GenSurg; Active Staff, Peterborough Civic & St. Joseph's Hosp's; Tel. 745-0581.

SMITH, Robert L.; 107B Carmarthen St., St. John, N.B.; Brookville, N.B. (res); Dal'53; Paed; **Active Staff, St. John Gen. Hosp. & St. Joseph's Hosp.; Tel. 657-2895.**

SMITH, Robert M.; McG'55; DiagRad; Staff, Royal Victoria Hosp., Montreal 2, P.Q.

SMITH, Robert S.; Qns '59; Res., Royal Victoria Hosp., Montreal 2, P.Q.

SMITH, Roger; Clarke City Hosp., Clarke City, P.Q.; Lav'42; MCGP; Med. Dir., Clarke City Hosp.; Med. Dir., Gulph Pulp & Paper Co.; Tel. 583-2507.

SMITH, Ronald B.; Ste. 630, 5025 Sherbrooke St. W., Montreal 28, P.Q.; McG '41; FACOG; Att'd. Staff (ObstGyn.), Queen Elizabeth Hosp.; Court. Staff, Catherine Booth Mothers Hosp.; Tel. 488-2622.

SMITH, Ronald M.; 1414 Drummond St., Montreal, P.Q.; 7530 de la Loire, Anjou (res); Wes '49; **Psy; Ass't. OPD (Psy), Mtl. Gen. Hosp.**; Tel. VI 4-7562.

SMITH, Royston R. W.; Balcarres, Sask.: Tor **'43; Dist. Coroner.; Tel. 334-2687.**

SMITH, Samuel G.; 10 Hillcrest St., Chatham, Ont.; Qns'59; Anaes.

SMITH, Sheelah B. (Cosgrove); 74 MacPherson Ave., Toronto 5, Ont. (res): Queen's U. (Belfast, N. Ire.) '45; D.P.H.: Dist. Phys., Riverdale Dist.

SMITH, Sheila; (See Mitchell, Sheila).

SMITH, Sherwood P.; Tor'65; Res., Royal Victoria Hospital, Montreal, P.Q.

SMITH, Stanley G.; Regina Medical Centre, 1847 Rose St., Regina, Sask; Trinity Coll. (Dublin, Ire)'60; MCGP; Staff, Regina Gen. & Regina Grey Nun's Hosp's; Tel. 522-6661.

SMITH, Stanley S.; Alb'65; Res., University Hosp., Edmonton, Alta.

SMITH, Stuart L.; McG '62; (Hons.), College of P. & S. (P.Q.) prize for Path & Med.; Jr. Intn., Montreal Gen. Hosp., Montreal 25, P.Q.

SMITH, Sydney A.; 3545 Cote des Neiges, Montreal, P.Q. (res); McG'48; IntMed; Part Time **Phys., Queen Mary Veterans' Hosp.; Staff, Reddy Memorial Hosp.; Tel. WE 5-2747.**

SMITH, T. Ormiston; 455 Avenue Rd., Toronto, Ont.; 6 Foxbar Rd. (res); Wes '22; M.C.G.P.; Med. Staff, Lambert Lodge; Tel. WA 2-0181.

SMITH, Verne P.; 3260 Edgemont Blvd., North **Vancouver, B.C.; UBC '58.**

SMITH, Vincent W.; 1139 Yates St., Victoria, B.C.; 160 Beach St., Qns '39; M.C.G.P.

SMITH, Wilfred D.; 430 Med. Arts Bldg., 170 St. George St., Toronto 5, Ont.; 288 Dawlish Ave. (res); Tor '33; F.A.C.S.; GenSurg; Staff (GenSurg), St. Michael's Hosp.; Teach, Staff (Surg.), U. of Toronto; Tel. 364-1527.

SMITH-WINDSOR, Morley H.; 325-21st St., Saskatoon, Sask.; 206-8th St. (res); Man '44; M.C.-G.P.; Staff, St. Paul's & University Hosp's; **Clin. Inst'r., (Med.) U. of Sask.**; Tel. 242-7991.

SMITHEN, Arthur H.; Dublin (Ire.) '56; Res., Kingston Gen. Hosp., Kingston, Ont.

SMOLARCZYK, Frank; 14 Pine St. S., Timmins, Ont.; 186-5th St. (res); Munich (Germ.) '49.

SMOLING, Leslie F.; 2196 Danforth Ave., Toronto 13, Ont.; Budapest (Hung.) '52; Tel. 694-9628.

SMOLKIN, Robert D.; 725 Churchill Ave., Ottawa, Ont.; Qns'61; AMCGP; Tel. 722-4566.

SMOLKIN, Samuel; 150 Metcalfe St., Ottawa, **Ont.; Qns '40; Tel. 235-8146.**

SMOUT, Marvin S.; 1553 McClure Dr., London, Ont.; Wes '53; DAB Path; Chief Pathol., Victoria Hosp.; Clin. Prof. Path.. U. of Western Ontario; Tel. 432-5261, Loc. 268.

SMUK, Avrillia H.; Sask'58; Res.. Royal Ottawa San., Ottawa 3, Ont.

SMULSKI, John; 303 Professional Bldg., 10830 Jasper Ave., Edmonton, Alta.; 4 Riverside Cres. (res); Alb '42; MCGP; Chmn. Bd. of Health, Edmonton; Tel. 424-1814.

SMYLIE, Donald T.; 224 King St. E., Brockville, Ont.; Qns '49; FRCS; Urol; Tel. DI 2-4476.

SMYLIE, Roderick T.; 170 Bloor St. W., Toronto, Ont.; Park Plaza Hotel, 4 Avenue Rd. (res); Tor '21; A.M.C.A.A.; Chest & All., St. Michael's **Hosp.; Tel. WA 1-3937.**

SMYLIE, Rodney D.; 16 Paget St., New Liskeard, Ont.; Qns '45.

SMYTH, John; Box 630, Leduc, Alta; Queen's (N. Ire.)'50; BAO; Tel. 446-3432.

SMYTH, John H.; 102 St. Francis St., Edmundston, N.B.; Qns'39.

SMYTHE, Clifford A.; 501 Med. Arts Bldg., 404-406 Graham Ave., Winnipeg 1, Man.; 66 Niagara St. (res); Tor '54; FRCS(C), Urol; Tel. 943-9878.

SMYTHE, Harold H.; 204 Medical Arts Bldg., 507 Baker St., Nelson, B.C.; 313 Silica St. (res); Alb '42; Dist. Coroner.

SMYTHE, Hugh A.; 130 Tor. Gen. Hosp., Toronto 2, Ont.; 2 Heathbridge Pk., Tor. 17 (res); Tor '50; FRCP(C), IntMed; Phys., Tor. Gen. Hosp.; Cons., Sunnybrook Hosp.; Tel. EM 6-8211.

SNARCH, Milton D.; 6591 Somerled Ave., Montreal, P.Q.; 4820 Mayfair Ave. (res); Qns '51; M.C.G.P.; Staff, Jewish Gen. Hosp. & Jewish Hosp. of Hope.

SNEATH, P. A. T.; OBE, CD; 29 Mark Ave. Apt. 9, Ottawa 2, Ont. (res); Tor '21; D.P.H., D.A.B.P.M. & P.H., PH; **Exec. Prof. Ass't. to Surg. Gen., Cdn. Forces Med Serv.; Tel. CE 2-**8211.

SNEDDEN, Frederick W.; Qns '31; D.Psy., Psy; Supt., Ontario Hosp., Hamilton, Ont.

SNELL, Arthur E.; 234 Rideau Terrace, Ottawa, Ont. (res); Tor '02.

SNELL, Bernard; University Hosp., Edmonton, Alta.; Glasgow (Scot.)'43; DPH(Edin.); MRCP (Ed.); FRCP(Ed.); MACHA; Exec. Dir., U. of Alberta Hosp.; Tel. 439-5911.

SNELL, Emanuel; 311 Norquay Bldg., 401 York Ave., Winnipeg 1, Man.; St. Mungo's Coll. (Glasgow, Scot.)'39; DPH; FAPHA; Dir. Prev. Med., Med. Cons. in Occup. Health & Radiation Health Authority, Prov Dept. of Health, Manitoba; Tel. WH 6-7721.

SNELL, F. Van; 66 Binscarth Rd., Toronto 5, Ont. (res); Tor '29; Anaes, IntMed; Ass't. Anaes., Hosp. for Sick Children, Toronto; Clin. Ass't. (Anaes), U. of Toronto; Tel. EM 6-7242.

SNELL, G. Douglas; 176 St. George St., Toronto, Ont.; 103 Blythwood Rd. (res); Tor '49; F.R.-C.S.(C), Otol; Clin. Ass't. Toronto Gen. Hosp.; Hon. Cons., Royal Victoria Hosp., Barrie; Clin. Teach., U. of Toronto; Tel. WA 2-4471.

SNELL, George C.; 176 St. George St., Toronto, Ont.; Leslie St., R.R. 1, Tedmorden (res); Tor '23; D.L.O., M.A.A.O., Otol; Sr. Surg., Toronto Gen. Hosp.; Assoc. (Otol.), U. of Toronto; Tel. WA 2-4471.

SNELLING, Charles E.; 235 Medical Arts Bldg., 170 St. George St., Toronto, Ont.; 3 St. Edmunds Dr. (res); Tor '27; Paed; Prof. Paed., U. of **Toronto; Phys., Sick Children's Hosp.; Tel. WA** 3-4774.

SNELLING, Charles F.; Tor'62; Res.. St. Joseph's Hosp., Toronto 3, Ont.

SNELLING, Walter W.; 196 E. Main St., Welland, Ont.; 194 Merritt St. W. (res); Tor '37; MCGP; Tel. 732-2486.

SNIDAL, Daniel P.; Man '52; IntMed; Staff, Respiratory Lab., St. Boniface Hosp., St. Boniface, Man.; Ass't. Prof. & Dir. Dept. of Cont. Med. Educ., U. of Manitoba; Tel. WH 3-0311.

SNIDER, Bernice E. (Znajda); Ste. 302, 200 St. Clair Ave. W., Toronto 7, Ont.; Tor '62; Tel. 921-2744.

SNIDER, Eugene P.; 223 College St., Toronto 2B, Ont.; Apt. 907, 19 Lascelles Blvd. Tor. 7 (res); Tor '36; Ass't. Dir., Gage Inst.; Tel. 924-2191.

SNIDER, James H.; Wes '62; Jr. Intn., St. Joseph's Hosp., London, Ont.

SNIDERMAN, A. D.; Tor'65; Res., Royal Victoria Hosp., Montreal 2, P.Q.

SNIDERMAN, Barry P.; Tor '65; Res., New Mount Sinai Hosp., Toronto 2, Ont.

SNIDERMAN, Harold R.; Ste. 406, 99 Avenue Rd., Toronto 5, Ont.; Tor '34; Ophth; Clin. Att. Ophth., Toronto Western Hosp.; Sr. Att. Ophth.. Mount Sinai Hosp.; Teach. Staff (Ophth.), U. of Toronto; Tel. WA 3-2830.

SNIDERMAN, Jacob B.; 483 George St. S., Peterborough, Ont.; Qns'64; Abroad.

SNIHUROWYCH, Melety; 3829 - 118th Ave., Edmonton, Alta.; Innsbruck (Aust.) '54; MCGP; Att'd. Staff, Edmonton Gen. Hosp.; Tel. GR 9-3318.

SNITMAN, Harry; 262 Wilson Ave., Downsview, Ont.; 613 Briar Hill Ave., Tor. 12 (res); Tor '40; Paed; Jr. Att'd. Paed., New Mount Sinai Hosp;. Tel. ME 6-2200.

SNOW, James T.; Kennetcook, Hants. Co., N.S.; Dal '57; Tel. 16.

SNOW, J. Murray; 5639 Spring Garden Road, Halifax, N.S.; Dal'54; AMCGP; Executive Director, Nova Scotia Alcoholism Research Foundation.

SNOW, Richard V.; 3 Park Ave., East Saint John, N.B.; Dal '59; AMCGP; Tel. 692-1133.

SNOW, Ronald E.; Dublin (Ire.) '60; Res. (Anaes.), Kingston Gen. Hosp., Kingston, Ont. Abroad.

SNOW, Sidney L.; Ott'63; Res., Royal Victoria Hosp., Montreal 2, P.Q.

SNOW, Vernon A.; Hampton, N.B.; McG '27; M.C.G.P.; Staff, St. Joseph's Hosp., St. John & Kings Co. Mem. Hosp., Sussex; Tel. WE 9-3720.

SNYDER, Richard E., Capt.; RCAMC Sick Bay, Halifax N.S.; Alb'65.

SO, Yan P.; 1102 Ridgway Avenue, New Westminster, B.C.; UBC'58; Att'd Staff, Royal Columbian Hosp.; Assoc. Staff, St. Mary's Hosp.; Tel. 939-3720.

SOANES, Eric P.; Medical Arts Bldg., 358 Reynold St. N. Oakville, Ont.; 8th Line N. (res); **Tor. '25; Chief of Staff, Oakville-Trafalgar Hosp.; Tel. VI 4-3201.**

SOANES, Stuart E.; Medical Arts Bldg., 358 Reynolds St. N., Oakville, Ont.; Tor '64.

SOBER, Stanley; 450 Central Ave., London, Ont.; 452 Victoria St. (res); London (Eng.) '47; DABN; FRCS(C), OrthSurg; Court. Staff, St. Joseph's & Victoria Hosp's.; Cons. Staff, Alexandra Hosp., Ingersoll; Tel. 432-4294.

SOBEY, Vernon W.; Med. Arts Clinic, 51-6th St. S.E., Medicine Hat, Alta.; 5 Huckvale Cres. S.W. (res); Dal '53; FACS; GenSurg; Staff, Medicine Hat Gen. Hosp.; Tel. JA 7-2281.

SOBRIAN, Jules; Omemee, Ont.; Tor '62. M.O.H Emily Twsp.; Tel. 799-5230.

SOBY, Harold W.; 214-6th Ave. W., Calgary, Alta.; 3044 - 1st St. S.W. (res); McG '26; Tel. AM 9-2710.

SOBY, W. H.; c/o Chief Medical Officer, Department National Health & Welfare, 61 Green St., London, W.1, England.

SOCHANIWSKYJ, Wolodymyr; 1208 Bloor St. W., Toronto 4, Ont.; 108 Ava Rd. Tor. 10 (res); Tor '57; Staff, O.P.D., St. Michael's & St. Joseph's Hosp's.; Tel. LE 1-6966.

SOCHOWSKI, J.; 1665 W. Broadway, Vancouver, B.C.; Qns. '44; Tel. 738-4033.

SOCOL, Harvey; 294 Bayview Plaza, Richmond Hill, Ont.; 465 North Taylor Mills Dr. (res); Tor'60; D.N.B.M.E.(U.S.A.); Pres. Med. Staff, York Central Hosp.; Tel. 884-4040.

SODERO, G. Watson; 558 Charlotte St., Sydney, N.S.; 201 S. Bentinck St. (res); Dal '34; FACS; GenSurg; Tel. 564-8146.

SODERO, Theodore C. C.; 548 Prince St., Truro, N.S.; 48 Duke St. (res); Dal '35; GenSurg.; Tel. 893-2915.

SODOMSKY, Martin E.; Man '61; Jr. Intn., University Hosp., Edmonton, Alta.

SOFFER, Hagi S.; Borden, Sask.; Bagdad (Iraq) '53; LRCP; MRCS;MCGP; Tel. 64.

SOGA, Kenichi K.; Irving Clinic, 74 W. Seymour St., Kamloops, B.C. 674 Brandon Ave. (res); UBC'58; MCGP.

SOICHER-RIPSTEIN, Riva B. — see **RIPSTEIN-SOICHER, Riva B.**

SOKOLOWSKA, Anna M.; 278 Friel St., Ottawa 2, Ont.; Edinburgh (Scot.)'46; Psy; Staff Phys., Royal Ottawa San.; Sr. Lect. Ottawa U.; Tel. 235-4244.

SOLANDT, Omond M.; O.B.E.; 36 Hawthorn Ave., Toronto 5, Ont.; Tor '36; FRCP (Lond.); D.Sc. (McGill, UBC, Dal, Lav, Man., St-Francis Xavier); Ll.D. (Dal., Toronto); FRSC; Retired.

SOLANZADEH, Amir; 396 Francis Rd., Richmond, B.C.; Tehran (Iran) '54; GenSurg; Tel. BR 7-7166.

SOLE, Joseph N.; 424 Main St. E., Hamilton. Ont.; Qns'63; Active Staff, Hamilton Civic & St. Joseph's Hosp's.; Tel. JA 8-4218.

SOLE, Nicholas; 424 Main St. E., Hamilton, Ont.; 175 Dalewood Cres. (res); Royal Hungarian Elizabeth U. (Hungary)'27; MCGP; Tel. JA 8-4218.

SOLLARS, Robert J.; Med. Arts Clinic, 2125-11th **Ave., Regina, Sask.; 13 Lamont Cr. (res); London (Eng.) '48; D.Obst.RCOG; FRCS(C); ObstGyn; Staff, Regina Grey Nuns & Regina Gen.** Hosp's. Tel. 523-0691.

SOLLBACH, Gerhard; 10104-124th St., Edmonton, Alta.; 12424-103rd Ave. (res); J. W. Goethe (Frankfurt, Germ.) '53; Tel. 488-4336.

SOLLBACH, W. Lilli (Herbst); 10104-124th St., Edmonton, Alta.; Marlburg (Germ.)'55; DiagRad; Staff, Royal Alexandra Hosp.

SOLLICH, William G.; 190 Ontario St., St. Catharines, Ont.; Innsbruck (Austria); '47; MCGP; Active Staff, St. Catharines Gen. Hosp.; Court. Staff, Hotel-Dieu Hosp.

SOLMES, James G.; Ste. 901, 1849 Yonge St., Toronto 7, Ont.; Tor '43; FRCS(C); ObstGyn; Staff, St. Michaels Hosp.; Clin. Teach., U. of Toronto; Tel. 483-1700.

SOLOMON, Barney W.; 301 Victoria Ave., Fort Frances, Ont.; Man '36; Med. Staff, Verendrye Hosp.; Dist. M.O., C.N.R.; Tel. 274-3287; Abroad.

SOLOMON, Edward B.; McG '64; Res., Jewish Gen. Hosp., Montreal 26, P.Q.

SOLOMON, Lawrence M.; Geneva (Switz) '59; FRCP(C), Derm; Staff, Jewish Gen. Hosp., Montreal, P.Q.; Tel. RE 5-3771, Loc. 275; Abroad.

SOLOMON, Martin L.; Qns'61; Psy; Staff, Hop. Ste. Justine, Montreal 26, P.Q.

SOLOMON, Morris; Ste. 360, 6000 Cote des Neiges Rd., Montreal 26, P.Q.; Lausanne (Switz.) '53; MCGP.

SOLOW, Halina R. (Rutkowska); 1369 Rometown Dr., Port Credit, Ont.; Beirut (Lebanon) '50; **Staff, Queensway Hosp.; Tel. CR 8-4728.**

SOLOWAY, Irving; 340 McLeod St., Ste. 407, Ottawa 4, Ont.; Qns'51; FACOG; ObstGyn; Staff, Civic & Grace Hosp's.; Cons., Kemptville Dist. Hosp.; Clin. Ass't., Ottawa U.; Tel. 233-6014.

SOLOWSKA, Vera; 10 Paulson Rd., Toronto 15, Ont.; Tor '49; Paed; Staff, Hosp. for Sick Children & **Northwestern Gen. Hosp's.; Tel. RO 7-1851.**

SOLTAN, Amir; 814 Cook Rd., Richmond, B.C.; '54; GenSurg.

SOLTICE, Norman J.; 8928-116th St., Edmonton, Alta. (res); Alb '55; FRCP(C), Anaes; Staff, University Hosp.; Tel. 439-5911.

SOLTYS, Sophie; Raxlen Clinic, 500 Parliament St., Toronto 5, Ont.; Ott. '61; Tel. WA 5-4381.

SOLURSH, Coleman B.; 2949 Bathurst St., Toronto 19, Ont.; Tor '31; MCGP; Cons. GP, New Mt. Sinai Hosp.; Tel. RU 2-7171.

SOLURSH, Lionel P.; Dept. of Psy., Toronto Western Hosp., Toronto, Ont.; Tor'59; D.Psy; FRCP(C), Psy; Active Att'd. Staff, Toronto Western Hosp.; Clin. Teach. (Depts. of Med. & Psy.), U. of Toronto; Tel. 369-5743.

SOLWAY, Albert J. L.; Ste. 304, 158 St. George St., Toronto, Ont.; 8 Dewbourne Ave. (res); **Tor '41; IntMed; Att'd. Phys., New Mount Sinai Hosp.; O.P.D. Staff, Toronto Western Hosp.; Tel. WA 2-8835.**

SOLWAY, Samuel D.; Ste. 101, 158 St. George St., Toronto 5, Ont.; 111 Glenayr Rd., Toronto 10 (res); Tor '36; M.Sc. (Med.); FACP; IntMed; Staff, New Mt. Sinai & Doctor's Hosp's.; Tel. WA 1-3484.

SOLWAY, S. H.; 384 Bloor St. W., Toronto 4, Ont.; 47 Wembley Rd. (res); Tor '38; Anaes; Staff Anaes., Mt. Sinai Hosp.; Tel. WA 2-8270.

SOLYMAR, Jeno; Ste. 510, 5300 Cote des Neiges Rd., Montreal 26, P.Q.; 3590 Ridgewood (res); Pazmany U. (Budapest, Hung.) '49; Gastroent (P.Q.); FRCP(C); IntMed; Jr. Clin. Ass't., St. Mary's Hosp.; Tel. 739-5249.

SOLYOM, Leslie; 1025 Pine Ave. W., Montreal 2, P.Q.; 1710 Norway Rd., Mtl. 9 (res); Budapest (Hung.) '50; D.Psy; Psy; Att'd. Staff, Royal Victoria Hosp.; Lect. McGill U.; Tel. 842-1251, Loc. 618.

SOMER, Kenneth G. R.; Wainwright Clinic, 401-10th St., Wainwright, Alta.; London (Eng.) '56; DObstRCOG; DCH; Staff, Wainwright Mun Hosp.; Tel. 842-3341.

SOMERLEIGH, Edward R.; Box 339, Nipigon, Ont.; Old Hudson's Bay Rd. (res); Qns '53; M.C.G.P.

SOMERTON, Kenneth F.; 262 Oxford St., Suite 105, London, Ont.; Wes'62; Courtesy Staff, St. Joseph's, St. Mary's, Victoria & Parkwood Hosp's.; Tel. 439-8021.

SOMERVILLE, A. Elwood; 110 Palisades, Saskatoon, Sask.; 230 Poplar Cr. (res); Qns '53; MRCP (Glas.); FRFPS (Glas.); FCCP; FAGS; FICA; FACA; FRCP(C), IntMed; Active Staff, University, St. Paul's, & Saskatoon City Hosp's. Clin. Assoc. (Med.), U. of Saskatchewan; Tel. 244-2977.

SOMERVILLE, Asbury; 11005 University Ave., Edmonton, Alta. (res); Man '24; D.P.H.; P.H.; Memb. U. of Alberta Hosp.; Retired.

SOMERVILLE, Glasier M.; Dal'60; Res., Toronto Gen. Hosp., Toronto 2, Ont.

SOMERVILLE, John C. W.; 185A Woolwich St., Guelph, Ont.; 25 Barber Ave. (res); Edinburgh (Scot.) '41; MRCOG; ObstGyn; Tel. TA 2-9652.

SOMLO, Agnes M. (Beer); Wes '59; Res. (Bact.), Dept. of Bact., McGill U., Montreal, P.Q.; Abroad.

SOMLO, Francois; 5300 Cote-des-Neiges Rd., Montreal 26, P.Q.; Italy '37.

SOMLO, Laszlo I.; Wes '59; Res. (Surg.Path.) McGill Pathol. Inst., Montreal, P.Q.

SOMMER, Felix; Graz (Austria)'54; Psy; Staff (Psy.), Verdun Protestant Hosp., Verdun, Montreal 19, P.Q.; Abroad.

SOMMERFREUND, Paul; 5025 Sherbrooke St. W., Montreal 28, P.Q.; 486 Victoria Ave., Westmount (res); Vienna (Austria) '37; F.C.C.P.; Staff, Montreal Gen. Hosp., & Royal Edward Chest Hosp.; M.O., C.N.R.; Dem., McGill U.; Tel. HU 1-7308.

SOMMERFREUND, Mrs. Stella (See Schiffman).

SOMMERS, Izzy; Tor '61; Jr. Intn., Toronto Gen. Hosp., Toronto 2, Ont.

SOMMERS, J.; 310 Bloor St. W., Toronto, Ont.; 637 Briar Hill (res); Tor '34; D & TRad.; Tel. WA 3-3638.

SOMMERVILL, Ronald P.; 427 Main St., Foam Lake, Sask.; McG '53; MCGP; Staff, Foam Lake Union Hosp.; Councillor, College of P. & S. Council; Precept., U. of Saskatchewan; Tel. 272-3533.

SOMMERVILLE, Robert J.; 5 Academy Med. Bldg., 1812 - 4th St., W. Calgary, Alta.; Alb '56; DABP; Paed; Staff, Calgary Gen., Holy Cross, Alberta Children's & Grace Maternity Hosp's.; Abroad.

SOMOGYI, Stephen H.; Ste. 501, 180 Metcalfe St., Ottawa, Ont.; Budapest (Hun.) '44.

SOMOS, Elemer S.; Park Ave. Med. Clinic, 5615 Park Ave., Montreal 8, P.Q.; Budapest (Hung.) '31; Staff, Lakeshore Gen. Hosp.

SONEA, Sorin; 4282 Badgley, Montreal, P.Q. (res); Bucharest (Rumania) '44; D.Hyg. (Paris); Bact; Prof. & Dir. (Bact.), U. of Montreal; Tel. RE 3-9951.

SONEDA, Margaret M.; Alb '60; Res., Vancouver Gen. Hosp., Vancouver, B.C.

SONG, Ki T.; Soeul (Korea)'50; GenSurg; Staff, Royal Victoria Hosp., Montreal 2, P.Q.

SONLEY, Marilyn J.; 88 Wellesley St. E.; Apt. 706, Toronto 5, Ont. (res); Tor '55; DABPaed; FRCP(C), Paed; Staff, Hosp. for Sick Children; Cons. Paed., Princess Margaret Hosp.; Clin. Instr., (Paed), U. of Toronto; Tel. EM 6-7242.

SOOD, Brijendra K.; Box 897, Banff Clinic, Banff, Alta.; Birmingham (Eng.) '54; M.B.; Ch.B., LRCP (Lond.); MRCS (Eng.); D.ObstRCOG; FRCS (Edin.); Staff, Minneral Springs Hosp.; Cons. to Park Ambulance Service; Tel. 762-2233.

SOODEEN, Tyrone; Leeds (Eng.)'63; Res., St. Boniface Hosp., Winnipeg 6, Man.

SOOKOCHOFF, Michael W.; 1940 Lonsdale Ave., North Vancouver, B.C.; UBC '58; Tel. YU 5-2060.

SOONG, Fang Y.; National North Western Med. School '44; Staff, Selkirk Mental Hosp., Selkirk, Man.

SOOTS, Marja L.; Tor'63; Res., Toronto East Gen. Hosp., Toronto 6, Ont.

SOPER, G. M.; Thamesville, Ont.

SOPER, Keith; 72 Yorkview Dr., Willowdale, Ont.; Tor '49; FRCS(C), OrthSurg.

SORBARA, V. James; 200 St. Clair Ave. W., Toronto 7, Ont.; 47 York Downs Dr., Downsview (res); Tor '47; ObstGyn; O.P.D. Staff, (Obst.Gyn.), St. Michael's Hosp.; Tel. WA 1-8252.

SORBIE, Charles; Etherington Hall, Queen's University, Kingston, Ont.; Glasgow (Scot.)'53; FRCS(Ed.); FRCS(C), OrthSurg; Att'd. Staff, Kingston Gen. Hosp.; Lect. (Surg.), Queen's University; Tel. 542-3688.

SOREMEKUN, S. O.; Tor '64; Res., University of Alberta Hosp., Edmonton, Alta.

SORENSEN, Cecil; Med. Arts Bldg., 420 East St. N., Sarnia, Ont.; 193 Queen St. (res), Wes '49; Paed; Tel. ED 7-2561.

SORMANY, Albert M.; C.P. 306, 44A Fraser Ave., Edmundston, N.B.; Lav '10; DA; D.Sc., Ll.D; Ph.D; DiagRad; Chief Cancer Clin.; MO, CNR; Prof. (Biol.), U. St.-Louis; Tel. RE 5-3743.

SORMANY, Armand; 53-34eme Ave., Edmunston, N.B.; Lav'40; MCGP; Med. Dir., Hotel-Dieu of St. Joseph; Tel. RE 5-5633.

SORMANY, Yvon; 1031 Desaulniers, Chicoutimi, P.Q. (res); Lav '42; Anaes; Anaes., Hotel-Dieu St. Vallier, Chicoutimi; Tel. 549-1452.

SOROKA, Morrell M.; Estevan Med. Assoc., Box 700, 1314 Third St., Estevan, Sask.; Man'56.

SOROKOLIT, Walter T.; 103 Med. Arts Bldg., 1 Young St., Hamilton, Ont.; Tor'59; FRCS(C), PlasSurg; GenSurg; Staff, Brant Mem. Hosp., Burlington, Chedoke Gen. & Children's Hosp., Hamilton, Hamilton Gen. Hosp. & St. Joseph's Hosp., Hamilton; Tel. 525-5462.

SOSA, Julio A.; Div. of Cardiol., Montreal Gen. Hosp., Montreal, P.Q.; McG'56; FRCP(C), IntMed; Cardiol.(P.Q.); Ass't. Phys. & Dir., Cardiac Catheterization Lab., Mtl. Gen. Hosp.; Lect. (Med.), McGill U.; Tel. 937-6011, Loc. 490.

SOTOLOV, L.; 200 Professional Bldg., 407 Graham Ave., Winnipeg, Man.; Man '52.

SOUCEK, Alfred, Sg. Lcdr; Regional Surg., Griesbach Barracks, Edmonton, Alta.; Vienna (Austria)'48; DPH.

SOUCIE, Guillaume; Kapuskasing Med. Centre, 29 Mundy, Kapuskasing, Ont.; Mon '34; M.O.H.; Dist. Coroner; Tel. 335-4138.

SOUCIE, Simon P.; Med. Clinic, Kapuskasing, Ont.; Ott '64; Jr. Staff, Sensenbrenner Hosp.; Tel. 335-4138.

SOUCY, Antoine J.; Gravelbourg, Sask.; Lav '13.

SOUCY, C. Andre; 3755 boul. St.-Martin, Chomedey, P.Q.; 61 ave. Verdi, Laval-des-Rapides (res); Mon '56; DABP; Paed; Staff (Paed), Hop. Ste.-Justine; Cons. (Paed), Hop. Gen.-des-Deux-Montagnes & Hop. Ste.-Rose-de-Laval; Med. Dir. St. Pie X Hop. pour Enfants Incurables; I/C Congen. & Urinary Infect. course, U. of Mtl.; Tel. MU 1-2633.

SOUCY, Donald; Lav'63; Res., Hop. Christ Roi, Montreal 19, P.Q.

SOUCY, Francois C.; 132 ave. Lowring, Drummondville, P.Q.; Lav'65.

SOUCY, Francois; San. St. Georges, Mont Joli, P.Q. Lav '34; Pulm. Dis. & TB (P.Q.); Chief, Serv., San. St. Georges, Mont Joli; Tel. 775-4632.

SOUCY, Gervais; Lav '53; Res., Hop. Notre-Dame, Montreal 24, P.Q.; Lav '53.

SOUCY, Maurice; Chandler, P.Q.; Lav '61. Abroad.

SOUCY-HIRTLE, Fernande; 847 Ernest Gagnon Ave., Quebec 6, P.Q.; Lav '60. Staff, Jeffery Hales Hosp.

SOULES, Melville H.; 32 Hurndale Ave., Toronto 6, Ont.; Tor '18; Semi-Spec. (Int. Med.); Orientist in Statistical Correlation; Tel. HO 6-8102.

SOURKAS, Shena, (Rosenblatt); 4645 Montclair Ave., Montreal 28, P.Q.; Tor'43; Staff, Lachine General Hospital; Tel. 488-5064.

SOUTER, Alexander W.; 42-2nd St., Kirkland Lake, Ont.; 33 Government Rd. E. (res); Aberdeen (Scot.) '37; MCGP; Chief of Anaes., Kirkland Distr. Hosp.; Anaes., Bingham Gen. Hosp., Mathieson; Tel. 567-5331.

SOUTHCOTT, Frederick R.; 159 Ridout St. S., London, Ont.; Wes '43; M.C.G.P.; Tel. 434-3733.

SOUTHCOTT, Thomas J.; Ott '54; Res., Winnipeg Gen. Hosp., Winnipeg, Man.

SOUTHERN, Robert F.; Main St., Shelburne, Ont.; Wes '62; Staff, Shelburne Dist. Hosp. & Dufferin Area Hosp.; Tel. 925-3110.

SOUTHERN-HOLT, Mary G. (Mrs. Herisson); 408 University Ave., Fredericton, N.B. (res); Cape Town (S. Africa) '44; M.B., Ch.B.; DCH (Lond.); Dir., Maternal & Child Health, Dept. of Health, New Brunswick; Tel. GR 5-7711. Abroad.

SOUTHWOOD, Keith J.; Suite 3, 1217 Oxford St. W., London, Ont.; Tor'52; AMCGP; Courtesy Staff, Victoria, St. Joseph's, St. Mary's & Parkwood Hosp's.; Tel. 471-6810.

SOVEREIGN, Arthur E.; Medical Clinic, 3009-31st Ave., Vernon, B.C.; Alb '53; Paed; Tel. 542-4321.

SOVILJ, Vladimir; 1125 E. Hastings St., Vancouver 6, B.C.; Zagreb (Yugoslavia) '54; Paed; Tel. 682-6681.

SOWA, Edward; Wes '56; D.Psy; Psy; Clin. Dir., Boys Village, 1651 Sheppard Ave. W., Downsview, Ont.; Tel. 633-0515.

SOWBY, F. David; Chelsea, P.Q. (res); Tor '51; Sr. M.O., Radiation Serv., Dept. of Nat. Health & Welfare.

SOWDEN, Kenneth A.; No. 1 4th Ave. S., Roxboro, P.Q.; London (Eng.) '46; M.D. (Lond.), D. PhysMed; FRCP(C), PhysMed & Rehab.; Physiatrist-in-Charge, Royal Victoria Hosp.; Med. Dir., Occup. Ther. & Rehab. Centre; Ass't. Prof., McGill U.; Tel. 684-3764.

SOYKAN, Nihat; Istanbul (Turk.); Staff, Riverview Hosp., Essondale, B.C.

SPACEK, Miroslav; Prague (Czech.) '46; Staff, Grand Manan Hosp., Grand Manan, N.B.

SPACKMAN, Edward V.; 1215-3rd Ave. S., Lethbridge, Alta.; 543-14th St. S. (res); Minnesota (USA) '28; MCGP; Tel. FA 7-3915.

SPACKMAN, Fred N.; Cardston, Alta.; Alb '49.

SPACKMAN, Geoffrey C.; 1111 Union St., Kitchener, Ont.; Cambridge (Eng.) '51; MRCS (Eng.), LRCP (Lond.); MCGP; Tel. SH 3-3122.

SPACKMAN, Leo F.; 214-6 Ave. W. Calgary, Alta.; 3128 Kil-Kenny Rd. (res); Alb '46; Urol; Head Urol. Dept., Calgary Holy Cross Hosp.; Cons (Urol.), Colonel Belcher & Calgary Gen. Hosp's.; Tel. AM 3-7120.

SPACKMAN, Roy R.; Cardston, Alta.; Alb '48; Anaes.

SPAKOWSKI, Walerian J.; 407 Canada Bldg., Windsor, Ont.; 2715 Virgina Pk. A. (res); Qns '55; Urol; Att. Staff, Windsor Area Hosp.; Tel. 256-4558.

SPANER, Sidney; Col. Mewburn Pavilion, University Hosp., Edmonton, Alta.; 9130 Valleyview Dr. (res); Alb '37; Psy; Active Staff, University Hosp.; Court. Staff, Royal Alexandra Hosp.; Cons. Psy., D.V.A. Hosp.; Clin. Prof., U. of Alberta Tel. GE 9-5911, Loc. 375.

SPANKIE, William E.; 608 Greyhound Bldg., Calgary, Alta; 234-26th Ave. W. (res); Qns '06.

SPARK, Derek H.; Med. Arts Bldg., Spring Garden Rd., Halifax, N.S.; 3423 Howe Ave. (res); Durham (Eng.) '53; Psy; Staff, Nova Scotia Hosp., Dartmouth; Lect. (Psy.), Dalhousie U.; Tel. 469-7500. Abroad.

SPARKES, John W.; 736 Granville St., Vancouver, B.C.; 6355 Marguerite St. (res); Tor '39; OrthSurg; Active Orth.Staff, St. Paul's & Children's Hosp's.; Clin. Instr., U. of British Columbia; Tel. MU 1-2742.

SPARKS, Balfour B.; 226 Roncesvalles Ave., Toronto 3, Ont.; 44 High Park Blvd. (res); Tor '31; IntMed; Med. Staff, St. Joseph's Hosp.; Tel. LE 6-6475.

SPARKS, Fred P.; Alb '33; D.P.H.; PathBact; Staff, Plummer Mem.Hosp., Sault Ste. Marie, Ont.

SPARLING, Douglas W.; 510 Seaforth Med. Bldg., 3550 Cote des Neiges Rd., Montreal 25, P.Q.; 3025 Glencoe Ave., Town of Mount Royal (res); Tor '30; FACS; FRCOG; MRCOG; FACOG; DABOG; ObstGyn; Assoc., Dept. ObstGyn., Montreal Gen. & Royal Victoria Hosp's. Ass't. Prof. (ObstGyn) McGill U.; Tel. 932-5007.

SPARLING, Frederick N.: 331 Sheddon Ave., Oakville, Ont.; Man '40; AMCGP; Tel. 844-3561.

SPARLING, James R.; Qns'65; Res., Royal Victoria Hosp., Montreal 2, P.Q.

SPARROW, Cecil J.; Reserve Mines, N.S.; Tor '01.

SPARROW, George R.; Apt. 5, 17 Tremont, St. Catharines, Ont.; Ann St., Port Dalhousie (res); Tor'31; FRCOG, FRCS(C), ObstGyn; Chief of Dept. Obst. Gyn., Hotel Dieu Hosp., St. Catharines; Tel. MU 4-4651.

SPASOFF, Robert A.; Sask'65; Res., Montreal General Hosp., Montreal 25, P.Q.

SPAULDING, William B.; Faculty of Medicine, McMaster University, Hamilton, Ont.; Tor'44; FACP; FRCP(C), IntMed; Prof. of Med., & Associate Dean; Tel. 522-4971, Loc. 426.

SPEAKMAN, George F.; 2525 Pine St., Vancouver 9, B.C., 1711 Drummond Dr., Van. 8 (res); Man '51; Ophth; Vis. Staff, Van. Gen., St. Paul's, St. Vincent's & Children's Hosp's.; Tel. RE 6-0401.

SPEAKMAN, John S.; 734 Med. Arts Bldg., 170 St. George St., Toronto 5, Ont.; 14 Vesta Dr., Tor. 10 (res); Tor '52; F.R.C.S.(C), Ophth; Staff, Toronto Gen. Hosp.; Assoc. Ophth., U. of Toronto; Tel. 928-8012.

SPEAKMAN, Thomas J.; Ste. 420, 8409 - 112th St., Edmonton, Alta.; 7441 Saskatchewan Dr. (res); Man'46; DABNS, FACS, FRCS(C), NeurSurg; Att'd. NeurSurg., Edmonton Gen. Hosp.; Ass't. Clin. Prof. (NeurSurg), U. of Alberta; Tel. 439-1124.

SPEARMAN, W. F.; 267 O'Connor St., Ottawa, Ont., Ste. 202; 1068 Chelsea Dr. (res); Ott '51; Ophth; Active Staff, Ottawa Gen., Riverside Hosp., & Cons. Staff, St. Louis-Marie-de-Montfort Hosp's.; Lect. (Ophth.), U. of Ottawa; Tel. 233-4149.

SPEARS, John C.; 170 St. George St., Toronto 5, Ont.; 25 Pricefield Rd. (res); Wes '57; FRCP (C); IntMed; Staff, Women's College Hosp.; Clin. Teach., Dept. of Med., U. of Toronto; Clin. Teach., Dept. of Therapeutics, U. of Toronto; Tel. 923-1941.

SPECKEN, John C.; Box 430, Cloverdale, B.C.; Sask. '57; Tel. 574-5619.

SPECTOR, Alvin R.; 98 Ridge Hill Drive, Toronto 10, Ont.; Tor '56; Anaes; Staff, Central Hosp.; Tel. WA 5-8991. Abroad.

SPECTOR, Leo; 400 Ellendale Med. Bldg., 5845 Cote-des-Neiges Rd., Montreal 26, P.Q.; 2216 Fulton Rd., Twn. of Mt. Royal (res); McG '31; GenSurg; Assoc. Surg., Jewish Gen. Hosp.; Tel. 735-3312.

SPEERS, Edgar A.; 106 Main St. W., Welland, Ont.; 216 Merritt W. (res); Tor '35; FRCS(C), GenSurg; Staff, Welland Co. Gen. & Port Colborne Gen. Hosp's.; Tel. RE 4-4551.

SPELLER, Stuart L.; Box 6, Bethany, Ont.; Dal '52; M.C.G.P.

SPENCE, Edward; 545 King St., London, Ont.; Wes '04; F.A.C.P., IntMed.; Tel. 439-8921.

SPENCE, Magnus; 1185 Avenue Rd., Toronto, Ont.; Tor'32; MCGP; Staff, Sunnybrook DVA & Grace Hosp's.; Court. Staff, Wellesley Hosp.; Dir., Ontario Cancer Soc.; Phys., Royal Winter Fair; Tel. 483-3213.

SPENCE, John B.; The Spence Clinic, 910 Ridgeway St., Fort William, Ont.; 403 South John St. (res); Tor '44; F.A.C.S., F.R.C.S.(C), GenSurg; Med. Staff, McKellar Gen. Hsop.; Tel. 622-5301.

SPENCE, John H.; 330 Queens Ave., London, Ont.; 545 King St. (res); Wes '42; Courtesy Staff, St. Joseph's & Victoria Hosp's.; Tel. 432-3142.

SPENCE, Margaret T. (Dewan); Ste. 507, 215 Victoria St., Toronto, Ont.; 529 St. Clements Ave. (res); Tor '51; Anaes; Teach. Staff, St. Michael's Hosp.; Retired.

SPENCE, Matthew W.; 2702 Baker St., Ville St. Laurent, P.Q. (res); Alb '59; Research, Mtl. Neurol. Inst.; Tel. VI 2-1251.

SPENCE, William J. E.; 430 Med. Arts Bldg., 170 St. George St., Toronto 5, Ont.; 228 Dunvegan Rd. (res); Qns '49; F.R.C.S.(C), GenSurg; Surg., Toronto Gen. Hosp.; Assoc. (Dept. of Surg.), & Lect., Schl. of Nursing, U. of Toronto; Tel. WA 4-9932.

SPENCER, Charles L.; 21 Pandora St. S., Kitchener, Ont.; Lemberg (Pol.) '32; M.D. (Poznan); Staff, Kitchener-Waterloo & St. Mary's Hosp's.

SPENCER, Earle W.; Man '31; DMR (Eng.); D&TRad; Staff, Digby Gen. Hosp., Digby, N.S.

SPENCER, Herbert W.; 116 W. 15th St., North Vancouver, B.C.; 161 E. Keith Rd., Ste. 303 (res); Tor '52; Tel. 988-1131.

SPENCER, John L.; Box 760, Shellbrook, Sask.; Sask '57; Staff, Shellbrook Union Hosp.

SPENCER, Jon R. L.; 367 Roehampton Ave., Toronto 12, Ont.; Tor'61; Ophth.

SPENCER, Louis R.; 772 Lawrence Ave. E., Don Mills, Ont.; Cambridge (Eng.) '49; M.R.C.S., L.R.C.P.; M.C.G.P.; Tel. HI 4-6151.

SPERBER, Gregory H.; 3039 Med. Sciences Bldg., U. of Alberta, Edmonton, Alta.; '56.

SPICER, Richard; 321 Yarrow Bldg., 645 Fort St., Victoria, B.C.; 1900 Ferndale Rd. (res); London (Eng.) '38; Tell. EV 5-4141.

SPICER, Sterling L.; U.E. Lodge, R.R. No. 2, Prescott, Ont.; Wes '11; Tel. Area 613; WA 5-2141.

SPICUZZA, Francesco; 78 Barton St. W., Hamilton, Ont.; Tel. JA 2-4633.

SPIELMANN, Victor; 3028 Mountain Hwy., N. Vancouver, B.C.; 364 Brand St. (res); Vienna (Aust.) '45; Tel. YU 8-0707.

SPIKA, Otto; 2031-33rd Ave. S.W., Calgary, Alta.; 3136 Kilkenny Rd. (res); Vienna (Aust.) '51; MCGP; Tel. CH 2-1188.

SPILSBURY, Bert W., Sg. Lt. Cdr; Tor '53; GenSurg; Staff, Toronto Military Hosp., Toronto 12, Ont.

SPIRO, Charles H.; 150 Metcalfe St., Ottawa, Ont.; 69 Orrin Ave. (res); McG '23; Ophth, Otol; Otol., Ottawa Civic Hosp.; Tel. 232-7633.

SPIRO, Harold M.; Ste. 412, 750 W. Broadway, Vancouver 9, B.C.; 6445 Churchill St. (res); Dal '42; B.Sc.; DiagRad; Tel. TR 2-7595.

SPITTEL, Wallace H.; 102 Briar Hill Ave., Toronto, Ont. (res); Tor '33; Ass't. Med. Dir., Canada Life Assurance Co., Toronto; Tel. 368-7432.

SPITZER, Mary L.; Tor'62; Res. (Ophth.), Illinois Eye & Ear Infirmary, Chicago, Ill., U.S.A.; Abroad.

SPITZER, Ralph W.; 1911 Knox Rd., Vancouver 8, B.C.; Man'57; MC Path; Ph.D.; Cons. Clin. Chem., Royal Columbian Hosp.; Assoc. Prof. (Path.), U. of British Columbia; Tel. LA 2-2771.

SPITZER, Walter O.; Tor'62; MHA; Exec. Dir., Christian Med. Soc. (International), 1122 Westgate, Oak Park, Ill., U.S.A.; Tel. 848-9510; Abroad.

SPIVAK, Manuel M.; 1849 Yonge St., Ste. 513, Toronto 7, Ont.; Tor '56; FRCS(C), ObstGyn; Staff, Toronto Gen. Hosp.; Tel. 485-4416.

SPOEREL, Wolfgang E.; 287 Queens Ave., London, Ont.; 420 Lawson Rd. (res); Frankfurt (Main, W. Germ.) '49; FRCP(C), Anaes; Clin. Prof. & Hd. Dept. of Anaes., U. of Western Ont.; Tel. GE 8-5143.

SPOHN, A. Howard; 3389 Pine Cres., Vancouver 9, B.C. (res); Tor '05; F.R.C.P.(C), Paed; Cons. Staff, St. Paul's & Children's Hosp's.; Tel. RE 3-3136.

SPOHN, Frederick J. D.; 1718 Marine Dr., West Vancouver, B.C.; 2950 Palmerston Ave. (res); Man '52; MCGP; Att'd. Staff, Lion's Gate Hosp.; Vis. Staff, St. Paul's Hosp.; Tel. WA 2-6164.

SPOHN, James D.; 571 Park St., Kitchener, Ont.; Tor'50; MCGP; Staff, Kitchener-Waterloo Hosp. & St. Mary's Hosp.; Tel. 742-8866.

SPOHN, Philip D.; 209 King St. S., Waterloo, Ont.; Tor '10.

SPOONER, C. Martin; 404 Toronto Western Medical Bldg., 25 Leonard Ave., Toronto 2B, Ont.; 194 Sandringham Dr. (res); Man '25; F.A.C.S.; FRCS(C), GenSurg; Urol; Ass't. Prof. (Surg), U. of Toronto; Urol.-in-Chief, Toronto Western Hosp.; Cons.(Urol), Princes Margaret Hosp.; Tel. EM 6-2080.

SPOONER, E. Gordon; Medical Arts Clinic, Regina, Sask.; 3001 Whitmore Ave. (res); Tor '36; Ophth, Otol.; Tel. 522-1651.

SPOONER, H. J.; Medical Arts Bldg., Regina, Sask.; 3037 Angus (res); Tor '32; OrthSurg.; Tel. 522-1651.

SPOONER, John D.; Thompson, Man.; Sask '61; Tel. 677-4521.

SPOONER, J. Stanley; 407 Canada Bldg., Windsor, Ont.; 1174 Devonshire Rd. (res); Tor '46; FACS; FICS; Urol; Active Staff (Urol.), Grace, Metropolitan & Hotel-Dieu Hosp's.; Cons. (Urol.), Riverview Hosp.; Tel. CL 6-4558.

SPOONER, Michael A.; Medical Arts Clinic, 2125-11th. Ave., Regina, Sask.; Tor '63; Tel. LA 2-1651.

SPOUGE, John D.; 6211 Wiltshire St., Vancouver 13, B.C.; (res); Sheffield (Eng.) '53; MDS; FDS; LRCP MRCS (Eng.) Assoc. Prof. (Oral Path.), U. of British Columbia.

SPRAGGE, J. William; 118 Simcoe St. N., Oshawa, Ont.; Tor '57; A.M.C.G.P.

SPRAGUE, J. D.; 968 Queen St. E., Sault Ste. Marie, Ont.; 29 Summit Ave. (res); Qns '38.

SPRAGUE, Percy H.; 521 Med. Arts Bldg., 11010 Jasper Ave., Edmonton, Alta.; 10334-130th St. (res); Alb '27; M.S.(Med.Minn.), F.A.C.P., D.A.B.I.M., M.C.A.A.; IntMed (Allerg.); Att'd. Staff, University & Royal Alexandra Hosp's.; Hon. Prof. (Med.), U. of Alberta; Retired.

SPRATT, E. H.; 940 Queen St., Sault Ste. Marie, Ont.; Tor '24.

SPRATT, Ernest H.; Wes '64; Res., Toronto Western Hosp., Toronto 2B, Ont.

SPRATT, Leslie M.; Tor '23; F.C.C.P.; IntMed (TB); Med. Dir., Beck Mem. Sanatorium; Clin., U. of Western Ont., London, Ont.; Tel. GE 2-2681.

SPRENGER, Robert A.; Box 87, Whitehorse, Y.T.; Man'48; Zone Dir., Chief M.O.H., Yukon.

SPRING, Morris H. R.; 988 Glencairn Ave., Toronto, Ont.; 602 Vesta Dr. (res); Tor '47; M.C.-G.P.; O.P.D., New Mt. Sinai & Northwestern Gen. Hosp's.; Tel. RU 2-1515.

SPRING, William B.; 99 Avenue Rd., Toronto 5, Ont.; 24 Viewmount Ave. (res); Tor '45; Urol; Jr. Att. Surg. (Urol.) Mt. Sinai Hosp.; Tel. WA 2-5790.

SPROAT, William C.; 52 Albert St., Stratford, Ont.; 386 William St. (res); Wes '26; F.A.C.S., GenSurg; Chief of Surg., Stratford Gen. Hosp.; Tel. 271-4050.

SPROAT, William R. E.; 407 Canada Bldg., Windsor, Ont.; 2196 Victoria Ave. (res); Wes '48; Urol; Staff, Div. Urol., Metropolitan, Hotel Dieu. & Grace Hosp's.; Tel. 256-4558.

SPROUL, R. Douglas; Ste. 105, 4900 Kingsway, S. Burnaby, B.C.; Man '52; D&TRad; Assoc. Rad., Burnaby Gen. Hosp.; Tel. HE 4-1345.

SPROUL, Robert F.; 234 Augustus St., Cornwall, Ont.; Tor'53; MCGP.

SPROULE, Brian J.; University Hosp., Edmonton, Alta.; Alb'51; M.Sc.; FCCP; FACP; FRCP(C), IntMed; Hd., Div. of Resp. Diseases, University Hosp.; Assoc. Prof. Med., U. of Alberta; Tel. GE 9-5911, Ext. 378.

SPROULE, Herman F.; 67 College St., Toronto 2, Ont.; Tor '39; Staff, Ontario Dept. of Health, T.B. Prevention.

SPROULE, W. Glenn; 425 Roselawn Dr., Windsor, Ont.; Ott'55; GenSurg; Tel. YO 9-4160.

SPROULL, Donald M.; 136 Simcoe St. N., Oshawa, Ont.; Glasgow (Scot.) '50; DABS; FACS; GenSurg; Active Staff, Oshawa Gen. Hosp.; Cons. Staff, Mem. Hosp., Bowmanville & Ajax & Pickering Gen. Hosp's.; Tel. 728-7571.

SPROWL, David L.; 2 Maple Ave. N., Burford, Ont.; Tor '63; Tel. 449-2421.

SPUDAS, Alexander; 2300 Lawrence Ave. E., Scarborough, Ont.; Mainz (Germ.)'61; Courtesy Staff, Scarborough General Hospital; Tel. 751-0082.

SPRUENKEN, Johannes M.; Ste. 1118, 925 W. Georgia St., Vancouver 1, B.C.; Berlin (Germ.) '37; Otol. (Germ.); Vis. Staff, Vancouver Gen., St. Paul's, Mt. St. Joseph's & Children's Hosp's.; Tel. MU 1-7034.

SPRUNG, Elizabeth B.; 1068 Eyremont Dr., West Vancouver, B.C. (res); Alb '39; Pt-time, North Shore Union Bd. of Health.

SPURGEON, Charles H.; 570 Waterloo St., London, Ont.; Wes '52; M.C.G.P.; Dist. M.O., CNR.

SPURRELL, Pierce A.; 1 Campbell Ave., St. John's, Nfld.; Dal'53; FRCP(C), IntMed; Dir., Div. of Resp. Dis. & Diag. Endoscopy, Grace Gen. Hosp.; Tel. 579-1199.

SQUIRE, Donald A.; 632 Vanderburgh Dr., Burlington, Ont. (res); Bristol (Eng.) '40; M.B., Ch.B., Dip. Psy (Tor); Psy; Unit Dir., Ontario Hosp., Hamilton; Tel. NE 4-8148.

SQUIRE, James B.; 108-118 Med. Arts Bldg., 404 Graham Ave., Winnipeg 1, Man.; 621 South Dr., Wpg. 19 (res); Dal '41; D & T Rad; Cons. Rad., Deer Lodge Hosp.; Att. Staff (Rad.), Grace Hosp.; Tel. 943-7301.

SQUIRES, Arthur H.; 730 Med. Arts Bldg., Toronto 5, Ont.; 282 St. Leonard's Ave. Tor. 12 (res); Tor '35; F.R.C.P.(C), IntMed; Phys.-in-Chief, Wellesley Hosp.; Cons. (Med.), Sunnybrook DVA & Princess Margaret Hosp's.; Assoc. Prof., U. of Toronto; Tel. WA 2-8263.

SQUIRES, Bruce P.; Wes'58; Ass't. Prof., Dept. of Physiol., U. of Western Ont., London, Ont.; Tel. 679-3852.

SQUIRES, Franklin J.; 160 Gordon Rd., Willowdale, Ont.; Man '45; Tel. BA 1-7701.

SQUIRES, Wayne G.; 416 Souris Ave., Weyburn, Sask.; Sask'61; Active Staff, Weyburn Union Hosp.; Tel. 684-5202.

SQUIRES, William G.; Cottage Hosp., Stephenville Crossing, Nfld.; Dal'66.

SRETER, Frank A.; Dept. of Anat., U. of British Columbia, Vancouver, B.C.

STACEY, Cooper H.; 1390 Sherbrooke St. W., Ste. 35, Montreal 25, P.Q.; McG '49; FACP; FRCP(C), IntMed; Ass't. Phys., Royal Victoria Hosp.; Ass't. Prof. (Med.), McGill U.; Chief Med. Exam. Bank of Montreal & Royal Trust Co.; Tel. AV 8-2802.

STACEY, Donald L. 14 Lynn Dr., Dartmouth, N.S. (res); Dal '56; Psy; Unit Dir., Nova Scotia Hosp. Tel. 469-7500.

STACHEWITSCH, Andreas; 103 Bord-d'l'Eau, Ste-Dorothee, P.Q.; Freiburg (Germ.) '55; Haem (P.Q.); Paed; Staff, Montreal Children's Hosp.; Tel. WE 7-6011.

STACKHOUSE, John G.; 240 Algonquin Ave., North Bay, Ont.; Qns'60; GenSurg.

STACPOOLE-RYDING, Frank; 6319 Bowness Dr., Calgary, Alta.; London (Eng.) '52; MRCS (Eng.); LRCP (Lond); Tel. 288-2121; Abroad.

STAFFORD, C. Michael; Grenfell, Sask.; Cambridge (Eng.) '52; M.C.G.P.

STAFFORD-MAYER, George; Innisfail, Alta.; Cambridge (Eng.) '34; L.R.C.P., M.R.C.S., F.R.-C.S. (Eng.).

STAHL, Oscar J.; 434 St. Paul St., St. Catharines, Ont.; 10 Adam St. (res); Tor '26; F.R.-C.S. (Edin.); GenSurg; Assoc. Staff, GenSurg, Hotel Dieu & St. Catherine's Gen. Hosp.; Tel. MU 4-2326.

STALKER, Gordon B.; 364 Kerrybrook Dr., Richmond Hill, Ont.; Tor '11; Retired.

STALKER, H. Stewart; 700 W. 57th St., Vancouver, B.C.; 1122 W. 27th, Van. 9 (res); Man '28; FCCP; IntMed (TB); Med. Dir., Pearson TB & Polio. Hosp.; Tel. 321-3231.

STALKER, M. John; 137 Cedar St., Sudbury, Ont.; 2A Cobalt, Coppercliffe (res) Tor '54; IntMed; Tel. 674-7011.

STALKER, Merrill E.; Ormstown Med. Centre, Ormstown, P.Q.; McG'51; MCGP; IntMed(P.Q.); Staff, Barrie Mem. Hosp.; Tel. 829-2331.

STANCER, Harvey C.; Clarke Inst., 250 College St., Toronto 2B, Ont.; Tor'57; PhD; Psy; Staff, Clarke Inst.; Ass't. Prof., U. of Toronto; Tel. 924-6811.

STANCER, Samuel L.; Apt. 104, 320 Tweedsmuir Ave., Toronto 10, Ont.; Tor '53; Staff, Health Centre, Parliament Bldgs., Toronto; Tel. EM 3-1211.

STANDEN, James R.; 294 Westcourt Pl., Waterloo, Ont.; Tor'59; FRCP(C), DiagRad.

STANDING, Harold K.; Box 757, Thompson, Man.; Man'58; Tel. 677-4521.

STANDLEY, Jonathan M.; 1806 Jane St., Weston, Ont.; Cambridge (Eng.) '59.

STANDRET, Daniel T.; 1437 Tyandaga Pk. Dr., Burlington, Ont.; Tor'60; Ophth.

STANFIELD, Michael J.; 204 Professional Bldg. 407 Graham Ave., Winnipeg 1, Man.; Sheffield (Eng.) '58; Tel. 942-2431.

STANFORD, Gary B.; 303 Med. Centre, 906-8th Ave. S.W., Calgary, Alta.; Alb '61; Tel. 263-4685.

STANFORD, Ronald L.; 4500 Sherbrooke St. W., Montreal 6, P.Q.; St. Bruno (res); McG'43; Int-Med (Cardiol.); Phys.-in-Charge Cardiol., St. Mary's Hosp.; Ass't Phys., Royal Victoria Hosp.; Lect. (Med. & Clin. Med.), McGill U.; Tel. 933-7914.

STANLEY, Gerald N.; Qns '64; Res., Kingston Gen. Hosp., Kingston, Ont.

STANLEY, John C.; P.O. Box 266, Rothesay, N.B. (res); National U. (Ire.) '47; Psy; Med. Supt., Children's Hosp. School, Lancaster.

STANLEY, Paul; 3875 rue St-Urbain, Montreal 18, P.Q.; Mon '51; GenSurg (P.Q.); Tel. 842-3865.

STANLEY, Raymond F.; 149 Kenneth St., Duncan, B.C.; Gibbins Rd. (res); Alb '51; King's Daughters Hosp.; Tel. 478-8151.

STANLEY, Robert A.; Ste. 380, 5655 Cambie St., Vancouver 15, B.C.; 5075 Marguerite St. (res); Man '39; MCGP; Clin. Instr., UBC; Tel. 261-8155.

STANLEY, Willard H.; 118 Simcoe St. N., Oshawa, Ont.; 530 Brookside Dr. (res); Wes '34; F.I.C.S., GenSurg; Staff, Oshawa Gen. Hosp.; Tel. 723-2144.

STANNERS, James; Daysland, Alta.; Glasgow (Scot.)'47; MB; ChB.

STANSFIELD, Hugh; Ste. 1212, Fairmont Medical Bldg., 750 West Broadway, Vancouver 9, B.C.; 6551 Wiltshire St., Vancouver 14 (res); Alb'42; **D.I.M., IntMed.; (Cardiol); Att. Staff, Vancouver Gen. Hosp.; Clin. Instr. (Med.), U. of British Columbia; Tel. TR 2-1913.**

STANTON, Irving I.; 2600 Eglinton Ave. W., Toronto 15, Ont.; 559 Briar Hill Ave. (res); Tor '49; M.C.G.P.; Staff, New Mt. Sinai & North-western Gen. Hosp's.; Tel. RO 7-0723.

STANTON, John J.; Qns '41; D.P.H.; Adm., Dept. of Public Health, Halifax, N.S.; Telephone 422-7341, Loc. 551.

STANTON, Oliver L.; R.R. 1, Scott Rd., Ganges, B.C.; Tor'29; Hon. Staff, Lady Minto Gulf Islands Hosp.; Tel. 537-2898.

STANTON, Rodger C.; 17-11th Ave. S., Cranbrook, B.C.; UBC'56; FRCS(C); GenSurg; Tel. 426-2001.

STANULYTE, Ruta; Turbingen (Germ.)'54; Staff, Doctor's Hosp., Toronto 4, Ont.

STANWOOD, D. H.; 1654 Renfrew St., Vancouver 6, B.C.; 2705 E. 23rd Rd. (res); Wes '42; M.C.G.P.; Active Staff, Burnaby Gen. Hosp.; Tel. AL 3-8833.

STANYON, John H.; 260 Cedar St., Sudbury, Ont.; 1870 Ramsey View Crt., Apt. 616 (res); Tor '36; IntMed.; Chief of Med., Sudbury Gen. & Sudbury Mem. Hosp's.; Chief Phys., International Nickel Co.; Tel. 673-3695.

STAPLES, John C.; Drawer 390, Parsons Clinic, Red Deer, Alta.; 4406-43 Ave. (res); Alb'48; MCGP; Staff, Red Deer Municipal Hosp.; Tel. 346-2042.

STAPLES, Thomas E.; 399-10th St., Hanover, Ont.; Wes'56; MCGP; Active Staff, Hanover Mem. Hosp.; Assoc. Satff, Walkerton Hosp. & Owen Sound Gen. & Marine Hosp.; Tel. 364-2820.

STAPLETON, John G.; McGregor Clin., 250 Main St. E., Hamilton, Ont.; Wes'41; FACR; DABR; DiagRad; Dir. of Rad. & Chmn., Bd. of Governors, McGregor Clinic, Hamilton, Cons. Rad., D.V.A. & Ontario Hosp., Hamilton; Tel. JA 7-2711.

STAPLETON, John H.; 54 Nanaimo Ave. E., Penticton, B.C.; 813 Winnipeg St. (res); Man '42; Att'd. Staff, Penticton Hosp.; Tel. 492-2937.

STAPLETON, Joseph J. E.; 1323 South Park St., Halifax, N.S.; Sydney (Australia) '44; DR (Sydney); DMRT; TherRad; Hd. (TherRad), Victoria Gen. Hosp.; Assoc. Prof. (Rad.), Dalhousie U.; Tel. 422-7371. Abroad.

STAPLETON, Martin W.; Box 188, Seaforth, Ont.; Wes'37; MCGP.

STARCK, Gordon P.; 844 Autumnwood Dr., Winnipeg 6, Man.; Cambridge (Eng.); MRCS; LRCP; D.Obst; RCOG.

STARDY, A. W.; 8123—118 Ave., Edmonton, Alta.

STARINK, Adriann W.; Utrecht (Neth.) '52; Res., Kingston Gen. Hosp., Kingston, Ont.

STARK, Eric J.; 556 Medical Arts Bldg., Saskatoon, Sask.; 505 Lake Cres. (res); Tor '46; Otol; Head, Otol. Serv., Saskatchewan U. Hosp.; Ass't. Clin. Prof. Surg., U. of Saskatchewan; Tel. 652-5585.

STARK, Gordon D.; Edinburgh (Scot.) '60; Res., Grace Hosp., Winnipeg 10, Man.

STARK, Ronald B.; Kyle, Sask.; London (Eng.) '41; MRCS (Eng), LRCP (Lond.); Staff, Kyle-White Bear Union Hosp.; Tel. 50.

STARK, W. Berkeley; 170 St. George St., Toronto, Ont.; 213 Strathallan Wood (res); Tor '15; M.S. Otol. (Minnesota), D.A.B.Ot.; Retired.

STARKEY, D. Hugh; 465 Cote-St.-Antoine Rd., Westmount 6, Mtl. P.Q.; McG '31; Bact; Dir. of Labs., Queen Mary Vet's. Hosp.; Adviser, Lab. Serv., DVA; Tel. RE 8-9481.

STARKMAN, Seymour; 99 Avenue Rd., Toronto 5, Ont.; 16 Fraserwood Ave. (res); Tor '51; F.R.C.P.(C), Neurol; Att. Phys., New Mt. Sinai Hosp.; Tel. WA 3-7524.

STARKO, Marvin M.; 225 Professional Bldg., 10830 Jasper Ave., Edmonton, Alta.; Alb '57; Otol.

STARK-RUEFFEL, Liselotte A.; Heidelberg (Germ.)'49; Staff, Chest Clinic, Victoria Hosp., Prince Albert, Sask.; Staff, Saskatchewan Anti-T.B. League; Tel. 763-3266.

STARON, Natalie M.; see DYER, Natalie M.

STAROSTE, Karl H.; 186 Oakwood Ave., Toronto, Ont.; 401 Clinton St. (res); Bonn (Germ.) '51; M.C.G.P.; Staff, Northwestern Gen. Hosp.; Tel. 536-4685.

STARR, Isadore; 5354 St. Urbain St., Montreal, P.Q.; Mon '52; IntMed.

STARR, Joseph A.; Tor'64; Res., Toronto Gen. Hosp., Toronto 2, Ont.

STARRATT, Victor C.; 6291 Coburg Rd., Halifax, N.S.; 6059 Oakland Rd. (res); Dal '53; AMCGP; Tel. 423-7167.

STARRS, Robert A.; 263 Somerset St. W., Ottawa, Ont.; Qns '27; F.A.C.P., F.R.C.P.(C), IntMed; Cons. Staff, Dept. Med., Ottawa Civic Hosp.; Tel. 232-1345.

START, Richard K.; Brant Sanatorium, Brantford, Ont.; Qns '28; IntMed (TB).

STASIAK, Joseph; 8 Campbell Ave., St. John's, Nfld.; Kaunas (Lith.)'42; Urol; Active Staff, St. Clare's Mercy Hosp.; Assoc. Staff, Grace & General Hosp's.; Tel. 722-3193.

STASIUK, Peter; 54 Canary Cres., Willowdale, Ont. (res); Wes 54; Admin. Staff, Physician's Servs. Inc., Toronto; Tel. HU 7-3311.

STASIUK, Russell B.; Man'65; Jr. Int., St. Boniface Hosp., Winnipeg, Man.; Abroad.

STATTEN, Page; 200 St. Clair Ave. W., Toronto, Ont.; 269 St. Leonard's Ave. (res); Tor '42; Otol; Ass't. Surg., Dept. Otol., Sick Children's Hosp.; Cons., Ontario Crippled Children's Centre. Clin. Inst'r., Dept. Otol., Toronto U.; Tel. WA 1-8106.

STATTEN, Taylor; Tor'40; Paed; Psy; Chief Psy., Student Health Serv., U. of Toronto, Toronto 5, Ont.

STAUB, Ludvik; 637 College St., Toronto, Ont.; 20 Heathdale Rd. (res); Rome (Italy) '53; Tel. LE 3-2425.

STAUBLE, William J.; 49 Glenview Ave., Toronto 12, Ont.; McG'52; D.Psy; Psy; Dir. of Education & Sr. Psy., Clarke Inst. of Psych.; Dir. of Education & Assoc. Prof. Psy., U. of Toronto; Tel. 924-6811.

STAVRAKY, George W.; 7 Thornton Ave., London, Ont. (res); '32; Prof. of Physiol, U. of Western Ontario.; Tel. VI 4-6311.

STAVRAKY, Kathleen M.; 105 Grand Ave., London, Ont. (res); Wes '58.

STAVRAKY, Waldo K.; 382 Queen's Ave., London, Ont.; Wes'58; FRCS(C), GenSurg; PlasSurg; Staff, Westminster Hosp.; Tel. GE 2-6711.

STAVRIDES, Alexander; 403 Agnes St., New Westminster, B.C. (res); Thessaloniki (Gr.) '53; Path; Staff, Dept. of Path., Royal Columbian Hosp.; Tel. LA 2-2771.

STAYURA, Lois A.; Alb '59; FRCP(C), Paed; Staff, University Hosp., Edmonton, Alta.

STEAD, Llewellyn T.; Dal'52; Res., Victoria Gen. Hosp., Halifax, N.S.

STEAD, Stanley; 330 Medical-Dental Bldg., Regina, Sask.; 40 Gardiner Ave. (res); Manchester (Eng.) '51; Dip. Ophth; Ophth; Staff, (Ophth), Regina Gen. & Grey Nuns' Hosp's.; Tel. LA 2-3024.

STEADMAN, Page; 584 Jones Ave., Toronto 6, Ont.; Wales '62.

STEBNICK, Alfred O.; Ste. 205, 5780 Cambie St., Vancouver 15, B.C.; Lav '43; Otol; Active Staff, Vancouver Gen. Hosp.; Cons. Staff, Shaughnessy Hosp.; Vis Staff, St. Paul's, St. Vincents & Children's Hosp's.; Clin. Instr. (Surg.), U. of British Columbia; Tel. 321-0522.

STECHISHIN, Orest; 14012-90A Ave., Edmonton, Alta. (res); Alb '43; M.Sc. (Biochem.); Anaes; Staff Anaes., Edmonton Gen. Hosp.; Tel. HU 8-8181.

STEED, Barrie L.; 310 Med. Centre, 906-8th Ave. S.W., Calgary, Alta.; Alb'65.

STEED, Charles M.; Witwatersrand (S. Africa) '52; DiagRad; Assoc. Rad., Greater Niagara General Hosp., Niagara Falls, Ont.

STEEDMAN, John A.; 4400 W. Grandview, Douglas Hwy., North Burnaby, B.C.; Tor'57; DPM; Psy.

STEEDS, J. Leslie; 77 Upper Middle Rd., Cooks-ville, Ont.; Tor '46; FACOG; ObstGyn; Active **Staff, South Peel & Queensway Gen. Hosp's.; Assoc. Staff, Toronto Western Hosp.; Tel. 279-1741.**

STEEL, Doreen (See PATRICK, Doreen).

STEELE, Bernard J.; 1525 Oxford St., Halifax, N.S.; Ott '42; GenSurg; Tel. 422-5922.

STEELE, B. S.; 73 Queen St. E., Brampton, Ont.; Tor'65; Assoc. Staff Memb., Peel Memorial Hosp.

STEELE, Darryl N., Capt.; Ortona Barracks Mir., Oakville, Ont.; Tor'65.

STEELE, Donald C. 27 Church St., St. Catharines, Ont.; 136 Highland Ave. (res); Tor '56; GenSurg; Tel. MU 4-3832.

STEELE, Earl C.; 200 Douglas Dr., Toronto, Ont. (res); Tor '32; Commr., Workmen's Comp. Bd., Ont.; Tel. 362-3411.

STEELE, F. Hawthorne; 216 Medical Arts Bldg., 170 St. George St., Toronto, Ont.; 241 Inglewood Dr. (res); Tor '29; Otol; Staff, Toronto East Gen. & St. Michael's Hosp's.; Teach. U. of Toronto; Tel. WA 2-5857.

STEELE, Howard D.; 47 Copperfield Dr., Kingston, Ont.; Qns '44; Path; Assoc. Dir. Clin. Labs & Dir. of Blood Bank, Kingston Gen. Hosp.; Path., Cdn. Forces & St-Mary's-of-the-Lake Hosp's.; Ass't. Prof (Path.), Queen's U.; Tel. 546-3841.

STEELE, John B.; Dal'58; Res., Nova Scotia Hosp., Dartmouth, N.S.
STEELE, John C.; 157 Collier St., Toronto 5, Ont.; Tor'59; FRCP(C), Neur; Staff, Toronto Gen. Hosp.; Tel. EM 6-8211.
STEELE, J. Philip; 130 Elm E., Sudbury, Ont.; Tel. 673-7181.
STEELE, Phyllis L.; Balcarres, Sask.; Alb '34; M.C.G.P.
STEELE, Robert; 64 Traymoor Ave., Kingston, Ont.; Glasgow (Scot.)'52; LRCP, LRCP(Ed); LRFPS(Glas.); DPH(Ed.).
STEELE, Robert J.; 26 Church Ave., Willowdale, Ont.; Loma Linda (Calif.)'51.
STEENSON, Gordon W. D.; 1st Ave., Ashern, Man. (res); Man '49; M.C.G.P.; M.O.H., Grahamdale, Siglunes; Dist. Coroner.
STEEPE, C. A. D.; Inco Medical Centre; Sudbury, Ont.; 278 Wellington Heights (res); Wes '50.
STEER, Donald G.; Ste. 407, 450 Central Ave., London, Ont.; 1010 Harrison Ave. (res); Wes '34; F.R.C.S.(E); GenSurg; Court. Staff, St. Joseph's & Victoria Hosp's; Tel. 439-9311.
STEER, John C.; 832 Headley Dr., Oakridge Park, London, Ont.; Tor'34; D.Psy; MCGP.
STEEVES, Lea C.; Dalhousie Public Health Clinic, University Ave., Halifax, N.S.; McG '40; FACP; FRCP(C), IntMed; (Cardiol.); Assoc. Att'd. Phys., Victoria Gen. Hosp.; Med. Spec., Camp Hill DVA Hosp.; Prof. of Med. & Dir. P.G. Div. & Ass't. Dean, Dalhousie U.; Tel. 429-1420, Loc. 262.
STEEVES, Richard A.; Apt. 805, 1868 Main St. W., Hamilton, Ont.; Wes'61.
STEFANCIK, Jan; Box 250, Vegreville Clinic, P.O. Box 250, Vegreville, Alta.; Alb'57; Tel. 632-2234.
STEFANELLI, John; 815 Victoria St., Trail, B.C.; 1355-2nd Ave. **(res); Alb '48; GenSurg;** Tel. 364-1234.
STEFANI, Martin; 4179 Lakeshore Rd., Burlington, Ont.; Staff, Hamilton Gen. Hosp. '39.
STEFANIK, George; Box 190, Fort St. John, B.C. Alb '55; GenSurg. Abroad.
STEFANYK, Harry; 728 Professional Bldg., 10830 Jasper Ave., Edmonton, Alta.; 7908-143rd St. (res); Alb '56; FRCP(C); IntMed; Staff, Edmonton General Hosp.; Tel. 488-8181.
STEIDL, Pippa E.; 418 Sherbrooke E., Montreal 24, P.Q.; Vienna (Austria) '49; Ophth; Tel. AV 8-7829.
STEIMAN, Iser; 612 Fairmont Med. Bldg., 750 W. Broadway, Vancouver 9, B.C.; Man '24; MCGP; Lectr., U. of British Columbia; Tel. TR 9-6505.
STEIN, David H.; Mall Med. Bldg., 280 Osborne St. N., Winnipeg, Man.; 520 Oxford St. (res); Tor '47; F.R.C.P.(C), IntMed; Assoc. Staff, St. Boniface Hosp., & Cardiol Misericordia Hosp., Dem (Med), U. of Manitoba; Tel. SP. 4-2411.
STEIN, Denis; 2385 Perodeau, Quebec 6, P.Q.; Lav'45.
STEIN, Harold A.; 170 Bloor St. W., Toronto 5, Ont.; 3000 Lawrence Ave. E., Scarborough, Ont.; Tor'53; MS (Ophth) (Minn); D.O. (Lond.); FRCS(C), Ophth; Att'd Staff, New Mount Sinai Hosp. & Sunnybrook Hosp.; Chief of Ophth., Scarborough Gen. Hosp.; Tel. WA 1-2131 & 923-4117.
STEIN, Mark M.; 1437 Queen St. W., Toronto, Ont.; 65 Lyndhurst Ave. (res); Tor '41; D.A.B.-I.M., F.R.C.P.(C), IntMed; Jr Attend. Phys., New Mt. Sinai Hosp.; Dir. Metropolitan Private Hosp; Tel. LE 3-1432.
STEIN, Paul B.; 437 Hale St., London, Ont.; London (Eng.) '62; M.B., B.S.; AMCGP; Tel. 451-9880.
STEIN, Samuel; Sask'62; Res., Children's Hosp., Montreal 25, P.Q.
STEIN, Werner O.; 118 Young St., Kitchener, Ont.; Freiberg (Germ.) '29; Paed; Staff, Kitchener-Waterloo & St. Mary's Hosp's.; Tel. SH 5-9451.
STEINBERG, Jacob; Qns'62; Res., Banting Inst., 100 College St., Toronto, Ont.
STEINBERG, James; Man'59; Res., Toronto Gen. Hosp., Toronto 2, Ont.
STEINBERG, Samuel; 835 Henderson Hwy., E. Kildonan, Winnipeg, Man.; 346 McAdam Ave. (res); Man '54; Attend. Staff, Ger. Sec., Dept. of Med., Deer Lodge Hosp.; Tel. ED 4-1353.
STEINBERG, Sidney; 314 St. Clair Ave. W., Toronto 10, Ont.; 29 Forest Wood (res); Tor '46; DermSyph; Att'd. Staff, New Mt. Sinai, Baycrest & North York Branson Hosp's.; Court. Staff, Doctor's Hosp.; Tel. WA 1-0046.
STEINER, Betty W. (Morris); 507 Medical Arts Bldg., 170 St. George St., Toronto 5, Ont.; 98 Banbury Rd. Don Mills (res); Liverpool U. (Eng.) '42; D.Psy; Psy; Ass't. Dir., Psy Unit, Women's College Hosp.; Tel. WA 1-9500.
STEINER, George; UBC'60; FRCP(C), IntMed; Staff, Dept. of Med., Banting Inst., Toronto 2, Ont.
STEINER, Jan W.; 98 Banbury Rd., Don Mills, Ont. (res); Prague (Czech.) & Liverpool (Eng.) '43; FRCP(C), Path; Assoc. Dean Student Affairs & Prof. (Pathol.), U. of Toronto; Tel. WA 3-6611.
STEINHARDT, Marvin I.; 550 University Ave., Toronto 2, Ont.; Berne (Switz.) '56; D.M.R.; DiagRad; Radiol., New Mount Sinai Hosp.; Tel. EM. 6-7361.
STEINHART, Melvin; 47 Charleswood Dr., Downsview, Ont.; Wes'60; DiagRad.
STEINHAUER, Paul D.; 59 Strathearn Rd., Toronto 10, Ont.; Tor '57; Psy; Staff, Thistletown Hosp.; Tel. CH 6-7491.
STEINHOFF, Gerhard E.; 385 Hebert St., Port Arthur, Ont.; Qns '57; AMCGP; Tel. 344-8475.
STEINMETZ, Nicholas; McG '63; Res., Children's Hosp., Montreal 25, P.Q.
STEINS, Adolf; 33 King St., Bolton, Ont.; Riga (Latvia)'44; Staff, Dufferin Area Hosp., Orangeville; Tel. 857-1344.
STEINSON, E. Bruce; Ste. 206, 625-5th Ave., New Westminster, B.C.; UBC'59.
STELLOS, Apostolos G.; 600 Med. Arts Bldg., Montreal 25, P.Q.; 116 Willowdale Ave., Outremont (res); Athens (Gr.) '53; Urol; Staff, Reddy Mem. & Lachine Gen. Hosp's.; Tel. WE 2-9285.
STELZER, Elizabeth; 415 King St. E., Hamilton, Ont.; Tel. JA 2-2263.
STENICKA, Francis J.; 157 Westbrook Mall, Calgary S.W., Alta.; 3031 Roxboro Glen Rd. (res); National U. (Ire.) '52; LAH (Dublin); MCGP; Active Staff, Holy Cross, Calgary Gen., Grace Alberta Children's & Auxillary Hosp's. Tel. 249-0611.
STENSTROM, John D.; Medical Arts Bldg., 1105 Pandora Ave., Victoria, B.C.; 2460 Cardigan Rd. (res); McG '38; F.R.C.S.(C), F.R.C.S.(Ed.), D.A.B.S., GenSurg; Tel. EV 5-1614.
STENTAFORD, Thomas S. G.; Newfoundland Anaesthesia Associates, 95 Le Marchant Rd., St. John's, Nfld.; 11 Winter Ave. (res); Dal '38; Anaes; Chief Anaes., St. John's Gen. Hosp.; Vis. Anaes., St. Clare's Mercy, Grace Maternity, St. John's Mental Hosp's & T.B. San.; Tel. 578-7909.
STEPAN, Michel; 150 King St. W., Sherbrooke, P.Q.; 301 Blvd. Desaulniers (res); Louvain (Belgium) '39; Tel. 569-4762.
STEPHANSSON, Norman S.; P.O. Box 160, Flin Flon, Man.; Man '39; MCGP; Phys., Cdn. National Railways & HBMS Co. Ltd.; Tel. 7-7571.
STEPHEN, Alexander; 514 Queen St., Saskatoon, Sask.; 1008-11th St. E. (res); Aberdeen (Scot.) '41; Psy; Med. Dir., MacNeill Clin. for Psy. Serv.; Clin. Assoc. (Psy.), U. of Saskatchewan; Tel. 652-4640.
STEPHEN, Charles H.; Vanderhoof, B.C.; McG '57; MCGP.
STEPHEN, David H.; 688 Coxwell Ave., Toronto 13, Ont.; 127 Birchcliff Ave., Scarborough (res); Tor '59; Tel. 699-1601.
STEPHEN, Hugh M.; 2080 Fairbank Ave., Ottawa, Ont. (res); Qns '27; D.P.H.; Registrar, Med. Council of Canada, 77 Metcalfe St., Ottawa 4, Ont.; Tel. CE 5-0948.

STEPHEN, James D.; 18 Turnbull Place, Regina, Sask., (res); St. Andrews (Scot.) '43; M.D. (Minn.), Path; Dir. Labs., Regina Gen. Hosp.; Med. Dir., Regina Depot, Can. Red Cross Blood Trans. Serv.; Clin. Assoc. (Path.), U. of Saskatchewan; Tel. LA 2-1811.
STEPHEN, Lawrence J.; 31-3rd Ave., N.E., Dauphin, Man.; 308 River Ave. (res); Man '55; MCGP; Med. Staff, Dauphin Gen. Hosp.; Tel. 638-3730.
STEPHEN, Leonard J.; Provincial Bldg., 90 Charlotte St. St. John, N.B.; R.R. 2, Rothesay, N.B. (res); Dal '49; Chief, M.O., WCB; Tel. 692-0181.
STEPHEN, Malcolm T.; Shediac, N.B.; Dal '59.
STEPHEN, Wesley J.; 114 Carleton St., Saint John, N.B.; McG '48; GenSurg; Att. Surg. Staff, St. John Gen. Hosp.; Tel. 692-1432.
STEPHENS, Clinton A.; 170 St. George St., Toronto, Ont.; 68 Hillholme Rd. (res); Tor '42; F.R.C.S.(C) GenSurg; Surg. Staff, Hosp. for Sick Children Assoc. (Surg.), U. of Toronto; Tel. WA 3-4954.
STEPHENS, Clive W.; 2226 Greenlands Rd., Victoria, B.C.; Alb'30; MCGP.
STEPHENS, Gordon M.; Counselling Serv., Student Union Bldg., U. of Manitoba, Fort Garry, Man.; 37-361 Westwood Dr., Wpg. 22 (res); Man'31; Psy; Assoc. Prof. Psy., U. of Manitoba; Psy. Cons. Counselling Serv., U. of Manitoba, Fort Garry; Tel. 474-9495.
STEPHENS, Hazel G.; Medical Centre, Stettler, Alta.; London (Eng.)'58.
STEPHENS, Herbert H.; Aberhart Mem. San., Edmonton, Alta.; Alb'32; IntMed(TB); Med. Supt., Aberhart Mem. San.; Dir., Div. of T.B. Control, Prov. of Alta.; Lect. Med., U. of Alberta; Tel. GE 9-0051.
STEPHENS, James G.; 749 King St. W., Kitchener, Ont.; Wes '52; GenSurg; Tel. 742-9290.
STEPHENS, Overton E.; 4151 Sheppard Ave. E., Agincourt, Ont.; Tor '34; M.C.G.P.; Telephone AX 3-4189.
STEPHENS, Robert O.; 4805 Yonge St., Willowdale, Ont.; Tor'47; DTM&H; MCGP; Tel. 222-4521.
STEPHENS, William B.; 4857 Kingsway, Burnaby 1, B.C.; 5743 Ontario, Vancouver 16 (res); Qns '51; Staff, Burnaby Gen. Hosp.; Tel. HE 4-4211.
STEPHENSON, Bette M. (Mrs. G. A. Pengelly); 20 McKee Ave., Willowdale, Ont.; Tor '46; M.C.-G.P.; Chief, Dept. G.P., & Dir., O.P.D., Women's College Hosp., Toronto; Tel. BA 1-7100.
STEPHENSON, Charles; 1450 Hillside Ave., Victoria, B.C.; London (Eng.) '58; M.S., B.S.; MRCS (Eng.); LRCP (Lond.).
STEPHENSON, Donald G.; 742 King W., Kitchener, Ont.; McG '54; PlasSurg.; Tel. 742-1531.
STEPHENSON, Earl; 605 Medical Arts Bldg., Winnipeg, Man.; 1167 Grosvenor Ave. (res); Man '31; FRCS(Edin.), FRCS(C), FICS, Ch.M., Urol: Urol., Deer Lodge Vets' Hosp.; Chief Urol., St. Boniface Hosp.; Ass't. Prof. (Urol.), U. of Manitoba; Tel. WH 2-2841.
STEPHENSON, Gordon H.; 202-755 W. Broadway, Vancouver 9, B.C.; 793 W. 26th Ave. (res): Tor '43; Psy: Att'd. Staff, Van. Gen. & Cons Psy., Grace Hosp's.; Dir., Narcotic Research & Rehab., Oakalla Prison Farm; Tel. TR 6-5422.
STEPHENSON, John M.; McBirnie Cleland, Port Colborne, Ont.; 218 Catherine St. (res): Tor '46; Chief of Med., Port Colborne Gen. Hosp.; Tel. TE 4-3556.
STEPHENSON, P. Susan (Penford); London (Eng.)'60; Psy; Staff, Vancouver Gen. Hosp., Vancouver, B.C.; Abroad.
STEPHENSON, Robert G.; 897 McIntyre St. W., North Bay, Ont. (res); Tor '45; Psy: Ass't. Supt., Ont. Hosp.; Tel. GR 4-1200.
STERLIN, Carlo; Haiti '56; FRCP(C), Psy; Staff, Hop. des Laurentides, L'Annonciation, P.Q.
STERN, Antony M.; McG '62; **Jr. Intn., Montreal Gen. Hosp., Montreal 25, P.Q.**
STERN, Dennis J.; London (Eng.) '60; Staff, Riverdale Hosp., Rivers, Man.; Tel. 328-5305.
STERN, Karl; 3830 Lacombe Ave., Montreal, P.Q.; 3800 Grey Ave. (res); Frankfurt (Germ.) '32; Psy; Psy-in-Chief, St. Mary's Hosp;. Assoc. Prof. (Psy), U. of Montreal; Prof. (Psy), U. of Ottawa; Tel. RE 7-3944.
STERN, Leo; 2300 Tupper St., Montreal 25, P.Q.; Man'56; FRCP(C), Paed; Dir., Premature & Newborn Nursery, Montreal Children's Hosp.; Lect. (Paed.), McGill U.; Tel. WE 7-8511, Loc. 446.
STERN, Leslie E.; Man'64; Res., Neurological Inst., 3801 University, Montreal 2, P.Q.
STERN, Lloyd G.; Ste. 320, 6000 Cote des Neiges Rd., Montreal 26, P.Q.; McG '43; Psy; Ass't. Psy., Jewish Gen. Hosp.; Dem. (Psy.), McGill U.; Tel. RE 1-2394.
STERN, Sandor G.; 187 St. Clair Ave. W., Toronto 7, Ont.; Tor'61; AMCGP; Tel. 925-7412.
STERN, Sidney; Beechy, Sask.; Glasgow (Scot.) '57.
STERNBERG, Joseph; 359 Wiseman Ave., Outremont, Mtl., P.Q.; Bucharest (Roum.) '37; M.Sc., MACP; MRSM (Lond.); Prof. (Physiol. & Nuclear Med.), U of Montreal; Tel. RE 3-9951; 271-2255.
STERNS, Ernest E.; Etherington Hall, Queen's University, Kingston, Ont.; Qns '58; FRCS(C); GenSurg; Lect. (Surg.), Queen's U.
STERNS, Laurence P.; Ste. 550, 8409-112th St., Edmonton, Alta.; Qns'55; FRCS(C), Cardiovasc. & ThorSurg.
STERNTHAL, Edward; McG'64; Res., Queen Elizabeth Hosp., Montreal 28, P.Q.
STEVENS, Arnott H.; 19 Richards Dr., Dartmouth, N.S.; Tor '50; MOH I/C Halifax Dept. of National Health & Welfare.
STEVENS, Burnley W.; Fort William Clinic, 117 S. John St., Fort William, Ont.; R.R. No. 2, Fort William (res); Tor '32; F.R.C.S.(Eng.), **F.R.C.S.(C) GenSurg; Surg., McKellar Hosp.; Tel. MA 2-5363.**
STEVENS, Donald G. H.; 628 Davis Dr., Ste. 103, Newmarket, Ont.; Wes '59; Paed; Active Staff, York County Hosp.; Tel. 895-8151.
STEVENS, Estelle M. (Heakes); Tor '49; Staff, (Psy), Nova Scotia Hosp., Halifax, N.S.; Tel. 466-7411.
STEVENS, Eugene; Plattsville, Ont.; Tor '28; M.C.G.P.; Tel. 684-7452.
STEVENS, G. Cyril; 229 Medical Arts Bldg., Winnipeg, Man.; 313 Park Blvd., Tuxedo, Wpg. 29 (res); Man '30; M.C.G.P.; Tel. WH 2-4847.
STEVENS, Harry D.; 109 Med. Arts Bldg., Montreal 25, P.Q.; McG '50; FRCS(C), GenSurg; Assoc. Surg., Reddy Mem. Hosp.; Cons. Surg., Queen Mary Vets. Hosp.; Ass't. O.P.D., Surg., Royal Victoria Hosp.; Dem. (Surg.), McGill U.; Tel. WE 7-1968.
STEVENS, Ian H. K.; 625 South Dr., Fort Garry, Winnipeg, Man.; London (Eng.)'25; MRCP; MRCS; D.ObstRCOG; Retired.
STEVENS, Joaquin M.; 450 Dundas St., Woodstock, Ont.; 145 Vansittart Ave. (res); Tor '48; Retired.
STEVENS, Nora E.; Sutton West, Ont.; Wes'65.
STEVENS, Robert; 3236 Weston Rd., Weston, Ont.; Wales (U.K.)'55; MB; BCh; DCH(Eng.).
STEVENS, William B.; 4900 Kingsway, Burnaby, B.C.; 4027 Southwood (res); Qns '51; Staff, Burnaby Gen. Hosp.; Vis. Staff, Mt. St. Joseph & Grace Hosp's.; Tel. HE 1-6696.
STEVENSON, Cameron McK.; 1 Grenville Cres., Kingston, Ont. (res); Qns '55; Psy; Staff, Ont. Hosp.; Assoc. Staff, Kingston Gen. Hosp.; Chief Psy., Male Serv., Ont. Hosp.; Lect. Psy., Queen's U.; Tel. 546-1101.
STEVENSON, Colan M.; London (Eng.)'53; MA(Cantab); Res., Hosp. for Sick Children, Toronto, Ont.
STEVENSON, C. Keith; Martin St., Milton, Ont.; Queen St. (res); Tor '28; M.C.G.P.: Chief of Staff, Milton Dist. Hosp.; Dist. Coroner. Retired.
STEVENSON, E. M.; 3105—31st St., Vernon, B.C.; Wes '45; Tel. 542-5700.

STEVENSON, George H.; 1222 Harwood St., Vancouver, B.C. (res); Tor '18; Psy; Research Prof. in Psy., U. of British Columbia; Retired.

STEVENSON, Henry C., MBE; Box 625, Minnedosa, Man.; Man '45; D.G.O. (Trinity), L.M. (Rotunda); Dist. Coroner; Tel. 867-2722.

STEVENSON, Isabel C.; 801 Royal Ave., Calgary, Alta. (res); Alb '50; Anaes; Staff, Calgary, Gen. Hosp.; Tel. AM 6-7541.

STEVENSON, James A.; 346 South St., London, Ont.; 145 Wychwood Place (res); McG '42; Cons. (Research), Westminster DVA Hosp.; Ed., Cdn. Jrl. Physiology & Pharm.; Prof. & Hd., Dept. of Physiol., U. of Western Ont.; Tel. GE 9-1681.

STEVENSON, John D.; 1541 W. Broadway, Vancouver 9, B.C.; 718 Granville St.; 2184 W. Broadway; 530 Eastcot Rd., West Vanc. (res); Man'45; DiagRad; TherRad; DABR; Assoc. Dir. (Rad.), St. Paul's Hosp.; Tel. RE 1-5394.

STEVENSON, Lloyd G.; 573 Lansdowne Ave., Westmount, Montreal, P.Q.; Wes '44; Ph.D. (Med. Hist., Johns Hopkins U., U.S.A.); Prof. History of Med. & Dean, Faculty of Med., McGill U.; Tel. VI 4-6311.

STEVENSON, L. John; 42 Bayview Dr., Lancaster, N.B. (res); Dal '48; D.A.B.R., Rad, D& TRad; Assoc. Rad., Gen. Hosp., St. John, N.B.; Tel. 693-3351.

STEVENSON, Robert H.; Edinburgh (Scot.)'33; Industrial M.O., Shawinigan Chemicals Ltd., Box 330, Shawinigan, P.Q.

STEVENSON, Theodore K.; Ste. 508, 625-5th Ave., New Westminster, B.C.; 301-3rd St. (res); Man '48; FACS; GenSurg; Chief of Surg., St. Mary's Hosp.; Surg. Staff, Royal Columbian Hosp.; Cons., Surrey Mem. & Burnaby Mem. Hosp's.; Tel. LA 2-9808.

STEVENSON, William D.; Med. Arts Bldg., 5880 Spring Garden Rd., Halifax, N.S.; 19 Waegwoltic Ave. (res); Tor '37; M.S. (Tor.), F.R.C.S.(C), NeurSurg; GenSurg; NeurSurg., Victoria Gen. Hosp.; Cons. (NeurSurg) DVA, Halifax Children's & N.S. Hosp's.; Assoc. Prof. (NeurSurg), Dalhousie U.; Tel. 2-4406.

STEVENSON, W. Joly S/L; 450 Moorgate St., St. James 12, Winnipeg, Man.; Trinity Coll. (Dublin, Ire.) '53; MPH (Harvard); Reg. FL/Surg. & Deputy Reg. Surg., Prairie Med. Reg. H.Q.; Tel. VE 2-1311, Loc. 270.

STEWARD, David J.; London (Eng.)'58; M.B., B.S.; LRCP; MRCS; Res., Sunnybrook Hosp., Toronto 12, Ont.

STEWARDSON, Elmer R.; Moose Jaw Clinic, 200 Scott Bldg., Moose Jaw, Sask.; 1143 Redland Ave. (res); Man'36; MCGP; Dir., Moose Jaw Clinic; Tel. 692-2373.

STEWART, A. James; 610 Fairmont Med. Bldg., 750 W. Broadway, Vancouver, B.C.; 1708 Allison Rd. (res); McG '38; Ophth; Clin. Teach., Fac. of Med., U. of British Columbia; Tel. RE 1-3108.

STEWART, Alexander R.; Glasgow (Scot.) '58; D.ObstRCOG; DPM; Clin. Dir. & Cons. Psy., Saskatchewan Hosp., Weyburn, Sask. Tel. 842-5461.

STEWART, Alfred E.; 3095 Church St., South Windsor, Ont. (res); Tor '04; Retired.

STEWART, Andrew R.; 10004-105th St., Edmonton, Alta.; Alb'61; Paed.

STEWART, Bruce M.; Tor'58; FRCP(C), Neur; Staff, St. Michael's Hosp., Toronto, Ont.; Clin. Instr. (Neurol.), U. of Toronto; Tel. EM 2-4461, Ext. 403.

STEWART-BURTON, Ann; Ste. 905, 1849 Yonge St., Toronto 7, Ont.; UBC'58; FRCS(C), ObstGyn; Staff, Grace Hosp.

STEWART, Cameron C.; 803 Glenmanor Dr., Oshawa, Ont. (res); Qns '51; DPH; MOH, City of Oshawa; Tel. 725-1153.

STEWART, C. Burton; Winnipeg Clinic, Winnipeg, Man.; Man '28; FRCS(Ed.) FRCS(C), Urol; Hon. Cons., Wpg. Gen., Children's & Grace Hosp's.; Assoc. Prof. (Surg.), U. of Manitoba; Tel. 942-0551.

STEWART, Charles; 134 Spruce St., Elliot Lake, Ont.; McG '59; Tel. VI 8-7118.

STEWART, Charles A.; 287 Queens Ave., London, Ont.; Wes '33; Anaes; Staff, Victoria Hosp.; Instr. U. of Western Ont.; Tel. GE 8-5143.

STEWART, C. Gordon; 6 Tweedsmuir Pl., Deep River, Ont. (res); Tor '43; D.T.M.; Dir. Med. Div., Atomic Energy of Canada Ltd.; Tel. Pembroke 732-9911, Loc 462.

STEWART, Chester B.; 6008 Oakland Rd., Halifax, N.S. (res); Dal '38; FAPHA; Dr.PH; DPH; MPH(Johns Hopkins); FRCP(C); PH; Dean, Faculty of Med. & Prof. of Epidemiology, Dalhousie U.; Cons. Nova Scotia Dept. of Health; Tel. 422-1361-400.

STEWART, Daniel L.; Musgravetown, Nfld.; St. Mary's (London, Eng.)'49; AMCGP.

STEWART, David; 179 Brookfield Cr., Oakville, Ont.; Glasgow (Scot.)'48; LRCP&S; LRFPS (Glas.); DPH(Tor.).

STEWART, David G.; Crapaud, PEI; Dal '62; AMCGP; Tel. 36.

STEWART, Donald A.; Tor '43; Paed; Staff, Hosp. for Sick Children, Toronto 2, Ont.

STEWART, Donald H.; 307 Grosvenor N., Hamilton, Ont.; Qns '24; Tel. LI 4-3427.

STEWART, Donald R.; Campbell Clinic, 430 Mayor Magrath Dr., Lethbridge, Alta.; 1603-23rd St. S. (res); Sask. '59; Staff, St. Michael's & Lethbridge Mun. Hosp's.; Tel. FA 7-5737.

STEWART, Donald W.; 1935 W. Broadway, Vancouver 9, B.C.; 404-W.22nd St. (res); UBC '57; Tel. 731-7111.

STEWART, E. H. Friel; 1310 Ouellette Ave., Windsor, Ont.; 2072 Willistead Cres. (res); Wes '44; Tel. CL 2-0311.

STEWART, Earle W.; 605 Medical Arts Bldg.; Winnipeg, Man.; '25; Tel. WE 2-5813.

STEWART, Edith G.; 283 Metcalfe St., Ottawa 4, Ont.; 233 Powell Ave. (res); Aberdeen (Scot.) '51; AMCGP; Staff, Ottawa Civic & Grace Hosp's.; Tel. 236-0564.

STEWART, Elizabeth L.; 2 Sultan St., Toronto 5, Ont. (res); Tor '11; D&TRad; Retired.

STEWART, Frances E.; 452 Hunter St. W., Peterborough, Ont. (res); Tor '42; Part-time Public Health.

STEWART, Frances H.; 104 West Block, Medical Arts Bldg., 280 Bloor St. W., Toronto 5, Ont.; 37 Kilbarry Rd. (res); Tor '38; Ass't. Dir. (Women), University Health Serv.; Telephone WA 2-7537.

STEWART, Frederick W.; National Health & Welfare, Immigration Bldg., Halifax, N.S.; Queen's U. (Belfast, Ire.)'56.

STEWART, Gerald N.; The Knox Clinic, 1605 Glenmore St., Kelowna, B.C.; 2375 Abbott St. (res); UBC '56; MCGP; Tel. 762-2002.

STEWART, Gilbert L.; 688 Coxwell Ave., Toronto 13, Ont.; Wes'60; AMCGP.

STEWART, Glen G.; Box 1813, Courtenay, B.C.; Alb '56; GenSurg.

STEWART, Harold B.; 118 Base Line Rd E., London, Ont.; Tor '44; Prof. of Biochem., U. of Western Ontario; Tel. GE 9-3764.

STEWART, Harold P.; 224 Queen St., Charlottetown, P.E.I.; Dal '45; MCGP; Active Staff, P.E.I. Hosp.; Court. Staff, Charlottetown Hosp.; Tel. 894-9811.

STEWART, H. Leslie; Ste. 202, 6156 Quinpool Rd., Halifax, N.S.; 6021 Roxton Rd. (res); Dal '44; GenSurg; Staff, Victoria Gen. Hosp.; Teaching Staff (Surg), Dalhousie U.; Tel. 422-4545.

STEWART, Ian F.; Box 130, Salmo, B.C.; Glasgow (Scot.)'46; Tel. 357-2221 & 2222.

STEWART, Ian MacL.; 23 Johnson Ave., Charlottetown, P.E.I.; St. Mary's Hosp. (London, Eng.)'52; DPM; Psy; Cons. Psy., P.E.I., Charlottetown & Prince County Hosp's.; Dir. Adult O.P. Clinics, P.E.I.; Tel. 892-2904.

STEWART, Ian M.S.; 9308-147 St., Edmonton, Alta. (res); Aberdeen (Scot.) '44; D.P.H. (Aberdeen), D.T.M.&H. (Eng.) M.O., W.C.B., Tel. GA 2-7151.

STEWART, Irwin F.; Westminster Med. Bldg., 625-5th Ave., New Westminster, B.C.; UBC'56; DLO(Lond.); FRCS(C), Otol; Deputy Chief Otol., Royal Columbian Hosp.; Chief Otol., St. Mary's Hosp.; Cons. Otol., Shaughnessy, Surrey Mem. & Maple Ridge Hosp's.; Tel. 521-2424.

STEWART, J. Donald; 3465 Cote des Neiges Rd., Ste. 53, Montreal 25, P.Q.; McG'54; Psy(P.Q.); Sr. Psy., Douglas Hosp.; Clin. Ass't. O.P.D., Montreal Gen. Hosp.; Tel. WE 7-6802.

STEWART, J. Duncan; 1598 Ouellette Ave., Windsor, Ont.; 2020 Loraine Ave. (res); Tor '41; IntMed.; Chm. (Med.) & Pres. Med. Staff, Metropolitan Gen. Hosp.; Tel. CL 4-8819.

STEWART, John A.; 723 Fort St., Victoria, B.C.; 418 Beach St. (res); Qns '12, OphthOtol; Tel. EV 3-0921. Retired.

STEWART, John D.; 900 King St. W., Kitchener, Ont.; Tor'58; IntMed; Staff, St. Mary's Gen. & Kitchener-Waterloo Hosp's.; Tel. 744-0161.

STEWART, John F.; Tor '50; DTM&H; GenSurg; Med. Staff, Ontario Hosp. School, Smiths Falls, Ont.

STEWART, John M.; 287 Queens Ave., London, Ont.; R.R. 3 (res); Wes '43; Anaes; Instr. (Anaes), U. of Western Ont.; Tel. GE 9-1681.

STEWART, John T.; 156 St. Paul Cr., St. Catharines, Ont.; Glasgow (Scot.)'54; Tel. 684-8507.

STEWART, John T. R.; 327 Charlotte St., Peterborough, Ont.; 452 Hunter St. W. (res); Tor '40; F.A.C.S.; GenSurg; Surg. Staff, Peterborough Civic & St. Joseph's Hosp's.; Cons. Campbellford Mem. Hosp.; 1966-67 Pres., Cdn. Assoc. Med. Clinics; Tel. 743-2040.

STEWART, John W.; Dal'63; Res., Montreal Gen. Hosp., Montreal 25, P.Q.

STEWART, Joseph P.; La Scie, Nfld.

STEWART, Kenneth G.; 148 Frederick St., Kitchener, Ont.; 215 Pandora Cres. (res); Tor '36; M.C.G.P.; Staff, Kitchener-Waterloo & St. Mary's Hosp's.; Tel. SH 5-7635.

STEWART, K. Royal; 149 Cartier Ave., Pointe Claire, P.Q.; McG'51; FRCP(C), IntMed; MCGP; Tel. 695-2101.

STEWART, Lloyd N.; 72 Bowland Ave., Sudbury, Ont. (res); Tor '43; D. & TRad; Rad., Dept. of Rad., Sudbury Gen. Hosp.; Tel. OS 3-3601.

STEWART, Mary H.; 10 Brooke Ave., Toronto, 12, Ont. (res); Tor '36; Phys., Gage Inst.

STEWART, Neil A.; T.C.A. Vancouver Amf., Sea Island, B.C.; Alb '33; Anaes.

STEWART, Neil R.; 227 Yarrow Bldg., 645 Fort St., Victoria, B.C.; 3065 Beach Dr. (res); Edinburgh (Scot.) '41; M.R.C.P. (Ed.), IntMed; Act. & Cons. Staff, St. Joseph's & Victoria Veterans' Hosp's.; M.H.O., Mun. of Oak Bay; Tel. EV 3-2312.

STEWART, Olive J.; 396 Victoria St., London, Ont.; Wes '35; Psy; Staff, Victoria Hosp.; Cons. (Psy), Westminster & Parkwood Hosp's.; Lect. (Psy), U. of Western Ont.; Tel. GE 4-4024.

STEWART, Oscar W.; 3634 Lorne Cres., Apt. 5, Montreal, P.Q.; Tel. AV 8-9379.

STEWART, P. Brian, DFC; 42 Answorth Rd., Westmount, Montreal 6, P.Q. (res); Middlesex Hosp. London U. (Eng.)'50 MRCP(Lond.); Clin. Ass't. Royal Victoria Hosp.; Ass't. Prof. (Med.) McGill U.; Med. Dir. Pharma-Research Canada Ltd., Pointe Claire; Tel. RE 9-2351.

STEWART, R. Colin; Box 190, Stewiacke, Colchester Co., N.S.; Dal '56; Tel. 378-2484.

STEWART, Robert A.; 414 Main St. E., Hamilton, Ont.; Qns '34; Tel. JA 7-3033.

STEWART, Robert F.; Blairmore, Alta.; Man '24; Retired.

STEWART, Robert J.; 15206-76A Ave., Edmonton, Alta. (res); Alb '54; Anaes; Staff, Royal Alexandra Hosp.; Tel. GR 4-3431.

STEWART, Robert W. G.; 508 Upper Gage Ave., Hamilton, Ont.; Aberdeen (Scot.)'53; D.Obst RCOG; AMCGP; Active Staff, Henderson Gen. Hosp.; Assoc. Staff, St. Joseph's & Chedoke Gen. Hosp's.; Tel. 385-4025.

STEWART, Roger G.; 501 Krug St., Kitchener, Ont.; Wes'62; AMCGP.

STEWART, Roy M., S/L; Box 185, CFB Comox, B.C.; Guys H. (London, Eng.)'54; Tel. 339-2211, Loc. 213.

STEWART, Thomas H.M.; Ottawa Gen. Hosp., Ottawa, Ont.; Edinburgh (Scot.) '55; FRCP(C), IntMed; Dir. Clin. Radiosotope Unit.; Instr. U. of Ottawa; Tel. CE 6-4592.

STEWART, Thomas W.; 340 McLeod, Ottawa 4, Ont.; Wes'50; Psy.

STEWART, William B.; 165 Hedgewood Dr., Moncton, N.B. (res); Dal '52; FRCP(C), DiagRad; Ass't Chief Rad., Moncton City Hosp.; Tel. EV 4-4421.

STEWART, William C.; Ralston, Alta. (res); Qns '47; Hd., Physiol. Defence Research Bd., Suffield Experimental Station, Ralston; Tel. 201.

STEWART, William D.; 745 W. Broadway, Vancouver 9, B.C.; 940 Younette Dr., W. Van. (res); Washington (USA) '50; FRCP(C), IntMed; Derm; Att'd. Staff (OPD), Van. Gen. Hosp.; Clin. Instr. (Derm), U. of British Columbia; Tel. TR 4-8138.

STEWART, William D.; 315 Greyhound Bldg., 622-1st St. S.W., Calgary, Alta.; 2117-2nd Ave. N.W. (res); Alb '44; Otol; Staff, Calgary Gen., Col. Belcher, Children's & Holy Cross Hosp's.; Tel. AM 2-3139.

STEWART, W. Gordon; 350 Beech Ave., Toronto, Ont.; 14 Pine Cr. (res); Tor'36; MCGP; Med. Dir., Beach Clinic; Med. Dir., Medical Testing Lab.; Med. Supt., Birchcliff Nursery Home; Tel. OX 4-1126.

STEWART, William R.; 139 North River Rd., Charlottetown, P.E.I. (res); Dal '51; Dir. of O.P.D. Clinics, Dept. of Health; Cons. P.E.I. & Prince County Hosp's.; Ass't. Supt. Provincial San.; Tel. 894-3290.

STEWART, Wilma G. (Allison); 2068 Chalmers Rd., Ottawa 8, Ont.; Tor '43; Staff Off., Med. Sec. Defence Research Bd. H Q.

STEWART, W. W.; 514—6th Ave., New Westminister, B.C.; Qns '35; Tel. LA 2-4814.

STIBBS, D. Michael; 7171 King George Hwy., North Surrey, B.C.; 13076-Coulthard Rd., R.R. 1, Cloverdale (res); London (Eng) '55; Tel. 596-8311.

STIBBS, Philip A.; U.K. '55; Intn., Toronto Gen. Hosp., Toronto 2, Ont.

STICKLES, Lee E.; 206 Rookwood Ave., Fredericton, N.B.; 11 Tamarack Terr. (res); Dal '55; FAAP; Paed; Staff, Victoria Public Hosp. & Polio Clinic Health Centre; Tel. 475-7701.

STICKNEY, Margaret G. (Rendall); Fergus, Ont.; Tor '35; Dip.Psy (Tor.).

STILES, Esmond; 19 Union St., St. Stephen, N.B.; McG'34; Chief of Surg., Charlotte County Hosp. & Staff, Calais Regional Hosp., Calais, Me., U.S.A.; Tel. 466-1577.

STILES, Gerald B.; Medical Arts Bldg., 539 Cassells St., North Bay, Ont.; 351 Worthington St. E. (res); Dal '53; GenSurg; Tel. 472-3620. Abroad.

STILES, Jack H.; 17 Elwood Blvd., Toronto, Ont. (res); Tor '31; Ass't. Med. Dir., Physician's Services Inc.; Tel. HU 7-3311.

STILL, Hereford C.; 6178 Quinpool Rd., Halifax, N.S.; Cambridge (Eng.) '43; MA, MCGP; Ass't. Phys., Victoria Gen. Hosp.; Instr. (Med.), Dalhousie U.; Tel. 423-7003.

STILLER, Calvin R.; Sask'65; Res., Victoria Hosp., London, Ont.

STILLWATER, Richard B.; 814 Boyd Bldg., 388 Portage Ave., Winnipeg 1, Man.; Man '57; Otol; Att'd. Staff, St. Boniface & Children's Hosp's.; Court. Staff, Misericordia, Grace, Victoria & Man. Rehab. Hosp's.; Dem. (Otol.), U. of Manitoba; Tel. WH 3-3354.

STILLWELL, J. Bernard; Campbell Clinic, Lethbridge, Alta.; 1010-15th St. S. (res); London U. (Eng.) '55; D.Obst., RCOG; Tel. FA 7-5737.

STILMAN, Abraham; 525 Ellendale Med. Bldg., 5845 Cote-des-Neiges Rd., Montreal 26, P.Q.; 4949 Grosvenor Ave. (res); Mon '31; F.A.C.S., Urol; Urol., Jewish Gen. Hosp.; Tel. RE 1-9531.

STILWELL, Harold E.; Alb '59; DiagRad; Staff, Royal Alexandra Hosp., Edmonton, Alta.; Tel. GR 4-3431.

STINSON, David A.; Ste 332, 200 St. Claire Ave. W., Toronto 7, Ont.; 177 Bayview Hgts. Dr. (res); Tor '49; MSc., F.R.C.P.(C), IntMed; Staff, Toronto Gen. Hosp.; Cons. Cardiol, Sunnybrook (DVA) Hosp.; Spec. Lect. Schl. of Social Work & Clin. Instr., U. of Toronto; Tel. WA 5-1572.

STINSON, Dora A.; Wes '63; Int., Montreal Children's Hosp., Montreal 25, P.Q.

STINTON, Arthur W.; 32 Academy Med. Bldg., 1812-4th St. S.W., Calgary, Alta.; McG'49; Plant Phys., C.I.L.; Clin. Phys., Div. of Alcoholism, Dept. of Health; Tel. 263-7272.

STIPE, Reginald; Lake Ave., Manitou Beach, Sask.; 4 Watrous Ave. (res); Tor '06; Retired.

STIPEC, Joseph; 9562-120th St., North Surrey, B.C.; 11744 River Rd. (res); Tor '57; Tel. 581-6233.

STIRLING, Mary; 6389 Coburg Rd., Halifax, N.S.; Dal '59; MCGP.

STIRLING, Robin A.; Tor '58; Staff, Ontario Hosp., Woodstock, Ont.; Tel. 539-1251.

STIRLING, Roderick J.; 306 Royal Trust Bldg., 612 View St., Victoria, B.C.; McG'52; Tel. 382-5129.

STIRRAT, James H.; 203 Professional Bldg., 10830 Jasper Ave., Edmonton, Alta.; 601 Valleyview Manor, Jasper Ave. (res); Glasgow (Scot.) '38; M.D. (Path, Glasgow); FC (Path, Eng.); Path; Dir. of Labs., Misericordia Hosp.; Con. Path, Edmonton Gen., Grand Prairie Mun. & High Prairie Hosp's.; Advisor & Guest Lect., (Med.), Northern Alberta Inst. of Technology; Ass't. Prof. (Path), U. of Alberta; Tel. HU 8-0921.

STITT, Howard S.; 292 Oakdale Ave., St. Catharines, Ont.; 167 Riverview Blvd. (res); Tor '58; Active Staff, St. Catharines Gen. Hosp.; Tel. MU 2-8344.

STITT, John F.; 21 Ashmount Cres., Weston, **Ont. (res); Tor '48; Staff, TB Hosp., Weston; Tel. 769-1161.**

STITT, Robert B.; Tor'61; FRCS(C), GenSurg; Staff, Kingston Gen. Hosp., Kingston, Ont.

STITT, William D.; 456 Med. Arts Bldg., 750 Spadina Cr. E., Saskatoon, Sask.; Alb '56; Obst Gyn; Tel. 242-2429.

STIVER, Walter B.; 26 Alexandra Wood, Toronto 12, Ont. (res); Tor '32; D.P.H.; Med. Dir., Physicians' Services Inc., 2221 Yonge St., Toronto; Tel. HU 7-3311.

STOBIE, A. Malcolm; Med. Centre, 68 King St. E., Cobourg, Ont.; Oxford (Eng.)'51; DRCOG; Staff, Cobourg & Trenton Hosp's.

STOBIE, George H.; McG '50; F.R.C.S.(C), GenSurg; Staff, Hosp. for Sick Children, Toronto 2, Ont.; Tel. EM 6-7242. Abroad.

STOBIE, Stephen N.P.; 693 McCowan Rd., Scarborough, Ont.; 22 Richbourne Crt., Agincourt (res); St. Andrews (Scot.) '43; DPH(Edin.); D.Psy; Psy; Att'd. Psy., Scarborough Gen. Hosp.; Cons. Psy., Juvenile Court, 311 Jarvis St., Toronto; Tel. AM 7-4964.

STOCK, George W.; 805 Med. Arts Bldg., 170 St. George St., Toronto 5, Ont.; 132 Lawrence Cres., Tor. 12 (res); Tor '48; FRCP(C), IntMed; Staff, Phys. Toronto Gen. Hosp.; Cons. Phys.,

STOCK, John S.; 249 William St., Belleville, Ont.; Tor'52; MCGP; Staff, Belleville Gen. Hosp.; District Coroner; Tel. 962-4300.

Sunnybrook Hosp.; Assoc. (Med.), U. of Toronto; Tel. WA 1-8636.

STOCK, Marvin; 1573 Eglinton W., Toronto, Ont.; 436 Glengrove W. (res); Tor '47; M.C.-G.P.; Staff, Mt. Sinai, & Northwestern Gen. Hosp's.; Tel. RU 3-3314.

STOCKDALE, Edwin; 5607 Dunbar St., Vancouver 13, B.C.; 2930 W. 38th Ave. (res); Guy's Hosp. (London, Eng.) '57; Tel. 263-3555.

STOCKDALE, Elizabeth C.; (See MARTIN, Elizabeth C.).

STOCKINGS, George T.; 2446-22nd St., Saskatoon, Sask.; London (Eng.) '36; M.B., B.S., DPM (Lond.); Staff, (G.P.), St. Paul's Hosp.; Tel. 652-5511.

STOCKS, Allan G.; Brooklin Medical Centre, Brooklin, Ont.; Brooklin (res); Tor '51; M.C.-G.P., Staff, Oshawa Gen. Hosp. Tel. 655-3321.

STOCKTON, Harold; Ste 405, 1541 W. Broadway, Vancouver 9, B.C.; Tor '35; FAAP; Paed; **Hd. (Dept. of Paed.), St. Paul's Hosp.; Active Staff, Children's Hosp.; Sr. Paed.**; Catholic Children's Aid; Clin. Instr. (Paed), U. of British Columbia; Tel. RE 3-3412.

STOCKWELL, Henry P.; McG '61; Jr. Intn., Montreal Gen. Hosp., Montreal 25, P.Q.

STODDARD, Carl C.; 6533 Coburg Rd., Halifax, N.S. (res); Dal '38; F.A.C.A., F.I.C.A.; Anaes; Prof. Anaes., Dalhousie U; Chief Anaes, Victoria Gen. Hosp., Cons. Anaes; Camp Hill Vets; Children's & Nova Scotia Hosp's.; Armed Forces Medical Council; Tel. 2-4406.

STODDARD, Robert H.; 1359 Barrington St., Halifax, N.S.; Dal'16; FACS, Ophth, Otol; **Chief Ophth. Otol., Camp Hill Hosp., Halifax. Tel. 423-1371.**

STODDART, T. Glen; 238 Sherwood Dr., Ottawa 3, Ont. (res); Qns '34; F.A.C.R., D&TRad; Dir., Dept. of Rad., Ottawa Civic Hosp.; Dir., Ottawa Clinic, Ontario Cancer Fndn.; Clin. Prof. (Rad.), U. of Ottawa; Tel. 728-3745.

STODDART, Warren O.; 240 Oriole Pkwy, Toronto, Ont. (res); Tor '22; OrthSurg; GenSurg; Court. Staff, Tor. Gen. Hosp.; Tel. WA 1-1248.

STOFFELS, Henry H.; 4614 Kingston Rd., West Hill, Ont.; Cape Town (S. Africa)'51; Tel. 282-2282.

STOFFMAN, Isaac W.; 2309 W. 41st Ave., Vancouver 13, B.C.; 6089 Hudson St. (res); Man '39; MCGP; Staff, Van. Gen., St. Paul's & Grace Hosp's.; Tel. AM 1-6622.

STOGDILL, C. G.; 39 Lowther Ave., Toronto, Ont.; Tor '31; Psy; Assoc. (Psy), U. of Toronto. Chief Child Adjustment Serv., Bd. of Education.

STOICOIU, Traian; 318 Alberta Corner Bldg., 804-1st St. S.W., Calgary, Alta.; Cluj (Roum.) '35; GenSurg; Tel. 262-5003.

STOJAN, Frank J.; 9905-101st. Ave., Grande Prairie, Alta.; Qns'51; Tel. 532-5511.

STOKES, Aldwyn B., CBE; 250 College St., Toronto 5, Ont.; Oxford (Eng.) '32; DCH; DPM; FRCP(Lond.); FRCP(C); Psy; Psy.-in-Chief, Clarke Inst. of Psy.; Cons., Toronto General, Wellesley, Hosp. for Sick Children & Sunnybrook DVA Hosp's.; Prof. & Head., Dept. of Psy., U. of Toronto; Tel. 924-6811.

STOKES, Lorne S.; Hanover, Ont.; Tor '24; M.C.G.P.

STOKES, Ronald E.; Dept. of Reform Institutions, Queen's Park, Toronto, Ont.; Tor'51; D.Psy; Psy; Dir. of Psy., Dept. of Reform Inst.; Lect. (Psy.), U. of Toronto & Spec. Lect., School of Social Work, U. of Toronto; Tel. 365-4336.

STOLAR, Stanley H.; 212 James St. S., Hamilton, Ont.; Dal '58; DA (McGill); Anaes; Staff, St. Joseph's Hosp.; Tel. 528-8437.

STOLBERG, Harold O.; Vienna (Austria) '50; DMR; DABR; FCCP; FRCP(C), DiagRad; Dir. Dept. of Rad., Hamilton Gen. Hosp., Hamilton, Ont.; Tel. JA 7-0271, Ext. 222.

STOLMAN, Lewis P.; Qns'65; Jr. Int., Toronto Western Hosp., Toronto 2B, Ont.; Abroad.

STONE, Archibald C.; 168 Ontario St., St. Catharines, Ont.; R.R. 1, Holland Rd., Fonthill (res); McG'38; Chief, EEN & T Dept., St. Catharines Gen. Hosp.; Tel. MU 4-7406.

STONE, Bryan; 168 Essex St., Sarnia, Ont.; Birmingham (Eng.) '60.; AMCGP; Tel. ED 7-3356.

STONE, George H.; 161 Hughson St. S., Hamilton, Ont.; 152 E. 8th St. (res); Qns '49; D.Psy; Psy.; Active Staff, Hamilton Gen. & St. Joseph's Hosp's.; Hd. (Psy.), Joseph Brant Hosp.; Tel. 522-4693.

STONE, John R.; Ste. 619, 1207 Douglas St., Victoria, B.C.; Tor'47; Anaes; Tel. EV 3-0921.

STONE, Murray E.; 89 Thorndale Cr., Hamilton, Ont.; Qns'58; D. Psy.; Psy; Staff, St. Joseph's, Chedoke & Hamilton Gen. Hosp's.; Tel. JA 8-1654.

STONE, Oscar R.; Bridgetown, N.S.; Dal '22.

STONE, Patrick H.; 11 Fielding Ave., Kentville, N.S.; London (Eng.) '42; MRCS (Eng.); LRCP (Lond.); DMRD (Eng.); Staff, Blanchard-Fraser Mem. Hosp.

STONE, Robert M.; Qns'64; Res., Hosp. for Sick Children, Toronto 2, Ont.

STONKUS, Stasys; Esterhazy, Sask.; Kaunus (Lith) '34.

STORCER, Joseph; 9924 Richmond Ave., Grand Prairie, Alta.; Alb '52; Coroner.

STORDY, Stanford N.; McG '57; FRCP(C), IntMed; Staff, (Med.), St. Paul's Hosp., Vancouver, B.C.; Tel. MU 3-2211.

STOREY, David W.; 1631 Islington Ave. N., Rexdale, Ont.; Tor '51; MCGP; Sr. Active Staff, Humber Mem. Hosp.; Tel. 741-0410.

STOREY, Robert N.; 27 Third St., Collingwood, Ont.; 380 Ste. Marie St. (res); Wes '39; Dist. Coroner; Tel. 445-4111.

STOREY, Vernon H.; 104 Wellington, Bowmanville, Ont.; 64 Temperance (res); Tor '15; Part-time Indust. Phys., Goodyear Tire & Rubber Co.

STORK, Jack; 8 Lilywood Rd., Toronto 19, Ont.; Tor'59; Pt.-time Staff, U. of Toronto Health Serv.; Phys., Central Y.W.C.A.

STORRAR, William, M.B.E.; 3078 Trafalgar Ave., Montreal, P.Q. (res); Edinburgh (Scot.) '39; Med. Dir., Montreal Gen Hosp.; Lect. (Soc.), McGill U.; Tel. WE 7-6011.

STORRIE, V. Marie; Manitoba Clinic, 790 Sherbrook St., Winnipeg, Man.; 11 Florence Apts., 145 Arlington St. (res); Man'50; IntMed; Hon. Att'd. Staff, Wpg. Gen.; Dem. (Med.), U. of Man.; Tel. SP 4-6541.

STORY, A. Laird; 15 George St., Blenheim, Ont.; 17 George St. (res); Wes '27; MCGP; Staff, Chatham Public Gen. Hosp.; Tel. 676-5400.

STORY, Clinton F.; Tor '43; DPH.; D.Psy.; Psy.; Staff, Homewood Sanitarium, Guelph. Ont.; Tel. TA 4-1010.

STORY, Gladys S. (See Cunningham).

STOTHERS, Robert; 1541 W. Broadway, Vancouver 9, B.C.; Wes '54; DiagRad; Staff, Shaughnessy Hosp.; Tel TR 6-6767.

STOTT, Nelson W.; 7001 Mumford Rd., Halifax, N.S.; 62 Wedgewood Ave., Birch Cove, (res); Dal'53; MCGP; Tel. 455-3146.

STOUFFER, Katharine E.; (See Mirhady Katharine E.).

STOUT, Terence D.; 828 W. 10th Ave., Vancouver, B.C.; Man '50.

STOYKA, W. W.; Tor'65; Res., East Gen. Hosp., Toronto 13, Ont.

STRACHAN, Grace E. (Pachal); 116 Med. Arts Bldg., Fort William, Ont.; 1415 Ridgway St. (res); Man '33; Tel. 622-1016.

STRACHAN, James G.; R.R. 2, Little Current, Ont.; Tor '18; M.R.C.S., L.R.C.P., Otol.; Retired.

STRACHAN, Michael; 214-6th Ave. W., Calgary, Alta.; 1106 Frontenac Ave. (res); London (Eng.) '40; MRCS (Eng.); LRCP(Lond.); MCGP; Staff, Holy Cross, Calgary Gen. Grace Hosp's.; Tel. 263-7120.

STRACHAN, P. G.; Tor '64; Res., Hosp. for Sick Children, Toronto 2, Ont.

STRACHAN, R. Patricia; 396 Francis Rd., Richmond, B.C.; Man'62.

STRACHAN, Stewart A.; Ste. 437, 2184 W. Broadway, Vancouver, B.C.; Man '46.

STRADIOTTI, Maria; UBC'64; Res., Vancouver Gen. Hosp., Vancouver, B.C.

STRAIN, Frederick A.; Gore Bay, Ont.; Tor '25.

STRAJA, Alexandre M.; Bucharest (Roum.)'49; Res., Hop. Notre-Dame, Montreal, P.Q.

STRAKER, Manuel; Seaforth Med. Bldg., 3550 Cote des Neiges Rd., Montreal 25, P.Q.; 373 Lazard Ave., Town of Mount Royal (res); McG '44; D. Psy.; Psy.; FAPA; DABNP; Psy. (P.Q.); Assoc. Psy., Montreal Gen. Hosp.; Cons. Psy., DVA; Assoc. Prof., McGill U.; Tel. 935-8444.

STRANG, Archibald G.; Box 250, Chippawa, Ont.; Qns '27; Gen Surg; Staff, Greater Niagara Gen. Hosp., Plant Phys., Norton Co.; M.O.H., Village of Chippawa.

STRANG, Robert I.; 136 E. 14th St., North Vancouver, B.C.; UBC '57; FRCP(C); IntMed.

STRANG, William H.; Wes'63; Res., Toronto Western Hosp., Toronto 2B, Ont.

STRANGWAY, Donald W.; Tor'62; Res., Toronto Gen. Hosp., Toronto 2, Ont.

STRANGWAY, Jean E.; Tor'62; Res., Toronto East Gen. Hosp., Toronto 6, Ont.; Retired.

STRANKS, Gordon; Tor'46; Res., Sunnybrook Hosp., Toronto 12, Ont.

STRASBERG, Alex; 1396 St. Catherine W., Montreal, P.Q.; 6271 Mountain Sights (res); McG '22; Urol; **Assoc. Urol., Jewish Gen. Hosp.; Clin. Ass't. in Urol., Royal Victoria Hosp.; Dem. (Urol.), McGill U.; Tel. UN 6-5927.**

STRASBERG, Steven M.; Tor'63; Res., Sunnybrook Hosp., Toronto, Ont.

STRASHIN, Israel; 200 Danforth Ave., Toronto, Ont.; 572 St. Clements Ave. (res); Tor '40; M.C.-G.P.; Staff, New Mount Sinai Hosp.; Telephone HO 5-1171.

STRATFORD, Graham K.; Cobourg Clinic, 188 King St. W., Cobourg, Ont.; 154 Ontario St. (res); Wes '55; DA; Tel. FR 2-3323.

STRATFORD Joseph G.; Montreal Gen. Hosp.; Montreal, P.Q.; 50 Summit Circle, Mtl. 6. (res); McG '47; F.A.C.S., F.R.C.S.(C), NeurSurg; Dir. NeurSurg., Mtl. Gen. Hosp.; Assoc. Prof. (NeurSurg), McGill U.; Tel. WE 7-6011.

STRATH, F. J.; Man '59; Res., Hosp. for Sick Children, Toronto 2, Ont.

STRATHEARN, John K.; 92 Mary St., Orillia Ont.; 82 Jarvis St. (res); Tor '47; Dist. Coroner.

STRATHMAN, Irvin; 1386 Ouellette Ave., Windsor, Ont.; 2276 Victoria Ave. (res); Tor '46; FACS; FACOG; FRCS(C), ObstGyn; Chief (ObstGyn), Grace Hosp.; Sr. Staff (ObstGyn), Hotel-Dieu; Cons. Essex Co. San. & Riverview Hosp.; Tel. 256-5416.

STRATHMANN, Hildegard; Erlangen (Germ.) '50; Res. (Anaes.), Montreal Children's Hosp., Montreal, P.Q.

STRATTON, Donald P.; 14 E. Hanna, Windsor, Ont.; Wayne (U.S.A.) '51; D.A.B.R.; M.C.G.P.

STRATTON, Henry G.; 2085 Tecumseh Rd. E., Windsor, Ont.; 2080 Lorraine Ave. (res); Wes '37; DABP; D.Psy; Psy; Chief (Psy), Metropolitan Gen. Hosp.; Tel. 254-8425.

STRATTON, John R.; 405 Broadway Ave., Killarney, Man.; Man'49; MCGP; MOH, Turtle Mountain; Tel. 523-5411.

STRAUSS, Gerald Z.; 901 O'Connor Dr., Ste. 16, Toronto 16, Ont.; Tor '55; FRCS(C), GenSurg; Assoc. Surg., Toronto East Gen. Hosp.; Tel. 751-3858.

STRAUSS, Rubin; 546 Rockland Ave., Montreal, P.Q.; McG '35; M.C.G.P.; Tel. 684-4422.

STRAUTMANIS, Ingrida Z.; Cancer Foundation, 700 Bannatyne Ave., Winnipeg, Man.; Man '57; TherRad; Staff, Cancer Treatment & Research Foundation; Att'd. Staff, Wpg. Gen. Hosp.

STRAWBRIDGE, Harry T. G.; 550 University Ave., Toronto 2B, Ont.; Edinburgh (Scot.) '43; MRCP(E); MC Path; FRCP(C), Path; Dir. of Labs., New Mount Sinai Hosp.; Ass't. Prof. (Path.), U. of Toronto; Tel. EM 6-7361.

STRAWCZYNSKI, Hanna; Apt. 18, 5020 St. Kevin, Montreal 29, P.Q.; Warsaw (Poland)'52; Paed.

STREAN, George J.; 1538 Sherbrooke St. W., Montreal, P.Q.; McG'21; FICS, FACOG, FRCOG, MRCOG, FACS, FRCS(C), ObstGyn; Hon. Cons. (ObstGyn), Jewish Gen Hosp.; Ass't. Prof. (ObstGyn), McGill U.; Hon. Treas., Cdn. Reg. Council R.C.O.G.; Tel. WE 5-4434.

STREATER, J. David; Ott'65; Res., Ottawa Gen. Hosp., Ottawa 2, Ont.

STREBIG, Donald L. M.; 1217 Bayview Ave., Toronto 17, Ont.; Tor '26; MRCP & S; Clin. Phys., Dept. of PH, Toronto; Tel. HU 9-5066.

STREET, John D.; Galiano Island B.C.; McG '19; M.Sc.; Phys., Workmen's Comp. Bd. of B.C.

STREET, Richard W.; Box 160, Blyth, Ont.; Wes'51; AMCGP; Tel. 523-4433.

STREETS, Charles W.; 600 Central Ave., Fort Erie, Ont.; Tor'23; MRCS(Can); GenSurg; Dist. Surg., C.N.R. & Norfolk & Western Rlwys.; Coroner; Tel. 871-6661.

STRICKLER, Albert C.; 136 Islington Ave. S., Toronto 18, Ont.; 41 Reid Manor, Tor. 18 (res); Tor '58; Ass't. Prof. (Anat.), U. of Toronto; Tel. BE 9-6167.

STRILCHUK, Nicholas C.; Mundare, Alta.; Alb '26; Dist. Coroner; Tel. 322.

STRINGER, Donald W.; 6436 Laburnum St., Vancouver 13, B.C.; UBC'55.

STRINGER, E. Paul; Ste. 302, 452 Main St. E., Hamilton, Ont.; Qns'60; Ophth.

STRINGER, Robert M.; 124 Chedoke Ave., Hamilton, Ont.; Qns '29; F.I.C.A., Anaes; Chief (Anaes.), Hamilton Gen. Hosp.; Tel. JA 7-0271.

STROHHOFER-LeMarry, Joseph; Ponteix, Sask.; Greifswald (Germ.) '38; Tel. 625-3525.

STROMBERG, Oscar O.; 1116-100th St., North Battleford Sask.; 1441 York (res); McG '41; M.C.G.P.; Dist. Coroner.

STROME, William; Haig Clinic, 601—6th St., Lethbridge, Alta.; 417—14th St. S. (res); Alb '36; Lect. in Anaes., Galt & St. Michael's Schools of Nursing; Staff, St. Michael's Gen., & Lethbridge Municipal Hosp's.

STRONG, Cameron G.; Alb '58; Res., Hop. Hotel-Dieu, Montreal 18, P.Q.

STROTHER-STEWART, Cuthbert R.; Swift Current Clinic, Swift Current, Sask.; 107 Dufferin St. E. (res); Edinburgh (Scot.)'43; FICS; FRCS(Edin.); Chief, Dept. of Surg., Swift Current Union Hosp.; Cons. Rehab., Dept. of Health, Prov. of Sask.; Tel. 773-4681.

STROUBOULIS, John P.; 9803-111th St., Edmonton, Alta.; **Athens (Gr.) '48; Staff, Prov. Mental Hosp.; Tel. 7-0221.**

STROZ, Edward S.; 128 Islington Ave. S., Toronto 18, Ont.; Tor'60; MCGP.

STRUIVIG de GROOT, Hero B.; 277 King St., Trenton, Ont.; Utrecht (Neth.) '40; GenSurg (Neth.); FICS; GenSurg; Staff, Trenton Mem. & Campbellford Hosp's.; Tel. EX 2-4700.

STRULOVICI, Strul; 770A St. Clair Ave. W., Toronto 10, Ont.; '36.

STRUMINSKY, Roman; 6550-11th Ave., Rosemont, Montreal 36, P.Q.; Innsbruck (Austria) '39; Ass't. Surg., Saint-Luc Hosp.; Tel. RA 2-5141.

STRUTHERS, Ernest B.; 28 Moore Ave., Toronto 7, Ont. (res); Tor '12; DPH (Tor); DTM & H (Eng.); IntMed; Retired.

STRUTHERS, James D., Sr.; Box 484, Port Dover, Ont.; '11.

STRUTHERS, J. Douglas; 14 Chapman St., Port Dover, Ont.; Prospect Hill, Port Dover (res); Wes '44; Dist. Coroner; Tel. 583-1322.

STRUTHERS, Mary E.; (see McKim, Mary E.).

STRUTHERS, R. Gordon; 48 St. Andrews Gdns., Toronto, Ont. (res); Tor '14; D.P.H., PH; P.H. Admin., Dept. of Health, Prov. of Ontario.

STRUTHERS, R. Rolf; 2047 Mansfield St., Montreal, P.Q.; McG '18; FRCP(C), Paed; Staff, Mtl. Gen. Hosp.; Tel. WE 7-6011.

STRUTZ, Walter A.; 560 Professional Bldg., 10830 Jasper Ave., Edmonton, Alta.; Alb '50; DABS; FACS, FRSC(C), GenSurg; Att'd. Staff, Royal Alexandra & Misericordia Hosp's.; Sess. Instr. (Surg.), U. of Alberta; Tel. 429-3351.

STRZALKOWSKA, Alicja.; ....See ROGERS, Alicja J.

STUART, C. Keith; 1845 Rogers Rd., Streetsville, Ont. (res); Wes '35; F.A.C.P.; IntMed; Geriatric Research; 350 Christie St., Toronto 4, Ont.; Tel. LE 1-5771.

STUART, Edward M. W.; 76 Division St., Welland, Ont.; Queens U. (Belfast, Ire.) '52 M.B., B.Ch., BAO; ObstGyn; Court. Staff, Welland County Gen. Hosp.; Hon. Cons. Staff, Douglas Mem. Hosp., Fort Erie; Assoc. Cons. Staff, Port Colborne Gen. & Haldimand Co. Mem. Hosp., Dunnville; Tel. 732-2489.

STUART, Edwin A.; Apt. 25, 1390 Sherbrooke St. W., Montreal 25, P.Q.; 3472 Grey Ave., N.D.G. (res); McG '33; A.B. Otol.; F.R.C.S. (Ed.), F.R.C.S.(C) Otol; Otol., Royal Victoria, & Shriner's Hosp. for Crippled Children; Assoc. Prof. (Otol.), McGill U.; Tel. VI 2-1637.

STUART, Elmer A.; Room 319, 1207 Douglas St., Victoria, B.C.; 516 Newport Ave. (res); Qns '32 Tel. EV 5-8696.

STUART, Frank G; 3002 Cadboro Bay Rd., Victoria, B.C. (res); Man '41; DABR; DMRT; D & T Rad; Dir. (Rad.), St. Joseph's Hosp.; Tel. 384-1131.

STUART, Frank K.; 1 Buena Vista Ave., Lancaster, N.B. (res); Dal '45; M.O., Lancaster DVA Hosp.; Staff, Dept. of Veterans' Affairs; Tel. 4-2651.

STUART, Jas R.; 5025 Sherbrooke St. W., Westmount, P.Q.; 835 Berwick Cres., Montreal 16, P.Q.; McG '45; Ph.D. (Path); Path; Chief (Path), Queen Elizabeth Hosp; Tel. 482-5521.

STUART, Lionel M.; 157 King St., Dundas, Ont. (res); Tor '18; D.P.H.; Dir. & M.O.H., Halton Co. Health Unit, Milton, Ont.; Tel. 878-2808.

STUART, Robert D.; 8935-120th St., Edmonton, Alta. (res); Aberdeen (Scot.) '27; M.B., Ch.B M.D., DPH; D.Sc., FRFPS (Glas.); DPH; FRCP (Glas.); Bact., University Hosp.; Dir. Prov. Lab. of Public Health, Edmonton; Prof. (Med. Bact.), U. of Alberta; Tel. GE 3-5887.

STUART, Ronald D., Fl/Lt.; Dal'66; C.F.B. Hosp., Cold Lake, Alta.

STUART, Vere G.; 123 Yarrow Bldg., 645 Fort St., Victoria, B.C.; 960 Foul Bay Rd. (res); Tor '48; MCGP; Active Staff, St. Joseph's Hosp.; Tel. 383-5441.

STUBBING, R.; Department of National Health & Welfare, c/o Regional Superintendent, European Region, Abroad.

STUBBINGS, Ralph S.; Creemore, Ontario; Tor '38; DPH; MCGP; Staff, Collingwood Gen. & Marine Hosp.; Sec. Treas., Collingwood & Dist. Med. Society; Tel. 466-2500.

STUBBINS, Robert A.; 2676 Bayview Ave., Willowdale, Ont.; Tor '49; MCGP; Staff, North York Branson & Wellesley Hosp's.; Tel. 221-2500.

STUBBS, Jack G.; 221 Brant Ave., Brantford, Ont.; 67 Marvin Ave. (res); Guy's (London, Eng.) '41; M.R.C.S. (Eng.), L.R.C.P. (Lond.), M. Ch. (Orth—Liverpool); F.R.C.S. (Eng); OrthSurg; Tel. 752-4731.

STUBBS, Sydney; Man'65; Res., Winnipeg General Hosp., Winnipeg, Man.

STUBINGTON, David; 4500 Sherbrooke St. W., Montreal, P.Q.; 152 Vivian Ave., Mtl. 16 (res); London (Eng.) '49; IntMed(Cardiol, P.Q.); FRCP(C), IntMed; Ass't. Phys., Royal Victoria Hosp.; Cons. (Cardiol.), Queen Mary Vet's. Hosp. & Royal Edward Laurentian San.; Staff, St. Mary's Hosp. Ass't. Prof. (Med.), McGill U.; Tel. 933-5338.

STUCKLER, Jozef; 712 College St., Toronto 4, Ont.; 4 Chater Crt., Tor. 19 (res); Rome (Italy) 38; DDS; Otol; Chief, ENT, Doctors' Hosp.; Staff, OPD, Tor. Gen. Hosp.; Tel. LE 7-2555.

STUEBNER, Karl G.; 150 Ontario St., St. Catharines, Ont.; West Berlin U, (W. Germ.) '55; Tel. MU 4-7985.

STUMBOF, Angel V.; Ste. 2, 545 Danforth Ave., Toronto 6, Ont.; Istanbul (Turkey) '38; Tel. 463-5763.

STUPARYK, Michael; 297 Old Kingston Road, Highland Creek, Ont.; Tor'58; IntMed; Staff, Lockwood Clinic, Toronto; Cons. Staff, Ajax & Pickering Hosp.; Tel. 282-1119.

STURDY, Donald D.; 104 Med. Arts Bldg., Calgary, Alta.; 66 Cromwell Ave. N.W. (res); McG '44; Orth; Staff, Calgary Gen., Alberta Children's & Holy Cross Hosp's.; Tel. 269-1557.

STURDY, John H.; 4490 Angus Dr., Vancouver, B.C.; Alb '39; Path; Assoc. Dir. (Path), St. Paul's Hosp.; Asst. Prof., U. of British Columbia; RE 8-1310.

STURGEON, Alec W.; 9 Ennisclare Dr., Oakville, Ont. (res); **Tor '37; Chief M.O., Ford Motor Co. of Canada Ltd.; Staff Phys., Oakville Trafalgar Mem. Hosp.; Tel. 845-2511.**

STURGEON, Leland W. C.; Welland & Dist. Health Unit, King St. E. at Fourth, Welland, Ont.; 9 Laughlin Pl. (res); Tor '30; DABPN, DPH, FAPHA, PH; Dir. & MOH, Welland Dist. Health Unit; Spec. Lect. (PH), U. of Toronto; Tel. RE 5-5697.

STURGESS, John M.; Wes'58; Res., Vancouver Gen. Hosp., Vancouver 9, B.C.

STURGIS, Daniel E.; 153 Simcoe N., Oshawa, Ont.; 188 Glenwood Cres. (res); Wes '33; Surg. Staff, Oshawa Gen., Port Perry, Bowmanville & Ajax Hosp's.; Tel. 725-3153.

STURROCK, F. Lindsay; 6616 Lambert Cres., R.R. No. 1, North Surrey, B.C. (res); Edinburgh (Scot.) '52; Path; Assoc. Dir. of Labs., Royal Columbian Hosp., New Westminster, B.C.; Clin. Instr. (Path.), U. of British Columbia; Tel. LA 2-2771.

STRURTRIDGE, John W.; Sudbury Gen. Hosp., Sudbury, Ont.; Tor '50; FRCP(C), IntMed; Dir. of Radioisotope Unit, Sudbury Gen. Hosp.; Staff, Copper Cliff Hosp.; Tel. 673-3601, Loc. 377.

STUTT, Helen A.; (see Bean, Helen A.).

STUTZER, Igor M.; 367 Springbank Dr., Kensal Park, London, Ont.; 328 St. George St. (res); Berlin (Germ.) '45; Tel. 434-1039.

STUTZMAN, John C.; USA'56; Staff, Grenfell Mission Hosp., St. Anthony, Nfld.; Abroad.

SUDERMANN, Peter; 501 Medical Arts Bldg., 404-406 Graham Ave., Winnipeg 1, Man.; 391 Oak (res); Goettingen (Germ.) '50; FRCS(C); GenSurg; Tel. 943-5689.

SUDERSHAN, Saxena; Lucknow (India) '60; Res., Princess Margaret Hosp., Toronto 5, Ont.

SUFFEL, Priscilla S. H. (Khoo); 1103 Richmond St., London, Ont.; West China Union U. '46.

SUGARMAN, Harold; 410 Lake Cres., Saskatoon, Sask. (res); Man'33; **FACP; Active Staff, St. Paul's & University Hosp's.; Vis. Cons., City** Hosp.; Inst. (Med.), St. Paul's Hosp. Schl. of Nursing; Ass't. Clin. Prof. (Med.), U. of Saskatchewan; Tel. 242-0271.

SUGARMAN, Irwin; Ste. 329, 5757 Decelles Ave., Montreal 26, P.Q.; 595 Lansdowne Ave., Westmount (res); Qns '36; ObstGyn (P.Q.); Assoc. (ObstGyn.), Jewish Gen. Hosp.; Tel. RE 8-6556.

SUGARMAN, Lillian; (See Clark Lillian).

SUGIYAMA, Henry S.; 500 Parliament St., Toronto 4, Ont.; Man'52.

SUGIYAMA, Shigeru; 385 Wellington St. W., Chatham, Ont.; Wes'64; Tel. 354-5290.

SUH, Mathew C. K.; New Provincial Bldg., 110 Charlotte St., Saint John, N.B.; Seoul (Korea) '57; D.Psy; Psy; Med. Dir., Child Psychiatric Serv., Dept. of Health; Cons. Child Psy., Saint John Gen. Hosp. & N.B. Boys' Training School, Kingsclear; Tel. 692-0181.

SUIKER, Alice; Box 1109, Kitimat, B.C.; UBC'61; Tel. 1603.

SUKMAN, Steven N.; 1575 Dupont St., Toronto 9, Ont.; 97 The Kingsway (res); Tor '35; M.C.-G.P.; Assoc. Staff, St. Joseph's Hosp.; Tel. LE 5-1503.

SULEIMAN, Louis W.; Cedar Heights Plaza, 695 Markham Rd., Scarborough, Ont.; '44.

SULKOWSKI, J. Gunther; 17 East Ave. S., Hamilton, Ont.; 4 Everton Place (res); Breslau (Germ.) '37; MCGP; Tel. JA 9-1619.

SULLIVAN, Cyril F.; 331 Queens Ave., London, Ont.; Wes '31; M.Sc., F.R.C.S.(Ed.), ObstGyn; Staff, St. Joseph's, Victoria & Bethesda Hosp's.; Sr. Instr. Obst. Gyn., U. of Western Ontario; Cons. Obst. Gyn., Beck Memorial San.; Tel. GE 4-7113.

SULLIVAN, Herbert J.; Medical Arts Bldg., Hamilton, Ont.; 328 Mountain Brow Blvd. (res); Tor'39; FCCP, FRCS(C), GenSurg; Hd., Dept. of Cardiovasc. & ThorSurg., St. Joseph's Hosp.; Tel. JA 7-2577.

SULLIVAN, Herman A.; 115 Hazen St., Saint John, N.B.; 131 Donaldson St. (res); McG '57; Dip. Urol (McGill); FRCS(C); Urol; Att'd. Staff, St. John Gen., St. Joseph's & Lancaster DVA Hosp's.; Tel. 693-7771.

SULLIVAN, James D.; McG'62; Ass't. Res., Montreal Gen. Hosp., Montreal, P.Q.

SULLIVAN, J. Kenneth; 38 Wellington Row, Saint John, N.B.; McG'25; Urol; Cons. Staff, Saint John Gen. Hosp.; Urol., St. John T.B. Hosp. & Provincial Hosp.; Tel. 693-3432.

SULLIVAN, John B.; 303-5th Ave., Timmins, Ont.; Tor'53; FRCS(C), GenSurg; Staff, St. Mary's Hosp.; Tel. 264-9055.

SULLIVAN, John F.; 90 The West Mall, Etobicoke, Ont.; Qns'62.

SULLIVAN, Joseph A.; One Medical Place, 20 Wynford Dr., Don Mills, Ont.; Tor'26; MB, FRSM(Eng.); FRCS(C), Otol; Chief, Hard of Hearing Clin. & Auditory Research, St. Michael's Hosp.; Chief Cons. (Otol.), Armed Forces of Canada; Memb. Bd. of Governors, U. of Toronto; Senator, Government of Canada.

SULLIVAN, Joseph E.; Lockwood Clinic, 300 Bloor St. E., Toronto 5, Ont.; Tor '50; Tel. WA 1-2121.

SULLIVAN, Leonard J.; 200 St. Clair Ave. W., Toronto 2, Ont.; Tor '46; F.R.C.S.(C), Urol.; Tel. WA 2-4464.

SULLIVAN, Lorne D.; Sask'62; Res., Shaughnessy Hosp., Vancouver 9, B.C.

SULLIVAN, Terence J.; 224-13 Ave. S., Cranbrook, B.C.; **Alb '38; Dist. Coroner; Tel. 426-2201.**

SULLIVAN, Thomas J.; 522 Med. Arts Bldg., 1538 Sherbrooke St. W., Montreal 25, P.Q.; **3538 Cote-des-Neiges Rd. (res); McG '54; DABD, FRCP(C), DermSyph; Staff, Mtl. Gen. & Children's Hosp's.; Dem. (Derm.), McGill U.; Tel. WE 5-3755**

SULLIVAN, William E.; 955 Queen St. E., Sault Ste. Marie, Ont.; 31 Riverside Cres. (res); **Tor '53; M.C.G.P.; Dist. Coroner; Tel. AL 3-4071.**

SULMA, Vladas; Lumsden, Sask.; Kaunas (Lith.) '39; Tel. 485-2229.

SULMANIS, Lydia; Ste. 705, 1849 Yonge St., Toronto 7, Ont.; Germany '46; Te. 485-5184.

SULTMANIS, Richard; Ste. 705, 1849 Yonge St., Toronto 7, Ont.; Hamburgh (Germ.) '46; Staff, Doctor's Hosp.; Tel. 485-5184.

SUMMERBY, John H.; 870 Clearview Ave., London, Ont.; McG '51; D.Psy; Psy; Med. Spec. **(Psy), Westminster DVA Hosp.; Instr. (Psy), U. of Western Ont.; Tel. GE 2-6711.**

SUMMERER, Margo M. (Mrs. C. M. Campbell); Collishaw St., Moncton, N.B.; Heidelberg (Germ.) **'51; Med. Dir., TB Clinic, Moncton; Tel. 855-5428.**

SUMMERS, John J.; Ste. 16, 5763 Oak **St., Vancouver 13, B.C.; 829 W. 17th Ave., Vancouver 9 (res); Alb '54; Tel. AM 6-6264.**

SUMNER, John; 11743-8th Ave., Haney, B.C.; Durham (Eng.) '38; MCGP; Active Med. Staff, Maple Ridge Hosp.; Tel. 463-9161.

SUNDERLAND, Kenneth B.; North Brook, Ont.; Tor. '42.

SUNDERLAND, William F.; 701—3rd Ave., New Westminster, B.C. (res); R.C.P.S. (Ire.) '40: **L.R.C.S. & P., R.C.O.G., DP.H., DObst. (Lond); Tel. LA 2-3534.**

SUNGAILA, Joseph; 109 Riverwood Pkwy., Toronto 18, Ont. (res); Innsbruck (Austria) '47; DiagRad; Staff (DiagRad), St. Michael's Hosp.; Tel. 362-4461.

SUNLEY, John G.; Lamont Clinic, Lamont, Alta.; Man '60; Tel. 5519.

SUNOHARA, John M.; 396 Royal York Rd., Toronto 18, Ont.; Tor'65; Tel. CL 9-8182.

SUNSHINE, Stanley L.; 720 W. Broadway, Vancouver 9, B.C.; UBC'60; Vis. Staff, Vancouver Gen. & Grace Hosp's.; Tel. TR 9-5271.

SUPPAL, Sushil K.; 399 King St., Bridgewater, N.S.; Calcutta (India)'55.

SURAN, Roland R.; 99 Avenue Rd., Toronto 5, Ont.; 1654 Bathurst St., Apt. 201 (res); Tor '39; ObstGyn; Adjunct, Dept. ObstGyn, New Mt. Sinai Hosp.; Clin Ass't., Gyn-Endocrine O.P.D., Toronto Gen. Hosp.; Tel. WA 3-3678.

SURANYI, Nicholas; 5651 Park Ave., Montreal, P.Q.; Bologna (Italy) '39.

SURCHIN, Hyman; 550 Seaforth Med. Bldg., 3550 Cote des Neiges Rd., Montreal 25, P.Q.; 645 Grosvenor Ave., Westmount (res); McG '44; FRCP(C); Paed; Clin. Ass't., Children's Mem. & Jewish Gen. Hosp's.; Assoc. (Med.), Reddy Mem. Hosp.; Dem. (Paed.), McGill U.; Tel. WE 7-1593.

SURES, Pearl; (See Driemen Pearl).

SURETTE, George D.; 15 Alma St., Moncton, N.B.; Ott'65.

SURKAN, Metro; 206 Med. Bldg., Prince Albert, Sask.; 425-24th St. W. (res); Alb '50; MCGP; Active Staff, Victoria Mun. & Holy Family Hosp' Tel. 763-6401.

SURKIS, Max; Anti Costi Island, Port Menier, P.Q.; Roumania'39.

SURPHLIS, William R.; Qns '58; D.Psy; Psy; Dir. Psy. Div., Sudbury Algoma San., Sudbury, Ont.: Tel. 675-8351.

SUSINI, Luciano; Genoa (Italy) '54; Box 10, Provincial Hosp., Campbellton, N.B.

SUSSET, Jacques G.; 261 Chemin de la Cote Ste-Catherine, Montreal 8, P.Q.; Paris (Fr.) '53; F.R.C.S.(C), Urol; Staff, Royal Victoria Hosp.; Cons. (Urol.) Royal Edward Laurentian San. & Rehab. Inst.; Lect.; (Surg.) McGill U.; Tel. CR 3-8761.

SUSSET, Veronique; 261 Cote-Ste-Catherine, Montreal 8, P.Q.; Paris (Fr.) '53; PhysMed & Rehab; Staff, Rehab. Inst.; Tel. 273-8922.

SUSSEX, Robert J.; Main St., Florence, Ont.; Wes '46; MCGP; Dist. Coroner.

SUSSMAN, Arthur H.; 345 Bloor St. W., Toronto 4, Ont.; Wes '44; F.A.A.A., FACA; D.A.B.I.M.; M.C.A.A., IntMed; Jr. Attend. Staff, New Mt. Sinai Hosp.; Attend. Staff OPD, Toronto Western Hosp.; Tel. WA 3-4348.

SUTCLIFFE, Charles K.; Sheffield (Eng.)'53; Staff, Ontario Hosp., Brockville, Ont.

SUTHERLAND, Arthur L.; 103 Charlotte St., Sydney, N.S.; 189 King's Rd. (res); Dal '32; M.C.G.P.

SUTHERLAND, D. Lawrence; Med. Arts Bldg., Empire Ave., St. John's, Nfld.; Dal '48; DABNS, MCNS, AMAAN; NeurSurg; Staff, St. John's Gen., Pepperell Children's & Grace Hosp's.; Con. Staff, Hosp. for Mental & Nervous Dis. & St. John's San.; Court. Staff, St. Clare's Mercy Hosp.; Tel. 579-4283.

SUTHERLAND, Donald F.; 115 Hazen St., Saint John, N.B.; 550 Lewin Ave., Lancaster (res); Dal '43; ObstGyn; Tel. 692-4532.

SUTHERLAND, Donald J.; Tor'61; Res., Montreal Gen. Hosp., Montreal 25, P.Q.

SUTHERLAND, Eleanor W. (Miller); 654 Highland Ave., Ottawa 13, Ont.; Alb '53.

SUTHERLAND, Frank D.; 100th St., Tisdale, Sask.; Man '30.

SUTHERLAND, Gerald W.; Tor '58; Res., Toronto East Gen. Hosp., Toronto 6, Ont.

SUTHERLAND, Gordon O.; 445 Oriole Parkway, Toronto 7, Ont. (res); Tor '46; DiagRad; Chief Rad., Orthopead. & Arthritic Hosp., 43 Wellesley St., Toronto.; Tel. 921-4611.

SUTHERLAND, Grant Q.; 170 Metcalfe St., Guelph, Ont.; 196 St. Andrew St., Fergus (res); Tor'33; CPH, DPH, PH; Med. Off of Health, Guelph; Tel. TA 4-2820.

SUTHERLAND, Harvey F.; Bank of Commerce Bldg., Sydney, N.S.; 539 Esplanade St. (res); Dal '33

SUTHERLAND, Ira R.; Sandy Cove, Digby Co., N.S., Dal '25.

SUTHERLAND, J. Barthelemy; 450 Elm Ave., Westmount, Montreal 6, P.Q. (res); McG '50; D.Anaes; F.R.C.P.(C), Anaes; Assoc. Anaes., Mtl. Gen. Hosp.; Ass't. Prof. (Anaes.), McGill U.; Tel. 937-1732.

SUTHERLAND, Joan (See Gilmour)

SUTHERLAND, John B.; Man '60; Staff, Atomic Energy of Canada, Pinawa, Man.

SUTHERLAND, John B.; Dal'58; GenSurg; Staff, Victoria Gen. Hosp., Halifax, N.S.

SUTHERLAND, Lawrence M.; 231 Victoria St., Kamloops, B.C.; 625 Penzer St. (res); Oregon (U.S.A.) '51; ObstGyn; Chief ObstGyn., & Instr., Nurses Training Schl., Royal Inland Hosp.; Tel. 372-5522.

SUTHERLAND, L. J.; 854—1st Ave. W., Owen Sound, Ont.; 664—2nd Ave. W. (res): Tor '25; IntMed; Staff, Gen. & Marine Hosp.; Tel. FR 6-3026.

SUTHERLAND, Leslie G.; 91 Tudhope St., Espanola, Ont.; Tor'50; GenSurg; Staff, Espanola Gen. Hosp.; Tel. 869-2620.

SUTHERLAND, Lynette E.; Room 8520, Hosp. for Sick Children, Toronto 2, Ont.; Tor'59.

SUTHERLAND, Ralph W.; 732 Fraser, Ottawa 13, Ont.; Alb'52; DHA (Tor); Staff, Dept. of National Health & Welfare, Ottawa, Ont.

SUTHERLAND, R. Bruce; Apt. 703, 9 Deer Park Cr., Toronto 7, Ont.; Qns'39; DPH; DIH; Dir., Environmental Health Branch, Ontario Dept. of Health; Assoc. Prof. Dept. of Physiol. Hygiene, School of Hygiene, U. of Toronto.

SUTHERLAND, Robert L.; 806 Med. Centre Bldg., 8th Ave. & 8th St. S.W., Calgary, Alta.; Alb'54; FRCS(C), Ophth; DAB(Ophth); Chief, Div. of Ophth., Foothills Gen. Hosp.; Tel. 263-3820.

SUTHERLAND, Roy A.; 1721 Hillside, Victoria, B.C.; UBC'57; MCGP; Tel. EV 5-8696.

SUTHERLAND, William H.; Ste. 380, 5780 Cambria St., Vancouver 15, B.C.; McG'41; FRCS(C), GenSurg; Assoc. Prof., (Surg.), U. of British Columbia; Tel. RE 3-0411.

SUTHERLAND, Winston A.; 103 Main St., Waterford, Ont.; Wes '29; M.C.G.P.; Staff, Norfolk Gen. Hosp.; Dist. Coroner; Tel. 443-5741.

SUTTER, Benjamin D.; 401-1st St. S., Souris, Man.; Man '45; MCGP; Chief of Staff, Souris Dist. Hosp.; Hon. Staff, Assiniboine Hosp.; Tel. 291.

SUTTER, Mary A.; 710 Seymour St., Vancouver 2, B.C.; UBC'60; ObstGyn.; Clin. Phys., B.C., V.D. Control; Tel. MU 4-1511.

SUTTER, Morley C.; Man'57; PhD(Pharmacol.); Ass't. Prof. Pharm., Dept. of Pharmacology, U. of British Columbia, Vancouver 8, B.C.

SUTTIE, Boyd; 37 Topsail Rd., St. John's, Nfld.; St. Andrew's (Scot.)'50; DMSA(Ed.); Med. Cons., Health Ins., Dept. of Health, St. John's; Tel. 579-51577.

SUTTON, David M.; Qns'63; Res., Toronto Western Hosp., Toronto 2B, Ont.

SUTTON, Geoffrey V.; Canora, Sask.; London (Eng.) '52.

SUTTON, Gerald L.; P.O. Box 268, Ormstown, P.Q.; McG '36; MCGP; Chief of Obst., & Member Med. Bd., Barrie Mem. Hosp.; Tel. 829-2331.

SUTTON, Harold C.; Cooksville, Ont.; Tor '14; Tel. 277-1151.

SUTTON, Isaac; 2116 Portage Ave., Winnipeg, Man. (res); Qns '30; Dip. Psy., Dip. Hosp. Admin.; Psy; Supt., Deer Lodge Hosp.; Tel. TU 8-4861.

SUTTON, Joan S. (See Thomson)

SUTTON, J. Carl; 720 Seaforth Med. Bldg., 3550 Cote des Neiges Rd., Montreal 25, P.Q.; 326 Geneva Cres., Mount Royal (res); McG '28; FACS; DABS; GenSurg; Cons. Phys., Ayerst, McKenna & Harrison Ltd. & Dominion Oil Cloth & Linen Co.; Tel. WE 2-6906.

SUTTON, Marilyn D.; Wes'61; Res., Toronto Gen. Hosp., Toronto 2, Ont.

SUTTON, Melvin R.; Ste. 109, 688 Coxwell Ave., Toronto 13, Ont.; Tor'53; MA; Urol; Adjunct. Surg., New Mount Sinai; Assoc. Staff, Tor. E. Gen. Hosp.; Tel. PL 9-1600.

SVARICH, Eugene W.; 7314 Ada Blvd., Edmonton, Alta. (res); Alb '33; Ass't. Med. Dir. Woodward's Sick Benefit Soc.

SVORCIK, Boris; 131 Frederick St., Kitchener, Ont.; 86 Talbot St. (res); Heidelberg (Germ.) '43; Wes '51; Tel. 742-3244.

SWAFFIELD, William R.; 306 Med. Bldg., Prince Albert, Sask.; 359-21st St. W. (res); Man '31; ObstGyn; Chief of ObstGyn., Holy Family Hosp.; Tel. 763-6401.

SWAIL, Shirley E. (See PARKER, Shirley E.).

SWAIN, Robert G.; Box 100, Eckville, Alta.; London (Eng.)'59; FRCS(Eng.); Med. Staff, Eckville Mem. Hosp.; Tel. 13.

SWAINE, Frederick M.; 4773 Sherbrooke St. W., Montreal 6, P.Q.; 655 Belmont Ave., Westmount; (res); McG '49; Ophth; Att. Staff, St. Mary's & Queen Mary's Vet's. Hosp's.; Tel. 932-4732.

SWAINE, Ralph L.; 117 Donegani Ave., Pte. Claire, Lachine, P.Q.; McG '54; Otol; Tel. 695-1811.

SWALES, David W.; McG'61; FRCP(C), DiagRad; Staff, Montreal Gen. Hosp., Montreal 25, P.Q.

SWALES, John O.; 503, 215 Victoria St., Toronto 1, Ont.; 274 Heath St. E. (res); Tor '48; FRCS (C), ObstGyn; Active Staff, St. Michael's Hosp.; Cons. (Gyn), Princess Margaret Hosp.; Clin. Fell., U. of Toronto; Tel. EM 6-4138.

SWALLOW, Gordon E.; 13506-100 Ave. Edmonton, Alta.; (res); Man'08; Paed.; Tel. 488-7442.

SWALLOW, Kathleen A.; 13506-100th Ave., Edmonton, Alta. (res); Alb '46; FAAP; Paed; Staff, University Hosp.; Ass't. Clin. Prof., U. of Alta; Tel. 439-5911. Abroad.
SWALLOW, Robert J.; 8407-75th Ave., Edmonton, Alta. (res); Alb '52; Path; Staff, Prov. Labs.; Ass't Prof. U. of Alta.; Tel. GE 9-8721.
SWALSKY, M.; 2425 St. Antoine St., Montreal PQ.; 4827 Grand Blvd (res); McG '40; Tel. WE 2-4838.
SWAN, Henry G.; Med. Arts Bldg., 121 Wellington St. W., Barrie, Ont.; Tor '35; Staff, Royal Victoria Hosp.; Tel. 728-5536.
SWAN, John A. C.; 318 Med. Arts Bldg., Winnipeg, Man.; 221 Montrose St. (res); Man '38; Schl. Med. Serv.; Ins. & Indus. Exam.; Tel. WH 2-5606.
SWAN, Matthew H.; 78 Roseberry St., Campbellton, N.B.; Dal '55.
SWAN, R. Alan; Sechelt, B.C.; Qns '53; Tel. 885-2257.
SWAN, William J.; Box 569, Walkerton, Ont.; Wes '56; MCGP.
SWANBURG, Angus R.; Haisla Med. Dental Bldg., Kitimat, B.C.; 21 Partridge (res); Dal '52; Tel. 1603.
SWANNIE, Edward M.; Oxford (Eng.) '56; MO, Bonne Bay Hosp., Norris Pt., St. Barbe, Nfld.
SWANSON, Arnold L.; McG '43; MHA; FACHA; Exec. Dir., Victoria Hosp., London, Ont.; Tel. 432-5261.
SWANSON, Gary E.; 215 Greyhound Bldg., 622-1st St. S.W., Calgary, Alta.; Man'60; DiagRad.
SWANSON, Harold A.; 48 Chinook Dr. S.W. Calgary, Alta; (res); Man '55; D.A.B.R.; DiagRad; Staff, Calgary Gen. & Alberta Children's Hosp's.; Tel. AM 2-2912.
SWANSON, John N.; 1849 Yonge St., Ste. 613, Toronto 7, Ont.; Edinburgh (Scot.) '42; FRCP (Ed.) IntMed; Dir. Arthritis Serv., Orthopaedic & Arthritis Hosp.; Vol. Ass't. Med., Toronto Gen. Hosp.; Tel. 489-1614.
SWANSON, Marjorie C.; Ste 908, 1849 Yonge St., Toronto 7, Ont.; 70 Heath St. W. (res); **Tor '55; MCGP; Staff, OPD Dept., St. Michael's** & Active Staff, Women's College Hosp's.; Tel. 487-0347.
SWANTON, Adrian L.; Fort San, Sask.; Man '27; Med. Supt., Fort Qu'Appelle San.; Tel. 332-5966.
SWARTZ, David; 332 Med. Arts Bldg., Winnipeg 1, Man.; 235 Park Blvd., Tuxedo (res); Man '28; FRCS(Ed.); FRCS(C), Urol; Staff, Deer Lodge Hosp. & Shriner's Hosp.; Tel. WH2-7144.
SWARTZ, Melville J.; Mall Med. Bldg., 280 Osborne St., Winnipeg 1, Man.; Qns'37; FICS; Urol; Chief of Urol., Misericordia Hosp.; Tel. SP 4-2411.
SWARTZLANDER, Frank C.; 415 Greyhound Bldg., Calgary Alta.; 446 Brunswick Ave. (res); Man '50; M.Sc (Proct.); DAPS; FAPS; Teach. Staff, Calgary Gen. Hosp.; Pres., Northwest Proct. Soc.; Tel. AM 2-3756.
SWAYE, Paul S.; Qns'65; Jr. Int., Toronto General Hosp., Toronto 2, Ont.; Abroad.
SWAYZE, A. G.; Mental Health Clinic, 514 Jarvis St., Toronto 5, Ont.; Tor'63.
SWAYZE, Claude R.; Tor '61; Jr. Intn., Toronto Western Hosp., Toronto 2B, Ont.
SWEENEY, Bernardin; Unite Sanitaire, 947 rue Principale, Richmond, P.Q.; Lav '53; DPH.
SWEENEY, Brendan; 3000 Lawrence Ave. E., Scarborough, Ont.; Tor'56; OrthSurg.
SWEENEY, John P.; Ste. 204, 450 Central Ave., London, Ont.; Wes'59; FRCS(C), GenSurg; Tel. GE 8-7118.
SWEENY, G. Patrick; 2057 Caroline St., Burlington, Ont.; McG '54; MCGP; Tel. NE 4-5391.
SWEET, Arthur H.; Islay, Alta.; McG '24; Dist. Coroner.
SWEET, George P.; 2492 Lake Shore Blvd. W., Toronto 14, Ont.; Tor'41; MCGP; Tel. 251-3833.
SWEET, Robert L.; 4680 Acadia Rd., Lachine, P.Q.; McG '50; GenSurg; Active Staff, Lachine Gen. Hosp.; Tel. 637-8277.
SWEET, Theodore A.; Tor '26; D.Psy., Psy; Ass't. Supt., Ontario Hosp., Whitby, Ont.; Tel. MO 8-5881.
SWEETING, Anthony M.; Shouldice Surgery, 618 Church St., Toronto 5, Ont.; Bristol (Eng.) **'51; Tel. WA 3-3507.**
SWEETING, Treleaven J.; Lampman, Sask.; **Cambridge (Eng) '60.**
SWENDROWSKI, Tadeusz; 2513 Edward St., Regina, Sask. (res); Poland '38; Staff, Munroe Wing, Regina Gen. Hosp.
SWENSSON-ROSENQUIST, Gerrard E.; Box 159, Williamsburg, Ont.; Alb '59; MCGP; Tel. KI 3-3194.
SWERDFEGER, Hugh S.; Ott'65; Res., Hamilton Civic Hosp., Hamilton, Ont.
SWISHER, Charles N.; McG'65; Res., Children's Hosp., Montreal 25, P.Q.
SWYER, Paul R.; 555 University Ave., Toronto 2, Ont.; Cambridge (Eng.) '43; MA(Cantab.); MRCP(Lond.); DCH(Eng.); Paed; Assoc. Phys., Hosp. for Sick Children; Ass't. Scientist, Research Inst., Hosp. for Sick Children; Assoc. (Paed.), U. of Toronto; Tel. EM 6-7242, Loc. 2157.
SYKES, Georges W.; Punnichy, Sask.; Leeds Eng.)'53; MRCS(Eng.), LRCP(Lond.); District Coroner; Tel. 63.
SYKES, Richard H. D.; 14 Sykes Blvd., Brandon, **Man.; Sheffield (Eng.) '51; DABR; DiagRad;** Radiol., Brandon Gen. Hosp.; Tel. PA 6-7421, Ext. 264.
SYLLING, Margaret F.; 1370 Queen's Ave., West Vancouver, B.C.; Tor'25; MCGP; Retired.
SYLVAIN, Albert; 253 Boischatel, Point Viau, Co. Laval, P.Q.; Lav '42; M.O., Unite Sanitaire, Montreal.
SYLVESTER, Allan B.; 156 Church St., Bowmanville, Ont.; Tor '54.
SYLVESTER, C. Edward; 386 Cambria St., Stratford, Ont.; 46 Birmingham St. (res); Tor '41; Chief, Anaes. Staff, Stratford Gen. Hosp.; **Phys., Perth County Gaol.; Tel. 271-7855.**
SYLVESTRE, Gaston; 285 Beaubien E., Montreal, P.Q.; 1205 St. Viateur O., Outremont (res); Mon '23. Retired.
SYLVESTRE, J. Ernest; Apt. 7, 410 Chemin-St.-Louis, Quebec 6, P.Q.; Mon '20; CPH(Boston), DPH, PH; Dir. Div. of Nutr., Maternal & Infant Hygiene, Dept. of Health (P.Q.); Assoc. Prof. Laval U.; Tel. LA 4-8411.
SYLVESTRE, Jacques; 451 Labarre, Sherbrooke, **P.Q. (res); Mon '51; DiagRad; TherRad; Staff,** St. Vincent de Paul Hosp.; Tel. LO 9-6381.
SYLVESTRE, Lucien; 4018 Delorimier Ave., Montreal, P.Q.; 915 Pratt (res); Mon '22; Tel. 272-1182.
SYLVESTRE, Marcel; C.P. 125, St. Andrews East, P.Q.; Mon '56.
SYLVESTRE, Norbert; 1011 Ouellette Ave., Windsor, Ont.; 72 Esdras Place, Riverside (res); Wes '26; OphthOtol; Staff, Metropolitan & Hotel Dieu Hosp's.; Tel. 256-7783; Retired.
SYLVESTRE, Robert; 11819 est rue Notre-Dame, Pointe-aux-Trembles, Montreal 5, P.Q.; 11812E., Notre Dame (res); Mon '52; Tel. 645-8323.
SYLVESTRE, Robert B.; Man '48; MCGP; Med. Dir., Grey Nuns Hosp., Regina, Sask.
SYLVESTRE, Rodrigue; 1255 Beaubien St. E., Montreal, P.Q.; Mon '24; Tel. 271-2868.
SYMINGTON, David C.; 338 Place Rd., Kingston, Ont.; Glasgow (Scot.)'51; D.PhysMed. (Eng.); DAB; PhysMed. & Rehab.
SYMINGTON, J. Bruce; 1088 Queen St. E., Sault Ste. Marie, Ont.; Tor '23; Rad., General Hosp., Sault Ste. Marie.
SYMINGTON, Kenneth D.; 4711 Coronation Dr. S.W. Calgary, Alta; (res); Wes '40; FACR; DiagRad; Dir., Rad., Calgary Gen. Hosp. & Alberta Red Cross Crippled Children's Hosp.; Tel. 262-1319.
SYMON, Hamish L.; Edinburgh (Scot.)'51; DRCOG; DPH; Dir., Central Vancouver Island Health Unit, Nanaimo, B.C.; Tel. 754-4441.
SYMONS, Francis A.; 30 Facendi Dr., Peterborough, Ont.; Tor'54; DiagRad.
SYNNOTT, Edmond; App. 3, 3890 ave Maplewood, Montreal, P.Q.; Mon '61; MAH; Med. Dir., Hop. Maisonneuve; Tel. 254-8341.
SYPHER, Frederick F.; Ste 611, 1849 Yonge St., Toronto 7, Ont.; Wes '41; FICS; FRCS(C), Orth-Surg.; Tel. 483-2433.

SYRENNE, Gaston; 2221 Keele St., Toronto 15, Ont.; Lav '59.
SYSLAK, Walter B.; 671 Centennial St., Winnipeg 9, Man.; Man'58; FRCP(C), Anaes.; Tel. HU 9-7640.
SZABO, Andrew J.; New York Med. Coll., 5th Ave at 106th St., New York, U.S.A.; McG '59; FRCP(C), IntMed; Abroad.
SZABO, Janos; Dept. of Anat., U. of Ottawa, Ottawa 2, Ont.; Pecs (Hung.)'55; Assoc. Prof. Neuroanat; Tel. 235-6751, Ext. 294.
SZABO, Leslie; 269 Huxley Ave. S. (res); Hamilton, Ont.; Wes '51; Tel. 549-8179.
SZABO, Zoltan L.; 21 Division St., Welland, Ont.; 16 ave. Place (res); Budapest (Hung.) '50; OrthSurg; Active Staff, Welland Co. Hosp.; Tel. RE 4-9434.
SZANT, Marvin; Tor '61; Jr. Intn., New Mount Sinai Hosp., Toronto 2, Ont.
SZASZ, George; 131 Stevens Dr. West, Vancouver, B.C. (res); UBC'55; MCGP; Tel. 985-5381.
SZASZ, Ivan J.; London (Eng.)'63; Res., Ottawa Civic Hosp., Ottawa 3, Ont.
SZASZ, John; 550 Ingersoll Ave., Woodstock, Ont.; Wes '54; Ophth; Staff, Woodstock Gen. Hosp.; Tel. 537-3871.
SZATMARI, Alexander; 288 St. Clair Ave. W., Toronto 7, Ont.; 219 Dunvegan Rd., Tor. 7 (res); Budapest (Hung.) '31; NeurSpsy; I/C EEG Dept., Ont. Hosp.; Clin. Instr. (Psy), U. of Toronto; Tel. 921-0556.
SZCZUCINSKI, Waclaw T.; 274 Linwell Rd., St. Catharines, Ont.; McG '48; Tel. 935-5131.
SZEGO, Peter L.; McG'65; Res., St. Mary's Hosp., Montreal 26, P.Q.
SZEKELY, Eugen; 308 Tegler Bldg., 10189-101 st St., Edmonton, Alta.; Budapest (Hung.) '35; MCGP; Tel. GA 4-6561.
SZEKELY, Peter E.; 798 Main St. E., Hamilton, Ont.; Budapest (Hung.) '22; Tel. LI 9-7911.
SZEKERES, Eva A.; Staff, Provincial Hosp., Campbellton, N.B. '40.
SZELENY, Frank L.; Budapest (Hung.) '50; Res., Victoria Hosp., London, Ont.
SZENAS, Paul; Basel (Switz.) '50; Res., Royal Victoria Hosp., Montreal 2, P.Q.
SZEPS, Jerzy; 274 King St. W., Chatham, Ont.; Dublin (Ire.) '56; LRCP; LRCS; LM(Ire.); FAGS; Active Staff, Ophth., Chatham Gen. & St. Joseph's Hosp's.; Tel. 354-5292.
SZERB, J. C.; 9 Ross St., Birch Cove, N.S. (res); Munich (Germ.) '50; Assoc. Prof. (Pharm.), Dalhousie U.; Tel. 455-1748.
SZESZYCKI, Leon W.; 293 Selkirk Ave., Winnipeg, Man.; 816 McDermot Ave. (res); Poznan (Poland) '35; Tel. JU 9-7145.
SZETLE, Anna A. M.; St.-Boniface Clinic, 343 Tache, Winnipeg 6, Man.; 1467 Wellington Cres., Wpg. 9 (res); Poznan (Poland) '47; Otol; Otol., St.-Boniface Hosp.; Tel. WH 7-1581.
SZIKLAS, Tibor; 720 Med. Arts Bldg., 1538 Sherbrooke St. W., Montreal 25, P.Q.; Budapest (Hung.) '53; Tel. 935-7149.
SZIROM, Stephen; St. Boniface, Clinic, 343 Tache Ave., St. Boniface, Man.; Budapest (Hung.) '52; AMCGP; Tel. 947-1581.
SZLAZAK, Jan P.; Med. Arts Bldg., Regina, Sask., 3116 Rae St. (res); Warsaw (Pol.) '34; PlasSurg; Hd. Plastics Maxillo Facial, Regina Gen. & Regina Grey Nuns Hosp's.; Tel. 523-0691.
SZLICHCINSKI, W.; 607 Tegler Bldg., Edmonton, Alta.; Ste. 8, 11933 Jasper Ave. (res); Poznan (Poland) '27; Tel. GA 4-2201.
SZOLLOSI, Sandor L.; Ste. 307, 99 Avenue Rd., Toronto 5, Ont.; 74 Spadina Rd., Tor 4 (res); Debrecen (Hung) '38; Assoc. Staff, Doctor's Hosp.; Tel. WA 2-2085.
SZOLLOSY, L. G. K.; 79 Sherman Ave. S., Hamilton, Ont.; Budapest (Hung.) '29; Tel. 549-5111.
SZORENYI-REISCHL, Michael; 14 Tillson Ave., Tillsonburg, Ont.; Pazmany Peter U. (Hung.) '45; Tel. VI 2-2242.
SZOTS, Francois; Lav '64; Res., Children's Hosp., Montreal 25, P.Q.
SZUCHEWYCZ, Bohdan; 317 Medical Dental Bldg., Rose St. & 11th. Ave., Regina, Sask.; Nat. U. (Ire.) '53; M.B., B.Ch., BAO; MCH; OrthSurg; Tel. 523-2634.
SZYBALSKI, Wlayslaw J.; 34 Jarvis St., Fort Erie, Ont.; 231 North St. (res); Lwow (Poland) '36; Active Med. Staff, Douglas Mem. Hosp.; Tel. 871-2341.
SZYMANSKI, Gregor; 312 Bathurst St., Toronto, Ont.; 1 Glenaden Ave. E., Toronto 18 (res); Lwow, (Pol.) '29; Tel. 366-3874.
SZYMONOWICZ-RUDNICKY, Halina; 4400 Prince of Wales Ave., Montreal 28, P.Q. (res); Phillips U. (Marburg, Germ.) '47; Court. Staff Anaes., Catherine Booth Mothers' Hosp.; Tel. 481-0431.
SZYRYNSKI, Victor; Ste. 423, 43 Bruyere St., Ottawa, Ont.; Warsaw (Poland) '38; Ph.D., FACP; FAPA; FBPsS (Lond.); FRCP(C), NeurPsy; Chief, Dept. of Psy., Ottawa Gen. Hosp.; Cons. Neurol. & Psy., St. Louis Marie de Montfort Hosp.; Cons. Ottawa Civic Hosp.; Prof. of Psy.; U. of Ottawa; Tel. 236-0333, Ext. 275.
TABAH, Edward J.; 1374 Sherbrooke St. W., Montreal 25, P.Q.; McG '42; FRCS(C), GenSurg; Att'd. Surg., Royal Victoria Hosp.; Cons. Surg., Reddy Mem. & Queen Mary Vet's. Hosp's.; Ass't. Prof. Surg., McGill U.; Tel. 842-7521.
TABESH, Ali R.; Tehran (Iran)'56; Anaes; Staff, St. Boniface Gen. Hosp., Winnipeg 6, Man.
TABIB, Negib; 53 John St., Sturgeon Falls, Ont.; Beirut (Lebanon) '46; GenSurg; Staff, St.-Jean-de-Brebeuf Hosp.; Tel. 753-2070.
TACHE, C. Robert; Mon'61; FRCS(C), PlasSurg; Staff, Hop. Maisonneuve, Montreal, P.Q.
TACK, Michael; Assoc. Med. Clinic, The Pas, Man.; London (Eng.) '53; MRCS; LRCP; Staff, St. Anthony's Hosp.; Tel. MA 3-3290.
TACKOOR, W. T.; 1277 York Mills Rd., Don Mills, Ont.; Tor '63.
TADROS, Peter; 4794A Joyce Ave., Powell River, B.C.; Sask'65.
TAGGART, James G.; Henderson Gen. Hosp., Hamilton, Ont.; Qns'56; Pathol., Henderson Gen. Hosp.; Tel. 389-4411, Ext. 261.
TAGUCHI, Yoshindri Y.; 5363 Van Horne Ave., Montreal 29, P.Q.; McG '59; FRCS(C), Urol; Staff, Royal Victoria Hosp.; Tel. 842-1251, Loc. 1698.
TAI, Joseph R.; Ott'65; Jr. Int., Victoria Hosp., London, Ont.; Abroad.
TAILLEFER, J. Bernard; Ste. 101, 428 Rideau St., Ottawa, Ont.; 1365 Dowler Ave. (res); Ott '54; FRCS(C) GenSurg; M.S. (Surg., Minn.); GenSurg; Clin. Ass't. (Surg.), U. of Ottawa; Tel. 235-2438.
TAILLEFER, Paul A.; 7229 St. Denis, Montreal, P.Q.; Lav '59; Ophth; Tel. 237-7944.
TAILLON, Armand P.; Lac-Etchemin, Cte Dorchester, P.Q.; Lav '56.
TAILLON, Claude; Lav '58; MCGP; Res., Hop. Hotel-Dieu, Montreal, P.Q.
TAILLON, Jean-Louis; 547 du-Domaine St. Jerom Co. Terrebonne, P.Q.; Mon '48; Med. Dir., Hosp.-Hotel-Dieu, St.-Jerome; Tel. GE 8-1317.
TAINSH, John M.; 5957 South St., Halifax, N.S.; London (Eng.) '43; MRCP; FRCS (Eng.); IntMed; Med. Supt., Halifax Mental Hosp.; Tel. 423-9173.
TAIT, Herbert M. S.; 216 St. Clair Ave. W., Toronto 7, Ont.; Tor'35; ObstGyn; Active Staff, Grace Hosp.; Vol. O.P.D., Toronto Gen. Hosp.; Court. Staff, Wellesley Hosp.; Tel. 921-7111.
TAIT, Wm. M.; 3195 Granville St., Vancouver 9, B.C.; 3655A The Kingsway (res); McG '39; DiagRad.; Tel. RE 1-5241.
TAKACS, Ernest S.; Alb'65; Res., Royal Alexandra Hosp., Edmonton, Alta.
TAKAHASHI, George Y.; 1500 Royal York Rd., Weston, Ont.; Tor'62; Court. Staff, Humber Mem. Hosp.; Tel. 249-2565.
TAKAHASHI, Joseph H.; Box 250, Picture Butte, Alta.; Alb'58; Tel. 732-4361.
TAKAHASHI, Paul K.; Tor'62; Res., Toronto East Gen. Hosp., Toronto 13, Ont.
TAKATS, Laszlo N.; Alb '63; Res., University Hosp., Edmonton, Alta.
TAKEDA, Misao; Yokohoma (Japan)'56; Staff & Lect. Path., Dept. of Pathol., University Hosp., Saskatoon, Sask.
TALAAT, Said; 1849 Yonge St., Toronto 7, Ont.; University Coll. Hosp. (London, Eng.)'44.

TALBOT, Charles A.; First St., Port McNicoll, Ont.; Tor '56.
TALBOT, Ernest J.; 52 Grande-Ile, Valleyfield, P.Q.; **4 Ewing (res); McG '39; MCGP; Staff Hop. Hotel-Dieu; Tel. 373-3212.**
TALBOT, Henri E.; 117 Ave. Ruel, Montmorency, P.Q. **119 Ave. Ruel (res); Lav '25; MCGP; Tel.** 663-9407; Abroad.
TALBOT, Jacques; Lav'65; Res., Institute Albert Provost, Montreal 9, P.Q.
TALBOT, Jean L.; Lav '37; Staff, Hop. Hotel Dieu, Gaspe, P.Q.; Tel. 502.
TALBOT, J. H. Bernard; 6300 Darlington Ave., Montreal 26, P.Q. App. 401, 3466 Aylmer (res); Lav '58; Phys. Med. & Rehab; Physiatrist, Inst. de Rehab.; Cons. Hop. Jean-Talon; Vis. Lect (Physiol.) Laval U.; Lect. Physiol., School of Rehab. & **Phys Med.; Staff (Med.), U. of Montreal; Tel. 735-3741.**
TALBOT, Roland; Armagh, Cte. Bellchasse, P.Q. **Lav '61; A.M.C.G.P.; Tel. 181.**
TALIBI, Talip; Istanbul (Turk.)'57; Staff, Royal Alexandra Hosp., Edmonton, Alta.
TALLAN, Zoltan; 1121 Yates St., Victoria, B.C. (res); Peter Pazmanny (Hung.) '41; **Phys-Med & Rehab; Staff, Royal Jubilee Hosp.; Tel. EV 6-3131.**
TALLON, John A.; 612—4th St. E., Cornwall, Ont.; 118-2nd St. E. (res); McG '19; F.A.C.S., **F.I.C.S., FRCS(C) GenSurg; MCGP; Chief of Staff, & Chief, Dept. of Surg., Hotel-Dieu Hosp.; Tel. WE 2-4630.**
TALLON, John B.; 742 King St. W., Kitchener, Ont.; McG '51; FRCS(C), OrthSurg; **Med. Advisory Bd., Rehab. Fdn., Prov. of Ont.; Tel. 745-**0251.
TALLON, Michael B.; 612 Fourth St. E., Cornwall, Ont.; Ott '59; Tel. WE 3-2114.
TALMEY, Richard C.; 686 No. 3 Rd., Richmond, Vancouver, B.C.; 830 Park Rd. (res); Wes '41; **MCGP; Tel. CR 8-8435.**
TALPASH, Orest S., Capt.; Nat. Defence Med. Centre, Ottawa 8, Ont.; Sask'63.
TAM, Ennio A.; Ste. 203, 1669 Victoria St., Prince George, B.C.; UBC'57; Tel. 564-6117.
TAM, Michael C.; Alb'63; Res., Toronto Western Hosp., Toronto 2B, Ont.
TAM, Teresa Y.; 536 Riverview Dr., Fort William, Ont.; Shangai (China) '48.
TAM, Y. Dick; 8431 Granville St., Vancouver 14, B.C.; London (Eng.)'64.
TAMAS, Andrew; 5845 Cote des Neiges Rd., Montreal 26, P.Q.; 159 Finchley Rd., Hampstead (res); Munich (Germ.) '51; TherRad; Ass't. Rad., Jewish Gen. Hosp.; Ass't. Rad., St. Mary's Hosp.; Tel. RE 1-8245.
TAMBOLINE, Beverley L.; UBC '60; Staff, Valley-view Hosp., Essondale, B.C.
TAMBURRO, Rocco A.; 697 Danforth Ave., Toronto 6, Ont.; 91 Cosburn Ave., Apt. 708 (res); **Tor '61; Tel. 466-5250.**
TAMMEMAGI, Voldemar; 147 Geneva St., St. Catharines, Ont. (res); **Tartu (Estonia) '41; M.C.G.P.; Tel. MU 2-1297.**
TAN, Kim H.; Hongkong (China) '46; DABR; D & TRad; Staff, Community Health Centre, 2363 McIntyre St., Regina, Sask.; Tel. 523-2880.
TAN, Mariano; 190 Tache, Winnipeg 6, Man.; Santo Tomas (Philipp.)'58; Assoc. Staff, St. Boniface Hosp.; Tel. CE 3-2394.
TAN, Richard; Tor'65; Res., Kingston Gen. Hosp., Kingston, Ont.
TAN, Siong K.; Apt. 525, 108 Isabella St., Toronto 5, Ont.; Indonesia '59; **DiagRad.**
TANAKA, Shuzo; 719 Upper James St., Hamilton, Ont.; Tor '55; Tel. FU 9-1933.
TANASICHUK, Murray A.; 3803-19th St. S.W., Calgary, Alta. (res); Man '52; Staff, Calgary Gen. Hosp.; Tel. 266-7451.
TANASIUK, Eli; Alb '54; Res., Royal Alexandra Hosp., Edmonton, Alta.
TANDAN, P. Janet; Leeds (Eng.) '61; Res., Toronto Gen. Hosp., Toronto, Ont.
TANENBAUM, Howard L.; McG'61; FRCS(C), Ophth; Dept. of Ophth., Queen's University, Kingston, Ont.
TANG, Marcos; 2915 Wyandotte W., Windsor, Ont.; Ott'60.
TANG, Peter S.; '55; Res., Winnipeg Gen. Hosp., Winnipeg, Man.
TANGUAY, Bernardin; Ste. 1, 132 Centre St., St. Thomas, Ont.; Lav'54.
TANGUAY, Fernand; 244 Heneker, Sherbrooke, P.Q. (res); Lav'43; Anaes; Med. Dir., & Chief Anaes., Hop. Gen. St-Vincent de Paul, 300 King St., Sherbrooke, P.Q.; Tel. 569-6492.
TANGUAY, Gervais; C.P. 280, 11 St-Louis, Princeville, Cte. Arthabaska, P.Q.; Lav '62.
TANGUAY, Hubert; 5647 Langelier, Montreal 5, P.Q.; Lav '51; Urol.; Tel. 254-6197.
TANGUAY, Jacques; 3253 est, rue Beaubien, Montreal 36, P.Q.; **Lav '54; GenSurg; Tel. 721-**6241.
TANGUAY, Leo; 19 Victoria St., Bagotville, Co. Chicoutimi, P.Q.; Lav '39; M.C.G.P.
TANGUAY, Nicole; Mon '62; Res. (Gyn.), Hotel-Dieu, Montreal, P.Q.
TANGUAY, Robert; Lav'63; Res., Hop. Maisonneuve, Montreal 36, P.Q.
TANNEN, Peter A.; 815 Victoria St., Trail, B.C.; 721 Eliot St. (res); London (Eng.) '53; Anaes; Staff, Trail Tadenac Hosp.; Tel. 364-1234.
TANNENBAUM, Isaac; 515 Ellendale Med. Bldg., 5845 Cote-des-Neiges Rd., Montreal 26, P.Q.; 17 **Briardale Rd., Hampstead, P.Q. (res); McG '46; M.C.G.P.; Clin. Ass't., Med., Jewish Gen. Hosp.;** Tel. RE 8-4163
TANNER, Arthur R.; Dept. of Health, 351 Legis**lative Bldg., Winnipeg, Man.;** 301 Cambridge St. (res); Man '37; Tel. WH 2-2139.
TANNER, Aubrey C.; Box 2054, Whitehorse, Y.T.; Seattle (U.S.A.) '51; FRCS(C), GenSurg; Tel. 7-2508.
TANNER, W. Reginald; 45 Academy Med. Bldg., 1812-4th S.W., Calgary, Alta.; 108 Eagle Ridge Dr. (res); UBC '54; Ophth; Cons. Ophth., Calgary Gen., **Alberta Children's, Holy Cross & Col. Belcher Hosp's.; Tel. 262-6221.**
TANOVICH, James; 846 Danforth Ave., Toronto 6, Ont.; Tor'62; Staff, St. Michael's & Toronto East Gen. Hosp.; Tel. HO 1-0785.
TANSER, Paul H.; Ott'62; Res., Dept. of Path., U. of Ottawa, Ottawa, Ont.
TANTON, Benjamin W.; 50 Hycroft Med. Bldg., 3195 Granville St., Vancouver, B.C.; 5650 Angus Dr. (res); McG '37; Otol; Assoc., Dept. of Surg., Sub. Dept. of Otol., Van. Gen. Hosp.; Vis. Staff, Children's Hosp.; Ass't. Prof., U. of British Columbia; Tel. RE 1-4625.
TANTON, Clare W.; 481 Dundas St. W., Belleville, Ont.; McG '41; Anaes.
TANTON, T. Muncey; Main St., Woodstock, N.B.; Broadway (res); McG '41; D.A.B.Ot.; **OphthOtol; Staff, Carleton Mem. Hosp.; Tel. 328-**3391.
TANZ, E. Mitchell; 215 Victoria St., Toronto 2, Ont.; Tor '53; FRCS(C); PlasSurg; Tel. EM 4-5325.
TANZER, H.; 160 Balmoral Ave., Toronto 7, Ont.; Tor '64; Abroad.
TANZER, Joseph; 158 St. George St., Toronto, **Ont.; 5 Glenarden Rd. (res); Tor '33; Tel. WA 2-2828.**
TANZER, Lionel I.; 158 St. George St., Toronto, Ont.; 24 Shallmar Blvd. **(res); Tor '48; F.R.C.S. (C), ObstGyn; Tel. WA 2-2828.**
TANZMAN, Joseph; 115 Hazen St., St. John, N.B.; 617 Sand Cove Rd., Lancaster (res); McG '27; ObstGyn; Chief (ObstGyn) St. Joseph's Hosp.; Att. ObstGyn., Saint John's & Provincial Hosp's.; Cons. (ObstGyn), Lancaster D.V.A. Hosp.; Tel. 692-6631.
TAORI, Girdharilal M.; Nagpur (India)'57; FRCP(C), Neur; Staff, Mtl. Neurological Inst., Montreal, P.Q.
TARANGER, Lawrence A.; Med. Arts Clinic, 51 Sixth St. S.E., Medicine Hat, Alta.; Alb '62; Staff, Medicine Hat Gen. Hosp.; Tel. 527-2281; Abroad.
TARANGLE, Steven G.; 12929-62nd St., Edmonton, Alta.; Loma Linda (Calif., U.S.A.)'64; DO; Tel. 476-5566.
TARANTINO, Achille M.; 2600 Eglinton Ave. W., Toronto 15, Ont.; Naples (Italy)'33; FICS; FACS; Assoc. Staff (Surg.), Toronto Western Hosp.; Tel. 651-5091.

TARANTINO, Leopold; 5325 Jean Talon, Montreal, P.Q.: Naples (Italy) '52; FRCS(C); Otol.
TARAS, Edward; Tor '58 Res., Jewish Gen. Hosp., Montreal, P.Q.
TARASOFSKY, Edward; Tor '58; Res., c/o 4734 Maplewood Ave., Montreal 26, P.Q.
TARASZCZUK, Paul; 3247 Bellechasse St., Montreal 36, P.Q.; Graz (Aust.) '27; Staff, Hop. Jean Talon; Tel. 727-8562.
TARDIF, Andre R.; Lav '60; Res., Hotel-Dieu Hosp., Quebec, P.Q.
TARDIF, Arthur; 415, rue Ste. Helene, Longueil, Que.; Lav '43; Tel. OR 4-6281.
TARDIF, Guy; Medical Centre, 55 Emerson St., Edmundston, N.B.; Lav '45; F.A.C.S., F.R.C.S. (C), GenSurg; Surg., Hop.-Hotel-Dieu; Tel. 735-5521.
TARDIF, Jacques; 460 2eme rue, Chibougamau, P.Q.; Mon'65.
TARDIF, J. Aristide; 595 E. Blvd. Charest, Quebec, P.Q.; 333 Grande Allee (res); Lav '25; Ophth Otol; Tel. 529-9721.
TARDIF, J. Bertrand; Lav '59; Cardiol (P.Q.); Staff, Hop. Youville, Noranda, P.Q.; Tel. 762-4135.
TARDIF, Luc; Ste. 103, 250 est, boul. St-Joseph, Montreal 14, P.Q.; Mon'59; DiagRad; Staff, Hop. Ste-Justine.
TARDIF, Marc; Lav '49; Exec. Med. Dir., Jewish Hosp. of Hope; Montreal, P.Q.; Tel. 352-3120.
TARI, Harjo; Ste. 132, 400 Walmer Rd., Toronto 10, Ont.; Tor'54; Staff, Doctor's Hosp.; Tel. 923-5411.
TARJAN, Georges; Unite Sanitaire, 3719 Boul. Levesque Chomedy, P.Q.; Budapest (Hung.)'51; PH(P.Q.).
TARRANT, Michael; 41 Chelsea St. N. W., Calgary, Alta.; Cambridge (Eng.) '61; Staff, Calgary Gen. & Grace Hosp's.; Tel. 289-1901.
TARTE, Paul D.; 607 Ste. Famille, Boucherville, P.Q.; Mon '43; IntMed (P.Q.), Gastroent (P.Q.).
TASCHEREAU, Dorion; 1069-6eme rue, Val D'Or, P.Q.; 83 rue Montcalm (res); Mon '48.
TASCHEREAU, J. T. de Montarville; C.P. 98, St.-Germain de Grantham, Cte. Drummond, P.Q.; Lav '33; Pres. Med. Staff, Hop. Ste.-Croix, Drummondville; Tel. 395-4545.
TASKER, Peter H.; 145 Wellington St., Sarnia, Ont.; Leeds (Eng.)'40; FRCS(Eng.); GenSurg; Chief of Staff, Sarnia Gen. Hosp.; Tel. 344-1201.
TASKER, Robert G.; The Cottage Hosp., Pembroke, Ont.; Cambridge (Eng.)'44; MRCS; LRCP; Am.Bd. Path; Dir. of Labs., Pembroke Cottage & Renfrew Victoria Hosp's.
TASKER, Ronald R.; Neurosurgical Unit, 11 CB, Toronto Gen. Hosp., 101 College St., Toronto 2, Ont.; 159 Collier St. (res); Tor '52; F.R.C.S.(C), NeurSurg; Ass't. Surg., Toronto Gen. Hosp.; Cons. NeurSurg., Sunnybrook Hosp. & Ont. Hosp. Schl., Orillia; Assoc. (Surg.), U. of Toronto; Tel. EM 6-8211, Loc. 2251.
TASS, David; Ste. 502, 1205 Grant Ave., Winnipeg 9, Man.; Man '33; Anaes; **Staff, St. Boniface &** Victor'a Hosp's.
TASSIN, John J.; 149 Ingram St., Duncan, B.C.; Quamichan Park Rd. (res); Louvain (Belg.) '40; MCGP; Tel. 746-4401.
TATARTCHEFF, Michel; 91 Pine St. S., Timmins, **Ont.**; Geneva (Switz.) '47; Tel. 264-6258.
TATE, Robert G.; 1315 Fairmont Med Bldg., 750 W. Broadway, Vancouver 9, B.C.; Qns '52; FRCS (C), OrthSurg; Assoc. Staff, Children's Hosp.; Vist. Staff, Vancouver Gen., St. Paul's, St. Vincent's & Burnaby Gen. Hosp's.; Staff, Health Centre for Children; Tel. 874-0614.
TATHAM, M. Ruth (Bell); Box 390; Listowel, Ont.; Qns '54; Retired.
TATLEMAN, Maurice; 21 Willowdale Ave., Montreal, P.Q.; McG '28; Clin. Ass't. (Med.), Jewish Gen. Hosp.; Tel. RE 8-7239.
TATLOW, W. F. Tissington; 660 Victoria Ave., Montreal 6, P.Q.; London (Eng.)'38; M.B., B.S. (Lond.), M.D. (Lond.), M.R.C.P. (Lond.); F.R.-C.P.(C), Neurol; **Assoc. Neurol., Montreal Gen.**; Ass't. Neurol., Montreal Neurol. Inst.; Dir. Neurol. Dept., Queen Mary Veterans' Hosp.; Neurol., Lakeshore Gen. Hosp.; Ass't. Prof. Neurol., McGill U.; Tel. 409-3318.
TATOR, Charles H.; Tor'61; PhD; Res., Neur-Surg., U. of Toronto, Toronto, Ont.
TATTERSALL, Evelyn (See Bateman).
TATTON, William G.; Alb'65; Res., Toronto General Hospital, Toronto 2, Ont.
TAUBE, Harold N.; 732 Spadina Ave., Toronto, Ont.; R.R. No. 1, Kleinburg, Ont. (res); Tor '31; DABIM, IntMed; Sr. Att. Staff, New Mt. Sinai Hosp.; Assoc. IntMed., Doctor's Hosp.; Tel. WA 2-2523.
TAUER, C.; 1538 Sherbrooke St., Montreal, P.Q.; **4822 Isabella (res); Tel. 935-6666.**
TAVENER, Roy H.; Box 9600, Selkirk, Man. (res); Man '50; Psy; Supt., Selkirk Mental Hosp.; Ass't. Prof. (Psy), U. of Manitoba; Tel. 482-3810.
TAVES, Iva R. (Sherk); 105 Union Blvd., Kit**chener, Ont. (res); Tor '52; Path; Dir. of Labs Kitchener-Waterloo Hosp.; Tel. SH 5-9451.**
TAYFEL, Roy S.; Qns'65; Res., Hotel Dieu Hosp., Kingston, Ont.
TAYLAR, Charles E.; Oxford (Eng.)'60; Psy; Staff, Mental Hosp., St. John's, Nfld.
TAYLOR, Addison; 1184 Mt. Pleasant Rd., Toronto 12, Ont.; Tor '14; Tel. HU 8-9974.
TAYLOR, Alan F.; 2115 Pelissier St., Windsor, Ont.; 600 Riverside Dr., St. Clair Beach (res); Tor '35; MCGP; Tel. 254-9294.
TAYLOR, Alan S.; 425 Sherring St., Preston, Ont. (res); Aberdeen (Scot.) '47; D.P.H.; Dir., Waterloo Co. Health Unit; Tel. 653-6168.
TAYLOR, Albert W.; 4 Weir Cr., St. John's, Nfld.; Dal'51; DHA (Tor); Med. Supt., General Hosp.; Tel. 578-0471.
TAYLOR, Alexander H.; 32 Caledonia Terr., Gode**rich, Ont. (res); Tor '10; GenSurg; I/C (Diag-Rad), Alexandra Marine & Gen. Hosp.**
TAYLOR, Andrew C. (O.B.E.); 812 Medical & Dental Bldg., Regina, Sask.; 3055 Angus St. (res); Tor '26; F.R.C.S.(Edin.), F.R.C.S.(C) GenSurg; D.T.M.; Chief, GenSurg, Serv., Regina Gen. Hosp.; Tel. LA 2-5629.
TAYLOR, B. Earle; 188 Main St., Picton, Ont.; Qns '54; GenSurg; Staff, Prince Edward Co. Mem. Hosp.; Tel. GR 6-5660.
TAYLOR, Bruce W.; 2302 Brooklawn Dr., Temple, Texas 76501, U.S.A.; UBC'60; FRCS(C), PlasSurg; Abroad.
TAYLOR, Carleton T.; Alb'65; Res., Misericordia Hosp., Edmonton, Alta.
TAYLOR, Carl L.; 323 Wentworth St. S., Hamil**ton, Ont.; Tor '43; M.C.G.P.; Tel. 383-3011.**
TAYLOR, Cecil H.; Mall Medical Bldg., Winnipeg, Man.; Man '28; Tel. SP 4-2411.
TAYLOR, Charles W.; 63 Academy Med. Bldg., 1812-4th St. S.W., Calgary, Alta.; Tor'40; MS; FRCS(C), NeurSurg; Chief, Div. of NeurSurg., Foothills Hosp.; Cons. NeurSurg., Calgary Gen., Holy Cross, Alberta Children's, Colonel Belcher, Banff Mineral Springs & St. Michael's Hosp., Lethbridge; Tel. 266-3952.
TAYLOR, Clifford C.; 43 Ridgemoor Ave., Scarborough, Ont.; McG '57; Tel. AM 1-4159.
TAYLOR, Clifford R.; 604 Brant St., Burlington, Ont.; Tor '55; ObstGyn; Active Staff, Joseph Brant Mem. Hosp.; Court. Staff, Hamilton Gen. & St. Joseph's Hosp's.; Tel. 637-2915.
TAYLOR, Cyril R.; 115 Hazen St., **Saint John, N.B.; Dal '53; GenSurg; Tel. 693-4416.**
TAYLOR, David A.; Qns '55; Staff, **Plant Hosp.,** Chalk River, Ont.
TAYLOR, Douglas S.; Edinburgh (Scot.)'62; Staff, Dept. of Pharm., McGill U., Montreal, P.Q.
TAYLOR, Edward; P.O. Box 249, Shaunavon Clinic, Shaunavon, Sask.; Dublin (Ire.) '51; M.B., B.Ch., B.A.O.; Med. Staff, Shaunavon Union Hosp.; Tel. 297-2625.
TAYLOR, Ellen F.; Man '19; Chief, Dept. of Infectious Dis., King George Hosp., Winnipeg, Man.
TAYLOR, G. Allan; Ott'62; DDS; Res., Toronto Gen. Hosp., Toronto 2, Ont.

TAYLOR, G. Douglas; 102 Med. Arts Bldg., 280 Bloor St. W., Toronto 5, Ont.; 566 Blythwood Rd., Tor. 12 (res); McG '28; IntMed; Chief, Arthritis Clin., Toronto Western Hosp.; Cons. Rheumatol., Queen Elizabeth Hosp. & Geriatric Centre, Dept. of Welfare, Ont. & Metropolitan Toronto; Tel. WA 2-7722.

TAYLOR, George O.; 2211 Riverside Dr., Ste. 207, Ottawa, Ont.; Ott'55; ObstGyn; Staff, Ottawa Civic Hosp. & Riverside Hosp.

TAYLOR, George W.; 114-10th St. W., Owen Sound, Ont.; 521-9th St. E. (res); Tor '34; Obst; Head of Obst., General & Marine Hosp.; Tel. FR 6-2354.

TAYLOR, Glen A.; Tor'61; GenSurg; Staff, Sunnybrook Hosp., Toronto 12, Ont.

TAYLOR, Graham C.; 1025 Pine Ave. W., Montreal, P.Q.; 1915 Laird Blvd., Twn. of Mt. Royal (res); McG '43; DABPN, Psy (P.Q.); Ass't. to Dir., Allan Mem. Inst.; Ass't. Psy., Royal Victoria Hosp.; Cons. Psy., Aluminum Co. of Canada; Ass't. Prof., McGill U.; Tel. 933-8236.

TAYLOR, Graeme M.; Qns'65; Res., Kingston Gen. Hosp., Kingston, Ont.

TAYLOR, Harlan G.; Raymond, Alta.; Alb '48; Staff, Raymond Municipal Hosp.; Tel. 752-3067.

TAYLOR, Harold E.; 6992 Churchill St., Vancouver, B.C. (res); Dal '36; MRCP(E); F.R.C.P. (Ed. & C.), Path Bact.; Exec. Dir., Dept. of Path., Vancouver Gen. Hosp.; Prof. & Head Dept. Path., U. of British Columbia; Tel. TR 6-3211.

TAYLOR, Harold M.; 24 Hope St. W., Tavistock, Ont.; Tor'29; MCGP; Staff, Stratford Gen. & Woodstock Gen. Hosp's.; Tel. 655-2322.

TAYLOR, Henry D.; Box 476, Windsor, Ont.; 473 Sunset (res); McG '18; Dist. Coroner.

TAYLOR, H. L.; Bolton, Ont.; Tor '41; Tel. 857-2265.

TAYLOR, Henry M.; 3000 Lawrence Ave. E., Scarborough, Ont.; 173 Sweeney Dr., Tor. 16 (res); Tor '57; DiagRad; Jr. Att'd. Staff, Scarborough Gen. Hosp.; Tel. 291-1121.

TAYLOR, Hugh; Manitoba Clinic, 790 Sherbrook St., Winnipeg 2, Man.; Man '57; Paed; Staff, Winnipeg Children's Hosp. & Wpg. Municipal Hosps.; Ass't. Prof. Paed., U. of Manitoba.

TAYLOR, James A.; 2965 Seaview Rd., Victoria, B.C. (res); Alb '36; DPH, FAPHA, DABPrevMed; PH; Deputy Min. of Health, Dept. of Health Serv. & Hosp. Ins., Parliament Bldgs., Victoria, B.C.; Tel. EV 2-6111.

TAYLOR, James A.; 73 Erie St. S., Leamington, Ont.; Wes '53; M.C.G.P.

TAYLOR, James E.; Golden, B.C.; Alb '51; M.C.G.P.; Dist. Coroner.

TAYLOR, James V.; UBC '54; FRCP(C), Anaes; Staff, Swedish Hosp., Seattle, Wash., U.S.A.; Abroad.

TAYLOR, John D.; Ste. 3, 244 Bloor St. W., Toronto 5, Ont.; Apt. 716, 108 Isabella St. (res); Tor '61; Tel. 921-7081.

TAYLOR, John K.; Ott '64; Jr. Int., Ottawa Civic Hosp., Ottawa 3, Ont.

TAYLOR, John L.; 22A Church St., Lennoxville, P.Q.; 43 Howard Ave. (res); McG '49; IntMed; Med. Staff & Chmn. Radio Active Isotope Commiss., Sherbrooke Hosp.; Tel. LO 7-7383.

TAYLOR, John R.; Qns'63; Res., Toronto Western Hosp., Toronto, Ont.

TAYLOR, J. Reid; Winnipeg Clinic, N.E. St. Mary's & Vaughan, Winnipeg, Man.; 306 Dromore Ave. (res); Man '45; Urol; Ass't. Urol., Winnipeg Gen. Hosp.; Cons. Urol., Municipal Hosp's.; Lect., in Urol., U. of Manitoba; Tel. WH 2-6441.

TAYLOR, Jean (See Nelson)

TAYLOR, Martin; Albany Clinic, 200 Danforth Ave., Toronto 6, Ont.; Wes '59; Staff, Toronto East Gen. Hosp., & Doctors Hosp.; Tel. 461-0761.

TAYLOR, Michael J. F/L; Dal '59; SMO, RCAF Station, Summerside, P.E.I.

TAYLOR, Norman B. G.; King High Dr., Concord, Ont.; Tor '42; Ph.D.; Hd. Physiol. Sec., Defence Med. Lab., Box 62, Postal Stn. "K", Toronto; Hon. Lect. (Med. Research), U. of Western Ont.

TAYLOR, Robert M.; 17 Green Valley Rd., Willowdale, Ont. (res); Tor '39; F.R.C.P.(C), IntMed.; Exec. Dir., Nat. Cancer Inst. of Canada; Exec. Vice Pres., Canadian Cancer Soc.: Cons., Princess Margaret Hosp.; Lect. Dept. Med. Biophysics & Clin. Teacher (Med.), U. of Toronto; EM 4-7483.

TAYLOR, Ross B.; 76 Hemlock St., Timmins, Ont.; McG '18.

TAYLOR, Russell F.; University Hosp., Edmonton, Alta.; McG'50; FRCP(C), IntMed; Ass't. Prof. Med., U. of Alberta.

TAYLOR, Thomas; Glasgow (Scot.)'51; D.Obst., RCOG; Res., Vancouver Gen. Hosp., Vancouver 9, B.C.

TAYLOR, Wilbur K.; Box 29, Ralston, Alta. (res); Dal '52; Staff, Suffield Experimental Stn., Suffield.

TAYLOR, William; 43 Pleasant Rd., Guelph, Ont.; Qns '51; IntMed; Staff, Homewood San.; Tel. TA 4-1010.

TAYLOR, William; 381 Patricia Blvd., Timmins, Ont. (res); Qns '33; F.C.C.P., IntMed (TB); Med. Dir., Miners' Chest Examining Station, Timmins.

TAYLOR, William A.; Apt. 401, 325 Giles Blvd. W., Windsor, Ont.; McG'45; Anaes; Chief of Anaes., Hotel-Dieu-Hosp.; Tel. 253-5492.

TAYLOR, William A.; Glasgow (Scot.) '45; Staff, Blanchard Fraser Hosp., Kentville, N.S.; Tel. 678-7381.

TAYLOR, William B.; 10 Farley Pl., St. Thomas, Ont. (res); McG '39; D & TRad; Dir., Roentgen. Dept., St. Thomas-Elgin Gen. Hosp., St. Thomas; Tel. ME 1-2020.

TAYLOR, William C.; 10941-89 Ave., Edmonton, Alta. (res); Aberdeen (Scot.) '45; DCH; FAAP; FRCP(C), Paed; Staff, University Hosp.; Assoc. Prof. (Paed.), U. of Alberta; Tel. GE 3-5747.

TAYLOR, William H.; Tor'61; Res., St. Michael's Hosp., Toronto 2, Ont.; Abroad.

TAYLOR, William I.; 30 Bloor St. W., Toronto 5, Ont.; 2692 Bayview Ave., Willowdale (res); Qns'35; Exec. Dir., Can. Council on Hosp. Accreditations; Guest Lect. (Hosp. Admin.), U. of Toronto, U. of Ottawa & HOM Students, C.H.A.; Tel. WA 3-1261.

TAYLOR, William J.; 360 Professional Bldg., 10830 Jasper Ave., Edmonton, Alta.; 8104-138th St. (res); Edinburgh (Scot.) '47; DMR(Tor); DiagRad; Staff, Edmonton Gen. Hosp.; Tel. 422-1390.

TAYLOR, W. J. Russell; 826 Med. Arts Bldg., 170 St. George St., Toronto 5, Ont.; 64 Admiral Rd., Toronto 5 (res); Man '56; MA; FCPC; Staff, Inst. of Aviation Med.; Research Assoc., Best Inst.; O.P.D. Teach Staff, Toronto Western Hosp.; Clin. Teach., (Therapeutics) U. of Toronto; Bd. of Directors Cdn. Premier Life Ins. Co.; Tel. 923-9182. Abroad.

TAYLOR, W. Keith; Ste. 903, 24 Queen St. E., Brampton, Ont.; Tor'56; AMCGP; Staff, Peel Mem. Hosp.; Tel. 451-2028.

TAYLOR, W. Ronald; 1005 Fairmont Med. Bldg., 750 W. Broadway, Vancouver 9, B.C.; 1738 Acadia Rd. (res); McG'36; D.A.B.Ot.; Otol; Hon. Cons. (Otol.), Vancouver Gen. Hosp.; Tel. TR 9-4012.

TCHANG, Pablo; 12774 ouest, boul. Gouin; Pierrefonds, P.Q.; Madrid (Spain) '55; GenSurg (P.Q.).

TCHANG, Stanley; Madrid (Spain) '54; DiagRad; Staff, University Hosp., Saskatoon, Sask.; Tel. CH 2-7641.

TCHOU, Chen-Shou; Bonn (W.Germ.)'60; Jr. Int., Halifax Children's Hosp., Halifax, N.S.

TCHOU, Ping K.; Hanoi (Vietnam)'52; FRCP(C), Derm; Staff, Hop. Hotel-Dieu, Quebec 4, P.Q.

TE, Leonard T.; Ste. 5, 6325 Fraser St., Vancouver 15, B.C.; Santo Tomas (Philipp.) '56; Anaes.

TE, Luis D.; Med. Arts Clinic, 2125-11th Ave., Regina, Sask.; Santo Tomas (Philipp.) '56; Tel. 523-0961.

TE, Pacita C.; Santo Tomas (Manila, Philippines) '56; Jr. Int'n., Ottawa Civic Hosp., Ottawa 3, Ont.

TEAGUE, P. E.; Tor'65; Res., Shaughnessy Hosp., Vancouver 9, B.C.

TEASDALE, Joyce, M.; Health Centre for Children, 715 W.—12th Ave., Vancouver 9, B.C.; Apt. 102, 5475 Yew St. (res); Leeds (Eng.) '49; D.C.H., Paed; Att. Staff (Paed.), Vancouver Gen. Hosp.; Assoc., Prof. (Paed.), U. of British Columbia; Tel. TR 6-3211.

TEASDALE, Sallie J.; 2 Ridgefield Rd., Toronto 12, Ont.; Tor'57; FRCP(C); Anaes., Staff, Toronto Gen. Hosp., Toronto, Ont.

TECSON, Miguel P.; Ste. 913, 925 W. Georgia St., Vancouver 1, B.C.; Santo Tomas (Philipp.) '54; Psy.

TECTOR, David J. C.; 112 St. Francis St., Lennoxville, P.Q.; McG'64.

TEDESCHINI, Mario I.; 308 Med. Arts Bldg., 11010 Jasper Ave., Edmonton, Alta.; 11520-134th St. (res); Alb '56; Paed; Staff, University Hosp.; Tel. 439-5911.

TEGLAS, Aloysius; 1684A Queen W., Toronto 3, Ont.; Tor '60; AMCGP; Tel. 535-5165.

TEICHMAN, Bernard; 158 St. George St., Toronto, Ont.; 26 Strathearn Rd. (res); Tor '44; F.R.C.S.(C), Ophth; Jr. Att. Ophth., New Mt. Sinai Hosp.; Att. Ophth., Toronto Western Hosp.; Cons. (Ophth.), D.V.A., Sunnybrook Vet's. Hosp.; Clin. Fell., U. of Toronto; Tel. 924-4282.

TEICHMAN, Jack G.; 262 Wilson Ave., Downsview, Ont.; 345 Bloor St. W., Toronto; 428 Glengrove W. (res); Tor '45; ObstGyn; Tel. ME 5-1011.

TEITELBAUM, Jacobo I.; 3950 Bellechasse, Montreal 36, P.Q.; Mon '54; DIM; Haem (P.Q.); FACP; FRCP(C), IntMed; Med. Dir. & Phys-in-Chief, Bellechasse Hosp.; Tel. 729-4371.

TEIXEIRA, Jose A. R.; Lisbon (Port.)'40; Psy; Staff, Hop. St. Charles, Joliette, P.Q.

TEJEDA, Priamo; Santo Domingo '56; Jr. Intn., Ottawa Gen. Hosp., Ottawa, Ont.

TELFER, Gordon W.; 171 King St., Trenton, Ont.; Qns '31; D.Psy.; Psy; Staff, Trenton Memorial Hosp.; Cons., Belleville Gen. Hosp.; Tel. EX 2-5432.

TELFER, Russell B.; 246 Brant Ave., Brantford, Ont.; Tor '50; Urol; Staff, Brantford Gen. & St. Joseph's Hosp's.; Tel. 759-2003.

TELFORD, Douglas; 103 Hycroft Medical Bldg., 3195 Granville St., Vancouver 9, B.C.; 1867 Knox Rd. (res); Tor '33; F.R.C.S.(Edin.), F.I.C.S., GenSurg.; Vis. Staff, Vancouver Gen., St. Paul's & St. Vincent's Hosp's.; Act. Staff, Children's Hosp.; Tel. RE 1-4260.

TELFORD, Kenneth M.; 103 Hycroft Bldg., 3195 Granville St., Vancouver, B.C.; 5807 Olympic St. (res); McG '40; IntMed; Ass't., O.P.D., Vancouver Gen. Hosp.; Tel. RE 1-2925.

TELLIER, Gilles; 241 Fleury W., Montreal 12, **P.Q.; 8619 rue St. Denis (res); Mon '56; AMCGP; Staff, Marie-de-Montford Hosp; Tel. DU 1-7281.**

TELLIER, Hermas; 3525 Durocher St., Apt. 84, Montreal, P.Q.; Mon '25; Psy; Ass't. Supt., Hop. St. Jean de Dieu; Tel. CL 4-5361.

TELLIER, Jacques; 3580 Northcliffe Ave., Montreal 28, P.Q.; Lav '52; Psy.; Tel. HU 6-9503.

TELLIER, Lambert A.; C.P. 80, 219, rue Ste.-Anne, Varennes, P.Q.; Lav '55; Tel. 254-4242.

TELMOSSE, Francois; 1656 Sherbrooke St. E., Montreal 24, P.Q.; 29 Ave Kelvin, Outremont (res); Mon '52; FACS; FRCS(C); GenSurg; ThorSurg; Ass't. Staff, Hop. Notre-Dame; Cons., Hop. St-Vincent de Paul, Hotel-Dieu & Hop. Bellechasse; Ass't. Prof. (Surg.), U. of Montreal; Tel. LA 6-3783.

TELMOSSE, Jules R.; Chambre 407, 3875 St-Urbain, Montreal 18, P.Q.; Mon '59; Otol.

TELNER, Paul P.; 490 Ellendale Med. Bldg., 5845 Cote-des-Neiges Rd., Montreal 26, P.Q.; 5201 Rosedale Ave. (res); Mon '38; FACP; FRCP (C), Derm; Sr. Derm. I/C Jewish Gen. Hosp.; Ass't. Derm., Royal Victoria Hosp.; Ass't. Prof., McGill U.; Tel. RE 1-9161.

TEMELCOFF, Emile E.; Tor '56; D. Psy; Psy; Staff, Lakeshore Psych. Clinic, Toronto 14, Ont.

TEMES, Samuel; 27 Meadowbrook Rd., Toronto 19, Ont.; Tor '24; Staff, Mount Sinai Hosp.

TEMPLE, Allen D.; McG '30; F.A.G.S., F.C.-C.P., IntMed; Head, Div. Pulm. Dis., Ste. Anne's Hop., Ste. Anne de Bellevue, P.Q.; Lect., Schl. of Rehab., U. of Mtl.; Tel. 453-3440; Loc. 317.

TEMPLE, George D.; 925 King St. W., Hamilton, Ont.; Tor '40; Staff, Hamilton Gen. & St. Joseph's Hosp's.; Tel. JA 9-1261.

TEMPLE, Jack J.; Box 190, Fort St. John, B.C.; Tor '52; Tel. 785-6677.

TEMPLETON, Donald Wm. A.; P.O. Box 740, Schumacher, Ont.; 338 Birch St. N. (res); Qns **'35; D.P.H.; M.C.G.P.; Staff, St. Mary's Hosp.; Indust. Phys., McIntyre Mines, Schumacher; Tel. AM 4-8181.**

TEMPLIN, Marian I.; 2090 Wyandotte St. E., Windsor, Ont.; 518 Chilver Rd. (res): Tor '22; D.P.H.; Ass't. M.O.H., Metropolitan Windsor Health Unit; Tel. 256-3416.

TENBY, Lionel; 873 No. One Road, Richmond, B.C.; London (Eng.)'55; MRCS; LRCP; Chmn., Richmond Gen. Hosp. Emerg. Commiss.; Tel. 277-7171.

Ten CATE, Adrian G.; Qns '62; Res., Kingston Gen. Hosp., Kingston, Ont.

TENCH, John F.; 440 Hinton Ave., Ottawa 3, Ont.; Tor '52; Anaes.; Tel. 722-3027.

TENDERENDA, Tadeusz; Box 441, 110 Ochterloney St., Dartmouth, N.S.; 10 Chestnut Lane, Woodlawn (res); Warsaw (Pol.)'34; DLO(Lond.), EENT Spec., Dartmouth Med. Centre; Tel. 466-2791.

TENEY, Heber F.; 328 Millwood Rd., Toronto, Ont.; Tor '26; Tel. HU 9-8583.

TENHUNEN, Aino E. (Koski); 1865 Paris St., Sudbury, Ont.; Tor '51; Retired.

TENHUNEN, Teuvo; 1865 Paris St., Sudbury, Ont.; Tor '48; Anaes; Staff, Sudbury Gen., Sudbury Mem. & St. Joseph's Hosp's.; Tel. OS 4-1718.

TENNEN, Allan B.; Tor'57; Res., Clarke Inst. of Psy., Toronto 2B, Ont.

TENNENT, Helen L.; Grace Anaes. Clinic, Winnipeg, Man.; 678 Wellington Cres., Wpg. 9 (res); Victoria U. (Manchester, Eng.) '48; DA (Lond.); Anaes; Active Staff, Grace Hosp.; Tel. SU 3-6732.

TEN PAS, Andrew; 8480 Waverly, Montreal 11, P.Q.; Utrecht (Neth.)'57; Haem(P.Q.); FRCP(C), IntMed; Staff, Royal Victoria Hosp.

TEODORO, Jose V.; Philippines'56; Res., St. Joseph's Hosp., Toronto 3, Ont.

TEOLIS, Jean P.; 6954-43eme Ave., Montreal 36, P.Q.; Mon'65.

TERLINGEN, H. A.; Tor'65; Jr. Int., St. Joseph's Hosp., Toronto 3, Ont.; Abroad.

TEPPERMAN, Isadore J.; 548 Palmerston Blvd., Toronto, Ont.; Tor '37; M.C.G.P.; Sr. Clin. Phys., O.P.D., New Mount Sinai Hosp.; Tel. LE 3-3411.

TERMANSEN, Paul E.; UBC'61; Psy; Staff, Vancouver Gen. Hosp., Vancouver 9, B.C.

TERNENT, Douglas F.; Box 322 Kinnaird, B.C.; McG '57.

TERRIEN, J. H. Jean; 1871 Rideau Garden Dr., Ottawa 1, Ont.; Lav'40; GenSurg, Gyn; Staff, Ottawa Gen. Hosp.; Courtesy Staff, St. Louis-Marie de Montfort & Grace Hosp's.; Lect. (Surg.), U. of Ottawa; Tel. CE 6-4592.

TERRY, E. N.; Germany '56; Staff, Pharma. Research Can. Ltd., 250 Hymus Blvd., Pointe Claire, P.Q.

TERSHAKOWEC, M. G.; Tor'65; Res., Banting Inst., Toronto 2, Ont.

TESHER, Martin S.; 1054A Wilson Ave., Downsview, Ont.; Qns'62; Staff, North York Branson Hosp.; Tel. ME 3-3711.

TESKEY, C. G.; 74 Queen St. N., Kitchener, Ont.; Qns '35.

TESKEY, Luke; 2221 Keele St., Toronto 15, Ont.; 17 Greenbrook Dr. (res); Tor '23; GenSurg; Hd. Dept. of Surg. Northwestern Gen. Hosp.; 247-6279.

TESKEY, Luke, Jr.; 2221 Keele St., Toronto 15, **Ont.; 168 Oakwood Ave., Toronto; 26 Greenbrook Dr. (res); Tor '49; F.I.C.S.;** GenSurg; Chief of Surg., Northwestern Gen. Hosp.; Tel. 247-6279; LE 6-5426.

TESKEY, William L.; 10 Marla Cres., London, Ont. (res); Qns '40; DiagRad; Rad., Westminster DVA Hosp.; Instr. (DiagRad), U. of Western Ont.; Tel. GE 2-6711.

TESSIER, Albert; 1150 est, Boul. St.-Joseph, Montreal 34, P.Q.; 6510 Chouinard (res); Lav '53; OphthOtol; Tel. LA 7-1241.

TESSIER, Bruno; Lav'51; Res., Hop. Notre-Dame, Montreal 24, P.Q.

TESSIER, Jean G.; Lav '55; D&TRAD; Staff, Hop. Lafleche, & Grand'Mere Gen. Hosp., Grand'-Mere, P.Q.

TESSIER, J. Emile; 255 Chemin River, Ottawa 7, Ont.; Lav '49; D&TRad; Staff, Hop-St-Louis-Marie-de-Montfort; Tel. SH 6-4621.

TESSIER, Jean L.; 17 ouest, Ste-Catherine, Longueuil, Cite-Jacques-Cartier, P.Q.; Lav '48; Ophth (P.Q.); Tel. 674-6001.

TESSIER, J. Horace; 165 Bonaventure, Trois Rivieres, P.Q.; Lav'36; Pulm. Dis. & TB (P.Q.); Staff, Cooke San.; Tel. FR 5-8571.

TESSIER, J. Robert; 505, boul Bastien, Neufchatel, P.Q.; Lav '56; Tel. 842-5462.

TESSIER, Jules L.; 665 - 3rd Ave., Val d'Or, P.Q.; Ott '64.

TESSIER, Leo J.; 1249 Blvd. St. Joseph E., Montreal 34, P.Q.; 1247 Blvd. St. Joseph E. (res); McG '31; Ophth,Otol; Ass't. Clin., Ophth. Otol., Hotel-Dieu Hosp.; Tel. 279-2283.

TESSIER, Paul E.; St. Casimir, Co. Portneuf, P.Q.; Lav '45.

TESSIER, Yves; Lav'65; Res., Hop. St. Sacrement, Quebec 6, P.Q.

TESSLER, Barry B.; Man'63; Res., Winnipeg Gen. Hosp., Winnipeg 3, Man.; Abroad.

TETRAULT, Paul; 834 Blvd. Ste. Croix, Ville St. Laurent, P.Q.; Mon '41; Tel. RI 7-2615.

TETREAULT, Adelard; 444 Laviolette, Trois Rivieres, P.Q.; 146 Bonaventure (res); Mon '25; Cardiol. (P.Q.); IntMed; Chief Dept. of Med., St. Joseph's Hop.; Assoc. Prof. Laval U.; Tel. FR 5-3823.

TETREAULT, Ernest R.; 73 A Ave., Pagnuelo, Montreal 8, P.Q.; Mon '49; Psy.

TETREAULT, Georges E.; 4304 St. Denis, Montreal, P.Q.; Mon '43; M.C.G.P.; Tel 842-6715.

TETREAULT, Harold I.; 3878 Ave. Kent, Montreal, P.Q. (res); Mon '36; Med. Supt., Hop St. Luc, Montreal; Tel. 861-7321.

TETREAULT, Julien; 1450 Gilford, Montreal, P.Q; Mon '28; Obst; Tel LA 2-9449.

TETREAULT, L. Leon; 11270 de St-Real, Montreal 12, P.Q. (res); Mon '58; M.Sc. (Pharm.) FCPC; Ass't. Prof., U. of Montreal; Tel. 331-2160.

TETU, Andre T.; 2415 Perodeau, Quebec 6, P.Q.; Lav '52; Cardiol (P.Q.); FRCP(C), IntMed; Staff, Hop. Christ-Roi.

TETU, Felix; 781 Marois, Quebec 6, P.Q.; 1632 Chemin Ste. Foy (res); Lav '20; IntMed (P.Q.), Cardiol (P.Q.); Tel. 681-4883.

TETU, Joseph L.; 3244 est Beaubien, Montreal 36, P.Q.; Lav'59; Tel. 729-1891.

TETZ, Wilford C.; Lacombe, Alta.; Coll. of Med. Evangelists, Loma Linda, Calif., U.S.A.'52; Tel. 782-3146.

TEVAARWERK, Gerald J.; Wes'65; Res., St. Joseph's Hosp., London, Ont.

TEW, William L.; Ste. 102, 450 Central Ave., London, Ont.; 1486 Stonybrook (res); Wes '53; LLD (Hon.); FACS; FRCS(C), ObstGyn; Teach. Staff, Victoria Hosp.; Court. Staff, St. Joseph's Hosp.; Instr., U. of Western Ont.; Tel. 433-0134.

TEW, W. Pelton; 102 Med. Dental Bldg., 450 Central Ave., London, Ont.; 657 Windermere Rd. (res); Tor '16; FRCOG, FRCS(Edin.), FACS, FRCS(C), ObstGyn; Emer. Prof. (ObstGyn), U. of Western Ont.; Tel. 434-6292.

THALER, A. Franklin; 558-10th Ave., Hanover, Ont.; Tor '26; MCGP.

THEAL, G. Irvine; 491 Cumberland Rd., Courtenay, B.C.; Qns '42; Staff, St. Joseph's, Comax; Tel. 334-2445.

THEMAN, A. Edward; 10022-103rd St., Edmonton, Alta.; 9623-148th St. (res); Man '43; FACS; FRCS(C), GenSurg; Treas., Misericordia Hosp.; Lect., U. of Alta.; Tel. 429-3781.

THEOBALD, Geoffrey M.; Uxbridge Med. Centre, Box 429, Uxbridge, Ont.; London (Eng.)'61; MRCS; LRCP; Tel. UL 2-3311.

THEOBALD, Joseph C.; 86 Bloor St. W., Toronto, Ont.; 20 Garfield Ave. (res); Tor '33; Tel. WA 2-5660.

THEOCHARIDES, Peter C.; 55 Church Ave., Montreal 19, P.Q.; Paris (Fr.)'55; FRCS(C), GenSurg; Staff, Verdun Gen. Hosp.; Tel. PO 8-8531.

THEODORE, Gene M.; Box 1180, Swan River, Man.; Man '64.

THEORET, John J.; 362 Wortley Rd., London, Ont.; Wes'60; MCGP; Tel. 438-3953.

THEORET, J. Rodrick; 88 ouest Blvd. S. Joseph, Montreal 14; P.Q.; Mon '41.

THERIAULT, Jean-Paul; 420 Melbourne, Town of Mt. Royal, Montreal, P.Q. (res); Mon '48; Path (P.Q.); Path., Hop. Gen. de Verdun; Tel. 766-8511.

THERIAULT, John C.; 76 Elizabeth Parkway, Kennebecasis Park, Saint John, N.B. (res.); Dal '49; Psy; Chief of Psy., St. John Gen. Hosp.; Con. DVA & St. Joseph's Hosp's.; Tel. 693-3351.

THERIAULT, Raymond; Lav '62; Res., Hop. Hotel-Dieu, Quebec, P.Q.

THERIAULT, Raymond; 392 Central Park W., Apt. 16M, New York, N.Y. 10025, U.S.A.; Lav'61; Otol; Abroad.

THERIEN, Bernard; Ste. 301, 825 sud, Belvedere, Sherbrooke, P.Q.; Mon '55; DABP; FAAP; FRCP (C); Paed; Hd., Dept. of Paed., Hotel-Dieu; Cons. (Paed.), Hop.-de-la-Providence, Magog; Vis. Cons. (Paed.), St-Vincent-de-Paul & Sherbrooke Hosp's.; Tel. 569-3945.

THERIEN, Rene; App 8, 7100, Bordeaux, Mont- real 35, P.Q. (res); Mon'22; Staff, Dept. of Health, Montreal; Abroad.

THERRIEN, A.; 1947 rue Dorion, Montreal, P.Q.; Mon '17; Staff, Dept. of Health, City of Montreal.

THERRIEN, Claude; Ott'61; IntMed(P.Q.); Staff, Hop. Laval, Quebec 10, P.Q.

THERRIEN, Elie; 10007 St. Denis, Montreal 12, P.Q.; Lav '50; Anaes (P.Q.) Tel. DU 9-2885;.

THERRIEN, Emile E.; 136 E. 15th St., North Vancouver, B.C.; 3172 Mathers Ave. W. Van. (res); Man '35; GenSurg; Chief of Staff, Lions Gate Hosp.; Tel. YU 8-8133.

THERRIEN, G. Emile; 17 de Lourdes, Rigaud, Co. Vaudreuil, P.Q.; Mon '50; MCGP; Tel. 238-5215.

THERRIEN, Laurier; 4647 Ave. Verdun, Montreal 19, P.Q.; Mon '65.

THERRIEN, Richard; Ste. 25, 220 Grand Allee, Quebec, P.Q.; 23 Ave. de la Tour (res); Lav'43; MCAA, All. (P.Q.); DermSyph; Ass't. Derm. Staff, Hop. Hotel Dieu; Cons. Derm. & All., Hop. Ste-Foy; Aux. Prof. in Derm., U. of Laval; Tel. 523-2104.

THERRIEN, Roger; 122 St. Jean, Drummondville, P.Q.; Mon '65.

THIBAUDEAU, **Jean;** 214 Ouest, rue King, Sherbrooke, P.Q.; Mon '61; Ophth.

THIBAUDEAU, Pierre; 2301 Jean Talon E., Montreal 35, P.Q.; 10442 Blvd. d'Auteuil (res); Mon '49; Tel. RA 9-5669.

THIBAUDEAU, Roland; 1195 ave-des-Erables, Quebec 6, P.Q.; Lav '32; F.A.A.P.; Paed; Hd. Dept. of Paed., Hop.-St.-Sacrement; Staff, Laval U.; Tel. 522-2310.

THIBAUDEAU, Yvan; 8415 St.-Denis, Montreal 11, P.Q.; 295 Querbes, Outremont (res); Mon '56; FRCP(C), IntMed; Hd. Dept. of Med., Hop. Jean-Talon; Tel. 381-5311.

THIBAULT, Alfred; Man '64; Res., Inst. Albert Prevost, Montreal 9, P.Q.

THIBAULT, **Antonio;** 831 Leprémont, Quebec 4, P.Q.; **Lav '57; D&TRAD; Staff, Hop. Hotel-**Dieu de Quebec.

THIBAULT, Arthur; 28 Blvd. Carignan, Victoriaville, P.Q.; Lav'34; Dist. Coroner; Tel. 752-2200.

THIBAULT, Eugene; 4000 Blvd. Lasalle, Verdun, Montreal 19, P.Q.; 4070 Blvd. Lasalle (res); Mon '27; IntMed (P.Q.); M.R.S.H., F.A.C.H.A.; Med. Dir., Hop.-Gen.-de-Verdun; Tel. 766-3551.

THIBAULT, H. Jacques; Lav '60; Res., Hop. L'Enfant Jesus, Quebec 3, P.Q.

THIBAULT, Jean; Ste. 12, Edifice Laure, Sept Iles, P.Q.; Lav'65.

THIBAULT, Jean; 180 St.-Denis, Arvida, P.Q.; Lav '58; Pt.-time Phys., Aluminum Co. & Simond's Canada Abrasive & Robervale Saguenay, Arvida; Tel. 548-4412.

THIBAULT, Jean; Ste. 12, Edifice Laure, Sept. Iles, P.Q.; Lav'65.

THIBAULT, J. Armand; 1670 ave Bardy, Quebec 3, P.Q. (res); Lav '52; Psy; Staff, Hop. St.-Michel-Archange; Tel. RA 2-2571.

THIBAULT, Jean P.; 39 Jacques Cartier, Valleyfield, P.Q.; 8 St.-Jean-Baptiste (res); Mon '55; FACOG; ObstGyn (PQ); Staff, Barrie Mem. Hosp., Ormstown; Tel. 373-7733.

THIBAULT, Jean P.; 285A rue St. Georges, St-Jerome, P.Q.; Lav '48; F.R.C.S.(C), GenSurg; Surg., Hop-Hotel-Dieu-de-St Jerome; Tel. GE 2-7722.

THIBAULT, Jean P.; 301 Mitchell St., Port Colborne, Ont.; Ott '53.

THIBAULT, Maurice; 858 Bellevue, Ste.-Foy, Quebec 10, P.Q.; Lav '53; F.R.C.P.(C), TherRad (P.Q.); Dir. Dept. of TherRad., Hotel-Dieu-Hosp.; Tel. 529-9151.

THIBAULT, Maurice; 5557 Queen Mary Rd., Hampstead, P.Q. (res); Mon '37; Supt., Queen Mary Vet's Hosp.; **Chief of Med. DVA Reg., Montreal**; Tel. 342-2320.

THIBAULT, Paul E.; 325 Blvd. St. Joseph, Roberval, P.Q.; Lav '40.

THIBAULT, Roger; App 5, 898 Puyjalon, Hauterive, P.Q.; Lav'54.

THIBEAULT, Jeanne-d'Arc; 14 Sarto, Repentigny Village, P.Q.; Mon'60; PH(P.Q.); Staff, Dept. of Health, Repentigny.

THIBERT, Florent; 1150 est Blvd. St.-Joseph, Montreal 34, P.Q.; 4075 Jauron, Mtl. 9 (res); Mon '54; Gastroent. (PQ); FRCP(C), IntMed; Ass't. (Med.), Hop. Maisonneuve; Ass't. Prof. (Med.), U. of Mtl.; Tel. LA 7-1241.

THIBERT, J. Roger; Ste. 302, 30 Blvd. St. Joseph E., Montreal 34, P.Q.; Apt. 1, 6074-44th Ave. (res); Mon'54; Otol; Staff (Otol.), Hop. Maisonneuve; Tel. LA 7-1241.

THIBERT, M. D'Arcy; 1150 est St. Joseph, Montreal 34, P.Q.; Mon'60; IntMed(P.Q.); Staff, Hop. Maisonneuve.

THIBERT, Norman E.; 605 Medical Arts Bldg., Windsor, Ont.; 436 Askin Blvd. (res); Wes '51; Int.Med.; Tel. 254-5991.

THIBERT, Roger; 30 est Boul. St. Joseph, Montreal 29, P.Q.; Mon'49; Path(P.Q.).

THIBODEAU, Alfred E.; 490 Brant St., Burlington, Ont.; 128 Atwood Crt. (res); Wes '56; Active Staff, Joseph Brant Hosp.; Tel. NE 4-2307

THIBODEAU, Ls. Phil.; 1150 est Blvd. St.-Joseph, Montreal 34, P.Q.; 7641 Pl. Daubigny, Ville-d'Anjou (res); Mon '51; Paed; Paed., Hop.-Maisonneuve; Tel LA 7-1551.

THIBODEAU, Raymond; Daveluyville, Cte., Arthabaska, P.Q.; Lav '61.

THIBODEAU, Yvon; Ste. Gregoire, Co. Nicolet, P.Q.; Lav '58.

THIBOUTAT, J. Art; 2307 Centre St., Montreal, P.Q.; 3531 Van Horne (res); Lav '22.

THICKE, Brian C.; 26 Rambler, Brampton, Ont.; Wes'56; MCGP; Tel. 451-5586.

THIEL, Chelsea J.; Wes '50; Anaes; Staff, NDMC, Ottawa 8, Ont; Tel. 992-2474.

THIELE, Isolde (May); Marburg (Germ.) '47; Staff, Alberta Hosp., Box 307, Edmonton, Alta.; Tel. 7-0221.

THIESSEN, Arnold E.; 9933 Elbow Dr., Calgary, Alta.; Man '62; Tel. 252-1168.

THIESSEN, Nicholas; 3379 Kingsway, Vancouver 16, B.C.; 7150 McBride St. (res); UBC '59; Tel. HE 1-3388.

THIFFAULT, Charles; Lav '62; Res., Hop. Hotel-Dieu, rue St.-Urbain, Montreal, P.Q.

THIFFAULT, Gilbert, Capt.; 1 Field Amb. Capo. 5050, Can. Armed Forces, Germany; Lav '65. Abroad.

THIVIERGE, Arthur; 1150 est Blvd. St. Joseph, Montreal 34, P.Q.; Lav'49; OrthSurg; Ass't. Chief (OrthSurg.), Hop. Maisonneuve; Tel. LA 7-1241.

THIVIERGE, Camille; Lav'64; Res., Dept. of Anaes., Hop. Notre-Dame, Montreal 24, P.Q.

THIVIERGE, Caroll; 4645 1ere Ave., Quebec 7, P.Q.; Lav '65.

THIVIERGE, Clement M.; 5 St. Joseph, Levis, P.Q.; Lav '43; IntMed (P.Q.); Staff, Int. Med. & Cardiol., Hop. Hotel-Dieu de Levis; Diag. Rad., Hop. Hotel Dieu de Montmagny; Tel. 837-9341.

THIVIERGE, Marcel; 44 B 2eme rue, Port Alfred, P.Q.; Lav '41.

THIVIERGE, Rolland E.; 1820 Blvd. St. Joseph E., Montreal 34, P.Q.; 2715 Darlington Pl., Apt. 100 (res); Mon '58; Tel. LA 3-3563.

THOM, Alexander T.; 4492 Sherbrooke St. W., Montreal 6, P.Q.; McG '37; PulmDist. & TB (P.Q.); IntMed; Cons. Phys. Mtl. Stat.; Tel. WE 5-3334.

THOM, Ian M.; Med. Arts Clinic, 2125-11th Ave., Regina, Sask.; 50 Martin St. (res); Edinburgh (Scot.)'52; M.B., Ch.B., D.Obst.RCOG; Staff, Regina Gen. & Grey Nun's Hosp's.; Tel. 523-0691.

THOMAN, Harry L.; 48 Balmoral St. S., Hamilton, Ont. Qns '39; Tel. LI 5-1373.

THOMAS, Alun L.; Ste. 360, 8409-112th St., Edmonton, Alta.; 11445 University Ave. (res); Edinburgh (Scotland)'32; Tel. GE 9-2868.

THOMAS, Alun P.; Irving Clinic, 74 W. Seymour St., Kamloops, B.C.; 602 Tunstall Cres. (res); Wales '50; DA (Eng.); Anaes; Anaes., Royal Inland Hosp. & St. Bart's., Lytton; Tel. 372-5251.

THOMAS, Barrie O.; 97 Charlotte St., Port Colborne, Ont.; London (England)'61; MCGP.

THOMAS, Bruce W.; Tor'62; Res., East Gen. Hosp., Toronto 13, Ont.

THOMAS, Carleton M.; Ramey Bldg., Portage la Prairie, Man.; 234 Crescent Rd. W. (res); Man '36; MCGP; Med. Staff, Portage Gen. Hosp.

THOMAS, Catherine E. (MacDonald); 150 Woodhaven Blvd., St. James, Wpg. 12, Man. (res); Man'45; M.Sc. (Bact.); Ass't. Prof. (Path.), U. of Manitoba; Tel. 786-3522.

THOMAS, Charles L.; Ste. 6, 2221 Keele St., Toronto 15, Ont.; Tor '33; FACS (Eng.), FCCP; Tel. 247-4111.

THOMAS, Edgar J.; 2471 Portage Ave., St. James, Wpg., Man.; 150 Woodhaven Blvd. (res); Man '45; IntMed; Staff DVA Deer Lodge & Mun. Hosp's.; Lect. (Med.), U. of Manitoba; Med. Dir. Manitoba Div., CARS; Tel. 837-1301.

THOMAS, Ferdinand A.; 650 Brimorton Dr., **Scarborough, Ont.; Dal '63; Tel. 282-4211.**

THOMAS, Gerald C.; 267 O'Connor St., Ottawa 4, Ont.; 2436 Georgina Dr. (res); Qns '50; Int-Med.; Att'd. Phys., Ottawa Civic Hosp.; Tel. 235-1133.

THOMAS, G. Keith; Med. Arts Bldg., 17 Dunedin St., Orillia, Ont.; 382 Highland Ave. (res); Queen's U., Belfast (Ire.) '45; F.R.C.S. (Eng.); F.I.C.S. GenSurg; Cons. Staff, Soldiers Mem. Hosp., Orillia & Bracebridge Mem. Hosp., Bracebridge; Tel. 326-7920.

THOMAS, Gordon W.; International Grenfell Assoc., S.t Anthony, Nfld.; McG '43; FACS; FRCS(C); ThorSurg; Surg-in-Chief, Grenfell Hosp. Port Phys., MOH; Supt., Int'l. Grenfell Assoc.

THOMAS, Gwyn S.; Calgary Assoc. Clinic, 214-6th Ave. W., Calgary, Alta.; London (Eng.) '40; M.B., B.S., M.R.C.S., L.R.C.P., F.R.C.O.G.; ObstGyn; Cons. ObstGyn., Holy Cross, Grace & Calgary Gen. Hosp's.; Tel. AM 3-7120.

THOMAS, Henry H.; 167 Oakwood Ave., Toronto, Ont.; 160 Glen Cedar (res); Tor '43; M.C.G.P.; Tel. LE 3-6961.

THOMAS, Howard B.; 1137 Royal York Rd., Islington, Ont.; McG'62; Ophth.

THOMAS, Jack R.; 751 King St. W., Kitchener, Ont.; Man'45; DiagRad; Staff, Kitchener-Waterloo Hosp., Kitchener, Ont.; Tel. SH 5-9451.

THOMAS, John P.; 7250 Arbutus Pl., W. Vancouver, B.C. (res); Dal '45; IntMed; Staff, Vancouver Gen. Hosp.; Clin. Ass't. Prof. (Micro-Anat.), U. of British Columbia; Tel. TR 6-3211.

THOMAS, Joseph C.; 925 W. Georgia St., Vancouver, B.C.; 1787 W. 49th Ave. (res); Tor '31; NeurPsy; Att. Staff, Vancouver Gen. Hosp.; Cons., Dept. of Attorney General of B.C.; Lect., U. of British Columbia; Tel. MU 1-8036.

THOMAS, J. Mervyn; 2490 Departure Bay Rd., Nanaimo, B.C. (res); Cambridge (Eng.)'45; MRCS, LRCP, MRCOG; ObstGyn; Tel. 753-4449.

THOMAS, Max Charles L.; Ste. 207, 2600 Eglinton Ave. W., Toronto 15, Ont.; Tor '33; F.R.C.S.(Eng.), F.R.C.P.(C), GenSurg; Staff, Northwestern Gen. Hosp.; Tel. RO 6-6371.

THOMAS, William D.; Bobcaygeon, Ont.; Tor '33; MCGP; Dist. Coroner & MOH; Tel. 738-2211.

THOMAS, William D.; Ste. 214, 3195 Granville St., Vancouver 9, B.C.; UBC'59; FRCS(C), ObstGyn.

THOMAS-CLINTON, Charles L.; see CLINTON-THOMAS, Charles L.).

THOMASON, Albert M.; Colorado (U.S.A.)'63; Res., Hop. du St-Sacrement, Quebec 6, P.Q.

THOMPSON, A. F.; 54 Blenheim, Galt, Ont.

THOMPSON, Alan G.; 1650 Cedar St., Room 947, Montreal 25, P.Q.; 492 Argyle St., Westmount (res); McG '43; DABS; FACS; FRCS(C); GenSurg; Sr. Surg., Montreal Gen. & Reddy Mem. Hosp's.; Att'd. Staff, Queen Mary Vets Hosp.; Assoc. Prof. McGill U.; Tel. 932-2093.

THOMPSON, Alfred L.; 6674 Fraser Ave., Vancouver, B.C.; New Zealand '45; M.B., Ch.B., Tel. FA 7-2326.

THOMPSON, Allen E.; 918 Hartland Ave., Montreal, P.Q. (res); McG '13; Retired.

THOMPSON, Asher B.; Manitoba Clinic, 790 Sherbrook St., Winnipeg 2, Man.; Man'60; FRCP(C), IntMed.

THOMPSON, Basil H.; 4026-W 40th Ave., Vancouver 13, B.C.; UBC '54; DiagRad; Tel. AM 6-0451.

THOMPSON, Benjamin L.; Ste. 400, 5300 Cote des Neiges, Montreal 26, P.Q.; McG'52; GenSurg.

THOMPSON, B. Gordon; Ormstown Med. Centre, Ormstown, P.Q.; McG'59; M.Sc. (Exper. Med.); Gen Surg(P.Q.); Att'd. Staff, Barrie Mem. Hosp.; Tel. 829-2331.

THOMPSON, C. Alan; 36 Main St., Georgetown, Ont.; Wes '54; MCGP; Chief of Staff, Georgetown & Dist. Mem. Hosp.; Tel. 877-4123.

THOMPSON, Chas. A.; 232 Queens Ave., London, Ont.; 114 St. James St. (res); McG '38; Ophth,Otol, Head, Dept. of Ophth., Westminster Hosp.; Staff, Ophth, Victoria Hosp.; Ass't. Prof. Ophth. U. of Western Ontario; Tel. GE 2-0351.

THOMPSON, Charles O.; 17 Church St., Brantford, Ont.; Wes'56; D.O.(Lond.); Ophth.

THOMPSON, Clifford S.; Box 460, Montreal, P.Q. (res); McG '25; FACS; GenSurg; Retired.

THOMPSON, Clive D.; Eastview Med. Clinic & Westpark Med. Clinic, Red Deer, Alta.; London (Eng.)'57; MB; BS; DRCOG; Staff, Red Deer Gen. Hosp.; Tel. 347-6601.

THOMPSON, Colin W.; 7375 Kingsway, Burnaby 3, New Westminster, B.C.; Birmingham (Eng.) '58.

THOMPSON, Donald A.; 210 St. George St., Bathurst, N.B.; 320 Parkside Dr. (res); Dal '33; F.A.C.S., F.R.C.S.(C), GenSurg; Chief of Staff, Hotel Dieu Hosp.; Phys., Bathurst Paper Co.; Tel. LI 6-4448 & LI 6-4449.

THOMPSON, Donald W.; 1979 Victoria Park Ave., Scarborough, Ont. (res); Tor '49; Path; Path., Dept. of Surg. Path., Toronto Gen. Hosp.; Cons. (Path.), Women's College Hosp.; Lect. (Path.), U. of Toronto; Tel. EM 6-8211.

THOMPSON, Douglas W.; 8 Brucedale Ave. E., Hamilton, Ont.; 75 W. 5th St. (res); Wes '49; MCGP; Active Staff, Hamilton Civic, Chedoke Gen. & Children's Hosp's.; Tel. FU 3-8951.

THOMPSON, F. F. Patrick; Medical Arts Bldg., 73 N. Cumberland St., Port Arthur, Ont.; 131 Winnipeg Ave. (res); Tor'34; MCGP; Staff, St. Joseph's Gen., & Port Arthur Gen. Hosp's.; Tel. 345-7232.

THOMPSON, F. G.; 41 Ontario St., Clinton, Ont.; Wes '24; Med. Attendant, Huron County Home for the Aged; Coroner, Huron Co.

THOMPSON, G. Douglas; Med. Arts Bldg., 1 Young St., Hamilton, Ont.; Qns'55; FAAP; FRCS(C), Urol; Chief Serv. Urol., St. Joseph's Hosp.; Court. Staff, Chedoke & Hamilton Civic Hosp's.; Tel. 525-1014.

THOMPSON, George A.; 1849 Yonge St., Ste 401, Toronto 7, Ont.; 23 Sandfield Rd. (res); Tor '41; FRCS(C); Ophth; Sr., Ophth., Toronto Gen. Hosp.; Cons. Ophth., Ont. Cancer Fdn.; Med. Dir., Eye Bank of Canada, Ont. Div.; Assoc. Dept. of Ophth., U. of Toronto; Tel. 483-1282.

THOMPSON, George H.; 1029 Douglas, Victoria, B.C.; 2980 Lansdowne Rd. (res); McG '47; Ophth; Staff, Royal Jubilee Hosp.; Cons. Staff, St. Joseph's Hosp.; Tel. EV 2-9611.

THOMPSON, G. Lloyd; Box 430, Selkirk, Man.; Man '52; GenSurg; Med. Staff, Selkirk Gen. Hosp.

THOMPSON, George R.; 108 Scott Blk., Moose Jaw, Sask.; 1113 Redland Ave. (res); Man '46; Gen Surg; Act. Staff, Moose Jaw Union, & Providence Hosp's.; Tel. 692-1827.

THOMPSON, G. Howard; 751 King St. W., Kitchener, Ont.; 207 Sherwood Ave. (res); Wes '54; M.C.G.P.; Staff, St. Mary's & Kitchener-Waterloo Hosp's.; Tel. 744-5257.

THOMPSON, Gordon B.; Ste. 711, Fairmont Med. Bldg., 750 W. Broadway, Vancouver 9, B.C.; 1408 W. 46th Ave., Van. 13 (res); McG'52; FRCS(C), NeurSurg; Chief & Hd. Div. of NeurSurg., Vancouver Gen. Hosp.; Clin. Assoc.; Prof. (Surg.), U. of British Columbia; Tel. 876-4313.

THOMPSON, Hamlet D.; 701 Amberley Ave., London, Ont.; Tor '06.

THOMPSON, Hugh H.; 117 Waterloo St. S., Stratford, Ont.; 152 Delamere Ave. (res); Wes '42; Tel. 271-5542.

THOMPSON, I. Maclaren; Dept. of Anatomy, University of Manitoba, Winnipeg, Man.; Edinburgh (Scot.) '20; F.R.S.C.(Eng); F.R.S.(E); Cons., Anat., Winnipeg Gen & Children's Hosp's.; Prof., & Chm. (Emer.) Dept. of Anat., U. of Manitoba; Retired.

THOMPSON, James; Queen's U. (Belfast, N. Ire.) '51; M.B., B.Ch., B.A.O.; Psy; Staff Psy., Alberta Hosp., Ponoka, Alta.; Tel. 783-3301.

THOMPSON, James S.; 7 Danville Dr., Willowdale, Ont.; Tor '45; Prof. (Anat.) U. of Toronto; Tel. 222-5854.

THOMPSON, John A. D.; 568 Lansdowne Ave., Calgary, Alta. (res); Alb '42; D.H.A.; Admin., Col. Belcher Hosp.; Tel. AM 6-7001.

THOMPSON, John E.; 2 Park Ave., Elmira, Ont.; 31 Second St. (res); Wes '54; MCGP; Active Staff, Kitchener-Waterloo & St. Mary's Gen. Hosp's.; Tel. MO 9-5471.

THOMPSON, John L.; 220 King St. E., Saint John, N.B.; 220 King St. E. (res); Tor '39; MAAA; AMCAA; Att'd. Phys. St. John's Gen. Hosp.; Tel. 693-2801.

THOMPSON, John M.; Wes'61; IntMed; Staff, St. Joseph's Hosp., London, Ont.

THOMPSON, John R.; Westlaw Bldg., 1920 Weston Rd., Weston, Ont.; Qns'59; IntMed; Cons. Staff, Humber Mem. Hosp.; Tel. 248-5158.

THOMPSON, Lloyd W.; 327 Charlotte St. Peterborough, Ont.; 456 Manorhill Ave. (res); Tor '30; F.C.C.P., F.R.C.P.(C), IntMed; Staff, Peterborough Civic & St. Joseph's Hosp's.; Tel. 743-2040.

THOMPSON, Margaret S.; 986 Ossington Ave., Toronto, Ont. (res); Tor '30; D.Psy.; Phys. Grade II, Ontario Hosp., Toronto.

THOMPSON, Murray C.; Ste. 211, 3000 Lawrence Ave. E., Scarborough, Ont.; Tor '50; Anaes; Tel. AX 3-8681.

THOMPSON, R. David; Dept. Nat. Health & Welfare, Rm. 607, 1110 W. Georgia, Vancouver 5, B.C.; Tor'36; DPH; Med. Dir. (Pacific Reg.), Med. Services Directorate; Tel. 682-7237.

THOMPSON, Robert B.; Minto, N.B.; Dal '59.

THOMPSON, Russell A.; Wellington, Ont.; Tor '24; Staff, Prince Edward County Hosp.; Dist. Coroner; Tel. 399-2055.

THOMPSON, Sevis F.; Port Dover, Ont.; Ott'65.

THOMPSON, Steinn O.; Riverton, Man.; Man '21.

THOMPSON, T. A. Main; 727 Main St. W., North Bay, Ont. (res); Tor '39; D.R., DiagRad; Rad., North Bay Civic & St. Joseph's Hosp's., North Bay.

THOMPSON, Trevor J.; c/o Bd. of World Mission, United Church of Canada, 85 St. Clair Ave. E., Toronto 7, Ont.; Qns '50; AMCGP. Abroad.

THOMPSON, Victor E.; 341 Ridge St., Ridgeway, Ont.; Tor '50; Staff, Port Colborne Gen. Hosp., Port Colborne; Tel. 869-2232.

THOMPSON, W. Allen; McG '59; AMCGP; Res., Montreal Gen. Hosp., Montreal 25, P.Q.

THOMPSON, W. Grant; Tor'60; FRCP(C), IntMed; Staff, Montreal Gen. Hosp., Montreal 25, P.Q.

THOMPSON, William J.; Ste. 10, 3195 Granville St., Vancouver 9, B.C.; Man'42; FRCS(C), OrthSurg; Chief of OrthSurg. Serv., Shaughnessy Hosp.; Ass't. Clin. Prof., Dept. of Surg., U. of British Columbia; Tel. 738-8727.

THOMPSON, Zonia R. (Thachuk); 13303-124th Ave., Edmonton, Alta.; Alb '58; Staff, Charles Campsell Hosp.; Sess. Instr., U. of Alberta.

THOMS, A. Edward; 70 Charles St., Brockville, Ont.; Qns'36; D.P.H.; Dir. & Sr. M.O.H., Leeds & Grenville Health Unit; Tel. 345-5685.

THOMSEN, Andreas E. T.; 117 East St., Napanee, Ont.; Amsterdam (Neth.)'50; FACS; GenSurg; Chief of Surg., Addington County Gen. Hosp.

THOMSON, Alexander; Box 1080, Drumheller, Alta.; Edinburgh (Scot.) '33; DPH; M.O.H., Drumheller.

THOMSON, Alexander; Pearl River, N.Y., U.S.A.; 1450 Palisade Ave., Palisade, N.J. (res); McG '51; DNB (USA); MCGP; Dir., Med. Advisory Dept., Lederle Labs.; Tel. 914-735-5000.

THOMSON, Allan W.; Watrous Med. Clin., Box 160, Watrous, Sask.; McG '52; Staff, Watrous Union Hosp.; Dist. Coroner; Tel. 946-3388.

THOMSON, Ashley E.; 100 Med. College, Bannatyne & Emily, Winnipeg 3, Man.; Man'45; M.Sc., FRCP(C), IntMed; Dir. Clin. Invest. Unit, Deer Lodge Hosp.; Ass't. Phys., Wpg. Gen. Hosp.; Ass't. Prof. (Med.), U. of Manitoba; Tel. 837-1301.

THOMSON, B. W.; Tor '63; Res., Princess Margaret Hosp., Toronto 5, Ont.

THOMSON, Donald M.; 180 Metcalfe St., Ottawa, Ont.; Man '35; F.R.C.S.(Eng.), F.R.C.S.-(C), GenSurg; Surg., Ottawa Civic & Grace Hosp's; Tel. 233-7911.

THOMSON, Douglas L.; 1650 Cedar Ave., Montreal 25, P.Q.; McG '54; FRCP(C), IntMed; Gastroent (P.Q.); Ass't. Phys., Montreal Gen. Hosp.; Clin. Ass't.; Prof. Med., McGill U.; Tel. WE 7-6011, Loc. 710.

THOMSON, Dugald H.; Victoria Hosp., South St., London, Ont.; Glasgow (Scot.)'47; DMRT (Eng.); TherRad; Sr. TherRad., London Clinic, Ontario Cancer Treatment & Research Fdn.; Cons. TherRad., St. Joseph's Hosp.; Clin. Assoc. Prof., U. of Western Ontario; Tel. 432-5261.

THOMSON, Edward G., Sg/Lcdr; PMQ, RCAF Station, Greenwood, N.S.; Edinburgh (Scot.)'58.

THOMSON, Frank B.; 750 W. Broadway, Vancouver, B.C.; Tor '39; F.R.C.S.(C), GenSurg; Clin. Instr., U. of British Columbia; Telephone TR 2-5461.

THOMSON, Harry S.; 201 Rideau Med. Dental Centre, 1711-4th St. S.W., Calgary, Alta.; 219 Malibou Rd. (res); McG '52; PlasSurg; Tel. 263-7076.

THOMSON, Hugh G.; Ste. 1120, 123 Edward St., Toronto 2, Ont.; Tor'54; FRCS(C), GenSurg; PlasSurg; Ass't. Surg., Hosp. for Sick Children; Clin. Inst. (Surg.), U. of Toronto; Tel. 364-3681.

THOMSON, I. Blake; Ste. 105, 1175 Cook St., Victoria, B.C.; Glasgow (Scot.) '48; Psy; Tel. 383-9912.

THOMSON, J. George; London (Eng.) '53; M.B., B.S., MRCS; LRCP; D.A.; Anaes; Staff, Grace Hosp., Winnipeg 10, Man.; Tel. SU 3-6732.

THOMSON, Joan S. (Sutton); 283 St. Clements Ave., Toronto 12, Ont. (res); Tor '51; D.Psy; Psy; Staff, Mental Health Clinic, 3131 Lakeshore Blvd. W., Tor. 14; Cons. Psy., U. of Toronto Health Serv. & Juvenile Family Court.

THOMSON, John; Box 2001, Essex, Ont.; Manchester (Eng.)'59.

THOMSON, John; Perth Med. Clinic, Perth, N.B., Glasgow (Scot.) '50.

THOMSON, John A.; Apt. 211A, 2055 Carling Ave. W., Ottawa 10, Ont.; Qns'41; MCGP; Tel. 233-3187.

THOMSON, John A. C.; Burris Clinic, 242 Victoria St., Kamloops, B.C.; 146 St. Paul St. W. (res); Tor '33; IntMed; Med. Staff, Royal Inland Hosp.; Tel. 372-3303.

THOMSON, John C.; Box 2001, Essex, Ont.; Otago (N. Zealand)'59; MB; ChB; MRCOG; Tel. 776-7394.

THOMSON, J. Niven; 2160 Weston Rd., Weston, Ont.; 1 Playdell Ct., Rexdale (res); Glasgow (Scot.) '55; Sr. Active Staff, Humber Mem. Hosp.; Tel. CH 4-5566.

THOMSON, Maurice J.; 11 Kirkland St., Kirk-Lake. Ont.; 74 Wishman St. (res); Tor '32; MCGP; Tel. 241.

THOMSON, Michael J.; Res., Psychiatric Inst., 75 Emily St., Winnipeg 3, Man.; London (Eng.) '51; Dip. Psychol. Med. (Eng.).

THOMSON, Peter G.; 250 St. Clair Ave. W., Toronto 7, Ont.; Durham (Eng.) '45; D.Psy.; Psy; Cons., Forensic Clin., Toronto Psychiatric Hosp.; Clin. Teach. (Psy.), U. of Toronto; Tel. WA 2-8101.

THOMSON, Robert K. C.; 510 Med. Arts Bldg., Edmonton, Alta.; 11804-91st Ave. (res); Alb '31; FACP; FRCP(C); IntMed; Psy; Chm., Advis. Bd., Alberta U. Hosp.; Dir., Div. of Arthritis, Dept. of PH, Prov. of Alberta; Clin. Prof., U. of Alta.; Memb. of Eugenics Bd., Prov. of Alb.; Tel. GA 2-6457.

THOMSON, Robert J.; 871 North Service Rd., Cooksville, Ont.; Tor '52; M.C.G.P.; Staff, St. Joseph's & Queensway Hosp's., Toronto & S. Peel Hosp., Pt. Credit; Tel. 277-1152.

THOMSON, Robert Mackay; 130 Elm St. E., Sudbury, Ont.; Tor'35; MCGP; Tel. 673-7181.

THOMSON, Stuart A.; 330 Medical Arts Bldg., 170 St. George St., Toronto, Ont.; 169 Dunvegan Rd. (res); Tor '31; GenSurg, OrthSurg; Surg., Hosp. for Sick Children; Assoc. Prof. (Surg.), U. of Toronto; Tel. WA 1-2035.

THOMSON, W. H. Montague; 574 Victoria St., London, Ont. (res); Wes '27; OphthOtol; Retired.

THORDARSON, Theodore T.; Ste. 14, 22707 Lougheed Hwy., Haney, B.C.; 12257-4th Ave. (res); UBC '56; MCGP; Chief of Staff, Maple-ridge Hosp.; Tel. 463-4102.

THORES, Orison A.; Aberdeen (Scot.)'60; DCH; D.Obst. RCOG; Res. (Paed.), Vancouver Gen. Hosp., Vancouver, B.C.

THORFINNSON, Patricia C.; Apt. 308, 48 Isabella St., Toronto 5, Ont.; McG '56; DiagRad; Staff, Sunnybrook Hosp.; Clin. Ass't. Rad., U. of Toronto; Tel. 485-8651.

THORKELSON, Grahame W.; 816 103rd. Ave., Dawson Creek, B.C.; Man '56.

THORLAKSON, Paul H. T.; Wpg. Clinic, St. Mary's & Vaughan Sts., Winnipeg, Man.; Man'19; LI.D., MRCS, LRCP, FACS, FRCS(C), GenSurg; Cons. Surg., Wpg. Gen. Hosp.; Dir., Wpg. Clinic; Commiss., Man. Hosp. Commission; Emer. Prof. Surg., U. of Manitoba; Tel. WH 2-6441.

THORLAKSON, Robert H.; Winnipeg Clinic, St. Mary & Vaughan, Winnipeg 1, Man.; Man '49; FRCS (Eng.); FACS; FRCS(C), GenSurg; Court. Staff, Misericordia, Grace, St. Boniface & Children's Hosp's.; Cons. Surg. Staff, St. Anthony's Gen. Hosp., The Pas; Ass't. Prof., U. of Manitoba; Tel. 942-0551.

THORLAKSON, Thorburn K.; Winnipeg Clinic, St. Mary & Vaughan, Winnipeg 1, Man.; 309 Montrose St., Wpg. 9 (res); Man '49; FACS; FRCS (Eng.); FRCS(C); GenSurg; Dir., Wpg. Clinic; Memb. Manitoba Hosp. Comm.; Prof., (Emer.), U. of Manitoba; Tel. 942-0551.

THORLEIFSON, Wilfred H.; 1541 W. Broadway, Vancouver 9, B.C.; Man'29; DABR; DiagRad; Tel. MU 1-0345.

THORN, J. Harrie; Ste. 103, 688 Coxwell Ave., Toronto 6, Ont.; Wes'58; FRCP(C), Anaes.; Staff, Toronto East Gen. & Orthopaedic Hosp's.; Tel. HO 5-7533.

THORNE, Edward L.; 2198 Gottingen St., Halifax, N.S.; 27 Connaught Ave. (res); Dal '41; Dist. M.O., CNR; Examin. Dept. of Transport; Sr. Examin., Prudential Life Assur. of London; Tel. 455-2144.

THORNER, Donald R.; 214 Margaret Ave., Wallaceburg, Ont.; 25 Martin Pk. Rd. (res); Wes '52; Tel. 627-2231.

THORNER, Lorne R.; 214 Margaret Ave., Wallaceburg, Ont.; 207 Lawrence Ave. (res); Wes '61; Tel. 627-2232.

THORNHILL, Mary E.; 715 Danforth Ave., Toronto 6, Ont.; 4 Butternut St., Tor. 6 (res); Tor '48; MCGP; Staff, Women's College Hosp.; Tel. HO 1-8811.

THORNTON, Kenneth R.; 2440 Sutton Rd., Victoria, B.C.; Leeds (Eng.) '50; Path.

THORNTON, Norman M.; Burris Clinic, Kamloops, B.C.; UBC'54; Anaes; Staff, Royal Inland Hosp.; Tel. 372-3131.

THORNTON, William B.; 200 St. Clair Ave. W., Toronto, Ont.; 7 Paddock Ct., Willowdale (res); Tor '37; InsMed; Chief M.O., Canada-Norwich Life Ins. Soc. & Canada Holland Life Ins. Soc.; Teach. Staff, O.P.D., Toronto Western Hosp.; M.O., Norwich Union Fire Soc., Att. Phys., Northern Electric Co. & Belmont Home for Aged; Staff (Med.), U. of Toronto; Telephone WA 3-9125.

THORP, Malcolm D.; 322 Wellington St., Sarnia, Ont.; 466 Maxwell (res); Dublin (Ire.) '37; M.C.G..P; Tel. ED 7-5414.

THORP, Robert H.; 3519 Mathers Ave., West Vancouver, B.C.; London (Eng.) '44; Anaes; Att'd. Staff, Lions Gate Hosp.; Vis. Staff, St. Paul's & St. Mary's Hosp's.; Tel. 922-7764.

THORPE, Ronald; Berwick Med. Centre, Berwick, N.S.; Dal'48.

THORSON, Stephen B.; 32 Academy Med. Bldg., Calgary, Alta.; Man'36; MS(Med); DABIM; FACP; Staff, Calgary Gen. & Holy Cross Hosp's.; Cons. Staff, Alta. Children's Hosp.; Dir., Calgary Prov. Arthritic Clinic; Governor (Alta.) Amer. College of Phys.; Med. Dir., Alta. Gas Trunk Line Co.; Tel. 263-7272.

THORSON, Stephen C.; Man '52; Res., Vancouver Gen. Hosp., Vancouver 9, B.C.

THOW, G. Bruce; Lockwood Clinic, 300 Bloor St. E., Toronto 5, Ont.; 18 Heathdale Rd., Tor. 10 (res); Tor '54; FRCS(C), GenSurg; DABS; Abroad.

THRASYBULE, Edner; 1384 est, Jean Talon, Montreal 35, P.Q.; 225 Champ Fleury, Duverney (res); Haiti '44; Otol; Staff (Oto-Rhino), Hop. Jean Talon; Tel. 274-5583.

THRELKELD, Agnes W. (De Mone); 6267 Quinpool Rd., Halifax, N.S.; Dal'50; MCGP; Assoc. Staff, Halifax Infirmary & Victoria Gen. Hosp.; Tel. 423-6701.

THRENDYLE, Kenneth L.; Corunna, Ont.; Wes '55; MCGP; Staff, St. Joseph's & Sarnia Gen. Hosp's.; Tel. TO 2-1155.

THUOT, Claude A.; Mon'65; Res., Verdun General Hosp., Montreal 19, P.Q.

THURBER, Donald S.; 36 Carleton Place, Baie Comeau, P.Q. (res); McG '25; Med. Dir., Quebec N. Shore Paper Co. & Boisvert Memorial Hosp.; M.O.H., Baie Comeau.

THURGAR, Ailsa M.; 5175 Rumble St., South Burnaby, B.C.; 2146 Yew St., Van. 9 (res); London (Eng.) '55; M.B., B.S.; Instr. (Paed.), U. of British Columbia; Tel. HE 3-2733.

THURLBECK, William M.; Cape Town (S. Africa)'53; MC (Path); Prof. of Path., McGill U., Montreal 2, P.Q.; Tel. 842-1251, Loc. 1723.

THURLOW, H. John; 247 Huron St., London, Ont.; Wes'61; MCGP; Lect. Dept. of PrevMed., U. of Western Ontario; Counsellor, Student Health Services.

THURSTON, Lyle M.; 110 W. 14th St., North Vancouver, B.C.; Sask'65.

THURSTON, Olin G.; Sask'58; FRCS(C), GenSurg.; Staff, University Hosp., Edmonton, Alta.

THURSTON, Willard G.; 42 W. 16th Ave., Vancouver 10, B.C.; McG '23; ObstGyn; Tel. TR 9-4857.

THUT, Henry W.; Wes'59; Res., Royal Victoria Hosp., Montreal 2, P.Q.

TIBBETTS, T. Michael; Box 980, Leduc, Alta.; London (Eng.)'54; MRCS(Eng.); LRCP(Lond.); D.ObstRCOG; DA(Eng.).

TIBBLES, John A. R.; 5750 South St., Halifax, N.S.; London (Eng.)'51; MRCP(Lond.); DCH; Paed; Neurol., Children's Hosp.; Lect. (Paed.), Dalhousie U.; Tel. 422-5821.

TICE, James W.; 516 Medical Arts Bldg., Hamilton, Ont.; Apt. 41, Herkimer Apts., 86 Herkimer St. (res); Tor '21; F.A.C.P.; IntMed.; Tel. JA 7-6515.

TICKETT, Fred W.; 11 Gorevale Ave., Toronto 3, Ont.; 51 Alexander St. (res); Tor '32; Ass't. Coroner for Toronto; Tel. EM 8-3754.

TICKTIN, Philip A.; 310 Bloor St. W., Toronto; Ont.; 15 Denton St. (res); Tor '28; Otol.; Tel. LE 1-9882.

TIDEY, Vernon L.; 33 Grant Blvd., Dundas, Ont.; Tor '43; DPH; M.O., Industrial Hygiene Branch, Ont. Dept. of Health.

TIDMARSH, Clarence J.; 1390 Sherbrooke St. W., Montreal 25, P.Q.; 2 Redpath Pl. (res); McG '24; Gastroent (P.Q.); F.A.C.P., D.A.B.I.M.; F.R.C.P.(C), IntMed; Attend. Staff, Royal Victoria Hosp.; Tel. VI 2-1311.

TIDMARSH, F. Wendell; 6 Richmond St., Charlottetown, P.E.I.; McG '14; Paed; Staff, Dept. of DVA; Tel. 894-5576.

TIDMARSH, William W.; 4700 Prince of Wales Ave., Montreal, P.Q.; 79 Percival Ave. (res); McG '43; Paed; Ass't. Phys., Montreal Children's Hosp.; Dem. McGill U.; Tel. HU 8-7044.

TIELENS, Raoul; Box 401, Langley, B.C.; Amsterdam (Neth.)'52; MCGP; Tel. 534-4214.

TIEMAN, Eugene E., OBE, CD; 104 Larkfield Dr., Don Mills, Ont.; Wes'35; DPH; Med. Dir., Toronto Depot, Cdn. Red Cross Blood Transfusion Serv.; Tel. 923-6692.

TIKKALA, Arne O.; Med. Arts Bldg., 121 Wellington St. W., Barrie, Ont.; Qns '56; Active Staff, Royal Victoria Hosp.

TILE, Marvin; 178 St. George St., Toronto 5, Ont.; Tor'57; FRCS(C), OrthSurg; Staff, St. Joseph's Hosp.; Cons., Sunnybrook Hosp.; Tel. 922-2593.

TILLER, William D.; 95 Lemarchant Rd., St. John's, Nfld.; Dal'66.

TILLEY, A. Ross, OBE; 200 St. Clair Ave. W., Toronto 7, Ont.; Tor'29; FACS; PlasSurg; Cons. (PlasSurg), Sunnybrook, Wellesley & Kingston Gen. Hosp., Kingston; Ass't. Prof. (PlasSurg.), Queen's U., Kingston, Ont.; Tel. WA 1-8606.

TILLEY, John V.; Box 460, 138-3rd St., Cochrane, Ont.; 189-7th Ave. (res); Tor '35; M.C.G.P.; Tel. 272-3226.

TILLMAN, William A.; 18 Chalmers St., London, Ont.; Wes '43; M.Sc., DABPN; Psy; Chief Psy., St. Joseph's Hosp.; Cons. Psy., St. Mary's Hosp.; Assoc. Prof. (Psy.), U. of Western Ontario; Tel. GE 9-1351 & GE 9-3271, Ext. 277.

TILSER, George; UBC'59; Res., St. Paul's Hosp., Vancouver 1, B.C.; Abroad.

TILTINS, Antonija; 5083 Chestnut St., Pierrefonds, P.Q. (res); Latvia '33; Staff, Hop-Ste-Justine, Montreal; Tel. RE 1-4931.

TILTINS, Mirdza; 955 Queen St. E., Sault Ste. Marie, Ont.; 127 McMeekin (res); Latvia '42.

TIMBOL, Jose V.; 138 Geneva St., St. Catharines, Ont.; Philippines '56; Tel. 685-0413.

TIMMONS, Terence J.; 610 Medical-Dental Bldg., Regina, Sask.; 10 Lakeview, Apt. 3 (res); Dublin (Ire.) '50; Tel. 522-0620.

TIMPSON, Ronald J.; Broadway Ave., Wawa, Ont.; 132 Churchill Ave. (res); Qns '60; Tel. UL 6-2231.

TINDALE, Robert M.; 672 Brant St., Burlington Ont.; Tor '51; ObstGyn; Chief, ObstGyn, Joseph Brant Mem. Hosp.; Court. Staff, Henderson Gen. Hosp.; Tel. 637-0222.

TINDALL, Jack B.; Box 174, Ripley, Ont.; Wes '38.

TING, David D.; Taiwan (Formosa) '58; Res., St. Boniface Hosp., St. Boniface, Man.

TING, Peter L.; Ott'65; Res., Queen Elizabeth Hosp., Montreal 28, P.Q.

TINMOUTH, Alan H.; McG'64; Res., St. John's Gen. Hosp., St. John's, Nfld.

TINNING, Robert A.; 1310 Ouellette Ave., Windsor, Ont.; 2050 Devonshire Ct. (res); Wes '48; FRCP(C), IntMed; Tel. CL 6-5384.

TIONGSON, Rodrigo V.; Apt. 15, 1027 Lucknow St., Halifax, N.S.; Santo Tomas (Philipp.)'58; IntMed.

TIPLER, Herbert A.; 199 Ontario St., St. Catharines, Ont.; Qns'57.

TIPPING, Clarence E.; 26 Herne Hill, Islington, Ont. (res); Tor '21; Anaes; Chief, Dept. of Anaes., St. Joseph's Hosp.; Tel. BE 1-8481.

TISCHLER, Bluma; 6210 Fremlin St., Vancouver 13, B.C.; Munich (Germ.)'48; Paed; Dir. of Paed. & Med. Serv., Woodlands School; Clin. Instr. (Paed.), U. of British Columbia.

TISCHLER, Isaak; Ste. 260, 5655 Cambie St., Vancouver 15, B.C.; Munich (Germ.)'48; Psy; Clin. Instr., U. of British Columbia.

TISDALE, C. Leroy; Medical Bldg., Prince Albert, Sask.; 420-21st St. W. (res); Man '34; Penitentiary Phys., Prince Albert; Tel. 763-6401.

TISDALE, James M.; 511 Lawrence Ave., Kelowna, B.C.; Wes'63; AMCGP; Tel. 762-0974.

TISDALE, John E.; 501 Medical Arts Bldg., Winnipeg, Man.; Man'06; Retired.

TISDALE, Paul K. E. D.; 501 Med. Arts Bldg., 404 Graham Ave., Winnipeg 1, Man.; 238 Kingsway Ave., Wpg. 9 (res); Man '38; FACP; Int-Med; Cons. (IntMed.), Deer Lodge, Grace & Victoria Hosp's.; Chmn., Dept. IntMed., Misericordia Gen. Hosp.; Lect., U. of Manitoba; Tel. 943-2935.

TISDALE, R. Walter, Jr.; P.Q. Box 520, 142 Church St., Delhi, Ont.; Tor '35; Staff, Norfolk Gen. Hosp., Simcoe, Ont.; Tel. 582-2780.

TISDALE, Terrance C.; McG '61; Res., Vancouver Gen. Hosp., Vancouver, B.C.

TISDALL, G. W.; Tor'64; Res., Clarke Inst. of Psy., Toronto 2B, Ont.

TISHLER, Jack M.; 1252 Mathers, Winnipeg 9, Man.; McG'61; FRCP(C), DiagRad.

TISSENBAUM, Ben; 460 Ellendale Med. Bldg., 5845 Cote-des-Neiges Rd., Montreal 26, P.Q.; 4620 Plamondon No. 10 (res); Mainz (Germ.) '60; MCGP.

TITCOMBE, Emerson P.; Thornbury, Ont.; Tor'43; MCGP; Staff, Meaford Hosp.; Coroner, Grey County; Tel. 599-3240.

TITCOMBE, Ruth (Whitfield); 23 Parent Ave., Ottawa, Ont.; Qns '49; Anaes; Anaesthetist, Ottawa Gen. Hosp.; Tel. CE 6-0333.

TITTEMORE, Delbert L.; Atkin Clin., Banff, Alta.; Alb '51; Dist. Coroner.

TITTLEY, J.-Rene; 11 ouest, blvd St-Joseph, Montreal 14, P.Q.; Mon '50; Obst (P.Q.); Staff, Hop. Ste-Justine; Tel. 273-7161.

TITUS, Arthur W.; 1970 Connaught Ave., Halifax, N.S.; Dal '47; MCGP; Med. Dir., Maritime Med. Care Inc.; Tel. 422-7641.

TJADEN, Robert J.; Man '62; Res., Winnipeg Gen. Hosp., Winnipeg, Man.

TKACHYK, S. John; Baker Clinic, 10004 105th St., Edmonton, Alta.; Alb'60; Paed.

TOBE, Allan D.; 917-750 W. Broadway, Vancouver 9, B.C.; Alb'59; FRCP(C), IntMed; Instr. Dept. of Med., U. of British Columbia; Tel. 872-5722.

TOBE, Barry A.; 250 Lawrence Ave. W., Toronto 12, Ont.; Tor '55; FRCP(C); IntMed.

TOBIN, Sidney M.; 99 Avenue Rd., Toronto 5, Ont.; Tor '46; FACS; FACOG; FRCS(C), ObstGyn; Att'd. Staff, Mt. Sinai Hosp.; Court. Staff, Toronto Gen. Hosp.; Tel. WA 3-9095.

TOD, D. Michael; Edinburgh (Scot.) '58; Int'n., University Hosp., Edmonton, Alta.

TODD, Iain A.; 2642 Eglinton Ave. E., Scarborough, Ont.; Cambridge (Eng.) '56; M.A., LRCP, MRCS, FRCS(C), GenSurg; Urol; Staff, Sunnybrook Hosp.; Att'd. Staff, Scarborough Gen. Hosp.; Tel. 293-8181.

TODD, Irvine M.; 297 Sunnyside Ave., Ottawa, Ont.; 3756 Revelstoke Dr. (res); Queen's (Belfast, N. Ire.) '50; MB, B.Ch., BAO; MCGP; Tel. 234-8952.

TODD, John E.; 460 Eglinton Ave. E., Toronto, Ont.; Tor'41; Staff, O.P.D. St. Michael's Hosp.; Staff, St. Michael's & Wellesley Hosp's.; Tel. HU 3-5134.

TODD, John K.; Durham (Eng.)'56; Staff, Calgary Gen. Hosp., Calgary, Alta.

TODD, Norman; 3 Gore Ave., Chilliwack, B.C.; London (Eng.) '58; Active Staff, Chilliwack Gen. & Coqualeeza Hosp., Sardis; Tel. 795-7211.

TODD, R. M.; 298 Lake Shore Rd. E., Port Credit, Ont.; Tor '51; Tel. CR 8-8611.

TODD, Thomas N. F.; White Clinic, 383 Ellis St., Penticton, B.C.; Queens U. (Belfast, N. Ire.) '49; FACA; Anaes; Tel. HY 2-3024.

TODOSIJCZUK, Demitrius; Karl-Frances (Graz, Austria) '51; Med. Dir., Royal Edward Laurentian Hosp., Ste.-Agathe-des-Monts, P.Q.; Tel. 326-4241.

TOES, Mary A.; 6 Masters Ave., Kentville, N.S.; London (Eng.)'52; D.ObstRCOG; Court. Staff, Blanchard Fraser Mem. Hosp.; Tel. 678-2818.

TOES, Norman A.; 6 Masters Ave., Kentville, N.S.; London (Eng.)'49; M.B., B.S.; MRCS (Eng.); LRCP (Lond.); DObstRCOG; Active Staff, Blanchard-Fraser Hosp.; Tel. 678-2818.

TOEWS, Cornelius J.; Dept. of Biochem., Queen's U., Kingston, Ont.; Man '63; Research Assoc., Muscular Distrophy Assoc. of Canada.

TOEWS, Helene A.; Man '61; Res., Winnipeg Gen. Hosp., Winnipeg, Man.

TOEWS, L. Jean, (Huntley); 117 Cassandra Blvd., Parkway South, Don Mills, Ont.; Qns '55; DMR; DiagRad; Staff, Women's College Hosp.

TOEWS, Rudolph R.; 2150 Valley Way, Niagara **Falls, Ont.; 626 Pettit Ave. (res); Tor '53; Ophth; Active Staff Gtr. Niagara Gen. Hosp.; Tel. EL 6-3311.**

TOFT, Bernard; UBC'62; Research Fell., Hosp. for Sick Children, Toronto, Ont.

TOGURI, Etsuko; 1274 Kennedy Rd., Scarborough P.O., Ont.; 37 North Hill Terr., Don Mills (res); Tor '51; M.C.G.P.; Tel. PL 7-1905.

TOLAN, J. Ronald; 2221 Keele St., Toronto 15, Ont.; Ott '52; DiagRad; Staff, Northwestern Gen. Hosp.; Tel. 249-1641.

TOLCZYNSKI, Borys; 5 Dunlop Blk., Yorkton, Sask.; 127-1st Ave. N., (res); Stefan Batory U. (Wilno, Poland) '31; Otol (Poland); Chm. (EN & T), Yorkton Union Hosp.; Tel. 783-3216.

TOLEDO-DIAZ, Jose M.; Madrid (Spain)'51; Res., Ottawa Gen. Hosp., Ottawa, Ont.

TOLEK, Ismail H.; Ankara (Turkey) '54; Staff, Union Hosp., Moose Jaw, Sask.; Cons. Psy., Providence Hosp.; Tel. 692-1841.

TOLGYES, Steven F.; 10 Grand Ave., London, Ont.; Budapest (Hung.)'29; Staff, Victoria & St. Joseph's Hosp's.; Tel. 432-1884.

TOLNAI, George; 1954 Lauder Ave., Ottawa 3, Ont.; Pecs (Hung.) '48; Path; Ass't. Prof. (Pathol.), U. of Ottawa; Tel. CE 5-6751.

TOLNAI, Susan; 1954 Lauder Dr., Ottawa 13, Ont.; Budapest (Hung.) '53; Ass't. Prof. (Med.), U. of Ottawa; Tel. CE 5-6751, Ext. 289.

TOLSON, Roger J.; London (Eng.)'57; MRCS (Eng.); LRCP(Lond.); D.ObstRCOG; IntMed; Staff, Toronto Western Hosp., Toronto 2B, Ont.

TOM, Mary I.; 701 Eglinton Ave. W., Apt. 308, Toronto, Ont. (res); Tor '22; Path; NeurPath., Tor. Gen. Hosp.; Assoc. Prof. of Neuropath., Banting Inst., U. of Toronto, 100 College St., Toronto; Retired.

TOMAS, John; Ott'64; Res., St. Michael's Hosp., Toronto 2, Ont.

TOMASHEWSKY, Edward E.; Box 416, Grand Forks, B.C.; Alb '39; M.C.G.P.; Dist. Coroner.

TOMIUK, Samuel; 370-44th Ave., Lachine, P.Q.; Ott '55.

TOMKA, Brian E.; Carruthers Clinic, 137 Wellington St., Sarnia, Ont.; Qns'65; Tel. 344-5261.

TOMLINSON, John W.; 2917 Bloor St. W., Toronto, Ont.; Tor '38; Tel. LE 3-0011.

TOMLINSON, Nelson F.; Claremont, Ont.; Tor '18; M.O.H., Pickering Twp.

TOMLINSON, William W.; Pickering, Ont. (Box 250); Wes '50; Active Staff, Ajax-Pickering, Oshawa Gen., & Toronto East Gen. Hosp's; Indus. Phys., Canadian Automotive Trim. Ajax; Dist. Coroner.

TOMM, Karl M., F/L; Alb '63; RCAF Station, Uplands, Ont.

TOMM, Gordon E.; 384 Tranquille Rd., North Kamloops, B.C.; 937 Renfrew Ave. (res); Alb '60; Tel. 376-3135.

TOMPKINS, Allan D.; Carson Blk., Vulcan, Alta.; Wes '43; Dist. Coroner; Tel. 485-2116.

TOMPKINS, James B.; Dominion, N.S.; Dal '51; M.C.G.P.

TOMPKINS, Jarvis W.; Box 1329, Quesnel, B.C.; Wes'48.

TOMPKINS, Kevin J.; 165 Plymouth Rd., Welland, Ont.; 39 Lillias St. (res); Dal '58; MRCOG; ObstGyn; Tel. 735-5710.

TOMPKINS, M. Gregor, Jr.; 5991 Spring Garden Rd., Halifax, N.S.; 5881 Chain Rock Dr. (res); Dal '49; FACOG; FRCS(C), ObstGyn; MCGP; Chief (ObstGyn), Halifax Infirmary; Assoc. Prof. (Gyn), Dalhousie U.; Tel. 423-8647.

TOMPSETT, David A.; 107 Vancouver Blk., 736 Granville St., Vancouver 2, B.C.; 1628 W. 28th Ave. (res); Man '12; Hon. Surg. Staff, Vancouver Gen. Hosp.; Tel. MU 3-2627.

TOMS, Albert A.; 32 Aylesbury Rd., Islington, Ont. (res); Man '43; Anaes; Staff, Queensway Gen. Hosp.

TOMS, Walter H.; Bonne Bay, Nfld.; Edinburgh (Scot.) '41; M.B., Ch.B.

TONI, Stephen S.; P.O. Box 240, Altona, Man.; Man '36; M.C.G.P.; M.O.H.

TONKEN, Harvey; 2915 Wyandotte St. W., Windsor, Ont.; Tor '55; Tel. 252-8283.

TONKIN, Roger S.; McG '62; Res., Montreal Children's Hosp., Montreal, P.Q.

TONNING, Daniel J.; 1354 Robie St., Halifax, N.S.; Dal '38; F.A.C.P., IntMed; Assoc. Phys., Victoria Gen. Hosp.; Assoc. Prof. of Med., Dalhousie U.; Tel. 423-7889.

TONNING, Henrik; 115 Hazen St., Saint John, N.B.; Dal'43; DABIM; FRCP(C), IntMed; Chief, Dept. of Med., Saint John Gen. & Lancaster DVA Hosp's.; Assoc. Prof. (Med.), Dalhousie U.; Med. Dir., N.B. Div. Cdn. Arthritis & Rheumatism Soc.; Tel. 692-5430.

TOOGOOD, John H.; 194 Hunt Club Dr., London, Ont.; Tor '46; Dip. IntMed (McGill); FCAA; FAAA; FRCP(C); IntMed; Dir., Allergy Lab., Victoria Hosp.; Ass't. Prof. (Med.), U. of Western Ontario; Tel. GE 2-5261, Loc. 491.

TOOLEY, Robert W.; 190 Belmont Ave., Ottawa 1, Ont.; London (Eng.)'52; MRCS; LRCP; DPH.

TOOMIK, Paul; Dominion Park, Lancaster, N.B.; Tartu (Estonia) '44; Staff Provincial Hosp.

TOONE, William M.; 2355 Richmond Rd., Victoria, B.C.; 5525 Parker Ave., (res); Tor '37; DTM & H; FACS; FICA; FRCS(Edin.); GenSurg; Chmn., Int. Comm. & Ass't. Chief of Surg., Veteran's Hosp.; Tel. EV 2-4221.

TOPLACK, Natale J.; 345 Victoria Ave., Chatham, Ont.; Wes '45; Path. & Dir. of Lab., Public Gen. Hosp.; Prov. Reg. Path.; Tel. EL 2-6400.

TOPP, James R.; Ste. 11, Toronto East Gen. Hosp., Toronto, Ont.; Ste. 534, Med. Arts Bldg., Toronto; Tor '51; FRCP(C), IntMed; Cons. Staff, Toronto East Gen. Hosp.; Tel. WA 2-9141.

TOPPING, F. O.; Medical Arts Bldg., Windsor, Ont.; 2431 Lincoln (res); Wes '37; Tel. 252-2281.

TORRANCE, Thomas L.; 31 Peter St. N., Orillia, Ont.; 273 Coldwater Rd. (res); Tor '32.

TORRES, Audomaro E.; 1119 Grant Ave., Ste. 24, Winnipeg 9, Man.; Nuevo Leon (Mexico)'62; Paed.

TORRIE, Alexander F.; Fredericton Med. Clinic, 206 Rookwood Ave., Fredericton, N.B.; Edinburgh (Scot.) '42; F.R.C.S. (Edin.), F.A.C.S.; OrthSurg; Chief of Orth Serv. Victoria Public Hosp.; Chief Surg., N.B. Poliomyelitis Hosp.; Tel. 475-4491.

TORRIE, Allan M.; Lake of the Woods Clinic, 112 Matheson St. S. Kenora, Ont.; Superior St., Keewatin (res); Man '51; M.C.G.P.

TOTH, Albert; Ste. 515, 5025 Cote des Neiges Rd., Montreal, P.Q.; 5675 Cote St. Luc Rd. (res); Budapest (Hung.) '52; ObstGyn; Clin. Fell., (ObstGyn.), Royal Victoria Hosp; Lect. McGill U.; Tel. HU 9-8070.

TOTH, Andrew I.; Woodland Plaza, Cooksville, Ont.; Wes '63.

TOTH, Joseph; Budapest (Hung.) '56; Res., Royal Victoria Hosp., Montreal 2, P.Q.

TOTH, Laszlo; Box 155, Vita, Man.; Budapest (Hung.) '51; Tel. 5-3313.

TOTTEN, Walter S.; 249 William St., Belleville, Ont.; Dal '54; IntMed; Tel. 962-7710.

TOUCHETTE, Louis; 2090 Chemin Ste. Foy, Quebec, P.Q. (res); Lav '54.

TOUGAS, Adrien; Clinique Medicale de Bedford, Place D'Estrie, Bedford, P.Q.; Lav '51.

TOUGAS, Gilles; 5586 Drake St., Montreal 20, P.Q. (res); Mon '53; Staff, Dept. Health, Montreal.

TOUGAS, Hubert W.; 4395 Verdun Ave., Montreal 19, P.Q.; 1220 Verdun (res); Mon '40; DABOt; Otol; Chief (Otol.), Hop. Gen.-de-Verdun; Dir. (Audiometrie), Queen Mary Vet's. Hosp.; Tel. PO 9-4471.

TOUGAS, J. Roger; 8 Prud'homme St., Ste-Philomene, P.Q.; Mon '61; Tel. 692-0171.

TOUGAS, Regis; 3521 Verdun Ave., Verdun, Montreal, P.Q.; 351 Regina (res); Mon '39; Tel. 768-4111.

TOUPIN, Henri M.; 217 Le Marchand Bldg., 116th St. & 100th Ave., Edmonton, Alta.; 603-12207 Jasper Ave. (res); Alb '49; DABN; NeurSurg; Att'd. Staff, General & Royal Alexandra Hosp's.; Tel. HU 8-7475.

TOUPIN, Jean N.; St. Maurice, Cte. Champlain, P.Q.; Lav '53; M.C.G.P.

TOURANGEAU, Ferdinand J.; 1570 St.-Hubert, Montreal, P.Q.; Mon '23; D.P.H. (Tor.); C.P.H. (Harvard); P.H. (P.Q.); Dir. Div. Industrial Hygiene.

TOURANGEAU, June A.; 2800 Lundy's Lane, Niagara Falls, Ont.; Ott'64.

TOURIGNY, Raymond; Lav '51; Path; (P.Q.); Staff, Hop. du-Christ-Roi, Quebec 8, P.Q.; Tel. MU 3-3607.

TOURILLON, Paule (Mrs. Jacques Gagnon); 62 Maplewood, Outremont, Montreal 8, P.Q.; Mon '53; DPH; Staff, (Prev Med.), City Health Serv.; Tel. 872-2255.

TOURVILLE, Yves; Lav'65; Res., Hop. Enfant Jesus, Quebec 3, P.Q.

TOUSIGNANT, Andre; App. 2, 1080 de l'Esperanto, Trois Rivieres, P.Q.; Lav'60.

TOUSIGNANT, Benoit; 874 Ste Julie, Trois Rivieres, P.Q.; Lav '57; IntMed (P.Q.); Cardiol (P.Q.); AMCGP; Staff, Hop. St. Joseph; Tel. FR 4-6211.

TOUSIGNANT, J. Pierre; Mon '57; Anaes; Staff, Hop. Maisonneuve, Montreal, P.Q.; Tel. 254-8341.

TOUSIGNANT, L. Yves; Clinique-Medico-Chirurgical, 2775 rue Bourdages, St.-Hyacinthe, P.Q.; Mon '55; Otol (P.Q.); Tel. PR 3-1000.

TOUSIGNANT, Michel; 163 est rue Laurier, Ottawa 2, Ont.; Lav '57; Anaes; Staff, Ottawa Gen. Hosp.; Tel. CE 6-4592.

TOVEE, E. Bruce; 1015 Medical Arts Bldg., Toronto 5, Ont.; 167 Old Yonge St., Willowdale (res); Tor '38; F.A.C.S., F.R.C.S. (Edin.), F.R.C.S.(C), GenSurg; Sr. Surg., Toronto Gen. Hosp; Chief Sur., Toronto Metropolitan Police Dept.; Assoc. Prof. (Surg.), U. of Toronto; Telephone WA 2-4377.

TOWELL, H. Vernon; UBC'51; Res., Vancouver Gen. Hosp., Vancouver, B.C.

TOWELL, Molly E.; Dept. ObstGyn., Vancouver Gen. Hosp., Vancouver, B.C.; London (Eng.)'52; MRCOG; FRCS(C), ObstGyn; Staff, Vancouver Gen. Hosp.; Tel. TR 6-3211.

TOWERS, Thomas L.; 219 St. George St., London, Ont. (res); Tor '08; Retired.

TOWN, James D.; Box 370, Mitchell, Ont.; Qns'64; AMCGP; Active Staff, Seaforth Commun. Hosp. & Stratford Gen. Hosp.; Tel. 348-8402.

TOWNSEND, Clary H.; Dal '64; Res., Victoria Gen. Hosp., Halifax, N.S.

TOWNSEND, Constance M.; 939 Lawrence Ave. E., Don Mills, Ont.; Tor'63; Tel. 445-5590.

TOWNSEND, Darryl E.; 500 Seaforth Med. Bldg., 3550 Cote des Neiges Rd., Montreal 25, P.Q.; 5686 Queen Mary Road (res); McG '55; FACOG; FRCS (C); ObstGyn; Ass't. ObstGyn., Mtl. Gen. Hosp.; Jr. Ass't. ObstGyn. & Post Med. Dir., Catherine Booth Hosp.; Dem., McGill U.; Tel. 932-5359.

TOWNSEND, F. Ralph; Earnscliffe Ave., Wolfville, N.S.; Westwood Ave. (res); Dal '49; Psy; Staff, Fundy Mental Health Centre; Tel. 542-2326.

TOWNSEND, H. J.; 185 Provost St., New Glasgow, N.S.; 248 Washington (res); Dal '30; M.C.G.P.; Med. Staff, Aberdeen Hosp; Tel. 752-4248.

TOWNSEND, Milton G.; 1261 Shearer St., Montreal 25, P.Q.; 4392 Western Ave., Westmount (res); McG '35; IntMed; Clin. Ass't., Dept. of Med., Montreal Gen. Hosp.; Lect., Dept. of Health & Social Med., McGill U.; Med. Dir., Northern Electric Co.; Tel. WE 3-6480.

TOWNSEND, R. Gordon; Ste. 10, Academy Bldg., 1812 4th St. S.W., Calgary, Alta.; 920 Sitton Blvd. (res); McG'29; FICS, FRCS(Edin.), OrthSurg; Chief (OrthSurg.), Alberta Crippled Children's Hosp.; Active Staff (OrthSurg.), Calgary Gen. & Holy Cross Hosp's.; Cons. (OrthSurg.), Baker Mem. San.; Memb. Senate, U. of Alberta; Tel. 263-1736.

TOWNSEND, Robert G.; Ste. 320, 1538 Sherbrooke St. W., Montreal, P.Q.; 331 Lansdowne Ave., Westmount (res); McG'41; M.Ch. (Orth), (Liverpool); FRCS (Edin.), FRCS(C) OrthSurg; Assoc. Surg. (Orth.) Royal Victoria & Shriners' Hosp. for Crippled Children; Cons. (Orth), Queen Mary Vets'., Queen Elizabeth & Grace Dart Hosp's.; Lect. (OrthSurg), McGill U.; Tel. WE 2-8955.

TOWNSEND, Stuart R.; 901-1414 Drummond St., Montreal, P.Q.; 570 Chester, Twn. of Mt. Royal, Mtl. 16 (res); McG '33; F.A.C.P.; IntMed; Haem(PQ); Sr. Phys. & Dir. Dept. of Haem. & Blood Bank, Mtl. Gen. Hosp.; Assoc. Prof. Med. & ClinMed., McGill U.; Tel. AV 8-3454.

TOWNSLEY, B. Reid; 4132 Virginia Cres., Vancouver, B.C. (res); Qns '43; Anaes; Staff, North Vancouver Gen. Hosp.; Tel. 876-3211.

TOWSON, Richard T.; 123 Sunrise Ave., Toronto, Ont.; Dublin (Ire.)'42; B.Ch., LM (Rotunda); BAO; FACCP; FCCP; Med. Dir., The Purdue Frederick Co. (Canada) Ltd.; Tel. 751-0780.

TRACK, Alan A.; Ste. 705, 99 Avenue Rd., Toronto 5, Ont.; 10 Silverwood (res); Tor '30; F.R.C.S.(Edin.); Sr. Surg., New Mt. Sinai Hosp; Tel. WA 2-6443.

TRACY, Francis L.; 233 Second St. E., Cornwall, Ont.; Ott'53.

TRAFF, Terence N.; 10951-124th St., Edmonton, Alta.; Alb'59; FRCS(C), ObstGyn; Assoc. Staff, Royal Alexandra Hosp.; Tel. 454-4551.

TRAFTON, W. D.; Department of National Health & Welfare, c/o Regional Superintendent, European Region; UBC '57. Abroad.

TRAHAN, Andre; 1381 rue Notre-Dame, St. Maurice, P.Q.; Lav'65.

TRAHAN, Maurice; 759, des Mille Iles, Ste. Therese en Haut, Cte Terrebonne, P.Q.; Lav'57; Anaes; Staff, Hop. Bellechasse.

TRAILL, Alexander C.; 4400 W. Grandview-Douglas Hwy., Burnaby 2, B.C.; 3565 Westmount Rd. (res); St. Andrews (Scot.) '47; DABPN; Spec. Mental Health Centre.

TRAIN, Louis; 9 Clintwood Gate, Don Mills, Ont.; Tor'62; AMCGP; Tel. 447-4712.

TRAIN, Wilma G.; 1884 Jane St., Weston, Ont.; 56 High Park Ave. (res); Tor'48; Tel. CH 1-3141.

TRAINOR, John M.; 1 Med. Arts Bldg., Winnipeg 1, Man.; Apt. 5A, 99 Roslyn Rd. (res); McG'55; DABP; Path; Assoc. Pathol., Grace Hosp.; Tel. WH 2-7928.

TRAMER, Egon; 413 Selkirk Ave., Winnipeg 4, Man.; Prague (Czechoslov.) '39; M.C.G.P.; Tel. JU 9-0002.

TRANQUIL, Jean; App. 211, 3250 Ellendale, Montreal 26, P.Q.; Mon '57; Staff, Dept. of Health.

TRANQUIL, Pierre; Ste. 514, 30 est Boul. St. Joseph, Montreal 14, P.Q.; L'ille (France)'64.

TRAPMAN, Johan L.; 2530 Jane St., Downsview, Ont.; Leiden (Neth.) '48; MCGP; Tel. CH 9-1341.

TRAPP, Ethlyn; 925 W. Georgia St., Vancouver, B.C.; 200 Keith Rd., W. Vancouver (res); McG '27; F.F.R., DiagRad; Cons. (RadTher.), B.C. Cancer Inst.; Hon. Lect. (RadTher.), U. of British Columbia; Retired.

TRAPP, Frederick W.; Man '53; Res., Deer Lodge Hosp., Winnipeg 12, Man.

TRAPP, William G.; 410 Fairmount Med. Bldg., 750 W. Broadway, Vancouver 9, B.C.; 1336 W. 57th Ave. (res); McG '39; FRCS(C), GenSurg; ThorSurg; Assoc. (ThorSurg), Van. Gen. Hosp.; Thor. Surg. (TB) Control, (BC); Cons. Thor-Surg., B.C. Cancer Inst.; Clin. Instr. (Surg.), U. of British Columbia; Tel. TR 9-5355.

TRASK, Beverley C.; Med. Arts Bldg., 336 Kings Rd., Sydney, N.S.; Dal '55; IntMed; Staff, St. Rita & City of Sydney Hosp's.; Cons. Staff, St. Elizabeth, New Waterford & Harbour View Hosp's.; DVA Cons.; Tel. 562-1202.

TRASK, Carl A.; 131 Main St., Lancaster, N.B.; Dal '61; Dept. of Public Health, V.D. Control; Tel. 694-7712.

TRASK, Carl R.; 341 Lancaster Ave., Lancaster, N.B. (res); Dal '38; D.P.H.; Dir., Saint John Gen. Hosp., Saint John, N.B.; Tel. 693-3351.

TRASK, N. B.; 271 Portland St., Dartmouth, N.S.; 127 Crichton Ave. (res); Dal '51.

TRAUB, Gordon E.; Alb'65; Jr. Int., Misericordia Hosp., Edmonton, Alta.

TRAUB, Paul; 71 Black Creek Blvd., Toronto 9, Ont.; Prague (Czech.) '46; M.O., W.C.B. Hosp. & Rehab. Centre, Downsview; Tel. 762-3756.

TRAUB, Sidney P.; Tor '48; DiagRad; Assoc. Prof. (Radiol.), U. of Saskatchewan, Saskatoon, Sask. Abroad.

TRAVELLI, Renato; 721-15th Ave. S.W., Calgary, Alta.; Rome (Italy)'57.

TRAVIS, A. Lawrence; Dryden Med. Clinic, Box 1090, Dryden, Ont.; Dal '58; MCGP; Tel. 223-2287.

TRAVIS, S. J.; Caramat, Ont.

TRAYNOR, A. Victor; 52 Water St. N., Kitchener, Ont.; Wes '24; M.C.G.P.; Tel. SH 5-7523.

TRAYNOR, J. Alan; 3195 Granville St., Vancouver, B.C.; 1260 Netley Pl. W. (res); Tor '40; F.R.C.P.(C), IntMed; Med. Cons., Shaughnessy D.V.A. Hosp.; Active Staff, St. Paul's Hosp. & Clin. Instr., U. of British Columbia; Tel. RE 8-6911.

TREANOR, James J.; 136 Simcoe St. N., Oshawa, Ont.; Glasgow (Scot.) '53.

TREBILCOCK, Karl H.; 712 Main St. E., Hamilton, Ont.; Qns '29; M.C.G.P.; Chief of Staff, Dept. of Gen. Practice, Hamilton Gen. Hosp.; Tel. LI 4-4247.

TREDGER, Cecil N.; Ste. 402, 625-5th Ave., New Westminster, B.C.; Alb'43; OrthSurg.

TREDGER, Enid N.; 5397 Buckingham Ave., Burnaby 2, B.C. (res); Alb '43; Part-time Metro Health Unit, Vancouver.

TREFFRY, Charles J.; Ste. 202, 3195 Granville St., Vancouver 9, B.C.; Ste. 101 1430 Maple St., Van. 9 (res); Tor '39; Paed; Active Staff (Paed), St. Paul's Hosp.; Clin. Ass't. U. of British Columbia; Tel. RE 3-1223.

TREILONS, Svetlana (Baltins); Box 40, Sudbury Algoma San., Sudbury, Ont.; Latvian U. (Riga) '42.

TREISSMAN, David A.; 39 Leisure Lane, Richmond Hill, Ont.; London (Eng.)'57; Anaes.

TRELEAVEN, Richard B.; 226 Hunt Club Dr., London, Ont.; (res); Wes '47; DABR; DiagRad; AMCGP; Assoc. Rad., Victoria Hosp.; Cons. Rad., Wingham Dist. Hosp.; Instr. Rad., U. of Western Ont.; Tel. GE 2-5261.

TRELFORD, John D.; 907 Med. Arts Bldg. 170 St. George St., Toronto 5, Ont.; 192 Cold Stream Ave., Tor. 12 (res); Tor '56; FRCS(C), Obst Gyn; Tel. WA 3-1221.

TRELOAR, E. James; Ste. 303, 750 West Broadway, Vancouver 9, B.C.; UBC'55; Anaes.; MCGP; Tel. TR 2-5844.

TREMBATH, James H.; 13665—96th Ave., North Surrey, B.C.; Tor'52; MCGP; Tel. 581-4212.

TREMBATH, Margaret L.; 13665-96th Ave., North Surrey, B.C. (Part-time practice); Tor '47.

TREMBLAY, Adrien; 1895 Ave. Monument, Quebec 5, P.Q.; Lav '35.

TREMBLAY, Adrien; 4114 rue St. Hubert, Montreal, P.Q.; Mon '30; Obst(P.Q.); Ass't. Obst., Hop. St. Luc.; Tel. AL 2-3834.

TREMBLAY, Bernard M.; 316 St.-Georges, St.-Jerome, P.Q.; 531 rue-du-Palais (res); Mon '44; MCGP; Ass't. Anaes., Hotel-Dieu de St.-Jerome.

TREMBLAY, Bertrand; 50 rue Jacques-Cartier, Valleyfield, P.Q.; Lav'61; Paed.

TREMBLAY, Camille; St. Gedeon, Co. Lac-St-Jean, P.Q.; Lav '60.

TREMBLAY, Claude; Lav'65; Res., Hop. St. Francis d'Assise, Quebec 3, P.Q.

TREMBLAY, Fidele; Lav'51; DiagRad; Staff, Royal Victoria Hosp., Montreal 2, P.Q.

TREMBLAY, Francois; Lav'62; Res., Hop. Ste. Justine, Montreal 26, P.Q.

TREMBLAY, Gaston; 698 ave Royale, Quebec 5, P.Q.; Lav '51; Tel. 663-6496.

TREMBLAY, Gaston; Lav '61; FRCP(C), Anaes; Staff, Hop. St-Joseph, La Tuque, P.Q.; Tel. 523-4581.

TREMBLAY, G. Claude; 97 St-Marcellin, Les Escoumains, Cte. Saguenay, P.Q.; Lav '53; Med. Dir., Hop. St-Alexandre.

TREMBLAY, Georges-P.; 178 Price Ouest, Chicoutimi, P.Q.; Lav '36.

TREMBLAY, George W.; 627 est Jacques Cartier, Chicoutimi, P.Q.; 427 Blvd. St.-Sacrement (res); Lav '20; Ophth,Otol; Staff, Hop.-Hotel-Dieu-St.-Vallier; Tel. 549-0292.

TREMBLAY, Gerard; Laurierville, Co. Megantic, P.Q.; Lav '51; Dist. Coroner.

TREMBLAY, Gerard; 838 est, Jacques-Cartier, Chicoutimi, P.Q.; Lav '32; PulmDis. & T.B. P.Q.; Tel. 549-2435.

TREMBLAY, Gerard M.; 1395 Montpellier, Montreal 9, P.Q.; Mon'60; Cardiol(P.Q.).

TREMBLAY, Gilles; 733 Hartland Ave., Montreal, 8, P.Q.; Mon '53; Path (P.Q.); Staff, Hop. Hotel-Dieu; Tel. VI 4-0161.

TREMBLAY, Guy; St. Zephirin de Courval, Co. Yamaska, P.Q.; Lav'51; Tel. 564-2133.

TREMBLAY, Jacques; 1028 des Erables, Quebec 6, P.Q.; 912 Ave. Bon-Air, Ste.-Foy, Quebec 10, P.Q. (res); Lav'34; Tel. 681-6424.

TREMBLAY, Jacques; Centre Medical St.-Urbain, 3875 St.-Urbain, Montreal 18, P.Q.; Place-d'Aiguillion, Cartierville (res); Mon '44; IntMed (PQ), Gastroent. (PQ); Staff, Hotel-Dieu Hosp.; Assoc. Prof., U. of Mtl.; Tel. 844-3615.

TREMBLAY, J. Albert; 471 rue Montfort, Jonquiere, P.Q.

TREMBLAY, J. Charles; 4018 Delorimier Ave., Montreal, P.Q. 744 Hartland (res); Mon '22; Tel. LA 2-1555.

TREMBLAY, Jean M.; Sacre-Coeur, Cte., Saguenay, P.Q.; Lav '54.

TREMBLAY, Jean M.; 235 Proulx, Quebec 8, P.Q.; Lav '42; DPH; Tel. 527-2268.

TREMBLAY, Jean M.; 72 du Roi, Sorel, P.Q.; Ste. Anne de Sorel (res); Lav '34; PH (P.Q.); M.O.H., Sorel.

TREMBLAY, Jean P.; 410 Ontario St., Sherbrooke, P.Q. (res); Lav '51; Path; Staff, Hop. St. Vincent-de-Paul; Tel. LO 9-6381.

TREMBLAY, Jean R.; 34 Beaumont, La Tuque, P.Q.; 339 rue Kitchener (res); Lav '53.

TREMBLAY, J. H. Gilles; 399 L'Assomption Chicoutimi, P.Q. (res); Lav '40; OrthSurg (P.Q.); Ass't. Med. Dir., Hotel-Dieu-St. Vallier; Tel. 549-1452.

TREMBLAY, J. Yves; 18 Ouimet, Laval-des-Rapides, P.Q.; Mon '54; MCGP; Vis. Staff, Hop. Sacre-Coeur; Tel. 669-0915.

TREMBLAY, Lambert; Lav'64; Res., Montreal Gen. Hosp., Montreal 25, P.Q.

TREMBLAY, Laureat; 359 Marie-Rollet, Chicoutimi, P.Q. (res); Lav '54; F.R.C.S.(C), Urol; Urol., Hotel-Dieu-St. Vallier; Tel. 549-2440.

TREMBLAY, Leonidas; 200 Ave. des Bernieres, Quebec, P.Q. (res); Lav '43; D&TRad; Chief Rad., Hop. Laval & Anti-T.B. League; Tel. 653-5251.

TREMBLAY, Lionel; 3840 Ave. Wilson, Montreal 28, P.Q.; Mon '51; Anaes (P.Q.).

TREMBLAY, Louis J.; Qns '52; Path; Staff, Belleville Gen. Hosp., Belleville, Ont.; Reg. Pathol., County of Hastings; Tel. WO 8-5511.

TREMBLAY, Louis M.; 395 Collard, Alma, P.Q.; Lav'55; Paed.

TREMBLAY, Majella; 291 de la Couronne, Quebec, P.Q.; 138 de la Couronne (res); Lav '36; Tel. 524-1708.

TREMBLAY, Marc A.; 284 McDougall, Montreal 8, P.Q.; Mon '59.

TREMBLAY, Marcel; Lav'59; MCGP; Res., Hop. Notre Dame, Montreal 24, P.Q.

TREMBLAY, Maurice; 475 Blvd. Talbot, Chicoutimi, P.Q.; 584 Blvd. Talbot (res); Lav '49; Dip.Paed (Paris, Fr.); Paed; Chief (Paed.) Hotel-Dieu St. Vallier; Tel. 549-0090.

TREMBLAY, Michel; Lav '63; Res. (Path.), Hop. Hotel-Dieu, Quebec, P.Q.

TREMBLAY, Napoleon J.; 1570 rue St. Hubert, Montreal 24, P.Q.; 6635-33e. Ave., Rosemount (res); Lav '37; FCCP; PulmDis & TB (P.Q.); Ass't. Dir. Hosp. Ins. (P.Q.), Mtl. Div. & Dir. Mtl. Dept. of Health; Tel. VI 9-9371.

TREMBLAY, Normand A., Capt.; CFB Military Hosp., Summerside, P.E.I.; Ott'65.

TREMBLAY, Paul E.; Lav '55; OrthSurg; Staff, Hotel-Dieu Christ-Roi, Alma, P.Q.; Tel. 662-3421.

TREMBLAY, Paul R.; Lav '58; AMCGP; Res., Hop. Hotel-Dieu, Quebec 4, P.Q.

TREMBLAY, Pierre; 29 East Gables Ct., Beaconsfield, P.Q. (res); Mon '31.

TREMBLAY, Pierre; 2375 Perodeau, Quebec 6, P.Q. (res); Lav'55; DABR; D & T Rad; Staff, Hop. Hotel-Dieu, Levis; Tel. 837-9341.

TREMBLAY, P. Coursolles; Royal Victoria Hosp., Montreal 2, P.Q.; Ott '51; FACS; FRCS(C), ObstGyn; Ass't. ObstGyn., Royal Victoria Hosp.; Lect., McGill U.; Tel. VI 2-2311.

TREMBLAY, Rene; 579 rue St-Hubert, Jonquiere, P.Q.; Lav '54; A.M.C.G.P.

TREMBLAY, Rene G.; 1840 rue St-Marc, Shawinigan, P.Q.; 144 Terrace Cascade (res); Lav '56; FRCS(C); GenSurg; Tel. LE 6-3403.

TREMBLAY, Rodolphe; 87 3eme rue, Rimouski, P.Q.; Lav '58; GenSurg; Tel. 724-4546.

TREMBLAY, Roland; 3065 de Louvigny, Quebec 10, P.Q.; Lav'64.

TREMBLE, G. Edward; 1374 Sherbrooke St. W., Montreal, P.Q.; McG '21; D.L.O. (Eng.); F.R.C.P. (C), Otol; Assoc. Otol., Royal Victoria Hosp.; Ass't. Prof., McGill U.; Tel. VI 2-1411.

TREMBLETT, Hilda; McG '55; Path; Staff, St. Elizabeth Hosp., North Sydney, N.S.; Tel. 794-4725.

TREMEER, Doris C. (Foster); R.R. 1, Claremont, Ont.; Tor'30; IntMed(TB).

TREMPE, Andre C.; 11824 Alexandre-Lacoste, Montreal 12, P.Q.; Mon '60; Anaes; Staff, Hop. Jean-Talon; Tel. 334-2891.

TREMPE, Florian; 1050 Chemin-Ste-Foy, Quebec 6, P.Q.; Apt. 6, 960 Raymond-Casgrain (res); Lav '25; GenSurg; Prof. (Clin.Surg.), Hop.-St.-Sacrement & Prof. Laval U.; Tel. 527-3461.

TREMPE, Lorraine; 355 ave. Kensington, Westmount, P.Q.; Mon '51; Staff, Hop. Mont-Providence, Riviere des Prairies; Tel. 935-0895.

TREMPE, Roger; 11 rue St-Pierre, St. Alexis des Monts, P.Q.; Mon '33.

TRENHOLME, William A.; Med. Arts Bldg., 1105 Pandora Ave., Victoria, B.C.; 3200 Midland Rd. (res); Alb '33; Active Staff, Royal Jubilee Hosp.; Assoc. Staff, St. Joseph's Hosp.; Tel. 382-1515.
TREPANIER, Armand; 3479 Grey Ave., N.D.G., Montreal, P.Q. (res); Mon '49; D&TRad; Ass't. Rad., Notre Dame Hosp.; Tel. LA 5-6363.
TREPANIER, Yves; Lav'65; Res., Hop. Enfant Jesus, Quebec, P.Q.; Abroad.
TREVOR-SMITH, Edward S.; Ste. 460, 2184 W. Broadway, Vancouver 9, B.C.; 2145-W. 2nd Ave. (res); UBC'61; AMCGP; Tel. RE 6-5565.
TREWIN, R. Bruce; 6 Sunplains Cr., Etobicoke, Ont. (res); Tor '52; Ass't. Med. Dir., Ontario Hydro, 620 University Ave., Toronto; Tel. 368-6767.
TRIANTAPHYLLOPOULOS, Demetrios C.; 7303-156th St., Edmonton, Alta. (res); Athens (Greece) '46; Internal Med. (Greece); Ass't. Prof. (Physiol), U. of Alberta. Abroad.
TRIAS, Antoni; Medical Arts. Bldg., 5880 Spring Garden Rd., Halifax, N.S.; Barcelona (Spain) '52; DABOS; FICS; FRCS(C); OrthSurg; Act. Staff, Victoria Gen., Children's & Camp Hill DVA Hosp's.; Ass't. Prof. (OrthSurg.), Dalhousie U.; Tel. 423-7581.
TRIMBLE, Alan S.; Toronto Gen. Hosp., 101 College St., Toronto, Ont.; Tor '56; FRCS(C), Cardiovasc. & ThorSurg; Surg., Cardiovasc. Unit, Toronto Gen. Hosp.; Research Assoc., Ontario Heart Fdn.; Clin. Teach. Surg., U. of Toronto; Tel. EM 6-8211.
TRINCHAN, Angel; 541A College St., Toronto 4, Ont.; 5 Elm Ave., Apt. 401 (res); Zaragoza U. (Spain) '54; Derm; Tel. WA 5-7532.
TRITES, Albert E. W.; 7085 Wiltshire St., Vancouver 14, B.C.; McG '54; Path; Chief of Path. Serv., Shaughnessy Hosp.; Clin. Ass't. Prof. (Path.), U. of British Columbia.
TRIVEDI, Bhanumati; Bombay (India)'53; Staff, Eastern Shore Mem. Hosp., Sheet Harbour, N.S.
TROBRIDGE, Geoffrey F.; Laurentian University, Ramsey Lake Rd., Sudbury, Ont.; Birmingham (Eng.)'48; MRCP(Ed); Cardio-Pulm. Physiol., Sudbury Mem. Hosp.
TROENSEGAARD-HANSEN, Erling; Gull Lake, Sask.; London (Eng.) '32; FRCS (Eng.); Tel. 672-3575.
TROFIMOFF, Terence N. (See TRAFF, Terence N.).
TROINI, Rudy; Mon'63; Res., Hop. Maisonneuve, Montreal 36, P.Q.
TROSSMAN, Bernard; 517 Pine Ave. W., Montreal 2, P.Q.; 5160 Coronation Ave. (res); McG '57; Psy.
TROSSMAN, Marshall; 7655 Querbes Ave., Montreal, P.Q.; 6300 Lennox Ave. (res); McG '50; MCGP; Clin. Ass't., Med., Reddy Mem. & Queen Mary Vets' Hosp's.; Tel. 279-8725.
TROSTER, M.; Ste. 210, 305 Finch Ave. N., Willowdale, Ont.; Tor'65; Tel. 221-5544.
TROTIER, Guy; Lav'50; Res., Hop. Hotel-Dieu, Quebec 4, P.Q.
TROTT, Alvin W.; Box 169, Golden, B.C.; Alb '45; FACCP; MCGP; Tel. 344-2741.
TROTTER, Gordon K.; 48 Wellington St. N., Woodstock, Ont.; 459 Devonshire Ave. (res); Qns '39; M.C.G.P.; Staff, Woodstock Gen. Hosp.; Phys., Standard Tube and T.I.; Tel. 537-7851.
TROTTER, Merrill C.; 75 William St., Kingston, Ont.; 76 Macdonnell St. (res); Qns '42; M.C.-G.P.; Assoc. Staff, Kingston Gen. & Hotel Dieu Hosp's.; Precept. (PrevMed.), Queen's U.; Tel. 548-7242.
TROTTIER, Leon; P.O. Box 219, St. Paul, Alta.; Alb '53; Tel. 645-3311.
TROTTIER, Michel; 485 Ellendale Med. Bldg., 5845 Cote des Neiges Rd., Montreal 26, P.Q.; Mon '60; Ophth.; Assoc. Staff, Ophth., Hop. du Sacre-Coeur; Tel. 731-3696.
TROTTIER, Richard; 9 Ste-Marie, Montreal Est, P.Q.; Mon '59; Tel. 642-2911.
TROUP, Wallace; 49 Powell Ave., Ottawa 1, Ont. (res); Qns '24; Retired.
TROUP, Wallace J.; 340 McLeod St., Ottawa, Ont.; Qns'54; FRCP(C), IntMed.; Chief, Dept. of Med., Riverside Hosp.; Cardiol., Ottawa Civic Hosp.; Tel. CE 4-5959.
TROUT, Ellen E.; 241 Queens Ave., London, Ont.; 21 McKenzie Ave. (res); Wes '43; Paed; Sr. Teach. Fell. (Paed), U. of Western Ont.; Tel. GE 4-4343.
TROW, Emerson J., Jr.; 207 Medical Arts Bldg., Toronto 5, Ont.; Tor '42; F.R.C.P.(C), Derm-Syph; Cons. (Derm.), Sunnybrook Hosp.; Sr. Phys., Toronto Gen. Hosp.; Assoc. Prof. Derm., U. of Toronto; Tel. WA 2-3417.
TROWBRIDGE, Edmund B.; 305-1541 W. Broadway, Vancouver, B.C.; 6010 Cartier St. (res); Alb '32; ObstGyn; Head, Dept. of Obst. Gyn., St. Paul's Hosp.; Tel. RE 8-6120.
TROWSDALE, Wanda; Durham (Eng.) '55; DCH; DRCOG; Staff, Alberta School Hosp., Box 580, Red Deer, Alta.; Tel. 346-5466; Abroad.
TRSIC, Jugoslav M.; Belgrade (Yugo.); Staff, Hop. des Laurentides, L'Annonciation, P.Q.
TRUDEAU, Charles H.; 7175 rue Christophe-Colomb, Montreal, P.Q.; Mon '22; Reg. Ass't. Derm., Hop. Ste. Justine.; Tel. 271-7233.
TRUDEAU, Eugenè A.; 3465 Place Decelles, App. 404, Montreal, P.Q.; OrthSurg(P.Q.).
TRUDEAU, Georges; 268 Churchill, Greenfield Pk., Cite-Jacques-Cartier, P.Q.; Mon '55.
TRUDEAU, Gerald; Mon '62; Res., Hop. Notre-Dame, Montreal 24, P.Q.
TRUDEAU, Hector; 4033 Dorchester St. W., Montreal, P.Q.; Mon '10; Retired.
TRUDEAU, Jean G.; Mon'65; Res., Hop. Notre-Dame, Montreal 24, P.Q.
TRUDEAU, Leon; 8415 St-Denis, Montreal 11, P.Q.; 6968 Chambord (res); Mon '54; ObstGyn (Geneva, Switz.); Active Staff, Hop.-Notre-Dame-de-l'Esperance, St. Laurent; Cons. Staff, Hop.-Ste-Justine) Hop. Fleury & Hop. Belle Chasse Tel. RI 7-4771.
TRUDEAU, Leon A.; 214 King St. W., Sherbrooke, P.Q.; 92 rue Peel (res); Mon '22; Ophth, Otol; Med. Dir., Hotel-Dieu Hosp.; Retired.
TRUDEAU, Louis A.; 211 l'Esperance St., St. Lambert, P.Q.; Mon '23.
TRUDEAU, Louis R.; Mon'65; Res., Hop Notre-Dame, Montreal 24, P.Q.
TRUDEL, Andre; 825 sud, Belvedere, Sherbrooke, P.Q.; Lav '54; ObstGyn.
TRUDEL, Andre J.; 22707 Lougheed Hwy., Haney, B.C.; Lav '50; M.O., Haney Correctional Inst.; Phys., Oakalla Alcohol Rehab. Unit; Tel. 463-8134.
TRUDEL, Hermile; 1990 Rachel St. E., Montreal, P.Q.; 5645 Ave., Woodbury (res); Mon '49; Paed (P.Q.); Tel. LA 2-1873.
TRUDEL, Jacques; Mon'58; FRCP(C), IntMed; Staff, Hop. St. Luc, Montreal 18, P.Q.; Teach. Fell., U. of Montreal.
TRUDEL, Jean-J.; 100 Great Western Bldg., 356 Main St., Winnipeg 1, Man.; 204 Lawndale Ave., Norwood Grove (res); Lav '13; Tel. GL 2-5307.
TRUDEL, Jules; Mon'61; FRCP(C), GenSurg.; Staff, Hop. St.-Luc, Montreal 18, P.Q.; Abroad.
TRUDELLE, J. Bernard; 1010 McCallum Hill Bldg., 1874 Scarth St., Regina, Sask.; Sask '51; Anaes.
TRUELOVE, Leslie H.; Manitoba Rehab. Hosp., 800 Sherbrook St., Winnipeg 2, Man.; Oxford (Eng.)'46; D.PhysMed; MRCP(Lond.); PhysMed. & Rehab; Chief of Med. Serv., Manitoba Rehab. Hosp.; Dir. School of Med. Rehab., U. of Manitoba; Cons. Phys. Med., Wpg. Gen., Shriner's, Deer Lodge & Victoria Hosp's.; Phys. I/C Dept. of PhysMed., Children's Hosp.; Ass't. Prof. Med., U. of Manitoba; Tel. SP 5-0181.
TRUEMAN, Douglas H. Sg/Lt.; Dal '65; HMCS Cornwallis, Cornwallis, N.S.
TRUEMAN, E. G. Tess; 214-6th Ave. W., Calgary, Alta.; Alb'53; FRCS(C), ObstGyn.; Staff, Holy Cross & Foothills Hosp's.; Tel. AM 3-7120.
TRUEMAN, Gordon E.; Ste. 505, 750 W Broadway, Vancouver, B.C.; 4211 Cyprus St. (res); Man '39; DiagRad; Ass't Dir. Dept. of Rad., Vancouver Gen. Hosp.; Clin. Instr., U. of British Columbia; Tel. TR 9-4177.

TRUEMAN, Kenneth R.; Wpg. Clinic, St. Mary's & Vaughan, Winnipeg, Man.; 179 Oxford St. (res); Man '34; FACS; GenSurg; Assoc. Surg., Winnipeg Gen. Hosp.; Ass't. Prof. (Surg.), U. of Manitoba; Tel. 942-0551.
TRUMPER, Michael B.; Box 1210, Stettler, Alta.; Cambridge (Eng.) '56.
TRUNKEY, Franklin M.; McG '60; Jr. Int'n., Montreal Gen. Hosp., Montreal, P.Q.
TRUPP, Howard C.; Ste. 11, 358 Reynolds Ave., Oakville, Ont.; Tor '53; D. Psy.; Psy.; Tel. 844-9021.
TRUSCOTT, D. Ross; 607 Chinook Prof. Bldg., 6100 MacLeod Trail, S.W., Calgary, Alta.; Alb'55; Paed; Active Staff, Holy Cross, Calgary Gen. & Alberta Children's Hosp.; Tel. 252-6651.
TRUSCOTT, Paul W.; 2969 Kingston Rd., Scarborough, Ont.; 3744 St. Clair E. (res); Tor '62; AMCGP; Tel. 261-3675.
TRUSLER, George A.; Ste. 1225, 123 Edward St., Toronto 2, Ont.; 138 Douglas Dr. (res); Tor '49; M.S.(Tor); FACS; FRCS(C); GenSurg; Ass't. Surg., Hosp. for Sick Children; Clin. Instr., U. of Toronto; Tel. 363-7021.
TRUSLER, William C.; 178 Hunt Club Dr., London, Ont. (res); Tor '54; D.M.R. (Tor.); **D.A.-B.R.; DiagRad; Assoc. Rad., Victoria Gen.** Hosp.; Instr. (DiagRad.), U. of Western Ont.; **Tel. GE 2-5261.**
TRYLINSKI, Zygmunt; North Battleford Med. Bldg., 1255 100th St., North Battleford, Sask.; Man'52; ObstGyn.; Tel. 445-8146.
TSAI, Luke S.-L.; Ste. 108, 1175 Cook St., Victoria, B.C.; St. John's U. (Shanghai, China) '42; **DO** (Lond.); Ophth; **Tel.** 385-0811.
TSAI, Shu; 2363 McIntyre St., Regina, Sask.; Taiwan (Formosa) '61; Tel. 527-0641.
TSANG, Hoi C.; National Defence Med. Centre Taiwan (Formosa)'65; Staff, Paddon Mem. Hosp., Happy Valley, Labrador.
TSANG, Randolph C.; Dal'61; Staff, Cottage Hosp., Placentia, Nfld.
TSE, Fong H.; 410 Hammond Bldg., 310 Main St. N., Moose Jaw, Sask.; Manila (Philipp.)'56; Tel. 693-3661.
TSE, Kam S.; 17-11th Ave. S., Cranbrook, B.C.; Sask'61; Tel. 426-2201.
TSE, Yat T.; 129 Dundas St. W. & Toronto Prof. Bldg., 123 Edward St., Toronto, Ont.; **92 College View Ave., Tor. 7 (res); Lingnan (Canton, China) '43; DPH; Staff (OPD), St. Michael's Hosp.; Tel. EM 3-8961.**
TSEGA, Edemariam; McG'65; Res., Montreal General Hosp., Montreal 25, P.Q.
TSITOS, Anas; 777 Nottingham Ave., Winnipeg, Man. (res); Istanbul (Turk.) '57; Staff, Psychopathic Hosp.; Dem. (Psy.) U. of Manitoba; Tel. SP 4-6511; Abroad.
TUASON, Vicente B.; Box 39, North Battleford, **Sask.; Santo Tomas (Philippines) '55; DABPN;** Psy; Sr. Psy., Saskatchewan Hosp.; Tel. 445-2421; Abroad.
TUCHTIE, Michael D.; 2 Surrey Pl., Toronto 5, Ont.; 5 Governor's Rd., (res); Qns '35; D.Psy; Psy-I/C Forensic Inpatient Serv., Tor. Psy. Hosp.; Lect. (Med. Jurisprudence) & Clin. Inst., Dept. of Psy., U. of Toronto; Tel. WA 5-6371.
TUCKER, Allan G.; Apt. 407, 108 Isabella St., Toronto 5, Ont. (res); Tor '57; Staff, Sunnybrook Hosp.; **Tel. 485-8561.**
TUCKER, Desmond K., Major; St. Bart's (London, Eng.)'47; DPH(Tor); MRCS(Eng.); LRCP (Lond.); Staff, Sunnybrook Hosp., Toronto 12, Ont.
TUCKER, Elrie C.; McG'61; FRCS(C), ObstGyn; Staff, Royal Victoria Hosp., Montreal 2, P.Q.
TUCKER, Frederick G.; 828 W. - 10th Ave., Vancouver, B.C.; London (Eng.) '39; M.Sc.; Psy; Deputy Dir. Mental Health Serv., B.C. Ass't. Clin. Prof., U. of British Columbia; Tel. 874-2331.
TUCKER, F. Robert; Dept. of Surg., Medical College, 750 Bannatyne, Winnipeg, Man.; Man'36; MCH, Orth. (Liverpool); FRCS (Edin.); FRCS(C), OrthSurg; Chief of OrthSurg., Children's Hosp.; Dir. of Teach. & Research, Wpg. Gen. Hosp.; Cons. (OrthSurg.), St. Boniface Hosp., Deer Lodge & Shriner's Hosp's.; Prof. & Hd. (OrthSurg.), U. of Manitoba; Tel. 786-3574.
TUCKER, H. Harold; 5991 Spring Garden Rd., Halifax, N.S.; Dal'51; FACS; FRCS(C), NeurSurg; Assoc. Staff, Victoria Gen. Hosp.; Cons., Halifax Infirmary, Children's Hosp., Halifax Convalescent, Cdn. Forces Hosp., Grace Maternity & Camp Hill D.V.A. Hosp's.; Tel. 423-7015.
TUDOR, John; 2271 King St. E., Kitchener, Ont.; London (Eng.)'57; MRCS(Eng.); LRCP(Lond.); D.ObstRCOG.
TUFFNELL, Peter G.; 26 Governors Rd., Toronto 5, Ont. (res); Sheffield (Eng.) '48; Dip. (Bact.); Hd. (Microbiol.), Dept. of Labs., Tor. Gen. Hosp., Toronto 2, Ont.; Tel. EM 6-8211.
TUFFORD, Walter H.; 290 Wellington St., Sarnia, Ont.: 771 Cathcart Blvd. (res); Wes '43; **Psy.; Tel. ED 7-5671.**
TUFTS, William B.; Man '28; Med. Dir. Workmen's Compensation Bd., 1840 Lorne St., Regina, Sask.; Tel. LA 7-1681.
TULCHINSKY, Theodore H.; Tor '61; Res., University Hosp., Saskatoon, Sask.; Abroad.
TULK, George D.; P.O. Box 197, Bishop Falls, Nfld.; Dal '36; Anaes., Botwood Cottage Hosp.; Active Staff, Central Nfld., & Grand Falls Hosp's.; M.O.H., Bishops Falls.
TULK, Helen C. (Spurr); Bishops Falls, Nfld.; Dal '38; Staff, Central Nfld. Hosp.; Public Health Well-Baby Clinic.
TULLE, L. Kenneth; Dal. 58; MCGP; Res., Ottawa Civic Hosp., Ottawa 3, Ont.
TULLIS, David C. H.; Box 158, St. Catharines, Ont. (res); St. Andrew's (Scot.) '45; Chest Phys., Niagara Pen. San.; Tel. CA 7-3731.
TULLOCH, Arthur M.; 294 Aylmer St., Peterborough, Ont.; Edinburgh (Scot.) '59; Anaes.; Staff, Peterborough Civic & St. Joseph's Hosp's.; Tel. 745-1122.
TULLOH, Marchant E.; 11250-84th Ave., Edmonton, Alta.; 8911-117th St. (res); Durham (Eng.) '53; DMRT; Cons. Rad., University & Royal Alexandra Hosp's.; Chief Radiother., Edmonton Cancer Clinic; Sess. Instr., U. of Alberta; Tel. GE 9-5911.
TUPLING, George D.; 3260 Edgemont Blvd., **North Vancouver, B.C.; UBC '58; Tel. YU 7-9361.**
TUPPER, Carl; Medical Arts Bldg., 5880 Spring Garden Rd., Halifax, N.S.; 7 Rogers Dr. (res); Dal '43; F.I.C.S., F.A.C.S., F.A.C.O.G.; **Obst-**Gyn; Prof. & Hd. Dept. of ObstGyn., Dalhousie U.; Tel. 423-7780.
TURCHIN, Roy; Tor '59; DiagRad; Staff, St. Joseph's Hosp., Toronto, Ont.
TURCOT, Georges H.; 1016 Medical Arts Bldg., 1538 Sherbrooke St., Montreal 25, P.Q.; Mon **'48; Psy.; Tel. WE 7-2416.**
TURCOT, Jacques; 35 rue Ste-Ursule, Quebec 4, P.Q.; 1339 Lemoine, Sillery 6 (res); Lav **'40; FACS; FRCS(C), GenSurg; Surg., Hotel-Dieu; Ass't. Prof. (Surg.), U. of Laval; Tel. 522-7670.**
TURCOT, Roland; 1500-18eme rue, Quebec 3, P.Q.; Lav'43; Paed(P.Q.); Staff (Paed.), Hop. de l'Enfant Jesus; Staff, Laval U.
TURCOTTE, Adelard N.; 449-3eme Ave., Quebec, P.Q.; 46 ave. de la Falaise, Beauport (res); Lav '20; Tel. 529-4258.
TURCOTTE, Antoine; 651 rue Lindsay, Drummondville, P.Q.; Lav '29; Obst (P.Q.).
TURCOTTE, Bernard; 2051 rue Brulart, Quebec 6, P.Q.; Lav'56; D&TRad (P.Q.).
TURCOTTE, Denis; Lav'61; FRCS(C), OrthSurg; Staff, Hop. Sacre-Coeur, Montreal 9, P.Q.
TURCOTTE, Hector; 1572 ave du Ruisseau, Sillery, Quebec 6, P.Q.; Lav '35; PathBact; Staff, Laval U.; Tel. LA 9-4511.
TURCOTTE, Jean M.; 31 rue Principale, Ste-Anne-de-la-Perade, P.Q.; Lav '65.
TURCOTTE, Leon; 46 Ave. de la Falaise, Beauport, Quebec, P.Q.; Lav '56; D&TRad.
TURCOTTE, Lorenzo A.; 615 Blvd. Bedard, Lachute P.Q. (res); Lav '37; D.P.H., PH (P.Q.); Dir. Argenteuil Health Unit, Lachute; Tel. LO 2-5045.
TURCOTTE, Maurice; 1090 Parc Thornhill, Quebec 6, P.Q. (res); Lav '39; IntMed (P.Q.) FBLIM; Chief (Med.), Hop Enfant Jesus; Med. Dir., Industrial Assur. Co.; Tel. 527-2581.

TURCOTTE, Raymond; 10130 Basile Routhier, Montreal 12, P.Q.; Mon '60.

TURGEON, Andre; 274 McNaughton, Sudbury, Ont.; Mon '57; FRCP(C), IntMed; Chief of Med., St. Joseph's Hosp.; Tel. 673-6461.

TURGEON, Charles A.; 910 Duchesneau, Quebec 10, P.Q. (res); Lav '37; Staff, Dept. of Health, (Quebec).

TURGEON, Elie; 787 Chevremont, Quebec, P.Q.; Lav '48; D&T Rad; Assoc. Rad., Hop. St.-Francois d'Assise; Tel. 529-7311.

TURGEON, Fernand; 5720 Parkhaven, Cote-St-Luc, Montreal 29, P.Q.; Mon '58; M.Sc. (Bact.); FRCP(C); Bact; Bact., Hop. St. Luc.; Cons Bact., Hop. Pasteur; Ass't. Prof., U. of Montreal; Tel. 489-4347.

TURGEON, Jean; Lav'65; Res., Hotel-Dieu St. Vallier, Chicoutimi, P.Q.

TURGEON, Pierre A.; 837 Cherrier, Montreal 24, P.Q.; 200 Normandy Dr. (res); Mon '43; Derm; Sr. Staff, Hop. Notre-Dame; Cons. Queen Mary Vet's. & Hop. Ste-Anne-de-Bellevue; Prof., U. of Mtl.; Pres., Mtl. Derm. Soc.; Tel. LA 2-1105.

TURGEON, P. L.; 148 St. Georges, Levis, P.Q.; Lav '36.

TURGEON, Raymond; Pont Rouge, Co. Portneuf, P.Q.; Lav '58.

TURGEON, Robert; 116 Church, Buckingham, P.Q.; Lav'65.

TURGEON-KNAACK, Claire; Mon '55; DABPath; Path; Staff, Hop. Ste-Justine, Montreal, P.Q.; Tel. RE 1-4931, Loc. 568.

TURKO, Michael; Hycroft Med. Bldg., 3195 Granville St., Vancouver 9, B.C.; 6037 Marguerite St., Van. 13 (res); Tor '47; ObstGyn; Sr.-I/C Gyn & Att'd. Staff, Vancouver Gen. Hosp.; Assoc. Staff, Grace Hosp.; Cons. (ObstGyn), Langley Mem. Hosp.; Clin. Ass't. Prof. U. of British Columbia; Tel. RE 3-1193.

TURKO, Roman; 952 Rocky Bluff Terr., Lancaster, N.B. (res); Lvov (Ukraine) '34; DiagRad; Rad., Lancaster DVA Hosp.; Tel. 694-6877.

TURKOGLU, Huseyin A.; Instanbul, (Turkey) '47; Jr. Intn., Regina Gen. Hosp., Regina, Sask.

TURKOWSKA, Irena D.; 424 Main St. E., Hamilton, Ont.; National U. (Ire.) '53.

TURLIUK, Nicholas; Tor'57; Res., Sunnybrook Hosp., Toronto, Ont.

TURMEL-DORION, Louise; 1032 ave des Erables, Quebec 6, P.Q.; Lav '58; Med. Research, Cardiol. Lab., Hotel-Dieu Hosp.

TURMEL, Eusebe; 450 St. Pierre, Drummondville, P.Q.; Lav '35.

TURMEL, Gerard; 224 Royale, Chateau Richer, P.Q.; Lav '43.

TURMEL, Jacques; 1500-18eme rue, Quebec 3, P.Q.; Lav'53; Psy; Staff, Hop. Enfant Jesus; Tel. 529-7130.

TURMEL, Jean J.; 190 rue Wolfe, Levis, P.Q.; Lav'55; FRCS(C), ObstGyn.; Staff, Hotel-Dieu; Tel. 837-9697.

TURMEL, J. T.; 110 ave. Des Erables, Quebec, P.Q.; 1034 Ave. Des Erables (res); Lav '26; Admin. Hop. Ste. Foye; Tel. 683-4821.

TURMEL, Nelson; 1500-18eme rue. Quebec 3, P.Q.; Lav'64.

TURMEL, Willie; 1087 Route-de-l'Eglise, Quebec 10, P.Q.; Lav '41; GenSurg; MCGP; Tel. 653-9444.

TURMEL, Yvon; 2969 Soissons, Montreal 26, P.Q.; Mon'61; Anaes.

TURNBULL, Alan D.; McG'61; Res., Queen Mary Vets Hosp., Montreal 26, P.Q.

TURNBULL, Alexander; Tor'21; NeurPsy; Pt.-time Staff, Ontario Hosp., London, Ont.; Tel. 455-5110.

TURNBULL, Andrew; 211-925 W. Georgia St., Vancouver, B.C.; 6150 Carnarvon St., Van. 13 (res); Man '29; M.S., FFR(Eng.), FACR, D & T Rad; Chief of Serv. (Rad.), Shaughnessy DVA Hosp., Powell River, Prince Rupert, Terrace & Kitmat Hosp's.; Tel. MU 4-4177.

TURNBULL, A. Ross; 158 Dunlop St. E., Barrie, Ont.; 16 Peel St. (res); McG '39; M.C.G.P. Tel. PA 8-2535.

TURNBULL, D. Ian; McG '62; Res., Victoria Hosp., London, Ont.; Abroad.

TURNBULL, Frank A.; Fairmount Med. Bldg., 750 W. Broadway, Vancouver 9, B.C.; 4649 Beverley Cres. (res); Tor '28; DABNS; FRCS(C), NeurSurg; Sr. Surg., I/C NeurSurg., Van. Gen. Hosp.; Assoc. Clin. Prof. (Surg.), U. of British Columbia; Tel. 874-1413.

TURNBULL, Ian M.; UBC'57; FRCS(C), NeurSurg; Staff, Dept. of Surg., Vancouver Gen. Hosp., Vancouver 9, B.C.; Instr., U. of British Columbia; Tel. TR 6-3211.

TURNBULL, James M.; London (Eng.) '61; LRCP; MRCS; Res., Vancouver Gen. Hosp., Vancouver 9, B.C.

TURNBULL, John B.; Medical Arts Clinic, 2125-11th Ave., Regina, Sask.; 3114 Assiniboine Ave. (res); Man '54; Ophth; Tel. LA 2-1651.

TURNBULL, Kenneth E.; Moose Jaw Clinic, 200 Scott Bldg., Moose Jaw, Sask.; 285 Fairford East (res); Wes '55; FRCS(C); ObstGyn; Tel. 692-2373.

TURNBULL, Wilfred L.; 2025 W. Broadway, Vancouver 9, B.C.; 6788 Adera St., Vancouver 14 (res); Wes '33; Ass't. Dir. of Med. Servs., Med. Servs. Assoc.; Tel. AM 6-4633.

TURNBULL, William; Ste. 440, 5 Place Ville Marie, Montreal, P.Q.; 1385 Dumfries Rd., Mt. Royal (res); McG '43; D.A.B.O., Ophth (P.Q.); Ass't. Ophth, Royal Victoria Hosp.; Cons. Ophth., C.N.R.; Lect'r., McGill U.; Tel. VI 9-9962.

TURNBULL, William; 146 Wellesley St. E., Toronto 5, Ont.; Durham (Eng.)'49.

TURNEL, Jean; 62 rue Wolfe, Levis, Quebec 6, P.Q.; Lav '55; Res., Hop. Notre Dame.

TURNER, A. Franklin; Wes '54; Sr. M.O., R.C.-A.F. Station, Moose Jaw, Sask.

TURNER, Alfred S.; 814 Cook Rd., Richmond, B.C.; Alb '37.

TURNER, Arthur M.; 707 Charlotte St., Peterborough, Ont.; 1500 Windermere Ave., (res); Tor '55; IntMed; Staff (IntMed.), Peterborough Civic Hosp.; Chief of Med. Serv., St. Joseph's Hosp.; Tel. 742-3871.

TURNER, Barbara F.; Lakeview Med. Centre, 63rd Ave. & 24th St. S.W., Calgary, Alta.; 2864 Lionel Cres. S.W. (res); Leeds (Eng.) '56; Staff, Holy Cross Hosp.; Tel. 242-1716.

TURNER, Cecil H.; 340 Brunswick St., Fredericton, N.B.; McG '32; GenSurg; Staff, Victoria Public Hosp.; Dir., Polio Clinic & Health Centre Fredericton; Chief Clin., Cancer Clinic, U.P.H.; Tel. 475-5201.

TURNER, David A.; U.S.A.'52; Staff, Hosp. for Sick Children, Toronto 2, Ont.; Tel. 366-7242.

TURNER, Edward J.; 507 Professional Bldg., Edmonton, Alta.; 9908½-11th St. (Res); U. of Malta '52; MMSA; DRCOG; DCH; FAAP; Paed; Paed., Royal Alexandra, Edmonton Gen. & Misericordia Hosp's.; Instr. (Paed) U. of Alberta; Tel. 422-8556.

TURNER, Frank W.; 316 Medical Arts Bldg., 11010 Jasper Ave., Edmonton, Alta.; Edinburgh (Scot.)'59; FRCS(C); GenSurg.; MSc(Exp.Surg.); Staff, University Hosp.; Clin. Instr., Dept. of Surg., U. of Alberta; Tel. 422-4246.

TURNER, Garnett W.; 60 Stannus St., Windsor, Ont.; Dal'41; Chief of Staff, Payzant Mem. Hosp.; Tel. 798-3221.

TURNER, Gene Anne (Stewart); 62 Glenvale Blvd., Toronto 17, Ont. (res); Tor '51; Public Health (Part-time).

TURNER, Geneva (Dye); 476 Arrowhead Rd., Port Credit, Ont. (res); George Washington U. (Washington, D.C.) '33; Clin. Ass't. Women's College Hosp., Toronto.

TURNER, George E.; 567 Lincoln Rd., Windsor, Ont.; 2281 Victoria Ave. (res); McG '33; Tel. 254-3449.

TURNER, G. R.; 1 Brentwood Rd. N., Toronto 18, Ont.; Tor'65.

TURNER, J. A. Peter; 250 Lawrence Ave. W., Toronto 12, Ont.; Tor'43; FCCP; Paed; Assoc. Phys. & Phys-in-charge Chest Clin., Hosp. for Sick Children; Ass't. Prof. Paed., U. of Toronto; Tel. 789-1321.

TURNER, J. Gilbert; 1535 Summerhill Ave., Montreal 25, P.Q. (res); McG '32; M.Sc (Col.); F.A.C.H.A.; Exec. Dir., Royal Victoria Hosp., Montreal; Lect., McGill U. & U. of Mtl.; Tel. VI 2-1251.

TURNER, John J.; Tor'62; Res., Sunnybrook Hosp., Toronto 12, Ont.

TURNER, J. Patrick; London (Eng.)'52; Staff, Alberta Hosp., Ponoka, Alta.

TURNER, Katherine; 10102 - 101st. St., Grande Prairie, Alta.; Tor '57.

TURNER, Kenneth P.; 19 Weber St. E., Kitchener, Ont.; R.R. No. 2 (res); Tor '44; IntMed; Chief of Med., Kitchener-Waterloo Hosp.; Tel. SH 5-9011.

TURNER, Lary J.; 910 Ridgeway St., Fort William, Ont.; Tor'60; FRCP(C), IntMed.

TURNER, Michael R.; Cambridge (Eng.)'59; FFARCS(Eng.); FRCP(C), Anaes; Staff, Vancouver Gen. Hosp., Vancouver, B.C.

TURNER, Neil S.; Edinburgh (Scot.)'62; Res., Royal Victoria Hosp., Montreal 2, P.Q.

TURNER, R. Edward; Clarke Inst. of Psy., 250 College St., Toronto 2B, Ont.; Tor'52; D.Psy; FAPA; Psy; Sr. Psy., Forensic Serv., Clarke Inst. of Psy.; Ass't. Prof. Psy., U. of Toronto; Tel. 924-6811.

TURNER, Ronald G. B.; Hanna Assoc. Clinic, Centre St., Hanna, Alta.; Glasgow (Scot.)'56; Staff, Hanna Mun. Hosp.; Tel. 854-3351-2.

TURNER, W. A.; 4 Perreault W., Rouyn, Co. Temiscamingue P.Q.; 71 Tremoy Rd., Noranda, P.Q. (res).

TURNER, William A.; Dal'57; Res., Victoria Gen. Hosp., Halifax, N.S.

TURNER, William P.; 264 Wellington St. W., Chatham, Ont.; Tor '39; Tel. 354-2500.

TURNER-DERNO, Edward J.; 507 Professional Bldg., 10983 Jasper Ave., Edmonton, Alta.; Royal **U. of Malta '52; Ph.C., MMSA (Lond.), DRCOG,** DCH, DABP, FAAP, Paed; Teach. Staff, Dept. of Paed., U. of Alberta; Staff, Misericordia, Edmonton Gen. & Royal Alexandra Hosp's.; Med. Dir., Cdn. Cystic-Fibrosis Fdn.; Tel. 422-8556.

TURNIER, Hugues; 5740 Ave. Northmount, Montreal, P.Q., (res); Port-au-Prince (Haiti) **'50; Anaes; Staff, Hop.-Ste-Justine, Montreal, P.Q. Tel. RE 1-0225.**

TURPEL, William N.; 51 Mary St., Picton, Ont.; R.R. No. 4 (res); McG'25; DPH; Dir., **Prince Edward Co. Health Unit; Tel. GR 6-3472.**

TURPIN, J. Hartley; 904B, Brunette St., New Westminster, B.C.; UBC '56. Abroad.

TURSKI, Marian; P.O. Box 42, Ste-Anne-de-Bellevue, P.Q. (res); Poznan (Poland)'35; Psy.; Staff, Hop. Ste-Anne-de-Bellevue; & Cons. **Queen Mary Vet's.; Dem. (Psy.), McGill U.; Tel.** 453-3440.

TURTON, Matthew, R.; Ste. 104, 1940 Lonsdale Ave., N. Vancouver, B.C.; 409 Eastcot (res); Tor **'53; Paed; Att'd. Staff, Van. Gen. Hosp.; Chief Paed; Lion's Gate Hosp.; Teach Staff, U. of British Columbia; Tel. YU 5-1636.**

TURVEY, John W.; 17 Martin Street, Milton, Ont.; Edinburgh (Scot.) '61.

TURVEY, Samuel E. C.; 301-1030 W. Georgia St., Vancouver 5, B.C.; 6280 McClury St. (res); Man '29; MRCP, FACP, FRCP(C), IntMed; Neur; Staff (IntMed & Neur), Van. Gen. Hosp.; **Vol. Research Assoc., U. of British Columbia;** Tel. MU 3-8494.

TUSZEWSKI, Marian S.; 203 Rideau Med. Centre, 1711-4th St. S.W., Calgary, Alta.; 5116 Grovehill Rd. (res); Durham (Eng.) '52; GenSurg; **Active Staff, Calgary Gen., Holy Cross & Alberta** Children's Hosp's.; Tel. 262-4035.

TUTERS, Kaspars; 603 Sherbourne St., Toronto 5, Ont.; Tor '63; O.P.D. Staff, St. Michael's Hosp.; Tel. WA 1-4478.

TUTERS, Laila M.; 603 Sherbourne St., Toronto 5, Ont.; Tor '59.

TUTTLE, Morley J.; 609 Earl Grey Cres., Calgary, Alta. (res); Alb '37; FCCP; FRCP(C), IntMed; Chief, Dept. of Med., Colonel Belcher Hosp., Calgary; Tel. AM 6-7001.

TUTTLE, Robert J.; 1429 Tyandaga Park Dr., Burlington, Ont.; Wes'56; FRCP(C), DiagRad.

TUTTON, Donald; 255 Hess St., Hamilton, Ont.; Wales '43; Tel. JA 5-0598.

TUZUN, Ilhan M.; Regina Med. Centre, 1847 Rose St., Regina, Sask., Ankara (Turk.) '57; Abroad.

TWEDDELL, John T.; 122 Wellington St., Kingston, Ont.; 369 Union St. W. (res); Qns '31 FACP; IntMed; Path; MCGP; Ass't. Prof. (Prev Med.) (Occup. Med.) & Lect. Med. & Med. Jurisprudence, Queen's U.; Med. Dir., Kingston Works, Dupont Co. of Canada; Tel. 548-3767.

TWEDDELL, Thos. N.; 41 William St., Kingston, Ont.; 25 Hillcroft Dr. (res); Qns '36; FACS, FICS, GenSurg; MCGP, Att. Staff, Hotel Dieu Hosp.; Assoc. Staff, Kingston Gen. Hosp.; Tel. 548-4232.

TWEED, William A., Sg./Lt.; Nat. Defence Med. Centre, Ottawa, Ont.; Man '64.

TWEEDIE, Frederick J.; 2-1390 Sherbrooke St. W., Montreal 25, P.Q.; 56 Kindersley Ave., Twn. of Mt. Royal (res); McG '40; FRCS(C), ObstGyn; ObstGyn., Royal Victoria Hosp.; Cons. Gyn. Mtl. Children's Hosp.; Assoc. Prof. (ObstGyn), McGill U.; Tel. VI 2-9791.

TWEEDIE, James W.; Drummond & Foster Sts., Perth, Ont.; 40 Drummond St. E. (res); Qns '55 Coroner, Lanark Co.; Tel. 267-1200.

TWEEDIE, Thomas; 196 George St., Hamilton, Ont.; 99 Paisley Ave. N. (res); Wes '35; M.C.-G.P.; Staff, Med., St. Joseph's Hosp.; Dep. Chief (Med.) O.P.D., Hamilton Gen. Hosp.; Tel. JA 7-1545.

TWEEDIE, Thomas E.; 196 George St., Hamilton, Ont.; Wes '62; AMCGP; Tel. JA 7-1545.

TWEEDLE, Lois E.; Box 10, 346 Cornell Dr., Midland, Ont.; Wes'31; FACCP; IntMed(T.B.); Travelling Chest Phys., various Ontario Hosp's.; Tel. 526-6956.

TWELVES, John E.; 1554 Main St. E., Hamilton, Ont.; 62 Pinehurst Dr. (res); Wes '53; MCGP; Active Staff (ObstGyn), Hamilton Civic Hosp.; Med. Cons., Multiple Sclerosis Soc.; Tel. 549-8863.

TWIDLE, Robert S. H.; Main St. W., Stevensville, Ont.; Sheffield (Eng.) '56; MCGP; Tel. 382-3511.

TWIDDY, E. Warren; Caledon E., Ont.; Qns '55; Tel. 584-2351.

TWISS, Donald J.; 4 Shasta Dr., Thornhill, Ont.; Wes '36; M.C.G.P.; Med. Cons., Ont. Hosp. Servs. Comm., Toronto.

TWOHIG, Michael J.; 610 Med. Dental Bldg., Regina, Sask.; 3051 Quinn Dr. (res); National U. (Ire.) '45; FRCS(Ed.); GenSurg; Surg. Staff, Grey Nuns & Regina Gen. & Hosp's.; Tel. 523-7681.

TWOMEY, Hugh M.; Water St., Botwood, Nfld. (res); Ire '46; M.C.G.P.; Supt. Botwood Hosp.

TWOREK, Edward J.; 421 Professional Bldg., 10830 Jasper Ave., Edmonton, Alta.; Alb'58; FRCS(C), GenSurg; Staff, Edmonton Gen. Hosp.; Tel. 424-9243.

TY, Manuel; Ste. 433, Med. Arts Bldg., 750 Spadina Cr. E., Saskatoon, Sask.; Philippines '52; FRCS (C), Urol; **Active Staff, University & St. Paul's** Hosp's.; Assoc. Surg. Staff, Saskatoon City Hosp.; **Clin. Assoc. Surg., U. of Saskatchewan; Tel. 652-**5757.

TYBER, Murray A.; 1456A Danforth Ave., Toronto 6, Ont.; 8 Longwood Dr., Don Mills (res); Tor '58; Clin. Ass't (Rheumat.) & Assoc. Staff, Tor. E. Gen. Hosp.; Tel. 461-6252.

TYE, Derek M. S/L; H.M.C.S. "Naden," Esquimalt, B.C.; UBC '63.

TYE, P. L.; Milverton, Ont.; Tor '07; M.O.H., Village of Milverton, Twsp. of Mornington. Tel. 62.

TYERS, G. Frank; UBC '62; Jr. Intn., Vancouver Gen. Hosp., Vancouver 9, B.C.

TYHURST, Libuse; Dept. of Psy., Vancouver Gen. Hosp., Vancouver 9, B.C.; Charles U. (Prague, Czech.)'47; Psy; **Clin. Ass't. Prof.,** Dept. of Psy., U. of British Columbia; Tel. 876-3211, Loc. 3132.

TYL, Johannaes W.; 560 Finch Ave. W., Willowdale, Ont.; 197 Newton Dr. (res); Groningen (Neth.) '51; Anaes; Assoc. Staff, North York Branson Hosp.; Tel. ME 5-1943.

TYNDEL, Milo; 316 Lytton Blvd., Toronto 12, Ont.; Vienna (Austria) '33; Ph.D. (Vienna); Neur Psy; Psy., Alcoholism & Drug Addiction Research Fdn.; Clin. Ass't. (Med.), Toronto Gen. Hosp.; Research Assoc. (Med.), U. of Toronto; Tel. 483-8833.

TYRRELL, J. Douglas; 1051 Mohawk Rd., Ancaste., Ont. (res); Tor '24; IntMed; Med Dir., Proctor & Gamble Ltd.; Hon. Staff, Hamilton Civic Hosp's.; Tel. MI 8-4379.

TYSDALE, Albert T.; R.R. 3, Dundas, Ont.; Tor'58; Psy.

TYSOE, F. William; 1008 Fairmont Med. Bldg., 750 W. Broadway, Vancouver 9, B.C.; 7375 Angus Dr. (res); Alb '45; ObstGyn; Att'd. Staff, Vancouver Gen. Hosp.; Clin. Instr., U. of British Columbia; Tel. TR 9-5533.

TYSCOE, John F.; 306 Royal Trust Bldg. 612 View St., Victoria B.C. 3380 Upper Terr. (res); Alb '43; MCGP; Tel. EV 2-5129.

TYSON, John E.; 205 Norfolk St. N., Simcoe, Ont.; Wes'60; FRCS(C), ObstGyn; Abroad.

TYTANECK, William N.; 7 Welland Ave., St. Catherines, Ont.; 195 Ontario St. (res); Tor '57; D.D.S.; Tel. MU 4-8555.

TYZEK, Theodor; Gimli Commercial Bldg., Gimli, Man.; Lwow (Poland)'38; Tel. JU 9-1929.

UCHIDA, M.; 193 East Hastings St., Vancouver, B.C., Tor '26; Tel. MU 4-7723.

UDEN, David Elliot F/L; R.C.A.F. Station, Rockcliffe, Ottawa 7, Ont.; McG '62 Med. Officer, Rockcliffe Station & National Defence Med. Centre Tel. 9932-174.

UEBERSCHAR, Karl H.; 306 Med. & Dental Bldg., Regina, Sask.; 124 Connaught Cres. (res); Muenster (Germ.) '49; DiagRad; Staff, Grey Nun's Hosp.; Tel. LA 3-7653.

UFFELMANN, R. Frederick; 749 King St. W., Kitchener, Ont.; Wes '49; F.R.C.S.(C), ObstGyn; Chief (ObstGyn), Kitchener-Waterloo Hosp.; Tel. SH 3-3162.

UGNAT, F. Antoine; CP 1420, 164 Maclaren, Buckingham, P.Q.; Istanbul (Turk.)'47; IntMed.

UGRAY, Eva; 10 Alexandra St., Oshawa, Ont.; Peter Pazmany U. (Budapest, Hung.) '51.

UGRAY, Imre K.; 10 Alexandra St., Oshawa, Ont.; 625 Brookside Dr. (res); P. Pazmany U. (Budapest, Hung.) '46; Urol; Staff, Oshawa Gen. Hosp.; Tel. 728 3761.

UGURALP, Aydin; Ankara (Turkey) '50; Staff, Saskatchewan Hosp., North Battleford, Sask.; Tel. 5-2421.

UHTHOFF-SCHUETTE, Annegrette L.; 498-38th Ave., Ville-La Salle, P.Q.; Freiburg (Germ.) '55; Anaes; Tel. DO 6-4465.

UHTHOFF, Hans K.; 498-38th Ave., Ville-La Salle, P.Q.; Marburg (Germ.) '51; F.R.C.S.(C), OrthSurg; Staff (OrthSurg), Verdun Gen. Hosp.; Tel. PO 6-3551.

UILENBERG, Catharina; Netherlands'53; Paed; Staff, Royal Alexandra Hosp., Edmonton, Alta.

UJEJSKA, Sophia; 30 est, boul. St-Joseph, Montreal 14, P.Q.; Cracovie (Ukraine) '37.

ULAN, Orest A.; Alb '57; AMCGP; Res., Hosp. for Sick Children, Toronto 2, Ont.

ULAN, Raymond A.; Alb'61; FRCP(C), IntMed; Staff, University Hosp., Edmonton, Alta.

ULDUKIS, J.; Fort San, Sask.; Kaunas (Lith.) '36.

ULECKAS, Maria J. - see - **ARSTIKAITIS**, Maria J.

ULEHLA, Boris; 1604 Danforth Ave., Toronto 6, Ont.; Yugoslavia '49; Staff, Doctors' Hosp.; Tel. HO 3-9163.

ULGEN, Aytekin; Ankara, (Turkey) '56; Jr. Intn., University Hosp., Saskatoon, Sask.

ULRICH, Donald G.; Ste. 508, 625-5th Ave., New Westminster, B.C.; Alb'46; FRCS(C), GenSurg.

ULRICH, T. Marianne; Copenhagen (Denmark) '55; Paed; Staff, Dept. of Paed., Queen's U., Kingston, Ont.

UMMAN, Cahit; Istanbul (Turk.)'50; Staff, Jordan Mem. San., The Glades, N.B.

UNDERHILL, A. Stanley; 1635 Abbott St., Kelowna, B.C.; 2210 Abbott St. (res); Man '26; Tel. 762-2740.

UNDERWOOD, W. John; 120 Gouldburn Ave., Ottawa 2, Ont.; Qns'60; Teach. Fell. Anat., U. of Ottawa.

UNGER, Albert G.; Box 1178, Maple Creek, Sask.; Sask'65.

UNGER, Frank J.; 402 Main St., Melfort, Sask.; Vienna (Austria)'32; MCGP; Tel. 752-2876.

UNGER, Ivan R.; Sask'64; Res., Saskatoon City Hosp., Saskatoon, Sask.

UNRUH, Cornelius J.; 110-2nd St., Morden, Man.; Park Apts. (res); Man'57; MCGP; Tel. 822-4474.

UNRUH, Henry A.; 2258 Irwin Ave., Rossland, B.C. (res); Qns '51; G.P. Staff, C. S. Williams Clinic, Rossland; Dep. Coroner.

UNSWORTH, Alexander D.; 10 Wellwood St., Hamilton, Ont. (res); Tor '04; IntMed; Retired.

UNWIN, John R.; 1025 Pine Ave. W., Montreal 2, P.Q.; Queensland (Australia)'56; DPM; D.Psy; Psy; Att'd. Staff, Royal Victoria Hosp.; Sr. Instr. (Psy.) McGill U.; M.R.C. Research Fell., Dept. of Psy., McGill U.; Lect. Psy., McGill U. School of Phys. Med. & O.T.; Dir., Adoles. Psy., Allan Mem. Inst.; Tel. 842-1251.

UPENIEKS, Eduard; 537 College St., Toronto 4, Ont.; 31 Hillcrest Dr., Tor. 4 (res); Salamanca (Spain) '53; Tel. WA 1-0455.

UPENIEKS, Ludwig; 85 Mill Rd., Etobicoke, Ont.; Cologne (Germ.) '54; M.O., Dept. of National Health & Welfare; Tel. 621-3253.

UPHOFF, Dean F.; McG'62; Res., Montreal Gen. Hosp., Montreal 25, P.Q.

UPMALIS, I. Henry; Ste. 104, 900 King St. W., Kitchener, Ont.; 133 Ripplewood Cr. (res); Wes '55; FRCS(C); GenSurg; Surg. Staff, St. Mary's & Kitchener-Waterloo Hosp's.; Cons. Freeport San.; Tel. 245-2272.

UPPER, S. Boyd; Qns'53; Chief M.O. & Dir., Associated Med. Services, 615 Yonge St., Toronto 5, Ont.

UPTHEGROVE, William E.; 301 Canada Bldg., Saskatoon, Sask.; Wes '30; Anaes; Anaes., St. Paul's Hosp.; Ass't. Clin. Prof. (Anaes), U. of Saskatchewan; Tel. 242-0353.

UPTON, Donald H.; Students Health Service, Union St., Kingston, Ont.; R.R. 3 Collins Bay (res); Qns '57; D.Psy; Psy; Cons. Psy., Kingston Gen. Hosp.; Dir., University Health Service & Ass't. Prof. Psy., Queens U.; Tel. 546-1731, Loc. 692.

URBACH, Gerald; 1027 St. Clair Ave. W., Toronto 10, Ont.; Tor '58; FACOG; FRCS(C), ObstGyn; Research Fell., Princess Margaret Hosp.; Abroad.

URBACH, Gordon; 732 Spadina Ave., Toronto 4, Ont.; Tor'58; Anaes; Staff, New Mount Sinai Hosp.; Tel. WA 1-9585.

URBACK, Percy G.; 99 Avenue Rd., Ste. 708, Toronto 5, Ont.; 88 Burnaby Blvd., Tor. 12 (res); Tor '53; FRCP(C), IntMed; Att'd. Phys., New Mt. Sinai Hosp.; Assoc. Phys., Doctor's Hosp.; Research Fell., Sunnybrook DVA Hosp.; Tel. WA 5-8011.

URBAITIS, Joseph; 1796 Bloor St. W., Toronto 9, Ont.; 1796 Bloor St. W. (res); Lithuania '40; Tel. RO 6-6791.

URBAN, Albin S.; 10207-57th St., Edmonton, Alta.; Alb'59; FRCS(C), OrthSurg; Staff, W.C.B.; Tel. 466-3350.

URBAN, Janusz R.; 848 Fennell Ave. E., Hamilton, Ont.; National U. (Eire) '55; Active Staff, St. Joseph's Hosp.; Court. Staff, Hamilton Gen. & Chedoke Hosp's.; Tel. FU 5-5614.

URBANEK, Zdenek; 1110—736 Granville St., Vancouver, B.C.; 570 Esquimalt Ave., West Vancouver (res); Oxford (Eng.) '43; M.D. (Czech.); Phys. (Part-time), T.B. Control, Dept. of Health & Welfare of B.C.; Tel. MU 1-1757.

URBANSKY, W. Alex; Ste. 514, 30 boul. St. Joseph E., Montreal 14, P.Q.; Poznan (Poland) '51; Staff, Hop. St. Jeanne d'Arc; Tel. 845-4035.

URE, Jean A.; 575 Quebec St., Prince George, B.C.; 1499-6th Ave. (res); UBC '55.

UREN, David M.; 277 Scarboro Cr., Scarborough, Ont.; Tor'52; Att'd. Staff, Scarborough Gen. Hosp.; Tel. AM 1-7211.

URIE, George N.; 84 Carling Ave., Ottawa 1, Ont. (res); Qns '13; Med. Adviser Royal Can. Legion, B.E.S.I.; Tel. CE 4-2834.

URIE, Matthew; Box 220, Parksville, B.C.; Glasgow (Scot.) '38; LRCP&S (Edin.); Staff, Nanaimo Reg. Gen. Hosp.; Tel. 248-3133.

URIE, Norman B.; 2400 Rosewood Ave., Ottawa 13, Ont. (res); Qns '51; D.A.; Anaes; Staff, Ottawa Civic Hosp.; Tel. PA 9-2511.

URIE, Percy R.; Watford, Ont.; Qns '19; Dist. Coroner.

UROWITZ, M.B.; Tor '63; Res., Sunnybrook Hosp., Toronto 12, Ont.; Abroad.

URQUHART, James L.; 44 Victoria, Aurora, Ont.; Tor '23; Tel. 727-5051.

URQUHART, Malcolm J.; Ste 105, 121 Nymark Ave., Willowdale, Ont.; Tor'56; Abroad.

URQUHART, Robert R.; UBC'60; FRCP(C), IntMed; Staff, Vancouver Gen. Hosp., Vancouver, B.C.; Abroad.

URQUHART, R. W. Ian; Apt. 1111-2, 141 Erskine Ave., Toronto 12, Ont. (res); Tor '24; Int Med; Chm. Ont. Hosp. Serv. Comm., 2195 Yonge St.; Tel. 487-1711; Retired.

URSCHEL, John W.; 13416-109th Ave., Edmonton, Alta.; Wes'55; Psy.

USHER, Barney; 917 Medical Arts Bldg., 1538 Sherbrooke St. W., Montreal, P.Q.; 7 Renfrew Ave., Westmount (res); McG '22; D.A.B.D., Derm.; DermSyph; Ass't. Prof., McGill U.; Assoc. Montreal Gen. & Jewish Gen. Hosp's.; Tel. WE 5-1354.

USHER, Michael; McG'62; Res., Children's Hosp., Montreal 25, P.Q.

USHER, Robert H.; 4116 Melrose Ave., Montreal, P.Q. (res); McG '54; Research Assoc. Paed., Jewish Gen. Hosp.; Clin. Ass't. Med., Royal Victoria Hosp.; Assoc. Med. Research Council; Lect. (ObstGyn. & Paed.) McGill U.

USHER, Saul J.; 4437 King Edward Ave., Montreal 28, P.Q.; McG '21; Paed; Tel. HU 1-8703; Semi-Retired.

UY, Isaac N.; Mitchell Apt. A 1, Park St., Saint John, N.B.; **Santo Tomas (Phillip.)'56**; Anaes.; Staff, Gen. Hosp.

UYGUR, Alli; Fort Smith, N.W.T.; Istanbul (Turk.) '50.

UZANS, Silvija; 52 Linsmore Cres., Toronto, Ont.; Latvia '31; Paed (Latvia); Tel. HU 5-2892.

UZICANIN, Richard R.; Terrace Bay, Ont.; Graz (Aust.) '46.

UZSAY, Vecoi; Istanbul (Turkey) '48; Staff, Sask. Training Schl., Moose Jaw, Sask.; Tel. 692-6491.

UZSOY, Namik K.; Istanbul (Turk.) '48; Staff, Gagetown Station Hosp., Oromocto, N.B.; Abroad.

UZUPIS, Aldona M. (Statkeviciute); 345 Kennedy Ave., Toronto 9, Ont.; Kaunas (Lith.) '39; Tel. 767-4461.

VACAFLOR, Luis A. R.; Tucuman (Argentine) '57; Psy; Staff, Douglas Hosp., Verdun, P.Q.

VACHON, Andre; Mon'62; Res., Hop. Maisonneuve, Montreal 36, P.Q.

VACHON, Claude; 16-23eme rue, Ville St-George E., Cte. Beauce, P.Q.; Lav'53; GenSurg; Tel. 228-4221.

VACHON, Clement; 262-13ème rue, Quebec, P.Q.; GenSurg(P.Q.).

VACHON, Georges; Noelville, Ont.; Mon '27.

VACHON, Louis; Mon '58; Res., Inst. Albert Prevost, Montreal, P.Q.

VACHON, Malcolm; 240 St. Jean, Quebec 4, P.Q.; 14 des Remparts (res); Lav '39; IntMed; (P.Q.); Ass't. Med., Hop. de l'Enfant Jesus; Ass't. Anti-T.B. League; Clin. Prof., Laval U.; Tel. 523-6757.

VACHON, Paul E.; 199 Canipco, Gatineau, P.Q.; Lav '51.

VACHON, Robert; 30 est, boul. St-Joseph, Montreal 14, P.Q.; Lille (France) '63.

VACHON, Rosaire; 122 St. Jean, Drummondville, P.Q.; 201 Chemin du Golf (res); Lav '54; AMCGP; Tel. 478-0787.

VADAS, George J.; Ott'62; Res., Path. Inst., McGill U., Montreal 2, P.Q.

VADAS, Joseph S.; 8 Neyer St., Hamilton, Ont.; Wes'63; Med. Staff, St. Joseph's Hosp.; M.O., HMCS Patriot & Star; Tel. 389-4312.

VADEBONCOEUR, Roland; 5200 Cote des Neiges, Montreal 26, P.Q.; 1630 Lucerne Rd. (res); Mon '52; Obst. (P.Q.); Ass't. (Obst. Med.), Hop. de la Misericordia; Tel. RE 8-0511.

VADNIS, Edgar J.; St. Denis sur Richelieu, P.Q. (res); Mon '24; Tel. 787-3017.

VAFIADAKIS, Michel; 400 est, rue Sherbrooke, Montreal 24, P.Q.; '55; Tel. AV 8-5833; Abroad.

VAGYI, Michael; Box 110, Chase, B.C.; Budapest (Hung.) '54; Tel. 2.

VAID, Vedbrat S.; '55; Res., St. Joseph's Hosp., Toronto 3, Ont.

VAIL, William J.; 202 Med. Arts Bldg., 628 Davis Dr., Newmarket, Ont.; Ott '52; FRCS(C); GenSurg; Staff, York County Hosp.; Tel. 895-6412.

VAIL, R. Viola; (see ROSE, R. Viola).

VAILE, Ivan R.; 384 Bloor St. W., Toronto, Ont.; 255 Cortleigh Blvd. (res); Tor '24; Otol.; Tel. WA 2-2343.

VAILE, Sigmund J.; Ste. 918, 1849 Yonge St., Toronto 7, Ont.; Tor'55; Ophth; Staff, New Mount Sinai, Scarborough Gen. & Toronto Gen. Hosp's.; Tel. 481-4433.

VAILLANCOURT, de Guise; 1414 Drummond St., Montreal 25, P.Q.; 341 Chester Ave., Town of Mt. Royal (res); Mon '47; D.Sc. (Med.); FACP; FRCP(C), IntMed; Att'd. Phys., Hotel-Dieu Hosp.; Ass't. Prof. (Med.), U. of Mtl.; Ass't. Dean & Dir. P.G. Med. Educ., U. of Montreal; Tel. VI 4-6972.

VAILLANCOURT, Francis W.; 690 Goldew Ave., **Ottawa 13, Ont.; Ott '53; DiagRad; Staff, Ottawa Civic Hosp.; Tel. 722-5214.**

VAILLANCOURT, Henri; 495 rue Pasteur, Jonquière, P.Q. (res); Lav'34; GenSurg (P.Q.); Chief, Surg. Staff, Hop. **Notre Dame de l'Assomption**; Tel. 547-3651.

VAILLANCOURT, J. Roland; 49 Elgin St. N., Sudbury, Ont.; Lav '45; Otol (P.Q.); Tel. 673-8798.

VAILLANCOURT, Paul E.; 6 rue St. Pierre, Quebec, P.Q.; 1227 Ave. William, Sillery (res); **Lav '51; Tel. 523-2527.**

VAILLANCOURT, Pierre; 30 est Boul. St. Joseph, Montreal 14, P.Q.; Mon'47; PlasSurg.

VAILLANCOURT, Roger; Ste. Dorothee, Co. Laval, P.Q.; Lav '43.

VAILLANCOURT, Roland; Lav '55; DiagRad; Staff, Hop. St-Joseph, Rimouski, P.Q.

VAIR, C. Donald; 180 Portland St., Dartmouth, N.S.; 3 Lawnsdale Dr. (res); Dal '51; MCGP; M.O., HMCS "Scotian"; Tel. 466-7471.

VAIR, Douglas H.; 249 Main St. N., Brampton, Ont.; Wes '64; Tel. 451-1937.

VAISRUB, Samuel; 203 Edmonton St., Winnipeg 1, Man.; 822 Campbell St. (res); Man '32; MRCP, Lond.). FACP, FRCP(C), Intmed; Staff, St. Boniface & Deer Lodge Hosp's; Ass't. Prof. (Med.), U. of Manitoba; Editor, Manitoba Med. Review; Tel. WH 2-5647. Abroad.

VALADKA, Aleksas; 1081 Bloor St. W., Toronto, Ont.; 43 Baby Pt. Cres. (res); Kaunas (Lith.) '43; M.C.G.P.; Tel. LE 1-2933.

VALAITIS, Ona; 57 Burris St., Hamilton, Ont.; **Kaunas (Lith.) '41; Tel. LI 4-5115.**

VALBERG, John D.; 267 O'Connor St., Ste. 307, Ottawa 4, Ont.; 1603 Aninsley Dr. (res); Qns '57; M.Sc. (Med); Ophth; Assoc. Staff, Ottawa Civic Hosp.; Cons. Ophth., National Defence Med. Centre; Tel. CE 6-0854.

VALBERG, Leslie S.; 55 Earl St., Kingston, Ont. (res); Qns '54; M.Sc., F.R.C.P.(C), IntMed; Ass't. Prof. (Med.), Queen's U.; Tel. 546-1731.

VALCOURT, Jean P.; Medico-Legal Labs., 443 St. Vincent, Montreal, P.Q.; Mon'53; Path(P.Q.); Medico-Legal Ass't.; Tel. UN 1-9311.

VALDERRAMA, Antonio; Riverview Hosp., Essondale, B.C.

VALDEZ, Romulo C.; Apt. 1, 63 Alma St., Moncton, N.B.; Manila (Philippines) '56; Tel. 389-9846.

VALE, Bruce W.; 622 Medical Arts Bldg., Toronto, Ont.; 6 Donlea Dr., Leaside (res); Tor '38; O.P.D., Toronto Western & Sunnybrook Hosp's.; Tel. WA 2-5381.

VALE, Joan M. (Mrs. Forman); 507 Med. Arts Bldg., 170 St. George St., Toronto 5, Ont.; 45 Glengowan Rd. (res); Tor '49; F.R.C.P.(C), IntMed; Assoc. Chief (Med.) Women's College Hosp.; Assoc. (Med.), U. of Toronto; Tel. 921-6027.

VALENS, William L.; 2408 Nottingham Rd., Victoria, B.C.; Alb '30; D.A.B.P.N. (Psy) & **D.A.B.Chi.P.; NeurPsy; Court. Staff, Royal Jubilee & St. Joseph's Hosp's; Tel. EV 5-4320.**

VALENTINE, G. Howard; The War Mem. Children's Hosp., 392 South St., London, Ont.; Bristol (Eng.)'42; DCH, MRCS(E); LRCP, MRCP (Lond.), FRCP(C), Paed; Ass't. Supt., War Mem. Children's Hosp.; Assoc. Prof. (Paed.), U. of Western Ont.; Tel. GE 2-5261, Loc. 602.

VALIAHO, Arvo J.; 261 Wembley Dr., Sudbury, Ont.; Tor '60; DiagRad.

VALIQUETTE, Chas. A.; 200 Rue Labelle, St. Jerome, Co. Terrebonne, P.Q.; Mon '52.

VALIQUETTE, G. Jean; Mon '64; Res., Hop. Maisonneuve, Montreal 36, P.Q.; Abroad.

VALIQUETTE, Jean; Lesage, Co. Terrebonne, P.Q.; Mon '58.

VALLANCE, Maelor; Glasgow (Scot.) '58; Psy; Staff, Riverview Hosp., Essondale, B.C.

VALLEE, Arthur F.; 170 Boul. Dorchester Est, Montreal 18, P.Q.; Lav '39; D&TRad; Dir., Dept. of Rad., Hop. St. Luc.; Assoc. Prof. (Rad.), U. of Montreal, Tel. 878-2220.

VALLEE, Guy; 2385 Jolicoeur, Montreal 20, P.Q.; Lav'58.

VALLEE, Henri; 68 Place des Acacias, Candiac, Cte. Laprairie, P.Q.; Lav'59; GenSurg (P.Q.); FRCS(C), PlasSurg.

VALLEE, Jacques: 3871 est, Belanger, Montreal 36, P.Q.; Mon '64; Tel. 729-5231.

VALLEE, Jean-G.; Ste. 510, 30 St.-Joseph Blvd. E., Montreal, P.Q.; 5401 ave Brodeur (res); Lav'55; FACS; DABS, FRCS(C), GenSurg.; Assoc., Ste.-Jeanne-d'Arc; Tel. 845-4241.

VALLEE, Louis-Ivan; 631 ave. Rockland, Montreal 8, P.Q.; Lav '40; D&TRad; PhysMed (P.Q.); **Rad.-in-charge, Hop. Pasteur, Inst. of Rehab. &** Doctor's Hosp.; Tel. 272-7041.

VALLEE, Roger; 55 Ave. de l'Eglise, Verdun, Montreal 19, P.Q.; 4080 Harvard Ave. Mtl. 28 (res); Lav '40; D&TRad; Chief Rad., Verdun **Gen. Hosp.; Tel. PO 8-1240.**

VALLIERE, Louis; 15 Begin Ave., Levis, P.Q.; 27 Verdun Ave. (res); Lav '58; Paed; Tel. 837-3167.

VALLIERES Andre; 1000 Chemin, Ste.-Foy, Quebec 6, P.Q.; Lav '56; FRCS(C), Urol; Staff, Hop St.-Sacrement; Tel. 681-5385.

VALLIERS, Guy; 1634 d'Argenteuil, Ste.-Foy, Quebec 10, P.Q.; Lav'53; Cons., Hop. du St. Sacrement; Tel. 653-7844.

VALLILLO, Luciano; Regina Med. Centre, 1847 Rose St., Regina, Sask.; Rome (Italy) '57.

VALLIS, Derek G.; Box 338, Greenwood, B.C.; UBC '59.

VALOIS, Antoine B.; Rm. 300, 700 Craig St. E., Annexe-Viger, Montreal, P.Q.; 3181 rue Tremblay (res); Mon '35; M.P.H.; PH; Ass't. Dir., Montreal Health Serv.; Prof., School of Hygiene, U. of Montreal; M.O.H., Verdun; Tel. RE 3-9951.

VALOIS, Gaetan; 168 Charlotte St., Ottawa, Ont.; 249 Glin Ave (res); Ott '51; Ass't. Supt., St. Vincent Hosp.; Clin. Ass't., Dept. of Med., U. of Ottawa; Tel. 232-8092.

VAN ALSTYNE, William B.; McG '59; DiagRad; Staff, Hotel-Dieu Hosp., Kingston, Ont.; Clin. Ass't. Rad., Queen's U.; Tel. 546-1151.

VANASSE, J. Edgar; 1635 Boul. St.-Louis, Trois-Rivieres, P.Q.; Lav '30; ObstGyn (P.Q.).

VANASSE, Rene; 205 Henecker, Sherbrooke, P.Q. (res); Lav '49; Path (P.Q.); Dir. of Labs., Hotel Dieu de Sherbrooke; Tel. 562-3487.

VAN BELKUM, Jacobus A. M.; Med. Arts Clinic, 51-6th St. S.E., Medicine Hat, Alta.; Johannesburg (S. Africa) '46; MRCOG; FACS; ObstGyn; Staff, Medicine Hat Gen. Hosp.; Tel. 527-2281.

VAN BELKUM, Joan; Medical Arts Clinic, 51-**6th St. S.E., Medicine Hat, Alta.; 730-7th St.** S.W. (res); London (Eng.) '47; M.R.C.P. (Eng.), **L.R.C.P. (Lond.); M.R.C.S.; Paed; Tel. 527-2281.**

VAN-BELLE, Johanna H. (Praamsma); 484 Soudan Ave., Toronto 7, Ont.; Tor '61; Staff, (G.P.), Toronto East Gen. Hosp.

VAN CAMPENHOUT, Jacques; Louvain (Belgium) '58; FRCS(C), ObstGyn; Staff, Hop. Notre-Dame, Montreal 24, P.Q.

VAN COTT, Glendon F.; Qns'55; Res., Kingston Gen. Hosp., Kingston, Ont.

VANDAL, Leo; 158 ouest, Prince, Chicoutimi, P.Q.; Lav '54; MCGP.

VAN de GUCHTE, Maarten P.; 444 Professional Bldg., 10830 Jasper Ave., Edmonton, Alta.; 14-002-101A (res); Amsterdam (Netherlands) '57; Memb. Med. Advisory Bd., Canadian Diabetic Assoc., Alberta Div.; Tel. 422-4693.

VAN de LEUR, Johannes; 576 Quebec St., Prince George, B.C.; Utrecht (Neth.) '45.

VAN DE MARK, Thorpe B.; Brunswick Diag. Group, 25 Brunswick Ave., Toronto 4, Ont.; Tor '59.

VAN DEN BERG, B.L.; Med. Supt., Fisher River Indian Hosp., Hodgson, Man.

van der BENT, David W.; 9 Mill St. W., Acton, Ont.; Tor'61.

VAN DER BENT, David W.; 9 Mill St. W., Acton, Ont.; Tor'61; Staff, Guelph Gen. & St. Joseph's Hosp's.; Tel. 853-2180.

VANDERBURG, Donald L.; Wes '62; Res., Kingston Gen. Hosp., Kingston, Ont.

VANDERBURGH, Jack R.; Tor '61; Res., St. Michael's Hosp., Toronto 2, Ont.

VANDERBURG, L. L. C.; 1268 Main St. E., **Hamilton, Ont.; Qns '21; Tel. LI 4-0985.**

Van der FLIER Robert W.; Port Arthur Clinic, 194 North Court St., Port Arthur, Ont.; 121 Winnipeg Ave. (res); Tor '49; IntMed; Tel. DI 4-7271.

VAN der HOEVEN, Ellen M. (Conlan); Box 375, R.R.1, Kingston, Ont.; National U. (Ire.) '54; M.B., B.Ch., BAO; Path; Bact; Staff, Hotel-Dieu Hosp; Ass't. Prof. (Microbiol. & Immunol.), Queen's U.

VANDERMAAS, Alan; 10 Norris Place, St. Catharines, Ont.; Leiden (Netherlands) '52; MCGP; Vice-Pres., Active Med. Staff, St. Catharines Gen. Hosp.; Tel. 682-9324.

van der MINNE, Dirk; 11747-8th Ave., Haney, B.C.; Edinburgh (Scot.)'60; Tel. 463-6613.

VANDEWATER, Stuart L.; 37 Lakeland Point Dr., Kingston, Ont.; Tor'47; ABA; FACA; FRCP(C); Anaes; Anaes-in-Chief, Kingston Gen. & Hotel-Dieu Hosp's.; Cons., Cdn. Armed Forces Hosp.; Prof. & Hd. Anaes., Queen's U.; Tel. 546-3841.

VANDOR, Frank; 80 King St. W., Welland, Ont.; Pecs (Hung.)'54.

VAN GOOR, John H.; Calgary Assoc. Clinic, 214-6th Ave., Calgary, Alta.; Alb'65; Tel. 263-7120.

van HOOGENHUIZE, William H.; 350 Christina St. N., Sarnia, Ont.; 1633 McGee (res); Wes '57; Active Staff, Sarnia Gen. Hosp.; Pt-time Phys., Imperial Oil Ltd.; Tel. ED 7-7531.

van HUSEN, Josephine E.; 14 Sandridge Rd., Ottawa 7, Ont '46; Tel. 746-1002.

VANLEEUWEN, James J.; Leiden (Neth.) '61; Psy; Staff, Toronto Psychiatric Hosp., Toronto 5, Ont.

VAN LOON, Glen R.; Tor'65; Res., Royal Victoria Hosp., Montreal, P.Q.

VANN, Earle K.; 126 Medical Arts Bldg., Winnipeg, Man.; 214 Overdale St. (res); Man '46; **FRCS(C), Urol; Dem. (Urol.), U. of Man.; Tel.** WH 2-3086.

VANNER, George A.; Main St., Palmerston, Ont.; Ott '52; MCGP; Staff, Palmerston Gen. Hosp.; Court. Staff, Gen. & St. Joseph's Hosp's., Kitchener-Waterloo & St. Mary's Hosp's., Kitchener; Tel. 140.

VAN NOORT, Alex; Leiden (Neth.) '49; AMC-GP; Res., St. Joseph's Hosp., London, Ont.

VAN NORDEN, Herman J.; 2021 E. 49th Ave., Vancouver 16, B.C.; 1438 Devonshire Cres. (res); Amsterdam (Neth) '47; MCGP; Vis. Staff, Vancouver Gen., St. Paul's, Grace, St. Vincent's & Mt. St. Joseph's Hosp's; Assoc. Staff, Burnaby Gen. Hosp.; Tel. FA 5-3818.

VAN NORDEN, Julia; 2021 E. 49th Ave., Vancouver 16, B.C.; 1438 Devonshire Cres. (res); Utrecht (Neth.) '49; MCGP; Tel. FA 5-3818.

VAN NORSTRAND, A. W. Peter; Tor '59; Res. (Path.), Toronto Gen. Hosp., Toronto, Ont.

VAN NOSTRAND, Frederick H.; Vandorf, Ont., via R.R. 1 Gormley; Tor '27; NeurPsy; Cons. Psy., W.C.B. of Ontario & Rehab. Centre, Downsview; Tel. 727-4380.

VAN ORMAN, Alan G.; Cardston Clinic, Cardston, Alta.; Alb '59; M.O.H., Cardston; Tel. 840.

VAN ORMAN, F. Lorne; 3331 Bloor St. W., Toronto 18, Ont.; 141 Kenollie Ave., Port Credit (res); Tor '48; FRCS(C), GenSurg; Staff (Surg.), Queensway Gen. & South Peel Gen. Hosp's.; Tel. BE 3-7601

VAN PATTER, Hugh; 74 Glencairn Ave., Toronto, Ont. (res); McG '49; Path; Ass't. Path., St. Michael's Hosp.; Dem., U. of Toronto; Tel. 362-4461.

VAN PRAAGH, David R.; 332 Sheldlrake Blvd., Toronto 12, Ont.; Tor '54; Paed; Staff, Hosp. for Sick Children; Tel. EM 6-7242.

VAN ROOYEN, Clennel E.; 5800 University Ave., Halifax, N.S.; Edinburgh (Scot.)'31; DSC(Edin); MRCP(Lond.); FC(Path); FRCP(C), Bact; Cons. Bact., Victoria Gen. Hosp., Camp Hill & Cdn. Forces Hosp's.; Cons. Bact., Cdn. Forces Med. Council, D.N.D., Ottawa; Prof. & Hd., Dept. of Bact., Dalhousie U.; Tel. 422-7371.

VAN STOLK, Jan B.; Capetown (S. Africa) '54; Psy; Staff, Guidance Clinic, 11120-102nd St., Edmonton, Alta.; Dir., Alberta Guidance Clin.; Lect., U. of Alberta.

VANT, J. Ross; 11010 Jasper Ave., Ste. 311, Edmonton, Alta.; 11626 Edinboro Rd. (res); Man '28; FACS; FACOG; FRCOG; FRCS(C); ObstGyn; Att'd. Staff, U. of Alberta Hosp.; Prof. (Emer.), U. of Alberta; Tel. GA 2-2217.

VAN TILBURG, Embert; Amsterdam (Neth.)'53; Med. Dir., St. Joseph's Hosp., Victoria, B.C.

van UCHELEN, Paul A.; 4027 E. Hastings St., North Burnaby, B.C.; 6340 Kitchener St. (res); Amsterdam (Neth.) '57; Tel. CY 9-2677.

VAN VEEN, Kaspar J.; 167 Talbot St. S., Essex, Ont.; Amsterdam (Neth.)'53; Tel. 776-7394.

VAN VIERSSEN TRIP, Agatha C.; (BONGA, Agatha C.).

VAN VIERSSEN TRIP, Hector L.; Manitowaning, Ont.; Groningen (Neth.)'31; M.O. Health, Dept. of Nat. Health & Welfare.

VAN VLIET, G. Alan., Lt. Col.; Hd. Dept. of Anaes., National Defence Med. Centre, Alta Vista Dr., Ottawa 8, Ont.; McG'50; FACA; Anaes.; Clin. Ass't. Surg., U. of Ottawa; Tel. 733-6600, Ext. 447.

VAN WART, A. D.; Tor '64; Res., Shaughnessy Hosp., Vancouver 9, B.C.

VAN WART, Arthur F.; 141 York St., Fredericton, N.B.; Tor'21; GenSurg; IntMed; MCGP; Tel. GR 5-6521.

VAN WEEL (See Cowan, Davina M.).

Van WIJHE, Marten; 145 Lindsay St.; Winnipeg 9, Man. (res); Leiden (Holland) '53; Path; Ass't Path., St. Boniface Hosp.; Lect. (Path.), U. of Man.; Tel. WH 3-0311.

VAN WYCK, Donald J.; 714 Med. Arts Bldg., 170 St. George St., Toronto 5, Ont.; 66 Rowanwood Ave. (res); Tor '42; FRCS(C), ObstGyn; Ass't., Dept. of ObstGyn., Toronto Gen. Hosp.; Clin. Instr. (ObstGyn), U. of Toronto; Tel. WA 2-6007.

VARADI, David P.; Tor '60; Jr. Int'n., Toronto Gen. Hosp., Toronto 2, Ont.

VAREY, Douglas H.; 250 Lawrence Ave. W., Toronto 12, Ont.; Tor'31; Tel. 787-5002.

VARGA, Anthony T.; Ste. 904, 24 Queen St. E., Brampton, Ont.; Tor'58; FRCS(C), GenSurg; Surg. Staff, Peel Mem. Hosp.

VARGA, Eugene A.; Tavistock Med. Group, Tavistock, Ont.; Qns '61; AMCGP.

VARGA-TOTH, Istvan; 41 Royal Rd. N., Portage La Prairie, Man.; Budapest (Hung.) '50; LRCP; LRCS; LRFPS (Glas); Tel. 857-6227.

VARGA, Gabriel; 2160 Eglinton Ave. W., Toronto, Ont.; 100 Portage Ave. Weston (res); Tor '53; Staff, Northwestern Gen. Hosp.; Tel. RU 3-9845.

VARGHA, Csaba O.; Caledon, Ontario; Budapest (Hung.)'56; Tel. 927-5271.

VARIBEAU, Leo; Gentilly, Co. Nicolet, P.Q.; Lav '59.

VARIN, Noel; 1808 Lake Breeze, St.-Eustache-sur-le-lac, P.Q. (res); Mon '48; MCGP; Med. Dir., St. Eustache Gen. Hosp.; Tel. 627-0501.

VARIN, Raymond; 5400 Cote de Liesse, Montreal 9, P.Q.; Mon '50; Ass't. Med. Dir., Abbott Laboratories; Tel. 735-2411.

VARLEY, John C.; 686 No. 3 Rd., Richmond, Vancouver 14, B.C.; 819 Westminster Hwy. (res); Tor '53; MCGP; Tel. CR 8-8435.

VARNAM, Gerald S.; Med. Dir., Bristol Laboratories, 100 Industrial Blvd., Candiac, P.Q.; Man '51; FACP; FRCP(C), IntMed.

VARNAM, Kenneth D.; 6543 Victoria Dr., Vancouver 16, B.C.; 5217 Clinton Ave., South Burnaby (res); Man '51; Vis. Staff, Vancouver Gen., Grace & St. Vincent's Hosp's.; Pt.-time, School Med. Officer, Metropolitan Health Committee; Div. Surg., St. John's Ambulance; Tel. FA 1-0604.

VARNAM, Russell I.; London (Eng.) '63; Staff, Coaldale Med. Clinic, Coaldale, Alta. Abroad.

VARSAMIS, Ioannis; Alexandria (Egypt) '57; FRCP(C), Psy. Staff, Psychiatric Inst., 75 Emily St., Winnipeg 3, Man.

VARSANYI, Endre I.; Budapest (Hung.) '50; Staff, Alberta Hosp., Ponoka, Alta.

VARTY, Earle J.; 455 Windemere Ave., Toronto, Ont.; 24 Thompson Ave., Toronto 18 (res); Tor '47; AMCGP; Assoc. Staff, Toronto Western Hosp.; Tel. RO 6-4550.

VARTY, Hilliard H.; 168 Annette St., Toronto, Ont.; 46 Halford Ave. (res); Tor '41; M.C.G.P.; O.P.D., Toronto Western Hosp.; Tel. RO 9-3430.

VARUGHESE, George; Calcutta (India) '55; FRCS(C), NeurSurg; Staff, Ottawa Civic Hosp., Ottawa, Ont.

VARVERIKOS, Emmanuel D.; Medical Arts Bldg., Sherbrooke St. W., Montreal, P.Q.; 5640 Somerled (res); Lav '44; ObstGyn; Tel. WE 5-1019.

VARVIS, Christopher J.; 10951-124th St. & 109A Ave., Edmonton, Alta.; Alb '53; M. Sc. (McG); FCCP; IntMed; Active Staff & Med. Advisor, Inhalation Therapy Dept., Royal Alexandra Hosp.; Instr. (Med.), U. of Alta.; Tel. 454-4551.

VAS, Magdalene (Raditz); 160 Stillview Rd., Pointe Claire, P.Q.; Budapest (Hung.)'52; Dip. IntMed(McG); Haem(P.Q.); Lect., McGill U.; Tel. 695-1310.

VAS, Stephen I.; 3775 University St. W., Montreal, P.Q.; Budapest (Hung.) '50; Bact; Assoc. Prof., McGill U.; Tel. 842-1251; Loc. 703.

VASCONCELOS, Jose A.; Brazil'56; Res., Children's Hosp., Winnipeg 3, Man.

VASQUEZ-CRUZ, Julio; Box 186, Station Outremont, Montreal, P.Q.; Paris (France) '39; Mon '43; NeurPsy (P.Q.); Staff, Inst. Albert Provost; Tel. 733-4111.

VASSAL, Kenneth P.; 106 Toronto Western Medical Bldg., 25 Leonard Ave., Toronto 2B, Ont.; 34 Edenbridge Dr., Islington, Ont. (res); Qns '52; D.M.R.; DiagRad; Att'd. Staff, Toronto Western Hosp.; Clin Teach. (Rad.), U. of Toronto; Tel. EM 3-1197.

VASSAR, Philip S.; London (Eng.) '55; M.R.C.S. (Eng.), L.R.C.P. (Lond..), F.C.A.P.; Res. (Path), Vancouver Gen. Hosp., Vancouver, B.C.; Assoc. Prof. (Path), U. of British Columbia; Tel. CA 4-1111

VASUDEVAIAH, Yshnavara; 720 McDermot Ave., Winnipeg, Man.; Mysore (India)'58; GenSurg.

VATANASUCHART, C.; Bangkok (Thailand) '53; Jr. Intn., Dept. of Psy., U. of Toronto, Toronto 5, Ont.

VAUCLAIR, Rene; Mon '60; FRCP(C), Path; Staff, Dept. of Anat., Hop. Notre-Dame, Montreal 24, P.Q.; Tel. 525-6363.

VAUGHAN, Charles E.; 793 Main St. E., Hamilton, Ont.; Tor '35; D.A.B.R., F.A.C.R., F.I.C.S., D&TRad; Cons. Rad, Hamilton Mountain San. & Hamilton D.V.A.; Tel. 547-0141.

VAUGHAN, E. Garth; Box 651, 33 Albert St., Windsor, N.S.; Dal '55; GenSurg; Tel. 3301.

VAUGHAN, Frank W.; 2851 Foul Bay Rd., Victoria, B.C.; UBC '56; Tel. EV 5-8522.

VAUGHAN, J. Avery; 471 Clifton Ave., Windsor, N.S.; Dal '47; GenSurg; Chief of Surg., Payzant Mem. Hosp.; Tel. 798-3123.

VAUGHAN, K. Diane (Sawyer); 1564 Cedarglen Rd., Victoria, B.C.; UBC '56; Pt-time Lect. (Physiol.), Victoria College.

VAUGHAN, Peter; P.O. Box 8100, 935 Lagauchetiere St. W., Montreal, P.Q.; 231 Stanstead Ave., Mtl 16 (res); McG '43; D.P.H., D.I.H., D.A.B.OccMed; F.A.C.PrevMed; Chief M.O., C.N.R. & Air Canada; Tel. 877-5742.

VAUGHAN, Robert L., F/L; Qns'63; Staff, British Military Hosp., Iserlohn, Germany; Abroad.

VAUGHAN, William A.; Whissell Clinic, Westlock, Alta.; Sask'60.

VAUGHAN, William C.; Tor'62; Res., Hosp. for Sick Children, Toronto 2, Ont.

VAVRUSKA, George W.; 1414 Drummond St., Montreal, P.Q.; 15 Granville Rd. (res); Prague (Czech.) '47; DermSyph; Staff, St. Mary's & Queen Elizabeth Hosp's.; Tel. VI 5-2336.

VAZ, Timothy T.; 212 Burrows Block, Swift Current, Sask.; Bombay (India)'59.

VEALE, William T. J.; King St., Harrow, Ont.; McAffee Ave. (res); Tor '24; M.O.H.; Tel. RE 8-2331.

VEASEY, H. Barrydale; Port Renfrew, B.C.; London (Eng.)'62.

VECES, Hanna; Geneva (Switz.) '51; Staff, Unite Sanitaire, 334 Lafontaine, Riviere du Loup, P.Q.

VECHTER, Max; Central Med. Bldg., 1105 Carling Ave., Ottawa 3, Ont.; 780 Byron Ave. (res); Qns'47; OrthSurg.; Staff OrthSurg., Ottawa Civic Hosp.; Clin. Instr. OrthSurg., U. of Ottawa; Tel. PA 9-8642.

VEDOVA, Joseph D.; 173 Main St. W., Welland, Ont.; Naples (Italy)'53; IntMed.

VEENHUIZEN, Pieter A.; 209 Medical Centre, 8th Ave. & 8th St. S.W., Calgary, Alta.; Amsterdam (Neth.) '56; Tel. 263-4690.

VEGA-JACOMBE, Carlos; Colombia (S. America) '58; Staff, Dept. of Microbiol., U. of Montreal, Montreal, P.Q.

VEIDLINGER, Otto; 117 Chaplin Cr., Toronto 7, Ont.; Tor'60; FRCP(C), Neur; Active Staff, Women's College Hosp.; Tel. 483-4264.

VEILLEUX, Claude; 3105 Montee St-Hubert, St-Hubert, P.Q.; Lav '65.

VEILLEUX, Herve, Capt.; 1 Field Amb. CAPO 5050, Can. Armed Forces, Germany; Lav '65. Abroad.

VEILLEUX, Jean; 40 Ave. Labmontagne, Quebec 3, P.Q.; Lav '56; F.R.C.P.(C), IntMed; Staff, Hop.-St. Francoie d'Assise; Tel. 522-7334.

VEILLEUX, Jean; 1491 Blvd. des Forces, Trois Rivieres, P.Q.; Lav '41; M.A.C.R., D&TRad; Dir., Dept. of Rad., Hop. Ste-Marie, Trois Rivieres, Hop. Cloutier Cap-de-la-Madeleine, & Hop. Comto's, Louiseville; Tel. FR 7721.

VEILLEUX, Joseph A. R.; 208 King St., Sherbrooke, P.Q.; Lav '28; Anaes.; Tel. 569-1810.

VEILLEUX, Paul H.; 1820 rue Jean Nicolet, Trois-Rivieres, P.Q. (res); Lav '41; DiagRad; Staff. Hop.-Ste. Marie; Tel. FR 7721.

VEILLEUX, Rene; Ste. Monique, Cte. Nicolet, P.Q.; Lav '53; Tel. 289-2861.

VEILLEUX, Roger; Ste. Felicite, Co. Matane, P.Q.; Lav '59.

VEITCH, Graeme R.; Glasgow (Scot.) '57; D.Obst. R.C.O.G.; Ass't. M.O., Walwyn Hosp., Come-By-Chance, Nfld.

VELDHUIS, Keimpe; Qns'65; Res., Victoria Hosp., London, Ont.

VENECEK, Danica; (Dousova); Ste. 321, 1396 St. Catherine St. W., Montreal 25, P.Q.; Charles U. (Prague, Czech.)'60; Neurol; Ass't. Reg. Mtl. Neurologic Hosp.; Clin. Ass't. Phys., St. Mary's Hosp.; Tel. 866-6052.

VENECEK, Ladislav; Ste. 510, 5025 Sherbrooke St. W., Montreal 28, P.Q.; Charles U. (Prague, Czech.) '50; FACOG; ObstGyn; Att'd. Staff (ObstGyn), Queen Elizabeth, Reddy Mem., Santa Cabrini & Catherine Booth Hosp's.; Tel. 488-7225.

VENIOT, Clarence J.; 229 King Ave., Bathurst, N.B.; Mon '10; FRCS(C), GenSurg; Retired; Senator, Gov't. of Canada.

VENIS, Stanley B.; Bloor Med. Clin., 609 Bloor St. W., Toronto 4, Ont.; Tor '57; M.C.G.P.; Staff, Doctors' Hosp.; Tel. LE 4-4214.

VENNE, Jean P.; Ste. 11, 222 Henri Bourassa E., Montreal 12, P.Q.; 10855 Esplanade (res); Lav'45; F.R.C.S.(C), GenSurg, ThorSurg (P.Q.); Surg., Hop. du Sacre-Coeur, Cartierville; Tel. 389-1305.

VENNE, Julien; 415 Ste-Helene, Longueuil, P.Q. Mon '62; Tel. 674-4052.

VENNE Louis; 5263 rue Brebeuf, Montreal, P.Q.; Mon '48; PlasSurg (P.Q.); Chief PlasSurg., Hop. Sacre Coeur; Ass't. Prof. (Anat.), Montreal, U.; Tel. LA 1-1261.

VENNEMA, Alje; 2120 Wellington Ave., Burlington, Ont.; McG'62.

VENNER, Albert; Box 790, Jasper, Alta.; London (Eng.) '42; MRCS; MRCP; IntMed; M.O.H., Jasper National Park; Dist. M.O., C.N.R.; Staff, Seton Hosp.; District Coroner; Tel. 852-3434.

VENTERS, D. Brian; Davidson, Sask.; Alb '54; Tel. 567-2104.

VENTURA, Joaquin C.; 5689 Blvd. Rosemont, Montreal, P.Q.; 11211 Joseph Casavant (res); Seville (Spain) '52; Ph.D. (Mont.); FRCP(C); Path; Staff, Hop. St. Joseph de Rosemont; Tel. CL 6-2681.

VERBEEK, Edmond O.; Beiseker, Alta.; Alb'60; Tel. 547-3257.

VERBEEK, Johannes H.; Qns'63; Res., Dept. of Path., Queen's U., Kingston, Ont.

VERBRUGGE, Magnus; Suite 202, 720 W. Broadway, Vancouver 9, B.C.; Amsterdam (Neth.) '45; Urol; Tel. TR 2-2344.

VERBRUGGE, Magdalenus; 1575 W. 28th Ave., Vancouver 9, B.C.; Amsterdam (Neth; '42; Urol Tel. RE 1-1664.

VERDICCHIO, A.; Mont Laurier, Co. Labelle, P.Q.; McG '41.

VERDY, Maurice B.; 3875 St-Urbain, Montreal 18, P.Q.; Mon '56; FRCP(C); IntMed; Staff, Hop. Hotel-Dieu; Tel. 733-0214.

VERESHACK, Paul; Tor '63; Fell. (Psy.), U. of Toronto, Toronto 5, Ont.

VERGE, Ernest; 1379 Maguire Ave., Quebec, P.Q.; Lav '41; GenSurg; Tel. 527-3314.

VERGE, Wylie; 34 Pleasant St., Dartmouth, N.S.; 27 Valley Field Rd., Woodlawn (res); Dal '55; M.C.G.P.

VERHULST, Jan; 160 Underhill Dr., Don Mills, Ont.; Leiden (Neth.)'49; D.Psy; Psy; Tel. 447-9092.

VERINDER, David; 706-14th Ave., Brandon, Man. (res); Sheffield (Eng.) '55; Staff, Hosp. for Mental Diseases; Tel. PA 6-2321.

VERITY, George E.; 17 William St., Brantford, Ont.; Tor '28; Otol; Tel. 752-2121.

VERMA, Santosh K.; Medical Arts Clinic, Swift Current, Sask.; Ireland'60; Assoc. Staff, Swift Current Union Hosp.; Tel. 773-4636.

VERMES, Gyorgy; 605 Bloor St. W., Toronto 4, Ont.; '51; Tel. WA 2-0962.

VERMETTE, H. Bernard; 805 Laurier Ave. E., Montreal 34, P.Q.; 4050 Blvd. Edouard Montpetit (res); Mon '54; GenSurg.; Tel. 272-9940.

VERMETTE, L. Normand; Centre Commercial, Ste-Adele, P.Q.; Ott '58; A.M.C.G.P.

VERMETTE, Rheal; 490-17eme rue, Grand'Mere, P.Q.; 921-12eme ave (res); Mon '54; GenSurg (P.Q.); Tel. LE 8-9070.

VERMEULEN, Henry; 511 Med. Arts Bldg., Edmonton, Alta.; 14724-91st Ave. (res); Gottingen (Germ.) '34; M.C.G.P.; Derm. & Ven. Dis. (Germ.); D.T.M. (Hamburg); School M.O., City of Edmonton; Tel. GA 4-2634.

VERNEREY, Roger; 1960 Arvida, St-Bruno, Cte Chambly, P.Q.; Mon'58; ObstGyn.

VERNIER, Leonard; 157 Avenue Rochette, Ste. Foy, Quebec 10, P.Q. (res); Lav '53; F.R.C.P.-(C), Path; Staff, Hop. Hotel Dieu, Quebec; Tel. 529-9151.

VERNON, C. Peter; 702 Medical Arts Bldg., 170 St. George St., Toronto 5, Ont.; Tor '54; FRSM; FRCS(C); ObstGyn; Assoc. (ObstGyn.), Toronto Gen. Hosp.; Cons. (Gyn.), Ont. Cancer Inst. & Princess Margaret Hosp.; Clin. Instr. (ObstGyn.), U. of Toronto; Tel. WA 3-5000.

VERNON, Elizabeth J. (Andrews); 1243 Clarkson Rd. N., Clarkson, Ont.; Wes '51; M.C.G.P.; Staff, Oakville & South Peel Hosp's.; Telephone TA 2-1351.

VERNON, Howard E.; 1243 Clarkson Rd. N., Clarkson, Ont.; 1265 Clarkson Rd. (res); Wes '50; MCGP; Staff, Oakville-Trafalgar Hosp.; Tel. TA 2-1351.

VERNON, Maurice A.; 214-6th Ave. W., Calgary, Alta.; McG'51; MCGP; Tel. 263-7120.

VERNON, Ross T. J.; 1574 Ouellette Ave., Windsor, Ont.; 1911 Riverside Dr., Riverside (res); Tor '49; D.M.R., D.A.B.R.; DiagRad; Att. Rad., Hotel Dieu Hosp.; Tel. CL 6-4914.

VERNY, Thomas; Tor'61; Psy; Staff, Clarke Inst. of Psy., 250 College St., Toronto 2B, Ont.

VERONNEAU, Suzanne; Ste. 220, 30 est Boul. St. Joseph, Montreal 14, P.Q.; Mon'57; FRCS(C), Ophth; Ass't. Serv. (Ophth.), Hop. Maisonneuve; I/C Basic Science Courses (Ophth.), affil., U. of Montreal; Tel. 845-0274.

VERRAULT, Jean M.; 6325 Ave Cairns, Ville d'Anjou, Montreal 5, P.Q. (res); Lav '53; Path; Staff (Path), Hop-St-Luc; Tel. UN 1-7261.

VERREAU, E. J.; 9629-111th Ave., Edmonton, Alta.; 11622-127th St. (res); Alb '26.

VERREAULT, Daniel; 78 Notre Dame S., Thetford Mines, P.Q.; Lav '59; Tel. 335-3553.

VERREAULT, Denis; 1500-18eme rue, Quebec 3, P.Q.; Lav '64.

VERREAULT, Raymond; C.P. 1538, Port-Cartier, Cte Saguenay, P.Q.; Lav '59.

VERRET, Simon; Lav'65; Res., Hop. Enfant Jesus, Quebec 3, P.Q.

VERSCHELDEN, Guy; 5360 Roi Rene, Ville d'Anjou, P.Q.; Mon'61; FRCS(C), ObstGyn.

VERSCHELDEN, Marcel; 5689 Blvd. Rosemount Montreal, P.Q. (res); Mon '33; F.C.C.P.; Pulm. Dis. & TB (P.Q.); Med. Dir, Hop. St-Joseph de Rosemount; Tel. CL 6-2681.

VERSCHELDEN, Noel; 2610 Desmoreaux St., **Montreal, P.Q.; Mon '33; Tel. CL 5-4242.**

VERSTEEG, Elmyre M.; Apt. 204, 3440 Place Decelles, Montreal 26, P.Q.; Ott'64; Ass't. Med. Dir., Hoechst Pharmaceutics, Montreal.

VERSTER, Arnoldus J.; 68 Main St. E., Grimsby, Ont.; Groningen (Neth.) '46; MCGP; Staff, West Lincoln Mem. Hosp.; Tel. 945-4922.

VERVILLE, Gilbert; 280 Montreal Rd., Ottawa 7, Ont.; Ott '58; MCGP; Tel. SH 6-0407.

VERVILLE, Henry W.; Box 234, 126 Sydney St., Cornwall, Ont.; Man '44; Derm.

VESSA, Giacomino; 5325 Jean Talon est, Montreal 36, P.Q.; Naples (Italy) '44; D&TRad; Staff, Santa Cabrini Hosp.

VEY, Albert G.; 210 Medical Arts Bldg., 1105 Pandora Ave., Victoria, B.C.; 2709 Cadboro Bay (res); Qns '47; MCGP; Tel. EV 4-9613.

VEY, David J.; Ste. 310, 1175 Cook St., Victoria, B.C.; Otago U. (N. Zealand) '57; Tel. EV 5-7122.

VEZINA, Andre; 701 rue du Couvent, Montreal, P.Q.; Lav'40; MCGP; Med. Staff, O.P.D. Psy., Hop. Notre-Dame; Tel. WE 2-5237.

VEZINA, Bernard; St-Basile, Cte. Portneuf. P.Q.; Lav '61.

VEZINA, Clement; 118 ave. Ruel, St-Gregoire, Quebec 5, P.Q.; Lav '63.

VEZINA, Gilles; 115-1ere rue, St. Fabien, P.Q.; Lav'65.

VEZINA, Henri; 1398, Laviolette, Trois-Rivieres, P.Q.; Lav '64.

VEZINA, Jean A.; 6900 rue Jean Bourdon, Montreal 9, P.Q.; Lav'54; D&TRad.

VEZINA, Jean J., Capt.; CFB, MIR, Longue Pointe, Montreal 5, P.Q.; Mon'65.

VEZINA, Jean L.; 5600 Stirling, Montreal 26, P.Q.; Lav '54; DiagRad; Staff, Royal Victoria Hosp.; Dem., McGill U.

VEZINA, Jean P.; Lav'57; ObstGyn(P.Q.); Staff, Hop. Enfant Jesus, Quebec 3, P.Q.

VEZINA, L. Rene; 1150 Holland, Quebec, P.Q. (res); Lav'22; DPH; PH; Retired.

VEZINA, Norbert; 557 rue Cherrier, Montreal 24, P.Q.; 793 Wilder, Outremont (res); Mon '38; **Court. Staff, Paed., Hop. Maisonneuve; Tel. AV 8-0361.**

VEZINA-VOYER, Jacqueline; Lav'62; Anaes; Staff, Hop. St. Joseph, Beauceville Ouest, P.Q.

VIALLET, Andre; 4041 Marcil, Montreal 28, P.Q.; Mon '57; FRCP(C), IntMed; Staff, Hop. St.-Luc; Tel. UN 1-7261.

VIAU, Andre; Ste. 212, 12245 Grenet, Montreal 9, P.Q.; Mon'65.

VIAU, Gerard; 9666 Hochelaga St., Montreal, P.Q.; Mon '59; Tel. CL 6-3455.

VIAU, Horace R.; 195 rue Laurier E., Ottawa, Ont.; 224 Island Pk. Dr. (res); Mon '28; Paed; Chief Paed., St. Louis de Montfort Hosp.; Tel. CE 4-2240.

VIBERT, James C.; 916 Prince St., Truro, N.S.; 70 Smith Ave. (res); Dal '51; M.Sc. (Surg.) (Minn.); FRCS(C), GenSurg; Chief Surg., Colchester Co. Hosp.; Tel. 893-7366.

VICAS, Emile; 960 Boul. Ste-Croix, Montreal 9, P.Q.; Cluj (Roum.)'37; FRCS(C), OrthSurg.

VICKERS, Kenneth W.; Med. Centre, 420 Lock St. W., Dunnville, Ont.; Tor '46; MCGP; Tel. 774-7541.

VICTOROS, Constantine; Athens (Greece)'59; Staff, James Paton Mem. Hosp., Gander, Nfld.

VIDAL, Joseph Avila; 389 E. Boul. St. Joseph, Montreal 14, P.Q.; 576 McEachran, Outremont (res); Lav '11; Pulm. Dis & TB (P.Q.); FACP; FRCP(C), IntMed; Pres. Spec. Comm. (TB), (PQ); Tel. VI 5-2624.

VIDINLI, Mustafa; 1705 Corydon Ave., Winnipeg 9, Man.; Ankara (Turk.)'49; Pt.-time Staff, Deer Lodge Hosp., Tel. 489-8228.

VIENS, Gilles; 1705 Girouard, St. Hyacinthe, P.Q.; Mon '61; Tel. PR 4-7062.

VIENS, Lucien; 2630 Louis Veuillot St., Montreal, P.Q.; 2608 Louis Veuillot St. (res); Mon '35; Tel. CL 5-1900.

VIERKOETTER, Hildegarde M. E. (Legresley); 932 Royal York Rd., Toronto 18, Ont.; Tor '48; Staff, Bell Telephone Co. (Part-time); Staff, University Health Serv. (Part-time).

VIETS, Celia A.; 305 Thorald Rd., Rockcliffe Park, Ottawa, Ont.; London (Eng.)'55; DCH; Paed; Staff, Baby Clinics, Ottawa; Clin. Ass't. (Paed.), University of Ottawa.

VIG, Kartar S.; Ste. 11, 725 McGee St., Winnipeg 3, Man.; Dublin (Ire.)'61; LAH(Dublin, Ire.); LRCP(I); LM; LRCS(I) & LM.

VIGEANT, J. H. Emilien; 350 Blvd. St. Joseph, Montreal, P.Q.; 22 Ave. Simcoe, Mont Royal (res); Mon '27; GenSurg (P.Q.); Surg., Hop. Ste. Justine; Tel. RE 1-4931.

VIGEANT, Jacques; 55 de l'Eglise, Montreal 19, P.Q.; Mon '58; FRCS(C), ObstGyn.

VIGEANT, Marcel; Mon'65; Res., Hop. Hotel-Dieu, Montreal 18, P.Q.

VIGER, Roland J.; Seaforth Med. Bldg., 3550 Cote des Neiges Rd., Montreal 25, P.Q.; 1524 Summerhill Ave. (res); Mon '37; DABO; FACS; Ophth; Senior Ophth. & Dir., Glaucoma Clinic, Montreal Gen. Hosp.; Cons., St. Mary's & Queen Elizabeth Hosp's.; Ass't. Prof., McGill U.; Tel. 935- 8338.

VIGH, Sandor G.; 631 Commissioner's Rd., London, Ont.; 709 Riverside Dr. (res); Budapest (Hung.) '50; GenSurg; Tel. 433-3865.

VIGNA, Victor; Wes'65; Res., War Mem. Children's Hosp., London, Ont.

VIGNAULT, J. Maurice; 1010 Chemin St-Roch, Tracy, P.Q.; Lav '53; FRCS(C); GenSurg.

VIGNEAU, Jean; 230 Mercille Ave., St. Lambert, Montreal 23, P.Q.; Mon '42; F.A.C.A., **Anaes; Staff (Anaes), Verdun Gen. Hosp.; Tel. PO 6-3551.**

VIGNEAU, Paul; 55 Ave. Church, Verdun, Montreal 19, P.Q.; Mon'42; OrthSurg (P.Q.); Staff, Verdun Gen. Hosp.; Cons., Hop. St. Joseph Lachine; Tel. 766-4901.

VIGNEAULT, Germain; St. Gedeon, Cte. Frontenac, P.Q.; Lav '61.

VIGNEAULT, Gilles; 825 sud rue Belvedere, Sherbrooke, P.Q.; Mon'61; Otol.

VIGNEAULT, Maurice; Lav'62; Path(P.Q.); Staff, Hop. St. Vincent De Paul, Sherbrooke, P.Q.

VIGNEAULT, Moise; App. 302, 5100 boul. Pie IX, Montreal 36, P.Q.; Lav'43; GenSurg.

VIGNEAULT, Patrice; 11470 rue Drouart, Montreal 12, P.Q.; Lav '55; Anaes (P.Q.); Staff, Hop.-Sacre-Coeur; Tel. FE 4-1210.

VIGRASS, Howard G.; 402 Main St., Melfort, Sask.; Sask'62; MCGP; Tel. 752-2876.

VIHVELIN, Hugo; 548 Lewin Pk., Lancaster, N.B. (res); Estonia '35; Staff, Provincial Hosp.

VIK, Knut E.; 9108A-142nd St., Edmonton, Alta.; 14016-Buena Vista Rd. (res); Alb '57; Tel. 488-0777.

VIKTOR, Eva (See UGRAY, Eva.).

VILLARD, Henri P.; Mon '58; MCGP; Res., Inst. Albert-Prevost, 6555 ouest, boul Gouin, Montreal 9, P.Q.

VILLANUEVA, Marcos P.; Box 1419, 825 Cliffe Ave., Courtenay, B.C.; Santo Tomas (Phillip.)'56.

VILLANUEVA, Rosendo R.; Manila (Philip.) '57; Staff, Saskatchewan Hosp., Box 7000, Weyburn, Sask. Tel. VI 2-3812.

VILLAROMAN, Malaya; Manila (Philip.) '55; Jr. Intn., St. Boniface Gen. Hosp., Winnipeg 6, Man.

VILLEMAIRE, J. A. Bernard; 390 rue Morin, Ste-Adele-en-Haut, P.Q.; Mon '45; Res. Phys., Hotel-Dieu-de-St.-Jerome, St. Jerome; Cons. Phys., Rolland Paper Co.; Tel. WE 3-3681.

VILLEMURE, Bruno; 55 ave. de l'Eglise, Montreal 19, P.Q.; Lille (France) '61; Tel. 768-4702.

VILLEMURE, R.; 987 St. Prosper, Trois Rivieres, P.Q.; 572 Bonaventure (res); Lav '49; M.C.G.P.

VILLENEUVE, Andre; 1665 Cote du Verger, Sillery, Quebec 6, P.Q.; Lav'58; MSc; Psy(P.Q.); Abroad.

VILLENEUVE, Bernard; Quartier Beauchesne, Roberval, P.Q. (res); Lav '56; Med. Dir., Hop. Hotel Dieu, St. Michel; Tel. 1290.

VILLENEUVE, Bertrand; Lav'62; Haem(P.Q.); Staff, Hop. St-Sacrement, Quebec, P.Q.

VILLENEUVE, David E.; 325-66th rue E., Charlesbourg, P.Q.; Lav '59; Tel. 623-0575.

VILLENEUVE, Jean M.; 3100 Laforest, Quebec 10, P.Q.; 27337 Montarville (res); Lav'45; Tel. 653-0363.

VILLENEUVE, Louise; 2529 Cote Ste. Catherine, Montreal 26, P.Q.; Lav'58.

VILLENEUVE, Paul M.; Lav'54; Psy(P.Q.); Staff, Clinique Roy Rousseau, Quebec 5, P.Q.

VILLENEUVE, Philippe J.; 278 Friel St., Ottawa 2, Ont.; 136 Powell (res); Ott '55; Cons. Students Health Serv.; Clin. Ass't. U. of Ottawa; Tel. CE 6-5689.

VILLENEUVE, Robert; 2157 Est rue Fleury, Montreal 12, P.Q.; 11485 Frigon (res); Mon '54; ObstGyn (P.Q.); Cons. Hop. Misericorde; Cons. Hop. St. Joseph de Rosemont; Chief, ObstGyn, Hop. Fleury; Tel. DU 1-2581.

VILLENEUVE, Victor P.; Ott'65; Res., Ottawa Gen. Hosp., Ottawa, Ont.

VILLEUX, Gabriel; St. Gedeon, Co. Frontenac, P.Q.

VINCE, Dennis J.; 455 Gordon Ave., West Vancouver, B.C.; Tor '54; FRCP(C), Paed; Staff, Children's Health Centre, 715 W. 12th Ave., Van. 9; Assoc. Prof. Paed. & Hd. Sect. of Paed. Cardiol., U. of British Columbia; Tel. TR 6-3211, Loc. 2696.

VINCENT, Arthur A.; Victoria St., Stevensville, Ont.; Bristol (Eng.)'26; Staff, Niagara Falls Gen. Hosp.; Tel. 382-3123.

VINCENT, B.; St. Germain (Drummond), P.Q.; Lav '55; A.M.C.G.P.

VINCENT, Jacques; 2040 Boul. Rosemont, Montreal 35, P.Q.; Mon'59; ObstGyn(P.Q.).

VINCENT, John E.; 209 Broughdale Ave., London, Ont.; 493 Victoria St. (res); Qns '49; FAAP; AMCAA; Paed; Staff Phys & Chief Of Paed. Allerg. Clin., Victoria Hosp.; Staff, St. Joseph's Hosp.; Lect. (Paed.), U. of Western Ont.; Tel. 439-2211.

VINCENT, Merville O.; 151 Delhi St., Guelph, Ont.; Dal '55; DABIM; FRCP(C), Psy; IntMed; Ass't. Med. Supt., Homewood San.; Cons. Staff, Guelph Gen. & St. Joseph's Hosp's.; Tel. TA 4-1010.

VINCENT, Pierre; Lav'65; Res., Hop. St-Michel Archange, Quebec, P.Q.; Abroad.

VINCENT, Pierre R.; 17 Fusey, Cap-de-la-Madeleine, P.Q.; Lav '64.

VINCENT, Roland; 8072 St. Denis St., Montreal, **P.Q.; Mon '25; Tel. DU 8-0920.**

VINE, Glenervon D.; Strathroy, Ont.; Tor '25; **M.C.G.P.; Tel. 245-0030.**

VINEBERG, Arthur M.; 3170 De Lavigne Rd., Montreal 6, P.Q.; McG'28; PhD.; FACS; GenSurg; ThorSurg(P.Q.); Cardiac Surg., Royal Victoria Hosp.; Cons. Cardiac. Surg., Montreal Inst. of Cardiol & Queen Mary Vet's Hosp.; Assoc. Prof. Surg., McGill U.; Tel. AV 8-9337.

VINER, Norman; 1425 Bishop St., Montreal, P.Q.; McG '05; NeurPsy; Cons., Montreal Gen., Jewish Gen. & Verdun Protestant Hosp's., & Montreal Neurological Inst.; Teach. Staff, McGill U.; Tel. VI 4-6311.

VINES, Norman M.; Ste. 3, 1452 Bishop St., Montreal, P.Q.; McG'24; Phys., Gazette Printing Co., B. F. Goodrich Rubber Co., Smith Transport Co., Boyds Express, Cdn. Broadcasting Corp. & 25 Life Insurance Companies; Tel. 849-3001.

VINGE, Lorne N.; Sask'58; Res., University Hosp., Saskatoon, Sask.

VINGILIS, Jerome J.; 1 Beaverbrook Ave., Islington, Ont.; Kaunas (Lith.) '43; Tel. BE 1-1310.

VINING, Joseph A.; 123 Edward St., Toronto 2, Ont.; 129 Burbank Dr. Willowdale (res); Tor '39; Anaes; Anaes-in-Chief, St. Michael's Hosp.; Assoc. in Anaes., U. of Toronto; Tel. EM 8-3439.

VIOLETTE, B. R. James; McG'43; Station M.O., Air Canada Clinic, Montreal Airport, Montreal, P.Q.; Tel. 636-2994.

VIPOND, Claude H.; Oshawa Clinic, 117 King St. E., Oshawa, Ont.; 642 Brookside Dr. (res); Qns '43; FRCS (Edin.); GenSurg; Surg. Staff, Oshawa Gen., Ajax-Pickering & Bowmanville Mem. Hosp's.; Tel. 728-1661.

VIRGIN, William J.; 250 Lawrence Ave. W., Toronto 12, Ont.; 19 Phyn Ave. Tor. 6 (res); Tor '33; M.Ch.(Orth, Liverpool); F.R.C.S. (Edin.); OrthSurg; Surg., Orthopaed. Hosp.; Staff, Bethesda Hosp.; Tel. 782-9741.

VIRICK, M. Singh; 63 Charlotte St., Sydney, N.S.; Christian Med. Coll. (India) '61.

VIROLLE, Pierre; 2385 Parc Garneau, Montreal, **P.Q.; Mon '45; Tel. PO 8-0551.**

VIRTUE, John A.; Suite 515, Medical Arts Bldg., Hamilton Ont.; 60 Auchmar Rd. (res); **Tor '43; F.R.C.S.(C), Otol; Staff Otol., St. Joseph's & Hamilton Gen. Hosps.; Tel. JA 9-8588.**

VISHWAKARMA, P. P.; Patna (India) '51; Ph.D. (Cinn., U.S.A.); Ass't Prof., Pharm., Queen's U., Kingston, Ont.

VISSER, Andrew H.; 30 Willow Ave., Westmount, Montreal 6, P.Q. (res); McG '43; M.O., Shawinigan Water & Power Comm.; Tel. LE 7-6616.

VITOU, Constantine K.; 2101 Graham Blvd., Montreal 16, P.Q.; McG'50; Tel. 735-0241.

VITOU, Suzanne; 2101 Graham Blvd., Montreal 16, P.Q.; Ott'56.

VITYE, Barna; 1140 Jean Talon E., Montreal 10, P.Q.; Mon'55; IntMed (P.Q.); MCGP; Tel. 274-3272.

VIVIAN, R. Percy; 6000 Fielding Ave., Montreal 29, P.Q.; Tor '26; Med. Cons., Protestant School Bd. of Gtr. Montreal; Tel. 482-6000.

VOADEN, M. E. Carol; 2135 Avenue Rd., Ste. 200, Toronto 12, Ont.; Tor'60; AMCGP; Assoc. Staff, Women's College Hosp.; Court. Staff, Grace Hosp.; Tel. 489-0040.

VOELKER, Philip A.; 36 Young St. W., Waterloo, Ont.; Tor '38; MOH, City of Waterloo; Tel. 745-8782.

VOGEL, Anne M.; Box 1429, Creston, B.C.; Dal '58.

VOGEL, Max J.; Ste 405, 1640-16th Ave. N.W., Calgary, Alta.; 2131 Victoria Ave. (res); Qns '42; MCGP; Staff, Calgary Gen., Grace, Holy Cross & Alberta Children's Hosp's.; Tel. 282-4577.
VOGELFANGER, Isaac J.; Central Med. Bldg., 1105 Carling Ave., Ottawa 3, Ont.; 86 Irving Pl. (res); John Casimir U. (Lwow, Poland) '34; FICS, M.Sc.D., FACS; GenSurg; Assoc. Prof. (Surg.), U. of Ottawa; Hd. Surg. Research, Ottawa Civic Hosp.; Tel. PA 8-3563.
VOGELSANG, Arthur; 305 Oxford St., London, Ont.; 10 Clenray Pl. (res); Wes '38; FAGS, FICA; Tel. GE 4-2922.
VOGHEL, Bertin; Res., Hop. Sacre-Coeur, Montreal 9, P.Q.; Mon '55.
VOGHEL, Donat; 300 St. Louis Sq., Montreal, **P.Q.; 1902 Van Horne (res); Mon '32; Tel. VI** 4-4301.
VOGT, Peter A.; Winkler Clinic, Winkler, Man.; Man'65.
VOISARD, Roland A.; 3414 Parc Ave., Montreal **18, P.Q.; Mon '44; Otol; Tel. 844-7731.**
VOISINE, Claude; Lav'65; Res., Hop St-Michel Archange, Quebec, P.Q.; Abroad.
VOITK, Andrus J.; Tor'65; Res., Montreal General Hosp., Montreal 25, P.Q.
VOKES, Fred A.; Medical Arts Bldg., Hamilton, Ont.; Qns '29.
VOKES, H. Arnold; Dungannon, Ont.; Tor '25; Tel. 529-7959.
VOLLMER, Helmut; 195 Simcoe St N., Oshawa, **Ont.; R.R. No. 1 (res); Munich (Germ.) '37; Tel.** 723-1171.
VOLPE, Aaron G.; 503 Markhom St., Toronto 4, **Ont.; Tor '22; IntMed; Tel. LE 1-7016.**
VOLPE, Robert; Toronto Wellesley Hosp., Toronto, Ont.; Tor'50; FRCP(C), IntMed; FACP; Active Staff, Wellesley Hosp.; Ass't. Prof. Med., U. of Toronto; Tel. 966-6947.
von HOCHSTETTER, Arthur H. C.; 458 Tecumseh Ave., London, Ont. (res); Vienna (Austria) **'43; Assoc. Prof. (Anat.), U. of Western Ontario;** Tel. GE 9-1681.
von KOENIGSLOEW, Erich O.; 332 le Marchand **Mansions, Edmonton, Alta.; Bonn (Germ.) '38; Tel. 488-9949.**
VON ONDARZA, U. Edgar; Ste. 505, 5025 Sherbrooke St. W., Montreal 28, P.Q.; Berlin (Germ.) '38.
VON RAFFLER, Werner; Thompson, Man.; Keil (Germ.)'52.
von ROSEN, Else; Ste. 101, 1541 W. Broadway, Vancouver 9, B.C.; 702-1260 Harwood St. (res); UBC '60; Tel. 6-6343.
VONTSO, Valfrid H.; Tartu (Estonia) '37; F.A.C.C.P.; Ass't. Med. Supt., Saint John Tuberculosis Hosp.; East Saint John, N.B.; Dir., St. Stephen T.B. Clin.; Memb. Cons. Staff, Saint John Gen. Hosp.; Tel. 693-6551.
VOSBURGH, John W.; Box 165 Sechelt B.C.; Alb '31; DABDR; DiagRad.; Staff, St. Mary's Hosp.
VOST, Alan; University Med. Clinic, Montreal Gen. Hosp., Montreal 25, P.Q.; Glasgow (Scot.) '58; FRCP(C); IntMed.
VOTH, Abraham B.; 356 Med. Arts Bldg., Saskatoon, Sask.; 1331-13th St. E. (res); Man '53; Staff, City & St. Paul's Hosp's.; Tel. 652-5454.
VOTH, Abraham R.; 3379 Kingsway St., Vancouver, B.C.; Man '56; MCGP; Tel. HE 1-3388.
VOWLES, Patricia; Bristol (Eng.) 51; Staff, Cariboo Health Unit, Williams Lake, B.C.; Med. Dir., Cariboo Health Unit.
VOYER, Armand; 41 St-David, Magog, P.Q.; Mon '27.
VOYER, D'Argenson; 605 Rockland, Montreal 8, P.Q.; Lav'53; Dip. Psychoanal. (Paris, Fr.)'53; **Psy(P.Q.); Staff, Hop. Sacre-Coeur; Tel. 334-1210.**
VOYER, Jean G.; Lav '63; Res., Hop. Hotel-Dieu, Quebec 4, P.Q.
VOYER, Jean P.; Lav'62; GenSurg(P.Q.); Staff, Hop. St. Joseph, Beauceville Ouest, P.Q.
VOYER, Louis; Room 904, 30 est Boul. St. Joseph, Montreal 14, P.Q.; Lav'55; Psy(P.Q.).
VOYER, Rosaire; 4 Taschereau, Hull, P.Q.; 20 Lacasse (res); Lav '49; FACS; FRCS(C); GenSurg; Tel. 771-8121.
VOYER, Victorin; 30 Est. Boul. St. Joseph, Montreal 14, P.Q.; Lav'43; Psy(P.Q.); Staff, Inst. Albert Prevost.
VOZIS, Dimitrina (Beshkowa); Ste 710, 1849 Yonge St., Toronto 7, Ont.; 257 Lawrence Ave. E., Tor. 12 (res); Sofia (Bulgaria) '49; Tel. 489-6615.
VOZIS, Gregory; Ste 710, 1849 Yonge St., Toronto 7, Ont.; Sofia (Bulgaria) '48; ObstGyn; Tel. 489-6615.
VOZORIS, Agathocles; 131 Bloor St. W., Toronto 5, Ont.; Athens (Greece) '52; Tel. 925-2895.
VOZORIS, Demosthenes S.; 1421 Danforth Ave., Toronto 6, Ont.; Nat. U. (Athens, Greece) '52; GenSurg; Staff, Toronto Gen. Hosp.
VRANIC-PETRICK, Margda; '58; Staff, Women's College Hosp., Toronto 5, Ont.; Tel. WA 3-7381.
V. TAPPEINER, Monika E. (See Kasserra).
VUCKOVIC, Vukasin; Main St., Caughnawaga, P.Q.; Strasbourg (Germ.) '23.
VULPE, Michael; Sask'58; Neur(P.Q.); Med. Adviser, Ciba Co. Ltd., 200 Metropolitan Blvd., Dorval, P.Q.; Staff, Mt. Providence Hosp.
VYAS, Vishnuprasad; Baroda (India) '55; Res., Queen Mary Vet's., Hosp., Montreal, P.Q.
WACHNA, Anthony T.; 1520 Ottawa St., Windsor, Ont.; 2030 Riverside Dr., Riverside (res); Man '37; M.C.G.P.; Surg. Staff, Hotel Dieu & Grace Hosp's; Tel. 253-9393.
WACHTER, Blair T.; 4602 W. 7th Ave., Vancouver, **B.C. (res); UBC '60; A.M.C.G.P.**
WACKENRODER, Henry; 718 Granville St., Vancouver, B.C.; 6161 St. **Georges Cres. (res); Man '24; GenSurg; Tel. MU 3-2722.**
WADA, Juhn A.; Med. Science Bldg., U. of British Columbia, Vancouver, B.C.; 4729 W. 7th Ave., Van. 8 (res); Hokkaido Imperial U. **(Japan) '46; Ph.D. (Neurphysiol.); Neur; Active** Vis. Staff (Neurol. & EEG), Van. Gen. Hosp.; Assoc. Prof. & Chief of Labs. of EEG & Neur-Physiol.), U. of British Columbia; Vis. Staff, St. Paul's Hosp.; Tel. 228-2556 & 228-3260.
WADDEL, Gabriel; 12 rue Blainville est, Ste. Therese, **P.Q.; Mon '48.**
WADDELL, James M.; 402 Rideau Medical Centre 1711-4th St. S.W., Calgary, Alta.; Qns '38; IntMed; District Coroner; Tel. 269-4842.
WADDELL, John T.; 606 Broder Bldg., Regina, Sask.; No. 1 Clifton Ct. (res); Man '16; MRCS (Eng.), LRCP(Lond.); Retired.
WADDELL, Robert W.; Qns '64; Res., Royal Victoria Hosp., Montreal, P.Q.
WADDELL, Walter G.; Ottawa Gen. Hosp., Ottawa, Ont.; Qns'53; FRCS(C), GenSurg; Gen-Surg., Ottawa Gen. Hosp. & Ottawa Civic Hosp.; Ass't. Prof. & Research Assoc., Experimental Surg., U. of Ottawa; Tel. 233-7377 & 236-0333.
WADDELL, William R.; 305 Med. Arts Bldg., 1011 Ouellette Ave., Windsor, Ont.; 2504 Lincoln Rd. (res); Qns '24; FRCP(C), IntMed; Tel. CL 6-6824.
WADDELL, William R.; Qns'60; IntMed; Staff, **Kingston Gen. Hosp., Kingston, Ont.**
WADDINGTON, Harrison; 1551 Bathurst St., Toronto 10, Ont.; 196 Montclair Ave., Tor. 10 (res); Tor '26; MCGP; Assoc. Toronto Western Hosp.; Phys., American Standard Products of Canada; Tel. LE 2-2500.
WADE, John C. L.; 402 Rideau Medical Centre, 1711-4th Street S.W., Calgary, Alta.; London Univ. (Eng.)'45; IntMed; Cons. Staff, Calgary Gen. Hosp.; Tel. AM 6-1954.
WADE, Mervin A.; Wetaskiwin Med. Clinic, Wetaskiwin, Alta.; 125 Spatinow Dr. (res); Alb '57; MCGP; Tel. 352-2242.
WADE, Robert C.; Apt. 108, 412 Highland Rd., Peterborough, Ont.; Tor'32; DPH; MCGP.
WADE, William W.; The Medical Centre, 68 King St. E., Cobourg, Ont.; 218 King St. E. (res); Qns'30; Tel. FR 2-5494.
WADMAN, Hamilton G.; 1008 Fairmont Med. Bldg,. 750 W. Broadway, Vancouver 9, B.C.; 1392 W. 46th Ave. (res); McG '50; F.R.C.S.(C), ObstGyn; Att'd. Staff, Vancouver Gen. Hosp.; Clin. Instr., U. of British Columbia; Tel. TR 9-5510.

WADUP, Rex S.; 149 Bonaccord St., Moncton, N.B.; Dal '52; Staff, Moncton Hosp.; Court. Staff, Hotel Dieu Hosp.; Tel. EV 2-6427.

WAGAR, H. Gerald; Qns'53; Psy; Staff, Hop. Hotel-Dieu, Kingston, Ont.

WAGG, H. Ovas; 2031-33rd Ave. S.W., Calgary, Alta.; Chinook Professional Bldg., Calgary; Qns'54; ObstGyn; Att'd. Staff, Calgary Gen., Holy Cross & Grace Hosp's.; Tel. 242-5176 & 255-6056.

WAGMAN, Benjamin B.; 293 Christie St., Toronto, Ont.; 109 Mona Dr. (res); Tor '41; M.C.-G.P.; Outdoor Staff, Mt. Sinai Hosp.; Tel. LE 3-3155.

WAGNER, Garth A.; Sask'64; Res., Sunnybrook Hosp., Toronto 12, Ont.

WAGNER, George; 1241-104th St., North Battleford, Sask.; National U. (Ire.)'56; D.Obst(Lond.); FRCS(C), GenSurg.

WAGNER, Gerhard H.; 455 Avenue Rd., Toronto, Ont.; 10 Tichester Rd. (res); Prague (Czech.) '35; Tel. WA 3-8627.

WAGNER, Gertrude F. (See Sleeva).

WAGNER, Jean P.; St. Paul, Cte. Montmagny, P.Q.; Lav'65.

WAGNER, John C.; 505 Professional Bldg., Red Deer, Alta.; Man '57; GenSurg.

WAGNER, Kenneth R.; UBC'62; Res., Vancouver Gen. Hosp., Vancouver 9, B.C.

WAGNER, Mildred; 18 Weber St. E., Kitchener, Ont.; 28 Maynard Ave. (res); Wes '32; Obst.; Tel. SH 5-5331.

WAHL, Otto E.; Box 490, Ocean Falls, B.C., Man '49; Tel. 289-3532.

WAIGHT, Peter J.; Med. Arts Clinic, 2125-11th Ave., Regina, Sask.; London (Eng.)'57; Tel. 523-0691.

WAINWRIGHT, David O.; Tor '62; Res., Kingston Gen. Hosp., Kingston, Ont.

WAINWRIGHT, Richard M.; 611 Upper James St., Hamilton, Ont.; Cambridge (Eng.) '56; B.Chir; DRCOG; Tel. 383-8454.

WAINWRIGHT, Ruth E.; 611 Upper James St., Hamilton, Ont.; London (Eng.) '58; DRCOG; Tel. 383-8454.

WAIT, Frederick E.; 323-6th Ave. N., Saskatoon, Sask.; McG '23; GenSurg; Retired; Tel. 244-7889.

WAIT, John H.; Apt. 41, 101 Lawton Blvd., Toronto 7, Ont.; Tor'60; FRCS(C), GenSurg; Staff, Hosp. for Sick Children; Tel. EM 6-7242.

WAIT, Richard H.; 1004-105th St., Edmonton, Alta.; McG'57; FRCP(C); IntMed; Assoc. Staff, Royal Alexandra Hosp.; Clin. Dem., U. of Alberta; Tel. 424-2121.

WAITE, Mary (see Spitzer)

WAITE, Robin C. H.; 68 Shrewsbury St., Stratford Ont. (res); Wes '56; Staff, Stratford Gen. Hosp.; Tel. 271-2120.

WAITE, Wilford I.; 105 Wellington St., Brantford, Ont.; R.R. 1 Paris (res); Wes '31; MCGP; Memb., Brant County Med. Soc.; Staff (G.P.), Brantford Gen. Hosp.; Tel. 752-1722.

WAKEFIELD, George E.; 6510 Lime St., Vancouver, B.C. (res); Man '41; IntMed; Ass't. Med. Dir., Vancouver, Gen. Hosp.; Tel. AM 1-7027.

WAKEFIELD, John K.; Alb '61; Res., University Hosp., Edmonton, Alta.

WAKEFORD, John; UBC'64; Res., Vancouver Gen. Hosp., Vancouver 9, B.C.

WALASEK, Joseph; Box 93, Base Borden, Ont.; Ott'60; Tel. 424-1881.

WALCOTT, David B.; Ste. 301, 4900 Kingsway, South Burnaby, B.C.; McG'49; FRCS(C), GenSurg; Clin. Instr., U. of British Columbia; Tel. 434-1211.

WALCOTT, John M. L.; 153 Pinnacle St., Belleville, Ont.; Man'50; ABOphth; Ophth; Chief Dept. of Ophth., Belleville Gen. Hosp.; Staff, Trenton Mem. Hosp.; Tel. 962-1296.

WALDEN, L. Paul; 69 Joseph St., Clinton, Ont.; Wes'49; FRCS(C), GenSurg; Active Staff, Clinton Public Hosp., South Huron Hosp., Exeter & Wingham & Dist. Hosp., Wingham; Tel. 482-6698.

WALDIE, Adam C.; 4326 W. 10th Ave., Vancouver 8, B.C.; Alb '48; MCGP; Att'd. Staff, Van. Gen. & Clin. Instr. (Prev. Med.), U. of British Columbia; Tel. CA 4-1355.

WALDIE, Bruce S.; 2461 Bloor St. W., Toronto 9, Ont.; 15 Edgevalley Dr., Islington (res); Wes '51; F.R.C.S.(C), ObstGyn; Staff, St. Joseph's Hosp.; Assoc. Staff, Queensway Gen. Hosp.; Tel. 763-5911.

WALDMAN, Sidney; Ste. 308, 736 Granville St., Vancouver 2, B.C.; 6875 Cypress St. (res); Beirut (Leb) '41; Tel. MU 5-7839.

WALDMAN, Hans K.; Island Highway, Parksville, B.C.; Hamburg (Germ.) '48; DiagRad; Staff, West Coast Gen. Hosp., Port Alberni; St. Joseph's Gen. Hosp., Comox, Cumberland Gen. Hosp., Cumberland, & Campbell River Dist. Gen. Hosp., Campbell River; Tel. 752-9515.

WALDMANN, Klara; 268 Larch St., Sudbury, Ont.; Tel. 674-2592.

WALDMANN, Stephen; 268 Larch St., Sudbury, Ont.; Budapest (Hung.) '51; FRCP(C); IntMed; Staff, Sudbury Gen., Mem. & St. Joseph's Hosp's.; Tel. 674-2592.

WALDON, Harold V.; 343 Bonner Ave., Winnipeg 16, Man.; Man '25; Tel. ED 4-4466.

WALDORF, Verne R.; Oakville Cytol. Service, 129 Reynolds St., Oakville, Ont.; Dal '53; Path; Dir. of Labs., Oakville Trafalgar Mem. Hosp.; Cons. Path., Milton Dist. Hosp., Milton; Tel. 845-5357.

WALDRON, Brian A.; Box 400, Canmore, Alta.; London (Eng.) '60; MRCS; LRCP; DRCOG; DA; Tel. 678-5511.

WALDRON, John J.; National U. (Ireland)'55; DPM; Psy; Staff, Ontario Hosp., Kingston, Ont.; Clin. Ass't. (Psy.), Queen's U.

WALES, William F.; The Westlaw Bldg., 1920 Weston Rd., Weston, Ont.; Tor'39; FRCS(C), GenSurg; Chief of Surg., Humber Mem. Hosp.; Tel. 247-2551.

WALFISH, Paul G.; 550 University Ave., Toronto 2, Ont.; Tor '58; FRCP(C), IntMed; Adjunct. Att'd. Staff, Dept. of Med., New Mount Sinai Hosp.; Research Scholar, Med. Research Council of Canada; Clin. Teach. (Med.), U. of Toronto; Tel. EM 6-7361, Loc. 401.

WALI, Mohammed N.; 4687 MacKenzie St., Montreal 26, P.Q.; Punjab (India) '58; Otol.

WALK, Franz; Goettingen (Germ.)'45; MCGP; Res., Toronto Gen. Hosp., Toronto 2, Ont.

WALKE, Lacey; McG '62; Jr. Intn., Kingston Gen. Hosp., Kingston, Ont.

WALKER, Agnes M. (Young); 31 Alexander St., Apt. 1508; Toronto 5, Ont. (res); Tor '16; D.P.H., IntMed (TB); Clin., Div. TB Prev., Ont. Dept. of Health; Retired.

WALKER, Alan J.; Drumheller Clinic, 376 Centre St., Box 508, Drumheller, Alta.; 421-5th St. E. (res); London (Eng.)'40; MRCS, LRCP, FACS, FRCS(Eng.), FRCS(C), GenSurg; Chief Surg., Drumheller Mun. Hosp.; Dist. M.O., CNR; Tel. 823-3345.

WALKER, Alfred J.; Box 1300, Regional Health Office, Rosetown, Sask.; London (Eng.)'39; MRCP(Lond.); MRCS(Eng.); LRCP(Lond.); DTM&H(Eng.); DPH(Lond.).

WALKER, Benjamin R.; Kapuskasing; Tor '55.

WALKER, Cecil E.; 193 Wilson St., Ancaster, Ont.; 54 Jerseyville Rd. W. (res); Tor '41; Tel. MI 8-4462.

WALKER, Evelyn (See Webster).

WALKER, Francis W.; 287 Queens Ave., London, Ont.; Wes'59; Anaes.; Staff, Victoria Hosp., London, Ont.; Tel. 432-5261.

WALKER, Frank N.; 218 Inglewood Dr., Toronto, Ont.; Tor '18; Retired.

WALKER, George F.; 225 Metcalfe St., Ste 502, Ottawa 4, Ont.; 69 Delong Dr. (res); Alb '56; FRCS(C); PlasSurg; Active Staff, Ottawa Gen. Hosp.; Cons. Staff, St. Vincent's Hosp. & National Defence Med. Centre; Hon. Cons. Staff, Sacred Heart Hosp., Hull; Vis. Staff, St. Louis de Montfort Hosp.; Lect. PlasSurg., U. of Ottawa; Tel. 232-1667

WALKER, George R.; 289 Cedar St., Sudbury, Ont.; 306 Stewart Dr. (res); Tor '41; M.S. (Tor.), DABS, FACS, FRCS(C), GenSurg, ThorSurg; Surg., Sudbury & Algoma San.; Chief of Staff Sudbury Mem. Hosp.; Staff, Sudbury Gen. Hosp.; Tel. 673-8447.

WALKER, George R.; 65 Victoria Ave., Chatham, Ont.; Wes '58; MCGP; Tel. EL 2-4705.
WALKER, Harold C., F/L; Tor '64; Staff, Sunnybrook Hosp., Toronto 12, Ont.

WALKER, Hilda M. (Dickey); Box 820, Fort MacLeod, Alta.; Dublin (Ire.) '51; BAO; MCGP; Tel. 234-3351.

WALKER, J. A. Leo; Ste. 300, 5300 Cote des Neiges Rd., Montreal 26, P.Q.; 4 Caron Point, Baie d'Urfe (res); McG '31; DABOS, FACS, FAAOS; FRCS(C), OrthSurg.; Hon. Cons., Mtl. Gen. & St. Mary's Hosp's.; Cons. (OrthSurg.), Queen Mary Vets'. Hosp.; Lect. (OrthSurg.), McGill U.; Tel. RE 1-7191.

WALKER, J. Harris; Raymond, Alta.; McG '43; Dist. Coroner.

WALKER, John B.; 403 Medical Dental Bldg., 450 Central Ave., London, Ont.; 380 Grosvenor St. (res); Wes '53; M.R.C.P. (Lond.), AFACC; FRCP(C), IntMed; Staff (Med.), Victoria Hosp.; Clin. Lect. (Med.) U. of Western Ontario; Ass't. Med. Dir., London Life Ins. Co.; Tel. GE 8-3498.

WALKER, John E.; Ste. 426, 925 W. Georgia St., Vancouver, B.C.; 1861 Tolmie St. (res); Tor '25; IntMed; Cons. in Med., Shaughnessy Hosp. D.V.A., Sr. in Med., Vancouver Gen. Hosp.; Clin. Ass't. Prof. of Med., U. of British Columbia; Tel. MU 1-7188.

WALKER, John H.; 484 William St., London, Ont.; 553 Dufferin Ave. (res); Wes '43; F.A.C.S., F.R.C.S.(C), GenSurg; Cons. Surg., Westminster & St. Joseph's Hosp's.; Instr. (Surg.), U. of Western Ontario; Tel. 432-4101.

WALKER, Kenneth F.; Medical Arts Bldg., Niagara Falls, Ont.; Niagara Rivr Pkwy., R.R. 1, Chippewa (res); Harvard U. (Boston, Mass., U.S.A.) '50; ObstGyn; Cons., Gyn., N.F. Gen. Hosp. & Douglas Mem., Ft. Erie; Tel. LE 8-3472.

WALKER, Lyman A.; Box 340, 151 Victoria St. E., Alliston, Ont.; Tor '36; Med. Staff, Stevenson Mem. Hosp.; Tel. 435-6282.

WALKER, Michael F. C.; 837 Princess St., Kingston, Ont.; Oxford (Eng.)'43; MRCS; LRCP; M.O., House of Providence & Prison for Women; Staff M.O., Ontario Hosp.

WALKER, Norman L.; Qns '28; Staff, Ontario Hosp., Brockville, Ont.; Retired.

WALKER, P. Janet; 23 King St. W., Stoney Creek, Ont.; Leeds (Eng.) '61; Tel. 662-8535.

WALKER, P. Reed; Alb '58; Anaes; Staff, University Hosp., Edmonton, Alta.; Abroad.

WALKER, Ralph H.; 65 Victoria Ave., Chatham, Ont.; Wes'24; MCGP; Staff, Public Gen. & St. Joseph's Hosp's.; Coroner, Kent. Co.; Home Phys., Thamesville Lodge Home for the Aged; Tel. EL 2-4075.

WALKER, Robert D.; Man'65; Res., Children's Hosp., Winnipeg 3, Man.

WALKER, Robert E.; Port Arthur Clinic, 194 Court St. N., Port Arthur, Ont.; Durham (Eng.) '55.

WALKER, Robert H.; 310 Medical Centre, 8th Ave. & 8th St. S.W., Calgary, Alta.; McG '48; FRCS(C), GenSurg; Tel. 263-4685.

WALKER, R. J.; 20 Church St. W., Smith's Falls, Ont.; Tor '23; Tel. 283-2222.

WALKER, Robert P.; Leeds & Grenville Health Unit, 70 Charles, Brockville, Ont.; Qns'23; Ass't. M.O.H., Leeds & Grenville Health Unit; Active Staff, St.-Vincent-de-Paul Hosp.; Tel. 345-5685.

WALKER, Sidney J. M.; Aberdeen (Scot.) '42; D.I.H.; (Soc. Apoth., Lond.); Clin. Div. Indus. Hygiene, Parliament Bldgs., Toronto, Ont.; Tel. 365-4075.

WALKER, Thomas J.; Box 820, Fort MacLeod, Alta.; Dublin (Ire.) '53; M.B., B.Ch., BAO; MCGP; Staff, Municipal Hosp.; Tel. 234-3351.

WALKER, Thomas L. B.; 41 Grand Ave. W., Chatham, Ont.; R.R. 1 (res); Tor '52; MCGP; Tel. EL 2-3210.

WALKER, W. Allan; 50 Sheppard Ave. E., Willowdale, Ont.; 156 Sheppard Ave. W. (res); McG '52; Paed; Clin. Ass't. Hosp. for Sick Children; Tel. BA 1-6200.

WALKER, William G.; McG'48; Res., Shaughnessy Hosp., Vancouver 9, B.C.

WALKER, W. John; 250 Main St. E., Hamilton, Ont.; Qns '46; IntMed; Court. Staff, Chedoke Hosp.; Staff, Hamilton Gen. & St. Joseph's Hosp's.; Tel. JA 7-2711.

WALKER, William T.; 212 Rideau Med. Dental Centre, 1711-4th. St. S.W., Calgary, Alta.; 105 President Apt's. (res); Man '52.

WALKO, Zbigniew S. (Bartkiewicz); 277 Powell Ave., Ottawa 1, Ont.; Beirut (Lebanon)'45; Tel. 233-8518.

WALL, Charles B.; 225 McIntyre St. W., North Bay, Ont.; 1214 Cedar Gr. Dr. (res); Wes '53; MCGP; Tel. 472-8419.

WALL, Mark B.; 404 Norlyn Bldg., 309 Hargrave St., Winnipeg 2, Man.; Man'45; FACOG; FICS; ObstGyn; Hd. Dept. of Obst., Victoria Gen. Hosp.; Active Staff, ObstGyn., St. Boniface & Misericordia Hosp's.; Tel. WH 3-8961.

WALLACE, A. Cameron; 1057 Waterloo St., London, Ont.; Wes'48; Path; Pathol., Westminster Hosp.; Prof. & Hd. Dept. of Path., U. of Western Ontario.

WALLACE, Ada I. (Wilson); 5890 Dunbar St., Vancouver 13, B.C.; Man '22.

WALLACE, Albert W.; 2435 McDonald St., Vancouver 8, B.C.; 6630 Churchill St. (res); Man '42; M.C.G.P.; Att. Staff, Vancouver Gen. Hosp.; Dem., U. of British Columbia; Tel. RE 8-0134.

WALLACE, Cecil A.; Box 71, Elora, Ont.; Wes '44.

WALLACE, Charles J.; Box 100, Zurich, Ont. London (Eng) '55; Tel. 232.

WALLACE, Donald S.; 214-6th Ave. S.W., Calgary, Alta.; Alb '54; FRCP(C); IntMed.

WALLACE, Gerald M.; 333 Ferguson St., North Bay, Ont.; R.R. No. 2, Lakeshore Rd., Corbeil (res); Tor '41; GenSurg; Phys., Dupont of Canada (Nipissing Wks.); Tel. GR 4-3010.

WALLACE, G. Scott; 1520 Fairfield Rd., Victoria, B.C.; Edinburgh (Scot.) '52; D.ObstRCOG; Active Staff, Royal Jubilee Hosp.; Court. Staff, St. Joseph's Hosp.; Tel. 382-0274.

WALLACE, Harold M.; 333 Ferguson St., North Bay, Ont.; 773 Scollard St. (res); Tor '42; GenSurg; Staff, Civic & St. Joseph's Hosp's; Surg. Cons., R.C.A.F. Stn., North Bay; Tel. GR 4-3010.

WALLACE, Harry C.; 1124-4th Ave. Wainwright, Alta. (res); Qns '11; Memb. of Council, College of P & S., Alta.; Retired.

WALLACE, James B.; New Medical Bldg., Prince Albert, Sask.; 1825-1½ Ave. W. (res); Alb '44; F.R.C.S.(C) GenSurg; Tel. 763-2681.

WALLACE, J. Douglas; Alb'40; MACH; MCGP; Ass't. Dir., Toronto Gen. Hosp., Toronto, Ont.; Tel. EM 6-8211.

WALLACE, J. W.; Goderich, Ont.; 9 Wellington St. (res); Tor '29.

WALLACE, Sallie J. — see TEASDALE, Sallie J.

WALLACE, William B.; 250 Lawrence Ave. W., Toronto 12, Ont.; 38 Wychwood Pk. (res); Tor '39; F.R.C.S.(C), Otol; Clin. Ass't. (Otol.), Hosp. for Sick Children; Cons., Sunnybrook Hosp. & Wellesley Hosp.; Clin. Instr., U. of Toronto; Tel. RU 1-2600

WALLAR, Durrand E.; Ste. 201, 2741 Portage Ave., Winnipeg 12, Man.; Qns'51; MCGP; Jr. Memb. Anaes. Assoc., Wpg. Gen. Hosp.; Pt.-time Staff, Public Health, Well Baby Clinic, St. James; Tel. 837-5881.

WALLAT, Gunter E.; Cape Town (S. Africa)'57; Anaes; Staff, Rockey Gen. Hosp., Calgary, Alta.

WALLBRIDGE, Peter H.; 21-23 Cedar N., Timmins, Ont.; 22 Lebel St., Kirkland Lake; Tor '52; GenSurg; Urol; Urol., Kirkland Lake Dist. Hosp. & St. Mary's Hop., Timmins; Tel. 267-3400, & 567-6263.

WALLER, Charles; 183 James St. S., Hamilton, Ont.; 44 Colquhoun Cres. (res); Edinburgh (Scot.) '48; DA; Anaes; Anaes., Chedoke Hosp.; Tel. JA 9-8875.

WALLER, Derek J. S/L; Guys Hosp. (London, Eng.) '53; Sr. M.O., RCAF Station, Uplands, Ottawa, Ont.

WALLER, Douglas F., Capt.; Z M 12183, Northwest Europe Bases, Germany; Alb'65; Abroad.

WALLING, Florence M.; 216 Park Victoria, South Park St., Halifax, N.S.; St. Andrews (Scot.)'53.
WALLING, Keith E.; St. Andrews (Scot.)'56; DPH; DLO; Res., Victoria Gen. Hosp., Halifax, N.S.
WALLINGFORD, Felix M.; 615 Main, Buckingham, P.Q.; Tor '33; M.C.G.P.; Cons. Phys., James McLaren Co.
WALLINGFORD, Wilson W.; Beardmore, Ont.; Tor '36.
WALLIS, Herbert B.; 290 Wellington St., Sarnia, Ont.; Toronto '40; Chief M.O., Dow Chemical of Canada; Chief of Med. Staff, St. Joseph's Hosp.; Tel. KI 2-5121.
WALLIS, Hugh M.; Ste. 24, 2221 Keele St., Toronto 15, Ont.; 9 Circle Ridge (res); Tor '44; FRCS (Eng.), FRCS(C), GenSurg; Staff Surg., Northwestern Gen. Hosp.; Tel. 247-8754.
WALLIS, W. Gerald; Ste. 608, 1405 Douglas St., Victoria, B.C.; St. Andrews (Scot.) '56; M.B., B.Ch., D.Psy; Psy; Tel. 384-4273.
WALLRAP, Albert A.; 5891 Arbutus Ave., Powell River, B.C.; Wes'61; Active Staff, Powell River Gen. Hosp.; Tel. 483-3852.
WALLS, Robert W.; 69 Margaret Ave. N., Waterloo, Ont.; 201 Vermont St. (res); Wes '54; MCGP; Staff, Kitchener-Waterloo & St. Mary's Gen. Hosp's.; Tel. 744-3397.
WALMSLEY, Douglas P.; 179 Bronte Rd., **Oakville, Ont.; Man. '51; MGCP; Tel. VA 7-3461.**
WALMSLEY, James B.; Queens U. (Belfast, Ire.)'60; Res., Royal Alexandra Hosp., Edmonton, Alta.
WALMSLEY, Joseph F. S.; 3500 Eglinton Ave. W., Toronto 15, Ont.; 19 Queen Mary Dr., Tor. 18 (res); Tor '39; DPH (Tor.); Comp. Phys., Cdn. Kodak Co. Ltd.; Tel. 766-8233, Loc. 401.
WALMSLEY, J. H.; 340 Main, Picton, Ont.; 344 Main (res); Qns '14; Tel. GR 6-5881.
WALPOLE, Joy C. (See Longley).
WALSH, A. Cyril; 214-6th Ave. W., Calgary, Alta.; 3817-9th St. S.W. (res); Man '39; OrthSurg; Att. OrthSurg., Calgary Gen. & Crippled Children's Hosp's., Head Orth. Div., Holy Cross Hosp.; Tel. AM 3-7120.
WALSH, Cyril J.; St. Lawrence, Nfld. (res); Dal '44; Staff, Lawrence Mem. Hosp.
WALSH, Edwin M.; 880 Adelaide St., London, Ont.; 769 Queens Ave. (res); Wes '53; Active Med. Staff, St. Mary's Hosp.; Tel. 434-8613.
WALSH, Frederick D.; 1499 Pharmacy Ave., Scarborough, Ont.; 51 Doonan Dr., Don Mills (res); Tor '56; MCGP; Staff, Scarborough Gen., St. Michael's & East Gen. Hosp's.; Tel. HI 4-4466.
WALSH, George C.; 5780 Cambie St., Vancouver 15, B.C.; 1344 W. 45th Ave. (res); McG '42; FACP, FRCP(C), IntMed; Att'd. Staff, Shaughnessy DVA & St. Vincent's Hosp's.; Clin. Instr., U. of British Columbia; Tel. FA 5-5123.
WALSH, J. Frazier; 294 Waterford Bridge Rd., **Box 4810, St. John's, Nfld. (res); Queen's U. (Belfast, N. Ire.) '45; Ment. Hosp. Admin. (APA); Psy; Supt., Hosp. for Mental & Nervous Diseases; Dir. Psy. Educ. Nfld.; Tel. 9-5061.**
WALSH, John; Nat. U. (Ire.) '33; DPM (Eng.); Staff, Valleyview Hosp., Port Coquitlam, B.C.; Tel. LA 1-1911.
WALSH, John A.; Manuels, Nfld.; U.K. '31; M.C.G.P.
WALSH, John E.; 33 Smithville Cres., St. John's, Nfld.; UK '46; Tel. 579-1712.
WALSH, Michael J.; Dal '58; Staff, Royal Victoria Hosp., Barrie, Ont.
WALSH, Neil F.; 21 Farm, Corner Brook, Nfld. (res); Ire. '43; D.M.R.D.; Cons. Rad., Western Memorial Hosp.
WALSH, Patric B. Capt.; Manchester (Eng.) '59; CFPO, 5050, Cdn. Armed Forces, Europe, Abroad.
WALSH, Paul J.; 121 Wellington St. W., Barrie, Ont.; Wes '57; Ophth; Active Staff, Royal Victoria Hosp.; Tel. 728-5951.
WALSH, Penelope E.; Qns '63; Res., Mtl. Gen. Hosp., Montreal 25, P.Q.; Retired.

WALSH, Robert L.; Assoc. Med. Dir., Pfizer Company Ltd., 50 Place Cremazie, Montreal 11, P.Q.; Edinburgh (Scot.) '40; DPH; MCGP; Tel. 381-9331.
WALSH, Stanley Y.; 324 Rubidge St., Peterborough, Ont.; 317 Margaret Ave. (res); Tor '15. Tel. 745-4715.
WALSH, Thomas E.; 1705 Wyandotte St., Riverside, Ont.; Wes '44; Tel. 945-2072.
WALSH, William J.; 217 James St. S., Hamilton, Ont.; 11 Oakwood Pl. (res); Wes '48; FACP; FRCP(C), IntMed; Cons. (Med.), St. Joseph's & Hamilton Civic Hosp's; Ass't. Dean (Med.), McMaster U.; Tel. 522-1182.
WALSHE, Flannan B.; Theodore, Sask.; Nat. U. (Ire.) '52.
WALTER, Arthur B., ED.; 377 Lawrence St., **Lancaster, N.B.; McG '12; FACP; FRCP(C), IntMed; Retired.**
WALTER, Dennis E.; 3418 Hill Ave., Regina, Sask.; London (Eng.) '60; MRCS (Eng.); LRCP (Lond.).
WALTER, Edward P.; 115 Hazen St., Saint John, N.B.; 170 Mt. Pleasant Ave. (res); McG '50; IntMed; Att'd. Staff, St. John Gen. & St. Joseph's Hosp's.; Cons. (Med.), Lancaster DVA & Prov. Hosp's.; Tel. Area 506; 692-8746.
WALTER, John B.; London (Eng.) '46; Staff, Dept. of Path., Banting Inst., Toronto, Ont.
WALTER, Magda M.; 713 Morin St., Ottawa 7, Ont.; Ott '61; Tel. 749-1019.
WALTERS, C. H. Austin; 126 Bridge St. E., Belleville, Ont.; Qns '30; GenSurg; Surg. Staff, Belleville Gen. Hosp.; Industrial Surg., Northern Electric Co. Ltd., & C.P.R.; Tel. WO 2-3565.
WALTERS, F. H.; 320 Regent St., London, Ont.; Wes'28; Retired.
WALTERS, Jack H.; 450 Central Ave., London, Ont.; Wes'51; MRCOG, FACS, FACOG, FRCS(C), ObstGyn; Chief (ObstGyn) & Dir. Cytol Unit, St. Joseph's Hosp.; Cons. (Gyn.), Ontario Cancer Fdn., London Clinic; Assoc. Prof. (ObstGyn.), U. of Western Ont.; Tel. GE 8-3363.
WALTERS, J. Allan; 922 Medical Arts Bldg., 170 St. George St., Toronto, Ont.; 104 Cluny Dr. (res); Tor'33; DPM(Eng.), FACP, FRCP(C), NeurPsy; Sr. Phys., Toronto Gen. Hosp.; Assoc. Prof. (Med.) & Assoc. Prof. (Psy.), U. of Toronto; Tel. WA 1-1013.
WALTERS, Kathleen J.; 104 Cluny Dr., Toronto, Ont. (res); Man '28; Psy; Retired.
WALTERS, Lawrence A.; Nipawin, Sask.; Sask '59; Staff, Nipawin Union Hosp.; Tel. 2633.
WALTERS, Lawrence G.; 1871 King St. E., Hamilton, Ont.; McG'62; AMCGP; Active Staff, Hamilton Civic Hosp.; Court. Staff, St. Joseph's & Chedoke Hosp's.; Tel. 545-3003.
WALTERS, Max B.; 750 W. Broadway, Vancouver 9, B.C.; 1092 W. 47th Ave. (res); Man '44; FACC; FACP; FRCP(C); IntMed; Staff, Shaughnessy Hosp.; Lect. (IntMed.), U. of British Columbia; Tel. TR 4-2012.
WALTERS, William C.; McG '53; IntMed; Staff, Lancaster Hosp., Saint John, N.B.; Tel. 694-2651.
WALTERS, William R.; Mildmay, Ont.; Tor '55.
WALTERS, W. Ross; 305 Main St., Toronto 13, Ont.; 320 Glen Manor Dr. (res); Tor '23; Obst-Gyn; Tel. OX 4-1400.
WALTHER, E.; 4614 Kingston Rd., West Hill, Ont.; '52.
WALTHER, Garth L.; McG '49; Path; Staff, St. Joseph's Hosp., Victoria, B.C.; Tel. 384-1131.
WALTON, Charles H.A. Ed.; Winnipeg Clinic, St. Mary & Vaughan Sts., Winnipeg 1, Man.; 2398 Portage Ave. (res); Man '32; FACP; FAAA; MCAA; IntMed; Chief of Med., Winnipeg Clinic; Phys., Winnipeg Gen. Hosp.; Cons. Allergy Children's & Misericordia Hosp's.; Assoc. Prof. (Med.), U. of Manitoba; Tel. 942-0551.
WALTON, Frederick A.; 713 Columbia St., New Westminster, B.C.; 827 Cherry St. (res); Man '33; Anaes; Anaes. Staff, Royal Columbia Hosp.; Tel. LA 2-4241.
WALTON, John H.; Box 669, Castlegar, B.C.; UBC '63; Tel. 365-6412.

WALTON, Richard J.; 154 Oak St., Winnipeg 9, Man. (res); New Zealand '39; D.M.R., D.M.R.T.; Dir., Dept. of TherRad., Winnipeg Gen. Hosp.; Assoc. Prof. (Rad.), U. of Manitoba; Exec. Dir., Manitoba Cancer Treatment & Research Fdn.; Tel. SP 4-6511; Abroad.

WALTON, Robert S.; The Pas, Man.; Liverpool (Eng.) '56; MRCS (Eng.); LRCP(Lond.).

WAN, Bang H.; Box 280, Uranium City, Sask.; Taiwan (Formosa)'62.

WANAMAKER, Frank D.; 62 Coburg St., Saint John, N.B.; Pielton Rd., Sandy Pt. (res); Dal'41* FACS, FACOG; ObstGyn; Sr. ObstGyn., Saint John Gen. Hosp.; Tel. 657-2293.

WANG, Catherine S.; Ste. 906, 1414 Drummond St., Montreal 25, P.Q.; Sask '58; Paed (P.Q.); Tel. 288-7318.

WANG, Stephan; 1663 Dufferin St., Toronto 4, Ont.; 763 Briar Hill Ave. (res); Florence (Italy) '39; Tel. LE 2-0459.

WANKLING, William J.; 26 Main St. S., Kenora, Ont.; Man'61.

WANLESS, Harold L.; 749 King St. W., Kitchener, Ont.; Tor'38; FACS; DABU; Staff, St. Mary's & Kitchener-Waterloo Hosp's.; Tel. 744-0731.

WARBURTON, E. Gilbert; Manchester (Eng.) '52; MRCP(Ed.); M.C. Path. (Eng.) Path; Dir. of Labs., York County Hosp., Newmarket, Ont.

WARCUP, Lloyd W.; 607 Fairmont Med. Bldg., 750 W. Broadway, Vancouver 9, B.C.; Tor '44; FRCS(Edin.), FRCS(C), GenSurg; Tel. 872-1123.

WARD, Clifford V.; Apt. 53, 3940 Cote des Neiges Rd., Montreal, P.Q.; McG'26; FACOG, FACS, FRCOG, FRCS(C), ObstGyn; Chm. Dept. **Obst. Gyn., Montreal Gen. Hosp.; Assoc. Prof. (Obst. Gyn.), McGill U.; Tel. WE 7-6011.**

WARD, C Stewart; 420 Oxford St., London, Ont.; 890 Clearview Ave. (res); Wes '34; Cons. Phys., Weston Enterprises & Gen. Motors; Tel. GE 3-0811.

WARD, Edward; Ott'61; Res., Toronto Western Hosp., Toronto 2B, Ont.

WARD, Francis J.; Associate Clinic, 4820 Gaetz Ave., Red Deer, Alta.; National U. (Ire.) '47; M.B., B.A.O., M.Ch, FR.CS(I); Tel. 346-2057.

WARD, John A.; Tor '55; Res., Ontario Hosp., Toronto, Ont.

WARD, John F.; UBC'60; Res., Toronto General Hosp., Toronto 2B, Ont.

WARD, Joseph H.; 189 Henderson Hwy., Winnipeg 5, Man.; 165 Scotia St. (res); Cambridge (Eng.) '36; MRCS; LRCP; MCGP; Court. Staff, St. Boniface Hosp.; Active Staff, Concordia Hosp.; **Tel. 533-6670.**

WARD, Kenneth A.; 109 Cedar St., Sudbury, Ont.; 234 Wembley Dr. (res); Wes '46; F.A.C.S., F.R.C.S.(C), GenSurg; Active Surg. Staff, Sudbury Gen., St. Joseph's & Sudbury Mem. Hosp's.; Tel. 673-9524.

WARD, Nicholas; Room 203, Riverside Med. Centre, Ottawa 8, Ont.; Oxford (Eng.)'52; Psy; MCGP; Staff Psy., Royal Ottawa San.

WARD, Pierre H.; 222 Victoria St., St. Lambert, P.Q.; Mon '54.

WARD, R. Vance; 630 Sherbrooke St. W., Montreal 2, P.Q.; 3787 Cote-des-Neiges, Apt. 507 (res); McG '24; FRCP(C), IntMed; Chief Med. Adviser, Montreal Life Ins. Co.; Tel. VI 2-9151.

WARD, Samuel L.; 845 Denman St., Vancouver, B.C.; Man'32; FICS, FRCS(Edin.), FRCS(C) GenSurg.; Tel. MU 4-2043.

WARD, Thomas F.; Thistledown Hosp., Rexdale, Ont.; Tor '54; Psy; Cons. Psy., Sacred Heart Children's Village; Cons. Metro Toronto Separate School Bd., Tel. 741-1210.

WARDILL, James C.; Ste. 201, 161 Larch St., Sudbury, Ont.; Cambridge (Eng.) '49; M.B., B.Ch., FRCS(Ed); FRCS(C), OrthSurg; Tel. 673-7131.

WARDILL, William R.; Main St., Geraldton, Ont.; Cambridge (Eng.) '46; M.R.C.P. (Lond.), M.R.C.S. (Eng.); Coroner, Dist. of Thunder Bay.

WARDROP, Dorothea M.; 11230-131st. St., Edmonton, Alta. (res); Man '39; Anaes; Retired.

WARENYCIA, Miroslaw; Germany '45; Staff, Alberta Hosp., Box 307, Edmonton, Alta.; Tel. 7-0221.

WARKENTIN, Abram P.; 315 Medical Arts Bldg., Winnipeg, Man.; 125 Riverbend Cres., St. James (res); Man '41; MCGP; Tel. WH 2-6174.

WARKENTIN, David E.; 4204 Sheppard Ave., Agincourt, Ont.; 24 Malamute (res); Tor '59; AMCGP; Tel. 293-4121.

WARKENTIN, John D.; 18 Jupiter Bay, Winnipeg 19, Man.; Wes '56; Path; Staff, St.-Boniface Hosp.; Dem. (Path.), U. of Manitoba; Tel. WH 3-0311.

WARMA, Sushil K.; Calcutta (India) '54; FRCS (Eng); GenSurg; Staff, Flin Flon Clinic, Flin Flon, Man.; Staff Flin Flon Gen. & Assoc. Hosp's.; Tel. 687-7571.

WARNE, J. W.; 1645 Commercial Dr., Vancouver, B.C.; 1994 Ogden Ave. (res); Wes '47; M.C.G.P.; Staff, St. Vincent's Hosp.; Treas., Vancouver G.P. Assoc.; Tel. AL 3-2688.

WARNER, Charles R.; London (Eng.)'42; Res., Saskatchewan Hosp., North Battleford, Sask.

WARNER, David M.; Ste. 1402, 750 W. Broadway, Vancouver 9, B.C.; London (Eng.)'51; MB; BS; Ophth; Research Assoc., U. of British Columbia.

WARNER, Donald L.; 136 E. 15th N. Vancouver, B.C.; UBC '54; MCGP; Tel. YU 7-1414.

WARNER, H. Alfred; 3550 Cote des Neiges Rd., Ste. 430, Montreal 25, P.Q.; 360 Kensington Ave. (res); McG '55; FRCP(C); IntMed (Gastroen.); Jr. Ass't. Phys., Montreal Gen. Hosp.; Chief Med. Cons., Verdun Protestant Hosp.; Dem. (Med.), McGill U.; Tel. 935-9175.

WARNER, Harry M.; 221 King St. E., Kingston, Ont.; 14 Macdonnell St. (res); McG '36; F.R.C.S.(C) GenSurg; Surg. Cons., D.V.A. & D.N.D.; Ass't. Prof. (Surg.), Queen's U.; Tel. 548-7444.

WARNER, Peter; 368 Wildwood Park, Fort Garry 19, Man. (res); London (Eng.)'44; M.R.C.S. (Eng.), L.R.C.P. (Lond), M.D. (Path, Gold Med.); Ph.D. (Lond. Virus Dis.), F.R.S.M. (Path); F.C. Path; Dir. (Dept. of Bact), Winnipeg Gen. Hosp.; Assoc. Prof. (MedBact), U. of Manitoba; Tel. SP 4-6511.

WARNER, Renate M.; 4697 Belmont Ave., Vancouver, B.C.: Queen's U. (Belfast, Ire.)'53.

WARNES, Hector; Tucuman '57; Psy; Staff, Verdun Protestant Hosp., Verdun P.Q.; Tel. 766-8511.

WARNICA, John K.; Tor '59; Res., Sunnybrook Hosp., Toronto 12, Ont.

WARNOCK, Mary D. B. (Macquistan); 1940 Lonsdale Ave., North Vancouver, B.C.; 153 West Balmoral Ave. (res); Manchester (Eng.) '50; MRCS; LRCP; Retired.

WARR, G. Owen; 314 Kerr St. N., Oakville, Ont.; 137-8th Line N. (res); Dal '50; Tel. 845-4213.

WARREN, Alfred J.; 710—925 W. Georgia St., Vancouver, B.C.; 4185 Angus Dr. (res); Man '36; D.P.M. (Lond.), F.A.P.A., Neur, Psy; Att. Staff (Psy.), Vancouver Gen. Hosp.; Clin. Instr. (Psy.). U. of British Columbia; Tel. MU 3-6144.

WARREN, Carmi M.; 105 Yonge Blvd., Toronto 12. Ont.; Tor '29; MCGP; Court. Staff, St. Michael's Hosp. & Bethesda Hosp.; Exec. Sec., Ontario Chapter College of G.P. of Canada; Tel. HU 8-9734.

WARREN, Donald A.; 221 Jackson St. W., Hamilton, Ont.; Tor '12; F.I.C.A., Anaes; Cons. Anaes., Hamilton Gen. Hosp., & Mountain San.; Dist. Coroner; Tel. JA 9-1808.

WARREN, Donald P.; Ste. 10, 285-17th St., West Vancouver, B.C.; Tor'60; FRCP(C), IntMed; Tel. 926-2622.

WARREN, Douglas R.; 168 Essex St., Sarnia, Ont.; Tor '41; DPH (Tor); MCGP; Staff, Sarnia Gen. & St. Joseph's Hosp's.; Med. Dir., Occupational Health Assoc. (Canada), Cabot Carbon of Canada Ltd., Catalytic Construction of Canada Ltd., & Ethyl Corp. of Canada Ltd.; Sarnia Cons. in Occupat. Health for: Allied Chemicals Canada, Bell Telephone Co. of Canada, Canadian Badger Co. Ltd., DuPont of Canada Ltd., Hudson's Bay Co., Mueller Ltd., Ralph E. Parsons Construction of Canada Ltd., Shell Canada Ltd., Sun Oil Operations & Union Gas Co. of Canada Ltd.; Tel. 337-3243.

WARREN, Gerald W.; 11 East Valley Rd., Cornerbrook, Nfld. Dal '61.

WARREN, James D.; 170 Med. Arts Bldg., 1105 Pandora Ave., Victoria, B.C.; Man '57; M.Sc. (Anat.); FRCS(C), OrthSurg.

WARREN, MacDonald R.; 900 Arthur St., Fort William, Ont.; 607 Rosewood Cres. (res); Tor '52; D.P.H.; Dir. & M.O.H., Fort William & Dist. **Health Unit; Tel. 322-5367.**

WARREN, Peter L.; 712 Canada Bldg., Saskatoon, Sask; Mon '22; M.C.G.P.; Tel. 242-3882.

WARREN, Ralph E.; Qns'61; FRCP(C), IntMed; Staff, Kingston Gen. Hosp., Kingston, Ont.; Abroad.

WARREN, Rupert F.; 1639B Bayview Ave., Toronto 17, Ont.; 9 Fleming Cres. (res); Tor '43; FICS, FRCS(C), GenSurg; Chief of Surg., Bethesda Hosp., & Active Staff, Branson Hosp., Willowdale; Tel. 485-2024.

WARREN, Stanley L.; Ste 309, 99 Avenue Rd., Toronto 5, Ont.; 31 Arrowstook Rd., Willowdale, (res); Tor '58; AMCGP; Staff, Doctor's Hosp.; Tel. LE 6-5551.

WARREN, Sydney A.; 2804 Bathurst St., Toronto, Ont.; 131 Dalemount (res); Tor '43; D.A.B.P.; **MCAA; Paed; Paed. Staff & Aller. Clin., New** Mt. Sinai Hosp.; Tel. 781-4323.

WARREN, W. Donald; 348 Simcoe St. N., Oshawa, Ont.; Tor '48; DIH; FACPM; DAB (Prev. Med.); Tel. 725-5274.

WARREN, William J.; Elnora, Alta.; Tor '27; Med. Staff, Elnora Mun. Hosp.

WARREN William P.; Dal'61; FRCP(C), IntMed; Staff, Victoria Gen. Hosp., Halifax, N.S.

WARRIAN, William G.; Man'65; Res., Deer Lodge Hosp., Winnipeg 12, Man.

WARRICK, Hubert J.; Medical Arts Bldg., Empire Ave., St. John's, Nfld.; St. Mary's H. (London, Eng.) '55; MCGP; Act. Staff, St. Clare's, Mercy, St. John's Gen. & Chief, Dept. of G.P., Grace Hosp's.; Editor, Nfld. Med. Assoc. Newsletter; Tel. 9-1171.

WARRINGTON, Alfred M.; 645 Fort St., Victoria, **B.C.;** 855 Pemberton Rd. (res); London (Eng.) '53; M.B., B.S.(Lond.); MCGP; Active Staff, St. Joseph's Hosp.; Court. Staff, Royal Jubilee Hosp.; Tel. 385-4511.

WARSHAW, H. L.; 403 Blvd. St. Joseph W., Montreal, P.Q.; McG '19; Tel. 271-5616.

WARSHWASKI, Edward; 163 Queenston St., St. Catharines, Ont.; Alb'52; PlasSurg; Tel. 685-0233 & 685-0291.

WARSHAWSKI, Herman; 403 St. Joseph Blvd. W., Montreal 8, P.Q.; McG'17.

WARSHAWSKI, Stanley J.; 103 LeMarchand **Bldg., Edmonton, Alta.;** 48 St. George's Cr. (res); **Alb '43; Otol; Tel. 488-7766.**

WARWARUK, Allan S.; 1428 Ouellette Ave., Windsor, Ont.; Sask'61; FRCS(C), ObstGyn.

WARWICK, O. Harold; 1642 Gloucester Rd., London, Ont. (res); McG '40; MRCP (Lond.); **FACP; Vice-Pres., Health Sciences, U. of Western Ontario; Tel. 679-3811.**

WARWICK, William E.; 1020 Victoria Ave., Fort William, Ont.; Qns'51.

WASHBURN, Herbert H.; 135 Union St., Simcoe, Ont.; Wes '36; DPH; Dir. & Med. Officer, Norfolk County Health Unit; Tel. 426-6170.

WASHBURN, Robert E.; 166 Douglas St., Sudbury, Ont.; Dal '47; R. T. (Can.); M. T. (ASCP); MCGP.

WASILEWSKA, Julia; 61 Lesperance St., St. Lambert, Montreal 23, P.Q.; Warsaw (Poland) **'27; Tel. OR 1-7059.**

WASMAN-CUNNINGHAM, Helen; Box 126, 233 Champlain St., Beloeil Station, P.Q.; Tor '47.

WASS, Norman H.; Sanatorium Residence, West Coast San., Corner Brook, Nfld.; Queen's U. (Belfast, N. Ire.)'39; Dir., West Coast San.; Tel. NE 4-4951.

WASSER, David A.; 1380 Kingsway, New Westminster, B.C. (res); Tor '48; Staff, Crease Clinic, Essondale, B.C.

WASSERMAN, David; 18 Barton Ave., Toronto, Ont.; Vienna (Austria)'23; Derm. Syph.; Tel. LE 1-1233.

WASSERMAN, John M.; Mall Medical Bldg., Winnipeg, Man.; 1123 Grosvenor Ave. (res); Qns '44; Assoc. (Med.), Miscordia Hosp.; Clinic **Ass't. (Med.), Children's Hosp.; Tel. SP 4-6581.**

WASTY, G. Husain; Adelaide (Aust.)'61; Res., Shaughnessy Hosp., Vancouver 9, B.C.

WASYLENKI, Alexander J.; 606 Med. Dental Bldg., Rose St. & 11th Ave., Regina, Sask.; Tor '42; MCGP; Tel. 527-2651.

WASYLENKI, Eugene W.; Tor '62; Jr. Intn., Toronto Western Hosp., Toronto, Ont.

WASYLENKI, Joseph M.; 606 Medical & Dental Bldg., Regina, Sask; 94 Langley St. (res); Ott '57; MCGP; Tel. 527-2651.

WASYLENKI, Morris; 46 Ontario Ave., Elliot Lake, Ont.; 1 Brown Rd. (res); Tor '53; DABS, FACS, FRCS(C), GenSurg; Chief of Surg., St. Joseph's Hosp.; Tel. VI 8-7176.

WASYLENKO, John; 1 Foxley St., Toronto 3, Ont.; 3 High Park Blvd. (res); Tor '32; M.C.-G.P.; Tel. 922-8657.

WATANABE, Hiroko; McG '64; Res., Royal Victoria Hosp., Montreal 2, P.Q.; Abroad.

WATANABE, Satoru; 157 Westcliffe Ave., Pointe Claire, Montreal 33, P.Q. (Res.); McG '44; Path. (P.Q.); Pathol., Queen Elizabeth Hosp., Montreal; Tel. HU 8-2311.

WATELLE, Hubert; Lorrainville, P.Q.

WATERLOW, Doreen E.; 619 Forrest Dr., Trail, B.C.; McG'49; Staff, Trail Tadanac Hosp.; Court. Staff, Mater Misericordia Hosp., Rossland; Tel. 368-5454.

WATERMAN, Robert A.; 1538 Foster St., White Rock, B.C.; 1501 High (res); Alb '52; MCGP; Tel. 531-5575.

WATERS, W. Reid; Winnipeg Clinic, St. Mary & Vaughan, Winnipeg, Man.; 745 Niagara St. (res); McG '55; FRCS(C); PlasSurg; Ass't. Surg., Winnipeg Gen. Hosp.; Att'd. Surg., Winnipeg Children's Hosp. & Misericordia Hosp.; Lect. (Surg.), U. of Manitoba; Tel. 942-0551.

WATKIN, G. S.; Tor'64; Res., New Mount Sinai Hosp., Toronto 2, Ont.

WATKINS, David B.; 249 Main St. W., Brampton, Ont.; Eng '61; Tel. 451-1937.

WATKINS, George B.; Ste. 108, 404 Graham Ave., Winnipeg 1, Man.; Sydney (Aust.) '47; M.B., B.S.; DMRD (Eng.), DiagRad.

WATKINS, Gillian M.; 66 Academy Med. Bldg., 1812-4th St. S.W., Calgary, Alta.; Aberdeen (Scot.) **'56; M.B., ChB; Paed; Tel. AM 9-2371.**

WATKINS, Robert T.; Kimberley, B.C.; Man '42.

WATKINSON, Ernest A.; Health Serv. Branch, Dept. of National Health & Welfare, 1138 Brooke Claxton Bldg., Ottawa, Ont.; Qns'39; DPH(Tor); Dir., General Health Serv.; Tel. 992-7376.

WATSON, Alexander G.; 267 O'Connor St., Ottawa, Ont.; 50 Lyttleton Gdns., Rockcliffe Pk. (res); St. Andrew's (Scot.) '44; A.B. Ophth; F.R.C.S.(C), Ophth; **Staff, Ottawa Gen. Hosp;** Ass't. Prof. (Ophth), Ottawa U.; Tel. CE 6-5548.

WATSON, Alvin B.; 101 Med. Dental Bldg., 10504-10th St., Dawson Creek, B.C.; 10405-13th St. (res); **Man '44; MCGP; Dist. Coroner; Tel. ST 2-3133.**

WATSON, Andrew R.; Edinburgh (Scot.) '43; DiagRad; Staff, Consolidated Hosp., New Waterford, N.S. & Sydney City Hosp., Sydney.

WATSON, Charles A.; 3460 Bonair Pl., Victoria, B.C. (res); McG '23; Supt., Veterans' Hosp., Victoria; Retired; Tel. EV 2-4221.

WATSON, Clifford H.; 520 Medical Arts Bldg., 170 St. George St., Toronto, Ont.; **Tor '21; F.R.-C.S. (Edin.), F.R.C.S.(C) GenSurg; Staff, St. Michael's Hosp.; Cons. in Surg., Sunnybrook Hosp.; Assoc. Prof., U. of Toronto; Tel. WA 2-1393.**

WATSON, C. Maurice; 13603-81st Ave., Edmonton, Alta. (res); Dublin (Ire.) '50; Anaes; Staff, Royal Alexandra Hosp.; Tel. HU 8-0805.

WATSON, Derek; London (Eng.) & Melbourne (Aust.) '48; Staff, Dept. of Labs., Royal Columbian Hosp., New Westminster, B.C

WATSON, Earle M.; 427 Regent St., London, Ont. (res); **Wes '19; F.A.C.P., F.R.C.P.(Edin.),** F.R.C.P.(C), IntMed; Semi-retired; Tel. 432-1510.
WATSON, E. E.; 1478 Kingston Rd., Scarborough, **Ont.; Tor '41; MCGP; Tel. OX 1-1572.**
WATSON, George F.; 11 Weber St. W., Kitchener, Ont.; 244 Stanley Dr. (res); Tor '21; Tel. 745-5873.
WATSON, Gerald L.; 2025 W. Broadway, Vancouver 9, B.C.; 6343 Granville St., Vanc. 13 (res); Man '34; Dir. of Med. Serv., Med. Serv. Assoc.; Tel. RE 8-3238.
WATSON, Harry N.; Ste. 304, 625-5th Ave., New Westminster, B.C.; 313 Queen's Ave., New Westminster (res); McG '48; M.C.G.P.; Teach., Nurses Training, Royal Columbian Hosp.; Dir., B.C. Med. Plan; Tel. LA 1-7535.
WATSON, Hector L.; 2933-5th Ave., Regina, Sask.; Qns '38; Tel. 523-6473.
WATSON, J. H. LT/COL; Sub. Reg. Surg., Western Ont. Med. Sub. Reg., Wolseley Barracks, London, Ont.; Dal '42; DPH (Tor); Pt-time Clin. Ass't. Prof. (PrevMed.), U. of Western Ontario.
WATSON, J. Ian; McG'60; FRCP(C), IntMed; Staff, Royal Victoria Hosp., Montreal 2, P.Q.
WATSON, Melville C.; 518 Medical Arts Bldg., 170 St. George St., Toronto, Ont.; 20 Thornwood Rd. (res); Tor '22; ObstGyn; Staff, Toronto Gen. Hosp.; **Cons., Sunnybrook Hosp. Ass't. Prof. (ObstGyn.); U. of Toronto; Tel. WA 2-4484.**
WATSON, Paul A.; 116 W. 15th St., North Vancouver, B. C.; UBC '62.
WATSON, Peter M.; Med. Arts Bldg., 121 Wellington St. W., Barrie, Ont.; Tor '56; Tel. 728-2476.
WATSON, R. E. L.; 3800 St. Patrick St., Montreal, P.Q.; 1680 Athlone Rd. Mtl. 16 (res); McG '34; Med. Dir., Crane Ltd.; Cons., Cdn. Potteries Ltd. & Warden & King Ltd.; Tel. RE 8-9106.
WATSON, Robert J.; 11 Adelaide St. N., Lindsay, Ont.; 27 Elgin St. (res); Tor '54; FACS; FRCS (C); GenSurg; Staff, Ross Mem. Hosp.; Tel. 324-6159 & 324-6150.
WATSON, Roland; Box 217, Frontier, Sask.; Liverpool (Eng.)'38.
WATSON, Ronald K.; Winnipeg Clinic, St. Mary's & Vaughan, Winnipeg 1, Man.; Man '53; **Otol; Dem. (Otol.), U. of Man.; Tel. WH 2-6441.**
WATSON, Stanley H.; 2401-22nd Ave. S., Lethbridge, Alta. (res); McG '55; Path; Path Staff Lethbridge Mun. & St. Michael's Hosp's.
WATSON, Thomas A.; 391 South St., London, Ont.; 484 Huntingdon Dr. (res); New Zealand '37; FACR; DMR (Eng.); TherRad; Hd. Dept. of TherRad., Victoria Hosp.; Dir., Ont. Cancer Fdn., London Clinic; Clin. Prof. & Hd. Dept. of TherRad., U. of Western Ont.; Tel. GE 2-5261, Loc. 380.
WATSON, Thomas P.; General Delivery, Duncan, B.C.; McG '40.
WATSON, Wayne R.; Group Health Assoc., 240 McNabb St., Sault Ste. Marie, Ont.; Wes'65.
WATSON, William E.; CFMS Clinic, 1107 Avenue Rd., Toronto, Ont.; Glasgow (Scot.)'44; DPH; DHA; M.O., RCAMC; Tel. 633-6200.
WATT, Adrien N.; Box 124, Uxbridge, Ont.; London (Eng.)'51; MRCS; LRCP; Dip. Anaes; Staff, Uxbridge & Perry Hosp's.; Tel. 852-6326.
WATT, Alan C.; Assoc. Med. Clinic, Westlock, Alta.; Aberdeen (Scot.)'58; Active Staff, Immaculata Hosp.; Tel. 342-3341.
WATT, Arthur J.; Tor '34; F.C.C.P., IntMed (TB); Staff Phys., Beck Memorial San., London, **Ont.; Instr. (Med.), U. of Western Ontario;** Tel. 471-1440.
WATT, David L.; 711 Med. Arts Bldg., 170 St. George St., Toronto 5, Ont.; Tor '54; FRCP(C), IntMed (Cardiol.); Staff, Toronto Gen. Hosp.; Cons. (Cardiol.), Sunnybrook DVA Hosp.; Clin. Teach., U. of Toronto; Tel. WA 3-4866.
WATT, G. Leslie; 711 Med. Arts Bldg., 170 St. George St., Toronto 5, Ont.; 16 Garfield Ave., Tor. 7 (res); Tor '26; ObstGyn; Sr. ObstGyn., Toronto Gen. Hosp.; **Assoc. Prof. (ObstGyn), U. of Toronto; Tel. WA 1-7641.**
WATT, H. James; 730 Med. Arts Bldg., 170 St. George St., Toronto 5, Ont.; 98 Lytton Blvd., Tor. 12 (res); Tor '53; FRCP(C), IntMed; Staff, St. Joseph's Hosp.; Cons. (Haem.), South Peel Hosp., Queensway & Humber Mem. Hosp's.; Clin. Dem. Med., U. of Toronto; Tel. WA 2-1275.
WATT, James C.; Apt. 221, The Clifton, 11 Elm Ave., Toronto 5, Ont. (res); Tor '10; Prof. Emeritus, U. of Toronto; Retired.
WATT, James G.; 205 Toronto Western Med. Bldg., 25 Leonard Ave., Toronto 2B, Ont.; 295 **Inglewood Dr. (res); Tor '41; FACP; FRCP(C), IntMed; Att'd. Phys., Toronto Western Hosp.;** Assoc.-in-Med., U. of Toronto; Director, The Carling Brewereies Ltd.; Cons., Cdn. Breweries; Tel. EM 6-2067.
WATT, John G.; Ste. 60, 3195 Granville St., Vancouver 9, B.C.; UBC '56; FRCS(C), OrthSurg; Vis. Staff, Vancouver Gen., St. Vincent's, St. Paul's & Burnaby Gen. Hosp's; Att'd. Staff, Shaughnessy Hosp.; Tel. RE 1-4611.
WATT, John S.; Box 679, Redwater, Alta; Aberdeen (Scot.) '56; MCGP; Chief of Med. Staff, St. Joseph's Hosp., Radway; Tel. 735-3649.
WATT, Lindsay O.; 190 MacLaren St., Ottawa 4, Ont.; 499 Island Park Dr. (res); Qns '36; M.R.-C.O.G., F.R.C.S. (Eng.), F.R.C.S.(C), ObstGyn; Staff, ObstGyn, Ottawa Civic Hosp.; Staff, Grace Hosp.; Clin. Ass't. (ObstGyn), U. of Ottawa; Tel. 236-1901.
WATT, W. Donald; 6762 Cypress St., Vancouver 14, B.C.; Tor '50; MCGP; Supt. of Hospitals, Board of Home Missions, The United Church of Canada; Tel. 266-5426.
WATT, W. Gordon; Oshawa Clinic, 117 King St. E., Oshawa, Ont. 348 Masson St. (res); Qns '29; Paed.; Tel. 728-1661.
WATT, William; 38 Bathgate Bay, Fort Garry, Man. (res); Aberdeen (Scot.) '42; DPH; Med. Dir., CARE Serv., Prov. of Man.; Tel. 942-6313.
WATT, William N.; St. Andrew's (Scot.)'38; Staff, Camp Hill Hosp., Halifax, N.S.
WATTERS, Gordon V.; 795 Goulding St., Winnipeg, Man. (res); Man '57; FRCP(C), Neur; Paed; Staff, Children's Hosp.; Lect. U. of Manitoba; Tel. SP 5-8311. Abroad.
WATTERS, Neil A.; Ste. 607, 1849 Yonge St., Toronto 7, Ont.; Tor '44; FACS; FRCS(C); GenSurg; Surg-in-Chief, Wellesley Hosp.; Assoc. Prof. (Surg.), U. of Toronto; Tel. 485-3242.
WATTERS, Robert; Fairhaven Rd., Hudson, P. Q. (res); Tor '53; MCGP; Med. Dir., Horner Pharmaceuticals Ltd., 5485 Ferrier St., Montreal; Tel. RE 1-3931.
WATTERS, Wendell W.; 3485 Atwater Ave., Montreal 25, P.Q.; Dal '53; Psy; Staff, Mtl. Gen. Hosp.; Tel. WE 7-6011.
WATTERS, William N.; 53 St. Patrick St., Goderich, Ont.; Wes '40.
WATTERSON, Donald J.; 611 Fairmont Med. Bldg., 750 W. Broadway, Vancouver 9, B.C.; Cambridge (Eng.) '36; M.D. (Cantab.); DPM (Lond); Psy; Att'd. Phys., Vancouver Gen. & St. Paul's Hosp's.; Cons. Psy., U. Health Service; Ass't. Prof., U. of British Columbia; Tel. 876-5111.
WATTS, A. Reginald, F/L; CFB Edmonton, Lancaster Park, Alta.; Alb'63.
WATTS, George O.; 825 Coxwell Ave., Toronto 6, Ont.; 54 Rykert Cres. (res); Tor '40; F.R.-C.P.(C), NeurPsy; Cons. Neur., Sunnybrook Hosp.; Tel. HO 1-1500.
WATTS, Henry M.; 194 Princess St., Saint John N.B.; 42 Cliff St. (res); Bologna (Italy) '39; IntMed; Chief of Med., St. Joseph's Hosp.; Att. Phys., St. John's Gen. Hosp.; Tel. 693-2700.
WATTS, Philip R.; 9367 Kingsway, Burnaby, B.C.; Alb'64; Tel. 434-8781.
WATTS, Terrence G.; Qns'62; Res., General Hosp., St. John's, Nfld.
WATTS, William G.; 550 Burnhamthorpe Rd., Etobicoke, Ont.; 23 Hernshaw Cres. (res); Qns '43; D.P.H.; M.O.H., Etobicoke.
WATTY, Edward I.; 68 Broadpath Rd., Don Mills, Ont.; Aberdeen (Scot.)'50; Path.

WAUD, Russell A.; 493 Baker St., London, Ont.; Wes'21; Ph.D., FACC (Card.); Assoc. Med. Dir., C. R. Will Pharmaceuticals, (Div. of Cdn. Duphar); Tel. 433-3951.

WAUGH, Douglas; Boulderwood, Armdale, N.S. (res); McG '42; M.Sc. (Path); Ph.D. (Path); FRCP(C), Path; Prof. & Hd., Dept. of Path., Dalhousie U. & Pathology Inst.; Tel. 422-1361, Ext. 306.

WAUGH, E. Harrison; 137 Wellington St., Sarnia, Ont.; Man '51; GenSurg; Assoc. Staff Surg., St. Joseph's & Sarnia Gen. Hosp's.; Tel. DI 4-5261.

WAUGH, Frederick P.; Man '53; Winnipeg Clinic, St. Mary's & Vaughan, Winnipeg, Man.

WAUGH, George A.; 625 Med. Arts Bldg., Winnipeg, Man.; 150 Wildwood Park (res); Man '43; FRCS(C), GenSurg; Surg. Staff, Wpg. Gen. & Deer Lodge Hosp's.; Ass't. Prof. (Surg.), U. of Manitoba; WH 3-8579.

WAUGH, Ian G., Drayton Valley, Alta.; Oxford (Eng.) '45; Tel. 542-3475.

WAUGH, Jack A.; 232 Medical Arts Bldg., Winnipeg, Man.; 60 Cordova St. (res); Man '38; **M.C.G.P.; Tel. WH 3-5495.**

WAUGH, Janet M. (See McGOEY).

WAX, Sydney L.; 609 Bloor St. W., Toronto 4, Ont.; 1 Model Ave., Downsview (res); Tor '52; M.C.G.P.; D.N.B.M.E.; Att'd. Phys., Jewish Home for the Aged; Jr. Clin. Phys., New Mt. Sinai Hosp.; Vis. Staff, Baycrest & Doctor's Hosp's.; Tel. LE 4-4214.

WAY, Roland C.; McG'58; FRCP(C), Paed; Staff, I.G.A. Hosp., St. Anthony, Nfld.; Abroad.

WAYE, Roma I. (Merritt); Workmen's Compensation Board, 90 Harbour St., Toronto, Ont.; Tor'42; Tel. 362-3411.

WAYNE, David L.; Calgary Assoc. Clinic, 214-6th Ave. S.W., Calgary, Alta.; 3152 Leduc Cres. (res); McG '53; DABR; MACR; DiagRad; Ass't. Rad., Holy Cross Hosp.; Tel. AM 3-7120.

WAYNE, Irving; Tor'42; Res., Ontario Hosp., 999 Queen St. W., Toronto 3, Ont.

WEARE, Maxwell K.; Box 398, Smithers, B.C.; Wes '50.

WEARE, William G.; 2150 Valley Way, Niagara Falls, Ont.; Tor '41; OrthSurg.

WEARING, Morris P.; 289 Dufferin Ave., London, Ont.; 14 Grosvenor St. (res); Wes '42; FACOG; ObstGyn; Clin. Ass't. Prof. (ObstGyn), U. of Western Ont.; Tel. 432-6151.

WEATHERILT, Joseph L.; Lamont, Alta.; Alb '43; IntMed; Staff, Archer Mem. Hosp.

WEATHERSTON, Charles E.; Medical Arts Bldg., 121 Wellington St. W., Barrie, Ont.; Qns '56; FRCS(C); ObstGyn; Tel. 728-5311.

WEAVER, E. Gwendolen; 90 Queen St., St. Catharines, Ont.; 4 Vergorda Circle (res); Tor '33; Active Staff, (Paed.), St. Catharines & Hotel-Dieu Hosp's.; Tel. 685-7431.

WEAVER, Howard G.; 750 W. Broadway, Vancouver 9, B.C.; 6248 Balaclava St. (res); Qns **'41; MCGP; Att'd. Staff, Vancouver Gen. Hosp.; Tel. TR 4-2820.**

WEAVER, Kenneth S.; 818-9th Ave. N., Port Alberni, B.C.; 411 Mar St. (res); Man '45; GenSurg.; Tel. 723-2111.

WEAVER, Morley A.; 88 Wentworth St. S., Hamilton, Ont.; Qns '42; DOMS (Eng.); Ophth; Chief of Ophth., St. Joseph's Hosp.; Active Staff, Hamilton Civic Hosp's.; Cons. Staff, Joseph Brant Hosp.; Court. Staff, Chedoke Gen. Hosp.; Tel. 522-3563.

WEAVER, Richard T.; 307 Medical Arts Bldg., Hamilton, Ont.; 39 Homewood Ave. (res); Tor '24; FRCS(C), ObstGyn; Tel. JA 7-4224.

WEAVER, S. Armand; Box 639, Medical Centre, Ponoka, Alta.; Alb'43; MCGP; Tel. 783-3306.

WEAVER, Wilber A.; 1470 Ontario St., Burlington, Ont.; 432 Brant St. (res); Qns '14; Phys., Niagara Brand Spray; Lect. (Anat.), St. Joseph's Hosp., Hamilton; District Coroner; Tel. NE 4-4833.

WEAVER, William W.; 27 Marmora St., Trenton, Ont.; Tor '51; MCGP; Active Staff, Trenton Mem. & Belleville Gen. Hosp's.; Tel. EX 2-3887.

WEBB, Donald A.; 1940 Lonsdale Ave., North Vancouver, B.C.; 615 King Georges Way, West Vanc. (res); Alb '51; ObstGyn; Active Staff, Lions Gate & North Vancouver Gen. Hosp's.; Vis. Staff, St. Paul's & Grace Hosp's.; Tel. YU 5-3233.

WEBB, Eric; 829 W. Broadway, Vancouver, B.C.; 1512 Acadia Rd. (res); Wes '40; D.A., Anaes; Att. Staff, Anaes., Vancouver Gen. & Children's Hosp's.; Clin. Instr. in Anaes., U. of British Columbia; Tel. TR 6-3211. Abroad.

WEBB, G. Allen; 360 Devonshire Ave., Woodstock, Ont.; **347 Light St. (res); Wes '37; Head, Dept. of Anaes., Woodstock Gen. Hosp.; Tel. 537-2527.**

WEBB, Jean F.; 1833 Riverside Dr., Ottawa, Ont. (res); McG'42; DPH, Paed; Chief, Div. of Child & Maternal Health, Dept. of Natl. Health & Welfare, Ottawa; Spec. Lect., Schl. of Hygiene, U. of Tor.; Tel. 922-2909.

WEBB, Marian L.; Alb '58; Med. Supt., Indian Hosp., North Battleford, Sask.; Tel. 445-4461.

WEBB, Stanley; Seeley's Bay, Ont.; Qns'53; Phys. (Pt.-time), Joyceville Penitentiary; Tel. 124.

WEBB-LEWIS, H. Barbara; 1610 Pine Ave. W., **Montreal 25, P.Q.; 5 Mercier St., Dollard-des-Ormeaux (res); McG '60; Tel. WE 7-4659.**

WEBBER, Stuart C.; 4349 E. Hastings St., North Burnaby, B.C.; McG '50; Chief of Staff, Burnaby Gen. Hosp.; Tel. CY 9-4388.

WEBBER, William A.; UBC'58; Assoc. Prof., Dept. of Anat., U. of British Columbia, Vancouver, B.C.

WEBER, Clifton R.; Dept. of Health, 2090 Wyandotte St., E., Windsor, Ont.; Tor '26; IntMed (TB) Dir., T.B. Control, Metro Windsor-Essex County; Tel. 254-4705.

WEBER, James L.; 440 Browns Line, Toronto 14, Ont.; Wes '55; FRCP(C); Paed; Clin, Ass't., Hosp. for Sick Children; Cons. (Paed.), Princess Margaret Hosp.; Clin. Teach., U. of Toronto; Tel. CE 1-7251.

WEBER, John J.; Tor '30; F.A.C.C.P., F.A.P.A., IntMed. (TB), Psy; Med. Supt., Ontario Hosp., Woodstock, Ont.; Retired.

WEBER, Robert K.; Tor'58; AMCGP; FRCP(C), Anaes; Staff, Toronto Gen. Hosp., Toronto 2, Ont.

WEBER, Walter H.; Tor'27; D.Psy; Psy; Pt.-time Staff, Ontario Hosp., Hamilton, Ont.

WEBSTER, Anthony C.; 172 Emma St., Guelph, Ont.; Leeds (Eng.)'52; FFA; Anaes.

WEBSTER, A. Rae; Kingston, N.S.; Dal '58; Ass't Med. Exam. (Prov.), W. King's Co. Dist.

WEBSTER, Desmond M.; 236 King St. W., Brockville, Ont.; London (Eng.)'50; Psy; Dir. Pt.-time Mental Health Clinic; Tel. 342-9427.

WEBSTER, Donald R., O.B.E.; 565 Roslyn Ave., Westmount, Montreal, P.Q.; **Dal '23; Ph. D.** (McG), FACS, FRCS(C), GenSurg; **Prof. of Surg. & Dir. Experimental Labs., McGill U.; Att'd. Surg., Royal Victoria Hosp.; Tel. VI 4-7697.**

WEBSTER, Evelyn (Walker); 19 Summerhayes Cr., R.R. No. 6, Brantford, Ont.; Leeds (Eng.) '55; M.B., Ch.B.; Retired.

WEBSTER, Harry W.; Port Alberni Med. Bldg., 818-9th Ave. N., Port Alberni, B.C.; UBC '54; MCGP; Tel. 723-2111.

WEBSTER, John; Notukeu Clinic, Vanguard, Sask.; Liverpool (Eng.)'60; M.B., Ch.B.; DObst-RCOG; Tel. 61.

WEBSTER, John Alexander; 12 Parade St., Yarmouth, N.S.; P.O. Box 327 (res); Dal '38; F.A.-C.S., GenSurg; Chief of Surg., Yarmouth Reg. Hosp.; Tel. 742-4121.

WEBSTER, J. Russell; 487 Edison Ave., Ottawa 13, Ont. (res); Tor '27; GenSurg; Pres., College of Physicians & Surgeons of Ont.; Tel. 722-3114.

WEBSTER, Kenneth; Man'63; Res., Child Guidance Clinic, Winnipeg 3, Man.

WEBSTER, Marion (See Morgan).

WEBSTER, Mary E. (Wimpory); 31 Southwick St., St. Thomas Ont.; 31 Southwick St. (res); Wes '41.

WEBSTER, W. Grant; 31 Southwick St., St. Thomas, Ont.; Wes '41; Staff, Ontario Hosp.

WEBSTER, William R.; 336 Main St. E., Hamilton, Ont.; Wes'37; Active Staff, St. Joseph's Hosp.; Phys., Bell Telephone Co.; Tel. JA 2-1700.
WECKOWICZ, Thaddeus E.; Polish Schl. of Med. (Edinburgh, Scot.) '45; DPM (Leeds); Psy; Staff, (Psy), University Hosp.; Ass't. Prof. (Psy & Psychol.), U. of Alberta; Tel. GE 9-4951.
WEDDELL, John A.; 4826 Ross St., Red Deer, Alta.; 4532 Waskasoo Cres. (res); Tor '40; MCGP; Staff, Red Deer Mun. Hosp.; Cons. Staff, Eckville Mun. Hosp.; Tel. 346-2042.
WEDDERSPOON, David K.; 4 Briarfield Cr., St. Catharines, Ont. (res); Tor '53; DiagRad; Staff, Hotel Dieu Hosp.; Tel. 684-9201.
WEDER, Carman H.; 656 Med. Arts Bldg., Saskatoon, Sask.; 505 Garrison Cres. (res); Alb '43; F.A.C.S., F.R.C.S.(C), GenSurg; Staff, University, **City & St. Paul's Hosp's.; Assoc. Prof.** (Surg.), & Lect. (Anat.), U. of Saskatchewan; Tel. 653-3366.
WEDLOCK, William; 319 Boswell Ave., Peterborough, Ont.; Qns'49; Active Staff, St. Joseph's & Peterborough Civic Hosp's.; Tel. 742-6311.
WEE, Roberto L.; Philipp. '64; Jr. Int., Winnipeg Gen. Hosp., Winnipeg, Man.
WEEDEN, Richard P.; 208 Mary St., Chilliwack, B.C.; 46163 Sycamore Pl. (res); UBC '58; Active Staff, Chilliwack Gen. Hosp.; Tel. SY 2-9441.
WEEKES, William E.; Ste. 101, 6455 West Boulevard, Vancouver 13, B.C. (res); Wes '20; M.O., D.V.A.
WEEKS, E. Leslie; Broadway Med. Clinic, Regina, Sask.; 628 Douglas Park Cr. (res); Man '56; Staff, Regina Gen. & Grey Nuns Hosp's.; Tel. 527-3793.
WEEKS, John L.; 54 Alexander Ave., Pinawa, Man.; St. Thoma's Hosp. (London, Eng.) '53; DIH; DRCOG; Supt., Health & Safety Br., Whiteshell Nuclear Research Establishment; Hon. Prof., U. of Manitoba; Tel. 753-2311, Ext. 233.
WEHNER, Raymond; Man'57; D. Psy; Staff, Hosp. for Mental Diseases, Selkirk, Man.
WEI, Patrick T.; Hong Kong (China) '58; **Jr.** Int'n., Hosp. for Sick Children, Toronto 2, Ont.
WEIDMAN, Martin L.; 805 Boyd Bldg., Winnipeg, Man.; **203-2300 Portage Ave., St. James (res); Man '54; Paed; Active Staff (Paed), Wpg. Children's & Misericordia Gen. Hosp's; Dem. (Paed.), U. of Man.; Tel. WH 3-0641.**
WEIGAND, Robert P.; 222 est Boul. Henri-Bourassa, Montreal, 12, P.Q.; 315 Ave. Lockhart, Mtl. 16 (res); Strasbourg (Fr.) '50; GenSurg; Anaes; Surg., Hop.-Sacre-Coeur; Tel. DU 8-3452.
WEIH, Gerd P.; 202 Northgate Bldg., Edmonton, Alta.; Frankfurt (Germ.) '51; Tel. GA 2-1184.
WEIL, Joseph M.; 150 The East Mall, Islington, Ont.; Zurich (Switz.)'56.
WEIL, Paul G.; 687 Pine Ave. W., Montreal, P.Q.; 3638 Lorne Cres. (res); McG '34; Haem (P.Q.); M.Sc., Ph.D. (Experim. Med.); FACP; IntMed; Dir. Transfusion Serv. & Ass't. Phys., Royal Victoria Hosp; Cons. (Med.), Queen Mary Vet's & Grace Dart Hosp's; Cons. (Transfus.), Queen Elizabeth & Royal Edward Laurentian Hosp's.; Phys-in-Charge, Montreal Protestant Hosp.; Lect., McGill U.; Tel. VI 2-1251, Loc. 482 & 227.
WEIL, Robert J.; 5770 South St., Halifax N.S.; 2 Burns Dr., Armdale (res); Prague (Czecho Slov.) '33; **Psy; Cons. Psy., D.V.A.; Assoc. Prof.,** Dept. of Psy., Dalhousie U.; Tel. 423-7931.
WEIN, Howard P.; Ste. 204, 586 Ouellette Ave., Windsor, Ont.; Man'58; Tel. 254-1385.
WEIN, Stanley E.; 586 Ouellette Ave., Windsor, Ont.; Man'60.
WEINBERG, Fred; 262 Wilson Ave., Wilson Med. Centre, Downsview, Ont.; 280 Glencairn Ave., Toronto 12 (res); Tor '44; F.A.A.P., Paed; Clin. Staff, Hosp. for Sick Children & New Mt. Sinai Hosp.; Tel. ME 3-2330.
WEINBERG, J. Murray; 1271 Dundas St. W., (Toronto, Ont.; Tor '43; M.C.G.P.; Phys., Parkdale Med. Clin.; Tel. LE 5-6300.
WEINBERG, Maurice B.; 1271 Dundas St. W., Toronto, Ont.; 66 DeQuincy Blvd., Wilson Heights (res); Tor '49; M.C.G.P.; Assoc. Staff, New Mount Sinai Hosp.; Tel. LE 5-6300.
WEINBERG, Reuben; Ireland'56; Res., University Hosp., Edmonton, Alta.
WEINBERG, Victor; 25 Brunswick Ave., Ste. 302, Toronto 4, Ont.; 131 Bloor St. W. (res); Tor '51; FRCS(C); ObstGyn; Chief, Dept. of ObstGyn., Doctor's Hosp.; Court. Staff, Queensway Gen. Hosp.; Tel. 923-1042.
WEINER, Hyman; 517 Davaar Ave., Montreal, P.Q.; McG '34; F.A.A.P., Paed; Ass't Paed., **Jewish Gen. Hosp.; Tel. 271-4200.**
WEINLOS, Harry C. W.; 401 Birks Bldg., Edmonton, Alta.; 10143-123rd St. (res); Alb '31; F.R.C.S.(C), GenSurg; Clin. Inst'r., Surg., U. of **Alberta; Tel. GA 2-2286.**
WEINLOS, Morris; Weinlos Clinic, 10022-103rd St., Edmonton, Alta; 13802 Ravine Dr. (res); Alb '28; F.R.C.S. (Edin.), F.R.C.S.(C), GenSurg; Chief of Surg., Misericordia Hosp; Ass't. Prof., Clin. Surg. & Pathol., U. of Alberta; Tel. 429-3781.
WEINS, Abram T.; 1726 Broadway W., Vancouver, B.C. (res); Man '35; D.A.B.R.
WEINSTEIN, Lionel J.; Qns '64; Res., Hosp. for Sick Children, Toronto 2, Ont.
WEINSTEIN, Ralph; 635 Bloor St. W., Toronto, Ont.; Basel (Switz.) '35; M.C.G.P.; Tel. LE 1-2622.
WEINSTEIN, Wilfred M.; Qns '64; Res., Royal Victoria Hosp., Montreal 2, P.Q.
WEINSTOCK, John W.; 32 Giles Blvd. E., Windsor, Ont.; Wes '34; Anaes.
WEINTRUB, Isadore W.; 665 Ellendale Med. Bldg., 5845 Cote-des-Neiges Rd., Montreal 26, P.Q.; McG'52; FRCP(C), IntMed (Gastroent); Hd., Gastroent. Lab., Dept. of Med., Jewish Gen. Hosp.; Tel. RE 1-8121.
WEIR, Alastair; Moose Jaw Clinic, 200 Scott Bldg., Moose Jaw, Sask.; Glasgow (Scot.)'64; Tel. 692-2373.
WEIR, Bryce K.; 518 Sanford Ave., St. Lambert, Cite Jacques Cartier, P.Q. (res); McG'60 FRCS(C), NeurSurg; Research, Montreal Neurological Inst., Montreal.
WEIR, Donald A.; 180 Portland St., Dartmouth, N.S.; Dal'56; MCGP; Precept., Dalhousie U.; Tel. 466-7471.
WEIR, J. Allister; 21 Upper Middle Rd., Cooksville, Ont.; Tor '50; Active (G.P.) Staff, South Peel Hosp.; Civil Aviation Exam., Dept. of Transport.
WEIR, James R.; Smith Clinic, Box 3830, Camrose, Alta.; 4408-52nd St. **(res); Alb '53; IntMed. Tel. 672-4166.**
WEIR, Norman W.; 10022-103rd St., Edmonton Alta.; 9531-148th St. (res); Queen's U. (Belfast, N.Ire.) '49; BAO; MRCOG; ObstGyn; Clin. Instr., (ObstGyn), U. of Alberta; Tel. 429-3781.
WEIR, Ormond A.; 231 Victoria St., Kamloops, B.C.; 638 Regina Ave., N. Kamloops (res); Qns '51; FRCS(C), GenSurg; Staff, Royal Inland Hosp.; Tel. 372-3221.
WEISBAUM, S. David; 927 Liverpool Rd., **Bay Ridges, Pickering, Ont.; Oxford (Eng.) '58; Tel. 839-1133.**
WEISBERG, H. Maurice; Ste. 15, 5757 Decelles Ave., Montreal 26, P.Q.; Mon '28; FICS; FACS; FACOG; ObstGyn; Assoc., Dept. of Obst. Gyn., Reddy Memorial Hosp.; Chief (ObstGyn), Doctor's Hosp.; Tel. RE 1-6500.
WEISBROD, Gerald I.; 1692 St. Clair Ave. W., Toronto 9, Ont.; 10 Model Ave., Downsview (res); Tor'51; Active Staff, Doctor's Hosp.; Adjunct Clin. Ass't., New Mount Sinai Hosp.; Tel. RO 7-4645.
WEISER, William J.; 609 Bloor St. W., Toronto 4, Ont.; Tor'64; AMCGP; Staff, New Mount Sinai & Doctor's Hosp's.; Tel. LE 4-4214.
WEISNAGEL, John; 960 Boul. Ste-Croix, Montreal 9, P.Q.; Mon '58; Allergy (P.Q.); Paed (P.Q.).
WEISS, Gabrielle C. (Lowenfeld); 1057 Vincent Massey, Chomedey, Mtl., P.Q.; 3051-8th St. (res); McG '55; Psy; Staff, Mtl. Children's Hosp.; Tel. 681-2386.
WEISS, Helene; 1 Harvie Ave., Toronto 10, **Ont.; Roumania '49; Tel. LE 6-7096.**

WEISS, Marcus H.; Northgate Med. Centre, Albert St., Regina, Sask.; Bristol (Eng.)'47; Staff, Regina Gen. & Grey Nun's Hosp's.; Tel. 568-2257.
WEISZ, Samuel; Weinlos Clinic, 10022-103rd St., Edmonton, Alta.; 13511-115th Ave. (res); Alb '56; FRCP(C), IntMed; Tel. GA 4-8076.
WEITZ, Annemarie (See Doenne).
WEIZEL, Harold A.; Doctor's Hosp. Med. Centre, 25 Brunswick Ave., Toronto 4, Ont.; Tor'47; DABS, FACS; FRCS(C), GenSurg.; Assoc. Chief of Surg. & Dir. Med. Educ. & Research, Doctor's Hosp.; Att'd. Surg., OPD, Tor. Western Hosp.; Tel. 927-3041.
WELBOURNE, Robert W.; 110 Med. Arts Bldg., 73 Cumberland St. N., Port Arthur, Ont.; Qns '57; FRCS(C); PlasSurg.
WELCH, Herbert C.; 140 Wallace St., Nanaimo, B.C.; 711 Arbutus Ave. (res); U. of Oregon (U.S.A.) '51; M.S.(Med., Minn); IntMed; Staff, Nanaimo Reg. Gen. Hosp.; Tel. SK 4-7531.
WELCH, Robert H.; 174 St. George St., Toronto 5, Ont.; 36 Old Bridle Path (res); Tor '42; Staff OPD, St. Michael's Hosp.; Clin. Ass't. (Med.), U. of Toronto; Tel. 924-2306.
WELD, Charles B.; 6550 Waegwoltic Ave., Halifax, N.S.; Tor '29; MA, FRSC, Prof. (Physiol.), Dalhousie U.; Tel. 2-4406.
WELDHEN, John W.; Beverly St., St. George, **Ont.; Wes '46; Staff, Brantford Gen. Hosp.; Tel. 448-1322.**
WELDON, Isaac T.; 309 King St., Midland, Ont.; 260-5th St. (res); Tor '39; M.C.G.P.; Staff, St. Andrews Hosp.; Dist. Coroner.
WELDON, J. Dale; Ste. 403A, 1105 Carling Ave., Ottawa 3, Ont.; McG'54; Psy.
WELLINGTON, James L.; Ste. 201, 10 Montreal St., Kingston, Ont.; Qns'59; FRCS(C), GenSurg; Court. Staff, Kingston Gen. & Hotel-Dieu Hosp's.; Tel. 548-3132.
WELLMAN, A. L.; 3201 King St. E., Kitchener, Ont. (res); Tor '12; Retired.
WELLMAN, I. Victoria; Tor '32; Staff, Ontario Hosp., Cobourg, Ont.; Tel. FR 2-3341.
WELLMAN, John M.; Dal'64; Res., Montreal Gen. Hosp., Montreal 25, P.Q.
WELLMAN, Marvin; c/o Naval Secretary, Office of Medical Director, Dept. of Nat. Defence, Ottawa, Ont.; Tor '31; Psy.
WELLS, Alice M.; Pelee Island, Ont.; Tor '21; M.C.G.P.; Anaes.
WELLS, Andrew M.; Cornwall Clinic, 325 Hamilton Ave., St. John's, Nfld.; R.C.P.S. (Ire.) '49.
WELLS, Bruce S.; 331 Sheddon Ave., Oakville, Ont.; Tor'44; FRCS(C) GenSurg.; Surg. Staff, Oakville-Trafalgar Mem. Hosp.; Tel. VI 5-1431.
WELLS, Carden M.; Dingwall Med. Group, Dryden, Ont.; Lakeshore Dr. (res); Tor '43; GenSurg; Staff, Dryden Dist. Gen. Hosp.; Tel. 223-2258.
WELLS, Gordon; Pelee Island, Ont.; Tor '22.
WELLS, Jean P.; 475 boul. Talbot, Chicoutimi, P.Q.; Lav'59; **IntMed.**
WELLS, John P.; 74 Hughson St. S., Hamilton, Ont.; Wes '31; DPH; Deputy, M.O.H.
WELLS, Leslie A.; Box 460, Carbonear, Nfld.; **Dublin (Ire.) '49; FRCS(Eng.); GenSurg; Surg.** Carbonear Red Cross Mem. Hosp.; Tel. 5018.
WELLS, L. Stewart; 2304 Howard Ave., Windsor, Ont.; 2128 Pelissier St. (res); Wes '45; Tel. 252-4182.
WELLS, Nicole; Lav '58; GenSurg (P.Q.); Staff, Hotel-Dieu-St-Vallier, Chicoutimi, P.Q.
WELLS, Thomas J.; 20 Clough St., Lennoxville, P.Q.; McG '22; M.C.G.P.
WELLWOOD, John P.; 32 Begbie St., New Westminster, B.C.; 221 Third Ave. (res); Alb '38; M.C.G.P.; Staff, Royal Columbian & St. Mary's **Hosp's.; Coroner City of New Westminster & Prov. of B.C.; Tel. LA 2-0741.**
WELPY, William R.; Manitoba Clinic, 790 Sherbrook St., Winnipeg 2, Man.; London (Eng.)'35; MRCS(Eng.); LRCP(Lond.); FRCS(Eng.); Sr. OrthSurg., **Grace Hosp.; OrthSurg., Children's,** Deer Lodge DVA, Wpg. Gen. & Manitoba Rehab. Hosp's.; Lect. & Examiner, U. of Manitoba; Vice Pres., Manitoba Medico-Legal Soc.; Vice Chmn., Wpg. Gen. Hosp., Med. Staff; Tel. 774-6541.
WELSH, Donald R. J.; Shouldice Clinic, 618 Church St., Toronto 5, Ont.; 41 Sandringham Dr., Tor. 12 (res); Tor '50; GenSurg; Staff Surg., **Shouldice Surgery; Tel. WA 3-3507.**
WELSH, James R.; Ste. 103, 77 Upper Middle Rd. Cooksville, Ont.; Glasgow (Scot.) '50; DRCOG.
WELSH, Mervin R.; 11216-58th Ave., Edmonton, Alta.; Alb '60; Anaes.
WELSH, W. Keith (O.B.E.); 903 Medical Arts Bldg, 170 St. George St., Toronto, Ont.; 453 Lytton Blvd. (res); Tor '26; F.A.C.S., F.R.C.S. **(Eng.), F.R.C.S.(C); GenSurg; OrthSurg; Surg.**-in-Chief, St. Michael's Hosp.; Prof. of Surg., U. **of Toronto; Tel. WA 1-8997.**
WELSH, W. T. Oscar; 1338 College Ave., Regina, Sask.; Man '08; Staff, Regina Grey Nuns' & **Regina Gen. Hosp's.; Dist Coroner; Tel. 522-8215.**
WENER, Joseph; 425 Ellendale Med. Bldg., 5845 Cote-des-Neiges Rd., Montreal 26, P.Q.; McG'41; DABIM, FACP, FACC; IntMed; Cardiol (PQ); Ass't. Phys., Jewish Gen. & Royal Victoria Hosp's.; Cardiol., Maimonides Hosp. for Aged; Lect. Med., McGill U.; Tel. RE 1-9381.
WENGEL, Aldis E.; 703 Wolseley Ave., Winnipeg, Man.; 353 Elm St. (res); Man '33; Tel. SP 4-9716.
WENGEL, Roman B. W.; 703 Wolseley Ave., **Winnipeg, Man.; 353 Elm St. (res); Man '30; Tel. SU 3-4012.**
WENGER, Heinz H.; 212-4th St., N.E., Calgary, **Alta.; Cologne (Germ.) '54; Tel. 269-3257.**
WENNING, Andrew S.; 5880 Chain Rock Dr., Halifax, N.S.; Dal '50; Anaes; Staff Anaes., Children's Hosp.; Instr. (Anaes), Dalhousie U.
WENSEL, Ronald H.; 505 Med. Arts Bldg., 11010 Jasper Ave., Edmonton, Alta.; Alb. '56; FRCP(C), IntMed; Att'd. Staff, U. of Alberta Hosp.; Instr. (Med.), U. of Alberta; Tel. 422-4804.
WENSLEY, A. Cameron; 502 Queen St. Med. Bldg., Saskatoon, Sask.; Tor'32; **FRCOG; FACOG;** FICS; FACS; ObstGyn; Hd. Dept. of ObstGyn., Saskatoon City Hosp.; Clin. Assoc., U. of Saskatchewan; Tel. 242-1293.
WENSLEY, James A.; 17 Dunedin St., Orillia, **Ont.; Tor'53; IntMed; Chief of Med., Soldier's** Hosp.; Cons., Royal Victoria Hosp., Barrie, St. Andrew's Hosp., Midland & Ontario Hosp's., Orillia & Penetang; Tel. 325-2101.
WENTWORTH, Paul; Cardiff (Wales) '60; M.B., Ch.B., MRCS (Eng.); LRCP (Lond); DObst-RCOG; Ass't. Path., Hosp. for Sick Children, Toronto 2, Ont.
WENTZELL, Robert A.; 30 Tacoma Dr., Dartmouth, N.S.; Dal '52; Urol; Tel. 466-1511.
WERDEN, Lloyd H.; 189 King St., St. Catharines, Ont. (res); Edinburgh (Scot.) '13; D.P.H.; Retired.
WERMENLINGER, Pierre; Mon '55; Path (Anat.) (P.Q.); Staff, Dept. of Path., U. of Montreal, Montreal, P.Q.
WERMUTH, E. G.; 718 Waterloo St., London, **Ont.; Vienna (Austria) '37; M.C.G.P.; Tel. 439-5241.**
WERMUTH, Ralph E.; Wes'65; Res., Westminster Hosp., London, Ont.
WERNER, Nathan H.; 404 Norlyn Medical Bldg., 309 Hargrave St., Winnipeg, Man.; 500 Renfrew St. (res); Man '53; D.A.B.Oph; F.A.A.O.O.; Ophth; Clin. Ass't. Winnipeg Gen. Hosp.; Tel. WH 3-7640.
WERNER, Robert P., S/L; Nat. Defence Med. Centre, Ottawa 8, Ont.; Dal '56.
WERNICK, Howard B.; 2390 Eglinton Ave. E., Scarborough, Ont.; 1725 Lawrence Ave. E. (res); Tor '58; AMCGP; Court. Staff, New Mt. Sinai, Grace, Tor. E. Gen. & Scarborough Gen. Hosp's.; Tel. 757-2854.
WERRY, Ernest E.; Queensway Gen. Hosp., Toronto, Ont.; Tor '59; FRCS(C), GenSurg; Court. Staff, St. Joseph's Hosp.
WERRY, John S.; 359 Montcalm Ave., Chateauguay, P.Q. (res); New Zealand '55; M.B., B.Sc., FRCP(C); Psy; Clin. Ass't. Montreal Children's Hosp.; Tel. WE 7-8511. Abroad.

WERSHOF, Eliot; 421 Tegler Bldg., Edmonton, **Alta.; 10340-121 St. (res); Man '17; Tel. 422-7410.**
WERTHENBACH, Frederick E.; Ste. 42, 11620—79th Ave., Edmonton, Alta. (res); Alb '30.
WERTMAN, Abraham M.; 702 Dollard Blvd., Montreal 8, P.Q. (res); Tor '32; MCGP; Staff, Jewish Gen. Hosp.; Part-time Indust. Phys.; Tel. 272-0668.
WESLEY, Robert H.; Ste. 406, Toronto Western Med. Bldg., 25 Leonard Ave., Toronto 2B, Ont.; 14 Ardmore Rd. (res); Tor '42; F.R.C.S.(C), ObstGyn; Staff, Toronto Western Hosp.; Clin. Instr. (ObstGyn), U. of Toronto; Tel. EM. 3-1764.
WESLEY, William R.; 8188 Yonge St., Thornhill, Ont.; Thornbank Rd. (res); Qns '33.
WESLEY-JAMES, Oliver; 250 Main St. E., Hamilton, Ont.; London (Eng.) '49; FRCS (Eng. & Edinburgh); GenSurg; Staff, Chedoke Gen., Hamilton Gen. & St. Joseph's Hosp's.; Tel. JA 7-2711.
WESOLOWSKI, Mathew J.; 8808-92nd St., Edmonton, Alta; 9623-86th St. (res); Alb '49; M.C.-**G.P.; Tel. 466-3731.**
WEST, Chris A. Sq./Cdr; Canadian Forces **Hosp., Halifax, N.S.; Tor '49; IntMed; Chief of Med., Cdn. Forces Hosp.; Assoc. Prof. Dalhousie U.**
WEST, G. Roger, Sg/Lt.; Box 10, RCAF Station, Holberg, B.C.; Alb'64.
WEST, Margaret H.; Halifax Health Centre, University Ave., Halifax, N.S.; Tor '42; Dir. of Health Serv.; Tel. 422-8571.
WEST, Michael H.; 350-955 Queen St. E., Sault Ste. Marie, Ont.; 125 Simpson St. (res); London (Eng.)'42; MRCS, LRCP, MRCP(Lond.), M.D. (Lond.), IntMed; Staff, Plummer & Gen. Hosp's.; Dist. Coroner; Tel. AL 3-6031.
WEST, William G.; 552-1st St., Chippawa, Ont. (res); Tor '31; Plant Phys., Welland Plant, North American Cyanamid Ltd., Niagara Falls, Ont.; Tel. EL 4-1621.
WEST, W. Therence; Brantford Clinic, 54 Brant Ave., Brantford, Ont.; 266 Dufferin Ave. (res); Tor '39; MCGP; Staff, Dept. of Surg., Brantford Gen., St. Joseph's Hosp's.; Willett Hosp., Paris, & Norfolk Gen. Hosp., Simcoe; Tel. 756-6333.
WESTBURY, Robert C.; 41 Chelsea St., Calgary, Alta.; 4012 Comarche Rd. (res); Cambridge (Eng.) '60; Tel. AV 9-1901.
WESTCOTT, Donald B.; Hawk Junction, Ont.; Tor '24; MCGP; Surg., Algoma Central Rlwy; Dist. Coroner.
WESTE, Ilse; 19 Pleasant St., Dartmouth, N.S.; Freiburg (Germ.) '40; Lect., Dalhousie U.; Tel. 2-4406.
WESTE, Ulrich A.; 91 Pleasant St., Dartmouth, **N.S.; Freiburg (Germ.) '42; Paed; Lect'r. (Dept.** of Paed.) Dalhousie U.; Tel. 2-4406.
WESTENBERG, H. H.; 115 Lower Union St., Kingston, Ont.; Amsterdam (Neth.) '60; DRS; M.O.H., Queen's U.; Clin. Ass't. Queen's U.; Tel. 542-7095.
WESTGATE, Archibald; 10022-103rd St., Edmonton, Alta.; Otago (N. Zealand)'53; MRCOG; FRCS(C), ObstGyn; Assoc. Staff, Misericordia Hosp.; Tel. 429-3781.
WESTGATE, F. Gordon; Ste. 708, 925 W. Georgia St., Vancouver 1, B.C.; 2406 Eddington Dr., Van. 8 (res); Tor'45; FACS, FRCS (Eng. & C), GenSurg; Surg., St. Paul's **& Van. Children's Hosp. & BC Cancer Inst.; Tel. MU 1-5632.**
WESTMAN, Gilbert B.; 177 Oxford St., Ingersoll, Ont.; McG '54.
WESTON, Agnes (Black); 6957 Laburnum St., Vancouver 14, B.C. (res); Glasgow (Scot.) '33; DPH; PH; Ass't. MOH, Metropolitan Health Services, Van.; Tel. TR 2-2511.
WESTON, Iain; Gerard Bldg., 101st St., North Battleford, Sask.; Edinburgh (Scot.) '60; Tel. 445-4422.
WESTON, Neville E.; 2300 Lawrence Ave. E., **Scarborough, Ont.; Tor '60; Tel. 757-1847.**
WESTON, R. Leonard; 46 George Henry Blvd., Willowdale, Ont.; Wes '50; Anaes; Staff, Toronto Western Hosp.; Clin. Teach. (Anaes.), U. of Toronto.
WESTON, Roy B.; 1746 Jane St., Weston, Ont.; National U. (Dublin, Ire.)'56; Anaes; Staff, Humber Mem. Hosp.; Tel. 249-5681.
WESTON, W. Wayne; 24 Hope St. W., Tavistock, Ont.; Tor'64; MCGP; Active Staff, Stratford Gen. Hosp.; Tel. 655-2322.
WESTOVER, Gary; Fort St. John, B.C.; Alb '55.
WESTWOOD, John C. N.; Dept. of Bact., U. of Ottawa, Ottawa, Ont.; Cambridge (Eng.)'42; MRCS; LRCP; Dip. Bact. (Eng.); Cons. Virol., Ottawa Civic Hosp.; Bact., Ottawa Gen. Hosp.; Cons., Defence Research Bd.; Memb. Defence Research Advisory Bd.; Prof. & Hd. Dept. of Bact., U. of Ottawa; Tel. 235-6751, Ext. 286.
WETSELAAR, Henri; 815 Park Road, Richmond, **B.C.; 585 Forsythe Cr. (res); Amsterdam (Neth.) '52; MCGP; Tel. 277-3167.**
WEVRICK, Noah; 790 Rockland Ave., Outremont, P.Q.; Mon '29; **Staff, Jewish Gen. Hosp., Montreal.**
WEWIORSKI, Kazimierz; 7372 Somerled Ave., Montreal 29, P.Q.; Innsbruck (Austria)'15; Tel. 486-1478.
WEXLER, George W.; 917 ave. Abitibi, Val-d'Or, P.Q.; Mon '55; Urol.; Tel. 824-6444.
WEXLER, Marvin J.; McG'65; Res., Royal Victoria Hosp., Montreal 2, P.Q.
WEYLIE, D. Ralph; 1 Kerr St., Cayuga, Ont.; Wes '36; MCGP; Active Staff, West Haldimand Gen. Hosp., Hagersville; M.O.H., Cayuga & North Cayuga Twnsp.; Tel. 722-3841.
WEYMAN, Stephen H.; 115 Hazen St., Saint John, N.B.; 22 Rocky Terrace (res); McG '45; Paed; Att. Paed., Saint John Gen. & St. Joseph's Hosp's.; Tel. 692-2741.
WEYMAN, S. John; 300 Laurentian Blvd., Montreal 9, P.Q.; McG'51; Med. Dir., Smith Kline & French Inter-American Corp.; Tel. 747-6565.
WHALEN, John S.; 94 Princess Anne Cres., Islington, Ont. (res); Tor '43; Anaes; Anaes. Staff, Hosp. for Sick Children; Clin. Ass't. **(Anaes), U. of Toronto; Tel. EM 6-7242.**
WHALEY, David W.; 16 Roy St., Kitchener, Ont.; Tor '26; D.A.B.P., Paed; Staff, Kitchener-Waterloo & St. Mary's Hosp's; Tel. SH 5-9753.
WHALEY, James B.; 526 Medical Arts Bldg., 170 St. George St., Toronto 5, Ont.; 22 The **Kingsway (res); Tor '30; D.L.O.(Eng.), Otol;** Chief of Otol., Hosp. for Sick Children; Ass't. **Prof. Otol., U. of Toronto; Tel. WA 2-5962.**
WHALEY, W. John; 9 Margaret Ave., Kitchener, Ont.; 328 Glasgow St. (res); Qns '55; Paed; Active Staff, Kitchener-Waterloo, & St. Mary's Gen-Hosp's.; O.P.D., Staff, Hosp. for Sick Children, Toronto; Tel. SH 3-1486.
WHAN, J. H.; 3111 Sheppard Ave. E., Agincourt, Ont.; Tor'63.
WHANG, Tai Y.; Blind River, Ont.; China '38.
WHAUN, June M.; UBC '60; FRCP(C), Paed; Clin. Research Fell., Dept. of Path., Hosp. for Sick Children, Toronto 2, Ont.
WHEATLEY, Michael L.; 31 James St., Parry **Sound, Ont.; 25 Wanbeck (res); London (Eng.)** '50; MCGP; Tel. RI 6-2133.
WHEATON, Robert R.; 508 **Med. Arts Bldg.,** Saskatoon, Sask.; Sask '57; AMCGP; **Staff (Obst-**Gyn), St. Paul's **& City Hosp's.;** Clin. **Fell. (Re-**habMed). University Hosp.; Tel. 652-6066.
WHEELDON, Peter J.; Tofino, B.C.; Birming-**ham, Eng. '60; AMCGP; Tel. 725-3282.**
WHEELER, Barry R.; 916 Prince St., Truro, N.S.; London (Eng.) '54; MRCS; LRCP; D.Obst-RCOG; Staff, Colchester Hosp.; Tel. 893-7161.
WHEELOCK, Gordon H.; 7 Halls Rd., Armdale, Halifax Co., N.S. (res); **McG '40; M.O., O.P.D.,** Treatment Centre, Camp Hill DVA Hosp.
WHEELWRIGHT, David A.; 3551 Charleswood **Dr., Calgary, Alta.; 3236 Conrad Dr. (res); Oxford (Eng.) '57; M.A.(Oxon); LMSSA (Lond.); Active Med. Staff, Calgary Gen., Holy Cross, Alberta Children's & Grace Hosp's.; Tel. 282-3944.**
WHELAN, Donald T.; McG'61; Paed; Staff, Montreal Children's Hosp., Montreal, P.Q.

WHELAN, Patrick J.; 31 Queens Rd., St. John's, Nfld.; 10 Bonaventure Ave. (res); Dal '49; GenSurg; Surg., St. Clare's, Grace & Gen. Hosp's.; Tel. 578-3994.

WHELEN, Warren S.; 360 Queen's Ave., London, Ont.; 314 Grosvenor St. (res); McG '53; Paed; Teach. Staff U. of Western Ontario; Tel. GE 9-1431.

WHELER, Ewart G.; 2357 Queen St. E., Toronto, Ont.; Tor '20; Tel. OX 1-3459.

WHELER, R. James; 1631 Islington Ave. N., Rexdale, Ont.; Tor '57; Assoc. Staff, Humber Mem. Hosp.; Tel. 741-0410.

WHERRETT, Brian A.; Qns '58; Paed; Med. Dir., Home Care Prog., & Clin. Ass't., Montreal Children's Hosp., Montreal 25, P.Q.; Tel. WE 7-8511.

WHERRETT, George J.; 164 Acacia Ave., Ottawa, Ont.; Man '24; MRCP (Lond.), FRCP(C), IntMed (TB); Dir. of Research & Spec. Projects, Cdn. TB Assoc.; Cons. Cdn. Pen. Comm. & Dept. Nat. Health & Welfare; Tel. CE 3-4167.

WHERRETT, John R.; 49 Farnham Ave., Toronto 7, Ont. (res); Qns '55; FRCP(C); Neurol; Staff, Neurol. Unit, Toronto Gen. Hosp.; Clin. Teach., U. of Toronto; Tel. EM 6-8211, Ext. 2741.

WHETHAM, John C.; Qns'65; Res., Toronto Gen. Hosp., Toronto 2, Ont.

WHETTER, Reginald W.; 12 College St., Chilliwack, B.C.; 16 Williams Rd. N. (res); Man '32; M.C.G.P.; Staff, Chilliwack Gen. Hosp.; Tel. 795-5727.

WHILLANS, James A.; 505 O'Connor St., Ottawa, Ont.; 153 Heath St. (res); Qns '44; Paed; Staff "A." Ottawa Civic Hosp.; Lect. (Clin-Paed), U. of Ottawa; Tel. CE 2-5761.

WHILLANS, Morley G.; Defence Research Bd., Dept. of Nat. Defence H.Q., Ottawa, Ont.; 21 Lakeside Ave. (res); Tor '35; Ass't. Chief Scientist, Dir., Biosciences Research; Tel. CE 2-8211.

WHILLANS, P. C.; Tor'64; Res., Toronto East Gen. Hosp., Toronto 13, Ont.

WHISSELL, George L.; Whissell Clinic, Main St., Westlock, Alta.; Mon '32; Chief of Staff & Chief of Surg., Immaculata Hosp.

WHISTON, Geoffrey J.; Edinburgh (Scot.) '53; Ophth; MO, RCAF; Staff, Mtl. Gen. Hosp., Montreal, P.Q.

WHISTON, Herbert G.; 27 Kennebecasis Park Torryburn, Kings Co., N.S. (res); Edinburgh (Scot.) '54; DMRT; TherRad; Ass't. Rad., St. John's Gen. Hosp., Saint John; Tel. 693-3351.

WHITAKER, Lorne; R.R. No. 3 St. Catharines, Ont. (res); Wes '32; PathBact; Path., St. Catharines Gen., West Lincoln Mem., Grimsby Haldimand War Mem., Dunneville & Niagara **(Niagara-on-the-Lake) Hosp.; Cons. Ont. Dept. of Health; Tel. MU 4-7271.**

WHITBREAD, David H.; 1737 Pandosy St., Kelowna, B.C.; 3082 Meikle Rd. (res); Alb '55; Att'd. Staff, Kelowna Gen. Hosp.; Tel. 762-4212. Abroad.

WHITBREAD, John L.; 1947 Cook St., Victoria, B.C.; 3030 Devon Rd. (res); Man '34; D.P.H. (Eng.); PH; Sr. M.O., Greater Victoria Metropolitan Bd. of Health; Tel. 384-0571.

WHITBY, David; 300 Waterford Bridge, St. John's, Nfld.; London (Eng.)'56; FRCP(C), Psy; Staff, Hosp. for Mental & Nervous Dis.

WHITE, Alan; Box 21, Sundre, Alta.; Durham (Eng.) '52.

WHITE, A. W. M.; "White Pines", R.R. No. 1, Maple, Ont. (res); Tor '26; F.R.C.S. (Edin.), F.R.C.S.(C), GenSurg; OrthSurg; Staff, Workmen's Comp. Bd., 115 Torbarrie Rd., Downsview, Ont.; Lect. (Surg.), U. of Toronto; Tel. 244-1761.

WHITE, Bruce M.; 2629 Wyandotte St., Riverside, Ont.; 824 Howard (res); Wes '52; AMCGP; Tel. 945-2610.

WHITE, Campbell; 116 Elm St. E., Sudbury, Ont.; Tor '50; OrthSurg.

WHITE, Clark A.; 3434 Lakeshore Rd., Toronto 14, Ont.; 1550 Stavebank Rd., Pt. Credit (res); Tor '33; MCGP; Staff, Queensway Gen. Hosp.; Tel. 251-2161.

WHITE, David F.; 20 Killerton Ave., London, Ont. (res); Wes '59; FRCP(C), IntMed; Phys., Ontario Cancer Fdn., London Clinic; Tel. GE 2-5261, Ext. 383; Abroad.

WHITE, D. Naldrett; Etherington Hall, Queen's University, Kingston, Ont.; Cambridge (Eng.)'40; MA; MD(Cantab.); MRCP(Lond.); FACP; FRCP(C), Neur; IntMed; Psy; Cons., Neurol., Kingston Gen. & Ottawa Civic Hosp's.; Dir. EEG Depts., Kingston Gen. & Ontario Hosp's at Kingston & Smiths Falls; Electroenceph., Ottawa Civic Hosp.; Tel. 548-7243.

WHITE, Douglas S.; Wainwright Clinic, Wainwright, Alta.; Edinburgh (Scot.)'51; MCGP; Staff, Wainwright Gen. & Wainwright-Provost Aux. Hosp's.; Coroner; Phys., C.N.R. & Camp Wainwright Mil. Hosp.; Tel. 842-3341.

WHITE, E. Perry; 199 Brock St., Kingston, Ont.; 67 College St. (res); Qns '34; FRCS(Edin.) Urol; Chief, Dept. of Urol., Hotel-Dieu; Ass't. Prof. Urol., Queen's U.; Tel. 542-1201.

WHITE, Ernest J.; 77 Westmount Rd., Guelph, Ont.; 8 Oriole Cr. (res); Dal '59; OrthSurg; Surg. Staff, Guelph Gen. & St. Joseph's Hosp's.; Tel. TA 2-6910.

WHITE, Emery L.; 114 St. George St., Bathurst, N.B.; Mon '50; GenSurg; Tel. LI 6-4516.

WHITE, George E.; 504 Medical Arts Bldg., 1011 Ouellette Ave., Windsor, Ont.; 748 Devonshire (res); Tor '13; D.A.B.P., Paed; Hon. Cons., Paed., Metropolitan Hosp.; Att. Staff, Fred Adam's Hosp.; Att. Paed., Children's Hosp., Detroit, Mich.; (Emer.); Active Staff, Children's Dept., Metro Health Unit; Retired.

WHITE, George M.; 42 Wellington Row, Saint John, N.B.; McG '24; FRCOG, FACS, FRCS(C), ObstGyn; MRCOG (Eng.), FIMA; Emeritus Chief, Dept. Obst. & Gyn., St. John Gen. Hosp.; Vis. Staff, St. Joseph's Hosp.; Gyn & Obst. Cons., St. John's T.B. & Provincial Hosp's.; Tel. 693-3083. Retired.

WHITE, Gordon B.; 87 Clarence St., Port Colborne, Ont.; 239 Sugarloaf St. (res); Tor '27 F.I.C.S., D.O.M.S., OphthOtol; Chief of Staff, Chief Ophth. Otol., Port Colborne Gen. Hosp.; Cons., Welland Co. Hosp. & Douglas Mem. Hosp., **Fort Erie; Tel. TE 4-3313.**

WHITE, Harry E.; 4794-A Joyce Ave., Powell River, B.C.; Alb '38.

WHITE, Hubert C.; 274 King St. W., Chatham, Ont.; 160 Llydican Ave. E. (res); Tor '56; FRCS(C), GenSurg; Staff, St. Joseph's & Public Gen. Hosp's.; Tel. EL 4-3460.

WHITE, James C.; 160 Brant Ave., Brantford, Ont.; Wes'53; FRCS(C), ObstGyn; Staff (ObstGyn), Brantford Gen. & St. Joseph's Hosp's.; Tel. 756-5313.

WHITE, Jermaine V.; Room 203, 825 Granville St., Vancouver 2, B.C.; 2910 W. 47th Ave. (res); Tor '43; FIAP; Tel. MU 1-1522.

WHITE, J. Graham; 54 Brant Ave., Brantford, Ont.; 49 Hillier Cres. (res); Wes '32 Ophth., **Brantford Gen. & St. Joseph's Hosp.; Tel. PL 6-6333.**

WHITE, John C.; Richmond Health Dept., 691 No. 3 Rd., Richmond, B.C.; Dublin (Ire.)'40; DPH (Tor.); Ass't. Health Officer, Van.; MOH, Richmond; Tel. CR 8-5511.

WHITE, John F.; Markham Med. Centre, 254 **Main St., Markham, Ont.; 44 Albert St. (res); Tor '57; MCGP; Staff, Scarborough Gen. Hosp.; Tel. 294-2290.**

WHITE, John G.; 142 Judith Cr., Ancaster, Ont. (res); Wes'50; D.Psy; Psy; Dep. Supt., Ontario **Hosp., Hamilton; Tel. 385-5361.**

WHITE, John J.; McG '57; Res., Royal Victoria Hosp., Montreal 2, P.Q.

WHITE, John L.; 165 Plymouth Rd., Welland, Ont.; 20 Colbeck Dr. (res); Tor '52; M.C.G.P.; Staff Phys., Welland Co. & Pt. Colborne Gen. **Hosp.; Tel. RE 2-3087.**

WHITE, Kathryn A.; 1506 Briarwood Cres., Oakville, Ont.; Qns '63; Part-time Practice. Temporarily Retired.

WHITE, Lawrence; Lav'49; DiagRad(P.Q.); Staff, Hop. Cloutier, Cap. de la Madeleine, P.Q.

WHITE, M. Patricia (Armstrong); 66 Bessborough Dr., Toronto 17, Ont. (res); Tor '47; MA; Psy; Staff, U. of Toronto Health Service; Tel. 928-2451.

WHITE, Norman F.; McG'62; Res., Jewish Gen. Hosp., Montreal 26, P.Q.

WHITE, Oliver J.; 83 Alma St., Moncton, N.B.; Man '45; OrthSurg; Co-Ordinator, Orth. Surg., Moncton Gen. & Hotel Dieu Hosp's; Cons., Moncton T.B. Hosp.; Tel. 389-1759.

WHITE, Paul D.; 342 Queen St. S., Kitchener, Ont.; Wes '59; Ophth; Active Staff, St. Mary's & Kitchener-Waterloo Gen. Hosp's.; Tel. 744-4951.

WHITE, Philip K. B.; 129 Academy Park Rd., Regina, Sask.; University Coll. (London, Eng.) '51; D.PhysMed; MRCS; LRCP; Spec. PhysMed., Physical Restoration Centre; Cons. PhysMed. Regina Geriatric Centre; Hon. Cons., Regina Gen. & Grey Nun's Hosp's.; Tel. 536-1011.

WHITE, R. Arthur; 1625 Oak Bay Ave., Victoria, B.C.; Man'44; MCGP; Tel. 383-2856.

WHITE, Reginald A.; 344 Ferguson St., North Bay, Ont.; Tor '27; Staff, St. Joseph's & Civic Hosp's.; Tel. 474-1110.

WHITE, Roy A.; 750 W. Broadway, Vancouver 9, B.C.; 2474 W. 35th Ave. (res); Washington (U.S.A.) '50; GenSurg; Vis. Staff, Vancouver Gen. Hosp.; Tel. 876-5313.

WHITE, T. E.; Medical Arts Bldg., Hamilton, Ont.; Old Sanatorium Rd. (res); Tor '16; Dist. Coroner; Tel. JA 7-4242.

WHITE, William H.; 383 Ellis St., Penticton, B.C.; 702 Winnipeg St. (res); McG '36; GenSurg; Coroner (Prov. App't.); Tel. 492-3024.

WHITE, William J.; 289 Cedar St., Sudbury, Ont.; Tor '43; MCGP; Tel. 674-3131.

WHITE, W. R.; 50 Yonge St. N., Richmond Hill, Ont.; Tor '64.

WHITEFIELD, Ruth; (See TITCOMBE, Ruth).

WHITEFORD, James W.; 510 Medical Arts Bldg., Winnipeg, Man.; 106 Middlegate (res); Man '44; GenSurg; Hon. Att. Staff, Div. of Surg., Children's & Deer Lodge Hosp's; Lect. Surg., U. of Manitoba; Tel. WH 2-6153.

WHITEHEAD, Edward; Edinburgh (Scot.) '61; Res., Tor. Gen. Hosp., Toronto, Ont.

WHITEHEAD, Frederick L.; East Riverside, King's County, N.B. (res); Dal '35; Exec. Sec., New Brunswick Med. Soc. & Prince Edward Island Med. Soc., East Riverside; Tel. 847-7353.

WHITEHEAD, Harry Y.; 14 Caithness E., Caledonia, Ont.; Tor '32; Tel. RO 5-2755.

WHITEHEAD, Robert G. D.; 841 Collinson St., Victoria, B.C.; 3850 Synod Rd. (res); Man '41; Anaes; Staff, Dept. of Anaes., St. Joseph's Hosp. Tel. EV 4-5622.

WHITEHEAD, V. Michael; 4 Redpath Place, Montreal 25, P.Q.; McG'59; Haem(P.Q.); FRCP(C), IntMed; Staff, Royal Victoria Hosp.; Tel. 842-1251.

WHITEHURST, Neville (O.B.E.); 49 Rutland Gate, London S.W. 7, Eng. (res); St. Bartholomews (Eng.) '29; M.R.C.S., L.R.C.P.; Dir. Med. Serv., Bowater Paper Corp'n., Corner Brook, Nfld.; Tel. 634-5151.

WHITELAW, D. MacKay; McG '39; FRCP(C); FACP; IntMed; Staff, B.C. Cancer Inst., 2656 Heather St., Vancouver 9, B.C.; Chief of Med. Shaughnessy Hosp.; Prof. (Med.), U. of British Columbia; Tel. TR 4-9321.

WHITELAW, John W.; 750 W. Broadway, Vancouver, B.C.; 5760 Marguerite (res); McG '41; Paed; Assoc. Staff, Vancouver Gen. Hosp.; Clin. Assoc. & Prof. Paed., U. of British Columbia; Tel. TR 9-4564.

WHITELAW, Marion M. (See Henderson)

WHITEMAN, Gabriel; 5025 Sherbrooke St. W., Ste 205, Westmount, P.Q.; 435 Strathcona Ave., Westmount (res); Tor '47; DABR; D&TRad; Rad-in-Chief, Queen Elizabeth Hosp.; Tel. 482-0681.

WHITESIDE, John H.; 16 Mann Ave., Toronto 7, Ont.; Tor'57; FRCS(C), ObstGyn; Staff, Women's College Hosp.

WHITESIDE, John H.; 408 Belmont Ave., Peterborough, Ont. (res); Tor '42; M.Sc.; Path; Pathol. & Dir. of Lab., Civic Hosp.; Tel. RI 2-3831.

WHITESIDE, Richard D.; Annan, Ont. (res); Tor '52; D.Psy; Psy; Supt., Ont. Hosp., Owen Sound; Cons., Gen. & Marine Hosp.; Tel. FR 6-6130.

WHITESIDE, W. Carleton; 415 Medical Arts Bldg., 1105 Pandora Ave., Victoria, B.C.; Alb'28; FACS, DABTS, FICS, FRCS(C), GenSurg, ThorSurg; Tel. EV 5-4512.

WHITESIDE, William H.; Wes '51; GenSurg; Staff; MO, Dept. of Nat. Health & Welfare, Marine Hosp.; Sydney, N.S.; Tel. 564-6122. Abroad.

WHITFIELD, Joan A.; Qns'65; Res., Hosp. for Sick Children, Toronto 2, Ont.

WHITFIELD, William A.; Alb'65; Jr. Int., Royal Alexandra Hosp., Edmonton, Alta.; Abroad.

WHITING, John E.; Tor '37; Med. Supt., Wrinch Mem. Hosp., Hazelton, B.C.; Tel. 11.

WHITING, M. Lloyd; 214 Jarvis St., Fort Erie, Ont.; 225 Highland (res); Tor'43; Active Staff, Douglas Memorial Hosp.; Tel. 871-2060.

WHITING, R. Harvey; 10004-105 St., Edmonton, Alta.; 9031 Saskatchewan Dr. (res); McG '42; F.A.C.P., F.R.C.P.(C), IntMed; Chief of Med., Royal Alexandra Hosp.; Court. Staff, University of Alta. Hosp.; Assoc. Clin. Prof., U. of Alberta; Tel. GA 4-2121.

WHITLA, John C.; 29 Dickson St., Galt, Ont.; 194 Main St. E. (res); Tor '33; A.M.C.G.P.

WHITLEY, Donald M.; 240 Medical Arts Bldg., 1105 Pandora Ave., Victoria, B.C.; 3775 Mystic Lane (res); Man '42; F.R.C.S. (Edin.), GenSurg; Chief of Staff, Royal Jubilee Hosp.; Assoc. Staff, St. Joseph's Hosp.; Tel. EV 3-8932.

WHITMAN, Herbert B.; Main St., Westville, N.S.; North Main St. (res); Dal'28; AICS; MCGP; Staff, Aberdeen Hosp., New Glasgow; Tel. 396-5161.

WHITMAN, Roderick L.; 710 Seymour St., Vancouver, B.C.; 3098 Paisley Rd. (res); McG '39; D.P.M., Psy; Att. Staff, Vancouver Gen. Hosp.; Clin. Inst., U. of British Columbia; Tel. MU 4-1511.

WHITMAN, Rodger A.; 218 Kenilworth Ave. S., Hamilton, Ont.; Wes'48; MCGP; Tel. 545-6395.

WHITMORE, G. Donald; Ste. 207, 100 Bonnie Doon Shopping Centre, Edmonton, Alta.; 9611-81st St. (res); Alb '51; MCGP; Active Staff, Misericordia Hosp.; Court. Staff, Edmonton Gen. & Royal Alexandra Hosp's.; Tel. HO 6-0791.

WHITNEY, Joan D. (Mrs. A. J. Moore); 4819 Inverness St., Vancouver 10, B.C. (res); Qns '53; Part-time, Vancouver Gen. Hosp.

WHITTAKER, Arthur T.; Med. Centre, Barrhead, Alta. Tor '57. GenSurg; Tel. 674-2246.

WHITTAKER, John N.; 985 Kingsway Dr., Burlington, Ont.; Liverpool (Eng.)'60; LRCP; MRCS; Tel. 945-4922.

WHITTAKER, John S.; 59 Fairmeadow Ave., Willowdale, Ont. (res); Edinburgh (Scot.)'50; Staff Phsy., Ont. Crippled Children's Centre; Tel. 487-5311. Ext. 219.

WHITTAKER, Keith W. B.; 3147 Kingsway, Vancouver 16, B.C.; 3551 Kingsway (res); Wes '32; Tel. 433-7636.

WHITTAKER, Michael R.; South Pelham St., Fonthill, Ont.; Manchester (Eng.)'60; Staff, Welland County Gen. Hosp.; Tel. 892-6333.

WHITTAKER, Richard; C.P. 280, Cap Chat, P.Q.; Mon '49.

WHITTAKER, William G.; 31 Centre St. S., Brampton, Ont.; Tor '50; FRCS(C), ObstGyn; Cons. (ObstGyn.), Peel Mem. & Georgetown & Dist. Mem. Hosp's.; Tel. 459-1881.

WHITTAL, J. Kenneth; 3823 W. 10th Ave., Vancouver 8, B.C. (res); Wes '44; D.P.H.; Anaes; Dir. Health Unit 2, Metropolitan Health Committee; Staff, Vancouver Gen. Hosp.; Tel. TR 6-3211.

WHITTEMORE, N. Blair; 160 Northview Ave., Montreal West, P.Q.; McG'60; FRCP(C), IntMed; Staff, Montreal Gen. Hosp.; Abroad.

WHITTIER, Catherine L.; Upper Rawdon, Hants Co., N.S.; Tor'26.

WHITTIER, Donald P.; 55 Sydenham St., Dundas, Ont.; Qns '51; M.C.G.P.; Tel. MA 8-6441.

WHITTINGDALE, Anne M.; Bristol (Eng.)'62; Res., Shaughnessy Hosp., Vancouver 9, B.C.

WHITTINGHAM, David S.; 18 Fairfax Ave., Ottawa 3, Ont.; Tor '50; D&TRad; Staff, Rad., Ottawa Civic Hosp.; Assoc. Rad., Radiology Assoc. of Ottawa; Tel. PA 9-2511, Loc. 327.

WHITTLE, Charles H., Sg. Lt.Cdr.; 891 Innswood Dr., Ottawa 13, Ont. (res); Tor '52; Ass't. Med. Dir., Surg. Gen. Staff, NDHQ; Tel. 232-8211, Ext. 24398.

WHITTLE, Edward; Ott '57; M.O., CNR Clinic, 151 Front St. W., Toronto 2, Ont.; Tel. EM 6-9011.

WHITTON, Thomas H.; 3014 Eva Dr., Burlington, Ont.; FRCP(C), Anaes.

WHITTY, Goldie T.; 643 Campbell Ave., Windsor, Ont.; Qns '24; Tel. 253-1922.

WHITTY, Robert J.; 1428 Ouellette Ave., Windsor, Ont.; 2234 Victoria (res); Wes '52; D.A.B.S., FACS; FICS; GenSurg; Active Staff (Surg.), Grace, I.O.D.E., Metropolitan & Hotel-Dieu Hosp's.; Tel. CL 6-7671.

WHYTE, Catherine (McGuigan); P.O. Box 239, Bedford, N.S. (res); Edinburgh (Scot.)'46; Tel. 835-2139.

WHYTE, Don W.; 495 Picadilly Ave., Ottawa 3, Ont.; Qns '40; Anaes; Chief Anaes., Ottawa Civic Hosp.; Lect. (Clin. Anaes), U. of Ottawa; Tel. PA 9-2511.

WHYTE, Francis; Lower Sackville, N.S.; U.K. '49.

WHYTE, J. Clinton; Qns '30; FACOG; FRCOG; FRCS(C), ObstGyn; Chmn., Div. of ObstGyn., Ottawa Civic Hosp.; Prof. (ObstGyn.), U. of Ottawa; Tel. 729-2511, Loc. 573.

WHYTE, W Donaldson; The Medical Centre, Peterborough, Ont.; 548 Weller St. (res); Man '33; F.R.C.S. (Edin.), GenSurg; Surg Staff, St. Joseph's & Peterborough Civic Hosp's.; Tel. RI 2-3871.

WHYTE, W. Robert; St. Catharines Med. Centre, 292 Oakdale Ave., St. Catharines; Ont.; Qns '55.

WHYTEHEAD, Lawrence L.; 790 Sherbrooke, St., Winnipeg 2, Man.; 275 Yale Ave. (res); Oxford (Eng.) '38; F.R.C.S. (Eng.); Ass't. Surg. (Thor. Surg.), Winnipeg Gen. Hosp.; Lect., Dept. of Surg., U. of Manitoba; Tel. SP 4-6541.

WHYTOCK, Arthur B.; 701 St. Clair Ave., Niagara Falls, Ont.; Qns '16; MRCS(Eng.), LRCP(Lond.), FACS, FICS, GenSurg; Dist. Coroner; Tel. EL 4-6414.

WHYTOCK, Karen J.; Tor '64; Res., Hosp. for Sick Children, Toronto 2, Ont.; Abroad.

WIANCKO, Kenneth B.; The Medical Centre, 10006-149th St., Edmonton, Alta.; Alb '57; FRCS(C), GenSurg; Staff, Univ. Hosp.; Tel. 439-5911.

WICKETT, John C., AFC., G/C; 13 Linden Terr., Ottawa, Ont. (res); Wes '50; M.Sc. (Biochem.); AviaMed; Dir. of Biochem., Surg. Gen. Staff, NDHQ; Tel. 992-2392.

WICKETT, William A.; 383 Ellis St., Penticton, B.C.; 689 Winnipeg St. (res); Alb '49; MCGP; Tel. 492-3024.

WICKHAM, Thomas; Ladysmith, B.C.; UBC'59; MCGP.

WICKS, Clarence A.; Tor '30; FCCP; IntMed (T.B.); Med. Supt., Toronto Hosp., Weston; Tel. RO 9-1161.

WICKWARE, Douglas M.; Qns '46; D.Psy., Psy; Med. Supt., Ontario Hosp., London, Ont.; Inst'r., Psy., U. of Western Ontario; Tel. 455-5110.

WICKWARE, John P.; 267 O'Connor St., Ottawa, Ont.; Tor'50; DiagRad; Active Cons., National Defence Med. Centre; Tel. 232-9629.

WICKWIRE, James A.; 1428 Ouellette Ave., Windsor, Ont.; Dal'57; DiagRad.

WICKWIRE, John C.; Liverpool, N.S.; Main St. (res); Dal '27; M.C.G.P.; Staff, Queens Gen. Hosp.

WIEBE, Bernhard B.; Box 999, Taber, Alta; Alb '62.

WIEBE, Cornelius W.; Winkler Clinic, Winkler, Man., Box 920 (res); Man '25; M.C.G.P.; Public Health Off.; Tel. 325-4312.

WIEBE, Harold J.; Alb'65; Res., Royal Alexandra Hosp., Edmonton, Alta.

WIEBE, Harvey L.; 21 Upper Middle Rd., Cooksville, Ont.; Alb'54; Ophth; Staff, South Peel Hosp.; Tel. 277-3554.

WIEBE, Heinz H.; 350 King St. W., Kitchener, Ont.; 158 John Blvd., Waterloo (res); Frankfurt (Germ.) '37; Tel. 742-6665.

WIEBE, James H.; 2091 Knightsbridge Rd., Ottawa 13, Ont.; Man '45; M.P.H. (Johns Hopkins); Regional Dir. Eastern Reg. Med. Serv., Dept. of National Health & Welfare; Tel. PA 2-1878.

WIEBE, Jerry P.; Medical Clinic, Fort Churchill, Man.; Sask'65.

WIEBE, John H.; 616 South Dr., Winnipeg 9, Man.; Man '50; (N.P.).

WIEBE, R. Herbert; Estevan, Sask.; Sask'62.

WIEGAND, Frederick M.; Box 2455, Campbell River, B.C.; McG'60; GenSurg.

WIEGAND, W. John; 30 Queen St. E., Galt, Ont.; 72 Blair Rd. (res); Tor '41; M.C.G.P.; Staff, South Waterloo Mem. Hosp.; Assoc. Staff, St. Mary's Hosp., Kitchener; Tel. 621-2560.

WIEGERINCK, Angeline T. (Vermaas); Miller & Ross Clinic, Elk Point, Alta.; Man '22; M.O.H. Elk Point; Tel. 724-3955.

WIELHORSKI, W. Alexander; 79 Cornwall Ave., Town of Mount Royal, P.Q.; Edinburgh (Scot.) '45; D.A.B.A., F.A.C.A., Anaes; Anaes., Maisonneuve Hosp., & Montreal Inst. of Cardiol; Ass't. Prof. (Anaes.), U. of Mtl.; Tel. RE 9-6006.

WIENER, Fred; 5140 Victoria, Montreal 26, P.Q.; 6210 Clanranald, Mtl. 29 (res); McG '43; FAAP; Paed; Ass't. Jewish Gen. & Mtl. Children's Hosp's.; Lect., (Health & Soc. Med.), McGill U.; Tel. 737-6687.

WIENS, A. Thomas; 1726 W. Broadway, Vancouver, B.C.; 1675 W. 58th St. (res): Man '35; DABR, DiagRad; Tel. RE 8-5118.

WIENS, Cornelius W.; Assiniboine Clinic, N. E. Booth & Lodge, Winnipeg, Man.; Man'65.

WIENS, Harold A.; Box 180, Coaldale, Alta.; Man'64.

WIGBY, Stephen B.; Box 157, Wells, B.C.; Tor '50; Staff, Gold Quartz Hosp.; Tel. 994-3313.

WIGDERSON, Arthur; Brunswick Diagnostic Group, 25 Brunswick Ave., Toronto 5, Ont.; Tor '53; IntMed; Staff, Doctor's Hosp.; Tel. 924-9741.

WIGGIN, Norman J. B.; Box 62, Station K, Toronto 12, Ont.; 172 Owen Blvd., Willowdale (res); Qns '44; M.Sc. (Med.), Ph.D. (Cambridge); Chief Supt., Defence Research Med. Labs.; Tel. 633-4240.

WIGGINS, Reginald H.; 664 Huron St., Toronto, Ont.; McG '24.

WIGGINS, R. Lawrence; 723 Fort St., Victoria, B.C.; 1118 D'Arcy Lane, R.R. 4 (res); Alb '45; D.M.Sc. (USA); DABO; FRCS(C), Ophth; Tel. 386-1451.

WIGHT, Douglas C.; 236½ King St. W., Brockville, Ont.; Qns'60; Court. Staff, St. Vincent de Paul & Brockville Gen. Hosp's.; Tel. 342-0233.

WIGHT, Eli W.; Qns'62; M.A., Ph.D.; Assoc. Admin. (Med. Dir.), St. John's Gen. Hosp., St. John's, Nfld.

WIGHT, G. Earle; O.B.E., C. St. J.; 640 Seaforth Med. Bldg., 3550 Cote des Neiges Rd., Montreal 25, P.Q.; 4698 Roslyn Ave. (res); McG '25; FAM; IntMed; Cons. Staff, Montreal Gen. Hosp.; Lect. (Med.), McGill U.; Chief of Med. Services, C.P.R.; Tel. 935-2831.

WIGHT, Norman J.; 200 Greyhound Bldg., 622-1st St. S.W., Calgary, Alta.; Alb'51; Tel. AM 3-5030.

WIGHTMAN, Keith J. R.; Private Patients Pavilion, Toronto Gen. Hosp., Toronto, Ont.; 181 Glencairn Ave., Tor. 12 (res); Tor '37; FACP, FRCP(C), IntMed; Phys.-in-Chief, Toronto Gen. Hosp.; Prof. & Chm., Dept. of Med., U. of Toronto; Tel. EM 6-8211; Loc. 2398.

WIGHTMAN, Patricia A. (Pickard); 408 Lamont Blvd., Winnipeg, Man.; Man'56.

WIGHTMAN, R. Clive; Assiniboine Clinic, 633 Lodge, Winnipeg 12, Man.; Man'53; FRCS(C), GenSurg; Active Staff, Grace Hosp.; Assoc. Staff, Misericordia Hosp.; Tel. 837-8361.

WIGLE, Douglas St. J.; Medical Arts Bldg., Windsor, Ont.; 4283 Riverside Dr. (res); Tor '22; F.R.C.S.(Edin.), GenSurg; Sr. Surg., Grace & Hotel Dieu Hosp's.; Tel. CL 2-8291. Retired.
WIGLE, E. Douglas; 83 Brooke Ave., Toronto 12, Ont. (res); Tor '53; FRCP(C); FACP; IntMed; Att'd. Phys., (Cardiovas.Unit.) Toronto Gen. Hosp.; Clin. Instr., U. of Toronto; Tel. EM 6-8211, Ext. 2284.
WIGLE, Ronald D.; Qns'65; Res., Kingston General Hosp., Kingston, Ont.
WIGLE, William D.; 875 Bay St., Toronto 5, Ont.; Tor '51; FRCP(C), IntMed; Dir. Div. of T.B. Prevention, Dept. of Health, Ontario; Tel. 365-2301.
WIGLE, William W.; Ste. 1110, 141 Laurier Ave. W., Ottawa 4, Ont.; Qns'43; MCGP; Pres., Pharmaceutical Manufacturers Assoc. of Canada; Tel. 233-9397.
WIGLESWORTH, Frederick W.; 344-41st Ave., Lachine, P.Q. (res); Man '31; D.A.B.P.; F.C.(Path); PathBact; Dir, Dept. of Path., Montreal Children's Hosp.; Prof. (Path), McGill U.; Tel. WE 7-8511, Loc. 353.
WIGMORE, Ernest W.; Fort Churchill, Man.; Sask'65.
WIGMORE, Frederick H.; Moose Jaw Clinic, 200 Scott Bldg., Moose Jaw, Sask.; 1148 Redland Ave. (res); Dal '35; F.A.C.S., F.R.C.S.(C), GenSurg; Dist. M.O., C.P.R.; Tel. 692-2373.
WIGNALL, Norman; St. Vincent's Hosp., Vancouver 9, B.C.; Liverpool (Eng.)'52; Path; Pathol., Grace Hosp.; Tel. 876-7171.
WILANSKY, Douglas L.; 445 Ellendale Med. Bldg., 5845 Cote-des-Neiges Rd., Montreal 26, P.Q.; 4050 Cote-Ste-Catherine Rd. Atp. 5 (res); Dalhousie '51; F.R.C.P.(C), IntMed (Metab. & Endocrin.); Biochem. (P.Q.); Clin. Fell., Dept. of Research & Jr. Clin. Ass't. (Med.), Jewish Gen. Hosp.; Tel. RE 3-3327.
WILBEE, Godfrey S.; 1284-56th St., Ladner, B.C.; 5065-6th Ave. (res); UBC '57; MCGP; Tel. 943-2712.
WILBUSH, Joel; 7113-106th St., Edmonton, Alta. (res); Sheffield (Eng.) '43; MB, Ch.B., MRCOG (Lond.); Tel. 477-5355.
WILBY, A. G.; Loring, Ont.; Qns '33; Tel. 757-2850.
WILCHESKY, Isaac L.; Room 305, 50 Place Cremazie, Montreal, P.Q.; Geneva (Switz.) '61; Tel. 388-9312.
WILCOCK, George F.; 200 Med. Arts Bldg., Calgary, Alt.; R.R. No. 4 (res); Qns '34; Active Staff, Calgary Gen., Grace & Alta Children's Hosp's.; Tel. 263-7626.
WILCOCK, Peter F.; 418 Medical Arts Bldg., 11010 Jasper Ave., Edmonton, Alta.; McG '59; FRCP(C), Paed.
WILCOX, Charles F.; 209 Medico-Dental Bldg., 150 Metcalfe St., Ottawa 4, Ont.; 716 Parkdale Ave. (res); Tor '34; Tel. 235-6084.
WILCOX, L. DeWitt; 719 Waterloo St., London, Ont.; Wes '29; F.R.C.P.(C) IntMed; Sr. Assoc. in Med., U. of Western Ontario; Tel. GE 4-5313.
WILDER, Edmund M.; 624-6th St., New Westminster, B.C.; 822 York St. (res); Man '34; MCGP; Active Staff, Royal Columbian Hosp; Tel. LA 2-0688.
WILDERSPIN, Kenneth; London (Eng.)'55; DMRD(Eng.); Staff, Henderson Gen. Hosp., Hamilton, Ont.
WILENIEC, M. John; Box 86, Qu'Appelle, Sask.; M.C.G.P.
WILENSKY, Beryl A. (See Chernick).
WILENSKY, Hyman M.; 311 Medical-Dental Bldg., 450 Central Ave., London, Ont.; 1017 Waterloo St. (res); Wes '30; F.C.C.P., A.M.-C.A.A., IntMed (TB); Tel. 432-8440.
WILEY, Alan M., M.B.E.; 306 Toronto Western Med. Bldg., 25 Leonard Ave., Toronto 2B, Ont.; 82 Poplar Plains Cres. Tor. 7 (res); Trinity Coll. (Dublin, Ire.) '48; M.Ch., FRCS(Eng.), FRCS (C), OrthSurg; Att'd. Surg., Toronto Western Hosp.; Lect., U. of Toronto; Tel. EM 8-2012.
WILEY, Elizabeth (Weiser); Ste. 201, Medical Arts Bldg., 280 Bloor St. W., Toronto 5, Ont.; 531 Blythwood Rd. (res); Prague (Czech.) '30; FAGS; GenSurg; ObstGyn; Cons. (ObstGyn.), Women's College Hosp.; Tel. 924-1949.
WILEY, James J.; 178 Laurier Ave. E., Ottawa, Ont.; 73 Marlow Cr. (res); Ott '55; FRCS(C); OrthSurg; Staff, Ottawa Gen. Hosp.; Cons. St. Vincent's Hosp.; Clin. Ass't. U. of Ottawa; Tel. 236-0586.
WILFONG, Dorothy E. W.; 126 Emerald St. S., Hamilton, Ont. (res); Wes '35; Retired.
WILFONG, James H.; Moose Jaw Clinic, 200 Scott Bldg., Moose Jaw, Sask.; 68 Oxford St. W. (res); Wes '35; GenSurg; Chief of Surg., Providence Hosp.; Tel. 692-2373.
WILFORD, Agatha; 415 Princess W., Chilliwack, B.C. (res); Tor '45; Not practising.
WILFORD, E. John; 299 Main St., Chilliwack, B.C.; 415 Princess W. (res); Tor '45; MCGP; Active Staff, Chilliwack Gen. Hosp.; Tel. 792-1908.
WILFORD, William L.; 510 Wellington St., Wallaceburg, Ont.; 208 William St. (res); Wes '54.
WILHELMSON, Marius; 146 Wellesley St. E., Toronto 5, Ont.; 2 Red Oaks Cres., Tor. 17 (res); Tor '33; MCGP; Court. Staff, Western, Wellesley & Grace Hosp's.; Tel. 924-7455.
WILK, Edward J.; 5 Elderidge Ave., Toronto 18, Ont.; Tor'59; FRCS(C), ObstGyn; Staff, St. Joseph's Hosp., Toronto 3, Ont.; Tel. 534-9531.
WILKE, Albert A.; 70-8th St. N.W., Medicine Hat, Alta.; Alb '62; Tel. 527-5256.
WILKES, L. Barry; 110 Yonge St. S., Aurora, Ont.; Tor'65; Staff, York County Hosp., Newmarket; Tel. 727-4245.
WILKES, James R.; Tor '56; Res., Sunnybrook Hosp., Toronto, Ont.
WILKENS, Claus H.; 1961 Gerrard St. E., Toronto 8, Ont.; Germ '56; Tel. OX 4-5051.
WILKEY, William D.; Med. Arts Bldg., 550 Ingersoll Ave., Woodstock, Ont.; 264 Victoria St. N. (res); Wes '46; M.Sc., MRCP(Lond.); FRCP (C), IntMed; Hd. Dept. of Med., Woodstock Gen. Hosp.; Cons. (IntMed), Ont. Hosp.; Tel. 537-8662.
WILKIE, Adam M.; Ste. 508, 1849 Yonge St., Toronto 7, Ont.; Edinburgh (Scot.) '57; MCGP.
WILKIE, Archibald L.; 3480 Cote des Neiges Rd. Montreal, P.Q. (res); F.R.C.S.(C), GenSurg; Staff, Royal Victoria Hosp.; Tel. VI 2-1251.
WILKIE, John S.; Sask'64; Res., Vancouver Gen. Hosp., Vancouver 9, B.C.
WILKIE, Theodore F.; Ste. 100, 755 W. Broadway, Vancouver 9, B.C.; Man'52; FACS; FRCS(C); PlasSurg; Tel. 874-3130.
WILKINS, A. Ralph; 631 Med. Arts Bldg., Toronto, Ont.; 219 Strathallan Wood (res); Tor '24; Anaes; Tel. WA 2-7495.
WILKINS, George D.; Hanna, Alta.; Wes '45; M.C.G.P.; Staff, Hanna Mun. Hosp.; Dist. Coroner; Tel. 854-3341.
WILKINS, Graeme E.; UBC'65; Res., Vancouver Gen. Hosp., Vancouver 9, B.C.
WILKINS, R. Dennis; London (Eng.)'40; FRCS (Eng.); FRCS(Edin.); M.O. I/C, Grand Bank Hosp., Grand Bank, Nfld.; Tel. 962.
WILKINS, Warren W. J.; Ste. 103, Medical Dental Bldg., 450 Central Ave., London, Ont.; Qns '43; D.M.R., D.A.B.R., F.R.C.P.(C), D & T Rad; Staff St. Joseph's Hosp.; Lect. (Rad.), U. of Western Ont.; Tel. 433-2841.
WILKINSON, Alexander A.; Box 213, Neilburg, Sask.; Cambridge (Eng.)'56; Tel. 823-4373.
WILKINSON, Allan A.; Dal'45; Staff, Old Perlican Hosp., Old Perlican, Nfld.
WILKINSON, David; 13916-86th Ave., Edmonton, Alta. (res); London (Eng.) '53; M.B., B.S.; Paed; Staff, Chas. Camsell Hosp.; Instr., U. of Alberta; Tel. GL 5-7141.
WILKINSON, Derek B.; Community Clinic, 8th Ave. & 1st St. E., Prince Albert, Sask.; Liverpool (Eng.) '48; Tel. 763-6466.
WILKINSON, Frank W.; 54 Golfdale Rd., Toronto 12, Ont.; Tor '21; Tel. HU 3-9751.

WILKINSON, Gordon W.; 416 Avenue Bldg., Saskatoon, Sask.; 306 Lake Cres. (res); Tor '46; F.R.C.S.(C), GenSurg; Staff, University, Saskatoon City & St. Paul's Hosps.; Tel. 244-6779.
WILKINSON, James A.; 31 Centre St. S., Brampton, Ont.; Tor '58; FRCS(C), GenSurg; Tel. 459-2106.
WILKINSON, Ralph D.; Royal Victoria Hosp., Montreal 2, P.Q.; Qns'56; FRCP(C), Derm.; Clin. Ass't. Med. & Dir., Derm. Research Unit, Royal Victoria Hosp.; Lect. Med., McGill U.; Tel. VI 2-1251, Loc. 1722.
WILKINSON, Robert H.; Toronto Western Med. Bldg., 25 Leonard Ave., Toronto 2B, Ont.; Tor '55; FRCS(C), GenSurg; Att'd. Surg., Toronto Western Hosp.; Clin. Teach., U. of Toronto; Tel. 366-4462.
WILKS, Washington E.; 851 Bidwell St., Vancouver, B.C.; (res); London (Eng.) '08; FRCS (Eng.); Retired.
WILL, Peter K.; Ste 305, 4900 Kingsway, Burnaby, B.C.; London (Eng.) '56; M.B., B.S., MRCS (Eng.); LRCP (Lond.); DRCOG; Paed; FRCP(C), Paed.
WILL, Ralph E.; 219 Med. Arts Bldg., 170 St. George St., Toronto, Ont.; 1392 Centre Rd. (res); Tor '37; F.R.C.P., IntMed.; Tel. WA 2-4240.
WILLANS, Martin; Ste. 10, 11440 60th Ave., Edmonton, Alta.; Alta'61.
WILLARD, Garry L.; Qns '63; Res., Toronto Western Hosp., Toronto 2B, Ont.
WILLETT, Alex W.; 76 Jane St., Toronto, Ont.; Tor '30; MCGP; Assoc. Staff, Toronto Western Hosp.; Tel. 762-2689.
WILLIAMS, Alfred D.; 4 Lake St., St. Catharines, Ont.; 15 Hillcrest (res); Tor '37; GenSurg; Staff, St. Catharines Gen., Hotel Dieu, & Niagara Falls Gen. Hosp's.; Tel. MU 5-5670.
WILLIAMS, A. Ralph; Box 730 Salmon Arm, B.C.; Man '53; Att'd. Staff, Shuswap Lake Gen. Hosp.; Tel. TE 2-2191.
WILLIAMS, B. D.; Bracebridge, Ont.; Tor'65.
WILLIAMS, C. D. G.; 2917 Bloor St. W., Toronto, Ont.; 38 King George's Rd. (res); Tor '32; F.R.C.S.(Edin.), GenSurg; Staff (Orth.), St. Joseph's Hosp.; Tel. RO 7-8778.
WILLIAMS, Christopher N.; Bay Despoir, Nfld.; London (Eng.)'60; Tel. St. Albans 3511.
WILLIAMS, Clair C.; Tor'63; Res., Toronto Gen. Hosp., Toronto 2, Ont.
WILLIAMS, Claude V.; R.R. 1, Georgetown, Ont.; Tor'22; MCGP; Retired.
WILLIAMS, Clement E.; 299-24th St., West Vancouver, B.C.; 1281-20th St. (res); Qns'60; MCGP; Tel. 922-5450.
WILLIAMS, Dita M. (Evans); 219-5th Ave. E., Hanna, Alta. (res); **Aberdeen (Scot.) '57; DPH; M.O., Big Country Health Unit.**
WILLIAMS, David R.; 223 Doris Ave., Willowdale, Ont.; 12 Sumner Hgts. Dr. (res); Tor '57; Staff, Branson & Grace Hosp's.; Tel. BA 1-8333.
WILLIAMS, Donald H.; 301 Wesbrook Bldg., U. of British Columbia, Vancouver, B.C.; 6187 Macdonald St. (res); Man '31; DABD; DermSyph; Hd., Dept. of Cont. Med. Educ., Van. Gen. Hosp.; Prof. & Hd., Dept. of Cont. Med. Educ., U. of British Columbia; Tel. CA 4-1111.
WILLIAMS, Eldon S. V.; 7529 Earle Rd., Cote St-Luc, Montreal, P.Q.; McG'60; GenSurg.
WILLIAMS, Floyd G.; 595 Newdale Rd., West Vancouver, B.C.; Alb'52; Anaes.
WILLIAMS, Garnet W.; 58 Wellington E., Aurora, Ont.; Tor '08; Dist. Coroner.
WILLIAMS, Getchel D.; 23 Applewood Village, **Ste. 3, Cooksville, Ont.; Man '50; FRCS(C), Urol;** Chief of Med. Staff, South Peel Hosp.; Tel. 277-3231.
WILLIAMS, Gordon E.; Box 25, 1725 Lakeshore Hwy. W., Clarkson, Ont.; 2043 Hindhead Rd. (res); Tor '59; Active Staff, Oakville-Trafalgar Mem. Hosp.; Court. Staff, South Peel Hosp., Cooksville.; Tel. 822-9161.
WILLIAMS, Harold A.; 38 Jane St., Toronto, Ont.; 10 Strath Ave. (res); Tor '33; D.C.H. (Eng.); Paed; Clin. Ass't., O.P.D., Hosp. for Sick Children; Tel. RO 9-8996.
WILLIAMS, H. Bruce; 430 Seaforth Med. Bldg., 3550 Cote des Neiges Rd., Montreal 25, P.Q.; McG'55; FRCS(C); PlasSurg; Ass't. Surg., Montreal Children's & Montreal Gen. Hosp's.; Dem. (Surg.), McGill U.; Tel. 933-7730.
WILLIAMS, Henry I.; Courtenay, B.C.; Comox (res); McG '39; M.C.G.P.
WILLIAMS, Henry T.; 1819 Saskatchewan Dr., Edmonton, Alta.; Liverpool (Eng.)'48; FRCS (Eng.), FRCS(C), FACS; GenSurg; Att'd. Surg., U. of Alberta Hosp.; Ass't. Prof. (Surg.), U. of Alberta; Tel. GA 2-6956.
WILLIAMS, Hugh R.; 1621 Harbour Dr., New Westminster, B.C.; Man'57.
WILLIAMS, Ignace K.; 194 Salaberry Rd., Chateauguay Basin, Que.; **Mon '30; Dist. Coroner;** Tel. 692-9222.
WILLIAMS, Ivor H.; Yellow Point Rd., R.R. 1, Ladysmith, B.C.; Cambridge (Eng.) '51; DABA; Anaes; Active Staff, Nanaimo Reg. Gen. Hosp.; Tel. 753-4229.
WILLIAMS, J. Collis; Harriston, Ont.; Qns '28; Staff, Palmerston Gen. & St. Joseph's Hosp's.; Guelph; Tel. 42.
WILLIAMS, John A.; Alb '55; MCGP; Res., Vancouver Gen. Hosp., Vancouver 9, B.C.
WILLIAMS, John G.; Med. Arts Bldg., Empire Ave., St. John's, Nfld.; 7 Osbourne St. (res); Dal '50; Psy; Staff, Grace & St. Clare's Mercy Hosp's.; Assoc. Staff, St. John's Gen. Hosp.; Electroenceph. & Epileptogest., Hosp. for Mental **& Nervous Dis. & Nfld. Dept. of Health; Tel. 578-5359.**
WILLIAMS, John P.; 7 Cashin Ave., St. John's, Nfld. (res); National U. (Ire.) '56; M.B., B.Ch.; BAO; Path; Staff, St. John's Gen., St. Clare's Mercy & Grace Hosp's.; Tel. 8-0471.
WILLIAMS, John V.; 852 Somerville Ave., Oshawa, Ont. (res); Qns '15; Staff, Oshawa Gen. Hosp.; Indus. Phys., General Motors of Canada Ltd.; Retired.
WILLIAMS, Kenneth J.; 4 Durham St. N., Sudbury, Ont.; 83 Regent St. S. (res); Qns '28; Active Staff, St. Joseph's Hosp.; M.O.H. Hagar Twnp.; Tel. 675-8466.
WILLIAMS, Kenneth J.; 270 Aberdeen Ave., Hamilton, Ont. (res); Man '49; MPH(Yale); MACHA; FAPHA; MCGP; Med. Dir., St. Joseph's Hosp.; Cons. Commiss. on Professional & Hosp. Activities, Ann Arbor, Mich.; Surveyor, Canadian Counicl on Hosp. Accreditation; Tel. 522-4949, Ext. 418; Abroad.
WILLIAMS, Kibben; Ste. 1314, 750 W. Broadway, Vancouver 9, B.C.; UBC'64.
WILLIAMS, Leonard J.; Ste. 404, Birks Bldg., 718 Granville St., Vancouver 2, B.C.; 1320 Mathers Ave. W. Vanc. (res); Tor '35; GenSurg; Vis. Staff, Vancouver Gen. Hosp., Sick Children's & Grace Hosp's.; Tel. MU 5-5528.
WILLIAMS, Leslie R.; 1006 Fairmont Med. Bldg., 750 W. Broadway, Vancouver 9, B.C.; 2626 Bellevue Ave. (res); McG '35; F.R.C.S.(Edin.), F.R.C.S.(C), Urol; Cons. (Urol.), Shaughnessy Hosp.; Assoc. Surg., Div. Urol., Dept. of Surg., Vancouver Gen. Hosp.; Clin. Ass't. Prof. U. of British Columbia; Tel. 876-5566.
WILLIAMS, Malcolm F.; 930 Simcoe St., Niagara Falls, Ont.; Tor '38; GenSurg; Surg. Staff, Greater Niagara Gen. Hosp.; Tel. EL 4-4242.
WILLIAMS, Mervyn P.; Alb'64; Res., Shaughnessy Hosp., Vancouver 9, B.C.
WILLIAMS, Milton D.; 86 Queen St., Kitchener, Ont.; Wes '35; Phys., Dominion Electrohome Ind. Ltd.
WILLIAMS, Murray G.; Ste. 1202, 123 Edward St., Toronto 2, Ont.; Man '49; MRCP(Ed.); Derm; Staff, Toronto Gen. Hosp.; Staff, U. of Toronto.
WILLIAMS, Norman; 14 Calder Cres., Regina, Sask. (res); London (Eng.) '47; M.R.C.S. (Eng.), L.R.C.P. (Lond.), D.P.H., D.I.H., Occup. Med (A.B.Prev.Med.); Dir. of Occup. Health, Prov. of Sask., Dept. of Public Health; Lect. (Soc. & Prev. Med.), U. of Saskatchewan; Tel. LA 3-0661.
WILLIAMS, Percy E.; 193 James S. Hamilton, Ont.; 506 Scenic Dr., (res); Tor '28; F.A.A.P., Paed; Tel. JA 8-1173.

WILLIAMS, Ralph C.; 659 Hamilton Rd., London, Ont.; Wes '61; Tel. 455-2850.
WILLIAMS, Robert G.; 210 Medical Centre, 8th Ave. & 8th St. S.W., Calgary, Alta.; Alb'43; FACS; FRCS(Ed.); FRCS(C), GenSurg; Att'd. Surg., Calgary Gen., Holy Cross & Alberta Children's Hosp.; Tel. 263-5453.
WILLIAMS, Robert L.; 91 King St. E., Kingston, Ont.; Qns'62; Research, Queen's U.; Abroad.
WILLIAMS, Robert T.; 3423 Utah Cr., Calgary, Alta.; Cardiff (S. Wales)'57; MRCS; LRCP; Anaes.
WILLIAMS, Seirol L.; 925 W. Georgia St., Vancouver, B.C.; 1457 W. 26th Ave. (res); Harvard (U.S.A.) '33; F.I.C.S., GenSurg; Staff, St. Paul's & Vancouver Gen. Hosp's.; Tel. MU 4-3449.
WILLIAMS, Sybella M.; Box 490, Ocean Falls, B.C.; Man '49.
WILLIAMS, Trevor W.; Rowell Clinic, Water St., Carbonear, Nfld.; Dublin (Ire.)'56; DPH; Paed; Paed-in-Chief, Carbonear Comm. Red Cross Hosp.; Tel. 5018.
WILLIAMS, Wilfrid O.; Box 276, Prescott, Ont.; Tor '24; Retired.
WILLIAMS, William; 133 de Touraine, Preville, P.Q.; London (Eng.)'51.
WILLIAMS, William G.; Wes '64; Res., Hosp. for Sick Children, Toronto 2, Ont.
WILLIAMS, W. W. Dickson; Ste. 4, Medical Bldg., 188 Prince St., Pembroke, Ont.; 278 William St. (res); Tor '31; M.C.G.P.; Staff, Cottage & Pembroke Gen. Hosp's.; Tel. RE 2-3841.
WILLIAMSON, D. Munro; Reg. Phys., Imperial Oil Ltd., Box 2356, 11140-109th St., Edmonton, Alta.; Alb'50; MCGP; Tel. 474-6421.
WILLIAMSON, E. Evelyn; 262 Dundas St. E., Belleville, Ont.; Qns'50; Tel. 968-6316.
WILLIAMSON, Elliot A.; 358 Reynolds St., Oakville, Ont.; Aberdeen (Scot.)'61.
WILLIAMSON, Frank M.; Box 1000, Blenheim, Ont.; Tor'25.
WILLIAMSON, George L.; 615 Tegler Bldg., Edmonton, Alta.; 10223-132nd St. (res); Tor '11; Tel. 422-2844.
WILLIAMSON, Harold F., DFC; 262 Dundas St. E., Belleville, Ont.; Qns '50; FRCS(C), GenSurg; Tel. WO 8-6316.
WILLIAMSON, John A.; Fredericton Med. Clinic, 206 Rookwood Ave., Fredericton, N.B.; 246 Parkhurst Dr. (res); McG '43.
WILLIAMSON, Norval L.; 267 O'Connor St., Ottawa 4, Ont.; 406 Huron St. (res); Qns '42; GenSurg, Att. Staff, Ottawa Civic Hosp.; Cons. (GenSurg), D.V.A.; Tel. CE 3-9464.
WILLIAMSON, Ralph D.; 4015 N. E. 104th St., Seattle, Washington, U.S.A.; Wes '60; Anaes.
WILLIAMSON, Samuel W.; 8 Vancouver St., Yarmouth, N.S.; Dal '96; Retired.
WILLINGS, Horace R.; Box 147, New Denver, B.C.; MRCS (Eng.); LRCP (Lond.).
WILLINSKY, Abraham I.; 120 Madison Ave., Toronto, Ont.; Tor '08; F.A.C.S., F.I.C.S., F.A.S. (M.A.O.), L.M. (Rotunda), F.R.C.S.(C), Urol.
WILLINSKY, Bernard; 604 Spadina Ave., Toronto 4, Ont.; 33 Gardiner Rd., Forest Hill (res); Tor '28; LDS, DDS, LRCP, MRCS, FRCS(Eng.), FICS, FRCS(C), GenSurg; Urol; Surg-in-Chief, New Mount Sinai Hosp. (Emer.); Tel. 922-1410 & 922-2431.
WILLINSKY, Jack M.; 240 McNabb St., Sault Ste. Marie, Ont.; 91 White Oak Dr. (res); Tor '44; Urol; DiagRad; Tel. AL 4-6421.
WILLIS, Diana M.; Wes'65; Res., Montreal General Hosp., Montreal 25, P.Q.
WILLIS, Howard; 175 Broadway E., Vancouver 10, B.C.; 3887 Cartier St. (res); Tor '20; Tel. TR 6-7731. Retired.
WILLIS, John S.; Medical Officer I/C, Dept. of National Health & Welfare, 3rd Floor, United Chinese Bank Bldg., 31-37 Des Voeux Rd., Central P.O. Box 183, Hong Kong, B.C.C.; Tor'45; Abroad.
WILLIS, Neil R.; Wes'65; Res., Victoria Hosp., London, Ont.
WILLIS, Pamela; 3114 Portage Ave., Kirkfield Pk., Winnipeg 12, Man.; Durham (Eng.) '54; M.B., B.S.
WILLISCROFT, Burton A.; 266-9th St. W., Owen Sound, Ont.; 883-7th Ave. E. (res); Tor '27.
WILLISTON, Donald H.; Box 460, Summerland, B.C.; Qns'45.
WILLISTON, John M.; Med. Centre, Maple Ave., New Glasgow, N.S.; 571 Willow Ave. (res); Dal'56; MCGP.
WILLITS, Reba E.; 563 Esquimalt Ave., West Vancouver, B.C.; Tor '31; DPH; PH; Dir. Med. Serv., City of Vancouver; Tel. MU 4-2377. Retired.
WILLMS, George G.; 1291 Ouellette Ave., Windsor, Ont.; 3405 Randolph (res); Wes '56; MCGP; Tel. 256-4100.
WILLMS, John; Ste. 304, 1669 Victoria St., Prince George, B.C.; UBC'55.
WILLOUGHBY, Charles J.; Burris Clinic, 242 Victoria St., Kamloops, B.C.; 133 Battle St. W. (res); Tor '16; GenSurg; Tel. 940.
WILLOUGHBY, Clark R.; 379 Hunter St., Woodstock, Ont.; 172 Light St. (res); Wes '42; Tel. 537-8335.
WILLOUGHBY, Donald V., Sg. Cdr.; 65 Wedgewood Ave., Birch Cove, N.S. (res); Tor '50; FRCS(C), GenSurg; Hd. Dept. of Surg., Cdn. Forces Hosp., Halifax; Ass't. Prof. Surg., Dalhousie U.
WILLOUGHBY, Henry W.; McG'62; PhD; Staff, Royal Victoria Hosp., Montreal 2, P.Q.
WILLOUGHBY, John A.; Burris Clinic, 242 Victoria St., Kamloops, B.C.; UBC '56; Paed; Staff, Royal Inland Hosp.; Tel. 372-3303.
WILLOUGHBY, Lawrence; Bristol (Eng.) '40; MRCOG; ObstGyn; Reg. M.O., Civil Aviation Med., Dept. of Nat. Health & Welfare, 750 Federal Bldg., 98th Ave. & 107th St., Edmonton, Alta.; Tel. 424-0251, Ext. 538.
WILLOWS, Ross L.; 523 Med. Arts Bldg., Winnipeg, Man.; 471 Kingston Cres. (res); Man '43; FRCS(C), ObstGyn; Hd. Dept. of ObstGyn., St. Boniface Hosp.; Ass't. Prof. (ObstGyn), U. of Manitoba; Tel. WH 3-5416.
WILLOX, G. Leslie; 504 Med. Arts Bldg., Edmonton, Alta.; 13911-91 Ave. (res); Alb '43; FACS; FRCS(C), GenSurg; Prof. (Clin.Surg.), U. of Alta; Tel. 422-6956.
WILLS, David G.; 101 Hersey St., Oromocto, N.B.; Dal'61; Tel. 357-8445.
WILLS, R. Roy; Lancaster Medical Centre, 131 Main St., Lancaster, N.B.; Dal'53; Assoc. Staff, Saint John Gen. & St. Joseph's Hosp's.; Tel. 694-5531.
WILLS, William J., W/C; 815 Fleming Ave., Ottawa 8, Ont. (res); Wes '46; M.Sc.(Path); Path; Ass't. Pathol., NDMC; Tel. 922-2474.
WILLSON, David A.; 38 Dorothy St., Welland, Ont.; 49 Weller Ave. (res); Wes '48; M.C.G.P. Tel. RE 4-9746.
WILLSON, Glenn N.; Box 160, Flin Flon Clin., Flin Flon, Man.; Man '42; M.C.G.P.; Anaes., Flin Flon Gen. Hosp. & Assoc. Hosp.; Dist. Coroner.
WILMSHURST, Amy A.; Box 1058, Langley, B.C.; McG '48; MCGP.
WILNER, Saul; 670 Ellendale Med. Bldg., 5845 Cote-des-Neiges Rd., Montreal 26, P.Q.; 759 Kenaston Ave., Twn. of Mt. Royal (res); McG '46; DABP; Psy; Assoc. Psy., Jewish Gen. Hosp.; Lect. (Psy), McGill U.; Tel. RE 1-9711.
WILO-NIRK, Maret M.; 357 Ellis Pk. Rd., Toronto 3, Ont.; Alexander U. (Erlangen, W. Germ.) '49; Tel. 766-0287.
WILSON, Ada (See Wallace, Ada).
WILSON, Addison E.; 406 Rideau Med. Bldg., 1711-4th St. S.W., Calgary, Alta.; 3903 Crestview Rd. (res); Alb '33; ObstGyn; Chief ObstGyn., Holy Cross Hosp.; Tel. 263-2736.
WILSON, Alexander S.; 2416 Portage Ave., Winnipeg 12, Man.; London (Eng.)'56; Tel. VE 2-2548.
WILSON, Alpheus M.; Barrington, N.S.; Dal '25.

WILSON, Andre; 2157 Fleury East, Montreal 12, P.Q.; 10610 Hague (res); Mon '54; Tel. DU 1-2581.

WILSON, Angus M.; 42 Albert St., Stratford, Ont.; 11 Dension St. (res); Tor '47; M.C.G.P. Tel. 271-0172.

WILSON, Arthur P.; 955 Ouellette Ave., Windsor, Ont.; R.R. No. 2, Harrow (res); Tor '43; D.A.B.D., DermSyph; Cons. Derm., Metropolitan Gen., Hotel Dieu & Grace Hosp's.; Tel. CL 2-8487.

WILSON, Bentley R.; Middleton, N.S.; Dal '43; MCGP.

WILSON, Bruce M.; 137 Cedar St., Sudbury, Ont.; Tor '43; FRCS(C), GenSurg; Chief of Surg., Sudbury Gen. Hosp.; Tel. OS 4-9641.

WILSON, C. Claire; Ste. 302, 625-5th Ave., New Westminster, B.C.; 920 Chestnut (res); Man '41; M.C.G.P.; Staff, Royal Columbian & St. Mary's Hosp's.; Tel. LA 2-7730.

WILSON, Charles L.; 3550 Cote des Neiges Rd., Ste. 700, Montreal, P.Q.; McG'40; FRCS(C), OrthSurg; Assoc. Surg., Montreal Gen. Hosp.; OrthSurg., Reddy Mem. Hosp.; Ass't. Prof. (Surg.), McGill U.; Tel. WE 5-8667.

WILSON, Clarence G.; Port Arthur Clinic, 194 North Court St., Port Arthur, Ont.; Man'37; Paed; Tel. DI 4-7271.

WILSON, Clifford S.; 159 Frederick St., Kitchener, Ont.; Conestogo (res); Qns '29; F.A.C.S., F.R.C.S.(C), GenSurg; Surg. Staff, Kitchener-Waterloo, St. Mary's & Freeport Hosp's.; Tel. SH 5-8183.

WILSON, David F.; Ste. 903, 24 Queen St. E., Brampton, Ont.; Wes'60.

WILSON, D. Laurence; Etherington Hall, Stuart St., Kingston, Ont.; Qns'44; MA(Tor); FACP; FRCP(C), IntMed; Att'd. Phys., Kingston Gen. Hosp.; Cons Med., DVA & Cdn. Forces Hosp.; Assoc. Prof. (Med.), Queen's U.; Tel. 546-9553.

WILSON, Donald H.; 221 Outremont Ave., Montreal 8, P.Q.; McG '56; Staff, Queen Mary Vet's Hosp.; Tel. 738-9481.

WILSON, Donald R.; 202 Toronto Western Med. Bldg., 25 Leonard Ave., Toronto 2B, Ont.; R.R. 3, Caledon, Ont. (res); Tor '42; FRCS(C), GenSurg; Hd. Cardiovasc Surg & Surg-in-Chief, Toronto Western Hosp.; Prof. of Surg., U. of Toronto; Tel. EM 4-7522.

WILSON, Donald R.; 9235-117th St., Edmonton, Alta. (res); McG '39; F.A.C.P., F.R.C.P.(C), IntMed.; Dir., Med. Serv., U. of Alberta Hosp.; Prof. & Chm. (Med.), U. of Alta.; Tel. 439-5911, Loc. 272.

WILSON, Douglas M., F/L; Nat. Defence Med. Centre, Ottawa 8, Ont.; Tor '64.

WILSON, Douglas R.; Tor '59; FRCP(C) IntMed; Staff, Toronto Gen. Hosp., Toronto 2, Ont.; Tel. EM 6-8211.

WILSON, Edward; Dublin (Ire.)'40; Supt., Henderson Gen. Hosp., Hamilton, Ont.

WILSON, Edward M.; St. Paul, Alb.; Alb'63; AMCGP.

WILSON, F. Lucille; 5033 Wesley Rd., R.R. No. 2, Royal Oak, B.C. (res); Tor '49; Path; Ass't. Path., & Dir. of Isotope Lab., Royal Jubilee Hosp., Victoria; Tel. EV 6-3131.

WILSON, Frank C. S.; 128 Robert St., Napanee, Ont.; Tor '04; Dist. Coroner.

WILSON, Frank D.; 5780 Cambie St., Vancouver 15, B.C.; 6187 Alma St. (res); Tor '47; M.S. (OrthSurg) (Tenn.); DABS; OrthSurg; Att'd. Staff, St. Vincent's & Children's Hosp's.; Tel. FA 7-1000.

WILSON, Frank L.; 901 Helena St., C. S. Williams Clinic, Trail, B.C.; 24 Hazelwood Dr. (res); McG '33; D. & TRad; Rad., Trail Tadanac, & Mater Misericordia Hosp's., & Dalhousie Clinic. Tel. 368-5211.

WILSON, G. Duff.; 850 King St. W., Kitchener, Ont.; Tor '29; DPH; M.O.H., Kitchener.

WILSON, George B.; 136 E. 15th St., North Vancouver, B.C.; 2749 Eastern Ave. (res); Man '45; IntMed; Active Staff, North Vancouver Gen. Hosp.; Tel. YU 8-0727.

WILSON, George S. M.; Medical Arts Bldg., 165 Plymouth Rd. Welland, Ont.; 133 Fitch St. (res); Edinburgh (Scot.) '37; M.B., Ch.B., F.R.C.S. (Edin.), F.R.C.S.(Eng.); D.L.O.; GenSurg; Urol; Staff, Welland County Gen. Hosp.; Tel. RE 2-2711.

WILSON, G. E. Pearson; 514 Medical Arts Bldg., 170 St. George St., Toronto, Ont.; 20 Chestnut Park Rd. (res); Tor '40; F.R.C.S.(C), GenSurg; Tel. WA 1-1938.

WILSON, Gerald C. H.; Med. Arts Bldg., 1105 Pandora Ave., Victoria, B.C.; 30 Beach Drive, (res); Manchester (Eng.)'54; DiagRad.; Staff, Royal Jubilee Hosp.; Tel. EV 3-6161.

WILSON, Gerald E.; 122 Sydney St., Cornwall, Ont.; 46 Bethune St., Long Sault (res); Tor '32; D.Psy; Psy; Staff Psy., Hotel-Dieu Hosp.; Psy., Cornwall Gen. Hosp.; Tel. WE 2-2168.

WILSON, Gerald L.; Ste. 110, 73 Cumberland St. N., Port Arthur, Ont.; Man'53; FRCS(C), ObstGyn.

WILSON, G. Lowen; Box 1147, Drumheller, Alta.; Belfast (Ire.)'59; BAO; MRCS; LRCP; Staff, Drumheller Gen. Hosp.; Tel. 823-3345.

WILSON, Gordon L.; Ste. 370, 8409 112th. St., Edmonton, Alta.; Alb '40; OrthSurg; Orth. Surg., U. of Alta., Edmonton Gen. & Royal Alexandra Hosp's.; Instr. in Orth. Surg., U. of Alta.

WILSON, Gordon McL; 511 Lawrence Ave., Kelowna, B.C.; R.R. 4 Sarsons Rd. (res); Tor '40; FICS; MCGP; Chmn., Med. Advisory Committ. & Chief of Staff, Kelowna Gen. Hosp.; Tel. 762-2005.

WILSON, Harry E.; 3250 W. 37th Ave., Vancouver, B.C. (res); Dal '37; Aviation Med.; Dist. M.O., C.P.R.; Ass't. Chief Med. Serv., C.P.A. Lines, Ltd.; Tel. MU 1-2212.

WILSON, Helen P. (Foulds); Banff, Alta.; London (Eng.) '54; Retired.

WILSON, Henry D.; 150 Elizabeth Dr., Gander, Nfld. (res); National U. (Galway, Ire.) '46; AB Rad; MACR; Radiol., James Paton Mem. Hosp.; Staff, The Grenfell Mission Hosp., St. Anthony.

WILSON, Hugh D.; 32 Esther Ann Dr., Orillia, Ont.; Wes '36; D.Psy.; Staff, Ontario Hosp. School, Orillia; Tel. FA 6-7361.

WILSON, Ian; Atkin Clin., Banff, Alta.; Trinity Coll. (Dublin, Ire.) '47; F.R.C.S.(Edin.) GenSurg; Pres. of Med. Staff, Mineral Springs Hosp.; Tel. PO 2-2155.

WILSON, Ian C.; 188 King St. W., Cobourg, Ont.; Wes'51; GenSurg.

WILSON, Irving W.; Alb '59; Res., Royal Alexandra Hosp., Edmonton, Alta.

WILSON, James A.; 1015 Med. Arts Bldg., 1538 Sherbrooke St. W., Montreal 25, P.Q.; Dal'48; FRCS(Ed.); FRCS(C), GenSurg; ThorSurg; Surg., Royal Edward Chest Hosp.; Cons. ThorSurg., Queen Mary Vet's Hosp.; Ass't. Surg., Queen Elizabeth & Reddy Mem. Hosp's.; Tel. WE 3-6903.

WILSON, James J.; 916 Prince St., Truro, N.S.; 44 Broad St. (res); Queen's (N. Ire.) '40; MB, BCh., BAO; Active Staff, Colchester Co. Hosp.; Tel. 893-7366.

WILSON, J. Marcel; 12774 ouest, boul Gouin, Pierrefonds, P.Q.; Mon '51; Tel. 626-5041.

WILSON, James W.; Ste. 505, 625-5th Ave., New Westminster, B.C.; McG'37; DABS; MS(Surg); FRCS(C), GenSurg; Chief of Surg., Royal Columbian Hosp.; Cons. Staff, Surrey Mem. Hosp., Surrey & Prov. Mental Hosp., Essondale; Staff, St. Mary's Hosp.; Clin. Instr., Surg., U. of British Columbia; Tel. 521-8432.

WILSON, John A.; 391 Merritt St., St. Catharines, Ont.; Tor'30; Tel. 684-4561.

WILSON, John C.; 360 Queen's Ave., London, Ont.; 274 Huron St. (res); Wes '49; F.R.C.S. (Eng.), F.R.C.S.(C), GenSurg; Tel. 438-1601.

WILSON, John C. S.; 176 Catherine St., Port Colborne, Ont.; 113 Tennessee Ave. (res); Qns '42; MCGP; Chief Dept. of G.P., Port Colborne Gen. Hosp.; Dist. Coroner Welland County; Tel. TE 4-3638.

WILSON, John K.; Ste. 1220, 123 Edward St., Toronto 2, Ont.; 83 de Vere Gds. (res); Tor '48; FRCP(C), IntMed; Staff Phys., St. Michael's Hosp;. Assoc. (Med.), U. of Toronto; Tel. EM 6-3629.

WILSON, John P.; 4 Church St. S., Richmond Hill, Ont.; Tor '11.

WILSON, John R.; Ste. 1215, 750 W. Broadway, Vancouver 9, B.C.; Qns '40; DABP; Psy; Att'd. Staff, Vancouver Gen. & Shaughnessy DVA Hosp's.; Lect. (Psy.), U. of British Columbia.

WILSON, John R.; 194 Court St. N., Port Arthur, Ont.; London (Eng.)'54; DTM&H; Med. Staff, St. Joseph's Gen., Port Arthur Gen. & Westmount Hosp's.; Tel. 344-7271.

WILSON, John R.; 3831 Albert St., Regina, Sask.; Edinburgh (Scot.)'49; Staff, Regina Gen. Hosp.; Tel. 536-0991.

WILSON, John T.; 1906 Como Lake Ave., Coquitlam, New Westminster, B.C.; Edinburgh (Scot.) '56; Tel. 936-4422.

WILSON, J. Sheldon; McG'50; DiagRad; Staff, Cariboo Mem. Hosp., Williams Lake, B.C.

WILSON, Katharine F.; (see Bradley, Katharine F.).

WILSON, K. Barrie; 32 Flamborough Dr., Toronto 15, Ont.; Qns '57; Anaes; Assoc. Staff, Northwestern Gen. Hosp.; Tel. 247-7003.

WILSON, Kenneth E.; Ste. 503, 267 O'Connor St., Ottawa, Ont.; 734 Island Park Dr. (res); McG '40; F.R.C.S.(C), GenSurg; Sr. Surg., Ottawa Civic Hosp.; Assoc. Prof. (Clin.Surg.), U. of Ottawa; Tel. CE 2-1817.

WILSON, L. Duane; 215 Cooper St., Suite No. 1, Ottawa, Ont.; 159 Clemow Ave. (res); Qns '28; F.I.C.S., GenSurg; Att. Surg., Ottawa Civic Hosp.; Ass't. Prof. & Clin. Surg., Queen's U.; Tel. CE 2-6608.

WILSON, Lucille; 5033 Wesley Rd., Victoria, B.C. (res); Tor '49; Path; Staff, Royal Jubilee Hosp.; Tel. EV 3-6161.

WILSON, Malcolm; 335 Pine St., New Westminster, B.C.; UBC'64.

WILSON, M. Muriel (Bannatyne); 361 Virginia Ave., Riverside, Ont. (res); Glasgow (Scot.) '50; Dir. of Med. Serv., Riverview Hosp., Windsor; Tel. CL 4-6426.

WILSON, Murray S.; Ste. 103, 153 St. George St., Toronto 5, Ont.; Tor '48; Psy.

WILSON, Orville B.; Box 99, Manotick, Ont.; Qns'52; MCGP; Active Med. Staff, Ottawa Riverside Hosp., Kemptville Dist. Hosp. & Grace Hosp., Ottawa; Tel. OX 2-3527.

WILSON, Phyllis M. Lee; 1424 Craig Rd., S.W., Calgary, Alta.; Dublin (Ire.) '50; M.B., B.Ch., B.A.O.; Retired.

WILSON, Pierre; Clinique Medicale d'Urgence, Mon '53; 1820 est, Boul. St.-Joseph, Montreal 34, P.Q.; Tel. 3-3563.

WILSON, R. Calvin; 318 Clemow Ave., Ottawa, Ont. (res); Qns '22; Med. Adv., Cdn. Pensions Comm.

WILSON, R. Donald; 10155—120th St., Edmonton, Alta.; 11104-85th Ave. (res); Alb '48; M.C.-G.P.; Tel. 488-7271.

WILSON, Reginald A.; 603-750 W. Broadway, Vancouver 9, B.C.; McG '34; F.R.C.P.(C), Paed; IntMed; Sr. Paed., Van. Gen. Hosp.; Assoc. Clin. Prof. (Paed), U. of British Columbia; Tel. TR 4-1411.

WILSON, Richard; 107 Valley Woods Rd., Apt. 120, Don Mills, Ont. (res); Tor '54; FRCS(C); ObstGyn; Staff, Private Patients Pavilion, Toronto Gen. Hosp.; Active Cons. Surg., Hosp. for Sick Children; Assoc. (ObstGyn.), U. of Toronto; Tel. EM 6-8211.

WILSON, Richard T.; 3800 Radisson St., Montreal 5, P.Q.; Paris (France)'53.

WILSON, R. John; 946 King St. W., Hamilton, Ont.; Qns '41; Tel. JA 9-1432.

WILSON, Robert C. D.; 42 Wharncliffe Rd. N., London, Ont.; 383 St. George St. (res); Aberdeen (Scot.) '56; AMCGP; ECFMG(U.S.A.); Tel. 432-6786.

WILSON, Robert D.; 10155-120th St., Edmonton, Alta.; Alb '48; Tel. 488-7271.

WILSON, Robert G.; C.M.A. (B.C. Div.), 1807 W. 10th Ave., Vancouver 9, B.C.; 4808 Paton St., Van. 8 (res); McG '51; MCGP; Att'd. Staff, Van. Gen. Hosp.; Clin. Instr. (Prev. Med.), U. of British Columbia; Exec. Sec. (BC) Div., CMA; Tel. 736-5551.

WILSON, Robert J.; Connaught Med. Research Labs., 1755 Steeles Ave. W., Willowdale, Ont.; Tor'42; MA; DPH; Ass't. Dir., Connaught Med. Research Labs.; Assoc. Prof. PH & PrevMed., U. of Toronto; Tel. 635-2622.

WILSON, Robert R.; Box 1180, Duncan, B.C.; Berkley St. (res); UBC '55; Tel. 746-4102.

WILSON, Roger; Ste. 804, 750 W. Broadway, Vancouver 9, B.C.; 1646 Laurier Ave. (res); McG '34; F.A.C.S., F.R.C.S.(Eng.), F.R.C.S.(C), GenSurg.; Att. Staff, Vancouver Gen. Hosp.; Cons. Surg., Shaughnessy Hosp. D.V.A.; Ass't. Clin. Prof.(Surg.), U. of British Columbia; Tel. TR 2-5288.

WILSON, Rolla E. (Freygood); Apt. 310, 1820 McGregor, Montreal 25, P.Q. (res); McG '53; D&T Rad.; Staff, Royal Victoria Hosp.; Dem., McGill U.; Tel. VI 2-1251.

WILSON, Ronald H.; Wes'63; Res., Toronto Gen. Hosp., Toronto 2, Ont.

WILSON, Thomas C.; 732 Professional Bldg., 10830 Jasper Ave., Edmonton, Alta; 13514-100th Ave. (res); Qns '37; Otol; Staff, Royal Alexandra, Edmonton Gen., & University of Alberta Hosp's.; Ass't. Prof. (Otol.), U. of Alta.; Tel. 422-4553.

WILSON, Thomas S.; 403 Medical Arts Bldg., Edmonton, Alta.; 11004—84 Ave. (res); Tor '41; F.A.C.S., F.R.C.S.(C), GenSurg; Clin. Prof. of Surg., U. of Alberta; Tel. GA 2-2767.

WILSON, Thomas V.; 245 St. David St., Fergus, Ont.; Tor '41; Tel. 843-1161.

WILSON, W. Andrew; 10523-100th Ave., Edmonton, Alta.; Alb'62.

WILSON, Wesley M.; Reg. Lab., 331 South St., London, Ont.; 162 Devonshire Ave. (res); Wes '28; Path, Bact; Dir., Reg. Lab., (Ont. Dept. of Health), London; Lect. (Path), U. of Western Ont.; Tel. GE 4-4547.

WILSON, Willard W.; 560 Finch Ave. W., Willowdale, Ont.; 16 Cavalier Cres., Thornhill (res); McG '43; Anaes; Chief of Anaes., North York Branson Hosp.; Tel. 633-9420.

WILSON, W. Everton; 5025 Sherbrooke St. W., Ste. 615, Westmount, P.Q.; McG'53; MSc (Exp. Surg.); FRCS(C), OrthSurg; GenSurg; Ass't. Surg., Royal Victoria Hosp.; Cons., Queen Mary Vet's Hosp.; Ass't. Prof. Surg., McGill U.; Tel. 631-9983.

WILSON, William E. C.; Med. Arts Bldg., Hamilton, Ont.; 81 Dromore Cr. (res); Qns '58; FRCP (C), IntMed.

WILSON, William H.; 173 Glenrose Ave., Toront, Ont.; Tor '24; Tel. HU 9-4609.

WILSON, William McC.; Box 700, Hanna, Alta.; Dublin (Ire.) '51; Coroner.

WILSON, Wm. M.; 608 Med. Arts Bldg., 1 Young St., Hamilton, Ont.; 45 Braemar Pl. (res); Tor '55; FRCP(C); Paed; Active Staff, Chedoke Gen., Children's & St. Joseph's Hosp's.; Dir., Cystic Fibrosis Clin., Chedoke, Children's & Gen. Hosp's.; Court. Staff, Gen. & Joseph Brant Mem. Hosp's.; Tel. JA 7-8655.

WILSON, William M.; Box 729, High River, Alta.; Dublin (Ire.) '51; AMCGP.

WILSON, William M.G.; 3195 Granville St., Vancouver 9, B.C.; 5638 Chancellor Blvd. (res); Tor '35; Ophth; Att'd. Staff, Vancouver Gen. Hosp.; Vis. Staff, Children's & St. Vincent's Hosp's.; Clin. Assoc. U. of British Columbia; Tel. RE 3-2028.

WILSON, W. Semple; 1394 Kingsway, Vancouver 10, B.C.; Glasgow (Scot.) '32; Tel. 874-7113.

WILSON, W. John; Ste. 204, 1849 Yonge St., Toronto 7, Ont.; 280 Bessborough Dr. (res); Tor '37; Phys., Hosp. for Sick Children; Clin. Ass't., U. of Toronto; Tel. 488-8876.

WILSON, W. Robert S.; 193 Frederick St., Kitchener, Ont.; Tor '41; D.Psy.; Tel. SH 4-8771.

WILT, John C.; 336 Oxford St., Winnipeg, Man.; Man '45; DABPath; DABClinPath; FACP; Path, Bact; Virol., Wpg. Gen. Hosp.; Prof. & Hd. Dept. of Bact & Immun., U. of Manitoba; Tel. GR 4-9110.

WILTON, Bruce W., Capt.; CFB, Adastral Park, Clinton, Ont.; Qns'65.

WIMPORY, Mary F.; (See WEBSTER, Mary F.).

WINBAUM, Edward S.; 1027 Ottawa St., Windsor, Ont.; 3715 Victoria Blvd (res); Tor '45; Paed; Chief (Paed.), Metropolitan Hosp.; Active Paed. Staff, Hotel-Dieu & Grace Hosp's.; Court. Teach. Staff, Children's Hosp., Detroit, Michigan; Tel. CL 4-4221.

WINBIGLER, Hugh C.; 4431 W. 10th Ave., Vancouver 8, B.C.; 1312 Acadia Rd. (res); Ohio State U. (U.S.A.) '29; Tel. CA 4-1636.

WINCH, Guy C.; 1904 Lonsdale Ave., North Vancouver, B.C.; St. Andrews (Scot.) '52; DRCOG; FRCS(C), ObstGyn; Cons. Staff, Lionsgate Hosp.; Clin. Instr. ObstGyn., U. of British Columbia; Tel. YU 8-3322.

WINCHESTER, Euphemia D.; 32 Alexandra Blvd., Toronto 12, Ont. (res); Tor '32; ObstGyn; Staff, Ontario Hosp., Toronto; Tel. LE 3-8501.

WINCOTT, V. Leigh; 305 Sarah Ave., Chippawa Ont. (res); Tor '36; Anaes. Staff, Gtr. Niagara Gen. Hosp.; Tel. 295-4716.

WINDELER, E. C. H.; 1448 Tecumseh Rd. E., Windsor, Ont. 3550 Church (res); Tor '14; Staff Paed. & Lect. to Nurses, Hotel Dieu, Grace & Metropolitan Hosp's., Windsor; Staff Paed., Children's Hosp. of Michigan, Detroit; Tel. CL 3-1033. Retired.

WINDER, John S.; Ste. 1, 361 Princess Ave., London, Ont.; 1597 Gloucester Rd., R.R. 2 (res); Wes'42; MCGP; Med. Dir., London Life Ins. Co.; Tel. GE 9-5821.

WINDISCH, Marie C.; 10318 ave de l'Esplanade, Montreal 12, P.Q.; Mon '64; Research, U. of Montreal.

WINDLE, Stanley C.; 105 Northgate Bldg., Edmonton, Alta.; Man'50; DABR(D); DiagRad; Chief of Rad., Royal Alexandra Hosp.; Ass't. Clin. Prof., U. of Alberta; Tel. 429-2508.

WINE, H. G.; Tor '64; Res., Royal Victoria Hosp., Montreal, P.Q.

WINE, Norman A.; 513 Boyd Bldg., 388 Portage Ave., Winnipeg 1, Man.; Sask'59; Ophth; Tel. 942-6651.

WINE, Stanley J.; Tor'65; Jr. Int., New Mount Sinai Hosp., Toronto 2, Ont.; Abroad.

WINEMAKER, Jules; 103 Rockford Rd., Richmond Hill, Ont.; Tor'52; Anaes.

WINESANKER, Harry; 459 Bloor St. W., Toronto 4, Ont.; 24 Croydon Rd. (res); Tor '33; Anaes; Sr. Att. Phys. in Anaes., New Mount Sinai Hosp.; Tel. WA 2-4432.

WINESTOCK, Aaron J.; 1835 Portage Ave., St. James, Winnipeg, Man.; 141 Elm St. (res); Man '37; MCGP; Ass't. Prof. Anat., Manitoba U.; Tel. TU 8-1996.

WINGATE, Martin B.; Med. Arts Clinic, 2125-11th Ave., Regina, Sask.; London (Eng.)'48; FRCS (Ed.); MRCS (Eng.); LRCP; MRCOG; ObstGyn.

WINKLER, Israel; Ste. 415, Ellendale Med. Bldg., 5845 Cote des Neiges Rd., Montreal 26, P.Q.; 4850 Cote St. Luc Rd., Apt. 38 (res); McG '39; DABIM; FACP; FCCP; IntMed; PulmDis & TB (P.Q.); Assoc. Phys., Jewish Gen. Hosp.; Phys., Royal Edward Chest Hosp.; Cons. Phys., Mt. Sinai Hosp., Ste-Agathe des Monts; Dem. (Med.), McGill U.; Tel. 731-8123.

WINKLER-PRINS, Vincent; Gronigen (Neth) '48; Staff, Channel-Port-Aux-Basques Hosp., Channel, Nfld.

WINNITOY, Nicholas W.; 3000 Lawrence Ave. E., Scarborough, Ont.; 21 Bendale Blvd. (res); Tor '42; ObstGyn; Staff, Scarborough Gen. Hosp.; Tel. 291-0991.

WINRAM, Robert G.; 601 Boyd Bldg., 388 Portage Ave., Winnipeg, Man.; 615 Oak St. (res); Man '43; FICS; GenSurg; Assoc. Staff, Misericordia Gen. Hosp.; Court. Staff, (GenSurg), St. Boniface, & Wpg. Gen. Hosp's.; Tel. WH 3-9528.

WINROB, Harry; 2364 W. 4th Ave., Vancouver 9, B.C.; Man '51; Tel. RE 8-4213.

WINSOR, A. E. Lacey; Church St., Norton, N.B.; Qns'29; MCGP; Tel. 839-2300.

WINSOR, Gordon M.; Dal'56; Res., Sunnybrook Hosp., Toronto. Ont.

WINTEMUTE, Robert W.; 216 Med. Arts Bldg., Calgary, Alta.; 231 Wildwood Dr. (res); Alb '52; DABOG; FACOG; ObstGyn; Dir. (ObstGyn), Ass't. Calgary Gen. Hosp.; Cons. (ObstGyn), Holy Cross, Grace & Foothills Hosp's.; Tel. 262-4321.

WINTER, Eric H.; 401 Laurel St., Preston, Ont.; Tor '64; Tel. 653-3852.

WINTER, Eugene C.; 401 Laurel St., Preston, Ont.; Leipzig (Germ.) '25; Ph.D.; Staff, South Waterloo Mem. Hosp., Galt.; Vis. Staff, Kitchener-Waterloo & St. Mary's Hosp's., Kitchener; Tel. 653-3852.

WINTER, John H.; Arichat, N.S.; Vienna (Austria) '49.

WINTER, Richard W.; 10004-105th St., Edmonton, Alta.; Dal'58; FACOG; FRCS(C), ObstGyn; Active Staff, Royal Alexander Hosp.; Clin., Edmonton Cancer Clinic; Tel. 424-2121.

WINTLE DES RUISSEAUX, Paul; 2497 Chemin St. Louis, Quebec, P.Q.; Ott '57.

WINTON, Lawrence; Qns '55; Res., Montreal Gen. Hosp., Montreal, P.Q.

WINTROB, Benjamin; 194 Wilson Ave., Toronto, Ont.; Tor'35; Tel. HU 3-7855.
Tor '35; Tel. HU 3-7855.

WIOR, George A.; 1538 Sherbrooke St. W., Montreal, P.Q.; 3570 Ridgewood (res); Paris (Fr.) '39; Ophth; Tel. WE 3-9312.

WIRGES, H. Georges; Ste 214, 1320-5th Ave., Prince George, B.C.; Sask '63; Tel. 564-4356.

WIRKKUNEN, R. Allan; Nelson St., Box 727, Meaford, Ont.; Tor'55; MCGP; Active Staff, Meaford Gen. Hosp.; Tel. 538-3101.

WISE, David K.; Brunswick Diagnostic Clinic, 25 Brunswick Ave., Toronto 4, Ont.; 21 Silverwood Ave., Forest Hill (res); Tor '38; IntMed; Staff, Doctor's & New Mt. Sinai Hosp's.; Tel. 924-9741.

WISE, Harold B.; Community Clinic, 8th St. & 1st Ave. E., Prince Albert, Sask. Tor '61; Tel. 763-6466.

WISE, H. Douglas; St. Lawrence St., Merrickville, **Ont.; Sydney (Australia) '41; Chief of Med., Smith Falls Public Hosp. & St. Francis Gen. Hosp.; Tel. 269-4955.**

WISE, Melvin B.; 620-5300 Cote-des-Neiges Rd., Montreal 26, P.Q.; 4660 Kensington Ave. (res); Wes '54; Paed; Staff, Mtl. Children's, Royal Ed. Laurentian & Jewish Gen. Hosp's.; Dem. McGill U.; Tel. RE 1-5048.

WISE, Sydney; 3089 Bathurst St., Toronto 19, Ont.; Tor'39; Staff, New Mt. Sinai Hosp.; Tel. RU 1-0878.

WISEBORD, Nathan; Ste. 1601, 1400 Pine Ave. W., Montreal 25, P.Q.; Mon '57; Psy.

WISELBERG, Dorothy; 407 Medical Arts Bldg., 1538 Sherbrooke St. W., Montreal, P.Q.; McG'32; Pulm. Dis. & TB (P.Q.); FCCP; IntMed; Phys., Royal Edward Laurentian Hosp.; Clin. Ass't., Jewish Gen. & Reddy Mem. Hosp's.; Dem., McGill U.; Tel. 935-5612.

WISEMAN, Carl; Aberdeen (Scot.)'61; Staff, Hosp. for Mental Diseases, Brandon, Man.

WISEMAN, Fred; Wes '64; Res., Children's Hosp., Montreal 25, P.Q.

WISEMAN John; 1 Hopecrest Cres., Scarborough, Ont.; Manchester (Eng.) '45; MRCS(Eng.), LRCP(Lond.); MCGP; Staff, Scarborough Gen. Hosp.; Tel. AM 1-9360.

WISEMAN, Lester J.; Apt. 1, 1400, Winding Trail, Cooksville, Ont.; Dal'58; Anaes.

WISEMAN, Max; 205 Ste. Catherine Rd., Outremont, Montreal, P.Q.; Lav '07; Obst.

WISHART, Francis B.; Chapel, Woodstock, N.B.; Dal'36; MCGP.

WISHART, Franklyn O.; 56 Servington Cresc., Toronto, Ont. (res); Tor '31; D.P.H., Bact. PH; Prof. of Microbiol., School of Hygiene, U. of Toronto; M.O., Connaught Med. Research Labs.; Tel. 928-2744.

WISHART, James M.; 294 Aylmer St. N., Peterborough, Ont.; Tor '43; Anaes; Staff (Anaes.), Peterborough Civic & St. Joseph's Hosp's.; Pres., Peterborough County Med. Soc.; Tel. 745-1122.

WISHLOW, Nicholas F.; 127 Church Ave., Chilliwack, B.C.; 631 Riverside (res); Man '44; DABOphth, FAAOO; Staff, Dept. of Ophth, Otol., Chilliwack Gen. Hosp.; Tel. 792-1951.

WISINGER, Hans J.; 210 Cuthbertson Block, Fort William, Ont.; Germany '45.

WISMER, Harold St. C.; 1124 The Parkway, London, Ont.; Wes '14; M.A.C.R., D&TRad; Court. Staff, St. Thomas-Elgin Gen. Hosp.; Semi-Retired.

WISNIEWSKI, Czeslaw; Paris (France)'55; GenSurg; Staff, Indian Hosp., Moose Factory, Ont.

WISS, F. Rene; 96 Larch St., Sudbury, Ont.; Haiti (W. Indies) '52; Ophth; Att'd. Ophth., Sudbury Gen., Sudbury Mem., St. Joseph's & Copper Cliff Hosp's.; Tel. 673-6680.

WISWELL, Gordon B., MC; 1322 Robie St., Halifax, N.S.; Dal '14; FAAP, FRCP(C), Paed; Hon. Cons., Children's Hosp.; Prof. Emer. (Paed.), Dalhousie U.; Retired.

WITKOV, Hyman R.; 1396 St. Catherine St. W., Ste. 316, Montreal, P.Q.; 840 Notre-Dame, Lachine; Mon'42; **FAADS; DermSyph; Active Cons., St.** Joseph's, Lachine Gen., Lakeshore Gen., **Jewish Gen., Lasalle Gen. & Mt. Sinai Hosp.;** Prefontaine; Tel. 866-7497.

WITNEY, Joan D.; (Mrs. Moore); Community Health Serv., 411-413 Avenue Bldg., 220-3rd Ave. S., Saskatoon, Sask.; Qns '53.

WITNEY, Michael R.; Hearts Content, Trinity South, Nfld.; London (Eng.) '50.

WITT, Hans A.; 292 Oakdale Ave., St. Catharines, Ont.; Wes'65.

WITT, Simon; 75 Woolwich St., Guelph, Ont.; 23 Waverley Dr. (res); London (Eng.) '39; FRCS (Edin.), MRCS, LRCP; GenSurg; Active Staff, Guelph Gen. & St. Joseph's Hosp's; Tel. TA 4-7700.

WITTERICK, Gordon H.; 8 Eastwood Ave., Scarborough, Ont.; Tor'54; MCGP; Att. Staff, Toronto East Gen. Hosp. & Treas., Dept. of G.P.; Court. Staff, Scarborough Gen. Hosp.; Tel. OX 8-1684.

WITTICK, Milton A.; Burks Falls, Ont.; Wes '18; M.O.H.; Burks Falls, Magnetawan Twps; Dist. Coroner.

WITTIG, Joseph E.; 15 East Ave., Kitchener, Ont.; Wes '46; ObstGyn; Chief of Staff, St. Mary's Gen. Hosp.; Active Staff, Kitchener-Waterloo Hosp.; Tel. 743-7351.

WITTKOWER, Eric D.; 1025 Pine Ave. W., Montreal, P.Q.; 363 Clarke Ave., Westmount, Mtl. 6 (res); Berlin (Germ.) '24; LRCP; LRCS; LRFPS (Glas); Psy; Cons. Psy., Mtl. Gen.; Assoc. Psy., Royal Victoria Hosp.; Prof. (Psy), McGill U.; Tel. VI 2-1251, Loc. 212.

WITTON, Thomas H.; 4052 New St., Burlington, Ont.; Tor'49; Anaes; Staff, Hamilton Civic Hosp., Hamilton, Ont.

WITZEL, Samuel H.; 204 Medical Arts Bldg., 300 King St. W., Oshawa, Ont.; R.R. 1, (res); Tor '50; Ophth; Staff, Oshawa Gen. Hosp. & Vol. Ass't. Toronto Gen. Hosp.; Tel. 723-9101.

WLODEK, George K.; 540 Seaforth Medical Bldg., 3550 Cote des Neiges Rd., Montreal 25, P.Q.; Qns'56; M.Sc.; FRCS(C), GenSurg.; Ass't. Surg., Montreal Gen. Hosp.; Cons. Surg., Douglas Mem. Hosp.; Teach. Fell., McGill U.; Tel. 932-2275.

WOBICK, Leroy; 2523 St. Johns St., Port Moody, B.C.; Alt '53.

WODEHOUSE, George E., MC; University Health Serv., 256 Huron St., Toronto 5, Ont.; 30 **Chestnut Pk. Rd., Tor. 5 (res); Tor '40; MRCP-(Lond.), FRCP(C), IntMed; Court. Staff, Toronto Gen. Hosp.; Dir. U. Health Serv., U. of Toronto; Hon.-Treas., CMA.; Tel. WA 2-2469.**

WOELBER, Werner; 32 Reid St., Chateauguay, **P.Q.; Berlin (Germ.) '47; Paed; Clin. Ass't., Mtl.** Children's Hosp.; Tel. OX 2-0343.

WOHLFARTH, Werner; Box 446, Melville, Sask; 124—10th Ave. W. (res); London (Eng.) '40; MRCS, LRCP; Staff, St. Peter's Hosp.; Tel. 728-5774.

WOJCICKI, Henryk M.; 323 LeMarchand Mansions, 116th St. & 100th Ave., Edmonton, Alta.; 13604 Ravine Dr. (res); Edinburgh (Scot.) '42; **MD (NeurPsy) (Ed.); Psy; Staff Psy., U. of Alta.** Hosp.; Cons., Misericordia & Royal Alexandra Hosp's. & Family & Child Welfare; Instr. (Psy), U. of Alberta; Tel. HU 8-5545.

WOLAN, Casimir T.; 433 Med. Arts Bldg., Saskatoon, Sask.; 508 Garrison Cres. (res); Man '41; FACS; F.R.C.S.(C); Urol; Active Staff University, St. Paul's & Saskatoon City Hosp's.; Clin. Assoc. Dept. of Surg. (Urol.), U. of Saskatchewan; Tel. 652-5757.

WOLANSKYJ, Bohdan; Reddy Mem. Hosp. (Dept. of Path.), 4039 Tucker St., Westmount, Montreal 6, P.Q.; 1028 J.J. Joubert, Duvernay, Laval-des-Rapides (res); Berlin (Germ.) '45; Path; Tel. WE 5-9641.

WOLFBERG, Maurice; Apt. 6, 139 Woodward Ave., Cochenour, Ont.; U.K. '53.

WOLFE, Aubie E.; 780 Seaforth Med. Bldg., 35-50 Cote des Neiges Rd., Montreal 25, P.Q.; Tor'46; ObstGyn.; FACOG; Ass't. ObstGyn., Reddy Mem. & Jewish Gen. Hosp's.; Tel. 937-4107.

WOLFE, Jean G.; 3606 de la Concorde, St-Vincent-de-Paul, P.Q.; Mon '62.

WOLFE, Leonhard S.; Neurol Inst., 3801 University Ave., Montreal 2, P.Q.; Wes'58; MSc (Surg.); PhD(Cantab); Neurochem-in-Charge, Donner Lab of Experimental Neurochem., Mtl. Neurological Inst.; Assoc. Prof. Neurol., McGill U.; Med. Research Assoc., Med. Research Council of Canada; Tel. 842-1251, Loc. 454.

WOLFE, Pierre M.; 2311 Oak Bay Ave., Victoria, B.C.; Qns '46; M.C.G.P.; Staff, Royal Jubilee Hosp.; Court. & Visit. Staff, St. Joseph's Hosp.

WOLFE, Samuel; Community Health Serv., Med. Clinic Group, Avenue Bldg., Saskatoon, Sask.; Tor'50; MPH; DPH(Columbia); Med. Dir., Community Health Serv., Med. Group; Tel. 652-0300.

WOLFE, William J.; 1132-100th St., North Battleford, Sask.; 1492 Queen St. (res); Trinity College (Dublin, Ire.) '42; MB, B.Ch., BAO; DRCOG; Tel. 3756.

WOLFISH, Arthur H.; 542 Oakwood Ave., Toronto 10, Ont.; 28 Glenayr Rd., Tor. 10 (res); Tor'36; Chief, Dept. of G.P., Northwestern Gen. Hosp.; Tel. RU 2-3605.

WOLFISH, Martin G.; 1543 Victoria Pk Ave., Scarborough, Ont.; 15 Donwoods Grove, Tor. 12 (res); Tor '49; F.R.C.P.(C), D.A.B.P.; Paed; Assoc. Phys., Hosp. for Sick Children, Tor.; Clin Instr, U. of Toronto; Tel. PL 5-3629.

WOLFMAN, Jean R. (Wasserman); 95 Chinook Dr., Calgary, Alta.; Tor '55; Staff, Calgary Gen. & Holy Cross Hosp's.; Tel. AL 5-4843.

WOLIN, Leo; 391 St. Clarence Ave., Toronto 4, Ont.; Moscow (U.S.S.R.)'48; Staff, Central Hosp.; Tel. LE 4-2108.

WOLKENSTEIN, Christopher F.; 407 Southport Blvd., Winnipeg 29, Man.; Melbourne (Aust.)'47; Anaes; Assoc. (Anaes.), Winnipeg Gen. Hosp.; Lect. (Anaes.), U. of Man.; Tel. HU 9-8009.

WOLLIN, Delbert G.; 74 Johnson St., Kingston, Ont.; 1206 Johnson St. (res); **Wes '39; DiagRad; Rad., Kingston Gen. Hosp.; Assoc. Prof. (Rad.),** Queen's U.; Tel. 542-2791

WOLOCHOW, Donald A.; Ste. 207, 291 Dundas St., London, Ont.; Qns '57; IntMed; Cons. G.I. Clinic Westminster Hosp.; Att'd. Phys., St. Joseph's Hosp.; Fell.(Med.), U. of Western Ontario; Tel. 434-2683; Abroad.

WOLOCHOW, Manley S.; 1105 Fairmont Med. Bldg., 750 W. Broadway, Vancouver 9, B.C.; Tor'52; MCGP; Vis. Staff, Vancouver Gen., Grace, St. Paul's, St. Vincent's & Children's Hosp's.; Tel. 872-7544.

WOLOCHOW, Michael; 720 W. Broadway, Ste. 102, Vancouver 9, B.C.; Alb'44; GenSurg; MCGP; Att'd. Staff, Vancouver Gen. Hosp.; Tel. 879-5271.

WOLOCHOW, Paul; Ste. 4, 11949 Jasper Ave., Edmonton, Alta.; Man '16; Retired.

WOLOSCHUK, Eugene; 284 Bathurst St., Toronto 2B, Ont.; Lav '53; ObstGyn.

WOLOSCHUK, Ostap; 284 Bathurst St., Toronto 2B, Ont.; Mon'57; GenSurg; Assoc. Staff, Doctor's Hosp. & Toronto Western Hosp.; Tel. 363-7711.

WOLOSZCZUK, Andrew; St. Barbara's Med. Bldg., 266 Bathurst St., Toronto 2B, Ont.; Poznan (Poland) '36; GenSurg; Tel. 366-3134.

WOLSTEIN, Edward; Ste. 307, 267 O'Connor St., Ottawa, Ont.; 69 Ruskin St. (res); McG '32; D.O.M.S. (Eng.), Ophth; Sr. Ophth., Ottawa Civic Hosp.; Tel. 236-0854.

WOLVERTON, Harold A.; 395 W. 49th Ave., Vancouver 15, B.C. (res); Tor '14; Retired.

WONG, Andrew, W-H.; Montreal Neurol Inst., 3801 University St., Montreal 2, P.Q.; Qns '59; FRCS(C), NeurSurg.

WONG, Bennet R.; 714-750 W. Broadway, Vancouver 9, B.C.; 894 Margaree Pl., W. Vanc. (res); Alb '55; Psy; Att'd. Staff, Vancouver Gen. Hosp.; Cons. B.C. Correctional; Cons. Central City Mission & Langley School Bd. & Big Brothers; Clin. Instr., U. of British Columbia; Tel. 874-9828.

WONG, Christopher K.; 1199 Austin Ave., Coquitlam, B.C.; Sask '63; Tel. 939-7345.

WONG, Chung N.; 12051 Haney Plaza, Haney, B.C.; Taiwan (China)'59.

WONG, Edgar D.; 21 Maynard Ave., Apt. 211, Toronto 3, Ont.; Qns '54; DABPN; Psy; Dir. of Mental Health, Dept. of Public Health; Tel. 367-7416.

WONG, Edward Y.; Tor '63; Res., St. Michael's Hosp., Toronto 2, Ont.

WONG, Ernest; 714 Fairmont Med. Bldg., 750 W. Broadway, Vancouver 9, B.C.; 6626 Ash St., Van. 14 (res); Man '57; Psy; Att'd. Staff, Van. Gen. Hosp.; Cons. Psy., Rehab. Fdn. of B.C.; Clin. Instr. (Psy.), U. of British Columbia; Tel. 879-2526.

WONG, Fook N.; Man'65; Jr. Int., St. Boniface Hosp., Winnipeg, Man.

WONG, Francis Chu-YN; 136 St. John St., Riverside, Ont.; Ott '60; Anaes.

WONG, Frank; Man'65; Res., Winnipeg Gen. Hosp., Winnipeg 3, Man.

WONG, George L.; 303 Med. Dental Bldg., 450 Central Ave., London, Ont.; Alb '48; DABOtol; Otol; Staff, St. Joseph's & Public Gen. Hosp's.; Instr. (Otol.), U. of Western Ont.; Tel. GE 9-4311.

WONG, Gerald S.; Tor'62; Res., Toronto General Hosp., Toronto, Ont.

WONG, Jock M. H.; 193 E. Hastings St., Vancouver, B.C.; Edinburgh (Scot.)'48; Paed.; Tel. MU 3-5230.

WONG, John; Ste. 109-110, 645 Fort St., Victoria, B.C.; 363 Foul Bay Rd. (res); UBC '56; Otol.; Tel. 385-7207.

WONG, John; Taiwan (Formosa)'64; Staff, Cottage Hosp., Old Perlican, Nfld.

WONG, John W.; 369 Marathon Ct., Coquitlam, New Westminster, B.C. (res); Man '59; Staff, Prov. Mental Hosp., Essondale; Tel. LA 1-1911.

WONG, Ken; UBC'64; Res., Shaughnessy Hosp., Vancouver 9, B.C.

WONG, Kenneth K. S.; National U. (Taiwan, China)'61; Res., Children's Hosp., Halifax, N.S.

WONG Lei Ching; 2125-11th Ave., Regina, Sask.; 114 Langley St. (res); Hsiang Med. Coll. (China) '48; Paed; Sr. Paed., Regina Gen. & Grey Nuns Hosp's.; Tel. 522-1651.

WONG, Marcus Y.; McG '64; Res., Montreal Gen. Hosp., Montreal 25, P.Q.

WONG-MARK, Mary; 109 Lincoln Rd., Beaconsfield, Ste Anne-de-Bellevue, P.Q.; Wes '37; ObstGyn; Obst. Staff, Lakeshore Gen. Hosp., Pointe Claire; Tel. 695-3319.

WONG, Paul W. K.; Children's Hosp., Winnipeg, Man.; HongKong (China) '58.

WONG, Shek-Leung; 13620 Grosvenor Rd., North Surrey, B.C.; UBC'65.

WONG, Thomas; 7 King St. N., Frankford, Ont.; Ott'64.

WONG, William A.; 420 East St. N., Sarnia, Ont.; 1264 Glen Douglas Dr. (res); Wes '43; M.Sc.; IntMed; Chief of Med. Sarnia Gen. Hosp.; Tel. ED 7-9224.

WONG, Wing Y.; 221 Main St., Vancouver 4, B.C.; 4044 Granville St. (res); Qns '34; Tel. MU 1-4709.

WOO, Arthur K.; McG '61; Intn., Queen Elizabeth Hosp., Montreal 28, P.Q.

WOO, George H. K.; UBC'65; Res., Shaughnessy Hosp., Vancouver 9, B.C.

WOOD, A. Eleanor C. (Riggs); 22 Edgehill Rd., Westmount, P.Q. (res); Tor '35; DPH; Teach. Staff, Dept. of Bac., McGill U.; Special Research Staff, Royal Edward Laurentian Hosp.; Tel. VI 4-6311.

WOOD, Angus E.; Ste. 408, 625-5th Ave., New Westminster, B.C.; Man'56; ObstGyn.

WOOD, Betty J.; Vancouver Gen. Hosp., Vancouver, B.C.; Man '54; Paed; DiagRad; Asst. Rad. Vancouver Hosp. & Health Centre for Children; Clin. Ass't. Prof., Paed. U. of British Columbia; Tel. TR 6-3211.

WOOD, Donald E.; 297 Yonge Blvd., Toronto 12, Ont.; Tor '56; FRCP(C), IntMed; Ass't. Phys., & Hd. Div. of Nuclear Med., Toronto Gen. Hosp.; Clin. Teach., U. of Toronto; Tel. EM 6-8211.

WOOD, Donald S.; 297 Yonge Blvd., Lindsay, Ont.; Qns '53; Tel. 324-5913.

WOOD, Edward H.; 151 Metcalfe St., Ottawa, Ont.; 101 Rustein Ave. (res); Qns '14; F.A.C.S., GenSurg; Hon. Cons. Surg., Ottawa Civic & St. Vincent's Hosp's.; Tel. CE 2-4645.

WOOD, George; 4920 Grosvenor Ave., Montreal, P.Q.; McG '37; GenSurg (P.Q.); Tel. 482-5508.

WOOD, George A.; Box 39, Grand Centre, Alta.; Aberdeen (Scot.)'49; Staff, John Neil Hosp., Cold Lake; Tel. 248-3529.

WOOD, Harold G.; Box 70, Lewisporte, Nfld.; McG '45.

WOOD, Ian A.; Rose Valley, Sask.; Sheffield (Eng.) '52; M.C.G.P.; Phys. & Surg., Rose Valley Med. Centre.

WOOD, James K.; 1539-8th St. E., Saskatoon, Sask.; Sask'65.

WOOD, John A.; 350 Albert St.. Nanaimo, B.C.; Aberdeen (Scot.)'55; DObst.RCOG; MRCOG; ObstGyn; Tel. 753-3431.

WOOD, J. Norman; Ste. 207, 131 Ontario St., St. Catharines, Ont.; 110 Marsdale Dr. (res); Wes '48; ObstGyn; Chief ObstGyn., St. Catharines Gen. Hosp.; Active Staff, Hotel-Dieu Hosp.; Tel. 684-8396.

WOOD, John B.; High Prairie, Alta.; Alb '37; MCGP.

WOOD, Lorne G.; 915 Fairmont Med. Bldg., 750 W. Broadway, Vancouver 9, B.C.; 5338 Laburnum St. (res) Alb '35; FRCS(C); Urol; Active Staff, Vancouver Gen. & St. Vincent Hosp's.; Tel. TR 4-6838.

WOOD, Marcia; 114 Queens Ave., New Westminster, B.C.; Man '50; Anaes.

WOOD, Margaret I.; 6 Northolt Court, Islington, Ont.; Tor'49; Paed; Ass't. Clin., Sick Children's Hosp.; Tel. WA 1-1902.

WOOD, Margaret M.; 398 Hollywood Ave., Willowdale, Ont. (res); Witwatersrand (Jo'burg, S. Africa) '49; Staff, Workmen's Comp. Bd., Toronto; Tel. 222-4377.

WOOD, Rayfield G. A.; 138 Lincoln St., Lunenburg, N.S.; Dal '32; GenSurg.; MCGP.

WOOD, Robert W.; Tor '53; Staff, Dept. of National Health & Welfare, Brooke Claxton Bldg., Tunney's Pasture, Ottawa, Ont.; Tel. 232-8211, Loc. 2-4885.

WOOD, Thomas E.; Wes'61; IntMed(P.Q.); Staff, Royal Victoria Hosp., Montreal 2, P.Q.

WOOD, William C.; 21 Woodward Cr., Rockingham, N.S.; Dal'52.

WOOD, William J.; Apt. 524, 840 Springland Cr., Ottawa 8, Ont.; Man '22; DPH; Retired.

WOOD, William S.; 320-925 W. Georgia St., Vancouver 1, B.C.; McG '51; FRCP(C), Derm; Att'd. Staff (Med.), Van. Gen. Hosp.; Clin. Instr., U. of British Columbia; Tel. MU 5-9456.

WOODALL, Gordon, Sg/Lcdr; CFPO 5055, RCAF 3 Wing, Belleville, Ont.; Man'57; Ophth; Chief of Ophth., No. 1 Air Div. RCAF.

WOODBURY, John F.; Medical Arts Bldg., 5880 Spring Garden Rd., Halifax, N.S.; 1920 Bloomingdale Terr. (res); Dal '43; IntMed; Ass't. Att'd. Phys., Victoria Gen. Hosp.; Assoc. Prof. (Med.), Dalhousie U.; Cons., Children's, Camp Hill & Halifax Infirmary Hosp's.; Tel. 423-7761.

WOODCOCK, D.; Royal Bank Bldg., Lethbridge, Alta.; 413—12th St. (res); Iowa State (U.S.A.) '07; Ophth, Otol; Local Staff App'ts.; Retired.

WOODGER, John B.; 77 Westmount, Guelph, Ont.; Tor'60.

WOODHEAD, Brian H.; Workmen's Comp. Bd., 7123-119th St., Edmonton, Alta.; Alb'61; Phys Med & Rehab.

WOODHOUSE, Catharine F.; 338 Mount Pleasant Rd., Toronto 7, Ont. (res); Tor '10; D.P.H., PH; Retired.

WOODHOUSE, Donald H.; 274 Sun Life Bldg., Montreal, P.Q.; 6 Lancaster Dr., Pointe Claire (res); Wes '41; F.R.C.P.(C); IntMed; (Cardiol, P.Q.); Assoc. Phys., Montreal Gen. Hosp.; Med. Dir., Sun Life Assce. Co. of Can.; Lect. (Med.), McGill U.; Tel. UN 6-6411.

WOODLEY, Thomas I.; 100 Queen St., Belleville, Ont.; 228 Foster Ave. (res); Qns '50; MCGP Chief of Staff, Belleville Gen. Hosp.; Tel. WO 8-7574.

WOODLEY, W. Robert; Box 129, Vernon, B.C.; Ott '52; DiagRad; Cons. Staff, Vernon Jubilee, Enderley & Dist. Hosp's.; Tel. 542-7526.

WOODMAN-FOX, Evelyn M. (Woodman); 1427 Albatross Ave., Kitimat, B.C.; Part-time Phys., Alcan; Tel. 452.

WOODMAN, James C.; Sunderland, Ont.; Qns '47.

WOODMAN, Kenneth J.; Brandon Clinic, Brandon, Man.; Man'56; IntMed; Active Staff, Brandon Gen. & Assiniboine Hosp's.; Tel. PA 9-6441.

WOODROOFE, Edward K.; Chester, N.S.; Tor '31.

WOODROW, Robert; 701-3rd St. E., Prince Albert, Sask.; Edinburgh (Scot.) '31; DPH; Reg. M.O., Prince Albert Health Serv.; Tel. 764-4208.

WOODROW, W. Arthur; 5 William St. N., Lindsay, Ont.; 20 Russell St. E. (res); Tor '34; Ophth, Otol; Tel. 324-3771.

WOODROW, Walter H.; 54 Coldwater St., Orillia, Ont.; Tor'23; OphthOtol.; Tel. 325-5522.

WOODRUFF, Frederick W.; Durham (Eng.) '53; M.B., B.S.; M.O., Notre Dame Mem. Hosp., Twillingate, Nfld.

WOODS, Alvin R.; 269 King St. W., Dundas, Ont.; Tor '31; M.C.G.P.; M.O.H., Dundas; Dist. Coroner; Tel. MA 8-6031.

WOODS, Barry M.; 103 Med. Arts Bldg., 300 King St. W., Oshawa. Ont.; 843 Glencairn St. (res); Qns '45; D.A.B.R., D.M.R., DiagRad; Assoc. Rad., Oshawa Gen. Hosp.; Rad., Uxbridge Cottage & Port Perry Mem. Hosp's.; Tel. 728-3691.

WOODS, B. J.; 70 Cedar St., Sudbury, Ont.; Tor '35; Tel. 675-8386.

WOODS, Desmond G. Sg. Cdr; National U. (Ire.) '47; DiagRad; Staff, R.C.N. Hosp., H.M.C.S. Naden, Esquimalt, B.C.

WOODS, Hyman L.; 3105 Van Horne, Montreal, P.Q.; 64 Finchley Rd., Hamstead (res); Ott '51; MCGP; Staff, Reddy Mem. Hosp.; Tel. RE 7-2212.

WOODS, John H.; 2564 Montrose Ave., Abbotsford, B.C.; UBC'54; Tel. 853-1563.

WOODS, John M.; 821 Coxwell Ave., Toronto 6, Ont.; 5 Danrose Cres., Don Mills (res); Man '50; FACS; FRCS(C), GenSurg; Att'd. Surg., Tor. E. Gen. Hosp.; Vis. Surg., St. Michael's Hosp.; Tel. HO 6-2443.

WOODS, June, (See Cowen, June).

WOODS, Lawrence W.; St. Michael's Hosp., Toronto 2, Ont.; Man'56; FRCP(C), Psy; Clin. Teach. Psy., U. of Toronto; Tel. 362-4622.

WOODS, Melville L.; Box 190, Treherne, Man.; London (Eng.)'58; M.O.H., South Norfolk Mun. & Village of Treherne; Staff, Treherne Hosp., St. Claude's, Lorne Mem., Balder & Glenborough Hosp's.; Tel. 28 ring 2.

WOODS, Philip E.; Ste 314, 1669 Victoria St., Prince George, B.C.; Birmingham (Eng.)'53; Tel. 564-2288.

WOODS, Thomas E.; Wes '61; Jr. Int'n., St. Joseph's Hosp., London, Ont.

WOODS, William A.; 151 London Rd., Sarnia, Ont.; National U. (Dublin, Ire.) '47; OrthSurg; OrthSurg., St. Joseph's & Sarnia Gen. Hosp's.; Tel. DI 4-7577; ED 6-6121; DI 4-3661.

WOODSIDE. Murray A.; 105 Adelaide St. W., Toronto 1, Ont.; 57 Bunty Lane, Willowdale (res); Tor'42; FRCP(C), IntMed; Med. Dir., North American Life Assur. Co., Toronto; Tel. EM 2-6011.

WOODSWORTH, Ralph S.; 4638 Pine Cres., Vancouver 9, B.C.; Man '35; Anaes; Staff, Van. Gen. Hosp.; Clin. Instr. (Anaes), U. of British Columbia; Tel. RE 3-8756.

WOODWARD, George E.; Tor'59; DHA; Ass't. Supt. Med., Hamilton Gen. Hosp., Hamilton, Ont.

WOODWARD, John B.; 689 E. 49th Ave., Vancouver 15, B.C.; 4875 Yew St. (res); UBC '58; MCGP; Tel. FA 5-5295.

WOODWARD, Ross; 3543 Upper Middle Rd., Cooksville, Ont.; Tor'50; DTM&H; Staff, South Peel Hosp.; Tel. 277-1433.

WOODWARK, George M.; Med. Arts Bldg., 1105 Pandora Ave., Victoria, B.C.; 2795 Seaview Rd. (res); Cambridge (Eng.) '47; M.A., M.R.C.P. (Lond.), L.R.C.P. (Lond.), M.R.C.S. (Eng.); IntMed.; Tel. EV 6-1942.

WOOKEY, Harold W.; 4 Glengowan Rd. (res); Tor '13; FRCS(Eng.), FRCS(C), GenSurg; Cons. Surg., Tor. Gen. Hosp.; PG Lect. (Surg.), U. of Toronto; Tel. HU 3-4624; Retired.

WOOLDRIDGE, David B.; 1920 37th St. S. W., Calgary, Alta.; Manchester (Eng.) '54; DObstRCOG; Tel. 242-4411.

WOOLEVER, Charles A.; 1538 Sherway Dr., Cooksville, Ont.; Wes'47; FRCS(C), ObstGyn.

WOOLF, Colin R.; Cardio-respiratory Lab., Toronto Gen. Hosp., Toronto 2, Ont.; 23 Birchwood Ave., York Mills (res); Capetown (S. Africa) '47; MRCP(Lond.), FRCP(C), IntMed; Ass't. Phys., Tor. Gen. Hosp.; Att'd. Phys., Sunnybrook DVA Hosp.; Clin. Instr., U. of Toronto; Research Assoc., Ont. Heart Fdn.; Tel. EM 6-8211, Loc. 2855.

WOOLF, Cyril I.; Mall Med. Group, 280 Memorial Blvd., Winnipeg 1, Man.; 304 Bower Blvd., Tuxedo (res); London (Eng.) '52; FRCS (Eng.); FRCS(Ed.); DLO; Otol; Active Staff (Otol.), St. Boniface Gen. & Children's Hosp's.; Instr., (Otol.) U. of Manitoba; Tel. SP 4-2411.

WOOLF, Stephen M.; New Waterford, N.S.; London (Eng.)'61.

WOOLFE, Clifford G.; Erindale Woodland Plaza, 3353 Credit Woodlands, Cooksville, Ont.; Tor'60; Med. Staff, South Peel Hosp.; Memb., South Peel Med. Soc., Branch of O.M.A.; Tel. 277-2842 & 277-4491.

WOOLFORD, Bernard J.; 136 Simcoe St. N., Oshawa, Ont.; London (Eng.)'61; MRCS(Eng.); LRCP(Lond.); DCH(Eng.); DObstRCOG.

WOOLFREY, Ivan R.; Dal'65; AMCGP; Ass't. MO, Botwood Cottage Hosp., Botwood, Nfld.

WOOLFSON, Solomon J.; 2 Evanston Dr., Downsview, Ont.; Tor '23.

WOOLHOUSE, Frederick M.; 1650 Cedar Ave., Montreal, P.Q.; 1190 Dunvegan Rd., Town of Mount Royal (res); McG '36; F.R.C.S.(C), GenSurg, PlasSurg; Dir. of Reparative & Traumatic Unit, Montreal Gen. Hosp.; Dir. of PlasSurg., Montreal Children's Hosp.; Cons. PlasSurg., Queen Mary Vet's, Catherine Booth & Jewish Gen. Hosp's.; Tel. 935-7880.

WOOLLACOTT, Paul J. V.; Haisla Med. Centre, Kitimat, B.C.; 111 Omenica (res); Tor. '52; MCGP; Staff, Kitimat Gen. Hosp.; Tel. 1246.

WOOLLEY, H. Ewart; Ste. 1109, 750 W. Broadway, Vancouver 9, B.C.; UBC'60; FRCS(C), ObstGyn; Staff, Vancouver Gen. Hosp.

WOOLNER, James M.; 902 King St. E., Hamilton, Ont.; 420 Mountain Park Ave. (res); Wes '46; Paed; Paed, Staff, Hamilton Gen., & St. Joseph's Hosp's.; Tel. LI 4-5732.

WOOLNER, Wm. S.; Bow Island, Alta.; Dal '33; M.R.C.S.
WOOLSEY, Robert G.; Tor '23; Staff, Ontario Hosp., Hamilton, Ont.
WOOLSTENCROFT, Robert; 9901-108th St., Edmonton, Alta.; London (Eng.) '37; MRCS(Eng.); LRCP (Lond.); MCGP; Exec. Sec., C.M.A. (Alta Div.); Deputy Registrar, College of Phys. & Surg. of Alta.; Tel. 422-6184.
WOOLVERTON, Edgar F.; 169 Chapel St., Woodstock, N.B.; Tufts (U.S.A.) '18; GenSurg; Pres. Med. Staff, Carleton Memorial Hosp.
WORD, E. France; Box 1719, Quesnel, B.C.; Oklahoma (U.S.A.) '41; GenSurg; Urol; FACS; FICS; FRCS(C); Tel. 992-5508.
WORDEN, Ernest M.; 1414 Drummond St., Ste. 906, Montreal, P.Q.; 111 Lazard Ave., Mount Royal (res); Tor '36; D.A.B.P., Paed; Phys.-in-Chief, Alexandra Hosp. & Phys., Shriners' Hosp. for Crippled Children; Ass't. Paed., Montreal Children's & Royal Victoria Hosp.; Assoc. Prof. McGill U.; Tel. AV 8-1081.
WORKMAN, Donald G.; Box 70, Amherst View, Ont.; Qns'60; AMCGP.
WORKMAN, E. Walter; 608 Med. Arts Bldg., 1538 Sherbrooke St. W., Montreal, P.Q.; 330 Brookfield Ave. (res); McG '27; F.A.C.S., GenSurg; Ass't. in O.P. Surg., Royal Victoria Hosp.; Hon. Att'd., Surg., Reddy Memorial Hosp.; Hon; Lect. in Anat., McGill U.; Tel. WE 5-2300.
WORLING, Robert V.; Tor'54; D.Psy; Res., Toronto Gen. Hosp., Toronto, Ont.
WOROBETZ, Stephen; 533 Med. Arts Bldg., Saskatoon, Sask., 405 Lake Cres. (res); Man '40; GenSurg; Clin. Assoc., U of Saskatchewan; Tel. 244-6665.
WORRAL, Joseph D.; 452 Main St. E., Hamilton, Ont.; Qns'38; Otol; Active Staff, Hamilton Gen., Chedoke, Children's & St. Joseph's Hosp's.; Tel. JA 8-1747.
WORRALL, Henry C.; 65 Academy Medical Bldg., 1812-4th St. S. W., Calgary, Alta.; 3917 Edison Cr., (res); Edinburgh (Scot.) '41; F.R.C.S. (Edin.), F.R.C.S.(C), GenSurg; Surg., Holy Cross, Alberta Children's & Calgary Gen. Hosp's.; Tel. 262-1013.
WORRALL, Kathleen M.; 65 Academy Medical Bldg., 1812-4th St. W., Calgary, Alta.; 3917-3rd St. W. (res); Edinburg (Scot.) '41; M.R.-C.O.G.; Tel. 262-1013.
WORRELL, John C.; 331 Sheddon Ave., Oakville, Ont.; 253 Allan St. N. (res); Dal '41; ObstGyn; Active Staff, Oakville-Trafalgar Mem. Hosp.; Court. Staff, Hamilton Gen. & Mountain Hosp's.; Tel. 845-7751.
WORSLEY, Geoffrey H.; Apt. 28, 4780 Cote des Neiges, P.Q.; Liverpool (Eng.)'54; MB, Ch.B.; DRCOG; IntMed; Clin. Ass't. (O.P.D.), Montreal Gen. Hosp.; Med. Advisor, (Boehringer), Geigy (Canada); Tel. 739-2711.
WORSLEY, Gordon H.; 511-713 Columbia St., New Westminster, B.C.; 830 Austin St., Coquitlam (res); Man '38; Anaes; Chief of Anaes., Royal Columbian Hosp.; Tel. LA 2-4241.
WORSLEY, Robert T. C.; The Bashaw Clinic, Bashaw, Alta.; London (Eng.) '55; MRCS (Eng.) LRCP (Lond.); Med. Staff, Bashaw Gen. Hosp.; Assoc. Staff, St. Mary's Hosp., Camrose; Tel. 372-3721.
WORTH, Ann J.; Ste. 1200, 1350 Broughton St., Vancouver 5, B.C. (res); UBC '55; FRCP(C), Path; Path., B.C. Cancer Inst.; Clin. Inst. (Path.) U. of British Columbia; Tel. TR 6-3211.
WORTH, Harry M.; 1245 Beach Ave., Vancouver 5, B.C.; London (Eng.) '25; MRCS, LRCP, FFR, DMRE (Eng.), DABR, LDSRCS (Eng.), FRC-P(C), D&TRad; Spec. Lect. U. of Toronto; Staff, Blanchard-Fraser Mem. Hosp., Retired.
WORTHYLAKE, M. Grant; Park Med. Bldg., 150 Park St., Kentville, N.S.; 34 King St. (res); Dal '54; Staff, Blanchard-Fraser Mem. Hosp.; Tel. 678-4113.
WORTZMAN, George; 101 College St., Toronto 2, Ont.; 26 Montressor Dr., Willowdale (res); Man '50; DABR; DiagRad; Ass't. Rad., Tor. Gen. Hosp.; Assoc. (Rad), U. of Toronto; Tel. EM 6-8211.
WOYCHUK, Walther; 230 Falconbridge Rd., Garson, Ont.; 1560 Gemmell St., Sudbury (res); Tor '59; Tel. OX 3-2321.
WOYSHYSHYN, John; 423 Bronson Ave., Ottawa 4, Ont.; Ott '57; MCGP; Tel. 232-1531.
WOYWITKA, Nicholas W.; 204 Northgate Bldg., Edmonton, Alta.; 8714-116 St. (res); Alb '41; Ophth; Staff, U. of Alberta, Misericordia, Edmonton Gen., & Royal Alexandra Hosp's.; Tel. GA 2-2743.
WRATHALL, Ernest L.; 23 Queen St., Port Hope, Ont.; 84 Victoria St. S. (res); Tor '40; MCGP; Dist. Coroner; MO., HMCS 'Skeena"; Pres. Med. Soc. & Med. Rep. The Hosp. Trust; Tel. 885-2611.
WRAY, D. B.; Workmen's Comp. Board, Edmonton, Alta.; Alb '48; Temp. Retired.
WRAY, George C.; 15 London St. S., Hamilton, Ont.; Tor '37; Anaes; Staff Anaes., Hamilton Gen. Hosp.; Tel. 527-0271.
WRAY, Richard G.; Box 910, Olds, Alta.; Alb'54; Tel. 226-3355.
WRAZEJ, W. John; 440 Minton Ave., Ottawa 3, Ont.; Ott'59; Anaes; Tel. 722-3027.
WREN, Henry J.; 671 Lansdowne Ave., Toronto 4, Ont.; Ott '60; Tel. 534-6379.
WREN, Simon F.; McG '63; Int., Shaughnessy Hosp., Vancouver, B.C.
WREN, Walter W.; 24 Lansdowne, Harrow, Ont.; Gwen Rd., (res); Wes '52; MCGP; Active Staff, Grace, Metropolitan & Hotel-Dieu Hosp's., Windsor; Tel. RE 8-4121.
WRIDE, Gordon E.; 899 Hemlock Rd., Ottawa, Ont. (res); Wes '33; D.P.H., PH; Prin. Med. Off., & National Health Grant Admin., Dept. Nat. Health & Welfare; Tel. CE 2-8211.
WRIDE, Reginald J.; 414 Yarrow Bldg., 645 Fort St., Victoria, B.C.; Ste. 4, 1558 Beach Dr. (res); Wes '25; GenSurg; Staff, Royal Jubilee Hosp.; Cons. Staff, St. Joseph's Hosp.; Tel. 383-2512.
WRIGHT, Alan R.; 109E Plains Rd. W., Burlington, Ont. Tor '42; Tel. NE 4-9866.
WRIGHT, Alex; Box 807. Nipawin, Sask.; Man'26.
WRIGHT, Alexander M.; Ste. 615, 5025 Sherbrooke St. W., Montreal 6, P.Q.; McG'50; DABOS; FACS; FRCS(C); OrthSurg; Att'd. Staff, Shriner's Crippled Children's, Reddy Mem. & Queen Elizabeth Hosp's.; Cons. OrthSurg., Royal Edward Chest & Queen Mary Vets Hosp's.; Instr. (OrthSurg.), McGill U.; Tel. HU 8-2636.
WRIGHT, Allen S.; 23 Academy Medical Bldg., 1812-4th St. S.W., Calgary, Alta.; 1317-9th St. N.W. (res); Alb '49; M.C.G.P.; Staff, Calgary, Gen., Holy Cross, Grace Maternity & Crippled Children's Hosp's.; Tel. 262-6432.
WRIGHT, Amos J. L.; 57 James St., Parry Sound, Ont.; 24 Waubeek St. (res); Tor '35; District Coroner; Tel. 746-2181.
WRIGHT, Blake N.; 710 Seymour St., Vancouver 2, B.C.; UBC'65.
WRIGHT, Caroline C.; Clarke Inst. of Psy., 250 College St., Toronto 2B, Ont.; Tor'60.
WRIGHT, C. Burton; 200 Greyhound Bldg., 622-1st St. S.W., Calgary, Alta.; McG'29; Staff, Calgary Gen. Hosp.; Alberta Dist. M.O., C.P.R.; Retired.
WRIGHT, Charles S.; 71 Hillhurst Blvd., Toronto 12, Ont.; Dal'48; DABOS; Admin., Arthritic & Orthopaed. Hosp.; Tel. 924-4611.
WRIGHT, Clarence F.; 101 Rosemount Avenue, Weston, Toronto 15, Ont.; Wes '13; M.C.G.P.; Staff, Humber Memorial Hosp.; Tel. CH 1-1421.
WRIGHT, David E.; Box 2001, 351 Talbot St., Essex, Ont.; 123 Fairview Ave. (res); London (Eng.)'50; AMCGP; Tel. PR 6-7347.
WRIGHT, Donald L.; 91 Talbot St. E., Aylmer West, Ont.; 22 Rutherford St. (res); Man '48; M.C.G.P.
WRIGHT, Earle S.; McG '58; Res., St. Mary's Hosp., Montreal 26, P.Q.
WRIGHT, Edward N.; Medical Arts Bldg., Port Arthur, Ont.; 607 Red River Rd. (res); McG '29; Ophth. Otol; Instr. Nurses (Otol.), St. Joseph's & Port Arthur Gen. Hosp's.; Tel. DI 5-5732.

WRIGHT Frederick J.; 183 James St., Hamilton, Ont.; Qns '57; FRCP(C), Anaes; Staff, Hamilton Civic Hosp.; Tel. 648-6298.

WRIGHT, Gerald A.; 501 Hunt Bldg., Lethbridge, Alta.; 1508-17th Ave. S. (res); Wales '41; M.R.C.P., IntMed; Staff, St. Michael's & Municipal Hosp.; Tel. 327-3184.

WRIGHT, Ian W. M.; London (Eng.)'50; FRCS(Ed); Res., University Hosp., Edmonton, Alta.

WRIGHT, Isobel L.; 1414 Drummond St., Montreal, P.Q.; 3010 Westmount Blvd., Apt. A12 (res); Tor '38; Paed; Assoc. Phys., Montreal Children's Hosp.; Phys., Royal Edward Inst.; & Alexandra Hosp.; Dem., Dept. of Paed., McGill U.; Tel. VI 5-2713.

WRIGHT, Jack C.; 2006-8th Ave., New Westminster, B.C.; 481 Karman Ave., S. Burnaby (res); Tor '53; MCGP; Tel. LA 2-1742.

WRIGHT, James A.; 228 King St., St. Catharines, Ont.; Tor'61; AMCGP; Tel. 685-5381.

WRIGHT, James M.; St. Peters, N.S.; Dublin (Ire.)'53; MCGP; Med. Staff, St. Anne's Hosp., Arichat; Tel. 131.

WRIGHT, John A. E.; R.R. No. 4, Galt, Ont. (res); Wes '24; Retired.

WRIGHT, John B.; Dublin (Ire.)'58; DPM (Lond.); Staff, Saskatchewan Hosp., Weyburn, Sask.

WRIGHT, John S.; 236 St. George St., Moncton, N.B.; 213 Havelock St., Riverview (res); Dal '43; F.A.C.S.; GenSurg; Active Surg. Staff, Moncton Hosp.; Cons. Staff, Hotel-Dieu; Tel. EV 2-1106.

WRIGHT, J. W.; Millbrook, Ont.; Tor'29; MCGP; Dist. Coroner.

WRIGHT, Lloyd A.; 1050 Beaver Hall Hill, Montreal, P.Q.; 224 Stonehenge Dr., Beaconsfield (res); Tor '48; AB Prev Med (Occ. Med.); DABPM; Area Med. Dir., Montreal Area, Bell Telephone Co. of Canada.; Tel. 870-8603.

WRIGHT, Mary Anna; (see Nicholson, Mary Anna).

WRIGHT, R. Barry; Oshawa Clinic, 117 King St. E., Oshawa, Ont.; Wes'62.

WRIGHT, Ralph N.; 715 Scarlett Rd., Weston, Ont.; Tor '44; Tel. CH 1-2761.

WRIGHT, Robert D.; P.O. Box 1000, Tisdale, Sask., Mon '41; Tel. 2151.

WRIGHT, Robert G.; Elmsdale, N.S.; Dal'40; Staff, Grace Maternity, Halifax Infirmary & Colchester Hosp's.; Tel. 883-2216.

WRIGHT, Robert P., C.M.G., D.S.O., Croix-de-Guerre; 4 Cedar Ave., Pete. Claire, P.Q.; F.R.C.S.(C); Hon. Att'd. Staff, Montreal Gen. Hosp.; Retired

WRIGHT, Thomas A.; 376 Centre St., Drumheller, Alta.; 370—2nd St. E. (res); Alb '43; MCGP; Dist. Coroner.

WRIGHT, Thomas A.; Ste. 101, 25 Leonard Ave., Toronto 2B, Ont.; Tor '56; FRCS(C); OrthSurg; Staff, Toronto Western Hosp.

WRIGHT, Vern C.; 40 Homestead Cr., London, Ont.; Wes'60; FRCS(C), ObstGyn.

WRIGHT, Victor W.; 11250-84 Ave., Edmonton, Alta.; Man'09; Dir., Alberta Gov't. Cancer Services, Edmonton; Tel. 488-5080.

WRIGHT, Virginia J.; UBC'65; Res., Dept. of Paed., University of B.C., Vancouver, B.C.

WRIGHT, Walter F.; 30 George St. N., Galt, Ont.; Tor '47; D.Psy; Psy; IntMed; Dir. of Psy., Dept. of Reforms, Prov. of Ont.; Cons. Med., South Waterloo Mem. Hosp.; Med. Staff, Kitchener-Waterloo Gen. Hosp.; Tel. 623-1904.

WRIGHT, Walter W.; 170 St. George St., Toronto, Ont.; 2 Lamport Ave. (res); Tor '04; D.Ophth., Ophth; Prof. Emeritus, Ophth., U. of Toronto; Cons., Canadian National Inst. Blind, Toronto Gen. Hosp. & Hosp. for Sick Children; Retired.

WRIGHT, Wayne J.; Alb'64; Res., University Hosp., Edmonton, Alta.

WRIGHT, William D.; Sask'65; Res., St. Paul's Hosp., Saskatoon, Sask.

WRIGHT, W. James; Bracebridge, Ont.; Wes '56; MCGP; Tel. 645-4457.

WRIGHT, W. Ross; Fredericton Med. Clinic, 206 Rookwood Ave., Fredericton, N.B.; 48 Alexandra St. (res); Dal '34; F.A.A.O.O., OphthOtol; Staff, Victoria Public Hosp.; Tel. 475-7701.

WRIGLEY, Frederic R.; 7421 Bayard St., Montreal 16, P.Q. (res); London (Eng.) '49; M.B., B.S., M R.C.S. (Eng.), L.R.C.P. (Lond.), D.R.C.O.G., D.A., F.R.C.P.)C), Anaes; Assoc. Anaes., Royal Victoria Hosp.; Lect. (Anaes.), McGill U.; Tel. 739-3839.

WRONG, Harry A.; 2180 Main St., Niagara Falls, Ont.; Tor '22; Anaes; Staff, Gtr. Niagara Gen. Hosp.; Court. Staff, Mem. Hosp., Niagara Falls, N.Y.

WRONG, Norman M.; 604 Med. Arts Bldg., 170 St. George St., Toronto 5, Ont.; 128 Buckingham Ave. (res); Tor '27; F.R.C.P.(C), DermSyph; Sr. Att'd. Phys., Tor. Gen. Hosp.; Act. Cons., Hosp., for Sick Children; Cons. (Derm.), Sunnybrook DVA Hosp.; Graduate Lect. (Med.), U. of Toronto; Tel. WA 2-5882.

WRONSKI, Bernard A.; 105 Grantbrook St., Willowdale, Ont. (res); Polish School of Med., Edinburgh (Scot.) '42; GenSurg; Staff, Workmen's Comp. Bd., Downsview; Tel. 242-1761.

WUERTH, Felix; Apt. 5, 6 Forest Hill Dr., Guelph, Ont.; Vienna (Austria) '49; Anaes.; Tel. 824-5310.

WUERTH, Walter J.; 459 Bloor St. W., Toronto, Ont.; 1601 Liveoak Dr., Port Credit (res); Wuertzberg (Germ.) '31; GenSurg; Staff, Doctor's & Central Hosp's.; Tel. WA 1-2552.

WUIDART, Yves Henri Raymond; 617 Bloomfield, Outremont, Montreal 8, P.Q.; Paris (France) '46; AMCGP.

WURM, Karl; 119 Christina St., Sarnia, Ont.; Munich (Germ.) '38; Derm.; Staff, Sarnia Gen. & St. Joseph's Hosp's.; Tel. ED 7-8188.

WYANT, Gordon M.; 522 Copland Cr., Saskatoon, Sask. (res); Bologna (Italy) '38; DA (Eng.), DABA, FACA, LRCP, LRCS (Edin.), LRFPS (Glasgow); FFARCS (Eng.), FICA, FRCP(C), Anaes; Vis. Cons. (Anaes.), Saskatoon City Hosp.; Prof. & Chief of Dept. of Anaes., U. of Saskatchewan & University Hosp.; Lt. Col. C.O. Med. Coy, RCAMC(M); Tel. 652-8221.

WYANT, John D.; McG '62; Res., Royal Victoria Hosp. Montreal 2, P.Q.

WYATT, Donald E.; Med. Arts Bldg., Empire Ave., St. John's, Nfld.; Dal'63; DNBME; AMCGP; Assoc. Staff, Grace & St. Clare's Hosp's.; Tel. 579-9673.

WYATT, E. Rix; 2 Park Ave., Elmira, Ont.; 25 Bobolink Pl. (res); McG '44; MCGP; Active Staff, Kitchener-Waterloo & St. Mary's Hosp's; Pres., Coll. of Phys. & Surgeons of Ontario; Tel. MO 9-5471.

WYATT, John K.; 301 Victoria Bldg., 111 Waterloo St., London, Ont.; Wes'54; F.R.C.S.(C), GenSurg; Urol; Fell. (Surg.), U. of Western Ont.; Cons. (Urol.), Westminster DVA Hosp.; Tel. GE 8-8835.

WYATT, John P.; Man '38; PathBact; Staff, Dept. of Path., Manitoba Med. College, Winnipeg 3, Man.; Tel. 786-3537.

WYATT, William J.; 70 Hartley St., Brockville, Ont. (res); McG '45; FCAP; Path; Dir. of Labs., St.-Vincent-de-Paul & Brockville Gen. Hosp's.; Cons. Path., St. Francis Gen. & Smiths Falls Hosp's.; Reg. Pathol., Dept. of Justice; Tel. DI 2-7884.

WYCHERS, John; 40 George St. N., Galt, Ont.; 15 Havill St. (res); Groningen (Neth.) '40; M.C.G.P.; Staff, South Waterloo Mem. Hosp. Tel. 621-6974.

WYLDE, Edmund; 311 3rd St., New Westminster, B.C.; McG'31; DPH; Dir., Simon Fraser Health Unit, New Westminster, B.C.

WYLIE, Alan R.; Wes '58; MCGP; Int., Hamilton Gen. Hosp., Hamilton, Ont.

WYLIE, Bernice (Russell); 150-5780 Cambie St., Vancouver, B.C.; 1032 W. 46th Ave., (res); Tor '54; F.R.C.P.(C), IntMed; Att'd. Staff, Shaughnessy DVA & Van. Gen. Hosp's.; Med. Coordinator, Holy Family Hosp.; Vis. Staff, St. Vincent's Hosp.; Tel. FA 1-3713.

WYLIE, Gordon B.; Thorold Rd., St. Catharines, Ont.; 512 Scott St. (res); Glasgow (Scot.) '49; F.R.C.S. (Edin.), Otol.

WYLIE, H. Laird; 17-11th Ave. S., Cranbrook, B.C.; 202-15th Ave. (res); Man'41.

WYLIE, Kenneth O.; 190 Tache Ave., St. Boniface 6, Man.; Man '52; Paed; Active Med. Staff, Children's Hosp. Winnipeg, & St. Boniface Hosp's; Cons. Paed. (Retarded Children), St. Boniface San.; Lect. (Paed.), U. of Manitoba; Tel. CE 3-2493.

WYLIE, Richard E.; Wes'64; Res., Dept. of Surg., U. of Western Ont., London, Ont.

WYLIE, Walter A.; 127 Riverhead Dr., Rexdale, Ont. (res); Tor '24; Retired.

WYLLIE, A. Kenneth; Box 728, 159 Wellington St., Kingston, Ont.; 252 Park St. (res); Qns'55; **FRCS (Ed.); FRCS(C); PlasSurg; Att'd. Staff, Kingston Gen. & Hotel-Dieu Hosp's.; Cons. Cdn. Forces Hosp.; Lect. Queen's U.; Tel. 548-8871.**

WYLLIE, John; 53 Kensington Ave., Kingston, Ont. (res); Glasgow (Scot.) '20; D.P.H. (Eng.); PH; Emeritus Prof. PH & Prev. Med. Queen's U.; Retired.

WYLLIE, John C.; 229 Westdale Ave., Kingston, Ont. (res); Qns '52; Path; DiagRad; Ass't. Prof. Path., Queens U.; Tel. 546-1731.

WYNANDS, John E.; 687 Pine Ave. W., Montreal 2, P.Q.; 22 Fairfield Cres., Mtl. W. 28 (res); McG '54; DA; Anaes; Ass't. Anaes., Royal Victoria Hosp.; Lect. (Anaes), McGill U.; Tel. VI 2-1251, Loc. 530.

WYND, Peter B.; Qns'65; Res., Hotel Dieu Hosp., Kingston, Ont.

WYNNE, Frederick; Berwyn, Alta.; Alb '39; Dist. Coroner.

WYNNE, John B.; 50 Yonge St. N., Richmond Hill, Ont.; Tor'52; AMCGP; Staff, York Central Hosp.; Tel. 884-1154.

WYNNE, John R. W. W/C; London (Eng.) '55; M.B., B.S., MRCS; LRCP; Sr. M.O., RCAF Hosp., Cold Lake, Alta.; Tel. 248-3311.

WYNNE-JONES, Megan; 22 Hillhurst Blvd., Toronto 12, Ont.; Tor '48; Staff, OPD, Women's College Hosp.; Research Ass't., Lyndhurst Lodge Hosp.; Tel. HU 3-7655.

WYNN-WILLIAMS, Robert N.; CTR Okanagan Med. Assoc., 1737 Pandosy St., Kelowna, B.C.; Liverpool (Eng.)'61.

WYNRIB, Morris; Wellington, B.C. (res); Paris (France) '34; Staff, Indian Hosp., Nanaimo, B.C.

WYNTER, Roderick A.; Aberdeen (Scot.) '58; DCH (Lond.); Res., Hosp. for Sick Children, Toronto, Ont.

WYSE, Carl W.; Wes'62; Res., Toronto Gen. Hosp., Toronto 2, Ont.

WYSE, Derek M.; 749 King St. W., Kitchener, Ont.; 697 Glasgow Rd. (res); McG '48; DIM; FRCP(C), IntMed; Tel. 743-4623.

WYSHYNSKI, Peter E.; Tor'61; Res., Hosp. for Sick Children, Toronto 2, Ont.

XENOS, John B.; 5315 Est. Jarry, St. Leonard De Port, Maurice, P.Q.; McG'63; Staff, Santa Cabrini Hosp., Montreal; Tel. 277-0115.

YABLON, Isadore; Tor'58; FRCS(C), OrthSurg; Staff, Royal Victoria Hosp., Montreal 2, P.Q.

YABLSLEY, Reginald H.; Apt. 312, 150 Maplehurst Ave., Willowdale, Ont.; Dal'60; FRCS(C), Orth Surg; Staff, Toronto Gen. Hosp.; Tel. EM 6-8211; Abroad.

YACHNIN, Irving; 817 Medical Arts Bldg., 1538 Sherbrooke St. W., Montreal 25, P.Q.; Mon '56; IntMed; Ward Serv., Reddy Mem. Hosp.; Tel. WE 2-9441.

YADAV, Daya R.; 606 Med. Dental Bldg., Regina, Sask.; Lucknow (India)'56; **AMCGP.**

YADAV, Vasant; Nagpur (India)'56; Res., Children's Hosp., Halifax, N.S.

YAEGER, Harold L.; 1140 Osler St., Saskatoon, Sask.; Tor '33; Dist. Coroner; Tel. 653-0695.

YAFFE, S. Adrian; 412 Med. Arts Bldg., Hamilton, Ont.; 1 St, James Pl. (res); **Qns '36;** MRCP (Lond.); FACC; IntMed; Cons., Hamilton Civic, **St. Joseph's, Lincoln & Dist., Oakville-Trafalgar Mem. Hosp's. & DVA Cardiac Cathet. Team., Ham. Gen. Hosp.; Tel. JA 7-1815.**

YAHOLNITSKY, Michael; 5A-3rd Ave., Yorkton, Sask.; 69-3rd Ave. (res); Man '37; Tel. 783-2884.

YAHOLNITSKY, Richard; 5A Third Ave., Yorkton, Sask.; 132 Third **Ave. (res); Alb '43; F.R.C.S. (Edin.); Tel. 783-2884.**

YAHOLNITSKY, Sam; 111A-8th Ave. S.W., Calgary, Alta.; Man '37; Tel. 269-6004.

YAK, John; 1949 Beach Ave., Vancouver 5, B.C. (res); McG '23; Retired.

YAKE, Wallace W.; Ste. A, 14230-85th Ave., Edmonton, Alta.; Alb '53; MCGP; Tel. 488-0670.

YAKIMETS, Walter W.; University of Alberta Hosp., Edmonton, Alta.; Alb'59; FRCS(C), GenSurg; Ass't. Prof. Surg., U. of Alberta; Tel. 439-5911.

YAKYMECHKO, Mary (Sushko); 5629-111th Ave., Edmonton, Alta.; Ludwigs-Maximillian (Munich, Germ.) '56; Staff, Alberta Hosp.

YAM, Diana E.; Qns'65; Jr. Int., St. Joseph's Hosp., Victoria, B.C.

YAMAN, Hasan F.; Box 335, Noranda, P.Q.; Istanbul (Turkey)'52; Abroad.

YAMANAKA, George J.; Box 368, Ladner, B.C.; UBC '57; Tel. FA 5-6936.

YAMKA, Edward M.; 11 Kirkland St., Kirkland Lake, Ont.; Tor'64; Staff, Kirkland & Dist. Hosp.; Tel. 567-3217.

YANCOFF, Vasil Y.; 162A O'Connor Dr., Toronto 6, Ont.; Tor '53; Tel. HO 5-6671.

YANDEL, Michael; Tor '56; MCGP; Res. (Orth-Surg.), University Hosp., Saskatoon, Sask.

YANG, Cheng-Chao; Ste. 210 ,814 Cook Rd., Richmond, B.C.; Taiwan (China)'57; FRCS(C), ObstGyn; Staff, Grace Hosp.

YANG, George; Listowel Clinic, Box 938, Listowel, Ont.; Cheelos (China)'42; FACS; FCCP; GenSurg; Staff, Listowel Mem. Hosp. & Wingham & Dist. Hosp., Wingham; Staff, Palmerston Gen. Hosp., Palmerston; Tel. 291-4200.

YANG, John T.; 243 Loch Lomond Road, St. John, N.B.; Dal '63; MCGP; Tel. 657-3920.

YANKOU, Chris J.; 701 Danforth Ave., Toronto 6, Ont.; Wes '55; Tel. HO 1-1932.

YANKOWSKY, M. Orest; 289 Cedar St., Sudbury, Ont.; Tor'56.

YANOVER, Philip; 1234 Main St. W., Hamilton, Ont.; Qns '58; Tel. JA 9-3211.

YAO, James; Philippines '58; Res., Hosp. for Sick Children, Toronto 2, Ont.

YAO, Jose P.; Box 597, Grand Falls, N.B.

YAO, Ming; 35 Fern Ave., Toronto, Ont. (res); Tor '42; F.A.C.A.

YAP, Victor U.; O'Mara Martin Bldg., Military Rd., St. John's, Nfld.; Manila (Philipp.) '57.

YAREMKO, Daphne; (see Patrick, Daphne).

YAREY, O. B.; 4687 Yonge St., Willowdale, Toronto, Ont.; Tor '48; M.C.G.P.; Tel. BA 1-6565.

YARN, James C.; 11 East Valley Rd., Corner Brook, Nfld.; Dal '60; Tel. 634-7676.

YARROW, Alex R.; Ste. 1103, 750 W. Broadway, Vancouver 9, B.C.; Tor'54; Psy.

YASAYKO, Jack F.; 110 W. 14th Ave., North Vancouver, B.C.; Alb'62; Tel. 987-2810.

YATES, Denis E.; Box 730, Virden, Man.; London (Eng.)'43; MRCS; LRCP; Tel. 461.

YATES, Douglas E.; 383 Ellis St., Penticton, B.C.; Tor '51; GenSurg.; Tel. HY 2-3024.

YATES, George R.; 8584 Granville St., Vancouver 14, B.C.; UBC '54; MCGP; Tel. 266-8010.

YATES, Maxwell; 619 Scollard Bldg., 1207 Douglas St., Victoria, B.C.; 2783 Somass Dr. (res); Alb '42; Anaes; Tel. EV 3-3261.

YATES, Paul; 1530 Albion Rd., Rexdale, Ont.; Wes'50; Abroad.

YATES, Thomas H.; Tor '60; DiagRad; Staff, Toronto Gen. Hosp., Toronto, Ont.

YAUNISKIS, Alphonse A.; 306 Boyd Bldg., 388 Portage Ave. Winnipeg 1, Man.; 555 Montague Ave. (res); Cardiff (Wales) '43; MCGP; Tel. 943-9162.

YAWORSKY, Raymond G.; Qns'57; FRCP(C), Path; Staff, St. Joseph's Hosp., Hamilton, Ont.; Tel. 522-4941.
YAWORSKY, Walter; 290 Giles Blvd. E., Windsor, Ont.; Psy; Tel. 253-2671.
YCAS, Jonas; 14 High Park Ave., Toronto 9, Ont.; Frankfurt (Germ.) '47; M.C.G.P.; Tel. RO 2-2221.
YEATES A. M.; 229 King St. W., Hamilton, Ont.; Wes '13; Tel. JA 2-8143.
YEATES, George R.; 1307 S.W. Marine Dr., Vancouver 14, B.C.; UBC '54.
YEE, George E.; Metropolitan Gen. Hosp., Windsor, Ont.; Man'60; Path; Assoc. Path., Leamington Dist. Mem. Hosp., Leamington; Tel. 256-3461, Ext. 63.
YEGOROV, Alexandra; 302 Evelyn Ave., Toronto 9, Ont.; Alb '40; Staff, City Welfare Dept.; Tel. RO 2-3023.
YEH, Hsu C.; Nat. Taiwan (Formosa); Staff, Soldier's Mem. Hosp., Campbellton, N.B.
YEH, Hui E.; China '58; Staff, Grace Dart Hosp., 6085 Sherbrooke St. E., Montreal 5, P.Q.
YELLAND, A. Colin, W/C; Transport Bldg., Rideau St., Ottawa, Ont.; Glasgow (Scot.)'50; LRCP; LRCS; FACA.
YELLAND, H. Max, E.D.; 707 Charlotte St., Peterborough, Ont.; 18 Charles St. (res); Tor '11; F.I.C.S.; F.R.C.S.(C), GenSurg; Surg. Staff, Peterborough Civic & St. Joseph's Hosp's.; Tel. 742-1210.
YELLAND, Leslie W.; Ste. 203, 625-5th Ave., New Westminster, B.C.; U.K.'50.
YELLE, Ernest F.; Calwood Clinic, 11816-124th St., Edmonton, Alta.; 14412-88th Ave. (res); Alb '48; MCGP; Tel. 454-6571.
YELLER, R. Michael; Capetown (S. Africa) '45; M.B., Ch.B., DPH; Reg. M.O., Yorkton-Melville Health, Reg. No. 10, Yorkton, Sask.; Tel. 783-3647; Abroad.
YENAL, Affan S.; 108 Medical Arts Bldg., 404 Graham Ave., Winnipeg 1, Man.; Istanbul (Turkey) '45; DiagRad; Staff, Deer Lodge & Grace Hosp's.; Tel. WH 2-3521.
YENDT, Edmund R.; Clinical Invest. Unit, Toronto Gen. Hosp., Toronto, Ont.; Tor'48; FRCP(C), IntMed; Sr. Phys., Toronto Gen. Hosp.; Research Assoc. Med. Research Council of Canada; Assoc. Prof. Med., U. of Toronto; Tel. EM 6-8211, Loc. 2830.
YEO, Harold E.; 193 Prince St., Charlottetown, P.E.I.; McG '37; Tel. 4-8212.
YEO, Thomas A.; Man '62; Jr. Intn., Winnipeg Gen. Hosp., Winnipeg, Man.
YERGEAU, Frank; Upton, P.Q.; Mon '18; Staff, Dept. of Health.
YESSAYAN, Garabed L.; 790 Sherbrook St., Winnipeg 2, Man.; 805 Sherbrook (res); Beirut (Lebanon) '56; FRCP(C), Paed; Active Staff, Children's Hosp.; Tel. SP 4-6561.
YEUNG, Jai Y.; Box 100, Eastend Med. Clinic, Eastend, Sask.; Sun-Yat-Sen (Canton, China)'52.
YEUNG, Yin-Chin; 696 Bessborough Dr., Oshawa, Ont. (res); Sun-Yat-Sen U. (Canton, China) '52; D.A.; Staff, Oshawa Gen. Hosp.; Tel. 723-1677.
YEWCHUK, Paul; Box 510, Lac La Biche, Alta.; Alb'60; Staff, St. Catharines Hosp.; Tel. 623-4421.
YIELDING, T. Edward; 277 Scarboro Cres., Scarborough, Ont.; 27 Chestermere Blvd. (res); Tor '58; MCGP; Tel. 267-9551.
YIP, K. Ghim; 536 Main St., Vancouver, B.C.; 2536 E. 15th Ave. (res); Qns '27; Tel. MU 1-1716.
YIP, Simm W.; 5224 Kingsway, South Burnaby, B.C.; UBC'61.
YIP, Suzanne; Sask'60; Res., University Hosp., Saskatoon, Sask.
YOELL, Barry J.; Dal'65; Staff, Bonne Bay Cottage Hosp., Norris Point, Nfld.
YOERGER, Russell G.; C.N.R. Station, 1150 Station St., Vancouver, B.C.; Ste. 11, 1485 W. 13th St. (res); Qns '22; F.I.C.S., F.A.C.S., GenSurg; Chief of Staff, & Surg. Att. Staff, St. Vincent's Hosp.; Vis. Staff, Vancouver Gen. & St. Paul's Hosp's.; Dist. M.O., C.N.R.; Tel. MU 4-0171.
YONEDA, Yoshitaro; 211 Med. Arts Bldg., Edmonton, Alta.; 7242-112th St. (res); Alb '44; F.A.C.S., F.R.C.S.(C), ObstGyn; Staff, U. of Alberta Hosp.; Lect., U. of Alta.; Tel. GA 4-6748.
YONEYAMA, Misao — see **FUJIWARA, Misao.**
YONG, Yu S.; Nat. U. (Taiwan)'61; Res., Deer Lodge Hosp., Winnipeg, Man.
YONGE, Keith A.; 10406 Connaught Dr., Edmonton, Alta. (res); McG '48; D.P.M., (Lond.); Psy; Dir. Dept. of Psy., U. of Alberta Hosp.; Prof. and Head, Dept. of Psy., U. of Alberta; Chief (Psy.), D.V.A.; Tel. 439-5911; Loc. 276.
YOON, Shu Hyun; Soel (Korea)'56; Urol; Staff, Provincial Hosp., Saint John, N.B.
YORK, J. Edward; 178 St. George St., Toronto, Ont.; London (Eng.)'52; DA(Eng.); FRCP(C), Anaes; Clin. Teach. Anaes., U. of Toronto; Lect. Med., Dental Fac., U. of Toronto; Tel. 923-1154.
YORK, Samuel E.; Victoria Gen. Hosp., Halifax, N.S.; Dal'59; FRCP(C), IntMed; Lect. Med., Dalhousie U.; Tel. 422-7371, Loc. 664.
YORKE, Zoltan G.; Budapest (Hung.) '37; Ophth. (Hung.); Staff, Ontario Hosp. School, Cedar Springs, Ont.
YOSHIDA, Samuel H.; Tor'61; Res., Dept. of Surg., U. of British Columbia, Vancouver, B.C.
YOSHIOKA, John M.; 331 Sheddon St., Oakville. Ont.; 369 Morrison Rd. (res); Tor '49; Anaes Staff, Oakville-Trafalgar Mem. Hosp.; Tel. VI 5-2571.
YOUNG, Alan E.; 1357 Mt. Pleasant Rd., Toronto, Ont.; Tor '29; D.P.H.; P.H.; Dir. TB Div., Dept. of P.H., City of Toronto; Tel. 366-8411.
YOUNG, Andrew B.; Ste. 110, 299 Main St., Chilliwack, B.C.; UBC '59; MCGP; Tel. 795-9161.
YOUNG, Archibald D.; 299 Main St., Chilliwack, B.C.; McG '51; MCGP; Active Staff, Chilliwack Gen. Hosp.; Tel. 795-9161.
YOUNG, Arthur F.; Moose Jaw Clinic, 200 Scott Bldg., Moose Jaw, Sask.; 1035 Alder Ave. (res); Man'45; FACS, FRCS(C), GenSurg; Staff, Union & Providence Hosp's.; Cons., Sask. Training School Hosp.; Tel. 692-2373.
YOUNG, Arthur L.; 23 Wildwood Blvd., Dartmouth, N.S.; London (Eng.)'36; MRCS; LRCP; FCCP.
YOUNG, Arthur W.; 4523 Kensington Ave., Montreal 28, P.Q. (res); McG '20; F.R.C.P.(C), Neur Psy; Retired.
YOUNG, Bruce H.; Crippled Children's Centre, 350 Rumsey Rd., Toronto 17, Ont.; Qns'40; Phys-Med. & Rehab; Ass't. Med. Dir., Ontario Soc. for Crippled Children & The Ontario Crippled Children's Centre; Tel. 487-5311.
YOUNG, Bryce G.; Guidance Centre, 11120-102nd St., Edmonton, Alta.; Glasgow (Scot.)'61; M.B., Ch.B.; Psy.
YOUNG, Cecil; 210 St. Clair Ave. W., Toronto 7, Ont.; 123 Glenrose Ave. (res); Tor '19; M.R.-C.P., IntMed; Cons. Med. Staff, Toronto Western Hosp.
YOUNG, Clifford T.; 2279 Queen St. E., Toronto 13, Ont.; Tor '35; N.I.P.
YOUNG, Connear; Carmel Med. Clin., 124-1st Ave. N.W., Swift Current, Sask.; St. Andrew's (Scot.)'59.
YOUNG, Crossman H.; 5 Cleveland Cres., Dartmouth, N.S.; Dal '41; IntMed; Active Staff (Med.), Hlfx. Infirm. & Camp Hill DVA Hosp's.; Med. Cons., N.S. Hosp., Dartmouth; Lect. (Med.), Dalhousie U.; Tel. 466-2269.
YOUNG David R.; Box 510. Fort Saskatchewan, **Alta.; Alb '54; MCGP.**
YOUNG, D. Murray; Apt. 1, 41 Spadina Rd., Toronto 4, Ont.; Tor '50; Ph.D.; Dir of Labs. & Staff Phys., Toronto Gen. Hosp.; Ass't. Prof. (Path.), & Assoc. in Med., U. of Toronto; Tel. EM 6-8211, Ext. 2108.
YOUNG, Donald A.; 232 Metcalfe St., Ottawa, 500 Kenwood St. (res); McG '35; GenSurg; Staff, Ottawa Civic Hosp.; Tel. CE 2-0177.
YOUNG, Donald F.; Young St., St. Jacobs, Ont.; Tor'36; Active Staff, St. Mary's & Kitchener-Waterloo Hosp's., Kitchener; Court. Staff, Freeport San.; **Tel. 664-2271.**

YOUNG, **Donald R.**; Drawer 60, Emo, Ont.; Wes '16; M.O.H., Emo; Coroner, Dist. of Rainy River. Retired.
YOUNG, **Doreen A.**; Ste. 7, 901 O'Connor Dr., Toronto 16, Ont.; 24 Presteign Ave. (res); Wes '59; MCGP; Staff (G.P.), Toronto East Gen. Hosp.; Tel. 759-9073.
YOUNG, Douglas R.; 35 Charlotte St., Brantford, Ont.; 74 Ridgewood Dr. (res); Wes '58; Tel. 752-2632.
YOUNG, **Du L.**; 14819-108th Ave., North Surrey, B.C.; National U. (Taiwan) '63.
YOUNG, **Edgar J.**; 84 Heathview Ave., Willowdale, Ont.; Tor'32; DPH; Phys. I/C, Northern Ont. Public Health Serv., Ontario Dept. of Health.
YOUNG, **Elizabeth G. L.**; 715 Danforth Ave., Toronto, Ont.; Tor '34; Staff (Obst.), Women's College Hosp.; Tel. HO 5-7717.
YOUNG, **Ernest M.**; 191 Holland Ave., Ottawa, Ont.; 628 Keenan Ave. (res); Qns. '30; Tel. PA 8-3533.
YOUNG, **Francis L. D.**; East Lawrencetown, Halifax Co., N.S.; Guys Hosp. (London, Eng.)'40; DPM; Sr. Clin. Psy., Nova Scotia Hosp.; Tel. 422-4206.
YOUNG, **Frank M.**; 504 Main St. E., Hamilton, Ont.; 20 Inverness Ave. W. (res); Qns '41; M.A.C.R., D.A.B.R., D.M.R. (Tor), DiagRad; Cons. Rad, D.V.A.; Tel. JA 8-1466
YOUNG, **Fred A.**; 558 Stradbrooke Ave., Winnipeg, Man.; Tor '99.
YOUNG, George E.; 15 Lorne St., Chapleau, Ont.; Qns '42; M.O.H.; District Coroner; Chief of Staff, Lady Minto Hosp.; Tel. 156.
YOUNG, **Gerard**; Edinburgh (Scot.)'49; Path; Staff, Children's Hosp., Winnipeg 3, Man.
YOUNG, G. Wright; 631 Medical Arts Bldg., 170 St. George St., Toronto, Ont.; 65 Colin Ave. (res); Tor '31; IntMed.; Tel. WA 1-4131.
YOUNG, H. Gordon; Moose Jaw Clinic, 200 Scott Bldg., Moose Jaw, Sask.; 320 Grant Hall Hotel (res); Tor'16; GenSurg; **Staff, Moose Jaw Gen.** Hosp.; Tel. 692-2373.
YOUNG, H. N. M.; 305 Stewart St., Peterborough, Ont.; Qns '26; M.C.G.P.; Dist. Coroner. Tel. 745-7752.
YOUNG, **Horace O.**; McG'62; Res., Mtl. Children's Hosp., Montreal, P.Q.
YOUNG, Hugh M.; 108 Scott Blk., Moose Jaw, Sask.; 1124 Clifton Ave. (res); Qns '12; F.A.C.S.; ObstGyn; Retired.
YOUNG, **Hugh V.**; 108 Scott Blk., Moose Jaw, Sask.; Man'50; Active Staff, Moose Jaw Union & Providence Hosp's.; Tel. 692-1827.
YOUNG, **J. Alexander**; 34 High St., Pictou, N.S.; Dal '36; Tel. 5-5101.
YOUNG, **James D., F/L**; Man'64; RCAF Station, St. Hubert, P.Q.
YOUNG, **J. C.**; 341½ Charlotte St., Sydney, N.S.; 112 Castle Drive (res); McG '36.
YOUNG, J. C. Gordon, M.B.E.; 640 Seaforth Med. Bldg., 3550 Cote des Neiges Rd., Montreal 25, P.Q.; 3111 Westmount Blvd. (res); McG '41; DIM; DABIM; FACP; Gastroent (P.Q.); IntMed; Ass't. Phys., Montreal Gen. Hosp.; Gastroscopist, Queen Mary Vet's Hosp.; Clin. Teach (Med.), McGill U.; Tel. 937-3260.
YOUNG, **J. Fraser**; 34 High St., Pictou, N.S.; Dal'36.
YOUNG, John H.; Smith Clinic, Camrose, Alta.; 4701-51st St., (res); Alb '41; Hon. Coroner.
YOUNG, **John K.**; 1640 16th. Ave. N.W., Calgary, Alta.; Alb '54; FRCS(C); GenSurg; Active Staff, all Calgary Hosp's.; Tel. 282-6005.
YOUNG, **John W. J. F. G/C**; National Defence Med. Centre, Smyth Rd. & Alta Vista Dr., Ottawa, Ont.; London & Cambridge (Eng.) '34; MRCS; LRCP; DPH; Pension Med. Examiner, Cdn. Pension Comm.; Tel. RE 3-6600, Ext. 277.
YOUNG, **J. Stuart**; 301 Canada Bldg., Windsor, Ont.; 825 Kildare Rd. (res); Qns '38; FRCS(Ed.), FACS, FRCS(C), GenSurg; Active Surg. Staff, Metropolitan Gen. & Grace Hosp's.; Tel. 254-3011.
YOUNG, **Leighton N.**; 807 Portage Ave., Winnipeg 10, Man.; Man'57; Paed.; Staff, Children's Hosp.; Lect., U. of Manitoba; Tel. 772-9777.
YOUNG, Lionel D.; Community Clinic, 113-3rd Ave. E., Biggar, Sask.; 416-7th Ave. E. (res); Dublin (Ire.) '56; M.B., B.Ch., BAO; MCGP; Tel. 948-3378.
YOUNG, **MacLean K.**; 10004-105th St., Edmonton, Alta.; 8711 Saskatchewan Dr. (res); Alb '40; IntMed; Att. Staff, U. of Alberta & Royal Alexandra Hosp's.; Court. Staff, Edmonton Gen. Hosp.; **Clin. Inst'r. (Med.), Alberta U.; Tel. GA 4-2121.**
YOUNG, **Mary E.** (Escott-Beal); 64 Eldomar Ave., Brampton, Ont.; Wes '39; Retired.
YOUNG, **Mary I. (Sanderson)**; 887 Victoria Ave., Windsor, Ont.; Tor '36; MCAA; Allerg. Cons., Hotel-Dieu & Grace Hosp's.; Tel. 252-9811.
YOUNG, Maurice D., C.D., Q.H.S.; Health Centre for Children, 715 W. 12th Ave., Vancouver, B.C.; 3181 Thompson Pl. (res); Cambridge (Eng.) '36; MRCS, LRCP, MRCP, FAAP; FRCP(C), Paed; Sr. Att'd. Staff, Van. Gen. Hosp.; Assoc. Prof. (Paed.), U. of British Columbia; Tel. TR 6-3211, Loc. 2667.
YOUNG, M. H. Vincent; 680 Seaforth Med. Bldg., 3550 Cote des Neiges Rd., Montreal 25, P.Q.; 435 Simcoe Ave., Town of Mount Royal (res); McG '41; FRCOG; FACS; FRCS(C); ObstGyn; Chief ObstGyn. Lakeshore Gen. Hosp.; Assoc. ObstGyn., Royal Victoria Hosp.; Clin. Ass't. (ObstGyn.), Montreal Gen. Hosp.; **Ass't. Prof., McGill U.** Tel. 937-3545.
YOUNG, **Michael K.**; Dal'65; Staff, Lakeshore Psy. Hosp., Toronto 14, Ont.
YOUNG, M. Isabel; Tor '47; Staff, Sudbury Al-goma San., Sudbury, Ont.
YOUNG, **Morley A. R.**; Lamont, Alta.; McG '21; F.A.C.S., F.R.C.S.(C) GenSurg; Chief of Surg., & Med. Supt., Archer Memorial Hosp.; Dist. Coroner; **Tel. H-18.**
YOUNG, Percival M.; Box 358, 135 Main St., Sturgeon Falls, Ont.; Wes'35; MCGP; Staff, St. Jean de Brebeuf Hosp.; Tel. 753-0860.
YOUNG, **Peter W.**; Ste. 205, 628 Davis Dr., Newmarket, Ont.; Tor'57; Ophth.
YOUNG, **Ralph A.**; 64 Eldomar Ave., Brampton, Ont. (res); Tor '40; Staff, Hosp. & Rehab. Centre, W.C.B., **Downsview, Ont.; Tel. 244-1761.**
YOUNG, **R. Clarence**; 34 High St., Pictou, N.S.; Dal'42; IntMed; Cons. in Cardiol., Aberdeen Hosp., New Glasgow; Tel. 485-5101.
YOUNG, **Robert J.**; 234 Romaine St., Peterborough, Ont.; **385 Stewart St. (res); Qns '32;** Tel. RI 2-4247.
YOUNG, **Robert N.**; 1625 Oak Bay Ave., Victoria, B.C.; 2555 Chelsea Pl. (res); UBC '56; MCGP; **Active Staff, Royal Jubilee Victoria & Vet's. Hosp.; Court. Staff, St. Joseph's Hosp.; Tel. EV 2-7281.**
YOUNG, Robert W.; 1 Campbell Ave., St. John's, Nfld.; Dal'58; FRCP(C); IntMed; Dir., Div. of Clin. Cardiol., Grace Gen. Hosp.; Tel. 579-1199.
YOUNG, Ronald G.; Ste. 2, Cinema Theatre Bldg., Swift Current, Sask.; Sask '59; Tel. PR 3-6074.
YOUNG, **S.**; Medical Arts Bldg., Regina, Sask.; 127 Angus Cres. (res); McG '40; GenSurg; Surg. Staff, Grey Nun's & Gen. Hosp's.; Surg. Cons., Sask. Cancer Comm.; Chief of Surg., D.V.A., Regina; Tel. LA 2-1651.
YOUNG, **Somerville B.**; 3437 W. 36th Ave., Vancouver, B.C.; Man '52; DiagRad.; Tel. 266-7955.
YOUNG, **William A.**; 1081 Burrard St., Vancouver, B.C.; **6451 Elm St. (res); Qns '43; FRCP (C)**; IntMed; Dir. Pulmonary Lab., St. Paul's Hosp.; Cons. Pulm. Dis., Shaughnessy Hosp.; Clin. Instr., (Med.), **U. of British Columbia**; Tel. 682-2344.
YOUNG, William E.; 123 Edward St., Toronto 2, Ont.; Apt. 706, 170 Jameson Ave. (res); Tor '57; FRCP(C); Anaes; Staff, St. Michael's Hosp.; Tel. 362-4461.
YOUNG, **William O.**; Box 2378, Kitimat, B.C.; London (Eng.) '53; M.R.C.S. (Eng.), L.R.C.P. (Lond.), D.Obst.R.C.O.G.; Staff, Kitimat Gen. Hosp.; Tel. 741.
YOUNGER, Ian; 503 Professional Bldg., Red Deer, Alta.; Alb'45; DABOt., Otol.; Active Staff, Red Deer Gen. Hosp.; Tel. 346-3683.

YOUNGHUSBAND, Omar Z.; 176 King St., St. Catharines, Ont.; 200 Queenston St. (res); **Qns** '43; F.R.C.P.(C) IntMed; Chief of Med., St. **Catharines Gen. Hosp.; Tel. MU 2-8638.**
YOUSUF, A. K.; India'62; Res., Grace Hospital, Winnipeg, Man.
YOVANOVICH, Lazar—see **JOVANOVIC, Lazar.**
YOVANOVICH, Lazar; 1210 Erie St. E., Windsor, Ont.; Rome (Italy)'47; MCGP; Tel. 253-9006.
YU, Yuk-C; 1655 W. 11th Ave., Ste. 201, Vancouver, B.C.; Man'60; Paed.
YUE, James K.; 240 McNabb St., Sault Ste. Marie, Ont.; Man'60; Active Staff, Plummer Mem. & Sault Ste. Marie Gen. Hosp's.; Tel. 254-6421.
YUE, Ka-Ping; UBC '62; Res., Vancouver Gen. Hosp., Vancouver 9, B.C.
YUE, King Y.; Freiburg (Germany); Jr. Int., Camp Hill Hosp., Halifax, N.S.
YUE, Kwok W.; 3108 Oak St., **Vancouver 9,** B.C.; China '44; Berne (Switz.) '48; Urol; Tel. RE 1-8264.
YULE, Waldo M.; Box 669, **Castlegar, B.C.;** Man '56.
YULE, Robert F.; 11927 Maplewood Ave., Haney, B.C.; Man '20.
YUN, Daniel D.; Yon-Sei **'58; Staff, Paddon Mem.** Hosp., Happy Valley, Labrador.
YUNG, Stephen W.; Fort McMurray. Alta.; Alb '62.
YURKOVICH, Anthony; 814 Cook Rd., Richmond, B.C.; UBC '55; MCGP.
YURTCU, Aydin; Ankara (Turk.) '57; Staff, Hop. Des Laurentides, L'Annonciation, P.Q.
YUSUF, Nasim; Punjab (Pakistan)'58; Jr. Int., Lakeshore Gen. Hosp., Pointe Claire, P.Q.
YUZPE, Abraham A.; Wes'64; Res., St. Joseph's Hosp., London, Ont.
YVON, Drolet C.; 401 St. S., **Cowansville, P.Q.;** 224 Bernard (res); Ott '53.
ZABOROWSKA, Janina (Bromirska); 443 Reynolds St. N., Oakville, Ont.; 234 Watson Ave. (res); St. Andrew's (Scot.)'49; MCGP; Tel. VI 4-3281.
ZACHARIAS, Abe; Man'63; Res., Royal Victoria Hosp., Montreal 2, P.Q.
ZACHARUK, Steven W.; Associated Med. Clinic, Prince Albert, Sask.; Sask '64; Tel. 763-6401.
ZACK, John J.; 2493 Commercial Dr., Vancouver 12, B.C.; 1755 W. 59th Ave. (res); Alb **'45; MCGP; Tel. TR 4-8919.**
ZACKS, Louis; 397 Reid St., Peterborough, Ont.; 477 Gordon Ave. (res); Qns '38.
ZADE, Kenneth J.; 1466 Ouellette Ave., Windsor, **Ont.; Ott'64.**
ZADRA, Modesto C.; St. Simeon, Co. Charlevoix, P.Q.; McG '29; Staff, St. Joseph's Hosp., La Malbaie; Tel. 638-2274.
ZADVORNY, Zenon G.; Tor '56; Staff, Anaes; Royal Alexandra Hosp., Edmonton, Alta.; Tel. GR 4-4341.
ZADVORNY, Zunowie G.; 2914-14th Ave., Saskatoon, Sask.; Tor '56; Anaes.
ZADYKO, Jerry; 168 Annette St., Toronto 9, Ont.; Tor '62; Tel. 762-8673.
ZAHARUK, Walter V.; 162 Cathcart St., Sault-Ste-Marie, Ont.; Wes'53; MCGP; Tel. 253-4011.
ZAHORUK, R. M.; Tor'65; Res., St. Michael's Hosp., Toronto 2, Ont.
ZAIDI, Saiyid M.; 126 King St., New Waterford, N.S.; Karachi (India) '57.
ZAITZEFF, V.; Port Arthur Clinic, Port Arthur, Ont.
ZAJAC, Andy S.; Clarke Inst. of Psy., 250 College St., Toronto 2B, Ont.; Tor'59; Psy.
ZAJCEW, Wasyl; 1329 Waller Ave., Winnipeg 19, **Man.; Berlin (Germ.) '43; Tel. GR 5-0513.**
ZALESKI, Ludmila A.; Edinburgh (Scot)'48; Staff, Sask. Training School, Moose Jaw, Sask.
ZALESKY, Christine A.; Tor'62; Res., University Hosp., Edmonton, Alta.
ZALESKI, Witold A.; Box 1300, Sask. Training School, Moose Jaw, Sask. (res); **Edinburgh** (Scot.)'46 DPM (Dublin); **Psy; Clin. Dir., Sask.** Training School; Vis. Cons., **University Hosp. &** Clin. Instr., U. of Saskatchewan, Saskatoon; Tel. 692-6491.
ZALESKY, Nicolas; 11309-130th St., Edmonton, Alta. (res); Prague (Czech.)'26; Pt.-time Staff, Charles Camsell Hosp.; Lect., Clin. Med., U. of Alberta; Tel. 455-3733.
ZALTZ, Charles; Wes'61; Res., Toronto Gen. Hosp., Toronto, Ont.
ZALTZ, Maurice M.; 221 Brant Ave., Brantford, Ont.; 3 Golfdale Rd. (res); Wes '46; Active Staff, Brantford Gen. & St. Joseph's Hosp.; Tel. 753-8666.
ZAMANSADEH, Djavad; Tabriz (Iran)'60; Staff, Hop. des Laurentides, L'Annonciation, P.Q.
ZAMORA, Emile N.; Qns '60; Psy; Staff, Ontario Hosp., Hamilton, Ont.; Tel. 385-5361.
ZAMORA, Steve P.; 72-No. 20 Hwy, Stoney **Creek, Ont.; Qns '58; MCGP; Active Staff, St. Joseph's & Hamilton Gen. Hosp's., Hamilton; Plant Phys., Cyanamid of Canada Ltd.; Tel. 664-4653.**
ZARETSKY, Ruth; Tor'64; 120 Overbrooke Pl:, Downsview, Ont.; Tor'64.
ZARFAS, A. Jean; 2412 Robin Dr., R.R. 2, Clarkson, Ont.; Qns '52.
ZARFAS, Donald E.; 2412 Robin Dr., R.R. 2, Clarkson, Ont.; Qns '52; Psy; Dir. Mental Retardation Serv., Mental Health Branch, Parliament Bldgs., Toronto.
ZARITSKY, Alexander; 5041 Park Ave., Montreal, P.Q.; 1311 Mount Royal Blvd. (res); McG **'29; Paed; Ass't. Paed., Reddy Mem. Hosp.; Tel. 277-7700.**
ZARITSKY, Michael; 7 Welland Ave., St. Catharines, Ont.; 11 Oakmount Dr. (res); Tor '40; In**dus. Phys., Thompson Products; Tel. MU 4-8555.**
ZARSADIAS, Romy G.; Santo Tomas (Philipp.) '58; Staff, Saskatchewan Hosp., Weyburn, Sask.
ZARZOUR, Ernest J.; 586 Ouellette Ave., Windsor, Ont.; Wes '59; Ophth.
ZATELNY, William; 3535 Lake Shore Blvd. W., **Toronto 14, Ont.;** Tor **'52;** Staff, St. Joseph's & Queensway Gen. Hosp's.; Tel. 259-3611.
ZAWADZKI, Jan; 96 Dewborne Ave., Toronto 10, **Ont.; Warsaw (Poland) '32; Tel. RU 3-6396.**
ZBEETNOFF, Peter; Langenburg, Sask.; Box 100 (res); Man '53.
ZBIGNIEW, G.; 11151—78th Ave., Edmonton, Alta. (res); Louvain (Belg.) '46; Radiol. (Belgium); Rad, X-Ray Dept., Edmonton Cancer Clin., 11250—84th Ave.
ZEAVIN, Samuel A.; 504 Boyd Bldg., Winnipeg, Man.; 390 Cordova St. (res); Alb '31; M.C.G.P.
ZED, Welmore M.; 75 Coburg St., St. John, N.B.; Tor '45; Tel. 693-3455.
ZEGLEN, Stanley T.; Toronto Professional Bldg., 123 Edward St., Toronto 1, Ont.; 16 Stormont Ave. (res); Tor '49; Anaes; Staff Anaes., St. Michael's Hosp.; Clin. Teach. (Anaes.), U. of Toronto; Tel. EM 8-3439.
ZEGLINSKI, Diane J.; 385 River Ave., Winnipeg 13, Man.; Man'64; Tel. 452-8142.
ZEILIG, Lauren V.; Ste. B, 1500 Royal York Rd., Weston, Ont.; Tor'62.
ZELCER, Morris; 500 College St., Toronto, Ont.; Strasbourg (France) '37; Tel. WA 1-3580.
ZELDENRUST-de-Vries, Brita G.; Southey, **Sask.; Amsterdam (Holland) '53; Tel. 163.**
ZELDIN, A. Joel; 56 Ontario St., St. Catharines, **Ont.; Tor '41; Otol.; Tel. MU 2-7269.**
ZELDIN, John; 99 Avenue Rd., Toronto 5, Ont.; 7 York Valley Cr., Willowdale (res); Tor '51; FRCS(C), OrthSurg; OrthSurg., New Mt. Sinai **& North York Branson Hosp's.;** Cons (OrthSurg.) **Humber Mem. Hosp.; Tel. WA 5-1951.**
ZELDOWICZ, Henry C.; Ste. 1112, 750 W. Broadway, Vancouver 9, B.C.; 1730 Knox Rd. (res); Rome (Italy) '31; Psy; Con. Psy. Shaughnessy D.V.A. Hosp.; Part-time Lectr. School of Social **Work & Clin. Assoc. Prof. Psy., U. of British Columbia Tel. 879-5165.**
ZELDOWICZ, Ludmila R.; Ste. 1112, 750 W. Broadway, Vancouver 9, B.C.; 1730 Knox Rd. (res); **Warsaw (Poland) '30; Neur;** Staff, Vancouver Gen. Hosp., **Lectr. in NeuroAnat. & Clin. Neur., U. of British Columbia; Tel. TR 2-5311.**

ZELITT, Irving J.; 1156 Brimley Rd., Scarborough, Ont.; Tor'58; MCGP; Active Staff, Scarborough Gen. Hosp.; Court. Staff, Toronto East Gen. Hosp.; Tel. 759-4241.

ZEMAN, Helen B.—see AIKENS, Helen B.

ZEMEL, R.; Tor '58; FRCS(C), GenSurg; Staff, Royal Victoria Hosp., Montreal, P.Q.

ZENDER, Robert J.; The Medical Centre, Stettler, Alta.; Alb '40; Staff, Stettler Municipal Hosp.; Dist. Coroner; Tel. 742-3441.

ZENNER, Lotar; 166 Main St., St. Catharines, Ont.; 398 Martindale Rd. (res); Free U. (Berlin, Germ.) '55.

ZEPS, Genovefa N.; 21 Whittaker Cr., Willowdale, Ont. '57.

ZERNY, John Cedric; Med. Arts Bldg., 121 Wellington St. W., Barrie Ont.; Guy's Hosp. (London) '43; MRCP; M.D. (London); IntMed; Cons. Staff, Royal Victoria Hosp.; Court. Cons. Staff, Midland, Penetanguishene & Orillia Soldier's Mem. Hosp's.

ZETTER, Gerald R.; 8225-105th St., Edmonton, Alta.; 9834-78th Ave. (res); Alb '59; Tel. 433-1402.

ZEVILLE, Matthias; Health Reg. No. 3, 5 Railway Ave., Weyburn, Sask.; Beirut (Lebanon)'45; DPH; DIH.

ZIEGENBEIN, Margaret; (see Boeske, Margaret).

ZIEGLER, Alfred; 76 Roncesvalles Ave., Toronto, Ont.; Tel. LE 2-3054.

ZIEGLER, David O., Sg/Lt.; Wes '63; Staff, National Defence Med. Centre, Ottawa, Ont.

ZIEGLER, M. Leopold; 4889 Mackenzie, Montreal **26. P.Q.; Munich (Germ.) '42; Tel. RE 3-1670.**

ZIEGLER, Wilfred H.; Youbou, B.C.; UBC '60; Tel. 321. Abroad.

ZIELINSKI, Lech K.; P.O. Box 13, Kensington, P.E.I.; Beirut (Lebanon) '45; MCGP; Active Staff, Prince County Hosp., Summerside; Tel. 267-3422.

ZIELONKA, Bronislaw G.; 7 Woodland Hgts. Toronto 3, Ont.; Marburg (Germ.) '50; Anaes; Staff, St. Joseph's Hosp.; Tel. LE 4-9531.

ZIELONKO, Walter; 68 Pleasant Rd., Guelph, Ont.; Wes '57; Psy; Staff, Homewood San.; Tel. 824-6285.

ZIKMAN, Jerrold; McG'65; Res., Jewish General Hosp., Montreal 26, P.Q.

ZILBERMAN, Joseph; 590 College St., Toronto 4, Ont.; '52; Tel. 531-7753.

ZIMBERG, Leslie L.; Ste. 22, 1944 Main St., Winnipeg, Man. (res); Man '57.

ZIMICH, Leonard; Ste. 203, 625-5th St., New **Westminster, B.C.; 1619 London St. (res); Trinity College (Dublin, Ire.) '55; Tel. LA 1-2515.**

ZIMMERMAN, B.; Tor'65; Res., Toronto General Hosp., Toronto 2, Ont.

ZIMMERMAN, Elfriede (See Schuh).

ZIMMERMAN, Harold W.; 4027 E. Hastings N., **Burnaby, B.C.; UBC '55; Tel. CY 9-2677.**

ZIMMERMAN, Ulrich A.; 1541 W. Broadway, Vancouver 9, B.C.; UBC '61; Tel. RE 3-6343.

ZINCK, Russell C.; Lincoln St., Lunenburg, N.S.; **McG '24; Staff, Dept. of Health & Welfare; Tel. 634-2221.**

ZINGG, Walter; 555 University Ave., Toronto 2, Ont.; 92 Highbourne Rd., Tor. 7 (res); Zurich (Switz.) '48; M.Sc. (Med.); FACS; FRCS(C); GenSurg; Research Assoc., Hosp. for Sick Children; Assoc. Scientist, Research Inst.; Cons., Crippled Children's Centre; Ass't. Prof. Surg., U. of Toronto; Tel. 366-7242, Loc. 2161.

ZINKANN, Russell W. J.; 227 King St. S., Waterloo, Ont.; 737 King St. W., Kitchener (res); Tor '33; C. Life Ins. Med.; Vice-Pres. & Med. Dir., Mutual Life Assur. Co. of Canada; Tel. SH 5-6181.

ZIPURSKY, Alvin; 536 Niagara St., Winnipeg 9, Man. (res); Man '53; F.R.C.P.(C), Paed; Staff, **Children's Hosp. & U. of Manitoba; Ass't Prof. (Paed.), U. of Man.; Tel. SP 5-8311.**

ZISKROUT, Isaac; 2528 Montrose Ave., Abbotsford, B.C.; 2303 McKenzie Rd. (res); Tor '45; M.C.G.P.; Staff, Matsqui-Sumas-Abbotsford Gen. Hosp., Tel. 853-1622.

ZITER, Michael J.; 3945 Tecumseh St. E., Windsor, Ont.; 2346 Rossini St. (res); France '47; AMCGP; Tel. 945-8111.

ZITSOW, Bernard S.; Man'64; Res., Toronto Western Hosp., Toronto 2B, Ont.

ZIVOT, B. A.; Sardis, B.C.; Vedder Rd. (res); Man '23.

ZNAJDA, James P.; 584 Jones Ave., Toronto 6, Ont.; 81 Mallory Cr., Apt. 4. (res); Qns '62; Tel. 461-9211. Abroad.

ZNAMIROWSKI, Roman; 391 Holland Ave., Ottawa, Ont. (res); National U. (Dublin, Ire.) '53; Assoc. Prof. (Bact.), U. of Ottawa; Tel. CE 5-6751.

ZOERB, Dale L.; Sask '60; Res., University Hosp., Saskatoon, Sask.

ZOLTAN, G.; 742 Stuart Ave., Outremont, Mtl., **P.Q.; Geneva (Switz.); Dermat (Hung.); Med.** Adviser., Poulenc Ltd.; Tel. DU 1-3961.

ZOWNIR, Jerry R.; 584 Jones Ave., Toronto 6, Ont.; Wes '64.

ZSOTER, Thomas T.; Budapest (Hung.)'47; FACP; FRCP(C), IntMed; Staff, Toronto Western Hosp., Toronto 2B, Ont.; Assoc. Prof. Pharm., U. of Toronto.

ZUARDI, P.; Buenos Aires (Argentina) '55; Staff, Hop. St-Charles, Joliette, P.Q.

ZUCK, Victor; 363 Markham Rd., Richmond Hill, Ont.; Birmingham (Eng.) '49; D.Obst; DRCOG; MCGP; Tel. TU 4-1008.

ZUCKER, Bernard B.; 2 St. Clair Ave. W., Toronto, Ont.; Tor'57; FRCS(C), Ophth; Att'd. Staff, Toronto Western & Scarborough Gen. Hosp's.; Research Assoc., Banting Inst.; Clin. Teach., U. of Toronto; Tel. 927-2023.

ZUKER, Gilbert A.; 20 Wynford Dr., Don Mills, Ont.; Tor'59; FRCS(C), GenSurg.; Court. Staff, Central Hosp.; Tel. 429-1283.

ZUCKERMAN, Arthur D.; 64-66 Vaughan Rd., Toronto 10, Ont.; Apt. 201, 740 Eglinton (res); Qns '40; MCGP; Tel. 535-1143.

ZUFELT, William E.; 11 Coldwater St., Orillia, Ont.; 51 Colborne St. E. (res); Qns'57; AMCGP; Tel. 325-2271.

ZURITSKY, Michael; 7 Welland Ave., St. Catharines, Ont.; 11 Oakmount Dr. (res); Tor '40.

ZUROWSKA, M. Christina A.; 134 Larch St., Sudbury, Ont.; Lwow (Poland) '30; M.C.G.P.; Tel. 674-1107.

ZWETTER, Gerald R.; Alb '59; Jr. Int'n., Edmonton Gen. Hosp., Edmonton, Alta.

ZYLBERBERG, Bernard; 316 St. Clair Ave W., Toronto 7, Ont.; Witwatersrand (S. Africa) '54; Tel. 922-6012.

ZYLBERSZAC, Bernard; 6 Chomedy Medical Centre, 4375 Notre Dame Blvd., Chomedy, P.Q.; Brussels (Belgium) '57.

ZYWINA, Paul R.; Qns'62; Res., Hosp. for Mental Diseases, Selkirk, Man.

section 2

CANADIAN MEDICAL DIRECTORY 1967

PHYSICIANS BY TOWN

Alberta

ACME
(328)
Fowler, W. G.

ATHABASCA
(1,492)
Brown, Josephine M.
Cousineau, C. R.
Kiltz, H.
Mackey, L. W.
Wright, E. K.

BANFF
(3,429)
Alexander, R. I.
Costigan, P. G.
Fleming, R. W.
MacQuarrie, A. W.
Sood, B. K.
Tittemore, D. L.
Wilson, I., GenSurg

BARRHEAD
(2,287)
Giles, J. P.
Godberson, C. V.
Horner, H. M.
Keir, W. R.
McIntosh, G. A.
McIntosh, Mary G.
Newell, P. J.
Whittaker, A. T., GenSurg

BASHAW
(612)
Gorman, B. J.
Worsley, R. T.

BASSANO
(813)
Faminow, W. S.
Shydlowski, W.

BEAVERLODGE
(893)
Young, W. A.

BEISEKER
(353)
Verbeek, E. O. M.

BENTLEY
(588)
Ardouin, G. J.

BERWYN
(342)
Wynne, F

BLACK DIAMOND
(1,042)
Lander, D.

BLAIRMORE
(1,978)
Aiello, E.
Amundsen, L. R.
Russell, W. F.

BONNYVILLE
(1,736)
Brosseau, B. E.
Bugeaud, J. P.
Chan, N. Y.
Cheng, Patricia

BOW ISLAND
(1,122)
Carr, S. F.
Nikaido, H.
Woolner, W. S.

BOYLE
(342)
Keys, J. H.

BRETON
(428)
Bhavnani, M. J.
Scott, W.

BROOKS
(2,827)
Bond, A. F., GenSurg

Hilborn, D. J.
Kasdorf, W.
MacLeod, B. M.
Medway, J. G.
Papadopoulas, D. F., IntMed
Reynar, J. A.

CALGARY
(323,000)
Aiken, J. B. IntMed
Aikenhead, J. F., Ophth, Otol.
Allan, L. C.
Anderson, J. O. Anaes
Asp, D. M., Path.
Atkins, E. L., IntMed
Atkinson, H. H.
Attariwala, G. S., Ophth
Austin, M.
Baker, J. B., DiagRad
Banks, B. W.
Barlass, J. L., NeurSurg.
Barnes, Priscilla
Barrett, K. A.
Bazant, F. J., OrthSurg
Beauchemin, L. O.
Belkin, A., IntMed
Bellamy, J. G.
Bercov, H. A.
Berry, R. J. OphthOtol.
Bertrand, N. R., ObstGyn
Binstead, A. H.
Birrell, J. D., Paed
Bishop, D. S.
Black, H. H.
Blair, D. C., PhysMed & Rehab
Blake, Roy M., Paed.
Blenkinsop, Jean
Blenkinsop, P. R., Otol
Bliek, A. J.
Blumes, A. B.
Boyar, W. T., GenSurg
Boyd, H. N. J., Path.
Boyd, R. P.
Brady, H.
Brayton, M J.
Brodie, I. H.
Brody, H., ObstGyn
Brown, H. M.
Brown, J. S., Otol
Brown, P S., Aanes.
Buchanan, D. R., ObstGyn
Buie, W. J., GenSurg
Bullard, J.
Cadger, D., IntMed
Calvert, K. G.
Cameron, J. A. M., GenSurg
Campbell, J. D., Otol
Carnat, M., Psy
Carpenter, W. B.
Carscallen, W. F.
Cassidy, D. M.
Cassin, S. B.
Chablani, G. P., Psy.
Chandler, C. R.
Chipperfield, W. G. GenSurg.
Chisholm, W. M.
Chuelos, N., Psy.
Clapperton, J. A.
Clapperton, Joyce C.
Cody, A. C., Paed
Cody, D. B.
Cohen, P. W.
Colwell, M. C., Paed
Conway, P. F., Psy.
Corbet, R. C. B., Paed
Corcoran, T. V.
Corley, J. B.
Costantini, W. A., OrthSurg
Cottrell, J. D., IntMed.
Craig, J. M., ObstGyn
Craig, J. S.
Cranston, T. R.
Crawford, J. S., Anaes.
Crichton, Erica P., Path.
Croft, J. H., Anaes
Crooks, W. L., OrthSurg
Crosbie, P. D.
Crossfield, P. O., IntMed
Cruse, P. J. E., GenSurg
Culver, R. W., Ophth,Otol
Currie, B. M.
Dahl, R. G.
Dale, C. C., Otol.
Davis, M. L.
Dawson, J. W., IntMed
De Haas, W. G., OrthSurg.
Denton, Daphne F., Anaes.
Diamond, E. G., Anaes
Dingle, W. T. ObstGyn, D & TRad
Dixon, A. A. DermSyph
Dixon, J. H. GenSurg
Dobbs, E. H. Anaes
Dobry, J. J.
Dodd, Norma
Donald, W. A. GenSurg
Donaldson, H. V., Anaes
Douglas, R. P. Anaes
Dowling, H. E. Ophth,Otol
Duff, Anne M.
Duff, F. GenSurg
Duffin, J. D. PathBact
Duggan, H. E., D&TRad
Duncan, A. G. DermSyph
Dunlop, I. H.
Durcan, D. J.
Dwan, D.
Dyke, J. L.
Edwards, G. E., OrthSurg
Elliott, Kathleen DiagRad
Etele, J.
Etzkorn, K. R.
Ewert, G. W.
Fair, J. W., Psy
Fairbairn, L. M. GenSurg
Fairbanks, C. J., OrthSurg
Farnalls, R. B., Psy
Fayerman, J., Otol
Ferguson, T. B., DiagRad.
Ferrier, R. A.
Fish, E. L.
Fisher, B. K., Derm
Florendine, D. G. D & TRad
Follett, A. V.
Forsyth, C. W.
Forward, J. D.
Foster, N. E. Anaes
Foster, P.
Fowlow, S. Beatrice
Fowlow, W. A., PlasSurg
Francis, J. R. GenSurg
Freigang, B., Paed
Fyvie, J. N.
Galbraith, F. O., GenSurg
Gallie, H. R. GenSurg
Gardner, J. S. GenSurg
Gavelin, G. E., PlasSurg.
Gee, E. M.
Gelfand, A. S.
Gibson, H. E. GenSurg
Gimbel, H. V., Ophth
Gimbel, H. W.
Gogan, I.
Gonsalves, C. G.
Goor, J. H. V.
Gorrell, D. S. Ophth,Otol
Graham-Brown, W. D.
Grainger, R. S.
Gregory, B. P.
Gretton, A. H.
Grinstein, M.
Gunn, I. M.
Gurevitch, R.
Hamman, H. A.
Hankins, G. W., GenSurg
Hanslip, A. R.
Hantho, J. A.
Hardy, G. E.
Harris, K. S., DiagRad
Harris, P. W.
Hatfield, C. B. IntMed
Hatfield, R. E., IntMed.
Hayes, A. C.

* Population not separately available.

Heimbach, M., Paed
Hemstock, J. R., Anaes
Hepburn, A. L. NeurSurg
Herman, I. H.
Herring, S. F.
Heuchert, C. H.
Higgin, J. R., ObstGyn.
Higgins, G. K. IntMed
Calgary (Cont'd.)
Hilderman, F. A.
Hill, C. G. IntMed
Hill, F. W. Anaes
Hill, G. H.
Hill, G. R.
Hill, W. F.
Hofmann, R.
Holloway, S. H.
Horne, M. M., Psy
Horne, N. C.
Howard, D. L. IntMed
Howarth, B. G.
Hudson, A., Path
Humphrey, Barbara M.
Hunter, J. M., OrthSurg
Ingram, W. E. GenSurg
Ishii, M., Anaes
Ivie, L. G.
Jackson, N. J., GenSurg.
Jenkins, Eunice K.
Jennings, H. N., IntMed.
Johns, W. S., Anaes.
Johnson, E. A., Ophth
Johnston, J. C.
Junkin, E. R. GenSurg
Kavanagh, A. J., Paed
Keil, A. M., Anaes
Keith, R. G.
Kenmuir-Evans, A. J.
Kereszturi, J., DiagRad.
Ketcheson, R. B., ObstGyn
Keys, D. N.
Kindrachuk, W. H. OrthSurg
Kirkebeck, E. Anaes
Kohut, C. D.
Kohut, D. R.
Kwong, Min K.
Laing, W. V.
Lam, A. K.
Lawrence, J. H. Anaes
Leblanc, L. C.
Letts, G. D. J., Psy.
Leweke, H. S.
Lindsay, D. S. Psy
Livingstone, E. S.
Logan, L. IntMed
Loginotto, M. B., Ophth, Otol.
Lorenz, M. A.
Loughrey, T. L.
Love, J. W.
Lundy, F. E. Anaes
Lynch, R. F. Psy.
MacDonald, M. H., GenSurg ThorSurg.
MacDonald, R.
MacDonald, W. J. ThorSurg
MacGougan, M. K. Ophth,Otol
MacGregor, D. J. ObstGyn
MacKinnon, A. H.
MacKinnon, N. D.
MacQueen, D. G. GenSurg
Magner, R. G.
Maguire, Nancy S.
Mahon, J. D. GenSurg
Malloy, L. P., ObstGyn
Main-Son-Hong, C. T., Neur.
Maquera, A. G.
Marshall, G.
Mason, V. T. ObstGyn
Mathieson, W. A., DiagRad
Maxwell, G. A.
Mazzolani, L.
McAllister, J. E. ObstGyn
McArthur, M. J.
McCowan, C. W.
McCulloch, C. F. GenSurg
McEwen, D. C., IntMed
McEwen, H., IntMed
McFadden, K. A.
McGarry, G. G.
McGeachy, W. G.
McKenna, P. B., DiagRad.
McKercher, L. A.
McKinley, W. H.
McLatchie, L. D. PathBact
McLean, R. I., IntMed
McLean, W. N. A.
McLeod, S. H.
McManus, F. R. GenSurg
McNeil, D. L. IntMed
McQuitty, G. D.
Melgrave, A. P. Anaes
Melling, T.
Melvie, O. A.
Mercer, J. E., GenSurg
Miller, G. E. ThorSurg
Miller, M. S. Ophth,Otol
Mills, J. G.
Milne, J. D.
Milner, Macey
Mitchell, L. I. Urol
Mitchell, M. D.
Moore, M. B., Psy
Mores, G. P. Anaes
Morgan, H. V. GenSurg
Morgan, J. C. IntMed
Moriarty, J. E.
Morrish, H. F., D & T Rad.
Morrison, A. E.
Motta, J. A., ObstGyn
Mudry, W. J.
Muldoon, A. D. IntMed
Mullen, L. M. IntMed (TB)
Mulloy, W. H.
Murphy, B. J. DiagRad
Murphy, V. J., OrthSurg
Mydland, W. E. GenSurg
Nation, E. W. IntMed
Naylor, G. A.
Newell, J. E., Path
Newlands, W. J.
Nip, Y. C., Anaes
Nixon, J. R. GenSurg
Noakes, J. A. Urol
Norys, W. J., Psy.
Oborne, H. G. Obst
O'Keefe, J. M.
Oko, J. K.
O'Neil, A. A. Anaes.
O'Neil, Agnes, PH
Ostry, E. I. ObstGyn
O'Sullivan, J. G. ObstGyn
Parker, D., Ophth
Pearce, K. I., Psy.
Pearson, Margaret G. Paed
Peintner, I.
Phin, J. M.
Pillow, W. M., Anaes.
Porter, J. J., D & TRad
Potts, D. A.
Pow, R. E. GenSurg
Price, H. W. Paed
Price, R D.
Prieur, G. O. Paed
Proudfoot, W. A.
Purkin, N.
Radford, C. J., Ophth.
Ramsay, D. W. GenSurg
Ramsay, F. W.
Reich, C. J., IntMed
Reynolds, H A. Path.
Richardson, D. Shirley
Richardson, J. W. GenSurg
Richardson, S. R.
Richardson, T. A. OrthSurg
Ridge, J. M., Path.
Robb, W. A. GenSurg, Urol
Robbins, G. E. Ophth
Robertson, Maryon
Robertson, R. B. Anaes
Robutka, L. P.
Ross, J. B.
Rothwell, A.
Rothwell, W. O. GenSurg
Rowat, F. L.
Ryder, J.
Ryll, H.
Sartorelli, A.
Saunders, T. C.
Scarlett, E. P. IntMed
Scott, G. W., GenSurg
Secter, M. B. IntMed
Selby, R. C.
Settle, J. R.
Shafto, C. M. Ophth
Shalom, M. S.
Shewchuk, H W. IntMed.
Shore, A. E. Ophth,Otol
Shute, D.
Sidebotham, R. E.
Simon, J. B.
Skinner, B. S., Anaes.
Slowick, O. J., Psy.
Smith, E. R. TherRad
Smith, L W.
Soby, H. W.
Spackman, L. F. Urol
Spankie, W. E.
Stackpoole-Ryding, F.
Stanford, G. B.
Steed, B. L.
Stenicka, F. J.
Stevenson, I. C. M. Anaes
Stewart, W. D. Otol IntMed
Stoicoiu, T., GenSurg
Sturdy, D. D. OrthSurg
Sutherland, R. L., Ophth
Swanson, G. E., DiagRad.
Swanson, H. A. DiagRad
Swartzlander, F. C.
Symington, K. D. DiagRad
Tanasichuk, M. A.
Tanner, W. R., Ophth
Tarrant, M.
Taylor, C. N.
Taylor, C. W. NeurSurg
Thiessen, A. E.
Thomas, G. S. ObstGyn
Thompson, J. A.
Thomson, H. S. PlasSurg
Thorson, S. B.
Todd, J. K.
Townsend, R. G. OrthSurg
Travelli, R.
Trueman, E. Tess ObstGyn
Truscott, D. R., Paed
Tuttle, M. J. IntMed
Tuszewski, Marian, GenSurg
Van Goor, J. H.
Veenhuizen, P. A.
Vernon, M. A.
Vogel, M. J.
Waddell, J. M. IntMed
Wade, J. C. IntMed
Wagg, H. O. ObstGyn
Walker, W. T.
Wallace, D. S. IntMed.
Wallat, G. E., Anaes.
Walsh, A. C. OrthSurg
Watkins, Gillian
Wayne, D. L. DiagRad
Weisz, S.
Westbury, R. C.
Wheelwright, D. A.
Wight, N. J.
Wilcock, G. F.
Williams, J. A.
Williams, R. G. Jr. GenSurg
Williams, R. T., Anaes.
Wilson, A. E. ObstGyn
Wintemute, R. W. ObstGyn
Wolfman, Jean R.
Wooldridge, D. B.
Worrall, H. C.
Worrall, Kathleen M.
Wright, A. S.
Wright, C. B.
Yaholnitsky, S.
Yegorov, Alexandra

* Population not separately available.

Calgary (Cont'd.)
Young, J. K., GenSurg
Younger, L. I. Otol

CAMROSE
(6,939)
Andrucson, V. M.
Baker, D. B. IntMed
MacInnis, F. H. IntMed
MacQuarrie, Jeannette
MacQuarrie, K. T.
Murray, D. J., ObstGyn
Peterson, A. D.
Reikie, R. D.
Siwak, W. J., GenSurg
Smith, C. H.
Smith, F. M.
Weir, J. R., IntMed
Young, J. H.

CANMORE,
(1,736)
Miltins, A.
Waldron, B. A.

CARDSTON
(2,803)
Larson, B. J., GenSurg
Spackman, F. M.
Spackman, R. R. Anaes
VanOrman, A. G.

CARMANGAY
(295)
Hwozdecki, R. M.

CARSTAIRS
(669)
O'Hea, T. P.
Prowse, W. C.

CASTOR
(1,019)
Foster, G. E.
Kaye, P. P.
Miller, M. K.

CEREAL
(190)
Baker, E. J.

CLARESHOLM
(2,149)
Cornish, S. J.
Hodgson, W. M.
Lloyd, J. E.
Rose, G. B.

COALDALE
(2,589)
Oshiro, J.
Palmer, G. R.
Wiens, H. A.

COLD LAKE
(1,307)
Allan, G. G., ObstGyn
Dunfield, J. C., GenSurg
Hodgkinson, J. R.
McLean, Janette
Savage, E. Margaret
Wood, G. A.

COLEMAN
(1,713)
Krebes, A. J.
Martinez, V.

CONSORT
(552)
Knight, C. P.

CORONATION
(864)
Anglin, J. V., GenSurg
O'Brien, J. C.

DAYSLAND
(541)
Stanners, J.

DEVON
(1,412)
Cherry, R. R.

DIDSBURY
(1,252)
Casey, R. J.
MacDonald, R. L.

Miller, Ian H.
Read, P. R.

DRAYTON VALLEY
(3,854)
Eustace, T. H.
Lewis, D. J.
Maclure, H. L.
Waugh, I. G.

DRUMHELLER
(2,931)
Aiello, A. L. Anaes
Julson, K. I.
Nahornick, B. A.
Thomson, A.
Walker, A. J. GenSurg
Wilson, G. L.
Wright, T. A.

EAST COULEE
(1,003)
Walton, R. S.

ECKVILLE
(578)
Swain, R. C.

EDMONTON
(385,000)
Aaron, T. H. IntMed
Adamson, D. N.
Adamson, M. C.
Albert, M., OrthSurg
Alexander, N. E. GenSurg
Allard, C. A. GenSurg
Allen, P.B., NeurSurg
Allin, E. S. GenSurg
Allin, G. E., GenSurg.
Alton, J. M., GenSurg, PlasSurg
Amerongen, L. J.
Anderson, D. L., Ophth.Otol.
Anderson, W. S. GenSurg
Ansari, A. H., ObstGyn.
Anselmo, J. E., GenSurg
Archibald, W. S. GenSurg
Armstrong, F. B.
Armstrong, H. B. Paed
Armstrong, W. S., Otol
Ashford, D. R., Path.
Ayers, T. N., GenSurg.
Aylesworth, J. A.
Ayotte, L. G., ObstGyn.
Babiuk, M. E.
Babiuk, M. J.
Bacon, H. M., Psy.
Bailey, R. A. Neursurg.
Bain, G. O. Path
Baker, K., ObstGyn.
Baker, Kathleen
Bako, E. E.
Ball, G. H.
Ball, N. J.
Barker, H. M., Psy
Barr, J. S. ObstGyn
Barton, M. C.
Beauchamp, L. E. Paed
Beck, R P., ObstGyn
Begg, H. N. C.
Bell, D. M. IntMed
Bell, D. M. ObstGyn
Bell, G. I. IntMed
Bell, H., Path
Bell, R. E.
Berner, C. A.
Bertram, L. I.
Besney, M., GenSurg.
Bissel, E. W. PlasSurg
Black, W. R., IntMed
Blunden, A. G.
Bobey, W.
Bode, O. R., IntMed
Boeske, Margaret
Boileau, G. R., GenSurg
Boissoneault, E.
Bondar, G. F., GenSurg
Boulanger, M. J.
Bouwman, H. W., OrthSurg

Bow, M. R. PH
Bowen, P., IntMed
Bowman, G. R.
Boyd, J. A. ObstGyn
Boyd, M. E., ObstGyn.
Boyd, T. A. Ophth
Bradley, J. E.
Bramley-Moore, W.
Brand, M. H.
Brett, H. B.
Brindle, M. J., DiagRad.
Brinsmead, A. N.
Broome, T. P., IntMed
Brown, G. D. IntMed
Brown, Helen, IntMed
Brown, I. S.
Brown, L. B. ObstGyn
Bryk, W. S.
Buchanan, D. I.
Buchanan, D. M., ObstGyn
Buchanan, I.
Bugis, J. ObstGyn
Bulajic, B.
Buoninsegni, F.
Burckak, E. C.
Burkhardt, Lore
Bursewiez, Anne M.
Bury, R. J. GenSurg
Bustillo, J. L., Ophth.Otol.
Butler, G. C.
Butler, K. F.
Bykowski, O. M.
Cairns, A. IntMed
Calarsu, F. R.
Calder, J. Paed
Callaghan, J. C. GenSurg. ThorSurg
Cameron, D. F. Anaes
Cameron, G. W. OrthSurg
Campbell, V. J. IntMed
Cantor, M. M. IntMed
Carson, G. D. Psy
Catterall, S., Psy.
Chappelle, G. F.
Charlesworth, G. S. Obst
Chen, R., Paed
Chepeha, N.
Chrzanowski, Z. P.
Clare, R. M. D & TRad
Clarke, K. A., Otol.
Clarke, K S., PlasSurg.
Clarke, Margaret E.
Clarke, T. R. ObstGyn
Clein, L. J., NeurSurg.
Cochrane, W. H., Anaes
Coglon, R. B., IntMed
Collip, J. B.
Colter, D. R., OrthSurg
Conradi, G. Paed
Conroy, F. D. Urol
Cookson, F. B.
Cormack, G. N.
Cornish, D. R.
Corrigan, C.
Costopoulos, L. B., DiagRad.
Couillard, T. J.
Coulter, H. B., Anaes.
Couves, C.M. GenSurg, ThosSurg,Cardiovasc.)
Cowan, Lorraine
Cranz, H. G. A., DiagRad.
Creurer, M.
Crockford, P. M., IntMed
Crooks, H. J., ObstGyn
Culver, R. L.
Cuthbertson, A. N. GenSurg
Dafoe, Charlotte S., Anaes
Dafoe, C. S. ThorSurg
D'Agata, V. P.
Daly, P. H.
Daly, T. Ophth
Daniels, R. K.
Davey, P. W. Path
Davis, R. G. GenSurg
Davison, G. R. IntMed
Day, F. G. OrthSurg

* Population not separately available.

Edmonton (Cont'd.)
Day, J. C., ObstGyn.
Day, R. A., ObstGyn
De Coutere, I. A., Psy.
de Jongh, H .J., Anaes.
Devine, S. W., ObstGyn
Dick, D. A., TherRad.
Diduch, L. T., Otol
Dimock, H. C.
Dobson, C. R. GenSurg
Dolgoy, M.
Donald, E. F. IntMed
Dorsey, F. R. J. ObstGyn
Dougall, R. H. IntMed
Douglas, R. G.
Downs, W. J. IntMed (TB)
Drummond, G., Anaes.
Duggan, J. W. Ophth
du Heaume, B.
Duncan, G. B.
Duncan, N. F. Paed
Duncan, R. A.
Dushinski, L. M.
Dvorkin, J. IntMed
Dyer, T. M.
Eadie, W. W.
Easton, D. R. Psy
Easton, Jessie K., PhysMed & Rehab
Eddy, G. E., Paed
Edwards, A. M. IntMed
Edwards, F. J., Psy.
Eid, T. C. Urol
Eidem, R. N., IntMed.
Elliott, J. F. IntMed
Ellis, C. N., Urol.
Elton, C. D. Anaes
Emery, M. A., OrthSurg
England, H. H. Anaes
Eritsland, O. B.
Evans, B. V., DiagRad
Falconer, W. L.
Farley, J. F. Anaes
Farrehi, C., IntMed
Fawcett, D. M.
Fehn, F.
Ferguson, J. H.
Ferguson, W. F. ObstGyn
Fink, A.
Fitzgerald, M.
Fivie, J. N.
Fletcher, C. M. Anaes
Fong, A.
Fowler, J. R. T. PhysMed & Rehab.
Foy, E. Ophth
Francis, G. T.
Francis, R. R. Urol
Fraser, R. S. IntMed
Frew, W. D. ObstGyn
Freidman, M. H., GenSurg
Friedman, M. W.
Fuerst, H. J., Psy
Gain, E. A. Anaes
Gal, S. I.
Galanti A, DiagRad.
Galbraith, J. D., IntMed(TB)
Gander, T. A. Paed
Gans, L. J. ObstGyn
Garcia, E.
Gauk, E. W. Paed.
Geddes-Smith, Elizabeth M.
Gendron, J. E., GenSurg
Genser, A., ObstGyn
Gibbs, J. T., Psy.
Gilbert, J. A. L. IntMed
Gilchrist, D. A., Anaes
Gillespie, J. C.
Gillison, N. B.
Giroux, L. L. Urol
Glasgow, R. R.
Gobius, R. J., Paed
Gold, Marjorie E.
Goldsand, G., IntMed.
Goodwin, J. W., ObstGyn
Gorman, A. A.
Gort, J., OrthSurg
Goulden, Leila, DiagRad.
Graham, W. H. Anaes
Gray, G. C. OrthSurg
Grebneff, G. A., IntMed.
Greenberg, C.
Greenhill, B.J., OrthSurg
Greenhill, G. E.
Greenhill, S. E. IntMed
Greenidge, A. H.
Gregory, L. J.
Grisdale, L. C. Paed
Grobman, J. S.
Gross, R. C., Ophth.
Grover, S. D., GenSurg.
Guild, J. Psy
Gulley, J. L. OrthSurg
Gutter, Z. D & TRad
Hackett, R. M. GenSurg
Hafso, Alice K.
Hagen, E. Odette
Hagen, J. M., Anaes.
Haley, F. C., Anaes
Halinen, Maire M.
Hall, A. S.
Hall, W. F. M. GenSurg
Hallgren, R. A.
Hamilton, K. A., IntMed, Psy
Hamilton, Rosemary
Hamilton, T. R.
Hanley, E. J.
Hanson, S. PathBact
Hardin, I. DermSyph
Hardy, A. W. GenSurg
Hassard, D. T., OphthOtol.
Haynes, E. R.
Haynes, H. G.
Hebb, H. D. GenSurg
Hellon, C. P., Psy.
Henderson, I. N.
Henderson, R. S. OrthSurg
Hendin, I. D., DiagRad
Hepburn, H. H. GenSurg, NeurSurg.
Herbert, F. A., IntMed
Hergott, C. W.
Hill, Elizabeth
Hill, J. R., Path
Hitchin, E., GenSurg
Hnatko, S. I., Bact
Hoar, Z. Anaes
Hoe, G. K. Anaes
Hohn, E. O.
Holmes, C. E., D & T Rad.
Holubitsky, N. D.
Hooper, J. B.
Hopkyns, J. C. IntMed
Horner, R. H. ObstGyn
Hraber, S.
Hsu, Lillian C. DiagRad.
Huckell, J. R. OrthSurg
Huckell, R. G. OrthSurg
Husel, D. H. ObstGyn
Hutchison, H. M.
Hutchison, J. H.
Hutton, M. M. ObstGyn
Hutton, W. K.
Hwang, Frances L.
Hyde, H. A. GenSurg
Hyndman, C. F. DiagRad
Irving, D. W. IntMed.
Irwin, J.
Isaacsen, Ruth
Iwanec, W.
Jackson, F. I., PH, DiagRad.
Jackson, F. L.
Jacobs, H., Neurol
Jamieson, R. C.
Jampolsky, N. A., DermSyph
Jesperson, R. E. GenSurg
Jimenez, J., PhysMed&Rehab
Johnson, Diane W.
Johnston, D. C., OrthSurg
Johnston, E. E., ObstGyn.
Johnston, R. J., GenSurg
Jordan, F. B. Psy
Judge, D. L. IntMed
Justik, J. C.
Kasper, T. A., Path
Kato, J. G.
Kaufman, V. S.
Kelemen, A.
Kelly, D.
Kelly, J. R.
Kennedy, G. G. GenSurg
Kennedy, R. J.
Keogh, R. K., DiagRad
Keohane, J. T., Otol
Khoo, E. E. C., IntMed.
Kidd, E. G. IntMed
Kimmitt, P. J. Paed
Klajn, R. P.
Kling, S. GenSurg
Kornell, S., IntMed
Kowalewski, K. IntMed
Koziak, P. H. Ophth
Kredenster, B., ObstGyn.
Kushniruk, M.
Kyle, W. D. Anaes
LaKey, W. H., Urol
Laskin, M. M. GenSurg
Laverman, J. M.
Lavallee, Marguerite O.
Law, F. F.
Leacock, A. M., Anaes.
Leber, S. M.
Leduc, Ishbel
Lee, S. J., IntMed
Leeder, J. R. ObstGyn
Leeson, T. S.
Lefebvre, C. E.
Legerski, R.
Leitch, D. B. Paed
Lekisch, E.
Le Riche, Jean
Leriche, L. H.
Letts, H. W. Path.
Letts, T. B.
Letwin, E., GenSurg
Lewis, M. J., Anaes.
Liesemer, E. J.
Links, H. GenSurg
Lipinski, J. J.
Liston, W. P. DiagRad
Little, A. S. IntMed
Little, G. M. PH
Lloyd, H. A.
Lobsinger, A. J. GenSurg
Loewen, G.
Long, G. S.
Louie, W. L.
Lunn, D. F. Anaes
Lynch, S. H.
Lynne-Davies, Patricia, IntMed.
MacAuley, M. G. Ophth
MacBeth, R. A. GenSurg
MacDonald, L. V. NeurSurg
MacDonald, W. A.
MacGregor, J. W. Path
Mackay, J. A., Anaes
MacKenzie, W. C. GenSurg
MacLean, W. A. GenSurg
MacLennan, R. A. ObstGyn
MacPhail, H. R. Anaes
MacPhee, D. M.
MacPherson, A. D. Psy
MacPherson, A. M., DiagRad
MacPherson, J. C.
Makaroff, R.
Makins, D. J.
Maksymiuk, Lore
Mallen, R. W. Otol.
Mallett, L. L. DiagRad
Mallett, M. DiagRad
Margolus, B. D. GenSurg
Marko, J., ObstGyn.
Marshall, F. C., Urol
Marshall, Gladys D.
Marshall, M. R. Ophth
Martin, J. K. Paed
Martyniuk, A.
Marynowski, B.

* Population not separately available.

Mason, J. T., DiagRad
Matas, M.
Mather, C. E.
McAllister, N. J.
McAlpine, D. G.
McCalla, R. I., Anaes
McCallum, M. G. PH
McCarten, A. B. GenSurg
McConnell, Aileen P., IntMed.
McConnell, F., DiagRad.
McDonald, A. D.
McGugan, A. C.
McIntyre, J. W. Anaes
McKenzie, A. H. OrthSurg
McLeod, L. E. IntMed
McLellan, W.
McManus, J. P.
McMillan, D. W., Ophth
McMillan, M. L.
McNaught, D. R., OrthSurg.
McPhail, W. G.
MacWilliam, Margaret Begg, IntMed.
Melling, P.
Melnyk, D.
Meltzer, H. ThorSurg
Mendes, P. C., IntMed
Metcalfe, J. O. Urol
Michalyshyn, B. GenSurg
Michle, T. C., Psy
Mielke, B. W., Path
Milbank, R. J.
Miller, J. D. M., Anaes.
Miller, J. D. R., DiagRad.
Miller, M. J.
Mitchell, M., Paed
Miyauchi, D. K., Psy.
Modi, S.
Moffat, D. J. Anaes
Monckton, G. Neur
Moonie, G. T. Anaes
Moreau, J. P. OrthSurg
Morrish, W. DiagRad
Mortis, E. A.
Morton, G. K. NeurSurg
Moyer, D. J. ObstGyn
Murenbeeld, W. H.
Murray, K. W.
Muttit, E. L., IntMed, (Allerg)
Myers, H. A. GenSurg
Myers, Violet
Myles, J. M., Anaes
Neaman, M. P. DiagRad
Nelson, C. L.
Nelson, Jean, Paed
Nelson, T. R. ObstGyn
Newson, Dora
Newton, J. B.
Niewchas, W. S.
Nix, H. L.
Nix, N. W. Anaes
Oakley, A. R. H.
O'Brien, J. A.
Okamura, Y.
Omelchuck, A.
Ordman, J. A., OrthSurg
O'Rooney, P.
Ostolosky, R. J. ObstGyn
Owen-Flood, J. H.
Paez, P. N.
Paletz, S. G. Anaes
Paproski, K. R.
Parish, J. G., PhysMed & Rehab.
Parker, W. R. DiagRad
Parlee, S. S.
Parney, F. S., Anaes.
Pascoe, H. Psy
Paterson, J. L. Psy
Patrick, A. Ophth.
Patrick, Doreen
Pawluk, W., GenSurg
Payne, P. F., Psy.
Pearce, J. W.
Pearson, C. L.
Peers, A. L.
Penny, C. G.
Perera, F. A., IntMed
Perreault, J. C.
Phillips, A. F. TherRad
Piche, J. A.
Pisesky, W., GenSurg
Poirier, R. Paed
Pollack, H.
Popowich, J. W.
Pourbaix, W. E., IntMed
Pribram, H. F. DiagRad
Pritchard, R. E.
Quehl, E. B. ObstGyn
Quinlan, P. T. Otol
Ramage, H. C. Urol
Ramanowski, E.
Ramsay, F. G.
Ramsay, F. W., Neurol
Ramsey, C. G. IntMed
Rangachari, S., Cardiovasc & ThorSurg
Rapier, D. O., Psy
Rawlinson, H. E.
Raynham, F.
Read, J. G.
Reid, D. W., ObstGyn
Rensaa, Margaret A., Anaes.
Rentiers, P. L. DermSyph
Rety, N. A.
Richard, H. L. GenSurg
Richards, M. T.
Riddle, W. J.
Ridgway, C. R., Ophth
Ringrose, C. D., ObstGyn
Ritchie, D. C. ObstGyn
Robertson, R. F.
Rodin, A. E. Path
Rodman, F. S. B. IntMed
Romanowski, E.
Rose, P. B.
Ross, C. A. ThorSurg
Ross, H. G., ObstGyn.
Ross, J. D.
Rossall, R. E. IntMed
Rostrup, O. OrthSurg
Rudnick, A.
Ruether, B. A., IntMed.
Ryan, J. M. IntMed
St. Clair, J. D. Anaes
St. Clair, W. R. IntMed
Salmon, P. A.
Samuell, C. N.
Sanderson, Moira, IntMed
Sarko, M. M.
Scales, J. J. Anaes
Schacter, M.
Schaefer, O., IntMed
Schmaltz, S. M.
Schmidt, Brenda, Paed.
Schmidt, K. E. GenSurg
Schrag, A. R. Psy
Schulze, W., ObstGyn
Schwatz, H. A.
Schwab, E. M., Psy
Schweda, N.
Scott, Flora, Psy
Scott, J. W. IntMed
Scragg, R. D. Anaes
Segall, M. L. J.
Selby, G. W.
Selinger, Z. Psy
Semchisen, O. M., DiagRad
Sereda, M. M.
Sewchuk, H. W.
Shandro, W. A. GenSurg, Urol
Shea, D. R.
Sherbaniuk, R. W., IntMed
Sherman, L. IntMed
Shimizu, H. J., PlasSurg
Shnitka, T. K. Path
Siegenberg, J., GenSurg
Siemens, H. PH
Siluch, K. A., Urol.
Singh, S., OrthSurg
Smith, A. S., GenSurg.
Smith, Elizabeth
Smulski, J.
Snell, B.
Snihurowych, M.
Sollbach, Lilli W.
Soltice, N. J., Anaes
Spaner, S. S. Psy
Speakman, T. J. NeurSurg
Sperber, G. H.
Sprague, P. H. IntMed
Sproule, B. J., IntMed
Starko, M. M., Otol.
Stayura, Lois A., Paed
Stechishin, O. Anaes
Stefanyk, H., IntMed
Stephens, H. H. IntMed (TB)
Sterns, L. P., Cardiovasc. & ThorSurg.
Stewart, A. R., Paed.
Stewart, I. M.
Stewart, R. J., Anaes
Stirrat, J. H., Path
Strouboulis, J. P.
Strutz, W. A. GenSurg
Stuart, R. D., Bact (Glas.)
Svarich, E. W.
Swallow, G. E. Sr. Paed
Swallow, R. J., Path
Szekely, E.
Szlichcinski, W.
Talibi, T.
Tarangle, S. G.
Taylor, C. T.
Taylor, R. F., IntMed
Taylor, W. C. Paed
Taylor, W. J., DiagRad
Tedeschini, M. I., Paed
Theman, A. E., GenSurg
Thiele, I.
Thomas, A. L.
Thompson, J. S.
Thompson, Zonia R.
Thomson, R. K. C., Psy
Thurston, O. G., GenSurg
Tkachyk, S. J.
Toupin, H. M. Neur
Traff, T. N., ObstGyn
Tulloh, M. E.
Turner, E. J. Paed
Turner, F. W., GenSurg
Tworek, E. J.
Uilenberg, Catharina, Paed.
Ulan, R. A., IntMed.
Urban, A. S., OrthSurg.
Urschel, J., Psy.
Vant, J. R. ObstGyn
Verchomin, J.
Van de Guchte, M. P.
Van Stolk, J. B., Psy
Vermeulen, H. H.
Vik, K. E.
von Koenigsloew, E.
Wait, R. H., IntMed
Wallace, J. D. Anaes
Warenycia, M.
Warschawski, S. J. Otol
Watson, C. M. Anaes
Wechowicz, T.
Weih, G. P.
Weinlos, C. H. W. GenSurg
Weinlos, M. GenSurg
Weir, N. W. ObstGyn
Weisz, S., IntMed
Welsh, M. R., Anaes
Wensel, R. H., IntMed
Wershof, E.
Werthenbach, F.
Wesolowski, M. J.
Westgate, A., ObstGyn.
Weston, R. B.
Whiting, R. H. IntMed
Whitmore, G. D.
Wiancko, K. B., GenSurg
Wilbush, J.
Wilcock, P. F., Paed
Wilkinson, D., Paed

* Population not separately available.

Willans, M.
Williams, H. T. GenSurg
Williamson, D. M.
Williamson, G. L.
Willoughby, L., ObstGyn
Willox, G. L. GenSurg
Wilson, D. R. IntMed
Wilson, G. L. OrthSurg
Wilson, R. D.
Wilson, T. C., Otol
Wilson, T. S. GenSurg
Wilson, W. A.
Windle, S. DiagRad
Winter, R. W., ObstGyn
Wojcicki, H. M.
Wolochow, P.
Wood, J. B.
Woodhead, B. H., PhysMed. & Rehab.
Woolstencroft, R.
Woywitka, N. W. Ophth
Wray, D. B.
Wray, R. G.
Wright, V. W.
Yake, W. W.
Yakimets, W. W., GenSurg
Yakynechko, Mary
Yelle, E. F.
Yoneda, Y. ObstGyn
Yonge, K., Psy
Young, B. G., Psy.
Young, M. K. IntMed
Zalesky, N.
Zbigniew, G.
Zetter, G. R.

EDSON
(3,198)
Brooks, D. H.
Brown, J. M.
Crawford, J. E.
Lee, A. P. N.
Lewis, I. H.
Macdonald, Allison, R.

ELK POINT
(694)
Miller, F. G.
Miller, K. C.
Ross, A. G.

ELNORA
(213)
Warren, W. J.

EMPRESS
(405)
Fraser, J. M.

EVANSBURG
(451)
Goba, H. K.

FAIRVIEW
(1,506)
Garrison, T. W.
Kratz, Hanna
Kratz, J. C.

FALHER
(741)
Campbell-Fowler, C.
Paine, W. A.

FORESTBURG
(678)
Carnaghan, W. C.

FORT MACLEOD
(2,490)
Adler, K.
Grynoch, R. L. GenSurg
MacLean, A. D.
Walker, Hilda M.
Walker, T. J.

FORT McMURRAY
(1181)
Nicholson, A. J.
Yung, S. W.

FORT SASKATCHEWAN
(2,978)
Bauld, E. D.

Ritchie, J. H.
Scarth, A. G.
Sheppard, L. D.
Young, D. R.

FORT VERMILION
(768)
Malone, G. M., GenSurg
Strouboulis, J. P.

GALAHEAD
(237)
Myles, P. J.

GARDEN BAY
*
Paetkau, E. J.

GLENDON
(320)
Ginzberg, L.
Lewis, W. S.
Mokuena, J. M.

GRAND CENTRE
(1493)
Wood, G. A.

GRANDE PRAIRIE
(8,352)
Backus, W. O.
Collins, A. L.
Cottrell, D. G.
Dobson, H. L.
Hoogewerf, P. E.
Matheson, D. T.
Murray, A. R.
Pagan, R. T.
Pitt-Payne, B.
Stillwell, H. E., DiagRad
Storcer, J.
Turner, Catherine

GRIMSHAW
(1,099)
Marjanovich, Katarina D.

HANNA
(2,645)
Donald, J. P.
Evans, D. M.
Knox, F. W.
Turner, R. G.
Wilkins, G. D.
Williams, Dita M.

HIGH PRAIRIE
(1,758)
Lewis, R. D.
Maxwell, J. B.
McFarland, I. W. A. GenSurg
McKendrick, W. H.

HIGH RIVER
(2,277)
Blayney, E. B.
Blayney, M. M.
Blayney, Y.
Cramer, J. E.
Ellis, A. C.
Rowland, E. M.
Wilson, W. M.

HINTON
(3,529)
Fraser, R. M.
Murray, D.
Reid, Anne M.
Reid, Ian W.

HOLDEN
(554)
Calo, R.

HYTHE
(449)
Glas, A. P.

INNISFAIL
(2,273)
Beardsworth, J. H.
Beckett, D. P.
Cope, R. A.
Galloway, W. R.
Graham, J. K.
Perry, J. W.
Stafford-Mayor, G.

ISLAY
(125)
Ryan, P. J.
Sweet, A. H.

JASPER
(2,360)
Betkowski, J. P. GenSurg
McFadyen, E. H., ObstGyn
Venner, A. IntMed

KEG RIVER
*
Jackson, M. P.

KILLAM
(548)
Amin, T. C.
McLeod, H. R.
Patel, D. G.

LAC LA BICHE
(1,314)
Bouvier, D. D.
Cadgow, W. J.
Cosentino, F. V.
Yewchuk, P.

LACOMBE
(3,029)
Haworth, G. C.
Henry, W. A.
Malone, M. C.
McFetridge, J. D.
McKibbin, J.
Tetz, W. C.

LAMONT
(705)
Armstrong, R. F.
Dobson, A., GenSurg
Preston, D. R.
Sunley, J. G.
Weatherilt, J. L. IntMed
Young, M. A. R. GenSurg

LANCASTER PARK
*
Bernier, J., DiagRad.

LEDUC
(2,356)
Griffiths, A. L.
Griffiths, G. Audrey
Jensen, J. K.
Kempton, A. R.
Nixon, A., GenSurg
Smyth, J.
Tibbetts, T. M.

LETHBRIDGE
(35,454)
Ainscough, G. A.
Arnold, H. A. IntMed
Bainborough, A. R. Path
Balfour, G. S. IntMed
Bassett, T. H.
Baster, N., PH
Bell, O. Gwyneth
Bennett, R.
Bigelow, J. K.
Black, B. C. DiagRad
Bower, J.
Brown, T. E.
Byrne, A. A.
Cairns, E. A. M. Paed
Campbell, D.
Chorley, G. E., Anaes.
Christie, F. M.
Cornock, W. Y. GenSurg
Craddock, A. B.
Craddock, Shirley R.
Cranley, W. J.
Crawford, W. S.
del Valle, R.
Dillabough, C. .D
Driedger, G., OrthSurg
Dunlop, D. L., ObstGyn.
Etherington, E. M.
Etherington, J. S.
Gore-Hickman, F. G. Paed
Gray, G. S. IntMed

* Population not separately available.

Lethbridge (Cont'd.)
Gray, W. A.
Gregory, S. J.
Haig, A. A. GenSurg
Haig, T. B., GenSurg.
Haig, W. R. GenSurg
Hall, R. G. ObstGyn
Hase, H.
Hepworth, Sheina
Hovan, N. A.
Hunt, H. B. GenSurg
Hunt, J. W.
Ive, F. A.
Johnson, F. L. Anaes.
Johnson, R. L. GenSurg.
Johnston, L. W. ObstGyn.
Kikinday, L.
King-Brown, R. IntMed.
Kotkas, L. J.
Leong, S. T. Ophth
Livingstone, A. G. Urol
Lowings, K. L.
Marshall, M. DiagRad.
Martin-Smith, B.
McCutcheon, J. D.
McLean, F. J.
McNally, J. A.
McPherson, D. F. Paed
McTavish, J. A.
Melling, M. T.
Morgan, J. E. ObstGyn.
Nicas, J. A.
Noble, J. H. GenSurg.
Okamura, Y., ObstGyn
Palmer, G. R.
Penner, E. P.
Pomahac, A.
Poulsen, E. R.
Preston, F. T.
Prokopishyn, H., GenSurg.
Rice, D. A.
Richards, T. J.
Roy, D. G.
Ruddell, J. S. Anaes
Schindler, Q. R. Ophth,Otol
Searby, B.
Seitz, H., IntMed
Spackman, E. V.
Stewart, D. R.
Stillwell, J. B.
Strome, W.
Walters, B. H.
Watson, S. H., Path
Wright, G. A. IntMed

MAGRATH
(1,334)
Dahl, R. M.

MANNING
(893)
Branigan, D. W.
Cullen, E. S.
Ogg, Marie

MANNVILLE
(629)
Hasinoff, D.

MAYERTHORPE
(665)
Cannon, P. J.
Jaglalsingh, L. H.
Scales, E. J.
Vermeulen, H.

McLENNAN
(1,074)
Fish, H. W.
Harvey, R. F.

MEDICINE HAT
(24,484)
Armitage, J.
Campbell, W. C.
Clementi, K. J.
Cowan, J. M., GenSurg
Cranston, J. A.
Davis, M., ObstGyn
Dillabough, C. D.
Dyer, A. M.
Edwards, J. L., IntMed.
Ferguson, I. A., ObstGyn.
Gershaw, F. W. GenSurg
Hassett, N.
Heslip, P. G.
Hobson, A. C., IntMed
Hunt, T.
Lawrason, D. M., DiagRad.
Lewis, D. F. IntMed
Lewis, L.
MacCharles, E. D. GenSurg
MacInnes, A.
McKenzie, H. F. TherRad.
Penrose, G. S., Anaes.
Phillips, L. J., Otol
Racette, Lois J.
Racette, P. C., Path
Sinton, E. J., Ophth
Skinner, E. G. F.
Sobey, V. W. GenSurg
Van Belkum, J. A. ObstGyn
Van Belkum, Joan, Paed
ObstGyn.
Wilke, A. A.

MILK RIVER
(801)
Finch, J. A.
Goretz, E. P.
Klassen, L.

MORINVILLE
(928)
Clark, G. N.

MULHURST
*
Melling, J.

MUNDARE
(603)
Strilchuk, N. C.

MYRNAM
(440)
Cholod, S.

NANTON
(1,047)
Little, A. W.

OKOTOKS
(1,046)
Gibson, Janet B.
Gibson, W. M.
Maltby, J. R.
McKenzie, R. E.

OLDS
(2,433)
Burland, G. R. GenSurg
Paasuke, R. T.
Wray, R. G.

OYEN
(774)
McCracken, J. A.

PEACE RIVER
(2,546)
Douchet, G. L.
Kozub, P.
Lawrie, S. W.
Schropp, J. H.
Sgro, G.
Skeephek, S. V.

PENHOLD
(317)
Seguin, H. L.

PICTURE BUTTE
(977)
Crapnell, V. E.
Takahashi, J. H.

PINCHER CREEK
(2,968)
Collins, L. B.
Collins, Rhonda M.
Hodgson, M. R.
Kerfoot, D. A.
Kraft-Goddard, D. G.
McCrimmon, J. R.
McLean, F. J.
Medlicott, H. G.

PONOKA
(3,937)
Backus, A. B.
Bradley, Katharine F.
Bradley, R. C.
Byers, J. M. Psy.
Byers, J. N. C.
Byers, S. J.
Chesney, D. D.
Elliott, A. J. K.
Gibbon, J. E.
Horsey, Mary E.
Karvellas, Penelope
Lall, H. D.,
MacLean, R. R., Neur-Psy
McAleer, J.
Mountain, T. C.
O'Sullivan, M. A., GenSurg.
Phillips, D. L., Psy
Runions, E. J.
Schofield, R.
Thompson, J., Psy
Turner, J. P.
Valle-Carero, C.
Varsanyi, E. J.
Weaver, S. A.

PROVOST
(1,022)
Acton, W. C.
Harper, H. E.
Harper, Patricia
Hnatuik, J. N.

RADWAY
(177)
Constantini, G.
Crossley, S. G.
Glasgow, R. M.

RALSTON
(600)
Lipp, J. A.
Stewart, W. C.
Taylor, W. K.

RAYMOND
(2,365)
Kotkas, L. J., Psy.
Low, J. S.
Norton, C. H.
Taylor, H. G.
Walker, J. H.

REDCLIFF
(2,226)
Fairbairn, R. F.

RED DEER
(19,612)
Bazzard, P. M.
Binding, D. G.
Boake, H. K.
Burt, R. K., ObstGyn
Carter, W. A.
Chadwick, R., IntMed
Coley, C. E.
Cooper, R. C.
Craig, C. G.
Craigie, A.
Cumming, J. D.
Haigh, J. B., Psy
Hancock, G. R.
Holmes, I. H., IntMed
le Vann, L. J.
March, R. J.
Marriott, R. D., GenSurg
McLuhan, W. J.
Merriam, R. K., D & T Rad
Miller, E.
Mitchell, J. E., GenSurg
More, C. G.
Onerheim, W. O. GenSurg.
Parkinson, T. J. Paed
Parsons, R. M., GenSurg
Parsons, W. B., DiagRad
Patterson, L. J.
Ritzen, A. A.
Scott, I. S.
Simpson, W.

* Population not separately available.

Red Deer (Cont'd.)
Staples, J. C.
Taylor, Coletta
Thompson, C. D.
Wagner, J. C., GenSurg.
Weddell, J. A.
Younger, L. I., Otol

REDWATER
(1,133)
Mirlen, W.
Watt, J. S.

RIMBEY
(1,269)
Boorman, G. C.
Cable, R. M.
Hedges, F. H.
More, J. H.

ROCKY MOUNTAIN HOUSE
(2,360)
Hay, R. L.
Hein, S. S.

ST. ALBERT
(4,059)
Downie, D. M.
Gomm, Audrey
Mirlin, W.
Skrobot, W.

ST. PAUL
(2,823)
Ashforth, I.
Decosse, F. R., OrthSurg.
Shewciw, Z.
Trottier, L.
Wilson, E. M.

SEDGEWICK
(653)
Pereira, C. J.

SEXSMITH
(531)
McCrum, J. R.

SHERWOOD PARK
(2,923)
Brooks, T. H.
Casper, G. F.
Ferrari, R. L.
Higgins, G. L.
Shea, D. R., Paed.

SLAVE LAKE
(467)
Rutt, J. M.

SMOKY LAKE
(621)
Lobay, F.

SPIRIT RIVER
(893)
Block, E. W.
Laventure, A. R.
Law, F. M.
Pawlovich, J.

STANDARD
(257)
Fletcher, D. A.

STETTLER
(3,638)
Berezan, D.
Dobson, D.
Fegler, J. G.
MacKay, D.
Malcolm, J. M.
Stephens, Hazel G.
Trumper, M. B.
Zender, R. J.

STONEY PLAIN
(1,311)
Brown, H. M.
Kritzinger, V.
Nicholson, C. G.
Paterson, J. C.
Ringham, M. C.

STRATHMORE
(916)
Giffin, J. W.

SUNDRE
(858)
Miller, C. A.
White, A.

SYLVAN LAKE
(1,387)
Cookson, T. S.
Mahaffy, Charlotte E. P. H.
Rowell, P. F.

TABER
(3,951)
Campbell, R. D.
Dick, C. J. W. GenSurg
Gibbings, J. S.
Jenkins, Elaine
Plimbley, W. R.
Sawada, K.
Wiebe, E. H.

THORHILD
(309)
Bostock, D.

THORSBY
(491)
Hankin, M.

THREE HILLS
(1,486)
Cumming, W. T.
Haigh, G.

TOFIELD
(900)
Freebury, W. H.
Price, G. M.

TROCHU
(670)
Hay, A. J. S.

TWO HILLS
(827)
Chonko, M. E.

VALLEYVIEW
(1,077)
Bell, J. F.
Lapointe, J. J.

VEGREVILLE
(2,908)
Couillard, A.
Edmunds, L. M.
Kuzyk, N.
Leslie-Spinks, A. J.
Lukenchuk, J. J.
Reid, J. F., GenSurg
Stefancik, J.

VERMILION
(2,449)
Attenborough, R. G.
Covill, F. J.
King, A. B.

VIKING
(1,047)
Caldwell, A. E.
Klein, A.

VILNA
(406)
Frobb, P. W.

VULCAN
(1,310)
Almond, W. W.
Koziol, M. E.
Lakins, Jill E.
Lakins, J. P.
Tomkins, A. D.

WAINWRIGHT
(3,353)
Bourke, G. J.
Evans, C. E.
McGechen, J. A., GenSurg.
Middlemass, J. G.
Sawchuk, V. N.
Somer, K. G.
Wallace, H. C.
White, D. S.

WARBURG
(284)
Fife, Brenda

WESTLOCK
(1,838)
Cobban, A. C.
Deacon, J. K.
Dumaine, L. D., GenSurg
Faulconbridge, A. J.
Gokiert, J. G.
Lam, S. P., IntMed.
Little, R. D.
Pritchard, R. E.
Vaughan, W. A.
Watt, A. C.
Whissell, G.

WETASKIWIN
(5,300)
Bellamy, R. P.
Casey, S. P.
Drolet, T. A.
Dykes, R. M.
Fairfield, F. M.
Ghitter, E. I.
Gramlick, E.
Johnson, L. E.
Wade, M. A.

WHITECOURT
(1,054)
Hayhurst, R. J.

WILLINGDON
(434)
Lazaruk, W. G.

British Columbia

ABBOTSFORD
(893)
Alberts, J. J.
Barkman, B. G.
Blanchard, K. R.
Boulton, K. A.
Buirs, E. J.
Cannon, H. E.
Fast, I. M.
Gibson, A. G.
Giesbrecht, W. R.
Pauls, H., GenSurg
Woods, J. H.
Ziskrout, I.

AGASSIZ
(600)
Booth, G. H. H.

ALBERNI
(4,616)
Anderson, J. L.
Burnett, D. J.
Clifford, D. J.
Johns, E. R.
Koszegi, B. S.
Pitreman, M. C.
Pitts, W. C.
Webster, H. W.

ALDERGROVE
(357)
Findlay, S. P., Anaes.
Mout, R.

ALERT BAY
(825)
MacLaren, L. B.
Pickup, H. J.

ARMSTRONG
(1,292)
Haugen, R.

ASHCROFT
(875)
Lynnes, H. M.
Ross, L. E.

BELLA BELLA
*
Chisholm, J. I.
Dalton, Roberta D.

* Population not separately available.

BELLA COOLA
*
Crosby, D. R.
Cuthill, J. D.
King, H. F.
Page, R. H.

BRALORNE
(613)
Young, P. W.

BRENTWOOD BAY
*
Ellis, J. P.

BURNABY
(See Vancouver)

BURNS LAKE
(1,041)
Battersby, G. S.
Mann, A. D.

CAMPBELL RIVER
(3,737)
Chen, L. T.
Chen, Patricia P.
Depew, J. G.
Duncan, K. B.
Gordon, R. B.
Graham, J. M.
Hall, A. A.
Hall, N. B.
Hancock, A. K.
Kirk, D. E.
Margets, P. G., GenSurg
Murphy, R.
Riley, G. T.
Ross, J. R.
Wiegand, F. M., GenSurg.

CASSIAR
(432)
Navin, S. J.

CASTLEGAR
(2,253)
Fowler, C. S.
Hall, J. V.
Johnson, A. D.
Walton, J. H.
Yule, W. M.

CHASE
(903)
Dagyi, M.

CHEMAINUS
(1,518)
Dick, R. N.
Fenton, L. G.
Heydon, G. K.
Philippson, G. J.

CHILLIWACK
(8,259)
Arneil, A. S.. PH
Borschneck, A. G.
Brachman, E. F.
Bryan, L. E.
Chouinard, C. J., DiagRad
Cram, G. A., ObstGyn.
de Montigny, J. P.
Dubois, P. F.
Dyck, V. J.
Enns, G. F.
Evans, G. E., Paed
Gibson, G. J.
Gorchynski, O.
Grandy, J. D.
Johnsen, H. V.
Klassen, B. G.
Klassen, D., Otol
Lane, R. F.
MacLeod, R. B.
Madill, F. M.
Marlatt, D. C., IntMed (T.B.)
McMahon, J. M.
Miki, P. Y., DiagRad
Moore, J. D.
Muth, K. L.
Pauls, H.
Phelps, A. H., **GenSurg**
Roberts, G. A. C.
Saviskey, M. F., Ophth.
Todd, N.
Weeden, R. P.
Whetter, R. W.
Wilford, E. J.
Wishlow, N. F.
Young, A. B.
Young, A. D.

CLEARBROOK
(1,964)
Krahn, J. J.

CLOVERDALE
(569)
Forster, J. M.
Kornder, L. D.
Markowski, E. G.
Murphy, Mary
Specken, J. C.

COMOX
(1,756)
Fairley, J.
Mooney, H. A.
Power, P. G.

COQUITLAM
see Port Quitlam

COURTENAY
(3,486)
Coleman, D. C.
Gibson, G. A., PH
Graham, H. M., Ophth, Otol
Lunam, J. B.
McCann, J. A.
Miller, D. M.
Stewart, G. G., GenSurg
Theal, G. I.
Villaneuva, M. P.
Williams, H. I.

COWICHAN LAKE
see Lake Cowichan

CRANBROOK
(5,545)
Askey, A. W.
Brockington, C. W. M.
Green, W. O.
Hatch, L. R.
Hengel, L. M.
Hopper, J. M.
Hsu, C. L., D. & T. Rad.
Mugan, J. F. M.
Sheppard, E. J.
Stanton, R. C., GenSurg.
Sullivan, T. J.
Tse, K. S.
Wylie, H. L.

CRESTON
(2,463)
Miller, J. S.
Murray, J. V.
Nelson, J. W.
Smith, G. L.
Vogel, Anne

CUMBERLAND
(1,303)
Cubbage, J. S.
Hicks, E. R.
Montgomery, C. B.

DAWSON CREEK
(10,948)
Archibald, W. S.
Boorman, S. T., **GenSurg**
Claremont, P. F., **DiagRad**
Galliford, B. W.
Gilmour, D. M.
Irvine, J. W., GenSurg
Jackson, T. E.
O'Brien, H. J.
Thorkelson, G. W.
Watson, A. B.

DUNCAN
(3,726)
Beevor-Potts, C. H.
Callbeck, G. R. M.
Coleman, G.
Coleman, J. U., GenSurg
Gloster, O. C.
Goodbrand, J. S.
Gunn, D., DiagRad
Hossein, E. V.
Janes, W. C. B., GenSurg
McCauley, W. D.
Norell, M. V.
Pawlowski, **J.**
Postuk, P.
Smith, D. M.
Stanley, R. F.
Tassin, J. J.
Thorkelson, G. W.
Watson, T. P.
Wilson, R. R.

ENDERBY
(1,075)
Dixon, A. E.
Kope, J. H.
Sawatzky, H. J.

ESPERANZA
*
Gereluk, Madeline
McLean, H. A.

ESQUIMALT
(10,174)
Schinbrin, J. E., GenSurg
Spilsbury, B. W., GenSurg
Woods, D. G. DiagRad

ESSONDALE
(500)
Adler, H. G., Psy
Ahmad, S.
Arenas, A. A.
Bryson, B. F.
Creamer, Alice, Psy
Dainard, R. B.
Dulay, J. R.
Gear, G. L.
Ghaed-Sharafy, M. A., Psy.
Grenier, A.
Hasselbach, I.
Hildebrand, H., GenSurg.
Jackson, J. M., Psy
Johnston, A. F., Psy.
Joneja, R. P., Psy.
Kabir, M. A.
Kontaxopoulos, G.
Kovacs, A., Psy.
McFarlane, W. J., Psy
Mellor, E.
Middleton, T. M., Psy
Muthanna, K. C.
Nicolson, G. A., Path
Parkinson, R., Psy
Prime, F. M.
Ramos, F. B.
Ramos, Virginia, G.
Rebbeck, Patricia M., GenSurg.
Richards, Frances M., Psy
Roa, Sylvia G.
Savran, N.
Schlichter, W.
Schwarz, C. J. Psy.
Sinclair, Olive
Valderrma, A.
Vallance, M., Psy

FERNIE
(2,661)
Baerg, D. J.
East, W. H. S.
Leroux, G. W.
McRitchie, M.

FORT LANGLEY
(501)
Neilson, J. M.
Neilson, G.

FORT NELSON
(1,607)
Forbes, W. D.
Kenyon, A.
Metten, D.
Robinson, D. C.

* Population not separately available.

FORT ST. JOHN
(3,619)
Erickson, L. M.
Haugen, O. D.
Kearney, G. H.
Kindrachuk, J.
Miller, T. D., GenSurg.
Stefanick, G., GenSurg
Temple, J. J.
Westover, G.

FRUITVALE
(1,033)
Jones, A. R.
Mackay, J. A.
Regan, G.

GANGES
(400)
Dixon, E. R.
Francis, A.
Jansch, Marjorie E.
Jansch, T. L.
Jarman, E. A.
Stanton, O. L.

GARDEN BAY
*
Masterson, T. L., GenSurg

GIBSON'S
(1,091)
Johnson, D. L.

GOLDEN
(1,782)
Braul, W.
Taylor, J. E.
Trott, A. W.

GRAND FORKS
(2,347)
Ahamad, S.
Payne, E. N.
Perley, D. A.
Salaruddin, A.
Tomashewsky, E. E.

GREENWOOD
(931)
Vallis, D. G.

HANEY
(2,117)
Arber, S. R.
Capling, L. C.
Firckser, B.
Gallagher, D. J. P.
Lusk, J. G.
Rhodes, R. C.
Schlagintweit, H. E.
Skaling, J. H.
Sumner, J.
Thordarson, T. T.
Trudel, A. J., Path
Van Der Minne, D.
Wong, C. N.
Yule, R. F.

HAZELTON
(410)
Whiting, J. E.

HOPE
(2,751)
Asche, G. A.
Asche-Quinte, Ursula
Juba, E.
Morrison, R. D.
Murakami, E. K.
Penner, L.

HUDSON HOPE
(70)
Haramia, J.
Jack, K. D.
Jones, G. G., Paed, IntMed

INVERMERE
(742)
Coy, F. P.
Duthie, G. A.
Martin, J. M.
Ostrander, A. B., GenSurg

KAMLOOPS
(10,076)
Beesley, J. B.
Bennett, G., Ophth
Boon, D. A., Otol.
Boucher, L. A.
Brownell, A. K.
Burns, O. G.
Burris, D. S., ObstGyn
Burris, H. L.
Chin, W. C., Paed
Davies, G. R., GenSurg
Dewar, J. W.
Dovey, B. D.
Edworthy, J. M., Paed.
Fellenz, K. P., Paed
Findlay, I. D., PH
Fournier, E.
French, W. E., GenSurg.
Hauser, W., Path.
Hunter, D. R., Psy.
Kolkind, T. K.
Lansdall, F. C. Urol.
Louie, R. A.
MacDonnell, J. K., DiagRad
MacKay, B. K., IntMed
Maher, L. A., Otol
Martin, G. M. Path
McDougall, A. D.
McKeen, J. L.
McLaren, W. J. GenSurg
Murray, H. O. GenSurg; IndustMed.
Nixon, L. H.
O'Neill, J. J.
Osborne, D. F. ObstGyn
Orr, A. M.
Poulsen, J. B.
Rose, I. R. L.
Sennewald, G.
Smillie, I. G.
Soga, K. K.
Sutherland, L. M., ObstGyn
Thomas, A. P. Anaes
Thomson J. A. C., IntMed
Thornton, N. M., Anaes
Tomm, G. E.
Weir O. A., GenSurg
Willoughby, J. A. Paed.
Willoughby, J. C. M., GenSurg

KASLO
(651)
Besecker, L. D.

KELOWNA
(13,188)
Anderson, W. F.
Athans, G. D.
Bennett, J. S., ObstGyn
Bowers, D., IntMed.
Brown, A. W. Ophth
Burran, E. L., Ophth
Campbell, J. S., DiagRad.
Carruthers, E. P., IntMed
Cave, W. S., GenSurg
Clarke, D. A., PH
Dick, A.
Dukelow, J. B., ObstGyn
Ellis, R. D., IntMed
Ferguson, R. B.
Found, N. P., Otol
France, K. A.
Harland, J. H. Anaes
Henderson, C. B., Paed
Holmes, C. B. Derm, IntMed
Holmes, J. A., IntMed
Huitema, P. A., GenSurg
Innes, D. M., Path.
Janzen, A.
Knox, W. J.
Lim, D. W., Ophth
McIntosh, A. D.
McNair, F. E., Psy
Moir, J. B.
Moir, J. H., GenSurg
Morrow, D. F., Path
Moss, C. B., DiagRad.

O'Donnell, W. J. GenSurg
O'Neil, T. J.
Pollock, F. D.
Rankine, J. A., GenSurg
Sherrin, Adrienne
Sherrin, D. A., GenSurg
Stewart, G. N.
Tisdale, J. M.
Underhill, A. S.
Wilson, G. M. A
Wynn-Williams, R. N.

KIMBERLEY
(6,013)
Backman, K. M.
Finch, P. G.
Johnston, D. R.
Lang, D. W.
Neve, C. R., GenSurg
Quenville, N. F.
Shaw, J. M.
Watkins, R. T.

KINNAIRD
(2,123)
Ternent, D. F.

KITIMAT
(8,000)
Baker, B. L.
Duncan, J. D.
Dundee, D. J.
Dundee, Yvonne E.
Kraft, B. P., Anaes
Mack, D. J.
Shimizu, K.
Suiker, Alice
Swanburg, A. R.
Woodman-Fox, Evelyn M.
Wollacott, P. J.
Young, W. O.

LADNER
(2,000)
Anderson, R. N.
Kanee, L.
Maguson, D.
Wilbee, G. S.
Yamanaha, G. J.

LADYSMITH
(2,173)
Bowker, H. A., GenSurg
Cantor, H.
Mitchell, P. J.
Neville, J. W.
Wickham, T.
Williams, I. H., Anaes.

LAKE COWICHAN
(2,146)
Lam, K. C.
Mewhort, C. W.
Morrow, J. J.
Semkuley, M.
Watts, P. R.

LANGLEY
(2,365)
Brown, H. I., DiagRad.
Ceresney, F. P.
Gilham, R. E.
Nataros, H. S.
Robinson, D. A.
Rutz, H.
Smart, J. M.
Tielens, R.
Wilmshurst, Amy A.

LILLOOET
(1,313)
Clark, M. D.
Levine, E. C.

LYTTON
(441)
Edwards, K. N.

McBRIDE
(593)
Ryall, D. B.

* Population not separately available.

MERRITT
(3,039)
Brant, D. J.
Carlson, G. C.
Carlson, Margaret
Hewson, R. T.
Klass, W. A.
Newhouse, A. L.
Sears, C. F.

MICA CREEK
*
Babin, C. E.

MICHEL
(524)
Luzod, E. R.

MISSION CITY
(3,251)
Balkany, A. F.
Black, D., PH
Erichson, E. H.
Graham, R. E.
Greham, A. J.
Humes, H. G.
Lee, D. B.
Marcellus, J. A.
Marshall, R. E.
Rayson, J. H.
Robson, P. A.

NAKUSP
(992)
Maxfield, F. B.

NANAIMO
(14,135)
Baldwin, J. H.
Bennett, N. T.
Blott, G. R.
Boulding, J. E., Psy.
Browne, C. C.
Campbell, D. R.
Chambers, P. J.
Chisholm, A. R.
Clarke, R. S., Path
Cooper, E., GenSurg
David, C. M.
Dekker, A. G. A.
Dudley, J. H.
Fumerton, J. L., Paed.
Gamble, C. S.
Gawthorp, P. C.
Giovando, L.
Good, W. C., GenSurg.
Gosling, R. E. Otol.
Grant, S. M., Path
Hall, A. B.
Hamilton, J. A., GenSurg
Hanley, J. L.
Horner, B. A., IntMed.
Horner, Frances, Derm.
Howden, G. D., Ophth
Howey, J. R. ObstGyn
Jensen, S. E. Psy
Johnson, J. E.
Latham, H. O.
Levell, G. W., DiagRad.
Little, W. F.
Lynch, J. B. Anaes
Mackenzie, C. J., PH
Maclean, R. B. Anaes.
Marsh, P. E.
McConnell, Doreen, Paed
McKerricher, D. E., Ophth
Miller, A. P.
Nuttall-Smith, J. C., Paed
Philcox, H. A., OrthSurg
Pollett, H. F.
Radcliffe, Patricia, ObstGyn
Radcliffe, R. W., ObstGyn
Roque, N. G., OrthSurg
Routley, J. V.
Scott-Kerr, M. T.
Smart, M. J., DiagRad
Symon, H. L.
Thomas, M. J., ObstGyn
Welch, H. C. IntMed.
Wood, J. A., ObstGyn.

Wynrib, M.

NELSON
(7,074)
Barrett, G. R.
Beauchamp, A. J.
Bitnum, S., Paed.
Brummitt, R. B.
Carpenter, J. C.
Geissinger, M. E., GenSurg
Hartley, J. M.
Kokan, P.
Massey, W. K. DiagRad
McMurchy, J. G. M.
Miller, R. E.
Morrison, N. E.
Shaw, R. B.
Smart, M. R., DiagRad
Smythe, H. H.

NEW DENVER
(566)
Willings, H. R.

NEWTON
(178)
Macdonald, R. L.

NEW WESTMINSTER
(33,654)
Allan, M. L., ThorSurg.
Angus, Elizabeth
Antonik, L.
Armstrong, C. A., GenSurg
Arrowsmith, R. C., Psy
Atnikov, M. G. Anaes
Barnes, G. W. Anaes
Barwell-Clarke, I. F., PlasSurg, GenSurg.
Beaudoing, R. J.
Bentz, J. B.
Bland, J. S., Psy.
Bowles, A. W., Ophth Otol
Brewster, W. R.
Brooks, H. J., Paed.
Brown, D. N., NeurSurg
Bruehler, G.
Bryson, B. F.
Bus, M.
Calverley, M. O. Psy.
Caunt, T. G. B., Psy
Chipperfield, L. S.
Chisholm, D. M.
Civkin, S. W., Otol
Coady, C. J., Path
Cook, E. G., Paed
Cote, Pacita
Couldwell, W. J., Ophth
Coursley, G., GenSurg., Cardiovasc & ThorSurg.
Crofton, F. D., DiagRad.
Dale, J. P. B., Ophth
Deane, L. S., ObstGyn
Debenham, P. A., Anaes
deRoos, T.
Dunn, R. W., ObstGyn
Edworthy, M. A.
Efford, R. J., IntMed
Fairbank, W. H.
Foulkes, R. G.
Foxwell, R. B., OrthSurg
Fraser, J., DiagRad.
Friesen, W. G.
Frinton, E., DiagRad.
Fyffe, G. T., Anaes.
Gain, D. B.
Gaudin, F. H. A., Paed
Gaudin, M. L., ObstGyn
Gavanski, M. S., Psy.
Gibson, J. A. Anaes.
Gill, G. S.
Graham, J. E., IntMed
Graham, W. C., PlasSurg
Green, K.
Gregson, W. A.
Greiner, A. IntMed.
Hakstian, A. IntMed (T.B.)
Hallowell, Mary, Paed
Hamilton, H. S. Ophth

Harder, D. H.
Harder, F. A.
Harrington, R. W.
Harris, D., Ophth
Harrison, C. P., DiagRad
Helgason, R. E., Psy.
Herberts, L. T., Urol
Hill, K. C., OrthSurg.
Hosein, L.
Hough, E. K.
Hughes, Pauline, Psy
Hutchins, J. D.
Ireland, J. R., Urol
Jaques, N.
Kamburoff, T. D.
Kelsey, H. A., ObstGyn
Kennedy, J. S. Urol
Kennedy, Ruth, Psy
Keogh, J. H., DiagRad
Kergin, A. J., GenSurg
Kinsey, F. E., ObstGyn
Kirkpatrick, F.
Klassen, P. W., Anaes
Laudan, J. C., DiagRad.
Laughland, W. W.
Lawson, J. T.
Lee, A. H.
Lehmann, Elsa
Lesack, B. J., GenSurg
Lesk, L.
Logan, R. I., Anaes
Lougheed, L. E., NeurSurg.
MacLean, J. R.
MacLean, J. R.
MacLean, N. B., Urol
MacNeill, R. D., ThorSurg, GenSurg.
Macrander, H.
Mandeville, A. F.
Mandeville, Audrey M.
Marsh, R. J., GenSurg
McCannel, J. A., DiagRad.
McDonald, D. M., OrthSurg
McLean, D.
McLean, P. M., OrthSurg
McLennan, J. A.
McNeill, R. D.
McPhee, J. G. D & TRad
Meth, B.
Millar, Irene, Anaes
Miller, R. J.
Mirabel, L., IntMed
Mitchell, R. E., DiagRad
Nazif, A., Psy.
Neilson, T. H.
Nelson, J. D., DiagRad
Nelson, R. A. C.
Olson, C. J.
Outerbridge, R. C., OrthSurg
Pedlow, A. L., DiagRad.
Pepper, V. W., ObstGyn
Piercy, G. I.
Pontifex, A. H. Path.
Prasloski, P., Ophth
Quayle, J. T. PlasSurg.
Radford, H. W.
Richards, A. G., IntMed
Richards, Frances M. F., Psy.
Rivers, I.
Robertson, J. G., Ophth, Otol
Rothwell, G. S.
Sackville, G. A.
Sadler, Olive, TherRad
Samaroo, L. L.
Satanove, A., DermSyph.
Schaffrin, Miriam
Schloss, S. M.
Sinclair, J. A.
Sinclair, W.
Skully, H. J.
So, Y. P.
Spitzer, R. W.
Stavrides, A., Path
Steinson, E. B.
Stevenson, T. K., GenSurg

*** Population not separately available.**

New Westminster (Cont'd.)
Stewart, I. F., Otol
Stewart, W. W.
Sturrock, F. L., Path
Thompson, C. W.
Tischler, Bluma, Paed
Tredger, C. M., OrthSurg
Tredger, Enid N.
Turpin, J. H.
Ulrich, D. G., GenSurg
Walton, F. A., Anaes
Watson, H. N.
Weir, E. F., IntMed
Wellwood, J. P.
Wilder, E. M.
Williams, H. R.
Wilson, C. C.
Wilson, J. T.
Wilson, J. W., GenSurg
Wilson, M.
Wong, C.
Wong, J. W.
Wood, A. E., ObstGyn
Wood, D. M.
Worsley, G. H. Anaes
Wright, J. C.
Wylde, E. W.
Yelland, L. W.
Zimich, L.

NORTH BURNABY
(Dist. of Vancouver)
Arthur J. F.
Buell, A. L.
Davis, C. J.
Davis, R. N. Psy.
Fitton, J. H.
Helgason, R. E., Psy.
Kirkwood, W. K.
Krause, D. A.
Lovegrove, W. M.
Macaulay, C. J., ObstGyn
MacDonald, J. A.
McKean, J. D.
Murphy, T. J.
Reid, E. M.
Robb, G. M., GenSurg.
Smith, G. L., GenSurg
Steedman, J. A., Psy.
Van Uchelen, P. A.
Walker, W. G.
Watson, D.
Webber, S. C.
Worsley, G. H., Anaes

NORTH KAMLOOPS
(6,456)
Allen, M. E.
Lazarchuk, M., GenSurg
Lazarchuk, O.

NORTH SURREY
(Dist. of New Westminster)
*
Beaton, J. M.
Brown, P. B.
Carney, L. R.
Cates, B. A., GenSurg
Das, J.
De Groot, W. P.
Dombsky, V.
de Rooy, G.
Ekaireb, S. Y., Paed
Emanuels, E. J.
Finley, G. R.
Flather, B. C.
Forbes, D. E.
Foxwell, R. B., OrthSurg
Fyffe, G. J., Anaes.
Harper, R. R.
Hartley, E. L.
Horniman, E. A.
Koch, C. A.
Law, J. T.
MacAskill, A. D., Ophth
Macdonald, D. C. Ophth Otol.
Mason, L. V.
McGregor, J. C.
Moore, P. S., Paed
Parker-Sutton, G. A.
Roffman, Ruth
Russell, E. N.
Schmok, A. C.
Shacklock, H. T.
Smailes, C. L.
Stibbs, D. M.
Stipec, J.
Trembath, J. H.
Trembath, Margaret
Wong, S. L.
Young, D. L.

NORTH VANCOUVER
(23,656)
Alderman, P. M.
Allan, M. L., ThorSurg
Anderson, L. S.
Arber, F. W., GenSurg
Armitage, T. F. H., IntMed
Bartlett, L. H., OrthSurg.
Berghuis, S.
Black, D. M., PH
Blackstock, R. E.
Bonham, G. H., PH
Breen, H., Psy.
Broman, R. D.
Campbell, F. M.
Corbett, W. J.
Coupe, R. L., Derm
Coupland, D. C. T.
Cousins, J. A.
Cragg, G. E.
Davis, R. N., Psy
Didcott, P. R.
Ditchburn, F. G.
Ferries, J. M., Ophth
Flather, V. D.
Gardner, W., Psy
Gelpke, N. H. OrthSurg.
Glass, L. S., ObstGyn
Greene, T. E., DiagRad
Hamilton, J. D.
Hassan, M. L.
Hughes, H. V., Anaes; Otol.
Hunt, B. M.
Jensen, W. G.
Jones, N. C., PlasSurg
Jurcic, P. J., Ophth
Klimczynski, J., Psy
Latham, C. F.
Lee, G. G., GenSurg
Litherland, O. K., IntMed
MacDonald, A. E.
MacGillivray, R. A.
MacLean, Catriona D., Paed
Madill, N. S.
Manning, R. Elizabeth
Marioni, P.
Matheson, D. C., Ophth
Mathieson, D. W.
Mathieson, Joan
McAdam, R., IntMed
McFarlane, W. T., G., Psy
McGregor, N. R.
McLaughlin, G. A., GenSurg
McNeill, C. G.
Meihuizen, S. H.
Mitarewski, W. W., Psy.
Morrall, A. B.
Morrall, S. F.
Morris, H. V.
Morrison, C. G. Ophth.
Mott, G. H., PH
Murray, D. G., Path
Norwell, D. M.
Osborne, J. C., GenSurg
Padwick, P. H., Paed
Parker, J. E., Paed
Parkinson, R. Psy.
Parson, J. V.
Pennet, R. C.
Pollak, J., Rad
Puddicombe, R. T., DiagRad
Richardson, N. L., Psy
Rinfret, P. C.
Smith, H. A., GenSurg., Urol.
Smith, V. P.
Sookochoff, M. W.
Spencer, H. W.
Spielmann, V.
Strang, R., IntMed.
Therrien, Emile E., GenSurg
Thurston, L. M.
Townsley, B. R., Anaes
Tupling, G. D.
Turton, M. R., Paed
Van Uchelen, P. A.
Warner, D. L.
Warnock, Mary D.
Watson, P. A.
Webb, D. A., ObstGyn
Wilson, G. B., IntMed
Winch, G. C., ObstGyn
Yasayko, J. F.

OCEAN FALLS
(3,056)
McDaniel, B. M.
Wahl, O.
Williams, Sybella M.

OLIVER
(1,774)
Ball, N. J.
Bridgman, M. C.
Champion, G.
Hospes, D. E.
Rousseau, P. W.

ONE-HUNDRED-MILE HOUSE
(327)
Bilbey, D. L. J.
Nixon, R. T. H.

OSOYOOS
(1,022)
Cornell, J. M.
Kristjanson, Kristjan
Shepherd, G. H.

OYAMA
(587)
McAnulty, J.

PARKSVILLE
(1,187
Morrison, K. J.
Peterson, D. M.
Urie, M.
Waldman, H. K., DiagRad.

PENTICTON
(13,859)
Barr, H. P.
Barry, M. L., GenSurg
Boyd, D. C.
Emanuele, H.
Foerster, D. K., IntMed
Garrioch, H. G. GenSurg
Gibson, J. J.
Houston, W. B.
Lowden, A. G.
McGregor, H. B.
Nyhus, T. P.
Plecash, M., Urol
Rowe, W. J. Ophth
Selwood, M.
Shiers, J. A., DiagRad
Sloan, S. E. M.
Stapleton, J. H.
Todd, T. N., Anaes
White, W. H. GenSurg
Wickett, W. A.
Yates, D. E., GenSurg

PORT ALBERNI
(11,560)
Bearden, W. A.
Begg, D. C.
Chisholm, W. L.
Garner, R. W. GenSurg
Helem, E. V.
Helem, G. B.
Helem, J. P.
Jones, N. H. GenSurg
Keddis, Erna
Laing, W. B.
Martin, W. E., IntMed.

* Population not separately available.

Miller, A. P.
Pendleton, R. L.
Weaver, K. S. GenSurg

PORT COQUITLAM
(8,111)
Angus, M. F. GenSurg
Baird, J. A.
Batty, D. M.
Cornish, A. L.
Ellis, Mildred
Fisher, F.
Heffeltinger, R. M.
King, A.
Richmond, R. G.
Rigby, F. M.
Shaw, H.
Sinclair, W.
So, Y. P.
Walsh, J.
Wong, C.

PORT HAMMOND
(1,267)
Vander Minne, D.

PORT HARDY
(606)
Gross, H. S.

PORT MOODY
(4,794)
Berkeley, J. A.
Cook, Arlen
Williams, H. R.
Wobick, L.

PORT NELSON
(*)
Nicholson, H. M., Otol

PORT RENFREW
(279)
Veasey, H. B.

POUCE COUPE
(664)
Aylward, B. Z.
Hollies, E. G.

POWELL RIVER
(9700)
Bredo, G. A.
Browett, R. J.
Collins, D. R.
Cookson, W. H., GenSurg
Cunningham, A. J., PH
Fisher, R. E., GenSurg
Gillanders, D. A.
Hobson, G. C., GenSurg.
Lees, M. Anne
MacLeod, J. L.
Perera, F. A., IntMed
Reynolds, P. J.
Wallrap, A. A.
White, H. E.

PRINCE GEORGE
(13,877)
Agnew, T. J.
Braaten, V. F., Paed
Brown, R. E.
Buska, E. S.
Carson, P. J.
Chambers, A. L., GenSurg
Chen, W. T.
Clark, D. M.
Dawkins, W. A., Path
DeRosario J. O., GenSurg
Ewert, R. A., GenSurg
Falk, W. M., Anaes
Hagen, B. A.
Heine, C.
Henry, E. W., IntMed
Horton, T. B.
Jaron, P. W.
Johnson, V. A.
Khare, U.
Killoh, J .A., Ophth
Kinahan, P. J.
Konrad, A. W.
Lee, E. E., ObstGyn
Lim, C. W., DiagRad
Maxwell, L. T., GenSurg
McKellar, J. M.
McKenzie, J. G.
Miller-Tait, R., DiagRad
Moody, D. L., Psy
Pirquet, A. S.
Plummer, P.
Pyper, Joanna F.
Robinson, J. M.
Tadros, P.
Tam, E. A.
Willms, J.
Wirges, H. G.
Woods, P. E.

PRINCE RUPERT
(11,989)
Chun, W. C.
Currie, G.
Ellis, D. G.
Fiddes, G. W. J.
Greene, L. M. GenSurg
Hick, W. B.
Holmes, R. G.
Hussain, S.
Kergin, W. S. GenSurg
Large, R. G. GenSurg
Luck, D., P.H.
Mitchell-Banks, W. H.
Oakley, D.
Schinbein, J. E., GenSurg

PRINCETON
(2,163)
Burr, L. H.
Hicks, A. R.
Roderique, E. M.

QUALICUM BEACH
(759)
de Candole, C. A.
Devito, W. B., DiagRad.
Livingston, P. C., Ophth
MacDonald, A. G.
MacDonald, J. A.
Waldman, H. K., DiagRad

QUEEN CHARLOTTE (CITY)
(283)
Henderson, R. B.
MacKenzie, K. S.
Uptigrove, O.

QUESNEL
(4,673)
Appleby, L. M.
Barber, N. C.
Havens, J. R.
Holley, D. A., GenSurg
Konkin, F.
Maile, J. K.
McGhee, G. D.
McIntyre, W J
Simpson, J. C., GenSurg
Tompkins, J. W.
Word, E. F. GenSurg. Urol.

REVELSTOKE
(3,624)
Armstrong, W. T.
Hamer, H. E.
MacKay, H. J.

RICHMOND
*
Bolduc, W. L.
Brown, B. J.
Campbell, J. M.
Cathcart, L. M.
Charnobay, W.
Clement, D. B.
DeKoven, P.
Doughty, W.
Durity, Joyce V.
Emery, A. W.
Evans, G. H., DiagRad.
Fisher, K. J., Psy
Gilbert, C.
Hodgins, Gladys
Jamieson, A., GenSurg
Kim, P. W.
Lee, H. J.
Lehmann, Elsa
Livingston, M. C.
MacLachlan, R. G. OrthSurg.
Murray, J. R.
Percival-Smith, R. K.
Puetz, Irene M.
Purcell, W. B., Ophth.
Soltanzadeh, A.
Strachan, R. Patricia
Talmey, R. C.
Tamboline, Beverley L.
Tenby, L.
Thompson, A. L.
Turner, A. S.
Varley, J. C.
Watt, J. G., OrthSurg
Wetselaar, H.
White, J. C.
Yang, C. C., ObstGyn.
Yarrow, A. R., Psy
Yurkovich, A.

ROSSLAND
(4,355)
Muth, H. J.
Unruh, H. A.

RUTLAND
(1,495)
Druitt, A. W. N.

SALMO
(894)
Carpenter, J. C.
Norris, P. L.
Pendry, Margaret A.
Stewart, I. F.

SALMON ARM
(1,506)
Barnhouse, L. Dorothy
Bennett, S. Z.
Cundy, R. R.
Deakin, B.
Gulliford, Eve
Henderson, J. R.
Lipsett, W. B.
Lundgren, F. M.
Marits, M.
Masterson T. L., GenSurg.
Williams, A. R.

SARDIS
(898)
Farewell, Anna E. B., Paed
Gordon, Mary E.
Graham, J. G.
Law, C. L.
Meuwissen, H.
Murie, J. J.
Zivot, B. A.

SEA ISLAND
*
Stewart, N. A. Anaes

SECHELT
(492)
Hobson, J. D.
Masterson, T. L., GenSurg
Paetkau, E. J.
Swan, R. A.
Vosburgh, J. W., DiagRad.

SHUSWAP
*
Williams, A. R.

SICAMOUS
(588)
Hemming, F. O.
Hemming, Sarah L.

SIDNEY
(1,558)
Chang, K. H.
Groves, J. S.
Hemmings, C. H.
Meekinson, W. D.
Moffoot, A. G., GenSurg
Ross, D. R. GenSurg
Urena, U.

* Population not separately available.

SMITHERS
(2,487)
Moore, D.
Ryon, Doreen B.
Weare, M. K.

SOOKE
(1,121)
Perry-Whittingham, B. D.
Rotgans, Sheila

SORRENTO
*
Drummond, W. A.

SOUTH BURNABY
Dist. of Vancouver
Baldwin, W. F. ObstGyn
Banno, M.
Blair, W. H. Anaes
Bloemhof, B., Otol
Chan, E. S.
Chu, D. Q. IntMed
Denny, D. A.
Devlin, J. D., IntMed.
Fassaert, H. A.
Fletcher, J. D.
Flint, J. R.
Ford, Joan
Gibson, S. W. Ophth
Gottschling, K. N.
Halliday, R. Psy
Hanna, R. J.
Harlos, R. E.
Heinrichs, P. D.
Martin, W. R., Ophth
Mate, Maria J. Anaes
Matheson, D. C., Ophth.
Matrick, L. E., Psy
McEachren, R. A.
McGill, K. J., ObstGyn
McKee, G. H.
Miller, L. L.
Neufeld, W. P.
Playfair, J. A.
Poole, J. K. Paed
Quirk, L. A.
Rees-Davies, E. Mary
Rideout, C. F.
Robertshaw, A. M.
Robertson, A. L.
Ross, D. A.
Siddall, J. R. Ophth
Siefenpiper, S. H.
Smylie, R. D.
Sproul, R. D. D&TRad
Walcott, D. B. GenSurg
Wallis, W. G., Psy
Watts, P. R.
Yip, S. W.

SQUAMISH
(1,558)
Kindree, L. C.
MacEwen, H. B. Anaes.
Rimmer, A. H. M.
Slade, S. E.

STEVESTON
(2,207)
Graves, C. A.

STEWART
(323)
Kennedy, A.

STILLWATER
(167)
Paine, G. C.

SUMMERLAND
(3,893)
Moss, Barbara A., Paed.
Williston, D. N.

TAHSIS
(504)
Calleia, Sarah G.

TAPPEN
*
Barnhouse, L. Dorothy, Anaes.

TERRACE
(4,682)
Boyd, G.
Chiasson, M.
Christensen, K. H.
Galizia, E. J.
Hicks, R. B.
Lee, R. E., GenSurg
Nicholson, J. R., ObstGyn.

TOFINO
(441)
McDiarmid, H. R.
Wheeldon, P. J.

TRAIL
(11,580)
Alvarez, A. F. GenSurg
Berno, E.
Brockway, E. N. OrthSurg
Campbell, H. C.
Christie, H. R. ObstGyn
Clark, R. F. Anaes
Colbert, J. G.
Crawford, D. J. M. IntMed
Daly, J. S. IntMed
D'Appolonia, G. L.
Dimock, H. B. IntMed
Dorgelo, G. H., Paed
Endicott, W. J.
Friesen, G., GenSurg
Gnass, J. E., Path
Graham-Marr, J. H. ObstGyn
Harrigan, J. R.
Love, R. A., IntMed
Mackenzie, C. J.
Mansfield, G. R. Psy
Mason, J. T. DiagRad
Muth, H. A., IntMed
Nicol, W. G., Ophth
Royle, N. D. ObstGyn
Simonetta, L. R.
Schmitt, M. PH
Stefanelli, J. GenSurg
Tannen, P. A.
Waterlow, Doreen
Wilson, F. L. D & TRad
Wrinch, L. B.

VALEMOUNT
(382)
Thompson, A. L.

VANCOUVER
(850,000)
Acheson, T. W.
Adilman, P. H.
Adler, H. G., Psy.
Adler, K.
Adrian, A.
Adrian, J. J.
Agnew, G. A.
Akins, K. B., Psy
Aldis, Pamela W.
Alexander, E. H. Ophth,Otol
Alexander, J. D. F. GenSurg
Allen, C. S. OrthSurg,
GenSurg.
Allen, P. GenSurg, ThorSurg
Amar, J. C., IntMed
Anderson, D. O., IntMed
Anderson, J. C.
Anderson, J. L.
Andrews, L. G., PhysMed& Rehab, Paed.
Angelomatis, S. G.
Ankenman, G. J. Urol
Appleby, K. G.
Appleby, L. H. GenSurg
Arbuckle, J. W. Jr. Urol.
Arena, U.
Arnold, C. R. IntMed
Asano, K.
Ashby, R. M.
Ashmore, P. G., GenSurg,
ThorSurg
Aspinall, R. J., Path Bact
Atkins, A. S. IntMed.
Atkinson, K. G., GenSurg
Attridge, F. R. Otol.
Auckland, N. L. D. Neur.
Austin, W. E. GenSurg.
Avery, J. F.
Avery, L. E., GenSurg.
Babatzanis, J., Psy
Bachop, D. M.
Badger, G. A. Otol.
Badre, E. J. P. GenSurg,
PlasSurg
Bagnall, A. W. IntMed.
Bain, T. D.
Baird, M. M. IntMed.
Baird, R. M., GenSurg
Baker, H. Paed.
Baker, H. G. IntMed
Baker, L. K.
Baker, S. W.
Baker-Thomas, Shirley M.
Baldwin, S. G. ObstGyn
Balfour, J. Urol.
Ballantyne, Gwyneth J.
Balmer, I. A.
Barber, P. A.
Barclay, W. S. IntMed (T.B.)
Barnbrook, R. B., Anaes
Barner, H. D.
Barnett, R. D.
Baron, P. J., GenSurg.
Basco, Vivian E., TherRad
Beach, D. W.
Bebb, D. E.
Becher, J. C.
Beck, R. E. IntMed
Beckett, M. C.
Beiser, M.
Bell, D. N.
Bell-Irving, P. IntMed
Bell-Irving, R. W. IntMed
Bell, J. N., Path.
Bensimon, J. R., Paed
Berger, B. Ophth
Belten, M. K., Anaes.
Berry, K., Neur
Berry, Marion, Anaes
Bezeredi, T., Psy.
Bickle, J. A.
Bie, W. F., ObstGyn.
Bigelow, H. M.
Birkbeck, J. A., Paed
Bismanis, J. Bact.
Bisson, R. D.
Bjarnason, A. E.
Black, I., Path
Black, J. H.
Blair, E. Murray. ObstGyn.
Blair, N. J. Otol
Blair, W. H.
Blanchard, J. D.
Blundell, S. F.
Bogoch, A. IntMed.
Bogoch, M. A., Paed.
Boland, Kathrine E.
Bolton, D. M.
Bonnell, R. R. DiagRad
Bonnell, S.
Boucher, H. H. OrthSurg.
Boulter, W. L. ObstGyn
Bowie, I. A.
Bowlsby, C. S. DiagRad
Bowmer, E. J. Bact
Boxall, E. A. IntMed.
Boxer, A.
Boyd, J. R. ObstGyn
Boyd, R. W. D & TRad
Boyes, D. A., ObstGyn,
TherRad.
Brand, T. M. IntMed
Bratty, P. J. Neurol.
Braun, W.
Bridge, H. W., Psy.
Bridge, T., DiagRad
Britten, S. E.
Brooke, H. H. W. D & TRad
Broughton, Florence E., Psy.
Brown, A. P.

*** Population not separately available.**

Vancouver (Cont'd.)
Brown, D. A., GenSurg
Brown, D. A.
Brown, W. T., Psy.
Browne, J. K., OrthSurg.
Browne, N. L. Psy
Brummitt, J. R., Paed
Brumwell, C. A.
Brunton, L. J., PhysMed. & Rehab.
Bryans, F. E. ObstGyn
Buck, H. W., Derm
Buckler, W. St. J.
Burke, G. L. OrthSurg.
Burmeister, R. F.
Burnes, J. S. D. GenSurg
Burwell, W. K., ObstGyn.
Busheikin, T. M., ObstGyn.
Cairns, A. R., IntMed
Cairns, J. A., Ophth.
Cambon, Eileen S., Ophth
Cambon, K. G. Otol
Cameron, D. M., DiagRad.
Campbell, A.
Campbell, C. A., DiagRad
Campbell, D. A.
Campbell, K. A., Paed.
Campbell, N. J., Anaes.
Caple, H. H. ObstGyn.
Carballo, A. S., Anaes.
Card, L. W. B. D & TRad.
Carlson, R. J.
Carpenter, C. W., ObstGyn
Carroll, J. J. Anaes.
Carruthers, B. M., IntMed
Cashmore, A .A.
Cathcart, L. M.
Caturay, G.
Cave, G. D., GenSurg
Cawker, C. A. M. Urol
Chambers, H. L. H. Urol.
Chan, E. J., Derm.
Chan, G. H.
Chan, T. S.
Chang, J. Anaes
Chang, S. K.
Chang, T. Y. GenSurg.
Charlton, W. J. GenSurg.
Chase, W. H. Path
Chepesuik, M. W. IntMed
Cherkezoff, A.
Chisholm, H. A. GenSurg.
Chiu, W. G.
Chodos, Hedwige, Ophth
Chodos, J. B., Ophth
Chong, H.
Chou, L. Y., Paed.
Christensen, H. F.
Christensen, R. M., GenSurg.
Christie, D. IntMed.
Christie, R. G., Psy
Christensen, R. M. GenSurg.
Christopherson, E. IntMed
Chu, F. S.
Chung, M. H. ObstGyn
Chung, W. B. GenSurg
Claman, A. D. ObstGyn.
Clark, G. F., Anaes.
Clark, N. H.
Clay, M. G., GenSurg
Clement, G. H. GenSurg.
Clokie, J. K. A.
Cluff, J. W. NeurSurg.
Coburn, W. A.
Cockcroft, W. H., Bact.
Coddington, R. D. GenSurg
Cody, P. C., OphthOtol.
Cohen, A. Ophth.
Cohen, L. G.
Coles, J. M., Psy
Colley, R. Q., Ophth.
Collison, D. B. ObstGyn
Coltart, J. L.
Connolly, J. F., ObstGyn.
Cook, C. E. OrthSurg.
Cooper, H. G. Urol
Cope, G. W.
Copp, D. H.
Corbett, W. J.
Cork, J. F.
Costello, J. B. ObstGyn
Coulson, G. M.
Courtemanche, A. D., PlasSurg
Coverton, C. C. IntMed
Cowan, R. J. GenSurg., PlasSurg
Cox, A. R., IntMed
Cox, K. G.
Cox, Margaret
Coy, P., TherRad.
Crawford, C. S. GenSurg
Crawford, G. M. TherRad
Crawford, Lois D. Anaes
Crawford, W. A.
Crichton, J. V., Paed.
Cronhelm, C. H. ObstGyn
Cserepes, A. O., GenSurg.
Cull, J. S. PH
Cuylits, M. Helen
Dalrymple, T.
Dalzell, R. T., Path.
D'Amico, Rina M.
Danto, J. L. DermSyph.
David, C. J.
Davidson, A. E. Psy
Davidson, A. M. DermSyph.
Davidson, G. A. NeurPsy.
Davidson, J. R. GenSurg
Davidson, K. DermSyph
Davies, C. E. Ophth.
Davies, E. Mary, PhysMed. & Rehab.
Davies, L. E. C.
Davies, Lois E., Anaes.
Davis, H. R. L.
Davis, T. W., IntMed
Day, E. E. Ophth,Otol.
Dean, J. Paed
Deane, Diane H.
Deane, L., ObstGyn.
Debenham, P. A., Anaes.
de Groot, L. C., Paed.
DeKaban, A. S.
deMaria, F. J., ObstGyn
Dennis, J. W. Anaes
DesBrisay, H. A. IntMed.
Devlin, J. D., IntMed.
Dewick, Betty C.
Dibaji, S. N., GenSurg.
Dick, J. IntMed.
Dickey, M. R. DiagRad.
Dickinson, J. H. ObstGyn
Dlin, B. M. Psy.
Dobrey, A. N., Anaes
Dodd, W. A. H., Derm.
Dodds, W. A. Anaes
Dodek, M.
Doll, W. A., Anaes
Dolman, C. E. Bact.
Dolman, Clarisse Path
Donnelly, C. W.
Donnelly, K. R.
Donnelly, T. H.
Donovan, E. G. DiagRad
Dorman, J. G.
Dorrance, W. J. GenSurg
Dower, G. E.
Dowsley, G. A.
Doyle, P. J., Otol.
Drache, V. GenSurg.
Drance, S. M., Ophth
Duffield, Anne, Anaes
Dumont, H. Anaes
Duncan, A. C. GenSurg.
Duncan, R. GenSurg
Dunham, B. T.
Dunn, H. G. Paed
Dunn, W. L., Path
Dunnett, I. P., ObstGyn
DuVernet, E. O. Anaes.
Dwyer, C. H.
Dyakowski, S.
Earle, M. R., ObstGyn.
Eden, J.
Edgar, M. L.
Elliot, A. J., Ophth
Elliot, G. R. F. PH
Elliot, J. A. F. GenSurg.
Elliot, S. G. Otol
Elliott, F. W.
Elliott, G. B., Path
Ellis, Mildred G.
Ellison, Lucille G.
Emmons, W. F., Neur., NeurSurg.
Engen, E. S.
English, R. A., Path
Epp, D. L.
Epp, F. L.
Esdale, W. L. Anaes
Evans, A. M. TherRad
Evans, S. E. ObstGyn.
Evelyn, K. A. IntMed
Ewasew, L. M.
Ewasew, W. T.
Fahrni, B. M. IntMed
Fahrni, G. S. GenSurg.
Fahrni, W. H. OrthSurg.
Faigen, M., Derm
Farish, J. R. GenSurg.
Farquhar, D. J.
Farquharson, R. A., GenSurg
Fast, C. W., IntMed.
Fayerman, J. W., Otol
Feir, T. C., Psy
Fenwick, J. B. IntMed.
Fidler, H. K. Path
Fishault, S. H.
Fishman, S., IntMed
Fitterman, H. N., Ophth
Fitzosborne, D. J.
Fleck, Elizabeth B.
Fleming, J. P., PlasSurg
Fleming, K. O. Ophth.
Forbes, W. D., GenSurg.
Ford, D. K., IntMed.
Ford, Joan J.
Forseng, E. G., Anaes
Forward, A. D., GenSurg
Fournier, C. J. DermSyph
Fowler, W. J. NeurSurg.
Fox, M.
Foxgord, R. N.
Frackson, S. H.
Francis, G. H. Otol.
Fraser, Christina A., D & T Rad.
Fraser, G. D.
Fratkin, L. B. GenSurg.
Friedman, S. M.
Friesen, L. V. C.
Frinton, E., DiagRad
Frkovich, G. GenSurg
Froese, D. W.
Frost, A. C., ObstGyn
Frost, H. M. ObstGyn
Frost, J. W. GenSurg.
Fulton, J. B. Anaes
Funk, E. H. GenSurg
Gaerber, B. J. Psy.
Galbraith, C. L.
Gale, H. V. B.
Ganshorn, J. A. GenSurg.
Gardiner, D. M. C., Anaes.
Garner, F. R. PH
Garner, Mary K.
Garrow, Barbara M., Neur
Garrow, D. G. DiagRad
Gayman, G. R. Paed.
Gayton, J. L. PH
Gee, Evelyn A. PathBact
Gell, G. W.
Gerein, A. N., ThorSurg.
Gerrie, R. G.
Ghabrial, S. L., Paed.
Gibbons, A. K. Anaes
Gibson, J. M. W., TherRad.
Gibson, T. C.
Gibson, W. C. NeurPsy.

* Population not separately available.

Vancouver (Cont'd.)
Gilchrist, R. A.
Gillespie, H. S. OrthSurg.
Gillies, G. E., GenSurg.
Gillis, J. G. IntMed
Gilmour, J. L., GenSurg
Goel, Devendra P., GenSurg
Goertzen, G.
Gofton, J. P. IntMed
Goldie, J. S.
Goldman, W. P. GenSurg.
Gomel, V., ObstGyn
Goodman, B. GenSurg
Goodman, G. B., TherRad
Gordon, A. A., IntMed.
Gordon, G.
Gordon, G.
Goresky, Dorothy
Goresky, W. V. Psy
Gorkin, M.
Gould. C. E. G. Neur
Gould, G. A.
Gourlay, R. H. ThorSurg, GenSurg
Govan, W. R. GenSurg
Graham, B. D., Paed.
Graham, D. C., IntMed.
Graham, K. S.
Grant, J. A. C.
Grant, J. H. B. Paed.
Grantham, P. R.
Grasset, A. V.
Grauer, F. W. GenSurg, Orth Surg.
Graves, H. B. Anaes.
Gray, D. W.
Gray, E. J., GenSurg
Gray, G. R., Path
Gray, T.
Greaven, W. F.
Green, P. D.
Greenberg, A. B.
Greig, J. H. DiagRad
Griffiths, M. E. M. Anaes
Griggs, F. C.
Grimson, J. C.
Groves, K. P., GenSurg
Grzybowski, S., IntMed.
Gundry, C. H. Psy.
Gung, E. B.
Gunn, S. W., GenSurg
Guntscheff, N.
Gurjar, M.
Halak, J.
Hall, M. E. GenSurg.
Hall, R. M. DiagRad
Hall, W. M. Anaes.
Halliday, R.
Hancock, R. J., GenSurg
Hankinson, H. W.
Hanley, F. W. Psy
Hardie, M. J.
Harold, T. C.
Hardin, E. D., Psy
Hardwick, D. F., Path
Hardyment, A. F. Path
Harris, G. S., Ophth
Harrison, C. P., DiagRad
Harrison, G. S.
Harrison, J. E. ObstGyn.
Harrison, R. C., GenSurg.
Harrison, W. E. GenSurg, ThorSurg.
Harry, B. H.
Hart, R. G.
Hartwell, L. W.
Hatfield, W. H. IntMed
Hawkes, V. S.
Hay, M. C.
Hayes, R. M.
Henry, A. T. GenSurg.
Hepworth, R. G., Urol
Herberts, E. D. Urol.
Herstein, A. ObstGyn.
Hertzman, V. O. IntMed.
Hiddleston, J. M., Anaes
Hignell, B.
Hill, A. E., IntMed
Hill, K. C., OrthSurg.
Hill, R. H., Paed
Hingston, Etheline E.
Hingston, J. Paed
Hirt, N. B. Psy
Ho, F. C.
Ho, W. C., GenSurg.
Hobbs, F. S. ObstGyn.
Hofmann, W. G.
Holt, Danica M.
Holubitsky, I. B., GenSurg
Honey, J. W.
Hooper, P. W., ObstGyn., GenSurg.
Horan, J. D., IntMed
Horii, A.
Hornung, Alisa
Hornung, Judith
Hornung, L.
Hotti, A. R.
Hseih, Y. S., ObstGyn
Hsu, S. H., Anaes
Huckvale, W. S.
Hudson, P. W. Anaes
Hugill, J. T. Anaes.
Hunt, A. L., ObstGyn.
Hunter, C. W.
Hunter, J. G. IntMed
Hurlburt, F. W. B. IntMed.
Hutton, G. H. Psy.
Ibbott, J. W. IntMed
Inglis, A. M. OrthSurg
Ingram, G. D., ObstGyn.
Ireland, J. A. DiagRad
Irish, R. H.
Ironside, J. J. GenSurg
Irvine, W. G.
Irving, J. A. Ophth
Irving, R. T., GenSurg
Iseli, H.
Israels, M. G., IntMed
Israels, S. IntMed; Paed.
Izatt, Jean A.
Jacks, Q. D. Otol
Jackson, C. C.
Jackson, P. P. GenSurg.
Jacobsen, A. K.
Jain, K. K. NeurSurg
James, A. W., Path
James, E. S. Paed
Jamison, C. A., DiagRad.
Jeffries, R. C., IntMed
Jenkins, L. C. Anaes
Jenkner, Sarah M.
Johnson, A. M. IntMed.
Johnson, E. A.
Johnson, Elizabeth M., Paed
Johnson, Gwendolyn O.
Johnson, H. W., Urol
Johnston, A. C.
Johnston, Margaret M., Derm.
Johnstone, F. R. GenSurg
Jones, D. P. Neur
Jones, E. A.
Jones, R. A. Anaes
Jones, R. C. GenSurg
Judd. A. B. IntMed
Kaleal, I. S.
Kalla, F. P.
Kamburoff, Tonka D.
Kane, E. W.
Kanee, B. DermSyph.
Kaplan, S.
Karjala, R. J., IntMed
Karme, A. B., Psy.
Kavanagh-Gray, Doris M. IntMed.
Kaye, C. H.
Kazun, W. J.
Keen, W. H., DiagRad.
Kemp, W. N. Anaes.
Kennedy, H. K., PH
Kennedy, W. W.
Kenny, P. N. Anaes
Kent, I. H., Psy.
Kepkay, P. H. IntMed
Kerr, R. B. IntMed.
Kerridge, J. H., IntMed
Kester, H. A., Anaes.
Kettyls, G. D., PH
Khairat, O.
Kidd, H. M.
Killett, J. R.
Kincade, G. F. IntMed (TB)
King, D. M.
Kirby, O. E. Ophth, Otol
Kirk, D. K.
Kirkbride, R. A. IntMed
Kirkpatrick, G. J. A. GenSurg
Kirkpatrick, G. M. Psy
Klady, A.
Klassen, P. W., Anaes.
Kliffer, E.
Kliman, M. R. GenSurg
Knickerbocker, W. J., DiagRad
Knott, N. D. IntMed.
Knudsen, A. M.
Kolotyluk, K.
Kolotyluk, W.
Komar, L.
Kong, G. P., Otol
Koop, W. H.
Korec, V.
Krause, M. E.
Kringhaug, O.
Krisman, A. M., ObstGyn
Krivel, H. Paed.
Kromar, L.
Laidlaw, R. A.
Laimon, H., GenSurg
Lake, J. R.
Langley, G. E.
Langston, R. G. PlasSurg, GenSurg
Large, G. C. Otol.
Lauener, R. W., IntMed
Laundy, P. W.
Lawler, A. W. IntMed
Layng, J. M.
Lazorko, W.
Leamy, P. J.
Lederman, J. A.
Ledgerwood, E. F.
Lee, A., Paed.
Lee, Flaviana S.
Lehmann, E. C. H. OrthSurg.
Lehmann, P. O. NeurSurg.
Leighton, K. M.
Leishman, J. D., Urol.
Leroux, J. A. IntMed
Leung, J.
Leung, S. W.
Levene, D. L.
Leviczky, Bella E.
Levine, M.
Levson, H.
Levy, L. A.
Lewchuk, Wm.
Lewis, T. H. C., IntMed.
Lewison, E. Otol.
Leyland, E. E., Psy
Liaw, W. C.
Lin, W.
Lindenfeld, B.
Lindenfeld, Elda, Psy
Lindsay, J. H.
Lipinski, E., Psy.
Lirenman, D. S., IntMed.
Litherland, H. K., GenSurg
Litherland, O. K. IntMed
Little, G. E.
Little, Shauna, Psy
Livingstone, C. S. Paed
Lockhart, H. B. Otol
Lockie, J. G.
Loh, G.
Longley, J. D. DiagRad
Longley, Joy
Longpre, L. F. Urol
Loo, L.
Lowry, R. B., Paed

* Population not separately available.

Lu, L. C.-T., Path.
MacAskill, A. D. Ophth
MacCrostie, M. W. Anaes.
MacDonald, A. A.
MacDonald, D. A., Urol
MacDonald, D. C. Psy.
MacDonald, D. K.
Macdonald, R. J.
MacDonald, W. C., IntMed
MacDougall, J. A. GenSurg.
MacEwan, W. R. ObstGyn.
MacFadyn, D. J., Neurol
MacKay, Doris E., Anaes, Phys Med & Rehab
MacKay, G. GenSurg.
MacKay, R. D.
MacKechnie, H. A. DermSyph
Mackenzie, F. D. GenSurg
Mackenzie, I. D.
MacKenzie, J. C.
MacKenzie, T. C.
MacKenzie-Sawers, V. Lois Paed.
MacKinnon, G. L. ObstGyn.
MacLaren, R. D.
MacLean, B., Anaes
MacLean, C. A. IntMed
MacLean, J. R. Paed
MacLennan, Jean M. Paed.
MacMillan, J. A.
MacNeil, H. C., OrthSurg
MacNutt, L. W.
MacPherson, M. M. GenSurg.
MacPherson, R. I., DiagRad.
Maddin, W. S. DermSyph.
Madill, J. S. D & TRad.
Maguire, W. T.
Maisonville, P. S. Ophth
Makaroff, R. P.
Mallek, H. Ophth.
Mallek, J. IntMed.
Manning, W. L.
Manson, A. B., GenSurg
Marcus, A. M., Psy
Margetts, E. L. Psy
Markham, W. G.
Marsden, J.
Marshall, R. H. GenSurg
Marteinsson, B. T. H. GenSurg.
Marshall, R. H. GenSurg
Mason, L. V.
Masterson, T. L. GenSurg.
Mather, J. M. PH
Matheson, D. Anaes
Mathisen, A. K. IntMed
Matthews, C. A.
Maybee, T. K., IntMed.
McAmmond, E. N. C. GenSurg.
McCaffrey, F. W. Anaes.
McCaffrey, R. P.
McCall, W. J.
McCallum, W. M.
McClure, W. G.
McColl, D. T.
McConkey, A. S. OrthSurg.
McConnell, J. A., Anaes
McCoy, E. C.
McCreary, J. F. Paed
McCreery, R. G., Ophth
McCurrach, A. C. D & TRad
McDonagh, J. E. ObstGyn.
McDonald, H. D.
McDonnell, C. E., IntMed
McDougall, G. M., Psy
McFetridge, S. A. GenSurg
McGhee, J. J., GenSurg
McGivern, E. A.
McGraw, R. W., OrthSurg.
McGreer, P. L.
McIntosh, H. D., Psy
McIntosh, H. W. IntMed.
McKechnie, R. E. GenSurg.
McKee, W. M.
McKenna, L. B.
McKenzie, A. D. GenSurg.
McKinlay, W. D. Ophth.
McKinnon, R. C. PhysMed & Rehab.
McLean, J. A. Ophth.
McLeod, E. C.
McLeod, W. A., Derm.
McMaster, E. Susan PH
McMillen, N. R. J. Anaes
McNab, J. A. Anaes
McNair, A. Y. IntMed, PathBact.
McNaughton, R. H. ObstGyn
McPherson, G. D., OrthSurg
McPhillips, A. S. G.
McTaggart, A. N., Psy
Meloche, L. Anaes.
Mercer, E. N., IntMed.
Merler, C., GenSurg
Merler, T.
Meuwissen, H.
Milbrandt, W. E.
Milburn, H. H.
Millar, J. W. ObstGyn
Millar, R. D. Anaes.
Millar, T. P., Psy
Miller, H. S. OrthSurg
Miller, J. M.
Miller, S. D & TRad.
Mills, F. G., Psy
Milne, D. R. S.
Milne, G. D.
Minnes, J. F. Ophth
Minorgan, G. A. Psy
Minovitz, O. IntMed
Mirabel, L. IntMed
Mirhady, F. Paed
Mirhady, Katharine E.
Mitchell, J. C. DermSyph
Mitchell, W. J.
Moffatt, C. D.
Moffatt, D. W.
Moghadam-Kazrini, H., PH
Moir, I. S.
Moir, R. S., Anaes
Moghadam, H. K. Paed
Molaro, A. L., IntMed
Moloney, P. J., Urol.
Monteith, J. S.
Moody, D. L., Psy
Moore, A. H. GenSurg.
Moore, P. S. Paed
Morrison, J. E.
Morrison, M.
Morris, D.
Morse, P. W. IntMed
Mortimer-Lamb, C.
Morton, J. W. IntMed
Morton, K. S. OrthSurg
Morton, W. A. GenSurg.
Morton, W. R., Ophth
Moscovich, B. B., IntMed
Moscovich, J. IntMed.
Mowat, D. IntMed.
Moyes, A.
Moyes, P. D., NeurSurg
Muirhead, W. R.
Mullinger, Margaret, Paed
Munroe, D. S. IntMed.
Munroe, J. P., Anaes
Munroe, J. D.
Murdoch, F. T.
Murdoch, G. W.
Murdoch, J. H.
Murdoch, Monica E. M., Psy.
Murphy, H. O. IntMed
Murray, A. A. GenSurg
Murray, A. D., Paed
Murray, D. G. Path
Musgrove, J. E. GenSurg
Naden, J. R. OrthSurg.
Nanson, G. L.
Nelles, T. R. B.
Nelson, A. J. PH
Nestman, J. M.
Neufeld, W. P.
Newman, R. L., Psy
Newstone, J. M.
Ney, P. G., Psy
Nichka, B. A., Otol
Nichol, H., Psy
Nicholson, M. A.
Nickerson, K. G. ObstGyn
Nixon, J. C.
Nixon, J. E. Anaes
Noble, R. L.
Norton, G. I. D & TRad.
Novak, Sylvia
Oakey, R.
O'Donnell, J. P. Anaes.
Olacke, F. A., DiagRad
Orchard, D. D.
Orlaw, R. G.
Osberg, E. A., DiagRad.
Osborne, J. A. IntMed
Osler, T. R. GenSurg.
Paige, B. F. IntMed.
Paine, R. J. Ophth.
Palmer, R. A. IntMed.
Panton, W. D.
Paris, R. P., Paed
Parkinson, R., Psy
Parks, J.
Parmley, J. R.
Parnell, J. L. IntMed.
Patrick, W. H. L.
Paterson, I. S., Anaes
Patterson, F. P. OrthSurg.
Patterson, L. A.
Patterson, W. J. Otol
Pedlaw, A. L.
Percheson, P. B. Anaes.
Peretz, D. I., IntMed
Perie, G. E., Paed
Perlman, I.
Perrett, T. S. GenSurg.
Petriw, J.
Piderman, J. P.
Piercy, Dorothy
Pinkerton, A. C. PhysMed
Pinkerton, E. K.
Pirie, G. E.
Piters, J. Paed.
Pitts, H. H. PathBact.
Pitts, H. H., Jr. Otol.
Poland, Betty J. ObstGyn
Poole, J. C. Anaes.
Posener, L. J. Paed
Potts, D. W.
Pow, C. G. PlasSurg.
Powell, H. C.
Powell, T. E. Anaes
Pratt-Johnson, J. A., Ophth
Preston, F. C. GenSurg, OrthSurg.
Price, G. E., IntMed
Price, J. D., IntMed
Prosterman, D. B. OrthSurg
Pump, K. K. IntMed.
Purkis, R. S.
Rad, S. F., GenSurg
Rae, M. V. PathBact
Ragan, J. D. Ophth
Ragan, T. M., Otol
Ragona, P.
Rally, C. R. IntMed
Randall, H. S. Anaes.
Randall, J. D.
Ranta, L. E. PH, Bact
Raynor, E. F. Ophth,Otol
Read, A. M.
Read, W. R., Psy.
Rees-Davies, P. E. GenSurg.
Reed, R. H. B. OrthSurg.
Reid, J. A. G. Cardiol, IntMed
Rennie, C. S. IntMed.
Richards, J. S. F., Ophth.
Rigg, J. M., Paed
Ritch, Elsie, Anaes
Ritchie, J. G., Anaes
Rivers, W. A.
Roach, C. J. Anaes.
Robb, G. M. L., GenSurg

* Population not separately available.

Roberts, F. J., Path
Roberts, H. E.
Robertshaw, A. M.
Robertson, C. E., Path
Robertson, D.
Robertson, G. D.
Robertson, R. GenSurg, Orth Surg., ThorSurg.
Robins, R. E. GenSurg.
Robinson, Barbara L.
Robinson, C. E. G. IntMed.
Robinson, E. G.
Robinson, E. S.
Robinson, G. L. Anaes.
Robinson, G. C. F. Paed
Robinson, H. S. IntMed
Roburn, M., Psy.
Rogers, R. H.
Ronan, Alice. Anaes
Rosenblatt, J.
Rosenfeld, M. W.
Ross, H. M.
Ross, J. E. ObstGyn
Roy, B. R.
Rubin, M.
Rush, R. D.
Rushton, Shirley J.
Rutherford, T. F., Path.
Ryan, C. A. OrthSurg.
St. Louis, H. E.
Salsbury, C. R. GenSurg
Salvador, H. S., ObstGyn.
Sandilands, J. IntMed
Sands, C. A. Anaes.
Sandy, J. T. GenSurg
Sarjeant, T. R. GenSurg.
Saunders, F. E. ObstGyn.
Saunders, W. G.
Sawers, V. Lois Paed
Saxton, G. D. GenSurg
Schaffer, L.
Schilder, G. IntMed.
Schofer, R. C., Anaes
Schom, C.
Schultz, M. H. Anaes
Schulzer, Gerza
Schulzer, M.
Schwartzkopff, O. M.
Schwarz, C. J., Psy
Scott, H. IntMed.
Scott, R. F. Path
Screech, G. Anaes
Secter, J. J.
Segal, S. Paed
Seraglia, M., IntMed
Sereno, L. R.
Shaker, G. T.
Shallard, B. T. IntMed.
Shaw, J. M.
Shaw, M. H. IntMed
Shaw, W. F.
Shea, M. B. B. Anaes.
Shepherd, W. E., Path
Sherkat, A., DiagRad
Shier, A. A.
Shier, J. W.
Shim, S. S., OrthSurg
Shimokura, H. M.
Shuman, B. Paed.
Sigal, C., Derm.
Sigurdson, F. T.
Simpson, C.
Simpson, D. G. Ophth.
Simpson, R. E. Anaes
Simpson, W. W. IntMed.
Sinanan, E. G., Otol.
Singleton, A. B.
Singleton, Jean A.
Skinner, F. L. IntMed.
Skwarok, E. W. NeurSurg.
Skwarok, R. L. Psy
Slade, H. C., IntMed., Psy.
Sladen, J. G., GenSurg
Slakov, R., Psy
Sleath, G. E. Anaes
Sleath, G. W.
Sleigh, A. D., Psy
Sloan, W. L. D & TRad.
Smaill, W. D. GenSurg.
Smith, E. L. Ophth
Smith, G. G. ObstGyn.
Smith, H. A. GenSurg. Urol
Smith, J. D., Obst
Smith, J. H.
Sochowski, J.
Soloniuk, V. J.
Soltan, A., GenSurg.
Sovilj, V., Paed
Sparkes, J. W. OrthSurg.
Speakman, G. F. Ophth
Spiro, H. M. DiagRad.
Spitzer, R. W.
Spohn, A. H. Paed
Spouge, J. D.
Spruenken, J. M.
Sreter, F. A.
Stalker, H. S. IntMed (TB)
Stanley, R. A.
Stansfield, H. IntMed
Stanwood, D. H.
Stebnick, A. O., Otol
Steiman, I.
Stephenson, G. H. Psy
Stevens, W. B.
Stevenson, J. D. D & TRad
Stewart, A. J. Ophth
Stewart, D. W.
Stewart, W. D. Derm, IntMed
Stockdale, E.
Stockton, W. H. S. Paed.
Stoffman, I. W.
Stothers, R. J., DiagRad
Stout, T. D.
Strachan, S. A.
Strang, R.
Stordy, S. M., IntMed
Stringer, D. W.
Sturdy, J. Path
Summers, J. J.
Sutherland, W. H. GenSurg
Sutter, Mary Alice, ObstGyn
Sutter, M. C.
Sylling, Margaret F.
Symington, D. C., IntMed
Tait, W. M. DiagRad
Tam, Y. D.
Tamboline, Beverley L.
Tanton, B. W. Otol.
Tate, R. G., OrthSurg
Taylor, H. E. PathBact.
Taylor, W. R. Otol.
Te, L. T., Anaes
Teasdale, J. Mavis, Paed
Tecson, M. P., Psy
Telford, D. GenSurg.
Telford, K. M. IntMed.
Termansen, P. E., Psy.
Thiessen, N.
Thomas, J. C. NeurPsy.
Thomas, W. D., ObstGyn.
Thompson, A. L.
Thompson, B. H., DiagRad
Thompson, G. B. NeurSurg
Thompson, R. D.
Thompson, W. J. OrthSurg.
Thomson, F. B. GenSurg.
Thorleifson, W. H. D & TRad.
Thurgar, A. M.
Thurston, W. G. ObstGyn
Tischler, I., Psy.
Tobe, A. D., IntMed
Tompsett, D. A.
Traill, A.
Trapp, E. TherRad
Trapp, W. G., GenSurg; ThorSurg
Traynor, J. A. IntMed.
Tredger, Enid
Treffry, C. J. Paed
Treloar, E. J., Anaes
Trevor-Smith, E. S.
Trites, A. E. W. Path
Trowbridge, E. B. ObstGyn
Trueman, G. E. DiagRad.
Tucker, F. G. Psy
Turko, M. ObstGyn.
Turnbull, A. D & TRad.
Turnbull, F. A. NeurSurg
Turnbull, I. M., NeurSurg.
Turnbull, W. L.
Turner, M. R., Anaes.
Turvey, S. E. C. IntMed, Neur.
Twohig, M. J., GenSurg
Tyhurst, J. S. Psy
Tyhurst, L.
Tysoe, F. W. ObstGyn.
Uchida, M.
Urbanek, Z.
Van Norden, H. J.
Van Norden, Julia
Van Rosen, Elsie
Varnam, K. D.
Verbrugge, M. Urol.
Verbrugge, Magdalenus, Urol
Vince, D. J. Paed
Voth, A. R.
Wackenroder, H. GenSurg
Wada, J. A., NeurSurg
Wadman, H. G. ObstGyn
Wakefield, G. E. IntMed.
Waldie, A. C.
Walker, Elspeth
Walker, J. E. IntMed
Wall, M. D.
Wallace, A. W.
Walsh, G. C. IntMed.
Walters, M. B. IntMed.
Warcup, L. W. GenSurg.
Ward, S. L. GenSurg.
Warne, J. W.
Warner, D. M., Ophth
Warner, R. M.
Warren, A. J. NeurPsy
Wassar, P. S.
Watson, G. L.
Watt, J. G.
Watt, W. D.
Weaver, H. G.
Webber, W. A.
Weekes, W. E.
Weir, M. C.
Westgate, F. G. GenSurg.
Weston, Agnes. PH
White, J. C.
White, J. V.
White, R. A. GenSurg
Whitelaw, D. M. IntMed
Whitelaw, J. W. Paed.
Whitman, R. L. Psy
Whittaker, K. W. B.
Whittal, J. K. Anaes
Wiens, A. T. DiagRad
Wignall, N. Path
Wilkie, T. F., PlasSurg
Wilks, W. E.
Will, P. K., Paed
Williams, C. E.
Williams, D. H. DermSyph
Williams, K.
Williams, L. J. GenSurg.
Williams, L. R. Urol.
Williams, S. L. GenSurg.
Willis, H.
Willits, Reba, PH
Wilson, F. D. OrthSurg
Wilson, H. E.
Wilson, J. R. Psy.
Wilson, R. A. IntMed, Paed
Wilson, R. GenSurg.
Wilson, R. G.
Wilson, W. M. G. Ophth
Wilson, W. S.
Winbigler, H. C.
Winch, G. C., ObstGyn
Winrob, H.
Wolochow, M. GenSurg.
Wolverton, H. A.
Wong, B. R., Psy

* Population not separately available.

Vancouver (Cont'd.)
Wong, E., Psy
Wong, J. M. H., Paed
Wong, W. Y.
Wood, Betty, Paed, DiagRad
Wood, L. G. Urol.
Wood, W. S. DermSyph
Woodward, J. B.
Woolley, H. E., ObstGyn
Worth, Ann, Path
Worth, H. M., D & TRad
Wright, B. N.
Wylie, Bernice IntMed
Yarrow, A. R., Psy
Yates, G. R.
Yip, K. G.
Yoerger, R. G. GenSurg.
Young, M. D. GenSurg
Young, S. B., DiagRad
Young, W. A., IntMed
Yu, Y-C., Paed.
Yue, K. W., Urol
Zack, J. J.
Zeldowicz, H. C. Psy.
Zeldowicz, L. Neur.
Zimmerman, U. A.

VANDERHOOF (1,457)
Edmund, E.
Hockly, G.
Khare, U.
Mooney, A. W. GenSurg
Mullin, G. M.
Stephen, C. H.

VERNON (10,250)
Alexander, H. J. GenSurg.
Barr, J. A.
Boggie, A.
Campbell-Brown, H. I.
Cunningham, W. J.
Dobry, E. J., Ophth
Fischer, H. R. DiagRad
Gilchrist, H. A.
Hartley, F. C., GenSurg.
Hilton, D. R.
Jordan, L. T. ObstGyn
Lattey, R. M.
McMurtry, T. S. IntMed
McRoberts, A. F.
O'Brien, E. G., GenSurg
Philip, I. J.
Prokopetz, G. V.
Rook, L. A. Ophth
Scarrow, H. G. GenSurg
Sovereign, A. E. Paed
Smart, M. R., P.H.
Smith, J. R. GenSurg
Woodley, W. R. DiagRad

VICTORIA (154,152)
Adams, D. G.
Adams, R. E.
Alcorn, D. E. NeurPsy
Allen, A. B.
Allen, E. A., IntMed
Amyot, G. F.
Anderson, J. B.
Anderson, J. L. M.
Anderson, J. W., GenSurg
Anderson, R. C. OrthSurg
Andrews, J. L. Anaes.
Aranas, A.
Argue, S. E., GenSurg
Aylward, G. F. Anaes
Baichwal, K. S., ThorSurg.
Bailey, N. L., Ophth
Bailey, T. J.
Balcer, W. E., Otol.
Ballam, C. F.
Banks, P. J. IntMed
Bapty, L. GenSurg
Bassett, L. W.
Beattie, A. N.
Bell, J. M.
Bell, W. J.
Benson, K. I., PH
Bigelow, G. B. Anaes.
Billung-Meyer, W.
Bonnell, F. H. D & TRad.
Borsman, C. H. ObstGyn
Boyd, D. M. Paed.
Brown, B. C.
Brown, C. Y. IntMed
Buffam, G. B.
Carlow, D. R.
Carruthers, H. C. Anaes
Carter, H. R. OrthSurg
Chapman, G. W., Anaes
Clearihue, Joyce G., Derm.
Coke, W. L.
Conn, R. S.
Cook, N. C. Otol
Cooper, J. W.
Cooper, M. A.
Cornelius, L. R.
Courtenay, P. H. E., OrthSurg.
Cox, G. E.
Cragg, B. E. Anaes.
Critchley, J. D.
Cruise, J. T. Ophth
Cupples, J. F. B.
Davidson, K.
Davidson, R. W.
Destrube, Ilse
D'Estrube, P. F., Psy
Dick, K. D.
Dickson, J. H., ObstGyn.
Duxbury, J. H., Urol
Edmison, H. M. D & TRad
Edmison, J. N., DiagRad.
Edwards, W. F.
Elder, T. R.
Elkington, E. H. W. Ophth
Elliott, M. R., PH
Emery, E. D. Ophth.
Evans, G. P., P.H.
Falk, W. A.
Felix, C. H.
Fiddess, J.
Flanagan, J. R.
Ford, H. S. GenSurg.
Forgie, R. R.
Fortye, R. A. Anaes.
Foster, W.
Fraser, W. A. Urol.
French, D. L.
Gale, R. A.
Gareau, U. P., PlasSurg
Gaudin, D. A. OrthSurg
Gelling, B. M.
Gillespie, A. E., Paed
Gough, H. M. ObstGyn
Gouws, F. B., GenSurg
Graham, M. D., Otol
Graham, W. GenSurg
Grant, G. H. GenSurg.
Grant, R. N. OrthSurg
Gray, A. G. GenSurg
Gray, T. W. A.
Green, J. W., Anaes
Greenwood, K. DermSyph
Gregory, C., Psy
Grieve, H. G. Ophth,Otol.
Hale, Helena B., Psy.
Hamdi, F. A., NeurSurg.
Harvey, J. E. NeurSurg
Harvey, J. M. GenSurg
Hay, J. A.
Hay, W. B., Path
Heard, F. S.
Heffernan, J. L.
Heimlich, H. J.
Henderson, C. B.
Henry, E. R. Anaes
Henry, H. G., DiagRad.
Higgins, J. F
Homer, G. F. GenSurg
Hopkins, J. A. Urol
Horne, L. E. ObstGyn
Horton, D. R.
Hosie, R. T., GenSurg
Hough, J. D. GenSurg
Houston, G. F.
Hughes, E. N., Anaes
Hunt, J. W. E.
Hunter, R. A. IntMed
Hutchison, J. A., Anaes
Ingram, H. G.
Ireland, L. C.
Irish, R.
Jackh, H. DiagRad
Johnston, Patricia
Kendrick, W. W., Urol
Kenning, I. S. Psy.
Kenning, S. G. IntMed
Kenning, S. P., IntMed.
Knapp, B. E.
Krayenhoff, J. J.
Lane, J. S.
Lane, R. M. IntMed
Larsen, A. A., P.H.
Lee, Anathalie W. DiagRad.
Lee, D. H. T. DiagRad
Le Huquet, J. R.
Leith, Mary P.
Lewis, H. J. Derm
Lockyer, N. S. TherRad
Loftus, L. J.
Longridge, D. M. N.
Lott, G. G., GenSurg
Lucas, O. C.
Lythgoe, Leyda
Maccartney, H. H., Anaes
MacDonell, J. A., D & TRad
MacGregor, A. J.
Mackay, M. I. GenSurg
MacLean, J. R.
Malcolm, G.
MacWilliam, H. D. Otol
Mahaffy, Charlotte, PH
Mair, C. M. H. ObstGyn
Marsh, Margaret
Marshall, W. D. ObstGyn
Matiko, R.
May, G. A.
McElmoyle, W. A. GenSurg
McGill, A. F. GenSurg
McHaffie, D. S.
McIlveen, Jean E.
McKenzie, G. J. Paed
McMahen, W. J. Urol
McNeely, R. G. D. Path
McNiven, E. L.
Mellor, N.
Milligan, F. D., IntMed.
Mitchell, W. E. M. GenSurg
Moore, C. H. Ophth
Moore, J. H. GenSurg
Morgan, R.
Morrison, J. H.
Morrison, M. G., ObstGyn
Muir, D. M. DiagRad
Mulholland, A. B., Anaes.
Nash, A. B. ObstGyn
Nash, E. T. W.
Newton, W. E. GenSurg
Nishioka, H., NeurSurg
North, D. P. Ophth
Nyhof, A.
O'Reilly, J. J. Ophth,Otol
Page, G. B., Otol
Paine, D. L. Ophth
Patriarche, M. Elizabeth
Parizeau, P.
Patterson, J. G.
Paul, G. M.
Peet, R. M. Neur
Peet, T. A.
Penn, M. J.
Perry, A. W. IntMed
Peterson, J. E.
Phillips, J. E.
Piper, A. V.
Portelance, H. J.
Powell, Elinor D. V., IntMed.
Prevost, E. C. ObstGyn
Pronger, R. C. Otol

* Population not separately available.

Victoria (Cont'd.)
Ptak, L. L.
Purdon, D. H.
Ransford, P. M. Paed
Rasmussen, G.
Reid, A. N. GenSurg, OrthSurg
Reilly, G. L.
Reilly, N. B.
Revell, D. G. Anaes
Rich, C. B. IntMed
Roach, M.
Roberts, J. B., D & TRad
Roberts, L. N., IntMed
Robson, G. W. ObstGyn
Roe, J. A.
Rogers, H. D.
Rogers, V. A., Anaes
Rose, T. F. IntMed
Roseborough, G. F., Ophth
Ross, M. A.
Ross, W. C.
Roxburgh, D. B. PathBact
Ruebsaat, H. J.
Ruskin, S. G.

Scott-Moncrieff, R. Otol
Semenchuk, P. W. IntMed
Semmewald, L. F.
Shorting, D. M.
Simpson, G. Paed
Sinclair, A. B. Urol
Sinclair, J. M. IntMed
Sinclare, R. G.
Singh, C. P., Urol.
Singh, G. S., NeurSurg.
Slakov, R.
Smith, R. B.
Smith, R. C., ThorSurg
Smith, V. W.
Spicer, R.
Stenstrom, J. D. GenSurg
Stephens, C. W.
Stephenson, C.
Stewart, J. A. Ophth,Otol
Stewart, N. R. IntMed
Stirling, R. J.
Stone, J. R. Anaes
Stuart, E. A.
Stuart, F. G. D & TRad
Stuart, V. G.
Sutherland, R. A.
Symington, D. C., PhysMed & Rehab

Tallan, Z., PhysMed & Rehab
Taylor, J. A. PH
Thompson, G. H. Ophth
Thomson, I. B., Psy
Thornton, K. R., Path
Toone, W. M. GenSurg
Trenholme, W. A.
Tsai, L. S.-L., Ophth
Tysoe, J. F.

Valens, W. L. NeurPsy
Vantilburg, E.
Vaughan, F. W.
Vaughan, K. Diane
Vey, A. G.
Vey, D. J.

Wallace, G. S.
Wallis, W. G., Psy
Walther, G. L., Path
Warren, J. D., OrthSurg
Warrington, A. M.
White, R. A.
Whitehead, R. G. D., Anaes
Whitley, D. M., GenSurg
Wiggins, R. L., Ophth
Wilson, G. C.
Wilson, Lucille, Path
Wolfe, P. M.
Wong, J., Otol
Woodwark, G. M., IntMed
Wride, R. J., GenSurg
Yates, M., Anaes
Young, R. M.

WELLINGTON
(504)
Boan, D. B.

WELLS
(459)
Wigby, S. B.

WESTBANK
(361)
Finnemore, B. I.

WEST SUMMERLAND
(3,893)
Evans, W. G.
Guttormsson, P. B., GenSurg.
Guttormsson, V. J.
MacInnis, F. C.
Munn, W. H. B.

WEST VANCOUVER
(Dist. of Vancouver)
Andersen, R. G.
Anthony, A. R., Ophth
Baker, H. G., IntMed
Barker, A. J.
Bell, J. N., Path
Bell-Irving, R. W., IntMed
Bennett, R. B.
Boothroyd, L. S., GenSurg, Urol.
Boyce, K. C., IntMed.
Buckler, W. J.
Bunton, P., Psy.
Calder, Norma M.
Calder, T. L.
Challenger, N. E.
Clark, G. F., Anaes
Crawford, Lois D., Anaes.
Davies, K. J., Psy
Davis, R. N. Psy
De Boissiere, V. R., Otol
Frazee, J. L., Psy
Grassett, A. V.
Guard, M. C.
Hall, E. R., Anaes.
Harmon, T. P.
Harmon, T. R. PathBact
Hunt, C. L., IntMed
Hunt, J. A.
Janz, L. B.
Johnson, T. C.
Johnston, T. A., GenSurg
Johnstone, D. W.
Kent, G. E., Anaes
Laird, R. R.
Langston, Kathleen W., Anaes.
Lugsdin, J. G.
Mashal, J. Paed
McCall, W. J.
McDaniel, E. S.
McKim, A., IntMed
McLean, C. C.
McPhee, J. G., D & T Rad
McQueen, Roberta, Psy
M'Gonigle, A. C., GenSurg.
Mills, F. G., Psy
Morton, J. W.
Nicol, W. G.
Onhauser, C. M.
Osborne, J. C. GenSurg
Paramonoff, A. DiagRad
Peacock, E. G. S.
Peacock, K. A.
Peretz, A. W.
Peretz, D. I.
Phillips-Wolley, C. J. F.
Rice, H. V.
Richardson, N. L. Psy
Screech, G.
Sharp, W. L., IntMed
Spohn, F. J.
Sprung, Elizabeth
Stewart, G. G.
Thomas, J. P., IntMed
Thompson, R. D.
Thorp, R. H., Anaes
Warren, D. P., IntMed
Webb, D. A.ObstGyn

Williams, C. E.
Williams, F. G., Anaes.

WHITE ROCK
(6,453)
Biro, L.
Blades, T. R.
Heinrichs, E.
Hogg, R. J. A.
Lamont, K. A., GenSurg
MacDonald, J. H., Ophth
Middleton, K. R.
Narod, Mairi M.
Narod, P.
Waterman, R. A.

WILLIAMS LAKE
(2,120)
Atwood, H. K.
Beblis, I.
Dormaar, N. G.
Kureshi, A-H., Paed
Lee, H. C. GenSurg
MacLean, D.
Manning, G.
Ringwood, J. B., GenSurg
Vowles, Patricia
Wilson, J. S., DiagRad.

WINFIELD
(358)
Dobson, M. C.

YARROW
(1,318)
Mertens, G. A., Path

YOUBOU
(1,153)
Ziegler, W. H.

Manitoba

ALTONA
(2,026)
Gutowski, W. D.
Loewen, W.
Toni, S. S.

ARBORG
(811)
Mowczan, I.

ASHERN
(374)
Steenson, G.

BALDUR
(550)
Hanks, G.

BEAUSEJOUR
(1,772)
Adam, B. H.
Giesbrecht, R.
Robbie, S. J.

BENITO
(424)
Bernier, L. J.
Maharaj, C. R.

BIRCH RIVER
(273)
Boon, A. H.

BIRTLE
(844)
Edwards, H. L.
Isitt, C. L.
Mohamed, G. E.
Petrinack, N. F.

BOISSEVAIN
(1,303)
Bird, F. V.
McPhail, D. M.
McPhail, Ethel M.

BRANDON
(28,166)
Aidun, J. S., Urol.
Alexander, J. F.
Andrews, R. H.
Arfai, E. K.
Bigelow, W. A., GenSurg

* Population not separately available.

Bristow, M. E., Psy
Camrass, H. P., Anaes
Cromarty, R. P., GenSurg
Cziller, Elizabeth
Dalling, J.
Elliott, A. J., IntMed
Evans, H. S., GenSurg
Farquhar, D. I.
Findlay, J. A., ObstGyn
Fjeldsted, F.
Gemmill, D. L.
Guy, W. D.
Hay, A. W. S., Psy.
Hendry, J., Path
Hirsch, W. P., ObstGyn
Hunter, H. B.
Ireland, D. J., Otol
Joe, B. K.
Johnson, D. L.
Joubert, Doreen
Joubert, N. Y.
Kanter, Y. C., Ophth.
Kelly, C. L.
Kunyckyj, T. G.
Lambert, R. C., IntMed
Lapko, A. P., Path.
Lockie, J. M.
Lopez, J.
Matheson, J. M., GenSurg
McDiarmid, R. O., Ophth, Otol
McIntosh, D., Psy
McQueen, R. C.
Millette, L., GenSurg
Mirzai, M.
Moyes, A.
Myers, R. F. M., Paed
O'Brien-Moran, S., Anaes
Ozman, I.
Parker, R. H.
Polo, R. F.
Povah, A. H.
Purdie, F. J. E., GenSurg
Pyun, K. W.
Rose, L. C.
Rowlands, J., GenSurg
Scott, J. H. Ophth.
Seifer, R.
Shahariw, W.
Sharpe, H. S., OrthSurg
Sharpe, V. J. H., IntMed
Skafel, E J.
Sykes, R. H., DiagRad
Verinder, D.
Woodman, J. K.

CARBERRY
(1,113)
Beveridge, T. F.
Jaremko, Lois M.
Morrison, T.

CARMAN
(1,930)
Cunningham, E. K.
North, H. W. C.

CARTWRIGHT
(483)
Davidson, D. A.

CHARLESWOOD
*
Lay, R. A. Q.
Welpy, W. R., OrthSurg

CHURCHILL
see Fort Churchill

CRYSTAL CITY
(541)
Irving, D. G.

DAUPHIN
(7,373)
Brandt, M. K.
Brinkop-Little, Hanna
Carleton, B. M.
Corbett, B. N.
Dicks, R. E.
Grant, T. P.
Jonat, L. V.
Little, H.
Lysack, A., GenSurg
Marshall, W.
Mulligan, G. W.
Potoski, M.
Ritchie, W. G.
Stephen, L. J.

DELORAINE
(920)
Bonar, J. G.
Malyska, W.

DOMINION CITY
(583)
Artes, W. E.

DUNREA
(202)
Lommerse, P. G.

EAST KILDONAN
(See Winnipeg)

ELIE
(368)
Champagne, R.

ELKHORN
(669)
Gardner, L. G.

EMERSON
(934)
Ferre, A. F.

ERICKSON
(526)
Donnelly, J. B.

ERIKSDALE
(260)
Archibald, D. W.

FISHER BRANCH
(637)
Bereznay, I.

FLIN FLON
(11,104)
Bailey, R. A.
Bland, R. C.
Caneilla, P. A.
Cockburn, D. G.
Johnson, P., GenSurg
Kilby, T. H.
Laschiazza, D.
Molaro, A. L.
Nicol, T.
Panikkar, M.
Premachuk, P. G.
Shnider, M.
Smithen, A. H.
Stephansson, N.
Warma, S. K., GenSurg.
Willson, G. N.

FORT CHURCHILL
*
Black, L. M.
Harvey, J. P.
Husain, S.
Molberg, C. L.
Monahan, G. J., IntMed
Wiebe, J. P.
Wigmore, E. W.

FORT GARRY
(1,485)
Asselstine J. L., Psy
Cadoret, R. J.
McPherson, V. A., GenSurg
Neal, W. S.
Watt, W.

GILBERT PLAINS
(855)
Franks, F. J.
Kinash, E. T.

GIMLI
(1,841)
Johnson, J. G.
Scribner, C. R.
Scribner, F. E.
Tyzek, T.

GLADSTONE
(944)
Jenkins, J. R.
Rahaman, A. R.

GLENBORO
(794)
Jemson, J. A.
McCulloch, K. C.

GRAND RAPIDS
(986)
McLean, D. R.

GRANDVIEW
(1,056)
Enns, J. W.
Leahy, D. W.

GRETNA
(575)
Boreskie, J. P.

HAMIOTA
(776)
Cashmore, P.
Hudson, J. E.

HARTNEY
(594)
Singh, S.

HODGSON
(600)
Eng, A.
Nenadkevich, A.
Pan, W. M.

HOLLAND
(361)
Ostapovitch, W. H.

KENTON
(126)
Hames, W. K.

KILLARNEY
(1,729)
Dow, G. E.
Marshall, W.
Stratton, J. R.

LAC DU BONNET
(564)
Beaumont, Margaret
Opie, C. H.

LUNDAR
(647)
Paulson, G.

LYNN LAKE
(1,881)
Lazarus, S. S.
McMahon, J. M.
Perry, J. R.

MANITOU
(864)
Dick, V.

McCREARY
(365)
Dirauf, J.
Miller, C., GenSurg.

MELITA
(1,036)
Kaye, H. A.
Singh, D. C.

MINNEDOSA
(2,211)
Bright, R. C.
Hinch, R. O.
St. John, Valerie E.
Stevenson, H. C.
Turkula, W.

MORDEN
(2,799)
Colert, W. M.
McRuer, Enid E.
Menzies, J. C.
Regehr, J. I.
Unruh, C. S.

MORRIS
(1,370)
Griggs, G. B.

* Population not separately available.

NEEPAWA
(3,197)
Dobson, T. B.
Domegan, P. R.
Hutchinson, H. H.
Jakobson, B. B.
Johnson, K. I.
Munro, A. T.
Sicotte, J.

NINETTE
(160)
Hernando, H. M.
Paine, A., LeR., ThorSurg
Reilly, Ruth

NORWAY HOUSE
(447)
Hermann, J. D. GenSurg., ThorSurg.
Manion, R. A.

NORWOOD
(Dist. of St. Boniface)
Currie, R. S.
Howden, R. L., Anaes
Wilt, J. C., Path

NOTRE DAME DE LOURDES
(400)
Delaquis, H

OAK LAKE
(436)
Scherz, M.

OAK RIVER
(175)
Gellatly, T. H.

OAKVILLE
(377)
Harsanji, I.

PILOT MOUND
(802)
Cohoe, C. E.

PINAWA
(*)
Beaumont, H. W.
Petkau, A.
Sutherland, J. B.

PINE FALLS
(1,244)
Geer, P.
Siddall, E. R.

PIPESTONE
(251)
Cairns, J. W.

PORTAGE LA PRAIRIE
(12,388)
Black, G. M., GenSurg
Chowhary, B. L.
Cheng, H.
Collier, K. J.
Fairfield, G. C.
Ford, E. R.
Gallinger, A.
Gibson, R.
Hamlin, G. H.
Kang, S. S.
Kent, T.
Kim, H. S.
Lowther, G. H.
MacNeil, J. D.
Rae, D. W.
Rennie, J. C.
Thomas, C. M.
Varga-Toth, I.

RAPID CITY
(467)
Bruser, H. H.

RESTON
(516)
Klotzek, J. S.

RIVERS
(1,574)
Heddle, R. W.
Lidster, D. K.

Lovell, B. A.
Stern, D. J.

RIVERTON
(808)
Thompson, S. O.

ROBLIN
(1,368)
Dorran, B. W.
Layng, J. L.

ROSSBURN
(588)
Head, P. W.

RUSSELL
(1,264)
Brownlee, T. I.
Lange, H. N.
Lim-Lu, Margaret
Lu, K. L.

STE ANNE DES CHENES
(720)
Doyle, **F. P.**
Gobeil, J. G.
Lafreniere, R. E.

ST. BONIFACE
(37,600)
Albi, F. Derm
Albi, W. N.
Blight, W. J.
Davies, H. L., Paed
De Pape, A. J., Paed
Desautels, J. L.
Deshaye, J. V.
French, W. G.
Grewar, D. A., Paed
Guyot, H.
Gyde, M. C., Otol
Hamonic, M.
Howden, R. L., Anaes
Huot, J. M.
Isabey, Amedee P.
Jacob, C. V., GenSurg.
Jonasson, H. D.
Jacques, R. A.
Kristof, A. C.
Lavoie, C. J. A.
L'Heureux, P., PH
Liu, E. T.
Medina, E. S.
Rich, P. J., GenSurg
Sabourin, G. A.
Sheedy, F. T.
Sinclair, A. C., ThorSurg
Snidal, D. P., IntMed
Szirom, S.
Ting, D.
Van Wijhe, M., Path
Warkentin, J. D., Path
Young, S. B.

ST. CLAUDE
(300)
Champagne, F. A.

ST. JAMES
(33,977)
Bowen, M. D.
Derbach, B.
MacDonell, J. A., IntMed
MacDonnell, Josefina A.
McMillan, J. D.
Rafuse, E. R.
Rosenberg, A.
Snell, E.
Thomas, E. J., IntMed
Wallar, D. E.

ST. JEAN BAPTISTE
(521)
Boucher, J. H.

ST. PIERRE, JOLYS
(857)
Cantin, P. R.
Gamez-Ruiz, D.

STE ROSE DU LAC
(790)
Gendreau, R. L.
Prefontaine, R.

ST. VITAL
*****
Braustein, D.
Truelove, L. H., PhysMed &Rehab.

SELKIRK
(8,576)
Anghelis, B.
Creasy, G. J.
Easton, W. I.
Frihagen, L. M.
Hollo, J. B.
Johnson, E.,, GenSurg
Kovacs, M. C., Psy
Kreyes, W., Psy.
Mann, Margaret
Nakielny, W.
Reid, I. L., GenSurg
Reid, W. S.
Roberton, R. O. ObstGyn
Rogers, R. D.
Rozecki, W. A.
Smith, D. J.
Soong, F. Y.
Tavener, R. H., Psy
Thompson, G. L., GenSurg
Wehner, R.
Zywina, P. R.

SHOAL LAKE
(766)
Bardal, S.
Prus, R. D.

SNOW LAKE
(659)
Millington, M.

SOMERSET
(540)
Mabon, G.

SOURIS
(1,846)
Grant, A. M.
Knight, L. W.
Letian, F. A.
Sinhanan, K.
Sutter, B. D.

STEINBACH
(3,739)
Choate, J. F.
Dick, J. B.
Giesbrecht, D. R.
Khodadadeh, M.
Penner, L.
Peters, P. F.
Propp, A. G.

STONEWALL
(1,420)
Gonty, J.
McQueen, B. M.
Przibislowsky, L.

STRATHCLAIR
(245)
Khan, N. A.
MacKenzie, J. E. G.

SWAN LAKE
(332)
Young, G.

SWAN RIVER
(3,163)
Cameron, A. P.
Doyle, P. E.
Honig, J. L.
Jonsson, B.
Maharaj, G. R.
Malcolm, T. F.
Theodore, G. M.
Young, G.

TEULON
(756)
Bishop, Beryl

* Population not separately available.

Teulon (Cont'd.)
Bishop, M. L.
Goodwin, J. M.

THE PAS
(4,671)
Abbott, R. T.
Cotton, A.
Lopez-Perez, J.
Millar, L.
Rolfe, H. C.
Seifer, R.
Tack, M.
Walton, R. S.
Wisinger, H. J.

THOMPSON
(3,418)
Johnston, J. B.
Reiner, D. H.
Spooner, J. D.
Standing, H. K.
Von Raffle, W.

TRANSCONA
(14,248)
Crawford, D. C.
Egan, B. J.
Grace, M. K.
Jamieson, H. S.
Law, G. A.
Markovits, S. L.
Marsh, D. W.

TREHERNE
(572)
Woods, M. L.
Welpy, W. R.

VIRDEN
(2,708)
Coals, J. T., GenSurg.
Harris, R. S.
McNeill, G. T.
Yates, D. E.

VITA
(404)
Toth, L.

WASKADA
(295)
Blanck, J. A.

WAWANESA
(459)
Kester, N. M.

WHITEMOUTH
(385)
Bilynski, W.

WINKLER
(2,529)
Khan, F.
Penner, H. U.
Vogt, P. A.
Wiebe, C. W.

WINNIPEG
(490,000)
Abbott, A. C., GenSurg, Urol.
Abbott, C. E., GenSurg
Abbott, W. E., ObstGyn
Abbott, W. F., ObstGyn
Adams, P. V., ObstGyn
Adamson, G. L., NeurPsy
Adamson, J. D., Psy.
Adhikari, P. K., IntMed
Ahsam, A., OrthSurg
Albi, F. J.
Albi, W. N.
Alcock, A. J., IntMed.
Alexander, W., Ophth, Otol
Allison, F. G., IntMed., Cardiol.
Allison, Gerda E., Psy
Alvi, A. W., IntMed.
Amann, E. W.
Anderson, J.
Andison, A. W., ObstGyn
Anhalt, A. W., DermSyph.
Anhalt, E. F., Ophth
Anthony, G. P., Anaes
Armstrong, Ida M.
Arnott, Janet E., Path
Asselstine, J. L., Psy.
Avren, M.
Bachynski, V. F.
Baird, D. A., GenSurg, PlasSurg.
Bala, R. M., IntMed
Bankier, R. G., Psy
Baragar, F. D., IntMed
Barker, W. E., OrthSurg
Barnes, P. H., ObstGyn
Barsky, M., GenSurg
Barsky, P., Paed
Bartlett, L. C., GenSurg
Barwinsky, J., GenSurg, ThorSurg.
Battershill, J. H., IntMed
Beamish, R. E., IntMed
Beazley, G. G.
Bebchuk, W., Psy
Beckman, I. H., Ophth, Otol
Beckstead, J. L., IntMed
Beighton, T. E.
Bell, L. G., IntMed
Bellan, S.
Bendor-Samuel, J. E., Ophth
Bennett, E. J.
Bennett, J. E., TherRad
Bennett, Marjorie R., Anaes
Bennett, W. J., IntMed
Benoit, C. F.
Berbrayer, P.
Bergal, J.
Berger, M., Paed
Berger, S., DermSyph
Bertalanffy, F. D.
Besant, D. F., Paed
Best, B. D., ObstGyn
Bigelow, D. R., OrthSurg.
Bigornia, G. V., Anaes
Birt, A. R., DermSyph
Black, B.
Black, E. F. E., ObstGyn
Black, W. A.
Blanchaer, M. C.
Bleeks, Cherry K., ObstGyn
Blouw, D.
Blumenthal, S., IntMed
Book, N. A., Ophth
Booth, D. H.
Bosley, Eliska M.
Bottomley, H. W., IntMed Allerg.
Boult, G. F. D. & TRad
Bourgouin, J. J., Urol
Bowden, D. H., Path
Bowden, N.
Bowen, M. D.
Bowles, H. E.
Bowman, J. M., Paed
Bowman, W. D., Paed
Boyd, S. A., Paed
Boyd, W. J.
Bracken, A. D., Ophth
Bradford, C. R., ObstGyn
Bradley, L. O.
Brereton, D. C., IntMed
Briggs, J. N., Paed
Brock, W. G., DermSyph
Broder, M. H., GenSurg
Brodovsky, D. M., Otol
Bronstein, G.
Brotman, E. H.
Brown, J. D.
Brown, J. H., Psy.
Brown, K. R.
Brown, R. P.
Brownell, E. G., IntMed
Bruser, D. M., GenSurg, OrthSurg.
Bruser, M., ObstGyn
Buchok, R. W.
Burch, J. E., Psy
Burgess, F. J., IntMed
Burgoyne, F. H., Path
Burke, M. E.
Burns, C. M., GenSurg
Burns, C. W., GenSurg.
Burrell, R. O., GenSurg
Cadham, R. G., PH
Cadoret, R. J.
Cameron, W. M., IntMed
Caminetsky, S.
Campbell, A. A.
Campbell, M. H.
Caplan, B. Urol
Carleton, M.
Carr, W. G. L., Paed.
Carroll, J.
Carter, S. A.
Cera, A. E.
Cera, L. J., IntMed
Chalmers, A. C.
Cham M., Anaes
Chang, I. W., ObstGyn
Cherniack, L., IntMed
Cherniack, R. M., IntMed
Chernick, V.
Childe, A. E., DiagRad
Chochinov, H., GenSurg
Chown, B., Paed.
Christie, K. A., Paed
Clark, C. W., GenSurg
Cleave, R. J.
Cleghorn, G. M., DiagRad
Coffey, O. F.
Cohen, M., GenSurg
Coke, L. R., IntMed
Colliou, L. L.
Connelly, P.
Constantinidis, P.
Coodin, F. J., Paed
Coodin, P.
Cooke, R. L.
Cooper, R. H.
Coppinger, H.
Corne, N. I.
Corne, R. A., IntMed.
Corrigan, C. E., GenSurg
Crisbin, J. S., GenSurg.
Croll, L. D., OrthSurg
Crowson, C. N., Path
Cruickshank, L. F. G., Anaes
Crust, J. H.
Cuddy, T. E., IntMed Cardiol.
Culligan, J. D., Anaes
Cumming, G. R., IntMed
Curran, Christina A., Paed.
Czubaty, W.
Daglish, G. H.
Dandenault, A. G.
Daniels, J. H., Anaes
Danzinger, R.
Davidson, A. L., GenSurg
Davies, J. E.
Davis, R. A., Derm
Davison, R. C., Otol
Deacon, A. E., OrthSurg
Decter, P. H., OrthSurg
DeKoven, M. J.
Derksen, C.
Desmarais, M. H.
Diehl, G.
Dirks, H. T.
Domke, O.
Donin, J. F., Ophth
Dorfman, Sheila
Dougan, J. M., Psy
Doupe, Nona, Psy
Dowling, S. O.
Downey, J. L. IntMed.
Downs, A. R., GenSurg
Dunlop, Monique L.
Drulak, S. L. Anaes
Duncan, C. W.
Duval, F. W., GenSurg
Dwyer, E.
Dyck, J., GenSurg
Eadie, J. A.
Earn, A. A., ObstGyn
Easton, S.
Edward, J. F.
Eggertson, S. H. O.

* Population not separately available.

Winnipeg (Cont'd.)
Ehrlich, B.
Erlich, S. K.
Elias, J. C.
Elliott, W. J., D & T Rad.
Ellis, C. D.
Elvin, N. L., Ophth
Enns, P.
Erenberg, M.
Eshoo, H. Anaes
Ethans, C. T., Anaes.
Ewart, W. B., IntMed
Fahrni, G. P., GenSurg
Fainman, J., ObstGyn
Falardeau, Ivy F.
Farr, J., GenSurg
Fast, B. B., IntMed.
Fattal, G. A., Path
Ferguson, C. A., GenSurg.
Finkel, K. C., Paed
Fleming, S. T., IntMed
Fletcher, H. W. IntMed.
Flett, R. O.
Ford, K. J., Psy
Fox, J. G., Path
Frain, J. B., IntMed
Friesen, P. H.
Friesen, R. F., ObstGyn
Friesen, W. J., ObstGyn
Froese, B. J.
Fryer, I. O.
Fyles, T. W., IntMed
Gagliano, E.
Galbraith, P. A., IntMed
Card, M., Anaes.
Garfield, H. D., DiagRad
Garwood, J. S.
Gaskell, P.
Gedgaudas, E., DiagRad
Gellman, D. D., IntMed
Gellman, Vera, Paed
Gemmell, J. I. P. IntMed
Gemmell, N.
Giles, R., Anaes.
Gilmour, Joan
Glassco, W. G., Psy
Goldberg, I. L., Paed
Goldenberg, G. J.
Goldstein, A.
Goldstein, A. S., GenSurg
Goidstein, A. V.
Goldstein, P., GenSurg
Golfman, S.
Gonsalves, C. T., Psy
Goodhand, T. K., GenSurg
Goodwin, A. M., ObstGyn
Gordon, A. R.
Gorrie, W. A.
Goudie, Margaret M.
Goudges d'Agincourt, R. L. A. GenSurg.
Gowron, A. T.
Graf, E.
Graf, J., Paed
Graham J. C., GenSurg
Grahame, G. R., IntMed.
Grahame, Ruth E.
Grant, H. G., Psy
Grant, I. M.
Grant, K. G.
Grant, W., Paed, Psy
Green, D. H. Ophth
Green, P. T., IntMed
Green, S. S.
Greenberg, L., GenSurg
Greer, R. G.
Grewar, D. A., Paed
Grogono, B. J. S., OrthSurg
Guenther, H., Psy.
Guest, H. A.
Guest, Sheena G.
Guest, W. C. Ophth
Guslits, S. S.
Guttman, A. P., OrthSurg
Habib, G. G.
Hagen, V. J.
Hall, C. W., DiagRad
Hall, Dorothy L.
Hamilton, G. F.
Handford, R. G., IntMed
Hanks, G. A., GenSurg
Hardy, G.
Harrop, A. H.
Hart, W. J.
Hastings, D. J.
Hawirko, L.
Haworth, J. C., Paed
Hay, R. K., NeurSurg.
Hayakawa, J., Anaes
Hayter, F. W., DiagRad
Hayter, R. R. PhysMed. & Rehab.
Haywood, G. S.
Heinisch, G.
Hellmuth, F. H., TherRad.
Henderson, A. G.
Henderson, Marion
Hendrie, H. C.
Henneberg, C. C.
Henteleff, P. D.
Hershfield, C. S.
Hershfield, E. S., IntMed
Hershfield, H.
Hershfield, L. S.
Hershfield, N. B., IntMed.
Hildes, J. A., IntMed.
Hill, N. C., NeurSurg
Hillsman, J. A., GenSurg
Hitesman, R. J.
Ho, C., GenSurg
Hogg, Georgia R., Path
Holland, T. E., GenSurg
Hollenberg, C., OrthSurg
Hollenberg, Dorothy M. O.
Hollenberg, J., GenSurg
Hollenberg, J.
Hollenberg, M. S., IntMed
Hollenberg, M. W., Ophth.
Holm, A. W., Anaes
Homik, A. M.
Hoogstraten, J.
Hope, B. K., DiagRad
Houston, A. B., IntMed
Howden, R. L.
Hrushovetz, S. B.
Huebert, H. T.
Huggins, D. M. H., Anaes
Hughes, J. F. S., IntMed
Hunzinger, W. W., Psy
Hurley, N.
Hurst, H. G., DermSyph
Hutchison, H. C., Anaes
Hynes, J. A., IntMed
Innes, I. R.
Isaac, J. E., GenSurg
Israels, Esther D.
Israels, L. G., IntMed
Jackson, D. C., DiagRad
Jackson, J. W., Otol
Jacobsen, L. W., PlasSurg
James, E. S., OrthSurg
James, R. A., GenSurg
Jamieson, F. L.
Janzen, M. H., ObstGyn.
Johannesson, T., Anaes
Johnson, E. E., Psy
Johnson, G.
Johnson, H. M.
Johnson, R. J.
Jolly, T. G.
Kagan, J. M., GenSurg
Kahanovitch, M. E.
Kantor, S., Anaes
Karasick, H. D., ObstGyn
Karlinsky, W., IntMed
Karsgaard, A. T., Ophth
Kasian, P.
Katz, P.
Kaufman, B. J., IntMed
Kaufman, R. IntMed
Kay, S., GenSurg.
Keenberg, A. A.
Kellock, Marie G.
Kennedy, E. J.
Kent, Elspeth
Kent, E. T.
Kernahan, D. A., PlasSurg
Kerr, D. L., Paed
Kettner, J.
Khan, H. U., Paed.
Kiernan, M. K., D & TRad
Kilgour, J. M., IntMed
Kiors, A.
Kippen, D. L., IntMed
Kirk, B., IntMed
Kitchen, H. D., IntMed.
Klass, A. A., GenSurg
Kobrinsky, L.
Kobrinsky, S.
Kocsis, L. F.
Kolesnichenko, Elizabeth
Kovacs, L.
Kovacs, S. F.
Kowall, M. H., Paed
Kowalson, Bella
Kozin, F.
Krahn, H. P., Urol
Kramer, S.
Krause, R. G.
Kristjansson, G.
Krolman, G. M., Ophth
Krywulak, W.
LaFleche, J. G. M.
Laing, I. M., GenSurg
Lamberd, W. G., Psy
Lambertsen, G.
Lambie, R. S., Anaes
Lamond, D. E.
Lamontagne, H.
Lander, J. J.
Lansdown, L. P., Bact
Large, W. A., Psy
Lauchlan, S. C., Path
Law, G. A.
Lawler, R. H., Psy
Lebbetter, T. A., Urol
Lebbetter, T. A., IntMed
Ledger, J. L., Psy
Lees, C. D.
Lehmann, M. J., GenSurg
Lenson, F. W.
Lerner, A. I., GenSurg
Lerner, M.
Lertzman, M., IntMed
Letienne, G. J. E., Ophth
Levin, M. B., GenSurg
Levin, S. R., Anaes
Lim, D. S., IntMed.
Lim, J. S.
Lind, J. F., GenSurg
Lindsay, J. H. Psy
Ling, C. H., Ophth.Otol.
Lippmann, H. H., Urol
Little, G. A., Psy
Llewellyn, Anne
Loadman, A. Evelyn, Paed.
Loadman, B. E. OrthSurg
Loban, L., Anaes
Loewen, Margaret, Anaes
Lubinski, G. A.
Lucy, J. D., Psy
Ludwig, J. A.
Lunn, J. T.
Lyons, B. H., IntMed
Lyons, R., ObstGyn
MacCharles, M. R.
MacDonald, D. G.
MacDonald, H.
MacDougall, J. T., GenSurg
MacEwan, D. W., D & T Rad.
Macfarland, M. T.
Mackey, L. R., Urol
MacKinnon, W. B., OrthSurg
MacLaughlin, J. P., DiagRad
MacLean, D. J. C.
MacLean, I. S.
MacLean, J. P., IntMed
MacLeod, I. .D, GenSurg & Urol

*** Population not separately available.**

MacNeil, F. A., Ophth
Macneil, J. D.
MacNeil, R. W., Paed
Macoomb, R. K., OrthSurg
Macpherson, R. A., D & TRad
Magee, D. R., Ophth
Magian, V. de C., Otol
Majury, A. S. ObstGyn (Eng.)
Malkin, S.
Malyska, Elizabeth
Mandelstam, Jocelyn, Anaes
Maniar, A.
Margolis, J., Ophth
Margolis, N.
Markovits, Molly H.
Mari, P.
Marlatt, H. M., Paed
Marmar, M.
Martin, J. H., IntMed
Matas, H.
Matas, J., Psy
Mather, J. H.
Mathewson, F. A. L., IntMed
Matuk, N.
Matwichuk, Z.
Maxwell, I., IntMed
Maxwell, J. B. W.
May, W., Ophth
Mayba, I., GenSurg
Mazer, I. H., Otol
McAlpine, K. W.
McBeath, J. H., Urol
McCaughey, T. J., Anaes
McCawley, J. C., ObstGyn
McCord, W. J., ObstGyn
McCreath, N. D.
McCulloch, A. W., DiagRad
McDonald, L. T., Paed
McDowell, J. D., IntMed
McEwen, D. S., IntMed
McFarlane, C. Jean, ObstGyn
McFarlane, R. H., IntMed
McGarry, P. M., Anaes
McGibbon, K. C., OrthSurg
McGoey, J. E., Otol
McGoey, J. S., ThorSurg
McGowan, A.
McGregor, Mary
McInnes, J. S., GenSurg.
McInnes M. F., IntMed
McInnis, A. C., ObstGyn
McIntyre, D. F.
McIntyre, D. N. C.
McKenty, J. S., Ophth Otol.
McKenty, Mary
McKenty, V. J.
McKenzie, K. D.
McKinna, C.
McLandress, M., Paed
McMorris, L. S., Path
McNicol, H. L., GenSurg
McNulty, P. H., GenSurg
McQuaig, K. D.
McQueen, D., GenSurg, OrthSurg.
McRae, K. N., Paed.
McTavish, W. B.
Medd, D.
Medovy, H., Paed
Meikle, A. L., TherRad
Meindl, A. G.
Mendelson, J., Ophth
Merkeley, N. P., GenSurg, PlasSurg.
Meszaros, G.
Michaels, L., IntMed
Mierau, P. H.
Mikolojewski, J., Psy
Milanese, C. A., Ophth
Milicevic, J.
Millan, V. G.
Miller, J. A., GenSurg
Miller, Josephine W.
Mills, T. J., OrthSurg
Milner, R. W.
Minuck, M. Anaes
Mitchell, J. R., ObstGyn
Mitchell, Rosslyn B., ObstGyn
Mitchell, R. G.
Mogle, B. P.
Mohamed, J. K., Urol.
Molgat, A., GenSurg
Montgomery, W. G.
Moon, I., IntMed
Mooradian, Anaid S.
Moorehouse, J. A.
Morgan, R. A.
Morison, J. B.
Morris, J. E., IntMed
Morris, R. N.
Morrow, I. M., DiagRad
Mosher, G. E.
Movafagh, P., Paed
Muczij, T.
Murphy, C. H.
Murray, J. B.
Muruve, G., Paed
Musgrove, W. M.
Mutchnik, A.
Mymin, D.
Nagy, Katrina
Naimark, A., IntMed
Nash, R. M.
Natsuk, A. W., Anaes
Nelko, S. L.
Neufeld, N. J.
Neumann, A. L.
Newman, D. E.
Newman, M. J., IntMed, Neurol
Newman, W. G.
Nickerson, M.
Nigam, K. K., Paed
Nigam, S., Paed
Normandeau, G.
Oatway, R. D., GenSurg
O'Dea, Mary
Ohrt, H. A., DiagRad
O'Keefe, J. M.
Osborne, J. A., GenSurg.
Otke, E.
O'Toole, J. W.
Owens, Audrey M., Paed
Owens, M.
Pakian, A.
Pan, A., IntMed
Paraskeya, S. F.
Parker, G. H., GenSurg.
Parker, Shirley, Bact
Parker, W. L. Path
Parkinson, D. NeurSurg
Patton, Donna
Pauls, L. A.
Pearlman, D.
Pearson, F. B.
Peever, I. C., ObstGyn
Peikoff, S. S. GenSurg
Penner, D. W. Path
Penner, E. H.
Percheson, Anne C.
Percheson, P. T.
Perry, W. F.
Peterkin, F. D.
Peters, Ella L.
Peters, J., Paed
Picard, J.
Pickard, E. W. PlasSurg
Pickard, H. T.
Pierce, M. M. Otol
Pincock, J. G. A. IntMed
Pincock, T. A. Psy
Pirnazar, R.
Podkomorska, Danuta, Otol
Polson, R. A. IntMed
Porritt, P. N., OrthSurg
Port, Muriel
Prosen, H. Psy
Provis, H. S.
Pyle, I. R., DiagRad
Rabkin, F. B.
Rabson, L. R. GenSurg
Ramsay, R. M. Ophth
Randle, Donna L.
Ranosky, M. J.
Rath, O. J.
Reddy, S. R..
Reed, H. N. Ophth
Rennie, J. W. R. GenSurg
Revie, Maureen
Reyes, C., Path.
Reznowski, L. W.
Richardson, R. W. GenSurg
Riddell, D. M., OrthSurg
Riese, K. T., GenSurg
Riml, O. G. N.
Ritchie, G. W. DiagRad
Robinson, R. T.
Rodgers, D. D., Psy
Roe, B. V. Anaes
Rogers, A. G. IntMed
Romeyn, J. A., Bact
Rosenberg, S.
Rosenfield, M. **GenSurg**
Rosenfield, V. L.
Ross, E. L. IntMed (T.B.)
Ross, H. M. Path
Ross, R. T. Neur
Ross, W. J.
Roulston, T. M. ObstGyn
Rubin, J. A. Otol
Rubin, L. ObstGyn
Rusen, S. D. IntMed
Russell, J. R.
Russell, Mary
Russell, W. H.
Rutledge, E. J.
Ryan, G. H. OrthSurg
Rybak, F. A.
Saunders, M. G.
Scatcliff, J. N.
Schacter, B. A.
Schludermann, E. F.
Schmidt, O. A. ObstGyn
Schoemperlen, C. B. IntMed
Schwartz, B.
Scott, D. L. IntMed (T.B.)
Sebghati, M., Anaes
Semelka, Donna L., DiagRad.
Semelka, G. Anaes
Shapera, G. H. Paed
Shaw, E. C.
Shell, B. Anaes
Shelton, P. J., GenSurg
Sheps, S. G. IntMed
Shnider, M.
Shojania, A. M., Paed
Shwartz, I.
Sigurdson, J. F. P., OrthSurg
Sigurdson, L. A.
Simpson, C. A., Neur
Simpson, J. W. DiagRad
Sinclair-Hall, A. H.
Sirett, M. A.
Sirett, Nancy
Sirkis, H.
Sisler, G. C. Psy
Smith, F. H. IntMed
Smith, G. J., Psy.
Smith, I. S.
Smith, M. Anne
Smith, N. K.
Smythe, C. A., Urol
Soper, K.
Squire, J. B. D & TRad
Stanfield, M. J.
Starck, G. P.
Stein, D. H. IntMed
Steinberg, S.
Stephens, G. M. Psy
Stephenson, E., Urol
Stevens, G. C.
Stevens, I. H. K.
Stevenson, W. J.
Steward, D. J.
Stewart, C. B. Urol
Stewart, E. W.
Stillwater, R. B., Otol
Storrie, V. Marie, IntMed
Strautmanis, Ingrida, TherRad

* Population not separately available.

Sudermann, P., GenSurg
Sutton, I. Psy
Swan, J. A. C.
Swartz, D. Urol
Swartz, M. J. Urol
Syslak, W. B., Anaes
Szeszycki, L. W.
Tabesh, A. R., Anaes.
Tan, M.
Tanner, A. R.
Tass, D. Anaes
Taylor, C. H.
Taylor, E. F.
Taylor, H. Paed
Taylor, J. R. Urol
Tennant, Helen Anaes
Thomas, Catherine
Thomas, E. J., IntMed
Thompson, A. B., IntMed.
Thompson, I. M. Anat
Thomson, A. E. IntMed
Thomson, J. G., Anaes.
Thomson, M. J.
Thorlakson, P. H. GenSurg
Thorlakson, R. H. GenSurg
Thorlakson, T. K., GenSurg
Tisdale, J. E.
Tisdale, P. K. IntMed
Tishler, J. M., DiagRad.
Torres, A. E., Paed.
Tramer, E.
Trainor, J. M., Path
Trudel, J. J.
Truelove, L. H., PhysMed & Rehab
Trueman, K. R. GenSurg
Tucker, F. R. OrthSurg
Vaisrub, S. IntMed
Vann, E. K. Urol
van Wijhe, M.
Varsamis, I., Psy
Vasudevaiah, Y., GenSurg.
Vidinli, M.
Vig, K. S.
Waldon, H. V.
Wall, M. B. Z. ObstGyn
Walton, C. H. A. IntMed
Ward, J. H.
Warkentin, A. P.
Warner, P. T.
Waters, W. R., PlasSurg
Watkins, G. B., DiagRad.
Watson, R. K., Otol
Watt, W.
Watters, G. V., Paed. Neur
Waugh, F. P.
Waugh, G. A. GenSurg
Welply, W. R., OrthSurg (Eng.)
Wengel, A. E.
Wengel, R. B. W.
Werner, N. H., Ophth
Weidman, M. L., Paed
Whiteford, J. W. GenSurg
Whytehead, L. L. ThorSurg (Eng.)
Wiens, C. W.
Wightman, Patricia
Willis, Pamela
Willows, R. L. ObstGyn
Wilson, A. S.
Wilt, J. C. PathBact
Wine, N. A., Ophth.
Winestock, A. J.
Winram, R. G., GenSurg
Wistnger, H. J.
Wolkenstein, C. F., Anaes
Wood, W. J.
Woodman, K. J., IntMed
Woolf, C. I., Otol
Wyatt, J. P., PathBact
Wylie, K. O., Paed
Yauniskis, A. A.
Yenal, A. S. DiagRad
Yessayan, G. L. Paed
Young, G., Path.
Zajcew, W.
Zeavin, S.
Zeglinski, Diane J.
Zipursky, A. Paed

WINNIPEGOSIS
(978)
Bashucky, W.
Shay, G. D. P.

New Brunswick

ALBERT
(250)
MacKay, A. M.

BATH
(895)
Lockhart, J. A.
MacInnis, J. A.
Nugent, T. E.

BATHURST
(5,494)
Billard, A. C., GenSurg.
Caron, J., Anaes
Carson, J. D.
Comeau, Adeline E.
Densmore, L. D., GenSurg
Duguay, J. E.
Eddie, E.
Hennessy, R. D.
Keating, D. W. DiagRad
Langis, J. G.
Orser, W. B.
Rodgers, Christine A.
Thompson, D. A. GenSurg
White, E. L. GenSurg

BAYFIELD
(*)
Hetherington, H. G.

BELLEDUNNE
(125)
Smith, R. D.

BLACK'S HARBOUR
(1,546)
Dimock, G. K.
Jordan, Z. A.
Saunders, R. O.

BOIESTOWN
(225)
Patrick, M. C.

BRISTOL
(698)
Burley, J. S.

BUCTOUCHE
(1,536)
LeBlanc, P. E.

BURTT'S CORNERS
(389)
Morehouse, O. E.

CAMPBELLTON
(9,873)
Alcantara, E. N., Path.
Boulay, J. R. ObstGyn
Choi, S. M., Psy.
Comeau, R.
Doucet, C. GenSurg
Dumont, F.
Eaton, R. C. Psy
Filip, J.
Gallant, J. A.
Giray, S.
Juretic, P.
Lagace, V., OrthSurg(P.Q.)
Lee, D. H., Path
Letourneau, R., Paed
Lo, M. C., Urol
MacLennan, D. A. GenSurg
MacPherson, W. J., IntMed.
McGaughey, H. R.
Nadeau, N. Ophth,Otol
Pamir, T. A.
Renault, C. G.
Rice, J. M. GenSurg
St. Laurent, F. X. DiagRad
St. Pierre, M. G.
Salgado, I., GenSurg
Stevenson, C.
Susini, L.
Swan, M. H.
Szekeres, Eva
Toth, J.
Yeh, H. C.

CARAQUET
(1,214)
Lebouthillier, P.
Savoie, Isabelle
Savoie, R.

CHATHAM
(7,109)
Aube, L. A.
Blanchard, A. C.
Duffy, J. C.
Losier, E. B.
Losier, P. J.
Moar, J. D.
Ozcan, E.

CHIPMAN
(1,490)
Burley, M. P.

CLAIR
(500)
Rioux, E.

DALHOUSIE
(5,856)
Bujold, E.
Daigle, M. J.
Fleck, W. W. GenSurg
Landry, E. L.
Pothier, B. E. GenSurg
Potter, J. M.

DOAKTOWN
(1,064)
Hamilton, J. B.

EAST RIVERSIDE
*
Whitehead, F. L.

EDMUNDSTON
(12,788)
Albert, D. J. D & TRad
Berube, M.
Bourque, J. C., Psy
Cloutier, B. GenSurg
Fournier, R.
Fouron, P., Ophth.
Gaudreau, C. GenSurg
Gaudreau, J. B.
Gauvin, G., IntMed(T.B.)
Guerrette, R., Anaes
Harrigan, J. F.
Johnson, C. H.
Laporte, P. C. GenSurg
LeBlanc, L. E. Paed
Levesque, G-H., IntMed
Padget, J. P., Path
Pelletier, R., Otol
Pichette, L. P. Ophth,Otol
Renault, C. G.
St. Pierre, C. E., DiagRad.
Savoie, B. G., GenSurg
Savoie, G.
Smyth, J. H.
Sormany, A. H.
Sormany, A. M. DiagRad
Stein, L
Tardif, G. GenSurg

FREDERICTON
(19,683)
Acker, J. C., Jr.
Baird, R. D. GenSurg
Bergh, R. M., Paed
Black, W. W., Psy
Bonnell, G. E. Urol
Brooks, D. H., Phys Med. & Rehab
Cabatu, M. D.

* Population not separately available.

Fredericton (Cont'd.)
Chalmers, G. E. GenSurg
Chalmers, R. H. ObstGyn
Clayden, G. R., D & TRad
Dolan, R. J.
Feindel, J. R.
Fekete, J. F., Path
Good, H. G., ObstGyn
Hurley, R. C.
Jamieson, W. E.
Jewett, B. L. GenSurg
Jewett, Marie, A. C.
Kelly, C. W.
Khazen, R. S.
LeBlanc, R. F.
Likely, J. C. Otol
Loane, Anna L., ObstGyn.
Lythgoe, C.
MacAulay, W. D.
MacDonald, A. G.
MacSween, H. M.
Magtibay, L. Z.
McCannel, J. S.
MacIntosh, R. A. GenSurg
Mackay, J. E., ObstGyn
McElman, G. W.
McInerney, A. J.
McInerney, J. F. Anaes
Melanson, J. A. PH
Moffatt, G. M. IntMed
Palmer, M. F., GenSurg
Patrick, M. C.
Petrie, E. A., Anaes.
Price, J., Anaes
Prosser, R. R. Psy
Robinson, Barbara J. Paed
Rowan, A. A. Otol
Saint-Pierre, G. J.
Southern-Holt, Mary
Stickles, L. E. Paed
Torrie, A. F. OrthSurg
Turner, C. H., GenSurg
VanWart, A. F. GenSurg IntMed
Williamson, J. A.
Wright, W. R. OphthOtol

GAGETOWN
(549)
Jenkins, W. M.

GRAND FALLS
(3,983)
Chiasson, E.
Corbin, E. N.
Gorayer, E. J., GenSurg.
Yao, J. P.

GRAND MANAN
(585)
Cyr, J. G.
Gorayeb, E. J. GenSurg
Nowlan, B. E.
Spacek, M.

HAMPTON
(435)
Macpherson, L.
Snow, V. A.

HAMPTON STATION
(580)
Leatherbarrow, A. T.
Robb, D. M.

HARDINGS POINT
*
Collins, R. J.

HARTLAND
(1,022)
Chestnut, W. O.

HARVEY STATION
(587)
Fletcher, G. E.

HATFIELD POINT
(180)
Brooks, R. W.

HILLSBOROUGH
(848)
Oxley, P. L.

KEDGWICK
(956)
Boulay, R.

KESWICK
see Mouth of Keswick

KINGHURST
(78)
Abel, R. B.

LAMEQUE
(997)
Lacroix, E. B.

LANCASTER
(13,848)
Aronson, A.
Aydin, M.
Baird, K. A. DermSyph.
Bashaw, Lynn E., PhysMed & Rehab.
Baxter, W. J. GenSurg
Branch, E. A. G. Path Bact
Chablani, G. V., Psy
Clark, S. D.
Edgar, A. B.
De Freitas, A.
Gregory, R. A. NeurPsy
Guner, A.
Hatfield, G. G. Psy
Kapkin, I. A.
Kelly, A. C.
Keyes, S. A.
Khakee, A. G.
Kotlowski, K., Psy
MacDonald, P. M.
Mainville, Lodois L.
Rasheed, A.
Riives, J., Neur
Robertson, Robina
Stuart, F. K.
Suh, C. K., Psy
Tiongson, R. V., IntMed
Toumik, P.
Trask, C. A.
Trask, C.. R.
Vihvelin, H.
Wills, R. R.
Walter, A. B. IntMed

LEWISVILLE
(3094)
Crandall, R. G., Psy.

LOWER SOUTHAMPTON
(130)
Bramstrup, P. A.

McADAM
(2,570)
Brown, C. B.

MEMRAMCOOK
(393)
Melanson, Jeane L.

MINTO
(1,549)
Gardiner, H. M.
Lawson, G. E.
Thompson, R. B.

MONCTON
(55,768)
Allanach, W. G. Urol
Arranz, C. C., Anaes.
Auffrey, P. E.
Bastarache, A. Path
Baxter, C. R. GenSurg
Beaulieu, R. P., DiagRad
Boillat, Joyce E. L.
Bourgeois, C. M.
Bourgeois, R. C. Ophth
Britton, H. E. GenSurg
Brown, R. J., PH
Clarke, A. M., IntMed(TB) PH
Cormier, D. C., ObstGyn
Cormier, E. J.
Daigle, J. E., Anaes.
Delaney, J. A. ObstGyn
Dennis, W. F.
D'Entremont, P. GenSurg
Dobson, J. A. Anaes
Dobson, J. W. GenSurg
Doiron, L.
Doyle, C. E. GenSurg
Dysart, R. M. IntMed, GenSurg
Eaton, R. B. GenSurg
Edgett, J. T. IntMed
Ewart, E. W. OrthSurg
Fitch, R. H. Paed
Fownes, J. A., IntMed
Gaudet, L. J.
Gautreau, B., OrthSurg(P.Q.)
Gillis, W. R.
Girouard, J. E. GenSurg
Goodridge, L. A. Otol
Grondin, J. G. GenSurg
Hache, A. G.
Hay, H. B.
Herman, M.
Hong, C. Y.
Hopper, S. A. Paed, IntMed
Hunter, J. O., DiagRad
Ibbotson, C. D & TRad
Jennings, K. H. Anaes
Landry, R. D.
Le Blanc, H. C. J.
Leger, E.
Leger, F. E.
Leger, G. C.
Leger, J. E. GenSurg
Leighton, C. M. Paed
Levitan, E. D.
Lyons, G. GenSurg
Lyons, P. GenSurg
MacDonald, W. D., Otol
MacKenzie, K. W. GenSurg
MacLean, H. M. GenSurg
MacLellan, D. I., OrthSurg.
MacLennan, I. A. PathBact
Majka, M.
Matthews, V. M.
Maurice, R., Otol
McCrea, J. C.
McKenna, R. I.
McLaughlin, V. D. ObstGyn
McLeod, D. A., Urol.
Melanson, H. P. GenSurg
Melanson, Jean
Michel, P., Psy
Minshull, F. A.
Murphy, A. P.
Murphy, F. G. GenSurg
Murphy, Hazel
Murphy, R. M.
Myers, R.
Noonan, J. S.
Oatway, W. A., Anaes
Parsons, G. F. Anaes
Prosser, R. R. Psy
Pugh, P. A. ObstGyn
Pullin, W. A. Ophth
Ramsay, E. L. Otol
Rich, J. H., GenSurg
Richard, L., Ophth
Ripley, H. R. D & TRad
Ross, A. W. Ophth,Otol
Senn, D. K.
Stewart, W. B., DiagRad
Summerer, Margo
Surette, G. D.
Valdez, R.
Wadup, R. S.
White, O. J. OrthSurg
Wright, J. S. GenSurg

MOUTH OF KESWICK
(270)
Bonga, Agatha C.

NASHWAAKSIS
(3,702)
Christy, G. B.

NEWCASTLE
(5,236)
Creaghan, M., GenSurg
Giovanetti, J. L.
Howatt, W. B. DiagRad

* Population not separately available.

Newcastle (Cont'd.)
Keays, J. F.
MacKay, W. W.
MacMillan, J. A.
McKenzie, R. B.
Morrissy, R. H.

NORTON
(830)
Winsor, A. L.

OROMOCTO
(12,170)
Byrne, A. J.
MacRae, E. E.
Miller, J. L.
Murchland, C. A.
Prosser, R. G.
Randell, O. T., GenSurg
Rioux, M.
Talpash, O. S.
Wills, D. G.

PERTH
(706)
Earle, R. W. L.
McCauley, M. M.
Moore, G. F. GenSurg
O'Neil, F. B.
Thomson, J.

PETITCODIAC
(900)
Caldwell, R. J.
Mellish, H. L.
Richardson, A. L.

PETIT ROCHER
(500)
Desjardins, C.

PLASTER ROCK
(1,403)
Frenette, F. F.
Rabatich, S.
Reid, E. C.

PORT ELGIN
(658)
Hill, G. V.
Winter, R. W.

REXTON
(668)
Graham, M. B.
Kenney, F. W.

RICHIBUCTO
(1,695)
Allaire, J.
Allard, J. T.
Boucher, A. J.

ROTHESAY
(782)
Branch, E. A. G., PathBact
Caskey, J. A., TherRad.
King, J. B.
Kirkland, A. S. D & TRad
Peat, G. B., ObstGyn
Peters, O. R.
Stanley, J. C., Psy

SACKVILLE
(3,038)
Andrews, T. C.
Barnhill, B. E. W.
Ferguson, G. G.
Gass, G. IntMed
Hirtle, W. E.
McFarlane, G. M.
Moorehouse, D. J.
Wrinch, J. H.

ST. ANDREWS
(1,534)
McGonigle, R. H.
Rigby, J. E.
Smith, D. W.

ST. BASIL
*
Cyr, H. Anaes
Kreyes, W.
Retfalvi, A.

ST. GEORGE
(1,125)
Allen, J. R. A.

SAINT JOHN
(95,563)
Alexander, C. J.
Allen, Irene V., IntMed(T.B.)
Arditti, J.
Baird, K. A., DermSyph
Bate, G. W., GenSurg
Baxter, W. J., GenSurg.
Bewick, J. B. IntMed
Bird, H. A. Path
Bonner, K. J. GenSurg
Boudreau, J. D.
Boulos, A. N., GenSurg
Brown, A. A. R., Anaes.
Brueckner, J. B.
Burditt, Anna M.
Bustin, H. B.
Caskey, J. A. TherRad
Cheesman, F. J. GenSurg
Chesley, A. E. Urol
Connell, F. R., Anaes.
Cooper, W. L., Ophth.
Cornelis, J. M., PlasSurg.
Craig, R. T.
Cram, E. T.
Creamer, T., ObstGyn
Davidson, V. D. GenSurg
Davis, E. R. Anaes
Donovan, A. L. IntMed
Duffy, D. A.
Evans, O. B. GenSurg
Fanjoy, R. W. Otol
Findley, J. A. GenSurg
Flood, H. J., DiagRad
Foster, T. A. ObstGyn
Freedman, L. H.
George, F. H. IntMed
Gibbon, A. D. Paed
Grant, N. C.
Grant, T. E. GenSurg
Guravich, J. L. IntMed
Handforth, J. R.
Hayes, R. T. OphthOtol
Higgins, D. J.
Higgins, R. B. GenSurg
Higgins, W. J.
Ingraham, D. R. GenSurg
Jennings, D. C. Anaes
Johnson, W. L.
Kanter, Y. C.
Karrel, I. A. IntMed
Keddy, G. W. A. GenSurg
Kelly, Allison C., Anaes.
Lea, R. H.
Leavitt, P. M.
Lee, R. W. IntMed
Lorimer, A., Path
Lund, G. E.
Lunney, E. W., Anaes
Lunney, T. E. Anaes
MacDonald, R. G. Paed
MacDougall, J. A. Anaes
MacKinnon, B. L.
MacLean, J. G. DermSyph
MacLennan, J. A., PathBact.
MacMillan, C. C., Ophth
Macpherson, R. T.
MacRae, D. R. Ophth,Otol
Maddison, G. E. PH
Malcolm, D. A.
Massie, R. A. Anaes
McInerney, J. P. GenSurg
McLean, J. D., Psy.
McLeese, Ruth V., DiagRad.
McLellan, N. W. IntMed Bact
Miller, W. D. GenSurg
Milrod, S. GenSurg
Mockler, G. R.
Moir, J. D.
Morgan, L. I.
Morse, L. R. Urol
Murphy, H. B. D & TRad
Murphy, W. J. IntMed
Nixon, M. D.
Nugent, J. R. GenSurg
Oake, C. M.
Orser, W. B.
Paraskevopoulos, G .Y., Paed
Parlee, H. B.
Pendrigh, R. M. GenSurg
Petrie, E. A. D & TRad
Pike, R. D.
Polowin, M. I. GenSurg
Pond, J. C., IntMed; Path
Randon, M. C.
Robertson, A. R.
Rodger, K. C. IntMed
Rosen, H. J. NeurSurg
Seaman, K. OrthSurg
Silivask, H.
Silver, S. Ophth,Otol
Simao, A. A., DiagRad
Simon, L. M.
Skinner, G. F. GenSurg, ThorSurg
Skinner, N. S. IntMed DiagRad
Smith, G. D. TherRad
Smith, R. L., Paed
Snow, P. V.
Stephen, L. J.
Stephen, W. GenSurg
Stevenson, L. J. DiagRad
Sullivan, H. A., Urol
Sullivan, J. K. Urol
Sutherland, D. F. Obst Gyn
Tanzman, J. ObstGyn
Taylor, C. R.
Theriault, J-C., Psy
Thompson, J. L.
Thompson, W. E.
Tonning, H. IntMed
Turko, R., DiagRad
Uy, I. N., Anaes
Vontso, V. H.
Walter, E. P. IntMed
Walters, W. C. IntMed
Wanamaker, F. D. ObstGyn
Watson, L. A.
Watts, H. M. IntMed
Weyman, S. Paed
Whiston, H. G., TherRad
White, G. M. ObstGyn
Yang, J. T.
Yoon, S. H., Urol.
Zed, V. M.

ST. LEONARD
(1,666)
Lapointe, G.
Mazerolle, D.

ST. MARTINS
(444)
Cooper, W. L. Ophth

ST. QUENTIN
(1,935)
Savoie, B.

ST. STEPHEN
(3,380)
Acker, M. I., IntMed, Anaes
Brownrigg, L. W. GenSurg
Everett, H. S. GenSurg
Johnston, E. B.
Lee, E. R. DiagRad
Stiles, E.

SALISBURY
(608)
Atkinson, T. E.

SHEDIAC
(2,159)
Gallant, O. J.
Inglis, D. S.
Renault, B.
Stephen, M. T.

SHIPPEGAN
(1,637)
Gauthier, J. D.
Mazerolle, A.

* Population not separately available.

STANLEY
(300)
Garnhum, D. G.

SUSSEX
(3,457)
Bryant, H. R.
Connolly, L. J.
Davidson, C. R.
O'Rafferty, E. P.
Reynolds, E. N.
Rideout, D. A.
Sharpe, H. H. Ophth

THE GLADES
*
Adams, A. R. F.
Blennerhassett, G. H.
Humman, M. J.

TORRYBURN
*
Knoll, F. G., Obst

TRACADIE
(1,651)
Anawati, N. K., Urol
Bourgeois, U. J.
Gaudet, P. E.
Le Blanc, V.
Leger, L. P., DiagRad.
Paulin, J. E.
Paulin, J. R.
Robichaud, A. GenSurg

VALLEE LOURDES
*
Nalbantoglu, H.
Porter, D. F. Paed

WESTFIELD
(80)
McLaughlin, J. A.

WOODSTOCK
(4,305)
Allanach, J. R.
Belyea, G. N., GenSurg.
Depow, C. W., GenSurg
Epstein, H. H., IntMed
Gibbons, T. G. DiagRad
Goodine, F. S.
Kee, C. G.
MacKinnon, M. H.
Margison, M. E.
Olmstead, G. A.
Tanton, T. M., Ophth Otol
Wishart, F. B.
Woolverton, E. F. GenSurg

Newfoundland & Labrador

AGUATHUNA
(134)
Biskupski, J. S.

AVONDALE
(798)
Conlon, M. P.

BAIE VERTE
(704)
Black, D. P.
Butt, D. F.
Devlin, J. T.
Drew, G. W.
Payne, D. E.

BAY d'ESPOIR
(*)
Rodriguez, C.
Williams, C. N.

BAY L'ARGENT
(210)
Aude, S.

BAY ROBERTS
(1,331)
Mallam, W. W.
Ploughman, R.

BELLEORAM
(570)
Forster, E. D.
Molineux, R. R.
Templeman, W.

BELL ISLAND
*
Lathouris, G.
Lewis, J.

BISHOP'S FALLS
(4,099)
Tulk, G. D. Anaes.
Tulk, Helen C.

BONAVISTA
(4,186)
Heath, J. W.

BONNE BAY
*
Ricketts, T. G.
Ross, J. M.
Toms, W. H.

BOTWOOD
(3,678)
Frecker, R. C.
Miguelino, O. M.
Steinmetz, N.
Woodfrey, R. I.

BRIGUS
(754)
Jones, E. D.

BROOKFIELD
*
Kelly, R.
McDonald, M. E.
Oliver, D. C.
Rolfe, H. C.

BURGEO
(1,454)
Calder, Aileen
Calder, C. M.

BURIN
(1,144)
Daya, F.
Hughes, P.

CARBONEAR
(4,234)
Bessell, J. A.
Kennedy, G. E.
Murray, P. J.
Rowe, A. T.
Wells, L. A.
Williams, T. W., Paed

CARMANVILLE
(764)
Igoe, J. M.

CHANNEL-PORT-AUX-BASQUES
(4,145)
Barnes, A. G.
Chung, H.
Le Grow, C. L.
Morrison, G. C.
Winkler-Prins, V.

CLARENVILLE
(1,543)
Barton, R. C.
Day, R. J., Anaes.
Horner, G. H.

COME-BY-CHANCE
(159)
Anderson, K.
Dingle, D. M.
Katz, M.
Leung, F.
MacSearraigh, E. S.
O'Neil, D. O.

CORNER BROOK
(25,188)
Bugden, R. L.
Butler, R. H. GenSurg
Butt, R. M., GenSurg
Cant, D. GenSurg, ThorSurg.
Conden, C., Anaes.
Cruz, A. A.
Davis, A. J., Paed
Delahunty, J. M.
Dove, R. F. GenSurg.
Farrell, T. C.
Forbes-Winslow, V. F.
Graham, J. S.
Harley, B. J. IntMed
Kerins, T. A.
Kerrigan, A. J.
King, J. H. Otol
Lees, B.
Magat, E.
Monaghan, T. T. GenSurg
Murphy, N. F.
Murphy, P. V.
O'Brien, B. J.
Parsons, K. W.
Peters, E. S. IntMed.
Pullin, L. B.
Rowe, W. D.
Simpson, I. M.
Warren, G. W.
Wass, N. H.
Yarn, J. C.

CURLING
(3,750)
Murray, B. V.
O'Connor, D. A.

DEER LAKE
(3,993)
Kennedy, A. M.
MacDonald, D. D.
Shaw, T. W.

DOYLES
(175)
Goulem, Y. L.

EASTPORT
(950)
Maret, E. P.
Stewart, D. L.

FERRYLAND
(656)
Foster, A. D.

FOGO
(1,154)
Medina, G.
Wilke, C.

GAMBO
(600)
Murphy, J. E.

GANDER
(5,725)
Blackie, P. B.
Boyle, P. J.
Brown, R.
Coxon, M. G.
Golding, D. R.
Gough, J.
Horner, G. S., Path.
Saver, J. J.
Victoros, C.
Wilson, H. D.

GLOVERTOWN
(1,193)
Parsons, M.

GOOSE BAY
(3040)
Devilly, D. J.

GRAND BANK
(2,703)
Burke, J.
Crawshaw, E. D.
Drake, H. M.
Wilkins, H. D.

GRAND FALLS
(6,064)
Alexander, A.
Black, J. H. S.
Brown, J. F.

* Population not separately available.

Grand Falls (Cont'd.)
Crosbie, J. C., Paed
Epstein, B. J., ObstGyn.
Fisher, J. E.
Galutira, J. B.
Harvey, M. L., Psy
Lee, J. R., IntMed
Martin, R. L.
O'Driscoll, R. F., GenSurg
Ricketts, T. G.
Shedden, D. A.

GREEN'S HARBOUR
(695)
Brett, F.
Sykes, G. W.

HAMPDEN
*
Misik, C.
Weeks, J.

HAPPY VALLEY
(2,861)
Ross, R. A.
Tsang, H. C.
Yun, D. D.

HARBOUR BRETON
(1,071)
Baimakos, D. G.
O'Neill, D.
Southcott, T. J.

HARBOUR GRACE
(2,654)
Kearney, D. D
McMcgrath, J. J., Anaes
Saltman, K.

HEART'S CONTENT
(646)
Hicks, D. O.

HERMITAGE
(395)
Moore, C. E.
Watson, C. P.

JEFFREY'S
*
Bugden, C.
King, D. L.

LABRADOR CITY
(Labrador)
(631)
Miller, R. H.
Paradis, M.

LA SCIE
(702)
Stewart, J. P.

LEWISPORTE
(2,702)
McVicker, M. A.
Pollock, A. W. L.
Wood, H. G.

LOURDES
(798)
McCann, K.

MANUELS
(522)
Butler, J. F.
Walsh, J. A.

MARKLAND
*
Newhook, W. H.

MARYSTOWN
(1,688)
Harris, C.
Remartinez, F. C.

MOUNT PEARL
(2,789)
Atkinson, P. I.

MUSGRAVETOWN
(570)
Stewart, D. L.

NORRIS POINT
(659)
Yoell, B. J.

NORTH WEST RIVER
(Labrador)
(563)
Brocklehurst, J.
Catling, Joy
Cormack, J. L.
Elkington, A. R.
Paddon, W. A.

OLD PERLICAN
(646)
Steele, P. R.
Wilkinson, H. H.
Wong, J.

PLACENTIA
(1,603)
Hogan, M. W.
Ross, J. M.
Russell, G. F.
Sabel, Barbara

PORT-AU-PORT
(214)
McCann, K.

ROSE BLANCHE
(627)
Carden, R. D.

ST. ALBAN'S
(1,334)
O'Callaghan, J.
O'Neill, D.

ST. ANTHONY
(1,820)
Beattie, Lillian M., ObstGyn.
Child, B.
Fish, Marjorie D.
Gray, J. M.
Korhonen, Annie E.
Purdell-Lewis, J. G.
Smith, A. J.
Thomas, G. W. ThorSurg

ST. BARBE
(*)
Swannie, E. M.

ST. GEORGE'S
(966)
Johnson, D. A.
Kilbane, M.
Murphy, D. P.

ST. JOHN'S
(90,838)
Acklie, Daphne W.
Allfree, A. J.
Anderson, T. G. Paed.
Andrade, E. M., ObstGyn.
Arjona, M. Q.
Baird, J. D. B. GenSurg
Battcock, G. W. GenSurg
Blackler, A. W. J. Ophth,Otol
Blackwell, H. J. GenSurg
Boddie, C. A., Psy
Bostock, D.
Boulos, J. B.
Brennan, J. C.
Brownrigg, G. M. GenSurg
Buckingham, G. A.
Buist, T. A.
Canilang, E. P.
Collingwood, W. P.
Collins, Bridget M.
Collins, J. F., Paed
Collins, T. M.
Colohan, A. B.
Cowan, J. E., OrthSurg
Coyle, J. V.
Craig, J.
Cremmell, E. H.
Cruz, Amelia M.
Daly, N., ObstGyn
Dickson, J., Anaes
Dominic, R. G., Paed.
Drover, W. H.
Duff, F. P., OrthSurg.
Duffy, R. A.
Elphinstone, Norah, Paed

Fahey, P. J., Urol.
Fanning, W. J.
Firme, F. N.
Forbes, R. A.
Fraser, J. O.
Frayworth, E. A.
Frechette, G., Psy
Frecker, G. A.
Freeman, E. O'B. Psy
Gough, D. W.
Gould, C. G.
Green, O.
Griffin, Jean
Guy, A.
Hanna, H. M., GenSurg.
Henderson, C. U., Anaes.
Henegan, W. D. D & TRad
Hicks, D. V., Psy
Higgins, W. J.
Ho, C. V.
Horan, P. J.
House, A. M., Neurol.
Ingram, D. W., IntMed.
Janes, A. W.
Josephson, J. E. IntMed, Path Bact
Joy, C. J. Paed
Kean, C. D. Anaes
Kean, G. T., ObstGyn.
Kennedy, B. J.
Kennedy, R. GenSurg
Knowling, Eithne
Knowling, T. A. IntMed (T.B.)
Land, J. Ophth,Otol
Landells, D. G. OrthSurg
Lawton, L. E.
Lawton, R. D. Ophth
Leclerc, R.
Lewis, A. S. GenSurg
Linegar, K. L. Paed
Lockwood, P.
Lopez, B.
Loveys, N. C.
Lush, N. J., Neur.
Lynch, J. G. OphthOtol
MacDonald, R. Anaes
Malone, E. W., DiagRad
Mangan, M. A.
Marshall, K. H. A.
McConn, Sheila
McDermott, A.
McGrath, J. M. F. PH
McKeever, R. W., Anaes.
McKilligin Helen R., Paed
McNamara, J. A.
McNicholas, P. J., Ophth
Mercer, A. R. Urol
Miller, A. B., ObstGyn
Miller, L. A. PH
Moores, E. F. GenSurg
Morris, C. A.
Morris, J. M., Psy
Murphy, G. M., IntMed.
Murphy, H. B. D & T Rad
Neary, A. J. GenSurg
O'Brien, G. J. Psy
O'Brien, K. J.
O'Dea, F. L.
O'Flaherty, W. J.
Parsons, Daphne
Parsons, W. D. IntMed
Paulse, D. T., Psy
Payne, W. J.
Peckham, G. B., IntMed
Peddle, D. B.
Peisley, Hazel N., Anaes
Pike, E.
Pillar, P. P.
Pottle, C. H. Psy
Quinlan, E. J.
Randell, Mary
Rho, Y. M.
Rice, D. M.
Roberts, H. D. GenSurg
Roberts, J. B. IntMed
Ross, J. B., Derm.

* Population not separately available.

St. John's (Cont'd.)
Russell, G. F.
Rusted, I. E. IntMed
Rusted, N. F. S. GenSurg
Ryan, Catherine
Scott, J.
Seary, J. M.
Severs, D.
Seviour, G. R.
Seviour, J. F., ObstGyn
Shapter, A. E. OrthSurg
Simms, D. C. Paed
Simms, R. J. IntMed
Sinclair, R. M.
Slowik, D. M.
Smith, Clare, Paed
Smith, J. T. GenSurg
Spurrell, P. A., IntMed
Stasiak, J., Urol
Stentaford, T. S. G. Anaes
Sutherland, D. L., NeurSurg
Taylar, C. E., Psy.
Taylor, A. W.
Tiller, W. D.
Walsh, J. E.
Walsh, J. F. Psy
Warrick, H. J.
Wells, A. M.
Whelan, P. J., GenSurg
Whitby, D., Psy
Wight, E. W.
Williams, J. G. Psy.
Williams, J. P., Path
Wyatt, D. E.
Yapp, V. U.
Young, R. W. IntMed

ST. JOSEPH'S
*
Seide, J.

ST. LAWRENCE
(2,095)
Hollywood, B. C.
Li, T. T.
Walsh, C. J.

ST. STEPHEN
(3380)
Brownrigg, L. W., GenSurg.

SPRINGDALE
(1,638) 6
Briffett, R. L.
Evans, W. M.
Tsang, R. C.

STEPHENVILLE
(6,041)
Grant R. Carroll
Malviya, D.

STEPHENVILLE CROSSING
(2,208)
Murphy, D. P.
Scott, A. F.
Squires, W. G.

TRINITY BAY
(639)
Brett, F.
Carr, M.

TWILLINGATE
(994)
Dennison, A. H.
Olds, J. M. GenSurg
Price, Carmen S.
Woodruff, F. W.

WABANA
(8,023)
Derjanecz, Brenda
Derjanecz, J. J., GenSurg

WABUSH (Labrador)
(151)
Armstrong, H. A.
Repo, R. U.

North West Territories

FORT SIMPSON
(495)
Black, L. M.
James, N. B.

FORT RAE
*
Martin, J. D.

FORT SMITH
(1,591)
Cass, Emily E.
Litwin, J.
Uygur, A.

FROBISHER BAY
(351)
Box, D. E.
Lacourciere, Helene

HAY RIVER
(1,338)
Covert, E. L.
Myrholm, G. S.

INUVIK
(1,248)
Habgood, Mary E.
Fleming, S. R.
MacNay, K. R.
Rooks, J.

NORMAN WELLS
(183)
Goyer, P.
Hackman, M. A.
King, G.
Nieboer, L. P.

YELLOWKNIFE
(3,100)
Ballard, E. J.
O'Donoghue, P. GenSurg
Powell, L. G.

NOVA SCOTIA

ADVOCATE HARBOUR
(338)
Kryski, T.

AMHERST
(10,788)
Ali, S., Ophth.
Brown, D. C.
Christie, H. E. IntMed
Coates, W. O. GenSurg
Donachie, J. P.
Drury, D.
Glen, N. G.
Kelley, E. G.
Langille, J. A. Ophth, Otol
Lawrence, G. A., GenSurg.
McCully, J. A.
McKendrick, A. J.
Morrison, W. R.
Myers, H. A. GenSurg
Ryan, E., Psy
Saunders, G. M. GenSurg

ANNAPOLIS ROYAL
(800)
Kerr, J. R.
Lawrence, J. A.

ANTIGONISH
(4,344)
Carroll, J. J.
Chou, W-H., Path
Donigiewicz, S., Anaes
Dunphy, A. E. GenSurg
Fraser, R. H.
George, J. A., DiagRad
Gorman, T. W. GenSurg
Greening, J. R., ObstGyn
Griffin, R. C.
MacCormick, J. A.
MacDonell, J. E. IntMed
MacDougall, D. A.
MacIntosh, C.
Murphy, P. N., Psy
Murphy, T. B.
Sers, Phyllis
Sers, R.

ARICHAT
(657)
Herbin, C. A.
Winter, J. H.

ARMDALE
(See Halifax)

AYLESFORD
(738)
Cogswell, D. L.
Kinsman, P. E.
Richardson, J.

BADDECK
(825)
MacDonald, C. S.
O'Brien, J. V.

BARRINGTON
(266)
Wilson, A. M.

BARRINGTON PASSAGE
(381)
Dalby, C.
Mears, T. S.

BASS RIVER
(325)
Elmik, A.

BEAR RIVER
(1,142)
Brennan, D. S.

BEDFORD
(2,025)
Atlee, H. B., ObstGyn
Fraser, J.
Fuller, S. C.
LeBrun, G. J., GenSurg
MacMurdo-MacMillan, Margaret
Schwartz, H. W., Ophth, Otol
Whyte, Catherine
Wilks, Helen M.

BERWICK
(1,288)
Cogswell, L. E.
Henshaw, J. D.
MacArthur, E. D
Moreash, R. A., GenSurg
Thorpe, R.

BIRCH COVE
(See Halifax)

BOUTILIERS POINT
(414)
Neilson, D. B., Path

BRIDGETOWN
(1,038)
Annand, R. T.
Mahaney, G. R.
Stone, O. R.

BRIDGEWATER
(4,499)
Bari, M. A.
Bennett, W. W.
Bent, W. I.
Biechl-O'Neill, Anna
Campbell, D. A.
Delory, M. E., GenSurg
Griffiths, A. J. DiagRad
Keller, E. S., Path.
Longden, D. E.
Marcus, S.
Prince, F. W.
Rowter, R. M.
Scantlebury, T. H.
Short, E. J.
Suppal, S. K.

CALEDONIA
(404)
Kavanagh, P. J.

* Population not separately available.

CANNING
(619)
Foley, H. A.
CANSO
(1,151)
Bland, H. J.
NYANZA
*
Cox, R. H
CHESTER
(1,064)
Jollymore, G. C.
Woodroofe, E.
Zwicker, D. W. N.
CHETICAMP
(1,107)
Bourdreau, G.
Ratchford, H. A., GenSurg
Samson, H. A.
CHEVERIE
(200)
Hines, A.
Hines, C. H.
CLARK'S HARBOUR
(950)
Corbett, J. R.
Sheehan, D. B.
CORNWALLIS
*
Gerlitz, J. H., Psy
DARTMOUTH
(46,966)
Akhtar, S. N.
Anselmo, R. S.
Badenoch, A G.
Barteaux, J .W.
Barton, F. J., GenSurg
Beazley, R. W.
Bentley, C. H.
Bessonette, J.
Bhattacharyya, A.
Bistevins, Rita
Brennan, M. D., GenSurg
Brown, J. R.
Bugden, C. W.
Cameron, J. R.
Cole, W. S.
Coskun, N.
Cunningham, Helen M.
Cunningham, R. M. D&TRad
Fahmy, H.
Ferguson, P. D.
Ferguson, P. J
Fisher, W. J., Neur, Psy
Fraser, G. M.
Gladwin, K. D.
Gordon, A.
Hanko, F.
Hansen, A. R.
Holland, Lieselotte, Psy.
Johnson-MacLeod, G. Enid, Anaes.
Johnston, D. W., ObstGyn
Johnston, S. R., D & TRad
Kovacs, Edith
Kovacs, L. L., Psy.
Lamplugh, A. N
MacDonald, G.
MacDonald, M. S.
MacKay, R. W. M., Psy
MacKeigan, D. S., GenSurg
MacLeod, A. G.
MacRae, A. E. C.
Malcolm, F. F.
Mathur, P. S., GenSurg.
McCann, G. T.
Measham, A. R.
Moore, E. A.
Moores, A. A., GenSurg.
Morris, M. U.
Morris, D. E., GenSurg
Muir, J. R.
Pace, G. C.
Parkin, R. P., Psy
Poulos, H. P., Psy.
Pudymaitis, O. J.
Richardson, J.
Ritchie, R. G.
Rosere, L. A.
Samad, A.
Sanders, D. H.
Savage, J. P.
Smith, E. A.
Spark, D. H.
Stacey, D. L., Psy.
Stevens, A. H.
Stevens, Estelle
Tenderenda, T.
Trask, N. B.
Tucker, W. G.
Vair, C. D.
Verge. W.
Weir, D. A.
Weste, Ilse
Weste, U. A., Paed
Young, A. L.
Young, C. H., IntMed
Young, F. L
DIGBY
(2,306)
Armstrong, R. A.
Black, D. G.
Lewis, D. E.
McCleave, J. R., GenSurg
Spencer, E. W., D & TRad
DOMINION
(2,994)
Tompkins, J. B.
EASTERN PASSAGE
(682)
Causing, S. S.
ELMSDALE
(535)
Burris, J. M.
Wright, R. G.
FAIRVIEW
(1,550)
Snow, J. M.
FREEPORT
(438)
Birsel, N.
Ming, P. H.
GLACE BAY
(24,186)
Appel, B.
Calder, A., IntMed (T.B.)
Fultz, W E., Ophth
Green, S. A., GenSurg
Gursahani, L.
Haq, B. Z.
Khalifa, A. M.
MacNeil, J. R.
Maxwell, B. R., DiagRad
McDonald, J. A.
McNeil, J. O , GenSurg
Nicholson, W. M.
Patodia, G. L.
Patton, W. W.
Rajani, M. R., GenSurg.
GLEN MARGARET
(*)
Sheenann, D. B.
GREAT VILLAGE
(498)
Johnson, A. E.
GUYSBOROUGH
(490)
Hall, K. A.
HALIFAX
(183,946)
Acker, J. C., OrthSurg
Acker, T. B., OrthSurg
Aikens, R. L., IntMed
Ali, M.
An, S. H.
Anderson, R. N., IntMed
Anderson, T. A., Anaes
Asuncion, J.
Aterman, K.
Auld, C. R. B., GenSurg
Bachmann, F.
Baker, C. H. L., Anaes
Ballem, R. W. M., Anaes
Barton, F. J., GenSurg.
Beckwith, C. J. W., IntMed T.B), PH
Bedwell, S. F., Neur
Bethune, C. M., Anaes
Bethune, G. W., GenSurg
Boudreau, J. F.
Brady, A. J. R
Brander, J. A., DiagRad.
Brown, D. C. S., OrthSurg.
Brown, H. J.
Brown, R. L.
Buhr, A. J., OrthSurg
Burnstein, M. E.
Cahill, J. F.
Cairns, J. M., IntMed
Cantwell, J. F
Carr, C. W., Anaes.
Carver, J. B.
Casey, M. T. GenSurg
Chandler, B. M. D., IntMed
Chandler, Margaret R.
Charman, J. H., GenSurg
Chipman, C. D., Path
Coady, B. K., GenSurg
Cochrane, W. A., Paed
Cole, P. A
Colford, H. B.
Colwell, G. J., PhysMed
Condy, W. A.
Constable, W. C.
Constantinides, S., GenSurg
Cooper, J. H., Path
Corston, J. M. ObstGyn
Coward, N. B., Paed
Crosby, A. B.
Crosby, Joan M , Paed
Cudkowicz, L.
Cudmore, D. W., ObstGyn.
Cunningham, R. M. D&TRad
Davis, G. E., DiagRad
Davis, M. M., ObstGyn
Delahunt, J. A.
Destounis, N.
Deveau, G. R.
Dhalla, S. H., GenSurg.
Dickson, R. C , IntMed
Dimitriades, G.
Dincsoy, H. P., Path.
Dincsoy, M. V., Paed
Doane, B. K.
Dolan, F. G., GenSurg
Dressler, J. A.
Drysdale, A. A., Anaes
Duncan, M.
Dunsworth, F. A.
Dussault, L., GenSurg (P.Q.)
Eagles, E. L., PH.
Elwood, T N.
Erdogan, M., OrthSurg
Ernst, W. A., Urol.
Feindel, J. H. Anaes
Filbee, J. F., TherRad
Fleming, R. A. P., Anaes
Flight, G. H., ObstGyn
Flynn, P., Psy
Fogo, E. M
Folkins, D. F., IntMed.
Fort, T. C., Otol.
Fraser, F. M.
Fullerton, S. G. B.
Fyfe, F. W.
Ganguli, A. K., GenSurg.
George, K. P., GenSurg
Gillespie, C. T., Paed.
Gillis, D. A., GenSurg
Glenister, E. I , Ophth
Glube, M. R., Anaes
Glynn, J. J.
Goldberg, H. I., DermSyph

* Population not separately available.

Halifax (Cont'd.)
Gordon, C. A., IntMed
Gordon, P. C., PH
Gorelick, M. M.
Gosse, C. L., Urol, GenSurg
Gosse, N. H., GenSurg.
Goulding, G. L., Anaes
Graham, C. H., GenSurg
Graham, D. V, Anaes
Grant, D. M.
Grant, K. M., ObstGyn
Grant, R. S., Paed
Grantmyre, E. B., DiagRad
Granville, E. T.
Green, L., IntMed
Green, S., GenSurg
Guptill, G. A.
Haldane, J. H.
Hall, H. K., Psy
Halley, L. J.
Hameed, K., Path.
Hammerling, Anne F.
Hammerling, J. S.
Hand, R. F., OphthOtol
Harlow, C M.
Hastings, James R. T., DiagRad.
Hayes, J. K.
Hayes, K. P.
Hines, S. D.
Hirsch, Doris, Psy
Hirsch, S., Psy
Hirtle, L. R.
Holland, C. W, IntMed
Holland, L. G., Ophth, Otol
House, W. K., GenSurg
Howell, D. R. S., DermSyph
Huestis, S., Neur.
Hunter, H. M. Paed
Ing, V. W-K., IntMed
Jakubovicz, A. A.
James, R. H.
Johnson, E. B.
Johnston, Lilia A.
Jones, C. M., D & TRad
Jones, R. O., Psy
Judah, J. I.
Keating, W J.
Keays, C. F., Ophth.
Keet, Sylvia, J.
Kendell, D.
Kerenyi, N. A., Path
Ketene, V.
Kilpatrick, Elizabeth
Kingston, W. B.
Kinley, C. E., GenSurg
Kirk, T. E.
Kitz, Alice D.
Knodell, H. L.
Korth, V. H., Anaes
Krause, V. W., Path
Landrigan, P. L. IntMed
Lane, R. A.
Lang, H. B, Path
Langdon, R. L.
Langley, G. R., IntMed
Laufer, S. T., IntMed.
Lee, D. T., ObstGyn.
Lewis, A. J., Path
Lucis, O. J.
Lynch, D. O., Psy
MacDonald, C. J., GenSurg
MacDonald, C. J.
MacDonald, H. N., Neur.
MacDonald, M. R. PH
MacDonald, P. M.
MacDonald, R. M., IntMed
MacGregor, H. J.
MacGregor, P. A., IntMed
MacIntosh, J. W., IntMed
MacIntosh, O. C., Path.
Mack, F. G., Urol.
MacKeen, A. D. DiagRad
MacKeigan, D. S., GenSurg
MacKenzie, A.
MacKenzie, D. J
MacKinnon, C. G., Anaes
MacKinnon, H. H., IntMed.
Maclean, T. R.
MacLeod, A. J., IntMed
McLeod, I. M., D & Trad
MacLeod, S. C., ObstGyn
MacPherson, Enid
MacPherson, I. G.
MacRae, D. M., Ophth, Otol
MacRae, W. M.
Macsween, J.
Mahabir, R. N., IntMed
Manchester, J. S., D & TRad
Marshall, A. M.
Marshall, C., NeurPsy
Maxwell, I. D., Path
McCaw, I. F.
McCurdy, D. J.
McDougall, Ruth, PH
McKiggan, J.J., IntMed
Millard, O. H., Urol
Miller, B. F, OrthSurg
Miller, J. E. H.
Mirchandani, G. R.
Mitra, A. K.
Molloy, J. H., Ophth
Moore, E. A., Psy
Moores A. A., GenSurg
Morehouse, C. N.
Morton, A. R. PH
Morton, B. S., Paed
Murphy, A. L., GenSurg
Murphy, R. S., Otol
Murray, A E., GenSurg
Murray, D. K., Ophth
Murray, W. A., IntMed
Myrden, J. A., GenSurg
Napier, R.
Neilson, D. B.
Nelson, R. F.
Nemethy, N. I., Derm
Nicholas, W. C. IntMed
Nicholson, D. M., GenSurg
Nicholson, J. F., Psy
Nigam, P. S.
Noble, J. A., GenSurg.
Nonamaker, E. P., ThorSurg, GenSurg
Norvell, S. T., GenSurg
Nugent, J. M.
O'Brien, D. B., Ophth
Orr, W. L.
Ozere, R. L., Paed
Pasquet, A. F., Anaes
Pereira, Ethel, ObstGyn
Perlin, I. A., ObstGyn
Phillips, H. R.
Phillips, W. C.
Pineo, G. F., IntMed.
Pollett, W. E., GenSurg
Prentice, R. S. A., Path
Pugh, R. E.
Purkis, I. E., Anaes
Purves, J. K., GenSurg
Quigley, H. G.
Quigley, J. H., Ophth
Rahman, F.
Read, H. C., IntMed
Reardon, C. H.
Reid, B. L.
Reid, B. S.
Reid, E. L.
Reid, J. W., IntMed
Ritchie, R. M., Paed
Robbins, J. H.
Roberts, T. M., PlasSurg.
Robertson, J. S., PH
Robinson, S. O, ObstGyn
Ross, Elizabeth, Paed
Ross, E. F., GenSurg
Ross, H. B., Paed
Ross, J. F., GenSurg
Roy, D. L., IntMed
Sabean, H. B., DiagRad
Sanghi, J. K.
Sarkar, Nellie N.
Sarkar, S. C., Paed
Saunders, S. C.
Saxon, R. D.
Scammell, H. L.
Scott, K. E., Paed.
Service, Gwendolyn
Shane, A. G., Otol
Shane, A. M., Psy
Shane, S. J., IntMed
Shannon, M. P., DiagRad
Shaw, A. J., DiagRad
Shaw, G. B.
Shears, A. H., Phys Med & Rehab.
Shephard, D. A., Anaes.
Shlossberg, R. S., Ophth, Otol
Sidorov, J. J., IntMed
Sigsworth, P. D., Paed
Simms, G. G., PH
Simpson, A. A.
Sinclair, A. M., OrthSurg
Slayter, J H.
Slipp, L. B.
Smith, C. B.
Smith, D. F., ObstGyn
Song, K. T., GenSurg
Sorger, K., Path
Stanton, J. J.
Stapleton, J. E, TherRad
Starratt, V. C.
Steele, B. J., GenSurg
Steeves, L. C., IntMed
Stevenson, W. D., NeurSurg, GenSurg
Stewart, C. B., PH
Stewart, F. W.
Stewart, H. L., GenSurg
Still, H. C.
Stirling, M.
Stoddard, C. C., Anaes
Stoddard, R. H., Ophth, Otol
Stott, N. W.
Sutherland, J. B., GenSurg.
Tainsh, J. M,, IntMed
Thorne, E. L.
Threlkeld, Agnes W.
Tibbles, J. J.
Tiongson, R. V., IntMed.
Titus, A. W.
Tompkins, M. G., Jr. ObstGyn
Tonning, D. J., IntMed
Trias, A., OrthSurg
Tucker, H. H., NeurSurg
Tupper, W. R. C., ObstGyn
Van Rooyen, C. E., PathBact
Walling, F. M.
Warren, W. P., IntMed.
Watt, W. N.
Waugh, D., Path
Weil, R. J., Psy
Weld, C. B.
Wenning, A. S., Anaes
West, Margaret
Wheelock, G. H
Whitby, D.
Wiswell, G. B., Paed
Woodbury, J. F. L., IntMed
York, S. E., IntMed

HANTSPORT
(1,385)
Kenny, G. E.
Smith, G. K.

HUBBARDS
(418)
Cole, P A.
Slipp, L. B.

INVERNESS
(2,109)
Lawley, A. M.
Maclean, C. B.
Maclean, N. J.
Risk, A.

KENNETCOOK
(328)
Snow, J. T.

* Population not separately available.

KENTVILLE
(4,612)
Anand, S.
Anand, S., GenSurg.
Buntain, J. H.
Crosson, E. W.
Forbes, G. R
Giffin, A. A.
Healy, R. W.
Hiltz, J. E., IntMed (T.B.)
Holden-Quinlan, Helen M., IntMed.
Kirkpatrick, D. H.
Kloss, G. A.
Laretei, A.
Lindsay, A., Ophth
McGrath, J. P., Ophth, Otol
Misener, F. J.
Quinlan, J. J., ThorSurg
Rostocka, M.
Sanghi, J. K., OrthSurg
Schaffner, V. D., GenSurg
Seaman, D. M.
Stone, P. H.
Taylor, W. A.
Toews, Mary A.
Toews, N. A.
Worthylake, M. G.

KINGSTON
(1,434)
Archibald, D , McD
Webster, A. R.

LAKE ECHO
*
Barlow, W. R.

LAWRENCETOWN
(509)
Morse, F. W., GenSurg

LITTLE BRAS D'OR
(1,131)
Gouthro, A. C.

LITTLE BROOK
(423)
Gaudet, L.
LeBlanc, P. H.

LIVERPOOL
(3,714)
Bell, F. G
Bird, S. B.
MacDonald, F. D.
MacLeod, L. A.
Wickwire, J. A.

LOCKEPORT
(1,235)
Robbins, S.

LOUISBOURG
(1,417)
Mosher, D. T.

LOUISDALE
(736)
Boffa, N.

LOWER SACKVILLE
(1,017)
Whyte, F.

LOWER SAULNIERVILLE
*
Pothier, H. J.

LUNENBURG
(3,062)
Cantelope, D. C.
Creighton, H. A., GenSurg
Hetherington, R. N., Anaes
Hewat, W A.
Keddy, D. B.
MacIntyre, K. R.
Saunders, R. M.
Wood, R. G. A., GenSurg
Zinck, R. C.

MAHONE BAY
(1,109)
Donaldson, G. D., Anaes
Keedy, D. B.
Langille, D. C.

MARGAREE FORKS
(361)
MacIsaac, W., Otol

METEGHAN
(842)
Belliveau, R. P.

MIDDLE MUSQUODOBOIT
(741)
Earle, T H.
Marshall, A. C.

MIDDLETON
(1,921)
Cable, R., DiagRad
Feener, J. R., GenSurg
Kelley, H. E.
Munro, R. E.
Wilson, B. R.

MONASTERY
(200)
Rostant, L. A.

MOSER'S RIVER
(230)
Parkin, R. P.

MULGRAVE
(1,149)
Layden, J. M.

MUSQUODOBOIT HARBOUR
(500)
Jardine, P. R.
Mackenzie, E A.

NEIL'S HARBOUR
*
Maharaj, D. T.
Munroe, R. G.

NEW GERMANY
(623)
Crowe, J. B.
Din, G.

NEW GLASGOW
(9,782)
Campbell, A. C.
Douglas, G. R., GenSurg
Felderhof, H. H.
FitzGerald, M. F.
Grieves, J K.
Harries, C. G.
Henderson, E. E., DiagRad
Hyslop, W. A.
Jakeman, W. A.
Locke, H. A.
MacKay, H. F.
MacQuarrie, N. A.
Mathur, K. C.
Miller, R. B., DiagRad
Munroe, R. G , GenSurg
Park, J. N.
Skinner, E. B.
Townsend, H. J.
Williston, J. M.

NEW WATERFORD
(10,592)
Chisholm, M. J.
Goldberg, A. H.
Mahboob, S.
Nathanson, D. S., GenSurg
Miller, C. P.
Roach, J. A.
Watson, A. R., DiagRad
Woolf, S. M.
Zaidi, S. M.

NORTH SYDNEY
(8,657)
Gardner, P S., ObstGyn
Kirkpatrick, P. H.
McKenzie, L. D.
Meech, L. R., GenSurg
Munro, J. S.
Nichol, P. R.
Skinner, L. A.
Tremblett, Hilda, Path

NYANZA
(52)
Cox, R H.

OXFORD
(1,465)
Athley, P. A.
Davies, D. R.
Hashmi, S.

PARRSBORO
(1,834)
Kernohan, D.

PICTOU
(4,534)
Dunn, S. D.
Smith, C. B.
Young, J. A F.

POINT EDWARD
(Cape Breton)
*
Muir, D. M.

PORT HAWKESBURY
(1,345)
Guzdziol, W.
Sharma, S. R.
Siddall, W. R.

PORT HOOD
(472)
Murphy, M.

PORT WILLIAMS
(805)
Milton, G. L.

PORTERS LAKE
(383)
Gangoli, A. K.

PUBNICO
(331)
Clark, A. M.

PUGWASH
(519)
Gass, K. V.

RAWDON
*
MacLellan, R. A.

RESERVE MINES
(2,789)
Sparrow, C. J.

RIVER HEBERT
(1549)
Boodoosingh, R. S.

RIVER JOHN
(526)
Lewis, J. W.

ROCKINGHAM
(1,451)
Aquino, A., TherRad.
Cullen, F. R., Anaes
Evans, E. H.
Kingston, M. B., ObstGyn.
Perry, R. A.
Wood, W. C.

ROSE BAY
*
Barss, Allison H.
Barss, G. A.

ST. PETER'S
(762)
Digout, J H.
Wright, J. M.

SANDY COVE
(400)
Sutherland, I. R.

SEABRIGHT
*
Cudkowicz, L.

SHAD BAY
(244)
Robertson, W. M. D.

SHEARWATER
*
Davis, Pamela M.
Knight, C. J.
McNeill, S. R.

* Population not separately available.

SHEET HARBOUR
(1,073)
MacMillian, D.
Potter, S. W.
Trivedi, B.

SHELBURNE
(2,408)
Campbell, D. R.
Campbell, Margaret
Cooper, M. T.
Jeffrey, W. H.
Markus, F.

SHERBROOKE
(324)
Silver, G. L.

SHUBENACADIE
(812)
Jones, J. T.
MacInnis, D. F.
MacInnis, D. R.

SOUTH OHIO
*
MacWilliam, J. V.

SPRINGHILL
(5,844)
Burden, R. A.
Davies, D. R.
Fisher, D. H.
Murray, J. C.

SPRYFIELD
(*)
Deyoung, G. G.
Gonsalves, R. C.
MacWhirter, R. B.
Mirchandani, G. R.
Smith, K. P.
Smith, Marjorie

STELLARTON
(5,327)
Cameron, S. H.
Hamm, J. F.
MacDonald, J. B.
MacKay, I. E., Anaes
Parker, V. H. T.

STEWIACKE
(1,045)
Havey, H. B.
Stewart, R C.

SYDNEY
(33,617)
Allen, L. S., GenSurg
Aquino, Lilia
Archibald, D. B., Urol
Blaikie, W. D.
Brennan, C. F., ObstGyn
Calder, A.
Corbett, H. R., DiagRad
Cormier, J. G., Ophth, Otol
Cunningham, A. L.
Davidson, H. J.
Devereux, H. J
D'Intino, C. A.
Donovan, C., Psy
Earle, Anne
Earle. B. V.
Ellerker, A. R.
Finch, G. C.
Gaum, A., GenSurg
Gaum, D.
Gouthro, P. J.
Gyorfi, A. W.
Intino, C. A. D.
Kelley, F. J., GenSurg
Kelly, P A.
Krzyski, T. K.
Land, H. D., Ophth, Otol
Lynch, J. G.
Macaulay, M. J.
MacDonald A. A., IntMed
MacDonald, C. A.
MacDonald, F. B
MacDonald, G. C.
MacDonald, H. S.
MacDonald, J. P.
MacGuire, G. F.
MacKenzie, D. E., IntMed
MacKenzie, D. H., GenSurg
MacLellan, C. L.
MacLennan, N. K., ObstGyn
Macneill, N. F.
Marsh, G. S.
Mason, D. R.
Mathieson, R.
McDonagh, Christina, Psy
McLellan, J. R., Ophth
McPhail, J. A.
McQuade, G. W.
Muir, D. M.
O'Neil F.
Ormiston, A. W.
Osyany, Bela G.
Pariagh, K.
Raz, V. M., OrthSurg.
Riley, C.
Robb, D. S.
Ross, H. R.,GenSurg
Simpson, R G.
Singh, V.
Sodero, G. W., GenSurg
Sutherland, A. L
Sutherland, H. F.
Thomas, O.
Trask, B. C., IntMed
Virick, M. S.
Whiteside, W. H., GenSurg
Young, J. C.
Young, R. C., IntMed

SYDNEY MINES
(9,122)
Danak, M. T.
Fraser, K
Lamond, W. J.
Martin, H. J.
McKeough, L. L., GenSurg
McKeough, T J.
Shaikh, M. A.
Sustring, J.

SYDNEY RIVER
(1954)
Jackson, P. D.
Mian, M. A.

TATAMAGOUCHE
(581)
Creighton, A. M

TRURO
(12,421)
Bruce, M. M.
Cook, G. H., GenSurg
Giffen, C. C., Psy
Handforth, C. P., Path
Karrel, B. D.
Lavers, H. D
Little, P. R.
MacDonald, W. J.
MacDonald, W. J., GenSurg
MacFayden, D. A.
MacKenzie, S. G., GenSurg
Martenstyn, H. R., DiagRad
McKean, H. R
Moore, D. S.
Morrison, N. A.
Peel, H. R.
Reid, J. B.
Royal, H. O.
Shephard, K. B
Smith, C. H.
Sodero, T. C. C., GenSurg
Starratt, V. C.
Vibert, J. C., GenSurg
Wheeler, B. R.
Wilson, J. J. S

TUSKET
(331)
Charlwood, R. R.
Lupin, J. A.

UPPER MUSQUODOBOIT
(475)
Kavanagh, P. J.

UPPER ROWDON
(*)
Whittier, Catherine L.

UPPER STEWIACKE
*
Bell, M. C.

WAVERLEY
(1,142)
Clark, D. S.

WESTMOUNT NORTH
(886)
Prossin, A. J.

WESTVILLE
(4,159)
Fraser, J. H.
Whitman, H. B.

WEYMOUTH
(584)
Doucet, F. J.
Erjavec, J.
Minc, R. H.

WINDSOR
(3,823)
Akin, F L.
Kryszek, S. H.
Morris, D. J.
Roby, H. R., DiagRad
Smith, G. M.
Smith, J. A.
Turner, G. W.
Vaughan, A , GenSurg
Vaughan, E. G.

WOLFVILLE
(2,413)
Beveridge, J. M.
Cleveland, E. J., Psy
Davison, D. L.
Denton, G. D., IntMed
Kirkpatrick, H. W., Ophth. Otol.
Nicholls, J. H.
Rice, W. C., GenSurg
Simms, H. N.
Townsend, F. R., Psy

YARMOUTH
(8,636)
Angus, G. A.
Balmanno, J. T., GenSurg
Belliveau, G. D.
Bergmann-Porter, Eleonore
Bruce, I. F.
Burton, G V. Jr.
Caldwell, R. M.
Cassells, Irene
Cassells, M. J., Path
Churchill, Margaret E., Paed
Fuller, C. K., Ophth, Otol
MacDonald, D. F., IntMed
MacDonald, G. M.
MacDonald, W. J.
Mallett, J. J
Melanson, F. J., GenSurg
Morse, W. I., IntMed.
Morton, L. M., GenSurg
O'Brien, M. W.
O'Brien, W. C.
Ozvegy, F. S., DiagRad
Phinney, W. M.
Ramsay, E L., Ophth
Rideout, V. K.
Siddall, A. M.
Webster, J. A., GenSurg
Williamson, S. W.

* Population not separately available.

Ontario

ACTON
(4,150)
Buckner, R. D.
Garrett, D. A
Hutchison, J. C.
Kenny, W. G.
Moore, T. B.
Ven der Bent, D. W.

AGINCOURT
(1,738)
Appleby, Shirley **V.**
Borland, K. R.
Coomey, E. J.
Datzeff, G. A.
Doney, E. H.
Fair, M. A.
Farquharson, C. D., IntMed., PH.
Greiger, Linda M.
Grogan, D. R.
Hood, D. C.
McClure, P.D., Paed
Moran, E. J.
Noble, A. J., Path.
Palmer, J. G.
Peters, A.
Prowse, G. G.
Raisbeck, W. A.
Robinson, R. E.
Stephens, O. E. A.
Stobie, S. N. P.
Warkentin, D. E.
Whan, J. H.
Wight, E. W.

AILSA CRAIG
(555)
Meredith, A. R.

AJAX
(7,759)
Bosch, J. W.
Davidson, H. D.
Gove, D. I.
Noble, D. M.
McIlveen, G. N.

ALDERSHOT
(2459)
Blodgett, A. L. N.

ALEXANDRIA
(2,590)
Bourdeau, Y.
Dolan, D. J.
Markson, M.
Roman, L.

ALFRED
(1,188)
Pinard, H. E.

ALLISTON
(2,881)
Baxter, R.
Charters, J. E.
Derjanecz, Brenda
Derjanecz, J., GenSurg.
Flower, C. D.
Gripper, N. D.
Irwin, T. G.
Marx, R., ObstGyn
Walker, L. A.

ALMONTE
(3,273)
Bach, R. K.
Fraser, J. R., ObstGyn.
King, J. K.
Schulte-Steinberg, O.

ALVINSTON
(664)
Clysdale, E. S.

AMHERSTBURG
(4,454)
Harris, E. C.
Holmes, A. B.
Hutchinson, E. B.
Hutchinson, E. D.
James, R. N.
Ladouceur, E. C.
Leonard, J. G.
McPherson, G. R.
Patt, N. L., DiagRad
Shelley, R. P.

AMHERST VIEW
(2,000)
Workman, D. G.

ANCASTER
(1,710)
Bethune, R. D.
Bradford, J. G.
Dean, T. W., D & TRad
Jepson, T. E.
McCurlie, J. M.
McHarg, R. G.
Middlemass, I. B., DiagRad
Robinson, D. C., ObstGyn
Roderick, J. H.
Ruland, N. W.
Tyrrell, J. D., IntMed
Walker, C. E.
White, J. G., Psy

ANGUS
(1101)
Cruickshank, J. W.

ANSONVILLE
(3,080)
Coates, G.
Mertens, D. J.

APPLE HILL
(394)
McDonald, G. V.

APSLEY
(298)
MacMillan, R. N.

ARKONA
(504)
Griffiths, Dorothy E.
Mesbur, K. H.

ARNPRIOR
(5,474)
Bonell, J. D., GenSurg
Box, J. H.
Cha-Chu, C. B.
Cooper, B. J.
Dauphinais, J. L.
Giberson, H. R.
Gregory, A. G., IntMed.
McCreary, R. H., Paed
Mesbur, K. H.
Parsons, C. J.
Roy, R. L.

ARTHUR
(1,200)
Hogg, J. S.

ATIKOKAN
(6,674)
Adey, A. B.
Grayson, W. R.
Kristjanson, G. V.

ATWOOD
(469)
Bigelow, W. L.

AURORA
(8,795)
Beveridge, K.
Diamond, A. W.
Faudemer, W. A.
Knowles, Betty
Knowles, J.
Rice, A. L.
Rose, C.
Rose, C. C.
Urquhart, J. L.
Wilkes, L. B.
Williams, G. W.

AVONMORE
(287)
Pollock, J. M.

AYLMER (west)
(4,705)
Beveridge, G.
Miller, M. M.
Poots, A. V.
Sinclair, D. W.
Wright, D. L.

AYR
(1,015)
Holland, J. B

AYTON
(500)
Hergott, J. J.

AZILDA
(2,929)
Huneault, G.
Leclair, J. E.

BADEN
(977)
Barton, R. W.

BALA
(499)
Krawetz, M.

BALMERTOWN
(710)
Delaney, F. G.

BANCROFT
(2,615)
Anderson, O. W.
Johnson, H. S.
Lehinant, V.
Lumb, S. S.

BARRIE
(21,169)
Aikins, J. A.
Asquith, R., Paed
Bailey, W. J.
Beaton, Anita, Anaes
Beaton, E. J., GenSurg
Bigelow, L. H.
Case, J. R., IntMed.
Clark, D. B., Psy.
Clinton-Thomas, C. L., GenSurg
Crossland, A., GenSurg
Delaney, R. J., GenSurg
Dick, J. J.
Doidge, W. A.
Farrington, W. C.
Forbes, R. I.
Friedrich, S. K.
Gray, A. D.
Hicks, J. P.
Hope-Gill, H. F.
Hopwood, G. M.
Ideson, R. S.
Laurie, N. M.
Little, W. C.
MacPherson, R. N.
McLoughlin, D. P., DiagRad.
Moodie, G. E.
Nelson, R. J., GenSurg
Phillips, J. R.
Postnikoff, J. I.
Quackenbush, H. A.
Ravenscroft, A. K.
Reid, R. F.
Renton, G. E.
Scott, P. A.
Seymour, G. C.
Shannon, F.
Smith, F. B.
Smith, J. H. N.
Swan, H. G.
Tikkala, A. O.
Turnbull, A. R.
Walsh, M. J.
Watson, P. M.
Weatherston, C. E., ObstGyn
Zerny, C. J., IntMed

* Population not separately available.

BARRY'S BAY
(1,439)
Chapeskie, A. H.
Smith, P. C.

BATH
(692)
Burleigh, H. C.

BATTERSEA
*
Freeman, N. V.

BAY RIDGES
*
Corbin, M. F.
Gahny, F.
Levy, R. A.
Ritchie, R. S.
Rotstein, M. I.

BEACHBURG
(544)
Murtagh, A. P.

BEAMSVILLE
(2,541)
Barnard, J. E.
Latham, H. D.
Russell, W. A. M.

BEARDMORE
(998)
Wallingford, W. W.

BEAVERTON
(1,217)
Ames, H. D.
Jardine, K.

BELLE RIVER
(1,860)
Poisson, T. C.

BELLEVILLE
(30,655)
Allore, R. L. W. ObstGyn
Asregadoo, E. R.
Bateman, J. H. GenSurg
Bateman, R.
Bates, W. F.
Beattie, W. B.
Birchard, J. R., ObstGyn
Blakslee, V.
Brearley, G. G.
Conn, E. B., Psy
Cronk, G. S. GenSurg
Cronk, L. B. IntMed
Dempsey, Ethel A., Anaes.
Douglas, K. M. GenSurg
Empson, J. D.
Forrester, J. H. Ophth,Otol
Gibson, R. S. Anaes
Hartt, J. N.
Hipwell, W. T.
Horne, S. D.
Lenk, C., PH.
Locke, A. C. Ophth,Otol
Loder, P. G. DiagRad
Loynes, J. S.
Macleod, D. E., Ophth
MacDonald, E. M.
Manderville, E. A.
McKenna, A. C.
McSherry, J. B.
Miles, A. E.
Morphy, R. S. Urol
Nelles, J. E. Paed
Patterson, R. K.
Pearce, G. A.
Peterkin, Edith, K. Paed
Potter, R. T.
Ross, F. R.
Rota, A. N. Path
Scott, J. R.
Scott, P. A., GenSurg
Stevenson, M., Urol
Stobie, G. H., GenSurg
Stock, J. S.
Tanton, Clare W., Anaes
Totten, W. S., IntMed
Tremblay, L. J. Path
Walcott, J. M. L. Ophth
Walters, A. GenSurg
Williamson, E. E.
Williamson, H. F. GenSurg
Woodley, T. I.

BELMONT
(649)
MacIntyre, H. I.
Marchuk, P.

BETHANY
(294)
Speiler, S. L.

BINBROOK
(295)
Bell, D.

BLENHEIM
(3,150)
Forde, J. D.
Graham, J. M.
Green, A. C.
Griffith, Idris M.
Huffman, A. S.
Rees, H. J.
Story, A. L.
Williamson, F. M.

BLIND RIVER
(4,098)
Hamill, F. C.
McCendie, R. G.
Pigeon, J.
Whang, T. Y.

BLYTH
(720)
Street, R. W.

BOBCAYGEON
(1,210)
Moran, F. J.
Thomas, W. D.

BOLTON
(2,104)
Bronstein, S.
Steins, A. M.
Taylor, H. L.

BOTHWELL
(821)
Scott, M. A.

BOURGET
(769)
Gendron, M.

BOWMANVILLE
(7,398)
Anfossi, H. C.
Austin, C. J.
Ewert, E. L.
Ferguson, H.
Hubbard, E. D.
Rundle, H. B.
Slemon, K. W.
Storey, V. H.
Sylvester, A. B.

BRACEBRIDGE
(2,927)
Baxter, K L.
Bennett, W. H.
Black, W. L.
Craymer, W. J.
Drake, R. M.
Eaton, D. E.
Henry, T. R.
Manketlow, R. T.
Monk, W. S., GenSurg.
Williams, B. D.
Wright, W. J.

BRADFORD
(2,342)
Blackwell, G. L.
Evans, J. C.
Hecking, S. J.

BRAMALEA
(1,251)
Armstrong, A. H.
Dales, M.
Diesch, R.
Hutchings, H. R.
Kristal, L.
Neeson, G. B.
Pederson, B. A. T.
Petrie, I. B.

BRAMPTON
(18,467)
Allan, W. K. G.
Allman, R. G., IntMed
Armitage, G. C.
Ashley, Mary Jane
Bartlett, W. W.
Bowyer, J. H., Paed
Braham, T. K., Psy
Caldwell, W. S.
Carroll, J. R.
Chamberlain, D. W.
Coop, C. W. A.
Cowen, June
Cowen, R. H., GenSurg
Dennis, S. M.
Diack, Helen
Douglas, E. S.
Eagleson, W. M., GenSurg
Freed, B. D.
Furness, A.
Hall, H. D.
Hall, Mary C.
Heggie, D. C.
Hetherington, H. H.
Huber, W. A.
Inglis, J. E.
Jarvis, G. J., Ophth.
Kellam, Shirley
Kerr, N. D.,ObstGyn
Khanna, R., GenSurg.
Korentager, H.
Kummel, G. E., GenSurg,
Longfield, G. M.
MacDonald, D. G. H., PH
Marshall, D. G.
McClure, J. D.
McQuibban, G. A.
Mech, Z. R., Psy
Miller, D.
Powell, M. G.
Quirk, J., Urol.
Rudis, L. A., GenSurg
Steele, B. S.
Thicke, B. C.
Vair, D. H.
Varga, A. T., GenSurg.
Watkins, D. B.
Whittaker, W. G., ObstGyn
Wilkinson, J. A., GenSurg
Wilson, D. F.
Young, Mary

BRANTFORD
(56,741)
Barber, G. S., GenSurg.
Buller, W. K., GenSurg
Calder, J. R., Anaes
Campbell, K. D., ObstGyn
Carson, J. E.
Carson, J. H.
Chiang, T. H.
Clarke, F. D.
Cleary, T. E., Paed
Cole, M. S., GenSurg
Craven, A. J., GenSurg
Croal, A. E., Path
Crysler, W. E., D & T Rad.
Diack, Helen
Digby, J. R., GenSurg
Douglas, R. W.
Drysdale, I. A.
Dunton, Aenid
Dwyer, W. F.
Eddy, R.
Elliot, A. W., DiagRad
Evans, D. T., GenSurg
Farley, R. G.
Farley, R. W.
Finlayson, A., Psy
Finlayson, A. J., ObstGyn
Gallego, M.

* Population not separately available.

Brantford (Cont'd.)
Garland, J. M. B., Anaes.
Greig, J. D., ObstGyn
Hadley, D. K., GenSurg.
Hagan, J. N., Psy.
Halliday, J. A., Ophth
Hazen, J. S.
Henry, B.
Henry, R. T.
Honeyman, D. G. GenSurg
Hutton, A. L.
Jennings, G. H. Anaes
Jentz, L. A. Path
Johnston, H. D., Otol
Kidd, T. W.
Knight, R. W., GenSurg DiagRad
Kruspe, R. C.
Lamon, C. B. DiagRad
Langley, R. K. Ophth
Langs. E. R.
Lathourias, N. G.
Lesser, A., Psy
Lind, J. A.
Lindsay, G. E., DiagRad
Longfield, G. M.
Lugsdin, G. H. Psy
Marin, G. A., OrthSurg
Marquis, J. A. D. IntMed
McFadzean, W. T.
McGill, W. L. C. GenSurg
Naiken, V.
Newell, A. N. IntMed
Olenski, S.
Overholt, A. A.
Overholt, B. M.
Pascoe, M. G. D.A.B.P.
Pedley, W. H.
Quinlan, J. J.
Richter. Katherine, E.
Riddell, A. D.
Roddick, J. E.
Rodgers, C. L. Paed
Rolland, W. GenSurg
Rose, A.
Rose, R. Viola, Psy
Rustige, L. R.
Skolnick, M., Derm
Skrypuch, J.
Start, R. K., IntMed (T.B.)
Stubbs, J. G., OrthSurg
Telfer, R. B. Urol
Thompson, C. O., Ophth.
Verity, G. E., Otol
Wagman, G. F., Path
Waite, W. I.
Warburton, E. G., Path
Webster, Evelyn
West, W. T.
White, J. C., ObstGyn
White, J. G.
Young, D. R.
Zaltz, M.

BRIGDEN
(620)
Gates, R. T.

BRIGHTON
(2,403)
Elliott, W. O.
Presutti, H. J.

BROCKVILLE
(17,744)
Amy, J. V.
Armstrong, I.
Baugh, C. W., IntMed
Bell-Smith, D., Psy.
Bird, G. S. Paed
Boss, M. M.
Brannen, R. E. DiagRad
Chadsey, L. C.
Code, T. G.
Cooke, J. F., ObstGny
Czigler, P.
Davis, C. B.
Deegan, F. K., GenSurg
Dunn, A. A.
Goodison, T. J.
Gransden, G. M., Ophth
Hoogenraad, A.
Judson, A. H. GenSurg
Kolche, E.
Kort, K.
Lanthier, J. C., DiagRad
Loughrey, R. S.
Lynch, T. J.
MacLeod, F. H. GenSurg
Matheson, D. I.
McAvoy, J. R. GenSurg
McDougall, J. W.
McGuire, M. G.
Miller, R. P. Psy
O'Connell, J. J. Psy
Page, J. IntMed
Palmer, Mary
Perrin, D. R. GenSurg
Perrin, Jyneen G., Ophth.
Perrin, W. H.
Preston, H. E. ObstGyn
Preston, J. H.
Raymond, G. H. GenSurg
Shanks, J. A., ObstGyn
Smylie, T. D., Urol
Sutcliffe, C. K.
Thoms, A. E.
Walker, R. P.
Webster, D. M., Psy
Wight, J. D.
Wyatt, W. J. Path

BRONTE
(2,029)
Walmsley, D. P.

BROOKLIN
(1,531)
Baldwin, W. W.
Cowman, D. R.
Grant, W. G. Y.
McKinney, J. H.
Price, R. M.
Stocks, A. G.

BURFORD
(1,075)
Judge, G. A.
McIntyre, N. R.
Sprowl, D. L.

BURK'S FALLS
(926)
Hallam, B. H. B.
Wittick, M. A.

BURLINGTON
(47,008)
Aikenhead, D. C. Anaes
Aldis, J. S. W.
Anderson, J. S. E.
Barker, L. K.
Best, D. W. S. Anaes
Bodkin, W. A. T.
Boswell, J. C.
Bower, C. M.
Bull, A. F.
Burrows, D. C., DiagRad
Campaigne, Margaret Y.
Costin, T. B.
Culverhouse, J. K., Anaes
Davidson, H. A.
Dean, T. W., D & TRad
De Jong, P.
Dingle, R. T.
Dyckhoff, Pauline R., Anaes
Foster, H. L. PathBact
Fowler, V. P., Path
Friend, W. D., DiagRad
Green, O. R., DiagRad
Gryfe, A., Path.
Haggar, R. Path
Hay, W. I.
Henderson, M. C., OrthSurg
Hodson, D S.
Hopmans, C. C., GenSurg., OrthSurg.
Hughes, R. A., NeurSurg.
Hunt, E. H.
Inglis, J. G.
Johnson, W. H., Ophth
Johnston, W. M., ObstGyn
Jones, S. F.
Kafato, K., Psy.
Kaminer, M., Anaes
Kendall, J. M., IntMed
Kenny, W. B.
Korhonen, P. A.
Langford, W. W.
Lapp, F. H., Anaes
Lepinskie, F. F.
MacArthur, A.
MacFarlane, G. N. GenSurg
MacFarlane, J. W.
Mackrell, Estelle
Malcolmson, C. H., Paed
Mann, Dorothy M. K. ObstGyn
Martin, J. W., GenSurg
McClenahan, C. A.
McCrae, W. H., Urol
McCullagh, M. S.
McIntyre, D. I., OrthSurg
McNabb, M. W. ObstGyn
McNeel, R. W. Paed
Milawski, W.
Mitchell, N. H.
Muir, A. P.
Neilson, J. B.
Nielsen, H. S.
Noonan, W. E.
Perrin, D. R., GenSurg
Poole, J. K.
Preston, W. H.
Procter, W. C.
Quarry, J. G.
Redfearn, D. S.
Redfearn, R. G.
Reininger, S. M. M. T.
Renton, A. J., Psy.
Roberts, J. A.
Rutherdale, J. A.
Scott, H. W.
Sereda, L. E.
Shepherd, I. L.
Sibly, J. C. A., IntMed
Slade, R. H.
Stafani, M.
Standret, D. T., Ophth.
Sweeny, G. P.
Taylor, C. R., ObstGyn
Thibodeau, A.
Tindale, R. M.
Tuttle, R. J. D., DiagRad.
Vennema, A.
Whittaker, J. N.
Witton, T. H., Anaes
Wright, A. R.
Yaworsky, R. G., Path

BURWASH
(616)
Ivanic, V.
Popov, C.

BYRON
(3,327)
Marth, E. A.
Robinson, H. C.

CALABOGIE
(300)
Hobson, W. J.

CALEDON
(301)
Twiddy, E. W.
Vargha, C. O.

CALEDONIA
(2,198)
Baillie, M. M.
Carter, I. E.
Whitehead, H. Y.

CAMPBELLFORD
(3,481)
Baker, W. W.
Burgess, D. W.
Cunningham, T. A.
Kaufmann, A. F.
Kirkwood-Hackett, T. J.

* Population not separately available.

CAMP BORDEN
*
Boyle, B. P., GenSurg
Walasek, J.

CANNINGTON
(1,023)
Nancekievill, I. W.

CAPREOL
(3,003)
McGowan, D. A.
Shields, G. H.

CARDINAL
(1,944)
Allen, A. S., GenSurg., Pulm. Dis. & T.B.(P.Q.)
Mustard, H. A., GenSurg.

CARLETON PLACE
(4,794)
Dobb, C. A.
Ferguson, D. H.
Ferrill, C. W.
Hanham, Wm. J.
Johnston, J. A.
MacDowall, C. R.
McEwen, J. A.
Roy, W. A.

CARP
(498)
Daykin, C. E.

CASSELMAN
(1,280)
Grenon, R. G.
Ladouceur, F.

CAYUGA
(900)
Marshall, T. D.
Ryan, G. V.
Weylie, D. R.

CEDAR SPRINGS
(100)
Scott, Grace
Truax, F. D.
Yorke, Z. G.

CHALK RIVER
(1135)
Evans, D. W.
Taylor, D. A.

CHAPLEAU
(3,386)
Young, G. E.

CHATHAM
(29,826)
Akkerman, O. S.
Baird, C. D., Ophth
Barlow, H. S.
Barlow, R. B.
Beattie, G. E. S.
Brown, E. G.
Callaghan, J. L. DiagRad
Charteris, R. W.
Coulter, P. T. Urol
Ferguson, J. S.
Foex, H. E. GenSurg
Glen, W. F.
Graham, A.
Griffith, G. T., IntMed.
Holmes, Shirley M. Ophth
Jenkin, J. R.
Johnston, W. H.
Keeley, C. D. GenSurg
Keevil, R. F., DiagRad
Lee, W. J. Paed
MacDonald, A.
MacDonald, S. A.
MacLennan, M. R., DiagRad
MacWilliam, J. C.
McKay, M. H.
Oestreicher, D. L. IntMed
O'Neill, J. D. ObstGyn
Packham, J. S.
Palanek, F. G.
Parry, J. C. Anaes
Patterson, D. M. GenSurg
Patterson, T. D., Path
Pearce, Lois C.
Peco, H. C.
Pierson, R. V.
Rees, H. J.
Roe, J. A., ObstGyn
Scott, M.
Shepley, J. M.
Shepley, L. J.
Smith, S. G., Anaes.
Sugiyama, H. S.
Szeps, J.
Toplack, Natale J.
Turner, W. P.
Walker, G. R.
Walker, R. H.
Walker, T. L.
White, H. C., GenSurg

CHATSWORTH
(419)
Chamberlain, G. E.
McDougall, A. A.
Mountain, H. E., Anaes.

CHELMSFORD
(2,561)
Sarabia, L. G.

CHESLEY
(1,691)
Dawson, K.
Divis, B. O.
Naidu, P.

CHESTERVILLE
(1,242)
Justus, H. W.

CHIPPAWA
(3,258)
Bidwell, P. A.
Dallimore, S. T.
Strang, A. G., GenSurg
West, W. G.
Wincott, V. L.

CLAREMONT
(544)
Tomlinson, N. F.
Tremeer, Doris C., IntMed. (P.Q.)

CLARKSBURG
(478)
Allin, R. W.

CLARKSON
(1,450)
Bolland, P. G.
Brown, D. C., DiagRad
Dales, J. W., Anaes.
Dennis, L. R.
Fisher, P. W.
Hooper, R. L., Anaes.
Horne, J. S., GenSurg
Mariz-Fernandez, S., Path.
Nichini, A.
Smith, J. D. GenSurg
Vernon, Elizabeth J.
Vernon, H. E.
Williams, G. E.

CLIFFORD
(537)
Creighton, K. J.

CLINTON
(3,491)
Addison, J. A.
Flowers, R. W., IntMed
Griffiths, Helen
Newland, F. M.
Oakes, W. A. GenSurg
Thompson, F. G.
Walden, L. P. GenSurg

COBALT
(2,209)
Dunning, H. A.

COBDEN
(941)
MacKercher, D. A.
Pye, E. C.

COBOCONK
(528)
Jamieson, R. E.

COBOURG
(10,646)
Barrie, M. D. L., Psy.
Blackwell, F. N.
Ford, B. F.
Gear, D. H.
Horner, Charlotte M.
Lawson, F. L., GenSurg
Leeson, J. F.
Mikel, D. E.
Moorhouse, H. C., Psy
Page, W. E.
Richards, W. H., DiagRad
Robertson, F. G.
Scott, R. S.
Shaw, I. M.
Stobie, A. M.
Stratford, G. K.
Wade, W. W.
Wellman, Victoria
Wilson, I. C., GenSurg.

COCHENOUR
(710)
Scott, Alice
Scott, G. B., GenSurg
Weinstein, J.

COCHRANE
(4,521)
Bernstein, P. H.
Karam, N. A.
Moore, J. A.
Peramaki, R. T.
Richardson, P., GenSurg.
Tilley, J. V.

COLBORNE
(1,333)
Eberlie, W. J.
Pember, F. R.

COLDWATER
(723)
Brown, R. F.
Hall, G. W.
Prior, J. D.

COLLINGWOOD
(8,385)
Harvie, D. A.
Irving, I. F.
MacLean, J., GenSurg
McGillivray, J. W., GenSurg
McKay, D. H., GenSurg
McKay, F. L.
Mitchell, W. B.
Paul, D. J.
Smith, L. A. E.
Storey, R. N.

COLLINS BAY
(491)
More, R. H., Path
Upton, D. H., Psy
Young, B. H., PhysMed

COMBER
(608)
Knister, C. E.

CONISTON
(2,689)
Kosar, E. W.
Kurdyak, Ruth

COOKSTOWN
(1,025)
McFarland, D. W.

COOKSVILLE
(1,800)
Abell, N. H., OrthSurg.
Black, C. R., Otol
Borgiel, A. E. H.
Brander, Margaret R.
Brayley, J. L., ObstGyn
Brown, D. C., DiagRad
Brown, E. W., Psy
Brunsdon, D. F. V., Path
Clement, G. F., Anaes

* Population not separately available.

Cooksville (Cont'd.)
Cochen, A. R., ObstGyn
Davies, E. G.
Dodds, J. K.
Frankling, S. R., Ophth
Fraser, Bridget, Anaes
Gonder, L. J.
Henderson, J. C.
Hooper, R. L., Anaes
Irwin, P.
Johnson, R. M., Paed
Kent, W. R., GenSurg
Knight, M. R., DiagRad
Koladich, S., Psy
Lalor, T. P., DiagRad
Ling, Grace
Lockwood, T. M., GenSurg
Ma, A., GenSurg
McBroom, G. L., IntMed
McGuire, J. H.
McKeown, T. J.
McLean, J. D.
Miller, J. E.
Murphy, E. G., Paed
Nessim, R.
Nero, R. P., ObstGyn
Palmer, B. K.
Patzauer-Votsch, Anna, IntMed
Perkin, R. L.
Platt, J. C.
Prouse, F. H., OrthSurg.
Rawling, E. G., GenSurg
Reid, J. D., ObstGyn
Robinson, G. E., GenSurg
Robison, D. L.
Sarne, A. J.
Schmidt-Malo, Hildegarde, Psy
Sims-Cochen, Sandra, J., Anaes
Sluzar, R. L., Anaes
Smith, Ann
Smith, J. D., GenSurg
Smith, P. E., Otol
Steeds, J. L. L., ObstGyn
Sutton, H. C.
Thompson, R. J.
Weir, J. A.
Welsh, J. R.
Wiebe, H. L., Ophth.
Williams, G. D., Urol
Wiseman, L. J., Anaes.
Woodward, R.
Woolever, C. A., ObstGyn.
Zarfas, A. Jean
Zarfas, D. E., Psy

COPPER CLIFF
(3,600)
Bennett, S. R., OphthOtol.
Blain, C. A.
Ferguson, C. R., GenSurg.
Grosso, R.
Hazelwood, B. F., GenSurg
Jacques, W. M.
Jones, J. H. L.
Prince, D. A.
Sturtridge, J. W., IntMed
Weeks, J.

CORNWALL
(43,639)
Aber, S.
Anderson, A. J. Urol
Aubin, R., GenSurg
Babineau, M. J. Paed
Baird, J. T. Ophth
Bateman, G. L.
Bateman, H. E. D.
Burns, J. H.
Caldwell, L. A. GenSurg
Cameron, G. J.
Chodyniecki, C. P.
Clarke, H. D.
Corbeil, C.
Crewson, A. L. Ophth,Otol
Daigneault, L. R.
Deslauriers, S. D.
Elliott, W. H., NeurSurg.
Emard, E. ObstGyn
Emard, L. M.
Fraser, S. B.
Gardner, A. J.
Gorecki, Z. ThorSurg
Gourley, I. M. Paed
Hebert, H. J. L.
Irwin, K. M., ObstGyn
Irwin, Patricia
Kelly, M. A.
Lalonde, C. F., ObstGyn.
Lavigne, R.
MacPhee, A. E. R. IntMed
McGillivray, A. M. DiagRad
McGillvary, J. I., Anaes
McGuire, J. A.
McKeown, J. GenSurg
McLean, A. J. GenSurg
Milligan, W. A.
Paiement, J. G.
Parisien, R. S.
Peachey, A. B.
Pender, C. B. Paed
Quesnel, L. A.
Randlett, R. P. GenSurg
Renner, W. D&TRad
Shannon, Jane C.
Shannon, W. J. Path
Tallon, J. A. GenSurg
Tallon, M. B.
Thomson, J. A.
Toth, A. I.
Tracy, F. L.
Verville, H. W., Derm
Wilson, G. E., Psy

CORUNNA
(1,942)
Cruikshank, G. H.
Threndyle, K.

COTTAM
(520)
Horton, H. R.

COURTRIGHT
(537)
Henrich, O. A.

CREEMORE
(853)
Stubbings, R. S.

CREIGHTON MINES
(1,792)
McGruther, W. J. B.

CRYSLER
(498)
McMillan, G. D.

CUMBERLAND
(360)
Kennedy, I. F.

DALKEITH
(165)
Munroe, A. T.

DASHWOOD
(411)
Gulens, V.

DEEP RIVER
(5,377)
Gasmann, H. C.
Goad, F. D. GenSurg
Robertson, D. S.
Skelly, W. R.
Stewart, C. G.
Weeks, J.

DELAWARE
(466)
Kasza, L.
McGregor, J. S.

DELHI
(3,427)
Gerhard, B. L.
Knipf, J.
McCallum, R. F.
Tisdale, R. W. Jr.

DELTA
(336)
Jacobs, H. E.

DESERONTO
(1,797)
McVicker, D. C.

DIXIE
(551)
Salkus, A. D.

DON MILLS
(District of Toronto)
Alexander, R. L., Ophth.
Anchelson, A. A.
Bain, Joan E.
Bain, S. T.
Baker, G. A., Psy
Bakker, J. P.
Barrington, T. W., OrthSurg
Barsony, P., Psy.
Bendeth, B. S.
Binns Smith, M., Path
Bird, B. L., DiagRad.
Box, T. R., IntMed
Boyle, E. J., GenSurg
Bradford, N. W.
Braudo, M,. Paed
Carlsen, L. N., PlasSurg
Cecutti, A., ObstGyn
Chernick, V.
Clark, W. N., Paed
Coderque, J. A., Otol
Coggins, B. H., Anaes
Cornet, J. W.
Crapper, D. R., Neur.
Dix, G. W., Anaes
Doran, T. A. ObstGyn
Drillis, G. L.
Ehrenreich, K. A.
Evans, D. C., OrthSurg
Evans, J. G., OrthSurg
Evans, R. J., GenSurg.
Farivar, J., Paed.
Francoeur, J.
Gooderham, M. E.
Grant, R. J.
Gustainis, Ona D., Anaes
Haber, H. N.
Hart, G. D., IntMed
Henderson, H. W., Psy
James, R. T.
James, W. A., Anaes.
Ing, R. Y. K., Paed.
Jones, G. E.
King, P. A. H., IntMed.
Lansdown, E. L., DiagRad
Leeson, Helen J., Paed.
Lunderville, C. W., Anaes
Mae, A.
Marks, C. P.
Masson, E. L.
McAskile, K., Otol
McCulloch, D. J., Psy
McEnnan, T. A., GenSurg
McGoey, P. F., OrthSurg
McGrail, J. C.
McIntosh, R. W., Anaes.
McLeod, D. L., Paed
Medhurst, J. O.
Mekdeci, A.
Meligrana, F., IntMed
Moran, D. B., IntMed (Cardiol)
Muir, R. K.
Murray, J. D. M., Paed
Napraua, T., ObstGyn
O'Heany, T. M., ObstGyn
O'Sullivan, P. M., IntMed
Pantalony, D., Path
Patterson, T. A.
Phillips, M. J., Path
Ponesse, D. J.
Pos, R., Psy
Renwick, W. A., Anaes
Robertson, C. M.
Rowland, E. M.
Russell, Ruth
Ryder, D. E., Path
Sakran, B. F.
Sheehan, Margaret M., Anaes
Sidgwick, Mary

* Population not separately available.

Don Mills (Cont'd.)
Smith, J. K. B., Urol.
Smith, L., ObstGyn
Smith, M. W. J.
Spencer, L. R.
Steward, D. J.
Sullivan, J. A., Otol.
Tackoor, W. T.
Tkachyk, S. J., Paed
Toews, L. Jean, DiagRad
Townsend, Constance
Trimble, A. S.
Verhulst, J., Psy
Watt, E. I., Path.
Wensel, R. H., IntMed
Wightman, R. C., GenSurg
Yates, T. H., DiagRad
Zealand, G. W.
Zuker, G. A., GenSurg.

DORCHESTER
*
Burk, L. A.

DOWNSVIEW
*
Abramson, H., IntMed
Alter, C., IntMed
Beder, E.
Bendreth, B. A.
Birenbaum, S. J.
Birnbaum, J.
Boothroyd, W. E., Psy.
Borg, F. X., Anaes
Cardello, P. J., GenSurg.
Cass, I. M., Path
Citron, S. P.
Coates, K. J.
Cohen, G. S.
Colman, H., GenSurg., Urol.
Dworatzek, L. G.
Ellison, N. P.
Esser, I. O.
Fines, S. G.
Gray, L. M.
Highman, S., GenSurg
Howitz, B., ObstGyn.
Jessel, L.
Kelly, N. H.
Kennard, A. B.
Kinash, B. R.
Laytner, B. D., Paed
Leneck, C. M.
Leventhal, A., Paed
Leventhal, J. I.
MacKenzie, J. K.
Malcho, T. J.
McNeely, D. T., IntMed
Mekler, B. S.
Meyer, E. G., GenSurg., Urol.
Miller, D.
Mitsui, K. K., IntMed.
Morrow, N.
Morton, A. E. W., DiagRad
Posen, O.
Puffer, A. D.
Reed-Davis, R.
Rice, M. C.
Rose, M.
Rosen, L. J. Paed, Allerg.
Rosen, S. I. Paed
Rubenzahl, S.
Rudnick, L. R.
Sandler, A.
Silverstein, H. PhysMed
Smith, H. M.
Snitman, H., Paed.
Solursh, L. P., Psy.
Sowa, E., Psy.
Steinhart, M., DiagRad.
Sutherland, G. W.
Taylor, J. D.
Teichman, J. G.
Tesher, M. S.
Trapman, J. L.
Van Norstrand, F. H., Neur Psy
Weinberg, F. Paed
White, A. W., OrthSurg, GenSurg.
Woolfson, J. S.
Young, R. A.
Zaretsky, Ruth

DRAYTON
(648)
Jones, H.

DRESDEN
(2,348)
Gibbs, P. L.
Moorhead, P. B.
Payne, L. G.
Ruttle, J. A.

DRYDEN
(5,728)
Bilsbarrow, G.
Cameron, W. G.
Daniel, E.
Dingwall, D. G.
Ford, S. E.
Hodkinson, E. S.
Potts, J. L.
Robinson, W. G.
Travis, A. L.

DUART
(157)
MacPherson, J. A.

DUNBARTON
*
Schmitz-Hertzberg, F. S.

DUNDALK
(845)
Lindsay, R. W.

DUNDAS
(12,912)
Bates, C. L.
Elliott, R.
Gow, J. A.
Guyatt, B. F.
Harvey, M. R.
Johnston, M. A.
Lynch, J. F., Path.
Malcolm, D. I.
McCoy, H. D.
Renton, A. J., Psy
Robinson, J.
Tysdale, A. T., Psy.
Whittier, D. P.
Woods, A. R.

DUNGANNON
(435)
Vokes, H. A.

DUNNVILLE
(5,189)
Blott, R. D.
Dunlop, P. E.
Greene, Carrol
Harrison, J. P. Ophth
Hesler, R. F.
Marshall, A. H.
McInnis, D. B.
McInnis, E. L.
Mills, W. C. B.
Mustard, K. I. GenSurg.
Rigg, F. D.
Vickers, K. W.

DURHAM
(2,179)
Burnett, R. R.
Jamieson, D. M.
Lowe, Anne
Mellor, K. V.

DUTTON
(815)
Campbell, D. C.

EASTVIEW
(24,555)
Dufour, T. T.
Nadon, A.
Nichols, E. B.
Robert, M.
Sneath, Paul, L. T. PH
Tessier, E. D & TRad

EGANVILLE
(1,545)
Reeves, R. L.

ELGIN
(330)
Kerr, N. W.

ELLIOT LAKE
(9,950)
Antochin, M. D.
Cassar, L.
Fairchild, W. G.
Guest, A. B.
Hunt, J. D.
McMillan, N. L.
Moody, J. P.
Stewart, C.

ELMIRA
(3,343)
Cserhalmi, E. D.
McCullough, J. T.
Thompson, J. E.
Wyatt, E. R. S.

ELMVALE
(961)
MacKenzie, J. W.
Patchell, D. J.

ELORA
(1,481)
O'Brien, J. H.
Wallace, C. A.

EMERYVILLE
*
Schisler, J. E.

EMO
(653)
O'Sullivan, J. L.
Young, D. R.

EMSDALE
(180)
Pocock, W. T.

ENGLEHART
(1,783)
Gibbon, G. W.
Higgins, J. I.
King, M. R.

ERIN
(1,005)
O'Connor, J. P.
Steer, J. C.

ERINDALE
(*)
Large, G. E.
Macmillan, R. V.
Woolf, C. G.

ESPANOLA
(5,358)
Eaton, G. D.
Harvie, H. H. GenSurg
Iversen, P. J.
Morand, J. C.
Robitaille, J. N.
Sutherland, L. G., GenSurg

ESSEX
(3,428)
Foster, D. D.
Hamilton, J. D., GenSurg
Rogers, G. W.
Thomson, J.
Van Veen, K. V.
Wright, D. E.

ETOBICOKE
(District of Toronto)
(155,358)
Ali, O. U.
Baker, R. S., Anaes.
Bremner, J. E., Path.
Buckridan, L.
Codrington, W. R.
Crowell, D. E.
Dale, G. G., OrthSurg.
Goodhall, Patricia O., Anaes.
Keenleyside, J. G., DiagRad

* Population not separately available.

Etobicoke (Cont'd.)
Kelly, Beverley, Psy.
Koch, E. A.
Little, W. M., DiagRad.
Menetrez, Gerda, Anaes
Prior, B. C.
Trewin, R. B.
Upenieks, L.

EXETER
(3,047)
Ecker, D. A.
Fletcher, M. C. G.
Gans, M.
Read, R. W.

FENELON FALLS
(1,361)
Graham, W. M.
Johnstone, G. C.

FENWICK
(264)
Dowd, J. E.

FERGUS
(3,831)
Bismillah, A. H.
Blinkhorn, D. H.
Cassimjee, M. I., ObstGyn
Russell, T. F.
Stickney, Margaret G.
Wilson, T. V.

FIELD
(733)
Patenaude, N. H.

FINCH
(390)
MacLeod, J. G.

FLESHERTON
(515)
Robinson, J. D.

FLORENCE
*
Sussex, R.

FONTHILL
(2,319)
Frohwein, G. E.
Jordan, G. B.
Matheson, W. A.
Whittaker, M. R.

FOREST
(2,192)
Calder, A. M.
Jay, H. J. D.

FORT ERIE
(9,027)
Brown, J. E.
Coshan, A. W., GenSurg
Derbyshire, W. J. B.
Klisowsky, A.
McGregor, J. K.
O'Mulvenny, T. W.
Reid, R. L.
Streets, C. W. GenSurg
Szybalsky, W. J.
Whiting, M. L.

FORT FRANCES
(9,481)
Boyle, W. G.
Challis, A. H. W.
Harvey, D. C.
Johnson, R. GenSurg
Johnstone, Audrey K.
Johnstone, B.
Kalkman, J. W.
Lo, L. Y.
Mohamed, J. K.
Moulton, R.

FORT WILLIAM
(93,251)
Augustine, J. R. IntMed
Bever, J. G.
Blouw, H.
Browne, R. C. Paed
Bull, A., ObstGyn
Bull, R. C.
Burrows, J. W., IntMed
Cain, D. R., Urol.
Cameron, C. G. IntMed
Campbell, J. S., Ophth.
Chan, N. T., Psy.
Clark, G. C., Anaes
Dodick, C.
Dubsky, F.
Fryer, A. I.
Gordon, A. C.
Hogarth, Barbara E.,
Hogarth, R. W. Urol
Hogarth, W. P. Urol
Hughes, H. J. Obst-Gyn
Jaseviciute, Emily
Juvshik, A.
Kane, T. J. IntMed
Koblenzer, P., Paed
Lopez, P. J.
Lower, A. H.
Lucas, G. R. J.
Lyon, W. R.
MacGillivray, P. C., Paed
Machan, J. R., IntMed
MacKenzie, R. N., DiagRad
MacLeod, B. A., ObstGyn
Magwood, Kathleen M.
Malloy, J. J., ObstGyn
Markham, J. D., IntMed
McIntosh, J. D.
McIntyre, H. M., DiagRad
McLeod, N. S.
Morrison, G. H., IntMed
Moulson, R. A.
Murphy, H. R.
Myhal, B.
Nancekivell, H. K., GenSurg
Neelands, P. J., Paed
O'Brien, F. F., Path
Okurmura, R. T., OrthSurg.
Park, R. J., ObstGyn
Pogonowski, S.
Rathbone, E. D.
Rayner, D. C., Path
Remus, L. A., GenSurg
Scott, G. A.
Scrimgeour, J. W., ObstGyn
Setterington, Eleanor, Path
Sewell, I. M., GenSurg
Skinner, J. H.
Spence, B. J., GenSurg
Stevens, B. W., GenSurg
Strachan, Grace E.
Tam, Teresa Y.
Turner, L. J., IntMed.
Warwick, W. E.

FRANKFORD
(1,646)
Beach, J. K.
McMullen, D.
Wong, T.

FREELTON
(276)
Kasserra, Monika
Kasserra, W.
Kellington, W. T.
Rifaat, M. R.

GALT
(27,830)
Bell, W. R., D. & TRad
Bergen, P. C.
Berkeley, K. H.
Bonney, W. R., IntMed
Caspers, A. P., Derm
Chant, G. N.
Clark, R. G.
Currie, R. E.
De Roche, J. E., Urol
Fayle, B. W., DiagRad.
Fisk, M. K., ObstGyn
Fleming, K. F., GenSurg
Foster, H. E., GenSurg
Fraser, W. P.
Gibson, G. A.
Goal, B. S., Anaes.
Goe, J. N., Ophth.
Grapes, B. G., GenSurg
Harvey, J. M., ObstGyn
Horn, A. A., Path
Howarth, R. B., Paed
Howell, J. H., Anaes
Howson, F. R.
MacLean, S. K., GenSurg
McNichol, J. F.
Mertens, G. A., Path
Midgley, G. H.
Moffat, J. H., GenSurg
Parratt, F. C., DiagRad
Richardson, W. F.
Rodger, W. A.
Seward, F. W.
Thomson, A. F.
Whitla, J. C.
Wiegand, W. J.
Wright, W. F., Psy IntMed.
Wychers, J.

GANANOQUE
(5,096)
Bird, H. G., IntMed
Davis, T. G.
Gray, K. C.
Jenkins, J. G.
Mabee, K. W.
Miller, B. C.
Miller, G. T.

GARSON
(3,786)
Woychuk, W.

GEORGETOWN
(10,298)
Ashenhurst, A. W.
Chamberlain, J. H.
Englebrecht, R. O.
Englebrecht, Florence M.
MacIntosh, A. E.
Martin, J. P.
McAllister, A.
O'Dwyer, M. G., GenSurg
Panabaker, J. P.
Williams, C. V.

GERALDTON
(3,375)
Malcolm, A. H.
Wardill, W. R.

GLENBURNIE
*
Medley, A. J.

GLENCOE
(1,156)
Gerrard, A. B.
Hicks, F. C.
Lockwood, C. A.
Sanders, M. R.

GODERICH
(6,411)
Jackson, N. C., GenSurg
Lambert, K. C., GenSurg
Leitch, J. R.
McCosh, R. A.
McGeough, V. C.
Mills, G. F.
Taylor, A. H., GenSurg
Wallace, J. W.
Watters, W. M.

GORE BAY
(720)
Strain, F. A.

GRAND BEND
(928)
McMaster, E. A.

GRAVENHURST
(3,078)
Boughen, F. L.
Chittick, W. J.
Fisher, M. M.
Goodwin, J. G.
Lindenfield, C. E.
O'Dell, J. H.
Ross, C. B., IntMed (TB)

* Population not separately available.

GRIMSBY
(5,148)
Bartley, A. H.
Bowers, N. S.
Dolson, E.
King, J. K., GenSurg
Koslowski, W.
Mackenzie, W. F.
MacMillan, J. H.
McBain, R. W., DiagRad
McLennan, D. W.
Polak, Danuta
Psutka, D. A.
Read, W. W.
Rowland, C. C.
Schroeder, W. E.

GUELPH
(39,838)
Barnaby, H. C., Otol
Barton, E. L., PathBact
Bending, G. C., Ophth
Brewster, O. M., GenSurg
Brown, J. J., Paed
Burchill, W. C., IntMed
Burton, G. S., Psy
Campolongo, J. T.
Cardillo, P. J., GenSurg
Carere, R. P.
Case, G. L., DiagRad
Caspers, A. P.
Clemes, I. L., GenSurg
Cobb, G. M., Ophth
Cray, J. F.
Crispin, E.
Dale, B. T.
Duthie, C. S.
Eaglesham, D. C., D & TRad
Farmer, H. F., GenSurg
Fernandez, E. M., Path.
Fraser, D. G.
Garrett, D. A.
Gelb, R. H., ObstGyn
Geoghegan, J. J., Psy
Gort, G. H., Psy.
Greenhow, D. E.
Haayen, P. J.
Hobson, K. W., GenSurg
Hoffman, Shirley G.
Howitt, C. W. E.
Hughes, J. F.
Hutchinson, G. M., Otol
Hutchison, W. G., Ophth.
Kilpatrick, C. D.
Kirby, J. W. GenSurg
Kirvan, F. J.
Labelle, B.
LeBlanc, L. P., GenSurg
Leggett, L. H., GenSurg
Little, Flora G.
Loree, L. A.
Loudoun, J. R.
MacKinnon, A. L., Psy
MacKinnon, A. M.
MacRae, A. I., IntMed
Marcinkovsky, E.
Martin, Elizabeth C.
Mellow, G. A.
Mutrie, E. T.
Nunez, M., Psy
Palmerston, D. G.
Parker, C. W., GenSurg
Phillips, J. N., Urol.
Piper, G. A.
Proud, J. D., ObstGyn
Raffan, H. M., IntMed
Reed, C. E.
Savage, D. C., Ophth
Scott, J. A. L., GenSurg
Scott, W. A., GenSurg
Secord, G. V. C.
Somerville, J. C., ObstGyn
Storey, C. F., Psy
Sutherland, G. Q., PH
Taylor, W., IntMed
Vincent, M. O., IntMed, Psy
Webster, A. C., Anaes.
White, E. J., OrthSurg
Witt, S., GenSurg
Woodger, J. B.
Wuerth, F., Anaes
Zielonka, W.

HAGERSVILLE
(2,080)
Awde, C. M.
Huschilt, N. P., GenSurg
Powell, W. C. D.
Salem, I.

HAILEYBURY
(2,638)
Arnold, W. C.
Erickson, E. R., Path.
Joyal, J. A. H.
Joyal, P.

HALIBURTON
(983)
Carroll, L. H.
Good, H. E.

HAMILTON
(431,000)
Adams, M. B.
Adamson, D. L., ObstGyn
Adamson, D. P.
Agro, C. F.
Aitchison, D. B., GenSurg
Andry, H. P., Anaes
Appleford, R. D.
Armstrong, A. R., Bact
Arro, E.
Arthurs, J. E.
Ashworth, E. J., Anaes
Atyeo, R. D., ObstGyn
Awrey, W. R.
Bagshaw, Elizabeth
Bagshaw, J. I.
Balinson, R. H.
Barnbrook, D. H., GenSurg
Barnes, W. H., GenSurg
Barry, R.
Bazoian, M., Anaes
Beacock, C. G., Psy
Beattie, H. W., GenSurg
Beattie, Nancy M.
Beatty, E. G., Path
Beck, C. Adeline
Bell, D.
Bell, J. D.
Bender, F. J., IntMed.
Bendkowski, B.
Bennetto, F. R., Ophth, Otol
Bianchi, F. A., IntMed
Biezuner, J. J.
Bingham. J. M., Psy
Birchard, Edna L., Paed
Board, H. K., Urol
Boccaccio, J. G.
Bolton, P. S., Derm
Boone, F. H., Paed
Born, G., PlasSurg
Bota, W., Anaes
Bowman, B., DermSyph
Bowman, F. B., Proct
Boyd, D. L., Anaes.
Boyd, J.
Bracalenti, I. A.
Brillinger, H. R., Psy
Brough, W. J.
Brown, E. J., ObstGyn
Browne, R. A., Anaes
Buck, J. D.
Bullford, H. E.
Burgess, Beverley A.
Burgess, G. W., OrthSurg.
Butson, A. R. C., GenSurg
Butt, R. B.
Byrne, E. H.
Cameron, G. S., GenSurg
Campbell, D. D., GenSurg
Card, J. R. J., DermSyph
Carr, M., Paed
Carroll, J. J., GenSurg
Catton, D. V., Anaes
Cauley, A. A.
Cecilioni, V. A.
Chapman, D. DiagRad
Charters, J. W.
Church, A. C.
Clare, W. H., Psy
Clark, T. C., Paed
Cohen, H.
Colling, K. G., DermSyph
Connell, G. F.
Connell, W. S. T.
Cooper, E. G., GenSurg, OrthSurg.
Cornett, R. W., IntMed
Cowan, L. H.
Crabb, A. M., Ophth
Crack, I. E.
Cranston, J. R., Otol
Crewson, W. L., Ophth
Dain, I., Psy
Davey, J. E.
Davidson, J. D.
Day, F. E. H.
Denfield, A. S.
Denney, W. S.
Detwiler, R. C., OrthSurg
Devenyi, P.
Dillane, J. G., Ophth
Dillane, W. E., DermSyph.
Dingwall, M., Paed
Doerffer, F. R., ObstGyn
Dolan, R. A., NeurSurg
Dorsey, D. M., Ophth.
Dorsey, M. C. C., Ophth, Otol
Downes, W. P.
Draganic, R.
Draper, D. C., GenSurg
Dutton, W. A., ObstGyn
Dvali, A.
Dwyer, D. E., IntMed.
Dyer, H. F.
Eaton, A. T., GenSurg
Eggleton, G. F. E.
Einhorn, R., Neur
Ellingham, F. H.
Elliott, H. R., Urol
Ellis, V. G.
Empey, R. L.
Enkin, M. W., ObstGyn
Evans, J. R., IntMed
Ewart, H. T.
Eydt, J. N., IntMed
Faris, J. W.
Farmer, R. H. D., PlasSurg
Farrell, Jean C.
Farrell, W. J., Anaes
Fawcett, J. P., ObstGyn
Feyerer, E. J., Urol
Filipich, R. L.
Finkelstein, B.
Finlayson, R. A., Psy
Finn, W. P., GenSurg
Fletcher, M.
Foote, R. E.
Forsyth, D. A.
Foster, H. L., PathBact
Foster, H. L., Anaes.
Frank, F. W.
Freitag, L.
Frid, J. I., IntMed
Friend, W. P., DiagRad.
Fyshe, T. G., GenSurg
Galloway, J. D.
Gauld, E. N., IntMed
Gauthier, G. J.
Gawman, W. G., DiagRad
Genyk-Berezowski, Daria O.
Genyk-Berezowski, J.
Geremias, M. T., Urol.
Gibson, T. C.
Gillrie, R. B.
Goldberg, W. M., IntMed
Grafton, I. G.
Greaves, K. W.
Green, L. S., D & TRad
Green, O. R., DiagRad

*** Population not separately available.**

Hamilton (Con'td.)
Green, W. G., ObstGyn
Griffiths, E. A., Ophth.
Groves, J. T., Path
Gryfe, A., Path.
Guest, W. A., Psy
Guyatt, J. M.
Guyatt, R. E.
Habros, R. E.
Haddon, R. A., Otol
Haggar, R. A. J., Path
Hall, J. G., Psy
Halpern, G. I. J.
Hamilton, F. B., GenSurg.
Harper, J. F.
Harris, G. W.
Harrison, R. M., GenSurg, OrthSurg
Hart, A. G., Paed.
Harvey, G. L.
Helt, A.
Helt, Marcia C.
Henderson, M. C., OrthSurg
Henning, J. N., Path.
Henry, G. G. GenSurg.
Hess, C. D., D & TRad
Hind, D. H.
Hitch, D. A. J., Otol
Hodge, K. E., DiagRad
Hogg, W. F., Psy.
Holbrook, R. H., Anaes
Hopkins, D. H.
Hopmans, C. C., GenSurg, OrthSurg
Hotz, H., Paed
Houston, F., Psy
Houston, J. F.
Hudecki, S. M., GenSurg, OrthSurg
Hughes, R. A., NeurSurg
Hughes, R. F.
Hurley, C. G., DiagRad
Hyde, D. Margaret
Iachelli, C.
Inch, F. A. B., Ophth.
Ingham, G. K., IntMed
Isbister, E. G., Urol
Jackson, W. O., IntMed
Jeremias, G., OrthSurg.
Jeremias, M. T., Urol.
Jewell, Marion C.
Johns, D. R.
Johnson, D. M.
Johnson, F. L., ObstGyn
Johnson, J. M., Psy
Jones, D. R.
Jones, G. C., Psy
Kaczanowski, Maria B., Psy
Kapur, P. L., DiagRad
Kelly, G. C., GenSurg, OrthSurg
Kennedy-Jackson, Irlma, NeurP
King, D., TherRad.
Kiss, Z., GenSurg.
Kitching, D. C.
Kitching, J. S., PH
Kneale, H. A., Psy
Koudouris, S. D.
Koziol, J. K.
Krar, F., ObstGyn
Kyles, J. N., Anaes
Lamb, E. R.
Lamont, J. A.
Lamont, W. E., Obst.
Lane, G. A., GenSurg
Lapp, P., Otol
Lee, H. H.
Lehoczky, L.
Lenog, W.
Lepinskie, F. F., Anaes
Levine, M. H., Ophth, Otol
Levinskas, L.
Levy, D., Neur
Levy, F.
Levy, I.
Lichtblau, S. I.
Liston, A. J.
Little D. C., IntMed
Lloyd, M. H.
Lockhart, J. O.
Lofthouse, R. N., OrthSurg, GenSurg
Lotimer, L. E., ObstGyn
Love, W. R., Otol
Lucke, H. H., Path
Lymburner, R. M., IntMed
Lynch, J. F., Path
Lynes, F. S., ObstGyn
MacFarlane, A. L.
Macfarlane, E. B., Ophth, Otol
MacIntyre, M. W.
MacLaren, R. G., TherRad
Maclennan, J. G.
MacMillan, A. B., Paed
Macmillan, A. H., OrthSurg
Madronich, J. S., Ophth
Malcolm, D. I.
Malpass, A. J.
Mann, Dorothy, M. K., ObstGyn
Marson, F. G., IntMed
Martin, H. S.
Martin, Laura, DermSyph
Martin, R. H.
Martins, A. W., Psy
Martyn, G. E., Urol
Martyniuk, F. J.
Matsusak, H.
Matthews, J. A.
Matthews, W. R., GenSurg.
Maynard, H. C.
McAlister, H. R., IntMed
McAuley, R. G.
McConnachie, T., Anaes
McCracken, W. J., GenSurg
McFarlane, A. H.
McGhie, A. G., IntMed
McGillivray, D. W., Ophth
McLean, D. W.
McLean, J. L.
McLellan, T. A.
McMillan, W. R.
McMorland, G. H., Anaes
McNabb, A. R., IntMed
McNichol, J. W., PlasSurg
Mepham, T. E.
Michalski, A.
Middlemass, I. B., DiagRad
Mighton, A. K., GenSurg
Minden, J. H., GenSurg
Minich, J.
Mink, L. M., Path
Mirehouse, O. J., PlasSurg
Miron, Rose, Anaes.
Mironowicz, Halina
Miya, R. T.
Moffat, R. G., D & T Rad.
Moore, C. A.
Moore, J. D., IntMed
Morgan, Deane K., Anaes
Morgan, H. R., ObstGyn
Morgan, Marion W., Anaes
Morphet, J. A. M.
Morris, J.
Morrison, J. S.
Morrison, R. E.
Motke, A. W., ObstGyn
Muirhead, W., TherRad
Munroe, D. H., Urol
Murray, J. K. P., GenSurg
Murray, M. E., ObstGyn
Nancekivell, E. W.
Narine, Toolsie
Nash, T. W.
Nathan, M. T., Paed
Neubauer, E.
Newhouse, M., IntMed
Nicholson, G. M.
Nicholson, R. E., GenSurg
Nixon, R. D., Psy
Noonan, W. E.
Numbers, A. A., IntMed
O'Brien, S. E., GenSurg
O'Brien, S. H.
Olivieri, F. A., Paed
Olmstead, A. I.
O'Malley, B. P., DiagRad.
Onhauser, J. B.
Opie, J. E.
Orr, F. R., IntMed
Osbaldeston, G. J.
Osbaldeston, J. B.
O'Sullivan, A. B.
Overend, F. B.
Page, E. L., IntMed
Paikin, H.
Pain, A. M., ObstGyn
Palmer, L.
Pamukoff, N.
Parisi, A., GenSurg
Parisi, I.
Pase, P.
Patterson, M. C., Path
Pazaratz, B.
Peacock, H. A., IntMed
Peart, H. E., IntMed (T.B.)
Peller, J. A., IntMed
Perkins, S. H.
Piper, W. A.
Podedworny, W. M., Ophth
Politi, V. L., Anaes
Premi, J. N.
Price, N. E.
Probert, R. I., Anaes
Pryce, H. A.
Purdy, Mary E., IntMed
Pylypuik, J. A.
Quigley, G. J., ObstGyn
Rabinowitz, Mabel
Rabinowitz, P., Otol
Rado, I. P., Anaes
Raja, K. D., GenSurg.
Rajnovich, E.
Ranalli, J. P.
Redfearn, D. S.
Reed-Davis, R., OrthSurg
Renshaw, H. V., PlasSurg
Reichenfeld, H.
Reid, J. C.
Reininger, S. M. M. T.
Rhamey, L. E., Psy
Ricci, E. E.
Richter, R. R., OrthSurg
Richards, B. A.
Ritchards, Jo-Anne
Ritchards, T. A., GenSurg
Roberts, R. W., Anaes
Robinson, D. C., ObstGyn
Robinson, H. C.
Robinson, J. G., IntMed
Rogers, D. B., DiagRad
Romeo, M. A.
Rosenthal, D., Derm.
Roukema, J.
Rudnick, K. V.
Ruff, H.
Ruff, P.
Ruston, F. G., Anaes
Rymal, L. C.
Sansone, A. J.
Scime, C.
Scime, I., IntMed
Scudamore, June
Senn, J. N., Psy
Shapiro, F.
Shekter, J. J.
Short, H. A., ObstGyn
Siegel, T.
Siksay, R. N. E.
Sim, D., Psy
Sincerbox, G. A.
Singh, I.
Slater, J., Ophth
Smith, Florence M.
Snedden, F. W., Psy
Sole, J. N.
Sole, N.
Sorokolit, W. T., GenSurg., PlasSurg.
Spaulding, W. B., IntMed.

* Population not separately available.

Hamilton (Cont'd.)
Spicuzza, F.
Squire, D. A., Psy
Stapleton, J. G., DiagRad
Steeves, R. A.
Stelzer, Elizabeth
Stewart, D. H.
Stewart, R. A.
Stewart, R. W.
Stolar, S. H., Anaes
Stolberg, H. O., DiagRad
Stone, G. H., Psy
Stone, M. E., Psy
Stringer, E. P., Ophth.
Stringer, R. M., Anaes
Sulkowski, J. G.
Sullivan, H. J., GenSurg
Szabo, L.
Szekely, P. E.
Szollosy, L. G.
Taggart, J. G.
Tanaka, S.
Tasker, R. G., Path
Taylor, C. L.
Temple, G. D.
Thoman, H. L.
Thompson, D. W.
Thompson, G. D., Urol
Tice, J. W., IntMed
Tidey, V. L.
Tindale, R. M., ObstGyn
Trebilcock, K. H.
Turkowska, Irene D.
Tutton, D.
Tweedie, T.
Tweedie, T. E.
Twelves, J. E.
Tyrrell, J. D., IntMed
Urban, J. R.
Vadas, J. S.
Valaitis, O.
Vanderburg, L. L. C.
Van Vierssen Trip, H. L.
Vaughan, C. E., D & TRad
Veidenheimer, M. C., GenSurg
Virtue, J. A., Otol
Vokes, F. A.
Wainwright, R. M.
Wainwright, Ruth E.
Walker, W. J., IntMed
Waller, C., Anaes
Walsh, W. J., IntMed
Walters, L. G.
Warren, D. A., Anaes
Weaver, M. A., Ophth
Weaver, R. T., ObstGyn
Webber, W. H., Psy.
Webster, W. R.
Wells, J. P.
Wesley-James, O., GenSurg
White, J. G., Psy
White, T. E.
Whitman, R. A.
Wilderspin, K.
Williams, P. E., Paed
Wilson, P. E.
Wilson, R. J.
Wilson, W. M., Paed
Witton, T. H., Anaes.
Woodward, E. G.
Woolner, J. M., Paed
Woolsey, R. G.
Worral, J. D., Otol
Wray, G. C., Anaes
Wright, F. J.
Wylie, A. R.
Yaffe, S. A., IntMed
Yanover, P.
Yaworsky, R. G., Path
Yeates, A. M.
Young, F. M., DiagRad
Zamora, E. N., Psy
Zamora, S. P.

HANNON
(*)
Moore, P. C.

HANOVER
(4,401)
Ballagh, R. G.
Ross, T. H.
Staples, T. E.
Stokes, L. S.
Thaler, A. F.

HARRIETSVILLE
(175)
McIntyre, Helen I.

HARRISTON
(1,630)
Clunas, D. E.
Williams, J. C. B.

HARROW
(1,789)
McCormick, R. W.
Veale, W. T. J.
Wren, W. W.

HASTINGS
(896)
Campbell, Janet, Paed
Campbell, W. N.
Fahey, J. J.
Patterson, L. D.

HAVELOCK
(1,261)
Holdcroft, D. J.
Pritchard, R. B.

HAWKESBURY
(8,661)
Auger, E.
Charbonneau, J. P.
Dubois, J. M.
Hunter, A.
Imrie, Elisabeth P.
Imrie, G. G.
Kirby, R. C.
Lafrance, C. E.
Maynard, G.
McLeman, D.
Noble, J. G.
Perrier, A.
Smith, H. D., GenSurg
Smith, I. T.

HAWK JUNCTION
(375)
Westcott, D. B.

HEARST
(2,373)
Blank, T., ObstGyn
Polnicky, T.
Samson, L. M.

HENSALL
(919)
Goddard, J. C.

HERON BAY SOUTH
*
Seamans, K. B.

HESPELER
(4,524)
Erb, R. G.
Gammie, R. B.
Middleton, R. J.

HIGHGATE
(379)
Macpherson, J. R.

HIGHLAND CREEK
(1,512)
Roy, L. V.
Stuparyk, M., IntMed.

HORNEPAYNE
(1,692)
Skinner, J. H.

HORNING'S MILLS
(311)
Shier, S. G.

HUNTSVILLE
(3,189)
Ascah, G. M.
Cloutier, E. J.
Johnston, K. D.
Jones, J. D.
Salmon, R. W.
Sarjeant, H. Lynn

ILDERTON
(289)
Meredith, A. R.

INDIAN RIVER
(65)
Devlin, R. J.

INGERSOLL
(6,874)
Bland, S. S.
Emery, G. H.
Kaboli, K. S.
Kellner, J.
Lawson, J.
Rowson, J. W.
Westman, G. B.

IROQUOIS
(1,136)
Marcellus, C. R.
Miller, J. R.
Monaghan, T. G.

IROQUOIS FALLS
(1,687)
Hall, H. B.
Haskins, C. D. R.

ISLINGTON
*
(District of Toronto)
Bremner. R. G.
Crawford, J. S., IntMed, PhysMed & Rehab.
Crompton, C. P., Anaes.
Dale, G. G., OrthSurg.
Deeth, J. H.
Dodds, D. J.
Dyer, Natalie M.
Fenton, D B.
Glatt, B. S., Paed.
Groshaw, R. E., Ophth
Hallett, W. M., IntMed
Harrison, H. M.
Imrie, R. J., Paed
Jones, E. E., DiagRad
Kneeshaw, R. S., Anaes
Kozner, Alice, Paed
Kucherepa, J. W.
MacKenzie, A. L., GenSurg
MacMillan, C.
Moore, R. F.
Mottrain, L. E.
Nedlski, M. M., IntMed.
O'Reilly, J. A., PhysMed
O'Reilly, Kathleen S., Anaes
Perry, V. R.
Piercey, W. D.
Richardson, R. N.
Romanick, Natalia
Sakamoto, K. K.
Shostack, B.
Sullivan, J. F.
Tolan, J. R., DiagRad
Thomas, H. B., Ophth.
Toms, A. A., Anaes
Vingilis, J. J.
Weil, J. M.
Wood, Margaret I., Paed.

JAMESTOWN
(See Wawa)

JARVIS
(787)
Lyons, A. A.

JASPER
(228)
Brennan, M.

JORDAN STATION
(248)
Smith, G. H.

KAPUSKASING
(6,870)
Asselstine, A. P.

* Population not separately available.

Kapuskasing (Cont'd.)
Davis, R. E.
Jacques, L. A., GenSurg
Lacroix, J. R., GenSurg.
Latimer, J. W.
McTavish, S.
Paterson, J. E., DiagRad.
Pineau, A. J.
Soucie, G.
Soucie, S. P.
Walker, B. R.
Wright, J. W.

KEENE
(310)
Ford, W. H.

KEEWATIN
(2,195)
Baker, W. A.

KEMPTVILLE
(1,959)
Beamish, O. F.
Flay, W. J.
Haythornthwaite, J. C., ObstGy
Jones, D. H.

KENORA
(10,907)
Bryngelson, E. S.
Burris, S. M.
Delamere, P. M.
Edie, J. C.
Johnson, J. H., Otol
King, H. F.
Leckie, G. B.
Molle, A., DiagRad
Pan, P. D. K-T., Path
Paton, J. P.
Playfair, P. F.
Torrie, A. M.
Wankling, W. J.

KESWICK
(847)
Mahon, W. S.

KILBRIDE
*
McDonald, H. R.

KILLALOE
(927)
Eggert, F. W.
Wallbridge, P. H., GenSurg

KINBURN
(174)
Dowd, W. R.

KINCARDINE
(2,847)
Couch, A. E. H.
Gurbin, G. M.
Helliwell, M. R.
Milne, D. A. D.

KING
(1,864)
Hardy, Q. A.
McPhee, J. A.
Saunders, J. A.
Van Norstand, A. P.

KINGSTON
(63,419)
Abrahams, Vivian
Adams, K. M.
Alexander, D. S., Paed
Amodeo, W.
Armstrong, L. N., Ophth, Otol
Basmajian, J. V.
Batstone, H. L., Psy
Beattie, W. H., DiagRad
Beck, I. T., IntMed., Gastroent(P.Q.)
Bencosme, S. A.
Benians, Mary E., Psy
Berry, J. W.
Billings, R. M., Psy
Bingham, D. L. C., GenSurg
Binhammer, H. E.
Bird, C. E., IntMed
Biro, G. P.
Blenkinsop, G. W.
Boston, R. W., Paed.
Botterell, E. H., GenSurg, NeurSurg
Boucher, D. W., GenSurg
Boyd, E. M.
Braden, D. H., Psy.
Briggs, R. F., Psy
Bruce, A. W., Urol
Bryans, A. M., Paed
Burr, R. C., D & TRad
Campbell, H. M.
Campbell, W. A., Anaes
Carmichael, J. A., ObstGyn.
Caverhill, J. W., Psy.
Cays, F. A., Ophth, Otol
Chadwick, P.
Challis, T. W., GenSurg, DiagRa
Chiong, M. A., IntMed.
Choi, J. H.
Clough-Ormiston, M. W.
Clow, L. R., ObstGyn
Colwell, B. T., D & T Rad.
Connell, W. F., IntMed, (Cardiol
Connolley, J. G., Urol
Cooper, H. G., Psy
Coppolino, H. G., Psy.
Corbett, W. E. N., Path
Cumming, H. W.
Curtis, A. C., DiagRad
Daicar, A. O., ObstGyn
Danby, C. W. E., DermSyph
Danilov, G.
Day, H. C.
Delahaye, D. J., Paed
Delahaye, J. S., Paed
Delva, P. L., Paed
Dingwall, R. W., IntMed
Dinsdale, H. B., Neurol.
Douglas-Murray, G. M., ObstGyn
Dunlop, H. W., GenSurg
Dupuis, R., IntMed
Edwards, K. F., Anaes
Egan, C., Anaes.
Einarson, D. W., Anaes.
Elgie, R. G., NeurSurg.
Ettinger, G. H.
Fay, J. E., IntMed
Firstbrook, J. B., IntMed
Fisher, J. H., Psy.
Forrest, W. J.
Forward, R. B.
Frame, J., TherRad
Fransman, S. L., DiagRad
Frayn, D. H.
Friday, W. H., Paed.
Galbraith, P. R., IntMed
Galbraith, Ruth
Geiger, D. W., Paed
George, S. W., ObstGyn
Ghent, W. R., GenSurg
Gibson, J. D.
Gibson, J. E., IntMed
Gorecki, Irena A., DiagRad.
Graham, J. R., Psy
Greenlaw, R. K.
Grennell, H. J., Anaes
Haden, P., Psy
Hagen, P. B.
Hatcher, J. D.
Haust, H. L.
Haust, Maria, Path
Hay, W. D., PathBact
Hazlett, J. W., OrthSurg
Henderson, J. C., Anaes
Hetherington, R. F., NeurSurg
Hinton, N. A., Bact
Hoaken, P. C., Psy
Hooper, D. G., Otol.
Hopkins, B. H., IntMed (TB)
Horne, G. R., Anaes
Houston, S. W., GenSurg
Houtman, S. G., Psy
Huang, S. N., Path
Hughes, R.
Hunter, R.C.A., Anaes.
Ives, G. A., Psy.
James, E. A., Psy
James, M. M.
James, R. N.
Jantz, J.
Jarzylo, S. V., DiagRad
Jennings, D. B.
Jones, W. A., D & TRad
Keenleyside, D. W.
Kelly, H. G., IntMed.
Kelly, R. A.
Kerr, J. W., GenSurg
Kinsman, J. L.
Kipkie, G. F., PathBact
Koster, B. M., GenSurg
Koval, A., IntMed
Kraicer, J.
Kumar, G., IntMed.
Lajos, T. Z., GenSurg.
Laurenson, R. D.
Laverty, S. G., Psy
Leacy, J. W.
Leeson, C. R.
Lewis, R. S.
Lindsay, G. C.
Livesey, R. J.
Low, J. A., ObstGyn
Lynn, R. B., ThorSurg
Lyons, G. M.
Mabee, H. C.
Mabee, K. W.
MacGregor, R. R., Paed
Mackie, K. W., DiagRad
MacPherson, G. B., Ophth, Otol.
Mahood, J. H., Anaes
Malloy, J. J., ObstGyn
Marshall, K. G., Path
Masotti, R. E., Paed
Maxwell, Maureen P., Paed.
Mayer, G. A.
McAuley, R. D., Psy
McBroom, J. G., Ophth, Otol
McCaldon, R. J., Psy
McConville, B. J., Psy.
McCorriston, J. R., GenSurg
McCuaig, C. H., Psy
McElligott, T. F.
McGaughey, H. R., Paed
McIntyre, R. W.
McKnight, R. D.
McMahan, J. S.
McLeod, P. A., ObstGyn
Medline, N., Path.
Melvin, W. J. S., OrthSurg
Merry, G. M.
Millard, W. E.
Milliken, J. A., IntMed
Milne, R. T. G.
Mohan, L. M.
More, R. H., Path
Morgan, J. F., Ophth
Morrin, P. A., IntMed
Mulligan, Mona
Mylks, G. R. W., Jr. ObstGyn
Naismith, J. T.
Neill, R., Anaes
Neily, H. H., Anaes
Nekus, V. A., Anaes
Neuman, H. W., GenSurg
Nickoloff, B. J., Anaes
Norris, A. S., Psy
O'Connor, F. J., Sr. Obst
O'Connor, F. J., Jr. Paed
O'Connor, F. X.
O'Connor, L. N., ObstGyn
O'Neill, T. O.
Padhi, R. K., GenSurg
Paloschi, G. B. G., GenSurg
Parker, J. O., IntMed
Parrot, K. B., DiagRad
Partington, M. W.
Patterson, W. S., ObstGyn
Pinkerton, R. M. H., Opth.
Pinto, B.
Power, G. R., DiagRad

* Population not separately available.

Kingston (Cont'd.)
Powles, W. E., Psy.
Pratten, J. S., Psy.
Prioreschi, P.
Purvis, J. R., Otol
Rajput, A. H., Neur.
Read, J. H., Paed
Regan, K. J.
Reid, J. D., Paed
Robertson, D. M., Path
Robertson, E., ObstGyn
Robinson, S. S.
Robinson, W. E., Psy.
Rosen, D., Ophth
Rublee, J. D., PathBact
Russell, E. S., Anaes
Rutherford, T. F., Ophth, Otol
Ryan, M.
Ryan, Valerie P.
Sada, M., IntMed
Santos, A. S.
Scott, G. D., Psy
Shaffer, H.
Simurda, M. A., OrthSurg
Singleton, F. B., Anaes
Sloane, R. B., Psy
Smith, P. M.
Sommerville, A. E.
Sorbie, C., OrthSurg.
Steele, H. D., Path
Steele, R.
Sterns, E. E., GenSurg.
Stevenson, C. M., Psy
Stitt, R. B., GenSurg.
Stringer, E. P., Ophth
Symington, D. C., PhysMed. & Rehab.
Tanenbaum, H. L., Ophth.
Thomson, J. A.
Toews, C.
Travill, A. A.
Trotter, M. C.
Tweddell, J. T., IntMed, Path
Tweddell, T. N., GenSurg
Ulrich, T. Marianne, Paed.
Valberg, L. S., IntMed
Van Alstyne, W. B. III, DiagRad.
VanCott, G. F.
Van der Hoeven, Ellen M. PathBact.
Vanderwater, S. L., Anaes.
Waddell, W. R., IntMed.
Wagar, H. G., Psy.
Waldron, J. J., Psy.
Walker, M. F.
Warner, H. M., GenSurg
Wellington, J. L., GenSurg.
West, R. O.
Westernberg, H. H.
White, D. N., IntMed, NeurPsy
White, E. P., Urol
Williams, R. L.
Wilson, D. L., IntMed
Wilson, K. B. Anaes.
Wilson, W. E. C., IntMed
Wollin, D. G., DiagRad.
Wyllie, A. K., PlasSurg
Wyllie, J., PH
Wyllie, J. C.

KINGSVILLE
(3,045)
Ablenas, V.
Baltrusaitis, V. P.
Bruner, G. W.
Jenner, L. C.

KIRKFIELD
(211)
Knowles, J. A.

KIRKLAND LAKE
(15,366)
Armstrong, T. W.
Brebner, C. N., GenSurg
Bryant, W. E.
Clegg, J. W.
Harris, C. S.
Harris, E. R., PH
Kozlik, T. J.
LeBlond, J. M.
Messenger, D. B.
Middlemiss, K. C., D & TRad
Rumball, W. C.
Rumball, W. J. S., GenSurg
Souter, A. W.
Thomson, M. J.
Wallbridge, P. H., GenSurg, Urc
Yamka, E. M.

KITCHENER
(154,864)
Adelberg, J. L.
Archibald, W. M., Anaes
Armstrong, W. J., PathBact
Austrup, Margaret J., ObstGyn.
Baird, R. P., Ophth
Barnes, D. S., Psy
Bastedo, D. L. A., Paed
Bean, D. E.
Bean, D. M., GenSurg
Beckham, L. M., Anaes
Belyea, C. C.
Bergman, B. J., Path
Brown, E. Earl, IntMed
Bruder, A.
Bryant, Marie, Paed
Bryant, W. H.
Cameron, D. A.
Cameron, D. J., GenSurg.
Campbell, A. D., Anaes.
Campbell, J. M.
Carlisle, R. V.
Christ, G. J.
Clarke, G. L., ObstGyn
Coppolino, A. G., Psy
Corrigan, V. A., Urol
Cowan, R., GenSurg
Cserhalmi, E. D.
Davidson, C. R. S.
de Aragon, J. M.
Demary, R. F.
Diamond, M. J., Anaes
Downie, F. J.
Dundon, C., GenSurg, Urol
Ernst, D. S., ObstGyn
Ewing, D.. ObstGyn
Farrell, W. A., D & TRad
Fisher, J. G.
Fojcik de Aragon, Hilary A.
Friday, W. H., Paed
Gibb, R. B., ObstGyn
Gibb, R. B.
Glaister, Deborah
Gordon, R. I., Ophth, Otol
Grant, D. J., Derm
Grant, R. A.
Hagmeier, J. E.
Hain, Irene
Hartford, J. J., Psy
Harvey, M. C., GenSurg
Harvey, W. H.
Hawkins, S. J., IntMed (TB)
Hay, G. M. D. GenSurg
Henderson, H. H.
Henderson, R. H., OphthOtol.
Holland, Eleonor
Holland, W. G., Anaes.
Holland, W. H.
Hopkins, D. P., IntMed.
Iwan, S. R., NeurSurg
Johns, W. R., Anaes
Keresztes, Sylvia
Kilborn, R. M., Anaes
Kinsman, G. W., Anaes
Krumins, Janis
Kulis, Dorothea, Psy.
Lackner, H. A., GenSurg
Lang, L. V.
Lansky, G. S., GenSurg
Leavine, D. F., Derm
Liang, D. V., ObstGyn.
Lippert, G. G., GenSurg
Longmore, A. J., IntMed
Lynne-Davis, G.
MacDonald, W. G.
MacEachern, W. N., Derm
MacGregor, L. S.
MacKenzie, C. G., Psy
MacLean, D. R.
McAdam, W. M.
McCallum, A. G., Otol
McCrystal, F.
McFadden, D. G., OrthSurg
McKenna, A. C.
McLean, J. W., Otol.
McMillan, D. B.
McMurchy, R.
McQuay, N. W., IntMed
Merei, L., Otol
Mickelson, C. H., Psy
Moogk, D. H., Psy
Morrison, N. A.
Moule, J. W.
Nichols, J. S., ObstGyn
O'Connell, C. L., GenSurg
Pequegnat, H. M.
Pidgeon, T. V.
Pizans, A.
Preston, A. Mary
Querengesser, E. I., Ophth
Rambough, W. G., Ophth
Reive, W. G. M., Anaes
Rhodes, J. R., DiagRad
Riddell, A. R. Jr, Anaes
Rockel, A. C.
Ross, J. A.
Ross, J. G.
Row, R. K.
Scheurlen, M. W., GenSurg
Schultz, E. B.
Schwager, P. G., IntMed
Sehl, J. R., ObstGyn
Sharkey, P. J., Obst
Shoniker, T. J., Path
Simpson, A. W., Anaes
Singleton, F. B., Anaes
Smart, R. W.
Spackman, G. C.
Spencer, C. L.
Spohn, J. D.
Stein, W. O., Paed
Stephens, J. G., GenSurg
Stephenson, D. G., PlasSurg
Stewart, J. D., IntMed.
Stewart, K. G.
Stewart, L. N.
Stewart, R. G.
Svorcik, B.
Tallon, J. B., OrthSurg
Teskey, C. G.
Thomas, J. R., DiagRad
Thompson, H.
Traynor, A. V.
Tudor, J.
Turner, K. P., IntMed
Uffelmann, R. F., ObstGyn
Upmalis, I. H., GenSurg
Wagner, M., Obst
Wanless, J. L.
Watson, G. F.
Whaley, D. W., Paed
Whaley, W. J., Paed
White, P. W., Ophth.
Wiebe, H. H.
Williams, M. D.
Wilson, C. S., GenSurg
Wilson, G. E. D.
Wilson, W. R. S.
Wittig, J. E., ObstGyn
Wyse, D. M., IntMed
Zinkman, R. W. J.

KLEINBURG
(227)
Balmer, H. C., Anaes.

LAKEFIELD
(2,172)
Fraser, A. A.
Gastle, H. E.
Reid, L. T.
Sherin, J. P.

* Population not separately available.

LAMBETH
(2,293)
Colling, J. F. C.
Merritt, J. O.

LANARK
(918)
Holmes, E.

LANGTON
(368)
Carnahan, C. J.
Loney, E. M.

LANSDOWNE
(490)
Bildfell, J. A.

LARDER LAKE
(2,030)
MacPhail, A. S.

LA SALLE
(2,703)
MacKinnon, M. A.
McKinnon, J. R., GenSurg

LEAMINGTON
(9,030)
Brewer, L. M., IntMed
Collyer, J. A.
Froese, A. D.
Garwood, G.
Kelly, F. P., GenSurg
Koch, Katharina
Lawrence, H. J., GenSurg
Lyon, E. K., GenSurg
Mathes, E. J.
McGirr, R. E.
Morrow, B. M.
Newman, H. E.
Nicklin, H. R.
Setterington, M. J., IntMed
Shotton, J. A.
Taylor, J. A.

LEVACK
(3,178)
Jessop, C. P.

LINDSAY
(11,399)
Arnup, W. B., IntMed
Blackwell, W. C.
Broadfoot, T. W. L.
Cosgrave, J. J.
Crowe, W. R.
Davies, H. R.
Gill, J. R. P., GenSurg
Gill, Nora D.
Gorman, M. E., GenSurg
Hollows, R. K.
Konyer, C.
Lindsay, J. G.
Ormerod, M .J.
Pitt, D. C., DiagRad
Service, C. W. M., GenSurg
Shier, L. V.
Watson, R. J., GenSurg
Wood, D. S.
Woodrow, W. A., Ophth, Otol

LINWOOD
(503)
Hain, G. R.

LION'S HEAD
(417)
Hopkinson, M. A.
Hopkinson, Nora

LISTOWEL
(4,002)
Conners, C. E.
Hay, F. E. J.
Munn, D. J.
Munn, W. D.
Yang, G., GenSurg

LITTLE BRITAIN
(300)
Hall. G. C. R.

LITTLE CURRENT
(1,527)
Bailey, J. F.
Henry, J. A.

LITTLE LONG RAPIDS
*
Rogers, S.

LIVELY
(3,211)
Bayly, P. L.
Carscadden, T. R.
Marlow, J. N.

LONDON
(196,000)
Abdelnour, G. M., Path
Aberhart, W. R.
Agnos, J. W., DiagRad.
Ahuja, S. P.
Aikenhead, D. E., IntMed
Aitken, Elizabeth H. P., Anaes
Aitken, R. R., Anaes
Albers, H. J., Derm.
Allcock, J. M., DiagRad
Allen, H. H., ObstGyn
Alway, A. E., IntMed
Annett, R. K.
Babb, J. W., Otol
Bailey, W. H., GenSurg., OrthSurg.
Bain, J. A. Anaes
Baird, A. G.
Ballantyne, J. F., Ophth,
Balogh, L.
Banerjee, P., TherRad
Barr, H. W., NeurSurg.
Barr, M. L.
Bartelink, D. L.
Barton, W. B., IntMed
Bartram, E. A., IntMed
Bean, S. J. T.
Beattie, J. H.
Berdusco, A. S., Otol.
Berry, R.
Bickle, G. S.
Blachford, J.
Bloomfield, M. A., DiagRad
Bocking, D., IntMed
Bondy, D. C., IntMed
Bowen, R. J.
Boyce, R. M., Psy
Boylan, T. M.
Brien, F. S., IntMed
Brieskorn, H. H.
Brubacher, L. E.
Bruce, S. B., Ophth
Bruckschwaiger, O., GenSurg, Urol
Buchanan, C. A., Ophth
Buck, Carol W.
Buck, R. C.
Bugg, W. J. F., GenSurg
Burnett, W. H., Otol.
Burns, S.
Busby, S. M., Urol
Butlin, J. R., Anaes.
Butson, F. J.
Calder, G. A.
Cameron, H., Anaes
Cameron, H. S., GenSurg, Orth Surg
Cameron, M. G. P., IntMed., PhysMed. & Rehab.
Cameron, W. J. M., IntMed
Campbell, Jean F., ObstGyn.
Campbell, Margaret K., Paed
Campsall, E. W. R.
Carr, D. H.
Carroll, S. E., GenSurg
Carscallen, H. B., Psy
Chapman, Marion, Psy
Chrzan, B. G.
Clancy, P. R., Anaes
Clark, G. A.
Cline, C. A.
Coles, J. C., GenSurg, ThorSurg
Collins, H. A.
Collyer, J. E.
Collyer, R. T., Ophth
Copeland, G. G., ObstGyn
Copestake, G. G., DiagRad
Copp, A. G. B.
Copp, W. F.
Coppinger, W. W., ObstGyn.
Coulter, W. K., IntMed
Cram, D. M., Paed
Curtis, F. W.
Dare, N.
DasVarma, R. L., IntMed.
Davies, Eleanor, Path
Deadman, A. C. OrthSurg
Deane, W. J. ObstGyn
De Beaupre, E. J.
Deinum, Eleanor, Psy
Denison, A. G. Paed
Dennis, Marion E.
de Veber, L. L., Paed
Dillon, M. T.
Donisch, E. W.
Donisch, Valentina
Douglas, J. H. C. IntMed
Downe, W. N. Psy
Drake, C. G. NeurSurg
Dubois, J. R.
Duncan, I. B. Bact
Dyson, C. W. Ophth
Eck, C. A. B.
Edgar, H. W., DiagRad
Elliott, D. W.
Ellyatt, W. G.
England, N. J. IntMed
Ewener, W. A.
Faulds, G. E.
Ferguson, D. B
Ferguson, K. G., IntMed.
Ferguson, R. S.
Fergusson, E. A. GenSurg
Fetterley, J. C. TherRad
Fischer, R. M.
Fisher, C. F. S. IntMed
Fisher, J. H. PathBact
Fitch, F. F.
Fitz-James, P. C.
Fletcher, H. G.
Foucar, H. O. GenSurg, PlasSurg.
Fowler, W.
Frei, J. V., Path(P.Q.)
Frischette, W. A.
Fry, W. R.
Galbraith, D. A., Psy.
Galbraith, H. C., Psy.
Gambrill, R. B.
Gardner, Elizabeth K.
Gatfield, P. D., Psy
Gay, K. E. IntMed
Gergely, N. F., Cardiovasc & ThorSurg
Gettas, P. G. Otol
Gibson, L. M. GenSurg
Gillick, R. H.
Gillman, R. G., GenSurg
Girvan, G. R. ObstGyn
Glennie, G. D. Anaes
Goddard, E. S. Psy
Goldberg, B., Psy
Gordon, B. A.
Grace, H. B.
Grebezs, J. P.
Greenway, R. E. Otol
Growse, J. M. Anaes
Gunton, R. W.
Haines, M.
Hale, G. C., IntMed.
Haley, F. W.
Hall, G. E.
Hall, I. M.
Harding, P. G., ObstGyn
Hardman, Anna B.
Harrison, Elizabeth Q. Ophth
Harth, M. M., IntMed.
Hartog, J. H., ObstGyn.

* Population not separately available.

London (Cont'd.)
Harwood, R. A., DiagRad.
Haryett, L. E.
Haslett, W. R. T. GenSurg
Hauch, P. P. DiagRad
Heagy, F. O.
Heard, H. S.
Henry, S. G.
Hersey, L. W., Anaes.
Hession, B. L. IntMed
Hill, M. B. DiagRad
Hinton, G. G., Paed
Hobbs, G. E. NeurPsy
Hodgins, B. A.
Hoover, M. P.
Hostetler, H. W.
Hudson, A. J. Neur
Hunter, A. T.
Hutchison, D. A.
Jaco, N. T., Paed.
Jamieson, W. G., GenSurg
Janauskas, A.
Jeffery, E. S.
Jeffs, J. I.
Jenkins, G. E. Psy
Jepson, G. L., Anaes
Johnson, F. G., Psy
Johnston, D. W. B. GenSurg
Johnston, E. E. D & TRad
Johnston, K. A.
Johnston, W. S. Anaes
Jory, T. A., GenSurg
Jurans, V. Psy
Kandel, Patricia F.
Kaveckas, A.
Keenleyside, H. B. Anaes
Keidan, H.
Keil, W., Psy
Kennedy, J. C. GenSurg, Orth Surg
Kimber, R. W., IntMed
Kinch, R. A. ObstGyn
King, M. F.
Kirk, C. J.
Knowlton, R. J., PlasSurg.
Lamont, K. G., ObstGyn.
Langdon, W. A., Paed
Lapp, C. A.
Leboldus, G. M., Otol.
Lefcoe, N. M. IntMed
Leitch, Sheila, Psy
Lepine, E. F.
Letts, A. E.
Lewis, F. N., Path.
Lewis, J. A. IntMed
Lewis, R. A.
Linsdell, F. J., DiagRad
Loudon, J. L., IntMed
Loughlin, E. I. ObstGyn
Loughlin, H. J. Paed
Lovatt, G. E., IntMed
Love, E. J., ObstGyn
Lovegrove, T. D.
Luce, Anna L.
Luciani, D., Psy
Luney, F. W. PathBact
MacDonald, A. C., Path, DiagRad.
MacKenzie, D. A. GenSurg
MacLachlan, D. O., IntMed
Macpherson, K. D.
Maddeford, W. R.
Maguire, F. P.
Maidenberg, R. O.
Majka, M.
Manners, D. O., ObstGyn
Manning, G. W., IntMed
Marshall, D. G. GenSurg
Matthews, W. H.
Max, P., Psy
Maynard, M. D.
Mayr, H. O.
Maziliauskas, E.
McAlpine, H.
McAlpine, K. L. Paed
McAninch, L. N. Urol
McCausland, A. Sr. NeurPsy
McCredie, J. A. GenSurg
McCue, D.
McCutcheon, O. E.
McDonald, Harriet
McDonald, Ida
McDonald, J. W.
McFarlane, D. C., Ophth
McFarlane, R. M. GenSurg, PlasSurg
McGugan, R. G.
McInnis, W. P.
McKenzie, F. A., Psy
McKercher, A. E. Psy
McKim, J. S., Paed
McLachlin, A. D. GenSurg, OrthSurg.
McLachlin, Sheilah Anaes
McLarty, T. D., GenSurg
McLeish, J. C. Psy
McNeil, J. R.
McNeil, M. R.
Meads, G. E., GenSurg.
Meltzer, D. B. IntMed
Metcalfe, E. V. Psy
Middleton, W. W. IntMed (TB)
Miller, G. E., TherRad.
Mills, D. V. M., Path
Mills, D. W., Ophth
Milner, F. J.
Montgomery, H., Path
Moore, L. H.
Morris, A. G. Anaes
Mosbaugh, M. M.
Mountain, H. E., Jr., Psy
Mowry, A. E. ObstGyn
Moyer, A. A. IntMed
Mularchy, K. E. S., Ophth.
Murray, R. G. E.
Myers, Lois M. TherRad
Napoli, V. M.
Naftolin, L. Z.
Nassr, D. G., Psy.
Neufeld, A. H. BioChem (P.Q.)
Newberry, P. D.
Nicholson, J. R. Paed
Nicol, D. A. D & TRad
Nielsen, J. S., Anaes
Noble, S.
Norry, H. T. Anaes
Ollerhead, W. W. OrthSurg (Eng.)
Orchard, J. W.
Osterhuis, J.
Pace, W. E. DermSyph
Palmer, R. B., Psy.
Parker, J. M.
Parthenis, A.
Patchell, R. D.
Paterson, J. C. PathBact
Patten, J. F.
Penikett, E. J.
Pennecott, C. W.
Pennington, P. W.
Pentland, E. S.
Pickard, H. A. IntMed
Pivnick, B. E. Psy
Platt, J. C.
Platt, M. A., ObstGyn
Plunkett, E. R.
Pozsonyi, J.
Pratt, G. E.
Price, I. C. DermSyph
Prueter, G. W. ObstGyn
Quinn, W. R.
Ragula, B.
Rai, J.
Rajic, D. S. D & TRad
Ramsay, A. G., IntMed
Rangecroft, R. G.
Rathbun, J. C. Paed
Reason, W.
Rechnitzer, P. A. IntMed
Reese, L. Urol
Richardson, K. R. Anaes
Roach, Margot R., IntMed
Roberts, J. V., DiagRad
Robinow, C. F.
Robinson, H. C.
Robinson, J. B. C. IntMed
Robinson, M. L., ObstGyn
Rochman, H. Psy
Rose, F. L.
Ross, C. C. GenSurg, OrthSurg.
Rossiter, Helen M.
Rossiter, R. J.
Rounthwaite, F. J. Ophth
Russell, N. C.
Sales, J. L., GenSurg, Urol
Schram, E. L. R. ObstGyn
Scoffield, Mary E. DermSyph
Sears, G. A. IntMed
Seleny, F. L., Anaes
Sexton, G. B. DermSyph
Seymour, R. J.
Sharpe, W. C. IntMed (TB)
Shaw, D. B.
Shaw, K. S.
Shute, E. V. ObstGyn, GenSurg
Silinsky, J.
Sills, H. L.
Simpson, H. M., GenSurg
Sivilotti, E. U.
Skinner, H. A.
Slinger, R. P., Path
Smeeton, F. R.
Smith, D. R. IntMed
Smith, Elizabeth A.
Smith, H. Dorothy
Smout, M. S. Path
Sober, S., OrthSurg
Somerton, K. F.
Southcott, F. R.
Southwood, K. J.
Spence, E. IntMed
Spence, J. H.
Spoerel, W. Anaes
Spratt, L. M. IntMed (TB)
Spurgeon, C. H.
Stavraky, G. W.
Stavraky, W. K., GenSurg., PlasSurg.
Steer, D. G. GenSurg
Steer, J. C.
Stein, P.
Stevenson, J. A. F.
Stewart, C. A. Anaes
Stewart, H. B.
Stewart, J. M. Anaes
Stewart, O. J. Psy
Stutzer, I. M.
Suffel, Priscilla
Sullivan, C. F. ObstGyn
Summerby, J. H., Psy
Swanson, A. L.
Sweeney, J. P., GenSurg
Teskey, W. L. DiagRad
Tew, W. L., ObstGyn
Tew, W. P., ObstGyn
Theoret, J. J.
Thompson, C. A. OphthOtol
Thompson, H. D .
Thompson, J. M., IntMed.
Thomson, D. H. TherRad
Thurlow, H. J.
Tolgyes, S.
Toogood, J. H. IntMed
Treleaven, R. B., DiagRad
Trout, Ellen E. Paed
Trusler, W. C. DiagRad
Turnbull, A., NeurPsy
Valentine, H. Paed
Vigh, S. G., GenSurg
Vincent, J. E. Paed
Vogelsang, A. B. F.
von Hochstetter, A.
Walden, L. P. GenSurg
Walker, F. W., Anaes
Walker, J. B. IntMed
Walker, J. H. GenSurg
Wallace, A. C., Path
Walsh, E. M.

* Population not separately available.

London (Cont'd.)
Walters, F. H.
Walters, J. H. ObstGyn
Ward, C. S.
Warwick, O. H.
Watson, E. M. IntMed
Watson, T. A., TherRad
Watt, A. J. IntMed (TB)
Waud, R. A.
Wearing, M. P. ObstGyn
Wermuth, E. G.
Whelen, W. S. Paed
White, D. F., IntMed
Wickware, D. M. Psy
Wilcox, L. D. IntMed
Wilensky, H. M. IntMed (TB)
Wilkins, W. W. DiagRad
Williams, R. C.
Wilson, J. C. GenSurg
Wilson, R. C.
Wilson, W. M. PathBact
Winder, J. S.
Wismer, H. St. C. D & TRad
Wong, G. L. Otol
Wright, V. C., ObstGyn.
Wyatt, J. K., GenSurg, Urol

LONG BRANCH
(11,039)
(District of Toronto)
Murray, L. L.
Noble, Alison, E.
White, C. A.
Zatelny, W.

LONGLAC
(1125)
Mainman, E. R.

LONG SAULT
(600)
Macaulay, J. D., Path.
Macaulay, Margaret H.

L'ORIGINAL
(1,194)
Laviolette, R.

LORING
*
Wilby, A. G.

LUCAN
(987)
Anderson, E. J.
George, C. H.

LUCKNOW
(1,030)
Corrin, M. H.
McKim, J. C.

LYNDEN
(533)
Cunningham, H. P.
Langs, E. R.

MADOC
(1,348)
Beatty, S. R.
Derry, C. C.
Mullin, G. L.

MALTON
(2,148)
(District of Toronto)
Bulmer, H. R., PH
Carroll, J. R.
Killikelly, Eva T.
Killikelly, H.
Korentager, H.
McNeilly, K. A.
O'Reilly, J. A. PhysMed & Rehab
Prentice, A. W.

MANITOUWADGE
(3500)
Robb, Diana
Rowed, R. B., GenSurg

MANITOWANING
(726)
Haywood, R.
Van Vierssen-Trip, Hector

MANOTICK
(485)
Laidlaw, R. G.
Leach, W. J.
Wilson, O. B.

MAPLE
(1,552)
Bigford, R. A.
Birkett, C. W.
Granger, M. P.
McAtter, F. M.
Perkin, G. W.
Sabo, G.
White, A. W. OrthSurg, GenSurg.

MARATHON
(2,400)
Arscott, A. G.
Bozyk, A. L.
Graham, S. S.
Reason, C. J. GenSurg

MARKDALE
(1,089)
Breakwell, W. G.
Gray, W. G., ObstGyn

MARKHAM
(4,294)
Burkholder, J. N.
Fleming, J. M.
Macdonald, I. M. Ophth
Outred, J. T.
Scott, J. R.
Seaver, R.
White, J. F.

MARLBANK
(350)
Hunt, D. A.
Hunt, G. G.

MARMORA
(1,378)
Burrows, J. F.
Parkin, H. E.

MASSEY
(1324)
Bebensee, D. L.

MATHESON
(856)
Chong, P. C. L.
Killingbeck, R. N

MATTAWA
(3,314)
Caron, J. M.
Monestine, S

MAXVILLE
(804)
Mutch, J.

MEAFORD
(3,834)
Eagles, A. M.
Finley, J. C.
Robinson, D. C.
Wirkkunen, R. A.

MERLIN
(595)
McLean, J. A.

MERRICKVILLE
(944)
Wise, H. D.

MIDLAND
(10,000)
Brasher, Irene M.
Brasher, P. H. GenSurg
Cardwell, R. J.
Carlson, K. M.
Grise, E. A.
Kettle, W. W.
Kiefer, H.
Moore, J.
Neale, W. F.
Pinchin, A. H.
Small, J.

Tweedle, Lois E., IntMed., Pulm Dis & T.B.(P.Q.)
Weldon, I. T.

MILDMAY
(849)
Walters, W. R.

MILLBROOK
(891)
Hobbs, M. E.
Wright, J. W.

MILTON
(5,629)
Aikenhead, D. H.
Edwards, R. B.
Hiltz, C. W.
Hunter, I. A.
Legate, W. S., GenSurg.
Mackay, R. A.
McCutcheon, J. W.
Stevenson, C. K.
Stuart, L. J.
Syer, G. E.
Taylor, A. S.
Turvey, J. W.

MILVERTON
(1,111)
Tye, P. L.

MIMICO
(District of Toronto)

MINDEMOYA
(356)
McQuay, J. B.

MINDEN
(658)
Fitz-Gerald, B. P. M., GenSurg.
Griffiths, F. E.
Koval, R. J.

MITCHELL
(2,246)
Moore, J. B.
Pridham, W. E.
Town, J. D.

MONKTON
(422)
Bower, H. L.

MOOSE FACTORY
(689)
Gilchrist, F. I.
Jonat, G. H.
Purser, Margaret J.
Wisniewski, C., GenSurg.

MORRISBURG
(1,820)
Dawson, P. S.
Lambert, E. H. N.
Robertson, D. M.
Shannette, A. T.

MOUNT ALBERT
(561)
Carruthers, W. L.
Cooper, F. C. T.
Singerland, J. O.

MOUNT BRYDGES
(1,036)
Pardy, W. V. V.

MOUNT FOREST
(2,624)
Demmer, H. T.
McPherson, R. H.
Smith, J. A.

MOUNT HOPE
(807)
Leeds, J. H.
Ridge, J. W.
Ridge, R. W.
Ridge, W. W.

NAKINA
(500)
McKillip, T. H.

* Population not separately available.

NAPANEE
(4,500)
Bergstome, B. E.
Burke, N. F.
Burns, W. E.
Duffett, W. H.
Ellicott, E. R.
McKinney, J. C.
McLellan, R. A.
Mounce, A. R.
Paul, E. B.
Thomsen, A. E., GenSurg.

NEWBURGH
(568)
Paidra, J.

NEWCASTLE
(1,270)
Miklos, L. S.

NEW HAMBURG
(2,185)
Kirkpatrick, C.
Lichtenheldt, J. E.
Row, R. K.

NEW LISKEARD
(4,896)
Barte, P.
Beland, A.
Bullen, A. E.
Farlinger, A. F.
Ross, J. T.
Smylie, R. D.

NEWMARKET
(8,932)
Arkinstall, Margaret
Arkinstall, W. C., GenSurg.
Blackwell, G. L.
Boulding, C. R.
Case, G. E.
Cock, J. G.
Edwards, J. C. R., GenSurg.
Farber, E. P., PlasSurg, GenSurg
Fearon, J. D.
Gordon, J. A., IntMed.
Greaves, P. C. W., Anaes.
Hughes, W. Psy
Hutchins, D., IntMed
Jackson, H. M., ObstGyn
Lennox, B. M.
Le Page, B. C.
Levers, P. E., Urol
McClintock, W. D., GenSurg
Mortimer, N. W., GenSurg
Murdoch, D. A.
Peever, G. M.
Perry, P. E., Psy
Ritchie, J. A., GenSurg
Schofield, C. C.
Scully, L. T.
Stevens, D. G., Paed
Young, P. W., Ophth.
Zealand, G. W.

NEW TORONTO
(13,382)
(District of Toronto)
Blazic, C. Psy
Burgess, R. M. Psy
Gunn, D. R. Psy
Kalb, S., Psy
Moorhouse, H. C. Psy
Simpson, R. T.
Schofield, T. E.
Stolove, M. A.

NIAGARA FALLS
(54,649)
Afrukhteh, D.
Ainslie, R. D.
Ainslie, W. H., GenSurg
Armstrong, T. K.
Beadsworth, B. J.
Baer, R. A., Urol
Bickle, Margaret E., DiagRad.
Bidwell, P. A.
Booth, J. F. Path
Brown, C. J. ObstGyn
Campbell, D. L.
Clark, J. W. GenSurg
Clark, Lillian S. Paed
Clement, H. F., GenSurg
Cooper, W. E. IntMed
Costanzo, J. F.
Cox, Felicity C.
Cullimore, Dora (Polynchuk) Paed
Davidson, J. P.
Davidson, J. H. Obst
Dickinson, T. E.
Duggan, R. S.
Dwyer, J., DiagRad
Eager, R. F. Otol
Fielding, E. M. V. Anaes
Fisher, A. A., ObstGyn
Fisher, S. A. GenSurg
Hadley, G. L. IntMed
Hanniwell, D. B., ObstGyn
Higgins, J. E.
Hoag, S. R. R.
Hood, E.
Hope-Gill, E. D., Otol.
Howatson, D. G., Path
Howe, W. A.
Howes, M. E.
Hulke, F. P. DiagRad
Humeniuk, R. B.
Jamieson, T. A. B.
Johnston, D. R. ObstGyn
Kelly, M. A., Otol.
Kyle, C. A. GenSurg
Kyle, J. L. Ophth
Le Masters, G. S.
Lewis, G. H. Ophth
Lewitzky, G.
Locke, C. J.
Mahoney, J. L.
Martin, W. J.
McGarry, G. C., IntMed.
McGarry, H. H. Paed
McGarry, J. R. ObstGyn
McIntyre, G. J.
Minnes, A. G.
Murphy, D. K. GenSurg
Nestler, H. A., GenSurg
Niesen, W. C., Urol
Overholt, B. M.
Pohran, N.
Powell, G. W.
Prime, R. L., Anaes.
Sahin, A. F., Urol.
Shoemaker, B. W.
Steed, C. M., DiagRad.
Toews, R. R., Ophth
Tourangeau, June A.
Walker, K. F. ObstGyn
Weare, W. G., OrthSurg
Whytock, A. B. GenSurg
Williams, M. F. GenSurg
Wrong, H. A. Anaes

NIAGARA-ON-THE-LAKE
(2,712)
Rigg, C. B.
Rigg, F. J.

NIPIGON
(2,105)
Harvey, T. J.
Somerliegh, E. R.
Wells, C. M. GenSurg

NOELVILLE
(250)
Vachon, G.

NORTH AUGUSTA
(247)
Davis, C. B.

NORTH BAY
(41,102)
Armstrong, W. F.
Asselstine, K. M., GenSurg
Ball, R. E.
Baltrusaitis, J.
Biron, P. E.
Bowers, N. H.
Boyd, W. T.
Brennan, E. J.
Brown, K. B. GenSurg
Butler, W. S. GenSurg
Coombes, W. N. GenSurg OrthSurg
Crowe, L. L.
de Grosbois, P. S.
Diren, G., Paed
Fazzari F. Paed
Girard, P. M.
Gravel, R. A.
Griffin, J. E.
Grose, P. S.
Guest, G. F. Ophth,Otol
Hancharyk, G.
Houghtling, W. J., IntMed
Hunter, R. D.
Jackson, G. A.
Jackson, R. M. GenSurg
Jamieson, J. S., Ophth Otol
Karnauchow, P. N. Path
Keech, W. A.
Lemasters, G. S.
Lowrey, H. E. D. GenSurg
Marks, M. M.
McIntyre, G. J.
McKinnon, F. A., GenSurg
McMurchy, A. D.
Menard, J. V.
Milne, P. L.
Pace, A. M., ObstGyn
Paine, D. GenSurg, Urol
Ranger, C. J., Psy.
Rendell, W. B., IntMed
Rivet, M. G.
Rochefort, J. M.
Ross, G. T.
Runnalls, K. W. Psy
Sauks, A. A.
Scappatura, A. R.
Schryer, M. J. P., Path
Sinclair, J. D.
Sinclair, R. A.
Stackhouse, J. G., GenSurg.
Stephenson, R. G. Psy
Thompson, M. DiagRad
Wall, C. B.
Wallace, G. M. GenSurg
Wallace, H. GenSurg
White, R. A.

NORTH BROOK
*
Sunderland, K. B.

NORWICH
(1,703)
Hall, R. M.
Price, F. E.

NORWOOD
(1,064)
Atkinson, A. R.

OAK RIDGES
(1864)
McBurney, D. A.

OAKVILLE
(10,366)
Aldridge, D., GenSurg
Alexander, J. C., Ophth
Alexander, Sara K.
Anderson, W. L.
Annis, R. V.
Base, G. S. Anaes
Birkett, Barbara M., Derm
Bow, L. W. D. Psy
Brandt, P. U.
Burke, D. T. DiagRad
Burke, W. D., DiagRad
Bustard, V. W., ObstGyn
Bykerk, H.
Campbell, D. B. ObstGyn
Cartwright, D. B.
Ciprick, W. J., Anaes.
Clark, J. M., Anaes.

* Population not separately available.

Oakville (Cont'd.)
Couch, J. H., GenSurg., OrthSurg.
Cranfield, H. V. PhysMed
Dixon, D. H.
Dubelstein, P. A.
Fowler, J. L. A. IntMed
Fujino, D. S., Anaes
Gear, J. R.
Gee, E. M.
Graham, M. E., Paed
Harley, H. C.
Harsanyi, I.
Haynes, J. D. GenSurg
Haynes, Thora, IntMed
Hayward, R. S.
Hines, R. M.
Homonylo, M., GenSurg, Urol
Horne, S. J., GenSurg.
Hunt, N. E.
Isaak, V. H.
Kilshaw, M. F.
Kober, Dorothy, S.
Kunica, R. D.
Langmuir, R. M.
Lawson, F. S., Psy.
Leslie, D.
MacArthur, W. J. C. GenSurg
McCarney, J. R. GenSurg
McCrae, W. H., Urol.
McCulloch, M. A.
McGovern, M. G. Paed
McHugh, J. J. IntMed
McKie, J. G.
McNeely, D. T., IntMed.
McRae, W. H., Urol
Milne, P. L.
Munroe, G. G. A. Anaes
Olson, R. M.
Owen, J. G.
Patterson, M. C., Path
Phillips, G. K.
Prince, W. R., Urol
Rawling, E. G., GenSurg
Roberts, F. B., Paed
Ross, A. E.
Ross, A. L.
Rouse, F. V.
Rowsell, P. W.
Sandford, J. R., Otol.
Selmeci, T. G.
Soanes, E. P.
Soanes, S. E.
Sparling, F. N.
Stewart, D.
Sturgeon, A. W.
Trupp, H. C., Psy.
Tuttle, R. T.
Walmsley, D. P.
Warr, G. O.
Wells, B. S. GenSurg
White, Kathryn, A.
Williamson, E. A.
Worrell, J. C. ObstGyn
Yoshioka, J. M. Anaes
Zaborowska, J.

OHSWEKEN
*****
Dobrinoff, M.
Nicholas, G. J.

OMEMEE
(809)
Sobrian, J.

ONAPING
*****
Jalkotzy, H.
Jalkotzy, Martha
Ockenden, K. A.

ORANGEVILLE
(4,593)
Austin, R. A.
Davison, D. H.
Henderson, W. E.
Hill, G. U.
Love, W. R.
McBurney, R. J.
McGee, R. B.
Moran, L.
Scott, D. J., GenSurg

ORILLIA
(15,345)
Armbrust, Nancy E.
Baillie, A. C.
Barton, F. C.
Binnington, Vera I., Paed.
Brandl, T., GenSurg
Buckley, G. F., Path
Costley, S. R.
Craymer, W. J.
Donevan, W. J.
Edmonds, E. P.
Edwards, J. M.
Galloway, C. A.
Green, E. T.
Hall, H. J.
Handy, B. H.
Harvie, C. A., GenSurg.
Hill, J. C.
Hipwell, R. E. ObstGyn
Hopwood, G.
Ironside, Nancy, Anaes
Irwin, H. J.
Jamieson, Agnes L.
Jones, F. C. Psy
Kiff, R. D., Ophth
Leeson, P. F.
McLennan, T. M. DiagRad
Meredith, J. T.
Pelletier, R. M.
Richardson, D. A.
Rynard, P. B.
Sansom, Kathleen E. J.
Scott, M. B.
Sinclair, J. N., GenSurg
Strathearn, J. K.
Thomas, G. K. GenSurg
Torrance, T. L.
Welch, J. D.
Wensley, J. A., IntMed
Wilson, H. D.
Woodrow, W. H. Ophth,Otol
Zufelt, W. E.

ORONO
(860)
McKenzie, A. F.

OSGOODE
(390)
Dowd, R. A.

OSHAWA
(80,913)
Anderson, J. O. ObstGyn
Antonevych, D. V. Anaes
Bayne, J. R.
Beaton, B. W.
Beckett, R. F., ObstGyn
Bell, R. G.
Blair, W. K.
Bowerman, D. Ophth
Brown, B. A.
Campbell, C. S. GenSurg
Cherewaty, T. W.
Chmara, J.
Clark, D.
Clark, R. M. Path
Culp, E. M.
Cummings, R. H., IntMed
Dekany, Eva, Ophth
Dicesare, J. N., DiagRad.
Dillon, J. J. Anaes
Doherty, B. G.
Ellis, P. M.
Fekete, Z. C., Derm
Ferrier, C. W.
Fulton, A. P. GenSurg
Gardner, C. C. GenSurg
Gilchrist, W. L., Paed
Gill, R. A. GenSurg, OrthSurg
Gillen, G. R.
Glazier, E.
Grant, W. G. IntMed
Guselle, R. D. W.
Halam-Andres, A. S.
Hall, H. C.
Harding, A. W. Ophth,Otol
Helson, K. G., DiagRad
Irwin, R. S.
Kimmerly, R. J.
King, A. E.
Kowalsky, N.
Kutzner, W.
Kwak, J., GenSurg
Kwan, C. Y.
Lee, I. N., Otol
Loos, A. J. R. DiagRad
Lovell, D. M.
Lowes, J. N.
MacDonald, A. J. GenSurg
MacPherson, W. C.
Madgwick, K. S.
Manax, W.
Mankiewicz, S., Urol
Maroosis, J. P. G.
McIlveen, C. E.
McKay, W. G. ObstGyn
McLean, D. J.
Miller, R. K. ObstGyn
Mills, D. G., GenSurg
Mills, O. G. IntMed
Morgan, C. A.
Morris, M. L.
Morrison, H. G.
Munt, P. W.
Murray, J. F.
Orton, T. H.
Ostafichuk, N.
Oxenham, L. W.
Patterson, J. A. IntMed
Pickering, J. W. Otol
Raskin, N. Psy
Richmond, H. A., GenSurg, Urol.
Rogers, D.
Ross, R. C. ObstGyn
Rowsell, H. R. IntMed
Rudnick, A.
Rundle, F. W., Otol
Rundle, G. A. Paed
Rundle, J. E.
Sanderson, H. M.
Scott, A. F.
Shaw, W. M. IntMed
Smith, D. E. IntMed
Spragge, J. W.
Sproull, D. M., GenSurg
Stanley, W. H. GenSurg
Stewart, C. C.
Sturgis, D. E.
Treanor, J. J.
Ugray, I. K., Urol
Vipond, C. H., GenSurg
Vollmer, H.
Warren, W. D.
Watt, W. G. Paed
Williams, J. V.
Witzel, S. H. Ophth
Woolford, B. J.
Woods, B. M. DiagRad
Wright, R. B.

OTTAWA
(482,000)
Abbatt, J. D.
Abelson, S. J. Psy
Acres, S. E.
Adam, J. E., Derm.
Adams, B. R., Paed.
Allen, J. D. Ophth
Allen, R. H.
Anderson, G. H., Path
Archambault, J. R., DiagRad.
Armstrong, G. W. OrthSurg
Armstrong, G. W., OrthSurg.
Armstrong, R. A.
Atack, E. A. Neur
Atkinson, J. W., Anaes
Atkinson, W. L.

*** Population not separately available.**

Ottawa (Cont'd.)
Auer, R. J.
Auns, Z.
Bagnall, H J. NeurSurg
Baker, J. E.
Banister, P. G., Paed.
Bard, M. G., Anaes.
Barends, H. A. Anaes
Barnes, H. M.
Barnes, R. R., ObstGyn
Baron, R. H., IntMed.
Barr, J. R., Path
Barr, Margaret, Anaes
Barron, R. D.
Bates, J. F. GenSurg
Batol, Z. G.
Beach, M. A.
Beardall, P. J., ObstGyn
Beattie, H. A.
Beattie, W. G. GenSurg
Beairsto, A.
Beaudoin, J. E., ObstGyn.
Bedford, R. F.
Beggs, J. A. ObstGyn
Belanger, J. E.
Belanger, L. F.
Belanger, P. B. GenSurg
Belcourt, C. L., DiagRad
Bell, D. N. Anaes
Bell, R. C.
Bellamy, K. E.
Benson, R. A. IntMed (TB)
Beresford, J. M., ObstGyn.
Berkman, Emily, ObstGyn.
Berkman, F. IntMed
Berry, J. V. Urol
Besley, J. K., GenSurg.
Best, E. W. PH
Beswick, J. A., Ophth
Beznak, Margaret.
Bhargava, U.
Bigras, J. M.
Bird, R. L.
Bishop, J. W.
Black, G. A. IntMed
Blair, W. A. Psy
Blais, A. M., Psy.
Blake, Barbara
Bociek, R. C., D & TRad
Bohatirckuk, F.
Bohlig, G. K.
Bonfield, J. P. Anaes
Bonfield, J. P., GenSurg
Borgaonkar, R. D., IntMed.
Bouchard, A. J. G., GenSurg.
Bourque, H. Paed
Box, D.E.
Boyd, C. E.
Boyd, W. J.
Brand, L. M.
Bresnahan, T. J. IntMed
Bright, H. J.
Britton, W. A., Ophth
Brooks, D. W., IntMed
Brown, B. R.
Brown, C. M., DiagRad.
Brown, D. R. GenSurg
Brown, F. N. GenSurg
Brown, G. M., IntMed
Brown, L. W. IntMed
Brown, M., IntMed
Brown, R., Psy
Brown, R. D.
Brown, T. M. D., IntMed.
Brown, W. F. IntMed
Brunet, A. J.
Brunet, E. Sr.
Brunet, J. E. D.
Burch, J. L.
Burdett, L. H.
Burke, J. P.
Burke, Margaret, Psy
Burton, P. M.
Butler, G. C.
Butler, K. C.
Caldwell, J. D. GenSurg
Caldbick, G. G. D., Derm.
Cameron, E. G. ObstGyn
Cameron, G. D. W.
Campbell, E. O. F., IntMed
Campbell, J. S., Path.
Campbell, R. W.
Capello, P., GenSurg.
Cargill, R. E. D. ObstGyn
Carlisle, J. S.
Carr, G. R.
Carson, G. T. ObstGyn
Cathcart, J. P. S., NeurPsy
Catterson, A. G., Psy.
Catton, G. E. TherRad
Caven, W. H. GenSurg
Chalke, F. C. Psy
Charbonneau, E.
Charbonneau, L. P. Otol
Chatterjee, K., Anaes
Chaudhuri, A. K., ObstGyn.
Chen, T. Y., TherRad.
Chew, C. K., IntMed.
Choi, O. S., IntMed.
Clancey, I. L., Psy
Clark, J. C. GenSurg
Clinckett, F. R. Ophth
Coburn, J. B.
Cockburn, D. W. D & TRad
Cohen, G. IntMed
Cole, R. H., Anaes.
Collins, S. B.
Collins, W. E., Urol
Conklin, F. J., ObstGyn.
Connelly, W. J. PH
Connolly, J. F.
Connolly, V. P. Derm.
Conway, D. J. Paed
Cormier, W. F. Pulm. Dis. & T.B. (P.Q.)
Corriveau, A. R. Ophth,Otol
Cosman, H. H. IntMed
Cote, F. H. GenSurg, Gyn
Coupal, J. L., Ophth, Otol
Courtenay, H. D. Ophth,Otol
Couture, E. Obst
Couture, R. A., IntMed.
Cowan, W. E. GenSurg
Cox, A. D.
Craig, R. H. GenSurg
Craig, W. F.
Crawford, J. N. Paed
Crepeau, G. A., ThorSurg (Card.) OrthSurg (P.Q.)
Crook, A. F. TherRad
Cross, J. P.
Cross, J. S.
Crummey, A. S., Otol.
Csont, L.
Cullinan, L. V., Anaes.
Cumming, R. K. Anaes
Curran, D. D. GenSurg
Curtis, R. B., Psy
Dale, A. D.
Danby, S. L. E. GenSurg
Dardick, I.
DaSilva, T. GenSurg
Davies, G. L.
Davies, J. W.
Davies, W. F. A.
Day, J. J.
de Bellefeuille, P. Paed
de la Bastide, Y. H., Otol
Delahay, J. R., Otol
Delaney, T. F.
Dennery, J. M., NeurSurg
Dennery, Mona, Path.
Dent, L. R.
Desai, U.
de Saint Victor, H. R. ObstGyn
Desjardins, D., OrthSurg
de Villiers, A. J.
Devitt, J. E. GenSurg
Diaz, J. M.
Don, C. J. DiagRad
Dooley, R. J.
Dorion, Marie M., PH (P.Q.)
Doubek, L.
Douglas, L. H.
Douville, E. L., ThorSurg
Dover, M. R., GenSurg
Doyle, J. A., Paed
Doyle, P. E. IntMed
Dreyfus, M. A.
Driemen, Pearl M.
Drouin, J. P., GenSurg.
Dube, F. J.
Ducharme, F. A. OrthSurg
Dufresne, J. A. Anaes
Duggan, F. A., Anaes.
Dunning, G. W. GenSurg
Dupont, J. A.
Dupuy, J. E., Anaes.
Durocher, Juliette, Anaes
Dworschak, F.
Dziuba, R. J.
Earle, F. E.
Edmison, R. E.
Edwards, G. K., Ophth
Edwards, W. S. ObstGyn
Elder, R. H., Bact
Elliot, W. J., Ophth
Elliott, R. C., GenSurg
Ellis, C. F. G., OrthSurg.
Embree, G. H., Neur
Evans, S. C. IntMed
Ewing, J. B. GenSurg
Farmer, G. R. D.
Faught, K. A., Paed
Featherston, H.
Feller, J. IntMed
Ferguson, R. H. Anaes
Ferre, N. J.
Fidler, A. IntMed
Fielding, J. F., PlasSurg
Fireman, H. H. IntMed
Fish, Margaret I.
Fisher, T. L. IntMed
Fletcher, J. P., Paed
Forgues, Laura, Psy
Forrester, J. A.
Fortier, J. A. B.
Fortin, P. H. Otol
Fournier, P. W., Path
Fraser, J. T. M. IntMed
Fraser, W. F. Ophth
Fraser, W. G. Ophth
Frost, L. J.
Frost, W. H.
Furesz, Eva
Furesz, J.
Fuzi, A.
Fyfe, J. G.
Gagne, R.
Galway, H. P., Paed
Gamble, D. E.
Gamble, J. E. D.
Gaukrodger, W. T. Ophth
Gaulin, P. Urol
Gauthier, J. E. R., Ophth.
Gay, B. C. GenSurg
Gencher, M., Psy.
Gendreau, L. P. Psy
Gilhooly, J. P. Ophth,Otol
Gillies, R. R., IntMed
Glass, I. H., Paed
Gluck, M., ObstGyn
Goldstein, A.
Gordon, A. S. P. Paed
Goyette, R.
Graham-Cumming, G.
Graham, J.
Graham, J. H. IntMed
Graham, M. D.
Grahovac, Z., DiagRad
Gray, D. G., DiagRad.
Gray, R. C. V.
Green, G. R.
Green, J. E. Anaes
Greenblatt, J. IntMed
Griffin, F. J.
Grimes, S. E. DermSyph
Grondin, G. E.

* Population not separately available.

Ottawa (Cont'd.)
Grove, J. H.
Guest, W. A. IntMed
Guillemette, M. E., Paed
Guiou, N. M. GenSurg, Gyn
Guthrie, J. S. GenSurg
Haight, Rachel K., IntMed.
Hamel, J. F. IntMed
Hamlin, J. H.
Hampson, L. M., Anaes
Hanna, H. E.
Hardman, A. C.
Harris, E. R., DiagRad.
Harris, W. C.
Heaton, P. B.
Hefferman, Angela, Psy
Heggtveit, H. A.
Henry, A. F.
Heringer, R., GenSurg
Hill, D. P.
Hill, R.
Hilton, J. H. B. IntMed
Hoffman, O.
Hoggarth, W. B.
Holden, J. P. N.
Hooper, G. D. GenSurg, ThorSurg
Hooper, G. V. GenSurg, Gyn
Horovitch, R. M., IntMed.
Houston, E. P., Psy.
Howard, M. J.
Howe, J. B.
Howe, W. D.
Hrnchiar, A., Psy
Humphreys, J. C., GenSurg
Hunt, Barbara J.
Hurley, J. D., DiagRad
Hurteau, C. A. D. G., ObstGyn
Hurteau, G., Obst.
Hurteau, J. L. A.
Hurtig, A. GenSurg
Irvine, A. H. Urol
Irwin, G. E. GenSurg
Jackson, J. R. Path
Jackson, R. DermSyph
Janik, J.
Javorsky, V.
Jaworwski, Z. F., IntMed
Jeanes, C. W.
Jeffrey, F. W. Paed
Jeffrey, J. I. OrthSurg
Jessamine, A. G.
Johnson, D. S. DiagRad
Jones, G. H., Ophth, Otol
Jost, H. T. Anaes
Julien, L.
Kadziora, M. B. ObstGyn
Kastner, A.
Katz, M.
Kawulu, L., Obst.
Kay, Elspeth S. Paed
Kay, H. T. Anaes
Kay, K. K.
Kealey, O. J., IntMed
Kellam, H. I. J. GenSurg, OrthSurg.
Kelley, C. W. GenSurg
Kendall, W. T.
Kennedy, R. A.
Kenney, A. S. Paed
Kilgour, J. A., IntMed
Kimm, G. E.
Kingma, H. DermSyph
Kitchen, S. F.
Klotz, M. O., Path., Bact.
Knapp, N. S.
Kniewasser, A. V.
Koch, B. R., IntMed
Kohli, J. D.
Kozakiewicz, M.
Kronick, S. ObstGyn
Krupa, Silvia A.
Kubilius, V.
Kubryk, D.
Kuwayti, K., IntMed
Lacroix, J. R.
Ladouceur, J., ObstGyn.
Laframboise, G. E. Ophth, Otol
Laframboise, G. G. Otol
Laframboise, J., GenSurg
Laidlaw, J. H., PathBact.
Lamberti, A. J., Psy
Lapointe, Marielle
La Rocque, J. A. Gyn
Laurier, J. J. Pulm. Dis. & T.B.(P.Q.)
Law, D. T., Anaes.
Law, Maureen M.
Law, W. B.
Laws, J. E., DiagRad.
Layton, B. D. B. PH
Leach, J. E. K. DermSyph
Leadman, T. P. GenSurg
Leblanc, L.
Lebrun, C. J., Otol
Lee, E. H.
Lee, S. B., GenSurg.
Lefebvre, B. M., GenSurg
Legare, L.
Legzdins, Alexandria
Lemay, P. M., ObstGyn.
Lenis, G. J.
Leslie, W. L.
Lettau, H. Frances
Liberty, G. L. GenSurg
Lidington, E. W.
Liepa, E. V. Path
Little, L. N. Otol
Liver, J. A., DiagRad.
Loeb, L. J. IntMed
Lossing, E. H.
Louden, C. G.
Lowi, R. Naomi
Lu, F. C.
Luna, S. P., IntMed.
Lussier, J. J.
Lydon, M. J., IntMed
MacAulay, A. F.
MacCharles, C. W.
MacKenzie, R. G., Anaes.
Mackey, A. G.
MacKinnon, A. G.
Maclaren, Mary C.
MacLeod, J. W., IntMed
Magner, D. E. O. Path
Mainville, M.
Major, E. J.
Malek, D. L.
Maley, S. C.
Malo, R. F.
Maloney, P. J. Paed
Mantha, L., IntMed
Mar, P. G.
Marion, G. Paed
Marier, L. P., Anaes
Marois, M., PhysMed & Rehab
Martin, M. G., Psy
Martin-Villar, J.
Maziec, K.
McCarthy, T. F.
McCunn, P. D., Ophth
McDermot, Rebecca, TherRad
McEwen, B. B.
McIntosh, W. C.
McIver, J. R., DiagRad
McKay, D. E., Urol.
McKee, Elisabeth F.
McKee, J. A., Paed
McKendry, J. B. R. IntMed
McKercher, D. D. Otol
McKerracher, F.
McLean, C. M., Ophth
McPherson, V. A., GenSurg
McSweyn, N. F. A. ThorSurg
Megill, A. H. GenSurg
Mehl, J. F. Otol
Mercantini, E. S., Derm
Mercer, S. GenSurg
Mercier, J. IntMed
Metcalfe, H. G. Urol
Michalkoff, M.
Michaud, R. J., D & TRad
Mickelson, W. P.
Mills, D. K., Psy.
Minnes, H. E. GenSurg
Mirsky, S. IntMed
Misener, C. C.
Moffatt, T. I. Obst
Moghal, A. N., GenSurg.
Moineau, A.
Moir, D. M.
Momose, K. J. D & TRad
Monagle, J. E.
Montgomery, D. C. DermSyph
Moore, P. E. PH
Moores, D. E., Urol.
Morin, G. D., Psy
Morin, L. Paed
Morin, T. J.
Moritz, D. V. Paed
Morrice, C. P. C., Paed.
Morrow, C. E. L.
Morton, Vyvian, Anaes
Mouldey, R. G., Psy.
Moulds, G. G. S.
Mount, H. T., GenSurg
Murphy, J. B.
Murphy, P. G., Urol
Myers, G. R.
Nadon, A.
Nagler, T. P. O.
Napke, E.
Neelin, W. E. E.
Neri, L. C.
Niblett, D. H.
Nichol, J. T., TherRad
Nixon, J. C.
Nodwell, G. R.
Noel, M.
Northover, R. J., PH
Nuven, A. J. J., ObstGyn.
O'Brien, B., Psy.
O'Brien, J. R.
O'Brien, Mary S.
O'Meara, B. B.
Orizaga, M., Path
Pace, F. C.
Paiement, R., OrthSurg
Panneton, M.
Parent, Paul E.
Park, J. M., Paed
Pataki, J. I., IntMed
Paterson, W. P., Jr., ObstGyn
Patterson, R. J., DiagRad
Patterson, T. H.
Patton, J. O., Path
Pearlman, L. N., Paed
Pekelsky, K.
Pelletier J. R., Psy
Pennock, G. M.
Perras, J. R., Obst (P.Q.)
Perrault, R. A.
Peterson, E. W., NeurSurg
Petrie, C. B., GenSurg
Pett, L. B., PH
Philips, T. B., D&TRad
Pilon, L. D.
Plenderleith, I. H., IntMed.
Pollock, P., IntMed
Pollonetsky, Elizabeth
Potvin, L., IntMed
Powell, Anne M.
Powell, T. J.
Powers, A., IntMed (TB)
Poznanski, W. J., IntMed
Procter, H. A.
Prowse, W. A.
Prud'homme, P.
Puddicombe, P. G.
Pugsley, E. B. M.
Purchase, E. C. R., IntMed
Pushman, D. R., Psy
Quarrington, A. J.
Quastel, M. R.
Radoiu, N.
Raine, R. J.
Rand, C. G., IntMed
Rashid, A., IntMed.

* Population not separately available.

Ottawa (Cont'd.)
Rea, D. H.
Ready, N. H., Anaes
Reardon, F. L.
Reid, S. I., ObstGyn
Renwick, Cynthia
Renwick, G. J.
Resnick, M.
Richard, A. L., GenSurg, Gyn
Richardson, H. J.
Riley, J. M.
Rioux, M.
Ritchie, K. S.
Roberts, Maureen H., Paed
Robertson, H. E., IntMed (TB)
Robertson, H. J. F., DiagRad.
Robertson, R. W.
Robichon, J., OrthSurg
Robillard, J. O.
Robinson, A. C., Otol
Robinson, L. K.
Robinson, P-M., IntMed.
Roche, J. W.
Roger, J. D., IntMed, DiagRad
Romero-Sierra, C.
Rosenberg, H. D.
Rossignol, J. P., Anaes
Rouleau, R.
Roussel, L.
Rowan-Legg, C. K., Paed
Rowswell, A. C.
Roy, D. E. IntMed.
Saar, Hilja
Sabetta, V.
Sachs, H. J., GenSurg., ThorSurg (Card.)
Saleh, W. S., GenSurg.
Samis, J. C., GenSurg
Sarda, P.
Sauer, J.
Sauve, G.
Sauve, N., Anaes
Scharf, R. F., GenSurg, OrthSurg.
Schecter, N., IntMed
Schenker, Marianne
Schryer, K. R.
Schuler, G. T.
Scobie, D. H., GenSurg
Scobie, T. K., GenSurg
Scott, A. C., Urol
Scott, Caroline
Sehgal, N. N., ObstGyn
Shapiro, C. E.
Shapiro, E. I., GenSurg
Sharpe, Anna E., Paed
Shatford, R. C.
Shaw, L. B.
Shenket, M.
Shirley, S. Y., Ophth
Shomody, S. H.
Shute, W. B., ObstGyn
Silverman, M., Psy
Simms, J. G.
Simo, J.
Sims, H. A., IntMed
Singh, H., Psy
Smart, R. E., Ophth
Smiley, R. K., IntMed
Smith, H. G., ObstGyn
Smolkin, R. D.
Smolkin, S.
Snell, A. E.
Sokolowska, Anna M., Psy
Soloway, I., ObstGyn
Spearman, W. F., Ophth
Spiro, C. H., Ophth, Otol
Sponsel, G. L.
Starrs, R. A., IntMed
Stephen, H. M.
Stewart, E. G.
Stewart, T. H. M., IntMed
Stewart, T. W., Psy
Stewart, Wilma G.
Stockdale, E.
Stoddart, T. G., D & T Rad
Sutherland, Eleanor W.
Sutherland, R.
Szyrynski, V., Neur, Psy
Taillefer, J. B. GenSurg.
Taylor, G. O., ObstGyn.
Tench, J. F., Anaes.
Terrien, J. H. J., GenSurg
Tessier, J. A. E., D & TRad
Thiel, C. J., Anaes
Thomas, G. C., IntMed
Thomson, D. M., GenSurg
Thomson, J. A.
Todd, I. M.
Tolnai, G., Path
Tooly, R. W.
Tousignant, M., Anaes
Troup, W.
Troup, W. J., IntMed
Uden, D. E.
Underwood, W. J.
Urie, G. M.
Urie, N. B., Anaes
Valberg, J. D., Ophth.
Vaillancourt, F. W. J., DiagRad.
Van Husen, Josephine
Varughese, G., NeurSurg
Vechter, M., OrthSurg
Verville, G.
Viau, H. R., Paed
Viets, Celia A., Paed.
Villeneuve, P. J.
Vogelfranger, I. J., GenSurg
Waddell, W. G., GenSurg
Walker, F. G., PlasSurg
Walko, Z. S., GenSurg
Walter, Magda
Ward, N., Psy
Watson, A. G., Ophth
Watt, L. O., ObstGyn
Webb, J. F., Paed
Webster, J. R., GenSurg
Weldon, J. D., Psy.
Wherrett, G. J.
Whillans, J. A., Paed
Whittingham, D. S., D & T Rad
Whyte, D. W., Anaes
Whyte, J. C., ObstGyn
Wickware, J. P., DiagRad
Wiebe, J. H.
Wigle, W. W.
Wilcox, C. F.
Wiley, J. J., OrthSurg
Williamson, N. L., GenSurg
Willis, J. S.
Wills, W., Path
Wilson, K. E. G., GenSurg
Wilson, L. D., GenSurg
Wilson, R. C.
Winfield, G. A., Urol
Wolstein, E., Ophth
Wood, E. H., GenSurg
Wood, R. W.
Woodruff, W. A., Psy
Woychyshyn, J.
Wrazej, W. J., Anaes
Wride, G. E.
Yao, M. C.
Young, D. A., GenSurg
Young, E. J.
Young, E. M.
Znamirowski, R.

OTTERVILLE
(682)
Batson, H. H.
Downing, G. M.

OWEN SOUND
(17,421)
Annis, L. H., DiagRad
Birkett, D. P.
Brewster, J. M., IntMed
Brewster, J. M., GenSurg
Campbell, C. G., Anaes
Eagles, G.
French, G. S., D & TRad
Gaviller, E. A.
Groustra, F. N.
Handford, S. L.
Harvey, W.
Hauch, C. Y., GenSurg
Howes, J. M., GenSurg.
Hughes, S. J., Otol
Jackson, I.M.
Keeling, C. J., IntMed.
Kindree, W. A.
Lumsden, W. F., GenSurg
Macivor, J., Ophth
MacLean, B. L.
McConachie, D.
McKee, Beverly W.
Middleboro, J. G.
Middlebro, A., Anaes
Middlebro, J. P., GenSurg
Penny, S. F., PathBact.
Pollock, A. D., GenSurg
Quirk, K. C.
Richards, F.
Shaw, R. A.
Sutherland, L. J., IntMed
Taylor, G. W., Obst
Warnica, J. K.
Whiteside, R. D.
Williscroft, B. A.

PAISLEY
(754)
Milne, D. H.

PALMERSTON
(1,552)
Graham, G. A., Psy
Graham, R. K., GenSurg
O'Donnell, M.
Razeck, A.
Riddell, J. R., GenSurg
Vanner, G. A.

PARIS
(5,820)
Dunton, A. S.
Foote, W. S.
Gregory, J. D.
Jarrott, T. R., Obst
Riddolls, W. E.
Williams, J. C.

PARKHILL
(1,171)
Boyes, F. F. R.
Scrimgeour, W. G.

PARRY SOUND
(6,004)
Aziz, Y., GenSurg
Culliton, Elsie
Curry, F. D., DiagRad
Daley, D. R.
Denholm, K. A.
Lepard, S. F.
MacKay, J. P.
Malkin, E.
McLaren, D. K.
Randell, O. T., GenSurg
Rublee, J. D., Path.
Roundhill, A.
Scott, P. F.
Wheatley, M. L.
Wright, A. J. L.

PELEE ISLAND
(644)
Wells, Alice, Anaes
Wells, G.

PEMBROKE
(16,791)
Bobra, S. T.
Bower, R. R.
Cashman, T.
Coombes, A. C.
Foohey, J. O.
Gilfillan, R. R., GenSurg
Gilfillan, Veronica J.
Hermitte, G. L.
Matzinger, Karl E.
McCluskey, L. U., GenSurg
McEwen, R. B., GenSurg
Munro, C. B.
Peters R. V.

* Population not separately available.

Pembroke (Cont'd.)
Reid, L. G.
Reinke, E. E.
Siegmund, K., GenSurg
Tasker, R. G.
Williams. W. W. D.

PENETANGUISHENE
(5,340)
Binkley, W. E.
Boyd, B. A., Psy
Darby, G. H.
Lauzon, R.
MacKenzie, A. D.
MacVittie, J. A.
McKnight, C. K., Psy
Orchard, B. C., Psy.
Snow, G. A.

PERTH
(5,360)
Boss, M. M.
Church, C. B. G.
Craig, D. O.
Fowler, A. C.
Kidd, J. A.
Noonan, J. F.
Ryan, I. G.
Tweedie, J. W.

PETAWAWA
(4,509)
Dominguez, A.
Dooley, P. E.

PETERBOROUGH
(49,902)
Aitken, D. W., Anaes
Anderson, J. R.
Belch, W. W., GenSurg
Bell, R. H.
Blastorah, W. D. J., GenSurg
Butt, J. A., ObstGyn
Cahill, C. F.
Calvert, L. J., GenSurg, Urol
Campbell, I. P.
Chenoweth, R. S., GenSurg
Clark, D. R., Paed
Clark, J. R.
Clarkson, M. F., IntMed
Cole, P., Otol
Cragg, C. E., Ophth
Currier, T. E., IntMed
Curtis, D. D.
Dalton, J. B., IntMed
Deacon, C. B., Paed, Derm
Deyo, G. M.
Dobson, H. V., IntMed
Doyle, P. J.
Dutkevich, E., Path
Eaton, R. D.
Elliott, A. M.
Epping, J. R.
Fitzpatrick, W. S., Paed
Flak, E. A., Otol
Flak, Ludmila
Forster, W., Psy
Fraser, J. H., ObstGyn
Frid, J. G., Paed
Gamble, W. J. W.
Gordon, W. J.
Gow, W. S., IntMed
Harterre, D. J.
Heine, H. X.
Howes, J. E., GenSurg
Hyatt, B. W.
Kelly, A., GenSurg
Kelly, D. B., IntMed
Kempff, J. G., DiagRad
Levy, A. H., GenSurg
Lewis, G. A., ObstGyn
Lundquist, A. S., Anaes
MacDougall, C. H.
MacIsaac, C. A.
MacKay, H. V.
MacLean, W. R., Paed
Magee, E. L., Anaes
Magee, R. K., GenSurg, OrthSur Urol
Martin, Alice
Martyn, J. W., GenSurg
Matthews, R. M., Paed
McCartney, H. J., Ophth
McKone, B.
McNeill, J. A.
Milne, K. W., DiagRad
Mitchell, H. A., IntMed
Moffat, Agnes K., Anaes, Paed
Morgan, J. R. E., IntMed
Must, C. J.
Neville, J. J.
Nott, R. F., Obst
Nugent, E. A., GenSurg.
Pfeifer, J. R.
Richardson, O. B., Ophth
Ross, S. R., GenSurg.
Rumball, W. G., Otol
Russell, K. T.
Rutledge, S. L., GenSurg
Sams, N. H.
Scott, C. M.
Scott, G. R., ObstGyn
Scott, N. A., Anaes
Sheppard, T. J., ObstGyn
Smith, Marcia, Paed
Smith, R. L., GenSurg.
Stewart, F. E.
Stewart, J. T. R., GenSurg
Symons, F. A., DiagRad.
Thompson, L. W., IntMed
Tulloch, A. M., Anaes
Turner, A. M., IntMed
Wade, R. C.
Walsh, S. Y.
Wedlock, W.
Whiteside, J. H., Path
Whyte, W. D., GenSurg
Wishart, J. M., PH, Anaes
Yelland, H. M., GenSurg
Young, H. N. M.
Young, R. J.
Zacks, L.

PETROLIA
(3,708)
Dougall, D. R.
Dougall, Marion
Fraleigh, S. B.
MacCallum, A. P.
Shabsove, H. B.

PICKERING
(1,758)
Atkinson, Joan
Morrison, Irene
Tomlinson, W. W.
Weisbaum, S. D.

PICKLE CROW
(341)
Hudson, H. D. L.

PICTON
(4,862)
Allison, G., GenSurg
Anderson, J. E.
Caughey, G. C.
Dockrill, L. G.
Hart, S. W. D.
McQueen, K. E.
Millar, K. G.
Murphy, F. W.
Pearce, J. P.
Publow, C. A., Ophth, Otol
Richmond, C. R.
Sarles, Sally
Taylor, B. E., GenSurg
Walmsley, J. H.

PLANTAGENET
(729)
Gaboury, H.
Larocque, E.

PLATTSVILLE
(459)
Stevens, E.

POINTE AU BARIL
*
McLaren, D. K.

PORT ARTHUR
(93,251)
Anten, E. V.
Appen, Ursula J.
Arnott, D. C., PhysMed & Rehal
Arnott, Ruth M.
Baker, C. E., GenSurg
Ballantyne, P. M., GenSurg
Bentz, P.
Best, C. N., IntMed
Bickford, F. L.
Bull, A. I., ObstGyn.
Burnford, D. W., Paed
Castor, W. R., D & T Rad.
Chapman, H. L., ObstGyn
Clark, G. C., Anaes
Coates, W. R., Psy.
Colquhoun, J. T.
Coulson, D. B. M.
Dawosyr, Irene
Dennis, F. T., Anaes
Diggins, W. L.
Falckh, R. C., Ophth
Falk, R. C.
Ferguson, G. C., IntMed
Ferrier, G. C., Psy
Garson, R. D.
Gooding, J. T., GenSurg
Gwozdecky, G.
Hargan, W. A., D & TRad
Harold, R. L., Obst
Hawkins, A. R.
Heringer, T. M.
Hoffman, D. V.
Howitt, J. R., Psy
Huang, E. P., DiagRad; Paed
Johnson, L. O.
Johnston, C. M., ObstGyn
Kajander, Ruth, Psy
Kent, H. A.
Koehler, B. E.
Kyle, V. N., Urol.
Leach, C. E., Psy
Lechow, B.
Lewkin, D., Psy
Lone, F. J., Path
MacKenzie, R. N., DiagRad
Merreck, A., Anaes.
McComb, C. R., GenSurg, Urol
McCutcheon, J. E., Anaes
Montemuro, T. J., IntMed
Morch, J. E.
Parry, J. D.
Patrick, E.
Pearson, J. C., GenSurg
Pietilainen, E. K., GenSurg
Powell, C. E., Ophth
Riches, J. V., GenSurg
Ritchie, K. C.
Rohr, E. A.
Salonen, O.
Schiewe, S. N.
Schmidt, P. P., GenSurg
Simonsen, L. E., Anaes
Smith, H. J., IntMed.
Steinhoff, G. E.
Thompson, F. F. P.
Van de Flier, R. W., IntMed
Walker, R. E.
Welbourne, R. W., PlasSurg.
Wilson, C. G., Paed
Wilson, G. L., ObstGyn.
Wilson, J. R.
Wright, E. N., Ophth, Otol
Zaitzeff, V.

PORT BURWELL
(777)
Leatherdale, C. L.

PORT CARLING
(528)
Archdekin, F. F.

PORT COLBORNE
(14,886)
Cockcroft, D., DiagRad
Cow, D. N.

* Population not separately available.

Port Colborne (Cont'd.)
Dewar, J. D.
Hall, J. S.
Hurst, D. W., GenSurg.
Longford, U. D.
Mackenzie, E. A. Sr.
May, J. R.
McAvoy, A. V., GenSurg
McBirnie, J. E., GenSurg
Morgan, W. B.
O'Brien, M. W.
Pariser, M.
Peacock, P. M.
Pedley, E.
Pettigrew, R. W. DiagRad.
Pond, R. A.
Stephenson, J. M.
Thibault, J. P.
Thomas, B.
White, G. B., Ophth, Otol
Wilson, J. C. S.

PORT CREDIT
(7,203)
Baker, A. R.
Barker, J. H.
Bell, J. W., PathBact
Boyd, K. D.
Brasch, H. A.
Brunsdon, D. F. V., Path
Campbell, D.
Cook, G. T., Urol
Copping, J. D.
Copping, Winona M.
Coulas, L. G., Ophth
Dunn, D. H.
Farkas, E. J.
Fleming, P. C.
Fooks, J. A.
Gagliano, A., Anaes
Giardine, F. P., ObstGyn
Grant, W. M.
Homonylo, M., GenSurg, Urol
Hutson, R. E., Path.
Jaffe, F. A., Path
Kolia, A.
MacKenzie, E. A.
MacLennan, D. S.
McCrae, W. H., Urol
McKillop, A. N., GenSurg
Manuel, F. R.
Morrison, A. L.
Mowat, H. F., GenSurg
Nero, R. P., ObstGyn
Nichol, W. W.
Platt, J. C.
Porter, R. H.
Prelipp, Joan B., Anaes
Prietz, H.
Reid, J. D., ObstGyn
Rennie, J. A.
Richardson, C. A., DiagRad.
Rix, E. J.
Shute, W. E.
Solow, H. R.
Steeds, J. L., ObstGyn
Todd, R. M.

PORT DOVER
(3,062)
Hynscht, R. O.
Struthers, J. D. Jr.
Struthers, J. D. Sr.
Thompson, S. F.

PORT ELGIN
(1,631)
Earl, T. J.
Fraser, J. E.
Nelles, J. V., IntMed (TB)

PORT HOPE
(8,091)
Benson, J. B.
Harrison, A. G.
Hunt, E. A.
Kelly, C. B.
Mack, B. H. R.
McDerment, R.
Robertson, J. A.
Wrathall, E. L.

PORTLAND
(250)
Harper, B. H.

PORT McNICOLL
(1,055)
Talbot, C. A.

PORT PERRY
(2,258)
Diamond, J.
Kandel, S. P.
Rennie, G. M.

PORT ROWAN
(788)
Archibald, D. A.
Reid, W. H.

PORT STANLEY
(1,461)
Bell, C. A.

POWASSAN
(1,063)
Aiyede, A. O.
Dillane, J. E.

PRESCOTT
(5,366)
Coffey, P. G., GenSurg.
Gray, F. R.
McPherson, C. F. S.
Pelton, D. A.
Peters, W. G.
Skelhorne, G. P.
Smellie. T. H.
Spicer, S. L.
Williams, W. O.

PRESTON
(11,577)
Borden, H. A.
Harding, W. G.
King, K. C., GenSurg
McCafferty, W. J.
McLagan, C.
Powers, C. G.
Taylor, A. S.
Winter, E. C.
Winter, E. H.

PRICEVILLE
(231)
Doenne, Annemarie

PRINCE ALBERT
*
Surkan, M

PRINCETON
(450)
McCaul, H. C.

RAINY RIVER
(1,168)
Bulloch, C.
Fraser, J. S. G.

RED LAKE
(2,051)
Andrew, R. F.
Gloster, M. E.
Hunt, P. K.

RED ROCK
(1,275)
Sittlinger, G.

RENFREW
(8,935)
Brown, W. A.
Burwell, G. B.
Burwell, W. B.
Guest, D. B.
Handford, E. Y.
Handford, H. L.
Mackie, A. T.
Mickevicius, V. A.
Mulvihill, L. J.

REXDALE
*
(District of Toronto)
Alladin,H. U.
Amies, C. R.
Ashley, E. P.
Ashley, H. I.
Bayens, J. H.
Blayney, R. Y.
Brail, J. N.
Chiang, J. B.
Cross, H. C., IntMed.
Davidson, W. E.
Fink, S.
Hacker, A. H.
Hodes, H.
Jones, E. E. DiagRad
Kalb, S., Psy.
Kavelman, D. A., GenSurg
Kirsh, E.
Kuolas, L. R.
Levine, H. H., GenSurg
MacLaren, D. B., GenSurg
MacTavish, J. N., Psy.
McCracken, E. C.
McIlraith, J. B.
Pelletier, G. J.
Pereszlenyi, A.
Scougall, K. H. L.
Ward, T. F., Psy
Wheler, R. .J
Wylie, W. A.

RICHARD'S LANDING
(300)
Sayles, Una J.

RICHMOND HILL
(16,446)
Abrams, M. J.
Arai, A. T., GenSurg.
Bate, J. T., ObstGyn.
Blakely, J. A., IntMed
Bloom, L. A., OrthSurg
Clemenger, A. K.
Cowan, W. C.
Farber, E. P., PlasSurg., GenSu
Fullerton, Kathleen A., Paed.
Granton, B. W.
Guthrie, D., Path.
Kerr, J. I., GenSurg
Kovacs, J. S.
Langstaff, J. R.
Levers, P. E., Urol.
McAteer, F. M.
McBurney, D. A.
McGregor, D. F.
Mogan, J. F.
Murphy, D. E., ObstGyn.
Nirenberski, J.
Philippidjis, P. J., Urol.
Nirenberski, Z.
Robson, D. B., GenSurg
Smith, A. J.
Socol, H.
Treissman, D. A., Anaes.
White, W. R.
Winemaker, J., Anaes.
Wynne, J. B.
Zuck, V.

RIDGETOWN
(2,603)
Button, J. R.
Malloy, L.
Orr, W. H.

RIDGEWAY
(1,871)
Docherty, D. F.
Green, F. A.
Legris, A. J.
Macey, H. P.
Rutherford, S. N.
Thompson, V. E.
Yewdall, Mary

RIPLEY
(469)
Tindall, J. B.

RIVERSIDE
(18,090)
Andrew, R. B., GenSurg
Bartlett, O. R., Anaes.

* Population not separately available.

Riverside (Cont'd.)
Demers, P. T., IntMed
Dodick, J.
Feore, D., DiagRad.
Ing, T. G., Ophth.
Linton, F. D.
Liu, Lillian, Paed
Scarff, M. A., Path.
Walsh, T. E.
White, B. M.
Wong, F. C-Y., Anaes

ROCKCLIFFE PARK
(2,082)
Davey, E. L., PH
Forrester, J. A.

ROCKLAND
(3,041)
Corbeil, J.
Powers, Annie

RODNEY
(1,036)
McCann, H. D.

ROSLIN
*
Hosein, A. A.

RUSSELL
(600)
Kinnaird, F. A.

RYCKMANS CORNERS
*
Roukema, J.

ST. CATHARINES
(95,577)
Aguirre-Ferro, J.
Aikens, Helen B.
Alexandroff, M.
Alvarez, G.
Anderson, C. L., Anaes
Anderson, T. W.
Armstrong, A. I., Psy.
Ball, J. C., Ophth
Ballard, J. H.
Ballyk, D. D.
Bandura, W. P., GenSurg
Bell, J. K.
Belton, J. H., ObstGyn
Black, J. D., GenSurg
Blair, E. J., OrthSurg
Blue, W. W., NeurSurg
Borsi, M. R.
Brook, J. R.
Brosnan, M. L., Otol
Brown, A. T., Anaes
Bryson, W.
Campion, G. F.
Coholan, F. G.
Connolly, B. M.
Csoka, Alice
Cumming, G. A.
Cunningham, A. I.
Cunningham, W. H.
Dalla-Vedova, G., IntMed
Dalrymple, S. J. V.
Daugavietis, H. E., IntMed
Davies, Helen, Psy
Dickson, R. R., IntMed
Dobson, J. B., Paed
Donevan, D. F., ObstGyn
Donnelly, A., Urol
Donworth, J. J., Anaes.
Drummond, J. C., OrthSurg
Dyck, H. H.
Elderkin, R. E., GenSurg
Evans, D. M. K.
Ewert, A., GenSurg
Ewert, Gertrude
Feitelsohn, Madaleine L.
Ferro, J. A.
Fraser, D. M.
Fujimagari, T., DiagRad
Gebbie, D. M.
Gillen, C. W., DiagRad
Gillen, D. H.
Gossen, C. M.
Grant, P. M., Psy
Gregor, W. M.
Grehan, J. F.
Gwassalia, Schotha
Hamilton, I. S.
Hardman, J. G., Paed
Hawthorne, K. O.
Healy, C. J. M.
Heide, A. R., GenSurg
Heitner, A.
Hill, N. P., Anaes
Hunt, D. E.
Johnston, K. M.
Johnston, R. E., Psy
Kanovsky, S., GenSurg
Keay, C. C., OrthSurg.
Karra, A. W.
Kister, E., Ophth
Krekorian, G. D.
Kunyk, M. B. J.
Lambert, H. F.
Langley, H. G.
LaPierre, A. P., Paed
Lewis, J. A. R.
Lewkowitz, I.
Lorenzen, D. I.
Lorimer, D. G.
Macdonald, W. D., GenSurg
MacGillivray, L. F., Paed
MacKenzie, C. R., ObstGyn
MacLean, C. P.
MacSween, G. B.
Maend, A.
Maguire, W. L.
Malcolmson, A. S.
Marriott, F. G., Ophth.
Mason, D. M., Path
McCormack, J. T., ObstGyn
McIlwraith, W.
McMain, P. B., Paed.
McMurtry, S. A., Ophth
McPhillips, B., D & TRad
Merritt, L. E.
Merritt, R. I., ObstGyn.
Mitchell, D. G., Ophth
Mitchell, W., DiagRad
Moodie, C. A., Path
Ord, T. W.
Orlik, E. G., IntMed
Orr, W. J., GenSurg
Peer, E. T.
Penton, R. B.
Pestri, T.
Petrowski, I.
Playfair, F. D., IntMed
Poirier, J. L.
Prokopetz, V., ObstGyn
Quinlan, H. F.
Quinn, M. H., GenSurg
Richman, N. A., GenSurg
Robinson, R. B., GenSurg
Rogers, F. J., DermSyph
Rogers, K. E., GenSurg
Sabia, M. J., GenSurg
Salton, W.
Shaver, C. G., IntMed (TB)
Sheahan, J.
Sheppard, R. D., Otol
Sheppard, R. J., Ophth, Otol
Sherk, B. E., GenSurg
Slesar, S. J., IntMed
Sollich, Wm. G.
Sparrow, G. R., ObstGyn
Stahl, O. J., GenSurg
Steele, D. C., GenSurg
Stewart, J. T.
Stitt, H. S.
Stone, A. C.
Stuebner, K. G.
Szczucinski, W.
Tammemagi, V.
Timbol, J. V.
Tipler, H. A.
Tytaneck, W. N.
Vandermass, A.
Warshawski, E., PlasSurg.
Weaver, E., Gwendolen
Wedderspoon, D. K., DiagRad
Whitaker, L., PathBact
Whyte, W. R.
Williams, A. D., GenSurg
Willinsky, J., DiagRad; Urol
Wilson, J. A.
Witt, H. A.
Wood, J. N., ObstGyn
Wright, J. A.
Younghusband, O. Z. IntMed
Zaritsky, M.
Zeldin, A. J., Otol
Zenner, L.
Zuritsky, M.

ST. DAVID'S
(480)
Lowrey, A. V.

ST. GEORGE
(569)
Pickett, C. H.
Weldhen, J. W.

ST. JACOB'S
(669)
Kulis, Dorothy F., Psy.
Young, D. F.

ST. MARY'S
(4,487)
Davis, W. J.
Hackney, J. C.
Hiscock, R. J.
Humphrys, M. H.
Latimer, R. H.
McInnis, T. J.
Munro, D. C.
Scott, F. G. E.

ST. THOMAS
(22,469)
Adilman, B., Path
Babiak, W., Psy
Balsdon, L. A.
Bandeen, J. Catherine, ObstGyn
Berry, A. G.
Bice, W. K.
Bloomer, E.
Bristow, R. J., GenSurg
Brown, E. L.
Burger, E. G.
Clark, K. L., IntMed
Cleland, C. A., Psy
Curtis, J. F.
Deinum, E. Jeanne, Psy
Dolan, J., Psy.
Duncanson, D. A.
Elliott, L.
Farley, R. O., GenSurg
Floyd, R. J.
Gliddon, E. C., GenSurg
Graham, C. A.
Hagerman, E. S., IntMed
Harris, B. P.
Henderson, Smilja, Psy
Kaufman, J. J., Psy
Kierluk, E. W., GenSurg
King, W. E., Psy
Livermore, M. L., Psy
Livingstone, F.
MacKenzie, C. R.
Mann, W. H., Ophth, Otol
McCallum, A. B.
McGregor, K. M., Psy
McLachlin, J. A., GenSurg
McManus, J. J.
Peart, J. A. Anaes
Porter, J. G. M., GenSurg
Post, A. R., GenSurg
Ryckman, M. B.
Scott, G. M.
Taylor, W. B., D & TRad
Webster, Mary F.
Webster, W. G.

SARNIA
(61,293)
Abraham, A. J., PlasSurg, Orth Surg

* Population not separately available.

Sarnia (Cont'd.)

Anderson, G. L. S., PH
Annear, W. C., GenSurg
Bennett, M. F., D & TRad
Biehn, J. T., Ophth, Otol
Biehn, J. T.
Bojko, M.
Borrowman, A. M., ObstGyn
Bradley, B. M., Ophth
Brajac, J.
Brown, H. M.
Bruce, J. D. C.
Butler, H. R.
Carruthers, Grace
Carruthers, W. B., IntMed
Clift, A. M.
Cook, B. W., Urol.
Coulter, J. G., DiagRad
Cross, D. F., Paed
Curtin, J. J., Psy
Dean, J. F.
di Profio, C. F., Path
Dobrowolski, K.
Duncan, D. GenSurg.
Duncan, Lucy
Dunseath, B.
Ferguson, H., ObstGyn
Ferreira, B. E., ObstGyn.
Gamula, S.
Gibson, G. P., Psy.
Gibson, J. H., GenSurg
Gladdy, P. V., ObstGyn
Gray, W. A., GenSurg
Harris, G. E., GenSurg
Hay, M. D.
Herdman, J. P., GenSurg
Hill, M.
Hill, M. G., IntMed
Hodgins, T. E., GenSurg
Hogg, W. A.
Hollands, W. W., PathBact
Hollinger, D. M., ObstGyn
Houston, A. C., IntMed
Johnston, T. C., Urol.
Jost, H. M., Urol
Keith, D.
Kennedy, D. W., Paed
Kinch, K. E., IntMed
Kindrachuk, W.
Kingsley, D. J., ObstGyn
Kohlmeier, A. C., ObstGyn
Lomax, W. W., ObstGyn
Lynch, J., DiagRad
MacEachern, D. A. G., GenSurg
MacIntyre, I. D., ObstGyn
Mackenzie, J. R.
MacKinlay, A. K.
MacKinlay, R., GenSurg
MacKinlay, R. D.
Mahony, J. B. O.
Mann, I. W., Anaes
Massig, E., Path
McCutcheon, C. W. V., GenSurg
McDowell, M. F., IntMed
McGarrity, P. B., GenSurg
Miles, F. T., D & TRad
Mosser, H. A., Path
Mulyk, I.
Murphy, J. P., IntMed.
Muskovitch, Z. F.
McLeod, Janey, Derm
O'Mahoney, J. B.
Panton, Frances
Panwar, K. M., Anaes
Partingdon, C. N., Path
Perchanok, M. R., IntMed
Perl, A. F., IntMed
Pritchard, R. W.
Richardson, C. D.
Roberts, J. F., GenSurg
Robinson, Margaret
Rounthwaite, H. L., GenSurg.
Rutherford, Isobel, Path
Rutherford, W. B., D & TRad
Scarrow, G. R., DiagRad
Schultz, A. G.
Shortreed, R. D., Otol
Sidenburg, R. E.
Sidenburg, S. H.
Sinclair, J. D., D & TRad
Sinkins, J. M., ObstGyn
Sorensen, C., Paed
Stone, B.
Tasker, P. H.
Thorp, M. D.
Tomka, B. E.
Tufford, W. H., Psy
Van Hoogenhuize, W. H.
Wallis, H. B.
Warren, D. R.
Waugh, E. H., GenSurg
Wong, W. A., IntMed
Wurm, K., Derm

SAULT STE. MARIE (43,088)

Aleixandre, L. E.
Algie, G. H. DiagRad
Armstrong, J. K. GenSurg
Baar, F. GenSurg
Bell, M. E., Adeline
Black, T. H.
Brereton, W. J.
Breton, T. A.
Casselman, B. W.
Cole, Anne Paed
Cowan, D. K.
Eaid, C. R. M.
Elgie, R. W.
Ferrier, T. A.
Fleming, D. M.
Fogg, N. W.
Friedman, L.
Fyfe, P. R., OrthSurg.
Gibson, J. W. IntMed
Golesic, S., Ophth.
Gould, D. H., IntMed.
Govoni, A. F., DiagRad
Greco, E. J. M.
Greig, C. H., GenSurg., OrthSurg., Urol.
Hackett, A. A.
Hall, J.
Hamilton, R. W., GenSurg.
Hutchinson, W. E. GenSurg
Hutton, W. F., ObstGyn
Kelly, M. J., ObstGyn
Kelly, W. J. GenSurg
Knirsch, A. K.
Kovac, A. J.
Kovac, Eleonora I., Paed.
Kowaliscin, P., Urol.
Lalonde, A. J. G. H., GenSurg
Lalouette, J., ObstGyn.
Leahy, W. H.
Luus, G. J.
MacArthur, F. C.
MacIntosh, J. F. Anaes
Marinker, S., GenSurg
Marcolin, L.
Martin, R. G., ObstGyn.
Mengebier, R. A.
Miller, N. E. ObstGyn
Minc, P. H.
Mosser, H. A.
Newbigging, D. K. Otol
O'Neill, J. P., Otol.
Prag, J. J.
Robertson, W. J. Paed
Rundle, L. G. IntMed
Sagle, L. A.
Schwartzkopff, O. M.
Schwarzl, J. L., Psy
Sevensma, J.
Shamess, S. H. Ophth
Shaver, C. H.
Sinclair, A. B. GenSurg
Sparks, F. P. Path, Bact
Sprague, J. D.
Spratt, E. H.
Sullivan, W. E.
Symington, J. B.
Tiltins, M.
Watson, W. R.
West, M. H. IntMed
Williams, J., DiagRad; Urol
Willinsky, J. M., Urol, DiagRad
Woods, W. A. OrthSurg
Yue, J. K.
Zaharuk, W. V.

SCARBOROUGH TOWNSHIP
(139,083)

Abbott, E. V.
Adderley, F. G.
Aitken, D. A.
Allison, J. C.
Appleby, J., Psy.
Arshawsky, Pearl R.
Azzopardi, P., Paed
Bahmann, H. J.
Balkissoon, M.
Bendeth, B. S.
Bentham, W. H., Anaes
Beverstein, J.
Blatchford, Ellen, Anaes
Breuls, A. M.
Brisby, J. M.
Brodie, R. B.
Bull, J. A.
Burak, M. A.
Bush, A. J., ObstGyn.
Cameron, C. G., IntMed
Campbell, J. D.
Carlsen, L. N., PlasSurg
Charlebois, P. A.
Chrom, Vivian
Cosens, C. G., GenSurg
Cranston, G. P.
Cromby, J. W.
Cserepka, Margaret I.
Das, Esmaralda
Deck, J. H.
Dickinson, O. B., GenSurg
Diniz, A. T.
Dobson, R. A., GenSurg
Donsky, H. J.
DuBoulay, M. R.
Durnin, R. A.
Edson, I.
Ehrlich, B.
Elder, A. M., DiagRad
Elder, L. J.
Enright, T. J., Psy
Farquharson, C. D. PH; IntMed
Fejer, I. F.
Fekete, Z. C., Derm
Fischell, Eve
Fox, J. E., Anaes
Fox, T. W., IntMed
Freedman, R. E., DiagRad
Futerman, B. R.
Gardiner, W. A.
Garvock, W. B.
Gerlach, H. J., Otol
Gerstein, M. C., Paed
Giblon, B. I.
Greenberg, H. J.
Guest, R. G.
Haber, H. N.
Halkiewicz, T. J., Anaes
Hardy, B. C., GenSurg.
Hargrave, R., Anaes
Hartley, B. M.
Harvey, J. H., Derm
Haw, B. G.
Helston, R. H.
Herriot, R. A.
Hofstader, E. L., IntMed
Hofstader, Sophie
Horn, G. M., Anaes
Horne, S., DiagRad.
Horning, C. M.
Hunter, D. D., Anaes.
Hutchins, E. K.
Isaac, G. H.
Jan, R.
Jansen, J. H., Otol
Jay, H.
Johnston, B.

* Population not separately available.

Scarborough Township (Cont'd.)
Kaminker, A., IntMed
Kapsos, J .E., ObstGyn
Kassay, G. I.
Kawa, M. Z., Otol
Keijzer, J. J.
Kelly, F. O., Urol
Kilty, H. C.
King, E. P.
Kramloc, N.
Kucharska, Wanda M.
Kucharski, J. W.
Kyle, Joan
Laforest, R. A., Paed
Laughton, J. S., GenSurg
Lee, R. B.
Lindsay, W. R., PlasSurg
Lipcsei, J.
Loney, E. M.
Loren, P.
Low, G. A., IntMed
Lukss, L.
MacKay, R. J., Path
MacMillan, J. C.
Magder, J. H.
Magee, D. E.
Marsh, J. K.
Masson, E. L.
Mathieson, D. I., Anaes
Matzko, P.
Mayer, G. P.
Mayer, J. M. GenSurg
Maynes, E. A.
McBrien, G. E.
McGarry, P., ObstGyn
McMillen, G. R.
Millar, O. .B, DiagRad
Moffatt, A. J.
Morris, W. G.
Morrow, A. M.
Munkley, F. H., ObstGyn
Murphy, W. J.
Murray, E. J.
Ower, R. C., PlasSurg
Parrot, R.
Pitt, P. L.
Pollock, F. H.
Powell, Marion G.
Pozner, S. N., ObstGyn
Prowse, G. G.
Prucha, Z.
Ralph-Edwards, E. S., GenSurg
Redman, J. A.
Richards, W. H. A.
Roach, K. E., IntMed
Roos, J. O.
Rowley, J. C.
Rowley, S. C.
Ryan, E. A., GenSurg
Sahay, U.
Salmon, J. D., GenSurg
Sedhev, H. S.
Shepley, D. J.
Sher, N., Paed
Shier, D. J.
Silfrer, A.
Silveira, C. J.
Singer, E. B.
Sipos, L.
Skorbinski, A. W., GenSurg
Smith, I. J.
Spudas, A.
Stein, H. A., Ophth
Stobie, S. N. P., Psy
Suleiman, L. W.
Sweeney, B., OrthSurg.
Thomas, F. A.
Thompson, M. C., Anaes
Todd, I. A., GenSurg, **Urol**
Toguri, E.
Truscott, P. W.
Uren, D. M.
Walsh, F. D.
Walther, E.
Watson, E. E.
Wernick, H. B.
Winnitoy, N. W., **ObstGyn**

Wiseman, J.
Witterick, G. H.
Wolfish, M. G., Paed
Yielding, T. E.
Zelitt, I. J.
Zucker, B. B., Ophth

SCHOMBERG
(500)
Jones, H. T.

SCHREIBER
(2,050)
Searles, G. K.

SCHUMACHER
(3017)
Templeton, D. W.

SCOTLAND
(444)
Shaver, J. E.

SEAFORTH
(2,262)
Brady, P. L.
Flewelling, W. H.
Gorwill, J. A.
Malkus, E.
Mann, C. H.
Stapleton, M. W.

SEBRINGVILLE
(710)
Sinclair, A.

SEELEY'S BAY
(285)
Webb, S.

SHEDDEN
(209)
Monteith, D. A.

SHELBURNE
(1,245)
Johnston, E. G.
Smith, H. H.
Southern, R. F.

SIMCOE
(8,754)
Forster, D. S.
Hare, R. B. GenSurg
Harker, J. R.
Jackson, A. B.
Jenkins, J. C.
Johnston, J. G.
Kursell, P. O.
Loudon, I. T.
Marshall, G. M.
McGavin, K. R.
McGuire, W. B.
McIntosh, J. D.
McIntosh, K. M.
Mull, J. D., Path
Parker, R. G. GenSurg
Peters, J. A., GenSurg
Shepherd, E. D.
Sihler, J. C. T.
Washburn, H. H.

SIOUX LOOKOUT
(2,452)
Allen, H. W.
Bernstein, A. D.
Dowd, J. A.
Kirkbride, J.
Krasins, Berta
Mallick, S.
Millar, J.
Simard, Camille
Van Volkingburgh, D. R.
Wesley-James, O., GenSurg

SMITH'S FALLS
(9,603)
Ashwell, T. O.
Barkauskas, A.
Brennan, M.
Erlich, B.
Fergusson, Roslyn M.
Frank, H., NeurPsy.
Hamilton, H. G. GenSurg
Hewitt, W. J.

Hogan, J. J. Anaes
Kerr, A. L.
Lloyd, H. H.
McCarley, J. S.
McGuire, J. J.
Murphy, A. B.
Murphy, W. O. GenSurg
Pasley, F.
Prytulak, W.
Schutt, C. Psy
Smith, M. S.
Stewart, F., GenSurg
Walker, R. J.

SMITHVILLE
(865)
Bond, A. W.
Uzicanin, R.

SMOOTH ROCK FALLS
(1,131)
Hurtubise, F. A.
Jobin, A.
Mizbah, G., GenSurg

SOUTHAMPTON
(1,818)
Flock, M. A.
MacDonald-Lawson, Jean, ObstGyn.
Mercer, D. D.

SOUTH PORCUPINE
(5,144)
Anderson, E. S.
Baines, Heather
Johnston, D.
Robinson, J. D.

SOUTH RIVER
(1,041)
Dawson, L. E.
Laing, R. R.

STAYNER
(1,673)
Ives, R. E.
Ives, W. G.

STEVENSVILLE
(640)
Twidle, R. S.
Vincent, A. A.

STIRLING
(1,315)
Briggs, P. D.

STITSVILLE
(1503)
Igel, W.
Watkinson, E. A.

STONEY CREEK
(6,043)
Burgess, Beverley A.
Chagnon, E. C.
Fulthorpe, G. H.
Gasewicz, S.
Green, L. S., D & T Rad.
Heddle, M. S.
Janack, E. S.
Kemp, C. R.
Laurimaa, I.
Mellow, R. C.
Pase, P. R. P.
Reid, J. C.
Robinson, F. T.
Smith, R. B.
Tandan, P. Janet
Zamora, S. P.

STOUFFVILLE
(3,189)
Brodie, D. W.
Button, F. J.
Freel, H. B.
Graham, G. A.
Mitchell, R. B.
Petrie, D. J.
Smith, D. H.

* Population not separately available.

STRATFORD
(20,467)
Aldis, R. M.
Allan, D. J. ObstGyn
Allan, Margaret D.
Bissonnette, R. N.
Campbell, B. A. GenSurg
Duffin, D., DiagRad
Fitzgerald, D. P.
Fitzpatrick, D. P.
Forster, F. J. R. Ophth,Otol
Gemmell, D.
Gilmore, W. M. D & TRad
Harris, Mabel J., Anaes.
Hazell, H. C.
Ingham, G. H. Ophth,Otol
Jarrott, G. C. ObstGyn
Kenner, H. B. GenSurg
Lindsay, I. GenSurg
McCaul, Evelyn K.
McDermott, J. G. GenSurg
McKenzie, A. W.
McWilliam, R. S.
Moore, J. B.
Overbeeke, C. J.
Penistan, J. L. Path
Pyper, J. E. Ophth
Quinlan, V. P., IntMed
Roberts, P. C.
Rowe, A. R. Otol
Schuh, Elfriede
Schuh, O. W. Anaes
Schulthies, L. G.
Scratch, N. W. F. IntMed
Sproat, W. C. GenSurg
Sylvester, C. E.
Thompson, H. H.
Waite, R.
Wilson, A. M.

STRATHROY
(5,150)
Butler, W. E.
Crowley, P. C. GenSurg
Fletcher, M. D.
Hauffe, H. W.
Marshall, Ann
McFadden, G. F.
Newton, O. R.
Sharpe, M. D.
Vine, G. D.

STREETSVILLE
(5,056)
Dodds, J. K.
MacDonald, K. G.
McIsaac, E. R.
Montemurro, G. A.
Olson, G. P.
Stuart, C. K. IntMed

STURGEON FALLS
(6,288)
Cholette, J. R.
Larocque, J. G.
Marengere, O. G.
Orr, K. F.
Tabib, N. GenSurg
Young, P. M.

SUDBURY
(110,694)
Andrews, P., Otol
Bonin, R., Path.
Bowers, J. D.
Bromley, K. J., Anaes
Bruce-Lockhard, P. ObstGyn
Buschlen, W. J.
Butto, A. S.
Cameron, J. D. Anaes
Cawthorpe, Harriet, A., Anaes
Cazabon, A. A.
Cecutti, A. G.
Comptois, J. B. Anaes
Cook, F. A.
Cook, J. B. PH
Crang, C. L. DiagRad
Crang, D. F., DiagRad
Crawford, Elsie M. H.
Cullen, P. J., DiagRad
D'Aloisio, J. F., Urol.
Desbrisay, W. M.
de-la-Rive, R.
Desmarais, G. Gyn
Desmarais, J. N. D & TRad
Dixon, F. O. Paed
Dixon, T. P. Psy
Doherty, C. J.
Ducharme, G. P. ObstGyn
Dunn, R. E.
Edington, R. F., ObstGyn.
Evans, C. C. ObstGyn
Farrell, P. J. ObstGyn
Field, P., GenSurg., Cardiovasc. & ThorSurg.
Foerster, A. R.
Fostiak, M.
Fyfe, J. W. Anaes
Ghent, R. D.
Giffen, A. B., ObstGyn
Greco, F. L.
Haddad, J. W.
Haddad, N. N.
Harrop, J., Path(P.Q.)
Helie, G. GenSurg
Hellat, A.
Henderson, J. W., IntMed
Hennessy, J. P. Paed
Hippolyte, R. GenSurg
Ho, E. C.
Hooey, L.
Jones, G. R.. GenSurg
Kelly, M. J., Anaes
Kirk, J. L.
Kosar, S. J.
Kusnierczwk, R. G.
Kyle, P. R., ObstGyn
Lafond, J. Y.
Lapchinski, E. S.
Lawler, W. R. GenSurg
Lee, A. J.
Levesque, F. H., GenSurg
Longmore, R. D.
MacLeod, E. C., Psy
Mador, M. L. Urol
Maloney, J. A., ObstGyn
Marechaux, E. W.
Marechaux, Susanne
McCullough, D. W. Ophth
McCullough, J. F. GenSurg
McCuskey, K. A., OrthSurg
McDonald, J. O. GenSurg
McInnes, J. D.
McKay, B. J.
Michaels, L., Path
Michaud, J. R. GenSurg
Mitchell, R. M. GenSurg
Moga, T. J.
Morgan, R. E.
Myatt, D. G. GenSurg
Mysak, J.
Newell, Edith C.
Noel-de-Tilley, B.
Orange, R. Anaes
Pancaro, L., GenSurg
Parraga, R.
Pearsall, H. E. Otol
Piasecki, A. J.
Pidutti, J. A.
Pogonowski, S.
Polack, S. S. Gyn. GenSurg
Poole, R. W. GenSurg
Power, F. L. GenSurg
Prevost, M. J., GenSurg
Prince, D. A.
Rinne, H. H. Derm
St. Denis, R. A.
Scott, Flora, Psy
Scott, J. G.
Seddall, H. R.
Shaw, R. S. Paed
Skinner, J. H.
Stalker, M. J., IntMed
Stanyon, J. H. IntMed
Steele, J. P.
Stewart, L. N. D & TRad
Sturtridge, J. D., IntMed
Surphlis, W., Psy.
Tanguay, H., Urol.
Tenhunen, T.
Trobridge, G. F.
Turgeon, A., IntMed
Thomson, R. M.
Vaillancourt, J. R.
Valiaho, A. J., DiagRad
Waldmann, Klara
Waldmann, S., IntMed.
Walker, G. R. GenSurg, ThorSu[r]
Wallrap, A. A.
Ward, K. A. GenSurg
Wardill, J. C.
Washburn, R. E.
White, C., OrthSurg
White, W. J.
Williams, K. J.
Wilson, B. M. GenSurg
Wiss, R., Ophth
Woods, B. J.
Yankowsky, M. O.
Young, M. Isabel
Zurowska, M. Christina

SUNDERLAND
(565)
Woodman, J. C.

SUNDRIDGE
(760)
Copeman, W. J.
Davis, F. G.

SUTTON WEST
(1,466)
Burrows, G. M.
Douglas, Mary
Knupp, G. C.
Noble, C. S.
Stevens, N. E.

SYDENHAM
(550)
Davis, G. W.
Rybak, S. E.

TAVISTOCK
(1,233)
Fisher, J. K.
Fuller, D. B.
Gibson, E. S.
Halliday. B.
Taylor, H. M.
Varga, E. A.
Weston, W. W.

TECUMSEH
(4,475)
Hemond, C. J.
McCabe, P. C.
Medine, S. M., ObstGyn
Potter, S. W.
Quenneville, P.

TEESWATER
(919)
Leahy, P. J.

TERRACE BAY
(1,901)
McCausland, D. J. M.
Uzicanin, R. R.

TERRA COTTA
*****
Jaquith, L. E.

THAMESFORD
(1,107)
Kosmal, R. J.
Powers, O. C.

THAMESVILLE
(1,060)
Lamont, C. T.
Sales, J. L., GenSurg, Urol
Soper, G. M.

THEDFORD
(751)
MacDonald, M. M.

* Population not separately available.

THESSALON
(1,731)
Beacock, P. R.
Fisher, W. F.

THISTLETOWN
(1,496)
Alderton, H. R. Psy
Atcheson, J. D., Psy.
Braham, J. K., Psy
Broder, Elsa A., Psy
Rich, E. J.
Shaw, W. H., Paed
Steinhauer, P. D.
Storey, D. W.

THORNBURY
(1,097)
Cargill, L. G.
Titcombe, E. P.

THORNDALE
(290)
Green, C. R.

THORNHILL
(1,135)
Belch, L. A., ObstGyn
Blakely, J. A., IntMed.
Ede, W. O.
Ferguson, J. K. W.
Glassey, D. W.
Fotheringham, J. B., Psy
Glassow, F. S. GenSurg
Lovett-Doust, J. W., Psy.
Morse, P. G.
Norheim, N. G.
Obney, N.
Pamenter, E. J.
Robson, D. B. GenSurg
Wesley, W. R.

THOROLD
(8,633)
Anderson, A. M.
Caira, E. G., GenSurg.
Conley, A. E.
Debenham, G., GenSurg
Fraser, J. J., ObstGyn
Longo, T. N.
Malcolmson, S. A.
McMillan, D. A.
McMillan, W. H.
Myers, D. S.
Orr, R. K.
Ralph, G. L.
Rose, R. C.

TILBURY
(3,029)
Macpherson, D. M.
Richardson, J. F.
Ruby, R. A.

TILLSONBURG
(6,600)
Alexander, H. J.
Dalby, R. W.
Ferrie, A. S.
Hevenor, D. W.
Lee, C. C.
McDermid, J. M.
McLeod, N. D.
Ort, R.R., GenSurg
Quintyn, E. A. GenSurg
Rankin, R. W.
Richards, C. A.
Szorenyi, M. R.

TIMMINS
(40,121)
Barry, J. E. GenSurg, ObstGyn
Bergeron, J. A.
Cooper, A. J.
Day, E. A. F.
Dobson, E. A. GenSurg
Dymond, R. F.
Estrella, F. I. GenSurg
Francis, M. A.
Giardine, J. R.
Hamerski, H. W.
Harrigan, E. R. D & TRad
Hope, J. D.
Jessel, S. J.
Kreiner, H. O.
Lane, G. B. IntMed (T.B.)
Lewis, J. E. Ophth
Little, R. M.
MacKechnie, G. S. GenSurg
McClinton, J. B. GenSurg
O'Shaughnessy, B. D.
Revelle, I. E.
Shaw, R. E.
Smolarczyk, F.
Sullivan, J. B., GenSurg
Tatartcheff, M.
Taylor, R. B.
Taylor, W. IntMed (T.B.)

TODMORDEN
*
Pugsley, H. E. IntMed

TORONTO
(2,066,000)
(See Don Mills, Etobicoke, Islington, Long Branch, Malton, Mimico, New Toronto, Rexdale, Scarborough, Willowdale, Weston)
Abbott, Caroline M.
Abbott, D.
Abbott, M. M. Int Med
Abbott, S. F.
Abraham, J. A.
Abramson, H., IntMed
Acker, M. S., PH.
Adderley, F. G.
Adler, O. J.
Adler, W.
Adlof, Inges
Agbebiyi, A. B.
Agnew, H. G.
Aguzzi, G.
Aikenhead, J. Wm.
Ainslie, J. D., GenSurg, Urol
Aitchison, Wm. S., PH
Aitken, J. A.
Akriotis, D. J.
Alaton, A.
Alaton, I., Ophth
Albelda, J. L., ObstGyn.
Albertson, M. E. Ophth
Aldis, J. S. W
Aldridge, H. E., IntMed
Alexander, H. D. GenSurg, ObstGyn
Alison, Ruth E. IntMed
Alladin, H. U.
Allan, B. E. M. Neur Psy
Allemang, W. H. ObstGyn
Allen, M. S. GenSurg
Allin, J. D. ObstGyn
Allison, J. C.
Allman, R. G. G. IntMed
Allodi, F. A., Psy.
Allt, W. E. TherRad
Alt, K.
Alter, C. IntMed
Alter-Kowalewski, J. E.
Alyanak, N. O.
Amann, E. W.
Amies, C. R.
Amoruso, F. F. GenSurg
Anchelson, A. A.
Anderson, A. J. GenSurg
Anderson, D. N. Psy
Anderson, H. M., Psy.
Anderson, J. R.
Anderson, J. S.
Anderson, R. M.
Anderson, T. W.
Anderson, W., Path
Andrachuk, J. J.
Angel, N.
Angelopoulos, T. M.
Anglin, A. F. W., IntMed
Anglin, C. S., Paed
Angus, R. J.
Anthony, L.
Appell, A. A., GenSurg
Appleby, J., Psy
Appleton, S. S., Psy
Appleyard, H. E., IntMed
Apted, Wm. E., ObstGyn
Archibald, A. M.
Archibald, G. W.
Argue, F. J.
Armour, W. E.
Armstrong, J. B., IntMed
Armstrong, J. D., Psy
Armstrong, R. D., DiagRad
Arnold, R. A.
Arnott, J. H., IntMed.
Arstikaitis, Maria J., Ophth
Arthurs, J.
Arthurs, R. G. S., Psy
Ash, C. L., D & TRad
Ashenhurst, A. E.
Ashley, Evelyn
Ashworth, M. A.
Atack, Mary H. G.
Atcheson, J. D., Psy
Atin, H. L., IntMed
Atkins, J. L., Otol
Auger, W. J.
Awad, S. A., Urol.
Awais, J. (G.), ObstGyn.
Awerbuck, B. G., DiagRad
Axelrod, A. A.
Axelrod, H. I., Anaes
Axmith, D.
Ayer, Isabel, ObstGyn
Azzopardi, P., Paed.
Babb, I. L., GenSurg
Babyn, R., OrthSurg
Bacon, T. N.
Baggs, C. R., Urol
Baglieri, J. A., ObstGyn
Baida, M., GenSurg
Bailey, J. D., Paed
Bailey, M.
Bailey, P., Anaes
Baillie, J. H., P.H.
Baillie, W. H.
Bain, H. W., Paed.
Baird, R. J., GenSurg
Cardiovasc & Thorsurg
Baitz, T., IntMed.
Bak, Z., Anaes
Baker, A. A., Otol
Baker, C. B., GenSurg, ThorSurg. (Cardiovasc.)
Baker, E. F. W., Psy
Baker, G .A., Psy
Baker, H. E.
Baker, S. E.
Balfour, G. R., Anaes
Balis, G. U., Psy
Balkany, M., ObstGyn
Ball, H. D.
Ball, R. B.
Ball, W. M.
Balmer, H. C., Anaes.
Balshin, B., Path
Banting, Henrietta, ObstGyn
Barber, H. O., Otol
Barclay, J. A., GenSurg.
Bardawill, C. J.
Bardins, P.
Barker, E. T., Psy
Barkin, M., Urol.
Barnes, L. S., Ophth, Otol
Barnes, W. B.
Barnett, H. J. M., Neur
Barr, A. S.
Barr, D. A.
Barr, Elizabeth B.
Barrett, Ann
Barrie, H. J., Path.
Barrington, T.W., OrthSurg
Barron, R. O.
Bartlett, G. S., GenSurg
Bartha, J.

* Population not separately available.

Toronto (Cont'd.)
Baryluk, V.
Basian, H., GenSurg
Bassett, A. A., GenSurg
Basta, D.
Bastedo, G. M., GenSurg
Bastow, D. C., Anaes
Basu, P. K.
Bateman, Evelyn, Anaes
Bateman, J. E., OrthSurg
Bateman, W. E., ObstGyn
Bateman, W. R.
Bates, G.
Bates, K.
Bates, R. W., IntMed.
Baumal, A., Derm
Bauman, L., DiagRad
Baxter, K. R.
Bayley, T. A., IntMed
Beale, F. A., TherRad
Beale, Lillias
Bean, J. L., ObstGyn
Beanlands, D. S., IntMed
Beaudry, R., IntMed.
Beauregard, W. L., GenSurg
Beazley, G. P.
Beck, H. O.
Beckett, T. R., Anaes.
Bedard, G.
Beesley, Mary, Psy
Beirne, P. F., ObstGyn
Belch, L. A., ObstGyn
Belcourt, R. J., Bact
Bell, A. G.
Bell, D. E.
Bell, H. M., OrthSurg
Bell, J. S., PH
Bell, R. D., Otol
Bell, T. J.
Bell, W. P.
Bellman, A. M.
Ben, J. H.
Bennett, I. M. F.
Bennett, K. T. F.
Bennett, W. D.
Bensley, Sylvia H.
Benson, C. K., GenSurg
Bentzon, Johanne W., Paed
Berg, M. D.
Berger, D. M., Psy.
Bergsagel, D. E.
Berlin, S.
Berman, B., Urol
Berner, G.
Berner, M., Barbara
Bernstein, A., ObstGyn
Berris, B., IntMed
Berry, B. H.
Berry, H., Neurol., IntMed.
Best, C. H., DSc
Bhalla, S. K., GenSurg.
Bhavakula, K., Anaes.
Bianco, M., Anaes
Bigelow, W. G., GenSurg
Billings, R. F., Psy.
Bilski, S. T.
Bingham, J. R., IntMed
Birch, J. R., PlasSurg.
Birchwood, Barbara
Bird, B. L., DiagRad
Bird, G. S., DiagRad
Bird, Josephine N., IntMed
Birnbaum, F. M.
Biro, G.
Birrell, R. G.
Bissylas, S. J., D & TRad
Black, D., Ophth
Black, L. W., GenSurg, OrthSur
Bladek, R., IntMed
Blair, J. H., Anaes
Blake, J. D.
Blanchard, R.
Blanchet, G. L.
Blatchford, Ellen H., Anaes
Blau, A., IntMed
Blazic, C., Psy
Blejer, H.
Blevis, L. S., Path
Blois, G. M.
Bloom, H. W., IntMed
Bloomfield, R. C., Otol
Blumenstein, J.
Blye, R. A.
Bobechko, W. P., OrthSurg
Bochner, M. K., Ophth
Boddington, G. D. M., Anaes
Bodrug, A.
Bohnen, D. R., GenSurg
Bond, I. K., Psy
Bond, S. C.
Bonkalo, A. Psy
Bonner, K. P., DiagRad
Boone, J. E., Paed
Booth, L., Isabel, Paed
Booth, Patricia M.
Boothroyd, W. E., Psy
Borins, Elaine F.
Borland, N. Joan
Borowy, Z. J., GenSurg
Borrajo, C. P., Paed.
Borron, R. W. J., DiagRad
Borsch, R. N., Psy.
Borsook, Dorothy H., ObstGyn
Bowen, H. M., Ophth, Otol
Bower, D.
Box, T. R., IntMed.
Boyd, A. R. J., PH
Boyd, E. A.
Boyd, J. A., DiagRad.
Boyd, W. K.
Boyden, R. W.
Boyes, H. W., Anaes
Boyle, E. J., GenSurg
Bradford, N. W.
Brady, F. A.
Braiden, R. S.
Brander, J. W. E., GenSurg
Bratina, Gloria
Braudo, M., Paed
Breithaupt, D. J., IntMed
Bremner, W. V., Neur Psy
Brennan, J. H. L., IntMed (TB)
Brennan, J. W., GenSurg
Brent, H. P., Ophth
Brereton, O. H.
Brereton, F. W.
Breslin, R. H.
Brettler, A., Urol
Briant, T. D., Otol
Brickenden, A. W.
Briggs, Alice, IntMed
Briggs, J. A., DiagRad
Brink, G. C., IntMed (TB)
Britt, Beverley, Anaes.
Broder, I., IntMed
Brodey, A.
Brodey, J. B., Psy
Brodie, Elizabeth, Psy
Bromley, A. J.
Brooks, A. J., DiagRad
Brooks, E. F., IntMed, Neur
Brooks, H. C.
Brooks, J. S.
Brossard, B. L.
Brown, C. B., IntMed
Brown, C. C.
Brown, E. W., Psy
Brown, J. R.
Brown, K. A., GenSurg
Brown, K. W., IntMed
Brown, M. H., PH, Bact
Brown, P. B.
Brown, T. C., Path
Brown, W. A., GenSurg, PlasSur
Brown, W. G., PH
Browne, A. F.
Brownlee, J. G.
Bruce-Robertson, A.
Bruce, W. R.
Bruckovsky, N. N.
Brummitt, W. M., Anaes
Brunton, J. E.
Bryan, C. G., Anaes
Bryant, E. C., ObstGyn
Bryant, M. E., ObstGyn
Bryce, D. P., Otol
Brzezina-Shkimba, Jeanie
Buck, C. A., Psy
Buckridan, L.
Buda, V.
Buick, R. J., DiagRad
Bull, R. C., GenSurg.
Bullock, B. J.
Bulmer, F. M. R.
Bulmer, H. R., PH
Bunker, M. L., ObstGyn
Bunt, D. G.
Burgess, G. H.
Burgess, R. M., Psy
Burke, C. L.
Burke, D. T., DiagRad.
Burnett, H. A., IntMed
Burnfield, C.R.
Burnie, Ruth M.
Burns, J. L., Ophth
Burton, Blanche E.
Burton, C. R., IntMed
Burton, Dorothy
Burwell, R. B., IntMed.
Butcher, J. J.
Butler, K. R., IntMed
Butler, P. O., Psy
Butler, V. J., Psy.
Butt, W. Anaes
Butt, W. D., PlasSurg
Butt, W. P., DiagRad
Byrnes, M. C., Psy.
Cahoon, E. B., Psy
Cain, M. C.
Calarco, J. A., Anaes
Caldwell, D. Y., Anaes
Callahan, G. A.
Callahan, W. P., Ophth
Cameron, D. S.
Cameron, H. C., Paed
Cameron, W. R.
Camil, V.
Campbell, B. A.
Campbell, D. B.
Campbell, E. B., GenSurg
Campbell, G. E.
Campbell, H. H., PlasSurg
Campbell, J. M., Anaes
Campbell, S. M., Anaes
Campbell, W. D., Anaes
Canavan, B.
Cannell, D. E., ObstGyn
Cantelon, J. F., IntMed
Caplan, J., Psy
Caplin, Doreen F., Anaes
Capon, A. W., IntMed
Cappe, S.
Cappon, D., Psy
Card, L. C.
Cardarelli, G.
Cardish, A. A.
Carlen, S. A., IntMed
Carleton, G. W.
Carlsen, L. N., PlasSurg.
Carpenter, L. E., Psy
Carrie, A. W., GenSurg
Carrow, G. W., GenSurg
Carruthers, J., Path
Carscadden, W. G., GenSurg
Carson, J. D.
Carson, M. M.
Carson, P. S.
Carter, G. W.
Carveth, R. W.
Casella, L., IntMed.
Cass, Elie
Cass, I. M., Path
Cassidy, F. R., IntMed
Caswell, C. B.
Caudwell, G. G., GenSurg
Caven, W. R., IntMed
Cawson, Helen A.

* Population not separately available.

Toronto (Cont'd.)
Cernavskis, Velta J.
Chaikof L., GenSurg
Chaikoff, J. S., Anaes
Chaikoff, R. H., IntMed
Challis, E. B.
Chambers, G. B., ObstGyn
Chambers, G. L.
Chambers, H. R.
Chambers, Margaret C., Anaes
Chan, P. L.
Chan, S-F., IntMed.
Chaplin, R. A., Anaes
Charlebois, P. A., Anaes
Charles, W. B., IntMed
Charron, K. C.
Charron, R. C., IntMed.
Chase, Lillian A., IntMed
Chase, N. D.
Chen, C., GenSurg.
Chepesiuk, M. W.
Cheskes, A., Ophth.
Chesnie, J. J., IntMed
Chetwynd, J. B., DiagRad
Chisholm, A. W., IntMed
Chisholm, L. D., Ophth
Chlebus, A., Paed, D & TRad
Chovil, A. C.
Chris, S., GenSurg
Christie, P., Psy
Chu, J. T.
Chute, A. L., Paed
Citry, E., Psy
Clark, R. D., GenSurg
Clark, R. M., TherRad.
Clark, S. K., IntMed
Clarke, E. Aileen
Clarke, W. T. W., IntMed
Clayton, J. K., Psy
Clifford, E. J., IntMed.
Clute, K. F., Paed
Coad, R. L.
Coates, D. B., Psy
Cochen, Sandra, Anaes
Cochrane, R. C., Psy
Cockfield, R. L.
Coderque, J. A., Otol
Coggins, B. H., Anaes
Cohanim, M.
Cohen, G. S.
Cohen, Minnie W.
Colantonio, A. F., DiagRad.
Colapinto, R. F., DiagRad
Colapinto, V., GenSurg, Urol
Cole, A. H., Anaes
Cole, A. R. C., Paed
Cole, C. E. C., IntMed
Cole, J. E. C., IntMed
Cole, L. J., IntMed
Coleman, H. M. OrthSurg
Coleman, Isobel, M.
Collins-Williams, C., Paed
Colman, H., GenSurg, Urol
Colwill, J. C., OrthSurg.
Conen, P. E., Path
Conn, A. W., Anaes
Conn, G. S., OrthSurg
Contway, M. A. A., GenSurg
Conway, B. B., Paed
Cook, C. T.
Cookson, B. A., Psy
Cooper, R. M.
Cooperman, E. M., Paed.
Copland, G. M., IntMed
Copley, D. R.
Copp, J. C.
Corbin, M. F.
Corcoran, M. C.
Cormack, G. D., Psy.
Cosbie, W. G., ObstGyn
Costain, W. A., GenSurg
Cotnam, H. R.
Cottrell, L. G., Psy.
Coulter, G. F.
Coulter, S. G.
Cowan, D. H., IntMed
Cowan, R.
Cowle, J. E.
Cox, M. A., Paed
Craig, C. B.
Crassweller, P. O., Urol, GenSurg
Crawford, J. S., Ophth
Crawford, J. S.
Crisp, A. G., NeurPsy
Crocker, Audrey N.
Crompton, C., Urol
Crompton, C. P., Anaes
Crookston, J. H.
Croome, R. R., GenSurg
Cross, E. G., IntMed
Cross, W. H.
Crotin, A. M., Otol.
Crowell, D. E., Anaes
Crowther, T. A., IntMed
Crozier, D. N., Paed
Crummey, C. B.
Cryderman, W. J., DiagRad
Cummings, E. A., Anaes
Cunningham, J. N., IntMed
Cunningham, Stella
Curkowskyj, R. N., OrthSurg
Currie, D. J., GenSurg
Currie, E. A.
Curry, B. H. G., OrthSurg
Curry, R. H., Path.
Curtin, A. Ann
Curtis, J. E., Anaes
Cutler, Judith H.
da Costa, G. A., Psy.
Dafoe, W. A., ObstGyn
d'Agata, G.
Dale, G. M., OrthSurg
Dales, C. W.
Daley, Dorothy E.
Dalgleish, P. D.
Daniel, Susan, Anaes
Daramola, Florence
Darte, J. M. M., Paed, TherRad
Dauphinee, J. A., IntMed
Davey, J. F., IntMed
Davidson, A. S., Psy
Davidson, J. W., DiagRad.
Davidson, R. E.
Davidson, W., Paed
Davies, J. H.
Davies, J. S., GenSurg
Davies, L. S., OrthSurg
Davis, F. H., Psy.
Davis, G. A., Paed
Davis, G. E. D., Psy
Davis, Marjorie I., GenSurg
Davis, Ruth M.
Davis, S.
Dawson, J. C., Obst
Day, C. S., GenSurg
Deacon, A. S.
Deadman, J. C., Psy
De Andrade, J. R., OrthSurg.
Debera, V.
DeBuda, Y. D. G.
Deck, Josephine
Deck, J. H. N., Path.
Deeth, J. H.
Defries, R. D., PH, Bact
Delarue, N. C., GenSurg., ThorSurg.
Demauele, F.
Denne, A. J.,
Denne, Doris H.
Dent, O. V., IntMed (T.B.)
Desmond, J. W., Anaes
Deveber, G. A., IntMed.
Detweiler, H. K., IntMed
Devlin, H.
Devlin, H. E., Anaes
Dewan, J. G., NeurPsy
Dewar, F. P., OrthSurg, GenSurg
Diamand, S.
Dick, J. J.
Dicker, R.
Dickinson, G. T.
Dickson, A. D.
Dickson, D. H.
Dickson, G. D.
Dickson, J. T.
Dickson, L. C.
Dickson, M. Elizabeth
Digby, J. W., IntMed
Dike, Anna I.
Dilisi, J.
Dimitroff, D. C.
Diosy, A., IntMed
Disenhaus, E. I.
Disler, Elizabeth
Dixon, G. D., Anaes
Dobai, B.
Dobbin, M. C., Ophth
Dobbs, K.
Dobson, Claire W., Otol.
Docrat, K.
Dodds, D. J.
Doerr, R. S.
Donnell, Margaret M.
Donohue, W. L., Path, Bact
Doran, T. A., ObstGyn.
Douglas, L. G.
Douketis, J.
D'ovidio, V.
Dowd, E. C., GenSurg
Dowd, J. R., ObstGyn.
Doyle, A. M., NeurPsy.
Doyle, H. S.
Drillis, G. L.
Drucker, W. R.
Drummond, Mable
Drutz, M. G.
Dryer, Ellice A., Anaes
Drysdale, I. O., Ophth.
Duckworth, D. A. Urol
Duckworth, G. S.
Duckworth, J. W. A.
Dudar, W. J.
Duffy, Mary H.
Dukszta, J., Psy
Duncan, A. H.
Dunham, H. S.
Dunlop, T. C.
Dunn, A. J., Anaes
Dunsmore, J. M., DiagRad
Dworkin, H. J.
Dyer, C. W., GenSurg
Dyer, D. W.
Dyer, J.
Dymond, M. B.
Eason, M.
East, H. M.
Easton, N. L., Psy
Ebbs, J. H., Paed
Eckert, L. A., GenSurg
Eddis, Mary J.
Edey, R. B.
Edmeads, J. G., Neur
Edmonds, W. B., Neur
Edwards, H. E., Paed
Egier, A. I., ObstGyn
Ehlers, E. O.
Ehrenreich, K. A.
Ehrlich, R. M., Paed
Eisen, A., ObstGyn
Eisen, D.
Eisen, Isadore M., ObstGyn
Eisen, S. M., Anaes
Elder, L. J.
Elek, M.
Elek, Susanne
Elkerton, L. E., Bact
Elliott, C. M.
Elliott, H. N
Elliott, J. T.
Ellis, G. H.
Emery, J. E., PlasSurg
Emmett, J. C.
Eng, F. W. H. T.
Enright, T. J., Psy
Epstein, A. A., D & TRad
Epstein, M.
Epstein, N., Paed

* Population not separately available.

Toronto (Cont'd.)
Epstein, S. W., IntMed.
Erb, J. T.
Erb, L. Jean
Erdei, A., IntMed
Erenst, M. M., GenSurg
Ernest, M., Path
Esperanca, M. J., Paed
Evans, D., Anaes
Evans, G., DiagRad
Evans, J. A.
Evelyn, S. J., Anaes
Evis, F. A.
Ezrin, C., IntMed
Fader, W. H.
Fainstein, S. B., Ophth
Fairhurst, K. W., Anaes.
Fairley, H. B., Anaes
Falconer, J. G., IntMed
Fallis, F. B.
Fallis, J. C., GenSurg
Farber, R., Paed
Farkashidy, J., Otol.
Farmer, A. W., GenSurg OrthSurg, PlasSurg
Farmer, R. A.
Farr, R. H.
Farrar, C. B., NeurPsy.
Farrell, M. J., ObstGyn.
Farrow, G. A., Urol.
Fearon, B. W., Otol
Feasby, W. R., IntMed
Fedder, J., ObstGyn
Fedyna, A.
Fee, G. A., Otol
Fehrmann, Anne
Feinman, S. V., IntMed
Feld, R.
Feldman, E. D. A.
Feldman, S., Psy
Felix, J. L.
Feness, J. Z.
Fenigstein, H.
Fenn, J. E., ObstGyn
Fenn, W. E., GenSurg
Fenton, J. A.
Ferguson, C. G.
Ferguson, J. G.
Ferns, J. M.
Ferrie, K. E., IntMed
Ferrier, G. J.
Ferris, P. W. H., Anaes
Feuer, S. I.
Fialkov, G. J., Otol
Fielden, E. C., PathBact
Fielden, R. H., OrthSurg
Fields, H., IntMed
Fine, B. N.
Fine, H., IntMed
Finlay, J. M., IntMed
Finlayson, D. C., Anaes
Finlayson, D. M., IntMed
Fiorine, G.
Fischer, Elsbeth
Fischer, M. A., Psy
Fischer, Phyllis V., Path
Fish, E. B., GenSurg
Fishbein, G. D.
Fishbein, Silvia
Fitzgerald, G. W., Neurol.
Fitzgerald, J. D. L., IntMed
Fitzhenry, E. M. J., Otol
Fitzpatrick, P. J., TherRad
Flatt, W. D., ObstGyn
Fleming, Adelaide L., Paed.
Fleming, J. R., NeurSurg
Fleming, P. C.
Fleming, Shirley A., Anaes.
Fletcher, G. M.
Fletcher, W. R., Obst
Flett, R. H., Urol
Flommerfelt, T. E., GenSurg
Florence, J., IntMed
Florence, R., Derm.
Flor-Henry, P.

Fogel, B.
Foldes, E. G.
Forbath, N. F., IntMed
Forbath, P. G., Paed
Forbes, M. Elizabeth, DiagRad
Forgiel, W. J.
Forman, D. M., IntMed
Forman, E. T.
Forrest, S. J., IntMed
Forrester, R. A.
Forstner, G. G., IntMed.
Foster, A. D., ObstGyn
Foster, D. L., Anaes
Foster, E. A.
Fotheringham, J. B., Psy
Found, N.
Fowler, R. S., Paed
Fox, T. W., IntMed
Frackowiak, J. T., GenSurg, Urol
Francis, W. G., ObstGyn
Francoeur, J.
Francombe, W. H., IntMed
Frank, F. J.
Frank, W.
Franks, W. L., PhysMed. & Rehab.
Franks, W. R.
Fraser, D., Paed
Fraser, Freida H., Bact, PH
Fraser, J. G., IntMed
Fraser, J. L., ObstGyn
Fraser, N. L.
Freedman, H. B., Psy
Freeman, K. I., DermSyph
Freeman, S. J., Psy.
Fremes, I. A., Paed
French, D. B., Otol
French, E. T., GenSurg
Freund, Gertrude E., Anaes
Fried, T.
Friede, H., NeurPsy
Friedlich, T. L.
Frieri, A.
From, G. L., IntMed.
Frost, L. J.
Fryer-Manacki, Ruth
Fujiwara, M. W., Paed
Fujiwara, Misao, ObstGyn.
Fullerton, Kathleen, Paed.
Fulton, J. R. W., GenSurg
Fyfe, P.R., OrthSurg
Gallie, J. G.
Galloway, R. J. M., GenSurg, OrthSurg
Galszechy, J. C.
Garbe, W., DermSyph
Garbutt, C. T. P.
Garcia, Martin A., GenSurg
Gardiner, J. H., Paed, DiagRad
Gardiner, W. J., PhysMed
Gardner, W. P.
Gare, J. D., ObstGyn
Gartha, I. V.
Gartha, Susan, Paed
Gauld, Dorothy M., Psy
Gedz, W.
Geisler, W. O., IntMed, Phys Med & Rehab
Gelbloom, A. J., Path
Geleff, T.
Gendron, J. E., GenSurg.
Geneen, B., Psy
Genesove, L. J.
Georgiouski, A.
Gerred, R. F., IntMed
Gerstein, M. C., Paed.
Giardine, F. P., ObstGyn
Gibson, D. A., OrthSurg
Giddens, S. W., Paed
Gilbert, J. A.
Gilchrist, J. W.
Gilchrist, M. M., Paed
Gill, J. M.
Gillan, J. G., Ophth

Gillespie, J. W.
Gillies, J. D. M., ObstGyn
Gillies, J. Z.
Gimbert, Shanna B.
Ginsberg, S.
Ginzberg, L.
Givan, Kathleen F., Bact
Gladstone, N.
Glassman, M., GenSurg
Glassman, M. M.
Glatt, B. S.
Glawdan, Helena
Glazman, B.
Glick, D.
Glover, T. J.
Godden, J. O., IntMed
Godfrey, C. M., PhysMed & Rehab.
Godfrey, J. G., Psy.
Godwin, T. F., IntMed.
Gokulanathan, K. S., Paed
Golab, S.
Gold, G.
Gold, S. S., Paed
Golden, I. M.
Goldenberg, H., IntMed
Goldberg, J.
Goldberg, L., DiagRad
Goldenberg, L., Paed
Goldenberg, L. M., DermSyph
Goldhar, A., ObstGyn
Goldie, J. H., IntMed.
Goldman, I., ObstGyn.
Goldthorpe, W. G.
Gollish, I.
Gollom, J., Otol
Gonsik, Helena
Gonzalez, V.
Gooderham, M. E.
Goodman, A. W., DiagRad.
Goodman, J. M., DermSyph
Goodman, W. E., Otol
Goodman, W. S., Otol
Goodwin, N. L.
Gopaul, H.
Gordon, D. IntMed
Gordon, Elisabeth A.
Gordon, R. A., Anaes
Gordon, S. D., PlasSurg, GenSu
Gordon, S. G., Urol
Gorman, C. K., IntMed
Gossage, C. D.
Gourlay, D. E.
Gow, G. A., IntMed
Gower, G. F., Psy
Goyo, G. C.
Goyo, M.
Gracie, J. P.
Grader, J., Ophth.
Graham, A. F. IntMed
Graham, C. B., IntMed
Graham, D., IntMed
Graham, R. T.
Graham, R. W., IntMed
Grant, D. K.
Grant, J. C. B.
Grant, J. P., Psy
Grant, R. J.
Gray, Alice E. W., PathBact
Gray, C. C., IntMed
Gray, H. M., IntMed
Gray, J. C., GenSurg
Gray, K. G., Psy
Gray, O. V., GenSurg
Greben, S. E., Psy
Green, A. H.
Green, D. Otol
Green, Mildred
Green, N., IntMed
Greenaway, A.C.
Greenbaum, G. H., Psy
Greenberg, H. J.
Greenwood, W. F., IntMed, (Cardiol)
Greer, K. C., Psy.
Greey, P. H., Bact

* Population not separately available.

Toronto (Cont'd.)
Griffin, B. M.
Griffin, J. D. M., Psy
Griffith, M. N.
Grimshaw, Isobel, Anaes.
Grimshaw, W. L.
Grobin, W., IntMed
Grodzinski, J., Psy
Grondin, Carol
Groshaw, R. E., Ophth
Grossman, H. J., GenSurg
Grotell, D.
Grunblatt, L.
Grundy, E. C., GenSurg
Guest, Joan E.
Gurrin, P. M., Anaes
Gurrin, Teresa M., Anaes.
Gustainis, Ona-Danute, Anaes
Guthrie, D., Path
Haber, A., DiagRad
Haber, J.
Haberfellner, Helga
Haberman, H. F., DermSyph
Hadley, D. K., GenSurg
Hafezi, D. M.
Haffey, M. J., Otol
Hahn, Charlotte E., IntMed.
Haidasz, S.
Hain, C. W.
Hair, H. C., Dermsyph
Haist, R. E.
Haldenby, D. A., Otol.
Hale, C.
Hall, F. M., IntMed.
Hall, H. G., IntMed
Hall, J. E., OrthSurg
Hall, J. Leo, ObstGyn
Hall, M. C., OrthSurg
Hall, M. R., D & TRad
Hall, W. E., IntMed
Hallam, H. T., GenSurg
Halmagyi, A. F., GenSurg.
Halmos, Veronica, IntMed
Halpern, I.
Ham, A. W.
Hamblin, G. P., Paed
Hamill, A. S., IntMed
Hamilton, F. C., IntMed
Hamilton, J. R., Paed.
Hamilton, J. D., PathBact
Hamilton,-Smith, B.
Haniford, E.
Hanley, E. G., Anaes
Hanley, Phillis E.
Hanley, T. R., Anaes
Hanley, W. B., Paed
Hanna, R. J. E.
Hannah, J. A., Path
Hannah, W. J., ObstGyn
Haraszthy, D., ObstGyn
Harbinson, D. J.
Harcourt, J. A. A.
Hardie, C. D.
Hardman, R. D.
Hardy, B. C., GenSurg
Hardy, E. B.
Harkins, E. B., Paed
Harkins, J. L., ObstGyn
Harnick, L. R., D & TRad —
Harper, D. W., Ophth
Harper, J. A., ObstGyn
Harris, C. W., GenSurg
Harris, F.
Harris, J. E., IntMed
Harris, L. J., ObstGyn
Harris, W. H., ObstGyn.
Harris, W. R., OrthSurg
Harrison, A. W., GenSurg.
Harrison, D. C., IntMed
Harrison, Elizabeth E.
Harrison, Joan
Harshman, J. P., Ophth
Hart, G. D., IntMed
Hart, J.
Hart, P. F.
Hart, R. A., IntMed.
Hartroft, W. S.
Harvey, W. F., Urol.
Harvie, J. N., DiagRad
Harvie, R. M.
Harwood, W. L., D & T Rad
Hassard, C. E. A.
Hasselback, R. C., IntMed
Hastings, D. E., OrthSurg.
Hastings, J. E., PH
Hauch, J. T., IntMed
Haugh, C. H.
Hausler, H. R., Ophth
Havelkova, M., Psy
Hawke, W. A., NeurPsy
Hawkings-Fink, Elma M.
Hawkins, N. V., TherRad
Hawks, G. H., Bact
Hayes, Ethel
Hayley, Margaret
Hazlett, Barbara, IntMed
Hazlett, J. M.
Healy, D. E. L., Otol
Heathcote, A. G. S.
Hebb, A. R., IntMed.
Hector, R. I., Psy
Heimbecker, R. O., GenSurg
Heller, E. M., IntMed
Heller, J. M.
Hellings-Evans, B. M.
Hellmann, K.
Henderson, D. N., ObstGyn
Henderson, H. W., Psy.
Henderson, M. H., IntMed
Henderson, R. D., GenSurg.
Hendrick, E. B., NeurSurg
Henry, G. A., Otol
Henry, Violet I. E.
Herman, M. L.
Hernando, H. M.
Herold, W. E., Ophth
Heron, J. S., Anaes
Hersak, E.
Herst, M.
Herst, Roslyn
Heslin, J. D., DiagRad.
Hess, F. W., ObstGyn
Hetenyi, Caroline, IntMed
Hetenyi, G. J.
Hethrington, H., IntMed
Heywood, P. M., IntMed
Higgins, H. P., IntMed
Hilditch, J. R.
Hill, A. G.
Hill, C. E., Ophth
Hill, F. Marguerite, IntMed
Hill, Jean M.
Hill, J. C., Ophth
Hill, J. G.
Hill, J. W.
Hill, Marian E., Neur.
Hill, Muriel, ObstGyn
Hilliard, I. M., IntMed
Hilliard, J. R., IntMed.
Hills, W. H.
Hiltz, J. W. Ophth
Himel, C.
Himel, H. A. IntMed
Hiraki, G. Y. GenSurg
Hiscox, P. E., Ophth.
Ho, J., DiagRad.
Ho, Yau Cheung
Hoare, D. S. Paed
Hobbs, Carolynne A., Psy.
Hodgkiss, W. R.
Hoebrechts, P. M. NeurSurg
Hoffman, C. M.
Hoffman, H. J., NeurSurg
Hogarth, F. S.
Hogarth, W. Jean IntMed
Hogg, F. R. DiagRad
Holbrook, J. D.
Holling, F. S.
Holmes, R. B. D & TRad
Holmes, S. J. Psy
Holt, Ann R.
Homonylo, W. H.
Hood, A. M. Psy
Hooey, Mary A., IntMed
Hopkins, P. D.
Hopwood, G. M.
Horn, H. I., IntMed.
Horowitz, B. ObstGyn
Horsey, W. J. GenSurg
Horwitz, A. N., ObstGyn
Houpt, J. B., IntMed
Howell, H. Doris PathBact
Howes, E. W. OrthSurg
Hubbs, D. H. IntMed
Hudson, A. L. DermSyph
Huffman, Janice, DiagRad
Hume, R. G. D.
Humeniuk, R. B.
Humphrey, J. G., Neurol
Humphrey, J. N.
Humphry, A. DiagRad
Hunt, T. M., Paed
Hunter, A.
Hunter, J. M.
Hunter, Margaret I. Paed
Hunter, Mary, Anaes
Hunter, W. S., Ophth
Hutchison, A. D.
Hyland, H. H. NeurPsy
Ibberson, Olive GenSurg
Iles, J. D.
Imirie, R. J., Paed.
Ing. M. C.
Innocenti, G.
Invidiata, F. P.
Ireland, F. A. DermSyph
Ireland, P. E. Otol
Ireton, H. J.
Irwin, R. N.
Iscove, A.
Istran, E. J., ObstGyn.
Ivanans, P.
Iwackniuk, Nadia R.
Jacks, W. G.
Jackson, E. J. Anaes
Jackson, Mary V. Psy
Jackson, R. W., OrthSurg
Jackson, S. G.
Jacobs, A. A.
Jacobs, J. A., Anaes
Jacobs, W. F.
Jacobsen, J. R. Anaes
Jaffe, F. A., Path
Jakiwczyk, N.
Jalil, S. M., GenSurg.
James, F. G.
Jamieson, R. A., Cardiol, IntMe
Jamieson, W. D. S.
Jansen, Margaret
Jansen, M. G.
Jarvis, G. J., Ophth.
Jastrzebski, Z. M.
Jedwab, S. J. Psy
Jeffs, R. D. Urol
Jeney, L., Psy.
Jeney, Piroska
Jenkin, R. D., TherRad
Jessel, L.
Jewell, T. C. ObstGyn
Job, Carla F., Anaes
Johnson, C. C. R. Paed
Johnson, D. H.
Johnson, E. W.
Johnson, M. D., IntMed
Johnson, R. H. Paed
Johnston, A. E., Anaes
Johnston, B.
Johnston, F. T. GenSurg
Johnston, H. W. J. ObstGyn
Johnston, J. F. A. Ophth
Johnston, J. L. GenSurg
Johnston, M. W., IntMed
Johnston, R. E.
Johnston, W. G. GenSurg
Johnston, W. H. Paed
Johnston, W. V.
Johnstone, C. G.
Jolly, R. D.

* Population not separately available.

Toronto (Cont'd.)
Jones, A. L. Psy
Jones, J. A., DiagRad
Jones, N. S.
Jones, R. A. GenSurg
Jones, W. F. IntMed
Jones, W. M. Anaes
Jones, W. W.
Jordan, D. A. Paed
Joslyn, M.
Josy, I., Derm.
Josy, Anna
Jousse, A. T. PhysMed
Joynt, G. H. C. GenSurg, IntMed
Jubb, E. Dawne, ObstGyn
Judge, R. H.
Jurk, V., PhysMed. & Rehab.
Kadysiewicz, M. M.
Kalant, H.
Kalinowski, M. R.
Kalow, Brigitte D. Anaes
Kalow, W.
Kaminker, A. IntMed
Kane, L. A. Otol
Kaplan, S. R.
Kapsos, J. E., ObstGyn
Kapusta, M.
Karabanow, O., Psy
Karaszthy, D. L., ObstGyn.
Karger, P. Paed
Karols, J. Y.
Karpati, L.
Kasari, L.
Kasari, V.
Kasler, D. IntMed
Kasten, S. L., Psy
Katz, A., Path
Katz, Deborah, IntMed
Katz, S., Urol
Kauffman, P. P.
Kaufman, P. M. DiagRad
Kavanagh, G. J.
Kavanagh, T.
Kay, G. D. OrthSurg
Kay, H. E.
Kay, M. S.
Kay, R. B., Psy
Kazdan, J. J., Ophth.
Kazdan, L. Ophth
Kazdan, M. S., Ophth
Kearns, H. J.
Keeler, W. R. Psy
Keenleyside, E. A.
Keenleyside, J. G., DiagRad
Keith, J. D. Paed
Keith, W. S. NeurSurg
Kelly, A. D.
Kelly, F. O., Urol
Kelly, Peter
Kelly, R. G. C. Ophth
Keltz, M.
Kemp, A. E.
Kemper, F. D., IntMed
Kendrick, G. B. Ophth, Otol
Kennedy, Sylvia
Keon, W. J., GenSurg.
Kerbel, G. A., Derm
Kerbel, N. C., IntMed
Keresteci, A. G., Urol
Kergin, F. G. GenSurg
Keri, J.
Kerr, H. T.
Kerr, J. H., Anaes
Kerr, W. H., GenSurg
Kerr, W. K. Urol
Kerwin, A. J. IntMed, (Cardiol)
Ketchum, Katherine D.
Kettles, J. S.
Kettlewell, J. W.
Key, J. A. GenSurg
Keyl, Anne
Khan, A. Y.
Khan, D-i-K., Derm
Kidd, B. S.
Kidd, L.
Kilgour, G. S. PlasSurg
Kincaide, C. M., Anaes
Kingstone, H.
Kingstone, R. A.
Kingstone, S. I.
Kirkham, F. R.
Kirshner, A. W.
Kiss, A.
Kitchen, G. H. GenSurg
Kleiman, H. J., D & TRad
Klein, A. V.
Kline, H.
Kline, H. J.
Klotz, P. G. Urol
Knapp, J. E.
Kneeshaw, R. S. Anaes
Knowlton, C. E. GenSurg
Knowlton, T. G. ObstGyn
Knox, J. E.
Knutson, G. H., PlasSurg.
Koegler, S. J., Paed.
Kofman, O. Neur
Kohari, J., GenSurg
Koladich, Carol J.
Koladich, S., Psy.
Kopytek, S.
Korman, I. A., IntMed.
Korsak, Christina M.
Korwan, G. J. W., DiagRad
Kosowsky, M.
Kosoy, M., Paed.
Kosta, Sophia
Kovacs, E.
Kovacs, Ida
Koven, I. H. GenSurg
Kowalewski, J. E. A.
Koyl, L. F. IntMed
Krajbich, G. P.
Kramolc, N.
Krasins, Berta
Krestow, M., Anaes.
Kruyff, E., DiagRad
Kryt, Maria, Anaes
Kucherepa, J. W.
Kuczmenda, S.
Kugler, M., OrthSurg
Kula, E. D.
Kurdyak, V. B., ObstGyn.
Kushevich, Z. A.
Kussner, J.
Kussner, N.
Kutasy, W.
Kuwabara, E. H.
Kuzminski, D. J.
Kyne, W. P., Psy
LaCroix, W. R. DiagRad
Lacy, E. ObstGyn
Laidlaw, J. C. IntMed
Laidlaw, W. R., Psy
Lailey, W. W.
Laing, L. P.
Laird, R. C. GenSurg OrthSurg, ThorSurg
Landis, N.
Lang, A. P.
Lang, S. R.
Langer, B. GenSurg.
Langford, E. R.
Lansdown, E. L., DiagRad
Lanskail, J. C. GenSurg
Laski, B. Paed
Laufer, O.
Lauks, Anna
Lawee, D.
Lawson, G. A. PhysMed
Lazarou, L. P., DiagRad
Lazarovits, S.
Lazenby, F. S. DermSyph
Leath, N. TherRad
Leckey, R. G. GenSurg
Lee, G. G.
Lee, Jane
Lee, J. Y.
Leers, W. D., Bact
Leeson, Helen J., Paed.
Leibel, B. S.
Leizner, H.
LeMesurier, A. B. OrthSurg, GenSurg
Lenczner, M. M. IntMed
Lenkei, Susan, C. IntMed (Cardiol)
Le Riche, W. H.
Leslie, S. W.
Lester, M. G., Derm
Leventhal, A. Paed
Levin, R. C.
Levinne, N. N.
Lewin, O.
Lewin, P. K.
Lewis, Beverly, Path
Lewis, C. H. Psy
Lewis, F. I.
Ley, Dorothy, C. H., IntMed
Librach, M. M.
Librach, S. ObstGyn
Liddy, B. F. S., Ophth.
Liebe, H. K.
Lind, J. R.
Lindsay, W. K. PlasSurg
Lindsay, W. R. N., PlasSurg
Lindzon, M.
Linell, E. A.
Linton, W. T., Derm
Lipa, M., Path.
Lipson, M. H.
Liquornik, Clara
Lister, J. G., Psy
Little, A. H., IntMed.
Little, B. J., Neur
Little, J. A. IntMed
Little, L. G.
Little, M. H., Anaes.
Little, W. M., DiagRad
Litzenberger, D.
Liu, Sim Fay, IntMed
Lively, F. M.
Liverpool, J. A.
Lizewski, W. J.
Llewellyn-Thomas, E. R.
Lloyd, Lois, Ophth
Loach, L. F. W., IntMed
Lobb, R. A. D & TRad
Lobley, P. G.
Locke, H. W. B., Urol.
Lockwood, A. L. GenSurg.
Loeb, J. A. GenSurg
Lofchy, A. N.
Lofft, T. F., Psy.
Logel, R.
Logothetopoulos, J.
Lome, Lillian T.
Long, J. E.
Longo, A. J.
Lorimer, W. R., Anaes
Lorinc, J., Path
Lotto, W. M., GenSurg; OrthSurg
Loudon, Esther, Gyn.
Lougheed, G. W. IntMed PathBact
Lougheed, J. U. R., Anaes.
Lougheed, W. M. NeurSurg,
Loukras, C.
Lovering, J. H. D.
Lovett-Doust, J. W., Psy
Low, D. M. ObstGyn
Lowrey, S. R. Urol
Lowrie, H. A.
Lucas, J. P.
Ludwig, B. ObstGyn
Luke, W. R. F. Ophth
Lukowski, Maria, Anaes
Lumsden, W. F., GenSurg.
Lunan, M. D. Otol
Lunderville, C. W. P., Anaes.
Luttor, C. ObstGyn
Lynch, M. J., Path
Lyon, R. K., GenSurg
Lyon, Sheila M.
Macaulay, D. N.
MacBean, E.

*** Population not separately available.**

Toronto (Cont'd.)
MacConnachie, H. F., Path
MacDonald, A. E. Ophth
MacDonald, D. K. Ophth
MacDonald, E. S. ObstGyn
Macdonald, Eva W. Bact
Macdonald, I. B. GenSurg
MacDonald, J. A., GenSurg
MacDonald, J. C., GenSurg
MacDonald, R. E., Otol
MacDonald, R. I. IntMed
MacDonald, R. K. Ophth
MacDougall, C. S. Otol
MacEwen, K. F. DiagRad
MacGowan, G. A.
MacIntosh, D. L. OrthSurg
MacIsaac, C. J.
MacKay, Elizabeth N. PH
Mackay, I. D., GenSurg.
MacKay, I. M. Anaes
MacKay, J. Psy
Mackay, J. S., Path
MacKay, K. H. ObstGyn
MacKay, R. C. IntMed
MacKenzie, A. L. GenSurg
MacKenzie, D. J. IntMed
MacKenzie, J. K.
MacKenzie, R. G.
MacKenzie, W. F.
MacLaren, D. B., GenSurg
MacLaren, Mary Anaes
MacLean, D. L. PH.
MacLean, J. A. Paed
MacLeod, C.
MacLeod, D. R. E. Bact
MacMillan, J. C.
MacMillan, R. L., IntMed
MacNab, I., OrthSurg.
Macnamara, H. O.
MacNeill, J. J., PlasSurg
MacNicoll, W. T.
MacPherson, B. E.
MacPherson, G. W.
MacRae, D.
Macrae, H. M. Ophth
Madely, Patricia M.
Madigan, J. L.
Machle, W. M.
Magwood, S. J. N. ObstGyn
Magyar, A.
Magyar, S.
Mahon, M. A.
Mahon, W. A., IntMed.
Mahoney, L. J. GenSurg
Mainprize, G. J.
Makhan, B. A.
Malcolm, A. I., Psy
Malkin, A.
Malkin, Dina G.
Male, R. W.
Maloney, G. C. ObstGyn
Malowney, V. C.
Maltby, E. J. IntMed
Maltby, Lila F. Psy
Malyon, M. H., IntMed
Malyon, R. H.
Manace, B. A. IntMed, All.
Manace, G. Paed
Manacki, J. A.
Mandell, H.
Mann, J. J.
Mann, R. W.
Marchant, P. Anaes
Marcolongo, V.
Margolian, J. GenSurg
Margulies, A. I., Psy
Mariz-Fernandez, S., Path
Mark, F. G.
Mark, I.
Markham, W. J., Anaes
Markens, I. J.
Markowitz, J.
Marks, L. IntMed
Markson, C. A. IntMed
Markson, E. R. Psy
Markson, S. S. Psy
Markus, N., DiagRad
Marmina, J. V.
Marotta, J. Neur
Marshall, B. M. Anaes
Marshall, E. B.
Martin, A. G.
Martin, D., Psy
Martin, G. K.
Martin, J. L.
Martin, R. F., OrthSurg.
Martyn, D. M. ObstGyn
Marwood, L. R.
Maryanka, Eva
Masson, E. L.
Mastromatteo, E.
Mathe, C. J.
Mathews, R. E., GenSurg
Matthews, R. L. Anaes
Mattimoe, P. F.
Mautner, L. S. PathBact
Maxmen, M. D. GenSurg
Maxwell, J. B. Urol
Mayer, J. A. NeurSurg
Mayer, J. M., GenSurg
Mayers, J. R.
Maynes, E. A.
McAskile, K. Otol
McBride, R. L., ObstGyn.
McBrien, G. E.
McBroom, W. T.
McCann, Maureen
McCann, N.
McCarthy, D. D & TRad
McCarthy, D. D.
McCausland, Joan
McClelland, J. C. Urol
McClintock, H. T.
McClure, P. D., Paed
McCollum, J. L. Urol
McConney, F. S. IntMed
McCormack, O. L.
McCormick, C. P. GenSurg
McCormick, W. J.
McCracken, G. NeurSurg
McCulloch, A. E.
McCulloch, E. A. IntMed
McCulloch, J.
McCulloch, J. C. Ophth
McCurdy, Margaret
McDonald, D. J., Ophth
McDonald, D. J., ObstGyn.
McDonald, G. A. OrthSurg, GenSurg
McDonald, H.
McDonald, J. L. OrthSurg, GenSurg
McDougall, E. P., GenSurg PlaSurg.
McDowell, H. C. T.
McEachern, K. D. IntMed
McEachern, Margaret A. Otol
McFarlane, D. V., DiagRad
McGee, A. R. D & TRad
McGee, D. A., Neur.
McGoey, Janet
McGreal, D. A. Neur
McGuigan, J. P.
McIlroy, W. J., Neur
McInnis, F. P. ObstGyn
McIntosh, Anna M. H.
McIntyre, D. H. Anaes
McIntyre, D. I., OrthSurg.
McIntyre, J. A. GenSurg
McIntyre, J. L., DiagRad
McJannet, W. A., Anaes.
McKay, A. L. PH
McKay, J. B. PathBact
McKee, D. C.
McKee, M. Elizabeth, Otol
McKellar, J. C. ObstGyn
McKelvey, A. D. IntMed
McKendry, J. B. J. Paed
McKenna, A. C.
McKenzie, L. E.
McKinley, Helen I. Paed
McKinnon, N. E. Path. PH
McKnight, C. K., Psy.
McLaren, D. K.
McLaren, K. A.
McLean, C. R. Path
McLean, D. B.
McLean, D. M.
McLennan, J. D. IntMed (T.B.)
McLennan, T. A.
McLeod, A. M. Otol
McLeod, D. L. Paed
McNeel, B. H. Psy
McNeilly, W. E.
McPhedran, H. IntMed
McPhedran, N. T. GenSurg
McPhedran, R. S., NeurPsy.
McQuade, Margaret Psy
McRae, C. A.
McRae, D. S.
McTavish, D. R.
McTavish, W. A. IntMed
Meakin, J. W., IntMed
Meehan, J. E.
Meema, H. E., DiagRad
Meiklejohn, H., R. B. ObstGyn
Meindok, H., IntMed
Mekedci, A.
Mele, V. L.
Meligrana, F., IntMed
Mellows, F. S., Paed.
Melnyk, F.
Melville, P. H. Psy
Melvin, R.
Mendelson, M., Anaes
Menzies, F. H.
Meredith, R. H. Anaes
Merrick, B. W.
Messecar, C. R.
Mester, Z., GenSurg
Metcalfe, M.
Metzler, W. S., IntMed
Meyer, E. G. Urol, GenSurg
Michaels, L.
Michalovsky, L.
Microys, Gisele I.
Middleboro, J. G.
Mileiko, W.
Milford, D. M.
Millar, H. A.
Millar, J. C.
Millar, O. B. D & TRad
Miller, A. Psy
Miller, G. W. PH
Miller, I. E.
Miller, J. H.
Miller, M.
Miller, M. E., Psy
Miller, W. R. A.
Mills, D. G., GenSurg
Mills, E. J.
Mills, J. R. F. GenSurg, OrthSurg, ThorSurg
Millson, J. W. ObstGyn
Milne, M. N.
Milton, Margaret
Mingie, P. G., Psy
Mink, M. M.
Misumi, Y. D.
Mitchell, C. Helen
Mitchell, D. R. Urol
Mitchell, E. W., GenSurg
Mitchell, H. D., Psy
Mitchell, J. GenSurg
Mitchell, Mary E.
Mitchell, R. I., GenSurg
Mitis, L. H. Psy
Mittler, N.
Miyagishima, R. T.
Moes, C. A. F. D & TRad
Moffat, J. F. ObstGyn
Moffat, J. G., GenSurg.
Moffat, W. W., GenSurg
Moffatt, W.
Mohacsy, J.
Moldofsky, H., Psy
Moldofsky, J., Psy

* Population not separately available.

Toronto (Cont'd.)
Moller, E. S.
Molony, T. J. Otol
Monagle, J. E.
Monkman, E. J.
Montfort, F. G.
Montgomery, D. B., IntMed
Montgomery, E.
Montgomery, R. C.
Moody, F. J.
Moore, D. C., ObstGyn
Moore, Jean
Moore, Marjorie, ObstGyn
Moore, P. C. F., Psy
Moore, R. F.
Mora, J.
Moran, J., Anaes
Morch, J. E., IntMed
Morgan, A. L. Ophth
Morgan, Ethel A. M. PathBact
Morgan, E. A. Paed
Morgan, E. L. D.
Morgan, J. E., ObstGyn
Morgan, J. F.
Morin, C., Paed(P.Q.)
Morin, J .D., Ophth
Morley, T. P. NeurSurg
Morphy, G. P.
Morris, C. W. PH
Morris, Sylvia
Morrison, J. K.
Morrow, J. D. IntMed
Morrow, W. N.
Mortimer, C. B., Ophth.
Mortimer, D. C.
Mortimer, N. W. GenSurg
Morton, P. L., Ophth
Moscarello, M. A.
Moscarello, Rebeka, Psy
Mosley, W. PH
Moss, G. W. O.
Mott, F. D., PH.
Movat, H. Z. Path
Mowat, H. F., GenSurg
Mueller, L. H.
Muir, D.
Mullens, J. E. GenSurg
Munkley, F. H. ObstGyn
Munn, J. D. D & TRad
Murby, W. H. ObstGyn
Murnaghan, D. P. IntMed
Murphy, D. E., ObstGyn
Murray, C. V. Psy
Murray, G. D. W. Surg
Murray, J. F. GenSurg, PlasSu
Murray, J. G. Anaes
Mustard, R. A. GenSurg
Mustard, W. T. OrthSurg
Mutrie, R. R., GenSurg, OrthSurg
Mycyk, M. D.
Myers, D. S.
Myers, E. D. Proct. GenSurg
Myers, L. Ophth
Mysak, J.
Nabeta, S. S., Anaes
Nadasdi, M.
Naguchi, A.
Nagy, Z. GenSurg
Naidoo, D., Psy
Nash, M.
Nash, S. S. ObstGyn
Naumoff, P.
Nedilski, M. M. IntMed
Neweduk, M. W.
Newton, R. A., PlasSurg
Ngai, S. K.
Nichka, B. A., Otol
Nicholas, W. C.
Nicholls, Doris M.
Nicholls, G. W.
Nichols, Florence, Psy
Nichols, G. B.
Nicholson, J. K.
Nikolajevich, V.
Niksac, Vera
Nishikawa, F. S.
Nishikawa, R.
Noble, A. J., Path
Noble, E. C.
Noble, E. J., IntMed
Nodwell, R. J.
Noguchi, A., Anaes
Nolan, W. J.
Noonan, W. T. ObstGyn
Norman, H. R. C. GenSurg
Norman, Margaret G., Path
Noronha, A. J., GenSurg; PlasSurg
Norris, J. R. ObstGyn
Norris, S. ObstGyn
Norwich, K. H.
Noyek, A. M., Otol.
Nunez, J.
Oakes, W. H., GenSurg.
Obney, N.
O'Brien, D. F.
O'Brien, M. J. Paed
Ocana, A.
O'Connor, M. J.
Ogryzlo, M. A. IntMed
O'Hara, J. G.
O'Hara, P. J. ObstGyn
O'Heany, Jean M.
Ohlke, R. F., Anaes
Oille, W. A. Cardiol, IntMed
O'Kelly, F., Urol
O'Leary, D. A., Paed
Olin, J. S. IntMed
Oliva, F. G.
Oliver, Elizabeth, Anaes
Omarali, U.
Ord, J. V. R. PlasSurg, GenSu
O'Reilly, Kathleen Anaes
Organ, L. W.
Ormsby, H. L. Ophth
O'Rourke, S. J. Anaes
Ortved, W. E. Urol
Osborn, N. J.
Osoba, D., IntMed.
Ostime, M.
O'Sullivan, P. M. IntMed
Oswald, J. M.
Ozkan, A., Path.
Pacevicius, A.
Pacevicius, S.
Pahapill, R.
Page, N. A. IntMed
Palacios, E.
Palij, B.
Palmer, C. R., GenSurg
Paloc, E.
Paloc, S. G., Derm
Pangalos, C., DiagRad
Pantalony, D., Path.
Papsin, F. R., ObstGyn
Park, A. M. Neur
Park, N. S. Anaes
Parker, G. M., DiagRad.
Parker, G. P. IntMed
Parker, J. A., Ophth.
Parkin, A.
Parks, A. E. IntMed
Parks, W. R.
Parliament, D. R.
Parliament, W. J.
Parmenter, Ellice, Anaes
Parrish, R. N.
Partington, M. W.
Pascal, O. DiagRad
Pascoe, W.
Pashby, T. J. Ophth
Patel, H., Paed.
Paterson, J. F. IntMed
Patt, N. L., DiagRad
Patterson, T. A.
Patzauer-Votsch, Anna, IntMed
Paul, M. M.
Paul, W. M., ObstGyn
Pawlowski, G.
Peacock, J. J., Neur.
Pearce, Joclyn, DiagRad
Peart, A. F. W. PH
Peat, R. S. PH
Pedler, J. A.
Pelton, D. A., Anaes
Pennal, G. F. OrthSurg
Penney, G. R.
Penney, R. H. IntMed
Pequegnat, L. A. PH.
Percival, J. A.
Pereszlenyi, A.
Perfect, K. E.
Periti, G. C.
Perkins, J. R.
Peters, M. Vera TherRad
Peterson, C. P.
Peterson, J.
Peterson, Natalie
Petropoulakis, A.
Pflug, M., IntMed
Phair, W. B. IntMed
Phillips, G. C.
Phillips, K. G. Paed
Phillips, M. J., Path
Piercey, W. D.
Pietz, C.
Pilkey, R. M. ObstGyn
Pinilla, J. V.
Pinto, R., Psy.
Piotrowski, A.
Piper, G. A.
Piper, S. A. DiagRad
Piyapongse, M., Anaes.
Platts, Marjorie, Path
Playfair, P.
Plewes, F. B. GenSurg
Plewes, W. F.
Plumb, L. M. Psy
Pohlman, E. R., Path
Polak, J. M.
Poland, Betty J. ObstGyn
Pollack, J.
Pollock, Ira J.
Pollock, J. O.
Pollock, M. A. IntMed
Polymenakos, L. G.
Porter, F. T.
Porter, J. M.
Porter, R. H.
Pos, R. B. Psy
Powell, A. .B, GenSurg
Pozner, S. N. ObstGyn
Pratt, H. H.
Pratt, K. E.
Preece, C. G., IntMed
Prendergast, W. F.
Preston, A. J., Psy
Preston, D. N.
Preston, Helen, Psy
Pretty, G. C.
Price, D. K., Anaes
Price, G. F.
Price, Vera, Derm
Prichard, J. S. Neur
Priddle, W. W. IntMed
Prince, G. E.
Prior, B. C. DiagRad
Procunier, C. W.
Prokipchuk, E. J., IntMed (Gastroent)
Puffer, D. S. PH
Pugh, D. S.
Pugh, E. C.
Purdy, A. D. T. ObstGyn
Purkis, R. S. A. IntMed
Purvis, W. M.
Quentin, M. R., Paed
Rabinovich, S., Path
Racz, F.
Radd, I C, IntMed
Rado, K.
Rado, P. P.
Rae, J. M. Psy
Ralley, D., Psy
Ralph, R. E.
Ramphal, P. J.
Rance, C. P. Paed

* Population not separately available.

Toronto (Cont'd.)
Ranking, G. N. Urol
Rapoport, A. IntMed
Rapson, L. M.
Rapp, C. R. GenSurg
Rapp, M. S., Psy.
Rappaport, A. M.
Rappaport, Rosa K. Derm
Raschka, L.
Rastogi, P N., Paed.
Rauf, M. N.
Raxlen, B. Anaes
Rayman, P.
Raymers, M. P. ObstGyn
Rebhan, A., Paed
Reese, L. W.
Reichert, J. N.
Reid, G. W.
Reid, J. D. ObstGyn
Reid, R. G. DiagRad
Reilly, Mary M.
Reine, J. W., Anaes
Reingold, A. A.
Reingold, M. M. ThorSurg, GenSurg
Reininger, S. M. M. T.
Rekai, J.
Rekai, P.
Relle, A. Anaes
Relton, J. E. S., Anaes
Renaud, R. E., PhysMed & Rehab
Renecker, G. T., Psy
Renouf, J. H.
Renwick, W. A. Anaes
Rewa, T.
Rhodes, A. J. Bact
Rice, D. I.
Rice, M.
Rich, E. J.
Richards, R. N.
Richardson. C, A.
Richardson, H. F., GenSurg
Richardson, J. C. NeurPsy
Richardson, O. B. Ophth
Richardson, R. B. NeurPsy
Rickart, J. H. IntMed
Ridley, C. M.
Risdon, E. F. PlasSurg
Ritcey, E. L., IntMed
Ritchie, A. C., Path
Ritchie, R. C., Path
Ritz, I. Urol
Roach, Margot
Roadhouse, R. C.
Robbins, F. C.
Roberts, C. A., Psy
Roberts, K. A.
Roberts, P. W.
Robertson, C. T. GenSurg
Robertson, D. C., GenSurg, Ph Surg
Robertson, Elizabeth C. Paed
Robertson, G. L., IntMed
Robertson, G. R.
Robertson, J. D.
Robertson, H. F. GenSurg
Robertson, Mary E., IntMed.
Robertson, S. F.
Robinson, C. E. Psy
Robinson, D. Roberta
Robinson, Eleanor M. IntMed
Robinson, J. G. Anaes
Robinson, J. M.
Robinson, Koraishia, ObstGyn
Robinson, L. IntMed
Robson, C. H. Anaes
Robson, C. J. Urol
Rockman, J. B.
Roebuck, M. J., Anaes
Rogers, Alicja
Rogers, H. P.
Rogers, J. R. GenSurg
Rogers, J. W. ObstGyn
Rogers, S. DermSyph
Rogoman, Edith, Anaes.
Rombough, W. G.
Romney, D. IntMed
Ronald, A. C., IntMed
Rorabeck, C. H.
Rose-Bernstein, Vera, Paed.
Rose, M.
Rose, R.
Roseborough, Jane F.
Rosen, E. J. Psy
Rosen, G. P., Otol
Rosen, I. E., DiagRad.
Rosen, I. GenSurg
Rosen, L. J., Paed, Allergy
Rosen, P. S. IntMed
Rosenblatt, A.
Rosenrouch, S.
Rosol, T.
Ross, C. S.
Ross, Janet K.
Ross, J. R. Paed
Ross, J. W. GenSurg
Ross, L. H.
Ross, Marion Bact
Ross, Peggy
Ross, R. C. Path
Ross, R. J., GenSurg
Rosset, M. DermSyph
Rossitter, F. P. Anaes
Rotenberg, C. D & TRad
Rotenberg, M. Anaes
Roth, F. B.
Rother, I. IntMed
Rotman, H. H.
Rotstein, M. I.
Rotstein, M. L. ObstGyn
Rotstein, M.
Rowan, J.
Rowland, W. A. IntMed
Rowley, J. C., DiagRad
Roy, T. E. PathBact
Roy, W. M. D & TRad
Rudd, M. S. GenSurg (Eng.)
Rudd, W. W., GenSurg.
Ruderman, R. L. GenSurg
Rumball, N. H. IntMed
Russell, C. S., ObstGyn
Russell, J. L. GenSurg, Urol
Russell, W. G.
Russell, W. H. GenSurg
Rutherford, R. W. IntMed
Ruttan, H. R., Derm
Ryan, P. A. (All) IntMed
Ryder, D. E.
Ryley, T. G., ObstGyn
Rzadki, E. I.
Saask, L., Psy
Sachis, J. H.
Sadowski, P. D.
Saez, A. J.
Sager, H. S. Psy
Sahey, P. A.
Saiphoo, C. S-A., IntMed.
Salama, Y. A., Paed
Salmon, J. D., GenSurg
Salter, R. B. OrthSurg
Samad, I. A., IntMed.
Samis, T. T. Ophth
Samis, W. D., Ophth.
Samu, D. Derm
Sanchez, A., Paed
Sand, N.
Sanders, B. M. DermSyph
Sanders, D. E. DiagRad
Sandhu, M. S.
Sansone, D.
Sarjeant, D. A.
Saunders, Sarah J.
Sauret, P.
Savage, H. G. Paed
Sawyer, G. I.
Sazant, M.
Scala, S.
Scandiffio, M. A.
Schachter, I. B., NeurSurg
Schachter, R. K. DermSyph
Schatz, D. L., IntMed
Schatz, S. W., NeurSurg
Schatzker, J., OrthSurg.
Scheffler, Hilda
Schick, R. J.
Schiffer, I.
Schimanek, T. A.
Schofield, T. E., Psy.
Schneider, R.
Schnider, K.
Schulte-Steinberg, O.
Sephton, R. B.
Schubert, J. F.
Schwab, J. A.
Schwab, W.
Schwenger, C. W.
Scott, Florence A. Psy
Scott, J. G., IntMed.
Scott, J. W.
Scott, T. B. DermSyph
Seelig, G. M. ObstGyn
Seeman, J.
Sekiguchi, S.
Selby, D. A., IntMed.
Sellers, A. H. PH
Sellers, E. A.
Selznick, M. W. ObstGyn
Senn, J. S. IntMed
Sepp, A. Path
Sereny, G. IntMed
Sexsmith, E. L.
Seymour, B. A. S. Anaes
Shack, L. Paed
Shafran, M. IntMed
Shandling, B., GenSurg
Shannon, E. H. D & TRad
Shanoff, H. M. IntMed
Shapiro, B. J. D & TRad
Shapiro, I. OrthSurg
Shapley, J. M. Anaes
Shardt, A.
Sharp, A. S. IntMed
Sharp, F. B.
Sharpe, J. E. Psy
Sharpe, N. C. PathBact
Sharpe, S. S. DermSyph
Shaul, D. L. ObstGyn
Shaver, E. R.
Shaw, A. E.
Shaw, A. G. GenSurg
Shaw, R. A.
Shaw, W. H., Paed; Psy
Shea, J. B. DiagRad
Shea, M. Ophth
Sheffman, E. J., Anaes
Shenken, E., Ophth.
Shephard, R. J.
Sheppard, Dorothy, ObstGyn
Sheppard, Mabel L.
Sheppard, R. H. IntMed
Shepherd, J. T.
Sheriton, J. E., ObstGyn
Shewchuk, A. R.
Shields, H. J. Anaes
Shields, Y. P.
Shier, C. B. ObstGyn
Shilletto, M. D.
Shime, J.
Shinobu, R. R., Psy
Shleser, I. H. IntMed
Shneidman, Nina
Shone, J. D., Paed
Shortreed, R. D., Otol
Shouldice, E. B.
Shugar, G., Psy.
Shukyn, D.
Shulman, M. P.
Shulman, P. N.
Shusterman, M. Ophth
Shykoff, H J. Anaes
Sidlofsky, S., GenSurg
Siegel, E. J.
Siefrer, A. G.
Sifton, J. A.
Sifton, J. S.
Silberman, M. Paed
Sildvee, O.

* Population not separately available.

Toronto (Cont'd.)
Silver, H. L. PlasSurg
Silver, H. D.
Silver, M. N.
Silverberg, J. G. DermSyph
Silverberg, L. R.
Silverman, B., Psy
Silversides, J. L. IntMed Neur
Silverstein, E. A., OrthSurg
Silverstein, H. PhysMed & Rehi
Silverthorne, L. N. Paed
Simmons, E. H. GenSurg, Orth Surg
Simon, F.
Simon, L.
Simor, I. DiagRad
Simpson, J. F.
Simpson, J. S. Jr., GenSurg
Simpson, W. J. K. IntMed & TherRad
Sims, S. D. ObstGyn
Sinclair, G. A. IntMed
Sinclair, J. C. IntMed
Singer, H. N., Urol.
Singh, W. S. A., Paed
Singleton, A. C. D & TRad
Sipos, L.
Sirek, Anna
Sisson, B. V.
Skain, F. J., ObstGyn
Skala, G. K.
Skorbinski, A. W.
Sky, R. C.
Slater, R. J. Paed
Slatt, B., Ophth
Slavens, J. J. Paed
Slemon, H. V. GenSurg
Sloan, I. A., Anaes
Small, A. A. DermSyph
Smith, A. G.
Smith, A. O. C. Anaes
Smith, C. G.
Smith, D. R. F.
Smith, E. S. O., P.H.
Smith, F. Anaes
Smith, F. A.
Smith, G. E.
Smith, G. W. IntMed
Smith, H. A. W. IntMed
Smith, I.
Smith, J. D.
Smith, J. K. B. Otol
Smith, L. ObstGyn
Smith, L. M.
Smith, M. B.
Smith, M. W. J.
Smith, P. E., Otol
Smith, R. L., Psy
Smith, Sheelah B.
Smith, T. O.
Smoling, L. F.
Smythe, H. A. IntMed
Snell, F. V. V. Anaes, IntMed
Snell, G. D. Otol
Snell, G. E. Otol
Snelling, C. E. Paed
Snider, Bernice
Snider, E. P.
Sniderman, H. R. Ophth
Sochaniwskyj, W.
Solandt, O. M.
Solmes, J. G. R. ObstGyn
Solowska, Vera Paed
Soltys, Sophie
Solursh, C. B.
Solway, A. J. L. IntMed
Solway, S. L. D. IntMed
Solway, S. H. Anaes
Sommers, J. D & TRad
Sonley, Marilyn, Paed
Sorbara, V. J. ObstGyn
Soules, M. H.
Sparks, B. B. IntMed
Speakman, J. S. Ophth
Spears, J. C., IntMed
Spector, A. R., Anaes
Spence, J. M.
Spence, W. J. GenSurg
Spencer, J. R. L., Ophth.
Spittel, W. H.
Spivak, M. M., ObstGyn
Spooner, C. M. GenSurg, Urol
Spring, M. H. R.
Spring, W. B. Urol
Sproule, H. F.
Squires, A. H. IntMed
Stancer, H. C., Psy
Stancer, S. L.
Stanton, I. I.
Stanulyte, Ruta
Starkman, S. Neurol
Staron, Natalie M.
Staroste, K. H.
Statten, P. Otol
Statten, T., Paed., Psy.
Staub, L.
Stauble, W. J., Psy
Steadman, P.
Steele, E. C.
Steele, F. H. Otol
Steele, J. C., Neur.
Stein, H. A. Ophth
Stein, M. M. IntMed
Steinberg, S. DermSyph
Steiner, Betty Psy
Steiner, G., IntMed.
Steiner, J. Path
Steinhardt, M. I., DiagRad
Steinhauer, P. D., Psy
Stephen, D. H.
Stephens, C. A. GenSurg
Stephens, R. O.
Stern, G. S.
Stewart, B. M., Neur.
Stewart, D. A., Paed
Stewart, F. H.
Stewart, G. L.
Stewart, J. F., GenSurg
Stewart, Mary H.
Stewart-Burton, Marjorie, ObstGyn
Stewart, W. G.
Stiles, J. H.
Stinson, D. A. IntMed
Stiver, W. B.
Stobie, G. H., GenSurg
Stobie, S. N., Psy
Stock, G. IntMed
Stock, M.
Stoddart, W. O. GenSurg, OrthSurg
Stogdill, C. G. Psy
Stokes, A. B. Psy
Stokes, R. E., Psy
Stork, J.
Strasberg, S. M.
Strashin, I.
Strauss, G. Z., GenSurg
Strawbridge, H. T. G., Path
Strebig, D. L.
Strickler, A. C.
Stroz, E. L.
Strulovici, S.
Struthers, E. B., IntMed
Struthers, R. G. PH
Stuckler, J. Otol
Stumbof, A. V.
Stuparyk, M., IntMed
Sugiyama, H. S.
Sukman, S. N.
Sullivan, J. A. Otol
Sullivan, J. E.
Sullivan, J. F.
Sullivan, L. J. Urol
Sultmanis, Lydia
Sultmanis, R.
Sumohara, J. M.
Sungaila, J. DiagRad
Suran, R. R. ObstGyn
Sussman, A. H. IntMed
Sutherland, G. O. DiagRad
Sutherland, Lynette E.
Sutherland, R. B. PH
Sutton, M. R. Urol
Swales, J. O. ObstGyn
Swan, H. G.
Swanson, J. N. IntMed
Swanson, Marjorie C.
Sweet, G.
Sweeting, A. M.
Swyer, P. R. Paed
Symons, F. A., DiagRad
Sypher, F. F., OrthSurg
Szatmari, A. NeurPsy
Szollosi, S. L.
Szymanski, G.
Tait, H. M. S. ObstGyn
Talaat, S.
Tamburro, R. A.
Tan, S. K., DiagRad
Tanovich, J.
Tanz, E. M. PlasSurg
Tanzer, H.
Tanzer, J.
Tanzer, L. I. ObstGyn
Tasker, R. R. NeurSurg
Taube, H. N. IntMed
Taylor, A.
Taylor, C. C.
Taylor, G. A., GenSurg.
Taylor, G. D. IntMed
Taylor, H. M., DiagRad
Taylor, J. D.
Taylor, W. I.
Taylor, W. J. R.
Teglas, A.
Teichman, B. Ophth
Teichman, J. G. ObstGyn
Temelcoff, E. E., Psy
Temes, S.
Teney, H. F.
Tepperman, I. J.
Teskey, L. GenSurg
Theobald, J. C.
Thomas, B.
Thomas, C. L. GenSurg
Thomas, F. A.
Thomas, H. H.
Thompson, G. A. Ophth
Thompson, J. R., IntMed
Thompson, Margaret S.
Thompson, T. J.
Thomson, H. G. GenSurg
Thomson, Joan, Psy
Thomson, J. N.
Thomson, P. G. Psy
Thomson, S. A. OrthSurg, GenSurg
Thorfinnson, Patricia, DiagRad
Thorn, J. H. Anaes
Thornhill, Mary E.
Thornton, W. B.
Tickett, F. W.
Tickton, P. A. Otol
Tieman, E. E.
Tile, M., OrthSurg
Tilley, A. R. PlasSurg
Tipping, C. E. Anaes
Tobe, B. A., IntMed
Tobin, S. M. ObstGyn
Todd, I. A., GenSurg, Urol
Todd, J. E.
Tolan, J. R. DiagRad
Tolson, R. J., IntMed.
Tom, Mary I. Path
Tomlinson, J. W.
Topp, J. R., IntMed
Tovee, E. B. GenSurg
Towson, R. T.
Track, A. GenSurg
Traub, P.
Trelford, J. D., ObstGyn
Trewin, R. B
Trimble, A. S., ThorSurg (Card)
Trinchan, A., Derm
Trow, E. J. Jr. DermSyph
Trusler, G. A. GenSurg
Tse, Y. T.

* Population not separately available.

Toronto (Cont'd.)
Tuchtie, M. D., Psy
Tucker, A. G.
Tuffnell, P. G.
Turchin, R., DiagRad
Turner, D. A.
Turner, J. A. Paed
Turner, G. Anne
Turner, G. R.
Turner, Geneva M.
Turner, R. E. Psy
Turofsky, H. A.
Tuters, K.
Tuters, Laila
Tyber, M. A.
Tyl, W. J., Anaes
Tyndel, M. NeurPsy
Ulehla, B.
Upenieks, E.
Upper, F. B.
Urbach, G.
Urbach, G. M., Anaes
Urback, P. G. IntMed
Urbaitis, J.
Urquhart, R. W. I. IntMed
Uzans, Silvija
Uzupis, Aldona
Vaile, I. R. Otol
Vaile, S. J., Ophth
Valadka, A.
Vale, B. W.
Vale, Joan, IntMed
Van-Belle, Johanna H.
Van de Mark, T. B.
Vanderlinden, R. G.
Vandewater, S. L. Anaes
Vang, G., GenSurg
Van Leeuwen, J. J., Psy.
Van Orman, F. L. GenSurg
Van Patter, H. T. Path
Van Praagh, D. R., Paed
VanWyck, D. J. ObstGyn
Varey, D. H.
Varga, A. T., GenSurg
Varga, G.
Varty, E. J.
Varty, H. H.
Vassal, K. P. DiagRad
Veidlinger, O. F., Neur.
Venis, S. B.
Verhulst, J.
Vermes, G.
Vernon, C. P. ObstGyn
Verny, T., Psy.
Verville, G.
Vierkotter, Hildegarde M.
Vining, J. F. A. Anaes
Virgin, W. J., OrthSurg
Voaden, Carol M.
Volpe, A. G. IntMed
Volpe, R. IntMed
Vozis, D. B.
Vozis, G. G., ObstGyn
Vozoris, Agathocles
Vozoris, D. GenSurg
Vranic-Petrick, Margada
Waddington, H.
Wainwright, D. O.
Wagman, B. B.
Wagner, G. H.
Wait, J. H., GenSurg
Waldie, B. S. ObstGyn
Waldmann, I. M., IntMed
Waldman, S., IntMed
Walker, A. M. IntMed (TB)
Walker, L. A.
Walker, S. J.
Walker, W. A., Paed
Wallace, W. B. Otol
Wallis, H. M. GenSurg
Walmsley, J. F.
Walsh, F. D.
Walsh, P. J., Ophth
Walter, J. B.
Walters, J. A. NeurPsy
Walters, W. R. ObstGyn
Wang, S.
Ward, J. F.
Warren, C. M.
Warren, R. F. GenSurg
Warren, S. L.
Wasserman, D. DermSyph
Wasylenko, J.
Watson, C. H. GenSurg
Watson, D. G. Paed
Watson, J. D., Anaes.
Watson, M. C. ObstGyn
Watt, G. D. L. IntMed
Watt, H. J. IntMed
Watters, N. A. GenSurg
Watts, G. O. NeurPsy
Watts, W. G.
Wax, S. L.
Waye, R. I.
Weber, J. L., Paed
Weber, R. K., Anaes.
Weinberg, J. M.
Weinberg, M. B.
Weinberg, V. ObstGyn
Weinstein, R.
Weisbrod, G. I.
Weiser, W. J.
Weiss, Helene
Weizel, H. A. E. GenSurg
Welch, R. H.
Welsh, D. R. J. GenSurg
Welsh, W. K. GenSurg, OrthSu
Werry, E. C., GenSurg
Wesley, R. H. ObstGyn
Weston, N. E.
Weston, R. L., Anaes
Whalen, J. S. Anaes
Whaley, J. B. Otol
Whaun, June M., Paed
Wheler, E. G.
Wherrett, J. R., Neur
White, A. W. M. GenSurg OrthSurg
White, E. J., OrthSurg
White, Mary P., Psy
Whiteside, J. H., ObstGyn
Whittaker, J. S.
Whittle, E
Widgerson, A., IntMed
Wiggin, N. J.
Wight, E. W.
Wightman, K. J. R. IntMed
Wightman, R. C., GenSurg
Wigle, E. D., IntMed
Wigle, W. D., IntMed
Wilcock, P. W., Paed.
Wiley, A. M. OrthSurg
Wiley, Elizabeth GenSurg, ObstGyn
Wiley, J. J., OrthSurg
Wilhelmson, M.
Wilk, E. J., ObstGyn.
Wilkens, C. H.
Wilkes, J. R.
Wilkie, A. M.
Wilkins, A. R. Anaes
Wilkinson, F. W.
Wilkinson, J. A., GenSurg
Wilkinson, R. H., GenSurg
Will, R. E. IntMed
Willett, A. W.
Williams, C. D. G. GenSurg
Williams, H. A. Paed
Williams, M. G. Derm
Willinsky, A. I. Urol
Willinsky, B. GenSurg, Urol
Wilo, M.
Wilson, D. R., IntMed
Wilson, D. R. GenSurg
Wilson, G. E. P. GenSurg
Wilson, J. K. IntMed
Wilson K. B., Anaes
Wilson, M. S., Psy
Wilson, R., ObstGyn
Wilson, W. H.
Wilson, W. J. Paed
Winchester, Euphemia ObstGyn
Winesanker, H. Anaes
Wintrob, B.
Wise, D. K. IntMed
Wise, S.
Wishart, F. O. Bact. PH
Wodehouse, G. E. IntMed
Wolfish, A.
Wolin, L.
Woloschuk, E. ObstGyn
Woloschuk, O., GenSurg
Woloszczuk, A. GenSurg
Wong, E. D., Psy
Wood, D. E., IntMed
Wood, Margaret I. Paed
Woods, J. M. GenSurg
Woods, L. W., Psy
Woodside, M. A. IntMed
Woodward, E. G.
Wookey, H. W. GenSurg
Woolf, C. R. IntMed
Woolfe, C. G.
Wortzman, G. DiagRad
Wren, H. J.
Wright, C. S. OrthSurg
Wright, T. A., OrthSurg
Wright, W. W. Ophth
Wrong, N. M. DermSyph
Wronski, B. A. GenSurg
Wuerth, Walter GenSurg
Wynne-Jones, M.
Yabsley, R. H., OrthSurg
Yancoff, V. Y.
Yankou, C. J.
Yankowsky, M. O.
Yates, P.
Yaworsky, W., Psy
Ycas, J.
Yegorov, A.
Yendt, E. R. IntMed
York, J. E., Anaes
Young, A. E. PH
Young, B. H., Phys Med & Rehab
Young, C. O. IntMed
Young, D. M.
Young, Doreen A.
Young, Elizabeth G.
Young, E. J.
Young, G. W. IntMed
Young, M. K.
Young, W. E., Anaes
Zadyko, J.
Zajac, A. S., Psy
Zateny, W.
Zawadzki, J.
Zeglen, S. T. Anaes
Zeldin, J. OrthSurg
Ziegler, A.
Zilberman, J.
Zingg, W., GenSurg
Zownir, J. R.
Zsoter, T., IntMed.
Zuckerman, A. D.

TORRANCE
(203)
Martin, W. E., Anaes

TRENTON
(13,183)
Alexander, W. H., DiagRad.
Bailey, W. S.
Beecroft, J. D.
Bishop, M. A.
Byrne, J. V.
Campbell, D. E. M.
Dow, E. W.
Dow, E. W. Jr.
Farley, J. W.
Flynn, K.
Griffiths, W. L.
Hutchison, H. ObstGyn
Johnston, J. G.
Lafarga, A. M., Path.
McDonald, W. A. L. GenSurg
Nugent, B. O.
Struivig-de-Groot, H. B., GenSur
Telfer, G. W. Psy

* Population not separately available.

Trenton (Cont'd.)
Weaver, W. W.
Zeps, G. N.

TWEED
(1,791)
Allen, A. G.
Berry, R. S.
McCue, F. J.

UNION
(*)
King, W. E., Psy.

UXBRIDGE
(2,316)
Lennox, T. E.
McIntyre, J. A. GenSurg
St. John, J. R.
Theobald, G. M.
Watt, A. N.

VAL CARON
(1751)
Fernandez, G.

VANDORF
*
Van Nostrand, F. H. NeurPsy

VANKLEEK HILL
(1,737)
MacIntyre, G. D.
Manouvrier, F. F.

VERONA
(275)
Day, H. G.

VINELAND
(1,082)
Campbell, W. G.
Dobson, W. G.
Hurlburt, W. E.

VIRGIL
(574)
Czerevko, J. Z.
Dawe, G. A.
Eden, J. D.
Elltoft, J. D.
Nowoselecki, P.

VIRGINIATOWN
(2,009)
Hagerman, G. E.

WALKERTON
(3,851)
Allen, D. R.
James, C. W.
O'Toole, G. W. K.
Robinson, J. T. H.

WALKERVILLE
*
(Dist. of Windsor)
Swan, W. J.

WALLACEBURG
(7,890)
Barg, P.
Booth, M. L.
Brooksbank, R. C.
Cathcart, B. C.
Holmes, J. R. IntMed
Lamont, T. W. GenSurg
Lauber, R. W.
MacKay, D. H. DiagRad
Ralling, A. GenSurg
Richardson, S. A.
Thorner, D. R.
Thorner, L. R.
Wilford, W. L.

WARKWORTH
(658)
Joliffe, R. F.

WATERDOWN
(1,848)
Berneske, G. M.
Robertson, K.
Smart, J. E.

WATERFORD
(2,221)
Lucas, S. I.
Procunier, F. A.

WATERLOO
(21,366)
Atkinson, R. D.
Austrup, R. H.
Beckham, L. M., Anaes
Boettger, R. F.
Cheeseman, N. H.
Clarke, June M., Psy.
Gagnon, R. F., D & TRad
Geiger, D. W. Paed
George, M. B. D & TRad
Gordon, Helen E., Anaes.
Hay, J. M. D., GenSurg
Holland, W. G., Anaes
Kayler, T. D.
Lawson, D. A.
Little, Hanna B. TherRad
MacKenzie, C. G. Psy
MacLean, D. R.
Mathies, H. D.
McQuay, N. W., IntMed
Mickleson, C. H. Psy
Moore, M. G.
Morlock, F. J. DiagRad
Reesor, Helen L.
Riddell, A. R., Anaes
Schumm, B. J.
Sehl, W. A., ObstGyn
Shantz, W. L.
Simpson, A. W.
Spohn, P. D.
Standen, J. R., DiagRad.
Taves, Iva, Path
Voelker, P. A.
Walls, R. W.

WATFORD
(1,293)
Price, D. K.
Urie, P. R.

WAWA
(4,040)
Czuba, T.
Lee, R. J.
Meade, Judith
Timpson, R. J.

WELLAND
(36,079)
Alexanda, Eileen
Bedard, J. E.
Briant, T. E. Ophth, Otol
Cardwell, H. A., Psy
Creighton, J. O.
Danziger, H. G. Path
Deyell, J. A. GenSurg
Dubois, J. D.
Ennis, J. M. Paed
Griffin, J. H.
Holmes, F. R.
Hulke, F. P. DiagRad
Keffer, G. W.
Kiss, A.
Kuharik, L.
Leon, J. M., IntMed
MacDonald, M. P., GenSurg
MacNeill, D. C. DiagRad
Melillo, E.
Pakozdy, S. P.
Patry, J. M.
Purdon, A. L., Anaes
Pylypuk, E. S., GenSurg
Railton, R. H., GenSurg
Railton, S. V., GenSurg
Renaud, M. A.
Rice, A. D.
Sanders, C. B., IntMed
Sikora, S.
Singer, H. O.
Snelling, C. F.
Snelling, W. W.
Speers, E. A., GenSurg
Stuart, E. M., ObstGyn

Sturgeon, L. W. C., PH
Szabo, Z. L.
Tompkins, K. J., ObstGyn
Vandor, F.
Vedova, G. D., IntMed.
White, J. L.
Willson, D. A.
Wilson, G. S. M., GenSurg, Urol.

WELLAND PORT
(250)
MacLean, K. T.

WELLESLEY
(750)
Finn, J. H.
Sellers, C. S.

WELLINGTON
(1,062)
Murie, J. J.
Thompson, R. A.

WESTBROOK
(see Kingston)

WESTHILL
*
Bonser, F. H.
Charlton, R. W.
Corson, J. A.
Jacobsen, P. A.
Lathe, F. E.
McDonald, H. A.
Schunk, H. K.
Schunk, Jane
Stoffeis, H. H.
Towson, R. T.
Walther, F.

WEST LORNE
(1,066)
Cantelon, C. B.
McKishnie, Eunice
McKishnie, J.

WESTON
(9,715)
Anderson, D. N., Psy.
Axmith, K.
Bailey, L. O.
Balmer, H. C., Anaes.
Brereton, F. W.
Brown, A. S.
Brown, Laurie M., Anaes.
Bull, R. C., GenSurg
Cameron, W. H.
Cameron, W. K.
Campioni, E. C.
Charlton, W. H. M.
Cheung, O. T.
Chlebus, A., D & TRad, Paed
Christie, R. J.
Coulthard, H. S., IntMed (TB)
Cromarty, R., Path
Cruickshank, D. A.
Cruickshank, F. D.
Cruickshank, Jane E.
Culnan, G. F., GenSurg
Davidson, J. W., Anaes
Deitcher, J.
Devlin, H. E., Anaes
Dirnberger, W., Anaes
Duckworth, D. A., Urol.
Everist, W. C.
Fowler, R. N.
Gale, G. L.
Garrett, D. R., IntMed (TB)
Groshaw, R. E., Ophth.
Hammond, A. A.
Harris, L. D.
Holtzman, J. H.
Homburger, Helene
Horwitz, A. N., ObstGyn
Jakab, L.
Jones, E. R.
Kaplan, S. R.
Kannard, A. B.
King, F. G., ObstGyn
Macpherson, B.

* Population not separately available.

Weston (Cont'd.)
MacRae, D.
Mair, G. T., GenSurg
McCutcheon, W. M., DiagRad
McMillan, R. S.
McRae, J. R., PhysMed & Rehab
Milburn, C. W.
Misumi, Y. D.
Moffat, F. L., GenSurg
Murray, J. L.
Murray, R. K.
Nathan, S. N.
Nehra, Narendra N.
Parliament, D. R.
Peters, A.
Pilo, L.
Rice, M. C.
Rodgerson, J. S.
Roe, A. A.
Ronald, A. C.
Rosen, M. S.
Shack, L., Paed
Shubert, S.
Sillers, D. E., Ophth
Sinclair, J. D.
Singh, H., Anaes
Standley, J. M.
Stevens, R.
Stitt, J. F.
Takahashi, G. Y.
Theoret, J. J.
Thompson, J. R., IntMed.
Train, W. G.
Wales, W. F., GenSurg
Ward, T. F., Psy.
Weston, R. B., Anaes.
Wicks, C. A., IntMed (T.B.)
Wilkinson, R. H., GenSurg
Wright, C. F.
Wright, R. N.
Zeilig, L. V.
Zielonka, B. G., Anaes

WESTPORT
(713)
Goodfellow, F. M.

WHEATLEY
(1,365)
Edsall, M. C.
McLean, E. M.

WHITBY
(14,685)
Ash, L. C.
Balis, G. U., Psy
Barton, R. S., Psy
Braund, Margaret R.
Butts, M. W.
Citry, E., Psy
Clements, D. A.
Cuddy, F. A.
Enright, T. J., Psy
Fejer, I. F.
Greszczyszyn, E. R.
Hebert, A. J. B.
Hobbs, K. C.
Jaciw, G. A.
Jennings, M. M.
Just, R., Psy
Kaczanowski, G., Psy
Kassay, G. L.
Keon, T. P.
Khan, N. A.
Lamplugh, C. M.
Lindsey, G. W.,
Liswornik, H.
Lynes, P. G., Psy
Milian, E. Z.
Richards, A. R., GenSurg
Ruddy, J. O.
Russell, C. D.
Schramm, W. D.
Sargeant, E. J.
Stobie, S. N., Psy
Sweet, T. A., Psy

WIARTON
(2,138)
Leeson, J. L.
Rae, P. L.

WILLIAMSBURG
(442)
Swensson-Rosenquist, G. E.

WILLOWDALE
(Dist. of Toronto)
Ainslie, E. H., Anaes, IntMed.
Alderton, H. R., Psy
Andrews, A. J., DiagRad
Armstrong, D. J.
Armstrong, J. D., Psy.
Armstrong, R. D., DiagRad.
Augustt-Moffatt, S. E., ObstGyn.
Bain, H. W., Paed
Bates, R. W., IntMed
Basior, R.
Bauckham, J. F.
Beanlands, D. S., IntMed
Beck, H. O., ObstGyn
Belcourt, R. J. P., Bact
Bell, R. G.
Blair, W. E., Anaes
Blake, J. D.
Blevis, L. S., Path
Booth, Patricia M.
Boyd, W., Path.
Brown, H. A.
Brown, T. L.
Brummitt, W. M., Anaes.
Burrel, A. P.
Burrington, J. D., GenSurg.
Buxton, Elmira M.
Buxton, N. A.
Cairns, J. D., ObstGyn
Catenacci, Victoria M.
Charendoff, M. D., OrthSurg.
Cogan, R.
Collins, S.
Copland, G. M., IntMed.
Coulson, E. G., DiagRad
Crane, H. G., Psy.
Crawford, E. A., ObstGyn
Davey, L. M.
Disenhouse, R. B., Paed
Dolman, R. S.
Duff, B. R., GenSurg.
Dunlop, T. C.
Edington, J. C., D & T Rad.
Emery, G. N., IntMed.
Fitzpatrick, P. J., TherRad.
Fremes, N. E., IntMed
Fujiwara, M. W., Paed
Harper, I., Anaes
Harrison, A.
Harrison, A. W., GenSurg
Heaslip, D. S.
Heathcote, A. G.
Henry, L.
Henry, L. W.
Hilderbrand, A. F., Anaes
Hill, C. E.
Horsley, J. I.
Humphrey, A., DiagRad.
Johns, G. J., Psy
Johns, R. P.
Johnson, J. E.
Johnston, A. E., Anaes
Johnston, F. T., GenSurg
Keller, H. W.
Keltz, I.
Kerbel, N. J.
Krieger, E. Paed
Kruyff, Elizabeth, IntMed., DiagRad.
Kurtz, J. A.
Langer, B., GenSurg
Levine, J. D., DiagRad
Linton, H., GenSurg
Lovett-Doust, J. W., Psy
MacFarlane, E. J., OrthSurg.
Magee, G. L.
Margulies, A. J., Psy.
Martin, G. K.
McAteer, D. K.
McDougall, J. A.
Mester, Z., GenSurg.
Miller, G. W., PH
Milton, Margaret
Mitchell, R. I., GenSurg
Mohacsy, J.
Moore, B. P.
Mudie, L. H.
Murray, E. J.
Murray, J. D., Paed.
Nicholis, Doris
Nicolson, D. N.
Norheim, N. G.
Ogryzlo, M. A., IntMed
Parchment, A. R.
Parliament, W. J.
Patrick, D.
Pengelly, G. A.
Pierce, Anna C.
Porter, F. T.
Porter, J. S.
Poznan, Z.
Prefontaine, R.
Pugsley, H. E., IntMed
Rein, A.
Revich, S. J.
Richards, A. J., D&TRad
Robertson, D. P., GenSurg.
Rojko, A., Anaes.
Rorabeck, C. H.
Ross, Marion, Bact
Ross, Peggy L.
Russel, B.
Rutter, P. E.
Scheffler, Hilda
Schatz, D. L., IntMed
Schatz, S. W., NeurSurg
Shandling, B., GenSurg
Sharpe, N. C., PathBact
Sheffman, E. J., Anaes
Shulman, P. N.
Silverstein, E. A., OrthSurg
Simor, I. S., DiagRad
Sleeva, A. N.
Sless, P.
Smith, A. O. C., Anaes
Soper, K. C., OrthSurg
Squires, F. J.
Stasiuk, P.
Steele, R. J.
Stephens, R. O.
Stephenson, Bette M.
Stubbins, R. A.
Taylor, R. M. IntMed
Thompson, J. S.
Troster, M.
Walfish, P. G., IntMed
Walker, W. A., Paed.
Walsh, F. D.
Warren, S. L.
Weston, R. L., Anaes.
Williams, D. R.
Wilson, W. W., Anaes
Yarey, O. B.
Young, E. J.
Zeps, Genovefa N.

WILSON HEIGHTS P.O.
*****
(District of Toronto)

WINCHESTER
(1,431)
Barton, H. G.
Byers, W. M.
Dyke, E. E.
Justus, D. W., GenSurg

WINDSOR
(206,000)
Adams, J. F., GenSurg
Alewick, N. A.
Anderson, C. D., IntMed
Anderson, R. E. C., Urol
Anderson, T. A.
Andrachuk, W. W.
Andrew, R. B., GenSurg.
Asa, M., GenSurg, ThorSurg

* Population not separately available.

Windsor (Cont'd.)
Asselstine, H. S., PathBact
Asselstine, S. M., IntMed, Path Bact.
Barber, J. R., OrthSurg
Barnby, T. I.
Bell, R.
Berkeley, J. PhysMed
Berks, G.
Bernstein, G. I. OrthSurg
Bernstein, M. Ophth
Best, R. G. Ophth
Beuglet, E. Otol
Boley, J. P. Ophth
Boyd, N. O.
Boyer, D. E., Anaes.
Bradshaw, Phyllis E.
Breault, H. J. Paed
Bricker, J. D. DiagRad
Brien, W. P.
Brisson, D. A., Otol
Brisson, J. E.
Broadwell, D. J.
Brown, D. R.
Brown, L. M.
Brownlee, R. W.
Bull, M. H.
Butt, E. G. DiagRad
Campbell, S. H.
Cantelon, G. W. Psy
Carom, D. P.
Carreno-Segura, L., GenSurg.
Carter, A. K.
Cashman, E. F., ObstGyn
Chan, W. S.
Chatters, O. P.
Chesler, A. L., DiagRad
Clare, W.
Cooper, D. A., IntMed
Corr, J. J.
Craig, C. R.
Crassweller, H. GenSurg
Crowe, F.
Crozier, P. G.
Daniel, A.
Daniel, M. A.
Davidson, D. A.
Davidson, W. R. Otol
DeMarco, F. F.
Dignan, J. G.
Dionne, J. D.
Dixon, A. L.
Doherty, J. M.
Dolan, J., Psy
Draisey, T. F., Path.
Drkulec, V.
Duffin, G. W.
Dunn, B. H. Path
Durocher, E.
Dziubanowsky, T.
Echlin, T. H.
Efthimiou, H.
Elek, D.
Fachnie, H. L.
Farkas, N., Anaes
Feore, D. R., DiagRad
Flock, G. M.
Foster, K. H.
Fraser, G. A. Paed
Fraser, R. L., OrthSurg.
Freemesser, G. F.
Freier, A. A., ObstGyn
Fretz, N. A., Psy
Fry, J. ObstGyn
Gascon, Pauline M.
Gatfield, W. T. Paed
Gawenda, A. W.
George, G. G.
Girard, L. J.
Glass, B. S.
Goldenberg, S. GenSurg
Gorman, J. E. Anaes
Goyeau, F. R.
Grieser, F.
Guindon, Noemi
Habros, J. S.
Haliburton, R. A., GenSurg.
Hasnain, S. A.
Heckadon, R. G., PlasSurg.
Henderson, G. L. Urol
Henkel, G. G.
Hennecke, Thea, Otol
Hersey, M. L.
Higgins, L. M., ObstGyn.
Horne, W. I., Path
Hough, H. B. GenSurg
Howie, J. PH
Hulka, L.
Hume, W. E. GenSurg
Hutton, D. V. Paed
Irwin, M. E.
Jacks, N. B.
Jacques, A. J.
James, K. W. Derm
Janssen, Gesina, Anaes
Jasey, M. G., ObstGyn
Jeffery, G. S., IntMed (TB)
Jerace, J. R., ObstGyn.
Johnson, R. W., IntMed
Jones, J. R.
Kalman, G. S. ObstGyn
Kaspardlov, M., DiagRad.
Keith, W. E. Anaes
Kelly, J. M.
Ketchum, J., ObstGyn.
Khan, A. C.
Kleider, V. NeurSurg
Klimkowski, E. J.
Kopstein, J. B., Derm
Lager, L. H.
Laing, C. A. GenSurg
Lamos, S.
Lanspeary, W. D.
Larocque, R. D. GenSurg
Laszla, T. A., Paed.
Lawson, J. B.
LeBlanc, A. E.
Lees, H. H. Anaes
Le Fave, L. R.
Lengyel, G.
Letourneau, A. G., Psy
Lever, M. A. DiagRad
Lewis, G. F.
Lithgow, A. D.
Liu, Lillian, Paed
Luborsky, B.
MacDonald, J. D.
MacDonald, N. GenSurg
MacLennan, J. A.
Macleod, R. K., ObstGyn
MacPhail, I. A.
MacVicar, A. A. Psy
Mandel, L. IntMed
Markkanen, V. W.
Marshall, N. L. GenSurg
Mason, R. J., Psy
Master, W. M.
Mattis, Martha
Maus, J. H. TherRad
McCabe, J. GenSurg
McCormick, G. R., GenSurg
McCormick, N. A. GenSurg, DiagRad
McCormick, W. K.
McDonald, J. C., DiagRad
McGavin, M. F.
McGrath, W. P. Ophth
McKay, A. R., GenSurg.
McKay, Berta E.
McKenna, F. E.
McKenzie, T. R. Ophth
McLister, J. C. TherRad
McTague, G. A.
Messer, V. R.
Michaud, A. J.
Milburn, L. H.
Millen, D. B. GenSurg
Mills, C. V.
Milos, P., IntMed
Miskew, J.
Mok, G. C., TherRad
Morand, J. C.
Morgan, P. J.
Morris, E. J.
Morton, G. M., GenSurg
Munholland, R. J.
Munholland, W. L.
Murray, I. H.
Needham, W. L.
Nesseth, M. E.
Newman, M. Jean
Oleksiuk, S., Otol
Papp, G.
Parent, J. P.
Parker, G. M.
Parla, A. N.
Pearce, C. F., Urol.
Percival, W. L., GenSurg
Peterson, O. L. GenSurg
Phin, K. G.
Poirier, L. T.
Poisson, P.
Powell, W. G. GenSurg
Priebe, V. H., DiagRad
Prince, J. E. IntMed
Pyle, W. IntMed (T.B.)
Quinn, M. H., GenSurg; OrthSurg
Radin, S., GenSurg
Raeder, H. A.
Raphael, S. S., Path
Rider, R. C. OrthSurg, GenSurg
Robson, T. B. ObstGyn
Rock, W. K.
Roemmele, E. A.
Romano, W. L., DiagRad
Rosenfeld, J.
Rubenstein, A. I.
Rutherford, D. D.
Rutherford, S. E.
St. Pierre, G. L
Sacharoff, M.
Sadowski, S.
Saikewich, P.
Sanborn, C. S., Otol
Sanborn, D. Kathleen
Sargeant, E. J.
Scarfone, F. P.
Schaffer, H.
Schiller, H.
Schincariol, E. A.
Schlappner, O. L.
Schulde, J. M. GenSurg
Schumacher, Eleonore
Schumacker, J. M., ObstGyn
Seymour, B.
Shackleton, H. O.
Shepherd, G. H.
Shier, K. J., Path
Shuren, A., Otol
Sirilotti, E. U.
Smeeton, F. R.
Smith, E. H. N., Ophth
Smith, H. B.
Spakowski, W. J., Urol
Spooner, J. S. Urol
Sproat, W. R. E. Urol
Sproule, W. G., GenSurg
Stewart, E. H. F.
Stewart, J. D. IntMed
Strathman, I., ObstGyn
Stratton, D. P. DiagRad
Stratton, H. G. Psy
Sylvestre, N., Ophth Otol.
Tang, M.
Taylor, A. F.
Taylor, H. D.
Taylor, W. A. Anaes
Templin, M. I.
Thibert, N. E. IntMed
Tinning, R. A. IntMed
Tonken, H.
Topping, F. O.
Turner, G. E.
Vaughan, E. G., GenSurg
Vernon, R. T. DiagRad
Wachna, A. T.
Waddell, W. R. Gastroent IntMed

* Population not separately available.

Windsor (Cont'd.)
Warwaruk, A. S. ObstGyn
Weber, C. R. IntMed (T.B.)
Wein, H. P.
Wein, S. E.
Weinstock, J. W., Anaes
Wells, L. S.
White, G. E. Paed
Whitty, G. T.
Whitty, R. J. GenSurg
Wickware, J. A., DiagRad.
Wigle, D. S. GenSurg
Willms, G. G.
Wilson, A. P. DermSyph
Wilson, Mary
Winbaum, E. S. Paed
Windeler, E. C. H.
Wyner, S. F. DiagRad
Yonanovich, L.
Yaworsky, W.
Yee, G. E., Path
Young, J. S. GenSurg
Young, Mary I.
Zade, K. J.
Zarzour, E. J., Ophth
Ziter, M.
Zurowska, M. Christina

WINGHAM
(2,922)
Corrin, B. N.
Crawford, W. A.
Klahsen, A. W.
McKibbon, W. A.

WINONA
(294)
Aitken, H. E.
Joynt, R. L.
Roland, C. C.

WOODBRIDGE
(2,315)
Berry, W. E.
Garriock, J.
Ostime, M. J.

WOODSTOCK
(20,486)
Adams, C. R. GenSurg
Allen, A. G. Psy
Blackwood, J. R.
Brown, I. D.
Brown, I. Patricia
Burt-Gerrans, N. E.
Butt, W. J.
Chan, G. A.
Clark, E. A., Psy.
Dietrich, M., Path
Evans, E. C. IntMed
Fenton, G. M.
Fournier, F. E.
Granger, H. P. IntMed (T.B.)
Hall, G. R.
Hawkins, A. R.
Jackson, J. E.
Johnson, Diana M., Psy
Kee, C. G.
Kruger, G. W. DiagRad
Kryn, S. L.
LeMoine, Menna
Lindsay, P. B. Anaes
Lockwood, C., IntMed
MacKenzie, J. R. Path
MacKenzie, K. B.
Massey, L. W. IntMed
Matukas, A.
McPherson, A. C. GenSurg
Minielly, H.
Munnoch, N. M
Palmer, J. E.
Patience, C. R. Ophth,Otol
Plant, J. S. DiagRad
Poole, J. B.
Prytulak, W. Psy
Ramsay, T. O.
Reid-Smith, E. A. M., DiagRad.
Sedgewick, W. S.
Simpson, W. R. GenSurg
Smith, E. N.
Smith, J. D., GenSurg
Stirling, R. A.
Szasz, J., Ophth
Trotter, G. K.
Webb, G. A. C.
Weber, J. J. Psy, IntMed (TB)
Wilkey, W. D. IntMed
Willoughby, C. R.

WOODVILLE
(401)
Anderson, E. J.
Cramer, J. B.

WYOMING
(873)
Norris, R. L.
Price, J. K.

ZURICH
(728)
Wallace, C. J.

Prince Edward Island

ALBERTON
(856)
Hellmich, H. S.
Shea, W. A.

BEDEQUE
*
Bonnell, J. C.

BONSHAW
*
MacLeod, A. A.

CHARLOTTETOWN
(18,318)
Aquino, A. D.
Beck, M. N. Psy
Berdalda, J.
Burge, J. L. F.
Burke, F. A.
Coady, C. A.
Cox, L. S. GenSurg
Craig, J.
Curtis, O. H.
Drysdale, R. D. IntMed
Farmer, T. L.
Forsythe, R. G.
Found, E. M.
Giddings, E. S. ObstGyn
Grant, A. R.
Grant, K. C., GenSurg
Green, E. G., Otol
Hooper, W. T., TherRad
Houston, G. G. Otol
Howatt, B.
Irwin, J. K. L. ObstGyn
Kennedy, R. D.
Killorn, L. H.
Laidlaw, T. A. GenSurg
Lantz, J. B.
Lantz, J. P. Ophth, Otol
Lea, R. G.
Leon, W. H.
MacDonald, D. A. Anaes
MacDonald, S.
MacDonald, W. L. D & TRad
MacLelland, J. A., DiagRad
MacMillan, C. I.
MacMillan, F. A.
MacMillan, H. A.
Maloney, J. H. ObstGyn
McMillan, J. A.
Moreside, J. W. Ophth
O'Hanley, J. H. Paed
Parker, K. R., Paed
Pierce, H. H. Obst
Powell, Eva G., Psy.
Prowse, L. E. Anaes
Putnam, M. GenSurg
Rachmel, I.
Roberts, A. L.
Sinnott, J. C.
Saunders, A. L.
Shea, W. A.
Stewart, H. P.
Stewart, W. R.
Tidmarsh, F. W., Paed
Yeo, H. E.

CRAPAUD
(198)
Stewart, D. G.

ELDON
*
Gillis, J. M.
MacKenzie, D. W. Jr. GenSurg

GEORGETOWN
(744)
Kennedy, A.

HUNTER RIVER
(236)
Ellis, K. G.

KENSINGTON
(885)
Auld, R. W.
Clark, M. R.
Zielinski, L. K.

MONTAGUE
(1,130)
Inman, G. S.
McIntyre, P. GenSurg

MOUNT STEWART
(427)
Sheppard, G. G.

MURRAY RIVER
(504)
Bonnell, L.

NEW GLASGOW
*
Brown, C. M.

O'LEARY STATION
(757)
Bruvels, N.
Dewar, C. M.
Dewar, L. G.

SOURIS
(1,537)
Kassner, E.

SUMMERSIDE
(8,611)
Beer, J. K. GenSurg
Callaghan, W. E.
Cameron, S. R.
Downing, J. B. IntMed
Gallant, G. J.
Jodrey, J. F.
Lee, G. H.
Mackay, W. A.
McNeill, H. B.
Moore, T., ObstGyn
Moyse, H. W.
Saunders, J. L.
Simpson, J. C. GenSurg

TYNE VALLEY
(200)
Robinson, G. E.

WELLINGTON
(1,062)
Reid, R. A.

Quebec

ABITIBI EAST
(*)
Arsenault, M.

ACTON VALE
(3,960)
Auger, L. D. PH(P.Q.)
Gauthier, R.
Laliberte, L.

* Population not separately available.

ALBANEL
(920)
St Cyr, R.

ALMA
(13,309)
Allary, B., PH(P.Q.)
Aube, L. R.
Auger, A.
Bouchard, R.
Couture, G. M., GenSurg.
Dorion, R.
Dube, Y., Anaes.
Fortin, R.
Gagnon, J., Otol(P.Q.)
Gagnon, M.
Gagnon, P. P., Otol
Gervais, G.
Jean, L. Anaes
Larouche, R., IntMed., Cardiol(P.Q.)
Michaud, A. GenSurg
Morin, B. Otol (P.Q.)
Noel, G., IntMed (Gastro) (P.Q.)
Perron, M.
Tremblay, L. M., Paed.
Tremblay, P. E., OrthSurg

AMOS
(6,086)
Bernier, A. G.
Berube, R., PH (P.Q.)
Chiasson, A., GenSurg(P.Q.)
Cossette, Jacquelin
Derome, L.
Dion, J.
Doyon, M., GenSurg
Fortin, R.
Godard, R.
Letendre, J., OrthSurg(P.Q.)
Richard, M.

AMQUI
(3,659)
Arsenault, L. J. A., GenSurg.
Blouin, L. C.
Boudreau, M. A.
Bourgeois, D., GenSurg
Guerette, G. E.
Roy, P. E.

ANCIENNE LORETTE
(3,956)
(Sub. P.O. of Quebec City)
Cote, R.
Coulombe, Giselle
Darveau, R.
Drouin, B.
Perretier, L.
Robataille, J. M

ANSE-ST.-JEAN
(Cte. Chicoutimi)
*****
d'Entremont, F.

ARMAGH
(914)
Talbot, R.

ARTHABASKA
(2,983)
Becotte, Jean Marie GenSurg
Gagne, J. G., Anaes.
Langelier, L. P. D & TRad
Larouche, G., IntMed (P.Q.)
Nguyen, D., DiagRad.
Piche, G. Anaes
Royer, J-L-L., Ophth

ARUNDEL
(350)
Henry, R. B.

ARVIDA
(14,460)
Belzile, A.
Dumont, P. M., ObstGyn.
Gagnon, R. GenSurg (P.Q.)
Gilbert, H. H. GenSurg (P.Q.)
Lacerte, M.
Letourneau, P. E.
Raymond, G.
Thibault, J.

ASBESTOS
(11,083)
Bachand, L.
Boux, P.
Carignan, L.
Gilbert, C. A.
Granger, T. R.
Paul, W. R. GenSurg
Roberge, J. P.

ASTON JUNCTION
(401)
Rancourt, D.

AURIGNY
*
Arsenault, M.
Labrie, E.
Leboursdais, P. E.

AYER'S CLIFF
(743)
Pettigrew, J.

AYLMER EAST
(6,289)
Cavanagh, J. V. A.
Chagnon, J. P.
Gompf, J. E.
Lebel, G. A.
Lecours, R. H.

BAGOTVILLE
(5,629)
Claveau, C.
Gagnon, A. J.
Gagnon, R.
Simard, C. E.
Tanguay, L.

BAIE COMEAU
(7,956)
Beaudry-Remillard, Janine
Beaumont, E. J.
Di Gaspari, J.
Leclerc, C.
Lemay, R.
MacNeil, J. J. PlasSurg
Poole, N. L., GenSurg
Provencher, J.
Simard, G.
Simard, R.
Thurber, D.

BAIE DES SABLES
(735)
Jean, P.

BAIE D'URFE
(See Ste. Anne de Bellevue)

BAIE ST. PAUL
(4,674)
Allard, E.
Desgagnes, J. R.
Fiset, A.
Gaudreault, J. R.
Gilbert, H.
Jean, B., Psy

BAIEVILLE
(558)
Lemire, A.

BARRAUTE
(1,196)
Plourde, J.

BATISCAN
(231)
Lacasse, F.

BEACONSFIELD
(See Ste. Anne de Bellevue)

BEAUCEVILLE
(3,571)
Bernard, R.
Dallaire, R. R. D.
Fontaine, L.
Pomerleau, A.
Roy, A.
Tremblay, P.
Vezina-Voyer, Jacqueline, Anaes.
Voyer, J. P., GenSurg(P.Q.)

BEAUHARNOIS
(8,701)
Bonhomme, P. E.
Carignan, L.
Dubuc, G.
Marchand, L. J.

BEAUPORT
(9,195)
Chabot, M.
Cote, R. M.
Lalonde, R.
Marcoux, G.
Turcotte, L. B., D & TRad

BEAUPRE
(2,587)
Cote, J.
Renaud, G.

BEAUREPAIRE
(See Ste. Anne de Bellevue)

BEAURIVAGE
(518)
Nadeau, A.

BEDARDVILLE
(See Cite de Jacques Cartier)

BEDFORD
(2,860)
Boileau, H. J.
Messier, A.
Tougas, A.

BEEBE
(1,366)
Lapierre, G.

BELOEIL
(6,283)
Bachand, R.
Beaule, J. L.
Bergeron, J. C., DiagRad (P.Q.)
Campeau, A.
Cote, R.
Dansereau, R.
Dowd, A. H

BERTHIERVILLE
(3,708)
Denis, B.
Gendron, O. M.
Gervais, G.
Laferriere, U. PH (P.Q.)

BIC
(1,176)
Plante, L. J.

BIENVILLE
*****
Bourget, J. O. R.

BLACK LAKE
(4,185)
Fortier, C.
Lecours, H.

BOIS DES FILLON
(2,499)
Poirier' G.

BOLDUC
(1,176)
Begin, M.

BONAVENTURE
(804)
Boudreau, R.
Levesque, R.

BOUCHERVILLE
(7,408)
Auger, M.
Dagenais, F.
Jamharian, J., Anaes(P.Q.)
Lajoie, J. L.
Lamarre, P.
Michaud, C., Ophth
Raymond, R.
Tarte, P. D. Gastroent (P.Q.)

*** Population not separately available.**

BOURLAMAQUE
(3,344)
Lapointe, H., PhysMed. & Rehab.

BROMPTONVILLE
(2,722)
Caron, P.
Cloutier, A.

BROSSARD
(3,786)
Dyrda, I.
St-Denis, J. A., Paed.

BROUGHTON
(287)
Grenier, L.

BROWNSBURG
(3,617)
Cote, A. R.
Daigle, G. E.
Morin, J. R.

BUCKINGHAM
(7,421)
Begin, G-L., GenSurg
Belisle, P. E.
Coupal, J. P., Paed
Drouin, J. E.
Joubert, J. GenSurg (P.Q.)
Lemieux, R.
MacLachlan, P. N., GenSurg (P.Q.)
Turgeon, R.
Ugnat, F. A., IntMed.
Wallingford, F. M.

CABANO
(2,694)
Beaulieu, O.
Fortin, G.
Latulippe, L.

CACOUNA
(832)
Rioux, H.

CAMP VALCARTIER
(*)
Juneau, C.

CANDIAC
(1,053)
Desjardins, R.
LePage, J. M.
Vallee, H., PlasSurg, GenSurg (P.Q.)
Varnan, G. S., IntMed

CAP-AUX-MEULES
(761)
Brochu, O., GenSurg (P.Q.)
Huard, I.

CAP CHAT
(2,032)
Miville, D.
Pelletier, J. E.
Whittaker, R.

CAP D'ESPOIR
*
Gaudreault, Y.

CAP DE LA MADELEINE
(26,930)
Aubry, A., ObstGyn
Beaudet, M., GenSurg (P.Q.)
Bellemare, J. L.
Bisson, Lise, Anaes.
Cossette, A., Anaes, (P.Q.)
Coutu, G., Psy(P.Q.)
Gagnon, B.
Hubert, R. P.
Jacob, R.
Lafontaine, G.
Marchand, A. Cardiol (P.Q.)
Marcotte, G.
Michaud, L. V.
Normandin, A., Pulm.Dis.&T.B. (P.Q.)
Vincent, P. R.
White, L., DiagRad(P.Q.)

CAP ST-IGNACE
(1199)
Brochu, D.

CARLETON-SUR-MER
(138)
Leblanc, J. M.

CARTIERVILLE
(see Montreal)

CAUGHNAWAGA
(2,240)
Vuckovic, V.

CAUSAPSCAL
(3,463)
Bergeron, J. A.
Grenier, J.
Lavoie, R.

CHAMBLY
(3,737)
Barrette, A.
Laverge, D.
Ladouceur, J.
Lapierre, C.
St-Onge, P.

CHAMPLAIN
(754)
Bordeleau, N. J.
Hebert, G.
Lachance, R.

CHANDLER
(3,406)
Bessette, M. GenSurg (P.Q.)
Czitrom, A.
Daigneault, G.
David, D.

CHAPAIS
(2,363)
Pelletier, F. E.

CHAPEAU
(546)
Keon, C. H.

CHARETTE
(488)
Cossette, H.

CHARLEMAGNE
(3,072)
Mercure, J.

CHARLESBOURG
(See Quebec City)

CHARNY
(4,194)
Alarie, Sylva
Gervais, G.
Gilbert, P. GenSurg (P.Q.)
Grondin, G.

CHATEAUGUAY
(7,593)
Boyer, C.
Desrochers, G.
Labarre, G.
Laberge, J. R.
Lafleur, J.
Pilan, L. J.
Preville, G., Anaes(P.Q.)
St. Onge, F.
Sauve, J.
Woelber, W.

CHATEAUGUAY BASIN
(7,573)
Williams, I. K.

CHATEAU RICHER
(1,837)
Mathieu, C.
Turmel, G.

CHELSEA
(310)
Sowby, F. D.

CHENEVILLE
(740)
Lenoir, E.

CHIBOUGAMAU
(8,200)
Brisson, B. P.
Lamarre, J. P.
Menard, C., GenSurg(P.Q.)
Morel, R.
Tardif, J.

CHICOUTIMI
(105,009)
Angers, B., IntMed., Cardiol(P.Q.)
Aubin, G., Paed
Beaudry, L. E., GenSurg
Belanger, G., Ophth
Belanger, M., Path (P.Q.)
Belisle, G.
Bergeron, C., GenSurg, Gyn (P.Q.)
Bertho, E. M. GenSurg
Blais, P. E. Anaes
Boivin, R. Anaes (P.Q.)
Boudreault, G. IntMed (P.Q.) Cardiol (P.Q.)
Brassard, R., Anaes.
Brisson, F. GenSurg (P.Q.)
Bruneau, J. Path (P.Q.)
Carrier, H. OrthSurg (P.Q.)
Charbonneau, A., ThorSurg (P.Q.) GenSurg (P.Q.)
Claveau, J. C. Paed
Claveau, R., IntMed, Haem (P.Q.)
Claveau, R.
Comtois, G. Anaes (P.Q.)
Deschenes, A., Ophth.
De Varennes, P. H. D&TRad
Dugas, A., Anaes
Duhaime, J. H. L. Ophth,Otol
Fernet, P. Y., Path
Fortin, B. PH (P.Q.)
Fortin, J. P., DiagRad (P.Q.)
Gadbois, J.
Gagne, E.
Gagnon, F., IntMed, (Cardiol)
Gagnon, G., GenSurg(P.Q.)Thor Surg (P.Q.) Gyn (P.Q.)
Gagnon, J. B. IntMed (P.Q.)
Gagnon, J. L., Anaes.
Gagnon, J. L., GenSurg
Gaudreault, L. PH (P.Q.)
Gauthier, G. A.
Gauthier, G. T., Ophth., Otol(P.Q.)
Gauthier, M.
Genest, L. E., D & TRad
Gosselin, J. L. IntMed
Guimond, R., PhysMed & Rehab
Guimond, V. ObstGyn
Guimont, A., OrthSurg
Jean, J. D., Cardiovasc (P.Q.)
Jourdain, Camille DermSyph
Lachance, J. C.
Lachance, W., PathBact, Haem (P.Q.)
Laperriere, V. OrthSurg
Lapointe, G. IntMed
Lapointe, G. A. Ophth
Lapointe, M.
Lapointe, V. D&TRad
Larochelle, J., Paed
Larouche, D.
Lavoie, J. C. Otol
Lavoie, R., Otol
Leblanc, G. L., NeurSurg
LeBlond, S. IntMed
Lemieux, H., Gastroent(P.Q.)
Lessard, Alphee, IntMed (P.Q.)
Levesque, L. M.
Madore, F. ObstGyn (P.Q.)
Masson, R.
Nadeau, D.
Plourde, Camille, Psy
Pouliot, P. E., Path(P.Q.)
Prive, L.
Provencher, B., Allerg (P.Q.)

* Population not separately available.

CHICOUTIMI (Cont'd)
Rainville, B.
St.-Cyr, J., PhysMed & Rehab
Saint-Pierre, Claire
Saucier, R. Psy (P.Q.)
Savard, L.
Simard, F. X., Anaes
Simard, J. E. GenSurg
Simard, L. P. Urol
Sormany, Y. Anaes
Tremblay, G. OrthSurg (P.Q.)
Tremblay, G. C.
Tremblay, G. O. Pulm. Dis. & T.B. (P.Q.)
Tremblay, G. P.
Tremblay, G. W., Ophth, Otol
Tremblay, L. Urol
Tremblay, M. Paed
Vandal, L.
Wells, J. P., IntMed.
Wells, N., IntMed., GenSurg (P.Q.)

CHOMEDY
(30,445)
(Dist. of Montreal)
Cabana, J. E., GenSurg
Choquette, J. L.
Cohen, S., Paed
Dery, P. R.
Giguere, P. H., Paed.
Grenier, Jocelyn
Gruffy, M. E.
Guilbault, G. H.
Hemond, B. G.
Kutschera, J. N.
Legresley, L. P., Path.
Mandor, E.
Morin, P. A.
Schiettekatte, F.
Tarjan, G., PH(P.Q.)
Zylberszac, B.

CITE DE JACQUES CARTIER
(40,807)
Achim, R.
Alaby, A. G., Otol
Allard, R., PhysMed(P.Q.)
April, J., Paed(P.Q.)
Arbour, J. C. DiagRad
Arbour, P., Otol.
Archambault, R.
Ast, Helga, Psy (P.Q.)
Aubry, U., Anaes
Beaudoin, R.
Beland, G. A., GenSurg (P.Q.) Urol.
Bergeron, C., GenSurg., Gyn(P.Q.)
Bernard, J. A.
Bessette, J., Anaes
Blais, J. M.
Blais, M.
Blanchard, P. L., ObstGyn.
Boisvert-Theoret, Suzanne, Path (PQ)
Boulais, C., ObstGyn
Brown, E. C.
Canakis, A. I. P., OrthSurg
Cange, R., IntMed., Cardiol(P.Q.)
Cassidy, L. E., IntMed (P.Q.)
Chalut, P. GenSurg
Chaput, N.
Charest, G. A.
Chartrand, G.
Cop-Hodjera, Branislava M., Anaes
Cote, L.
Cyr, R.
Daigle-Lock, Rita, Paed
De Serres, G.
Deslippe, P. A., Anaes
Desmarais, G., ObstGyn
Dupuis, M., PhysMed & Rehab.
Durand, L.
Dussault, F.
Dussault, G.
Ferron, J.
Ferron, L. P., Psy (P.Q.)
Flint, Clare
Gaudet, A. OrthSurg
Gingras, P.
Girard, R.
Gravel, R.
Graveline C., TherRad (P.Q.)
Harpin, D.
Helle, S. J., IntMed
Huot, R. E.
Jodoin, P.
Joly, J. G.
Lackey, A. A.
Lamarre, F.
Lamarre, R.
Lamothe, A., Obst (P.Q.)
Lanctot, J.
Laurin, G., GenSurg (P.Q.)
Leblanc, J. L. Paed
Legault, M.
Legault, P., Cardiol (PQ)
Legendre, J.
Letellier, E. H.
Liard, J., Psy (P.Q.)
Marchessault, J. H. V. Paed
Marcil, R.
Mathieu, J. E. GenSurg
McNally, L. B.
Menard, A. E.
Michaud, J. B.
Millette, H.
Mongeau, S.
Morissette, G., Paed
Ouellet, Camille, Anaes
Patry, B.
Payette, H.
Peltier, J. A.
Perreault, H., Anaes
Perreault, J. P., DiagRad
Phaneuf, M., GenSurg.
Phillips, J. N.
Pinault, A., Anaes.
Plamondon, R.
Plante, G.
Randall, M. T. Clare, Paed
Reesal, M. R.
Renzi, N., IntMed (P.Q.)
Rioux, P., Anaes(P.Q.)
Roberge, J. J.
Rochon, J. L.
Rolland, P. E.
Roux, R.
Samson, L. M.
Shackleton, Monica
Shooner, F., Anaes
Tardif, A.
Tchang, P., GenSurg (P.Q.)
Tessier, J. L. Ophth (P.Q.)
Trudeau, G.
Trudeau, L. A.
Venne, J.
Vigneau, J. Anaes
Wasilewska, Julia
Williams, W.

CLARKE CITY
(834)
Smith, R.

CLERMONT
(3,114)
McNicoll, A.
Ouellet, L.

COATICOOK
(6,906)
Caron, R.
Germain, G.
Samson, A.
Samson, G. A. GenSurg (P.Q.)

COMO
(806)
Elliott, N. W., NeurSurg
Johnston, K. B., Ophth.

COMPTON
(536)
Berube, M.

CONTRECOEUR
(2,007)
Brunet, G.
Coallier, J. A.
Desmaris, M.

COOKSHIRE
(1,412)
Bourdrias, J.
Lepine, A. M.

COTEAU DU LAC
(699)
Marcotte, M.

COTE ST. MICHEL
(Dist. of Montreal)

COURCELLES
(498)
Groslouis, L.

COURVILLE
(4,675)
Pouliot, C.
Roy, J. C.

COWANSVILLE
(7,055)
Bisson, G. E., GenSurg.
Daigle, J. M.
Desmeules, J.
Duprat, G. E. GenSurg
Langlois, Y.
Monast, N. E.
Mooney, M. C., GenSurg
Pincott, R. S.
Roy, P. E.

CROYDON
(See Cite de Jacques Cartier)

DANVILLE
(2,563)
Johnston, H. A.
Letendre, G.
Proulx, L.
Roy R.

DAVELUYVILLE
(732)
Thibodeau, R.

DELISLE
(See St. Coeur de Marie)

DELSON
(2,075)
Pie, L.

DESBIENS
(1,969)
Lachance, V.

DESCHAILLONS
(1,697)
Lemay, R.

DESCHAMBAULT
(1,058)
Gignac, A. B. PH (P.Q.)

DEUX MONTAGNES
(7276)
Letondal, P., Paed
Roberge, Y.
Varin, N.

DISRAELI
(3,077)
Dubreuil, R. PH (P.Q.)
Langis, L. J.
Plante, J. M.
Rochette, L.

DOLBEAU
(6,052)
Bergeron, D.
Cote, G.
Dionne, J. M.
Lauzier, L. GenSurg
Lou, P. GenSurg
Maltais, B.
Morin, N.
St. Cyr, L.
Tremblay, L.-M., Paed

*** Population not separately available.**

DOLLARD-DES-ORMEAUX
(1,248)
Borzecki, Julita, Anaes
Genender, L. J., GenSurg.
Hemmings, L. M., GenSurg. (P.Q.)
Lorant, D., Paed(P.Q.)
Paradis, J. D., ObstGyn.

DONNACONA
(4,819)
Cantin, R.
Cauchon, R.
Huot, A.

DORION
(4,999)
Clement, M.
Cuillerier, J. F.
Edwards, P. A. Pulm. Dis. & T.B. (P.Q.)
Gendron, O.
Sauve, C.

DORVAL
(See Lachine)

DRUMMONDVILLE
(39,307)
Allaire, A., OrthSurg(P.Q.)
Arsenault, G.
Beauchesne, G., Ophth, Otol (P.Q.)
Blouin, C.
Carrier, J. G.
D'Argencourt, G. GenSurg, ObstGyn
Gendron, A.
Goyer, M. Anaes
Grondin, C.
Houle, N. J., IntMed
Lamoureaux, J. PH (P.Q.)
Leblanc, M., D & T Rad.
Lemaire, J. G. GenSurg (P.Q.)
Masse, L. GenSurg (P.Q.)
Melancon, W. GenSurg
Milette, R., Anaes (P.Q.)
Millet, R.
Morin, J. M., Ophth, Otol(P.Q.)
Paille, G., GenSurg
Paille, J. B., GenSurg
Pelletier, N.
Pion, P. P.
Quintal, J. F.
Rodrigue, G. D & TRad
St. Onge, L. F. G. Paed (P.Q.)
Saint-Pierre, H. L. IntMed
Soucy, F. C.
Therrien, R.
Turcotte, A. Obst (P.Q.)
Turmel, E.
Vachon, R.

DUVERNAY
(See Montreal)

EAST ANGUS
(4,759)
Guerette, O.
Larose, M.
Levesque, L.

EAST BROUGHTON STATION
(1,136)
Groleau, V. E.

ESTCOURT
(737)
Savard, R.

FABREVILLE
(5,213)
Berankova, Vera
Kaufmann, N. R.
Lesperance, J., D & TRad
Menard, J. A.
Perreault, G.

FARNHAM
(6,354)
Beaudin, R.
Cardin, J. L.
Clouarte, A.
Gerin-Lajoie, G.

Jacques, E.
LaRoche, G.
Lavigne, J.

FERME-NEUVE
(1,969)
Paquette, J. C.

FORESTVILLE
(1,529)
Ouellet, J. G.
Rheaume, D.

FORT CHIMO
(480)
Bourdua, S.

FORT COULONGE
(1,823)
Laycock, H. E.
Rabb, H. R.

FORTIERVILLE
(559)
Laliberte, J.

GAGNON
(1,900)
Harvey, G. H.
Lemieux, G., GenSurg.

GAMELIN
*
Dubois, J. M., Psy
Julien, F.

GARTHBY
(502)
Menard, A.

GASPE
(2,603)
Albert, G., IntMed.
Aparicio, C., DiagRad(P.Q.)
Beaudet, P. E.
Coffin, E., ObstGyn (P.Q.)
Cotton, O., GenSurg (P.Q.)
Duguay, G. H., Otol.
Fortier, A. G., GenSurg
Grenier, P. E., PulmDis & T.B. (P.Q.)
Pelletier, L., GenSurg
Pouliot, M. A., Paed (P.Q.)
Rioux, J. E., GenSurg
Roy, P. A., Path (P.Q.)
Talbot, J. L.

GATINEAU
(13,022)
Coupal, J. P., Paed
Cousineau, J.
Desrosiers, B.
Simurda, J., GenSurg
Vachon, P. E.

GATINEAU POINTE
(8,857)
Lemay, G.
Robinson, H., Paed

GIFFARD
(see Quebec City)

GRACEFIELD
(676)
Blais, R.
Martin, P.

GRANBY
(31,463)
Auger, P.
Blais, N., GenSurg (P.Q.)
Bonin, R.
Brown, B. S. W.
Bruneau, R. F.
Brunelle, S.
Cote, S. G.
Derome, A.
Desparts, F.
Dube, Marie J.
Dube, R.
Duchesne, A., Anaes (P.Q.)
Dumouchel, J. P., D & TRad
Dupont, R.
Gagnon, J. M. Cardiol (P.Q.)
Guertin, J.

Labranche, D. A.
Lavigne, A., ObstGyn (P.Q.)
Leclerc, L.
Lecoq, J. P. A.
Noiseux, M.
Pearl, H.
Picard, H.
Quenneville, E.
Rochon, G., Ophth, Otol (P.Q.)
Rodrigue, M.
St. Jean, C., GenSurg

GRANDE BAIE
*
Gobeil, L. J.

GRANDE RIVIERE
(1,181)
Clapperton, G.
Duguay, C.

GRAND'MERE
(15,806)
Beaudet, A.
Bedard, P., Anaes
Brassard, V. N., Anaes
Brunet, D.
Buisson, J.
Busque, D.
Cossette, R., GenSurg.
Croteau, L.
Dessureault, R., Path (P.Q.)
Frenette, L. A., GenSurg
Gagnon, J. B., GenSurg
Hooper, H. S., GenSurg
Lavallee, J. G., ObstGyn
Lemieux, J. R.
Lupien, M.
Mondor, L., Anaes (P.Q.)
Morin, B.
Normand, D., GenSurg (P.Q.)
Poisson, A.
Poulin, N.
Robert, R., IntMed(P.Q.)
Tessier, J. G., D&TRad
Turgeon, C. A.
Vermette, R., GenSurg (P.Q.)

GRANDE VALLEE
(824)
Melanson, E. R.

GREENFIELD PARK
(see Cite de Jacques Cartier)

GRENVILLE
(1,330)
Bowes, G. C.
Dupont, C. A.

GRINDSTONE (Magdalen Islands) see AURIGNY, P.Q.

HAM NORD
(573)
Frenette, R.

HARRINGTON HARBOUR
(479)
Hodd, D. G.

HAUTERIVE
(5,980)
Allard, A., GenSurg (P.Q.)
Bouffard, M.
Chasse, R.
Larouche, N.
Martel, R., GenSurg
Morissette, Y. C.
Pruneau, C.
St.-Pierre, P.
Thibault, R.

HAVRE ST. PIERRE
(2,407)
Cote, L., GenSurg (P.Q.)

HEBERTVILLE
(1,604)
Potvin, L.

HEMMINGFORD
(778)
Abram, A. J.
Belanger, P. R.

*** Population not separately available.**

HENRYVILLE
(711)
Saindon, D.
HUBERDEAU
(605)
Rondeau, G.
HUDSON
(1,668)
Barrette, G.
Johnson, C. A.
Runnells, G. W.
HUDSON HEIGHTS
(1539)
Black, K. D., GenSurg.
HULL
(56,929)
Amours, O. D., Pulm. Dis. & T.B. (P.Q.)
Barrette, M.
Bartulica, N.
Bedard, G., GenSurg
Beznak, N. L.
Bisson, J. R.
Bouchard, J. P., Psy (P.Q.)
Brisson, G., GenSurg.; ObstGyn (P.Q.)
Brisson, J. M., Otol
Bundock, B.
Charette, H., D & TRad
Coupal, J.-P., Paed
Coutu, N., GenSurg (P.Q.)
D'Amours, O., PulmDis & T.B. (P.Q.)
Demers, M. A., ObstGyn
Desjardins, E. L.
Despins, C., Haem (P.Q.)
Dion, R. M., GenSurg
Douville, E. L., ThorSurg
Faubert, G. C., OrthSurg (P.Q.)
Fortier, C., D & TRad
Gagne, A. A., Anaes
Gagne, G., GenSurg (P.Q.)
Gariepy, J. J.
Gay, G.
Gosselin, F. D., PH (P.Q.)
Gregoire, B., Ophth.
Harnois, G., Psy.
Hebert, L., Paed (P.Q.)
Isabelle, G.
Jolicoeur, G., IntMed
Jules, D. R.
Labelle, P. E.
Lachance, R., Pulm Dis & T.B. (P.Q.)
Lacoursiere, A.
Laferriere, R., DiagRad.
Lair, R. H
Lambert, B., Ophth, Otol (P.Q.)
Lamont, J. E., Paed.
Lamothe, L.
Larose, C. L., Allergy (P.Q.), IntMed (P.Q.)
Leblanc, J. J., Anaes
Leboeuf, J. L.
Lessard, P.
Letarte, A., Paed (P.Q.)
Martin, J. H.
Meilleur, P. A.
Morissette, J. G., OrthSurg (P.Q.)
Panneton, M.
Parent, B. D&TRad
Parent, J., OrthSurg (P.Q.)
Pepin, A.
Pepin, G., Obst (P.Q.)
Petcovitch-Panneton Leposova
Pichette, J. L., GenSurg (P.Q.)
Pilon, H., Anaes
Plouffe, D.
Robinson, P-M., IntMed
Roy, J. D., IntMed (Cardiol) (P.Q.)
Sheridan, B. B., Ophth
Simard, J. C.
Sirois, J. L., Path
Sirois, P. E., Anaes
Slater, S. Urol
Voyer, R., GenSurg
HUNTINGDON
(3,134)
Cameron, K. G.
Lefebvre, G. T. G.
McCrimmon, F. G., GenSurg.
IBERVILLE
(7,588)
Bedard, G.
Ethier, F.
Lacasse, J., Anaes
Laflamme, H., IntMed
Pare, H.
ILE PERROT
(1,344)
Lavoie, B.
ISLE VERTE
(1,517)
Drapeau, N.
Plowde, J. L.
JOLIETTE
(18,088)
Aall-Jilex, Louise M., Psy.
Acked, E.
Amyot, R.
Bohemier, J. A., Ophth, Otol (P.Q.)
Bonin, G., GenSurg
Boulard, G., DiagRad
Boyer, C. M.
Chevrette, G. A.
Chiasson, J. P., Psy (P.Q.)
Desrosiers, H., Path (P.Q.)
Dhaiti, J. J. G., IntMed.
Ducharme, A.
Dufresne, Y.
Ferland, L.
Ferland, S., GenSurg (P.Q.)
Forest, J. E., GenSurg (P.Q.)
Gauthier, M.
Gauthier, Y., OrthSurg
Gautreau, R. M., OrthSurg (P.Q.)
Geoffroy, A.
Gervais, P.
Harnois, M.
Henault, P. E.
Jilek, W., Psy.
Joly, R.,
Lafortune, C., GenSurg.
Lafortune, J. A., Anaes (P.Q.)
Lanoie, J. M., IntMed (Cardiol) **(P.Q.)**
Laporte, J.
Laporte, L. P., Urol (P.Q.)
Laporte, S.
Magnan, R.
Masse, R., GenSurg (P.Q.)
Mireault, J. P.
Nobert, A.
Perales, A.
Piette, J. E., GenSurg
Poulin, R.
Preville, R.
Quenneville, R.
Rajotte, P., Psy
Regaudie, B., Paed.
Roberto, Sarah
Roussin, C. A.
Schnurr, Ilona
Teixeira, J. A. R., Psy.
Zuardy, P.
JONQUIERE
(105,009)
Beaudoin, G., GenSurg
Belanger, H., ObstGyn
Bouchard, G. R., Otol (P.Q.)
Boucher, D.
Boucher, R., DiagRad
Brassard, J. E.
Crepeau, M., OrthSurg
Delisle, R., IntMed.
Gagnon, J. S., GenSurg.
Groleau, F., Path (P.Q.)
Houde, J. A., IntMed, Cardiol (P.Q.)
Lambert, Y.
Lapointe, A., Anaes.
Lapointe, A., Paed (P.Q.)
Lemay, Y., GenSurg
Marchand, P., Paed
Munger, L. P.
Paquet, P. P., Anaes
Plamadon, G.
Poirier, F., Anaes
St-Georges, F.
Simard, R. Paed (P.Q.)
Tremblay, J. A.
Tremblay, R.
Vaillancourt, H., GenSurg (P.Q.)
KAZABAZUA
(200)
Kearns, J. A., GenSurg
KENOGAMI
(11,816)
Caron, G.
Fortin, J. P.
Laliberte, L. A.
Marchand, J. E.
KILDARE—see St. Ambroise de Kildare
KILMAR
(116)
Dunn, E. V.
KNOWLTON
(1,392)
Douglass, A. S.
Miller, C. H.
Skeet, H. J.
L'ABORD A PLOUFFE
(see Montreal)
LABELLE
(1,230)
Bergeron, R., GenSurg
Dufour, F.
Huapaya, L. V.
L'Allier, P.
LAC-AU-SAUMON
(1,552)
Martin, R.
LAC-AUX-SABLES
(857)
Girard, G. H.
LAC BEAUPORT
*
Raymond, W. J. A.
LAC BOUCHETTE
(911)
Beland, L.
LAC EDOUARD
(250)
Descarreaux, G., IntMed (T.B.)
Pelletier, J. J.
Rousseau, L., IntMed (T.B.)
LAC ETCHEMIN
(2,299)
Dugre, J. R.
Perron, M.
Poirier, J. A.
Rodrique, B.
Taillon, A. P.
LACHEVROTIERE
(126)
Mayrand, L.
LACHINE
(38,630)
Adams, K. W., Ophth
Albert, J. R., IntMed., Haem (P.Q.)
Amalraj, S., IntMed.
April, J., Paed (P.Q.)
Archambault, P., DiagRad.
Bachand, A.
Barron, L. R., ObstGyn
Barnabe, G.

*** Population not separately available.**

LACHINE (Cont'd)
Beauchemin, J. M.
Beaudreau, C., Gastroent(P.Q.)
Beaulieu, R. W.
Berkson, N., GenSurg
Bonnier, J. G., PH (P.Q.)
Bourbonnais, A.
Brennan, R. L.
Brennand, Shirley, Paed
Brown, E. J., GenSurg
Cageorge, J. D.
Champoux, M.
Chaput, N.
Charters, J. S., Paed
Chartrand, J. L.
Cirkovic, M., Anaes
Cooper, B. M.
Cousineau, L. E., Haem(P.Q.)
Crawford, E. M., D & TRad
Daoust, P.
Decary, C., IntMed (P.Q.)
Dixon, W. G., ObstGyn
Dubois, J. M., Psy
Duplantis, F., Neur.
Emanuel, E., Psy
Emo, R. G., IntMed.
Farkouh, E. F., GenSurg.
FitzGerald, P. J., DiagRad
Fortie, R. Y.
Galeam, J., Path(P.Q.)
Garon, N., Obst (P.Q.)
Gatien, L. H., Anaes
Gaudet, O. P.
Gauron, J. G.
Gerard, O.
Gordon, R.
Goulet, G., DiagRad.
Grant-Whyte, I.
Gulyas, Julia, Paed
Hamel, C. J. C., Paed.
Hamel, P. C., GenSurg (P.Q.)
Harkness, J. J., GenSurg
Haslam, L. C.
Hay, J.
Hemmings, M. L., GenSurg (P.Q.)
Hewitson, A. G., Paed
Houle, J. A., OrthSurg.
Hyndman, W. W. B., GenSurg (P.Q.)
Jasmin, A.
Lachance, M., GenSurg(P.Q.)
Lamoth, M.
Landry, J. J.
Laporte, J., Psy(P.Q.)
Larocque, A., GenSurg (P.Q.)
Larocque, A.
Laurendeau, P., Otol(P.Q.)
Lavallee, B. W.
Leblanc, J. L., Paed
Leduc, A. M.
Lefebvre, A.
Lefebvre, J. A. F.
Lefebvre, R., Path (P.Q.)
Leith, A. B., Ophth
Lewis, J. W.
Linkletter, A. M., ObstGyn
Luke, J. C., GenSurg.
Lussier, C., GenSurg (P.Q.)
MacDonald, J. F.
McDougall, H. A., GenSurg (P.Q.)
McDowell, W.
Maheu, J. O., PH(P.Q.)
Marksfield, W. C., GenSurg
Martin, J., GenSurg (P.Q.)
McMillan, G. C., Path
Moore, F. C., IntMed
Morris, L. C., IntMed
Moyle, A. H.
Murphy, C. W.
O'Regan, K. B.
Paquin, H., GenSurg (P.Q.)
Parent, J. F.
Parent, J. G.
Perron, L., IntMed.
Poirier, J. P., Paed
Preville, G., Anaes (P.Q.)
Pringle, D. F.
Ranger, H., Anaes
Richter, H. A., Anaes.
Rochon, J. L.
Rotman, L., GenSurg
Roy, G. T.
St. Martin, R. W., Paed (P.Q.)
Sanchez-Arroyo, E., DiagRad (P.Q.)
Saucier, C.
Scherer, G.
Schiffman, Stella
Shamsie, S. J., Psy.
Sharp, J. D., Paed
Shepherd, R. W.
Simmons, S. P.
Smith, N. E., ObstGyn
Soicher, R. B.
Stewart, R. R., IntMed.
Swaine, R. L.
Sweet, R. L., GenSurg
Terry, E. M.
Uhthoff, A. L., Anaes
Vigeant, J., ObstGyn
Vulpe, M., Neur(P.Q.)
Watanabe, S., Path (P.Q.)
Wiglesworth, F. W., PathBact

LACHUTE
(7,568)
Bissonnette, M. X., GenSurg
Christie, J. E.
Lavigne, R.
MacKimmie, J. C.
MacKimmie, Suzanne S.
Middleton, L. A.
Papineau, M.
Percival, R.
Prevost, P.
Saindon, Z.
Sauve, A.
Turcotte, L., PH (P.Q)

LAC MEGANTIC
(7,016)
Aubut, J. E., Anaes (P.Q.)
Durand, G. E.
Grenier, R.
Huard, J.
Lamond, R.
Michaud, R. C.
Noel, G.
Roy, B. J. E.

LACOLLE
(1,191)
Belisle. L. G. G
Desgroseilliers, Irenee
Langlois, Y.

LA GUADELOUPE
(1,734)
Roy, L.

LA MALBAIE
*
Bergeron, J. B.
Jean, C., PH(P.Q.)
Lacoursiere, V.
Lambert, J.
Rochette, M., Ophth, Otol(P.Q.)

LAMBTON
(701)
Chabot, J. E.

LANDRAIE (Co. Berthierville)
(*)
Lacourse, M.

L'ANGE GARDIEN
(1,543)
Levesque, G. H.

L'ANNONCIATION
(1,046)
Cartier, J.
Cartier, J., Jrn.
Groh, G. J.
Kalayci, N.
Koryak, D. T.
Rizza, Marta
Sterlin, C., Psy
Trsic, J. M.
Yurtcu, A.
Zamansedeh, D.

LANORAIE
(1,060)
Mongeau, J. G.

L'ANSE ST. JEAN
(250)
Masson, R.

LA PATRIE
(518)
Cabana, M.

LA POCATIERE
(3086)
Bastarache, Marie S.
Bastarache, W., GenSurg.
Dallaire, G.
Dumais, J.
Mercier, A.
Ouellet, B.
Raymond, R. M.

LAPRAIRIE
(7328)
Belanger, A.
Clermont, A.
Daigneault, B.
Deslippe, G.
Gouin, L.
Hebert, J. G.
Lamarche, J. J.

LA SALLE
(see Lachine)

LA SARRE
(3,944)
Balthazard, Y.
Belanger, R.
Belleau, L. P. G.
Bernier, J. M. W.
Paradis, J., GenSurg.
Racicot, M.
Rheault, G.

L'ASSOMPTION
(4,448)
de Grace, M.
Gascon, L. P.
Gauthier, J. B.
Payette, L.

LATERRIERE
(650)
Cote, G., PH (P.Q.)

LA TUQUE
(13,023)
Beaulieu, D.
Bergeron, P.
Crete, C.
Gregoire, C. J. A., GenSurg.
L'Heureux, J. A.
Loiselle, G., IntMed., Cardiol (P.Q.)
Michaud, L. J., GenSurg
Potvin, V., GenSurg
Rivard, P. L., GenSurg
Tremblay, G. A., Anaes

LAURENTIDES
See St. Lin

LAURIERVILLE
(877)
Tremblay, G.

LAUZON
(11,533)
Bard, J. L.
Chabot, F.
Guay, L. P., DiagRad (P.Q.)
Morin, R. M.

LAVAL DES RAPIDES
(19,225)
Albert-Gravel, C. Y.
Bourret, A.
Dozois, J.

* Population not separately available.

LAVAL DES RAPIDES (Cont'd)
Frenette, H. C.
Gagnon, M.
Gareau, S. DiagRad.
Gauthier, D.
Gauthier, P. E., Pulm. Dis. & T.B.(P.Q.)
Gervais, J.
Gouin, M.
Gravel, H.
Harel, C., Anaes (P.Q.)
Harris, J .G.
Lasnier, R.
Lett, G.
Liboiron, G.
Mauriello, G.
Mayrand, Y., DiagRad(P.Q.)
Nadeau, G., Paed(P.Q.)
Pontbriand, R.
Racine, R., Psy (P.Q.)
Reeves, A., Haem (P.Q.)
Regimbald, A.
Savoie, P.
Tessier, B.
Tremblay, J. Y.

LAVAL OUEST
(5,440)
Maisonneuve, J.

LAVAL SUR-LE-LAC
(619)
Brunet, J. M.

LAVALTRIE
(1,034)
Lavallee, G.

LEMIEUX
(250)
Blanchette, O.

LENNOXVILLE
(3,692)
Dougan, A. A., Anaes
Klinck, W. J., GenSurg
Murray, J. C.
Taylor, J. L., IntMed
Tector, D. J. C.
Wells, T. J.

L'EPIPHANIE
(2,660)
Bourassa, M.
Desmarais, R.
Germain, C. E., PH(P.Q.)

LESAGE
(229)
Valiquette, J.

LES CEDRES
(426)
Clement, A. B.
Paquin, P. P.

LES EBOULEMENTS
(520)
Freve, L.

LES ESCOUMAINS
(1,607)
Tremblay, G. C.

LES SAULES
(4,096)
Caron, R. R.

LEVIS
(15,112)
Auger, S.
Belanger, A., Paed (P.Q.)
Belzil, B., Ophth, Otol (P.Q.)
Breton, J. P., PH(P.Q.)
Cadrin, G., ObstGyn(P.Q.)
Corrireau, R. A.
Corriveau, G.
Couture, J. P., Anaes(P.Q.)
Daigle, G. H., OrthSurg
Dube, J., PhysMed & Rehab.
Dussault, J. F.
Fafard, J. A., Ophth Otol
Gamache, A., Psy.
Gauthier, M., GenSurg
Gelinas, J. C., Ophth, Otol(P.Q.)
Genest, J. P.
Guay, R. M., Otol
Halle, M., Gastroent(P.Q.)
Houle, J. G., Urol(P.Q.)
Lamonde, J., ObstGyn
Lapointe, F.
Lemay, R., Paed (P.Q.)
Lessard, F.
Mercier, M., Ophth
Morin, R. M.
Morisset, J., Anaes
Nadeau, A.
Paradis, Y., PulmDis & T.B. (P.Q.), Cardiol (P.Q.)
Parent, R. J., Psy.
Potvin, R., Psy (P.Q.)
Powers, R., GenSurg (P.Q.)
Racicot, J., GenSurg
Racicot, P., GenSurg
Roy, L., GenSurg (P.Q.)
Roy, M., GenSurg (P.Q.)
Roy, R., Path (P.Q.)
Saucier, C.
Thivierge, C. M., IntMed (P.Q.)
Turgeon, P. L.
Turmel, J., ObstGyn
Valliere, L., Paed

LINIERE
(1,264)
Groleau, Y.

L'ISLET
(818)
Courcy, G.
Leclerc, L. P.

L'ISLETVILLE
(1,185)
Cote, J. M.
Jean, R.

LONGUEUIL
(see Cite de Jacques Cartier)

LORETTEVILLE
(6,520)
Boisvert, M. J., Anaes
Desrosiers, J. R. F., GenSurg
Drolet, H., Anaes (P.Q.)
Gignac, F.
Jean, G.
Lajeunesse, C.
Larochelle, L.
Paquet, E., IntMed
Pouliot, L., IntMed
Pronovost, R.
Rivard, J.
Savard, M.
Sirois, E.
Turgeon, C. A.

LORRAINE
(197)
Gregoire, H., DiagRad.

LOUISEVILLE
(4,140)
Bastrash, N.
Beland, G.
Dalcourt, A.
Latourelle, R., PH (P.Q.)
Marchand, M.
Mayrand, L.
Morinville, Y.
Plante, L.

LOURDES DU BLANC SABLO
(412)
Marcoux, Camille

LUCEVILLE
(1,423)
Gendreau, L.

LYSTER
(912)
Leblanc, P. E.

MACAMIC
(1,616)
Balthazard, L.
Drolet, G. P.
Gagnon, Camille
Vergati, A.

MAGOG
(13,139)
Beaudry, R., GenSurg (P.Q.)
Bergeron, J. L.
Blouin, R. H., GenSurg (P.Q.)
Boily, J.
Bryant, J. A.
Bureau-Blouin, Liliane
Goulet, J. P., IntMed(P.Q.)
Guertin, R.
Larue, V., Cardiol (P.Q.)
Monette, Lucie, Paed
Pellerin, W., Anaes (P.Q.)
Peloquin, L. P.
Rochefort, J., DiagRad (P.Q.)
Roy, A. D.
Scott, J. A.
Voyer, A., GenSurg (P.Q.)

MALARTIC
(6,992)
Dargis, G.
Roberge, J. P.

MANICOUAGAN
*****
Aube, M.
Laflamme, M.

MANIWAKI
(6,349)
Bresner, C.
Francoeur, J. A.
Gauthier-Leblanc, Terese
Genest, P.
Hetu, J.
Le Blanc, W. L.
L'Ecuyer, J. T.
Poliquin, L. P.

MANSEAU
(846)
Proulx, A.

MANSONVILLE
(463)
Jarema, M.

MARIA
(500)
Gagnon, A. J., GenSurg (P.Q.)
Gauthier, J-P., DiagRad(P.Q.)
Langis, J. C., Otol(P.Q.)
Langlais, J. C.
Martin, J. M. B., GenSurg(P.Q.)
Poirier, P. E., IntMed (P.Q.)

MARIEVILLE
(3,804)
Beauregard, L.
Mayer, J. L.
Poirier, H. W.

MASCOUCHE
(1,152)
Cantin, G.

MASKINONGE
(896)
Berneche, R.
Caron, F.
Hebert, P.

MASTAI
*
Blais, A.
Bouchard, M., Psy
Desrochers, G., NeurPsy.
Drolet, C., Psy
Magnan, J. A.
Martin, C. A., Psy, NeurPsy. (P.Q.)
Paradis, G.
Patry, L., Psy
Samson, M., DiagRad

MATAGAMI
(*)
Landry, R.

* Population not separately available.

MATANE
(9,190)
Ahier, A., Ophth, Otol (P.Q.)
Fradette, A.
Gagnon, J. R.
Gauthier, R.
Gosselin, J., GenSurg.
Langis, E.
Leclerc, M., GenSurg
Nolin, G. H.
Piuze, J. M.
Poitras, J. P.
Sarrasin, P., OrthSurg (P.Q.)

MATAPEDIA
(1,100)
Leblanc, P.

METABETCHOUAN
(1,962)
Brassard, G. R., Anaes
Lamy, F.
Plourde, A.

MISTASSINI
(3,461)
Audet, J. C.
Berard, P. E.

MONTEBELLO
(1,494)
Menard, M.

MONT JOLI
(6,178)
Beaulieu, F. X., PulmDis&T.B. (P.Q.)
Belanger, L., PulmDis & T.B. (P.Q.)
Boucher, D., PulmDis & T.B. (P.Q.)
Gauthier, H., IntMed(TB), Pulm. Dis. & TB(P.Q.)
Jean, L.
Kimpton, A. J., IntMed (TB) (P.Q.)
Langlais, J. C., PH(P.Q.)
Lemieux, L.
LePage, R. A.
Levesque, P. A.
Reid, H., PulmDis & TB (P.Q.)
Soucy, F., PulmDis&T.B.(P.Q.)

MONT LAURIER
(5,860)
Labelle, C.
Labelle, Jacqueline
Lachapelle, G.
Lachapelle, P.
Lemieux, J. E., GenSurg(P.Q.)
Ouelette, A. J.
Paquette, J. A.
Reid, G.
Roy, C. G.
Verdicchio, A.

MONTMAGNY
(6,850)
Darveau, J. C.
Dupuis, P. C., IntMed (P.Q.)
Gauthier, C., GenSurg
Laforest, M. G.
Lessard, R.
Plante, G.
Plourde, P., Anaes
Prevost, A. R.
Richard, A.

MONTMORENCY
(see Quebec City)

MONTREAL
(2,321,000)
Abbe, R. L., D & T Rad.
Abou-Shabanah, E. H.
Abramovitch, H., IntMed
Achong, E. H., Psy.
Achpise, A., GenSurg
Ackman, C .F. D., Urol(P.Q.)
Ackman, F. D., GenSurg, ThorSurg (P.Q.)
Adamkiewicz, Lidia M., IntMed (P.Q.)
Adams, G. T., DiagRad
Adams, K. W., Ophth
Adams, L. J., IntMed
Adams, S. T., Ophth
Addleman, W., IntMed., Gastroent(P.Q.)
Aerichide, N., IntMed (Cardiol) **(P.Q.)**
Agras, W. S., Psy
Aguayo, A. J., Neur
Ahad, V.
Alarie, R.
Albert, J. R., IntMed., Haem(P.Q.)
Alcindor, J. A., Path
Aldous, N. R., Psy
Alexander, B., Ophth
Alexander, W. J., DiagRad
Alexandris, A., Psy.
Allaire, J. N., DiagRad
Allan, C. M., GenSurg
Allard, A.
Allard, R., PhysMed (P.Q.)
Allard, R., Anaes
Allen, A.
Almuderia, M.
Amir-Jahed, A. K., GenSurg
Amos, E. A., Opth
Amyot, G., Obst
Amyot, L.
Amyot, R., NeurPsy.
Andermann, F., Neurol
Andrukaitis, E., Neur
Angel, A., IntMed.
Angioli, G., Gyn(P.Q.)
Anjilvel, G. M., GenSurg
Anthonisen, N. R.
Anthony, A.
Antic, B., Paed.
Antonuk, P., ObstGyn, (P.Q.)
Archambault, A. D., Anaes
Archambault, J., Anaes
Archambault, J. P. E.
Archambault, L. F.
Archambault, L. G., GenSurg
Archambault, L.
Archambault, P.
Archambault, P. A.
Archambault, P. R., IntMed (TB) Pulm Dis & TB(P.Q.)
Archambault, R.
Archambault, R. A., Paed(P.Q.)
Archambault, R. J., DiagRad.
Archambault, V.
Armstrong, B. P.
Aronoff, A., IntMed., Pulm. Dis. & TB(P.Q.)
Aronovitch, M., IntMed
Arronet, G. H., ObstGyn
Arsenault, A., Otol
Ashkenazy, W.
Asselin, J. P., GenSurg.
Attendu, C. A., Obst
Auclair, P.
Audet-Lapointe, J., Ophth., Otol
Audet-Lapointe, P., ObstGyn.
Audet, W.
Aufreiter, G., Psy (P.Q.)
Aufreiter, J., Psy (P.Q.)
Auger, H. R., PulmDis & T.B. (P.Q.)
Auld, P. A., Paed
Aumont, G.
Aumont, M.
Autotte, E. E., Paed (P.Q.)
Avon, I. C., DiagRad(P.Q.)
Ayllon-Galvin, R.
Ayre, W. B.
Azim, H., Psy
Azoulay, L.
Bacal, H. L., Paed, Aller(P.Q.)
Bachand, A., Haem(P.Q.)
Bachand, M., ObstGyn
Backer, D. R.
Badeaux, G.
Badeaux, J., Otol (P.Q.)
Bailey, G. M., ObstGyn (P.Q.)
Baillargon, B., IntMed
Baillargeon, J., IntMed, Gastroent (P.Q.)
Baillargeon, Y., DermSyph(P.Q.)
Bailly, R.
Bajusz, E.
Bakish, M.
Balangero, E. F., GenSurg
Ballem, C. M., IntMed., Gastroent(P.Q.)
Ballon, D. H., Otol
Ballon, H. C., GenSurg
Ballon, J. D., IntMed
Balthazard, J. G., Otol
Ban, T. A., Psy
Banerjee, S., OrthSurg
Banfill, S. M.
Banville, P.
Barbeau, A., Neur.
Barbeau, E., Anaes
Barcelo, R. IntMed
Bardari, A., GenSurg (P.Q.)
Baril, E., Paed (P.Q.)
Barker, C. S., IntMed
Barkun, H.
Baron, H. A., ObstGyn
Barrette, J. A., Ophth
Barron, L. R., ObstGyn
Barry, P. P., Anaes
Barry, T. L. J.
Barskey, S., IntMed, Card(P.Q.)
Barza, D., IntMed
Barza, S., Psy
Basecqz, G.
Bassett, B. C.
Bastien, G. P., GenSurg (P.Q.)
Bastien, J. C.
Bastien, M.
Bastien, P.
Bastomsky, C. H.
Batalion, H.
Bates, D. V.
Batshaw, Anne T.
Battersby, L. H.
Baxter, D. W., Neurol
Baxter, H. A., PlasSurg,GenSurg.
Baxter, J. D., Otol
Baxter, R. G., IntMed (P.Q.)
Bayne, R. D., IntMed
Bayrokal, S.
Bazin, A. R., GenSurg
Bazinet, D., Anaes
Bazinet, H. P., Paed
Beardmore, H. E.
Beaubien, F.
Beaubien, J. F., Psy (P.Q.)
Beaubien, Miriam F., Psy (P.Q.)
Beauchamp, M., GenSurg (P.Q.)
Beauchemin, J.
Beauchemin, J. C., GenSurg.
Beauchemin M., Anaes
Beaudet, A., Anaes (P.Q.)
Beaudoin, E.
Beaudoin, G. L.
Beaudoin, G., Psy (P.Q.)
Beaudoin, L. A., GenSurg
Beaudoin, L. P.
Beaudoin, R.
Beaudry, C., IntMed
Beaudry, J. M., PH(P.Q.)
Beaudry, P. E.
Beaudry, P. H., Paed
Beaulac, Gisele, Paed, (P.Q.)
Beaulieu, E. E. J., DiagRad.
Beaulieu, R. ClinPath (P.Q.)
Beaulnes, Aurele
Beaupre, J.
Beauregard, P., GenSurg
Beauvilliers, J., PH (P.Q.)
Beauvilliers, R. P.H. (P.Q.)
Bechard, M. Ophth (P.Q.)

* Population not separately available.

Montreal (Cont'd.)
Beck, J. C. IntMed
Becklake-McGregor, Margaret R. Pulm Dis & TB(P.Q.)
Bedard, E. Anaes
Bedard, P., GenSurg.
Begin, B. G. ThorSurg (P.Q.)
Beique, C., Paed (P.Q.)
Beique, L. GenSurg
Belair, A. Urol
Beland, J. E., Path (P.Q.)
Belanger, G., NeurSurg (P.Q.)
Belanger, G. A.
Belanger, J. E.
Belanger, J. F.
Belanger, J. M. GenSurg
Belanger, P. M. Urol
Belanger, R., D&TRad
Belanger, Y.
Belcourt, D. GenSurg (P.Q.)
Beldavs, J. T. Anaes
Belisle, F.
Belisle, L. G., Psy.
Belisle, L. P., DiagRad.
Belisle, M. IntMed
Beliveau, D. GenSurg (P.Q.)
Beliveau, L., Psy (P.Q.)
Bellemare, G. Derm, Syph (P.Q.)
Bellemare, H., IntMed
Bellemare, J. A.
Belliveau, N. J. GenSurg
Belmonte, Mimi Paed
Belque, C., Aller(P.Q.)
Belzile, M. J. B., Otol.
Benfey, J. G.
Benierakis, C., Psy
Benjamin, P., Paed
Bennetts, R. C. IntMed
Benoit, I.
Benoit, J.
Benoit, J., IntMed.
Benoit, M.
Benoit, R. H. Paed
Bensley, E. H. IntMed
Bentley, Dorothy C., IntMed (P.Q.)
Berard, M. J., ObstGyn.
Berard, R.
Bercovici, J. T. Otol
Bercovitch, D. D., IntMed.
Berdnikoff, G. Path
Berdnikoff, Katherine, Paed
Berger, D., D & TRad
Bergeron, L. GenSurg
Bergeron, O.
Berkman, P.
Berman G., Psy
Bernard, A. IntMed, Cardiol (P.Q.)
Bernard, G., Obst (P.Q.)
Bernard, L., GenSurg, Gyn(P.Q.)
Bernard, P. L. GenSurg (P.Q.)
Bernath, J., Cardiol(P.Q.)
Berne, M. Otol (P.Q.)
Bernier, G., ObstGyn.
Bernier, J. IntMed
Bernier, M.
Bernier, P. E.
Bernstein, F. IntMed (P.Q.)
Berthiaume, C. A. Ophth, Otol
Berthiaume, J., Anaes (P.Q.)
Berthiaume, L.
Berthiaume, M. Psy
Bertrand, C.
Bertrand, C., NeurSurg
Bertrand, G. G. P. NeurSurg
Bertrand, J. A., Bact.
Bertrand, L. R.
Bertrand, M.
Bertrand, P. Pulm. Dis. & T.B. (P.Q.)
Bertrand, P., OrthSurg
Bertrand, P. E., Urol
Bertrand, R. A., Otol.
Bertrand, R. L., DiagRad
Bessette, G. D & TRad

Better, N., GenSurg
Bettez, P., Path.
Bews, D. C.
Bhambhani, M. D., Anaes.
Biely, G. G., Psy
Bien, E.
Bigras, J., Psy.
Bikadoroff, S., Psy
Bilodeau, R., Obst
Binda, A.
Binda, J.
Binet, E. E.
Birks, R. S.
Birmingham, L. W. GenSurg
Biron-Beaudry, Pauline Anaes
Biron-Sutto, Madeleinc
Biron, P.
Bisset, J. G., Ophth
Bisson, B., DiagRad
Bisson, C. GenSurg
Bisson, D. R.
Bisson, F. R. Psy
Bissonnette, G.
Bissonnette, J.
Bissonnette, R. G., GenSurg
Bitenc, I. A. OrthSurg
Blackburn, G., Path.
Blahey, P. R. ObstGyn
Blain, E. Ophth
Blain, G.
Blain, R.
Blais, E. R. DermSyph (P.Q.)
Blais, J. A. IntMed (P.Q.)
Blais, J. C.
Blais, R. Otol
Blais, R.
Blake, J. M.
Blanchard, B., OrthSurg
Blanchard, G. A., OrthSurg.
Blanchard, G. A. Ophth, Otol (P.Q.)
Blanchard, H., GenSurg.
Blanchet, J., ObstGyn
Blanchet-Patry, Madeline, PH (P.Q.)
Bliss, J. O.
Blondal, H.
Bloom, J. DiagRad (P.Q.)
Bloomberg, M. L., GenSurg
Blouin, R.
Bloyard, G. J.
Blumer, H. M., IntMed
Blundell, J. E., Neur(P.Q.)
Blundell, P. E., ThorSurg
Blustein, J. E., Psy.
Bluteau, P., Path
Boctor, Z. N., Urol
Bodnar, S. A., ObstGyn
Bogert, J. R., Anaes, GenSurg (P.Q.)
Bohemier, A. IntMed (P.Q.)
Boileau, G.
Boileau, J. G.
Boileau, P. A., Obst
Boileau, W. ClinPath (P.Q.)
Bois, M. A., Cardiol (P.Q.)
Bois, P.
Boisvert, M. Psy
Boisvert, M.
Boivin, Y., Path(P.Q.)
Bolte, E., IntMed(P.Q.)
Bombardier, J. P. Paed (P.Q.)
Bombardier, R.
Bonaccorsi, Maria T., Psy
Bonin, A., Path(P.Q.)
Bordeleau, J. M., Psy(P.Q.) Int **Med (P.Q.)**
Borduas, J. L. Cardiol (P.Q.)
Boretsky, P.
Boright, H. A., IntMed (P.Q.)
Boright, R. R. Anaes
Bos, C. G. Psy
Bosco, F.
Bosse, J., Psy(P.Q.)
Bosse, J-P., PlasSurg
Bouchard, J. D & TRad

Bouchard, L.
Boucher, G. H.
Boucher, J. R., Anaes
Boucher, R.
Boudriau, A.
Boulais, F. DermSyph
Boulanger, J. B., Psy, NeurPsy (P.Q.)
Boulanger, M. L., Anaes
Boulay, L. GenSurg (P.Q.)
Boulet, R.
Bourassa, M. G., IntMed, Cardiol (P.Q.)
Bourassa, R.
Bourassa, Y., Cardiol(P.Q.)
Bourbonnais, A. J. H.
Bourgault, J. M.
Bourgault, N. R. Ophth, Otol
Bourgeau, D., OrthSurg
Bourgeau, P. E.
Bourgeois, Jeanne, Path(P.Q.)
Bourgeois, P. Urol, GenSurg
Bourget, J. E.
Bourgie, B. Obst (P.Q.)
Bourgouin, M. R.
Bourne, F. M. IntMed
Bourne, H. B. ObstGyn
Bourne, R. A. Ophth
Bourne, R. H., IntMed, Gastroent (P.Q.)
Bournival, J. Otol
Bourque, J. C.
Bourque, J. M. GenSurg (P.Q.)
Bourque, R.
Bourret, R.
Bousquet, J. E., ThorSurg(P.Q.) IntMed(T.B.), GenSurg(P.Q.), Pulm Dis & TB(P.Q.)
Bousquet, J. P.
Boussens, J., Otol
Boutin, J. R.
Boutin, R., Psy(P.Q.)
Bouziane, N. R., Bact, Haem (P.Q.)
Bowman, Helen, Anaes
Boxer, L. Ophth
Boyaner, D. Ophth
Boyer, J. A.
Boyer, L.
Boyer, R., GenSurg(P.Q.)
Boyle, E. S.
Brabander, J. O. W. IntMed
Brahy, J. Ophth, Otol
Brais, E. P. IntMed (P.Q.)
Branch, C. L.
Brandovacky, E.
Brandt, J. L.
Bratjakin, Anna A., IntMed (P.Q.)
Brattmen, D. P., DiagRad
Brault, J. P. Urol
Brault, J. Ophth, Otol
Brault, T.
Braunstein, M. M.
Breitman, R. OrthSurg
Brent, F. D. P.H. (P.Q.)
Breton, F.
Brickman, Helen F. Paed
Briere, J., GenSurg
Briere, J. P., Physiat(P.Q.)
Brindle, G. F. Anaes
Brisebois, M.
Brisebois, R. C. Psy (P.Q.)
Brisset Des Nos, A. L.
Brodeur, J.
Brodeur, P. Paed
Brodie, H. R. Paed (P.Q.)
Brodkin, E., Path
Brodrick, R. J. IntMed
Bromage, P. Anaes
Brosseau, A.
Brosseau, B. L. P.
Brosseau, M. Psy
Brosseau, R.
Brosseau, W. Obst (P.Q.)
Brotman, H. L. GenSurg

* Population not separately available.

Montreal (Cont'd.)
Broughton, R. J.
Brouillet, J.
Brouillette, G.
Brousseau, J. G.
Brow, G. R., IntMed, Cardiol (P.Q.)
Browman, M. GenSurg (P.Q.)
Brown, B., St. J., DiagRad, TherRad.
Brown, H. A., Anaes
Brown, Lyla I.
Brown, N.
Brown, N. M., D & TRad; Ophth Otol (P.Q.)
Brown, T. A. IntMed
Browne, J. S. IntMed
Bruneau, I. E.
Bruneau, J., GenSurg, ThorSurg (P.Q.)
Bruneau L., GenSurg (P.Q.)
Brunelle, J.
Brunelle, J. P. Anaes
Brunelle, P. Otol (P.Q.)
Brunet, J. C., OrthSurg(P.Q.)
Brunet, J. L. Anaes
Brunet, J. P. E., Psy.
Brunet, M. R. P., Ophth.
Brunet, Suzanne, Paed
Brunette, J. R., Ophth
Brunton, L., IntMed, Haem (P.Q.)
Bruyere, R., ObstGyn
Brytow, Praxeda
Buckiewicz, L. P.
Buies, R., Psy (P.Q.)
Buka, N. J., ObstGyn
Burfoot, M. F., Anaes
Burgen, A. S.
Burgess, J. H., IntMed, Cardiol (P.Q.)
Burke, H. E., IntMed(T.B.), Pulm Dis & TB(P.Q.)
Bussiere, H, C., Paed(P.Q.)
Bussieres, J. D., Otol(P.Q.)
Butas, C., Bact (P.Q.)
Butas, N.
Butler, A. A. OrthSurg
Byk, A. A. Anaes
Cabana, J. E. GenSurg
Cadieux, A.
Cadieux, J. P., IntMed(P.Q.)
Cadieux, R.
Cadieux, R.
Cadotte, J. M., Path(P.Q.)
Cadotte, M. L. C.
Cahill, C. F., Psy (P.Q.)
Cahn, C. H. Psy
Cailloux, R. Obst (P.Q.)
Caisse, J. G. OrthSurg
Callegarini, U., Paed (P.Q.)
Calloc'h, J. P
Cameron, D. E. Psy
Cameron, D. G., IntMed, Haem (P.Q.)
Campbell, A. D. ObstGyn
Campeau, L., IntMed., Cardiol. (P.Q.)
Campeau, P.
Candlish, H. M.
Cange, R., IntMed(P.Q.) Cardiol **(P.Q.)**
Cantero, A., IntMed., Gastroent (P.Q.)
Cantin, A.
Cantin, J., GenSurg.
Cantin, M. P.H. (P.Q.)
Cantlie, G. S. D., IntMed.
Cantlie, Helene
Cape, D. G. M., Anaes.
Capello, P. J., GenSurg
Caplan, H. Otol
Caplan, H. Psy
Capombassis, P., Ophth **(P.Q.)**
Carignan, A. P.
Carignan, G., Anaes
Carle, A.
Carle, J. A.
Carle, L.
Carle, R., Paed(P.Q.)
Caron, G.
Caron, M., Pulm Dis & T.B. (P.Q.)
Caron, P., IntMed
Caron, P., Anaes
Caron, R.
Caron, R. Anaes
Caron-Smith, Ginette
Carriere, J. S., IntMed
Cartier, G. E. GenSurg
Cartier, P., Cardiovasc Surg (P.Q.)
Cartier, T. D. Anaes
Casgrain, G. Aller (P.Q.)
Casselman, Juanila
Casselman, W. B.
Cassidy, J. G. IntMed
Castonguay, B.
Castonguay, D.
Castonguay, E. J.
Castonguay, M., ObstGyn
Castonguay, Y. R., ThorSurg (P.Q.), GenSurg(P.Q.)
Caswell, L. A. IntMed
Catterill, T. B., ObstGyn
Caumartin, A., GenSurg (P.Q.)
Caumartin, P. GenSurg (P.Q.)
Caux, M. Ophth, Otol (P.Q.)
Cayouette, P. E., Psy (P.Q.)
Cerat, J.
Chabot, M., IntMed
Chagnon, G. G.
Chagnon, J. Paed
Chalut, F.
Champagne, E. B.
Champeau, J. Obst
Champoux, G.
Champoux, H. P.
Champoux, R., GenSurg.
Chander, V., Anaes
Chang, T. M.
Chapados, R., Anaes
Chapdelaine, A., IntMed
Chapman, N. H., ObstGyn(P.Q.)
Chaput, Y., IntMed, Gastroent (P.Q.)
Charbonneau, J. Urol
Charbonneau, J. H. Paed
Charbonneau, P. E. GenSurg
Charbonneau, R., Ophth., Otol (P.Q.)
Charbonneau, R., IntMed., Pulm Dis & TB(P.Q.)
Charbonneau, R., Psy
Charbonneau, R.
Charest, F. NeurSurg
Charest, G., PH (P.Q.)
Charest, Y. Otol (P.Q.)
Charette, D. GenSurg
Charette, J. J.
Charette, R., Psy(P.Q.)
Charghi, A., Urol
Charland, R. A. Otol
Charlebois, B.
Charles, L., Anaes
Charron, J., Urol
Chartier, A.
Chartier, J.
Chartier, M. G. IntMed.
Chartrand, F.
Chartrand, J. L.
Chartrand, R.
Chartrand, Y. GenSurg
Chasse, A., Paed(P.Q.)
Chaurette, G., IntMed
Cheng, M. C. Anaes
Chenier, R. Gyn (P.Q.)
Cherniak, M. M. Paed
Chesney, L. P.
Chevalier, L. M., Paed (P.Q.)
Chevrefils, P. E.
Chevrette, L., Ophth.
Chicoine, F. L. Paed
Chicoine, P. E.
Chicoine, R. E. Paed
Cholette, A. M.
Cholette, C. GenSurg
Cholette, G. GenSurg
Cholette, J. P. GenSurg
Choquet, J. Gyn (P.Q.)
Choquette, G. Cardiol (P.Q.), In Med (P.Q.)
Choquette, G.
Choquette, R.
Choquette, S.
Choras, P. T., Psy(P.Q.)
Christie, R. V.
Christin, R.
Chu, D. Q. IntMed
Chughtai, M. S., GenSurg.
Cianflone, C. G., DiagRad
Ciotola, G. J.
Clamen, M. IntMed
Cleghorn, J. M., Psy
Cleghorn, R. A. IntMed, Psy (P.Q.)
Clement, J.
Clermont, J., GenSurg(P.Q.)
Cleroux, A. IntMed (P.Q.)
Clogg, D. K. Paed
Cloutier, A. M., PlasSurg(P.Q.)
Cloutier, F., Psy.
Cloutier, G. E. PlasSurg
Cloutier, G.
Cloutier, J. M., OrthSurg.
Cloutier, L. P.
Cloutier, R. Ophth
Coallier, G.
Coallier, R.
Coffey, J. E., ObstGyn
Cohen, A., Otol
Cohen, H. GenSurg
Cohen, M. S. DermSyph
Cohen, M. Anaes
Cohen, S.. Paed
Cohen, W. IntMed
Coiteux, C.
Colin, Anne Marie
Collin, P. P. GenSurg (P.Q.)
Colonnier, M. L.
Colpron, G.
Comeau, M., IntMed & Pulm. Dis. & TB(P.Q.)
Compton, S. F.
Comtois, M.
Comtois, M.
Connor, T. P., DiagRad
Conroy, J. B. Ophth
Cook, M. S.
Cooke, W. A., ObstGyn
Cooper, B. A. IntMed
Cooper, S. R. IntMed
Cooperberg, A. A., IntMed, Haem (P.Q.)
Cop-Hodjera, Branaslava M., Anaes
Copping, G. A. IntMed
Corbeil, J. ObstGyn
Corber, A. A.
Cordeau, Claire ObstGyn
Cordeau, J. P.
Cordeau, L. J., Psy
Cormier, A. A. ObstGyn
Cormier, B. M. Psy (P.Q.)
Cormier, W. F. IntMed (P.Q.) PulmDis & T.B. (P.Q.)
Corrigan, J. A.
Corsilli, M.
Cosgrove, J. B. Neur
Cossette, G., Anaes
Costin, P. A.
Costin, S. J.
Costom, D. IntMed (P.Q.)
Cote, A. L.
Cote, C. A.
Cote, F. Psy, NeurPsy (P.Q.)
Cote, G. A., Psy
Cote, P.

* Population not separately available.

Montreal (Cont'd.)
Cote, Y.
Coulombe, L.
Coupal, J. A.
Couper, W. M. GenSurg
Courteau, R. Urol
Courtemanche L.
Courtois, G. A. Neurol
Cousineau, G. Anaes
Cousineau, G.
Cousineau, G. G. Ophth (P.Q.)
Cousineau, M.
Coutu, A. GenSurg
Coutu, L. Paed
Coutu, L. L. IntMed
Couture, J. P., IntMed(P.Q.)
Couturier, A. OrthSurg
Cowan, Barbara W.
Cowan, T. A. Paed
Cox, Phoebe L.
Craft, G.
Craig, G. E. DermSyph
Craythorne, N. W., Anaes
Crepeau, A., Anaes
Crevier, P. H. NeurSurg (P.Q.)
Croisetiere, F., OphthOtol(P.Q.)
Cronin, R. F. P., IntMed (Cardiol.)
Croteau, J. R.
Cruess, R. L., OrthSurg
Cruickshank, W. H. PH
Cullen, W. G. Anaes
Cumberland, June R., Psy
Cusson, A. H. OrthSurg (P.Q.)
Cusson, L.
Custeau, P., Anaes.
Cynberg, D. IntMed (P.Q.)
Cyr, Claire, Ophth
D'Abadie, F. A., IntMed, Cardiol(P.Q.)
Dagenais, G., Anaes.
Dagenais, M.
Dagenais-Perusse, P.,Paed(P.Q.)
Dagenais, Y. M. IntMed
Daigle, R. C.
Dallaire, L.
Dalpe, C.
Dancey, T. E. Psy
Dandurand, J. E.
Daniel, G. A., GenSurg
D'Anna, A.
Dansereau, A. Obst (P.Q.)
Dansereau, J., PlasSurg
Dansereau, M.
Daoust, J. P., IntMed
Daoust, L. C., Psy
Darche, J. H. GenSurg (P.Q.)
Dargis, J., PH (P.Q.)
Darragh, J. H. IntMed
DaSilva, G. Psy (P.Q.)
DaSylva, N. P.
Daunais, G.
Daunais, J. A., GenSurg (P.Q.)
Davenport, H. T., Anaes
David, A., IntMed, Cardiol(P.Q.)
David, C., GenSurg
David, P. C., Neur
David, P. P. IntMed, Cardiol (P.Q.)
David, P. P.
David, P. R., IntMed. Cardiol(P.Q.)
Davignon, A., Paed. Cardiol (P.Q.)
Davis, B. A. ObstGyn
Davis, P. L., Ophth.
Dawson, H. L., GenSurg
Dawson, K. G., IntMed
Day, A.
Day, J. A.
Dayal, V. S., Otol
Dayal, Susheela, ObstGyn.
Daze, F. IntMed (P.Q.)
Decarie, L. IntMed
Decarie, M., NeurSurg(P.Q.)
Decarie, P. A.
Decarie, R. GenSurg
Decary, P. Psy, Anaes (P.Q.)
de Domenico, I. J., Urol
DeGrandpre, R.
de Guise, C. P.H. (Johns Hopkins)
Dejaiffe, G. S., Psy.
DeJong, D. IntMed
Delaquerriere, Liliane
deLeeuw, Nannie, IntMed, Haem (P.Q.)
Delisle, Andree E., Anaes(P.Q.)
Delorme, P. J. IntMed, Aller (P.Q.)
Delporte, G. A. D.
Delvecchio, M. DiagRad
Demers, A. Ophth
Demers, J. P., Ophth
Demers, P. A.
Demers, P-E., Ophth(P.Q.)
Demers, R. IntMed
Demirsar, A.
Denhez, J., PH (P.Q.)
Denis, G.
Denis, J. Aller (P.Q.), IntMed (P.Q.)
Denis, J. P. R., Anaes.
Denis, M.
Denton, R. L., Paed, Haem (P.Q.)
Depocas, P.
Derby, A. C., GenSurg
Derome, A., IntMed
Derome, A., OrthSurg
Derome, G. ObstGyn
Derome, L. IntMed
Derry, D. M.
Dery, A.
Dery, L. ObstGyn (P.Q.)
Desaulniers, R. I. IntMed
Desaultels, S., IntMed, Cardiol (P.Q.)
Descarries, L., Neur.
Descary, L.
Deschenes, L., Paed
Descormiers, A. GenSurg
Descoteaux, W.
DeSeve, A.
Desforges, A. DermSyph
Deshaies, B., GenSurg
Desilets, R. G. GenSurg
DesJardins, A. E., Urol
DesJardins, A.
Desjardins, B.
Desjardins, E. GenSurg
Desjardins, J. E., GenSurg
Desjardins-McMillan, Helene
Desjardins, P., ObstGyn.
Desjardins, R., Otol
Deslauriers, J. A.
Deslauriers, J. J.
Deslippe, P. A., Anaes
Desloges, A., Ophth.
Desmarais, B.
Desnoyers, Y., Anaes.
Desrochers, J. B.
Desrochers, J. L., Neurol, Neur Psy (P.Q.)
Desrochers, L. P.
Desrochers, Y. Cardiol (P.Q.)
Desroches, F.
Desroches, J. M.
Desrosiers, G.
Desrosiers, G.
Desrosiers, H. Anaes
Desrosiers, J., ObstGyn
Desrosiers, J. L. Paed
Desrosiers, L. Obst
Desrosiers, P.
Des Rosiers, St. J. Gastroent (P.Q.)
Dessureault, P. Urol
des Trois Maisons, R. Ophth Otol (P.Q.)
de Tavel, F. E.
De Torregrosa, N. C. GenSurg
Deutsch, L., Psy(P.Q.)
De Verteuil, R. L. Psy (P.Q.)
De Vries, Joan A., Bact(P.Q.)
Deziel, J., GenSurg
Dickison, J. C. GenSurg
Diez, P.
Dimitrov, S. I., GenSurg
Dinan, J. J. GenSurg
Dinelle, J.
Dion, M., Anaes
Dion, M. A., PlasSurg
Dion, Y., GenSurg (P.Q.)
Dionne, A.
Dionne, J. GenSurg (P.Q.)
Dionne, J. A., ObstGyn (P.Q.)
Dionne, P. Bact (P.Q.)
Dionne, P. E.
Dionne, W. L. R. GenSurg
Dirks, J. H., IntMed.
Disher, I. S., Psy.
Divic, J.
Dixon, Margaret J., Anaes.
Dixon, M. E., IntMed.
Dobell, A. R., GenSurg., ThorSurg.
Dobija-Domaradzki, Maria Bact (P.Q.)
Dodds, J. R. ObstGyn
Dolan, H. S. GenSurg
Dolovich, J., IntMed.
Dominique, A., Ophth Otol
Domingue, G., DiagRad
Don, H. F., Anaes
Donahoe, J. E. GenSurg (P.Q.)
Donato, G.
Donevan, R. E., IntMed, Pulm Dis & TB (P.Q.)
Donnelly, Grace C. ObstGyn
Dontigny, G.
Dontigny, P. IntMed (P.Q.)
Doray, B. H. Paed
Doray, J. E., GenSurg, PlasSurg
Doray, M., PulmDis&TB(P.Q.) Cardiol (P.Q.)
Dorian, W., IntMed
Dorr, H. P., ObstGyn
Dorrance, F. S.
Dossetor, J. B. IntMed
Doubilet, S. I. Paed
Doucet, L. P., Psy.
Douglas, F. G. V., IntMed.
Dowd, K. E.
Doyle, G., TherRad(P.Q.)
Doyon, D., Psy.
Drake, L. J., GenSurg
Drapeau, P., Psy.
Drouin, J., Psy(P.Q.)
Drouin, R., Anaes
Drummond, J. A. PlasSurg
Drummond, K. N., Paed
Dube, E.
Dube, J., IntMed
Dubeau, J. A. M. Anaes
DuBerger, P.
Dubicinac, S. T.
Dubois, G.
Dubow, H. I., OrthSurg
Dubreuil, L. P.H. (P.Q.)
Dubuc, C. Y.
Dubuc, G. OphthOtol (P.Q.)
Dubuc, H. Ophth, Otol
Ducharme, G. Obst (P.Q.)
Ducharme, J. C., GenSurg
Ducharme, J. R. Paed (P.Q.)
Duchastel, Y. J., Neur (P.Q.)
Duchesne, L.
Duckett, G., D & TRad
Duclos, G. Ophth
Dufault, Camille, IntMed
DuFeutrelle, H.
Duff, J. H., GenSurg
Duffy, St. C. GenSurg (P.Q.)
Dufour, J., Psy(P.Q.)
Dufresne, J. A.

*** Population not separately available.**

Montreal (Cont'd.)
Dufresne, M. H., Urol., GenSurg.
Dufresne, M. R.
Dufresne, M. R. D & TRad
Dufresne, O. D & TRad, PhysMed (P.Q.)
Dugas, Y., Anaes (P.Q.)
Duguay, M. R., Psy
Duhaime, Constance
Duhaime, M., OrthSurg(P.Q.)
Duhamel, H.
Dukay, A. C.
Dumais, B. G. Cardiol (P.Q.)
Dumais, G., Derm
Dumas, C. F., NeurPsy.
Dumas, J., Ophth
Dumas, P. IntMed
Dumont, A., Path(P.Q.)
Dumont, G., IntMed, Cardiol (P.Q.)
Dunbar, J. S., D & T Rad.
Duncan, H. A. G. Ophth
Dundas, J. B., Paed
Dunkley, E. M., Anaes
Dunn, F. W. IntMed
Dunn, P. R., IntMed., Gastroent(P.Q.)
Dupal, Marie-F., Paed
Duplessis, L. G.
Duplessis, J. Paed (P.Q.)
Dupont, C. G., GenSurg., PlasSurg.
Dupont, Denyse
Dupont-Legault, Micheline
Dupre, J., IntMed(P.Q.)
Dupre-Strachan, Suzanne
Dupuis, G.
Dupuis, G.
Dupuis, R. L. GenSurg
Dupuis, R. GenSurg
Duquette, J. IntMed (P.Q.)
Durand, G. A.
Durand, L.
Durivage, J. IntMed (P.Q.)
Durost, H. B. Psy
DuSablon, G.
Dussault, Jeanne M.
Dussault, R., IntMed, Haem (P.Q.)
Duval, L., GenSurg
Duval, P. C., Anaes (P.Q.)
Duvenci, J.
Dworkin, S. IntMed
Dyble, R. H.
Dyer, W. J.
Eakin, W. W., IntMed., Cardiol(P.Q.)
Echenberg, I.
Edelstein, E.
Edgell, P. G. Psy
Edwards, P. A., Pulm Dis & TB(P.Q.)
Egeli, C. N., ObstGyn
Eibel, P. OrthSurg
Eidinger, S. L., IntMed., Pulm Dis & TB(P.Q.)
Eidinger, S. L. Aller (P.Q.)
Eisdorfer, M.
Eisen, A.H., Paed Allergy (P.Q.
Eitchis, Sara
Elder, J. M. Paed
Elias, G. L., GenSurg
El-Khatib, A., GenSurg(P.Q.)
Elkin, D. PlasSurg
Ellenberger, H. F.
Elliott, H. W., NeurSurg.
Ellis, C. F., OrthSurg
Ellison, Gladys N. Anaes
Elnes, N. R.
Elvidge, A. R. NeurSurg
Emond, G. V.
Emond, M., IntMed.
Enesco, M., IntMed
Engels, W. D., Psy
Entin, M. A. PlasSurg, Psy
Epstein, N. B. Psy
Ereaux, L. P. DermSyph
Essig, K. H.
Estrada, R. L. GenSurg
Ethier, J. L.
Ethier, J. P.
Ethier, R. DiagRad
Etziony, M. IntMed (P.Q.)
Faille, R. GenSurg
Falardeau, M., GenSurg.
Farah-Lajoie, C.
Farfan, H. F. OrthSurg
Faribault, C. D&TRad
Farley, L. V. IntMed
Farley, W. J., Anaes
Farmer, L., Paed.
Farmer, R. Path, Anat (P.Q.)
Farrell, H. S., GenSurg.
Faucher, G. L., ObstGyn.
Fauteux, G. M., IntMed (P.Q.
Fauteux, J. P. GenSurg
Fauteux, P., DiagRad
Favreau, J., Derm.
Favreau, J. C. OrthSurg
Favreau, R., ObstGyn
Favreau-Ethier, M. F. DiagRad
Fawcett, J. S., Path(P.Q.)
Feeney, N., IntMed., Cardiol. (P.Q.)
Feher, P. J., Derm.
Feindel, W. H. NeurSurg
Fejes, D.
Feldman, A., Paed(P.Q.)
Feldman, R. B., Psy
Feldman, R. M.
Feldman, S., IntMed
Feldman, W., Paed.
Ferguson, K. R. Psy
Ferguson, R., Anaes
Ferland, H., Anaes
Ferland, J. A.
Ferland, M.
Ferron, G.
Ferron, M. Obst (P.Q.)
Fieldman, J. D.
Figlioli, G., Psy
Filiatrault, J. M. PulmDis & T.B. (P.Q.)
Filion-Laporte, Liliane
Filteau, M., Anaes.
Findlay, D.
Finkelstein, M. N.
Finkelstein, P. M.
Finlayson, M. H., Neur, Path
Finley, A. H. Paed
Firth, J. D. A. Anaes
Fisk, G. H. PhysMed
Fitzhardinge, Pamela, Paed
Fleming, D. S., Bact, PH
Fleury, P. H.
Flint, Anna, DermSyph
Flood, F. P. GenSurg
Foisy, J. P., DermSyph
Fontaine, A., DiagRad.
Fontaine, J., Bact
Fontaine, R.
Fontaine, R.
Foote, W. R. ObstGyn
Forbes, D. B., OrthSurg
Forbes, F.
Forbes, Patricia A., Paed
Ford, R. M., NeurSurg.
Foreman, J. A. Ophth
Forest, J. P. Gyn (P.Q.)
Forget, J. P.
Forgues, R., GenSurg
Forrest, J. R.
Forse, R. A. GenSurg
Forsey, R. R. P. DermSyph
Fortier, J. Obst
Fortier, Lise ObstGyn
Fortier, L. IntMed
Fortier, M. OrthSurg
Fortier, M. OrthSurg
Fortin, A. Neurol
Fortin, G., Anaes.
Fortin, J.
Fortin, J., PhysMed & Rehab (P.Q.)
Fortin, J. M.
Fortin, J. N. Psy
Fortin, R.
Foucher, A.
Foucher, E.
Fournelle-LeBuis, F., TherRad.
Fournier, L.
Fournier, L. E. Urol
Fournier, M.
Fowler, A. F. IntMed
Fox, G. S., Anaes
Francois, G., IntMed.
Frank, H., IntMed Pulm Dis & TB (P.Q.)
Frappier, A. Bact
Frappier-Davignon, Lise
Frappier, J.
Frappier, J. R.
Fraser, D. C. IntMed (P.Q.)
Fraser, F. C.
Fraser, R. G., D & T Rad
Fraser, W. D. ObstGyn
Frederick, A.
Freedman, A. N., GenSurg
Freedman, Giselle, ObstGyn.
Freedman, N., Obst (P.Q.)
Freedman, N. B. GenSurg (P.Q.)
Freedman, S. O., IntMed, Allergy (P.Q.)
French, A. D., DiagRad.
Frenette, L.
Frenette, U. OrthSurg
Friedman, R., Ophth(P.Q.)
Friedman, S.
Friefield, H.
Friesen, H. G., IntMed.
Frigon, J. L.
Frohlich, L. I.
Fugere, P., ObstGyn
Fulford, R. A., OrthSurg.
Fullerton, C. W. IntMed
Fung, R.-H., Paed
Fyfe, R. M.
Fyles, Shirley H., Neurol
Gabor, A.
Gaboury, J., GenSurg
Gadbois, A. GenSurg (P.Q.)
Gagnan-Brunette, Michelle, Paed.
Gagne-Desrosiers, Rita, Anaes
Gagne, R.
Gagnier, L. A. D & TRad
Gagnier, M Obst (P.Q.)
Gagnon, A. P.
Gagnon, A., Ophth, Otol
Gagnon, C.
Gagnon, C.
Gagnon, E. D., GenSurg., ThorSurg.
Gagnon, G., Psy
Gagnon, G., Cardiol(P.Q.)
Gagnon, J. A. Path (P.Q.)
Gagnon, J. H., DiagRad.
Gagnon, J. J. GenSurg (P.Q.)
Gagnon, J. N. Obst (P.Q.)
Gagnon, J. O. Gastroent (P.Q.)
Gagnon, J. R. P.
Gagnon, M., IntMed.
Gagnon, M. G., Obst
Gagnon, N. B., Otol.
Gagnon, P. A. OrthSurg
Gagnon, P-A., OrthSurg.
Gagnon, R.
Gagnon, R. GenSurg
Gagnon, R. Anaes
Gagnon, R., Ophth
Gaillard, C. GenSurg (P.Q.)
Galipeau, V.
Gallai, Z.
Gandkin, J.

* Population not separately available.

Montreal (Cont'd.)

Garand, A., Anaes
Garber, H. Otol
Garceau, E., DermSyph.
Gareau, J.
Gareau, R.
Gareau, R. IntMed (P.Q.) Gastroent (P.Q.)
Gareau, R. J., Path(P.Q.)
Gareau, S., DiagRad.
Gariepy, L. H. IntMed
Gariepy, R. OrthSurg
Garneau. G. IntMed (P.Q.), Cardiol (P.Q.)
Garneau, J. F., Anaes
Garneau, N., Psy.
Garon, G. IntMed (P.Q.)
Garretson, H. D.
Gascon, B.
Gascon, J., IntMed
Gascon, R.
Gatien, R.
Gattereau, A., IntMed
Gaudette, J. P., PlastSurg(P.Q.)
Gault, M. H. IntMed
Gauthier, A.
Gauthier, B. OrthSurg
Gauthier, G., Gyn (P.Q.), Haem. (P.Q.)
Gauthier, G. A.
Gauthier, G. E., Urol (P.Q.)
Gauthier, J., Gyn(P.Q.), Haem(P.Q.)
Gauthier, L. J. Paed (P.Q.)
Gauthier, P. E., PulmDis&T.B. (P.Q.)
Gauthier, P. G.
Gauthier, P. J. Gyn
Gauthier, P.
Gauthier, R.
Gauthier, R. Otol (P.Q.)
Gauthier, V. PulmDis & T.B. (P.Q.)
Gauthier, Y., Psy(P.Q.)
Gautier, E.
Gauvin, P., Ophth.
Gavsie, W. H. Paed
Gazinsky, W.
Geddes, A. K. Paed (P.Q.)
Gelber, H., Psy
Gelber, Sheila P.
Gelfand, M. M. ObstGyn
Gelinas, A., Pulm Dis & TB P.Q.), IntMed(TB)
Gelinas, C., Otol
Gelinas, Georgette P. Paed PH (P.Q.)
Gelinas, H., IntMed (P.Q.)
Gelinas, J. P.
Gelinas, M.
Gelinas, M., Cardiol (P.Q.)
Gelinas-MacKay, Claire Path (P.Q.)
Gelinas, R. A. IntMed
Gendreau, C.
Gendron, C. P., Haem (P.Q.)
Gendron, J. L.
Gendron, L.
Gendron, R.
Genest, A. PlasSurg
Genest, J. IntMed
Genest, P., IntMed.
Genest, R. NeurPsy
Geoffrion, Louise
Geoffroy, M., D & TRad
Geoffroy, Y. G., Neur (P.Q.)
Gerlache, F.
Germain, G. IntMed
Gerrie, J. W., PlasSurg, Otol
Gerstein, W., Derm
Gertler, M. M.
Gervais, G. A., DiagRad(P.Q.)
Gervais, H., DiagRad
Gervais, J.
Gervais, L., Psy
Gervais, M. GenSurg (P.Q.)
Gervais, R., Anaes
Gervais, R.
Getzler, N. A., DermSyph(P.Q.)
Ghamande, A. R., IntMed.
Ghys, R., Ther Rad
Gialloretto, O. P., Cardiol(P.Q.)
Giannotti, R., ObstGyn(P.Q.)
Giard, N., Neur
Giasson, C.
Gibbard, B. A., Psy.
Gibbons, J. E. Cardiol (P.Q.)
Gibeault, H. Obst
Gibson, J. D. DiagRad
Gignac, G.
Gilbert, A., GenSurg.
Gilbert, G. Cardiol (P.Q.), IntMed (P.Q.)
Gilbert, J. PH
Gilbert, R. G. B. Anaes
Gillies, Deirdre M., Anaes.
Gingras, G., PhysMed & Rehab.
Girard, A. OrthSurg
Girard, D., Anaes (P.Q.)
Girard, F.
Girard, M. DiagRad
Girard, M.
Girard, Y. M., ObstGyn.
Girardin, G. M. Paed (P.Q.)
Giroux, J. C., NeurSurg.
Giroux, J. M., Derm
Giulianelli, L. S., IntMed
Glay, A., D & TRad
Gledhill, R. B., OrthSurg.
Glickman, I., ObstGyn
Gloor, P.
Godin, P. E. A., Ophth, Otol
Godron, Eleonore R.
Gokcen, M. I., Psy
Gold, A., IntMed
Gold, M., IntMed, Cardiol(P.Q.)
Gold, P., IntMed.
Gold, S., ObstGyn
Gold, S.
Goldberg, E. H.
Goldberg, J.
Goldberg, Karolina
Goldberg, N. J., IntMed
Goldbloom, A., Paed
Goldbloom, R. B., Paed
Goldbloom, V. C., Paed
Golden, C., Paed
Goldenberg, M. H., DiagRad.
Goldfarb, H. P.
Goldman, H., Paed
Goldman, S. E., OrthSurg
Goldstein, E., IntMed (P.Q.)
Goldstein, S. E., Psy
Golfman, M.
Golt, M.
Gomberg, C. L., IntMed
Gonda, A., IntMed.
Goodall, R. G., GenSurg
Gordon, A., Paed
Gordon, A. L., IntMed
Gordon, E., Ophth (P.Q.)
Gordon, L.
Goresky, C. A., IntMed
Gosselin, B. Y., Haem (P.Q.)
Gosselin, G., Biochem(P.Q.)
Gosselin, G., IntMed (P.Q.) Haem (P.Q.)
Gosselin, J., Bact (P.Q.)
Gosselin, R. A.
Gosselin, W.
Gougoux, J. C. J., PulmDis & T.B. (P.Q.)
Goulet, C., Cardiol(P.Q.)
Goulet, F.
Goulet, M., OrthSurg(P.Q.)
Goulet, R., Paed (P.Q.)
Goulet, T. G., DiagRad.
Goulet, Y., IntMed, Cardiol(P.Q.)
Gourdeau, R., Paed, Haem(P.Q.)
Graham, B. F., Neurol.
Grainger, F. A., D & TRad
Grandbois, C., Paed.
Grant, P. D.
Gratton, A., IntMed
Gratton-Amyot, Monique
Gratton, J. D., Cardiol (P.Q.)
Grauer, H., Psy
Gravel, H.
Gravel, Y., Anaes.
Green, B. L., OrthSurg
Greenwood, F. A., OrthSurg
Gregoire, F. S., IntMed
Gregoire, G.
Gregoriou, G., Psy
Gregory, A. J.
Greig, D. H., Otol.
Grenier, A.
Grenier, L. R.
Grenier, R.
Griffin, M. B.
Griffith, H. R., Anaes
Griffith, J. J., GenSurg
Grignon, C. E., IntMed
Grignon, J., IntMed
Grignon, R., GenSurg (P.Q.)
Grimard, M.
Groleau, F.
Grondin, P., GenSurg., ThorSurg.
Grondin, R., D & TRad
Groom, R. H.
Grossman, A. A., Otol
Grossman, B. M.
Grossman, Sheila
Groszman, M.
Groulx, A., PH
Groulx, R., Gyn
Gruner, P. H.
Grymaloski, Martha R., DiagRad
Guay, J., Urol
Gubbay, E. R., IntMed; Cardiol (P.Q.)
Guenette, E.
Guenette, P. J.
Guertin, C.
Guertin, P., Otol.
Guevin, R. M., IntMed
Guilbeault, J. A., Paed
Guilbert, P. W., Paed (P.Q.)
Guillet, M. A., IntMed.
Guilmete, C., GenSurg.
Guimond, J. J. Paed
Guindon, M., OrthSurg(P.Q.)
Gurd, F. N., GenSurg
Gurrin, Teresa, Anaes.
Gutelius, J. R., GenSurg, ThorSurg
Guttman, F. M., GenSurg
Guy, R., Path (P.Q.)
Guzman, D. A., Neur.
Hackett, J. D., Psy
Haffke, S., DiagRad (P.Q.)
Haimson, J.
Hajdu, A.
Hakstian, R. W., PlasSurg
Hale, B. B., D & TRad
Hale, T. R., IntMed, Cardiol (P.Q.)
Halpenny, G. W., IntMed
Halperin, D., Otol
Halpern, N. N., Urol
Hamann, Christa
Hamel, A. O., Psy (P.Q.)
Hamel, E.
Hamel, G.
Hamel, J.
Hamel, M.
Hamel, P. C.
Hamelin, L., D & T Rad.
Hamelin, M., IntMed (P.Q.)
Hamelin, P. E., PH (P.Q.)
Hamilton, J. D.
Hampson, L. G., GenSurg
Handcock, K. A., Psy
Handfield, G. Y.

* Population not separately available.

Montreal (Cont'd.)
Handfield, R. H., GenSurg (P.Q.) Gyn (P.Q.)
Handfield, Therese
Hanrahan, G. E., Psy
Hansebout, R. R., NeurSurg (P.Q.)
Haque, A. W., DiagRad.
Hara, V.
Harbeck, M.
Harbert, R. G. M.
Hardy, J., NeurSurg
Harel, C., DiagRad (P.Q.)
Harel, P., Haem (P.Q.)
Hariton, N.
Harpur, Eleanor R. M., PathBact
Harris, B. R., Psy
Harris, C., Haem (P.Q.)
Harris, D. P., Psy
Harris, Marguerite, Psy
Harris, M. E.
Haslam, L. C.
Hatcher, G. H., PH.
Hawthorne, A. B., Urol
Hazel, B., IntMed (P.Q.)
Hazel, J. J., TherRad.
Heath, E. S., Psy.
Hebert, A., Urol
Hebert, C. E., GenSurg
Hebert, E., Gyn (P.Q.)
Hebert, F., PulmDis&TB (P.Q.)
Hebert, F., DiagRad
Hebert, G., IntMed
Hebert, G., Gyn (P.Q.)
Hebert, G.
Hebert, H.
Hebert, J. G., PlasSurg
Hebert, J. G., IntMed
Hebert, J. P.
Hebert, L., GenSurg
Hebert, L.
Hebert, P. E.
Heffez, A., GenSurg
Helle, S. J., IntMed
Heller, B. P., DermSyph
Heller, I. H., Neurol
Heller, L., OrthSurg
Heller, N., IntMed
Hellstrom, J. G., IntMed
Helman-Zalewska, Maria
Henault, G.
Hendelman, M. ObstGyn
Henderson, I. W., GenSurg
Henderson, J. A., IntMed
Henderson, R. W., Otol (P.Q.)
Henry, F., Ophth, Otol
Henry, J. S., Sr. ObstGyn
Henry, J. S., ObstGyn
Herba, M. J. W., Diag Rad
Herlich, S.
Herscovitch, O.
Heseltine, G. F., Psy
Heslam, R. M.
Heynemand, R.
Hickey, M. A., IntMed., Pulm. Dis. & TB (P.Q.)
Hidvegi, R. S., DiagRad
Hierz, O., ObstGyn.
Hier, D., GenSurg
Hill, R. O., D & T Rad.
Hill, W. H. P., IntMed
Hillman, D. A., Paed (P.Q.)
Hillman, Elizabeth, Paed
Hinchey, E. J., GenSurg
Hisey, L. G., Psy (P.Q.)
Hoffman, M. M., IntMed (P.Q.)
Hogan, T. G., ObstGyn.
Hogue, G.
Holland, G. A., GenSurg
Hollenberg, C., IntMed
Hollinger, H. Z., IntMed
Hollo-Zeliger, Agnes M., Paed
Holowski, F. B.
Hood, A. B., IntMed, Haem (P.Q.)
Hooper, G., GenSurg
Hooper, J. E., GenSurg
Horowitz, I.
Hospodarewska, Sophie
Houde, L., Psy
Houle, G. L., Anaes.
Houle, J.
Houle, J. A., OrthSurg (P.Q.)
Howett, D. A.
Howie, M. F.
Howlett, J., IntMed
Hradecky, R. A.
Hreno, A., GenSurg
Huard, G., Paed (P.Q.)
Huard, J. A., Psy
Huard, L. G.
Hudon, R., Anaes
Hughes, R. A., IntMed (P.Q.)
Hunt, B. R., Psy.
Hunter, Margaret, Paed
Hout, L., DiagRad
Huot, L. A., Otol
Hurley, G. A. P., ThorSurg., GenSurg.
Hurtubise, J. M., DiagRad
Hutchison, G. A., GenSurg
Hutchison, I. E., IntMed
Hutchison, J. L., IntMed
Hyams, B. B., Urol
Hyde, R. W., Otol
Hymovitch, I. V.
Ibberson, J. R.
Illievitz, A. B.
Inglis, F. G., GenSurg
Ingram, R. F.
Inman, Fay, IntMed
Irving, R. W.
Isomura, S.
Ittkin, P. Otol
Iutcovish, F.
Jackson, L. G.
Jacob, M., Anaes
Jacques, P. E.
Jarry, G., PulmDis & TB (P.Q.)
Jarry, L., OrthSurg
Jarry-Laporte, Jocelyne
Jasmin, F.
Jasmin, G.
Jasper, H. H.
Javicoli, A., IntMed (Gastro) (P.Q.)
Jean, A., Path (P.Q.)
Jean, J. P., D & TRad
Jean, P.
Jegier, Wanda, Paed
Jegyud, A. T.
Jeliu, Gloria, Paed
Jepson, Joanne
Jette, J.
Jette, M. C.
Jette, Y.
Joannette, J. P.
Jobin, D. G., PhysMed & Rehab.
Jobin, M.
Johnson, A. L., Cardiol (P.Q.), IntMed.
Johnson, L. G., IntMed.
Johnson, R., IntMed., Cardiol (P.Q.)
Johnson, T. E., GenSurg.
Johnston, K. B., Ophth.
Jolicoeur, G., Otol
Jolivet, G. Y., Paed
Joly, J. P., Obst
Joncas, F., IntMed (P.Q.)
Joncas, J. H., Paed.
Jones, A. F., GenSurg
Jones, F. M.
Jorizzo, A. O., Path.
Joron, G. E., IntMed
Joubert, L.
Journet, L., Obst (P.Q.)
Joyal, A. C., Anaes
Joyal, J. F., Urol (P.Q.)
Joyce, C. R.
Julien, F., Psy (P.Q.)
Julien, L., GenSurg (P.Q.)
Julien, P. P., IntMed
Junger, P. W. F., Paed
Jutras, A., D & TRad
Jutras, M.
Kadish, M. E., DiagRad.
Kahn, A. IntMed
Kahn, D., PathBact
Kahne, H. M., Paed
Kakos, A., IntMed
Kalant, N., IntMed
Kaludi, P. M., IntMed
Kalz, F., DermSyph
Kalz, Gertrude G., Bact
Kapusta, M. A., IntMed.
Karam, D. B.
Karn, G. M., GenSurg
Kasyapan, M. D., NeurSurg
Kato, L.
Katz, A. H., Ophth
Katz, E., Otol
Katz, M., Psy.
Kaufmann, M. I. H., Ophth (P.Q.)
Kaufmann, N. R.
Kaye, M., IntMed
Kerri-Szanto, M., Anaes
Kelen, L.
Keller, J., Obst (P.Q.)
Keller, Rhona J.
Kelly, J. J., Anaes.
Kendall, A. G., IntMed, Haem (P.Q.)
Kennedy, J. E.
Kennedy, W. R., IntMed
Kerenyi, A. B., Psy
Kerner, Ilona, Path
Kerrin, H. F., IntMed
Kerwood, L. A., Psy.
Kessler, J. I., IntMed., Gastroent (P.Q.)
Khan, I., Anaes.
Khera, S. A. K., Paed
Khobreh, M., GenSurg
Kindy, A., Psy (P.Q.)
Kindy, D., DiagRad
Kingstone, E., Psy
Kinnear, D. G., IntMed
Kinsella, T. D., IntMed
Kirsch, A.
Kirschberg, L. S., Ophth
Kiss, J., DiagRad
Kiteala, J., Paed.
Klassen, G. A., IntMed., Cardiol (P.Q.)
Klein, D., Paed
Klemchuck, S. E., Otol
Knight, A., IntMed
Knox, S. H.
Kober, W. R.
Kobernick, D.
Kohlhepp, H.
Kolber, B.
Komaromi, G., IntMed
Koranyi, E., Psy
Korenberg, L. J., IntMed (P.Q.) Cardiol (P.Q.)
Korenberg, M., IntMed (P.Q.)
Korman, D., Anaes
Korman, H., GenSurg
Kovacs-Bimbi, Agnes E., Paed.
Kovacs, Eva M.
Kovacs, L. L., IntMed
Kovalik, M., IntMed (P.Q.)
Kozlowski, F. B.
Kral, Katherine, Ophth.
Kral, V. A., NeurPsy
Kravitz, H., Psy
Kristof, F. E., Psy
Krohn, H. S.
Krygier, J.
Kucharyszin, M.
Kulcsar, D., ObstGyn
Kunstler, W. E., ThorSurg, GenSurg
Kunstler-Meyer, M. S., Paed PulmDis & TB (P.Q.)

* Population not separately available.

Montreal (Cont'd.)
Kupferszmidt, Irena
Kurkji, H., GenSurg
Kushner, A. G., Ophth
Kwitko, M. L., Ophth
L'Abbe, P., Psy (P.Q.)
L'Abbe, R., D & TRad
Labelle, A.
Labelle, A. R., Ophth, Otol(P.Q.)
Labelle, E.
Labelle, P. H., OrthSurg
Laberge, E., Paed (P.Q.)
Laberge, I., Urol
Laberge, J., D & TRad
Laberge, Marie J., PulmDis & T (P.Q.)
Laberge-Nadeau, Claire
Laberge, P., Psy(P.Q.)
Labossiere, M., PulmDist & TB (P.Q.)
Labrecque, B., Anaes.
Labrecque, C.
Labrecque, J. P., Psy (P.Q.)
Labrecque, P. GenSurg
Labrecque, R., Paed
Lachaine, G. A., IntMed(P.Q.) Cardiol (P.Q.)
Lachance, J. Y.
Lachance, P., D & T Rad
Lachance, R. E., IntMed
Lachance, R. R.
Lacharite, H., D & TRad, PhysMed (P.Q.)
Lacombe, M., IntMed, Haem (P.Q.)
Lacroix, J. P.
Ladouceur, L.
Lafave, W. J., ObstGyn (P.Q.)
Laferriere, R.
Lafleche, L. R., ThorSurg, GenSurg (P.Q.)
Lafleur, F., Anaes.
Lafleur, L., D & T Rad(P.Q.)
Lafleur, Lucette, Bact
Lafond, G., OrthSurg.
Lafontaine, R., Neur (P.Q.)
Laforest, B., ObstGyn
Laforest, M. G., IntMed(P.Q.)
Lafortune, G. O., Anaes
Lafortune, L. L., GenSurg.
Lafortune, J. O.
Lafortune, P. E.
Lafrance, A., Derm.
Lafrance, R., GenSurg
Lagace, R.
Lagarde, J. P., PulmDis & TB (P.Q.)
La Haie, E. M.
Lahaise-Levesque, F. D., Psy
L'Heureux, J.
Lai, Suke-Y., Gen Surg.
Laing, W. A. R., IntMed.
Lal, L., Otol
Lalande, E.
Lalande, R.
L'Allier, R., Anaes
Lalonde, C. E.
Lalonde, J. B., Cardiol(P.Q.)
Lalonde, J. L., NeurSurg.
Lalonde, W.
Lamarche, A.
Lamarche, L.
Lamarre, C., OrthSurg
Lamarre, G., IntMed (P.Q.)
Lamarre, L., PulmDis & TB (P.Q.)
Lambert, B., ObstGyn
Lambert, D.
Lambert, J. A., DermSyph.
Lambert, J., PulmDis & TB (P.Q.)
Lambert, J., GenSurg.
Lambert, J. J., Anaes.
Lamer, L., Ophth
Lamonica, J., GenSurg(P.Q.)
Lamontagne, C. H., Psy (P.Q.)
Lamantagne, R., Cardiol(P.Q.)
Lamothe, F.
Lamoureux, C., Path.
Lamoureux, E.
Lamoureux, J.
Lamoureux, L., Anaes
Lamoureux, M., GenSurg.
Lamquin, R.
Lamy, J. L., GenSurg., ThorSurg(P.Q.)
Lamy, R. L.
Lande, J.
Landreville, J. A., PH (P.Q.)
Landriault, G.
Landriault, R.
Landry, A.
Landry, H. J., IntMed(P.Q.)
Landry, J. P., OrthSurg
Landry, P., PulmDis&TB(P.Q.)
Langevin, E., Ophth, Otol(P.Q.)
Langevin, H., Psy
Langevin, J.
Langevin, P., Paed
Langevin, R., OrthSurg
Langevin, S.
Langevin, Suzanne
Langlois, C., IntMed., Allergy(P.Q.)
Langlois, C. A., D & T Rad (P.Q.)
Langlois, C. H., IntMed
Langlois, J. D., PulmDis & TB (P.Q.)
Langlois, J. L., Psy (P.Q.)
Lannon, S. G., Urol
Lanthier, A., IntMed
Lanthier, H. J.
Lantier, R., PhysMed & Rehab
Lapalme, R., Urol
Laperriere, J.
Lapierre, A.
Lapierre, A. A.
Lapierre, B.
Lapierre, C.
Lapierre, J.
Lapierre, L., IntMed(P.Q.)
Lapierre, R.
Lapin, A., Cardiol(P.Q.), IntMed.
Lapin, I.
Lapin, L., IntMed
Laplante, A. E., GenSurg
Laplante, J. P.
Laplante, M., Gyn.
Lapointe, Carol
Lapointe, Constance K.
Lapointe, J. A., OphthOtol.
Lapointe, J. L., Psy
Lapointe, L., IntMed, Cardiol (P.Q.)
Lapointe, M. A.
Lapointe, M. L.
Lapointe, R., ObstGyn
Lapointe, R., Ophth, Otol
Laporte, A. F.
Laporte, G.
Laporte, J., Anaes
Laporte, J. M.
Laporte, J. M.
Laporte, J. N., PH (P.Q.)
Laporte, L. J., GenSurg
Laporte, L. M., GenSurg (P.Q.)
Laporte, M.
Laporte, R.
Laramee, A., Psy (P.Q.)
Laramee, B., Obst (P.Q.)
Laramee, F., PulmDis & TB (P.Q.), IntMed (P.Q.)
L'Archeveque, A., Paed
L'Archeveque, M.A., Obst (P.Q.)
Larichelliere, R., OrthSurg(P.Q.)
Larini, G. P., D & TRad
Larivee, L.
Lariviere, P., NeurPsy
Lariviere, P. M., Paed
Larking, E. W., Anaes.
LaRoche, G.
LaRoche, N., Urol (P.Q.)
LaRochelle, G., Psy
LaRochelle, R., ObstGyn
Larocque, H.
Larocque, J. J., Obst (P.Q.)
Larose, M.
Larouche, J., DiagRad
Larue, P., IntMed., Pulm. Dis. & TB (P.Q.)
LaSalle, G.
LaSalle, R., Paed
Laskaris, M. A.
Laszlo, Clara E.
Latour, G. L., D & T Rad.
Latour, J. P. A., ObstGyn
Latour, P.
Latraverse, V., Otol.
Laufer, F.
Laurence, G. C., IntMed
Laurendeau, F., GenSurg.
Laurier, R., PulmDis & TB(P.Q.) IntMed(P.Q.)
Laurin, A., DiagRad(P.Q.)
Laurin, Camille, Psy (P.Q.)
Laurin, C., OrthSurg
Laurin, J. G., Haem (P.Q.)
Laurin, P. E., PathBact
Laurin, R.
Laurin, Suzanne T.,Haem(P.Q.)
Lauze, S., Path (P.Q.)
Lauzer, R., GenSurg
Lauzier, J. M.
Lauzon, G., GenSurg., PlasSurg(P.Q.)
Lauzon, M.
Lauzon, R.
Lavallee, A., Urol
Lavallee, J-L., Ophth.
Lavallee, J. P., Anaes
Lavallee, M.
Lavallee, M., IntMed & Haem (P.Q.)
Lavergne, P. H., PulmDis&TB **(P.Q.)**
Lavigne, L. R.
Lavinge, P., OrthSurg(P.Q.)
Lavigne, R.
Lavoie, D., GenSurg
Lavoie, G. P., GenSurg
Lavoie, H., ObstGyn(P.Q.)
Lavoie, J. G., Anaes
Lavoie, Lucie
Lavoie, M.
Lavoie, P., GenSurg.
Lavoie, R. J., Paed.
Laws, H. W., Ophth
Lawson, R. N., GenSurg
Lawton-Gregory, Michelle V.
Lazar, G.
Lazure, D., Psy
Leavitt, J., Anaes
Lebeau, R., Anaes
Lebel, Etiennette, Anaes
Lebel, G., Paed (P.Q.)
Lebel, J., Obst (P.Q.)
Lebel, J. E., TherRad(P.Q.)
Lebel, L. L., IntMed (Cardiol) (P.Q.)
Lebeuf, J., Psy (P.Q.)
LeBlanc, C., GenSurg
LeBlanc, P., GenSurg, NeurSurg. (P.Q.)
Leblanc, R., Paed.
Leblanc, W.
Leblond, C. P.
Leboeuf, B., IntMed
Leboeuf, Y.
LeBrun, J. A.
Leclair, P. E., Cardiol (P.Q.)
Leclair, R. B.
Leclerc, G., DermSyph
Leclerc, L.
Leclerc, M. Y., Anaes
Leclerc, Therese
Lecoq, H.

*** Population not separately available.**

Montreal (Cont'd.)
Lecours, A., GenSurg.
Lecours, J. R., IntMed (P.Q.)
L'Ecuyer, M., OrthSurg(P.Q.)
Lederer, L.
Ledoux, L., OrthSurg
Ledoux, R., DiagRad
Leduc, A., Bact (P.Q.)
Leduc, C. Anaes
Leduc, G., PulmDis&TB(P.Q.)
Leduc, G., Psy
Leduc, G. G., IntMed (P.Q.), Cardiol (P.Q.)
Leduc, J. M.
Leduc, J. R.
Leduc, L. J., Anaes
Leduc, P. E., IntMed (P.Q.)
Lee, D. H., Path(P.Q.)
Lefebvre, A.
Lefebvre B. A.
Lefebvre, E.
Lefebvre, G. A., Anaes.
Lefebvre, J.
Lefebvre, J. A.
Lefebvre, P., Psy (P.Q.)
Lefebvre, P., Psy.
Lefebvre, R., IntMed (P.Q.), Cardiol (P.Q.)
Lefebvre, Y., ObstGyn
Legare, A., DiagRad.
Legare, A. M., PlasSurg
Legare, M., Anaes
Legare, Marguerite
Legault, G.
Legault, J. P., Urol
Legault, L., Anaes
Legault, R., Psy
Legault, R.
Legendre, J. H., IntMed
Leger, A.
Leger, F., IntMed
Leger, Hugette, IntMed.
Leger, J., IntMed (P.Q.), Aller (P.Q.)
Leger, J. L., D & TRad
Leger, L. P., DiagRad
Leger, Y., Psy
Legrand, J. H., Ophth, Otol
Legresley, L. P., Path
Lehman, G. W., GenSurg
Lehmann, H. E., Psy (P.Q.)
Leith, A. B., Ophth
Leith, J. D. F.
Leith, W., IntMed, Aller(P.Q.)
Leitman, H. R. R.
Lekie, R.
Lemaire, R., OrthSurg
Lemay, C.
Lemay, C. A.
Lemay, J.
Lemieux, R.
Lemieux, R. R., Psy (P.Q.)
Lemire, A.
Lemire, Claire, Anaes
Lemire, P. G., DiagRad.
Lemire, Y., Cardiol (P.Q.)
Lemyre, R.
Leonard, C., Paed (P.Q.)
Leonard, F., Psy
Leonard, G., Obst (P.Q.)
Leonard, G. J.
Lepage, A. J., Psy
Lepage, C. C., Anaes
LePage, G., ThorSurg
Lepage, P. M., IntMed (P.Q.)
Lepine, C., PulmDis&TB(P.Q.)
Lepine, E., OrthSurg
Lepine, H., Anaes(P.Q.)
Lepine, R.
Leroux, H., GenSurg(P.Q.)
Leroux, O.
Leroy, A., Obst
LeRoy, M. J.
Lesage, E., IntMed (P.Q.)
Le Sage, J. B., GenSurg
Lesage, M.
Lessard, C.
Lessard, J. M., PhyMed (P.Q.)
Lessard, P. A., Anaes (P.Q.)
Lester, Evangeline, Psy
Letendre, P., IntMed, Gastroent. (P.Q.)
Letendre, S., Gyn (P.Q.)
L'Etoile, M., Anaes
Letourneau, J., TherRad
Levac, A., Anaes (P.Q.)
Levac, Therese, Neur (P.Q.)
Leveille, A., Paed (P.Q.)
Leveille, B. A.
Leveque, C. P.
Levesque, H. P., DiagRad
Levin, D. C., Psy
Levin, H.
Levine, A. H., GenSurg (P.Q.)
Levine, B., IntMed
Levine, R. M., GenSurg
Levinson, E. D., Psy
Levitan, B. A., IntMed, Cardiol (P.Q.)
Levitsky, P., IntMed Gastroent (P.Q.)
Levitt, M. N., Otol (P.Q.)
Levitz, A., Anaes
Levy, Edith
Levy, H. H., ThorSurg (Cardiol)
Levy, L., Psy
Lewis, D. J., Psy
Lewis, D. S., IntMed
Lezonoff, A., IntMed, Allergy (P.Q.)
L'Heureux, J.
Libman, I., Neurol
Lieblich, B. A.
Liefmann, R.
Light, A. W., D & T Rad.
Limoges, J. E.
Limougelli, F. M., GenSurg.
Lin, D. T. W., GenSurg (P.Q.)
Lin, Sylvia J-P., Paed.
Lindsay, C. C., ObstGyn
Lingard, W. F., Urol
Lipowska, Barbara
Lipowski, Z., Psy(P.Q.)
Lithe, W.
Little, G. D., GenSurg
Little, J. G., Ophth
Little, J. M., Ophth(P.Q.)
Lizotte, A. J.
Lizotte, P.
Lloyd-Smith, D., Neur
Lloyd-Smith, W. C., GenSurg
Locke, J. C., Ophth
L'Oddo, G.
Lohrenz, J. G., Psy
Loignon, G., Psy
Long, L., IntMed (P.Q.) & ClinPath (P.Q.)
Long, R. C., GenSurg
Longpre, D., Paed
Longtin, J., IntMed, Pulm Dis & TB (P.Q.), Cardiol (P.Q.)
Longtin, L., Anaes
Longtin, M., D & TRad
Lorange, G. C., PulmDis & TB (P.Q.) Int-Med. (P.Q.)
Lorrain, J., ObstGyn
Lortie, E., Anaes
Lortie, G., Psy(P.Q.)
Lortie, M.
Lough, J. O., Path
Lougheed, M. N., D&TRad
Loungnarath, V., GenSurg.
Lowenstein, L., IntMed, Haem (P.Q.)
Lowy, F. H., Psy
Lozinski, E., IntMed
Lubinski, H. H., Bact
Lundell, F. W., Psy
Lupien, J. E., Anaes
Lupu, G. H., Paed
Lussier, A., IntMed (P.Q.)
Lussier, Gisele, DiagRad
Lussier, J., IntMed (P.Q.)
Lussier, M., Ophth
Lussier, R., Anaes (P.Q.)
Luthe, W.
Lynch, L., PulmDis&TB(P.Q.)
Lyon, H. T.
Maaloux, Hanna, GenSurg
Macarthur, J. L., ObstGyn
MacCallum, E. A., ObstGyn
MacDermot, P. N., Paed, PulmDis & TB (P.Q.)
MacDonald, A. D., IntMed
Macdonald, C. C., IntMed
MacDonald, D. O.
MacDonald, F. R., DiagRad
MacDonald, R. N., IntMed., Haem(P.Q.)
MacDonald, S. A., Urol
MacDougal, J. R.
MacDougall, D. A.
MacDougall, J. I., IntMed.
Macfarlane, J.
MacFarlane, K. T., ObstGyn
Machabee, G.
MacHabee, Y.
MacIntosh, D. J., IntMed
MacIntosh, Nadine
MacIsaac, S. G., Urol.
MacKay, A., IntMed
MacKay, D. G.
MacKay, J. R., Psy
MacKenzie, D. E., IntMed
MacKenzie, J. R., GenSurg
MacKenzie, K. R., IntMed (P.Q.)
MacKenzie, M. B., Path (P.Q.)
MacKinnon, K. J., Urol
Macklem, P. T., IntMed
MacLean, J. T., Urol
MacLean, L. D.
MacLeod, A. W., Psy
MacMillan, C. W., PH
MacNaughton, E. A., GenSurg, ThorSurg (P.Q.)
MacPhail, F. L., ObstGyn(P.Q.)
MacPherson, R. I., DiagRad
MacWatt, D. J., Anaes
Madore, P., GenSurg, Thor-Surg (P.Q.)
Madore, P. R., TherRad.
Magder, H., Ophth
Mageau, G.
Magill, F., IntMed(P.Q.)
Magnan, L. A., ObstGyn
Maguire, G. H., D&TRad
Maguire, J. G., Psy
Maheux, P., Path (P.Q.)
Mailhot, M.
Maille, J. G. Anaes
Maille, G., OrthSurg
Maille, R., PH (P.Q.)
Mailloux, J. L. J.
Mailloux, L.
Mailloux, L., Ophth, Otol
Majeau, G.
Major, W., Paed (P.Q.)
Mally, Martha C.
Malo, Muriel, P.H.(P.Q.)
Malo, R. A.
Malouf, H., GenSurg.
Maltais, R., DiagRad
Mancuso, F.
Mancuso, S.
Mandavia, M. G.
Mandel, B., Paed (P.Q.)
Mandeville, H-P., DiagRad
Mankiewicz, E.
Mann, A. M., Psy
Mann, H. B.
Manseau, J. A., Obst (P.Q.)
Manseau, P., PulmDis & TB (P.Q.)
Marc-Aurele, J., IntMed(P.Q.)
Marceau, M., Otol.
Marchand, J.
Marchand, L., Otol (P.Q.)

* Population not **separately available.**

Montreal (Cont'd.)
Marchildon, A. IntMed (P.Q.), Ophth
Marchildon, P. A., GenSurg
Marcotte, J. E. A., Psy
Marcoux, A.
Marcoux, G.
Marcoux, R.
Marcoux, R.
Marcus, D. M., IntMed
Marien, B., GenSurg
Marin, C. E., Psy (P.Q.)
Marineau, J. M.
Marinier, M., Obst (P.Q.)
Marion, D., Obst (P.Q.)
Marion, J. E.
Marion, J.
Marion, P. G., IntMed (P.Q.), Cardiol (P.Q.)
Markus, A. J., Paed
Markarian-Demers, A., Ophth (P.Q.)
Maroun, F. B., NeurSurg
Marsan, R. G.
Marsolais, A., Anaes
Martel, F.
Martel, J. A., Paed
Martel, J. C., GenSurg (P.Q.)
Martel, P. G., Psy
Martel-Jutras, Therese
Martimbeau, E., Anaes (P.Q.)
Martin, G.
Martin, G., PhysMed & Rehab
Martin, J. R., IntMed
Martin, P., PathBact
Martin, S. A., Psy
Martin, S. J., GenSurg
Martineau, B., Bact (P.Q.)
Martineau, J. E.
Martineau, M.
Martineau, R., Obst (P.Q.)
Martineau, Y., GenSurg
Martinez, S. N., NeurSurg
Mason, W. E., IntMed
Masse, J.
Masse, M.
Massicotte, P., Paed
Masson, Anne M.
Masson, C. L., Ophth, Otol
Masson, J. A. R., DiagRad
Mastropasqua, C. A., Anaes.
Mathews, W. H., Path Bact
Mathieson, G.
Mathieu, E.
Mathieu, G., Psy (P.Q.)
Mathieu, J., IntMed
Mathieu, M., Ophth
Matton, J.
Matzko, A., IntMed, Anaes
Mauffette, J.
Maughan, G. B., ObstGyn
Maugile, D., Psy
Mauriello, A. H.
Mauriello, V., Psy
Maurins, Janis
Mayer-Carre, M. Alaine
Mayman, A. B.
Mazaide, P. I.
Mazur, J., DiagRad(P.Q.)
McCallum, L., IntMed
McClean, Jeannette
McCory, T. P.
McCoy, R. H., Otol
McCrimmon, D. R., Paed
McCutcheon, R. M., Anaes.
McDonald, A. W., Anaes
McDonald, F. R., DiagRad
McDonald, J. C.
McDonald, R. C.
McEvoy, J. V.
McGovern, J. E., GenSurg
McGraw, J. Y., GenSurg (P.Q.)
McGregor, F. R.
McGregor, M.
McHugh, H. E., Otol
McIlquham, M. C.
McIntosh, C. A., GenSurg, ThorSurg (P.Q.)
McIntyre, J. M., OrthSurg
McKay, Y., Path(P.Q.)
McKenna, R. D., IntMed (P.Q.)
McKenty, F. E.
McKenzie, J. M., IntMed.
McKenzie, J. R., GenSurg
McKeown, R. A., ObstGyn
McKibbin, G. T., GenSurg(P.Q.)
McKiernan-Lavoie, Clarice M., Anaes
McKim, L. H., GenSurg
McKinna, A. J., Ophth
McLaughlin, P., Anaes
McLean, A. P., GenSurg.
McLean, L. D., GenSurg
McLellan, W. G., IntMed (P.Q.) Aller (P.Q.)
McLeod, C. K., GenSurg
McMartin, J. W.
McMartin, W. F., IntMed
McMillan, R. M., Otol
McMurty, Shirley O.
McNally, W. J., Otol
McNaughton, F. L., NeurPsy
McNeill, A., Obst
McRae, D. L., D & TRad
Meakins, J. F., IntMed, Pulm Dis & TB (P.Q.)
Mehra, Y. N., Otol
Meilleur, R.
Melancon, D., DiagRad(P.Q.)
Melancon, J., IntMed.
Melhado, G. C., ObstGyn
Melillo, C.
Mellor-Fricker, Mary D., IntMed.
Meloche, B., NeurSurg
Meloche, R.
Melville, K. I.
Menard, B. S., Psy
Menard, E., IntMed
Menard, J. C., GenSurg (P.Q.)
Mendelson, H. I.
Mendelson, J., Bact(P.Q.)
Meng, M.
Menticoglou, K.
Mercier, J., Urol (P.Q.)
Mercier, L. ObstGyn
Mercier, R. J.
Mercure, C., Paed
Mergler, L., Psy
Messier, C. A.
Messinger, M. J., IntMed., Aller. (P.Q.)
Meszaros, A. F., Psy
Methot, J. P., Anaes (P.Q.)
Methot, Y., D & TRad
Metrakos, Katherine
Meunier, A., DiagRad
Meunier, P. E., Gyn
Meunier, R. C.
Meyers, J. F., GenSurg(P.Q.)
Mher-El-Saadi, A-H., DiagRad.
Michaud, C., Ophth
Michaud, R., Psy
Michaud, R., IntMed Cardiol (P.Q.)
Michon, J. B., ObstGyn
Midgley, R. D., GenSurg., PlasSurg.
Mignault, G., Anaes
Mignault, J., Cardiol (P.Q.)
Mikelsons, Velta K., Anaes (P.Q.)
Millar, J. K., DiagRad
Miller, A., IntMed
Miller, Carol
Miller, F.
Miller, J. E., OrthSurg.
Miller, M. C., IntMed
Miller, M. J.
Millette, J. E.
Milne, I. G., IntMed, Cardiol (P.Q.)
Milot, J. P., PulmDis TB(P.Q.)
Milot, P. E.
Minde, K. K., Psy
Mingie, W. J. E.
Miron, D.
Mitchell, D. S., DermSyph
Mitchell, H. S., IntMed
Mitchell, N. S., OrthSurg(P.Q.)
Mitmaker, B., GenSurg
Mitton, C. C., Anaes.
Mizgala, H. F., IntMed, Cardiol (P.Q.)
Mlynaryk, P., IntMed, Gastroen (P.Q.)
Mode, G. S.
Moisan, A., IntMed
Moise, A. L., Anaes.
Moll, A. E., Psy
Monaghan, E. D., GenSurg
Mondor, A., Anaes (P.Q.)
Mondor, E.
Mondoux, G.
Monfette, C. B., Ophth, Otol (P.Q.)
Mongeau, J-G., Paed.
Mongeau, M., PhysMed
Monks, H. T. J., DermSyph
Montgrain, P., IntMed(P.Q.) Gastroent(P.Q.)
Montgomery, L. C., IntMed
Montour, J.
Montpetit, J., Psy(P.Q.)
Montpetit, V. J. A., Path(P.Q.)
Montreuil, F., Otol
Monty, L. A.
Monty, P.
Moon, C. S., DiagRad.
Mooney, J. K., IntMed (P.Q.)
Moore, C. A., Urol
Moore, J .R., GenSurg
Moore, S., Path
Moors, D. E., Urol
Moralejo, R. V., GenSurg
Moreau, A., GenSurg
Moreau, F. A.
Moreault, P., Psy
Morehouse, D. D., Urol
Morf, G., Psy (P.Q.)
Morgentaler, H.
Moriarity, A. J.
Morin, C., IntMed
Morin, G., Paed
Morin, G., IntMed
Morin, G. M., Bact.
Morin, L., Psy
Morin, P., IntMed
Morin, P. A.
Morin-Gonthier, Mariette
Morisset, R.
Morissette, A.
Morissette, G., Paed
Morissette, J.
Moros, G. P.
Morris, Mary, Anaes
Morrissette, L., IntMed (P.Q.), Haem (P.Q.)
Morrow, Mary M., Neur (P.Q.)
Morton, A., Neur (P.Q.)
Morton, A. C.
Morton, H. S., GenSurg ObstGyn (P.Q.)
Moseley, H. F., GenSurg, OrthSurg
Mousseau, Jean Marie
Mousseau, P.
Mulclair, J. G., ObstGyn
Muller, A. K.
Muller, H. F., Psy
Mulligan, G. W., GenSurg (P.Q.)
Mungall, A. N., Anaes
Munio, Natalie
Munro, D. D., ThorSurg (P.Q.)
Murphy, Beverley
Murphy, D. R., Path
Murphy, G. R., OrthSurg

* Population not separately available.

Montreal (Cont'd.)
Murray, W. A.
Musgrave-McConnell, Aileen, IntMed
Nadeau-Jodoin, Marie
Nadeau, L. H., IntMed
Nadeau, P., IntMed
Pulm Dis & TB (P.Q.)
Nadeau, R. A., IntMed
Nadeau, Roger
Nadiak, Olga, Anaes(P.Q.)
Nadler, N.J., IntMed (P.Q.)
Naihouse, M.
Naiman, J., Psy
Naimark, A. P., DiagRad(P.Q.)
Nancekivell, A. F., IntMed
Nantel, A.
Nantel, M.
Nash, P. H.
Nathens, M. S., DiagRad
Neaga, A., Path
Nearing, T. N., Urol
Negrete, J. C., Psy.
Neilson, W. I., Anaes (P.Q.)
Neiman, G. M., IntMed
Nelligan, L. P., GenSurg
Nerman, Y., Psy
Nestel, M. B.
Neubauer, E.
Neuman, A. A., ObstGyn
Neuman, Alice
Neumann, P. Z., Paed
Nicholaides, T.
Nicholls, J. V. V., Ophth
Nickerson, G. H., Paed
Nicolle, F. V., PlasSurg
Niloff, P. H., GenSurg
Noble, A. B., Anaes
Noel, J. M., ObstGyn (P.Q.)
Nogrady, Bernadette, DiagRad
Nogrady, G. L., Bact
Nogrady, Marie, DiagRad
Noiseaux, J., Ophth
Nolin, P. G., Paed
Normandin, J., Anaes(P.Q.)
Notkin, L. J., IntMed
Notkin, M., IntMed
Novella, C., Psy
Novick, W. H., Otol
Nucci, C., ObstGyn
Nutik, H. L., GenSurg
Nutik, O., ObstGyn
Obrenovitch, Milena, Psy
O'Brien, J. R., ObstGyn
Ogilvie, R. I., IntMed.
Ogilvy, W. L., GenSurg
O'Gulnik, F. V.
Ohri, H. R., Psy
Oldfield, F. S. J., Path.
Olesker, N. H.
Oliver, J. A., Urol
Oliver, J., Path Bact
Olney, G. P., GenSurg (P.Q.)
O'Neill, J. H., Paed
Orlando, M. P., GenSurg
Ortenberg, S. L., IntMed
Osmolsky, E., Anaes
Ostapovitch, J. J., GenSurg (P.Q.)
Ostiguy, G. L., IntMed., Pul. Dis. & TB (P.Q.)
Ostiguy, G., ObstGyn
Ostiguy, J. P.
Ostiguy, L., Anaes (P.Q.)
Ostiguy, M., Ophth, Otol
Ostro, S.
Oszadszky, S., DiagRad
Otton, P. E., Anaes
Ouellet, C., Anaes
Ouellette, G.
Ouimet, C., Gyn (P.Q.)
Ouimet, Denise, D & TRad
Owen, H. F., GenSurg
Oxorn, H., ObstGyn
Pace-Floridia, A. P., Anaes
Page, A. A., GenSurg
Page, J. U.
Page, L., Paed (P.Q.)
Pager, R. Ophth
Paiement, P. A.
Pakes, E. H., Psy.
Palardy, R.
Palayew, M. J., DiagRad
Palmer, J. D., GenSurg
Palmer, W. H., IntMed
Panaccio, L., Psy (P.Q.)
Panaccio, V., DermSyph
Panet-Raymond, J. A., NeurPsy **NeurSurg**
Panneton, A., Paed
Panneton, A., OphthOtol
Papamtheaki-Lester, E.
Papich, D. F., GenSurg
Papillon, L. P.
Papillon, R.
Papineau, L., GenSurg,OrthSurg
Pappalardo, C., PlasSurg
Paquet, A. E., Paed
Paquet, B.
Paquet, J.
Paquet, J. E.
Paquette, C. J., GenSurg
Paquette, G.
Paquin, Antonine
Paquin, C. A.
Paquin, J. G.
Pare, C., Paed (P.Q.)
Parent, B.
Parent, J. D.
Parent, J. H., OrthSurg (P.Q.)
Parent, J. M., GenSurg
Parent, M.
Parenteau, A., NeurSurg(P.Q.)
Parenteau-Carreau, Suzanne
Parrin, M., ObstGyn.
Pasquale, M., GenSurg (P.Q.)
Parsons, R. M., ObstGyn
Patenaude, E. S., PH
Patenaude, J. S. E.
Pateras, V. R., IntMed
Patoine, L.
Patoine-Laporte, M.
Patrick, J. W., ObstGyn
Pattee, C. J., IntMed (P.Q.)
Patton, H. B.
Patton, Jocelyn
Paulette, R. E., GenSurg, ThorSurg, P.Q.
Paul-Hus, G. A., Psy
Paulin, C., IntMed
Paulin, R., GenSurg, ThorSurg (P.Q.)
Pavilanis, V., Bact ,P.Q.)
Payette, Y.
Payne, H.
Pearl, G. J., GenSurg.
Pearman, R. W., Ophth
Pearson, G., Bact (P.Q.)
Pedvis, S., Paed, Aller (P.Q.)
Peirce, C. B., D & TRad
Pelchat, C.
Pellerin, R., Ophth, Otol
Pelletier, Helene E.
Pelletier, J. O. A.
Pelletier, J. P., Cardiol (P.Q.), IntMed (P.Q.)
Peloquin, A.
Peloquin, A. B., GenSurg
Peloquin, A. P.
Peloquin, R.
Peltier, A. J. E., NeurSurg
Penfield, W., NeurSurg
Percival, Eleanor S., ObstGyn
Percy, E. C., OrthSurg
Perey, B. J., GenSurg
Perot, P. L., Jr.
Perras, Colette, PlasSurg(P.Q.)
Perras, Loyola L., Anaes
Perras, P., DiagRad
Perrault, R., GenSurg
Perreault, G., IntMed (P.Q.) Gastroent (P.Q.)
Perreault, H., Anaes
Perreault, J. P., Obst (P.Q.)
Perreault, L., Anaes (P.Q.)
Perreault, R.
Perreault, W., GenSurg
Perrier, R.
Perrigard, G. E., GenSurg
Perron, L., Ophth, Otol
Perron, L., IntMed
Perron, M.
Perron, P., Anaes
Perron, S.
Pesant, G. L.
Pesant, P.
Peterfy, G., Psy
Petrasek, A., Anaes
Petrella, N. J.
Petrie, A. H., IntMed.
Petrie, J. G., OrthSurg
Phaneuf-Filion, Gisele
Phaneuf, I. A., Anaes
Phelps, L. E., ObstGyn
Phills, J. A.
Philpott, N. W., ObstGyn
Phoenix, P., Psy
Piasecki, G., IntMed
Picard, J. L., Paed
Piche, B., Psy (P.Q.)
Piche, C. G., Path
Piche, L. G.
Pichette, L. P., IntMed., Gastroent (P.Q.)
Pick, C. A., IntMed, Haem(P.Q.)
Piette, J., Paed (P.Q.)
Piette, Y., IntMed
Pigeon, G., IntMed (P.Q.)
Pillet, J. V.
Pilon, A., NeurPsy
Pilon, B., GenSurg
Pilon, J. L., PulmDis & TB (P.Q.)
Pilote, L., GenSurg
Pinault, A., Anaes
Pinsonneault, G., D & TRad, PhysMed (P.Q.)
Pintar, K.
Pirozynski, W. J., Path
Piuze, Y. E., Anaes (P.Q.)
Pivnicki, D., Psy.
Place, R. E. F., IntMed
Plamondon, G.
Plante, A.
Plante, C., Psy (P.Q.)
Plante, C. A., OrthSurg
Plante, G. C., Psy
Plante, R., GenSurg
Plouffe, A.
Poirier, F., Neur
Poirier, G.
Poirier, J. R., Ophth
Poirier, L.
Poirier, P., Derm
Poirier, R.
Poirier, R., Paed
Poirier, R.
Poison, J. S., IntMed
Poisson, R. C., GenSurg
Poitevan, N.
Polan, W. D., ObstGyn
Pollak, B., PulmDis&TB(P.Q.)
Pollalis, S., Ophth
Pomerantz, D.
Pomerantz, H. Z., IntMed
Pompa, C.
Pontbriand, R.
Popov, T.
Portnuff, J. C., ObstGyn
Pothier, G., GenSurg (P.Q.)
Potvin, P., OrthSurg
Poulin, O.
Poulin, R.
Pouliot, G. E., Ophth (P.Q.)
Pouliot, M. R.
Poupart, G., PulmDis & TB (P.Q.)
Powel-Smith, C. J., TherRad

* Population not separately available.

Montreal (Cont'd.)
Power, D. J.,Anaes
Power, M. R. H., ObstGyn
Power, R. H., Jr., ObstGyn
Prat, Alain, IntMed
Prados, M., Psy
Prefontaine, G., Bact (P.Q.)
Pretty, H. G., GenSurg
Prevost, J. H., IntMed
Prevost, M., Urol.
Prevost, Y., GenSurg, PlasSurg
Pridham, G. R.
Primeau, B., PH (P.Q.)
Primeau, R., IntMed(P.Q.)
Primrose, T., ObstGyn
Prince, J., GenSurg (P.Q.)
Prince, J. B., GenSurg(P.Q.)
Prince, R. H., Psy
Prissick, F. H., Bact
Pritchard, J. F., PathBact
Proulx, A., IntMed,Cardiol(P.Q.)
Proulx, J. L. C., Paed.
Provost, A., Obst (P.Q.)
Provost, G., IntMed, Pulm Dis & TB (P.Q.)
Provost, J. G.
Provost, L.
Provost, M., Gyn (P.Q.)
Prud'homme, C.
Prud'homme, G. Anaes(P.Q.)
Prud'homme, G.
Prud'homme, Hortense, Anaes (P.Q.)
Prud'homme, J., IntMed
Quan, P., Anaes
Quastel, J. H.
Que, M.
Quenneville, J. G., IntMed
Quenneville, J. H.
Quesnel, B., Paed
Quinn, L. J., ObstGyn
Quintal, D.
Rabin, E. Z., IntMed.
Rabinovitch, B.
Rabinovitch, I.
Rabinovitch, P.
Rabinovitch, S., IntMed
Racine, Eva C., IntMed
Racine, J., DiagRad
Racine, L., OrthSurg
Radacovici, C. E., GenSurg (P.Q.)
Radhakrishnan, M., Anaes.
Raff, D., IntMed (P.Q.)
Raff, M. J., Otol (P.Q.)
Raginsky, B. B., IntMed, Psy (P.Q.)
Rainville, N. S.
Rakoff, Vivian M., Psy
Ram, A., Otol
Ramos, A.
Ramsey, R. B., Ophth
Ramsey, S., Ophth
Randall, M. T. Clare, Paed.
Rasmussen, T., NeurSurg
Ratelle, Germaine, D & TRad
Ratner, J., IntMed, Gastroent (P.Q.)
Ravary, P. Q.
Raymond C., GenSurg
Raymond, G.
Raymond, O., DiagRad (P.Q.)
Raymond, R.
Raynauld, P., Obst
Recester, T.
Reed, R. W., Bact (P.Q.)
Reed-Daoust, Lise, IntMed
Reesal, M. R., Path.
Regnault, Paule, PlasSurg
Reich, S., DiagRad
Reid, A.
Reid, E. A. S., IntMed,
Reid, E. C., Urol
Reid, R. G., Urol
Reilly, D. H., IntMed
Reisler, H., IntMed, Cardiol (P.Q.)
Remillard, B.
Remillard, P. E., GenSurg(P.Q.)
Remington, J. H.
Remy, M., ObstGyn
Renaud, P. E., GenSurg., OrthSurg(P.Q.)
Rennert, C.
Renzi, G., IntMed, Pulm Dis & TB (P.Q.)
Requena, C.
Rhea, L. D., ObstGyn
Rheault, F.
Rheault, J., Anaes
Rheault, M., GenSurg (P.Q.)
Ricard, A., Obst
Ricard, G.
Ricard, H., Obst
Ricard, J., Obst (P.Q.)
Ricard, J. P. M., ThorSurg(P.Q.)
Ricard, R. C., PlasSurg
Richard, F. S., GenSurg
Richard, J. B. L.
Richardson, Anne B., Anaes
Richardson, R. L.
Richardson, S. L., IntMed, Cardiol(P.Q.)
diol (P.Q.)
Richer, C.
Richer, P. A.
Richer, P. F.
Richer, S. L., Psy
Richter, M.
Rinfret, G. G. F., NeurSurg
Rinfret, L.
Riopelle, J. L., PathBact
Rioux, A., Anaes
Rishikof, J. R.
Rivard, G.
Riven, D. J.
Rivest, R.
Rivest, S. P., D & TRad
Rivest, Y.
Rivet, R.
Robb, J. P., Neur
Robbins, Evelyn E., IntMed
Roberge, Y.
Robert, A. H., IntMed
Robert, A., Bact
Robert, A.
Robert, Francoise, Path (P.Q.)
Robert, Giselle, Psy
Robert, P., IntMed (P.Q.)
Roberts, P. H., ObstGyn
Robertson, H. R., GenSurg
Robichaud, E.
Robichaud, P. A.
Robillard, E.
Robillard, F. A., Anaes
Robillard, G., DiagRad
Robillard, J. M., Anaes (P.Q.)
Robillard, J. R., Neur
Robillard, R., IntMed
Robillard, R., TherRad
Robson, N. G., IntMed.
Rocheleau, J. F.
Rochette, Madeline, Paed(P.Q.)
Rochman, S., Paed
Rochon, J. C.
Roden, R. G.
Rodger, N. W., IntMed
Rodrique, F.
Rogers, B. T., IntMed
Rolland, G., GenSurg
Rolland, R.
Romagnoli, A., Anaes (P.Q.)
Rona, Agnes
Rona, G., Path
Rona-Revesz, Clara
Rona, S.
Root, H. S.
Roper, P. L., Psy
Rosales, J. K., Anaes
Rose, B., IntMed, Aller (P.Q.)
Rosenberg, G., IntMed
Rosenbaum, P., Ophth
Rosenfeld, H.
Rosensweig, J., GenSurg, ThorSurg
Rosenthall, L., D & TRad
Ross, A. S., Paed
Ross, H. G.
Ross, M. M.
Ross, S. G., Paed
Ross, Winnifred, ObstGyn, TherRad.
Rossi, S., ObstGyn (P.Q.)
Roth, E. M.
Rothbart-Fox, Zelda R., Paed.
Rothstein, B., IntMed
Rouleau, A., Otol (P.Q.)
Rouleau, G. A.
Rouleau, P.
Rouleau, Y., Cardiol (P.Q.), IntMed (P.Q.)
Rondeau, Y., Anaes
Rousse, G.
Rousseau, P. J., Anaes.
Rousseau, Therese M.
Roussel, J. M.
Routledge, J. H., ObstGyn
Roux, F. C., Urol(P.Q.)
Roux, J. R., GenSurg (P.Q.)
Roux, L.
Rovinescu, I. A., Urol.
Roy, A. PH (P.Q.)
Roy, C. E., Anaes
Roy, J., IntMed (P.Q.), Aller (P.Q.)
Roy, J. L., GenSurg (P.Q.)
Roy, P. B., Psy (P.Q.)
Roy, R., OrthSurg
Royer, J. A., Paed
Royer, P. H., DiagRad. (P.Q.)
Rubin, I. C.
Rubin, J. H., PulmDis & TB (P.Q.)
Rubin, S., IntMed (P.Q.)
Rubinyi, Lea, Anaes
Ruddick, D. W., GenSurg
Ruddick, W. W., GenSurg
Ruedy, J., IntMed.
Ruel, A. H., Gastroent (P.Q.)
Ruggeri, F.
Ruhman, W.
Russell, A.
Ryan, J. J., GenSurg (P.Q.)
Sabin, M., ObstGyn
Sagritalo, G. C.
Saibil, D., IntMed (P.Q.)
Saibil, M., IntMed
Saine, J.
Saint-Denis, J. A. P., Paed.
St. Georges, P.
St. Germaine, J. P.
St-Hilare, J. M., Neur
St. Jacques, A., DiagRad
St. Jean, A.
St. Jean, M.
Saint-Laurent, C., Psy
St. Laurent, J.
St-Laurent, J. Psy
St. Laurent, P. G., Paed, Haem (P.Q.)
St. Laurent, R., GenSurg
St. Martin, M., Bact
St. Onge, G., GenSurg
St. Pierre, J. G.
St. Pierre, L. J., PulmDis & TB **(P.Q.)**
Saint-Rome, G., Paed
Sakkal, K. A., GenSurg
Salter, Elizabeth, Paed.
Saltiel, J. J., D & TRad
Salvi, G. J.
Samson, G. H., Psy
Samson, J.
Samson, J. E., OrthSurg
Samson, R., OrthSurg
Sandborn, B. E.

*** Population not separately available.**

Montreal (Cont'd.)

Sanche, H., Obst
Sanche, P., Obst (P.Q.)
Sanchez, A., Psy(P.Q.)
Sangowicz, J.
Sansregret, A., DiagRad
Sansregret, D.
Sansregret, E., Obst
Sansregret, J., Obst (P.Q.)
Sansregret, V.
Sarwer-Foner, G. J., Psy
Saucier, Cossette
Saucier, J., NeurPsy
Saucier, J. F., Psy
Saunders, D. R., IntMed
Savard, G.
Savard, R. M., Cardiol (P.Q.)
Savoie, E., GenSurg
Savoie, M.
Sayegh, V., DiagRad
Scarlatesco, A. I.
Scharfe, E. E., Otol
Scheffer, Y.
Schickler, O.
Schiffman, Wanda, Neur
Schipper, H. L., GenSurg
Schirmer, K. E., Ophth
Schlesinger, I. A.
Schmidt, C. H.
Schneiderman, C., Urol
Schneiderman G., Psy
Schopflocher, Paula H., Derm
Schulte-Steinberg, O.
Schwartz, A., Neur
Schwartz, H. T., IntMed (P.Q.)
Schwartz, J. P., Haem (P.Q.)
Schwartz, M. H.
Schwartzman, J. C.
Scott, A.
Scott, B. H.
Scott, H. J., GenSurg, ThorSurg, (P.Q.)
Scott, H. M., IntMed.
Scott, W. C., Psy (P.Q.)
Scotti, R.
Scriver, C. R., Paed
Scriver, J. B., Paed
Scriver, W. De M., IntMed
Sebastien, G., PlasSurg
Sedlezki, I., D & TRad (P.Q.)
Segal, P. .M, Psy
Segall, H. N., IntMed
Segall, S. IntMed
Seguin, F., IntMed (P.Q.), Cardi (P.Q.)
Sequin, H., ObstGyn (P.Q.)
Seguin, R., DiagRad
Selye, H., Exper Med
Seamans, K. B., Neur.
Semogas, J., GenSurg
Senay, R. G.
Sendbuehler, J. M., Psy
Senecal, C.
Senecal, L., Path(P.Q.)
Senecal, P. M., Paed
Seng, M. I.
Seregerie, C.
Serres, R.
Shabanah, E.
Shamsie, S. J., Psy
Shane, R., Paed (P.Q.)
Shanks, J. A., IntMed
Shannon, J. G., OrthSurg
Shansie, S. J., Psy
Shapiro, E. K., Ophth
Shapiro, L., IntMed
Shapiro, S. B., Paed
Shaver, F. W., Otol (P.Q.)
Shaw, D. B.
Sheiner, N. M., ThorSurg (Cardio), GenSurg
Sheldon, H.
Shephard, D. A. E., Anaes.
Sheridan, C. A., Anaes
Sherman, E. D., IntMed
Sherwin, A. L., Neurol
Shibata, H. R., GenSurg.
Shimo-Takahara, G., Otol
Shippam, F., Paed
Shister, H. E., IntMed, Cardiol
Shooner, J. T. F.
Shortt, C. D.
Shragovitch, I., GenSurg
Shugar, J. L., OrthSurg
Shulman, A., IntMed
Shulman, R., IntMed
Shuster, S., IntMed (P.Q.)
Siahaan, C.
Sicard, A., Derm
Sieniewicz, D. J., D & TRad
Sigman, H. H., GenSurg
Siller, T. N., OrthSurg
Silva-Azaustre, J., PhysMed. & Rehab(P.Q.)
Silva, Y. J., GenSurg.
Silver, A.
Silver, M. D.
Silverberg, M., Paed
Silverman, B., Paed
Simard, F.
Simard, J. G., GenSurg
Simard, L. C., PathBact
Simard, P., Path (P.Q.)
Simard, P. R.
Simard, R. Gyn
Simard, R. P., GenSurg (P.Q.)
Simard, R., ObstGyn
Simard, V., GenSurg
Siminovitch, J., IntMed (P.Q.)
Siminovitch, M., Urol
Simon, A. V., Anaes
Simon, J. C.
Simon, M. A., PathBact
Simoneau, R., Psy(P.Q.)
Simoneau, R.
Simoneau, R. J. H., OrthSurg
Simons, S. P., Psy(P.Q.)
Simor, L.
Simpson, G. A., ObstGyn
Sinclair, G. M., Otol
Sinclair, H. A., IntMed (P.Q.)
Sinder, Slema
Sindon, A., Anaes.
Singer, O. P., Paed
Singh, C. R., Anaes
Sinha, S. P., Otol
Sinotte, L.
Sipos, J. K.
Skinner, G. B., DiagRad
Skitch, C. H., Psy
Skoryna, S. C., GenSurg (P.Q.)
Slapak, M., GenSurg.
Slater, H. M., Anaes
Slatkoff, W. R.
Sloman, L., Psy
Smart, I. H.
Smit, J. S., GenSurg
Smith, C. B.
Smith, C. C., Psy
Smith, D. A.
Smith, E. J., Otol
Smith, H. H., DermSyph
Smith, J. A.
Smith, L.
Smith, M., IntMed
Smith, P., GenSurg
Smith, R. B.
Smith, R. M., DiagRad.
Smith, S. A., IntMed
Snarch, M. D.
Solomon, M.
Solomon, M. L., Psy.
Solymar, J., IntMed, Gastroent (P.Q.)
Solyom, L., Psy
Somlo, F.,
Sommerfreund, P.
Somos, E.
Sonea, S. I. L., Bact
Sosa, J. A., IntMed., Cardiol(P.Q.)
Soucy, A., Paed
Sourkes, Shena
Sowden, K. A., PhysMed&Rehab.
Sparling, D. W., ObstGyn
Spector, L., GenSurg
Spence, M. W.
Stacey, C. H., IntMed
Stanford, R. L., IntMed
Stanley, P., GenSurg (P.Q.)
Starkey, D. H., Bact
Stattner, P.
Steidl, Pippa Ophth
Stellos, A., Urol
Stern, K., Psy
Stern, L., Paed
Stern, L. G., Psy
Sternberg, J.
Stevens, H. D., GenSurg
Stevenson, L. G.
Stewart, J. D., Psy (P.Q.)
Stewart, O. W.
Stewart, P. B.
Stilman, A., Urol
Storrar, W.
Straja, M.
Straker, M., Psy (P.Q.)
Strasberg, A., Urol
Stratford, J. G., NeurSurg
Strauss, R.
Strawczynski, Hanna, Paed
Strean, G. J., ObstGyn
Struminsky, R.
Struthers, R. R., Paed
Stuart, E. A., Otol
Stuart, J. R., Path
Stubington, D., IntMed
Sugarman, I., ObstGyn (P.Q.)
Sullivan, T. J., Derm
Sundaram, E. B., GenSurg
Surani, N.
Surchin, H., Paed
Susset, J. G., Urol
Susset, Veronique, PhysMed & Rehab
Sutherland, J. B. I., Anaes
Sutton, J. C., GenSurg
Swaine, F. M., Ophth
Swaine, R. L., Otol
Swales, D. W., DiagRad.
Swalsky, M.
Sylvain, A.
Sylvestre, G.
Sylvestre, L.
Sylvestre, Robert
Sylvestre, R.
Synnott, E.
Szenas, P.
Sziklas, T.
Szymonowicz-Rudnicky, Halina
Tabah, E. J., GenSurg
Tache, C. R., PlasSurg.
Taguchi, Y., Urol
Taillefer, P. A., Ophth
Talbot, B., PhysMed & Rehab
Tamas, A., D & TRad (P.Q.)
Tanguay, J., GenSurg
Tannenbaum, I.
Taori, G. M., Neur.
Taraszczuk, P.
Tardif, L., DiagRad.
Tardif, M.
Tatleman, M.
Tatlow, W., Neur
Tauer, C.
Taylor, D. S.
Taylor, G. C., Psy (P.Q.)
Tchang, S. P., DiagRad
Teitelbaum, J. I.
Tellier, G.
Tellier, H., Psy
Tellier, J., Psy
Telmosse, F., GenSurg, ThorSurg.
Telner, P. P., DermSyph
Ten Pas, A., IntMed., Haem (P.Q.)
Teolis, J. P.

* Population not separately available.

Montreal (Cont'd.)
Tessier, A., Ophth Otol
Tessier, L. J., Ophth, Otol
Tetrault, P.
Tetreault, E. R., Psy
Tetreault, G. E.
Tetreault, H. I.
Tetreault, J., Obst
Tetreault, L.
Tetu, J. L.
Theocharides, P., GenSurg
Theoret, R.
Theriault, J. P., Path (P.Q.)
Therrien, A.
Therrien, E., Anaes (P.Q.)
Therrien, L.
Thibaudeau, P.
Thibaudeau, Y., IntMed
Thibault, E., IntMed (P.Q.)
Thibault, M., TherRad (P.Q.)
Thibert, F., IntMed (Gastro) (P.Q.)
Thibert, J. R., Otol
Thibert, M. D'A., IntMed(P.Q.)
Thibert, R., Path(P.Q.)
Thibodeau, L. P., Paed
Thiverge, A., OrthSurg
Thivierge, R. E.
Thom, A. T., IntMed, PulmDis & TB (P.Q.)
Thompson, A. G., GenSurg
Thompson, B. L., GenSurg.
Thompson, C. S., GenSurg
Thompson, W. G., IntMed.
Thomson, D. L., IntMed, Gastroent (P.Q.)
Thrasybule, E., Otol
Thurlbeck, W. M.
Thut, N. W.
Tidmarsh, C. J., IntMed, Gastroent (P.Q.)
Tidmarsh, W. W., Paed
Tiltins, Antonija
Tissenbaum, B.
Tittley, J. R., Obst (P.Q.)
Tomiuk, S.
Toth, A., ObstGyn
Tougas, G.
Tougas, H. W., Otol
Tougas, R.
Tourangeau, F. J., PH (P.Q.)
Tourillon, Marie P.
Tousignant, J. P., Anaes
Townsend, D. E., ObstGyn
Townsend, M. G., IntMed
Townsend, R. G., OrthSurg
Townsend, S. R., IntMed
Tranquil, J.
Tranquil, P.
Tremblay, A., Obst (P.Q.)
Tremblay, F., DiagRad.
Tremblay, G.
Tremblay, G., Path (P.Q.)
Tremblay, G. M., Cardiol(P.Q.)
Tremblay, J. C.
Tremblay, J., IntMed (P.Q.) & Gastroent (P.Q.)
Tremblay, J. J., Gastroent
Tremblay, J. N., PulmDis & TB (P.Q.)
Tremblay, L., Anaes
Tremblay, M. A.
Tremblay, P. C., ObstGyn
Tremble, G. E., Otol
Trempe, A. Anaes
Trempe, L.
Trepanier, A., D & TRad
Trossman, B., Psy
Trossman, M.
Trottier, M., Ophth
Trottier, R.
Trudeau, C. H.
Trudeau, E. A., OrthSurg(P.Q.)
Trudeau, H.
Trudel, H., Paed (P.Q.)
Trudel, L.
Trudel, J., IntMed.
Tucker, E. C., ObstGyn.
Turcot, E. A.
Turcot, G. H., Psy
Turcotte, D., OrthSurg.
Turcotte, R.
Turgeon, F., Bact
Turgeon, P. A., DermSyph
Turgeon-Knaack, Claire, Path
Turmel, A., Anaes.
Turmel, Y., Anaes
Turnbull, W., Ophth (P.Q.)
Turner, J. G.
Turnier, H., Anaes
Tweedie, F. J., ObstGyn
Uhthoff, H. K., OrthSurg
Uhthoff-Schuette, Annegrette, Anaes
Ujejska, Sophia
Unwin, J. R., Psy
Urbanski, W. A.
Usher, B., DermSyph
Usher, R. H.
Usher, S. J., Paed
Vacaflor, L. A. R., Psy.
Vachon, R.
Vadeboncoeur R., Obst (P.Q.)
Valcourt, J. P., Path (P.Q.)
Vaillancourt, D. G., IntMed
Vaillancourt, P., Plas Surg
Vallee, A., D & TRad
Vallee, G.
Vallee, J.
Vallee, J. G., GenSurg
Vallee, L. I., D & TRad, PhysMed (P.Q.)
Vallee, R., DiagRad
Vallois, A. B., PH
Van Campenhout, J., ObstGyn
Varin, R. D.
Varkey, G. P., Anaes
Varverikos, E. D., ObstGyn (P.Q.)
Varvis, C. J., IntMed
Vas, Magdalene, Haem (P.Q.)
Vasquez-Cruz, J., NeurPsy(P.Q.)
Vauclair, R., Path
Vaughan, P.
Vavruska, G. W., DermSyph
Vega-Jacombe, C.
Venecek, Danica, NeurPsy
Venecek, L., ObstGyn
Venne, J. P., ThorSurg
Venne, L., PlasSurg (P.Q.)
Ventura, J. C., Path
Verdy, M. B., IntMed
Vermette, H. B., GenSurg
Veronneau, Suzanne, Ophth
Verrault, J. M., Path
Verschelden, G., ObstGyn
Verschelden, M., PulmDis & TB (P.Q.)
Verschelden, N.
Versteeg, E. M.
Vessa, G., D & TRad
Vezina, A.
Vezina, J. A., D & T Rad.
Vezina, J. L., DiagRad
Vezina, L. J.
Vezina, N.
Viallet, A., IntMed.
Viau, A.
Viau, A.
Vicas, E., OrthSurg
Vidal, J. A., IntMed TB, Pulm Dis & TB (P.Q.)
Vielleux, G., Anaes
Viens, L.
Vigeant, E., GenSurg (P.Q.)
Vigeant, J., ObstGyn
Viger, R. J., Ophth
Vigneau, P., OrthSurg (P.Q.)
Vigneault, M., GenSurg
Vigneault, Patrice, Anaes(P.Q.)
Villemune, B.
Villeneuve, Louise
Villeneuve, R., ObstGyn (P.Q.)
Vincent, J., ObstGyn (P.Q.)
Vincent, R.
Vineberg, A. M., GenSurg
Viner, N., Neur, Psy
Vines, N. M.
Violette, B. R. J.
Virolle, P.
Visser, A. H.
Vitou, C.
Vitye, B., IntMed (P.Q.)
Voghel, D.
von Ondarza, U. E.
Vost, A.
Voyer, d'A., Psy(P.Q.)
Voyer, L., Psy(P.Q.)
Voyer, Victoria, Psy (P.Q.)
Wali, M. N., Otol
Walker, J. A. L., OrthSurg
Walsh, R. L.
Wang, Catherine S., Paed(P.Q.)
Ward, C. V., ObstGyn
Ward, R. V., IntMed
Warner, H. A., IntMed
Warnes, H., Psy
Warshaw, H. L.
Warshawski, H.
Waters, W. R., PlasSurg
Watson, J. I., IntMed.
Watson, R. E. L.
Watters, R.
Watters, W. W., Psy
Webb Lewis, Barbara
Webster, D. R., GenSurg
Weigand, R. P., Anaes, GenSurg
Weil, P., IntMed, Haem (P.Q.)
Weiner, H., Paed
Weintrub, I. W., IntMed
Weir, B. K., NeurSurg.
Weisberg, H. M., ObstGyn
Weisnagle, J., Allergy (P.Q.), Paed (P.Q.)
Weiss, Gabrielle, Psy
Wener, J., IntMed
Wermenlinger, P., Path Anat (P.Q.)
Wertman, A. M.
Wevrick, N.
Wewiorski, K.
Whelan, D. T., Paed.
Wherrett, B. A., Paed (P.Q.)
Whiston, G. J.
Whitehead, V. M., IntMed., Haem(P.Q.)
Whiteman, G., D & TRad
Wielhorski, W. A., Anaes
Wiener, F., Paed
Wight, G. E., IntMed
Wilansky, D. L., IntMed., Biochem(P.Q.)
Wilchesky, I. L.
Wilkie, A. L., GenSurg
Wilkinson, R. D., Derm
Williams, E. S. V., GenSurg.
Williams, J. B., GenSurg
Williams, H. B., PlasSurg
Williams, M. E.
Wilner, S., Psy
Wilson, A.
Wilson, C. L., OrthSurg.
Wilson, D. H.
Wilson, J. A., GenSurg, Thor-Surg
Wilson, P.
Wilson, Rolla E., DiagRad
Wilson, R. T.
Wilson, W. E., GenSurg, OrthSur
Windisch, Marie C.
Winer, J.
Winkler, I., IntMed
Wintrob, R. N.
Wior, G. A., Ophth, Otol
Wise, M. B., Paed
Wisebrod, N., Psy

* Population not separately available.

MONTREAL Cont'd
Wiselberg, Dorothy, IntMed, Pulm Dis & TB (P.Q.)
Wiseman, M., Obst
Witkov, H. R., DermSyph
Wittkower, E. D., Psy
Wlodek, G. K., GenSurg
Wolanskyj, B., Path
Wolf, J. G.
Wolfe, A. E., ObstGyn
Wolfe, J. G.
Wolfe, L. S.
Wong, A-W-H., NeurSurg
Wong-Mark, Mary, ObstGyn
Wood, T. E., IntMed(P.Q.)
Woodhouse, D. H., IntMed
Wood, A. Eleanor
Wood, G.
Woods, H. L.
Woolhouse, F. M., GenSurg, PlasSurg
Worden, E. M., Paed
Workman, E. W., GenSurg
Worsley, G. H., IntMed
Wortzman, G., DiagRad
Wright, A. M., OrthSurg
Wright, Isobel L., Paed
Wright, L. A.
Wrigley, F. R., Anaes
Wuidart, Y. H. R.
Wynands, J. E., Anaes
Xenos, J. B.
Yablon, I., OrthSurg.
Yachnin, I., IntMed
Young, J. C. G., IntMed, Gastroent (P.Q.)
Young, M. H. V., ObstGyn
Zaritsky, A., Paed
Zemel, R., GenSurg
Ziegler, M. L.

MONTREAL NORD
(See Montreal)

MONTREAL SUD
(see Cite de Jacques Cartier)

MORIN HEIGHTS
(600)
Robertson, B. D.

MURDOCHVILLE
(2,951)
May, W. L.
Paje, A. Q., GenSurg.

NAPIERVILLE
(1,812)
Aumont, R.
Palardy, J.
Beaudin, J.
Ouimet, A.

NEUFCHATEL
*
Roy, P. E.
Tessier, J. R.

NEUVILLE
(802)
Angers, C. E.

NEW CARLISLE
(1,333)
Dube, Louisella, PH
Gillies, J. N.

NEWPORT
(540)
Joncas, R.

NEW RICHMOND
(411)
Boileau, J. R. E.
Gauvreau, A.
Gauvreau, A.
Lambert, F.
MacLean, A. C.

NICOLET
(4,441)
Auger, P.
Laperriere, A., PH (P.Q.)

Piche, P., GenSurg (P.Q.)
Porter, H.
Roy, G. E., GenSurg
Roy, R., OrthSurg
St. Onge, A.

NOMINIQUE
(741)
Mailly, G. A.

NORANDA
(11,477)
Bellegard, J. V.
Bernier, J. J., GenSurg (P.Q.)
Firlotte, R. W.
Germain, L. M., Paed.
Ibrahim, A.
Linklater, E. W., GenSurg
Lukeman, R., GenSurg
McArthur, J. E., GenSurg
Tardif, J. B., Cardiol (P.Q.)

NORMANDIN
(1,838)
Levasseur, M.
Simard, R.

NORMETAL
(2,284)
Parrot, C.

NOTRE DAME DES LAURENTIDES
*
Larose, G.
Roberge, R.

NOTRE-DAME DU LAC
(1,690)
Dube, J., GenSurg (P.Q.)
Lizotte, J. A.

NOTRE-DAME DU NORD
(493)
Simard, P.

NOTRE DAME DU SACRE COEUR
(see Cite de Jacques Cartier)

NOUVELLE
(350)
Maguire, E.

OKA
(1,243)
Giroux, A.
Guibault, C.

OLD CHELSEA
(181)
Miskelly, Lorna

ORMSTOWN
(1,529)
Davidson, J. A., GenSurg (P.Q.)
Francis-Kelen, Marian
Johnson, J. C.
Kelen, A., IntMed (P.Q.)
McCallum, J. A., GenSurg
Poliquin, R. W., GenSurg
Ruberto, C. H., Jr.
Stalker, M. E., IntMed(P.Q.)
Sutton, G. L.
Thompson, B. G., GenSurg (P.Q.)

ORSAINVILLE
(4,236)
Gagnon, F.
Massicotte, C.
Paquet, B., IntMed(P.Q.), PH(P.Q.)
Roy, M., DermSyph

OUTARDES QUATRE
*
Bergeron, H.
Leblanc, R.

OUTREMONT
(see Montreal)

PALMAROLLE
*
Thibault, R.

PASPEBIAC
(800)
Langevin, G. E.
Morin, P. G.
Pelletier, F. E.
Roy, P. E.

PETIT SAGUENAY
*
Gobeil, J.

PIERREFONDS
(see Cite Jacques Cartier)

PIERREVILLE
(1,557)
Ebacher, R.
Robert, L. P.

PINCOURT
(2,689)
Fournier, A., GenSurg(P.Q.)
Morin, J. M.

PLESSISVILLE
(6,570)
Boisvert, J.
Cantin, J.
Charron, R.
Giguere, G., GenSurg
Savoie, C. B.

POINTE-AU-PIC
(1328)
Leclerc, J. A., GenSurg(P.Q.)

POINTE AUX TREMBLES
(see Montreal)

POINTE CLAIRE
(see Lachine)

POINTE DU LAC
(934)
de Charette, L. G.
Dugre, J. R. GenSurg
Le Blanc, J. L.

POINTE GATINEAU
(see Gatineau Pointe)

PONT ROUGE
(2,982)
Gingras, G.
St. Louis, F.
Turgeon, R.

PONT VIAU
(see Montreal)

PORT ALFRED
(9,066)
Beaulieu, E.
Thivierge, M.

PORT CARTIER
(3,464)
Fortin, C.
Verreault, R.

PORT DANIEL
(233)
Quesnel, A. E.

PORT MENIER
(438)
Pelletier, F. E.
Surkis, M.

PORTNEUF
(1,372)
Cote, N.
Hudon, M.

PREVILLE
(see Cite de Jacques Cartier)

PRICE
(3,099)
Joubert, G. A.

PRINCEVILLE
(3,174)
Tanguay, G.

QUEBEC
(392,000)
Allard, E., Anaes
Allen, L. P., Gyn (P.Q.)
Alloucherie, Marthe, Neurol.

*** Population not separately available.**

Quebec (Cont'd.)
Anctil, M. A.
Amours, C. D., Path(P.Q.)
Asselin, J. N.
Aube, L. DiagRad.
Audet, J., Ophth, Otol
Audet, L., D & TRad
Auger, C. L., PathBact.
Auger, G. L., GenSurg
Auger, L. C., Path, Bact
Auger, P., GenSurg (P.Q.)
Auger, R., Anaes
Authier, R. (JR) Path
Barrette, E.
Beauchesne, A., PulmDis & TB
Beaudet, G.
Beaudet, H. J. A., GenSurg.
Beaudoin, J. L., IntMed., Cardiol. (P.Q.)
Beaudry, J., Anaes.
Beaudry, M., DermSyph
Beaule, A., GenSurg (P.Q.)
Beaulieu, M., ThorSurg
Beaulieu, R., Otol (P.Q.)
Beauregard, L., D & T Rad.
Bedard, A., Urol
Bedard, D.
Bedard, J. A.
Bedard, J. H.
Bedard, J. U.
Bedard, R.
Belanger, C., Neur
Belanger, J., Marie
Belanger, M., ObstGyn.
Belhumeur, J. M., ObstGyn
Belleau, P. E., IntMed.
Bellefeuille, F. L.
Bellemare, F. B., PH (P.Q.)
Bellemare, F., Ophth, Otol(P.Q.)
Bellemare, J.
Belley, M., Otol
Bergeron, A.
Bergeron, G. A., IntMed
Bergeron, J., IntMed (P.Q.)
Bergeron, L. G.
Bergeron, L.
Bergeron, R., GenSurg.
Bernier, L., Path
Bernier, R., D & T Rad.
Bertrand, G., Gastroent(P.Q.)
Bertrand, J. H.
Bertrand, P. E.
Bigonesse, P., Paed(P.Q.)
Bigue, P., Ophth, Otol (P.Q.)
Bilodeau, M.
Bissonnette, J. E.
Bissonnette, J. P., GenSurg (P.Q.)
Bissonnette, M.
Blagdon, G., ObstGyn(P.Q.)
Blanchet, G.
Boilard, C. A., ObstGyn(P.Q.)
Boiteau, G. M., Cardiol (P.Q.)
Bonenfant, J. L., Path
Bossinotte, A.
Bouaziz, A., GenSurg.
Bouchard, M., Paed
Bouchard, M., Biochem(P.Q.)
Boucher, B., IntMed (P.Q.)
Boucher, M. F., Anaes.
Boucher, M. H., Anaes(P.Q.)
Boudreau, A.
Boudreau, A. T.
Boulaine, R. J., D & T Rad
Boulanger, J., OphthOtol(P.Q.)
Boulay, J., IntMed., Haem (P.Q.)
Boulet, M.
Bourbeau, J. M.
Bourgoin, L. P., Psy.
Boutet, C.
Brault, R., ObstGyn (P.Q.)
Brissette, Yvette B.
Brochu, J., GenSurg (P.Q.)
Brochu, J. L.
Brochu, L. A.
Brochu, P., GenSurg (P.Q.)
Brochu, R.
Brosseau, C. R., IntMed, Haem
Brunet, C., GenSurg
Brunet, J., GenSurg (P.Q.)
Brunet, J. R., IntMed
Brunet, W., Jr.
Brunet, W. E.
Busque, L., Anaes.
Cantin, R.
Caouette, J. G., Otol
Caouette, M. G., ObstGyn
Caouette, R., IntMed
Caouette, Suzanne
Carbonneau, M., OrthSurg. (P.Q.)
Carbotte, M. N., ObstGyn(P.Q.)
Carette, L.
Caron, E. S., NeurPsy.
Caron, J., Anaes (P.Q.)
Caron, J., Otol
Caron, J. G.
Caron, M.
Caron, P., IntMed (P.Q.)
Caron, R.
Caron, W. M., GenSurg
Carrette, J. P., GenSurg.
Carrier, G. R., Biochem(P.Q.)
Carrier, C., Paed.
Carter, C. J. O.
Carter, G.
Cauchon, R., Urol, GenSurg (P.Q.)
Caux, M., Ophth, Otol (P.Q.)
Cayer, L., ObstGyn (P.Q.)
Chabot, C., Psy (P.Q.)
Chabot, J-A., Neur(P.Q.)
Chabot, J. A., PH
Charrois, Marie
Charrois, R., Urol.
Chenard, J. P., Path
Chenel, L.
Chouinard, J., Anaes
Chretin, L., GenSurg.
Claveau, P., PH
Clavet, M., Anaes
Cliche, P. A., GenSurg (P.Q.),
Clouthier, J. R. P., GenSurg.
Cojocaru, N., Urol.
Cole, L., GenSurg(P.Q.)
Corkran, R. G., GenSurg
Cormier, P. E., Psy
Cote, A.,Pulm Dis & TB (P.Q.)
Cote C. E., Ophth, Otol (P.Q.)
Cote, G.
Cote, J., GenSurg (P.Q.)
Cote, N.
Cote, Patrice
Cote, P. E., D & TRad
Cote, R., GenSurg
Cote, R., IntMed
Cote, R., Psy.
Couillard, E.
Couillard, J. M.
Coulombe, M., Psy
Coulombe, P., PlasSurg (P.Q.)
Coulonval, L. F., Urol
Courchesne, G. H., Anaes
Couture, F., IntMed, Cardiol (P.Q.)
Couture, J. G., GenSurg
Crepin, G., Paed.
Dallaire, H.
D'Amours, C., Path(P.Q.)
Darveau, R.
D'Auteuil, P., IntMed, Haem (P.Q.)
de Blois, P., Otol (P.Q.)
Dechene, L. E., Paed
DeHostos, G. A.
Delage, J., Psy
Delage, J. M., IntMed, Haem (P.Q.)
Delage, M., PhysMed
Delaney, W. L.
de Launiere, H.
Delgado, A.
Delisle, J. C.
Demers, F. X., ObstGyn
Demers, P. P., Paed
Dery, R., Anaes
Dery, T., Path (P.Q.)
de St. Victor, J., ObstGyn
Descharreaux, J.
Deschenes, L., GenSurg
Desmeules, R., IntMed TB (P.Q.
Despres, J. P., GenSurg., ThorSurg.
DesRochers, M., DiagRad(P.Q.)
Desrosiers, D., PH (PQ)
Desrosiers, R., Anaes.
Des Ruisseaux, P. W.
Deubrevil-Charrois, Marie
Dion, C., Psy
Dion, R., PulmDis & TB (P.Q.)
Dionne, G., DiagRad.
Dionne, L. J., GenSurg
Dombrowski, S., Anaes (P.Q.)
Donati, S.
Dorion, J. E.
Dorion, M., DiagRad.
Dorion, Marguerite, PH (P.Q.)
Dorval, C. H., PulmDis & TB (P.Q.)
Douville, G. J. T., Anaes (P.Q.)
Drolet, C., Psy
Drolet, M., D & TRad.
Drolet, M. J.
Drouin, C.
Drouin, G.
Drouin, G., ObstGyn(P.Q.)
Drouin, G., IntMed, Cardiol (P.Q.
Drouin, J. G.
Drouin, N. H.
Drouin, Patrice, Neur
Drouin, R., D & TRad
Dube, M., GenSurg(P.Q.)
Duchaine, P., ObstGyn (P.Q.)
Duchesne, R., Anaes
Dufour, A.
Dufour, F.
Dugal, J. P., IntMed, Aller (P.Q.) Gastroent (P.Q.)
Dugal, L.
Dugre, J., Ophth
Dumas, A., PH(P.Q.)
Dumont, R.
Dunne, R. F., IntMed (P.Q.)
Dupuis, P., GenSurg (P.Q.), ThorSurg (P.Q.)
Durand, H. A., Anaes
Dussault, J. O.
Elliott, J. M., GenSurg
Faucher, E., GenSurg (P.Q.)
Ferland, J. J., OrthSurg.
Fisher, J. G., Urol
Fleury, B.
Foley, A. R., PH
Fontaine, G.
Fortier, C.
Fortier, de la B. Paed.
Fortier, J. R., IntMed., Cardiol (P.Q.)
Fortier, P. E.
Fortin, C. L., GenSurg
Fortin, G., GenSurg (P.Q.)
Fortin, J. P.
Fortin, P., Path
Fortin, P. E. ObstGyn
Fortin, R. J., D & TRad.
Fournier, A.
Fournier, J., Anaes.
Foy, G.
Francoeur, J. ObstGyn
Fredette, J. M., PH(P.Q.)
Fugere, L. P., Anaes
Fugere, P. Otol
Gagne, L. F., Path.
Gagne, S. P., Cardiol(P.Q.)
Gagnon, A.
Gagnon, L.

* Population not separately available.

Quebec (Cont'd.)
Gagnon, L. F.
Gagnon, P. E.
Gagnon, P. P., PlasSurg, GenSurg (P.Q.)
Galibois, P. E. Anaes
Garant, L. D.
Garant, O. ObstGyn
Gareau, E. P., Pulm Dist & TB (P.Q.), Cardiol (P.Q.)
Garneau, R. Path
Gauthier, C. A. NeurPsy
Gauthier, J. PH(P.Q.)
Gauthier, J. C. A.
Gauthier, V. GenSurg ((P.Q.)
Gauvin, J., Anaes (P.Q.)
Gauvin, P-H., Anaes(P.Q.)
Gauvin, R. ObstGyn(P.Q.)
Gauvreau, L. Bact
Gelinas, J.
Gendron, D. GenSurg (P.Q.)
Genest, B.
Gerard, J. A.
Germain, C., DiagRad.
Gervais, R.
Giguere, A. GenSurg
Giguere, R., Neurol
Gilbert, A., OrthSurg.
Gingras, R.
Gingras, R. L. J., Biochem. (P.Q.)
Girard, G., GenSurg.
Girard, M., ObstGyn (P.Q.)
Giroux, M. PathBact
Godin, A.
Godin, P. E.
Gosselin, C., GenSurg
Gosselin, G.
Gosselin, J. Y. Psy
Goulet, L. R., OrthSurg(P.Q.)
Goulet, R.
Gourdeau, Y. S. Urol
Gourgue, R., Psy(P.Q.)
Grandbois, J. DermSyph
Grantham, H., Psy
Gravel, J. A. GenSurg, Thor Surg
Gregoire, C., IntMed, Allergy (P.Q.)
Gregoire, H. A., OrthSurg
Gregoire, J. PH (P.Q.)
Gregoire, L. PulmDis & T.B. (P.Q.)
Gregoire, Y. A.. Paed
Gregory, J.
Grenier, B. ObstGyn
Grenier, J., Psy
Grenier, M.
Grondin, Carrol, Bact(P.Q.)
Guay, J. M., Paed.
Guay, M. IntMed
Guillemette, L. P.
Guimond, J. C., Anaes (P.Q.)
Guimont, C., Paed(P.Q.)
Guimont, R.
Guthrie, D. G., DiagRad
Halle, J., Ophth, Otol
Hamelin, A., Anaes (P.Q.)
Hebert, C. D., Anaes
Heon, M. NeurSurg
Hivon, M.
Houde, J., Anaes.
Hould, F. Paed
Hubbard, A. R. F.
Hudon, F., Anaes
Huot, J. M.
Jacob, D., Paed
Jacques, A., Anaes
Jacques, G., D&TRad
Jacques, R., DiagRad
Jean, C., Path
Jobidon, A., Anaes
Jobin, F., IntMed.
Jobin, J., IntMed
Jobin, J. B., IntMed
Jobin, P., GenSurg(Hon.)
Johnson, G., Psy
Jolicoeur, A., GenSurg, PlasSurg (P.Q.)
Julien, J. M., IntMed, Pulm Dis & TB (P.Q.)
Kelly, J. W., GenSurg.
Koenig, Lucile
Kozak, P., Urol
Labbe, P., GenSurg
Laberge, M., GenSurg (P.Q.)
Laberge, R. J.
Labrecque, A., Anaes
Labrecque, B.
Labrecque, E., PulmDis & TB (P.Q.)
Labreque, M.
Labrie, F.
Labrie, G.
Labrie, J. M., Psy.
Lacerte, J., Ophth.Otol
Lacerte, M., IntMed (Gastroenet) **(P.Q.)**
Lachance, P. A., PhysMed & Rehab.
Lacroix, P.
Ladouceur-Dupuis, P.
Laflamme, C., IntMed
Laflamme, J.
Laflamme, R., IntMed
Lafond-Letarte, Therese
Lajeunesse, A., ObstGyn (P.Q.)
Laliberte, B.
Laliberte, C., IntMed (P.Q.)
Lamarche, G.
Lamarche, Y., Anaes
Lambert, J. J., Psy
Lambert, Suzanne, Bact(P.Q.)
Lamontagne, A., Anaes (P.Q.)
Lamontagne, C.
Lamontagne, G.
Lamontagne, J. M., Otol.
Langlais, L. D
Langlois, M., Psy
Lapierre, Jeanne
Lapointe, A., D&TRad
Lapointe, D., Paed
Laroche, F., DiagRad
Larochelle, J. L., OrthSurg
Larochelle, L. N., IntMed
Larochelle, P. R., Ophth,Otol
Larose, R.
Larue, A., Paed (P.Q.)
Larue, G. H., NeurPsy
La Rue, L., NeurPsy
Larue, R., PH (P.Q.)
Lateunesse, A., ObstGyn.
Lavergne, J. N., Urol (P.Q.)
Lavoie, J. V., Ophth,Otol
Lavoie, R., Otol
Lavoie, R. G., Ophth
LeBlanc, Irene E.
LeBlanc, J. A. R.
LeBlond, J.
Leblond, W., IntMed, Clin Path (P.Q.), Path Bact
Leclerc, J., GenSurg
Leclerc, J., OrthSurg
Leclerc, J. E., ObstGyn
Leclerc, L., OrthSurg.
Leclerc, L. P., GenSurg
Leclerc, R., Paed.
Lefebvre, J. L.. Ophth,Otol
Legare, B., ObstGyn
Legare, J. P.
Lehoux, L. M., Otol
Lemelin, F., Psy (P.Q.)
Lemieux, A., Psy
Lemieux, G.
Lemieux, J., OrthSurg (P.Q.)
Lemieux, J. M., ThorSurg, GenSurg
Lemieux, J. R., IntMed
Lemieux, L. H., Neur
Lemire, Suzanne, ObstGyn
L'Esperance, A., IntMed(TB), Pulm Dis & TB(P.Q.)
L'Esperance, P., GenSurg
Lessard, Andree
Lessard, Camile, Pulm Dis & TB (P.Q.)
Lessard, Francoise, PH(P.Q.)
Lessard, G., PhysMed & Rehab (P.Q.)
Lessard, J. M., OrthSurg
Lessard, L., GenSurg (P.Q.)
Lessard, Richard, IntMed, Cardiol. (P.Q.)
Lessard, R., Derm.
Lessard, R., D & T Rad.
LeTarte, F. J., Ophth,Otol
Letendre, G. A.
Letourneau, J.
Letourneau, J. L., GenSurg.
Levasseur, L. J., GenSurg
Levert, G.
Limoges, P.
Lizotte, L.
Loiselle, J. M.
Lou, W., GenSurg
Lussier, L.
MacMillan, D. W., Anaes (P.Q
MacRae, F. R., IntMed (P.Q.)
Magnan, J. A., Psy (P.Q.)
Maranda, E., Ophth, Otol
Marceau, G., GenSurg
Marceau, P., GenSurg
Marchand, R., Obst (P.Q.)
Marcoux, G.
Marcoux, G., GenSurg
Marcoux, H., PathBact
Marois, A., Cardiol (P.Q.)
Marois, M., Path (P.Q.)
Marquis, A. B., ObstGyn
Marquis, J., Anaes
Marquis, P. A., Psy.
Martel, A., IntMed
Martel, S. B., Paed(P.Q.)
Martineau, G. A., PH(P.Q.)
Martineau, J. A. G., GenSurg.
Martin, G.
Martin, W. W., Anaes (P.Q.)
Masson, V.
Matte, G.
Matte, R., Anaes(P.Q.)
McClish, A., Anaes
McGraw, J. Y.
McKinnon, I. A.
McKinnon, J. P.
Meilleur, R.
Meisels, A.
Mercier, A., Urol (P.Q.)
Mercier, G., IntMed & Cardiol (P.Q.)
Mercier, R.
Merler, C., GenSurg
Michaud, G.
Miller, G., Path
Mino, R.
Moisan, A., IntMed, Cardiol (P.Q.)
Moisan, F., PulmDis & T.B. (P.Q.)
Montgrain, N. H., Psy.
Montgrain, P., Gastroent(P.Q.)
Moreau, A., OphthOtol (P.Q.)
Morin, Jeanie, Path(P.Q.)
Morin, J. E., IntMed
Morin, Y. L., IntMed, Cardio (P.Q.)
Morissette, G.. OrthSurg
Nadeau, C., Cardiol (P.Q.)
Nadeau, J.
Naud, R., GenSurg
Normandeau, F. W.
Ouellet, J. A.
Ouellet, P.
Page, R., OrthSurg
Painchaud, C. A., Bact
Painchaud-Marcoux, C., Psy

* Population not separately available.

QUEBEC (Cont'd)
Painchaud, P., Otol
Paquet, A.
Paquet, B.
Paquet, J. P., Urol
Paradis, B., Anaes
Paradis, C., IntMed (P.Q.)
Paradis, G., Psy
Paradis, G., PulmDis & T.B. (P.Q.)
Paradis, R.
Parant, F., Anaes, Phys Med Rehab
Pare, G.
Parent, J. P., IntMed (Gastro) (P.Q.)
Parrot, P., PH (P.Q.)
Patoine, J. G., Anaes
Payeur, Leo, D&TRad, PhysMed (P.Q.)
Pelland, M., Neur
Pelletier, G.
Pelletier, J. A., NeurPsy
Pelletier, J. E., Ophth, Otol
Pelletier, J. N. J., Anaes
Pelletier, N., Paed
Periera, V. L., Paed.
Perron, J., Ophth
Petitclerc, R., Psy
Pettigrew, A., GenSurg
Philippon, P., GenSurg (P.Q.)
Pichette, R.
Pinault, P.
Pion, R., Psy
Plamondon, C. A., IntMed
Plamondon, J. L. M., Ophth
Plamondon, M., Anaes
Plante, N., Psy
Plante, R., Urol (P.Q.)
Poirier, G.
Poirier, L.
Poisson, J.
Poliquin, J., Anaes (P.Q.)
Poliquin, P. A., GenSurg
Pollack, S. L., ObstGyn (P.Q.)
Pomerleau, C., PH (P.Q.)
Pomerleau, P. A., GenSurg (P.Q.)
Pothier, P., Psy(P.Q.)
Potvin, A., Bact
Potvin, A. R., D&TRad
Potvin, P.
Potvin, R., IntMed, Cardiol (P.Q.)
Poudrier, C., PhysMed & Rehab.
Poulin, G., Otol (P.Q.)
Pouliot, J. C., Anaes
Pouliot, L. E., IntMed
Pouliot, M. J., Biochem(P.Q.)
Pouliot, P. E., GenSurg
Proulx, G. H.
Proulx, P.
Racine, G.
Rail, J. R.
Rainville, P. H.
Ramon-Moliner, O.
Rancourt, D.
Rayes, H., GenSurg(P.Q.)
Raymond, W. J. A.
Reid, L., ObstGyn
Reinhardt, G. H., NeurSurg (P.Q.)
Richard, J. E., Otol
Richard, M., Paed
Richard, R. V.
Rinfret, C.
Rinfret, L., Anaes
Rioux, A., ObstGyn
Rioux, E., IntMed(P.Q.), Haem (P.Q.)
Rioux, J. E., GenSurg
Rioux, Monique
Rivard, R., OrthSurg(P.Q.)
Riviere, L.
Roberge, A.
Roberge R., IntMed
Robert, A.
Robert, L.
Robitaille, J. C., D&TRad
Robitaille, L.
Rochette, E.
Rochette, M.
Roger, J. P., OrthSurg, ThorSur (P.Q.)
Rondeau-Rivard, Lucie
Rosen, L. J., Paed
Rouleau, Y., Psy
Rousseau, A. P., Ophth
Rousseau, C.
Rousseau, J., IntMed (P.Q.)
Rousseau, M., Paed (P.Q.)
Roussel, J.
Roy, C. C., Paed
Roy, C., TherRad
Roy, E.
Roy, E. P.
Roy, F.
Roy, J. C.
Roy, F., GenSurg
Roy, J. F.
Roy, J. P., ObstGyn (P.Q.)
Roy, L.
Roy, L., Psy(P.Q.)
Roy, L., GenSurg(P.Q.)
Roy, M., DermSyph
Roy, P-E., Path(P.Q.)
Roy, R.
Roy, R., Path
Royer, L., Otol
Royer, M., OrthSurg
Ruelland, R., Psy
Ruelland, Y.
St. Arnaud, G. Gyn
St. Cyr, L.
St. Martin, J.
St Pierre, J. P. E., GenSurg.
Salvi-Guillem, J.
Sampson, M., IntMed (Cardiol) (P.Q.)
Samson, A.
Samson, E., GenSurg
Samson, J.
Samson, J. W.
Samson, M., GenSurg (P.Q.)
Saucier, G., IntMed
Saucy, L. P.
Saulnier, G., IntMed, Card (P.Q.)
Savary, P., Otol
Savoie, J. R., GenSurg (P.Q.)
Savoie, M.
Scherrer, R., ObstGyn (P.Q.)
Simard, P., Otol
Simard, R., ObstGyn
Simard, R. M., ObstGyn (P.Q.)
Sirois, J., NeurSurg
Sirois, S., PH (P.Q.)
Stein, D.
Sylvester, J. E., PH
Talbot, H. E.
Tardif, A.
Tardif, J. A., Ophth, Otol
Tchou, P. K., Derm.
Tetu, A. T., IntMed, Cardiol (P.Q.)
Tetu, F., Cardiol(P.Q.), IntMed. (P.Q.)
Therrien, C., IntMed(P.Q.)
Therrien, R., DermSyph Aller (P.Q.)
Thibaudeau, R., Paed
Thibault, A., DiagRad, TherRad.
Thibault, J. A., Psy
Thivierge, G.
Touchette, L.
Tourigny, R., Path (P.Q.)
Tremblay, A.
Tremblay, G.
Tremblay, J.
Tremblay, J. M.
Tremblay, L., D&TRad
Tremblay, M.
Tremblay, P., DiagRad
Tremblay, R.
Trempe, F., GenSurg
Turcot, J., GenSurg
Turcot, R., Paed (P.Q.)
Turcotte, A. N.
Turcotte, B., D & T Rad(P.Q.)
Turcotte, H., PathBact
Turcotte, M., IntMed (P.Q.)
Turgeon, E., D&TRad
Turko, R.
Turmel-Dorion, Louise
Turmel, J. A., ObstGyn
Turmel, J., Psy
Turmel, J. T.
Turmel, N.
Turmel, W., GenSurg
Vachon, C., GenSurg(P.Q.)
Vachon, M., IntMed (P.Q.)
Vaillancourt, P. E.
Vallieres, A., Urol
Vaillieres, G.
Veilleux, J., IntMed
Verge, E., GenSurg
Verrehault, D.
Vezina, J-P., ObstGyn(P.Q.)
Vezina, R., PH
Vigeant, J. L., ObstGyn
Villeneuve, A., Psy(P.Q.)
Villeneuve, B., Haem(P.Q.)
Villeneuve, D. E.
Villeneuve, P. M., Psy(P.Q.)
Wintle Des Ruisseaux, P.

QUYON
(816)
Hudson, R. M.

RAWDON
(2,391)
Bailey, G.
Danais, S.
Godin, L.

REPENTIGNY
(9,139)
Beaulieu, J., DiagRad
Bettez, P., Path.
Carignan, R.
Desjardins, A.
Dupont, J. R.
Gravel, B. G., Psy
Lemire, J., Ophth.
Lanthier, Suzanne
Lussier, R.
Pesant, P., IntMed
Thibeault, Jeanne d'Arc, PH(P.Q.)

RICHELIEU
(1,612)
Coles, B. C.
Grenier, L. J. G.

RICHMOND
(4,072)
Chaput, M.
Dykeman, D. L.
Manning, C.
Sweeny, B.

RIGAUD
(1,989)
Plante, J. L.
Therrien, G. E.

RIMOUSKI
(17,739)
Bedard, G.
Belanger, R.
Bernier, A. H., ObstGyn
Berube, G., Otol, Ophth(P.Q.)
Berube, G.
Catellier, C., IntMed
Cote, F.
Dion, G., IntMed
Drapeau, J. O.
Filiatrault, C., Anaes
Filiatrault, J., GenSurg (P.Q.)
Forbes, G.
Fournier, M., Path(P.Q.)

* Population not separately available.

RIMOUSKI (Cont'd)
Gagnon, G. H.
Lamontagne, J. P.
Lamontagne, L., GenSurg.
Langis, N., Anaes (P.Q.)
Lavoie, R.
Leblanc, A.
Lepage, V., Ophth
Martel, C. R., Cardiol(P.Q.)
Martineau, G., OrthSurg
Masson, P., Paed
Morin, Yvon, OrthSurg
Moriset, J., Paed (P.Q.)
Ouellet, G.
Plourde, S., GenSurg
Poulin, J. C., Anaes
Quimper, A., PH (P.Q.)
Ringuet, J. H., GenSurg
Riviere, L., Path
Simard, D.
Tremblay, R.
Vaillancourt, R., DiagRad

RIVIERE AU RENARD
(1,772)
Rioux, L.
Roy, A.

RIVIERE BLEUE
(1,541)
Ouellet, T.

RIVIERE DES PRAIRIES
(10,054)
Masson, R. N.
Paquin, G.

RIVIERE DU LOUP
(10,835)
Cote, R., Jr.
Couturier, A., GenSurg, OrthSurg.
Daris, J. A., Gyn (P.Q.)
Desjardins, O.
Dion, C., Ophth, Otol
Dufour, L., Anaes (P.Q.)
Gagnon, D., Anaes.
Godbout, Y.
Landry, C.
Langford, A., GenSurg
Lessard, I., IntMed, Cardiol (P.Q.)
Paradis, A., GenSurg
Paradis, L., GenSurg
Ratte, V., PH(P.Q.)
Saindon, D., Anaes
Veces, Hanna

ROBERTSONVILLE
(1,158)
Cote, J. Marie

ROBERVAL
(7,739)
Audet, Irenee
Blanchette, C., Paed
Boudreault, W.
Boissoneault, Y., Anaes.
Bouchard, R., GenSurg.
Brassard, G., GenSurg (P.Q.)
Brassard, R., GenSurg
Brouchard, R., GenSurg
Desbiens, A.
Dube, G.
Fortin, C., OrthSurg
Gervais, S. J., Anaes (P.Q.)
Houde, R.
Latour, J. P., DiagRad
Plante, A., Ophth,Otol (P.Q.)
Sasseville, R., Otol(P.Q.)
Tetu, A. T., IntMed
Thibault, P. E.
Tourigny, R.
Villeneuve, B.

ROCK ISLAND
(1,602)
Bouchard, G.

ROSEMERE
(6,158)
Mongeau, J. A.

ROUGEMONT
(721)
Senecal, J. G.

ROUYN
(18,716)
Bergeron, G. H., DiagRad
Bernard, G.
Constantin, L., Paed
Duval, P. E., PulmDis & TB (P.Q.)
Germain, L. M., Paed
Juneau, A.
Juteau, Y., Anaes (P.Q.)
Kalabus, F., PH(P.Q.)
Kunkel, R. G.
Leblanc, J. A., PH (P.Q.)
Lemay, J. F., GenSurg(P.Q.)
Marcil, P. P., GenSurg
Paiement, L., **OrthSurg (P.Q.)**
Racine, P. A.
Turner, W. A.

ROXBORO
(6,298)
Chartrand, C.
Demers, G.
Hanslik, A. F.
Harrold, A. J.
Kinsella, T. D., IntMed
LeGault, G.
Lillie, J. B.
Phillmore, E. E.
Pamukoff, **Maria, Paed (P.Q.)**

ROXTON FALLS
(971)
Lefebvre, A.

SACRE COEUR
(400)
Tremblay, J. M.

STE. ADELE
(1,331)
Milot, C.
Vermette, L. N.

STE. ADELE EN HAUT
*
Alford, L.
Villemaire, B.

ST. ADELPHE de CHAMPLAIN
(699)
Couillard, F.

ST. AGAPIT
(1,117)
Pouliot, J. P.

STE AGATHE
(5,726)
Belanger, P.
Caron, R. E.
Daunais, G.
Giard, C., GenSurg.
Joannette, A., PulmDis & T.B. (P.Q.)
Kahana, L. M., PulmDis & TB (P.Q.)
Palacio, A.
Phelps, F. L., IntMed(T.B.)
Poulin, Y.
Todosijszuk, D.

STE. AGATHE DE LOTBINIER
(598)
McKinnon, J. A.

ST. AIME
(574)
Falardeau, J. J.

ST. ALBAN
(786)
Patry, S.

ST. ALEXIS DES MONTS
(1,964)
Giard, C., GenSurg(P.Q.)
Grignon, G.
Trempe, R.

ST. AMBROISE DE CHICOUTIMI
(1,581)
Blackburn, G. H.

ST-AMBROISE-DE-KILDARE
(450)
Gosselin, A.

ST. ANDRE AVELLIN
(1,070)
Bourgault, L.
Drouin, G.
St. Louis, H.

ST. ANDREWS EAST
(1,181)
L'Allier, P. A.
Sylvestre, M.

STE. ANGELE DE LAVAL
(484)
Levasseur, C. A.
Plante, C. U.

STE. ANNE DE BEAUPRE
(1,872)
Mayrand, P.
Patton, D. R.
Simard, A.

STE. ANNE DE BELLEVUE
(4,044)
Barron, L. R., ObstGyn
Brent, F. D., PH (P.Q.)
Chapdelaine, P.
Cop-Hodjera, Branislava M., Anaes
Davies, R.O.
Donnell, J. L.
Ferguson, J. M., GenSurg
Fortier, G. L.
Gossage, W.
Hackney, J. W.
Jordan, R. H., Neur(P.Q.)
Leblanc, L. G., IntMed (P.Q.)
Leger, A.
Lewis, G. A., Anaes (P.Q.)
MacDougal, J. R.
Macklem, P. T.
MacPherson, A. S., Psy
Marchildon, R. B., GenSurg (P.Q.)
Mark, Mary M., ObstGyn
Martin, W. S.
McCulloch, K. G., GenSurg
McGee, G. P., Paed
Newby-Good, F. W.
Osterreicher, Marianne
Papp, O. A., Cardiol(P.Q.)
Paquin, J. L.
Patton, G. O., Psy
Pochereva, W., GenSurg
Poitras, V. S.
Ripstein-Soicher, Riva B.
Robson, G. F.
Robson, J. G.
Scott, G. F.
Shepherd, R. W.
Stewart, K. R., IntMed
Swaine, R. L., Otol
Temple, A. D., IntMed
Turski, Marian Psy
Wright, L. A.

STE. ANNE DE LA PERADE
(1,179)
Touzin, J.
Turcotte, J. M.

STE. ANNE-DE-LA-POCATIER
(See La Pocatiere)

STE. ANNE DES MONTS
(1,906)
Goupil, J. L.
Lemire, G., GenSurg
Miville, J.

STE. ANNE DES PLAINES
(1,256)
Delorme, F.
Limoges, G.

ST. ANSELME
(1,136)
Pelletier, C.

* Population not separately available.

ST. APOLLINAIRE
(966)
LaFleur, J. C.
Lamontagne, J.

ST. AUGUSTIN
(550)
Petitclerc, L.

ST. BARNABE NORD
(600)
Grenier, G.

ST. BARTHELEMY
(620)
Chauveau, P.
Gelinas, M.

ST. BASILE
*
Chamberland, J. A.
Vezina, B.

ST BASILE-LE-GRAND
(1604)
Boisvert, L. P.

ST. BENOIT
(576)
Roux, A.

ST BERNARD
(498)
Laliberte, J. M.

ST. BONIFACE
(921)
Janelle, L. P.
Szettle, Anna, Otol

ST. BRUNO
(6,760)
Bonenfant, G.
Davis, J. F.
Donati, S.
Fournier, J. D.
Guerin, G., Anaes
Joncas, G., Paed (P.Q.)
Lanthier, A., IntMed
Matteau, P.
Mayrand, L.
Paierme, G. R., ObstGyn.
Perreault, J. G., DiagRad.
Thompson, W. A.
Vernery, R., ObstGyn.

ST. CAMILE-DE-BELLE CHASSE
(639)
Morin, W.

ST. CASIMIR
(1,926)
Tessier, P. E.

STE. CATHERINE
(893)
Archambault, H., DiagRad (P.Q.)
Pednault, J. R.

ST. CELESTIN
(368)
Laliberte, B.

STE. CESAIRE
(2,097)
Bherer, R.
Dupont, G. J. E.
Lemyre, G. E.

ST. CHARLES DE BELLECHASSE
(985)
Lemieux, G.
Nadeau, A.

ST. CHARLES DE CAPLAN
*
Dumais, J. A. R.

ST. CHRYSOSTOME
(970)
Hetu, M. A.

STE. CLAIRE
(1,322)
Beaudoin, H.
Chabot, J. A. N.
Leclerc, J. P.

STE. CLOTHILDE DE HORTON
(364)
Slater, G.

ST. COEUR DE MARIE
(1,302)
Gauthier, I. M.
Gauthier, J. I.

ST. COME
(525)
Cote, J. A.

ST. CONSTANT
(2,739)
Lapierre, J. L.
Plouffe, M.

STE. CROIX
(1,363)
Boucher, B.

ST. CUTHBERT
(308)
Boucher, J. L.

ST. CYPRIEN
(575)
Coulombe, P.
Martin, G.

ST. CYRILLE DE WENDOVER
(1,140)
Morin, P. A.
Pelissier, R.

ST. DAMIEN
(1,396)
Lachance, R.

ST. DAVID DE LEVIS
*
Dusseault, C. GenSurg (P.Q.)

ST. DENIS SUR RICHELIEU
(1,062)
Rondeau, J.
Vadnais, E. J.

STE. DOROTHEE
(5,297)
Beauchemin, A.
Laurier, C.
Stachewitsch, A., Paed, Haem (P.Q.)
Vaillancourt, R.

ST. EDOUARD
(500)
Carrier, O.

ST. ELEUTHERE
(1,033)
Raymond, P. E.

ST. EPHREM DE BEAUCE
(898)
Poulin, J.
Roberge, G.

ST. ESPRIT
(850)
Raymond, R.

ST. ETIENNE DES GRES.
(569)
St. Onge, R.

ST. EUSTACHE
(5,459)
Binette, C.
Bourgeois, J. G.
Corriveau, Y.
Hache, L., GenSurg
Jette, J. J.
Lacroix, R.
Laurent, G.
Milot, L., PH(P.Q.)

ST. EUSTACHE SUR LE LAC
(See Deux Montagnes)

ST. FABIEN
(1,466)
Cote, G.
Vezina, G.

STE. FAMILLE
(300)
Gaulin, R.

ST. FELICIEN
(5,133)
Banville, R.
Boily, L.
Dumas, W.
Gagnon, F.
Racine, J.

ST. FELICITE
(1,062)
Vielleux, R.

ST. FELIX DE VALOIS
(1,397)
Henault, P. E.
Mayrand, M.

ST. FERDINAND D'HALIFAX
(2,706)
Lamontagne, J.
Savoie, L.

ST. FLAVIEN
(610)
Caux, J. A., PH (P.Q.)
Hamel, J. B.

STE. FLORE
(622)
Gelinas, R.

STE. FOY
(Sub P.O. of Quebec)
(29,716)
Beaulieu, M., ThorSurg.
Bourque, R. A., GenSurg
Cardinal, G., Pulm Dis & TB(P.Q.)
Charlesbois, J.
Cormier, R. J., G. GenSurg, Urol.
Dechene, J. P., Anaes
Dery, T., Path (P.Q.)
Feuiltault, R., IntMed
Gagnon, O., IntMed(P.Q.), Gastroent(P.Q.)
Germaine, C.
Houde, P. J.
Julien, J.-M., IntMed
Labrie, F.
Legendre, J. A.
Lessard, C. PulmDis & T.B. (P.Q.)
Martineau, G. A., PH(P.Q.)
Masson, Victoria, Anaes
Montiminy, L. PulmDis & T.B. (P.Q.)
Morin, B., Otol (P.Q.)
Pelletier, N., Paed
Petitclerc, C., Haem(P.Q.)
Poulin, G.
Radoux, V. H.
Rousseau, A. P., Ophth
Sadler, B. G.
Thibault, M. TherRad
Turmel, W., GenSurg
Vallieres, A.
Vallieres, G.
Villeneuve, J. M.

ST FRANCOIS
(5,122)
Forest, L., Anaes

ST. FRANCOIS DU LAC
(982)
Bourgault, R.
Nadeau, G.

ST. FRANCOIS MONTMAGNY
(567)
Gervais, L.

ST. GABRIEL DE BRANDON
(3,422)
Boutet, L.
Lefebvre, J.
Roy, M.

ST. GEDEON
(887)
Tremblay, C.
Tremblay, P. E.
Veilleux, M.
Vigneault, Germaine

* Population not separately available.

STE. GENEVIEVE
(2,391)
Barette, R.
Brunet, T.
Marcotte, E., Cardiol (P.Q.), IntMed
Paiement, B., Anaes
Wilson, M.

ST. GEORGES
(1,776)
Bernard, R. M.
Chamberland, J. M.

ST. GEORGES DE BEAUCE
(4,086)
Cliche, F., Anaes.
Cloutier, L. V. IntMed (P.Q.)
Lavoie, J.
Maheux, R.
Morisset, P. IntMed (P.Q.)
Paquet, J. A.
Poulin, M.
Vachon, C., GenSurg

ST. GEORGES EAST
*
Bernard, J. G.
Desjardins, R., Otol (P.Q.)
Vachon, C., GenSurg

ST. GEORGES WEST
(4,754)
Caron, P., Anaes
Cliche, F., Anaes.
Fortin, R., ObstGyn (P.Q.)
Guimont, F.
Roy, G.

STE. GERMAINE
(275)
LaRue, P. A.

ST. GERMAIN DE GRANTHAM
(1,018)
Taschereau, J. T. D.
Vincent, B.

STE. GERTRUDE
(361)
Parent, Y.

ST. GERVAIS
(576)
Picard, C.

ST. GREGOIRE
(674)
Thibodeau, Y.

ST. GUILLAUME
(791)
Hivon, M.
McClure, R.
Pelletier, G.

STE. HENEDINE
(518)
Roberge, Marie

ST. HERMAS
(285)
Prager, A., IntMed

ST. HILAIRE
(2,911)
Deslauriers, G., TherRad
Paquin, P.
Phaneuf, J., Anaes

ST. HILAIRE STATION
*
Fortin, G., Anaes

ST. HONORE
(1,000)
Beaulieu, L.

ST HUBERT
(14,380)
Gibeault, R.
Poulin, F.
Veilleux, C.

ST. HUBERT DE TEMISCOUATA
(800)
Albert, P.

Langevin, B.
Pednault, J. R.

ST. HUGUES
(432)
Couture, R.

ST. HYACINTHE
(22,354)
Archambault, R., ObstGyn
Barnabe, G., Paed
Beauregard, G.
Benoit, L., Anaes
Bergeron, M., PH (P.Q.)
Blain, J.
Boisvert, P. R., Ophth (P.Q.), Otol
Boucher, Y., GenSurg.
Brodeur, G.
Brodeur, Y.
Campbell, R.
Chartier, M.
Daudelin, A.
Desmarais, O., Anaes
Fontaine, A.
Fortin, J. L., PulmDis & T.B., (P.Q.)
Gagnon, H. IntMed.
Germain, R. Path (P.Q.)
Gosselin, A.
Goulet, G., OrthSurg (P.Q.)
Hevey, G.
Hevey, J. G., GenSurg
Labrie, H., GenSurg (P.Q.)
Lafond, J. R.
Lague, P. A.
Lemire, C.
Lessard, A. L
Morin, P., GenSurg
Patry, R., Anaes
Peloquin, L.
Perrault, M.
Perreault, A., GenSurg
Phaneuf, G., IntMed (P.Q.) Cardiol (P.Q.)
Phaneuf, J., Anaes
Pothier, Y., Anaes (P.Q.)
Richard, J. P.
Roy, L.
St. Pierre, G.
Tousignant, L. Y., Otol (P.Q.)
Viens, G.

ST. ISIDORE
(728)
Metivier, P.

ST. ISIDORE LAPRAIRIE
(241)
Delorme, A.

ST. JACQUES
(2,037)
Lafortune, M.

ST. JANVIER
(1,811)
Leroux, H.
Kaufmann, N. R.

ST. JEAN
(34,576)
Archambault, G.
Archambault, L. P.
Baribeau, L., ObstGyn.
Bergeron, F.
Boutin, J. G., OrthSurg.
Choiniere, J. A., Path (P.Q.)
Cote, J. M.
Dufresne, J.
Fournier, J. M.
Girard, E. A., Paed (P.Q.)
Keroack, R.
Landry, J. G.
Lavoie, V.
Lemieux, G., IntMed (P.Q.)
Lessard, R.
Logier, P. E.
Marcoux, R.
Masson, R.

Messier, M., IntMed(P.Q.) Cardiol(P.Q.)
Moreau, M., GenSurg(P.Q.)
Normandin, J.
Papineau, L. J., GenSurg
Phaneuf, J., GenSurg
Phaneuf, J. G., Anaes
Phaneuf, P., GenSurg
Phenix, G.
Poirier, R.
Prince, G., Paed
Remillard, F. A.
Robert, T.
Savoie, L. P., GenSurg (P.Q.)
Senikas, J.
Simard, P. D., D & TRad

ST. JEAN DE DIEU
(1,177)
Gaudreau, N.

ST. JEAN DE MATHA
(1,016)
Lessard, H. P.

ST. JEAN PORT JOLI
(1,615)
Chasse, N J.
Lizotte, F.
Lizotte, R.
Raymond, L.
Roy, C.

ST. JEROME
(24,546)
Aubin, G.
Barrette, M., IntMed (Cardiol.) (P.Q.)
Blanchard, R., Paed
Boivin, J. C., Path
Castagner, J.
Chagnon, R., D & T Rad
Champagne, J., Obst (P.Q.)
Cloutier, P. E., PH(P.Q.)
Dore, B., Ophth, Otol (P.Q.)
Filteau, C., IntMed.
Forget, G., GenSurg
Garon, J.
Gilbert, P. E., Anaes
Hamel, M.
Jodoin, R.
Joly, J. R., Anaes (P.Q.)
Lamarre, C. OrthSurg
Lamoureux, A.
Laplante, A.
Laurence, M., ObstGyn.
Laurendeau, I., IntMed(P.Q.) Cardiol(P.Q.)
Leclerc, J. F.
Lemire, J. J., GenSurg
Leonard, C. E.
Lepine, I., Paed
Mailhot, P., OrthSurg(P.Q.)
Marcoux, P., Anaes.
Masson, J. A. R., DiagRad.
Mathieu, Y.
Nadon, A.
Pelletier, G. E., OphthOtol(P.Q.)
Pinard, R., DiagRad
Potvin, J. G.
Rochon, B.
Sadler, B. G., OrthSurg
St. Denis, J. A. M., Paed.
St. Pierre, P. M., GenSurg(P.Q.)
Taillon, J. L.
Thibault, J. P., GenSurg
Tremblay, B.
Valiquette, C. A.

ST. JOSEPH D'ALMA
(See Alma)

ST. JOSEPH DE BEAUCE
(2,484)
Bernard, F.
Legare, L.

ST. JOSEPH DU LAC
(442)
Bachand, L. J.

* Population not separately available.

ST. JOVITE
(2,696)
Dupre, R. N.
Lemieux, M., Psy (P.Q.)
Ouimet, M.
Proulx, M.
Robillard, P.

ST. JUDE
(700)
Beauregard, G.

ST. LAMBERT
(See Cite de Jacques Cartier)

ST. LAURENT
(See Montreal)

ST. LEONARD
(1,666)
David, J. R., DiagRad.
Fortin, L., Psy (P.Q.)

ST. LEON LE GRAND
(500)
Pelletier, T.

ST. LIBOIRE
(581)
Bousquet, H.

ST. LIN
(1,698)
Archambault, A.
Auger, P. C.
Desormiers, Y.
Frenette, R.

ST. LOUIS DE L'ISLE AUX COUDRES
*
Matte, G.

STE. MADELEINE
(965)
Lague, P. A.

SAINT MARC DES CARRIERE
(2,622)
Dussault, A. B.

STE. MARIE DE BEAUCE
(3,662)
Dionne, L. P.
Lessard, R.
Levesque, E.
St. Jacques, **J. A.**

STE MARTHE
(267)
Coulombe, **R.**

ST. MARTIN
(See Montreal)

STE.-MARTINE
(1,695)
Belanger, R.
Langis, **A., PH (P.Q.)**

ST. MAURICE
(604)
Toupin, J. N.
Trahan, A.

ST. MICHEL
(300)
Nadeau, A.

ST. MICHEL DE BELLECHASSE
(843)
Giguere, G., Anaes (P.Q.)

ST. MICHEL DES SAINTES
(1,737)
Gauthier, G.

STE. MONIQUE DE NICOLET
(232)
Veilleux, R.

ST. NARCISSE
(877)
Desrosiers, G.

ST. NAZAIRE
(95)
Girard, **J. M.**

ST. NICOLAS
(350)
Beaudet, J. C.
Masse, L. R.

ST. OURS
(711)
Cloutier, L.

ST. PACOME
(1,242)
Royer, A.

ST. PAMPHILE
(1,839)
Gagnon, J. A.

ST. PASCAL
(2,144)
Boulanger, L.

ST. PAUL DE MONTMINY
(793)
Wagner, J. P.

ST. PAULIN
(920)
Michaud, C.

ST. PAUL L'ERMITE
(2,935)
McDuff, R. E.

STE. PERPETUE DE L'ISLET
(674)
Bedard, C.
Bourget, P.

ST. PHILIPPE DE LAPRAIRII
(498)
Brossard-Daigneault, Paulette
Daigneault, B.
Deslippe, G.

ST. PHILIPPE DE NERI
(746)
Leclerc, L.

ST. PIE
(1,436)
Chaput, J. M.
Fournier, F.

ST. PIERRE D'ORLEANS
(380)
Vezina, C.

ST. PIERRE LES BECQUETS
(451)
Pouliot, L.

ST. PLACIDE
(336)
Roy, G. M.

ST. POLYCARPE
(560)
Filion, Y.

ST. PRIME
(658)
Taillon, C.

ST. PROSPER DE DORCHESTER
(1,277)
Reny, R.

ST. RAPHAEL BELLECHASSE
(1,135)
Roy, A.

ST. RAYMOND
(3,931)
Caron, G.
Denis, C.
Jinchereau, Y.
Lortie, C. B.
Moisan, O.

ST. REMI
(2,269)
Dubuc, L.
Ferdais, J. P.
Joly, J. J.
Labelle, A.

ST. ROCH DE L'ACHIGAN
(614)
Locat, W.

ST. ROCH DES AULNAIES
(350)
Mackay, J. C. G.

ST. ROMUALD D'ETCHEMIN
(5,183)
Chouinard, P. P.
Genest, J. P.
Lachance, J. W.
Lambert, G. A. Anaes (P.Q.)
Lapierre, Irene, Anaes.

STE. ROSE (LAVAL CO.)
(7,571)
Cyr, R.
Depot, R.
Frappier, G.
Hebert, R.
Lambert, M. J.
Nadeau, G.

STE ROSE DE LIMA
(2,965)
Lorrain, J.

STE. ROSE DU DEGELE
(1,943)
Chabot, C. E., **GenSurg (P.Q.)**
Lavoie, A.

ST. SAMUEL
(550)
Rodrigue, V.

ST. SAUVEUR DES MONTS
(1,702)
Desy, A.

STE. SCHOLASTIQUE
(833)
Choquet, M.
Paradis, J. L.

ST. SIMEON
(1,199)
Zadra, C. M.

ST. STANISLAS DE CHAMPLAIN
(589)
Douville, J.

ST. STANISLAS DE KOSTKA
(243)
Brosseau, E.

ST. SYLVESTRE
(650)
Dube, L. P.

ST. THECLE
(2,009)
Marchand, J. C.
Marchand, J. R

STE-THERESE-DE-BEAUPORTE
*
Cote, R. M.

STE THERESE DE BLAINVILLE
(11,771)
Borduas, A. G.
Bourbonniere, G.
Deschambault, J.
Desjardins, F. R.
Huot, Y.
Lamarche, C.
Larose, J. A.
Leduc, P.
Limoges, A.
Milot, J. J.
Waddel, G.

STE-THERESE-EN-HAUT
*
Cote, M., Anaes(P.Q.)
Couture, J. P.
Rondeau, Y., Anaes.
Trahan, M., Anaes.

ST. TIMOTHEE
(1,003)
Labrossiere, S. D.

* Population not separately available.

ST. TITE
(3,250)
Francoeur, L.
Francoeur, N.
Marchand, P.

ST. UBALD
(770)
Gauthier, J.

ST. ULRIC
(1,021)
Roy, V.

ST. URBAIN
(300)
Bouchard, J.

STE URSULE
(486)
Caron, F.
Nepveu, T.

ST. VICTOR
(179)
Savard, Y.

ST. VINCENT DE PAUL
(See Montreal)

ST. ZACHARIE
(1,367)
Robitaille, M.

ST. ZEPHIRIN
(247)
Tremblay, G.

ST. ZOTIQUE
(370)
Benoit, R.

SAN BEGIN
*
Brosseau, V., PulmDis & T.B. (P.Q.)

SAWYERVILLE
(784)
Lowry, C.

SAYABEC
(2,314)
Caron, L.
Gagnon, Irenee

SCHEFFERVILLE
(3,178)
Boies, E., GenSurg
Gelinas, R.M.

SCOTSTOWN
(1,033)
Blanchette, Roger

SENNETERRE
(3,246)
Bolduc, L. de G.
Fortin, G.
LaFleche, M.

SENNEVILLE
(See Ste. Anne de Bellevue)

SEPT ILES
(14,196)
Archambault, J., GenSurg P.Q.)
Banasse, J. E., ObstGyn(P.Q.)
Banville, R.
Beaulieu, G.
Chouinard, A. M.
Coupal, Y.
Drouin, J.
Flamank, J. P.
Laflamme, L. E.
Pelletier, U.
Plante, G.
Riverin, L.
Roy, L. J., GenSurg (P.Q.)
Roy, P. M.
Thibault, J.

SHAWINIGAN
63,518
Baillargeon, T-Ls.
Barrette, J. P. J., Gensurg (P.Q.)
Bellerive, R.
Bergeron, J. A., Paed
Bergeron, J. M., Anaes (P.Q.)
Bilodeau, H. P., Cardiol (P.Q.)
Blais, Y.
Brunelle, G.
Chabot, O.
Chretien, J. F. M., ObstGyn
Cossette, Y., Paed (P.Q.)
Damphousse, J. B A., GenSurg
Daneau, J., D&TRad
Dufresne, A.
Fauteux, H.
Fortin, J.
Francoeur, F.
Gelinas, C. L.
Jacques, R.
Julien, P. E., Ophth,Otol
Kaine, G.
Lamontagne, C. E.
Liddle, C. A.
Melancon, H., Otol (P.Q.)
Menard, J., Anaes
Michaud, C. E.
Noel, F.
Paradis, A., IntMed (P.Q.)
Pelletier, L. A.
Perron, J. M., DiagRad (P.Q.) Anaes
Pinsonneault, J. P., GenSurg
Smith, H. G.
Stevenson, R. H.
Tremblay, R. G., GenSurg

SHAWVILLE
(1,541)
Cowley, F. C.
Horner, E. B.
McDowell, S. E.

SHERBROOKE
(70,253)
Beaudry, G., ObstGyn
Beaudry, J. F.,ObstGyn (P.Q.)
Beauregard, J. M., IntMed.
Bedard, J. P., OrthSurg
Belle-Isle, J., Derm
Bernier, M., OrthSurg (P.Q.)
Bertrand, G. L., GenSurg
Besmargian, Marie J., Paed (P.Q.)
Berube, A., GenSurg(P.Q.)
Blackburn, R., D & T Rad.
Blais, L. E., GenSurg (P.Q.)
Blouin, Y., GenSurg(P.Q.)
Boisvert, R., PulDis&T. B. (P.Q
Boivin, Germain, PhysMed& Rehab
Boulay, G., IntMed (P.Q.)
Bourque, J., DiagRad
Brautt, N.
Breault, Y., Anaes(P.Q.)
Bruneau, E. F., GenSurg (P.Q.)
Bureau, J., GenSurg
Cadman, T. A., Otol (P.Q.)
Campbell, D. K.
Chevalier, P. A.
Cloutier, M., OrthSurg
Cooper, E. A., ObstGyn
Cote, B. M.
Cote, C. J. G., GenSurg
Cote, R., GenSurg (P.Q.)
Cote, Z.
Crepeau, J. J., IntMed, Cardiol (P.Q.)
Dagneau, C. J., GenSurg (P.Q.)
Darche, J. L.
Darche, L., Ophth, Otol
Decarie, J. O., ObstGyn (P.Q.)
deMargerie, J. M., Ophth.
Demers, L., GenSurg
Demers, L. P.
Deschenes, J. A.
Desroberts, Y.
d'Etcheverry, A., DiagRad
Dion, J. A., Gyn (P.Q.)
Dionne, P., GenSurg
Dougan, A. A., Anaes
Drapeau, B., Otol
Drolet, M., IntMed
Duberger, R. L., DiagRad
Dufresne, R., Gastroent(P.Q.)
Dumont, F., IntMed (P.Q.)
Einbinder, H.
Favreau, G. L.
Fletcher, H. B.
Fontaine, V., Bact(P.Q.)
Fortier, J. P., Ophth
Fortin, J. P.
Fortin, L. J.
Frenette, R. G., Urol (P.Q.)
Gadbois, Y., Ophth,Otol (P.Q.)
Gagner, R., ObstGyn
Gagnon, L.
Gagnon, P. M., Path.
Gaudet, R., GenSurg (P.Q.)
Gauthier, Patrice, OphthOtol (P.Q.)
Georgesco, M., IntMed (P.Q.) Haem (P.Q.)
Gladu, L. M., Anaes (P.Q.)
Gosselin, J. L., Bact (P.Q.)
Gregoire, R.
Hardy, R. D.
Hebert, A.
Hicks, M. W., Urol
Hill, A. C.
Kimoff, R.
Kintzen, Charlotte M.
Kintzen, W., Path
Laberge, L., Pulm Dis & TB (P.Q.)
Lachance, C. R.
Lachance, P. A.
Lachance, P. M., Derm
Lafond, R., (ObstGyn (P.Q.)
Lagasse, P., Urol
Lamarre, C. J., Psy.
Lamy, R., Anaes
Langis, R. L., Paed (P.Q.)
Langlois, L. E., Paed
Langlois, M., IntMed
Larouche, G. L., IntMed (P.Q.), Cardiol (P.Q.)
Lasalle, G.
Leclair, J. M., IntMed., Haem(P.Q.)
Ledoux, A., GenSurg (P.Q.)
Leduc, P.
Lefebvre, G.
Lefrancois, J., OrthSurg
Lejeune, L. P., GenSurg
Lemay, J. D., Anaes (P.Q.)
Levy, J.
Longpre, B., IntMed, Haem (P.Q.)
Loomis, G. B., GenSurg.
MacLeod, J. A., GenSurg (P.Q.
Maheux, Carol E.
Mailhot, R., GenSurg (P.Q.)
Marchand, R., Anaes(P.Q.)
Marin, R. Anaes
Marquis, M., Anaes(P.Q.)
Massey, D. G., IntMed., **Pulm.** Dis. & TB(P.Q.)
Massicotte, G., PlasSurg
Masson, G., IntMed (P.Q.)
McMahon, L. P., Anaes
Michaud, P.
Mignault, A. A., ObstGyn (P.Q
Mills, F. C., IntMed (P.Q.)
Mongeau, B.
Noel, J. O., Anaes
Page, L. A., Paed (P.Q.)
Panneton, A., Paed
Papageorges, C. J. S., Phys. Med. & Rehab.
Parenteau, G. R., OrthSurg (P.Q.)
Paris, J. P.
Paulette, R. E., GenSurg, ThorSurg (P.Q.)
Pepin, J. M., IntMed
Poisson, E.
Poulet, C. E.

* Population not separately available.

Sherbrooke (Cont'd.)
Quintin, T. J., IntMed
Reny, P.
Richard, M.
Ross, J. L., GenSurg
Saine, G.
Silny, J., D&TRad
Smart, Margaret C.
Stepan, M.
Sylvester, J., D&TRad
Tanguay, F., **Anaes**
Therien, B.
Thibaudeau, J. Ophth
Tremblay, **J. P., Path**
Trudel, A., **ObstGyn**
Vanasse, R., Path (P.Q.)
Veilleux, R., **Anaes**
Vigneault, G., Otol.
Vigneault, M., Path(P.Q.)
Vigneault, Mary

SILLERY
(See Quebec)

SOREL
(17,145)
Belanger, J., Anaes
Belanger, M., ObstGyn.
Ducharme, G.
Dupre, G. H.
Forgacs, P.
Frappier, S.
Gill, G., D & TRad
Grondin, L.
Lafleur, H., **Anaes (P.Q.)**
Lamonde, R.
Legere, H., DiagRad(P.Q.)
Montel, G. B., **GenSurg (P.Q.)**
Painchaud, C. A., **Bact,**
Haem (P.Q.)
Parent, R.
Peloquin, A.
Poissant, A.
Proulx, J., Path(P.Q.)
Roy, H.
Savignac, B.
Tremblay, **J. M., PH (P.Q.)**

SOUTH DURHAM
(437)
Chabot, M.

SQUATTECK
(1,088)
Arsenault. C.

STANDON
(*)
Desautels, P. G.
Robitaille, J. D.

STANSTEAD
(1,120)
Bonin, M.

STRATHMORE
*
Ricard, M.

SUTTON
(1,753)
Bedard, J. P.
Rioux, P.

SWEETSBURG
(957)
Brouillette, M., DiagRad
Hogan, J. T.
Mooney, M. C., **GenSurg**

TASCHEREAU
(1,000)
Lacombe. H.

TELLIER
*
Cormier, P. E., **Psy**

TEMISCAMING
(Temyscouta)
(2,521)
Church, J. P.
Laine, C. A.
Neagher, P. Y.

TERREBONNE
(6,207)
Anbin, J. M.
Lacroix, R.
Lefebvre, R., Anaes.
Lemire, A.
Macelin, A.
Paquin, F.
Parent, J. M.
Richer, G.
St. Armand, M.

THETFORD MINES
(21,618)
Andreiu, L., Otol (P.Q.)
Bertrand, G., IntMed.
Caron, J. M.
Cartier, P. H., Pulm Dis &
T.B.(P.Q.)
Delage, M., GenSurg (P.Q.)
Dubreuil, P., Paed(P.Q.)
Dussault, J. J., PulmDis & T.B.
(P.Q.)
Gagnon, R., DiagRad
Giguere, B.
Lambert, R. A., **GenSurg**
Laughrea, **P., Anaes**
Lauriault, Louise
Leblond, A., ObstGyn(P.Q.)
Lemieux, R.
Lessard, C.
Mercier, C.
Poulin, M., Path (P.Q.),
Haem (P.Q.)
Poulin, R.
Verreault, D.

THURSO
(3,306)
Lafreniere. R.
Page, G.
Veilleux, **R.**

TRACY
(8,176)
Bastarache, R., IntMed
Coulombe, C.
Doucet, N., GenSurg (P.Q.)
Gervais, P. B.
Gill, G., D & TRad
Guertin, C.
Leblanc, R.
Marcoux, J. R., Cardiol (P.Q.)
Vigneault, J. M., GenSurg

TRING JUNCTION
(1,213)
Beaulieu, J. C.

TROIS PISTOLES
(4,349)
Gamache, M.
Langlais, J. P.
Lebel, R.

TROIS RIVIERES
(83,659)
Albert, J., Anaes
Allen, M., Anaes
Baribeau, G., Haem (P.Q.)
Beaudet, J. P., Paed (P.Q.)
Aller (P.Q.)
Beaudoin, H., PulmDis & T.B.
(P.Q.)
Beaudry, J. L. Obst (P.Q.)
Bedard, L., GenSurg (P.Q.)
Beland, C., Paed (P.Q.)
Bellefeuille, P
Bellemare, M., GenSurg(P.Q.)
Bellemare, M., Ophth,Otol (P.Q
Berlinguet, L.
Bisson, M.
Boily, M. G., PhysMed & Rehab
Boivin, J. L., Anaes
Boucher, C.
Boucher, T., IntMed(P.Q.),
Pulm Dist & TB(P.Q.)
Bourque, R. C., IntMed.,
Cardiol(P.Q.)
Boyer, R., GenSurg.

Brouillette, J., OrthSurg
Campbell, J. C. M., IntMed.
Caron, R. A.
Cosette, R.
Damphouse, J. B. H., GenSurg
DeCharrette, B.
Demontigny, P. D.
Denoncourt, J. A., GenSurg,
OrthSurg
Desjarlais, E.
Dontigny, M. Y., ObstGyn(P.Q.)
Dostaler, A. P.
Dufresne, Jean P., DermSyph
Dugre, R., GenSurg
Dugre, Y.
Duhaime, M., GenSurg
Dumoulin, P. C., Paed (P.Q.)
Fournier, G. E.
Frechette, A., NeurSurg
Gagnon, R.
Garneau, J. J., DiagRad(P.Q.)
Gauthier, F., ObstGyn (P.Q.)
Gelinas-Desaulniers, A.
Gelinas, G., ObstGyn
Gelinas, J. J., IntMed.
Gendron, P., Anaes
Germain, L. A., GenSurg (P.Q.)
Gervais, L. M., Psy (P.Q.)
Gingras, J.
Gouin, J. A., ObstGyn (P.Q.)
Groulx, J. E. G., Path
Hamelin, P., Anaes
Hould, R., Anaes
Houle, P.
Lafond, A., IntMed
Lafreniere, J., ObstGyn
Lagace, G.
Lambert, P. E., Otol (P.Q.)
Lamoureux, C. E., OrthSurg
Lamoureux, J., Ophth,Otol
Langis, Camille, Gastroent(P.Q.)
Langlois, P. R., Otol
Lavallee, H., Paed
Lemaire, C.
Lemire, F., GenSurg
Letienne, L., OrthSurg
Letournneau, J. L., GenSurg
(P.Q.)
Lupien, L. C.
Malone, J. M. F., GenSurg
Marchand, M. A.
Martel, A., GenSurg
Martin, J. C.
Matteau, J. C., Gastroent(P.Q.)
Matteau, R., Urol (P.Q.)
Mayrand, G.
Michaud, M. R., OrthSurg(P.Q.)
Nadeau, C., Otol(P.Q.)
Neveu, M., Ophth
Normand, G., GenSurg (P.Q.)
Normand, H.
Normand, J. M.
Normand, Y., OrthSurg
Panneton, A., Ophth
Paquin, J. J., GenSurg (P.Q.)
Paquin, R.
Pellerin, C. G., Urol
Perigny, Y., GenSurg
Philibert, R. P., Path
Poitras, B.
Pothier, A., PulmDis & T.B.
(P.Q.)
Racicot, G. N., PulmDis&T.B.
(P.Q.)
Ringuet-Gagnon, Madeline
St-Amand, J., Anaes(P.Q.)
St. Pierre, R., PulmDis & T.B.
(P.Q.)
Sevigny, J.
Sicard, J.
Tessier, J. H., PulmDis & T.B.
(P.Q.)
Tetreault, A., IntMed
Tison, P. G.
Tousignant, A.
Tousignant, B., IntMed (P.Q.)

* Population not separately available.

TROIS RIVIERES (Cont'd)
Vanasse, J. E., ObstGyn
Veilleux, P. H.
Vezina, H.
Villemure, R.
UPTON
(822)
Hivon, J.
Yergeau, J. A. F.
VALCOURT
(848)
Marcoux, A.
VAL D'OR
(10,983)
Bigue, G., GenSurg
Fortin, M., GenSurg (P.Q.)
Giguere, J.
Gonzales, D. B.
Kingston, P. T., GenSurg
Lapointe, G.
Lessard, J. N., GenSurg (P.Q.)
Mercier, M.
Paquet, R.
Reid, C. D.
Taschereau, D.
Tessier, J. L.
Wexler, G. W., Urol
VALLEYFIELD
(29,849)
Bechard, J. B., GenSurg (P.Q.)
Bibaud, B., DiagRad (P.Q.)
Bourbonnais, E.
Boyer, J. M., Anaes (P.Q.)
Brassard, Y., DiagRad
Caza, M., GenSurg (P.Q.)
Dandenault, J. Y.
DeGrandpre, L.
Deom, P., Psy
Doucet, P., Cardiol(P.Q.)
Dube, C. B., OphthOtol (P.Q.)
Dumaine, M.
Eftihiades, T. D.
Gauthier, G., PH (P.Q.)
Hebert, H., OrthSurg (P.Q.)
Karkalas, Yani
Lavallee, G.
Leduc, A., Gyn
Nantel, J.
Poliquin, R. W., GenSurg.
Racicot, G., Paed
Roy, R.
St. Onge, C.
Sansoucy, J., DiagRad
Saulnier, A., GenSurg (P.Q.)
Seguin, G., Anaes (P.Q.)
Talbot, J. E.
Thibault, J. P.
Tremblay, B., Paed.
VALOIS
(3,500)
Currie, E. V.
Martineau, J. E.
VARENNES
(2,241)
Larose, H.
Tellier, L.
VAUDREUIL
(897)
Caille, J. J.
VERCHERES
(1,772)
Dupre-Strachan, **Suzanne**
Frenette, E., PH (P.Q.)
Gaudette, C. E.
Lapierre, R.
Paradis, V.
Petrin, P.
VERDUN
(See Montreal)
VICTORIAVILLE
(18,720)
Andersen, A., Otol (P.Q.)
Arseneault, R.
Carignan, A.
Caux, D., Otol.
Chagnon, G. E.
Cote, E., GenSurg
Cote, J. P., OrthSurg(P.Q.)
Dubois, G. H., Path
Duval, L., PH (P.Q.)
Gervais, J. G.
Jutras, R., Paed (P.Q.)
Leblanc, Marien
Martel, Therese
Massicotte, J. P. H.
Patry, J. C., OrthSurg
Patry, P. E., GenSurg
Plante, F.
Proulx, P. Y., IntMed
Provencher, J. P.
Roy, G. E.
St-Pierre, F., ObstGyn
Thibault, A.
VILLE D'ALMA
(See Alma)
VILLE D'ANJOU
(See Montreal)
VILLE JACQUES CARTIER
(See Cite de Jacques Cartier)
VILLE LEMOYNE
(See Cite de Jacques Cartier)
VILLE MARIE
(1,710)
Despins, R.
Gaboury, P.
Lalonde, E., GenSurg
Morin, L. P.
VILLE ST. JOSEPH
*
Dufresne, Irenee, D & T Rad.
VILLE ST. MICHEL
(See Montreal)
VILLE ST. PIERRE
(See Lachine)
VIMONT
(4,151)
Paiment, L.
Roy, J.
WAKEFIELD
(374)
Geggie, D. C.
Geggie, J. H. S.
Geggie, N. S.
Wilson, M. S., Psy.
WARWICK
(2,493)
Bechard, J. C.
Breton, L.
Lacourciere, Y.
Rousseau, J. M.
WATERLOO
(4,543)
Barcelo, M.
Blake, E. M.
Katz, M.
Larose, I.
Montminy, R.
Norris, C. K.
WEEDON
(1,426)
St-Pierre, Y.
WESTMOUNT
(See Montreal)
WINDSOR
(6,593)
Bilodeau, M.
Caux, R.
Frechette, G.
Gouin, R.
Houle, G. A., GenSurg (P.Q.)
YAMACHICHE
(1,185)
Lamy, P
YAMASKA
(454)
Hebert D.

Saskatchewan

ARBORFIELD
(583)
Baker, B.
ARCOLA
(561)
Fabrigar, Carmelo
Plaster, E. L.
ASSINIBOIA
(2,496)
Belak, Z. O.
Bridge, R. C.
Gallet, J. P.
McCutchion, A.
Robertson, K.
BALCARRES
(710)
Mortellaro, A.
Smith, R. R. W.
Steele, P. L.
BEECHY
(399)
de Los Santos, J. M.
BENGOUGH
(606)
Cunningham, Janet
Cunningham, J. B.
Jones, D. M.
BIENFAIT
(840)
Miller, J. E.
Rennie, R. T.
BIGGAR
(2,702)
Grapentine, W. L.
Heinrich, R. G.
King, B. M.
Mason, B. L.
Ormerod, B.
Rayman, M. R.
Young, L. D.
BIG RIVER
(907)
Oldroyd, K.
BIRCH HILLS
(531)
Jack, W.
Malhomme, B. E.
Marshall, M.
BORDEN
(209)
Soffer, H. S.
BROADVIEW
(1,008)
Campbell, A. H., GenSurg.
Kenny, K. J.
BROCK
(224)
Ritchie, R. E. C.
CABRI
(711)
Coneghan, Catherine
Davies, D. W.
Holden, G. P.
CANORA
(2,114)
Danylchuk, A.
Lee-Sing, M. S.
Lee-Sing, S.
Sutton, G. V.
CANWOOD
(811)
Blenkinsop, E. I.
CARLYLE
(978)
Harvey, E.
Jamieson, J.
Neil, A. J. B.
Neil, Christella

* Population not separately available.

CARNDUFF
(956)
Harding, H. G.

CARROT RIVER
(935)
Mandin, J. A.
McCullough, J. A.

CENTRAL BUTTE
(461)
Christ, Elly
Christ, L. W.
Mainprize, G. W.

CLIMAX
(428)
Meyer, J. H.

CORONACH
(395)
Calder, A. D.

CRAIK
(603)
McCaw, J. W

CUDWORTH
(626)
Kondzielewski, Z.
Opseth, M. O.

CUPAR
(577)
Haworth, D. H.

CUTKNIFE
(489)
Scratch, J. R.

DAVIDSON
(923)
Herman, M.
Venters, D. B.

DELISLE
(508)
Hayes, D. F.
Schacherl, U.

DINSMORE
(436)
Corner, F. D.

DODSLAND
(371)
Silbermann, O. H.

EASTEND
(764)
Millions, J. V.
Powell, A.
Yeung, J. Y.

EATONIA
(609)
King, Delores
McClure, D.

EDAM
(275)
Smith, I. M.

ELBOW
(401)
Drummond, K. L.

ELROSE
(580)
Richardson, D. S.

ELSTOW
(106)
Bicum, G.

ESTERHAZY
(1,109)
Chapman, E. F.
Kershaw, T. G.
McKenzie, W. G.
Prestage, P. T.
Stonkus, S.

ESTEVAN
(7,730)
Barnes, M. J.
Bastian, F. O.
Castaneda, J., DiagRad.
Eaton, J. L.
Inglis, R., ObstGyn
Keegan, D. L.
Lowson, C.
Samuels, N.
Soroka, M. M.
Wiebe, R. H.

ESTON
(1,698)
Fung, W. K.
Holmes, S. E.

FILLMORE
(342)
Quiggin, F. S.

FOAM LAKE
(931)
Ghatan, S.
O'Callaghan, J. J.
Sommervill, R. P.

FORT QU'APPELLE
(1,521)
Bimpeh-Segu, M.
Doyle, L. J., PulmDis & TB (P.Q.)
Fleming, R. A.
Hiliopoulos, D.
Matthews, A. R.
Mutch, J.
Porth, E. J.
Singh, G.
Smuk, A. H.

FORT SAN
*
Barnett, G. D.
Hardy, E. A.
O'Reilly, F. Joan
O'Reilly, H.
Swanton, A. L.

FOX VALLEY
(478)
Jain, R.

FRONTIER
(272)
Watson, R.

GAINSBOROUGH
(411)
Hobbs, W. G.

GLASLYN
(264)
Coghlan, R. O.

GOODSOIL
(241)
Barrit, D. S.
Schlagintweit, H. E. O.

GRAVELBOURG
(1,499)
LeBlanc, R. P.
Morin, R. E.
Sheer, W. T.
Soucy, A.

GRENFELL
(1,256)
Gilbert, M. J.
Stafford, C. M

GULL LAKE
(1,034)
Ko, H. Y.
Smith, D. M.
Troensegaard-Hansen, E.

HAFFORD
(511)
Nykiforuk, E.

HERBERT
(1,009)
de Vere, N. F
Goertz, O. P.
Gubuan, R. C.
Higgie, C. B.

HODGEVILLE
(381)
Lipitch, H. S.

HOLDFAST
(362)
Bruce, D. S.

HUDSON BAY
(1,601)
Else, D. G.
Ewing, R. D.
Silver, J. B.

HUMBOLDT
(3,245)
Davis, M. W.
Henning, E. T.
Junk, G. J.
Miller, P. J.
Radomski, T.
Ryall, P.

ILE A LA CROSSE
(570)
Hoffmann, M. W.

IMPERIAL
(550)
Kennedy, C.

INDIAN HEAD
(1,802)
Davies, A. J. M., GenSurg
Laxdal, A. T.

INVERMAY
(396)
McCormack, F.
McCormack, Mary A.

ITUNA
(839)
Connolly, J.
McCourt, J. F.

KAMSACK
(2,971)
Bishop, M. B.
Dutton, P. W.
Laevans, L. V.
Mallow, W. E.

KELLIHER
(466)
Johnston, D. B.

KELVINGTON
(883)
Hamilton, R. R.
McGettigan, J.

KERROBERT
(1,225)
Adams, M, D.
Clews, A. G.

KINCAID
(314)
Phillips, Eileen M.
Phillips, J. K.

KINDERSLEY
(2,990)
Gulka, O. N.
Hooge, P. D.
Howie, J. L.
Khosla, S. V.
Penner, L. U.

KINISTINO
(770)
Chan, W. Y.
Fahlman, J. J.
Louttit, R. T.

KIPLING
(777)
Camgoz, H. T.
Novotny, M. E.
Nowell, A. L.

KYLE
(533)
Stark, R. B.

LAFLECHE
(755)
Hennessy, D. B.
Morin, J. M.

LAMPMAN
(640)
Bowers, B. S.
Sweeting, T. J.

* Population not separately available.

LANGENBURG
(751)
Neilmeyer, C. L.
Zbeetnoff, P.

LANIGNAN
(515)
Allen, G. G.

LA RONGE
(707)
Bradley, R., PH

LASHBURN
(477)
Kernohan, H. R.

LEADER
(1,205)
Cousins, R. J.
Dusevic, J.

LEMBERG
(465)
Hughes, W. W.

LEOVILLE
(421)
Buckley, F. J.
Lambert, C. S.

LEROY
(514)
Korol, P.

LESTOCK
(412)
Cusack, C. A.

LLOYDMINSTER
(5,667)
Blitz, A. E.
Campbell, D. I.
Cooke G. L.
Daly, P. J.
Dickout, J. M.
Doherty, Elisabeth M.
Hemstock, J. W.
Mitchell, J.
Nattress, J. R.
Reimer, J.
Sherstan, J. H., GenSurg.
Skene, J. S.
Smith, E. L. J.

LOON LAKE
(335)
Scott, F.

LUCKY LAKE
(426)
Bennett, I.

LUMSDEN
(689)
Sulma, V.

LUSELAND
(664)
Graham, E. R.
Harry, J. E.

MACKLIN
(688)
Eid, F. L., GenSurg
Johnsrude, R. L.

MAIDSTONE
(580)
Marfleet, T. L.

MANKOTA
(480)
Murphy, P. J.

MAPLE CREEK
(2,293)
Charles, D., ObstGyn
Smith, H. G.
Unger, A. G.

MARYFIELD
(474)
Mackie, A. A.

MAYMONT
(238)
Scratch, J. A.

MEADOW LAKE
(2,805)
Al-Katib, F.
Dixon-Warren, **B. C.**
Haight, K. R.
Heine, H. X.
Kotwall, A. N.
Kuckertz, Berta
Kuckertz, H. W.
Martine, R.
Wisinger, H. J.

MELFORT
(4,039)
Golumbia, J. E.
Green, H. C.
Hutton, C. F.
Kolke, R. H.
Lavoie, A. L.
Pannell, R. W.
Unger, F. J.
Vigrass, H. G.

MELVILLE
(5,196)
Brennan, F. J.
Leszczynski, J.
Millette, O. J.
Wohlfarth, W.

MIDALE
(641)
Halliday, F.
Mainprize, W. G.

MILDEN
(394)
Fern, B. J.

MONTMARTE
(475)
Painchaud, L. A.
Prefontaine, L. L.

MOOSE JAW
(33,206)
Amies, D. R., IntMed
Beddie, A. J.
Belcourt, L. E.
Bennett, W. E. J., GenSurg
Berry, F.
Betzner, N. E.
Bray, L. G., Paed
Bromley, A. T.
Bryce, J. C., Psy.
Chang, C. A., Anaes
Colpitts, G. A., Path.
Cox, A. J.
Crimp, L. H., Urol
Drzewicka-Kubinski, Halina
Dunn, J. F.
Dunn, N. E., DiagRad
Enta, T., Derm.
Ewart, D. M., Anaes.
Fitzgerald, J. J.
Franklin, Yvette
Galambos, M.
Garner, H. L. C., IntMed
Gass, D. A.
Hanson-Dunse, S.
Heal, F. C., IntMed
Hourigan, J. M.
Johnston, H. J., Anaes.
Kao, H., PhysMed & Rehab
Kubinski, Z .T. Anaes
Lacny, J.
Lowden, A. G.
Lowe, T.
MacDonald, C. E.
Matheson, J. A., GenSurg
McCarroll, J. G., ObstGyn
McIntyre, H. R., GenSurg
Menyasz, L., Otol
Miller, R.
Morris, F. R., GenSurg
Murphy, J.
Nairnsey, C.
Oakes, R. G.
Olgac, S.
O'Reilly, P. O., Psy
Parvaresh, G. A.
Probert, L. A., Ophth
Pugh, R. F.
Read, R. M.
Reynaud, E.
Rubinski, Helena M.
Rudd, D. R.
Skeet, B. J.
Stewardson, E. R.
Thompson, G., GenSurg
Tolek, I. H.
Tse, F. H.
Turnbull, K. E., ObstGyn
Weir, A.
Wigmore, F. H., GenSurg
Wilfong, J. H., GenSurg
Young, A. F., GenSurg
Young, H. G., GenSurg
Young, H. M., ObstGyn
Young, H. V.
Zaleski, W. A., Psy

MOOSOMIN
(1,777)
Chestnut, H. W., GenSurg
Davidson, B. D.
McHugh, B.

MOSSBANK
(574)
Baker, K. A.
Miller, J. E.

NEILBURG
(332)
O'Sullivan, P.
Wilkinson, A. A.

NEUDORF
(408)
Black, M.
Shepherd, J. K.

NIPAWIN
(3,836)
Christiansen, H
Couper, E. H.
Fitton, H.
Gale, A. R.
Jonat, P. G.
Jones, A. B., GenSurg
Jones, Betty
MacKenzie, H. N.
Mark, R. J.
Smith, A. R.
Tabili, T.
Walters, L. A
Wright, A.

NOKOMIS
(558)
Magnus, V. J.
Nunan, T.

NORQUAY
(498)
Scholtz, M. K.

NORTH BATTLEFORD
(11,230)
Acheson, H. F.
Bradley, J., Ophth
Breton, G. J., GenSurg
Chan, P. S.
Chou, C. L.
Dalal, A., IntMed
Daly, P. J.
Das, K. C.
Dayap, F. D.
del Rosario, P. G.
Demay, M., Psy
Docherty, J. A
Eaton, R. D.
Gonor, A. B.
Gormley, M. A.
Hames, C. F., W., PH
Houston, W. H.
Imperial, B. S., Psy
James, R. D., GenSurg.
Jedlicki, S. M.
Johnston,, R. V.
Kerpel, Martha
Lowe, F. C. F.

* Population not separately available.

North Battleford (Cont'd.)
Lukas, Martha
Lukas, W. J., D & T Rad.
MacDonald, D. C., **Ophth,Otol**
Maningas, C. S., Paed
Marjerrison, G. L., Psy
Matheu, H.
McPhail, Mary K.
Mejia, M. S.
Nikiforuk, W. J.
Oktem, N.
Onel, J.
Pearce, K. L.
Podilsky, M.
Prasard, L.
Saldivar, E.
Sen, Susanta
Simpson, E. R.
Stromberg, O. O.
Trylinski, Z., ObstGyn
Uguralp, A.
Wagner, G., GenSurg.
Webb, Marian L.
Weston, I.
Wolfe, W. J.

OGEMA
(467)
Allaire, L. R. E.

OUTLOOK
(1,335)
McBride, G. A.
Neufeld, B.
Siemens, P.

OXBOW
(1,360)
Drummond, K. A.
Galloway, G. D.

PANGMAN
(256)
Gibson, S. M.

PARADISE HILL
(277)
Graham, H.

PONTEIX
(886)
Strohofer-LeMarry, J.

PORCUPINE PLAIN
(706)
Bain, J. A.
Derechin, W.
Kalyana-Sundaram, K.

PREECEVILLE
(924)
Bisset, J. M. C., GenSurg
Forshner, R. S.
Gray, L. N.

PRELATE
(618)
Daly, P.
Fennessy, T. J.

PRINCE ALBERT
(24,168)
Alford, M.
Andrews, C. H., **OphthOtol**
Bailey, Mamie, Path
Chipperfield, D. V.
Craigen, D.
de Kenedy, G. L., Urol
Dyker, G. R., IntMed
Edes, A. O., IntMed
Finlayson, C. M., Urol
Fry, W. H., ObstGyn.
Galambos, M.
Green, G. H.
Green, R. G.
Hall, H. H.
Hammond, K. C.
Hart, Susan E., GenSurg
Hjertaas, O. K.
Ho, T. J., DiagRad
Hynes, A. M., Urol
Irwin, A. C.
Jenkins, R. E., Psy

Johnston, J. J.
Johnston, R. K.
Kim, C. H., DiagRad
Kirkby, R. W., IntMed (T.B.)
Korvin, C.
Lane, O. G., Path
Lim, R.
MacDonald, T. S.
Martinson, H. A.
May, M. J.
Maynard, H. C.
McIntosh, H. A., IntMed
Nelson, G. F., Psy
Ormerod, R. O.
Palmer, C. F.
Pollock, Ilse, Paed.
Powles, G. P S.
Rich, P. J., GenSurg
Roberts, M.
Shenouda, G-Z., GenSurg.
Smith, L. W.
Stark-Rueffel, Liselotte
Surkan, M.
Swaffield, W. R., **ObstGyn**
Tisdale, C. L.
Tsai, L., Ophth
Wilkinson, D. B.
Wallace, J. B.. GenSurg
Wise, H. B.
Woodrow, R.
Zacharuk, S. W.

PUNNICHY
(415)
Sykes, G.

QU'APPELLE
(562)
Wileniec, M. J

QUILL LAKE
(534)
Cross, J.

RABBIT LAKE
(193)
Crux, N. W.

RADVILLE
(1,071)
Fernando, B. A.
Smith, M. S.

REDVERS
(644)
Hamwee, C. M.
McConnachie, C. C.

REGINA
(112,141)
Adhikari, K. C., IntMed.
Aftahi, F., Paed
Albertson, D. B., NeurSurg
Allan, N. J., ObstGyn.
Allan, W. S.
Almeida, J. G.
Alport, P. Jill, Anaes.
Alport, W. E. H.
Alvarez, E., PlasSurg
Anderson, J. D., Ophth, Otol
Armit, J. C.
Asquith, E.
Babchuk, R. B.
Bachynski, B., **OrthSurg**
Bailey, A. J.
Bakos, L. D., DiagRad
Barclay, T. H. C.
Barootes, E. W., Urol
Barry, M. P., DiagRad
Bawden, J. W., TherRad.
Beaglehole, P.
Bean, Helen A., TherRad
Bean, I. W.
Best, S. C., Paed.
Bishop, J. R.
Black, T. M., **ObstGyn**
Borcenca, Herminia C.
Bowering, M. W., **Anaes**
Boyd, T. A. B., GenSurg., ThorSurg.
Bradley, G. C.

Brown, J. A., ObstGyn
Brown, J. D.
Brown, W. G., DiagRad.
Brownridge, T.
Bryant, A. J. S., TherRad IntMed
Bugg, T. E.
Campbell, J. S., Urol
Carnduff, D. W., **GenSurg**
Cartmill, T., Otol
Cawsey, L. A.
Chacko, J. C., GenSurg.
Chatwin, J. C.
Chernenkoff, R. M.
Chiao, J. T.
Christie, T. A., **Anaes**
Clarkson, J. G.
Cohen, S.
Comrie, C. L., **IntMed**
Coneghan, J. L.
Cowan, L. E.
Crook, R. A., Otol.
Crosby, C. H., **GenSurg ThorSurg**
Cunning, C. L.
Cutler, N. M., GenSurg
Dakin, W. A., Urol.
D'Almeida, J. G.
Danby, J. H.
Darke, T. V.
Dehnel, M. K.
Dewaji, V. R.
Dexter, D., Path
Dillenberg, H. O.
Dobie, F. C., GenSurg
Dogan, K.
Duncan, B. P., Paed
Duncan, E. H., GenSurg
Eistetter, A. E., ObstGyn
Ellenburgh, N., GenSurg
Elliott, G. F.
Ewing, G. H., IntMed
Ficke, K. H., DiagRad
Ficzycz, N.
Finkelstein, M.
Flint, W. F.
Fraser, M. M., GenSurg
Froggatt, J. R., OrthSurg.
Gautama, V. B.
Geist, Susanna
George, H. C., IntMed
Glaisher, I. L.
Goldthorpe, A. M.
Good, J. D.
Good, P. H., Urol
Goodfellow, Alice, Paed
Gordon, D. F., ObstGyn
Gorman, F. J., GenSurg
Gregory, I. L., GenSurg.
Griffith, G. S.
Grocott, H. C., Paed.
Grunberg, F., Psy.
Gudgeon, A. B.
Hanna, L. M., PH
Hashi, J. I. O.
Harvey, J. P.
Haughton, T. J., Otol
Heasman, G. A., Psy
Hendrie, J.
Hewat, C. M.
Hill, I. R.
Hodgins, K. W.
Hoffmann, N. L.
Hsu, Nora
Hubar, M.
Hudec, A. V. J.
Husain, I. S., OphthOtol.
Huston, A. F., PhysMed&Rehab.
Hutchison, Patricia, Paed
Jackson, F. I., PH
James, E. H., NeurSurg
Jamieson, D.
Janczur, S., IntMed
Jones, E. A., OrthSurg
Jones, R. H. T., Paed.
Jow, Eleanor P., IntMed

* Population not separately available.

Regina (Cont'd.)
Jowsey, J. W., OrthSurg
Juckes, A. W., GenSurg
Kalla, G.
Kenny, M. M., DiagRad
Kerster, G. G., ObstGyn
Kim, J. H. K., Anaes.
Kim, J. P., OrthSurg
Kitchen, B.
Klassen, W.
Kobrynski, B., IntMed
Komjathy, C. A.
Kovach, J. C., GenSurg
Krause, C. C., Urol
Kuan, P. W.
Kumar, K., NeurSurg
Kumar, Kamla, Paed.
Kumar, S. D., IntMed.
Kurtze, W. L., GenSurg
Larsen-Lung, Violet A., Anaes.
Laxdal, O. E., Paed
Laycraft, G. H., **Anaes**
LeBlond, J. W. R.
LeBoldus, J. M.
Lee, T.
Loguinoff, J. B.
Loken, J. D.
MacDougall, W. G., IntMed
MacInnes, I.
MacIntosh, J. H. M.
MacRae, W. D., GenSurg
Marcellus, D. F.
Marioni, P.
Martin, D. T., Otol
Martin, M. G., Psy
Massig, H., Path
Matthews, A. M.
McAlpine, D. F., **Anaes**
McCannel, N. B.
McFetridge, J. G., IntMed
McFetridge, J. G., GenSurg
McGillivray, J. A. S.
McGregor, J. A., Anaes.
McLaughlin, J. H.
McLean, C. S.
McLurg, J. J. A., **Psy**
McLurg, R. J.
McMichael, L. A.
Merry, C. C.
Mesbur, J. B.
Moffit, Kathleen, Paed
Mohagerin, A. H.
Molnar, R. R.
Murphy, J. K., ObstGyn
Murray, H. M.
Muttitt, E. L., IntMed
Ng, A. C., DiagRad
Nicholl, J. O., Bact
Nowosielski, T.
Oktem, M. R.
O'Reilly, Julia
Orford, T. J.
Orteza, Josefina M.
Paveley, G. E.
Penman, D.
Perry, A. E., **D&TRad**
Philips, H. H., DiagRad
Pickles, A. C.
Pomeroy, J. K.
Poulakakis, G. M.
Powers, N.
Preston, K.
Preston, Margaret
Quinto, M. G., Paed
Rad, M. J.
Rafaat, M., Paed
Ramsay, J. D.
Rathana-Nakintara, T.
Rayman, M. R.
Rejskind, M. D., Psy
Ring, E. D., IntMed
Road, D. A.
Rodger, D. E., IntMed
Rodko, E. A., DiagRad
Roy, A. K., DermSyph
Rublack, A. E., GenSurg
Rusnak, C. H., GenSurg.
Russel, A.
Russon, G. W., **Psy**
Ryan, G. C., Anaes
Sanchez, Yolanda
Sauer, E. K., **GenSurg**
Schwann, P. G.
Shelinger, D. J.
Simon, S. A.
Sinclair, A. S.
Sinclair, G. E., IntMed
Skinner, L. C., **Anaes**
Smith, N. S. H.
Smith, S. G.
Sollars, R. J,. ObstGyn
Sommerville, R. J., Paed
Spooner, E. G., Ophth.Otol
Spooner, H. J., OrthSurg
Spooner, M. A.
Stead, S., Ophth
Stephen, J. D., Path
Swendrowski, T.
Szlazak, J., PlasSurg
Szuchewycz, B. OrthSurg
Sylvestre, R. M.
Tan, K. K. H., D&TRad.
Taylor, A. C., GenSurg
Te, L.
Thom, I. M.
Thomson, H. S.
Timmons, T. J.
Trudelle, J. B.
Tsai, S.
Tufts, W. B.
Turnbull, J. B., Ophth
Ueberschar, K. H., DiagRad
Vallillo, L.
Waight, P. J.
Walter, D. E.
Warwick, W. E.
Wasylenki, A. J.
Wasylenki, J. M.
Watson, H. L.
Weeks, E. L.
Weiss, M. H.
Welsh, W. T. O.
Westgate, A., ObstGyn
White, P. B.
Williams, N.
Wilson, J. R.
Wingate, M. B., ObstGyn.
Wong, L. C., Paed.
Yadov, D. R.
Young, S., GenSurg

ROCANVILLE
(496)
Saunders, M. H.

ROCKGLEN
(484)
Evans, H. S.

ROSETOWN
(2,453)
Buentipo, B. V., Jr, GenSurg
Giles, C. R.
Ositis, A.
Salmon, H. A.
Walker, A. J.

ROSE VALLEY
(625)
Wood, I. A.

ROSTHERN
(1,255)
Friesen, H. E.
Hesse, H. B.
Janzen, H. W.
Janzen, J. F.
Nichel, J. A.

ST. WALBURG
(693)
Gibbons, R. R.
Mowat, C. W.

SASKATOON
(95,526)
Adams, J. W., Path
Allen, W. A.
Alms, M., OrthSurg
Altschul, R.
Amoozegar-Fard, E., Psy.
Anderson, J. F. C., IntMed
Anderson, R. C., IntMed
Andres, D. J.
Ash, D. D.
Ashenhurst, E. M., Neurol
Aw, C. F., Path.
Baergen, E. H.
Bailey, A. A., NeurPsy
Baker, F. W. Paed.
Balaton, J.
Baltzan, Betty
Baltzan, D. M., IntMed
Baltzan, M. A., IntMed
Baltzan, R. B., IntMed
Barry, Gladys N.
Barsony, Bela, Anaes.
Bauer, B. Iris
Bayatpour, M.
Beall, G. M.
Beck, R. N., IntMed
Becker, A., D&TRad
Begg, R. W.
Berg, C. D., GenSurg
Biro, C., GenSurg
Block, H. J., Path
Blue, G. D., **Urol**
Bobyn, P.
Bolton, C. F., Neurol.
Boughton, H. C., IntMed(TB)
Boyd, D. M., GenSurg
Bray, G., DiagRad
Bremner, R. M., **DermSyph**
Brook, J.
Brook, M. H.
Brown, A. B., ObstGyn
Brown, Esther M., TherRad
Buchan, D. J., IntMed
Burkell, C. C., **TherRad**
Burrell, R. H., Psy.
Bury, J. D.
Campbell, J. M., **Urol**
Cates, G. W., Path
Chasmar, L. R., GenSurg, PlasSurg.
Chernenkoff, W.
Chertkow, G., IntMed
Chorney, J. K., **Path**
Cipywnyk, D.
Clark, R. F.
Clementson, C. A. B., ObstGyn.
Coburn, F. E., Psy.
Cockings, E. C., Anaes
Collins, H. M.
Cowan, D. M.
Cowan, G. A., **TherRad**
Cram, R. W., **GenSurg**
Crocker, K. M., **ObstGyn**
Cumming, J. F.
Cunningham, T. A., IntMed, Path
Dalgleish, H. D., GenSurg
Dangor, A. I.
Dantow, M., PH
Darja, Maria
Daunt, I. E.
Dempster, G.
Denson, R., Psy
Dick, A. A., GenSurg
Dick, J. A.
Dickie, A. W.
Dimililer, I.
Doig, J. N.
Donegan, E. A., Ophth.
Dosman, J. A.
Duggleby, H. E.
Dwersteg, E. V. C., Otol
Dyck, F., ObstGyn
Emson, H. E., Path
Ervilmag, K.
Esher, E. J.
Estey, H. W., Urol
Ewing, C. C., Ophth
Fee, D. A., TherRad

* Population not separately available.

Saskatoon (Cont'd.)
Firor, W. B., Cardiovasc & ThorSurg.
Flegel, Helen M.
Fogel, S.
Fritsche, W.
Garson, J. E.
Garson, J. Z.
Genereux, A. G., OphthOtol.
Genereux, G. P., DiagRad.
Gerrard, J. W., Paed
Gold, R. J.
Goluboff, L.
Goluboff, N., Paed
Groenendyk, J.
Guanzon, A. Z., Anaes
Hardy, L. W., Paed.
Hargarten, B. W.
Harris, A. L.
Hart, H. D.
Heichman, W. J.
Hathway, W. W.
Hawes, E. G., IntMed
Hayton, R. C., IntMed
Hazen, G. M., OphthOtol
Hickerty, J. C., DiagRad.
Hindmarsh, A. W.
Hirte, W. E., IntMed
Hodgson, R. O., OphthOtol
Hoffer, A., Psy
Holden, F. A.
Holmes, W. S., Obst
Hooge, A. A.
Hopper, P. W., ObstGyn, GenSurg
Horlick, L., IntMed
Horn, H.
Hosking, D. J.
Houston, C. S., DiagRad
Hunt, T. E., IntMed, PhysMed & Rehab.
Irvine, G. T.
Ivan, L. P., NeurSurg
Ives, Elizabeth J., Paed
Jackson, B. A., GenSurg
Jen, I.
Jones, Eloise M., Psy.
Katty, V. S., GenSurg
Kavanagh, N. W.
Kent, H. P., DiagRad
Khalil, E. F., Paed.
Kilduff, C. J., Anaes
Kinnear, W. S., Paed
Kirby, A. R.
Kirkaldy-Willis, W. H., OrthSurg.
Klaassen, D. J., IntMed.
Knight, C. R., PlasSurg
Knowles, V. R., Ophth
Korn, G. W., ObstGyn
Kost, W.
Kostick, E. L.
Krishnayya, K. V.
Krochak, M. B.
Kunkel, M. G., OrthSurg
Kushniruk, W., Derm
Landa, S.
Landells, D. G., OrthSurg.
Langer, M. H., GenSurg
Leakos, J., Otol
Leckie, G. G.
Leddy, J. E., GenSurg
Lesche, K. M.
Lindsay, W. S., PathBact
Loewen, L. M.
Logie, F. A.
Lopez, J. F., IntMed
Low, E. W.
Ma, H. F.
MacDonald, W. B., Anaes
MacDonnell, A. B., D&TRad
MacFadyen, R. D.
MacKenzie, J. W. A., Paed
MacLachlan, T. B., ObstGyn
MacPherson, R. H., ObstGyn
Mahood, Margaret, Psy
Mallouh, G. E., ObstGyn
Mann, J. A.
Marciniak, J. L., IntMed
Marian, J. J., GenSurg, Cardiovasc & ThorSurg, Urol
Marshall, Mary E., Psy
Matthews, V. L., PH.
McAlister, S. L.
McCorkell, W. J.
McDonald, I. M., Psy
McFadden, D., GenSurg
McFarland, J. D., Anaes.
McGowan, D. G.
McIntyre, R. W.
McKenna, B. F., OrthSurg.
McKerracher, D. G., Psy
McPherson, A. R., IntMed(T.B.)
McSheffrey, J. B., Paed.
Merriman, J. E.
Mitchell, D. M., IntMed
Monks, J. G., DiagRad
Moore, D. F., PathBact
Moss, M. S.
Mowbray, J. A.
Mowbray, J H., IntMed
Muir, J. M., Anaes.
Murphy, F. A., Path
Murray, F. S., Psy
Murray, R. G., Ophth
Myers, C. A.
Nanson, E. M., GenSurg
Noble, J. G., OrthSurg
Oberdieck, K. E., Psy.
O'Keefe, J. F., ObstGyn
Orchard, C. B., GenSurg
Orchard, S. A.
O'Regan, J. B., Psy
Paine, K. W., NeurSurg
Palko, P. D.
Park, I. H.
Paul, J. A. D.
Peacock, G. W.
Peterson, E. R., GenSurg
Petkovich, N. J., IntMed.
Pettigrew, M.
Pimblett, D. T., Anaes
Piper, G. W.
Polisiuk, A.
Pollock, A., GenSurg
Posner, Hertha
Postma, K. J.
Pritchard, R. E.
Pugh, R. F., Anaes.
Rafi-Zadeh, E., IntMed
Rao, S. V. K., DiagRad
Renpenning, H. J.
Richards, A. G.
Richards, Elizabeth
Robertson, A.
Robertson, C. L., GenSurg
Robertson, D. E., OrthSurg
Rosher, F. W
Rozdilsky, B., Path
Russell, E. A., ObstGyn
Sada, M., IntMed
Sadro, T.
Salisbury, Gladys
Scharf, A. A., OphthOtol
Senensky, E. R.
Schmidt, E. W.
Schulman, I.
Schulman, L.
Scott, R. M.
Seddon, T. T.
Sellers, F. J., Paed
Sheridan, P. A.
Silver, W. A.
Slobodzian, M. S.
Smith, C. M., Psy
Smith, E. W., Ophth
Smith, M. J.
Smith-Windsor, M. H.
Somerville, A. E., IntMed
Spencer, E. W., D&TRad
Stark, E. J., Otol
Steele, R.
Stephen, A., Psy
Stitt, W. D., ObstGyn
Stockings, G. T.
Sugarman, H.
Syrenne, G.
Takeda, M.
Tchang, S., DiagRad
Ty, M., Urol
Upthegrove, W. E., Anaes
Voth, A. B.
Voth, C. G.
Wait, F. E., GenSurg
Warren, P. L.
Watson, T. A., TherRad
Weder, C. H., GenSurg
Wensley, A. C. H., ObstGyn
Wheaton, R. R.
Wilkinson, G. W., GenSurg
Witney, Joan
Wolan, C. T., Urol
Wolfe, F.
Wood, J. K.
Worobetz, S., GenSurg
Wyant, G. M., Anaes
Yaeger, H. L.
Yip, Suzanne
Zadvorney, Z. G., Anaes

SEDLEY
(385)
Parent, C. E.

SEMANS
(386)
Shapero, G. D.

SHAUNAVON
(2500)
Adamson, J. W.
O'Dea, J. J.
Taylor, E.

SHELLBROOK
(1,038)
Dobson, D.
Spencer, J. L.

SOUTHEY
(478)
Zeldenrust-de-Vries, Brita

SPAULDING
(415)
Scott, C. R.

SPIRITWOOD
(551)
Michaud, J. R

STOUGHTON
(616)
Markov, B. H.
Markova, T.
Mowbray, J. H.

STRASBOURG
(628)
Hitsman, E. H.

SWIFT CURRENT
(12,186)
Adolph, J., Path.
Armanious, F., IntMed.
Beare, M. S.
Boyd, M. S.
Burroughs, R. B.
Carreras, P.
Falkingham, J. P.
Hare, A.
Henry, A. P.
Huang, S. H.
Iffy, L., ObstGyn
Irwin, N. T., ObstGyn.
Irwin, O. M., GenSurg
Irwin, R. W., GenSurg
Jacobs, C. Gloria
Jacobs, R., GenSurg
Johnston, D.
Keene, J. D., Anaes
Krahn, A.
Likar, I.
Little, R. B., DiagRad
Lontok, R. M.

* Population not separately available.

SWIFT CURRENT (Cont'd)
McKerrell, D. M.
Miller, K. R., Paed
Mizrahi, A. M., Psy.
Retzer, O. D., GenSurg
Sabry, E.
Sood, B. K.
Strother-Stewart, C. R.
Verma, K. S.
Young, C.
Young, R. G.

THEODORE
(446)
Walshe, F. B.

TISDALE
(2,402)
Amundson, C.
Falkner, C. F.
Kinman, H. L.
Sutherland, F D.
Wright, R. D.

TURTLEFORD
(352)
Gelson, J.
MacGill, R. D.
Richards, J. M.

UNITY
(1,902)
Davies, A. J.
Doyle, W. J.
James, C. V.

URANIUM CITY
(1,665)
Gray, J. C.
Wan, B. H.

VAL MARIE
(448)
Aichroth, P. M

VANGUARD
(433)
Webster, J.

VONDA
(233)
Lemiszka, J.

WADENA
(1,311)
Baird, J. C.
Rollins, N.

WAKAW
(972)
Cenaiko, F. T.
Nickorick, Elsie

WATROUS
(1,466)
Heseltine, Jean M.
Heseltine, J. R.
Thomson, A. W.

WATSON
(910)
Rogstad, V. S

WAWOTA
(456)
Murphy, J. P.

WEYBURN
(9,101)
Burrell, R. H., Psy
Camunais, E. R.
Caparas, Virginia P.
Choi, J. K.
Colledge A. D.
Decter, O.
Dimarucot, Avelina
Eaglesham, F. C. F.
Fong, W. C. P.
Herjanic, Barbara L.
Herjanic, M., Psy
Horbaczewski, J., IntMed
Kargas, A. K.
Kuhbacher, F. G.
Little, M. W., GenSurg
March, B. W., Psy
Mizrahi, A. M.
Nagy, F.
Nicolas, Monica T.
Nicolos, T. D.
Ross, H. F., Psy
Segovia, C. G.
Squires, W. G.
Stewart, A.
Villaneuve, R.
Wright, J. B.
Zarsadias, I. G.
Zeville, M.

WHITEWOOD
(900)
Adams, W. E.

WILKIE
(1,612)
Hermesh, Irmgard
Mera, Z.

WOLSELEY
(1,031)
Isman, G. B.

WYNYARD
(1,690)
Haver, J. V.
Polec, E. M.

YORKTON
(9,996)
Andrews, W. N., Psy.
Battle, F. G.
Brennan, K. S.
Chatterjee, Maureen
Chu, M.
Conway, D. F.
Copas, D. E.
Crossley, H.
El Deiry, S. K.
Flatman, J. G., DiagRad
Gabel, F. E.
Houston, C. J., GenSurg
Houston, Sigga C.
Junek, D. V.
MacIntyre, J. A.
Nieuwenhuizen, M., Psy
Novak, M. C.
Portnuff, H. A. L.
Potoski, Stephanie
Potoski, P.
Ridsdel, W. B.
Sequeira, H.
Skoll, L. S.
Tolczynski, B.
Yaholnitsky, M.
Yaholnitsky, R.

ZENON PARK
(382)
Konik, W.

Yukon

DAWSON
(886)
Constantine, R. R.

ELSA
(395)
Kirk, D. E.

MAYO
(342)
Clark, J. V.

WHITEHORSE
(5,031)
Doran, M. L.
Dutta, P. C., IntMed.
Helm, A. R.
Hibbard, J. C.
Kinloch, D. R.
Scrogger, D. G.
Sprenger, R. A.
Symon, H. L.
Tanner, A. C., GenSurg

* Population not separately available.

section 3

CANADIAN MEDICAL DIRECTORY 1967

GENERAL INFORMATION

PHYSICIAN'S OATH

I swear by Apollo the physician, by Aesculapius, Hygeia, and Panacea, and I take to witness all the gods, all the goddesses, to keep according to my ability and my judgment the following Oath:

To consider dear to me as my parents him who taught me this art; to live in common with him and if necessary to share my goods with him; to look upon his children as my own brothers, to teach them this art if they so desire without fee or written promise; to impart to my sons and the sons of the master who taught me and the disciples who have enrolled themselves and have agreed to the rules of the profession, but to these alone, the precepts and the instruction. I will prescribe regimen for the good of my patients according to my ability and my judgment and never do harm to anyone. To please no one will I prescribe a deadly drug, nor give advices which may cause his death. Nor will I give a woman a pessary to procure abortion. But I will preserve the purity of my life and my heart. I will not cut for stone, even for patients in whom the disease is manifest; I will leave this operation to be performed by practitioners (specialists in this art). In every house where I come I will enter only for the good of my patients, keeping myself far from all intentional ill-doing and all seduction, and especially from the pleasure of love with women or with men, be they free or slaves. All that may come to my knowledge in the exercise of my profession or outside of my profession or in daily commerce with men, which ought not to be spread abroad, I will keep secret and will never reveal. If I keep this oath faithfully, may I enjoy my life and practice my art, respected by all men and in all times; but if I swerve from it or violate it, may the reverse be my lot.

—HIPPOCRATES

CONTENTS

GENERAL

MEDICAL M.P.'s. M.P.P.'s AND SENATORS

SENATORS:

F. W. GERSHAW, M.D.
FREDERIC A. McGRAND, M.D.
JOSEPH SULLIVAN, M.D.
CLARENCE J. VENIOT, M.D.

MEMBERS OF PARLIAMENT:

LEWIS M. BRAND, M.D.
STANLEY HAIDASZ, M.D.
HARRY HARLEY, M.D.
HUGH M. HORNER, M.D.
WILLIAM D. HOWE, M.D.
GASTON ISABELLE, M.D.
PHILIP BERNARD RYNARD, M.D.

MEMBERS OF PROVINCIAL PARLIAMENTS:

Alberta
Hon. J. D. ROSS, M.D., Minister of Health

British Columbia
P. L. McGEER, M.D.

Manitoba
Hon. GEORGE JOHNSON, M.D., Minister of Education

Ontario
Hon. MATTHEW B. DYMOND, M.D., Minister of Health

Quebec
Hon. ROCH BOIVIN, M.D., Minister without portfolio.
ANTONIO AUGER, M.D., Memb., Legislative Council
Hon. FERNAND LIZOTTE, M.D., Minister of Transport & Communication
J.-ARTHUR-GUY FORTIER, M.D.
GUY GAUTHIER, M.D.
VICTOR CHARLES GOLDBLOOM, M.D.
JOSEPH-ROBERT-EDOUARD LUSSIER, M.D.
ZOEL SAINDON, M.D.
GASTON TREMBLAY, M.D.

Newfoundland
JAMES M. McGRATH, M.D., B.M., B.Ch.
CLIFTON JOY, M.D.
NOEL MURPHY, M.D., O. St. J.

New Brunswick
Hon. GEORGES DUMONT, M.D., Minister of Health
G. E. CHALMERS, M.D.
J. F. McINERNEY, M.D.

Nova Scotia
PAUL KINSMAN, M.D.
JAMES A. LANGILLE, M.D.
NORMAN J. MacLEAN, M.D.
C. L. MacMILLAN, M.D.
THOMAS McKEOUGH, M.D.
H. J. POTHIER, M.D.

Prince Edward Island
M. LORNE BONNEL, M.D.
LLOYD G. DEWAR, M.D.
HUBERT B. McNEILL, M.D.

MEDICAL COUNCIL OF CANADA

The Medical Council of Canada was established in 1912 by the Canada Medical Act to examine candidates for medical registration sent forward by the provincial medical licensing bodies. It employs a Main Board of Examiners who set and mark the written papers, and local boards of oral and clinical examiners at the various centres of examination. Members of Council do not themselves act as examiners.

Address all communications to The Registrar, The Medical Council of Canada, 77 Metcalfe Street, Ottawa 4, Canada. Tel. 235-0948.

Officers 1966-1967

President	1st Vice-President	2nd Vice-President
Dr. A. L. Richard	Dr. V. A. Snow	Dr. R. B. Kerr

Representing the Governor in Council

Dr. R. S. Duggan St. David's, Ont.	Dr. A. M. House St. John's, Nfld.	Dr. R. M. Dysart Moncton, N.B.

MEDICAL COUNCIL (*Cont'd*)

The Provincial Medical Councils

Newfoundland	— Dr. J. A. Davis, Corner Brook — Dr. J. E. Josephson, St. John's
Prince Edward Island	— Dr. J. B. Downing, Summerside — Dr. J. M. Gillis, Eldon
Nova Scotia	— Dr. J. F. Macneil, Glace Bay — Dr. G. J. LeBrun, Bedford
New Brunswick	— Dr. V. A. Snow, Hampton — Dr. J. P. McInerney, Saint John
Quebec	— Dr. A. Roy, Montreal — Dr. L. Coutu, Montreal
Ontario	— Dr. J. C. C. Dawson, Toronto — Dr. A. R. Turnbull, Barrie
Manitoba	— Dr. A. R. Birt, Winnipeg — Dr. C. H. A. Walton, Winnipeg
Saskatchewan	— Dr. E. W. Barootes, Regina — Dr. E. G. Hawes, Saskatoon
Alberta	— Dr. W. Bramley-Moore, Edmonton — Dr. L. C. Grisdale, Edmonton
British Columbia	— Dr. R. G. Langston, Vancouver — Dr. W. E. Harrison, Vancouver

The Universities

Dalhousie	— Dr. L. C. Steeves, Halifax	**Toronto**	— Dr. R. I. Macdonald, Toronto
Laval	— Dr. G. A. Bergeron, Quebec	**W. Ontario**	— Dr. O. H. Warwick, London
Montreal	— Dr. P. Nadeau, Montreal	**Manitoba**	— Dr. L. G. Bell, Winnipeg
McGill	— Dr. G. E. Joron, Montreal	**Saskatchewan**	— Dr. R. W. Begg, Saskatoon
Ottawa	— Dr. A. L. Richard, Ottawa	**Alberta**	— Dr. D. F. Cameron, Edmonton
Queen's	— Dr. J. B. Firstbrook, Kingston	**Br. Columbia**	— Dr. R. B. Kerr, Vancouver

The Homoeopathic Practitioners

Dr. J. J. Griffith, Westmount, P.Q.

N.B. Every provincial medical council elects two members.

PROVINCIAL REGISTRARS

Dr. Cluny Macpherson,
Registrar,
Newfoundland Medical Board, P.O. Box 5279,
St. John's, Newfoundland — Tel. 726-8546.

Dr. R. G. Lea,
Registrar,
Medical Council of P.E.I.,
170 Fitzroy St.,
Charlottetown, P.E.I. — Tel. 7325.

Dr. John R. Nugent,
Registrar.-Treasurer,
Medical Council of New Brunswick,
112 Carleton St.,
Saint John, N.B. — Tel. Area 506 ; 693-2266.

Dr. M. R. Macdonald,
Registrar,
Prov. Medical Board of Nova Scotia,
Victoria Gen. Hosp.,
Halifax, N.S. — Tel. 422-7371.

Dr. Augustin Roy,
Registrar,
College of Physicians & Surgeons of the
Province of Quebec.
1896 Dorchester West,
Montreal, P.Q. — Tel. 935-2591.

Dr. J. C. C. Dawson,
Registrar.-Treasurer,
The College of Physicians & Surgeons of Ontario,
64 Prince Arthur Ave.,
Toronto 5, Ont. — Tel. 924-2577.

Dr. M. T. Macfarland,
Registrar,
The College of Physicians & Surgeons of Manitoba,
Second Floor, 201 Kennedy St.,
Winnipeg 1, Man. — Tel. 947-0424.

Dr. G. W. Peacock,
Registrar,
College of Physicians & Surgeons of Saskatchewan,
932 Spadina Cres. E.,
Saskatoon, Sask. — Tel. 244-7355.

Dr. W. Bramley-Moore,
Registrar,
College of Physicians & Surgeons of Alberta,
9901 - 108th St., Edmonton, Alta., — Tel. 422-6184.

Dr. W. G. McClure,
Registrar,
College of Physicians & Surgeons of British Columbia,
1807 W. 10th Ave.,
Vancouver, B.C. — Tel. 736-5551.

THE ROYAL COLLEGE OF PHYSICIANS AND SURGEONS OF CANADA

74 Stanley St., Ottawa 2, Ont. — Tel. SH 6-8177.

President	Dr. Robert B. Kerr, Vancouver, B.C.
Immediate Past-President	Dr. Walter C. MacKenzie, Edmonton, Alta.
Vice-President — Division of Medicine	Dr. Donald R. Wilson, Edmonton, Alta.
Vice-President — Division of Surgery	Dr. Edouard D. Gagnon, Montreal, P.Q.
Honorary Treasurer	Dr. F. J. Tweedie, Montreal, P.Q.
Secretary	Dr. James H. Graham, Ottawa, Ont.
Honorary Assistant Secretary	Dr. W. Gordon Beattie, Ottawa, Ont.

Members of Council

Division of Medicine

Dr. Ronald V. Christie, Montreal, P.Q.
Dr. Lea Steeves, Halifax, N.S.
Dr. Jacques Genest, Montreal, P.Q.
Dr. John P. Gemmell, Winnipeg, Man.
Dr. William M. Goldberg, Hamilton, Ont.
Dr. Jean Grandbois, Quebec, P.Q.
Dr. James B. Hilton, Ottawa, Ont.
Dr. Robert B. Kerr, Vancouver, B.C.
Dr. Donald F. Moore, Saskatoon, Sask.
Dr. Ian E. Rusted, St. John's Nfld.
Dr. K. J. R. Wightman, Toronto, Ont.
Dr. Donald R. Wilson, Edmonton, Alta.

Division of Surgery

Dr. Frederick E. Bryans, Vancouver, B.C.
Dr. Eric C. Nanson, Saskatoon, Sask.
Dr. Charles G. Drake, London, Ont.
Dr. Colin C. Ferguson, Winnipeg, Man.
Dr. Edouard D. Gagnon, Montreal, P.Q.
Dr. Fraser N. Gurd, Montreal, P.Q.
Dr. Frederick G. Kergin, Toronto, Ont.
Dr. Robert C. Laird, Toronto, Ont.
Dr. W. Douglas Miller, Saint John, N.B.
Dr. Walter C. MacKenzie, Edmonton, Alta.
Dr. E. P. Nonamaker, Halifax, N.S.
Dr. Jacques Turcot, Quebec, P.Q.

THE CANADIAN MEDICAL ASSOCIATION

Secretarial and Editorial Offices — 150 St. George St., Toronto 5, Ontario

General Secretary
A. F. W. PEART, M.D.

Assistant Secretary — R. G. Prefontaine, M.D., D. M. Aitken, M.D.

Executive Secretary — Mr. B. E. FREAMO

Secretary, Public Relations — Mr. K. C. CROSS

President — DR. R. K. C. THOMSON, Edmonton

President-Elect — DR. N. J. BELLIVEAU, Montreal

Immediate Past President — DR. R. O. JONES, Halifax

Chairman of the General Council and Chairman of the Executive Committee
R. D. ATKINSON, M.D., Waterloo

Honorary Treasurer — DR. J. H. MALONEY, Charlottetown

Editor, C.M.A. Publications (The Canadian Medical Association Journal,
The Canadian Journal of Surgery) — DR. G. T. DICKINSON, Toronto

Managing Editor — A. D. KELLY, M.B., Toronto

Associate Editors — DR. J. O. GODDEN, Toronto; DR. J. R. ANDERSON, Toronto; DR. L. R. RABSON, Toronto

Secretaries of the Provincial Divisions

BRITISH COLUMBIA — E. C. McCOY, 1807 W. 10th Ave. Vancouver 9, B.C.

ALBERTA — Wm. BRAMLEY-MOORE, M.D., CMA Alberta House, 9901-108th St., Edmonton, Alta.; Tel. 422-6184.

SASKATCHEWAN — G. W. PEACOCK, M.D., 932 Spadina Cres. E., Saskatoon, Sask,; Tel. CH 4-7355.

MANITOBA — Mr. R. P. H. SPRAGUE, Exc. Dir., 201 Kennedy St.-2nd Floor, Winnipeg, Man.; Tel. 947-0421.

ONTARIO — GLENN I. SAWYER, M.D., 244 St. George St., Toronto 5, Ont; Tel. WA. 5-3264

QUEBEC — de GUISE VAILLANCOURT, M.D., 2115 Drummond St., Ste. 33, Montreal 25, P.Q.; Tel. 849-5773.

NOVA SCOTIA — C. J. BECKWITH, M.D., Dalhousie Public Health Clinic, University Ave., Halifax, N.S.,; Tel. 423-8848.

NEW BRUNSWICK — F. L. WHITEHEAD, M.D., East Riverside, King's County, N.B.

PRINCE EDWARD ISLAND — DR. JOHN CRAIG, 48 St. Claire Ave., Charlottetown.

NEWFOUNDLAND — W. D. PARSONS, M.D., O'Mara Martin Bldg., Rawlins Cross, St. John's, Nfld.

ASSOCIATION DES MEDECINS DE LANGUE FRANCAISE DU CANADA

Secrétariat — 5064, avenue du Parc, Montréal 8, P.Q. — Tél. 273-2321—273-3881

OFFICIERS

Directeur Général
Dr Emile Blain
Adjoint au Directeur Général
Dr André Leduc

Secrétaire-Trésorier Général
Dr E.-Rolland Blais
Adjoint au Secrétaire-Trésorier Général
Dr Raymond Caron

EXECUTIF

Dr. Emile Blain (Montréal)
Dr. André Leduc (Montréal)
Dr. Paul David (Montréal)
Dr. Wilfred-M. Caron (Québec)
Dr. E.-Rolland Blais (Montréal)
Dr. Raymond Caron (Montréal)
Dr. Henri R. de Saint Victor (Ottawa)
Dr. Richard Lessard (Québec)
Dr. Jacques Léger (Montréal)

Directeur des Relations Extérieures
Dr. Antonio Lecours

Directeur des Expositions
Dr. B. G. Bégin

Comité Provincial de la Nouvelle-Ecosse .... Philippe-H. LeBlanc
Comité Provincial du Nouveau-Brunswick .... Calixte Doucet
Comité Provincial du Québec .... Jacques Léger
Comité Provincial de l'Ontario .... Armand Dufresne
Comité interprovincial de l'Ouest .... J.-P. Moreau

---

CANADIAN MEDICAL PROTECTIVE ASSOCIATION

Office Address: Suite 115, 26 Nepean St., Ottawa 4, Canada. Tel. 237-4830

The Canadian Medical Protective Association is a mutual defence union of Canadian doctors organized for the protection of its members from suits for malpractice or negligence. Members are eligible for advice, legal aid, and the payment of costs and damages should they be awarded. The Association has been in existence since 1901 and now has a membership of over half the doctors in Canada.

President .... JAMES H. B. HILTON, M.D., Ottawa

Executive Committee

Hon. Life President .... **GEORGE W. ARMSTRONG, M.D., Ottawa.**
1st Vice-President .... J. C. THOMAS, M.D., Vancouver.
2nd Vice-President .... N. J. BELLIVEAU, M.D., Montreal.
Secretary-Treasurer .... T. L. FISHER, M.D., Ottawa.
Assistant-Secretary-Treasurer .... F. NORMAN BROWN, M.D., Ottawa.

Elected Members of Council: W. F. Connell, M.D., Kingston; G. A. Copping, M.D., Montreal; E. B. Tovee, M.D., Toronto; W. E. Collins, M.D., Ottawa; J. L. Coupal, M.D., Ottawa; G. W. **Dunning, M.D., Ottawa; George Hooper, M.D., Ottawa; R. G. Mackenzie, M.D., Ottawa; R. E.** Smart, M.D., Ottawa; T. G. Stoddart, M.D., Ottawa.

General Counsel: Messrs. Gowling, MacTavish, Osborne & Henderson, Ottawa.

Provincial Advisory Committees

Alberta:
A. R. Bainborough, M.D., Lethbridge; H. L. Dobson, M.D., Grande Prairie; **Howard McEwen, M.D., Calgary; W. B. Parsons, M.D., Red Deer; J.B.T. Wood, M.D., High Prairie.**

British Columbia:
G. R. Barrett, M.D., Nelson; J. A. Elliot, M.D., Vancouver; H. B. Graves, M.D., Vancouver; D. M. King, M.D., Vancouver; J. A. C. Thomson, M.D., Kamloops; J. F. Tysoe, M.D., Victoria; D. M. Whitelaw, M.D., Vancouver.

Manitoba:
A. R. Birt, M.D., Winnipeg; W. J. Boyd, M.D., Winnipeg; C. E. Corrigan, M.D., Winnipeg; E. Johnson, M.D., Selkirk; M. T. Macfarland, M.D., Winnipeg; Ross Mitchell, M.D., Winnipeg.

New Brunswick:
H. E. Britton, M.D., Moncton; H. O. Tonning, M.D., Saint John; A. F. Van Wart, M.D., Fredericton.

Newfoundland:
W. D. Parsons, M.D., St. John's.

Nova Scotia:
A. Calder, M.D., Glace Bay; H. A. Creighton, M.D., Lunenburg; S. R. Johnston, M.D., Halifax; S. G. MacKenzie, M.D., Truro; L. A. MacLeod, M.D., Liverpool.

Ontario:
F. S. O'Brien, M.D., London; G. E. Cooper, M.D., Hamilton; W. E. Keith, M.D., Windsor; J. C. Pearson, M.D., Port Arthur; W. A. Oille, M.D., Toronto; J. W. Sturtridge, M.D., Copper Cliff.

Prince Edward Island:
J. A. McMillan, M.D., Charlottetown; J. C. Simpson, M.D., Summerside.

Quebec:
J. A. Denoncourt, M.D., Trois Rivieres; G. W. Halpenny, M.D., Montreal; **P. P. Julien. M.D., Montreal; Richard Lessard, M.D. Quebec City; Arthur Powers, M.D., Ottawa; W. deM. Scriver, M.D., Montreal.**

Saskatchewan:
J. M. Campbell, M.D., Saskatoon; H. D., Dalgleish, M.D., Saskatoon; C. J. Houston, M.D., Yorkton; C. L. Tisdale, M.D., Prince Albert; S. Young, M.D., Regina.

SPECIALIST SOCIETIES

Allergy	**The Canadian Academy of Allergy (L'Academie Canadienne d'Allergie)**—Dr. Francois Léger, 3766 Queen Mary Rd., Montreal, P.Q.
Anaes.	**Canadian Anaesthetists' Soc.**—Dr. S. M. Campbell, Sec., 178 St. George St., Toronto 5, Ont.; Tel. WA 3-1154.
Anat.	**Canadian Assoc. of Anatomists**—Dr. J. V. Basmajian, Dept. of Anat., Queen's U., Kingston, Ont.; Tel. LI 6-1731.
Arth.	**Canadian Arthritis & Rheumatism Soc.**—Mrs. John Dottridge, Sec., 45 Charles St. E., Toronto 5, Ont.; Tel. 924-0766.
Bact.	**Canadian Association of Med. Bacteriologists—(Association Canadienne des Medecins Bacteriologistes)**—Dr. I. B. R. Duncan, Sec.-Treas., Dept. of Microbiol., St. Joseph's Hosp., London, Ont.; Tel. GE 9-3271, Ext. 225.
Biochem.	**Canadian Biochemical Soc.**—Dr. H. D. Branion, Sec., Faculty of Graduate Studies, University of Guelph, Guelph, Ont.; Tel. TA 4-4120.
Biol.	**Canadian Federation of Biological Societies—(Constituent Societies include): The** Canadian Assoc. of Anatomists; The Canadian Biochemical Soc.; The Canadian Physiological Soc.; The Pharmacological Soc. of Canada; The Nutrition Soc. of Canada; Dr. A. H. Neufeld. Hon. Sec., Faculty of Med., U. of Western Ont., London, Ont.; Tel. 432-5261, Loc. 270.
Card.	**Canadian Cardiovascular Soc. (Societe Canadienne de Cardiologie)**—Dr. R. E. Beamish, Sec., 100 Medical College, Winnipeg 3, Man.; Tel. 774-6541.
Chest.	**Canadian Thoracic Society**—Dr. C. W. L. Jeanes, Sec., 343 O'Connor St., Ottawa 4, Ont.; Tel. 237-1208. **Canadian T.B. Assoc.**—Dr. C. W. L. Jeanes, Sec., 343 O'Connor St., Ottawa 4, Ont.; Tel. 237-1208.
Clin. Chem.	**Canadian Soc. Clinical Chemists—(La Societe Canadienne des Clinico-Chemistes)**—Dr. D. Michener Schatz, Sec., Dept. of Labs., Toronto Gen. Hosp., Toronto, Ont.; Tel. 248-3184.
Clin. Invest.	**Clinical Research Soc. of Toronto**—Dr. A. Bruce-Robertson, c/o Princess Margaret Hosp., 500 Sherbourne St., Toronto 5, Ont.; Tel. WA 4-0671.
Dietetic	**The Canadian Dietetic Assoc.**—Miss Joan E. Brown, Gen. Sec., 1393 Yonge St., Toronto 7, Ont.; Tel. WA 1-7704.
Gastroent.	**Canadian Assoc. of Gastroenterology (L'Association Canadienne de Gastroenterologie)**—Dr. J. M. Finlay, Ste. 426, 170 St. George St., Toronto 5, Ont.
Hosp.	**Canadian Hosp. Assoc.**—Mr. George McCracken, Sec., 25 Imperial St., Toronto 7, Ont.; Tel. HU 1-2244. **National Sanitarium Assoc.**—Mr. F. D. Beauchamp, B.A., C.A., 130 Rosedale Valley Rd., Apt. 308, Toronto 5, Ont.; Tel. 924-6936. **Catholic Hosp. Assoc. of Canada**—Rev. A. L. M. Danis, O.M.I., Exec. Dir., 312 Daly Ave., Ottawa 2, Ont.; Tel. 233-6836.
Indust. Med.	**Industrial Med. Assoc. of the Province of Quebec (L'Association de Medecine Industrielle de la Province de Quebec)**—Dr. Lloyd A. Wright, Sec., Rm. 930, 1050 Beaver Hall Hill, Montreal, P.Q.; Tel. 870-1511.
Lab. & Rad. Tech.	**Canadian Soc. of Laboratory Technologists**—Mr. A. R. Shearer, Exec. Sec., 99 Wentworth St. S., Hamilton, Ont.; Tel. JA 8-8642.
Med. Ident.	**Canadian Medic-Alert Fdn. Inc.**—Miss Ada Adamson, Sec., 176 St. George St., Toronto 5, Ont.; Tel. 923-5393 (24 Hr. Member Emergency Serv.)
Med. Lib.	**Canadian Assoc. of Med. Record Librarians**—Mrs. Janet Milner, R.R.L., Exec. Sec., 770 Glenforest St., Oshawa, Ont.; Tel. 728-9743. **Canadian Library Assoc. Committee on Med. Science Libraries**—Mrs. Mary Galt, Medical Library, U. of Toronto, Toronto, Ont.
Mult. Scler.	**Multiple Sclerosis Society of Canada**—Mrs. D. Konradis, Exec. Sec., 76 Avenue Rd., Toronto 5, Ont.; Tel. 922-6065.
Musc. Dys.	**Muscular Dystrophy Assoc. of Canada**—Mrs. Audrey Mundell, Exec. Sec., Room 511, 160 Bay St., Toronto 1, Ont.; Tel. 925-2914.
Neur.	**Canadian Neurological Soc.**—Dr. H. J. M. Barnett, Sec., 170 St. George St., Toronto 5, Ont.
Nurs.	**L'Association des Infirmieres Catholiques du Canada**—Mlle. H. Turcotte, 401 St-Cyrille ouest, Quebec 6, P.Q. **Canadian Nurses' Assoc.**—50 The Driveway, Ottawa 4, Ontario; Tel. 237-2133. **Victorian Order of Nurses for Canada**—Miss Jean Leask, Dir.-in-Chief, 5 Blackburn Ave., Ottawa 2, Ont.; Tel. 233-5694.
Nutr.	**The Canadian Dietetic Assoc.**—Miss Joan E. Brown, Gen. Sec., 1393 Yonge St., Toronto 7, Ont.; Tel. WA 1-7704.
Obst. Gyn.	**Society of Obstetricians & Gynaecologists of Canada**—Dr. J. L. Harkins, Sec., Ste. 537, Med. Arts Bldg., Toronto 5, Ont.; Tel. WA 3-2171.
Occ. Ther.	**The Canadian Assoc. of Occupational Therapists**—331 Bloor St. W., Toronto 5, Ont.; Tel. 922-3701.
Ophth.	**Canadian Ophthamological Soc.**—Dr. R. G. C. Kelly, Sec., Ste. 902, 1849 Yonge St., Toronto 7, Ont.
Orthopaed.	**Canadian Orthopaedic Assoc.**—Dr. C. A. Laurin, 3875 St. Urbain, Montreal, P.Q.

SPECIALIST SOCIETIES (*Cont'd*)

Otol.	**Canadian Oto-Laryngological Soc.**—Dr. D. P. Bryce, Sec., 320 Med. Arts Bldg., Toronto 5, Ont.; Tel. WA 2-7676.
Paed.	**Canadian Paediatric Soc. (Sociéte Canadienne de Pediatrie)**—Dr. J. H. V. Marchessault, Sec., 14 Green Ave., St. Lambert, Montreal 23, P.Q.; Tel. 671-0555.
Path.	**Canadian Association of Pathologists**—Dr. D. W. Penner, Sec., Dept. of Path., Winnipeg Gen. Hosp., Winnipeg 3, Man.; Tel. SP 2-7487.
Pharm.	**Canadian Pharmaceutical Assoc. Inc.**—Mr. J. C. Turnbull, B.S.P., Exec. Dir., 175 College St., Toronto 2B, Ont. **Pharmaceutical Manufacturers Assoc. of Canada**—Mr. Guy Beauchemin, Exec. Sec., 1110 Gillin Bldg., 141 Laurier Ave. W., Ottawa 4, Ont.; Tel. 236-9993.
Phys. Med.	**Canadian Assoc. of Phys. Med. & Rehab.**—Dr. W. O. Geisler, Sec., FRCP(C), 153 Lyndhurst Ave., Toronto 4, Ont.; Tel. WA 3-0928. (Div. of Cdn. Fed. Biol. Soc.) **Canadian Physiotheraphy Assoc.**—Mrs. Curtis Millar, Exec. Sec., 64 Avenue Rd., Toronto 5, Ont.; Tel. WA 3-1318.
Psy.	**Canadian Psychiatric Assoc.—Association des Psychiatres du Canada**—Dr. W. A. Blair, Sec., Ste. 103, 225 Lisgar St., Ottawa 4, Ont.; Tel. 234-6644, Area Code 613.
Pub. Health	**Canadian Public Health Assoc.**—Dr. G. W. O. Moss, Sec., 1255 Yonge St., Toronto 7, Ont.; Tel. 925-2271.
Rad.	**Canadian Assoc. of Radiologists**—Dr. Maurice Dufresne, Hon. Sec.-Treas., 1555 Summerhill Ave., Ste. 511, Montreal 25, P.Q.; Tel. WE 2-9782. **The Canadian Soc. of Radiological Technicians**—Mrs. E. I. Hood, R.N., R.T., Sec., 2175 W. 16th Ave., Vancouver 9, B.C.; Tel. 733-6230.
Retard.	**The Canadian Assoc. for Retarded Children**—Dr. G. Allan Roeher, Ph.D., Exec. Dir., 87 Bedford Rd., Toronto 5, Ont.; Tel. 922-3104.
Rheum.	**The Canadian Arthritis & Rheumatism Soc.**—Mrs. John Dottridge, Sec., 45 Charles St. E., Toronto 5, Ont.; Tel. 924-0766. **Canadian Rheumatism Assoc.—Sociéte Canadienne de Rheumatologie**—Dr. Phillip Rosen, Sec., Ste. 402, 99 Avenue Rd., Toronto 5, Ont.; Tel. WA 1-4912.
Urol.	**Canadian Urological Assoc.**—Dr. Kenneth J. MacKinnon, Sec., Royal Victoria Hospital, Montreal 2, P.Q.; Tel. VI 2-1251, Loc. 479.

COLLEGE OF GENERAL PRACTICE OF CANADA

Secretaries Office - - 1260 Bay St., Toronto 5, Ont. — Tel. 923-7367

Executive Director	Dr. D. I. Rice, Toronto, Ont.
Past President	Dr. G. R. Diehl, Winnipeg, Man.
President	Dr. D. E. Hunt, St. Catharines, Ont.
President-Elect	Dr. W. E. H. Alport, Regina, Sask.
Honorary Treasurer	Dr. J. A. D. Brunet, Grand'Mère, P.Q.
Chairman of Board of Directors	Dr. J. J. Zack, Vancouver, B.C.
Member at Large	Dr. H. I. MacGregor, Halifax, N.S.

BOARD OF DIRECTORS

Representative: Dr. J. C. Mackenzie, Vancouver, B.C.; Dr. J. B. Corley, Calgary, Alta.; Dr. D. A. Gass, Moose Jaw, Sask.; Dr. R. A. Jacques, St. Boniface, Manitoba; Dr. P. L. Brady, Seaforth, Ont.; Dr. A. T. Hunter, London, Ont.; Dr. J. P. Genest, Lévis, P.Q.; Dr. M. D. Snarch, Montreal, P.Q.; Dr. S. G. B. Fullerton, Halifax, N.S.; Dr. W. E. Hirtle, Sackville, N.B.; Dr. H. A. MacMillan, Charlottetown, P.E.I.; Dr. M. L. W. Parsons, Glovertown South, Nfld.

Alternates to Board: Dr. L. M. Cathcart, Richmond, B.C.; Dr. H. H. Black, Calgary, Alta.; Dr. S. A. Orchard, Saskatoon, Sask.; Dr. J. D. McMillan, Winnipeg, Man.; Dr. H. H. Hetherington, Brampton, Ont.; Dr. L. M. Mudie, Willowdale, Ont.; Dr. G. Courcy, L'Islet, P.Q.; Dr. Isaac Tannenbaum, Montreal, P.Q.; Dr. H. C. Still, Halifax, N.S.; Dr. N. C. Grant, Saint John, N.B.; Dr. H. Stewart, Charlottetown, P.E.I.

WORKMEN'S COMPENSATION PROVINCIAL BOARDS

WORKMEN'S COMPENSATION BOARD—B.C.—707 W. 37th Ave., VANCOUVER 13, B.C.
Tel. 266-0211

Chairman of the Board .... J. E. Eades, Q.C.
Commissioner .... E. V. Ablett
Commissioner .... H. Wright
Executive Secretary .... R. M. Bagshaw, C.A., F.C.I.S.
Chief Medical Officer .... J. R. Davidson, M.D.

WORKMEN'S COMPENSATION BOARD—ALBERTA—10048-101A AVE., EDMONTON, ALTA., TEL. 422-7151

Chairman .... C. M. Macleod, Q.C.
Commissioner .... I. Casey
Commissioner .... C. R. Gilbert
Secretary .... R. D. Ross, C.A., F.C.I.S.
Comptroller .... D. J. Duncan, C.A.
Chief Medical Officer .... W. F. Hall, M.D., F.R.C.S.(C), F.A.C.S.
Chief Claims Officer .... J. H. Adams

WORKMEN'S COMPENSATION BOARD—SASKATCHEWAN—1840 LORNE ST., REGINA, SASK., TEL. LA. 7-1681 — Area Code—306

Executive Secretary .... G. Begg
Chief Medical Officer .... Wm. B. Tufts, M.D.

WORKMEN'S COMPENSATION BOARD—MANITOBA—333 MARYLAND ST., WINNIPEG 10, MAN., Tel. SP. 4-5593

Chairman .... D. Elliott Wilson, Q.C.
Commissioner .... D. Harry Young
Commissioner .... Peter McSheffrey
Chief Medical Officer .... C. D. Lees, M.D.
Secretary .... R. G. Jones

WORKMEN'S COMPENSATION BOARD—ONTARIO—90 HARBOUR ST., TORONTO 1, ONT. TEL. 362-3411 — Area Code 416

Chairman .... B. J. Legge, Q.C.
Vice-Chairman .... John F. Cauley
Commissioner .... Earl C. Steele, M.D.
Executive Director .... George R. Poole, B.A.
Director, Medical Services .... Dr. A. B. Powell
Chief, Medical Department .... Dr. H. F. Richardson
Medical Director, Hosp. & Rehab. Centre .... B. H. G. Curry, M.D., FRCS(C)

WORKMEN'S COMPENSATION COMMISSION—QUEBEC—225 GRANDE ALLEE E., QUEBEC 4, P.Q.; Tel. 693-5850

President .... Judge Joseph Marineau
Vice-President .... Roger Mathieu
Commissioner .... Bertrand Bellemare, M.D., F.A.A.C.M.
Commissioner .... H.-Conrad LeBrun
Commissioner .... St-Georges White, C.A.

General Secretary .... Euclide Bisson, Q.C.
Executive Director .... Emile Gignac, R.I.A.
Special Adviser .... Romeo Depeyre, M.D., LL. L.
Comptroller .... Paul Pare
Chief Accountant .... Henri Belanger
Technical Adviser .... Albert Paquet
Assistant Secretary .... Roland Champoux

Treasurer .... L.-P. Pelletier
Chief of Claims Service .... Joseph Delage
Chief of Assessment Division .... H. Gingras
Chief of Audit Division .... J.-A. Morency
Chief of Collection Division .... J.-R. Paquet
Chief of Social Rehabilitation Division .... L.-P. Tessier

Medical Director .... Dr. Henri Bedard
Medical Officer .... Dr. Louis-A. Brochu
Medical Officer .... Dr. Leo Bergeron
Medical Officer .... Dr. Louis Lessard
Medical Officer .... Dr. Marcel Rochette
Medical Assistant Director .... Dr. Irenee Leblanc
Medical Officer .... Dr. Maurice Jacques
Medical Officer .... Dr. Dollard Garant
Chief of Medical Aid Division .... J.-E. Raoul Demers
Medical Officer .... Romeo Goulet
Medical Officer .... Paul Lacroix
Medical Officer .... Antoine Fiset
Physiatrist .... Dr. Maurice Delage
Physiatrist .... Dr. Guy Lessard
Medical Officer .... Dr. Napoléon Côté
Medical Officer .... Léon Chenel
Medical Officer .... Sauveur Patry

WORKMEN'S COMPENSATION PROV. BOARDS (*Cont'd*)

WORKMEN'S COMPENSATION BOARD—NEW BRUNSWICK—PROVINCIAL BLDG., CHARLOTTE ST., P.O. BOX 160, SAINT JOHN, N.B., TEL. 692-0181

Chairman	Robert G. Jones
Vice-Chairman	J. Michel Fournier
Commissioner	J. Harold Farthing
Secretary	Donald Ayer
Chief Medical Officer	Leonard J. Stephen, M.D.

WORKMEN'S COMPENSATION BOARD—NOVA SCOTIA—P.O. BOX 1150, JOHNSTON BLDG., COR. PRINCE & GRANVILLE STS., HALIFAX, N.S. TEL. 422-7341; 423-7965 (AFTER 6:00 P.M.)

Chairman of the Board	W. T. Hayden, Q.C.
Executive Sec. & Comptroller	S. E. Watt
Chief Medical Officer	D. M. Grant, M.D.
Commissioner	Robert Murrant
Commissioner	W. W. Downie
Medical Officer	A. G. MacLeod, M.D.

WORKMEN'S COMPENSATION BOARD—P.E.I.—76 GREAT GEORGE ST., CHARLOTTETOWN, P.E.I. Tel. 894-8555

Chairman	J. W. McAleer
Vice-Chairman	J. M. McAlduff
Commissioner	E. A. Keeping
Board Medical Officer	J. L. F. Burge, M.D.

WORKMEN'S COMPENSATION BOARD—NEWFOUNDLAND—CONFEDERATION BLDG., ST. JOHN'S NFLD., TEL. PBX-95011

Chairman	Irving Fogwill
Vice-Chairman	John J. Maddigan
Commissioner	Clarence V. Hancock
Secretary	Roland H. Baggs
Administrative Officer	Richard A. Fagan
Medical Officers	C. U. Henderson, M.D.
	L. E. Lawton, M.D.
	W. D. Parsons, M.D.

WORLD MEDICAL ASSOCIATION, INC.

10 Columbus Circle, New York 10019, N.Y., U.S.A.

Officers 1965-1966

President	Sir Clement Price-Thomas, KCVO, 69 Harley St., London, W.1, England
President-Elect	Dr. Jesus V. Tamesis, Clinica Tamesis, 42 Quezon Blvd. Ext., Quezon City, Philippines
Treasurer	Dr. Ernst Fromm, Arztehaus, An der Alster 48, Hamburg 1, Germany
Chairman of Council	Dr. Leonard W. Larson, 221 Fifth Street, Bismarck, North Dakota
Vice-Chairman of Council	Dr. J. Joncheres, P.B. 83, Saintes (17), France
Secretary General	Dr. Alberto Z. Romualdez, 10 Columbus Circle, New York, N.Y. 10019
Secretary, Africa	Dr. J. K. M. Quartey, Korle Bu Hospital, Box 29F, Accra, Ghana
Secretary Asia	Dr. A. P. Mittra, 26 Curzon Road, New Delhi 1, India
Secretary Europe	Dr. M. Poumailloux, 14 Avenue Bosquet, Paris VIIe, France
Secretary Latin America	Dr. Hector Rodriquez Casilla 394, Santiago, Chile
Secretary North Pacific	Dr. J. C. Denoga, 1850 Taft Avenue, Manila, Philippines
Secretary, South Pacific	Dr. C. J. Ross-Smith, 77-79 Arundel St., Glebe, N.S.W., Australia

Members of Council — 1966

Dr. O. K. Harlem Inkognitogt 26, Oslo, Norway
Dr. L. W. Larson, 221 Fifth Street, Bismarck, North Dakota, U.S.A.
Dr. Antonio Spinelli, Catona, Calabre, Italy
Dr. A. H. Tonkin, 35 Wale Street, Cape Town, South Africa

Members of Council — 1967

Dr. R. Castellanos, Plaza Bellas Artes, Los Chaguaramos, Caracas, Venezuela
Dr. J. Joncheres, P.B. 83, Saintes (17), France
Mr. J. R. Nicholson-Lailey, Orchard Rise, Trull, Taunton, Som., England

Members of Council — 1968

Dr. Gerald D. Dorman, 51 Madison Avenue, New York, New York
Dr. Ernst Fromm, An der Alster 48, Arztehaus 2, Hamburg 1, Germany
Dr. A. P. Mittra, 26 Curzon Road, New Delhi 1, India
Dr. T. G. Swinburne, 158 Mont Albert Road, Canterbury, Melbourne, Victoria, Australia

Council Emissaries

Dr. E. R. Annis, 2121 Biscayne Blvd., Miami, Florida, U.S.A.
Dr. Austin Smith, Parke Davis & Co., P.O. Box 118 GPO, Detroit, Michigan 48232
Dr. Felix Worre, 24 Grand rue, Luxembourg

Executive Editor

Dr. S. S. B. Gilder, White Gables, Copperkins Lane, Amersham, Bucks, England

W.M.A., (*Cont'd*)

Associate Editors

Dr. J.-R. Gosset, 37 rue de Bellefond, Paris IX, France
Dr. F. Giannetto, Sindicato Medico del Uruguay, Colonia 1938, 20 piso, Montevideo, Uruguay

Committee Chairman

International Liaison: Dr. Jean Maystre, 108 Chemin de Ruth, Geneva, Switzerland; **Medical Education: Dr. L. W. Larson, 221 Fifth Street, Bismark, North Dakota, U.S.A.;Medical Ethics:** Dr. Antonio Spinelli, Catona, Calabre, Italy; **Planning:** Dr. L. W. Larson, 221 Fifth Street, Bismark, North Dakota, U.S.A.; **Socio-Medical Affairs:** Sir Clement Price-Thomas, KCVO, 69 Harley Street, London, W.1, England; **Finance:** Dr. E. Fromm, An der Alster 48, Arztehaus 2, Hamburg 1, Germany

Non-Council Committee Members

Dr. Charles Jacobsen, 12 Kristianiagade, Copenhagen, Denmark
Dr. R. Schlogell, Haedenkampstrasse 3, Koln-Lindenthal, Germany

THE DECLARATION OF GENEVA

Adopted by the General Assembly of the World Medical Association at Geneva, Switzerland, Sept. 1948. At the Time of Being Admitted as Member of the Medical Profession:

I SOLEMNLY PLEDGE myself to consecrate my life to the service of humanity;
I WILL GIVE to my teachers the respect and gratitude which is their due;
I WILL PRACTISE my profession with conscience and dignity;
THE HEALTH OF MY PATIENT will be my first consideration;
I WILL RESPECT the secrets which are confided in me;
I WILL MAINTAIN by all the means in my power the honour and the noble tradition of the medical profession;
My COLLEAGUES will be my brothers;
I WILL NOT PERMIT considerations of religion, nationality, race, party politics or social standing to intervene between my duty and my patient;
I WILL MAINTAIN the utmost respect for human life from the time of conception; even under threat. **I will not use my medical knowledge contrary to the laws of humanity.**
I MAKE THESE PROMISES solemnly, freely and upon my honour.

WORLD HEALTH ORGANIZATION

AVENUE APPIA
Geneva, Switzerland

Elected Officers

President of the Nineteenth World Health Assembly, May 1966:
Dr. Arnold Sauter (Switzerland)

Vice-Presidents of the Assembly:
Dr. B. N'Dia Koffi (Ivory Coast)
Dr. A. Roldos Garcès (Ecuador)
Dr. A. Sushila Nayor (India)

Chairman, Committee on Programme and Budget:
Dr. Ahmad Nabulsi (Jordan)

Chairman, Committee on Administration, Finance and Legal Matters:
Sir William Refshauge (Australia)

Chairman, WHO Executive Board:
Dr. Karl Evang (Norway)

Vice-Chairmen, WHO Executive Board:
Dr. Hurustiati Subandrio (Indonesia)
Dr. Ousmane Keita (Guinea)

Staff Members

Director General: Dr. M. G. Candau (Brazil) ....WHO, Avenue Appia, Geneva, Switzerland
Deputy Dir. Gen.: Dr. P. Dorolle (France) ....WHO, Avenue Appia, Geneva, Switzerland
Ass't. Dir. Gen.: Dr. T. Karefa-Smart (Sierra Leone) ....WHO, Avenue Appia, Geneva, Switzerland
Ass't. Dir. Gen.: Dr. N. F. Izmerov (USSR) ....WHO, Avenue Appia, Geneva, Switzerland
Ass't. Dir. Gen.: P. M. Kaul (India) ....WHO, Avenue Appia, Geneva, Switzerland
Ass't. Dir. Gen.: Mr. M. P. Siegel (USA) ....WHO, Avenue Appia, Geneva, Switzerland

Dir. WHO Regional Office for Europe ....Dr. P. J. J. van de Calseyde (Belgium)—WHO Regional Office for Europe, 8 Scherfigsvej, Copenhagen, Denmark.

Dir. WHO Regional Office for Africa ....Dr. A. Quenum (Dahomey)—WHO Regional Office for Africa, P.O.B. 6, Brazzaville, Africa.

Dir. WHO Regional Office for the Western Pacific ....Dr. I. C. Fang (China)—WHO Regional Office for the Western Pacific, P.O.B. 2932, Manila, Philippine Islands.

Dir. PASB/WHO Regional Office for the Americas ....Dr. A. Horwitz (Chili)—PASB/WHO Regional Office for the Americas, 525, 23rd Street N.W., Washington, D.C., 20037.

Dir. WHO Regional Office for South-East Asia ....Dr. C. Mani (India)—WHO Regional Office for South-East Asia. World Health House, Indraprastha Estate, Ring Road, New Delhi-I, India.

Dir. WHO Regional Office for the Eastern Mediterranean ....Dr. A. H. Taba (Iran)—WHO Regional Office for the Eastern Mediterranean, P.O.B. 1517, Alexandria, Egypt.

DEPARTMENT OF NATIONAL DEFENCE

Medical Officers of Canadian Forces Medical Service

SG RADM	Elliot, WJ, CD, QHS
Brig	Barr, JWB, CD
A/C	Nelson, DGM, CD, QHP
G/C	Barclay, IH, CD
Col	Barron, RD, MC
G/C	Beach, AM, DFC, CD
Col	Besley, JK, CD
Col	Croskery, WHR, CD
Col	Cullen, FR, CD
Col	Edwards, LH, CD
Col	Fitch, M, CD
SG CAPT	Fleming, JH, CD
G/C	Hampson, KW, CD
SG CAPT	Irwin, RB, DFM
G/C	Jackson, JR, CD
Col	Kerr, AL, CD
G/C	Leach, WG, CD
SG CAPT	MacHattie, FGW, CD
SG CAPT	Maciver, DA
Col	McLaren, AG, CD
Col	McNally, NH, CD
G/C	Murray, JH, CD
G/C	Orr, WL, CD
G/C	Powell, TJ, CD
Col	Reed, WA, CD
SG CAPT	Roberts, RH, CD
G/C	Robinson, HC, CD
Col	Robitaille, JAR, CD
SG CAPT	Rogers, JW, CD
G/C	Wade, NSG, CD
G/C	Wickett, JC, AFC, CD
A/Col	Elliott, RC, CD
A/Col	Greenidge, HW, CD
A/Col	Hitsman, JS, MBE, CD
A/Col	Johnston, JL, CD
W/C	Baker, JRD, CD
Lt Col	Bennett, WLL, CD
Lt Col	Beswick, JA, CD
W/C	Carter, YK, DFC, CD
Lt Col	Chapman, GW, CD
Lt Col	Coleman, WR, CD
SG CDR	Connolly, VPL
Lt Col	Crawford, WM, CD
Lt Col	Davidson, AM, CD
Lt Col	Edwards, JK, CD
Lt Col	Evans, JF, CD
Lt Col	Fitzgerald, EK, CD
W/C	Fitzgibbon, GM, CD
W/C	Gazley, LA, CD
W/C	Hobbs, WK, CD
Lt Col	Holden, CP, CD
Lt Col	Ives, HMP, CD
W/C	Jackson, RF, CD
Lt Col	Jaffey, BD, MBE, CD
SG CDR	Kidd, DJ, CD
Lt Col	Leclaire, Y, CD
Lt Col	Lizotte, A, CD
W/C	MacFie, DD, CD
Lt Col	Malcolm, F, CD
W/C	Marriott, IA, CD
W/C	McElroy, J, CD
Lt Col	McQuaig, KD, CD
Lt Col	Morgan, BE, CD
W/C	O'Brien, JM, CD
SG CDR	Oliver, HD, CD
W/C	Rassell, JA, CD
Lt Col	St Arnaud, L, CD
SG CDR	Simpson, JS, CD
Lt Col	Smillie, RA, MBE, CD
Lt Col	Thiel, CJ, CD
Lt Col	VanVliet, GA, CD
Lt Col	Watson, JH, CD
SG CDR	West, CA, CD
SG CDR	Willoughby, DV, CD
W/C	Wills, WJ, CD
SG CDR	Woods, DG, CD
W/C	Wynne, JRW, CD
W/C	Yelland, AC, CD
A/Lt Col	Guthrie, DG
Major	Adamson, J
S/L	Allan, CG, CD
S/L	Anderson, IH, CD
S/L	Anderson, TS
S/L	Andrews, JWH
S/L	Anholt, LM
Major	Babineau, G, CD
Major	Beland, C
S/L	Benoit, JJGS
S/L	Bergin, MB
Major	Bernier, J
S/L	Berry, AJ
S/L	Bisset, JG, CD
S/L	Blake-Knox, PEA, CD
S/L	Boxall, LBH
S/L	Brown, R, CD
S/L	Bruce, TA
S/L	Bryan, AC, CD
S/L	Burden, CA
Major	Byrne, AJ
Major	Campbell, AN, CD
S/L	Carey, TM
S/L	Carriere, NJ, CD
S/L	Carrigan, EP, CD
Major	Chiasson, JD, CD
S/L	Clayton, AJW
Major	Cocker, WJB
Major	Cumming, ARS, CD
Major	Daigle, RC
SG LCDR	Davis, MJ
S/L	de la Bastide, YH, CD
S/L	Despatis, JGA
S/L	Desrochers, JPE
Major	Doyle, BP, CD
SG LCDR	Dubois, GG
Major	Dunfield, JC, CD
Major	Dupuis, R
Major	Evans, FJ, CD
Major	Fink, NRT, CD
SG LCDR	Flegg, KR, CD
S/L	Forgie, RE
S/L	Gamache, JGP, CD
S/L	Garrity, J
S/L	Gauthier, JER
SG LCDR	Gerlitz, JH
S/L	Gill, GAT
S/L	Grace, BW
Major	Green, EA, CD
S/L	Greenlaw, WE
Major	Haley, JF, CD
Major	Harrison, JF, CD
Major	Hatfield, JG
S/L	Haworth, GL, CD
SG LCDR	Holmes, GR, CD
S/L	Howlett, LN, CD
S/L	Hryciuk, N
SG LCDR	Keirstead, ER, CD
S/L	Kenny, JG, CD
SG LCDR	Knight, CJ
S/L	Knowles, RJ
Major	Korth, VH
Major	Kreutz, DM
SG LCDR	Kuder, GR
Major	Lacasse, JOPH
Major	Laflamme, AM
Major	Langlais, IM
SG LCDR	Lawrie, TR, CD
Major	Leduc, JHGJ, CD
Major	Letourneau, G
Major	Levis, WH, CD
Major	Liddy, BFS, CD
S/L	Lilley, K
S/L	Little, JKL
Major	Lounder, JH, CD
S/L	Low, RWD
SG LCDR	Lydon, MJ
S/L	Mallam, AS
Major	Mazewski, SM, CD
Major	Mazurek, L

DEPT. OF NAT. DEFENCE (*Cont'd*)

SG LCDR	McCulloch, TAH CD
Major	McFarland, HM, CD
S/L	McNab, J
Major	McPherson, VA, CD
S/L	McVicar, AS, CD
Major	Monahan, GJ, CD
S/L	Morgan, JF, CD
Major	Morrissette, JPAG
S/L	Neily, HH, CD
S/L	Newberry, PD, CD
S/L	Niblett, DH, CD
S/L	Novotny, GM
Major	Oldfield, DL
SG LCDR	Page, GB
Major	Pellerin, JCR
S/L	Penny, JA
Major	Perron, JJLE
S/L	Phillips, BAA
S/L	Power, GRI, CD
S/L	Pritchard, R
Major	Rail, JR
Major	Reid, JY, CD
S/L	Roberge, JGWJ
Major	Robertson, A
Major	St Pierre, PE
Major	Scharf, RF
S/L	Seguin, JHL, CD
Major	Slavik, RJ
SG LCDR	Soucek, A
SG LCDR	Spilsbury, BW
S/L	Stevenson, CM
S/L	Stevenson, WJC, CD
SG LCDR	Thomson, EG
Major	Tucker, DK, MBE, CD
Major	Vezina, JP
S/L	Waller, DJ, CD
Major	Watson, WE
S/L	Werner, RP
S/L	Whiston, GJ, CD
SG LCDR	Whittle, CH
SG LCDR	Wood, WC, CD
SG LCDR	Woodall, GP
A/SG LCDR	Bruyere, JC
A/Major	Giard, JJB
A/Major	Harris, WC
A/S/L	Kinghorn, MGC
A/Major	Lafleche, FLJPR
A/Major	McLean, JFL
A/S/L	Murray, AS
A/SG LCDR	Scott, DJ
A/S/L	Stewart, RM
Capt	Alarie, JJGS
Capt	Allard, JEP
Capt	Armstrong, RP
F/L	Arnot, GR
Capt	Baars, CM
SG LT	Bateman, CL
Capt	Beauregard, JDCG
Capt	Belanger, JRM
F/L	Bendall, A
F/L	Benoit, BG
SG LT	Berube, GJ
F/L	Blizzard, SVA
SG LT	Boisvert, RG
Capt	Boulianne, JC
Capt	Bourque, JJ
Capt	Bouthillette, JSM
Capt	Bowen, RA
Capt	Brooks, CH
Capt	Budzinski, MG
F/L	Burns, JAGM
F/L	Campbell, CM
Capt	Carlyle, RW
SG LT	Cartier, JJ
F/L	Chadwick, JA
Capt	Chagnon, JLJ
Capt	Chatterton, RT
Capt	Clement, JPA
Capt	Cloutier, JGD
F/L	Cody, MC
F/L	Conly, DB
F/L	Connery, MA
F/L	Connop, PJ
F/L	Cork, SB
Capt	Cote, JHG
F/L	Cumming, RA
Capt	Dallison, FL
F/L	Dantow, JED
Capt	Davis, LA
Capt	Demers, JEG
Capt	Demers, JROJ
F/L	Deslauriers, JM
F/L	Dolan, JD
Capt	Donald, PJ
Capt	Dumont, AL
Capt	Dunster, BJ
Capt	Dupont, JAG
F/L	Enns, PS
Capt	Evenson, LG
Capt	Farr, JA
F/L	Florent, JDVH
F/L	Fontaine, LJ
Capt	Fortin, JZ
Capt	Gencsy, L
Capt	Gervais, JJG
F/L	Gervais, JP
Capt	Giddings, CR
F/L	Gillis, FG
Capt	Gladman, DJ
F/L	Godbout, JJR
SG LT	Gowette, JG
Capt	Graham, DN
Capt	Grant, DJ
Capt	Gray, JN
Capt	Grenier, JPJP
Capt	Griffiths, PAG
Capt	Groves, TD
Capt	Hansen, NH
SG LT	Hansen, WB
F/L	Harpur, GD
Capt	Harvey, JS
Capt	Haywood, GL
F/L	Heroux, JRCG
F/L	Hickey, MC
F/L	Higley, AJ
Capt	Hillson, RF
SG LT	Hogan, JD
F/L	Hogg, JC
Capt	Hogg, NA
SG LT	Holland, RGL
SG LT	Hollingsworth, WJ
Capt	How, RK
Capt	Hudon, JE
SG LT	Hudson, H
F/L	Hulyk, MR
Capt	Humphreys, GR
F/L	Hunter, JDW
Capt	Jamieson, GG
Capt	Jean, JIM
Capt	Jefferson, JC
Capt	Joss, SS
F/L	Kanjilal, N
Capt	Kardera, EP
Capt	Keeler, HSG
Capt	Kidd, JCA
Capt	King, DWF
F/L	Kowalsky, NB
Capt	Lajoie, JYR
F/L	Lambert, JCRJJ
Capt	Lambert, JJCA
F/L	Lamontagne, JLG
Capt	Lanctot, JJ
F/L	Landry, JJG
Capt	Lapierre, YDJ
Capt	Leclair, JLC
Capt	Lefebvre, JMC
Capt	Lemay, JMG
F/L	Letourneau, EG
F/L	Letts, RM
F/L	Livingstone, DA
F/L	Louie, NV
SG LT	Maberley, AL
F/L	MacDougall, JA
F/L	MacKenzie, AD
F/L	MacKenzie, J
Capt	MacKenzie, RA
Capt	Mahon, KW
SG LT	Mahoney, PR
F/L	Manara, AMAEGAF

DEPT. OF NAT. DEFENCE (*Cont'd*)

Capt	Marcoux, JAHM
F/L	Marston, JG
F/L	Martens, RG
Capt	Maryniak, OM
F/L	Matheson, GM
F/L	Mathieu, JGL
F/L	McClure, JA
Capt	McCrudden, BEV
F/L	McGhie, TG
Capt	McLean, AR
SG LT	McNeill, SRC
F/L	Merrick, HK
F/L	Meyer, D
F/L	Michevicius, VA
F/L	Moffatt, AJ
SG LT	Monforton, FL
SG LT	Moody, AD
Capt	Morin, JMC
Capt	Morrissette, JPJJ
F/L	Murray, TM
F/L	Nicol, J
SG LT	O'Dwyer, MPT
F/L	O'Hara, WJHA
F/L	Olsen, PP
F/L	Orbeck, WK
Capt	O'Reilly, FL
F/L	Paquin, JFM
Capt	Paradis, JWR
Capt	Park, D
F/L	Patel, DJ
F/L	Paterson, HH
SG LT	Patrick, TR
SG LT	Perrault, RA
F/L	Poulin, JGJ
Capt	Prosser, RG
F/L	Quesnel, JLGE
SG LT	Quigley, MP
Capt	Quirion, JRR
F/L	Raby, JLP
SG LT	Raine, RJ
F/L	Reid, EP
Capt	Rioux, JEM
Capt	Robb, KI
SG LT	Roberts, DG
Capt	Robin, JPLP
F/L	Ross, JB
F/L	Rousseau, JJMR
Capt	Ruel, JRJM
Capt	Russell, DB
F/L	Russell, JE
Capt	St Germain, JJJ
SG LT	St Hilaire, GA
SG LT	Saxon, DR
SG LT	Seland, TP
F/L	Shaw, MG
F/L	Shearer, RS
Capt	Sheremata, WA
Capt	Simard, JHN
F/L	Smillie, HAG
Capt	Snyder, RE
Capt	Steele, DN
Capt	Stuart, RD
Capt	Talpash, OS
Capt	Thiffault, JNG
F/L	Thores, OA
F/L	Tomm, KM
Capt	Tremblay, NAG
SG LT	Trueman, DH
SG LT	Tweed, WA
SG LT	Tye, DM
F/L	Uden, DE
F/L	Vaughan, RL
Capt	Veilleux, JAH
Capt	Vezina, JFG
F/L	Walker, HCG
Capt	Waller, DF
Capt	Walsh, PB
F/L	Watts, AR
F/L	Webber, OH
Capt	Webster, RD
SG LT	West, GR
F/L	Whitfield, WA
F/L	Wilson, DMC
Capt	Wilton, BW
F/L	Young, JD
F/L	Younge, BR
SG LT	Ziegler, DO
Capt	Zywina, PR

Medical Staff, Defence Research Board

Caldbick, G.D., M.D., C.M., D.P.H.
Stewart, W. C., M.D.
Stewart, Wilma, G., M.D.
Taylor, N. Burwell, M.D., Ph.D.
Whillans, Morley G., M.D.
Wiggin, Norman, M.D., Ph.D.

Defence Medical Association of Canada

HEAD OFFICE

Dr. Robert W. Wood, Sec.-Treas., c/o Medical Services, Dept. of National Health and Welfare, Room 1066, Brooke Claxton Bldg., Ottawa.

Lt.-Col. P. J. Maloney, Assistant Secretary, 267 O'Connor Street, Ottawa, Canada.

EXECUTIVE AND COUNCIL

Colonel J. E. H. Miller,
President,
596 Young Avenue,
Halifax, N.S.

Wing Commander C. H. Weder,
Past-President,
656 Medical Arts Building,
Saskatoon, Sask.

Lieutenant-Colonel H. Stansfield,
1st Vice President,
750 W. Broadway,
Vancouver 9, B.C.

Wing Commander N. W. Bradford,
2nd Vice President,
148 Underhill Drive,
Don Mills, Ontario.

Surgeon Commander D. H. Starkey,
3rd Vice President,
465 Cote St. Antoine Road,
Westmount, Montreal 6, P.Q.

Colonel Paul Martin,
351 Querbes,
Outremont, Montreal, P.Q.

Colonel I. M. MacKay,
230 Rosedale Heights Drive,
Toronto 7, Ont.

Lt.-Col. E. J. Bowmer,
1919 Linden Road,
Vancouver 13, B.C.

Lt.-Col. D. P. Snidal,
c/o University of Manitoba,
Medical Buildings,
Winnipeg 3, Man.

Major P. Ryan,
229 St. Clair Ave. W.,
Toronto 7, Ont.

Surgeon Lieutenant Commander H. D. J. McCoy,
8 Sydenham Street,
Dundas, Ontario.

BRANCHES

PRESIDENT	SECRETARY-TREASURER
B,C, Lt.-Col, E, J. Bowmer, 1919 Linden Road, Vancouver 13, B.C.	Surg. Lt. Cmdr. K. G. S. Davidson, 925 W. Georgia St., Vancouver 1, B.C.
Alberta Surg. Lt. Cmdr. D. M. Williamson, 11816 - 124th St., Edmonton, Alta.	Lt.-Col. G. M. Wyant, 522 Copland Crescent, Saskatoon, Sask.
Saskatchewan Colonel R. W. Begg, c/o College of Medicine, University of Saskatchewan, Saskatoon, Sask.	
Manitoba-Lakehead Dr. G. R. Diehl, 332 Medical Arts Bldg., Winnipeg 1, Man.	
Western Ontario Lieutenant-Colonel L. Reese, 450 Central Avenue, London, Ontario.	Major J. C. Bryce, 152 Wychwood Park, London, Ontario.
Central Ontario Colonel I. M. MacKay, 230 Rosedale Heights Dr., Toronto, Ontario.	Surg. Lt. Cmdr. J. W. Copeman, 262 Essex Avenue, Richmond, Hill, Ont.
Eastern Ontario Lieutenant-Colonel D. Kubryk, c/o Emergency Health Services, Dept. of National Health & Welfare, Ottawa, Canada.	Major P. C. M. Ladelpha, 447 Sussex, Ottawa, Canada.
Western Quebec Major Maurice Thibault, c/o Queen Mary Veteran's Hospital, Montreal, P.Q.	Major J. Y. McGraw, 3011 Cedar Avenue, Montreal 25, P.Q.
Nova Scotia Captain H. C. Read, 151 Inglis Street, Halifax, N.S.	Major S. H. Kryszek, Box 612, Windsor, N.S.
New Brunswick Lieutenant-Colonel F. George, C.D., 101 Carleton Street, St. John, N.B.	
Prince Edward Island Captain J. L. F. Burge, 123 Kent Street, Charlottetown, P.E.I.	

DEPARTMENT OF VETERANS AFFAIRS

Head Office ...... Veterans Affairs Bldg., Ottawa

Tel. CE 2-8211

Minister	The Honourable Roger Teillet, P.C., M.P.
Deputy Minister	Paul Pelletier, B.A.
Departmental Secretary	C. F. Black, C.D., B.A.
Assistant Deputy Minister	F. T. Mace, C.D., C.A.
Chief of Information and Business Manager, Medical Services Journal, Canada	G. S. Way, C.D.

Treatment Services Branch

Director General	K. S. Ritchie, B.A., M.D., C.M.
Director, Hospital Administration	
Director, Admission Services	C. C. Misener, B.A., M.D.
Director, Hospital Accommodation, Medical Research, Education	A. J. Brunet, B.A., M.D., C.M.
Director, Dental Services	D. M. Tanner, M.B.E., D.D.S., B.Sc.D., F.I.C.D.
Consultant, Nursing Services	Miss G. E. Johnson, B.Sc., R.N.
Consultant, Dietary Services	Miss J. C. Macdiarmid, B.H.S., R.P.Dt.

Welfare Services Branch

Director, Veterans' Welfare Services and Supt. Veterans Insurance	E. J. Rider, M.B.E., B.A.

Veterans' Land Administration Branch

Director, Veterans' Land Act	R. W. Pawley, B.S.A., P.Ag.

Veterans' Bureau

Chief Pensions Advocate	P. E. Reynolds, E.D., B.A., LL.B.

Administrative Services

Director, Engineering, Accommodation and Transport	A. W. Davison, B. Arch., M.R.A.I.C.
Director, Finance, Purchasing and Stores	J. E. Walsh, C.A.
Director, Legal Services	P. E. Reynolds, E.D., B.A., LL.B.
Director of Personnel Administration	R. D. Boyd

ASSOCIATED BOARDS AND COMMISSIONS

Canadian Pension Commission

Chairman	T. D. Anderson
Chief Medical Adviser	W. F. Brown, M.D., F.R.C.P. (Edin.)

War Veterans Allowance Board

Chairman	W. T. Cromb, D.S.O., E.D.
Medical Adviser	G. R. D. Farmer, C.B.E., E.D., M.B.

Commonwealth War Graves Commission (Canada)

Secretary-General	C. B. Fuller

The Department of Veterans Affairs administers the legislation under which veterans receive treatment, war service gratuities and re-establishment credits, land settlement and home construction assistance, training, veterans insurance and veterans welfare benefits.

The Canadian Pension Commission administers the Pension Act, Parts I to X of the Civilian War Pensions and Allowances Act, and the Flying Accidents Compensation Order, and is responsible for the adjudication of claims under any.

The War Veterans Allowance Board directs the administration of the War Veterans Allowance Act and of Part XI of the Civilian War Pensions and Allowances Act.

The Commonwealth War Graves Commission (Canada) is responsible for the marking and maintenance of the graves in North America of British Commonwealth servicemen who died during World Wars I and II, and for the erecting of memorials to commemorate those who have no known graves.

The Treatment Services Branch provides free treatment to veterans for their pensionable disabilities, and to veterans who are in receipt of war veterans allowances. Eligible veterans with limited resources may be given hospitalization free or with the charges reduced according to their incomes and resources, providing beds are available; and any veteran may be admitted to a DVA hospital for treatment if accommodation is available and if he agrees to pay the cost of hospitalization. Domiciliary care may be provided to older veterans under certain conditions.

Where treatment is given for non-pensioned conditions to insured persons, the Department recovers the cost of the insured services from the provincial insurance hospital plan concerned.

The Department also provides treatment to other persons who are the responsibility of other departments and other governments, at the request and expense of the authority concerned.

To carry out its responsibilities, the Branch operates 11 active treatment hospitals and three institutions for long term care with a total rated capacity of 8,823 beds as at March 31, 1965. The active treatment hospitals have been approved by the Royal College of Physicians and Surgeons for postgraduate training in internal medicine and surgery, and the majority of them have been approved for advance postgraduate teaching in many of the specialties.

The Department is actively engaged in clinical research. The largest single field of research concerns the older veterans and studies are in progress on the problems of the aging veteran generally.

CANADIAN PENITENTIARIES

Justice Bldg., Wellington Street, Ottawa 4, Canada

Tel. 232-8211

Commissioner	A. J. MacLeod, Q.C.
Deputy Commissioner	J. R. Stone
Director Medical Services	L. P. Gendreau, M.D., Psychiatrist

DORCHESTER PENITENTIARY
Dr. W. E. Hirtle (Physician)
Dr. P. Michel (Psychiatrist)
Dr. R. G. Crandall (Psychiatrist)

SPRINGHILL INSTITUTION
Dr. D. H. Fisher (Physician)

BLUE MOUNTAIN
Dr. Robb (Physician)

ST. VINCENT DE PAUL PENITENTIARY
Dr. J. G. Lefebvre (Physician)
Dr. R. Simard (Surgeon)
Dr. B. Cormier (Psychiatrist)

FEDERAL TRAINING CENTRE and LECLERC INSTITUTION
Dr. J. G. Harris (Physician)

VALLEYFIELD
Dr. M. Boyer (Physician)

GATINEAU
Dr. N. S. Geggie (Physician)

COWANSVILLE
Dr. Noel E. Monast (Physician)

KINGSTON PENITENTIARY
Dr. W. Amodeo (Physician)
Dr. H. Neuman (Surgeon)
Dr. G. D. Scott (Psychiatrist)
Dr. R. J. McCaldon (Psychiatrist)

JOYCEVILLE INSTITUTION
Dr. S. Webb (Physician)

COLLIN'S BAY PENITENTIARY
Dr. J. E. Gibson (Physician)

PRISON FOR WOMEN
Dr. M. Walker (Physician)

BEAVER CREEK CORRECTIONAL CAMP
Dr. C. E. Lindenfield (Physician)

MANITOBA PENITENTIARY
Dr. N. Bowden (Physician)
Dr. S. Schultz (Psychiatrist)

DRUMHELLER, ALBERTA
Dr. T. A. Wright (Physician)

SASKATCHEWAN PENITENTIARY
Dr. C. L. Tisdale (Physician & Surgeon)

BRITISH COLUMBIA PENITENTIARY
Dr. A. C. Ross (Physician & Surgeon)
Dr. D. C. MacDonald (Psychiatrist)

WILLIAM HEAD INSTITUTION
Dr. H. J. Portelance (Physician)

AGASSIZ CORRECTIONAL CAMP MOUNTAIN PRISON
Dr. A. C. Ross (Physician & Surgeon)

MATSQUI INSTITUTION
Dr. H. E. Cannon (Physician)
Dr. D. Craigen (Psychiatrist)

DEPARTMENT OF NATIONAL HEALTH AND WELFARE
Ottawa

Minister of National Health and Welfare	The Honourable Allan J. MacEachen, P.C., M.P.
Parliamentary Secretary	Mrs. Margaret Rideout, M.P.
Deputy Minister of National Health and Welfare (Health)	J. N. Crawford, M.B.E., E.D., M.D., LL.D.
Principal Medical Officer, International Health	B. D. B. Layton, M.D., M.P.H.
Principal Medical Officer, Special Projects	J. B. Bundock, O.B.E., M.D., M.R.S.H.
Deputy Minister of National Health and Welfare (Welfare)	J. W. Willard, M.A., M.P.A., A.M., Ph.D.

HEALTH BRANCH

Director General, Health Services Directorate	E. A. Watkinson, M.D., C.M., D.P.H.
Deputy Director General	L. B. Pett, Ph.D., M.D., C.P.H.
Consultant and Advisory Services	
Aerospace Medicine and Safety, Consultant	W. A. Prowse, M.D., C.M., D.P.H., D.I.H.
Child and Maternal Health Division, Chief	Jean F. Webb, B.Sc., M.D., D.P.H.
Dental Health Division, Chief	R. A. Connor, D.D.S., D.D.P.H., F.I.C.D.
Emergency Health Services Division, Chief	W. S. Hacon, M.B.B.S., D.C.H., D.H.A.
Epidemiology Division, Chief	E. W. R. Best, M.D., D.P.H.
Health Education, Consultant	M. E. Palko, B.A., M.P.H.
Laboratory of Hygiene, Chief	E. T. Bynoe, Ph.D.
Medical Rehabiiitation Division, Chief	O. Hoffman, M.D.
Mental Health Division, Chief	M. G. Martin, M.D., M.Sc.
Nursing Advisory Service, Consultant	Miss D. M. Percy, R.R.C., Reg. N.
Nutrition Division, Chief	J. E. Monagle, M.D.
Occupational Health Division, Chief	T. H. Patterson, M.D., C.M., D.P.H., M.P.H.
Planning and Evaluation, Consultant	G. H. Josie, Ph.D.
Public Health Engineering Division, Chief	W. R. Edmonds, P.Eng., M.A.Sc.
Radiation Protection Division, Chief	P. M. Bird, M.Sc., Ph.D.
Research Development Division, Consultant	R. W. Tooley, M.R.C.P., L.R.C.S., D.P.H.
Director General, Health Insurance and Resources Directorate	E. H. Lossing, M.D., C.M., M.P.H.
Deputy Director General	
Hospital Insurance, Director	
Assistant Director	R. B. Goyette, M.D., D.P.H.
Health Grants, Director	G. E. Wride, M.D., D.P.H.
Assistant Director	J. A. E. Dupont, M.D., D.P.H.
Health Facilities Design, Chief	G. W. Peck, B.Arch., M.Sc., M.R.A.I.C.
Health Resources Fund, Director	
Assistant Director	
Medical Care, Director	
Assistant Director	
Director General, Medical Services Directorate	H. A. Procter, D.S.O., Ph.D., M.D.
Medical Staff Officer	J. E. Gompf, M.D., D.P.H.
Medical Liaison Officer	G. Graham-Cumming, M.B., Ch.B., D.P.H., D.T.M.
Senior Medical Advisor, Public Health	W. H. Frost, M.D., C.M., D.P.H.
Senior Treatment Officer	R. A. Armstrong, M.D.
Civil Service Health, Civil Aviation Medicine, Advisor	E. L. Davey, M.D., D.P.H.
Immigration Medical, Advisor	R. W. Wood, M.D.
Quarantine, Advisor	R. W. Robertson, M.D.
Director General, Food and Drug Directorate	R. A. Chapman, B.S.A., M.Sc., Ph.D.
Deputy Director General	L. I. Pugsley, B.A., M.Sc,, Ph.D.
Assistant Director General (Drug Control)	M. G. Allmark, M.A.
Assistant Director General (Food Control)	D. G. Chapman, B.S.A., M.Sc., Ph.D.
Research Laboratories, Director	J. A. Campbell, Ph.D.
Bureau of Scientific Advisory Services, Director	A. C. Hardman, M.D.
Bureau of Operations, Director	A. Hollett, M.Sc.
Narcotic Control Division, Chief	R. C. Hammond, Phm.B.
Administrative Services, Chief	A. B. Tennenhouse, B.S.A., M.Sc.

DEPARTMENT OF NATIONAL HEALTH & WELFARE (*cont'd*)

CENTRAL SERVICES

Research and Statistics Division, Director	J. E. E. Osborne, M.A., D.H.A.
Information Services Division, Director	H. W. Adams
Legal Advisor	R. E. Curran, Q.C., B.A., LL.B.

ADMINISTRATION BRANCH

Director General, Administration	W. B. Brittain, D.F.C., B.Sc.
Financial Administration, Director	D. R. Aitchison, A.C.W.A.
Personnel Administration, Director	E. J. Preston, B.A., M.A.
Departmental Librarian	Miss M. D. Morton, B.H.Sc., B.L.S.
Management Services Division, Chief	G. H. Aubut, B.Comm.
Materiel Management Division, Chief	
Office and Secretarial Services Division, Chief	F. E. Goudge, C.P.A.
Registry Services, Chief	G. E. Logan

HEALTH BRANCH FIELD OFFICES
FOOD AND DRUG

Food and Drug Laboratories

Ottawa, Ont., Tunney's Pasture
Halifax, N.S., Ralston Building
Montreal, P.Q., Customs House, 400 Youville Sq.
Toronto, Ont., 55 St. Clair Avenue East
Winnipeg, Man., 310 Federal Building
Vancouver, B.C., Federal Building

Food and Drug Offices

Ottawa, Ont., Tunney's Pasture
Halifax, N.S., Ralston Building
Charlottetown, P.E.I., Dominion Building
Saint John, N.B., 517 New Customs Building
Sydney, N.S., Federal Building
St. John's, Nfld., Sir Humphrey Gilbert Building
Quebec, P.Q., Gare Maritime Champlain
Montreal, P.Q., 400 Youville Square
Sherbrooke, P.Q., 315 King Street
Hull, P.Q., Federal Building
Trois Rivieres, P.Q., Post Office Building
Toronto, Ont., 55 St. Clair Avenue East
Belleville, Ont., New Federal Bldg., Pinnacle St.
Hamilton, Ont., National Revenue Building
Kitchener, Ont., Federal Building
London, Ont., Dominion Public Building
Cornwall, Ont., Federal Building
Windsor, Ont., Dominion Public Building
Sudbury, Ont., New Federal Building
Port Arthur, Ont., 33 Court Street South
Winnipeg, Man., Federal Building
Brandon, Man., Federal Building
Saskatoon, Sask., 307 London Building
Regina, Sask., 312 Motherwell Building
Calgary, Alta., Customs Building
Edmonton, Alta., 541 Federal Building
Kamloops, B.C., 317 Seymour Street
Vancouver, B.C., Federal Building
Victoria, B.C., 805 Government St., Belmont Bldg.

MEDICAL SERVICES
Regional and Zone or Area (*) Offices and Clinics

EASTERN REGION, Ottawa, Ont.	Kenson Bldg., 233 Metcalfe St.
Saint John's, Nfld.	Federal Bldg., North Duckworth St.
Sydney, N.S.	North Charlotte St.
*Halifax, N.S.	Immigration Bldg. Annex Pier 21
Halifax, N.S.	Immigration Bldg., Pier 21
St. John, N.B.	Immigration Bldg., Pier 9
*Montreal, (Quebec)	685 Cathcart Street
Quebec City, Que.	Rm. 594, Champlain Harbour Stn.
Montreal, Que.	150 St. Paul's Street
Dorval, Que.	Montreal International Airport
*Ottawa, Ont. (S. Ontario)	Kenson Bldg., 233 Metcalfe St.
Malton, Ont.	Toronto International Airport
*Ottawa, Ont. (N. Ontario)	Kenson Bldg., 233 Metcalfe St.
Manitowaning, Ont.	
*Moose Factory, Ont. (James Bay)	Moose Factory Indian Hospital
CENTRAL REGION, Winnipeg, Man.	705 Commercial Building, 169 Pioneer Avenue
Winnipeg, Man.	Commercial Building, 169 Pioneer Avenue
*Sioux Lookout, Ont. (N. Western Ont.)	Sioux Lookout Indian Hospital
*Norway House, Man. (Central Man.)	Norway House Indian Hospital
*The Pas, Man. (N. Man.)	Post Office Bldg., Fischer Ave.
*Winnipeg, Man. (S. Man.)	Immigration Bldg., 83 Maple St.
SASKATCHEWAN REGION, Regina, Sask.	735 Motherwell Building
*Regina, Sask. (Sask. North-East)	735 Motherwell Building
Prince Albert, Sask.	Immigration Building
*Regina, Sask. (Sask. South)	735 Motherwell Building
*North Battleford, Sask. (Sask. North)	North Battleford Indian Hospital
ALBERTA REGION, Edmonton, Alta.	11344 - 128th Street
Edmonton, Alta.	Federal Building, 9820 - 107th Street
*Edmonton, Alta. (N. Alberta)	11344 - 128th Street
Hobbema, Alta.	
*Calgary, Alta. (S. Alberta)	404 Customs Building

DEPT. OF NATIONAL HEALTH & WELFARE (*cont'd*)

NORTHERN REGION, Edmonton, Alta.	12702 - 114th Avenue
***Edmonton, Alta. (S. & North-East MacKenzie District)**	12702 - 114th Avenue
Fort Smith, N.W.T.	
Rae, N.W.T.	
Fort Simpson, N.W.T.	
***Whitehorse, Y.T. (Yukon)**	Riverdale St., P.O. Box 87
***Churchill, Man. (Keewatin Dist.)**	Fort Churchill General Hospital
***Frobisher Bay, N.W.T.**	Frobisher Bay General Hospital
***Inuvik, N.W.T. (N. West MacKenzie District)**	Inuvik General Hospital
PACIFIC REGION, Vancouver, B.C.	1110 West Georgia Street
***Vancouver (S. West B.C.)**	Canadian Immigration Building, Ft. of Burrard Street
Victoria, B.C.	816 Government Street
***Nanaimo, B.C. (Western B.C.)**	Nanaimo Indian Hospital
***Sardis, B.C. (Southern B.C.)**	Coqualeetza Indian Hospital
Williams Lake, B.C.	
Alexis Creek, B.C.	
***Prince Rupert, B.C.**	P.O. Box 488, Miller Bay Indian Hospital
EUROPEAN REGION, London, England	38 Grosvenor Street, W1
IMMIGRATION MEDICAL OFFICE, Hong Kong, B.C.C.	United Chinese Bldg., 31-37 Des Voeux Road, Central
OTTAWA, Ont. (C.S. Health and Civil Aviation Medicine)	No. 3 Temporary Building

PUBLIC HEALTH ENGINEERING DIVISION FIELD OFFICES

Moncton, N.B.	Federal Building, P.O. Box 86
Montreal, P.Q.	150 St. Paul Street West
Winnipeg, Man.	2nd Floor, Postal Station "B", Magnus Avenue at Main Street
Edmonton, Alta.	Room 541, Federal Building
Vancouver, B.C.	Room 605, 1110 West Georgia St.

The first federal Department of Health was established by an Act of Parliament in 1919. Authority for the present Department of National Health and Welfare is provided by the Department of National Health and Welfare Act, 1944-45, c. 22 (R.S. 1952), c. 74).

The Health Branch comprises the Directorates of Health Services, Health Insurance and Resources, Medical Services and Food and Drugs.

The Health Branch administers the General Health Grants and Hospital Construction Grants Rules under which grants are made available to the Provinces for the improvement and extension of health services and is responsible for the administration of the federal aspects of the Hospital Insurance and Diagnostic Services Act. Its officers participate in the work of the International Joint Commission in regard to air pollution and the pollution of boundary waters between the United States and Canada; through the Laboratory of Hygiene, it provides a national public health reference laboratory service; it is responsible for the health aspects of the federal Emergency Measures program and its Radiation Protection Division carries out a program designed to protect Canadians from the harmful effects of radiation. Technical advisory and consultant services in these and other special health areas are provided to provincial health departments and to other departments of the Federal Government. It acts as an advisor to the Government and associated agencies in connection with problems relating to the health, safety and comfort of aviation personnel and air passengers.

The Health Services Directorate carries responsibilities, also, arising out of Canada's role in the international health field and its membership in the World Health Organization and other specialized agencies of the United Nations.

The Food and Drug Directorate is responsible for the administration of the Food and Drugs Act, the Narcotic Control Act and the Proprietary or Patent Medicine Act. The Narcotic and Controlled Drug Division of the Directorate administers the Narcotic Control Act and the Controlled Drug Part of the Food and Drugs Act. A member of the Directorate represents Canada on the United Nations Commission on Narcotic Drugs. The Directorate functions as a central clearing house for the Canadian Poison Control Centres and operates a drug adverse reaction reporting program.

The Medical Services Directorate is responsible for administering a health services program to Indians and Eskimos and residents of the Northwest and Yukon Territories. It is also responsible for the administration of the Quarantine Act; Part V of the Canada Shipping Act dealing with sick Mariners and those sections of the Immigration Act dealing with the medical examination of immigrants. Again, it is responsible for the provision of a health program for Federal Civil Servants and acts as advisor to the Department of Transport on the physical standards for licensed aviation personnel.

A number of federal-provincial committees act in an advisory capacity to the Department on health matters. The most important of these is the Dominion Council of Health, composed of the Deputy Minister of National Health acting as Chairman, the Deputy Minister or Chief Health Officer of each province and five persons appointed by the Governor-in-Council. Various Federal-Provincial committees of a technical or advisory nature supplement the activities of the Council.

CANADIAN PENSION COMMISSION

Ottawa — Canada

Tel. CE 2-8211

Medical Staff

Commissioners

Blier, Dr. U.
Forrester, Dr. J. A.
Fyfe, Dr. J. G.
Thompson, Dr. J. L.

Medical Advisers (Ottawa)

Bedford, Dr. R. F. H.
Bird, Dr. R. L.
Brown, Dr. L. W.
Brown, Dr. W. F. (Chief Medical Adviser)
Campbell, Dr. R. W.
Gray, Dr. R. C. V.
Laurin, Dr. J. B.
Lee, Dr. E. H.
Lenis, Dr. G. J.
MacKinnon, Dr. A. G.
McKee, Dr. D. B.
Pilon, Dr. L. J.
Pollonetsky, Dr. E.
Richardson, Dr. H. J.
Rosenberg, Dr. H. D.
Shatford, Dr. R. C.
Terrien, Dr. J. H. J.

Medical Examiners (Other Centres)

Aberhart, Dr. W. R., London
Booth, Dr. D. H., Winnipeg
Carette, Dr. L., Quebec
Christie, Dr. D., Vancouver
Coles, Dr. B. C., Toronto
Copley, Dr. D. R., Toronto
Croome, Dr. R. R. M., Toronto
Donnelly, Dr. T. G., Vancouver
Ellingham, Dr. F. H., Hamilton
Evans, Dr. E. H., Victoria
Fowler, Dr. W., London
Fry, Dr. W. R., London
Greenberg, Dr. C., Edmonton
Hemming, Dr. J. H., Hamilton
Hill, Dr. A. E., Vancouver
Homik, Dr. A. E., Vancouver
Knoll, Dr. F. G., Saint John, N.B.
Laing, Dr. W. R. V., Calgary
Lefebvre, Dr J. F. A., Montreal
MacDonald, Dr. S., Charlottetown
McKenty, Dr. V. J., Winnipeg
McLeod, Dr. J. G., Regina
Moore, Dr. A. H., North Bay
Myers, Dr. C. A., Saskatoon
Payette, Dr. H., Montreal
Peloquin, Dr. G., Montreal
Procunier, Dr. C. W., Toronto
Reardon, Dr. F. L., Ottawa
Robbins, Dr. J. H. L., Halifax
Rowland, Dr. E. M., Toronto
Shultz, Dr. V. C., Vancouver
Walsh, Dr. J. E., St. John's, Nfld.
Watt, Dr. W. N., Halifax

DEANS
CANADIAN SCHOOLS OF PHARMACY

B.C.
Dr. A. W. Matthews,
Dean, Faculty of Pharmacy,
University of British Columbia,
Vancouver, B.C.

ALB.
Dr. M. J. Huston,
Dean, Faculty of Pharmacy,
University of Alberta,
Edmonton, Alta.

SASK.
Dr. W. C. MacAulay,
Dean, College of Pharmacy,
University of Saskatchewan,
Saskatoon, Sask.

MAN.
Dr. J. R. Murray,
Director, School of Pharmacy,
University of Manitoba,
Winnipeg, Man.

ONT.
Dean F. N. Hughes,
Faculty of Pharmacy,
University of Toronto,
25 Russell St.,
Toronto 5, Ont.

P. Q.
Dr. A. Archambault,
Dean, Faculty of Pharmacy,
University of Montreal,
Montreal, P.Q.

Prof. J. A. Marquis,
Director, School of Pharmacy,
Laval University,
Quebec, P.Q.

N.S.
Dr. J. Gordon Duff,
Dir. of College of
Pharmacy, Dalhousie U.,
Halifax, N.S.

DEPARTMENT OF HEALTH, NEWFOUNDLAND

Confederation Bldg., St. John's, Nfld.

Tel. 9-5011

Minister of Health .... THE HONOURABLE JAMES McGRATH

Administration

Deputy Minister .... Leonard Miller, M.D.
Ass't. Deputy Minister .... T. A. Knowling, M.B.
Adm. of Health Services .... T. C. Sellars
Adm. Officer .... G. E. Cummings
Sr. Adm. Assistant .... L. G. Vey
Adm. Assistant .... Douglas Whitten

Medical Services

Chief Medical Health Officer .... David Severs, B.M., B.Ch.
Dir. of Laboratory Services .... J. E. Josephson, M.D.
Dir. of Tuberculosis Control .... E. S. Peters, M.D., C.M.
Consultant, Treatment Services .... Wm. P. Collingwood, M.B.
Director, Mental Health Services .... C. H. Pottle, M.D.
Dir. Departmental Nurses .... Miss Jean Lewis, S.R.N.

Hospital Services

St. John's General Hosp.—Supt., Albert W. Taylor, M.D.; Dir. of Nurses, Miss Janet Story, B.N., R.N.
St. John's Tuberculosis San. — Supt., A. B. Colohan, M.B.; Dir. of Nurses, Miss M. Chard, R.N.
Hospital for Mental and Nervous Diseases—Supt., J. Frazier Walsh, M.B.; Dir. of Nurses, Miss Mary Maloney, R.N.

Special Services

Med. Consultant Hospital Insurance .... B. Suttie, M.B.
Director, Hospital Ins. Div .... R. J. Burnell
Registrar, Vital Statistics .... C. H. Tobin
Chief Health Inspector .... D. A. Strong, C.S.I. (C)
Regional Health Inspector, Corner Brook .... Melvin Graham, C.S.I. (C)
Director Health Education .... Mrs. Daphne House, B.A.
Nutritional Adviser .... Olga Anderson, M.S.P.H.

NOTIFICATION TO CORONERS (Newfoundland)

Attention is directed to the following wording used in the Summary Jurisdiction Act, chapter 117 of the Revised Statutes of Newfoundland, 1952 as amended in 1953 and in this present year.

Section 116 provides that in all cases of persons slain, drowned, suddenly dead, having committed suicide, or dead in prison a magistrate in whose jurisdiction the death occured shall, except in the case of a person suddenly dead where a registered medical practitioner certifies that death was solely from natural causes, hold an enquiry into the death. In the excepted case the magistrate may hold an enquiry, but if he does not the Attorney General may order an inquiry.

Section 116A reads as follows:

"116A. — (1) A magistrate may, by order in writing, at anytime when he deems it necessary so to do, direct that an autopsy be held or that any other post mortem examination be made for the purpose of ascertaining the cause of the death of any person, and for that purpose may order any constable to take possession of the remains of the deceased and to disinter the remains, and a constable acting under any such order may for the purpose of executing it enter any place and do such acts and things as are reasonably necessary to enable him to carry out the order.

(2) Where a magistrate orders an autopsy to be held or a post mortem examination to be made under subsection (1) the autopsy or post mortem examination shall be held or made under the supervision of a medical practitioner named in the order.

(3) A magistrate may cancel or amend any order made under this section or make an order in substitution thereof."

DEPARTMENT OF HEALTH PRINCE EDWARD ISLAND

Box 3000, Charlottetown, P.E.I.

Tel. 892-1293

Minister of Health .... THE HONOURABLE H. W. WEDGE

Administration

Deputy Minister of Health	O. H. Curtis, M.D., D.P.H.
Ass't. Deputy Minister & Health Officer	Burton Howatt, M.D., D.P.H.
Director, Division of Cancer Control	W. T. Hooper, M.D.
Director of Dental Public Health	B. J. O'Meara, D.D.S., D.D.P.H.
Staff Dentist	R. J. Romcke, D.D.S.
Director, Division of Laboratories	John Craig, M.B., C.H.B.
Pathologist	Andres Aquino, M.D.
Bacteriologist	F. W. Jelks, Ph.D.
Director, Division of Mental Health	R. G. Forsythe, M D.
Director of Child Guidance Clinics	M. N. Beck, M.D.
Psychiatrist	I. Stewart, M.B.
Director, Division of Public Health Nursing	Bernice Rowland, B.N.
Director, Division of Sanitary Engineering	Donald Champion, B.Sc., P.Eng.
Veterinarian, Div. of San. Eng.	J. E. Sterns, D.V.M., D.V.P.H.
Director, Division of T.B. Control	E. M. Found, M.D., F.C.C.P.
Director of Field Services, Division of T.B. Control	W. R. Stewart, M.D.
Med. Dir., Rehabilitation Centre	Todor Gencheff, M.D.
Director, Division of Venereal Disease Control	VACANT
Director, Division of Vital Statistics	John MacAleer

NOTIFICATION TO CORONERS

(Prince Edward Island)

9. (1) When a Medical Examiner is informed that a dead body of a person is lying within his jurisdiction, and such person has died, or there is reasonable cause to suspect that such person has died
- (a) as a result of violence, misadventure, or unfair means; or
- (b) as a result of negligence or misconduct or malpractice on the part of others; or
- (c) from any cause other than disease or under such circumstances as may require investigation; or
- (d) a sudden death of which the cause is unknown: or
- (e) in a prison, a jail, reformatory, industrial farm or lock-up; or
- (f) within 24 hours after admission to a hospital; or
- (g) in a hospital during an operation; or
- (h) under such circumstances as to require an inquest, in pursuance of any Act; or
- (i) having been admitted to a hospital suffering injuries as a result of negligence, misconduct or malpractice on the part of others and without being discharged from the hospital

the Medical Examiner, whether the cause of death arose within his jurisdiction or not, shall, as soon as practicable, issue his warrant to take possession of the body and shall view the body and make such further investigation as may be required to enable him to determine whether or not an Inquest is necessary.

DEPARTMENT OF HEALTH NEW BRUNSWICK

P.O. Box 760, Fredericton, N.B.

Tel. GR 5-7711

Minister of Health	The HON. G. L. DUMONT, M.D.
Deputy Minister of Health Fredericton, N.B.	C. W. Kelly, M.D.
Public Health Services Co-ordinator	Guy St. Pierre, M.D., D.P.H.
Administrative Management Director	A. F. B. Knight
Dir. of Tuberculosis Control, Saint John, N.B.	G. E. Maddison, M.D., D.P.H.
Dir. of Health Planning Services, Dept. of Health, Fredericton, N.B.	C. W. Kelly, M.D.
Reg. Gen. & Official Committee of the Estates of Patients at the Provincial Hospitals, Dept. of Health, Fredericton, N.B.	A. E. Wilby, B.C.L.
Director, Prov. Laboratories (Saint John Gen. Hosp.).	I. A. MacLennan, M.D.
Director Regional Laboratory, Moncton Hosp.	Alfred Bastarache, M.D.
Director, Regional Laboratory, Victoria Public Hospital, Fredericton, N.B.	J. Fekete, M.D.

NEW BRUNSWICK DEPT. OF HEALTH (*Cont'd*)

Director Regional Laboratory, Provincial Hospital Campbellton, Campbellton, N.B. ....

Dir. Regional Laboratory, Hotel-Dieu Hosp., Edmunston, N.B. .... J. P. Paget, M.D.

Dir. Cancer & Communicable Disease Control Div., Dept. of Health, Fredericton, N.B. .... J. R. Feindel, M.D., D.P.H.

Dir. Maternal & Child Health, Dept. of Health, Fredericton, N.B. .... R. S. Khazen, M.D.

Dir. Mental Health Serv., Dept. of Health, Moncton, N.B. .... R. R. Prosser, M.D.

Dir. Dental Health, Dept. of Health, Fredericton, N.B. .... **R. S. Langstroth, D.D.S., D.D.P.H.**

Dir. Public Health, Nursing, Dept. of Health, Fredericton, N.B. .... **Apolline Robichaud, R.N.**

Prov. Sanitary Engineer, Dept. of Health, Fredericton, N.B. .... A. J. Cameron, B.Sc.

Accountant, Dept. of Health, Fredericton, N.B. .... H. A. O'Donnell

Information Writer .... **A. A. Maillet**

Dir. Rehabilitation Div., Dept. of Health, Fredericton, N.B. .... Yvon Melanson

Dir. Hosp. Services Div., Dept. of Health, Fredericton, N.B. .... R. F. LeBlanc, M.D.

Dir. Alcohol Educ. & Community Services Dept. of Health, Fredericton, N.B. .... J. E. Carten

---

Hospital Services

Children's Hospital School, Lancaster, N.B. — Supt. John C. Stanley , M.B., B.Ch.

Provincial Hospital, Campbellton, N.B. — Supt., J. A. Gallant, M.D.

Provincial Hosp., Lancaster, N.B. — Supt., R. A. Gregory, M.D.

Jordan Memorial Sanatorium, The Glades, N.B. — Supt. G. H. Blennerhassett, M.D.

Polio Clinic and Health Centre, Fredericton, N.B. — Med. Dir., C. H. Turner, M.D.

Dist. Medical Health Off., Woodstock, N.B. .... J. R. Allanach, M.D., D.P.H.

Dist. Medical Health Off., 400 Collishaw St., Moncton, N.B. .... R. D. Landry, M.D., D.P.H.

Dist. Medical Health Off., 2 Mecklenburg St., Saint John, N.B. .... Stephen Clark, M.D., (acting)

Dist. Medical Health Off., Sussex, N.B. .... E. F. O'Rafferty, M.D., D.P.H.

Dist. Medical Health Off., Dalhousie, N.S. .... W. W. Fleck, M.D.

Dist. Medical Health Off., Edmundston, N.B. .... Euclide Rioux, M.D. (acting)

Dist. Medical Health Off., Campbellton, N.B. .... Richard Comeau, M.D., (acting)

Dist. Medical Health Off., St. Stephen, N.B. .... H. S. Everett, M.D., (acting)

NOTIFICATION TO CORONERS (New Brunswick)

Attention is drawn to the following Vital Statistics Regulation under the Health Act: Whenever it shall appear to any sub-deputy registrar that reasonable cause exists, notwithstanding any certificate of cause of death that may be given in the case, that the body of a deceased person should not be buried in or removed from his registration area before further investigation be had relative to the cause of death, he shall not issue such burial or removal permit, but shall at once notify a Coroner, and no burial or removal permit shall issue until permission for burial be obtained from said Coroner.

It is advisable to notify a Coroner of:

(1) Any person who dies without the attendance of a medical practitioner;

(2) Any person who dies as the result of gun shot wounds;

(3) Any person who dies as the result of an accident at work — Industrial accidents;

(4) Any person who dies as the result of being struck or run over by a Railway Train;

(5) Any person who dies as the result of being struck by an automobile;

(6) Any person who dies as the result of an abortion;

(7) Any person who dies where there is any suspicion of foul play;

(8) Any person who dies during or within 24 hours following surgical procedure;

(9) Any person who dies within 24 hours of hospital admission.

DEPARTMENT OF HEALTH NOVA SCOTIA

Hollis St., Halifax, N.S.

Tel. 422-7341

Minister of Public Health .... THE HONOURABLE R. A. DONAHOE, LL.B., Q.C.

Administration

Deputy Minister .... J. S. Robertson, M.D.
Administrator, Health Unit Services .... J. J. Stanton, M.D.
Administrator, Mental Health Services .... Clyde Marshall, M.D.
Administrator, Tuberculosis Control Services .... J. E. Hiltz, M.D.
Administrator, Consultation Services .... D. G. McCurdy, M.D.
Director, Maternal & Child Health and Communicable Diseases Control Division .... H. B. Colford, M.D.
Director, Dental Health Division .... W. C. King, D.D.S.
Director, Public Health Nursing Division .... Miss P. J. Lyttle, R.N.
Director, Environmental Hygiene Division .... R. D. McKay, P. Eng.
Director, Nutrition Division .... Miss Jessie Rae
Director, Registration Services .... H. E. Naugler
Inspector of Humane Institutions .... Clyde Marshall, M.D.
Co-ordinator of Rehabilitation .... Frank Wellard
Director of Office Services .... G. E. Gregoire
Director, Emergency Health Services .... S. H. Kryszek, M.D.

Central Laboratories — **Halifax**

Head, Department of Pathology .... D. O. W. Waugh, M.D.
Administrator, Dept. of Pathology .... J. H. Cooper, M.D.
Director, Division of Anatomical Pathology .... N. A. Kerenyi, M.D.
Director, Division of Clinical Chemistry .... A. MacKenzie, M.D.
Director, Division of Haematology .... H. C. Read, M.D.
Head, Department of Bacteriology .... C. E. van Rooyen, M.D.
Director, Div. of Clinical Bacteriology .... William Henderson, M.D.
Director, Div. of Public Health Bacteriology .... R. S. Martin, Ph.D.

Hospital Services

Victoria General Hospital, Halifax, N.S. — C. M. Bethune, M.D., Supt.

Nova Scotia Hospital (Mental), Dartmouth, N.S. — Murray MacKay, M.D., Supt.

Nova Scotia Sanatorium (Tb.), Kentville, N.S. — J. E. Hiltz, M.D., Administrator, Tuberculosis Services

Point Edward Hospital (Tb.), Sydney, N.S. — D. S. Robb, M.D., Supt.

The Province operates three Travelling Dental Units and one Travelling Hearing Test Unit

NOTIFICATION TO MEDICAL EXAMINERS
(Nova Scotia)

The Fatality Inquiries Act requires that a Medical Examiner conduct an inquiry where it appears that

(a) there is reasonable cause to suspect that a person died by violence, undue means or culpable negligence, or

(b) a person died in a place or under circumstances requiring an inquest under any statute, or

(c) the cause of death is undetermined, or

(d) the person died in jail or in prison.

It is advisable to notify the Medical Examiner in all such cases and, without restricting the generality of these classifications, the Medical Examiner should be advised where any person dies of gunshot wounds, as a result of a railway or motor vehicle accident, as a result of an abortion, by drowning, or in cases of apparent suicide.

DEPARTMENT OF HEALTH QUEBEC

930, St-Foy Rd., Quebec City
Tel. 693-6303

Minister of Health .... Hon. Eric Kierans
Deputy Minister of Health .... Jacques Gélinas, M.D.
Associate Deputy Minister .... Laurent Lizotte, M.D.

Chiefs of Division with Offices in Quebec

Demographer .... Paul Parrot, M.D.
Emergency Health Service .... Rodolphe Gervais, M.D.
Epidemiologist .... Adrian-Roger Foley, M.D.

QUEBEC DEPT. OF HEALTH (*Cont'd*)

Health Units	Paul Claveau, M.D.
Nutrition & Child Health	Lucile Koenig, M.D.
Psychiatric Services	**Dominique Bédard, M.D.**
Public Charities and Assistance	Charles-A. Turgeon, M.D.
Hospital Insurance	Jean-Paul Marcoux, C.A.
Industrial Hygiene and Sanitary Engineering Services	Jean-A. Roy, Eng. M.Sc.
Information & Publicity	Charles-G. Denis
Administrative Services	Raymond Gendron
Material and Acc'n Services	Pierre-Henri Côté

Chiefs of Division with Offices in Montreal, 1570 St. Hubert St.

Ass. Chief Hospital Insurance Montreal area	J. Napoléon Tremblay, M.D.
Laboratories	Arnold J. Drapeau
Venereal Diseases	L. P. Des Rochers, M.D.

NOTIFICATION TO CORONERS (Quebec)

Attention is directed to the following wording used in Chapter 22 revised statuts of Quebec 1942 and the pertinent section of that act are sections 16, 20 and 21 which read as follows:

"16. The Coroner may himself investigate the circumstances which preceded or accompanied the death of any person when he has good reason to believe that the deceased came to his death not from natural causes or from mere accident of mischance, but from violence, or negligent or culpable conduct of some other person, under circumstances such as might subsequently require the holding of a Coroner's inquest.

The Attorney General may also, when ever he deems it expedient in the public interest, direct the Coroner to make an investigation into the circumstances which have preceded or accompanied the death of any person.

The Coroner shall give a burial permit when it is established by his investigation, that the deceased came to his death from natural causes or from mere accident or mischance. R.S. 1925, c. 153, s. 16.

"20". Whosoever may learn or know that a person has died of violent or sudden death, or a death due to causes which do not appear to be natural, or which are unknown or of a suspiscious nature, shall immediately and as quickly and as inexpensively as possible, give notice of such facts to the Coroner of the district, or to his deputy".

It shall be the special duty of the persons living in the vicinity of the place where such death occured to give the notice required by this section. R.S. 1925, ch. 153, s. 20."

"21" On the death of a person confined in a penitentary, prison, house of correction or detention, or in a lunatic asylum, it shall be the duty of the warden, jailor, superintendant or person in charge of such institution to immediately notify the Coroner having jurisdiction, giving the details of all the circumstances connected with such deaths, R.S. 1925, c153, s. 21."

DEPARTMENT OF HEALTH ONTARIO

Parliament Buildings, Ontario

Minister of Health	THE HON. MATTHEW B. DYMOND, M.D.
Deputy Minister	K. C. Charron, M.D.
Assistant to the Deputy Minister	W. B. Nichols, M.A., C.P.H.
Executive Director, Financial and Administrative Services	G. S. Tattle
Director of Legal Services	C. Walker, Q.C., B.A.
Executive Director, Public Health Division	G. K. Martin, M.D., D.P.H.
Nurse Consultant, Special Assignments	Dorothy G. Riddell, Reg.N.
Director, Local Health Services Branch	VACANT
Senior Consultant, Public Health Dentistry	F. A. Kohli, D.D.S., D.D.P.H.
Senior Consultant, Public Health Education	John J. Keays, M.P.H.
Senior Consultant, Public Health Inspection	VACANT
Senior Consultant, Public Health Nursing	VACANT
Chief, Northern Ontario Public Health Service	E. J. Young, M.D., D.P.H.

ONTARIO DEPT. OF HEALTH (*Cont'd*)

Director, Special Health Services Branch	G. E. Large, M.D., D.P.H.
Chief, Medical Rehabilitation and Chronic Care	VACANT
Chief, Emergency Health Service	VACANT
Chief, Epidemiology	J. S. Bell, M.D., D.P.H.
Chief, Maternal and Child Health	VACANT
Chief, Tuberculous Prevention	C. H. Rorabeck, M.D.
Officer-in-Charge, Nutrition Service	Barbara Broadfoot, M.A.
Officer in-Charge, R.N.A. Schools	Helen McCallum, Reg.N.
Officer in-Charge, Drug and Biologics Program	VACANT
Director, Environmental Health Branch	R. B. Sutherland, M.D., D.P.H.
Chief, Air Pollution Control	W. B. Drowley, P.Eng.
Chief, Civil Service Employee Health Service	W. E. O'Hara, M.D.
Chief, Environmental Health Laboratories	R. G. Elson
Chief, Occupational Health	E. Mastromatteo, M.D., D.P.H.
Chief, Public Health Engineering	W. M. Walkinshaw, M.A.Sc., P.Eng.
Chief, Radiation Protection	L. B. Leppard, Ph.D.
Officer-in-Charge, Pesticides Control	W. L. Smith
Officer-in Charge, Stuffed Articles	J. MacDougall
Director, Laboratories Branch	L. E. Elkerton, M.D., D.P.H.
Associate Director	J. W. A. Percy, M.A.
Chief, Bacteriology	C. R. Amies, M.D., M.R.C.P.(L)
Chief, Biochemistry	R. G. Reynolds, B.Sc.A.
Chief, Pathology	J. B. McKay, M.D.
Chief, Serology	H. B. Smith, B.Sc., Dip.Bact.
Chief, Virology	N. A. Labzoffsky, D.V.M., D.V.Sc.
Executive Director, Mental Health Division	H. W. Henderson, M.D.
Director, Professional Services Branch	B. H. McNeel, M.D.
Director, Mental Hospitals Branch	VACANT
Director, Mental Retardation Branch	D. E. Zarfas, M.D.
Director, Hospital Management Services Branch	R. A. Farmer, M.D.
Executive Director, Research and Planning Branch	VACANT
Assistant Director	A. H. Sellers, M.D., D.P.H.
Principal Nurse Consultant	Isabel Black, Reg.N., B.S., M.A.

*Community Mental Health **Services. Details are set out in a separate publication which is available** from the Mental Health Branch.

Other Services

Ontario Hospital Services Commission, 2195 Yonge Street, Toronto 7
Ontario Cancer Treatment and Research Foundation, 69 Bloor Street East, Toronto
Alcoholism & Drug Addiction Research Foundation Clinic, 24 Harbord Street, Toronto

NOTIFICATION TO CORONERS
(Ontario)

7. Every person who has reason to believe that a deceased person died:
   (a) as a result of,
      (i) violence,
      (ii) misadventure,
      (iii) negligence,
      (iv) misconduct, or
      (v) malpractice;
   (b) by unfair means;
   (c) **during pregnancy** or **following pregnancy in circumstances that might reasonably be attributable** thereto;
   (d) suddenly and unexpectedly;
   (e) from disease or sickness **for which he was not treated by a duly qualified medical practitioner;**
   (f) from any cause other than disease, or
   (g) under such circumstances as may require **investigation,**

shall immediately notify a coroner **of the facts and circumstances relating to the death. 1960-61,** c.——, s.3.

DEPARTMENT OF HEALTH MANITOBA

Legislative Bldg., Broadway Ave., Winnipeg 1, Man.

Tel. WH 6-7207

Minister of Health .... **The Honourable C. H. Witney**

Administration

Deputy Minister of Health	M. R. Elliott, M.D.
Dir. Medical Insurance Services	A. R. Tanner, M.D.
Departmental Accountant	W. H. Benabo
Recorder of Vital Statistics & Records	D. W. Matheson
Dir. Health Education	D. F. McLean
Dir. Rehabilitation Services	W. N. Boyd, M.S.W.
Dir. Health Services	J. B. Morison, M.D.
Dir. Local Health Services	J. C. Elias, M.D.
Dir. Dental Services	C. H. McCormick, D.D.S.
Dir. Northern Health Services	H. C. Rolfe, M.D.
Med. Dir. Care Services	W. Watt, M.D.
Asst. Med. Dir. Care Services	E. L. Peters, M.D.
Dir. Preventive Medical Services	E. Snell, M.D.
Dir. Venereal Disease Control	J. A. Eadie, M. D.
Dir. Public Health Nursing Services	Miss J. I. Williamson, R.N.
Dir. Environmental Sanitation	L. A. Kay, M.A. (Sc.)
Dir. Public Health Engineering	J. N. Warrener
Dir. Food Control	A. G. McLeod
Industrial Hygiene Laboratory	W. Ward
Dir. Laboratory Services	J. G. Fox, M.D.
Dir. Psychiatric Services	E. Johnson, M.D.
Supt. Brandon Hosp. for Mental Diseases	A. H. Moyes, M.D.
Supt. Selkirk Hosp. for Mental Diseases	R. H. Tavener, M.D.
Supt. Manitoba School for Retardates	G. H. Lowther, M.D.
Supt. Psychiatric Institute & Community Mental Health	E. Johnson, M.D.
Med. Dir. Greater Winnipeg Child Guidance Clinic	J. Asselstine, M.D.
Chairman, Manitoba Hospital Commission	Gordon W. Holland, B. Commerce

NOTIFICATION TO CORONERS
(Manitoba)

Attention is drawn to the following quotations from the Vital Statistics Act:

subsection (4) of section 14: Where a death occurs without medical attendance . . . the funeral director shall forthwith notify a coroner having jurisdiction . . . or a legally qualified medical practitioner designated by the coroner . . . who shall thereupon inquire into the facts and shall complete the medical certificate. . .

subsection (6) of section 14: . . . where there is reason to believe that a person has died (a) as a result of violence of misadventure: (b) by unlawful means: (c) as a result of negligence or misconduct on the part of others; or (d) under circumstances that require investigation; no acknowledgement of registration of the death and no burial permit shall be issued by the division registrar unless (e) the body has been examined by the coroner and investigation has been made into the circumstances of the death, as provided by The Coroners Act: (f) the coroner has signed the medical certificate of the cause of death. .

DEPARTMENT OF HEALTH SASKATCHEWAN

Health & Welfare Bldg., Regina

TEL. LA 3-0661

Minister of Public Health .... The Honourable D. G. Steuart

Administration

Deputy Minister	J. G. Clarkson, M.B., M.P.H.
Director, Health and Safety Education Division	
Director, Provincial Laboratories	H. E. Robertson, Ph.D.
Dir., Admin. Services Branch	Mr. C. P. Feader
Dir., Research & Planning	J. D. Ramsay, M.B., Ch.B., D.P.H.
Dir. Div. Vital Statistics	Mr. W. C. N. Reed
Dir. Psychiatric Services Branch	
Deputy Director Psych. Services	Mr. C. J. Jillings, M.A.
Supt. Sask. Hospital, Weyburn	H. G. Lafave, B.A., M.D.

SASKATCHEWAN DEPT. OF HEALTH (*Cont'd*)

Supt. Sask. Hospital, North Battleford	M. Demay, M.D.
Supt. Training School, Moose Jaw	A. J. Beddie, M.B., Ch.B.
Supt. Sask. Training School, Prince Albert	Mr. D. G. Rice, B.Ed.
Dir. Munroe Wing, Gen. Hosp., Regina	M. Resjkind, M.D.
Dir. Mental Health Clinic, Gen. Hosp., Regina	M. Resjkind, M.D.
Dir. MacNeill Clinic, Saskatoon	A. Stephen, M.B.
Dir. Adult Outpatient Service, Saskatoon	Dr. I. H. Park
Dir. Mental Health Clinic, M. J. Union Hospital, Moose Jaw Dir. Psychiatric Dept., M. J. Union Hospital	P. O. O'Reilly, M.B., D.Ch., B.A.O.
Dir. Mental Health Clinic, Swift Current	A. M. Mizrahi, M.B., B.Ch.
Dir. Mental Health Clinic, Prince Albert	R. A. Jenkins, M.D., D.P.M.
Dir. Psychiatric Centre, Yorkton	G. A. Ives, M.D., D.P.M.
Dir. Psychiatric Research Unit, University Hospital, Saskatoon	A. Hoffer, Ph.D., M.D.
Dir. Regional Health Services Branch	S. L. Skoll, M.B., Ch.B.
Dir. Child Health Div.	
Dir. Maternal Health	
A/Dir. Commun. Disease Control Div.	Mr. C. J. Goss
Dir. Dental Health Div.	H. A. Grimsrud, D.D.S., D.D.P.H.
Dir. Nursing Services Div.	Miss E. L. Miner, R.N., M.P.H.
Dir. Nutrition Div.	Mrs. Alice L. Jenner, B.Sc., H.E., D.I.N.
Dir. Sanitation Div.	Mr. M. H. Prescott, B.Sc.
A/Dir. Venereal Disease Control Div.	Mr. C. J. Goss
Dir. Hospital Branch	F. Grunberg, M.D.
Supt. Air Ambulance Service	Mr. D. N. Campbell
Med. Dir. Med. Services Div.	
Dir. Med. Services Div.	Mr. W. J. Totten, B.S.P.
Admin. Dir. Physical Rehabilitation Div.	Mr. D. F. Clark, B.E.D., M.A.
Med. Dir. Physical Rehabilitation Centre, Regina	A. F. Huston, M.B., B.S.
Ex. Dir. Sask. Hosp. Services Plan	Mr. J. C. Sangster
Dir. Occuptional Health Services	N. Williams, M.D., D.P.H., D.I.H.
Dir. Emergency Health Services	J. H. McLaughlin, M.B., Ch.B., D.P.H.

Saskatchewan Cancer Commission

Chairman	F. H. Wigmore, M.D., F.A.C.S., F.R.C.S.(C) 200 Scott Blk., Moose Jaw
Dir. Cancer Services for Sask.	Cancer Clinic, Saskatoon, Sask
Secretary	Mr. O. H. Pratt, Allan Blair Mem. Cancer Clinic, Grey Nuns' Hosp., Regina
Dir. Saskatoon Cancer Clinic	C. C. Burkell, B.Sc., M.D., D.M.R.(T)
Dir. Allan Blair Mem. Cancer Clinic, Grey Nuns' Hosp., Regina, Sask.	A. J. S. Bryant, M.D., D.M.R.(T)

Saskatchewan Anti-Tuberculosis League

Med. Dir. & Gen. Supt., Sanatorium, Fort Qu'Appelle	G. D. Barnett, M.D.
Supt. Fort Qu'Appelle San.	A. L. Swanton, M.D.
Supt. Saskatoon San.	E. H. Fieguth, M.D.

NOTIFICATION TO CORONERS
(Saskatchewan)

Attention is drawn to the following wording used in subsection 5, (a), (b), (c) & (d) of the Vital Statistics Act being Chapter 44 R.S.S. 1953.

5. (a) as a result of violence or misadventure or by unfare means;
(b) from any cause other than disease or sickness;
(c) as a result of negligence or misconduct or mal practice on the part of others; or
(d) under such circumstances as require investigation;

DEPARTMENT OF HEALTH, ALBERTA

Administration Bldg., Edmonton, Alta.
Tel. 229-3443

Minister of Health	The Honourable J. D. Ross, M.D.

Administration

Deputy Minister	M. G. McCallum, M.D.
Assistant Deputy Minister	H. E Homan
Dir. of Vital Statistics	J. Colville
Dir. of Local Health Services	E. S. O. Smith, M.D.
Dir. of Public Health Nursing	(Mrs.) Janet C. Bailey, R.N.

ALBERTA DEPT. OF HEALTH (*Cont'd*)

Dir. of Dental Health Services	A. T. Salter, D.M.D.
Dir. of Health Education	(Miss) Amy M. Elliott
Dir. of Entomology & Vector Control and Poison Control Services	J. H. Brown, M.Sc.
Dir. of Nutrition Services	(Miss) Elva Perdue, B.Sc.
Dir., Prov. Lab., Univ. of Alberta, Edmonton	R. D. Stuart, M.D.
Dir., Southern Branch Prov. Lab., Calgary	D. Shute, M.D.
Dir. of Social Hygiene	P. L. Rentiers, M.D.
Dir. of Sanitary Engineering	H. L. Hogge, B.Sc.
Dir. of Industrial Health	H. Siemens, M.D.
Dir. of Medical Services	P. B Rose, M.D.
Dir. of Emergency Health Services, E.M.O.	R. A. Duncan, M.D.
Dir. of Cerebral Palsy Clinics	G. P. Mores, M.D.
Dir. of Arthritis Services	R. K. Thomson, M.D.
Dir. of Cancer Services	A. S. Little
Dir. of Alcoholism	J. P. Matheson
Executive Director of Hospital Services	J. D. Campbell, M.Com., F.C.A.
Dir. of T.B. Control, Aberhart Memorial Sanatorium **Med. Supt., Aberhart Memorial Sanatorium**	H. H. Stephens, M.D.
Med. Supt., Baker Memorial Sanatorium, Calgary	J. Ryder, M.D.
Dir. of Mental Health	T. C. Michie, M.D.
Ass't. Dir. of Mental Health	A. R. Schrag, M.D.
Clinic Psychiatrist, Alberta Guidance Clinic, Edmonton	J. B. Van Stolk, M.D.
Clinic Psychiatrist, Alberta Guidance Clinic, Calgary	N. C. Horne, M.D.
Clinic Psychiatrist, Alberta Guidance Clinic, Ponoka	F. J. Edwards, M.D.
Clinic Psychiatrist, Alberta Guidance Clinic, Lethbridge	J. Bower, M.D.
Med. Supt., Alberta Hosp., Ponoka	J. M. Byers, M.D.
Med. Supt., Alberta Hosp., Edmonton	A. D. MacPherson, M.D.
Med. Supt., Alberta School Hosp., Red Deer **Clinic Psychiatrist, Alberta Guidance Clinic, Red Deer**	L. J. le Vann, M.D.

NOTIFICATION TO CORONERS

(Alberta)

Attention is directed to the following wording used in The Coroners Act for Alberta, Section 7, subsections 1 and 2.

7. (1) Any medical practitioner, undertaker, embalmer, any inmate of the house in which the deceased resided immediately before his death, any peace officer or other person who has reason to believe that a deceased person died

(a) as a result of violence, misadventure or by unfair means,
(b) from any cause other than disease or sickness,
(c) as a result of negligence or misconduct or malpractice on the part of others, or
(d) under circumstances that require investigation,

shall immediately give notice of the facts and circumstances of the death to a coroner who ordinarily has jurisdiction in the locality in which the body of the deceased person is found.

(2) Where a person dies in a hospital in the Province within thirty days after an operation upon him, the medical superintendent of the hospital shall immediately give notice of the details of the death to the coroner who ordinarily has jurisdiction in the locality in which the hospital is situate.

DEPARTMENT OF HEALTH BRITISH COLUMBIA

Parliament Buildings, Victoria, B.C.

Tel. EVergreen 2-6111

Health Branch

Parliament Buildings, Victoria, B.C.

Deputy Minister of Health and Provincial Health Officer	**J. A. Taylor, M.D., D.P.H.**
Assistant Provincial Health Officer and Director, Bureau of Local Health Services	K. I. G. Benson, M.B., ChB., D.P.H.
Director, Bureau of Administration	**A. H. Cameron, B.A., M.P.H.**
Director, Division of Epidemiology and Director, Emergency Health Services	A. A. Larsen, B.A., M.D., D.P.H., M.P.H.
Director, Division of Preventive Dentistry	F. McCombie, L.D.S., R.C.S., D.D.P.H
Director, Division of Public Health Engineering	**W. Bailey, B.Sc., Civil Eng. M.S. in Sanitary Eng.**
Director, Division of Public Health Nursing	**Miss M. Frith, R.N., B.A.Sc., M.P.H.**
Director, Division of Vital Statistics	**J. H. Doughty, B.Com., M.A.**
Director, Division of Public Health Education	
Chief Sanitary Inspector	**C. E. Stonehouse, C.S.I. (C)**
Consultant, Public Health Nutrition	
Departmental Comptroller	J. McDiarmid
Consultant, Sanitary Inspection	R. G. Scott, C.S.I.(C)

BRITISH COLUMBIA DEPT. OF HEALTH (*Cont'd.*)

Provincial Health Building,
828 West 10th Avenue, Vancouver 9, B.C.

Deputy Provincial Health Officer and Director, Bureau of Special Preventive and Treatment Services	G. R. F. Elliot, M.D., C.M., D.P.H.
Director Division of Tuberculosis Control	G. F. Kincade, M.D., C.M.
Director, Division of Veneral Disease Control and Director, Division of Occupational Health	J. H. Smith, M.D., D.I.H., D.P.H., PH.
Director, Division of Laboratories	E. J. Bowmer, M.D., Ch.B.
Director of Registry and Rehabilitation Services	C. L. Hunt, M.R.C.S., L.R.C.P.
Rehabilitation Coordinator	C. E. Bradbury

Hospital Insurance Service

Deputy Minister of Hospital Insurance	D. M. Cox, F.A.C.H.A., F.C.I., F.C.I.S.
Assistant Deputy Minister	W. J. Lyle, F.C.I.S.
Dir. of Hosp. Consultation, Development and Research	J. Mainguy, M.H.A.
Medical Consultant	C. F. Ballam, M.D.
Manager, Hospital Finance Division	N. S. Wallace, C.G.A.
Manager, Hosp. Construction and Planning Division	A. W. E. Pitkethley
Manager, Hosp. Consultation and Inspection Division	J. Bainbridge
Director, Research Division	D. S. Thomson, B.A.
Administrative Officer	K. G. Wiper

Information regarding the listing of personnel of the Mental Health Services Branch may be obtained by contacting Dr. A. E. Davidson, Deputy Minister of Mental Health Services, 828 West 10th Avenue, Vancouver 9, B.C.

NOTIFICATION TO CORONERS
(British Columbia)

Attention is directed to the following wording used in Subsection (4) of Section 14 of the "Vital Statistics Act":

> **"Where there is reason to believe that a person has died under circumstances that require an inquiry or inquest under the 'Coroners Act', no acknowledgment of registration of** the death and no burial permit shall be issued by the District Registrar unless an inquiry **has been made into the circumstances of the death or an inquest has been held under the 'Coroners Act' and the coroner has signed the medical certificate of the cause of death in accordance with Subsection (3), ..."**

Section 14 (3) (b) of the "Vital Statistics Act" permits a physician to sign the medical certificate of death "where the death occurs without medical attendance and under circumstances that do not require an inquiry or inquest under the 'Coroners Act'."

It is advisable for medical practitioners to notify the coroner of:

(1) any person who dies where there is any suspicion of foul play;
(2) any person who dies as the result of gunshot wounds;
(3) any person who dies as the result of an accident;
(4) any person who dies as the result of an abortion;
(5) any person who dies without the attendance of a medical practitioner except where the cause of death is clearly due to natural causes.

ORGANIZATIONS SUPPORTING MEDICAL RESEARCH

Medical research plays an increasing important role in the programme of Canadian universities, hospitals and other institutions. The costs of such research are borne in part by the institutions themselves; substantial additional funds are provided by government and "voluntary" agencies. Some of these agencies are listed below

Alberta Heart Foundations, 11046-83rd Ave., Edmonton, Alberta.

Alcoholism and Drug Addiction Research Foundation, 344 Bloor St. West, Toronto 5, Ont.
Executive Director: H. D. Archibald.

Atkinson Charitable Foundation, 80 King St. West, Toronto, Ont.

Banting Research Foundation, c/o Dept. of Medical Biophysics, University of Toronto, 500 Sherbourne St., Toronto 5, Ont.

B.C. Heart Foundation, 1956 West Broadway, Vancouver, B.C.

B.C. Medical Research Foundation, P.O. Box 4105, Vancouver, B.C.

Canadian Arthritis & Rheumatism Society, 45 Charles St. East, Toronto 5, Ont.
Executive Director: Edward Dunlop, O.B.E., G.M.

Canadian Association for Retarded Children, 87 Bedford Rd., Toronto 5, Ont.
Executive Director: Dr. G. A. Roeher.

Canadian Diabetic Association, 1491 Yonge St., Toronto 7, Ont.

Canadian Foundation for the Advancement of Therapeutics, P.O. Box 120, Lachine, P.Q.
Secretary: Dr. C. W. Murphy

Canadian Heart Foundation, 1130 Bay St., Toronto 5, Ont.
Executive Director: Dr. J. B. Armstrong.

Canadian Hemophilia Society, 122 Arlington, Montreal 6, P.Q.
President: Mr. Frank Schnabel.

Canadian Hemophilia Society, Ontario Chapter, 49 Belvedere Blvd., Toronto 18, Ont.
President: Mrs. J. Rosenthal.

Canadian Life Insurance Officers' Association, 302 Bay St., Toronto 1, Ont.

Canadian Mental Health Association, 52 St. Clair Ave. East, Toronto 7, Ont.
General Director: Dr. J. D. Griffin.

Canadian Rehabilitation Council for the Disabled, 263 McCaul St., Toronto 2B, Ont.
National Executive Director: Dr. K. S. Armstrong.

Canadian Tuberculosis Association, 343 O'Connor St., Ottawa 4, Ont.
Executive Secretary: Dr. C. W. L. Jeanes.

Charles H. Best Foundation, 112 College St., Toronto, Ont.
Director: Dr. C. H. Best.

Defence Research Board, Dept. of National Defence, Ottawa 2, Ont.
Head, Medical Research Section: Dr. G. C. Caldbick.

Department of National Health and Welfare, Ottawa, Ont.
Consultant, Research Development: Dr. R. W. Tooley.

Gairdner Medical Research Foundation, 73 Homewood Ave., Toronto 5, Ont.
Director of Research: Dr. G. D. W. Murray.

J. P. Bickell Foundation, 20 King St. East, Toronto, Ont.
Secretary of Foundation Committee: C. E. Alan Smith.

Manitoba Heart Foundation, 642 Somerset Bldg., Winnipeg, Man.

Medical Research Council, National Research Building M-58, Montreal Road, Ottawa 7, Ont.
Secretary: Dr. J. Auer.

Multiple Sclerosis Society, P.O. Box 1214, Postal Station "O", Montreal 9, P.Q.
Executive Secretary: A. Gordon Cleland.

Muscular Dystrophy Association of Canada, 160 Bay St., Toronto 1. Ont.
Executive Secretary: Mrs. A. S. Weldon.

ORGANIZATIONS CARRYING OUT RESEARCH (*Cont'd*)

National Cancer Institute of Canada, 790 Bay St., Toronto, Ont.
Executive Director: Dr. R. M. Taylor.

Ontario Cancer Treatment and Research Foundation, 69 Bloor St. East, Toronto, Ont.
Medical Director: Dr. D. E. Cannell.

Ontario Heart Foundation, 22 College St., Toronto, Ont.
Executive Director: M. H. Robertson.

Ontario Society for Crippled Children, 350 Rumsey Road, Toronto 17, Ont.
Executive Director: R. Auld.

Quebec Heart Foundation, 680 Sherbroke St. West, Montreal, P.Q.
Chairman, Medical Committee: Dr. Paul David.

Queen Elizabeth II Canadian Research Fund, National Research Building M-58, Montreal Road, Ottawa 7, Ont.
Secretary to the Board of Trustees: Dr. J. Auer.

R. S. McLaughlin Foundation, 217 Bay St., Toronto, Ont.

Saskatchewan Heart Foundation, 204 Grain Bldg., Saskatoon, Sask.

Traffic Injuries Research Foundation, 74 Stanley Ave., Ottawa, Ont.
Medical Director: Dr. E. Campbell.

MEDICAL RESEARCH COUNCIL

The Medical Research Council was established in November 1960 as a result of a recommendation to the Privy Council Committee on Scientific and Industrial Research by a Special Committee appointed to review extramural support of medical research by the Government of Canada.

The Medical Research Council is prepared to support research in the broad field of medical science. The support consists mainly of an extensive extramural programme of grants-in-aid of research proposed and carried out by staff members of the Canadian universities, hospitals and institutes, and of the provision of personnel support under the Fellowship, Scholarship and Associateship programmes.

Members of the Council are: Dr. G. Malcolm Brown, Chairman; Dr. C. Fortier, Vice-Chairman; Dr. J. Auer, Secretary; Dr. R. Gingras, Dean of Medicine, Laval University, Quebec, P.Q.; Dr. R. V. Christie, Dean of Medicine, McGill University, Montreal, P.Q.; Dr. J. P. Cordeau, Head of the Dept. of Physiology, University of Montreal, Montreal, P.Q.; Dr. P. B. Hagen, Head of the Dept. of Biochemistry, Queen's University, Kingston, Ontario; Dr. J. A. McCarter, Director, Cancer Research Unit, University of Western Ontario, London, Ontario; Dr. J. C. Wilt, Head of the Department of Bacteriology, University of Manitoba, Winnipeg, Manitoba; Dr. R. W. Begg, Dean of Medicine, University of Saskatchewan, Saskatoon, Saskatchewan; Dr. W. Paul, Head of the Department of Obstetrics and Gynecology, University of Toronto, Toronto, Ontario; Dr. J. C. Szerb, Head of the Department of Physiology, Dalhousie University, Halifax, N.S.; Dr. G. O. Bain, Department of Pathology, University of Alberta, Edmonton, Alberta; Dr. H. E. Taylor, Head of the Department of Pathology, University of British Columbia, Vancouver, B.C.; Dr. G. E. Connell, Head of the Dept. of Biochemistry, University of Toronto, Toronto, Ont.

CANADIAN TIME ZONES

Newfoundland .... 52° .5 W. Long. 3-h 30-m *slow of Greenwich*

Atlantic .... 60° W. Long. 4h *slow of Greenwich*

Eastern .... 75° W. Long. 5-h *slow of Greenwich*

Central .... 90° W. Long. 6-h *slow of Greenwich*

Mountain .... 105° W. Long. 7-h *slow of Greenwich*

Pacific .... 120° W. Long. 8-h *slow of Greenwich*

Yukon .... 135° W. Long. 9-h *slow of Greenwich*

DALHOUSIE UNIVERSITY

Halifax N. S.

Tel. 2-4406

Principal Officers

President	Henry D. Hicks
Registrar	Beatrice R. E. Smith
Comptroller	D. H. McNeill
Librarian	
Dean of Faculty of Medicine	C. B. Stewart, M.D.
Assistant Deans	L. B. Macpherson, Ph.D.
	L. C. Steeves, M.D.
Secretary of the Faculty of Medicine	S. J. Patrick, Ph.D.

Heads of Departments

Anaesthesia	C. C. Stoddard, M.D.
Anatomy	R. L. deC. H. Saunders, M.D.
Bacteriology	C. E. vanRooyen, M.D
Biochemistry	C. W. Helleiner, Ph.D.
Hospital Administration	C. M. Bethune, M.D.
Medicine	R. C. Dickson, M.D.
Obstetrics & Gynaecology	W. R. C. Tupper, M.D.
Otolaryngology	D. M. MacRae, M.D.
Ophthamology	J. S. Hammerling, M.D.
Paediatrics	W. A. Cochrane, M.D.
Pathology	D. O. W. Waugh, M.D.
Pharmacology	J. G. Aldous, Ph.D.
Physiology	J. C. Szerb, M.D.
Postgraduate Div.	L. C. Steeves, M.D.
Preventive Medicine	G. H. Hatcher, M.D.
Psychiatry	R. O. Jones, M.D.
Radiology	J. S. Manchester, M.D.
Surgery	I. Mackenzie, M.D.
Urology	C. L. Gosse, M.D.

In 1818, the Rt. Hon. George Ramsay, 9th Earl of Dalhousie, obtained approval from the Prince Regent to establish a college of higher learning to be founded on the principles of "religious toleration and whose doors would be open to worthy students regardless of creed." Two years later, in 1820, the cornerstone was laid of the first structure, where the City Hall now stands. In spite of high hopes, Dalhousie did not function as a University until 1838 and a few years later, activity declined until in 1845, teaching was suspended. Efforts toward a revival were begun in 1848, and 1863 Dalhousie was permanently established as a Provincial University. In 1868 the Faculty of Medicine was inaugurated and continued until 1875. In that year, the Halifax Medical College, affiliated with Dalhousie, took over its responsibilities which it bore until 1911, when Dalhousie resumed the teaching of Medicine.

Present Course

The present course of medicine covers five years, and the final year is one of internship. The degree conferred by the University is Doctor of Medicine (M.D.).

Postgraduate Courses

The Dalhousie Refresher Course is held annually and is now entering its 40th year. This is an intensive course of one week for the general practitioners of the four Atlantic Provinces and consists of clinics, clinical demonstrations and lectures. The average attendance is about 200 physicians.

For the past 12 years an enlarged programme of postgraduate medical education has been carried on for general practitioners as follows:

A. Individual speakers or teams from the Faculty of Medicine visit local Medical Societies and Hospitals, presenting short courses, or single lectures.

B. Short courses in specific subjects are held in Halifax and other Provincial Centres. Full details of such courses may be obtained from the Director of the Postgraduate Division.

McGILL UNIVERSITY

Montreal P. Q.

Tel.: Gen. - 844-6311

Principal of the University	H. Rocke Robertson, M.D., F.A.C.S., F.R.C.S.(C)
Vice-Principal (Academic)	H. Noel Fieldhouse
Registrar	C. M. McDougall
Dean of the Faculty of Medicine	R. V. Christie, M.D.
Vice Dean of the Faculty of Medicine	E. H. Bensley, M.D.
Assoc. Dean (Admissions)	S. M. Banfill, M.D.
Assoc. Dean (Graduate Studies and Research)	D. V. Bates, M.D.
Assist. Dean (Professional Relations)	G. E. Joron, M.D.
Exec. Sec., of Faculty of Medicine	J. G. Hampson, B.Com.
Administrative Assistant	Merle Peden, B. Com.

Departmental Heads

Anaesthesia	R. G. B. Gilbert, M.D.
Anatomy	C. P. Leblond, M.D.
Microbiology and Immunology	R. W. Reed, M.D.
Biochemistry	K. A. C. Elliott, Ph.D.
Epidemiology and Health	J. C. McDonald, M.D.
History of Medicine	D. G. Bates, M.D.
Investigative Medicine	J. S. L. Browne, M.D.
Medicine	D. G. Cameron, M.D.
Neurology & Neurosurgery	T. Rasmussen, M.D.
Obstetrics & Gynaecology	G. B. Maughan, M.D.
Ophthalmology	John C. Locke, M.D.
Otolaryngology	H. E. McHugh, M.D.
Paediatrics	Alan Ross, M.D.
Pathology	G. C. McMillan, M.D.
Pharmacology	K. I. Melville, M.D.
Physiology	B. D. Burns, L.R.C.P., M.R.C.S.
Psychiatry	R. A. Cleghorn, M.D.
Radiology	J. Bouchard, M.D.
Surgery	F. N. Gurd, M.D.

The Faculty of Medicine of McGill University, now in its 135th year, is the outcome and continuance of a teaching body known as the Montreal Medical Institution. This institution was organized as a medical school in 1823 by four doctors who had received training at the University of Edinburgh, Scotland, and who formed the medical staff of the Montreal General Hospital, established four years earlier.

In 1829 the Montreal Medical Institution was invited by the Governors of McGill to become the Faculty of Medicine of the University. The medical school is thus the oldest Faculty of McGill and the first university degree, a medical one, was conferred in 1833. Except for a period of three years, 1836-39, when political disturbances interrupted, the Faculty of Medicine has continued its teaching and about 8,000 men and women have graduated.

The undergraduate course is four years — preclinical subjects are taught during First and Second years; clinical instruction begins during the Second Year and graduation is at the end of the Fourth year, when the degree of M.D., C.M. (Doctor of Medicine, Master of Surgery) is conferred. However a graduate must interne for at least one year in an approved hospital before being permitted to take examinations required to obtain a licence to practice medicine. There is also a double course in science and medicine for a limited number of students.

Graduate education is conducted in two types of courses. If a graduate wishes advanced training, then a pre-clinical or clinical department may be able to accommodate him while registered in the Faculty of Graduate Studies, working towards an M.Sc. or Ph.D. degree. The other alternative is provided by some of the clinical departments which have courses leading to University Diplomas. Such courses require 4-5 years of resident training at the University or in approved appointments elsewhere. Candidates seeking such graduate training are considered in an individual manner in the competition for the limited opportunities available.

LAVAL UNIVERSITY

Quebec P. Q.

Tel. 681-9611

Official Visitor and High Chancellor	His Eminence Cardinal Maurice Roy
Rector	Monsignor Louis-Albert Vachon
Vice-Rector	Monsignor Alphonse-Marie Parent
Vice-Rector	Doctor Louis-Philippe Bonneau
Vice-Rector	Reverend Lorenzo Roy
Secretary General	Mr. Paul A. Laberge
Administrator	Reverend Fernand Gingras
Public Relations	Mr. André Barnard
Director of Students	Mr. Jean Charles Bouffard
Dean of the Faculty of Medicine	Dr. Rosaire Gingras
Assistant Dean	Dr. Jean-Baptiste Jobin
Assistant Dean	Dr. Georges-A. Bergeron
Secretary	Dr. Gérard Girard
Librarian	Mr. Andras K. Kirchner

Departmental Heads

Anatomy	Dr. Pierre Jobin
Anesthesiology	Dr. Fernando Hudon
Biochemistry	Dr. Louis Birlinguet
Surgery	Dr. Wilfrid Caron
Medicine	Dr. Renaud Lemieux
Microbiology	Dr. Léo Gauvreau
Obstetrics and Gynaecology	Dr. René Simard
O.R.L. and Ophthalmology	Dr. Paul Painchaud
Pathology	Dr. Carlton Auger
Paediatrics	Dr. Donat Lapointe
Pharmacology	Dr. C. Radouco-Thomas
Physiology	Dr. Claude Fortier
Psychiatric	Dr. Charles A. Martin
Radiology	Dr. Henri Lapointe

The School of Medicine was established in the Fall of 1853, less than a year after the foundation of Laval University. In 1847, a medical school had been incorporated by the city of Quebec and in 1850 twenty students were registered. In 1852 some of the teachers were invited to become the first Professors of the new Faculty, and they were officially granted the degree of Doctor of Medicine by Lord Elgin, then Governor General of Canada.

With the years many hospitals were affiliated for clinical teaching. Presently we count seven general hospitals and five specialized hospitals.

Due to the increase in students and the expansion of the different departments the Board of Directors of Laval University decided the erection of a new Medical School, which was officially inaugurated on September 20th 1957.

Present Course

The medical course at Laval University covers four years, and students with a B.A. or B.Sc. may be admitted to the first year. The first two years of the course are devoted primarily to acquiring a knowledge of the preclinical medical sciences. At the beginning of the 2nd year, instruction is transferred in part to some of the teaching hospitals.

The 3rd and 4th years of the course are designed to bring the students into contact with patients and to develop the essentials of modern treatments. It is to be noted that all the lectures are given in French; those who wish to write the examinations in English may do so.

The degree of Doctor of Medicine is granted at the end of the 4th year. Those who obtain 90% on their final examinations graduate Magna Cum Laude and with 80% Cum Laude.

UNIVERSITY OF MONTREAL

Montreal P. Q.

Tel. 733-9951

High Chancellor	**His Eminence Cardinal Paul-Emile Leger**
Rector	Roger Gaudry, D.Sc.
Vice-Rector	**Lucien PICHE, Ph.D.**
General Treasurer	**Mr. Paul Huot.**

Faculty of Medicine

Dean and Director of Studies	**Lucien L. COUTU, M.D.**
Vice-Dean	**Eugene Robillard, M.D.**
Secretary	**François Archambault, M.D.**
Assistant to the Dean and Registrar	**Jean Frappier, M.D.**
Assistant to the Dean in charge of post-graduate studies	de Guise Vaillancourt, M.D.

Departmental Heads

Bacteriology	Sorin Sonea, M.D.
Biochemistry	Walter Verly M.D.
Experimental Medicine and Surgery	Hans Selye, M.D.
Obstetrics-Gynecology	Michel Berard, M.D.
Anatomy	Pierre Bois, M.D.
Medicine	Jacques Genest, M.D.
Physiology	Jean-Pierre Cordeau, M.D.
Pathology	Gilles Tremblay, M.D.
Pediatrics	Albert Royer, M.D.
Pharmacology	Aurèle Beaulnes, M.D.
Psychiatry	Gerard Beaudoin
Radiology	Jean-Louis Leger, M.D.
Surgery	Maurice Parent, M.D.

The present Faculty of Medicine of the University of Montreal was first established in Montreal and was incorporated in 1845 under the name of School of Medicine and Surgery of Montreal. Later on, in 1877, it became the Montreal Branch of Laval University Faculty of Medicine. This agreement was approved by the Legislature in 1891 and the School received the privilege of its autonomy in 1920. Thereafter by an Act of the Quebec Legislature, the School of Medicine and Surgery of Montreal was granted its independence and became the Faculty of Medicine of the University of Montreal. In 1925 the Faculty of Medicine was officially classed "A" by the American Medical Association.

General Information

The minimum period of professional training required by the University of Montreal as a qualification for a M.D. degree is 4 years. In order to get his licence, the student has to complete one-year rotating internship in hospitals approved by the College of Physicians and Surgeons of the Province of Quebec.

The medical curriculum includes instruction and laboratory cources in basic medical sciences at the University building, and clinical teaching in affiliated hospitals. There are four sessions of thirty-two weeks exclusive of examination periods. The sessions begin on the Tuesday following Labor Day.

Application for admission to the Faculty of Medicine must be made upon the regular application form which may be obtained from the Registrar.

Other Degrees

A course in Dietetics leading to a B.Sc(Nut'r.) and a programme of graduate work leading to M.Sc. and Ph. D. degrees are also provided by the Faculty of Medicine.

Technical Schools Administered by the Faculty

The Faculty of Medicine includes a School of Medical Technology (Director: Roger Beaulieu, M.D.) and a school of Rehabilitation, comprising two sections: A section of Physiotherapy, Occupational Therapy, and a section of Orthophony and Audiology (Director: Gustave Gingras, M.D.).

SHERBROOKE UNIVERSITY

Sherbrooke P. Q.

Tel. 569-7431

Dean	Dr. Gérald LaSalle
Vice-Dean	Dr. J.-M. Beauregard
Director of basic sciences	Dr. L.-Paul Dugal
Director of clinical sciences	Dr. Maurice LeClair
Director of social medicine	Dr. Roger Dufresne

General Information

The Faculty of Medicine of the University of Sherbrooke has been established in March, 1961. It is the first new Faculty of Medicine to be organized in the Province of Quebec since 1853.

The objectives of the Faculty of Medicine are to graduate practitioners of the best quality, to promote research and to raise the standards of the practice of medicine in the region of the Eastern Townships. The four-year Medical School is planned to be a part of an University Medical Center. The University Hospital will be a referral hospital serving the entire region.

The Faculty has accepted its first contingent of 24 students for September 1966.

SCHOOL OF HYGIENE
UNIVERSITY OF TORONTO, TORONTO, ONTARIO

Tel. 928-2741

Director	**A. J. Rhodes, M.D., F.R.C.P. (Edin), F.R.S.C.**
Associate Director	**M. H. Brown, O.B.E., M.D., B.Sc., D.P.H.**
Secretary	**D. L. MacLean, O.B.E., M.D., B.Sc., D.P.H.**
Assistant Secretary	**E. R. Langford, M.D., C.M., D.P.H.**

The School of Hygiene offers courses leading to the following diplomas: Diploma in Public Health; Diploma in Industrial Health; Diploma in Hospital Administration; Diploma in Dental Public Health; Diploma in Veterinary Public Health; Diploma in Bacteriology; Diploma in Nutrition; Certificate in Public Health.

Facilities are also provided for advanced graduate work leading to the following research degrees: Master of Applied Science, Master of Science, Doctor of Philosophy.

The School also provides instruction for undergraduates in Microbiology, Public Health and Preventive Medicine, Physiological Hygiene and Nutrition.

SCHOOL OF HYGIENE
UNIVERSITY OF MONTREAL, MONTREAL, P.Q.

Tel.: 733-9951

Dean	Maurice Panisset, Dr. V., D.M.V., F.R.C.S.
Vice Dean	Gilbert Blain, M.D., M.A.H.
Secretary	J. Denhez, M.D., D.H.P.

The School of Hygiene offers to French speaking students courses leading to the following diplomas: Diploma in Public Health, Diploma in Dental Public Health, Diploma in Veterinary Public Health, Master in Hospital Administration, Bachelor in Physical Education, Certificate in Public Health, Licence in Hygiene (Sanitary Education).

Facilities are also provided in the Department of Environmental Health, for work leading to the following degrees: Master of Science, Hygiene (environment), Doctor of Sciences, Hygiene (environment).

QUEEN'S UNIVERSITY

Kingston **Ont.**

Tel. 546-3871

Chancellor	J. B. Stirling, B.A., B.Sc., D.Sc., LL.D.
Principal and Vice-Chancellor	J. A. Corry, LL.B., B.C.L., LL.D., F.R.S.C.
Rector	L. W. Brockington, C.M.G., Q.C., D.C.L., LL.D.
Dean of the Faculty of Medicine	E. H. Botterell, O.B.E., M.D., M.S., F.R.C.S.(C.)
Associate Dean	J. B. Firstbrook, M.D., Ph.D.
Director of Continuing Education	H. G. Kelly, M.D., C.M., F.R.C.P.(C.)

Departmental Heads

Anaesthesiology	S. L. Vandewater, M.D., F.R.C.P.(C.)
Anatomy	J. V. Basmajian, M.D.
Biochemistry	P. B. Hagen, M.D., B.S.
Diagnostic Radiology	S. L. Fransman, M.D., F.R.C.P.(C.)
Medicine	W. F. Connell, M.D., C.M., F.R.C.P.(C.)
Microbiology and Immunology	N. A. Hinton, M.D., C.M., M.Sc.(Med.)
Obstetrics and Gynaecology	J. A. Low, M.D., F.R.C.S.(C.)
Opthalmology	D. A. Rosen, B.Sc., M.D., C.M., F.R.C.S.(C.)
Otorhinolaryngology (Acting)	J. R. Purvis, M.D., C.M.
Paediatrics	A. M. Bryans, M.D., F.R.C.P.(C.)
Pathology	R. H. More, M.D., M.Sc., F.R.C.P.(C.)
Pharmacology	E. M. Boyd, M.A., M.D., C.M.
Physiology	J. D. Hatcher, M.D., Ph.D.
Psychiatry	R. C. A. Hunter, M.D., C.M.
Public Health and Preventive Medicine	J. H. Read, B.Sc., M.D., C.M., D.P.H.
Rehabilitation Medicine	To be appointed
Surgery	J. R. McCorriston, B.A., M.D., C.M., M.Sc., F.R.C.S.(C.)
Therapeutic Radiology	R. C. Burr, M.D., C.M., F.R.C.S.(C.)
Urology	A. W. Bruce, M.B., Ch.B., F.R.C.S.(C.)

Queen's University owes its origin to the efforts of the Synod of the Presbyterian Church in Canada to found a college at Kingston along the lines of the Scottish National Universities. On October 16, 1841, a Royal Charter was issued and the first classes were opened at Kingston in March, 1842. The Faculty of Medicine was established in 1854. In 1866, it was reorganized as the Royal College of Physicians and Surgeons in affiliation with the University, but, in 1891, the original status was resumed.

The Medical Course

The course consists of two premedical and four medical years leading to the degree of Doctor of Medicine. Students are admitted to the first premedical year on completion of Senior Matriculation requirements. A number of places in the first medical year are available to candidates who have credit for two or three years of university work beyond Senior Matriculation, including at least two years of Chemistry (General and Organic), one year of Physics, and one year of Biology. Preference is given to candidates with university degrees. Further information may be obtained from the Office of the Dean, Faculty of Medicine.

Courses for Graduates

In co-operation with the School of Graduate Studies, courses are offered leading to the degrees of Master of Science and Doctor of Philosophy. Diploma courses in Anaesthesiology, Radiology, and Surgery are also offered. In the clinical departments, training is provided to meet the requirements for certification and fellowship of the Royal College of Physicians and Surgeons of Canada.

Continuing Education

An active program of continuing medical education for physicians includes weekly lectures, special courses, and decentralized clinics.

UNIVERSITY OF OTTAWA

Ottawa **Ont.**

Tel. 235-6751

Rector	Very Rev. Roger Guindon, O.M.I., B.A., L.Ph., D.Th.
Dean of the Faculty of Medicine	**J. Jacques Lussier, M.D., Ph.D.**
Associate Dean	Joseph Auer, M.D., D.Sc.
Assistant Dean	**R. Kennedy Smiley, M.D., C.M., F.R.C.P.(C).**
Secretary of the Faculty Council	**J. J. Day, M.D., C.M., D.P.H.**
Assistant Treasurer	**Reverend F.-X. Lefebvre, o.m.i., L.Ph., L.Th.**
Medical Librarian	Maurice Alarie, B.A., B.L.S.

Departmental Heads

Anatomy	**Joseph Auer, M.D., D.Sc.**
Bacteriology	John C. N. Westwood, B.A., M.B., B.Ch., M.R.C.S., L.R.C.S.
Biochemistry	A. D'Iorio, Ph.D.
Gynacology & Obstetrics	Arthur L. Richard, M.D.
History of Medicine	**to be named**
Histology & Embryology	**Léonard-F. Bélanger, M.D., M.A.Med.Sc.**
Medicine	R. Kennedy Smiley, M.D., C.M., F.R.C.P.(C)
Ophthalmology (Acting)	Donald Allen, M.D., C.M.
Otolaryngology (Acting)	Guy Laframboise, B.A., M.D.
Paediatrics	Dominick J. Conway, M.D.
Pathology	Desmond Magner, M.D., B.Sc.Med.
Pharmacology	George M. Ling, B.A., M.A., Ph.D.
Physiology	Margaret Beznak, M.D.
Psychiatry	F. C. R. Chalke, M.D., M.Sc. (Exec. Dir.)
Preventive Medicine	John J. Day, M.D., C.M., D.P.H.
Radiology	C. J. Don, M.B., B.S.
Surgery	J. Burke Ewing, M.D., C.M.

Established in September, 1945, the Faculty of Medicine of the University of Ottawa now offers the complete undergraduate course. Its first graduates received their doctorate in Medicine on May 26th, 1951.

Requirements

The Faculty of Medicine limits each pre-medical year registration to forty students who are selected on the basis of their qualifications. Applications for admission or requests for information are to be addressed to the Dean. Applications for admission to the pre-medical years will be accepted until August 15th. Applications for admission to the medical years should be completed before July 1st.

Medical Course

The course consists of two years of premedical work and four years of medicine.

Graduate Training

Facilities are available for a limited number of graduate students to work towards the M.Sc. of the Ph.D. degree in the basic sciences. Requests for information should be addressed directly to the Head of the Department concerned.

The Ottawa General Hospital and the Ottawa Civic Hospital, the main teaching hospitals of the Faculty, have also been approved by the Royal College of Physicians and Surgeons for graduate training in the various medical specialties.

Research Funds

Arrangements may be made to carry on research in the departments of the Medical School.

UNIVERSITY OF TORONTO

Toronto **Ont.**

Tel. 928-2710

President	C. T. BISSELL, M.A., Ph.D., D.Litt., LL.D., FRSC.
Registrar & Director of Student Services	R. ROSS, M.B.E., M.A.,
Dean of the Faculty of Medicine	A. L. CHUTE, M.A., M.D., Ph.D., FRCP(C)
Associate Deans	Ian MacDonald, FRCP (Lond.), FRCP(C), FACP F. G. Kergin, M.A. (Oxon), M.D., M.S., FRCS (Eng.), FRCS(C), FACS E. A. Sellers, M.D., Ph.D. J. W. Steiner, M.D.
Executive Assistant to the Dean	R. O. Benson, B. Comm.
Secretary of the Faculty	Miss M. L. Cassidy, B.A.

Departmental Heads

Anaesthesia	R. A. Gordon, M.D.
Anatomy	J. S. Thompson, M.A., M.D.
Biochemistry	G. E. Connell, B.A., Ph.D.
Bacteriology	P. H. Greey, M.D.
Medical Biophysics	H. E. Johns, Ph.D., Ll.D.
Medicine	K. J. R. Wightman, M.D.
Obstetrics & Gyn.	W. M. Paul, M.D.
Ophthalmology	J. C. McCulloch, M.D.
Otolaryngology	D. P. Bryce, M.D.
Paediatrics	
Pathological Chemistry	A. G. Gornall, B.A., Ph.D.
Pathology	A. C. Ritchie, M.B., Ch.B., D.Phil.
Pharmacology	W. Kalow, M.D.
Physiology	R. E. Haist, M.D., Ph.D.
Psychiatry	A. B. Stokes, B.M., B.Ch.
Radiology	R. B. Holmes, M.D., M.Sc.
Surgery	W. R. Drucker, B.S., M.D.
Therapeutics	
Art as applied to Medicine	Miss Nancy Joy
Div. of Rehabilitation Medicine	A. T. Jousse, M.D.
Div. of Postgraduate Medical Education	Ian MacDonald, M.D.
Banting & Best Department of Medical Research	C. H. Best, M.D.

The school was founded in 1843 as the Medical Faculty of King's College, discontinued in 1853 and re-established in 1887. The medical faculty of Victoria University became affiliated with this faculty in 1902, and the medical faculty of Trinity University in 1903.

The course consists of two premedical years and four professional years, at the end of which the degree of Doctor of Medicine is conferred. A student who has a degree in Arts or Science may be admitted to the first professional year and complete the course in four years.

Affiliated teaching hospitals are: Toronto General Hospital, Toronto Western Hospital, St. Michael's Hospital, Toronto Psychiatric Hospital, Hospital for Sick Children, Sunnybrook Hospital, Women's College Hospital, Wellesley Hospital, Princess Margaret Hospital, New Mount Sinai Hospital, Lyndhurst Lodge.

Other Degrees

The degree of Bachelor of Science (Medicine) may be conferred for special work or investigation, as a graduate degree, or under certain circumstances for an extra year's work as an undergraduate.

The degree of Master of Surgery may be conferred on graduates who have completed three years' postgraduate training in surgery beyond a general interneship, and one further year's training in the teaching hospitals of the University of Toronto, during which time they must be registered in the School of Graduate Studies of the University.

The degree of Doctor of Clinical Science is offered in the School of Graduate Studies. Candidates must be graduates in Medicine and have had one year of hospital internship. The four year course includes study and investigation in both a basic science and a clinical department.

The following courses leading to a Diploma are offered by the Faculty:

Diploma in: Industrial Health; Psychiatry; Medical Radiology; Anaesthesia.

Organized graduate courses in Medicine, Surgery, Obstetrics & Gynaecology, Ophthalmology, Oto-Laryngology, Anaesthesia, Psychiatry are offered by the Faculty in conjunction with the affiliated teaching hospitals. (Address enquiries to the Secretary, Div. of Postgraduate Medical Education, University of Toronto.)

UNIVERSITY OF WESTERN ONTARIO

London, Ont.

Tel. 679-2111

Official Visitor	W. Earl Rowe, P.C., Lieutenant-Governor of Ontario
Chancellor	Verschoyle P. Cronyn, A.F.C., E.D.
President & Vice-Chancellor	G. Edward Hall, M.S.A., M.D., Ph.D., LL.D., Des S., F.R.S.C.
Vice-President	Ross Baxter Willis, M.A.
Vice-President (Health Sciences)	Orlando Harold Warwick, M.A., M.D., C.M., LL.D., Mt. Allison
Comptroller	Robert Ross Glover, B.A.
Registrar	J. Keith Watson, M.A., Ph.D.

Faculty of Medicine

Dean	Douglas Bocking, M.D., F.R.C.P.(C), F.A.C.P.
Medical Librarian	M. Anne Seheult, B.A., New Brunswick, B.L.S., McGill

Departmental Heads

Anaesthesia	Wolfgang Eberhart Gottfried Alfred Spoerel, M.D., F.R.C.P.(C)
Anatomy	Murray Llewellyn Barr, B.A., M.Sc., M.D., LL.D., Queen's and Toronto, F.R.S.C., F.R.C.P.(C), F.A.C.P., F.R.S.C.
Bacteriology & Immunology	Robert George Everitt Murray, B.A., Cantab., M.A., Cantab., M.D.C.M., F.R.S.C.
Biochemistry	Harold Brown Stewart, M.D., Toronto, Ph.D., ibid, Ph. D. (Cantab.)
Biophysics	Alan Chadburn Burton, M.B.E., B.Sc.(Lond.), M.A., Toronto, Ibid., Ph.D., L.L.D., Alberta, F.R.S.C.
Medical Research (Acting Head)	Kenneth Kitchener Carroll, B.Sc., New Brunswick, M.Sc., ibid., M.A., Ph.D. Toronto
Medicine	Ramsay Willis Gunton, M.D., D.Phil. (Oxon), F.R.C.P.(C), F.A.C.P.
Obstetrics & Gynaecology	Robert Arthur Hugh Kinch, M.R.C.S.(Eng.), L.R.C.P.-(Lond.), M.B., B.S., M.R.C.O.G., F.R.C.S.(C)
Ophthalmology	Charles Dyson, M.D., D.Oph.
Otology, Rhinology & Laryngology	Robert Edward Greenway, M.D., F.R.C.S.(C).
Paediatrics	John Campbell Rathbun, M.D., F.R.C.P.(C), F.A.A.P.
Pathological Chemistry	Abram Herman Neufeld, B.Sc., Manitoba, M.Sc., Ph.D., M.D., C.M., McGill, F.C.I.C.
Pathology	Alexander Cameron Wallace, B.A., M.D.
Pharmacology	Charles Willis Gowdey, B.A., M.Sc., D.Phil. (Oxon)
Physical Medicine & Rehabilitation	Malcolm Gair Peter Cameron, M.D., F.R.C.P.(C).
Physiology	James Alexander Franklin Stevenson, B.A., McGill, M.A., ibid., M.D.C.M. ibid.
Psychiatry & Preventive Medicine	George Edgar Hobbs, B.A., M.D., M.P.H., F.R.C.P.(C)
Radiology, Diagnostic	Gerald Goodall Copestake, B.A. (Cantab.), M.R.C.S. (Eng.), L.R.C.P. (Lond.), D.M.R.D. (Edin.).
Radiology, Therapeutic	Thomas Alastair Watson, M.B., Ch.B., D.M.R., M.D., Saskatchewan, F.A.C.R.
Surgery	Angus Duncan McLachlin, M.D., M.Sc., D.Phil.(Oxon.), M.S., F.R.C.S.(C), F.R.C.S.(Eng.), F.A.C.S.

The Medical Course at The University of Western Ontario covers four years, and students may be admitted to the first year in the Faculty of Medicine from a variety of educational backgrounds, provided that the minimum requirements for scientific subjects are satisfied.

Applicants from outside this University should apply to the Registrar for the necessary entrance requirements.

Graduate Training in Clinical Specialties

Facilities are available through the University and Affiliated Hospitals for training in the Departments of Anaesthesia, Internal Medicine, Surgery, Paediatrics, Obstetrics and Gynaecology, Ophthalmology, Otology, Rhinology and Laryngology, Psychiatry, Pathology, Diagnostic Radiology, and Therapeutic Radiology. The details of the training in the various specialties can be obtained from the Heads of the Departments concerned. The courses have been devised to meet the requirements of The Royal College of Physicians and Surgeons, either for Certification of Specialists or Fellowship examination.

Applications will be received from graduates who are taking or who have taken their junior interneship.

Graduates in Medicine, who have completed the required postgraduate training in a clinical department of the Faculty of Medicine, are eligible for the Degree of Master of Clinical Science (M.Cl.Sc.) provided that they have passed the Examinations for Fellowship in the Royal College and have presented and defended a thesis on original work.

Interested graduates should consult the Calendar of the Faculty of Graduate Studies for further details.

UNIVERSITY OF MANITOBA

Winnipeg Man.

Tel. GR 4-9110

President	H. H. SAUNDERSON, M.Sc., Ph.D., LL.D., F.C.I.C.
Dean, Medical Faculty	Lennox G. BELL, M.B.E., M.D., LL.D., F.R.C.P.(C) & (Lond.), F.A.C.P.
Associate Dean, Medical Faculty	T. W. Fyles, M.D., M.Sc. (Man.), F.R.C.P.(C), F.A.C.P.

Departmental Heads

Anatomy	Keith L. Moore, B.A., M.Sc., Ph.D. (W. Ont.)
Bacteriology & Immunology	J. C. Wilt, M.D., M.Sc., F.A.C.P.
Biochemistry	M. C. Blanchaer, B.A., M.D., C.M.(Queens).
Medicine	J. P. Gemmell, M.D., M.R.C.P.(Lond.) F.R.C.P.(C).
Obstetrics & Gynaecology	T. M. Roulston, M.B., B.Ch., B.A.O.(Queen's U. Belfast), F.R.C.O.G.
Ophthalmology	G. M. Krolman, B.Sc., M.D., D.O., F.R.C.S., (Ed. & C.)
Otolaryngology	W. A. Alexander, M.D.
Paediatrics	Harry Medovy, B.A., M.D., F.R.C.P.(C).
Pathology	J. P. Wyatt, M.D.
Pharmacology	M. Nickerson, M.D.(Utah), A.B.(Linfield), ScM.(Brown), Ph.D(Johns Hopkins)
Physiology & Medical Research	J. Doupe, M.D., M.R.C.P. (Lond.) F.A.C.P.
Psychiatry	G. C. Sisler, M.D., F.R.C.P.(C).
Radiology	D. W. MacEwan, B.Sc., M.D., C.M., (McGill), F.R.C.P.(C)
Social & Preventive Med.	Roper G. Cadham, M.D., D.P.H.
Surgery	Colin C. Ferguson, M.D., F.R.C.S.(C), F.A.C.S., A.B.S.

In 1883 thirteen physicians applied to the local legislature for a charter to form Manitoba Medical College. Dr. James Kerr was the Dean and Dr. James Patterson, Registrar. Dr. Kerr delivered an introductory lecture on November 15th, 1883, and the first lectures of the medical course were given in the Central Collegiate Building on November 21st. The first practical work was done in a cottage on Isabel Street. With funds entirely furnished by members of the Faculty, a building was erected on the corner of McDermot and Kate Streets, and was utilized for teaching purposes during the second session. The College from its beginning, was affiliated with the University of Manitoba and the first graduating class of six students received their degrees from the University in May, 1886.

Present Course

The present medical course at the University of Manitoba is of four years' duration, and full details may be secured from the Registrar. Application for admission should be made before April 30th.

Degrees Offered

The degrees offered are Doctor of Medicine (M.D.), Bachelor of Science in Medicine (B.Sc.Med.), Master of Science (M.Sc.), and Doctor of Philosophy (Ph.D.).

Post Graduate Courses in Medicine

Special Tutorial Courses planned as preparations for examination and certification by the Royal College of Physicians and Surgeons of Canada have been arranged as occasion arises. If there are requests for similar courses, it is likely that they will be offered. The Departments of Psychiatry and Surgery offer comprehensive four-year graduate training programmes, approved by the Royal College of Physicians and Surgeons of Canada, for specialty examination qualifications in psychiatry, surgery and Anaesthesia. Details may be obtained at the Dean's office. Graduate training is under the Faculty of Graduate Studies and Research. Courses may be arranged with various Departments.

UNIVERSITY OF SASKATCHEWAN

Saskatoon **Sask.**

Tel. CH. 2-7671

President	J. W. T. Spinks, M.B.E., Ph.D., D.Sc., F.R.S.C.
Registrar	N. K. Cram, B.A., B.Ed.
Dean of the Faculty of Medicine	R. W. Begg, M.D., C.M., D.Phil., F.R.C.P.(C).

Departmental Heads

Anaesthesia	G. M. Wyant, M.D.
Anatomy	S. Fedoroff, Ph.D.
Bacteriology	G. Dempster, M.B., Ch.B., M.D.
Biochemistry	C. S. McArthur, Ph.D.
Cancer Research	J. F. Morgan, Ph.D.
Diagnostic Radiology	H. P. Kent, M.B., B.Chir.
Medicine	A. A. Bailey, M.D.
Obstetrics and Gynecology	A. B. Brown, M.D.
Ophthalmology	R. G. Murray, M.D.
Paediatrics	J. W. Gerrard, B.M., B.Ch., D.M.
Pathology	D. F. Moore, M.D.
Physiology and Pharmacology	L. B. Jaques, Ph.D.
Psychiatry	D. G. McKerracher, M.D.
Rehabilitation Medicine	T. E. Hunt, M.D.
Social and Preventive Medicine	V. L. Matthews, M.D.
Surgery	E. M. Nanson, M.B., Ch.B.
Therapeutic Radiology	C. C. Burkell, M.D.

The University prepares students for entrance to medicine and dentistry and offers a full medical course. The affiliated University Hospital opened with 550 beds in January, 1955. Instruction is carried out also in St. Paul's and Saskatoon City Hospitals and the Saskatoon Sanatorium, as well as the Regina General and Grey Nuns' Hospitals in Regina.

For students completing at least two years of Medicine who wish to undertake additional study in one or more of the basic medical sciences, a course is offered leading to the degree of Bachelor of Science in Medicine—B.Sc. (Med.).

Admission

The number of students admitted to the first year of the medical course is limited to 50. Of this number approximately ten percent may come from outside the province. The selection will depend upon university records, selected references, interviews and general qualifications, as well as the scores of the Medical College Admission Test, which must be taken previously.

Applications for admission should be made in writing to the Dean of the College of Medicine before February 15th.

The regulations governing admission and the required classes of the premedical year will be found in the Calendar of General Information.

Registration

Registration first and second-year students will be September 20, 21, — third and fourth year students will register on August 30.

UNIVERSITY OF ALBERTA

Edmonton **Alta.**

Tel. GE 9-8721

President	**W. H. Johns, B.A., Ph.D**
Registrar	**A. D. Cairns, B.A.**
Bursar	**J. M. Whidden, B.Com.**
Dean of the Faculty of Medicine	W. C. MacKenzie, M.D.
Associate Dean	D. F. Cameron, M.D.

Departmental Heads

Anaesthesiology	E. A. Gain, M.D.
Anatomy	**T. S. Leeson, M.D.**
Bacteriology	F. L. Jackson, M.D.
Biochemistry	J. S. Colter, Ph.D.
Medicine	D. R. Wilson, M.D.
Obstetrics and Gynaecology	W. Paul, M.D.
Paediatrics	J. K. Martin, M.D
Pathology	J. W. Macgregor, M.D.
Pharmacology	E. E. Daniel, Ph.D.
Physiology	M. Schacter, M.D.
Preventive Medicine	S. Greenhill, M.D.
Psychiatry	K. A. Yonge, M.D.
Radiology	F. McConnell, M.D.
Surgery	R. A. Macbeth, M.D.

The Faculty of Medicine of the University of Alberta was founded in 1913. The principal course offered leads to the M.D. degree. The number of candidates accepted for entrance into the first year of the programme is restricted. All students who wish to enter are required to make application to the Registrar, University of Alberta by April 1st each year.

The course leading to the degree of M.D. is a four year programme following a minimum of 2 years University work.

Other Degrees

A Bachelor of Science in Medicine, degree programme, is available to Medical Students or graduates who have not obtained a previous Bachelor's degree and who take one year special training in one of the departments of the medical faculty with the approval of the Faculty of Medicine.

The degrees of M.Sc. and Ph.D. are obtainable in certain departments of the Faculty. Candidates for these degrees are under the jurisdiction of the Faculty of Graduate Studies, University of Alberta.

A full programme of graduate training in all clinical specialties is available under the direction of a Faculty Committee on Graduate Training.

Continuing Medical Studies

An active programme in Continuing Medical Education, is conducted by the faculty in co-operation with the College of Physicians & Surgeons of Alberta.

Allied Training

A course in Medical Laboratory Science leading to a B.Sc., M.L.S., degree is conducted under the jurisdiction of the Faculty of Medicine. The Faculty of Medicine is in close co-operation with a School of Nursing and a School of Rehabilitation Medicine.

UNIVERSITY OF BRITISH COLUMBIA

Vancouver B. C.

Tel. CA 4-1111

Visitor	**Major-General The Honourable George R. Pearkes, V.C., P.C., C.B., D.S.O., M.C., LL.D., Lieutenant-Governor of British Columbia**
Chancellor	**Phyllis G. Ross, C.B.E., M.A., LL.D.**
President	**John B. Macdonald, D.D.S., M.S., Ph.D., A.M., LL.D. (Man.), F.A.C.D.**
Dean, Medical Faculty	**John F. McCREARY, M.D.**
Associate Dean	Donald C. Graham, M.D.

Departmental Heads

Anatomy	Sydney M. Friedman, M.D.
Biochemistry	Marvin Darrach, Ph.D.
Cancer Research Centre	Robert L. Noble, M.D., Director
Continuing Med. Education	Donald H. Williams, M.D.
History of Medicine & Science	William C. Gibson, M.D.
Medicine	Robert B. Kerr, O.B.E., M.D
Obstetrics & Gynaecology	Fred E. Bryans, M.D.
Paediatrics	**Sydney Israels, M.D.**
Pathology	Harold E. Taylor, M.D.
Pharmacology	James G. Foulks, M.D.
Physiology	D. Harold Copp, M.D.
Psychiatry	James S. Tyhurst, M.D
Preventive Medicine	G. R. F. Elliot, M.D. (Acting)
School of Rehabilitation Medicine	Brock M. **Fahrni, M.D.,** Director
Surgery	Cameron Harrison, M.D.

The medical course extends through four academic sessions and leads to the degree of Doctor of Medicine (M.D.). The purpose is to provide graduates with the basic knowledge required for the modern practice of medicine.

The first two years of the course are devoted primarily to acquiring a knowledge of the preclinical medical sciences, and for the most part are given on the campus of the University. At the beginning of the Second Year, instruction is transferred in part to the Vancouver General Hospital, Shaughnessy Hospital and St. Paul's Hospital.

The Third and Fourth Years of the course are designed to bring the student into contact with patients and to develop, not only a knowledge of the natural history of diseases and how to recognize them, but also the essentials of modern treatment. In addition to the hospitals previously mentioned, during the clinical years the facilities of the Children's Hospital, Grace Hospital, the Provincial Mental Hospital, and G. F. Strong Rehabilitation Centre are also utilized for clinical teaching.

Classes entering the First Year of Medicine are limited to sixty students. All entrants are required to have completed a minimum of 3 years in a Faculty of Arts and Science beyond Grade XII.

In British Columbia, the College of Physicians and Surgeons requires that in addition to holding the certificate of the Medical Council of Canada an applicant must have served a one-year rotating interneship in an approved hospital before being eligible for a licence to practice.

Courses for Graduate Students

In co-operation with the Faculty of Graduate Studies, courses are offered in the preclinical departments leading to the degrees of Master of Arts or Master of Science and Doctor of Philosophy. In the department of Psychiatry, courses are offered leading to the degree of Master of Science. In the clinical departments, training is available directed towards Certification and Fellowship of the Royal College of Physicians and Surgeons of Canada.

GRADUATES IN MEDICINE 1966

Dalhousie University

Ali, Muntaz
Archambault, John L.
Baker, David A.
Beck, C. Adeline
Bessonnette, John R. W.
Blackie, Peter B.
Bloom, Harold R.
Brake, Robert J.
Caines, L. William
Cameron, Mary F.
Canfield, M. Joyce
Casey, Joan I.
Christie, Garth B.
Covert, Mrs. Kersti
Covert, William H. N.
Crocker, John F. S.
Duncan, Jeanne R.
Dunn, J. Michael
Edstrom, Henry W.
Finch, Graham C.
Frecker, Richard C.
Freedman, Melvin H.
Gailiunas, Vytautas R.
Graham, Michael R.
Harvey, Neil G.
Hong, Kim E.
Inglis, Douglas S.
Jamieson, W. R. Eric
Leavitt, P. M.
Macdonald, Alexander G.
MacDonald, G. Vernon A.
MacKay, W. Allan
MacKenzie, B. Ross
MacSween, H. Miller
Martin, Robert H.
Miller, J. Lance
Nichols, Peter R.
Paster, Robert H.
Piper, W. Archibald A.
Pollett, Harry F. L.
Roberts, Robert
Rushton, Donald K.
Sanders, David H.
Sapp, George A.
Scantlebury, Thomas H.
Smith, Frances M.
Squires, William G.
Strober, Morton
Stuart, Ronald D.
Sutherland, Doris Y.
Tiller, William D.
Tong, Q. L. Raymond
Velcoff, Shirley M.
Webster, Russell D.
Wight, Harold G.
Yoell, Barry J.

Laval University

Angers, Jocelyn
Bastarache, Edouard
Beaulieu, Jean-Pierre
Beaupre, Andre
Bedard, Robert
Belanger, Claude
Bergeron, Jacques
Bernard, André
Bessette, Réal
Bilodeau, Gilles
Biron, Roger
Blanchet, Michel
Boivin, Georges
Borgeat, Francois
Bouchard, Jean-Guy
Bouchard, Remi
Bouchard, Victor
Boucher, Jean-Guy
Bourassa, Gérard
Bournival, Bertrande
Boutet, Jacques
Boutin, Rodrigue
Brassard, André
Brousseau, Yves
Cormier, Gilles
Dagneault, Yves
D'Anjou, Guy
Demers, Georges
Denault, Yves
Desjarlais, Nicole
Dorion, Pierre
Dorval, Jean
Doucet, Paul
Drolet, Pierre
Dufour, André
Dugal, Paul
Dumont, Jacques
Dumont, Yves
Dupuy, André
Drapeau, Gaston
Fournier, André
Gagnon, Raymonde
Gamache, Alain
Gerin-Lajoie, Jean
Gilbert, Marcel
Girard, Claude
Goulet, Claude
Grenier, Réjean
Grondin, Gaétan
Hamel, Jean-Yves
Houde, Jacques
Hudon, Jacques
Hudon, Marcel
Jolicoeur, Claude
Keighan, Leslie
Laberge, Jean-Guy
Labonte, André
Laflamme, Marc
Lagace, Réal
Lainesse, André
Lajoie, Yvon
Laliberte, Jean
Lamonde, Denis
Lamontagne, René
Landry, René
Langis, Louis
Laperriere, Pierre
Larochelle, Réal
Larouche, Léon-M.
Laverdiere, Jacques
Lavoie, Claude-André
Lebel, Marcel
Leclerc, André
Leclerc, Jean-Louis
Lemaire, Jean-René
Lemire, Guy
Lemire, Yvon
Lepage, Michel
Letendre, Jacques
L'Heureux, Guy
Litalien, Albert
Malenfant, Mario
Malouin, Georges
Mathon, Gilles
Mercier, Gilles
Morin, Gilles
Morissette, Pierre
Nadeau, Richard
Naud, Yvon
Ouellet, Henri
Painchaud, Georges
Paquin, Jacques
Pelletier, Jean-Guy
Petitclerc, Michel
Petitclerc, Micheline
Poirier, Gérard
Poitras, André
Poulin, Pierre
Proulx, Roland
Rheault, Michel
Roberge, Louis
Robitaille, Guy
Robitaille, Raymond
Rochon, Jean
Rodrigue, Jean-Marie
Rodrigue, Pierre
Roy, Jacques
Saint-Hilaire, Richard
Samson, Jean
Samson, Pierre
Soucy, Jacques
Soucy, Paul-Eugéne
Talbot, Jean
Tanguay, Bernadette
Theriault, Gilles
Thivierge, Jean-Claude
Tremblay, Normenn
Turcotte, Giles
Turcotte, Jean-Jacques
Villeneuve, Claude

GRADUATES IN MEDICINE — 1966 *(cont'd.)*

University of Montreal

Allard, Michel
Archambault, Jacques
Baillargeon, Marielle
Beauregard, Hugues
Bergeron, Zotique
Boileau, Camille (Mlle)
Boutin, Guy
Bovo, Michel-Ange Pierre
Brais, Maurice
Breton, Claude
Brodeur, André
Brosseau, André
Brossoit, Jacques
Brunet, Robert
Cardinal, Jean
Choquet, Yves
Clement, Claude
Cote, Pierre
D'Amour, Monique
Desaulniers, Denis
Desjardins, Gilles
Desjardins, Louis-Philippe André
Drainville, Yvon
Dube, Michel B.
Dussault, Gilles
Ferland, André
Forget, Pierre L.
Fortier, Robert
Gaboury, Jean
Gagnon, Jean
Gagnon, Roger
Galarneau, Pierre
Gelinas, Marcien
Gendron, Jean-Paul
Gingras, Jean-Marie
Girard, Robert
Giroux, Pierre Francois
Grand'Maison, Yvon
Helie, Robert
Jodoin, Marcel
Lafortune, Michel
Lafreniere, Bernard
Lalumiere, Robert
Lanctot-Bedard, Ghislaine
Landry, Madeleine
Langevin, Michel
Lapierre, Yves
Larochelle, Yves
Lassonde, Jean
Lassonde, Robert
Latreille, Bernard
Latrielle, Jean-Marie
Lavallee, Paul
Lavallee, Pierre
Lavigueur, Jean
Leblanc, Claude
Leblanc, Jude
Leclaire, Richard
Leduc, Maurice
Leger, Serge
Lemay, Jacques
Lemlin, Pierre
L'Esperance, Pierre
Levesque, Jacques Pierre
Maillette, Jean-Clément
Malo, Jacques
Marin, Pierre
Martimbeau, Pierre
Masse, André
Meloche, Jacques
Menard, Guy
Messier, Réal
Mital, Bernard
Monday, Jacques
Monier, Danielle
Montplaisir, Jacques
Montplaisir, Serge
Morazain, Louis
Myre, Maurice
Nobert, Léo
Noel de Tilly, Ferdinand
Poitras, Robert
Potvin, Claude
Prescott, Lise
Provost, Jacques
Rajotte, Jacques
Raymond, Gilles
Raymond, Yvon
Rheault, Bernard
Rioux, André J. A.
Robert, Jean-Luc
Robitaille, Yvon
Rochon, Marcel
Rollin, Pierre
Rossignol, Jean-Serge
Roy, Jean-Guy
Royer, Marie
Spire, Jean-Paul Charles
St-Georges, Guy
Stebenne, Rodrigue
Sullivan, Normand
Teasdale, Francois
Thibault, Maurice
Trempe, Germain
Trempe, Jocelyne
Trudeau, Adéle
Turcotte, Fernand
Turgeon, J-Maurice
Vallee, Arthur Claude
Viger, Pierre

McGill University

Aikman, Robert H.
Barnes, Alan J.
Belman, David A. J.
Ber, Abram
Bishop, Ralph M.
Boloten, Sidney M.
Bruneau, Charles D.
Burggraf, Gary W.
Chandler, Stephen G.
Chiu, Kevin K.
Cohen, Lorne
Cole, Andrew T.
Cook, P. Joan
Courey, Norman L.
Csordas, James E.
Doyle, Brian B.
Eastman, Harvey W.
Fewer, Derek
Freeman, Joel B.
Geggie, Peter H. S.
Gelfand, Erwin W.
Gilday, David L.
Girey, George J. D.
Golde, David W.
Greer, Thomas
Hall, Gordon W.
Hall, Susanne
Hayes, Hamilton R.
Humphreys, Peter
Jaggassar, Theo A.
Jamison, James C.
Johnson, Richard A.
Jones, Barry H.
Killam, Donald A.
Kleinberg, Frederic
Kraus, Paul A.
Lacoursiere, Roy B.
Lander, Philip H. F.
Lefcoe, Michael S.
Louey, Julian P.
Lutz, Harold P.
McEwen, Diane M.
McGuire, Peter F.
MacKenzie, Richard G.
MacLean, William C.
MacLeish, M. Heather
Macko, Irene
Matlin, Arnold H.
Mauer, S. Michael
Meldrum, Donald A. N.
Messenger, Orville J.
Millington, Vivian B.
Mitchell, Richard W.
Morse, Frank P.
Morton, Brian C.
Moscovitz, Walter
Moseley, Colin F.
Navach, Joseph H.
Ng, Raymond C. W.
Ogilvy, Caroline G.
Orr, Robert D.
Osborne, Raymond L.
Owens, Milton L.
Parker, Lewis P.
Peckhold, John C.
Peterson, Perry A.
Popkin, David R.
Portner, Oliver T.
Portnoy, Joseph
Price, Lawrence A.
Rogala, Eugene J.
Ross, David M.
Shapera, Ronald M.
Shuster, David N.
Silver, Hulbert K. B.
Silverberg, Harvey H.
Somerville, Gordon W.
Spaulding, Stephen W.
Straker, Norman L.
Sue, David W.
Sutton, J. Carl
Tessler, Irving
Thirlwell, Michael P.
Trimingham, J. Lock
Uhrich, Philip C.
Van Nimwegan, Donald
Vargas, Roberto F.
Vinger, Irving
Wainger, Susan
Weller, Sydney L.
Whelchel, Lynn W.
Zidulka, Arnold
Zimmerman, C. Benjamin

GRADUATES IN MEDICINE — 1966 *(cont'd.)*

University of Ottawa

Alexander, C. J.
Alexis, H. C.
Ambis, R. J. S.
Ballon, L. L.
Beaudry, C. J.
Benoit, P. J.
Biro, J. E.
Camirand, P.
Cartier, P. F.
Cochrane, B. M.
Comerford, T. A. M.
Damanka, E. S. K.
DePetrillo, D. A.
Falzarano, J. S.
Fleming, C. L.
Gershon, S.
Gittens, R. O.
Govan, W. R.
Griswold, J. F.
Gyurik, C. E.
Hanny, T. A.
Hauser, D. J.
Hyde, B. M.
James, Mary Ann
Johnston, B. G.
Kunkel, A. B.
Lapine, T. J.
Landry, S. G.
Lazar, M. L.
Lebel, J. S.
Lemire, J. G.
Lemoine, G. T.
Lewis, R. J.
Low, G.
Mazerolle, B.
Noonan, A. P.
O'Driscoll, R. G.
Patry, M.
Polomeno, R.
Pouliot, M.
Regoli, R. L.
Rémillard, G. M.
Rock, W. J.
Schwarz, G.
Smith, Mary
Tazzeo, J. J.
Tétreault, C. M.
Trempe, C.

Queen's University

Armstrong, Paul Wayne
Batley, William James
Baumber, John Scott
Biggar, William Douglas
Bobechke, Peter Edward
Chambers, Robert Tully
Chang, Keith Ronald
Clugston, Keith Lloyd
Connor, Calvin Wendell
Cormode, Edward James
Daly, Donald Stuart
Delaney, William Sandford
Dobkin, Martin Lyon
Dorey, James Michael Francis
Fellows, George Fraser
Ferguson, Ronald Allan
McWalters, Dorothy Linda (Fisher)
Fejer, Thomas Peter
Gilbert, Helen Anne Frances (Macdonald)
Gleeson, Thomas Richard
Golomb, Philip Nathan
Gosse, Gordon David
Graham, Anthony Francis
Greene, Mitchell Dale
Gregory, Walter
Hirst, Roger Derek
Houze, George E.
Humphries, Paul Wellington
Johnson, Donald Hugh
Lester, Frances Thelma
Lockett, Lawrence John
Loewen, Dale Raymond
Lukinuk, Morris George
Maartense, Cornelius Peter
Macdonald, Ian Laidlaw
MacLean, John Dick Fleming
Malby, Frederick Charles
Manning, Robert Frederick
Marshall, Lynn Margaret
Maxwell, Thomas Murray
McCallum, Beverley Faye
O'Grady, Terrence Thomas
Patton, John MacMillan Stevenson
Rathburn, James Broatch
Sands, William James
Scott, Alexander Victor Ferguson
Scott, Shirley Agnes
Shanks, Gavin Lauchlan
Smith, Susan Clair
Staebler, Robin Jacob
Sutherland, William Alexander
Trebilcock, Robert George
Watson, Robert Douglas
Watt, Gordon Lindsay Drayton
Went, John Harvey
Whitfield, Margaret Diana
Wiebe, Edward John
Wynd, Henrietta Dorothea

University of Western Ontario

Armitage, Kathleen Jean
Assad, Norman Abraham
Bate, Larry Robert
Borre, Adrian Joseph
Brannan, Dennis Leslie
Carmichael, Avid Gabriel
Carter, Robert Paul
Chambers, Norman Donald
David, Lawrence Samuel
De Jonge, Christina
Dreimanis, Mara
Edmonds, Merrill Walter
Edwards, Dale Virginia
Edwards, Mohammed Avard
Epstein, David Henry
Franczak, Edwin John
Girvan, David Pugsley
Glaister, Joseph Tertius Drysdale
Green, Peter Calder
Grieser, Gerhard M. (Gary)
Hobbs, Barry Brandon
Holliday, Ronald Leonard
Homer, Joseph James Annesley
Howell, Wayne Alexander
Jenkins, George Edward
Johns, Charles Henry
Jones, Kelly Oliver
Keene, Dennis Michael
Keevil, Louise Ann
Lamont, John Allan
Loopstra, Lawrence William
Love, Robert Russell
Ludwig, Rainer Ernst Georg
McCraw, David Bruce
McElroy, James Ross Charles
Meakins, Jonathan Larmonth
Moore, Andrew Jenkins
Musclow, Catherine Elizabeth
Myers, Michael Francis
Newell, Emilie Novak
Newell, Joseph Paul
Patel, Yezdi Jehangirje
Rempel, Jacob (Jack)
Richards, Larry Marshall
Rowed, David Watson
Schen, Sanford Elliott
Sharpe, James Arthur
Steinbach, Andrew Maxwell
Thatcher, Robert Frederick
Weisler, Marvin
Wigle, Donald Theodore
Will, Bruno O.
Wilson, Paul Elliott
Wong, Kai-Lai (Colin)

GRADUATES IN MEDICINE — 1966 *(cont'd.)*

University of Toronto

Achiume, Mrs. P. M.
Ambus, U.
Angell, W. F.
Apps, R. C.
Baker, M. A.
Ballantyne, D. P.
Bavington, W. J.
Bernstein, S. K.
Berry, W.
Boughton, K. G.
Boyce, F. G.
Boyce, J. R.
Braaten, E. P.
Burke, E.
Burton, J. R.
Busse, E. W.
Butler, S. H.
Campbell, T. A.
Cattran, D. C.
Chintu, C. R. T.
Couper, C. E.
Culbert, P. S.
Daniels, N. J.
Davison, Miss C. E.
Debow, G.
Dellandrea, D. A.
Dick, E. W.
Douglas, G. J.
Eckler, H. B.
Edwards, M. O.
Ellis, D. A. F.
English E.
Erlick, Miss G. G.
Falletta, J. S. A.
Fear, D. W.
Fenton, W. J.
Ferris, F. Z.
Forrest, P. R.
Fradette, K. P.
Fremont, L. E.
Frimer, M. L.
Fruitman, S.
Gadacz, I.
Gayle, B. A.
Gear, Miss J. S.
Gertzbein, S. D.
Grant, Miss D. J.
Grover, L. F. L.
Gryniewski, Mrs. H.
Hachinski, V.
Hardin, S.
Helmel, G. A.
Hoffman, B. F.
Horwich, J. P.
Howes, W. J.
Hudson, R. W.
Innanen, V. T.
Inouye, Miss S. T.
Isenberg, G. N.
Johnson, T. F.
Johnston, K. W.
Jones, A. E.
Juzych, M. S.
Kee, N. G.
Kelly, A. G.
Kidman, H. L.
King, C. G.
King, D. S.
Kivi, R.
Kurtz, B. C.
Kutcy, R. R.
Langer, H. M.
Law, Miss M.K-H.
Levitt, R.
Levy, Miss D. E.
Ling, C-K
Link, R. E.
Lofsky, S.
Logan, A. G.
Lutley, Miss E. R.
MacKenzie, M. T.
McLean, Mrs. J. A. G.
McLeod, P. K.
MacMurray, S. B.
Magee, G. C.
Mahon, J. A. G.
Marshall, A. B.
Melnyk, I.
Mildon, Miss M. J. F.
Miller, H. B.
Milne, Miss S. J.
Minarik, P. B.
Mittleman, M. A.
Mohindra, B. K.
Moore, N. J.
Mueller, J. C.
Munro, T. G.
Myers, S.
Nelems, J. M.
Nelson, J. W.
Newbigging, P.
Ouchterlony, D. P.
Palazij, R.
Pearson, B. W.
Perz, Miss Z. M.
Pierce, Miss S. J.
Presant, S. B.
Quraishi, M. Z.
Richardson, D. W.
Richardson, J. D.
Roseborough, Miss A. H.
Rozkalns, Miss B.
Salmon, E. A. T.
Salsberg, B. B.
Scandiffio, R. J.
Schillinger, J. F.
Scholtz, A. P.
Shafir, Mrs. M. S.
Shields, C. B.
Shulman, H. S.
Sider, R. C.
Sinclair, R. B. I.
Skory, G. M.
Slater, Miss H. J.
Smith, E. E.
Smuckler, R. H.
Soboloff, M. J.
Sole, M. J.
Steciw, I.
Steinberg, W. M.
Stewart, Mrs. J. E. F.
Stewart, S. J.
Strub, D.
Swackhammer, W. B.
Szecsen, A.
Thompson, Mrs. C. L. P.
Thompson, M. G. G.
Tilly, W. A.
Toi, A.
Trent, J. K. T.
Trent, Miss M.
Trotman, J. S.
Trusler, M. B.
Turley, Miss J. J. E.
Tyrrell, J. B.
Van Ast, W. J.
Vidins, Miss E. I.
Vidrih, V. E.
Von Baillou, Miss A.
Wallace, Mrs. A. A. E. J.
Watson, C. P. N.
Waugh, D. C.
Wells, C. C.
Wheeler, R. R.
Wuerth, F.
Young, H. D.
Zizzo, A. J.

University of Manitoba

Ali, Jameel
Andrew, Hugh C.
Aoki, Fred Y.
Armstrong, John D.
Auger, Raymond G.
Ayotte, Brian J. S.
Bland, Chas. Sheldon
Bracken, John
Bracken, Robert Bruce
Bubis, Perry
Callender, Irvin
Capp, Robert E.
Douglas, Gordon R.
Dyck, Donald R.
Findlay, Leslie I. (Miss)
Finkel, Annette
Frankelson, Elliott N.
Gold, Robert E.
Gorchynski, M. Zenon
Harrison, Ross E.
Heppenstall, Ron Bruce
Johnson, Garth E.
Kussin, Dennis J.
LeBoldus, Leonard A.
Long, Kathleen L.
Luce, John T.
Lukie, Bryan E.
Mackie, G. Gary
MacLaughlin, Eithne F. (Miss)
MacLeod, John Neil
McIver, Douglas Keith
McKiernan, Bernard
Meloff, Keith L.
Meloff, Phyllis R. (Mrs.)
Moggey, Doreen E.
Paterson, Donald
Perkins, Russell M.
Schroeder, Maria-Louise
Sigmundson, Harold Keith
Sigurdson, Wilfred F.
Speirs, Harvey R.
Stent, Raymond M.
Tanner, John R.
Toews, Melvin R.
Van Horne, Wayne A.
Warnica, Wayne J.
Waters, John R.
Wood, David J.
Wood, Larry H.
Zarowny, Donald P.

GRADUATES IN MEDICINE — 1966 *(cont'd.)*

University of Alberta

Akpata, M. O.
Amy, R. W. M.
Bilan, L. J.
Bochinski, B.
Brown, F. A. C.
Cassils, J. G.
Chornell, J. G.
Chue, P. W. Y.
Davidman, M.
Deane, J. A.
Donnelly, P. J.
Dutton, E. W.
Enns, G. D.
Florkowski, Joanne M.
Forsyth, R. D.
Harris, F. W.
Hutchinson, J. C.
Janzen, V. D.
Krynen, W. A. G.
Kulak, L. L.
Lampard, J. D.
McBride, R. G.
McMillan, Marilyn E.
McMurtry, G. J.
Mah Poy, G. L.
Makar, R. T.
Marfleet, B. R.
Nash, P. A.
Nelson, D. A.
Olekshy, J. A.
Orr, F. W.
Peters, R.
Quandt, P. L. F. K.
Rawlinson, D. G.
Reese, R. H.
Reist, Marilyn Y.
Remington, B. K.
Rentiers, Paul K.
Sereda, W. M.
Kass, Carol A.
Shubert, E. E.
Simichak, H.
Steward, W. W.
Stuart, W. A.
Sunohara, P. T.
Voloshin, P. J.
Vos, C.
Wharton, D. J.
Whidden, P. G.
Whitla, J. M.
Wiebe, Diana H. (nee Fischer)
Wiebe, G.
Willans, G. W.
Woodman, J. C.
Wright, J. E.
Yasayko, H. H. M.
Zuege, R.

University of Saskatchewan

Beckie, Gerald Victor Frederick
Bowman, Doreen Virginia
Burke, David Lionel
Cook, Bernard Geoffrey
Edwards, James Hugh
Epp, Carl Henry
Ernst, Alfred Henry
Goluboff, Lanny Gerald
Gordon, Philip Harry
Griffith, William Roger
Johnsrude, Theodore Eugene
Letkeman, Jacob Aaron
Lewke, Margareta
MacKay, Maralyn Joan
MacLean, George William Arthur
Malfair, Theodore Lucien
Mayhew, Duane George
McKinstry, Errol Ernest
Morrison, Murray Douglas
Opsal, James Orville
Perzow, Sydney Michel
Peto, David Alan
Petrich, Lucille, Carol
Salter, Eden Robert
Slywka, Brian Howard
Thompson, Barry Vincent
Thompson, Robert Pinder
Turanski, James Julias
Voth, Arnold John

University of British Columbia

Aceman, Paul J.
Arundell, Geoffrey
Bard, Leon
Barre, Paul E.
Batt, Nathan
Benedet, Lawrence J.
Bertoia, Wayne A.
Bjarnason, David F.
Blanchard, Joy R.
Bostic, Oswald
Brownlee, Lawrence
Blair, (Burt) Jacqueline
Chan, Kai
Chow, Bill
Chung, David
Clare, Sanford
Clement, John
Crowley, James
De Levie, Melvin
Evans, Robert
Fast, Richard
Friedman, Samuel
Gable, Eric
Gant, Thomas
Geen, David
Hestrin, Morris
Grant, Igor
Hiller, Ronald
Hunter, Marlene
Jack, Robert
McDonald, Earl
McDonald, Thomas
McInnis, Joseph B.
MacPherson, Ronald
Michas, Constantine
Mundel, Hans
Neumeyer, Alvin
Orlik, Herbert
Paget, John
Pankratz, Edgar
Paton, Walter
Patterson, Brian
Patterson, Richard
Schloss, Melvin
Scriver, Frederick
Shortt, David
Sivucha, Walter
Stanley, Robert
Stockdill, Peter
Sutherland, Donald
Tolman, Keith
Tredwell, Stephen
Trueman, Mark
Wale, Norman
Winslow, Edward

PROVINCIAL RADIATION THERAPY CLINICS

BRITISH COLUMBIA:

(1) **The British Columbia Cancer Institute, 2656 Heather Street, Vancouver 9**
Director: DR. A. M. EVANS
(2) **The Victoria Cancer Clinic, Royal Jubilee Hospital, Victoria**
Director: DR. N. S. LOCKYER

ALBERTA:

(1) **The Edmonton Cancer Clinic, 11250 - 84th Avenue, Edmonton**
Director: Dr. A. S. Little
(2) **The Calgary Cancer Clinic, Holy Cross Hospital, Calgary**
Associate Director: DR. T. MELLING
(3) **The Lethbridge Cancer Clinic, Lethbridge**
Associate Director: DR. D. A. RICE

SASKATCHEWAN:

(1) **Saskatoon Cancer Clinic, University Hospital, Saskatoon**
Director: DR. C. BURKELL
(2) **Allan Blair Memorial Cancer Clinic, Grey Nuns' Hospital, Regina**
Director: DR. A. J. S. BRYANT

MANITOBA:

(1) The Radiotherapy Dept., **Winnipeg General Hospital, Winnipeg**
Director: DR. R. J. WALTON
(2) The Radiotherapy Dept., **St. Boniface Hospital, Winnipeg**
Director: DR. R. J. WALTON

ONTARIO:

(1) **The Ontario Cancer Institute, The Princess Margaret Hospital, 500 Sherbourne Street, Toronto**
Director: DR. C. L. ASH
(2) **The Ontario Cancer Foundation, London Clinic, Victoria Hospital, London**
Director: DR. T. A. WATSON
(3) **The Ontario Cancer Foundation, Hamilton Clinic, Hamilton General Hospital, Hamilton**
Director: DR. L. S. GREEN
(4) **The Ontario Cancer Foundation, Kingston Clinic, Kingston General Hospital, Kingston**
Director: DR. R. C. BURR
(5) **The Ontario Cancer Foundation, Windsor Clinic, Metropolitan General Hospital, Windsor**
Director: DR. J. H. MAUS
(6) The Ontario Cancer Foundation, Ottawa Clinic
Ottawa Civic Hospital Division, Ottawa
Ottawa General Hospital Division, Ottawa
Director: DR. T. G. STODDART
(7) The Ontario Cancer Foundation, Thunder Bay Clinic
General Hospital of Port Arthur, Port Arthur
Director: DR. W. A. HARGAN
(8) Sarnia Auxiliary Radiotherapy & Follow-up Clinic, St. Joseph's Hospital, Sarnia
Director: DR. F. T. MILES

QUEBEC:

The treatment of cancer by radiation in the Province of Quebec is undertaken in hospitals with qualified radiation therapists.

NEW BRUNSWICK:

(1) Saint John Cancer Clinic, **Saint John General Hospital, Saint John**
Director: DR. J. A. CASKEY
(2) Moncton Cancer Clinic, **The Moncton Hospital, Moncton**
Director: DR. H. R. RIPLEY
(3) Fredericton Cancer Clinic, **Victoria Public Hospital, Fredericton**
Director: Dr. G. R. Clayden

NOVA SCOTIA:

(1) **Nova Scotia Tumour Clinic, Victoria General Hospital, Halifax**
Director: DR. J. A. MYRDEN

PRINCE EDWARD ISLAND:

(1) **Div. of Cancer Control, Dominion Building, Charlottetown**
Director: DR. W. T. HOOPER

NEWFOUNDLAND:

(1) **St. John's Cancer Clinic, St. John's General Hospital, St. John's**
Director: DR. H. B. MURPHY

Provinces which have a specially appointed Provincial Group responsible for the treatment of cancer are as follows: British Columbia — The British Columbia Cancer Foundation; Saskatchewan — Saskatchewan Cancer Commission; Manitoba — Manitoba Cancer Treatment and Research Foundation and Ontario — Ontario Cancer Treatment and Research Foundation.

We are indebted to the National Cancer Institute of Canada for the above information.

HOSPITALS

Hospitals and Nursing Homes are listed by province and town. Name of institution, street, address, number of beds and telephone numbers where available are shown; all correspondence may be directed to the Superintendent.

Abbreviations

Alc.—Alcoholic
Bas.—Bassinet
Cont.—Contagious
Dom.—Domicilary
Emer.—Emergency
Epil.—Epilepsy
Gen.—General
Ger.—Geriatric
Isol.—Isolation
Mat.—Maternity
Ment.—Mental
Neur.—Neuroses
Orth.—Orthopaedic
Paed.—Paediatric
Psy.—Psychiatric
Rehab.—Rehabilitation
TB—Tuberculosis

British Columbia

ABBOTSFORD
Cottage Private Hosp.; 2219 McCallum Rd.; Infirm 32; Tel. 853-1333.
Matsqui-Sumas-Abbotsford Gen. Hosp.; McCallum Rd., P.O. Box 940: Gen. 87; Tel. 853-2201.
Menno Hosp.; Marshal Rd., R.R. 5; Gen. 75; Tel. 859-8221.

AGASSIZ
Glenwood Priv. H., 7257 McDonald Rd., P.O. Box 410; Inf. 20; Tel. 796-2511.

ALERT BAY
St. George's Hosp.; P.O. Box 223; Gen. 82; Tel. 974-5221.

ALEXIS CREEK
Red Cross Outpost Hosp.; Gen. 4; Tel. 2R.

ARMSTRONG
Armstrong-Spallumcheen Hosp.; P.O. Box 460; Gen. 21; Tel. LI. 6-2266.

ASHCROFT
Lady Minto Hosp.; P.O. Box 488; Gen. 38; Tel. 453-2211.

ATLIN
Red Cross Outpost Hosp.; Gen. 2; Tel. AN 352.

BAMFIELD
Red Cross Outpost Hosp.; Gen. 4; Tel. 9.

BELLA BELLA
R. W. Large Memorial Hosp.; Campbell Island P.O.; Gen. 36.

BELLA COOLA
Bella Coola Gen. Hosp.; P.O. Box 225; Gen. 28; Tel. 7T.

BLUE RIVER
Red Cross Outpost Hosp.; Gen. 4; Tel. 1R.

BRALORNE
Bralorne Mines Hosp.; P.O. Box 305; (Priv.); Gen. 20; Tel. 65.

BURNS LAKE
Burns Lake & Dist. H.; 9th & Centre St., Box 479; Gen. 43; Tel. 232.

CAMPBELL RIVER
Campbell River & District Gen. Hosp.; Birch & 2nd Ave., P.O. Box 1120; Gen. 83; Psych.; Tel. 287-7111.

CASSIAR
Cassiar Private Hosp.; Gen. 9; Tel. 23.

CASTLEGAR
Castlegar & District Hosp.; P.O. Box 790: Gen. 49: Tel. 365-7711.

CEEPEECEE (See Esperanza)

CHEMAINUS
Chemainus Gen. Hosp.; P.O. Box 499; Gen. 42; Tel. CH 6-3212.

CHILLIWACK
Chilliwack Gen. Hosp.; 45550 Hodgins Ave.; Gen. 173; Tel. 795-7211.
Valleyhaven Hosp.; 310 Hodgins Street, P.O. Box 270; Gen. 38

COBBLEHILL
Salvation Army Mary Moore Home & H.; P.O. Box 274; Chron. 21; Tel. 743-2512.

COMOX
Fort Private Hosp.; P.O. Box 579; Infirm 30; Tel. 339-3131.
St. Joseph's Gen. Hosp.; Box 580, Vancouver Island; Gen. 85; Tel. 339-2242.

CRANBROOK
St. Eugene Hosp.; St. Joseph St., P.O. Box 820; Gen. 93; Tel. JU 6-2241.

CRESTON
Creston Valley Hosp.; 500 - 15th Ave., P.O. Box 430; Gen. 43; Tel. EL 6-2545.

CUMBERLAND
Cumberland Gen. Hosp.; Windermere Ave., P.O. Drawer 400; Gen. 47; Tel. 336-2211.

DAWSON CREEK
St. Joseph's Gen. Hosp.; 11100—13th St., Gen. 126; Tel. ST 2-8501.

DUNCAN
King's Daughters Hosp.; Jubilee St., P.O. Box 368; Gen. 127; Tel. 746-4141.

EDGEWOOD
Red Cross Outpost Hosp.; Gen. 4; Tel. 2J.

ENDERBY
Enderby & District Memorial Hosp.; 500 George St., P.O. Box 29; Gen. 28; Tel. TE 8-7400.

ESPERANZA
Esperanza Gen. Hosp.; Gen. 26.

ESQUIMALT (See Victoria)

ESSONDALE (See Vancouver)

FERNIE
Fernie Memorial Hosp.; Dalton Ave., P.O. Box 670; Gen. 50; Tel. 123.

FORT LANGLEY
Simpson Private Hosp.; 8838 Glover Rd., P.O. Box 40; Infirm 31; Tel. 534-6112.

FORT NELSON
Fort Nelson Gen. Hosp.; P.O. Box 60; Gen. 39; Tel. 774-3271.

FORT ST. JOHN
Providence Hosp.; 9820 100th Ave.; Gen. 95; Tel. 875-6611.

GANGES
Lady Minto Golf Islands Hosp.; Gen. 26; Tel. 537-5545.

GOLDEN
Golden & District Gen. Hosp.; River St., P.O. Box 230; Gen. 28; Tel. 344-2710.

GRAND FORKS
Boundary Hosp.; P.O. Box 189; Gen. 33; Tel. 442-8211.

HAMMOND
Parkridge Priv. H.; 11483 2nd Ave., P.O. Box 292; Int. 54; Tel. 467-4611.

HANEY
Alouette Private Hospital; 14th Ave. & 32nd Rd., R.R. 1; Chron. 22; Tel. IN 5-8411.
Maple Ridge Hosp.; 3rd Ave. & Lougheed Hwy., P.O. Box 5000; Gen. 82; Tel. 463-4111.

HAZELTON
Wrinch Memorial Hosp.; P.O. Box 8, Gen. 57; Tel. 11.

HOPE
Fraser Canyon Hosp.; 7th Ave. & Hope Princeton Hwy., P.O. Box 1090; Gen. 35; Tel. 869-5656.

INVERMERE
Windermere District Hosp.; P.O. Box 160; Gen. 30; Tel. 342-6115.

KAMLOOPS
Mount Paul Priv. H.; 313 McGowan Ave. N.
Royal Inland Hosp.; 311 Columbia St.; Gen. 208; Tel. 372-3131.

KASLO
Victorian Hosp. of Kaslo; P.O. Box 607; Gen. 30; Tel. 353-2211.

HOSPITALS & CONVALESCENT HOMES — B.C.

KELOWNA
Kelowna Gen. Hosp.; 2268 Pandosy St.; Gen. 173; **Rehab. 8; Psy. 7; Tel. PO 2-4000.**
Still Waters Priv. H.; 1450 Vernon Rd., Infirm. 75; Tel. PO 2-0555.
KIMBERLEY
Kimberley & District Gen. Hosp.; McDougal Heights, Box 6000; Gen. 63; **Tel. 427-2215.**
KITIMAT
Kitimat Hosp.; Haisla and Lahakas, P.O. Box 1700; (Priv.); Gen. 101; **Tel. 1100.**
KYUQUOT
Red Cross Outpost Hosp.; Gen. 4.
LADNER
Delta Private Hosp.; 9321 Burns Dr., R.R. 3; Chron. 41; **Tel. 946-2737.**
LADYSMITH
Ladysmith Gen. Hosp.; 4th & Symonds Sts., P.O. Box 10; Gen. 48; **Tel. CH 5-3341.**
LILOOET
Lilooet District Hosp.; P.O. Box 249; Gen. 29; **Tel. 33.**
LYTTON
St. Bartholomew's Hosp.; P.O. Box 99, Main St.; Gen. 42; **Tel. 455-2221.**
MASSET
Red Cross Outpost Hosp.; Gen. 4; **Tel. 3.**
McBRIDE
McBride & District Hosp.; P.O. Box 128; Gen. 29; **Tel. LO 9-2663.**
MERRITT
Nicola Valley Gen. Hosp.; 2125 Priest Ave., P.O. Box 129; Gen. 47; **Tel. 378-2242.**
MICHEL
Michel Hosp.; Gen. 17; Tel. 425-6212.
MISSION CITY
Mission Memorial Hosp.; 5th St., P.O. Box 1120; Gen. 49; **Tel. PR 2-2651.**
MURRAYVILLE
Langley Memorial Hosp.; 22051 Trans Canada Hwy., Box 10; Gen. 105; **Tel. 534-4121.**
NAKUSP
Arrow Lakes Hosp.; 820 Broadway St.; P.O. Box 87; Gen. 16; **Tel. 265-3212**
NANAIMO
Nanaimo Indian Hosp.; Gen. 70; T.B. 30; **Tel. SK 3-4321.**
Nanaimo Regional Gen. Hosp.; 1200 Dufferin Cresc.; Gen. 209; Psy. 10; Rehab. 8; **Tel. SK 4-2141.**
NELSON
Kootenay Lake Gen. Hosp.; 3 View St.; Gen. 119; **Tel. 352-3111.**
Mount St. Francis Infirmary; Gordon Rd., P.O. 8, Infirm 98; **Tel. 352-3531.**
Willowhaven Private Hosp.; R.R. 1; Infirm. 75; **Tel. 352-2411.**
NEW DENVER
Slocan Community Hosp.; Kildare St., P.O. Box 129; Gen. 31; **Tel. 358-2411.**
NEW WESTMINSTER
See VANCOUVER
NORTH SURREY
See VANCOUVER
NORTH VANCOUVER
See VANCOUVER
OCEAN FALLS
Ocean Falls Gen. Hosp.; Lewthwaite Ave, P.O. Box 640; Gen. 39; **Tel. 289-3325.**
OLIVER
St. Martin's Hosp.; 4th Ave. W., P.O. Box 730; Gen. 55; **Tel. HY 8-2422.**
PENTICTON
Penticton Hosp.; Carmi Ave.; Gen. 153; **Tel. HY 2-4000.**
PORT ALBERNI
West Coast Gen. Hosp.; 814—8th Ave. N.; Gen. 137; **Tel. 723—2135.**
PORT ALICE
Port Alice Private Hosp.; P.O. Box 240; Gen. 22; **Tel. 284-3412.**
POUCE COUPE
Pouce Coupe Community Hosp.; P.O. 98; Gen. 30; **Tel. ST 6-5433.**
POWELL RIVER
Powell River Gen. Hosp.; 5871 Arbutus St., P.O. Box 130; Gen. 139; **Tel. 483-3211.**
PRINCE GEORGE
Prince George Regional H.; 2001 - 13th St., Gen. 231; **Tel. LO 4-4411.**
Simon Fraser Priv. H.
PRINCE RUPERT
Miller Bay Indian Hosp.; P.O. Box 488; Gen. 92; **Tel. 624-1821.**
Prince Rupert Gen. Hosp.; 551—5th Ave. E.; Gen. 127; **Tel. 624-2171.**
PRINCETON
Princeton Gen. Hosp.; Vernon Ave., P.O. Box 610; Gen. 42; **Tel. 25.**
QUEEN CHARLOTTE CITY
Queen Charlotte Islands Gen. Hosp.; P.O. Box 9; Gen. 27; **Tel. 7-4411.**
QUESNEL
G. R. Baker Memorial Hosp.; Front St.; P.O. Box 4000; Gen. 93; **Tel. 992-2181.**
REVELSTOKE
Queen Victoria Hosp.; 510—1st St. W., Box 160; Gen. 49; **Tel. 837-2131.**
ROSSLAND
Mater Misericordia Hosp.; 1961 Georgia St., P.O. Box 1239; Gen. 53; **Tel. 362-7344.**
SALMON ARM
Shuswap Lake Gen. Hosp.; P.O. Box 520; Gen. 66; **Tel. TE 2-2182.**
SARDIS
Coqualeetza Indian Hosp.; Vedder Rd.; Gen. 55; Rehab. 10; TB 85; **Tel. 858-3321.**
SECHELT
St. Mary's H.; P.O. Box 10; Gen. 54; **Tel. 885-2224.**
SIDNEY
Rest Haven Hosp.; 10465 Rest Haven Drive; Gen. 66; **Tel. 656-1121.**
SMITHERS
Bulkley Valley District Hosp.; 8th Ave., P.O. Box 370; Gen. 81; **Tel. 847-3321.**
SQUAMISH
Squamish Gen. Hosp.; 4674 Clarke Drive, P.O. Box 498; Gen. 30; **Tel. 892-5211.**
STEWART
Stewart Gen. Hosp.; Brightwell St., P.O. Box 8; Gen. 0; **Tel. 23L.**
SUMMERLAND
Summerland Gen. H.; R.R. 1; Gen. 32; Tel. 494-2426.
TERRACE
Mills Memorial Hosp.; Tetrault and Ferry Sts.; P.O. Box 1297; Gen. 78; **Tel. VI 3-2211.**
Skeenaview H.; P.O. Box 1030; Gen. 306; **Tel. VI 3-2265.**
TOFINO
Tofini Gen. Hosp.; Neil St.; P.O. Box 50; Gen. 23; **Tel. 725-3212.**
TRAIL
Trail-Tadanac Hosp.; 1200 Hospital Bench; Gen. 206; **Tel. 368-3311.**
TRANQUILLE
Tranquille Schl.; Ment. 576 (Adults); Inf. 10; **Tel. 376-3361.**

VANCOUVER
Alexandra Private Hosp.; 3890 Alexandra St., **Zone 9; Infirm. 15; Tel. RE 1-6214.**
Altamont Private Hosp.; 1675—27th St., West Vancouver; Chron. 56; **Tel. Wa 2-5620.**
Amherst Priv. H.; Albert St. and 59 Ave.; **Inf.** 75.
Arbutus Private Hosp.; 6650 Arbutus St.; Inf. 75.
Avalon Private Hosp.; 2545 W. 1st Ave., Zone 9; Infirm. 18; **Tel. RE 3-1944.**
Bayview Private Hosp.; 2320 W. 1st Ave.; Infirm 23. **Tel. RE 3-5432.**
Bonnie Lynn Priv. H.; 2774 W. 1st St.; **Inf.** 18, **Tel. RE 3-3233.**
Braddan Private Hosp.; 2450 W. 2nd Ave., Zone 8; **Chron. 45; Tel. RE 8-1535.**
British Columbia Cancer Fdn.; 2656 Heather St., Zone 9; (Priv); Cancer 54; **Tel. TR 4-9321.**

HOSPITALS & CONVALESCENT HOMES — B.C.

Burnaby Gen. Hosp.; 3800 Ingleton Ave., Zone 1; Gen. 311; Tel. HE 4-4211.
Cambie Private Hosp.; 2836 Ash St., Zone 9; Orth. 32; Tel. TR 6-9323.
Canadian Red Cross Soc. (B.C. Division); 1235 W. Pender St.
Carlsbad Private Hosp.; 2423 Cornwall St., Zone 9; Infirm 17; **Tel. RE 3-7133.**
Cedarhurst Private Hosp.; 7279 152nd St.; North Surrey; Infirm 33; Tel. 596-8811.
Children's Hosp.; 250 West 59th Ave., Zone 15; Paed. 88; Tel. FA 7-1101.
Como Lake Private Hosp. & Nursing Home; 657 Gatensbury St., Pt. Coquitlam; Infirm 75; Tel. 939-9277.
Edith Cavell Hosp.; 2855 Sophia St., Zone 10; (Priv); Chron. 52; **Tel. TR 4-7131.**
Fellburn Priv. H.; 6650 Hastings St. E.
Florence Nightingale Private Hosp.; 13453-111A Ave. N. Surrey; Inf. 75; Tel. 581-3388.
George Derby Health & Occupational Centre (Now George Derby Wing Unit of Shaughnessy Hosp.)
G. F. Strong Rehabilitation Centre; 900 W. 27th Ave., Zone 9; Rehab. 53; **Tel. RE 1-3111.**
Glen Brae Priv. H.; 1690 Matthews Ave., Chron. 18; **Tel. RE 3-7828.**
Glen Hosp. Ltd.; 1036 Salsbury Dr.; Infirm 86.
Grace Hosp.; 26th Ave. & Heather St.; Gen. 159; Tel. TR 4-3454.
Grandview Hosp. & Nursing Home Ltd.; 1090 Victoria Dr., Zone 6; (Priv); Chron. 61; **Tel. AL 3-2255.**
Hawthorne Private Hosp.; 2665 Point Grey Rd., Zone 9; Chron. 18; **Tel. 713-4213.**
Hollywood Hosp.; 515—5th Ave., New Westminster; (Priv); Gen. 73; **Tel. LA 2-8621.**
Holy Family Hosp.; 7801 Argyle St., Zone 15; Rehab. 52; Tel. 321-2661.
Inglewood Priv. H.; 725 Inglewood Ave.; Inf. 75; **Tel. 922-9394.**
Kensington Priv. Hosp.; 750 W. 41st Ave.
King George Highway Priv. H.; King George Hwy. & Townline Rd.; Inf. 75; Tel. 5816161.
Kitsiliano Private Hosp.; 2336 W. 3rd Ave., Zone 9; Infirm 18; Tel. RE 3-5443.
Larwood Private Hosp.; 1847 **Larch St., Zone 9; Chron. 18; Tel. RE 3-3141.**
Lindross Private Hosp.; 6907 Elwell St., Burnaby; Chron. 30; Tel. LA 1-4951.
Lion's Gate H.; 230 E. 13th St.; N. Van., Gen. 387; Tel. YU 8-3131.
Lonsdale Private Hosp.; 151 E. 12th St., North Vancouver; Infirm 25; Tel. 987-1343.
Mahon Park Private Hosp.; 351 W. 19th St., North Vancouver; Infirm 18; Tel. YU 7-3911.
Mary Hill Private Hosp.; 2050 Mary Hill Rd.; Port Coquitlam; Infirm 23; Tel. WH 2-8311.
McKay Private Nursing Home; 6335 McKay Ave., South Burnaby; Infirm 31; Tel. HE 3-8311.
Medical-Dental Hosp. Unit; 925 W. Georgia St., Zone 1; Gen. 21; **Tel. MU 5-9231.**
Melrose Park Private Hosp.; 1621—6th Ave., New Westminster; Chron. 73; Tel. LA 2-4433.
Mount St. Joseph's Hosp.; 3080 Prince Edward Zone 10; Gen. 104, Chron. 64; Tel. TR 4-1141.
Normandy Priv. H.; 4505 Valley Drive.
Oakherst Nursing Home; 7430 Oak St., Zone 14; Infirm 41.
Park Lane Priv. H.; 950 W. 58 Ave.
Pearson Hosp.; 700 W. 57th Ave., Zone 14; TB. 132; Polio 41; Chron 132; **Tel. FA 1-3231.**
Princess Margaret Children's Village; (See Sunny Hill Hosp. for Children.)
Richmond Private Hosp.; 611 Minoru Blvd., Richmond; Infirm. 75; **Tel. Crestwood 8-9595.**
Riverview Hosp., Essondale; Psy. 3066; Tel. 521-1911.
Royal Columbian Hosp.; 330 E. Columbia St., New Westminster; Gen. 485; **Cont. 12; Tel. LA 2-2771.**
St. Mary's Hosp.; 220 Royal Ave., New Westminster; Gen. 201; **Tel. LA 1-1811.**
St. Paul's Hosp.; 1081 Burrard St., Zone 1; Gen. 586; Orth. 115; Tel. 682-2344.
St. Vincent's Hosp.; 33rd Ave. & Heather St., Zone 9; Gen. 233; Tel. TR 6-7171.
Scenic View Hosp.; 3071 Pacific Hwy., Cloverdale; Infirm. 29; **Tel. 574-4231.**
Shaughnessy Hosp. (DVA); 30th Ave. & Laurel St., Gen. 544; Psy. 44, Chron. 368; Dom. 211; **Tel. 876-6767.**
Southpines Private Hosp.; 325 W. 59th Ave. **Zone 15; Chron. 33; Tel. FA 1-0214.**
Steadman Private Hosp.; 1238 Cardero St.; Infirm 18; **Tel. MU 3-4638.**
Strathcona Private Hosp.; 2646 Yukon St., Zone 10; Infirm 18.
Sunnyhill Hosp. for Children; 2755 E. 21st Ave., Zone 12; Gen. 70; **Tel. HE 4-1331.**
Sunnyside Private Hosp.; 2190 Argyle Ave., West Vancouver; Infirm 16; **Tel. WA 2-8331.**
Surrey Memorial Hosp.; 13750—96th Ave., Gen. 120; Tel. 581-3311.
University Health Service; Wesbrook Bldg., U. of B.C., Zone 8; Gen. 22, Cont. 4; **Tel. 224-5650.**
Valleyview Hosp.; Essondale; Ger. 791; **Tel. LA 1-1911.**
Vancouver Gen. Hosp.; 12th Ave. W., Zone 9; Gen. 1500; Cont. 64; Orth. 109; Psy. 40; Inf. 244; **Tel. TR 6-3211.**
Willingdon Priv. H.; 4435 Grange St., Burnaby.
Willow Chest Centre; 2647 Willow St., Zone 9; TB 93; **Tel. TR 4-2331.**
Woodlands School; 9 E. Columbia St., P.O. Box 70; New Westminster; Ment. 1375; **Tel. LA 1-2611.**
Worthington Private Hosp.; 2635 W. 1st Ave., Zone 8; Infirm 18; Tel. RE 8-2635.

VANDERHOOF

St. John Hosp.; River Rd.; Gen. 64; **Tel. 567-2211.**

VERNON

Dellview H.; 31st St.; Ger. 239; Tel. 542-3011.
Vernon Jubilee Hosp.; 32nd St.; Gen. 130; Tel. LI 2-4000.

VICTORIA

Belmont Private Hosp.; 1023 Belmont Ave.; Infirm 13.
Cedars Private Hosp.; 130 Menzies St.; Chron. 45; Tel. EV 3-9011.
Chinese Community Hosp.; 555 Herald St.; (Priv); Chron. 24; **Tel. EV 4-5243.**
Clovelly Private Hosp.; 1196 Clovelly Terrace; **Infirm 42; Tel. EV 3-7814.**
Glengarry Priv. Hosp.; 1780 Fairfield Rd.
Glenwarren Private Hosp.; 1430 Balmoral Rd.; **Chron. 63; Tel. EV 3-2323.**
Gorge Road Hosp.; 63 Gorge Rd. E.; Gen. 97; **Tel. EV 6-2464.**
Macauley Lodge Ltd.; 1037 Lyall St.; Inf. 29; **Tel. 385-6122.**
Manor Private Hosp.; 338 Foul Bay Rd.; Infirm 20; Tel. 382-6522.
Mount St. Mary Hosp.; 999 Burdett Ave.; Chron. 145; **Tel. EV 4-7158.**
Oak Lodge Private Hosp.; 4036 Quadra St.; Infirm 39; **Tel. GR 9-2151.**
Pemberton Road Private Hosp.; 840 Pemberton Rd.; **Infirm 12; Tel. EV. 2-1513.**
Queen Alexandra Solarium for Crippled Children; 2400 Arbutus Rd., P.O. Box 600; Orth. 80; Tel. GR 7-1826.
Richmond Heights Priv. H.; 3690 Richmond Rd.
Rockland Priv. H.; 1617 Rockland Ave.; Inf. 18; Tel. EV 3-6902.
Royal Canadian Navy Hosp.; Esquimalt RCN Barracks; Gen. 100.
Royal Jubilee Hosp.; 1900 Fort St.; Gen. 502; Psy. 43; Cont. 29; Ophth. 20; **Tel. EV 6-3131.**
Royal Oak Private Hosp.; 4353 Glanford, R.R. 3; Infirm 42; **Tel. GR 9-1641.**

HOSPITALS & CONVALESCENT HOMES — B.C. & ALTA.

St. Joseph's Hosp.; 841 Collinson St.; Gen. 486; Tel. EV 4-1131.
St. Mary's Priory H.; 567 Goldstream Ave.; Ext. Care 24; Tel. 478-1721.
Sandringham Priv. H.; 1648 Fort St.; Inf. 75; Tel. 386-2928.
Veterans' Hosp. (DVA); 2355 Richmond Rd.; Gen. 235; Ger. 65; Tel. EV 2-4221.
Wayside House; 550 Foul Bay Rd., P.O. Box 636; Infirm 18; Tel. EV 4-7420.
West Bay Private Hosp.; 531 West Bay Terrace; Infirm 45; **Tel. EV 5-0130.**
WELLS
Gold Quartz Hosp. Ltd.; P.O. Box 132; (Priv); Gen. 15; Tel. 994-3217.
WHITE ROCK
Burkley Priv. Hosp.; 15455 Russel Ave.
White Rock District Hosp.; 15520 North Bluff Ave.; Gen. 57; **Tel. 531-5512.**
WILLIAMS LAKE
Cariboo Memorial Hosp.; P.O. Box 4300; Gen. 106; **Tel. EX 2-4411.**

Alberta

ATHABASCA
Athabasca Municipal Hosp.; P.O. Box 240; Gen. 65; Tel. 5-2183.
BANFF
Mineral-Springs Hosp.; Spray Ave., P.O. Box 1050; Gen. 60; **Tel. PO 2-2222.**
BARRHEAD
St. Joseph's Hosp.; 51 N. 49th St., Box 880; Gen. 80; Tel. 674-2221.
BASHAW
Bashaw Gen. Hosp.; P.O. Box 449; Gen. 37; Tel. 372-3731.
BASSANO
Bassano General Hosp.; P.O. Box 120; Gen. 37; Tel. 472-3520.
BEAVERLODGE
Beaverlodge Municipal Hosp.; No. 32, 422—10A St., P.O. Box 480; Gen. 40; **Tel. 354-2136.**
BENTLEY
Bentley Municipal Hosp.; No. 43, 3834—52 Ave., P.O. Box 30; Gen. 21; Tel. 22.
BERWYN
Berwyn Municipal Hosp.; P.O. Box 154; Gen. 26; Tel. 364.
BLAIRMORE
Crows Nest Pass Municipal Hosp.; P.O. Box 510; Gen. 78; Tel. 562-2333.
BONNYVILLE
Duclos Hosp.; P.O. Box 98; Gen. 18; **Tel. 136.**
St. Louis Hosp.; P.O. Box 68; Gen. 71; Tel. 826-3311.
BOW ISLAND
Bow Island Municipal Hosp.; P.O. Box 399; Gen. 30; Tel. 545-2588.
Boyle Gen. Hosp.; Box 190; Gen. 37.
BRETON
Breton Gen. Hosp.; P.O. Box 340; Gen. 37; Tel. 696-3742.
BROOKS
Brooks Gen. H.; 315—3rd St. W.; Gen. 73; Tel. 362-3411.
CALGARY
Alberta Children's Hosp.; 1820 Richmond Rd.; **Paed 44; Orth 84; Tel. CH 4-2111.**
Ashlewood Priv. H.; 1712 13th Ave. S.W.; Inf. 12; Tel. CH 4-1225.
Baker Memorial San.; P.O. Box 72; T.B. 267; Ment. Def. 90; Tel. BU 8-2311.
Bengtsson Nursing Home; 607—23rd Ave. S.W.; Infirm 12.
Bethany Auxiliary Hosp.; 1918 8th Ave. N.W.; Chron. 100; **Tel. 289-2531.**
Blunt's Kenwood Nursing Home; 1520—8th Ave. N.W.; Inf. 94; Tel. 289-0236.
Calgary Gen. Hosp.; Centre Ave. & 8th St. S.E. Gen. 980, **Psy. 42, Rehab. 41; Tel. AM 6-7541.**
Colonel Belcher Hosp. (DVA); 12th Ave. & 4th St. W.; Gen. 185; Inf. 125; Dom 75; Psy 15; Tel. AM 6-7001.
Cross Bow Aux. H.; Centre Ave. & 10th St. N.E.; Cron. 100; Tel. 255-8171.
Foothills Provincial Gen. Hosp.; 29th St. & 16th Ave. N.W., Station B; Gen. 702, Psy. 70, Rehab. 76, Cont. 35; Tel. 283-0751.
Glenmore Park Aux. Hosp.; 1609—14th St. S.W.; Chron. 200; Tel. 255-8171.
Grace Hosp.; 1402—8th Ave. N.W.; Gen. 78; Tel. AV 9-5541.
Hilltop Rest Home; 1705—25th Ave. S.W.; Infirm 37.
Holy Cross Hosp.; 2nd St. S.W. & 22nd Ave.; Gen. 421; Tel. AM 6-7231.
Mount Royal Private Nursing Home; 1730—10A **St. S.W.; Chron. 18; Tel. CH 4-0355.**
Rundle Lodge; 12th Ave. & 6th St. S.E.; Ger. 50; Tel. AM 2-7662.
Sarcee Aux. Hosp.; 29th St. S.W.; Chron. 100; Tel. 255-8171.
Sunset Lodge; 1302—8th Ave. N.W.; Infirm 60; **Tel. AV 9-7546.**
Windsor Nurs. Home; 720 - 16th St. W.; Infirm. 18; Tel. AM. 2-2065.
Windsor Nursing Home; 529A—13th Ave. W.; Inf. 11; Tel. AM 2-2334.
CAMROSE
Bethany Chron. H.; 45th Ave., P.O. Box 1390; Gen. 50; Inf. 60; Dom. 56; **Tel. 672-2358.**
Rosehaven Hosp.; Psy. & Ger. 510; Tel. 672-2544.
St. Mary's Hosp.; P.O. Box 1090; Gen. 120; **Tel. 672-4401.**
CANMORE
Canmore Municipal Hosp.; P.O. Box 130; Gen. 18; **Tel. 678-5400.**
CARDSTON
Blood Indian Hosp.; 95—1st Ave. W., P.O. Box 490; Gen. 49; **Tel. 653-3351.**
Cardston Municipal Hosp.; 150—1st Ave. W., P.O. Box 310; Gen. 53; Inf. 22; **Tel. 653-4512.**
CARMANGUAY
Little Bow Municipal Hosp.; P.O. Box 160; Gen. 19; **Tel. 643-3511.**
CASTOR
Our Lady of the Rosary Hosp.; Young St.; Gen. 34; Tel. 882-3930.
CEREAL
Cereal Municipal Hosp.; P.O. Box 37; Gen. 15; Tel. 19.
CLARESHOLM
Alberta Hosp.; P.O. Box 490; Gen. 353; **Tel.** 235-3696.
Claresholm Municipal Hosp.; P.O. Box 610; Gen. 48; Tel. 235-3344.
Willow Creek—Claresholm Aux. H.; P.O. Box 700; Gen. 50; **Tel. 235-3577.**
COALDALE
Coaldale Community Hosp.; P.O. Box 358; Gen. 30; **Tel. DI 5-3777.**
COLD LAKE
John Neil Hosp.; P.O. Box 128; Gen. 41; **Tel.** 347-3021.
CONSORT
Consort Municipal Hosp.; P.O. Box 310; Gen. 30; **Tel. 7.**
CORONATION
Coronation Municipal Hosp.; P.O. Box 250; Gen. 31; **Tel. 125.**
DAYSLAND
Providence Hosp.; Jackson St., P.O. Box 27; Gen. 37; **Tel. 7.**
DESMARAIS
St. Martin's Hosp.; Gen. 16.
DEVON
Devon Civic Hosp.; 6 Columbia Ave. W., P.O. Box 400; **Gen. 23; Tel. 447-3401.**
DIDSBURY
Didsbury Lodge; 2102—22nd Ave.; Ger. 11.
Didsbury Municipal Hosp.; P.O. Box 130; Gen. 43; Tel. 335-3414.
Mountain View-Kneehill Auxiliary Hosp.; Chron. 50.
DRAYTON VALLEY
Drayton Valley Municipal Hosp.; P.O. Box 838; Gen. 45; Tel. 542-3922.

HOSPITALS & CONVALESCENT HOMES—ALTA.

DRUMHELLER
Drumheller Aux. H.; Riverside Drive, P.O. Box 1434; Gen. 30; **Tel. VA. 3-3034.**
Drumheller General Hosp.; Riverside Dr., P.O. **Box 450; Gen. 125; Tel. VA 3-2657.**
ECKVILLE
Eckville Municipal Hosp.; P.O. Box 130; Gen. 42; **Tel. 10R2.**
EDMONTON
Aberhart Memorial San.; 114th St. & University Ave., Zone 20; TB 295; Tel. GE 9-0051.
Alberta Hosp.; Box 307; Psy. 1351; T.B. 125; Tel. 7-0221.
Allen Gray Aux. Hosp.; 7510 89th St.; Chron. 50; Tel. 469-4584.
Bonnie Doon Eventide H.; 9310—82nd Ave.; Dom. 46; **Tel. 466-2706.**
Charles Camsell Hosp.; 1412—128th St.; Gen. 267; T.B. 201; **Tel. GL 5-7141.**
Edmonton Gen. Hosp.; Jasper Ave. & 111th St.; Gen. 440; Tel. HU 8-8181.
Elizabeth House; 11717—93 St., Ger. 14; Tel. 479-3562.
Glenrose Prov. Gen. Hosp.; 10230-111th Ave.; Gen. 260; Tel. 474-2451.
Good Samaritan Hosp.; 97th St. & 71st Ave.; **Chron. 174; Tel. 439-6381.**
Misericordia Hosp.; 9830—111th St.; Gen. 386; **Tel. HU 8-0921.**
Norwood Aux. Hosp.; 11135—105th St.; Ger. 172; Tel. 474-5441.
Provincial Mental Inst.; Box 307; Psy. 1351, TB 125; Tel. 70221.
Royal Alexandra Hosp.; 10240 Kingsway Ave.,; Gen. 872; Orth. 56; Psy. 20; Tel. GR 4-3431.
St. Joseph's Hosp.; 107th St. & 82nd Ave.; Chron. 200; Tel. GE 3-5831.
Sunset Lodge; 11034—124th St.; Ger. 50; Tel. GL 4-5484.
University of Alberta Hosp.; 84th Ave. & 112 St.; Gen. 1138; Ger. 78; Rehab. 33; Polio 28; Tel. **439-5911.**
Venta Nursing Home; 13525—102nd. St.; Inf. 55.
Veteran's Home; 12845 102nd Ave. P.O. Box 640; Dom. 76; **Tel. HU 8-4244.**
West Haven Lodge; 16349 Stoney Plain Rd., Jasper Place; Infirm. 55; Tel. HU 9-1252.
EDSON
St. John's Hosp.; 4710—5th Ave. E.; P.O. Box 1810; Gen. 44; **Tel. 723-3331.**
ELK POINT
Elk Point Municipal Hosp.; Gen. 65; Tel. 724-3847.
ELNORA
Elnora Municipal Hosp.; P.O. Box 589; Gen. 21: **Tel. 638-3636.**
EMPRESS
Empress Municipal Hosp.; P.O. Box 159; Gen. 20; Tel. 26.
FAIRVIEW
Fairview Municipal Hosp.; P.O. Box 520; Gen. 60; **Tel. 835-2201.**
FORT CHIPEWY
Fort Chipewy Nursing Stn.; Gen. 5.
FORT MACLEOD
MacLeod Municipal Hosp.; 26th St., P.O. Box 520; Gen. 43; **Tel. 234-4024.**
FORT McMURRAY
St. Gabriel Hosp.; Box 240; Gen. 31; Tel. 743-**2349.**
FORT SASKATCHEWAN
Agnes Forbes Lodge; 10111—108 St.; Ger. 20; Tel. 543-2110.
FORT VERMILION
St. Theresa Hosp.; P.O. Box 128; Gen. 48; Tel. 3272.
GALAHAD
St. Joseph's **Hosp.; P.O. Box 85; Gen 46; Tel. 34.**
GLEICHEN
Blackfoot Indian Hosp.; P.O. Box 100; Gen. 21; Tel. 159.

GLENDON
Glendon Municipal Hosp.; P.O. Box 180; Gen. 24; Tel. 15.
GRANDE PRAIRIE
Grande Prairie Aux. H.; 10409—98th St.; Chron. 50; Tel. 532-7711.
Grande Prairie Municipal Hosp.; 10409—98th St.; Gen. 157; **Tel. 532-7711.**
Pioneer Lodge; Richmond Ave. E.; Dom. 52.
GUNN
Gunn Welfare Centre; Dom. 80; Tel. X702.
HABAY
Hay Lake Nursing Station; Gen. 6.
HANNA
Hanna General Hosp.; P.O. Box 730; Gen. 65; **Tel. 854-3623.**
HARDISTY
St. Anne's Hosp.; P.O. Box 58; Gen. 36; Tel. 388-3626.
HIGH PRAIRIE
Providence Hosp.; Gen. 85. **Tel. 3-3341.**
HIGH RIVER
High River Municipal Hosp.; P.O. Box 430; Gen. 78; **Tel. 652-2311.**
HINTON
Hinton Municipal Hosp.; P.O. Box 40; Gen. 37; Tel. 865-2239.
HYTHE
Hythe Municipal Sub. Hosp.; P.O. Box 207; Gen. 19; Tel. 21.
INNISFAIL
Innisfail Municipal Hosp.; P.O. Box 250; Gen. 46; Tel. 227-3444.
ISLAY
Islay Municipal Hosp.; P.O. Box 55; Gen 16; **Tel. 19.**
JASPER PARK
Seton Hosp.; Robson St., P.O. Box 310; Gen. 37; Tel. UL 2-3142.
KILLAM
Flagstaff-Beaver Aux. Hosp.; P.O. Box 100; Chron. 50; **Tel. 385-3741, Ex. 31.**
General Hosp.; Gen. 37; Tel. PABX8.
Killam Gen. Hosp.; Gen. 37; Tel. PABX 385-3741.
LAC-LA-BICHE
St. Catherine's Hosp.; MacKenzie Ave., P.O. Box 507; Gen. 91; **Tel. 632-4404.**
LACOMBE
Lacombe General Hosp.; P.O. Box 1450; Gen. 72; **Tel. 782-3656.**
LAMONT
Archer Memorial Hosp.; Gen. 84; **Tel. 54-56.**
Lamont-Smoky Lake Auxiliary Hosp.; P.O. Box 14; Chron. 50; **Tel. 199.**
LEDUC
Leduc Municipal Hosp.; P.O. Box 550; Gen. 43; **Tel. 446-2231.**
LETHBRIDGE
Galt Rehabilitation Centre; 5th Ave. S.: Chron. 70; Tel. FA 8-3351.
Lethbridge Auxiliary Hosp.; 935—17th St. S., Gen. 100; **Tel. 328-5571.**
Lethbridge Municipal Hosp.; 9th Ave. S.; Gen. 251; Tel. FA 7-8591.
Lethbridge Nursing Home; 204—5th Ave. S.; Inf. 23; Tel. 327-4623.
St. Michael's Gen. Hosp.; 9th & 13th St. S.; Gen. 225; **Tel. FA 7-1531.**
LINDEN
Linden Nursing Home; P.O. Box 36; Inf. 37; Tel. Acme R 2615.
LLOYDMINSTER
Lloydminster Aux. H.; 4200—56th Ave.; Chron. 50;
MAGRATH
Magrath Municipal Hosp.; P.O. Box 550; Gen. 34; **Tel. 758-3214.**
MANNING
Manning Mun. H.; 2nd Ave. N., P.O. Box 250; Gen. 30; **Tel. 836-3391.**

HOSPITALS & CONVALESCENT HOMES — ALTA. & SASK.

MANNVILLE
Mannville Municipal Hosp.; P.O. Box 180; Gen. 22; Tel. 763-3621.
MAYERTHORPE
Mayerthorpe Municipal Hosp.; P.O. Box 80; Gen. 26; **Tel. 786-2030.**
McLENNAN
Sacred Heart Hosp.; P.O. Box 240; Gen. 84; **Tel. 188.**
MEDICINE HAT
Baptist Haven of Rest; P.O. Box 877; Infirm 90; **Tel. JA 6-2002.**
Dr. Dan MacCharles Aux. Hosp.; 4th St. & 6th Ave. S.W., P.O. Box 998; Gen. 100; **Tel. 527-1181.**
Medicine Hat General Hosp.; 5th St. S.W., P.O. Box 134; Gen. 261; **Tel. JA 7-2211.**
St. Joseph's Home for the Aged; 156—3rd St. N.E.; Dom. 75.
MIDNAPORE
Father Lacombe Nursing Home; Chron. 100; **Tel. 255-0181.**
MILK RIVER
Border Counties Gen. Hosp.; P.O. Box 90; Gen. 37; **Tel. 647-3500.**
MUNDARE
Mary Immaculate Hosp.; P.O. Box E; Gen. 28; **Tel. 319.**
MYRNAM
Myrnam Municipal Hosp.; P.O. Box 220; Gen 33; Tel. 72.
OLDS
Olds Municipal Hosp.; P.O. Box 398; Gen. 54; **Tel. 226-3150.**
Sherwood Old Folk's H.; P.O. Box 734; Dom. 24; Tel. 226-3565.
OYEN
Oyen Municipal Hosp.; P.O. Box 150; Gen. 29; **Tel. 664-3553.**
PEACE RIVER
Peace River Fairview Aux. Hosp.; Gen. 50; **Tel. 664-2551.**
Peace River Municipal Hosp.; P.O. Box 400; Gen. 86; **Tel. 624-2551.**
PICTURE BUTTE
Picture Butte Mun. H.; P.O. Box 430; Gen. 30; **Tel. RE 2-4339.**
PINSCHER CREEK
St. Vincent's Hosp.; 696 Kettles St.; P.O. Box 968; **Gen. 70; Tel. 627-3333.**
PONOKA
Alberta Hosp.; P.O. Box 1000; Ment. 1268; **Tel. 783-3301.**
Ponoka Gen. Hosp.; 50th St., P.O. Box 699; Gen. 61; Isol. 2; **Tel. 783-3864.**
PROVOST
Provost Municipal Hosp.; P.O. Box 270; Gen. 40; **Tel. 403-753-2153.**
RADWAY
St. Joseph's Hosp.; P.O. Box 70; Gen. 20; Tel. 12.
RAYMOND
Alberta Hosp.; P.O. Box 260; Psy. 125; **Tel. 752-3049.**
Raymond Municipal Hosp.; P.O. Box 388; Gen. 34; Tel. 752-3007.
RED DEER
Alberta School Hosp.; P.O. Box 580; Ment. 946; **Tel. 346-2760.**
Deerhome H.; P.O. Box 698; Psy. 1375; **Tel. 347-2522.**
Dr. Richard Parsons Auxiliary Hosp.; 3929—52nd Ave.; Chron. 100; **Tel. 347-3326.**
Red Deer General Hosp.; 3942—50A Ave.; Gen. 182; **Tel. 346-3321.**
Twilight Lodge; 4820—33rd St.; Dom. 48; **Tel. 346-4942.**
RIMBEY
Rimbey General Hosp.; P.O. Box 440; Gen. 40; **Tel. 843-2101.**
The Three Way Aux. Hosp.; 5409-50th St., P.O. Box 680; Chron. 32; **Tel. 643-2004.**
ROCKY MOUNTAIN HOUSE
Rocky Mountain House Municipal Hosp.; 5016—52nd Ave.; **P.O. Box 940; Gen. 44; Tel. 845-3100.**
ST. PAUL
St. Theresa Hosp.; P.O. Box 880; Gen. 95; **Tel. MI 5-3331.**
SMOKY LAKE
George McDougall Memorial Hosp.; P.O. Box 340; Gen. 30; **Tel. 72.**
SPEDDEN
Goodfish Lake Nursing Station; Gen. 4.
SPIRIT RIVER
Holy Cross Hosp.; Gen. 58; P.O. Box 339; Tel. 93.
STETTLER
Stettler Aux. Hosp.; P.O. Box 1148; Chron. 50; **Tel. 742-3776.**
Stettler Municipal Hosp.; 50th Ave., P.O. Box 909; Gen. 70; **Tel. RI 2-2334.**
STONY PLAIN
Stony Plain Mun. Hosp.; P.O. Box 300; Gen. 37; **Tel. 777-2241.**
SWALWELL
Linden Nursing Home; (Priv); Infirm. 37; Tel. AC 2615.
TABER
Taber Gen. Hosp.; 5011—49 Ave., P.O. Box 939; Gen. 89; **Tel. 223-3511.**
THREE HILLS
Prairie Bible Inst. Infirmary; (Priv); Inf. 40; Tel. 443-5515.
Three Hills Municipal Hosp.; 749—2nd St. N., P.O. Box 340; Gen. 33; **Tel. 443-5232.**
TOFIELD
Tofield Municipal Hosp.; P.O. Box 300; Gen. 49; **Tel. 662-3311.**
TROCHU
St. Mary's Hosp.; P.O. Box 100; **Gen. 37; Tel. 126.**
TURNER VALLEY
Turner Valley Municipal Hosp.; Gen. 30; **Tel. 625.3311.**
TWO HILLS
Two Hills Municipal Hosp.; P.O. 160; Gen. 48; Isol. 2; **Tel. 657-2838.**
VALLEYVIEW
Valleyview Gen. H.; P.O. Box 358; Gen. 37; Tel. 524-3356.
VEGREVILLE
Minburn-Eagle Aux. H.; P.O. Box 959; Gen. 50; **Tel. 632-2871.**
St. Joseph's Gen. Hosp.; 5125—41st St., P.O. Box 490; Gen. 80; **Tel. 632-2811.**
VERMILION
Vermilion Municipal Hosp.; Vermilion Heights, P.O. Box 1050; Gen. 66; **Tel. 853-3784.**
VIKING
Viking Municipal Hosp.; P.O. Box 60; Gen. 47; **Tel. 336-3316.**
VILNA
Our Lady's Hosp.; P.O. Box 160; Gen. 21; Tel. 10.
VULCAN
Vulcan Municipal Hosp.; P.O. Box 299; Gen. 44; **Tel. 485-2206.**
WAINWRIGHT
Wainwright General Hosp.; 6th Ave., P.O. Box 820; Gen. 66; **Tel. PBX 842-3326.**
Wainwright Provost Aux. Hosp.; 6th Ave., P.O. Box 910; Chron. 50; **Tel. 842-4406.**
WESTLOCK
Barhead-Thorhild-Westlock Aux. Hosp.; P.O. Box 987; Chron-Conv. 50; **Tel. 342-3306.**
Immaculata Hosp.; P.O. Box 70; Gen. 109; **Tel. 342-3301.**
WETASKIWIN
Eventide Home; 5402—54 St. & 47 Ave., P.O. Box **1389; Ger. 16; Tel. EL 2-2155.**
Green Acres Nursing Home Ltd.; 5211—54th St., P.O. Box 1718; Dom. 50; **Tel. 352-3328-9.**
Wetaskiwin Municipal Hosp.; 5505—50th Ave., P.O. Box 1808; Gen. 106; **Tel. 352-3371.**

WHITELAW
Hotel Dieu of St. Joseph Auxiliary H.; P.O. Box 149; Chron. 42; **Tel. 835-6786.**
WILLINGDON
Mary Immaculate Hosp.; P.O. Box 179; Gen. 31; **Tel. 367-2318.**
YOUNGSTOWN
Pleasant View Home; P.O. Box 9; Dom. 60; Tel. 17.

Saskatchewan

ARBORFIELD
Arborfield Union Hosp.; P.O. Box 117; Gen. 14; Tel. 769-8722.
ARCOLA
Brock Union Hosp.; P.O. Box 87; Gen. 27; Tel. 455-2344.
ASSINIBOIA
Assiniboia Union Hosp.; 5th Ave. E., P.O. Box 940; Gen. 55; Tel. 642-3350.
BALCARRES
Balcarres Union Hosp.; Gen. 41; Tel. 334-2636.
BATTLEFORD
Salvation Army Eventide Home; Drawer 9; Dom. 47.
BEECHY
Beechy Union Hosp.; P.O. Box 68; Gen. 12; Tel. 69.
BENGOUGH
Bengough Union Hosp.; P.O. Box 456; Gen. 25; **Tel. 70.**
BIENFAIT
Bienfait Coalfields Union Hosp.; P.O. Box 189; Gen. 20; **Tel. 388-2232.**
BIGGAR
St. Margaret's Hosp.; 7th Ave. W., P.O. Box 130; Gen. 49; **Tel. 948-3323.**
BIG RIVER
Big River Union Hosp.; P.O. Box 100; Gen. 29; **Tel. 32.**
BIRCH HILLS
Birch Hills Memorial Union Hosp.; P.O. Box 249; Gen. 19; **Dom. 6; Tel. 749-3331.**
BORDEN
Borden Municipal Hosp.; P.O. Box 90; Gen. 20; Tel. 90.
BROADVIEW
St. Michael's Hosp.; Nina St., P.O. Box 100; Gen. 20; **Tel. 696-2441.**
BUFFALO NARROWS
Buffalo Narrows Outpost Hosp.; P.O. Box 40; Gen. 5; **Tel. 235-4344.**
CABRI
Cabri Union Hosp.; Gen. 24; **Tel. 587-2623.**
CANORA
Canora Union Hosp.; P.O. Box 749; Gen. 86; Tel. 563-5621.
CARROT RIVER
Carrot River Union Hosp.; Box 396; Gen. 27; Tel. 768-2722.
CENTRAL BUTTE
Central Butte Union Hosp.; P.O. Box 40; Gen. 36; Tel. 112.
CLIMAX
Climax-Bracken-Union Hosp.; P.O. Box 60; Gen. 16; Tel. 16.
CORONACH
Coronach Union Hosp.; Box 150; Gen. 19; Tel. 26.
CRAIK
Craik Community Hosp.; P.O. Box 208; Gen. 12; **Tel.** 734-2288.
CUDWORTH
St. Michael's Hosp.; 6th St., P.O. Box 268; Gen. 26; Tel. 256-3443.
CUMBERLAND HOUSE
Cumberland House Outpost Hosp.; Gen. 5.........
CUPAR
Cupar Union Hosp.; P.O. Box D; Gen. 21; Tel. 723-4646.

CUT KNIFE
Cut Knife Union Hosp.; P.O. Box 220; Gen. 11; Tel. 398-2262.
DALMENY
Dalmeny Home for the Aged; P.O. Box 83; Dom. 30.
DAVIDSON
Davidson Union Hosp.; P.O. Box 460; Gen. 27; Tel. 567-2801.
DELISLE
Delisle Union Memorial Hosp.; P.O. Box 119; Gen. 17; **Tel. 493-2323.**
DINSMORE
Dinsmore Union Hosp.; P.O. Box 219; Gen. 14; Tel. 44.
DODSLAND
Dodsland Union Hosp.; P.O. Box 215; Gen. 20; Tel. 29.
EARL GREY
Mrs. Pennock's Nursing Home; (Priv); Inf. 2.
EASTEND
Eastend Union Hosp.; Box 456; Gen. 17; **Tel.** 295-3202.
EATONIA
Eatonia Union Hosp.; P.O. Box 327; Gen. 25; Tel. 967-2212.
EDAM
Lady Minto Union Hosp.; P.O. Box 1; Gen. 18; **Tel. 397-2221.**
ELROSE
Elrose Union Hosp.; P.O. Box 99; Gen. 19; Tel. 378-2202.
ESTERHAZY
St. Anthony's Hosp.; Gen. 31; **Tel. 745-3973.**
ESTEVAN
St. Joseph's Gen. Hosp.; 1401—1st St.; Gen. 120; **Tel. 634-3604.**
ESTON
Eston Union Hosp.; Main St., P.O. Box 760; Gen. 31; **Tel. 926-3667.**
FILLMORE
Fillmore Union Hosp.; Gen. 23; Tel. 36.
FOAM LAKE
Foam Lake Union Hosp.; P.O. Box 190; Gen. 29; **Tel. 272-3737.**
FORT QU'APPELLE
Qu-Appelle Indian Hosp.; P.O. Box 220; Gen. Gen. 58; TB 41; **Tel. 332-5550.**
FORT SAN
Fort Qu'Appelle San.; Gen. 178; **Tel. 332-5785.**
FRONTIER
Frontier Municipal Hosp.; P.O. Box 150; Gen. 13; **Tel. 23.**
GAINSBOROUGH
Gainsborough Union Hosp.; P.O. Box 276; Gen. 25; **Tel. 55.**
GOODSOIL
Goodsoil Union Hosp.; P.O. Box 58; Gen. 18; Tel. 28.
GRAVELBOURG
St. Joseph's Hosp.; P.O. Box 520; Gen. 47; Dom. 50; **Tel. 648-2450.**
GREEN LAKE
Red Cross Nursing Station; Emer. 1, Bas. 1.
GRENFELL
Grenfell Union Hosp.; Gen. 26; Tel. 697-2585.
GULL LAKE
Gull Lake Union Hosp.; P.O. Box 300; Gen. 22; **Tel. 672-3337.**
HAFFORD
Hafford Union Hosp.; P.O. Box 130; Gen. 32; Tel. 48.
HERBERT
Herbert Invalid Home; P.O. Box 520; Infirm 25; Tel. 784-2466.
Herbert-Morse Union Hosp.; P.O. Box 220; Gen. 33; **Tel. 784-2202.**
HUDSON BAY
Hudson Bay Union Hosp.; P.O. Box 97; Gen. 22; Tel. 865-2644.

HOSPITALS & CONVALESCENT HOMES — SASK.

HUMBOLDT
St. Elizabeth's Hosp.; P.O. Box 10; Gen. 101; Tel. 682-2611.
ILE A LA CROSSE
St. Joseph's Hosp.; Gen. 41.
IMPERIAL
Imperial Union Hosp.; P.O. Box 180; Gen. 16; Tel. 60.
INDIAN HEAD
Indian Head Union Hosp.; P.O. Box 340; Gen. 34; Tel. 695-2272.
INVERMAY
Invermay-Canora Union Hosp.; P.O. Box 160; Gen. 15; Tel. 50.
ITUNA
Ituna Union Hosp.; P.O. Box 39; Gen. 25; Tel. 795-2622.
KAMSACK
Kamsack Union Hosp.; 507—2nd St., P.O. Box 429; Gen. 65; Tel. 542-2635.
KELVINGTON
Kelvington Union Hosp.; P.O. Box 70; Gen. 29; Tel. 327-4711.
KERROBERT
Kerrobert Union Hosp.; P.O. Box 320; Gen. 41; Tel. 834-2733.
KINCAID
Kincaid Union Hosp.; P.O. Box 186; Gen. 19; Tel. 31.
KINDERSLEY
Kindersley Union Hosp.; Main St. N., P.O. Box 1180; Gen. 54; Tel. 463-2613.
Sunset Lodge Ltd.; 800—1st St. W., P.O. Box 1179; Ger. 36; Tel. 463-2382.
KINISTINO
Kinistino Union Hosp.; Gen. 23; Tel. 864-2525.
KIPLING
Kipling Memorial Union Hosp.; P.O. Box 420; Gen. 34; Tel. 736-2553.
KYLE
Kyle-White Bear Union Hosp.; P.O. Box 170; Gen. 15; Tel. 375-2251.
LAFLECHE
Lafleche Union Hosp.; P.O. Box 159; Gen. 19; Tel. 472-5230.
LA LOCHE
St-Martin's Hosp.; Gen. 15.
LAMPMAN
Lampman Union Hosp.; Gen. 19; Tel. 51.
LANGENBURG
Langenburg Union Hosp.; P.O. Box 570; Gen. 40; Tel. 743-2661.
LANIGAN
Lanigan Union Hosp.; Gen. 19; Tel. 365-2022.
LA RONGE
Lac La Ronge Hosp.; P.O. Box 69; Gen. 30; Tel. 3541.
LASHBURN
Lashburn & District Union Hosp.; Gen. 16; Tel. 124 & 72.
LEADER
Leader Union Hosp.; P.O. Box 129; Gen. 44; Tel. 628-3343.
LEOVILLE
Leoville Union Hosp.; Gen. 17; Tel. 73.
LEROY
Leroy Union Hosp.; P.O. Box 9; Gen. 25; Tel. 286-3331.
LESTOCK
St. Joseph's Hosp.; P.O. Box 90; Gen. 41; Tel. 80.
LLOYDMINSTER
Lloydminster Hosp.; P.O. Box 860; Gen. 107; Tel. 875-2211.
LOON LAKE
Loon Lake Union Hosp.; P.O. Box 69; Gen. 24; Tel. 57.
LUCKY LAKE
Lucky Lake Union Hosp.; P.O. Box 9; Gen. 17; Tel. 70.
MACKLIN
St. Joseph's Hosp.; P.O. Box 190; Gen. 33; Tel. 15.
MAIDSTONE
Maidstone Union Hosp.; P.O. Box 160; Gen. 23; Tel. 893-2544.
MANKOTA
Mankota Union Hosp.; P.O. Box 277; Gen. 16; Tel. 478-2200.
MAPLE CREEK
Maple Creek Union Hosp.; Block 28, P.O. Box 1330; Gen. 60; Tel. 667-2611.
MARYFIELD
Maryfield Memorial Union Hosp.; P.O. Box 98; Gen. 15; Tel. 47.
MEADOW LAKE
Meadow Lake Union Hosp.; Centre St., P.O. Box 670; Gen. 57; Tel. 236-5656.
MELFORT
Melfort Union Hosp.; P.O. Box 1480; Gen. 107; Tel. 752-2811.
Provincial Geriatric Centre; Bemister Ave. E., P.O. Box 1330; Ger. 150; Tel. 752-2767.
MELVILLE
St. Paul's Lutheran Home; 940—9th St. W., P.O. Box 1390; Inf. 112; Tel. 728-5041.
St. Peter's Hosp.; 718 Manitoba St.; Gen. 93; Tel. 728-5407.
MIDALE
Midale Union Hosp.; P.O. Box 29; Gen. 16; Tel. 69.
MILDEN
Milden Union Hosp.; P.O. Box 70; Gen. 15; Tel. 69.
MONTMARTRE
Montmartre Union Hosp.; P.O. Box 206; Gen. 15; Tel. 63.
MOOSE JAW
Ina Grafton Gage Home; 200 Iroquois St. E.; Infirm. 86; Tel. OX 2-4882.
Moose Jaw Union Hosp.; Fairford St. E.; Gen. 280; Tel. 692-1841.
Providence Hosp.; Lillooet St. E.; Gen. 183; Tel. 692-6471.
St. Anthony's Home; 525—7th Ave. S.E., P.O. Box 1000; Ger. 150; Tel. OX 2-7874.
Saskatchewan Training School; P.O. Box 1300; Ment. 1109; Tel. 692-6491.
Williams Nursing Home; 1091—3rd Ave. N.E.; Infirm 10.
MOOSOMIN
Moosomin Union Hosp.; P.O. Box 400; Gen. 59; Inf. 10; Tel. 435-3303.
MOSSBANK
Sutton-Lake Johnston Union Hosp.; P.O. Box 69; Gen. 21; Tel. 354-2344.
NEILBURG
Neilburg & District Union Hosp.; P.O. Box 7; Gen. 17; Tel. 823-4262.
NEUDORF
Neudorf Union Hosp.; Main St., P.O. Box 40; Gen. 16; Tel. 748-2515.
NIPAWIN
Bethel Haven Rest Home; 4th St. E., P.O. Box 2043; Infirm. 32; Tel. 2254.
Nipawin Union Hosp.; P.O. Box 2104; Gen. 76; Tel. 2633.
NOKOMIS
Nokomis Union Hosp.; 2nd Ave., P.O. Box 98; Gen. 22; Tel. 59.
NORQUAY
Norquay-Canora Union Hosp.; Gen. 19; Tel. 41.
NORTH BATTLEFORD
North Battleford Indian Hosp.; P.O. Box 730; Gen. 68; Tel. 445-4461.
Notre Dame Hosp.; 1080—107th St.; Gen. 190; Tel. 445-2411.
Saskatchewan Hosp.; P.O. Box 39; Psy. 1352; Tel. 445-2421.
OUTLOOK
Outlook Union Hosp.; Conquest Ave., P.O. Box 309; Gen. 36; Tel. 867-8676.
OXBOW
Oxbow Union Hosp.; P.O. Box 268; Gen. 29; Tel. 483-2366.

PANGMAN
Pangman Union Hosp.; P.O. Box 90; Gen. 16; Tel. 32.
PARADISE HILL
Paradise Hill Union Hosp.; P.O. Box 179; Gen. 20; Tel. 34.
PELICAN NARROWS
Pelican Narrows Nursing Station; Gen. 4.
PONTEIX
Gabriel Hosp.; P.O. Box 119; Gen. 16; **Tel. 306-**625-3355.
PORCUPINE PLAIN
Porcupine-Carragana Union Hosp.; P.O. Box 70; Gen. 24; Tel. 13.
PREECEVILLE
Preeceville Union Hosp.; Gen. 43; Tel. 547-2102.
PRELATE
Prelate Union Hosp.; P.O. Box 40; Gen. 20; Tel. 3.
PRINCE ALBERT
Holy Family Hosp.; 675—15th St. W.; Gen. 174; Tel. 763-2605.
Mount St. Joseph; 125—25th St. E., P.O. Box 187; Ger. 90; **Tel. 763-7322.**
Saskatchewan Training Schl.; P.O. Box 1240; Ment. 315; **Tel. 763-7401.**
Victoria Union Hosp.; 49—18th St. W.; Gen 181; Cont. 17; **Tel. 306-763-7481.**
QU'APPELLE
Qu'Appelle Memorial Hosp.; P.O. Box 37; Gen. 24; Tel. 699-2243.
QUILL LAKE
Quill Lake Union Hosp.; P.O. Box 188; Gen. 16; **Tel. 306-383-2266.**
RABBIT LAKE
Rabbit Lake Union Hosp.; P.O. Box 176; Gen. 14; **Tel. 9R3.**
RADVILLE
Marion Home; P.O. Box 310; Dom. 50; Tel. 869-2711.
Radville Community Hosp.; P.O. Box 310; Gen. 33; Tel. 869-2224.
REDVERS
Redvers Union Hosp.; P.O. Box 30; Gen. 30; Tel. 453-3553.
REGINA
Canadian National Inst. for the Blind; 2550 Broad St., P.O. Box 1845; Dom. 31; **Tel. 522-5575.**
Canadian Red Cross Society (Sask. Division); 2571 Broad St.; Tel. LA 3-4601.
Eventide Home; 2505 Victoria Ave.; Ger. 76; **Tel. 523-7935.**
Grace Haven; 3304 Dewdney Ave.; Mat. 24; Dom. 33; Tel. JO 9-1630.
Martha House; 1915—2nd Ave. N.; Gen. 17; **Tel. 569-5855.**
Provincial Geriatric & Rehab. Centre; Legislative **Grounds, P.O. Box 1095; Chron.** 194, Rehab. 50; Dom. 60; **Tel. 536-4114.**
R. C. M. P. Post Hosp.; R.C.M.P. Depot Division; Box 650; Infirm. 18; **Tel. JO 9-5481.**
Regina Gen Hosp.; 14th Ave. & St. John St.; Gen. 677, Cont. 48, Psy. 34, Orth. 47; **Tel. LA 2-1811.**
Regina Grey Nuns' Hosp.; 7 Dewdney Ave.; Gen. 520; **Tel. 527-9641.**
ROCKGLEN
Rockglen Union Hosp.; P.O. Box 90; Gen. 14; **Tel. 9.**
ROSETOWN
Rosetown Union Hosp.; P.O. Box 850; Gen. 45; **Tel. 882-2672.**
ROSE VALLEY
Rose Valley Union Hosp.; P.O. Box 310; Gen. 26; **Tel. 87.**
ROSTHERN
Mennonite Youth Farm Invalid Home; P.O. Box 370; Infirm 77; **Tel. 232-4377.**
Rosthern Mennonite Home for the Aged; Carroll St., P.O. Box 442; Dom. 45; **Tel. 232-4353.**
Rothern Union Hosp.; P.O. Box 309; Gen. 46; **Tel. 232- 4422.**

ST. WALBURG
St. Walburg Union Hosp.; P.O. Box 339; Gen. 16; **Tel. 248-3355.**
SALTCOATS
Saltcoats & District War Memorial Hosp.; P.O. Box 78; Gen. 11; **Tel. 744-2232.**
SANDY BAY
Sandy Bay Outpost Hosp.; Gen. 5.
SASKATOON
Bethany Hosp. and Home; 802 Queen St.; Mat. 12; Dom. 20; **Tel. CH 4-6758.**
Lutheran Sunset Home; 1212 Osler St.; Ger. 125; **Tel. 652-8566.**
Oliver Lodge; 1405 Faulkner Cres.; Dom. 56; Tel. 244-5884.
Riverview Nursing Home; 508 Saskatoon Cres.; Infirm. 34.
St. Ann's Home; 1220 Alberta Ave.; Ger. 64; Tel. CH 4-4414.
St. Paul's Hosp.; 1702—20th St. W.; Gen. 368; **Tel. 652-8220.**
Salvation Army Eventide Home; 311—20th St. E.; Ger. 49; Tel. CH 2-2491.
Saskatoon City Hosp.; Queen St. & 7th Ave.; **Gen. 364; Cont. 20; Tel. CH 2-6681.**
Saskatoon Convalescent Home; 101—31 St. W.; Dom. 60; Tel. CH 4-6956.
Saskatoon San.; 1 Wellington Park, P.O. Box 1241; TB 161; **Tel. OL 2-5282.**
Saskatoon Veterans' Home (DVA); 2109 Preston Ave., Dom. 75; **Tel. 374-4747.**
University Hosp.; Gen. 510; Rehab. 57; Psy 39; **Tel. CH 2-7641.**
SHAUNAVON
Shaunavon Union Hosp.; 632—2nd St. E., P.O. Box 789; Gen. 46; **Tel. 7-2644.**
SHELLBROOK
Shellbrook Union Hosp.; P.O. Box 70; Gen. 38; **Tel. 747-2505.**
SMEATON
Smeaton Union Hosp.; P.O. Box 22; Gen. 15; **Tel. 14.**
SPALDING
Spalding Union Hosp.; 2nd Ave. S., P.O. Box 220; Gen. 18; Tel. 5R11.
SPIRITWOOD
Spiritwood Union Hosp.; P.O. Box 89; Gen. 24; **Tel. 16.**
STONY RAPIDS
Stony Rapids Outpost Hosp.; Gen. 5.
SWIFT CURRENT
Provincial Geriatric Centre; 440 Central Ave. S.; Ger. 120; **Tel. 773-8307.**
Swift Current Union Hosp.; 4th Ave. N.E.; Gen. 179; **Tel. 773-4641.**
THEODORE
Theodore Union Hosp.; P.O. Box 70; Gen. 22; **Tel. 55.**
TISDALE
St. Therese Hosp.; 102nd St., Box 700; Gen. 83; Tel. 306-2621.
TURTLEFORD
Riverside Memorial Union Hosp.; P.O. Box 58; Gen. 25; **Tel. 98.**
TUXFORD
Tuxford Nursing Home; Ger. 24; Tel. 693-2778.
UNITY
Unity Union Hosp.; P.O. Box 741; Gen. 42; **Tel. 228-2666.**
URANIUM CITY
Municipal Hosp.; Gen. 46; **Tel. 8411 or 4221.**
VANGUARD
Vanguard Union Hosp.; P.O. Box 9; Gen. 25; **Tel. 62.**
WADENA
Wadena Union Hosp.; P.O. Box 10; Gen. 54; Tel. 8-2515.
WAKAW
Wakaw Union Hosp.; 1st St. N., P.O. Box 309; Gen. 28; Tel. 233-4433.
WATROUS
Watrous Union Hosp.; P.O. Box 130; Gen. 44; Tel. 946-3341.

HOSPITALS AND CONVALESCENT HOMES — SASK., Y.T., N.W.T.. & MAN.

WATSON
Watson Union Hosp.; P.O. Box 220. Gen. 27; **Tel. 287-3366.**
WAWOTA
Wawota Memorial Union Hosp.; P.O. Box 58; Gen. 21; **Tel. 739-2244.**
WEYBURN
Mount St. Mary's Home; 10th Ave. S.E., P.O. Box 97; Ger. 47; **Tel. VI 2-2661.**
Saskatchewan Hosp.; P.O. Box 1056; Ment. 663; **Tel. 842-5461.**
Weyburn Union Hosp.; 301—1st Ave. N.E.; Gen. 113; **Tel. VI 2-2611.**
WHITEWOOD
Joan of Arc Home; P.O. Box 15; Inf. 92; **Tel. 735-2997.**
Whitewood-Moosomin Union Hosp.; Lalonde St., P.O. Box 58; Gen. 17; **Tel. 735-2688.**
WILKIE
Wilkie Union Hosp.; 404—7th Ave. E., P.O. Box 429; Gen. 39; Tel. 843-2644.
WILLOW BUNCH
Willow Bunch Union Hosp.; P.O. Box 338; Gen. 18; **Tel. 59.**
WOLSELEY
Provincial Geriatric Centre; P.O. Box 10; Ger. 100; **Tel. 698-2393.**
Wolseley Memorial Union Hosp.; Ruimer St.; Gen. 29; **Tel. 698-2515.**
WYNYARD
Wynyard Union Hosp.; P.O. Box 670; Gen. 30; Isol. 2; **Tel. 4-2353.**
YORKTON
Yorkton Union Hosp.; Bradbrooke Dr.; Gen. 211; Psy. 148; **Tel. 783-2401.**
ZENON PARK
Notre Dame de l'Assomption; P.O. Box 187; Gen. 21; **Tel. 26.**

Yukon & Northwest Territories

AKLAVIK
Aklavik Nursing Station; Gen. 4.
BAKER LAKE
Baker Lake Nursing Station; Gen. 4.
CAMBRIDGE BAY
Cambridge Bay Nursing Station; Gen. 7.
CAPE DORSET
Cape Dorset Nursing Station; Gen. 4.
CHESTERFIELD INLET
Ste-Therese de l'Enfant-Jesus Hosp.; via Churchill; Gen. 20.
COPPERMINE
Coppermine Nursing Station; Gen. 4.
CORAL HARBOUR
Coral Harbour Nursing Station; Gen. 4.
DAWSON, Y.T.
St. Mary's Hosp.; Front St., P.O. Box 310; Yukon Territory; Gen. 14; Dom. 15; **Tel. 3331.**
ESKIMO POINT
Eskimo Point Nursing Stn.; Gen. 6.
FORT FRANKLIN
Fort Franklin Nursing Station, Gen. 5.
FORT GOOD HOPE
Fort Good Hope Nursing Station; Gen. 4.
FORT LAIRD
Fort Laird Nursing Station.
FORT McPHERSON
Fort McPherson Nursing Station; Gen. 4.
FORT NORMAN
Fort Norman Nursing Station; Gen. 4.
FORT RAE
Faraud Hosp.; Gen. 32; Tel. 6121.
FORT RESOLUTION
St-Joseph's Hosp.; Gen. 15; **Tel. 2381.**
FORT SIMPSON
St. Margaret Hosp.; Gen. 32; **Tel. 2211.**
FORT SMITH
St. Anne's Gen. Hosp.; Gen. 67; **Tel. 3281.**
FROBISHER BAY
Frobisher Bay Gen. H.; P.O. Box 580; Gen 26; Tel. 231.
HALL BEACH
Foxe Nursing Station, Gen. 4.
HAY RIVER
H.H. Williams Memorial Gen. Hosp.; P.O. Box 280; Gen. 22; **Tel. 2412.**
INUVIK
Inuvick Gen. H.; Box 1070; Gen. 77; TB 32; **Tel. 2431.**
MAYO Y.T.
Mayo Gen. Hosp.; P.O. Box 98; Gen. 20; Tel. 3271.
NORMAN WELLS
Norman Wells Hosp.; (Priv); Gen. 14.
OLD CROW, Y.T.
Old Crow Nursing Stn.; Gen. 5.
PANGNIRTUNG
St. Luke's Hosp.; c/o Eastern Arctic Patrol R.M.S., Ottawa, Ont.; **Gen. 17, TB 15.**
RANKIN INLET
Rankin Inlet Nursing Station; Gen. 2.
SPENSE BAY
Spense Bay Nursing Station; Gen. 5.
TUKTOYAKTUK
Tuktoyaktuk Nursing Station; Gen. 4.
WATSON LAKE, Y.T.
Watson Lake Nursing Station; Gen. 4.
WHITEHORSE Y.T.
Whitehorse Gen. Hosp.; Riverdale St.; P.O. Box 87; Gen. 150; **Tel. 667-2561.**
YELLOWKNIFE
Stanton Yellowknife H.; P.O. Box 10; Gen. 50; Tel. 4667.

Manitoba

ALTONA
Altona District Hosp.; P.O. Box 660; **Gen. 48; Tel. 324-6607.**
ARBORG
Arborg Mem. Hosp.; P.O. Box 10; Gen. 24; Tel. 376-2272.
ASHERN
Siglunes Med. Nursing Unit; P.O. Box 110; Gen. 17; **Tel. 79.**
BALDUR
Baldur District Hosp.; P.O. Box 128; Gen. 19; **Tel. 141.**
BEAUSEJOUR
Beausejour Hosp.; 150 First St., P.O. Box 178; Gen. 34; Tel. 107.
BERENS RIVER
Berens River Hosp.; (Priv); Gen. 21.
BIRCH RIVER
Birch River Med. Nursing Unit; Victoria Ave; Gen. 16; **Tel. AD 6-4301.**
BIRTLE
Birtle Dist. Hosp.; P.O. Box 10; Gen. 33; Tel. 842-3493.
BISSETT
San Antonio Gold Mines Hosp.; P.O. Box 138; (Priv); Gen. 7; **Tel. 12.**
BOISSEVAIN
Boissevain, Morton and Minto Mem. Hosp.; P.O. Box 899; Gen. 23; **Tel. 534-6368.**
BRANDON
Assiniboine Hosp.; 10th St. S.; Chron. 198; **Tel. PA 9-6451.**
Brandon Gen. Hosp.; 150 McTavish Ave. E.; Gen. 268; **Tel. PA 6-7421.**
Brandon Hosp. for Mental Diseases; P.O. Box 420; Psy. 1200; **Tel. PA 6-2321.**
Fairview Home; 1331—13th St.; Dom. 167; **Tel. PA 6-4782.**
CARBERRY
Fox Mem. Hosp.; Gen. 36; **Tel. 473.**
CARMAN
Carman Mem. Hosp.; 75 O'Brien Ave., P.O. Box 610; Gen. 55; **Tel. SH 5-2021.**
CARTWRIGHT
Cartwright Dist. Hosp.; Division St., P.O. Box 118; Gen. 11; Tel. 78.

HOSPITALS & CONVALESCENT HOMES — MAN.

CLEARWATER
See The Pas.
CROSS LAKE
Cross Lake Nursing Stn.; Gen. 4.
CRYSTAL CITY
Crystal City Mem. Hosp.; Machray Ave., P.O. Box 86; Gen. 22; Tel. 78.
DAUPHIN
Dauphin Gen. Hosp.; 624—3rd St. S.W.; Gen. 117; Chron. 35; **Tel. 638-3010.**
DELORAINE
Deloraine Mem. Hosp.; Kellet St., P.O. Box 447; Gen. 28; **Tel. 446.**
ELKHORN
Elkhorn Med. Nursing Unit; P.O. Box 170; Gen. 12; **Tel. 35.**
EMERSON
Emerson Medical Nursing Unit; P.O. Box 68; Gen. 17; Tel. 18.
ERICKSON
Erickson Med. Nursing Unit; P.O. 124; Gen. 18; Tel. 636-2521.
ERIKSDALE
Elizabeth M. Crowe Mem. Hosp.; P.O. Box 130; Gen. 24; **Tel. 88.**
FISHER BRANCH
Fisher Branch Med Nursing Unit; P.O. Box 40; **Gen. 21; Tel. 372-6321.**
FLIN FLON
Flin Flon Gen. Hosp.; 3rd St. P.O. Box 158; Gen. 130; Cont. 2; Ortho. 2; **Tel. 687-3474.**
Hudson Bay Mining Employees' Health Assoc. Hosp.; P.O. Box 160; (Priv); Gen. 23; **Tel. 687-3987.**
FORT CHURCHILL
Fort Churchill Gen. Hosp.; Gen. 61; Tel. 141.
GILBERT PLAINS
Gilbert Plains Dist. Hosp.; Gen. 26; Tel. 140.
GIMLI
Johnson Mem. Hosp.; 7th Ave.; P.O. Box 250; Gen. 49; **Tel. 642-5225.**
GLADSTONE
Gladstone Dist. Hosp.; P.O. Box 250; Gen. 29; Tel. 60.
GLENBORO
Glenboro Med. Nursing Unit; Murray Ave., Box 310; Gen. 21; Tel. 52.
GOD'S LAKE
God's Lake Narrows Nursing Stn.; Gen. 4.
GRANDVIEW
Grandview Dist. Hosp.; Rose Ave., P.O. Box 8; Gen. 28; Tel. 1.
HAMIOTA
Hamiota Dist. Hosp.; P.O. Box 190; Gen. 33; Tel. 6.
HARTNEY
Hartney Medical Nursing Unit; River Ave., P.O. Box 280; Gen. 9; **Tel. 91.**
HODGSON
Fisher River Indian Hosp.; Gen. 37; Tel. 1003.
ISLAND LAKE
Garden Hill Nursing Station; Gen. 4.
KILLARNEY
Killarney & District Gen. Hosp.; Park St., P.O. Box 400; Gen. 39; **Tel. 523-4697.**
LITTLE GRAND RAPIDS
Little Grand Rapids Nursing Station; Gen. 4.
LYNN LAKE
Lynn Lake Nursing Station; Gen. 4.
Sherritt Gordon Mines Hosp.; (Priv); Gen. 16; Tel. FL 6-2241.
MacGREGOR
North Norfolk MacGregor Medical & Nursing Unit; P.O. Box 250; Gen. 13; **Tel. 110.**
MANITOU
Pembina-Manitou Hosp.; Mary St., P.O. Box 268; **Gen. 16; Tel. 11.**
McCREARY
McCreary Dist. Hosp.; P.O. Box 250; Gen. 24; Tel. 46.
MELITA
Wilson Memorial Hosp.; P.O. Box 459; Gen 32; Tel. 522-3403.
MIDDLECHURCH
Middlechurch Home of Winnipeg; Infirm. 125; Tel. ED 9-1957.
MINNEDOSA
Minnedosa District Hosp.; 3rd St. S.W., P.O. Box 960; Gen. 37; Tel. 867-2736.
MORDEN
Morden District Gen. Hosp.; P.O. Box 190; Gen. 62; Tel. 882-4411.
Tabor Home for the Aged; 9th St., P.O. Box 879; Inf. 35; **Tel. 822-4848.**
MORRIS
Morris Gen. Hosp.; Railroad Ave., P.O. Box 209; Gen. 53; Tel. 270.
NEEPAWA
Neepawa District Memorial Hosp.; Hospital St., P.O. Box 70; Gen. 42; Tel. 148.
NELSON HOUSE
Nelson House Nursing Station; Gen. 4.
NINETTE
Manitoba San.; TB 171; Tel. 3322.
NORWAY HOUSE
Norway House Indian Hosp.; P.O. Box 40; Gen. 45; **Tel. 6242.**
NOTRE DAME DE LOURDES
Notre Dame Medical Nursing Unit; P.O. Box 90; Gen. 14; **Tel. 62.**
OXFORD HOUSE
Oxford House Nursing Station; Gen. 4.
PILOT MOUND
Pilot Mound Medical Nursing Unit; P.O. Box 61; Gen. 15; **Tel. 175.**
PINAWA
Pinawa Hosp.; Vanier Ave.; P.O. Box 220; Gen. 23; **Tel. 753-2334.**
PINE FALLS
Pine Falls Gen. Hosp.; P.O. Box 70; Gen. 61; Tel. 367-2241.
PORTAGE LA PRAIRIE
Holiday Retreat; 550 Portage Ave. S.; Inf. 47; **Tel. 7-6386.**
Manitoba School for Retardates; Main St. N., P.O. Box 1190; Ment. Def. 1134; **Tel. 7-3403.**
Portage Gen. Hosp.; 524 Broadway St. S.; Gen. 120; Tel. 857-3471.
PUKATAWAGAN
Pukatawagan Nursing Station; Gen. 4.
RESTON
Reston Community Hosp.; First St.; P.O. Box 208; Gen. 22; **Tel. 3331.**
RIVERS
Riverdale Hosp.; 6th & Quebec, P.O. Box 428; Gen. 28; **Tel. 501.**
ROBLIN
Roblin District Hosp.; P.O. Box 740; Gen. 38; Tel. 180.
ROSSBURN
Rossburn Medical Nursing Unit; 4th St., P.O. Box 40; Gen. 26; **Tel. 14.**
RUSSELL
Sacred Heart Hosp.; Assiniboine Ave., P.O. Box 550; Gen. 44; **Tel. 30.**
STE. ANNE
Ste. Anne Medical Nursing Unit; P.O. Box 10; Gen. 20; Tel. GA 2-5345.
ST. CLAUDE
St. Claude Hospital; Roy St.; Gen. 17; **Tel. 30.**
SAINT PIERRE
Desalaberry District Hosp.; P.O. Box 320; Gen. 30; **Tel. 46.**
STE. ROSE DU LAC
Ste. Rose Gen. Hosp.; Gen. 81; Tel. 1.
STE. THERESE'S POINT
Ste. Therese's Point Nursing Station; Gen. 4.
SELKIRK
Hosp. for Mental Diseases; P.O. Box 9600; Psy. 902; **Tel. 482-3810.**
Selkirk Gen. Hosp.; Idell Ave., P.O. Box 5000; Gen. 88; **Tel. 482-5800.**
SHOAL LAKE
Shoal Lake District Hosp.; Jane St.; Gen. 32; Tel. 27.

HOSPITALS & CONVALESCENT HOMES — MAN. & ONT.

SNOW LAKE
Hudson Bay Mining Employees' Health Assoc. Hosp.; P.O. Drawer 10; (Priv); Gen. 10; Tel. 358-2300.
SOURIS
Souris District Hosp.; P.O. Box 638; Gen. 44; Tel. 188.
SPLIT LAKE
Split Lake Nursing Station; Gen. 4.
STEINBACH
Bethesda Hosp.; Hospital St., P.O. Box 939; Gen. 79; Tel. DA 6-6411.
Rest-Haven Nursing Home; 299 Kroeker; P.O. Box 820: Inf. 64; Tel. DA 6-2206.
STONEWALL
Doctor Evelyn Memorial H.; P.O. Box 220; Gen. 24; Tel. 231.
SWAN LAKE
Lorne Memorial Nursing Unit; Gen. 22; Tel. 88.
SWAN RIVER
Swan River Valley Hosp.; 9th Ave. S., P.O. Box 1450; Gen. 72; Tel. 405.
TEULON
Hunter Memorial Hosp.; 3rd St.; P.O. Box 89; Gen. 31; Tel. 11.
THE PAS
St. Anthony's Gen. Hosp.; 67 1st St., P.O. Box 240; Gen. 127; Tel. MA 3-3411.
THOMPSON
Thompson Hospital; (Priv.); Gen. 49; Tel. 677-2381.
TREHERNE
Victoria South Norfolk Treherne Hosp.; Kelly Ave. W., P.O. Box 130; Gen. 32; Tel. 160.
VIRDEN
Virden District Hosp.; 480 King St. E., P.O. Box 400; Gen. 43; Tel. 91.
VITA
Vita District Hosp.; First Ave., P.O. Box 39; Gen. 22; Tel. 5-3222.
WAWANESA
Wawanesa Medical Dist. Nursing Unit; P.O. Box 179; Gen. 12; Tel. 148.
WHITEMOUTH
Whitemouth Medical Nursing Unit, River Drive, P.O. Box 187; Gen. 17; Tel. 348-2316.
WINKLER
Bethel Hosp.; 133 - 6th St., P.O. Box 1070; Gen. 69; Tel. 325-4354.
WINNIPEG
All Saints Nursing Home; 15 Osborne St., Zone 13; Infirm 46; Tel. GR 5-1003.
Arcadia Nursing Home; 1 Mayfair Pl., Zone 13; Infirm 40; Tel. GL 2-3610.
Baron Nursing Home; 66 Smith St., Zone 1; Infirm 40; Tel. WH 2-5628.
Brandon's Nursing Home; 15 Roselyn Rd., Zone 13; Infirm 40; Tel. GR 5-1443.
Central Tuberculosis Clinic; 668 Bannatyne Ave., Zone 3; TB 64; Tel. SP 5-0181.
Children's Hosp. of Winnipeg; 685 Bannatyne Ave., Zone 3; Paed. 232; Infirm. 4; Tel. 775-8311.
Concordia Hosp.; 400 Desalaberry Ave.; Gen. 101; Tel. JU 6-8005.
Conquist Nursing Home Ltd.; 1776 Pembina Hwy., Zone 9; Inf. 60; Tel. 475-0358.
Convalescent Home of Winnipeg; 276 Hugo St., Zone 9; Infirm. 60; Tel. GR 5-1987.
Curran Nursing Home; 29 Roslyn Rd., Zone 13; Infirm 38.
Deer Lodge Hosp. (DVA); 2109 Portage Ave., Zone 12; Gen. 420; Chron. 184; Dom. 10; Tel. 837-1301.
Easton Nursing Home; 530 Stradbrook Ave.; Infirm. 18; Tel. GL. 3-3556.
Grace Hosp.; 200 Arlington St., Zone 10; Gen. 286; Tel. SU 3-7271.
Holy Family Nursing Home; 165 Aberdeen Ave., Zone 4; Infirm. 140; Tel. JU 9-4305.
Jewish Old Folks' Home; 146 Magnus Ave. E.; Zone 4; P.O. Box 3537; Ger. 174; Tel. JU 2-5583.
Manitoba Rehabilitation Hosp.; 800 Sherbrook St., Zone 2; Rehab. 158; Tel. SP 5-0181.
Melvin Nursing Home; 160 Mayfair Ave.; Infirm 21.
Misericordia Gen. Hosp.; 99 Cornish Ave., Zone 1; Gen. 428; Cont. 14; Psy. 20; Tel. SP 4-6581.
Moore Nursing Home; 165 Maryland St.; Ger. 28.
Nebylowich Nursing Home; 651 Redwood Ave., Zone 4; Infirm 20; Tel. JU 2-6158.
Nightingale Nursing Home; 123 Mayfair Ave.; Zone 13; Infirm 48; Tel. GR. 5-6065.
Osborne Nursing Home; 12 Osborne St., Zone 13; Infirm 31; Tel. GL 3-1505.
Rehill Nursing Home; 92 Maryland St.; Infirm 12.
Riverside Nursing Home; 21 Roslyn Rd.; Infirm 26.
St. Boniface Gen. Hosp.; Tache Ave.; Gen. 715; Tel. WH 3-0311.
St. Boniface San.; Lot 55, Greendel Ave., Zone 8, St. Vital; Ext. Treat. 148; Ret. Child. 167; Tel. AL 3-1311.
St. Joseph's Residence; 160 Salter St., Zone 4; Ger. 115; Tel. JU 6-1090.
St. Michael's Nursing Home; 36 Roslyn Rd.; Infirm 30.
Shriners' Hosp. for Crippled Children; 633 Wellington Cres., Zone 9; (Priv); Orth. 50; Tel. GL 2-4311.
Stradbrook Nursing Home; 499 Stradbrook Ave., Zone 13; Infirm. 21; Tel. GI 3-4276.
Sunset Lodge; 2281 Main St. N., R.R. 1; Ger. 57; Tel. ED 4-1822.
Tache Hospice; 500 Tache Ave., St. Boniface; Inf. 392; Tel. CE 3-1411.
Victoria Gen. Hosp.; 424 River Ave., Zone 13; Gen. 167; Tel. GL 2-3511.
Walsh Nursing Home; 60 Roslyn Rd.; Infirm 27.
Winnipeg Gen. Hosp.; 700 William Ave., Zone 3; Gen. 984; Psy. 115; Tel. SP 4-6511.
Winnipeg Municipal Hosps.; Morley Ave. E., Zone 13; Chron. 386; Cont. 22; Polio 37; Tel. GL 2-3411.
Winnipeg Psychiatric Institute; 75 Emily St., Zone 3; Psy. 56; Tel. SP 4-6511.
WINNIPEGOSIS
Crerar Hosp.; 34 Bridge St., P.O. Box 280; Gen. 36; Tel. OL 6-4431.

Ontario

AGINCOURT
Florence Nightingale Home; 2606 Midland Ave.; Ger. 18.
Shepherd Lodge; 3760 Sheppard Ave. E., Box 70; Dom. 104; Tel. AX 3-8241.
AJAX
Ajax & Pickering Gen. Hosp.; Harwood Ave. & 3rd St., P.O. Box 370; Gen. 134; Chron. 18; Tel. WH 2-2320.
ALEXANDRIA
Glengarry Memorial Hosp.; Highway 43, P.O. Box 514; Gen. 52; Tel. 980.
ALLISTON
Stevenson Memorial Hosp.; 40 Fletcher Cres.; Gen. 93; Tel. HE 5-6281.
ALMONTE
Almonte Gen. Hosp.; 75 Spring St., P.O. Box 750; Gen. 51; Tel. 256-2500.
ARNPRIOR
Arnprior & District Memorial Hosp.; 17 John St., P.O. Box 940; Gen. 82; Tel. 623-3166.
ATHENS
Austen-Barclay Nursing Home; Wellington St., P.O. Box 57; Dom. 7; Tel. 924-2167.
Leeds & Grenville Counties Home; P.O. Box 100; Ger. 40; Tel. 924-2696.
ATIKOKAN
Atikokan Gen. Hosp.; 24 Hematite Ave., P.O. Box 970; Gen. 44; Tel. 4216.
ATTAWAPISKAT
St. Mary's Hosp.; via Moosonee, Gen. 19.
ATWOOD
Maple Crest Rest Home; John St., P.O. Box 106; Dom. 14; Tel. 356-2862.
AURORA
Aurora Resthaven Nursing Home; 50 Tyler St., Infirm 14; Tel. PA 7-4091.

HOSPITALS & CONVALESCENT HOMES — ONT.

Cobblestone House; 121 Yonge St. S.; Chron. 12; **Tel. PA 7-5705.**
Ontario Hosp.; P.O. Box 130; Gen. 258; Dom. 60; Tel. PA 7-4291.
AYLMER
Aylmer Nursing Home; 258 Talbot St., P.O. Box 1107; Inf. 22; **Tel. 773-3423.**
BANCROFT
Red Cross Hosp.; P.O. Box 157; Gen. 34; Tel. 30.
BARRIE
Burton Lodge Nursing Home; 67 Burton Ave.; Inf. 20; **Tel. 726-8905.**
Inniswood Private Hosp.; R.R. 4, Hwy. 11; Chron. 25; **Tel. PA 8-4268.**
I.O.O.F. Home; 93 William St.; Ger. 80; Tel. PA 8-2364.
Royal Victoria Hosp.; 76 Ross St.; Gen. 248; **Tel. PA 8-5951.**
BARRY'S BAY
St. Francis Mem. Hosp.; P.O. Box 129; Gen. 42; Tel. 218
BEAMSVILLE
Nipponia Home; R.R. 3; Ger. 30; **Tel. LOGAN 3-8312.**
BEARDMORE
Red Cross Hosp.; Gen. 18; **Tel. 875-2058.**
BEETON
Simcoe Manor; Ger. 115; **Tel. 10.**
BELLEVILLE
Belleville Gen. Hosp.; East Dundas St., P.O. Box 428; Gen. 370; **Tel. WO 8-5511.**
Hastings County Home; P.O. Box 390; Ger. 218.
BIG TROUT LAKE
Big Trout Lake Nursing Station; Via Sioux Lookout; Gen. 4.
BLENHEIM
Golden Acres Nursing Home; R.R. 6; Inf. 18; **Tel. 676-2929.**
BLIND RIVER
St. Joseph's Gen. Hosp.; Lakeside Ave., P.O. Box 970; Gen. 77; **Tel. EL 6-2265.**
BOBCAYGEON
Hillcroft Private H.; P.O. Box 40; Gen. 18; Tel. 738-2551.
BOLTON
Bolton Nursing Home; 28 Ann St.; Dom. 15; **Tel. 857-3413.**
BOWMANVILLE
Marnwood; 26 Elgin St., P.O. Box 404; Inf. 30; **Tel. 623-5731.**
Memorial Hosp.; Liberty St. S., P.O. Box 820; Gen. 124; Chron. 31; **Tel. 623-3331.**
Strathaven Nursing Home Ltd.; 264 King E.; Inf. 31; **Tel. 623-5555.**
BRACEBRIDGE
South Muskoka Mem. Hosp.; 75 Anne St., P.O. Box 1570; Gen. 61; Chron. 14; **Tel. 645-4404.**
The Pines; District of Muskoka, P.O. Box 877; Dom. 105.
BRADFORD
Martingate Villa; 136 Barrie St.; Dom. 36; **Tel. 775-2305.**
BRAMPTON
Peel County Manor; P.O. Box 809, Main St. N.; Dom. 240; **Tel. GLendale 1-2150.**
Peel Memorial Hosp.; 20 Lynch St.; Gen. 274; Psy. 21 **Tel, GL 1-1710.**
Tullamore Nursing Home Ltd.; 133 Kennedy Rd. S.; Dom. 149; **Tel. 459-2324.**
BRANTFORD
Bethel Nursing Home; 130 Park Ave.; Infirm 19; Tel. PL 3-1421.
Brantford Gen. Hosp.; Terrace Hill St.; Gen. 421; Cont. 36; Psy. 34; Chron. 62; **Tel. 752-7871.**
Brantford Widow's Home; 6 Sheridan St.; Ger. 18.
Brant San.; T.B. 23; Chron. 28; Cribs 71; **Tel. PL 3-2658.**
Golden Years Rest Home; 104 Brant Ave.; Infirm 40; Tel. 752-5059.
John Noble Home; Mount Pleasant Rd.; Ger. 291.
Rouleau Nursing Home; 76 Brock St.; Infirm 14.
St. Joseph's Hosp.; 97 Park Rd. N.; Gen. 191; **Tel. 753-8641.**
BROCKVILLE
Brockville Gen. Hosp.; 122 Pearl St. E.; Gen. 208; Chron. 40; **Tel. DI 5-5645.**
Ontario Hosp.; P.O. Box 1050; Ment. 1416; **Tel. DI 5-1461.**
St. Vincent de Paul Hosp.; Pine & Garden Sts.; Gen. 131; **Tel. 613-342-4461.**
BRUSSELS
Callander Nursing Home; P.O. Box 112; Inf. 29; **Tel. 271.**
BURFORD
Bellview Private Hosp.; 54 King St. E., P.O. Box 217; Gen. 11; **Tel. HI 9-2431.**
BURK'S FALLS
Red Cross Hosp.; Gen. 34; **Tel. 382-2927.**
BURLINGTON
Joseph Brant Memorial Hosp.; 1230 North Shore Blvd.; Gen. 271; **Tel. 637-2361.**
Schenkel's Nursing Home; 271 West Plains Rd.; Inf. 10; **Tel. JA 7-2887.**
CAMPBELLFORD
Campbellford Memorial Hosp.; 146 Oliver Rd.; Gen. 77; Chron. 10; **Tel. 653-1140.**
CARLETON PLACE
Bartlett Nursing Home; 179 Lake Ave.; Dom. 38.
Carleton Place & District Memorial Hosp.; Lake Ave. E., P.O. Box 670; Gen. 45; **Tel. 257-2000.**
CASSELMAN
Casselman Nursing Home Ltd.; Inf. 49; **Tel. 764-2933.**
CEDAR SPRINGS
Ontario H. Schl.; R.R. 1, Blenheim, P.O. Box 1000; Retd. Child. 1046; **Tel. OR 6-5431.**
CHAPLEAU
Lady Minto Hosp.; 10 Queen St., P.O. Box 757; Gen. 80; Tel. 864-1520.
CHATHAM
Public Gen. Hosp.; 106 Emma St.; Gen. 271, Chron. 40; **Tel. EL 2-6400.**
St. Joseph's Hosp.; King St. W.; Gen. 230; Tel. EL 2-2500
Thamesview Lodge Kent County Home; Dom. 134.
Victoria Home; 190 Stanley Ave.; Ger. 88; **Tel. EL. 4-0610.**
CHESLEY
Chesley & District Memorial Hosp.; Mill St., P.O. Box 297; Gen. 32; **Tel. 363-2340.**
McCulligh Nursing Home; River St.; Dom. 18; **Tel. 363-2702.**
Parkview Manor Nursing Home; Adolph St.; Inf. 35; **Tel. 363-3309.**
Spruce Lawn Nursing Home; Second Concession St.; Inf. 22; **Tel. 363-2625.**
CHIPAWA
Margaret Clare Rest Home; P.O. Box 599; Inf. 15; **Tel. AX 5-4464.**
CLAREMONT
Claremont Vill. Nursing Home; P.O. Box 17; Inf. 15; **Tel. 649-2107.**
CLARKSBURG
Hillcrest Haven; Hillcrest Dr., P.O. Box 8; Chron. 12; **Tel. 150.**
CLARKSON
Pines Nursing Home; Sayers Rd.; P.O. Box 201; Chron. 40; **Tel. TA 2-0491.**
CLINTON
Clinton Public Hosp.; Shipley St., Gen. 72, Chron. 8; **Tel. HU 2-3447.**
Huronview; P.O. Box 219; Ger. 235; **Tel. HU 2-3451.**
COBOURG
Cobourg District Gen. Hosp.; Chapel St.; P.O. Box 340; Gen. 131; **Tel. FR 2-5451.**
Kent Cottage; 130 Bay St.; Dom. 4; **Tel. 372-3663.**
Northumberland & Durham Counties Home; P.O. Box 248; Ger. 150.

HOSPITALS & CONVALESCENT HOMES — ONT.

Ontario Hosp.; 78 University Ave.; P.O. Box 110; Ment. 536; **Tel. 372-3341.**
Sidbrook Private Hosp.; 411 King St. E.; Chron. 38; **Tel. FR 2-3411.**
COCHENOUR
Margaret Cochenour Memorial Hosp.; P.O. Box 160; Gen. 34; **Tel. 3281.**
COCHRANE
Cochrane Nursing Home; 221 Railway St.; Inf. 60; **Tel. 705-272-4144.**
Lady Minto Hosp.; 8th St., P.O. Box 660; Gen. 104; Chron. 10; **Tel. 272-4246.**
COLDWATER
Jay-Haro Rest H.; 3 Reinbird St., Dom. 17; **Tel. 686-3307.**
COLLINGWOOD
Cara Villa Nursing Home; 150 Cedar St.; Inf. 27; **Tel. 445-4191.**
General & Marine Hosp.; 67 Moberly St.; Gen. 131; Chron. 10; **Tel. 705-445-2550.**
Glen Moore Nursing H.; 50 St. Paul St., Inf. 12.
Green Gables Rest Home; 104 Hume Street; Dom. 5; **Tel. 445-1613.**
COOKSVILLE
South Peel Hosp.; 100 Upper Middle Rd., Gen. 382; **Tel. 279-7330.**
The Willows Nursing Home; 2116 Dixie Rd.; Dom. 15; **Tel. 277-2863.**
COPPER CLIFF
Inco Hosp.; 38 Granite St., P.O. Box 647; (Priv); Gen. 37; **Tel. MU 2-4421.**
CORNWALL
Cornwall Gen. Hosp.; 510—2nd St. E.; Gen. 209; Chron. 46; **Tel. WE 2-3300.**
Glen Stor Dun Lodge; Stormont, Dundas & Glengarry Counties; Ger. 237.
Hotel Dieu Hosp.; McConnell Ave. N., P.O. Box 939; Gen. 315; **Tel. WE 2-4630.**
MacDonell Memorial Hosp.; 211 Water St. W., P.O. Box 489; Chron. 118; **Tel. 613-4911.**
Megan Nursing Home; 128 Marlborough St.; Dom. 18; **Tel. WE 3-1154.**
Nixon Nursing Home; 219 Hoople St.; Dom. 3; **Tel. WE 2-4428.**
Payment Nursing Home; 511 Amelia St.; Inf. 12; **Tel. WE 3-2196.**
St. Lawrence San.; East Front St., TB 47; **Tel. WE 3-4975.**
COTTAM
Cottam Nursing Home; P.O. Box 59; Dom. 11; **Tel. 839-4834.**
DEEP RIVER
Deep River Hosp.; Moncton St., P.O. Box 307; (Priv); Gen. 40; **Tel. JU 4-3333.**
DELAWARE
Delaware Nursing Home; River Rd.; Inf. 58; **Tel. 652-3483.**
DRUMBO
Drumbo Nursing Home; P.O. Box 10; Dom. 15; **Tel. 463-5400.**
DRYDEN
Dryden District Gen. Hosp.; Van Horne Ave., P.O. Box 1360; Gen. 81; Chron. 12; **Tel. 223-4845.**
DUNDAS
House of Providence; Governor's Rd., Ger. 133;
Wentworth Lodge; Ger. 155.
DUNNVILLE
Grand View Lodge; P.O. Box 710; Ger. 104; **Tel. 531.**
Haldimand War Memorial Hosp.; John St., P.O. Box 100; Gen. 100; **Tel. 774-7431.**
DURHAM
Durham Memorial Hosp.; Chester & College Sts.; Gen. 84; Chron. 6; **Tel. 369-2340.**
St. Raphael's Nursing Home; 31 Durham Rd. E.; Dom. 49; **Tel. 369-3741.**
Watson Nursing Home; 134 Garafraxa N.; P.O Box 140; Inf. 12; **Tel. 369-3315.**
DUTTON
Bobier Convalescent Home; Inf. 30; **Tel. 762-2417.**
ELLIOT LAKE
St. Joseph's Gen. Hosp.; Spine Rd.; Gen. 142; Tel. 818-7181.
ELMIRA
Elmira Private Hosp.; 11 Herbert St., P.O. Box 729; Chron. 17; **Tel. MO 9-2921.**
EMBRO
Rosedale Nursing Home; John St.; Inf. 21; Tel. 475-4015.
EMO
Red Cross Hosp.; Gen. 23; Tel. 324.
ENGLEHART
Englehart & District Hosp.; Riverside Dr., P.O. Box 69; Gen. 42; **Tel. LI 4-2355.**
ERINDALE
Carmel Heights; Springbank Rd. & Dundas Hwy.; Ger. 63.
ESPANOLA
Espanola Gen. Hosp.; 79 Tudhope St., P.O. Box 10; **Gen. 52; Tel. 420.**
EVERETT
Smith Nursing Home; P.O. Box L; **Dom. 7; Tel.** 435-5024.
EXETER
Exeter Nursing Home; 20 Sanders; **Inf. 13; Tel.** 235-0810.
South Huron Hosp.; 24 Huron St. W., P.O. Box 700; Gen. 61; Chron. 8; **Tel. 235-2700.**
FERGUS
Groves Memorial Community Hosp.; 235 Union St. E., P.O. Box 520; Gen. 74; Chron. 20; **Tel. 843-2010.**
St. Andrew's Nursing Home; 487 St. Andrew St. W.; P.O. Box 583; Ger. 13; **Tel. 626.**
Wellington County Home; R.R. 1; Ger. 94; Tel. 33.
FORT ALBANY
Ste. Anne Indian Hosp.; via Moosonee; Gen. 25.
FORT ERIE
Douglas Memorial Hosp.; 230 Bertie St.; Gen. 93; **Tel. 871-6600.**
Tradewoods Manor Nursing Home; Niagara Blvd.; Dom. 37; **Tel. 871-1250.**
FORT FRANCES
La Verendrye Hosp.; 110 Victoria Ave.; Gen. 141; **Tel. 274-3261.**
Rainycrest; 450 Home St., P.O. Box 249; Dom. 174; **Tel. BR 5-6842.**
FORT GEORGE
Ste-Therese de l'Enfant-Jesus; Gen. 39; **Tel. 31.**
FORT WILLIAM
Grandview Lodge; Lillie St.; Dom. 199; **Tel. MA 2-7793.**
Fort William San.; 300 N. Lillie St., TB 150; Ret. 54; **Tel. MA 3-7493.**
McKellar Gen. Hosp.; Ridgeway St.; P.O. Box 3; Gen. 322; **Tel. MA 3-6471.**
Westmount Hosp.; Cedar St.; Chron. 100; Conv. 50; **Tel. MA 3-0416.**
FRASERDALE
Hydro Electric Power Commission Hosp.; Emer. 2.
GALT
Cavell Convalescent Home; 201 Hespler Road; Inf. 25; **Tel. 623-0411.**
Hilltop Manor; 20 Elliott St.; Dom. 30; **Tel. 621-3067.**
Marsdale Manor; 25 Linwood Ave.; **Inf. 34; Tel. 621-8154.**
Salvation Army Eventide Home; 255 St. Andrew's St.; Infirm 129; **Tel. 621-1881.**
St. Jerome's Nursing Home; 20 Elliott St.; Infirm. 26; **Tel. 621-3067.**
South Waterloo Memorial Hosp.; Coronation Blvd.; Gen. 310; **Tel. 621-2330.**
GEORGETOWN
Georgetown & Dist. Mem. Hosp.; Princess Anne Drive; Gen. 84; **Tel. TR 7-2294.**
GERALDTON
Geraldton District Hosp.; Hogarth St.; Gen. 59; **Tel. 854-1862.**
GODERICH
Alexandra Marine & Gen. Hosp.; Napier St., P.O. Box 1510; Gen. 87; Chron. 16; **Tel. JA 4-8323.**
Maitland-Manor Ltd.; 15 Bennett W.; Inf. 42; **Tel. 524-7324.**

Ontario Hosp.; Hwy. 21, P.O. Box 71; Psy. 300; **Tel. 524-7331.**

GORE BAY

Red Cross Health Centre; Emer. 1; Tel. 234.

GRAND VALLEY

Walker's Nursing Home; Gier St.; Inf. 12; **Tel. 928-2171.**

GRIMSBY

Kilean Lodge; 83 Main St. E.; Inf. 28; **Tel. Whitehall 5-5846.**

West Lincoln Memorial Hosp.; Main St. E.; Gen. 74; Tel. WH 5-2253.

GUELPH

Cambridge Lodge; 86 Cambridge St.; Inf. 22; Tel. TA 2-7810.

Elim Lodge; 143 Norfolk St.; Inf. 16; **Tel. 822-6195.**

Elliott Home; 170 Metcalfe St.; Dom. 82. **Tel. 2-0491.**

Ellis Nursing Home; 211 Liverpool St., Dom. 12; Tel. 822-2736.

Guelph Gen. Hosp.; Delhi St.; Gen. 203; **Tel. TA 2-5350.**

Homewood San. of Guelph; 150 Delhi St.; P.O. Box 602; (Priv); Psy. 225; **Tel. TA 4-1010.**

Ontario Reformatory Hosp.; P.O. Box 600; Gen. 40; Psy. 25; **Tel. TA 2-0020.**

St. Joseph's Home; Edinburgh Road; Inf. 132; **Tel. TA 4-2620.**

St. Joseph's Hosp.; 80 Westmount Rd.; Gen. 237; Chron. 109, Dom. 121; **Tel. TA 4-2620.**

Salvation Army Eventide Home; 24 Clark St. W.; Ger. 44; **Tel. TA 2-8021.**

HAGERSVILLE

Hendriks Nursing Home; 24 King St. W.; Inf. 17.

West Haldimand Gen. Hosp.; King and Parkview; Gen. 74; **Tel. 768-3311.**

HAILEYBURY

Misericordia Hosp.; Georgina Ave.; Gen. 124, Chron. 86; **Tel. OS 2-3315.**

HALIBURTON

Red Cross Hosp.; Gen. 15; **Tel. 270.**

HAMILTON

Brow Infirmary; P.O. Box 590; Chron. 75; Conv. 20; Tel. 385-5341.

Central Park Lodge; Arkledun Ave.; Inf. 106.

Chedoke Gen. & Children's Hosp.; P.O. Box 590; Gen. 214; Tel. 385-5341.

Clarion Nursing Home; 120 Hunter St. W.; Inf. 23; **Tel. 522-7911.**

Edgewood Hall; 1686 Main St. W. (C.N.I.B.); Ger. 61.

Hamilton and District Rehab. Hosp.; P.O. Box 590; Gen. 64; **Tel. 385-5341.**

Hamilton Gen. Hosp.; Barton St. E.; Gen. 561; Psy. 30; **Tel. 527-0271.**

Hamilton Nursing Home; 125 Wentworth St. S.; Gen. 30; **Tel. 527-1482.**

Henderson Gen. Hosp.; Concession St.; Gen. 817; Chron. 102; Rehab. 88; **Tel. 389-4411.**

"Idlewyld" Women's Home; 449 Sanatorium Rd.; Ger. 96.

Lady Patricia Nursing Home; 265 Bay St. S.; Dom. 19; **Tel. 522-0784.**

Macassa Lodge; Upper Sherman Ave.; Ger. 358; **Tel. FU 5-5311.**

MacKenzie Retreat; 7 Blake St.; Inf. 25; Tel. LI 9-2511.

Mountain San.; P.O. Box 590; T.B. 43; **Tel. 385-5341.**

Ontario Hosp.; Ment. 1800; **Tel. 385-5361.**

Pine Lodge; 93 Emerald St.; Inf. 24; **Tel. JA 9-0741.**

Rest Haven Private Hosp.; 83—85 Emerald St. S.; Chron. 34; Tel. JA 7-0403.

St. Elizabeth Home; 307 John St. S.; Inf. 108; Tel. 529-3589.

St. Joseph's Hosp.; 50 Charlton Ave. E.; Gen. 771; **Tel. 522-4941.**

St. Peter's Infirmary; 88 Maplewood Ave.; Chron. 200; **Tel. LI 9-6561.**

West Willow Nursing Home; 27 Mountain Ave.; Infirm. 33; **Tel. JA 9-8323.**

HANOVER

Densmore Faith Nursing Home; 326 E. 12th St.; P.O. Box 128; Inf. 22; **Tel. 364-3700.**

Hanover Memorial Hosp.; 101—10th St., P.O. Box 220; Gen. 73; Chron. 2; **Tel. 364-2340.**

HARRISTON

Beth-Shan Rest Home; Thomas & Union Sts.; **Tel. 129.**

Pleasant Haven Nursing Home; William & Thomas Sts.; Inf. 7; **Tel. 166.**

Whitehouse Nursing Home; King St.; Dom. 8; **Tel. 331.**

HAWKESBURY

Notre-Dame Hosp.; 340 rue William, C.P. 1120; **Gen. 40; Tel. ME 2-2724.**

Pleasant Rest Nursing Home; Wankleek Hill Rd.; Inf. 23.

St-Coeur-de-Marie Hosp.; 342 rue McGill; Gen. 61; Tel. ME 2-7031.

Smith Hosp.; 144 Main St. W., P.O. Box 1509; (Priv); Gen. 58; **Tel. ME 2-2711.**

HEARST

Notre-Dame Hosp.; Alexandria St., P.O. Box 850; Gen. 98; **Tel. 362-4211.**

HENSALL

Spruce Haven Lodge; 260 Guelph Rd.; Inf. 37; **Tel. 658-2761.**

HESPELER

Spruce-Haven Lodge; Guelph Rd., P.O. Box 910; Inf. 26; **Tel. 658-2761.**

HORNEPAYNE

Hornepayne Community Hosp.; Front St. P.O. Box 190; Gen. 17; **Tel. 690-9192.**

HUNTSVILLE

Huntsville District Memorial Hosp.; Mill St., P.O. Box 1150; Gen 59; Chron. 22; **Tel. 789-2311.**

INGERSOLL

Alexandra Hosp.; Noxon St.; Gen. 77; Chron. 15; **Tel. 485-1700.**

Faith Haven Rest Home; Culloden Rd., R.R. 1; Inf. 28; **Tel. 485-3920.**

King Merritt Nursing Home; 140 Merritt St.; Inf. 17; **Tel. 485-0960.**

Pinecrest Nursing Home; 189 Thames St. N.; Inf. 25; **Tel. 485-3776.**

IROQUOIS FALLS

Anson Gen. Hosp.; 8th St., P.O. Box 370; Gen. 58; **Tel. 258-3272.**

KAPUSKASING

Sensenbrenner Hosp.; 10 Drury St.; (Priv); Gen. 102; Chron. 6; **Tel. 335-2305.**

KEMPTVILLE

Kemptville District Hosp.; P.O. Box 759; Gen. 39; **Tel. 258-3435.**

Oxford Private Hosp.; Oxford Mills Rd., R.R. 5; (Priv); Gen. 18; Dom. 7; Tel. 258-3301.

KENORA

Kenora Gen. Hosp.; R.R. 1, Tunnel Island; Gen. 120; **Tel. HO 8-9861.**

Pinecrest Home for The Aged; 1220 Valley Dr., P.O. Box 460; Dom. 207; **Tel. HO 8-9696.**

St. Joseph's Hosp.; R.R. 1, Ocean Ave.; Gen. 65; **Tel. HO 8-9836.**

KINCARDINE

Kincardine Gen. Hosp.; R.R. 5; Gen. 69; Tel. 71.

KINGSTON

Canadian Forces Hosp.; Camp Barriefield; Gen. 125; **Tel. 8-3060.**

Hotel Dieu Hosp.; Sydenham St.; Gen. 364; **Tel.** 546-1151.

House of Providence; 115 Ordnance St.; Ger. 213; Tel. Liberty 8-4479.

Institute of Psychotherapy; 113 Lower Union St., (Priv); Psy. 18; Tel. LI 6-3116.

Kingston Gen. Hosp.; 24 Stuart St.; Gen. 629; Psy. 36; Tel. 546-3842.

Ongwanada San.; 790 Princess St.; TB 134; Tel. LI 8-4417.

Ontario Hosp.; King St., P.O. Box 603; Ment. 797; Inf. 782; Tel. 546-1101.

Quinte St-Lawrence Hall (CNIB); 466 Union St. W.; **Ger. 28.**

Rideaucrest Home for the Aged; 362 Montreal St., Ger. 152; Tel. LI 8-4901.
St. Mary's Of The Lake Hosp.; 355 King St. W.; Gen. 214; **Tel. LI 8-3304.**
Winters Nursing Home; 229 Alfred Street; Inf. 6; Tel. Liberty 8-3587.

KIRKLAND LAKE
Kirkland & District Hosp.; 2nd St., Gen. **165,** Chron. 19; **Tel. 567-5251.**
Teck Pioneer Residence; Churchill Drive & Fourth Ave.; Ger. 77.

KITCHENER
A. R. Goudie Eventide; 369 Frederick St.; Dom. 71.
Belvedere Lodge; R.R. 4; Inf. 12; **Tel. 743-6449.**
Central Park Lodge; 290 Queen St. S.; Inf. 132.
Freeport San.; R.R. 3; TB 45; Chron. 80; Conv. 15; Tel. 742-5891.
Kitchener-Waterloo Hosp.; 835 King St. W.; Gen. 371; Chron. 110; **Tel. SH 5-9451.**
St. Mary's Gen. Hosp.; 911B Queen's Blvd.; Gen. 432; **Tel. 744-3311.**
Sunnyside; 247 Franklin Ave.; Ger. 256.

LAC SEUL
Lac Seul Nursing Station; via Souix Lookout; Gen. 4.

LAKEFIELD
Armstrong Nursing Home; R.R. 1; Dom. 6; **Tel.** 657-8544.
Harborne Nursing Home; Queen St.; Inf. 21; Tel. 652-3241.
Lakefield Private Hosp.; Chron. 11; Tel. OL 2-3421.
Peterborough County Home; Ger. 87.

LANSDOWNE HOUSE
Nursing Station; Gen. 4.

LEAMINGTON
Leamington District Memorial Hosp.; Talbot St. W.; Gen. 114; Tel. FA 6-6131.
Leamington Mennonite; 22 Garrison Ave.; Ger. 44.
Sun Parlor Home for Senior Citizens; Talbot St. E.; Dom. 175; **Tel. FA 6-5221.**

LIMOGES
St. Viateur Nursing Home; Inf. 22; **Tel.** Casselman 764.

LINDSAY
Douglas Waterman Private Hosp.; 51 Adelaide St. N.; Chron. 14; Tel. 324-3796.
Lindsay Private Hosp.; 11 Ridout St.; Gen. 23; Tel. 324-5121.
Ross Memorial Hosp.; Kent St. W.: Gen. 174; **Tel. 324-6111.**
Spruce Lawn Private Hosp.; 245 Kent St. W.; Infirm 14; **Tel.** 324-5125.
Victoria County Home; R.R. 2; Dom. 111.

LION'S HEAD
Red Cross Hosp.; Gen. 17.

LISTOWEL
Listowel Memorial Hosp.; Elizabeth St.; P.O. Box 160; Gen. 84; Tel. 291-3120.

LITTLE BRITAIN
Starr-Haven Nursing Home; P.O. Box 27; Inf. 16; Tel. 30.

LITTLE CURRENT
St. Joseph's Gen. Hosp.; Meredith St., P.O. Box 250; Gen. 66; Tel. 685.
Little Long Rapids Ont. Hydro H., (Priv.); Gen. 10.

LONDON
Beck Memorial San.; Sanatorium Rd.; TB 124; **Tel. 471-1440.**
Bethesda Hosp.; 54 Riverview Ave.; (Priv); Mat. 17; Dom. 26; **Tel. 438-8371.**
B-Rra Mor Villa; 711 Waterloo St.; Inf. 26; **Tel. GE 9-8162.**
Bruceside Convalescent Home; 79 Rideout St. S.; Dom. 7; **Tel.** 433-2941.
Central Park Lodge; 279-273 Horton St.; Inf. 147.
Children's Psychiatric Research Institute; P.O. Box 2460, Terminal A.; Gen. 117; **Tel.** 471-2540.
Dearness Home for Elder Citizens; R.R. 10; Dom. 359; **Tel. GE 4-2183.**
Egerton Private Hosp.; 266 Egerton St.; Chron. 17; **Tel. GL 1-0300.**
Greenwood Nursing Home; 551 Hale St.; Inf. 32; **Tel.** 451-8322.
Grandview Rest Home; 153 Rideout St. S.; Dom. 7; **Tel.** 434-6405.
Malvine Nursing Home; 578 Colborne St., Inf. 12.
Marian Villa; 200 College Ave.; Ger. 215.
Mason Villa Hosp. Ltd.; 201 Mount Pleasant Ave.; (Priv); Chron. 60; Tel. GE 8-7422.
McCormick Home For Aged People; 1050 Richmond St.; Dom. 97; Tel. GE 4-6194.
Ontario Hosp.; P.O. Box 2532, Terminal A.; Psy. 1010; **Tel.** 455-5110.
Parkwood Hosp.; 81 Grand Ave.; Chron. 193; Tel. GE 2-3408.
St. Joseph's Hosp.; Richmond St. N.; Gen. 670; Psy. 44; **Tel. GE 9-3271.**
St. Mary's Hosp.; 35 Grosvenor St.; Chron. 211; Tel. GE 8-6185.
Sher Park Nursing Home; R.R. 9; Inf. 10.
Tweedsmuir Hall (CNIB); 96 **Ridout St. S., P.O.** Box 443; Ger. 38.
Victoria Hosp.; 375 South St.; Gen. 927; Cont. 35; Psy. 49; **Tel. GE 2-5261.**
War Memorial Children's Hospital; (Unit of Victoria Hosp.) Paed. 170.
Westminster Hosp.; (DVA); 777 Base Line Rd., P.O. Box 2337; Gen. 409; Psy. 605; Dom. 334; **Tel.** 432-6711.

L'ORIGINAL
Prescott & Russell Counties Home; Ger. 94; **Tel.** 674-4696.

LUCKNOW
Pinecrest Manor Nursing Home; Gough St., P.O. Drawer 220; Inf. 31; **Tel. 528-2136.**

MANITOUWADGE
Manitouwadge Gen. Hosp.; Gen. 43; **Tel. TA 6-3251.**

MARATHON
Wilson Memorial Hosp.; Gilbert St., P.O. Box 550; (Priv); Gen. 25; **Tel. 229-0141.**

MARKDALE
Centre Grey Gen. Hosp.; Isle St., P.O. Box 249; Gen. 50, Chron. 12; **Tel. 40.**
Grey County Home; Ger. 85.

MARKHAM
Markham Nursing Home; 5 George St.; Inf. 10; **Tel.** 294-2811.
Markhaven Inc.; 176 Main St. N.; Dom. 15; **Tel.** 294-2233.

MATACHEWAN
Red Cross Health Centre; Emer. 1; Tel. 43.

MATHESON
Bingham Memorial Hosp.; 8th Ave., P.O. Box 70; Gen. 39; Isol. 1; **Tel. 16.**

MATTAWA
Mattawa Gen. Hosp.; 2nd St., P.O. Box 70; Gen. 50; Tel. 744-5511.

MEAFORD
Meaford Gen. Hosp.; Nelson St., P.O. Box 340; Gen. 62; **Tel. 520.**

MERRICKVILLE
Hilltop Rest Home; St. Lawrence St.; Inf. 25; **Tel. 269-4707.**

MIDLAND
St. Andrew's Hosp.; Dominion Ave. E.; Gen. 102; Chron. 15; **Tel. 526-5411.**

MILLBROOK
Fairweather Nursing Home; King St.; Inf. 14; Tel. 932-2932.

MILTON
Halton Centennial Manor; 147 Ontario St. S.; **Ger. 226; Tel. TRiangle 8-4451.**
Milton District Hosp.; 10 Side Road; **P.O. Box** 1209; Gen. 69: **Tel. TR 8-2383.**
Lakeshore Nursing Home; 197 Royal York Rd.; Inf. 25; **Tel.** 251-2641.

MINDEMOYA
Red Cross Hosp.; Gen. 24; **Tel. 2-R-2.**

MINDEN
Red Cross Hosp.; Gen. 13; **Tel. 107.**

HOSPITALS & CONVALESCENT HOMES — ONT.

MITCHELL
Braeside Rest Home; 32 Huron St.; **Tel. 348-8861.**
Riverside Nursing Home; 89 St. Andrew St.; P.O. Box 340; Inf. 29; Tel. 348-8903.
MOOSE FACTORY
Moose Factory Indian Hosp.; Gen. 69, TB 90; **Tel. 336-4500.**
MOOSONEE
Assumption Private Hosp.; Box 38; Gen. 32; **Tel. 336-2341.**
MOUNT ALBERT
Cedar Haven; R.R. 1; Dom. 8; Tel. 473-2742.
Cooper's Nursing Home; Centre St.; Inf. 25; Tel. 473-2440.
MOUNT FOREST
Louise Marshall Hosp.; Dublin St., P.O. Box 190; Gen. 41; Tel. 32.
MOUNT PLEASANT
Bracefield Manor (Home for Aged); Ger. 12.
NAPANEE
Lennox & Addington County Gen. H.; P.O. Box 1450; Gen. 90; **Tel. 354-3301.**
McDonald Nursing Home Ltd.; 118 Robinson St.; Dom. 21; Tel. 354-5270.
NEWCASTLE
The Lodge Nursing Home; King St. W.; Inf. 22; Tel. 987-4252.
NEW LISKEARD
New Liskeard & District Hosp.; Hessle Ave., P.O. Box 340; Gen. 58; **Tel. 647-4361.**
Northdale Manor; 130 Lakeshore Rd.; Ger. 35.
NEWMARKET
Cooper's Nursing Home; 329 Eagle St., Inf. 28; Tel. 895-5187.
Greenacres Home for the Aged; 194 Eagle St.; Ger. 630; Tel. TW 5-2381.
Martin Manor Nursing Home; 266 Prospect St.; Inf. 44; Tel. 895-9453.
York County Hosp.; 596 Davis Dr.; Gen. 270; Dom. 24; Psy. 22; Tel. 895-4521.
York Manor; Ger. 168.
NIAGARA FALLS
Clifton Villa Nursing Home; 809 Clifton Ave.; Inf. 23; Tel. 4-3128.
Greater Niagara Gen. Hosp.; 1546 Portage Rd.; Gen. 353; **Tel. EL 8-3611.**
Salvation Army Eventide Home; 1050 Jepson St.; Dom. 173; **Tel. EL 6-1221.**
Sunrise Rest Haven; 972 Jepson St.; Inf. 15; Tel. 354-9133.
NIAGARA-ON-THE-LAKE
Niagara Hosp.; 176 Wellington St., P.O. Box 300; Gen. 34; **Tel. HO. 8-3261.**
NIPIGON
Nipigon District Memorial Hosp.; 98 Churchill St., P.O. Box 37; Gen. 33; **Tel. 887-3136.**
NORTH BAY
Cassellholm; 400 Olive St.; Dom. 192; **Tel. 474-4250.**
North Bay Civic Hosp.; 750 Scollard St.; Gen. 121; **Tel. GR 2-2700.**
Ontario Hosp.; Hwy. 11N., P.O. Box 1010; Psy. 843; Tel. 474-1200.
St. Joseph's Gen. Hosp.; 720 McLaren St.; Gen. 255; **Tel. GR 2-6100.**
OAKVILLE
Oakville-Trafalgar Memorial Hosp.; 327 Reynolds St.; Gen. 369; **Tel. VI 5-2571.**
OHSWEKEN
Lady Willingdon Hosp.; Gen. 41; Tel. HI 5-2251.
ORANGEVILLE
Dufferin Area Hosp.; 32—1st St., Gen. 156; Tel. 941-2410.
Marquardt Nursing Home; 1 Hillside Dr.; Inf. 40; **Tel. 941-1960.**
ORILLIA
Cedar Brae Nursing Home; 190 Laclie St.; Inf. 29; Tel. 5-1782.
Hannaford Nursing Home; 327 Old Muskoka Road; Inf. 23; Tel. 326-6038.
Hillcrest Lodge; 86 Cedar St.; Ger. 13; Tel. Fairview 4-3181.
Ontario Hosp. School; P.O. Box 1000; Ment. 2956; Bas. 2; Tel. 326-7361.
Orillia Soldiers' Memorial Hosp.; Colborne St. W.; Gen. 215; Chron. 35; **Tel. 325-2201.**
Salvation Army Sunset Lodge; 127 Peter St. N.; **Ger. 33.**
ORONO
Lyntonhurst Manor; Centre St.; Inf. 9.
OSHAWA
Hillsdale Manor; 185 Hillsdale Ave.; Ger. 304.
Oshawa Gen. Hosp.; 24 Alma St.; Gen. 576; Chron. 42; Tel. 723-2211.
Sunnybrae Nursing Home; R.R. 3; Inf. 30; Tel. 725-2330.
OTTAWA
Bronson Home 81 Bronson Ave.; Dom. 40; Tel. CE 2-0959.
Belair Nursing Home; 176 Brinson Avenue; Inf. 18; **Tel. 235-0773.**
Carleton Lodge; Carleton County Home; Dom. 130.
Central Park Lodge; Carling Ave. & Edgeworth; Inf. 147.
Grace Hosp., The Salvation Army; 1156 Wellington St., Zone 3; Gen. 132; **Tel. PA 8-4611.**
Hartington Private Hosp.; 66 Cartier St.; Zone 4; Chron. 32; **Tel. CE 2-4743.**
Hillel Lodge; 125 Wurtemburg St.; Ger. 23.
Island Lodge and Geriatric Centre; Porter's Island, Ottawa 2; Dom. 173.
Mary Jane Manor; 297 First Ave.; Inf. 18; **Tel. 237-0954.**
May Court Club Convalescent Home; 114 Cameron Ave., Dom. 41.
National Defence Medical Centre; Smyth Road; Zone 8; Gen. 320; **Tel. RE 3-6600.**
New Orchard Lodge; 99 New Orchard Ave.; Dom. 100; Tel. 728-3551.
Ottawa Civic Hosp.; Carling Ave., Zone 3; Gen. 1171; **Tel. PA 9-2511.**
Ottawa Gen. Hosp.; 43 Bruyere St.; Zone 2, Gen. 618; Orth. 36; Psy. 38; **Tel. CE 6-0333.**
Ottawa Home and Welfare Centre; 398 O'Connor St.; (C.N.I.B.) Dom. 27; **Tel. 233-8471.**
Perley Hosp.; 2 Barton St., Zone 1; Chron. 218; **Tel. CE 6-7171.**
Protestant Home for the Aged; 954 Bank St., Zone 1; Dom. 32; **Tel. CE 4-5533.**
Rideau Health & Occupational Centre (DVA); 363 Smyth Rd., Billings Bridge, Zone 8; Chron. 116, Dom. 44; **Tel. RE 3-6600.**
Rockwood Nursing Home; 2 Rockwood St.; Inf. 22; Tel. 235-6963.
Royal Ottawa San.; 1145 Carling Ave., Zone 3; TB 94; Psy. 100; **Tel. PA 2-6521.**
St. Charles Home; 159 Bruyere St., Zone 2; Dom. 242; **Tel. CE 3-9371.**
Saint Louis-Marie-de Montfort Hosp.; Chemin Montreal, Zone 7; Gen. 276; **Tel. SH 6-4621.**
St. Patrick's Home; 2865 Riverside Dr.; Dom. 181.
St. Vincent Hosp.; 60 Cambridge St., Zone 4; Chron. 456; Conv. 49; **Tel. CE 3-4041.**
St. Michels Nursing Home; 37 Beechwood; Inf. 47; Tel. 749-9807.
Zonta House; 15 Delaware Ave.; Dom. 11; **Tel. 232-8044.**
OWEN SOUND
Greystone Nursing Home; 1731—8th Ave. E.; Inf. 12; **Tel. 376-4204.**
Hillview Nursing Home; 956 6th Ave. E.; Inf. 7; Tel. FR 6-8897.
Justice Nursing Home; 1121—4th Ave. E.; Inf. 9; Tel. 276-5285.
Ontario Hospital; Box 600; **Psy. 300; Tel. FR 6-6130.**
Owen Sound Gen. & Marine Hosp.; 1201—6th Ave. W.; Gen. 243, Chron. 34; **Tel. FR 6-2121.**
White Manor Nursing Home; R.R. 2; Inf. 22; **Tel. FR 6-6376.**
OXFORD MILLS
Greenhaven Rest Home; P.O. Box 77; Inf. 24; **Tel. 258-3542.**

HOSPITALS & CONVALESCENT HOMES — ONT. (*Toronto*)

PALMERSTON
Barnes Nursing Home; York St.; Dom. 14; **Tel. 491.**
Midwestern Regional Children's Centre; P.O. Box 330; **Tel. 694.**
Myrtle Lodge Nursing Home; Main St.; Dom. 12; **Tel. 317.**
Palmerston Gen. Hosp.; Main St., P.O. Box 130; Gen. 53; **Tel. 694.**
PARIS
Broadway Manor Nursing Home; 54 Broadway St. W.; Inf. 36; **Tel. 442-2442.**
Willett Hosp.; Grand River St. N., P.O. Box 520; Gen. 79; **Tel. HI 2-2251.**
PARKHILL
Green Gables Nursing Home; Main St.; Inf. 27; **Tel. 294-6342.**
PARRY SOUND
Parry Sound District Home; Ger. 103.
Parry Sound Gen. Hosp.; 26 James St., P.O. Box 1450; Gen. 149; **Tel. 746-9321.**
St. Joseph's Gen. Hosp.; 116 Church St., P.O. Box 1300; Gen. 59; **Tel. RI 6-2111.**
PEMBROKE
Cottage Hosp.; Cecilia St.; Gen. 165; **Tel. 735-6851.**
Marianhill; 695 MacKay St.; Ger. 137; **Tel. RE 2-8612.**
Pembroke Gen. Hosp.; 705 MacKay St.; Gen. 192; **Tel. RE 2-2811.**
PENETANGUISHENE
Beechwood Private Hosp.; 55 Church St., P.O. Box 609; Chron. 20; **Tel. 549-7792.**
Georgian Manor; Robert St.; P.O. Box 676; Dom. 101; **Tel. KI 9-7676.**
Ontario Hosp.; Church Street; P.O. Box 698; Psy. 561; **Tel. 549-7437.**
Penetanguishene Gen. Hosp.; 35 Jeffrey St., P.O. Box 670; Gen. 87; **Tel. 549-7442.**
PERTH
Four Winds Hosp.; 19 Isabella St.; P.O. Box 730; Gen. 23; **Tel. 267-1523.**
Great War Memorial Hosp. of Perth District; Drummond St. W., P.O. Box 300; Gen. 110; **Tel. 267-1500.**
Tayview Home of Lanark County; R.R. 4; Dom. 63; **Tel. 139.**
Wiseman's Private Hosp.; 67 Drummond St., P.O. Box 159; Conv. 18; **Tel. 424.**
PETERBOROUGH
Anson House; 36 Anson St.; Ger. 34; **Tel. Riverside 3-3272.**
Balmoral Lodge; 293 London St.; Inf. 33; **Tel. 742-4861.**
Fairhaven Home; Langton St., Inf. 175; **Tel. RI 3-4265.**
Kawartha Nursing Home; 303 Brock St.; Inf. 33; **Tel. 742-4761.**
Marycrest; 200 St. Luke Ave.; Dom. 144; **Tel. 743-4744.**
Peterborough Civic Hosp.; Gen. 335; Psy. 26; Chron. 72; **Tel. 743-2121.**
St. Joseph's Gen. Hosp.; 348 Roger St.; Gen. 263; **Tel. RI 3-4251.**
PETROLIA
Adams Private Nursing Home; 421 Princess St.; P.O. Box 399; Inf. 29; **Tel. 882-0620.**
Charlotte Eleanor Englehart Hosp.; Greenfield St., P.O. Box 220; Gen. 75; **Tel. 882-1170.**
Lambton Twilight Haven; Lambton County Home; Ger. 175.
Petrolia Rest Home; 419 King St., P.O. Box 81; Inf. 20; **Tel. 882-1300.**
PICKLE CROW
Pickle Crow Gold Mines Private Hosp.; Gen. 7; **Tel. 3551.**
PICTON
Happy Life Nursing Home; Ontario St.; Dom. 33; **Tel. 476-5671.**
Prince Edward County Home; R.R. 6; Ger. 64; **Tel. GR 6-5824.**
Prince Edward County Mem. Hosp.; Main St. E., P.O. Box 90; Gen. 95; Chron. 20; **Tel. GR. 6-2181.**
Rest Haven Nursing Home; 9 Hill St.; Inf. 48; **Tel. 476-6140.**
PIKANGIKUM
Pikangikum Nursing Station; via Red Lake; Gen. 4.
PLAINFIELD
Ontario Homes for Mentally Retarded Infants Inc.; P.O. Box 100; Ment. Ret. Child. 65; **Tel. Thurlow 477-2440.**
PORT ARTHUR
Cumberland Hall (CNIB); 499 N. Cumberland St.; Dom. 31; **Tel. DI 5-6252.**
Dawson Court; North Algoma St., P.O. Box 478; Ger. 247; **Tel. DI 4-7241.**
Gen. Hosp. of Port Arthur; 460 N. Court St.; Gen. 314; **Tel. DI 4-6621.**
Ontario Hosp.; 580 North Algoma St. P.,O. Box 930; Gen. 727; **Tel. DI 4-3571.**
St. Joseph's Gen. Hosp.; 35 N. Algoma St.; Gen. 169; **Tel. DI 4-2431.**
PORT COLBORNE
Belvedere Nursing Home; 171 Killaly St. W.; Inf. 10; **Tel. 834-3659.**
Port Colborne Gen Hosp.; 260 Sugarloaf St.; Gen. 165; **Tel. TE 834-4501.**
Port Convalescent Home; 240 Clarence St.; Infirm 10; **Tel. TE 4-4624.**
PORT HOPE
Dorset Nursing Home; 66 Dorset St. E.; Inf. 9; **Tel. 885-4722.**
Hope Haven Rest Home; 65 Ward St.; Inf. 70; **Tel. 885-6367.**
Port Hope and District Hosp.; Wellington St.; Gen. 71; Chron. 15; **Tel. 885-6371.**
PORT LORING
Red Cross Hosp.; Gen. 10; **Tel. 757-2830.**
PORT PERRY
Community Memorial Hosp.; P.O. Box 179; Lilla St.; Gen. 40; **Tel. 985-7321.**
POWASSAN
Parry Sound District Home; Ger. 33.
PRESTON
Fairview Mennonite Home; 799 Concession Rd.; Ger. 76.
Golden Years Nursing Homes Ltd.; 704 Eagle St. N.; Dom. 50; **Tel. 653-5493.**
Preston Springs Gardens; Fountain St.; Ger. 76; **Tel. 653-4241.**
PUCE
McPherson Nursing Home; R.R. 1, Belle River; Dom. 13; **Tel. 727-3343.**
PUSLINCH
Morrison Nursing Home; R.R. 2; Inf. 14; **Tel. TA 2-9219.**
QUEENSBOROUGH
Queensboro Nursing Home; Inf. 16; **Tel. 473-2224.**
QUEENSVILLE
Queensville Nursing Home; P.O. Box 67; Inf. 29; **Tel. 478-4251.**
RAINY RIVER
Red Cross Hosp.; Gen. 22; **Tel. 852-3232.**
RED LAKE
Red Cross Hosp.; Gen. 28; **Tel. 315.**
RENFREW
Bonnechere Manor; 782 Raglan St., P.O. Box 309; Ger. 277; **Tel.. HE 2-4873.**
Renfrew Victoria Hosp.; 499 Raglan St. N.; Gen. 119; **Tel. HE 2-4851.**
Renfrew Victoria H. Rehab Centre; 720 Raglan St. S.; Chron. 35; **Tel. HE 2-4851.**
REXDALE
Thistletown Hosp.; 1800 Islington Ave. N.; Paed.-Psy. 64; **Tel. 741-1210.**
RICHARD'S LANDING
Red Cross Hosp.; Gen. 13; **Tel. 66.**
RICHMOND HILL
York Central Hosp.; Maple Side Rd.; Gen. 166; **Tel. 884-1171.**
RIDGWAY
Maple Bray Lodge Nursing Home; 415 Ridge St.; Inf. 17; **Tel. 869-2150.**

HOSPITALS & CONVALESCENT HOMES — ONT. (*Toronto cont'd*)

RIPLEY
Thompson Nursing Home; Malcolm St.; Inf. 13; Tel. 183-R.
ROCKLAND
St. Joseph Nursing Home; Laurier St.; Inf. 66; Tel. 762-4974.
ROSEBANK STATION
Rosebank Con. Home; Inf. 41; Tel. 284-1628.
ROUGE HILLS
Rouge Hills Villa; Altona Rd. & Old Highway No. 2; Inf. 23; Tel. 282-5556.
ST. CATHARINES
Hotel Dieu Hosp.; 155 Ontario St.; Gen. 328; Tel. 682-6411.
Ingleside Nursing Home Ltd.; 164 Geneva St.; Inf. 15; Tel. 682-9489.
Linhaven; Ontario St., P.O. Box 580; Ger. 250; Tel. WE 4-3364.
Linwell Hall (CNIB); 211 Queenston St.; Dom. 61.
Mount Carmel Home; 78 Yates St.; Ger. 48.
Niagara Ina Grafton Gage Home; 413 Linwell Rd.; Dom. 46; Tel. WE 5-6822.
Niagara Peninsula San.; P.O. Box 158; Gen. 25; Chron. 34; T.B. 107; Tel. CA 7-3731.
St. Catharines Gen. Hosp.; 142 Queenston St., Gen. 451, Chron. 68; Psy. 22; Tel. MU 4-7271.
Salina Nursing Home; 9 Salina St.; Inf. 14; Tel. 685-5514.
ST. JACOBS
Brubacher's Rest Home; Young St.; Dom. 8; Tel. 664-2034.
Likeholme Lodge; P.O. Box 86; Inf. 19; Tel. MO 4-2871.
ST. MARY'S
Kingsway Lodge; P.O. Box 777; Inf. 25-30; Tel. 284-2921.
St. Mary's Memorial Hosp.; P.O. Box 940; Queen St.; Gen. 68; Tel. 284-1330.
ST. THOMAS
Alma Nursing Home; 22 Alma St.; Dom. 11; Tel. 633-0860.
Elgin Manor; Dom. 85.
Ontario Hosp.; R.R. No. 4, P.O. Box 204; Psy. 1702; Gen. 273; Tel. ME 1-8510.
St. Thomas-Elgin Gen. Hosp.; Elm St., P.O. Box 2007; Gen. 363; Chron. 87; Tel. ME 1-2020.
Thomas Williams Home; 57 Walnut St.; Ger. 27.
Willson Nursing Home; 58 St. George St.; Inf. 64; Tel. ME 1-6496.
ST. WILLIAMS
Rest Haven Nursing Home; Main & Queen Sts.; Inf. 27; Tel. 586-3331.
SALEM
Short Nursing Home; George St.; Inf. 14; Tel. 846-9821.
SANDY LAKE
Sandy Lake Nursing Station; via Favourable Lake; Gen. 4.
SARNIA
Pioneer Nursing Home; 1183 Confederation St.; Inf. 22; Tel. 337-6113.
St. Joseph's Hosp.; 286 N. Russell St.; Gen. 392; Tel. ED 6-6121.
Sarnia Gen. Hosp.; 220 Mitton St. N.; Gen. 302; Psy. 23; Chron. 29; Tel. DI 4-3661.
Whitfield Nursing Home; 126 Martin; Inf. 10; Tel. 344-6704.
SAULT STE. MARIE
F. J. Davey Home for the Aged; Algoma District, R.R. 2; Ger. 210; Tel. AL 6-5101.
Gen. Hosp.; 941 Queen St. E.; Gen. 252; Psy. 20; Chron. 60; Tel. AL 4-5181.
Plummer Memorial Public Hosp.; 969 Queen St. E.; Gen. 246; Chron. 21; Tel. 254-5161.
SEAFORTH
Kilbarchan Nursing Home; Church St.; Inf. 22; Tel. 527-0860.
Seaforth Manor; James & Wilson Sts., Inf. 36; Tel. 527-0030.
Scott Memorial Hosp.; Goderich St. E., P.O. Box 99; Gen. 48; Tel. 527-1650.
SEELY'S BAY
Rideau House; P.O. Box 104; Inf. 24; Tel. 101.
SHELBURNE
Bakers Nursing Home; Owen Sound St.; Inf. 23; Tel. 925-3746.
Dufferin Oakes; Inf. 70.
Shelburne District Hosp.; First Avenue, P.O. Box 190; Gen. 39; Tel. 925-3340.
SIMCOE
Colborne Nursing Home; 121 Colborne St.; Dom. 26; Tel. 426-0786.
Norfolk Gen. Hosp.; West St.; Gen. 162; Tel. GA 6-0750.
Norview Norfolk County Home; Hwy. 3 W., P.O. Box 340; Ger. 130; Tel. GA 6-0902.
SIOUX LOOKOUT
Sioux Lookout Gen. Hosp.; 5th Ave. S., P.O. Box 909; Gen. 50; Tel. 737-3700.
Sioux Lookout Indian Hosp.; 7th Ave., P.O. Box 1500; Gen. 75; Tel. 737-3030.
SMITHS FALLS
Ontario Hospital School; P.O. Box 2000; Ment. Ret. (Children) 2350; Tel. 283-2990.
St. Francis Gen. Hosp.; 170 Elmsley St. N.; Gen. 80; Chron. 26; Tel. 283-2330.
Smiths Falls Public Hosp.; Elmsley St. S.; Gen. 117; Tel. 283-1200.
SMOOTH ROCK FALLS
Smooth Rock Falls Hosp.; 105—2nd Ave.; Gen. 25; Tel. 338-2515.
SOMBRA
Riverside Rest Home; Water St.; Dom. 14; Tel. 892-3951.
SOUTHAMPTON
Saugeen Memorial Hosp.; High St., P.O. Box 310; Gen. 50; Tel. 797-3230.
SOUTH MOUNTAIN
Montgomery Rest Home; P.O. Box 78; Inf. 6; Tel. 989-2031.
SOUTH PORCUPINE
Porcupine Gen Hosp.; Bruce Ave., P.O. Box 850; Gen. 6; Tel. 235-3377.
STAYNER
Sunnidale Nursing Home; P.O. Box 194; Dom. 10; Tel. 428-3039.
STOUFFVILLE
Brierbush Private Hosp.; Main St., P.O. Box 940; Gen. 28; Tel. 640-2111.
Green Gables Manor; Whitchurch Twnp., R.R. 2; Inf. 19; Tel. 640-3061.
Parkview Home; P.O. Box 90; Ger. 62.
STRATFORD
Biggin Nursing Home; 220 Albert St.; Inf. 12; Tel. 271-1430.
Calcott Nursing Home; 198 Mornington St.; Infirm. 18; Tel. 271-4440.
Hillside Nursing Home; R.R. 5; Ger. 39; Tel. 393-6116.
Spruce Lodge; Ger. 69.
Stratford Gen. Hosp.; Gen. Hospital Dr.; Gen. 248; Chron. 103; Tel. 271-2120.
STRATHROY
Dubs Rest Home; 64 High St., P.O. Box 356; Inf. 15; Tel. 245-2080.
Merry Hill Nursing Home; 336 Carrie St.; Dom. 61; Tel. 245-0181.
Strathmere Lodge; Albert St.; Gen. 170; Tel. 245-2540.
Strathroy Middlesex Gen. Hosp.; 395 Carrie St.: Gen. 129; Tel. 245-1550.
STREETSVILLE
Glen Ridge Convalescent Home; 84 Main St.; Inf. 30; Tel. 277-0419.
STURGEON FALLS
St. Jean de Brebeuf Hosp.; 145 Main St., P.O. Box 940; Gen. 116; Tel. 753-2300.
West Nipissing Dist. Home; Dom. 104.
SUDBURY
Cambrian Hall (CNIB); 303 York St.; Dom. 37.
Pioneer Manor; 296 Notre Dame Ave.; Ger. 212.
St. Joseph's Hosp.; Mackenzie St.; Gen. 228; Tel. OS 4-3101.

HOSPITALS & CONVALESCENT HOMES — ONT. (*Toronto cont'd*)

Sudbury-Algoma San.; 680 Kirkwood Dr., P.O. Box 40; TB 82; Psy. 37; Tel. OS 5-8351.
Sudbury Gen. Hosp. of the Immaculate Heart of Mary; Paris St.; Gen. 365; Psy. 31; Tel. 705-673-3601.
Sudbury Memorial Hosp.; Regent St. S.; Gen. 246; Chron. 24; **Tel. OS 3-8421.**

TARA
Tara Manor Nursing Home; Yonge St.; Inf. 18; Tel. 934-2950.

TEMAGAMI
Red Cross Health Centre; Emer. 1, Bas. 1; Tel. 4551.

TERRACE BAY
Terrace Bay Private Hosp.; Kenogami Rd.; Gen. 30; Tel. TA 5-3627.

THAMESVILLE
The Clayton Nursing Home; Victoria St., P.O. Box 357; Inf. 22; Tel. 692-3967.

THESSALON
Red Cross Hosp.; Gen. 20; Tel. 842-2238.

THORNHILL
Shouldice Surgery; 7750 Bayview Ave.; (Priv.); Unit of Shouldice Surgery, Toronto; **Tel. AV 5-1125.**
Villa Private Hosp.; P.O. Box 490; N. Bathurst St.; Chron. **38; Tel. AV 5-4931.**

THORNTON
The Five Maples Nursing Home; Barrie St.; Inf. 11; Tel. 458-4804.

THOROLD
Maple Hurst Private Hosp.; 14 St. David's St. W.; Chron. 30; **Tel. CA 7-2301.**

TILLSONBURG
Stonecrest Lodge; 48 Bidwell St.; Inf. 26; Tel. 842-4953.
Tillsonburg District Memorial Hosp.; 167 Ralph St., P.O. Box 310; Gen. 123; **Tel. 519-842-3611.**

TIMMINS
Golden Manor; 481 Melrose Blvd.; Ger. 171; **Tel. AM 4-5375.**
St. Mary's Hosp.; 41 Pine St. N.; Gen. 199; Tel. AM 4-1211.
Porcupine Villa; 205 Birch St. S.; Inf. 35; **Tel.** 264-9475.

TORONTO
Addiction Research Foundation of Ont.; 24 Harbord St.; Alch. 20; Narc. 3; **Tel. 365-4545.**
Aged Men's and Women's Homes; 53 Belmont St.; Ger. 249.
Andrea Villa; 2541 Lakeshore Blvd.; Dom. 29; Tel. 259-4060.
Baycrest Hosp.; 3560 Bathurst St., Zone 19; Chron. 87; Tel. RU 1-3501.
Bel-Air Nursing Home; 525 Sherbourne St., Zone 5; Inf. 22; Tel. WA 2-9535.
Bendale Acres Home for the Aged; 2920 Lawrence Ave. E., Scarborough; Inf. 326.
Bethesda Gen. Hosp.; 325 Sheppard Ave. W., Willowdale; (Priv); Gen. 22; **Tel. 225-8801.**
Beverley Private Hosp.; 230 Beverley St., Zone 2B; Chron. 18; **Tel. WA 1-6215.**
Birchcliff Nursing Home; 1673 Kingston Rd., Scarboro; Inf. 61; **Tel. OX 9-3245.**
Blake Nursing Home; No. 1, Sand Beach, Zone 14; Dom. 6; Tel. 259-7925.
Bloorview Children's Hosp.; 278 Bloor St. E., Zone 5; Chron. (Children) 48; **Tel. WA 3-7365.**
Canadian Mothercraft Hosp.; 616 Avenue Rd., Zone 7, Conv. (Child.) 18; **Tel. 481-7277.**
Cedarcrest Nursing Home; 20 Maynard Ave., Zone 3; Inf. 20; Tel. 1-4904.
Central Park Lodge; 10 William Morgan Drive, Thorncliffe; Dom. 192; **Tel. 425-3722.**
Central **Park** Lodge; Jane St. & Queen's Drive; Dom. 169.
Central Hosp.; 331 Sherbourne St., Zone 2; Gen. 84; **Tel. WA 5-8991.**
Church Home for the Aged; 87 Bellevue Ave.; Ger. 43.
Clarke Inst. of Psychiatry; 250 College St.; Psy. 205; **Tel. 924-6811.**
Clarkewood; 1929 Bayview Ave.; Ger. 125, **Tel. HU 5-9476.**
Crawford Nursing Home; 15 High Park Gardens; **Tel. RO 7-1354.**
Dalmeny Private Hosp.; 8 May St., Zone 5; Psy. 40; **Tel. WA 3-4637.**
Dewson Private Hosp.; 47 Dewson, Zone 4; Chron. 29; Tel. LE 6-5009.
Doctor's Hosp.; 45 Brunswick Ave., Zone 4; (Priv); Gen. 352; Tel. WA 3-5411.
Dowling Manor Rest Home; 143 Dowling Ave.; Inf. 17; **Tel. LE 4-5386.**
Emerald Nursing Home; 3309 Kingston Rd.; Inf. 21; **Tel. 266-2068.**
Eveleigh Nursing Home; 486 Jarvis St., Zone 5; **Infirm 29; Tel. WA 2-8449.**
Fairhaven House; 123 Isabella St.; Dom. 23; **Tel. WA 2-0023.**
Fleming Nursing Home; 9 Glebe Rd. E.; Infirm 9; Tel. HU 9-0969.
Foxbar Nursing Home; 26 Foxbar Rd.; Inf. 18; Tel. WA 4-5272.
Fred Victor Mission, Older Men's Home; 139 Jarvis St.; Ger. 65.
Garden Court Rest Home; 2523 Lakeshore Rd., **Zone 14; Dom. 40; Tel. CL 9-6172.**
Glebe Rest Home Ltd.; 17 Glebe Rd. W., Zone 7; Infirm 20; Tel. HU 7-5251.
Grace Hosp.; 650 Church St., Zone 5; Gen. 198; **Tel. WA 5-2251.**
Happy Life Nursing Home; 2507 Dundas St. W.; Dom. 25; Tel. 762-2518.
Hillcrest Convalescent Hosp.; 47 Austin Terrace, **Zone 4; Conv. 120; Tel. 537-3421.**
Hill Top Acres; 1098 Davenport Rd., Zone 4; **Ger. 200; Tel. LE 1-5771.**
Hosp. for Sick Children; 555 University Ave., **Zone 2; Paed. 713; Comm. 97; Tel. EM 6-7242.**
Humber Memorial Hosp; 200 Church St., Zone 15, Weston; Gen. 377; **Tel. 249-8111.**
Ina Grafton Gage Home; 2 O'Connor Dr., Zone 6; Ger. 52; Tel. HO 3-5919.
Institute of Traumatic, Plastic & Restorative Surgery; 215 Victoria St., Zone 2; (Priv); Surg. **4; Tel. 364-5325.**
Isabel & Arthur Meighen Lodge; 100 Davisville Ave., Zone 7; Ger. 166; **Tel. HU 7-1271.**
Jewish Home for Aged; 3560 Bathurst St., Zone 19; Ger. 200; **Tel. RU 1-3501.**
Julia Greenshields Memorial Home; 586 University Ave.; Ger. 28; **Tel. EM 4-2732.**
Katharine McTear Nursing Home; 57 Oriole Rd., Zone 7; Dom. 6; **Tel. 924-5581.**
Kipling Acres; 1575 Kipling Ave. N., Rexdale; Ger. 382; Tel. CH 6-6601.
Lakeshore Psyc. H.; 3131 Lakeshore Blvd. W.; Ment. 450; Inf. 12; Dom. 287; **Tel. 259-8291.**
Lambert Lodge; 350 Christie St., Zone 4; Ger. 710; Tel. LE 1-5771.
Laughlen Lodge; 87 Elm St.; Ger. 188; Tel. EM 3-0715.
Leisure World Nursing Home; 2 Sandown Ave.; Inf. 65; Tel. 267-9600.
Lockwood Clinic; 300 Bloor St. E., Zone 5; Gen. 43; **Tel. WA 1-2121.**
Lyndhurst Lodge Hosp.; 153 Lyndhurst Ave., Zone 4; Paraplegic 50; Tel. WA 3-0928.
MacLean Nursing Home; 19 Bales Ave.; Inf. 7; Tel. 225-4947.
Maple Grove Nursing Home; 102 Craiglee Dr.; Inf. 20; **Tel. AM 7-3173.**
Martin's Nursing Home; 268 High Park Ave.; Dom. 3; **Tel. RO 6-3643.**
Mayfair Private Hospital; 682 Broadview Ave., Zone 2; Gen. 16; **Tel. HO 6-8143.**
Montgomery Nursing Home; 80 Wychwood Park; Infirm 15; Tel. LE 3-3617.
New Mount Sinai Hosp.; 550 University Ave., Zone 2; Gen. 446; Tel. EM 6-7361.
Northwestern Gen. Hosp.; 2175 Keele St., Zone 15; Gen. 327; **Tel. 762-3641.**

HOSPITALS & CONVALESCENT HOMES — ONT. & P.Q.

North York Branson Hosp.; 555 Finch Ave. W., Willowdale; Gen. 222; **Tel. 633-9420.**
Ontario Crippled Children's Centre; 350 Rumsey Rd., P.O. Box 1700, **Zone 17;** Rehabs 105; **Tel. 487-5311.**
Ontario Hosp.; 999 Queen St. W., Zone 3; P.O. Box 14; Psy. 750; Inf. 200; Dom. 200; **Tel. LE 3-8501.**
Orthopaedic & Arthritic Hosp.; 43 Wellesley St. E.; Orth. and Arth. 96; **Tel. 924-4611.**
Our Lady of Mercy Hosp.; 100 Sunnyside Ave., Zone 3; Chron 300; **Tel. LE 3-9457.**
Princess Margaret Hosp.; 500 Sherbourne St., Zone 5; Cancer 120; Tel. 924-0671.
Providence Hosp.; 3276 St. Clair Ave. E., Scarborough; Gen. 122; Tel. 759-9321.
Providence Villa; 3276 St. Clair Ave. E., Scarborough; Inf. 525; Tel. 759-9321.
Queen Elizabeth Hosp.; 130 Dunn Ave., Zone 3; Chron. 523; Tel. LE 4-7513.
Queensway Gen. Hosp.; Sherway Dr., **Zone 18;** Gen. 356; Dom. 21; Psy. 20; Tel. CL. 9-6671.
Redwing Convalescent Home; 501 Broadview Ave.; Inf. 36; **Tel. HO 3-1339.**
Riverdale Hosp.; St. Mathews Rd., Zone 8, Chron. 503; Conv. 409; **Tel. 461-8251.**
Rose Nursing Home; 27-29 Rose Ave.; Dom. 19; **Tel. 923-5264.**
Roulet Nursing Homes Ltd.; 31 Walmer Rd.; Infirm. 61; **Tel. WA 3-3628.**
Runnymede Hosp.; 274 St. John's Rd.; Zone 9; Chron. 130; **Tel. RO 2-1167.**
St. Bernard's Convalescent Hosp.; 685 Finch Ave. W., Willowdale; (Priv); Conv. 61; Tel. ME 5-8422.
St. John's Convalescent Hosp.; Newtonbrook, 285 Cummer Ave., Willowdale; Conv. 208; **Tel. BA 5-8871.**
St. Joseph's Hosp.; 30 The Queensway, **Zone 3;** Gen. 721; Cont. 26; Tel. 534-9531.
St. Joseph's Inf.; 3377 Bayview Ave.; Inf. 35; **Tel. 222-1101.**
St. Michael's Hosp.; 30 Bond St., Zone 2; Gen. 993; Psy. 30; **Tel. 362-4461.**
St. Paul's Nursing Home; 140 Close Ave.; Inf. 16; **Tel. 537-5481.**
St. Raphael's Nursing Home; 141 Springhurst Ave.; Inf. 17; **Tel. LE 1-4371.**
Salvation Army Eventide Home; 248 Dufferin St.; Ger. 57.
Scarborough Gen. Hosp.; 3050 Lawrence Ave. E.; Gen. 448; **Tel. AX 3-8181.**
Shouldice Surgery; 618 Church St., Zone 5; (Priv); Hern. 62; **Tel. WA 3-3507.**
Strachan Houses; 790 Queen St. W.; Ger. 38.
Sunnybrook Hosp. (DVA); Bayview Ave., Zone 12; Gen. 739; Psy. 66; Neur. 90; Arth. 90; Chron. 463; **Tel. 485-8651.**
Sunnyside Private Hosp.; 1437 Queen St. W.; Psy. 12; Tel. LE 7-1000.
Toronto East Gen. & Orthopaedic Hosp.; Coxwell & Sammon Ave., Zone 6; Gen. 761; **Tel. 461-8272.**
Toronto Eye Institute; 88 Warren Rd., Zone 7; (Priv); **Eye Surg. 14; Tel. 924-8368.**
Toronto Gen. Hosp.; 101 College St., Zone 2; Gen. 1036; Others 384; **Tel. EM 6-8211.**
Toronto Hosp.; 82 Buttonwood Ave., Weston P.O. Box 4, Zone 15; Chron. 150; TB 464; **Tel. RO 9-1161.**
Toronto Military Hosp.; c/o Sunnybrook Veterans' Hosp., Bayview Ave.; Gen. 94.
Toronto Western Hosp.; 399 Bathurst St., Zone 2B; Gen. 790; Psy. 31; Ger. 44; Tel. 368-2581.
Tweedle Nursing Home; 257 Beech Ave.; Inf. 16; **Tel. OX 9-2168.**
Ukrainian Home for the Aged; Ivan Franko Home; 35 High Park Gdns; Dom. 22.
Victoria Nursing Home; 57 Myrtle Ave., Zone 8; Infirm 18; Tel. HO 5-2448.
Village Nursing Home; 344 Spadina Rd.; Inf. 21; **Tel. 923-5360.**
Wellesley Hosp.; 160 Wellesley St. E., Zone 5; Gen. 355; **Tel. WA 1-4111.**
Willowdale Hosp.; 15 Horsham Ave., Willowdale; (Priv); Alc. 9; **Tel. BA 1-9331.**
Women's College Hosp.; 76 Grenville St., Zone 5; Gen. 369; Psy. 20; Tel. WA 3-7381.
W. C. B. Hosp. & Rehabilitation Centre; 115 Torbarrie Rd., **Downsview; Rehab. 180;** Dom. 340; **Tel. 244-1761.**

TRENTON
Green Acres Nursing Home; R.R. 2; Inf. 30; **Tel. EX. 2-4786.**
Trenton Memorial Hosp.; 242 King St. W.; Gen. 166; **Tel. EX 2-3526.**

TROUT CREEK
Stonehouse Nursing Home; Inf. 18; **Tel. 723-5232.**

UXBRIDGE
Cottage Hosp.; Campbell Dr.; Gen. 38; **Tel. UL 2-3341.**

VINELAND
Fairhaven Rest Home; P.O. Box 64; Ger. 10; Tel. LO 2-4523.
United Mennonite Home for the Aged; 2nd St. E., P.O. Box 120; Ger. 63.

VIRGIL
Medical Centre Hosp.; P.O. Box 10; (Priv); Gen. 10; **Tel. 468-3275.**

WALKERTON
Bruceiea Haven; Drawer 100; Ger. 92; **Tel. 68.**
County of Bruce Gen. Hosp.; McGivern St., P.O. Box 30; Gen. 109; **Tel. 881-1220.**
Walkerton Rest Home; 515 Colborne St., P.O. Box 540; Inf. 16; **Tel. 881-0822.**

WALLACEBURG
Lapointe-Fisher Nursing Home; 427 Nelson St.; Infirm. 45; **Tel. 627-2751.**
Sydenham District Hosp.; Margaret Ave., P.O. Box 130; **Gen. 112; Tel. 627-3325.**

WARDSVILLE
Beattie Haven; R.R. 1; Ger. 46.

WATERLOO
Bast Rest Home; 391 Bridgeport Rd.; Dom. 10; **Tel. 742-4188.**
Parkwood Manor; 79 Cardinal Cr., Dom. 56.
Pinehaven Nursing Home; 229 Lexington Rd.; Inf. 21; **Tel. 743-2461.**

WATFORD
Maplehurst Home; Erie St.; Dom. 8; **Tel. 876-3019.**
Parker Nursing Home; P.O. Box 215; Inf. 35; **Tel. 876-2520.**

WAWA
Lady Dunn Hosp.; Station Rd., **P.O.** Box 179; **Gen. 26; Tel. UL 6-2335.**

WELLAND
Sunset Haven; 1st Ave. N.; Ger. 347; **Tel. RE 4-3722.**
Welland County Gen. Hosp.; Third St.; Gen. 310; Chron. 79; **Tel. RE 2-6111.**

WEST HILL
Open Gate Nursing Home; Inf. 37; **Tel. 282-2832.**

WHITBY
Fairview Lodge; Dundas St. W.; P.O. Box 1300; Ger. 235; **Tel. MO 8-5851.**
Ontario Hosp.; P.O. Box 1270; Ment. 1623; **Tel. MO 8-5881.**

WIARTON
Bruce Peninsula & District Memorial Hosp.; Mary St.; P.O. Box 359; Gen. 32; **Tel. 534-1260.**

WINCHESTER
Winchester District Memorial Hosp.; P.O. Box 427; Gen. 109; **Tel. 774-2420.**

WINDSOR
Alexander Hall (CNIB); 230 Strabane Ave.; Dom. 30; **Tel. WH 5-2321.**
Grace Hosp.; 339 Crawford Ave.; Gen. 209; **Tel. CL 6-2361.**
Hotel-Dieu of St. Joseph; 1030 Ouellette Ave.; Gen. 540; Psy. 34; **Tel. CL 2-3631.**

Huron Lodge; 1475 Huron Line; Inf. 163; Tel. CL 2-5747.
I.O.D.E. Mem. Hosp. and Essex County San.; 1453 Prince Road; Gen. 142, Psy. 37, T.B. 42; Tel. CL 2-2771.
Metropolitan Gen. Hosp.; 1995 Lens Ave.; Gen. 369, Cont. 9; Psy. 30; Tel. 256-3461.
Riverview Hosp.; 3177 Riverside Dr. E.; Chron. 262; Tel. CL 4-6426.
Villa Maria; 2856 Riverside Dr. W.; Ger. 120; Tel. CL 6-3174.
WINGHAM
Wingham Gen. Hosp.; Carling Terrace, Gen. 107; Tel. 357-3210.
WOODSTOCK
Millway Nursing Home; 241 Mill St.; Inf. 14; Tel. LE 7-2108.
Ontario Hosp.; P.O. Drawer 310; Epil. 539; TB 853; Tel. LE 9-1251.
Oxford County Home; P.O. Box 112; Ger. 47; Tel. LE 7-2711.
Sutherland's Nursing Home; 768 Lawrason St.; Inf. 11; Tel. LE 7-2506.
Woodstock Gen. Hosp.; 270 Riddell St.; Gen. 220; Tel. LE 7-5511.
Woodstock Private Hosp.; 369 Huron St.; Chron. 16; Tel. LE 7-8162.

Quebec

ACTON VALE
Hop. St. Andre; 1151 rue St. Andre; Gen. 9; Tel. 546-2781.
ALMA
Hotel Dieu d'Alma; 245 rue Champlain; Gen. 274; Tel. 662-3421.
AMOS
Hotel-Dieu d'Amos; rue Youville; C.P. 3000; Gen. 241; Chron. 20; Tel. 732-3341.
AMQUI
D'Amqui, Hosp.; Co. Matapedia; Gen. 150; Tel. 651.
Vieillards, Hospice de; rue St. Charles; C.P. 554; Dom. 11; Tel. 573.
ARTHABASKA
Hotel-Dieu d'Arthabaska; 5 rue Quesnel; C.P.-DD; Gen. 248; Tel. 357-2031.
ARVIDA
Saguenay Gen. Hosp.; Deschene River Rd., P.O. Box 306; Gen. 84; Tel. LI 8-8231.
ASBESTOS
Canadian Johns-Manville Hosp.; 149 Jeffrey St.; P.O. Box 1500, (Priv.) Gen. 17; Tel. 879-5471.
Hop Saint Luc; 55 rue du-Roi; Mat. 41; Tel. 879-5401.
ATHELSTAN
Levers Home; Herdsman's Corner; Dom. 4; Tel. CO 4-5873.
AUSTIN
Cecil Butters Memorial Hosp.; R.R. 1; Ment. 400; Tel. VI 3-5212.
AYERS CLIFF
Blake Nursing Home; Pleasant St., P.O. Box 98; Conv. 6; Tel. 838-4966.
AYLMER
Hop. St. Isadora; 8 rue Bancroft; Dom. 27; Tel. MU 4-6355.
St. Paul Hosp.; 67 Rue Albert, C.P. 730; Gen. 12; Tel. MU 4-5522.
AYLMER EAST
Dublin Private Hosp.; 73 Notre Dame; (Priv); Alcoh. 8, Dom 2; Tel. MU 4-5014.
BAIE COMEAU
Boisvert Memorial Hosp.; Carleton Place, P.O. Box 310; (Priv); Gen. 36; Tel. 584-2261.
BAIE DES SABLES
Foyer de l'Assomption; C.P. 1000; Dom. 34; Tel. 772-4429.
BAIE ST-PAUL
Hop. Ste-Anne; 44 Blvd. Fafard; Ment. 1156; Tel. 435-2005.
BEAUCEVILLE-OUEST
Hop. St-Joseph; C.P. 50; Gen. 70; Dom. 98; Tel. 1090.
BEAUHARNOIS
Therien, Foyer; 256 Blvd. Maple Grove; Conv. 9; Tel. CO 8-4835.
BEAUPORT
Maison du Fargy; 700 Blvd. des Chutes; C.P. 5; Dom. 65; Tel. 663-9934.
Maison St. Laurent; 172 rue Pie XII; Inf. 25; Tel. MO 1-2167.
BEDFORD
Hop. Notre-Dame du Rosaire; 14 rue du Couvent, C.P. 567; (Priv); Gen. 44; Tel. CH 8-3393.
BELOEIL
Barry Nursing Home; 196 Richelieu Dr.; Inf. 18.
St-Mathieu de Beloeil; 221 Rue Brunelle; C.P. 97; (Priv); Chron. 54; Tel. FO 7-3356.
BERNIERVILLE
Hop. St-Julien; via St. Ferdinand, C.P. 250; Gen. 1323; Psy. 25; Tel. 428-3771.
BERTHIERVILLE
Hop. Chateau de Berthier; 235 Frontenac, C.P. 240; (Priv); Gen. 40; Tel. TE 6-4013.
BLANC SABLON
Notre Dame Hosp.; rue Lourdes du Blanc Sablon; Gen. 44.
BOLTON CENTRE
Twin Mountain Home; Ment. 40; Tel. Waterloo 705J3.
BOUCHERVILLE
Parilion Marie Goretti; 695 Marie Victorian.
BRISTOL
Ade Mem. Hosp.; Chron. 16.
BUCKINGHAM
Hop. St-Michel; 155 rue MacLaren, C.P. 310; Gen. 125; Tel. YU 6-3341.
CAP AUX MEULES
Clinique Brochu.
CAP DE LA MADELEINE
Hop. Cloutier; 155 rue Toupin, C.P. 218; Gen. 130; Tel. FR 4-6261.
CAUGHNAWAGA
Kateri Memorial Hosp.; P.O. Box 10; Gen. 49; Tel. ME 7-3121.
CHANDLER
Hop de la Providence; C.P. 190; Gen. 104; Tel. 516.
CHAPAIS
Opemiska Gen. Hosp.; P.O. Box 10; (Priv); Gen. 19; Tel. 5511.
CHAPEAU
Chapeau Community Hosp. Inc.; (Priv); Gen. 9; Tel. 689-2565.
CHARLESBOURG
Maison de Convalescence; 7185—3c. Ave., C.P. 204; Inf. 5; Tel. 626-2258.
CHARNY
Hop. Notre-Dame; 562—10eme rue; C.P. 430; Gen. 70; Tel. 832-2981.
Pension Charney; 803—17e rue, C.P. 299; Dom. 11.
CHATEAUGUAY
Davidson Nursing Home; 459 Salaberry Blvd.; Inf. 12; Tel. OX 2-9221.
CHICOUTIMI
Hotel-Dieu St.-Vallier; C.P. 1006; Gen. 663; Psy. 44; Cont. 50; Tel. 549-2195.
CHOMEDEY
Riviera Hosp.; 3860 boul. Levesque; Inf. 15; Tel. MU 1-7721.
CLARKE CITY
Clarke City Hosp.; Spruce St.; (Priv); Gen. 10; Tel. 583-2507.
COATICOOK
Hop. Ste. Catherine Laboure; 138 rue Jeanne Mance, C.P. 340, Gen. 84, Dom. 30; Tel. VI 9-2761.
COUTEAU LANDING
Notre-Dame Hosp.; 261 rue Principale; Chron. 41; Tel. 267-3370.
COURVILLE
St-Augustin Hosp.; 2135 rue Terrasse Cadieux; Chron. 150; Tel. 661-3746.

COWANSVILLE
Pine Gables Nursing Home; P.O. Box 760; Inf. 15; Tel. 1482.
DISRAELI
Foyer Ste-Luce; 770 rue Gregoire; C.P. 526; Ment. 300; **Tel. 400.**
DOLBEAU
Hotel-Dieu du Sacre-Coeur de Jesus; Boul. Sacre-coeur; Gen. 105; **Tel. 276-1420.**
DRUMMONDVILLE
Foyer St-Paul; 255 rue Brock; Inf. 104; Tel. GR 2-6454.
Ste-Croix; 570 rue Heriot; Gen. 218; Tel. GR 8-1381.
ENTRY ISLAND
Red Cross Nursing Station; Magdalen Islds.
FABREVILLE
Fabreville Nursing Home; 943-40th Ave.; Dom. 29; Tel. NA 7-3572.
FARNHAM
Farnham Convalescent Home; 6 St. Alphonse St., P.O. Box 219; Inf. 14; **Tel. AX 3-6903.**
Hospice Ste-Elizabeth; rue St-Paul, C.P. 150; Dom. 120; **Tel. 3-4303.**
FORT CHIMO
Fort Chimo Nursing Station; Gen. 4.
FRAMPTON
Hop. Ste-Famille; R.R. 2, Dorchester; Inf. 20. Tel. 479-2166.
FRESNIERE
Ste. Cecile Hosp.; (Priv); Mat. 6.
GAGNON
Gagnon, Hop. de; lere Rue; Gen. 31; **Tel. 532-6331.**
GAMELIN
St-Jean-de-Dieu Hop.
GASPE
Hotel-Dieu de Gaspe; Gaspe Harbour; Gen. 142; **Tel. 400.**
Sanatorium Ross; C.P. 800; T.B. 85; Chron. 84; Psyc. 120; Dom. 42; **Tel. 215.**
GATINEAU
Hop. Notre-Dame; 176 rue Brian, C.P. 309; Gen. 54; **Tel. 663-5346.**
GRANBY
Notre-Dame de Granby Hosp.; 363 Notre-Dame; Chron. 16; **Tel. FR 8-5194.**
Orchard Manor Convalescent & Nursing Home; 89 Drummond St.; **Inf. 12.**
Hop. Saint-Joseph; 205 Blvd. Leclerc; Gen. 170; **Tel. FR 2-5491.**
GRANDE ENTREE
Red Cross Nursing Station; Magdalen Islands.
GRAND'MERE
Grand Mere Gen. Hosp.; 601 First Ave., P.O. Box 450; Gen. **32; Tel. LE 8-8635.**
Hop. Lafleche; 1650-6eme ave., C.P. 270; Gen. 162; Tel. LE 8-3381.
GRAND METIS
Refuge pour Vieillards; R.R. 1, Co. Matane; Ger. 12; Tel. 775-3797.
GREAT WHALE RIVER
Great Whale Nursing Station; Gen. 4.
HAM-NORD
Ste-Anges, Foyer; rue Principale; Inf. 30; **Tel. 52.**
HARRINGTON HARBOUR
Harrington Hosp.; Co. Saguenay; Gen. 29.
HAUTERIVE
Hotel-Dieu de Hauterive; C.P. 219; Gen. 200; Tel. 589-3701.
HAVRE-ST PIERRE
Hop. St-Jean-Eudes; C.P. 190; Gen. 114.
HEMINGSFORD
Duquette Boarding House; Inf. 4; Tel. CH 7-2027.
HULL
Centre Medical de Hull Enrg.; 142 rue Champlain; (Priv); Gen. 5; **Tel. PR 1-6239.**
Clinique Labelle; 4 rue Montclair; (Priv); Gen. 5; Tel. PR 7-5811.
Montcalm Centre Medical; 31 rue Montcalm; Tel. PR 1-5881.
Notre Dame de Hull Hosp.; 41 rue Front; **Tel. 771-5853.**

Pierre Janet H.; 20 rue Pharand; T.B. 20; Tel. 777-5245.
Sacre-Coeur, Hop. de; 230 Blvd. Gamelin; **Gen.** 409; **Tel. PR 7-2721.**
HUNTINGDON
Huntingdon County Hosp.; 198 Chateaugay St., P.O. Box 370; Gen. 38; **Tel. CO 4-5133.**
Patterson Nursing Home; 72 Wellington St., P.O. Box 112; Inf. 10; **Tel. CO 4-5472.**
Riverview Terrace Convalescent Centre; Infirm. 15; Tel. CO 4-5049.
IBERVILLE
Pavillon Iberville; 3—8ieme Ave.; (Priv.); Chron. 21; Tel. FI 7-3987.
ILE BIZARD
Lidstone Convalescent Home; 376 Cherier.
ILE D'ANTICOSTI
Anticosti Hosp.; Port Menier; (Priv); Gen. 7; **Tel. 0920.**
ISLES DE LA MADELEINE
Notre-Dame-de-la-Garde Hop.; Cap-aux-Meules; Gen. 138, Chron. 20, Dom. 63; **Tel. 6-2121.**
JOLIETTE
Hop. St-Charles de Joliette; 1000 Boul. Ste. Anne, C.P. 450; Psy. 1291; **Tel. 756-1681.**
Hop. Saint-Eusebe; 585 Blvd. Manseau; C.P. 560; Gen. 225; Inf. 140; Dom. 60; **Tel. PL 6-8041.**
JONQUIERE
Hotel-Dieu Notre-Dame de l'Assomption; 450 rue de l'Hopital; C.P. 610; Gen. **243**; **Tel. 547-3651.**
LAC BRULE
L'Accueil Guay; Dom. **21**; **Tel. 326-2085.**
LAC EDOUARD
San. du Lac Edouard; TB 105.
LAC ETCHEMIN
San Begin; T.B. 27; Psy. 249; Chron. 135; **Tel. 3-1011.**
LACHUTE
Argenteuil Hop.; Chemin Brownsburg; C.P. 310; Gen. 80; **Tel. LO 2-5211.**
Hop. Notre-Dame-du-Sourire; 181 rue Bethany; (Priv); Conv. 10; **Tel. LO 2-6470.**
LAC MEGANTIC
Frere Andre Hosp.; 29 rue Champlain, C.P. 219; Gen. 46; **Tel. 583-0350.**
Hop St. Joseph; rue Laval; C.P. 430; Gen. 130; **Tel. 583-0330.**
LAFLECHE
Regina Hosp.; 2042 Blvd. Marie; Chron. 67; **Tel. OR 1-5596.**
LA MALBAIE
Hop. St-Joseph; 303 rue St-Etienne, C.P. 160; **Gen. 80; Tel. MO 5-3711.**
L'ANNONCIATION
Hop. des Laurentides; 11 Co. Labelle; Psy. 780; **Tel. 275-2118.**
LA SARRE
Hop. St. Francois d'Assise; Chemin Macamic; Gen. 148; **Tel. FE 3-2311.**
LA TUQUE
Hop. St. Joseph; 885 Boul. Ducharme; Gen. 250, Chron. 25; **Tel. LA 3-4581.**
LENNOXVILLE
Grace Christian Home; P.O. Box 700; Inf. 33; **Tel. LO 9-0546.**
LES EBOULEMENTS
Dr. Freve, Hop. du; C.P. 210; Mat. 6; **Tel. 635-2444.**
LES ESCOUMINS
Hop. St-Alexandre; C.P. 400; Gen. 51, **Tel. 233-2931.**
LEVIS
Hotel-Dieu de Levis; 143 rue Wolfe; Gen. 360; **Tel. 837-9341.**
St-David Hosp.; 362 rue St-Laurent; Chron. 18; Tel. TE 9-8077.
St-Joseph-de-la Delivrance Inst.; 93 rue St-Louis; C.P. 86; Dom. 115; **Tel. 837-4987.**
Ste-Marie Foyer; 51 rue Commerciale Bienville; Dom. 10; **Tel. 837-1007.**
LORETTEVILLE
Hop. St-Ambroise de Loretteville; 29 de l'Hopital; Gen. 150; **Tel. 842-3651.**

HOSPITALS & CONVALESCENT HOMES — P.Q. (*Montreal cont'd*)

LOUISEVILLE
Hop. Comtois; Blvd. Comtois, C.P. 1360; Gen. 100; **Tel. CA 8-2731.**
MACAMIC
San. St-Jean; Chron. 128; TB 72; **Tel. 747-3662.**
MAGOG
Hop de la Providence; 50 rue St. Patrice est; Gen. 121; Dom. 109; Tel. VI 3-3381.
MALARTIC
Hop. Lemieux; 610 rue Wolfe, C.P. 906; Mat. 2.
Hop. Renaud; 514 rue Jacques-Cartier, C.P. 1178; (Priv); Mat. 8; Tel. 176.
MANICOUGAN
Manicougan Hosp.; C.P. 490; Gen. 38; **Tel. 588-2307.**
MANIWAKI
St-Joseph de Maniwaki; boul. Desjardins; Gen. 93.
MARIA
Hop. Notre-Dame de Chartres; C.P. 40; Gen. 148; Tel. 443.
MARIEVILLE
Ste-Croix H.; 141 rue Edmond Guillet; C.P. 40; Dom. 358; Tel. LU 9-7912.
MATANE
Hop. du St. Redempteur; 2 rue Thibault, C.P. 1390; Gen. 150; Tel. 562-3135.
METABETCHOUAN
Notre-Dame de la Presentation Hop.; 40 rue Ste-Croix; Chron. 200; **Tel. 349-2861.**
MONT JOLI
Notre-Dame du Rosaire; 157 rue Aubin, C.P. 236; (Priv); Gen. 56; **Tel. PR 5-4535.**
Ste-Bernadette Foyer; 220 Blvd. Jacques Cartier N.; C.P. 248; Inf. 27; **Tel. 775-3407.**
San. St-Georges; T.B. 187; Ment. 358; Chron. 202; Tel. PR 5-4355.
MONT-LAURIER
Hop. Notre-Dame de Ste-Croix; rue Mont-Laurier; C.P. 504; Gen. 120; Tel. 623-1234.
MONTMAGNY
Hospice St-Thomas; Dom. 160.
Hotel-Dieu de Montmagny; R.R. 1; Gen. 155; Tel. 248-0360.
MONTREAL
Aide A La Femme, L'; 2375 due Aird, Zone 4; Chron. 247; Dom. 20; Tel. CL 5-4088.
Alexandra Hosp.; 230 Charron St., Zone 22; Cont. 90; T.B. 52.
Archambault Hosp.; 7163 Blvd. Churchill, Verdun; Gen. 15; Tel. 767-5351.
Bayview Nursing Home; 27 Lakeshore, Pte. Clair; Chron. 29; **Tel. OX 5-9384.**
Beaulac Hop.; 800 est rue Sherbrooke, Zone 24; (Priv); Gen. 28; Tel. LA 6-3381.
Belanger Clinique Medicale; 3871 rue Bellanger est; Zone 36; Gen. 22; Tel. RA 9-5231.
Belisle Nursing Home; 9099 Lasalle Blvd., Zone 32, Ville LaSalle; **Inf. 17.**
Bellechasse Hosp.; 3950 rue Bellechasse, Zone 36; Gen. 219; **Tel. 729-4371.**
Bellevue Hop.; 3836 Parc Lafontaine, Zone 24; (Priv); Mat. 15; Tel. LA 3-3737.
Bernadette Foyer; 12355 Rue Parent, Pte-aux-Trembles; Inf. 36; **Tel. MI 5-9884.**
Bourget Hosp.; 11570 rue Notre Dame est, Pte-aux-Trembles; Inf. 85; **Tel. MI 5-1673.**
Bruchesi de Montreal Institut; 2225 est rue Rachel, Zone 34; **Tel. LA 4-6825.**
Bussey Chronic H.; 2069 St. Joseph St., Lachine; Inf. 40; Tel. 637-3981.
Cardiologie de Montreal, Institut; 5415 Blvd. de l'Assomption, Zone 36; Card. 46; **Tel. 254-8341.**
Catherine Booth Hosp.; 4375 Montclair, Zone 28; Gen. 155; **Tel. HU 1-0431.**
Champlain Conval. Hosp.; 585 Fortune St.; Inf. 15; Tel. WE 2-4752.
Cherrier, Hop.; 916 rue **Cherrier, Zone 24; (Priv); Gen. 4.**
Christ-Roi de Verdun, H. Gen. du; 4000 Blvd. LaSalle, Zone 19, Verdun; Gen. 489; Tel. PO 6-3551.
Crescent Hop.; 2165 rue Crescent; Gen. 37; Tel. VI 9-4501.
De L'Est, Clinique Medicale; 30 Blvd. St. Joseph est; Zone 34; Gen. 31; Tel. 845-4241.
Doctors' Hosp. Inc.; 6733 Cote des Neiges Rd., Zone 26; (Priv); Gen. 70; **Tel. RE 9-7771.**
Douglas Hosp.; 6875 LaSalle Blvd.; Gen. 155; Ger. 413; Psy. 1281; **Tel. 766-8511.**
Dr. Dance Memorial Nursing Home; 17112 St. Mary Rd., Ste. Genevieve; R.R. 2; Infirm 10; Tel. OX 5-2293.
Eastern Hosp.; 3800 **Radisson St., Zone 5; Gen.** 46; **Tel. 254-3581.**
Echo Nursing Home; 5918 Jeanne Mance, Zone 8; Infirm 12; Tel. CR 7-0450.
Ellis Rowe Nursing Home; 7011 rue Champagneur; Chron. 3; **Tel. CR 2-7806.**
Father Dowd Memorial Home; 481 W. Lagauchetiere St. W., Zone 1, Dom. 110; Tel. UN 6-5717.
Fleury Gen. Hosp.; 2180 est rue Fleury, Zone 12; Gen. 310; Tel. DU 1-9311.
Gamelin, Hospice; 1440 rue Dufresne, Zone 24; Dom. 238; Tel. LA 2-6640.
Gauvin, Hop.; 13540 Notre-Dame est, Pointe-aux-Trembles; Inf. 45; **Tel. MI 5-8583.**
Glenelg Rest Home; 8705 LaSalle Blvd., Ville La Salle; Zone 32; Infirm 32.
Grace Dart Hosp.; 6085 Sherbrooke St. E., Zone 5; Chron. 128; Tel. 256-9021.
Hasle Nursing Home; 3794 Cote des Neiges Rd., Zone 25; Inf. 20.; Tel. WE 5-8043.
Helling's Rest Home; 317 Claremont, Westmount; Zone 6.
Hotel-Dieu de Montreal; 3840 rue St. Urbain; Zone 18; Gen. 712; **Tel. VI 4-0161.**
Jeanne-Mance Hosp.; 1640 rue Tillemont; (Priv); Gen. 42; **Tel. RA 9-6371.**
Jean Talon, Hop.; 1385 est rue Jean Talon, Zone 35; Gen. 418; **Tel. CR 3-5151.**
Jewish Gen. Hosp.; 3755 Cote St. Catherine Rd., Zone 26; Gen. 418; **Psy. 35; Tel. 735-3771.**
Jewish Hosp. of Hope; 7745 Sherbrooke St. E., Zone 5; Chron. 137; **Tel. 352-3120.**
Julius Richardson Convalescent Hosp.; 5425 Bessborough Ave., Zone 29; Chron. 90; Tel. HU 1-0461.
Kateri Pavillion; 26 Strathyre Ave., Zone 32; C.P. 32; **Inf. 12; Tel. DO 6-9090.**
Lachapelle Convalescent Home; 3570 St-Joseph Blvd., **Zone 32, Lachine; Infirm 8.**
Lachine Gen. Hosp.; 3320 Notre Dame St., **Zone** 32; Lachine; Gen. 158; **Tel. ME 7-1161.**
Lakeshore Gen. Hosp.; 160 Stillview Rd., Pte. Claire; Gen. 325; Psy. 30; **Tel. 695-1310.**
Larichelliere Clinique du Dr R; 80 ouest Blvd. St-Joseph, **Zone 14; (Priv.); Foot Disorders 6;** Tel. 849-5890.
LaSalle Convalescent Home, Registered; 9125 LaSalle Blvd., Zone 32, Ville LaSalle; (Priv); Chron. 36; **Tel. DO 6-5790.**
LaSalle Gen. Hosp.; 8585 Terrasse Champlain 1; Gen. 171; **Tel. DO 5-1510.**
Lefebvre, Foyer; 16056 Blvd. Gouin Ouest, Ste-Genevieve-de-Pierrefonds; Infirm 10; Tel. NA 6-5467.
Lincoln Convalescent Home; 2020 St. Marc, Zone 25; Inf. 24; WE 2-6671.
Lochart Residence; 1724 Cedar Ave.; Zone 25; **Inf. 6; Tel. WE 2-7372.**
Longueuil Hop.; 311 Blvd. Quinn; Gen. 23; Tel. OR 7-5243.
MacGregor, House of; 1540 Church St., Zone 9, Ville St-Laurent; Infirm 14; Tel. RI 7-1207.
MacKenzie Nursing Home; 7401 Churchill St. **Verdun; Infirm 55.**
Maimonides Hosp. & Home for the Aged; 4373 Esplanade, Zone 18; **Inf. 141; Tel. 845-2105.**
Maison du Sourire, La; 1410 9e Ave.; Pte. aux Trembles.
Maison du Sourire Hosp.; 63 Blvd. St-Joseph ouest; **(Priv); Inf. 9; Tel. 276-5922.**
Maisonneuve, Hop.; 5415 Blvd. de l'Assomption, Zone 36, Rosemont; Gen. 496; Psy. 39; Tel. 254-8341.

HOSPITALS & CONVALESCENT HOMES — P.Q. (*Montreal cont'd*)

Marida Hosp.; 3377 Blvd. Rosemont; Inf. 36; **Tel. 725-9525.**
Marie-Claret Hosp.; 3345 rue Henri-Bourassa; Chron. 78; Tel. DA 2-4380.
Marie Enfant Hosp.; 5200 rue Belanger est; Zone 36; Ped. 170; Tel. RA 7-2844.
Mayfair Hosp. 1311 Pine Ave. W., Zone 2; **(Priv)**; Gen. 35; **Tel. AV** 8-9176.
McFadden's Boarding Home; 0646 Charlevoix; Zone 22; Dom. 6; Tel. WE 2-9951.
Misericorde, Hop. General de la; 1051 rue St-Hubert, Zone 24; Gen. 364; **Tel.** VI 2-7181.
Mont Providence, Hop.; 7200 Blvd. Gouin, est, Zone 39; Psy. 1100; Tel. 665-4971.
Montreal Children's Hosp.; 2300 Tupper St., Zone 25; Paed. 310; Psy. 32; Cont. 27; Tel. WE 7-8511.
Montreal Chinese Hosp.; 7500 St. Denis; Gen. 49; Tel. 273-9154.
Montreal Convalescent Hosp.; 3001 Kent Ave., Zone 26; Conv. 213; Tel. RE 7-3661.
Montreal Gen. Hosp.; 1650 Cedar Ave., Zone 25; Gen. 794; Tel. WE 7-6011.
Montreal Neurological Inst.; 3801 University St., Zone 2; Neur. 135; **Tel. VI 2-1251.**
Montreal Nord. des Convalescents, H.; 3351 Blvd. Gouin est, Montreal-Nord; Inf. 37; **Tel. DA** 2-9170.
Montreal Protestant Homes; 5150 St. Catherine E., Zone 4; Inf. 130.
Montreal Protestant Hosp.; 5155 St. Catherine St. E., Zone 4; Gen. 146; Tel. 255-2833.
Morin, Résidence; 6365 rue St-Vallier, Zone 10; Infirm 66; **Tel. 277-7860.**
Mount Royal Hosp.; 4351 Esplanade, Zone 18; (Priv); Gen. 8; Tel. VI 4-2200.
Nord, Hop. du; 7225 St-Denis, Zone 10; (Priv); Gen. 11; **Tel. 274-6472.**
Notre-Dame Hosp.; 1560 rue Sherbrooke est, Zone 24; Gen. 1104; **Tel.** LA 5-6363.
Notre-Dame-de-Grace; 12051 rue L'Archevesque Nord; Inf. 18; **Tel. DA 2-1810.**
Notre-Dame de l'Esperance, Hop.; 1275 Cote Vertu, Zone 9, Ville St-Laurent; Gen. 124; Tel. **RI 7-4771.**
Notre-Dame-de-Lourdes, Hop.: 1870 Blvd. Pie IX, Zone 34; Chron. 238; **Tel. 527-4595.**
Notre-Dame-de-la-Merci, Hop.; 555 Blvd. Gouin ouest, Zone 12; Chron. 485; **Tel. 331-2320.**
Notre-Dame-du-Rosaire, Hop.; 7003 rue Boyer, Zone 10; (Priv); Mat. 62; Tel. CR 1-3533.
Notre-Dame-du-Sacre-Coeur, San.; 701 Claremont Ave., Zone 28; Infirm 38.
Ouellette Nursing Home; 1180 Bishop, Zone 25; Infirm. 28; **Tel. UN 1-6043.**
Pasteur, Hop.; 3095 est rue Sherbrooke, Zone 4; Cont. 286; Rehab. 48; Tel. LA 3-1173.
Pointe-Aux-Trembles, H. Gen. de; 501 6th Ave., Zone 5; Pointe-Aux-Trembles; Gen. 22; **Tel. MI 5-8841.**
Prefontaine Hop.; 4820 rue Adam, Zone 4; (Priv.); Mat. 16; Tel. CL 9-5943.
Prevost, Institut Albert; 6555 ouest Blvd. Gouin, Zone 9, Cartierville; Psy. 152; **Tel. FE 4-2440.**
Queen Elizabeth Hosp. of Montreal; 2100 Marlowe Ave., Zone 28; Gen. 252; Isol. 4; Dom. 36; Tel. HU 8-2311.
Queen Mary Veterans' Hosp. (DVA); 4565 Queen Mary Rd., Zone 26; Gen. 700; Tel. 342-2320.
Radium, Institut du; 4120 rue Ontario Est., Zone 4; Cancer 18; **Tel. LA 3-3151.**
Reddy Memorial Hosp.; 4039 Tupper St., Zone 6; Gen. 161; Tel. 933-7531.
Regina Hosp.; 2042 Blvd. Marie, La Fleche; Inf. 85; **Tel. OR 1-2222.**
Rehabilitation Inst. of Montreal; 6300 Darlington Ave., Zone 26; Rehab. 111; **Tel. 735-3741.**
Resthaven Convalescent Home; 99 Pointe-Claire Ave., Zone 33; Infirm 8.
Rosemont Hosp.; 1970 Blvd. Rosemont, Zone 35; (Priv.); Gen. 43; **Tel. CR 4-2511.**
Royal Edward Chest Hosp.; 3650 St. Urbain St., Zone 18; Gen. 100; T.B. 24; **Tel. VI 9-5201.**
Royal Victoria Hosp.; 687 Pine Ave. W., Zone 2; Gen. 1004; Psy. 129; **Tel. VI 2-1251.**
Rutherford Rest Home; 1510 Woodland Ave., Zone 20; Inf. 13; **Tel. PO 9-0457.**
Sacre-Coeur, Hop. du; 5400 boul. Gouin ouest, Cartierville; Gen. 687; T.B. 110; **Tel. 334-1210.**
Ste-Anges, Hop.; 394—44th Ave., Zone 32, Lachine; (Priv); Mat. 23; **Tel. 637-6756.**
St-Albert Le Grand, Hop.; 4357 rue Charlemagne, Zone 36; (Priv); Chron. 20; **Tel.** 259-6905.
Ste-Anne, Hop.; 5829 Ave. du Parc, Zone 8; (Priv); Mat. 4.
St. Anton Private H.; 4120 55th St., St. Michel; Inf. 37; Tel. DA 1-3696.
St-Benoit, Retraite; 8050 est rue Notre-Dame, Zone 5; Ment. 145; Chron. 173; Tel. 254-3526.
Saint-Charles-Borromee, Hop.; 66 est rue Dorchester, Zone 18; Chron. 430; **Tel. UN 1-8591.**
St-Denis Hop.; 2870 Blvd. Rosemont; Chron. 21; **Tel. 721-1663.**
St. Edouard Foyer; 5605 rue Beaubien est, Zone 36; Dom. 260; **Tel. CL 9-0625.**
St.-Enfant Jesus Foyer; 817—15eme Ave., Pointe-aux-Trembles; Inf. 24; Tel. 645-8753-54.
St-Felix Hop.; 292 Chemin Chambly, Longueuil; (Priv.); Chron. 74; Tel. OR 7-5253.
St.-Francois Hosp.; 3879 Blvd. Tachereau, Lafleche; Inf. 40; **Tel. OR 6-4101.**
St-Francois d'Assise, Creche; 3601 rue de la **Rousselire, Zone 5,** Pointe-aux-Trembles; Dom. 325; Tel. MI 5-1620.
Ste-Germaine Cousin H.; 14241 rue Victoria, Pointe-aux-Trembles; Inf. 47; Tel. MI 2-5341.
Ste-Gertrude des Convalescents, Hop.; 4895 Blvd. Gouin E., Zone 12; Inf. 8; **Tel. DA** 2-2920.
St-Jean de Dieu, Hop.; rue Hochelaga, Gamelin, Zone 5; Psy. 4467; Gen. 80; Tel. 254-8381.
St-Jean des Convalescents, Hop.; 3595 rue Papineau; Inf. 10; **Tel. LA 6-7352.**
Ste-Jeanne d'Arc, Hop.; 3570 rue St-Urbain, Zone 18; Gen. 446; Psy. 7; **Tel. 842-6141.**
St-Joseph H.; 11379 3eme rue, Riviere des Prai-ries; Inf. 12; **Tel. MO 5-4141.**
St-Joseph, Hop.; 650-16eme Ave., Zone 32; La-chine; Gen. 197; **Tel. 637-2351.**
St. Joseph Artisan Hop.; 4585 rue Berri, **Zone** 34; Inf. 35; **Tel. 524-1924.**
St-Joseph de la Providence Hop.; 11844 rue **Bois de Boulogne, Zone 12, Bordeaux; Chron. 168; Tel. FE 4-3120.**
St-Joseph de Rosemont, Hop.; 5689 Blvd. Rosemont, Zone 36; Gen. 166; TB 306; **Tel. CL. 6-2681.**
St-Jude de Laval, Hop.; 14 Blvd. Marois, Zone 12, Laval des Rapides; Inf. 40; **Tel. 681-2100.**
Ste-Justine, Hop.; 3175 Chemin Ste-Catherine. Zone 26; Gen. 835; Cont. 54; Psy. 14; **Tel. RE 1-4931.**
St-Louis des Convalescents, Hop.; 5995-11e Ave., Rosemont, Zone 36; Inf. 26; Tel. RA 7-2885.
St-Luc, Hop.; 1058 rue St-Denis, Zone 18; Gen. 452; **Tel. 861-7321.**
St. Margaret's Home; 51 W. Sherbrooke St., Zone 18; Inf. 63.
Ste-Marie des Convalescents H.; 4045 rue Prieur est; Inf. 30; **Tel. DA 2-0650.**
St. Mary's Memorial Hosp. of Montreal; 3830 Lacombe Ave.; Zone 26; Gen. 396; **Tel. 735-3511.**
St-Michel, Hop.; 8040 9th Ave., Zone 38, St. Michel; Gen. 313; **Tel.** 722-2571.
St. Pierre Hospice; 12051 rue L'Achevesque; Chron. 18; **Tel. 322-1022.**
Ste-Rita, Hop.; 1287 Parc Lafontaine, Zone 34; Infirm 26; **Tel. 525-3369.**
Ste-Therese Hop.; 307 Carre St-Louis, Zone 18; (Priv); Chron. 13; Tel AV 8-1022.
Ste-Therese des Convalescents; 11129 rue Ethier, Montreal Nord; Dom. 34; **Tel. DA 1-3211.**
St. Vital H.; 3295 Blvd. Gouin E., Zone 12; Infirm 30; **Tel. DA 2-0450.**
Santa Cabrini Hosp.; 5655 est rue St. Zotique: Zone 36; Gen. 409; **Tel. CL 4-8311.**

HOSPITALS & CONVALESCENT HOMES — P.Q.

Shriners' Hosp. for Crippled Children; 1529 Cedar Ave., Zone 25; Orth. 60; **Tel. VI 2-4464.**
Suzanne Memorial Home; 131—2nd Ave., Ville LaSalle; Dom. 11.
Tres St. Redempteur Hop. du; 3591; rue Ste Catherine est; Zone 4; Chron. 16; **Tel. LA 2-2257.**
Villa Maria, Hop.; 6027 rue Dolorimier; (Priv); Gen. 40; **Tel. RA 9-4351.**
Villa Medica; 225 Sherbrooke St. E.; Conv. 200; Tel. 288-8201.
Visitation, Hop. La.; 161 ouest rue Henri-Bourassa; Zone 12, Gen. 46; **Tel. 331-2220.**
West-End Convalescent Clinic; 6201 Beaulieu St.: Zone 20; (Priv.); Conv. 20; **Tel. PO 9-3811.**
West End Inc. Hosp.; 6935 Hamilton St., Ville Emard, Zone 20; Gen. 70; **Tel. PO 9-3811.**
Wheeler Convalescent Home; 210 Salaberry S., Chateauguay Centre, Inf. 30; **Tel. OX 2-2151.**
Woodlawn Chronic Hosp.; 1391 College St., St. Laurent, Zone 9; Chron. 13; **Tel. RI 7-1433.**
Woodpine Village Convalescent Home; 4501 Radisson Ave., **Zone 5;** Inf. 10; **Tel. CL 5-5329.**
Zion Garden Convalescent Home; 557 Des Prairies Blvd., Zone 12, Laval des Rapides; Infirm 26; Tel. MU 1-4422.

MURDOCHVILLE
Murdochville, Hop. de; 600 Ave. est; C.P. 1090; Gen. 29; Tel. 2561-62.

MUTTON BAY
Mutton Bay Nursing Station; Gen. 5.

NEW GLASGOW
Kelly Nursing Home; Kilkenny Rd., Infirm 13; **Tel. GE 8-8118.**

NICOLET
Christ-Roi, Hop. du; 675 rue St-Jean-Baptiste; Gen. 123; **Tel. 293-4473.**
Foyer de Nicolet (Hotel-Dieu); 175 Ave. d'Youville; Dom. 165; **Tel. 293-4714.**
Sacre Coeur, Hop. du; 251 rue St. Jean Baptiste; Gen. 40; Inf. 20; Dom. 45; **Tel. 293-4461.**

NORANDA
Youville, Hop.; 9eme Rue; Gen. 261; **Tel. RO 2-2301.**

NOTRE-DAME-DES-LAURENTIDES
Pavillon St. Joseph; 536 Notre-Dame C.P. 23; Dom. 33; **Tel. VI 9-3625.**

NOTRE DAME DU LAC
Notre-Dame-Du-Detour, Hop.; C.P. 215 Cte. Temiscouata; Gen. 85; **Tel. 899-6751.**
Repos du Viellard, Le; 109 rue Commercial; Dom. 68; **Tel. 899-6725.**

ORMSTOWN
Barrie Mem. Hosp.; Gale St., P.O. Box 200; Gen. 69; **Tel. 829-2321.**
Ormstown Convalescent Home; 2 Church Street; Inf. 17; Tel. 829-2261.

ORSAINVILLE
Mont St-Aubert; 400 rue lere, C.P. 71; Dom. 55; **Tel. 842-1925.**

PAINT HILLS
Paint Hills Nursing Station; Gen. 4.

PLESSISVILLE
Notre-Dame des Champs, Hop.; (Priv); Rehab. 75.
Sacre-Coeur, Hop. du; 1353 rue St-Calixte, Gen. 102; Tel. 362-7351.

PORT HARRISON
Port Harrison Nursing Station; Gen. 4.

POVUNGNITUK
Povungnituk Nursing Station, Gen. 4.

PRINCEVILLE
St-Hilaire de Princeville Hop.; 145 rue St-Jacques, C.P. 190; (Priv) Gen. 25; **Tel. 364-5656.**

QUEBEC CITY
Bigue Chinique du Dr.; 449 3eme Ave; Gen. 5; Tel. LA 9-1765.
Centre Antituberculeux de Quebec; 261 St-Vallier ouest; Tel. LA 9-4121.
Centre Hospitalier Notre-Dame du Chemin; 510 Ste-Foy; Chron. 54; **Tel. 681-7882.**
Centre Hospitalier St-Francois; 1604 lere Ave; Chron. 30; **Tel. 524-6033.**
Christ-Roi; 300 Blvd. Wilfrid Hamel; **Zone 8;** Gen. 265; **Tel. 681-7331.**
Civique, Hop.; 2480 Chemin de la Canardiere, Zone 3; Cont. 86; **Tel. 663-3518.**
Couillard Hospital; 797 Chemin Ste-Foy, Chron. 29; **Tel. 683-9482.**
De Beauport Clinique Medicale; 550 ave Royale; Chron. 18; **Tel. 667-2562.**
Dufrost Pavillon; Mastai.
Enfant Jesus, Hop. de l'; 1401-18eme Rue, Zone 3; Gen. 602; **Tel. 529-8711.**
Fleur De Lys Hop.; 220 rue Sapiniere-Dorion, Zone 3; Inf. 31; **Tel. 623-1690.**
Hotel-Dieu de Quebec; 11 Cote du Palais, Zone 4; Gen. 576; **Tel. 529-9151.**
Hotel-Dieu du Sacre-Coeur de Jesus; Ave. du Sacre-Coeur, Zone 8; Chron. 47; Epil. 206; **Tel. 529-6851.**
Jeffery Hale's Hosp.; 1250 Ste. Foy Rd., Zone 6; Gen. 193; Chron. 9; **Tel. 683-4471.**
Laval, Hop.; 2725 Chemin Ste-Foy, Zone 10; TB 232; Gen. 273; **Tel. 653-5251.**
Madeleine de Vercheres, Hop.; 1640 Chemin Ste-Foy; Infirm 21; **Tel. MU 3-0011.**
Mallet—Maison Mere; 945 rue St-Olivier, Zone 4; Dom. 168; **Tel. LA 9-2586.**
Mastai, San.; Zone 5, Mastai; Alc. 50; **Tel. 661-7781.**
Maternite Privee Laroche, Hop.; 194 Blvd. Pierre Bertrand, **Zone 8, Mat. 3.**
Misericorde, Hop. de La; 1212 Chemin Ste-Foy, Zone 6, C.P. 999; Gen. 54; **Telephone 681-6281.**
Notre-Dame de L'Esperance, Hop.; 383 Chemin Ste-Foy, **Zone 6; Gen. 73; Tel. MU 3-4911.**
Petites Franciscaines de Marie, Les; 330 Chemin Ste-Foy, **Zone 6;** Infirm 30.
Quebec Clinic; Champlain Harbour Stn., Wolfe's Cove; **Tel. 522-7029.**
Quebec, Hop. General de; 260 Blvd. Langelier, Zone 8; Dom. 245; Inf. 218; **Tel. 529-0931.**
Quebec Military Hosp.; 2705 Laurier Blvd., c/o Ste. Foy Veterans' Hosp., Gen. 75.
Roy-Rousseau, Clinique; Chemin de la Canardiere, **Zone 5, Mastai;** NeurPsy. 174; **Tel. 661-7735.**
Saint-Antoine, Hospice; 560 rue St-Francois E., Zone 2; Inf. 132; **Tel. 525-8882.**
St. Brigid's Home; 80 Grande Allee est, Zone 4; Inf. 130; **Tel. 525-4478.**
Ste. Foy Hosp. (DVA); 2705 Laurier Blvd., Zone 10; Gen. 283; Dom. 42; **Tel. 653-7201.**
Saint Francois d'Assise, Hop.; 1605-lere Ave., Zone 3; Gen. 415; **Tel. 529-7311.**
St. Joseph de Bellevue; 750 Chemin, Ste Foy; Zone 6; Gen. 35; **Tel. 683-4434.**
Saint-Michel-Archange, Hop.; rue de la Canardiere, Zone 5; Psy. 4800; **Tel. 661-7781.**
Saint-Paul Hop.; 2115 rue Richer, Ste-Foy, Zone 10; Chron. 26; **Tel. 681-0558.**
St.-Sacrament Foyer; 1165 Chemin Ste Foy, Zone 6; Inf. 60; **Tel. 527-4836.**
St. Sacrement Hop. du; 1050 Chemin Ste-Foy, Zone 6; Gen. 511; **Tel. 681-7211.**
St-Vincent-de-Paul Creche; 1210 Chemin Ste-Foy, Zone 6, C.P. 999; Dom. 500; **Tel. 638-3655.**

RAWDON
Heather Hosp.; 687-3rd Ave., P.O. Box 400, Chron. 38; **Tel. 834-2512.**

REPENTIGNY
Le Gardeur, H. 141 rue Ethier; Gen. 82; **Tel. 581-3020.**

RICHMOND
Wales Home, The; Infirm. 200; **Tel. 826-3266.**

RIMOUSKI
St-Joseph, Hop.; rue Rouleau; Gen. 459; **Tel. 723-7851.**

RIPON
Notre-Dame Hosp.; Inf. 48; **Tel. 614R13.**

RIVIERE-AU-RENARD
St-Martin, Clinique; C.P. 190, Co. Gaspe; (Priv); Mat 8; **Tel. 144.**

RIVIERE-DU-LOUP
St-Joseph du Precieux Sang, Hop.; 28 rue Joly; Gen. 118; Dom. 53; Tel. UN 2-3541.

HOSPITALS & CONVALESCENT HOMES — P.Q. & N.B.

ROBERVAL
Hotel-Dieu-St-Michel; Blvd. St-Joseph; Gen. 256; Chron. 84; TB 160; **Tel. 275-0110.**
Ste-Elizabeth Hosp.; Blvd. Marcotte; Gen. 764; **Tel.** 275-1081.
St-Michel, San.; Blvd. St-Joseph; TB 213; **Tel. 275-0110.** (part of Hotel-Dieu St. Michel).
ROUYN
Le Foyer; 80 rue Mgr. Tessier est; Infirm 29; **Tel. RO 2-6559.**
RUPERT'S HOUSE
Rupert's House Nursing Station; Gen. 4.
STE-ADELE-EN-BAS
Notre-Dame des Monts, San.; 131 rue Notre Dame; Gen. 20; **Tel. CA 9-2044.**
STE-ADELE-EN-HAUT
Villa du Repos; 381 rue Lesage; Infirm 14; Tel. CA 9-3348.
STE. AGATHE DES MONTS
Mount Sinai Hosp.; P.O. Box 1000; TB 52; Chest Diseases 55; **Tel. 326-2303.**
Laurentian Chest Hosp.; St. Vincent St., P.O. Box 400; TB 144; **Tel. 326-4241.**
Ste-Agathe, Hop. de; rue Prefontaine, C.P. 939; Gen. 49; Tel. 326-3551.
ST. ALEXANDRE
Foyer Villa Maria, Hop. du; C.P. 129; Gen. 20; Tel. 492-2914.
ST. ANDREWS EAST
Foyer Long-Sault; rue Principale; C.P. 142; Inf. 15.
STE. ANNE-DE-BEAUPRE
Notre-Dame-du-Sacre-Coeur, Hop.; 10034 rue Royale; Gen. 33; Tel. 263-3787.
Sainte-Anne-de-Beaupre, Hop.; 9974 rue Royale; Gen. 36; **Tel. 263-3727.**
STE. ANNE DE BELLEVUE
Ste Anne's Hosp. (DVA); Gen. 220; Psy. 453; TB 45; Chron. 382; **Tel. 453-3440.**
STE. ANNE DE LA POCATIERE
Notre-Dame de Fatima, Hop.; 6ieme Ave., C.P. 326; Gen. 134; **Tel. 856-3540.**
STE. ANNE DES MONTS
Ste-Anne-des-Monts, Hop.; Co. Gaspe-N., C.P. 57; Gen. 154; Cont 5; **Tel. 117.**
STE-ANNE-DE-YAMACHICHE
Providence Ste-Anne Hosp.; St-Maurice; C.P. 128; Dom. 37; **Tel. 80.**
ST-CELESTIN
St-Anne, Foyer; rue Hauld; Inf. 60; **Tel. 21.**
ST-DENIS SUR RICHELIEU
St. Denis des Convalescents H.; rue Ste. Catherine, C.P. 1; Inf. 65.
ST-DIDACE DE MASKINONGE
Maison de Convalescence St. Marcel Enrg.; rue Principale, Conv. 13; **Tel. 604-R32.**
ST-ELEUTHERE
St-Joseph-du-Lac, Hop.; C.P. 70; Gen. 63; **Tel. 22.**
ST-ETIENNE DES GRES
Maison de Convalescence; Dom. 14; **Tel. 537-0957.**
ST-EUSTACHE
St-Eustace, H. Gen. de; 520 Blvd. Paul Sauvé; Gen. 122; **Tel. 473-6811.**
ST-EUSTACHE-SUR-LE-LAC
Deux-Montagnes, Hop. des; 2700 Chemin Oka; Inf. 31; **Tel. 473-5111.**
ST-FELIX DE VALOIS
Convalescents, H.; des, rue Principale; Inf. 25; Tel. 205.
ST-GEORGES EST
Maison de Repos; 728 2eme Ave. est.; **R.R. 3; Inf. 22; Tel. 1113.**
Repos, Foyer Du; R.R. 3; Beauce; Inf. 14; **Tel. 8-4550.**
ST-GEORGES-OUEST
Hotel-Dieu Notre-Dame de Beauce; C.P. 370. Gen. 195; **Tel. 228-4831.**
Pouponniere Doyon; 360 rue 20ieme; C.P. 365; Bas. 24; **Tel. 228-2432.**
ST-HENRI DE LEVIS
Maison, Mon Repos; Dom. 17; **Tel. 292W.**
ST-HILAIRE
Dieppe House, Foyer; 75 Laurier Blvd., Gen. 160; **Tel. FO 7-4412.**
ST-HONORE BEAUCE
St.-Honore Foyer; rue Gobin; Dom. 38; Tel. 163.
ST-HYACINTHE
Hotel-Dieu-de-St.-Hyacinthe; 1800 rue Dessaules; Chron. 430; Paed. 134; **Tel. PR 4-6495.**
Providence, Hop. La; 1285 St. Pierre; (Priv); Gen. 13; **Tel. PR 3-1466.**
St. Hyacinthe, H. Gen. De; 2750 rue Laframboise; Gen. 230; **Tel. 774-6495.**
ST-JEAN
Saint-Jean, Hop.; 217 rue Longueuil; Gen. 212; Dom. 46; **Tel. 6-6871.**
ST-JEAN-PORT-JOLI
St-Jean-Port-Joli, Hop.; C.P. 9; Gen. 42; **Tel. 303.**
ST-JEROME
Hotel-Dieu de Saint-Jerome; 290 rue Montigny; Gen. 262; Orth. 49; Cont. 4; **Tel. GE 2-9711.**
St-Georges, Clinique; 683 rue St. Georges; (Priv); Gen. 9; **Tel. GE 2-7373.**
ST-JOVITE
St-Paul Hosp.; 1004 rue Ouimet; (Priv); Gen. 18; **Tel. 425-2741.**
STE. JULIENNE
Ste. Julienne, H.; rue Albert; Inf. 10; **Tel. 839-3636.**
ST-LAMBERT
St-Lambert, Hop.; 831 Notre-Dame; Gen. 182.
ST-LIBOIRE
St-Liboire, Foyer; rue St. Patrick; Dom. 7; **Tel. 3651.**
ST-LIN DES LAURENTIDES
Providence St-Antoine de Padoue; 521 rue St-Joseph; Dom. 116; **Tel. 223-2213.**
STE-MARIE-DE-LA-BEAUCE
Notre-Dame-de-Protection, Hop.; rue de l'Hopital; C.P. 99; Dom. 80; **Tel. 387-5228.**
ST. METHODE
Valin, Foyer; C.P. 60; Dom. 90; **Tel. 61-S-2.**
ST-MICHEL-DE-BELLECHASSE
Lourdes, de H.; rue St-Michel; Inf. 80; **Tel. 884-2811.**
ST. PAUL d' ABBOTSFORD
Abbotsford Nursing Homes.
ST-RAPHAEL
St-Raphael, Foyer; C.P. 11; Inf. 19; **Tel. 70.**
ST-RAYMOND
St. Raymond, Hop.; C.P. 850; Gen. 44; **Tel. 384-2266.**
STE-ROSE
St-Etienne, Hosp.; 29 rue Venise, C.P. 4; Inf. 6; **Tel. NA 5-3578.**
Ste. Rose de Laval H.; 240 rue Roy du Nord. C.P. 219; Gen. 34; **Tel. NA 5-6907.**
ST-SCHOLASTIQUE
St-Scholastique, Hop.; C.P. 134; (Priv); Infirm 26; **Tel. 258-3451.**
STE-SOPHIE
St Jude's Pension; Co. Terrebonne; Inf. 6; **Tel. GE 8-1524.**
ST-VINCENT DE PAUL
Rose Gardens Convalescent and Nursing Home; 371 Bellevue Ave.; Conv. 30; **Tel. 1-2323.**
SAYABEC
Saindon, Clinique; (Priv); Mat. 28; **Tel. 45.**
SCHEFFERVILLE
Schefferville, Hop.; Pearce Lake Road; P.O. Box 1450; Gen. 45; **Tel. 585-2446.**
SENNETERRE
Senneterre Clinique H de; C.P. 130; Gen. 33; **Tel. 7-2291.**
SEPT-ILES
Sept-Iles, H. des; 45 rue Pere Divet; Gen. 209; **Tel. 942-9761.**
SHAWINIGAN
Joyce Memorial Hosp.; 1161 Maple Ave.; Gen. 40; **Tel. LE 7-6661.**
Ste-Therese, Hop.; 1705 rue Georges; Gen. 199; **Tel. LE 6-4446.**
SHAWVILLE
Pontiac Community Hosp.; P.O. Box 280; Gen. 64; **Tel. 647-2214.**

SHERBROOKE
Hotel-Dieu de Sherbrooke; 580 Bowen Sud, Sub. P.O. 8; Gen. 408; **Tel. LO 9-2551.**
St-Francois, San.; 585 rue Murray, Sub. P.O. 8; TB 60; **Tel. LO 9-2551.**
St-Vincent-de-Paul, Hop. General; 300 rue King Est; Gen. 301; **Tel. LO 9-6381.**
Sherbrooke Hosp.; 375 Argyle St., Gen. 170; **Tel. LO 9-3661.**
Youville, Hop. d'; 1036 rue Belvedere Sud; Chron. 293; Dom. 134; **Tel. LO 9-9041.**
SOREL
Hop. General; 151 rue Georges; Chron. 160; Inf. 25; **Tel. RI 3-3303.**
Hotel-Dieu de Sorel; 400 Ave. Hotel-Dieu; C.P. 250; Gen. 190; **Tel. RI 3-5521.**
Richelieu, Hop.; 89 rue Prince, C.P. 354; Gen. 63; **Tel. RI 3-5569.**
SOUTH STUKELY
Courville Nursing Homes Inc.; P.O. Box 10; Inf. 20; **Tel. 297-2864.**
STANSTEAD
Hetherington Rest & Convalescent Home; 19 Park St., P.O. Box 149; Infirm 7; **Tel. TR 6-2442.**
SWEETSBURG
Brome-Missisquoi Perkins Hosp.; Main St., P.O. Box 70; Gen. 95; **Tel. 263-1333.**
Regal Nursing Home; 68 Main St., P.O. Box 119; Infirm 14; **Tel. 263-1797.**
St-Louis Hop.; rue Larouche; C.P. 118; Inf. 31; **Tel. 263-2220.**
TEMISKAMING
Temiskaming Hosp.; Thorne Ave., P.O. Box 440; (Priv); Gen. 28; **Tel. 327-3260.**
TERREBONNE
St-Louis de Terrebonne Hop.; 27 Boul. des Braves, C.P. 580; (Priv); Gen. 27; **Tel. NO 6-8755.**
Shelling Hosp.; 3885 Cote Terrebonne; Infirm 17; **Tel. NO 6-8004.**
THETFORD MINES
Hop. St-Joseph; rue Notre Dame nord; Gen. 170; **Tel. 335-2971.**
Sainte-Croix Hospice; 45 Notre Dame Sud; C.P. 96; Inf. 43; **Tel. FE 5-6565.**
TROIS-RIVIERES
Cooke, Hop.-San.; rue Ste. Marguerite; Gen. 140; T.B. 130; **Tel. FR 5-7713.**
St-Joseph, Hop.; 731 rue Ste-Julie; Gen. 326; **Tel. 4-6211.**
Sainte-Marie Hop.; 1991 Blvd. du Carmel; Gen. 318; Neuro 15; Orth. 20; Psy. 10; **Tel. FR 5-7721.**
VAL-DAVID
Sanatorium des Soeurs; Inf. 26.
VAL D'OR
Providence, Hop.; 83 rue Montcalm; (Priv): Gen. 36; **Tel. VA 4-6828.**
St. Sauveur, H.; 725 5ieme rue; Gen. 142; **Tel. 824-3663.**
VALLEYFIELD
Hotel-Dieu de Valleyfield; 245 rue Salaberry; Gen. 187; **Tel. FR 3-3360.**
St-Vincent de Paul Providence; 18 rue de la Fabrique; Dom. 108; **Tel. FR 3-4013.**
VARENNES
Lajammerais, Foyer la; 2 rue Youville; Inf. 34; Berc. 98; **Tel. OL 2-2642.**
VICTORIAVILLE
Ste. Anne Hop.; R.R. No. 2; Gen. 49; **Tel. PL 2-2281.**
St. Joseph Ermitage; Ave de l'Ermitage; Inf. 300; **Tel. 752-5562.**
VILLE BROSSARD
Preville Ltee H.; 2370 boul. Lapiniere; Chron. 213; Psy. 17; **Tel. OR 6-1838.**
VILLE LES SAULES
Ste-Monique, H.; boul. Hamel; Chron. 54; **Tel. 527-4759.**
VILLE-MARIE
Sainte-Famille, Hop.; 51 rue Notre Dame; C.P. 20; Gen. 130; **Tel. 421.**
WAKEFIELD
Gatineau Memorial Hosp.; P.O. Box 158; Gen. 39; **Tel. 459-2895.**
Waterloo Enr, H.; Hillside St.; Gen. 35; **Tel. 539-1333.**
WINDSOR
Hop. St-Louis de Windsor; 23 rue Dearden, C.P. 1100; Gen. 71; **Tel. VI 5-2751.**

New Brunswick

ALBERT
Albert County Hosp. Inc.; Gen. 22; **Tel. 123-122.**
BAKER BROOK
Foyer Ste. Elizabeth; Dom. 60; **Tel. 258-3332.**
BATH
North Carleton H.; Box 99; Gen. 51; **Tel. 278-5231.**
BATHURST
Foyer St-Camille de Lellis; 1250 St-Peter Ave.; Dom. 63; **Tel. LI 6-4654.**
Hotel-Dieu Annex; Vallee Lourdes; Mat. 30; Paed. 38; Chron. 12; **Tel. LI 6-4408.**
Hotel-Dieu de Saint-Joseph; 665 Murray Ave., Gen. 104; **Tel. LI 6-4471.**
Notre-Dame de Lourdes San.; Vallee Lourdes; TB 92; **Tel. 546-6551.**
BLACK'S HABOUR
Fundy Hosp.; Gen. 40; **Tel. 456-3325.**
CAMPBELLTON
Hotel-Dieu St. Joseph; 6 Arran St.; Gen. 234; **Tel. PL 3-3301.**
Provincial Hosp.; Hospital Rd., P.O. Box 10; Psy. 775; **Tel. 753-4461.**
Restigouche & Bay Chaleur Soldiers' Memorial Hosp.; 38 Arran St., P.O. Box 396; Gen. 115; **Tel. PL 3-4451.**
CAMPOBELLO
Red Cross Nursing Station.
CANTERBURY
Red Cross Nursing Station.
CARAQUET
L'Enfant Jesus Hop. de; Gen. 73; **Tel. 727-2880.**
CHATHAM
Hotel Dieu; 53 Lobban Ave., P.O. Box 260; Gen. 145; **Tel. PR 3-4405.**
Mount Saint Joseph Hosp.; Lobban Ave.; Dom. 80; **Tel. PR 3-3122.**
DALHOUSIE
Saint Joseph Hosp.; Victoria St.; Gen. 132, **Tel. SK 4-3391.**
EDMUNDSTON
Hotel-Dieu de Saint Joseph; 54—21st Ave.; Gen. 248; **Tel. RE 5-3361.**
FREDERICTON
Forest Hill Rehabilitation Centre Inc.; Woodbridge St., P.O. Box 265; (Priv); Rehab. 20; **Tel. GR 5-3309.**
Municipal Home; York St., P.O. Box 130; Dom. 32; **Tel. GR 5-8056.**
Polio Clinic & Health Centre; 71 Brunswick St.; Orth. 69; **Tel. 475-9944.**
Victoria Public Hosp.; Woodstock Rd.; Gen 309; **Tel. GR 5-3351.**
GRAND FALLS
Grand Falls Gen. Hosp.; rue Main, C.P. 130; Gen. 75; **Tel. 113.**
Grand Falls Hosp.; Main St., P.O. Box 600; Gen. 35; **Tel. 640.**
GRAND MANAN
Grand Manan Hosp.; North Head, P.O. Box 219; Gen. 18; **Tel. Castalia 154.**
HARVEY STATION
Harvey Community Hosp.; Gen. 24; **Tel. 366-2812.**
JUNIPER
Red Cross Nursing Station.
LAMEQUE
Hotel-Dieu de St. Joseph; rue Lameque; Gen. 54; **Tel. 344-2261.**
McADAM
McLean Memorial H.; Saunders Rd.; Gen. 31; **Tel. 784-3300.**

MILLTOWN
Red Cross Nursing Station.
MINTO
Minto Hosp.; Gen. 29; Tel. 327-3353.
MISCOU CENTRE
Red Cross Nursing Stn.
MONCTON
Eventide Home for Men; 245 Church St.; Dom. 55; Tel. EV 2-5572.
Green Acres; R.R. 8; Dom. 16; Tel. 2-7559.
Hotel-Dieu de L'Assomption; rue Providence; Gen. 215; Tel. 382-3351.
Mills Nursing Home; 12 Dufferin St.; Infirm 10.
Moncton Hosp.; MacBeath Ave.; Gen. 407; Psy. 22; Tel. 855-1600.
Moncton Hosp. Annex; Collishaw St.; Chron. 85.
Thompson Rest Home; 85 Cameron St.; Inf. 13; Tel. EV 4-8439.
NEWCASTLE
Miramichi Hosp.; King George Hwy., P.O. Box 240; Gen. 133; Tel. MA 2-1341.
PAQUETVILLE
Red Cross Nursing Stn.
PERTH
Hotel Dieu of St. Joseph; P.O. Box 345; Gen. 53; Tel. 341.
PLASTER ROCK
Tobique Valley Hosp.; R.R. 2; Gen. 36; Tel. 356-2615.
REXTON
Kingston Hall Community Hosp.; Gen. 19; Tel. 523-4441.
ST. BASILE
Hotel-Dieu St-Joseph; Ger. 105; Tel. 263-5561.
San. Saint Joseph; R.R. 2; TB 126; Tel. 263-5561.
SAINT JOHN
Canadian Red Cross Soc. (N.B. Division); 64-66 Prince William St., P.O. Box 39.
Lancaster Hosp. (D.V.A.); Prince St., P.O. Box 1406; Gen. 193; Psy. 32; Chron. 51; Tel. 694-2651.
Mater Misericordiae Home; 133 Waterloo St.; Ger. 107; Tel. 692-2681.
Provincial Hosp.; 281 Lancaster Ave., P.O. Box 20; Ment. 1300; Tel. 694-4481.
Saint John Gen. Hosp.; Waterloo St.; Gen 496; Neuro. 25; Rad. 18; Chron. 51; Psy. 24; Tel. 693-3351.
Saint John Tuberculosis Hosp.; Bayside Drive, East Saint John; TB 235; Tel. 693-6551.
St. Joseph's Hosp.; Bayard Dr.; Zone 8; Gen. 252; Tel. OX 2-2621.
Sunset Manor; Bayside Drive; Dom. 48; Tel. 693-2249.
St. John Clinic; 89 Canterbury St.; Tel. 657-1583.
Sunset Manor, Bayside Dr.; Dom. 48; Tel. 693-2249.
Turnbull Home; 240 Wentworth St.; Inf. 34; Tel. 693-3915.
ST. LEONARD
Foyer Notre Dame; Ger. 65; Tel. GA 3-6457.
ST. QUENTIN
Hotel Dieu de St. Joseph; R.R. 1; Gen. 51; Tel. 271.
ST. STEPHEN
Charlotte County H.; Prince William St.; Gen. 141; Tel. 466-1140.
Marie F. Ganong Old Folks Home; 28 Union St.; P.O. Box 670; Dom. 24; Tel. 466-1471.
SACKVILLE
Sackville Memorial Hosp.; 135 West Main St., P.O. Box 1170; Gen. 67; Tel. 536-1200.
Tantramer Haven; 111 East Main St., P.O. Box 300; Dom. 27; Tel. 536-0682.
SHEDIAC
Providence St-Joseph; 215 rue Main; Inf. 163; Tel. KE 2-3209.
Saint Joseph Hosp.; Main St.; P.O. Box 490; Gen. 27; Tel. 532-6108.
STANLEY
Stanley Memorial Hosp.; P.O. Box 248; Gen. 16; Tel. 94.
SUSSEX
Kings County Memorial Hosp.; Gen. 77; Tel. 433-3100.
THE GLADES
Jordan Memorial San.; Ger. 119; Tel. 756-3355.
TRACADIE
Hotel-Dieu de Saint Joseph; Gen. 116; Tel. 395-2261.
WOODSTOCK
Carleton Memorial Hosp.; Main St., P.O. Box 400; Gen. 101; Tel. 328-3391.
N.B. Women's Institute Home; Chapel St., P.O. Box 1148; Ger. 20; Tel. 328-2148.
YOUNG'S COVE
Bethel Home for The Aged; Queens County, Youngs' Cove Rd.; Inf. 80; Tel. 120.

Nova Scotia

ADVOCATE HARBOUR
Bayview Mem. Hosp.; Cumberland Co.; Gen. 19; Tel. 15.
AMHERST
Highland View Hosp.; 88 Charles St.; Gen. 135; Tel. 667-3361.
ANNAPOLIS ROYAL
Annapolis Gen. Hosp.; St. George St.; Gen. 26; Tel. 532-2381.
ANTIGONISH
St. Martha's Hosp.; 30 Bay St., Gen. 191; Psy. 14; Tel. 863-2830.
ARCADIA
Yarmouth Municipal Home; Yarmouth Co.; Dom. 34.
ARGYLE
Argyle Municipal Home; Yarmouth Co.; Infirm. 22; Tel. 3-20.
ARICHAT
St. Ann Hosp.; Gen. 30; Tel. 22.
BADDECK
Alderwood Home; Inf. 20; Tel. 111.
Victoria County Memorial Hosp.; P.O. Box 220; Gen. 28; Tel. 102.
BARRINGTON
Barrington Municipal Home; Shelburne Co.; Crowells P.D.; Dom. 18; Tel. 186.
BERWICK
Spicer's Rest Home; Box 40; Inf. 30; Tel. 743.
Western Kings Memorial Hosp.; P.O. Box 190; Gen. 60; Tel. 511.
BRIDGETOWN
Annapolis County Municipal H.; Church Street; Ment. 58; Tel. 665-4566.
Annapolis County Municipal Home; Church Rd., R.R. 1; Dom. 36; Tel. 665-4393.
BRIDGEWATER
Dawson Memorial Hosp.; 197 Dufferin St., P.O. Box 229; Gen. 56; Tel. 543-2411.
Lunenburg Municipal Hosp.; R.R. 3; Ment. 220; Tel. 543-4197.
CALEDONIA
North Queens Cottage Hosp.; Queens Co., P.O. Box 39; (Priv); Gen. 16; Tel. 28.
CANSO
Eastern Memorial Hosp.; School St., P.O. Box 97; Gen. 15; Tel. 83.
CHETICAMP
Sacred Heart Hosp.; Gen. 54; Tel. 19.
COLE HARBOUR
Halifax County Hosp.; R.R. 1; Dartmouth; Ment. 540; Tel. 466-7456.
DIGBY
Digby Gen. Hosp.; Warwick St., Gen. 112; Tel. 245-2501.
EASTERN PASSAGE
Ocean View Home; Dom. 80; Tel. 466-7646.
GLACE BAY
Glace Bay Gen. Hosp.; Brookside St.; Gen. 153; Tel. 849-5511.
Mack's Nursing Home; Inf. 9.
St. Joseph's Hosp.; 197 Main St., Zone E.; Gen. 166; Tel. 849-5531.

HOSPITALS & CONVALESCENT HOMES — P.E.I. & NFLD.

GUYSBOROUGH
Guysborough Mem. Hosp.; P.O. Box 136; Gen. 21; Tel. 13.
HALIFAX
Basin View Home; 1250 Gottingen St.; Dom. 139; Tel. 455-4287.
Camp Hill Hosp. (DVA); Robie St.; Gen. 225; Psy. 22; Ger. 163; **Tel. 423-1371.**
Canadian Forces Hosp.; HMCS Stradacona; Gen. 150; Tel. 3-1161.
Children's Hosp.; University Ave.; Paed 217; **Tel. 422-8441.**
Flinn Mem. Home; 84 Morris St.; Inf. 28; **Tel. 423-9445.**
Grace Maternity Hosp.; 5821 University Ave.; Mat. 235; Tel. 422-6501.
Halifax Convalescent Hosp.; 5938 University Ave., Conv. 53; Tel. 422-1731.
Halifax Infirmary; 1335 Queen St.; Gen. 595; Psy. 22; Tel. 422-1511.
Halifax Mental Hosp.; 5957 South St., Ment. 200; Tel. 423-9173.
Home of the Guardian Angel; 6109 Quinpool Rd.; Dom. 10; **Tel. 422-7964.**
Nova Scotia Hosp.; P.O. Box 1004; Dartmouth, Psy. 615; Tel. 469-7500.
Nova Scotia Rehabilitation Centre; 5950 University Ave.; Rehab. 20; Tel. 422-6567.
Old Ladies' Home; 528 Gottingen St.; Ger. 47; **Tel. 454-2115.**
Salvation Army Bethany Home; 980 Tower Rd.; Inf. 35; Tel. 422-5900.
Victoria Gen. Hosp.; 1240 Tower Road; Gen. 534; Psy. 24; Tel. 422-7371.
Vincentian Home; 371 Brunswick St.; Ger. 40; Tel. 455-7670.
Willow Nursing Home; 5538 Inglis St.; Inf. 46; **Tel. 423-8667.**
INVERNESS
Inverness County Memorial Hosp.; James St.; Gen. 42; Tel. 241.
St. Mary's Hosp.; Railway St., P.O. Box 100; Gen. 45; Tel. 8.
KENTVILLE
Blanchard-Fraser Memorial Hosp.; 186 Park St.; Gen. 139; Tel. 678-7381.
Nova Scotia San.; TB 192; **Tel. 678-3251.**
LIVERPOOL
Fahie's Nursing Home Ltd.; School St., R.R. 1, Queens Co.; Inf. 25; Tel. 354-4144.
Queen's Gen. Hosp.; School St., P.O. Box 370; Gen. 69; Tel. 354-3436.
LUNENBURG
Fishermen's Memorial Hosp.; High St., P.O. Box 490; Gen. 83; Tel. 634-8801.
METEGHAN CENTRE
Clare Municipal Home; Digby Co.; P.O. Box 28; Dom. 26; **Tel. 65.**
MIDDLEFIELD
Queens County Municipal Home; Ger. 35; **Tel. 2-32.**
MIDDLE MUSQUODOBOIT
Musquodoboit Valley Memorial Hosp.; Gen. 15; Tel. 53.
MIDDLETON
Soldiers' Memorial Hosp.; Main St.; P.O. Box 610; Gen. 90; Tel. 825-3411.
MUSQUODOBOIT HARBOUR
Twin Oaks Mem. Hosp.; Gen. 15; **Tel. 20-1.**
NEIL'S HARBOUR
Buchanan Memorial Hosp.; Victoria Co. Gen. 23; Tel. 76-3.
NEW GLASGOW
Aberdeen Hosp.; East River Rd.; Gen. 268; **Tel.** 752-8311.
NEW WATERFORD
New Waterford Consolidated Hosp.; Upper King St., P.O. Box 100; Gen. 106; **Tel. 862-6411.**
NORTH SYDNEY
Saint Elizabeth Hosp.; Purves St., Gen. 180; Tel. 794-4725.
PARRSBORO
South Cumberland Memorial Hosp.; Western Ave., P.O. Box 308; Gen. 17; Tel. 161.

PICTOU
Sutherland Memorial Hosp.; Denoon St., P.O. Box 1059; Gen. 40; **Tel. 485-4381.**
PUGWASH
North Cumberland Memorial Hosp.; R.R. 1; Gen. 21; Tel. 243-2521.
Sunset Nursing Home; Box 130; Inf. 120; **Tel.** 243-2571.
SHEET HARBOUR
Eastern Shore Memorial Hosp.; Halifax Co.; Gen. 27; Tel. 55.
SHELBURNE
Roseway Hosp.; Sandy Point Rd.; Gen. 40; **Tel. 480.**
SHERBROOKE
St. Mary's Memorial Hosp.; Gen. 17; Tel. 8.
SOUTH MAITLAND
East Hants Municipal Home; Infirm 70; Tel. 4-3.
SPRINGHILL
All Saints' Springhill Hosp.; 10 Princess St.; P.O. Box 470; Gen. 80; **Tel. 597-3773.**
STELLARTON
Pictou County Hosp. & Home; R.R. 1; **Ment.** 245; Tel. 752-7163.
SYDNEY
Cape Breton County Hosp.; Sydney River, P.O. Box 515; Ment. 500; Tel. 564-6382.
Dosco Emergency Hosp.; (Priv); Gen. 5; **Tel.** 564-6292.
Medical Services Clinic; 63 Charlotte St.; **Tel.** 564-6122.
Point Edward Hosp.; P.O. Box 608; TB 146; **Tel. 564-5531.**
St. Anthony's Home; 51 York St.; P.O. Box 323; Dom. 60; **Tel. 564-4242.**
St. Rita Hosp.; 409 King's Rd.; Gen. 190; **Tel. 539-3740.**
Sydney City Hosp.; Hospital St.; Gen. 234; **Tel.** 564-5507.
SYDNEY MINES
Harbour View Hosp.; Brown St., P.O. Box 510; Gen. 100; **Tel. 736-6283.**
TATAMAGOUCHE
Lillian Fraser Memorial Hosp.; Main St.; P.O. Box 40; Gen. 27; **Tel. 153.**
TRURO
Colchester County Home; R.R. 1; Dom. 23; **Tel.** 893-9101.
Colchester County Hosp.; Willow St.; Gen. 159; **Tel. 893-9425.**
Nova Scotia Training School; P.O. Box 460; Dom. 228; Inf. 4; **Tel. 893-9593.**
Weirs Nursing Home; East Prince St.; Inf. 31.
WATERVILLE
Kings County Hosp.; Ment. 270; Tel. Berwick 566.
Mountain View Home; Inf. 65; Tel. 401-3.
WINDSOR
Payzant Memorial Hosp.; Wiley St.; Gen. 103; Tel. 798-8351.
WOLFVILLE
Eastern Kings Memorial Hosp.; 23 Earnscliffe Ave., P.O. Box 880; Gen. 37; **Tel. 542-2266.**
Elmhurst Home for Aged & Convalescent; Infirm 16.
YARMOUTH
Yarmouth Hosp.; Vancouver St.; Gen. 197; Tel. 742-3541.

Prince Edward Island

ALBERTON
Western Hosp.; Poplar St., P.O. Box 10; Gen. 57; Chron. 9; **Tel. 24.**
CHARLOTTETOWN
Beach Grove; P.O. Box 3500; Ger. 160; Tel. 6222.
Charlottetown Hosp.; Haviland St.; Gen. 195; Tel. 894-5561.
Livingston & McArthur Nursing Home; 6 Centennial Dr.; Conv. 14; **Tel. 7729.**
Prince Edward Island Hosp.; Brighton Rd.; Gen. 201; Tel. 894-8532.
Provincial Home for the Aged
Provincial San.; McGill Ave.; TB 70; **Tel. 4-7331.**
Rehabilitation Centre; McGill Ave.; Orth. 30; **Tel. 892-1225.**

HOSPITALS & CONVALESCENT HOMES — P.E.I. & NFLD.

Riverside Hosp.; Sherwood; P.O. Box 4000; Psy. 350; Tel. 894-5581.
Sacred Heart Home; 13 Haviland; Ger. 130; Tel. 894-6414.
Salvation Army Sunset Lodge; 78 Walthen Dr.; Dom. 30; Tel. 4-7214.
Sherwood Hosp.; P.O. Box 4000; Ment. Ret. Chil. 21; Tel. 894-8856.
Wood Convalescent Home Ltd.; 9 Grafton St.; Inf. 18; Tel. 894-9372.
MONTAGUE
Kings County Memorial Hosp.; Main St., P.O. Box 328; Gen. 50; Tel. 838-2152.
O'LEARY
O'Leary Community Hosp.; Gen. 32; Tel. 175.
SOURIS
Souris Hosp.; P.O. Box 339; Gen. 29; Tel. 198.
SUMMERSIDE
Golden Years Nursing Residence; 150 Belmont St.; Inf. 12; Tel. 436-5372.
Prince County Hosp.; Beattie Ave., P.O. Box 1630; Gen. 132; Chron. 16; Tel. 436-9131.
Summerset Manor; 205 Lefurgey Ave.; Inf. 70; Tel. 436-9261.
TYNE VALLEY
Stewart Memorial Health Centre; Gen. 18; Tel. 20-2.

Newfoundland

BAIE VERTE
M. J. Boylen Hosp.; Gen. 56; Tel. 2281.
BELL ISLAND
Bell Island Hosp.; Gen. 53; Dom. 6; Tel. 2821.
BONAVISTA
Bonavista Hosp.; Gen. 26; Tel. 7883.
BONNE BAY
Bonne Bay Cottage Hosp.; Norris Point; Gen. 32; Tel. 2211.
BOTWOOD
Botwood Cottage Hosp.; Gen. 65; Tel. 2833.
BROOKFIELD
Brookfield Cottage Hosp.; Bonavista Bay; Gen. 50. Tel. 2161.
BUCHANS
Buchans Hosp. Gen. 26; Tel. 3305.
BURGEO
Burgeo Cottage Hosp.; Gen. 19.
BURIN
Burin Cottage Hosp.; Gen. 30; Tel. 112.
CARBONEAR
Carbonear Community Hosp.;
P.O. Box 160; Gen. 57; Tel. 5004.
CARTWRIGHT
Lady MacLay Nursing Stn.; Labrador; Gen. 23.
CHANNEL
Channel Cottage Hosp.; Gen. 42.
COME-BY-CHANCE
Come-By-Chance Cottage Hosp.; Gen. 37. Tel. 2121.
CONCHE
Conche Nursing Station; Gen. 10.
CORNER BROOK
Western Memorial Hosp.; Hospital Hill; Gen. 247. Psy. 15; Tel. 4-5101.
ENGLEE
Englee Nursing Station; Gen. 9.
FLOWER'S COVE
Flower's Cove Nursing Station; Gen. 20.
FOGO
Fogo Cottage Hosp.; Gen. 23; Tel. 2222.
FORTEAU
Forteau Nursing Station; Labrador; Gen. 12.
GANDER
James Paton Mem. Hosp.; Trans Canada Hwy.; P.O. Box 5000; Gen. 155; Tel. 3961 .
GARNISH
Garnish Nursing Station; Fortune Bay; Inf. 2.
GOOSE BAY
R.C.A.F. Hospital; Labrador; Gen. 45; Tel. 896-2971.
GRAND BANK
Grand Bank Cottage Hosp.; Gen. 38; Tel. 3042.
GRAND FALLS
Central Newfoundland Hosp.; Union St., P.O. Box 397; Gen. 166, Tel. 2123.

HAPPY VALLEY
"Harry L. Paddon Mem. Hosp."; Labrador; Gen. 26; Tel. 896-2413.
HARBOUR BRETON
Harbour Breton Hosp.; Gen. 31; Tel. 2301.
HARBOUR DEEP
Harbour Deep Nursing Station; Gen. 4 .
HOPEDALE
Hopedale Nursing Stn.; Labrador; Gen. 4.
JACKSON'S ARM
Jackson's Arm Nursing Station; Inf. 2.
LABRADOR CITY
Capt. William Jackman Mem. H.; P.O. Box 1790; Gen. 76; Tel. 944-2632.
LASCIE
Lascie Nursing Stn.; (Prov. Govt.)
MAKKOVIK
Makkovik Nursing Stn., Labrador; Gen. 4.
MARKLAND
Markland Hosp.; Gen. 22; Tel. 177.
MARY'S HARBOUR
Mary's Harbour Nursing Station; Labrador; Gen. 20.
NAIN
Nain Nursing Station; Labrador; Gen. 12.
NORTHWEST RIVER
Grenfell Mission Hosp.; Labrador; Gen. 38; T.B. 6; Tel. 243.
OLD PERLICAN
Old Perlican Cottage Hosp.; Gen. 57; Tel. 21.
PLACENTIA
Placentia Cottage Hosp.; Gen. 49; Tel. 2013.
PORT SAUNDERS
Port Saunders Nursing Stn.; Gen. 4.
RODDICKTON
Roddickton Nursing Station; Gen. 14.
ST. ANTHONY
St. Anthony Hosp.; Gen. 94; TB 22; Orth. 6; Cont. 3; Tel. 709-2501.
ST. BRIDES
St. Brides Nursing Station; Inf. 2.
ST. JOHN'S
Grace Hosp.; LeMarchant Rd.; Gen. 239; Tel. 579-1181.
Hayles Home for the Aged; Portugal Cove Rd.; Inf. 225.
Hopedale Sunset Lodge! 11 Circular Rd.; Dom. 32; Tel. 8-5516.
Hosp. for Mental & Nervous Diseases; Waterford Bridge Rd.; P.O. Box 4810; Ment. 826; Tel. 579-5061.
International Grenfell Ass'n; Bus. Office.
88 Metcalfe St., Ottawa 4, Ont.
St. Clare's Mercy Hosp.; LeMarchant Rd.; Gen. 266; Tel. 578-0421.
St. John's Gen. Hosp.; Forest Rd., P.O. Box 5355 Gen. 343; Cont. 45; Orth. 120; Chron. 30; Inf. 5; Tel. 8-0471.
St. John's San.; Topsail Rd.,; T.B. 278; Tel. 579-2081.
St Luke's Homes; Topsail Rd.
St. Patrick's Mercy Home; Elizabeth Ave.; Inf. 180; Tel. 9-2031.
Salvation Army Glenbrook Girls' Home; Torbay Rd., P.O. Box 716; (Priv); Dom. 33; Tel. 579-1099.
Sunshine Camp Children's Rehab. Centre; Thornburn Rd., P.O. Box 1403; Rehab. Children 32; Tel. 9-2070.
Waterford Hall; Waterford Bridge Rd.; Dom. (Infants).
ST. LAWRENCE
U.S. Memorial Hosp.; Gen. 26; Tel. 232.
SPRINGDALE
Springdale Cottage H.; Gen. 44; Tel. 6912.
STEPHENVILLE CROSSING
Stephenville Crossing Hosp.; Gen. 78; Tel. 646-2542.
TREPASSEY
Trepassey Nursing Station; Inf. 3.
TWILLINGATE
Notre Dame Bay Memorial Hosp.; P.O. Box 9; Gen. 98; Dom. 2; Tel. 2214.

CANADIAN SCHOOLS OF NURSING

AND UNIVERSITY SCHOOLS OF NURSING

BRITISH COLUMBIA	
Kamloops	Royal Inland Hospital, Miss C. E. Mary Rowles, Director of Nursing.
Westminster	Royal Columbian Hospital, Miss Norah M. Fisher, Director of Nursing.
Vancouver	St. Paul's Hospital, Miss Roberta J. Cunningham, Director, School of Nursing.
Vancouver	Vancouver General Hospital, Miss Mary L. Richmond, Director of Nursing.
Vancouver	University of British Columbia, Miss Evelyn Mallory, Director.
Victoria	Royal Jubilee Hospital, Miss Muriel E. Thompson, Director of Nursing.
Victoria	St. Joseph's Hospital, Reverend Sister Mary Doris, Director, School of Nursing.
ALBERTA	
Calgary	Calgary General Hospital, Miss Eileen E. Jameson, Director of Nursing Education.
Calgary	Foothills Provincial General Hospital, Mrs. J. Tronningsdahl, Director of Nursing.
Calgary	Holy Cross Hospital, Rev. Sister M. Letourneau, Director of Nursing Education.
Edmonton	Edmonton General Hospital, Rev. Sr. Cecile Leclerc, Director of Nursing Education.
Edmonton	Misericordia Hospital, Rev. Sister St. Dephina, Director, School of Nursing.
Edmonton	Royal Alexandra Hospital, Miss Georgia Nobles, Assistant Director of Nursing.
Edmonton	University of Alberta, Miss Ruth E. McClure, Director.
Edmonton	University of Alberta Hospital, Miss M. Geneva Purcell, Director of Nursing.
Lamont	Archer Memorial Hospital, Lamont School of Nursing, Miss Ethel C. James, Director of Nursing.
Lethbridge	Lethbridge Municipal Hospital, Galt School of Nursing, Miss Claudia Tennant, Director of Nursing.
Lethbridge	St. Michael's Hospital, Rev. Sister M. Beatrice, Director of Nursing.
Medicine Hat	Medicine Hat General Hospital, Miss Winnifred M. Day, Director of Nursing Education.
Ponoka	Alberta Hospital, Miss Edith D. Kemp, Director of Nursing.
Vegreville	St. Joseph's General Hospital, Rev. Sister Madeleine Beaulieu, Director of Nursing Education.
SASKATCHEWAN	
Humboldt	St. Elizabeth Hospital, Rev. Sister M. Rufina, Director, School of Nursing.
Moose Jaw	Moose Jaw Union Hospital, Miss C. Louise Bartsch, Director of Nursing.
Moose Jaw	Providence Hospital, Rev. Sister Mary Fanchea, Director, School of Nursing.
Prince Albert	Holy Family Hospital, Rev. Sister M. Jane Frances, Director of Nursing.
Prince Albert	Victoria Union Hospital, Miss V. E. Parker, Assoc. Dir. of Nursing Education.
Regina	Regina General Hospital, Mrs. M. E. Magdalin, Acting Director of Nursing.
Regina	Regina Grey Nuns' Hospital, Rev. Sister T. Castonguay, Director, School of Nursing.
Saskatoon	St. Paul's Hospital, Rev. Sister Fernande Dussault, Director, School of Nursing.
Saskatoon	Saskatoon City Hospital, Miss Orma J. Smith, Director of Nursing.
Saskatoon	University of Saskatchewan, Miss Hazel B. Keeler, Director, School of Nursing.
	University of Saskatchewan Hospital, Miss Hazel B. Keeler, Director, School of Nursing.
Yorkton	Yorkton Union Hospital, Miss Kathleen G. Wood, Director of Nursing Education.
MANITOBA	
Brandon	Brandon General Hospital, Miss M. E. Jackson, Director of Nursing.
Winnipeg	Children's Hospital of Winnipeg, Miss Patricia Scorer, Director of Nursing.
Winnipeg	Salvation Army Grace Hospital, Captain Eleanor P. Johnson, Director of Nursing.
Winnipeg	Misericordia General Hospital, Rev. Sister St. Odilon, Director of Nursing.
Winnipeg	University of Manitoba, Dr. Margaret E. Hart, Director.
Winnipeg	Victoria General Hospital, Miss Dorothy M. Dick, Director of Nursing Education.
Winnipeg	Winnipeg General Hospital, Miss Margaret E. Cameron, Assistant Administrator.
St. Boniface	St. Boniface General Hospital, Rev. Sister A. Fleury, Director of Nursing Education.
ONTARIO	
Barrie	Royal Victoria Hospital, Miss E. Joyce Ardiel, Director of Nursing.
Belleville	Belleville General Hospital, Mrs. Madge Flindall, Director of Nursing Education.
Brantford	Brantford General Hospital, Miss Olive L. Plumstead, Director of Nursing.
Brockville	Brockville General Hospital, Miss Vera J. Preston, Director of Nursing.
Brockville	Ontario Hospital, Miss Ena M. Orr, Director of Nursing.
Chatham	Public General Hospital, Miss Sheila M. Creeggan, Director of Nursing Education.
Chatham	St. Joseph's Hospital, Rev. Sister M. Eunice, Director of Nursing.
Cornwall	Cornwall General Hospital, Mrs. Marlene A. Wert, Director of Nursing.
Cornwall	Hotel-Dieu Hospital, Rev. Sister Mary MacKenzie, Director, School of Nursing.
Fort William	McKellar General Hospital, Miss Carmel D. Connelly, Acting Director of Nursing Education.
Galt	South Waterloo Memorial Hospital, Miss E. J. Wearring, Dir. of Nursing Education.
Guelph	Guelph General Hospital, Miss Lois Campbell, Director of Nursing.
Guelph	St. Joseph's Hospital, Rev. Sister M. St. John, Director of Nursing.
Hamilton	Hamilton Civic Hospitals, Miss Merle E. Smith, Director of Nursing.

SCHOOLS OF NURSING — (ONTARIO & P.Q.)

Hamilton	Hamilton and District School of Nursing, Box 590, Miss Elizabeth M. Maus, Director.
Hamilton	St. Joseph's Hospital, Rev. Sister M. Celestine, Director of Nursing.
Hamilton	McMaster University, Miss Alma Reid, Director.
Kingston	Kingston General Hospital, Miss Sylvia M. Burkinshaw, Director of Nursing.
Kingston	Hotel-Dieu Hospital, St. Joseph's School of Nursing, Rev. Sister Mary A. Higgins, Director, School of Nursing.
Kingston	Ontario Hospital, Miss Herta M. Zarins, Director of Nursing Education.
Kingston	Queen's University, Miss Jenny M. Weir, Director.
Kitchener	Kitchener-Waterloo Hospital, Miss Rahno M. Beamish, Director of Nursing.
Kitchener	St. Mary's General Hospital, Rev. Sister M. Bonaventure, Director of Nursing.
London	St. Joseph's Hospital, Rev. Sister M. St. Roch, Director of Nursing.
London	University of Western Ontario, Miss R. Catharine Aikin, Dean, School of Nursing.
London	Victoria Hospital, Miss Dorothy Morgan, Director of Nursing.
Niagara Falls	Greater Niagara General Hospital, Miss Evelyn Paul, Director of Nursing.
North Bay	St. Joseph's General Hospital, Rev. Sister St. Louis, Director, School of Nursing.
Orillia	Orillia Soldiers' Memorial Hospital, Miss B. M. Jones, Director of Nursing.
Oshawa	Oshawa General Hospital, Miss Gladys E. Hill, Assoc. Dir. of Nursing Educ.
Ottawa	Ottawa Civic Hospital, Miss Dorothy Starr, Director of Nursing Education.
Ottawa	Ottawa General Hospital, Rev. Sister St. Albert, Director of Nursing Education.
Ottawa	St. Louis Marie de Montford Hospital, Sister Laurette de la Ste-Face, Director, School of Nursing.
Ottawa	University of Ottawa, Rev. Sister Francoise de Chantal, Director, School of Nursing.
Owen Sound	Owen Sound General & Marine Hospital, Miss Alma E. Patterson, Director of Nursing.
Pembroke	Pembroke General Hospital, Lorrain School of Nursing, Rev. Sister Mary Rena, Director, School of Nursing.
Peterborough	Peterborough Civic Hospital, Miss L. E. Fay Rutledge, Director of Nursing.
Peterborough	St. Joseph's Hospital, Rev. Sister M. Benedicta, Director, School of Nursing.
Port Arthur	General Hospital of Port Arthur, Miss Beverley R. McIntyre, Director of Nursing Education.
Port Arthur	St. Joseph's General Hospital, Rev. Sister M. Barbara, Director of the School of Nursing.
St. Catherines	St. Catherines' Hospital, The Mack Training School of Nurses, Mrs. J. Elizabeth Porteous, Director of Nursing.
St. Thomas	St. Thomas-Elgin General Hospital, Miss H. Bernice Lewis, Director of Nursing.
Sarnia	Sarnia General Hospital, Miss Una L. Ridley, Director, School of Nursing.
Sault Ste. Marie	Sault Ste. Marie General Hospital, St. Mary's School of Nursing, Rev. Sister St. Leonard, Director of Nursing.
Sault Ste. Marie	Plummer Memorial Public Hospital, Mrs. M. Dennison, Principal.
Stratford	Stratford General Hospital, Miss Mary F. Philpott, Director of Nursing Education.
Sudbury	St. Joseph's Hospital, St. Elizabeth School of Nursing, Sister Paul-Armand, Director of Nursing Education.
Sudbury	Sudbury General Hospital, Rev. Sister Mariam, Director, School of Nursing.
Timmins	St. Mary's Hospital, Miss Evelyn McKey, Director, School of Nursing.
Toronto	Toronto Western Hospital, Atkinson School of Nursing, Miss Grace Paterson, Director of Nursing.
Toronto	The Hospital for Sick Children, Miss Elsbeth Geiger, Director of Nursing.
Toronto	The Nightingale School of Nursing, 2 Murray Street, Mrs. Blanche Duncanson, Director.
Toronto	The Quo-Vadis School of Nursing, 38 Sunnyside Avenue, Miss Margaret Mackenzie, Director.
Toronto	Ryerson Polytechnical Institute, 50 Gould Street, Dr. H. H. Kerr Principal, Miss Dorothy Rowees, Supervisor of Nursing Course.
Toronto	St. Michael's Hospital, Rev. Sister M. de Sales, Director, School of Nursing.
Toronto	St. Joseph's Hospital, Rev. Sister Mary Herbert, Director of Nursing.
Toronto	Toronto East General Hospital and Orthopaedic Hospital, Mrs. Ruth Couse, Director of Nursing.
Toronto	Toronto General Hospital, Miss M. Jean Dodds, Director of Nursing.
Toronto	University of Toronto, Dr. Helen M. Carpenter, Director.
Toronto	Wellesley Hospital, Miss E. Dorothy Arnot, Director of Nursing.
Toronto	Women's College Hospital, Miss Irene Norton, Director of Nursing Education.
Whitby	Ontario Hospital, Mrs. R. Marguerite Steffler, Acting Director of Nursing and Nursing Education.
Willowdale	Branson Hospital, Miss Patricia H. Okimi, Director.
Windsor	Hotel Dieu of St. Joseph, Rev. Sister G. Trudell, Director of School of Nursing.
Windsor	Metropolitan General Hospital, Miss Kathleen Moderwell, Director of School of Nursing.
Windsor	Salvation Army Grace Hospital, Mrs. Shirley B. Gault, Director of Nursing Education.

SCHOOLS OF NURSING — (QUEBEC, N.B., N.S., P.E.I. & NFLD.)

Windsor	University of Windsor, Miss Florence M. Roach Dean, School of Nursing.
Woodstock	Woodstock General Hospital, Miss Phyllis C. Bluett, Director of Nursing.

QUEBEC

Alma, Lac St-Jean	Hôtel-Dieu d'Alma, Rév. Soeur Ste-Marie, Directrice.
Arthabaska	Hôtel-Dieu, 44 ave des Erables, Rév. Soeur Cécile Mercier, Directrice.
Chicoutimi	Hôtel-Dieu St-Vallier, Rév. Soeur Jean de l'Eucharistie, Directrice.
Drummondville	Hôpital Ste-Croix, 750 rue Hériot, Rév. Soeur L. Mongrain, Directrice.
Gaspé	Hôtel-Dieu de Gaspé, Rév. Soeur St-Jean-Eudes, Directrice.
Hull	Hôpital du Sacré coeur, 230 boul. Gamelin, Rev. Soeur Marie-Victoire, Directrice.
Joliette	Hôpital St. Eusèbe, 585 boul. Monseau, Rév. Soeur Louis de la Providence, Directrice.
Lévis	Hôtel-Dieu, 143 rue Wolfe, Rév. Soeur Saint-Paul, Directrice.
Mastai	Hôpital St-Michel-Archange, Rév. Soeur Ste-Marie de Magdala, Directrice.
Montréal 24	Hôpital de la Miséricorde, 1051 rue St-Hubert, Rév. Soeur Maris Stella, Directrice.
Montréal 9	Hôpital du Sacré Coeur, 5400 ouest, boul. Gouin, Rév. Soeur Jean-Rémi, Directrice.
Verdun, Montréal 19	Hôpital Général de Verdun, 3922 boul. Lasalle, Rév. Soeur Marie-Albini, Directrice.
Montréal 36	Hôpital Maisonneuve, 5415 boul. L'Assomption, Rév. Soeur Claire Jeannotte, Directrice.
Montréal 24	Hôpital Notre-Dame, 2205 rue Maisonneuve, Rév. Soeur Cécile Labonté, Directrice.
St-Laurent, Montréal 9	Hôpital Notre-Dame de l'Espérance, 1275 Cote Vertu, Rév. Soeur Gemma, Directrice.
Montréal 18	Hôpital Ste-Jeanne d'Arc, 3597 rue St-Urbain, Mlle Pierrette Lemay, Directrice.
Montréal 26	Hôpital Ste-Justine, 3180 Ellendale, Rév. Soeur Marie Bernard du Divin Coeur.
Montréal 18	Hôpital St-Luc, 264 est, boul. Dorchester, Mlle Pauline Crevier, Directrice de l'Ecole des Infirmières.
Montréal 18	Hôtel-Dieu de Montréal, 3880 rue St-Urbain, Rév. Soeur Thérèse Robert, Directrice.
Montreal	Institut Marguerite Youville, Rev. Sister Denise M. Lefèbvre.
Montreal	McGill University, Miss Elizabeth Logan, Director.
Montréal	St. Mary's Hospital, Rév. Sister Mary Felicitas, Director, School of Nursing.
Montréal	Jewish General Hospital, Miss Joan M. Gilchrist, Director of Nursing.
Montréal	Montréal General Hospital, Mrs. A. Isobel MacLeod, Director of Nursing.
Montréal	Queen Elizabeth Hospital of Montreal, Miss Floranna D. Bryant, Director of Nursing.
Montréal	Royal Victoria Hospital, Miss Helene M. Lamont, Director & Principal of School of Nursing.
Montreal	University of Montreal, Miss Alice Girard, Dean.
Noranda	Hôpital Youville, Rév. Soeur André-du-Sauveur, Directrice.
Québec 3	Hôpital de l'Enfant-Jésus, 1410-18e rue, Rév. Soeur Thérèse des Buissonnets, Directrice.
Québec 6	Hôpital du St-Sacrement, 1051 Chemin Ste-Foy, Rév. Soeur Claire du St-Sacrement Directrice.
Québec City	Jeffrey Hale's Hospital, Miss Kathleen Marshall, Director of Nurses.
Québec 3	Hôpital St-François d'Assise, 1605-1ère avenue, Rév. Soeur Suzanne Lafleur, Directrice de l'Ecole des Infirmières.
Québec 4	Hôtel-Dieu de Québec, 11 Côte du Palais, Rév. Soeur St-Thomas d'Aquin, Directrice.
Québec	Laval University, Miss Noëlla Bertrand, Directrice.
Rimouski	Hôpital St-Joseph, Rév. Soeur Ste-Thérèse du Sauveur, Directrice.
Rivière-du-Loup	Hôpital St-Joseph du Precieux-Sang, Rév. Soeur Hélène Augustine Directrice.
St-Georges-Ouest	Hôtel-Dieu Notre-Dame de Beauce, C.P. 370, Rév. Soeur St.-Augustin, Directrice.
St-Hyacinthe	Hôpital St-Charles, 2750 rue Laframboise, Rév. Soeur Thérèse-du-Lisieux, Directrice.
St-Jean	Hôpital St-Jean, 217 est Longueuil, Rév. Soeur Claire Gagnon, Directrice.
St-Jérôme, Cte Terrebonne	Hôtel-Dieu de St-Jérôme, Rév. Soeur Thérèse Perreault, Directrice de l'Ecole.
Shawinigan	Hôpital Ste-Therese, 1705 rue Georges, Rév. Soeur Marie-Léonille, Directrice.
Sherbrooke	Hôtel-Dieu, 580 Bowen Sud, Rév. Soeur Ste-Véronique, Directrice de l'Ecole.
Sherbrooke	Hôpital St-Vincent-de-Paul, 300 rue King est, Mlle Pauline Provençal, Directrice.
Sherbrooke	Sherbrooke Hospital, Miss Clara R. Aitkenhead, Director of Nursing.
Trois-Rivières	Hopital St-Joseph, 731 rue Ste-Julie, Rév. Soeur Laurent, Directrice.

NEW BRUNSWICK

Bathurst	Hotel-Dieu of St. Joseph, Rev. Sr. Térèse Haché, Director of Nursing.
Campbellton	Hotel-Dieu de St. Joseph, Rev. Soeur Céline Doucet, Director of Nursing Education.
Chatham	Hotel-Dieu de St. Joseph, Rev. Sister Clora Skidd, Director of Nursing Education.
Edmundston	Hotel-Dieu de St. Joseph, Rev. Sister Imelda Roy, Director of Nursing Education.
Fredericton	University of New Brunswick, Dr. Katherine MacLaggan, Director.

SCHOOLS OF NURSING—(Quebec, N.B., N.S., P.E.I. & Nfld)

Moncton	University of — Sr. Jacqueline Bouchard, Dir.
Fredericton	Victoria Public Hospital, Miss Jean Anderson, Director of Nursing.
Moncton	Hotel-Dieu de l'Assomption, Soeur Marie Fidelis, Director of Nursing Education.
Moncton	The Moncton Hospital, Mrs. Katherine Wright, Director of Nursing.
Newcastle	Miramichi Hospital, Mrs. Anna M. Allison, Director of Nursing.
Saint John	Saint John General Hospital, Miss M. Jane Stephenson, Director of Nursing.
Saint John	St. Joseph Hospital, Rev. Sister Helen Marie, Director of Nursing.
St. Stephen	Charlotte County Hospital, Miss E. Irene Rumsey, Director of Nursing.
Woodstock	Carleton Memorial Hospital, Mrs. Adeline Dunbar, Director of Nursing.
NOVA SCOTIA	
Antigonish	St. Martha's Hospital, Rev. Sister Marie Barbara, Director of Nurses.
Antigonish	St. Francis Xavier University, Rev. Sister Marie Barbara, Director of Nurses.
Dartmouth	Nova Scotia Hospital, Miss Eleanor C. Purdy, Director of Nursing.
Glace Bay	Glace Bay General Hospital, Miss Gladys Smith, Director of Nursing.
Glace Bay	St. Joseph's Hospital, Rev. Sister Clare Marie, Director of Nurses.
Halifax	Children's Hospital, Mrs. Margaret M. Ross, Director of Nurses.
Halifax	Dalhousie University, Miss E. A. Electa MacLennan, Director.
Halifax	Halifax Infirmary, Rev. Sister Catherine Peter, Director of Nursing.
Halifax	Mount Saint Vincent College, Rev. Sister Jean Eudes, Dir. Nursing Education.
Halifax	Victoria General Hospital, Miss Florence B. Gass, Director of Nursing.
New Glasgow	Aberdeen Hospital, Miss Mary J. Ross, Director of Nursing.
North Sydney	St. Elizabeth Hospital, Rev. Sister Francis Joseph, Director of Nursing.
Sydney	St. Rita Hospital, Rev. Sister Mary Donald, Director of Nursing.
Sydney	Sydney City Hospital, Miss M. Blanche Anderson, Director of Nursing.
Windsor	Payzant Memorial Hospital, Miss Marilyn Riley, Director of Nursing.
Yarmouth	Yarmouth Hospital Training School, Mrs. Dorothy E. Allan, Director of Nursing.
PRINCE EDWARD ISLAND	
Charlottetown	Charlottetown Hospital, Rev. Sister Mary Irene, Director of Nursing.
Charlottetown	Prince Edward Island Hospital, Miss Ella B. MacLeod, Director of Nursing.
Summerside	Prince County Hospital, Miss Mary E. Murphy, Associate Director of Nursing Education.
NEWFOUNDLAND	
St. John's	Memorial University, Miss Joyce Nevitt, Director, School of Nursing.
St. John's	St. Clare's Mercy Hospital, Rev. Sister M. Xaverius, Director of Nursing.
St. John's	St. John's General Hospital, Miss Janet E. Story, Director of Nursing.
St. John's	Salvation Army Grace Hospital, Major Elsie Hill, Director of Nursing.

V. D. REGULATIONS

Venereal diseases, under the existing Legislation, are reportable directly to the Provincial Departments of Health rather than to the office of the local medical officer of health, as in the case of other communicable diseases. Registration cards, for this purpose, are available from the Division of Venereal Disease Control of the Provincial Department of Health.

POISON CONTROL CENTRES CANADA

The following Poison Control Centres have been established through the co-operation of the Canadian Paediatric Society, The Food & Drug Directorate of the Department of National Health & Welfare, the Provincial Health Departments and the Canadian Medical Association.

It is suggested that when needed, doctors consult the Emergency Department of the listed hospitals or if specific information is desired, the doctor named as Consultant for the Poison Control can be directly contacted.

NEWFOUNDLAND

LABRADOR CITY
Capt. Wm. Jackman Memorial Hospital ....
Capt. W. Hammond

CORNER BROOK
Western Memorial Hospital **634-5232**
Mr. Karapita, A.D., Administrator.

GANDER
James Paton Mem. Hosp. ....
Mr. G. Gover, Administrator.

GRAND FALLS
Central Newfoundland Hospital 2123
Mr. R. D. Moore, Administrator.

ST. ANTHONY
The Internat. Grenfell Association ....
Mr. D. P. Fish, Administrator.

ST. JOHN'S
St. John's General Hospital **578-0471**
Dr. E. W. Wight, Administrator.
Grace Hospital **578-3021**
Mrs. Charlotte Pomeroy, R.N.

ST. JOHN'S
The Children's Hospital Pleasantville ....
Mr. D. E. J. Kelland, Administrator.

PRINCE EDWARD ISLAND

CHARLOTTETOWN
Charlottetown Hospital **894-5561**
Dr. J. H. O'Hanley.
Prince Edward Island Hospital **894-8532**
Dr. K. Ross Parker.

MONTAGUE
Kings County Memorial Hospital 27
Dr. John Bonnell.

SUMMERSIDE
Prince County Hospital **436-2246**
Dr. Sheldon Cameron.

NOVA SCOTIA

HALIFAX
Halifax Children's Hospital 422-8441
Dr. R. L. Ozere.

NEW BRUNSWICK

CAMPBELLTON
Hotel-Dieu Hospital 753-3301
Dr. R. Le Tourneau

EDMUNDSTON
Hôtel-Dieu de St-Joseph **735-3361**
Dr. L. E. LeBlanc.

FREDERICTON
Polio Clinic and Health Centre 475-9944
Dr. L. E. Stickles & Dr. R. M. Bergh

MONCTON
Moncton Hospital 384-4421
Dr. C. M. Leighton.

SAINT JOHN
Saint John General Hospital 692-8708
Dr. S. H. Weyman.

QUEBEC

BEAUCE
Hotel-Dieu, Notre Dame de Beauce, ...
Dr. Francois Cliche

GASPE
Hôtel-Dieu de Gaspé **400**
Dr. Marc-André Pouliot.

HULL
Hôpital du Sacré-Coeur .... **PR 7-2721**
Dr. André Letarte.

JONQUIERE
Hotel-Dieu Notre-Dame de L'Assomption
Dr. Pierre Marchand

MONTREAL
Hôpital Sainte-Justine .... **RE 1-4931**
Dr. Luc Chicoine.
Montreal Children's Hospital .... **WE 7-8511**
Dr. E. S. Hillman.

NORANDA
Hôpital Youville ....
Dr. J. O. V. Bellegarde.

QUEBEC
Hôpital de l'Enfant-Jésus **529-8711**
Dr. Roland Turcot.
Jeffery Hale Hospital **683-4471**
Dr. Clarence Rosenhek

RIMOUSKI
Hôpital St-Joseph **723-7851**
Dr. Jean Morisset.

SHAWINIGAN
Joyce Memorial Hospital .... **LE 7-6661**
Dr. A. H. Moyle.

SHERBROOKE
Hôtel-Dieu de Sherbrooke .... **LO 9-2551**
Dr. Adrien Pagé.
Sherbrooke Hospital .... **LO 9-3661**
Dr. R. Kimoff

SWEETSBURG
Brome-Missisquoi Perkins Hospital **263-1333**
Dr. Robert S. Pincott.

TROIS-RIVIERES
Hôpital St-Joseph .... **FR 4-6211**
Dr. J. P. Beaudet

ONTARIO

BARRIE
Royal Victoria Hospital .... **PA 8-5951**
Dr. Roy Asquith.

BELLEVILLE
Belleville General Hospital .... **WO 8-5511**
Dr. James E. Nelles.

BRANTFORD
Brantford General Hospital **752-7871**
Dr. C. L. Rodgers.
St. Joseph's Hospital .... **PL 3-3461**
Dr. T. Emmet Cleary.

BURLINGTON
Joseph Brant Memorial Hospital **637-2361**
Dr. H. Davidson.

POISON CONTROL CENTRES — (ONT. *cont'd*)

FORT WILLIAM
McKellar General Hospital .... MA 3-6471
Dr. P. C. MacGillivray.

GUELPH
St. Joseph's Hospital .... TA 4-2620
Dr. J. J. Brown.

HAILEYBURY
Misericordia Hospital .... OS 2-3315
Dr. W. J. Houghtling.

HAMILTON
Hamilton General Hospital .... JA 7-0271
Dr. M. T. Nathan.
Chedoke General & Children's Hospital 385-5341
Dr. A. B. MacMillan.

KINGSTON
Kingston General Hospital .... LI 2-2821
Dr. J. H. Read.

KIRKLAND
Kirkland and District Hospital 136
Dr. D. G. Howatson.

KITCHENER
Kitchener-Waterloo Hospital .... SH 5-9451
Dr. J. H. Finn.
St. Mary's General Hospital 744-3311
Dr. W. H. Friday.

LONDON
Victoria Hospital .... GE 2-5261
Dr. J. C. Rathbun.

OTTAWA
Ottawa Civic Hospital .... PA 9-2511
Dr. I. H. Glass.
Ottawa General Hospital .... CE 6-4592
Dr. P. de Bellefeuille

PICTON
Prince Edward Memorial Hospital ...... GR 6-2181
Dr. Gerald Allison.

PORT ARTHUR
Port Arthur General Hospital .... DI 4-6621
Dr. J. V. Riches.

ST. CATHARINES
St. Catharines General Hospital .... MU 4-7271
Dr. A. T. Brown.

SARNIA
Sarnia General Hospital .... DI 4-3661
St. Joseph's Hospital .... ED 6-6121
Dr. Morris Perchanok.

SAULT STE-MARIE
Plummer Memorial Public Hospital ...... AL 4-5166
Dr. W. J. Robertson.

SIMCOE
Norfolk General Hospital 426-0750
Dr. K. R. McGavin.

SUDBURY
St. Joseph's Hospital .... OS 4-3101
Dr. F. O. Dickson.
Sudbury General Hospital .... OS 3-3601
Dr. J. B. Hennessy.

TORONTO
East General & Orthopaedic Hospital 461-8272
Dr. Hugh C. Cameron.
Hospital for Sick Children .... EM 6-7242
Dr. Robert J. Imrie.

WALLACEBURG
Sydenham District Hospital 627-3325
Dr. J. R. Holmes.

WINDSOR
Hotel-Dieu de St-Joseph .... CL 2-3631
Dr. H. J. Breault.

MANITOBA

WINNIPEG (Provincial Hdqts. for Program)
Winnipeg Children's Hospital 775-8311
Dr. Vera Gellman.

BIRTLE
Birtle District Hospital 44
Mr. S. B. Labovich, Adm.
Birtle-Shoal Lake Health Unit 27
Dr. H. Cheng.

BRANDON
Brandon Hospital .... PA 6-7421
Dr. Jim Hendry.

CHURCHILL
Fort Churchill Hospital ....

DAUPHIN
Dauphin General Hospital 638-3010
Mr. Harvey House.

FLIN FLON
Northern Local Health Unit 687-3459
Mrs. L. Klassen.

GIMLI
Stonewall Health Unit 465
Dr. J. Gonty.

MORDEN
Morden Hospital 822-4411
Miss Van Dongen.

MORRIS
Morris Hospital 270
Mr. R. J. Bartlette, (Pharm.)

NEEPAWA
Neepawa Health Unit 200
Mrs. Marie Salway.

PORTAGE LA PRAIRIE
Dr. John C. Elias, P.O. Box 187 857-6788

ST. BONIFACE
St. Boniface Hospital .... WH 3-0311
Dr. Ken Wiley.

SWAN RIVER
Swan River Valley Hospital ....

THE PAS
Northern Health Services .... MA 3-2251
Dr. Peter Lommerse.

VIRDEN
Virden Hospital 91
Mrs. L. Walton.

SASKATCHEWAN

REGINA
Regina General Hospital .... LA 2-1811
Dr. M. D. Heimback.

SASKATOON
University Hospital 242-7641
Dr. J. W. Gerrard & Dr. N. Goluboff.

ALBERTA

MAIN CENTRES

There is a Poison Treatment Centre in the Emergency Service of every active Treatment Hospital in Alberta (110)

CALGARY
Calgary General Hospital .... AM 6-7541

EDMONTON
University Hospital .... GE 9-5911

BRITISH COLUMBIA

ALERT BAY
St. George's Hospital 974-5221

BURNABY
Burnaby General Hospital 434-4211

CAMPBELL RIVER
Campbell River General Hospital 287-6221

CHILLIWACK
Chilliwack General Hospital 792-3411

COURTENAY-COMOX
St. Joseph's General Hospital 339-2242

CRANBROOK
St. Eugene Hospital 426-2241

DAWSON CREEK
St. Joseph's General Hospital 782-8501

DUNCAN
King's Daughters' Hospital 746-4141

GANGES
Lady Minto Hospital 9

KAMLOOPS
Royal Inland Hospital 372-3131

KELOWNA
Kelowna General Hospital 762-4000

POISON CONTROL CENTRES — (B.C. *cont'd*)

KEMANO
Kemano Hospital

KITIMAT
Kitimat General Hospital 1100

LADYSMITH
Ladysmith General Hospital 245-3341

MISSION
Mission Memorial Hospital 772-2651

NANAIMO
Nanaimo General Hospital 754-2141

NELSON
Kootenay Lake General Hospital 352-3111

NEW WESTMINSTER
Royal Columbian Hospital 522-2771

PRINCE RUPERT
Prince Rupert General Hospital 1821

PENTICTON
Penticton General Hospital 492-4000

PORT ALBERNI
West Coast General Hospital 723-2135

POWELL RIVER
Powell River General Hospital 483-2275

QUESNEL
Baker Memorial Hospital 246

PRINCE GEORGE
Prince George and District Hospital 564-4411

REVELSTOKE
Queen Victoria Hospital 837-3000

ROSSLAND
Mater Misericordiae Hospital 363-7344

SALMON ARM
Salmon Arm Hospital 832-2182

SMITHERS
Bulkley Valley Hospital 847-3312

TERRACE
Terrace and District Hospital 843-2211

TOFINO
Tofino General Hospital 725-3414

TRAIL
Trail-Tadanac Hospital 368-3311

VANCOUVER
Vancouver General Hospital (Main Centre) 876-3211
North Vancouver General (Lions Gate) 983-3131
St. Paul's Hospital 683-2211

VANDERHOOF
St. John's Hospital 181

VERNON
Vernon Jubilee Hospital 542-4000

VICTORIA
Royal Jubilee Hospital (Main Centre) EV 6-3131
St. Joseph's Hospital 384-1131

WHITE ROCK
White Rock District Hospital 531-5512

LAND AREA AND POPULATION, CANADA, 1961

Canada is composed at present of ten provinces and two territories so called, each having local government operating within designated bounds. Their respective names, seats of government, areas and populations (1961 census)* are as follows:

	Seat of Government	Land Area in sq. miles	Pop. 1961 Census
NEWFOUNDLAND, INCLUDING LABRADOR	St. John's	143,045	457,853
PRINCE EDWARD ISLAND	Charlottetown	2,184	104,629
NOVA SCOTIA	Halifax	20,402	737,007
NEW BRUNSWICK	Fredericton	27,835	597,936
QUEBEC	Quebec City	523,860	5,259,211
ONTARIO	Toronto	344,092	6,236,092
MANITOBA	Winnipeg	211,775	921,686
SASKATCHEWAN	Regina	220,182	925,181
ALBERTA	Edmonton	248,800	1,331,944
BRITISH COLUMBIA	Victoria	359,279	1,629,082
YUKON	Whitehorse	205,346	14,628
NORTHWEST TERRITORIES	Ottawa	1,253,438	22,998
CANADA (Total)		3,560,238	18,238,247

* Preliminary figures subject to revision.

NECROLOGY

Doctors Deceased Since 1966 Edition, Canadian Medical Directory

Aberhart, Carl, Toronto, Ont.
Allin, Albert E., Fort William, Ont.
Anderson, Winfred G., Medicine Hat, Alta.
Annett, Robert L., London, Ont.
Archambault, Francois, Montreal, P.Q.
Ayotte, Pierre F., Battleford, Sask.
Bastien, C. H., Vancouver, B.C.
Beaumier, Joseph A., Montreal, P.Q.
Bebenek, Bernard J., Georgetown, Ont.
Belanger, J. Cleophas, Hull, P.Q.
Bell, C. H. C., Vancouver, B.C.
Bellemare, J. Onias, St.Jean-Baptiste-Rouville, P.Q.
Belliveau, Pierre E., Meteghan, N.S.
Bennett, C. F., Moose Jaw, Sask.
Bernard, Leonce, Charlesbourg, P.Q.
Boileau, Jacques R., Ottawa, Ont.
Boivin, Jean-M, Alma, P.Q.
Bond-Nichols, Roberta, Halifax, N.S.
Borthwick-Leslie, Kathleen V., Winnipeg, Man.
Boucher, Romeo, Montreal, P.Q.
Boulva, R. M., Prince Albert, Sask.
Boyer, G. F., Toronto, Ont.
Bradley, Basil V., Toronto, Ont.
Brand, C. W., Toronto, Ont.
Brereton, Thomas C., Winnipeg, Man.
Brien, J. Wilbert, Windsor, Ont.
Bruck, Elmer, Hamilton, Ont.
Bryan, Herman R., Port Arthur, Ont.
Buktenica, N. F., Toronto, Ont.
Burton, G. W., St. Stephen, N.B.
Cade, John P., Prince Rupert, B.C.
Cameron, H. M., Ottawa, Ont.
Campbell, Bartley D., Verona, Ont.
Caron, Maurice, Quebec, P.Q.
Carrier, Leonard, Montreal, P.Q.
Cartier, Come, L'Annonciation, P.Q.
Case, Mayes, Saint John, N.B.
Casgrain, Gerard, Montreal, P.Q.
Cawthorpe, Joseph F., St. Thomas, Ont.
Chabot, Edouard, Thetford Mines, P.Q.
Cherington, Frederick J., Winnipeg, Man.
Chirico, Frank, North Bay, Ont.
Clark, D. A., Victoria, B.C.
Clark, Norman S., Toronto, Ont.
Clegg, Frank R., London, Ont.
Cloutier, G. A., St. Leonard, N.B.
Code, Douglas B., Brockville, Ont.
Collyer, Gerald R., London, Ont.
Colquhoun, John D., London, Ont.
Comtois, Jos., St. Barthelemy, P.Q.
Corbet, Gordon A., Ottawa, Ont.
Cotnam, Ira D., Pembroke, Ont.
Couture, Antoine, Quebec, P.Q.
Cragg, Bertram H., Peterborough, Ont.
Crowley, Joseph, St. John's, Nfld.
Curry, W. Allan, Halifax, N.S.
David, Gordon E., Toronto, Ont.
Day, Allan, Edmonton, Alta.
Dean, Keith C., Caledonia, Ont.
Dechene, Gaston M., Sherbrooke, Ont.
Delorme, Emile G., Montreal Nord, P.Q.
Dennison, J. Hoyle, Fort William, Ont.
Dinsmore, James D., Port Clyde, N.S.
Domingue, Charles, Montreal, P.Q.
Douglas, Lennox H., Galt, Ont.
Doupe, Joseph, Winnipeg, Man.
Dowd, Peter J., Sussex, N.B.
Drouin, Louis P., Montreal, P.Q.
Duggan, Lawrence, Regina, Sask.
Dumont, Georges L., Campbellton, N.B.
Dunaj, Zygmunt, Toronto, Ont.
Dunlop, William R., Vancouver, B.C.
Durocher, Ulysses J., Windsor, Ont.
Dyck, Harold F., Winkler, Man.
Dyma, Bronislaw, Winnipeg, Man.
Earle, W. Purvis, Kirkland Lake, Ont.
Ellis, Edward G., Bracebridge, Ont.
Enman, J. R., Taber, Alta.
Evans, Edward G., Vermillion, Alta.
Ferguson, Farquhard C., London, Ont.
Finlay, Francis S., Halifax, N.S.
Fischer, Lavern C., Kitchener, Ont.
Fisher, Kenneth J., Vancouver, B.C.
Fisher, Richard S., Hagersville, Ont.
Floren, Samuel A., Hamilton, Ont.
Fowler, Jordan M., Victoria, B.C.
Gagnon, Arthur, Charny, P.Q.
Gagnon, U. J., Yamaska, P.Q.
Gauthier, Claude, Montreal, P.Q.
Gauthier, Pierre P., Montreal, P.Q.
Geggie, Harold, Wakefield, P.Q.
Gendron, Vincent, Campbellton, N.B.
Germain, Marcel, St. Prosper, P.Q.
Giard, Thomas, Montreal, P.Q.
Gibson, Thomas F., Gainsborough, Sask.
Gillanders, H. Edwin, Mansonville, P.Q.
Girard, J. A., Quebec, P.Q.
Goodchild, Sandford F., Toronto, Ont.
Gowland, Marshall M., Point Edward, Ont.
Grabis, Eric L., Hamilton, Ont.
Graham, Gordon D., Winnipeg, Man.
Grant, A. Roy, Summerside, P.E.I.
Gregory, Alexander W., Lambeth, Ont.
Greig, Fraser M., Bracebridge, Ont.
Groleau, Maurice, St. Jerome, P.Q.
Groner, Paul, Toronto, Ont.
Hamilton, J. Gregory, Westport, Ont.
Hamilton, Reg. C. M., Baie d'Urfe, P.Q.
Hammond, Archie S., Fort Erie, Ont.
Hardiman, Benjamin C., Fort William, Ont.
Hare, Jack H., St. Thomas, Ont.
Harris, Robert I., Toronto, Ont.
Hassard, F. R., Toronto, Ont.
Haszard, John F., Kimberley, B.C.
Hartman, Clare C., Olds, Alta.
Haubrich, Theresa, Downsview, Ont.
Henderson, Charles S., Parrsboro, N.S.
Henderson, David A., Bala, Ont.
Hillary, Norman L., Windsor, Ont.
Hilliard, W. L., Waterloo, Ont.
Hilton, G .E. M., Vancouver, B.C.
Hjalmarsson, Numi, Lundar, Man.
Hopkins, Herbert E., Toronto, Ont.
Houston, William G., White River, Ont.
Huggard, L. Roy, Vancouver, B.C.
Hume, Rowena G., Toronto, Ont.
Hutcheson, Herwald O., Melfort, Sask.
Janes, Ernest C., Hamilton, Ont.
Janes, Robert M., Toronto, Ont.
Jenner, Harley D., Regina, Sask.
Joyner, J. H., Pembroke, Ont.
Jupp, Jas. B., Woodstock, Ont.
Kennedy, Richard H., Tignish, P.E.I.
Khattar, Thomas J., Glace Bay, N.S.
Kinsella, Malcolm D., Toronto, Ont.
Kinsey, Harold I., Toronto, Ont.
Kinsey, Peter A., Toronto, Ont.
Kirk, James G., Listowel, Ont.
Kuegle, Reinhold, Hamilton, Ont.
Lariviere, P. E., Valleyfield, P.Q.
Latchford, J. K., Ottawa, Ont.
Lauzon, Albert, Montreal, P.Q.
Lawrence, R. Grant, Vancouver, B.C.
Leatherdale, Donald G., Tillsonburg, Ont.
Leboldus, Michael W., Montreal, P.Q.
Leclerc, Arthur, Quebec, P.Q.
Leduc, Philippe A., Granby, P.Q.
Leggett, W. Grant, Kingsville, Ont.
Le May, J. Albert, Ottawa, Ont.
Levesque, Felix A., Trois Rivieres, P.Q.
Levesque, Ruben, Montreal, P.Q.
Levy, James M., Calgary, Alta.

DOCTORS DECEASED SINCE 1966 C.M.D. *(cont'd.)*

Lewin, George W., Niagara Falls, Ont.
Lewis, Gordon A., Oil Springs, Ont.
Lindsay, Lionel M., Montreal, P.Q.
Lochead, John R., Montreal, P.Q.
Lockhart, Wm. T., Salt Springs Island, B.C.
MacDonald, A., Regina, Sask.
MacFarlane, Joseph A., Toronto, Ont.
MacKenzie, Ian, Halifax, N.S.
Macklim, J. E., Calgary, Alta.
MacPherson, Cluny, St. John's, Nfld.
MacPherson, Fuller S., Edmonton, Alta.
MacPherson, John J., Campbellton, N.B.
Malyska, Marvin M., Winnipeg, Man.
Manning, Frederick W., Amherstburg, Ont.
Margulius, Jack, New Westminster, B.C.
Mathieson, Lily F., Belleville, Ont.
Mayer, Jean-Louis, Marieville, P.Q.
McArthur, J. A., Blackstock, Ont.
McCaffrey, John A., Vancouver, B.C.
McDonnell, Eugene D., Brockville, Ont.
McGeachy, Jessie A., Ottawa, Ont.
McGreer, C. G., Winnipeg, Man.
McIntosh, John F., Montreal, P.Q.
McKittrick, Edward A., South Porcupine, Ont.
McLandress, Kenneth W., Mitchell, Ont.
McLean, Thomas, Humboldt, Sask.
McNaughton, George A., Toronto, Ont.
Metcalfe, Herbert G., Lindsay, Ont.
Millette, Edouard, Ste-Adele-en-Bas, P.Q.
Moffatt, W. A., Vancouver, B.C.
Moreau, R. Laurent, St. Jean, P.Q.
Morgan, George S., Montreal, P.Q.
Morison, H., Winnipeg, Man.
Morrison, Clarence N., Halifax, N.S.
Morrison, R. Lindsay, Toronto, Ont.
Morse, Harry D., Winnipeg, Man.
Murray, Ronald B., Newmarket, Ont.
Nicholls, R. Frederick, Edmonton, Alta.
Oliver, J. H., Sunderland, Ont.
O'Neil, Hugh P., St. Andrew's, N.B.
Ower, R. Campbell, Scarborough, Ont.
Panneton, Auguste, Trois-Rivieres, P.Q.
Paquette, J. P., Montreal, P.Q.
Paterson, William P., Ottawa, Ont.
Perkins, Reginald J., Hamilton, Ont.
Perry, Florence, Vancouver, B.C.
Pettman, Frank E., Vernon, B.C.
Plouffe, Romeo, Montreal, P.Q.
Post, Gilbert C., Whitney, Ont.
Puddicombe, John F., Ottawa, Ont.
Purdie, Peter B., South Porcupine, Ont.
Rae, C. A., Toronto, Ont.
Rainville, Rosaire, Quebec, P.Q.
Reeve-Newson, F. A. R., Thornbury, Ont.
Reid, Fred I., Chatham, Ont.
Reid, F. L., Kingston, Ont.
Rochon, P. E., Montreal, P.Q.
Rolph, A. H., Weston, Ont.
Roome, Norman W., Toronto, Ont.
Roy, Joseph J., Quebec, P.Q.
Roy, Louis P., Quebec, P.Q.
Saint Pierre, Damien, Ottawa, Ont.
Sarjeant, Percy A., Toronto, Ont.
Schram, John S., London, Ont.
Schwalm, F. G., Blubber Bay, B.C.
Schwartz, Hugh W., Halifax, N.S.
Scott, Donald M., Belleville, Ont.
Shaw, William T., Petrolia, Ont.
Shillabeer, J. C., Vancouver, B.C.
Simpson, Robert A., Vancouver, B.C.
Smith, David, Stratford, Ont.
Smith, Ralph L., Halifax, N.S.
Sommerville, Andrew N., Winnipeg, Man.
Spearing, Frederick, Beeton, Ont.
Stalker, Malcolm, Toronto, Ont.
Stevenson, A. R., Peterborough, Ont.
Stevenson, R. H., Danville, P.Q.
Stevenson, Wm. O., Hamilton, Ont.
Stewart, Roy J., Winnipeg, Man.
Strickland, Randolph W., Sydney Mines, N.S.
Swan, Richard C., Montreal, P.Q.
Sweeney, Denis, Regina, Sask.
Sweeney, John P., Charlottetown, P.E.I.
Tait, Archibald C., St. John's, Nfld.
Tardif, J. Alexandre, Rimouski, P.Q.
Templeman, Walter, Bell Island, Nfld.
Tisdale, R. W., Sr., Delhi, Ont.
Townsend, Murray P., Oshawa, Ont.
Tweedie, William C., Rockland, Ont.
Vanasse, S. F., Ferme Neuve, P.Q.
Vandanaigue, Isaac, Montreal, P.Q.
Van Geyn, Jacobus, Port Renfrew, B.C.
Wace, Cyril, Victoria, B.C.
Wallbridge, Cecil T., Killaloe, Ont.
Waller, Kenneth B., Rockwood, Ont.
Warren, J. G., Hamilton, Ont.
Webb, Fred E., Barrie, Ont.
Weston, Rene E., Tillsonburg, Ont.
Wilkin, Wyllie I., Warman, Sask.
Williamson, George S., Ottawa, Ont.
Wilson, Charlemagne, Montreal, P.Q.
Wilson, Wallace A., Vancouver, B.C.
Wilson, William M., Windsor, Ont.
Wlodkowski, Wladyslaw K., Toronto, Ont.
Wood, Laurence E., Galt, Ont.
Workman, Harold C., Port Colborne, Ont.
Wright, Edwin K., Athabasca, Alta.
Wrinch, Leonard B., Trail, B.C.
Yarmey, William J., Toronto, Ont.
Yeo, Ira J., Charlottetown, P.E.I.
Yuan, Shu-Lung, Vancouver, B.C.
Young, William A., Beaverlodge, Alta.
Zillman, Heinz D., Montreal, P.Q.
Zinchesin, William J., Toronto, Ont.

NARCOTIC CONTROL ACT AND PART III OF THE FOOD AND DRUGS ACT

The Narcotic Control Act 1961, formerly the Opium and Narcotic Drug Act, is administered by the Department of National Health and Welfare, Ottawa, under the supervision of Mr. R. C. Hammond, Chief of the Division of Narcotic Control.

A complete list of drugs which come under the Narcotic schedule is included with the copy of the Act, which may be obtained from the Department of National Health and Welfare, Ottawa. This list includes all drugs ruled internationally as Narcotics, including Codeine.

In addition, Part III of the Food and Drug Act was proclaimed by Parliament in September 1961. Special measures of control over the groups of drugs known as Barbiturates and Amphetamines were provided by this legislation. These drugs are designated as "Controlled Drugs" and Schedule "G" of the Food and Drugs Act was created. The administration and enforcement of the Regulations made under this Act have been assigned to the Division of Narcotic Control.

VOLUNTARY HEALTH AGENCIES

ACCIDENTS

Canadian Highway Safety Council, 30 Driveway, Ottawa 4, Ontario; Tel. 235-5157
W. Arch Bryce, Exec. Dir.; Tel. 235-7866.
Industrial Accident Prevention Assoc. Inc., 90 Harbour St., Toronto 1, Ont.; Tel. 363-0051.

ARTHRITIS AND RHEUMATISM

Canadian Arthritis and Rheumatism Society, 45 Charles St. E., Toronto 5, Ont.; Tel. 924-0766.

BLINDNESS

Association Canadienne-Francaise des Aveugles, 900 Beaubien E., Montreal, P.Q.; Tel. 276-2588.
Canadian Council of the Blind, 96 Ridout St. S., London, Ont.
Canadian Federation of the Blind Inc., 1172 St. Mathew St., Montreal, P.Q.; Tel. 932-3439.
Canadian National Institute for the Blind, Bakerwood, 1929 Bayview Ave., Toronto 17, Ont.; Tel. 485-8644.

CANCER

Canadian Cancer Society, 790 Bay St., Toronto 2, Ont.; Tel. EM 4-7483.
National Cancer Institute of Canada, 790 Bay St., Toronto 2, Ont.; Exec. Dir., Dr. R. M. Taylor; Tel. EM 4-7483.

CRIPPLED CHILDREN (DISABLED)

Canadian Rehabilitation Council for the Disabled, 263 McCaul St., Toronto 2B, Ont.; Tel. 368-1817.

CYSTIC FIBROSIS

Canadian Cystic Fibrosis Fdn., 263 McCaul St., Toronto 2B, Ont.; Tel. 368-1817.

DEAFNESS

Canadian Assoc. of the Deaf Inc., 485 McDonnel St., Peterborough, Ont.; R. E. McBrien, Pres.
The Canadian Hearing Society, 60 Bedford Rd., Toronto 5, Ont.; Tel. 922-1118.
Canadian Federation for the Hard of Hearing, 5 Lawlor Ave., Toronto 13, Ont.; Mrs. H. F. Turner, Pres.

DIABETES

Canadian Diabetic Assoc., 1491 Yonge St., Toronto 7, Ont.; Tel. 927-5861.

DISASTER RELIEF

Disaster Services, Canadian Red Cross Society, 95 Wellesley St. E., Toronto 5, Ont.; Tel. 923-6692.

FIRST AID

St. John Ambulance Assoc., 321 Chapel St., Ottawa, Ont.; Tel. 232-2495.

FITNESS AND RECREATION

British Empire & Commonwealth Games Assoc., 3449 Vendome Ave., Montreal 28, P.Q.
Correspondence to be addressed to the President, Lt.-Col. John W. Davies at above address. Sec., N. J. Farrell.
Canadian Association for Health, Physical Education & Recreation, 703 Spadina Ave., Toronto 4, Ontario. Pres., Mr. Jack Passmore; Exec. Dir., C. R. Blacklock.
Canadian Olympic Assoc., Ste. 224, 12 Richmond St. E., Toronto 1, Ont.; Pres., J. Worrall, Tel. EM 3-0177; Sec. Treas.; E. Howard Radford, 67 Melborne Ave., Montreal 16, P.Q.; Exec. Dir., H. W. Hoppner, 3562 Northcliffe Ave., Montreal 28, P.Q.
Canadian Amateur Sports Fed., 1833 Riverside Drive, Ottawa, Ont.; Sec., Mrs. D. Forsythe.

HAEMOPHILIA

Canadian Hemophilia Soc., 263 McCaul St., Toronto 2B, Ont.

HEALTH (GENERAL)

Canadian Assoc. for Health, Physical Education and Recreation, 703 Spadina Ave., Toronto 4, Ont.; Pres., Jack Passmore; Exec. Dir., C. R. Blacklock.
Canadian Public Health Assoc., 1255 Yonge St., Toronto 7, Ont.; Tel. 925-2271.
Health League of Canada, 111 Avenue Rd., Toronto, Ont.; Tel. WA 3-8405.

HEART

Canadian Heart Fdn., 1130 Bay St., Toronto 5, Ont.; Dr. John B. Armstrong, Exec. Dir.; Tel. 924-1411.

HOSPITALS

Canadian Hospital Assoc., 25 Imperial St., Toronto 7, Ont.; Tel. HU 1-2244.
Catholic Hospital Assoc. of Canada, 312 Daly St., Ottawa, Ont.; Tel. 233-6836.
National Sanitarium Assoc., 223 College St., Toronto 2B, Ont.; Tel. 924-2191.
Canadian Council on Hosp. Accreditation, 150 St. George St., Toronto, Ont.; Tel. WA 3-1261.

MEDICAL

Association des Medicins de Langue Francaise, 5064 Ave. du Parc, Montreal 8, P.Q.; Tel. 273-2321.
Canadian Medical Assoc., 150 St. George St., Toronto 5, Ont.; Tel. 924-0751.
Federation of Medical Women of Canada, 727 South Dr., Winnipeg, Man., or C.M.A. House, 150 St. George St., Toronto 5, Ont.
The Medical Council of Canada, 77 Metcalfe St., Ottawa, Ont.; Tel. 235-0948.
Royal College of Physicians and Surgeons of Canada, 74 Stanley St., Ottawa, Ont.; The Registrar, Tel. 746-8177.

MEDICAL IDENTIFICATION (Re: Ident discs for diabetics, allergies, epileptics, etc.)

Canadian Medic-Alert Fdn., 176 St. George St., Toronto 5, Ont.; Mr. F. E. Finkle, Pres.; Tel. 923-5393.

VOLUNTARY HEALTH AGENCIES (*cont'd.*)

MENTAL

Canadian Assoc. for Retarded Children, 87 Bedford Rd., Toronto 5, Ont.; Tel. 923-3104.
Canadian Mental Health Assoc., 52 St. Clair Ave. E., Toronto 7, Ont.; Tel. 925-4264.

MOTHERCRAFT

Canadian Mothercraft Society, 217 Poplar Plains Rd., Toronto 7, Ont.; Tel. 923-9872.

MULTIPLE SCLEROSIS

The Multiple Sclerosis Society of Canada, 1505 Decelles Street, Montreal, P.Q.; Tel. 747-9956.

MUSCULAR DYSTROPHY

The Muscular Dystrophy Assoc. of Canada, Rm. 307, 160 Bay St., Toronto 1, Ont.; Tel. EM 6-7618.

NURSES

Victorian Order of Nurses for Canada, 5 Blackburn Ave., Ottawa, Ont.; Tel. 233-5694.

PARAPLEGIC

Canadian Paraplegic Assoc., 153 Lyndhurst Ave., Toronto 4, Ont.; Tel. WA 3-2954.

POLIOMYELITIS (See Disabled)

RED CROSS

Canadian Red Cross Society, 95 Wellesley St. E., Toronto 5, Ont.; Tel. 923-6692.
Canadian Junior Red Cross Society, 95 Wellesley St. E., Toronto 5, Ont.; Tel. 923-6692.
Traffic Injury Research Fdn. of Canada, 74 Stanley Ave., Ottawa 2, Ont.; Tel. 746-8177.

TRAFFIC

Traffic Injury Research Fdn. of Canada, 74 Stanley Ave., Ottawa 2, Ont.; Tel. 746-8177.

TUBERCULOSIS

Canadian Tuberculosis Assoc., 343 O'Connor St., Ottawa, Ont.; Dr. C. W. L. Jeanes, Exec. Sec.; Tel. 237-1208.

WAR AMPUTATIONS

War Amputations of Canada, 140 Merton St., Toronto 7, Ont.; Tel. HU 8-7957.

THE CANADIAN HEART FOUNDATIONS

RESEARCH AWARDS

The Canadian Heart Foundations give notice of the following types of Research Award, normally tenable in Canada.

A. FELLOWSHIP PROGRAMME

Awards for the support of persons engaged in cardiovascular research may be in the form of:

Senior Research Fellowships — $7,000.00-13,000.00
Research Fellowships — $3,000.00 - 8,000.00

Each applicant must arrange for his admission to a recognized Institution, and submit a statement of acceptance from the Departmental or other Head. An application for the Award of Research Associate must made by the Institution on behalf of a person.

B. GRANTS IN AID OF RESEARCH

Awards for the support of projects of an experimental nature in cardiovascular research will be on an annual basis.

The Fellowship Programme will be the responsibility, in the main, of the Canadian Heart Foundation. The Grants In Aid will be the responsibility of the Provincial Heart Foundations. These terms will not be mutually exclusive but all applications are to be forwarded to the Provincial Heart Foundation, by October of any year, to become tenable, usually, on July 1st of the year following.

The addresses of the Provincial Heart Foundations are:

The Alberta Heart Foundation,
Room 2, 108A-8th Avenue S.W.,
Calgary, Alberta.

British Columbia Heart Foundation,
1956 West Broadway,
Vancouver 9, B.C.

Manitoba Heart Foundation,
642 Somerset Building,
Winnipeg, Manitoba.

Ontario Heart Foundation,
247 Davenport Rd.,
Toronto 5, Ontario.

Quebec Heart Foundation,
Room 432, 1500 Stanley St.,
Montreal, Quebec.

Saskatchewan Heart Foundation,
511 Canada Building,
Saskatoon, Saskatchewan.

The following divisions in the Atlantic Provinces: New Brunswick Division, Canadian Heart Foundation, 2 Germaine Street, Saint John, New Brunswick. Newfoundland Division, Canadian Heart Foundation, Room 16, Board of Trade Building, Water Street, St. John's, Newfoundland. Nova Scotia Division, Canadian Heart Foundation, 406 Roy Building, Halifax, Nova Scotia.

Application Forms and Regulations may be obtained from any of the above Provincial Heart Foundations or from the Canadian Heart Foundation, 1130 Bay St., Toronto 5, Ontario.

MEDICAL CARE PLANS

Alberta Blue Cross Plan — 10025-108 St., Edmonton, Alta.; Mr. J. A. Monaghan, Ex. Dir.; Tel 424-0871.

Associated Medical Services Inc. — 615 Yonge St., Toronto 5, Ont.; Mr. K. W. Atcheson, Sec.-Treas.; Tel. 921-4193.

British Columbia Govt. Employees Medical Services Assoc. — Parliament Bldgs., Victoria, B.C.; Mr. G. A. Stewart, Sec.-Treas.; Tel. EV 2-6111, Loc. 3215.

British Columbia Medical Services Inc. — 2045 W. Broadway, Vancouver 9, B.C.; Mr. J. N. Gibson, Asst. Ex. Dir.; Tel. 736-9811.

Canadian Council of Blue Cross Plans — 10025-108 St., Edmonton, Alta.; Mr. J. A. Monaghan, Sec.; Tel. 424-0871.

Canadian Health Ins. Assoc. — 1303 Yonge St., Toronto 7, Ont.; Mr. R. R. Rowlands, Ex. Asst.; Tel. 924-1467.

Capital Co-operative Ltd. — Box 145, Fredericton, N.B.; Mr. W. S. McKay, Asst. Mgr.; Tel. 472-4456.

Christian Reformed Church Co-operative Med. & Hosp. Soc. — Box 473, Hamilton, Ont.; Mr. John VanderVliet, Sec.; Tel. 383-7044.

Co-operative Farm Services Ltd. — Box 872, Moncton, N.B.; Mr. D. F. MacDonald, Gen. Mgr.; Tel. EV 4-9657.

Co-operative Medical Services Federation of Ontario — 35 Oak St., Weston, Ont.; Mr. E. Schofield, Prov. Sec.; Tel. 247-9121.

Brant Medical Co-operative — 1 King St. West, Burford, Ont.; Mrs. E. M. Weir, Sec.-Mgr.

Bruce Co-operative Medical Services — Paisley, Ont.; Mr. Lorne B. Evans, Mgr. and Sec.-Treas.

Carleton Co-operative Medical Services — 1266 Stanton Rd., Ottawa 5, Ont.; Mrs. Margaret A. Collier, Sec.-Treas.; Tel. 828-5531.

Dufferin Co-operative Medical Services — P.O. Box 94, Shelburne, Ont.; Mr. W. McCarthy, Sec.; Tel. 925-2044.

Durham County Co-operative Medical Services — Orono, Ont.; Mr. R. G. Moffat, Sec.

Elgin Medical Co-operative — 44 Elgin St., St. Thomas, Ont.; Mr. L. R. Hoag, Sec.-Mgr.

Essex County Medical Co-operative — Woodslee, Ont.; Mr. Norman Knight, Pres.

Grey Co-operative Medical Services — R.R. #1, Meaford, Ont.; Mr. R. Boyes, Sec.-Treas.

Haldimand Co-operative Medical Services — R.R. #3, Caledonia, Ont.; Mrs. G. Ridley, Sec.-Treas.

Halton Co-operative Medical Services — P.O. Box 474, Milton, Ont.; Mrs. R. Coulter, Sec.-Treas.

Huron Co-operative Medical Services — P.O. Box 256, Clinton, Ont.; Miss C. E. Plumtree, Asst. Mgr.; Tel. 482-9751.

Kawartha Co-operative Medical Services — 326 Water St., Peterborough, Ont.; Miss Olive Bell, Sec.-Treas.; Tel. 745-5184.

Kent Co-operative Medical Services — 27½ Market Square East, Chatham, Ont.; Mr. W. G. McCoig, Sec.-Mgr.; Tel. EL 4-1320.

Lambton Co-operative Medical Services — Corunna, Ont.; Mr. W. A. Bradshaw, Sec.-Mgr.; Tel. TO 2-1125.

Lanark Co-operative Medical Services — R.R. #4, Almonte, Ont.; Mrs. J. V. Kellough, Sec.-Mgr.

Leeds Co-operative Medical Services — P.O. Box 307, Brockville, Ont.; Mr. Connor Pyke, Mgr.; Tel. 342-6003.

Lincoln Co-operative Medical Services — R.R. #1, Smithville, Ont.; Mrs. G. H. Railton, Mgr.; Tel. 957-3948.

Middlesex Co-operative Medical Services — 505 Talbot St., London, Ont.; Mr. E. W. Howlett, Sec.-Mgr.; Tel. 433-0031.

Norfolk Co-operative Medical Services — 60 Main St. North, Waterford. Ont.; Mrs. D. Murton, Sec.-Treas.

Ontario (County) Co-operative Medical Services — R.R. #1, Locust Hill, Ont.; Mrs. I. L. McLean, Sec.-Treas.; Tel. Ajax 942-3787.

Peel Co-operative Medical Services — Caledon, Ont.; Mr. Charles Barrett, Sec.-Mgr.; Tel. 927-5058.

Perth Co-operative Medical Services — Poole, Ont.; Mrs. J. E. Chalmers, Sec.-Treas.

Quinte Co-operative Medical Services — 247 Coleman St., Belleville, Ont.; Mr. Clare B. Horton, Sec.-Treas.; Tel. WO 8-7188.

Renfrew Co-operative Medical Services — Adamston, Ont.; Mr. J. D. Campbell, Mgr.; Tel. HE 2-3926.

Simcoe Co-operative Medical Services — 259 Innisfil St., Barrie, Ont.; Mrs. L. B. Parr, Sec.-Treas.

Stor-Dun-Glen Co-operative Medical Services — 36 Lefebvre Ave., Cornwall, Ont.; Mr. Wm. Legault, Sec.-Mgr.; Tel. WE 2-6921.

Waterloo Co-operative Medical Services — 347 Lancaster St. West, Kitchener, Ont.; Mr. R. R. Mills, Sec.-Mgr.; Tel. SH 5-7709.

Welland (County) Co-op Medical Services — 479 Portage Rd., Niagara Falls, Ont.; Mr. C. W. Hyde, Treas.-Mgr.

Wellington Co-operative Medical Services — Drayton, Ont.; Mrs. T. E. McClanaghan, Sec.-Mgr.; Tel. 20W.

Wentworth Co-operative Medical Services — 915 Barton St. E., Hamilton, Ont.; Mr. C. H. Magee, Mgr.; Tel. LI 5-4134.

York Co-operative Medical Services — 31 Yonge St. N., Richmond Hill, Ont.; Mr. A. Wadsworth, Mgr.

MEDICAL CARE PLANS (*Cont'd*)

Creston Valley Sick Benefit Assoc. — P.O. Box 1171, Creston, B.C.; Mr. A. R. Speers, Sec.; Tel. EL 6-2140.

C.U. & C. Health Services Society — Room 21, 96 E. Broadway, Vancouver 10, B.C.; Mr. C. G. Dean, Controller.

Cumba Co-operative Health Services — 32 Front St. West, Toronto 1, Ont.; Mr. T. R. Rowe, Off. Mgr.; Tel. 362-1623.

Cunningham-Western Drug Sick Benefit Assoc. — 2780 E. Broadway, Vancouver 12, B.C.; Miss M. Stonely, Dir.; Tel. AL 5-1166.

Fraser Valley Med. Services Soc. — 604 Blackford St., New Westminster, B.C.; Mr. D. F. Fairweather, Public Relations Officer; Tel. LA 2-0626.

Group Medical Services — 1942 Hamilton St., Regina, Sask.; Mr. R. V. Johnston, Sec.-Mgr.; Tel. 523-7638.

Hants County Co-operative Health Association — Newport, Hants Co., Brooklyn, N.S.; Mr. D. Fillmore, Sec.-Treas.

Health Insurers Association — Derrick Bldg., 2431-11th Ave., Regina, Sask.; Mr. R. D. Sprague, Mgr.; Tel. 523-8512.

Les Services de Santé du Québec — C.P. 3339, Québec 2, P.Q.; M. Jacques de la Chevrotiere, Dir. Gen.; Tel. 529-3701.

Manitoba Medical Service — 599 Empress St., Winnipeg 10, Man.; J. C. McMaster, M.B., Exec. Dir.; Tel. SP 5-8371.

Maritime Hospital Service Assoc. — P.O. Drawer 220, Moncton, N.B.; Mr. T. L. Doyle, Exec. Dir.; Tel. 389-9621.

Maritime Medical Care Inc. — P.O. Box 428, Halifax, N.S.; Mr. D. H. Waller, Office Mgr.; Tel. 422-7461.

Medical Services (Alberta) Inc. — 10169 - 104 St., Edmonton, Alta.; Dr. S. M. Schmaltz, Ex. Dir.; Tel. 429-1731.

Medical Services Assoc. — 2025 W. Broadway, Vancouver 9, B.C.; Mr. H. W. Jones, Ex. Dir.; Tel. 733-8141.

Medical Services Inc. —516-2nd Ave. N., Saskatoon, Sask.; Mr. M. J. Cooney, Accountant.

Ontario Co-operative Medical Services Federation (See Co-operative above)

Ontario Hospital Association — 24 Ferrand Drive, Don Mills, Ont.; Mr. W. E. Cannon, Dir.; Tel. 421-0660.

Oxford Co-operative Medical Services — 527 Dundas St., Woodstock, Ont.; Miss A. L. Austin, Sec.; Tel. 537-2931.

Physicians' Services Inc. — 2221 Yonge St., Toronto 7, Ont.; Mr. W. S. Major, Gen. Mgr.; Tel. HU 7-3311.

Pontiac County Co-operative Med. Services — Box 479, Shawville, Que.; Mrs. Gladys D. Ely, Sec. Mgr.; Tel. 647-2568.

Prescription Services Inc. — 541 University Ave. W., Windsor, Ont.; Mr. W. A. Wilkinson, Pres.; Tel. CL 6-9662.

Provincial Teachers' Medical Services — 1815 W. 7th Ave., Vancouver 9, B.C.; Mr. W. E. Whatmough, Sec.-Treas.; Tel. RE 1-8121.

Quebec Hospital Services Assoc. — 550 Sherbrooke St. W., Montreal 2, P.Q.; Mr. H. W. Brown, Vice-Pres.; Tel. 844-3781.

Rossland-Trail Sick Benefit Assoc. — 1410 Bay Ave., Trail, B.C.; Mr. L. A. Read, Sec.-Treas.; Tel. 368-3633.

Sault-Ste-Marie & Dist. Group Health Assoc. — 240 McNabb St., Sault-Ste-Marie, Ont.; Mr. F. H. Griffith, Admin.; Tel. 254-6421.

Scotsburn Co-operative Services Ltd. — Scotsburn, N.S.; Mr. T. C. MacDonnell, Mgr.

Telephone Employees' Med. Services Assoc. of B.C. — 768 Seymour St., Vancouver 2, B.C.; Miss Mary Grantham, Sec.; Tel. 662-8191.

Trans Canada Medical Plans — 150 St. George St., Toronto 5, Ont.; Mr. C. Howard Shillington, Ex. Dir.; Tel. WA 2-0945.

United Health Insurance Corporation Ltd. — P.O. Box 1046, Winnipeg, Man.; J. C. MacMaster, M.B., Vice-Pres. and Gen. Mgr.; Tel. SP 5-8371.

Vancouver School Teachers' Med. Serv. Assoc. — 1815 W. 7th Ave., Vancouver 9, B.C.; Mr. N. L. Ornes, Sec.-Treas.; Tel. RE 1-8121.

Windsor Medical Services Inc. — 1427 Ouellette Ave., Windsor, Ont.; Mr. C. S. Day, Sec.; Tel. CL 6-7861.

MEDICAL JOURNALS

CANADIAN

ACADEMY OF MEDICINE (Toronto) BULLETIN OF—288 Bloor St. W., Toronto 5, Ont. (Off. Pub.); Dr. F. C. Hamilton, Editor; Monthly; $3.00 a yr.

ALBERTA MED. BULLETIN—Pub. by College of Physicians & Surgeons, 9901-108th St., Edmonton, Alta.; Dr. S. E. Greenhill, Editor; Quarterly (Members & Libraries only.)

APPLIED THERAPEUTICS—Seccombe House, 443 Mount Pleasant Rd., Toronto 7, Ont.; Terence W. Anderson, M.D., Editor; Monthly; (Controlled circ.); Canada: $12.00 1 yr.; $22.00 2 yrs.; $30.00 3 yrs.; U.S.A.: $15.00 1 yr.; $27.00 2 yrs.; $36.00 3 yrs.; Gt. Britain: $15.00 1 yr.; $27.00 2 yrs.; $36.00 3 yrs.

BULLETIN OF THE CANADIAN TUBERCULOSIS ASSOC. (Off. Pub.)—343 O'Connor St., Ottawa 4, Ont.; (Miss) Anne R. Grant, Editor; Quarterly; Included in Annual Membership Fee of $1.00.

BULLETIN OF THE CATHOLIC HOSPITAL ASSOC. OF CANADA—312 Daly Ave., Ottawa, Ont. (Off. Pub.); A. L. M. Danis, O.M.I., Editor; Monthly (Free to members).

BULLETIN OF THE CANADIAN ASSOC. OF MED. RECORD LIBRARIANS—(Off. Pub.); c/o Mrs. Janet Milner, R.R.L., 770 Glenforest Rd., Oshawa, Ont.; Pub. by Maracle Press Ltd., 1156 King St. E., Oshawa; Miss Joan Marshall, R.R.L., R.N., Editor; Quarterly; $5.00 a yr. non members.

CANADIAN ANAESTHETISTS' SOC. JOURNAL—178 St. George St., Toronto 5, Ont.; (Off. Pub.); Dr. R. A. Gordon, Editor; Bi-monthly; $10.00 a yr.

CANADIAN DOCTOR—Pub. by National Business Publications Ltd., Gardenvale, P.Q.; A. W. Dancey, Pub. Mgr., Ross Warren, Editor; Monthly; $5.00 a yr., free to registered practising physicians & surgeons in Canada.

CANADIAN HOSPITAL—Pub. by Can. Hosp. Assoc., 25 Imperial St., Toronto 7, Ont. (Off. Pub.); Dr. B. L. P. Brosseau, Editor; Published Monthly; $6.00 a yr. U.S. & Canada; Each additional Sub. if sent to same address $3.00 per issue; U.K. & Foreign $10.00 a yr.

CANADIAN HOSPITAL DIRECTORY—25 Imperial St., Toronto 7, Ont.; (Off. Pub., Can. Hosp. Assoc.); Mr. Peter Smith, Editor; Annual; $3.00 a yr.

CANADIAN JOURNAL OF MED. TECHNOLOGY—99 Wentworth St. S., Hamilton, Ont.; (Off. Pub., Can. Soc. of Lab. Technologists); Mr. L. D. Mellor, Editor; Bi-monthly; $5.00 a yr.

CANADIAN JOURNAL OF OCCUPATIONAL THERAPY—57 Bloor St. W., Toronto 5, Ont.; (Off. Pub., Cdn. Assoc. of Occ. Ther.); Miss Joan Crosby, O.T. Reg., Editor; Quarterly; $2.50 a yr.

CANADIAN JOURNAL OF PHARMACEUTICAL SCIENCES—175 College St., Toronto 2B, Ont.; M. J. Hunter, Scientific Editor & A. V. Raison, Managing Editor; Quarterly; $10.00 a yr.; $7.50 a yr. to members of Can. Pharm. Assoc. & Can. Pharmacy Students.

CANADIAN JOURNAL OF PODIATRIC MEDICINE—Secretary, A. M. Goldman, D.S.C., 151 Eglinton Ave. W., Toronto, Ont.; (Off. Pub. Can. Podiatric Assoc.); D. J. Clemow, D.S.C., Editor; Published quarterly; $3.00 a yr.

CANADIAN JOURNAL OF PSYCHOLOGY—225 Lisgar St., Ste. 210, Ottawa 4, Ont.; (Off. Pub. Can. Psych. Assoc.); Pub. by U. of Toronto Press; Dr. P. L. Newbigging, Editor; Bimonthly; $10.00 a yr.

CANADIAN JOURNAL OF PUBLIC HEALTH—1255 Yonge St., Toronto 7, Ont.; (Off. Pub. Can. Public Health Assoc.); W. G. Brown, M.D., Editor; Monthly; $10.00 a yr.

CANADIAN JOURNAL OF SURGERY—150 St. George St., Toronto 5, Ont.; (Off. Pub. C.M.A.); Dr. G. T. Dickinson, Editor; Quarterly; $10.00 a yr.

CANADIAN MED. ASSOC. JRL.—150 St. George St., Toronto 5, Ont.; (Off. Pub.); Dr. G. T. Dickinson, Editor; Weekly; $15.00 a yr.

CANADIAN PAEDIATRIC DIRECTORY—14 Green Ave., Montreal 23, P.Q.; (Off. Pub., Can. Paed. Soc.)—A membership directory only.

CANADIAN PHARMACEUTICAL JRL.—175 College St., Toronto 2B, Ont.; (Off. Pub., Can. Pharm. Assoc.); A. V. Raison, Editor; Monthly; $4.00 a yr.—Canada; $5.00 a yr.—U.S.A., British & Commonwealth $6.00 a yr.—Foreign.

CANADIAN PSYCHIATRIC ASSOC. JRL.—LA REVUE DE L'ASSOCIATION DES PSYCHIATRES DU CANADA—Ste. 103, 225 Lisgar St., Ottawa 4, Ont.; (Off. Pub., Can. Psy. Assoc.); Dr. F. C. R. Chalke, Editor; Bi-monthly; $10.00 a yr.

FEDERATION NEWS & PROCEED., CDN. FED. BIOL. SOC'S.—Dr. K. K. Carroll, Editor, U. of Western Ont., London, Ont.; Annually (Memb. only).

HEALTH MAGAZINE—Pub. by Health League of Canada, 111 Avenue Rd., Toronto, Ont. (Off. Pub.); Dr. Gordon Bates, Editor; 6 times yearly; Non-members $1.00 a yr.

JRL. OF THE CANADIAN ASSOC. OF RADIOLOGISTS—1555 Summerhill Ave., Ste. 511, Montreal, P.Q.; (Off. Pub.); Dr. J. Scott Dunbar, Editor; Quarterly; $5.00 a yr.

JRL. OF THE CANADIAN DIETETIC ASSOC.—1393 Yonge St., Toronto 7, Ont.; (Off. Pub.); Mrs. Helen J. Morningstar, Editor; Published Intermittently.

JRL. OF THE CANADIAN PHYSIOTHERAPY ASSOC.—c/o Mrs. C. Millar, 64 Avenue Rd., Toronto 5, Ont. (Off. Pub.); Mrs. Joan Mergler, Editor; Quarterly; $2.50 a yr.

JRL. OF THE COLLEGE OF GEN. PRACTICE OF CANADA—Printed by Harpell's Press Cooperative, Gardenvale, P.Q. (Off. Pub. College of Gen. Practice of Canada—1260 Bay St., Toronto 5, Ont.); Monthly; (Controlled circ.)

LAVAL MEDICAL—BULL., DE LA SOC. MEDICALE DES HOPS. UNIVERSITAIRES LAVAL—Pub. by Fac. of Med., Laval U., Quebec, P.Q. (In French); Dr. George A. Bergeron, Editor; Monthly, except July & Aug.; $10.00 a yr.

L'UNION MEDICALE DU CANADA—Pub. by Therien Freres, 8125 St. Lawrence St., Montreal 11, P.Q.; (Off. Pub. Assoc. des Medicines de Langue Francais du Canada); Dr. Roma Amyot, Editor; Monthly; $15.00 a yr.

MANITOBA MEDICAL REVIEW—Pub. by Manitoba Med. Assoc., 201 Kennedy St., Winnipeg 1, Man.; (Off. Pub.); Dr. P. Warner, Editor; Monthly (except June-July-and-Aug.-Sept., which are combined); $10.00 a yr.

MD OF CANADA—Pub. by MD Publications (Canada) Ltd.; Editor-in-Chief, Felix Mari-Ibanez, M.D., 1310 Greene Ave., Westmount 6, P.Q.; Monthly; Controlled Circ.—free to all physicians & surgeons; $7.50 a yr. to those in allied professions; $10.00 a yr. to all others.

MEDECINE MODERNE DU CANADA—Seccombe House, 443 Mount Pleasant Rd., Toronto 7, Ont.; John W. Digby, M.D., Editor; Monthly (controlled circ.); pub. in French; Medical Students and R.N.'s in Canada may subscribe at $4.00 per annum. To others: Canada, British Isles & U.S.A., $5.00 a yr.; Foreign, $6.00 a yr.

PROFESSIONAL JOURNALS (*cont'd.*)

MED. SERVICES JRL., CANADA—Pub. by the Queen's Printer, Ottawa, Canada; (Off. Pub., Med. Jrl. of the Gov't. of Canada); J. B. Bundock, OBE, MD, FRSH; B. R. Brown, CD, BSc, MD, MIH, FACPM, & Colonel R. C. Elliott, CD, Associate Editors; Monthly; $5.00 a yr.—Canada, U.S. & Mexico; $6.00 a yr. others.
MENTAL RETARDATION—(Off. Pub., Can. Assoc. for Retarded Children); Secretary, 87 Bedford Rd., Toronto 5, Ont.; Quarterly; $1.00 a yr.
MODERN MEDICINE OF CANADA—Seccombe House, 443 Mount Pleasant Rd., Toronto 7, Ont.; John W. Digby, M.D., Editor; Monthly (controlled circ.); Medical Students and R.N.'s in Canada may subscribe at $4.00 per annum. To others: Canada, British Isles & U.S.A. $5.00 a yr. Foreign $6.00 a yr.
MONTREAL MEDICAL—Pub. by students of Med., U. of Montreal; Cdn. Agent—Seg. Publications Services Ltd., 3305 Masson St., Montreal 36, P.Q. (Off. Pub.); Andre Bellavance, Editor; Monthly during Academic Yr.; $5.00 a yr.
MUSCULAR DYSTROPHY REPORTER—160 Bay St., Toronto 1, Ont.; (Off. Pub.); Mrs. D. W. Mundell, Editor; Quarterly; Circ. members.
NEWS LETTER OF CDN. ASSOC. OF PATHOL.—(Off. Pub.); Dr. D. W. Penner, Editor; Dept. of Path., Winnipeg Gen. Hosp., Winnipeg, Man.; Monthly; Free to Members.
NOVA SCOTIA MED. BULLETIN—Pub. by Med. Soc. of Nova Scotia—c/o Dalhousie Public Health Clinic, University Ave., Halifax, N.S.; Ian Purkis, M.B., Editor; Monthly; $6.00 a yr.
ONTARIO MED. REVIEW—Pub. by Ontario Med. Assoc. (Div. of C.M.A.), 244 St. George St., Toronto 5, Ont.; Dr. G. Sawyer, Editor; Mr. R. E. Brownridge, Assoc. Editor; Mr. R. Gary Cooper, Advertising Manager; Monthly; $5.00 a yr.
PROCEEDINGS OF THE CANADIAN FED. OF BIOL. SOC. (CDN. FED. NEWS)—Dr. K. K. Carroll, Editor, U. of Western Ont., London, Ont.; Annually; (members only).
THE BULLETIN OF CATHOLIC NURSES' ASSOC. OF CANADA—312 Daly, Ottawa, Ont. (Off. Pub. Assoc. of Catholic Nurses of Canada). Quarterly; $1.00 a yr.
THE CDN. PSYCHOLOGIST—225 Lisgar St., Ste. 210, Ottawa 4, Ont.; Editor, Dr. W. H. Coons; (Off. Pub., Cdn. Psychol. Assoc.); Quarterly; $7.00 a yr.
UNIVERSITY OF TORONTO MED. JRL.—Pub. by Med. Soc. of the U. of Toronto, 109 Med. Bldg., Toronto 5, Ont.; S. MacLeod & K Pritzker, Co-editors; Monthly (Nov.-Apr.) $4.50 a yr.
UNIVERSITY OF WESTERN ONT. MED. JRL.—Pub. by Undergraduates of the U. of Western Ont., Health Sciences Center, London, Ont.; Harold Watts, Editor; Quarterly; $5.00 a yr.

GENERAL

AMERICAN MEDICAL DIRECTORY (24th Ed. 1967)—Pub. by American Med. Assoc., 535 N. Dearborn St., Chicago, Ill. 60610, U.S.A.; (Off. Pub.); U.S. Poss., Canada & Mexico $60.00; All other countries $65.00 (Complete set consists of 3 parts—2 hard bound and 1 paper bound book).
AMA NEWS—Pub. by American Med. Assoc., 535 N. Dearborn St., Chicago, Ill. 60610, U.S.A.; (Off. Pub.); Marvin L. Rowlands, Jr., Editor; Weekly; $5.00 a yr.; $7.50 2 years. (U.S. Poss., Canada & Mexico).
MODERN MEDICINE—Pub. by Modern Medicine Publications Ltd., 65th at Valley View Rd., Southdale Park, Minneapolis, Minn. 55435, U.S.A.; Irvine H. Page, M.D., Editor; Alternate Mondays; $10.00 a yr. U.S. and Canada.
JOURNAL OF THE AMERICAN MEDICAL ASSOC. (JAMA)—Pub. by American Med. Assoc., 535 N. Dearborn St., Chicago, Ill. 60610, U.S.A.; (Off. Pub.); John H. Talbott, M.D., Editor; Weekly; $18.00 a yr.; $27.00 2 yrs. (U.S. Poss., Canada & Mexico).
JOURNAL OF THE ROYAL COLLEGE OF PHYSICIANS OF LONDON; Pub. by Pitman Medical Publishing Co. Ltd., 46 Charlotte St., London W.1., England. Quarterly; $12.00 a yr. (In Canada: J. B. Lippincott Company of Canada Ltd., 60 Front St. W., Toronto 1, Ont.). A. Stuart Mason, M.D., FRCP, Editor.
POSTGRADUATE MEDICINE—Pub. by IPMA Pub. Co., 4015 W. 65th St., Minneapolis 35, Minn., U.S.A.; Dr. C. W. Mayo, Editor-in-Chief; Sylvia Covet, Exec. Editor; Monthly; $10.00 a yr.—Interns & Residents $5.00 a yr.
THE NEW ENGLAND JOURNAL OF MED.—(Can. Agents)—McAinsh & Co., 1835 Yonge St., Toronto 7, Ont. & 730 W. Broadway, Vancouver 9, B.C.; Joseph Garland, M.D., Editor; Weekly; $9.90 a yr.; Internes $6.60 a yr.
TODAY'S HEALTH—Pub. by American Med. Assoc., 535 N. Dearborn St., Chicago, Ill. 60610, U.S.A.; (Off. Pub.); Elliott H. McCleary, Editor; Monthly; $4.00 a yr.; $6.00 2 yrs. (U.S. Poss., Canada & Mexico).
WORLD MED. JRL.—Pub. by WMA, Inc., 10 Columbus Circle, New York, N.Y. 10019; (Off. Pub.); (Can. Agents) C.M.A., 150 St. George St., Toronto 5, Ont.; Dr. S. S. B. Gilder, Editor; Bi-monthly; $3.00 a yr.

ALLER. — **THE JRL. OF ALLERGY**—Pub. by C. V. Mosby Co., 3207 Washington Blvd., St. Louis 3, Mo., U.S.A.; (Off. Pub. Am. Acad. of Allergy); Dr. David W. Talmage, Editor; Monthly; $16.00 a yr.

ANAES. — **ANESTHESIOLOGY**—The Jrl. of the American Soc. of Anes., Inc.—Pub. by J. B. Lippincott, Co., E. Washington Sq., Philadelphia 2, Pa., U.S.A.; (Off. Pub.); (J. B. Lippincott Company of Canada Ltd., 60 Front St. W., Toronto 1, Ont.; Canadian Agents); Leroy D. Vandam, M.D., Editor; Bi-monthly; $12.00 a yr.
ANESTHESIA & ANALGESIA—Current Researches—(Off. Pub. of International Anesthesia Research Soc.); Secretary, 3645 Warrensville Center Rd., Cleveland, Ohio 44122, U.S.A.; Editor, T. H. Seldon, M.D.; Bi-monthly; $15.00 a yr.
CANADIAN ANAESTHETISTS' SOC. JOURNAL—178 St. George St., Toronto 5, Ont.; (Off. Pub.); Dr. R. A. Gordon, Editor; Bi-monthly; $10.00 a yr.

BIOL. — **PROCEEDINGS OF THE CANADIAN FED. OF BIOL. SOC. (CDN. FED NEWS)**—Dr. K. K. Carroll, Editor, U. of Western Ont., London, Ont.; Annually; (members only).

PROFESSIONAL JOURNALS (*cont'd.*)

CANCER	**CANCER**—Pub. by J. B. Lippincott Company of Canada Ltd., 60 Front St. W., Toronto 1, Ont.; (Off. Pub. American Cancer Soc.); Wendell G. Scott, M.D., Editor; Monthly; $21.50 a yr.
CARD.	**AMERICAN HEART JRL.**—Pub. by C. V. Mosby Co., 3207 Washington Blvd., St. Louis 3, Mo., U.S.A.; Dr. George E. Burch, Editor; Monthly; $15.00 a yr.
	CIRCULATION—Pub. by American Heart Assoc. Inc., 44 East 23rd St., New York, N.Y. 10010, U.S.A.; Howard B. Burchell, M.D., Editor, 200 First St. S.W., Rochester, Minn. 55902; (Off. Pub.); Monthly; $16.00 a yr.
	CIRCULATION RESEARCH—Pub. by Amer. Heart Assoc. Inc., 44 East 23rd St., New York, N.Y. 10010, U.S.A.; Julius H. Comroe, Jr., M.D., Editor, Cardiovasc. Research Inst., U. of California Med. Center, San Francisco, Calif. 94122; (Off. Pub.); Monthly; $16.00 per yr.
	CARDIOVASCULAR NURSING—Pub. by American Heart Assoc. Inc., 44 E. 23rd St., New York, N.Y. 10010, U.S.A.; (Off. Pub.); Maurice R. Chassin, M.D., Editor & Marie S. Andrews, R.N.; Published Bi-monthly; Available by application to Canadian Heart Assoc.
	MODERN CONCEPTS OF CARDIOVASCULAR DISEASE—Pub. by American Assoc. Inc., 44 E. 23rd St., New York, N.Y. 10010, U.S.A.; (Off. Pub.); Dr. Edward S. Orgain, Duke University Med. Centre, Durham, North Carolina 27706, Editor; Monthly; (available by application to Can. Heart Assoc.).
	THE AMERICAN JOURNAL OF CARDIOLOGY—Pub. by The Reuben H. Donnelley Corp., 466 Lexington Ave., New York, N.Y. 10017, U.S.A.; (Off. Pub. Amer. Coll. of Card.); Simon Dack, M.D., F.A.C.C., Editor; Monthly; $15.00 a yr.
CHEST	**DISEASES OF THE CHEST**—Pub. by the American College of Chest Physicians, 112 E. Chestnut St., Chicago, Ill. 60611, U.S.A.; (Off. Pub.); Dr. J. Arthur Myers, Editor; Monthly; $18.00 a yr.
DERM.	**ARCHIVES OF DERMATOLOGY**—Pub. by American Med. Assoc., 535 N. Dearborn St., Chicago, Ill. 60610, U.S.A.; (Off. Pub.); Walter C. Lobitz, Jr., M.D., Chief Editor; Monthly; $12.00 a yr.; $18.00 2 yrs.; (U.S. Poss., Canada & Mexico).
	DERMATOLOGICA TROPICA—Pub. by J. B. Lippincott Company of Canada Ltd., 60 Front St. W., Toronto 1, Ont.; (Off. Pub. Int'l. Soc. of Trop. Derm.), 19 E. 80th St., New York, N.Y. 10021, U.S.A.; Quarterly; $9.00 a yr.; Single Copies—$2.50 each.
DIAB.	**DIABETES—THE JRL. OF THE AMERICAN DIABETES ASSOC.**, 18 East 48th St., New York, N.Y. 10017, U.S.A.; (Off. Pub.); Harvey C. Knowles, Jr., M.D., Editor; Monthly; $14.00 a yr.
E.E.N.T.	**ARCHIVES OF OPHTHAMOLOGY**—Pub. by American Med. Assoc., 535 N. Dearborn St., Chicago, Ill. 60610, U.S.A.; (Off. Pub.); David G. Cogan, M.D., Chief Editor; Monthly; $12.00 1 yr.; $18.00 2 yrs. (U.S. Poss., Canada & Mexico).
	ARCHIVES OF OTOLARYNGOLOGY—Pub. by the American Med. Assoc., 535 N. Dearborn St., Chicago, Ill. 60610, U.S.A.; Geo. E. Shambaugh, Jr., M.D., Chief Editor; Monthly; $12.00 1 yr.; $18.00 2 yrs. (U.S. Poss., Canada & Mexico).
	INVESTIGATIVE OPHTHALMOLOGY—Pub. by C. V. Mosby Co., 3207 Washington Blvd., St. Louis 3, Mo., U.S.A. (Off. Pub., Assoc. for Research in Ophth.); Dr. B. Becker, Editor; Bi-monthly; $19.00 a yr.
	SIGHT-SAVING REVIEW— 16 E. 40th St., New York, N.Y. 10016, U.S.A. (Off. Pub., Nat. Soc. for the Prevent. of Blindness, Inc.); Dr. J. W. Ferree, Editor-in-Chief; Quarterly; $3.50 a yr.
	THE EYE, EAR, NOSE AND THROAT MONTHLY—Pub. by The Professional Press, Inc., 5 N. Wabash Ave., Chicago, Ill. 60602, U.S.A.; A. R. Hollender, M.D., Editor; Monthly; $3.00 a yr.
	THE LARYNGOSCOPE—Editorial Office, 517 South Euclid, St. Louis, Mo. 63110; (Off. Pub.); Business Office, 222 Pine Lake Rd., Collinsville, Ill. 62234, U.S.A.; Dr. T. E. Walsh, Editor; Monthly; $19.00 a yr.
ENDO.	**ENDOCRINOLOGY**—Pub. by J. B. Lippincott Company of Canada Ltd., 60 Front St. W., Toronto 1, Ont.; (Off. Pub., Endocrine Soc.); Frederick G. Hofmann, M.D., Editor; Monthly; $27.00 a yr.
	THE JRL. OF CLIN. ENDOCRINOLOGY & METABOLISM—Pub. by J. B. Lippincott Company of Canada. Ltd., 60 Front St. W., Toronto 1, Ont.; (Off. Pub., Endocrine Soc.); Nicholas P. Christy, M.D., Editor; Monthly; $27.00 a yr.
ENVIR. HEALTH	**ARCHIVES OF ENVIRONMENTAL HEALTH**—Pub. by Amer. Med. Assoc., 535 N. Dearborn St., Chicago, Ill. 60610, U.S.A.; (Off. Pub.); Katharine R. Boucot, M.D., Chief Editor; Monthly; $12.00 1 yr.; $18.00 2 yrs. (U.S. Poss., Canada & Mexico).
GER.	**GERIATRICS**—Pub. by Lancet Publications Ltd., 65th at Valley View Rd., Southdale Park, Minneapolis, Minn. 55435, U.S.A.; Walter C. Alvarez, M.D., Editor Emer.; John F. Briggs. M.D., Editor; Monthly; $6.00 a yr.
HAEM.	**TRANSFUSION**—Pub. by J. B. Lippincott Company of Canada Ltd., 60 Front St. W., Toronto 1, Ont.; (Off. Pub., Am. Assoc. of Blood Banks); Dr. Tibor J. Greenwalt, Editor; Bi-monthly; $11.00 a yr.
	VOX SANGUINIS—Pub. by S. Karger, Basel, Switzerland, (J. B. Lippincott Company of Canada Ltd., 60 Front St. W., Toronto 1, Ont., Can. Agents); Dr. J. J. Van Loghem, Jr., Amsterdam, Holland, Chairman; (Off. Pub., Int. Blood Transfusion Soc., Pub. in collab. with Int. Red Cross, Geneva, Switzerland); Monthly; $25.00 a yr.

PROFESSIONAL JOURNALS (*cont'd.*)

LAB. & CLIN. **THE JRL. OF LABORATORY & CLIN. MED.**—Pub. by C. V. Mosby Co., 3207 Washington Blvd., St. Louis 3, Mo., U.S.A.; (Off. Pub. for Central Soc. for Clinical Research); Dr. Wm. H. Daughaday, Editor; Monthly; $19.00 a yr.

MED. **ANNALS OF INTERNAL MED.**—Pub. by the American College of Physicians, 4200 Pine St., Philadelphia, Pa. 19104, U.S.A.; (Off. Pub.); J. Russell Elkinton, Editor; Monthly; $10.00 a yr.

ARCHIVES OF INTERNAL MEDICINE—Pub. by American Med. Assoc., 535 N. Dearborn St., Chicago, Ill. 60610, U.S.A.; (Off. Pub.); Wm. B. Bean, M.D., Chief Editor; Monthly; $12.00 a yr.; $18.00 2 yrs.; (U.S. Poss., Canada & Mexico).

DISEASES OF THE COLON & RECTUM—Pub. by J. B. Lippincott Company of Canada Ltd., 60 Front St. W., Toronto 1, Ont.; (Off. Pub. Amer. Proct. Soc.); Louis A. Buie, Sr., M.D., Editor-in-Chief; Bi-monthly; $13.50 a yr.

JOURNAL OF THE AMERICAN MEDICAL ASSOC. (JAMA)—Pub. by Amer. Med. Assoc., 535 N. Dearborn St., Chicago, Ill. 60610, U.S.A.; (Off. Pub.); John H. Talbott, M.D., Editor; Weekly; $18.00 a yr.; $27.00 2 yrs. (U.S. Poss., Canada & Mexico.)

JOURNAL OF THE ROYAL COLLEGE OF PHYSICIANS OF LONDON: Pub. by Pitman Medical Publishing Co. Ltd., 46 Charlotte St., London W. 1, England. Quarterly; $12.00 per yr.; (In Canada: J. B. Lippincott Company of Canada Ltd., 60 Front St. W., Toronto 1, Ont.); A. Stuart Mason, M.D., FRCP, Editor.

MEDICAL CARE—Pub. by Pitman Med. Pub. Co. Ltd.; (Cdn. Agents—J. B. Lippincott Company of Canada Ltd., 60 Front St. W., Toronto 1, Ont.); Editor, Dr. Abraham Marcus, 46 Charlotte St., London W. 1, Eng.; Quarterly; $10.00 per year.

MEDECINE MODERNE DU CANADA—Seccombe House, 443 Mount Pleasant Rd., Toronto 7, Ont.; John W. Digby, M.D., Editor; Monthly (controlled circ.); pub. in French; Medical Students and R.N.'s in Canada may subscribe at $4.00 per annum. To others: Canada, British Isles & U.S.A., $5.00 a yr.; Foreign $6.00 one yr.

MODERN MEDICINE—Pub. by Modern Medicine Publications Ltd., 65th at Valley View Rd., Southdale Park, Minneapolis, Minn. 55435, U.S.A.; Irvine H. Page, M.D., Editor; Alternate Mondays; $10.00 a yr., U.S. and Canada.

MODERN MEDICINE OF CANADA—Seccombe House, 443 Mount Pleasant Rd., Toronto 7, Ont.; John W. Digby, M.D., Editor; Monthly (Controlled Circ.); Medical Students and R.N.'s in Canada may subscribe at $4.00 per annum. To others: Canada. British Isles & U.S.A., $5.00 one yr.; Foreign $6.00 one yr.

MD OF CANADA—Pub. by MD Publications (Canada) Ltd.; Editor-in-Chief, Felix Mari-Ibanez, M.D., 1310 Greene Ave., Westmount 6, P.Q.; Monthly; Controlled Cir.—free to all physicians & surgeons; $7.50 a yr. to those in allied professions; $10.00 a yr. to all others.

POSTGRADUATE MEDICINE—Pub. by IPMA Pub. Co., 4015 W. 65th St., Minneapolis 35, Minn., U.S.A.; Dr. C. W. Mayo, Editor-in-Chief, Sylvia Covet, Exec. Editor; Monthly; $10.00 a yr.—Interns & Residents $5.00 a yr.

THE AMERICAN JOURNAL OF MEDICINE—Pub. by the Reuben H. Donnelly Corp., 466 Lexington Ave., New York, N.Y. 10017, U.S.A.; Alexander B. Gutman, M.D., Editor; Monthly; $17.00 a yr.

THE JOURNAL-LANCET—Pub. by Lancet Publications, Inc., 65th at Valley View Rd.. Southdale Park, Minneapolis, Minn. 55435, U.S.A.; (Off. Pub. North Dakota State Med. Assoc., Etc.); J. A. Myers, M.D., Editor; Monthly; $5.00 a yr.

THE NEW ENGLAND JOURNAL OF MED.—(Can. Agents)—McAinsh & Co., 1835 Yonge St., Toronto 7, Ont. & 730 W. Broadway, Vancouver 9, B.C.; Joseph Garland, M.D., Editor; Weekly; $9.90 a yr.; Internes $6.60 a yr.

MED. ED. **JRL. OF MED. EDUCATION**—Pub. by Assoc. of American Med. Colleges, 2530 Ridge Ave., Evanston, Ill.; (Off. Pub.); Dr. J. A. D. Cooper, Editor; Monthly; $15.00 a yr.

MED. ILL. **MEDICAL RADIOGRAPHY & PHOTOGRAPHY**—Pub. by Eastman Kodak Co., 343 State St., Rochester. N.Y. 14650, U.S.A.; (distributed in Can. by Can. Kodak Co., Ltd., Toronto 15); T. E. Callear, Editor; Quarterly; gratis.

MED. TERM. **CURRENT MED. TERMINOLOGY**—Pub. by Amer. Med. Assoc., 535 N. Dearborn St., Chicago, Ill. 60610, U.S.A.; (Off. Pub.); Burgess Gordon, M.D., Editor; $4.00 each, U.S. Poss., Canada & Mexico.

NEUR. **ARCHIVES OF NEUROLOGY**—Pub. by Amer. Med. Assoc., 535 N. Dearborn St., Chicago, Ill. 60610, U.S.A.; (Off. Pub.); H. Houston Merritt, M.D., Chief Editor; Monthly; $12.00 a yr.; $18.00 2 yrs. (U.S. Poss.. Canada & Mexico).

CONDITIONAL REFLEX—Pub. by J. B. Lippincott Company of Canada Ltd., 60 Front St. W., Toronto 1, Ont.; Editor, W. Horsley Gantt, M.D.; Quarterly; $11.00 a yr.

NEUROLOGY—Pub. by Lancet Publications Inc., 65th at Valley View Rd., Southdale Park, Minneapolis, Minn. 55435, U.S.A.; (Off. Pub. American Acad. of Neurol.); Russell N. DeJong, M.D., Editor; Monthly; $12.00 a yr.

NURS. HOMES **NURSING HOMES**—Pub. by Professional Publications Inc., 65th at Valley View Rd., Southdale Park, Minneapolis, Minn. 55435, U.S.A.; (Off. Pub. Amer. Nursing Home Assoc.); Wendell Weed, Editor; Monthly; $10.00 a yr.

PROFESSIONAL JOURNALS (*cont'd.*)

OBST. GYN.	**AMERICAN JRL. OF OBSTETRICS & GYNECOLOGY**—Pub. by C. V. Mosby Co., 3207 Washington Blvd., St. Louis 3, Mo., U.S.A. (Off. Pub. Am. Gyn. Soc,, Am. Assoc. of ObstGyn., Central Assoc. of ObstGyn., etc.); Howard C. Taylor, M.D., John I. Brewer, M.D., & Allan C. Barnes, M.D., Editors; Semi-Monthly; $20.50 a yr., Canada.
	SURGERY, GYNECOLOGY & OBSTETRICS—Pub. by the Franklin H. Martin Mem. Fdn., 55 E. Erie St., Chicago, Ill. 60611, U.S.A.; (Off. Pub., Amer. Coll Surg.); Loyal Davis, M.D., Editor; Monthly; $15.00 a yr.
PAED.	**AMERICAN JRL. OF DISEASES OF CHILDREN**—Pub. by Amer. Med. Assoc., 535 N. Dearborn St., Chicago, Ill. 60610, U.S.A.; (Off. Pub.); A. Ashley Weech, M.D., Chief Editor; Monthly; $12.00 a yr.; $18.00 2 yrs.; (U.S. Poss., Canada & Mexico).
	CANADIAN PAEDIATRIC DIRECTORY—14 Green Ave., Montreal 23, P.Q.; (Off. Pub., Can. Paed. Soc.)—A membership directory only.
	CLINICAL PAEDIATRICS—Pub. by J. B. Lippincott, Company of Canada Ltd., 60 Front St. W., Toronto 1, Ont.; Irving J. Wolman, M.D., Editor; Monthly; $11.00 a yr.
	PEDIATRICS—Pub. by American Acad. of Pediatrics Inc., P.O. Box 1034, Evanston, Ill. 60204, U.S.A.; (Off. Pub.); Dr. Clement A. Smith, Editor; Monthly; $12.00 a yr.
	THE JOURNAL OF PEDIATRICS—Pub. by C. V. Mosby Co., 3207 Washington Blvd., St. Louis 3, Mo., U.S.A.; Dr. Waldo E. Nelson, Editor; Monthly; $16.50 a yr.
PATH.	**ARCHIVES OF PATHOLOGY**—Pub. by American Med. Assoc., 535 N. Dearborn St., Chicago, Ill. 60610, U.S.A.; (Off. Pub.); D. Murray Angevin, M.D., Chief Editor; Monthly; $12.00 a yr.; $18.00 2 yrs.; (U.S. Poss., Canada & Mexico).
PHARM. THER.	**APPLIED THERAPEUTICS**—Seccombe House, 443 Mount Pleasant Rd., Toronto 7, Ont.; Terence W. Anderson, M.D., Editor; Monthly; (Controlled circ.); Canada $12.00 1 yr.; $22.00 2 yrs.; $30.00 3 yrs.; U.S.A. $15.00 1 yr.; $27.00 2 yrs.; $36.00 3 yrs.; Great Britain $15.00 1 yr.; $27.00 2 yrs.; $36.00 3 yrs.
	CANADIAN JOURNAL OF PHARMACEUTICAL SCIENCES—175 College St., Toronto 2B, Ont.; M. J. Hunter, Scientific Editor & A. V. Raison, Managing Editor; Quarterly; $10.00 a yr.; $7.50 a yr. to members of Can. Pharm. Assoc. & Can. Pharmacy Students.
	CANADIAN PHARMACEUTICAL JRL.—175 College St., Toronto 2B, Ont.; (Off. Pub. Can. Pharm. Assoc.); A. V. Raison, Editor; Monthly; $4.00 a yr.—Canada; $5.00 a yr.—U.S.A., British & Commonwealth $6.00 a yr.—Foreign.
	CLINICAL PHARMACOLOGY & THERAPEUTICS—Pub. by C. V. Mosby, 3207 Washington Blvd., St. Louis 3, Mo., U.S.A.; (Off. Pub. Am. Therapeutics Soc.); Dr. Walter Modell. Editor; Bi-monthly; $18.50 a yr.
	HOSPITAL PHARMACY—Pub. by J. B. Lippincott Company of Canada Ltd., 60 Front St. F., Toronto 1, Ont.; Editor, Sidney Kahn; Monthly; $11.00 a yr.
POD.	**CANADIAN JOURNAL OF PODIATRIC MEDICINE**—Secretary, A. M. Goldman, D.S.C., 151 Eglinton Ave. W., Toronto, Ont.; (Off. Pub., Can. Podiatric Assoc.); D. J. Clemow, D.S.C., Editor; Published Quarterly; $3.00 a yr.
PSY.	**AMERICAN JRL. OF ORTHOPSYCHIATRY**—Pub. by Amer. Orthopsy Assoc., 1790 Broadway, New York, N.Y. 10019, U.S.A.; (Off. Pub.); Dr. Leon Eisenberg, Editor; 5 issues; $12.50 a yr. (U.S. Funds).
	AMERICAN JOURNAL OF PSYCHIATRY—Pub. by American Psychiatric Assoc., 1700-18th St. N.W., Washington 9, D.C., U.S.A.; (Off. Pub., American Psych. Assoc.); Francis J. Braceland, M.D., Editor; Monthly; $12.00 a yr.
	ARCHIVES OF GENERAL PSYCHIATRY—Pub. by Amer. Med. Assoc., 535 N. Dearborn St., Chicago, Ill. 60610, U.S.A.; (Off. Pub.); Roy R. Grinker, Sr., M.D., Chief Editor; Monthly; $12.00 1 yr.; $18.00 2 yrs. (U.S. Poss., Canada & Mexico).
PSYCHIATRY	**JRL. FOR THE STUDY OF INTERPERSONAL PROCESSES**—Pub. by Wm. Alanson White, Psychiatric Fdn., Inc., 1610 New Hampshire Ave. N.W., Washington, D.C. 20009; (Off. Pub.); Dr. Donald L. Burnham, Editor; Quarterly; $10.80 a yr.
	PSYCHOSOMATICS—Pub. by Bruce Pub. Co., 2642 University Ave., St. Paul, Minn., U.S.A.; (Off. Pub. Acad. of Psychosom. Med.); Wilfred Dorfman, M.D., FACP, Editor; 1921 Newkirk Ave., Brooklyn 26, N.Y., U.S.A.; Bi-monthly; $10.00 a yr.
RAD.	**INVESTIGATIVE RADIOLOGY**—Pub. by J. B. Lippincott Company of Canada Ltd., 60 Front St. W., Toronto 1, Ont.; Bi-monthly; $15.75 a yr.
RHEUM.	**BULLETIN OF RHEUMATIC DISEASES**—Pub. by Arthritis Fdn., Jock Wyckert, M.D., Editor; Monthly (Sept.-May); free on request—The Canadian Arthritis & Rheumatism Soc., 45 Charles St. E., Toronto 5, Ont.
SCIENCE	**SCIENCE PROGRESS**: Pub. by Blackwell Scientific Publications Ltd., 5 Alfred St., Oxford, England. (Can. Agents—J. B. Lippincott Company of Canada Ltd., 60 Front St. W., Toronto 1, Ont.); Quarterly; $14.00 a yr.
SURG.	**AMERICAN SURGEON**—Pub. by J. B. Lippincott Company of Canada Ltd., 60 Front St. W., Toronto 1, Ont.; (Off. Pub. S. Eastern Surgical Congress); Dr. G. H. Yeager, Editor; Monthly; $15.50 a yr.
	ANNALS OF THE ROYAL COLLEGE OF SURGEONS OF ENGLAND—Pub. by the Royal College of Surgeons of England, Lincoln's Inn Fields, London, W.C. 2, Eng.; (Off. Pub.); Sir Cecil Wakeley, Bt., KBE, CB, LLD, FRCS, Editor; Monthly; $8.13 a yr.

PROFESSIONAL JOURNALS *(cont'd)*

ANNALS OF SURGERY—Pub. by J. B. Lippincott Company of Canada Ltd., 60 Front St. W., Toronto 1, Ont.; (Off. Pub. Am. Surg. Assoc., Philadelphia Acad. of Surg., Southern Assoc. & New York Surg. Soc.); John H. Mulholland, M.D., Chm. Edit. & Advisory Bd.; Monthly; $19.50 a yr.

ARCHIVES OF SURGERY—Pub. by Amer. Med. Assoc., 535 N. Dearborn St., Chicago, Ill. 60610, U.S.A.; (Off. Pub.); J. Garrott Allen, M.D., Chief Editor; Monthly; $12.00 1 yr.; $18.00 2 yrs. (U.S. Poss., Canada & Mexico).

BULLETIN OF THE AMERICAN COLLEGE OF SURGEONS—(Non-Scientific) —Pub. by American College of Surgeons, 55 E. Erie St., Chicago, Ill. 60611, U.S.A.; (Off. Pub.); Laura Louise Kuhl, Editor; Bi-monthly; (Controlled Circ.).

REVIEW OF SURGERY—Pub. by J. B. Lippincott Company of Canada Ltd., 60 Front St. W., Toronto 1, Ont.; Henry N. Harkins, M.D., Editor-in-Chief; Lloyd N. Nyhus, M.D., Editor; Bi-monthly; $12.00 a yr.

SURGERY—Pub. by C. V. Mosby Co., 3207 Washington Blvd., St. Louis 3, Mo., U.S.A.; (Off. Pub., Soc. of University Surgeons & Soc. for Vascular Surg.); Dr. Alton Ochsner & Dr. Owen H. Wangensteen, Editors; Monthly; $19.00 a yr.

SURGERY, GYNECOLOGY & OBSTETRICS—Pub. by the Franklin H. Martin, Mem. Fdn., 55 E. Erie St., Chicago, Ill. 60611, U.S.A.; (Off. Pub., Amer. Coll. Surg.); Loyal Davis, M.D., Editor; Monthly, $15.00 a yr.

THE AMERICAN JRL. OF SURGERY—Pub. by Reuben H. Donnelly Corp., 466 Lexington Ave., New York, N.Y. 10017, U.S.A.; R. M. Zollinger, M.D., Editor; Monthly; $16.00 a yr.

THE BRITISH JOURNAL OF SURGERY—Pub. by John Wright & Sons Ltd., The Stonebridge Press, Bath Rd., Bristol 4, England; (Can. Agents, The Macmillan Co. of Canada Ltd., 70 Bond St., Toronto 2, Ont.); Sir Cecil Wakeley, Editor; $21.45 per yr.

THE JRL. OF THORACIC & CARDIOVASCULAR SURGERY—Pub. by C. V. Mosby Co., 3207 Washington Blvd., St. Louis 3, Mo., U.S.A.; (Off. Pub. Am. Assoc. for Thoracic Surg. & Soc. of Thoracic Surgeons of Gt. Britain & Ireland); Dr. Brian Blades, Editor; Monthly; $26.50 a yr.

VET. SCIENCE

RESEARCH IN VETERINARY SCIENCE—A journal of the British Veterinary Assoc. Pub. by Blackwell Scientific Publications Ltd., 5 Alfred St., Oxford, England (Can. Agents—J. B. Lippincott Company of Canada Ltd., 60 Front St. W., Toronto 1, Ont.); Scientific Editor, D. L. Hughes; Quarterly; $20.00 a yr.

FELLOWSHIP AND POSTGRADUATE TRAINING

Full details with regard to study abroad may be obtained from Index Generales in the University Medical Libraries or by writing National Medical Authorities.

General

World Health Organization — Palais des Nations, Geneva, Switz. Fellowships financed from the WHO regular budget, UNICEF and the funds of the Technical Assistance Programme for Economic Development.

a) Individual fellowships for post-graduate study, observation of practices and techniques, research & the facilitating of the exchange of personnel.

b) fellowships to attend a group training programme (course, symposium, seminar) organized by WHO or assisted by WHO.

Fields of Study — Public Health & Preventive Medicine (public health administration, nursing, sanitation, control of communicable diseases, maternal & child health, etc.; Basic and Clinical Medical Sciences. Applications addressed to — Health Dept. of candidate's own government.

The Commonwealth Fund — Robert Jordan, Sec., Fellowship Comm., The Commonwealth Fund, 1 E. 75th St., New York 21, N.Y.

Embassies — Correspondence may be directed re foreign medical training to the Embassies of France, Italy, Norway, Sweden, etc. — Ottawa, Canada.

International Children's Centre — Chateau de Longchamp, Carrefour de Longchamp, Bois de Boulogne, Paris 16, France.

Fields of Study — Problems of School Hygiene; Social Paediatrics; Maternity & Child Welfare; Rearing Premature Children. Applications addressed to — Education Dept. of International Children's Centre, or the Ministry of Health or the Ministry of Social Welfare in candidate's own Country.

United Kingdom and Ireland

British Institute of Radiology — 32 Welbeck St., London, W.1. Hon. Sec., John Blewett, M.D.

British Postgraduate Medical Federation (University of London) — Dir., Prof. Sir James Patterson Ross, Bt., KCVO, 18 Guilford St., London, W.C.1. Full details of Postgraduate Courses in Great Britain.

Cambridge University — Elmore Medical Research Studentship. Apply Regius Prof. of Physic, Dept. of Med., U. of Cambridge, Cambridge.

Empire Rheumatism Council — Faraday House, 8-10 Charing Cross Rd., London, W.C.2.

Henderson Trust Grants — Kenneth Walker, Esq., Sec. to the Trustees, 190 West George St., Glasgow C. 2, Scotland.

Institute of Accident Surgery — Birmingham Accident Hospital, Bath-row, Birmingham 15, England.

Institute of Cancer Research — Royal Cancer Hospital — Dir., Royal Marsden Hospital, Fullham R., London, S.W.3.

Lister Institute of Preventive Medicine — Chelsea Bridge Rd., London, S.W.1. Chm., Sir Henry H. Dale.

London School of Hygiene & Tropical Medicine — Keppel St (Gower St.), London, W.C.1. — Dir., Dr. Charles Wilcocks.

Medical Research Council — 20 Park Cres., London, W.1. Dir., Nat. Institute for Medical Research, The Ridgeway, Mill Hill, London, N.W. 7, Sir Charles Harington.

Oxford University — Apply The Secretary, Medical School, Osler House, Woodstock Rd., Oxford, Eng.

Postgraduate Medical School of London — For details of courses, apply the Secretary, Postgraduate Medical School of London, Ducane Rd., London, W.12.

Royal College of Obstetricians and Gynaecologists — The Hon. Sec., 58 Queen Anne St., London, W.1.

Royal College of Physicians of London — Sec., 12 Pall Mall E., London S.W.1.

Royal College of Surgeons of London — Secretary, Lincoln's Inn Fields, London, W.C. 2.

Royal Institute of Public Health & Hygiene — 28 Portland Pl., London, W.1. S. Sec., A. R. Horsham, F.C.I.S., F.C.C.S.

Royal Society — The Assistant Secretary, Royal Society, Burlington House, Picadilly, London W.1.

Royal Society of Health — 90 Buckingham Palace Rd., London, S.W. 1. Sec., P. Arthur Wells.

Royal Society of Medicine — Secretary, Royal Society of Medicine, 1 Wimpole St., London, W.1, Eng.

St. Bartholomew's Hospital Medical College — Courses leading to specialization and degree of F.R.C.S. Apply Sub-Dean, St. Bartholomew's Hosp. Medical College, West Smithfield, London, E.C. 1.

Society of Apothecaries of London — D.I.H. (Dip. in Industrial Health) and D.M.J. (Dip. in Med. Jurisprudence). For regulations, apply Registrar, Apothecaries Hall, Black-Friars Lane, London, E.C.4.

Strangeway Research Laboratory — Wort's Causeway, Cambridge.

Tavistock Institute of Human Relations — 3 Devonshire St., London, W.I.

University of London — The Academic Registrar, U. of London, Senate House, London, W.C.1.

— The Registrar, Imperial College of Science and Technology, U. of London, South Kensington, London, S.W.7, Eng.

— The Secretary St. Mary's Medical School, Paddington London, W.2.: prior to April 30.

FELLOWSHIP AND P.G. TRAINING (*cont'd.*)

— The Secretary, Institute of Neurology, The National Hospital, Queen's Square, London, W.C.1.: by June 30.
— The Secretary, Royal Free Hospital School of Medicine, 8 Hunter St., London, W.C.1.: by May 1.
The Institute of Orthopaedics, Royal Nat. Orthopaedic Hosp. — Apply the Dean, 234 Great Portland St., London, W. 1.
Wright-Fleming Institute of Microbiology. For details apply St. Mary's Hospital Medical School, Norfolk Pl., London, W. 2.

Scotland

Aberdeen University — The Registrar, Faculty of Medicine, Aberdeen, Scotland.
Edinburgh Postgraduate Board for Medicine — Courses in Medical Sciences, Basic Sciences and Internal Medicine. Apply, Dir., P.G. Studies, Surgeon's Hall, Edinburgh 8, Scotland.
Royal College of Physicians of Edinburgh — Sec., 9 Queen St., Edinburgh, Scotland.
Royal College of Surgeons of Edinburgh — Sec., Surgeon's Hall, Edinburgh.
Royal College of Physicians & Surgeons of Glasgow — Hon. Sec., 242 St. Vincent St., Glasgow, C. 2, Scot.
University of St. Andrews — Apply for Courses, The Dean, U. of St. Andrews, St. Andrews, Scotland.
University of Edinburgh — For information concerning research scholarships and fellowships — Apply, The Dean, Faculty of Medicine, U. of Edinburgh, South Bridge, Edinburg 8, Scotland. (By April 30.)
University of Glasgow — Courses in General Medicine, General Surgery and the Specialties — Applications to The Dean, Faculty of Medicine, U. of Glasgow, Glasgow, Scotland.

Ireland

Medical Research Council of Ireland — 50 Merrion Square, Dublin 2, Ire. Chmn., Prof. J. F. Cunningham.
Queen's University (Belfast) — The Dean, Faculty of Medicine, Queen's U., Belfast, Northern Ireland.
Royal College of Surgeons of Ireland — Primary Fellowship Courses — The Registrar 123 St. Stephens Green, Dublin, Ire.

Wales

University of Wales — Cathays Park, Cardiff, Wales. (1) Ewen Maclean Research Scholarship (ObstGyn). (2) Cecil Prosser Research Scholarship (TB). Apply to Registrar, U. of Wales, Cardiff, Wales.

United States of America

A. E. Bennett Neuro Psychiatric Foundation — Secretary, Society of Biologic Psychiatry, 2010 Wiltshire Blvd., Los Angeles, Calif.
Alton Ochsner Medical Foundation — 3503 Prytania St., New Orleans, La.
Alfred P. Sloan Foundation — 630 Fifth Ave., New York 20, N.Y. Exec. Dir. Sec., James F. Kenney.
American Academy of Arts and Sciences — Chm., Permanent Science Fund Committee, American Acad. of Arts & Sciences — 280 Newton St., Brookline Stn., Boston 46, Mass.: by Feb. 1 and Sept. 1.
American Academy of Paediatrics — 1801 Hinman Ave., Evanston, Ill.
American Association of Psychiatric Clinics for Children — Miss Sylvia Lurie, Administrative Asst., Amer. Assoc. Psych. Clinics for Children, 250 W. 57th St., New York 19, N.Y.
American Board of Obstetrics & Gynaecology — Sec., Robert L. Faulkner, M.D., 2105 Adelbert Rd., Cleveland 6, Ohio.
American College of Chest Physicians — 112 East Chestnut St., Chicago 11, Ill.
American College of Gastroenterology—33 W. 60th St., New York 23, N.Y.
American College of Physicians — 4200 Pine St., Philadelphia, Penn.
American College of Surgeons — 40 East Erie St., Chicago 1, Ill.
American Institute of Psychoanalysis — 329 E. 62nd St., New York 21, N.Y.
American Otological Society — Dr. Philip E. Meltzer, Sec., The Central Bureau of Research, Amer. Otol. Soc. Inc., 285 Commonwealth Ave., Boston 16, Mass.
Aviation Medicine — (1) Ohio State University, Columbus. Ohio. (2) Harvard School of Public Health, Boston, Mass. (3) Johns Hopkins Medical School of Postgraduate Studies, Baltimore 5, Md. Specialized advanced courses.
Brandeis University — Chm., Dept. of Microbiology, Brandeis U., Waltham 54, Mass.
Child Development Centre — 120 W. 57th St., New York 19, N.Y.
Child Study Centre — Institute of the Pennsylvania Hospital — 110 N. 48th St., Philadelphia 39, Penn. Foreign Student Training Programme.
Columbia University — The Dean, Columbia University College of Physicians and Surgeons, 630 W. 168th St., N.Y. 32, N.Y.
Committee on P.G. Activities — California Medical Association, 693 Sutter St., San Francisco 2, Calif.
Cook Co. Graduate School of Medicine — 707 S. Wood St., Chicago 12, Ill.
Damon Runyon Memorial Fund for Cancer Research, Inc. — 55 E. 55th St., New York 22, N.Y.
Dept. of the Army — Office of the Surgeon General, Education and Training Division, Washington 25, D.C. Course at Walter Reed Army Med. Centre, Washington 12, D.C.
Emory University — School of Medicine Fellowships Committee, 201 Woodruff Memorial Building, Emory U., Georgia.
Endocrine Soc. — The Secretary, 1200 N. Walker St., Oklahoma City, Okla., U.S.A.
Frank E. Bunts Educational Institute — The Registrar, 2020 East 93 Street, Cleveland 6, Ohio, U.S.A.

FELLOWSHIP AND P.G. TRAINING (*cont'd.*)

U.S.A. (cont'd.)

Foundations Fund for Research in Psychiatry — Research Fellowships & Grants in Psychiatry, etc. Address: Foundations Fund for Research in Psy., 251 Edward St., New Haven 11, Conn.

Gray Pharmaceutical Co. Inc. — Dr. James Cummins, Scientific Dept., Gray Pharm. Co. Inc., 50 Hunt St., Newton 58, Mass.

Gorgas Memorial Institute of Tropical & Preventive Medicine, Inc. — 1835 Eye St., N.W., Washington 6, D.C.

Graduate School of Medicine — U. of Pennsylvania, Philadelphia, Penn.

Harvard Medical School for Graduates — 25 Shattuck St., Boston 15, Mass.; Ass't. Dean.

Hitchcock Foundation — Executive Director, Hitchcock Fdn., Hanover, New Hampshire, U.S.A.

Indiana University School of Medicine — 1100 West Michigan St., Indianapolis, Ind.

Industrial Hygiene Foundation of America Inc. — 4400 Fifth Ave., Pittsburgh 13, Pa. Man. Dir., C. Richard Walmer, M.D.

Institute of Physical Medicine & Rehabilitation — New York University Bellevue Medical Centre, 400 East 34th St., New York 16.

Johns Hopkins University School of Medicine — Baltimore 5, Md.

Joint Committee on Postgraduate Education — 1313 Bedford Ave., Brooklyn 16, New York.

Lahey Clinic — The Administrator, Lahey Clinic, 605 Commonwealth Ave., Boston 15, Mass.

Lalor Foundation — Lalor Fdn., 4400 Lancaster Pike, Wilmington 5, Del.; by Jan. 14.

Leukemia Research Grants — Leukemia Society Inc., 405 Lexington Ave., New York 17, N.Y.

Life Insurance Medical Research Fund — The Scientific Director, Life Ins. Med. Research Fund, 1030 E. Lancaster Ave., Rosemont, Pa.

Loma Linda University — 1720 Brooklyn Ave., Los Angeles 33, Cal.

Mayo Foundation — Rochester, Minn.

Medical Research Institute — Michael Reese Hospital, Chicago 16, Ill.

Memorial Sloan-Kettering Cancer Centre — 444 East 68th St., New York, N.Y.

National Council to Combat Blindness, Inc. — 41 W. 57th St., New York 19, N.Y.

National Foundation for Infantile Paralysis, Inc. — 301 East 42nd Street, New York 17, N.Y. Exec. Dir., Raymond H. Barrows.

National Psychiatric Reform Institute — Star Route, Altamont, N.Y.

National TB Association — 1790 Broadway, New York 19, N.Y. Sec., Mrs. Morrell DeReign.

New York University—Bellevue Medical Centre — The Director, International Training Program, Institute of Physical Medicine & Rehabilitation, 400 East 34th St., New York 16, N.Y.

New York Polyclinic Medical School — 345 West 50th St., New York, N.Y. Courses in the Specialties.

New York University Postgraduate Medical School — 550 First Ave., New York, N.Y. Courses in the Specialties.

Northwestern University Medical School — 303 East Chicago Ave., Chicago 11, Ill.

Oak Ridge Institute of Nuclear Studies — Box 117, Oak Ridge, Tenn., U.S.A.

Ohio State University — Dean of the Graduate School, Ohio State U., Columbus 10, Ohio; by March 1.

Postgraduate Centre for Psychotherapy — 218 East 70th St., New York, N.Y.

Postgraduate Education—U.S.A.—Apply Dir., Council on **Medical Education & Hospitals, c/o American Medical Association, 535 North Dearborn St., Chicago 10, Ill.**

Postgraduate Medical Institute—22 Fenway, Boston 15, Mass.

Postgraduate Inst., N. Charles Gen. Hosp., Charles at 28th St., Baltimore 18, Md.

Public Health—Accredited Schools of Public Health leading to degree M.P.H.—(1) U. of California, Berkeley 4, Cal. (2) Columbia U., New York 32, N.Y. (3) Harvard U., Boston 15, Mass. (4) Johns Hopkins U., Baltimore 5, Md. (5) U. of Michigan, Ann Arbor, Mich. (6) U. of Minnesota, Minneapolis 14, Minn. (7) U. of North Carolina, Chapel Hill, N.C. (8) U. of Pittsburgh, Pittsburgh 13, Pa. (9) Tulane U., New Orleans 12, La. (10) Yale U., New Haven, Conn.

Clinical Centre of the National Institutes of Health—Bethesda 14, Md.—The Research arm of the Public Health Service in the Dept. of Health, Education & Welfare. Highly specialized institution serving the seven National Institutions of Health. (a) National Institution of Arthritis & Metabolic Diseases. (b) National Cancer Institute. (c) National Institute of Dental Research. (d) National Health Institute. (e) National Institute of Mental Health. (f) National Institute of Allergy & Infectious Diseases. (g) National Institute of Neurological Diseases & Blindness. Dir. of Clinical Centre, Jack Masur, M.D. Dir., National Institutes of Health, James A. Shannon, M.D.

Rockefeller Institute—66th St. and York Ave., New York 21, N.Y.

Rutgers University—The Dean of the Graduate School, Rutgers U. of N.J., New Brunswick, N.J.

St. Louis University—1402 S. Grand Blvd., St. Louis 4, Mo.

Society for Paediatric Research—Sec., Dr. C. West, Children's Hosp., Cincinnati 29, Ohio.

Society for the Study of Development & Growth—Sec., Dr. R. O. Erickson, Botanical Labs., U. of Pennsylvania, Philadelphia 4, Pa.

Society of Medical Jurisprudence—New York Academy of Medicine, 2 East 103rd St., New York, N.Y. Sec., Edward B. Willing, 22 West First St., Mount Vernon, N.Y.

Stritch School of Medicine—706 Wolcott Ave., Chicago, Ill.—Courses in Psychiatry & Neurology.

U.S.A. (cont'd.)

Temple University School of Medicine—3400 North Broad St., Philadelphia 40, Pa.

Training Programme in the Biochemistry of Steroids—Sponsored by National Cancer Institute—Address: Dr. Kristen Eik-Nes, Dept. of Biochemistry, U. of Utah, Salt Lake City, Utah.

Tufts University School of Medicine—Postgraduate Division, 171 Harrison Ave., Boston, Mass.

University of Buffalo School of Medicine—3435 Main St., Buffalo, New York.

University of California (Berkeley)—Chm. of Dept., U. of California, Berkeley 4, Calif., U.S.A.

University of California School of Medicine—San Francisco 22, Calif.

University of Chicago—Admissions Counselor, Office of Admissions, U. of Chicago, Chicago 37, Ill.

University of Colorado Postgraduate Medical School—4200 East 9th Ave., Denver, Col.

University of Illinois College of Medicine—1853 West Polk St., Chicago 12, Ill.

University of Michigan Medical School—Dept. of Postgraduate Medicine, 1610 University Hospital, Ann Arbor, Mich. Dir., John M. Sheldon, M.D. Courses in the Specialties.

University of Minnesota—Dean of the Graduate School, 316 Johnston Hall, U. of Minnesota, Minneapolis 14, Minn.; by Feb. 15.

University of Missouri—The Dean of Graduate School, U. of Missouri, Columbia, Mo.

University of Nebraska—The Dean, U. of Nebraska College of Medicine, Omaha 5, Nebraska.

University of Pittsburgh—Pittsburgh 13, Pa., U.S.A.—Committee on Education Exchange—Teaching and/or Research Assistantships.

University of Southern California Post-Graduate Medical School—2025 Zonal Ave., Los Angeles 33, Cal.

University of Texas Postgraduate School of Medicine—Texas Medical Centre, Houston 25, Texas.

University of Vermont—Chm. of Dept., U. of Vermont, Burlington, Vt.: in Sept. or Oct. of year preceding award.

University of Virginia—Dean, Medical School, U. of Virginia, Charlottesville, Virginia.

Vanderbilt University—Nashville, Tenn., in Sept. or Oct. in year preceding award.

Wayne State University—The Dean, College of Medicine, Wayne State U., 1401 Rivard St., Detroit 7, Mich.

Western Reserve University—The Dean, School of Medicine, Western Reserve U., 2065 Adelbert Rd., Cleveland 6, Ohio.

William Alanson White Institute of Psychiatry—12 East 86th St., New York 28, N.Y.

Yale University School of Medicine—New Haven, Conn.

Canada

Canadian Arthritis & Rheumatism Society—900 Yonge St., Toronto 5, Ont. Clinical Fellowship in Internal Medicine (special emphasis on Rheumatology).

Canadian Cancer Society—790 Bay Bay St., Toronto, Ont. Medical Studies related to cancer—available to medical graduates resident in Canada. Allan Blair Memorial Fellowship.

Canadian Heart Foundation of Canada—501 Yonge St., Toronto, Ont. Fellowship and Research Programmes. Exec. Dir., Dr. J. B. Armstrong.

Canadian Inst. of Psychoanalysis—Dir. Dr. J. B. Boulanger, 1637 Sherbrooke W., Montreal 25, P.Q.

Canadian Orthopaedic Association—Dr. R. J. Harris, Chm. of Committee on Exchange Fellowships, Can. Orth. Assoc., 609 Medical Arts Bldg., Toronto 5, Ont.

Canadian Society for Study of Diseases of Children—Montreal Children's Hospital, Montreal, P.Q. Sec., Dr. R. L. Denton.

Canadian TB Association—343 O'Connor St., Ottawa 4, Ont. Exec. Sec., Dr. C. W. L. Jeanes.

Dept. of National Defence—Defence Medical & Dental Service Advisory Board. Dr. P. A. T. Sneath, Exec. Sec.

Jas. Picker Fdn.—Fellowships in Radiological Research available for tenure in Canada. Cdn. Sel. Comm., National Research Bldg., Sussex Dr., Ottawa 2, Ont.

Medical Research Council of Canada—Research in Medical Sciences. Available to Canadians resident in Canada, age limit 35. Must have M.D. or Ph.D. degree and capacity for medical research. Address: Sussex St., Ottawa, Ont. Chm.: Dr. R. F. Farquharson.

Nuffield Fdn.—Travelling Fellowships (Med.) for Cdn. doctors' training in U.K. Cdn. Sel. Comm., National Research Bldg., Ottawa 2, Ont.

Ontario Research Foundation—43-47 Queen's Park, Toronto 5, Ont. Chm., H. M. Turner.

Public Health—Public Health Subjects—Courses leading to diplomas in Canadian Schools of Hygiene as listed elsewhere—see index.

Queen Elizabeth II, Cdn. Research Fund—Fellowships for Research in Diseases of Children. Bd. of Trustees, National Research Bldg., Sussex Dr., Ottawa 2, Ont.

R. Samuel McLaughlin Foundation—Dr. W. E. Gallie, Trustee, McLaughlin Foundation, 607 Medical Arts Bldg., Toronto 5, Ont.

Royal College of Physicians & Surgeons of Canada—For details of requirements for certification in the specialties, write: Sec., Dr. J. H. Graham, 74 Stanley Ave. Ottawa 2, Ont.

University Medical Schools—Details of Postgraduate Courses may be obtained by writing the Dean of Medicine at any of the Provincial Universities, fully listed elsewhere in the Canadian Medical Directory.

GENERAL INFORMATION

The Minister of National Health and Welfare for Canada

The Hon. Allan J. MacEachen

Official Medical Bodies

The Medical Council of Canada—77 Metcalfe St., Ottawa, Canada
Provincial Registrars are listed in detail as noted in the index.

The Royal College of Physicians and Surgeons of Canada—74 Stanley St., Ottawa, Ont. Application forms for certification in the specialties may be obtained by addressing requests to the Honorary Secretary at this address:

MEDICAL SPECIALISTS—Anaesthesia; Bacteriology; Dermatology and Syphilology; Internal Medicine; Neurology; Paediatrics; Pathology; Physical Medicine; Psychiatry; Public Health; Diagnostic Radiology; Therapeutic Radiology.

SURGICAL SPECIALTIES—General Surgery; Neurosurgery; Obstetrics and/or Gynaecology; Ophthalmology; Orthopaedic Surgery; Otololaryngology; Plastic Surgery; Thoracic Surgery; Urology.

National Research Council of Canada—Sussex Dr., Ottawa 2, Canada.

Associations:

Association des Medecins de Langue Francaise du Canada—5064, Ave. du Parc, Montreal 8, P.Q.

Canadian Medical Association—150 St. George St., Toronto 5, Ontario.

Canadian Medical Protective Association—Suite 115, 26 Nepean St., Ottawa, Ont.

ETHICS—The formal Code of Ethics *of* the Canadian Medical Association, may be obtained on written request to the secretarial offices at 150 St. George Street, Toronto 5, Ontario.

REGISTRATION TO PRACTICE MEDICINE—Details of regulations governing licensure to practice medicine in Canada may be obtained by writing the Medical Council of Canada—77 Metcalfe Street, Ottawa, Ontario or the Provincial Registrars listed elsewhere in this Directory.

(For more detailed information—see General Index).

THE LARGEST CITIES OF THE WORLD

CITIES OF WORLD HAVING OVER 500,000 INHABITANTS

Figures supplied through the courtesy of the International Statistical Institute, The Hague

City	Approximate Population	Date of Census
Addis Ababa	500,000	1957
Adelaide	562,500	1959
Ahmedabad	1,047,000	1960
Alexandria	1,352,300	1960
Algiers	800,000	1960
Amsterdam	868,043	1963
Ankara	646,151	1960
Anshan	805,000•	1957
Antwerp (Greater)	637,600	1960
Athens	565,084	1951
Baghdad	656,399	1957
Baku	636,000	1959
Baltimore	939,024	1960
Bandung	941,564	1959
Bangalore	1,269,000	1960
Bangkok	1,330,153	1960
Barcelona	1,553,258	1960
Belgrade	587,900	1961
Belo Horizonte	583,019	1960
Berlin (East)	1,076,445	1960
Berlin (West)	2,170,596	1963
Birmingham	1,105,651	1961
Bogota	1,188,200	1960
Bombay	4,132,600	1961
Boston	697,197	1960
Bremen	576,767	1963
Brisbane	567,000	1959
Brussels (Greater)	1,014,632	1960
Bucharest	1,225,507	1960
Budapest	1,820,000	1960
Buenos Aires	3,767,887	1958
Buffalo	532,759	1960
Cairo	3,027,600	1960
Calcutta	3,040,000	1960
Cali	645,410	1959
Canton	1,840,000	1957
Cape Town	739,600	1960
Caracas	1,136,000	1959
Casablanca	960,812	1960
Changchung	975,000	1957
Changsha	703,000	1957
Chengchow	766,000	1957
Chengtu	1,107,000	1957
Chicago	3,550,404	1960
Chungking	2,121,000	1957
Cincinnati	502,550	1960
Cleveland	876,050	1960
Cologne	830,252	1963
Copenhagen	725,250	1960
Dairen-Port Arthur (see Lu-ta)		
Dallas	679,684	1960
Delhi	1,672,000	1960
Denver	520,500	1956
Detroit	1,670,144	1960
Djakarta	2,814,210	1959
Dnepropetrovsk	660,000	1959
Dortmund	649,076	1963
Dublin	539,476	1956
Duisburg	500,859	1963
Dusseldorf	705,994	1963
Durban	655,370	1960
Erevan	509,000	1959
Essen	731,494	1963
Foochow	616,000	1957
Frankfurt	688,605	1963
Fukuoka	632,000	1959
Fushun	985,000	1957
Genoa	768,520	1960
Glasgow	1,049,115	1963
Gorki	942,000	1959
Guadalajara	734,346	1960
Hamburg	1,847,584	1963
Hangchow	784,000	1957
Hanover	573,578	1963
Harbin	1,552,000	1957
Havana	785,455	1953
Hongkong	2,340,000	1955
Houston	938,219	1960
Hyderabad	1,050,000	1960
Instanbul	1,924,912	1960
Johannesburg	1,096,541	1960
Kanpur	874,000	1960
Karachi	1,916,000	1961
Kawasaki	572,000	1959
Kazan	643,000	1959
Kharkov	934,000	1959
Kiev	1,104,000	1959
Kirin	568,000	1952
Kobe	1,113,900	1960
Kuibyshev	806,000	1959
Kunming	880,000	1957
Kweiyang	504,000	1957
Kyoto	1,284,800	1960
Lahore	849,476	1951
Lanchow	699,000	1957
Leeds	510,597	1961
Leipsig	589,850	1960
Leningrad	2,888,000	1959
Lima	1,262,107	1960
Lisbon	911,200	1960
Liverpool	747,490	1961
Lodz	707,400	1960
London (Greater)	8,171,902	1961
Los Angeles	1,479,015	1960
Lucknow	549,000	1960
Lu-ta (Dairen and Port Arthur)	1,200,000	1953
Lyon	528,535	1962
Madras	2,208,000	1960
Madrid	2,062,349	1960
Madurai	532,000	1960
Manchester	661,041	1961
Manilla	1,145,723	1960
Marseilles	778,071	1962
Medellin	578,940	1959
Melbourne	1,831,100	1960
Mexico	2,697,994	1960
Milan	1,523,583	1960
Milwaukee	741,324	1960
Minneapolis	551,000	1956
Minsk	509,000	1959
Molotov	538,000	1956
Monterrey	600,609	1960
Montevideo	860,000	1955
Montreal	1,191,062	1961
Montreal (Metro.)	2,109,509	1961
Moscow	5,032,000	1959
Mukden (see Shenyang)		
Munich	1,149,810	1963
Nagoya	1,591,900	1960
Nanchang	508,000	1957
Nagpur	651,000	1960
Nanking	1,419,000	1957
Naples	1,160,255	1960
New Orleans	627,525	1960
New York	7,781,984	1960
Novosibirsk	887,000	1959
Odessa	667,000	1959
Omsk	579,000	1959
Osaka	3,011,600	1960
Palermo	601,324	1960
Paris	3,733,545	1962
Peking	4,010,000	1957
Perm	628,000	1959
Philadelphia	2,002,512	1960
Phnom-Penh	500,000	1956
Pinchiang	1,163,000	1953
Pittsburgh	604,332	1960
Poona	798,000	1960
Porto Alegre	553,051	1959
Prague	998,690	1960
Pusan	1,097,000	1958
Rangoon	774,676	1958
Recife	765,305	1959
Riga	605,000	1959
Rio de Janeiro	3,123,984	1959
Rome	2,019,514	1960
Rosario	561,637	1958
Rostov-on-Don	597,000	1959
Rotterdam	731,899	1963
Saigon-Cholon	1,383,000	1959
St. Louis	750,026	1960
Salvador	571,101	1959
San Antonio	587,718	1960
San Diego	573,224	1960
San Francisco	740,316	1960
Santiago de Chili	1,699,711	1959
Sao Paulo	3,674,373	1960
Saratow	581,000	1959
Seattle	557,087	1960
Seoul	2,444,883	1960
Shanghai	6,900,000	1957
Shenyang	2,411,000	1957
Shikiachwang	598,000	1957
Sian	1,310,000	1957
Singapore	992,500	1959
Sofia	686,738	1960
Soochow	633,000	1957
Stalingrad	591,000	1959
Stalino	699,000	1959
Stockholm	807,200	1960
Stuttgart	642,356	1963
Surabaya	1,146,641	1959
Suchow	676,000	1957
Sverdlovsk	777,000	1959
Sydney	2,098,490	1960
Tashkent	911,000	1959
Taegu	511,000	1958
Taipei	854,061	1959
Taiyuan	1,020,000	1957
Tangshan	800,000	1957
Teheran	1,838,982	1960
The Hague	604,888	1963
Tientsin	3,220,000	1957
Tiflis	694,000	1959
Tokyo	8,302,565	1960
Toronto	672,407	1961
Toronto (Metro)	1,824,481	1961
Tchaljabinsk	688,000	1959
Tsinan	862,000	1957
Tsingtao	1,121,000	1957
Tsitsihar	668,000	1957
Turin	963,188	1960
Tsepo	806,000	1957
Ufa	546,000	1959
Valencia	574,939	1960
Vancouver (Metro)	790,165	1961
Vienna	1,625,952	1959
Warsaw	1,136,000	1960
Washington	763,950	1960
Wuhan	2,146,000	1957
Wusih	613,000	1957
Yokohama	1,375,700	1960

IF YOUR LISTING IS INCORRECT

Please complete a temporary form of questionnaire containing the following information and return to The Editor, Canadian Medical Directory, Seccombe House, 443 Mount Pleasant Rd., Toronto 7, Canada.

SURNAME ....

FIRST NAME & INITIALS ....

OFFICE ADDRESS ....

TELEPHONE NO. ....

CITY/TOWN ....

RESIDENCE ADDRESS ....

NAME & LOCATION OF
UNIVERSITY OF GRADUATION
IN MEDICINE .... YEAR ....

OTHER MEDICAL DEGREES INCLUDING CERTIFICATION ....

....

....

SPECIALTY PRACTICE IN: ....Full Time ( ); Part Time ( )

RETIRED FROM PRACTICE? ....Yes ( ) ....No ( )

IN WHICH CANADIAN PROVINCES ARE YOU REGISTERED FOR PRACTICE? ....

APPOINTMENTS NOW HELD (include internship, residency, hospital, teaching, industrial, public health or administrative posts only.

Please reserve a copy of the 1968 C.M.D. and invoice me later ( ).

Name.. Address ....

City .... Date ....

CONVENTIONS AND INTERNATIONAL MEDICAL MEETINGS - 1967

General

AMERICAN MED. ASSOC.—Annual Meeting — June 18th-22nd, 1967 — Atlantic City, N.J., Exec. Vice Pres., F. J. L. Blasingame, M.D., 535 N. Dearborn St., Chicago 60610, Ill.

AMERICAN MED. ASSOC.—Clinical Convention — Nov. 26th-29th, 1967 — Houston, Texas. Exec. Vice Pres.: F. J. L. Blasingame, M.D., 535 N. Dearborn St., Chicago 60610, Ill.

BRITISH MED. ASSOC.—Annual Clinical Meeting, Londonderry, Northern Ireland. April 13th-16th. Info.: Secretariat, British Med. Assoc., Tavistock Square, London, W.C. 1, England.

BRITISH MED. ASSOC.—Annual Scientific Meeting — Bristol, England. July 10th-14th. Info: Secretariat, British Med. Assoc., Tavistock Square, London, W.C. 1, England.

CANADIAN MED. ASSOC.—Annual Meeting — Montreal, P.Q. June 18th-23rd. Gen. Sec., Arthur F. W. Peart, M.D., 150 St. George St., Toronto 5, Ont.

COLLEGE OF GENERAL PRACTICE OF CANADA—Annual Meeting — July 10th-13th. Vancouver Hotel, Vancouver, B.C. Exec. Dir., Dr. D. I. Rice, 1260 Bay St., Room 531, Toronto 5, Ont.

ONTARIO MED. ASSOC.—Annual Meeting — Royal York Hotel, Toronto, Ont. May 8th-12th. Sec., Dr. Glenn Sawyer, 244 St. George St., Toronto 5, Ont.

ALLERG.

AMERICAN ACADEMY OF ALLERGY, (E), Holiday Inn-Riviera, Palm Springs, Calif., Feb. 18-22nd. Exec. Sec.: James O. Kelley, 756 N. Milwaukee St., Milwaukee 53202.

AMERICAN COLLEGE OF ALLERGISTS (E), The Roosevelt, New Orleans, March 19-24th. Exec. Vice-Pres.: Mr. Eloi Bauers, 2160 Rand Tower, Minneapolic, Minn. 55402.

CANADIAN ACADEMY OF ALLERGY, ACADEMIE CANADIENNE D'ALLERGIE, Queen Elizabeth Hotel, Montreal, P.Q., June 18th. Sec.: Francois Leger, 3766 Queen Mary Rd., Montreal, P.Q.

ANAES.

AMERICAN SOCIETY OF ANESTHESIOLOGISTS, (E), Las Vegas, Nev., Sept. 30-Oct. 4th. Exec. Sec.: J. W. Andes, 515 Busse Hwy., Park Ridge, Ill. 60608.

CANADIAN ANAESTHETISTS' SOCIETY, Montreal, P.Q., June 24-30th. Sec.: S. M. Campbell, M.B., 178 St. George St., Toronto 5, Ont.

INTERNATIONAL ANESTHESIA RESEARCH SOCIETY, (41st Congress), Americana Hotel, Bal Harbour, Fla., March 5-9th; Exec. Sec.: B. B. Sankey, M.D., 3645 Warrensville Center Rd., Cleveland.

ANAT.

AMERICAN ASSOCIATION OF ANATOMISTS, Hotel Muehlebach, Kansas City, Mo., April 4-7th. Exec. Sec.: Russell T. Woodburne, The University of Michigan East Medical Bldg., Ann Arbor, Mich. 48104.

CANADIAN ASSOCIATION OF ANATOMISTS, McGill University, Montreal, P.Q., July, 1967. Sec.: Dr. J. V. Basmajian, Dept. of Anatomy, Queen's University, Kingston, Ont.

AVIA. MED.

AEROSPACE MEDICAL ASSOCIATION, The Washington Hilton Hotel, Washington, D.C., April 10-13th. Exec. Vice Pres.: William J. Kennard, M.D., Washington National Airport, Washington, D.C. 20001.

BIOCHEM.

CANADIAN BIOCHEMICAL SOCIETY, McGill University, Montreal, P.Q., June 5-7th. Sec.: Dr. H. D. Branion, Faculty of Graduate Studies, University of Guelph, Guelph, Ontario.

BIOL.

CANADIAN FEDERATION OF BIOLOGICAL SOCIETIES, McGill University, Montreal, P.Q., July 5-7th. Hon. Sec.: Dr. A. H. Neufeld, University of Western Ontario, London, Ont.

CARD.

AMERICAN COLLEGE OF CARDIOLOGY, (E), Washington Hilton Hotel, Washington, D.C., Feb. 15-19th. Exec. Dir.: William D. Nelligan, 9650 Rockville Pike, Washington, D.C. 20014.

AMERICAN HEART ASSOCIATION, Hilton Hotel, San Francisco, Oct. 20-24th. Exec. Dir.: Rome A. Betts, 44 E. 23rd St., New York 10010.

CANADIAN CARDIOVASCULAR SOCIETY—SOCIETE CANADIENNE DE CARDIOLOGIE, Montreal, P.Q., Oct. 23-28th. Sec.: Dr. R. E. Beamish, 100 Medical College, Winnipeg, Man.

ONTARIO HEART FDN. & UNIVERSITY OF WESTERN ONTARIO, INTERNATIONAL SYMPOSIUM ON ELECTRICAL ACTIVITY OF THE HEART, London, Ontario, Canada. May 24th-26th. Info: Dr. G. W. Manning, Victoria Hosp., London, Ont., Canada.

CEREB. PALSY	**AMERICAN ACADEMY FOR CEREBRAL PALSY,** San Francisco-Hilton Hotel, San Francisco, Dec. 10-13th. Exec. Sec.: J. D. Russ, M.D., 1520 Louisiana Ave., New Orleans 70115.
CHEST	**AMERICAN COLLEGE OF CHEST PHYSICIANS, (E),** Atlantic City, N.J., June 15-19th. Exec. Dir.: Murray Kornfeld, 112 E. Chestnut, Chicago 60611. **AMERICAN COLLEGE OF CHEST PHYSICIANS** (Interim Clinical Meeting), Houston, Nov. 25-26th. Exec. Sec.: Murray Kornfeld, 112 E. Chestnut St., Chicago 60611. **AMERICAN THORACIC SOCIETY, (E),** Penn-Sheraton Hotel, Pittsburgh, May 21-24th. Exec. Sec.: Frank W. Webster, 1790 Broadway, New York 10019. **CANADIAN THORACIC SOCIETY,** Quebec, P.Q., May 30-June 2nd. Sec.: Dr. C. W. L. Jeanes, 343 O'Connor St., Ottawa 4, Ont. **CANADIAN TUBERCULOSIS ASSOC.**—Quebec, P.Q., May 30th-June 2nd. Sec.: Dr. C. W. L. Jeanes, 343 O'Connor St., Ottawa 4, Ont.
CLIN. INVEST.	**AMERICAN SOCIETY FOR CLINICAL INVESTIGATION,** Chalfonte-Haddon Hall, Atlantic City, N.J., April 30-May 3. Sec.-Treas.; Grant W. Liddle, M.D., Vanderbilt University School of Medicine, Nashville, Tenn. 37203.
CLIN, PHARM.	**AMERICAN COLLEGE OF CLINICAL PHARMACOLOGY & CHEMOTHERAPY.** Chalfonte-Haddon Hall, Atlantic City, April 26-28th. Exec. Sec.: Duncan Hutcheon, M.D., 7 E. 82nd St., New York 10028.
CYTOL.	**AMERICAN SOCIETY OF CYTOLOGY (Joint Program with District VIII of the American College of Obstetricians & Gynecologists), (E),** Denver-Hilton Hotel, Denver, Oct. 21-23rd. Sec.-Treas.: Warren R. Lang, M.D., 1012 Walnut St., Philadelphia 19107.
DERM.	**AMERICAN ACADEMY OF DERMATOLOGY, (E),** Palmer House, Chicago, Dec. 2-7th. Sec.-Treas.: Stanley E. Huff, M.D., 636 Church St., Evanston, Ill. **AMERICAN DERMATOLOGICAL ASSOCIATION, (M),** Broadmoor Hotel, Colorado Springs, Colo., May 28-June 1st. Exec. Sec.: Robert R. Kierland, M.D., Mayo Clinic, 200 First St. S.W., Rochester, Minn. 55901. **BRITISH ASSOC. OF DERMATOLOGY,** London, England. July 20th-23rd. Exec. Sec.: Stephen Gold, M.D., 149 Harley St., London, W. 1, England.
DIET.	**AMERICAN DIETETIC ASSOCIATION,** Chicago, Aug. 15-18th. Exec. Sec.: Ruth M. Yakel, 620 N. Michigan Ave., Chicago. **THE CANADIAN DIETETIC ASSOCIATION,** Chateau Laurier Hotel, Ottawa, Ont., June 14-16th. Sec.: (Miss) Joan E. Brown, 1393 Yonge St., Toronto 7, Ont.
E.E.N.T.	**AMERICAN ACADEMY OF OPHTHALMOLOGY & OTOLARYNGOLOGY, (E, M),** Palmer House, Chicago, Oct. 29-Nov. 3rd. Exec. Sec.: William L. Benedict, M.D., 15 Second St. S.W., Rochester, Minn. 55901. **AMERICAN CLEFT PALATE ASSOCIATION,** Palmer House, Chicago, April 13-15th. Sec.-Treas.; Kenneth R. Bzoch, Phd., Dept. of Communicative Disorders, College of Health Related Professions, University of Florida, Gainesville, Fla. 32603. **AMERICAN LARYNGOLOGICAL ASSOC.,** Quebec, P.Q., May 15th-16th. Exec. Sec.: Dr. Lyman Richards, 12 Clevelly Rd., Wellesley Hills 81, Mass. **AMERICAN LARYNGOLOGICAL, RHINOLOGICAL & OTOLOGICAL SOC.,** Montreal, P.Q., May 21st-23rd. Sec.: Victor R. Alfaro, M.D., 916 19th St. N.W., Washington, D.C. **AMERICAN OPHTHALMOLOGICAL SOCIETY, (M),** The Homestead, Hot Springs, Virginia, May 29-31st. Exec. Sec.: S. D. McPherson, Jr., M.D., 1110 W. Main St., Durham, N.C. **AMERICAN OTOLOGICAL SOC.,** Quebec, P.Q., May 17th-18th. Exec. Sec.: James A. Moore, M.D., 525 E. 68th St., New York 21, N.Y. **CANADIAN OPHTHALMOLOGICAL SOCIETY,** Quebec, P.Q.; June 24th-28th. Sec.: Dr. R. G. C. Kelly, 1849 Yonge St., Ste. 902, Toronto 7, Ont. **CANADIAN OTOLARYNGOLOGICAL SOCIETY,** Quebec, P.Q.; June 11th-14th. Sec.: Dr. D. P. Bryce, 320 Med. Arts Bldg., Toronto, Ont.
ENDO.	**ENDOCRINE SOCIETY,** American Hotel, Miami Beach, Fla., June 15-17th. Exec. Sec.: Mrs. Nona Lee Mattox, 1200 N. Walker, Oklahoma City 73103.
ELECTRO-ENCEPH.	**AMERICAN ELECTROENCEPHALOGRAPHIC SOCIETY,** Atlantic City, N.J., June, Sec.: Dr. Robert J. Ellingson, Nebraska Psychiatric Institute, 602 S. 44th Ave., Omaha 68105.
GASTRO	**AMERICAN COLLEGE OF GASTROENTEROLOGY,** Biltmore Hotel, Los Angeles, Oct. 29-Nov. 1st. Exec. Dir.: Daniel Weiss, 33 W. 60th St., New York 10023. **AMERICAN GASTROENTEROLOGICAL ASSOCIATION, (E),** Broadmoore Hotel, Colorado Springs, Colo., May 25-27th. Sec.: David Cayer, M.D., 2240 Cloverdale Ave., Winston-Salem, N.C. 27103. **AMERICAN SOCIETY FOR GASTROINTESTINAL ENDOSCOPY,** Broadmoor Hotel, Colorado Springs, Colo., May 24. Exec. Sec.: B. H. Sullivan, Jr., M.D., 2020 E. 93rd St., Cleveland 44106. **CANADIAN ASSOCIATION OF GASTROENTEROLOGY — L' ASSOCIATION CANADIENNE DE GASTROENTEROLOGIE,** Quebec City, Quebec, June 11-15th. Sec.: J. M. Finlay, M.D., Ste. 426, 170 St. George St., Toronto 5, Ont.
GER.	**AMERICAN GERIATRICS SOCIETY, (OS),** Claridge Hotel, Atlantic City, N.J., June 16-17th. Exec. Dir.: Edward Henderson, M.D., 10 Columbus Circle, Room 1405, New York 10019.
HAEM.	**AMERICAN ASSOCIATION OF BLOOD BANKS, (E),** Americana Hotel, New York, Oct. 21-24th. Info: Lois J. James, 30 N. Michigan Ave., Chicago 60602.
HEALTH	**AMERICAN COLLEGE HEALTH ASSOCIATION,** Mayflower Hotel, Washington, D.C., March 28-31st. Exec. Sec'y: Lee D. Stauffer, M.P.H., P.O. Box 9117, University of Miami Branch, Coral Gables, Fla. 33124.

A.M.A. NATIONAL CONGRESS OF ENVIRONMENTAL HEALTH MANAGEMENT, Hotel Americana, New York, April 24-26th. Info: A.M.A. Department of Environmental Health, 535 N. Dearborn St., Chicago 60610.

HOSP. AMERICAN HOSPITAL ASSOCIATION, (E), Palmer House, Chicago, Aug. 21-24th. Exec. Vice Pres.: Edwin L. Crosby, M.D., 840 N. Lake Shore Dr., Chicago 60611.

CANADIAN HOSPITAL ASSOC., May 10th-12th, 1967. Mount Royal Hotel, Montreal, P.Q.; Sec.: Mr. George McCracken, 25 Imperial St., Toronto 7, Ont.

HYPNOSIS AMERICAN SOCIETY OF CLINICAL HYPNOSIS, New York Hilton, New York, Oct. 18-23rd. Info: F. D. Nowlin, 800 Washington Ave. S.E., Minneapolis 55414.

IMMUNOL. AMERICAN ASSOCIATION OF IMMUNOLOGISTS, Chicago, April 17-21st. Sec.-Treas.: Dr. Sheldon Dray, 9650 Wisconsin Ave., Washington, D.C. 20014.

INDUST. MED. INDUSTRIAL MEDICAL ASSOCIATION, Americana Hotel, New York, April 10-13th. Managing Dir.: Clark D. Bridges, 55 E. Washington St., Chicago 60602.

THE INDUSTRIAL MEDICAL ASSOCIATION OF THE PROVINCE OF QUEBEC —L'ASSOCIATION DE MEDECINE INDUSTRIELLE DE LA PROVINCE DE QUEBEC, Hotel Champlain, Montreal, P.Q., Oct. 12-14th. Sec.: Dr. Lloyd A. Wright, Room 930, 1050 Beaver Hall Hill, Montreal, P.Q.

INT. MED. AMERICAN SOCIETY OF INTERNAL MEDICINE, (E), St. Francis Hotel, San Francisco, April 7-9th. Exec. Dir.: Albert V. Whitehall, 3410 Geary Blvd., San Francisco 94118.

LAB. TECH. CANADIAN SOCIETY OF LABORATORY TECHNOLOGISTS, Chateau Frontenac, Quebec City, P.Q., June 18-22nd. Exec. Sec.: Mr. A. R. Shearer, 99 Wentworth St. S., Hamilton, Ont.

MED. AMERICAN ACADEMY OF GENERAL PRACTICE, (E), Dallas, Tex., Sept. 15-23rd. Exec. Dir.: Mac F. Cahal, J.D., Volker Blvd. at Brookside, Kansas City 12, Mo.

AMERICAN COLLEGE OF PHYSICIANS, (E, M), Fairmont Hotel, San Francisco, April 10-14th. Exec. Dir.: Edward C. Rosenow, Jr., M.D., 4200 Pine St., Philadelphia 19104.

AMERICAN MED. ASSOC.—Annual Meeting — June 18th-22nd, 1967 — Atlantic City, N.J. Exec. Vice Pres.: F. J. L. Blasingame, M.D., 535 N. Dearborn St., Chicago 60610, Ill.

AMERICAN MED. ASSOC.—Clinical Convention—Nov. 26th-29th, Houston, Texas. Exec. Vice Pres.: F. J. L. Blasingame, M.D., 535 N. Dearborn St., Chicago 60610, Ill.

ASSOCIATION OF AMERICAN PHYSICIANS, Haddon Hall, Atlantic City, N.J., May 2-3rd. Exec. Sec.: Eugene Stead, Jr., M.D., Duke Hospital, Durham, N.C.

BRITISH MED. ASSOC.—Annual Clinical Meeting, Londonderry, Northern Ireland. April 13th-16th. Info: Secretariat, British Med. Assoc., Tavistock Square, London, W.C. 1, England.

BRITISH MED. ASSOC.—Annual Scientific Meeting — Bristol, England — July 10th-14th. Info.: Secretariat, British Med. Assoc., Tavistock Square, London W.C. 1, England.

CANADIAN MED. ASSOC.—Annual Meeting — Montreal, P.Q., June 18th-23rd. Gen. Sec.: Arthur F. W. Peart, M.D., 150 St. George St., Toronto 5, Ont.

COLLEGE OF GENERAL PRACTICE OF CANADA—Annual Meeting — July 10th-13th. Vancouver Hotel, Vancouver, B.C. Exec. Dir.: Dr. D. I. Rice, 1260 Bay St., Room 531, Toronto 5, Ont.

NATIONAL MEDICAL ASSOCIATION, Hilton Hotel, St. Louis, Aug. 12th. Exec. Sec.: John T. Givens, M.D., 2400 Corprew Ave., Norfolk, Va.

ONTARIO MED. ASSOC.—Annual Meeting — Royal York Hotel, Toronto, Ont. May 8th-12th. Sec.: Dr. Glenn Sawyer, 244 St. George St., Toronto 5, Ont.

MED. CLIN. AMERICAN ASSOCIATION OF MEDICAL CLINICS, The Drake, Chicago, Sept. 21-23rd. Exec. Dir.: Edwin P. Jordan, M.D., P.O. Box 58, Charlottesville, Va. 22902.

MED. COLL. ASSOCIATION OF AMERICAN MEDICAL COLLEGES, Detroit, Oct. 23-27th. Exec. Sec.: Richard H. Young, M.D., 303 E. Chicago Ave., Chicago 60611.

MED. & DENT. CAMDA (Canadian-American Medical and Dental Association), Vail, Colo., March 4-11th. Sec.-Treas.: Tony Trapasso, M.D., 816 Ashmum St., Sault Ste. Marie, Mich. 49783.

MED. HIST. AMERICAN ASSOCIATION FOR THE HISTORY OF MEDICINE, New Haven, Conn., April 27-29th. Sec.: John B. Blake, Ph.D., National Library of Medecine, Bethesda, Md. 20014.

MED. LIB. AMERICAN ASSOCIATION OF MEDICAL RECORD LIBRARIANS, Los Angeles, October. Exec. Dir.: Mrs. Mary-J. Waterstraat, R.R.L., 840 N. Lake Shore Dr., Chicago 60611.

CANADIAN ASSOC. OF MED. RECORD LIBRARIANS—The Holiday Inn, Montreal, P.Q.; Sept. 3rd-5th. Sec.; Mrs. J. Milner, R.R.L., 770 Glenforest St., Oshawa, Ont.

MEDICAL LIBRARY ASSOCIATION, (E), Americana Hotel, Miami, Fla., June 11-16th. Exec. Sec.: Mrs. Helen Brown Schmidt, 919 N. Michigan Ave., Chicago 60611.

MED. WOMEN AMERICAN MEDICAL WOMEN'S ASSOCIATION, Denver, June. Exec. Dir.: Mrs. Gertrude F. Conroy, 1790 Broadway, New York 10019.

AMERICAN MEDICAL WOMEN'S ASSOC., (M), Atlanta, Nov. 29-Dec. 3rd. Exec. Dir.: Mrs. Gertrude F. Conroy, 1790 Broadway, New York 10019.

MED. WRITERS AMERICAN MEDICAL WRITERS ASSOCIATION, Palmer House, Chicago, Sept. 21-24th. Exec. Sec.: James E. Bryan, 2000 P. St. N.W., Washington, D.C. 20036.

MENTAL HEALTH AMERICAN ASSOCIATION ON MENTAL DEFICIENCY, Denver-Hilton Hotel, Denver, May 15-20th. Exec. Sec.: John J. Noone, Ed.D., 5201 Connecticut Ave. N.W., Washington, D.C.

MICROBIOL. **AMERICAN SOCIETY FOR MICROBIOLOGY,** New York Hilton Hotel, New York, April 29-May 4th. Exec. Sec.: R. W. Sarber, 115 Huron View Blvd., Ann Arbor, Mich. 48103.

MULT. SCLER. **NATIONAL MULTIPLE SCLEROSIS SOCIETY,** New York, Feb. 28th. Exec. Dir.: Sylvia Lawry, 257 Park Ave. S., New York 10010.

NEUROL. **AMERICAN ACADEMY OF NEUROLOGY,** San Francisco Hilton Hotel, San Francisco, April 24-29th. Exec. Sec.: Thomas D. Swedien, 7100 France Ave. South, Minneapolis 55410.

AMERICAN NEUROLOGICAL ASSOCIATION, (ES), Claridge Hotel, Atlantic City, June 12-14th. Sec.-Treas.: Melvin D. Yahr, M.D., 710 W. 168th St., New York 10032.

NUC. MED. **SOCIETY OF NUCLEAR MEDICINE,** Olympic Hotel, Seattle, June. Exec. Sec.: Samuel N. Turiel, 33 N. Michigan Ave., Chicago.

NURS. **VICTORIAN ORDER OF NURSES FOR CANADA**—Chateau Laurier Hotel, Ottawa, Ont.; May 4th-5th. Dir.-in-Chief: Miss Jean Leask, 5 Blackburn Ave., Ottawa 2, Ont.

OBST. GYN. **AMERICAN ASSOCIATION OF OBSTETRICIANS & GYNECOLOGISTS, (M),** Homestead, Hot Springs, Va., Sept. 7-9th. Sec.: Robert B. Wilson, M.D., 200 First St. S.W., Rochester, Minn.

AMERICAN COLLEGE OF OBSTETRICIANS & GYNECOLOGISTS, (E), Hilton Hotel, Washington, D.C., April 16-20th. Sec.: Harold A. Kaminetsky, M.D., 1129 Rossell, Oak Park, Ill. 60302.

AMERICAN GYNECOLOGICAL SOCIETY, Arizona Biltmore Hotel, Phoenix, Ariz., May 4-6th. Sec.: Gordon W. Douglas, M.D., 550 First Ave., New York 10016.

SOCIETY OF OBSTETRICIANS & GYNAECOLOGISTS OF CANADA—Manoir Richelieu, Murray Bay, Quebec. Sec.: Dr. John Harkins, 537 Med. Arts Bldg., Toronto 5, Ont.

OCC. MED. **AMERICAN ACADEMY OF OCCUPATIONAL MEDICINE,** San Francisco Hilton Hotel, San Francisco, Feb. 8-10th. Sec.: Bertram D. Dinman, M.D., Dept. of Industrial Health, University of Michigan, Ann Arbor, Mich. 48104.

CONGRESS ON OCCUPATIONAL HEALTH, The Regency Hyatt House, Atlanta, Sept. 25-26th. Info: A.M.A. Dept. of Occupational Health, 535 N. Dearborn St., Chicago 60610.

OCC. THER. **AMERICAN OCCUPATIONAL THERAPY ASSOCIATION,** Americana Hotel, Boston, Oct. 15-20th. Exec. Dir.: Frances Helmig, 250 W. 57th St., New York 10019.

ORTHOPAED. **AMERICAN ACADEMY OF ORTHOPAEDIC SURGEONS, (E),** Civic Auditorium, San Francisco, Jan. 14-19th. Exec.-Sec.: Mr. John K. Hart, 29 E. Madison St., Chicago 60602.

AMERICAN FRACTURE ASSOCIATION, (E), Sheraton-Chicago Hotel, Chicago, Oct. 28-Nov. 2nd. Sec.-Gen.: H. W. Wellmerling, M.D., 626 Griesheim Bldg., Bloomington, Ill. 61701.

AMERICAN ORTHOPAEDIC ASSOCIATION, Homestead, Hot Springs, Va., June 26-29th. Exec. Sec.: Sam W. Banks, M.D., 29 E. Madison St., Chicago 60602.

THE CANADIAN ORTHOPAEDIC ASSOC.—June 18th-23rd. Montreal, P.Q. Sec.: Dr. C. A. Laurin, 3875 St. Urbain, Montreal, P.Q.

PAED. **AMERICAN ACADEMY OF PEDIATRICS,** Hilton Hotel, San Francisco, April 3-5th. Exec. Dir.: E. H. Christopherson, M.D., 1801 Hinman Ave., Evanston, Ill. 60204.

AMERICAN ACADEMY OF PEDIATRICS, (E), Washington Hilton Hotel, Washington, D.C., Oct. 21-26th. Exec. Sec.: E. H. Christopherson, M.D., 1801 Hinman Ave., Evanston, Ill. 60204.

AMERICAN PEDIATRIC SOCIETY, Seaside Hotel, Atlantic City, N.J., April 27-28th. Sec.-Treas.: Charles D. Cook, M.D., 333 Cedar St., New Haven, Conn. 06510.

CANADIAN PAEDIATRIC SOCIETY—Toronto, Ont.; Sept. 3-9th; Sec.: Dr. Victor Marchessault, 14 Green Ave., St. Lambert, P.Q.

PATH. **AMERICAN ASSOCIATION OF PATHOLOGISTS & BACTERIOLOGISTS, (E),** Sheraton-Park Hotel, Washington, D.C., March 10-15th. Sec.-Treas.: J. Lowell Orbison, M.D., University of Rochester School of Medicine & Dentistry, 260 Crittenden Blvd., Rochester, N.Y. 14620.

AMERICAN SOCIETY OF CLINICAL PATHOLOGISTS, Palmer House, Chicago, Sept. 22-29th. Adminis. Sec.: Martha Damron, 445 N. Lake Shore Dr., Chicago 60611.

AMERICAN SOCIETY FOR EXPERIMENTAL PATHOLOGY, (E), Chicago, April 17-21st. Sec.-Treas.: Thomas D. Kinney, M.D., Duke University Medical Center, Durham, N.C. 27706.

CANADIAN ASSOC. OF PATHOLOGISTS—Quebec, P.Q.; June 11th-17th. Sec.: Dr. D. W. Penner, Dept. of Path., Winnipeg Gen. Hosp., Winnipeg 3, Man.

COLLEGE OF AMERICAN PATHOLOGISTS, (E, M), Palmer House, Chicago, Sept. 22-29th. Exec. Dir.: Oliver J. Neibel, Jr., 230 N. Michigan Ave., Chicago 60601.

PHARM. **CANADIAN PHARMACEUTICAL ASSOCIATION**—Toronto, Ont.; August 13th-17th. Sec.: J. C. Turnbull, 175 College St., Toronto 2B, Ont.

PHARMACEUTICAL MANUFACTURERS ASSOC. OF CANADA—Chateau Champlain, Montreal, P.Q.; May 29th-31st; Exec. Sec.: Mr. Guy Beauchemin, 1110 Gillin Bldg., 141 Laurier Ave. W., Ottawa 4, Ont.

PHYSIOL. **AMERICAN PHYSIOLOGICAL SOCIETY (Spring Meeting),** Conrad Hilton Hotel, Chicago, April 16-21st. Exec. Sec.: Dr. Ray G. Daggs, 9650 Rockville Pike, Bethesda, Md. 20014.

AMERICAN PHYSIOLOGICAL SOCIETY (Fall Meeting), Howard University, Washington, D.C., Aug. 23-26th. Exec. Sec.: Dr. Ray G. Daggs, 9650 Rockville Pike, Bethesda, Md. 20014.

PHYS. MED. & REHAB.	**AMERICAN CONGRESS OF PHYSICAL MEDICINE & REHABILITATION, (E, M)**, Americana Hotel, Miami Beach, Fla., Aug. 27-Sept. 1st. Exec. Dir.: Creston C. Herold, 30 N. Michigan Ave., Ste. 922, Chicago 60602. **CANADIAN ASSOC. OF PHYSICAL MED. & REHAB.**; Winnipeg, Man.; August 1967 (dates unknown). Sec.. Dr. Wm. O. Geisler, 153 Lyndhurst Ave., Toronto, Ont.
PREV. MED.	**AMERICAN COLLEGE OF PREVENTIVE MEDICINE**, Fontainebleau Hotel, Miami Beach, Fla., Oct. 22-23rd. Exec. Sec.: Robert E. Coker, Jr., M.D., P.O. Box 1263, Chapel Hill, N.C. **AMERICAN COLLEGE OF PREVENTIVE MEDICINE**, Fontainbleau Hotel, Miami Beach, Fla., Nov. 22-23rd. Exec. Sec.: Dr. Robert E. Coker, Jr., P.O. Box 1263, Chapel Hill, N.C. 27514.
PROCT.	**AMERICAN PROCTOLOGIC SOCIETY**, Jung Hotel, New Orleans, April 17-19th. Adminis. Sec.: James A. Ferguson, M.D., 320 W. Lafayette, Detroit 48226.
PSY.	**ACADEMY OF PSYCHOANALYSIS**, Cobo Hall, Detroit, May 6-7th. Sec.: Alfred H. Rifkin, M.D., 125 E. 65th St., New York 10021. **ACADEMY OF PSYCHOSOMATIC MEDICINE**, Diplomat Hotel, Miami Beach, Fla., Oct. 16-18th. Exec. Sec.: Edwin Dunlop, M.D., 150 Emory St., Attleboro, Mass. 45. **AMERICAN COLLEGE OF PSYCHIATRISTS**, Annual Meeting, Detroit, May 6th. Sec. Gen.: J. Martin Myers, M.D., 111 N. 49th St., Philadelphia 19139. **AMERICAN ORTHOPSYCHIATRIC ASSOCIATION**, Hilton Hotel, Washington, D.C., March 22-25th. Exec. Sec.: Marion F. Langer, Ph.D., 1790 Broadway, New York 10019. **AMERICAN PSYCHIATRIC ASSOCIATION**, Cobo Hall, Detroit, May 7-12th. Sec.: Robert S. Garber, M.D., The Carrier Clinic, Belle Mead, N.J. 08502. **AMERICAN PSYCHOANALYTIC ASSOCIATION**, Statler-Hilton Hotel, Detroit, May 5-8th. Exec. Sec.: Mrs. Helen Fischer, One E. 57th St., New York 10022. **AMERICAN PSYCHOANALYTIC ASSOCIATION**, Waldorf-Astoria Hotel, New York, Dec. 15-17th. Exec. Sec.: Mrs. Helen Fischer, One E. 57th St., New York 10022. **AMERICAN PSYCHOSOMATIC SOCIETY**, Jung Hotel, New Orleans, April 7-9th. Sec.-Treas.: Herbert Weiner, M.D., 265 Nassau Rd., Roosevelt, N.Y. 11575. **CANADIAN PSYCHIATRIC ASSOCIATION—ASSOCIATION DES PSYCHIATRES DU CANADA**—Hotel des Laurentides, Quebec, P.Q.; June 14th-17th. Sec.: Dr. W. A. Blair, Ste. 103, 225 Lisgar St., Ottawa 4, Canada.
PH.	**AMERICAN ASSOCIATION OF PUBLIC HEALTH PHYSICIANS**, Miami Beach, Fla., Oct. 23-27th. Exec. Sec.: John S. Neill, M.D., P.O. Box 1731, Tampa, Fla. 33601. **AMERICAN PUBLIC HEALTH ASSOCIATION, (E)**, Hotel Fontainebleau, Miami, Fla., Oct. 23-27th. Exec. Dir.: Berwyn F. Mattison, M.D., 1790 Broadway, New York 10019. **CANADIAN PUBLIC HEALTH ASSOC.**—Chateau Laurier Hotel, Ottawa, Ont.; April 24th-27th. Sec.: Dr. G. W. O. Moss, 1255 Yonge St., Toronto 7, Ont.
RAD.	**AMERICAN ROENTGEN RAY SOCIETY, (E)**, Washington Hilton Hotel, Washington, D.C., Sept. 26-29th. Exec. Sec.: C. Allen Good, M.D., Mayo Clinic, Rochester, Minn. 55901. **CANADIAN SOC. OF RADIOLOGICAL TECHNICIANS**—Banff School of Fine Arts, Banff, Alta.; June 26th-30th. Sec.: Mrs. E. I. Hood, R.N., R.T., 2175 W. 16th Ave., Vancouver 9, B.C.
RAILWAY SURG.	**AMERICAN ASSOCIATION OF RAILWAY SURGEONS**, The Drake, Chicago, April 13-15th. Exec. Dir.: Dr. Carl Y. Werelius, Ill. Central Hospital, 5800 Stony Island Ave., Chicago 60637.
REPROD.	**AMERICAN SOCIETY FOR THE STUDY OF STERILITY**, Washington, D.C., April. Exec. Sec.: Herbert H. Thomas, M.D., 944 S. 18th St., Birmingham, Ala.
RHEUM.	**AMERICAN RHEUMATISM ASSOCIATION**, New York Hilton, New York, June. Exec. Sec.: Gerard W. Speyer, 1212 Avenue of the Americas, New York.
SCIENCE	**ASSOCIATION OF CLINICAL SCIENTISTS**—Meeting on "The Latest Advances in Clinical Science," Robert Meyer Motor Inn, Orlando, Fla., May 4-7th. Sec.-Treas.: Dr. Robert P. MacFate, 300 N. State St., No. 5322, Chicago 60610. **ASSOCIATION OF CLINICAL SCIENTISTS**, International Inn, Washington, D.C., Oct. 19-22nd. Sec.: Dr. Robert P. MacFate, 300 N. State St., No. 5322, Chicago 60610.
SURG.	**AMERICAN ACADEMY OF FACIAL PLASTIC & RECONSTRUCTIVE SURGERY**, Annual Meeting, Montreal, P.Q. May 25th-27th. Sec.: Jack R. Anderson, M.D., 1111 Tulane Ave., New Orleans 70112. **AMERICAN ASSOCIATION FOR SURGERY OF TRAUMA**, Drake Hotel, Chicago, Sept. 28-30th. Sec.: Sawnie B. Gaston, M.D., 180 Ft. Washington Ave., New York 10032. **AMERICAN ASSOCIATION FOR THORACIC SURGERY**, Americana Hotel, New York, April 17-19th. Admin. Ass't.: Ada Hanvey, 311 Carondelet Bldg., West 7730 Carondelet Ave., St. Louis 63105. **AMERICAN ASSOCIATION OF GENITOURINARY SURGEONS, (E)**, Westchester Country Club, Rye, N.Y., May 24-26th. Exec. Sec.: Harry M. Spence, M.D., 4105 Live Oak St., Dallas 75221. **AMERICAN ASSOC. OF PLASTIC SURGEONS**, Royal York Hotel, Toronto, Canada, May 18-21st. Sec.: Clarence W. Monroe, M.D., 715 Lake St., Oak Park, Ill. 60301. **AMERICAN COLLEGE OF SURGEONS**, Arizona Chapter, Arizona Inn, Tucson, Ariz., Jan. 20-21. Info: Bernard W. Simons, Jr., M.D., 3131 E. Second St., Tucson, Ariz.

AMERICAN COLLEGE OF SURGEONS, (E), Conrad Hilton, Chicago, Oct. 2-6th. Dir.: John Paul North, M.D., 55 E. Erie St., Chicago 60611.

AMERICAN SOCIETY FOR ARTIFICIAL INTERNAL ORGANS, (E), Sheraton-Chicago Hotel, Chicago, April 15-16th. Exec. Sec.: Dr. Pierre M. Galletti, Dept. of Physiology, Emory University, Atlanta.

AMERICAN SOCIETY FOR SURGERY OF THE HAND, Jack Tar Hotel, San Francisco, Jan. 13-14th. Sec.-Treas.: Raymond M. Curtis, M.D., 2947 St. Paul St., Baltimore 21218.

AMERICAN SOCIETY OF ABDOMINAL SURGEONS, (E), Sheraton Park Hotel, Washington, D.C., April 8-12th. Exec. Sec.: Blaise F. Alfano, M.D., 675 Main St., Melrose, Mass. 02176.

AMERICAN SOCIETY OF PLASTIC & RECONSTRUCTIVE SURGEONS, (E, M), Waldorf-Astoria, New York, Nov. 5-9th. Gen. Sec.: Paul P. Pickering, M.D., 2850 Sixth Ave., Ste. B, San Diego, Calif. 92103.

AMERICAN SURGICAL ASSOCIATION, (M), Broadmoor Hotel, Colorado Springs, Colo., May 11-14th. Exec. Sec.: Harris B. Shumacker, Jr., 1100 W. Michigan St., Indianapolis 46207.

CONGRESS OF NEUROLOGICAL SURGEONS, San Francisco Hilton Hotel, San Francisco, Oct. 25-28th. Sec.: John M. Thompson, M.D., 1955 Blossom Way South, St. Petersburg, Fla. 33712.

ROYAL COLLEGE OF PHYSICIANS & SURGEONS OF CANADA, Royal York Hotel, Toronto, Ont., Jan. 18-20th, 1968. Sec.: Dr. James H. Graham, 74 Stanley, Ottawa, Ont.

SOCIETY FOR SURGERY OF THE ALIMENTARY TRACT, Holiday Inn, Atlantic City, N.J., June 17-18th. Exec. Sec.: John Van Prohaska, M.D., 950 E. 59th St., Chicago 60637.

SOCIETY OF THORACIC SURGEONS, (E), Muehlbach Hotel, Kansas City, Mo., Jan. 23-25th. Exec. Sec.: Francis X. Byron, M.D., City of Hope Medical Center, 1500 E. Duarte Rd., Duarte, Calif. 91010.

T.B. **ACADEMY OF TUBERCULOSIS PHYSICIANS,** Atlantic City, N.J., June 17. Sec.: George P. Bailey, M.D., 1295 Clermont, Denver 20.

CANADIAN TUBERCULOSIS ASSOCIATION, Quebec, P.Q., May 30-June 2nd. Sec.: Dr. C. W. L. Jeanes, Canadian Tuberculosis Association, 343 O'Connor St., Ottawa 4, Ont.

THERAPEUT. **AMERICAN THERAPEUTIC SOCIETY,** Atlantic City, N.J., June 15-18th. Exec. Sec.: Dr. Alan Frank Kreglow, 1801 Eye St. N.W., Washington, D.C.

THYROID **AMERICAN THYROID ASSOCIATION,** Michigan Union, Ann Arbor, Mich., Sept. 14-16th. Sec.: Theodore Winship, M.D., 110 Irving St. N.W., Washington, D.C. 20010.

TOXICOL. **SOCIETY OF TOXICOLOGY,** Marriott Hotel, Atlanta, March 23-25th. Sec.: Mr. Carrol S. Weil, Mellon Institute, 4400 Fifth Ave., Pittsburgh 15213.

TROP. MED. **AMERICAN SOCIETY OF TROPICAL MEDICINE & HYGIENE, (E),** Benjamin Franklin Hotel, Philadelphia, Nov. 7-10th. Exec. Sec.: Dr. G. M. Jeffrey, P.O. Box 295, Kensington, Md. 02795.

UROL. **AMERICAN UROLOGICAL ASSOCIATION, (E),** New York Hilton Hotel, New York, May 29-June 1st. Exec. Sec.: William P. Didusch, 1120 N. Charles St., Baltimore 21201.

CANADIAN UROLOGICAL ASSOC.—Queen Elizabeth Hotel, Montreal, P.Q.; June 4th-7th. Sec.: Dr. Kenneth J. MacKinnon, Royal Victoria Hospital, Montreal 2, P.Q.

Printed by
GENERAL PRINTERS LTD.
57 Simcoe St. S.,
Oshawa, Ont.
Toronto Office: 432 Church St., Tel. WA 5-4424